Addiction Medicine

Addiction Medicine

Science and Practice

2ND EDITION

Bankole A. Johnson, DSc, MD, MB, ChB, MPhil, DFAPA, FRCPsych, FACFEI, ABDA

Founder and Executive Chairman
The Global Institutes on Addictions and the Hyperion Institute
Miami, Florida
Founder and Chairman of Board of Directors
Adial Pharmaceuticals, Inc.
Charlottesville, Virginia
Professor of Anatomy and Neurobiology
Professor of Medicine
Professor of Neurology
Professor of Pharmacology
Professor of Psychiatry
University of Maryland School of Medicine
Baltimore, Maryland
Former Dr. J Irving Taylor Professor and Chairman of Psychiatry
University of Maryland
Former Alumni Professor and Chairman of Psychiatry and Neurobehavioral Sciences
University of Virginia

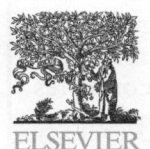

ELSEVIER

Elsevier
1600 John F. Kennedy Blvd.
Ste 1600
Philadelphia, PA 19103-2899

ADDICTION MEDICINE: SCIENCE AND PRACTICE:
SECOND EDITION

ISBN: 978-0-323-75440-8

Chapter 16, "Neurobiological Basis of Drug Reward and Reinforcement" by David M. Lovinger, is in the public domain.

Previous edition copyrighted © 2011 by Springer Science+Business Media.

ISBN: 978-0-323-75440-8

Senior Acquisitions Editor: Joslyn T. Chaiprasert-Paguio
Senior Content Development Specialist: Joanie Milnes
Publishing Services Manager: Catherine Albright Jackson
Senior Project Manager: Doug Turner
Designer: Brian Salisbury

Printed in the United States

Last digit is the print number: 9 8 7 6 5 4 3 2 1

Working together
to grow libraries in
developing countries

www.elsevier.com • www.bookaid.org

For the phenomenal Alexander and the amazing Julian,
My wonderful boys, now and for all of time.

About the Editor

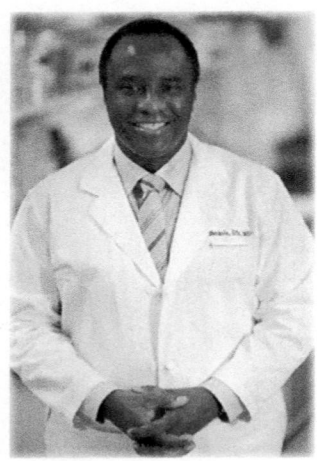

Professor Bankole A. Johnson, DSc, MD, MB, ChB, MPhil, DFAPA, FRCPsych, FACFEI, ABDA, is one of the leading neuroscientists in the world. He was the Dr. J Irving Taylor Professor and Chairman of Psychiatry at the University of Maryland. Professor Johnson coordinated all brain science activities at the University of Maryland. He is a Professor of Anatomy and Neurobiology, Medicine, Neurology, Pharmacology, and Psychiatry. He is licensed as a physician and board certified as a psychiatrist. He has been listed among the *Best Doctors in America* for decades. In addition to his qualifications in medicine and neuroscience, Professor Johnson is a renowned expert in forensic psychiatry, which is a subspecialty that seeks to understand the mental processes associated with criminal acts or behaviors. He is also one of the world's leading experts in addiction medicine.

Professor Johnson's primary area of research expertise is the psychopharmacology of medications for treating addictions. He is internationally recognized for his work on ion channels as they pertain to the actions of the serotonin system in the brain. An important part of his discoveries was to combine that knowledge with molecular genetics to develop a method of treating individuals with alcohol use disorder, using the medication ondansetron. This treatment modality requires no rehab—just an emphasis on taking the tablets and about 10 minutes of follow up a week. That's it!

Professor Johnson also is well known in the field for his discovery that topiramate, a gamma-aminobutyric acid (GABA) facilitator and glutamate antagonist, is an effective treatment for alcoholism.

To further Professor Johnson's work on novel treatments in addiction, he founded a company called Adial Pharmaceuticals and has been the Chairman of the Board of Directors since its inception, which has grown tremendously and is now listed on the Nasdaq exchange (see more later). This is a very important achievement as it shows a path from the scientific setting to the bedside and into the community. Rarely do scientists champion the development of their ideas into a nationally recognized pharmaceutical company.

Biography

Professor Johnson was born on 5 November 1959 in Nigeria. Johnson attended King's College in Lagos, Nigeria, and received his diploma in 1975. He then went on to Davies' College in Sussex, England, followed by the Institute Catholique de Paris (now the Catholic University of Paris) in Paris, France. Johnson graduated from the University of Glasgow in Scotland in 1982 at the age of 22 years with a *Medicinae Baccalaureum et Chirurgie Baccalaureum* degree. He went on to train in psychiatry at the Royal London Hospital, the Maudsley Hospital, and the Bethlem Royal Hospital and in research at the Institute of Psychiatry (University of London). In 1991, Johnson graduated from the University of London with a Master of Philosophy degree in neuropsychiatry. Johnson conducted his doctoral research at Oxford University and obtained a doctorate degree in medicine, *Medicinae Doctorem*, from the University of Glasgow in 1993. Most recently, in 2004, Johnson earned his *Doctor of Science degree in medicine* from the University of Glasgow—the highest degree that can be granted in science by a British university. These advanced degrees are for his research in neuroscience, neuropharmacology, neuroimaging, and molecular genetics.

Honors and Awards

Professor Johnson has received many awards. Notable among them are the following:

1. The 2001 Dan Anderson Research Award from the Hazelden Foundation for his "distinguished contribution as a researcher who has advanced the scientific knowledge of addiction recovery"
2. The 2002 Distinguished Senior Scholar of Distinction Award from the National Medical Association
3. Induction into the Texas Hall of Fame for Science, Mathematics, and Technology in 2003
4. The 2006 American Psychiatric Association Distinguished Psychiatrist Lecturer Award for outstanding achievement in the field of psychiatry as an educator, researcher, and clinician
5. The 2009 Solomon Carter Fuller Award by the American Psychiatric Association, which honors a black citizen who has pioneered in an area that has significantly improved the quality of life for black people
6. The 2013 Jack Mendelson Award from the National Institutes of Health for his outstanding scientific work that has

transformed our understanding of how abnormalities in the brain can promote addiction

7. The 2019 R. Brinkley Smithers Distinguished Scientist Award from the American Society of Addiction Medicine

In addition, Professor Johnson has an i10-index of 150 and an h-index of 57 (https://en.wikipedia.org/wiki/H-index); his work has been cited by other scientists more than 16,000 times. His h-index places him as one of the leading scientists in the world, which is also reflected in his many international awards for his scientific work.

Coat of Arms

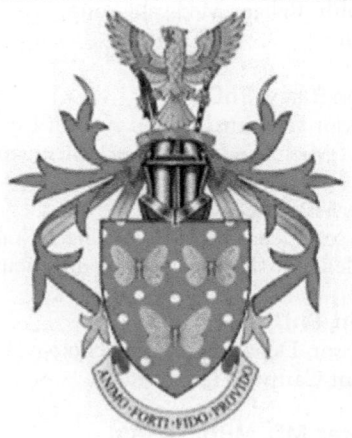

Professor Bankole Johnson was granted a coat of arms by Her Majesty Queen Elizabeth II. As seen here, the coat of arms depicts the butterflies associated with Psyche, pills to show a relationship with the development of medicines, a quill for higher learning and scholarship, and a javelin, symbolic of his noble African ancestry. Indeed, the markings on the javelin come from his Yoruba roots and depict the symbol of *Adimu*, which is traditional to the Eyo ceremony in Nigeria. The eagle is a representation of his affiliation with the United States, which is overlaid with the Cross of St. George, the traditional symbol of England in its flag. The motto, *Animo forti fido provido*, describes the drive to strive to provide and help others.

Media

Professor Johnson's discoveries have generated tremendous press interest. He has been featured on all the major networks and in several press outlets, including Reuters, MSNBC, CBS, ABC, CNN, Fox News, USA Today, and the Associated Press. The HBO series *Addiction,* which featured some of his work and has been watched by an estimated 30 million people, won prestigious Governors Award, a special Emmy Award, from the Academy of Television Arts and Sciences.

More About Adial Pharmaceuticals Inc.

Adial Pharmaceutics (https://www.adialpharma.com) is listed on the Nasdaq (Ticker: ADIL). Adial seeks to bring personalized treatments for alcohol use disorder and other addictions. Personalized treatments, now better known as precision medicine, offer the potential to reduce the variability in medication response by targeting individuals through their genetic profile, increasing the likelihood that a patient will respond to a particular modality of treatment. If you have interest in learning more about Adial Pharmaceuticals, please contact David Waldman at the following:

Crescendo Communications, LLC
Tel: 212-671-1021
Email: dwaldman@crescendo-ir.com

Conflict of Interest Disclosure: Professor Johnson is the Chairman of the Board of Directors of Adial Pharmaceuticals and a significant shareholder in the company.

About the Global Institutes on Addictions (GIA)

The GIA (www.gia.miami), which was founded to deliver the best evidence-based translation of addiction science to clinical practice, aims to be at the forefront of substance abuse treatment. The GIA deploys innovative treatment programs using a combination of personalized neuropharmacological approaches, molecular genetic techniques, and neurostimulation, accompanied by deep behavioral phenotyping and targeted psychobehavioral support. Synergizing with the GIA is the Hyperion Institute, which will offer one of the world's only direct-to-practice higher degrees in addiction medicine, and shall shepherd the latest discoveries in addiction science to clinical practices and industry for the benefit of all.

Contributors

Ashley Acheson, PhD
Associate Professor, Department of Psychiatry and Behavioral Sciences, Director, Program on the Translational Science of Drug Abuse, University of Arkansas for Medical Sciences, Little Rock, Arkansas

Giovanni Addolorato, MD
Assistant Professor, Department of Internal Medicine and Gastroenterology, Catholic University of Rome, Alcohol Use Disorder and Alcohol Related Disease Unit, Department of Internal Medicine and Gastroenterology, Fondazione Policlinico Universitario A. Gemelli IRCCS Research Hospital, Rome, Italy

Mariangela Antonelli, MD
Internal Medicine Specialist, Department of Internal Medicine and Gastroenterology, Catholic University of Rome, Alcohol Use Disorder and Alcohol Related Disease Unit, Department of Internal Medicine and Gastroenterology, Fondazione Policlinico Universitario A. Gemelli IRCCS Research Hospital, Rome, Italy

Bachaar Arnaout, MD
Assistant Professor, Department of Psychiatry, Yale School of Medicine, Veterans Affairs Connecticut Healthcare System, West Haven, Connecticut

David L. Atkinson, MD
Assistant Professor, Department of Psychiatry, The University of Texas Southwestern Medical Center at Dallas, Dallas, Texas

Jeffrey N. Baldwin, PharmD, RPh, FAPhA, FASHP
Emeritus Professor of Pharmacy Practice and Science, College of Pharmacy, University of Nebraska Medical Center, Omaha, Nebraska

Peter A. Baldwin, PhD
Postdoctoral Fellow, School of Psychology, New South Wales University, Sydney, New South Wales, Australia

Michael T. Bardo, PhD
Professor, Department of Psychology, University of Kentucky, Lexington, Kentucky

Iris M. Balodis, PhD
Assistant Professor, Department of Psychiatry and Behavioral Neurosciences, Peter Boris Centre for Addictions Research, DeGroote School of Medicine, McMaster University, Hamilton, Ontario, Canada

Danielle Barry, PhD
Behavioral Health, Reliant Medical Group, Worcester, Massachusetts

Kristen Lawton Barry, PhD
Research Professor Emeritus, Department of Psychiatry, University of Michigan, Ann Arbor, Michigan

Robert Beech, MD, PhD
Assistant Professor, Department of Psychiatry, Yale University School of Medicine, New Haven, Connecticut

Amit Bernstein, PhD
Associate Professor, Department of Psychology, University of Haifa, Mount Carmel, Haifa, Israel

Michael F. Bierer, MD, MPH, FASAM
Physician, Division of General Medicine, Department of Medicine, Massachusetts General Hospital, Assistant Professor, Harvard Medical School, Boston, Massachusetts

David S. Black, PhD, MPH
Assistant Professor, Departments of Preventive Medicine and Psychology, Institute for Health Promotion and Disease Prevention Research, Keck School of Medicine, University of Southern California, Alhambra, California

Derek Blevins, MD
Postdoctoral Fellow, Department of Psychiatry, Columbia University/New York State Psychiatric Institute, New York, New York

Frederic C. Blow, PhD
Professor and Director, U-M Addiction Center, Department of Psychiatry, University of Michigan, Research Scientist, Center for Clinical Management Research, Department of Veterans Affairs, Ann Arbor, Michigan

Marcel O. Bonn-Miller, PhD
Assistant Professor, National Center for PTSD and Center for Innovation to Implementation, VA Palo Alto Health Care System, Menlo Park, California, Center of Excellence in Substance Abuse Treatment and Education, Philadelphia VA Medical Center, Department of Psychiatry, University of Pennsylvania Perelman School of Medicine, Philadelphia, Pennsylvania

Marc D. Breton, PhD
Associate Professor, Department of Psychiatry and Neurobehavioral Sciences, University of Virginia School of Medicine, Charlottesville, Virginia

Kirk J. Brower, MD
Professor, Department of Psychiatry, University of Michigan, Ann Arbor, Michigan

Qiana L. Brown, PhD, MPH, LCSW
Assistant Professor, The Substance Use Research, Evaluation, and Maternal and Child Health Group, Center for Prevention Science, School of Social Work, Rutgers University, New Brunswick, New Jersey, Department of Urban-Global Public Health, School of Public Health, Rutgers University, Piscataway, New Jersey, TrendologyIT Corporation, Baltimore, Maryland

Eliza Buelt, MD
Instructor, Department of Psychiatry, Yale School of Medicine, New Haven, Connecticut

Fabio Caputo, MD, PhD
Internal Medicine Specialist, Department of Internal Medicine, SS Annunziata Hospital, Cento, Italy

Jacqueline C. Carter, DPhil, RPsych
Professor, Department of Psychology, Memorial University of Newfoundland, St. John's, Newfoundland, Canada

Joy Chang, MD
Assistant Professor, Division of Addiction Research and Treatment, Department of Psychiatry, University of Maryland School of Medicine, Baltimore, Maryland

Joseph F. Cheer, PhD
Professor, Department of Psychiatry, University of Maryland School of Medicine, Baltimore, Maryland

Shih-Fen Chen, PhD
Hualien Tzu Chi Hospital, Buddhist Tzu Chi Medical Foundation, Hualien, Taiwan

Paul M. Cinciripini, PhD
Professor and Chair, Department of Behavioral Science, The University of Texas MD Anderson Cancer Center at Houston, Houston, Texas

H. Westley Clark, MD, JD, MPH
Dean's Executive Professor of Public Health, Public Health Program, Santa Clara University, Santa Clara, California

Leon G. Coleman, Jr., MD, PhD
Research Assistant Professor, Department of Pharmacology, Bowles Center for Alcohol Studies, University of North Carolina School of Medicine, Chapel Hill, North Carolina

Gregory T. Collins, PhD
Assistant Professor, Department of Pharmacology, The University of Texas Health Science Center at San Antonio, San Antonio, Texas

Catherine Corno, PhD
Psychology Postdoctoral Fellow, Trauma Recovery Program, VA Maryland Health Care System, Baltimore, Maryland

Dan P. Covey, PhD
Assistant Professor, Department of Anatomy and Neurobiology, University of Maryland School of Medicine, Baltimore, Maryland

Fulton T. Crews, PhD
John Andrews Distinguished Professor, Professor of Pharmacology and Psychiatry, Director, Bowles Center for Alcohol Studies, School of Medicine, University of North Carolina at Chapel Hill, Chapel Hill, North Carolina

Karen L. Cropsey, PsyD
Conatser Turner Endowed Professor of Psychiatry, University of Alabama at Birmingham, Birmingham, Alabama

Anita Cservenka, PhD
Assistant Professor, School of Psychological Science, Oregon State University, Corvallis, Oregon

Leon Cushenberry, MD
Public Health Psychiatry Fellow, University of Pennsylvania, Staff Psychiatrist, Philadelphia, Pennsylvania

Cristina d'Angelo, MD
Specialist in Internal Medicine and Psychotherapy, Gli Angeli di Padre Pio, Fondazione Centri di Riabilitazione Padre Pio Onlus, San Giovanni Rotondo, Italy, Alcohol Use Disorder and Alcohol Related Disease Unit, Department of Internal Medicine and Gastroenterology, Fondazione Policlinico Universitario A. Gemelli IRCCS Research Hospital, Rome, Italy

Hannah M. Dantrassy, BA
Department of Psychology, University of Maryland, College Park, College Park, Maryland

Caroline Davis, PhD
York University, Faculty of Health Sciences, Center for Addiction and Mental Health, Toronto, Ontario, Canada

Matt Davis, BA
Santa Clara University, Santa Clara, California

Nancy Diazgranados, MD
Deputy Clinical Director, National Institute on Alcohol Abuse and Alcoholism, National Institutes of Health, Bethesda, Maryland

David A. Deitch, PhD
Professor Emeritus of Clinical Psychiatry, Department of Psychiatry, University of California, San Diego, San Diego, California

Carlo C. DiClemente, PhD
Professor Emeritus, Department of Psychology, University of Maryland, Baltimore County, Baltimore, Maryland

Tommaso Dionisi, MD
Internal Medicine Attending Physician, Department of Internal Medicine and Gastroenterology, Catholic University of Rome, Alcohol Use Disorder and Alcohol Related Disease Unit, Department of Internal Medicine and Gastroenterology, Fondazione Policlinico Universitario A. Gemelli IRCCS Research Hospital, Rome, Italy

Brian M. Dodge, PhD
Professor, School of Public Health-Bloomington, Indiana University, Bloomington, Bloomington, Indiana

Liliane Drago, MA, CASAC, MAC
Director, Outreach Training Institute, Richmond Hill, New York

Linda P. Dwoskin, PhD
Professor, Department of Pharmaceutical Sciences, University of Kentucky College of Pharmacy, Lexington, Kentucky

Gloria D. Eldridge, PhD
Professor, Department of Psychology, University of Alaska, Anchorage, Alaska

†Ahmed Elkashef, MD
Vice President, Clinical Development, Insys Pharmaceuticals, Chandler, Arizona

Troy W. Ertelt, PhD
Clinical Psychologist, Department of Psychology, University of North Dakota, Grand Forks, North Dakota

Karin M. Eyrich-Garg, PhD
MSW Program Director and Associate Professor, School of Social Work, College of Public Health, Temple University, Philadelphia, Pennsylvania

Samantha G. Farris, PhD
Assistant Professor, Department of Psychology, Rutgers University, New Brunswick, New Jersey

Francisco Fernandez, MD
Professor, Department of Psychiatry, The University of Texas Rio Grande Valley, Harlingen, Texas

Anna Ferrulli, MD, PhD
Internal Medicine Specialist, Department of Endocrinology and Metabolism, IRCCS Policlinico San Donato, San Donato Milanese, Italy, Alcohol Use Disorder and Alcohol Related Disease Unit, Department of Internal Medicine and Gastroenterology, Fondazione Policlinico Universitario A. Gemelli IRCCS Research Hospital, Rome, Italy

Alyssa A. Forcehimes, PhD
Assistant Professor, Department of Psychology, University of New Mexico, Albuquerque, New Mexico

Shauna Fuller, PhD
Psychologist, Trauma Recovery Services, Post-Deployment Clinical Team, Outpatient Behavioral Health, Clement J. Zablocki Veterans Affairs Medical Center, Milwaukee, Wisconsin

Antonio Gasbarrini, MD, PhD
Professor and Chief, Department of Internal Medicine and Gastroenterology, Catholic University of Rome, Alcohol Use Disorder and Alcohol Related Disease Unit, Department of Internal Medicine and Gastroenterology, Fondazione Policlinico Universitario A. Gemelli IRCCS Research Hospital, Rome, Italy

Michael H. Gendel, MD
Medical Director Emeritus, Colorado Physician Health Program, Denver, Colorado

Lisa R. Gerak, PhD
Assistant Professor, Department of Pharmacology, The University of Texas Health Science Center at San Antonio, San Antonio, Texas

Brett C. Ginsburg, PhD
Assistant Professor, Department of Psychiatry, The University of Texas Health Science Center at San Antonio, San Antonio, Texas

Cassandra D. Gipson, PhD
Assistant Professor, Department of Psychology, Arizona State University, Tempe, Arizona

Paul E.A. Glaser, MD, PhD
Professor, Department of Psychiatry, Washington University School of Medicine, St. Louis, Missouri

David Goldman, MD
Senior Investigator, Laboratory of Neurogenetics, National Institute on Alcohol Abuse and Alcoholism, National Institutes of Health, Bethesda, Maryland

Karl Goodkin, MD, PhD, DLFAPA, FACPsych, FRSM
Professor, Department of Psychiatry and Behavioral Sciences, Quillen College of Medicine, East Tennessee State University, Johnson City, Tennessee

Jon E. Grant, MD, JD, MPH
Professor, Department of Psychiatry and Behavioral Neuroscience, University of Chicago, Chicago, Illinois

Meagan Graydon, PhD
Department of Psychology, University of Maryland, Baltimore County, Baltimore, Maryland

Jessica R. Grisham, PhD
Professor, School of Psychology, New South Wales University, Sydney, New South Wales, Australia

Marc Grifell Guàrdia, MD
Research Scholar, Department of Psychology, Columbia University, New York, New York, Clinical Researcher, Hospital del Mar Medical Research Institute (IMIM), CIBERSAM, Barcelona, Doctoral Student, Department of Psychiatry and Legal Medicine, Universitat Autònoma de Barcelona, Cerdanyola del Vallés, Barcelona, Spain

John H. Halpern, MD
Assistant Professor, Department of Psychiatry, Harvard Medical School, Boston, Massachusetts, Laboratory for Integrative Psychiatry, Alcohol and Drug Abuse Research Center, Division of Alcohol and Drug Abuse, McLean Hospital, Belmont, Massachusetts

† Deceased.

Emily R. Hankosky, PhD
Postdoctoral Fellow, Department of Pharmaceutical Sciences, University of Kentucky College of Pharmacy, Lexington, Kentucky

Carl L. Hart, PhD
Ziff Professor of Psychology (in Psychiatry), Departments of Psychology and Psychiatry, Columbia University, Research Scientist, New York State Psychiatric Institute, Department of Psychiatry, College of Physicians and Surgeons, New York, New York

Deborah Hasin, PhD
Professor, Departments of Psychiatry and Epidemiology, Columbia University, New York State Psychiatric Institute, New York, New York

Angela Hawken, PhD
Professor of Public Policy, Marron Institute, New York University, New York, New York

Scott E. Hemby, PhD
Professor, Department of Basic Pharmaceutical Sciences, Fred Wilson School of Pharmacy, High Point University, High Point, North Carolina

Meredith A. Holmgren Shaw, PhD
Assistant Professor of Psychiatry, The University of Texas Southwestern Medical Center at Dallas, Dallas, Texas

M. Christina Hove, PhD
PTSD/SUD Liaison, Staff Psychologist, Trauma Recovery Services, Outpatient Behavioral Health, Clement J. Zablocki Veterans Affairs Medical Center, Milwaukee, Wisconsin

Hanyun Huang, PhD
Associate Professor, School of Journalism and Communication, Xiamen University, Xiamen, China

Pedro E. Huertas, MD
Department of Psychiatry, Harvard Medical School, Boston, Massachusetts, Laboratory for Integrative Psychiatry, Alcohol and Drug Abuse Research Center, Division of Alcohol and Drug Abuse, McLean Hospital, Belmont, Massachusetts

Gary K. Hulse, PhD
Professor of Addiction Medicine, Division of Psychiatry, University of Western Australia, Crawley, Western Australia, Australia

Kent E. Hutchison, PhD
Professor, Department of Psychology and Neuroscience, University of Colorado at Boulder, Boulder, Colorado

Karen S. Ingersoll, PhD
Professor, Department of Psychiatry and Neurobehavioral Sciences, University of Virginia School of Medicine, Charlottesville, Virginia

Dorothy O. Jackson
Consortium for Substance Abuse Research and Training Program, Department of Psychology, University of Alabama, Birmingham, Alabama

Jack E. James, PhD
Professor, Department of Psychology, Reykjavík University, Reykjavík, Iceland

Martin A. Javors, PhD
Professor, Department of Psychiatry and Behavioral Sciences, The University of Texas Health Science Center at San Antonio, San Antonio, Texas

Bankole A. Johnson, DSc, MD, MB, ChB, MPhil, DFAPA, FRCPsych, FACFEI, ABDA
Founder and Executive Chairman, The Global Institutes on Addictions and the Hyperion Institute, Miami, Florida, Founder and Chairman of Board of Directors, Adial Pharmaceuticals, Inc., Charlottesville, Virginia, Professor of Anatomy and Neurobiology, Professor of Medicine, Professor of Neurology, Professor of Pharmacology, Professor of Psychiatry, University of Maryland School of Medicine, Baltimore, Maryland

Jeannette L. Johnson, PhD
Professor, School of Social Work, University of Buffalo, Buffalo, New York

Raja Kadib, MPsych (Clin)
Clinical Psychologist, School of Psychology, New South Wales University, Sydney, New South Wales, Australia

Maher Karam-Hage, MD
Professor of Psychiatry, Department of Behavioral Science, The University of Texas MD Anderson Cancer Center, Houston, Texas

Asaf Keller, PhD
Professor and Chair, Department of Anatomy and Neurobiology, Program in Neuroscience, University of Maryland School of Medicine, Baltimore, Maryland

Steven F. Kendell, MD
Department of Psychiatry and Behavioral Sciences, Quillen College of Medicine, East Tennessee State University, Johnson City, Tennessee

George A. Kenna, PhD
Center for Alcohol and Addiction Studies, Brown University, Providence, Rhode Island

Therese E. Kenny, MSc
Department of Psychology, Memorial University of Newfoundland, St. John's, Newfoundland, Canada

Katherine Keyes, PhD
Associate Professor, Department of Epidemiology, Co-Director, Psychiatric Epidemiology Training Program, Columbia University, New York, New York

Surbhi Khanna, MD
Medical Director, Gladstone Psychiatry and Wellness, Columbia, Maryland

Thomas S. King, PhD
Professor, Department of Cellular and Structural Biology, The University of Texas Health Science Center at San Antonio, San Antonio, Texas

Daniel Knoblach, PhD
Psychology Fellow, VA Medical Center, Baltimore, Maryland

George F. Koob, PhD
Director, National Institute on Alcohol Abuse and Alcoholism, Rockville, Maryland

Boris P. Kovatchev, PhD
Professor, Department of Psychiatry and Neurobehavioral Sciences, University of Virginia School of Medicine, Charlottesville, Virginia

Jonathan D. Kulick, PhD
Senior Research Scholar, Marron Institute, New York University, New York, New York

Karol L. Kumpfer, PhD
Professor, Department of Health Promotion and Education, University of Utah, Salt Lake City, Utah

Howard I. Kushner, PhD
Nat C. Robertson Distinguished Professor Emeritus, Center for the Study of Human Health, Emory University, Atlanta, Georgia

Kathy Lancaster, BA
Research Consultant, Neuropsychiatric Research Institute, Fargo, North Dakota

Kirsten J. Langdon, PhD
Professor, Department of Psychiatry and Human Behavior, Warren Alpert Medical School of Brown University, Providence, Rhode Island

Noeline C. Latt, MB BS, MPhil, MRCP, FAChAM
Former Senior Staff Specialist, Northern Sydney Drug and Alcohol Services, Royal North Shore Hospital, St. Leonards, Sydney, New South Wales, Australia

William B. Lawson, PhD, MD, DFAPA
Adjunct Professor, Department of Psychiatry, University of Maryland, Emeritus Professor (retired), Howard University, Silver Spring, Maryland

Nicole Lee, PhD, BSc(Hons)
Professor, National Drug Research Institute, Curtin University, Perth, Western Australia, Australia

Lorenzo Leggio, MD, PhD, MSc
Senior Investigator and Chief, Section on Clinical Psychoneuroendocrinology and Neuropsychopharmacology, National Institute on Alcohol Abuse and Alcoholism and National Institute on Drug Abuse, National Institutes of Health, Bethesda, Maryland, Associate Director for Clinical Research, Medication Development Program, National Institute on Drug Abuse, National Institutes of Health, Baltimore, Maryland, Senior Medical Advisor to the Director, National Institute on Alcohol Abuse and Alcoholism, National Institutes of Health, Rockville, Maryland, Adjunct Professor, Brown University, Providence, Rhode Island

Louis Leung, PhD
Professor, Department of Journalism and Communication, Hong Kong Shue Yan University, Hong Kong, China

Shaul Lev-Ran, MD, MHA
Deputy Director, Lev Hasharon Medical Center, Associate Professor, Department of Psychiatry, Sackler Faculty of Medicine, Tel Aviv University, Tel Aviv, Israel

David C. Lewis, MD
Professor Emeritus, Center for Alcohol and Addiction Studies, Brown University, Providence, Rhode Island

Teresa M. Leyro, PhD
Assistant Professor, Department of Psychology, Rutgers University, New Brunswick, New Jersey

Mary Kay Lobo, PhD
Associate Professor, Department of Anatomy and Neurobiology, University of Maryland School of Medicine, Baltimore, Maryland

David M. Lovinger, PhD
Laboratory for Integrative Neuroscience, National Institute on Alcohol Abuse and Alcoholism, National Institutes of Health, Rockville, Maryland

Jason B. Luoma, PhD
Psychologist, Cofounder, Portland Psychotherapy Clinic, Research, and Training Center, Portland, Oregon

Wendy J. Lynch, PhD
Associate Professor, Department of Psychiatry and Neurobehavioral Sciences, University of Virginia School of Medicine, Charlottesville, Virginia

Robert Malcolm, MD
Associate Dean for Continuing Medical Education, Professor, Department of Psychiatry and Behavioral Sciences, Medical University of South Carolina, Charleston, South Carolina

Joanna M. Marinoa, PhD
Clinical Psychologist, Potomac Behavioral Services, Arlington, Virginia

Gabrielle Marzani, MD
Associate Professor, Department of Psychiatry and Neurobehavioral Sciences, University of Virginia School of Medicine, Charlottesville, Virginia

Kimberly R. McBride, PhD
Assistant Professor, School of Population Health, College of Health and Human Services, University of Toledo, Toledo, Ohio

Jennifer Minnix, PhD
Assistant Professor, Department of Behavioral Science, The University of Texas MD Anderson Cancer Center at Houston, Houston, Texas

Antonio Mirijello, MD, MSc
Internal Medicine Specialist, Department of Medical Sciences, IRCCS Casa Sollievo della Sofferenza General Hospital, San Giovanni Rotondo, Italy, Alcohol Use Disorder and Alcohol Related Disease Unit, Department of Internal Medicine and Gastroenterology, Fondazione Policlinico Universitario A. Gemelli IRCCS Research Hospital, Rome, Italy

James E. Mitchell, MD
Professor Emeritus, Neuropsychiatric Research Institute, Fargo, North Dakota

Rudolf H. Moos, PhD
Professor Emeritus, Center for Innovation to Implementation, Stanford University School of Medicine and Department of Veterans Affairs Health Care System, Menlo Park, California

Carolina Mosoni, MD
Internal Medicine Resident, Department of Internal Medicine and Gastroenterology, Catholic University of Rome, Alcohol Use Disorder and Alcohol Related Disease Unit, Department of Internal Medicine and Gastroenterology, Fondazione Policlinico Universitario A. Gemelli IRCCS Research Hospital, Rome, Italy

Clayton Neighbors, PhD
John and Rebecca Moores Professor, Director of Social Psychology Program, Department of Psychology, University of Houston, Houston, Texas

Tanseli Nesil, PhD
Research Scientist, Department of Psychiatry and Neurobehavioral Sciences, University of Virginia School of Medicine, Charlottesville, Virginia

Carol S. North, MD
Nancy and Ray L. Hunt Chair in Crisis Psychiatry, Professor, Departments of Psychiatry and Emergency Medicine, The University of Texas Southwestern Medical Center, Dallas, Texas

M. Foster Olive, PhD
Professor, Department of Psychology, Arizona State University, Tempe, Arizona

Asher Ornoy, MD
Professor Emeritus of Medical Neurobiology, Department of Medical Neurobiology, Hebrew University-Hadassah Medical School, Jerusalem, Israel

Gabriela Pachano, MD
Assistant Professor, Department of Psychiatry and Neurobehavioral Sciences, University of Virginia School of Medicine, Charlottesville, Virginia

Torsten Passie, MD, PhD
Professor, The Laboratory for Neurocognition and Consciousness, Department of Psychiatry, Social Psychiatry and Psychotherapy, Hannover Medical School, Hannover, Germany

J. Kim Penberthy, PhD
Chester F. Carlson Professor, Department of Psychiatry and Neurobehavioral Sciences, University of Virginia School of Medicine, Charlottesville, Virginia

J. Morgan Penberthy, BA
Office of CE Sponsor Approval, American Psychological Association, Washington, District of Columbia

Daena L. Petersen, MD, MPH, MA
Psychiatric Services Director of HIV Psychiatry and Gender and Sexuality, South Carolina Department of Mental Health, Staff Psychiatrist, Berkeley Community Mental Health Center, Moncks Corner, South Carolina

Ismene L. Petrakis, MD
Professor, Department of Psychiatry, Yale School of Medicine, Veterans Affairs Connecticut Healthcare System, West Haven, Connecticut

†Nancy M. Petry, PhD
Professor, Department of Medicine, University of Connecticut Health Center, Farmington, Connecticut

Pallav Pokhrel, PhD
Associate Professor, Cancer Prevention in the Pacific Program, University of Hawaii Cancer Center, University of Hawaii, Honolulu, Hawaii

David E. Pollio, MSW, PhD
Distinguished Professor and Chair, Department of Social Work, University of Alabama, Birmingham, Alabama

Marc N. Potenza, PhD, MD
Professor, Department of Psychiatry, Child Study Center, Director, Center of Excellence in Gambling Research, Yale University School of Medicine, Connecticut Mental Health Center, New Haven, Connecticut

Maria Margherita Rando, MD
Internal Medicine Resident, Department of Internal Medicine and Gastroenterology, Catholic University of Rome, Alcohol Use Disorder and Alcohol Related Disease Unit, Department of Internal Medicine and Gastroenterology, Fondazione Policlinico Universitario A. Gemelli IRCCS Research Hospital, Rome, Italy

Lara A. Ray, PhD
Professor, Department of Psychology, University of California, Los Angeles, Los Angeles, California

Michael Reece, PhD, MPH
Lecturer, Department of Social and Public Health, Ohio University, Athens, Ohio

John A. Renner, MD
Professor of Psychiatry, Boston University School of Medicine, Associate Chief of Psychiatry, VA Boston Healthcare System, Boston, Massachusetts

---

†Deceased.

Nathaniel R. Riggs, PhD
Professor, Director, Prevention Research Center, Human Development and Family Studies, College of Health and Human Sciences, Colorado State University, Fort Collins, Colorado

John D. Roache, PhD
Hugo A. Auler Professor of Psychiatry, Department of Psychiatry and Behavioral Sciences, Department of Pharmacology, Chief, Psychiatry Division of Alcohol and Drug Addiction, Deputy Director, STRONG STAR Consortium to Alleviate PTSD, Director, FIRST Program of the Institute for the Integration of Medicine and Science, The University of Texaas Health Science Center at San Antonio, San Antonio, Texas

Daniel Rounsaville, PhD
Instructor, Harvard Medical School, Boston, Massachusetts, Brockton VA Medical Center, Brockton, Massachusetts

Richard Saitz, MD, MPH
Chair and Professor of Community Health Sciences, Department of Community Health Sciences\Boston University School of Public Health, Professor of Medicine, Clinical Addiction Research and Education Unit, Section of General Internal Medicine, Department of Medicine, Boston Medical Center and Boston University School of Medicine, Boston, Massachusetts

John B. Saunders, MA, MB BChir, MD, FRACP, FAChAM
Consultant Physician in Internal Medicine and Addiction Medicine, Center for Youth Substance Abuse Research, University of Queensland, Brisbane, Brisbane, Queensland, Australia, Professor, Faculty of Medicine, University of Sydney, Sydney, New South Wales, Australia

Samantha P. Schiavon, MA
Department of Psychiatry and Behavioral Neurobiology, University of Alabama School of Medicine, Birmingham, Alabama

Sidney H. Schnoll, MD, PhD
Vice President, Pharmaceutical Risk Management Services, Pinney Associates, Westport, Connecticut

Chamindi Seneviratne, MD
Assistant Professor, Department of Psychiatry, Division for Addiction Research and Treatment, Institute for Genome Sciences, University of Maryland School of Medicine, Baltimore, Maryland

Luisa Sestito, MD
Internal Medicine Resident, Department of Internal Medicine and Gastroenterology, Catholic University of Rome, Alcohol Use Disorder and Alcohol Related Disease Unit, Department of Internal Medicine and Gastroenterology, Fondazione Policlinico Universitario A. Gemelli IRCCS Research Hospital, Rome, Italy

Yu-Chih Shen, MD, PhD
Director, Department of Psychiatry, Hualien Tzu Chi Hospital, Buddhist Tzu Chi Medical Foundation, Associate Professor, School of Medicine, Tzu-Chi University, Hualien, Taiwan

Shiva M. Singh, PhD
Professor, Molecular Genetics Unit, Department of Biology, Western University, London, Ontario, Canada

Rajita Sinha, PhD
Professor, Department of Psychiatry, Yale University School of Medicine, New Haven, Connecticut

Rainer Spanagel, PhD
Professor, Department of Psychopharmacology, Central Institute of Mental Health, University of Heidelberg, Mannheim, Germany

Scott F. Stoltenberg, PhD
Associate Professor, Department of Psychology, University of Nebraska-Lincoln, Lincoln, Nebraska

Steve Sussman, PhD
Professor, Departments of Preventive Medicine and Psychology, Institute for Health Promotion and Disease Prevention Research, School of Social Work, Keck School of Medicine, University of Southern California, Alhambra, California

Joji Suzuki, MD
Assistant Professor of Psychiatry, Harvard Medical School, Director, Division of Addiction Psychiatry, Department of Psychiatry, Brigham and Women's Hospital, Boston, Massachusetts

Robert Tait, PhD
Senior Research Fellow, National Drug Research Institute, Faculty of Health Sciences, Curtin University, Perth, Western Australia, Australia

Nilesh S. Tannu, BDDS, MS
Department of Psychiatry and Behavioral Sciences, McGovern Medical School, The University of Texas Health Sciences Center at Houston, Houston, Texas

Claudia Tarli, MD
Internal Medicine Resident, Department of Internal Medicine and Gastroenterology, Catholic University of Rome, Alcohol Use Disorder and Alcohol Related Disease Unit, Department of Internal Medicine and Gastroenterology, Fondazione Policlinico Universitario A. Gemelli IRCCS Research Hospital, Rome, Italy

Faye S. Taxman, PhD
Professor, Center for Advancing Correctional Excellence!, George Mason University, Fairfax, Virginia

Christine Timko, PhD
Senior Research Career Scientist and Clinical Professor (Affiliated), Center for Innovation to Implementation, Stanford University School of Medicine and Department of Veterans Affairs Health Care System, Menlo Park, California

Nassima Ait Daoud Tiouririne, MD
Professor, Department of Psychiatry and Neurobehavioral Sciences, University of Virginia School of Medicine, Charlottesville, Virginia

J. Scott Tonigan, PhD
Professor, Department of Psychology, University of New Mexico, Albuquerque, New Mexico

Alison Trinkoff, RN, ScD, FAAN
Professor, Department of Family and Community Health, University of Maryland School of Nursing, Baltimore, Maryland

Raihan K. Uddin, PhD
Director, Undergraduate Lab Operations, Department of Biology, Western University, London, Ontario, Canada

Gabriele Angelo Vassallo, MD, PhD
Internal Medicine Specialist, Department of Internal Medicine, Barone Lombardo Hospital, Canicattì (AG), Italy, Alcohol Use Disorder and Alcohol Related Disease Unit, Department of Internal Medicine and Gastroenterology, Fondazione Policlinico Universitario A. Gemelli IRCCS Research Hospital, Rome, Italy

Michelle Vaughan, PhD
Associate Professor, School of Professional Psychology, Wright State University, Dayton, Ohio

Frank Vocci, PhD
President and Senior Research Scientist, Friends Research Institute, Inc., Baltimore, Maryland

Christopher C. Wagner, PhD
Associate Professor, Department of Rehabilitation Counseling, Virginia Commonwealth University, Richmond, Virginia

Michael F. Weaver, MD
Professor, Department of Psychiatry, John P. and Katherine G. McGovern Medical School, The University of Texas Health Science Center at Houston, Houston, Texas

Christopher Welsh, MD
Associate Professor, Division of Addiction Research and Treatment, Department of Psychiatry, University of Maryland School of Medicine, Baltimore, Maryland

Laurence M. Westreich, MD
Clinical Associate Professor, Division of Alcoholism and Drug Abuse, Department of Psychiatry, New York University School of Medicine, New York, New York

Alishia D. Williams, PhD
Conjoint Associate Professor, School of Psychology, New South Wales University, Sydney, New South Wales, Australia

Alicia Wiprovnick, MA
Department of Psychology, University of Maryland, Baltimore County, Baltimore, Maryland

Sarah Yacobi, PhD
Department of Neurobiology, Hebrew University-Hadassah Medical School, Jerusalem, Israel

Chelsie M. Young, PhD
Assistant Professor, Department of Psychology, Rowan University, Glassboro, New Jersey

L. Brendan Young, PhD
Associate Professor, Department of Communication, Western Illinois University, Moline, Illinois

Adnin Zaman, MD
Clinical/Research Fellow, Division of Endocrinology, Metabolism, and Diabetes, Department of Medicine, University of Colorado Anschutz Medical Campus, Aurora, Colorado

Michael J. Zvolensky, PhD
Professor, Department of Psychology and HEALTH Institute, University of Houston, Department of Behavioral Science, The University of Texas MD Anderson Cancer Center, Houston, Texas

Preface

"…The chimeric face of addiction medicine"

In Media Res

At the heart of the matter, as in Homer's *Odysseus,*[1] the motive to compile what hopefully represents the most comprehensive treatise on the fundamentals of addiction and its translation into practice was not based simply on a thirst for knowledge and the desire to learn every relevant shred of science-based information available from the contributors to this book, who are considered among the finest in the field. Rather, the real reason was even more fundamental, and perhaps intellectually curious. It was to dispel the present Socratic[2] argument, now ever present in popular consciousness, that the world is replete with experts on the treatment of addiction and that either true experts are not needed or what they know, either in form or substance, is esoteric and does not do much to alleviate the suffering of those who have the disease.

While shocking, the truth, these critics might say, is that the empirical knowledge that we have amassed in the neurobehavioral and psychosocial science is a far cry from what is delivered in clinical practice, which appears to be mostly unstandardized and not evidence driven. Indeed, how would you even begin a logical search for what are the best treatment centers, what is their actual success rate, and if, and by how much, is there a clear, metric-driven standard to provide the best quality of care?

Indeed, the argument might be, that you only need to pose the question to any layperson, What treatment you would suggest for someone who is an addict? Most of the time, you will get a detailed prescription for treatment and, for good measure, a prognosis that has a Kafkaesque spiral, as in the *Metamorphosis,*[3] toward further decline, repulsion, and hopeless decay. In contrast, that same layperson would not usually dare, or at least hesitate, to respond to a question about how to help someone with cancer or heart disease in the same way, and, most likely, would recommend that the afflicted person seek expert help. These layperson-advised treatments are often not well informed and seem united, as if in a Jung-like *Mandala,*[4] to profess a fixed, almost geometric, pattern of treating every person with an addiction in much the same way. This approach gives little consideration to the fact that addiction is one of the more complex diseases in medicine, with considerable interindividual variation in both presentation and treatment response. Simplistically, the inability to consistently translate neurobehavioral and psychosocial scientific knowledge into modern addiction practice has been the *metier* that has bedeviled the field, stalled progress, and promoted tolerance for poor clinical outcomes.

The addiction profession seems almost to need to wrestle with itself to dispel these misguided beliefs about the fundamental underpinnings of the disease before taking on the promulgation of the most modern and evidence-based approaches to treatment. Indeed, such misinformation has led to our current health care provider–driven opioid epidemic[5] in the United States, and as a consequence, to a plethora of expert panels and task forces designed to address the problem. Identifying the problems seem relatively easy while solutions seem to be ever more complicated, perhaps more than they need be, and costly in terms of time and resources.

In such an environment, true expertise in addiction medicine is not well practiced, and current information is dispersed neither properly nor effectively. Preconceptions and stigma abound, treatment delivery and outcomes are highly variable, and new information on successful evidence-based approaches is not highlighted, disseminated, or followed consistently.

This book presents a sharp retort to the earlier Socratic argument. It aims to demonstrate that the systematic accumulation of knowledge on the science and practice of addiction medicine can be used to arm all in the field with a renewed charge, with some lessons learned. This renewed charge will benefit the health care practitioner who, treating one client at a time, can dispense evidence-based treatment based on current neuropsychosocial knowledge and understanding, thereby promoting a platform to build a true standard of care for treatment.

From the Darkness Into the Light

Not that long ago, the field of addiction medicine was not considered by some authorities to be a part of medicine. Certainly, drugs of abuse were known to have medical consequences, but the "driver" of the disease was the set of behaviors that led to the initiation, maintenance, and progression of substance taking. Indeed, in many current spheres, even within current diagnostic criteria,[6,7] the substance-seeking behavior seems to define the disease in such a way that these nosological entities contain no actual measure of the amount of the substance taken.[8] This would be analogous to a tailor being asked to make a suit or a dress with no measuring tape and all we had to judge about the correctness of the suit or dress was whether or not the client liked it. Paradoxically, however, when it comes to measuring treatment outcome, the historical gold standard for defining success is the measurement of the amount of the substance taken, or rather the lack of it.

Fortunately, new research has shown that in many instances harm-reduction, or a dramatic diminution in the amount of the substance that is consumed, either as an end goal or a path toward eventual abstinence, also is a critical and important measure of success in treatment. Except in specific instances (e.g., pregnant women or individuals with the potential for a catastrophic exacerbation of a medical condition), harm reduction is becoming the focus of treatment for a growing group of experts due to its practicality and perhaps greater sustainability and ecological validity. Notably, these reductions in the consumption of substances that are being abused, perhaps best characterized for alcohol use disorder, have been shown to be associated with important general improvements in health.[9]

The study and application of addiction medicine has, therefore, to not only bridge the paradoxical concepts between its diagnostic criteria and the measurement of treatment outcome but also unite the various elements that form the constellation of the disease state at the level of the individual. This complex state of affairs requires that the underlying foundations of the disease—be they psychosocial or biomedical or a mixture of both—need to be understood firmly before the options for all modalities of treatment, either singly or combined, can be addressed properly.

New vistas to our basic biological understanding of the addiction disease that might apply directly to treatment, such as the fields of precision medicine, the exquisite and constantly growing evidence of diversity within neuronal populations, are featured prominently in this volume to alert the reader about the promising diagnostic and treatment options that are beginning to unfold.

New areas of science, such as vaccine development, are growing to become incorporated in our understanding and treatment of addictive diseases.

New and powerful tools that combine neuroimaging and neuropsychological assessment, such as the ABCD[10] and Healthy BCD studies,[11] will not only enable us to characterize more fully normal brain development—from birth to early adulthood—but might also enable us to fuse more specifically targeted psychosocial and neurobiological treatments.

Promising new information on the utility of transcranial magnetic stimulation and other brain stimulation approaches for addictive disorders, for those that are pharmacological or behavioral or both in nature, is on the near horizon and may offer the advantage of a more metered, portable, and reproduceable approach and effect of treatment.

Finally, the use of artificial intelligence to assist healthcare practitioners in delivering highly optimized patient care, and the deployment of advanced machine-learning technologies, fused with neurobiological information to perform and enhance the precision of neuropsychosocial diagnosis and treatment, may now be within our reach. Notably, even if an individual is presenting for treatment with an index disorder (e.g., alcohol use disorder), it is likely that the person might have other complicating mental disorders, such as anxiety or depression or a medical complication like hypertension. Consider now that groups of individuals with alcohol-use disorder also will likely have a gallimaufry of associated mental or medical conditions. Hence, determining the true diagnosis or diagnoses or the best algorithms for treatment for each individual, based on empirical information that will optimize outcomes, now becomes a complex heuristic exercise.

An Epidemic of Our Own Making Is Defining Us

This book dedicates much effort to detailing current knowledge on the present opioid crises in the United States, which claims about 70,000 lives each year, and the mortality statistic appears to be trending upward[12] despite the colossal medical, scientific, and legislative effort to curb it. For some, it would seem that this crisis is new, yet we know that a similar level of crisis occurred in Victorian England,[13] with even less being known about how to attenuate the epidemic. Yet, that epidemic was expunged through a multifaceted process of social re-engineering, physician education, and legislative action pertaining to the prohibition of opium dens.

We now possess all the tools needed to curb the current opiate epidemic; what is lacking is a consistent adherence to the tenants of an organized and algorithmic approach,[14,15] and several of these are critical. Rigorous and systematic education of current and future health care providers on prescribing medicines for pain relief needs to be provided in medical schools and reinforced as part of a continuing education program that requires the mandatory and regular recertification of all doctors. Doctors in practice need to be required to adhere to current standards of care published by many authorities, including SAMHSA.[16] Doctors prescribing and pharmacist dispensing pain medications need to be monitored in real-time through an organized database that immediately flags apparently excessive, simultaneous, or multi-sited prescriptions for individual clients. Other health care workers such as nurses, dentists, and general practitioners all need to be certified and recertified regularly with respect to pain relief and opiate management. Outcomes based on an agreed set of simple criteria will need to be published for all treatment facilities, with those that consistently fail to meet expectations receiving sanctions or closure. Emergency responders, including those not usually associated with direct health care such as the police and fire services, need to be trained to respond to an overdose and, ideally, have opiate antagonist medication readily available in their vehicles or on their persons while on duty. Coordinated services need to be developed not only in primary care but also in aftercare to maintain addicts in treatment. Legislative efforts should empower drug courts to adopt medication-assisted treatment for opiate addicts and, perhaps controversially, even among those incarcerated. Preventative efforts in schools need to be part of the curriculum, with the education of teachers and support staff to recognize, assess, and provide avenues for the receiving of intervention. If just a fraction of these approaches were delivered and monitored consistently, there would be a significant reduction in the mortality rate from opiate overdoses.[11] New technologies may be helpful, including the approval of efficacious nonopioid medicines and vaccines to both treat and prevent opiate addiction and overdoses, respectively. While we await these new strategies, there is no better time than the present for all health practitioners to be advocates for the best practice treatment of individuals with an addiction.

What's Old Is New Again?

Much of our primary neurotransmitters reside in our gut rather than just in our brains. While people casually talk about their "gut reaction," it is only because of our current understanding of neuronal signaling that we are beginning to appreciate how the microbiome may regulate emotion, a propensity to additive diseases or behaviors, and even their treatment. Admittedly, it is early in this book to elaborate on the promising early findings, but we expect this to be a part of this book in the future.

Diagnostically, there is a growing need for a more fundamental comprehension of the interconnectivity of disease states. Most addictive states overlap in presentation and are co-inherited, some with associated mental and physical disorders. Thus, our linear understanding of disease states will have to give way to a more multidimensional understanding of brain disorders. Indeed, our ability to arrive at reduced-error diagnoses in the addictions will require more rather than less complex insights, and outcomes will need to be understood within this wider concept of disease. That is, individuals may not have dual or triple diagnoses—using present linear terminologies—but a common or a set of associated multidimensional diseases, and the various outcomes simply emanate from disparate trajectories of disease outcome. If we are able to understand addictive diseases using such a conceptual approach, we may be able to bridge the gap of interindividual variation in treatment response and develop true and reduced-error diagnostic "fingerprints."

Back to the Future

This book brings some of the best minds in the field together into a comprehensive treatise that first lays the fundamentals of the scientific knowledge in the basic, translational, associated, and clinical sciences and then tackles how this affects treatments of various addictive diseases. By layering up from the elements of what is known, this book provides a systematic analysis for understanding addictive diseases. In contrast to the earlier Socratic arguments, this book demonstrates that there is no support for the assertion that nonexperts have greater skills in any fundamental aspect of disease understanding compared with experts. The real problem, it would seem, is that there is a tremendous gap between the amassed knowledge and its dissemination into evidence-based treatments. This is a complex problem, perhaps not based entirely on the science itself but on the lack of structure on how this knowledge is implemented. As always, there are multiple streams of solutions, but the more fundamental is the restructuring of the building blocks of the profession within the realm of brain disorders and an approach that fully integrates neuroscience and psychosocial and educational elements. The seeming and, in my view, artificial duality between brain function and behavior that permeates the field needs to be rejected in favor of integration. At a fundamental level, much of the expression of brain disorders, irrespective of severity, is in the manifest behavior, and trying to separate them out, as if they were unrelated, is pointless. Consequently, behavior needs to be understood in the context that it is part and parcel of the brain dysfunction, and both must be understood simultaneously. This is the basis of integrative treatments that include the modalities of both neuroscientific and psychosocial knowledge.

Res ipsa loquitur: Confutatio

In conclusion, this book should provide nourishment for those who thirst for new and integrated knowledge to understand the principles of addictive disease and their treatment. It has been written to be understandable, even to the nonspecialist, but detailed enough to be a reference text for certification in the specialty. Experienced clinicians should find that the chapters provide a practical guide to treatment approaches and associated expected outcomes. Much effort has been made to ensure clarity and to rely most firmly on what is known and to reduce speculative concepts that are still in emergence. With the specialty certifications now being widened to those without a background in the mental health sciences, this book provides the fundamentals to the state-of-the-art application of neurobehavioral as well as psychosocial concepts. Here, in this book, the assembled field of experts speak in one voice to deliver to you their knowledge for your consideration, and hopefully, edification.

Professor Bankole Johnson
Professor of Anatomy and Neurobiology
Professor of Medicine
Professor of Neurology
Professor of Pharmacology
Professor of Psychiatry
University of Maryland School of Medicine

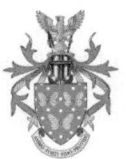

Letters Patent and Crest awarded to Professor Bankole Johnson by the Sovereign, Queen Elizabeth II.

References

1. https://en.wikipedia.org/wiki/Odysseus.
2. https://en.wikipedia.org/wiki/Socratic_method.
3. https://en.wikipedia.org/wiki/The_Metamorphosis#Lost_in_translation.
4. https://www.carl-jung.net/mandala.html.
5. Dasgupta N, Beletsky L, Ciccarone D. Opioid crisis: no easy fix to its social and economic determinants. *Am J Public Health*. 2018;108(2):182–186.
6. American Psychiatric Association. *Diagnostic and Statistical Manual of Mental Disorders*. 5th ed. Washington, DC: APA; 2013:5–25.
7. Johnson BA. FDA and EMA need homology on alcohol outcome measures—Semper: simplicitas est purius modum. *Alcohol Clin Exp Res*. 2017;41(7):1383–1384.
8. Johnson BA. Toward rational, evidence-based, and clinically relevant measures to determine improvement following treatment for alcohol use disorder. *Alcohol Clin Exp Res*. 2017;41(4):703–707.
9. Ritter A, Cameron J. A review of the efficacy and effectiveness of harm reduction strategies for alcohol, tobacco, and illicit drugs. *Drug Alcohol Rev*. 2006;25(6):611–624.
10. National Institutes of Health/National Institute of Drug Abuse. *Longitudinal Study of Adolescent Brain Cognitive Development (ABCD Study)*; 2019. Available at https://www.drugabuse.gov/related-topics/adolescent-brain/longitudinal-study-adolescent-brain-cognitive-development-abcd-study.
11. https://grants.nih.gov/grants/guide/rfa-files/RFA-DA-19-029.html.
12. National Institutes of Health/National Institute of Drug Abuse. *Overdose Death Rates*; 2019. Available at https://www.drugabuse.gov/related-topics/trends-statistics/overdose-death-rates.
13. Milligan B. The opium den in Victorian London. In: Gilman SL, Zhou, eds. *Smoke: A Global History of Smoking*. London: Reaktion Books; 2014:118–125. Available at https://corescholar.libraries.wright.edu/english/124/.
14. The Office of Lt. Governor Boyd K. Rutherford. *Meet Maryland's Heroin Task Force*; 2019. Available at https://governor.maryland.gov/ltgovernor/home/heroin-and-opioid-emergency-task-force/meet-marylands-heroin-task-force/.
15. Maryland Patient Safety Center. *The Governor's Heroin and Opioid Emergency Task Force Final Report Recommendations*; 2019. Available at http://www.marylandpatientsafety.org/documents/medication_safety/2016/cameron.pdf.
16. Substance Abuse and Mental Health Services Administration. *Federal Guidelines for Opioid Treatment Programs*. 2015. https://store.samhsa.gov/system/files/pep15-fedguideotp.pdf.

Contents

†Deceased.

†Deceased.

1

Emerging Health Perspectives

H. WESTLEY CLARK, DEBORAH BOATWRIGHT, AND MATT DAVIS

CHAPTER OUTLINE

Introduction

This chapter addresses a few issues that are emerging as critical health issues with substance use perspectives. First, there is a brief review of the epidemiology of substance use; this is linked to the growing problem of prescription drug abuse. Second, the issue of screening and brief intervention for substance use disorders

(SUDs) is addressed. Then the issue of new technologies as a vehicle for enhancing SUD services is reviewed. Finally, the issue of how to pay for SUD services is reviewed.

The epidemiology of substance use makes it quite clear that clinicians of any stripe will encounter patients or clients who use or misuse alcohol or psychoactive drugs. Therefore, the interrelationship between SUDs, brain function, and treatment outcome should be of interest to the clinician concerned with patient and client health.

Alcohol Use

The National Survey on Drug Use and Health (NSDUH) annually interviews nearly 68,000 persons to establish national estimates of substance use.[9] More than half of Americans 12 years or older report being current drinkers of alcohol in the 2016 NSDUH; this means that almost 127 million people have had at least one drink in the past month. Other than underage drinking, current drinking is not inherently problematic. However, more than one-fifth (24.2%) of persons 12 years or older admit to binge drinking, which the NSDUH defines as five or more drinks on a single occasion for males and four or more drinks for females. Binge drinking is associated with a number of acute adverse events, including motor vehicle accidents, trauma, domestic violence, assaults, homicides, child abuse, suicide, fires, boating accidents, alcohol poisoning, and high-risk activities that threaten the health and well-being of the consumers. Another confounding population of alcohol consumers is the heavy drinking population. It is estimated by the NSDUH that 16.3 million people, or 6.0% of the population, 12 years of age or older admit to heavy drinking (binge drinking on at least 5 days in the past 30 days).

Naturally, alcohol consumption rates vary by—among other things—age, gender, and race/ethnicity. Among young adults 18–25 years of age, consumption rates are the highest in the current use, binge drinking, and heavy alcohol use categories. This age range is also associated with higher risk-taking and the consequences associated with risk-taking. Thus physicians and other clinicians who provide primary and/or emergency room care, or college health care practitioners, are more likely to see patients in this age group for a variety of alcohol-related injuries or conditions.

Among adolescents and young adults under the age of 21, alcohol consumption rises fairly rapidly from 1.4% for those who are 12 or 13 to 39% for those who are between the ages of 18 and 20. Fig. 1.1 shows the various levels of alcohol consumption for individuals 12 years or older by age grouping. It is apparent

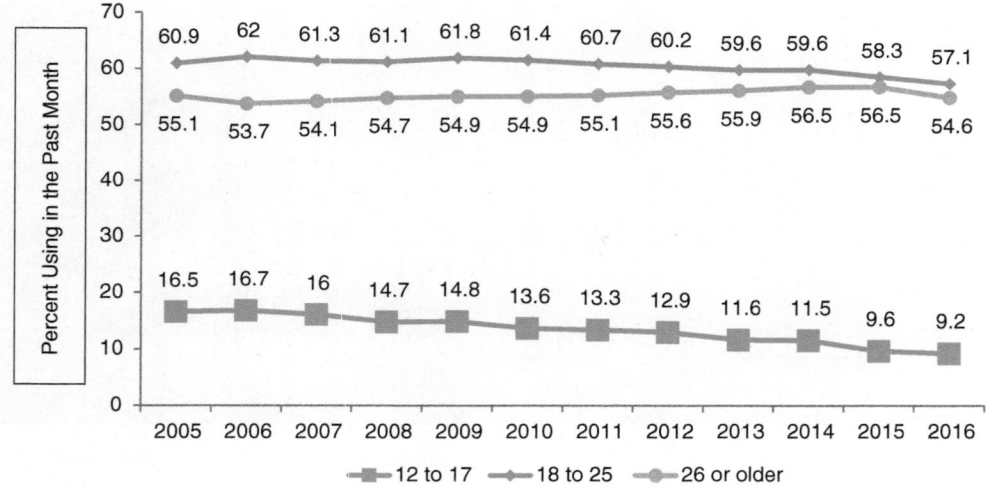

• **Fig. 1.1** Current alcohol use among persons age 12 or older: 2005–2016. (Data from SAMHSA, Center for Behavioral Health Statistics and Quality, National Survey on Drug Use and Health, 2002–2016.)

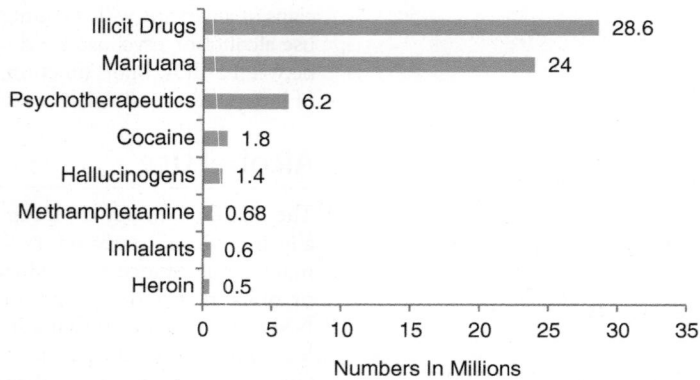

• **Fig. 1.2** Past-month use of specific illicit drugs among persons age 12 or older: 2016. (Data from SAMHSA, Center for Behavioral Health Statistics and Quality, National Survey on Drug Use and Health, 2002–2016.)

from these prevalence rates that late adolescents and young adults are likely to engage in substantial alcohol consumption. Knowing whether alcohol use is related to a presenting physical or psychiatric complaint should be helpful to the clinician. Although many young adults 18- to 25-years-old will visit a clinician for very limited purposes, such as a job- or school-related physical, the prevalence of alcohol use problems in this age range clearly offers the clinician an opportunity to address the issue of alcohol-related medical, social, or behavioral problems. Clinicians should take advantage of such opportunities. In addition, Fig. 1.1 reveals that current alcohol use among youth 12- to 17-years-old has progressively declined from 2006 to 2016.

Illicit Drug Use

In 2016 there were an estimated 28.6 million Americans age 12 or older who admitted to using at least one illicit drug in the past month according to the NSDUH. This represented an estimated 10.6% of the population 12 years or older. For the purposes of the survey, illicit drugs included marijuana/hashish, cocaine (including crack), heroin, hallucinogens, inhalants, or prescription-type psychotherapeutics used nonmedically. Marijuana is the most commonly used illicit drug by Americans, with 24 million people

admitting to past-month use. The second category of prevalent drug use is nontherapeutic or nonmedical use of prescription drugs (Fig. 1.2).

Specific categories of psychotherapeutics include a range of substances such as pain relievers, sedatives, tranquilizers, and stimulants. NSDUH data for persons age 12 or older reveal an elevation of nonmedical use of prescription pain relievers (Fig. 1.3).

It has been recognized that use of prescription opioids is associated with higher rates of abuse and dependence than use of other substances, as well as increased mortality.[26] The misuse of benzodiazepines in combination with therapeutic opioids can create problems with respiration and cardiac functioning, predisposing to respiratory depression or cardiac dysrhythmia, leading to death.

Age Variations

However, as with alcohol use and misuse, there are age variations in illicit drug use. NSDUH data indicate that there has been a progressive decline, with some fluctuation, in the prevalence of drug use among adolescents age 12–17 years of age since 2011 (Fig. 1.4A–B). NSDUH data are supported by the Monitoring the Future Data, with both surveys revealing the same basic trends.[33]

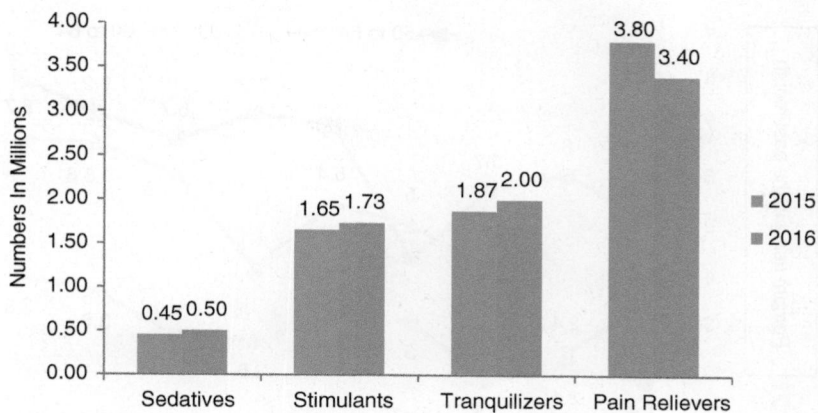

• **Fig. 1.3** Past-month nonmedical use of prescription drugs (psychotherapeutics) among persons age 12 or older: 2015–2016. (Data from SAMHSA, Center for Behavioral Health Statistics and Quality, National Survey on Drug Use and Health, 2002–2016.)

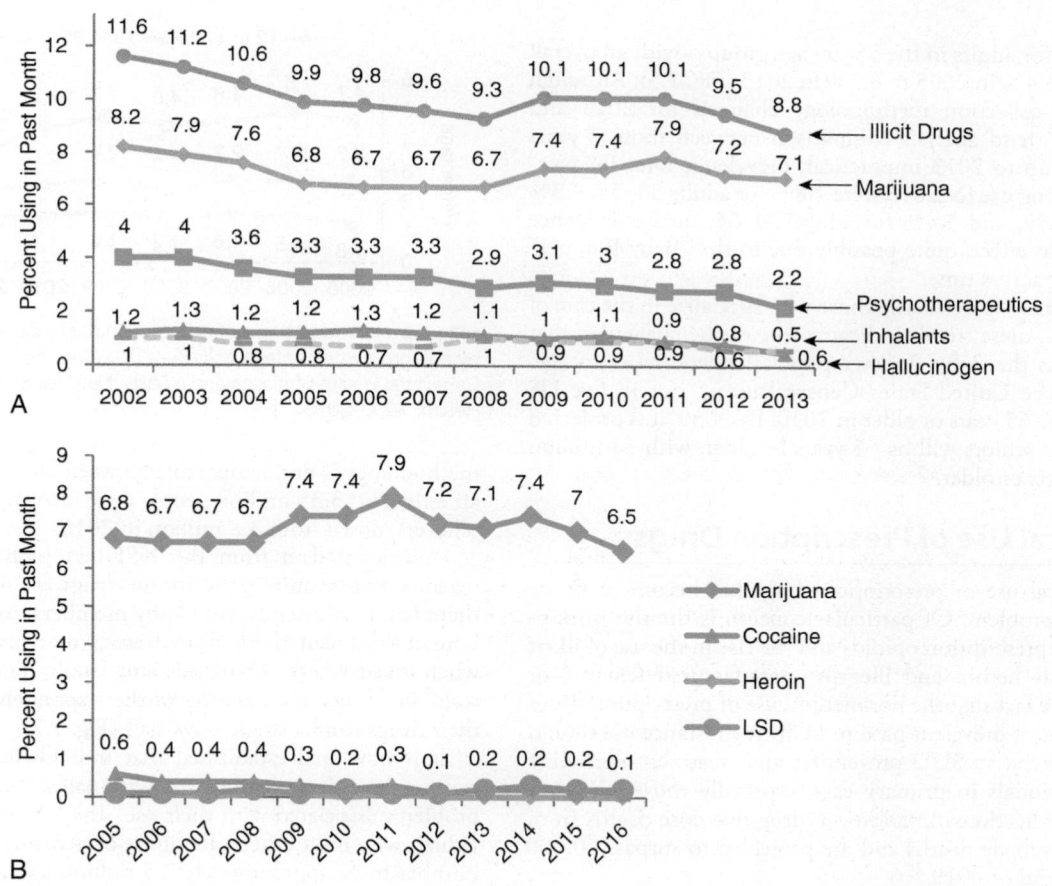

• **Fig. 1.4** Past-month use of selected illicit drugs among persons 12 years or older: percent, 2002–2013. (A) Data from SAMHSA, Center for Behavioral Health Statistics and Quality, National Survey on Drug Use and Health, 2002–2013. (B) Past-month use of selected illicit drugs among youths age 12–17: 2005–2016. (Data from SAMHSA, Center for Behavioral Health Statistics and Quality, National Survey on Drug Use and Health, 2002–2016.)

It is important for primary care clinicians to recognize that the progress being made in reducing substance use of adolescents has not resulted in an elimination of the problem of drug use. Although substantial progress has been made, much effort needs to be exercised to keep up the pressure to continue to reduce the use of such substances among adolescents.

Another interesting observation seen in the 2016 NSDUH data involves adults 50–59 years of age. According to the survey data, this age group showed an irregular increasing trend between 2005 and 2013 regarding current illicit drug use. For adults ages 50–54, illicit drug use (past month) increased from 5.2% in 2005 to 7.9% in 2013. There was a greater increase in past-month use

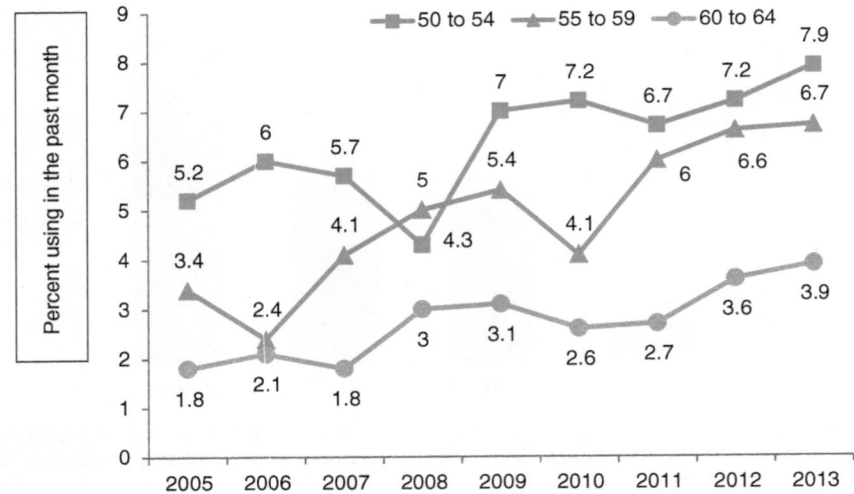

• **Fig. 1.5** Past-month illicit drug use among adults age 50–64: 2005–2013. (Data from SAMHSA, Center for Behavioral Health Statistics and Quality, National Survey on Drug Use and Health, 2002–2013.)

of illicit drugs for adults in the 55–59 age group—with an overall increase from 3.4% in 2005 to 6.7% in 2013 (Fig. 1.5). Although the NSDUH collection methodology changed for 2015 and 2016, making trend analysis comparison between those 2 years and the years up to 2013 impractical, prevalence rates for past-month illicit drug use for 2016 were 7.8% for adults 50–54, 9.3% for adults 55–59, and 5.4% for adults 60–64, further evidence of an important effect, quite possibly due to the "Baby Boomer" cohort moving across time.

For physicians—particularly those who specialize in the care of older patients—these trends indicate some of the challenges that may develop as the Baby Boomer population continues to age. According to the United States Census Bureau, one in five US residents will be 65 years or older in 2030. By 2050, it is projected that 84 million seniors will be 65 years or older, with 18 million of them 85 years or older.[65]

Nonmedical Use of Prescription Drugs

The nonmedical use of prescription drugs has become a major public health problem. Of particular concern is the rise in nonmedical use of prescription opioids and the rise in the use of illicit opioids such as heroin and illegally manufactured fentanyl or carfentanil. The fact that the nonmedical use of prescription drugs is the second most prevalent pattern of illicit substance use should be of great interest to SUD prevention and treatment specialists and to professionals in primary care, especially those who prescribe such medications. In addition, drug overdose deaths from exceed motor vehicle deaths and are projected to surpass 70,000 deaths by the end of 2019.[47]

As with alcohol misuse, there are age variations in the nonmedical use of prescription drugs. NSDUH data show a relatively stable rate in the nonmedical use of pain relievers in the past month, from 1.9% to 1.7% over 2005–2013. However, in young adults 18–25 years of age, there has been a gradual *decrease* in the nonmedical use of prescription drugs from 4.7% to 3.3% for the same period. Concomitantly, there has been a gradual increase for adults 26 or older from 1.3% to 1.5% during that period. In 2013 alone, an estimated 4.5 million individuals were currently misusing prescription pain relievers (Fig. 1.6). However, although the

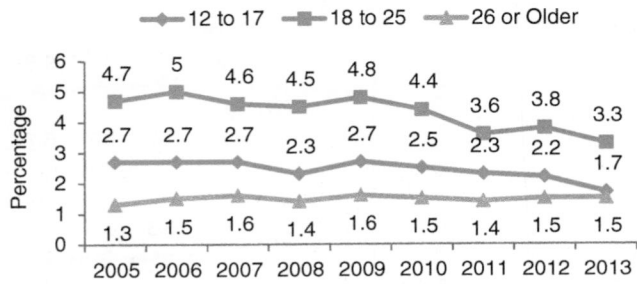

• **Fig. 1.6** Nonmedical use of prescription pain relievers in the past month, by age group: percentages, 2005–2013. (Data from SAMHSA, Center for Behavioral Health Statistics and Quality, National Survey on Drug Use and Health, 2002–2013.)

methodology is not comparable between 2013 and 2016, in 2016 an estimated 3.35 million people were identified as misusing pain relievers, down from 3.8 million in 2015.

Additional data from the NSDUH highlight that 40% of persons who acquire prescription drugs for nonmedical use get them free from friends and family members. Another 12.6% have bought or stolen them from friends or relatives. Furthermore, when asked where the friends and family members got the prescription drugs, the majority of the respondents reported getting their drugs from a single physician (Fig. 1.7).

It is now well established that individuals are not just consuming prescription drugs "recreationally." Many are developing problems associated with their use. The NSDUH looked at individuals who meet criteria for abuse or dependence and found that number to be approximately 2.5 million age 12 or older. Within the prescription drug category, prescription pain relievers account for 1.75 million of the individuals who meet criteria for abuse or dependence, making prescription drugs the second most common category of drugs of misuse and the second most common category of abuse and dependence.

Thus it is clear that the misuse of prescription drugs is a public health problem of importance. In 2011 the Centers for Disease and Prevention (CDC) declared prescription drug abuse an epidemic. In addition during the same year, the Office of National Drug Control Policy (ONDCP) released a report entitled "Epidemic:

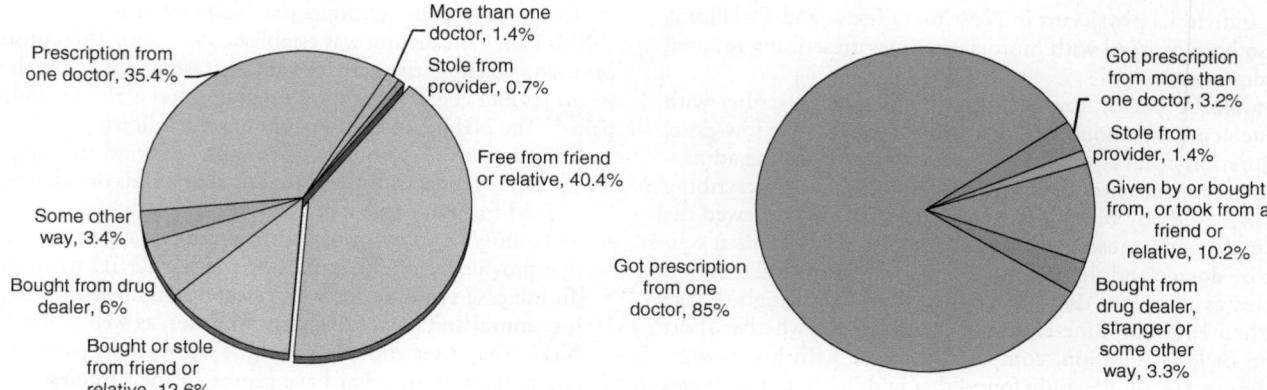

• **Fig. 1.7** Source where pain relievers were obtained for most recent nonmedical use among past-year users age 12 or older: 2016. Note: Totals may not sum to 100% because of rounding or because suppressed estimates are not shown. (Data from SAMHSA, Center for Behavioral Health Statistics and Quality, National Survey on Drug Use and Health, 2016.)

Responding to America's Prescription Drug Abuse Crisis"; the ONDCP also promulgated a Prescription Drug Abuse Prevention Plan, which focused on (1) education, (2) monitoring, (3) proper medication disposal, and (4) enforcement. However, the problem of misuse of prescription drugs is complicated by the therapeutic need for the various agents, especially pain relievers, for clinical purposes. There does not seem to be any question about the need to treat pain adequately. In fact, NSDUH data reveals that in 2016, 62% of those who misused prescription pain relievers in the past year used those medications in their last episode of misuse to relieve physical pain.[9] It is not clear whether this physical pain was associated with withdrawal or with the undertreatment of nonwithdrawal-related physical pain.

Among the implications of these findings are that prescribers of prescription drugs must assume some role in the education of patients or clients about the appropriate use of prescription drugs, and that the appropriate disposition of unused prescription drugs by patients and clients needs to be emphasized. Because prescription drug misuse is intimately tied to the therapeutic use of critical medications, strategies that simply address drug dealing, Internet sales, misprescribing clinicians, and doctor shopping are inadequate. Forty-nine US states and the District of Columbia have prescription drug monitoring program (PDMP) laws as a way of tracking the behavior of both patients and prescribers.[40] Missouri's governor, by executive order, created a statewide PDMP, making Missouri the last state to adopt a PDMP.[29]

PDMPs continue to evolve with information technology. Some programs are hampered because they are not operating in real time but promise to become real time in the future. Another limitation of PDMPs is that they are often limited to specific states and do little to address patient or physician behavior across state jurisdictional lines. Furthermore, PDMPs may not be as effective in reducing doctor shopping or reducing diversion of controlled substances as intended.[37] Nevertheless, it appears that PDMPs are associated with reductions in opioid use among disabled and older Medicare beneficiaries.[39]

As suggested earlier, the category of prescription drugs that ranks highest in abuse is that of analgesics, particularly pain relievers in the Controlled Substances Act (CSA) Schedules II and III.[16] The treatment of pain in American society is the fundamental basis for the use of controlled substances, and access to appropriate pain

medication is essential. Strategies designed to monitor the prescribing of pain relievers were historically not proffered as efforts to limit access to pain medication, but to discourage the misprescribing of pain medication. However, among prescribing practitioners the fear of legal consequences may have a "chilling" effect.

An older study by Goldenbaum et al. noted that only 725 physicians between 1998 and 2006 were criminally charged and/or administratively reviewed for offenses associated with the prescribing of opioid analgesics.[28] This represented only 0.1% of the estimated 691,873 patient-care physicians active in 2003. Furthermore, the study concluded that "Practicing physicians, including Pain Medicine specialists, have little objective cause for concern about being prosecuted by law enforcement or disciplined by state medical boards in connection with the prescribing of CS [controlled substances] pain medications."[28] However, times have changed.

Both state and federal prosecutors have brought charges against physicians and other prescribers for questionable pain management practices involving the use of opioid analgesics. In addition, attorneys general have filed claims against at least two pharmaceutical companies. Multiple state and local governments have sued Purdue Pharma, accusing it of deceptive marketing and of convincing physicians that oxycodone (OxyContin) had a low risk of addiction; as early as 2007 Purdue Pharma agreed to pay $634.5 million to resolve a US Department of Justice claim. In addition, in 2017, two companies, McKesson, a pharmaceutical drug distributor, and Mallinckrodt LLC, a pharmaceutical company, were required to pay the US government millions to settle claims that they violated provisions of the CSA and that they failed to design and implement effective systems to detect and report "suspicious orders" for controlled substances. McKesson agreed to pay $150 million and Mallinckrodt agreed to pay $35 million.[20,68]

Although Goldenbaum et al. concluded that physicians have little objective cause for concern, physicians are being held liable for misprescribing opioids and for the deaths of their patients who overdose on opioid analgesics.[28] An analysis of the National Practitioner Data Bank (NPDB), from 2011 to 2014, revealed that the United States Drug Enforcement Administration (DEA) has stepped up its actions against physicians; in 2011 there were 88 such cases, but in 2014, there were 371 cases.[74] Furthermore, in 2015, a California physician was convicted of murder for overprescribing opioid analgesics and sentenced to 30 years to life in prison. Individual physicians in New York, Texas, and Oklahoma have also been charged with murder after overprescribing resulted in overdose deaths.[17]

It should be noted, however, that the average prescriber with a routine acute care population with requirements for low-dose, short-duration opioids should have little to fear from the administrative and legal processes monitoring physician-prescribing behavior. A study by Blue Cross/Blue Shield (BCBS) reviewed the rate of patients diagnosed with opioid use disorders and their opioid use by dosage and duration in 2015, and they found substantial increases in opioid use diagnoses for those with high dosage (more than 100 morphine-equivalent daily doses), whether short duration or long duration, compared to those with low dosage. Furthermore, the BCBS study found that with high dosage, it was the duration of the prescription that produced the highest rate of diagnosed opioid use disorder (OUD); high-dose opioid prescriptions beyond 7 days produced the highest rates of OUDs.[7]

The policy discussion about pain and the use of controlled substances for the management of pain in patients is an important one. With an estimated 50–60 million people within the United States with chronic pain, and a larger estimate of the prevalence of various acute pain syndromes, the availability of appropriate treatment strategies is of critical importance.

The legitimate role of controlled substances in the treatment of the spectrum of pain-related conditions is often discussed. Clinicians are admonished to use clinical guidelines, transparent practices with documentation, and conservative strategies when monitoring patient compliance and dysfunctional patient behavior. Clinicians are also told to anticipate that some percentage of their patients or clients may develop SUDs associated with their treatment regimens or may present to treatment with preexisting SUDs or vulnerabilities.

Prescription opioid dependence is also associated with other psychiatric conditions. Depression and posttraumatic stress disorders are two DSM-5 (*Diagnostic and Statistical Manual of Mental Disorders, Fifth Edition*) diagnoses found to be related to OUDs. Managing co-occurring disorders and chronic pain conditions requires specific treatment strategies that take into account the full spectrum of the patient's conditions.

In 2016, the CDC issued the "CDC Guideline for Prescribing Opioids for Chronic Pain – United States, 2016."[19] These guidelines are recommendations for primary care clinicians who are prescribing opioids for chronic noncancer pain treatment; the guidelines are not for cancer treatment, palliative care, or end-of-life care. The guidelines focus on: "(1) when to initiate or continue opioids for chronic pain; (2) opioid selection, dosage, duration, follow-up, and discontinuation; and (3) assessing risk and addressing harms of opioid use."

In 2017, the Federation of State Medical Boards (FSMB) released an updated version of its "Guidelines for the Chronic Use of Opioid Analgesics."[24] The preamble of the FSMB Guidelines stated that the diagnosis and treatment of pain is integral to the practice of medicine. While noting that the FSMB Guidelines are not a specific standard of care for the safe and evidenced prescribing of opioids for the treatment of chronic, noncancer pain, the FSMB contends that the fact-specific totality of circumstances should govern the decision to use opioids over other pharmacological and nonpharmacological treatment of chronic noncancer pain.

In addition to the CDC and the FSMB, a number of states have promulgated their own guidelines for the use of opioid analgesics for the treatment of pain. Washington State,[71] Arizona,[2] Tennessee,[63] Ohio,[45] Indiana,[30] and Wisconsin[72] are just some examples.

To enhance pain research, the National Institutes of Health (NIH) Pain Consortium was established in 2006. This consortium promotes collaborative activities among researchers across the NIH institutes and centers that have programs and activities addressing pain.[42] The NIH Pain Consortium has the following goals:

- To develop a comprehensive and forward-thinking pain research agenda for the NIH—one that builds on what we have learned from our past efforts.
- To identify key opportunities in pain research, particularly those that provide for multidisciplinary and trans-NIH participation.
- To increase visibility for pain research—both within the NIH intramural and extramural communities, as well as outside the NIH. The latter audiences include our various pain advocacy and patient groups that have expressed their interests through scientific and legislative channels.
- To pursue the pain research agenda through public-private partnerships, wherever applicable. This underscores a key dynamic that has been reinforced and encouraged through the Roadmap process.

In addition to the NIH, the US Department of Health and Human Services (HHS) through the NIH established the Interagency Pain Research Coordinating Committee (IPRCC) to coordinate all pain research efforts within the HHS and across other federal agencies. The IPRCC was instrumental in 2016 in promulgating the National Pain Strategy, which outlined a coordinated plan for reducing the burden of chronic pain that affects millions of Americans. The Implementation of the National Pain Strategy includes such activities as (1) professional education and training, (2) public education and communication, (3) disparities, (4) prevention and care, (5) service delivery and payment, and (6) population research.[43]

Opioid Overdose Deaths

By the end of 2015, drug overdoses accounted for 52,404 deaths in the United States; this included 33,091 deaths (63.1%) that involved an opioid.[49] From 2014 to 2015, the death rate from synthetic opioids other than methadone, which includes fentanyl, increased by 72.2%, and heroin death rates increased by 20.6%.

The issue of the pain management and the appropriate use of opioids in a therapeutic context has been complicated by the advent of an increase in the use of illicitly manufactured fentanyl and carfentanil, in addition to heroin use. Fentanyl and its analog carfentanil were estimated to account for the single largest category of opioid overdose deaths in 2017, with an estimated 20,000 deaths, or 38% of all opioid deaths. The precursor to the wave of opioid overdoses and overdose deaths was thought to be the increase in prescribing of prescription opioids, which occurred even though there has been no change in the amount of pain experienced by people in the United States.[46]

The hue and cry about opioid overdoses resulted in actions by the US Congress discussed later in this chapter, and by the President of the United States. In 2017, President Trump appointed a Commission on Combating Drug Addiction and the Opioid Crisis. The Interim Report of that Commission called upon the President to declare a national emergency under either the Public Health Service Act or the Stafford Act.[46] In addition to calling for a National Emergency, the Interim Report called for, among other things to:

1. Rapidly increase treatment capacity. Grant waiver approvals for all 50 states to quickly eliminate barriers to treatment resulting from the federal Institutions for Mental Diseases (IMD) exclusion within the Medicaid program.

2. Mandate prescriber education initiatives with the assistance of medical and dental schools across the country to enhance prevention efforts. Mandate medical education training in opioid prescribing and risks of developing an SUD by amending the CSA to require all DEA registrants to take a course in proper treatment of pain. HHS should work with partners to ensure additional training opportunities, including continuing education courses for professionals.

3. Immediately establish and fund a federal incentive to enhance access to medication-assisted treatment (MAT). Require that all modes of MAT are offered at every licensed MAT facility and that those decisions are based on what is best for the patient. Partner with the NIH and the industry to facilitate testing and development of new MAT treatments.

4. Better align, through regulation, patient privacy laws specific to addiction with the Health Insurance Portability and Accountability Act (HIPAA) to ensure that information about SUDs be made available to medical professionals treating and prescribing medication to a patient.

5. Provide model legislation for states to allow naloxone dispensing via standing orders, as well as requiring the prescribing of naloxone with high-risk opioid prescriptions; we must equip all law enforcement in the United States with naloxone to save lives.

6. Prioritize funding and manpower to the Department of Homeland Security (DHS) Customs and Border Protection, the Department of Justice Federal Bureau of Investigation (FBI), and the DEA to quickly develop fentanyl detection sensors and disseminate them to federal, state, local, and tribal law enforcement agencies. Support federal legislation to staunch the flow of deadly synthetic opioids through the US Postal Service (USPS).

7. Provide federal funding and technical support to states to enhance interstate data sharing among state-based PDMPs to better track patient-specific prescription data and support regional law enforcement in cases of controlled substance diversion. Ensure federal health care systems, including veteran's hospitals, participate in state-based data sharing.

8. Enforce the Mental Health Parity and Addiction Equity Act (MHPAEA) with a standardized parity compliance tool to ensure that health plans cannot impose less favorable benefits for mental health and substance use diagnoses versus physical health diagnoses.

Notice how broad is the spectrum of efforts recommended to address the issue of opioid misuse and how focused are those efforts on engaging the medical establishment and changing its clinical behavior with regard to prescription opioids.

Naloxone and Opioid Overdose

As the President's Commission on Combating Drug Addiction and the Opioid Crisis observes, naloxone is a drug that can be used to reverse opioid overdose. The increase in opioid-related deaths has prompted the public health community to provide naloxone to at-risk individuals and their families. Community-based opioid-overdose prevention programs and first responders, such as police officers, have equipped themselves with naloxone in order to save the lives of individuals who have consumed opioids to the point of respiratory depression leading to coma. In 2014, the Substance Abuse and Mental Health Services Administration (SAMHSA) published an Opioid Overdose Prevention Toolkit that serves as a foundation for educating and training of (1) communities, (2) prescribers of opioid pain medications, (3) first responders, (4) patients who have been prescribed opioid medications, and (5) individuals and family members who have experienced an opioid overdose. Clinicians concerned about opioid overdose as a risk from prescribing opioids should access this overdose toolkit for themselves and their patients.[58]

Over the past decade, substantial research has been done to map out the dimensions of the prescription drug misuse problem. Clinical treatment strategies for patients with pain who require controlled substances will still need to be refined, whereas substance abuse prevention and treatment programs will need to develop targeted treatment protocols.

As previously mentioned, recent survey data indicate that approximately 40% of diverted pain relievers are obtained free from friends and family members. Another 12.6% of individuals either bought their pain relievers from a friend or a relative, or stole their pain relievers from a friend or relative. In short, almost 53% of individuals who admit to the nonmedical use of pain relievers got them from friends or family. This means that there is a substantial cultural component to prescription drug misuse. The attitudes and values of the community constitute a major component of the problem. This clearly means that public health and medical efforts need to be directed toward altering community attitudes as well as provider attitudes.

Clinicians, researchers, and others who are interested in the public health implications of prescription drug abuse should obviously focus more energy on addressing the social and behavioral features of the social network aspects of prescription drug transactions. An emphasis on appropriate prescribing, with minimal excess, and appropriate storage with limited access, should be incorporated into clinician-patient interactions. In addition, clinicians should advise patients or clients about the appropriate disposal of excess controlled substances; this enlists the patient further in accepting responsibility for the medication and enhances the awareness that controlled substances can be dangerous if misused. SUD specialists should also be aware of the increase in prevalence of prescription drug abuse, with a particular recognition that prescription opioids are a growing problem among individuals with abuse and dependence who might present for treatment.

Legislative, Regulatory, and Community Controls Over Opioid Prescribing

In the previous edition of this book, it was noted that clinicians in general should be aware that an ongoing problem of prescription drug misuse, particularly with narcotic analgesics, will produce calls for increased regulation and control of prescribing authority and patient access.

With one in four adults in the United States saying that they had a day-long bout of pain in the past month, and 1 in 10 saying that the pain lasted a year or more,[10] the issue of treatment of pain in this country is quite real. These numbers amount to 76 million people who have had a day-long bout of pain in the past month and 30.5 million who have had pain lasting a year or more. With 5.2 million people admitting to the nonmedical use of opioid pain relievers, the larger number of individuals potentially affected by legal or regular constraints of the prescription of controlled substances for therapeutic purpose would be those who have pain, not those who misuse or divert pain medications.

Common chronic pain complaints include headache, low back pain, cancer pain, arthritis pain, neurogenic pain (pain resulting from damage to the peripheral nerves or to the CNS itself), and psychogenic pain (pain not due to past disease or injury or any visible sign of damage inside or outside the nervous system). Whether all of these conditions require the use of specific opioid medications for any specific patient should be determined by research and clinical evidence. However, concerns have produced demands for change.

In 2012, the US Food and Drug Administration (FDA) published the extended-release (ER)/long-acting (LA) Opioid Analgesic Risk Evaluation and Mitigation Strategy (REMS). This was followed by the 2017 extension of REMS for immediate-release (IR) opioid analgesics.[70] The goal of this REMS is to reduce serious adverse outcomes resulting from inappropriate prescribing, misuse, and abuse of opioid analgesics while maintaining patient access to pain medications. Adverse outcomes of concern include addiction, unintentional overdose, and death. The REMS program requires health professional training in pain management, including the principles of acute and chronic pain management, nonpharmacologic treatments for pain, and pharmacologic treatments for pain (both nonopioid analgesic and opioid analgesic).

In 2014, the DEA rescheduled all hydrocodone combination products from Schedule III to Schedule II of the CSA; this action followed a public hearing that was required by Section 1139 of Public Law 112-144, the FDA Safety and Innovation Act (FDASIA) of 2012. In addition, the DEA put together its DEA 360 Strategy, which involves coordinated law enforcement operations targeting all levels of drug trafficking organizations and violent gangs that supply drugs to our neighborhoods; engaging drug manufacturers, wholesalers, practitioners, and pharmacists through diversion control to increase awareness of the opioid epidemic and encourage responsible prescribing practices, and use of opioid painkillers throughout the medical community; community outreach and partnership with local organizations following enforcement operations; and equipping and empowering communities to fight the opioid epidemic.[21]

Another strategy proposed by the DEA is to reduce the amount of controlled substance that may be manufactured in the United States. Schedule II opioid pain relievers such as oxycodone, hydrocodone, oxymorphone, hydromorphone, morphine, and fentanyl would be reduced by an average of 10% in 2019. Of interest, the DEA reports that the demand for these opioid medicines has dropped apparently as a result of state monitoring—using, among other things, PDMPs.[22,25]

Medication-Assisted Treatment Prescription Drug and Opioid Addiction Grant Program

In response to the growing opioid epidemic, in 2015, SAMHSA issued a grant program called the Medication-Assisted Treatment Prescription Drug and Opioid Addiction (MAT-PDOA) program. MAT-PDOA provides funding to states to:
- Enhance or expand their treatment service systems to increase access to MAT by building capacity.
- Provide MAT and recovery services that are accessible, effective, comprehensive, coordinated, and evidence-based.

Target populations include people with OUDs who are seeking or receiving MAT, with a particular focus on racial, ethnic, sexual, and gender-identity minority groups. Examples of some of these populations include pregnant and parenting women, people in the criminal justice system, veterans, and rural communities.[62]

The 2015 cohort of the MAT-PDOA grantees included only 11 states, which divided $12 million for this effort. The 2016 cohort of the MAT-PDOA grantees included another 11 states, with funding levels from $950,000 to $1 million.

Comprehensive Addiction and Recovery Act

In addition to the actions of the HHS to expand the number of patients that a physician can see, the Comprehensive Addiction and Recovery Act (CARA) of 2016, Public Law 114-198, made changes that were designed to respond to the opioid epidemic. CARA is a comprehensive authorization bill that ultimately got linked to a major appropriations bill, the 21st Century Cures Act discussed later.

CARA has nine titles that cover a wide range of issues: (1) Title I covers prevention and education; (2) Title II covers law enforcement and treatment; (3) Title III covers treatment and recovery; (4) Title IV covers a Government Accountability Office (GAO) Report on Recovery and Collateral Consequences; (5) Title V covers addiction and treatment services for women, families, and veterans; (6) Title VI covers state demonstration grants for comprehensive opioid abuse response; (7) Title VII covers miscellaneous provisions such as partial refills of Schedule II controlled substances and Good Samaritan assessments; (8) Title VIII deals with the protection of classified information in federal court challenges under the Foreign Narcotics Kingpin Designation Act; and (9) Title IX covers the Department of Veterans Affairs (VA) with four subtitles.[15]

Although the full act is too voluminous to cover here, there are several key provisions that are germane to the theme of this chapter. Section 101 of Title I authorized the creation of a Pain Management Best Practices Inter-Agency Task Force made up of a wide range of entities including representatives from the HHS, VA, the Department of Defense (DOD), the ONDCP, physicians, dentists, nonphysician prescribers, pharmacists, pain researchers, patient advocates, and patients; this task force has a 2-year term. A draft report describing preliminary recommendations of the Task Force will be finalized and submitted to Congress in 2019.

Section 107 of Title I, Improving Access to Overdose Treatment, authorized the Secretary of the HHS to award grants of up to $200,000 per year to federally qualified health centers (FQHCs), opioid treatment programs (OTPs), or any practitioner waivered to prescribe buprenorphine to establish a naloxone coprescription program, train health care providers on naloxone coprescribing, purchase naloxone, offset copayments for naloxone, or establish protocols to connect patients who have experienced an overdose with appropriate treatment.

Section 110 of Title I, Opioid Overdose Reversal Medication Access and Education program, authorized the HHS Secretary to make grants to states to implement strategies for pharmacists to dispense naloxone pursuant to a standing order and to develop naloxone training materials for the public.

Section 201 of Title II, Comprehensive Opioid Abuse Grant Program, authorized $103 million to the DOJ for a comprehensive opioid abuse grant program for alternatives to incarceration. Section 203 of Title II, Prescription Drug Take Back Expansion, authorized the expanding or making available disposal sites for unwanted prescription medications.

Section 301 of Title III, Evidence-based Prescription Opioid and Heroin Treatment and Interventions Demonstration, authorizes the HHS Secretary to award grants to state substance abuse agencies, local governments, and nonprofit organizations in areas with high rates of or rapid increases in heroin or other opioid use to expand the availability of MAT. It authorizes $25 million for each fiscal year between 2017 and 2021.

Section 302 of Title III, Building Communities of Recovery, authorizes the HHS Secretary to award $1 million to be used for grants to recovery community organizations to enable them to develop, expand, and enhance recovery services. However, the federal share of the costs of a program funded by the grant may not exceed 50%.

Section 303 of Title III, Medication-Assisted Treatment for Recovery from Addiction, makes several changes to the law regarding office-based opioid addiction treatment with buprenorphine. Specifically, it:

- Expands prescribing privileges to nurse practitioners (NPs) and physician assistants (PAs) for 5 years (until October 1, 2021). NPs and PAs must complete 24 hours of training to be eligible for a waiver to prescribe and must be supervised by or work in collaboration with a qualifying physician if required by state law. The HHS Secretary has 18 months to issue updated regulations governing office-based opioid addiction treatment to include NPs and PAs.
- Gives the HHS Secretary the authority to exclude from the patient limit those patients to whom medications are directly administered.
- Allows states to lower the patient limit and allows states to require practitioners to comply with additional practice setting, education, or reporting requirements. States may not lower the patient limit below 30.
- Directs the HHS Secretary to review every 3 years the provision of opioid addiction treatment services in the United States and to submit a report to Congress, including an assessment of whether there is a need to change the patient limit.

Section 501 of Title V, Improving Treatment for Pregnant and Postpartum Women, reauthorizes a grant program for residential opioid addiction treatment of pregnant and postpartum women and their children and creates a pilot program for state substance abuse agencies to address identified gaps in the continuum of care, including nonresidential treatment services.

Section 601 of Title VI, State Demonstration Grants for Comprehensive Opioid Abuse Response, authorizes the HHS Secretary to award grants to states to establish a response plan to the opioid epidemic. The plan may include:

- Education efforts related to opioid use, treatment, and addiction recovery, including education of medical students, residents, physicians, and other controlled substances prescribers.
- Establishing, maintaining, or improving a PDMP.
- Expanding the availability of prescription opioid addiction treatment.
- Developing, implementing, and expanding efforts to prevent opioid overdose deaths.
- Advancing education and awareness of the public regarding the dangers of opioid misuse, safe medication disposal, and detection of early signs of opioid addiction.

Although CARA authorizes a number of new and innovative programs, it is not an appropriations bill. Thus it was not until the 21st Century Cures Act was passed and made into law in December of 2016 that resources were genuinely available to foster change. However, with respect to buprenorphine, the inclusion of appropriate NPs and PAs into the ranks of qualified prescribers promises to expand the number of clinicians available to prescribe

the agent to those who need that medication. It should be noted that CARA only gave those NPs and PAs independent authority to prescribe buprenorphine in those jurisdictions where the right to practice independently existed and where the authority to prescribe Schedule II, III, or IV drugs was a part of that independent right.

21st Century Cures Act

The 21st Century Cures Act, Public Law 114-255, signed into law in December of 2016, is an important appropriations law that is divided into three divisions:

- Division A: 21st Century Cures
- Division B: Helping Families in Mental Health Crisis
- Division C: Increasing Choice, Access, and Quality in Health Care for Americans

Of the three divisions, several titles, and subtitles, while not discounting the importance of the other provisions, only several are of immediate interest to this chapter. Section 103 of Title I of Division A provides for an account for funding to the states. It provides for $1 billion over 2 years for grants to states to supplement opioid abuse prevention and treatment activities, such as improving PDMPs, implementing prevention activities, training for health care providers, and expanding access to opioid treatment programs. It provides for ensuring accountability without increasing burden on states by requiring grantees to report on activities funded by the grant in the substance abuse block grant report.[64]

Title VI of Division B of the 21st Century Cures Act, otherwise known as the Helping Families in Mental Health Crisis Act of 2016, focuses on the reorganization of the SAMHSA. Of note here is that it changes the top leadership of that agency from an administrator to an Assistant Secretary.

It requires the Assistant Secretary to, among other things:

- Work with relevant agencies of the HHS on integrating mental health promotion and SUD prevention with general health promotion and disease prevention, and integrating mental and SUD treatment services with physical health treatment services;
- Use by SAMHSA programs of evidence-based and promising best practices for prevention, treatment, and recovery support services for individuals with mental health and SUDs,
- Collaborate with the Secretary of Defense and the Secretary of Veterans Affairs to improve the provision of mental health and SUD services provided by the DOD and the VA to members of the Armed Forces, veterans, and the family members of such members and veterans, including through the provision of services using the telehealth capabilities of the DOD and VA;
- Advance, through existing programs, the use of performance metrics;
- Work with states and other stakeholders to develop and support activities to recruit and retain a workforce addressing mental health and SUDs.

CARA and the 21st Century Cures Act are important because they created the potential for an expanded substance abuse treatment system focusing on the opioid crisis. SAMHSA released funding for the first phase of the $1 billion appropriation under the 21st Century Cures in April of 2017. This initiative was called the State Targeted Response (STR) grant program. STR funding went to state authorities for subsequent programing involving community-based entities.

State-Targeted Response to the Opioid Crisis Grants (Short Title: Opioid STR)

SAMHSA, the Center for Substance Abuse Treatment (CSAT), and the Center for Substance Abuse Prevention (CSAP) accepted applications for fiscal year (FY) 2017 State Targeted Response to the Opioid Crisis Grants (Short Title: Opioid STR). The program aims to address the opioid crisis by increasing access to treatment, reducing unmet treatment need, and reducing opioid-related overdose deaths through the provision of prevention, treatment, and recovery activities for OUD (including prescription opioids as well as illicit drugs such as heroin). These grants were awarded to states and territories via formula based on unmet need for OUD treatment and drug-poisoning deaths.

Grantees are required to do the following: use epidemiological data to demonstrate the critical gaps in availability of treatment for OUDs in geographic, demographic, and service level terms; utilize evidence-based implementation strategies to identify which system design models will most rapidly address the gaps in their systems of care; deliver evidence-based treatment interventions including medication and psychosocial interventions; and report progress toward increasing availability of treatment for OUDs and reducing opioid-related overdose deaths based on measures developed in collaboration with the HHS.

The STR program supplements activities pertaining to opioids currently undertaken by the state agency or territory and supports a comprehensive response to the opioid epidemic using a strategic planning process to conduct needs and capacity assessments. The results of the assessments identify gaps and resources from which to build upon existing substance use prevention and treatment activities.

STR Grantees were required to describe how they would expand access to treatment and recovery. Grantees were also required to describe how they would advance substance misuse prevention in coordination with other federal efforts such as those funded by the CDC. Grantees must use funding to supplement and not supplant existing opioid prevention, treatment, and recovery activities in their state. Grantees were required to describe how they will improve retention in care, using a chronic care model. To the extent applicable, grantees should align STR prevention efforts with CDC's State's Opioid Program.[62]

Under the STR program, some states received as little as $2 million a year, whereas other states received substantially more. California, for example, received $44 million in extra funding, while Maine received $2 million. Abstracts from the funded STR grants can be found on the SAMHSA website.[62]

Most of the funds under the STR grant were for the use of medications. Thus narcotic treatment programs that use methadone and entities that use buprenorphine or naltrexone for the treatment of OUDs are playing a major role in addressing the opioid epidemic. Physicians and other prescribers will be mobilized to work under the auspices of the STR grant program.

Medication-Assisted Treatment

Methadone

The misuse of opioids can produce abuse and dependence that requires treatment. There are three treatment strategies: use of methadone, use of buprenorphine, and use of naltrexone. Methadone has been used for more than 40 years in the treatment of drug addiction. Its use for treatment of pain has increased in the last 5–10 years. Methadone can cause fatalities in individuals who have not developed any tolerance to opiates: children and adults who accidentally take methadone and those who experience fatal intoxications during the first weeks of treatment or as the result of adjusting a methadone dose. Several risk factors have been identified for methadone mortality: the concomitant use of benzodiazepines and other opioids, and/or alcohol; an elevated risk of some individuals for torsade de pointes; inadequate or erroneous induction dosing and monitoring by physicians, primarily when prescribing methadone for pain; and drug poisoning that occurs as a result of diversion of the drug and its nonmedical use.

It is important for the clinician to recognize that there are differences between prescribed methadone for pain and dispensed methadone for MAT. When methadone is used for pain treatment, no required risk management plan has been required. However, an FDA-required black box label cautions methadone prescribers about (1) addiction, abuse, and misuse; (2) life-threatening respiratory depression; (3) accidental ingestion; (4) life-threatening QT prolongation; (5) neonatal opioid withdrawal syndrome; (6) cytochrome P450 interaction; and (7) risks from concomitant use with benzodiazepines or other CNS depressants.[69] Prescribers who are unfamiliar with methadone should refer to the package insert and pay close attention to the black box warning.

When methadone is used for addiction treatment, the distribution is limited to certified, accredited, and registered programs. There are limits on the initial dose and restrictions on dispensing. The federal government, through SAMHSA, recognizes the following entities as accrediting bodies: Joint Commission on Accreditation of Health Care Organizations, Commission on Accreditation of Rehabilitation Facilities, Council on Accreditation, National Commission on Correctional Health Care, and the state authorities of Missouri and Washington. For detoxification and maintenance of opioid dependence, methadone should be administered in accordance with the treatment standards cited in 42 CFR Section 8, including limitations on unsupervised administration; these federal regulations govern the use of methadone for the treatment of opioid use disorders. In 2016, there are only about 1283 opioid treatment programs licensed by the federal government. Those programs treat approximately 345,443 individuals.

Another public health concern associated with the therapeutic use of opioids is the phenomenon of deaths associated with their use. The CDC reported that there has been a 9.1% decrease in methadone-related deaths between 2014 and 2015.[11]

Within the opioid treatment community, there is concern about the prolongation of the rate-corrected QT interval and its relationship with torsade de pointes, potentially leading to sudden death. As more methadone is being used for the treatment of pain, it has become clear that even in the treatment of opioid dependence some risk exists for patients. Special concern applies to patients who are being induced onto methadone.

SAMHSA's Center for Substance Abuse Treatment convened two expert panels over a 4-year period to examine etiologic factors related to methadone mortality. As a result of those reviews, it became clear that there were those in the medical community who believed that a routine preinduction electrocardiogram screening should occur for all patients to measure the QTc interval and a follow-up electrocardiogram should occur within 30 days and annually thereafter. Particular sensitivity should be exhibited for patients with histories of cardiac dysfunction.[34]

Although this advice is directed to opioid treatment programs, it applies to patients who are receiving methadone for the treatment of chronic pain. Such advice recognizes that there are clinical challenges in the use of opioid medications, such as methadone,

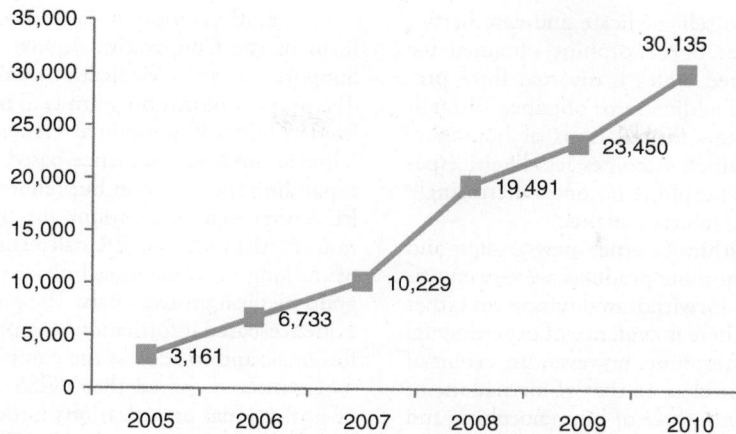

• **Fig. 1.8** Emergency department (ED) visits involving buprenorphine: 2005–2010. (From Substance Abuse and Mental Health Services Administration, Center for Behavioral Health Statistics and Quality. (January 29, 2013). The DAWN Report: Emergency Department Visits Involving Buprenorphine. Rockville, MD.)

that extend beyond the issue of abuse and dependence. A preoccupation with abuse and dependence may detract from the physiological phenomenon that results from the greater use of a class of medications that play a critical role in preserving the public health.

Buprenorphine

Under the Drug Addiction Treatment Act of 2000, qualified physicians can treat individuals addicted to heroin or prescription opioids under a waiver provision administered by SAMHSA and the DEA. To qualify, a physician must meet certain requirements (e.g., trained by a medical organization such as the American Psychiatric Association). Buprenorphine is the only FDA-approved opioid agonist that can be prescribed for this purpose.

In July 2005, Congress removed the 30-patient restriction on medical groups that prescribe buprenorphine for opioid dependence and addiction. The 30-patient limit was then applied to each physician's caseload, rather than to that of the entire clinic. The Office of National Drug Control Policy (ONDCP) Reauthorization Act of 2006 increased the number of individuals a physician can treat with buprenorphine to 100 if specific conditions are met. On July 6, 2016, the HHS issued a final rule that increased access to buprenorphine medications in the office-based setting as authorized under the Controlled Substances Act 21 U.S.C. 823(g)(2).270. The rule allows eligible practitioners to request approval to treat up to 275 patients under section 303(g)(2) of the CSA.

Although approximately 443,000 primary care physicians practice medicine in the United States, only slightly more than 30,000 have a buprenorphine waiver, and only about half of those are actually treating patients with an OUD.[52] By expanding the number of patients that a physician can have to 275, it is hoped that more patients will be seen, thereby compensating for the number of physicians who are actually seeing patients.

There are a number of issues associated with the increased use of buprenorphine. Foremost is the need for medical schools, internships, residencies, and fellowships to address the underlying issues of abuse and dependence of prescription opioids and/or heroin. Buprenorphine offers the primary care, specialist, or addiction medicine physician the opportunity to address opioid abuse or dependence at the patient level. However, training is a necessary precursor. An evolving twist in the practice of medicine is the use of buprenorphine for the treatment of pain. Of course, increased focus is also needed on those patients who have a pain condition and who have an addiction to opioids.

As buprenorphine has gained in popularity, it is inevitable that adverse event reports would increase in occurrence.[66] The increased use of buprenorphine magnifies the risk to children in homes in which it is used. Clinicians should remain vigilant for pediatric exposures.[27] Clinicians should *not* assume that because buprenorphine and naloxone combination are reasonably safe for adults, pediatric patients are not at risk for opioid toxicity.[8,50] The CDC estimates that there were 8136 buprenorphine/naloxone emergency department (ED) visits by children under the age of 6 between 2008 and 2015. Despite this, the CDC noted a decline in the rate of ED visits by children, from 28.2 ED visits per 100,000 in 2008–2010 to 9.8 visits per 100,000 during 2013–2015. It was also noted that unit-dose packaging increased to over 80%, suggesting that packaging/formulation changes might reduce pediatric ingestion. Buprenorphine tablets were available only until late 2010, when film strips in unit-dose, child-resistant packaging became available.[8]

Individuals receiving buprenorphine on an outpatient basis should be educated regarding steps they can take to ensure that the agent is not accessible to any young children in their homes.

In 2005, there were 3161 ED visits involving buprenorphine; by 2010 there were 30,135 ED visits involving buprenorphine (Fig. 1.8).

The increase in the number of physicians prescribing buprenorphine may be related to the increased access. Although there were 5656 physicians certified to prescribe buprenorphine in 2005, SAMHSA reports that there were 18,582 physicians in 2010. In addition, although there were an estimated 100,000 patients receiving buprenorphine in 2005, there were an estimated 800,000 patients receiving buprenorphine in 2010.[53] Not only is the number of patients increasing with time, the estimated number of buprenorphine prescriptions has nearly tripled from 2008 when there were 3.2 million prescriptions to 2015 when there were 9.1 million.[8]

The most common pattern of abuse used to involve crushing the sublingual tablets and injecting the resulting extract. When the agent is injected intravenously, addicts claim that buprenorphine effects are similar to equipotent doses of morphine or heroin. More than one-third of buprenorphine abusers reported that they took the drug in an effort to self-medicate and ease heroin withdrawal.[13] Indications are that buprenorphine obtained for nonmedical purposes in the United States is diverted from prescriptions written for treatment of addiction or obtained through "doctor shopping."[56] With the new formulations of buprenorphine, crushing the sublingual tablets becomes less likely, especially with the film. Still as buprenorphine becomes increasingly generic, the possibility of crushing tablets remains.[8]

Monitoring of discussions within Internet newsgroups and interviews found that the buprenorphine products are viewed primarily as medications to avoid or ease withdrawal symptoms rather than as a means of getting high. There is evidence of experimental use and illegal diversion of buprenorphine; however, the extent of abuse and diversion does not come close to that of methadone or oxycodone (OxyContin). Intravenous use of buprenorphine and naloxone or buprenorphine without naloxone appears to be rare, but it is evident from street interviews.[18]

A buprenorphine implant was approved by the FDA in 2016. This formulation may offer a partial solution to the diversion problem. In addition, the implant may help to facilitate medication adherence given that it delivers a steady-state level of buprenorphine for about 6 months.[32]

Physician Training

The Drug Addiction Treatment Act of 2000 (DATA 2000) prescribes a minimum of 8 hours of education for physicians not otherwise exempted. It became clear that additional support was needed for a number of practitioners new to the effort to provide care to those who abused or were dependent on opioids using buprenorphine. CARA prescribes 24 hours of education for NPs and PAs.

SAMHSA's CSAT created the Physician Clinical Support System for Buprenorphine (PCSS-B). In 2010, SAMHSA awarded this grant program to the American Academy of Addiction Psychiatry (AAAP); this public-private partnership permitted physicians who prescribe or dispense buprenorphine to contact the Physician Clinical Support System for information, support, or mentorship.

A second initiative launched in 2011, the Prescribers' Clinical Support System for Opioid Therapies (PCSS-O; now the Providers Clinical Support System) was awarded to AAAP with a coalition of primary care and specialty organizations. The purpose of this grant was to develop a free national mentoring network that would provide clinical support (e.g., clinical updates, consultations, evidence-based outcomes, and training) to physicians, dentists, and other medical professionals in the appropriate use of opioids for the treatment of chronic pain and opioid-related addiction. This initiative was to help SAMHSA address the nation's major concern about morbidity and mortality that have been caused by misuse/abuse and fatal drug interactions involving opioids used in the treatment of addiction and chronic pain. Levin et al. noted that the PCSS-O consortium of national professional organizations led by the AAAP, included the American Psychiatric Association (APA); the American Osteopathic Academy of Addiction Medicine (AOAAM); the American Medical Association (AMA); the American Dental Association (ADA); the American College of Physicians (ACP); the American Academy of Pediatrics (AAP); the American Academy of Neurology (AAN); the American Academy of Pain Medicine (AAPM); the International Nurses Society on Addictions (In-tNSA); and the American Society for Pain Management Nursing (ASPMN).[35] Levin et al. contend that the PCSS-O consortium and steering committee represent over 1 million health care professionals and other stakeholders.

The third iteration of the PCSS approach came in 2013 in the form of the Cooperative Agreement for the Physician Clinical Support System – Medication-Assisted Treatment (PCSS-MAT). The purpose of this program is to build on the current SAMHSA-funded PCSS-B, a national mentoring network offering support (clinical updates, evidence-based outcomes, and training) by expanding the focus on buprenorphine to include the other two FDA-approved medications for the treatment of opioid addiction, methadone and ER naltrexone, and increasing the amount of training for office-based physicians and opioid treatment program medical professionals. The program provides up-to-date and evidence-based information to support training of health care professionals and to address the complex issues of addiction.[61]

Levin et al. noted that PCSS-MAT comprises a consortium of professional organizations under the leadership of the AAAP, including four of the five DATA 2000 organizations (AAAP, ASAM, AOAAM, and APA); the Association for Medical Education and Research in Substance Abuse (AMERSA) and NIATx, a learning collaborative specializing in evaluation of systems and organizational change, also joined the initiative. This consortium developed a novel mentoring and training program for health care professionals to help them in identifying and treating OUDs.[35]

Since July 1, 2011, a total of 248 training modules and webinars have been held and 49,895 participants have been trained. Since August 2013, a total of 246 PCSS-MAT waiver trainings have been held and 4130 providers have received waiver training. AAAP has had over 2260 providers take its online course. Access to information about the PCSS-MAT can be acquired from the website: https://pcssmat.org/.

Utilization of Substance Abuse Treatment Services

The NSDUH presents findings about the utilization of substance abuse treatment services in addition to a comprehensive overview of substance use. In 2016, an estimated 20.1 million persons 12 years or older were classified with substance dependence or abuse in the past year; this represented 7.5% of the population. Of these, 2.3 million were classified with dependence on or abuse of both alcohol and illicit drugs, 1.9 million were dependent on or abused illicit drugs but not alcohol, and 15.1 million were dependent on or abused alcohol but not illicit drugs.

In 2016, only 3.8 million of the 20.1 million persons who met criteria for substance dependence or abuse received some form of treatment for a problem related to the use of alcohol or drugs. Treatment was reported to be received in a range of settings: self-help groups, outpatient rehabilitation, inpatient rehabilitation, outpatient mental health centers, hospital inpatient, private doctor's offices, emergency room, or prisons or jails. Looking beyond the full universe of treatment options and focusing only on hospital inpatient units, drug or alcohol rehabilitation facilities (inpatient or outpatient), or mental health centers as specialty substance abuse treatment settings, the NSDUH reported that only 2.2 million people 12 years or older who met criteria for substance abuse or substance dependence received treatment at an inpatient hospital, rehabilitation facility, or mental health center. What is striking about the findings is that 18.7 million people in 2016 who were classified as needing substance abuse treatment did not receive it from a specialty facility.

Of the 18.7 million people who met criteria for needing treatment but did not receive it, 95.5% did not feel that they needed treatment and made no effort to get treatment. Another 2.5% felt

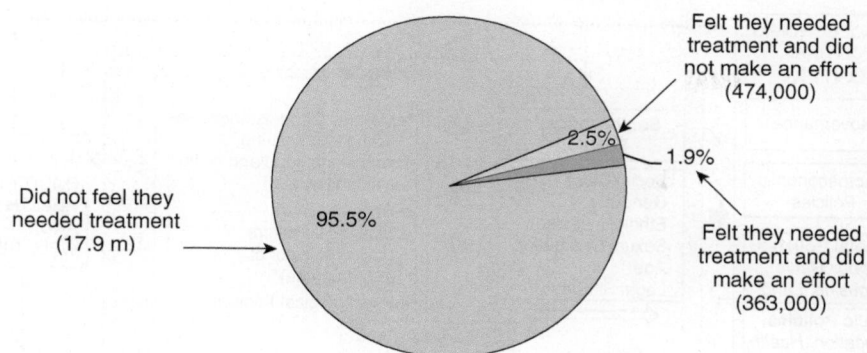

• **Fig. 1.9** Past-year perceived need for and effort made to receive specialty treatment among persons age 12 or older needing but not receiving treatment for illicit drug or alcohol use: 2016; 18.7 million needing but not receiving treatment for illicit drug or alcohol use. (Data from SAMHSA, Center for Behavioral Health Statistics and Quality, National Survey on Drug Use and Health, 2015 and 2016.)

that they needed treatment but did not make an effort to get it, whereas 1.9% or 363,000 people felt that they needed treatment, made an effort to get it, but did not receive it. In short, 98.1% of the 18.7 million people who met criteria for needing treatment made no effort to receive it.

These findings created the basis of two evolving concepts. The first is that the "true" waiting list is made up of only 363,000 people: the individuals who made an effort to get treatment but who were not successful. The second is that the overwhelming majority of individuals who meet criteria are not seeking treatment despite being symptomatic (Fig. 1.9). It is not clear why the overwhelming majority of individuals who meet criteria for needing treatment do not seek it. However, it is clear that these individuals must have some psychosocial decrements of function noticeable not only to themselves but to those in their environment. Environmental motivators can include family, employers, health care practitioners, law enforcement, faith leaders, friends, and associates. Therefore, from a public health perspective and a public safety perspective, it is important to determine the role of substances of misuse in the lives of individuals. It is also important to understand the developmental significance of alcohol and drugs to those in the 18- to 25-year age range, for these young adults account for the peak misuse of alcohol, traditionally illicit drugs, and now prescription drugs. The data above clearly show that our efforts to reach young adults need to be intensified.

Social Determinants of Health

There are many social determinants of health, with varying influence depending on the individual's unique condition (Fig. 1.10). The use of alcohol or drugs has many cultural, biological, and social precursors. The misuses, then, are similarly disposed. Why a substance is used beyond the obvious reality of the physiological and psychological effects remains a mystery. This is clearly seen among people who meet criteria for treatment but who do not seek assistance. The World Health Organization (WHO) has an established focus on the social determinants of health. The conceptual model depicted in Fig. 1.10 recognizes that there are structural determinants of health inequities coupled with intermediate determinants of health that influence the equity in health and well-being. The socioeconomic and political context of an individual's life plays a role in that individual's health. A modified version of the WHO's model includes drug laws and laws governing the use of alcohol. A person's socioeconomic position in society also contributes, with material circumstances, behavioral and biological factors, and

psychological factors figuring into access to a health care system and impacting on the health care system available to a person. Health does not occur in a vacuum. In addition, substance use and misuse do not occur in a vacuum. The issue of marijuana, either so-called "medical marijuana" or "recreational marijuana," captures the tension within the American culture. Thirty-three states and the District of Columbia currently have passed medical marijuana laws. In addition, 10 states and the District of Columbia have passed laws permitting adult use of marijuana for recreational purposes.[29a]

The CSA is still the law of the land and preempts state law; this means that despite state action, federal law still classifies marijuana as a Schedule I drug. The exception to this scheduling is the drug Epidiolex, which contains cannabidiol, a major component of cannabis. Epidiolex is classified as a schedule V drug and is the first FDA-approved drug to contain a purified extract from the marijuana plant. Thus, under federal law, the possession of marijuana is still illegal. This state's rights versus federal law dynamic captures the essence of the cultural ambivalence about marijuana in the United States. As indicated earlier, some 24 million people in the United States are current marijuana users, with 37.6 million past-year users and 118.5 million lifetime users. In short, 44% of Americans 12 or older admit to using marijuana at least once in their lifetime. In addition, those states that have legalized "recreational" marijuana may develop an economic interest in the commercialization of marijuana; Colorado, for example, collected $109 million in taxes, licenses, and fees in 2016.[14]

Perceived Risk of Harm With Substance Use

NSDUH data from 2016 reveal that 69.5% of persons 12–17 years of age perceive great risk of harm in smoking one or more packs of cigarettes per day; of the persons 18–25, 68.6%; and of persons 26 or older, 73.9% perceived great risk of harm. By contrast, only 40% of persons 12–17 years of age, 17.2% of those 18–25, and 36.1% of those 26 or older perceived smoking marijuana once or twice a week as a great risk of harm. Furthermore, 44% of persons 12–17 years of age, 37.1% of persons 18–25, and 45.6% of persons 26 or older perceived binge drinking once or twice a week as a great risk of harm.

The actions of the US government reflected in the 21st Century Cures Act is one strategy to address the needs of Americans who are dependent on opioids and who need treatment. The surge funding of over $1 billion over 2 years captures the urgency of addressing both the issues of opioid overdoses and overdose deaths and the issue of increasing access to treatment. However, the issue

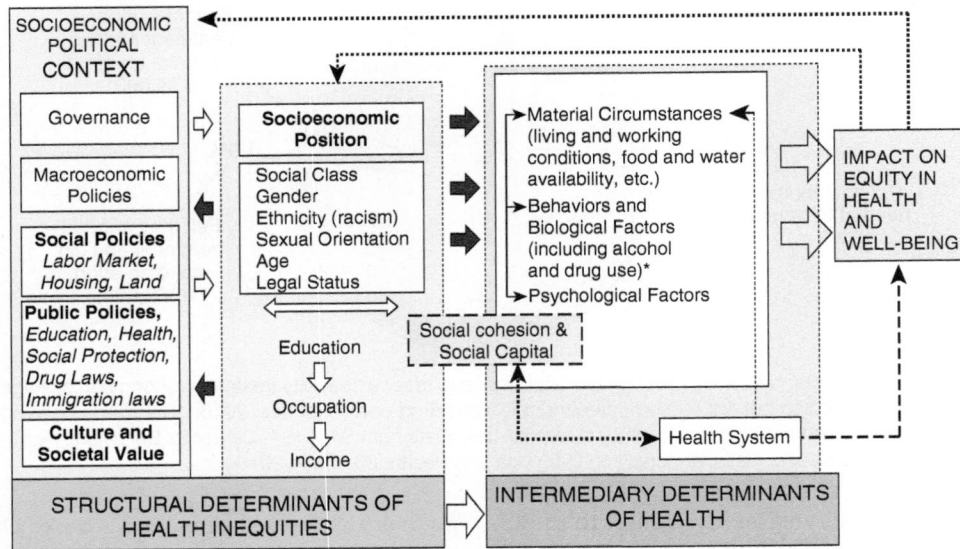

• **Fig. 1.10** The social determinants of health. (Adapted from the diagram in section V.9 on p. 48 of World Health Organization, Commission on Social Determinants of Health.[73])

of use and misuse of psychoactive substances covers a broader spectrum of substances. Consequently, after CARA was enacted and before the 21st Century Cures Act was passed, the Surgeon General released a seminal report.

Facing Addiction in America: The Surgeon General's Report on Alcohol, Drugs, and Health

The goal of the SG Report (Facing Addiction in America: The Surgeon General's Report on Alcohol, Drugs, and Health) is to inform policymakers, health care professionals, and the general public about effective, practical, and sustainable strategies to address the misuse of alcohol and other psychoactive drugs. The report is broken down into seven distinct chapters: an overview of the report, the neurobiology of substance misuse, prevention programs and policies, early intervention and treatment strategies, the various paths to recovery, the role of health care systems on recovery, and finally, the vision for recovery in the future, all from a public health perspective.

Each chapter of the SG Report explains in plain English the scientific and evidence-based findings. This report is an invaluable tool because it packs a lot of information under one useful umbrella. By going to the Surgeon General's website, each chapter can be downloaded separately and used accordingly (https://addiction.surgeongeneral.gov/).[67]

When it comes to initiating change for the future of SUD prevention, treatment, and recovery, the SG Report is an ideal means of addressing a broad range of psychoactive substances, both licit and illicit. By moving away from the harsh judgment of moral condemnation into the realms of neurobiology, trauma, and vulnerability, prevention can be enhanced, treatment facilitated, and recovery promoted. The SG Report lays the foundation for supporting individuals who enter treatment by addressing cultural and psychosocial barriers and by promoting the wealth of credible scientific and clinical evidence that prevention is possible, that

treatment works, and that there are many pathways to recovery. Although activities at the federal level are important, the activities in the general community and in the recovery community are the most important. By using the SG Report to inform local action agendas, rational and reasonable community-based strategies can be facilitated.

The SG Report reminds the reader that such services as transportation, child care, literacy training, self-help facilitation, recovery-based training and relapse prevention, assistance with the criminal justice system, transitional housing, and employment coaching are considered an integral part of the recovery process (Fig. 1.11).

The basis for recovery support services is predicated on the work of the National Institute on Drug Abuse (NIDA). The critical components of treatment are captured in the NIDA "Wheel." According to NIDA data, individuals without community or family supports are more vulnerable to relapse than those with such supports.

Screening, Brief Intervention, and Referral to Treatment

The second effort—Screening, Brief Intervention, and Referral to Treatment (SBIRT)—recognizes that most people in need of care are not presenting to specialty treatment programs, but are presenting at alternative sites of care, specifically trauma centers, community health centers, and other primary care venues (Fig. 1.12).

According to the NSDUH, the 17.9 million people who meet criteria for alcohol use disorders but perceive no need for treatment and are not receiving treatment, are not going to specialty care settings. Thus from a public health approach, if those affected by alcohol use disorders will not go to formal treatment, some form of treatment must go to them. Furthermore, as recently as a decade ago, it was recognized that drug-related ED visits are continuing to increase.[12] Consequently, such entities as the WHO, the United States Preventative Services Task Force, the Committee on Trauma of the ACS, and the Academic Emergency Department

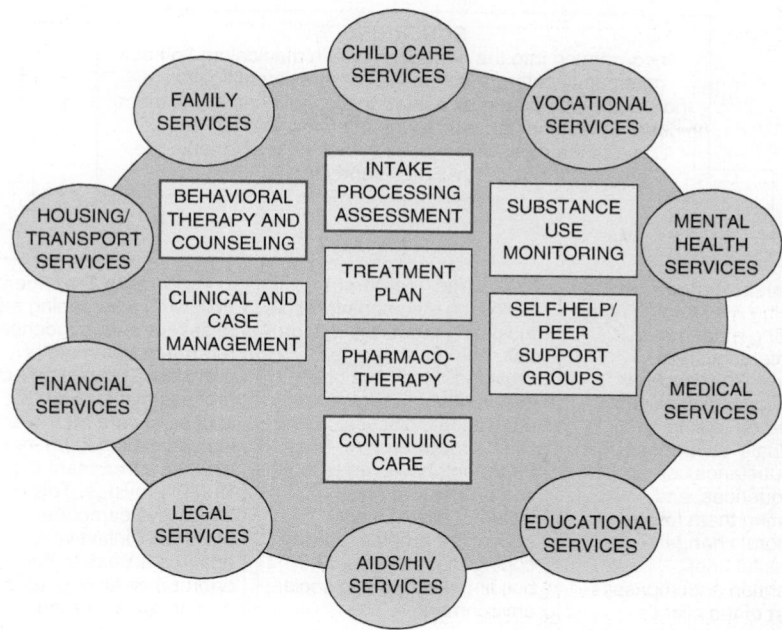

• **Fig. 1.11** Treatment services. (Reprinted from the National Institute on Drug Abuse.[41])

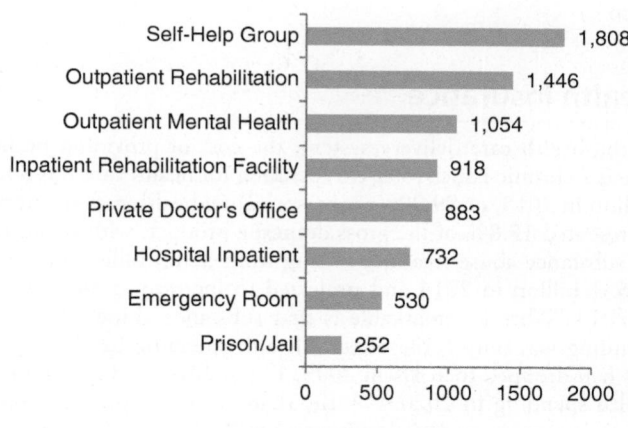

Location	Numbers in Thousands
Self-Help Group	1,808
Outpatient Rehabilitation	1,446
Outpatient Mental Health	1,054
Inpatient Rehabilitation Facility	918
Private Doctor's Office	883
Hospital Inpatient	732
Emergency Room	530
Prison/Jail	252

Numbers in Thousands

• **Fig. 1.12** Locations where past-year substance use treatment was received among persons 12+: 2016. (Data from SAMHSA, Center for Behavioral Health Statistics and Quality, National Survey on Drug Use and Health, 2015 and 2016.)

Screening, Brief Intervention, and Referral to Treatment Research Collaborative all recommend routine screening for alcohol problems in various health care settings.

It has long been known that screening for problem drinking and brief counseling by primary care providers is an effective approach to reducing alcohol consumption.[31] In fact, the United States Preventive Services Task Force recommends screening and behavioral counseling interventions to reduce alcohol misuse by adults, including pregnant women, in primary care settings.[51] Because it is recognized that a unique opportunity exists also to address illicit drugs in the primary health care setting, the question of whether it is practicable to screen for these substances has been raised.[1] At this point, the United States Preventive Services Task Force has concluded: "for adolescents, adults, and pregnant women, the evidence is insufficient to determine the benefits and

harms of screening for illicit drug use."[51] Nevertheless, the FSMB adopted a policy statement to develop "methods and/or modules of information to be used to educate medical students, residents and practicing physicians regarding the identification of substance use disorders, brief intervention and the proper prescribing of controlled substances."[24] In addition, the Centers for Medicare & Medicaid Services added to the Healthcare Common Procedures Coding System new Level II billing codes for screening and brief intervention for alcohol and/or drugs that went into effect on January 1, 2007.[44] The AMA also has added to its current procedural terminology codes two new codes covering services related to alcohol and drug abuse screening and treatment.[54]

Furthermore, researchers are exploring the utility of using screening and brief intervention as a tool to address more carefully the issue of drug abuse.[4-6] Use of substances such as marijuana, prescription drugs, and cocaine occurs with sufficient frequency to make them ideal targets for a screening effort. The epidemiology of a given community might elevate other substances of misuse to a level that makes screening in that community practical and feasible.

As noted, screening is not the only component of a process of detection and intervention. Screening, Brief Intervention, and Referral to Treatment is predicated on any of the three following strategies: brief intervention, brief treatment, or referral to treatment[57] (Fig. 1.13). It became clear to the federal government that one of the engines that drive the demand for drugs is the lack of perceived need for care. At the same time, people were being seen for injuries and conditions related to drug abuse and misuse. The challenge was how to take advantage of the opportunity to provide this population with at least brief intervention or treatment.

The CSAT of SAMHSA implemented a grant program in 2003 to encourage state jurisdictions and tribal organizations to initiate Screening, Brief Intervention, and Referral to Treatment programs in a variety of health care settings, including inpatient programs, EDs, ambulatory care settings, community health centers, and other primary care settings. Since 2003, SAMHSA has

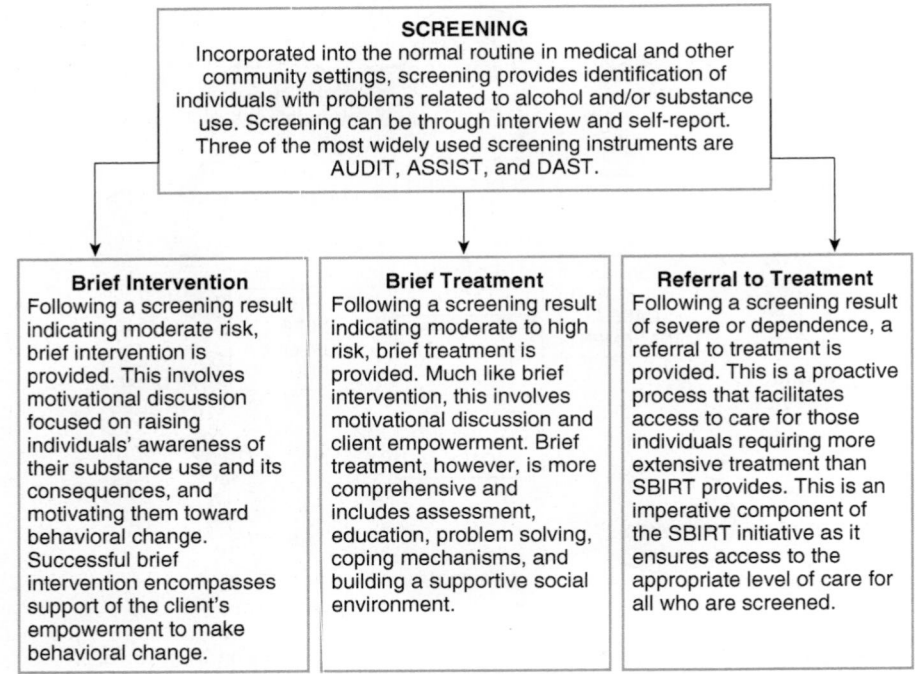

SCREENING
Incorporated into the normal routine in medical and other community settings, screening provides identification of individuals with problems related to alcohol and/or substance use. Screening can be through interview and self-report. Three of the most widely used screening instruments are AUDIT, ASSIST, and DAST.

Brief Intervention
Following a screening result indicating moderate risk, brief intervention is provided. This involves motivational discussion focused on raising individuals' awareness of their substance use and its consequences, and motivating them toward behavioral change. Successful brief intervention encompasses support of the client's empowerment to make behavioral change.

Brief Treatment
Following a screening result indicating moderate to high risk, brief treatment is provided. Much like brief intervention, this involves motivational discussion and client empowerment. Brief treatment, however, is more comprehensive and includes assessment, education, problem solving, coping mechanisms, and building a supportive social environment.

Referral to Treatment
Following a screening result of severe or dependence, a referral to treatment is provided. This is a proactive process that facilitates access to care for those individuals requiring more extensive treatment than SBIRT provides. This is an imperative component of the SBIRT initiative as it ensures access to the appropriate level of care for all who are screened.

• **Fig. 1.13** Screening, brief intervention, brief treatment, and referral to treatment. (Reprinted from the Substance Abuse and Mental Health Services Administration.[57])

funded 17 Medical Residency Cooperative Agreements, 32 State Cooperative Agreements, 12 Targeted Capacity Expansion Campus Screening and Brief Intervention (SBI) Grants, and 14 SBIRT Medical Professionals Training grants.[60]

SAMHSA offers a number of resources addressing SBIRT. For instance, in 2013, SAMHSA published a Technical Assistance Publication, TAP 33, "Systems-Level Implementation of Screening, Brief Intervention, and Referral to Treatment." In addition, on the SAMHSA SBIRT website, a number of SBIRT Grantee web links can be found.[59] SAMHSA grantees are pursuing SBIRT activity in community health centers, trauma care centers, schools and student assistance programs, occupational health clinics, and hospital EDs.

Recovery as a Holistic System

The SG Report notes that the process of change through which an individual achieves abstinence and improved health, wellness, and quality of life benefits from an integrated system of care that views the treatment agency as one of many resources needed to ensure the client's successful integration into the community. Just as each person's path toward substance misuse was different, the path to recovery will also look different for each client. The recovery system must be person-centered and self-directed, drawing on resources that meet the particular needs of the client. Hence, a recovery-oriented system of care model operates very much like the etiological model suggested by the model that the WHO promulgates about the social determinants of health. Chronic care approaches, including self-management, family supports, integrated services, and intensive case management, improve recovery outcomes. Integrated and collaborative care not only optimizes recovery outcomes but also improves cost-effectiveness.

Health Insurance

In the health care delivery system, the cost of providing health care is a chronic issue. Total US spending for health care was $3.2 trillion in 2015, or $9,900 per person. Total health care spending represented 17.8% of the gross domestic product, with spending on substance abuse treatment rising from $24.3 billion in 2009 to $31 billion in 2014 and projected to increase to $42 billion in 2014. What is remarkable is that substance abuse treatment spending was only 2.1% of total health spending in 1986, and this had dropped to 1.3% in 2003, 1% in 2014, and 1% of total health spending in 2020.[36,55] The share of SUD spending from public sources is predicted to increase to 71% for SUD treatment by 2020, up from 69% in 2009. This makes substance abuse disorder treatment unique in the pantheon of health expenditures.

In 2014, private insurers paid only 16% of the bill for substance abuse services, whereas state and local dollars paid for 28% of the bill for services; Medicaid paid for 25% of the substance abuse treatment services bill.[55] The burden on the public sector is demonstrably great, particularly at a time when state budgets are strained under the weight of deficits. Yet, as with health care in general, the question is: if substance abuse treatment is to continue, "Who will pay for it?"

There are two emerging movements that shifted substance abuse treatment services into a more contemporary payment scheme: health care parity and health care reform. How SUD treatment services are compensated clearly plays a role in what treatment options are available to an affected individual. Furthermore, the clinical algorithm employed by the clinician will also be influenced by the patient's or client's ability to pay for services or to get services provided.

Parity for SUD services was addressed in recent federal legislation, the Paul Wellstone and Pete Domenici Mental Health Parity and Addiction Equity Act of 2008.[48] In that law, which went into effect on January 1, 2010, health plans that offer mental health and SUD treatment benefits must do so on par with other health benefits. Under the law, insurance plans are not mandated to offer addiction and mental health benefits but plans that do have those benefits must provide them in a nondiscriminatory manner. Parity is also extended to coverage for out-of-network providers—increasing access to treatment for many insured individuals. Plans have the right to manage the benefit as they see fit and can decide which mental health and substance abuse treatment services they cover, as long as their decisions do not discriminate. However, they must provide to individuals and providers the medical necessity terms and conditions for any denials.[48]

The law also acknowledges that some states have already implemented parity laws, some of which may be stronger than the federal laws. In such cases, stronger state laws will not be preempted.

In short, the Wellstone/Domenici bill does not require the inclusion of SUD treatment services in a health insurance benefits plan; it only requires parity of benefit structure with other health benefits if the SUD treatment benefit is offered. However, the Affordable Care Act (ACA), with its essential health benefits requirement, compensated for the limitations of the Wellstone/Domenici bill.

The rising share of SUD public spending results from the ACA with its permitted expanded enrollment in Medicaid in those states that chose to expand eligibility. Furthermore, the ACA requires coverage of SUD screening and brief intervention for all insurance plans as a part of prevention services.

It is estimated that between 1.6 and 2.8 million people with SUDs gained access to insurance coverage as a result of the ACA.[3] Thus the ongoing debate about health care reform, centering on universal access to health care services, poses the greater challenge for those who require substance abuse treatment services, those who provide such services, and those who refer patients to such services. A repeal of the ACA without a parallel assurance that the SUD services would be included in its replacement would have a substantially negative impact on public health.

Critical themes in health care reform will continue be the issues of cost of services, the quality of the services provided, accountability for the provision of the services, and access to the services. Decision-making within the province of substance abuse treatment services will have to be transparent, with a clear view of the qualifications of the providers and assessment tools used to determine the various treatment components necessary for treatment, documentation of services provided through electronic health records, and the appropriate use of evidence-based practices with some evidence of fidelity to those practices and verification of acceptable outcomes in choosing the relevant practices.

References

1. Agency for Healthcare Research and Quality, U.S. Preventive Services Task Force. Screening for illicit drug use. 2008. https://www.uspreventiveservicestaskforce.org/Page/Document/RecommendationStatementFinal/drug-use-illicit-screening. Accessed 2 Oct 2017.
2. Arizona Opioid Prescribing Guidelines. 2014. http://www.azdhs.gov/documents/audiences/clinicians/clinical-guidelines-recommendations/prescribing-guidelines/az-opiod-prescribing-guidelines.pdf. Accessed 2 Oct 2017.
3. Bailey P. *ACA Repeal Would Jeopardize Treatment for Millions with Substance Use Disorders, Including Opioid Addiction, Center on Budget and Policy Priorities*; 2017. https://www.cbpp.org/sites/default/files/atoms/files/2-9-17health.pdf. Accessed 10/09/2017.
4. Bazargan-Hejazi S, Bing E, Bazargan M, et al. Evaluation of a brief intervention in an inner-city emergency department. *Ann Emerg Med.* 2005;46:67–76.
5. Bernstein E, Bernstein J, Levenson S. ASSERT: an ED-based intervention to increase access to primary care, preventive services, and the substance abuse treatment system. *Ann Emerg Med.* 1997;30:181–189.
6. Bernstein J, Bernstein E, Tassiopoulos K, et al. Brief motivational intervention at a clinic visit reduces cocaine and heroin use. *Drug Alcohol Depend.* 2005;77:49–59.
7. Blue Cross Blue Shield The Health of America Report. *America's Opioid Epidemic and Its Effect on the Nation's Commercially-Insured Population*; 2017. https://www.bcbs.com/sites/default/files/file-attachments/health-of-america-report/BCBS-HealthOfAmericaReport-Opioids.pdf. Accessed 2 Oct 2017.
8. Budnitz DS, Lovegrove MC, Sapiano RP, et al. Pediatric emergency department visits for buprenorphine/naloxone ingestion —United States, 2008–2015. *MMWR.* 2016;65(41):1148–1149.
9. Center for Behavioral Health Statistics and Quality. *2016 National Survey on Drug Use and Health: Detailed Tables*. Rockville, MD: Substance Abuse and Mental Health Services Administration; 2017.
10. Centers for Disease Control and Prevention, National Center for Health Statistics. *Health, United States, 2006, with Chartbook on Trends in the Health of Americans with Special Feature on Pain* (DHHS Publication No. 017-022-01602-8). Washington, DC: U.S. Government Printing Office; 2006.
11. Centers for Disease Control and Prevention, National Center for Health Statistics. *Provisional Counts of Drug Overdose Deaths, as of 08/6/2017*; 2017. https://www.cdc.gov/nchs/data/health_policy/monthly-drug-overdose-death-estimates.pdf. Accessed Oct 2, 2017.
12. Cherpitel CJ, Ye Y. Trends in alcohol- and drug-related ED and primary care visits: data from three US national surveys (1995–2005). *Am J Drug Alcohol Abuse.* 2008;34:576–583.
13. Cicero T, Inciardi J. Potential for abuse of buprenorphine in office-based treatment of opioid dependence. *N Engl J Med.* 2005;353:1863–1865.
14. *Colorado State "Marijuana Tax Data"*; 2017. https://www.colorado.gov/pacific/revenue/colorado-marijuana-tax-data. Accessed Oct 2, 2017.
15. *Comprehensive Addiction and Recovery Act of 2016*. https://www.congress.gov/bill/114th-congress/senate-bill/524. Accessed 2 Oct 2017.
16. Controlled Substances Act (1970). Drug enforcement administration. https://www.deadiversion.usdoj.gov/21cfr/21usc/index.html. Accessed 2 Oct 2017.
17. CNN. Doctors increasingly face charges for patient overdoses. http://www.cnn.com/2017/07/31/health/opioid-doctors-responsible-overdose/index.html. Accessed 2 Oct 2017.
18. CRS Associates LLC. *Surveillance Report, July 1 thru September 30, 2007.* [Reckitt Benickiser Pharmaceuticals, Inc. internal document; 2007.]
19. Dowell D, Haegerich TM, Chou R. CDC guideline for prescribing opioids for chronic pain-United States, 2016. *MMWR.* 2016;65(1):1–49.
20. Drug Enforcement Administration. McKesson Settlement: Pays $150 Million, Largest Fine in DEA History. https://www.dea.gov/divisions/det/2017/det011717a.shtml. Accessed 2 Oct 2017.
21. Drug Enforcement Administration. DEA 360 Strategy. (n.d.). https://www.dea.gov/prevention/360-strategy/360-strategy.shtml. Accessed 2 Oct 2017.
22. Drug Enforcement Administration. DEA proposes reduction to amount of controlled substances to be manufactured in 2018;2017. https://www.dea.gov/divisions/hq/2017/hq080417.shtml. Accessed 2 Oct 2017.
23. Reference deleted in review.
24. Federation of State Medical Boards. https://www.fsmb.org/Media/Default/PDF/Advocacy/Opioid%20Guidelines%20As%20Adopted%20April%202017_FINAL.pdf. Accessed 2 Oct 2017.

25. Federal Register (2017), Proposed Aggregate Production Quotas for Schedule I and II Controlled Substances and Assessment of Annual Needs for the List I Chemicals Ephedrine, Pseudoephedrine, and Phenylpropanolamine for 2018, Vol. 82, No. 150, August 7, 2017. Federal Register, Vol. 82, No. 150, August 7, 2017, pg. 36830.

26. Fingerhut LA. *Increases in Poisoning and Methadone-Related Deaths: United States, 1999–2005*. National Center; 2008. https://www.cdc.gov/nchs/data/hestat/poisoning/poisoning.pdf. Accessed 2 Oct 2017.

27. Geib AJ, Babu K, Ewald, et al. Adverse effects in children after unintentional buprenorphine exposure. *Pediatrics*. 2006;118:1746–1751.

28. Goldenbaum DM, Christopher M, Gallagher RM, et al. Physicians charged with opioid analgesic-prescribing offenses. *Pain Med*. 2009;9:737–747.

29. Greitens E. *Governor Eric Greitens Announces Statewide Prescription Drug Monitoring Program*; 2017. https://governor.mo.gov/news/archive/governor-eric-greitens-announces-statewide-prescription-drug-monitoring-program. Accessed 2 Oct 2017.

29a. Governing: *The States and Localities, State Marijuana Laws in 2019 Map*. 2019. https://www.governing.com/gov-data/safety-justice/state-marijuana-laws-map-medical-recreational.html. Accessed 21 May 2019.

30. Indiana State Medical Association. *Indiana Pain Management Prescribing Final Rule*; 2014. https://www.ismanet.org/pdf/legal/IndianaPainManagementPrescribingFinalRuleSummary.pdf. Accessed 2 Oct 2017.

31. Israel Y, Hollander O, Sanchez-Craig M, et al. Screening for problem drinking and counseling by the primary care physician-nurse team. *Alcohol Clin Exp Res*. 1996;20:1443–1450.

32. Itzoe ML, Guarnieri M. New developments in managing opioid addiction: impact of a subdermal buprenorphine implant. *Drug Des Devel Ther*. 2017;11:1429–1437.

33. Johnston LD, O'Malley PM, Miech RA, Bachman JG, Schulenberg JE. *Monitoring the Future National Survey Results on Drug Use, 1975-2016: Overview, Key Findings on Adolescent Drug Use*. Ann Arbor: Institute for Social Research, The University of Michigan; 2017.

34. Krantz MJ, Martin J, Stimmel B, et al. QTc interval screening in methadone treatment. *Ann Intern Med*. 2009;150:387–395.

35. Levin FR, Bisaga A, Sullivan MA, Williams AR, Cates-Wessel K. A review of a national training initiative to increase provider use of mat to address the opioid epidemic. *Am J Addict*. 2016;25(8):603–609.

36. Levitt KR, Kassed CA, et al. *Projections of National Expenditures for Mental Health Services and Substance Abuse Treatment 2004–2014*. Rockville, MD: Substance Abuse and Mental Health Services Administration Publication No. SMA; 2008. 08-4326.

37. Lin H, Wang Z, Boyd C, Simoni-Wastila L, Buu A. Association between statewide prescription drug monitoring program (PDMP) requirement and physician patterns of prescribing opioid analgesics for patients with non-cancer chronic pain. *Addictive Behaviors*. 2018;76:348–354.

38. McLellan AT, Turner B. Prescription opioids, overdose deaths, and physician responsibility. *JAMA*. 2008;300:2672–2673.

39. Moyo P, Simoni-Wastila L, Griffin BA, et al. Impact of prescription drug monitoring programs (PDMPs) on opioid utilization among Medicare beneficiaries in 10 US States. *Addiction*. 2017;112(10). 1784–179.

40. National Alliance for Model State Drug Laws. Compilation of Prescription Monitoring Program Maps. http://www.namsdl.org/library/CAE654BF-BBEA-211E-694C755E16C2DD21/. Accessed 2 Oct 2017.

41. National Institute on Drug Abuse. *Principles of Drug Addiction Treatment: A Research-Based Guide*. 3rd ed. NIH Publication No. 12–4180; 2012.

42. National Institutes of Health Pain Consortium. https://painconsortium.nih.gov/. Accessed 2 Oct 2017.

43. National Institutes of Health the Interagency Pain Research Coordinating Committee (IPRCC), https://iprcc.nih.gov/. Accessed 2 Oct 2017.

44. New Codes could encourage more screening and brief intervention. *Alcohol Drug Abuse Weekly*. 2006;18(37):1–6.

45. Ohio Governor's Opiate Action Team. *Ohio Guideline for the Management of Acute Pain Outside of Emergency Departments*; 2016.

46. President's Commission on Combatting Drug Addiction and the Opioid Crisis. *"Interim Report"*; 2017. https://www.whitehouse.gov/sites/whitehouse.gov/files/ondcp/commission-interim-report.pdf. Accessed 2 Oct 2017.

47. *ProCon.org, 29 Legal Medical Marijuana States and DC*; 2017. https://medicalmarijuana.procon.org/view.resource.php?resourceID=000881. Accessed 2 Oct 2017.

48. Public Law 110-343. *Paul Wellstone and Pete Domenici Mental Health Parity and Addiction Equity Act of 2008*; 2008. https://www.congress.gov/110/plaws/publ343/PLAW-110publ343.pdf. Accessed 2 Oct 2017.

49. Rudd RA, Seth P, David F, Scholl L. Increases in drug and opioid-involved overdose deaths-united states, 2010-2015. *MMWR*. 2016;65(50 & 51):1445–1452.

50. Schwarz K, Cantrell F, Vohra R, et al. Suboxone (buprenorphine/naloxone) toxicity in pediatric patients: a case report. *Pediatr Emerg Care*. 2007;23:651–652.

51. Screening and behavioral counseling interventions in primary care to reduce alcohol misuse: US Preventive Services Task Force recommendation statement. *Ann Int Med*. 2013;159(3):210–218.

52. Stein BD, Pacula RL, Gordon AJ, et al. Where is buprenorphine dispensed to treat opioid use disorders? The role of private offices, opioid treatment programs, and substance abuse treatment facilities in urban and rural counties. *Milbank Quarterly*. 2015;93(3):561–583.

53. Substance Abuse and Mental Health Services Administration. Center for Behavioral Health Statistics and Quality. Rockville, MD: The DAWN Report: Emergency Department Visits Involving Buprenorphine; 2013.

54. Substance Abuse and Mental Health Services Administration. *Coding for Screening and Brief Intervention Reimbursement*; 2017. https://www.samhsa.gov/sbirt/coding-reimbursement. Accessed 2 Oct 2017.

55. Substance Abuse and Mental Health Services Administration. *Projections of National Expenditures for Treatment of Mental and Substance Use Disorders, 2010–2020 HHS Publication No. SMA-14-4883*. Rockville, MD: Substance Abuse and Mental Health Services Administration; 2014.

56. Substance Abuse and Mental Health Services Administration. *Diversion and Abuse of Buprenorphine: A Brief Assessment of Emerging Indicators*; 2006. https://www.samhsa.gov/sites/default/files/programs_campaigns/medication_assisted/diversion-abuse-buprenorphine-final-report.pdf. Accessed 2 Oct 2017.

57. Substance Abuse and Mental Health Services Administration. *Medication-Assisted Treatment Prescription Drug and Opioid Addiction (MAT-PDOA) Grant Program 2016*. https://www.samhsa.gov/medication-assisted-treatment/mat-pdoa. Accessed 2 Oct 2017.

58. Substance Abuse and Mental Health Services Administration. Naloxone. (n.d.). https://www.samhsa.gov/medication-assisted-treatment/treatment/naloxone. Accessed 2 Oct 2017.

59. Substance Abuse and Mental Health Services Administration (2013) Systems-Level Implementation of Screening. *Brief Intervention, and Referral to Treatment (SBIRT), Technical Assistance Publication (TAP) Series 33. HHS Publication No. (SMA) 13-4741*. Rockville, MD: Substance Abuse and Mental Health Services Administration; 2013.

60. Substance Abuse and Mental Health Services Administration. *Screening, Brief Intervention, and Referral to Treatment (SBIRT) Grantees*; 2017. *https://www.samhsa.gov/sbirt/grantees https://www.samhsa.gov/sbirt/grantees*. Accessed 2 Oct 2017.

61. Substance Abuse and Mental Health Services Administration. *FY 2013 Cooperative Agreement for the Physician Clinical Support System-Medication Assisted Treatment (Short Title: PCSS-MAT)*; 2013. http://media.samhsa.gov/grants/2013/ti-13-003.aspx. Accessed 2 Oct 2017.

62. Substance Abuse and Mental Health Services Administration. *TI-17-014: State Targeted Response to the Opioid Crisis Grants (Opioid STR) Individual Grant Awards*; 2017. https://www.samhsa.gov/sites/default/files/grants/pdf/other/ti-17-014-opioid-str-abstracts.pdf. Accessed 2 Oct 2017.

63. Tennessee Department of Health. *Tennessee Chronic Pain Guidelines*; 2017. https://www.tn.gov/assets/entities/health/attachments/ChronicPainGuidelines.pdf. Accessed 2 Oct 2017. http://mha.ohio.gov/Portals/0/assets/Initiatives/GCOAT/Guidelines-Acute-Pain-20160119.pdf. Accessed 2 Oct 2017.

64. 21st Century Cures Act, Public Law 114-255. 2016. https://www.congress.gov/bill/114th-congress/housebill/34?q=%7B%22searc h%22%3A%5B%2221st+Century+Cures%22%5D%7D&r=3. Accessed 2 Oct 2017.

65. U.S. Census Bureau. *An Aging Nation: The Older Population in the United States*; 2014. https://www.census.gov/prod/2014pubs/p25-1140.pdf. Accessed 2 Oct 2017.

66. U.S. Department of Health and Human Services DAWN Live! [data file]. http://dawninfo.samhsa.gov/files/ED2006/DAWN2k6ED.htm. Accessed 2 Oct 2017.

67. U.S. Department of Health and Human Services (HHS), Office of the Surgeon General. Facing Addiction in America. *The Surgeon General's Report on Alcohol, Drugs, and Health*. Washington DC: HHS; 2016.

68. U.S. Department of Justice. *Mallinckrodt Agrees to Pay Record $35 Million Settlement for Failure to Report Suspicious Orders of Pharmaceutical Drugs and for Recordkeeping Violations*; 2017. https://www.justice.gov/opa/pr/mallinckrodt-agrees-pay-record-35-million-settlement-failure-report-suspicious-orders. Accessed 2 Oct 2007.

69. U.S. Food and Drug Administration. *Highlights of Prescribing Information of Dolophine Tablets*; 2016. https://www.accessdata.fda.gov/drugsatfda_docs/label/2016/006134s040s041lbl.pdf. Accessed 2 Oct 2007.

70. U.S. Food and Drug Administration. *Risk Evaluation and Mitigation Strategy (REMS) for Opioid Analgesics*; 2017.

71. Washington State Agency Medical Directors' Group. *Interagency Guideline on Prescribing Opioids for Pain*; 2015. http://agencymeddirectors.wa.gov/Files/2015AMDGOpioidGuideline.pdf. Accessed 2 Oct 2017.

72. Wisconsin Medical Examining Board. *Wisconsin Medical Examining Board Opioid Prescribing Guideline – November 16, 2016*; 2016. http://dsps.wi.gov/Documents/Board%20Services/Other%20Resources/MEB/20161116_MEB_Guidelines_v4.pdf. Accessed 2 Oct 2017. https://www.fda.gov/Drugs/DrugSafety/InformationbyDrugClass/ucm163647.htm. Accessed 2 Oct 2017.

73. World Health Organization, Commission on Social Determinants of Health. *A Conceptual Framework for Action on the Social Determinants of Health*; 2007. http://www.who.int/social_determinants/resources/csdh_framework_action_05_07.pdf. Accessed 2 Oct 2007.

74. Yang YT, Larochelle MR, Haffajee RL. Managing increasing liability risks related to opioid prescribing. *Am J Med*. 2017;130(3):249–250.

2

The Epidemiology of Alcohol and Drug Disorders

DEBORAH HASIN AND KATHERINE KEYES

What Is Epidemiology?

The field of epidemiology involves investigation of the distribution and determinants of health conditions in populations or population subgroups. Epidemiological investigations fall under two common domains: descriptive and analytic. Descriptive epidemiological studies provide estimates of the incidence and prevalence of illnesses or health behaviors. Incidence refers to the proportion of new cases of a particular health outcome during a specific period of time in a specific at-risk population (i.e., among individuals free of the outcome at the beginning of the time period). Prevalence refers to the proportion of a group or population affected with a health condition at a particular point in time. This includes new cases as well as chronic cases that began earlier and continued into the period of observation. Analytic epidemiological studies focus on identifying causes/risk factors (e.g., genetic variants, contextual circumstances) of illness, often through retrospective comparison of cases with noncases or prospective study of disease development among individuals exposed versus unexposed to a particular hypothesized causal factor.

This chapter covers the epidemiology of alcohol and drug abuse and dependence (referred to together as "substance use disorders" [SUDs]). From an epidemiological standpoint, SUDs have common as well as unique characteristics. This chapter identifies common characteristics of the epidemiology of alcohol and drug use disorders and highlights some important characteristics unique to specific substances.

Substance Use in the United States: Historical Overview and Recent Prevalence Trends

Alcohol Consumption

The use of substances to alter mood states has been a part of civilization from prehistoric through modern time periods. Archeological records document the conversion of sugar into fermented beverages for recreational use, as part of religious ceremonies, and as an analgesic or disinfectant as early at 10,000 BCE.[1,219] Alcohol remains incorporated in the fabric of many cultures for a variety of uses, including social and recreational use, as a part of religious ceremonies and secular festivities, and as a normative aspect of daily life. Furthermore, moderate consumption is associated with health and longevity, and is considered to be protective against several adverse health outcomes including cardiovascular disease.[14]

Long-term historical information on US alcohol consumption is available through per-capita alcohol consumption statistics derived from sales records. These records show that drinking levels in the United States varied greatly over time from the early days of the United States to the 21st century.[203,205] Per-capita

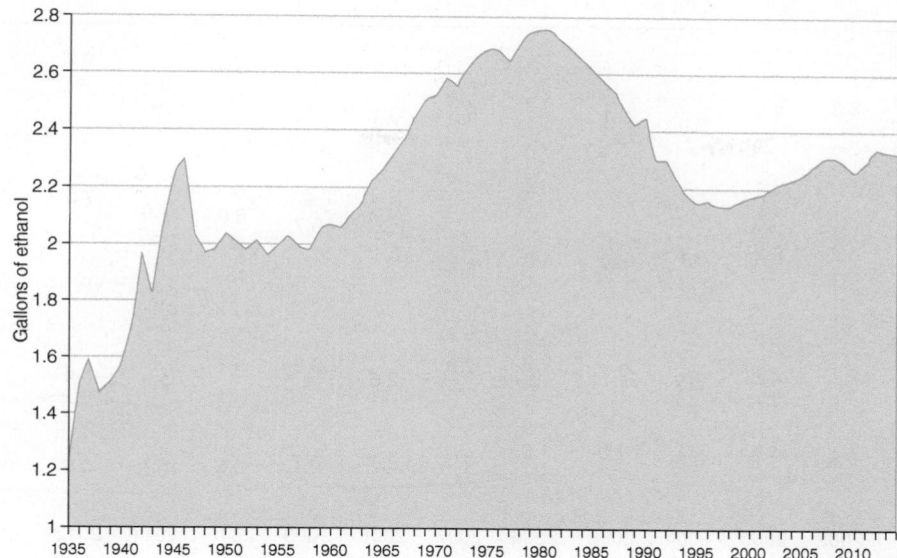

• **Fig. 2.1** Total per-capita ethanol consumption, United States, 1935–2014. (From Haughwout SP, LaVal-lee RA, Castle IJP. Surveillance report #104: apparent per capita alcohol consumption: national, state, and regional trends, 1977–2014. Rockville, MD: NIAAA, Division of Epidemiology and Prevention Research, Alcohol Epidemiologic Data System: March 2016.)

consumption ranged from extraordinarily high levels during the US colonial period (from an estimated 5.8 gallons per year per capita in 1790 to 7.1 gallons in 1830) to very low levels before and during Prohibition (from an estimated 1.96 gallons in 1916 to 0.97 gallons in 1934). Prohibition refers to the period during which the United States prohibited the manufacture, sale, and transportation of alcoholic beverages by the 18th Amendment to the US Constitution. This period began in 1920 and ended in 1933 with the repeal of the 18th Amendment by the 21st Amendment.

From 1935 until 1982, shown in Fig. 2.1, per-capita alcohol consumption increased steadily to a peak of nearly 2.8 gallons of ethanol per year in 1982.[203] After that, consumption declined until the late 1990s, and then began to increase again.

These data are generally consistent with US general population survey data from 2001–2002 to 2012–2013,[53] showing an increase in the prevalence of drinking, as well as volume and frequency of drinking and prevalence of at least monthly heavy episodic drinking among drinkers. Liver cirrhosis mortality statistics show similar variations over time, including an uptick in alcohol-related liver cirrhosis mortality since 2009, especially notable in young adults 25–34 years of age. [323]

Worldwide, alcohol consumption patterns vary considerably. Consumption is lowest in predominantly Muslim countries (e.g., individuals in Afghanistan and Pakistan consume 0.03 and 0.31 pure alcohol per capita, respectively) and eastern Mediterranean countries, and highest in eastern European countries (e.g., individual in Ukraine and the Russian Federation consume 15.58 and 15.23 L pure alcohol per capita, respectively) and western European countries such as France, Germany, and the United Kingdom.[322]

Alcohol consumption is also heterogeneous within countries. For example, about one-third of US adults do not drink, although US per-capita consumption is 2.32 gallons per year.[249,258] Abstainers are rare in Eastern Europe (including Russia and Ukraine), where per-capita consumption is the highest in the world.[249] After immigration, immigrants tend to retain the drinking levels of their country of origin rather than hanging onto the patterns of their new country, for example, Mexican immigrants in the United States[97] and Russian immigrants in Israel.[124,247]

Drug Use

Drugs such as cannabis, opium, and cocaine have been cultivated and used medicinally as well as recreationally for centuries. Opium poppies are believed to have been first grown in the region near modern-day Iraq as early as 3400 BCE. Opium was used primarily as an analgesic and anesthetic, but medical use did not become widespread until the development of the hypodermic needle in the early 1800s.[239] Historical analysis also indicates that marijuana was smoked recreationally and medically in ancient China as early as 2737 BCE.[230] In South America, societies have grown and consumed coca, the plant grown to create cocaine, for centuries. The most common mode of administration is to chew the leaves of the coca plant, or to mix the leaves into a tea. In the 20th century, innovations in pharmacological knowledge led to the development of synthetic drugs such as lysergic acid diethylamide, categorized as a hallucinogen, and methylenedioxymethamphetamine (or "ecstasy"), categorized as an amphetamine.

In Western countries prior to the 1960s, drug use was rare and the few studies that addressed prevalence focused on heroin, with widely varying results. Morphine is believed to have been prescribed often in the 19th and early 20th centuries mainly as a cough suppressant to ease the suffering of individuals with tuberculosis,[230] although no data are available to empirically estimate incidence and prevalence. During the Civil War, it is believed that more than 400,000 soldiers became dependent on morphine, as it was liberally prescribed for pain associated with battle wounds.

Systematic surveys of US drug use began in the 1960s with a series of national household surveys on drug use conducted by the National Institute on Drug Abuse (NIDA) and later by the Substance Abuse and Mental Health Services Administration (SAMHSA). These were originally known as the Household Surveys on Drug Use, and are now known as the National Survey on Drug Use and Health (NSDUH[234]). A series of three national surveys conducted by the National Institute on Alcohol Abuse and Alcoholism have also provided important information on US adult alcohol and drug use in the years 1991–1992, 2001–2002, and 2012–2013. The survey conducted in 1991–1992 is known

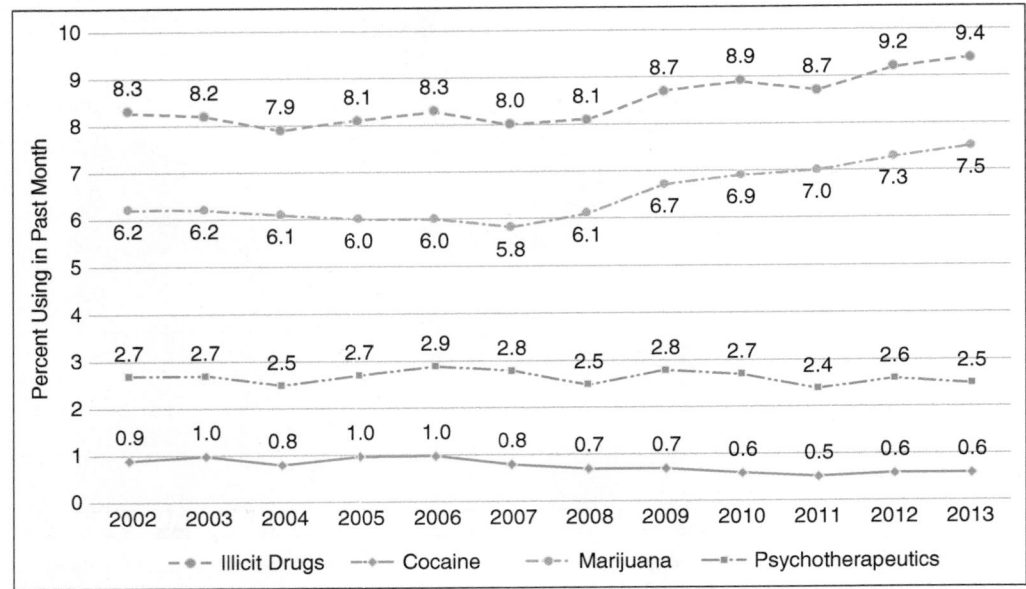

• **Fig. 2.2** Past month use of selected illicit drugs among persons aged 12 or older: 2002–2013. (Results from the 2013 National Survey on Drug Use and Health: Summary of National Findings, U.S. Department of Health and Human Services, Substance Abuse and Mental Health Services Administration Center for Behavioral Health Statistics and Quality, 2014.)

as the National Longitudinal Alcohol Epidemiologic Survey (NLAES[94,128]). The survey conducted in 2001–2002 is known as the National Epidemiologic Survey on Alcohol and Related Conditions (NESARC[98,99]). The third survey, conducted in 2012–2013, is known as the National Epidemiologic Survey on Alcohol and Related Conditions III (NESARC-III).

Earlier, Household Surveys on Drug Use surveys showed that illicit drug use, especially marijuana, increased greatly after the late 1960s. Heroin use also increased in the late 1960s, when the profile of users changed from "bohemians" to inner-city, unemployed males.

More recent NSDUH data on adults provides time trend information from 2002 to 2013 (Fig. 2.2). This shows that since about 2007, drug use has increased in the US general population, largely driven by increases in the use of marijuana. More detailed examination of NSDUH marijuana data shows increases in adults age 18 or older since 2007 in use, daily/near-daily use, and other cannabis indicators, with increases particularly concentrated within male users from lower income families The increases in marijuana use since the early 2000s are consistent with findings from the NESARC (2001–2002) and NESARC-III (2012–2013[103,106]), which also show marked increases in marijuana use among adults, including men, younger individuals, and those from lower-income households.

An area of illicit drug use that has become a source of much concern over the last 10 years is prescription opioids, largely fueled by an epidemic of unintentional fatal opioid overdoses, which became a leading cause of injury death and hospital admissions.[160] NSDUH data show increases in nonmedical use of prescription opioids up to about 2006, and a steadying in these rates among adults aged 26 or older, and some decline in the 12–17 and 18–25 age groups. NESARC data show that between 2001–2002 and 2012–2013, nonmedical opioid use increased among adults, as did heroin.[218] NSDUH data do not show overall increases in cannabis use in adolescents 12–17 years of age since 2002.

Another source of information on drug use among adolescents is the Monitoring the Future (MTF) series of annual national surveys of 8th, 10th, and 12th grade students. MTF data since 1991 show that in 1991, 44.1% of 12th graders had ever used an illicit drug, increasing to 54.3% in 1997, and decreasing to 48.9% in 2015. In 1991, 18.7% of 8th graders, 30.6% of 10th graders, and 44.1% of 12th graders had ever used an illicit drug. By 1997, these had increased to 29.4%, 47.3%, and 54.3%, respectively. In 2015, the prevalences were 20.5%, 34.7%, and 48.9%, respectively. By far the most commonly used drug was marijuana (15.5%, 31.4%, and 44.7% among 8th, 10th, and 12th graders in 2015).

Substance Use in the United States: A Public Health Problem

Although alcohol and drug use is common both in the United States and in many countries worldwide, excess alcohol consumption is estimated to be the third largest cause of US preventable mortality and the fifth largest cause of preventable disability worldwide.[73] Excess substance use and SUDs are associated with a broad range of adverse outcomes including but not limited to crashes and traffic fatalities, domestic violence, fetal alcohol syndrome and other prenatal and perinatal insults,[244] neuropsychological impairment,[13] poor medication adherence (e.g., HIV),[263] economic costs, lost productivity, psychiatric comorbidity,[22,137] and functional disability. Thus, prevention and intervention of excess substance use is an important public health priority.

When Does Use Become Pathological? Substance Abuse and Dependence

The *Diagnostic and Statistical Manual of Mental Disorders* of the American Psychiatric Association defines psychiatric disorders, including substance use disorders (or SUDs) within a common framework for individuals and groups with different

TABLE 2.1 **DSM-IV and DSM-5 Criteria for Substance Use Disorders (SUDs)**

	DSM-IV Abuse (≥1 criterion[a])	DSM-IV Dependence (≥3 criteria[b])	DSM-5 SUD (≥2 criteria[c])
Hazardous use	X	—	X
Social/interpersonal problems related to use	X	—	X
Neglected major roles to use	X	—	X
Legal problems	X	—	—
Withdrawal[d]	—	X	X
Tolerance	—	X	X
Used larger amounts/longer	—	X	X
Repeated attempts to quit/control use	—	X	X
Much time spent using	—	X	X
Physical/psychological problems related to use	—	X	X
Activities given up to use	—	X	X
Craving	—	—	X

[a]One or more abuse criteria within a 12-month period *AND* no dependence diagnosis; applicable to all substances except nicotine for which DSM-IV abuse criteria were not given.
[b]Three or more dependence criteria within a 12-month period.
[c]Two or more SUD criteria within a 12-month period.
[d]Withdrawal not included for cannabis, inhalant, and hallucinogen disorders in DSM-IV; cannabis withdrawal added in DSM-5.

training, experience, and interests. Users include medically and behaviorally trained clinicians, neuroscientists, geneticists, investigators conducting clinical trials, epidemiologists, policymakers, insurance companies, and others. The *Diagnostic and Statistical Manual of Mental Disorders, Fourth Edition* (DSM-IV[6]) was published in 1994, and was in use until the publication of *Diagnostic and Statistical Manual of Mental Disorders, Fifth Edition* (DSM-5[7]). Thus, although DSM-5 is more recent, the DSM-IV definitions of SUD were the basis of a very large body of research, including many of the references cited in this chapter.

Substance Disorders in the Diagnostic and Statistical Manual of Mental Disorders

For SUDs, DSM-IV provided diagnostic criteria for two disorders, dependence and abuse (Table 2.1), as well as symptoms for diagnosing substance-specific intoxication and withdrawal syndromes, and methods for diagnosing substance-induced psychiatric disorders. Note that DSM-IV-TR, published in 2000, provided updated text but did not change the diagnostic criteria.[7] The DSM-IV substance dependence criteria, shown in Table 2.1, are based on the alcohol dependence syndrome,[66] which was generalized to drugs in 1981. Dependence was considered a combination of physiological and psychological processes leading to increasingly impaired control over substance use in the face of negative consequences. Dependence was considered one "axis" of substance problems, and the consequences of heavy use (social, legal, medical problems,

hazardous use) considered a different axis of substance problems. This biaxial concept[66] led to the distinction between abuse criteria (social, role, legal problems, or hazardous use, most commonly driving while intoxicated) and dependence (tolerance, withdrawal, numerous indicators of impaired control over use).

The focus on *dependence* is based on its centrality in research and on its psychometric properties. DSM-IV defined dependence similarly to the definition found in the International Statistical Classification of Diseases and Related Health Problems, 10th Revision (ICD-10). These definitions had good to excellent reliability across samples and instruments,[a] with few exceptions (rare substances; hallucinogens). Dependence validity has also been shown to be good via several study designs. These include multimethod comparisons[b]; longitudinal studies[c]; latent variable analysis[17,115,231]; and construct validation.[120,134] Animal models of a syndrome of cocaine dependence symptoms (as distinct from use patterns)[56,255,301] lend credence to the dependence syndrome not only as a cross-cultural phenomenon, as suggested by a World Health Organization (WHO) study[46,122,246] but as a cross-species phenomenon as well.

Substance *abuse* was a different case. Contrary to clinical assumptions, abuse did not necessarily lead to dependence.[d] Furthermore, not all cases of alcohol or drug dependence manifested

[a] References 25, 27, 95, 122, 123, 125, 300.
[b] References 46, 91, 125, 132, 246, 259, 270.
[c] References 93, 121, 122, 127, 267, 269.
[d] References 93, 121, 127, 133, 267, 269.

abuse symptoms.[129,135] Dependence is more familial than abuse is.[121,118] DSM-IV–defined alcohol abuse was most often diagnosed in the general population based on one symptom, driving while intoxicated[119,120,183]; preliminary analyses of national data show this was also the case for drug abuse. The DSM-IV definition of abuse was problematic in that it depended on the availability of a car, while dependence was a heritable, complex condition.

Various psychometric analyses were conducted to examine the validity of the Edwards and Gross taxonomy of two distinct, correlated factors for substance abuse and dependence criteria prior to the start of the DSM-5 Substance-Related Disorders Workgroup (of whom one of the authors, DH, was a member). Confirmatory factor analysis on the alcohol abuse and dependence items provided mixed evidence; several studies show that a two-factor model best described abuse and dependence items[100,115,231,232] but with very high correlations between the factors, whereas several other studies found evidence of similar model fit for one- and two-factor models and selected the one-factor model on the basis of parsimony and high factor correlations.[216,245] Factor analyses of cannabis abuse and dependence items have generally found support for a one-factor model or similar fit of one- and two-factor models,[81,216,235,291] although results from a general population survey support a two-factor model.[17] Taken together, these studies showed some support for combining abuse and dependence, albeit with some evidence to the contrary. Differences across studies may also have occurred due to characteristics of the populations studied (e.g., general population versus community sample, adults versus adolescents).

One of the main issues for the DSM-5 Substance-Related Disorders Workgroup was how to address the distinction between abuse and dependence. Workgroup members and other investigators conducted many studies of the dependence and abuse criteria in different adolescent and adult samples and populations. These studies were based on Item Response Theory (IRT) analyses, which provide more nuanced information on the relationship of abuse to dependence symptoms than the factors analyses that had been done before. By the time DSM-5 criteria were finalized, studies on this issue had included more than 200,000 participants. Results were very consistent: abuse and dependence formed a single, unidimensional construct,[138] leading the DSM-5 Substance-Related Disorders Workgroup to eliminate the distinction between abuse and dependence, and combine most of the criteria into a single disorder (see Table 2.1). Additional changes of note in DSM-5 were the addition of a craving criterion, removal of the DSM-IV legal problems criterion, and addition of a withdrawal criterion for cannabis, since considerable evidence had accumulated since DSM-IV that a cannabis withdrawal syndrome existed.[138]

Substance Disorders: A Categorical or Dimensional Trait?

Recent psychometric analyses of the substance abuse and dependence criteria have suggested that these disorders are not categorical entities; instead, evidence supports an underlying continuum of alcohol severity across a variety of samples and populations.[e] Such information may be critical when statistical power is limited, as it often is in studies of gene-gene or gene-environment interaction. The DSM-5 addressed this issue by providing definitions of mild, moderate, and severe SUD: 2–3 criteria for mild, 4-5 criteria for moderate, and 6 or more criteria for severe.[138]

Descriptive Epidemiology: The Incidence and Prevalence of Substance Disorders

Prevalence and Incidence of Substance Disorders

The most comprehensive epidemiologic US information on the incidence, prevalence, and psychiatric comorbidity of alcohol and drug disorders comes from the two NESARC surveys. The NESARC was a longitudinal survey of 43,093 respondents 18 years or older conducted in 2001–2002[92,96] with a 3-year follow-up of 34,653 respondents. The NESARC-III was a survey of a fresh sample of 36,309 participants conducted in 2012–2013.[103,104] The diagnostic interview for both surveys was the Alcohol Use Disorder and Associated Disabilities Interview Schedule (AUDADIS), a structured interview for nonclinicians with high reliability and validity for SUDs.[f] The AUDADIS-IV was used to assess DSM-IV criteria for SUD and other disorders in the NESARC, and the AUDADIS-5 was used to assess DSM-IV and DSM-5 criteria for SUD in the NESARC-III, and DSM-5 criteria for other disorders.

In the NESARC, the prevalence of current (past 12 month) DSM-IV alcohol use disorder (abuse or dependence) was 8.5%,[137] whereas the prevalence of lifetime DSM-IV alcohol use disorder was 30.3%.[137] In the NESARC-III, the prevalence of current (past 12 months) DSM-5 alcohol use disorder was 13.3%,[104] whereas the prevalence of lifetime alcohol use disorder was 20.1%. Corresponding DSM-IV rates of current and lifetime alcohol use disorder (12.7% and 43.6% in NESARC-III) showed that substantial increases had occurred in the prevalence of alcohol use disorders in the more recent NESARC-III. Current and lifetime alcohol disorders were more prevalent in men than women in both surveys, and compared with individuals of white race/ethnicity, blacks, Hispanics, and Asians had a lower prevalence of current and lifetime alcohol disorders in both surveys. In both surveys, alcohol disorder prevalence is inversely related to age; persons in younger age groups are most likely to have an alcohol disorder. As shown in the Wave 2 follow-up interview for the NESARC, the incidence of alcohol dependence was 1.66 per 100 person-years,[99] meaning 1.66 cases per year of alcohol dependence for every 100 individuals without alcohol dependence at the beginning of that year. The incidence of alcohol abuse was slightly lower at 1.03 per 100 person-years.[99] In general, predictors of incidence were similar to predictors of prevalence.

Drug disorders were substantially less common than alcohol disorders. In the NESARC, the prevalence of current (past 12 months) DSM-IV drug use disorder (abuse and dependence) was 2% for any current drug use disorder, whereas the lifetime prevalence was 10.3%.[40] In the NESARC-III, the prevalence of current (past 12 months) DSM-IV drug use disorder (abuse and dependence) was 3.9% for any current drug use disorder, whereas the lifetime prevalence was 9.9%.[106] Using DSM-IV criteria in the NESARC-III survey, current and lifetime prevalence of DSM-IV drug use disorder were 4.1% and 15.6%, respectively,[41,90]

[e] References 136, 169, 197, 217, 245, 261.

[f] References 27, 95, 105, 125, 141, 142, 260, 300.

indicating substantial national increases in the prevalence of drug use disorders in the United States between the two surveys. Of the substances, cannabis use disorders were the most common in both surveys. The past-year prevalence of DSM-IV marijuana use disorder was 1.5% in the 2001–2002 NESARC and 2.8% in the 2012–2013 NESARC-III, a substantial and significant increase (P < .05) in prevalence.[140]

Current and lifetime drug disorders are more prevalent in men than in women in both surveys. Drug disorder prevalence is inversely related to age; persons in younger age groups are most likely to have a drug disorder. There was no consistent trend by race for drug disorders. In the NESARC, incidence of drug dependence was estimated at 0.32 per 100 person-years of observation[102]; incidence of drug abuse was slightly lower at 0.28 per 100 person-years. In general, predictors of incidence were similar to predictors of prevalence.

The Course of Substance Disorders

Initiation of alcohol consumption and drug use often occurs during adolescence. Onset of alcohol abuse and dependence is most likely among individuals 18–29 years of age, although 15% of alcohol dependence cases begin before age 18.[153] Often, substance disorders are not lifelong conditions. Indeed, a high rate of recovery has been documented in general population samples, even among individuals who have never sought treatment. Studies of alcohol disorders in the general population also show that a high proportion of recovered individuals return to moderate drinking as opposed to abstinence.[51,311] Data from the NESARC has indicated that approximately 75% of individuals diagnosed with alcohol dependence at some point in the past did not have a current (i.e., past year) diagnosis, but that only about 20% of these individuals were abstinent from alcohol.[51] Follow-up of this sample indicates that low-risk drinking represents a risk factor for relapse to an alcohol disorder compared with abstinence.[50] However, using WHO indicators of very high risk, high risk, moderate risk, and low risk drinking,[321] any shifts downward in WHO risk drinking levels from very high risk or high risk at baseline (2001–2002) to a lower level at the 3-year follow-up (2004–2005) was associated with a significant decrease in the likelihood of current alcohol dependence at follow-up.[130]

The transition to adulthood represents a key developmental phase in which alcohol disorders often remit, in a process termed "maturing out."[10,52] Major predictors of recovery include key lifestyle components, such as employment, marriage, and childbirth. Whether or not these factors have a causal influence on recovery or reflect common factors underlying the positive lifestyle components and the recovery remains unknown.

Despite substantial progress in the development of treatments for alcohol and drug disorders, only about one-fifth of those individuals with an alcohol disorder[39,137] and one-sixth of individuals with a drug disorder[40] seek treatment for the condition during their lifetime. Furthermore, the delay from onset of disorder to treatment is typically 8–10 years.[310] Finally, in contrast to sharp increases in treatment utilization for disorders such as depression between 1990 and 2003,[181] a corresponding increase in the proportion of individuals seeking treatment for alcohol and drug disorders did not occur during this period.[137] Data from NESARC-III continue to show poor rates of treatment for those with alcohol and drug use disorders.[104,106]

The path from first use to dependence to treatment also differs by gender. Women who use alcohol and drugs often start using later than men, have a faster progression from first use to dependence, and enter treatment sooner than men given equal ages of dependence onset,[242,248] although no such differences have been observed for crack-cocaine users.[60,204] This phenomenon has been termed "telescoping."

Evidence is accumulating that these well-documented gender differences in the course of alcohol disorders are converging. Studies of adolescent alcohol use have consistently shown a convergence in rates of alcohol and drug use initiation in younger birth cohorts, especially those born after World War II.[167,168] Furthermore, several genetically informative samples have researched gender differences in DSM-IV–defined alcohol and drug disorders over time, also finding support for such a convergence.[154,253] Similarly, large, representative cross-sectional studies in the United States support gender convergence in rates of DSM-IV–defined alcohol abuse and dependence.[109,182] Finally, evidence indicates that the traditional "telescoping" phenomenon whereby women exhibit later onset of use and disorder but earlier treatment and shorter course may be diminishing, as women are more closely approximating men in both onset and course of disorder.[155] Searches into the causes of these shifts are ongoing, but this evidence indicates increased social acceptability of alcohol use by women in younger generations.[108]

Analytic Epidemiology: The Etiology of Substance Disorders

SUDs have a complex etiology involving genetic and environmental factors. These occur along a continuum, ranging from the macro level consisting of broad social influences, to the micro level, consisting of molecular-level influences. These can be thought of as external to internal levels (Fig. 2.3). In the remainder of this chapter, we address these levels in turn. We begin with macro/external factors, including societal availability and desirability of the substances, geographic and temporal differences, pricing, laws, and advertising. We next consider externally imposed stress. Intermediate-level factors include religiosity and parental and peer social influences. Moving increasingly toward the micro and internal levels, we consider cognitive and personality variables, subjective responses to substances, and specific genetic risk variants.

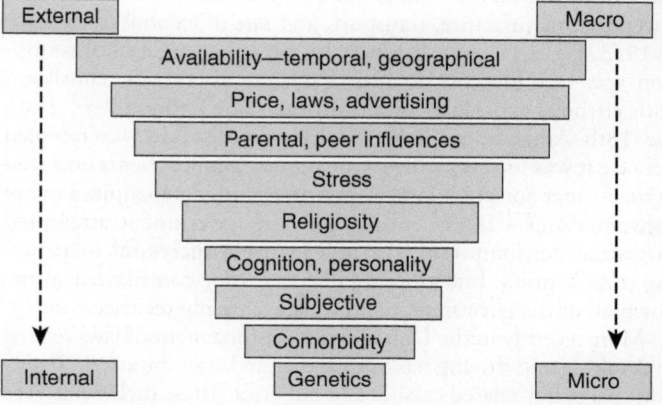

• **Fig. 2.3** Factors affecting substance use and substance use disorders.

Availability—Temporal and Geographical

Political Events

Political events, both local and global, influence the availability of substances and thus the risk of substance use and dependence. In 2004, for example, religiously motivated attacks on alcohol retailers in Iraq[14a] reduced the availability of alcohol locally for that region. After the Taliban government fell in Afghanistan in 2001, heroin production in Afghanistan increased greatly,[199] coinciding with increased heroin use among American teenagers.[289] Political instability in South American countries such as Bolivia and Colombia, especially in the 1970s, influenced the production of cocaine and increased the availability of cocaine in the United States.[286] Thus, political events at a great geographic distance may influence local substance use availability and patterns of use.

Outlet Density

Counties, cities or states with a higher density of alcohol outlets (places were alcohol is sold) have higher alcohol consumption and higher rates of alcohol-related problems, including hospital admissions, pedestrian injury collisions, and crashes and crash fatalities.[38,272,290,295,296] Ecologic and multilevel analysis controlling for individual level factors indicates that outlet density is related to higher mean group rates of consumption and drinking norms scores and to driving after drinking.[111,272] Community-based interventions to limit access to alcohol by reducing the density of outlets have been shown to reduce alcohol-related traffic injury and self-reported consumption.[156] Although information regarding outlet ("dealer") density is unavailable for drugs, the vigorous efforts of parents, schools, and law enforcement agencies to keep drug dealers away from schools are consistent with the same idea.

Pricing, Laws, and Advertising

Pricing

Alcohol taxation is the major determinant of state variation in the price of alcohol and is thus a government intervention. An inverse relationship exists between state-level price of alcohol and per-capita consumption or adverse consequences of drinking.[35] Furthermore, higher state-level beer tax is associated with lower prevalence of DSM-IV–defined alcohol dependence.[149] Outside the United States, cutting the tax on spirits has been followed by increased per-capita alcohol consumption.[147,257]

Laws and Law Enforcement: Alcohol

Laws and their enforcement also affect consumption patterns. In the United States, the 18th Amendment to the Constitution outlawed the manufacture, transport, and sale of alcohol from 1920 to 1933. Fig. 2.1 shows that in 1935, per-capita ethanol consumption was very low, but increased steadily afterwards, consistent with cirrhosis mortality rates from the same period.[204,323] Thus, the 18th Amendment achieved its purpose, but was repealed because it was unacceptable to the public. Similar events occurred in the former Soviet Union, an area of very high per-capita alcohol consumption.[322] In the mid-1980s, the government attempted to restrict consumption. The policies were successful in reducing consumption, but so unpopular that they contributed to the downfall of the government and were eventually reversed.[275]

More recently in the United States, enforcement of laws related to drinking and driving has been shown to be an important deterrent to alcohol-related crashes and fatalities. These include driver's license suspensions[172] and lowering the maximum legal blood alcohol concentration among drivers.[74,293,303] In addition, stricter driving-under-the-influence laws and their enforcement are consistently related to decreased hazardous use[212] and alcohol-related traffic fatalities.[8,303]

Minimum-age drinking laws influence the availability and acceptability of consumption among young people. Laws vary considerably by country both in scope and in minimum age.[322] For example, the minimum consumption age in the United States is 21, while in Cyprus it is 12. Israel did not have a minimum legal drinking age until 2004, but public concern about increased risky drinking among young adults led to the establishment of a national minimum drinking age (18 years) at that time.[282] Some countries have separate age restrictions for consumption and purchase. For example, in Greece, the minimum consumption age is 14, whereas the minimum purchase age is 17. In Italy, there is no age restriction on consumption in private but a minimum age requirement of 16 to drink in public.

Minimum drinking age laws have a positive effect on community health as well as the health and safety of adolescents. Research in the United States and other developed countries has indicated that minimum drinking age laws reduce traffic crash and fatality rates[75,276,303,305]; positive effects among adolescents include reducing alcohol consumption and high risk drinking.[238] In addition, several studies have documented an association between minimum drinking age laws and a reduction in youth suicide.[16,22]

State Distribution Policies

In the United States, states differ in the ways they control the availability of alcohol. Some states exert more control through the operation of state alcoholic beverage sales, whereas others exert less control through the licensing of alcohol outlets. This difference affects sales and consumption patterns.[304] Compared with "wet" counties, "dry" counties, where alcohol is not sold, have lower rates of alcohol-related accidents, driving-under-the-influence arrests, and cirrhosis mortality.[319] International studies corroborate these findings; in Norway, stringent alcohol regulations, such as mandatory closing on Saturdays, led to lower detoxification admissions.[257]

Grass-Roots Efforts

Mothers Against Drunk Driving (MADD) was started in 1980 by a group of women after a teenage girl was killed by a repeat-offense drunk driver. MADD, a very active organization, national since the early 1980s, has been highly effective in influencing state legislation pertaining to intoxicated driving, such as increasing the minimum drinking age from 18 to 21, and the enforcement of maximum-blood-alcohol-level laws among drivers.[113] In particular, a highly publicized media campaign called "Rate the State" in which states were graded A through D on driving-under-the-influence countermeasures, put pressure on legislators to increase the stringency of these laws, shown as an effective strategy in reducing alcohol-impaired driving.[277,302]

Alcohol Marketing and Advertising

Product development and marketing aim to increase sales and consumption.[32] Alcohol companies allocate substantial resources to researching consumer preferences, developing new products and promoting them.[165] For example, the alcohol beverage industry spent 696 million dollars on magazine advertising alone between 1997 and 2001, largely targeted to adolescents.[82] The alcohol industry does not publish the results of its marketing research, and resources necessary for definitive public health studies of advertising and other marketing effects are limited by comparison.

Public health concerns often focus on marketing that targets adolescents.[31,45] Existing data from longitudinal studies show associations between late childhood-early adolescent exposure to advertising and subsequent drinking initiation and frequency.[43,69,283]

Cross-sectional studies also show associations of various marketing and advertising strategies with positive attitudes about drinking and drinking frequency.[79,201] Furthermore, an imaging study of adolescent response to alcohol advertising indicated greater brain activation in areas linked to reward and desire among adolescents with alcohol use disorders than infrequent drinkers,[288] suggesting that advertisements are especially salient to vulnerable adolescents.

Laws and Law Enforcement: Drugs

The literature on government efforts to reduce illicit drug use overall by reducing availability is inconsistent. Some studies suggest that the strategies are ineffective,[18,312,320] while others find supply reductions efficacious.[54,313] Reducing the supply of specific illicit drugs can have unintended consequences, including increased use of other substances.[294] Data from US college studies, however, indicate that increased restrictions on alcohol use does not increase marijuana use, as has been hypothesized, but instead serves to decrease both alcohol and marijuana use.[317] Thus, the evidence is inconsistent on the efficacy of government attempts to limit illicit drug use through supply reduction via law enforcement.

The legal status of marijuana has undergone large-scale changes in the United States over the last two decades. Throughout this time, marijuana has been illegal at the federal level, where it is considered a Schedule I substance (high addiction potential, no evidence of medical efficacy or safety). However, 33 states and the District of Columbia have now passed laws legalizing the use of marijuana for medical purposes, beginning with California in 1996 (Table 2.2). Further, among the states that have passed medical marijuana laws (MMLs), 10 (see Table 2.2) have now passed laws legalizing use for recreational purposes (recreational marijuana laws [RMLs]).

Considerable attention has been paid to the potential for MMLs to increase marijuana use and have other unintended adverse consequences in the states in which MMLs were passed. With the use of cross-sectional designs, illicit marijuana use in adolescents[307] and adults[33] was shown to be higher in states with MMLs than in other states. However, using more informative pre-post designs that appropriately controlled for contemporaneous trends in non-MML states, studies of ours[139] and many others[264] have shown that within the states that passed these laws, post-MML increases in adolescent marijuana use did not occur. Only two studies have been done so far to address the effects of MMLs on adult illicit marijuana use using pre-post designs, one using NSDUH data from 2004 to 2013,[314] and a study of ours using NESARC survey data extending from 1991–1992 to 2012–2013.[131] Both of these studies showed post-MML increases in the adult prevalence of illicit cannabis use and DSM-IV cannabis use disorders, suggesting that MMLs were having an influence on rates of adult illicit marijuana use. Many questions remain to be answered about the effects of MMLs on other substances and on other potentially related outcomes.

Because RMLs have been passed so recently, little is known about their impact on adolescent and adult marijuana use and related consequences. One study addressing this among adolescents in the states of Colorado and Washington found post-RML increases in Washington but not Colorado.[34] Because recreational marijuana laws eliminate the need for medical personnel to authorize access to marijuana, such laws may have broader impacts on the use of marijuana and other substances than MMLs. Research on the effects of these laws will be needed as data accumulate after the laws have been passed.

TABLE 2.2	Changes in Marijuana Laws in US States	
State	**Year Passed** *Medical* **Law**	**Year Passed** *Recreational* **Law**
California	1996	2016
Alaska	1998	2014
Oregon	1998	2014
Washington	1998	2012
Maine	1999	2016
Colorado	2000	2012
Hawaii	2000	—
Nevada	2000	2016
Maryland	2003	—
Montana	2004	—
Vermont	2004	2018
Rhode	2006	—
New Mexico	2007	—
Michigan	2008	2018
Arizona	2010	—
New Jersey	2010	—
Delaware	2011	—
Connecticut	2012	—
Massachusetts	2012	2016
Illinois	2013	—
New Hampshire	2013	—
Minnesota	2014	—
New York	2014	—
North Dakota	2016	—
Arkansas	2016	—
Louisiana	2016	—
Florida	2016	—
Ohio	2016	—
Pennsylvania	2016	—
West Virginia	2017	—
Missouri	—	2018
Oklahoma	2018	—
Utah	2018	—

Parental and Peer Influences

Parental Modeling of Substance Use

Twin studies indicate that up to half the liability to alcohol dependence is environmental, and parental modeling has been proposed as one such environmental factor affecting subsequent substance use in their children.[72] Adoption studies do not support this, however, since rates of alcoholism in adopted children of alcoholics are not elevated.[158] One etiologic model with empirical support from twin studies posits that influential factors for substance use and the progression to dependence change over time; environmental and social factors mediate the initiation and use of substances in childhood and adolescence, whereas genetic factors become more influential in the adult substance use and dependence.[178]

Parenting Practices

Poor parental monitoring increases the association with substance-abusing peers,[144] a risk factor for alcohol misuse. Harsh, inconsistent parenting predicts earlier initiation of alcohol use, conduct problems, and poor regulatory competencies.[200,251] On the other hand, warm yet authoritative parenting styles protect adolescents from alcohol problems.[240]

Peers

Peer influence is a strong predictor of adolescent drug and alcohol use and problems.[170,284,306] Twin studies show that shared environmental influences such as peers have a significant effect on initiation of alcohol and any drug use.[185,252] Two models have been proposed to explain peer influence on adolescent substance use, social selection, and socialization.[171] The social selection theory proposes that young adolescents selectively "mate" with friends; those children who display deviant behavior as children will be prone to choose deviant friendships in adolescence.[78] This can lead to the initiation of drug use (especially marijuana use) and may be a factor in the transition to "heavier" drugs. It has been further proposed that an underlying trait such as sensation seeking (see later) influences both the selection of peers and substance use.[58] In contrast, the socialization theory proposes that adolescents can be influenced to use substances by peers in their environment[55] via modeling, offers, development of expectancies, and social norms.[19,271] Substance use by older siblings is also associated with individual substance use.[24,85,163,220] Studies that could examine these various environmental effects while controlling for genetic and other biological influences are needed to resolve the social selection/causation debate.

Peers may also be protective. Some US ethnic/immigrant groups use substances less than the norm.[97] Adolescents from these groups with ethnically homogeneous peers encounter less pressure to use substances.[23]

Stress

Drug disorders are often preceded and accompanied by disruptive behavior and conduct problems[202] that have a shared genetic vulnerability with drug disorders.[177] These behaviors evoke negative reactions from the environment, resulting in stressful life events that are not always independent of the individuals, making a causal direction between stress and disease onset difficult to discern. In animal studies where stress can be experimentally applied, cause and effect are clearer, as is also the case in studies of early stressful experiences in humans that antedate the onset of SUDs.

Animal Models

In animal studies, the timing of stress relative to normal development can be experimentally manipulated. In adult animals, substance use increases after exposure to physical stressors[86,243] and social stressors.[48,99,114,226]

Early life stressors also contribute to drug-using behaviors in animals. Neonatally isolated rats are more likely than handled rats to acquire stimulant self-administration behaviors[161,193,210] and show higher dopamine levels in response to cocaine, suggesting that early stress leads to greater cocaine reward.[21,194] Early life rearing stressors predict ethanol seeking in primates.[12] Isolated rearing led to increased drinking of morphine solution under various conditions.[5,214] Animal models of Δ9-tetrahydrocannabinol self-administration[20] may allow similar studies for cannabis.

Early Stressors and Drug Use in Humans

Childhood stressors, including parental separation, neglect, and abuse (physical and sexual) are associated with later substance use, problems, and dependence.[59,175,179] However, up to about 10 years ago, most studies had failed to control for parental history of substance abuse, a potential confounder given that substance abuse is associated with poor parenting.[206] Since then, many studies with appropriate controls for parental history of substance abuse have shown a relationship between childhood maltreatment and adult substance abuse problems,[g] and a recently published 30-year prospective study showed transmission of child abuse from one generation to the next.[315] One informative study showed that among adolescents with a substance-abusing parent, strong family cohesion (the opposite of neglect) protected against drug problems.[159] Twin studies allow the study of environmental stressors while controlling for genetic influences, and have shown that childhood sexual abuse is an environmental risk factor for SUDs.[176,236]

Religiosity

Religiosity has been called "one of the more important environmental factors that affect the risk for substance use and dependence."[173] An inverse relationship between religiosity and drinking is cross-cultural.[4,9,241] Longitudinal studies of adolescents and college and professional students show that religiosity protects against later heavy drinking.[11,213] Religiosity is strongly correlated within twin pairs due to shared environmental effects.[173,191,297] Heritability of drinking differs between religious and nonreligious twins, an example of gene-environment interaction.[192] In twins studied longitudinally,[281] religiosity predicted later drinking more than drinking predicted later religiosity, suggesting that religiosity is more likely to influence drinking than the reverse. These studies indicate that religiosity is largely environmental and protects against alcohol use disorders. Religiosity also protects against drug disorders,[36,229] although this literature is less extensive.

Cognition, Personality

Substance Expectancies and Motivations

Positive substance expectancies constitute an important risk factor for the development of alcohol dependence.[88,273] For example, alcohol expectancies are considered the beliefs that drinking alcohol will result in decreased negative emotions or enhanced positive emotions.[87,280] These expectancies can be derived from parents and peers, and are believed to be environmentally influenced rather than genetically influenced.[279] Motivations for drinking often fall under four main domains: (1) drinking to obtain social rewards or enhance social interactions; (2) drinking to enhance

---

[g] References 29, 70, 71, 77, 184, 186–190, 223, 233.

positive mood; (3) drinking to reduce negative mood; and (4) drinking to avoid social rejection and conform to social norms. Although individuals with alcohol disorders often rate all motivations highly, reduction of negative affect and enhancement of positive affect have been prospectively associated with heavy use and alcohol and drug disorders.[15,30,164]

Personality Traits

No single personality trait predicts alcoholism,[274] but traits associated with the development of alcohol use disorders include novelty seeking[37] and sensation seeking,[215,325], traits that are often associated.[63,318] The heritability of sensation seeking is unclear, with some twin studies suggesting that approximately half of the variance can be attributed to genetic factors,[145,148,162] and another suggesting a much weaker influence of genetic factors.[227] Additional personality traits related to alcohol use disorders, albeit less consistently, are neuroticism/negative emotionality,[324] impulsivity/disinhibition,[220] and extraversion/sociability.[151] Similar traits have been examined in relation to drug use disorders. For example, research has shown that impulsivity/inhibition is reliably lower among individuals with drug abuse/dependence,[44,221] whereas negative emotionality tends to be higher.[287,318]

Subjective Reactions

The level of response to alcohol indicates the quantity needed to obtain an effect. Individuals with a low level of response need to drink more to obtain an effect. This is a genetically influenced characteristic associated with enhanced risk for alcohol use disorders.[268] Level of response varies by ethnicity. Several groups at high risk for alcohol use disorders show low response, including children of alcoholics, Native Americans, and Koreans,[68,229,308] while high response is found among Jews,[268] a group with relatively low levels of alcohol disorders.[124,206] A low level of response predicts later onset of alcohol dependence in young adult males,[266] and may contribute to transition from lighter to heavier drinking in individuals in a heavy-drinking environment.[265] Several chromosomal regions have shown suggestive linkage results to level of response,[316] and an association with variations in the *ADH1B* gene (one of the genes that influences metabolism of alcohol in the liver) has been documented,[62] but replication is needed.

Subjective reactions can also be characterized by whether they are positive or negative. A stimulating (reinforcing), rather than sedating, effect of alcohol has been identified in moderate/heavy drinkers,[157] as well as untreated alcoholics.[292] In contrast, a flushing reaction to alcohol, found among Asians, includes unpleasant physical sensations.[150] A strong flushing reaction precludes drinking, while moderate flushing protects against alcohol dependence. Individuals also vary in their subjective responses to marijuana, and positive and/or negative responses are moderately heritable.[211]

Psychiatric Comorbidity

Individuals with SUDs exhibit higher rates of mood, anxiety, and personality disorders than the general population.[42,98,137,180,254] For example, national surveys indicate that individuals with an alcohol disorder are approximately 3.0 times more likely to be diagnosed with major depression; the association between drug disorders and major depression is even stronger, with odds ratios around 7.0.[40,117] A strong association has also been documented between substance disorders and personality disorders. For example, the NESARC data estimates that 39.3% and 72.4%

of individuals with antisocial personality disorder meet criteria for lifetime drug disorders and alcohol disorders, respectively.[89] Borderline personality disorder was also strongly associated with alcohol and drug disorders in the NESARC,[101] and antisocial, borderline, and schizotypal personality disorder were associated with persistent course of alcohol and drug use disorders at the 3-year follow-up interview of the NESARC.[76,126] New findings from the 2012–2013 NESARC-III replicate the strong relationships between SUDs and psychiatric comorbidity.[104,106,143,223]

The strong and consistent relationships between SUDs and other psychiatric disorders have prompted etiologic researchers to evaluate evidence for an underlying vulnerability to psychiatric disorders in general. Adult twin studies indicate at least moderate genetic heritability across disorders,[174,177,212] and some genetic studies have indicated specific genetic variants associated with the transmission of several psychiatric disorders in general, rather than particular disorders.[57,309] "Internalizing" and "externalizing" domains have been proposed as a means of organizing individual disorders into larger, more meaningful groups. Internalizing disorders are often characterized by the anxiety and depression domains, whereas externalizing disorders are often characterized by alcohol, drug, and antisocial personality disorders. Research into the validity and utility of broad versus narrow categorizations of disorders has been a major area of psychiatric research for decades,[251] and is ongoing.[64,195,196,198,256]

Genetics

Family and Twin Studies of Alcohol and Drug Dependence

Alcoholism[47,237] and drug disorders[222] are familial. Genetic epidemiology studies of heritability use twin samples to compare concordance for a disorder between monozygotic (identical) and dizygotic (nonidentical) twins. In these studies, significantly higher concordance in identical twins, who share 100% of their genes, compared with nonidentical twins, who share only an average of 50% of their genes, indicates genetic heritability for a disorder. Twin studies of alcohol dependence show substantial heritabilities (50%–60%).[146,252] Heritability estimates from studies of illicit drugs are more variable, perhaps due to more varied phenotypes (use, heavy use, abuse, and dependence); for drug dependence, heritability estimates are similar to those for alcohol dependence.[80,176,252] For all substances, environmental factors appear to influence initiation and continuation of use, whereas genetic factors move individuals from use to dependence. In addition, as noted previously, environmental and social factors mediate the initiation and use of substances in childhood and adolescence, whereas genetic factors become more influential in adult substance use and dependence.[178] Some twin studies investigating shared heritability of dependence on different substances showed high shared genetic variance between substances,[177,298] whereas other studies suggest that dependence on different classes of drugs is not genetically interchangeable.[298] Molecular genetics studies may be able to clarify these issues.

Genetics in Epidemiology Studies

Some genetic variants that affect the process of alcohol metabolism in the liver such as alcohol dehydrogenase 4 (*ADH4*) are related to both alcohol[65,112,207,208] and drug dependence.[207-209] Alcohol dehydrogenase 2 (*ADH2* or *ADH1B*) and aldehyde dehydrogenase (*ALDH2*) have also shown well-replicated relationships to alcohol phenotypes.[49] However, genetic linkage and candidate gene association studies, used for decades to map and characterize genomic loci and genes that underlie the genetic vulnerability to SUDs,[83,84] have been only moderately successful in identifying relevant genetic variants. Recently, genome-wide association (GWAS) studies have become a major tool for identifying genetic variants related to alcohol and drug use disorders[2,166] by examining correlations between millions of common single-nucleotide polymorphisms with diagnosis status or related underlying endophenotypes.[224,225] GWAS studies are just beginning to uncover novel biology.[250] However, although the functional significance of results remains a matter of extensive debate and uncertainty,[250] genetics remains an important field of study in the etiology of SUDs. The availability of a panel of genetic variants from over 20,000 participants in the NESARC-III may offer new information from a large sample that has been well characterized in terms of phenotypes and other characteristics.

Although twin studies show that genetic and environmental factors are both important, relatively few studies have addressed whether the relationship of specific genetic variants to alcohol and drug dependence is modified by environmental circumstances. Examples of this approach involving candidate genes are studies showing that exposure to childhood maltreatment interacts with a gene influencing stress reactions to predict early onset of drinking among adolescents,[172] and interacts with *ADH1B* on risk for alcohol phenotypes in Jewish Israeli drinkers.[223] GWAS studies remain to be conducted.

Studying the interaction between certain genes and specific environmental factors has important implications for the prevention and treatment of alcohol and drug use disorders. First, better knowledge in this area may help early identification of individuals who are unlikely to be able to use drugs or alcohol in moderation for early education, additional support, or supervision. Second, the knowledge may help identify individuals exposed to particular stressors who would particularly benefit from intervention. Finally, clearer knowledge of the interaction of environmental with genetic effects may suggest new lines of investigation to determine the biological mechanisms of protective or risk-enhancing environmental events or conditions, which may eventually aid in developing better treatments.

Conclusion

In summary, a number of factors influencing the risk for substance dependence have been identified. Through trans-disciplinary research, epidemiologists and others can work together in the future to address multi-level factors conjointly.

References

1. Acker CJ, Tracy SW. *Altering American Consciousness: Essays on the History of Alcohol and Drug Use in the United States, 1800–2000.* New York: University of Massachusetts Press; 2004.
2. Agrawal A, Edenberg HJ, Gelernter J. Meta-analyses of genome-wide association data hold new promise for addiction genetics. *J Stud Alcohol Drugs.* 2016;77(5):676–680.
3. Agrawal A, Lynskey MT. Does gender contribute to heterogeneity in criteria for cannabis abuse and dependence? Results from the National Epidemiological Survey on Alcohol and Related Conditions. *Drug Alcohol Depend.* 2007;88(2-3):300–307.
4. Aharonovich E, et al. Differences in drinking patterns among Ashkenazic and Sephardic Israeli adults. *J Stud Alcohol.* 2001;62: 301–305.
5. Alexander BK, et al. Effect of early and later colony housing on oral ingestion of morphine in rats. *Pharmacol Biochem Behav.* 1981;15:571–576.
6. American Psychiatric Association. *Diagnostic and Statistical Manual of Mental Disorders.* 4th ed. Washington, DC; 1994.
7. American Psychiatric Association. *Diagnostic and Statistical Manual of Mental Disorders.* 5th ed. Washington, DC: American Psychiatric Association; 2013.
8. Asbridge M, et al. The criminalization of impaired driving in Canada: assessing the deterrent impact of Canada's first per se law. *J Stud Alcohol.* 2004;65(4):450–459.
9. Azaiza F, et al. Patterns of psychoactive substance use among Arab secondary school students in Israel. *Subst Use Misuse.* 2008;43(11):1489–1506.
10. Bachman JG, et al. *The Decline of Substance Use in Young Adulthood: Changes in Social Activities, Roles, and Beliefs.* Mahwah, NJ: Lawrence Erlbaum; 2002.
11. Barnes GM, Farrell MP, Banerjee S. Family influences on alcohol abuse and other problem behaviors among black and white adolescents in a general population sample. *J Res Adolesc.* 1994;4:183–201.
12. Barr CS, et al. The use of adolescent nonhuman primates to model human alcohol intake: neurobiological genetic, and psychological variables. *Ann N Y Acad Sci.* 2004;1021:221–233.
13. Bates ME, Bowden SC, Barry D. Neurocognitive impairment associated with alcohol use disorders: implications for treatment. *Exp Clin Psychopharmacol.* 2002;10:193–212.
14a. BBC World News, July 22, 2004.
14. Bertelli AA. Wine, research and cardiovascular disease: instructions for use. *Atherosclerosis.* 2007;195(2):242–247.
15. Beseler CL, et al. Adult transition from at-risk drinking to alcohol dependence: the relationship of family history and drinking motives. *Alcohol Clin Exp Res.* 2008;32(4):607–616.
16. Birckmayer J, Hemenway D. Minimum-age drinking laws and youth suicide, 1970–1990. *Am J Pub Health.* 1999;89:1365–1368.
17. Blanco C, et al. The latent structure of marijuana and cocaine use disorders: results from the National Longitudinal Alcohol Epidemiologic Survey (NLAES). *Drug Alcohol Depend.* 2007;91(1): 91–96.
18. Blumenthal RN, et al. Collateral damage in the war on drugs: HIV risk behaviors along injection drug users. *Int J Drug Policy.* 1999;10:25–38.
19. Borsari B, Carey KB. Peer influences on college drinking: a review of the research. *J Subst Abuse.* 2001;13:391–424.
20. Braida D, et al. Delta9-tetrahydrocannabinol-induced conditioned place preference and intracerebroventricular self-administration in rats. *Eur J Pharmacol.* 2004;506:63–69.
21. Brake WG, et al. Influence of early postnatal rearing conditions on mesocorticolimbic dopamine and behavioral responses to psychostimulants and stressors in adult rats. *Eur J Neurosci.* 2004;19:1863–1874.
22. Brent DA. Risk factors for adolescent suicide and suicidal behavior: mental and substance abuse disorders, family environmental factors, and life stress. *Suicide Life Threat Behav.* 1995;25(suppl):52–63.
23. Brook JS, et al. Pathways to marijuana use among adolescents: cultural/ecological, family, peer, and personality influences. *J Am Acad Child Adolesc Psychiatry.* 37:759–766.
24. Brook JS, et al. Sibling influences on adolescent drug use: older brothers on younger brothers. *J Am Acad Child Adolesc Psychiatry.* 1991;30(6):958–966.
25. Bucholz KK, et al. Reliability of individual diagnostic criterion items for psychoactive substance dependence and the impact on diagnosis. *J Stud Alcohol.* 1995;56:500–505.
26. Caetano R, Nelson S, Cunradi C. Intimate partner violence, dependence symptoms and social consequences of drinking among white, black and Hispanic couples in the United States. *Am J Addict.* 2001;10(suppl):60–69.
27. Canino G, et al. The Spanish Alcohol Use Disorder and Associated Disabilities Interview Schedule (AUDADIS): reliability and concordance with clinical diagnoses in a Hispanic population. *J Stud Alcohol.* 1999;60:790–799.

28. Carliner H, et al. The widening gender gap in marijuana use prevalence in the U.S. during a period of economic change, 2002-2014. *Drug Alcohol Depend.* 2017;170:51–58.

29. Carliner H, et al. Childhood trauma and illicit drug use in adolescence: a population-based National Comorbidity Survey Replication-Adolescent Supplement study. *J Am Acad Child Adolesc Psychiatry.* 2016;55(8):701–708.

30. Carpenter KM, Hasin D. A prospective evaluation of the relationship between reasons for drinking and DSM-IV alcohol-use disorders. *Addict Behav.* 1998;23(1):41–46.

31. Casswell S. Alcohol brands in young peoples' everyday lives: new developments in marketing. *Alcohol Alcohol.* 2004;39:471–476.

32. Centers for Disease Control (CDC). Point-of-purchase alcohol marketing and promotion by store type—United States, 2000–2001. *MMWR.* 2003;52:310–313.

33. Cerda M, et al. Medical marijuana laws in 50 states: investigating the relationship between state legalization of medical marijuana and marijuana use, abuse and dependence. *Drug Alcohol Depend.* 2012;120(1–3):22–27.

34. Cerda M, et al. Association of state recreational marijuana laws with adolescent marijuana use. *JAMA Pediatr.* 2017;171(2):142–149.

35. Chaloupka FJ, Grossman M, Saffer H. The effects of price on alcohol consumption and alcohol-related problems. *Alcohol Res Health.* 2002;26(1):22–34.

36. Chen CY, et al. Religiosity and the earliest stages of adolescent drug involvement in seven countries of Latin America. *Am J Epidemiol.* 2004;159(12):1180–1188.

37. Cloninger CR, et al. Personality antecedents of alcoholism in a national area probability sample. *Eur Arch Psychiatry Clin Neurosci.* 1995;245(4-5):239–244.

38. Cohen DA, Mason K, Scribner R. The population consumption model, alcohol control practices, and alcohol-related traffic fatalities. *Prev Med.* 2002;34(2):187–197.

39. Cohen E, et al. Alcohol treatment utilization: findings from the National Epidemiologic Survey on Alcohol and Related Conditions. *Drug Alcohol Depend.* 2007;86(2-3):214–221.

40. Compton WM, et al. Prevalence, correlates, disability, and comorbidity of DSM-IV drug abuse and dependence in the United States: results from the National Epidemiologic Survey on Alcohol and Related Conditions. *Arch Gen Psychiatry.* 2007;64(5):566–576.

41. Compton WM, et al. Crosswalk between DSM-IV dependence and DSM-5 substance use disorders for opioids, cannabis, cocaine and alcohol. *Drug Alcohol Depend.* 2013;132(1-2):387–390.

42. Compton WM, et al. Marijuana use and use disorders in adults in the USA, 2002-14: analysis of annual cross-sectional surveys. *Lancet Psychiatry.* 2016;3(10):954–964.

43. Connolly GM, et al. Alcohol in the mass media and drinking by adolescents: a longitudinal study. *Addiction.* 1994;89(10):1255–1263.

44. Conway KP, et al. Personality, drug of choice, and comorbid psychopathology among substance abusers. *Drug Alcohol Depend.* 2002;65(3):225–234.

45. Cooke E, et al. Marketing of alcohol to young people: a comparison of the UK and Poland. *Eur Addict Res.* 2004;10(1):1–7.

46. Cottler LB, et al. Concordance of DSM-IV alcohol and drug use disorder criteria and diagnoses as measured by AUDADIS-ADR, CIDI and SCAN. *Drug Alcohol Depend.* 1997;47(3):195–205.

47. Cotton NS. The familial incidence of alcoholism: a review. *J Stud Alcohol.* 1979;40:89–116.

48. Covington HE, Miczek KA. Repeated social-defeat stress, cocaine or morphine. Effects on behavioral sensitization and intravenous cocaine self-administration "binges". *Psychopharmacology.* 2001;158(4):388–398.

49. Crabb DW, et al. Overview of the role of alcohol dehydrogenase and aldehyde dehydrogenase and their variants in the genesis of alcohol-related pathology. *Proc Nutr Soc.* 2004;63(1):49–63.

50. Dawson DA, Goldstein RB, Grant BF. Rates and correlates of relapse among individuals in remission from DSM-IV alcohol dependence: a 3-year follow-up. *Alcohol Clin Exp Res.* 2007;31(12):2036–2045.

51. Dawson DA, et al. Recovery from DSM-IV alcohol dependence: United States, 2001-2002. *Addiction.* 2005;100(3):281–292.

52. Dawson DA, et al. Estimating the effect of help-seeking on achieving recovery from alcohol dependence. *Addiction.* 2006;101(6):824–834.

53. Dawson DA, et al. Changes in alcohol consumption: United States, 2001-2002 to 2012-2013. *Drug Alcohol Depend.* 2015;148:56–61.

54. Day C, et al. Decreased heroin availability in Sydney in early 2001. *Addiction.* 2003;98(1):93–95.

55. Deater-Deckard K, Annotation. Recent research examining the role of peer relationships in the development of psychopathology. *J Child Psychol Psychiatry.* 2001;42(5):565–579.

56. Deroche-Gamonet V, Belin D, Piazza PV. Evidence for addiction-like behavior in the rat. *Science.* 2004;305(5686):1014–1017.

57. Dick DM, et al. A Systematic single nucleotide polymorphism screen to fine-map alcohol dependence genes on chromosome 7 identifies association with a novel susceptibility gene ACN9. *Biol Psychiatry.* 2008;63(11):1047–1053.

58. Donohew RL, et al. Sensation seeking and drug use by adolescents and their friends: models for marijuana and alcohol. *J Stud Alcohol.* 1999;60(5):622–631.

59. Dube SR, et al. Childhood abuse, neglect, and household dysfunction and the risk of illicit drug use: the adverse childhood experiences study. *Pediatrics.* 2003;111(3):564–572.

60. Dudish SA, Hatsukami DK. Gender differences in crack users who are research volunteers. *Drug Alcohol Depend.* 1996;42(1):55–63.

61. DuPont RL, Greene MH. The dynamics of a heroin addiction epidemic. *Science.* 1973;181(4101):716–722.

62. Duranceaux NC, et al. Associations of variations in alcohol dehydrogenase genes with the level of response to alcohol in non-Asians. *Alcohol Clin Exp Res.* 2006;30(9):1470–1478.

63. Earleywine M, et al. Factor structure and correlates of the Tridimensional Personality Questionnaire. *J Stud Alcohol.* 1992;53(3):233–238.

64. Eaton NR, et al. Transdiagnostic factors of psychopathology and substance use disorders: a review. *Soc Psychiatry Psychiatr Epidemiol.* 2015;50(2):171–182.

65. Edenberg HJ, Foroud T. The genetics of alcoholism: identifying specific genes through family studies. *Addict Biol.* 2006;11(3-4):386–396.

66. Edwards G. The alcohol dependence syndrome: a concept as stimulus to enquiry. *Br J Addict.* 1986;81(2):171–183.

67. Edwards G, Arif A, Hadgson R. Nomenclature and classification of drug- and alcohol-related problems: a WHO memorandum. *Bull World Health Organ.* 1981;59(2):225–242.

68. Ehlers CL, et al. Electroencephalographic responses to alcohol challenge in Native American Mission Indians. *Biol Psychiatry.* 1999;45(6):776–787.

69. Ellickson PL, et al. Does alcohol advertising promote adolescent drinking? Results from a longitudinal assessment. *Addiction.* 2005;100(2):235–246.

70. Elliott JC, et al. The risk for persistent adult alcohol and nicotine dependence: the role of childhood maltreatment. *Addiction.* 2014;109(5):842–850.

71. Elliott JC, et al. Childhood maltreatment, personality disorders and 3-year persistence of adult alcohol and nicotine dependence in a national sample. *Addiction.* 2016;111(5):913–923.

72. Ellis DA, Zucker RA, Fitzgerald HE. The role of family influences in development and risk. *Alcohol Health Res World.* 1997;21(3):218–226.

73. Ezzati M, et al. Selected major risk factors and global and regional burden of disease. *Lancet.* 2002;360(9343):1347–1360.

74. Fell JC, Voas RB. The effectiveness of reducing illegal blood alcohol concentration (BAC) limits for driving: evidence for lowering the limit to .05 BAC. *J Safety Res.* 2006;37(3):233–243.

75. Fell JC, et al. The relationship of underage drinking laws to reductions in drinking drivers in fatal crashes in the United States. *Accid Anal Prev.* 2008;40(4):1430–1440.

76. Fenton MC, et al. Psychiatric comorbidity and the persistence of drug use disorders in the United States. *Addiction.* 2012;107(3):599–609.

77. Fenton MC, et al. Combined role of childhood maltreatment, family history, and gender in the risk for alcohol dependence. *Psychol Med.* 2013;43(5):1045–1057.

78. Fergusson DM, Woodward LJ, Horwood LJ. Childhood peer relationship problems and young people's involvement with deviant peers in adolescence. *J Abnorm Child Psychol.* 1999;27(5):357–369.

79. Fleming K, Thorson E, Atkin CK. Alcohol advertising exposure and perceptions: links with alcohol expectancies and intentions to drink or drinking in underaged youth and young adults. *J Health Commun.* 2004;9(1):3–29.

80. Fu Q, et al. Shared genetic risk of major depression, alcohol dependence, and marijuana dependence: contribution of antisocial personality disorder in men. *Arch Gen Psychiatry.* 59(12):1125–1132.

81. Fulkerson JA, Harrison PA, Beebe TJ. DSM-IV substance abuse and dependence: are there really two dimensions of substance use disorders in adolescents? *Addiction.* 1999;94(4):495–506.

82. Garfield CF, Chung PJ, Rathouz PJ. Alcohol advertising in magazines and adolescent readership. *JAMA.* 2003;289(18):2424–2429.

83. Gelernter J, Kranzler HR. Genetics of alcohol dependence. *Hum Genet.* 2009;126(1):91–99.

84. Gelernter J, Kranzler HR. Genetics of drug dependence. *Dialogues Clin Neurosci.* 2010;12(1):77–84.

85. Gfroerer J. Correlation between drug use by teenagers and drug use by older family members. *Am J Drug Alcohol Abuse.* 1987;13(1-2):95–108.

86. Goeders NE, Guerin GF. Non-contingent electric footshock facilitates the acquisition of intravenous cocaine self-administration in rats. *Psychopharmacology (Berl).* 1994;114(1):63–70.

87. Goldman MS, Rather BC. Substance use disorders: cognitive models and architectures. In: Kendall P, Dobson KS, eds. *Psychopathology and Cognition.* Orlando, FL: Academic; 1993:245–291.

88. Goldman MS, et al. Alcoholism and memory: broadening the scope of alcohol-expectancy research. *Psychol Bull.* 1991;110(1):137–146.

89. Goldstein RB, et al. Antisocial behavioral syndromes and DSM-IV drug use disorders in the United States: results from the National Epidemiologic Survey on Alcohol and Related Conditions. *Drug Alcohol Depend.* 2007;90(2-3):145–158.

90. Goldstein RB, et al. Nosologic comparisons of DSM-IV and DSM-5 alcohol and drug use disorders: results from the National Epidemiologic Survey on Alcohol and Related Conditions-III. *J Stud Alcohol Drugs.* 2015;76(3):378–388.

91. Grant BF. DSM-IV, DSM-III-R, and ICD-10 alcohol and drug abuse/harmful use and dependence, United States, 1992: a nosological comparison. *Alcohol Clin Exp Res.* 1996;20(8):1481–1488.

92. Grant BF, Moore TC, Kaplan K. *Source and Accuracy Statement: Wave 1 National Epidemiologic Survey on Alcohol and Related Conditions (NESARC).* National Institute on Alcohol Abuse and Alcoholism; 2003.

93. Grant BF, Stinson FS, Harford TC. Age at onset of alcohol use and DSM-IV alcohol abuse and dependence: a 12-year follow-up. *J Subst Abuse.* 2001;13(4):493–504.

94. Grant BF, et al. Prevalence of DSM-IV alcohol abuse and dependence: United States, 1992. *Alcohol Health Res World.* 1992;18:243–248.

95. Grant BF, et al. The Alcohol Use Disorder and Associated Disabilities Interview schedule (AUDADIS): reliability of alcohol and drug modules in a general population sample. *Drug Alcohol Depend.* 1995;39(1):37–44.

96. Grant BF, et al. Co-occurrence of 12-month alcohol and drug use disorders and personality disorders in the United States: results from the National Epidemiologic Survey on Alcohol and Related Conditions. *Arch Gen Psychiatry.* 2004;61(4):361–368.

97. Grant BF, et al. Immigration and lifetime prevalence of DSM-IV psychiatric disorders among Mexican Americans and non-Hispanic whites in the United States: results from the National Epidemiologic Survey on Alcohol and Related Conditions. *Arch Gen Psychiatry.* 2004;61(12):1226–1233.

98. Grant BF, et al. Prevalence and co-occurrence of substance use disorders and independent mood and anxiety disorders: results from the National Epidemiologic Survey on Alcohol and Related Conditions. *Arch Gen Psychiatry.* 2004;61(8):807–816.

99. Grant BF, et al. Source and accuracy statement: Wave 1 National Epidemiologic Survey on Alcohol and Related Conditions (NESARC). [Website] http://www.niaaa.nih.gov. Accessed July 2, 2005.

100. Grant BF, et al. DSM-IV alcohol dependence and abuse: further evidence of validity in the general population. *Drug Alcohol Depend.* 2007;86(2-3):154–166.

101. Grant BF, et al. Prevalence, correlates, disability, and comorbidity of DSM-IV borderline personality disorder: results from the Wave 2 National Epidemiologic Survey on Alcohol and Related Conditions. *J Clin Psychiatry.* 2008;69(4):533–545.

102. Grant BF, et al. Sociodemographic and psychopathologic predictors of first incidence of DSM-IV substance use, mood and anxiety disorders: results from the Wave 2 National Epidemiologic Survey on Alcohol and Related Conditions. *Mol Psychiatry.* 2009;14(11):1051–1166.

103. Grant BF, et al. *Source and Accuracy Statement: National Epidemiologic Survey on Alcohol and Related Conditions-III (NESARC-III).* National Institute on Alcohol Abuse and Alcoholism; 2014.

104. Grant BF, et al. Epidemiology of DSM-5 alcohol use disorder: results from the National Epidemiologic Survey on Alcohol and Related Conditions III. *JAMA Psychiatry.* 2015;72(8):757–766.

105. Grant BF, et al. The Alcohol Use Disorder and Associated Disabilities Interview Schedule-5 (AUDADIS-5): reliability of substance use and psychiatric disorder modules in a general population sample. *Drug Alcohol Depend.* 2015;148:27–33.

106. Grant BF, et al. Epidemiology of DSM-5 Drug use disorder: results from the National Epidemiologic Survey on Alcohol and Related Conditions-III. *JAMA Psychiatry.* 2016;73(1):39–47.

107. Greene MH, Nightingale SL, DuPont RL. Evolving patterns of drug abuse. *Ann Intern Med.* 1975;83(3):402–411.

108. Greenfield TK, Room R. Situational norms for drinking and drunkenness: trends in the US adult population, 1979-1990. *Addiction.* 1997;92(1):33–47.

109. Grucza RA, et al. Correspondence between secular changes in alcohol dependence and age of drinking onset among women in the United States. *Alcohol Clin Exp Res.* 2008;32(8):1493–1501.

110. Grucza RA, et al. Declining prevalence of marijuana use disorders among adolescents in the United States, 2002 to 2013. *J Am Acad Child Adolesc Psychiatry.* 2016;55(6):487–494 e6.

111. Gruenewald PJ, Johnson FW, Treno AJ. Outlets, drinking and driving: a multilevel analysis of availability. *J Stud Alcohol.* 2002;63(4):460–468.

112. Guindalini C, et al. Association of genetic variants in alcohol dehydrogenase 4 with alcohol dependence in Brazilian patients. *Am J Psychiatry.* 2005;162(5):1005–1007.

113. Hamilton WJ. Mothers Against Drunk Driving--MADD in the USA. *Inj Prev.* 2000;6(2):90–91.

114. Haney M, et al. Social stress increases the acquisition of cocaine self-administration in male and female rats. *Brain Res.* 1995;698(1-2):46–52.

115. Harford TC, Muthen BO. The dimensionality of alcohol abuse and dependence: a multivariate analysis of DSM-IV symptom items in the National Longitudinal Survey of Youth. *J Stud Alcohol.* 2001;62(2):150–157.

116. Harwood R, Fountain D, Livermore G. *The Economic Costs of Alcohol and Drug Abuse in the United States, 1992.* National Institute on Alcohol Abuse and Alcoholism and National Institute on Drug Abuse; 1998.

117. Hasin D, Nunes E, Meydan J. Comorbidity of alcohol, drug, and psychiatric disorders: epidemiology. In: Kranzler HR, Tinsley JA, eds. *Dual Diagnosis and Psychiatric Treatment: Substance Abuse and Comorbid Disorders.* New York, NY: Marcel Dekker; 2004:1–34.

118. Hasin D, Paykin A. Alcohol dependence and abuse diagnoses: concurrent validity in a nationally representative sample. *Alcohol Clin Exp Res.* 1999;23(1):144–150.

119. Hasin D, Paykin A. Dependence symptoms but no diagnosis: diagnostic 'orphans' in a 1992 national sample. *Drug Alcohol Depend.* 1999;53(3):215–222.

120. Hasin D, Paykin A. DSM-IV alcohol abuse: investigation in a sample of at-risk drinkers in the community. *J Stud Alcohol.* 1999;60(2):181–187.

121. Hasin D, et al. Alcohol dependence and abuse diagnoses: validity in community sample heavy drinkers. *Alcohol Clin Exp Res.* 1997;21(2):213–219.

122. Hasin D, et al. Nosological comparisons of alcohol and drug diagnoses: a multisite, multi-instrument international study. *Drug Alcohol Depend.* 1997;47(3):217–226.

123. Hasin D, et al. The alcohol use disorder and associated disabilities interview schedule (AUDADIS): reliability of alcohol and drug modules in a clinical sample. *Drug Alcohol Depend.* 1997;44(2-3):133–141.

124. Hasin D, et al. The drinking of earlier and more recent Russian immigrants to Israel: comparison to other Israelis. *J Subst Abuse.* 1998;10(4):341–353.

125. Hasin D, et al. Diagnosis of comorbid psychiatric disorders in substance users assessed with the Psychiatric Research Interview for Substance and Mental Disorders for DSM-IV. *Am J Psychiatry.* 2006;163(4):689–696.

126. Hasin D, et al. Personality disorders and the 3-year course of alcohol, drug, and nicotine use disorders. *Arch Gen Psychiatry.* 2011;68(11):1158–1167.

127. Hasin DS, Grant B, Endicott J. The natural history of alcohol abuse: implications for definitions of alcohol use disorders. *Am J Psychiatry.* 1990;147(11):1537–1541.

128. Hasin DS, Grant BF. Major depression in 6050 former drinkers: association with past alcohol dependence. *Arch Gen Psychiatry.* 2002;59(9):794–800.

129. Hasin DS, Grant BF. The co-occurrence of DSM-IV alcohol abuse in DSM-IV alcohol dependence: results of the National Epidemiologic Survey on Alcohol and Related Conditions on heterogeneity that differ by population subgroup. *Arch Gen Psychiatry.* 2004;61(9):891–896.

130. Hasin DS, et al. (In press). Change in non-abstinent WHO risk drinking levels and alcohol dependence: a 3-year follow-up study in the United States general population. *Lancet Psychiatry.* 2017;4(6):469–476.

131. Hasin DS, et al. (In press). U.S. Adult Illicit Cannabis Use, Cannabis Use Disorder, and Medical Marijuana Laws: 1991-1992 to 2012-2013. *JAMA Psychiatry.*

132. Hasin DS, et al. Psychiatric Research Interview for Substance and Mental Disorders (PRISM): reliability for substance abusers. *Am J Psychiatry.* 1996;153(9):1195–1201.

133. Hasin DS, et al. Differentiating DSM-IV alcohol dependence and abuse by course: community heavy drinkers. *J Subst Abuse.* 1997;9:127–135.

134. Hasin DS, et al. The validity of DSM-IV alcohol dependence: what do we know and what do we need to know? *Alcohol Clin Exp Res.* 2003;27(2):244–252.

135. Hasin DS, et al. Co-occurring DSM-IV drug abuse in DSM-IV drug dependence: results from the National Epidemiologic Survey on Alcohol and Related Conditions. *Drug Alcohol Depend.* 2005;80(1):117–123.

136. Hasin DS, et al. DSM-IV alcohol dependence: a categorical or dimensional phenotype? *Psychol Med.* 2006;36(12):1695–1705.

137. Hasin DS, et al. Prevalence, correlates, disability, and comorbidity of DSM-IV alcohol abuse and dependence in the United States: results from the National Epidemiologic Survey on Alcohol and Related Conditions. *Arch Gen Psychiatry.* 2007;64(7):830–842.

138. Hasin DS, et al. DSM-5 criteria for substance use disorders: recommendations and rationale. *Am J Psychiatry.* 2013;170(8):834–851.

139. Hasin DS, et al. Medical marijuana laws and adolescent marijuana use in the USA from 1991 to 2014: results from annual, repeated cross-sectional surveys. *Lancet Psychiatry.* 2015;2(7):601–608.

140. Hasin DS, et al. Prevalence of marijuana use disorders in the united states between 2001-2002 and 2012-2013. *JAMA Psychiatry.* 2015;72(12):1235–1242.

141. Hasin DS, et al. Procedural validity of the AUDADIS-5 depression, anxiety and post-traumatic stress disorder modules: substance abusers and others in the general population. *Drug Alcohol Depend.* 2015;152:246–256.

142. Hasin DS, et al. The Alcohol Use Disorder and Associated Disabilities Interview Schedule-5 (AUDADIS-5): procedural validity of substance use disorders modules through clinical re-appraisal in a general population sample. *Drug Alcohol Depend.* 2015;148:40–46.

143. Hasin DS, et al. Prevalence and correlates of DSM-5 cannabis use disorder, 2012–2013: findings from the National Epidemiologic Survey on Alcohol and Related Conditions-III. *Am J Psychiatry.* 2016;173(6):588–599.

144. Hawkins JD, Catalano RF, Miller JY. Risk and protective factors for alcohol and other drug problems in adolescence and early adulthood: implications for substance abuse prevention. *Psychol Bull.* 1992;112(1):64–105.

145. Heath AC, Cloninger CR, Martin NG. Testing a model for the genetic structure of personality: a comparison of the personality systems of Cloninger and Eysenck. *J Pers Soc Psychol.* 1994;66(4):762–775.

146. Heath AC. Genetic influences on alcoholism risk: a review of adoption and twin studies. *Alcohol Health Res World.* 1995;19:166–171.

147. Heeb JL, et al. Changes in alcohol consumption following a reduction in the price of spirits: a natural experiment in Switzerland. *Addiction.* 2003;98(10):1433–1446.

148. Heiman N, et al. Investigating age differences in the genetic and environmental structure of the tridimensional personality questionnaire in later adulthood. *Behav Genet.* 2003;33(2):171–180.

149. Henderson C, et al. The effects of US state income inequality and alcohol policies on symptoms of depression and alcohol dependence. *Soc Sci Med.* 2004;58(3):565–575.

150. Higuchi S, et al. Alcohol and aldehyde dehydrogenase polymorphisms and the risk for alcoholism. *Am J Psychiatry.* 1995;152(8):1219–1221.

151. Hill SY, et al. Factors predicting the onset of adolescent drinking in families at high risk for developing alcoholism. *Biol Psychiatry.* 2000;48(4):265–275.

152. Hingson RW, Heeren T, Edwards EM. Age at drinking onset, alcohol dependence, and their relation to drug use and dependence, driving under the influence of drugs, and motor-vehicle crash involvement because of drugs. *J Stud Alcohol Drugs.* 2008;69(2):192–201.

153. Hingson RW, Heeren T, Winter MR. Age at drinking onset and alcohol dependence: age at onset, duration, and severity. *Arch Pediatr Adolesc Med.* 2006;160(7):739–746.

154. Holdcraft LC, Iacono WG. Cohort effects on gender differences in alcohol dependence. *Addiction.* 2002;97(8):1025–1036.

155. Holdcraft LC, Iacono WG. Cross-generational effects on gender differences in psychoactive drug abuse and dependence. *Drug Alcohol Depend.* 2004;74(2):147–158.

156. Holder HD, et al. Effect of community-based interventions on high-risk drinking and alcohol-related injuries. *JAMA.* 2000;284(18):2341–2347.

157. Holdstock L, King AC, de Wit H. Subjective and objective responses to ethanol in moderate/heavy and light social drinkers. *Alcohol Clin Exp Res.* 2000;24(6):789–794.

158. Hopfer CJ, Crowley TJ, Hewitt JK. Review of twin and adoption studies of adolescent substance use. *J Am Acad Child Adolesc Psychiatry.* 2003;42(6):710–719.

159. Hopfer CJ, et al. Family transmission of marijuana use, abuse, and dependence. *J Am Acad Child Adolesc Psychiatry.* 2003;42(7):834–841.

160. Hsu DJ, et al. Hospitalizations, costs, and outcomes associated with heroin and prescription opioid overdoses in the United States 2001–2012. *Addiction*. 2017.

161. Hu M, et al. Biological basis of sex differences in the propensity to self-administer cocaine. *Neuropsychopharmacology*. 2004;29(1):81–85.

162. Hur YM, Bouchard Jr TJ. The genetic correlation between impulsivity and sensation seeking traits. *Behav Genet*. 1997;27(5):455–463.

163. Irons DE, et al. Mendelian randomization: a novel test of the gateway hypothesis and models of gene-environment interplay. *Dev Psychopathol*. 2007;19(4):1181–1195.

164. Jackson KM, Sher KJ. Similarities and differences of longitudinal phenotypes across alternate indices of alcohol involvement: a methodologic comparison of trajectory approaches. *Psychol Addict Behav*. 2005;19(4):339–351.

165. Jackson MC, et al. Marketing alcohol to young people: implications for industry regulation and research policy. *Addiction*. 2000;95(suppl 4):S597–608.

166. Jensen KP. A review of genome-wide association studies of stimulant and opioid use disorders. *Mol Neuropsychiatry*. 2016;2(1):37–45.

167. Johnson RA, Gerstein DR. Initiation of use of alcohol, cigarettes, marijuana, cocaine, and other substances in US birth cohorts since 1919. *Am J Public Health*. 1998;88(1):27–33.

168. Johnston LD, et al. *Monitoring the Future National Survey Results on Drug Use, 1975–2003. Volume I: Secondary School Students*. National Institute on Drug Abuse; 2004.

169. Kahler CW, Strong DR. A Rasch model analysis of DSM-IV alcohol abuse and dependence items in the National Epidemiological Survey on Alcohol and Related Conditions. *Alcohol Clin Exp Res*. 2006;30(7):1165–1175.

170. Kandel D. Adolescent marihuana use: role of parents and peers. *Science*. 1973;181(4104):1067–1670.

171. Kandel DB. On processes of peer influences in adolescent drug use: a developmental perspective. *Adv Alcohol Subst Abuse*. 1985;4(3-4):139–163.

172. Kaufman J, et al. Genetic and environmental predictors of early alcohol use. *Biol Psychiatry*. 2007;61(11):1228–1234.

173. Kendler KS, Gardner CO, Prescott CA. Religion, psychopathology, and substance use and abuse; a multimeasure, genetic-epidemiologic study. *Am J Psychiatry*. 1997;154(3):322–329.

174. Kendler KS, Prescott CA. A population-based twin study of lifetime major depression in men and women. *Arch Gen Psychiatry*. 1999;56(1):39–44.

175. Kendler KS, et al. Childhood parental loss and alcoholism in women: a causal analysis using a twin-family design. *Psychol Med*. 1996;26(1):79–95.

176. Kendler KS, et al. Childhood sexual abuse and adult psychiatric and substance use disorders in women: an epidemiological and cotwin control analysis. *Arch Gen Psychiatry*. 2000;57(10):953–959.

177. Kendler KS, et al. Specificity of genetic and environmental risk factors for use and abuse/dependence of cannabis, cocaine, hallucinogens, sedatives, stimulants, and opiates in male twins. *Am J Psychiatry*. 2003;160(4):687–695.

178. Kendler KS, et al. Genetic and environmental influences on alcohol, caffeine, cannabis, and nicotine use from early adolescence to middle adulthood. *Arch Gen Psychiatry*. 2008;65(6):674–682.

179. Kessler RC, Davis CG, Kendler KS. Childhood adversity and adult psychiatric disorder in the US National Comorbidity Survey. *Psychol Med*. 1997;27(5):1101–1119.

180. Kessler RC, et al. Lifetime and 12-month prevalence of DSM-III-R psychiatric disorders in the United States. Results from the National Comorbidity Survey. *Arch Gen Psychiatry*. 1994;51(1):8–19.

181. Kessler RC, et al. Prevalence and treatment of mental disorders, 1990 to 2003. *N Engl J Med*. 2005;352(24):2515–2523.

182. Keyes KM, Grant BF, Hasin DS. Evidence for a closing gender gap in alcohol use, abuse, and dependence in the United States population. *Drug Alcohol Depend*. 2008;93(1-2):21–29.

183. Keyes KM, Hasin DS. Socio-economic status and problem alcohol use: the positive relationship between income and the DSM-IV alcohol abuse diagnosis. *Addiction*. 2008;103(7):1120–1130.

184. Keyes KM, Hatzenbuehler ML, Hasin DS. Stressful life experiences, alcohol consumption, and alcohol use disorders: the epidemiologic evidence for four main types of stressors. *Psychopharmacology (Berl)*. 2011;218(1):1–17.

185. Keyes MA, Iacono WG, McGue M. Early onset problem behavior, young adult psychopathology, and contextual risk. *Twin Res Hum Genet*. 2007;10(1):45–53.

186. Keyes KM, et al. Child maltreatment increases sensitivity to adverse social contexts: neighborhood physical disorder and incident binge drinking in Detroit. *Drug Alcohol Depend*. 2012;122(1-2):77–85.

187. Keyes KM, et al. Childhood maltreatment and the structure of common psychiatric disorders. *Br J Psychiatry*. 2012;200(2):107–115.

188. Keyes KM, et al. Stress and alcohol: epidemiologic evidence. *Alcohol Res*. 2012;34(4):391–400.

189. Keyes KM, et al. Exposure to the Lebanon War of 2006 and effects on alcohol use disorders: the moderating role of childhood maltreatment. *Drug Alcohol Depend*. 2014;134:296–303.

190. Kim JH, et al. Childhood maltreatment, stressful life events, and alcohol craving in adult drinkers. *Alcohol Clin Exp Res*. 2014;38(7):2048–2055.

191. Kirk KM, et al. Frequency of church attendance in Australia and the United States: models of family resemblance. *Twin Res*. 1999;2(2):99–107.

192. Koopmans JR, et al. The influence of religion on alcohol use initiation: evidence for genotype X environment interaction. *Behav Genet*. 1999;29(6):445–453.

193. Kosten TA, Miserendino MJ, Kehoe P. Enhanced acquisition of cocaine self-administration in adult rats with neonatal isolation stress experience. *Brain Res*. 2000;875(1-2):44–50.

194. Kosten TA, Zhang XY, Kehoe P. Chronic neonatal isolation stress enhances cocaine-induced increases in ventral striatal dopamine levels in rat pups. *Brain Res Dev Brain Res*. 2003;141(1-2):109–116.

195. Kramer MD, Krueger RF, Hicks BM. The role of internalizing and externalizing liability factors in accounting for gender differences in the prevalence of common psychopathological syndromes. *Psychol Med*. 2008;38(1):51–61.

196. Krueger RF, Eaton NR. Transdiagnostic factors of mental disorders. *World Psychiatry*. 2015;14(1):27–29.

197. Krueger RF, et al. Using latent trait modeling to conceptualize an alcohol problems continuum. *Psychol Assess*. 2004;16(2):107–119.

198. Krueger RF, et al. Linking antisocial behavior, substance use, and personality: an integrative quantitative model of the adult externalizing spectrum. *J Abnorm Psychol*. 2007;116(4):645–666.

199. Kulsudjarit K. Drug problem in southeast and southwest Asia. *Ann N Y Acad Sci*. 2004;1025:446–457.

200. Kumpfer KL, Bluth B. Parent/child transactional processes predictive of resilience or vulnerability to "substance abuse disorders". *Subst Use Misuse*. 2004;39(5):671–698.

201. Kuo M, et al. The marketing of alcohol to college students: the role of low prices and special promotions. *Am J Prev Med*. 2003;25(3):204–211.

202. Kuperman S, et al. Developmental sequence from disruptive behavior diagnosis to adolescent alcohol dependence. *Am J Psychiatry*. 2001;158(12):2022–2026.

203. Lakins NE, et al. *Surveillance Report #78: Apparent Per Capita Alcohol Consumption: National, State, and Regional Trends, 1977–2004*. NIAAA, Division of Epidemiology and Prevention Research. Alcohol Epidemiologic Data System; 2006.

204. Lejuez CW, et al. Risk factors in the relationship between gender and crack/cocaine. *Exp Clin Psychopharmacol*. 2007;15(2):165–175.

205. Lender ME, Martin JK. *Drinking in America: a History*. New York, NY: Free; 1982.

206. Locke TF, Newcomb M. Child maltreatment, parent alcohol and drug-related problems, polydrug problems, and parenting practices: a test of gender differences and four theoretical perspectives. *J Fam Psychol.* 2004;18(1):120–134.

207. Luo X, et al. ADH4 gene variation is associated with alcohol and drug dependence: results from family controlled and population-structured association studies. *Pharmacogenet Genomics.* 2005;15(11):755–768.

208. Luo X, et al. ADH4 gene variation is associated with alcohol dependence and drug dependence in European Americans: results from HWD tests and case-control association studies. *Neuropsychopharmacology.* 2006;31(5):1085–1095.

209. Luo X, et al. Recessive genetic mode of an ADH4 variant in substance dependence in African-Americans: a model of utility of the HWD test. *Behav Brain Funct.* 2008;4:42.

210. Lynch WJ, Mangini LD, Taylor JR. Neonatal isolation stress potentiates cocaine seeking behavior in adult male and female rats. *Neuropsychopharmacol.* 2005;30(2):322–329.

211. Lyons MJ, et al. How do genes influence marijuana use? The role of subjective effects. *Addiction.* 1997;92(4):409–417.

212. Maghsoodloo S, Brown DB, Greathouse PA. Impact of the revision of DUI legislation in Alabama. *Am J Drug Alcohol Abuse.* 1988;14(1):97–108.

213. Margulies RZ, Kessler RC, Kandel DB. A longitudinal study of onset of drinking among high-school students. *J Stud Alcohol.* 1977;38(5):897–912.

214. Marks-Kaufman R, Lewis MJ. Early housing experience modifies morphine self-administration and physical dependence in adult rats. *Addict Behav.* 1984;9(3):235–243.

215. Martin CA, et al. Sensation seeking, puberty, and nicotine, alcohol, and marijuana use in adolescence. *J Am Acad Child Adolesc Psychiatry.* 2002;41(12):1495–1502.

216. Martin CA, et al. Sensation seeking and symptoms of disruptive disorder: association with nicotine, alcohol, and marijuana use in early and mid-adolescence. *Psychol Rep.* 2004;94(3 Pt 1):1075–1082.

217. Martin CS, et al. Item response theory analysis of diagnostic criteria for alcohol and cannabis use disorders in adolescents: implications for DSM-V. *J Abnorm Psychol.* 2006;115(4):807–814.

218. Martins SS, et al. (In press). Changes in lifetime heroin use and heroin use disorder: United States 2001-2002 to 2012-2013. *JAMA Psychiatry.*

219. McGovern PE, et al. Fermented beverages of pre- and proto-historic China. *Proc Natl Acad Sci U S A.* 2004;101(51):17593–17598.

220. McGue M, Slutske W, Iacono WG. Personality and substance use disorders: II. Alcoholism versus drug use disorders. *J Consult Clin Psychol.* 1999;67(3):394–404.

221. McGue M, et al. Personality and substance use disorders: I. Effects of gender and alcoholism subtype. *Alcohol Clin Exp Res.* 1997;21(3):513–520.

222. Merikangas KR, et al. Familial transmission of substance use disorders. *Arch Gen Psychiatry.* 1998;55(11):973–979.

223. Meyers JL, et al. Childhood adversity moderates the effect of ADH1B on risk for alcohol-related phenotypes in Jewish Israeli drinkers. *Addict Biol.* 2015;20(1):205–214.

224. Meyers JL, et al. A genome wide association study of fast beta EEG in families of European ancestry. *Int J Psychophysiol.* 2016.

225. Meyers JL, et al. An endophenotype approach to the genetics of alcohol dependence: a genome wide association study of fast beta EEG in families of African ancestry. *Mol Psychiatry.* 2017.

226. Miczek KA, Mutschler NH. Activational effects of social stress on IV cocaine self-administration in rats. *Psychopharmacology (Berl).* 1996;128(3):256–264.

227. Miles DR, et al. A twin study on sensation seeking, risk taking behavior and marijuana use. *Drug Alcohol Depend.* 2001;62(1):57–68.

228. Mokdad AH, et al. Diabetes trends in the U.S.: 1990-1998. *Diabetes Care.* 2000;23(9):1278–1283.

229. Monteiro MG, et al. TSH response to TRH and family history of alcoholism. *Biol Psychiatry.* 1990;27(8):905–910.

230. Musto DF. *The American Disease: Origins of Narcotic Control.* New York: Oxford University; 1999.

231. Muthen BO, Grant B, Hasin D. The dimensionality of alcohol abuse and dependence: factor analysis of DSM-III-R and proposed DSM-IV criteria in the 1988 National Health Interview Survey. *Addiction.* 1993;88(8):1079–1090.

232. Muthen BO. Factor analysis of alcohol abuse and dependence symptom items in the 1988 National Health Interview Survey. *Addiction.* 1995;90(5):637–645.

233. Myers B, et al. Associations between childhood adversity, adult stressful life events, and past-year drug use disorders in the National Epidemiological Study of Alcohol and Related Conditions (NESARC). *Psychol Addict Behav.* 2014;28(4):1117–1126.

234. National Survey on Drug Use and Health. https://nsduhweb.rti.org/respweb/homepage.cfm.

235. Nelson CB, et al. Factor structures for DSM-IV substance disorder criteria endorsed by alcohol, cannabis, cocaine and opiate users: results from the WHO reliability and validity study. *Addiction.* 1999;94(6):843–855.

236. Nelson EC, et al. Association between self-reported childhood sexual abuse and adverse psychosocial outcomes: results from a twin study. *Arch Gen Psychiatry.* 2002;59(2):139–145.

237. Nurnberger Jr JI, et al. A family study of alcohol dependence: coaggregation of multiple disorders in relatives of alcohol-dependent probands. *Arch Gen Psychiatry.* 2004;61(12):1246–1256.

238. O'Malley PM, Wagenaar AC. Effects of minimum drinking age laws on alcohol use, related behaviors and traffic crash involvement among American youth: 1976-1987. *J Stud Alcohol.* 1991;52(5):478–491.

239. Musto DF, Korsmeyer P, Malucci TW, eds. *One Hundred Years of Heroin.* New York: Auburn House; 2002.

240. Patock-Peckham JA, et al. A social learning perspective: a model of parenting styles, self-regulation, perceived drinking control, and alcohol use and problems. *Alcohol Clin Exp Res.* 2001;25(9):1284–1292.

241. Perkins HW. Parental religion and alcohol use problems as intergenerational predictors of problem drinking among college youth. *J Sci Study Reli.* 1987;26:340–357.

242. Piazza PV, et al. Factors that predict individual vulnerability to amphetamine self-administration. *Science.* 1989;245(4925):1511–1513.

243. Piazza PV, et al. Stress- and pharmacologically-induced behavioral sensitization increases vulnerability to acquisition of amphetamine self-administration. *Brain Res.* 1990;514(1):22–26.

244. Potter DA, et al. Effect of follicular-phase cocaine administration on menstrual and ovarian cyclicity in rhesus monkeys. *Am J Obstet Gynecol.* 1998;178:118–125.

245. Proudfoot H, Baillie AJ, Teesson M. The structure of alcohol dependence in the community. *Drug Alcohol Depend.* 2006;81(1):21–26.

246. Pull CB, et al. Concordance between ICD-10 alcohol and drug use disorder criteria and diagnoses as measured by the AUDADIS-ADR, CIDI and SCAN: results of a cross-national study. *Drug Alcohol Depend.* 1997;47(3):207–216.

247. Rahav G, Hasin D, Paykin A. Drinking patterns of recent Russian immigrants and other Israelis: 1995 national survey results. *Am J Public Health.* 1999;89(8):1212–1216.

248. Randall CL, et al. Telescoping of landmark events associated with drinking: a gender comparison. *J Stud Alcohol.* 1999;60(2):252–260.

249. Rehm J, et al. The global distribution of average volume of alcohol consumption and patterns of drinking. *Eur Addict Res.* 2003;9(4):147–156.

250. Reilly MT, et al. Genetic studies of alcohol dependence in the context of the addiction cycle. *Neuropharmacology.* 2017.

251. Repetti RL, Taylor SE, Seeman TE. Risky families: family social environments and the mental and physical health of offspring. *Psychol Bull.* 2002;128(2):330–366.

252. Rhee SH, et al. Genetic and environmental influences on substance initiation, use, and problem use in adolescents. *Arch Gen Psychiatry.* 2003;60(12):1256–1264.

253. Rice JP, et al. Age and birth cohort effects on rates of alcohol dependence. *Alcohol Clin Exp Res.* 2003;27(1):93–99.

254. Robins LN, et al. Lifetime prevalence of specific psychiatric disorders in three sites. *Arch Gen Psychiatry.* 1984;41(10):949–958.

255. Robinson TE. Neuroscience. Addicted rats. *Science.* 2004;305(5686):951–953.

256. Rodriguez-Seijas C, Eaton NR, Krueger RF. How transdiagnostic factors of personality and psychopathology can inform clinical assessment and intervention. *J Pers Assess.* 2015;97(5):425–435.

257. Room R. Effects of alcohol controls: nordic research traditions. *Drug Alcohol Rev.* 2004;23(1):43–53.

258. Room R, et al. Drinking and its burden in a global perspective: policy considerations and options. *Eur Addict Res.* 2003;9(4):165–175.

259. Rounsaville BJ, et al. Cross system agreement for substance use disorders: DSM-III-R, DSM-IV and ICD-10. *Addiction.* 1993;88(3):337–348.

260. Ruan WJ, et al. The alcohol use disorder and associated disabilities interview schedule-IV (AUDADIS-IV): reliability of new psychiatric diagnostic modules and risk factors in a general population sample. *Drug Alcohol Depend.* 2008;92(1–3):27–36.

261. Saha TD, Chou SP, Grant BF. Toward an alcohol use disorder continuum using item response theory: results from the National Epidemiologic Survey on Alcohol and Related Conditions. *Psychol Med.* 2006;36(7):931–941.

262. Saha TD, et al. Nonmedical prescription opioid use and DSM-5 nonmedical prescription opioid use disorder in the United States. *J Clin Psychiatry.* 2016;77(6):772–780.

263. Samet JH, et al. Alcohol consumption and antiretroviral adherence among HIV-infected persons with alcohol problems. *Alcohol Clin Exp Res.* 2004;28(4):572–577.

264. Sarvet AL, et al. (Under review). Medical marijuana laws and adolescent marijuana use: a systematic review.

265. Schuckit MA. Biological, psychological and environmental predictors of the alcoholism risk: a longitudinal study. *J Stud Alcohol.* 1998;59(5):485–494.

266. Schuckit MA, Smith TL. An 8-year follow-up of 450 sons of alcoholic and control subjects. *Arch Gen Psychiatry.* 1996;53(3):202–210.

267. Schuckit MA, Smith TL. A comparison of correlates of DSM-IV alcohol abuse or dependence among more than 400 sons of alcoholics and controls. *Alcohol Clin Exp Res.* 2001;25(1):1–8.

268. Schuckit MA, Smith TL, Kalmijn J. The search for genes contributing to the low level of response to alcohol: patterns of findings across studies. *Alcohol Clin Exp Res.* 2004;28(10):1449–1458.

269. Schuckit MA, Smith TL, Landi NA. The 5-year clinical course of high-functioning men with DSM-IV alcohol abuse or dependence. *Am J Psychiatry.* 2000;157(12):2028–2035.

270. Schuckit MA, et al. A comparison of DSM-III-R, DSM-IV and ICD-10 substance use disorders diagnoses in 1922 men and women subjects in the COGA study. Collaborative Study on the Genetics of Alcoholism. *Addiction.* 1994;89(12):1629–1638..

271. Schulenberg J, et al. Getting drunk and growing up: trajectories of frequent binge drinking during the transition to young adulthood. *J Stud Alcohol.* 1996;57(3):289–304.

272. Scribner RA, Cohen DA, Fisher W. Evidence of a structural effect for alcohol outlet density: a multilevel analysis. *Alcohol Clin Exp Res.* 2000;24(2):188–195.

273. Shen S, Locke-Wellman J, Hill SY. Adolescent alcohol expectancies in offspring from families at high risk for developing alcoholism. *J Stud Alcohol.* 2001;62(6):763–772.

274. Sher KJ, Grekin ER, Williams NA. The development of alcohol use disorders. *Annu Rev Clin Psychol.* 2005;1:493–523.

275. Shkolnikov V, Nemtsov A. The anti-alcohol campaign and variations in Russian mortality. In: Bobadilla J, Costello C, Mitchell F, eds. *Premature Death in the New Independent States.* Washington, DC: National Academy; 1997.

276. Shults RA, et al. Reviews of evidence regarding interventions to reduce alcohol-impaired driving. *Am J Prev Med.* 2001;21(suppl 4):66–88.

277. Shults RA, et al. Association between state level drinking and driving countermeasures and self reported alcohol impaired driving. *Inj Prev.* 2002;8(2):106–110.

278. Singer M. The vitality of mythical numbers. *Public Interest.* 1971;4:3–9.

279. Slutske WS, et al. Genes, environment, and individual differences in alcohol expectancies among female adolescents and young adults. *Psychol Addict Behav.* 2002;16(4):308–317.

280. Smith GT. Psychological expectancy as mediator of vulnerability to alcoholism. *Ann NY Acad Sci.* 1994;708:165–171.

281. Sokol RJ, Delaney-Black V, Nordstrom B. Fetal alcohol spectrum disorder. *JAMA.* 2003;290(22):2996–2999.

282. Spivak B, et al. Effect of ADH1B genotype on alcohol consumption in young Israeli Jews. *Alcohol Clin Exp Res.* 2007;31(8):1297–1301.

283. Stacy AW, et al. Exposure to televised alcohol ads and subsequent adolescent alcohol use. *Am J Health Behav.* 2004;28(6):498–509.

284. Steinberg L, Fletcher A, Darling N. Parental monitoring and peer influences on adolescent substance use. *Pediatrics.* 1994;93(6 Pt 2):1060–1064.

285. Streatfeild D. *Cocaine: a Definitive History.* New York: Virgin Books; 2002.

286. Streatfeild D. *Cocaine: An Unauthorized Biography.* New York: Picador; 2003.

287. Swendsen JD, et al. Are personality traits familial risk factors for substance use disorders? Results of a controlled family study. *Am J Psychiatry.* 2002;159(10):1760–1766.

288. Tapert SF, et al. Neural response to alcohol stimuli in adolescents with alcohol use disorder. *Arch Gen Psychiatry.* 2003;60(7):727–735.

289. Tarabar AF, Nelson LS. The resurgence and abuse of heroin by children in the United States. *Curr Opin Pediatr.* 2003;15(2):210–215.

290. Tatlow JR, Clapp JD, Hohman MM. The relationship between the geographic density of alcohol outlets and alcohol-related hospital admissions in San Diego County. *J Community Health.* 2000;25(1):79–88.

291. Teesson M, et al. The structure of cannabis dependence in the community. *Drug Alcohol Depend.* 2002;68(3):255–262.

292. Thomas SE, et al. Following alcohol consumption, nontreatment-seeking alcoholics report greater stimulation but similar sedation compared with social drinkers. *J Stud Alcohol.* 2004;65(3):330–335.

293. Tippetts AS, et al. A meta-analysis of .08 BAC laws in 19 jurisdictions in the United States. *Accid Anal Prev.* 2005;37(1):149–161.

294. Topp L, Day C, Degenhardt L. Changes in patterns of drug injection concurrent with a sustained reduction in the availability of heroin in Australia. *Drug Alcohol Depend.* 2003;70(3):275–286.

295. Treno AJ, Gruenewald PJ, Johnson FW. Alcohol availability and injury: the role of local outlet densities. *Alcohol Clin Exp Res.* 2001;25(10):1467–1471.

296. Treno AJ, et al. The impact of outlet densities on alcohol-related crashes: a spatial panel approach. *Accid Anal Prev.* 2007;39(5):894–901.

297. Truett KR, et al. A model system for analysis of family resemblance in extended kinships of twins. *Behav Genet.* 1994;24(1):35–49.

298. Tsuang MT, et al. Co-occurrence of abuse of different drugs in men: the role of drug-specific and shared vulnerabilities. *Arch Gen Psychiatry.* 1998;55(11):967–972.

299. U.S. Department of Health and Human Services. 289.290. *Results from the 2013 National Survey on Drug Use and Health: Summary of National Findings*. Substance Abuse and Mental Health Services Administration Center for Behavioral Health Statistics and Quality; 2014.
300. Ustun B, et al. WHO Study on the reliability and validity of the alcohol and drug use disorder instruments: overview of methods and results. *Drug Alcohol Depend*. 1997;47(3):161–169.
301. Vanderschuren LJ, Everitt BJ. Drug seeking becomes compulsive after prolonged cocaine self-administration. *Science*. 2004;305(5686):1017–1019.
302. Voas RB, Tippetts AS, Fell J. The relationship of alcohol safety laws to drinking drivers in fatal crashes. *Accid Anal Prev*. 2000;32(4):483–492.
303. Voas RB, Tippetts AS, Fell JC. Assessing the effectiveness of minimum legal drinking age and zero tolerance laws in the United States. *Accid Anal Prev*. 2003;35(4):579–587.
304. Wagenaar AC, Holder HD. A change from public to private sale of wine: results from natural experiments in Iowa and West Virginia. *J Stud Alcohol*. 1991;52(2):162–173.
305. Wagenaar AC, Toomey TL. Effects of minimum drinking age laws: review and analyses of the literature from 1960 to 2000. *J Stud Alcohol*. 2002;Suppl(14):206–225.
306. Walden B, et al. Identifying shared environmental contributions to early substance use: the respective roles of peers and parents. *J Abnorm Psychol*. 2004;113(3):440–450.
307. Wall MM, et al. Adolescent marijuana use from 2002 to 2008: higher in states with medical marijuana laws, cause still unclear. *Ann Epidemiol*. 2011;21(9):714–716.
308. Wall TL, et al. Evaluation of the self-rating of the effects of alcohol form in Asian Americans with aldehyde dehydrogenase polymorphisms. *J Stud Alcohol*. 1999;60(6):784–789.
309. Wang JC, et al. Evidence of common and specific genetic effects: association of the muscarinic acetylcholine receptor M2 (CHRM2) gene with alcohol dependence and major depressive syndrome. *Hum Mol Genet*. 2004;13(17):1903–1911.
310. Wang PS, et al. Twelve-month use of mental health services in the United States: results from the National Comorbidity Survey Replication. *Arch Gen Psychiatry*. 2005;62(6):629–640.
311. Watson AL, Sher KJ. Resolution of alcohol problems without treatment: methodological issues and future directions of natural recovery research. *Clin Psychol: Sci Prac*. 1998;5:1–18.
312. Weatherburn D, Lind B. The impact of law enforcement activity on a heroin market. *Addiction*. 1997;92(5):557–569; discussion 611–613.
313. Weatherburn D, et al. Supply control and harm reduction: lessons from the Australian heroin 'drought. *Addiction*. 2003;98(1):83–91.
314. Wen H, Hockenberry JM, Cummings JR. The effect of medical marijuana laws on adolescent and adult use of marijuana, alcohol, and other substances. *J Health Econ*. 2015;42:64–80.
315. Widom CS, Czaja SJ, DuMont KA. Intergenerational transmission of child abuse and neglect: real or detection bias? *Science*. 2015;347(6229):1480–1485.
316. Wilhelmsen KC, et al. The search for genes related to a low-level response to alcohol determined by alcohol challenges. *Alcohol Clin Exp Res*. 2003;27(7):1041–1047.
317. Williams J, et al. Alcohol and marijuana use among college students: economic complements or substitutes? *Health Econ*. 2004;13(9):825–843.
318. Wills TA, Vaccaro D, McNamara G. Novelty seeking, risk taking, and related constructs as predictors of adolescent substance use: an application of Cloninger's theory. *J Subst Abuse*. 1994;6(1):1–20.
319. Wilson RW, Niva G, Nicholson T. Prohibition revisited: county alcohol control consequences. *J Ky Med Assoc*. 1993;91(1):9–12.
320. Wood E, et al. Impact of supply-side policies for control of illicit drugs in the face of the AIDS and overdose epidemics: investigation of a massive heroin seizure. *CMAJ*. 2003;168(2):165–169.
321. World Health Organization (WHO). *International Guide for Monitoring Alcohol Consumption and Related Harm*. Geneva, Switzerland: World Health Organization.
322. World Health Organization. *Global Status Report: Alcohol Policy*. WHO; 2004.
323. Yoon YH, Chen CM. *Surveillance Report #105: Liver Cirrhosis Mortality in the United States*. National Institute on Alcohol Abuse and Alcoholism, Division of Epidemiology and Prevention Research; 2016.
324. Zimmermann P, et al. Primary anxiety disorders and the development of subsequent alcohol use disorders: a 4-year community study of adolescents and young adults. *Psychol Med*. 2003;33(7).1211–1222.
325. Zuckerman M, Kuhlman DM. Personality and risk-taking: common biosocial factors. *J Pers*. 2000;68(6):999–1029.

3

United States Federal Drug Policy

ANGELA HAWKEN AND JONATHAN D. KULICK

Introduction

The United States federal government takes an active role in setting and implementing drug-control policy, directly and in concert with state and local authorities and with international partners—even as the other polities' policies may be widely at variance with federal policies. Over the last century, the government's formal policies, budgetary commitments, and actions reflect enduring tensions between different conceptions of the problem of drug abuse: civil liberties versus public order, public health versus criminal justice, use reduction versus harm reduction, and demand driven versus supply driven. Accordingly, the balance among the three pillars of treatment, prevention, and law enforcement has shifted with changes in drug use; public sentiment; external political, economic, and social forces; and research findings. Even so, the span of federal drug-control policy is best characterized as periods of perfervid law enforcement, driven by acute concern about the menace of particular drugs, alternating with periods of routine management of one of many social ills.

This chapter addresses the development of federal drug-control policy, and current policies and functions of the federal government. In particular, it considers the role of research in influencing policy. It is necessarily synoptic, and the interested reader is referred to more detailed source materials.

History

The use of some drugs that are now illicit, especially marijuana and opiates, was commonplace and uncontroversial in the United States before the late 19th century[62] (milestones in federal drug-control policy are outlined in Table 3.1). Opium appeared in many patent medicines, and the medical benefits were considered to outweigh the acknowledged harms.[5] Morphine and, later, heroin, were introduced in the 19th century, and were widely prescribed into the 1920s. Cocaine appeared first in beverages, and then in many prescription medicines around the turn of the century.[47]

The anti-alcohol temperance movement grew in force in the late 19th century, leading to calls for the prohibition of alcohol, but the movement leaders were not concerned with other drugs, which they did not regard as degrading to character.[76] Nonetheless, the success of the temperance movement established a precedent that "prohibition was the only logical or moral policy when dealing with such a great national problem."[48]

Until the turn of the century, the federal government had not exercised general police powers over public health. The rise of the progressive movement and public concerns about the depredations of the patent-medicine industry led to the passage of the Pure Food and Drug Act of 1906, which imposed labeling and purity requirements. Although it did not prohibit any ingredients, it is regarded as having reduced the rate of opiate addiction.[39]

The first federal prohibition against drug use addressed opium, driven by concerns about opium smoking by Chinese immigrants, by foreign-policy interests in China and the Philippines, and by the observation that merely restrictive laws had spurred smuggling without much reducing supply. A 1905 law that prohibited the import and sale of opium in the Philippines, then a US colony, was the first federal law to prohibit trafficking of a drug, although opium for smoking had been subject to a special duty since 1862.[27] The Smoking Opium Exclusion Act of 1909 prohibited the import of opium for smoking, but did not cover other forms of opium, which was widely used for medicine and recreation throughout the United States. The United States was also signatory to several international conventions restricting the trade in opium.

As opium smoking was associated with Chinese immigrants, so did cocaine use become associated with poor blacks around the turn of the century, even as whites dominated cocaine consumption.[83] Similarly, marijuana became associated with Mexican immigrants, and concern about its use was highest in the border regions where they were concentrated.[48]

The Harrison Narcotics Tax Act of 1914[28] was positioned as a revenue measure, rather than as prohibition, and as required for the United States to comply with the Hague Convention of 1912[34]; the congressional debate on the Act saw almost no mention of moral concerns. The Act required that any party involved

TABLE 3.1	Milestones in Federal Drug-Control Policy.	
Year	Measure	Effect or Goal
1906	Pure Food and Drug Act	Required medicines to have labels of ingredients.
1909	Smoking Opium Exclusion Act	Prohibited import of opium for smoking.
1912	Hague Convention	Required signatories to pass domestic legislation to combat international drug trade.
1914	Harrison Narcotics Tax Act	Regulated trade in opium and coca products; effectively prohibited their use.
1918	Rainey Committee	Found illicit drugs to be a serious threat; called for stricter law enforcement.
1919	Heroin Act	Prohibited trade and possession of heroin, even for medical purposes.
1922	Narcotics Drugs Import and Export Act	Prohibited nonmedical use of opiates and cocaine; established the Federal Narcotics Control Board.
1925	Linder v. United States	Allowed for prescription of illicit drugs for addiction treatment.
1928	Nigro v. United States	Upheld constitutionality of Harrison Act.
1929	Porter Act	Created Public Health Services Narcotics Division and prison hospitals for addicts.
1930	Federal Bureau of Narcotics	Created enforcement structure in Treasury Department, under a Narcotics Commissioner.
1932	Uniform State Narcotic Act	Encouraged state governments to control marijuana use in line with 1922 Act, in lieu of federal legislation.
1936	Reefer Madness	Documentary about the dangers of marijuana distributed by government.
1937	Marihuana Tax Act	Effectively criminalized distribution of marijuana.
1942	Opium Poppy Control Act	Prohibited growing opium poppies without a license.
1951	Boggs Act	Established mandatory-minimum prison sentences, with uniform penalties for opiates, cocaine, and marijuana.
1956	Narcotic Control Act	Increased penalties under the 1951 Boggs Act.
1960	Narcotics Manufacturing Act	Placed controls on legal manufacturers of opiates and cocaine.
1961	Single Convention on Narcotic Drugs	Consolidated earlier drug-control treaties, and added cannabis; superseded 1912 Hague Convention.
1963	President's Advisory Commission on Narcotics and Drug Abuse (Prettyman Commission)	Called for using all resources of federal government to combat trafficking.
1965	Drug Abuse Control Amendments	Placed controls on stimulants and depressants, and restricted research into hallucinogens.
1966	Narcotic Addict Rehabilitation Act	Diverted some addicts to treatment as an alternative to incarceration. Authorized support to states' rehabilitation programs.
1968	Bureau of Narcotics and Dangerous Drugs	Created from merger of Federal Bureau of Narcotics and Bureau of Drug Abuse Control.[a]
1969	Operation Intercept	Closed Mexican border and searched vehicles crossing it.
1970	Controlled Substances Act[b]	Consolidated many drug-control laws, placing all controlled drugs into one of five schedules. Addressed prevention and treatment, and interdiction. Repealed mandatory-minimum penalties.
1971	War on Drugs	Comprehensive policy announced by White House to combat domestic and international production, distribution, and use.
1972	National Commission on Marihuana and Drug Abuse	Federal study recommended marijuana decriminalization.[62]
	Drug Abuse Office and Treatment Act	Established national network of treatment programs. Created Special Action Office for Drug Abuse Prevention in Executive Office of the President.
	Drug Abuse Warning Network and National Household Survey on Drug Abuse	Surveys initiated under the Special Action Office for Drug Abuse Prevention.
1973	Methadone Control Act	Established federally funded clinics for prevention and treatment of heroin addiction.
	Heroin Trafficking Act	Increased penalties for drug traffickers and established strict bail procedures.
	Drug Enforcement Administration	Created to supersede the Bureau of Narcotics and Dangerous Drugs.

Continued

TABLE 3.1	Milestones in Federal Drug-Control Policy.—cont'd	
Year	Measure	Effect or Goal
	Alcohol, Drug Abuse, and Mental Health Administration	Created to oversee the National Institute of Mental Health, the National Institute on Drug Abuse, and the National Institute on Alcohol Abuse and Alcoholism.
	National Institute on Drug Abuse	Established as focal point for research, treatment, prevention, training, services, and data collection.
	National Drug and Alcohol Treatment Unit Survey	Initiated at the National Institute on Drug Abuse to characterize prevention and treatment programs.
1975	Monitoring the Future Survey	Initiated at the National Institute on Drug Abuse to measure use and attitudes in young adults.
1976	Comprehensive Alcohol Abuse and Alcoholism Prevention, Treatment, and Rehabilitation Act Amendments	Directed attention to prevention and treatment for women and youth.
1978	Drug Abuse Education Amendments	Coordinated state and federal education programs. Established Office of Alcohol and Drug Abuse Education in Department of Education.
1980	Drug Abuse Prevention, Treatment, and Rehabilitation Amendments	Encouraged foreign cooperation in eradication and interdiction. Strengthened federal leadership in prevention, education, treatment, and rehabilitation. Reimposed mandatory-minimum sentences.
1982	National Research Council marijuana-policy study[47]	Called for allowing states to decriminalize.
1986	Controlled Substances Analogue Enforcement Act	Established controls for enforcement of "designer drugs" (e.g., 3,4-methylenedioxymethamphetamine); allowed for immediate scheduling.
	Drug-Free Workplace	Executive order required federal agencies to institute urine-testing programs.
1988	Drug Free Workplace Act	Required federal contractors to institute urine-testing programs.
	Anti-Drug Abuse Act	Authorized funds for school-based prevention programs. Established different penalties for powder and crack cocaine.
	Office of National Drug Control Policy	Created in Executive Office of the President.
1991	National Commission on Acquired Immune Deficiency Syndrome	Report called for expansion of treatment and decriminalizing needle sale and possession.
1992	Substance Abuse and Mental Health Services Administration.	Established in the Department of Health and Human Services. Transferred the National Institute on Drug Abuse, the National Institute of Mental Health, and the National Institute on Alcohol Abuse and Alcoholism to the National Institutes of Health. Abolished the Alcohol, Drug Abuse, and Mental Health Administration.
1993	Departments of Labor, Health and Human Services, and Education FY 1994 Appropriations Act	Prohibited funding for sterile-needle programs.
	Domestic Chemical Diversion Control Act	Instituted Drug Enforcement Administration registration requirement for many precursor chemicals for controlled substances.
	International Counternarcotics Policy (Presidential Decision Directive 14)	Provided policy framework for international drug control.
1995	Heroin Control Policy (Presidential Decision Directive 44)	Provided policy framework for source-country eradication and trafficker-financing efforts.
1996	Methamphetamine Control Act	Established new controls over methamphetamine precursor chemicals, and increased penalties for their possession.
1997	Drug-Free Communities Act	Provided funds to community anti-drug coalitions.
1998	Drug-Free Workplace Act	Provided federal funds to small businesses for mandatory employee drug testing.
	Drug Free Media Campaign Act	Required the Office of National Drug Control Policy to conduct a national youth-targeted media campaign.
	Office of National Drug Control Policy Reauthorization Act	Expanded the Office of National Drug Control Policy's mandate and elevated it to cabinet status.
2000	Drug Addiction Treatment Act	Allowed physicians to provide opiates to addicts outside of drug-treatment clinics.

TABLE 3.1	Milestones in Federal Drug-Control Policy.—cont'd	
Year	Measure	Effect or Goal
	Ecstasy Anti-Proliferation Act	Increased penalties for trafficking in 3,4-methylenedioxymethamphetamine.
	Children's Health Act	Repealed the Narcotic Addict Rehabilitation Act. Waived parts of the Controlled Substances Act of 1970 to permit office-based treatment of opiate dependence. Authorized expansion of National Institute on Drug Abuse research on methamphetamine and 3,4-methylene-dioxymethamphetamine.
	Plan Colombia	Emergency Supplemental Act funded counter-drug activities of Government of Colombia.
2001	National Prevention Research Initiative	National Institute on Drug Abuse effort to promote science-based prevention strategies.
	National Research Council comprehensive federal policy study[53]	Found that data and research are "strikingly inadequate" to support policymaking.
2002	Vulnerability to Ecstasy Act	Provided for prosecution of owners and managers of facilities hosting drug use, trade, or manufacturing.
2004	Anabolic Steroids Control Act	Significantly expanded list of scheduled anabolic steroids.
2005	Combat Methamphetamine Epidemic Act	Regulated retail sales of medicines used in the manufacture of methamphetamine.
	Gonzales v. Raich	Upheld right of Congress to ban marijuana use, under the Commerce Clause.
2006	Organized Crime Drug Enforcement Task Force Fusion Center	Drug Enforcement Administration established center to fuse investigative and regulatory reporting.
2007	Merida Initiative	Counter-drug cooperation agreement with Mexico and Central American countries.
2009	End of War on Drugs	Office of National Drug Control Policy would not use "War on Drugs," which emphasizes incarceration over treatment.
2010	Fair Sentencing Act	Reduced sentencing disparity for crack and powder cocaine from 100:1 to 18:1.
	Affordable Care Act	Required insurance companies to cover treatment for addiction as for any chronic disease.
2011	Prescription Drug Abuse Prevention Plan	Multi-agency plan to address epidemic of prescription-drug overdoses.
2013	Cole Memorandum	Obama Administration would not challenge state-level recreational-marijuana legalization.
2014	Drug Guidelines Amendment	US Sentencing Commission reduced sentencing guidelines for most federal drug offenders.
2015	Presidential Memorandum Addressing Prescription Drug Abuse and Heroin Use	Obama Administration required federal agencies to provide prescriber training and improve access to treatment.

[a]Formerly the Federal Bureau of Narcotics had been responsible for heroin, cocaine, and cannabis, and the Bureau of Drug Abuse Control (in the Food and Drug Administration) had been responsible for depressants, stimulants, and hallucinogens.

[b]The Controlled Substances Act of 1970 was Part II of the Comprehensive Drug Abuse Prevention and Control Act.

in the distribution of opiates or coca products register with the federal government and pay a tax. It allowed for selling small quantities of the controlled drugs over the counter, and for larger sales authorized by a physician, so doctors (and the American Medical Association) did not feel that it threatened the practice of medicine.[48] Soon after passage, however, the Act was interpreted to prohibit a physician from supplying the controlled drugs to addicts (who at the time were not considered patients). Under this interpretation, federal agents arrested many physicians and made it clear that the government was not going to tolerate treatment of addicts who maintained their addiction.[18] The Narcotics Division of the Prohibition Unit of the Internal Revenue Service (Treasury Department) was given enforcement authority, which was transferred to the Prohibition Bureau in 1927.

There followed a series of committees to investigate the effects of the Harrison Act and the scope of the drug problem. A 1918 committee finding called for stricter law enforcement and greater coordination of state laws with federal statutes.[39]

Many court rulings on whether Congress had the power to regulate physicians and punish drug possession established federal authority by 1925,[6] and a 1928 Supreme Court ruling affirmed that the Harrison Act was constitutional.[54] Alcohol prohibition, established by the Eighteenth Amendment in 1919, was by this time hotly debated, but the Harrison Act occasioned little controversy, despite the fact that drug violations accounted for a greater number of federal prisoners than any other class of offenses.[54]

The growing scope of prosecutions under the Harrison Act spurred Congress to build an institutional structure to manage the consequences. The Porter Narcotic Farm Act of 1929 established two facilities where addicts could be held and treated. In 1930, the Federal Bureau of Narcotics was established in the Treasury Department, under the direction of Commissioner Harry J. Anslinger, who would go on to dominate federal drug-control policymaking and implementation for decades. (Anslinger was the nephew of the Treasury Secretary, Andrew J. Mellon; it is not apparent that Mellon shared what turned out to be his nephew's zeal for drug control.[64]) Initially, the Federal Bureau of Narcotics focused its efforts on heroin, and Anslinger publicly downplayed the threat from marijuana.[24] In the 1930s, advances in the processing of hemp fiber threatened powerful petroleum and timber interests, who lobbied Congress for the prohibition of hemp and used their influence in the newspaper business to demonize marijuana users.[62] (Because industrial hemp and marijuana are the same plant—albeit very different strains—it is difficult to distinguish between cultivation of the two in the law.)

The Federal Bureau of Narcotics responded to these pressures with the Marihuana Tax Act of 1937, and a media campaign to stir fears of marijuana use. The Act did not explicitly prohibit the possession or sale of marijuana, but rather imposed registration and transaction tax obligations on anyone trafficking in it, with heavy fines and prison terms up to 20 years. (The transfer tax was a contrivance, as a measure under treaty powers was infeasible and a revenue measure would be difficult to enforce.[83])

Drug use declined during World War II and rose again thereafter.[83] The wartime decline was due, in part, to supply reductions from countries embroiled in conflict. The shortage of legal supplies spurred the growth of the black market, especially for heroin.[38] In response to the growing public perception that marijuana use led to the use of opiates, and urged on by the Federal Bureau of Narcotics, Congress responded with reinforcements of the Harrison Act. The Boggs Act of 1951[7] was the first to impose mandatory-minimum sentences and to lump together marijuana, opiates, and cocaine, with uniform penalties.[63] National medical and legal associations questioned this stricter regime and called for a Congressional study of the government's drug policy. The Daniel Committee found that drugs posed a great threat to the country and recommended increased powers for the Federal Bureau of Narcotics and harsh measures, including denial of bail, making smuggling and heroin trafficking capital offenses, and the closing of treatment clinics.[38] The Narcotic Control Act of 1956[49] implemented these recommendations.

The Narcotics Manufacturing Act of 1960[50] established licenses and quotas for drug manufacturers to bring the United States into compliance with international conventions on the medical and scientific uses of natural and synthetic opiates and cocaine. By the language of the conventions, the following were not covered by the Act: barbiturates, amphetamines, and tranquilizers.[28]

As public concern over drug abuse (including prescription drugs) grew in the 1960s, the White House established the President's Advisory Commission on Narcotics and Drug Abuse (Prettyman Commission). Its 1963 report called for marshaling all the powers of the federal government to combat drug use and trafficking.[58] In particular, it recommended (1) that enforcement and investigative responsibilities be transferred to the Department of Justice, (2) a substantial increase in federal agents, and (3) extension of federal control over all drugs "capable of producing serious psychotoxic effects when abused."

Following on the report, the Drug Abuse Control Amendments of 1965 placed restrictions on the manufacture of prescription drugs with a potential for abuse, with the establishment of the Bureau of Drug Abuse Control in the Food and Drug Administration. As previous prohibitions had done for opiates, the Drug Abuse Control Amendments created shortages that drove up the street price (especially of amphetamine) and spurred the involvement of criminal organizations in manufacturing and trafficking.[18] In 1968 the Bureau of Drug Abuse Control was merged with the Treasury Department's Federal Bureau of Narcotics to form the Bureau of Narcotics and Dangerous Drugs in the Department of Justice.

Despite these efforts to control drugs (and similar measures in other countries), the use of marijuana and heroin continued to increase. Under President Nixon, the United States government redoubled its campaign against drug trafficking and abuse, formally declaring a "War on Drugs"; in 1971, President Nixon declared that drugs were "public enemy number one."[6] In 1969, the United States closed the border with Mexico and instituted searches of vehicles crossing the border. The National Commission on Marihuana and Drug Abuse was created in 1970.

The Controlled Substances Act of 1970[16] supplanted the Harrison Act as the basis of federal drug-control policy, and remains so today. Extant federal laws were reformulated under the federal power to regulate interstate commerce, and drugs were placed into five categories ("schedules") according to their medical utility and potential for abuse. (See Table 3.2 for a summary of the current schedules.) In earlier decades, courts had found that Congress did not have the authority to regulate the local production and distribution of drugs under its interstate-commerce powers, but opinions had shifted by the mid-1960s. Following the 1965 Drug Abuse Control Amendments model, the Controlled Substances Act of 1970 established administrative procedures for scheduling new drugs. The ongoing tension within the government over which agencies would have control over drug policy was evident in the drafting of the Controlled Substances Act of 1970. In the Senate version of the bill, the Attorney General was required only to "request the advice" of the Secretary of Health, Education, and Welfare (now Health and Human Services) and of a (nonbinding) scientific-advisory committee before amending the schedule. In the House version, which was finally adopted, the Attorney General was not allowed to override the Secretary's determination *not* to schedule a new drug, and he was required to accept the Secretary's recommendation regarding medical and scientific considerations.[65]

Drug control was a less visible priority under the Ford and Carter administrations. President Ford endorsed the findings of the Domestic Council Drug Abuse Task Force that the federal government could at most contain the problems of drug abuse and should not operate under the model of eliminating them.[26] President Carter went so far as to publicly entertain the notion of marijuana decriminalization, but this idea gained no traction in Congress and public sentiment was against it.[47]

The Drug Abuse Prevention, Treatment and Rehabilitation Act of 1979[19] reflected the latest, slight swing of the pendulum away from law enforcement. It imposed minimum requirements on the National Institute on Drug Abuse (NIDA) for spending on prevention, and identified high-risk populations to be targeted with intervention programs.

The 1980s saw another escalation of the War on Drugs. President Reagan created the position of the White House Drug Policy Advisor in 1982, which was supplanted by an even more powerful Director of the Office of National Drug Control Policy in 1988, under the National Narcotics Leadership Act. (These officials are commonly known as the "Drug Czars." The Director of the Office of National Drug Control Policy has held cabinet-level rank, until the appointment of Gil Kerlikowske by President Obama.[17] For a comparative assessment of the performance of the Drug Czars to 2008, see Moses.[45])

TABLE 3. 2   Schedule of Controlled Substances.

Schedule I

Criteria	• High potential for abuse • No currently accepted medical use in treatment in the United States • No safety for use under medical supervision
Major drugs	• Cannabis • Heroin • Gamma-hydroxybutyric acid • Lysergic acid diethylamide • 3,4-Methylenedioxymethamphetamine (Ecstasy) • Methaqualone (Quaalude) • Peyote[a] and mescaline • Psilocybin mushrooms

Schedule II

Criteria	• High potential for abuse • Currently accepted medical use in treatment in the United States • Abuse may lead to severe psychological or physical dependence
Major drugs	• Amphetamines • Barbiturates—short acting • Cocaine • Methamphetamine • Methylphenidate (Ritalin) • Opiates (e.g., methadone, morphine, oxycodone, fentanyl)

Schedule III

Criteria	• Potential for abuse less than in Schedules I and II • Currently accepted medical use in treatment in the United States • Abuse may lead to moderate or low physical dependence or high psychological dependence
Major drugs	• Anabolic steroids • Barbiturates—intermediate acting • Codeine • Ketamine • Synthetic tetrahydrocannabinol (Marinol)

Schedule IV

Criteria	• Low potential for abuse relative to Schedule III • Currently accepted medical use in treatment in the United States • Abuse may lead to limited physical dependence or psychological dependence relative to Schedule III
Major drugs	• Barbiturates—long acting • Benzodiazepines (e.g., Valium, Xanax)

Schedule V

Criteria	• Low potential for abuse relative to Schedule IV • Currently accepted medical use in treatment in the United States • Abuse may lead to limited physical dependence or psychological dependence relative to Schedule IV
Major drugs	• Codeine cough suppressant • Opiate anti-diarrheals

[a]Members of the Native American Church are allowed to use peyote in their rituals.

From Drug Enforcement Administration.

A series of measures increased federal penalties for many offenses, increased drug-control spending, and improved the coordination of federal drug-control efforts. The Comprehensive Crime Control Act of 1984[15] amended the Controlled Substances Act of 1970 to allow for fast-tracked scheduling of newly emerging "designer drugs" and when there exists an imminent public-safety hazard. Rising public concern about crack cocaine, catalyzed by the overdose death of a star college basketball player, led to the Anti-Drug Abuse Act of 1986,[2] which reinstated mandatory-minimum sentences for possession (large amounts were considered prima facie evidence of intent to distribute) and allowed for the death penalty for some offenses.

Sentencing requirements were based on weight (see Table 3.3), with crack and powder cocaine treated dramatically differently; Congress justified the 100:1 powder-to-crack ratio on the basis of the social harms associated with crack, despite the identical chemical composition of the two forms. Whatever the original intent of Congress, this sentencing distinction has had hugely disproportionate racial impacts, as the majority of offenders sentenced for crack have been black, and the majority sentenced for powder have been white.[37] Congress rejected repeated recommendations by the United States Sentencing Commission that the crack-powder distinction be eliminated, and let die in committee every bill that would reduce or eliminate sentencing disparities,[21] before passing the Fair Sentencing Act in 2010, which reduced the ratio to 18:1.[23]

The Anti-Drug Abuse Act of 1988[3] states that "it is the declared policy of the United States Government to create a drug-free America by 1995." It established the White House Office of National Drug Control Policy to be the principal architect of national drug-control strategy. The Act also requires some federal contractors and all grantees to meet requirements for providing a "drug-free workplace," and extends mandatory-minimum sentencing requirements to conspiracy convictions. Under the statute, the Office of National Drug Control Policy is to set priorities, implement a national strategy, and certify federal budgets. The strategy is to be comprehensive and research based, with measurable objectives. Subsequent executive orders, reauthorization bills, and other legislative initiatives have added to the Office of National Drug Control Policy's authority and responsibilities, to include media campaigns, grants to communities, and cabinet-department budget assessments.[74] Smarting from criticism that the office was politically driven and insufficiently evidence based, it asked the National Research Council to establish a Committee on Data and Research for Policy on Illegal Drugs, which found that:

> [N]either the data systems nor the research infrastructure needed to assess the effectiveness of drug control enforcement policies now exists. It is time for the federal government to remedy this serious deficiency. It is unconscionable for this country to continue to carry out a public policy of this magnitude and cost without any way of knowing whether and to what extent it is having the desired effect.[41]

The subsequent presidential administrations have seen smaller-bore legislative initiatives and less rhetorical emphasis on drugs, even as the War on Drugs has continued apace. At the same time, conflicts between federal law and state- and local-level statutes and enforcement have increased. In President Clinton's first term, he reduced the Office of National Drug Control Policy staff, appointed a low-key director, and made almost no mention

TABLE 3.3   Federal Penalties for Drug Trafficking.

Drug (Schedule)	Quantity	Penalties	Quantity	Penalties
Cocaine (II)	500–4999 g	1st Offense: 5–40 years. If death or serious injury, 20 years–life. ≤$5 M if an individual, $25 M if not. 2nd Offense: 10 years–life. If death or serious injury, life. ≤$4 M if an individual, $10 M if not.	≥5 kg	1st Offense: 10 years–life. If death or serious injury, 20 years–life. ≤$10 M if an individual, $50 M if not. 2nd Offense: 20 years–life. If death or serious injury, life. ≤$20 M if an individual, $75 M if not. 2 or More Prior Offenses: Life. ≤$20 M if an individual, $75 M if not.
Cocaine Base (II)	28–279 g		≥280 g	
Fentanyl (II)	40–399 g		≥400 g	
Fentanyl Analogue (I)	10–99 g		≥100 g	
Heroin (I)	100–999 g		≥1 kg	
Lysergic acid diethylamide (I)[a]	1–9 g		≥10 g	
Methamphetamine (II)	5–49 g		≥50 g	
Phencyclidine (II)	10–99 g		≥100 g	
Other Schedule I and II	Any	1st Offense: ≤20 years. If death or serious injury, 20 years–life. $1 M if an individual, $5 M if not. 2nd Offense: ≤30 years. If death or serious injury, life. ≤$2 M if an individual, $10 M if not.		
Schedule III	Any	1st Offense: ≤10 years. If death or serious injury, ≤15 years. ≤$500 k if an individual, $2.5 M if not. 2nd Offense: ≤20 years. If death or serious injury, ≤35 years. ≤$1 M if an individual, $5 M if not.		
Schedule IV (Other than 1+ gm Flunitrazepam)	Any	1st Offense: ≤5 years. ≤$250 k if an individual, $1 M if not. 2nd Offense: ≤10 years. ≤$500 k if an individual, $2 M if not.		
Schedule V	Any	1st Offense: ≤1 year. ≤$100 k if an individual, $250 k if not. 2nd Offense: ≤4 years. ≤$200 k if an individual, $500 k if not.		
Cannabis				
Marijuana	50–99 kg or plants	1st Offense: ≤20 years. If death or serious injury, 20 to life. ≤$1 M if an individual, $5 M if not. 2nd Offense: ≤30 years. If death or serious injury, life. ≤$2 M if an individual, $10 M if not.		
	100–999 kg or plants	1st Offense: 5–40 years. If death or serious injury, 20 years–life. ≤$5 M if an individual, $25 M if not. 2nd Offense: 10 years–life. If death or serious injury, life. ≤$8 M if an individual, $50 M if not.		
	≥1000 kg or plants	1st Offense: 10 years–life. If death or serious injury, 20 years–life. ≤$10 M if an individual, $50 M if not. 2nd Offense: 20 years–life. If death or serious injury, life. ≤$20 M if an individual, $75 M if not.		
Hashish	≤10 kg or 1 kg hashish oil	1st Offense: ≤5 years. ≤$250 k if an individual, $1 M if not. 2nd Offense: ≤10 years. ≤$500 k if an individual, $2 M if not.		
	>10 kg or 1 kg hashish oil	1st Offense: ≤20 years. If death or serious injury, 20 years–life. ≤$1 M if an individual, $5 M if not. 2nd Offense: ≤30 years. If death or serious injury, life. ≤$2 M if an individual, $10 M if not.		

[a]Lysergic acid diethylamide weights include the carrier medium (e.g., blotter paper).

From Drug Enforcement Administration.

of drugs, occasioning criticism even from Democratic officials.[4] President Clinton reversed these positions during his reelection campaign and appointed a very visible director.

In the same election season, voters in Arizona and California approved measures that legalized the use of marijuana for medical purposes, in direct contravention of the federal Controlled Substances Act. (Other state initiatives to allow for the medical use of marijuana date back to 1978 but were ineffective.[42]) Top administration officials vowed to enforce federal laws and sought to prosecute physicians who prescribed marijuana. The George W. Bush Administration continued to campaign against increasingly lenient state laws and local decisions to make marijuana arrests a low priority, and went after (locally legal) sellers of drug paraphernalia.[8]

Nonetheless, despite Drug Enforcement Administration raids on dispensaries, a few prosecutions of prescribing doctors, and a Supreme Court ruling upholding the federal government's authority to prohibit the use of marijuana,[29] medical marijuana has proved popular, and the Obama Administration announced that it would no longer prosecute marijuana dispensaries that were operating legally in the 13 states (now 33 plus Washington, DC) that allowed for them.[44]

Ten states (Colorado [2012], Washington [2012], Alaska [2014], Oregon [2014], California [2016], Massachusetts [2016], Nevada [2017], Maine [2018], Michigan [2018], Vermont [2018]) and Washington, DC (2014), have made legal the recreational use of marijuana, and have instituted a variety of mechanisms for the legal cultivation and sale of marijuana and marijuana products; marijuana remains an illegal, Schedule I drug, at the federal level. Nonetheless, in 2013, the U.S. Department of Justice announced that it would not thwart legalization efforts in states that enforce strong regulatory systems,[14] and the Obama administration demonstrated an increasing acceptance of the state-level reforms.[35] Even though the federal government has made its nonenforcement position clear, that marijuana remains illegal at the federal level creates many challenges for the emerging recreational marijuana industry in states where marijuana is now legal. Among the most pressing barriers is access to banking services.[31]

Beyond marijuana laws, states and localities have become laboratories for experimenting with reforms of drug policy, for example, with sentencing, needle-exchange programs, and diversion of offenders to treatment. An accurate understanding of drug policy *as practiced* in the United States requires closer attention to state and local drug policies.[59]

Federal Drug-Control Operations

The federal government budgets nearly 30 billion dollars to drug-control efforts, divided among 15 federal agencies with drug-control functions (unless otherwise noted, all budget figures are for fiscal year [FY] 2017). The lion's share of these resources is controlled by four cabinet departments: Health and Human Services, Justice, Homeland Security, and Defense (see Table 3.4). The Department of Health and Human Services has the largest share ($13.7 billion). It houses the National Institute on Drug Abuse (or NIDA), the largest supporter of drug-abuse and addiction research, and the Substance Abuse and Mental Health Services Administration (SAMHSA). Following the attacks of September 11, 2001, the drug-funds interception functions of the Department of Homeland Security were increased with the passing of the USA PATRIOT Act, which

gave the Department of Homeland Security and federal security agencies additional authority to investigate and preempt future terrorist activities.

The Department of Justice budget is $7.9 billion. The Department of Justice supports prison- and community-based drug treatment through the Bureau of Prisons; enforces federal illicit-substance laws and regulations through the Drug Enforcement Administration; targets drug-trafficking and money-laundering organizations through the Interagency Crime and Drug Enforcement account; and manages drug-control–strategy programs through the Office of Justice Programs.

The Department of State budget is $0.51 billion, for the Bureau of International Narcotics and Law Enforcement Affairs and the US Agency for International Development. Roughly two-thirds is for eradication and interdiction efforts, and one-third is for promoting alternatives to drug production in source countries.

The Department of Defense budget is $1.3 billion, used for drug-related threats to national security. The Department of Defense oversees interdiction and the disruption of illegal-drug flows toward the United States, collects and disseminates intelligence on drug activity, and trains American and foreign drug-enforcement agents (including foreign militaries). The Department of Defense's drug-control efforts include a demand-reduction program (random drug testing with sanctions, anti-drug education, and treatment) for the military.

Policymaking and Budgeting

Although drug-control policy is implemented in many agencies of the executive branch, it is directed from, and coordinated by, the White House Office of National Drug Control Policy (ONDCP). Responsibility for drug-control legislation is spread across many House and Senate subcommittees (see Table 3.5 for those subcommittees with principal responsibility, and Table 3.6 for bills introduced in recent sessions).

When the ONDCP was created in 1988, it was tasked with compiling a federal drug-control budget. Each year federal agencies submit drug-control–budget data to the ONDCP, which produces a single federal budget. The ONDCP has no budget-enforcement authority, so its budget is not prescriptive.

Federal agencies and the ONDCP have some discretion in what they identify as drug-control expenditures, so the federal budget (and the balance between demand- and supply-side control measures) is sensitive to assumptions about what constitutes drug control.[46] In 2004, the ONDCP changed its methodology for assembling the federal drug-control budget.[86] The ONDCP's stated purpose was to more directly measure efforts targeting drug use itself, rather than its consequences[68]—that is, to exclude expenditures that were considered ancillary to drug control. Critics of this revision regard it as a manipulation by the Bush Administration to hide the costs of the War on Drugs. Previously, the drug-control budget reflected consistent annual increases in spending, and a stable 2:1 ratio between supply- and demand-side expenditures over the years. The revised methodology yielded a much smaller drug-control budget, with 90% of the apparent reductions appearing on the supply side. The most significant change was the exclusion of costs associated with prosecuting and incarcerating drug users.[84] The methodology was changed again in 2012, to include more agencies that were found to have a drug-control nexus.[70]

TABLE 3. 4   Federal Drug-Control Fiscal Year 2017 Budget and Activities.

Agency	Drug-Control Programs and Functions	Budget ($ million)
Department of Health and Human Services	National Institute on Drug Abuse (drug-abuse and addiction research), Substance Abuse and Mental Health Services Administration (substance-abuse treatment and prevention), Indian Health Services (treatment and prevention), Centers for Medicare and Medicaid Services (screening and intervention for at-risk beneficiaries)	13,681.3
Department of Justice	Assets Forfeiture Fund, Criminal Division, Organized Crime Enforcement Task Force Program, US Attorneys, US Marshals Service, Drug Enforcement Administration, Interagency Crime and Drug Enforcement, Office of Justice Programs, Bureau of Prisons	7,929.4
Department of Homeland Security	Office of Counternarcotics Enforcement, Customs and Border Protection, Immigration and Customs Enforcement, Coast Guard	4501.6
Department of Defense	Interdiction, intelligence, state and local assistance, prevention, and treatment programs	1297.5
Department of Veterans Affairs	Veterans Health Administration	707.6
Department of State	Bureau of International Narcotics and Law Enforcement Affairs, US Agency for International Development	514.3
Department of Housing and Urban Development	Community Planning and Development	589.1
Office of National Drug Control Policy	High Intensity Drug Trafficking Area program, other federal drug control programs, salaries/expenses	314.2
Department of the Treasury	Internal Revenue Service	95.8
Department of Education	Office of Elementary and Secondary Education Safe and Drug-Free Schools and Communities Act programs	50.1
Court Services and Offender Supervision Agency for the District of Columbia		58.7
Department of Transportation	Federal Aviation Administration, National Highway Traffic Safety Administration	43.1
Department of the Interior	Bureau of Indian Affairs, Bureau of Land Management, National Park Service	18.1
Department of Agriculture	US Forest Service	17.9
Department of Labor	Employment and Training Administration	6.0
	Total	29,824.7

From Office of National Drug Control Policy.

The 1980s and 1990s saw a shift in spending from treatment to law enforcement. In real terms, the federal drug-control budget increased by 600% between 1981 and 2000, from about 3 to 18 billion dollars.[77] This increase was driven primarily by criminal-justice expenditures. The change in budgeting approach makes it difficult to track the federal budget over time. The ONDCP recalculated earlier budgets using their new methodology, but only as far back as 1996. Fig. 3.1 shows the federal drug-control budget from 1996 to 2015, which is the longest series for which consistent budget data are available (i.e., comparable budgeting methodologies were used). The federal drug-control budget increased steadily over this period (even after controlling for inflation). The two lowermost areas in Fig. 3.1 represent the total demand-reduction budget, with the three uppermost representing the total supply-reduction budget. In recent years, demand-reduction spending has seen a sharp increase in its share of the total, so that demand-reduction and supply-reduction spending are approximately equal.

Law Enforcement

The enforcement of federal drug laws entails the seizure of illicit drugs and the arrest, prosecution, and punishment of traffickers and users. In addition to targeting the drug-supply chain, federal law-enforcement agencies also seek to reduce ancillary harms of the drug trade through, for example, Project Safe Neighborhoods, a national program to reduce gun and gang violence. Supply-side strategies are predicated on the assumption that disrupting the supply chain increases the price of illicit drugs and reduces the quantity available for sale. Demand-side strategies target drug users by imposing consequences for purchasing drugs (through the probability of arrest and the severity of the sanction imposed). The federal government spends more than $15 billion (49.1% of the drug-control budget) on domestic and international law enforcement and interdiction.[72] These strategies target the entire supply chain, but federal agencies focus primarily on international and interstate actors.

TABLE 3.5   Congressional Subcommittees With Drug-Policy Oversight.

Subcommittee	Committee
Senate	
International Development and Foreign Assistance, Economic Affairs and International Environmental Protection	Foreign Relations
Western Hemisphere, Peace Corps, and Narcotics Affairs	Foreign Relations
Crime and Drugs	Judiciary
House of Representatives	
Early Childhood, Elementary and Secondary Education	Education and Labor
Health, Employment, Labor, and Pensions	Education and Labor
Western Hemisphere	Foreign Affairs
Border, Maritime, and Global Counterterrorism	Homeland Security
Crime, Terrorism, and Homeland Security	Judiciary
Criminal Justice, Drug Policy and Human Resources	Oversight and Government Reform
National Security and Foreign Affairs	Oversight and Government Reform
Research and Science Education	Science and Technology

From United States Senate and House of Representatives.

Domestic law enforcement accounts for 62.4% of enforcement and interdiction spending.[72] Under the revised budget methodology, the drug-control budget no longer includes the (substantial) cost of prosecuting and incarcerating drug offenders; 46.5% of federal inmates were sentenced on drug charges.[25] The costs of investigations, intelligence, assistance to state and local authorities, and law-enforcement research are included. The ONDCP highlights three programs that assist state and local authorities: the High Intensity Drug Trafficking Area (HIDTA) program, Organized Crime Drug Enforcement Task Force, and the Federal Law Enforcement Training Center.

The Director of the ONDCP has the authority to designate qualifying jurisdictions in the United States as HIDTAs, centers of production or distribution that have harmful effects on other areas. When a jurisdiction is identified as a HIDTA, federal resources are provided to facilitate investigations and information sharing across enforcement agencies and to fund strategic intervention initiatives to reduce the production and distribution of drugs and drug-related money laundering. As HIDTA initiatives are tailored to the needs of the jurisdiction, activities differ across sites. Each jurisdiction is responsible for developing and monitoring performance measures relevant to its HIDTA program.[71] The Organized Crime Drug

Enforcement Task Force (OCDETF) coordinates federal, state, and local efforts against high-value drug trafficking and money-laundering organizations (Consolidated Priority Organization Targets [CPOTs]), with the goal of disrupting the chain of command within these organizations. Key measures used to monitor the performance of the OCDETF are the number of organizations that are disrupted or dismantled, and the number of defendants convicted:

Between 2003 and 2011, OCDETF agencies dismantled 49 CPOT organizations and severely disrupted the operations of another 29. In addition, during FY 2003 through FY 2011, OCDETF disrupted or dismantled a total of 2115 CPOT-linked organizations—organizations working with or otherwise associated with a CPOT.[56] (p. 29)

Other domestic law-enforcement efforts include the Drug Enforcement Administration Mobile Enforcement Teams and the US Immigration and Customs Enforcement Border Enforcement Security Task Forces. The Drug Enforcement Administration focuses on major drug organizations involved in international and interstate trafficking. In 1995, Mobile Enforcement Teams were established to assist with lower-level enforcement efforts, by giving technical and investigative help to local law-enforcement agencies to fight traffickers and the violent crime related to trafficking, especially gang violence. Mobile Enforcement Teams are rapid-response teams, deployed in response to requests by local sheriffs, police, or district attorneys.

Border Enforcement Security Task Forces were established in response to the growing threat from trafficking across the Mexican border and drug-gang–related violence associated with the Mexican drug cartels. The Border Enforcement Security Task Forces facilitate information sharing among local, state, federal, and foreign law-enforcement agencies. Border Enforcement Security Task Forces have been responsible for many arrests and convictions, and seizures of drugs and weapons, equipment, and currency that support trafficking.[80]

Suppressing drug production and trafficking in other countries, and preventing illicit drugs from entering the United States, are top priorities of federal drug enforcement; 37.5% of the supply-reduction budget is for international programs and interdiction. The United States provides direct assistance to foreign countries (primarily through the Departments of State and Defense), as well as multilateral assistance through international organizations, such as the United Nations Office on Drugs and Crime.[78] US efforts have targeted the Andean region (Plan Colombia,[43] and the Andean Counterdrug Initiative,[81] for Bolivia, Peru, Ecuador, Brazil, and Panama), Iraq, and Afghanistan,[66] with small initiatives in Pakistan and Haiti. Increasing attention and resources are being devoted to Mexico as violence associated with the major Mexican drug cartels has spilled over the border.

Foreign assistance consists primarily of bolstering law enforcement and antitrafficking efforts, and crop eradication.[9] Relatively little emphasis is placed on alternative development and crop-substitution programs. Most illicit-drug crops are in poor countries, tended by peasant farmers; eradication programs have been criticized for leaving locals without alternative livelihoods, sometimes threatening state stability and reversing eradication successes, as with coca eradication in Bolivia in the 1990s.[25]

TABLE 3.6	Recent Congressional Bills.	
Bill Number	**Title**	**Purpose**
113th Congress		
S 1686	Saving Kids From Dangerous Drugs Act of 2013	To amend the Controlled Substances Act to provide enhanced penalties for marketing controlled substances to minors
S 2825	Ensuring Safe Access to Prescription Medication Act of 2014	To amend the Controlled Substances Act to treat as dispensing the delivery of a controlled substance to a practitioner, pursuant to a patient-specific prescription of the practitioner, under certain circumstances
HR 88	No More Tulias: Drug Law Enforcement Evidentiary Standards Improvement Act of 2013	To increase evidentiary standard required to convict a person for drug offenses, to require screening of law enforcement officers or others acting under color of law participating in drug task forces
HR 499	Ending Federal Marijuana Prohibition Act of 2013	To decriminalize marijuana at the federal level, to leave states a power to regulate marijuana
HR 689	States' Medical Marijuana Patient Protection Act	To provide for rescheduling of marijuana and for medical use of marijuana in accordance with the laws of the various states
HR 784	States' Medical Marijuana Property Rights Protection Act	To amend the Controlled Substances Act so as to exempt real property from civil forfeiture due to medical-marijuana-related conduct that is authorized by state law
HR 1635	National Commission on Federal Marijuana Policy Act of 2013	To establish the National Commission on Federal Marijuana Policy
HR 1930	Drug Testing Integrity Act of 2013	To prohibit manufacture, marketing, sale, or shipment in interstate commerce of products designed to assist in defrauding a drug test
HR 2130	Access to Substance Abuse Treatment Act of 2013	To amend the Public Health Service Act to provide grants for treating heroin, cocaine, methamphetamine, ecstasy, and PCP abuse
HR 2148	Synthetics are Dangerous Act of 2013	To amend the ONDCP Reauthorization Act of 1998 to increase public awareness of synthetic drug dangers
HR 2372	Fairness in Cocaine Sentencing Act of 2013	To amend the Controlled Substances Act and Controlled Substances Import and Export Act regarding cocaine-offense penalties
HR 3088	Major Drug Trafficking Prosecution Act of 2013	To concentrate federal drug prosecution resources on major offenses
HR 3510	Stopping Unfair Collateral Consequences from Ending Student Success Act	To amend the Higher Education Act of 1965 to repeal suspension of eligibility for grants, loans, and work assistance for drug-related offenses
HR 3969	PACT Act	To amend the Federal Food, Drug, and Cosmetic Act to prevent abuse of dextromethorphan
HR 4046	Unmuzzle the Drug Czar Act of 2014	To strike provisions prohibiting the Director of ONDCP from studying marijuana legalization and requiring the Director to oppose attempts to legalize marijuana
HR 4169	SOS Act	To prevent deaths occurring from drug overdoses
HR 4502	Stop Meth Labs and Enhance Patient Access Act of 2014	To authorize the AG to exempt certain products from the Controlled Substances Act section 310 (e)(3) if they are not practical to use in the illicit manufacture of methamphetamine
HR 4771/S 2012	Designer Anabolic Steroid Control Act of 2014	To amend the Controlled Substances Act to more effectively regulate anabolic steroids
114th Congress		
S 36	Protecting Our Youth from Dangerous Synthetic Drugs Act of 2015	To address the continued threat posed by dangerous synthetic drugs by amending the Controlled Substances Act relating to controlled-substance analogues
S 64	Drug Free Families Act of 2015	To amend title IV of the Social Security Act to require states to implement a drug-testing program for applicants for and recipients of assistance under the Temporary Assistance for Needy Families (TANF) program
S 134	Industrial Hemp Farming Act of 2015	To amend the Controlled Substances Act to exclude industrial hemp from the definition of marijuana, and for other purposes

TABLE 3.6   Recent Congressional Bills.—cont'd

Bill Number	Title	Purpose
S 348	PLANT Act	To impose enhanced penalties for conduct relating to unlawful production of a controlled substance on federal property
S 392	Stop Drugs at the Border Act of 2015	To combat heroin and methamphetamine trafficking across the southern border of the United States
S 483	Ensuring Patient Access and Effective Drug Enforcement Act of 2016	To improve enforcement efforts related to prescription-drug diversion and abuse, and for other purposes
S 636	Increasing Safety of Prescription Drug Use Act of 2015	To reduce prescription-drug misuse and abuse
S 1138	Reclassification to Ensure Smarter and Equal Treatment Act of 2015	To reclassify certain low-level felonies as misdemeanors, to eliminate the increased penalties for cocaine offenses where the cocaine involved is cocaine base
S 1327	SALTS Act	To amend the Controlled Substances Act relating to controlled-substance analogues
S 1333	Therapeutic Hemp Medical Access Act of 2015	To amend the Controlled Substances Act to exclude cannabidiol and cannabidiol-rich plants from the definition of marijuana
S 1392	Safer Prescribing of Controlled Substances Act	To require certain practitioners authorized to prescribe controlled substances to complete continuing education
S 1410	Treatment and Recovery Investment Act	To amend the Public Health Service Act to provide grants to improve the treatment of substance-use disorders
S 1431	Prescription Drug Abuse Prevention and Treatment Act of 2015	To provide for increased federal oversight of prescription opioid treatment and assistance to states in reducing opioid abuse, diversion, and deaths
S 1893	Mental Health Awareness and Improvement Act of 2015	To reauthorize and improve programs related to mental health and substance-use disorders
S 1984	Keeping out Illegal Drugs Act of 2015	To prevent Indian tribes and tribal organizations that cultivate, manufacture, or distribute marijuana on Indian land from receiving federal funds
S 2405	METH Disclosure Act	To require the disclosure of information concerning the manufacture of methamphetamine upon transfer or lease of covered housing
HR 43	Border Security, Cooperation, and Act Now Drug War Prevention Act of 2015	To provide for emergency deployments of U.S. Border Patrol agents and to increase the number of DEA and ATF agents along the international border of the United States to increase resources to identify and eliminate illicit sources of firearms into Mexico for use by violent drug-trafficking organizations
HR 920	Smarter Sentencing Act of 2015	To reduce the mandatory minimum sentencing for controlled-substance offenses and "couriers"
HR 953/S 524	Comprehensive Addiction and Recovery Act of 2015	To authorize the Attorney General to award grants to address the national epidemics of prescription-opioid abuse and heroin use
HR 1013	Regulate Marijuana Like Alcohol Act	To decriminalize marijuana at the federal level, to leave to the states a power to regulate marijuana that is similar to the power they have to regulate alcohol, and for other purposes
HR 1014	Marijuana Tax Revenue Act of 2015	To amend the Internal Revenue Code of 1986 to provide for the taxation of marijuana
HR 1252	Fair Sentencing Clarification Act of 2015	To apply reduced sentences for certain cocaine-base offenses retroactively for certain offenders
HR 1538/S 683	CARERS Act of 2015	To extend the principle of federalism to state drug policy, provide access to medical marijuana, and enable research into the medicinal properties of marijuana
HR 1635	Charlotte's Web Medical Access Act of 2015	To exclude cannabidiol and cannabidiol-rich plants from the definition of marijuana
HR 1774	Compassionate Access Act	To provide for the rescheduling of marijuana, the medical use of marijuana in accordance with state law, and the exclusion of cannabidiol from the definition of marijuana
HR 1940	Respect State Marijuana Laws Act of 2015	To amend the Controlled Substances Act to provide for a new rule regarding the application of the Act to marijuana
HR 2076/S 1726	Marijuana Businesses Access to Banking Act of 2015	To create protections for depository institutions that provide financial services to marijuana-related businesses

Continued

HR 2331	No Welfare for Weed Act of 2015	To amend the Food and Nutrition Act of 2008 to prohibit the use of benefits to purchase marijuana products, to amend part A of title IV of the Social Security Act to prohibit assistance provided under the program of block grants to states for temporary assistance for needy families from being accessed through the use of an electronic benefit-transfer card at any store that offers marijuana for sale
HR 2373	Legitimate Use of Medicinal Marijuana Act	To provide for the legitimate use of medicinal marijuana in accordance with the laws of the various states
HR 2536/S 1455	Recovery Enhancement for Addiction Treatment Act	To provide access to medication-assisted therapy
HR 2598	Lucid Act of 2015	To amend title 23, United States Code, to establish requirements relating to marijuana-impaired driving, to direct the Administrator of the National Highway Traffic Safety Administration to issue comprehensive guidance on the best practices to prevent marijuana-impaired driving
HR 2805/S 1134	Heroin and Prescription Opioid Abuse Prevention, Education, and Enforcement Act of 2015	To address prescription-opioid abuse and heroin use
HR 2872	Opioid Addiction Treatment Modernization Act	To amend the Controlled Substances Act to modernize the treatment of opioid addiction
HR 3010	Preserving Welfare for Needs Not Weed Act	To prohibit assistance provided under the program of block grants to states for temporary assistance for needy families from being accessed through the use of an electronic benefit-transfer card at any store that offers marijuana for sale
HR 3047	Drug Testing for Welfare Recipients Act	To require certain welfare programs to deny benefits to persons who fail a drug test
HR 3124	Clean Slate for Marijuana Offenses Act of 2015	To permit the expungement of records of certain marijuana-related offenses
HR 3250	DXM Abuse Prevention Act of 2015	To amend the Federal Food, Drug, and Cosmetic Act to prevent the abuse of dextromethorphan, and for other purposes
HR 3380/S 32	Transnational Drug Trafficking Act of 2015	To provide the Department of Justice with additional tools to target extraterritorial drug trafficking activity
HR3489/HR 3530	Mandatory Minimum Reform Act of 2015	To eliminate mandatory minimum sentences for all drug offenses
HR 3518	Stop Civil Asset Forfeiture Funding for Marijuana Suppression Act of 2015	To amend title 28, United States Code, to prohibit the use of amounts from the Asset Forfeiture Fund for the Domestic Cannabis Suppression/Eradication Program of the Drug Enforcement Administration
HR 3537	Synthetic Drug Control Act of 2015	To amend the Controlled Substances Act to clarify how controlled substance analogues are to be regulated
HR 3561	Fair Access to Education Act of 2015	To amend the section 484(r) of the Higher Education Act of 1965 to exclude certain marijuana-related offenses from the drug-related offenses that result in students being barred from receiving federal educational loans, grants, and work assistance
HR 3677	Opioid Abuse Prevention and Treatment Act of 2015	To reduce opioid misuse and abuse
HR 3680	Co-Prescribing to Reduce Overdoses Act of 2015	To provide for the Secretary of Health and Human Services to carry out a grant program for co-prescribing opioid-overdose-reversal drugs
HR 4183/S 2027	Stop Trafficking in Fentanyl Act of 2015	To increase the penalties for fentanyl trafficking

From GovTrack.us.

The many billions of dollars spent on international drug-law enforcement has yielded meager results; the mechanics of drug production and distribution militate against enforcement efforts bringing about lasting reductions in supply. Focused efforts that reduce drug production in one area are offset by increased production elsewhere. In addition, since most of the profits accrue to actors at the end of the supply chain, street prices are relatively insensitive to supply shocks, as retailers have latitude to adjust their profit margins.[24]

Prevention

Preventing the initiation of drug use precludes later physiological and social harms, and so may be cost-effective, but less than 5% of the federal drug-control budget goes to prevention programs. This is due, in part, to the difficulty of appropriately targeting these programs, and to the lack of documented success of those existing prevention programs. In 2015, an estimated 20.5% of 8th graders, 34.7% of 10th graders, and 48.9% of

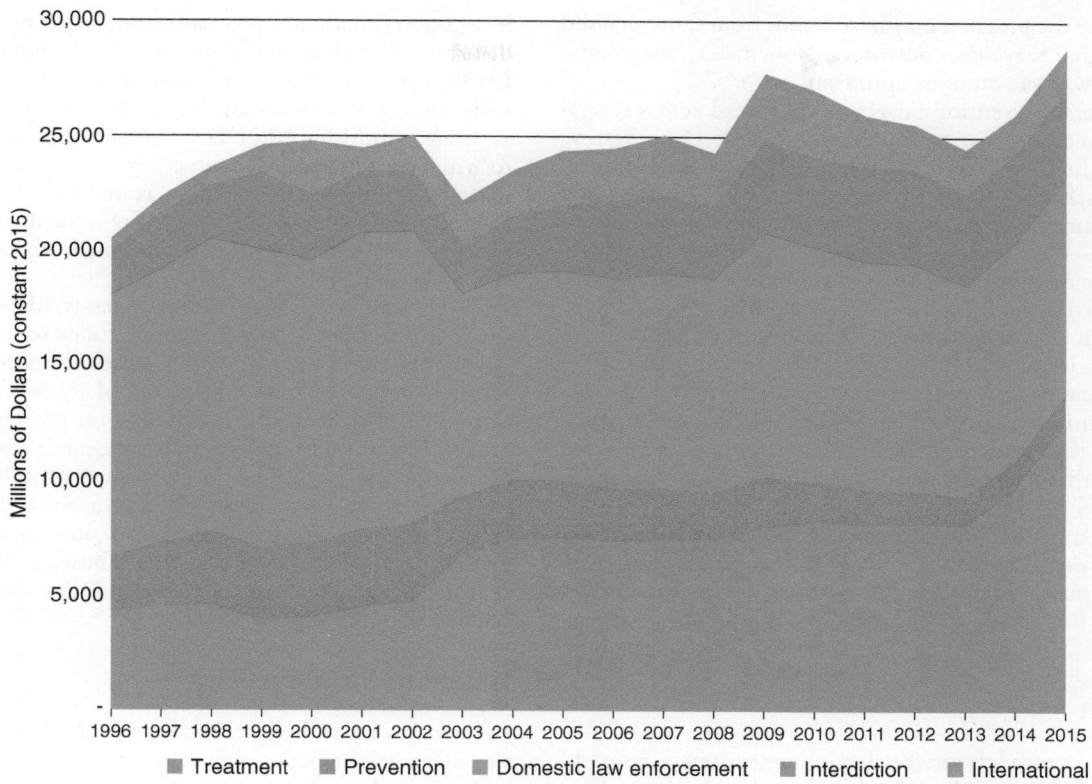

• **Fig. 3.1** Federal drug-control budget 1996–2015 (constant 2015 dollars). (Data for 1996–2001 are from The White House[69]. Data for 2002–2015 are from The White House[72]. All data reflect budgets using the revised Office of National Drug Control Policy methodology. To correct for changes in the purchasing power of the dollar, we have adjusted the data to constant 2015 dollars, using the Consumer Price Index.)

12th graders were using illicit drugs (according to NIDA's Monitoring the Future Survey and SAMHSA's National Survey on Drug Use and Health), making youth prime targets for prevention programs.

Among the better-known prevention programs are Drug Abuse Resistance Education (DARE) and school-based random drug testing. DARE involves a uniformed police officer visiting classrooms and educating students on how to resist drug use. Successive evaluations of DARE have found no meaningful differences in knowledge, attitudes, or drug use for those students participating, compared with those who did not.[36] When it became apparent that DARE was an ineffective use of drug-control resources, the program was "retooled" into what became the New-Drug Abuse Resistance Education (New-DARE) program.[60] New-DARE provides a more interactive curriculum, where students are exposed to brain imaging as proof of how drug use impairs brain functioning; provides data on actual levels of drug use among youth; and teaches refusal skills.[40] Evaluations of New-DARE fail to show any improvements over its predecessor.[1] The federal government has had a rocky relationship with DARE, and negative findings have led it to almost eliminate financial support for the program. In 2001, the Surgeon General identified DARE as a program that "Does Not Work,"[61] and, in 2003, the US Government Accountability Office concluded that DARE was potentially counterproductive in certain populations

(i.e., it was associated with *increased* drug use).[36] Remaining federal support for DARE is largely rhetorical; it continues to be listed as a model prevention program on the ONDCP website,[73] and President Obama declared a National Drug Abuse Resistance Education Day to celebrate the work of the program.[55]

The ONDCP directly manages two prevention programs: The National Youth Anti-Drug Media Campaign and the Drug Free Communities Support Program. The National Youth Anti-Drug Media Campaign was created by Congress in 1998 with the goal of preventing and reducing drug use through radio, television, and other media. NIDA-funded evaluations have shown that, while it has positively affected parents' beliefs and behaviors, there has been no measurable impact on initiation or reduced use among targeted youth.[57]

The Drug Free Communities Program, funded by Congress in 1997, supports local initiatives to address drug use. The Drug Free Communities Program is managed jointly by the ONDCP and SAMHSA, and the program currently supports 697 community coalitions. An ongoing evaluation suggests that communities receiving support through the Drug Free Communities Program have reduced drug use at a greater rate than nonrecipient communities.[32] There are many inherent difficulties in drawing conclusions about the causal effect of this type of program. As communities have to apply for Drug Free Communities Program support, selection bias can muddy findings: communities that opted into the program may be different from those that did not, in ways that may affect outcomes. Nonetheless, the evaluation findings warrant cautious optimism.

Other federal prevention programs are spread across several executive agencies.[73] For example, the Student Drug-Testing Institute in the Department of Education provides technical support for schools interested in establishing a school-based testing program. Random drug testing ostensibly serves a double function—it deters drug use and detects early drug involvement, thereby disrupting the path to addiction. By 2012, 59% of school districts had implemented drug-testing programs.[13] An assessment of school drug testing found no differences in student drug-use outcomes between schools with drug testing (whether for cause or at random) and those without.[85] A more-recent randomized controlled trial of school drug-testing programs found that students subject to random testing reported less drug use than comparable students in schools without random testing.[33]

Despite some troubling instances of persisting support for unproven or even discredited programs, there are federal government efforts to bring research-based evidence to bear on prevention.[12]

Treatment

In FY17, drug-treatment services (excluding treatment research) accounted for 43.7% of the federal drug-control budget (about $13.6 billion for treatment), and about 29% of services are provided through SAMHSA. Implementation is left mostly to the states, as 70% of SAMHSA's drug-treatment funding is distributed via block grants (lump sums allocated to states, with very few stipulations on how resources are to be spent). The Center for Substance Abuse Treatment within SAMHSA works with states and local groups to improve and expand effective treatment services provided under the block grants.

The remaining 30% of SAMHSA's funds are issued on a discretionary basis, under Programs of Regional and National Significance: capacity programs, which identify needed system changes and extend evidenced-based care and science and service programs, which identify practices that might improve services and disseminate information about these practices. The federal government has made strides toward promoting treatment practices that are grounded in evidence,[52] but the quality of the evidence based on "what works" remains weak, and the standards for considering a treatment program "evidence-based" are low.[22]

Research

Four percent of the budget (about 1.1 billion dollars) goes to research. Of this, about 65% goes to treatment and 35% to prevention. The National Institute on Drug Abuse (or NIDA), created in 1974, is the principal federal agency funding basic, clinical, and epidemiological research into drug abuse and addiction; the National Institute of Justice and the National Institute of Mental Health also fund research. NIDA-funded research has made major contributions to the science of addiction and has led to a number of innovations in drug treatment, including the clinical development of levo-α-acetylmethadol and naltrexone (medications used to treat opioid dependence). Despite being effective treatments for opioid addiction,

levo-α-acetylmethadol and naltrexone faced market barriers to distribution and were ultimately of little policy significance. Levo-α-acetylmethadol is no longer produced; for many years naltrexone was provided to few addicts[30] but is now regarded as more promising.[67] NIDA disseminates research findings to promote science-based practices and policies, through its *Research Monograph Series* (first issued in 1975) and the bimonthly newsletter *NIDA Notes* (first issued in 1985). NIDA accounts for some 85% of global biomedical research on drugs and addiction.[79]

NIDA's billion-dollar budget gives it high visibility, and the Institute has on occasion come under scrutiny for its role in shaping federal drug policy, through both the types of research it funds and the targeting of its research dissemination. The Institute has been criticized for promoting politically expedient research messages and a research agenda that reinforces the War on Drugs, to maintain its funding, while paying little attention to harm-reduction strategies.[55] However, Nora Volkow, a neuroscientist who was appointed director of the National Institute on Drug Abuse in 2003, maintains that its agenda is divorced from politics and is driven by science.[82]

Issues in Policymaking

In the next decade, budget constraints may yield a welcome scrutiny of federal drug-control policies and programs. If outcomes are to improve, federal drug-control policymakers will have to take resource allocation seriously and prioritize their efforts. What will this mean for federal drug control?

Picking Battles

Drug policymakers will need to pick their battles, which will require clearly elaborating the mission and goals of the federal drug-control strategy. This may entail focusing on particular drugs and drug-control activities.

The stated goal of the national drug-control policy is "curtail illicit drug consumption in America and improve the public health and public safety of the American people by reducing the consequences of drug abuse."[75]

It seems reasonable, then, that the strategy should focus on those drugs associated with the most severe crime, violence, and health consequences—and, further, that policymakers establish that the program's fiscal and social costs are outweighed by the benefits obtained. Under current law, alcohol—the costliest drug by far—is legal, while the scheduling of illicit and controlled substances is only loosely determined by social harms. Because alcohol is legal, it is usually divorced from the drug-policy debate. If public health is to be the driving principle, the policy for each drug should reflect its social costs.

Setting Minimum Standards for "Evidence"

Few people will object to a call for "evidence-based" practices; indeed, the ONDCP is required to "develop and implement a set of research-based principles" for drug-abuse–prevention programs.[51] But this desideratum compels stakeholders to justify their existence and continued funding by demonstrating that their programs "work," which may have the perverse effect of stifling progress. A low bar for "effectiveness" renders many ineffective programs "evidence-based," and makes it difficult to identify worthy programs. Good programs get lost in the mix, and weak programs persist. Clear, strict standards for the quality of evidence would shield policymaking from some of the malign influences of politics.[40]

The Obama administration's top drug-policy appointments were received with optimism by advocates of reform and were not identified as ardent drug warriors (although Vice President Biden has long been so). Although the many federal agencies implicated in drug policy were not necessarily aligned in their interests and orientation, federal drug policy has taken a turn toward harm reduction and away from prohibition and punishment.[10] Whatever their orientation, previous administrations have called for evidence-based policymaking, but the political process has trumped science and program evaluation. Should policymakers be committed to thoroughgoing reform, there is ample evidence to inform their efforts.

Appendix

The Controlled Substances Act of 1970 created five schedules under which drugs of abuse are classified.[a,20] Scheduling of a drug determines, in part, federal penalties for possession and distribution and the terms under which it may be prescribed.

The legislation created the initial listing, but the Drug Enforcement Administration and the Department of Health and Human Services determine adjustments to the schedules, based on a drug's potential for abuse, accepted medical use in the United States, and potential for dependence. The Drug Enforcement Administration begins or accepts petitions for investigations, and then passes its findings to the Department of Health and Human Services for a recommendation based on scientific and medical evaluations. The Drug Enforcement Administration then makes the scheduling decision.[b]

See Table 3.2 for the scheduling criteria and major scheduled drugs.

References

1. Alcohol Problems and Solutions. *DARE Still Fails to Reduce Alcohol and Drug Abuse*; 2008. http://www.alcoholproblemsandsolutions.org//.htm. Accessed 01 March 2016.
2. Anti-Drug Abuse Act of 1986(1987). *Pub Law 570, 99th Cong.*, approved 27 Oct.
3. Anti-Drug Abuse Act of 1988(1988). *Pub Law 690, 100th Cong.*, approved 18 Nov.
4. Bennett W, DiIulio J, Walters J. *Body Count: Moral Poverty and How to Win America's War Against Crime and Drugs*. New York: Simon and Schuster; 1996.
5. Bertram E, Blachman M, Sharpe K, Andreas P. *Drug War Politics: The Price of Denial*. Berkeley: University of California; 1996.
6. Bickel WK, DeGrandpre RJ. *Drug Policy and Human Nature: Psychological Perspectives on the Prevention, Management, and Treatment of Illicit Drug Abuse*. New York: Springer; 1996.
7. Boggs Act of 1951(1951). *Pub Law No. 255, 82nd Cong.*, approved 2 Nov.
8. Bulwa D. U.S. Raids Firms Selling Items used by Pot Smokers. *San Francisco Chronicle*; 2003:A4.
9. Bureau of International Narcotics and Law Enforcement Affairs. *Fiscal Year 2013 Program and Budget Guide*. Washington, DC: Department of State; 2012.
10. Castillo T. Harm reduction at a crossroads. *The Fix*. 2014. https://www.thefix.com//reduction-conference. Accessed 23 March 2016.
11. Center for Cognitive Liberty and Ethics. *US Nitrous Oxide Laws*; 2002. http://www.cognitiveliberty.org//_state_laws.htm. Accessed 01 March 2016.
12. Center for Substance Abuse Prevention. *Identifying and Selecting Evidence-Based Interventions*. Rockville, MD: Substance Abuse and Mental Health Services Administration; 2009.
13. Centers for Disease Control. *School Health Policies and Practices Study: Alcohol or Other Drug-Use Prevention*; 2012. Atlanta. http://www.cdc.gov//////_AlcoholOrOtherDrugUsePrevention_SHPPS2012.pdf. Accessed 23 March 2016.
14. Cole JM. *Guidance Regarding Marijuana Enforcement*. Washington, DC: Office of the Deputy Attorney General; 2013.
15. Comprehensive Crime Control Act of 1984(1984). *Pub Law No. 473, 98th Cong.*, approved 12 Oct.
16. Controlled Substances Act of 1970(1970). *Pub Law No. 513, 91st Cong.*, approved 27 Oct.
17. Cook D. New drug czar gets lower rank, promise of higher visibility. *Christian Science Monitor*; 2009. http://features.csmonitor.com/////drug-czar-gets-lower-rank-promise-of-higher-visibility. Accessed 01 March 2016.
18. Davenport-Hines R. *The Pursuit of Oblivion: A Global History of Narcotics*. New York: W.W. Norton; 2002.
19. Drug Abuse Prevention, Treatment and Rehabilitation Act of 1979(1980). *Pub Law 181, 96th Cong.*, approved 2 Jan.
20. Drug Enforcement Administration. *The Combat Meth Act of 2005*; 2005. http://www.deadiversion.usdoj.gov//q_a.htm. Accessed 01 March 2016.
21. Drug Policy Alliance. *Legislative Proposals for Reform of the Crack/Cocaine Disparity*; 2007. http://www.drugpolicy.org////_cocaine.cfm. Accessed 01 March 2016.
22. Eliason MJ. *Improving Substance Abuse Treatment: An Introduction to the Evidence-Based Practice Movement*. Los Angeles: SAGE; 2007.
23. Fair Sentencing Act of 2010 (2010). *Pub Law No. 220, 111th Cong.*, approved 22 Aug.
24. Falco MUS. Federal drug policy. In: Lowinson JH, Ruiz P, Millman RB, Langrod JG, eds. *Substance Abuse: A Comprehensive Textbook*. Philadelphia: Lippincott Williams & Wilkins; 2004:21–32.
25. Federal Bureau of Prisons. *Statistics*. Washington, DC: Department of Justice; 2016. https://www.bop.gov///_inmate_offenses.jsp. Accessed 24 Mar 2016.
26. Ford GF. *Statement on Receiving the Report of the Domestic Council Drug Abuse Task Force*; 1975. http://www.presidency.ucsb.edu//.php?pid=5325. Accessed 01 March 2016.
27. Gieringer D. *America's Hundred Years War on Drugs: Centennial of the 1st Congressional Anti-Drug Law prohibiting opium in the Philippines*; 2006. http://www.drugsense.org//.htm. Accessed 01 March 2016.
28. Gonzales M, McEnery K, Sheehan T, Mellody S. *America's Habit: Drug Abuse, Drug Trafficking, and Organized Crime: President's Commission on Organized Crime*. Derby, PA: DIANE; 1986.
29. Gonzales v. Raich; 2005. 545 U.S. 1 (2005) 352 F.3d 1222. http://www.law.cornell.edu///.ZS.html. Accessed 01 March 2016.
30. Goodman C, Ahn R, Harwood R, Ringel D, Savage K, Mendelson D, et al. *Market Barriers to the Development of Pharmacotherapies for the Treatment of Cocaine Abuse and Addiction: Final Report*. Washington, DC: Department of Health and Human Services; 1997.
31. Hill JA. Banks, marijuana, and federalism. *Case Western Reserve Law Review*. 2015;65:597–647.

[a] Some states impose controls on the sale and use of substances not covered under the federal schedules, such as nitrous oxide and amyl nitrite.[11] Pseudoephedrine is widely used in the manufacture of methamphetamine, and medicines containing pseudoephedrine are separately regulated under an amendment to the USA PATRIOT Act.[20]

[b] The scheduling procedure may be bypassed when an international treaty requires controlling a drug, or "to avoid an imminent hazard to the public safety."[2]

32. ICF International. *Drug-Free Communities Support Program: 2014 National Evaluation Report*. Virginia: Fairfax; 2015.

33. Institute of Educational Sciences National Center for Education Evaluation and Regional Assistance. *The Effectiveness of Mandatory-Random Student Drug Testing*. Washington, DC: Department of Education; 2010. https://ies.ed.gov/////.pdf. Accessed 24 Mar 2016.

34. International Opium Convention. *Translation 222*. The Hague: League of Nations; 1912. http://treaties.un.org/////%208/.pdf. Accessed 01 March 2016.

35. Kamin S. The battle of the bulge: the surprising last stand against state marijuana legalization. *Publius*. 2015;45(3):427–451.

36. Kanof ME. *Youth Illicit Drug use Prevention: DARE Long-Term Evaluations and Federal Efforts to Identify Effective Programs*. Washington, DC: General Accounting Office; 2003.

37. Kennedy R. *Race, Crime, and The Law*. New York: Pantheon Books; 1997.

38. King R. *The Drug Hang-Up, America's Fifty Year Folly*. Springfield, IL: Bannerstone House; 1972.

39. Kolb L, Du Mez AG. The prevalence and trend of drug addiction in the United States and factors influencing it. *Public Health Reports*. 1954;39(21):1179–1204.

40. MacCoun R, Reuter P. The implicit rules of evidence-based drug policy: a U.S. perspective. *Int J Drug Policy*. 2008;19(3):231–232.

41. Manski CF, Pepper JV, Petrie CV, eds. *Informing America's Policy on Illegal Drugs: What We Don't Know Keeps Hurting Us*. Washington, DC: National Academies Press; 2001:11.

42. Marijuana Policy Project. *State-By-State Medical Marijuana Laws: How to Remove the Threat of Arrest*. Washington, DC: Marijuana Policy Project; 2008.

43. Mejia D. *Plan Colombia: An Analysis of Effectiveness and Costs*. Washington, DC: Brookings Institution; 2015.

44. Meyer J, Glover S. U.S. Won't Prosecute Medical Pot Sales. *Los Angeles Times*; 2009.

45. Moses C. *Do Czars Matter? An Assessment of Effectiveness of Drug Czars*. Chicago: MPSA Annual National Conference; 2008.

46. Murphy P. *Keeping Score: the Frailties of the Federal Drug Budget*. Santa Monica: RAND Corp; 1994.

47. Musto DF. *The American Disease: Origins of Narcotic Control*. New York: Oxford University; 1999.

48. Musto DF. *The History of Legislative Control Over Opium, Cocaine, and their Derivatives*. n.d. http://www.druglibrary.org///.htm. Accessed 01 March 2016.

49. Narcotic Control Act of 1956(1956). *Pub Law No. 728, 84th Cong., approved 18 July*.

50. Narcotic Manufacturing Act of 1960(1960). *Pub Law No. 429, 86th Cong., approved 22 Apr*.

51. National Criminal Justice Reference Service. *Evidence-Based Principles for Substance Abuse Prevention*. Washington, DC: Department of Justice; 2003. http://www.ncjrs.gov////_based_eng.html. Accessed 01 March 2016.

52. *National Registry of Evidence-Based Programs and Practices*. Rockville, MD: Substance Abuse and Mental Health Services Administration; 2016. http://www.nrepp.samhsa.gov. Accessed 01 March 2016.

53. National Research Council. *Informing America's Policy on Illegal Drugs: What We Don't Know Keeps Hurting Us. Commission on Behavioral and Social Sciences and Education*. Washington, DC: National Academies; 2001.

54. Nigro v. U.S.; 1928:276. U.S. 332. http://www.druglibrary.org////.htm. Accessed 01 March 2016.

55. Office of the Press Secretary. *National D.A.R.E. Day*. Washington, DC: The White House; 2009. https://www.whitehouse.gov//ocuments/_prc1_final.pdf. Accessed 01 March 2016.

56. Organized Crime Drug Enforcement Task Forces. *FY 2013 Interagency Crime and Drug Enforcement: Congressional Budget Submission*. Washington, DC: Department of Justice; 2012.

57. Orwin R, Cadell D, Chu A, Kalton G, Maklan D, Morin C, et al. *Evaluation of the National Youth Anti-Drug Media Campaign: 2004 Report of Findings*. Bethesda, MD: National Institute on Drug Abuse; 2006.

58. Prettyman Commission. Report of the President's advisory commission on narcotics and drug abuse. H.R. Rep. No. 1444, 91st Cong., 2nd Sess. Cited In Gonzales M., McEnery K., Sheehan T., Mellody S., eds. *America's Habit: Drug Abuse, Drug Trafficking, and Organized Crime: President's Commission on Organized Crime*. Derby, PA: DIANE; 1986. 1963.

59. Sabet KA. The "local" matters: a brief history of the tension between federal drug laws and state and local policy. *J Global Drug Policy Prac*. 2007;1(4).

60. Sack JL. DARE anti-drug program to shift strategy. *Education Week*. 2001;20(23):1–2.

61. Satcher D. *Youth Violence: A Report of the Surgeon General*. Washington, DC: United States Public Health Service; 2001.

62. Schaller M. The federal prohibition of marihuana. *J Social History*. 1970;4(1):61–74.

63. Shafer RP. *Marihuana: A Signal of Misunderstanding*. Washington, DC: U.S. Government Printing Office; 1972.

64. Shulgin AT. *Controlled Substances: A Chemical and Legal Guide to the Federal Drug Laws*. Berkeley, CA: Ronin; 1988.

65. Sonnenreich MR, Roccograndi AJ, Bogomolny RL. *Handbook on the 1970 Federal Drug Act*. Springfield, IL: Charles C. Thomas; 1975.

66. Special Inspector General for Afghanistan Reconstruction. *Poppy Cultivation in Afghanistan: After a Decade of Reconstruction and Over $7 Billion in Counternarcotics Efforts, Poppy Cultivation Levels are at an All-Time High*. Washington, DC: SIGAR; 2014.

67. Substance Abuse and Mental Health Services Administration. *Federal Guidelines for Opioid Treatment Programs*; 2015. Rockville, MD.

68. The White House. *National Drug Control Strategy: FY 2004 Budget Summary*. Washington, DC: Office of National Drug Control Policy; 2003.

69. The White House. *National Drug Control Strategy: FY 2005 Budget Summary*. Washington, DC: Office of National Drug Control Policy; 2004.

70. The White House. *National Drug Control Strategy: FY 2012 Funding Highlights*. Washington, DC: Office of National Drug Control Policy; 2011.

71. The White House. *High Intensity Drug Trafficking Areas Program Report to Congress*. Washington, DC: Office of National Drug Control Policy; 2011.

72. The White House. *National Drug Control Budget: FY 2017 Funding Highlights*. Washington, DC: Office of National Drug Control Policy; 2011.

73. The White House. *Prevention Programs*. Washington, DC: Office of National Drug Control Policy; 2016. http://www.whitehousedrugpolicy.gov//.html. Accessed 30 Jan 2016.

74. The White House. *ONDCP Fact Sheets*; 2016. https://www.whitehouse.gov//fact-sheets. Accessed 24 Mar 2016.

75. The White House. *ONDCP National Drug Control Strategy*. Washington, DC: Office of National Drug Control Policy; 2016.

76. Timberlake JH. *Prohibition and the Progressive Movement, 1900–1920*. Cambridge, MA: Harvard University; 1963.

77. Timberlake JH, Lock ED, Rasinski KA. How should we wage the war on drugs? Determinants of public preferences for drug control alternatives. *Policy Studies J*. 2003;31(1):71–88.

78. United Nations Office on Drugs and Crime. *World Drug Report 2015: Advanced Briefing to Member Countries*. Vienna: United Nations; 2015.

79. United States Senate. *Senate Report 106–293. Departments of Labor, Health and Human Services, and Education and Related Agencies Appropriation Bill, 2001*; 1999.

80. *U.S. Immigration and Customs Enforcement Border Enforcement Security Task Forces Overview*; 2016. https://www.ice.gov/. Accessed 24 Mar 2016.

81. Veillette C. *Andean Counterdrug Initiative (ACI) and Related Funding Programs: FY 2006 Assistance.* Washington, DC: Congressional Research Service; 2009.

82. Volkow N. *Messages from the Director: Introduction.* National Institute on Drug Abuse; 2004. https://www.drugabuse.gov/nida/page/director///. Accessed 24 March 2016.

83. Walker WO. *Drug Control in the Americas.* Albuquerque: University of New Mexico; 1989.

84. Walsh JM. Fuzzy math: why the White House drug control budget doesn't add up. *Fas Drug Policy Analysis Bulletin.* 2004;10.

85. Yamaguchi R, Johnston LD, O'Malley PM. *Drug Testing in Schools: Policies, Practices, and Association with Student Drug Use.* Princeton: Robert Wood Johnson Foundation; 2003.

86. Zeese K. *Revising the Federal Drug Control Budget Report: Changing Methodology to Hide the Cost of the Drug War? Common Sense for Drug Policy;* 2002. Washington, DC. http://www.csdp.org//.pdf. Accessed 01 March 2016.

4

Historical Perspectives of Addiction

HOWARD I. KUSHNER

CHAPTER OUTLINE

Histories of Addiction

In the past quarter century, historians of addiction have focused on contextualizing the political, social, and cultural meanings of addiction. Building on Harry Gene Levine's classic 1978 article, "The Discovery of Addiction," historians have suggested that the classification of certain substances as illicit or licit tells us more about social norms and power relationships than about the psychopharmacological properties of the substances themselves.[32] Historians have contextualized the definitions of addiction, alerting us to the extent to which alcohol prohibition and the criminalization of narcotics and stimulants reflected dominant cultural values rather than robust scientific findings. These studies pose an intellectual challenge to the treatment and control of addiction. So far, however, they have made a less significant impact on addiction policy and treatment. In a recent article, I argued that historians of addiction should take biology seriously.[44] Here I hope to persuade addiction scientists and practitioners of the value of these recent histories for their research and practice.

Doing so requires an appreciation of historical methods. Academic historians are not simply engaged in telling a chronological story; nor, since the late 19th century have they assumed that they can uncover "facts" that recreate the past as it was. Rather, academic historians insist that historical sources do not speak for themselves, but are subjects of contested interpretations framed by current and past cultural and political contexts. From this perspective, there can never be one final "factual" reading of the past; today's landmark interpretation is regularly subjected to tomorrow's reinterpretation because, odd as it may sound to the nonacademic historian, the past is always subject to change as historians redefine the contexts in which events occur. The current scientific paradigm that addiction is a brain disease[56] is placed in social and cultural contexts. The implicit message is that, whatever the biological substrates of addiction, by acknowledging social, cultural, and political forces, addiction scientists, policymakers, and practitioners can develop more effective policies and interventions.

Brain Disease Redux

Often, writes historian Nancy Campbell, what has been learned in addiction science has been ignored in succeeding paradigms. More than a half century ago, Campbell found that addiction researchers Maurice S. Seever and Abraham Wikler had independently concluded that addiction was a chronic relapsing/remitting condition, a view presented in 2000 by then National Institute on Drug Abuse (NIDA) director, Alan Leshner, as novel.[48] Campbell also points to a rhetorical resilience of a traditional "moral lexicon" of addiction. Citing the work of current NIDA director, Nora Volkow, and her colleagues as exemplars, Campbell finds that their notion of "disrupted volition" parallels 19th century constructs of addiction "as a 'disease of the will' subject to voluntary control." Thus, writes Campbell, with "amnesiac gesture toward its own repressed past, the addiction enterprise comes full circle into the present."[12]

As Campbell suggests, the claims that addiction is a brain disease would sound familiar to 19th century neurologists. In many respects, current views resemble degeneration theory as expounded by the French physician Théodule Ribot in his 1883 study *Les Maladies de la Volonté* (which was reissued in 32 subsequent editions in French and English).[64] Degeneration theory offered a hereditarian explanation for a variety of disorders including retardation, depression, depravity, and sterility. Behaviors that today would include addictions such as alcoholism, diet, and sexual addictions were alleged to have a cumulative destructive impact on the nervous system that was inherited by succeeding generations.[24] Practitioners took extensive family histories and prepared elaborate pedigrees that sought to explain a current disorder by uncovering patterns of disease and behavior in a patient's family. Adherents sought to portray degeneration as organic, but much like addiction practices today, treatment revolved around an array of psychological and moral interventions under the rationale that alterations in habits had a direct physiological influence on the nervous system.[24,53,58,61]

Degeneration theory meshed with the views of the influential neurologist James Hughlings Jackson, whose "dissolution theory" was based on his claim that lesions in the neocortex reversed the evolutionary process in which the "higher" cortical structures restrained the "lower" emotive, limbic functions. Jackson's hydraulic theory reinforced the assumptions that addictions reflected a hijacking by these more primitive structures, often referred to as the "reptilian brain." Thus addiction was a brain disease because the behaviors were enabled by damage to cortical censors.[32] Because these behaviors appeared to run in families, it was a small step to connect Jackson's dissolution with degeneration.

Both degeneration and dissolution were translated into early 20th century popular scientific explanations of the physical effects of alcohol and other drugs. For instance, historian Susan Speaker writes of Richmond P. Hobson, a retired naval officer and three-term congressman from Alabama, who published *Alcohol and the Human Race* in 1919 and portrayed it as based on the best "evolutionary science" of the time.[35] Hobson, who founded the American Alcohol Education Association in 1921, wrote that alcohol was a toxin that paralyzed white blood cells, making them unable to "catch the disease germ" that was "devouring" the drinker. This led to the destruction of the "centers of the brain upon whose activities rest the moral sense," resulting in what Hobson labeled "retrograde evolution." For Hobson, "alcoholic beverages, even in moderation reverse the process of nature." Ninety-five percent of "all the acts of crime and violence committed in civilized communities," Hobson claimed, "are the direct result of men being put down by alcohol to the plane of savagery."[72]

Hobson's "science" both influenced and was influenced by early 20th century prohibitionist sentiments. With the end of Prohibition, a new science of alcoholism emerged. Americans, according to Speaker, ceased "demonizing alcohol after Prohibition, and chose to deal with its risks largely through regulation, education, and harm-reduction strategies." However, she writes, "they have resisted" treating users of most other psychoactive drugs in a similar manner.[72] What emerged were distinct attitudes, policies, and sciences that separated alcohol from other addictive substances. However, Speaker implies, these distinctions were based less on objective evidence than on the cultural, social, and economic attitudes toward alcohol and other mind-altering substances. I begin with historians' interpretations of the science of alcohol addiction and then move on to other substances.

Alcohol and Other Drugs

The federal government has created two separate divisions for addiction research: (1) the National Institute on Alcohol Abuse and Alcoholism, which has focused exclusively on alcohol, and (2) the National Institute on Drug Abuse, which has studied the use of all other addictive substances. Despite this official separation of alcohol from other drugs, in a recent collection, *Altering American Consciousness: The History of Alcohol and Drug Use in the United States, 1800–2000*, historians Sarah W. Tracy and Caroline Jean Acker argue that bringing alcohol and other addictive substances together is justified: "Despite the chasm created by law, which separates them into legal and illegal categories, all psychoactive drugs share important commonalities."[78] "America's drug habits cannot be understood, nor effective drug policy made," they insist, "until we have a clearer picture of the range of drugs used yesterday and today, and the ways in which specific historical circumstances have shaped their use and regulation."[78]

The theme that runs through *Altering American Consciousness* is best summed up by the historian Alan Brandt, who writes that although the addictive nature of nicotine may today be seen as an undisputed fact of its chemical properties, nicotine's classification as an addictive substance is rooted more in the history of attitudes toward smoking than in its neurochemical mechanisms.[7] Brandt believes that the history of nicotine provides a window to understanding the meaning of addiction. He rejects what he calls "universal, transhistorical approaches to the mechanisms of addiction" in favor of "specific historical contexts" that illuminate "the social processes by which addictions are created and experienced, categorized, and treated."[7]

The history of nicotine provides a context for the increased labeling of a variety of substance uses and behaviors—from carbohydrates and coffee to shopping and sex—as addictions. Perhaps this has occurred because, as William L. White[84] points out, there continues to be no consensus on the language and meaning of addiction itself.[37,69,83] "The rhetoric of addiction," White believes, "grew out of the multiple utilities" of the constituencies it served.[84] Deconstructing the various definitions of inebriety, intemperance, drunkenness, and alcoholism, White argues that the contested rhetoric of addiction served as "a means of staking out professional territory." At stake was which institutions and professions could claim "legitimate ownership of the problem."[84]

Taking White's view further, anthropologist Helen Keane's *What's Wrong With Addiction?* focuses on how addiction rhetoric is constituted in current discourses.[37] Like Brandt, Keane eschews a universalist view, arguing instead that what has become characterized as addiction "is tied to modernity, medical rationality and a particular notion of the unique and autonomous individual."[37] Although addiction has been portrayed as restricting freedom and individual autonomy, Keane argues that discourses of addiction have tended to limit freedom, as they have authorized the prohibitive power of the family, the state, and the corporation.

Keane's and White's claims are best examined in historical context. We begin with histories of alcohol use and then move on to other substances.

Alcohol: Predisposed or Culturally Determined

The histories of alcohol addiction have much in common with those of other drug addictions, but unlike illicit and (still) legal drugs such as nicotine, alcohol putatively poses a danger only to predisposed alcoholics. The prevailing view in America is that moderate consumption of alcohol by those without a predisposition is safe and not addictive. In contrast, the dominant media and scientific view today holds that, although some people are more prone to addictive behaviors than others, no predisposition is necessary for addiction to illicit substances and nicotine; any exposure potentially places any user at risk.[19,56]

Connected to the risk dichotomy is the widely accepted belief that alcoholism is a disease. Although a number of historians have pointed to a long genealogy supporting the notion that excessive and seemingly uncontrollable drinking was driven by forces beyond an individual's power, most agree with Griffith Edwards,[25] former chairman of the UK's National Addiction Centre, that the modern concept defining alcoholism as a disease comes from the work of the director of the Yale Center for Alcohol Studies, Elvin M. Jellinek, in the 1940s.[36] Not all experts have been persuaded by the disease paradigm. Two types of challenges emerged: the first questioned the almost universal belief that alcoholics must abstain from drinking for their entire lives, and the second was aimed at the validity of the disease construct.

In 1962, the renowned British psychiatrist D.L. Davies published a report of seven alcohol-dependent individuals who returned to normal drinking without reverting to alcoholism.[21,25] Edwards, who trained under Davies, followed these alcoholics and concluded that Davies' optimism was not sustained by their long-term behaviors.[25] In the 1970s, California psychologists Mark and Linda Sobell claimed that behavior modification could enable recovered alcoholics to return to what they called "controlled drinking."[70,71] The Sobells' research was the subject of a damning analysis published in the journal *Science* in 1982, which concluded that "a review of the evidence, including official records and new interviews, reveals that most of the subjects in the controlled drinking experiment failed from the outset to drink safely. The majority were hospitalized for alcoholism treatment within a year after discharge from the research project." In fact, a 10-year follow-up revealed that only one of the original 20 subjects could be classified as having met the criteria of controlled drinking; four had died of alcohol-related causes.[25]

When a number of studies attacking the construct of alcoholism as a disease appeared in the late 1980s and 1990s, the response of the alcohol research community was hostile. These critiques, including highly publicized ones written by Herbert Fingarette[28] and Stanton Peele,[60] have been the focus of sustained attacks from a wide range of alcohol researchers, and the authors have been marginalized and often stigmatized.

Although historians generally do not confront the controversy over controlled drinking, recent addiction histories can be read as providing support for the minority view, questioning the robustness of the claims that alcohol addiction is a disease. Building on the writings of Levine, they have concluded that the separation and classification of alcohol addiction as substantially different from other drug addictions is a cultural construct.

Earlier histories of alcohol use have detailed the battles between pro- and antiprohibitionists,[47] but sociologist Ron Roizen believes that this focus has obscured the more important story of the depoliticization of alcohol.[65] The construct of alcoholism as a disease, according to Roizen, meshed with the values of both the "spiritual orientation" of Alcoholics Anonymous and the "disinterestedness, objectivity, and empiricism" of contemporary science. Ironically, the notion that alcoholism was a disease "also offered destigmatization to the alcoholic and a measure of new symbolic legitimacy for [the] beverage alcohol itself." From the disease perspective, alcohol "harbored little more responsibility for alcoholism or alcohol related troubles than did sugar for the disease of diabetes."[65] The dominant belief remains that moderate drinking is safe for all but the potential and actual alcoholic. For Roizen, "the story of modern alcoholism" reveals "its strongly social-constructionist character and flimsy science base" and "invites our attention to the relationship between alcohol science and the wider society."[65] Roizen also has been particularly vocal in his opposition to what he sees as a new public health campaign to demonize alcohol.[27]

One of the linchpins for the notion of alcoholism as a disease is the widespread popular belief that Native Americans are genetically vulnerable to alcoholism. This view has been challenged by a number of recent studies. In 2000, in the *American Journal of Public Health*, John W. Frank and his colleagues emphasize that beyond obvious "risk factors in contemporary life," there is the need to consider the historical sources of Native American drinking problems. "In contrast to other explanatory factors," they write, "the role of history seems to have been underemphasized in the voluminous literature attempting to explain the problem of drinking among Native Americans." For instance, one must acknowledge "the extraordinary barrage of inducements to drink heavily in the early years after European contact. The harmful drinking patterns established during those years have largely persisted." Thus they conclude that "the cultural dimensions of Native American drinking must be considered far more important than the notion that Native Americans' propensity for heavy and dependant drinking is primarily genetic."[29]

Although the historian Peter C. Mancall does not cite Frank et al., he endorses their findings.[50] Mancall agrees that some individuals "seem to possess an inherited predisposition toward alcohol abuse," but he insists that "there is no convincing evidence suggesting that Indians as a group are more inclined to possess these traits than the general American population."[50] Historical research, according to Mancall, reveals that "there has been no single Native American response to liquor. Consumption patterns have differed over time by region and even in specific communities." They also have varied by age and gender. "Patterns of alcohol-related illness, disease … and trauma are not uniform within the Native American population today, and were not in past centuries either."[50] Europeans, Mancall reminds us, who had been exposed to alcohol for centuries, "had developed rules for its consumption." Nevertheless, they too experienced "periods of wide-spread alcohol-related problems," including the so-called gin craze in the mid-18th century, which "occurred in part because of wider availability of more potent alcohol during the early phases of the industrial revolution when the English and other Europeans drank more alcohol" in an attempt to "escape from the disorienting social changes of their everyday lives."[50] For Mancall then, like Frank et al., "history, not biology, holds the key to understanding Native American drinking patterns, just as history, not biology holds the key to understanding alcohol consumption in other American populations."[50]

Mancall's thesis is built on a number of studies,[41] including the 1969 cultural anthropology classic, *Drunken Comportment: A Social Explanation*, by Craig MacAndrew and Robert B. Edgerton, which explored variations in behaviors observed in different populations when they are drunk.[49] In relatively simple societies, people learn how they are supposed to behave when intoxicated; in more complex societies, the cultural expectations may vary, but the same principle holds. Edwards supports MacAndrew and Edgerton's anthropology. Acknowledging that "alcohol is a drug which has the inherent capacity to interfere with brain function and produce a state of intoxication," Edwards, nevertheless, argues that "intoxication is not, however, a fixed and monolithic state." Rather, based on narratives of South African and Bolivian drinking behaviors, Edwards explains behavioral reactions to alcohol intoxication as "plastic." By this he means that "drunkenness behavior can be molded by influences which include the immediate context, the way people react to drunkenness, the drinker's personality, and the expectations given by culture and society." From this perspective, "drunkenness is more like clay than concrete."[25]

The history of attempts to treat drunkenness suggests that clay was often mistaken for concrete. This response can be seen in historian Katherine A. Chavigny's discussion of 19th century drinking reform.[15] She focuses on the emergence—from the antebellum period to the 1880s—of a consensus among a group of individuals whom she labels as "inebriety physicians" that drunkards were suffering from an inherited disease. If the cause of drunkenness was a degenerative inheritance, "those persons who had inherited a constitutional weakness for alcohol had little chance of becoming sober without long-term quarantine from temptation." These physicians urged the construction and maintenance of facilities to house and treat the afflicted, many of whom were poor, homeless, and criminal. Legislatures were not persuaded, and other more traditional reformers rejected "hereditarian interpretations of inebriety," because they "believed that such views discouraged drunkards from trying to reform and provided them with a ready excuse for backsliding."[15] Nevertheless, the failure of inebriety physicians to persuade legislatures and other reformers that drunkenness was a disease was a temporary setback.

In contrast, historian Sarah Tracy's "Building a Boozatorium," examines a successful attempt to medicalize habitual drunkenness in turn-of-the-century Iowa.[76] Similar to the physicians discussed by Chavigny, Tracy's reformers relied on degeneration theory and its eugenic offspring. Unlike the experts in Chavigny's narrative, this cohort of clinicians, clergy, and social reformers persuaded the Iowa legislature to designate a facility for confinement and treatment of the disease of intemperance. Tracy connects this success to its context in wider Progressive social reform. "As much as any reform passed in turn-of-the-century Iowa," writes Tracy, "the creation of inebriate hospitals embodied a diversity of elements that characterized Progressivism in America: the search for order." These include "the rise of 'issue-focused coalitions,' the secular institution of Protestant moral values; the growth of an increasingly regulatory state with a well-articulated, efficiently organized, social reform mission; the maturation of the professions; and the expansion of scientific and medical authority."[76]

While Chavigny uncovers the roots of the contemporary triumph of the medicalization of alcoholism in the ideology of earlier reformers, Tracy finds a disconnect. A number of factors, writes Tracy, "worked against the wholesale adoption of the medical perspective" on alcohol abuse. Foremost was the failure of these institutions to demonstrate a robust cure rate. Moreover, these institutions "addressed a small percentage of the alcoholic population," and, as a result, medical care never was able to supplant the criminal justice system. "Prohibition and World War I cut short the medical efforts of physicians, drying up much of the political concern for the drunks."[76] Thus, "Iowa's efforts to medicalize habitual drunkenness were unsuccessful for as wide a range of reasons as they were initiated."[76]

Tracy's 2005 volume, *Alcoholism in America: From Reconstruction to Prohibition*, finds no medical consensus that alcoholism was a disease. However, like Chavigny, Tracy uncovers a persistent attempt by practitioners and social reformers to attach drunkenness to forces beyond individual choice.[77] Thus, reformers located the etiology of alcoholism in social forces, biological destiny, or some combination. Therefore, the current dominant discourse, in which alcoholism is considered a disease, has deep, if contested, historical roots.

Although, today, alcoholism is widely assumed to be organic, mid-20th century psychiatry focused on psychogenic etiologies, often tied to gender role confusion. Alcoholic males, writes Michelle McClellan, were characterized as effeminate with homosexual tendencies manifested by employment difficulties. In contrast, psychiatrists portrayed female alcoholics as displaying "masculine traits such as aggressiveness," and they "were often promiscuous or frigid" women and inadequate mothers.[52] Given the psychoanalytic paradigm that underpinned these views, gender identity and behavior issues were tied to childhood conflicts resulting from poor parenting. "Experts," according to McClellan, found that "many alcoholic women had displayed masculine and therefore deviant behavior as children—some had acted like tomboys, for example, while others exhibited unfeminine temper tantrums."[52] When later life stressors and emotional difficulties arose, particularly those tied to sexual and reproductive issues, these vulnerable women turned to alcohol.

Gendered assumptions, according to historian Lori E. Rotskoff, also informed psychiatric views about the role that sober wives played in their husbands' alcoholism.[66,67] Underlying many of these observations was the tension of postwar readjustment of gender role expectations, with returning males displacing working women. The task, seen by many psychiatrists and social workers in the 1940s and 1950s, was to reestablish traditional gender roles within the American family. A number of psychiatrists suggested that "wives had a vested interest in maintaining their husbands' incompetence."[67] Some practitioners suggested that a husband's alcohol abuse was triggered by his wife's neuroses, manifested in dominating their emasculated husbands. Others saw the domination as resulting from the stress of their husband's addiction. Nevertheless, both of these perspectives suggested that alcoholism was a "family illness" and that "the whole family would need to convalesce."[67] Thus, by the 1950s, psychiatrists and social workers advocated group therapy for alcoholics' wives. "Given the nation's deep psychological investment in marriage," Rotskoff concludes, "it is apt that alcoholism's deleterious effects would increasingly be measured in marital terms. In large part, the cultural construct of the 'recovering' alcoholic marriage—comprised of sober husbands and supportive wives—gained public acceptance because it reflected and reshaped familial values in American society at large."[67]

What these historians have shown is that the theories that informed these arguments, interventions, and policies—degeneration, psychoanalysis, and eugenics—reflected dominant social values in the guise of science. One might argue that current scientific claims about alcoholism as a disease rely on a completely different science, informed by neurobiology, biochemistry, and genetics.[9,59] However, having shown the culture-bound nature of earlier scientific theories supporting the idea that drunkenness is a disease, historians are skeptical of current scientific assertions that alcoholism is a disease.

Opiates and Other Illicit Drugs

The same science and psychiatry that have consistently viewed host predisposition as the trigger for alcohol addiction have, just as consistently, viewed opiates as posing an addictive risk for all who use them. According to Edwards, this is because alcohol intoxication "is remarkably susceptible to cultural prescriptions and proscriptions" and alcohol is "a widely accepted recreational drug," whereas, "in contrast, intoxication with crack cocaine, or injected amphetamines, or with a heavy dose of lysergic acid diethylamide (known more commonly as LSD), is not so easily shaped, and these are not drugs which society is ever likely to accord a licit recreational status."[25]

Alcohol prohibition was attempted, and, despite some revisionist arguments that it reduced drunkenness and alcohol addiction substantially,[11] Prohibition was a social and political failure.[46] The contrast between the rejection of alcohol prohibition and the expansion of opiate prohibition is underscored by the triumph of the belief that alcohol use had a wide range of possible individual effects, from benign to deadly. Where these effects fell on the spectrum was a consequence of host differences and excessive drinking. The refusal to accept a similar range of possibilities for opiates and other mind-altering substances, including marijuana, stimulants, and amphetamines, framed both the official response and individual behavior of users.[55] Nevertheless, there remains a deeply held belief that there is such a thing as an addictive personality that leads one to drugs. This concept, as we will see, has deep historical roots, often attached to an array of negative character traits. In contrast to the alcoholic, predisposition toward narcotic use became evidence that drug addicts were sociopaths. As a result, prohibition of drugs and punishment for dependence were framed by a combination of claims about the nature of the substances and that of the addicts.

In *Creating the American Junkie* (2002) and her subsequent publications, Caroline Acker traces this history of opiate prohibition through an examination of the experience of users as they negotiated a world in which opiate use increasingly became criminalized.[1] Acker's work reinforces David Courtwright's study, *Dark Paradise* (2001), which, using similar narratives, demonstrates that "what we think about addiction very much depends on who is addicted."[16] In the early 20th century, addicts could seek medical treatment that included prescriptions of maintenance doses. Beginning with the Harrison Narcotics Act in 1914, however, nonmedical use or purchase of cocaine and opiates was restricted and all narcotics sold or prescribed were required to be registered. As a result, physicians were no longer able to treat addicts through maintenance, and ceased treating them altogether. This shift, writes Acker, transformed the context of opiate use and "as the context for the use of opiates changed, so did the meanings for those who used them."[1] Thus, "addicts developed their own strategies for maintaining their addiction," which resulted in "a new form of addict identity as the behaviors to maintain addiction were criminalized."[1]

Courtwright has a slightly different take. With the decline of medical (iatrogenic) addiction in the late 19th century, "opiate addiction … began to assume a new form: it ceased to be concentrated in upper-class and middle-class white females and began to appear more frequently in lower-class urban males, often neophyte members of the underworld. By 1914 the trend was unmistakable." For Courtwright, "the trend toward criminalization … was well underway before the basic narcotic statutes were enacted."[16]

Part of that identity, according to historian Timothy Hickman, was the emergence of "a double meaning of addiction," in which some of the addiction was attributed to disease and some to hedonism and antisocial behavior.[34] "The addiction concept of habitual narcotic use was embedded in the early 20th century paradigm of professionalizing medical authority"[34] because it placed juridical addicts under medical authority and criminal addicts under criminal jurisdiction. Antinarcotic legislation, argues Hickman, reflected this dichotomy, and, by the early 1920s, "volitional addicts came to be defined as *criminals*" while "juridical addicts … were defined as innocent *patients*" because of their willingness to seek medical treatment.[34] Hickman does not distinguish between alcohol and narcotic use, but his evidence and the wider historical record indicate that the division between those who were considered diseased and those who were classified as criminal mirrored the division between alcoholics and drug addicts.

Although Hickman does not make the connection, his essay provides a context for the emergence of the psychoanalytic construct of the "addicted personality," which first appeared in Lawrence Kolb's 1925 article, "Types and Characteristics of Drug Addicts,"[38] and in his subsequent works.[39] Despite Kolb's insistence that addiction was a medical issue, federal officials adopted Kolb's construct as evidence of the general character defects of addicts and as justification to extend the criminalization of drug use.[16,78]

Speaker explains such results as almost inevitable given the rhetoric that informed drug addiction from the 1920s to the 1940s.[72] Acknowledging that "drug abuse is a significant and difficult public health problem," Speaker, nevertheless, points to accumulated evidence that suggests "that at least some persons can use drugs moderately without becoming abusers, that even heavy abuse may not be a lifelong pattern, and that many 'outbreaks' of drug abuse are self-limiting and fairly short-lived."[72] Illicit drugs and nicotine were demonized with similar, if not the same, adjectives and hyperbole that once framed alcohol prohibition campaigns: "The drugs in question are powerful, seductive, and rapidly addictive; that everyone is at risk for addiction; that drugs *by themselves* are sufficient to cause any imaginable deviant behavior and are directly responsible for most crime and violence."[72] Although, as Speaker asserts, with the end of Prohibition alcohol consumption was destigmatized, the use of other psychoactive drugs has not been. Indeed, made illicit, their use is not only illegal, but also considered immoral.[72]

As medical treatment for alcohol addiction became the norm in the mid-20th century, maintenance clinics for the treatment of narcotics addiction became illegal. From 1923 to the opening of the first methadone treatment center in 1965 in New York City, writes Jim Baumohl, "addicts were demonized, hounded, subjected to draconian criminal penalties, and never treated except in the confines of a hospital or jail." Aside from a very few wealthy private clients, "abstinence was the only legitimate goal of treatment."[5] By the 1930s, even the supporters of maintenance programs "believed most addicts to be incurable."[5]

It was in this context that in 1935 the U.S. Public Health Service established the Center for Drug Addiction at the federal prison hospital in Lexington, Kentucky.[12] Informally labeled as "Narco," the facility, which continued its addiction research until 1979, was designed to be a treatment hospital for incarcerated addicts. In 1948, the research unit became the first basic research laboratory of the newly formed National Institute of Mental Health, the Addiction Research Center. Inmates became voluntary participants in Addiction Research Center experiments that tested reactions to a wide variety of substances including alcohol, barbiturates, heroin, methadone, major and minor tranquilizers, and psychedelics. Campbell's *Discovering Addiction* examines the Center for Drug Addiction and Addiction Research Center in detail. She found that inmates often were readdicted and some of the information obtained "was used by pharmaceutical companies seeking to bring drugs to market."[12] Nevertheless, Campbell concludes that "the research program yielded broadly distributed benefits to persons from the addicted class."[12]

The Center for Drug Addiction's benign approach to addicts was an exception, but the venue for its research, a federal prison, reflected the policies of Henry Anslinger, the influential director of the Federal Bureau of Narcotics (1930–1962). With bipartisan support, Anslinger advocated incarceration as the only deterrent. It did not matter to Anslinger, writes Baumohl, whether addicts were confined to a jail or a hospital, but "the more like a jail, the better he liked the hospital."[5]

Anslinger's role in shaping and extending the criminalization of drug use policy, writes Rebecca Carroll, cannot be overestimated.[13,14] Anslinger "influenced Americans' attitudes toward narcotic drugs and drug users and sellers, depicting both users and sellers as criminals." This is evident in Anslinger's 1937 Congressional testimony in which he claimed that marijuana "is dangerous to the mind and body, and particularly dangerous to the criminal type, because it releases all of the inhibitions." It causes some individuals to "have an increased feeling of physical strength and power," which is dangerous because they "fly into a delirious rage, and they are temporarily irresponsible and may commit violent crimes."[4]

Although a number of influential experts, including leaders of the American Medical Association and the American Bar Association, argued for the medicalization and clinical treatment of addicts, Anslinger stifled their voices.[75] In 1944, at the urging of New York City Mayor Fiorella La Guardia, the New York Academy of Medicine conducted a study on the effects of marijuana, the findings of which contradicted Anslinger's claims. The commission found that cannabis did not cause violence and, despite Anslinger's insistence otherwise, concluded that marijuana could be medically beneficial. Anslinger denounced the report and instructed the Bureau of Narcotics agents to investigate the commission members' own drug use. Furthermore, he threatened prison sentences for anyone carrying out independent research on cannabis.

In the postwar era, Anslinger altered his views of marijuana's effect on its users but not his policy toward its use. Testifying in Congress in 1948, Anslinger claimed that cannabis caused the user to become peaceful and pacifistic; thus, the Communists were recruiting Americans into cannabis use as part of a plot to weaken their will to fight.[75]

Like Anslinger, those who continue criminalizing marijuana use in the United States today claim to base their views on scientific research, but, also like Anslinger, their antipathy toward marijuana use reflects deeper cultural values rather than robust science. A similar claim can probably be made about those who support unrestricted availability of marijuana. The point here, as much of recent addiction history reveals, is that the classification of substances as licit or illicit has less to do with science than with politics.

This political influence can be seen in attempts to control demand. Historian William B. McAllister's examination of international drug control shows that increasing regulation and criminalization of drugs has ended up pretty much as it began, with incarceration of drug users and a failure to stem the activities of suppliers.[51] What has changed, according to McAllister, is the "nature and scope" of antidrug efforts. "Governments and international agencies constructed massive bureaucracies, engaged in considerable legislative activity, and attempted to implement policies intended to change the behaviors of millions of individuals, with varying degrees of success."[51] Although McAllister finds that "since the late nineteenth century, the American drug experience has largely mirrored that of other Western industrialized nations," he notes that the United States "has acted as the center of demand" for all types of drugs and has been the greatest force of "regulatory activism." As a result, McAllister concludes, "policy-makers, legislators, and citizens of the United States, much like addicts, cannot escape their relationship to the global drug scene."[51] If, as a number of historians have indicated, the century-long activism failed to stem the drug addiction that it was aimed at curing,[73] the rhetoric surrounding drug use, combined with the increasing classification of substances as addictive, has exacerbated the problem.

In a recent book, Richard Davenport-Hines argues that the criminalization and prohibition of drugs have resulted in an epidemic of use and an exacerbation of fatal encounters. The almost paranoid response of puritanical American policymakers has, according to Davenport-Hines, led to a black market and growth in all types of criminal activity.[20] David Courtwright finds this argument unpersuasive: "What is unique about [Davenport-Hines']

The Pursuit of Oblivion is that it combines the simplification inherent to world history with the simplification peculiar to polemical exertion. The result is a book that, for all its length and erudition, is almost startlingly reductive: the story of a bad idea imposed upon a doubtful world by aggressive fools."[18]

Licit Mind-Altering Drugs

Neuroscientists typically attribute the heightened antidrug rhetoric to a more sophisticated understanding of how these substances work on the human brain, a view shared by historian turned bioethicist Steven Novak.[57] He finds that when it came to lysergic acid diethylamide (i.e., LSD), despite the desires and pressures from researchers, their pharmaceutical sponsors, and influential lay persons, clinical and neurobiological research determined its ultimate classification. LSD became suspect because research data revealed suicide risks, prolonged psychotic sequelae, and antisocial behaviors. Meanwhile, LSD was being used illegally for recreational purposes with many of the same dangerous effects. Although for some—Timothy Leary and his followers—it was LSD's mind-altering, liberating effect that spelled its doom, Novak's history suggests otherwise. The ongoing thalidomide revelations and resultant increased Congressional oversight led to legislation requiring prior U.S. Food and Drug Administration approval for all investigational drug trials, as well as a finding that a substance was safe and efficacious before it could be marketed. LSD met neither test and was eliminated from medical investigation, albeit with some resistance.[57] The importance of this history is that it was the biochemical action of LSD that determined its marginalization and eventual criminalization.[79]

In contrast to LSD is the history of antidepressants—often addictive, mind-altering, but licit, drugs. With the introduction of a new class of antidepressants in the late 1980s called selective serotonin reuptake inhibitors (SSRIs; fluoxetine hydrochloride [Prozac], paroxetine hydrochloride [Paxil], and sertraline hydrochloride [Zoloft]), antidepressant use has grown exponentially. Spurred on by massive advertising efforts in the late 1990s and Peter Kramer's best-selling book, *Listening to Prozac*,[40] SSRIs, according to psychiatrist Nicholas Weiss, have become "consumer products appropriate for wide usage or general lifestyle enhancement." Predecessors of SSRIs—monoamine oxidase inhibitors and tricyclic antidepressants—were viewed as "disease therapies to be kept strictly in the medical domain."[83] Why, asks Weiss, had "no one listened to [the tricyclic antidepressant] imipramine?"[83] His answer, like so much else connected to addiction, lies in the history of alcoholism.

The definition of "alcoholism" as a distinct disease affecting only a minority of drinkers, writes Weiss, has removed the blame for alcohol-related social problems from the substance to a subgroup of susceptible individuals. Thus, alcohol use, although not abuse (drunkenness), is socially acceptable. "This enabled the alcohol beverage industry to sell its product, despite widespread concerns about the dangers and evils of alcohol, as long as drinking was officially proscribed for that susceptible population."[83] The diagnosis of depression, according to Weiss, "functioned in an analogous, though inverse manner." A diagnosis of depression identified a susceptible group "who *should* become users, those with a current or potential medical depression"[83] (italics added). Therefore, dependence on SSRIs is authorized, even though they are mind-altering (and often addictive) substances, because depression has been constructed as a disease. The risks of SSRI use are downplayed because the condition that they treat is defined as illness, despite a spate of warnings about the hazards associated with SSRIs.[10,30,33]

Similarly, although Weiss does not make this connection, a diagnosis of attention-deficit/hyperactivity disorder authorizes placing individuals (mainly children) on addictive stimulant medications such as methylphenidate (Ritalin).[22] According to historian Nicholas Rasmussen, the current amphetamine epidemic should be viewed in the context of the medical use of stimulants to treat depressive disorders and how this resulted in a wider epidemic of stimulant use by the mid-20th century. Building on this history, Rasmussen connects the present methamphetamine epidemic to the earlier iatrogenic epidemic.[62,63] This history appears to be repeating itself as Ritalin and other stimulants prescribed for the treatment of attention-deficit/hyperactivity disorder become widely used as recreational drugs on American college campuses and beyond.

Recognizing how prescription medication use once again has morphed into recreational and self-medicating substance use and abuse has important implications for those who wish to understand and treat the current wave of addiction and substance abuse. For Rasmussen, these evolutions have resulted as much from changing populations who use stimulants as from the biological actions of these drugs. A similar argument has recently been made by psychologist Richard DeGrandpre in *The Cult of Pharmacology* (2006).[23]

In fact, for most illicit addictive substances, there is a companion licit substance, such as methylphenidate, the action of which mirrors that of the proscribed drug. As DeGrandpre points out, although Ritalin and cocaine act similarly on the brain, the former is widely prescribed for children while the use of cocaine is a felony. Similarly, the street drug ecstasy acts on the same serotonin receptors as SSRIs. Although far from controversial, the risk of addiction to mind-altering pharmaceuticals has been justified because of the putative benefit conferred by their consumption. This returns us to the tensions that exist regarding alcohol and nicotine use. Each has been sanctioned because of their alleged benefits and vilified because of their harms.

Smoking and Nicotine

As Alan Brandt points out, although the addictive potential of nicotine in tobacco was often noted long before the 1988 Surgeon General's report on nicotine and addiction,[82] attitudes toward cigarette smoking have a complex history. The prohibition of alcohol in 1919, writes Brandt, "had the effect of further legitimating the use of cigarettes. Cigarettes now assumed many of the positive cultural and social attributes previously associated with drinking—leisure, pleasure, and sociability—without the risks of intoxication with its consequent social and familial pathologies."[7] For the next several decades, moderate smoking was portrayed in the media, including in medical journals, as risk free and possibly beneficial to overall health. Smoking, Brandt argues, was contrasted with drug addiction and characterized as "a habit that could be broken without much trouble."[7] In fact, "often cigarettes were seen as a vehicle for assisting in breaking addictions to more dangerous substances like alcohol or opiates."[7] As late as 1964, the Surgeon General's advisory committee on the health consequences of smoking concluded that "the evidence indicates this dependence to be psychogenic in origin" and "the biological effects of tobacco, like coffee ... are not comparable to those produced by morphine, alcohol, barbiturates, and many other potent addicting drugs."[80] As a result of the dramatic decline of smoking

because of its associated health risks, its recategorization as addictive in the 1980s was, according to Brandt, "far less problematic than would have been the case a decade earlier." This was particularly so because smoking increasingly had become "associated with certain social groups—generally those less educated and of lower socioeconomic status," and, notes Brandt, "in a culture prone to stigmatize its poor and disfavored, changing perceptions about the 'average smoker' eased the growing attribution of addiction."[7]

In his recent book, *The Cigarette Century*, Brandt focuses more on the dangers associated with smoking, and, consonant with his role as an expert witness for the Justice Department in its prosecution of the tobacco industry, he focuses on the health risks associated with smoking.[8] Although Brandt remains sympathetic to those who continue to smoke, others have been less scrupulous in translating the justified demonization of the tobacco industry to smokers themselves.

In sequential media conferences hosted by the American Cancer Society in 1985 and the National Cancer Institute in 1988, strategies were adopted that were aimed at portraying the tobacco industry as illegitimate, deceptive, and criminal. The American Cancer Society's *Media Handbook, Smoke Signals*, suggested delegitimizing the industry by referring to them as "drug pushers," "profiteers from human misery," environmental polluters, and "death and disease merchants."[3] At the American Cancer Society meeting and its follow-up 1988 Media Advocacy Consensus Conference in Washington, DC, attendees were urged to shame the industry's allies and dependent community arts organizations into severing their ties with the tobacco industry.[3,81] Although both conferences warned "to be careful about blaming the victim,"[81] inevitably these attitudes spilled over to the smokers as well. The American Cancer Society's *Media Handbook* suggested that one response to claims of smokers' rights was: "your right to smoke stops where my nose begins and my lungs are exposed." Smokers were to be confronted with the dangers that they posed to children who are "more prone to bronchitis, pneumonia, and other respiratory problems." Children, smokers were to be reminded, deserved "fresh, clean, smoke-free air."[3] In the last two decades, the rhetoric has ratcheted up as accusations claiming deception and criminal activity by the tobacco industry have become the subject of seemingly endless lawsuits. Those who continue to smoke often find themselves collateral victims, increasingly ostracized and demonized. "There are," writes Brandt, "powerful currents in our culture that define smokers as weak-willed and ignorant, who abuse their own health and others,' while polluting the common environment."[7]

Despite these powerful forces and the health risks associated with smoking, many persist in the habit. Part of the reason for this persistence, according to Keane, is evident if one contrasts the immediate rewards of smoking with its long-term consequences.[37] For instance, Keane cites studies that suggest that smoking enables working-class women to cope with boring working conditions. However, as she points out, from a rhetorical perspective, smoking "is reduced to its potentially most undesirable outcomes, namely, various premature, painful, and protracted forms of death," whereas any potential benefits are dismissed as "illusory and excluded from the calculation of risk."[37] Given that those who smoke are, as Brandt points out, already socially marginalized, the benefits of smoking, like those who smoke, have become increasingly unattractive.

Speaker[72] argues that the prohibition of a substance is almost always preceded by a demonization of its producers and users. If this observation is correct, we may be well along the road to prohibiting smoking in North America.

Rhetoric and Reality

In combination, these new histories make a persuasive case for the cultural construct of drug classification and addiction. They illuminate the role of rhetoric in influencing legal statutes, court decisions, and the criminal justice system. The ambiguous attitude toward smoking and nicotine addiction provides an ongoing case study of how cultural values and legal structures evolve and interact, determining where on the spectrum of legitimacy a mind-altering substance and its users are located.

Despite the growth of restrictions, heightened rhetoric, and ratcheting up of penalties for many mind-altering drugs, the use of those drugs is either persistent or increasing. However, Courtwright warns against conflating drug policy with drug use. "When doing drug *policy* history, it pays to zoom in on details: What was the mix of regulations, taxes, and penalties governing access to this drug in this society at this time? When doing drug *use* history, it pays to zoom out, looking for broader connections among drugs and across cultures." Thus, writes Courtwright, "Opium smoking would not have taken root in China had it not been for the introduction and spread of tobacco, with which opium was first smoked. Marijuana smoking would not have taken such hold among Western youth had it not been for the antecedent cigarette revolution. Fewer alcoholics would have meant fewer narcotic addicts, the relief of hangover often inspiring the use of opiates. 'Licit' and 'illicit' categories obscure the indivisibility of drug history."[18]

If substances such as caffeine, chocolate, and carbohydrates are included, not to mention addictive behaviors including gambling, sex, and shopping, we either inhabit the most addictive society that ever existed or have failed to notice retrospectively how addictive human behaviors are. Alternatively, as the logic of the histories that are reviewed here suggests, a wide range of human consumption and behaviors have been (re)constructed as addictions.

Speaker asks to what extent the "characteristic rhetoric" toward addictive substances is a "reflection of genuine drug problems … and to what extent it is an expression of various social tensions—class struggles, demographic changes, racial and ethnic conflicts, etc.—or an expression of particular values and ideologies?" She also wonders "what accounts for the persistent use of these themes and images," and "to what extent … this popular rhetoric not only reflected but shaped public perceptions and drug policy itself during this century."[72] To these questions we may add what the histories of addiction reveal about the biological effects on the human brain and what these biological mechanisms reveal about the histories of addiction.

The skepticism of many addiction historians toward current scientific claims is rooted in the evidence that each successive psychiatric addiction paradigm has revealed more about the culture that enabled it than about the robustness of scientific findings. For many historians, portraying biology and the past sciences of addictions as culturally constructed appears to authorize ignoring current science altogether. However, the fact that science, like everything else, is socially constructed in no way diminishes its explanatory power any more than it limits the value of historical interpretations, such as those examined in this chapter, which—like all historical research and writing—are socially constructed and contingent.[42] In any case, an increasing number of historians of addiction have begun to engage rather than ignore current addiction science. Those historians have much to say that addiction scientists should consider.

Taking History Seriously

What does addiction history reveal about addictive behaviors? Can all this evidence be interpreted as culturally framed? According to Edwards, the answer is both yes and no. He suggests that histories of alcohol use lead to a deeper engagement with the putative organic mechanisms that have been attached to alcoholism. Such an approach opens up an alternative interpretation that brings together seemingly contradictory social constructionist and biologically reductionist claims. Alcoholism, according to Edwards, is "best approached through a framework of the dependence-syndrome concept," where "the dependent state is not a matter of all or nothing (addict or not addict), but something which can be experienced in varied and measurable degrees (more or less dependent)."[25] Edwards' insistence on the distinction between syndrome and disease is not trivial. Measles, polio, and Huntington are diseases because a tentative diagnosis based on signs and symptoms is confirmed or rejected through a laboratory test indicating infection by a pathogen or the presence of a genetic mutation. In contrast, the cause of a syndrome, such as schizophrenia, Tourette syndrome, or affective disorders (depressions), remains unknown.[45,74] The diagnosis of syndromes depends on the identification of a list of possible combinations of signs and symptoms displayed by an individual within a certain time period. This list of signs and symptoms is tentative, and disagreement often surfaces over which signs and symptoms are crucial to authorize a diagnosis.[31,43] As a result, identification of a syndrome often varies over time and by geographic location.[86]

As with pneumonia, a variety of routes can lead to alcohol dependence. Unlike pneumonia, but like most psychiatric syndromes, these include both cultural and/or biological factors in the enabling spectrum. Those who meet the criteria (in terms of signs and symptoms) for alcohol dependence experience real illness, even if the etiology and level of distress and particular path to dependence are not the same for every alcohol-dependent person. Recognition of the many routes to an alcohol dependence syndrome sanctions researchers and clinicians to craft a variety of interventions and policies that consider a spectrum of cultural and biological triggers. Such recognition must include, no matter what the trigger, the biological and social effects on the individual. This requires engagement with the accumulating evidence from recent research that substance dependence, including alcohol dependence, alters brain reward mechanisms, such as brain architecture and neurochemistry, sometimes permanently.[9,85] This seems true even when the addiction, such as gambling, is not attached to a substance. The question remains whether labeling nonsubstance behaviors as addictions is justified because they impact and alter the same brain reward systems (i.e., the ventral tegmental area) as do cocaine and heroin.[6,56,85] Because most behaviors have an impact on brain chemistry, how do we decide which of these are addictions and which are not? Many of the histories of addiction discussed in this chapter agree that what is considered and not considered an addiction reflects social and cultural values as much as it tells us a truth about the mechanisms of the brain.

Saying that does not, however, excuse trivializing the importance of biology to addiction. As Edwards writes in his discussion of the history of the failed controlled drinking experiments, the "belief that the troubled drinker can recover only through abstinence" was based on "accumulated personal testimony and front-line clinical experience." Dismissing these observations and experiences "as no more than repressive moralism" is "mistaken and ungenerous."[25] Effective treatment requires acceptance by uncontrolled drinkers and those around them that the alcoholism involves organic mechanisms. Such an admission in no way diminishes the reality that alcohol dependence includes both cultural causes and social consequences. Any understanding of the history of alcoholism requires such an integrative approach. The same claims may be made for all addictions—they are syndromes of dependence, informed and "enabled" by an interaction of culture and biology.

As with alcohol, nicotine acts differently on different hosts. It may be extremely addictive, but 50% of smokers have managed to cease smoking since the late 1960s. All smokers probably fit into some definition of addiction, but if we were to apply Edwards' notion of syndrome of dependence, we might develop better insights into who smokes, why some persist despite overwhelming evidence of negative health consequences, and why others are able to stop smoking.

As Tracy and Acker write, earlier scientific explanations for the mechanisms of addiction seem retrospectively quaint,[78] but there have been persistent observations of addictive predispositions, or what psychoanalysts used to label "addictive personalities." If previous theories of the mechanisms of addiction appear retrospectively tenuous, the existence of addictive personality types seems less so.

This returns us to Edwards' view that what we call addictions are actually syndromes of dependence that have multiple triggers and pathways, ranging from the cultural to organic, but are probably informed by a combination that we might label as "cultural biology." This cultural biology of substance dependence is based on centuries of observations. The science of each era has attempted to identify the mechanisms that underlay the observed behaviors. The fact that, in retrospect, these attempts reflect the dominant scientific paradigm of each era is not surprising; nor does it undercut the evidence that there are organic triggers for and biological effects from substance dependence. That these interact with cultural and social forces would not surprise any serious neuroscientist. Like Edwards, they would concede that current neurobiological hypotheses are by definition tentative, precisely because for a scientific claim to be robust, it must be testable (falsifiable) and replicable.

This interdisciplinary perspective allows us to consider the multiple meanings of the Tracy and Acker title, *Altering American Consciousness*. As Courtwright has shown in *Forces of Habit*, humans have attempted to alter their consciousness since time immemorial.[17] Evolutionary biologist Tammy Saah finds that "drug use and addiction seem to have been a part of mammalian society since ancient times." For Saah, "looking at drug addiction from an evolutionary perspective" is the best way to "understand its underlying significance and evaluate its three-fold nature: biology, psychology, and social influences."[68] Any persuasive interpretation of the history of addiction, insists Courtwright, must consider the impact of the biological action of drugs on human hosts. However, if it ignores history and culture, the impact of that biology will be missed.[17]

Western economies and culture, writes Courtwright, are built on the production, sale, and use of mind-altering drugs, including alcohol, tobacco, coffee, cocoa, tea, sugar, carbohydrates, and an array of prescription medications. This could not have happened without biological as well as cultural mechanisms. In *Dark Paradise*, Courtwright shows how addiction is exacerbated and enabled by the availability of and exposure to mind-altering substances.[16] Considering the neurobiological mechanisms of addiction, says Courtwright, can offer powerful clues for comprehending this drive to alter consciousness.

As Edwards reminds us, for much of human history, including our own era, most mind-altering substances have been consumed initially as a means of self-medication for a variety of ills, not least of all for disorders of consciousness, including major and minor psychiatric disorders.[25] That self-medication plays an important role in persistent substance use and abuse, despite awareness of potential harm, provides fertile ground for further historical research.[2,26,54] Self-medication, like the conditions it aims to treat, is rooted in culture and biology and cannot be understood apart from that interaction. Like all culturally mediated biological phenomena, each society responds to these human behaviors within the context and confines of larger social, political, and cultural constraints. From this perspective, addiction is one possible outcome of humans' drive to alter consciousness; what we label "addiction" might be understood as a *possible* consequence of the human desire to alter consciousness.

Taking history seriously would force addiction scientists to confront the reasons for failure of the abstinence policy. First and foremost, abstinence is a failed policy because it denies the historical evidence that humans in all societies and cultures have relied and continue to rely on substances to alter their consciousness. Addictive behaviors, rather than diminishing, have increased, spurred on in part by industries that manufacture and market consciousness-altering commodities. In the face of persistent human drives to alter consciousness and markets that cater to them, abstinence appears unattainable. Moreover, the pursuit of abstinence has led to a number of counterproductive policies. Among them is the assumption, writes Campbell, that restricting knowledge about the safe use of illicit drugs or about ways to reduce the harms associated with their use "is good because condoning drug use is bad." Yet, by denying illegal drug users information that could reduce risks, we ensure even worse outcomes. The histories of addiction indicate that abstinence is also a failed policy because, as both historians and brain researchers recognize, addiction is a chronic relapsing/remitting syndrome. From that perspective as well, any successful policy or intervention must include harm reduction. Historians of addiction, Campbell insists, "have a crucial role to play in shifting drug policy toward public health and harm reduction."[12] The history discussed in these pages supports that claim.

Acknowledgments

The research and writing of this article were partially supported by a grant from the National Institutes of Health, National Institute on Drug Abuse, entitled "Current Smokers: A Phenomenological Inquiry" (R01 DA015707–01A2) and a grant from the Engelhard Foundation, "Sophomore Year at Emory Living and Learning Experience: An Interdisciplinary Seminar Course/Internship in Addiction and Depression." Some of the material in this chapter appeared previously in Howard I. Kushner, "Taking Biology Seriously: The Next Task for Historians of Addiction?" *Bulletin of the History of Medicine* 80 (Spring 2006): 115–143. I thank Carol R. Kushner and Robert Cormier for editorial assistance.

References

1. Acker CJ. *Creating the American Junkie: Addiction Research in the Classic Era of Narcotic Control*. Baltimore, MD: Johns Hopkins University Press; 2002.
2. Allen TJ, Moeller FG, Rhoades HM, Cherek DR. Impulsivity and history of drug dependence. *Drug Alcohol Depend*. 1998;50: 137–145.

3. American Cancer Society. *Smoke Signals: The Smoking Control Media Handbook (Publication Developed on the Recommendation of the September 1985 International Summit of Smoking Control Leaders).* New York: American Cancer Society; 1987.

4. Anslinger H. Marijuana and violence. *Congressional Testimony.* Washington, DC: US Government Printing Office; 1937.

5. Baumohl J. Maintaining orthodoxy: the Depression Era struggles over morphine maintenance in California. In: Tracy SW, Acker CJ, eds. *Altering American Consciousness: the History of Alcohol and Drug Use in the United States.* Amherst, MA: University of Massachusetts Press; 2004:1800–2000.

6. Blaszczynski A, Nower L. A pathways model of problem and pathological gambling. *Addiction.* 2002;97:487–499.

7. Brandt A. From nicotine to Nicotrol: addiction, cigarettes, and American culture. In: Tracy SW, Acker CJ, eds. *Altering American Consciousness: the History of Alcohol and Drug Use in the United States.* Amherst, MA: University of Massachusetts Press; 2004:1800–2000.

8. Brandt AM. *The Cigarette Century: the Rise, Fall, and Deadly Persistence of the Product that Defined America.* New York: Basic Books; 2007.

9. Braun S. *Buzz: the Science and Lore of Alcohol and Caffeine.* New York: Oxford University; 1996.

10. Breggin P, Breggin GR. *Talking Back to Prozac: What Doctors Aren't Telling You About Today's Most Controversial Drug.* New York: St. Martin's; 1994.

11. Burnham JC. New perspectives on the prohibition 'experiment' of the 1920s. *J Soc Hist.* 1968;2:51–68.

12. Campbell ND. *Discovering Addiction: The Science and Politics of Substance Abuse Research.* Ann Arbor, MI: University of Michigan; 2007.

13. Carroll R. The Narcotic Control Act triggers the great nondebate: treatment loses to punishment. In: Erlen J, Spillane JF, eds. *Federal Drug Control: the Evolution of Policy and Practice.* Binghamton, NY: Pharmaceutical Products; 2004.

14. Carroll R. Under the influence: Harry Anslinger's role in shaping America's drug policy. In: Erlen J, Spillane JF, eds. *Federal Drug Control: the Evolution of Policy and Practice.* Binghamton, NY: Pharmaceutical Products; 2004.

15. Chavigny KA. Reforming drunkards in nineteenth-century America. In: Tracy SW, Acker CJ, eds. *Altering American Consciousness: The History of Alcohol and Drug Use in the United States.* Amherst, MA: University of Massachusetts Press; 2004:1800–2000.

16. Courtwright DT. *Dark Paradise: A History of Opiate Addiction in America.* Cambridge, MA: Harvard University; 2001.

17. Courtwright DT. *Forces of Habit: Drugs and The Making of the Modern World.* Cambridge, MA: Harvard University; 2001.

18. Courtwright DT. Drug wars: policy hots and historical cools. *Bull Hist Med.* 2004;78:440–450.

19. Dalgarno P, Shewan D. Reducing the risks of drug use: the case for set and setting. *Addict Res Theory.* 2005;13:259–265.

20. Davenport-Hines RPT. *The Pursuit of Oblivion: a Global History of Narcotics.* New York: Norton; 2002.

21. Davies DL. Normal drinking in recovered alcoholics. *Q J Alcohol Stud.* 1962;23:94–104.

22. DeGrandpre R. *Ritalin Nation: Rapid-Fire Culture and the Transformation of Human Consciousness.* New York: W.W. Norton; 1999.

23. DeGrandpre RJ. *The Cult of Pharmacology: How America Became the World's Most Troubled Drug Culture.* Durham, NC: Duke University; 2006.

24. Dowbiggin IR. *Inheriting Madness: Professionalization and Psychiatric Knowledge in Nineteenth-Century France.* Berkeley, CA: University of California; 1991.

25. Edwards G. *Alcohol: The World's Favorite Drug.* New York: St. Martin's; 2002.

26. Felitti VJ. Ursprünge des Suchtverhaltens—Evidenzen aus einer Studie zu belastenden Kindheitserfahrungen [The origins of addiction: evidence from the Adverse Childhood Experiences Study]. *Prax Kinderpsychol Kinderpsychiatr.* 2003;52:547–559.

27. Fillmore KM, Roizen R. The new manichaeism in alcohol science. *Addiction.* 2000;95:188–190.

28. Fingarette H. *Heavy Drinking: The Myth of Alcoholism as a Disease.* Berkeley, CA: University of California; 1988.

29. Frank JW, Moore RS, Ames GM. Historical and cultural roots of drinking problems among American Indians. *Am J Public Health.* 2000;90:344–351.

30. Glenmullen J. *Prozac Backlash: Overcoming the Dangers of Prozac, Zoloft, Paxil, and Other Antidepressants with Safe, Effective Alternatives.* New York: Diane; 2000.

31. Hacking I. *Rewriting the Soul: Multiple Personality and the Sciences of Memory.* Princeton, NJ: University Press; 1995.

32. Harrington A. *Medicine, Mind, and the Double Brain: a Study in Nineteenth-Century Thought.* Princeton, NJ: University Press; 1987.

33. Healy D. *The Antidepressant Era.* Cambridge, MA: Harvard University; 1997.

34. Hickman T. The double meaning of addiction: habitual narcotic use and the logic of professionalizing medical authority in the United States, 1900–1920. In: Tracy SW, Acker CJ, eds. *Altering American Consciousness: The History of Alcohol and Drug use in the United States, 1800–2000.* Amherst, MA: University of Massachusetts Press; 2004.

35. Hobson RP. *Alcohol and the Human Race.* Fleming H. New York: Revell Company; 1919.

36. Jellinek EM. *The Disease Concept of Alcoholism.* New Haven, CT: Hillhouse; 1960.

37. Keane H. *What's Wrong with Addiction?* New York: University Press; 2002.

38. Kolb L. Types and characteristics of drug addicts. *Ment Hyg.* 1925;9:300–313.

39. Kolb L. *Drug Addiction: A Medical Problem.* Springfield, IL: Thomas; 1962.

40. Kramer PD. *Listening to PROZAC.* New York: Viking; 1993.

41. Kunitz SJ, Levy JE. *Drinking Careers: Twenty-Five-Year Follow-Up of Three Navajo Populations.* New Haven, CT: Yale University; 1994.

42. Kushner HI. Beyond social construction: toward new histories of psychiatry (review essay). *J Hist Neurosci.* 1998;7:141–149.

43. Kushner HI. *A Cursing Brain? The Histories of Tourette Syndrome.* Cambridge, MA: Harvard University; 1999.

44. Kushner HI. Taking biology seriously: the next task for historians of addiction? *Bull Hist Med.* 2006;80:115–143.

45. Kushner HI, Turner CL, Bastian JF, Burns JC. The narratives of Kawasaki disease. *Bull Hist Med.* 2004;78:410–439.

46. Kyvig DE. *Repealing National Prohibition.* Chicago, IL: University of Chicago; 1979.

47. Lender ME, Martin JK. *Drinking in America: a History.* Revised and expanded ed. New York: Free, Macmillan; 1987.

48. Leshner A. *The science of Nicotine Addiction and Why We Should Care.* Paper presented at the 11th World Conference on Tobacco or Health: Chicago, IL;2000.

49. MacAndrew C, Edgerton RB. *Drunken Comportment: A Social Explanation.* Chicago, IL: Aldine; 1969.

50. Mancall P. 'I was addicted to drinking rum': four centuries of alcohol consumption in Indian country. In: Tracy SW, Acker CJ, eds. *Altering American Consciousness: The History of Alcohol and Drug Use in the United States.* Amherst, MA: University of Massachusetts Press; 2004:1800–2000.

51. McAllister WB. Habitual problems: the United States and international drug control. In: Erlen J, Spillane JF, eds. *Federal Drug Control: The Evolution of Policy and Practice.* Binghamton, NY: Pharmaceutical Products; 2004.

52. McClellan M. Lady tipplers: gendering the modern alcoholism paradigm. In: Tracy SW, Acker CJ, eds. *Altering American Consciousness: The History of Alcohol and Drug Use in the United States.* Amherst, MA: University of Massachusetts Press; 2004:1800–2000.

53. Micale MS. *Approaching Hysteria: Disease and its Interpretations.* Princeton, NJ: University Press; 1995.

54. Murphy JM, Horton NJ, Monson RR, Laird NM, Sobol AM, Leighton AH. Cigarette smoking in relation to depression: historical trends from the Stirling County Study. *Am J Psychiatry.* 2003;160:1663–1669.

55. Musto DF. *The American Disease: Origins of Narcotic Control.* New York: Oxford University; 1987.

56. Nestler EJ, Malenka RC. The addicted brain. *Sci Am.* 2004;290: 78–85.

57. Novak S. LSD before Leary, Sidney Cohen's critic of 1950s psychedelic drug research. In: Tracy SW, Acker CJ, eds. *Altering American Consciousness: The History of Alcohol and Drug Use in the United States.* Amherst, MA: University of Massachusetts Press; 2004:1800–2000.

58. Nye RA. *Crime, Madness, and Politics in Modern France: The Medical Concept of National Decline.* Princeton, NJ: University Press; 1984.

59. Oscar-Berman M, Marinkovic K. Alcoholism and the brain: an overview. *Alcohol Res Health.* 2003;27:125–133.

60. Peele S. *Diseasing of America: Addiction Treatment Out of Control.* Lexington: MA: Lexington Books; 1989.

61. Pick D. *Faces of Degeneration: A European Disorder.* Cambridge: MA: University Press; 1989:1848–1918. c.

62. Rasmussen N. America's first amphetamine epidemic 1929–1971: a quantitative and qualitative retrospective with implications for the present. *Am J Public Health.* 2008;98:974–985.

63. Rasmussen N. *On Speed: The Many lives of Amphetamine.* New York: University Press; 2008.

64. Ribot TR. *Les Maladies De La Volonté.* Paris, France: Félix Alcan; 1900.

65. Roizen R. How does the nation's 'alcohol problem' change from era to era?. In: Tracy SW, Acker CJ, eds. *Altering American Consciousness: The History of Alcohol and Drug Use in the United States.* Amherst, MA: University of Massachusetts Press; 2004:1800–2000.

66. Rotskoff LE. *Love on the Rocks: Men, Women, and Alcohol in Post-World War II America.* Chapel Hill, NC: University of North Carolina; 2002.

67. Rotskoff LE. Sober husbands and supportive wives: marital dramas of alcoholism in post-World War II America. In: Tracy SW, Acker CJ, eds. *Altering American Consciousness: The History of Alcohol and Drug Use in the United States.* Amherst, MA: University of Massachusetts Press; 2004:1800–2000.

68. Saah T. The evolutionary origins and significance of drug addiction. *Harm Reduct J.* 2005;2:8.

69. Schaffer HF. The most important unresolved problem in the addictions: conceptual chaos. *Subst Use Abuse.* 1997;32:1573–1580.

70. Sobell MB, Sobell LC. Alcoholics treated by individualized behavior therapy: one year treatment outcome. *Behav Res Ther.* 1973;11:599–618.

71. Sobell MB, Sobell LC. Second year treatment outcome of alcoholics treated by individualized behavior therapy: results. *Behav Res Ther.* 1976;14:195–215.

72. Speaker SL. Demons for the twentieth century: the rhetoric of drug reform, 1920–1940. In: Tracy SW, Acker CJ, eds. *Altering American Consciousness: The History of Alcohol and Drug Use in the United States.* Amherst, MA: University of Massachusetts Press; 2004:1800–2000.

73. Spillane JF. Building a drug control regime. In: Erlen J, Spillane JF, eds. *Federal Drug Control: the Evolution of Policy and Practice.* Binghamton, NY: Pharmaceutical Products; 2004:1919–1930.

74. Sutter MC. Assigning causation in disease: beyond Koch's postulates. *Perspect Biol Med.* 1996;39:581–592.

75. Toby N. *A History of the Killer Weed: the Violence Myth, Federal Bureaucracy, and American Society.* Master of Arts thesis submitted to the Faculty of the Graduate School of Emory University; 2005:1914–1951.

76. Tracy SW. Building a boozatorium: state medical reform for Iowa's inebriates, 1902–1920. In: Tracy SW, Acker CJ, eds. *Altering American Consciousness: The History of Alcohol and Drug Use in the United States.* Amherst, MA: University of Massachusetts Press; 2004:1800–2000.

77. Tracy SW. *Alcoholism in America: From Reconstruction to Prohibition.* Baltimore, MD: Johns Hopkins University; 2005.

78. Tracy SW, Acker CJ. *Altering American Consciousness: The History of Alcohol and Drug Use in the United States.* University of Massachusetts Press; 2004.

79. Ulrich RF, Patten BM. The rise, decline, and fall of LSD. *Perspect Biol Med.* 1991;34:561–578.

80. United States Public Health Service. *Office of the Surgeon General of the United States Surgeon General's Advisory Committee on Smoking and Health Smoking and Health: Report of the Advisory Committee to the Surgeon General of the Public Health Service.* Washington, DC: U.S. Department of Health, Education, and Welfare, Public Health Service; 1964.

81. United States Public Health Service. *Media Strategies for Smoking Control, From A Consensus Workshop Conducted by the Advocacy Institute for the National Cancer Institute (Published Pamphlet).* Washington, DC: U.S. Government Printing Office; 1988.

82. United States Public Health Service. Office of the Surgeon General of the United States. Center for Health Promotion and Education (U.S.). Office on Smoking and Health. *The Health Consequences of Smoking: Nicotine Addiction: A Report of the Surgeon General,* 1988. Washington, DC: U.S. Government Printing Office; 1988.

83. Weiss N. No one listened to imipramine. In: Tracy SW, Acker CJ, eds. *Altering American Consciousness: The History of Alcohol and Drug Use in the United States.* Amherst, MA: University of Massachusetts Press; 2004:1800–2000.

84. White WL. The lesson of language: historical perspectives on the language of addiction. In: Tracy SW, Acker CJ, eds. *Altering American Consciousness: The History of Alcohol and Drug use in the United States.* Amherst, MA: University of Massachusetts Press; 2004:1800–2000.

85. Wilson WA, Kuhn C. How addiction hijacks our reward system. *Cerebrum.* 2005;7:53–66.

86. Ziporyn T. *Nameless Diseases.* New Brunswick, NJ: Rutgers University; 1992.

5

Diagnosis and Classification of Substance Use Disorders

JOHN B. SAUNDERS AND NOELINE C. LATT

Introduction

Diagnosis and classification are ways in which we make sense of our clinical and epidemiological observations and help communicate our findings to others. These systems provide an important basis for the prevention of human disorders and for their management in people who develop them. This applies as much to substance use and other addictive disorders as to other conditions. Indeed, careful diagnosis and categorization are particularly important in the addictions, given the great variety of psychoactive substances (of different pharmacological and chemical classes), the wide spectrum of use and misuse of these substances, and the innumerable complications that arise from such use. Precision in diagnosis is clearly vital for clinical purposes, and epidemiological researchers

and health statisticians need valid and cross-culturally applicable diagnoses.

This chapter explores three distinct but overlapping areas. In the first section, there is a review of the nature of psychoactive substance use, misuse, and dependence. The alternative, indeed competing, conceptualizations of these disorders over the past century are discussed. There follows an account of how the present diagnostic and classification systems have been developed. The next section describes the main substance use diagnoses in the *Diagnostic and Statistical Manual of Mental Disorders* (DSM), currently in its Fifth Edition (DSM-5), and the previous Fourth Edition (DSM-IV), and the *International Classification of Diseases* (ICD), including the Tenth Revision (ICD-10) and the Eleventh Revision (ICD-11). This section includes DSM-5 Substance Use Disorder and ICD-10/11 Substance Dependence and Harmful Substance Use, and also hazardous or risky use and the main substance-induced disorders. The final section is an account of practical ways of making these diagnoses that are applicable to clinical practice.

The Nature of Substance Use Disorders

Given the many professional disciplines that have contributed to our understanding of psychoactive substances and their effects, it is not surprising that scientists and practitioners have drawn upon different traditions to explain the nature of the disorders related to substance use. In addition, there have been many lay interpretations. In the 19th century, a popular conceptualization of excessive alcohol and drug use was that it represented a failure of morals or character.[65] This notion, although superseded in the professional literature of the later 20th century, continues to influence community and political views as to the nature of substance use disorders and that of people with them.

Personality Disorder

In the First Edition of the DSM, published in 1952, substance misuse was included in the personality disorders.[1] Drug addiction was not specifically defined, but there was a statement that "Addiction is usually symptomatic of a personality disorder. The proper personality classification is to be made as an additional diagnosis." The Second Edition of the DSM, published in 1968,[2] still had substance use disorders classified within the personality disorders. No specific definitions or criteria were provided, and there was little description of the conditions, although the text included a statement that "the best direct evidence for alcoholism is the appearance of withdrawal symptoms" and that the diagnosis of drug dependence required "evidence of habitual use or a clear sense of a need for the drug."[2]

The Disease Concept

A different tradition saw substance misuse as reflecting a disease process, which was biologically determined, resulting in the individual having some type of idiosyncratic reaction to alcohol or a drug, and having a relatively predictable natural history. This conceptualization influenced and was subsequently embraced by the self-help movements, such as Alcoholics Anonymous. Jellinek developed the concept of the disease of alcoholism in the 1940s and 1950s,[30] although in his later work he increasingly recognized the role of environmental influences. Over many years in the latter half of the 20th century, the concept that substance misuse might represent a disease process was dismissed by many scientists and professionals. Likewise, the role of genetic predisposition was thought to be inconsequential, with the familial aggregation of substance misuse explained by cultural influences, role-modeling, or malfunction within families.

Epidemiological and Sociological Formulations

A third tradition may be described as the epidemiological and sociological one. Put simply, substance misuse and problems arise fundamentally because of the overall level of use of that particular substance in society. In the 1950s, Ledermann[40] proposed a relationship between the level of alcohol consumption in the community and the prevalence of alcoholism. The level of use is, in turn, influenced by the availability of alcohol, its manufacture and distribution, its price (importantly), and cultural traditions and sanctions. Inherent in these conceptualizations is that individual pathology is considered of secondary importance. The social constructionist school views substance use problems as disaggregated, with no special relationship among them. This school of thought was concerned about the stigma attributable to diagnostic labels and the potential of treatment as a form of social control.[58]

Learned Behavior

The 1970s saw the rise of social-cognitive theory[9] as an influential paradigm to explain the development and resolution of alcohol and drug problems. This school of thought teaches that the (many) influences that determine behavior in general apply to the uptake of substance use and the development of disordered use. Positive consequences encourage repeated use, and negative ones the opposite. Patterns of substance use behavior can become established in this way, but, equally, repetitive substance use can be "unlearnt." This led to the development of a range of cognitive behavioral therapies, some of which were aimed at moderated or "controlled" substance use.[70]

Clinical Syndrome

The need for an understanding of substance misuse that spanned these various discipline-bound conceptualizations and terms was largely met by the formulation of the concept of a "substance dependence syndrome" originally proposed with regard to alcohol dependence by Edwards and Gross in 1976.[21] The basis of the dependence syndrome was a clinical description of key clinical features in a way that was essentially atheoretical and was not based on any particular etiological understanding of the disorder, be it biological, behavioral, or sociological. Rather, certain experiences, behaviors, and symptoms related to repetitive alcohol use were identified as tending to cluster in time and to occur repeatedly. The advantage of a descriptive account of dependence is that it can accommodate etiological models but not be beholden to them.

The concept of the dependence syndrome has been very influential.[19] It has been shown to apply to many other psychoactive substances that have the potential for reinforcement of use, including benzodiazepines, illicit and prescribed opioids, cannabis, inhalants, psychostimulants such as cocaine and the amphetamines, nicotine, caffeine, and anabolic steroids.[a] It also may apply to repetitive behaviors that do not involve self-administration of a psychoactive substance. These include excessive gambling, excessive online (computer/Internet) gaming, and possibly excessive shopping and exercise.[32,33,51]

Until the development of the DSM-5, Substance Dependence was at the heart of the present classification systems of psychoactive substance use disorders.[65,69] It takes center stage in ICD-10[78] and ICD-11,[80] and it was the master substance use diagnosis in DSM-IV,[3] having been introduced into the *Diagnostic and Statistical* Manual *of Mental Disorders, 3rd Edition, Revised* (DSM-IIIR). However, it was removed as such from DSM-5, being replaced by Substance Use Disorder as the central diagnosis.[4] Eight of the 11 criteria are those of Substance Dependence.

---

[a]References 24, 42, 48, 50, 66, 70, 72.

Neurobiological Disorder

Arguably the most important developments in our understanding of the nature of substance misuse in recent years have been in neurobiological processes and especially the neurocircuitry of dependence/addiction.[34–36,73,74,76] This has been complemented by findings from genetic research[17,18,63] that supports what some term the "brain disease model" of addiction.[40]

There is now compelling evidence that repeated use of psychoactive substances leads to powerful and enduring changes in cortico-mesolimbic reward, stress, and control systems.[35,36,73,74] In turn, these result in reinforcement and perpetuation of such use. Repeated exposure to the substance may invoke both long-term potentiation in which transmission of signals increases, and long-term depression, in which signal transmission decreases. Neuroplastic changes have been found in the nucleus accumbens (a crucial brain-reward region), in the dorsal striatum (implicated in encoding of habits and routines), the amygdala (involved in emotions, stress, and desires), and the hippocampus (involved in memory).[74]

The key neurobiological changes that underpin dependence/addiction include:

1. Activation and then blunting of brain reward systems, particularly involving dopaminergic transmission and opioidergic transmission. This has the effect of resetting the reward systems such that larger amounts of the substance are needed to produce the desired effect. Natural rewards are not as reinforced because of the relatively low response from these systems.[73] During withdrawal, activation of the brain regions involved in emotion results in negative mood and enhanced sensitivity to stress.[76]
2. Recruitment of brain stress systems, including those subserved by glutamate neurotransmission and corticotropin-releasing factor (CRF)[35] and suppression or uncoupling of antistress systems.[25] Disruption of dopamine and glutamate systems and stress control systems are related to CRF and dynorphin.[74,76]
3. Alterations occur in the salience of the substance involved, with its climbing up the "ladder of priorities" in the person's life. This has the effect of relegating other interests, activities, and responsibilities to the periphery of the person's life.
4. Impairment of inhibitory control pathways from the prefrontal cortex to the mesolimbic systems, resulting in impaired decision-making capacity, and an inability to balance the strong desire for the substance with the will to abstain. This triggers relapse.[73,74]

Dopamine release leads to induction of neuronal plasticity,[35] which underpins associative learning and memories that result in repetitive substance use even though the original personal triggers and environmental influences have changed. Dependence/addiction may be construed as an "internal driving force"[67] that results from repeated exposure to a psychoactive substance and in turn leads to further repetitive substance use, which is now self-perpetuating and typically occurs even in the face of harmful consequences. Developments in neuroscience research into the mechanisms of addiction have been summarized in a monograph published by the World Health Organization (WHO)[79] and by Volkow, Koob, and colleagues from the US National Institutes of Health.[34–36,73,74,76]

Biological and Social Risk Factors

1. Investigations into possible genetic influences have accompanied this research on neural circuitry. Biometric genetic studies have shown that children born of parents with substance dependence are more likely to have substance dependence themselves[63] and that this is largely explained by genetic transmission rather than environmental factors.[17,18,41] Genomic analysis in human and laboratory animals has identified several areas of the genome where mutations are associated with increased risk of substance use disorders.[17,18]
2. Patients with certain mental illness such as mood disorders, trauma-related disorders, attention-deficit/hyperactivity disorder, psychotic disorders, and anxiety states are at higher risk of substance use disorders. A key finding in recent years has been the central role of abuse and trauma in childhood and adolescence. Social and environmental influences on substance use disorders include: poor familial and social supports, early exposure to substance use, risk taking, novelty seeking, peer pressure, socially stressful environments, easy availability of substance, and permissive attitudes to substance use.[67]

Achieving a Synthesis

It is clear that psychoactive substance use exists as a continuum in society, but it is equally clear that within this spectrum it is possible—and important—to define disorders that have a distinct set of physiological and behavioral features. Substance dependence is a syndrome that occurs in response to repeated and typically high-level alcohol or other substance use, is driven by a profound resetting of key neurobiological systems, is compounded by impaired executive control, and leads to continuing and damaging substance use. As indicated, it is a central diagnosis in the ICD system and is at the core of DSM-5 Substance Use Disorder.

Other forms of repetitive substance use seem not to have these neurobiological changes—at least not to the extent of dependence. They appear to be influenced primarily by factors that affect many types of repetitive human behavior.[9] These include expectations of a substance's effect, responding to learned associations with substance use, and many and varied environmental influences, including peer group pressure, ethnic and workplace culture, and the influences of availability and accessibility of alcohol and various drugs.

Separate from the dependence syndrome and nondependent forms of substance misuse are the multiple consequences of substance misuse. These may be physical, neurocognitive, mental, and social. They typically reflect the adverse effects of the substance, the mode and means of administration of the substance, and/or the implications of the dependence processes. They include disorders of the heart, lungs, gastrointestinal tract, liver, muscles, brain, and peripheral nerves.[8,24,57,59,77] Mental health complications include mood and anxiety disorders and various psychoses. Social complications encompass interpersonal, financial, occupational, and legal difficulties.

Substance Use Diagnoses in the DSM and ICD Systems

Although many different systems of diagnosis and classification have been proposed for substance use disorders over the years, two have international recognition and a third is in widespread use among specialist addiction services. The two internationally recognized systems are the *Diagnostic and Statistical Manual of Mental Disorders*, of which the current version is DSM-5,[4] and the International Classification of Diseases published by WHO, the current versions being the Tenth Revision (ICD-10),[78] and with the

Eleventh Revision (ICD-11) having been published in 2019[80] and scheduled for implementation in 2022. The International Classification of Diseases is a classification of all diseases, injuries, and causes of death. The DSM system specifically covers mental, substance use, and behavioral disorders. The third diagnostic system is that published by the American Society of Addiction Medicine (ASAM),[5,6] which has been endorsed in its essentials by the International Society of Addiction Medicine (ISAM).

Comparisons of DSM-IV, DSM-5, ICD-10, and ICD-11

There are substantial differences in the diagnostic entities that feature in DSM-5 compared with DSM-IV and also ICD-10, and there are comparable differences between DSM-5 and ICD-11.

The DSM and ICD systems have as primary subclassifications (1) the substance or group of substances implicated (Table 5.1) and (Table 5.2), the nature (type) of the disorder that is present (see, for example, Fig. 5.1, which depicts the structure of ICD-11). In DSM-5 are included 10 separate classes of substance, namely alcohol, caffeine, cannabis, hallucinogens, inhalants, opioids, sedatives and anxiolytics, stimulants, tobacco, and other substances. The DSM-IV diagnosis of "Polysubstance Dependence" has been eliminated (see Table 5.1). ICD-10 is similar in its coverage, but it subdivides psychostimulants into cocaine on the one hand, and other stimulants such as amphetamine-type compounds and caffeine on the other. Multiple drug use is combined with other psychoactive substances. ICD-11 has expanded the range and number of substance categories, reflecting its role as an international system for monitoring trends in substance use as well as a clinical manual (see Table 5.1). There are three separate psychostimulant categories, covering cocaine, amphetamines, and caffeine respectively, a separate category for empathogens such as methylenedioxy-methamphetamine (MDMA or "Ecstasy") and for dissociative drugs such as phencyclidine and ketamine. A recent development has been to include new psychoactive substances, namely synthetic cannabinoids and synthetic cathinones[50] in separate groups.

The range of disorders due to substance use can be subdivided conceptually into those that represent (1) the actual use of the substance, whether one-off or repeated, and its immediate effects, and (2) those which reflect its complications, including disease processes in the brain and the rest of the body (see Fig. 5.1). Among the former are the DSM-5 Substance Use Disorder, DSM-IV Substance Dependence, and ICD-10 and ICD-11 Substance Dependence. Substance dependence has at its core a psychobiological driving force to consume the substance. In DSM-5, a decision was made to combine (essentially) DSM-IV Substance Abuse and Substance Dependence into a broader diagnostic entity known as "Substance Use Disorder" (see Table 5.2).

As described above, the entity of substance dependence arose largely from the work of Griffith Edwards at the Maudsley Hospital in London from the mid-1970s onward.[20] It emphasizes a central syndromal grouping of features such as craving, impaired control over substance use, stereotyping of use, and prioritizing of substance use, together with physiological features of tolerance and withdrawal. This central syndrome replaced the much broader notions of alcoholism and addiction, which had typically incorporated some of the mental and social complications as well as externalizing behaviors and denial of the problem. The existence of substance dependence has been supported by numerous studies of its psychometric properties. Applied first to alcohol it became accepted as applying to prescribed medications such as

benzodiazepines and opioids and to a range of recreational and illicit drugs such as cannabis, heroin, and psychostimulants.

We now summarize the features and diagnostic criteria of the principal disorders due to substance use as appear in the four systems.

Substance Use Disorder (DSM-5)

In DSM-5, Substance Use Disorder is now the central diagnosis and represents essentially a combination of the diagnostic features of DSM-IV Substance Dependence and Substance Abuse (see Table 5.2), with one Substance Abuse criterion omitted and the ICD-10 criterion of craving added. This offers a simplified diagnostic system. In DSM-5, Substance Use Disorder is defined as a problematic pattern of substance use leading to clinically significant impairment or distress, manifested by at least two of the following 11 criteria occurring within a 12-month period:

1. The substance is often taken in larger amounts over a longer period than was intended
2. There is persistent desire or unsuccessful efforts to cut down or control substance use
3. A great deal of time is spent in activities necessary to obtain the substance, use the substance, or recover from its effects
4. Craving or a strong desire or urge to use the substance
5. Recurrent substance use resulting in a failure to fulfil major role obligations at work, school, or home
6. Continued substance use despite having persistent or recurrent social or interpersonal problems caused or exacerbated by the effects of the substance
7. Important social, occupational, or recreational activities are given up or reduced because of substance use
8. Recurrent substance use in situations in which it is physically hazardous
9. Continued substance use despite knowledge of having a persistent or recurrent physical or psychological problem that is likely to have been caused or exacerbated by that substance
10. Tolerance as defined by either of the following: (a) a need to markedly increase amounts of substance to achieve intoxication or desired effect, or (b) a markedly diminished effect with continued use of the same amount of substance
11. Withdrawal as manifested by either of the following: (a) the characteristic withdrawal syndrome for the substance or (b) the substance (or a closely related substance) is taken to relieve or avoid withdrawal symptoms.

The severity is graded on the number of criteria met viz mild: 2–3; moderate 4–5; severe: 6 or more (see Table 5.2).

This aggregation is supported by analyses of the components of the DSM-IV diagnoses of Substance Dependence and Substance Abuse, using item response theory (IRT) and similar analyses.[60,61] It also avoids what were termed "diagnostic orphans," persons who fulfilled only two of the DSM-IV Substance Dependence criteria.[21] The problem is that Substance Use Disorder is a very broad and heterogeneous condition for diagnosis. Indeed one can calculate that there are more than 2000 combinations of the diagnostic criteria that fulfill the requirements for Substance Use Disorder, which detracts from the concept that it is syndromal in nature. There is a risk of it being so broad and heterogeneous that it is a less useful entity than substance dependence was in terms of determining treatment. This change has occurred despite DSM-IV Substance Dependence being a psychometrically robust syndrome,[14,47,65,69,71] as identified in the research phase of the DSM-5 developmental process.[65,69] Two examples of these are the

TABLE 5.1 Coverage of Psychoactive Substance Groups in DSM-IV, DSM-5, ICD-10, and ICD-11.

Class	DSM-IV	DSM-5	ICD-10	ICD-11	Comments
CNS Depressants	Alcohol	Alcohol	Alcohol	Alcohol	
	Cannabis	Cannabis	Cannabinoids	Cannabis Synthetic cannabinoids	
	Inhalants	Inhalants	Volatile solvents	Volatile inhalants	
	Opioids*	Opioids*	Opioids*	Opioids*	
	Sedatives, hypnotics, or anxiolytics	Sedatives, hypnotics, or anxiolytics	Sedative-hypnotics	Sedatives, hypnotics, or anxiolytics	
	Nicotine	Tobacco	Tobacco	Nicotine	
CNS Stimulants	Caffeine	Caffeine	Other stimulants including caffeine	Caffeine	
	Amphetamines	Stimulants		Stimulants including amphetamines, methamphetamine, or methcathinone	The stimulants category in DSM-5 includes amphetamine-type substances, cocaine, and other or unspecified stimulants. For some diagnoses the type of substance can be specified.
				Synthetic cathinones	
	Cocaine		Cocaine	Cocaine	
Hallucinogens, Empathogens, and Dissociative Drugs	Hallucinogens	Hallucinogens	Hallucinogens	Dissociative drugs including ketamine and phencyclidine	In DSM-5 there are separate descriptions for phencyclidine and for other hallucinogens. MDMA is classified under other hallucinogens.
	Phencyclidine			Hallucinogens	
				MDMA and related drugs including MDA	
Polysubstance Use	Polysubstance		Multiple drug use and use of other psychoactive substances		The category Polysubstance Use does not appear in DSM-5 or ICD-11
Other and Unknown Substances	Other substances	Other or unknown substances		Other specified psychoactive substances	
				Unknown or unspecified psychoactive substances	There is no category for unknown or unspecified substances in DSM-IV

fact that dependence is required on heroin or other opiates for there to be justification in prescribing replacement opioid agonist therapy with methadone or buprenorphine. In a similar vein, alcohol pharmacotherapies such as naltrexone and acamprosate have been trialled among people with alcohol dependence rather than the broader entity that is alcohol use disorder.

Substance Dependence (ICD-10, ICD-11, and DSM-IV)

Substance dependence is the central disorder of repetitive substance use in ICD-10 and remains so in ICD-11.[78,80] It emphasizes a central syndromal grouping of features such as impaired control over substance use, craving, prioritizing of substance use, together with physiological features of tolerance and withdrawal. These features are found in DSM-5 Substance Use Disorder, but what is less emphasized in the latter's diagnostic criteria is the clustering and repeated experience of these central experiences. As described earlier, this central syndrome replaced broader notions of alcoholism and addiction that had typically incorporated some

of the mental and social complications as well as externalizing behaviors and denial of the problem.

The definitions and diagnostic guidelines in ICD-10 and ICD-11 are shown in Table 5.2. Substance Dependence in ICD-11 is described as:

A disorder of regulation of substance use arising from repeated or continuous use of that substance. The characteristic feature is a strong internal drive to use the substance, which is manifested by impaired ability to control use, increasing priority given to use over other activities and persistence of use despite harm or negative consequences. These experiences are often accompanied by a subjective sensation of urge or craving to use the substance. Physiological features of dependence may also be present, including tolerance to the effects of the substance, withdrawal symptoms following cessation or reduction in use of the substance, or repeated use of the substance or pharmacologically similar substances to prevent or alleviate withdrawal symptoms. The features of dependence are usually evident over a period of at least 12 months but the diagnosis may be made if substance use is continuous (daily or almost daily) for at least one month.[80]

TABLE 5.2   Diagnostic Criteria for Substance Dependence and Substance Use Disorder in DSM-IV, DSM-5, ICD-10, and ICD-11.

	DSM-IV Dependence	DSM-5 Substance Use Disorder	ICD-10 Substance Dependence	ICD-11 Substance Dependence
Stem	A maladaptive pattern of substance use, leading to clinically significant impairment or distress, as manifested by three or more of the following occurring at any time in the same 12-month period.	A problematic pattern of substance use leading to clinically significant impairment or distress, as manifested by at least two of the following occurring within a 12-month period	A cluster of physiological, behavioral, and cognitive phenomena in which the use of the substance takes on a much higher priority for a given individual than other behaviors that once had greater value. Three or more of the following [six] manifestations should have occurred together for at least 1 month, or occurred together repeatedly within a 12-month period.	A disorder of regulation of the substance use arising from repeated or continuous use of the substance. The characteristic feature is a strong internal drive to use the substance. The diagnosis requires two or more of the three central features to be present in the individual at the same time and to occur repeatedly over a period of at least 12 months or continuously over a period of at least 1 month.
1	No equivalent criterion mentioned in text	Craving or a strong desire or urge to use the substance	A strong desire or sense of compulsion to take the psychoactive substance (craving or compulsion)	1. Impaired control over substance use—in terms of the onset, level, circumstances, or termination of use, and often, but not necessarily, accompanied by a subjective sensation of urge or craving to use the substance.
2	There is persistent desire or unsuccessful attempts to cut down or control substance use	There is persistent desire or unsuccessful efforts to cut down or control substance use	No equivalent criterion but text states that the subjective awareness of compulsion is most commonly seen during attempts to stop or control substance use.	
3	The substance is often taken in larger amounts or over a longer period than was intended	The substance is often taken in larger amounts or over a longer period than was intended	Difficulties in controlling substance-taking behavior in terms of its onset, termination, or levels of use (loss of control)	
4	Important social, occupational, or recreational activities are given up or reduced because of drinking or psychoactive substance use.	Recurrent substance use resulting in a failure to fulfill major role obligations at work, school, or home	Progressive neglect of alternative pleasures and responsibilities because of psychoactive substance use, or increased amount of time necessary to obtain or take the substance or to recover from its effects.	2. Substance use becomes an increasing priority in life such that its use takes precedence over other interests or enjoyments, daily activities, responsibilities, or health or personal care. It takes an increasingly central role in the person's life and relegates other areas of life to the periphery. Substance use often continues despite the occurrence of problems.
5	A great deal of time is spent in activities necessary to obtain the substance, use the substance or recover from its effects.	A great deal of time is spent in activities necessary to obtain the substance, use the substance or recover from its effects	Subsumed in the above criterion.	
6.	The substance use is continued despite knowledge of having a persistent or recurrent physical or psychological problem that is likely to have been caused or exacerbated by the substance	Substance use is continued despite knowledge of having a persistent or recurrent physical or psychological problem that is likely to have been caused or exacerbated by that substance	Persisting with substance use despite clear evidence of overtly harmful consequences.	

TABLE 5.2   Diagnostic Criteria for Substance Dependence and Substance Use Disorder in DSM-IV, DSM-5, ICD-10, and ICD-11.—cont'd

	DSM-IV Dependence	DSM-5 Substance Use Disorder	ICD-10 Substance Dependence	ICD-11 Substance Dependence
7.	Tolerance: as defined by either (a) a need for markedly increased amounts of the substance to achieve the desired effects or (b) markedly diminished effect with continued use of the same amount of the substance.	Tolerance is defined by either of the following: (a) a need for markedly increased amounts of the substance to achieve intoxication or desired effect (b) a markedly diminished effect with continued use of the same amount of the substance	Tolerance: such that increased doses of the psychoactive substances are required to achieve effects originally produced by lower doses.	3. Physiological features (indicative of neuro-adaptation to the substance) as manifested by (i) tolerance, (ii) withdrawal symptoms following cessation or reduction in use of that substance, or (iii) repeated use of the substance (or pharmacologically similar substance) to prevent or alleviate withdrawal symptoms. Withdrawal symptoms must be characteristic for the withdrawal syndrome for that substance and must not simply reflect a hangover effect.
8.	Withdrawal as manifested by either (a) the characteristic withdrawal syndrome for the substance or (b) the same (or a closely related) substance is taken to relieve or avoid withdrawal symptoms.	Withdrawal is manifested by either (a) the characteristic withdrawal syndrome for the substance or (b) the substance (or a closely related substance) is taken to relieve or avoid withdrawal symptoms	A physiological withdrawal state when substance use has ceased or been reduced, as evidenced by the characteristic withdrawal syndrome for the substance; or use of the same (or a closely related substance) with the intention of relieving or avoiding withdrawal symptoms.	
9. Former DSM-IV abuse	Continued substance use despite having persistent or recurrent social or interpersonal problems caused or exacerbated by the effects of the substance (e.g., arguments with spouse about consequences of intoxication, physical fights)	Continued substance use despite having persistent or recurrent social or interpersonal problems caused or exacerbated by the effects of the substance.	To some extent subsumed in criterion no. 4.	To some extent subsumed in criterion no. 2.
10. Former DSM-IV abuse	Recurrent substance use in situations in which it is typically hazardous (e.g., drink driving)	Recurrent use in situations in which it is physically hazardous	No equivalent criterion	No equivalent criterion
11. Former DSM-IV abuse	Recurrent substance use which results in failure to fulfil major obligations at work, school or home	Important social, occupational or recreational activities are given up or reduced because of substance use	To some extent subsumed in criterion no. 4.	To some extent subsumed in criterion no. 2.
Former DSM-IV abuse, now omitted	Recurrent substance-related legal problems (e.g., driving an automobile or operating a machine when impaired by substance use)			

In DSM-5 the diagnosis of substance use disorder is further classified according to severity: Presence of 2–3 symptoms: mild; presence of 4–5 symptoms: moderate; presence of 6 or more symptoms: severe.

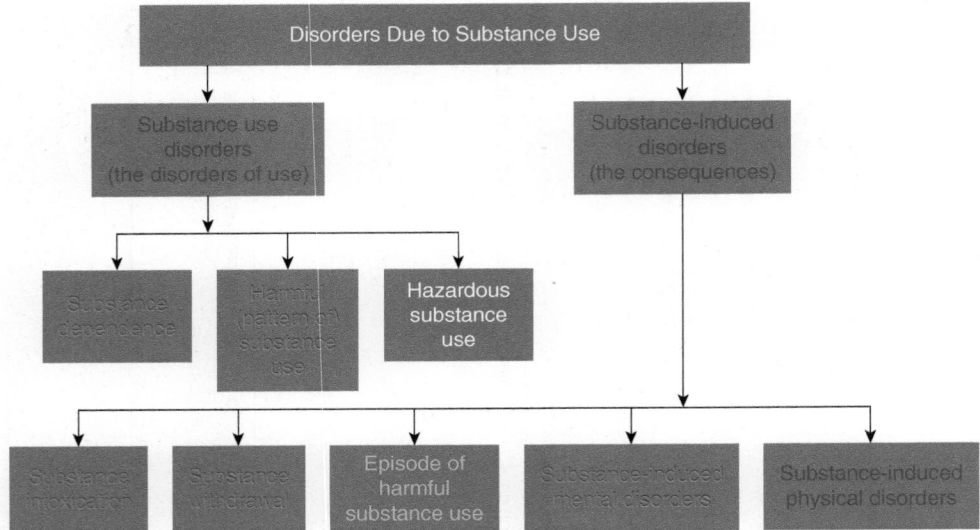

• **Fig. 5.1** Conceptual structure of substance-related conditions in ICD-11. *CVS*, Cardiovascular system; *GIT*, gastrointestinal tract.

Substance dependence in ICD-11 (see Table 5.1) requires the presence of two or more of the three diagnostic guidelines[52,64,65,69]:

1. **Impaired control over substance use**—in terms of the onset, level, circumstances, or termination of use, often but not necessarily accompanied by a subjective sensation of urge or craving to use the substance.

2. **Substance use becomes an increasing priority in life** such that its use takes precedence over other interests or enjoyments, daily activities, responsibilities, or health or personal care. Substance use takes an increasingly central role in the person's life and relegates other areas of life to the periphery. Substance use often continues despite the occurrence of problems.

3. **Physiological features** (indicative of neuroadaptation to the substance) as manifested by (i) tolerance, (ii) withdrawal symptoms following cessation or reduction in use of that substance, or (iii) repeated use of the substance (or pharmacologically similar substance) to prevent or alleviate withdrawal symptoms. Withdrawal symptoms must be characteristic for the withdrawal syndrome for that substance and must not simply reflect a hangover effect.

There are several reasons for retaining Substance dependence as a diagnostic entity, notably its excellent psychometric performance of ICD 10 Substance Dependence for all substance groups (reviewed in Saunders[65] and Saunders and Janca[69]). In addition, it gives guidance to clinicians as to when pharmacotherapies are appropriate, including agonist maintenance for opioid use disorders. The research evidence for anti-craving, relapse-prevention and agonist maintenance treatments is based on controlled trials of these treatments in patients diagnosed with substance dependence (or in some cases the equivalent diagnosis of alcoholism or drug addiction).

The simplified ICD-11 guidelines have been found to be in almost perfect agreement with the ICD-10 and DSM-IV classifications of dependence,[37] but not so much with DSM-5 Substance Use Disorder.[37] Early indications are that DSM-5 captures different individuals in other systems.[15,37] Initial data found that the moderate and severe subgroups of DSM-5 Substance Use Disorder (4–5 symptoms, and 6+ symptoms respectively) corresponded to DSM-IV and ICD-11 dependence, but there are emerging data that 5+ symptoms in DSM-5 might be the nearest equivalent to ICD-10 Substance Dependence.

The dependence syndrome applies to most psychoactive substances that have the potential for reinforcement of use (such as benzodiazepines, opioids, cannabis, psychostimulants, nicotine, caffeine, and anabolic steroids, as described earlier). However, elements of the syndrome are not necessarily applicable to all substances.

Typically substance dependence occurs in people who use large amounts of psychoactive substances repeatedly—for example, consuming alcohol in excess of 120 g/day (men) or 80 g/day (women). However, the diagnosis of substance dependence is not made primarily on the level of consumption.[61]

Addiction as a Disease (ASAM, ISAM)

The American Society of Addiction Medicine (or ASAM) introduced its own definition of substance use disorders, aimed primarily at its clinician members.[5,6] Reflecting its origins in regarding addiction as primarily a brain disease, its definition describes a severe, progressive disorder. Addiction is characterized as a primary, chronic disease of the brain reward, motivation, memory, and related circuits, with dysfunction in these circuits leading to characteristic biological, psychological, social, and spiritual manifestations. This is reflected in an individual pathologically pursuing reward and/or relief by substance use and other behaviors.

It is further defined by an inability to consistently abstain, impairment of behavioral control, craving, diminished recognition of significant problems with one's behaviors and interpersonal relationships, and a dysfunctional emotional response. Like other chronic diseases, addiction involves cycles of relapse and remission. Without treatment or engagement in recovery activities, addiction is progressive and can result in disability or premature death.[5,6] Other organizations have adopted this definition, including the International Society of Addiction Medicine (ISAM).

Harmful Substance Use (ICD-10 and ICD-11)

Repetitive substance use causing harm that does not fulfill the criteria for the dependence syndrome is referred to as "Harmful Substance Use" in ICD-10 and "Harmful Pattern of Use of a Substance" in ICD-11. It does not encompass substance use causing social problems, as the ICD system eschews the notion of a disorder that is defined by social criteria. Harmful substance use is a pattern of substance use that has caused damage to a person's physical or mental health or has resulted in behavior leading to harm to the health of others. The pattern of substance use is evident over a period of at least 12 months if substance use is episodic or at least 1 month if use is continuous (i.e., daily or almost daily). Harm to the health of the individual occurs due to one or more of the following: (1) behavior related to intoxication; (2) direct or secondary toxic effects on body organs and systems; or (3) a harmful route of administration. It does not fulfill the criteria for the dependence syndrome.[78,80]

The harmful effects may be acute or chronic. Examples of acute complications include fractures and other forms of trauma, acute gastritis, and acute psychotic symptoms following substance use. Chronic medical complications encompass liver disease (e.g., alcoholic liver disease or hepatitis C–induced liver disease following injecting drug use), cardiovascular diseases, respiratory diseases, various neurological sequelae, and many others. Examples of mental complications are depressive episodes secondary to heavy alcohol intake, and substance-induced psychosis. In what was a clear distinction from DSM-IV Substance Abuse, social consequences are insufficient by themselves to justify a diagnosis of Harmful Substance Use.[67,78,80] Where a diagnosis of Substance Dependence has been made, the diagnosis of Harmful Substance Use cannot be made for the same substance over the same time period.

In the ICD 11, the concept of Harmful Substance Use is expanded by including behavioral problems that cause harm to others.[80] These include any form of physical harm, including trauma, or mental disorder that is directly attributable to behavior related to substance intoxication.

A new diagnosis in ICD-11 is Episode of Harmful Substance Use. This would apply in situations where harm has been caused by use of a substance but there is no information about whether the person's consumption represents a pattern of repeated use or a one-off episode.[53,80]

Hazardous Substance Use and Related Conditions

The above diagnoses do not encompass the whole spectrum of repetitive, damaging (or potentially so) substance use and, therefore, pose limitations, especially for epidemiological purposes.[16,24,77] In the work of a World Health Organization Expert Committee in the 1970s, several other conditions characterized by repetitive substance use were proposed to complement the dependence syndrome.[19] However, only one, harmful substance use, survived to appear in ICD-10. Perhaps because of the breadth of the task, there have been few attempts to develop a classification system that encompasses the broad spectrum of substance use and misuse. The other condition that was introduced into WHO terminology and survived as a descriptive term but was not included in ICD-10 is "Hazardous Substance Use." This is now included in ICD-11 as a factor affecting health status, in a chapter separate from the Disorders due to Substance Use.

As an example, Hazardous Alcohol Use, otherwise known as "unhealthy," "at-risk," "risky," or "high-risk" use, is defined as use that increases the risk for health consequences, and has been operationalized in several countries.[12,46] For example, in the United States, hazardous or at-risk use is defined in men as consumption of five or more standard 13 gram drinks in a day (e.g., 1.5 oz of 80 proof liquor, 4–5 oz of wine of regular strength, 12 oz of regular strength beer) or more than 14 drinks per week on average.[46] Thresholds for women and for men 65 years or older, are four or more drinks in a day or more than seven in a week on average. A heavy drinking episode occurs whenever a person's alcohol consumption meets or exceeds the daily threshold of five drinks or more for men and four drinks or more for women and for men 65 years and older.[6,46,61] Heavy episodic drinking is defined as repeated heavy drinking episodes. Repeatedly consuming five or more (men) or four or more (women) US standard drinks (65 g and 50 g of alcohol, respectively) confers a risk of alcohol use disorders, acute and chronic illnesses, and injuries.[46,61] In Australia, hazardous or risky consumption is defined presently as repeated daily consumption of more than two Australian standard drinks (20 g of alcohol) for both men and women.[12] In other countries, it is variably defined[67]. Some authorities state that a person should have at least two alcohol-free days per week as well as keeping below a specified level. In some Asian countries, hazardous or risky drinking indicates consumption at levels that lead to intoxication twice a month or more.

The application of hazardous or risky use to other substances has been slower. For nicotine (tobacco), it can be argued that there is no nonhazardous level of use. Likewise, because of uncertainties as to whether there is truly a safe or low-risk level of use for other substances, the concept has not been applied widely to illicit drugs such as cannabis, the amphetamines, cocaine, or heroin, although research on quantifying and establishing the risk of low-level cannabis use is emerging.

Hazardous substance use appeared in early drafts of ICD-10 but was omitted from the published version following the results of field trials that revealed an interrater reliability (kappa) coefficient of only 0.4. Because of the difficulty in operationalizing it, the diagnosis was considered to be open to misuse. The decision to omit hazardous substance use was also influenced by whether it represented a disease process, which was considered by many to be a prerequisite for inclusion in a classification system of diseases. For epidemiological and public health purposes, having a term that defines various levels or patterns of substance use as conferring risk is advantageous. Indeed, data from the National Epidemiologic Survey of Alcohol and Related Conditions indicate that hazardous alcohol consumption (defined as the United States 5+/4+ standard drink criterion) exists within the continuum of abuse and dependence criteria.[61] As the frequency of this level of consumption increases, this experience moves along the severity continuum to overlap with dependence criteria.

In ICD-11, Hazardous Substance Use has been restored as a diagnostic entity. It is classified in a separate chapter as a "Factor influencing health status" and not included with the substance use disorders, which are in the chapter covering mental and behavioral disorders.[80] In ICD-11 it is defined as:

A pattern of psychoactive substance use that appreciably increases the risk of harmful physical or mental health consequences to the user or to others to an extent that warrants attention and advice from health professionals. The increased risk may be from the frequency of substance use, from the amount used on a given occasion, from risky behaviors associated with substance use or the context of use, from a harmful route of administration, or from a combination of these. The risk may be related to short-term effects of the substance or to longer-term cumulative effects on physical or mental health or functioning. Hazardous substance use has not yet reached the level of having caused harm to the physical or mental health of the user or others around the user. The pattern of substance use often persists despite awareness of increased risk of harm to the user or to others.[80]

In support of including hazardous use in a diagnostic system is the evidence that it can be defined and it responds to therapy, the evidence base for the effectiveness of interventions for hazardous alcohol consumption being particularly strong.[31] Thus in a comprehensive diagnostic system, there are grounds for having a dependence category, a nondependence disorder that is of clinical consequence, and a subthreshold disorder that indicates risk to individuals and populations.

The term "unhealthy alcohol use" has been introduced as an umbrella term that encompasses the whole range of disorders of alcohol use, including those at the severe end such as dependence through to alcohol use that poses a risk for the individual but where no harm has occurred.[62] This is a valuable concept and a practical means of grouping all the above diagnoses.

Substance Intoxication (DSM-IV, DSM-5, ICD-10, and ICD-11)

Substance Intoxication (Table 5.3) is defined in DSM-5 as a reversible substance-specific syndrome due to (a) recent ingestion of a substance, (b) clinically significant problematic behavioral or psychological changes that develop during, or shortly after use, and (c) the signs and symptoms are not attributable to another medical condition and are not better explained by another mental disorder, including intoxication with another substance. ICD-11 defines substance intoxication as:

a clinically significant transient condition that develops during or shortly after the consumption of a substance that is characterized by disturbances in consciousness, cognition, perception, affect, behavior, or coordination. These disturbances are caused by the known pharmacological effects of the substance and their intensity is closely related to the amount of the substance consumed. They are time-limited and abate as the substance is cleared from the body.[80]

Substance-specific features of intoxication are then listed. Substance intoxication may be graded as mild, moderate, or severe. In the case of intoxication with central nervous system (CNS) depressants such as alcohol, opiates, or sedative hypnotics, the patient may present with stupor, coma, or even death. In the case of intoxication with CNS stimulants, the patient may present with substance-induced psychosis, cerebrovascular accidents, or cardiovascular collapse.[67]

Substance Withdrawal (DSM-IV, DSM-5, ICD-10, and ICD-11)

Substance Withdrawal refers to a state when substance use is curtailed in individuals with substance dependence or have a

TABLE 5.3	Diagnostic Guidelines for Substance Intoxication (DSM-5, ICD-10, and ICD-11).		
	DSM-5	**ICD-10**	**ICD-11**
Primary definition	Acute intoxication is a transient condition following administration of a psychoactive substance resulting in disturbance of level of consciousness, cognition, perception, affect, or behavior or other psycho-physiological functions and responses. Symptoms of intoxication are substance specific and may produce different types of effect at different levels.	A transient condition following the administration of alcohol or other psychoactive substances, resulting in disturbances in level of consciousness, cognition, perception, affect, or behavior, or other psycho-physiological functions and responses.	Substance Intoxication is a clinically significant transient condition that develops during or shortly after the consumption of a substance that is characterized by disturbances in consciousness, cognition, perception, affect, behavior, or coordination. These disturbances are caused by the known pharmacological effects of the substance, and their intensity is closely related to the amount of the substance consumed. They are time-limited and abate as the substance is cleared from the body.
Additional guidelines and text	Acute intoxication is closely related to dose levels. Exceptions occur with certain underlying organic conditions such as renal or hepatic insufficiency where smaller doses may produce an intoxicating effect.	Acute intoxication is a transient condition. Intensity of intoxication lessens with time and effects eventually disappear in the absence of further use of the substance. Recovery is therefore complete except where tissue damage or another complication has arisen. Acute intoxication is usually closely related to dose levels. Exceptions may occur in individuals with certain underlying organic conditions. Disinhibition due to social context should also be taken into account.	Further guidelines describe it as a reversible substance-specific syndrome with requirements of: (A) Recent ingestion of a substance (B) Clinically significant problematic behavioral or psychological changes that develop during, or shortly after use, and that (C) The signs and symptoms are not attributable to another medical condition and are not better explained by another mental disorder, including intoxication with another substance. Substance Intoxication is common in those with a substance use disorder but may occur in individuals without a substance use disorder
Explanatory notes	*Note that substance-specific features of intoxication are listed under the primary criteria.*		*Note that substance-specific features of intoxication are listed under the primary definitions.*

physiological dependence on a psychoactive substance even though the diagnosis of Substance Dependence may not apply. It is an important manifestation of the neurobiological changes that underpin dependence. In general, the features of Substance Withdrawal are opposite to those of the acute pharmacological effects of the substance. In contrast to substance dependence, substance withdrawal varies appreciably according to the substance used. Psychostimulant withdrawal is very different from withdrawal from that due to, say, sedative-hypnotics.

Substance withdrawal is defined as a clinically significant cluster of symptoms specific to the known withdrawal state of that substance (Table 5.4). There is variable severity and duration of these symptoms, which occur following the absolute or relative withdrawal of a substance. The ICD system specifies that there has been repeated and usually prolonged and/or high-dose use of that substance. The withdrawal syndrome develops in a period from hours to a few days (or more rarely longer) after cessation or reduction in use. The DSM system requires that the signs or symptoms cause clinically significant distress or impairment in social, occupational, or other areas of functioning.

The specific criteria in these systems are listed in Table 5.4. The onset and course of the withdrawal state are time limited and are related to the type of substance and the dose being used immediately before cessation of use. For alcohol, three types of withdrawal are recognized, namely simple uncomplicated

withdrawal, withdrawal with convulsions, and withdrawal with delirium (Table 5.5).

Substance-Induced Mental Disorders (DSM-IV, DSM-5, ICD-10, and ICD-11)

Substance-related problems (or disabilities) were conceptualized by the WHO Committee as the *consequences* of repetitive substance use.[19,65,69] They include both acute (short-term) effects and chronic (long-term) ones.

In DSM-IV, DSM-5, ICD-10, and ICD-11, there are several substance-related mental disorders.[3,4,78,80] These are variable in severity, are usually temporary, but may persist over weeks or more rarely months. They include substance-induced mood disorders, anxiety disorder, sleep-wake disorder, sexual dysfunction, and for psychostimulants, substance-induced obsessive-compulsive disorder. Different syndromes are caused by different substances. Here we discuss just three of them: delirium, psychotic disorder, and amnesic syndrome.

Substance-Induced Delirium (DSM-IV, DSM-5, and ICD-11)

Substance-induced delirium may occur due to a variety of pathological processes. Recognized entities include Substance Intoxication with Delirium (DSM-IV), although it does not feature in

TABLE 5.4   Diagnostic Guidelines for Substance Withdrawal (DSM-5, ICD-10, and ICD-11).

	DSM-5	ICD-10	ICD-11
Primary definitions and criteria	(A) Characteristic withdrawal syndrome that develops within hours or a few days after the cessation of (or reduction in) heavy and prolonged substance use. (B) The development of two or more signs/symptoms specific to the substance, developing within hours to a few days after cessation or reduction in use. (C) The signs or symptoms cause clinically significant distress or impairment in social, occupational, or other areas of functioning.	A group of symptoms of variable clustering and severity occurring on absolute or relative withdrawal of a substance. For a diagnosis of withdrawal syndrome there should be clear evidence of recent cessation or reduction of substance use after repeated and usually prolonged and/or high dose use of that substance. A withdrawal state is one of the main indicators of the dependence syndrome.	A clinically significant cluster of symptoms, behaviors, and/or physiological features, varying in degree of severity and duration, that occurs upon cessation or reduction of use of a substance in individuals who have developed substance dependence or have used the substance for a prolonged period or in large amounts.
Additional guidelines		Symptoms and signs compatible with the known features of a withdrawal state from the particular substance or substances. Physical symptoms vary according to the substance being used. Psychological disturbances (e.g., anxiety, depression, sleep disorders) are also common features of withdrawal. Typically, the patient reports that withdrawal symptoms are relieved by further substance use. The features are not accounted for by a medical disorder unrelated to the substance use, and not better accounted for by another mental or behavioral disorder.	Physical symptoms vary according to the substance being used. Psychological disturbances (e.g., anxiety, depression, sleep disorders) also are common features of withdrawal. Typically, the patient reports that withdrawal symptoms are relieved by further substance use. Onset and course of the withdrawal state are time limited and are related to the type of substance and the dose being used immediately before abstinence. Less commonly, the withdrawal state is complicated by seizures. Substance-induced delirium includes withdrawal states that are complicated by delirium.
Explanatory notes	Note that substance-specific features of withdrawal are listed under the primary criteria.		Note that substance-specific features of withdrawal are listed under the primary definitions.

TABLE 5.5	Features of Delirium Tremens.

Prodromal symptoms:
- Insomnia
- Tremulousness
- Fear

Clinical features:
- Clouding of consciousness and confusion
- Vivid hallucinations and illusions affecting any sensory modality
- Marked tremor
- Delusions
- Agitation
- Insomnia or sleep cycle reversal
- Autonomic overactivity

ICD-10. ICD-11 defines Substance-Induced Delirium as an acute state of disturbed attention and awareness with specific features of delirium that develops during or soon after substance intoxication or withdrawal or during the use of the substance. The amount and duration of substance use must be capable of producing delirium.

More commonly, delirium is seen in those with severe substance withdrawal from alcohol or sedative-hypnotic drugs. The classical disorder is delirium tremens,[68] which is a severe and occasionally life-threatening toxic-confusional state with accompanying somatic disturbances, which lasts for 3 to 10 days. It usually is a consequence of absolute or relative cessation of alcohol in severely dependent drinkers with a long history of use. Its onset may be preceded by features of simple withdrawal and/or by withdrawal convulsions. A similar withdrawal delirium is seen after cessation of benzodiazepines and other sedative-hypnotics, although with less tremor.

Substance-Induced Psychotic Disorder (DSM-IV, DSM-5, ICD-10, and ICD-11)

Psychosis or psychotic symptoms occur in many people with substance use disorders. In some the psychosis is a consequence of drug use. In others it reflects an underlying independent disorder such as schizophrenia. Sometimes the etiology and mechanisms are unclear.

Substance-induced psychotic disorder is presented as an example of a mental disorder induced by substance use. It features in both the DSM and ICD systems.

DSM-5 sets out the following diagnostic criteria for Substance-Induced Psychotic Disorder:

1. The presence of one or both of the following symptoms: (a) delusions, (b) hallucinations.
2. Evidence that the symptoms developed during or soon after substance intoxication or withdrawal and the substance is capable of producing the symptoms.
3. The disturbance is not better explained by an independent psychotic disorder (not substance-induced), as evidenced by: (a) the symptoms preceded the onset of substance use; (b) the symptoms persist for a substantial period of time (e.g., about 1 month) after cessation of acute withdrawal or intoxication; and (c) there is no evidence of non–substance-induced disorder (e.g., history of recurrent non–substance-related episodes).
4. The disturbance does not occur exclusively during the course of a delirium.
5. The disturbance causes clinically significant distress or impairment in social, occupational, or other important areas of functioning.

ICD-10 defines Substance-Induced Psychotic Disorder as a phenomenon that occurs during or immediately after psychoactive substance use (usually within 48 hours) and is characterized by vivid hallucinations (typically auditory but often in more than one sensory modality), misidentifications, delusions, and/or ideas of reference (often of a paranoid or persecutory nature), psychomotor disturbances (excitement or stupor), and an abnormal affect, which may range from intense fear to ecstasy.[77] The sensorium is usually clear, but some degree of clouding of consciousness, although not severe confusion, may be present. The disorder typically resolves at least partially within 1 month and fully within 6 months. The diagnosis is excluded if the psychotic state is a manifestation of substance withdrawal syndrome. ICD-11 Substance-Induced Psychotic Disorder is characterized by psychotic symptoms (e.g., delusions, hallucinations, disorganised thinking, grossly disorganized behavior) that develop during or soon after intoxication with or withdrawal from a substance. The amount and duration of substance use must be capable of producing psychotic symptoms. The symptoms are not better explained by a primary mental disorder (e.g., schizophrenia, a mood disorder with psychotic symptoms) as might be the case if the psychotic symptoms preceded the onset of substance use, if the symptoms persist for a substantial period of time after cessation of substance use or withdrawal, or if there is other evidence of a preexisting primary mental disorder with psychotic symptoms (e.g., a history of prior episodes not associated with substance use).[80] The psychotic symptoms are in excess of the symptoms normally associated with substance intoxication or withdrawal.

For psychostimulants such as amphetamines and cocaine, there is a dose-response relationship, with psychosis occurring especially in those who have been using high doses and/or using the drug over a lengthy period. According to ICD-10, a diagnosis of psychotic disorder should not be made merely on the basis of perceptual distortions or hallucinatory experiences when substances having primary hallucinogenic effects (e.g., lysergic acid, mescaline, and cannabis in high doses) have been taken. In such cases, and also for confusional states, a possible diagnosis of Substance Intoxication should be considered.

Substance-Induced Amnesic Syndrome (DSM-IV, DSM-5, ICD-10, and ICD-11)

Amnesic (or amnestic) syndrome (Table 5.6) is an example of a substance-related disorder where there is anatomical brain damage, caused in this case by the combined effects of thiamine deficiency and toxicity of the substance, typically alcohol.[38] The most common chronic form is characterized by impairment of recent memory, with relative preservation of remote memory and with normal immediate recall. Disturbances of time sense and ordering of events are usually evident, as are difficulties in learning new material. Confabulation may be marked but is not invariably present and should not be regarded as a prerequisite for diagnosis. It is important to note that other cognitive functions are usually relatively well preserved; the amnesic defects are, therefore, out of proportion to other disturbances. Personality changes, often with apparent apathy and loss of initiative, and tendency toward self-neglect may be present but are not necessary for the diagnosis.

Substance-induced amnesic syndrome is classified in the DSM-5 within the Neurocognitive Disorders and not as a substance-induced mental disorder. The diagnostic criteria are those of Substance/Medication-Induced Neurocognitive Disorder, and

TABLE 5.6   Diagnostic Guidelines for the Amnesic Syndrome/Amnestic Disorder in DSM-5, ICD-10, and ICD-11.

	DSM-5	ICD-10	ICD-11
Explanatory notes	Amnesic syndrome is covered by the general criteria for Neurocognitive Disorders, which are listed below. They replaced criteria that were proposed specifically for the amnesic syndrome.		Substance-induced amnestic disorder is included within the general descriptions and guidelines for Neurocognitive Disorders.
Primary criteria and definitions	Evidence of significant cognitive decline from a previous level of functioning. The cognitive deficits interfere with independence in everyday activities. The cognitive deficits do not occur exclusively in the context of a delirium. The cognitive deficits are not better explained by another mental disorder. *Note that for substance/medication-induced disorders, the following additional criteria apply:* 1. The Neurocognitive impairments do not occur exclusively during the course of a delirium and persist beyond the usual duration of intoxication and acute withdrawal. 2. The involved substance or medication and duration and extent of use are capable of producing the neurocognitive impairment. 3. The temporal course of the neurocognitive deficits is consistent with the timing of substance or medication use and abstinence.	Amnesic syndrome is a syndrome associated with chronic prominent impairment of recent memory; remote memory is sometimes impaired, while immediate recall is preserved. Disturbances of time sense and ordering of events are usually evident, as are difficulties in learning new material. Confabulation may be marked but is not invariably present. Other cognitive functions are usually relatively well preserved and amnesic defects are out of proportion to other disturbances. Where this syndrome is produced by alcohol or other psychoactive substances, the following guidelines apply: 1. Memory impairment as shown in impairment of recent memory and learning of new material; disturbance of time sense (e.g., rearrangement of chronological sequence, telescoping of repeated events into one, etc.) 2. Absence of defect in immediate recall, impairment of consciousness, and of generalized cognitive impairment 3. History of objective evidence of chronic (and particularly high-dose) use of alcohol or drugs. Includes Korsakoff psychosis or syndrome, induced by alcohol or other psychoactive substance.	A severe memory impairment relative to the individual's age and general level of intellectual functioning that is disproportionate to impairment in other cognitive domains. It is manifest by a severe deficit in acquiring memories or learning new information or the inability to recall previously learned information, without disturbance of consciousness or generalized cognitive impairment. Recent memory is typically more disturbed than remote memory and immediate recall is usually preserved. The memory impairment is not attributable to substance intoxication or substance withdrawal, and is presumed to be attributable to an underlying neurological condition, trauma, infection, tumor, or other disease process affecting specific areas of the brain or to chronic use of specific substances or medications. For the substance-induced type, all definitional requirements for amnestic disorder should be met. There is evidence from history, physical examination, or laboratory findings that the disturbance is caused by the direct physiologic consequences of use of a substance or medication. If the specific substance inducing the amnestic disorder has been identified, it should be classified using the appropriate subcategory (e.g., amnestic disorder due to use of alcohol).

although an amnesic-type disorder seen with alcohol is noted, no specific criteria are included. In ICD-10, Substance-Induced Amnesic Syndrome is included in the substance disorders chapter, with a specific definition and diagnostic guidelines. However, in ICD-11, it is included in the Neurocognitive Disorders chapter within the section of Amnestic Disorders (and therefore distinct from the dementias) and under the heading of "Amnestic Disorder due to Psychoactive Substances including medications."

Substance-Induced Physical Disorders

Alcohol consumption can cause disease in virtually every organ system in the body and is also associated with a range of malignancies. Cannabis and tobacco use commonly induce respiratory disorders, with the latter being a major cause of bronchial and other cancers.[8,57]

Psychostimulant use can lead to stroke and myocardial infarction through their vasoconstrictive properties. Complications arising from repetitive substance use stem not only from (1) the pharmacological properties of a particular substance but also from (2) the unknown potency, purity, and sterility due to contaminants and adulterants with which the substance is prepared; (3) unsafe injecting practices; and (4) the associated lifestyle of the user. The spread of bacterial infections and viral infections, such as hepatitis C and HIV, and to a lesser extent hepatitis B, is important in this regard. The disinhibiting effect of alcohol and substance use also places users at risk of sexually transmitted diseases.

In the ICD system substance-induced physical disorders are not included with the main grouping of disorders due to substance use but are classified in the respective organ and body systems sections. For example, alcoholic cirrhosis of the liver is included as one of several forms of alcoholic liver disease in the section on diseases of the liver within the chapter "Diseases of the Digestive System." It should be noted that alcohol and certain other substances are risk factors for many physical disorders in addition to those for which they are a principal causal agent.

Substance-Related Social Problems

The adverse consequences of a substance use disorder are legion. Some will be the presenting problem(s) and will be uppermost in the patient's (or relative's) mind. Examples of social problems are:
- relationship problems
- interpersonal difficulties
- financial problems
- work-related problems/unemployment/prostitution
- legal/forensic problems such as drunk driving, assault, and criminal charges.

Practical Approaches to Diagnosis

The Distinction Between Research and Practice

The ways in which diagnoses are made vary considerably. For the research scientist, there are several well-validated diagnostic interview schedules, which allow diagnoses to be made from a systematic structured interview of the respondent. They include the Diagnostic Interview Schedule,[54,55] the Composite International Diagnostic Interview,[56] the Schedules for Clinical Assessment in Neuropsychiatry, and the Alcohol Use Disorder and Associated Disabilities Interview Schedule.[11,27] The constituent questions represent or inquire about the individual diagnostic criteria of the particular disorder. Algorithms are employed to establish whether the combination of responses fulfills these criteria and then to determine whether the number and combination of criteria that are required to fulfill the diagnosis are present. These questionnaires have sound psychometric properties; they have been subjected to rigorous testing of their reliability and validity,[11,14,47,72] and there is much information available on their cross-cultural applicability.[72] In addition to their use in research studies, the structured interview schedules have an important role in the training of psychiatrists, psychologists, and other health practitioners.

Making a diagnosis in clinical practice is usually less structured than this. The practitioner should have a clinical qualification, typically in medicine or psychology, and have undergone an appropriate training program, which includes experience with addictive disorders and supervision from a medical specialist or senior clinician, as appropriate. In most cases, the clinician will take a narrative history and there will be an assessment of the person's mental state and, in the case of internal medicine practitioners, the person's physical state. The information amassed is set against the known features and diagnostic criteria of the various disorders, and a decision is made as to whether the individual has a particular condition or not. Following completion of training, clinicians tend not to employ diagnostic schedules. However, some clinical services require completion of such a schedule or an alternative, such as the Addiction Severity Index (ASI),[44-46] to ensure consistency in the assessment of clients. Shorter screening and brief assessment questionnaires, such as the Alcohol Use Disorders Identification Test (AUDIT)[66] and the Alcohol, Smoking and Substance Involvement Screening Test (ASSIST),[81] also are employed in many services to facilitate assessment.

Much of the information obtained in clinical work is designed to identify experiences and problems that the person has had and that lead not only to a diagnosis but to a comprehensive understanding of the person's background, symptoms, problems, and difficulties.[67] Thus the information obtained in a clinical assessment is broad-ranging and has multiple purposes, of which only one, albeit a crucial one, is to make the diagnosis. In this final part of the chapter, we summarize the information that is relevant to collect in clinical practice and the extent to which this points to a diagnosis or is important ancillary information.

Approaches to the History

The great majority of diagnostic information relevant to substance use disorders is obtained from a careful and comprehensive history.[67] The accuracy of the information is highly dependent on the setting and context of the interview and the interactional style of the clinician. With an empathic approach and in a clinical (as opposed to a custodial) setting, a high level of accuracy can be obtained. Interrater and test-retest assessment indicates reliability coefficients of 0.8–0.9 for average daily alcohol consumption and the experience of dependence symptoms and problems.[13,42] Validity, as assessed by comparison with information provided and by a collateral source or from official statistical data, is also high, with intraclass coefficients of approximately 0.65–0.85.[42]

Among the approaches that enhance the quality and accuracy of the history are to:
1. show empathy and understanding,
2. establish a good therapeutic rapport with the client,
3. be non-judgmental, and
4. be sensitive to the client's cultural background.

Experienced practitioners sometimes employ what are termed "enhancement techniques", such as:

1. placing the onus of denial of substance use on the client,
2. suggesting high levels of intake, the "top high technique,"[67] and
3. being aware of diversionary tactics and not being diverted from the line of questioning.

These techniques should be employed only by experienced clinicians as their use may rebound on the practitioner and lead to termination of the interview.

In addition, collaborative information should be sought from family members, the family physician, and the client's medical records, with due care paid to ethical and privacy issues.

Presenting Problems

Patients may present with a variety of medical, psychiatric, social, legal or forensic complications of substance use. Symptoms of substance use disorders include those of intoxication, substance-induced mental disorders, physical complications of substance use, or withdrawal symptoms that may occur concurrently with an underlying mental disorder. Particular attention should be paid to the longitudinal history and duration of substance use and the duration of the mental disorder and their temporal relationship with each other. It is often difficult to differentiate a primary underlying mental disorder from a substance-induced mental disorder. In many cases the two may coexist (dual diagnosis or comorbidity) and require treatment as distinct entities.

Inquiry about social problems should focus on those typically associated with the substance in question. These can be grouped conveniently with the following domains:

- relationships
- interpersonal difficulties
- financial
- work-related/unemployment/prostitution
- legal/forensic—drunk driving, assault, and criminal charges.

After identifying the presenting problems, the clinician should cover three main domains: (1) intake, (2) dependence, and (3) consequences and harms for each major class of substance.

Substance Use History

Intake

Quantification of the amount of a substance used is a key aspect of the history. This is relatively easy with legal substances such as alcohol, tobacco, and prescribed medication but still is feasible with illicit drugs (Table 5.7).

Among the information that should be obtained for each substance of use is the following:

- quantity
- frequency
- cost
- duration
- pattern or variability
- mode of administration
- time of last use
- periods of abstinence
- precipitants of relapse.

TABLE 5.7	Quantification of Substance Use.
Substance	**Typical Measures**
Alcohol	Amount in milliliters, deciliters, or ounces of specified beverages Amount in grams Standard drinks Standard units
Tobacco	Number of cigarettes Ounces or grams of tobacco
Sedative-hypnotics	Dose (per tablet) Number of tablets per day
Cannabis	Number of joints Number of cones Amount in grams
Heroin	Amount in "street" grams Cost (e.g., dollars)
Amphetamines/ methamphetamine	Amount in points (0.1 g) or grams Cost (e.g., dollars)
MDMA	Number of tablets
Cocaine	Number of lines Amount in grams Cost (e.g., dollars)

The reliability and validity of such information obtained on illicit drug use is generally good, provided that there are no negative implications of supplying the information.[26,42,67]

In addition, current prescribed medications should be documented, for example, opioid analgesics (morphine, oxycodone, fentanyl, hydromorphone, codeine), sedative-hypnotic anxiolytics (benzodiazepines, z drugs), antidepressants, antipsychotics, and other medications including over-the-counter preparations.

Dependence

Although the quantity and frequency of substance use are important parameters, they do not in themselves indicate whether a person has a Substance Use Disorder (DSM-5) or Harmful Substance Use or Substance Dependence (ICD-10 and ICD-11). The experienced practitioner will, however, assess whether the history of substance use points to these diagnoses from information provided about the circumstances and intensity of use, whether this has continued despite harm, and the extent to which the person's life is shaped around the substance. Establishing whether an individual has (1) nondependent Harmful Substance Use (ICD-10 and ICD-11) or mild Substance Use Disorder (DSM-5) or (2) Substance Dependence (ICD-10 and ICD 11) or moderate-to-severe Substance Use Disorder (DSM-5) is the next step. The reader is referred to the relevant diagnostic criteria and guidelines set out in preceding text of this chapter.

Determining whether the patient has Substance Dependence (or its nearest DSM-5 counterpart) or a sub-dependence disorder enables management of patients under two broad streams, namely (1) brief therapy or counseling for nondependent harmful substance use/mild substance use disorder and for hazardous substance use; and (2) detoxification, consideration of pharmacotherapy, and/or a variety of relapse prevention therapies plus

TABLE 5.8   Sample Questions for Substance Use Disorder/Dependence Criteria.

Criterion	Sample Questions
Craving	Have you felt a strong desire or urge to use that you could not resist it?
Impaired control (DSM "Cut down") (DSM "Larger, longer")	Have you wanted to stop or cut down on your use but could not? Have you more than once tried unsuccessfully to stop or cut down on your use? Have you started using and found it difficult to stop (before you became intoxicated)? Have you used much more than you expected to when you began, or for a longer period than you intended to?
Salience (DSM "Give up") (DSM "Time spent") (DSM "Fail expect")	Have you given up or greatly reduced important activities in order to use? Like sports, work, or associating with friends and relatives? Is a great deal of time spent using a substance or getting over the effects of the substance? Has your substance use caused you not to fulfill obligations at work, school, or home?
Tolerance	Have you found that you need to use much more than before to get the same effect? Or that using the usual amount has less effect than before?
Withdrawal	Did stopping or cutting down use ever cause you problems such as (list expected withdrawal symptoms)? Have you ever used to keep from having problems or make any of these problems go away?
Continued use despite harm	Has substance use ever caused you any physical or psychological problems? (If yes, list the problem/s), and then ask: Did you continue to use after you realized that it caused you problems? Has substance use ever caused you any social or interpersonal problems? (If yes, list the problem/s), and then ask: Did you continue to use after you realized that it caused you problems?
Substance use in hazardous situations (DSM only)	Have you used the substance (specify what it is) when you have been in physically hazardous situations such as driving or working with machinery?

involvement with self-help fellowships for those with dependence/moderate-severe substance use disorders (see Fig. 5.1). Questions reflecting the individual diagnostic criteria for dependence are then asked. Sample questions and the criteria from which they derive are presented in Table 5.8.

Consequences and Harms

The adverse consequences of a substance use disorder are legion. At this stage in the interview, the practitioner will have identified several that are uppermost in the client's (or relative's) mind. Inquiry should continue on problems typically associated with the substance in question. These can be grouped conveniently with the following domains:

Physical Consequences/Harms
- Acute physical illnesses, for example, acute gastritis, pancreatitis, Wernicke encephalopathy, acute withdrawal syndrome, coma, intoxication, overdose
- Trauma
- Chronic physical disorders, for example, chronic liver disease, chronic pancreatic disease, cardiomyopathy, neuropathy, substance-induced brain damage

Psychiatric Consequences/Harms
- Anxiety
- Depression, suicidal ideation
- Psychotic disorders

Social Consequences
- Relationships
- Interpersonal difficulties
- Financial
- Work-related/unemployment/prostitution
- Legal/forensic—drunk driving, assault, criminal charges.

Antecedent Factors

Antecedent factors for alcohol and other substance use such as genetic factors, childhood abuse, personality traits, family history of substance use or mental health problems, social problems, and forensic issues should be inquired about and taken into account.[67]

Key Aspects of the Physical Examination

Physical examination is an integral part of a comprehensive medical assessment, but it is often omitted, in which case important diagnostic information can be missed. Signs on physical examination can, on occasion, point almost instantaneously to diagnoses, and a wealth of corroborative information is potentially available. In general, physical examination abnormalities are more apparent in individuals with alcohol use disorders and in injecting drug users. Physical abnormalities evident in the latter group include local complications at the site of injection, or systemic infections. Significant respiratory abnormalities also may be apparent in people who are tobacco or cannabis smokers.

Physical examination is routinely undertaken by internal medicine physicians and most addiction physicians. A focused examination is undertaken typically by family physicians. Physical examination is considered by many psychiatrists to interfere with the development of a therapeutic relationship, and there are readily apparent requirements for chaperoning, particularly when examining individuals of the opposite sex. These compose significant hurdles in a busy practice. Psychiatrists often refer patients to their general medical practitioner for physical examination. Attempts have been made to establish a minimum physical examination that is appropriate for psychiatric practice,[8] but there is no consistency nationally or internationally as to what an accepted minimum is.

Table 5.9 depicts some of the findings on physical examination that are commonly seen in substance use disorders in relation to the primary substance used. There are many more that stem from alcohol use disorders than any other substance class, reflecting the widespread tissue toxicity caused by alcohol misuse.[67]

Mental State Examination

The mental state examination is a vital component of the overall assessment. Emphasis should be placed on identifying common mental comorbidities and neurocognitive impairments. Patients may present with symptoms of substance use disorders, acute intoxication, substance-induced mental disorders, or withdrawal symptoms, which may occur concurrently with an underlying mental disorder.

Key components are the client's general appearance, his/her reaction to the interview, speech, mood, affect, speech, thought form, thought content, perception, presence of hallucinations, cognitive function, attention, concentration, orientation, memory (immediate recall, short-term memory, and long-term memory), intelligence, insight, and judgment.[67] Risk assessment (of suicidal ideation, intent and attempts, and of other forms of self-harm) is mandatory.

Establishing a Provisional Diagnosis

Based on the history covering the domains of (1) intake, (2) dependence, (3) consequences and harms, together with information on antecedents and co-occurring disorders, the practitioner should be in a position to make a diagnosis or identify several candidate diagnoses.

The central diagnosis should be listed, and this may be a Substance Use Disorder (DSM-5) or the ICD-10/11 diagnoses of Substance Dependence or Harmful Substance Use. Where DSM-5 Substance Use Disorder is diagnosed, there should be a statement as to whether this is mild (2–3 criteria fulfilled), moderate (4–5 criteria fulfilled), or severe (6+ criteria fulfilled). Although there is imperfect correspondence, moderate or severe DSM-5 Substance Use Disorder is considered to equate to ICD-10/11 Substance Dependence.

Other diagnoses may be particularly relevant to the patient's presentation, and these include Substance Intoxication and Substance Withdrawal. These may be made as sole diagnoses, or they may be additional diagnoses where DSM-5 Substance Use Disorder or ICD-10/11 Substance Dependence or Harmful Substance Use are made as well. In some settings, the primary diagnosis may be Episode of Harmful Substance Use or one of the substance-induced mental disorders. DSM-5 Substance Use Disorder and ICD-10/11 Substance Dependence and Harmful Substance Use require information about a maladaptive pattern of substance use. In contrast, the remaining diagnoses of Substance Intoxication, Substance Withdrawal, Episode of Harmful Substance Use, and the substance-induced mental disorders do not require detailed information of the pattern of substance use. It is perfectly in order to make diagnoses of substance-induced disorders as well as Substance Dependence and other disorders of use.

Laboratory Tests

The assessment of the client is complemented by undertaking relevant laboratory tests.[28,67,75] These include routine blood tests, urine drug screens (for drugs or metabolites), saliva analysis, breath analysis, and, less commonly, analysis of hair. Such samples can be examined for the presence of alcohol, nicotine, prescribed medications and illicit drugs, and their metabolites. When

TABLE 5.9	Findings on Physical Examination.
Alcohol	Alcohol on breath
	Features of intoxication or of withdrawal
	Facial/periorbital puffiness
	Facial flushing/telangiectasia
	Old scars
	Conjunctival injection
	Scleral jaundice
	Trauma and burns
	Head injury
	Signs of malnutrition
	Nystagmus - consider Wernicke encephalopathy
	Stigmata of chronic liver disease
	Clinical signs of pancreatitis
	Hypertension
	Atrial fibrillation
	Rib fractures
	Peripheral neuropathy
	Cognitive impairment
Tobacco	Nicotine-stained fingers
	Chronic airways disease
	Cardiovascular disease
Cannabis	Smell of marijuana
	Conjunctival injection
	Features of intoxication
Sedative-hypnotics	Drowsy, slurred speech (overdose)
	Anxious agitated (withdrawal)
Injecting drug users (unsafe injecting practices, associated lifestyle)	Malnutrition
	Poor self-care
	Needle track marks (fresh or old)
	Tattoos
	Jaundice (consider hepatitis C and B)
	Thrombophlebitis
	Cellulitis
	Infective endocarditis
	Skin abscesses
	Indurated skin
	Caries
	Mouth ulcers
	Pneumonia
	Septic arthritis
	HIV/AIDS and sexually transmitted infections
Heroin	Overdose or withdrawal
	Pupillary size:
	• pinpoint (overdose)
	• dilated (withdrawal)Low blood pressure
	Low respiratory rate
	Noncardiogenic pulmonary edema
Psychostimulants	Underweight and emaciated
	Pupil size—dilated
	Excoriations (formication)
	Clenched jaws (bruxism)
	Caries/broken teeth
	Repetitive stereotypic movements
	Nasal septal necrosis (cocaine)

clinically necessary, the American Society of Addiction Medicine (2019) recommends drug testing as a therapeutic tool as part of evidence-based addiction treatment (and not as a punitive measure). Patient informed consent is required, and the results should be confidential to the extent permitted by law.[7]

For alcohol there are numerous tests, termed "biological markers," which reflect a range of pathophysiological effects on blood, the liver, and other organs.[28,75] These physiological processes include:

- liver enzyme induction (gammaglutamyltransferase [GGT]);
- liver cell damage (aspartate aminotransferase [AST], alanine aminotransferase [AAT], GGT);
- impaired synthetic and excretory functioning (bilirubin, albumin, coagulation parameters);
- suppression of hematopoiesis (elevated MCV, thrombocytopenia);
- effects of alcohol's metabolites on transport proteins (carbohydrate-deficient transferrin (CDT)); and
- metabolic disturbances, such as hyperuricemia.

None of these abnormalities is specific to alcohol. The most specific test reflecting the biological effects of alcohol is the presence of abnormal isoforms of transferrin, collectively known as carbohydrate-deficient transferrin (or CDT). An elevated blood CDT level is found in 40%–70% of persons with alcohol dependence or harmful alcohol consumption. It is highly specific for these diagnoses (a specificity of 98% has been reported), with only a few uncommon inherited metabolic disorders and occasionally primary biliary cirrhosis and pregnancy resulting in abnormal levels.

Alcohol metabolites such as ethyl glucuronide (EtG) and ethyl sulfate (EtS) provide a longer window for detecting alcohol consumption than measuring the presence of alcohol only.[10] Table 5.10 summarizes some of the most commonly employed laboratory markers of alcohol use.[67,75]

Depending on the presentation, blood glucose levels, thyroid function tests, vitamin B_{12}/folate levels, C-reactive protein (CRP), cardiac enzymes (e.g., in cocaine use), and blood cultures help in assessing associated disorders. Serological tests for hepatitis B and C and HIV are important for those at risk of such infections and are essential in injecting drug users and their contacts. A check for sexually transmitted diseases is often appropriate.

Considerable effort has been devoted to the development of laboratory tests of substance use disorders. There remains a lingering concern by many researchers and clinicians about the validity of self-report despite the evidence for its accuracy in most circumstances. There is a desire for corroboration of self-report information, particularly in forensic settings or where there are significant implications for the individual for being diagnosed with a substance use disorder. In addition, there is a desire for tests to simplify or speed the diagnostic process. A test that reflects the biological processes of dependence would be a valuable addition to diagnostic capability but none such exist at present.

At present, no diagnostic test or procedure such as imaging directly points to a specific substance use disorder. Finding a high blood alcohol or drug level may support a diagnosis of substance intoxication but this is primarily based on clinical criteria. A high level in a person who shows no signs of intoxication (or any substance effect) may point to tolerance and a likely substance dependence or moderate-to-severe substance use disorder.

Imaging and Other Investigations

Depending on the clinical presentation, other investigations may include chest radiographs, electrocardiography (ECG),

TABLE 5.10	Biological Markers of Alcohol Misuse.
Laboratory Tests	
Urine or blood alcohol concentration >0.05%	Indicates recent alcohol intake. Does not distinguish between acute and chronic consumption of excess alcohol
Full blood count: • Macrocytosis	Detects heavy drinkers: 20%–30% in the community and 50%–70% in hospital inpatients
Liver function tests • Elevated gamma-glutamyl transferase	Detects heavy drinkers: 30%–50% in the community and 50%–80% in hospital inpatients
Carbohydrate-deficient transferrin	Carbohydrate-deficient transferrin >2.6% reflects heavy alcohol use in the past 2 weeks
Ratio of urinary 5-hydroxytryptophol to 5-hydroxyindole-acetic acid	Increased ratio of 5-hydroxytryptophol/5-hydroxyindoleacetic acid
Ethanol metabolites in the urine • Ethyl glucuronide • Ethyl sulfate	Helps to detect excess alcohol use when blood alcohol concentration is zero in the emergency department. It is raised when there has been alcohol consumed in the previous 1–3 days.
Ethanol metabolites in hair samples • Ethyl glucuronide • Fatty acid ethyl esters (FAEE)	Evidence of excessive drinking when: • >25 pg/mg • >1 ng/mg

echocardiography, and hepatic fibroscan.[30,48] The fibroscan has revolutionized the noninvasive diagnosis of alcoholic and hepatitis C and B–induced liver disease. It provides an index of fibrosis that can distinguish with good accuracy various stages of fibrosis and cirrhosis.

Standard neuroimaging procedures such computed tomography (CT) and magnetic resonance imaging (MRI) scanning of the brain are vital for diagnosis of many of the neurological and neurocognitive complications of substance use disorders.[22,67,82] CT scanning is widely available and is used primarily to identify space-occupying lesions such as skull fractures, intracranial hematomas, cerebral tumors, and marked general cerebral atrophy. MRI scanning is more expensive but is more precise and can demonstrate atrophy in specific brain areas such as the mamillary bodies (in Wernicke encephalopathy), cerebellar vermis (in truncal ataxia), and hypodense lesions (in multi-infarct dementia).

Functional neuroimaging techniques such as functional magnetic resonance imaging (fMRI), positron emission tomography (PET), and single-photon emission computerized tomography (SPECT) currently are illuminating some of the central neurobiological mechanisms of dependence. They are not part of routine clinical assessment, the reason being that although brain imaging findings from a group of subjects with a substance disorder clearly identify the areas of the brain that are activated or suppressed by exposure to a substance or to cues associated with that substance, there is considerable variation among individuals in their responses. This means that functional imaging for diagnostic purposes in the individual lacks the precision (sensitivity and specificity) necessary for clinical diagnosis. This may well change with greater experience using these techniques over the next decade.

Establishing the Final Diagnosis

When information is available from any laboratory tests or imaging procedures that have been undertaken, the practitioner is likely to be in the position of making a definitive diagnosis of the substance use disorders and relevant antecedent factors and co-occurring disorders that the patient has. Laboratory tests may, for example, point to an unexpected degree of chronic liver disease. CT or MRI brain scans may point to cerebral shrinkage or the unexpected presence of other intracranial pathology. The diagnoses should now be in a more refined state and should guide the practitioner to an appropriate plan of management to be discussed with the patient and the patient's family members as appropriate. Some diagnoses may not be evident for several more weeks and this applies particularly to comorbid and possible antecedent mental health disorders, which may be masked by the pharmacological and mental effects of the substance use for weeks or sometimes months. In the substance use disorders field, the practitioner needs to keep an open mind for other disorders that may be revealed with the passage of time. In this area, more than most, there is a need to have a longitudinal perspective to diagnosis where the disorders affecting the patient become clearer as time passes.

This should not, however, deviate the practitioner from establishing a management plan during the first assessment and to offer a plan of action to the patient, which at that time could be a powerful motivator to the patient to engage in treatment. The plan may include urgent measures such as detoxification and the administration of thiamine and other vitamins. During the first or subsequent consultations, the practitioner may, in conjunction with the patient, decide on referral to a professional colleague such as a psychiatrist, internal medicine physician, a psychologist, or therapist.

Acknowledgments

We thank Corinne Lim for her expert contribution to the literature and cross-checking of the citations to the literature.

References

1. American Psychiatric Association. *Diagnostic and Statistical Manual for Mental Disorders*. Washington, DC: American Psychiatric Association; 1952.
2. American Psychiatric Association. The Diagnostic and Statistical Manual for Mental Disorders, 2nd edn. American Psychiatric Association, Diagnostic and Statistical Manual for Mental Disorders, 4th edn. Washington, DC: American Psychiatric Association; 1968.
3. American Psychiatric Association. *The Diagnostic and Statistical Manual for Mental Disorders*. 4th ed. Washington, DC: American Psychiatric Association; 1994.
4. American Psychiatric Association. *The Diagnostic and Statistical Manual for Mental Disorders*. 5th ed. Washington, DC: American Psychiatric Association; 2013.
5. American Society of Addiction Medicine. *Public Policy Statement: Definition of Addiction*; 2011. (Available via https://www.asam.org/resources/definition-of-addiction.)
6. American Society of Addiction Medicine. *Public Policy Statement: Terminology Related to the Spectrum of Unhealthy Substance Use*; 2013. (Available via https://www.asam.org/advocacy/find-a-policy-statement.)
7. American Society of Addiction Medicine. *Public Policy Statement: The Ethical Use of Drug Testing in the Practice of Addiction Medicine*; 2019. (Available via https://www.asam.org/advocacy/find-a-policy-statement.)
8. Baigent M. Physical complications of substance abuse: what the psychiatrist needs to know. *Curr Opin Psychiatry*. 2003;16:291–296.
9. Bandura A. *Social Learning Theory*. Englewood Cliffs, NJ: Prentice-Hall; 1977.
10. Cabarcos P, Álvarez I, Tabernero MJ, Bermejo AM. Determination of direct alcohol markers: a review. *Ana Bioanalyt Chem*. 2015;407:4907–4925.
11. Chatterji S, Saunders JB, Vrasti R, et al. Reliability of the alcohol and drug modules of the alcohol use disorder and associated disabilities interview schedule–alcohol/drug revised (AUDADIS–ADR): an international comparison. *Drug Alcohol Depend*. 1997;47:171–185.
12. Commonwealth Department of Health and Ageing. *Australian Alcohol Guidelines: Health Risks and Benefits*. Commonwealth of Australia; 2012. Available via http://www.alcohol.gov.au/internet/alcohol/publishing.nsf/Content/guide-adult.
13. Conigrave KM, Degenhardt LJ, Whitfield JB, et al. CDT, GGT and AST as markers of alcohol use: the WHO/ISBRA Collaborative Project. *Alcohol Clin Exp Res*. 2002;26:332–339.
14. Connors GJ, Watson DW, Maisto SA. Influence of subject and interviewer characteristics on the reliability of young adults' self-reports of drinking. *J Psychopath Behav Assess*. 2005;7:365–374.
15. Cottler LB, Grant BF, Blaine J, et al. Concordance of DSM-IV alcohol and drug use disorder criteria and diagnoses as measured by AUDADIS-ADR, CIDI and SCAN. *Drug Alcohol Depend*. 1997;47:195–205.
16. Degenhardt L, Bruno R, Lintzeris N, et al. Agreement between definitions of pharmaceutical opioid use disorders and dependence in people talking opioids for chronic non-cancer (POINT) study. *Lancet Psychiatry*. 2015;2:314–322.
17. Degenhardt L, Hall W. Extent of illicit drug use and dependence, and their contribution to the global burden of disease. *Lancet*. 2012;379:55–70.
18. Ducci F, Goldman D. The genetic basis of addictive disorders. *Psychiatr Clin North Am*. 2012;35:495–519.
19. Edenberg HJ, Foroud T. Genetics and alcoholism. *Nat Rev Gastroenterol Hepatol*. 2013;10:487–494.
20. Edwards G, Arif A, Hodgson R. Nomenclature and classification of drug and alcohol-related problems: a WHO memorandum. *Bull World Health Org*. 1981;59. 255–242.
21. Edwards G, Gross MM. Alcohol dependence: provisional description of a clinical syndrome. *Br Med J*. 1976;1:1058–1061.
22. Eng MY, Schuckit MA, Smith TL. A five-year prospective study of diagnostic orphans for alcohol use disorders. *J Stud Alcohol*. 2003;64:227–234.
23. Ersche KD, Williams GB, Robbins TW, Bullmore ET. Meta-analysis of structural brain abnormalities associated with stimulant drug dependence and neuroimaging of addiction vulnerability and resilience. *Curr Opin Neurobiol*. 2013;23:615–624.
24. Feingold A, Rounsaville B. Construct validity of the dependence syndrome as measured by DSM-IV for different psychoactive substances. *Addiction*. 1995;90:1661–1669.
25. GBD 2016 Alcohol Collaborators. Alcohol use and burden for 195 countries and territories, 1990-2016: a systematic analysis for the Global Burden of Disease Study 2016. *Lancet*. 2018;392:1015–1035.
26. Gilpin NW, Misra K, Herman MA, et al. Neuropeptide Y opposes alcohol effects on gamma-aminobutyric acid release in amygdala and blocks the transition to alcohol dependence. *Biol Psychiatry*. 2011;69:1091–1099.
27. Gossop M, Best D, Marsden J, et al. Test re-test reliability of the severity of dependence scale. *Addiction*. 1997;92:352–354.
28. Grant BF, Goldstein RB, Smith SM, et al. The Alcohol Use Disorders and Associated Disabilities Interview Schedule-5 (AUDADIS-5): reliability of substance use and psychiatric disorder modules in a general population sample. *Drug Alcohol Depend*. 2015;148:27–33.
29. Hashimoto E, Riederer PF, Hesselbrock VM, et al. Consensus paper of the WFSBP task force on biological markers: biological markers for alcoholism. *World J Biol Psychiatry*. 2013;14:549–564.

30. Jellinek EM. *The Disease Concept of Alcoholism. Hillhouse.* New Brunswick; 1960.

31. Jiang T, Tian G, Zhao Q, et al. Diagnostic accuracy of 2D-Shear Wave Elastography for liver fibrosis severity: a meta-analysis. *PLoS One.* 2016;11(6):e0157219.

32. Kaner EFS, Beyer FR, Muirhead C, Campbell F, et al. Effectiveness of brief alcohol interventions in primary care populations. *Cochrane Database Syst Rev.* 2018;2:CD004148.

33. Kim NR, Hwang SS, Choi JS, et al. Characteristics and psychiatric symptoms of Internet Gaming Disorder among adults using self-reported DSM-5 criteria. *Psychiatry Investig.* 2016;13:58–66.

34. King DL, Delfabbro PH, Zwaans T, Kaptsis D. Clinical features and Axis comorbidity of Australian adolescent pathological Internet and video game users. *Aus New Zealand J Psychiat.* 2013;47:1058–1067.

35. Koob GF, Le Moal M. Plasticity of reward neurocircuitry and the dark side of drug addiction. *Nature Rev Neurosci.* 2005;8:1442–1444.

36. Koob GF, Le Moal M. Addiction and the brain antireward system. *Ann Rev Psychol.* 2008;59:29–53.

37. Koob GF, Volkow NB. Neurobiology of addiction: a neurocircuitry analysis. *Lancet Psychiatry.* 2016;3:760–773.

38. Lago L, Bruno R, Degenhardt L. Concordance of ICD 11 and DSM-5 definitions of alcohol and cannabis use disorders: a population survey. *Lancet Psychiatry.* 2016;3:673–684.

39. Latt N, Dore G. Thiamine in the treatment of Wernicke encephalopathy in patients with alcohol use disorders. *Inter Med J.* 2014;44:911–915.

40. Ledermann S. *Alcool, Alcoolism, Alcoolisation: Données Scientifiques De Caractère Physiologique, Économique et Social.* Paris: Presses Universitaires de France, Institut National d'Etudes Demographiques; 1960.

41. Leshner A. Addiction is a brain disease. *Iss Sci Tech.* 2001;17:75–80.

42. Lessov CN, Martin NG, Statham DJ, et al. Defining nicotine dependence for genetic research: evidence from Australian twins. *Psychol Med.* 2004;34:865–879.

43. Maisto SA, Sobell LC, Sobell MA. Corroboration of drug abusers' self-reports through the use of multiple data sources. *Am J Drug Alcohol Abuse.* 1982;9:301–308.

44. McLellan AT, Carise D, Coyne TH. *Addiction Severity Index.* 5th ed. Treatment Research Institute; 2012.

45. McLellan AT, Kushner H, Metzger D, et al. Addiction severity index. *J Subst Abuse Treatment.* 1992;9:199–213.

46. McLellan AT, Luborsky L, O'Brien CP, et al. An improved diagnostic instrument for substance abuse patients: the Addiction Severity Index. *J Nerv Ment Dis.* 1980;168:26–33.

47. National Institute on Alcohol Abuse and Alcoholism. *Helping Patients Who Drink Too Much: A Clinician's Guide.* Rockville. MD: National Institute on Alcohol Abuse and Alcoholism; 2005.

48. Nelson CB, Rehm J, Üstün TB, et al. Factor structures for DSM-IV substance disorders criteria endorsed by alcohol, cannabis, cocaine and opiate users: results from the WHO reliability and validity study. *Addiction.* 1999;94:843–855.

49. Nguyen-Khac E, Chatelain D, Tramier B, et al. Assessment of asymptomatic liver fibrosis in alcoholic patients using fibroscan: prospective comparison with seven non-invasive laboratory tests. *Alimen Pharmacol Therap.* 2008;28:1188–1198.

50. Park TW. *Benzodiazepine Use Disorder: Epidemiology, Pathogenesis, Clinical Manifestations, Course and Diagnosis. UpToDate.* Waltham, MA: UpToDate Inc; 2018. (Available via https://www.uptodate.com/home/content.)

51. Papaseit E, Farré N, Schifano F, Torrens M. Emerging drugs in Europe. *Curr Opin Psychiatry.* 2014;27:243–250.

52. Potenza MN. Should addictive disorders include non-substance related conditions? *Addiction.* 2006;101(s1):142–151.

53. Poznyak V. Alcohol use disorders: their status in the draft ICD 11. Presented at the Joint Congress of the Research Society on Alcoholism and the International Society for Biomedical Research on Alcoholism. Seattle, USA: 2014.

54. Poznyak V, Reed GM, Medina-Mora ME. Aligning the ICD-11 classification of disorders due to substance use with global service needs. *Epidemiol Psychiatr Sci.* 2018;27:212–218.

55. Robins LN, Helzer JE, Croughan J, et al. National Institute of mental health diagnostic interview schedule: its history, characteristics and validity. *Arch Gen Psychiatry.* 1981;38:381–389.

56. Robins LN, Helzer JE, Ratcliff KS, et al. Validity of the diagnostic interview schedule, version II: DSM III diagnoses. *Psychol Med.* 1982;12:855–870.

57. Robins LN, Wing J, Wittchen H-U, et al. The Composite International Diagnostic Interview: an epidemiologic instrument suitable for use in conjunction with different diagnostic systems and in different cultures. *Arch Gen Psychiatry.* 1988;45:1069–1077.

58. Roerecke N, Rehm J. Alcohol use disorders and mortality: a systematic review and meta-analysis. *Addiction.* 2013;108:1562–1578.

59. Room R. Drugs, consciousness and self-control: popular and medical conceptions. *Int Rev Psychiatry.* 1989;1:63–70.

60. Rehm J, Greenfield TK, Kerr W. Patterns of drinking and mortality from different diseases—an overview. *Contemp Drug Probl.* 2006;33:205–235.

61. Saha TD, Chou PS, Grant BF. Toward an alcohol use disorder continuum using item response theory: results from the National Epidemiologic Survey on Alcohol and Related Conditions. *Psychol Med.* 2006;36:931–941.

62. Saha TD, Stinson FS, Grant BF. The role of alcohol consumption in future classification of alcohol use disorders. *Drug Alcohol Depend.* 2007;89:82–92.

63. Saitz R. Unhealthy alcohol use. *N Engl J Med.* 2005;352:596–607.

64. Saunders JB. Alcoholism: new evidence for a genetic contribution. *Br Med J.* 1982;284:1137–1138.

65. Saunders JB. *Rationale for Changes in the Clinical Descriptions and Diagnostic Guidelines of Disorders Due to Substance Use and Related Conditions in the Draft ICD 11.* Madrid, Spain: Presented at the World Congress of the World Psychiatric Association; 2014.

66. Saunders JB. Substance use and addictive disorders in DSM-5 and ICD 10 and the draft ICD 11. *Curr Opin Psychiatry.* 2017;30:227–237.

67. Saunders JB, Aasland OG, Babor TF, et al. Development of the Alcohol Use Disorders Identification Test (AUDIT): WHO collaborative project on early detection of persons with harmful alcohol consumption II. *Addiction.* 1993;88:791–804.

68. Saunders JB, Conigrave KM, Latt NC, et al. *Addiction Medicine.* 2nd ed. Oxford: Oxford University Press; 2016. ISBN:978-0-19-871475-0.

69. Saunders JB, Janca A. Delirium tremens: its aetiology, natural history and treatment. *Curr Opin Psychiatry.* 2000;13:629–633.

70. Saunders JB, Peacock A, Degenhardt L. Alcohol Use disorders in the draft ICD-11, and how they Compare with DSM-5. *Curr Addict Rep.* 2018;5:257–264.

71. Sobell MB, Sobell LC. *Problem Drinkers: Guided Self-Change Treatment.* New York and London: Guilford; 1993.

72. Teesson M, Lynskey M, Manor B, et al. The structure of cannabis dependence in the community. *Drug Alcohol Depend.* 2002;68:255–262.

73. Üstün B, Compton W, Mager D, et al. WHO Study on the reliability and validity of the alcohol and drug use disorder instruments: overview of methods and results. *Drug Alcohol Depend.* 1997;47:161–169.

74. Volkow ND, Fowler JS, Wang GJ. The addicted brain viewed in the light of imaging studies: brain circuits and treatment strategies. *Neuropharmacology.* 2004;(47s):3–13.

75. Volkow ND, Koob G, Baler R. Biomarkers in substance use disorders. *ACS Chem Neurosci.* 2015;6:522–525.

76. Volkow ND, Koob GF, McLellan T. Neurobiologic advances from the brain disease model of addiction. *N Eng J Med.* 2016;374(4):363–371.

77. Walsham NE, Sherwood RA. Biomarkers of alcohol misuse. In: Wolff K, White J, Karch S, eds. *The SAGE Handbook of Drug and Alcohol Studies*. London: SAGE Publications; 2017.

78. Wood AM, Kaptoge S, Butterworth AS, Willeit P, et al. Risk thresholds for alcohol consumption: combined analysis of individual-participant data for 599 912 current drinkers in 83 prospective studies. *Lancet*. 2018;391:1513–1523.

79. World Health Organization. *The ICD-10 Classification of Mental and Behavioural Disorders: Clinical Descriptions and Diagnostic Guidelines*. Geneva: World Health Organization; 1992.

80. World Health Organization. *Neuroscience of Psychoactive Substance Use and Dependence*. Geneva: World Health Organization; 2004.

81. World Health Organization. *International Classification of Diseases 11th Revision (ICD-11)*. Geneva: World Health Organization; 2019. Available at https://icd.who.int/en/.

82. World Health Organization ASSIST Working Group. The alcohol, smoking and substance involvement screening test (ASSIST): development, reliability and feasibility. *Addiction*. 2002;97:1183–1194.

6

Drug Reinforcement in Animals

WENDY J. LYNCH, TANSELI NESIL, AND SCOTT E. HEMBY

CHAPTER OUTLINE

Introduction

Early demonstrations that drugs could serve as reinforcers, maintaining operant behavior in laboratory animals, led to the development of a model of human substance use disorder (Box 6.1). The traditional self-administration model was developed within a behavioral analysis conceptual framework that views drugs as reinforcers similar to other "natural" reinforcers such as food. The fundamental principle underlying behavioral analysis is that certain aspects of behavior are controlled by their consequences.[120] A drug is said to be functioning as a reinforcer if responding for it is maintained above responding for saline or other control conditions. The traditional model entails training an animal to self-administer a drug during a short daily session, typically 1–2 h. A low ratio requirement is typically used, such as a fixed ratio 1, where each response produces a drug delivery. Intake is stable under these conditions, which allows for the determination of the effects of pharmacological and environmental manipulations on a stable baseline.[132]

Although the rat is most often used in these studies, this model has been implemented with a variety of species including nonhuman primates, mice, dogs, cats, and baboons.[14,72,101,187,210] A variety of operant responses have also been used, and typically they depend on the species being studied. For example, a lever press or a nose poke response is typically used for rats and mice, whereas a panel press response is typically used for nonhuman primates. The most common routes of administration are intravenous and oral, but intracerebroventricular, intracranial, inhalation, intragastric, and intramuscular routes have also been used. Generally, these studies use the route of administration that is most similar to the route used in humans for that particular drug. For example, animal studies with alcohol typically use an oral route of administration, whereas an intravenous route is typically used for drugs that have a rapid onset in humans, such as cocaine, methamphetamine, heroin, and nicotine. There is also growing interest in the development and use of inhalation self-administration procedures for the latter type of drugs, since, unlike the intravenous route, this route would not require the use of an indwelling catheter. Such approaches have been used successfully in nonhuman primates,[150] with more recent work demonstrating its feasibility in rats[216] and mice.[110]

Historically, male animals have typically been used in drug self-administration studies. This focus was initially justified by higher rates of drug use and substance use disorder in men versus women.[10] However, gender differences have narrowed over time, and among current adolescent populations, rates of drug use and substance use disorder are often similar between males and females.[88-89,118] There are also important differences between men and women with respect to many aspects of substance use disorder, including initiation of use, the development of substance use disorder, and relapse and treatment.[151] In addition, sex differences are observed in animal models of substance use disorder, indicating a biological basis for the gender differences observed in humans.[186] Such differences also further support the need to include both sexes in studies on drugs as reinforcers and substance use disorder, a focus now mandated by the National Institutes of Health.[159]

Results from animal drug self-administration studies have revealed good correspondence between humans and animals; drugs abused by humans generally maintain responding in animals, whereas drugs that do not maintain responding in animals are typically not abused by humans, indicating this paradigm's utility for determining abuse liability.[1,46,91,107,163] In addition, similar patterns of drug intake have been reported in humans and animals for ethanol, opioids, nicotine, and cocaine self-administration.[90] These parallel results between the human and animal drug literature validate the animal model of drug self-administration and suggest that its use may lead to a better understanding of human drug-taking behavior and substance use disorder.

• BOX 6.1 | Definitions and Terms

This glossary of some of the terms used in studying drug reinforcement, drawn primarily from Iverson and Lattal,[106] is provided to aid in the reading of this chapter.

Acquisition: the process by which a new behavior, such as lever pressing for drug delivery, is added to the organism's behavioral repertoire.

Addicted phenotype: term used in preclinical studies to signify the development of one of more behavioral features believed to be analogous to features that are characteristic of human substance use disorder.[129] These features include an enhanced motivation for the drug, enhanced drug-seeking, and an enhanced choice for drug over nondrug rewards as compared to baseline or to short access controls. Compulsive use, or use despite negative consequences, has also been used to define its development.

Choice procedure: the allocation of one of two or more alternative, usually incompatible, responses.

Fixed-ratio schedule: a schedule in which a response is reinforced only after the animal has responded a specified number of times. For example, with a fixed-ratio 5 schedule of reinforcement, responding is reinforced after every five responses.

Incubation effect: a progressive increase, or incubation, of drug-seeking over abstinence, which is believed to model relapse vulnerability.

Operant behavior: emitted behavior that can be modified by its consequences (also termed instrumental behavior). This class of behavior is often referred to as purposeful or voluntary.

Progressive-ratio schedule: a higher-order schedule that requires the animal to emit an increasing number of responses for each successive reinforcer. For example, at the start of the session, the animal may be required to lever press once to receive a drug delivery, twice for the second drug delivery, four times for the third, eight times for the fourth, and so on.

Reinforcer: a stimulus event that strengthens the behavior that follows it.

Reinforcement: the *process* whereby a behavior is strengthened by the event that follows the behavior, and a *procedure* by which the contingencies between the reinforcers and behavior are arranged within a paradigm.

Reinforcing efficacy: the likelihood that a drug will serve as a reinforcer under various experimental conditions (also termed reinforcing strength). For example, a drug that is self-administered only when the work requirement to obtain a delivery is low (i.e., fixed-ratio 1) would be considered a weak reinforcer, whereas a drug that is self-administered under a variety of different experimental conditions and when the work requirement is high would be considered a strong reinforcer.

Reinstatement paradigm: a model of relapse whereby the animal is tested on responding on a lever that was formerly associated with the drug following reexposure to a small priming dose of the drug or the environmental stimuli associated with the drug. Stress also is often used as a trigger for drug-seeking behavior during reinstatement testing.

Self-administration: operant responding that directly produces drug deliveries.

Second-order schedule (higher-order schedule): a schedule that requires the completion of an individual component of the schedule that produces availability to the terminal event. A second schedule of reinforcement must then be completed to produce the terminal event. For example, under a second-order fixed-ratio 10 (i.e., fixed interval of 10 s) schedule of reinforcement, 10 successive fixed-interval schedules would have to be completed before a response is reinforced.

Substance use disorder (or addiction): defined in the *Diagnostic and Statistical Manual of Mental Disorders, Fifth Edition* (DSM-5)[8] as a disease resulting from use of a substance that the individual continues to take despite adverse consequences and characterized by impaired control over use of the drug, craving and urge to use the drug, and increased time spent seeking, using, and recovering from drug use.

In addition to screening drugs for abuse liability, the traditional self-administration procedure has been used to study, through biochemical and pharmacological manipulation, the neurobiological processes underlying the drug reinforcement process. For example, by demonstrating that lesions in some areas of the brain decrease or abolish self-administration behavior, we have developed an understanding of the neuroanatomical substrates for drug reinforcement (e.g., Wise and Bozarth[223]).

Assessing Reinforcing Efficacy

Despite the advances in our understanding of drug reinforcement in animals, reinforcing efficacy, or a drug's reinforcing strength, has been difficult to measure. The ability of a drug to support self-administration in laboratory animals under different experimental conditions is a measure of the drug's strength as a reinforcer.[21] Thus, a highly efficacious drug will be self-administered under a variety of experimental conditions such as low-dose conditions, conditions that require a large work effort, or enriched environmental conditions where other reinforcers are available as choices. In contrast, a weakly efficacious drug will be self-administered only under limited conditions such as food-restricted conditions, moderate- to high-dose conditions, conditions that require a low work effort, or impoverished environmental conditions where there are few or no other reinforcers available as choices. Such effects also depend on the route of drug self-administration. For example, under oral self-administration conditions, enriching the environment with toys or social peers can markedly reduce levels of opioid or psychostimulant drug intake,[6] whereas, under intravenous self-administration conditions, such environmental manipulations are much less effective.[23] Although it is generally believed that the reinforcing strength of a drug is related to its abuse liability, actually measuring reinforcing strength is not straightforward because factors other than the drug's reinforcing effects can, directly and indirectly, influence responding (i.e., satiating effects, direct effects on responding, and aversive effects).[132] The fixed-ratio schedule is typically used in studies investigating drug reinforcement in animals (e.g., 1–2 h sessions), and under these conditions, an inverted U-shaped relationship has been described between drug dose and rate of responding.[36,82,177–178] That is, as dose increases, responding initially increases (ascending limb) and then decreases (descending limb). At low doses, responding decreases and these doses may not maintain responding. However, doses on the descending limb, which would be presumed to be more efficacious than doses on the ascending limb, maintain quantitatively similar levels or even lower levels of responding than those maintained by doses on the ascending limb. This issue is problematic for the interpretation of changes in reinforcing efficacy in that it is difficult to determine the direction of the change.[132] A number of approaches have been taken to address this issue, including the use of rate-independent approaches such as the progressive-ratio schedule, the threshold procedure, second-order schedules, and choice procedures. Reinforcing efficacy is more readily determined using these approaches, and as such, they have been useful for determining changes as a result of pharmacological or environmental manipulation, or changes over time with the development of substance use disorder.

Progressive-Ratio Schedule

The progressive-ratio schedule is commonly used to evaluate the reinforcing strength of self-administered drugs, particularly psychostimulants. With this schedule, the ratio requirement to obtain a delivery progressively increases within a session, and the final ratio completed, or breakpoint, is believed to be a sensitive measure of motivation to obtain the drug (for a review, see Arnold and Roberts[11]). In contrast to the fixed-ratio schedule, the dose-effect curve under the progressive-ratio schedule is linear, whereby responding is directly related to reinforcer magnitude: an increase in the unit dose of the self-administered drug corresponds to an increase in breakpoint. This linear relationship allows for a more straightforward determination of the direction of change in reinforcing efficacy than is allowed by more traditional self-administration procedures. Other strengths are that responding for a particular dose of drug can be incredibly stable from day to day within subjects and that there are considerable individual differences in levels of responding between subjects. Sensitivity to pharmacological and environmental manipulations and to individual differences are thus strengths of the progressive-ratio schedule. Sex differences and hormonal influences on drug self-administration behavior are good examples of its sensitivity to individual differences in that under simple fixed-ratio schedules, sex differences and hormonal influences are generally not revealed, whereas, under progressive-ratio schedules, these factors robustly influence breakpoints (for a review, see Perry et al.[127]). Another advantage of this schedule is that it can be used reliably across different pharmacological classes of drugs including psychostimulants, nicotine, opiates, synthetic cathinones or "bath salts," and alcohol.[54,61,85,180,221] It has also been used successfully in several different species including rats, mice, and nonhuman primates[29,54,73] with parallel effects observed in laboratory studies in humans with substance use disorder.[203] However, as with the more traditional self-administration paradigms, the satiating and behavioral disruptive effects of drugs can also impact responding under a progressive-ratio schedule, particularly during earlier parts of the sessions, with high doses of the drug, and under low or slowly increasing progressive-ratio schedules.

Threshold Procedure

Recent studies have used the threshold procedure to disentangle reinforcing efficacy from satiating and behavioral disruptive effects. With this procedure, animals are given access to a descending series of drug doses under a fixed-ratio 1 schedule using either a between-session (i.e., dose progressively decreases with each successive daily session) or within-session approach (e.g., multiple doses are available each session with doses decreasing every 10 min[165,167,227]). The goal with either approach is to identify the lowest drug dose, or the threshold dose, that maintains self-administration. Each animal's motivation to obtain the drug and its preferred level of drug consumption are then determined using a behavioral economic analysis of the response/intake data.[20,167] For example, at suprathreshold doses, animals regulate their drug intake, presumably to a preferred level, such that as dose decreases, levels of responding increase. However, as dose further decreases and threshold is reached, the behavioral cost of maintaining the preferred level of intake exceeds the maximum acceptable price, and the animal stops responding.

The threshold procedure is similar to the progressive-ratio schedule in that the effort required to obtain drug (i.e., the price) progressively increases and allows for a sensitive measure of motivation for the drug. The two procedures appear to measure different aspects of motivation for drug in that one measures motivation to maintain a preferred level of drug intake (threshold), and the other measures motivation to obtain a particular dose of the drug (progressive-ratio). Like the progressive-ratio schedule, the threshold procedure appears to be sensitive to individual differences, pharmacological and environmental manipulations, and to changes over time within animals.[a] An added advantage of the threshold procedure is that it allows for an examination of effects on reinforcing efficacy versus consumption.[167] Although most studies using the threshold procedure have been conducted with cocaine, it has also been used successfully for remifentanil and nicotine self-administration.[86,87,182]

Second-Order Schedules

Second-order schedules have also been useful for minimizing issues of satiety and other rate-limiting effects of drugs on responding. Much of the early work using second-order schedules was conducted with nonhuman primates and focused on conditioned or secondary reinforcement (for a review, see Schindler et al. [193]). With this type of schedule, a nondrug stimulus, usually a light or a tone, takes on the characteristics of a reinforcer by its association with the drug delivery. Second-order schedules of drug delivery allow for the study of more complex behavioral sequences than do traditional self-administration procedures. Second-order schedules have also been used in studies with rats and mice,[57-58,119] and these studies have been useful for the investigation of drug-seeking behavior (i.e., responding for drug that occurs prior to drug availability or when the drug is no longer available) and its neurobiological mechanisms (e.g., Di Ciano[57] and Kumaresan et al.[117]).

Like the progressive-ratio schedule, second-order schedules minimize the descending limb of the dose-effect curve, allowing for determination of changes in reinforcing efficacy as a result of pharmacological or environmental manipulation. Another advantage is that high rates of behavior can be maintained by the conditioned reinforcer with relatively few actual primary reinforcers delivered. Nicotine is a good example of a drug that is robustly self-administered under second-order schedules, whereas, under simple fixed-ratio schedules, it has been more difficult to establish that it functions as a reinforcer.[83,96] In fact, even under more traditional self-administration paradigms, nicotine maintains more robust levels of responding when the drug deliveries are paired with a stimulus cue, such as a light.[28] However, one disadvantage of this approach is that it is often difficult to separate the reinforcing strength of the secondary reinforcer from that of the primary reinforcer.

Choice Procedures

Choice procedures are an increasingly popular tool for examining the reinforcing efficacy of drugs of abuse, particularly for work conducted in nonhuman primates (for review, see Banks,[15] Banks and Negus,[16] and Negus and Banks[160]). Early studies employing choice procedures showed that laboratory monkeys chose to self-administer a reinforcing drug over its vehicle.[109] The procedures used in choice experiments typically involve one of three types of experimental schedules: discrete trial schedules, concurrent

---

[a] References 32, 93, 112, 166, 195, 200, 227.

schedules, or concurrent chain schedules. Sessions typically begin with a sampling period during which the subject can respond to obtain each of the available reinforcers (i.e., a high versus a low drug dose or saline, or drug versus some other reinforcer, such as food). Animals then choose between the different reinforcer options in a series of trials by completing the response requirement on the lever associated with a particular reinforcer. Response allocation, rather than response frequency, provides a measure of the drug's reinforcing strength. This feature allows for the determination of reinforcing strength relative to behavior allocated toward an alternative reinforcer. As such, choice procedures are believed to mirror more directly the real-world situation where drug users allocate resources to obtain drugs rather than other nondrug reinforcers such as food and extracurricular activities.[155] Indeed, most self-administration studies conducted in humans with substance use disorder use choice procedures, where subjects choose between drug deliveries and a nondrug alternative such as money.[47]

Studies have shown that laboratory animals not only choose drug over saline deliveries, but also prefer higher doses of drugs. For example, Carroll[37] conducted a study in which monkeys chose between a standard dose of phencyclidine (0.25 mg/kg) or one of several other doses that were concurrently available (0.06, 0.12, 0.50, or 1.00 mg/kg), and found that subjects chose the large concentrations more often than the smaller ones. Similar results have been shown for a variety of other drugs including cocaine, ethanol, methadone, remifentanil, methylphenidate, and pentobarbital.[b] It is notable that larger doses have been shown to be preferred over lower doses even under conditions where the behavioral disruptive effects of the drug are apparent (i.e., conditions that allow for access to the moderate-to-high drug doses with relatively short interdose intervals[104]). One disadvantage with the choice procedure is that preference for high doses over lower ones and for drug versus nondrug rewards have been more difficult to show in rats,[35,103,123,217] with evidence suggesting that such effects may be restricted to a minority of vulnerable individuals.[3] However, recent work indicates that such preferences can occur in rats if they are given a drug-priming injection prior to the choice test[208,209,211,212,214] or if the delivery of the palatable alternative is delayed.[168] The likelihood of observing a preference for a large versus small drug dose or for drug versus nondrug reward can also be increased in rats following protracted abstinence from extended access self-administration[123] (see Cantin et al.[34]) indicating that such preferences may reflect the development of an addicted phenotype (see section on *Animal Models of Substance Use Disorder*). Such effects are also more likely to occur in female than in male rats, with results showing that female rats show a greater preference for drug versus nondrug rewards and show a greater increase in this preference over time as compared to male rats.[170]

Modeling Phases of Substance Use Disorder

The majority of the preclinical studies on substance use disorder have used the traditional self-administration paradigm or other conditions that limit drug intake—that is, maintenance conditions that produce stable and relatively low levels of self-administration. As such, the behavioral and neurobiological principles defined by these studies may be restricted to drug reinforcement and not necessarily characteristic of substance use disorder. Specifically, although the positive reinforcing effects of drugs are believed to be a primary mechanism mediating drug use during the early phases

of substance use disorder (i.e., during substance use initiation and maintenance), other characteristics appear to be critical for motivating drug use at later stages (i.e., following the development of substance use disorder, during relapse), such as a loss of control over use, compulsive use, and relief from craving. Several procedures have been developed to try to incorporate features of human substance use disorder that are not represented in more traditional procedures. These methods have focused on addressing critical questions regarding addiction, such as: "Why do some individuals develop substance use disorder but not others?" "What factors influence the transition from controlled or casual use to the development of substance use disorder?" and "What factors influence relapse or reinstatement of drug use?" The models that have been developed to address these questions are discussed below.

Animal Models of Drug Use Initiation

The reinforcing effects of a drug appear to be a primary determinant of vulnerability during the initiation or acquisition phase. Retrospective reports from individuals with substance use disorder reveal that the response to initial drug exposure varies from highly positive to negative,[78] and some evidence suggests that individual differences in sensitivity to drug reinforcement are predictive of later use.[50] Consistent with these clinical findings, there is considerable variability in laboratory animals in their propensity to self-administer drugs. Animal models of the acquisition phase have been developed to identify biological and behavioral factors underlying individual differences in vulnerability to the reinforcing effects of drugs of abuse that may apply to prevention efforts in humans (for a review, see Campbell and Carroll[33]). However, the acquisition phase is difficult to study because it is typically brief and is characterized by a sudden shift from low to high levels of intake. Thus, methods that slow the acquisition process and increase intersubject variability are necessary to observe this transitory period. For example, acquisition of drug self-administration is optimally investigated in drug- and experimentally-naive animals that are maintained under food-satiated conditions (e.g., food restriction serves as a stressor that can greatly accelerate the acquisition process and obscure individual differences) and tested under low dose conditions (e.g., high doses are associated with not only reinforcing effects but also direct effects and aversive effects that may interfere with responding). Under these conditions, individual differences are maximized, and some rats will acquire self-administration, whereas others will not; the question that is addressed is: "Which animals can detect the reinforcing effects of this low drug dose?"

A simple method of evaluating acquisition is to give an animal access to a drug during a daily experimental session, with deliveries available contingent upon an operant response (i.e., lever press; e.g., Davis et al.[51]). Another method that has been used to investigate individual differences in acquisition of drug self-administration is an autoshaping procedure. This procedure was adapted to the study of the acquisition of drug self-administration[38] from methods used to study the acquisition of food-reinforced responding.[27] With this method, daily sessions begin with a noncontingent drug administration component, wherein rats receive computer-automated infusions delivered on a random interval schedule that are paired with light cues and lever retraction. A self-administration component then follows wherein the lever remains extended and responses on it result in drug infusions. With both procedures, acquisition of drug self-administration is measured as the number of sessions needed to

---

[b]References 9, 104, 108, 116, 143, 153.

reach a criterion level of intake, which can be standardized and adjusted for dose and drug availability. The ratio of active to inactive lever-press responses is often used in conjunction with the intake criteria. All of the animals are included in the analyses, whether or not they acquire self-administration, and the focus is on how rapidly this process takes place and what percentage of each group of animals acquires drug-reinforced responding.

These acquisition methods have revealed a number of organismic and physiological factors that predict vulnerability to drug self-administration, such as genetic strain,[43,198,215] impulsivity,[22,173] exploratory behavior in a novel environment,[51,76,154,158] reactivity to stress,[52,66,176] innate saccharin preference,[84,171] dopamine release and receptor levels in brain regions associated with drug reward,[49,80–81,99,181] reactivity to injections of drugs[144,225] age,[94,196] and sex.[127] For example, we used an autoshaping procedure to train male and female rats to lever press for either cocaine infusions (0.2 mg/kg) or heroin infusion (0.015 mg/kg) under a fixed-ratio 1 schedule (i.e., one response per infusion[131]). Under these low-dose conditions, female rats acquired cocaine and heroin self-administration at a faster rate than male rats, and a greater percentage of female rats acquired cocaine self-administration than did male rats. Similar results of enhanced vulnerability in females have also been reported in several other studies for cocaine[41,102,128] and heroin,[41] and for other drugs including nicotine[61] and phencyclidine.[42] As mentioned previously, however, individual differences can be obscured under conditions that speed up the acquisition process. For example, a recent study showed that when rats are food restricted, which serves as a stressor and enhances rates of acquisition,[33] sex differences in rates of acquisition are reversed, and male rats acquire both cocaine and nicotine self-administration faster than female rats.[206]

Environmental factors, such as feeding condition, the presence of an alternative nondrug reinforcer, exercise, and drug history, can also greatly impact acquisition.[40,44,46,138] For example, several studies have reported that exercise via running in a wheel attenuates the acquisition of drug self-administration for numerous drugs of abuse including nicotine, cocaine, heroin, and methamphetamine (for review see Lynch et al.[135] and Lynch et al.[138]). The effects of exercise on acquisition are robust, and have been observed for both concurrent conditions, that is, when exercise is available during the self-administration session, and for nonconcurrent conditions, that is, when exercise precedes or follows the daily self-administration session, indicating that its effects extend beyond its ability to function as an alternative nondrug reinforcer. Rates of acquisition also vary widely as a function of drug dose, type of drug, and route of administration.[33] For example, under high-dose conditions with a drug that rapidly enters the brain after an intravenous infusion (i.e., cocaine), most, if not all, animals, will acquire self-administration rapidly. However, when lower intravenous doses of the drug are used, or an oral route of administration is used, fewer animals will acquire, and the rates of acquisition become much slower. Similarly, with drugs such as caffeine or alcohol, which are considered to have a less-intense or less-rapid onset of action, the acquisition process is slowed. With oral administration, the taste of the drug can also influence the probability and rates of acquisition (e.g., the acquisition of oral alcohol self-administration is relatively slow because animals typically have an aversion to the taste of unsweetened alcohol).

Although these studies provide insight on factors that influence the initial vulnerability to drug use and reinforcement, they do not necessarily reflect vulnerability factors for the development of substance use disorder. For example, in humans, although most

individuals have used drugs (i.e., greater than 90% if alcohol is included[204]), only a small percentage will develop a substance use disorder. Thus, recreational drug use does not invariably lead to the development of substance use disorder. This is also true for preclinical studies, with results suggesting that drug access conditions are critical for determining whether an animal will develop features characteristic of substance use disorder.

Animal Models of Substance Use Disorder

Two of the defining features of substance use disorder in humans—loss of control over drug use and the resulting excessive use of the drug—have been modeled in animals using several different methods (for a review, see Edwards and Koob,[64] Lynch,[129] and Roberts et al.[189]). For example, early studies showed that when nonhuman primates or rats were given unlimited 24-h/day access (i.e., each response is reinforced under a fixed-ratio 1 schedule) to intravenous infusions of psychostimulants such as cocaine, D-amphetamine, or methamphetamine, they self-administered high levels of the drug and displayed binge-abstinent patterns of intake with drug self-administration occurring erratically throughout each 24-h period.[24,53,109] Unlimited access to opiate drugs, such as heroin or morphine, also results in high levels of intake that increase, or escalate, rapidly over time.[24,53] Toxicity also develops rapidly under these conditions, particularly for psychostimulants and opiates, thus necessitating the use of procedures that limit access to these drugs in some way.

More recent studies have attempted to capture these features—excessive intake and a dysregulated or escalating pattern of drug use—but without serious signs of toxicity. For example, excessive drug intake with limited signs of toxicity has been observed under unlimited 24-h/day access conditions with low unit doses of drug[39] and under unlimited access conditions that restrict the number of hours of access each day (i.e., 6–12 h daily[4]) or each period of continuous access (i.e., 72 h[48,213]). The long access procedure developed by Ahmed and Koob[4] is probably the most well-established extended-access procedure. With this procedure, animals, typically rats, are given unlimited access (fixed-ratio 1) to intravenous infusions of a drug for 6–12 h/day. Toxicity is limited under these conditions, and animals self-administer high levels of the drug and show an escalating pattern of drug intake over time.[64] Escalation of intake has been observed under these conditions for numerous drugs of abuse including cocaine, methamphetamine, methylphenidate, heroin, fentanyl, oxycodone, and bath salts.[4,149,161,185,218] In addition, drug-use escalation has been observed in nonhuman primates and mice,[42,226] and for other routes of drug self-administration, including oral[42] and more recently, vapor self-administration of sufentanil.[216]

Another method that allows for extended access to the drug with limited toxicity is the discrete trial procedure, wherein animals are given 24-h access to drug infusions that are available in discrete 10-min trials.[71] With this method, excessive intake and binge-abstinent patterns of use are observed as access conditions increase. For example, under short-access conditions (1–2 discrete trials/h; 1 infusion/trial), rats consume low and stable levels of drug and show a diurnally regulated pattern of intake (i.e., intake occurs predominantly during the dark phase).[188] However, under extended-access conditions (i.e., four discrete trials/h, 1.5 mg/kg/infusion), rats self-administer high levels of drug in "binge-abstinent" patterns, taking nearly every infusion available for the first 1–2 days, followed by periods of self-imposed abstinence interspersed with periods of active drug use. Although most of the work conducted with this procedure has focused on cocaine self-administration, similar findings of high intake and binge-abstinent patterns of use have also been reported for heroin and the combination of cocaine and heroin self-administration.[148,220] A variation of this procedure was developed recently that allows multiple infusions within each trial, thus allowing animals to choose their preferred "dose."[227] With this model, the intermittent-access model, rats have unlimited fixed-ratio 1 access to cocaine or methylphenidate infusions within 5-min discrete trials that initiate every 30 or 60 min for up to 24-h/day.[7,30,31,32,200] Under these conditions, rats self-administer high levels of the drug in repeated binge cycles and show an escalation in total daily levels of drug intake as well as dose escalation within trials. One advantage of this procedure over the other methods is that it appears to induce both escalation of intake and binge-abstinent patterns of use.

It is important to note that other critical features of substance use disorder, including increased motivation for the drug, use despite negative consequences, and increased drug-seeking and relapse vulnerability, are also observed following extended-access self-administration, particularly when behavior is examined after an abstinence period.[74,75,77,129,217] For example, a history of escalating cocaine, methamphetamine, and heroin self-administration under the long-access procedure has been shown to lead to enhanced drug-seeking following protracted abstinence (i.e., 7 days or more) as compared to earlier time-points during abstinence or to short-access controls.[5,115,146,190] It also induces incubation of drug-seeking, or the progressive increase in drug-seeking over abstinence,[217] as well as persistent responding despite concomitant punishment (e.g., drug deliveries are paired with shock[77]), a feature believed to reflect use despite negative consequences.[202] Extended-access drug self-administration under the discrete trial procedure also induces high levels of drug-seeking and its incubation over abstinence, as well as an enhanced motivation for the drug.[c] Specifically, 10 days of access to cocaine under the discrete trial procedure (4 trials/h) resulted in a sustained increase from baseline levels of progressive-ratio responding for the drug when assessed following an abstinence period of 7 days or more.[62,125,157,183,184] Notably, when motivation is assessed at earlier time-points during abstinence, it is either decreased or not different from baseline or short-access controls,[141,156,188] indicating that, like drug-seeking behavior, motivation for drug may incubate over abstinence.

Other drugs, such as nicotine and ethanol, typically can be available under unlimited-access conditions with limited toxicity, and results from studies with these types of drugs have also revealed "addiction-like" behavioral phenotypes. For example, Wolffgramm and Heyne developed an animal model of this transitional phase for oral alcohol, etonitazene, and amphetamine self-administration in rats.[97,224] Their procedure entails long-term ad libitum self-administration (1–2 months) followed by an extended drug abstinence period (4–9 months). Subsequently, rats were retested on self-administration behavior, and those animals that developed escalating patterns of intake prior to abstinence, self-administered higher levels of intake compared with rats that did not show escalation. These animals were also resistant to punishment and continued to self-administer the drug even after it was adulterated with bitter-tasting quinine. Similar effects can also be observed under shorter-term self-administration conditions and following shorter periods of abstinence when access

conditions are cyclical and alternate between self-administration and abstinence.[45,95,100,201]

Access conditions, drug dose, route of administration, and the drug being self-administered are crucial factors for the observation of excessive and dysregulated patterns of self-administration and the subsequent development of an addicted phenotype.[4,114,129,132,188] The time-course for the development of certain features of substance use disorder also appears to differ between the different extended access procedures. For example, several recent studies have shown that extended access under the intermittent-access procedure reliably induces an enhanced motivation for the drug as soon as 18 h after the last self-administration session.[112] Seven days appears to be a threshold condition for the induction of this motivational shift following self-administration under the discrete trial procedure.[140,183,184] The time-course also appears to be prolonged following self-administration under the long-access procedure, with results from several studies showing that motivation is unchanged from baseline even when assessed after 5 or more days of abstinence.[125,156,166,188] This interpretation is also consistent with results showing that key molecular correlates for the incubation of drug-seeking emerge 3–4 weeks after self-administration under the long-access procedure.[126]

Individual differences during this transition phase also have been reported. For example, female rats require less drug exposure and/or shorter periods of abstinence than male rats to display an increased motivation for cocaine,[140] and in female rats, estradiol may be required for its development.[184] A high preference for sweets, level of anxiety, and level of reactivity to stress, drug injections, and novelty, as well as a preference for drug over food, have also been reported to predict a vulnerability for the development of an addicted phenotype including drug escalation/dysregulation, enhanced motivation, and drug-seeking behavior.[d] Notably, the underlying neurobiology associated with extended-access drug self-administration is different from the neurobiology associated with short-access drug self-administration.[e] Such differences may be critical from a medication development standpoint, since they indicate that it may be necessary to use self-administration models that induce an addicted phenotype to identify treatments for substance use disorder.

Animal Models of Relapse

Relapse, or recurrent resumption of drug use after abstinence, is one of the most challenging problems in the treatment of substance use disorder.[8] Various types of stimuli can precipitate relapse, including internal cues such as reexposure to small "priming" doses of the drug or stress and external cues such as specific people and places that were associated with drug use. Often, external stimuli lead to drug use, and then internal stimuli sustain relapse.[25] Animal models of relapse have been developed and have provided critical information on the neurobiological mechanisms underlying vulnerability to relapse.[60,121,197,217]

One model that has been used to investigate mechanisms underlying drug-seeking and relapse vulnerability over abstinence is the reinstatement paradigm.[111,217] With this procedure, animals are trained to self-administer a drug and, once stable, responding is extinguished by discontinuing drug delivery. After responding reaches some criterion of unresponsiveness (e.g., fewer than 10 responses/session or h), the ability of various stimuli to reinstate

---

[c] References 62, 125, 134, 140, 156, 183, 184.

[d] References 13, 64, 98, 122, 145, 170, 172.
[e] References 12, 19, 26, 62, 69, 79, 152, 183, 207.

drug seeking is determined under conditions of nonreinforcement (i.e., responding is no longer reinforced by the drug). Extinction and reinstatement testing typically occur following the self-administration component during abstinence either within a single session (e.g., six 1-h extinction sessions followed by a 1-h reinstatement session all run with 1-day[2,18]), or over multiple daily sessions (e.g., daily 1-h extinction sessions followed by a 1-h reinstatement session conducted on a separate day[147,164,194]). This sequence of events, self-administration, extinction, and reinstatement, can also occur all within a single session (e.g., de Wit and Stewart[55] and de Wit and Stewart[56]). Results from preclinical studies using the reinstatement procedure have revealed that, like in humans, in laboratory animals, multiple stimuli can trigger drug-seeking behavior including priming doses of the drug, stress, and drug-associated cues (for a review, see Katz and Higgins[111]). These parallel findings validate the reinstatement model, and indicate its utility for screening potential interventions for relapse prevention in humans as well as for studying factors influencing and mechanisms underlying relapse.

Although most of the early studies using the reinstatement paradigm determined effects following short-access self-administration, more recent work has focused on determining effects following extended-access self-administration, given that levels of drug-seeking are higher and involve different neurobiological mechanisms following extended versus short-access self-administration.[f] Current studies also focus predominantly on characterizing changes following protracted abstinence, when levels of drug-seeking are known to be high.[179,217] Specifically, numerous studies have shown that drug-seeking increases, or incubates, over a protracted period of abstinence. This effect has been reported in several species including rats, mice, and nonhuman primates,[22,92,162,222] as well as humans,[17,124,169,219] and for numerous drugs of abuse including cocaine, nicotine, methamphetamine, alcohol, and heroin self-administration.[179] Notably, several recent studies have shown that the incubation of cocaine, nicotine, and methamphetamine-seeking can be blocked through the use of exercise during abstinence.[g] The availability of nondrug rewards, such as saccharin, toys, or other environmental enrichments during abstinence, have also been shown to block the incubation of drug-seeking following protracted abstinence.[41,139,142,199]

A number of factors are known to predict a vulnerability to seeking drugs following abstinence from short-access self-administration including high preference for saccharin, high responsiveness to acute and chronic drug exposure and novelty, risky decision making, a pattern of drug intake prior to reinstatement testing, age, and sex.[67,68,128,172,205] Although less work has focused on identifying factors predictive of vulnerability following extended-access self-administration, results from the available studies indicate that similar factors are involved including saccharin preference, impulsivity, avoidance of a drug-paired taste cue, age, and sex.[59,63,105,172,185] Notably, there appear to be important interactions of cues used to trigger reinstatement responding and vulnerability factors. For example, although female rats show enhanced reinstatement responding compared with male rats following exposure to priming injections of a drug,[185] male and female rats have been reported to respond at similar levels following exposure to drug-associated cues.[127] Similar results have been reported in laboratory studies in men and women with substance use disorder (for a review, see Lynch et al.[137]), suggesting

that vulnerability to relapse may be due to a complex interplay of environmental and biological factors.

Conclusions

Traditional self-administration procedures have firmly established that drugs of abuse function as reinforcers in animals. Although the reinforcing effects of drugs are certainly important in the initiation of substance use disorder, it is becoming increasingly apparent that other factors are involved at later stages. The shift to focusing on vulnerability factors for substance use disorder and the use of models that mimic more closely characteristics of substance use disorder in humans is likely to advance our ability to understand the key factors involved and, ultimately, to identify potential pharmacological and environmental treatments.

References

1. Aarde SM, Taffe MA. Predicting the abuse liability of entactogen-class, new and emerging psychoactive substances via preclinical models of drug self-administration. *Curr Top Behav Neurosci.* 2017;32:145–164.
2. Adhikary S, Caprioli D, Venniro M, Kallenberger P, Shaham Y, Bossert JM. Incubation of extinction responding and cue-induced reinstatement, but not context- or drug priming-induced reinstatement, after withdrawal from methamphetamine. *Addict Biol.* 2017;22(4):977–990.
3. Ahmed SH. Trying to make sense of rodents' drug choice behavior. *Prog Neuropsychopharmacol Biol Psychiatry.* 2018. [Epub ahead of print].
4. Ahmed SH, Koob GF. Transition from moderate to excessive drug intake: change in hedonic set point. *Science.* 1998;282(5387):298–300.
5. Ahmed SH, Walker JR, Koob GF. Persistent increase in the motivation to take heroin in rats with a history of drug escalation. *Neuropsychopharmacology.* 2000;22(4):413–421.
6. Alexander BK, Beyerstein BL, Hadaway PF, Coambs RB. Effect of early and later colony housing on oral ingestion of morphine in rats. *Pharmacol Biochem Behav.* 1981;15(4):571–576.
7. Allain F, Bouayad-Gervais K, Samaha AN. High and escalating levels of cocaine intake are dissociable from subsequent incentive motivation for the drug in rats. *Psychopharmacology.* 2018;235(1):317–328.
8. American Psychiatric Association. *Diagnostic and Statistical Manual of Mental Disorders.* 5th ed. Washington, DC: American Psychiatric Association; 2013.
9. Anderson KG, Woolverton WL. Effects of dose and infusion delay on cocaine self-administration choice in rhesus monkeys. *Psychopharmacology.* 2003;167(4):424–430.
10. Anderson TL. Drug use and gender. Encyclopedia of criminology and deviant behavior. 2001;4(2):286–289.
11. Arnold JM, Roberts DC. A critique of fixed and progressive ratio schedules used to examine the neural substrates of drug reinforcement. *Pharmacol Biochem Behav.* 1997;57(3):441–447.
12. Backes E, Hemby SE. Discrete cell gene profiling of ventral tegmental dopamine neurons after acute and chronic cocaine self-administration. *J Pharmacol Exp Ther.* 2003;307(2):450–459.
13. Ball KT, Slane M. Tolerance to the locomotor-activating effects of 3,4-methylenedioxymethamphetamine (MDMA) predicts escalation of MDMA self-administration and cue-induced reinstatement of MDMA seeking in rats. *Behav Brain Res.* 2014;274:143–148.
14. Balster RL, Kilbey MM, Ellinwood EH Jr. Methamphetamine self-administration in the cat. *Psychopharmacologia.* 1976;46(3):229–233.
15. Banks ML. Utility of preclinical drug versus food choice procedures to evaluate candidate medications for methamphetamine use disorder. *Ann N Y Acad Sci.* 2007;1394(1):92–105.

---

[f]References 62, 70, 113, 115, 126, 146, 179, 190, 194.
[g]References 130, 136, 164, 174, 175, 191, 192.

16. Banks ML, Negus SS. Insights from preclinical choice models on treating drug addiction. *Trends Pharmacol Sci.* 2017;38(2):181–194.

17. Bedi G, Preston KL, Epstein DH, Heishman SJ, Marrone GF, Shaham Y, et al. Incubation of cue-induced cigarette craving during abstinence in human smokers. *Biol Psychiatry.* 2011;69(7):708–711.

18. Beiter RM, Peterson AB, Abel J, Lynch WJ. Exercise during early, but not late abstinence, attenuates subsequent relapse vulnerability in a rat model. *Transl Psychiatry.* 2016;6:e792.

19. Ben-Shahar O, Moscarello JM, Ettenberg A. One hour, but not six hours, of daily access to self-administered cocaine results in elevated levels of the dopamine transporter. *Brain Res.* 2006;1095(1):148–153.

20. Bentzley BS, Fender KM, Aston-Jones G. The behavioral economics of drug self-administration: a review and new analytical approach for within-session procedures. *Psychopharmacology.* 2013;226(1):113–125.

21. Bergman J, Paronis CA. Measuring the reinforcing strength of abused drugs. *Mol Interv.* 2006;6(5):273–283.

22. Bird J, Schenk S. Contribution of impulsivity and novelty-seeking to the acquisition and maintenance of MDMA self-administration. *Addict Biol.* 2013;18(4):654–664.

23. Bozarth MA, Murray A, Wise RA. Influence of housing conditions on the acquisition of intravenous heroin and cocaine self-administration in rats. *Pharmacol Biochem Behav.* 1989;33(4):903–907.

24. Bozarth MA, Wise RA. Toxicity associated with long-term intravenous heroin and cocaine self-administration in the rat. *JAMA.* 1985;254(1):81–83.

25. Bradizza CM, Stasiewicz PR, Maisto SA. A conditioning reinterpretation of cognitive events in alcohol and drug cue exposure. *J Behav Ther Exp Psychiatr.* 1994;25(1):15–22.

26. Briand LA, Flagel SB, Garcia-Fuster MJ, Watson SJ, Akil H, Sarter M, et al. Persistent alterations in cognitive function and prefrontal dopamine D2 receptors following extended, but not limited, access to self-administered cocaine. *Neuropsychopharmacology.* 2008;33:2969–2980.

27. Brown PL, Jenkins HM. Auto-shaping of the pigeon's keypeck. *J Exp Anal Behav.* 1968;11:1–8.

28. Caggiula AR, Donny EC, Chaudhri N, Perkins KA, Evans-Martin FF, Sved AF. Importance of nonpharmacological factors in nicotine self-administration. *Physiol Behav.* 2002;77(4–5):683–687.

29. Caine SB, Thomsen M, Barrett AC, et al. Cocaine self-administration in dopamine D3 receptor knockout mice. *Exp Clin Psychopharmacol.* 2012;20(5):352–363.

30. Calipari ES, Ferris MJ, Siciliano CA, Zimmer BA, Jones SR. Intermittent cocaine self-administration produces sensitization of stimulant effects at the dopamine transporter. *J Pharmacol Exp Ther.* 2014;349(2):192–198.

31. Calipari ES, Jones SR. Sensitized nucleus accumbens dopamine terminal responses to methylphenidate and dopamine transporter releasers after intermittent-access self-administration. *Neuropharmacology.* 2014;82:1–10.

32. Calipari ES, Siciliano CA, Zimmer BA, Jones SR. Brief intermittent cocaine self-administration and abstinence sensitizes cocaine effects on the dopamine transporter and increases drug seeking. *Neuropsychopharmacology.* 2015;40:728–735.

33. Campbell UC, Carroll ME. Acquisition of drug self-administration: environmental and pharmacological interventions. *Exp Clin Psychopharmacol.* 2000;8(3):312–325.

34. Cantin L, Lenoir M, Augier E, et al. Cocaine is low on the value ladder of rats: possible evidence for resilience to addiction. *PLoS One.* 2010;5(7):e11592.

35. Caprioli D, Zeric T, Thorndike EB, Venniro M. Persistent palatable food preference in rats with a history of limited and extended access to methamphetamine self-administration. *Addict Biol.* 2015;20(5):913–926.

36. Carney JM, Llewellyn ME, Woods JH. Variable interval responding maintained by intravenous codeine and ethanol injections in the rhesus monkey. *Pharmacol Biochem Behav.* 1976;5(5):552–577.

37. Carroll ME. Concurrent access to two concentrations of orally delivered phencyclidine: effects of feeding conditions. *J Exp Anal Behav.* 1987;47(3):347–362.

38. Carroll ME, Lac ST. Autoshaping i.v. cocaine self-administration in rats: effects of nondrug alternative reinforcers on acquisition. *Psychopharmacology.* 1993;110(1–2):5–12.

39. Carroll ME, Lac ST. Acquisition of i.v. amphetamine and cocaine self-administration in rats as a function of dose. *Psychopharmacology.* 1997;129(3):206–214.

40. Carroll ME, Lac ST, Nygaard SL. A concurrently available nondrug reinforcer prevents the acquisition or decreases the maintenance of cocaine-reinforced behavior. *Psychopharmacology.* 1989;97(1):23–29.

41. Carroll ME, Morgan AD, Lynch WJ, Campbell UC, Dess NK. Intravenous cocaine and heroin self-administration in rats selectively bred for differential saccharin intake: phenotype and sex differences. *Psychopharmacology.* 2002;161(3):304–313.

42. Carroll ME, Roth ME, Voeller RK, Nguyen PD. Acquisition of oral phencyclidine self-administration in rhesus monkeys: effect of sex. *Psychopharmacology.* 2000;149(4):401–408.

43. Chen H, Luo R, Gong S, Matta SG, Sharp BM. Protection genes in nucleus accumbens shell affect vulnerability to nicotine self-administration across isogenic strains of adolescent rat. *PLoS One.* 2014;9(1):e86214.

44. Childs E, Shoaib M, Stolerman IP. Cocaine self-administration in rats with histories of cocaine exposure and discrimination. *Psychopharmacology.* 2006;186(2):168–176.

45. Cohen A, Koob GF, George O. Robust escalation of nicotine intake with extended access to nicotine self-administration and intermittent periods of abstinence. *Neuropsychopharmacology.* 2012;37(9):2153–2160.

46. Collins RJ, Weeks JR, Cooper MM, Good PI, Russell RR. Prediction of abuse liability of drugs using IV self-administration by rats. *Psychopharmacology.* 1984;82:6–13.

47. Comer SD, Ashworth JB, Foltin RW, Johanson CE, Zacny JP, Walsh SL. The role of human drug self-administration procedures in the development of medications. *Drug Alcohol Depend.* 2008;96(1–2):1–15.

48. Cornett EM, Goeders NE. 96-hour methamphetamine self-administration in male and female rats: a novel model of human methamphetamine addiction. *Pharmacol Biochem Behav.* 2013;111:51–57.

49. Czoty PW, Gage HD, Nader SH, Reboussin BA, Bounds M, Nader MA. PET imaging of dopamine D2 receptor and transporter availability during acquisition of cocaine self-administration in rhesus monkeys. *J Addict Med.* 1(1):33–39.

50. Davidson ES, Finch JF, Schenk S. Variability in subjective responses to cocaine: initial experiences of college students. *Addict Behav.* 1993;18:445–453.

51. Davis BA, Clinton SM, Akil H, Becker JB. The effects of novelty-seeking phenotypes and sex differences on acquisition of cocaine self-administration in selectively bred high-responder and low-responder rats. *Pharmacol Biochem Behav.* 2008;90(3):331–338.

52. Deminiere JM, Piazza PV, Le Moal M, Simon H. Experimental approach to individual vulnerability to psychostimulant addiction. *Neurosci Biobehav Rev.* 1989;13(2–3):141–147.

53. Deneau G, Yanagita T, Seevers MH. Self-administration of psychoactive substances by the monkey. *Psychopharmacologia.* 1969;16(1):30–48.

54. Depoortere RY, Li DH, Lane JD, Emmett-Oglesby MW. Parameters of self-administration of cocaine in rats under a progressive-ratio schedule. *Pharmacol Biochem Behav.* 1993;45(3):539–548.

55. de Wit H, Stewart J. Reinstatement of cocaine-reinforced responding in the rat. *Psychopharmacology*. 1981;75(2):134–143.

56. de Wit H, Stewart J. Drug reinstatement of heroin-reinforced responding in the rat. *Psychopharmacology*. 1983;1:29–31.

57. Di Ciano P. Drug seeking under a second-order schedule of reinforcement depends on dopamine D3 receptors in the basolateral amygdala. *Behav Neurosci*. 2008;122(1):129–139.

58. Di Ciano P, Everitt BJ. Conditioned reinforcing properties of stimuli paired with self-administered cocaine, heroin or sucrose: implications for the persistence of addictive behaviour. *Neuropharmacology*. 2004;47(Suppl 1):202–213.

59. Doherty J, Ogbomnwan Y, Williams B, Frantz K. Age-dependent morphine intake and cue-induced reinstatement, but not escalation in intake, by adolescent and adult male rats. *Pharmacol Biochem Behav*. 2009;92(1):164–172.

60. Dong Y, Taylor JR, Wolf ME, Shaham Y. Circuit and synaptic plasticity mechanisms of drug relapse. *J Neurosci*. 2017;37(45):10867–10876.

61. Donny EC, Caggiula AR, Mielke MM, et al. Nicotine self-administration in rats on a progressive ratio schedule of reinforcement. *Psychopharmacology*. 1999;147(2):135–142.

62. Doyle SE, Ramôa C, Garber G, Newman J, Toor Z, Lynch WJ. A shift in the role of glutamatergic signaling in the nucleus accumbens core with the development of an addicted phenotype. *Biol Psychiatry*. 2014;76(10):810–815.

63. Economidou D, Pelloux Y, Robbins TW, Dalley JW, Everitt BJ. High impulsivity predicts relapse to cocaine-seeking after punishment-induced abstinence. *Biol Psychiatry*. 2009;65(10):851–856.

64. Edwards S, Koob GF. Escalation of drug self-administration as a hallmark of persistent addiction liability. *Behav Pharmacol*. 2013;24(5-6):356–362.

65. Edwards S, Baynes BB, Carmichael CY, et al. Traumatic stress reactivity promotes excessive alcohol drinking and alters the balance of prefrontal cortex-amygdala activity. *Transl Psychiatry*. 2013;3:e296.

66. Ewing Corcoran SB, Howell LL. Impact of early life stress on the reinforcing and behavioral-stimulant effects of psychostimulants in rhesus monkeys. *Behav Pharmacol*. 2010;21(1):69–76.

67. Fattore L, Piras G, Corda MG, Giorgi O. The Roman high- and low-avoidance rat lines differ in the acquisition, maintenance, extinction, and reinstatement of intravenous cocaine self-administration. *Neuropsychopharmacology*. 2009;34:1091–1101.

68. Ferland JN, Winstanley CA. Risk-preferring rats make worse decisions and show increased incubation of craving after cocaine self-administration. *Addict Biol*. 2017;22(4):991–1001.

69. Ferrario CR, Gorny G, Crombag HS, Li Y, Kolb B, Robinson TE. Neural and behavioral plasticity associated with the transition from controlled to escalated cocaine use. *Biol Psychiatry*. 2005;58(9):751–759.

70. Fischer KD, Houston AC, Rebec GV. Role of the major glutamate transporter GLT1 in nucleus accumbens core versus shell in cue-induced cocaine-seeking behavior. *J Neurosci*. 2013;33(22):9319–9327.

71. Fitch TE, Roberts DC. The effects of dose and access restrictions on the periodicity of cocaine self-administration in the rat. *Drug Alcohol Depend*. 1993;33(2):119–128.

72. Foltin RW. Food and cocaine self-administration by baboons: effects of alternatives. *J Exp Anal Behav*. 1999;72(2):215–234.

73. Freeman KB, McMaster BC, Roma PG, Woolverton WL. Assessment of the effects of contingent histamine injections on the reinforcing effectiveness of cocaine using behavioral economic and progressive-ratio designs. *Psychopharmacology*. 2014;231(12):2395–2403.

74. Galli G, Wolffgramm J. Long-term voluntary D-amphetamine consumption and behavioral predictors for subsequent D-amphetamine addiction in rats. *Drug Alcohol Depend*. 2004;73(1):51–60.

75. Galli G, Wolffgramm J. Long-term development of excessive and inflexible nicotine taking by rats, effects of a novel treatment approach. *Behav Brain Res*. 2011;217(2):261–270.

76. Gancarz AM, San George MA, Ashrafioun L, Richards JB. Locomotor activity in a novel environment predicts both responding for a visual stimulus and self-administration of a low dose of methamphetamine in rats. *Behav Processes*. 2011;86(2):295–304.

77. Gancarz-Kausch AM, Adank DN, Dietz DM. Prolonged withdrawal following cocaine self-administration increases resistance to punishment in a cocaine binge. *Sci Rep*. 2014;4:6876.

78. Gawin FH. Cocaine abuse and addiction. *J Fam Pract*. 1989;29(2):193–197.

79. George O, Mandyam CD, Wee S, Koob GF. Extended access to cocaine self-administration produces long-lasting prefrontal cortex-dependent working memory impairments. *Neuropsychopharmacology*. 2008;33:2474–2482.

80. Glick SD, Merski C, Steindorf S, Wang S, Keller RW, Carlson JN. Neurochemical predisposition to self-administer morphine in rats. *Brain Res*. 1992;578(1–2):215–220.

81. Glick SD, Raucci J, Wang S, Keller Jr RW, Carlson JN. Neurochemical predisposition to self-administer cocaine in rats: individual differences in dopamine and its metabolites. *Brain Res*. 1994;653(1–2):148–154.

82. Goldberg SR, Hoffmeister F, Schlichting UU, Wuttke W. A comparison of pentobarbital and cocaine self-administration in rhesus monkeys: effects of dose and fixed-ratio parameter. *J Pharmacol Exp Ther*. 1971;179(2):277–283.

83. Goldberg SR, Spealman RD, Risner ME, Henningfield JE. Control of behavior by intravenous nicotine injections in laboratory animals. *Pharmacol Biochem Behav*. 1983;19(6):1011–1020.

84. Gosnell BA, Krahn DD, Yracheta JM, Harasha BJ. The relationship between intravenous cocaine self-administration and avidity for saccharin. *Pharmacol Biochem Behav*. 1998;60(1):229–236.

85. Grasing K, Li N, He S, Parrish C, Delich J, Glowa J. A new progressive ratio schedule for support of morphine self-administration in opiate dependent rats. *Psychopharmacology*. 2003;168(4):387–396.

86. Grebenstein P, Burroughs D, Zhang Y, LeSage MG. Sex differences in nicotine self-administration in rats during progressive unit dose reduction: implications for nicotine regulation policy. *Pharmacol Biochem Behav*. 2013;114-115:70–81.

87. Grebenstein PE, Burroughs D, Roiko SA, Pentel PR, LeSage MG. Predictors of the nicotine reinforcement threshold, compensation, and elasticity of demand in a rodent model of nicotine reduction policy. *Drug Alcohol Depend*. 2015;151:181–193.

88. Greenfield SF, Back SE, Lawson K, Brady KT. Substance abuse in women. *Psychiatr Clin North Am*. 2010;33(2):339–355.

89. Greenfield SF, Manwani SG, Nargiso JE. Epidemiology of substance use disorders in women. *Obstet Gynecol Clin North Am*. 2003;30(3):413–446.

90. Griffiths RR, Bigelow GE, Henningfield JE. Similarities in animal and human drug-taking behavior. In: Mello NK, ed. *Advances in Substance Abuse*. CT: JAI; 1980:1–90.

91. Griffiths RR, Brady JV, Bradford LD. Predicting the abuse liability of drugs with animal drug self-administration procedures: psychomotor stimulants and hallucinogens. In: Thompson T, Dews P, eds. *Advances in Behavioral Pharmacology*. Vol. 2. New York: Academic; 1979:163–208.

92. Grimm JW, Hope BT, Wise RA, Shaham Y. Neuroadaptation. Incubation of cocaine craving after withdrawal. *Nature*. 2001;412(6843):141–142.

93. Groblewski PA, Zietz C, Willuhn I, Phillips PE, Chavkin C. Repeated stress exposure causes strain-dependent shifts in the behavioral economics of cocaine in rats. *Addict Biol*. 2015;20(2):297–301.

94. Hankosky ER, Westbrook SR, Haake RM, Marinelli M, Gulley JM. Reduced sensitivity to reinforcement in adolescent compared

to adult Sprague-Dawley rats of both sexes. *Psychopharmacology.* 2018. [Epub ahead of print].

95. Hauser SR, Deehan Jr GA, Knight CP, Toalston JE, McBride WJ, Rodd ZA. Parameters of context-induced ethanol (EtOH)-seeking in alcohol-preferring (P) rats: temporal analysis, effects of repeated deprivation, and EtOH priming injections. *Alcohol Clin Exp Res.* 2016;40(10):2229–2239.

96. Henningfield JE, Smith TT, Kleykamp BA, Fant RV, Donny EC. Nicotine self-administration research: the legacy of Steven R. Goldberg and implications for regulation, health policy, and research. *Psychopharmacology.* 2016;233(23-24):3829–3848.

97. Heyne A, Wolffgramm J. The development of addiction to d-amphetamine in an animal model: same principles as for alcohol and opiate. *Psychopharmacology.* 1998;140(4):510–518.

98. Homberg JR, Karel P, Verheij MM. Individual differences in cocaine addiction: maladaptive behavioural traits. *Addict Biol.* 2014;19(4):517–528.

99. Homberg JR, van den Akker M, Raasø HS, et al. Enhanced motivation to self-administer cocaine is predicted by self-grooming behaviour and relates to dopamine release in the rat medial prefrontal cortex and amygdala. *Eur J Neurosci.* 2002;15(9):1542–1550.

100. Hopf FW, Chang SJ, Sparta DR, Bowers MS, Bonci A. Motivation for alcohol becomes resistant to quinine adulteration after 3 to 4 months of intermittent alcohol self-administration. *Alcohol Clin Exp Res.* 2010;34(9):1565–1573.

101. Howell LL, Fantegrossi WE. Intravenous drug self-administration in nonhuman primates. In: Buccafusco JJ, ed. *Methods of Behavior Analysis in Neuroscience.* 2nd ed. Boca Raton (FL): CRC Press/Taylor & Francis; 2009:Chapter 9.

102. Hu M, Crombag HS, Robinson TE, Becker JB. Biological basis of sex differences in the propensity to self-administer cocaine. *Neuropsychopharmacology.* 2004;29(1):81–85.

103. Huynh C, Fam J, Ahmed SH, Clemens KJ. Rats quit nicotine for a sweet reward following an extensive history of nicotine use. *Addict Biol.* 2017;22(1):142–151.

104. Iglauer C, Llewellyn ME, Woods JH. Concurrent schedules of cocaine injection in rhesus monkeys: dose variations under independent and non-independent variable-interval procedures. *Pharmacol Rev.* 1975;27(3):367–383.

105. Imperio CG, Grigson PS. Greater avoidance of a heroin-paired taste cue is associated with greater escalation of heroin self-administration in rats. *Behav Neurosci.* 2015;129(4):380–388.

106. Iverson IH, Lattal KA. Experimental analysis of behavior. In: Huston JP, ed. *Techniques in the Behavioral and Neural Sciences.* Vol. 6. New York: Elsevier; 1991.

107. Johanson CE, Balster RL. A summary of the results of a drug self-administration study using substitution procedures in rhesus monkeys. *Bull Narc.* 1978;30:43–54.

108. Johanson CE, Balster RL, Bonese K. Self-administration of psychomotor stimulant drugs: the effects of unlimited access. *Pharmacol Biochem Behav.* 1976;4(1):45–51.

109. Johanson CE, Schuster CR. A choice procedure for drug reinforcers: cocaine and methylphenidate in the rhesus monkey. *J Pharmacol Exp Ther.* 1975;193(2):676–688.

110. Juarez-Portilla C, Kim RD, Robotham M, et al. Voluntary inhalation of methamphetamine: a novel strategy for studying intake non-invasively. *Psychopharmacology.* 2017;234(5):739–747.

111. Katz JL, Higgins ST. The validity of the reinstatement model of craving and relapse to drug use. *Psychopharmacology.* 2003;168(1–2):21–30.

112. Kawa AB, Bentzley BS, Robinson TE. Less is more prolonged intermittent access cocaine self-administration procedures incentive-sensitization and addiction-like behavior. *Psychopharmacology (Berl).* 2016;233:3587–3602.

113. Kippin TE, Fuchs RA, See RE. Contributions of prolonged contingent and noncontingent cocaine exposure to enhanced reinstatement of cocaine seeking in rats. *Psychopharmacology.* 2006;187(1):60–67.

114. Kitamura O, Wee S, Specio SE, Koob GF, Pulvirenti L. Escalation of methamphetamine self-administration in rats: a dose-effect function. *Psychopharmacology.* 2006;186(1):48–53.

115. Knackstedt LA, Kalivas PW. Extended access to cocaine self-administration enhances drug-primed reinstatement but not behavioral sensitization. *J Pharmacol Exp Ther.* 2007;322(3):1103–1109.

116. Koffarnus MN, Woods JH. Quantification of drug choice with the generalized matching law in rhesus monkeys. *J Exp Anal Behav.* 2008;89(2):209–224.

117. Kumaresan V, Yuan M, Yee J, et al. Metabotropic glutamate receptor 5 (mGluR5) antagonists attenuate cocaine priming- and cue-induced reinstatement of cocaine seeking. *Behav Brain Res.* 2009;202(2):238–244.

118. Lal R, Deb KS, Kedia S. Substance use in women: current status and future directions. *Indian J Psychiatry.* 2015;57(suppl 2):S275–285.

119. Lamb RJ, Pinkston JW, Ginsburg BC. Ethanol self-administration in mice under a second-order schedule. *Alcohol.* 2015;49(6):561–570.

120. Lattal. Scheduling positive reinforcers. In: Iversen IH, Lattal KA, eds. *Experimental Analysis of Behavior: Part I.* Amsterdam: Elsevier Science; 1991:87–130.

121. Lê A, Shaham Y. Neurobiology of relapse to alcohol in rats. *Pharmacol Ther.* 2002;94(1–2):137–156.

122. Legastelois R, Botia B, Coune F, Jeanblanc J, Naassila M. Deciphering the relationship between vulnerability to ethanol-induced behavioral sensitization and ethanol consumption in outbred mice. *Addict Biol.* 2014;19(2):210–212.

123. Lenoir M, Cantin L, Vanhille N, Serre F, Ahmed SH. Extended heroin access increases heroin choices over a potent nondrug alternative. *Neuropsychopharmacology.* 2013;38(7):1209–1220.

124. Li P, Wu P, Xin X, et al. Incubation of alcohol craving during abstinence in patients with alcohol dependence. *Addict Biol.* 2015;20(3):513–522.

125. Liu Y, Roberts DC, Morgan D. Effects of extended-access self-administration and deprivation on breakpoints maintained by cocaine in rats. *Psychopharmacology.* 2005;179(3):644–651.

126. Loweth JA, Tseng KY, Wolf ME. Adaptations in AMPA receptor transmission in the nucleus accumbens contributing to incubation of cocaine craving. *Neuropharmacology.* 2014;(76 Pt B):287–300.

127. Lynch WJ. Sex differences in vulnerability to drug self-administration. *Exp Clin Psychopharmacol.* 2006;14(1):34–41.

128. Lynch WJ. Acquisition and maintenance of cocaine self-administration in adolescent rats: effects of sex and gonadal hormones. *Psychopharmacology.* 2008;197(2):237–246.

129. Lynch WJ. Modeling the development of drug addiction in male and female animals. *Pharmacol Biochem Behav.* 2018;164:50–61.

130. Lynch WJ, Abel J, Robinson AM, Smith MA. Exercise as a sex-specific treatment for substance use disorder, part II. Special Edition, Current Addiction Reports: Women and Addictions, in press; 2018.

131. Lynch WJ, Carroll ME. Sex differences in the acquisition of intravenously self-administered cocaine and heroin in rats. *Psychopharmacology.* 1999;144(1):77–82.

132. Lynch WJ, Carroll ME. Regulation of drug intake. *Exp Clin Psychopharmacol.* 2001;9(2):131–143.

133. Reference deleted in review.

134. Lynch WJ, Mangini LD, Taylor JR. Neonatal isolation stress potentiates cocaine seeking behavior in adult male and female rats. *Neuropsychopharmacology.* 2005;30(2):322–329.

135. Lynch WJ, Peterson AB, Sanchez V, Abel J, Smith MA. Exercise as a novel treatment for drug addiction: a neurobiological and stage-dependent hypothesis. *Neurosci Biobehav Rev.* 2013;37(8):1622–1644.

136. Lynch WJ, Piehl KB, Acosta G, Peterson AB, Hemby SE. Aerobic exercise attenuates reinstatement of cocaine-seeking behavior and associated neuroadaptations in the prefrontal cortex. *Biol Psychiatry.* 2010;68(8):774–777.

137. Lynch WJ, Potenza MN, Cosgrove KP, Mazure CM. Sex differences in vulnerability to stimulant abuse: a translational perspective. In: Brady KA, Back SE, Greenfield SF, eds. *Women and Addiction: A Comprehensive Handbook*. New York, NY: Guilford Press; 2009:242–256.

138. Lynch WJ, Robinson AM, Abel J, Smith MA. Exercise as a prevention for substance use disorder: a review of sex differences and neurobiological mechanisms, Part I. Special Edition, Current Addiction Reports: Women and Addictions, in press; 2018.

139. Lynch WJ, Tan L, Narmeen S, Beiter R, Brunzell DH. Exercise or saccharin during abstinence block estrus-induced increases in nicotine-seeking. *Physiol Behav*. 2017;(17):pii: S0031-9384 30377–30373.

140. Lynch WJ, Taylor JR. Sex differences in the behavioral effects of 24-h/day access to cocaine under a discrete trial procedure. *Neuropsychopharmacology*. 2004;29(5):943–951.

141. Lynch WJ, Taylor JR. Decreased motivation following cocaine self-administration under extended access conditions: effects of sex and ovarian hormones. *Neuropsychopharmacology*. 2005;30(5):927–935.

142. Madsen HB, Zbukvic IC, Luikinga SJ, Lawrence AJ, Kim JH. Extinction of conditioned cues attenuates incubation of cocaine craving in adolescent and adult rats. *Neurobiol Learn Mem*. 2017;143:88–93.

143. Maguire DR, Gerak LR, France CP. Delay discounting of the μ-opioid receptor agonist remifentanil in rhesus monkeys. *Behav Pharmacol*. 2016;27(2-3 Spec Issue):148–154.

144. Mandt BH, Schenk S, Zahniser NR, Allen RM. Individual differences in cocaine-induced locomotor activity in male Sprague-Dawley rats and their acquisition of and motivation to self-administer cocaine. *Psychopharmacology*. 2008;201:195–202.

145. Mantsch JR, Ho A, Schlussman SD, Kreek MJ. Predictable individual differences in the initiation of cocaine self-administration by rats under extended-access conditions are dose-dependent. *Psychopharmacology*. 2001;157(1):31–39.

146. Mantsch JR, Yuferov V, Mathieu-Kia AM, Ho A, Kreek MJ. Effects of extended access to high versus low cocaine doses on self-administration, cocaine-induced reinstatement and brain mRNA levels in rats. *Psychopharmacology*. 2004;175(1):26–36.

147. Markou A, Li J, Tse K, Li X. Cue-induced nicotine-seeking behavior after withdrawal with or without extinction in rats. *Addict Biol*. 2018;23(1):111–119.

148. Martin TJ, Kahn W, Cannon DG, Smith JE. Self-administration of heroin, cocaine and their combination under a discrete trial schedule of reinforcement in rats. *Drug Alcohol Depend*. 2006;82(3):282–286.

149. Marusich JA, Beckmann JS, Gipson CD, Bardo MT. Methylphenidate as a reinforcer for rats: contingent delivery and intake escalation. *Exp Clin Psychopharmacol*. 2010;18(3):257–266.

150. Mattox AJ, Thompson SS, Carroll ME. Smoked heroin and cocaine base (speedball) combinations in rhesus monkeys. *Exp Clin Psychopharmacol*. 1997;5(2):113–118.

151. McHugh RK, Votaw VR, Sugarman DE, Greenfield SF. Sex and gender differences in substance use disorders. *Clin Psychol Rev*. 2018. [Epub ahead of print].

152. McIntosh S, Howell L, Hemby SE. Dopaminergic dysregulation in prefrontal cortex of rhesus monkeys following cocaine self-administration. *Front Psychiatry*. 2013;4:88.

153. Meisch RA, Lemaire GA. Oral self-administration of pentobarbital by rhesus monkeys: relative reinforcing effects under concurrent fixed-ratio schedules. *J Exp Anal Behav*. 1988;50(1):75–86.

154. Meyer AC, Rahman S, Charnigo RJ, Dwoskin LP, Crabbe JC, Bardo MT. Genetics of novelty seeking, amphetamine self-administration and reinstatement using inbred rats. *Genes Brain Behav*. 2010;9(7):790–798.

155. Moeller SJ, Stoops WW. Cocaine choice procedures in animals, humans, and treatment-seekers: can we bridge the divide? *Pharmacol Biochem Behav*. 2015;138:133–141.

156. Morgan D, Brebner K, Lynch WJ, Roberts DC. Increases in the reinforcing efficacy of cocaine after particular histories of reinforcement. *Behav Pharmacol*. 2002;13(5–6):389–396.

157. Morgan D, Roberts DC. Sensitization to the reinforcing effects of cocaine following binge-abstinent self-administration. *Neurosci Biobehav Rev*. 2004;27(8):803–812.

158. Nadal R, Armario A, Janak PH. Positive relationship between activity in a novel environment and operant ethanol self-administration in rats. *Psychopharmacology*. 2002;162(3):333–338.

159. National Institutes of Health. *Consideration of Sex as a Biological Variable in NIH-Funded Research*. 2015. Access January 24, 2018 at: http://grants.nih.gov/grants/guide/notice-files/NOT-OD-15-102.html.

160. Negus SS, Banks ML. Modulation of drug choice by extended drug access and withdrawal in rhesus monkeys: implications for negative reinforcement as a driver of addiction and target for medications development. *Pharmacol Biochem Behav*. 2018;164:32–39.

161. Nguyen JD, Grant Y, Creehan KM, Vandewater SA, Taffe MA. Escalation of intravenous self-administration of methylone and mephedrone under extended access conditions. *Addict Biol*. 2017;22(5):1160–1168.

162. Nugent AL, Anderson EM, Larson EB, Self DW. Incubation of cue-induced reinstatement of cocaine, but not sucrose, seeking in C57BL/6J mice. *Pharmacol Biochem Behav*. 2017;159:12–17.

163. O'Connor EC, Chapman K, Butler P, Mead AN. The predictive validity of the rat self-administration model for abuse liability. *Neurosci Biobehav Rev*. 2011;35(3):912–938.

164. Ogbonmwan YE, Schroeder JP, Holmes PV, Weinshenker D. The effects of post-extinction exercise on cocaine-primed and stress-induced reinstatement of cocaine seeking in rats. *Psychopharmacology*. 2015;232(8):1395–1403.

165. Oleson EB, Richardson JM, Roberts DC. A novel IV cocaine self-administration procedure in rats: differential effects of dopamine, serotonin, and GABA drug pre-treatments on cocaine consumption and maximal price paid. *Psychopharmacology*. 2011;214(2):567–577.

166. Oleson EB, Roberts DC. Behavioral economic assessment of price and cocaine consumption following self-administration histories that produce escalation of either final ratios or intake. *Neuropsychopharmacology*. 2009;34(3):796–7804.

167. Oleson EB, Roberts DC. Cocaine self-administration in rats: threshold procedures. *Methods Mol Biol*. 2012;826:303–319.

168. Panlilio LV, Secci ME, Schindler CW, Bradberry CW. Choice between delayed food and immediate opioids in rats: treatment effects and individual differences. *Psychopharmacology*. 2017;234(22):3361–3373.

169. Parvaz MA, Moeller SJ, Goldstein RZ. Incubation of cue-induced craving in adults addicted to cocaine measured by electroencephalography. *JAMA Psychiatry*. 2016;73(11):1127–1134.

170. Perry AN, Westenbroek C, Becker JB. The development of a preference for cocaine over food identifies individual rats with addiction-like behaviors. *PLoS One*. 2013;8(11):e79465.

171. Perry JL, Anderson MM, Nelson SE, Carroll ME. Acquisition of i.v. cocaine self-administration in adolescent and adult male rats selectively bred for high and low saccharin intake. *Physiol Behav*. 2007;91(1):126–133.

172. Perry JL, Morgan AD, Anker JJ, Dess NK, Carroll ME. Escalation of i.v. cocaine self-administration and reinstatement of cocaine-seeking behavior in rats bred for high and low saccharin intake. *Psychopharmacology*. 2006;186(2):235–245.

173. Perry JL, Nelson SE, Carroll ME. Impulsive choice as a predictor of acquisition of IV cocaine self-administration and reinstatement of cocaine-seeking behavior in male and female rats. *Exp Clin Psychopharmacol*. 2008;16(2):165–177.

174. Peterson AB, Abel JM, Lynch WJ. Dose-dependent effects of wheel running on cocaine-seeking and prefrontal cortex Bdnf exon IV expression in rats. *Psychopharmacology*. 2014l;231(7):1305–1314.

175. Peterson AB, Hivick DP, Lynch WJ. Dose-dependent effectiveness of wheel running to attenuate cocaine-seeking: impact of sex and estrous cycle in rats. *Psychopharmacology.* 2014;231(13):2661–2670.

176. Piazza PV, Maccari S, Deminière JM, Le Moal M, Mormède P, Simon H. Corticosterone levels determine individual vulnerability to amphetamine self-administration. *Proc Natl Acad Sci USA.* 1991;88(6):2088–2092.

177. Pickens R, Muchow D, DeNoble V. Methohexital-reinforced responding in rats: effects of fixed ratio size and injection dose. *J Pharmacol Exp Ther.* 1981;216(2):205–209.

178. Pickens R, Thompson T. Cocaine-reinforced behavior in rats: effects of reinforcement magnitude and fixed-ratio size. *J Pharmacol Exp Ther.* 1968;161(1):122–129.

179. Pickens CL, Airavaara M, Theberge F, Fanous S, Hope BT, Shaham Y. Neurobiology of the incubation of drug craving. *Trends Neurosci.* 2011;34(8):411–420.

180. Pickering C, Moreira T, Liljequist S. Delayed access to alcohol accelerates self-administration of alcohol on a progressive ratio schedule. *Basic Clin Pharmacol Toxicol.* 2007;100(2):109–114.

181. Pisanu A, Lecca D, Valentini V, et al. Impairment of acquisition of intravenous cocaine self-administration by RNA-interference of dopamine D1-receptors in the nucleus accumbens shell. *Neuropharmacology.* 2015;89:398–411.

182. Porter-Stransky KA, Bentzley BS, Aston-Jones G. Individual differences in orexin-I receptor modulation of motivation for the opioid remifentanil. *Addict Biol.* 2017;22(2):303–317.

183. Ramôa CP, Doyle SE, Lycas MD, Chernau AK, Lynch WJ. Diminished role of dopamine D1-receptor signaling with the development of an addicted phenotype in rats. *Biol Psychiatry.* 2014;76(1):8–14.

184. Ramôa CP, Doyle SE, Naim DW, Lynch WJ. Estradiol as a mechanism for sex differences in the development of an addicted phenotype following extended access cocaine self-administration. *Neuropsychopharmacology.* 2013;38(9):1698–16705.

185. Reichel CM, Chan CH, Ghee SM, See RE. Sex differences in escalation of methamphetamine self-administration: cognitive and motivational consequences in rats. *Psychopharmacology.* 223(4):371–380.

186. Riley AL, Hempel BJ, Clasen MM. Sex as a biological variable: drug use and abuse. *Physiol Behav.* 2018. [Epub ahead of print].

187. Risner ME, Goldberg SR. A comparison of nicotine and cocaine self-administration in the dog: fixed-ratio and progressive-ratio schedules of intravenous drug infusion. *J Pharmacol Exp Ther.* 1983;224(2):319–326.

188. Roberts DC, Brebner K, Vincler M, Lynch WJ. Patterns of cocaine self-administration in rats produced by various access conditions under a discrete trials procedure. *Drug Alcohol Depend.* 2002;67(3):291–299.

189. Roberts DC, Morgan D, Liu Y. How to make a rat addicted to cocaine. *Prog Neuropsychopharmacol Biol Psychiatry.* 2007;31(8):1614–1624.

190. Rogers JL, De Santis S, See RE. Extended methamphetamine self-administration enhances reinstatement of drug seeking and impairs novel object recognition in rats. *Psychopharmacology.* 2008;199(4):615–624.

191. Sanchez V, Moore CF, Brunzell DH, Lynch WJ. Effect of wheel-running during abstinence on subsequent nicotine-seeking in rats. *Psychopharmacology.* 2013;227(3):403–411.

192. Sanchez V, Moore CF, Brunzell DH, Lynch WJ. Sex differences in the effect of wheel running on subsequent nicotine-seeking in a rat adolescent-onset self-administration model. *Psychopharmacology.* 2014;231(8):1753–1762.

193. Schindler CW, Panlilio LV, Goldberg SR. Second-order schedules of drug self-administration in animals. *Psychopharmacology.* 2002;163(3–4):327–344.

194. Schwendt M, Rocha A, See RE, Pacchioni AM, McGinty JF, Kalivas PW. Extended methamphetamine self-administration in rats results in a selective reduction of dopamine transporter levels in the prefrontal cortex and dorsal striatum not accompanied by marked monoaminergic depletion. *J Pharmacol Exp Ther.* 2009;331(2):555–562.

195. Sciliano CA, Jones SR. Cocaine potency at the dopamine transporter tracks discrete motivational states during cocaine self-administration. *Neuropsychopharmacology.* 2017;42:1893–1904.

196. Shahbazi M, Moffett AM, Williams BF, Frantz KJ. Age- and sex-dependent amphetamine self-administration in rats. *Psychopharmacology.* 2008;196(1):71–81.

197. Shalev U, Grimm JW, Shaham Y. Neurobiology of relapse to heroin and cocaine seeking: a review. *Pharmacol Rev.* 2002;54(1):1–42.

198. Shoaib M, Schindler CW, Goldberg SR. Nicotine self-administration in rats: strain and nicotine pre-exposure effects on acquisition. *Psychopharmacology.* 1997;129(1):35–43.

199. Sikora M, Nicolas C, Istin M, Jaafari N, Thiriet N, Solinas M. Generalization of effects of environmental enrichment on seeking for different classes of drugs of abuse. *Behav Brain Res.* 2017;341:109–113.

200. Singer BF, Fadanelli M, Kawa AB, Robinson TE. Are cocaine-seeking "habits" necessary for the development of addiction-like behavior in rats? *J Neurosci.* 2018;38:60–73.

201. Skupio U, Sikora M, Korostynski M, et al. Behavioral and transcriptional patterns of protracted opioid self-administration in mice. *Addict Biol.* 2017;22(6):1802–1816.

202. Smith RJ, Laiks LS. Behavioral and neural mechanisms underlying habitual and compulsive drug seeking. *Prog Neuropsychopharmacol Biol Psychiatry.* 2017;(17):30354–33058:pii: S0278–5846.

203. Stoops WW. Reinforcing effects of stimulants in humans: sensitivity of progressive-ratio schedules. *Exp Clin Psychopharmacol.* 2008;16(6):503–512.

204. Substance Abuse and Mental Health Services Administration. *Overview of Findings from the 2006 National Survey on Drug use and Health.* MD: Office of Applied Studies; 2007.

205. Sutton MA, Karanian DA, Self DW. Factors that determine a propensity for cocaine-seeking behavior during abstinence in rats. *Neuropsychopharmacology.* 2000;22(6):626–641.

206. Swalve N, Smethells JR, Carroll ME. Sex differences in the acquisition and maintenance of cocaine and nicotine self-administration in rats. *Psychopharmacology.* 2016;233(6):1005–1013.

207. Tang W, Wesley M, Freeman WM, Liang B, Hemby SE. Alterations in ionotropic glutamate receptor subunits during binge cocaine self-administration and withdrawal in rats. *J Neurochem.* 2004;89(4):1021–1033.

208. Thomsen M, Barrett AC, Butler P, Negus SS, Caine SB. Effects of acute and chronic treatments with dopamine D2 and D3 receptor ligands on cocaine versus food choice in rats. *J Pharmacol Exp Ther.* 2017;362(1):161–176.

209. Thomsen M, Barrett AC, Negus SS, Caine SB. Cocaine versus food choice procedure in rats: environmental manipulations and effects of amphetamine. *J Exp Anal Behav.* 2013;99(2):211–233.

210. Thomsen M, Caine SB. Chronic intravenous drug self-administration in rats and mice. *Curr Protoc Neurosci Chapter.* 2005;9:20. Unit 9.

211. Thomsen M, Fink-Jensen A, Woldbye DP, et al. Effects of acute and chronic aripiprazole treatment on choice between cocaine self-administration and food under a concurrent schedule of reinforcement in rats. *Psychopharmacology.* 2008;201(1):43–53.

212. Thomsen M, Fulton BS, Caine SB. Acute and chronic effects of the M1/M4-preferring muscarinic agonist xanomeline on cocaine vs. food choice in rats. *Psychopharmacology.* 2014;231(3):469–479.

213. Tornatzky W, Miczek KA. Cocaine self-administration "binges": transition from behavioral and autonomic regulation toward homeostatic dysregulation in rats. *Psychopharmacology.* 2000;148(3):289–298.

214. Vandaele Y, Cantin L, Serre F, Vouillac-Mendoza C, Ahmed SH. Choosing under the influence: a drug-specific mechanism by which the setting controls drug choices in rats. *Neuropsychopharmacology.* 2016;41(2):646–657.

215. Vargas-Irwin C, van den Oord EJ, Beardsley PM, Robles JR. A method for analyzing strain differences in acquisition of IV cocaine self-administration in mice. *Behav Genet.* 2006;36(4):525–535.

216. Vendruscolo JCM, Tunstall BJ, Carmack SA. Compulsive-like sufentanil vapor self-administration in rats. *Neuropsychopharmacology.* 2018. [Epub ahead of print].

217. Venniro M, Caprioli D, Shaham Y. Animal models of drug relapse and craving: From drug priming-induced reinstatement to incubation of craving after voluntary abstinence. *Prog Brain Res.* 2016;224:25–52.

218. Wade CL, Vendruscolo LF, Schlosburg JE, Hernandez DO, Koob GF. Compulsive-like responding for opioid analgesics in rats with extended access. *Neuropsychopharmacology.* 2015;40(2):421–428.

219. Wang G, Shi J, Chen N, et al. Effects of length of abstinence on decision-making and craving in methamphetamine abusers. *PLoS One.* 2013;8(7):e68791.

220. Ward SJ, Läck C, Morgan D, Roberts DC. Discrete-trials heroin self-administration produces sensitization to the reinforcing effects of cocaine in rats. *Psychopharmacology.* 2006;185(2):150–159.

221. Watterson LR, Kufahl PR, Nemirovsky NE, et al. Potent rewarding and reinforcing effects of the synthetic cathinone 3,4-methylenedioxypyrovalerone (MDPV). *Addict Biol.* 2014;19(2):165–174.

222. Weerts EM, Goodwin AK, Kaminski BJ, Hienz RD. Environmental cues, alcohol seeking, and consumption in baboons: effects of response requirement and duration of alcohol abstinence. *Alcohol Clin Exp Res.* 2001;30:2026–2035.

223. Wise RA, Bozarth MA. Brain substrates for reinforcement and drug self-administration. *Prog Neuropsychopharmacol.* 1981;5(5–6):467–474.

224. Wolffgramm J, Heyne A. From controlled drug intake to loss of control: the irreversible development of drug addiction in the rat. *Behav Brain Res.* 1995;70(1):77–94.

225. Yamamoto DJ, Nelson AM, Mandt BH, et al. Rats classified as low or high cocaine locomotor responders: a unique model involving striatal dopamine transporters that predicts cocaine addiction-like behaviors. *Neurosci Biobehav.* 2013;37(8):1738–1753.

226. Zhang Y, Mayer-Blackwell B, Schlussman SD, et al. Extended access oxycodone self-administration and neurotransmitter receptor gene expression in the dorsal striatum of adult C57BL/6 J mice. *Psychopharmacology.* 2014;231(7):1277–1287.

227. Zimmer BA, Oleson EB, Roberts DC. The motivation to self-administer is increased after a history of spiking brain levels of cocaine. *Neuropsychopharmacology.* 2012;37:1901–1910.

7

Role of Human Laboratory Studies in the Development of Medications for Alcohol and Substance Use Disorders

JOHN D. ROACHE AND LORENZO LEGGIO

Introduction

The development of medications that are useful for the treatment of alcohol or substance use disorders requires the clinical and preclinical testing of existing and novel compounds in various experimental models useful for evaluating the mechanism, safety, and possible efficacy of the putative treatment.[131,156,215,283] Medication development research has sought to evaluate both existing medications already on the market for other indications as well as new, novel compounds never yet tested in humans. Regardless of the stage of development for any particular medication, experimental human studies in controlled environments (i.e., "human laboratory" studies) will be required at some step of the process for at least one of three possible reasons.

1. *Phase I Safety Testing of Novel Compounds*: For novel compounds not yet approved by the US Food and Drug Administration (FDA), Phase I clinical trials will be required to evaluate the safety and abuse liability of the new medications. Basic safety testing in healthy subjects is normally required for first-in-human studies but basic Phase I safety testing approaches will be required in the drug-using target population as well before the FDA will allow Phase II and III treatment trials to proceed.

2. *Phase I, II Safety Testing in the Target Population*: If the medication is already approved by the FDA for another indication, development of that medication for addiction treatment still will require safety testing in drug-using or addicted populations. Safety evaluation includes both the

biomedical safety of treatment in a drug-using population as well as an assessment of the abuse liability of the medication in a population likely to misuse substances. In addition, the FDA likely will require these studies to address the safety of the drug interaction between the treatment medication and the drug of abuse.[89,138]

3. *Evaluation of Pharmacokinetic and Pharmacodynamic Mechanisms*: Although Phase III treatment trials will be required to demonstrate efficacy, human laboratory studies also can be helpful to evaluate the clinical pharmacology (both kinetics and dynamics) of a medication. These studies can evaluate the possible behavioral or neurochemical mechanism(s) of action or use human laboratory models to estimate the possible efficacy of new medications.

For many human laboratory studies, subjects are research volunteers not engaged in treatment. However, individuals who are "in treatment" also may be tested under controlled human laboratory conditions. The purpose of this review is to identify and highlight the role of and contributions made by human laboratory studies in the development of new medication treatments for addictions.

Pioneering studies conducted in the 1950s, 1960s, and 1970s at the Addiction Research Center of the Public Health Service Hospital in Lexington, Kentucky, developed the basic experimental approaches useful for understanding the clinical pharmacology of alcohol and drug dependence, and their treatment.[72-74,184] In many cases, early development studies may require the administration of alcohol or drugs to human subjects who have the alcohol or drug use disorder. The National Advisory Council on Drug Abuse and the National Advisory Council on Alcohol Abuse and Alcoholism have both recommended guidelines for the ethical and safe study of, respectively, drugs and alcohol, given to human subjects (http://www.drugabuse.gov/Funding/HSGuide.html, https://www.niaaa.nih.gov/research/guidelines-and-resources/administering-alcohol-human-studies).[62,63,196] Broadly speaking, pharmacological approaches to the study of the behavioral effects of drug abuse and its treatment are characterized under the umbrella of abuse liability assessment.[15,16,83] Abuse liability assessment involves estimation of the likelihood that a substance will be used or self-administered and/or the liability or harmfulness of that use.[235,240] Thus, abuse liability assessment approaches to human laboratory studies encompass all aspects necessary to evaluate both the safety (i.e., abuse liability of the treatment agent and the harmfulness of the drug interaction) and possible efficacy (i.e., does it reduce the likelihood of using the drug of abuse) of medications useful for treating alcohol and drug dependence.

Role of the Human Laboratory in Evaluating the Abuse Liability of New Medications

When medications are developed for human use, the FDA or Drug Enforcement Administration may require an assessment of the abuse potential of the new agent and this generally will require human laboratory studies.[15,21,180] Typically, abuse liability assessment will be required when the medication under development shares pharmacological characteristics or planned indications with other drugs of known abuse potential. Broadly speaking, the abuse liability of a potential medication can be characterized in the human laboratory using one or more of three different behavioral approaches as described below.

To Characterize Adverse or Harmful Effects

Characterizing the effects of a new drug on various dimensions of physiological function and performance or other behavioral impairment can be valuable to understand how the drug might alter or impair important biobehavioral functions.[235] For example, drugs could be examined for how they alter cognitive, psychomotor, or other behavioral performance[43,44,113] or physiological functioning.[121,122,184] Characterization of drug effects on each of these dimensions provides valuable information to assess the potential *liability* or *harm* that can occur with drug use. In the context of drug abuse, it also is important to know about the safety of the drug interaction should the new medication be combined with the drug of abuse. For this reason, many studies have been devoted to assessing the potential interactions between the new medication and alcohol—the most common drug for which potentially dangerous interactions might occur.[7,8,89] The safety of drug interactions also is very important for FDA approval of potential treatments for alcohol or drug addiction because it is very likely that drug-dependent populations undergoing treatment with a medication will at some point at least sample their primary drug of dependence. Furthermore, the characterization of the drug interaction in the experimental laboratory may provide insight into the mechanism and possible effectiveness of that medication.

To Characterize Its Comparative Pharmacological Profile

The most common approach to abuse liability assessment is the pharmacological bioassay, which is a standard evaluation of the clinical and pharmacological profile of the new drug in comparison with another known drug from the same or similar pharmacological class.[15,83,240,256] Necessarily, pharmacological profiling means evaluating the pharmacodynamic effects of the drug on a variety of dimensions, which could include assessment of performance or physiological effects, but for abuse liability also includes assessment of subjective effects or euphoria. An adequate evaluation of pharmacological profile requires the testing of a range of doses to construct a dose-response curve because the testing of a single dose fails to provide information on the dose-responsiveness of observed effects and is fraught with the potential for false-negative findings. Comparison of the new drug with a standard drug of known abuse potential is an essential element in the pharmacological comparison approach for at least three reasons. First, use of the standard drug establishes the positive control level of response to drugs of abuse under the standard conditions employed by the experiment. This is particularly important given that false-positive or false-negative results may occur due to variations in the assessments, population, or other study conditions. Second, relative potency or relative effect-size comparisons between the novel drug and the standard drug of abuse provide the basis for the most meaningful interpretation of data. Thus, the new drug may differ in the dose-response slope, the maximum effect size, or the relative potency on different dimensions of effect. Each of these variables has a different implication for abuse liability. Third, for clinical advantage estimation purposes, the FDA and medical prescribers would like to know about the differential efficacy contrast of the new drug in comparison with a known drug, which may be a standard drug of abuse or a scheduled prescription medication that has known abuse potential.

To Evaluate Reinforcing Effects or Potential for Self-Administration

Numerous animal models of addiction studied across a wide variety of drugs and species have shown that drug taking is a drug-reinforced behavior controlled by operant contingencies and schedules of reinforcement.[84,244] The same also has been shown in humans, where several human laboratory models of drug reinforcement and self-administration have been established.[37,84,108,109,267] Ultimately, the behavior we are interested in understanding, predicting, and treating, is the likelihood that a drug/substance will be used or consumed in a pattern consistent with abuse or dependence. A yes/no decision whether or not the drug is self-administered by the subject population may not be sufficient here because the environment and the availability of alternatives influence choice behavior. For example, the likelihood that a sedative or stimulant drug will be self-administered is influenced by how stimulating the experimental environment is.[260,269] This phenomenon likely explains how even the sedating atypical antipsychotic quetiapine, with little intrinsic abuse liability, may become a highly preferred drug of abuse in a prison or psychiatric hospital environment where access to other drugs is limited.[155,276] Therefore, an all-or-none conclusion of whether or not a drug is self-administered under one set of conditions does not indicate much about its potential for self-administration under a different set of circumstances. Thus, studies of the potential for reinforcement or self-administration are limited by the range of conditions (dose, circumstance, population, etc.) under which they are tested.[83,240,256]

Issues in Human Laboratory Studies of Abuse Liability

There are several issues that need to be considered by any human laboratory study of abuse liability. The information below summarizes the issues that generally exist in the field and potentially limit any conclusions coming from human laboratory studies of medication effects on drugs of abuse.

Role of Subjective Effects

Since the earliest studies at the addiction research unit at the United States Public Health Service Hospital at Lexington, Kentucky, it has been observed that drugs of abuse as diverse as alcohol, barbiturates, opiates, and psychomotor stimulants all share a profile of psychoactive effects characterized as euphoria.[61,226,229] It is generally accepted that euphoria is at least a partial explanation of why these drugs are abused. Because of the subjective and unobservable nature of this psychoactivity, self-report questionnaires are used to assess these subjective effects. One of the early questionnaires developed to measure the subjective effects of drugs of abuse was the Addiction Research Center Inventory, a multi-item questionnaire completed by human subjects during drug intoxication.[91] Factor analysis was used to empirically derive subscales of items responsive to characteristic drugs of abuse including amphetamine, benzedrine, morphine, pentobarbital, alcohol, chlorpromazine, and lysergic acid diethylamide. Subsequently[72] the morphine-benzedrine groups were combined to represent an opiate or stimulant-type of "euphoria" scale, the pentobarbital-chlorpromazine-alcohol group a distinctly "sedative" scale, and the lysergic acid diethylamide scale as a "dysphoria" or unpleasantness

scale. It is important to recognize that these scales actually were derived to measure subjective mood changes induced by pharmacologically distinct drugs of intoxication and not euphoria per se.[72,83,240] The Profile of Mood States[191] is a multi-item questionnaire derived in the measurement of mood in normal healthy college students. Nonetheless, it has been used commonly to measure changes in depression-dejection, tension-anxiety, vigor, arousal, and other mood states by various populations under the influence of drugs.[45,60,61,296] Generalized mood measures are valuable to assess the pharmacological profile of a drug and are sometimes presumed to predict abuse potential under the assumption that positive mood states could reflect an increased potential while negative mood states could reflect a decreased potential. In alcoholism research, the biphasic alcohol effects scale[182] was derived to measure the positive and disinhibiting arousal that may occur during the ascending limb of the blood-alcohol curve and the sedative-inhibition that occurs on the descending limb of the curve. Actually there are many other factor-analyzed and single-item rating scales that have been used to evaluate the subjective effects of psychoactive drugs, and enumerating them is beyond the scope of this review.

The psychoactive effects of psychotropic drugs are studied in animals using discriminative stimulus procedures, where subjects are trained to discriminate the differences between drugs. Discriminative stimulus procedures also have been developed to train human subjects to discriminate the interoceptive stimulus effects of drugs.[53,124,225,229,270] Although subjective rating scales take advantage of the verbal capacity of human subjects to quantitatively report the qualitative characteristics of their subjective experience, the discriminative stimulus approach uses a qualitative analysis of same/different comparisons between drugs. There is reasonable correspondence between conclusions drawn from subjective effects and those from discriminative stimulus studies in humans.[53,229,270] Because of differential reinforcement of behavior during discriminative training, it is likely possible to gain a tighter level of discriminative control with this paradigm than with standard subjective questionnaires. However, the specificity and sensitivity of this procedure very much depend on the discrimination training conditions[125] and are achieved only through lengthy training procedures. Nonetheless, the ability to compare the human study results with the preclinical data using discriminative stimulus analyses is a distinct advantage of this procedure.[53,124] Although there is a good correspondence between "positive" subjective effects and the likelihood of drug self-administration, it is certainly not true that either positive or negative subjective effects alone explain the cause or the reason that drugs are or are not self-administered.[37,64,65].

Role of Subjective Euphoria

The cardinal subjective effect commonly assumed to be important to abuse potential is the experience of psychoactive drug effects that are pleasant, preferred, or "euphoric." A number of reviews of human abuse liability have discussed issues of drug-induced subjective euphoria and its measurement.[a] Actually, most drug users do not refer to "euphoria" but rather describe the drug intoxication as a "high." Although cocaine intoxication has been described as "intensely stimulating and pleasurable," or "orgasmic," it is clear that not all drugs of abuse produce such intense pleasurable sensations. For many drugs, including alcohol, the intoxication is more

---

[a] References 61, 64, 65, 83, 226, 229, 240.

often described as a "buzz," or "drunk," or "high" that has "good" features and that people report "liking." Consequently, most studies employ individual-item rating scales for subjects to rate the extent of "high" and "good" subjective effects and the extent to which subjects "like" the effect. There is no standard euphoria scale used by a majority of studies.

Importance of Measuring Self-Administration Behavior

Current conceptions of the disease condition recognize that the core feature of substance abuse or dependence is the pattern of drug self-administration that is harmful or compulsive.[12,215] Consequently, most studies of abuse liability seek primarily to predict the *likelihood* of drug self-use for nonmedical purposes. Ample previous research clearly has demonstrated that drugs of abuse maintain the self-administration behavior of both humans and animals through the process of operant reinforcement. Ever since the earliest studies at the Addiction Research Center observing heroin self-administration in a heroin addict,[297] a variety of different procedures have been developed to study self-administration behavior in human laboratory environments, and these have been described in previous reviews.[b] These reviews describe the effects of variations in self-administration procedures such as:

1. the specific drug reinforcer, its route of administration, and whether or not dose was varied (higher doses and more rapid increases in blood level are more reinforcing);
2. whether the drug reinforcer was administered immediately or after a time delay (immediate drug delivery is more reinforcing);
3. whether the self-administered dose was a high bolus dose or multiple smaller doses (multiple smaller doses result in more sensitive measures of reinforcement);
4. whether or not the drug reinforcer was "blinded" and placebo controls were employed (blinded procedures have greater validity);
5. whether the self-administration behavior was a verbal request or responses on a response instrument (responses on a manipulandum provide quantitative measures of behavior);
6. the extent to which behavioral "cost" was varied in the operant contingency (increasing "cost" decreases the probability of self-administration);
7. whether the self-administration procedure included choices among alternative reinforcers (choice between alternatives provides a better quantitative assessment of relative reinforcement); and
8. whether drug taking was quantified by measuring amount consumed versus the proportion of subjects responding (amount measures are more sensitive measures).

Thus validated operant models of drug reinforcement have been established for human laboratory studies, and these have become used increasingly over the last two decades. Although pleasant subjective effects are generally correlated with the tendency of subjects to self-administer drugs in the human laboratory,[c] drug-taking behavior does occur in the absence of measurable subjective effects.[168,239] At times, the needs to examine complete dose-response functions in making between-drug pharmacological comparisons[83] may preclude

self-administration studies.[240] Nonetheless, direct observations of drug-taking behavior generally are preferred over measures of subjective effects alone.[37]

Role of Environment and Cost in Controlling Self-Administration

Although this review does not discuss specific advantages and disadvantages of different self-administration procedures, variations in the procedure are likely to alter the sensitivity to change of the drug-taking measure.[267] In fact these procedural variables are likely to be important both in determining whether the drug is self-administered, as well as the sensitivity to change to show increases or decreases in drug-taking behavior. One of the variables that has an important influence on drug-taking behavior is the role of the internal or external stimulus environment and how that can increase or decrease the likelihood of self-use. For example, diazepam is not normally preferred by healthy controls[126] but preference increases under environmental conditions that increase anxiety.[106] In addition, sedative drugs are preferred over stimulants in sedentary environments while stimulants are preferred over sedatives when task performance contingencies require alertness.[260,269] A stimulating environment may decrease the reinforcing effects of a sedative but enhance the reinforcing effects of a stimulant likely because of behavioral cost and alternative reinforcement.[244,267] Understanding this phenomenon involves recognition of the behavioral economics of drug taking.[19,20] In behavioral economics, choice of the drug involves a behavioral cost and may occur at the expense of access to alternative reinforcers.[176] In human laboratory studies it is common to make monetary choices available as an alternative to drug taking,[39,111,194,267] wherein choices between increasing amounts of money versus drug result in reductions of drug self-administration. Griffiths and colleagues[85,86] exploited this phenomenon in creating the "Multiple Choice Procedure," a questionnaire wherein across a series of single-item questions, subjects choose between receiving the drug or a gradually increasing amount of money. To establish the questionnaire responses as a true measure of choice/preference for drug, one of the many item questions is selected at random and the subjects actually receive as a consequence the drug or the money amount they selected for that item.

Role of Subject Population Variables

One of the issues associated with subjective-effects assessment is that the extent to which subjective psychoactivity is considered pleasurable or "euphoric" varies across different populations and is shaped and influenced by experience. For example, early studies by Beecher[17] showed that normal healthy volunteers reported unpleasant experiences when given opiates or barbiturates while drug-experienced users reported those drug effects to be pleasant or euphoric. Balanced placebo research designs controlling subject expectations with *2 × 2* factorial experiments where subjects were either told or not told they were receiving drug under conditions where they actually did or did not receive drug have shown that the subjective reports of drug effects in normal populations are substantially influenced by expectation.[190] Of course expectations occur in drug-dependent populations as well. Compared with normal drinkers, heavy alcohol drinkers report greater expectations of euphoric responses and other positive or beneficial effects of alcohol.[29,40] It is likely that some of the differences between drug-experienced and drug-naive

b References 37, 84, 98, 106, 109, 244, 267.
c References 35, 45, 84, 126, 127, 229, 240.

populations are due to learned or acquired factors altering attribution or expectation. Generally, populations of normal subjects, who do not abuse drugs, do not report higher levels of liking drug effects or euphoric mood changes, and do not self-administer most drugs of abuse.[83,126,127,240,256] Strong evidence for the importance of drug abuse history and experience is seen in patient-controlled analgesia studies where opiate analgesics with known addiction potential can be given for medically ill populations to self-administer, and yet those without a substance abuse history do not become drug abusers or addicts.[112,295] Therefore, valid assessment of abuse liability must employ drug-experienced abuser populations in order to gauge what drug abusers will do with a drug of abuse.[83,240,256] This is not to say that certain drugs may not have some abuse liability even for normal healthy populations. In fact, studies of stimulant abuse liability[64,65] among normal college populations observe that amphetamines tend to be preferred over placebo while sedative benzodiazepines are not preferred.[45,126,127] Of course, caffeine clearly has reinforcing properties in healthy human populations worldwide.[87] For these reasons, valid inferences about relative changes in abuse liability have to include experimental controls showing base response rates of the study population and study procedures as a point of comparison.[83,240,256] For pharmacological studies comparing across drugs, the comparison drug may show greater or less abuse liability than a standard reference drug in the designated population under standard study conditions.

Population-related differences in drug response could be due in part to genetically controlled individual differences in innate sensitivity.[187] An example of this is found in Asian populations who commonly have the *ALDH2*2* allele for aldehyde dehydrogenase, which increases levels of the ethanol metabolite acetyl aldehyde, resulting in an unpleasant flushing response, which reduces the risks of experiencing alcohol-induced euphoria.[286,288] Another example of a population-related difference may be found in studies showing that young adult children of alcoholic parents may report greater euphoric response and lesser negative, sedative effects of alcohol than do children without a family history of alcoholism.[259]

Role of Craving

Many addicted individuals report that stimulus cues in the environment elicit powerful "cravings" and impulses to use drugs.[50,213,214] However, there has been much debate about the meaning of the term "craving" and what role it plays in the risk of drug use.[224,278] Early pioneering work in the human laboratory considered craving as a conditioned-withdrawal-like motivational state.[298,299] With the operant model of drug dependence, it has been argued that "craving" refers primarily to the urge or impulse to use.[164] Still others suggest that craving involves at least three dimensions: (1) withdrawal and negative affect–related escape motivation, (2) reward-related conditioned impulses/urges, and (3) obsessive thoughts and/or cognitive-control mechanisms.[51,278] Many human laboratory studies have studied cue-induced craving in addicted populations.[33,51,213,214] These studies provide visual, olfactory, auditory, and/or tactile stimuli historically associated with drug use; although tactile cue procedures of handling drug paraphernalia have been among the most effective stimulus cues.[13,246] Idiosyncratic script-driven mental imagery techniques also can be used to guide the cue exposure session.[262,263] Cue responses can be physiological (i.e., heart rate) or subjective (i.e., craving). Although there often is not a good correlation between

the physiological and subjective measures,[245] a meta-analysis[33] concluded that subject ratings of craving were the most reliable and selective reaction to drug cues and showed the largest effect size across studies. Multi-item factor scales have been used in the human laboratory to measure craving for alcohol,[23,257] marijuana,[105] or cocaine,[93] but many studies commonly use only graded analog scales of single item ratings such as "crave,"[120] "desire,"[47] "urge," or "want."[64,65,293] Craving ratings sometimes have been correlated with drug use in outpatient studies[103] and with risk of relapse in treatment seekers.[201] However, dissociation between craving ratings and drug-taking behavior has been demonstrated clearly in laboratory studies,[52,96,171,224] and the extent of cue-craving observed in the laboratory has not always correlated with relapse to alcohol drinking among alcohol-dependent individuals.[249] Thus, craving is neither a necessary nor sufficient precursor to drug use or relapse. Rather, it appears to reflect a parallel cognitive process as proposed by Tiffany[277,278] or a subjective state experienced as urge or impulse that is associated with drug-related environmental stimuli as suggested by a consensus panel.[224] On the other hand, cue-elicited craving procedures seem sensitive to medication response, for example, naltrexone reduces craving for alcohol.[201]

Human Laboratory Studies of Pharmacological Agonist and Antagonist Treatments

Human laboratory studies have been useful to help us understand the potential value of various pharmacological approaches to treatment. The potential of using pharmacological agonists or antagonists in the treatment of substance abuse is best illustrated through studies of opiate dependence as described below.

Utility of Evaluating Pharmacological Antagonist Treatments

Early studies of opiate antagonists at the Addiction Research Center showed that they could completely block the subjective and physiological effects of morphine[73,122,183] and precipitate withdrawal in dependent individuals.[121,122] Subsequent studies showed that oral naltrexone[2,194] blocked heroin self-administration and subjective effects in human laboratory models of drug taking. The robustness of the observed pharmacological antagonism and the nearly complete blockade of any behavioral effects or abuse liability of heroin observed in these studies strongly suggested efficacy for the antagonist approach. However, outpatient treatment effectiveness with antagonists like naltrexone is poor[161] because of poor medication compliance among heroin addicts who find it too easy to discontinue antagonist therapy so as to recover the heroin effect they seek. These findings suggest a significant weakness of human laboratory procedures to predict efficacy with antagonist approaches. Specifically, even perfect blockade of abuse potential does not predict treatment efficacy because medication noncompliance will nullify even complete pharmacological blockade. More recently, human laboratory studies again have evaluated the depot formulation of naltrexone[38,273] and shown that it will block heroin self-administration and subjective effects. Although there is reason to hope that depot formulations of naltrexone could improve the effectiveness of antagonist treatments, especially in conjunction with court-ordered treatment,[221] the outcome data do not yet exist to support it.[175,272] Notably, because of the diffuse mechanisms of action for alcohol, cocaine, and methamphetamine, direct, receptor-mediated pharmacological antagonists are unlikely to exist for those drugs. For nicotine dependence, human laboratory studies of the nicotinic antagonist mecamylamine have shown increased smoking[206] or increased intravenous nicotine self-administration,[251] which is consistent with a surmountable pharmacological blockade. However, another human laboratory study found no effect of mecamylamine,[294] and clinically, there is no evidence for treatment efficacy with nicotinic antagonists[30] in outpatient treatment. No efficacy trial has examined the use of the cannabinoid-1 antagonist, anandamide (rimonabant), for cannabis dependence, but early human laboratory studies have shown only partial or inconsistent blockade of the effects of smoked cannabis.[115]

Utility of Evaluating Pharmacological Agonist Replacement Approaches

A study at the Addiction Research Center[150] was the first human laboratory study showing that oral methadone produced dose-related decreases in the subjective effects, liking, and self-administration of hydromorphone. Thirty years later, a human laboratory study showed that short-term treatment with methadone doses of 50, 100, and 150 mg showed dose-related blockade of the subjective effects and self-administration of heroin.[48] The authors of this later study used their human laboratory data to argue that clinical tendencies to use lower methadone doses for maintenance are counterproductive. It is notable that these findings exactly parallel the dose equivalence and clinical experience with methadone maintenance treatment.[271] Previous reviews[21,121,226] have described human abuse liability testing with a variety of opiate agonists, partial agonists, and mixed agonists/antagonists that demonstrated unequivocally that agonist effects at the mu opiate receptor are responsible for the abuse potential of opiates. In the course of this work, human laboratory studies were critical to the ultimate development of buprenorphine as a partial agonist pharmacotherapy, with a reduced abuse potential.[37,123,289] Human laboratory studies were particularly important to demonstrate that buprenorphine reduced the reinforcing effects of heroin[193] and that small doses of naloxone could be added to buprenorphine to further reduce its abuse potential without precipitating withdrawal in morphine-dependent subjects.[195] These studies illustrate clearly a strong concordance between the human laboratory studies and clinical experience with buprenorphine. Furthermore, when compared with the studies and clinical experience with antagonist medications, they suggest that human laboratory studies seeking to antagonize the reinforcing effects of a drug of abuse might look for medications that have at least a partial agonist-like activity. Of course, nicotine-replacement strategies for tobacco dependence have been very successful[30] in reducing smoking behavior. Human laboratory studies have shown that smoking[223] and nicotine gum[207] pretreatments each decreased cigarette smoking. In addition, transdermal nicotine patches decreased cue-induced craving,[279] the discriminative stimulus and reinforcing effects of nicotine spray,[222] and the reinforcing effects of intravenous nicotine.[264] The partial nicotinic agonist, varenicline, is the first nicotinic agonist treatment for tobacco dependence approved by the FDA.[281] Varenicline's efficacy in smoking cessation has been confirmed by a recent meta-analysis.[31] Human laboratory studies showed that varenicline, as compared to placebo, reduced cigarette cue-elicited craving and produced parallel reductions in cigarette cue-elicited ventral striatum and medial orbitofrontal cortex responses assessed by functional magnetic resonance imaging (fMRI).[71] Another human laboratory study with smokers showed that varenicline reduced cigarette craving in a manner correlated with blood varenicline concentrations, suggesting that acute agonist administration produces temporary relief in cigarette craving.[231] A complex human laboratory study examined the effects of chronic varenicline treatment on self-administration of intravenous nicotine, intravenous cocaine, and intravenous nicotine and cocaine combined. Results showed that varenicline selectively attenuated the reinforcing effects of nicotine alone but not cocaine alone, and its effects on nicotine and cocaine combined were dependent on the dose of cocaine. Clearly, complex drug-drug interactions likely exist in this specific population with nicotine and cocaine use disorder comorbidity.[192]

Role of Human Laboratory Studies in Developing Medications for Alcohol Dependence

A brief review of medications that have been or are being developed for alcoholism treatment is used to illustrate how pharmacological mechanisms other than agonist replacement or direct pharmacological antagonism of the drug of abuse can be exploited in medication development. Currently, there are three medications approved by the FDA for the treatment of alcohol dependence. In addition, we discuss human laboratory studies conducted with other medications that have shown promise in clinical treatment trials.

Disulfiram

Disulfiram was the first medication approved by the FDA for the treatment of addiction. Human laboratory studies as well as preclinical studies of biochemistry and toxicology were included in the first report of the disulfiram-ethanol reaction that ensues upon alcohol exposure.[92] Over a period of more than 40 years, human laboratory studies have been important to characterize the nature, the safety, and the mechanism of the disulfiram-alcohol reaction.[34,128,230,253] These studies were instrumental in showing that inhibition of aldehyde dehydrogenase and the subsequent accumulation of the acetyl aldehyde metabolite is responsible for the unpleasant effects of the disulfiram reaction and that a hypotensive crisis is a serious medical risk. Either because of the way the disulfiram makes alcohol effects so unpleasant or because of the direct side effects of disulfiram itself, compliance with this medication is a serious problem limiting its utility and effectiveness for the treatment of alcohol dependence.[27,167] Consequently, there is little ongoing research in further development of disulfiram as a treatment for alcohol dependence.

Naltrexone

The opiate antagonist, oral naltrexone, was the second medication approved by the FDA for the treatment of alcohol dependence. Subsequently, an intramuscular naltrexone formulation was approved by the FDA for the treatment of alcohol dependence. A recent meta-analysis supports naltrexone efficacy in in alcohol-dependent individuals.[149] Based largely on preclinical studies showing that naltrexone reduced alcohol drinking in rodents, the first clinical trials[217,285] were Phase III outpatient efficacy trials of a medication that had already been approved for narcotic addiction. Subsequently, human laboratory studies were useful for demonstrating that naltrexone can reduce alcohol self-administration in some paradigms[50,218] but not others,[49] and has a mixed profile to reduce some of alcohol's positive subjective effects[160,275] and cue-reactive craving.[43,201,218,248] Naltrexone also has been shown to reduce the behavioral-activating effects of alcohol as measured by heart rate increases, subjective liking, and corticotropin (ACTH)/cortisol elevations.[189] This latter finding is interesting given that other studies have shown that parental family histories of alcoholism are associated with greater activation of the hypothalamic-pituitary-adrenal axis at baseline and in response to mu opioid receptor blockade by naloxone,[110] and that these differences may predict naltrexone response.[160,218] A study administered naltrexone versus placebo to 92 non–treatment-seeking, alcohol-dependent subjects for 6 outpatient days before bringing them into the human laboratory for a drink self-administration session.[166] Study findings showed that naltrexone reduced alcohol self-administration in subjects with a positive family history of alcoholism and may actually have increased drinking in subjects without a family history. More recently, the efficacy of naltrexone in alcohol cue-elicited craving and subjective effects of alcohol has been replicated in adolescent problem drinkers,[199] suggesting its potential use in underage populations with at-risk alcohol use. Although the genes associated with family history are not known, an earlier laboratory study identified a single nucleotide polymorphism of the mu-receptor conferring naloxone-reactive hypothalamic-pituitary-adrenal activation,[292] and this same polymorphism recently was shown to predict naltrexone treatment response in Project COMBINE.[6,11.] Albeit not without inconsistencies,[220] other studies have further confirmed these pharmacogenetic findings, including a human laboratory study that specifically enrolled Asian-American individuals.[232] It is also important to note that variability in medication responses may depend on several factors, such as participants' readiness to seek treatment, how alcohol is administered, and how these factors may interact with the medication itself. For example, a recent human laboratory study with treatment-seeking alcoholic inpatients indicated that naltrexone resulted in increased craving in response to cues and increased subjective effects of alcohol (feeling high and intoxicated) after an intravenous alcohol challenge.[266] Overall, these human laboratory studies have shown results consistent with the outpatient treatment trials, concluding that naltrexone is modestly effective in reducing some of the reinforcing but not the subjective effects of alcohol, and that this action may block the alcohol-seeking or craving that is primed or cued by the initial doses of alcohol consumed during a binge. Finally, a recent meta-analysis confirmed that, overall, naltrexone reduces alcohol self-administration and craving under well-controlled human laboratory conditions.[107]

Acamprosate

Based largely upon three European treatment trials,[165] the FDA approved the glutamate antagonist acamprosate as the third medication for the treatment of alcohol dependence. Prior to that approval, a human laboratory study examined the safety of the combination of acamprosate with naltrexone in alcohol-dependent subjects[138] as a prelude to the larger outpatient treatment trial known as Project COMBINE, which tested the efficacy of acamprosate and naltrexone alone and in combination.[10] Although

meta-analyses of several clinical trials have supported the efficacy of acamprosate at preventing relapse in alcohol-dependent individuals,[149,165,179] Project COMBINE did not demonstrate efficacy at reducing drinking in alcohol-dependent outpatients. Despite a large body of preclinical literature examining acamprosate's actions and mechanisms,[46] only two human laboratory studies have been reported. One study found that acamprosate reduced the heart rate response, but not the subjective craving induced by alcohol cues.[219] Another study administered repeated doses of acamprosate to non–treatment-seeking heavy drinkers in an outpatient setting and brought the subjects into a human laboratory where acamprosate was without effect to alter the subjective or behavioral responses to challenge doses of alcohol.[25]

Other Possible Medications for Alcohol Dependence

A few other medications have been reported to have efficacy in the outpatient treatment of alcohol dependence and to be examined in human laboratory studies evaluating possible mechanisms. The serotonin-3 antagonist ondansetron was initially reported to reduce the subjective effects of ethanol in social drinkers.[136,274] Subsequently, a large clinical trial showed efficacy of ondansetron in reducing alcoholic drinking, at least in Early Onset Alcoholics, but not Late Onset Alcoholics.[145] Serotonergic abnormalities in "biologically predisposed" individuals have been suggested as the mechanism of this differential efficacy.[130] A subsequent human laboratory study reported that the alcohol cue-induced craving of early onset alcoholics may differ as a function of genetic polymorphisms in the serotonin transporter.[1] More recently, both human laboratory studies with nontreatment seekers[157-159] and outpatient treatment clinical trials[134,147] have provided further evidence on the role of genetic polymorphisms in the serotonin transporter in the beneficial effects of ondansetron in reducing excessive alcohol drinking. Topiramate has been shown to have efficacy in reducing drinking in alcohol-dependent outpatients in two randomized controlled trials.[132,146] Two subsequent human laboratory studies further confirmed the role of topiramate in affecting alcohol drinking, craving, and subjective effects of alcohol.[197,198] Of special note, in order to reduce some of the adverse cognitive side effects of topiramate, these studies included a gradual dose-escalation period of more than 5 weeks during which subjects received placebo, or 200 or 300 mg per day during outpatient treatment before they were brought into the laboratory.

Hutchinson and colleagues have been studying olanzapine in the human laboratory and in the clinic as a medication having a mixed profile of actions as an antagonist at the D_2, D_4, and serotonin-2 receptors. An initial laboratory study of heavy social drinkers reported that 5 mg olanzapine reduced the urge to drink after exposure to alcohol cues and a priming dose of alcohol.[117] However, a treatment trial in alcohol-dependent outpatients failed to show efficacy of 10–15 mg olanzapine.[88] Subsequently, another laboratory study[116] showed that a functional polymorphism in the dopamine D_4 receptor (DRD4) gene mediates the cue-reactive effects of alcohol and that olanzapine really was only effective in reducing cue-reactivity[119] in the subgroup of subjects having the long (L) form of the variable number tandem repeat for the DRD4 gene. Finally, this investigative group studied a group of alcohol-dependent subjects given 2.5–5 mg olanzapine versus placebo during a 12-week treatment trial.[118] These subjects were brought into the human laboratory before and after 2 weeks of double-blind treatment and were tested in the cue-reactivity paradigm. The study showed that olanzapine was effective only in the L-carriers where it reduced cue-reactive craving observed in the laboratory, and also was effective in reducing alcohol drinking in the outpatient treatment component of the study.

Another medication studied in alcohol human laboratory settings is baclofen. Some treatment clinical trials but not others have suggested its efficacy for alcoholic patients, especially those with significant liver disease and/or higher severity of alcohol dependence.[169] Three alcohol human laboratory studies with baclofen have been conducted and converge to a similar conclusion that baclofen does not reduce alcohol craving even though it alters the subjective effects of alcohol.[57,59,170] The latter might represent a biobehavioral mechanism by which baclofen could reduce excessive alcohol drinking for some individuals.

Another promising medication, gabapentin, reported to be safe when combined with alcohol, did not alter alcohol effects[22] but delayed the onset to heavy drinking.[28] Consistent with a human laboratory study indicating that gabapentin may reduce alcohol cue-elicited craving,[185] outpatient treatment clinical trials support a role of gabapentin in reducing excessive alcohol use and craving,[9,186] especially in those patients with high baseline alcohol withdrawal symptoms.[9]

Role of the Human Laboratory in Evaluating Medications for Cocaine Dependence

Many different potential medications with a variety of different pharmacological mechanisms have been tested in Phase II and III efficacy trials looking for a medication to treat cocaine dependence.[54] Several recent reviews have described the different medications that have been evaluated for the treatment of cocaine dependence and so the reader is referred to those articles for further information.[41,76,79,265,284] Although there have been sporadic positive findings in some of these studies, no medications have yet been proven effective or approved by the FDA. Cocaine acts to inhibit monoamine transporters, although the mechanism of action related to addiction is believed to be primarily through actions on the dopamine transporter to enhance dopamine activity in brain reward neurocircuitry. Consequently, many pharmacological studies have targeted dopamine synthesis, receptors, and the reuptake transporter. In addition, other medications targeting other neurochemical modulators of the brain reward pathways also have been studied.

Evaluation of Dopamine Agonists and Antagonists for Cocaine Treatment

Several human laboratory studies have examined the ability of dopamine antagonists to reduce cocaine-induced subjective effects or self-administration. In cocaine-dependent individuals, haloperidol antagonized cue-elicited craving.[18] In subjects with cocaine abuse or dependence, risperidone[209] reduced the subjective effects of cocaine, but flupenthixol[58] had no effect on cocaine's subjective effects or self-administration. Again, in subjects with cocaine abuse or dependence, the $D_{1/5}$ antagonist ecopipam reduced cocaine's subjective effects acutely[250]; however, these effects were not replicated in a study employing repeated ecopipam dosing[204] or in a study of smoked cocaine where ecopipam actually increased the subjective and reinforcing effects of cocaine.[99] These results suggest that at best, dopamine antagonists produce variable and inconsistent reductions in positive subjective effects of cocaine. The overall conclusion from these and other studies do not support the utility of dopamine antagonist treatments.[37,79,81,284] Furthermore, they suggest that direct and potentially unpleasant side effects of treatment with dopamine antagonists could actually enhance the reinforcing effects of cocaine, which could explain the increase in cocaine use observed in an outpatient treatment study using olanzapine.[153]

Human laboratory studies also have examined the effects of direct-acting dopamine agonists. The D_2 agonist, bromocriptine, was shown to reduce the blood pressure elevations but enhance the heart rate effects of cocaine and it caused undesirable "fainting" without changing cocaine's subjective effects.[228] Another D_2 agonist pergolide[96] reduced the subjective effects but did not alter cocaine self-administration. The D_1 agonist ABT-431 was reported also to reduce the subjective effects and blood pressure but enhance the heart rate effects of cocaine without altering cocaine self-administration.[95] Two dopamine partial agonists also have been examined. Amantadine had no effect on the cardiovascular or subjective effects of cocaine or on cocaine self-administration,[36] and aripiprazole was actually reported to increase cocaine subjective effects[173] and self-administration.[97] Although not acting directly upon the dopamine receptor, but rather indirectly upon the dopamine transporter, bupropion was found only to produce slight alterations in cocaine-related subjective effects.[216] The general lack of positive results in these human laboratory studies is consistent with the lack of efficacy of dopamine agonists, partial agonists, and bupropion in the outpatient treatment of cocaine dependence.[79,287]

Evaluation of Stimulant-Replacement Strategies for Cocaine

In contrast to the disappointment with dopamine agonists and antagonist approaches, studies examining the use of psychomotor stimulants in a stimulant "replacement"-type of reproach[79,81,243] have been more encouraging. An intriguing 5-week inpatient human laboratory study showed that gradually increasing oral doses of cocaine (25–100 mg/kg, four times daily) produced modest reductions in the subjective effects of intravenous challenge doses of cocaine without potentiating the cardiovascular effects of cocaine.[290] Previous human laboratory studies have shown that cocaine binges are associated with substantial "acute" tolerance, whereas most of the subjective and cardiovascular effects of cocaine are seen with the initial dose and subsequent doses only serve to maintain the initial effect without adding additional effect.[3,66,69,70] When combined with data that speed of onset is an important determinant of euphoria,[205] the efficacy of the oral cocaine pretreatment is likely due to the lesser euphoria resulting from the oral pretreatment dose of cocaine coupled with cross-tolerance to the acute effects of the additional cocaine challenge doses. This is exactly analogous to what is believed to occur with methadone maintenance and is similar to that observed in a human laboratory study, where experimenter-administered doses of heroin given on top of methadone pretreatment show diminished responses.[48] Nonetheless, concerns about the ethics or social acceptance of cocaine-replacement approaches for cocaine addiction are likely to limit consideration of this approach. Thus, most studies of the agonist-like replacement approach[79,81,243] have examined dopamine reuptake inhibitors and stimulant drugs other than cocaine. Although human laboratory studies with cocaine have reported substantial tolerance to the cardiovascular acceleration that occurs within a cocaine binge,[66,69,70] there still are substantial cardiovascular safety concerns regarding the possible drug-drug interactions between cocaine and other stimulant drugs.

A double-blind, placebo-controlled efficacy trial examined the effects of placebo and two doses of oral dextroamphetamine as a treatment for cocaine-dependent outpatients.[78] That study included a human laboratory component that gave the outpatients their initial double-blind dose in a controlled environment as part of a safety assessment.[243] In the laboratory assessment component, dextroamphetamine showed characteristic stimulant effects including mild elevations of subjective effects and euphoria, and there were no limiting adverse events observed. Coupled with treatment findings showing dose-related increases in treatment retention and reduced cocaine use without evidence of abuse or diversion of dextroamphetamine, these data suggest that stimulant therapy for cocaine dependence may be a reasonable approach. In another study taking the same approach with methylphenidate, the human laboratory component found that methylphenidate produced adverse stimulant effects but not subjective euphoria in the cocaine-dependent population.[238] Of interest, methylphenidate also was not efficacious in the main outpatient treatment trial either.[80] Thus, these two studies conducted in treatment-seeking individuals show a good correspondence between the human laboratory findings and treatment outcome and further suggest that the positive subjective effects of dextroamphetamine may be an essential component of efficacy in the stimulant-replacement approach to treatment of cocaine dependence.[79,81,243] More recently, a human laboratory study indicated that choice to use cocaine was significantly lower during D-amphetamine maintenance, as compared to placebo.[252]

Still the question remains about the safety of the cocaine + stimulant drug interaction in cocaine-dependent populations. Several human laboratory studies have evaluated the cardiovascular safety and abuse liability of giving combinations of cocaine plus other stimulants. In one such study,[227] acute dosing with mazindol did not substantially alter the acute subjective effects of cocaine, but it significantly enhanced the blood pressure and heart rate elevations produced by intravenous cocaine leading the authors to suggest that mazindol would not be a desirable treatment. A follow-up clinical treatment trial in cocaine-dependent methadone maintenance participants did not find mazindol versus placebo differences in outcome,[181] although it is important to note that there was no evidence for harmful or countertherapeutic effects of mazindol either. Another study gave up to 30 mg oral dextroamphetamine in combination with up to 96 mg intranasal cocaine to non–treatment-seeking cocaine abusers and reported that there were no significant potentiating effects on cardiovascular measures[236,237,243]—a finding that was generally supported in the outpatient trial of dextroamphetamine for cocaine dependence.[78] In yet another study,[42] modafinil blunted several subjective effects and even the systolic blood pressure increases produced by intravenous cocaine infusion. This human laboratory study was followed up by the National Institute on Drug Abuse in a clinical treatment trial, which found that modafinil was superior to placebo in reducing cocaine use among the subgroup of individuals without a comorbid alcohol use disorder, but it was not effective among the subgroup of individuals who had a comorbid alcohol use disorder.[6] Following up on this trial, Kampman and colleagues[152] performed another treatment trial where they specifically excluded cocaine use disorder individuals with alcohol use disorder comorbidity and found that modafinil was significantly more effective than placebo in increasing cocaine abstinence. Although other treatment trials have been inconsistent in generating either positive[255] or negative[154,254] findings, overall, these human laboratory data clearly predicted that stimulant medications with lesser abuse potential than cocaine could be given safely to cocaine-dependent populations with a reasonable expectation that individuals would benefit from a stimulant-replacement approach to treatment.

Evaluation of Cocaine Treatments Affecting Other Neurochemical Systems

A number of other pharmacological approaches to treatment for cocaine dependence also have been evaluated in the human laboratory. Aside from dopamine, several studies have attempted to alter other monoamine neurotransmitter levels (i.e., norepinephrine and serotonin). Catecholamine depletion by means of consuming a tyrosine-depleting amino acid beverage was shown to reduce cue and low-dose cocaine-induced craving for more cocaine, but did not alter cocaine-induced euphoria or self-administration.[171] The monoamine oxidase-B inhibitor selegiline, which should increase catecholamine levels including dopamine, was reported to have no effect[90] or to reduce[114,208] the subjective effects of cocaine. Two studies[62,162] reported that the catecholamine reuptake inhibitor desipramine increased baseline blood pressures, decreased cocaine craving, and altered the positive subjective effects of cocaine without altering the high or self-administration of cocaine. Blockade of the serotonin transporter with fluoxetine was reported to reduce the subjective euphoria of cocaine in one study[291] but not another study.[100] These human laboratory studies indicate that, at best, medications that alter serotonin or norepinephrine activity in general do not have robust effects to alter cocaine euphoria or reinforcement, and so it is no surprise that outpatient treatment trials with these medications have not been positive either.[79,284] In cocaine-using research volunteers, the γ-aminobutyric acid reuptake inhibitor tiagabine had no effect on the subjective or reinforcing effects of oral cocaine,[172] and the γ-aminobutyric acid agonist gabapentin reduced the subjective effects but not self-administration in cocaine-dependent subjects.[102] Each of these pharmacological approaches has been evaluated in clinical trials and none have been found to be efficacious.[79,284] More recent work has explored the potential role of progesterone for cocaine use disorder. A human laboratory study did not find significant differences between progesterone and placebo on cocaine self-administration in women.[234] By contrast, a preliminary treatment trial with postpartum women indicated that progesterone was superior to placebo in reducing self-reported cocaine use, although no difference was found on free urine drug tests.[301] Neither a human laboratory study[24] nor two treatment trials[200,300] support the potential use of the 5-HT$_{1A}$ receptor partial agonist buspirone for cocaine use disorder. Finally, a human laboratory study testing low and high doses of intravenous cocaine indicated that topiramate, as compared to placebo, reduced cocaine craving and monetary value of high-dose cocaine; by contrast, monetary value of low-dose cocaine was increased in the topiramate group.[141] Consistent with this laboratory study, a treatment trial indicated the efficacy of topiramate, compared to placebo, in increasing cocaine-free days and cocaine-free urine tests and decreasing cocaine craving.[135]

Several human laboratory studies have examined the effects of antihypertensive calcium channel blockers in cocaine dependence. As cerebrovascular vasodilators, they have been suggested as possible treatments for vascular stroke and cognitive impairment related to cocaine dependence.[77,137] In this regard, isradipine was shown to reduce the ischemic effects of cocaine infusion.[129] In other laboratory studies in cocaine-dependent subjects, nifedipine,[203] nimodipine,[163] and isradipine[143] were shown to block the blood pressure–elevating effects of cocaine in subjects but not the stimulant or euphoric subjective responses. Following both acute[143] and repeated dosing[148] with isradipine, the reduction in cocaine-related pressor effects was also associated with an exacerbation of cocaine-related heart rate increases. In addition, repeated dosing with isradipine was shown to produce headaches and other unpleasant effects and to increase the positive and reinforcing effects of intravenous cocaine infusion.[241] Given these laboratory results as noted earlier, it is no wonder that a 12-week trial of amlodipine for the treatment of cocaine-dependent outpatients was plagued by high drop-out rates, and failed to reduce cocaine craving or cocaine use more than was seen with placebo treatment.[177]

Two other medications have shown efficacy in human laboratory and outpatient treatment studies but are not likely to be pursued as treatments for primary cocaine dependence for safety reasons. The mu-receptor partial agonist, buprenorphine, was shown in two studies to reduce cocaine self-administration. One study in intravenous heroin and cocaine users reported that buprenorphine decreased intravenous cocaine self-administration, but it also potentiated several subjective effects including euphoria and sedation.[67] Another study in cocaine-dependent methadone maintenance participants found that substitution to buprenorphine was superior to continued methadone maintenance to decrease desire ("I want") for cocaine and self-administration behavior without altering other subjective effects.[68] Despite these positive results, the abuse potential of buprenorphine coupled with its potential for physiological dependence make its use for primary cocaine dependence unlikely. Nonetheless, it still may be useful to decrease cocaine use in buprenorphine-maintenance therapy for opioid dependence.[202] A second medication, shown to have efficacy in the outpatient treatment of cocaine dependence,[32] is the alcoholism treatment agent disulfiram. Several human laboratory studies have shown that disulfiram inhibits cocaine metabolism and increases cocaine blood levels and its cardiovascular effects.[94,188] Although those initial studies reported no significant alteration of cocaine's subjective effects, a more recent study[14] reported that disulfiram decreased cocaine-induced subjective high. The putative mechanism for efficacy of disulfiram in the treatment of cocaine dependence is presumed to be its inhibition of dopamine beta-hydroxylase.[265] However, because of disulfiram's inhibition of cocaine metabolism and its side-effect profile, there are concerns about its safety as a treatment for primary cocaine dependence. Because alcohol may be consumed by a cocaine-intoxicated individual treated with disulfiram, the safety of a disulfiram-alcohol reaction was evaluated in subjects with cocaine abuse or dependence in a three-way drug interaction study.[242] That study found that alcohol administration was associated with clinically significant hypotension and increased heart rate in subjects given 5–7 days of disulfiram (250–500 mg) pretreatment. Intravenous infusion of 30 mg cocaine under these conditions counteracted the hypotension but tended to potentiate the heart rate effects. However, safety stop-point criteria prevented the administration of cocaine in two of three subjects who were hypotensive due to an disulfiram-alcohol reaction in subjects treated with 500 mg disulfiram. This human laboratory study illustrates the safety concerns of using disulfiram in the treatment of cocaine dependence. Nonetheless, a review of the safety data from a number of published studies administering disulfiram to cocaine-dependent outpatients and to patients with dual cocaine-alcohol dependence has concluded that it can be safely used for cocaine treatment.[178]

Human Laboratory Studies of Medications for Amphetamine or Methamphetamine

Evaluation of Dopaminergic Treatments for Methamphetamine

In normal healthy volunteers, acute doses of pimozide failed to reduce the subjective effects of amphetamine,[26] and neither haloperidol nor risperidone reduced the euphoric effects of methamphetamine.[287] In subjects with histories of amphetamine abuse or dependence, acute doses of haloperidol did reduce positive subjective effects of amphetamine,[258] as did repeated doses of chlorpromazine and to a lesser extent pimozide.[151] However, these mixed findings focusing on subjective effects are similar to those seen using dopamine antagonists for cocaine dependence. There is no reason to believe that dopamine antagonists will be any more successful for amphetamine or methamphetamine dependence than they have been for cocaine.[81] The partial D_2 receptor agonist, aripiprazole, has been evaluated in two human laboratory studies and in one outpatient treatment trial. In normal healthy subjects, acute doses of aripiprazole produced dose-related reductions in the discriminative stimulus, subjective effects, and cardiovascular increases produced by D-amphetamine.[268] In methamphetamine-dependent volunteers, 2 weeks of treatment with aripiprazole did not increase cue-induced craving for methamphetamine but did increase methamphetamine-induced stimulant and euphoric subjective effects, and increased baseline levels of desire for methamphetamine.[210] In a clinical treatment trial of amphetamine-dependent outpatients, a three-arm comparison study was stopped early in the trial because an interim analysis showed that aripiprazole increased amphetamine use relative to placebo, while methylphenidate was significantly better than placebo.[280] These data clearly indicate that dopamine agonist treatments may be countertherapeutic for the treatment of amphetamine/methamphetamine dependence. However, the one study with methylphenidate, and several with bupropion, suggest that dopamine reuptake inhibitors may be beneficial for the treatment of amphetamine/methamphetamine dependence. In methamphetamine-dependent research volunteers, a Phase I safety study showed that repeated oral doses of bupropion reduced both the cardiovascular pressor effects of methamphetamine as well as the subjective high and liking produced by intravenous infusion of moderate doses of methamphetamine.[211,212] Subsequent to this human laboratory study, an initial multisite treatment trial[56] found that bupropion was superior to placebo to reduce methamphetamine use in outpatients who used less frequently than daily, but not in frequent daily users. However, a subsequent clinical trial reported no difference between bupropion and placebo in enhancing methamphetamine abstinence in nondaily users.[5] Like for any clinical trial, and especially in the addiction field, medication compliance remains an issue. For example, a recent 12-week clinical trial indicated no difference between modafinil and placebo in methamphetamine use; however, the study was considered inconclusive due to the poor compliance to the study medication.[4] Finally, an 8-week trial found significant benefits of dextroamphetamine in reducing methamphetamine withdrawal and craving but not in reducing methamphetamine-negative urine tests.[75]

Evaluation of Methamphetamine Treatments Affecting Other Neurochemical Systems

In two human laboratory studies conducted in healthy volunteers, ondansetron was reported to produce modest reductions of positive subjective effects of amphetamine[82] or to reduce the amphetamine-induced decrease in hunger.[261] However, a treatment trial using varying doses of ondansetron in methamphetamine-dependent outpatients did not show evidence of efficacy.[134] The N-methyl-D-aspartate antagonist memantine was reported to alter the discriminative stimulus effects of methamphetamine in healthy subjects with limited histories of cocaine or amphetamine use.[101] It is notable that memantine also produced positive stimulant-like subjective effects of its own and did not reduce those produced by methamphetamine. In methamphetamine-dependent volunteers given intravenous methamphetamine, acute doses of topiramate produced sedative and undesirable side effects by itself, enhanced the positive subjective effects,[139] and reduced the perceptual-motor facilitating effects[140] of methamphetamine. These human laboratory studies are consistent with the findings of an outpatient treatment study where topiramate was not helpful to promote abstinence in methamphetamine users overall, although on secondary outcomes, topiramate decreased methamphetamine use and relapse rates in those patients who were already abstinent.[55] In healthy volunteers, acute doses of isradipine reduced some of the positive subjective effects produced by methamphetamine and increased ratings of "I could refuse."[144] In subjects with methamphetamine dependence, a within-subject crossover design found that repeated doses of isradipine reduced euphoria and positive subjective effects of methamphetamine but only when placebo treatment occurred first and not when isradipine treatment occurred first.[142] Although isradipine did reduce methamphetamine-induced blood pressure elevation, it also enhanced the heart rate effects.[148] No treatment study has been attempted to our knowledge; however, the potential for tachycardic interactions between isradipine and methamphetamine is considered a sufficient concern to preclude further development. Although not tested in a treatment trial, naltrexone and varenicline have been tested for methamphetamine in human laboratory studies. Compared to placebo, naltrexone decreased methamphetamine craving as well as subjective ratings of "stimulated" and "would like drug access,"[233] and varenicline significantly reduced methamphetamine-related ratings of "any drug effect," "stimulated," "high," "drug liking," and "good effects."[282]

General Conclusions Regarding Human Laboratory Studies

Methods to assess the abuse liability of multiple classes of drugs of abuse in human subjects tested in experimental laboratory environments are well established and validated. Increasingly, over the past decade, the human abuse liability assessment model has been used to examine the drug interaction of candidate medication treatments with opiates, alcohol, cocaine, and methamphetamine. This review illustrated the: (1) results with the agonist/antagonist approaches that have been the basis for the treatment of opiate and nicotine dependence; (2) mechanistic evaluation of approved and potential medications for alcohol dependence; and (3) numerous medications that have been evaluated as possible treatments for cocaine and methamphetamine dependence. Useful and important information from these studies has helped

to advance our understanding of the safety, mechanism, and possible efficacy of different pharmacological approaches to treatment and has contributed to the development of specific agents for treatment. Several general conclusions are possible from this review.

Human laboratory studies of direct pharmacological agonist or antagonist therapy mostly have been possible only in the study of opiate and nicotine dependence where opiates and nicotine act directly and selectively upon specific neurotransmitter systems. Here it is notable that human laboratory studies of the effects of agonist replacement therapy with nicotine replacement, methadone, and buprenorphine have played an important role to verify possible efficacy and understand the mechanism(s) involved in such drug-drug interactions. Conclusions from the human laboratory studies showing that agonist replacement produces cross-tolerance with commensurate reductions in euphoria and reinforcing effects are consistent with outpatient treatment trials showing efficacy with agonist replacement strategies for nicotine and opiate dependence. However, human laboratory studies with antagonist treatments generally have produced false-positive results because although a pharmacological antagonist shows perfect efficacy in the human laboratory, clinical experience reveals poor effectiveness of antagonist treatment due to poor medication compliance. Behavioral/legal contingencies may be useful to enhance compliance and efficacy of antagonist therapy; however, this is not a strategy that is generally available in community practice.

In the alcohol-related literature, the laboratory study results showing that disulfiram and naltrexone can reduce the euphoric and reinforcing effects of alcohol are generally consistent with the outpatient treatment literature. Again, although human laboratory studies did reveal the aversive and unpleasant effects of the disulfiram-alcohol reaction, it took clinical experience to recognize that this would be a limitation on effectiveness due to poor compliance. It also important to note that, although human laboratory studies represent an important cost-effective step toward medication development,[174] most studies have been conducted in nontreatment seekers, whereas larger efficacy trials are conducted in treatment seekers. This might explain the discrepancy sometimes observed between human laboratory studies and treatment trials. This is especially important in light of recent data suggesting differences between nontreatment versus treatment seekers in several factors (e.g., personality, impulsivity, trauma/stress, cognition, aggression, mood, and liver enzyme tests) beyond the quantity of alcohol consumption.[247]

Many different pharmaceutical approaches have been tried for cocaine and methamphetamine dependence treatment. Because none have proven generally useful or effective, it is difficult to gauge exactly the extent to which the human laboratory results have been helpful toward this objective. Nonetheless, this review has suggested that, in general, the results from the human laboratory studies have been consistent in the following ways. First, direct-acting dopamine agonists and antagonists generally have not been effective in either the human laboratory or in the outpatient clinical setting, and there is some evidence from both the laboratory and clinic that dopamine agonists may actually be countertherapeutic. Second, human laboratory experiments with agonist-like replacement strategies using stimulant medications have been valuable to show possible efficacy and the safety of this approach. These findings are consistent with the results of outpatient treatment trials showing efficacy with D-amphetamine, modafinil, or bupropion. Third, although there are some false-positive results from human laboratory studies showing treatment-related reductions in cocaine or methamphetamine effects, we conclude that many of these have limitations related to studying healthy volunteers rather than drug-dependent populations and/or because of a focus on craving/subjective effects rather than self-administration. Fourth, the human laboratory plays an indispensable role in enabling Phase I and II safety evaluations of medication effects in the target population both with and without the addition of the drug interaction between the treatment and cocaine/methamphetamine.

Finally, this review shows that when one recognizes the strengths and limitations of human laboratory methods in the medication development process, it is clear that these kinds of studies are valuable and will play an increasingly important role in the evaluation of the mechanism, safety, and possible efficacy of putative treatment agents for alcohol, cocaine, and methamphetamine. Indeed, not only do human laboratory studies hold the potential of a cost-effective approach toward medication development, but they also may shed light on personalized medicine approaches. The latter aspect may be achieved with several approaches, which include but are not limited to genetic analysis and/or neuroimaging techniques that may help identifying theragnostic biomarkers for personalized treatments.[104] Although it has not been discussed specifically, it is reasonable to suggest that human laboratory methodological approaches are useful to evaluate medication treatments for other drug dependencies as well.

Acknowledgments

Dr. Leggio's work is supported by National Institutes of Health (NIH) intramural funding ZIA-AA000218 (*Section on Clinical Psychoneuroendocrinology and Neuropsychopharmacology*), and jointly supported by the Division of Intramural Clinical and Biological Research of the National Institute on Alcohol Abuse and Alcoholism (NIAAA) and the Intramural Research Program of the National Institute on Drug Abuse (NIDA).

The authors would like to thank Vignesh Sankar, BSc, from the NIAAA/NIDA Section on Clinical Psychoneuroendocrinology and Neuropsychopharmacology for bibliographic assistance.

The content of this article is solely the responsibility of the authors and does not necessarily represent the official views of the NIH.

References

1. Ait-Daoud N, Roache JD, Dawes MA, et al. Can serotonin transporter genotype predict craving in alcoholism? *Alcohol Clin Exp Res.* 2009;33:1329–1335.

2. Altman JL, Meyer RE, Mirin SM, McNamee, McDougle HB. Opiate antagonists and the modification of heroin self-administration behavior in man: an experimental study. *Int J Addict.* 1976;11: 485–499.

3. Ambre JJ, Berlknap SM, Nelson J, Ruo TI, Shin SG, Atkinson AJ. Acute tolerance to cocaine in humans. *Clin Pharmacol Therap.* 1988;44:1–8.

4. Anderson AL, Li SH, Biswas K, McSherry F, et al. Modafinil for the treatment of methamphetamine dependence. *Drug Alcohol Depend.* 2012;120(1-3):135–141.

5. Anderson AL, Li SH, Markova D, et al. Bupropion for the treatment of methamphetamine dependence in non-daily users: a randomized, double-blind, placebo-controlled trial. *Drug Alcohol Depend.* 2015;150:170–174.

6. Anderson AL, Reid MS, Li SH, et al. Modafinil for the treatment of cocaine dependence. *Drug and Alcohol Dependence.* 2009;104: 133–139.

7. Anonymous. Alcohol and drugs: mixing can be risky. *Consumer Rep.* 2005;70:49.

8. Anonymous. National highway traffic safety administration (NHTSA) notes. Commentary: drugged driving—different spin on an old problem [comment]. *Ann Emergency Med.* 2000;35: 399–400.

9. Anton RF, Myrick H, Baros AM, et al. Efficacy of a combination of flumazenil and gabapentin in the treatment of alcohol dependence: relationship to alcohol withdrawal symptoms. *J Clin Psychopharmacol.* 2009;29(4):334–342.

10. Anton RF, O'Malley SS, Ciraulo DA, et al. (for the COMBINE Group). Combined pharmacotherapies and behavioral interventions for alcohol dependence: the COMBINE study: a randomized controlled trial. *J Am Med Assoc.* 2006;295:2003–2017.

11. Anton RF, Oroszi G, O'Malley S, et al. An evaluation of mu-opioid receptor (OPRM1) as a predictor of naltrexone response in the treatment of alcohol dependence: results from the Combined Pharmacotherapies and Behavioral Interventions for Alcohol Dependence (COMBINE) study. *Arch Gen Psychiatry.* 2008;65(2): 135–144.

12. APA. *Diagnostic and Statistical Manual of Mental Disorders Fourth Edition Text Revision (DSM-IV-TR).* Washington, DC: American Psychiatric Association; 2000.

13. Avants SK, Margolin A, Kosten TR, Cooney NL. Differences between responders and nonresponders to cocaine cues in the laboratory. *Addict Behav.* 1995;20:215–224.

14. Baker JR, Jatlow P, McCance-Katz EF. Disulfiram effects on responses to intravenous cocaine administration. *Drug Alcohol Depend.* 2007;87:202–209.

15. Balster RL, Bigelow GE. Guideline and methodological reviews concerning drug abuse liability assessment. *Drug Alcohol Depend.* 2003;70:S13–S40.

16. Barcelona Conference. Barcelona meeting on clinical testing of drug abuse liability: consensus statement and recommendations. *Br J Addict.* 1991;86:1527–1528.

17. Beecher HK. *Measurement of Subjective Responses: Quantitative Effects of Drugs.* New York: Oxford University; 1959.

18. Berger SP, Hall S, Mickalian JD, Reid MS, Crawford Cl, Delucchi K, et al. Haloperidol antagonism of cue-elicited cocaine craving. *The Lancet.* 1996;347:504–508.

19. Bickel WK, DeGrandpre RJ, Higgins ST. Behavioral economics: a novel experimental approach to the study of drug dependence. *Drug Alcohol Depend.* 1993;33:173–192.

20. Bickel WK, DeGrandpre RJ, Higgins ST. The behavioral economics of concurrent drug reinforcers: a review and reanalysis of drug self-administration research. *Psychopharmacology.* 1995;118: 250–259.

21. Bigelow GE. Human drug abuse liability assessment: opioids and analgesics. *Br J Addict.* 1991;86:1625–1628.

22. Bisaga A, Evans SM. The acute effects of gabapentin in combination with alcohol in heavy drinkers. *Drug Alcohol Depend.* 2006;83(1):25–32.

23. Bohn MJ, Krahn DD, Staehler BA. Development and initial validation of a measure of drinking urges in abstinent alcoholics. *Alcohol Clin Exp Res.* 1995;19:600–606.

24. Bolin BL, Lile JA, Marks KR, Beckmann JS, Rush CR, Stoops WW. Buspirone reduces sexual risk-taking intent but not cocaine self-administration. *Exp Clin Psychopharmacol.* 2016;24(3): 162–173.

25. Brasser SM, McCaul ME, Houtsmuller EJ. Alcohol effects during acamprosate treatment: a dose-response study in humans. *Alcohol Clin Exp Res.* 2004;28:1074–1083.

26. Brauer LK, de Wit H. High dose pimozide does not block amphetamine-induced euphoria in normal volunteers. *Pharmacol Biochem Behav.* 1997;56:265–272.

27. Brewer C. How effective is the standard dose of disulfiram: a review of the alcohol-disulfiram reactions in practice. *Brit J Psychiat.* 1984;144:200–202.

28. Brower KJ, Myra Kim H, Strobbe S, Karam-Hage MA, Consens F, Zucker RA. A randomized double-blind pilot trial of gabapentin versus placebo to treat alcohol dependence and comorbid insomnia. *Alcohol Clin Exp Res.* 2008;32(8):1429–1438.

29. Brown SA, Goldman MS, Christiansen BA. Do alcohol expectancies mediate drinking patterns of adults? *J Consulting Clin Psychol.* 1985;53:512–519.

30. Buchhalter AR, Fant RV, Henningfield JE. Novel pharmacological approaches for treating tobacco dependence and withdrawal: current status. *Drugs.* 2008;68:1067–1088.

31. Cahill K, Lindson-Hawley N, Thomas KH, Fanshawe TR, Lancaster T. Nicotine receptor partial agonists for smoking cessation. *Cochrane Database Syst Rev.* 2016;5:CD006103.

32. Carroll KM, Fenton LR, Ball SA, et al. Efficacy of disulfiram and cognitive behavior therapy in cocaine-dependent outpatients. *Arch Gen Psychiatr.* 2004;61:264–272.

33. Carter BL, Tiffany ST. A meta-analysis: meta-analysis of cue-reactivity in addiction research. *Addiction.* 1999;94:327–340.

34. Christensen JK, Moller IW, Ronsted P, Angelo HR, Johansson ZB. Dose-effect relationship of disulfiram in human volunteers. I: clinical studies. *Pharmacol Toxicol.* 1991;68:163–165.

35. Chutuape MAD, de Wit H. Relationship between subjective effects and drug preferences: ethanol and diazepam. *Drug Alcohol Depend.* 1994;34:243–251.

36. Collins ED, Vosburg SK, Hart CL, Haney M, Foltin RW. Amantidine does not modulate reinforcing, subjective or cardiovascular effects of cocaine in humans. *Pharmacol Biochem Behav.* 2003;76:401–407.

37. Comer SD, Ashworth JB, Foltin RW, Johanson ED, Zacny JP, Walsh SL. The role of human drug self-administration procedures in the development of medications. *Drug Alcohol Depend.* 2008;96:1–15.

38. Comer SD, Collins ED, Kleber HD, Nuwayser ES, Kerrigan JH, Fischman MW. Depot naltrexone: Long-lasting antagonism of the effects of heroin in humans. *Psychopharmacology.* 2002;159:351–360.

39. Comer SD, Collins ED, Wilson ST, Donovan MR, Foltin RW, Fischman MW. Effects of an alternative reinforcer on intravenous heroin self-administration by humans. *Eur J Pharmacol.* 1998;345:13–26.

40. Conners GJ, O'Farrell TJ, Cutter HSG, Thompson DL. Alcohol expectancies among male alcoholics, problems drinkers, and non-problem drinkers. *Alcohol Clin Exp Res.* 1986;10:667–671.

41. Czoty PW, Stoops WW, Rush CR. Evaluation of the "Pipeline" for development of medications for cocaine use disorder: a review of translational preclinical, human laboratory, and clinical trial research. *Pharmacol Rev.* 2016;68(3):533–562.

42. Dackis CA, Lynch KG, Yu E, et al. Modafinil and cocaine: a double-blind, placebo-controlled drug interaction study. *Drug Alcohol Depend.* 2003;20:29–37.

43. Davidson D, Palfai T, Bird C, Swift R. Effects of naltrexone on alcohol self-administration in heavy drinkers. *Alcohol Clin Exp Res.* 1999;23:195–203.

44. Deptula D, Pomara N. Effects of antidepressants on human performance: a review. *J Clin Psychopharmacol.* 1990;10:105–111.

45. de Wit H, Uhlenhuth EH, Johanson CE. Individual differences in the reinforcing and subjective effects of amphetamine and diazepam. *Drug Alcohol Depend.* 1986;16:341–360.

46. de Witte P, Littleton J, Parot P, Koob G. Neuroprotective and abstinence-promoting effects of acamprosate: elucidating the mechanism of action CNS *Drugs.* 19:517–537.

47. Donny EC, Bigelow GE, Walsh SL. Choosing to take cocaine in the human laboratory: effects of cocaine dose, inter-choice interval, and magnitude of alternative reinforcement. *Drug Alcohol Depend.* 2003;69:289–301.

48. Donny EC, Braser SM, Bigelow GE, Stitzer ML, Walsh SL. Methadone doses of 100 mg or greater are more effective than lower doses at suppressing heroin self-administration in opioid-dependent volunteers. *Addiction.* 2005;100:1496–1509.

49. Doty P, de Wit H. Effects of naltrexone pretreatment on the subjective and performance effects of ethanol in social drinkers. *Behav Pharmacol.* 1995;6:386–394.

50. Drobes DJ, Anton R, Thomas SE, Voronin K. A clinical laboratory paradigm for evaluating medication effects on alcohol consumption: naltrexone and nalmefene. *Neuropsychopharmacology.* 2003;28:755–764.

51. Drummond DC. Human models in craving research: what does cue-reactivity have to offer clinical research? *Addiction.* 2000;95(suppl):S129–S144.

52. Dudish-Poulsen SA, Hatsukami DK. Dissociation between subjective and behavioral responses after cocaine stimuli presentations. *Drug Alcohol Depend.* 1997;47:1–9.

53. Dykstra LA, Preston KL, Bigelow GE. Discriminative stimulus and subjective effects of opioids with mu and kappa activity: data from laboratory animals and human subjects. *Psychopharmacology.* 1997;130:14–27.

54. Elkashef A, Holmes TH, Bloch DA, et al. Retrospective analyses of pooled data from CREST I and CREST II trials for treatment of cocaine dependence. *Addiction.* 2005;100:91–101.

55. Elkashef A, Kahn R, Yu E, et al. Topiramate for the treatment of methamphetamine addiction: a multi-center placebo-controlled trial. *Addiction.* 2012;107(7):1297–1306.

56. Elkashef AM, Rawson RA, Anderson AL, et al. Bupropion for the treatment of methamphetamine dependence. *Neuropsychopharmacology.* 2008;33:1162–1170.

57. Evans SM, Bisaga A. Acute interaction of baclofen in combination with alcohol in heavy social drinkers. *Alcohol Clin Exp Res.* 2009;33(1):19–30.

58. Evans SM, Walsh SL, Levin FR, Foltin RW, Fischman MW, Bigelow GE. The effects of flupenthixol on the subjective and cardiovascular effects of intravenous cocaine in humans. *Drug Alcohol Depend.* 2001;64:271–283.

59. Farokhnia M, Schwandt ML, Lee MR, et al. Biobehavioral effects of baclofen in anxious alcohol-dependent individuals: a randomized, double-blind, placebo-controlled, laboratory study. *Translational Psychiatry (in press).* 2017.

60. Fischman MW. Relationship between self-reported drug effects and their reinforcing effects: studies with stimulant drugs. In: Fischman MW, Mellow NK, eds. *Testing For Abuse Liability of Drugs in Humans.* National Institute on Drug Abuse Research Monograph No. 92, DHEW Pub. No. (ADM) 89–163. Washington, DC: U.S. Government Printing Office; 1989.

61. Fischman MW, Foltin RW. Utility of subjective-effects in measurements assessing abuse liability of drugs in humans. *Br J Addict.* 1991;86:1563–1570.

62. Fischman MW, Foltin RW, Nestadt G, Pearlson GD. Effects of desipramine maintenance on cocaine self-administration by humans. *J Pharmacol Exp Ther.* 1990;253:760–770.

63. Fischman MW, Johanson CE. Ethical and practical issues involved in behavioral pharmacology research that administers drugs of abuse to human volunteers. *Behav Pharmacol.* 1998;9:479–498.

64. Foltin RW, Fischman MW. Assessment of abuse liability of stimulant drugs in humans: a methodological survey. *Drug Alcohol Depend.* 1991;28:3–48.

65. Foltin RW, Fischman MW. Methods for the assessment of abuse liability of psychomotor stimulants and anorectic agents in humans. *Br J Addict.* 1991;86:1633–1640.

66. Foltin RW, Fischman MW. Smoked and intravenous cocaine in humans: acute tolerance, cardiovascular and subject effects. *J Pharmacol Exp Ther.* 1991;257:247–261.

67. Foltin RW, Fischman MW. Effects of buprenorphine on the self-administration of cocaine by humans. *Behav Pharmacol.* 1994;5:79–89.

68. Foltin RW, Fischman MW. Effects of methadone or buprenorphine maintenance on the subjective and reinforcing effects of intravenous cocaine in humans. *J Pharmacol Exp Ther*. 1996;278:1153–1164.

69. Foltin RW, Fischman MW, Levin FR. Cardiovascular effects of cocaine in humans: laboratory studies. *Drug Alcohol Depend*. 1995;37:193–210.

70. Foltin RW, Ward AS, Haney M, Hart CL, Collins ED. The effects of escalating doses of smoked cocaine in humans. *Drug Alcohol Depend*. 2003;70:149–157.

71. Franklin T, Wang Z, Suh JJ, et al. Effects of varenicline on smoking cue–triggered neural and craving responses. *Arch Gen Psychiatry*. 2011;68(5):516–526.

72. Fraser HF, Jasinski DR. The assessment of the abuse potentiality of sedative/hypnotics (depressants): methods used in man. In: Martin WR, ed. *Drug Addiction I: Morphine, Sedative-Hypnotic and Alcohol Dependence. Handbook of Experimental Pharmacology*. Heidelberg: Springer; 1977;45:159–196.

73. Fraser HF, Van Horn GC, Isbell H. Studies on *N*-Allylnormorphine in man: antagonism to morphine and heroin and effects of mixtures of *N*-Allylnormorphine and morphine. *Am J Med Sci*. 1956;231:1–8.

74. Fraser HF, Van Horn GC, Martin WR, Wolbach AB, Isbell H. Methods for evaluating addiction liability. (A) "Attitude" of opiate addicts toward opiate-like drugs. (B) A short-term "direct" addiction test. *J Pharmacol Exp Ther*. 1961;133:371–387.

75. Galloway GP, Buscemi R, Coyle JR, et al. A randomized, placebo-controlled trial of sustained-release dextroamphetamine for treatment of methamphetamine addiction. *Clin Pharmacol Ther*. 2011;89(2):276–282.

76. Gorelick DA, Gardner EL, Xi ZX. Agents in development for the management of cocaine abuse. *Drug*. 2004;64:1547–1573.

77. Gottschalk PCH, Kosten TR. Isradipine enhancement of cerebral blood flow in abstinent cocaine abusers with and without chronic perfusion deficits. *Am J Addict*. 2002;11:200–208.

78. Grabowski J, Rhoades H, Schmitz J, et al. Dextroamphetamine for cocaine-dependence treatment: a double-blind randomized clinical trial. *J Clin Psychopharmacol*. 2002;21:522–526.

79. Grabowski J, Rhoades H, Stotts A, et al. Agonist-like or antagonist-like treatment of cocaine dependence with methadone for heroin dependence: two double-blind randomized clinical trials. *Neuropsychopharmacology*. 2004;29:969–981.

80. Grabowski J, Roache JD, Schmitz JM, Rhoades H, Creson D, Korszun A. Replacement medication for cocaine dependence: methylphenidate. *J Clin Psychopharmacol*. 1997;17:485–488.

81. Grabowski J, Shearer J, Merrill J, Negus SS. Agonist-like, replacement pharmacotherapy for stimulant abuse and dependence. *Addictive Behaviors*. 2004;29:1439–1464.

82. Grady TA, Broocks A, Canter SK, et al. Biological and behavioral response to d-amphetamine, alone and in combination with the serotonin3 receptor antagonist ondansetron, in healthy volunteers. *Psychiat Res*. 1996;64:1–10.

83. Griffiths RR, Bigelow GE, Ator NA. Principles of initial experimental drug abuse liability assessment in humans. *Drug Alcohol Depend*. 2003;70:S41–S54.

84. Griffiths RR, Bigelow GE, Henningfield JE. Similarities in animal and human drug-taking behavior. In: Mello NK, ed. *Advances in Substance Abuse*. 1. Greenwich, CT: JAI; 1980:1–90.

85. Griffiths RR, Rush CR, Puhala KA. Validation of the multiple-choice procedure for investigating drug reinforcement in humans. *Exp Clin Psychopharmacol*. 1996;4:97–106.

86. Griffiths RR, Troisi JR, Silverman K, Mumford GK. Multiple-choice procedure: an efficient approach for investigating drug reinforcement in humans. *Behav Pharmacol*. 1993;4:3–13.

87. Griffiths RR, Woodson PP. Reinforcing effects of caffeine in humans. *J Pharmacol Exp Ther*. 1988;246:21–29.

88. Guardia J, Segura L, Gonzalvo B, Iglesias L, Roncero C, Cardus M, et al. A double-blind, placebo-controlled study of olanzapine in the treatment of alcohol-dependence disorder. *Alcohol Clin Exp Res*. 2004;28:736–745.

89. Haass-Koffler CL, Akhlaghi F, Swift RM, Leggio L. Altering ethanol pharmacokinetics to treat alcohol use disorder: can you teach an old dog new tricks? *J Psychopharmacol*. 2017:269881116684338. https://doi:10.1177/0269881116684338. [Epub ahead of print] PubMed PMID: 28093021.

90. Haberny KA, Walsh SL, Ginn DH, et al. Absence of acute cocaine interactions with the MAO-B inhibitor selegiline. *Drug Alcohol Depend*. 1995;39:55–62.

91. Haertzen CA. Development of scales based on patterns of drug effects, using the Addiction Research Center Inventory (ARCI). *Psychol Rep*. 1966;18:163–194.

92. Hald J, Jacobsen E, Larsen V. The sensitizing effect of tetraethylthiuramdisulphide (Antabus) to ethylalcohol. *Acta Pharmacol*. 1948;4:285–296.

93. Halikas JS, Kuhn KL, Crosby R, Carlson G, Crea F. The measurement of craving in cocaine patients using the Minnesota cocaine craving scale. *Comprehensive Psychiatry*. 1991;32:22–27.

94. Hameedi FA, Rosen MI, McCance-Katz EF, et al. Behavioral, physiological, and pharmacological interaction of cocaine and disulfiram in humans. *Biol Psychiatry*. 1995;37:560–563.

95. Haney M, Collins ED, Ward AS, Foltin FW, Fischman MW. Effect of a selective dopamine D1 agonist (ABT-431) on smoked cocaine self-administration in humans. *Psychopharmacology*. 1999;143:102–110.

96. Haney M, Foltin RW, Fischman MW. Effects of pergolide on intravenous cocaine self-administration in men and women. *Psychopharmacology*. 1998;137:15–24.

97. Haney M, Hart CL, Reed SC, Vosburg SK, Foltin RW. *Aripiprazole Increases Cocaine Self-Administration in Humans*. Quebec City, Canada: Presented at International Study Group Investigating Drugs as Reinforcers. (ISGIDAR); 2007.

98. Haney M, Spealman R. Controversies in translational research: drug self-administration. *Psychopharmacology*. 2008;199:403–419.

99. Haney M, Ward AS, Foltin RW, Fischman MW. Effects of ecopipam, a selective D1 antagonist, on smoked cocaine self-administration by humans. *Psychopharmacology*. 2001;155:330–337.

100. Harris DS, Batki SL, Berger SP. Fluoxetine attenuates adrenocortical but not subject response to cocaine cues. *Am J Drug Alcohol Abuse*. 2004;30:765–782.

101. Hart CL, Haney M, Foltin RW, Fischman MW. Effects of the NMDA antagonist memantine on human methamphetamine discrimination. *Psychopharmacology*. 2002;164:376–384.

102. Hart CL, Ward AS, Collins ED, Haney M, Foltin RW. Gabapentin maintenance decreases smoked cocaine-related subjective effects, but not self-administration by humans. *Drug Alcohol Depend*. 2004;73:279–287.

103. Hartz DT, Frederick-Osborne SL, Galloway GP. Craving predicts use during treatment for methamphetamine dependence: a prospective, repeated-measures, within-subject analysis. *Drug Alcohol Depend*. 2001;63:269–276.

104. Heilig M, Leggio L. What the alcohol doctor ordered from the neuroscientist: theragnostic biomarkers for personalized treatments. *Prog Brain Res*. 2016;224:401–418.

105. Heishman SJ, Singleton EG. Assessment of cannabis craving using the marijuana craving questionnaire. *Methods Mol Med*. 2006;123:209–216.

106. Helmus TC, Tancer M, Johanson CE. Reinforcing effects of diazepam under anxiogenic conditions in individuals with social anxiety. *Exp Clin Psychopharmacol*. 2005;13:348–356.

107. Hendershot CS, Wardell JD, Samokhvalov AV, Rehm J. Effects of naltrexone on alcohol self-administration and craving: meta-analysis of human laboratory studies. *Addict Biol*. 2016. https://doi.org/10.1111/adb.12425. [Epub ahead of print].

108. Henningfield JE, Cohen C, Heishman SJ. Drug self-administration methods in abuse liability evaluation. *Br J Addict*. 1991;86:1571–1577.

109. Henningfield JE, Lukas SE, Bigelow GE. Human Studies of Drugs as Reinforcers. In: Goldberg SR, Stolerman IP, eds. *Behavioral Analysis of Drug Dependence*. Orlando, FL: Academic; 1986:69.

110. Hernandez-Avila CA, Oncken C, Van Kirk J, Wand G, Kranzler HR. Adrenocorticotropin and cortisol responses to a naloxone challenge and risk of alcoholism. *Biol Psychiatr*. 2002;51:652–658.

111. Higgins ST, Bickel WK, Hughes JR. Influence of an alternative reinforcer on human cocaine self-administration. *Life Sci*. 1994;55:179–187.

112. Hill HF, Chapman R, Kornell JA, Sullivan KM, Saeger LC, Benedetti C. Self-administration of morphine in bone marrow transplant patient reduces drug requirement. *Pain*. 1990;40:121–129.

113. Hindmarch I, Kerr JS, Sherwood N. The effects of alcohol and others drugs on psychomotor performance and cognitive function. *Alcohol Alcohol*. 1991;26:17–79.

114. Houtsmuller EJ, Notes LD, Newton T, et al. Transdermal selegiline and intravenous cocaine: safety and interactions. *Psychopharmacology*. 2004;172:31–40.

115. Huestis MA, Boyd SJ, Heishman SJ, et al. Single and multiple doses of rimonabant antagonize acute effects of smoked cannabis in male cannabis users. *Psychopharmacology*. 2007;194:505–515.

116. Hutchison KE, McGeary J, Smolen A, Bryan AD, Swift RM. The DRD4 VNTR polymorphism moderates craving after alcohol consumption. *Health Psychol*. 2002;21:139–146.

117. Hutchison KE, McGeary J, Smolen A, Wooden A. Craving after alcohol consumption: olanzapine and the DRD4 VNTR polymorphism. *Alcohol Clin Exp Res*. 2001;25:66a.

118. Hutchison KE, Ray L, Sandman E, et al. The effect of olanzapine on craving and alcohol consumption *Neuropsychopharmacology*. 31:1310–1317.

119. Hutchison KE, Wooden A, Swift RM, Smolen A, McGeary J, Adler L, et al. Olanzapine reduces craving for alcohol: a DRD4 VNTR polymorphism by pharmacotherapy interaction. *Neuropsychopharmacology*. 2003;28:1882–1888.

120. Jaffe JH, Cascella NG, Kumor KM, Sherer MA. Cocaine-induced cocaine craving. *Psychopharmacology*. 1989;97:59–64.

121. Jasinski DR. Assessment of the abuse potentiality of morphine like drugs (methods used in man. In: Martin WR, ed. *Handbook of Experimental Pharmacology*. New York: Springer; 1977:45:197–258.

122. Jasinski DR, Martin WR, Haertzen CA. The human pharmacology and abuse potential of N-Allylnormxoymorphone (Naloxone). *J Pharmacol Exp Ther*. 1967;157:420–426.

123. Jasinski DR, Pevnick JS, Griffith JD. Human pharmacology and abuse potential of the analgesic buprenorphine: a potential agent for treating narcotic addiction. *Arch Gen Psychiatry*. 1978;35:501–516.

124. Johanson C. Discriminative stimulus effects of psychomotor stimulants and benzodiazepines in humans. In: Glennon R, Jarbe T, Frankenheim J, eds. *Drug Discrimination: Applications to Drug Abuse Research*. Rockville, MD: National Institute on Drug Abuse; 1991;116:181–196.

125. Johanson CE, Lundahl LH, Lockhart N, Schubiner H. Intravenous cocaine discrimination in humans. *Exp Clin Psychopharmacol*. 2006;14:99–108.

126. Johanson CE, Uhlenhuth EH. Drug preference and mood in humans: diazepam. *Psychopharmacology*. 1980;71:269–273.

127. Johanson CE, Uhlenhuth EH. Drug preference and mood in humans: d-Amphetamine. *Psychopharmacology*. 1980;71:275–279.

128. Johansson B, Angelo HR, Christensen JK, Moller IW, Ronsted P. Dose-effect relationship of disulfiram in human volunteers. II: a study of the relation between the disulfiram-alcohol reaction and plasma concentrations of acetaldehyde, diethyldithiocarbamic acid methyl ester, and erythrocyte aldehyde dehydrogenase activity. *Pharmacology and Toxicology*. 1991;68:166–170.

129. Johnson B, Barron B, Fang B, et al. Isradipine prevents global and regional cocaine-induced changes in brain blood flow: a preliminary study. *Psychopharmacology*. 1998;136:335–341.

130. Johnson BA. Serotonergic agents and alcoholism treatment: rebirth of the subtype concept—an hypothesis. *Alcohol Clin Exp Res*. 2000;24:1597–1601.

131. Johnson BA. Update on neuropharmacological treatments for alcoholism: scientific basis and clinical findings. *Biochem Pharmacol*. 2008;75:34–56.

132. Johnson BA, Ait-Daoud N, Bowden CL, et al. Oral topiramate for treatment of alcohol dependence: a randomized controlled trial. *Lancet*. 2003;361:1677–1685.

133. Johnson BA, Ait-Daoud N, Elkashef AM, et al. A preliminary randomized, double-blind, placebo-controlled study of the safety and efficacy of ondansetron in the treatment of methamphetamine dependence. *Int J Neuropsychopharmacol*. 2008;11:1–14.

134. Johnson BA, Ait-Daoud N, Seneviratne C, et al. Pharmacogenetic approach at the serotonin transporter gene as a method of reducing the severity of alcohol drinking. *Am J Psychiatry*. 2011;168:265–275.

135. Johnson BA, Ait-Daoud N, Wang XQ, et al. Topiramate for the treatment of cocaine addiction: a randomized clinical trial. *JAMA Psychiatry*. 2013;70(12):1338–1346.

136. Johnson BA, Campling GM, Griffiths P, Cowen PJ. Attenuation of some alcohol-induced mood changes and the desire to drink by 5-HT3 receptor blockade: a preliminary study in healthy male volunteers. *Psychopharmacology*. 1993;112:142–144.

137. Johnson BA, Devous MD, Ruiz P, Ait-Daoud N. Treatment advances for cocaine-induced ischemic stroke: focus on dihydropyridine-class calcium channel antagonists. *Am J Psychiatry*. 2001;158:1191–1198.

138. Johnson BA, O'Malley SS, Ciraulo DA, et al. Dose-ranging kinetics and behavioral pharmacology of naltrexone and acamprosate, both alone and combined, in alcohol-dependent subjects. *J Clin Psychopharmacol*. 2003;23(3):279–291.

139. Johnson BA, Roache JD, Ait-Daoud N, et al. Effects of acute topiramate dosing on methamphetamine-induced subjective mood. *Int J Neuropsychopharmacol*. 2007;10:85–98.

140. Johnson BA, Roache JD, Ait-Daoud N, et al. Effects of topiramate on methamphetamine-induced changes in attentional and perceptual-motor skills of cognition in recently abstinent methamphetamine-dependent individuals. *Prog NeuroPsychopharm Biol Psychiat*. 2007;31:123–130.

141. Johnson BA, Roache JD, Ait-Daoud N, et al. Topiramate's effects on cocaine-induced subjective mood, craving and preference for money over drug taking. *Addict Biol*. 2013;18(3):405–416.

142. Johnson BA, Roache JD, Ait-Daoud N, et al. Effects of isradipine, a dihydropyridine-class calcium-channel antagonist, on d-methamphetamine's subjective and reinforcing effects. *Int J Neuropsychopharmacol*. 2005;8:203–213.

143. Johnson BA, Roache JD, Ait-Daoud N, Wells LT, Mauldin JB. Effects of isradipine on cocaine-induced subjective mood. *J Clin Psychopharmacol*. 2004;24:180–191.

144. Johnson BA, Roache JD, Bordnick PS, Ait-Daoud N. Isradipine, a dihydropryidine-class calcium channel antagonist, attenuates some of d-methamphetamine's positive subjective effects: a preliminary study. *Psychopharmacology*. 1999;144:295–300.

145. Johnson BA, Roache JD, Javors MA, et al. Ondansetron for reduction of drinking among biologically predisposed alcoholic patients. *J Am Med Assoc*. 2000;284:963–971.

146. Johnson BA, Rosenthal N, Capece JA, et al. Topiramate for treating alcohol dependence: a randomized controlled trial. *JAMA*. 2007;298:1641–1651.

147. Johnson BA, Seneviratne C, Wang XQ, Ait-Daoud N, Li MD. Determination of genotype combinations that can predict the outcome of the treatment of alcohol dependence using the 5-HT(3) antagonist ondansetron. *Am J Psychiatry*. 2013;170(9):1020–1031.

148. Johnson BA, Wells LT, Roache JD, Wallace C, Ait-Daoud N, Wang Y. Isradipine decreases the hemodynamic response of cocaine and methamphetamine: results from two human laboratory studies. *Am J Hypertension.* 2005;18:813–822.

149. Jonas DE, Amick HR, Feltner C, et al. Pharmacotherapy for adults with alcohol use disorders in outpatient settings: a systematic review and meta-analysis. *JAMA.* 2014;311(18):1889–1900. https://doi.org/10.1001/jama.2014.3628. Review. PubMed PMID:24825644.

150. Jones BE, Prada JA. Drug-seeking behavior during methadone maintenance. *Psychopharmacology.* 1975;41:7–10.

151. Jonsson LE. Pharmacological blockade of amphetamine effects in amphetamine dependent subjects. *Eur J Clin Pharmacol.* 1972;4:206–211.

152. Kampman KM, Lynch KG, Pettinati HM, et al. A double blind, placebo controlled trial of modafinil for the treatment of cocaine dependence without co-morbid alcohol dependence. *Drug Alcohol Depend.* 2015;155:105–110.

153. Kampman KM, Pettinati H, Lynch KG, Sparkman T, O'Brien CP. A pilot trial of olanzapine for the treatment of cocaine dependence. *Drug Alcohol Depend.* 2003;70:265–273.

154. Karila L, Leroy C, Dubol M, et al. Dopamine transporter correlates and occupancy by modafinil in cocaine-dependent patients: a controlled study with high-resolution PET and [(11)C]-PE2I. *Neuropsychopharmacology.* 2016;41(9):2294–2302.

155. Keltner N, Vance D. Incarcerated care and quetiapine abuse. *Perspectives Psychiatric Care.* 2008;44:202–206.

156. Kenna GA, Nielsen DM, Mello P, Schiesl A, Swift RA. Pharmacotherapy of dual substance abuse and dependence. *CNS Drugs.* 2007;21:213–237.

157. Kenna GA, Zywiak WH, McGeary JE, et al. A within-group design of nontreatment seeking 5-HTTLPR genotyped alcohol-dependent subjects receiving ondansetron and sertraline. *Alcohol Clin Exp Res.* 2009;33(2):315–323.

158. Kenna GA, Zywiak WH, Swift RM, et al. Ondansetron and sertraline may interact with 5-HTTLPR and DRD4 polymorphisms to reduce drinking in non-treatment seeking alcohol-dependent women: exploratory findings. *Alcohol.* 2014;48:515–522.

159. Kenna GA, Zywiak WH, Swift RM, et al. Ondansetron reduces naturalistic drinking in nontreatment-seeking alcohol-dependent individuals with the LL 5'-HTTLPR genotype: a laboratory study. *Alcohol Clin Exp Res.* 2014;38:1567–1574.

160. King AC, Volpicelli JR, Frazer A, O'Brien CP. Effect of naltrexone on subjective alcohol response in subjects at high and low risk for future alcohol dependence. *Psychopharmacology.* 1997;129:15–22.

161. Kirchmayer U, Davoli M, Verster Ad, Amato L, Ferri A, Perucci CA. A systematic review on the efficacy of naltrexone maintenance treatment in opioid dependence. *Addiction.* 2002;97:1241–1249.

162. Kosten T, Gawin FH, Silverman DG, et al. Intravenous cocaine challenges during desipramine maintenance. *Neuropsychopharmacology.* 1992;7:169–176.

163. Kosten TR, Woods SW, Rosen MI, Pearsall HR. Interactions of cocaine with nimodipine: a brief report. *Am J Addict.* 1999;8:77–81.

164. Kozlowski LT, Mann RE, Wilkinson, Poulos CX. "Cravings" are ambiguous: ask about urges or desires. *Addict Behav.* 1989;14:443–445.

165. Kranzler HR, Gage A. Acamprosate efficacy in alcohol-dependent patients: summary of results from three pivotal trials. *Am J Addict.* 2008;17:70–76.

166. Krishnan-Sarin S, Krystal JH, Shi J, Pittman B, O'Malley SS. Family history of alcoholism influences naltrexone-induced reduction in alcohol drinking. *Biol Psychiat.* 2007;62(6):694–697.

167. Kristenson H. How to get the best out of antabuse. *Alcohol Alcoholism.* 1995;30:775–783.

168. Lamb RJ, Preston KL, Schindler CW, et al. The reinforcing and subjective effects of morphine in post-addicts: a dose-response study. *J Pharmacol Exp Ther.* 1991;259:1165–1173.

169. Leggio L, Garbutt JC, Addolorato G. Effectiveness and safety of baclofen in the treatment of alcohol dependent patients. *CNS Neurol Disord Drug Targets.* 2010;9(1):33–44.

170. Leggio L, Zywiak WH, McGeary JE, et al. A human laboratory pilot study with baclofen in alcoholic individuals. *Pharmacol Biochem Behav.* 2013;103(4):784–791.

171. Leyton M, Casey KF, Delaney JS, Kolivakis T, Benkelfat C. Cocaine craving, euphoria, and self-administration: a preliminary study of the effect of catecholamine precursor depletion. *Behav Neurosci.* 2005;119:1619–1627.

172. Lile JA, Stoops WW, Glaser PEA, Hays LR, Rush CR. Acute administration of the GABA reuptake inhibitor tiagabine does not alter the effects of oral cocaine in humans. *Drug Alcohol Depend.* 2004;76:81–91.

173. Lile JA, Stoops WW, Hays LR, Rush CR. The safety, tolerability, and subject-rated effects of acute intranasal cocaine administration during aripiprazole maintenance II: increased aripiprazole dose and maintenance period. *Am J Drug Alcohol Abuse.* 2008;34:721–729.

174. Litten RZ, Falk DE, Ryan ML, Fertig JB. Discovery, development, and adoption of medications to treat alcohol use disorder: goals for the phases of medications development. *Alcohol Clin Exp Res.* 2016;40(7):1368–1379.

175. Lobmaier P, Kornor H, Kunoe N, Bjornal A. Sustained-release naltrexone for opioid dependence. *Cochrane Database Syst Rev.* 2008;2:Art. No.: CD006140. https://doi.org/10.1002/14651858.CD006140.pub.2.

176. MacKillop J. The Behavioral Economics and Neuroeconomics of Alcohol Use Disorders. *Alcohol Clin Exp Res.* 2016;40(4):672–685. https://doi.org/10.1111/acer.13004. Review. PubMed PMID: 26993151; PubMed Central PMCID: PMC4846981.

177. Malcolm R, LaRowe S, Cochran K, et al. A controlled trial of amlodipine for cocaine dependence: a negative report. *J Subst Abuse Treatment.* 2005;28:197–204.

178. Malcolm R, Olive MF, Lechner W. The safety of disulfiram for the treatment of alcohol and cocaine dependence in randomized clinical trials: guidance for clinical practice. *Expert Opinion Drug Safety.* 2008;7:459–472.

179. Mann K, Lehert P, Morgan MY. The efficacy of acamprosate in the maintenance of abstinence in alcohol-dependent individuals: results of a meta-analysis. *Alcohol Clin Exp Res.* 2004;28:51–63.

180. Mansbach RS, Feltner DE, Gold LH, Schnoll SH. Incorporating the assessment of abuse liability into the drug discovery and development process. *Drug Alcohol Depend.* 2003;70:S73–S85.

181. Margolin A, Avants SK, Kosten TR. Mazindol for relapse prevention to cocaine abuse in methadone-maintained patients. *Am J Drug Alcohol Abuse.* 1995;21:469–481.

182. Martin CS, Earleywine M, Musty RE, Perrine MW, Swift RM. Development and validation of the biphasic alcohol effects scale. *Alcohol Clin Exp Res.* 1993;17:140–146.

183. Martin WR, Jasinski DR, Manskey PA. Naltrexone, an antagonist for the treatment of heroin dependence. *Arch Gen Psychiatry.* 1973;28:784–791.

184. Martin WR, Sloan JW, Sapira JD, Jasinski DR. Physiologic, subjective, and behavioral effects of amphetamine, methamphetamine, ephedrine, phenmetrazine, and methylphenidate in man. *Clin Pharmacol Therap.* 1971;12:245–258.

185. Mason BJ, Light JM, Williams LD, Drobes DJ. Proof-of-concept human laboratory study for protracted abstinence in alcohol dependence: effects of gabapentin. *Addict Biol.* 2009;14(1):73–83.

186. Mason BJ, Quello S, Goodell V, Shadan F, Kyle M, Begovic A. Gabapentin treatment for alcohol dependence: a randomized clinical trial. *JAMA Intern Med.* 2014;174(1):70–77.

187. Mayfield RD, Harris RA, Schuckit MA. Genetic factors influencing alcohol dependence. *Br J Pharmacol.* 2008;154:275–287.

188. McCance-Katz EF, Kosten TR, Jatlow P. Disulfiram effects on acute cocaine administration. *Drug Alcohol Depend.* 1998;52:27–39.

189. McCaul ME, Wand GS, Stauffer R, Lee SM, Rohde CA. Naltrexone dampens ethanol-induced cardiovascular and hypothalamic-pituitary-adrenal axis activation. *Neuropharmacology*. 2001;25:537–547.

190. McKay D, Schare ML. The effects of alcohol and alcohol expectancies on subjective reports and physiological reactivity: a meta-analysis. *Addictive Behaviors*. 1999;24:633–647.

191. McNair DM, Lorr M, Droppleman LF. *Manual of the Profile of Mood States*. San Diego, CA: Educational and Industrial Testing Service; 1971.

192. Mello NK, Fivel PA, Kohut SJ, Carroll FI. Effects of chronic varenicline treatment on nicotine, cocaine, and concurrent nicotine+cocaine self-administration. *Neuropsychopharmacology*. 2014;39(5):1222–1231.

193. Mello NK, Mendelson JH. Buprenorphine suppresses heroin use by heroin addicts. *Science*. 1980;207:657–659.

194. Mello NK, Mendelson JH, Kuehnle JC, Sellers MS. Operant analysis of human heroin self-administration and the effects of naltrexone. *J Exp Ther*. 1981;216:45–54.

195. Mendelson J, Jones RT, Welm S, et al. Buprenorphine and naloxone combinations: the effects of three dose ratios in morphine-stabilized, opiate-dependent volunteers. *Psycho-pharmacology*. 1999;141:37–46.

196. Mendelson JH. Protection of participants and experimental design in clinical abuse liability testing. *Br J Addict*. 1991;86:1543–1548.

197. Miranda Jr R, MacKillop J, Monti PM, et al. Effects of topiramate on urge to drink and the subjective effects of alcohol: a preliminary laboratory study. *Alcohol Clin Exp Res*. 2008;32:489–497.

198. Miranda Jr R, MacKillop J, Treloar H, et al. Biobehavioral mechanisms of topiramate's effects on alcohol use: an investigation pairing laboratory and ecological momentary assessments. *Addict Biol*. 2016;21:171–182.

199. Miranda R, Ray L, Blanchard A, et al. Effects of naltrexone on adolescent alcohol cue reactivity and sensitivity: an initial randomized trial. *Addict Biol*. 2014;19(5):941–954.

200. Moeller FG, Dougherty DM, Barratt ES, Schmitz JM, Swann AC, Grabowski J. The impact of impulsivity on cocaine use and retention in treatment. *J Subst Abuse Treat*. 2001;21(4):193–198.

201. Monti PM, Rohsenow DJ, Hutchison KE, et al. Naltrexone's effect on cue-elicited craving among alcoholics in treatment. *Alcohol Clin Exp Res*. 1999;23:1386–1394.

202. Montoya ID, Gorelick DA, Preston KL, et al. Randomized trial of buprenorphine for treatment of concurrent opiate and cocaine dependence. *Clin Pharm Ther*. 2004;75:34–48.

203. Muntaner C, Kumor KM, Nagoshi C, Jaffe JH. Effects of nifedipine pretreatment on subjective and cardiovascular responses to intravenous cocaine in humans. *Psychopharmacology*. 1991;105:37–41.

204. Nann-Vernotica E, Donny EC, Bigelow GE, Walsh SL. Repeated administration of the D1/5 antagonist ecopipam fails to attenuate the subjective effects of cocaine. *Psychopharmacology*. 2001;155:338–347.

205. Nelson RA, Boyd SJ, Ziegelstein RC, et al. Effect of rate of administration on subjective and physiological effects of intravenous cocaine in humans. *Drug Alcohol Depend*. 2006;82:19–24.

206. Nemeth-Coslett R, Henningfield JE, O'Keeffe MK, Griffiths RR. Effects of mecamylamine on human cigarette smoking and subjective ratings. *Psychopharmacology*. 1986;88:420–425.

207. Nemeth-Coslett R, Henningfield JE, O'Keeffe MK, Griffiths RR. Nicotine gum: dose-related effects on cigarette smoking and subjective effects. *Psychopharmacology*. 1987;92:424–430.

208. Newton TF, Kalechstein A, Beckson M, Bartzokis G, Bridge TP, Ling W. Effects of selegiline pretreatment on response to experimental cocaine administration. *Psychiatry Res*. 1999;87:101–106.

209. Newton TF, Ling W, Kalechstein AD, Uslaner J, Tervo K. Risperidone pre-treatment reduces the euphoric effects of experimentally-administered cocaine. *Psychiatry Res*. 2001;102:227–233.

210. Newton TF, Reid MS, De La Garza R, et al. Evaluation of subjective effects of aripiprazole and methamphetamine in methamphetamine-dependent volunteers. *Int J Neuropsychopharmacol*. 2008;11:1037–1045.

211. Newton TF, Roache JD, De Le Garza R, et al. Safety of intravenous methamphetamine administration during treatment with bupropion. *Psychopharmacology*. 2005;182(3):426–435.

212. Newton TF, Roache JD, De La Garza R, et al. Buproprion reduces methamphetamine-induced subjective effects and cue-induced craving. *Neuropsychopharmacology*. 2006;7:1537–1544.

213. O'Brien CP, Childress AR, McLellan AT, Ehrman R. Classical conditioning in drug-dependent humans. *Ann NY Acad Sci*. 1992;654:400–415.

214. O'Brien CP, Childress AR, McLellan AT, Ehrman R, Ternes JW. Types of conditioning found in drug-dependent humans. In: Ray BA, ed. *Learning Factors in Substance Abuse*. NIDA Res Monogr; 1988;84:44–61.

215. O'Brien CP, Gardner EL. Critical assessment of how to study addiction and its treatment: human and non-human animal models. *Pharmacol Therap*. 2005;108:18–58.

216. Oliveto A, McCance-Katz FE, Singha A, Petrakis I, Hameedi F, Kosten TR. Effects of cocaine prior to and during bupropion maintenance in cocaine-abusing volunteers. *Drug Alcohol Depend*. 2001;63:155–167.

217. O'Malley SS, Jaffe AJ, Chang G, Schottenfeld RS, Meyer RE, Rounsaville B. Naltrexone and coping skills therapy for alcohol dependence: a controlled study. *Arch Gen Psychiatr*. 1992;49:881–887.

218. O'Malley SS, Krishnan-Sarin S, Farren C, Sinha R, Kreek MJ. Naltrexone decreases craving and alcohol self-administration in alcohol-dependent subjects and activates the hypothalamo-pituitary-adrenocortical axis. *Psychopharmacology*. 2002;160:19–29.

219. Ooteman W, Koeter MW, Verheul R, Schippers GM, van den Brink W. The effect of naltrexone and acamprosate on cue-induced craving, autonomic nervous system and neuroendocrine reactions to alcohol-related cues in alcoholics. *Eur Neuropsychopharmacol*. 2007;17:558–566.

220. Oslin DW, Leong SH, Lynch KG, et al. Naltrexone vs placebo for the treatment of alcohol dependence: a randomized clinical trial. *JAMA Psychiatry*. 2015;72(5):43–47.

221. Patapis NS, Nordstrom BR. Research on naltrexone in the criminal justice system. *J Subst Abuse Treat*. 2006;31:113–115.

222. Perkins KA, Fonte C, Meeker, White W, Wilson A. The discriminative stimulus and reinforcing effects of nicotine in humans following nicotine pretreatment. *Behav Pharmacol*. 2001;12:35–44.

223. Perkins KA, Grobe J, Fonte C. Influence of acute smoking exposure on the subsequent reinforcing value of smoking. *Exp Clin Psychopharmacol*. 1997;5:277–285.

224. Pickens RW, Johanson CE. Craving: consensus of status and agenda for future research. *Drug Alcohol Depend*. 1992;30:127–131.

225. Preston KL, Bigelow GE. Subjective and discriminative effects of drugs. *Behav Pharmacol*. 1991;2:293–313.

226. Preston KL, Jasinski DR. Abuse liability studies of opioid agonist-antagonists in humans. *Drug Alcohol Depend*. 1991;28:49–82.

227. Preston KL, Sullivan JT, Berger P, Bigelow GE. Effects of cocaine alone and in combination with mazindol in human cocaine abusers. *J Pharmacol Exp Ther*. 1993;267:296–307.

228. Preston KL, Sullivan JT, Strain EC, Bigelow GE. Effects of cocaine alone and in combination with bromocriptine in human cocaine abusers. *J Pharmacol Exp Ther*. 1992;262:279–291.

229. Preston KL, Walsh SL, Sannerud CA. Measures of interoceptive stimulus effects: relationship to drug reinforcement. In: Johnson BA, Roache JD, eds. *Drug addiction and its Treatment: Nexus of Neuroscience and Behavior*. Philadelphia: Lippincott-Raven; 1997:91–114.

230. Raby K. Investigations on the disulfiram-alcohol reaction. *Q J Stud Alcohol*. 1953;14:545–556.

231. Ravva P, Gastonguay MR, Faessel HM, Lee TC, Niaura R. Pharmacokinetic-pharmacodynamic modeling of the effect of varenicline on nicotine craving in adult smokers. *Nicotine Tob Res.* 2015;17:106–113.

232. Ray LA, Bujarski S, Chin PF, Miotto K. Pharmacogenetics of naltrexone in Asian Americans: a randomized placebo-controlled laboratory study. *Neuropsychopharmacology.* 2012;37(2):445–455.

233. Ray LA, Bujarski S, Courtney KE, et al. The effects of naltrexone on subjective response to methamphetamine in a clinical sample: a double-blind, placebo-controlled laboratory study. *Neuropsychopharmacology.* 2015;40(10):2347–2356.

234. Reed SC, Evans SM, Bedi G, Rubin E, Foltin RW. The effects of oral micronized progesterone on smoked cocaine self-administration in women. *Horm Behav.* 2011;59(2):227–235.

235. Roache JD. Performance and physiological measures in abuse liability evaluation. *Br J Addict.* 1991;86:1595–1600.

236. Roache JD. Human laboratory safety evaluations in cocaine-dependent patients. In: Harris LS, ed. *Problems of Drug Dependence 1998: Proceedings of the 60th Annual Meeting of the College on Problems of Drug Dependence, National Institute on Drug Abuse Research Monograph.* Washington, DC: U.S. Government Printing Office; 1999;179:38.

237. Roache JD, Creson DL, La Vergne C, Grabowski J. *Human Laboratory Evaluation of Cocaine and d-Amphetamine Drug Interactions.* San Antonio, TX: Presented at the Annual Scientific Meeting of the Texas Research Society on Alcoholism (TRSA); 1998.

238. Roache JD, Grabowski J, Schmitz JM, Creson DL, Rhoades HM. Laboratory measures of methylphenidate effects in cocaine-dependent patients receiving treatment. *J Clin Psychopharmacol.* 2000;20:61–68.

239. Roache JD, Griffiths RR. Diazepam and triazolam self-administration in sedative abusers: concordance of subject ratings, performance, and drug self-administration. *Psychopharmacology.* 1989;99:309–315.

240. Roache JD, Griffiths RR. Abuse liability of anxiolytics and sedative/hypnotics: methods assessing the likelihood of abuse. In: Fischman MW, Mello NK, eds. *Testing for Abuse Liability of Drugs in Humans. Nida Research Monograph,* Vol 92. DHEW Pub. No. (ADM) 89–163. Washington, DC: U.S. Government Printing Office; 1989:123–146.

241. Roache JD, Johnson BA, Ait-Daoud N, et al. Effects of repeated-dose isradipine on the abuse liability of cocaine. *Exp Clin Psychopharmacol.* 2005;13:319–326.

242. Roache JD, Kahn R, Newton TF, et al. A double-blind, placebo-controlled assessment of the safety of potential interactions between intravenous cocaine, ethanol, and oral disulfiram. *Drug Alcohol Depend.* 2011;119(1-2):37–45.

243. Roache JD, Kuhar MJ, Glowa JR, Grabowski J, Levin F, Walsh SL. Agonist-type approaches to the treatment of cocaine dependence. In: Harris LS, ed. *Problems of Drug Dependence 1998: Proceedings of the 60th Annual Meeting of the College on Problems of Drug Dependence. NIDA Research Monograph.* Washington, DC: U.S. Government Printing Office; 1999;179:37–39.

244. Roache JD, Meisch RA. Drug self-administration research in drug and alcohol addiction. In: Miller NS, ed. *Comprehensive Handbook of Drug and Alcohol Addiction.* New York: Marcel Dekker; 1991:625–638.

245. Robbins SJ, Ehrman RN, Childress AR, O'Brien CP. Relationships among physiological and self-report responses produced by cocaine-related cues. *Addict Behav.* 1997;22:157–167.

246. Robbins SJ, Ehrman RN, Childress AR, O'Brien CP. Comparing levels of cocaine cue reactivity in male and female outpatients. *Drug Alcohol Depend.* 1999;53:223–230.

247. Rohn MC, Lee MR, Kleuter SB, Schwandt ML, Falk DE, Leggio L. Differences between treatment-seeking and nontreatment-seeking alcohol-dependent research participants: an exploratory analysis. *Alcohol Clin Exp Res.* 2017;41(2):414–420.

248. Rohsenow DJ, Monti PM, Hutchison KE. Naltrexone's effects on reactivity to alcohol cues among alcoholic men. *J Abnorm Psychol.* 2000;109:738–742.

249. Rohsenow DJ, Monti PM, Rubonis AV, et al. Cue reactivity as a predictor of drinking among male alcoholics. *J Consult Clin Psychol.* 1994;62:620–626.

250. Romach MK, Glue P, Kampman K, et al. Attenuation of the euphoric effects of cocaine by the dopamine D1/D5 antagonist Ecopipam (SCH39166). *Arch Gen Psychiatry.* 1999;56:1101–1106.

251. Rose JE, Behm RM, Westman EC, Bates JE. Mecamylamine acutely increases human intravenous nicotine self-administration. *Pharmacol Biochem Behav.* 2003;76:307–313.

252. Rush CR, Stoops WW, Sevak RJ, Hays LR. Cocaine choice in humans during D-amphetamine maintenance. *J Clin Psychopharmacol.* 2010;30(2):152–159.

253. Sauter AM, Boss D, von Wartburg JP. Reevaluation of the disulfiram-alcohol reaction in man. *J Stud Alcohol.* 1977;38:1680–1695.

254. Schmitz JM, Green CE, Stotts AL, et al. A two-phased screening paradigm for evaluating candidate medications for cocaine cessation or relapse prevention: modafinil, levodopa-carbidopa, naltrexone. *Drug Alcohol Depend.* 2014;136:100–107.

255. Schmitz JM, Rathnayaka N, Green CE, Moeller FG, Dougherty AE, Grabowski J. Combination of modafinil and d-amphetamine for the treatment of cocaine dependence: a preliminary investigation. *Front Psychiatry.* 2012;3:77.

256. Schoedel KA, Sellers EM. Assessing abuse liability during drug development: changing standards and expectations. *Development.* 2008;83:622–626.

257. Schulze D, Jones BT. The effects of alcohol cues and an alcohol priming dose on a multifactorial measure of subjective cue reactivity in social drinkers. *Psychopharmacology.* 1999;145:452–454.

258. Sherer MA, Kumor KM, Jaffee JH. Effects of intravenous cocaine are partially attenuated by haloperidol. *Psychiat Res.* 1989;27:117–125.

259. Shuckit MA. Low level of response to alcohol as a predictor of future alcoholism. *Am J Psychiatr.* 1994;151:184–189.

260. Silverman K, Kirby KC, Griffiths RR. Modulation of drug reinforcement by behavioral requirements following drug ingestion. *Psychopharmacology.* 1994;114:243–247.

261. Silverstone PH, Johnson B, Cowen PJ. Does ondansetron attenuate amphetamine-induced behavior in human volunteers? *Psychopharmacology.* 1992;107:140–141.

262. Sinha R, Fuse T, Aubin LR, O'Malley SS. Psychological stress, drug-related cues and cocaine craving. *Psychopharmacology.* 2000;152:140–148.

263. Sinha R, Talih M, Malison R, Cooney N, Anderson GM, Kreek MJ. Hypothalamic-pituitary-adrenal axis and sympatho-adreno-medullary responses during stress-induced and drug cue-induced cocaine craving states. *Psychopharmacology.* 2003;170:62–72.

264. Sobel B-FX, Sigmon SC, Griffiths RR. Transdermal nicotine maintenance attenuates the subjective and reinforcing effects of intravenous nicotine, abut not cocaine or caffeine, in cigarette-smoking stimulant abusers. *Neuropsychopharmacology.* 2004;29:991–1003.

265. Sofuoglu M, Kosten TR. Novel approaches to the treatment of cocaine addiction. *CNS Drugs.* 2005;19:13–25.

266. Spagnolo PA, Ramchandani VA, Schwandt ML, et al. Effects of naltrexone on neural and subjective response to alcohol in treatment-seeking alcohol-dependent patients. *Alcohol Clin Exp Res.* 2014;38(12):3024–3032. https://doi.org/10.1111/acer.12581. PubMed PMID: 25581657; PubMed Central PMCID: PMC4293087.

267. Spiga R, Roache JD. Human drug self-administration: a review and methodological critique. In: Johnson BA, Roache JD, eds. *Drug Addiction and its Treatment: Nexus of Neuroscience and Behavior.* Philadelphia: Lippincott-Raven; 1997:39–71.

268. Stoops WW. Aripiprazole as a potential pharmacotherapy for stimulant dependence: human laboratory studies with d-amphetamine. *Exp Clin Psychopharmacol.* 2006;14:413–421.

269. Stoops WW, Lile JA, Fillmore MT, Glaser PE, Rush CR. Reinforcing effects of methylphenidate: influence of dose and behavioral demands following drug administration. *Psychopharmacology.* 2005;177:349–355.

270. Stoops WW, Lile JA, Glaser PE, Rush CR. Discriminative stimulus and self-reported effects of methylphenidate, d-amphetamine, and triazolam in methylphenidate-trained humans. *Exp Clin Psychopharmacol.* 2005;13:56–64.

271. Strain EC, Bigelow GE, Liebson IA, Stitzer ML. Moderate vs. high-dose methadone in the treatment of opioid dependence: a randomized trial. *J Am Med Assoc.* 1999;281:1000–1005.

272. Sullivan MA, Bisaga A, Mariani JJ, et al. Naltrexone treatment for opioid dependence: does its effectiveness depend on testing the blockade? *Drug & Alcohol Dependence.* 2013;133(1):80–85.

273. Sullivan MA, Vosburg SK, Comer SD. Depot naltrexone: antagonism of the reinforcing, subjective, and physiological effects of heroin. *Psychopharmacology.* 2006;189:37–46.

274. Swift RM, Davidson D, Whelihan W, Kuznetsov O. Ondansetron alters human alcohol intoxication. *Biol Psychiatry.* 1996;40:514–521.

275. Swift RM, Whelihan W, Kuznetsov O, Buongiorno G, Hsuing H. Naltrexone-induced alterations in human ethanol intoxication. *Am J Psychiatr.* 1994;151:1463–1467.

276. Tcheremissine OV. Is quetiapine a drug of abuse? Reexamining the issue of addiction. *Expert Opinion Drug Safety.* 2008;7:739–748.

277. Tiffany ST. A cognitive model of drug urges and drug-use behavior: role of automatic and non-automatic processes. *Psychol Rev.* 1990;97:147–168.

278. Tiffany ST, Conklin CA. Human models in craving research: a cognitive processing model of alcohol craving and compulsive alcohol use. *Addiction.* 2000;95(suppl):S145–S153.

279. Tiffany ST, Sanderson-Cox L, Elsah CA. Effects of trandermal nicotine patches on abstinence-induced and cue-elicited craving in cigarette smokers. *J Consulting Clin Psychol.* 2000;68:233–240.

280. Tiihonen J, Kuoppasalmi K, Fohr J, Tuomola P, Kuikanmaki O, Vorma H, et al. A comparison of aripiprazole, methylphenidate, and placebo for amphetamine dependence. *Am J Psychiat.* 2007;164:160–162.

281. Tonstad S. Varenicline for smoking cessation. *Expert Rev Neurotherapeutics.* 2007;7:121–127.

282. Verrico CD, Mahoney 3rd JJ, Thompson-Lake DG, Bennett RS, Newton TF, De La Garza 2nd R. Safety and efficacy of varenicline to reduce positive subjective effects produced by methamphetamine in methamphetamine-dependent volunteers. *Int J Neuropsychopharmacol.* 2014;17(2):223–233.

283. Vocci FJ, Acri J, Elkashef A. Medication development for addictive disorders: the state of the science. *Am J Psychiatr.* 2005;162:1432–1440.

284. Vocci FJ, Ling W. Medications development: successes and challenges. *Pharmacol Ther.* 2005;108:94–108.

285. Volpicelli JR, Alterman AI, Hayashida M, O'Brien CP Naltrexone in the treatment of alcohol dependence. *Arch Gen Psychiatr.* 1992;49:876–880.

286. Von Wartburg JP, Buhler R. Biology of disease: alcoholism and aldehydism: new disease concepts. *Lab Invest.* 1984;50:5–15.

287. Wachtel SR, Ortengren A, de Wit H. The effects of acute haloperidol or risperidone on subjective responses to methamphetamine in healthy volunteers. *Drug Alcohol Depend.* 2002;68:23–33.

288. Wall TL, Peterson CM, Peterson KP, et al. Alcohol metabolism in Asian–American men with genetic polymorphisms of aldehyde dehyrdrogenase. *Ann Intern Med.* 1997;127:376–379.

289. Walsh SL, Eissenberg T. The clinical pharmacology of buprenorphine: extrapolating from the laboratory to the clinic. *Drug Alcohol Depend.* 2003;70:S13–S27.

290. Walsh SL, Haberny KA, Bigelow BE. Modulation of intravenous cocaine effects by chronic oral cocaine in humans. *Psychopharmacology.* 2000;150:361–373.

291. Walsh SL, Preston KL, Sullivan JT, Fromme R, Bigelow GE. Fluoxetine alters the effects of intravenous cocaine in humans. *J Clin Psychopharmacol.* 1994;14:396–407.

292. Wand GS, McCaul M, Yang X, et al. The mu-opioid receptor gene polymorphism (A118G) alter HPS axis activation induced by opioid receptor blockade. *Neuropharmacology.* 2001;26:106–114.

293. Ward AS, Haney M, Fischman MW, Foltin RW. Binge cocaine self-administration in humans: intravenous cocaine. *Psychopharmacology.* 1997;132:375–381.

294. Weinberger AH, Sacco KA, Creeden CL, Vessicchio JC, Jatlow PI, George TP. Effects of acute abstinence, reinstatement, and mecamylamine on biochemical and behavioral measures of cigarette smoking in schizophrenia. *Schizophr Res.* 2007;91:217–225.

295. White PF. Use of patient-controlled analgesia for management of acute pain. *J Am Med Assoc.* 1988;259:243–247.

296. White TL, Lott DC, de Wit H. Personality and the subjective effects of acute amphetamine in healthy volunteers. *Neuropsychopharmacology.* 2006;31:1064–1074.

297. Wikler A. A psychodynamic study of a patient during experimental self-regulated re-addiction to morphine. *Psychiatric Q.* 1952;26:270–293.

298. Wikler A. Interaction of physical dependence and classical and operant conditioning in the genesis of relapse. In: Association for Research in Nervous and Mental Disease, ed. *The Addictive States: Proceedings of the Association.* New York, NY, 2–3 December 1966. Williams & Wilkins, Baltimore,1968;280–286.

299. Wikler A. Dynamics of drug dependence: implications of a conditioning theory for research and treatment. *Arch Gen Psychiat.* 1973;28:611–616.

300. Winhusen TM, Kropp F, Lindblad R, et al. Multisite, randomized, double-blind, placebo-controlled pilot clinical trial to evaluate the efficacy of buspirone as a relapse-prevention treatment for cocaine dependence. *J Clin Psychiatry.* 2014;75(7):757–764.

301. Yonkers KA, Forray A, Nich C, et al. Progesterone reduces cocaine use in postpartum women with a cocaine use disorder: a randomized, double-blind study. *Lancet Psychiatry.* 2014;1(5):360–367.

8
Conditioning of Addiction

M. FOSTER OLIVE AND CASSANDRA D. GIPSON

Introduction

Addiction to drugs of abuse is a chronically relapsing disorder characterized by a compulsion to take the drug, loss of control of intake, and the development of a negative emotional state when drug access is withheld.[108] Initiation of drug use typically includes a variety of influencing factors, including (but not limited to) social, biological, and emotional factors. It is widely held that drug use is initiated because of the ability of these substances to produce feelings of pleasure and well-being (i.e., euphoria). Over time, however, tolerance develops to the euphorigenic properties of many drugs of abuse, which perpetuates drug-seeking behavior by leading the user to increase the dose and/ or frequency of drug use in order to obtain the euphoria that was previously experienced (so-called chasing the dragon). With repeated drug use, the user begins to form associations between the subjective effects of the drug and environmental stimuli that are associated with the drug. These associations are formed by classical (Pavlovian) conditioning processes, and the types of stimuli or cues that become paired with drug use can be spatial, visual, auditory, tactile, olfactory, temporal, or interoceptive in nature. Of interest, and as discussed in more detail later, tolerance can develop that is conditioned to the stimuli associated with drug administration, and these stimuli become quite powerful in exerting control over the biological expression of tolerance. Examples of such stimuli include drug paraphernalia, the location in which the drug is repeatedly taken, the smell of alcohol or tobacco smoke, and the time of day. Because drug addicts do not typically live under conditions in which they are isolated from drug-associated cues (possible exceptions being an addict who has been incarcerated or placed in a residential-treatment program), active drug addicts typically encounter these drug-associated environmental stimuli on a daily basis. This repeated exposure to drug-associated stimuli can elicit expectation of drug availability or memories of previous euphoric experiences under the influence of a particular drug, which may in turn result in drug craving and drug-seeking behavior, leading ultimately to the perpetuation of drug self-administration and the addiction cycle.[37,71,108,111]

Most drugs of abuse are consumed in cyclic patterns consisting of active drug self-administration followed by abstinence. During the abstinence phase, the repeated emergence of withdrawal symptoms may result in conditioned associations between environmental stimuli and the negative affective state (i.e., depression, anxiety, and irritability) that typically manifest during withdrawal. As a result, withdrawal-associated environmental stimuli may also trigger drug-seeking behavior to alleviate the evoked negative affect via negative reinforcement processes (i.e., removal of withdrawal-induced dysphoria).

The neurobiological basis of conditioning in drug addiction has been advanced significantly by (1) the development of various animal models of drug-environment conditioning and (2) human imaging studies in which brain activity is monitored during exposure of an addict to drug-associated stimuli. In this chapter, we discuss the most widely used animal models of drug conditioning:

the conditioned place preference paradigm, cue-induced enhancement of drug-self administration, second-order schedules of reinforcement, and cue- and context-induced reinstatement of drug-seeking behavior. We also discuss additional processes of drug conditioning including incentive salience attribution and Pavlovian-instrumental transfer. We then summarize key findings from studies using these paradigms on the neural substrates of drug conditioning, in addition to results from human brain imaging studies. Finally, we highlight several recent studies using newer neurobiological methods to reveal novel neural substrates of drug conditioning and the mechanisms underlying cue-evoked relapse-related behaviors.

Methods for Assessing the Conditioned Effects of Drugs of Abuse in Laboratory Animals

Like human beings, laboratory animals including rats, mice, dogs, and nonhuman primates are able to form associations between environmental stimuli and appetitive rewards such as food, sweetened substances such as sucrose, and drugs of abuse. These species are also able to form similar associations between environmental stimuli and aversive events such as the presentation of an electric shock or the experience of drug withdrawal symptoms. The most notable experimental studies on this type of conditioning were conducted in the late 19th and early 20th centuries by noted Russian physiologist Ivan Pavlov.[77] Pavlov noted that experimental dogs began to salivate in anticipation of the presentation of food. Eventually Pavlov was able to elicit salivation in these dogs by presentation of a discrete environmental stimulus (the sounding of a bell) immediately before the presentation of food. These landmark studies, for which Pavlov was awarded the Nobel Prize in Physiology and Medicine, were the first to describe the phenomenon of classical or Pavlovian conditioning, where a previous neutral stimulus (i.e., the sound of a bell, serving as the conditioned stimulus) becomes associated with a naturally appetitive stimulus (i.e., food, the unconditioned stimulus). Eventually, with repeated conditioning, the organism learns to predict the availability of the unconditioned stimulus upon presentation of the conditioned stimulus, and thus the conditioned stimulus becomes motivationally salient.

In the context of drug addiction, classical conditioning is a widely prevalent phenomenon, such that during the course of repeated drug-taking behavior, environmental stimuli associated with the drug (i.e., the conditioned stimulus, such as the smell of tobacco smoke or the sight of a hypodermic syringe) become associated with and eventually predict the availability of the drug (i.e., the unconditioned stimulus). The chronic nature of drug addiction allows for numerous pairings of the conditioned stimulus and unconditioned stimulus, to the point that the conditioned stimulus becomes motivationally salient to the addicted individual. In the case of an individual attempting to abstain from drug use, encountering a conditioned stimulus can provoke intense drug craving, which leads to drug-seeking behavior and greatly increases the propensity for relapse.

The neural basis of classical conditioning has been studied for decades at the cellular and molecular levels from in vitro preparations to the behavioral analysis of animals and humans. Here, we briefly summarize four of the most commonly used behavioral paradigms in laboratory rodents that are designed to investigate the phenomenon of conditioning factors in drug addiction. These include the conditioned place preference paradigm, cue-induced enhancement of drug-self administration, second-order schedules of reinforcement, and cue-induced reinstatement of drug-seeking behavior. Although preclinical models of addiction processes are frequently used to examine the neurobiology of drug use and relapse, it is important to critically examine their predictive validity.[10,11,35,87,106] In addition, it is important to examine the translational value of the models, as effective treatment of drug use is the goal. However, it should be noted that relapse rates remain high, and thus although animal models have led to important advancements in our knowledge of the neurobehavioral underpinnings of addiction, there is more to uncover in our understanding of these processes.

Conditioned Place Preference

In the *conditioned place preference paradigm*, an animal learns to associate the effects of a passively administered substance with the environment in which the drug was received. A typical conditioned place preference apparatus is shown in Fig. 8.1, and consists of two compartments with unique tactile and visual characteristics (i.e., striped walls and mesh flooring in one compartment versus transparent or solid walls and metal bar flooring in the other). Occasionally, distinct olfactory cues are used in each compartment. These two conditioning compartments are connected by a neutral center start compartment. Each compartment is typically equipped with photobeams located just above the floor that can detect the presence of the animal and concurrent locomotor activity and record them via an interfaced computer.

In a typical conditioned place preference experiment, an animal undergoes baseline preference testing and habituation, whereby it is placed in the center start compartment and allowed free access to both conditioning chambers for a set amount of time (i.e., 30 min). This allows for the animal to habituate to the testing environment as well as for the experimenter to determine whether the animal exhibits any innate bias toward one of the two conditioning compartments. (An ideal conditioned place preference apparatus would produce no innate preferences for either compartment.) This first period of access to the conditioning compartment also serves as a preconditioning test, and the time spent in either compartment can later be compared against the same variable after conditioning with the drug. Following this habituation and preconditioning test, the animal is injected with a neutral substance (i.e., saline) and is then confined to one of the two conditioning compartments (using automated or manual guillotine-type doors) for a fixed period of time. On the following day, the animal is injected with the conditioning drug (e.g., morphine, cocaine, or amphetamine) and confined to the other conditioning compartment for the same amount of time. These conditioning trials are repeated in an alternating fashion (i.e., saline-drug-saline-drug-...) a number of times so that the animal learns to associate the unique physical characteristics of the drug-paired compartment with the subjective effects of the conditioning drug. Finally, on the test day, the animal is placed back in the center compartment in a drug-free state and is allowed free access to both conditioning compartments for the same amount of time as during the preconditioning test. If the animal spends significantly more time in the drug-paired compartment than in the saline-paired compartment, conditioned place preference has been established, reflecting the animal's association of the drug compartment with the subjective (presumably pleasurable or rewarding) effects of

Conditioning with neutral substance (e.g., saline) in one compartment

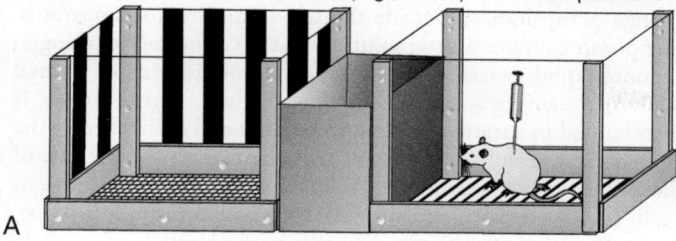

A

Conditioning with drug in opposite compartment

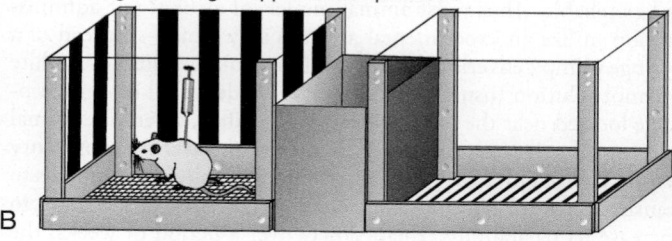

B

Place preference testing

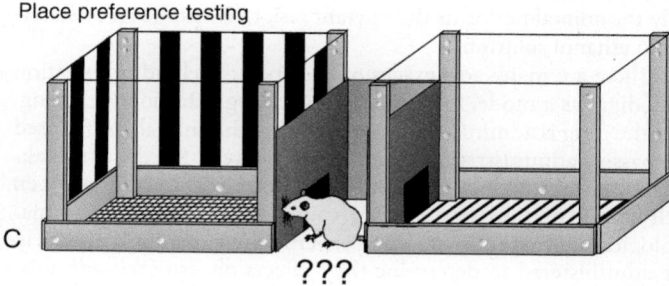

C

???

• **Fig. 8.1** The conditioned place preference paradigm. (A) Following a preconditioning test to habituate the animal to the conditioned place preference apparatus and to detect any innate bias toward one of the conditioning compartments, the animal is injected with a neutral substance, such as saline, and confined to one of the two contextually distinct conditioning compartments for a fixed amount of time. (B) After a period of several hours or on the following day, the animal is injected with a drug of abuse, such as cocaine, and confined to the other compartment for the same amount of time. (C) Following several days of conditioning, the animal is then placed in the center "start" compartment and is given the opportunity to enter either compartment at will (as indicated by *question marks* in the figure). Most abused drugs reliably produce a preference for the drug-paired environment over the saline-paired environment. The front wall of the start compartment in panel C is removed to show the location of the animal.

the drug. Conditioned place preference has been demonstrated in rodents for all drugs of abuse,[4,69,104] although the experimental procedures may vary by the drug and its individual pharmacokinetic properties. Conditioned place aversion is observed if the animal spends significantly less time in the drug-paired compartment than in the saline-paired compartment. Withdrawal from chronic drug exposure reliably produces conditioned place aversion. In addition, some drugs such as ethanol can also produce conditioned place aversion if the peak positive subjective effects of the drug are not timed and are paired correctly with the drug-conditioned compartment.[21,64,83]

One advantage of the conditioned place preference paradigm is that the experiments are relatively simple, inexpensive, and less time-consuming to conduct than more involved procedures

such as intravenous drug self-administration. In addition, conditioned place preference paradigms can be used to simulate various aspects of relapse. This is accomplished in one of two ways: (1) extinguishing an established conditioned place preference by repeatedly pairing the previously drug-paired compartment with saline, or (2) allowing the conditioned place preference to dissipate over a period of several weeks by repeated testing of place preference. Then drug priming or stress can be introduced to the animal to reinstate the original conditioned place preference, a phenomenon that has been hypothesized to model drug-seeking behavior.[4,64,69,104]

Despite its simplicity and ease of use, there are several disadvantages of the conditioned place preference paradigm. First and foremost, the animal subjects do not actively self-administer the drug; it is passively administered as a bolus injection by the experimenter. In addition to potential pharmacokinetic differences in plasma and brain levels of the drug between passive and active self-administration, a substantial amount of evidence has accumulated indicating that active versus passive drug administration produces significant differences in neurochemical, endocrine, and other responses to drugs of abuse.[34,52,56,101] These differences may underlie some of the discordant findings between studies using pharmacological or other experimental manipulations in the conditioned place preference paradigm and those utilizing active self-administration. In addition, the primary dependent variable measured in the conditioned place preference paradigm does not directly measure drug-seeking behavior but, rather, the motivation for drug-associated environments. Despite these limitations, the conditioned place preference paradigm undoubtedly has provided useful information on the neural substrates that underlie drug-environment conditioning and their contribution to addictive behaviors, as discussed later in this chapter.

Another important point to address is what exactly is learned in conditioned place preference? We know that temporal contiguity is necessary and sufficient for learning.[53,77] In conditioned place preference experiments, there tends to be a perfect predictive relationship between the context conditioned stimulus (CS) and administration of the drug. In addition, the drug unconditioned stimulus (US) and context CS always co-occur. Thus, the rules of temporal contiguity are met and learning occurs in this model. However, the CS is a complex, multimodal stimulus (a context) that includes distinct olfactory, visual, tactile, auditory, and spatial elements. Does each element of the stimulus enter into an independent association with the drug US, or do all of the distinct elements combine to form a single, configural stimulus that then becomes associated with the US?[4] These relationships are somewhat unclear; thus we really do not know how the context CS is neurally encoded. This is problematic for interpretation of the neurobiological underpinnings of drug conditioning in this model. In addition, drug self-administration is a model typically used to identify the reinforcing efficacy of drugs of abuse (see subsequent text). Is conditioned place preference isomorphic with self-administration? In some cases, drugs of abuse elicit place preference and are self-administered, but this is not always the case. Thus it appears that these two models might tap into different neurobiological systems that govern the ability of stimuli to elicit drug-motivated behavior.

Conditioned Tolerance

It has long been known that exposure to drugs of abuse can lead to biological changes that are governed by environmental stimuli.

Indeed, environmental stimuli that are contiguously and consistently paired with administration of drugs of abuse begin to take on value and become quite powerful in their ability to modulate the biological and behavioral effects of the drug.[70] When individuals with substance use disorders are asked to consider factors that contribute to relapse, environmental stimuli are identified as being equally or more powerful than other influences, including mood or impulsive choices.[51] One biological phenomenon that occurs is tolerance, in which repeated use of a drug over time results in a decreasing effect of the drug, and drug-associated stimuli elicit conditioned responses that attenuate the drug effect. For example, early studies have shown that tolerance to heroin can be conditioned to the environment in which the drug is normally consumed. If the drug is taken in a novel environment, this conditioned tolerance will not protect against a high dose of the drug, and overdose is likely to occur to a dose that would be tolerated in the conditioned environment.[96] This phenomenon can be modeled in animals. Specifically, rats were exposed to either heroin or placebo in a colony room or a noisy room, repeatedly for 30 days. Following this exposure, rats were given a high dose of heroin (15 mg/kg) on a test day either in the same room they had received the injections previously, or in a novel room in which they never received heroin exposure (either the colony or noisy room). Mortality rates of rats that received the high dose of heroin in the room in which they had previously received placebo were quite high (96%), whereas rats that received the high dose of heroin in the room in which heroin was previously administered had a relatively low mortality rate (32%).[96] This experiment demonstrates the power of environmental stimuli in governing the biological responses underlying drug use.

Conditioned Cue Enhancement of Drug Self-Administration

One of the most widely used paradigms to study drug addiction in animals is the intravenous self-administration paradigm (Fig. 8.2). In the case of rodents, a rat or mouse is surgically implanted with an indwelling intravenous catheter into the jugular or femoral vein, which exits the skin on the dorsal side of the animal and is connected to a vascular access port. Following recovery from surgery, the animal is placed in a self-administration apparatus chamber equipped with one or two levers that are interfaced with a computer and a syringe pump. In lieu of levers, some investigators utilize a nose-poke hole on the wall of the self-administration apparatus, whereby a nose-poke into the correct hole triggers the delivery of a reinforcer. A positive reinforcer is defined as a stimulus that increases the likelihood that the response will occur again in the future (e.g., an addictive drug), whereas a negative reinforcer is defined as a stimulus that decreases the likelihood that the response will occur again (e.g., an aversive stimulus such as an electric shock). To learn the operant task (i.e., lever-press or nose-poke), the animal is often initially trained to perform the task in order to receive a natural reinforcer such as a food or sucrose pellet. (The animal is mildly food-restricted to increase its motivation to seek food during initial training.) However, not all investigators use this initial food restriction and training, since it changes the nutritional and metabolic state of the animal. Instead, some investigators may choose to capitalize on the intrinsic exploratory nature of rodents, since over time the animal will eventually exert the correct operant response, receive an intravenous drug infusion, and, with repeated training sessions, learn that this correct response results consistently in the delivery of the drug solution.

The drug solution is delivered by a computer-controlled syringe pump located outside the self-administration apparatus. The pump contains a drug solution that is connected to a single-channel liquid swivel, which allows free rotation of the animal while maintaining a continuous flow of fluid. Plastic tubing is then housed in a stainless steel spring tether and is attached to the animal via a vascular access port implanted on the dorsal side of the animal, which is connected to the indwelling venous catheter.

In the case of alcohol, intravenous self-administration procedures are used less frequently, since this method lacks the face validity and pharmacokinetics of human oral alcohol consumption, and the ability of intravenous ethanol to function as a reinforcer is less reliable. Thus most animal models of alcohol self-administration utilize an experimental apparatus by which—instead of a syringe pump delivering the drug solution intravenously—a dilute ethanol solution (usually 8%–12% v/v) is delivered into a receptacle located near the lever or nose-poke orifice, where the animal can consume it orally. However, because of the aversive orosensory nature of ethanol, many researchers often initially train animals to consume alcohol solutions sweetened with sucrose or saccharin to increase its palatability. Then, slowly over a period of weeks, the concentration of the sweetener is gradually reduced until eventually the animal performs the operant task to consume an unsweetened ethanol solution.

There are many advantages of the operant self-administration paradigm as a model for human drug-taking behavior, including: (1) the drug is administered voluntarily by the animal (as opposed to passive administration by an experimenter); (2) the drug-taking behavior can be temporally examined within and between self-administration sessions; (3) candidate therapeutic pharmacological compounds or other experimental manipulations can be administered to determine their effects on drug self-administration; (4) the number of responses that must be exerted by the animal to receive the drug can be gradually increased (called a "progressive ratio") until the animal gives up and no longer performs the operant task (called the "breakpoint")—this method is used to measure the level of motivation to self-administer the drug as well as the efficacy of the reinforcer, and, finally; (5) the procedure is amenable to the study of relapse-like behavior (see "Cue- and Context-Induced Reinstatement of Drug-Seeking Behavior").

One additional advantage of operant self-administration procedures is their amenability to the study of the role of conditioned cues in the reinforcing effects of drugs of abuse. In addition to delivery of the drug, many researchers also use environmental cues such as the presentation of stimulus light, auditory tone, olfactory cue, or combinations thereof that are simultaneously paired with the intravenous delivery of the drug solution. Over successive self-administration sessions, the animal learns to associate these cues with the availability of the drug and its pharmacological effects. It should be noted that these cues act as conditioned reinforcers that are typically delivered contingent upon a lever press. Indeed, noncontingent conditioned reinforcers do not elicit an increase in motivated behavior.[50] Stimuli can also act as discriminative stimuli or occasion setters, which are noncontingent and involve the array of environmental stimuli that occur in conjunction with drug use. These types of stimuli modulate the response-eliciting ability of discrete conditioned stimuli paired with drug self-administration or serve a discriminatory function that predicts the availability of a drug of abuse upon the completion of a particular emitted response.[112,114] Studies have shown that, for most drugs of abuse, the presence of drug-associated cues greatly increases the number

Responding for drug reinforcement in the *absence* of drug-associated cues

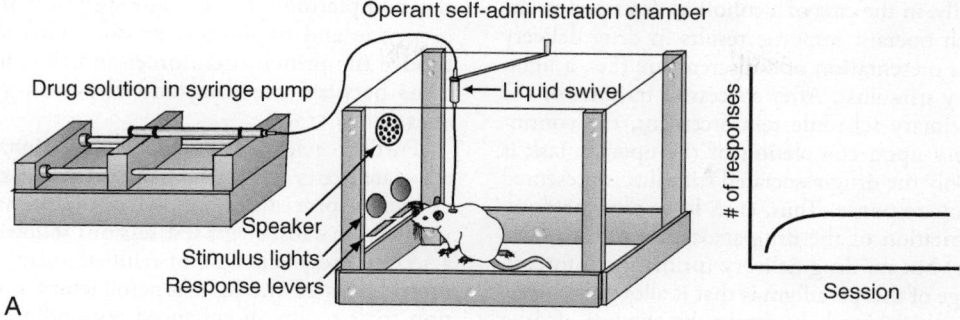

A

Responding for drug reinforcement in the *presence* of drug-associated cues

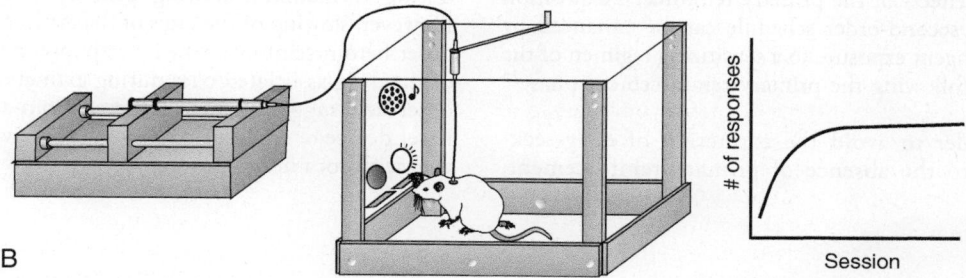

B

• **Fig. 8.2** Cue-induced enhancement of drug self-administration. (A) Animals trained to perform an operant task (such as a lever-press or nose-poke) in the absence of simultaneous presentation of any discrete cues (i.e., light, tone, or olfactory stimulus) show relatively low levels of responding for the drug alone. (B) In animals trained to self-administer the drug with concomitant presentation of discrete cues, responding for drug reinforcement is increased.

of operant responses exerted per test session, compared with when the drug is self-administered in the absence of such cues (see Fig. 8.2).[a] These findings suggest that in addition to the primary reinforcing effects of the drug itself, drug-associated stimuli (also termed secondary reinforcers or conditioned stimuli) regulate drug self-administration behavior, a phenomenon referred to by experimental psychologists as stimulus control of behavior. This stimulus control has also been demonstrated in human cocaine users in a laboratory setting.[75] In the case of psychostimulants, this enhancement of drug reinforcement by drug-associated cues has been hypothesized to be a result of the augmentation of the impact of sensory information caused by this class of drugs.[37]

The power of conditioned cues can also be seen in their ability to modulate intake of the drug itself in their presence or absence. Stimulus control, when instrumental behavior comes under control of a particular stimulus (e.g., a conditioned reinforcer such as a light or tone discrete stimulus), is evident by the ability of these stimuli to drive motivated behavior. Animals will respond one way in the presence of the stimulus and in a different way in the presence of another stimulus. This demonstrates the power of these stimuli to control behavior. In the self-administration model, animals are typically given short access (~12 hours/day) to take the drug. This is believed to model maintenance of drug use rather than the dysregulated intake that occurs in human addicts.[1] Ahmed and colleagues thus developed a model of escalated drug

use that was designed to capture this dysregulation in the spiral of addiction that occurs in humans. Although it is thought that this models dysregulated drug use behavior, these data typically show a plateau of intake within the sessions. If this truly models dysregulation, in theory it should never plateau. Thus, Beckmann and colleagues designed experiments to test whether it truly is dysregulation of intake, or rather a form of learning when animals are switched from short-access (1 hour/day) to long-access (6 hours/day) sessions. In these experiments, cocaine intake came under stimulus control when a house light was illuminated on 6-hour sessions, and not illuminated on 1-hour sessions, which alternated every other day. On long-access (6-hour) days, animals showed escalation of intake, and on short-access (1 hour) days, animals showed consistent levels of intake. These experiments not only showed that animals were simply acquiring a new form of temporal discrimination learning (thus modifying intake based on acquisition of the length of session), but also that escalation (dysregulated drug intake) of drug self-administration can come under stimulus control.[7] How can animals be dysregulated and regulated in their intake simultaneously? As well, how can dysregulated intake come under stimulus control if there is no learning mechanism involved?

Second-Order Schedules of Reinforcement

Another experimental paradigm that exemplifies the ability of drug-associated cues to exert stimulus control over behavior is

[a] References 17, 23, 38, 48, 54, 62, 73, 74, 80, 113.

the *second-order schedule of reinforcement*.[90,106] In this paradigm, animals are initially trained to self-administer a drug of abuse intravenously (or orally, in the case of alcohol) as described in the previous section; each operant response results in drug delivery and the simultaneous presentation of a discrete cue (i.e., a light, tone, and/or olfactory stimulus). After successful training of the animal under this primary schedule reinforcement, the contingency of drug delivery upon completion of the operant task is removed, such that only the drug-associated stimulus is presented following each operant response. Thus, each lever press or nose-poke results in presentation of the drug-associated cue stimulus (secondary reinforcer) but no drug delivery (primary reinforcer). The primary advantage of this paradigm is that it allows the investigator to examine drug-seeking behavior in the absence of drug delivery, similar to the cue- and context-induced reinstatement discussed in the next section. Thus, the effect of pharmacological or neurobiological manipulations on responding for the secondary reinforcer can be performed without the potential confound of the psychoactive effects of the primary reinforcer. Acquisition of responding on a second-order schedule can be enhanced by non–response-contingent exposure to a sensitizing regimen of the drug (i.e., cocaine) following the primary reinforcement phase[25] (Fig. 8.3).

However, in order to avoid the extinction of drug-seeking behavior due to the absence of primary reinforcement, a response-contingent delivery of the drug solution must be given at a fixed time interval (i.e., every 30 or 60 min) after the completion of a certain number of operant responses, or at the end of the test session. This allows the animal to receive the primary reinforcer and thus maintain the associations between the drug and responding for drug-associated cues.

Further evidence for the motivational salience of drug-associated cues lies in the fact that when animals are subject to extinction procedures (i.e., when the primary drug reinforcer is withheld in subsequent test sessions following responding under a second-order schedule of reinforcement), response-contingent presentation of the light/tone/olfactory stimulus during extinction trials results in enhanced responding and a slowing of the rate of extinction in rats trained to self-administer cocaine,[3] suggesting that the drug-associated cues maintain their motivational salience despite the fact that the primary drug reinforcer is no longer available. This phenomenon has also been demonstrated during extinction following primary drug reinforcement.[91,94] However, slowing of the rates of the extinction following second-order heroin reinforcement by response-contingent presentation of the drug-associated cues during extinction trials has not been observed,[2] suggesting that discrete heroin-associated cues exert a lesser degree of stimulus control over behavior than those associated with cocaine.

First-order schedule of drug reinforcement

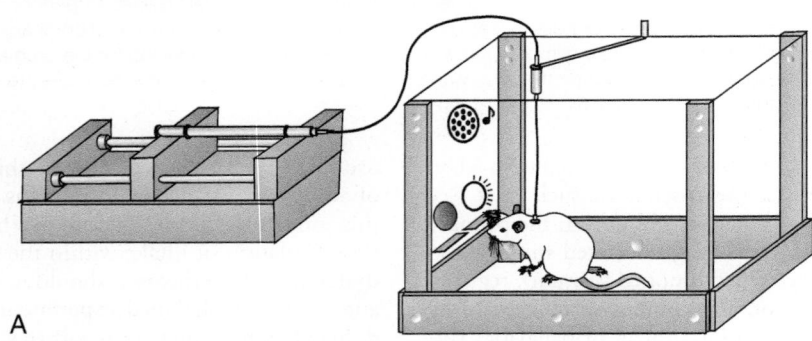

A

Second-order schedule of drug reinforcement

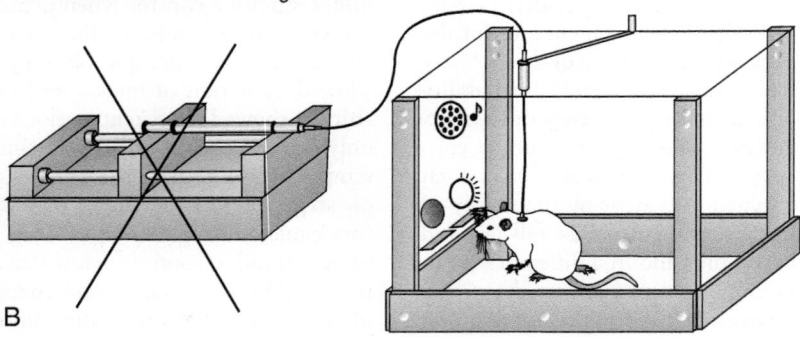

B

• **Fig. 8.3** First- and second-order schedules of reinforcement. (A) In a first-order schedule of reinforcement, each correct operant response (i.e., lever-press or nose-poke) results in the delivery of the drug solution as well as simultaneous presentation of discrete drug-associated stimuli. (B) Following sufficient training on a first-order schedule of reinforcement, a second-order schedule of reinforcement can be initiated whereby each correct lever response results in the presentation of the drug-associated cue, but infusion of the drug solution is withheld until a fixed time point or the end of the test session.

Cue- and Context-Induced Reinstatement of Drug-Seeking Behavior

Relapse is one of the most problematic aspects in the treatment of drug addiction, as it can occur months or years following the last episode of drug intake. Fortunately animal models have been developed that appear to mimic the phenomenon of relapse in humans. The most widely used animal model of relapse is the *reinstatement* paradigm.[b] In this paradigm, animals are trained to self-administer a particular drug of abuse as described in the section "Conditioned Cue Enhancement of Drug Self-Administration." Following stabilization of patterns of self-administration, animals are then subject to extinction training, where the operant response that previously resulted in drug delivery either has no consequences or results in the delivery of a non-reinforcing substance such as saline. During extinction training, the animal learns that the operant response no longer results in drug delivery and subsequently decreases the number of operant responses exerted. Once specific extinction criteria have been reached (for example, the number of operant responses performed during an extinction trial is less than 20% of those that were observed prior to the commencement of extinction training), the animal is then exposed to one of three types of stimuli that are known to trigger relapse in human addicts: brief exposure to the drug (drug priming), exposure to drug-associated cues, or stressors. The animal then exhibits a significant increase in the number of operant responses that previously resulted in drug delivery; in other words, drug-seeking behavior has been *reinstated*. It should be noted, however, that in the reinstatement model, performing the operant task does not actually result in drug delivery; the behavior is not reinforced by the drug, and, therefore, the reinstatement of drug seeking is relatively short-lived. Herein lies one of the fundamental (and often criticized) aspects of the reinstatement paradigm where it diverges from the human condition of relapse, since in humans drug-seeking behavior is usually followed by drug self-administration. In the reinstatement paradigm, execution of the operant response does not result in drug availability and self-administration. Nevertheless, the reinstatement paradigm offers a particularly unique method for studying the neural basis of relapse, since *drug-seeking* behavior is inherently parsed out from actual *drug-self-administration* behavior, and the behavior of the animal can be observed and recorded in the absence of psychomotor-altering effects of the drug itself.

With regard to the study of the influence of conditioned cues on drug-seeking behavior, the reinstatement paradigm offers the possibility of studying two distinct phenomena. First, if the discrete conditioned reinforcers (i.e., a tone, light, or olfactory stimuli) that were presented to the animal during each drug delivery prior to extinction procedures are reintroduced to the animal in a response-contingent manner, presumably the animal expects that the drug is now available and exerts a significant increase in the number of operant responses that previously resulted in drug delivery. Alternatively, some investigators present the drug-associated cues in a non–response-contingent manner (although this does not reinstate behavior[47,50]). Regardless, this phenomenon is known as *cue-induced reinstatement*, and has been used extensively to study the role of discrete drug-associated cues in the control over drug-seeking behavior (Fig. 8.4).

During the phase of the experiment where animals are actively self-administering the drug, the animal makes associations not only between the drug and the discrete cues presented upon its delivery but also between the drug and the physical environment in which the drug is self-administered. This is particularly relevant to drug addiction in humans, since drug-taking behavior is usually performed ritualistically in distinct physical locations (i.e., in the addict's bedroom, local crack house, and so on). The role of the physical environment in controlling drug-seeking behavior can be modeled in animals through what is known as *context-induced* or *contextual reinstatement*.[14,20] It should be noted that in this model, the stimuli typically act as discriminative stimuli in which they inform the animal of the availability of the drug. In this paradigm, animals are trained to self-administer the drug in a particular self-administration apparatus. However, subsequent extinction training is conducted in an apparatus that is contextually distinct from that where the active drug self-administration phase occurs (i.e., with different colored walls, different textured flooring, the presence of a different odor, and so on). After extinction criteria have been met, the animal is placed back in the original apparatus where the initial drug self-administration was performed. As a consequence of the drug-environment associations formed during active drug self-administration, the animal then displays a significant increase in the number of operant responses that previously resulted in drug delivery. (This phenomenon is sometimes referred to as a *renewal* effect.) Renewal of drug seeking, however, involves a behavioral mechanism different from reinstatement. It is notable that a behavior is *renewed* after extinction when it is tested and increased in a different context. This phenomenon shows that extinction processes are not permanent and is subject to changes in context.[16] Alternatively, a behavior is *reinstated* when a US is presented by itself before the CS is tested again.[15,82] It is important to note that in typical reinstatement procedures that are currently used to assess the ability of drug paired conditioned stimuli to elicit neurobiological changes (current models of relapse), these stimuli are presented contingently and independently of the US following extinction, in the context in which extinction learning took place.[35,47] In most models used currently, no drug is actually delivered as a result of the operant response, so as to provide a model of contextual influences over drug-seeking rather than drug self-administration behavior. If drug was presented with the CSs following extinction, this would be termed *rapid reacquisition*, where extinguished responding returns rapidly when it is again reinforced.[16]

Incentive Salience Attribution

Although the phenomenon of incentive salience attribution is not novel, it has recently become a frequently used preclinical model of addiction vulnerability.[8,39,41,84] In this model, the Pavlovian Conditioned Approach (PCA) is used to study the ability of cue-predictive rewards come to exert control over behavior. In PCA, a lever located next to a food receptacle is typically used to reliably predict a noncontingent food reward, and this tends to elicit differential responses in rodents.[6] In this model, two distinct behavioral phenotypes emerge: (1) sign tracking, when animals approach and engage with a cue that predicts reward; and (2) goal tracking, when animals approach the location where the reward will be delivered when a cue is presented, rather than approaching the cue itself. It has been shown that animals that primarily sign track acquire cocaine self-administration at a faster

---

[b] References 10, 11, 14, 35, 87, 106.

Acquisition and maintenance of drug self-administration

Extinction training

Cue-induced reinstatement of drug-seeking behavior

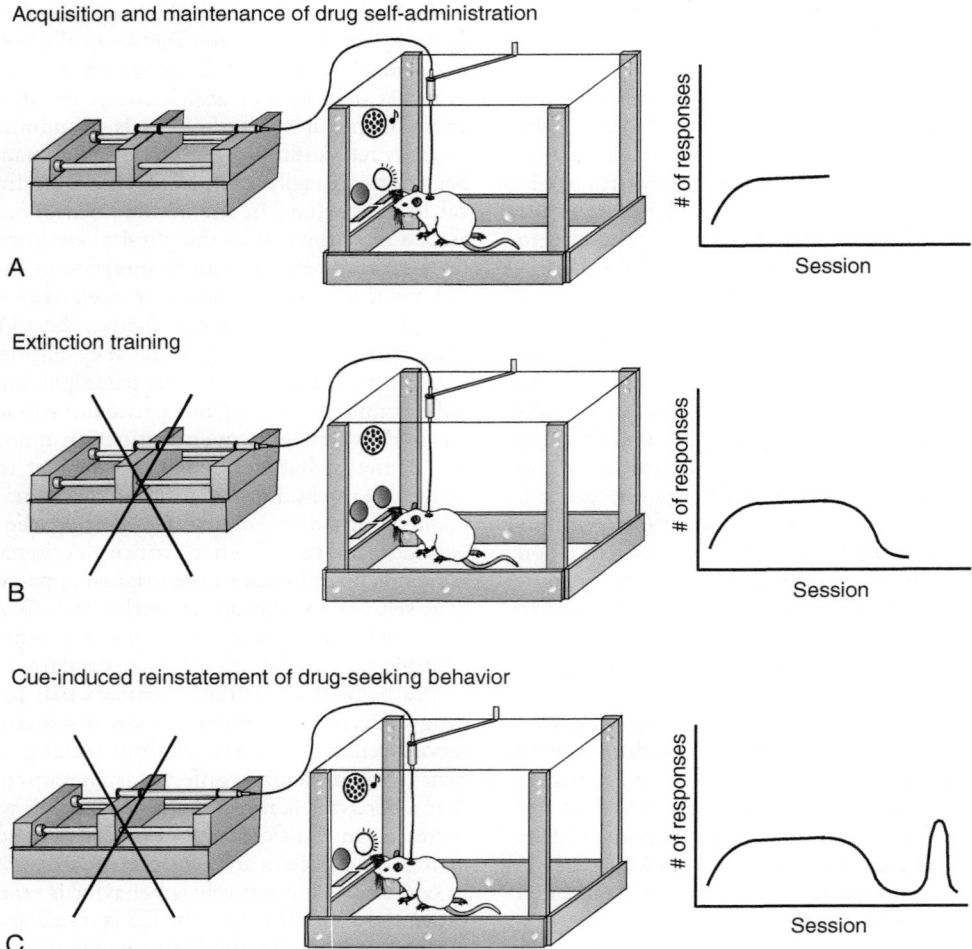

• **Fig. 8.4** Cue-induced reinstatement of drug-seeking behavior. (A) The animal is first trained to self-administer the drug solution under a standard first-order schedule of reinforcement in the presence of discrete drug-associated cues during drug delivery. This schedule of reinforcement is maintained until response patterns stabilize. (B) During extinction training, each correct operant response that previously resulted in drug delivery either results in infusion of saline or has no programmed consequences. Extinction training is performed until predefined extinction criteria have been met. (C) During cue-induced reinstatement testing, discrete cues that were previously paired with drug delivery are presented to the animal in a response-contingent or noncontingent manner. Most investigators conduct reinstatement testing in the absence of actual drug delivery so as to separate drug-seeking behavior from actual drug-self-administration behavior, as well as to avoid the potential confounds of psychomotor effects of the drug on operant performance.

rate,[8] thus it is thought that sign trackers have a predisposition toward drug addiction vulnerability.[39] It is notable that Robinson and colleagues showed in rodents that this procedure characterizes individual propensity to resist drug-associated cues prior to any exposure to a drug of abuse, and this may be a screening tool for addiction vulnerability prior to drug use.[84,88] Using this model, neurobiological substrates of incentive salience attribution have shown important advancements that seem to be in line with the different behavioral phenotypes.[40] Although underlying neurobiological substrates of sign versus goal tracking are mostly unknown, recent evidence suggests that differential responding (sign versus goal) in the PCA procedure engages differential patterns of dopaminergic signaling. Specifically, sign-tracking responses have been linked with more sensitive changes in dopamine signaling than goal-tracking responses.[40,89] These data suggest that the underlying neurobiological mechanisms governing these two response phenotypes may involve differential

recruitment of phasic dopamine signaling patterns, and that this may govern the incentive value attributed to a drug-paired stimulus within an individual.

Pavlovian-Instrumental Transfer

It is important to note that Pavlovian stimuli that become conditioned through repeated pairings with a drug of abuse can come to influence output of instrumental behavior. These CSs can impact instrumental responding toward the same or a different reward. In addiction models, Pavlovian-instrumental transfer (PIT) has shown that under certain conditions, CSs elicited increased responding previously maintained by a drug of abuse (e.g., ethanol[19,68] or cocaine[63,72]). Although there is evidence that Pavlovian stimuli can elicit increased instrumental responding that was previously maintained by drug reinforcers, it is unknown if these stimuli act as occasion setters or conditioned stimuli,

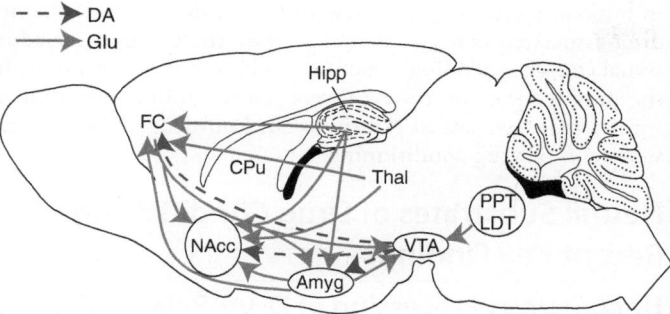

• **Fig. 8.5** Sagittal section of the rat brain showing the neural circuitry underlying conditioning processes in drug addiction. The ventral tegmental area *(VTA)* sends dopaminergic *(DA)* projections *(blue dashed lines)* to the nucleus accumbens *(NAcc)*, frontal cortex *(FC)*, and amygdala *(Amyg)*, and this pathway is believed to mediate the primary reinforcing effects of most drugs of abuse. These structures also receive substantial glutamatergic (Glu) input *(red solid lines)*. For example, the hippocampus *(Hipp)* and FC send glutamatergic projections to the FC, NAcc, and Amyg, while the thalamus *(Thal)* also innervates the NAcc and FC with glutamatergic input. Finally, the VTA receives glutamatergic input from many of the aforementioned regions as well as the pedunculopontine tegmentum *(PPT)* and laterodorsal tegmentum *(LDT)* in the brainstem. *CPu,* Caudate putamen.

where they either elicit behavior that makes drug taking more probable, or they increase motivation for drug taking. Depending on this relationship (modulatory or reinforcing), it could elicit very different neurobiological mechanisms. It should be noted that in most of the examples showing PIT with a drug CS, there is an explicitly unpaired stimulus as a control condition that is problematic, as these stimuli can come to predict nondelivery of the US.[81] Thus, it has been proposed that a truly random control procedure to control for other nonassociative conditioning is needed for parsing out the effects of a drug CS on increasing instrumental behavior.[60]

Neural Substrates of Drug Conditioning: General Neurochemical Circuitry

Studies utilizing the aforementioned animal models of drug conditioning have yielded a wealth of information regarding the neural mechanisms underlying the ability of drug-associated stimuli to control drug-seeking behavior in the absence of primary drug reinforcement. The results of these studies have identified several brain regions that subserve stimulus control over drug-seeking behavior, namely the amygdala, nucleus accumbens, dorsal striatum, hippocampus, frontal cortex, and ventral tegmental area, with both glutamatergic and dopaminergic transmission in many of these regions being implicated (Fig. 8.5). As will be discussed later, advances in imaging of the living human brain have also greatly added to our understanding of the neural basis of reactivity to drug-associated cues, and have particularly extended our understanding of the role of subregions of the frontal cortex.

Amygdala

The amygdala, or amygdaloid complex, is a small set of nuclei found in the temporal lobe that receives a considerable amount of input from cortical regions involved in sensory processing as well as other cortical, subcortical, and limbic structures. In turn, the amygdala provides efferent output to many of these same regions.

Using selective lesion methods, Everitt and colleagues were among the first to show that the basolateral portion of the amygdala is important for stimulus-reward associations utilizing natural rewards such as sucrose,[36] and later extended these findings to drugs of abuse by demonstrating that lesions of the basolateral amygdala reduced the ability of rats to respond for cocaine under a second-order schedule of reinforcement.[116] Numerous other studies have shown that lesions or inactivation of the basolateral amygdala also attenuate cue- and/or context-induced reinstatement of cocaine-seeking behavior,[43,65,93] and that cocaine-associated stimuli increase the expression of immediate early genes such as c-fos in the basolateral amygdala.[22,59,118] Additional studies using site-specific intracranial microinjections have revealed a distinct role of dopamine transmission, particularly D_1- or $D_{2/3}$-like receptors, as well as serotonergic transmission, whereas evidence for a role of glutamatergic transmission is less evident.[28,58,79,95]

Nucleus Accumbens

One of the most commonly studied brain regions with regard to drug addiction is the nucleus accumbens, located within the ventral striatum of the rostral forebrain. This region receives dense dopaminergic input from the ventral tegmental area of the midbrain as well as glutamatergic projections from the prefrontal cortex, hippocampus, amygdala, and thalamus. There appears to be subregion-specific roles of the nucleus accumbens in drug conditioning, as inactivation of the nucleus accumbens core, but not the shell subregion, selectively impair acquisition of second-order drug reinforcement and cue-induced or contextual reinstatement of drug-seeking behavior while having no effect on maintenance of responding.[31,32,44,55,85] However, unlike the amygdala, glutamatergic signaling in the nucleus accumbens may be more important than dopamine signaling in drug-conditioned stimulus control of behavior. Evidence for this comes from studies showing that blockade of α-amino-3-hydroxy-5-methylisoxazole-4-propionic acid (AMPA)/kainic acid–type glutamate receptors in the nucleus accumbens core reduces second-order responding for cocaine,[26,27] whereas blockade of D_3 receptors in the nucleus accumbens shell has no effect on second-order cocaine reinforcement.[24]

Dorsal Striatum

In addition to the nucleus accumbens, the dorsal striatum (particularly the dorsolateral region) plays a role in cue-controlled cocaine seeking,[32,42] with both dopamine and glutamatergic transmission being involved.[9,107] An elegant study by Di Ciano and Everitt demonstrated a functional interaction between the basolateral amygdala and the nucleus accumbens core in mediating drug seeking under a second-order schedule of reinforcement.[30] In this study, bilateral antagonism of dopamine but not AMPA receptors in the basolateral amygdala impaired second-order cocaine reinforcement, whereas the reverse was true when these manipulations were performed in the nucleus accumbens core. When unilateral injections on opposite sides of the brain were performed in a disconnection procedure, dopamine receptor blockade in the basolateral amygdala combined with blockade of AMPA receptors in the contralateral nucleus accumbens core produced the same effect as the bilateral injections. A similar disconnection procedure recently showed that unilateral dopamine receptor antagonism in the dorsal striatum combined with a unilateral lesion of the nucleus accumbens core impairs second-order cocaine responding.[9]

Ventral Tegmental Area

In addition to being the primary source of dopaminergic input to the nucleus accumbens, various studies have indicated that the ventral tegmental area, particularly glutamatergic input to this region, modulates the ability of drug-associated cues to influence drug-seeking behavior. For example, suppression of glutamate transmission in the ventral tegmental area by local infusion of a type 2/3 metabotropic glutamate receptor agonist or infusion of kynurenate attenuates contextual reinstatement of heroin- or cocaine-seeking behavior.[13,102] Likewise, temporary inactivation of the ventral tegmental area attenuates second-order responding for cocaine.[29] Thus, there is evidence to suggest that the ventral tegmental area controls both primary and secondary drug reinforcement.

Hippocampus

Another region involved in drug conditioning is the hippocampal formation, which is involved not only in episodic memory storage but also in spatial navigation and the influence of environmental contexts on behavior. Inactivation of the dorsomedial hippocampus attenuates contextual reinstatement of cocaine-seeking behavior,[43] whereas inactivation of slightly more ventral portions of the hippocampus reduces cue-induced reinstatement.[86] However, conflicting evidence exists over whether inactivation of ventral output regions of the hippocampal formation (i.e., the subiculum) mediates cue-induced reinstatement evoked by discrete drug-associated cues.[12,103] Nonetheless, the hippocampus appears to play a role in the ability of drug-associated contexts to influence drug-seeking behavior.

Prefrontal Cortex

Finally, there is overwhelming evidence that the prefrontal cortex and many of its subregions also play a significant role in drug conditioning and stimulus control of behavior. In nonhuman primates, lesions of the orbitofrontal cortex impair second-order responding for cocaine,[78] whereas in rodents, lesions of the medial prefrontal cortex actually increase responding for cocaine under a second-order schedule of reinforcement.[115] Inactivation of the dorsomedial/prelimbic, ventral prefrontal, and lateral orbitofrontal cortices attenuates cue- or context-induced reinstatement of drug-seeking behavior.[33,43,45,67]

Human Neuroimaging Studies

Imaging studies of the human brain support a pivotal role for the prefrontal cortex and other aforementioned brain regions in responsivity to drug-associate cues.[49,57,109,110,117] One advantage offered by human neuroimaging studies is delineation of subregions of the prefrontal cortex, which are less anatomically and functionally distinct in rodents. Presentation of cues associated with drug intake to subjects with a history of drug use activate forebrain regions such as the anterior cingulate, dorsolateral prefrontal, and orbitofrontal cortices; the insular cortex; and striatal and limbic regions such as the amygdala and nucleus accumbens (reviewed in Goldstein and Volkow,[49] Jasinska et al.,[57] Volkow and Morales,[108] Volkow et al.,[109,110] and Yalachkov et al.[117]). Many of these studies have revealed that activation of these brain regions is also highly correlated with drug craving. Due to methodological constraints inherent

to human neuroimaging, it remains to be determined whether drug-associated contextual cues activate these regions or additional context-encoding structures such as the hippocampus. In the next section, we review several recent animal and human studies that have added greatly to our knowledge of the neural substrates of drug conditioning.

Neural Substrates of Drug Conditioning: Recent Key Findings

Unconscious Processing of Drug-Related Cues

Many neuroimaging studies have utilized functional magnetic resonance imaging (fMRI) to reveal activation patterns of brain reward and associated limbic regions elicited by presentation of drug-associated cues. However, one recent study revealed the impact of drug-associated cues presented at an unconscious level, with the goal of elucidating the neural mechanisms of cue processing that occur outside of conscious awareness. In this study,[18] male subjects with a history of cocaine use were subjected to event-related fMRI procedures to assess neural responses to various cues presented in a backward-masked manner for a duration too short for conscious processing (33 msec). The cues presented were of a cocaine, sexual, aversive, or neutral nature, and subsequent reactivity was observed during an affective bias priming task. Results of this study showed that many limbic brain regions known to be activated by longer cue exposure were also activated by these unseen cues. However, additional increased activity was observed in a transition zone between the amygdala and ventral pallidum, suggesting that some regions of the brain are activated by drug-associated visual stimuli even when unseen at the conscious level 2 days after imaging. The authors suggested that these reward signals may represent a primordial signature of desire in the brain, and may reveal vulnerability to addictive and other impulse control disorders.

Reinstatement Induced by Novel Cues

Although reinstatement of drug-seeking behavior in animal models of addiction is frequently conducted by exposure to cues previously associated with drug availability or infusion, the effects of exposure to completely novel cues were largely unknown until a recent study by Bastle and colleagues.[5] In this study, male rats were trained to self-administer cocaine that was paired with either a light or a tone cue, followed by traditional extinction training. During reinstatement testing, however, rats were exposed to cues to which they were previously naive (i.e., the tone was presented to rats previously receiving cocaine infusions associated with the light stimulus and vice versa). A surprising finding was that not only did exposure to novel cues reinstate cocaine-seeking to the same magnitude as cocaine-associated cues but also increased c-fos expression in various brain regions, including the dorsal and ventral striatum and basolateral amygdala. However, some differences were noted, with the anterior cingulate showing selectivity for the cue modality presented (light versus tone), and the dorsomedial striatum where c-fos expression was correlated with responding only in the novel cue groups. In addition, the authors showed that novel cues could also elicit reinstatement of sucrose-seeking. These surprising findings reveal potential influences of novelty, action-outcome habits, and contextual effects on reward and reinforcement processes for both drugs of abuse and natural rewards.

Optogenetic Regulation of Cocaine Seeking

The field of optogenetics has largely revolutionized the field of neuroscience, where neurons can now be genetically engineered to express light-reactive proteins that allow for unprecedented levels of spatiotemporal and cell-type specificity control. Numerous recent studies have applied this technique to animal models of addiction. One such study by Pascoli and colleagues[76] found that cocaine seeking was correlated with rectifying (calcium-impermeable) AMPA responses and reduced AMPA/N-methyl-D-aspartate (NMDA) ratios in neurons projecting from the medial prefrontal cortex to D_1-expressing neurons in the nucleus accumbens shell, whereas the opposite was true for projections to these neurons arising from the ventral hippocampus. In addition, the authors were able to abolish this cocaine-induced plasticity in both sites via optogenetic stimulation, and region-selective behavioral effects were observed, with reversal at prefrontal inputs impairing response discrimination while reversal at ventral hippocampal inputs reduced the vigor of responding. These findings revealed new information on inputs to the nucleus accumbens arising from different brain regions that promote relapse. Additional studies utilizing optogenetic silencing techniques have confirmed a role for direct basolateral amygdala projections to the nucleus accumbens, indirect basolateral amygdala projections to the prelimbic subregion of the prefrontal cortex, prelimbic projections to the nucleus accumbens core, and nucleus accumbens projections to the ventral pallidum, in regulating cue-evoked drug-seeking behavior.[98-100]

Another study examined the effects of optogenetic activation (via cation-permeable channelrhodopsin) or inactivation (via anion-permeable halorhodopsin) of excitatory pyramidal cells in the ventromedial prefrontal cortex on the expression of a cocaine-conditioned place preference.[105] When performed within 1–2 days of cocaine conditioning (recent memory), optogenetic activation of the ventromedial prefrontal cortex was without effect, but facilitated the extinction of place preference assessed 3 weeks after conditioning (remote memory). In contrast, optogenetic inhibition of pyramidal cells impaired recall of the recent cocaine memory but was without effect on remote memory. However, inhibition of these cells inhibited extinction learning at the latter time point. These findings suggest a critical time-dependent switch in the role of ventromedial prefrontal pyramidal cells in regulating recall and extinction of cocaine-associated contextual memories.

Inhibition of Cue-Induced Cocaine Seeking by Synthetic Designer Receptors

In addition to the revolutionary technique of optogenetics, another approach to selectively modulating specific neural circuits is known as chemogenetics. In this method, designer receptors activated exclusively by designer drugs (DREADDs) have been engineered to be activated only by exogenous ligands, such as clozapine-N-oxide. Depending on the precise G-proteins coupled to this designer receptor, the exogenous ligand can either activate or inhibit cells in which it is expressed. Recently, Scofield and colleagues[92] utilized viral vectors to selectively express an excitatory (Gq-coupled) DREADD in astrocytes in the nucleus accumbens core of rats also trained to self-administer cocaine. Results showed that activation of this DREADD increased extracellular glutamate levels that were determined to be of glial origin, and inhibited cue-induced reinstatement of cocaine seeking. This effect was prevented by pharmacological blockade of Group II

mGluR2/3 receptors. This methodology may reveal novel information on the neuroanatomical and neurochemical substrates of drug conditioning.

Structural Plasticity Induced by Drug-Associated Cues

Drugs of abuse are known to produce both physiological synaptic plasticity (as evidenced by long-term potentiation and depression of synaptic function) as well as structural plasticity (as indicated by alterations in dendritic spine density, morphology, or other synaptic rearrangements). In our recent studies[46,97] we showed that both discrete cue and context-induced reinstatement of cocaine seeking results in enlargements of dendritic spine head diameter in the nucleus accumbens core medium spiny neurons at 15 minutes following reinstatement testing, but these effects were largely diminished just 45 minutes after this time point. In addition, contextual reinstatement of cocaine-seeking was without effect on dendritic spine density in this region, suggesting that cocaine-associated contextual cues induced subtle and transient changes in dendritic spine morphology. It should be noted, however, that with discrete cues, we found an increase in the AMPA-to-NMDA ratio in accumbens medium spiny neurons. This is interpreted as a functional readout of the structural changes reported in these studies; however the currents were recorded from the cell somas, whereas the dendritic spine morphological readouts were measured from distal dendrites. Thus the precise functional contribution of these structural changes to cocaine-seeking behavior is of great interest for future studies.

Conclusions

Although drug addiction is a chronic, multifaceted, relapsing disease that has numerous genetic, socioeconomic, and behavioral causes, one of its key features is an increased incentive salience of drug-associated stimuli and impaired executive inhibitory control of drug craving elicited by these cues. These manifestations of the addictive state are mediated by dysfunction of limbic and prefrontal-accumbens circuitry. Therefore, it is of clinical interest to restore the normal functioning of these circuits during the course of treatment of the addict so as to allow him or her to extinguish the motivational salience of drug-associated cues and regain inhibitory control of drug-seeking and drug self-administration behaviors. Clearly, more research is needed to parse out the neurobiological substrates of drug conditioning at the molecular, cellular, and systems levels, and how this conditioning can be reversed in the addicted state. It should also be noted that preclinical modeling of conditioning in drug addiction does not readily parse out the modulatory versus reinforcing relations of drug-associated stimuli, and pharmacotherapeutic advancements from these models have yielded inconsistent clinical success.[61,66] Thus, it is important to dissociate the roles these powerful stimuli play in the varied paths to addiction and relapse, in order to better tailor treatment to promote drug use cessation outcomes.

References

1. Ahmed SH, Koob GF. Long-lasting increase in the set point for cocaine self-administration after escalation in rats. *Psychopharmacology*. 1999;146:303–312.
2. Alderson HL, Robbins TW, Everitt BJ. Heroin self-administration under a second-order schedule of reinforcement: acquisition and maintenance of heroin-seeking behaviour in rats. *Psychopharmacology (Berl)*. 2000;153:120–133.

3. Arroyo M, Markou A, Robbins TW, et al. Acquisition, mainte-nance and reinstatement of intravenous cocaine self-administration under a second-order schedule of reinforcement in rats: effects of conditioned cues and continuous access to cocaine. *Psychopharma-cology (Berl)*. 1998;140:331–344.

4. Bardo MT, Bevins RA. Conditioned place preference: what does it add to our preclinical understanding of drug reward? *Psychophar-macology (Berl)*. 2000;153:31–43.

5. Bastle RM, Kufahl PR, Turk MN, et al. Novel cues reinstate cocaine-seeking behavior and induce Fos protein expression as effectively as conditioned cues. *Neuropsychopharmacology*. 2012;37:2109–2120.

6. Beckmann JS, Chow JJ. Isolating the incentive salience of reward-associated stimuli: value, choice, and persistence. *Learn Mem*. 2015;22:116–127.

7. Beckmann JS, Gipson CD, Marusich JA, et al. Escalation of cocaine intake with extended access in rats: dysregulated addiction or regu-lated acquisition? *Psychopharmacology (Berl)*. 2012;222:257–267.

8. Beckmann JS, Marusich JA, Gipson CD, et al. Novelty seeking, incentive salience and acquisition of cocaine self-administration in the rat. *Behav Brain Res*. 2011;216:159–165.

9. Belin D, Everitt BJ. Cocaine seeking habits depend upon dopa-mine-dependent serial connectivity linking the ventral with the dorsal striatum. *Neuron*. 2008;57:432–441.

10. Belin-Rauschent A, Belin D. Animal models of drug addiction. In: Belin D, ed. *Addictions - From Pathophysiology to Treatment*. InTech Open; 2012:21–64.

11. Belin-Rauscent A, Fouyssac M, Bonci A, et al. How preclinical models evolved to resemble the diagnostic criteria of drug addic-tion. *Biol Psychiatry*. 2016;79:39–46.

12. Black YD, Green-Jordan K, Eichenbaum HB, et al. Hippocampal memory system function and the regulation of cocaine self-admin-istration behavior in rats. *Behav Brain Res*. 2004;151:225–238.

13. Bossert JM, Liu SY, Lu L, et al. A role of ventral tegmental area glutamate in contextual cue-induced relapse to heroin seeking. *J Neurosci*. 2004;24:10726–10730.

14. Bossert JM, Marchant NJ, Calu DJ, et al. The reinstatement model of drug relapse: recent neurobiological findings, emerging research topics, and translational research. *Psychopharmacology (Berl)*. 2013;229:453–476.

15. Bouton ME, Bolles RC. Role of conditioned contextual stimuli in reinstatement of extinguished fear. *J Exp Psychol Anim Behav Pro-cess*. 1979;5:368–378.

16. Bouton ME, Winterbauer NE, Todd TP. Relapse processes after the extinction of instrumental learning: renewal, resurgence, and reacquisition. *Behav Process*. 2012;90:130–141.

17. Chaudhri N, Caggiula AR, Donny EC, et al. Operant respond-ing for conditioned and unconditioned reinforcers in rats is differentially enhanced by the primary reinforcing and reinforce-ment-enhancing effects of nicotine. *Psychopharmacology (Berl)*. 2006;189:27–36.

18. Childress AR, Ehrman RN, Wang Z, et al. Prelude to passion: limbic activation by "unseen" drug and sexual cues. *PLoS One*. 2008;3:e1506.

19. Corbit LH, Janak PH. Ethanol-associated cues produce general pavlovian-instrumental transfer. *Alcohol Clin Exp Res*. 2007;31: 766–774.

20. Crombag HS, Bossert JM, Koya E, et al. Context-induced relapse to drug seeking: a review. *Philos Trans R Soc Lond B Biol Sci*. 2008;363:3233–3243.

21. Cunningham CL, Fidler TL, Hill KG. Animal models of alcohol's motivational effects. *Alcohol Res Health*. 2000;24:85–92.

22. Dayas CV, Liu X, Simms JA, et al. Distinct patterns of neural acti-vation associated with ethanol seeking: effects of naltrexone. *Biol Psychiatry*. 2007;61:979–989.

23. Deroche-Gamonet V, Piat F, Le Moal M, et al. Influence of cue-conditioning on acquisition, maintenance and relapse of cocaine intravenous self-administration. *Eur J Neurosci*. 2002;15: 1363–1370.

24. Di Ciano P. Drug seeking under a second-order schedule of rein-forcement depends on dopamine D_3 receptors in the basolateral amygdala. *Behav Neurosci*. 2008;122:129–139.

25. Di Ciano P. Facilitated acquisition but not persistence of respond-ing for a cocaine-paired conditioned reinforcer following sensitiza-tion with cocaine. *Neuropsychopharmacology*. 2008;33:1426–1431.

26. Di Ciano P, Cardinal RN, Cowell RA, et al. Differential involve-ment of NMDA, AMPA/kainate, and dopamine receptors in the nucleus accumbens core in the acquisition and performance of pav-lovian approach behavior. *J Neurosci*. 2001;21:9471–9477.

27. Di Ciano P, Everitt BJ. Dissociable effects of antagonism of NMDA and AMPA/KA receptors in the nucleus accumbens core and shell on cocaine-seeking behavior. *Neuropsychopharmacology*. 2001;25:341–360.

28. Di Ciano P, Everitt BJ. Reinstatement and spontaneous recovery of cocaine-seeking following extinction and different durations of withdrawal. *Behav Pharmacol*. 2002;13:397–405.

29. Di Ciano P, Everitt BJ. Contribution of the ventral tegmental area to cocaine-seeking maintained by a drug-paired conditioned stimu-lus in rats. *Eur J Neurosci*. 2004;19:1661–1667.

30. Di Ciano P, Everitt BJ. Direct interactions between the basolateral amygdala and nucleus accumbens core underlie cocaine-seeking behavior by rats. *J Neurosci*. 2004;24:7167–7173.

31. Di Ciano P, Everitt BJ. Neuropsychopharmacology of drug seek-ing: insights from studies with second-order schedules of drug rein-forcement. *Eur J Pharmacol*. 2005;526:186–198.

32. Di Ciano P, Robbins TW, Everitt BJ. Differential effects of nucleus accumbens core, shell, or dorsal striatal inactivations on the persistence, reacquisition, or reinstatement of responding for a drug-paired conditioned reinforcer. *Neuropsychopharmacology*. 2008;33:1413–1425.

33. Di Pietro NC, Black YD, Kantak KM. Context-dependent pre-frontal cortex regulation of cocaine self-administration and rein-statement behaviors in rats. *Eur J Neurosci*. 2006;24:3285–3298.

34. Donny EC, Caggiula AR, Rose C, et al. Differential effects of response-contingent and response-independent nicotine in rats. *Eur J Pharmacol*. 2000;402:231–240.

35. Epstein DH, Preston KL, Stewart J, et al. Toward a model of drug relapse: an assessment of the validity of the reinstatement proce-dure. *Psychopharmacology (Berl)*. 2006;189:1–16.

36. Everitt BJ, Morris KA, O'Brien A, et al. The basolateral amygdala-ventral striatal system and conditioned place preference: further evidence of limbic-striatal interactions underlying reward-related processes. *Neuroscience*. 1991;42:1–18.

37. Everitt BJ, Robbins TW. Neural systems of reinforcement for drug addiction: from actions to habits to compulsion. *Nat Neurosci*. 2005;8:1481–1489.

38. Falk JL, Lau CE. Stimulus control of addictive behavior: persis-tence in the presence and absence of a drug. *Pharmacol Biochem Behav*. 1995;50:71–75.

39. Flagel SB, Akil H, Robinson TE. Individual differences in the attri-bution of incentive salience to reward-related cues: Implications for addiction. *Neuropharmacology*. 2009;56(suppl 1):139–148.

40. Flagel SB, Clark JJ, Robinson TE, et al. A selective role for dopamine in stimulus-reward learning. *Nature*. 2011;469: 53–57.

41. Flagel SB, Watson SJ, Akil H, et al. Individual differences in the attribution of incentive salience to a reward-related cue: influence on cocaine sensitization. *Behav Brain Res*. 2008;186: 48–56.

42. Fuchs RA, Branham RK, See RE. Different neural substrates medi-ate cocaine seeking after abstinence versus extinction training: a critical role for the dorsolateral caudate-putamen. *J Neurosci*. 2006;26:3584–3588.

43. Fuchs RA, Evans KA, Ledford CC, et al. The role of the dorso-medial prefrontal cortex, basolateral amygdala, and dorsal hip-pocampus in contextual reinstatement of cocaine seeking in rats. *Neuropsychopharmacology*. 2005;30:296–309.

44. Fuchs RA, Evans KA, Parker MC, et al. Differential involvement of the core and shell subregions of the nucleus accumbens in conditioned cue-induced reinstatement of cocaine seeking in rats. *Psychopharmacology (Berl)*. 2004;176:459–465.

45. Fuchs RA, Evans KA, Parker MP, et al. Differential involvement of orbitofrontal cortex subregions in conditioned cue-induced and cocaine-primed reinstatement of cocaine seeking in rats. *J Neurosci*. 2004;24:6600–6610.

46. Gipson CD, Reissner KJ, Kupchik YM, et al. Reinstatement of nicotine seeking is mediated by glutamatergic plasticity. *Proc Natl Acad Sci U S A*. 2013;110:9124–9129.

47. Gipson CD, Kupchik YM, Shen H, et al. Relapse induced by cues predicting cocaine depends on rapid, transient synaptic potentiation. *Neuron*. 2013;77:867–872.

48. Goldberg SR, Spealman RD, Kelleher RT. Enhancement of drug-seeking behavior by environmental stimuli associated with cocaine or morphine injections. *Neuropharmacology*. 1979;18:1015–1017.

49. Goldstein RZ, Volkow ND. Dysfunction of the prefrontal cortex in addiction: neuroimaging findings and clinical implications. *Nat Rev Neurosci*. 2011;12:652–669.

50. Grimm JW, Kruzich PJ, See RE. Contingent access to stimuli associated with cocaine self-administration is required for reinstatement of drug-seeking behavior. *Psychobiology*. 2000;28:383–386.

51. Heather N, Stallard A, Tebbutt J. Importance of substance cues in relapse among heroin users: comparison of two methods of investigation. *Addict Behav*. 1991;16:41–49.

52. Hemby SE, Co C, Koves TR, et al. Differences in extracellular dopamine concentrations in the nucleus accumbens during response-dependent and response-independent cocaine administration in the rat. *Psychopharmacology (Berl)*. 1997;133:7–16.

53. Hull C. *Principles of Behavior*. New York: Appleton-Century-Crofts; 1943.

54. Hyytia P, Sinclair JD. Stimulus-controlled responding for ethanol in AA and Wistar rats. *Alcohol*. 1991;8:229–234.

55. Ito R, Robbins TW, Everitt BJ. Differential control over cocaine-seeking behavior by nucleus accumbens core and shell. *Nat Neurosci*. 2004;7:389–397.

56. Jacobs EH, Smit AB, De Vries TJ, et al. Neuroadaptive effects of active versus passive drug administration in addiction research. *Trends Pharmacol Sci*. 2003;24:566–573.

57. Jasinska AJ, Stein EA, Kaiser J, et al. Factors modulating neural reactivity to drug cues in addiction: a survey of human neuroimaging studies. *Neurosci Biobehav Rev*. 2014;38:1–16.

58. Khaled MA, Pushparaj A, Di Ciano P, et al. Dopamine D$_3$ receptors in the basolateral amygdala and the lateral habenula modulate cue-induced reinstatement of nicotine seeking. *Neuropsychopharmacology*. 2014;39:3049–3058.

59. Kufahl PR, Zavala AR, Singh A, et al. c-Fos expression associated with reinstatement of cocaine-seeking behavior by response-contingent conditioned cues. *Synapse*. 2009;63:823–835.

60. Lamb RJ, Schindler CW, Pinkston JW. Conditioned stimuli's role in relapse: preclinical research on Pavlovian-Instrumental-Transfer. *Psychopharmacology*, in press. 2016.

61. Larowe SD, Kalivas PW, Nicholas JS, et al. A double-blind placebo-controlled trial of N-acetylcysteine in the treatment of cocaine dependence. *Am J Addict*. 2013;22:443–452.

62. Le Foll B, Goldberg SR. Control of the reinforcing effects of nicotine by associated environmental stimuli in animals and humans. *Trends Pharmacol Sci*. 2005;26:287–293.

63. LeBlanc KH, Ostlund SB, Maidment NT. Pavlovian-to-instrumental transfer in cocaine seeking rats. *Behav Neurosci*. 2012;126:681–689.

64. Liu Y, Le Foll B, Liu Y, et al. Conditioned place preference induced by licit drugs: establishment, extinction, and reinstatement. *Sci World J*. 2008;8:1228–1245.

65. Marchant NJ, Li X, Shaham Y. Recent developments in animal models of drug relapse. *Curr Opin Neurobiol*. 2013;23:675–683.

66. McClure EA, Gipson CD, Malcolm RJ, et al. Potential role of N-acetylcysteine in the management of substance use disorders. *CNS Drugs*. 2014;28:95–106.

67. McLaughlin J, See RE. Selective inactivation of the dorsomedial prefrontal cortex and the basolateral amygdala attenuates conditioned-cued reinstatement of extinguished cocaine-seeking behavior in rats. *Psychopharmacology (Berl)*. 2003;168:57–65.

68. Milton AL, Schramm MJ, Wawrzynski JR, et al. Antagonism at NMDA receptors, but not beta-adrenergic receptors, disrupts the reconsolidation of pavlovian conditioned approach and instrumental transfer for ethanol-associated conditioned stimuli. *Psychopharmacology*. 2012;219:751–761.

69. Napier TC, Herrold AA, de Wit H. Using conditioned place preference to identify relapse prevention medications. *Neurosci Biobehav Rev*. 2013;37:2081–2086.

70. O'Brien C, Childress AR, Ehrman R, et al. Conditioning mechanisms in drug dependence. *Clin Neuropharmacol*. 1992;15(suppl 1 Pt A):66A–67A.

71. O'Brien CP, Childress AR, McLellan AT, et al. Classical conditioning in drug-dependent humans. *Ann N Y Acad Sci*. 1992;654:400–415.

72. Ostlund SB, LeBlanc KH, Kosheleff AR, et al. Phasic mesolimbic dopamine signaling encodes the facilitation of incentive motivation produced by repeated cocaine exposure. *Neuropsychopharmacology*. 2014;39:2441–2449.

73. Panlilio LV, Weiss SJ, Schindler CW. Cocaine self-administration increased by compounding discriminative stimuli. *Psychopharmacology (Berl)*. 1996;125:202–208.

74. Panlilio LV, Weiss SJ, Schindler CW. Effects of compounding drug-related stimuli: escalation of heroin self-administration. *J Exp Anal Behav*. 2000;73:211–224.

75. Panlilio LV, Yasar S, Nemeth-Coslett R, et al. Human cocaine-seeking behavior and its control by drug-associated stimuli in the laboratory. *Neuropsychopharmacology*. 2005;30:433–443.

76. Pascoli V, Terrier J, Espallergues J, et al. Contrasting forms of cocaine-evoked plasticity control components of relapse. *Nature*. 2014;509:459–464.

77. Pavlov IP. *Conditioned Reflexes: an Investigation of the Physiological Activity of the Cerebral Cortex*. London: Oxford University Press; 1927.

78. Pears A, Parkinson JA, Hopewell L, et al. Lesions of the orbitofrontal but not medial prefrontal cortex disrupt conditioned reinforcement in primates. *J Neurosci*. 2003;23:11189–11201.

79. Pockros-Burgess LA, Pentkowski NS, Der-Ghazarian T, et al. Effects of the 5-HT$_{2C}$ receptor agonist CP809101 in the amygdala on reinstatement of cocaine-seeking behavior and anxiety-like behavior. *Int J Neuropsychopharmacol*. 2014;17:1751–1762.

80. Ranaldi R, Roberts DC. Initiation, maintenance and extinction of cocaine self-administration with and without conditioned reward. *Psychopharmacology (Berl)*. 1996;128:89–96.

81. Rescorla RA. Pavlovian conditioning and its proper control procedures. *Psychol Rev*. 1967;74:71–80.

82. Rescorla RA, Heth CD. Reinstatement of fear to an extinguished conditioned stimulus. *J Exp Psychol Animal Behav Process*. 1975;1:88–96.

83. Risinger FO, Cunningham CL, Bevins RA, et al. Place conditioning: what does it add to our understanding of ethanol reward? *Alcohol Clin Exp Res*. 2002;26:1444–1452.

84. Robinson TE, Yager LM, Cogan ES, et al. On the motivational properties of reward cues: individual differences. *Neuropharmacology*. 2014;76(Pt B):450–459.

85. Rogers JL, Ghee S, See RE. The neural circuitry underlying reinstatement of heroin-seeking behavior in an animal model of relapse. *Neuroscience*. 151:579–588.

86. Rogers JL, See RE. Selective inactivation of the ventral hippocampus attenuates cue-induced and cocaine-primed reinstatement of drug-seeking in rats. *Neurobiol Learn Mem*. 2007;87:688–692.

87. Sanchis-Segura C, Spanagel R. Behavioural assessment of drug reinforcement and addictive features in rodents: an overview. *Addict Biol.* 2006;11:2–38.

88. Saunders BT, Robinson TE. A cocaine cue acts as an incentive stimulus in some but not others: implications for addiction. *Biol Psychiatry.* 2010;67:730–736.

89. Saunders BT, Robinson TE. The role of dopamine in the accumbens core in the expression of Pavlovian-conditioned responses. *Eur J Neurosci.* 2012;36:2521–2532.

90. Schindler CW, Panlilio LV, Goldberg SR. Second-order schedules of drug self-administration in animals. *Psychopharmacology (Berl).* 2002;163:327–344.

91. Schuster CR, Woods JH. The conditioned reinforcing effects of stimuli associated with morphine reinforcement. *Int J Addict.* 1968;3:223–230.

92. Scofield MD, Boger HA, Smith RJ, et al. Gq-DREADD selectively initiates glial glutamate release and inhibits cue-induced cocaine seeking. *Biol Psychiatry.* 2015;78:441–451.

93. See RE. Neural substrates of cocaine-cue associations that trigger relapse. *Eur J Pharmacol.* 2005;526:140–146.

94. See RE, Grimm JW, Kruzich PJ, et al. The importance of a compound stimulus in conditioned drug-seeking behavior following one week of extinction from self-administered cocaine in rats. *Drug Alcohol Depend.* 1999;57:41–49.

95. See RE, Kruzich PJ, Grimm JW. Dopamine, but not glutamate, receptor blockade in the basolateral amygdala attenuates conditioned reward in a rat model of relapse to cocaine-seeking behavior. *Psychopharmacology (Berl).* 2001;154:301–310.

96. Siegel S, Hinson RE, Krank MD, et al. Heroin "overdose" death: contribution of drug-associated environmental cues. *Science.* 1982;216:436–437.

97. Stankeviciute NM, Scofield MD, Kalivas PW, et al. Rapid, transient potentiation of dendritic spines in context-induced relapse to cocaine seeking. *Addict Biol.* 2014;19:972–974.

98. Stefanik MT, Kalivas PW. Optogenetic dissection of basolateral amygdala projections during cue-induced reinstatement of cocaine seeking. *Front Behav Neurosci.* 2013;7:213.

99. Stefanik MT, Kupchik YM, Brown RM, et al. Optogenetic evidence that pallidal projections, not nigral projections, from the nucleus accumbens core are necessary for reinstating cocaine seeking. *J Neurosci.* 2013;33:13654–13662.

100. Stefanik MT, Kupchik YM, Kalivas PW. Optogenetic inhibition of cortical afferents in the nucleus accumbens simultaneously prevents cue-induced transient synaptic potentiation and cocaine-seeking behavior. *Brain Struct Funct*, in press. 2015.

101. Stefanski R, Ziolkowska B, Kusmider M, et al. Active versus passive cocaine administration: differences in the neuroadaptive changes in the brain dopaminergic system. *Brain Res.* 2007;1157:1–10.

102. Sun W, Akins CK, Mattingly AE, et al. Ionotropic glutamate receptors in the ventral tegmental area regulate cocaine-seeking behavior in rats. *Neuropsychopharmacology.* 2005;30:2073–2081.

103. Sun WL, Rebec GV. Lidocaine inactivation of ventral subiculum attenuates cocaine-seeking behavior in rats. *J Neurosci.* 2003;23:10258–10264.

104. Tzschentke TM. Measuring reward with the conditioned place preference (CPP) paradigm: update of the last decade. *Addict Biol.* 2007;12:227–462.

105. Van den Oever MC, Rotaru DC, Heinsbroek JA, et al. Ventromedial prefrontal cortex pyramidal cells have a temporal dynamic role in recall and extinction of cocaine-associated memory. *J Neurosci.* 2013;33:18225–18233.

106. Vanderschuren LJ, Ahmed SH. Animal studies of addictive behavior. *Cold Spring Harb Perspect Med.* 2013;3:a011932.

107. Vanderschuren LJ, Di Ciano P, Everitt BJ. Involvement of the dorsal striatum in cue-controlled cocaine seeking. *J Neurosci.* 2005;25:8665–8670.

108. Volkow ND, Morales M. The brain on drugs: from reward to addiction. *Cell.* 2015;162:712–725.

109. Volkow ND, Wang GJ, Fowler JS, et al. Addiction circuitry in the human brain. *Annu Rev Pharmacol Toxicol.* 2012;52:321–336.

110. Volkow ND, Wang GJ, Tomasi D, et al. Unbalanced neuronal circuits in addiction. *Curr Opin Neurobiol.* 2013;23:639–648.

111. Weiss F. Neurobiology of craving, conditioned reward and relapse. *Curr Opin Pharmacol.* 2005;5:9–19.

112. Weiss F, Ciccocioppo R, Parsons LH, et al. Compulsive drug-seeking behavior and relapse. Neuroadaptation, stress, and conditioning factors. *Ann N Y Acad Sci.* 2001;937:1–26.

113. Weiss F, Maldonado-Vlaar CS, Parsons LH, et al. Control of cocaine-seeking behavior by drug-associated stimuli in rats: effects on recovery of extinguished operant-responding and extracellular dopamine levels in amygdala and nucleus accumbens. *Proc Nat Acad Sci USA.* 2000;97:4321–4326.

114. Weiss F, Martin-Fardon R, Ciccocioppo R, et al. Enduring resistance to extinction of cocaine-seeking behavior induced by drug-related cues. *Neuropsychopharmacology.* 2001;25:361–372.

115. Weissenborn R, Robbins TW, Everitt BJ. Effects of medial prefrontal or anterior cingulate cortex lesions on responding for cocaine under fixed-ratio and second-order schedules of reinforcement in rats. *Psychopharmacology (Berl).* 1997;134:242–257.

116. Whitelaw RB, Markou A, Robbins TW, et al. Excitotoxic lesions of the basolateral amygdala impair the acquisition of cocaine-seeking behaviour under a second-order schedule of reinforcement. *Psychopharmacology (Berl).* 1996;127:213–224.

117. Yalachkov Y, Kaiser J, Naumer MJ. Functional neuroimaging studies in addiction: multisensory drug stimuli and neural cue reactivity. *Neurosci Biobehav Rev.* 2012;36:825–835.

118. Zhao Y, Dayas CV, Aujla H, et al. Activation of group II metabotropic glutamate receptors attenuates both stress and cue-induced ethanol-seeking and modulates c-fos expression in the hippocampus and amygdala. *J Neurosci.* 2006;26:9967–9974.

9

Overlapping Striatal Circuits and Molecular Mechanisms in Rodent Models of Addiction and Depression

MARY KAY LOBO

Overview of Striatal Circuits

The striatum is a major brain nuclei in the basal ganglia (BG) system. The BG consists of set of corticobasal ganglia-cortical loops, which are a series of parallel projection loops that convey limbic, associative, and sensorimotor information.[62] In this circuit, cortical neurons send input to striatum, which conveys output through various BG nuclei, relaying information to thalamus and then ultimately back to cortex.[30,31] The striatum consists of the dorsal striatum (dStr, caudate and putamen in humans), which regulates actions and habits, and the ventral striatum (a.k.a. nucleus accumbens [NAc]), which is involved in motivation and reinforcement.[21,73] These striatal areas have distinct projections through the BG output nuclei, consisting of two distinct pathways (often referred to as the direct and indirect pathways) and they were originally proposed to play antagonistic but balancing roles on BG output and behavior.[1,17,33] The two pathways can be resolved at a cellular level in the main projection neurons of the striatum. The projection neurons, which comprise 90%–95% of all neurons in the

striatum, are medium spiny neurons (MSNs), which are divided into two morphologically identical and heterogeneously distributed cell types.[30,31] The MSNs in striatum are subdivided into two subtypes based on their axonal targets. MSNs that are considered part of the direct pathway project to globus pallidus internal (GPi), ventral pallidum (VP), and midbrain regions including substantia nigra (SN) and ventral tegmental area (VTA); whereas the indirect pathway MSNs project to the globus pallidus external (GPe) and VP[31,68] (Fig. 9.1). However, it is important to note that MSN projections from dStr appear more segregated from those in NAc. The dStr MSN subtypes have distinct projections with minimal overlap to BG nuclei, whereas the NAc MSN subtypes both send input to VP. Thus this ventral BG circuit does not quite represent the classical direct and indirect pathways[14,49,68] (see Fig. 9.1). Due to this overlap in NAc MSN subtype projections, we refer to these two neuron subtypes based on their enrichment of dopamine receptors 1 versus 2, with D1-MSNs being part of the classical direct pathway and D2-MSNs part of the indirect pathway.[28] Although both D1-MSNs and D2-MSNs in NAc project to VP, the NAc D1-MSNs also send projections to classical direct pathway nuclei including GPi, SN, and VTA[25,49,68] (see Fig. 9.1).

Along with their enrichment of D1 versus D2 receptors, the two MSN subtypes are further distinguished by their differential expression of several other genes, most notably G-protein–coupled receptors and neuropeptides. D1-MSNs express muscarinic receptor 4, substance P, and dynorphin, whereas D2-MSNs express adenosine receptor 2a, G-protein–coupled receptor 6, and enkephalin[28,38,54] (Fig. 9.2). Through the two BG pathways the D1-MSNs versus D2-MSNs have been demonstrated to display differential behavioral output. Activity in the D1-MSNs is implicated in movement initiation, reinforcement, and reward seeking, whereas activity in the D2-MSNs antagonizes the D1-MSN pathway, thus inhibiting movement, promoting punishment or avoidance, and inhibiting reward seeking.[a] However, there are some studies that support a role for coordinated activity in these two neurons in actions and natural reward behaviors.[15,69] Studies on animal models of addiction and depression have demonstrated distinct roles of these MSN subtypes in striatal circuits in these motivational diseases. This chapter discusses these current findings and the overlap between these striatal circuits in addiction and depression.

---

[a]References 23, 25, 39, 46, 48, 52, 55.

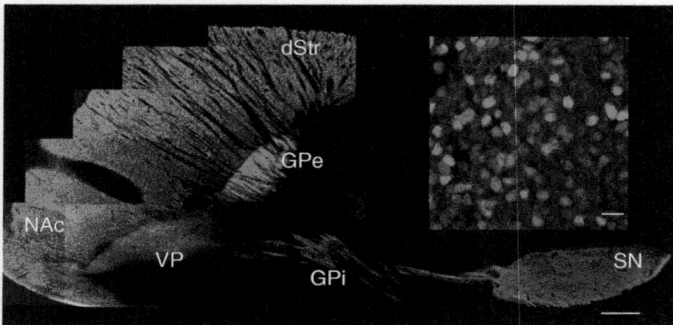

• **Fig. 9.1** D1-tdTomato/D2-GFP mouse demonstrates D1-MSNs *(red)* versus D2-MSNs *(green)* in dorsal striatum *(dStr)* or ventral striatum (nucleus accumbens *[NAc]*). These MSNs have distinct projections to BG output nuclei: globus pallidus external *(GPe)*, globus pallidus internal GPi), ventral pallidum *(VP)*, and substantia nigra *(SN)*. Scale bar 200 μm. Right inlay image shows little overlap in D1-MSNs *(red)* versus D2-MSNs *(green)*. Scale bar 20 μm.

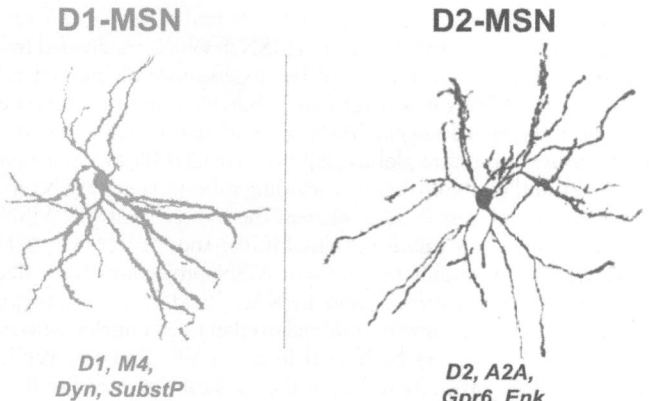

• **Fig. 9.2** Images of a D1-MSN *(green)* and D2-MSN *(purple)* and their respective enriched genes. D1-MSNs are enriched in dopamine 1 receptor *(D1)*, acetylcholine muscarinic receptor 4 *(M4)*, dynorphin *(Dyn)*, and substance P *(SubstP)*. D2-MSNs are enriched in dopamine 2 receptor *(D2)*, adenosine 2A receptor *(A2A)*, G-protein–coupled receptor 6 *(Gpr6)*, and enkephalin *(Enk)*.

Striatal Circuit Activity in Animal Models of Addiction and Depression

Striatal MSN Subtype Activity in Addictive Drug Exposure and Behavior

Much of the evidence for the differential roles of D1-MSNs and D2-MSNs in addiction is based on studies examining cocaine-induced behaviors in rodents, using neuron-subtype–specific techniques to activate or inhibit these MSN subtypes.[55,68] Enhanced activity in D1-MSNs underlies the reinforcing and sensitizing effects of cocaine. Likewise, blocking activity in D2-MSNs results in similar outcomes.[b] The first insight into MSN-subtype participation in psychostimulant-mediated behavior involved NAc D2-MSN ablation. Ablating these MSNs increased psychostimulant-induced conditioned place preference without altering normal locomotion.[20]

---

[b] References 8, 11, 23, 39, 52, 70.

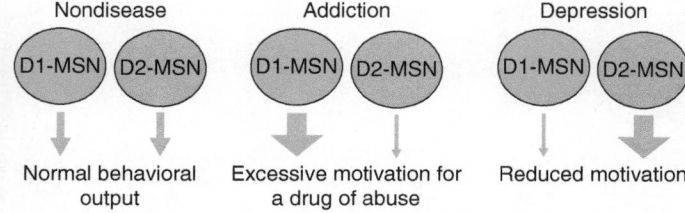

• **Fig. 9.3** Predicted model of MSN-subtype activity within the basal ganglia in addiction and depression. In a nondiseased brain the two MSN subtypes display balanced activity to produce normal behavioral output. In addiction, the D1-MSN pathway is overactive, while the D2-MSN pathway is suppressed, leading to excessive motivation for a drug of abuse. In depression the D1-MSN pathway is reduced, while the D2-MSN pathway is enhanced, leading to reduced motivation. *MSN*, Medium spiny neuron.

Subsequent studies demonstrated an opposite role for D1-MSNs versus D2-MSNs in psychostimulant-mediated behavior. Optogenetic stimulation, using the blue light–activated channelrhodopsin-2 (ChR2)[22] of NAc D1-MSNs enhances the rewarding properties of cocaine, and NAc D2-MSN optogenetic stimulation reduces this outcome.[52] In addition, after repeated exposure to cocaine the optogenetic activation of NAc D1-MSNs resulted in enhanced locomotor activity. This implicates that cocaine primes these MSN subtypes to display a sensitized response to other stimuli, in this case artificial activation. The selective blockade of neurotransmission in D1-MSNs reduces cocaine-induced locomotor sensitization and conditioned place preference.[39] Conversely, using optogenetics or chemogenetics, the latter using designer receptor activated by designer drugs (DREADDs), inhibition of D1-MSNs or activation of D2-MSNs reduces psychostimulant-induced locomotor sensitization, while the inhibition of D2-MSNs increases this behavior.[11,23] Furthermore, chemogenetic inhibition of D2-MSNs, in cocaine self-administration, enhanced the motivation to obtain cocaine, whereas optogenetic activation of D2-MSNs suppressed cocaine self-administration.[8] Finally, a recent study using in vivo fiber photometry with the calcium indicator, gCamp6f, confirmed the MSN subtype activity manipulation studies described above.[9] This study showed that acute cocaine exposure enhanced D1-MSN and suppressed D2-MSN activity, and that cocaine-induced D1-MSN activity is required for formation of cocaine–context associations. In addition, MSN subtype–specific signaling encodes contextual information about the cocaine environment such that increased D1-MSN activity precedes entry into a cocaine-paired environment, while decreased D2-MSN activity occurred after entering the cocaine-paired environment. Finally, inhibiting this D1-MSN calcium signal by DREADD inhibition blocked the cocaine-conditioned preference. Altogether, these findings show that a circuit imbalance of these D1-MSN versus D2-MSN pathways occurs upon cocaine exposure, leading to an enhanced D1-MSN pathway, thus promoting cocaine-seeking, intake, and sensitization behaviors (Fig. 9.3).

Electrophysiology studies examining psychostimulant-induced plasticity in the MSN subtypes corroborate with the activity studies described earlier. Excitatory synaptic potentiation occurs at D1-MSNs after repeated cocaine exposure or cocaine self-administration.[8] Of interest, mice that display poor cocaine intake display enhanced excitatory synaptic input at D2-MSNs. Consistent with this, increased dendritic spine remodeling occurs in D1-MSNs after repeated injections (i.p) of cocaine.[34,44,50] Evidence demonstrates that the increased spines in D1-MSNs are thin or immature spines, characterized as silent synapses, since they consist of

N-methyl-D-aspartate (NMDAR) receptors but lack α-amino-3-hydroxy-5-methyl-4-isoxazolepropionic acid receptor (AMPAR) receptors.[34] The silent synapses, which are typical throughout the immature brain, can either retract or develop into fully functional synapses to induce new neural circuits, after periods of cocaine withdrawal.[19] It is likely that these new neural circuits mediate enduring behaviors in response to cocaine, such as relapse behavior. Future studies examining MSN subtypes in relapse behavior will be important for understanding their role in the long-term effects of cocaine and the transition from early drug taking to the addictive state. Finally, examination into MSN subtype output in the VP, the one region receiving dense innervation from both MSN subtypes, demonstrates potentiated output of D1-MSNs but weakened output of D2-MSNs after repeated cocaine exposure.[14] This study further showed that optogenetic depotentiation of D1-MSN output to the VP abolished cocaine locomotor sensitization; however, restoring D2-MSN transmission to VP did not alter this behavior.

As described in the preceding text, much of the data examining the striatal MSN circuits in drug abuse are from studies performed with cocaine. However, a small number of studies examine striatal circuits in morphine-mediated behaviors. Similar to the cocaine studies, optogenetic activation of NAc D1-MSNs enhanced morphine-conditioned place preference, whereas optogenetic activation of NAc D2-MSNs blunted this behavior.[45] Of interest, examination of plasticity in these MSNs reveals a different outcome compared to cocaine, since silent synapses are induced in D2-MSNs after repeated morphine exposure.[34] Finally, examination of analgesic tolerance demonstrated that optogenetic activation of D1-MSNs facilitates the development of morphine tolerance, whereas activation of D2-MSNs did not affect the development of tolerance.[27] Additional studies examining these MSN subtypes in opiate-mediated behaviors are needed to uncover the mechanisms accounting for differences between cocaine and morphine.

Striatal MSN Subtype Activity in Depression-Like Behavior

There are sparse studies examining activity in MSN subtypes in animal models of depression. In contrast to the cocaine studies described earlier (which show enhanced excitatory synaptic input onto D1-MSNs and reduced input onto D2-MSNs), stress models, showing depression-like behavior, display reduced excitatory input onto D1-MSNs and/or enhanced input onto D2-MSNs.[25,51] The D2-MSN data are in line with those of previous studies demonstrating enhanced excitatory input onto MSNs, which correlates with increased mushroom-shaped spines in MSNs, using an animal model of stress-induced depression, chronic social defeat stress.[12] Use of optogenetics or DREADDs in mice that underwent chronic social defeat stress uncovered a bidirectional role for MSNs in depression-like behavior.[25] Repeated high-frequency optogenetic activation of D1-MSNs, in mice that display depression-like behavior to chronic social defeat stress, resulted in an antidepressant phenotype. In contrast, repeated DREADD inhibition of D1-MSNs in mice displaying resilient behavior (lack of depression-like behavior) after chronic social defeat stress shifted these mice to a susceptible, depression-like state. Altering activity in D2-MSNs after stress did not alter behavioral outcomes to chronic social defeat stress. However, priming D2-MSNs with repeated activity prior to stress induced a depression-like outcome to a subthreshold social defeat stress. These data are in line with the BG model of activity in D1-MSNs promoting reward, while activity in D2-MSNs promotes avoidance or punishment.[26,47,55]

Molecular Mechanisms in Striatal Circuits in Addiction

MSN Subtype Signaling Mechanisms in Addictive Drug Exposure and Behavior

D1-MSNs and D2-MSNs display different molecular adaptations in response to cocaine. This potentially occurs via differential signaling through dopamine receptors. Enhanced dopamine levels, occurring with exposure to drugs of abuse, can positively modulate excitatory glutamatergic input in D1-MSNs through activation of D1-receptor signaling via G_s or G_{olf}, which stimulate adenylyl cyclase, leading to increased protein kinase A (PKA) activity. In contrast, dopamine negatively modulates D2-MSNs through D2-receptor signaling via G_i and G_o, which inhibit adenylyl cyclase causing decreased PKA activity.[29,71] This can lead to differential phosphorylation of the dopamine- and cAMP-regulated neuronal phosphoprotein (DARPP-32) in MSN subtypes after cocaine exposure.[5] As a result, the deletion of DARPP-32 from D1-MSNs decreases cocaine-induced locomotion, while its deletion from D2-MSNs increases locomotion.[6] In addition, brain-derived neurotrophic factor (BDNF) signaling has been shown to exert opposing roles on MSN subtypes. Deletion of the BDNF receptor, tropomyosin receptor kinase B (TrkB), from D1-MSNs increases cocaine-conditioned place preference and locomotor sensitization, while TrkB deletion from D2-MSNs reduces these behaviors.[52] Of interest, the D2-MSN results are consistent with those of previous studies that used non-cell-type specific deletion of TrkB from NAc,[32] demonstrating that the main effects of cocaine on BDNF might be occurring through D2-MSNs. However, assessment of morphine-conditioned place preference in these TrkB MSN subtype lines showed enhanced morphine place preference with deletion in D1-MSNs but no altered behavior with deletion in D2-MSNs. Investigation of dopamine- and BDNF-signaling targets, with repeated cocaine exposure, demonstrated activate extracellular signal-regulated kinase (pERK) associated with a downregulation of its direct nuclear target mitogen- and stress-activated kinase-1 (pMSK1) in D1-MSNs exclusively.[7] Finally, the cell-type-specific silencing of p11 (S100A10), a protein linked with the transport of neurotransmitters and receptors to the plasma membrane, on D1-MSNs increases cocaine-conditioned place preference.[2]

Transcription Factors in MSN Subtypes in Addictive Drug Exposure and Behavior

Overall, molecular adaptations occur in both MSN subtypes in response to drugs of abuse, such as cocaine.[38] However, many experiments highlight major molecular alterations in the D1-MSN pathway, confirming its predominant role in cocaine-mediated behaviors.[55] This predominant role of D1-MSNs has been well documented with immediate early gene transcription factors. Early studies examining immediate early genes provided the first insight into how the MSN subtypes respond to psychostimulants. Previous studies, in rats, demonstrate c-Fos induction in both MSN subtypes when a psychostimulant is given in a novel environment.[24,3] Using D1-GFP and D2-GFP reporter mice, researchers demonstrate that c-Fos induction by cocaine in a novel environment occurs primarily in D1-GFP MSNs throughout striatum with a small induction in D2-GFP MSNs in dorsal striatum.[7] Isolation and molecular profiling of active striatal neurons in context-dependent cocaine locomotor sensitization, using a c-Fos reporter rat line, demonstrated that these neuronal ensembles express both D1-MSN and D2-MSN markers.[36] However, they express higher levels of a D1-MSN enriched gene, dynorphin, and lower levels of D2-MSN enriched genes, D2 and adenosine 2A receptor, suggesting a greater number of D1-MSNs in this population. c-Fos deletion in D1-MSNs, blunted cocaine-induced locomotor sensitization and MSN dendritic spine formation.[77] Of interest, c-Fos deletion in D1 neurons did not alter cocaine-conditioned place preference but it did prevent the extinction of this contextual association. These data illustrate a dynamic role for c-Fos induction in D1-MSNs; however, one cannot rule out the differential behavioral effects as being mediated by other brain regions that express the D1 receptor.

The immediate early gene (IEG), FosB, has been well studied in MSN subtypes in addiction. FBJ murine osteosarcoma viral oncogene homolog B (FosB) is induced in striatum by acute cocaine,[40] but the long-lasting ΔFosB, generated from the FosB primary transcript,[75] persistently accumulates after chronic psychostimulant exposure.[41] This long-lasting induction of ΔFosB by cocaine is dependent on D1-receptor signaling,[59] and use of a D1-GFP reporter lines confirmed that ΔFosB induction occurs primarily in D1-MSNs after chronic cocaine.[50,53] Consistent with these findings, FosB messenger RNA (mRNA) was induced in D1-MSNs with acute and chronic injection (i.p.) of cocaine using a ribosomal tagging approach.[10,38]

Initial studies using a transgenic line with preferential overexpression of ΔFosB D1-MSNs resulted in enhanced locomotor and conditioned place preference responses to cocaine.[43] In addition, this D1-MSN ΔFosB line shows facilitated acquisition to cocaine self-administration at low-threshold doses and enhanced effort to maintain self-administration of higher doses on a progressive ratio schedule of reinforcement.[13] These behaviors are occurring potentially through enhanced structural plasticity in D1-MSNs, since adenoassociated virus (AAV)–mediated ΔFosB overexpression in NAc enhances MSN structural plasticity.[56] Use of Cre-inducible herpes simplex virus (HSV) to overexpress ΔFosB in D1-MSNs in the NAc of D1-Cre mice confirmed the enhanced cocaine-mediated behavioral responses and showed that ΔFosB alone can enhance immature spine formation and reduce AMPAR/NMDAR ratios in D1-MSNs.[35] These structural and synaptic plasticity changes by ΔFosB are an indication of enhanced silent synapses, which are characteristic of cocaine effects on D1-MSNs.[34.] Thus, ΔFosB may set the stage for long-term cocaine abuse by regulating the establishment of silent synapses in D1-MSNs during the initial stage of drug exposure. Finally, investigation of ΔFosB overexpression in D2-MSNs had no effect on cocaine-induced behaviors or spine formation but did enhance AMPAR/NMDAR ratios,[34] suggesting that ΔFosB in these MSNs might play a role in mature spine formation. A mechanistic role of ΔFosB in promoting behavioral and structural plasticity after cocaine has been examined. The D1-MSN ΔFosB line displayed enhanced expression of GluR2 in NAc, and GluR2 overexpression in NAc enhances cocaine conditioned place preference.[43] In addition, ΔFosB increased *CAMKIIα* gene expression in NAc of the D1-MSN ΔFosB line and the enhanced cocaine-mediated behavioral and structural plasticity effects of ΔFosB in NAc are *CAMKIIα* dependent.[64] ΔFosB also transcriptionally regulates a number of genes in NAc by chronic cocaine.[58,63] Future studies using neuronal subtype chromatin immunoprecipitation to examine FosB enrichment on target genes can provide improved understanding into the MSN subtype transcriptional role of ΔFosB in cocaine action.

ΔFosB induction has been examined in other drugs of abuse including THC, ethanol, and opioids.[53] Similar to the cocaine studies, repeated THC and ethanol leads to increased ΔFosB in D1-MSNs. Of interest, chronic morphine and heroin self-administration resulted in increased ΔFosB in both MSN subtypes. This could reflect induction in D1-MSNs in response to the rewarding effects of morphine and induction in D2-MSNs during the aversive, withdrawal phase of opioids. However, the D1-MSN-specific ΔFosB line displayed enhanced place preference for morphine, reduced morphine analgesia, and accelerated morphine tolerance, whereas a D2-MSN-specific ΔFosB line did not show any altered behavioral responses to morphine.[76]

Another transcription factor examined is the early growth response (Egr) family member, Egr3. A modest decrease in Egr3 in total NAc tissue was observed after repeated cocaine exposure and cocaine self-administration. However, use of the RiboTag methodology[66] to isolate ribosome-associated mRNA from each MSN subtype, demonstrated an enrichment of Egr3 mRNA in D1-MSNs, with a decrease occurring in D2-MSNs. Overexpressing Egr3 in D1-MSNs and knocking down Egr3 in D2-MSNs enhanced cocaine-conditioned place preference and locomotor sensitization, while reducing Egr3 in D1-MSNs and enhancing it in D2-MSNs blunted these behaviors, confirming the opposing role of Egr3 in both MSN subtypes.[10] These results further support the predominant role for D1-MSNs in cocaine-mediated behaviors; however, the cell-type-specific study demonstrated that the molecular changes in D2-MSNs also account for critical aspects of the responses to cocaine. Taken together, the above studies show that changes in transcription factor regulation are pivotal in cocaine-related behaviors.

MSN Subtype Epigenetic and Posttranscriptional Modifications in Addictive Drug Exposure and Behavior

In recent years, a growing number of studies have evaluated epigenetic changes induced by cocaine. Repeated cocaine exposure can induce stable changes in gene expression that may underlie addiction. However, only a few studies examined cell-type-specific epigenetic changes after cocaine exposure. For instance, in D1-GFP versus D2-GFP mice, an increase in phosphorylation of histone 3 on Ser-10 was found after acute and chronic cocaine injections (i.p).[7] Using ribosome-associated mRNA profiling, a recent study found cocaine-induced decrease of G9a (a repressive histone methyltransferase) in both D1- and D2-MSNs. However, developmental knockout of G9a from D1-MSNs decreased cocaine-conditioned place preference and locomotor sensitization, while knockout from D2-MSNs had the opposite effect. Surprisingly, the G9a knockout from D2-MSNs induced a partial-phenotypic switch, making D2-MSNs more similar to D1-MSNs, providing insight on the epigenetic mechanisms, as well as potential developmental mechanisms contributing to cocaine abuse.[57] Recently the histone arginine methylation enzyme, protein-R-methyltransferase-6 (Prmt6), was examined in MSN subtypes after repeated cocaine exposure.[16] Ribosome-associated mRNA profiling revealed a downregulation of Prmt6 in D2-MSNs after repeated cocaine, which was consistent with reduced Prmt6 levels in total NAc in this condition. In contrast, Prmt6 was upregulated in D1-MSNs. The decreased Prmt6 levels led to a reduction of the repressive mark H3R2me2a on the Src kinase signaling inhibitor 1 (*Srcin1*) gene, which resulted in increased Scrin1 protein in NAc after repeated cocaine. Overexpression of Prmt6 in D2-MSNs or total NAc enhanced cocaine-conditioned place preference, while overexpression in D1-MSNs reduced this behavior. Consistent with reduced Prmt6 resulting in increased Srcin1, the overexpression of Srcin1 in D2-MSNs or total NAc reduced cocaine-conditioned place preference, with opposite effects observed with D1-MSN overexpression. These results suggest that the effects of reduced Prmt6 in D2-MSNs counteracts the rewarding effects of cocaine through enhancement of Srcin1 in these neurons. Srcin1 is an endogenous inhibitor that constrains the activity of the Src family of protein tyrosine kinases.[60] Further examination in this pathway in D2-MSNs could uncover improved information into the role of D2-MSNs in cocaine action. Other work has shown cell-type-specific and time-dependent epigenetic modifications after cocaine. For instance, H3K5 acetylation was steadily increased in D1-MSNs while only transiently in D2-MSNs, whereas H3K14 increased after acute cocaine in D1-MSNs and after chronic cocaine in D2-MSNs.[42] This type of study further points out the importance of examining cell-type-specific patterns of histone modifications, since epigenetic changes may differ with drug-exposure time and have distinct effects on gene transcription.

In addition to transcriptional and epigenetic studies in cocaine abuse, researchers are beginning to examine posttranscriptional adaptations. Reduction in Argonaute 2 (Ago 2), which plays a role in micoRNA (miRNA) generation and miRNA gene silencing, in D2-MSNs reduces the motivation to self-administer cocaine. Furthermore, this study demonstrated a number of miRNAs enriched in D2-MSNs after cocaine exposure that are also downregulated in Ago 2–deficient striatum.[67] Collectively, identifying transcriptional and posttranscriptional changes, such as chromatin modifications and miRNA functions, in striatal circuits in cocaine addiction will be important for better understanding of the complex molecular networks underlying addiction.

Molecular Mechanisms in Striatal Circuits in Stress and Depression-Like Behavior

Although there is a large body of work examining molecular mechanisms in MSN subtypes in addiction, there is a sparse number of studies examining these underlying mechanisms in depression. Much like drug abuse, significant research on the immediate early gene ΔFosB has demonstrated its role in resilience to stress. NAc ΔFosB expression is significantly reduced in human depressed patients.[72] In addition, NAc ΔFosB expression is significantly enhanced in NAc, specifically of mice that are resilient to chronic social defeat stress. This induction is specific to D1-MSNs, while D2-MSNs have enhanced ΔFosB in mice displaying depression-like behavior (susceptible) to chronic social defeat stress.[53] Furthermore, chronic social defeat stress mice treated with the common selective serotonin reuptake inhibitor (SSRI) fluoxetine display enhanced ΔFosB expression and enhanced resilience, and SSRI treatment in stress-naïve animals results in increased ΔFosB in D1-MSNs.[53,65] The D1-MSN-specific ΔFosB line[43] promotes resilience to social defeat stress, which is likely occurring through enhancement of glutamate ionotropic receptor AMPA-type subunit 2 (Gria2) expression.[72] Furthermore, a recent study using epigenetic editing of the *FosB* gene in MSN subtypes demonstrates that histone acetylation targeted to the *FosB* gene to increase its transcription, in D2-MSNs or histone methylation targeted to the *FosB* gene to reduce its transcription in D1-MSNs promotes susceptibility to social defeat stress.[37] The converse manipulation to reduce FosB transcription in D2-MSNs or enhance it in D1-MSNs promotes stress resiliency.

The WNT-DVL-β-catenin signaling cascade has been examined in MSN subtypes in stress. Disheveled (DVL1) activity

inhibition in the WNT-DVL-β-catenin signaling cascade promotes susceptibility to social defeat stress and DVL1 is found to be significantly downregulated in the NAc of human depressed patients. Pharmacological and dominant negative activity inhibition of the downstream inhibition target of DVL1, GSK3β, promotes resilience to chronic social defeat stress.[74] β-Catenin is activated by the nonphosphorylated form of GSK3β. β-Catenin expression in NAc D2-MSNs, but not in D1-MSNs, promotes resilience to chronic social defeat stress.[18] This effect was shown to be specific to expression of an miRNA synthesis-related protein, double-stranded RNA-specific endoribonuclease (Dicer1), which is downstream of β-catenin signaling. These data suggest that posttranscriptional regulation of a wide variety of mRNAs by β-catenin, in D2-MSNs, can mediate outcomes to social stress.

Although the preceding data pinpoint mechanisms occurring in both MSN subtypes in depression and antidepressant or resilient outcomes, there is a larger body of work focused on D1-MSNs in stress-induced depression. NAc D1-MSN-specific knockout of Cdk5 increases cAMP/PKA activity and promotes antidepressant outcomes.[60] This is in line with data demonstrating that enhanced G_i signaling, which reduces cAMP/PKA activity, in D1-MSNs causes depression-like outcomes in response to stress.[25] Finally, stress promotes central and peripheral adaptations in body systems susceptible to the hypothalamic-pituitary-adrenal (HPA) axis, which feeds back on the brain via release of corticosteroids.[61] The HPA axis may have effects in NAc through D1-MSNs, since deletion of the primary target of corticosterone, the glucocorticoid receptor, in NAc D1-MSNs promotes resilience to social defeat stress.[4] Overall this small body of work illustrates the importance of MSN subtypes, which make up these striatal circuits, in depression. However, further work is needed to understand the complex molecular processes occurring in these MSN subtypes and how they lead to cellular and circuit adaptations in these neurons, which ultimately underlie depressive-like behavior.

Conclusions

In the past decade a large body of work has provided insight into the role of striatal circuits in drug abuse, and a sparse number of studies give insight into these circuits in depression. Overall, the data support the D1-MSN pathway of promoting reward and reinforcement, since activity in this pathway promotes drug seeking, drug sensitization, and antidepressant or resilient behaviors to stress. In contrast, activity in the D2-MSN pathway results in reduced drug seeking, reduced drug sensitization, and increased depression-like behavior to stress, thus supporting the D2-MSN pathway in mediating aversive or avoidance behavior. In addition, molecules such as ΔFosB are induced in D1-MSNs, which mediates drug reward and stress-resilience behavior. Although ΔFosB in D2-MSNs does not alter drug reward, it does underlie depression-like behaviors associated with stress susceptibility. It will be important for the field to understand how transcription factors, epigenetic mechanisms, and signaling mechanisms ultimately underlie MSN-subtype cellular and circuit responses that lead to an imbalance in these BG circuits and ultimately alter reward or aversive behaviors. Although some of these studies support the opposing role of MSN subtypes within the BG in mediating behavioral output, it is challenging to reconcile these findings with comorbid addiction and depression disease. Future studies examining the striatal MSN subtypes in stress-induced addiction behavior can provide information on concurrent mechanisms occurring in these neurons in comorbid disease.

References

1. Albin RL, Young AB, Penney JB. The functional anatomy of basal ganglia disorders. *Trends Neurosci.* 1989;12(10):366–375.
2. Arango-Lievano M, et al. Cell-type specific expression of p11 controls cocaine reward. *Biol Psychiatry.* 2014;76(10):794–801.
3. Badiani A, et al. Amphetamine-induced behavior, dopamine release, and c-fos mRNA expression: modulation by environmental novelty. *J Neurosci.* 1998;18(24):10579–10593.
4. Barik J, et al. Chronic stress triggers social aversion via glucocorticoid receptor in dopaminoceptive neurons. *Science.* 2013;339(6117):332–335.
5. Bateup HS, et al. Cell type-specific regulation of DARPP-32 phosphorylation by psychostimulant and antipsychotic drugs. *Nat Neurosci.* 2008;11(8):932–939.
6. Bateup HS, et al. Distinct subclasses of medium spiny neurons differentially regulate striatal motor behaviors. *Proc Natl Acad Sci U S A.* 2010;107(33):14845–14850.
7. Bertran-Gonzalez J, et al. Opposing patterns of signaling activation in dopamine D1 and D2 receptor-expressing striatal neurons in response to cocaine and haloperidol. *J Neurosci.* 2008;28(22):5671–5685.
8. Bock R, et al. Strengthening the accumbal indirect pathway promotes resilience to compulsive cocaine use. *Nat Neurosci.* 2013;16(5):632–638.
9. Calipari ES, et al. In vivo imaging identifies temporal signature of D1 and D2 medium spiny neurons in cocaine reward. *Proc Natl Acad Sci U S A.* 2016;113(10):2726–2731.
10. Chandra R, et al. Opposing role for Egr3 in nucleus accumbens cell subtypes in cocaine action. *J Neurosci.* 2015;35(20):7927–7937.
11. Chandra R, et al. Optogenetic inhibition of D1R containing nucleus accumbens neurons alters cocaine-mediated regulation of Tiam1. *Front Mol Neurosci.* 2013;6:13.
12. Christoffel DJ, et al. IkappaB kinase regulates social defeat stress-induced synaptic and behavioral plasticity. *J Neurosci.* 2011;31(1):314–321.
13. Colby CR, et al. Striatal cell type-specific overexpression of DeltaFosB enhances incentive for cocaine. *J Neurosci.* 2003;23(6):2488–2493.
14. Creed M, et al. Convergence of reinforcing and anhedonic cocaine effects in the ventral pallidum. *Neuron.* 2016;92(1):214–226.
15. Cui G, et al. Concurrent activation of striatal direct and indirect pathways during action initiation. *Nature.* 2013;494(7436):238–242.
16. Damez-Werno DM, et al. Histone arginine methylation in cocaine action in the nucleus accumbens. *Proc Natl Acad Sci U S A.* 2016;113(34):9623–9628.
17. DeLong MR, Wichmann T. Circuits and circuit disorders of the basal ganglia. *Arch Neurol.* 2007;64(1):20–24.
18. Dias C, et al. beta-catenin mediates stress resilience through Dicer1/microRNA regulation. *Nature.* 2014;516(7529):51–55.
19. Dong Y, Nestler EJ. The neural rejuvenation hypothesis of cocaine addiction. *Trends Pharmacol Sci.* 2014;35(8):374–383.
20. Durieux PF, et al. D2R striatopallidal neurons inhibit both locomotor and drug reward processes. *Nat Neurosci.* 2009;12(4):393–395.
21. Everitt BJ, Robbins TW. From the ventral to the dorsal striatum: devolving views of their roles in drug addiction. *Neurosci Biobehav Rev.* 2013;37(9 Pt A):1946–1954.
22. Fenno L, Yizhar O, Deisseroth K. The development and application of optogenetics. *Annu Rev Neurosci.* 2011;34:389–412.
23. Ferguson SM, et al. Transient neuronal inhibition reveals opposing roles of indirect and direct pathways in sensitization. *Nat Neurosci.* 2011;14(1):22–24.
24. Ferguson SM, Robinson TE. Amphetamine-evoked gene expression in striatopallidal neurons: regulation by corticostriatal afferents and the ERK/MAPK signaling cascade. *J Neurochem.* 2004;91(2):337–348.
25. Francis TC, et al. Nucleus accumbens medium spiny neuron subtypes mediate depression-related outcomes to social defeat stress. *Biol Psychiatry.* 2015;77(3):212–222.
26. Francis TC, Lobo MK. Emerging role for nucleus accumbens medium spiny neuron subtypes in depression. *Biol Psychiatry.* 2017;81(8):645–653.
27. Gaspari S, et al. Nucleus accumbens-specific interventions in RGS9-2 activity modulate responses to morphine. *Neuropsychopharmacology.* 2014;39(8):1968–1977.
28. Gerfen CR, et al. D1 and D2 dopamine receptor-regulated gene expression of striatonigral and striatopallidal neurons. *Science.* 1990;250(4986):1429–1432.
29. Gerfen CR, Surmeier DJ. Modulation of striatal projection systems by dopamine. *Annu Rev Neurosci.* 2011;34:441–466.
30. Gerfen CR. The neostriatal mosaic: compartmentalization of corticostriatal input and striatonigral output systems. *Nature.* 1984;311(5985):461–464.
31. Gerfen CR. The neostriatal mosaic: multiple levels of compartmental organization. *Trends Neurosci.* 1992;15(4):133–139.
32. Graham DL, et al. Tropomyosin-related kinase B in the mesolimbic dopamine system: region-specific effects on cocaine reward. *Biol Psychiatry.* 2009;65(8):696–701.
33. Graybiel AM. The basal ganglia. *Curr Biol.* 2000;10(14):R509–511.
34. Graziane NM, et al. Opposing mechanisms mediate morphine- and cocaine-induced generation of silent synapses. *Nat Neurosci.* 2016;19(7):915–925.
35. Grueter BA, et al. FosB differentially modulates nucleus accumbens direct and indirect pathway function. *Proc Natl Acad Sci U S A.* 2013;110(5):1923–1928.
36. Guez-Barber D, et al. FACS identifies unique cocaine-induced gene regulation in selectively activated adult striatal neurons. *J Neurosci.* 2011;31(11):4251–4259.
37. Hamilton PJ, et al. Cell-type specific epigenetic editing at the Fosb gene controls susceptibility to social defeat stress. *Neuropsychopharmacology.* 2018;43(2):272–284.
38. Heiman M, et al. A translational profiling approach for the molecular characterization of CNS cell types. *Cell.* 2008;135(4):738–748.
39. Hikida T, et al. Distinct roles of synaptic transmission in direct and indirect striatal pathways to reward and aversive behavior. *Neuron.* 2010;66(6):896–907.
40. Hope B, et al. Regulation of immediate early gene expression and AP-1 binding in the rat nucleus accumbens by chronic cocaine. *Proc Natl Acad Sci U S A.* 1992;89(13):5764–5768.
41. Hope BT, et al. Induction of a long-lasting AP-1 complex composed of altered Fos-like proteins in brain by chronic cocaine and other chronic treatments. *Neuron.* 1994;13(5):1235–1244.
42. Jordi E, et al. Differential effects of cocaine on histone posttranslational modifications in identified populations of striatal neurons. *Proc Natl Acad Sci U S A.* 2013;110(23):9511–9516.
43. Kelz MB, et al. Expression of the transcription factor deltaFosB in the brain controls sensitivity to cocaine. *Nature.* 1999;401(6750):272–276.
44. Kim J, et al. Cell type-specific alterations in the nucleus accumbens by repeated exposures to cocaine. *Biol Psychiatry.* 2011;69(11):1026–1034.
45. Koo JW, et al. Loss of BDNF signaling in D1R-expressing NAc neurons enhances morphine reward by reducing GABA inhibition. *Neuropsychopharmacology.* 2014;39(11):2646–2653.
46. Kravitz AV, et al. Regulation of parkinsonian motor behaviours by optogenetic control of basal ganglia circuitry. *Nature.* 2010;466(7306):622–626.
47. Kravitz AV, Kreitzer AC. Striatal mechanisms underlying movement, reinforcement, and punishment. *Physiology (Bethesda).* 2012;27(3):167–177.
48. Kravitz AV, Tye LD, Kreitzer AC. Distinct roles for direct and indirect pathway striatal neurons in reinforcement. *Nat Neurosci.* 2012;15(6):816–818.

49. Kupchik YM, et al. Coding the direct/indirect pathways by D1 and D2 receptors is not valid for accumbens projections. *Nat Neurosci.* 2015;18(9):1230–1232.

50. Lee KW, et al. Cocaine-induced dendritic spine formation in D1 and D2 dopamine receptor-containing medium spiny neurons in nucleus accumbens. *Proc Natl Acad Sci U S A.* 2006;103(9):3399–3404.

51. Lim BK, et al. Anhedonia requires MC4R-mediated synaptic adaptations in nucleus accumbens. *Nature.* 2012;487(7406):183–189.

52. Lobo MK, et al. Cell type-specific loss of BDNF signaling mimics optogenetic control of cocaine reward. *Science.* 2010;330(6002):385–390.

53. Lobo MK, et al. DeltaFosB induction in striatal medium spiny neuron subtypes in response to chronic pharmacological, emotional, and optogenetic stimuli. *J Neurosci.* 2013;33(47):18381–18395.

54. Lobo MK, et al. FACS-array profiling of striatal projection neuron subtypes in juvenile and adult mouse brains. *Nat Neurosci.* 2006;9(3):443–452.

55. Lobo MK, Nestler EJ. The striatal balancing act in drug addiction: distinct roles of direct and indirect pathway medium spiny neurons. *Front Neuroanat.* 2011;5:41.

56. Maze I, et al. Essential role of the histone methyltransferase G9a in cocaine-induced plasticity. *Science.* 2010;327(5962):213–216.

57. Maze I, et al. G9a influences neuronal subtype specification in striatum. *Nat Neurosci.* 2014;17(4):533–539.

58. McClung CA, Nestler EJ. Regulation of gene expression and cocaine reward by CREB and DeltaFosB. *Nat Neurosci.* 2003;6(11):1208–1215.

59. Moratalla R, et al. D1-class dopamine receptors influence cocaine-induced persistent expression of Fos-related proteins in striatum. *Neuroreport.* 1996;8(1):1–5.

60. Okada M. Regulation of the SRC family kinases by Csk. *Int J Biol Sci.* 2012;8(10):1385–1397.

61. Pittenger C, Duman RS. Stress, depression, and neuroplasticity: a convergence of mechanisms. *Neuropsychopharmacology.* 2008;33(1):88–109.

62. Redgrave P, et al. Goal-directed and habitual control in the basal ganglia: implications for Parkinson's disease. *Nat Rev Neurosci.* 2010;11(11):760–772.

63. Renthal W, et al. Genome-wide analysis of chromatin regulation by cocaine reveals a role for sirtuins. *Neuron.* 2009;62(3):335–348.

64. Robison AJ, et al. Behavioral and structural responses to chronic cocaine require a feedforward loop involving DeltaFosB and calcium/calmodulin-dependent protein kinase II in the nucleus accumbens shell. *J Neurosci.* 2013;33(10):4295–4307.

65. Robison AJ, et al. Fluoxetine epigenetically alters the CaMKIIalpha promoter in nucleus accumbens to regulate DeltaFosB binding and antidepressant effects. *Neuropsychopharmacology.* 2014;39(5):1178–1186.

66. Sanz E, et al. Cell-type-specific isolation of ribosome-associated mRNA from complex tissues. *Proc Natl Acad Sci U S A.* 2009;106(33):13939–13944.

67. Schaefer A, et al. Argonaute 2 in dopamine 2 receptor-expressing neurons regulates cocaine addiction. *J Exp Med.* 2010;207(9):1843–1851.

68. Smith RJ, et al. Cocaine-induced adaptations in D1 and D2 accumbens projection neurons (a dichotomy not necessarily synonymous with direct and indirect pathways). *Curr Opin Neurobiol.* 2013;23(4):546–552.

69. Soares-Cunha C, et al. Activation of D2 dopamine receptor-expressing neurons in the nucleus accumbens increases motivation. *Nat Commun.* 2016;7:11829.

70. Song SS, et al. Optogenetics reveals a role for accumbal medium spiny neurons expressing dopamine D2 receptors in cocaine-induced behavioral sensitization. *Front Behav Neurosci.* 2014;8:336.

71. Surmeier DJ, et al. D1 and D2 dopamine-receptor modulation of striatal glutamatergic signaling in striatal medium spiny neurons. *Trends Neurosci.* 2007;30(5):228–235.

72. Vialou V, et al. DeltaFosB in brain reward circuits mediates resilience to stress and antidepressant responses. *Nat Neurosci.* 2010;13(6):745–752.

73. Voorn P, et al. Putting a spin on the dorsal-ventral divide of the striatum. *Trends Neurosci.* 2004;27(8):468–474.

74. Wilkinson MB, et al. A novel role of the WNT-dishevelled-GSK3beta signaling cascade in the mouse nucleus accumbens in a social defeat model of depression. *J Neurosci.* 2011;31(25):9084–9092.

75. Yen J, et al. An alternative spliced form of FosB is a negative regulator of transcriptional activation and transformation by Fos proteins. *Proc Natl Acad Sci U S A.* 1991;88(12):5077–5081.

76. Zachariou V, et al. An essential role for DeltaFosB in the nucleus accumbens in morphine action. *Nat Neurosci.* 2006;9(2):205–211.

77. Zhang J, et al. c-Fos facilitates the acquisition and extinction of cocaine-induced persistent changes. *J Neurosci.* 2006;26(51):13287–13296.

10

The Role of Endocannabinoids in Amphetamine-Driven Actions in Dopamine Neurons: Implications for Understanding and Treating Dysfunction in the Mesolimbic Circuit

HANNAH M. DANTRASSY, DAN P. COVEY, AND JOSEPH F. CHEER

CHAPTER OUTLINE

Introduction

Amphetamine (AMPH) and AMPH-type psychostimulants (e.g., methamphetamine, MDMA) are the second most widely abused illicit drug worldwide.[41] Prescription psychostimulants like d-AMPH (Adderall) and methylphenidate (Ritalin) remain widely prescribed for disorders such as attention-deficit/hyperactivity disorder (ADHD) and narcolepsy.[19,40] Because an increase in brain dopamine (DA) levels is the primary action mediating AMPH's psychostimulant and abuse-related properties, the mechanisms by which AMPH alters brain DA neurotransmission have been studied extensively.[39] Nevertheless, there remains no accepted or effective pharmacotherapy for AMPH abuse or addiction.[23] Recent work demonstrating novel mechanisms by which AMPH alters DA neuron function suggests that the endocannabinoid (eCB) system represents an important target for controlling AMPH effects on DA neurons and a potential target for treating AMPH abuse and addiction.

Mesolimbic Dopamine

Addiction—or the state of engaging in compulsive behaviors despite adverse consequences—is believed to occur as a result of long-lasting changes in neural circuitry associated with rewards that influence cognition, motivation, and learning.[1,13] Colloquially known as the "reward circuit," the mesolimbic pathway consists of DA neurons projecting from the ventral tegmental area (VTA) to the nucleus accumbens (NAc).[9,43] In the addictive state, these DA neurons exhibit increased activity specifically toward drug-related environmental triggers, with drugs of abuse engaging a variety of cellular processes. Numerous projections throughout the forebrain and midbrain nuclei modulate the activity of VTA DA neurons.[1,10] Among these inputs, cells releasing glutamate (Glu), γ-aminobutyric acid (GABA), acetylcholine (ACh), and noradrenaline bind to DA neurons to modulate activity and subsequent DA release in the NAc.[24,42]

Glutamatergic afferents from the prefrontal cortex (PFC), hypothalamus (HY), lateral habenula (LHb), and pedunculopontine (PPT), induce excitatory postsynaptic potentials through ionotropic N-methyl-D-aspartate (NMDA)/α-amino-3-hydroxy-5-methyl-4-isoxazolepropionic acid (AMPA) glutamate receptors. Subsequent depolarization opens voltage-gated Ca^{2+} channels (VGCC), which triggers a conformational change in calmodulin (a calcium-binding secondary messenger that binds to intracellular proteins), thereby increasing cellular activity. Metabotropic group I Glu receptors ($mGluR_{1/5}$) activate phospholipase C (PLC), an enzyme that catalyzes phospholipids. In this case, phosphatidylinositol 4,5-bisphosphate (PIP_2) is cleaved into the secondary messengers inositol trisphosphate (IP_3) and 1,2 diacyl glycerol (DAG). IP_3 initiates transport of Ca^{2+} from internal stores (e.g., endoplasmic reticulum) into the cytosol, wherein DAG is a precursor for 2-arachidonylglycerol (2-AG), the most prevalent eCB in the brain.[21]

Endocannabinoid Modulation of DA

The eCB system is composed of transmembrane receptors, lipid signaling molecules, and proteins that synthesize or degrade these molecules.[21] Following activation, PLC cleaves PIP_2 into DAG, which is then catalyzed by membrane-bound diacylglycerol lipase α (DGLα) into 2-AG. 2-AG is released "on demand," meaning release is initiated following depolarization, wherein VGCCs allow influx of Ca^{2+}, or following G-protein-induced IP_3 production, which Ca^{2+} increases from IP_3-induced depletion of internal stores.[34] DA neurons release 2-AG in retrograde fashion onto presynaptic inputs, reducing GABA and glutamatergic inputs by binding to G-protein-coupled CB_1 receptors. CB_1 receptors are coupled to inhibitory G-proteins that decrease the duration of excitatory potentials by potentiating inwardly rectifying K^+ channels. 2-AG is then degraded by monoacylglycerol lipase (MAGL).[6,20]

In this way, DA neurons release eCBs as retrograde messengers, modulating presynaptic inputs during periods of high activity by inhibiting GABAergic inputs (depolarization-induced suppression of inhibition) or inhibiting glutamatergic inputs (depolarization-induced suppression of excitation).[6] In fact, this retrograde signaling mechanism is necessary for reward-related DA signaling in the mesolimbic pathway.[4,25,49] CB_1-mediated suppression of GABA inputs in particular is hypothesized to allow addictive drugs or reward-associated stimuli to disinhibit DA neurons projecting to the NAc. Because CB_1 receptor blockade concurrently reduces reward seeking and DA transients evoked by reward-predicting cues, diminished phasic DA signaling may underlie the suppression of drug reward, reinforcement, and relapse by CB_1 receptor antagonists. Thus eCB-mediated modulation of phasic DA signaling appears to be a common mechanism in reinforcement, and an attractive target for treating drug abuse and addiction.

GABAergic afferents local to the VTA and originating from midbrain and forebrain nuclei—namely the rostromedial tegmentum (RMTg), ventral pallidum (VP), HY, and NAc—inhibit DA neurons through GABAR activation, hyperpolarizing DA neurons through Cl^- influx (GABA$_A$R) and K^+ efflux (GABA$_B$R). ACh released from brainstem nuclei—namely the pedunculopontine (or PPT) and laterodorsal tegmentum (LDT)—functions similarly to excitatory afferents, with depolarizing current flow through nicotinic ACh receptors (AChRs) and metabotropic AChR activation of PLC [14].

In contrast to other projections, noradrenaline (NA) afferents from locus coeruleus (LC) affect both DA neurons and presynaptic inputs. Metabotropic α_1 adrenergic receptors (ARs) located postsynaptically on DA neurons activate PLC, while α_2ARs are found on presynaptic inputs and are coupled to inhibitory G-protein cascades. Given that AMPH functions on the NA reuptake transporter similarly to DAT, extended NA release can serve to further extend PLC activation in DA neurons.[30]

With modulation from these various afferents, VTA neurons release DA in the NAc to drive reward-guided associative learning. How DA regulates the associative learning mechanisms that underlie drug-seeking behaviors depends on the temporal dynamics, location, and context of action potential-dependent DA release.[33,48] DAergic signaling operates on multiple time-scales including very rapid events in vesicular DA release (phasic signaling) riding on top of a low, slowly changing DA tone (tonic signaling).[32] Tonic signaling is thought to be predominantly maintained by low frequency cell firing, and may have an enabling influence on postsynaptic mechanisms. In contrast, phasic release is thought

to occur when DA neurons respond to motivationally significant stimuli with a rapid burst of spikes.[31] These signals are important for encoding temporally specific information such as associating cues with as well as approach behaviors directed at obtaining rewards.[26] Critical temporal requirements also exist for DA signaling to promote synaptic plasticity associated with learning at the cellular level similar to the precise timing requirements for learning on the basis of reinforcement.

Phasic DA signaling also plays an intricate role in addiction. Several abused substances, such as cocaine, nicotine, ethanol, and opioids directly elevate phasic DA release. In addition, phasic release occurs in response to cues indicating drug availability are time-locked to the operant response for drug self-administration[26]; and facilitate reinstatement of an extinguished instrumental response for drug reward. Moreover, the well-known ability of abused substances to preferentially increase DA in the NAc shell may be directly attributable to a selective increase in phasic release events in this region.

Amphetamine

AMPH and its many derivatives are a diverse group of synthetic compounds originating from the naturally occurring substance phenethylamine.[39] Modifications to the benzene ring or side chain of the phenethylamine compound produce a variety of powerfully active drugs such as AMPH, methamphetamine (METH), 3,4-methylenedioxy-N-methylamphetamine ("ecstasy", or MDMA), and methylphenidate (MPH). AMPHs produce feelings of euphoria, relief from fatigue, improved performance on some simple tasks, increased activity levels, and anorexia. After marijuana, AMPHs are the most widely used illicit drugs worldwide, nearly equaling the number of cocaine and heroin users combined (25 million vs. 28 million).[41] Nonetheless, the medical utility of AMPHs is unequivocal. AMPH's psychostimulant effects are clinically indicated for treating narcolepsy, attention-deficit/hyperactivity disorder, obesity, and traumatic brain injury. The widespread use and abuse of this powerful compound necessitates a further understanding of the mechanisms by which the AMPHs affect cognition and behavior.

Amphetamine at Dopamine Terminals

AMPH's reinforcing and behavioral properties arise from its ability to increase extracellular DA concentrations ($[DA]_{EC}$) at VTA terminals projecting to the striatum. Of particular relevance here, AMPH acts similar to other drugs of abuse and elicits relatively large increases in extracellular DA levels in the NAc. Drug-evoked alterations in DA neurotransmission are implicated in virtually all stages of addiction, from induction to maintenance and then to relapse after a period of abstinence.[16] Addictive drugs are a unique type of reward in that they generally lack rewarding sensory properties, but are rather rewarding due to their direct interactions with brain physiology. By greatly elevating brain DA, drugs of abuse are thought to usurp normal reward learning mechanisms, which promotes their relatively powerful arousing and incentive-learning properties compared to natural rewards.

AMPH has traditionally been thought to elevate brain DA levels through interactions with the plasma membrane DA transporter (DAT), located on DA neuron terminals (Fig. 10.1A). The DAT tightly regulates the duration and strength of DAergic neurotransmission through high-affinity uptake of released DA, thus terminating DA action at pre- and postsynaptic sites. DAT

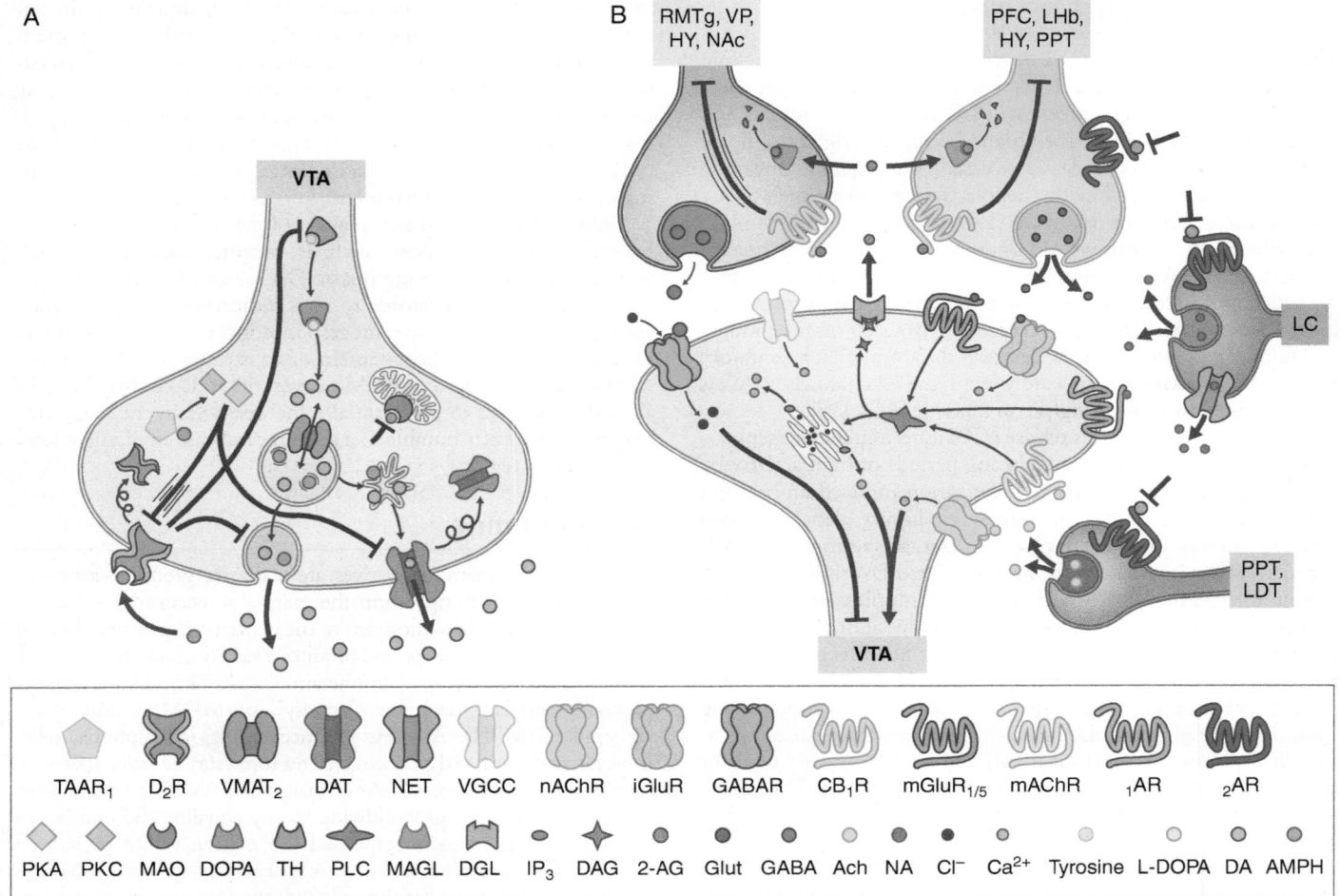

• **Fig. 10.1** Amphetamine (AMPH) mediated dysfunction in ventral tegmental dopamine (DA) neurons. (A) At the terminal, AMPH prevents monoamine oxidase (MAO) degradation of DA and increases the production of protein kinases A and C (PKA, PKC) by trace amine-associated receptor 1 (TAAR$_1$). Protein kinases phosphorylate DA transporter (DAT), disrupting reuptake, and D$_2$ autoreceptor, lowering the inhibition of intracellular processes governing DA production and vesicular release. Phosphorylated DAT reverses transport of DA (efflux), and both DAT and D$_2$R are eventually internalized. AMPH also hijacks vesicular monoamine transporter 2 (VMAT2) function by disrupting internal pH, resulting in internal content depletion into the cytosol, increasing DA available for DAT-driven efflux into the synapse. (B) VTA DA neurons receive numerous inputs that modulate intracellular activity and vesicular release of DA. G-protein-coupled glutamatergic ($_m$GlutR$_{1/5}$), cholinergic ($_m$AChR), and adrenergic (α_1AR) receptors increase PLC production, which leads to synthesis of the eCB 2-arachidonylglycerol (2-AG) and secondary messenger inositol 1,4,5-triphosphate (IP$_3$). Following Ca^{2+} increases, 2-AG works in retrograde fashion to inhibit presynaptic inputs by binding to inhibitory CB$_1$Rs, whereas IP$_3$ increases intracellular Ca^{2+} by inducing efflux from internal stores (e.g., endoplasmic reticulum). Following adrenergic (NA) activation, NA binds to inhibitory α_2ARs on presynaptic inputs. AMPH increases burst firing of DA neurons by antagonizing presynaptic α_2ARs, resulting in an increase of Glut, NA, and ACh transmission, driving eCB production and subsequent release onto presynaptic inputs.

functions by binding extracellular substrate along with Na$^+$ and Cl$^-$, which promotes translocation of substrate and a conformational change in the DAT, exposing the binding site to the intracellular milieu. By acting as a substrate for DAT, AMPH competitively inhibits DA reuptake, increasing inward Na$^+$ transport, and also extending the duration of DA signals. This promotes a reversal of DAT conformation leading to an increase in the proportion of inward-facing DAT. Intracellular DA and Na$^+$ are then able to bind DAT, which promotes DAT-mediated reverse DA release (efflux) through a facilitated exchange-diffusion mechanism that also induces an extended duration of DA neurotransmission. A channel-like transporter mechanism and/or rapid mobilization

of the DAT to and from the cell surface also appear to regulate AMPH's effects on DA uptake and efflux.

Extensive work demonstrates that AMPH also acts on mechanisms controlling DA neurotransmission including synthesis by tyrosine hydroxylase (TH), packaging by vesicular monoamine transporter 2 (VMAT2), and degradation by monoamine oxidase (MAO).[35,37,39] In addition, AMPH activates trace amine-associated receptor 1 (TAAR1), an intracellular G-protein-coupled receptor (GPCR) that increases levels of protein kinases (PKA, PKC) that phosphorylate DAT and D$_2$ receptors.[2,7,18,44,46] Phosphorylation induces downregulation and internalization of both receptors.[22]

Inside the cell, AMPH is also able to deplete vesicular stores through a weak base[38] or exchange diffusion mechanism. Depletion of vesicular stores has the effect of decreasing the amount of transmitter released per secretory vesicle fusion event (i.e., the "quantal size")[36] and increasing cytoplasmic concentrations of unpackaged DA available for reverse transport. AMPH may also promote a redistribution of certain vesicular populations away from the plasma membrane, but how this affects $[DA]_{EC}$ remains unclear. Uptake inhibition, reverse DA transport, and decreased exocytotic release were all simultaneously demonstrated with cyclic voltammetry recordings in mouse striatal slices following incubation with 10 μM AMPH. Collectively, these studies have established the primary mechanism of AMPH action as a functional switch from action potential-dependent vesicular release to a mode of transmission independent of normal presynaptic control and reliant on stimulation-independent DA efflux via DAT-mediated reverse transport.[12,35] Overall, these terminal effects result in increased baseline levels of DA, as AMPH reduces elimination and increases nonexocytotic release of DA into the extracellular space.[2,7,12,44,46]

Amphetamine at the Cell Body

In contrast to AMPH's classically defined mechanisms, which were all described in reduced preparations, recent in vivo work demonstrates that, rather than depleting releasable dopamine stores, AMPH main mode of action in an intact brain is to enhance vesicular release, supporting an increase in the peak concentration of phasic DA release events (Fig. 10.1B).[5,28]

Pharmacological investigations indicate that AMPH may primarily ramp up 2-AG-mediated disinhibition of DA neurons through the antagonism of the metabotropic α2 adrenergic receptor, which inhibits cyclic AMP and subsequent intracellular cascades.[8,15,17,29,47] In this way, inhibitory feedback onto Glu, ACh, and NA projections lessons, allowing excitatory inputs to become more active, and increasing depolarization of DA neurons. In a circular manner, 2-AG signaling disinhibits presynaptic inputs, leading to G-protein-coupled cascades, which further increase 2-AG production, proliferating this cycle and further ramping up phasic activity of DA neurons. In VTA projections to the NAc, AMPH increases phasic DA responding, and upregulation of TH and Glu levels are all disrupted by CB_1 receptor antagonism, supporting the idea that AMPH interacts with eCB modulation to influence DA signaling of drug-induced reward.[3,27]

Moreover, Covey et al.[3] showed that AMPH-evoked increases in NAc DA levels require midbrain DA cell firing, with Na^+ channel blockage using tetrodotoxin curtailing AMPH-evoked phasic signals.[3] These findings starkly contrast action potential–independent DA release as AMPH's primary mechanism of action. Thus AMPH alters DA signaling in a manner similar to that of drugs of abuse like cocaine. It is important to note that these findings indicate that, despite vastly different mechanisms of action and cellular targets, all classes of addictive drugs share augmentation of phasic DA signaling as a common cellular action. Furthermore, the generation of these phasic DA signals is implicated in drug reinforcement and can produce an addictive phenotype.

Endocannabinoids and Amphetamine

Covey et al.[3] extend this retrograde eCB mechanism in the VTA to AMPH's actions in DA neurons. Blocking CB_1 receptor activation during AMPH administration shows that 2-AG modulation of presynaptic inputs is necessary for drug-induced phasic DA activation, as it is with reward-induced DA activation. In addition, the effect is localized to the DA cell body, supporting the idea

that eCB-mediated feedback onto presynaptic inputs in the VTA is the cause behind amplified DA signaling, not AMPH-driven efflux at terminals in the NAc. Given these findings, Covey et al.[3] argue that eCB modulation of presynaptic inputs in the VTA may serve as a cornerstone for understanding and possibly developing pharmacotherapeutic avenues for drugs of abuse.

Consistent with the VTA as a likely target for drugs of abuse, intra-VTA CB_1 receptor blockade or inhibition of DGLα reduces cocaine-induced transient activation,[45] and CB_1 receptor drugs modify VTA DA neuron electrophysiology measured in slices,[45] supporting the idea of eCB modulation of local circuitry in the VTA. CB_1 receptor antagonism reduces phasic DA signaling evoked by cannabinoids, cocaine, nicotine, and ethanol as well as to food or brain stimulation reward (BSR).

However, this work indicates further complexity in CB_1 mediation of AMPH, particularly in relation to glutamate function. These authors found that CB_1R antagonism attenuated AMPH-driven action potentials through activation of mGluR_5. Freestone et al.[11] support these findings, albeit in substantia nigra in vitro, with observations of a glutamate spillover, wherein CB_1R blockade induced group I mGluR activation, resulting in subsequent inhibition exclusively of GABAergic transmission. These recent experiments highlight the multifaceted influence of the eCB system on AMPH's mechanisms in the mesolimbic system. Because AMPH acts in an action potential–dependent manner, retrograde signaling of 2-AG plays a significant role in AMPH's ability to influence DA signaling and provides therapeutic avenues through which AMPH's effects can be modulated and explored, for instance with the use of 2-AG synthesis inhibitors.

Conclusions

AMPH's effects on the mesolimbic pathway prove to be a fascinating subject for researchers given the increasingly complex relationship between VTA neurons and their modulatory afferents, which serve to increase and decrease phasic DA signaling of reward and reward-related stimuli. AMPH influences DA neurotransmission through mechanisms that are both action potential–dependent and action potential–independent, at cell bodies in the VTA and at terminals in the NAc, although its primary mode of action in vivo appears to be an action on DA neuron excitability. The eCB system emerges as a focal point for treatment of AMPH-driven dysfunction because 2-AG production fine-tunes presynaptic inputs onto VTA DA neurons. Through this review, we hope to bring attention to the need for exploration into these relationships, as well as the potential pharmacotherapies that may emerge from a more detailed understanding of these interactions.

References

1. Beier KT, Steinberg EE, DeLoach KE, et al. Circuit architecture of VTA DA neurons revealed by systematic input-output mapping. *Cell*. 2015;162(3):622–634.
2. Calipari ES, Sun H, Eldeeb K, et al. AMPH self-administration attenuates DA D2 autoreceptor function. *Neuropsychopharmacology*. 2014;39(8):1833–1842.
3. Covey DP, Bunner KD, Schuweiler DR, Cheer JF, Garris PA. AMPH elevates nucleus accumbens DA via an action potential–dependent mechanism that is modulated by endocannabinoids. *Eur J Neurosci*. 2016;43(12):1661–1673.
4. Covey D, Mateo Y, Sulzer D, Cheer JF, Lovinger DM. Endocannabinoid modulation of DA neurotransmission. *Neuropharmacology*. 2017.

5. Daberkow DP, Brown HD, Bunner KD, et al. AMPH paradoxically augments exocytotic DA release and phasic DA signals. *J Neurosci.* 2013;33(2):452–463.

6. Diana MA, Marty A. Endocannabinoid–mediated short–term synaptic plasticity: Depolarization–induced suppression of inhibition (DSI) and depolarization–induced suppression of excitation (DSE). *Br J Pharmacol.* 2004;142(1):9–19.

7. Eiden LE, Weihe E. VMAT2: a dynamic regulator of brain monoaminergic neuronal function interacting with drugs of abuse. *Ann N Y Acad Sci.* 2011;1216(1):86–98.

8. Elverdin JC, Fiszman ML, Stefano FJE, Perec CJ. Interaction between AMPH and α2–postsynaptic adrenoreceptors in the rat submaxillary gland. *Auton Autacoid Pharmacol.* 1987;7(3):199–204.

9. Everitt BJ, Robbins TW. Drug addiction: updating actions to habits to compulsions ten years on. *Annu Rev Psychol.* 2016;67:23–50.

10. Ferrada C, Sotomayor-Zárate R, Abarca J, Gysling K. The activation of metabotropic glutamate 5 receptors in the rat ventral tegmental area increases DA extracellular levels. *NeuroReport.* 2017;28(1):28–34.

11. Freestone PS, Guatteo E, Piscitelli F, Di Marzo V, Lipski J, Mercuri NB. Glutamate spillover drives endocannabinoid production and inhibits GABAergic transmission in the Substantia Nigra pars compacta. *Neuropharmacology.* 2014;79:467–475.

12. Freyberg Z, Sonders MS, Aguilar JI, et al. Mechanisms of AMPH action illuminated through optical monitoring of DA synaptic vesicles in Drosophila brain. *Nat Commun.* 2016;7.

13. Godino A, Jayanthi S, Cadet JL. Epigenetic landscape of AMPH and methamphetamine addiction in rodents. *Epigenetics.* 2015;10(7):574–580.

14. Holmstrand EC, Sesack SR. Projections from the rat pedunculopontine and laterodorsal tegmental nuclei to the anterior thalamus and ventral tegmental area arise from largely separate populations of neurons. *Brain Struct Funct.* 2011;216(4):331–345.

15. Inyushin MU, Arencibia-Albite F, Vázquez-Torres R, Vélez-Hernández ME, Jiménez-Rivera CA. Alpha-2 noradrenergic receptor activation inhibits the hyperpolarization-activated cation current (I h) in neurons of the ventral tegmental area. *Neuroscience.* 2010;167(2):287–297.

16. Koob GF, Volkow ND. Neurocircuitry of addiction. *Neuropsychopharmacology.* 2010;35(1):217.

17. Langer SZ, Dubocovich ML. Cocaine and amphetamine antagonize the decrease of noradrenergic neurotransmission elicited by oxymetazoline but potentiate the inhibition by alpha-methylnorepinephrine in the perfused cat spleen. *J Pharmacol Exp Ther.* 1981;216(1):162–171.

18. Leo D, Espinoza S. Trace Amine-Associated Receptor 1 Modulation of DA System. Trace Amines and Neurological Disorders: Potential Mechanisms and Risk Factors. 2016:125.

19. McHugh RK, Nielsen S, Weiss RD. Prescription drug abuse: from epidemiology to public policy. *J Subst Abuse Treat.* 2015;48(1):1–7.

20. Melis M, Pistis M, Perra S, Muntoni AL, Pillolla G, Gessa GL. Endocannabinoids mediate presynaptic inhibition of glutamatergic transmission in rat ventral tegmental area DA neurons through activation of CB1 receptors. *J Neurosci.* 2004;24(1):53–62.

21. Murataeva N, Straiker A, Mackie K. Parsing the players: 2–arachidonoylglycerol synthesis and degradation in the CNS. *Br J Pharmacol.* 2014;171(6):1379–1391.

22. Namkung Y, Sibley DR. Protein kinase C mediates phosphorylation, desensitization, and trafficking of the D2 dopamine receptor. *J Biol Chem.* 2004;279(47):49533–49541.

23. Padala PR, Bhatia SC. Stimulant Use and Addictive Disorder: AMPH, Cocaine and Other Stimulants. Substance and Nonsubstance Related Addiction Disorder: Diagnosis and Treatment. 2017:188.

24. Paladini CA, Williams JT. Noradrenergic inhibition of midbrain DA neurons. *J Neurosci.* 2004;24(19):4568–4575.

25. Parsons LH, Hurd YL. Endocannabinoid signalling in reward and addiction. *Nat Rev Neurosci.* 2015;16(10):579–594.

26. Phillips PE, Stuber GD, Heien ML, Wightman RM, Carelli RM. Subsecond dopamine release promotes cocaine seeking. *Nature.* 2003;422(6932):614–618.

27. Polissidis A, Chouliara O, Galanopoulos A, et al. Cannabinoids negatively modulate striatal glutamate and DA release and behavioural output of acute D-amphetamine. *Behav Brain Res.* 2014;270:261–269. Endocannabinoids mediate presynaptic inhibition of glutamatergic transmission in rat ventral tegmental area DA neurons through activation of CB1 receptors.

28. Ramsson ES, Howard CD, Covey DP, Garris PA. High doses of AMPH augment, rather than disrupt, exocytotic DA release in the dorsal and ventral striatum of the anesthetized rat. *J Neurochem.* 2011;119(6):1162–1172.

29. Ritz MC, Kuhar MJ. Relationship between self-administration of amphetamine and monoamine receptors in brain: comparison with cocaine. *J Pharmacol Exp Ther.* 1989;248(3):1010–1017.

30. Robertson SD, Matthies HJG, Galli A. A closer look at amphetamine-induced reverse transport and trafficking of the dopamine and norepinephrine transporters. *Mol Neurobiol.* 2009;39(2):73–80.

31. Schultz W. Predictive reward signal of dopamine neurons. *J Neurophysiol.* 1998;80(1):1–27.

32. Schultz W. *Reward. Scholarpedia.* 2007;2(3):1652.

33. Schultz W. DA reward prediction-error signalling: a two-component response. *Nat Rev Neurosci.* 2016;17(3):183–195.

34. Shonesy BC, Winder DG, Patel S, Colbran RJ. The initiation of synaptic 2-AG mobilization requires both an increased supply of diacylglycerol precursor and increased postsynaptic calcium. *Neuropharmacology.* 2015;91:57–62.

35. Sulzer D. How addictive drugs disrupt presynaptic dopamine neurotransmission. *Neuron.* 2011;69(4):628–649.

36. Sulzer D, Chen TK, Lau YY, Kristensen H, Rayport S, Ewing A. Amphetamine redistributes dopamine from synaptic vesicles to the cytosol and promotes reverse transport. *J Neurosci.* 1995;15(5):4102–4108.

37. Sulzer D, Cragg SJ, Rice ME. Striatal DA neurotransmission: regulation of release and uptake. *Basal ganglia.* 2016;6(3):123–148.

38. Sulzer D, Rayport S. Amphetamine and other psychostimulants reduce pH gradients in midbrain dopaminergic neurons and chromaffin granules: a mechanism of action. *Neuron.* 1990;5(6):797–808.

39. Sulzer D, Sonders MS, Poulsen NW, Galli A. Mechanisms of neurotransmitter release by amphetamines: a review. *Prog Neurobiol.* 2005;75(6):406–433.

40. Sweeney CT, Sembower MA, Ertischek MD, Shiffman S, Schnoll SH. Nonmedical use of prescription ADHD stimulants and preexisting patterns of drug abuse. *J Addict Dis.* 2013;32(1):1–10.

41. United UNODC. *Nations Office on Drugs and Crime: World Drug Report 2014*; 2014.

42. Velásquez-Martínez MC, Vázquez-Torres R, Rojas LV, Sanabria P, Jiménez-Rivera CA. Alpha-1 adrenoreceptors modulate GABA release onto ventral tegmental area DA neurons. *Neuropharmacology.* 2015;88:110–121.

43. Volkow ND, Morales M. The brain on drugs: from reward to addiction. *Cell.* 2015;162(4):712–725.

44. Wallace LJ. Trace Amine-Associated Receptor 1: Implications for Treating Stimulant Drug Addiction. *Trace Amines and Neurological Disorders: Potential Mechanisms and Risk Factors.* 2016:339.

45. Wang KH, Penmatsa A, Gouaux E. Neurotransmitter and psychostimulant recognition by the DA transporter. *Nature.* 2015;521(7552):322.

46. Wang Q, Bubula N, Brown J, Wang Y, Kondev V, Vezina P. PKC phosphorylates residues in the N-terminal of the DA transporter to regulate AMPH-induced DA efflux. *Neurosci Lett.* 2016;622:78–82.

47. Wei-Xing S, Chen-Lun P, Zhou Y. Psychostimulants induce low-frequency9 oscillations in the firing activity of DA neurons. *Neuropsychopharmacology.* 2004;29(12):2160.

48. Wise RA. Dual roles of DA in food and drug seeking: the drive-reward paradox. *Biol Psychiatry.* 2013;73(9):819–826.

49. Zlebnik NE, Cheer JF. Drug-induced alterations of endocannabinoid-mediated plasticity in brain reward regions. *J Neurosci.* 2016;36(40):10230–10238.

11

Pain and Negative Affect

ASAF KELLER

CHAPTER OUTLINE

Pain not only hurts. Pain can also lead to anxiety and depression, and patients with anxiety and depression experience pain more strongly and are more likely to develop chronic pain. Pain can impair cognitive function, and cognitive processes can modulate pain perception. Not surprisingly, these complex interactions are mediated by central nervous system substrates that are shared by nociceptive and affective processes. Recent discoveries and hypotheses on the interactions between pain and negative affect are revealing the pathogenesis of these comorbid conditions and are suggesting novel approaches for treating them.

Pain Is a Multidimensional Experience

Clinicians and those doing basic research have long recognized that pain is a multidimensional percept, composed of unpleasant sensory, affective, and cognitive experiences.[6,46,94,114,144] Although sensory characteristics of pain are tightly coupled to activation of nociceptors,[57] nociceptor activation does not always produce pain, and pain can occur without an identifiable nociceptive input.[141] This, and the fact that pain experience is affected by contextual and cognitive factors,[155] indicates that pain circuits within the central nervous system are an integral part of the experience of pain. These circuits represent a distributed neuronal network that includes parallel somatosensory, limbic, and other components.[93] Human and animal studies have shown that the different dimensions of the pain experience may arise from activity in different components of this matrix.[17] The "lateral system," including the somatosensory thalamus and cortex, is thought to be involved primarily in the sensory-discriminative dimension of pain; this dimension reports the location and intensity of pain. The "medial system"—including the mesolimbic structures, medial thalamic nuclei, and the anterior cingulate and the prefrontal cortex—is thought to be involved primarily in the affective-motivational-cognitive dimensions of pain. These relate to feelings of unpleasantness and emotions, and a determination of the appropriate or possible response in a particular situation.[116]

Thus, the conscious experience of pain represents an interpretation of nociceptive stimuli influenced by memories, and emotional, pathological, genetic, and cognitive factors.[142] This explains why the perception of pain cannot be predicted from an analysis of the nociceptive drive or input. Accordingly, the International Association for the Study of Pain (IASP) defines pain as "An unpleasant sensory and emotional experience associated with actual or potential tissue damage, or described in terms of such damage."[95]

Indeed, it is intuitive that pain perception is a multidimensional percept, involving sensory and affective components. Most individuals have experienced the effect of mood swings on their perception of pain or on their pain thresholds. Popular literature frequently refers to a "runner's high" that provides athletes not only with a sense of euphoria, but that can also suppress pain perception. The neurobiological mechanisms underlying such phenomena are beginning to be unraveled.[52] More exotic descriptions of dissociation between affective and sensory pain components include reports of yogi that can consciously modulate their pain perception; this behavioral feat is apparently associated with significant changes in brain activity.[111] The phenomenon of initial painlessness described by wounded soldiers is also often described.[12]

In a laboratory setting, subjects can readily dissociate the degree of unpleasantness from the perceived intensity of different noxious stimulus modalities.[119] Researchers have also showed that hypnotic suggestion can affect the perception of the affective component of pain, while leaving the perception of the intensity of pain constant.[118] In this condition, positron emission tomography reveals changes in the anterior cingulate cortex, but not in the primary somatosensory cortex, suggesting that these cortical areas are differentially involved in the affective and sensory components of pain, respectively. Related to this, other imaging studies suggest that the regions related to the affective components of pain, but not to its sensory-discriminative aspects, are crucial to the empathy for others' pain.[97,130] A dramatic demonstration of the fact that the affective and sensory components of pain are not only dissociable, but are subserved by different neuronal pathways, is a report that transecting the corpus callosum eliminates sensation in the cerebral hemisphere ipsilateral to the stimulus, while leaving intact in that hemisphere unpleasantness evoked by noxious stimuli.[135]

Chronic Pain and Negative Affect

The reciprocal influences between the affective and sensory components of pain are relevant to both acute and chronic pain, which are fundamentally and mechanistically different conditions. Acute pain is essential for survival, initiating immediate action by retreating from harm, or by suppressing movement to promote healing. Acute nociceptive pain, triggered by nociceptor activation, is a symptom of an underlying medical condition, tends to correlate with the severity of that condition, and ends with the termination of the medical condition.[43]

Chronic pain, on the other hand, has no obvious survival value. (The IASP recognizes that chronic pain arises from many different conditions, and, therefore, recommends flexibility in the definition of chronic pain.[95] In general, chronic pain is recognized as pain that persists past the normal time of healing,[15] or pain that persists beyond a particular length of time determined by common medical experience.) The transition from acute to chronic pain is difficult to define, but is thought to involve the engagement of central nervous system structures.[108]

Chronic pain affects over 100 million Americans—more than are affected by heart disease, cancer, and diabetes combined. Pain also costs the United States up to $650 billion/year in medical treatment and lost productivity.[75] Chronic pain is the most common complaint of patients in outpatient clinics.[146] Common chronic pain complaints include headache, low back pain, cancer pain, arthritis pain, and neurogenic pain, and can result from a variety of conditions and insults at any level of the peripheral and central nervous systems. In most patients, chronic pain starts within weeks or months after the original insult and includes increased pain with noxious stimulation (hyperalgesia) and pain in response to previously innocuous stimuli (allodynia).[3] Perhaps most debilitating is the presence, in nearly all patients, of tonic, or spontaneous pain, which occurs in the absence of a stimulus.[13,14,60]

Although the management and treatment of acute pain is reasonably good, the needs of chronic pain sufferers are largely unmet.[149] For example, analgesics, including opioids, are inefficient in about 70% of patients.[48,55] This failure is due to a convergence of obstacles, including scientific ignorance, skewed funding and health care priorities, and policy and political considerations. A scientific obstacle is that nearly all previous attempts to reveal the pathophysiology of chronic pain have focused on the lateral, sensory-discriminative system. This is despite the lack of success of this approach to lead to effective therapies, and despite emerging evidence that therapies that target the motivational-cognitive dimensions of pain might prove more promising.[6] Furthermore, there is increasing evidence that the negative affective, cognitive, and psychosocial state of chronic pain is universal in different chronic pain states.[63] Therefore, understanding the role of the affective-motivational pathways in chronic pain may lead to innovative therapies to treat these widespread conditions.

The Vicious Cycle of Pain and Negative Affect

The persistency of chronic pain, with its accompanying negative affective symptoms, may create a self-amplifying stressor, in which pain increases fear,[34] depression,[50] and catastrophizing,[117] and these negative affects, in turn, amplify pain perception.[43] Pain catastrophizing is an important construct, defined as a set of negative emotional and cognitive processes involving amplification of pain-related symptoms, rumination about pain, feelings of helplessness, and pessimism about pain-related outcomes.[42,136,137]

Pessimism about pain-related outcomes can strongly influence pain perceptions and negatively affect normal functioning. Fischerauer et al.[49] recently demonstrated that a threshold level of intolerance of uncertainty is required for the development of pain anxiety and its effect on function, and as intolerance of this uncertainty rises, the effect of pain on function goes from being independent of the anxiety to being more and more carried by and through anxiety about pain.

Indeed, pain can be modulated by emotional (fear and anxiety) and cognitive (attention, expectation, or memory) factors.[35,121,125] This pain amplification occurs even in newborns: Jones et al[79] recently measured nociceptive behavior, brain activity, and levels of physiological stress in newborn human infants, and found that infants with higher levels of stress exhibit larger-amplitude cortical nociceptive responses, but this this was not reflected in their behavior. This suggests that brain activity evoked by noxious stimulation is enhanced by stress, but this cannot be deduced directly from observation of pain behavior.

Clearly, of particular concern is the emotional tax from chronic pain that commonly results in life-altering events, including suicide.[26,45,59,64,72]

The influence of affect on pain perception may be immediately relevant for personalizing opioid treatment for patients with chronic pain. Burns et al.[23] demonstrated recently that, in patients with chronic low back pain, depressive symptoms and pain catastrophizing correlate significantly and positively with opioid-induced pain relief. Therefore, these markers may serve to identify individuals who benefit the most from opioid therapy. Of interest, their results suggest also that individuals with greater depressive symptoms, trait anxiety, pain catastrophizing, and perceived disability may have deficits in endogenous opioid function, which may serve as another predictor of enhanced response to opioid analgesics.

Estimating the prevalence of comorbidity of chronic pain and affective disorders is complicated by the fact that the clinical instruments designed to identify depression are often "contaminated" by measures—including sleep disturbances and headaches—that frequently occur in chronic pain.[91] Nevertheless, nearly all studies suggest that chronic pain increases the risk of depression, but data exist to support also that people with a history of depression are at a higher risk for chronic pain. However, the magnitude of this increased risk is thought to be modest—less than twofold—whereas other factors seem more important: Early life stressors, other psychiatric conditions, prior pain, and poor sleep are all stronger predictors of subsequent chronic pain.[91]

Of interest, neuropathic pain affecting the trigeminal system, in particular, is frequently associated with negative affective states, including a high incidence of depression, anxiety, and sleep disorders.[99,133,160] This suggests that trigeminal pain is a particularly painful condition, resulting in substantial psychosocial and affective burden.

The relationship between pain and affect has been confirmed also in animal studies aimed at understanding how anticipation and anxiety cause a heightened pain experience. Although these data are at times conflicting—demonstrating, for example, that anxiety can be either pro- or antinociceptive (depending on the animal model and the endpoints)—these studies demonstrate that animals' pain responses are emotion-specific, suggesting that higher brain centers may determine the behavioral response to the same noxious stimulus.[142]

Stress-induced analgesia is a form of adaptive pain suppression, an evolutionarily conserved response to stress that has survival value.[2,25,51] Stress-induced analgesia may be mediated by both opioid and nonopioid mechanisms, the latter including the endocannabinoid system.[69,104,147]

Neugebauer et al.[105] and Woodhams et al.[158] demonstrated that stress-induced analgesia is critically dependent on supraspinal sites, including the periaqueductal gray (PAG) and the rostroventral medulla (RVM), key components of the descending pain pathway. As discussed later, these regions are thought to be critically involved in mediating the interactions between affect and pain perception.

Stress and anxiety do not always suppress pain—they can also enhance nociception and exacerbate pain. This phenomenon is referred to as stress-induced hyperalgesia.[77] For example,[143] it has been demonstrated in rats that muscle inflammation followed by stress induces visceral hypersensitivity that persists for months, modeling these human comorbid pain conditions. This stress-induced hyperalgesia phenomenon was accompanied by increased activation of brain regions associated with the affective component of pain.[73] Visceral stress-induced hyperalgesia may involve the endocannabinoid system.[71] Chronic stress in rodent models results not only in visceral stress-induced hyperalgesia, but also in thermal and mechanical stress-induced hyperalgesia.[128] This form of stress-induced hyperalgesia also involves the endocannabinoid system.[87]

Thus stress can evoke both stress-induced analgesia and stress-induced hyperalgesia, and both phenomena appear to involve the endocannabinoid system and descending pain modulatory pathways. Neugebauer, Hohmann, and collaborators[158] proposed that endocannabinoid signaling in key components of the descending pain pathway mediates stress-induced analgesia, whereas a deficit in endocannabinoid signaling may underlie stress-induced hyperalgesia.

The relationship between stress and pain perception is likely related to the curious phenomenon of social transfer of pain. Langford et al.[84] showed that pairs of mice given identical noxious stimuli and tested together display increased pain behaviors, compared to being tested alone, or compared with mice that have not received the noxious stimulus. This "social modulation of pain" is dependent on visual cues. Similarly, mice housed for long periods in the same cage with mice that have peripheral nerve injury exhibit enhanced pain responses to acetic acid.[10] This behavior appears to represent stress-induced hyperalgesia, because the cage mates of the nerve-injured animals displayed anxiety-like behavior on elevated plus maze and the open-field tests. More recently, Smith et al.[134] reported that naïve, "bystander" mice housed and tested in the same room as mice subjected to inflammatory pain develop corresponding hyperalgesia. This form of social transfer of pain appears to be mediated by olfactory cues and appears to occur without affecting anxiety.[134] It is likely that social transfer of pain, as a social cue, provides a recognition of another's pain that can lead to the avoidance of harm or trigger empathy and caregiving behavior.[134]

Comorbidity

Indeed, affective, anxiety, and behavior disorders are early risk factors for developing chronic pain.[140] For example, patients with depression and anxiety, or who have a tendency to catastrophize,

report more intense pain experiences.[66,137] Similarly, chronic pain shows significant comorbidity with clinical depression.[7,8,24] The majority of patients with depression report at least one pain complaint, and depression is present in 5% to 85% (depending on the study setting) of patients with pain conditions.[7] Patients with chronic pain often have affective disorders, such as anxiety,[8,24] and anxiety is a risk factor for developing chronic pain.[24,37,61,62]

Several large studies of individuals, including twins, found a greater than chance association between chronic pain conditions—such as low back pain, joint pain, headaches, temporomandibular joint pain—and affective disorders, including major depression, panic attacks, and posttraumatic stress disorder, suggestive of a common etiology for these conditions.[80,123]

Fibromyalgia is a syndrome that is characterized by chronic widespread pain, muscle tenderness, and emotional distress.[1,164] The frequent comorbidity of fibromyalgia with stress-related disorders, such as chronic fatigue, posttraumatic stress disorder, irritable bowel syndrome, and depression, as well as the similarity of many CNS abnormalities, suggests at least a partial common substrate for these disorders. Despite the numerous cerebral alterations associated with it, fibromyalgia might not be a primary disorder of the brain but rather may be a consequence of early life stress or prolonged or severe stress affecting brain modulatory circuitry of pain and emotions in genetically susceptible individuals.[124]

The comorbidity of affective disorders and chronic pain often results in misdiagnosis of and treatment of depression and similar disorders. As Bair et al.[7] remind us, more than 75% of patients in primary care settings who have depression present exclusively with physical complaints, and their affective disorders are rarely diagnosed.[83,129]

Pain as a Negative Reward

There is a growing realization that pain, and in particular its affective facets, may be causally related to impaired reward and motivation functions.[11,38,96,100] As reviewed by Elman and Borsook,[43] the notion of unity of negative and positive rewards dates to the early Greek and Chinese scholars and physicians, and was later refined by Fichte and Hegel. Elman and Borsook also remind us that "Dostoevsky and Nietzsche expanded this concept to the holistic and indivisible pain-pleasure amalgamation, while Spinoza upheld the pain-pleasure continuum by designating them opposite anchors of the perfection scale." In this context, behaviors that result in pain relief, or in the prevention of painful states, are rewarding.

These rewarding behaviors appear to depend on dopamine transmission in mesolimbic centers, in particular in the nucleus accumbens (NAc). This nucleus is a key node in the reward circuitry, as it integrates inputs from mesencephalic dopaminergic neurons and from neurons in the ventral hippocampus, amygdala, and frontal cortical areas, all structures that process affective information.[19,21] Anatomical and functional changes in these reward/motivation circuits in chronic pain may lead to the comorbid affective and cognitive disorders observed in these patients.[101,105] NAc activity in humans appears to encode its predicted value and anticipates its analgesic potential on chronic pain.[9] In patients with fibromyalgia, for example, dopaminergic responses to pain appear to be abnormal[157]: Patients with fibromyalgia experience noxious stimuli as more painful than healthy controls do, and control subjects release dopamine in the basal ganglia during the painful stimulation, whereas patients with fibromyalgia do not. Hypersensitivity to pain and high rates of comorbid chronic pain are common in several disorders linked with deficits in dopamine system function, including disorders of mood and affect, substance abuse, and Parkinson disease. In contrast, hyposensitivity to pain is common in patients with schizophrenia, which is linked to excessive dopamine neurotransmission.[76]

Nerve injury, in either rats or mice, increases the excitability of NAc neurons, and this amplified activity appears to be causally related to injury-induced pain.[120] The NAc neurons, the activity of which is amplified, are known to drive descending pain modulatory pathways, and to regulate aversive responses. The activity of dopaminergic neurons is also profoundly affected by painful stimuli that depress the majority of mesolimbic dopamine neurons (value-coding neurons) and increase activity in a subset of neurons (salience-coding neurons).[18]

In rats with chronic pain, peripheral nerve block results in conditioned place preference (a positive-reward behavior) and evokes dopamine release in NAc.[103] Similar behavioral and neurochemical events occur after pharmacological pain relief.[161] The relief of ongoing pain requires opioid signaling in the cingulate cortex and subsequent downstream activation of dopamine activity in the NAc, mediating the reward of pain relief.[102] Indeed, dopamine release in the NAc may emerge as a biomarker of pain relief reward that reflects analgesic efficacy.[161]

Extensive evidence for an overlap in neuronal circuits subserving both pain perception and reward/motivation strongly supports the notion that pain may be related to impaired reward functions.[96,113] For example, brain areas involved in the reward-aversion neuronal circuitry that are important for decision-making are also implicated in pain processing: They respond to noxious stimuli and their activation or inhibition modulates the level of perceived pain.[13a,112a] Several lines of evidence suggest that chronic pain leads to a hypodopaminergic state that impairs motivated behavior.[139] The resulting decreased responsiveness to rewards may be related to the anhedonia and depression common with chronic pain. Thus, strategies to restore dopamine signaling may represent a novel approach to manage the affective sequelae of chronic pain.

That chronic pain involves impaired reward function relates directly to the epidemiological and mechanistic links between pain and addiction. Because addiction is driven by changes in reward pathways,[28,44,81,153] and because these same reward pathways are apparently involved in chronic pain (see preceding text), addiction should be considered, with negative affect and with chronic pain, as mutually reinforcing maladaptive mechanisms.

Chronic pain is linked to other addictions. For example, alcohol use disorder is highly comorbid with chronic pain.[162]

Shared Brain Circuits

The pathogenesis of chronic pain, as well as that of affective disorders, involves neuronal networks distributed throughout the nervous system. Similarly, the perception of both pain and negative affect involves distributed CNS networks. Therefore, it is unlikely that the reinforcing interactions of pain and negative affect will be restricted to a single locus. However, there exist several loci at which negative affect may amplify pain, and where pain may exacerbate affective disorders.

The Amygdala

The amygdala is one of the key sites for interactions between chronic pain and negative affect. It is well established that the amygdala has an important role in emotions and affective disorders.[90,110,112] Anatomical, neurochemical, electrophysiological, and behavioral studies support its role in the emotional–affective dimension of pain.[53,67,104,106,121] This almond-shaped brain area in the medial temporal lobe is closely associated with cortical and subcortical structures relevant to both pain processing and emotions. The amygdala affects the insular, orbital, and medial prefrontal cortex; basal forebrain nuclei; bed nucleus of the stria terminalis; and medial dorsal thalamus; as well as the hypothalamus and key brainstem areas.[16] The amygdala projects to key structures in the descending modulation of pain (described in subsequent text), including the PAG, parabrachial nucleus (PB), reticular formation, dorsal nucleus of the vagus, solitary tract nucleus, and ventrolateral medulla.[32,86,115]

Amygdala inputs to the medial prefrontal cortex are thought to provide emotion and value-based information to guide decision-making and behavior control.[70,85,92] A complex network of connections intrinsic to the amygdala regulates the outputs from this structure, thereby modulating emotional responses and pain-related outputs and behaviors.[105,106] Through interactions with cortical areas, the amygdala also contributes to cognitive aspects of the pain experience, such as pain-related decision-making deficits.[78] An example of the role of these amygdala-related interactions comes from findings demonstrating that activation of the amygdala differentiates fibromyalgia patients with and without major depression.[54]

Thus, the amygdala interacts with brain regions and systems involved in nociception and pain perception, fear and anxiety, attention and cognition, as well as autonomic function. Neugebauer and collaborators have promoted the hypothesis, and provided evidence to support it, that impaired cortical cognitive control leading to amygdalar disinhibition results in the persistence of pain and its affective dimension.[104,158]

Descending Pain Modulation

Pain perception is strongly influenced by cognitive factors, including attentional state, emotional context, attitudes, expectations, hypnotic suggestions, or anesthesia-induced changes in consciousness,[24,46,150] Cognitive influences on pain perception are attributed to cortical circuits whose descending outputs modulate information processing at spinal and brainstem levels.[4,142]

The most completely characterized descending pain modulating circuit is the periaqueductal gray–rostroventral medulla (or PAG-RVM) system.[39,46,67] These descending pathways exert bidirectional control over nociception; imbalance in this circuitry toward facilitation of postsynaptic targets may promote and maintain chronic pain.[109,148,163] The RVM includes the raphe magnus, nucleus reticularis gigantocellularis-pars alpha, and the nucleus paragigantocellularis lateralis.[47] It is the final common relay in the descending modulation of pain, integrating inputs from PAG and other subcortical and cortical structures to the spinal dorsal horn as well as the trigeminal nucleus caudalis (SpVc).[47,67] There is growing evidence that imbalance between facilitatory and suppressive outputs from RVM to spinal neurons contributes to chronic pain states (reviewed in Denk et al.,[36] Heinriche et al.,[67] and Ossipov et al.[109]).

Both the PAG and RVM are implicated directly in mediating negative affect, and in affective disorders. As mentioned earlier,

Hohmann, Neugebauer, and their collaborators[158] demonstrated that stress-induced analgesia is critically dependent on both the PAG and the RVM. In rats, prolonged electrical stimulation of PAG produces lasting and profound increases in measures of negative affect.[159] Buhle et al.[22] showed that two conditions known to elicit strong emotional responses—physical pain and negative image viewing—both enhance negative affect and PAG activity in humans.

Human imaging suggests that patients with fibromyalgia have significant disruptions in the functional connectivity of the PAG, particularly with brain regions implicated in negative affect, and that these reductions are associated with worse fibromyalgia impact scores. These findings suggest that the PAG is a site of dysfunction contributing to the clinical manifestations and pain.[29] In addition, human imaging studies reveal representation of aversive prediction errors in the PAG.[122]

"Social pain" is thought of as a painful perception elicited by impactful life experiences, such as romantic rejection. Koban et al.[82] recently compared, in human subjects, the effects of placebo treatment on both noxious (heat) stimuli and on social pain. Placebo treatment reduced both social and physical pain, and increased activity in the prefrontal cortex in both modalities. Placebo further altered the relationship between affect and both prefrontal cortex and PAG activity during social pain. Koban et al.[82] also demonstrated that the effects on behavior were mediated by a pathway connecting prefrontal cortex to the PAG. These findings suggest that placebo treatments reduce emotional distress by altering affective representations in frontal brainstem systems.

Corticotrigeminal Pathways

Besides these indirect pathways, the neocortex provides dense anatomical projections that directly target second-order neurons in the spinal cord and the trigeminal nuclei. Brodal et al.[20] provided one of the first descriptions of direct projections from cortical areas, in the cat, to sensory trigeminal nuclei. Subsequent work in cats showed direct inputs from primary somatosensory cortex (SI)[41] and the second somatosensory cortex (SII)[138] to the spinal subnucleus caudalis (or SpVc), the target of primary nociceptive afferents from the head and neck.[40] In rats, direct inputs to SpVc arise from SI, SII, and from the insula,[56,88,107,154,] and the inputs from SI are somatoscopically organized.[156] Efferents from SI and SII in the rat diverge to target overlapping regions in SpVc.[132] SI projects directly to trigeminal nuclei also in the mouse.[65]

That these corticotrigeminal pathways affect sensory processing was demonstrated more than a century ago.[68] Researchers showed that corticotrigeminal inhibitory influences may occur through both presynaptic and postsynaptic mechanisms.[31] We, and others, have shown that these influences strongly affect nociceptive processing in trigeminal nuclei, and thereby modulate pain perception.[27,56,89,154]

As discussed in the following section, cortical areas contributing—both directly (e.g. corticotrigeminal) or indirectly (via PAG/RVM)—to descending pain modulation are critically involved also in regulating affect. Therefore, these pathways are likely involved in interactions between pain and negative affect.

Thalamus and Cortex

Thalamocortical and corticothalamic interactions gate, modulate, and process information related to nearly all aspects of sensation, perception, affect, cognition, and motor control.[127] It is therefore not surprising to find evidence that thalamocortical-corticothalamic pathways are critically involved in pain-affect interactions. Neuroimaging studies demonstrate that nociceptive inputs almost always result in activation in SI and SII cortex, insular cortex, anterior cingulate cortex (ACC), and related thalamic nuclei. At the risk of phernological simplification, it can be stated that SI is associated with sensory-discriminative aspects of pain, SII has both sensory and affective/cognitive functions, and the insula and ACC are important for affective-motivational and certain cognitive aspects of pain, including anticipation, attention, and evaluation.[105] The medial prefrontal cortex (mPFC) has important interactions with both the amygdala and descending pain modulatory pathways—both described earlier—through which pain and affect can modulate each other.

Such interactions have been demonstrated in human imaging studies. These studies have shown, for example, that negative affect, pain, and cognitive control activate overlapping regions in the cingulate cortex.[126] Emotional states affect pain unpleasantness, and the magnitude of this effect often correlates with altered pain-evoked ACC activations.[151] In addition, combining imaging with a delayed-discrimination task in healthy volunteers[145] showed that brain regions involved in this working memory encoding process are dissociable, according to whether the stimulus was painful. The medial thalamus and the cingulate cortex were found to encode painful stimuli, and SI encoded innocuous stimuli. Furthermore, encoding of painful stimuli significantly enhanced functional connectivity between the thalamus and mPFC. Tseng et al.[145] also found that participants with higher anxiety levels showed significant performance advantages when encoding painful stimuli. It is notable that only during the encoding of pain were the interindividual differences in anxiety associated with the strength of coupling between medial thalamus and mPFC, which was furthermore related to activity in the amygdala.

A Brighter Future?

The other side of the coin of the chronic pain–affective disorders link is that treatments directed at one condition may alleviate the burden of the other. This notion is supported by several clinical studies. For example, Davis et al.[33] showed that, in depressed women with pain, improving mood ameliorates pain recovery. Thus interventions that address the negative affect of patients with chronic pain may help lessen pain.

Light therapy, which has been used effectively to control depression,[58,98] can also alleviate pain (at least in animals), possibly by acting through central opioid mechanisms and descending pain modulation.[74] More invasive interventions may also be appropriate in severe cases. Vagus nerve stimulation—an apparent panacea for a myriad of conditions[5]— may alleviate both pain and depression.[30]

There exist multiple anatomical substrates that provide for direct and potent interactions between pathways that process and modulate pain and affect. These interactions play a role in the amplification of pain perception by negative affect, and in the exacerbation of depression and anxiety that plagues patients with chronic pain. Yet, there is promise that a more complete understanding of the interactions between mechanisms related to pain and affective disorders will lead to novel approaches to treat these crippling conditions.

References

1. Abeles M, Solitar BM, Pillinger MH, Abeles AM. Update on fibromyalgia therapy. *Am J Med.* 2008;121(7):555–561.
2. Amit Z, Galina ZH. Stress-induced analgesia: adaptive pain suppression. *Physiol Rev.* 1986;66(4):1091–1120.
3. Apkarian AV, Baliki MN, Geha PY. Towards a theory of chronic pain. *Prog Neurobiol.* 2009;87(2):81–97.
4. Apkarian AV, Bushnell MC, Treede RD, Zubieta JK. Human brain mechanisms of pain perception and regulation in health and disease. *Eur J Pain.* 2005;9(4):463–484.
5. Attenello F, Amar AP, Liu C, Apuzzo ML. Theoretical Basis of Vagus Nerve Stimulation. *Prog Neurol Surg.* 2015;29:20–28.
6. Auvray M, Myin E, Spence C. The sensory-discriminative and affective-motivational aspects of pain. *Neurosci Biobehav Rev.* 2010;34(2):214–223.
7. Bair MJ, Robinson RL, Katon W. Depression and pain comorbidity: a literature review. *Arch Intern Med.* 2003;163(20):2433–2445.
8. Bair MJ, Wu J, Damush TM, Sutherland JM, Kroenke K. Association of depression and anxiety alone and in combination with chronic musculoskeletal pain in primary care patients. *Psychosom Med.* 2008;70(8):890–897.
9. Baliki MN, Geha PY, Fields HL, Apkarian AV. Predicting value of pain and analgesia: nucleus accumbens response to noxious stimuli changes in the presence of chronic pain. *Neuron.* 2010;66(1):149–160.
10. Baptista-de-Souza D, Nunciato AC, Pereira BC, Fachinni G, Zaniboni CR, Canto-de-Souza A. Mice undergoing neuropathic pain induce anxiogenic-like effects and hypernociception in cagemates. *Behav Pharmacol.* 2015;26:664–672 (7 Spec No).
11. Becker S, Gandhi W, Schweinhardt P. Cerebral interactions of pain and reward and their relevance for chronic pain. *Neurosci Lett.* 2012;520(2):182–187.
12. Beecher HK. Pain in men wounded in battle. *Ann Surg.* 1946;123(1):96–105.
13. Bennett GJ. What is spontaneous pain and who has it. *J Pain.* 2012;13(10):921–929.
13a. Becerra L, Breiter HC, Wise R, Gonzalez RG, Borsook D. Reward circuitry activation by noxious thermal stimuli. *Neuron.* 2001;32:927–946.
14. Boivie J. Central pain. In: Wall PD, McMahon SB, Koltzenburg M, eds. *Wall and Melzack's Textbook of Pain.* Philadelphia: Elsevier/Churchill Livingstone; 2006:1057–1074.
15. Bonica JJ. *The Management of Pain; with Special Emphasis on the Use of Analgesic Block in Diagnosis, Prognosis, and Therapy.* Philadelphia: Lea & Febiger; 1953.
16. Bourgeais L, Monconduit L, Villanueva L, Bernard JF. Parabrachial internal lateral neurons convey nociceptive messages from the deep laminas of the dorsal horn to the intralaminar thalamus. *J Neurosci.* 2001;21(6):2159–2165.
17. Bowsher D. Termination of the central pain pathway in man: the conscious appreciation of pain. *Brain.* 1957;80(4):606–622.
18. Brischoux F, Chakraborty S, Brierley DI, Ungless MA. Phasic excitation of dopamine neurons in ventral VTA by noxious stimuli. *Proc Natl Acad Sci U S A.* 2009;12:4894–4899.
19. Britt JP, Benalioued F, McDevitt RA, Stuber GD, Wise RA, Bonci A. Synaptic and behavioral profile of multiple glutamatergic inputs to the nucleus accumbens. *Neuron.* 2012;76(4):790–803.
20. Brodal A, Szabo T, Torvik A. Corticofugal fibers to sensory trigeminal nuclei and nucleus of solitary tract; an experimental study in the cat. *J Comp Neurol.* 1956;106(2):527–555.
21. Bromberg-Martin ES, Matsumoto M, Hikosaka O. Dopamine in motivational control: rewarding, aversive, and alerting. *Neuron.* 2010;68(5):815–834.
22. Buhle JT, Kober H, Ochsner KN, et al. Common representation of pain and negative emotion in the midbrain periaqueductal gray. *Soc Cogn Affect Neurosci.* 2013;8(6):609–616.
23. Burns JW, Bruehl S, France CR, et al. Psychosocial factors predict opioid analgesia through endogenous opioid function. *Pain.* 2017;158(3):391–399.
24. Bushnell MC, Ceko M, Low LA. Cognitive and emotional control of pain and its disruption in chronic pain. *Nat Rev Neurosci.* 2013;14(7):502–511.
25. Butler RK, Finn DP. Stress-induced analgesia. *Prog Neurobiol.* 2009;88(3):184–202.
26. Campbell G, Darke S, Bruno R, Degenhardt L. The prevalence and correlates of chronic pain and suicidality in a nationally representative sample. *Aust N Z J Psychiatry.* 2015;49(9):803–811.
27. Castro A, Raver C, Li Y, et al. Cortical regulation of nociception of the trigeminal nucleus caudalis. *J Neurosci.* 2017;37(47):11431–11440.
28. Cooper S, Robison AJ, Mazei-Robison MS. Reward circuitry in addiction. *Neurotherapeutics.* 2017;14(3):687–697.
29. Coulombe MA, Lawrence KS, Moulin DE, et al. Lower functional connectivity of the periaqueductal gray is related to negative affect and clinical manifestations of fibromyalgia. *Front Neuroanat.* 2017;11:47.
30. Craig AD. Human feelings: why are some more aware than others? *Trends Cogn Sci.* 2004;8(6):239–241.
31. Darian-Smith I, Yokota T. Corticofugal effects on different neuron types within the cat's brain stem activated by tactile stimulation of the face. *J Neurophysiol.* 1966;29(2):185–206.
32. Davis KD, Kwan CL, Crawley AP, Mikulis DJ. Functional MRI study of thalamic and cortical activations evoked by cutaneous heat, cold, and tactile stimuli. *J Neurophysiol.* 1998;80(3):1533–1546.
33. Davis MC, Thummala K, Zautra AJ. Stress-related clinical pain and mood in women with chronic pain: moderating effects of depression and positive mood induction. *Ann Behav Med.* 2014;48(1):61–70.
34. De Peuter S, Van Diest I, Vansteenwegen D, Van den Bergh O, Vlaeyen JW. Understanding fear of pain in chronic pain: interoceptive fear conditioning as a novel approach. *Eur J Pain.* 2011;15(9):889–894.
35. deCharms RC, Maeda F, Glover GH, et al. Control over brain activation and pain learned by using real-time functional MRI. *Proc Natl Acad Sci U S A.* 2005;102(51):18626–18631.
36. Denk F, McMahon SB, Tracey I. Pain vulnerability: a neurobiological perspective. *Nat Neurosci.* 2014;17(2):192–200.
37. Dimova V, Horn C, Parthum A, et al. Does severe acute pain provoke lasting changes in attentional and emotional mechanisms of pain-related processing? A longitudinal study. *Pain.* 2013;154(12):2737–2744.
38. DosSantos MF, Moura BS, DaSilva AF. Reward circuitry plasticity in pain perception and modulation. *Front Pharmacol.* 2017;8:790.
39. Dubner R, Ren K. Endogenous mechanisms of sensory modulation. *Pain.* 1999;(suppl 6):S45–S53.
40. Dubner R, Ren K. Brainstem mechanisms of persistent pain following injury. *J Orofac Pain.* 2004;18(4):299–305.
41. Dunn RCJ, Tolbert DL. The corticotrigeminal projection in the cat. A study of the organization of cortical projections to the spinal trigeminal nucleus. *Brain Res.* 1982;240(1):13–25.
42. Edwards RR, Smith MT, Kudel I, Haythornthwaite J. Pain-related catastrophizing as a risk factor for suicidal ideation in chronic pain. *Pain.* 2006;126(1-3):272–279.
43. Elman I, Borsook D. Common brain mechanisms of chronic pain and addiction. *Neuron.* 2016;89(1):11–36.
44. Elman I, Borsook D, Volkow ND. Pain and suicidality: insights from reward and addiction neuroscience. *Prog Neurobiol.* 2013;109:1–27.
45. Fegg M, Kraus S, Graw M, Bausewein C. Physical compared to mental diseases as reasons for committing suicide: a retrospective study. *BMC Palliat Care.* 2016;15:14.
46. Fields HL. Pain modulation: expectation, opioid analgesia and virtual pain. *Prog Brain Res.* 2000:122245–122253.

47. Fields HL, Basbaum AI, Heinricher MM. Central nervous system mechanisms of pain modulation. In: McMohan SB, Koltzenburg M, Tracey I, eds. *Wall and Melzack's Textbook of Pain*. Philadelphia: Elsevier; 2006:125–142.

48. Finnerup NB, Attal N, Haroutounian S, et al. Pharmacotherapy for neuropathic pain in adults: a systematic review and meta-analysis. *Lancet Neurol*. 2015;14(2):162–173.

49. Fischerauer SF, Talaei-Khoei M, Vissers FL, Chen N, Vranceanu AM. Pain anxiety differentially mediates the association of pain intensity with function depending on level of intolerance of uncertainty. *J Psychiatr Res*. 2017;97:30–37.

50. Fishbain DA, Cutler R, Rosomoff HL, Rosomoff RS. Chronic pain-associated depression: antecedent or consequence of chronic pain? A review. *Clin J Pain*. 1997;13(2):116–137.

51. Ford GK, Finn DP. Clinical correlates of stress-induced analgesia: evidence from pharmacological studies. *Pain*. 2008;140(1):3–7.

52. Fuss J, Steinle J, Bindila L, et al. A runner's high depends on cannabinoid receptors in mice. *Proc Natl Acad Sci U S A*. 2015;112(42): 13105–13108.

53. Gauriau C, Bernard JF. Pain pathways and parabrachial circuits in the rat. *Exp Physiol*. 2002;87(2):251–258.

54. Giesecke T, Gracely RH, Williams DA, Geisser ME, Petzke FW, Clauw DJ. The relationship between depression, clinical pain, and experimental pain in a chronic pain cohort. *Arthritis Rheum*. 2005;52(5):1577–1584.

55. Gilron I, Max MB. Combination pharmacotherapy for neuropathic pain: current evidence and future directions. *Expert Rev Neurother*. 2005;5(6):823–830.

56. Gojyo F, Sugiyo S, Kuroda R, et al. Effects of somatosensory cortical stimulation on expression of c-Fos in rat medullary dorsal horn in response to formalin-induced noxious stimulation. *J Neurosci Res*. 2002;68(4):479–488.

57. Gold MS, Gebhart GF. Nociceptor sensitization in pain pathogenesis. *Nat Med*. 2010;16(11):1248–1257.

58. Golden RN, Gaynes BN, Ekstrom RD, et al. The efficacy of light therapy in the treatment of mood disorders: a review and meta-analysis of the evidence. *Am J Psychiatry*. 2005;162(4):656–662.

59. Gray D, Coon H, McGlade E, et al. Comparative analysis of suicide, accidental, and undetermined cause of death classification. *Suicide Life Threat Behav*. 2014;44(3):304–316.

60. Greenspan JD, Ohara S, Sarlani E, Lenz FA. Allodynia in patients with post-stroke central pain (CPSP) studied by statistical quantitative sensory testing within individuals. *Pain*. 2004;109(3):357–366.

61. Gross C, Hen R. The developmental origins of anxiety. *Nat Rev Neurosci*. 2004;5(7):545–552.

62. Grupe DW, Nitschke JB. Uncertainty and anticipation in anxiety: an integrated neurobiological and psychological perspective. *Nat Rev Neurosci*. 2013;14(7):488–501.

63. Gustin SM, Wilcox SL, Peck CC, Murray GM, Henderson LA. Similarity of suffering: equivalence of psychological and psychosocial factors in neuropathic and non-neuropathic orofacial pain patients. *Pain*. 2011;152(4):825–832.

64. Hassett AL, Aquino JK, Ilgen MA. The risk of suicide mortality in chronic pain patients. *Curr Pain Headache Rep*. 2014;18(8):436.

65. Hattox AM, Nelson SB. Layer V neurons in mouse cortex projecting to different targets have distinct physiological properties. *J Neurophysiol*. 2007;98(6):3330–3340.

66. Haythornthwaite JA, Sieber WJ, Kerns RD. Depression and the chronic pain experience. *Pain*. 1991;46(2):177–184.

67. Heinriche MM, Tavares I, Leith JL, Lumb BM. Descending control of nociception: specificity, recruitment and plasticity. *Brain Res Rev*. 2009;60(1):214–225.

68. Hernandez-Peon R, Hagbarth KE. Interaction between afferent and cortically induced reticular responses. *J Neurophysiol*. 1955;18(1):44–55.

69. Hohmann AG, Suplita RL, Bolton NM, et al. An endocannabinoid mechanism for stress-induced analgesia. *Nature*. 2005;435(7045):1108–1112.

70. Holland PC, Gallagher M. Amygdala-frontal interactions and reward expectancy. *Curr Opin Neurobiol*. 2004;14(2):148–155.

71. Hong S, Fan J, Kemmerer ES, Evans S, Li Y, Wiley JW. Reciprocal changes in vanilloid (TRPV1) and endocannabinoid (CB1) receptors contribute to visceral hyperalgesia in the water avoidance stressed rat. *Gut*. 2009;58(2):202–210.

72. Hooley JM, Franklin JC, Nock MK. Chronic pain and suicide: understanding the association. *Curr Pain Headache Rep*. 2014;18(8):435.

73. Hubbard CS, Karpowicz JM, Furman AJ, da Silva JT, Seminowicz DA, Traub RJ. Estrogen-dependent visceral hypersensitivity following stress in rats: an fMRI study. *Mol Pain*. 2016;12.

74. Ibrahim MM, Patwardhan A, Gilbraith KB, et al. Long-lasting antinociceptive effects of green light in acute and chronic pain in rats. *Pain*. 2017;158(2):347–360.

75. Institute of Medicine. *Relieving Pain in America: A Blueprint for Transforming Prevention, Care, Education, and Research*; 2011.

76. Jarcho JM, Mayer EA, Jiang ZK, Feier NA, London ED. Pain, affective symptoms, and cognitive deficits in patients with cerebral dopamine dysfunction. *Pain*. 2012;153(4):744–754.

77. Jennings EM, Okine BN, Roche M, Finn DP. Stress-induced hyperalgesia. *Prog Neurobiol*. 2014;12:11–18.

78. Ji G, Sun H, Fu Y, Li Z, Pais-Vieira M, Galhardo V, et al. Cognitive impairment in pain through amygdala-driven prefrontal cortical deactivation. *J Neurosci*. 2010;30(15):5451–5464.

79. Jones L, Fabrizi L, Laudiano-Dray M, et al. Nociceptive cortical activity is dissociated from nociceptive behavior in newborn human infants under stress. *Curr Biol*. 2017;27(24):3846–3851.e3.

80. Kato K, Sullivan PF, Evengård B, Pedersen NL. Chronic widespread pain and its comorbidities: a population-based study. *Arch Intern Med*. 2006;166(15):1649–1654.

81. Keiflin R, Janak PH. Dopamine prediction errors in reward learning and addiction: from theory to neural circuitry. *Neuron*. 2015;88(2):247–263.

82. Koban L, Kross E, Woo CW, Ruzic L, Wager TD. Frontalbrainstem pathways mediating placebo effects on social rejection. *J Neurosci*. 2017;37(13):3621–3631.

83. Kroenke K, Jackson JL, Chamberlin J. Depressive and anxiety disorders in patients presenting with physical complaints: clinical predictors and outcome. *Am J Med*. 1997;103(5):339–347.

84. Langford DJ, Tuttle AH, Brown K, et al. Social approach to pain in laboratory mice. *Soc Neurosci*. 2010;5(2):163–170.

85. Laviolette SR, Grace AA. Cannabinoids potentiate emotional learning plasticity in neurons of the medial prefrontal cortex through basolateral amygdala inputs. *J Neurosci*. 2006;26(24):6458–6468.

86. LeDoux J. Fear and the brain: Where have we been, and where are we going? *Biological Psychiatry*. 1998;44(12):1229–1238.

87. Lomazzo E, Bindila L, Remmers F, et al. Therapeutic potential of inhibitors of endocannabinoid degradation for the treatment of stress-related hyperalgesia in an animal model of chronic pain. *Neuropsychopharmacology*. 2015;40(2):488–501.

88. Malmierca E, Chaves-Coira I, Rodrigo-Angulo M, Nuñez A. Corticofugal projections induce long-lasting effects on somatosensory responses in the trigeminal complex of the rat. *Front Syst Neurosci*. 2014;8:100.

89. Malmierca E, Martin YB, Nunez A. Inhibitory control of nociceptive responses of trigeminal spinal nucleus cells by somatosensory corticofugal projection in rat. *Neuroscience*. 2012;221:115–124.

90. Maren S. Synaptic mechanisms of associative memory in the amygdala. *Neuron*. 2005;47(6):783–786.

91. McCaffrey P. *Pain and Depression: A Comorbidity Conundrum*. Pain Research Forum; 2014.

92. McGaugh JL. The amygdala modulates the consolidation of memories of emotionally arousing experiences. *Annu Rev Neurosci*. 2004; 27:1–28.

93. Melzack R. From the gate to the neuromatrix. *Pain*. 1999;(suppl):6S121–6S126.

94. Melzack R, Casey KL. Sensory, motivational and central control determinants of pain. In: Kenshalo DR, ed. *The Skin Senses*. Springfield: Thomas; 1968:423–439.

95. Merskey H, Bogduk N. *Classification of Chronic Pain*. 2nd ed. 2012 (Revised).
96. Mitsi V, Zachariou V. Modulation of pain, nociception, and analgesia by the brain reward center. *Neuroscience*. 2016;338:81–92.
97. Morrison I, Lloyd D, di Pellegrino G, Roberts N. Vicarious responses to pain in anterior cingulate cortex: is empathy a multisensory issue. *Cogn Affect Behav Neurosci*. 2004;4(2):270–278.
98. Moscovici L. Bright light therapy for seasonal affective disorder in Israel (latitude 32.6 degrees N): a single case placebo-controlled study. *Acta Psychiatr Scand*. 2006;114(3):216–218; discussion 218.
99. Mousavi SH, Sekula RF, Gildengers A, Gardner P, Lunsford LD. Concomitant depression and anxiety negatively affect pain outcomes in surgically managed young patients with trigeminal neuralgia: Long-term clinical outcome. *Surg Neurol Int*. 2016;7:98.
100. Navratilova E, Morimura K, Xie JY, Atcherley CW, Ossipov MH, Porreca F. Positive emotions and brain reward circuits in chronic pain. *J Comp Neurol*. 2016;524(8):1646–1652.
101. Navratilova E, Porreca F. Reward and motivation in pain and pain relief. *Nat Neurosci*. 2014;17(10):1304–1312.
102. Navratilova E, Xie JY, Meske D, et al. Endogenous opioid activity in the anterior cingulate cortex is required for relief of pain. *J Neurosci*. 2015;35(18):7264–7271.
103. Navratilova E, Xie JY, Okun A, et al. Pain relief produces negative reinforcement through activation of mesolimbic reward-valuation circuitry. *Proc Natl Acad Sci U S A*. 2012;109(50):20709–20713.
104. Neugebauer V. Amygdala pain mechanisms. *Handb Exp Pharmacol*. 2015;227:261–284.
105. Neugebauer V, Galhardo V, Maione S, Mackey SC. Forebrain pain mechanisms. *Brain Res Rev*. 2009;60(1):226–242.
106. Neugebauer V, Li W, Bird GC, Han JS. The amygdala and persistent pain. *Neuroscientist*. 2004;10(3):221–234.
107. Noseda R, Constandil L, Bourgeais L, Chalus M, Villanueva L. Changes of meningeal excitability mediated by corticotrigeminal networks: a link for the endogenous modulation of migraine pain. *J Neurosci*. 2010;30(43):14420–14429.
108. Okubo M, Castro A, Guo W, et al. Transition to persistent orofacial pain after nerve injury involves supraspinal serotonin mechanisms. *J Neurosci*. 2013;33(12):5152–5161.
109. Ossipov MH, Morimura K, Porreca F. Descending pain modulation and chronification of pain. *Curr Opin Support Palliat Care*. 2014;8(2):143–151.
110. Paré D, Quirk GJ, Ledoux JE. New vistas on amygdala networks in conditioned fear. *J Neurophysiol*. 2004;92(1):1–9.
111. Peper E, Wilson VE, Gunkelman J, et al. 2006. Tongue piercing by a Yogi: QEEG observations. *Appl Psychophysiol Biofeedback*. 2006;31(4):331–338.
112. Phelps EA, LeDoux JE. Contributions of the amygdala to emotion processing: from animal models to human behavior. *Neuron*. 2005;48(2):175–187.
112a. Ploghaus A, Becerra L, Borras C, Borsook D. Neural circuitry underlying pain modulation: expectation, hypnosis, placebo. *Trends Cogn Sci*. 2003;7:197–200.
113. Potvin S, Grignon S, Marchand S. Human evidence of a supraspinal modulating role of dopamine on pain perception. *Synapse*. 2009;63(5):390–402.
114. Price DD. Psychological and neural mechanisms of the affective dimension of pain. *Science*. 2000;288(5472):1769–1772.
115. Price DD, Greenspan JD, Dubner R. Neurons involved in the exteroceptive function of pain. *Pain*. 2003;106(3):215–219.
116. Price DD, Verne GN, Schwartz JM. Plasticity in brain processing and modulation of pain. *Prog Brain Res*. 2006;157:333–352.
117. Quartana PJ, Campbell CM, Edwards RR. Pain catastrophizing: a critical review. *Expert Rev Neurother*. 2009;9(5):745–758.
118. Rainville P, Duncan GH, Price DD, Carrier B, Bushnell MC. Pain affect encoded in human anterior cingulate but not somatosensory cortex. *Science*. 1997;277(5328):968–971.

119. Rainville P, Feine JS, Bushnell MC, Duncan GH. A psychophysical comparison of sensory and affective responses to four modalities of experimental pain. *Somatosens Mot Res*. 1992;9(4):265–277.
120. Ren W, Centeno MV, Berger S, et al. The indirect pathway of the nucleus accumbens shell amplifies neuropathic pain. *Nat Neurosci*. 2016;19(2):220–222.
121. Rhudy JL, Williams AE, McCabe KM, Russell JL, Maynard LJ. Emotional control of nociceptive reactions (ECON): do affective valence and arousal play a role. *Pain*. 2008;136(3):250–261.
122. Roy M, Shohamy D, Daw N, Jepma M, Wimmer GE, Wager TD. Representation of aversive prediction errors in the human periaqueductal gray. *Nat Neurosci*. 2014;17(11):1607–1612.
123. Schur EA, Afari N, Furberg H, et al. Feeling bad in more ways than one: comorbidity patterns of medically unexplained and psychiatric conditions. *J Gen Intern Med*. 2007;22(6):818–821.
124. Schweinhardt P, Sauro KM, Bushnell MC. Fibromyalgia: a disorder of the brain? *Neuroscientist*. 2008;14(5):415–421.
125. Seminowicz DA, Davis KD. Pain enhances functional connectivity of a brain network evoked by performance of a cognitive task. *J Neurophysiol*. 2007;97(5):3651–3659.
126. Shackman AJ, Salomons TV, Slagter HA, Fox AS, Winter JJ, Davidson RJ. The integration of negative affect, pain and cognitive control in the cingulate cortex. *Nat Rev Neurosci*. 2011;12(3):154–167.
127. Sherman SM, Guillery RW. *Functional Connections of Cortical Areas : A New View from the Thalamus*. London, England ; Cambridge, Mass: The MIT Press; 2013.
128. Shi M, Qi WJ, Gao G, Wang JY, Luo F. Increased thermal and mechanical nociceptive thresholds in rats with depressive-like behaviors. *Brain Res*. 2010;1353:225–233.
129. Simon GE, VonKorff M, Piccinelli M, Fullerton C, Ormel J. An international study of the relation between somatic symptoms and depression. *N Engl J Med*. 1999;341(18):1329–1335.
130. Singer T, Seymour B, O'Doherty J, Kaube H, Dolan RJ, Frith CD. Empathy for pain involves the affective but not sensory components of pain. *Science*. 2004;303(5661):1157–1162.
131. Reference deleted in review.
132. Smith JB, Watson GD, Alloway KD, Schwarz C, Chakrabarti S. Corticofugal projection patterns of whisker sensorimotor cortex to the sensory trigeminal nuclei. *Front Neural Circuits*. 2015;9:53.
133. Smith JG, Elias LA, Yilmaz Z, et al. The psychosocial and affective burden of posttraumatic neuropathy following injuries to the trigeminal nerve. *J Orofac Pain*. 2013;27(4):293–303.
134. Smith ML, Hostetler CM, Heinricher MM, Ryabinin AE. Social transfer of pain in mice. *Sci Adv*. 2016;2(10):e1600855.
135. Stein BE, Price DD, Gazzaniga MS. Pain perception in a man with total corpus callosum transection. *Pain*. 1989;38(1):51–56.
136. Sullivan MJ, Rodgers WM, Kirsch I. Catastrophizing, depression and expectancies for pain and emotional distress. *Pain*. 2001a;91(1-2):147–154.
137. Sullivan MJ, Thorn B, Haythornthwaite JA, et al. Theoretical perspectives on the relation between catastrophizing and pain. *Clin J Pain*. 2001b;17(1):52–64.
138. Tashiro T, Matsuyama T, Higo S. Distribution of cells of origin of the corticotrigeminal projections to the nucleus caudalis of the spinal trigeminal complex in the cat. A horseradish peroxidase (HRP) study. *Exp Neurol*. 1983;80(1):178–185.
139. Taylor AM, Becker S, Schweinhardt P, Cahill C. Mesolimbic dopamine signaling in acute and chronic pain: implications for motivation, analgesia, and addiction. *Pain*. 2016;157(6):1194–1198.
140. Tegethoff M, Belardi A, Stalujanis E, Meinlschmidt G. Comorbidity of mental disorders and chronic pain: chronology of onset in adolescents of a national representative cohort. *J Pain*. 2015;16(10):1054–1064.
141. Tracey I. Getting the pain you expect: mechanisms of placebo, nocebo and reappraisal effects in humans. *Nat Med*. 2010;16(11):1277–1283.

142. Tracey I, Mantyh PW. The cerebral signature for pain perception and its modulation. *Neuron.* 2007;55(3):377–391.

143. Traub RJ, Cao DY, Karpowicz J, et al. A clinically relevant animal model of temporomandibular disorder and irritable bowel syndrome comorbidity. *J Pain.* 2014;15(9):956–966.

144. Treede RD, Apkarian AV, Bromm B, Greenspan JD, Lenz FA. Cortical representation of pain: functional characterization of nociceptive areas near the lateral sulcus. *Pain.* 2000;87(2):113–119.

145. Tseng MT, Kong Y, Eippert F, Tracey I. Determining the neural substrate for encoding a memory of human pain and the influence of anxiety. *J Neurosci.* 2017;37(49):11806–11817.

146. Upshur CC, Luckmann RS, Savageau JA. Primary care provider concerns about management of chronic pain in community clinic populations. *J Gen Intern Med.* 2006;21(6):652–655.

147. Valverde O, Ledent C, Beslot F, Parmentier M, Roques BP. Reduction of stress-induced analgesia but not of exogenous opioid effects in mice lacking CB1 receptors. *Eur J Neurosci.* 2000;12(2):533–539.

148. Vanegas H, Schaible HG. Descending control of persistent pain: inhibitory or facilitatory. *Brain Res Brain Res Rev.* 2004;46(3):295–309.

149. Vardeh D, Mannion RJ, Woolf CJ. Toward a mechanism-based approach to pain diagnosis. *J Pain.* 2016;17(suppl 9):T50–69.

150. Villemure C, Bushnell MC. Cognitive modulation of pain: how do attention and emotion influence pain processing? *Pain.* 2002;95(3):195–199.

151. Villemure C, Bushnell MC. Mood influences supraspinal pain processing separately from attention. *J Neurosci.* 2009;29(3):705–715.

152. Reference deleted in review.

153. Volkow ND, Morales M. The brain on drugs: from reward to addiction. *Cell.* 2015;162(4):712–725.

154. Wang J, Li ZH, Feng B, et al. Corticotrigeminal projections from the insular cortex to the trigeminal caudal subnucleus regulate orofacial pain after nerve injury via extracellular signal-regulated kinase activation in insular cortex neurons. *Front Cell Neurosci.* 2015;9:493.

155. Wiech K, Tracey I. Pain, decisions, and actions: a motivational perspective. *Front Neurosci.* 2013;7:46.

156. Wise SP, Murray EA, Coulter JD. Somatotopic organization of corticospinal and corticotrigeminal neurons in the rat. *Neuroscience.* 1979;4:65–78.

157. Wood PB, Schweinhardt P, Jaeger E, et al. Fibromyalgia patients show an abnormal dopamine response to pain. *Eur J Neurosci.* 2007;25(12):3576–3582.

158. Woodhams SG, Chapman V, Finn DP, Hohmann AG, Neugebauer V. The cannabinoid system and pain. *Neuropharmacology.* 2017;124:105–120.

159. Wright JS, Panksepp J. Toward affective circuit-based preclinical models of depression: sensitizing dorsal PAG arousal leads to sustained suppression of positive affect in rats. *Neurosci Biobehav Rev.* 2011;35(9):1902–1915.

160. Wu TH, Hu LY, Lu T, et al. Risk of psychiatric disorders following trigeminal neuralgia: a nationwide population-based retrospective cohort study. *J Headache Pain.* 2015;16:64.

161. Xie JY, Qu C, Patwardhan A, et al. Activation of mesocorticolimbic reward circuits for assessment of relief of ongoing pain: a potential biomarker of efficacy. *Pain.* 2014;155(8):1659–1666.

162. Yeung EW, Craggs JG, Gizer IR. Comorbidity of alcohol use disorder and chronic pain: genetic influences on brain reward and stress systems. *Alcohol Clin Exp Res.* 2017;41(11):1831–1848.

163. You HJ, Lei J, Sui MY, et al. Endogenous descending modulation: spatiotemporal effect of dynamic imbalance between descending facilitation and inhibition of nociception. *J Physiol.* 2010;588(Pt 21):4177–4188.

164. Yunus MB. Central sensitivity syndromes: a new paradigm and group nosology for fibromyalgia and overlapping conditions, and the related issue of disease versus illness. *Semin Arthritis Rheum.* 2008;37(6):339–352.

12

Genetic Vulnerability to Substance Use Disorders

CHAMINDI SENEVIRATNE AND BANKOLE A. JOHNSON

CHAPTER OUTLINE

Introduction

Genetic influences on addictive substance use vary across developmental stages of life. When an individual initiates substance use (i.e., experiments with drugs), environmental factors have a greater impact on his or her substance use patterns.[15,48,76] Access to drugs, peer pressure, and socioeconomic factors are all crucial determinants of an individuals' substance use patterns.[21,54,82] Environmental factors are especially important in adolescents, as more of their activities are under monitoring of authority figures (parental).[14,63] As an individual moves along the trajectory of continued heavy use, genetic influences become more prominent, and individual differences can be explained by the unique environmental conditions that interact with genetic factors.[37] Unlike in other complex psychiatric disorders, substance use disorders (SUDs) require exposure to and ingestion of the substance as an obligatory environmental component for the development of SUDs and related phenotypes.[3] Since the observation that the family history of substance use is a crucial component in developing SUDs,[24,50,66] the exploration of specific genetic loci contributing to the moderate to high heritability has become the goal of many genetic analyses in the addiction genetics field. This chapter discusses basic concepts utilized in the quest to find genes for SUD vulnerability and the most replicated findings to date, with an emphasis on biological relevance and dynamic changes of gene expression when exposed to the abused substances.

Heritability (*h²*) of SUDs

Heritability Based on Family, Adoption, and Twin Genetic Studies

The first empirical evidence for a genetic basis of SUDs comes from family, adoption, and twin studies carried out in the pre-genomic era. The traditional family studies were observational studies that reported familial aggregation of addictive phenotypes.[7,36,64,65] First-degree relatives of individuals with a SUD were reported to be at two times or more risk of developing a substance use problem compared with siblings of non–drug-dependent relatives.[56,83] These observational studies were, however, not designed to examine whether the familial clustering of addictive phenotypes were due to the environment, genes, or their interaction. Adoption and twin study designs were employed to tease apart genetic from environmental effects on addiction vulnerability.

Adoption study design compares the similarity in SUDs or patterns between adopted children and their biological parents with the adopted children and their adoptive parents or between adopted sibling pairs and biological sibling pairs. Several well-powered studies conducted in the United States and Europe in the 1970s and 1980s showed that the risk for developing an alcohol use disorder (AUD) was much greater in the offspring of alcoholics, even when children were raised by nonalcoholic foster parents.[9,28,62] The risk of developing an AUD was shown to be about four times greater in sons of alcoholics compared to sons of nonalcoholics adopted by nonalcoholic foster parents.[11] Furthermore, rearing by an alcoholic parent had a greater influence on alcohol abuse but not on alcohol dependence in the offspring, which suggested a strong genetic influence on dependence as a phenotype.[55] Similarly, the risk for nicotine dependence also was reported to be greater between biological siblings but not the adopted siblings, and the sons and their nicotine-dependent biological mothers.[30] The age at adoption is an important confounder of genetic effects in adoption studies, as early environmental exposures can overestimate genetic influences.[61]

Twin studies compare the agreement in the behavior between monozygotic (MZ) or identical twins who are genetically identical, and dizygotic (DZ) or fraternal twins who share on average 50% of their genetic makeup. The term *concordant* is used if both twins engage in the same behavior (e.g., they both drink heavily). A higher rate of concordance in MZ than DZ twins suggest that genetics likely contributes to addiction vulnerability in addition to environmental factors. Heritability of a phenotype is estimated statistically by modeling the percentage of variation in the phenotype that is explained by genes (heritability), experiences shared by family members (shared environment), and experiences unique to the individual (nonshared environment). Twin studies assume that both twins are exposed to equal environmental influences that affect their substance use behavior. If MZ twins are exposed to more similar environments than DZ twins are, twin studies provide inflated estimates of genetic influences on the phenotype.

The heritability estimates from family, adoption, and twin studies for addictive substances range from 40% to 70%, with lowest rates for hallucinogens and highest for cocaine addiction.[17] In addition to addiction, substance initiation and heaviness of use also are heritable phenotypes.[20] Some studies have suggested gender and race differences in heritability of SUDs,[51,58,84] but the replicability of these findings are not consistent across studies.[19,35] Notably, adoption and early twin studies are suggestive of genetic effects but do not imply any specific genetic loci for addiction vulnerability. Furthermore, data from these large twin registries also can be used to compare how one twin's dependence on a substance influences his/her co-twin becoming dependent on a different class of substances. In addition, there is only a modest amount of family data available to compare concordance in first- versus second-degree relatives. The existing evidence does not, however, support less concordance in second-degree relatives than we would anticipate based on the observed concordance in first-degree relatives.

SNP-Based Heritability (h^2_{SNP})

Estimation of heritability in traditional family, adoption, and twin studies relied on data from closely related individuals. The recent developments in the molecular genetics field allow estimation of heritability in unrelated individuals by using the variance explained by all single nucleotide polymorphisms (SNPs) used in genome-wide association (GWA) array—defined as h^2_{SNP}.[67,85] The definition for h^2_{SNP} is now extended to include variance explained by any set of SNPs, whether they are a set of candidate SNPs or all SNPs from whole-genome sequencing (WGS). Generally, heritability estimates captured by common SNPs (frequency >1%) for many substances are much lower than their initial estimates from classical genetic studies. A comparison of published twin study–based and SNP-based estimates of heritability for the five most widely used addictive substances in the United States (excluding prescription drugs) and related phenotypes are presented in Table 12.1. Possible reasons for the discrepancies between heritability estimates derived from twin and SNP-based methodologies are discussed further discussed in the section Missing Heritability.

TABLE 12.1	A Comparison of SNP-Based (h^2_{SNP}) and Twin Study–Based Heritability (h^2) Rates.	
SUDs and Related Phenotypes	h^2 [references]	h^2_{SNP} [references]
Alcohol use disorders	40–60[49,74]	33–40[49,79]
Problem drinking	43–50[13]	13–26[10,79]
Intoxication frequency	50[84]	
Nicotine use disorders	27–60[46,71]	38[79]
Number of cigarettes per day (CPD)	45–86[8,41]	0.68[6]
Smoking initiation	50–75[8,42,46]	15[6]
Tolerance	73[6]	29[6]
Withdrawal	9–53[6,57]	67[6]
Cannabis use disorders	51–72[39,75]	21[2]
Cannabis-use initiation	40–59[20,75]	6–25[53,75]
Opiate use disorders	23–54[38,72]	
Opiate-use initiation	58[20]	
Cocaine use disorders	42–79[38,72]	>80[a,70]
Cocaine-use initiation	14[20]	

[a]Heritability for a continuous variable created by summing up the number of positive responses to the seven DSM-IV cocaine dependence criteria with equal weights.
SNP, Single nucleotide polymorphisms; *SUDs*, substance use disorders.
All heritability estimates are given as percentiles and represent estimates in both genders.

Genetic Architecture of Addiction Vulnerability

Based on molecular genetic studies from the past few decades, we now know that the genetic architecture of vulnerability to developing an SUD using legal or illegal addictive substances in the population is polygenic and is influenced by variants in individual genes, and that each contributes modest amounts to this overall phenotypic variability. Most of the known genetic variations increase the risk for development, progression, and severity of SUDs. Although a few of the risk or protective genetic influences are specific to one class of substance, most of them influence neurobiological mechanisms common to SUDs regardless of the class of abused substance.

Mapping Genetic Loci Influencing Vulnerability to SUDs

Mapping of specific genetic loci that correlate with phenotypes/traits began with mapping DNA markers to chromosomes in affected family members of extensive pedigrees. This locus-driven linkage mapping approach identified chromosomal regions or loci containing many genes that cosegregated with several SUDs.

The first linkage analysis in AUD was carried out by the Collaborative Study on the Genomics of Alcoholism (COGA). This multisite study initially enrolled 10 nuclear and multigenerational families with 987 individuals. Findings of the first genome-wide linkage scan identified chromosomes 1 and 7 as conferring risk and chromosome 2 as being suggestive of protective effects for developing Diagnostic and Statistical Manual of Mental Disorders, Fourth Edition (DSM-IV) Alcohol Dependence. A follow-up study confirmed these loci and provided evidence of additional linkage to chromosome 3. The linkage locus on chromosome 4p harbors the *GABRA2/B1* cluster and was detected in early linkage analyses of both Southwestern Indian and Caucasian populations. Similarly, strong linkage signals are detected for nicotine addiction on chromosome 9q22 that harbors *GABRB1*. Many reviews are available on findings from other well-powered linkage analyses to identify chromosomal locations associated with vulnerability to develop nicotine, opioid, cocaine, and cannabis use disorders.[a]

The next stage of genetic mapping is highlighted by the search to identify specific alleles associated with SUDs. Genetic association studies are a form of linkage analyses based on alleles, rather than loci that consist of multiple genes. Four different association analyses approaches have been used to identify specific alleles: (1) fine mapping of chromosomal loci from linkage analyses; (2) hypothesis-driven candidate gene approaches; (3) GWAs using SNP arrays; and (4) GWAs based on DNA sequencing. A limited number of large studies were performed with samples collected from individuals with SUDs and their family members. The majority of association studies were performed with unrelated individuals from racially diverse populations with and without a diagnosis of SUDs. The statistical power to detect an association between a specific genetic variant affecting a complex phenotype such as SUD depends on: (1) the effect size of a genetic variant (mutation) affecting some aspect of SUD; (2) how many times the phenotype-affecting variant segregates in the studied population; (3) the number of such phenotype-affecting variants detected in the studied population; (4) the studied sample size; (5) heterogeneity of the trait being studied; and (6) coverage of the genetic panel used in the genome-wide association studies (GWAS) or candidate-based analyses to screen for variants.

Candidate Gene Analyses

Hypothesis-driven small-to-medium scale candidate gene analyses have been reported on a wide range of SUD-related phenotypes and analyzed in populations of different racial and geographic origins. Candidate gene analyses have now covered genes within almost all of the neurotransmitter systems, including γ-aminobutyric acid (GABA), serotonin, dopamine, and glutamate. Other candidate analyses have looked at substance-specific metabolic pathways, and neuroimmune, neuroendocrine, and cell-adhesion pathways.

Genome-Wide Association Results for Addiction

All analyses exploring genotype-phenotype associations with genetic data covering the entire genome can essentially be termed genome-wide association studies (or GWAS), irrespective of whether the acquisition of genotypes was based on sequencing or array-based technology. Application of GWAS in SUDs is now at least 10 years old. GWAS was initially designed as an experimental method to identify SNPs spanning the entire genome that contribute to complex disorders, especially those with polygenic genetic bases. That is, those derived from effects at many gene loci, each with modest effects through their interactions with environmental elements. To date, nearly 10,000 robust SNP-trait associations have been discovered by GWAS for complex traits across all areas of biomedical sciences that reach genome-wide statistical significance level of 5×10^{-8}.[78,81]

SNP Array-Based GWAS

Early GWAS in SUD focused mainly on SNP associations with the DSM-IV diagnosis of *substance dependence* as a trait. These early array-based GWAS compared allelic differences for SNPs in those who did not meet or who met any three of the seven DSM-IV criteria for substance dependence. The lack of precision of the phenotype is now being viewed as one of the reasons that led to *disappointing* results in the early GWAS era in addiction research. As the field of addiction genetics evolved, focus has shifted more toward quantitative and qualitative intermediate phenotypes or endophenotypes that constitute the broader phenotype of dependence. These secondary endophenotypes include the age at initiation of substance use, and the degree of substance use such as cigarettes per day or standard drinks per day. Individual studies have analyzed arrays consisting of about 2 million SNPs in Asian, African, and European populations of up to 20,000.

GWAS, as well as smaller candidate genotyping analyses, to date rely on the correlation structure, that is, linkage disequilibrium (LD) estimates that exist between variants in the human genome that process a causal effect on the trait and the genotyped variants in an experimental panel. This is one of the reasons that the commercially available SNP arrays are not yet powerful enough to capture the effects of causal rare variants. Apart from these conceptual issues, relatively smaller sample sizes to detect rare genetic effects and other technical limitations of SNP arrays have contributed to a lack of variant discovery in these studies. There are a number of excellent articles that discuss limitations of early GWAS studies in depth.[29,33,77] A commonly used strategy to gain some of the missed information from SNP array genotyping is to statistically infer (i.e., impute) the ungenotyped variants from haplotypes observed in a fully sequenced reference panel. Reference panels for European, African, and Asian ancestry human genomes are publicly available through large-scale population genome sequencing projects such as 1000 Genomes Project, International HapMap Project, and the Personal Genome Project Korea (http://opengenome.net/).

Sequencing-Based GWAS

The main difference between relatively cheaper SNP array based and whole genome sequencing (WGS) based is that the WGS association analyses provide a much larger coverage of the density of variations in the genome from very rare to common SNPs and other DNA variations that are several base pairs in length. Sequencing of large-scale samples is new to the addiction field and the data will provide evidence for the missing heritability.

Interactions Between Genetic and Environmental Factors

Analyses of twin studies for vulnerability to SUDs do not account for the possibility of large interactions between genetic and environmental effects (G×E interactions). Such large interactions may reduce the additive genetic and environmental contributions to addiction vulnerabilities. There are several types of G×E interactions described in the literature. One classification group's gene-environment influences into G×E *correlations* versus *interactions*.[16] G×E correlations occur when the genotype correlates (r) with the probability of exposure to an environmental factor to influence a disease phenotype. Whereas, G×E interactions are defined as occurring when the effect of the environmental exposure on an outcome is modified by genotype. The serotonin transporter (*SLC6A4*) variants contributing to interindividual differences in stress resilience is an example of a G×E interaction.[32]

Another classification is passive versus active versus reactive G×E.[34] A passive correlation occurs when parents transmit both genetic and environmental influences on a trait. Active G×E

---

[a]References 1, 22, 31, 43, 68, 73, 86.

correlation occurs when subjects of a certain genotype actively select environments that are correlated with that genotype. Reactive G×E correlation occurs when an individual's genotype provides different reactions to stimuli that come from the environment. Small values for c^2 influences of common environments shared by members of sib pairs appear to provide evidence against passive G×E correlations. Active and reactive G×E correlations remain possible.

Large interactions between genetic and environmental components would likely lead to differences in estimates of heritability from samples obtained in different environments and to differences in molecular genetic findings in individuals from different environments. As we have noted, data from studies of twins who were sampled from a number of different environments are nevertheless similar. Such convergence supports relatively modest G×E interactions between genetic and environmental influences on addiction vulnerability, at most. Modest G×E influences also are consistent with GWA molecular genetic results that identify substantial overlaps between the molecular genetics of vulnerability to dependence on illegal substances in samples from substantially different environments, such as the United States and Asia (see subsequent text).

Missing Heritability

The concept of missing heritability implies that better scrutiny of DNA sequence variations is required in thousands of more people to unearth more associations with addiction phenotypes.[25,47] The common variant associations detected in large-scale genotype-phenotype association studies have failed to explain all the heritability for addiction phenotypes. Many studies in the post-GWAS era have embarked on exploring the missing heritability employing various methodologies. These include (1) screening for rare variations of the DNA sequence; (2) polygenic risk score assessments; and (3) identifying epistatic effects.

Rare Variations of the DNA Sequence

Several rare variants also explain significant fractions of the genetic vulnerability for addiction that can modulate its effects. Advancements in genome sequencing have enabled the discovery of thousands of rare variations.[48] Although a few individuals are necessary to discover novel genetic variations, thousands of individuals are required to establish associations between rare variants and complex phenotypes such as addiction that present with a high individual variability. In fact, many more individuals are required to establish associations compared with common genetic variations. Even with the reducing costs of genome sequencing, it is still not cost-effective to sequence sample sizes powerful enough to detect rare variants associated with common phenotypes. Rare-variant genotyping chips are available as cheaper alternatives. A recent approach adopted in other fields of common phenotypes is to deconstruct the phenotypes into relatively homogeneous subgroups and explore rare variations within these extreme phenotype subcategories.

Assessing Polygenetic Risk Scores (PRS)

Polygenetic risk scores (PRS) sum statistically insignificant allelic effects of all variants within a gene or a genetic locus for a given trait. PRS is a particularly strong method for identifying unique environmental conditions under which the collective genetic effects are stronger. Currently, PRS has been applied to only a few SUD studies. One of the few studies showed that smoking and PRS increased with increased number of traumatic events.[52] Another study showed that lower parental knowledge was associated with low PRS and higher alcohol consumption.

Findings From SUD Genetic Studies

Genetic Contributions Specific to Substances

Notably, the effect sizes of genetic variants on phenotypic variation is modest, as would be expected for any complex disorder. Several large-scale consortia have done meta-analyses of GWAS data on the vulnerability to develop SUD and related substance use behaviors.

Genetics of alcohol use: Variations within genes for the enzymes involved with alcohol's metabolism are, by far, the most consistently replicated genetic associations with alcoholism phenotypes. Indeed, they have shown the largest effect size for the genetic contribution to alcohol addiction and use. Large-scale early linkage studies first reported a risk locus on chromosome 4q.[40,45] Successive analyses[18,26] found this region to harbor the alcohol dehydrogenase (*ADH*) gene cluster on chromosome 4q23.

Genetics of smoking-related traits: The strongest signals for smoking-related traits are detected in genes coding for the nicotine receptor subunits. Meta-analyses of GWAS have identified SNPs in the *CHRNA3*, *CHRNA5*, *CHRNA6*, *CHRNB3*, and *CHRNB4* genes. Genes coding for the enzymes involved in the nicotine metabolism pathway also were reported to confer risk for smoking in cytochrome P450 (CYP)2A6–CYP2B6.

Genetics of cannabis use–related phenotypes: Cannabis is the most widely used illicit substance worldwide. Frequent use can progress to addiction, with physical, psychological, and adverse social outcomes. The frequency of cannabis use is a heritable trait.[2] The International Cannabis Consortium was established with the goal of identifying specific genetic variants that conferred risk for increased use. That Consortium did meta-analyses of genomes from over 30,000 cannabis users. Even with the large sample size, researchers failed to identify any single SNP associated with cannabis use at a genome-wide significance level. Polygenic risk scores did, however, reveal four genes—*NCAM1*, *CADM2*, *KCNT2*, and *SCOC*—that were associated with lifetime cannabis use. These genes are not unique to cannabis use. Previous studies have identified that they also are associated with alcohol and nicotine use disorders as well as conduct disorders. For example, the association between the neuronal adhesion molecule 1 with nicotine dependence has been reported by many research groups.[4,5,23]

Many of the genetic influences on addiction vulnerability appear common to dependence on multiple different substances, although others appear to be substance-specific. These features suggest that many of the genetic influences on vulnerability to addiction are more likely to be related to underlying brain mechanisms that are common to addictions, and that fewer may be specific to the primary pharmacological properties of specific drugs, such as aspects of absorption, distribution, metabolism, or excretion.

Elsewhere we have suggested levels of analysis for pharmacogenomics and pharmacogenetics: (1) primary pharmacogenomics that describe the genetics of individual differences in the adsorption, distribution, metabolism, and/or excretion of a drug; (2) secondary pharmacogenomics that describe individual differences in drug targets, such as the G-protein-coupled receptors, transporters, and ligand-gated ion channels that are the primary targets of opiates, psychostimulants, and barbiturates, respectively; and (3) higher order pharmacogenomics that provide individual differences in post-receptor drug responses. Such postreceptor drug responses are more likely to be common to the actions of abused substances that come from several different chemical classes and act at distinct primary receptor or transporter sites in the brain. Based on the data for twins that are available currently, we posit that much of the human genetics of addiction vulnerability represents higher order pharmacogenomics.

Genetic Contributions Common to Behavioral Phenotypes Underlying SUDs

There are a few careful studies of the ways in which most human addiction vulnerabilities move through families (e.g., segregation analyses). No such study indicates a major gene effect on addiction vulnerability in most current populations. There is an exception: the flushing syndrome, whereby variants at the ALDH loci in Asian individuals do provide genes of major effect in this population. Individuals with these gene variants are at lower risk of becoming dependent on alcohol compared with individuals with other genotypes in the Chinese, Korean, Japanese, and other populations. Homozygous *ALDH2*2* individuals are strongly protected from alcohol dependence. Thus, this locus provides a good example of primary pharmacogenomics, although in a restricted population.

Quantity-frequency data for smoking also provide evidence for a replicable secondary pharmacogenomic effect of moderate magnitude. Markers in the chromosome 15 gene cluster that encodes the α3, α5, and β4 nicotinic acetylcholine receptors display different allelic frequencies in heavy versus light smokers in each of several studies. This chromosome 15 locus is likely to provide a good example of secondary pharmacogenomics, since it has not been associated reproducibly with dependence on other substances.

Linkage-based analyses for addiction vulnerabilities would be expected to reproducibly identify many of the genes whose variants exerted major influences on human addiction vulnerability. Existing linkage data for human dependence on alcohol, nicotine, and a number of other substances do, however, fail to provide any highly reproducible results that would support any major gene locus. These results appear to point to a negative conclusion: that no locus individually contributes a large fraction of the vulnerability to dependence on any addictive substance in most individuals. There are caveats. Many of these data come from subjects with largely European ethnic/racial backgrounds. Rare variants might well contribute disproportionate amounts to the vulnerability of individuals within a relatively few pedigrees. Nevertheless, as with many complex human disorders in which initial hopes for an easier (e.g., oligogenic, caused by variants in only a few genes) underlying genetic architecture supported the use of linkage approaches, the linkage peaks that are identified in each individual study may be more likely to arise on other bases when the underlying architecture is, in fact, polygenic.

Phenotypes That Might Have Contributed to Balancing Selection of Addiction-Related Alleles

It is tempting to speculate about the phenotypes that may have provided the basis for balancing or other selective processes for the common allelic variants that are observed in several current populations and influence vulnerability to substance dependence in current environments. Heritable, interrelated influences on cognitive abilities and brain volumes, especially of the frontal lobe,

provide interesting examples of such phenotypes. Both of these phenotypes are substantially heritable in data from twin studies. The heritability of both of these phenotypes is substantially correlated in twin study data. Samples of substance dependent individuals, although of modest size, reproducibly display smaller frontal lobes and poorer performance on tests of cognitive function. It is easy to see how cognitive function might have provided a selective pressure. When we consider the substantial mortality that cephalopelvic disproportion is likely to have caused in the environments in which our distant ancestors lived, it is easy to develop a plausible balancing selection hypothesis.

We have identified substantial, reproducible data for both of these phenotypes from GWA datasets, and identified large overlaps between the genes identified on the basis of cognitive abilities versus the genes identified on the basis of frontal lobe brain volumes, as expected.

Of interest, there also is significant overlap, more than expected by chance, between these sets of genes and those identified in comparing addicted versus control samples.

Personality traits that display substantial evidence for heritability are also found in substance-dependent individuals at rates different from those in the general population. A GWA dataset for the most addiction associated personality feature, neuroticism, displays highly significant overlap with data for substance dependence as well.

Psychiatric and Neurologic Comorbidity

Data for the highly heritable psychiatric diagnosis, bipolar disorder, is now available from four largely independent samples from European ancestries. Our clustering analyses for these datasets provide ample evidence of overlap between the results for bipolar disorder. Of interest, these data also overlap with the molecular genetic results for substance dependence to extents greater than chance.

Success in Smoking Cessation

Studies involving twins support the idea that an ability to successfully quit at least one of the major addictive substances, tobacco smoking, is substantially heritable. Much of this heritability apparently is not the same as the heritability for vulnerability to substance dependence, although some does overlap. We have recently reported GWA analyses of three datasets of smokers who were successful versus unsuccessful in quitting smoking in the context of a clinical trial. These results display gratifying convergence with each other and more modest, but still significant, overlap with results from vulnerability to become substance dependent, as would have been predicted by the results of classical genetic studies.

Failure of Control Experiments to Support Alternative Hypotheses for the Observed Genome-Wide Association Results

There also is no evidence that many of the clustered, reproducibly positive SNPs identified in these data cited earlier and a number of control comparisons, included controls for occult racial/ethnic differences and assay noise within each comparison group.

An Evolutionary Perspective on Genetic Architecture of Addiction

In line with the common disease-common allele model, which holds that complex diseases can be accounted for by a large number of common variants with individually small effects, most of the allelic variants detected in candidate and GWAS currently reported in addiction vulnerability are common and are thus likely to be old in an evolutionary sense.[44] Data indicating that such variants can be identified in diseased individuals from European, African, and Asian genetic backgrounds also point, in general, to variants of substantial age.

Our current understanding of human history increasingly points to long periods when most humans lived in Africa in relatively small groups that remained in relative genetic isolation from each other for many millennia. Such small groups can be viewed as competing with each other to provide the ancestry of most modern humans within and outside Africa. In thinking about how genetic selection might act on common functional allelic variants, it is thus important to consider how selective processes might act in early African environments of small groups of humans. No study of these early environments finds any strong evidence for the presence of any potent addictive substance. We, therefore, need to consider the ways in which selective processes might have operated in the absence of both addictive substances and in the absence of selective evolutionary pressures that can be attributed to use of addictive substances. As one starting point, it is conceivable that some currently common allelic variants could exert polygenic influences on addiction vulnerability without exerting any significant positive or negative selective effects during lengthy evolutionary histories. However, most such neutral variants would be expected to display evidence for genetic drift and related stochastic mechanisms that would provide fixation for their alleles long before current human populations were born (e.g., one allele would disappear on stochastic grounds).

Seemingly, many allelic variants that influence addiction vulnerability must have provided balancing selection. Balancing selection provides one of the few theoretical means for maintaining common allelic variants over extended periods. "In the era of molecular population genetics … balancing selection (refers to) loci (that display) levels of nucleotide polymorphism that exceed neutral expectation." We think of balancing selection as providing influences that are favorable in some individuals or organs or circumstances and unfavorable in other individuals or organs or circumstances.

Thinking about such balancing selection could have several consequences. First, the biology of some genes might allow for common, functional allelic variants that could escape selective pressures or exert balancing selection over many generations. By contrast, other genes might not be able to harbor such allelic variations without engendering selective pressures that would reduce the frequency of all but one of the allelic variants in the population over time. Common allelic variants that are able to influence addiction vulnerability are thus likely to be restricted to a subset of the genes whose products are involved in the addictive processes. An important consequence of this logic follows: If a gene fails to display variants that influence vulnerability to addiction, the gene's products are not at all excluded from involvement in addiction.

Second, the nature of balancing selection suggests strongly that addiction vulnerability alleles that display great evolutionary ages were likely to experience both positive and negative selection pressures that balanced based on their effects on other phenotypes, not addiction. Below, we summarize some of the current evidence that many addiction-vulnerability allelic variants might provide pleiotropic influences on a variety of related, heritable phenotypes.

In the context of this evolutionary discussion, balancing selection thus requires that an allelic variant influence a phenotype that can be subjected to balancing selection pressures in the absence of addictive substances. Put another way, convincing data that implicate a gene's common variants in addiction should prompt us to consider mechanisms whereby such variants might provide balancing (e.g., both positive and negative) selective influences in the differing environments through which the ancestors of current human populations have passed.

It is important to note that this logic is different from the logic of many other brain disorders that: (1) are also influenced by complex genetic determinants, but (2) which lead to reduced fertility in current populations and are thus likely to have provided substantial negative selection pressures in older environments. Such logic would lead to the conclusion that more newer allelic variants would be identified for these disorders.

How does this discussion of common disease/common allele hypotheses relate to the postulates of genetic heterogeneity noted earlier? None of the preceding discussions about common alleles and common variants preclude (or even reduce the likelihood of) contributions of rarer (or even "private") allelic variants, including those that have arisen more recently in evolutionary time. Recently arising variations would be much more likely to persist for a number of generations in the face of even moderately negative influences on survival or fertility. Indeed, based on experience with other genetic disorders, it may be worthwhile to actively search for effects of rarer phenocopy variants in genes that are initially identified based on common (and evolutionarily older) allelic variants. A rarer copy number variant might contribute to addiction vulnerability by altering expression levels of a gene that also contains more common allelic variants that alter expression via SNPs in other gene elements, for example. Such considerations support searches within identified loci for molecular genetic heterogeneity relevant to addiction.

The Genetic Architecture for Substance Dependence in Individuals

At a population level, a polygenic architecture describes a trait influenced by the small effects of many genes. When applied to individuals, this means that each individual with an SUD will carry several genetic variants (alleles) that increase and/or decrease the risk of developing a drug use problem at some point following the first exposure to a drug. Hence, the number of different unique combinations of these variants in a population can be in the hundreds, each affecting different aspects of drug addictive behavior or varying severity of a trait.

Both between-locus heterogeneity and within-locus heterogeneity are likely. Polygenic models for addiction vulnerability imply that each dependent individual might even display a nearly distinct set of risk-elevating or risk-reducing allelic variants. As an illustrative example, we might postulate that (1) an individual must display at least 75 risk alleles to significantly elevate his likelihood of acquiring a substance dependence disorder and (2) there are 300 genes that contain common allelic variants that can augment addiction risk. Under such circumstances, it is easy to see that the exact genetic recipe for addiction vulnerability found in one addicted individual might be replicated in only a relatively few other addicted individuals. Such an underlying genetic architecture would be consistent with the failure of linkage-based methods to provide reproducible results in addictions, since linkage relies on identifying consistent patterns in the ways that specific DNA markers and phenotypes move through many families that display high densities of the disorder.

As noted above, the best documented genetic heterogeneity for addictions comes from the chromosome 4 major gene effects found in poorly alcohol-metabolizing (flushing) Asian individuals. The best documented substance-specific influence comes from the chromosome 15 nicotinic acetyl cholinergic receptor gene cluster. There are likely to be other examples of between-locus genetic heterogeneity and of genes whose variants exert substance-specific effects on use and/or dependence that have yet to be elucidated.

We also postulate that within-locus heterogeneity is likely, although not yet clearly documented in addiction, to our knowledge. Many common Mendelian disorders and rarer Mendelian phenocopies of common disorders display substantial heterogeneity within their pathogenic loci. Evidence for within-locus heterogeneity in complex disorders is just beginning to be accrued; such evidence now includes data from neurexin gene family variants in autism.

Epigenetics and Individual Differences in SUDs

The term *epigenetics* was conceived by Conrad Waddington in the 1940s[80] by integrating concepts of epigenesis and genetics to define gene-environment interactions that influence embryological growth and differentiation. As the field of biochemistry advanced, the classical definition of epigenetics has moved toward emphasizing the importance of genetic and nongenetic factors in controlling gene expression downplaying developmental processes.[12,69] More recent definitions of epigenetics emphasize "...the study of any potentially stable and, ideally, heritable change in gene expression or cellular phenotype that occurs without changes in Watson Crick base-pairing of DNA."[27]

In the context of this chapter, heritable epigenetic influences are most relevant. One example of a classical, heritable epigenetic influence is imprinting. Imprinting conveys information from parent to child through mechanisms that include DNA methylation or histone acetylation. These mechanisms retain the primary DNA sequence but can dramatically alter function of specific genes. DNA methylation at CpG sequences in the promoter regions of genes can profoundly alter gene transcription. Since methylation during the course of maternal oocyte (or paternal sperm) development is key to this process, familial patterns of gender-specific transmission can provide evidence for this subset of heritable epigenetic influence.

The modest quality of current family datasets for addiction renders them a relatively weak basis for any strong inferences concerning parent-of-origin effects. Nevertheless, there is no segregation data of which we are aware that supports strong parent-of-origin effects on substance dependence. Thus, although there are obvious and large roles for nonheritable epigenetic influences in the biology of addiction, there is no current compelling evidence that there are any strong effects of overall heritable epigenetic influences, as classically defined. We nevertheless need to be alert for such influences as we unravel the effects of variants in specific genes.

Ethical Issues in High-Density Genotyping of Individuals With Substance Use Disorders

Individuals who are genotyped in relationship to addiction and related phenotypes are subject to a number of potential risks. Current SUD research is focused mainly on finding disease susceptibility variants and variants that are predictive of response to treatment or pharmacogenetics. Ethical issues in genetic studies can arise both during the conduct of research and in the manner in which the results are interpreted and used. Maintaining a healthy balance between gathering data and biological information while protecting the privacy and confidentiality of participants is imperative during the conduct of research. General measures such as employing appropriate consent procedures and obtaining federal confidentially certificates that can protect sensitive genetic data from legal subpoena are measures that apply to all human subject research, including addiction genetics research, to ensure participant privacy. More up-to-date information on these procedures is available on the NIH website (https://grants.nih.gov/policy/humansubjects/coc.htm; https://www.genome.gov/about-genomics/policy-issues/Informed-Consent).

The emergence of large-scale biobanks of samples and data and the use of electronic medical records (EMR) is another set of challenges that requires robust privacy measures. Current US regulations require de-identification to protect the confidentiality and privacy of research participants. Adequacy of de-identification is generally established by institutional review boards (IRBs).[11a] De-identification makes re-identification more difficult, but not impossible. For example, it has been shown that individuals can be identified with 30 to 80 statistically unlinked SNPs.[9a] This is an evolving topic that is increasingly discussed in the literature.

Another important ethical consideration is the cautious interpretation of genetic findings from individuals with SUDs. Individuals with SUDs are often socially and/or psychologically impaired and stigmatized by the society. Many of them suffer from low socio-economic and educational status, as well as psychological and physical comorbidities. While the general expectation among the scientific community is that the discovery of disease acceptability variants would help prevent SUDs in substance users, genetic literacy in the general public is limited. Most people believe that a single gene can alter specific human behaviors.[9b] Misconceptions such as the idea that the individuals with SUDs are biologically abnormal and incurable can negatively influence populations that are already vulnerable. It is extremely important that the researchers carefully communicate that SUDs are a product of complex interactions between genetic factors and various environmental conditions. Individual contributions of these genetic factors are small, and their functions depend on environmental conditions that the individuals are exposed to.

Summary and Conclusions

The rapid emergence of -omics data from thousands of individuals with substance use problems facilitates the unraveling of the contribution of genetics to the complexity of development and progression of SUDs at an ever-increasing pace. Findings from GWA analyses for dependence and related endophenotypes clearly indicate a striking convergence of genetic factors underlying different classes of addictive substances. The specific genetic variants detected to confer risk or protective effects in racially and geographically diverse populations to date are mostly common or prevalent in more than 1% of the population. Common allelic variants are evolutionarily old that they are present in members of each major racial population. These data, together with the results from smaller candidate association and linkage-based studies, support a polygenic genetic architecture for addiction with a substantial contribution of common allelic variants. Hence, the common disease/common variant (CD-CV) hypothesis on genetic architecture of complex disorders[59] holds true at least partially for SUD vulnerability. Such a genetic architecture is consistent with data from family, adoption, and twin classical genetic studies.

Recent *big data* generating efforts such as the NIH Big Data to Knowledge (BD2K) program, have also significantly advanced genetic discovery.[60] Many researchers have cautioned over the propensity to empiricism in big data mining over research based on theoretical frameworks. In this regard, secondary analyses performed on genome-wide big datasets that are accessible to the scientific community through resources such as *dbGAP*, have already begun to demonstrate how the genetic and environmental complexity uniquely captured in big datasets enables the generation and testing of new theoretical frameworks for neurobiologically defining the clinical construct termed SUD. The availability of data on thousands of genes from each individual enrolled in large-scale studies affords the testing of perturbations within networks of genes caused by drug use. At the time of the writing of this chapter, that characterizing of drug-induced perturbations within gene networks is at an initial stage. Few genome-wide gene expression studies have been conducted to date using blood cells in living individuals and postmortem brains from addicts. Furthermore, most of these analyses were performed with microarrays rather than newer RNA sequencing technology with isoform-level quantification.

Identification of addiction-associated variants in genes that are likely to alter underlying pathophysiology provides a first step toward defining a new neurobiology for the underpinnings of specific diseases and phenotypes. For many of these diseases and phenotypes, only little current research focuses on the direct study of brain connections. The connectivity constellation concepts that we introduce here support studies that develop and use current and novel means for assessing the qualities and quantities of brain connections, especially in the contexts in which they assess their functional properties. We have identified contributions of connectivity constellation genes to volumes of the same brain regions in which many of these genes are expressed. This convergence may provide new insights into data that documents individual differences in frontal lobe volume and/or in function, detected by volumetric, deoxyglucose positron emission tomography, and/or functional magnetic resonance imaging, for virtually all of the connectivity constellation phenotypes or disorders noted here.

The addiction vulnerability genes identified in this work contribute to the growing body of data that implicate cell adhesion and related memory-like and other cognitive processes in addiction. Studies that alter reconsolidation and other memory-related processes using knockout mice, protein synthesis inhibitors, and/or pharmacologic treatments demonstrate powerful influences on addictions. This empirical evidence enriches theoretical work that increasingly recognizes memory-like features for addiction and work that implicates memory-associated brain regions in relapse to addiction. Such work also complements clinical observations that document that the enhanced vulnerabilities of addicts to substance abuse relapse can persist for decades after their last use of addictive substances.

There is also substantial evidence for generalization of these results from addiction. This evidence comes from the significant overlaps between the molecular genetics of addiction and the molecular genetics of a number of related phenotypes and disorders. Overlap with bipolar disorder provides one of several likely psychiatric diagnoses for which shared genetic influences are likely a priori, based on the substantial heritabilities of both addiction and the high frequency of addiction/bipolar disorder comorbidity. This same logic suggests that abundant shared genetics may well also underpin the frequent comorbidities between addictions and antisocial personality/conduct disorders. Less-compelling evidence points to overlaps with other depressive, anxiety, and schizophrenic disorders as well.

We have sought evidence for genetic influences that are shared between addiction and (1) frontal lobe brain volumes and (2) cognitive function. Hypotheses about such shared genetic influences are based, in part, on initial observations that so many of the genes that we and others have identified in addiction GWA relate to cell connections. These molecularly based hypotheses were reinforced by the evidence for substantial, complex genetic components to each of these phenotypes. These hypotheses were strengthened by evidence, although often from small samples, that appears to document (1) small frontal lobe volumes in samples of addicts, (2) lower performance levels on tests of cognitive and executive function in samples of addicts, and (3) large roles of heritability versus little role for the drug exposure itself in determining the cognitive abilities of twin pair members who are discordant for cannabis use. These hypotheses are further reinforced by twin data that document strong shared genetic influences on frontal brain volumes and cognitive function measures.

Disease-associated markers both within and between genes can begin to allow us to assess individual differences in vulnerability to addiction based on profiles of genotypes. In settings in which prevention of addiction is sought, addiction vulnerability genomic profiles could help to target more (or different) prevention resources to individuals who are at the most (or at different) genetic risk. When a therapeutic opiate is being considered as therapy for chronic, noncancer pain, for example, the costs of engendering substance dependence are likely to be sufficient to justify genotyping even if the results provide only partial information about risk assessment and minimization for prescribing physicians. When treatment for an established dependence on nicotine, opiates, or alcohol is being contemplated, a number of different therapeutic options with different pharmacological mechanisms of action are now available. Subsets of the SNPs that we have associated with success in quitting smoking appear to provide selective influence on success in responding to bupropion, while others appear to provide selective influences on success in response to nicotine replacement. Replication and extension of these observations to treatments for alcohol, opiates, and other addictive substances will make it more and more likely that SNP markers will increasingly aid personalization of antiaddiction therapies within the near future, in ways that are now impacting the design of clinical trials in this area.

This work, taken together, supports the idea that the heritable brain bases for individual differences in addiction vulnerability lie squarely in the midst of the repertoire of common complex determinants of individual differences that are manifested in many heritable complex brain disorders and phenotypes. Such conclusions place the biology of addictions squarely in the midst of important biologies of a number of brain phenotypes and disorders, hopefully in ways that will benefit them all. Translation of genetic data into prevention and treatment: Knowing how the presence of certain genetic variations alters the expression of certain genes that affect biological pathways in ways that may result in chemical imbalances when exposed to drugs can identify candidates for targeted treatment. Knowing genetic variants that predispose individuals to risk-taking behaviors can be useful to improve preventative interventions. Deeper collaborations are needed.

Glossary

A priori: Existing in the mind prior to and independent of experiments.

Balancing selection: A natural process that results in the survival and reproductive success of individuals or groups best adjusted to their environment and that leads to the perpetuation of genetic qualities best suited to that particular environment.

Between-locus heterogeneity: A single disorder, trait, or pattern of traits caused by mutations in genes at different chromosomal loci.

Common disease and common allele model: The illness results from the cumulative impact of multiple common small-effect, genetic variants, interacting with environmental exposures to exceed a biological threshold.

Complex genetic phenotype (polygenic and multifactorial traits): Any *phenotype* that results from the effect of multiple *genes* at two or more loci, with possible environmental influences too.

Epigenetic: Changes in the regulation of the expression of gene activity without alteration of DNA sequence.

Epistasis: A mutation in one gene masks the expression of a different gene.

Genetic heterogeneity: A single disorder, trait, or pattern of traits caused by genetic factors in some cases and nongenetic factors in others.

Genetic selection: Differential and nonrandom reproduction of different genotypes operating to alter the gene frequencies within a population.

Genome-wide association study: Any study of genetic variation across the entire human genome that is designed to identify genetic associations with observable traits (such as blood pressure or weight), or the presence or absence of a disease or condition.

Linkage: The tendency for genes or segments of DNA closely positioned along a chromosome to segregate together at meiosis and therefore be inherited together.

Linkage analysis: Study of chromosomal segments that co-segregate with a disease phenotype through families.

Linkage disequilibrium: In a population, co-occurrence of a specific DNA marker and a disease at a higher frequency than would be predicted by random chance.

Pharmacogenetics: The study focused on specific genes, such as drug-metabolizing enzymes.

Pharmacogenomics: The study of how an individual's genomic system affects the body's response to drugs.

Pleiotropy: Multiple, often seemingly unrelated, physical effects caused by a single altered gene or pair of altered genes.

Segregation analysis: The determination of the number of progeny that have inherited distinct and mutually exclusive phenotypes.

Susceptibility gene: A gene mutation that increases the likelihood that an individual will develop a certain disease or disorder. When such a mutation is inherited, development of symptoms is more likely but not certain.

Transitive: Passing over to or affecting something else.

Within-locus heterogeneity: A single disorder, trait, or pattern of traits influenced by several different variants at a single chromosomal locus.

References

1. Agrawal A, Lynskey MT. The genetic epidemiology of cannabis use, abuse and dependence. *Addiction.* 2006;101(6):801–812.
2. Agrawal A, Lynskey MT, Bucholz KK, et al. DSM-5 cannabis use disorder: a phenotypic and genomic perspective. *Drug Alcohol Depend.* 2014;134:362–369.
3. American Psychiatric Association. *Diagnostic Criteria from DSM-IV-TR.* Washington, D.C.: American Psychiatric Association; 2000.
4. Bidwell LC, McGeary JE, Gray JC, Palmer RH, Knopik VS, MacKillop J. NCAM1-TTC12-ANKK1-DRD2 variants and smoking motives as intermediate phenotypes for nicotine dependence. *Psychopharmacology (Berl).* 2015;232(7):1177–1186.
5. Bidwell LC, McGeary JE, Gray JC, Palmer RH, Knopik VS, MacKillop J. An initial investigation of associations between dopamine-linked genetic variation and smoking motives in African Americans. *Pharmacol Biochem Behav.* 2015;138:104–110.
6. Bidwell LC, Palmer RH, Brick L, McGeary JE, Knopik VS. Genome-wide single nucleotide polymorphism heritability of nicotine dependence as a multidimensional phenotype. *Psychol Med.* 2016;46(10):2059–2069.
7. Bowers Jr MB. Family history and early psychotogenic response to marijuana. *J Clin Psychiatry.* 1998;59(4):198–199.
8. Broms U, Silventoinen K, Madden PA, Heath AC, Kaprio J. Genetic architecture of smoking behavior: a study of Finnish adult twins. *Twin research and human genetics : the official journal of the International Society for Twin Studies.* 2006;9(1):64–72.
9. Cadoret RJ, Cain CA, Grove WM. Development of alcoholism in adoptees raised apart from alcoholic biologic relatives. *Arch Gen Psychiatry.* 1980;37(5):561–563.
9a. Chapman AR, Carter A, Kaplan JM, Morphett K, Hall W. Ethical guidelines for genetic research on alcohol addiction and its applications. *Kennedy Inst Ethics J.* 2018;28(1):1–22.
9b. Christensen KD, Jayaratne TE, Roberts JS, Kardia SL, Petty EM. Understandings of basic genetics in the United States: results from a national survey of black and white men and women. *Public Health Genomics.* 2010;13(7-8):467–476.
10. Clarke TK, Adams MJ, Davies G, et al. Genome-wide association study of alcohol consumption and genetic overlap with other health-related traits in UK Biobank (N=112 117). *Mol Psychiatry.* 2017;22(10):1376–1384.
11. Cotton NS. The familial incidence of alcoholism: a review. *J Stud Alcohol.* 1979;40(1):89–116.
11a. Dankar FK, Ptitsyn A, Dankar SK. The development of large-scale de-identified biomedical databases in the age of genomics-principles and challenges. *Hum Genomics.* 2018;12(1):19.
12. Deans C, Maggert KA. What do you mean, "epigenetic"? *Genetics.* 2015;199(4):887–896.
13. Derks EM, Vink JM, Willemsen G, van den Brink W, Boomsma DI. Genetic and environmental influences on the relationship between adult ADHD symptoms and self-reported problem drinking in 6024 Dutch twins. *Psychol Med.* 2014;44(12):2673–2683.
14. Dick DM. Gene-environment interaction in psychological traits and disorders. *Annu Rev Clin Psychol.* 2011;7:383–409.
15. Dick DM. The Genetics of Addiction: Where Do We Go From Here? *J Studies Alcohol Drugs.* 2016;77(5):673–675.
16. Ducci F, Goldman D. Genetic approaches to addiction: genes and alcohol. *Addiction.* 2008;103(9):1414–1428.
17. Ducci F, Goldman D. The genetic basis of addictive disorders. *Psychiatr Clin North Am.* 2012;35(2):495–519.
18. Edenberg HJ, Xuei X, Chen HJ, et al. Association of alcohol dehydrogenase genes with alcohol dependence: a comprehensive analysis. *Hum Mol Genet.* 2006;15(9):1539–1549.

19. Ehlers CL, Gizer IR, Vieten C, et al. Age at regular drinking, clinical course, and heritability of alcohol dependence in the San Francisco family study: a gender analysis. *Am J Addict*. 2010;19(2):101–110.
20. Ehlers CL, Wall TL, Corey L, Lau P, Gilder DA, Wilhelmsen K. Heritability of illicit drug use and transition to dependence in Southwest California Indians. *Psychiatr Genet*. 2007;17(3):171–176.
21. Fang L, Barnes-Ceeney K, Lee RA, Tao J. Substance use among Asian-American adolescents: perceptions of use and preferences for prevention programming. *Soc Work Health Care*. 2011;50(8):606–624.
22. Gelernter J, Kranzler HR. Genetics of drug dependence. *Dialogues Clin Neurosci*. 2010;12(1):77–84.
23. Gelernter J, Yu Y, Weiss R, et al. Haplotype spanning TTC12 and ANKK1, flanked by the DRD2 and NCAM1 loci, is strongly associated to nicotine dependence in two distinct American populations. *Hum Mol Genet*. 2006;15(24):3498–3507.
24. Giancola PR, Parker AM. A six-year prospective study of pathways toward drug use in adolescent boys with and without a family history of a substance use disorder. *J Stud Alcohol*. 2001;62(2):166–178.
25. Girirajan S. Missing heritability and where to find it. *Genome Biol*. 2017;18(1):89.
26. Gizer IR, Edenberg HJ, Gilder DA, Wilhelmsen KC, Ehlers CL. Association of alcohol dehydrogenase genes with alcohol-related phenotypes in a Native American community sample. *Alcohol Clin Exp Res*. 2011;35(11):2008–2018.
27. Goldberg AD, Allis CD, Bernstein E. Epigenetics: a landscape takes shape. *Cell*. 2007;128(4):635–638.
28. Goodwin DW, Schulsinger F, Moller N, Hermansen L, Winokur G, Guze SB. Drinking problems in adopted and nonadopted sons of alcoholics. *Arch Gen Psychiatry*. 1974;31(2):164–169.
29. Hall FS, Drgonova J, Jain S, Uhl GR. Implications of genome wide association studies for addiction: are our a priori assumptions all wrong? *Pharmacol Ther*. 2013;140(3):267–279.
30. Hall W, Madden P, Lynskey M. The genetics of tobacco use: methods, findings and policy implications. *Tobacco Control*. 2002;11(2):119–124.
31. Han S, Gelernter J, Luo X, Yang BZ. Meta-analysis of 15 genome-wide linkage scans of smoking behavior. *Biol Psychiatry*. 2010;67(1):12–19.
32. Hariri AR, Mattay VS, Tessitore A, et al. Serotonin transporter genetic variation and the response of the human amygdala. *Science*. 2002;297(5580):400–403.
33. Hart AB, Kranzler HR. Alcohol Dependence Genetics: Lessons Learned From Genome-Wide Association Studies (GWAS) and Post-GWAS Analyses. *Alcohol Clin Exp Res*. 2015;39(8):1312–1327.
34. Jaffee SR, Price TS. Genotype-environment correlations: implications for determining the relationship between environmental exposures and psychiatric illness. *Psychiatry*. 2008;7(12):496–499.
35. Jang KL, Livesley WJ, Vernon PA. Gender-specific etiological differences in alcohol and drug problems: a behavioural genetic analysis. *Addiction*. 1997;92(10):1265–1276.
36. Kartikeyan SK, Chaturvedi RM, Bhalerao VR. Role of the family in drug abuse. *J Postgrad Med*. 1992;38(1):5–7.
37. Kendler KS, Chen X, Dick D, et al. Recent advances in the genetic epidemiology and molecular genetics of substance use disorders. *Nat Neurosci*. 2012;15(2):181–189.
38. Kendler KS, Karkowski LM, Neale MC, Prescott CA. Illicit psychoactive substance use, heavy use, abuse, and dependence in a US population-based sample of male twins. *Arch Gen Psychiatry*. 2000;57(3):261–269.
39. Kendler KS, Ohlsson H, Maes HH, Sundquist K, Lichtenstein P, Sundquist J. A population-based Swedish Twin and Sibling Study of cannabis, stimulant and sedative abuse in men. *Drug Alcohol Depend*. 2015;149:49–54.
40. Kennedy JL, Basile VS, Macciardi FM. Chromosome 4 workshop summary: sixth world congress on psychiatric genetics, bonn, Germany, October 6-10, 1998. *Am J Med Genet*. 1999;88(3):224–228.
41. Koopmans JR, Slutske WS, Heath AC, Neale MC, Boomsma DI. The genetics of smoking initiation and quantity smoked in Dutch adolescent and young adult twins. *Behav Genet*. 1999;29(6):383–393.
42. Li MD. The genetics of smoking related behavior: a brief review. *Am J Med Sci*. 2003;326(4):168–173.
43. Li MD, Burmeister M. New insights into the genetics of addiction. *Nat Rev Genet*. 2009;10(4):225–231.
44. Lin YL, Pavlidis P, Karakoc E, Ajay J, Gokcumen O. The evolution and functional impact of human deletion variants shared with archaic hominin genomes. *Mol Biol Evol*. 2015;32(4):1008–1019.
45. Long JC, Knowler WC, Hanson RL, et al. Evidence for genetic linkage to alcohol dependence on chromosomes 4 and 11 from an autosome-wide scan in an American Indian population. *Am J Med Genet*. 1998;81(3):216–221.
46. Maes HH, Sullivan PF, Bulik CM, et al. A twin study of genetic and environmental influences on tobacco initiation, regular tobacco use and nicotine dependence. *Psychol Med*. 2004;34(7):1251–1261.
47. Maher B. Personal genomes. The case of the missing heritability. *Nature*. 2008;456(7218):18–21.
48. Mayfield RD, Harris RA, Schuckit MA. Genetic factors influencing alcohol dependence. *Br J Pharmacol*. 2008;154(2):275–287.
49. Mbarek H, Milaneschi Y, Fedko IO, et al. The genetics of alcohol dependence: Twin and SNP-based heritability, and genome-wide association study based on AUDIT scores. *Am J Med Genet B Neuropsychiatr Genet*. 2015;168(8):739–748.
50. McCaul ME, Turkkan JS, Svikis DS, Bigelow GE, Cromwell CC. Alcohol and drug use by college males as a function of family alcoholism history. *Alcohol Clin Exp Res*. 1990;14(3):467–471.
51. McGue M, Pickens RW, Svikis DS. Sex and age effects on the inheritance of alcohol problems: a twin study. *J Abnorm Psychol*. 1992;101(1):3–17.
52. Meyers DG, Neuberger JS, He J. Cardiovascular effect of bans on smoking in public places: a systematic review and meta-analysis. *J Am Coll Cardiol*. 2009;54(14):1249–1255.
53. Minica CC, Dolan CV, Hottenga JJ, et al. Heritability, SNP- and gene-based analyses of cannabis use initiation and age at onset. *Behav Genet*. 2015;45(5):503–513.
53a. Mitchell-Olds T, Willis JH, et al. Which evolutionary processes influence natural genetic variation for phenotypic traits? *Nat Rev Genet*. 2007;8:845–856.
54. Monnat SM, Rigg KK. Examining rural/urban differences in prescription opioid misuse among US adolescents. *J Rural Health*. 2016;32(2):204–218.
55. Newlin DB, Miles DR, van den Bree MB, Gupman AE, Pickens RW. Environmental transmission of DSM-IV substance use disdorders in adoptive and step families. *Alcohol Clin Exp Res*. 2000;24(12):1785–1794.
56. Niu T, Chen C, Ni J, et al. Nicotine dependence and its familial aggregation in Chinese. *Int J Epidemiol*. 2000;29(2):248–252.
57. Pergadia ML, Heath AC, Martin NG, Madden PA. Genetic analyses of DSM-IV nicotine withdrawal in adult twins. *Psychol Med*. 2006;36(7):963–972.
58. Pickens RW, Svikis DS, McGue M, Lykken DT, Heston LL, Clayton PJ. Heterogeneity in the inheritance of alcoholism. A study of male and female twins. *Arch Gen Psychiatry*. 1991;48(1):19–28.
59. Reich DE, Lander ES. On the allelic spectrum of human disease. *Trends Genet*. 2001;17(9):502–510.
60. Reilly MT, Noronha A, Goldman D, Koob GF. Genetic studies of alcohol dependence in the context of the addiction cycle. *Neuropharmacology*. 2017;122:3–21.
61. Rutter M, Pickles A, Murray R, Eaves L. Testing hypotheses on specific environmental causal effects on behavior. *Psychol Bull*. 2001;127(3):291–324.
62. Samek DR, Keyes MA, Hicks BM, Bailey J, McGue M, Iacono WG. General and specific predictors of nicotine and alcohol dependence in early adulthood: genetic and environmental influences. *J Stud Alcohol Drugs*. 2014;75(4):623–634.
63. Scarr S, McCartney K. How people make their own environments: a theory of genotype greater than environment effects. *Child Dev*. 1983;54(2):424–435.
64. Schuckit MA, Gunderson EK, Heckman NA, Kolb D. Family history as a predictor of alcoholism in U.S. navy personnel. *J Stud Alcohol*. 1976;37(11):1678–1685.

65. Sher KJ, Gotham HJ, Erickson DJ, Wood PK. A prospective, high-risk study of the relationship between tobacco dependence and alcohol use disorders. *Alcohol Clin Exp Res.* 1996;20(3):485–492.

66. Sher KJ, Walitzer KS, Wood PK, Brent EE. Characteristics of children of alcoholics: putative risk factors, substance use and abuse, and psychopathology. *J Abnorm Psychol.* 1991;100(4):427–448.

67. Speed D, Cai N, Consortium U, Johnson MR, Nejentsev S, Balding DJ. Reevaluation of SNP heritability in complex human traits. *Nat Genet.* 2017;49(7):986–992.

68. Stallings MC, Corley RP, Hewitt JK, et al. A genome-wide search for quantitative trait loci influencing substance dependence vulnerability in adolescence. *Drug Alcohol Depend.* 2003;70(3):295–307.

69. Stotz K, Griffiths P. Epigenetics: ambiguities and implications. *Hist Philos Life Sci.* 2016;38(4):22.

70. Sun J, Kranzler HR, Bi J. Refining multivariate disease phenotypes for high chip heritability. *BMC Med Genomics.* 2015;8(suppl 3):S3.

71. Treur JL, Boomsma DI, Lubke GH, Bartels M, Vink JM. The predictive value of smoking expectancy and the heritability of its accuracy. *Nicotine & tobacco research : official journal of the Society for Research on Nicotine and Tobacco.* 2014;16(3):359–368.

72. Tsuang MT, Lyons MJ, Meyer JM, et al. Co-occurrence of abuse of different drugs in men: the role of drug-specific and shared vulnerabilities. *Arch Gen Psychiatry.* 1998;55(11):967–972.

73. Uhl GR, Drgonova J, Hall FS. Curious cases: Altered dose-response relationships in addiction genetics. *Pharmacol Ther.* 2014;141(3):335–346.

74. Verhulst B, Neale MC, Kendler KS. The heritability of alcohol use disorders: a meta-analysis of twin and adoption studies. *Psychol Med.* 2015;45(5):1061–1072.

75. Verweij KJ, Zietsch BP, Lynskey MT, et al. Genetic and environmental influences on cannabis use initiation and problematic use: a meta-analysis of twin studies. *Addiction.* 2010;105(3):417–430.

76. Vink JM. Genetics of Addiction: Future Focus on Gene x Environment Interaction? *J Stud Alcohol Drugs.* 2016;77(5):684–687.

77. Visscher PM, Brown MA, McCarthy MI, Yang J. Five years of GWAS discovery. *Am J Hum Genet.* 2012;90(1):7–24.

78. Visscher PM, Wray NR, Zhang Q, et al. 10 Years of GWAS Discovery: Biology, Function, and Translation. *Am J Hum Genet.* 2017;101(1):5–22.

79. Vrieze SI, Feng S, Miller MB, et al. Rare nonsynonymous exonic variants in addiction and behavioral disinhibition. *Biol Psychiatry.* 2014;75(10):783–789.

80. Waddington CH. *Organisers & Genes.* Cambridge Eng.: The University Press; 1940.

81. Welter D, MacArthur J, Morales J, et al. The NHGRI GWAS Catalog, a curated resource of SNP-trait associations. *Nucleic Acids Res.* 2014;42:D1001–1006 (Database issue).

82. Whitesell M, Bachand A, Peel J, Brown M. Familial, social, and individual factors contributing to risk for adolescent substance use. *J Addict.* 2013;2013:579310.

83. Whitlock FA. Alcoholism: a genetic disorder? *Aust N Z J Psychiatry.* 1975;9(1):3–7.

84. Wu SH, Guo Q, Viken RJ, Reed T, Dai J. Heritability of usual alcohol intoxication and hangover in male twins: the NAS-NRC Twin Registry. *Alcohol Clin Exp Res.* 2014;38(8):2307–2313.

85. Yang J, Benyamin B, McEvoy BP, et al. Common SNPs explain a large proportion of the heritability for human height. *Nat Genet.* 2010;42(7):565–569.

86. Yang J, Li MD. Converging findings from linkage and association analyses on susceptibility genes for smoking and other addictions. *Mol Psychiatry.* 2016;21(8):992–1008.

13

The Assessment and Treatment of Addiction: Best Practices in a Direct-to-Consumer Age

NANCY DIAZGRANADOS AND DAVID GOLDMAN

CHAPTER OUTLINE

Introduction

Addictions are a constellation of complex and chronic illnesses that affect multiple domains in a patient's life, primarily for the worst. Nosologically, they are defined by use of an addictive agent and effects, rather than process, in contrast to many other diseases that are not defined primarily by chief complaint, but by etiology. As with other recurrent illnesses, multidisciplinary assessment and therapy improve chances of recovery, but perhaps no other diseases pose a greater variety of challenges, are met with more diverse and even opposite therapies, and are more neglected. Increasingly, people are reliant on web-based tools, direct-to-consumer self-help books and websites, and portable electronic devices when seeking solutions for lifestyle-related problems and health problems and risks that lie along a contiuum of risk factor to disease. Here, we propose a medically centered, generalized framework for the treatment of addictions, which can incorporate such new tools to deliver better assessment and interventions. We target multiple domains, which frequently involve severe, complex, and intractable problems that require a multidisciplinary team of expert providers. The treatment team integrates new measures and new interventions—some enabled by new technology and most not—that will hopefully be based on the pathophysiology of addictions. Individuals at risk, users, individuals with use disorder, and recovering patients represent different stages of the disease process, requiring assessments and interventions targeted to the stage. Multiple domains of vulnerability, use, addiction process, and consequence require evaluation and integration into a comprehensive treatment plan. Dramatic progress in the treatment of other chronic diseases for which etiologic-specific treatments are wanting, including cystic fibrosis and diabetes, indicates that a comprehensive approach, expensive though it may be, and incorporating appropriate technologies for at-home testing and intervention, can greatly improve the current prevalence and relapse statistics for addictions, which are diseases whose expense and impact on lives and communities justify the cost.

The Assessment

As with any medical evaluation, a detailed History and Physical (H&P) remains essential. One may ask why. For example, screening questionnaires such as the Fagerstrom (smoking) and Michigan Alcohol Screening Test (MAST) can ascertain most smokers and alcoholics. Furthermore, any heavy user of an addictive agent—be it a drug, gambling, or the Internet—is more than likely addicted and this can be readily ascertained by direct or indirect observation of use, and, for example, a blood alcohol level, or the reading from an electronic monitoring device.

DOMAINS	At-risk cases	Heavy users without a diagnosis	Substance use disorder patients	Patients in recovery
			STAGES	
Genetics	⊕⊕	⊕	⊕⊕	⊕⊕
Physiological interface	⊕	⊕	⊕⊕	⊕
• End-organ damage		⊕	⊕⊕⊕	⊕⊕
• Allostatic changes		⊕	⊕⊕	⊕
• Neurocognitive functioning	⊕	⊕	⊕⊕⊕	⊕⊕
Family interface	⊕⊕		⊕⊕⊕	⊕⊕
Work and vocational interface	⊕		⊕⊕⊕	⊕⊕
Community interface and legal problems	⊕		⊕⊕⊕	⊕⊕
Hedonic and recreational interface	⊕		⊕⊕⊕	⊕
Spiritual interface	⊕		⊕⊕	⊕

• **Fig. 13.1** Relevance of the domain for this stage: minimal, moderate, and substantial.

A person may enter mood or craving scores into an electronic device, or the information might be directly collected, for example, by recording their movements or changes in facial expression over time. However, such observations are insufficient to define a *Diagnostic and Statistical Manual of Mental Disorders*, Fifth Edition (DSM-5),[1] Use Disorder, and diagnosis of a DSM-5 Use Disorder represents only a starting point for understanding causes, process, and consequences of a patient's addiction, and the beginnings of therapeutic engagement—the deep partnership that must be formed between patient and the multidisciplinary team. Fig. 13.1 highlights some of the key domains of addictions that need to be included in an H&P. All should be evaluated during the initial assessment to stage severity. It is important to understand the individual events that led a patient to this point in disease progression. This process will create the full clinical problem list, help to identify resources for recovery, and help to establish for the patient that their problems are of concern. This begins a therapeutic process, which includes the patient appreciating the relationship of their addiction to other causes and consequences. In line with a process-oriented conceptualization of addiction, this scheme includes at-risk individuals, understanding that addiction medicine needs to address its identifiable "precancerous lesions," which may include escalating use or signs of progression to full disease; for example, in the way that physicians do not disregard infection or metabolic syndrome until a patient is actually septicemic or in renal failure. The complexity of initial assessment will only increase as new tools become available from multiple disciplines ranging from neuroimaging and genetics[24] to electronic monitoring of substance use and emotional state. For example, in the domain of *genetics*, the heritability of addictions has been well established, suggesting that more clinically useful genetic variants in addition to *ALDH2* (alcoholism/flushing/upper gastrointestinal [GI] cancer) and *CHRNA5* and *CYP2D6* (smoking, lung cancer) will be found.[16,34] Many people are already receiving such genetic results direct-to-consumer, and websites devoted to the *Asian flush*, and inappropriate and potentially harmful treatments, have proliferated. For example, in the domain of addiction neuroscience, psychophysiological differences in executive cognition, emotion, and reward are being identified.[44] Such measures offer the prospect of identifying at-risk individuals and offering early interventions. However, and actually as required by the diversity of assessments that may be required following whatever screening methods that may have been used, the true starting point of assessment is not an individual test—be it genetic, neuropsychologic, or behavioral—but the detailed H&P.

The Stages of Addiction

Addictions are chronic relapsing and remitting diseases, and although they are diverse, assessment will vary according to stage.

At-Risk Individuals

These individuals are not easily identified, except in the broader and more pessimistic sense that the population as a whole is at moderate-to-high risk of one addiction or another. Addiction medicine needs to move toward prevention and early intervention, and one component of that is identification of those at highest risk. Critically, addictions are common such that a large fraction of the population have either an addictive disorder or are at risk. For example, some 29.1% of adults in the United States meet criteria for Lifetime Alcohol Use Disorder according to the National Epidemiologic Survey on Alcohol and Related Conditions (NESARC) household survey of more than 36,000 people.[13] Approximately 15% of Americans smoke cigarettes and most who do are addicted to nicotine. Easy availability of potent opioids such as oxycodone and fentanyl; legal tetrahydrocannabinol (THC)–enhanced marijuana; and gambling in many forms ranging from state-sponsored lotteries and casinos to sports-league–sponsored daily fantasy gambling, often delivered on handheld devices, will successfully addict larger segments of the population—addiction being an inherent component of the success of several of these products on the basis that addicts consume 50% or more of the product.[25,26] Increasingly, it may be more useful to identify protective factors; for example, the *ALDH2* polymorphism that protects against alcoholism via flushing,[8] information about which is available by direct-to-consumer testing, as an experience in self-knowledge, and other nonmedical contexts such as testing of incoming university freshman, as a learning experience. On the other hand, genetic risk, as measured via specific genotypes or by family history, and environmental risk, in particular early life trauma, can be incorporated into risk assessment, and could be useful in many scenarios; for example, to assess addiction risk, and plan the tapering of the drug, when a patient requires an opioid over several weeks for pain management, or even to assess occupational hazards such as being a bartender or a physician.

Heavy Users Who Do Not Meet Criteria for Substance Use Disorders

As illustrated by the opioid epidemic initiated by heavy prescribing of oxycodone, any heavy user of an addictive agent is at high risk even if that person is innately resilient and under the care of a physician. Repetitive use of addictive substances and other addictive agents such as gambling create tolerance and allostatic changes that in some cases lead to "physiological" or "psychological" dependence.[11] Following withdrawal, there will in many cases be no functional repercussions, and indeed, it can be conceded that in many cases a person's life may have been enhanced by the experience be it a wine-tasting, relief of pain, or a horse race. The ability of a person to use an addictive agent heavily without some severe adverse outcome will be determined not only by factors and processes internal to them but by external factors: their employment, general health and nutrition, and social relationships, and by luck.

Patients with substance use disorder represent most of the individuals counted in studies and statistics. They are the cases where the use of a substance causes functional impairments such that they meet the criteria of a DSM-5 substance use disorder. In contrast to individuals at risk, patients with substance use disorder are easily identifiable and will occasionally ask for help. As has been well studied, only a minority of patients seek treatment and even fewer receive a therapy that has evidence of effectiveness. About 13.5% of Drug Use Disorder patients with a diagnosis in the last 12months received any form of treatment.[14] For patients with a lifetime diagnosis of alcohol use disorder, only 19.8% were ever treated.[13] Following the DSM-5 scheme, their substance use disorder (SUD) can be classified as mild (2–3 criteria), moderate (4–5 criteria), or severe (6–11 criteria). Traditionally we call the severe cases "dependent," implying that it is difficult for the patients to make changes in their behavior without supervised care. Of the criteria for alcohol use disorder, two—#10 and #11—are related to tolerance or dependence: "Had to drink much more than you once did to get the effect you want? Or found that your usual number of drinks had much less effect than before?" and "Found that when the effects of alcohol were wearing off, you had withdrawal symptoms, such as trouble sleeping, shakiness, restlessness, nausea, sweating, a racing heart, or a seizure? Or sensed things that were not there?."[1] However, tolerance and dependence are insufficient to define a "Use Disorder" and they only imply some of the etiological changes that we need to better understand. In total there are 1024 combinations of 6 or more DSM symptoms that can define a patient as "Severe."

Patients in Recovery

Due to predisposing factors (e.g., genetics and early life trauma) and brain changes, most patients in recovery are at high risk for relapse. Some live with severe sequelae even if they maintain sobriety. End-organ damage, cancer, chronic infections, legal problems, unemployment, social dislocation and alienation, and stigma shape the lives of many patients in recovery. Recovery is not always equivalent to rehabilitation. We need to aim for higher functioning in the recovery group to achieve real rehabilitation. As ambitious as sobriety can be, due to the high percentage of relapses to different substances, and the potential for harm reduction even with failure to achieve abstinence, sobriety is insufficient as a marker for success in treatment.[46]

The Domains

Genetics

Multiple genes have been identified as protective or risk factors for developing addictions and their complications. With advances in genetics, the identification of some of these genes in an individual at risk or with an SUD should become a standard practice. They can guide therapeutic approaches, from early intervention to pharmacotherapy, and relapse prevention. For example, at any stage of addiction to alcohol, any of 500 million people carrying the *ALDH2* Lys 487 Asian flush allele can know that moderate alcohol consumption, with or without antihistamine drugs that can block flushing (and whose use is advocated on websites) would expose them to high risk of upper GI and other cancer risks.[4]

Physiological Interface

As has been discussed, the repetitive behavior or use of a substance with addictive potential will change the brain, making the absence of this behavior or substance ego-dystonic. The changes in the body are not limited to the brain depending on the substance used. The continued use of a substance despite adverse consequences is a characteristic and symptom of an addiction.[21]

End-Organ Damage

Traditionally the main area of assessment and treatment for addiction medicine has been limited to allostatic changes in brain physiology and their behavioral presentation. For some substances (primarily alcohol and tobacco) there has been detailed study of their effects on other systems (e.g., hepatic and pulmonary function). Nevertheless, treatments, when they exist, have targeted the brain. Changes in the reward circuitry, cue conditioning, and negative salience can be modified by medications or psychotherapeutic approaches like Cognitive Behavioral Therapy (CBT) and Motivational Interviewing (MI). Most patients would require a team of doctors, as many of our patients will have complications from their SUDs. Addiction medicine physicians frequently consult with dentists, cardiologists, hepatologists, infectious diseases specialists, and physiatrists.[32,36,41]

Allostatic Changes

In an attempt to maintain functioning, the brain and other organs exposed to addictive substances gradually modify their baseline parameters, adjusting to the presence of the substance. If the substance is withheld, acute withdrawal may follow. Allostatic change also produces long-lasting deficits beyond the horizon of acute withdrawal such that a subsequent exposure to a specific cue or nonspecific stress can lead to relapse and rapid reinstatement to the highest levels of use. A classic example are the γ-aminobutyric acid (GABA)ergic and glutamatergic changes present in alcohol dependence, with benzodiazepine drugs capable of alleviating acute withdrawal, and long-lasting activations of the brain stress axis with changes in corticotropin-releasing factor (CRF) expression, and that thus far we do not know how to alleviate or reverse.[20]

Neurocognitive Functioning

The brain is the main organ changed by addictive substances and behaviors, and addictions are diseases caused by changes in neuronal circuits. Some predisposing characteristics are seen in at-risk groups. However, SUDs have toxic consequences ranging from neuronal damage to changes in neuronal systems. From impulsivity and aggression to dementia, brain functioning changes with substance use. Some of these changes are postulated as the reason for the rapid reinstatement and reescalation of substance use once a patient relapses after a period of sobriety. Progress in characterizing neurocognitive functioning in addiction is likely to be rapid; such measures of function can guide and directly measure the effects of treatments, whether direct neurofeedback therapies and pharmacotherapies or indirect cognitive and behavioral therapies, that aim to modify the neurocircuitry of addiction and restore the addicted brain.[12,23,35,42]

Family Interface

Addictions frequently disintegrate families, especially the relationships between close relatives who bear the brunt. The behavior of the patient, which may be erratic, aggressive, neglectful, criminal, or abusive, as well as the general deterioration of house and home, and economy, estrangement, loss, and accidents, all create difficult situations for dependents who may themselves to be at higher genetic risk. Via the family, addictions are transmitted both horizontally, and—in a transgenerational fashion—vertically. It is important to recognize that the addicted patient, who may have been initially ineffective and is now hampered by neurocognitive changes, can fail at ordinary family roles, even if the family is not estranged. Absent overt abuse or aggression toward loved ones, deficits in attention, reward, and motivation cause addicted individuals to neglect family duties and the needs of partners and dependents.[3,19,27]

Work and Vocational Interface

Changes in the reward system alter productivity and engagement with work and other activities that give purpose and satisfaction. As addiction progresses, patients disengage from other passions, finding reward and pleasure only in the addictive agent of choice. As they develop tolerance, relief of withdrawal symptoms becomes their primary, and more immediate, goal. The need to prevent withdrawal leads to use while at work, or absenteeism. Negative work consequences are frequent, as are unemployment and underemployment. Some industries have a higher frequency of substance use due to exposure to trauma and stress (e.g., military, health care), exposure to addictive substances (e.g., bartender and other service industries), or in some cases the expectation of substance use as part of the job (e.g., sales, lobbying). For some patients, sobriety means restarting or rebuilding their professional life.[17,39]

Community Interface and Legal Problems

Due—in part—to the punitive approach to SUDs and the stigma of addiction, legal consequences are common. Community support other than peer support groups (e.g., Alcoholics Anonymous [AA], Narcotics Anonymous [NA], Smart recovery) is rare for patients with SUDs. This leads to marginalization of our patients and obstacles to vocational, family, and social recovery. It is also important to recognize that many or most psychoactive addictive agents impair judgment and motor control, leading directly to aggression, bad decisions, and accidents that draw the attention of the criminal justice system.[2,9,43]

Hedonic and Recreational Interface

For patients with addictions, finding recreational opportunities without their addictive agent of choice can be a challenge. In many cases, friends, loved ones, and even acquaintances use the same agent, making abstinence difficult. Alcohol is ubiquitous in most cultures and it can be difficult for some patients to even imagine having fun without it. Young Asian flushers may therefore use antihistamines to block alcohol-induced flushing but not the genotoxic effects. Because the reward system is modified by these substances, it might be difficult for some patients to reengage with earlier pleasures and passions when a facilitating substance or addictive agent has been removed from the equation.[38,40]

Spiritual Interface

For many patients addiction is a sin or disgrace. For some, their system of values chastises use of addictive substances, creating negative connotations and shame. In some cases, shame leads to voluntary isolation or ostracism. However, it can also enlist the intervention of spiritual leaders and counselors. Many patients only seek help from religious figures because they see their illness as a "character defect" or "sin." This has led to many support communities within religious establishments (e.g., most AA groups take place in churches or temples). Training on substance use counseling is a common skill for religious figures. Spiritual or religious practices like mindfulness have evolved into therapeutic approaches. Reintegration into religious communities can be a therapeutic tool in many cases.[28,30]

The Treatment

A multidisciplinary team that includes one or more physician, nurse, psychologist, counselor, nutritionist, social worker, vocational therapist, recreational therapist, spiritual guide, and peers (with whatever level of training) can be useful to target all the domains affected by addictions. Depending on the stage of the illness and the substance used, different combinations of these health providers are required.

At-Risk Individuals

For cases at-risk the primary physician can provide the treatment needed with the aid of social workers and vocational therapists. Education about the risks predicted by genetic profiles and environmental exposures is an ongoing process that should happen at different stages of an individual's development. Identifying patients with early life trauma and providing treatment and protection is key for many areas of mental health. Understanding that these patients are at-risk for substance use and providing education, supervision, and support could improve the current statistics on addiction. However, there is still a gap in our knowledge about preventive medicine in addictions. More studies to assess different early interventions are needed.[34]

Heavy Users Who Do Not Meet Criteria for Use Disorders

Because this group is unlikely to seek help, they need to be identified by screening at primary care offices. Most primary care physicians use a few screening questions about alcohol, tobacco, and illicit drug use while their patients sit in the waiting room. The screens can help identify patients needing referral and at-risk individuals who use addictive agents but have no functional impairment or need for a multidisciplinary approach. The screens can lead to interventions and education about the risks they are taking. These patients can also learn the early signs of developing a use disorder. Studies of the efficacy of therapeutic and preventive interventions in this group are also needed.

Use Disorder Patients

According to the severity of illness (mild, moderate, or severe) and the substance of choice, the team of providers should vary. All use disorder patients need supervised care by health care professionals. A full assessment to determine the extent of end-organ damage and comorbidities is needed. Depending on the substance of choice, a supervised detox that requires pharmacological interventions and constant monitoring can improve the rates of abstinence and even survival. Because multiple needs and complications are frequent, multiple providers are needed. In some cases, due to comorbidities and complications of SUDs, other medical consultants are required. Pharmacotherapy to help maintain sobriety is always recommended if available.[16,18,31,33] A therapist that can identify thought distortions and help patients move forward with their resolve toward sobriety is critical.[6,35] Peer support groups are common and very helpful for some patients who feel isolated or shamed by their illness.[43] We recommend vocational and recreational therapy consultants to aid in the hedonic and social functional rehabilitation.[17,40] As stated earlier, many patients need to create or rebuild a career. Social work to help with sober housing options, family counseling, and individual therapy is a key service.[3,9] We also recommend working with a spiritual advisor according to the preference of the patient to change some of the religious negative constructs around addictions and to learn relaxation, meditation, and prayers that can help them take their minds off their addictive agent of choice. This multidisciplinary team can be a transitional community when patients decide to move away from a system that enables or encourages addiction. As they learn skills and maintain sobriety, patients will build new safer communities around them. Some of the parts of this team of providers have more evidence than others. Studies to determine vocational rehabilitation in addictions are needed. Controversy around peer support groups are frequent. Because anyone in this group is formally diagnosed with a mental illness we strongly believe that health care professionals, not peers or direct-to-consumer options, need to lead the treatment.

Patients in Recovery

Patients in recovery are at high risk for relapse. Some of the team members that helped them achieve abstinence will be needed for them to maintain abstinence. If there is a pharmacotherapy approved as a maintenance treatment it should be offered. As discussed earlier, many patients are also living with the sequelae or complications from their SUD. In these cases, a team of medical consultants is required. Social, vocational, family, and community functioning need to be assessed to determine further needs and decrease risk of relapse.

New Frontiers

Addictions research and clinical practice are exciting areas of work due to the extensive need for services and knowledge and a rapidly changing technological environment in which consumers have many alternatives to medical care. We need to move into an etiological diagnostic system and develop better early interventions and preventative measures.[44] Advances in genetics, neuroimaging, and neurocognitive assessments might help us identify at-risk individuals and provide targeted interventions to prevent the development of addictions. In the era of eHealth, geographical and ecological momentary assessment make real-time interventions possible.[10] Multinational collaborations in imaging and genetics make big data a reality and a source of knowledge that we are only starting to exploit. Better imaging biomarkers such as real-time functional magnetic resonance imaging (fMRI) neurofeedback[15] have allowed us to better assess the effectiveness of our therapeutic interventions. Moreover, with the understanding that addictions are primarily brain illnesses, we are now moving into neuromodulation with the knowledge acquired from neuroimaging. Neurocircuit-based interventions are an ongoing area of research with great potential.[7,37,42] Vaccine research and novel therapeutics that target neurobiological processes will change the pharmacologic treatment of addiction.[22] Finally, advances in genetics and epigenetics, in some cases making genetic testing routine, will facilitate individualized therapy.[34] As we start the study of the epigenome, we are gaining understanding of novel potential preventive and therapeutic interventions.[5,47] Optogenetics research and the potential for other genetic therapeutics are expanding the field, allowing for neurocircuit interventions that can be more precisely delivered.[29,45] Addictions treatment needs to expand, and we have many potential avenues for this, each one adding exiting new areas of study.

References

1. American Psychiatric Association. *Diagnostic and Statistical Manual of Mental Disorders*. 5th ed. Arlington, VA: American Psychiatric Publishing; 2013.
2. Bassuk EL, Hanson J, Greene RN, Richard M, Laudet A. Peer-delivered recovery support services for addictions in the united states: a systematic review. *J Subst Abuse Treat*. 2016;63:1–9.
3. Bisetto Pons D, Gonzalez Barron R, Botella Guijarro A. Family-based intervention program for parents of substance-abusing youth and adolescents. *J Addict*. 2016:4320720.
4. Brooks PJ, Enoch MA, Goldman D, Li TK, Yokoyama A. The alcohol flushing response: an unrecognized risk factor for esophageal cancer from alcohol consumption. *PLoS Med*. 2009;6(3):e50.
5. Cecil CA, Walton E, Viding E. Epigenetics of addiction: current knowledge, challenges, and future directions. *J Stud Alcohol Drugs*. 2016;77(5):688–691.
6. Choi SW, Shin YC, Kim DJ, et al. Treatment modalities for patients with gambling disorder. *Ann Gen Psychiatry*. 2017;16:23.
7. Diana M, Raij T, Melis M, Nummenmaa A, Leggio L, Bonci A. Rehabilitating the addicted brain with transcranial magnetic stimulation. *Nat Rev Neurosci*. 2017;18(11):685–693.
8. Ducci F, Goldman D. The genetic basis of addictive disorders. *Psychiatr Clin North Am*. 2012;35(2):495–519.
9. Dutra L, Stathopoulou G, Basden SL, Leyro TM, Powers MB, Otto MW. A meta-analytic review of psychosocial interventions for substance use disorders. *Am J Psychiatry*. 2008;165(2):179–187.
10. Epstein DH, Tyburski M, Craig IM, et al. Real-time tracking of neighborhood surroundings and mood in urban drug misusers: application of a new method to study behavior in its geographical context. *Drug Alcohol Depend*. 2014;134:22–29.
11. George O, Le Moal M, Koob GF. Allostasis and addiction: role of the dopamine and corticotropin-releasing factor systems. *Physiol Behav*. 2012;106(1):58–64.
12. Goldman D, Barr CS. Restoring the addicted brain. *N Engl J Med*. 2002;347(11):843–845.
13. Grant BF, Goldstein RB, Saha TD, et al. Epidemiology of DSM-5 alcohol use disorder: results from the national epidemiologic survey on alcohol and related conditions III. *JAMA Psychiatry*. 2015;72(8):757–766.

14. Grant BF, Saha TD, Ruan WJ, et al. Epidemiology of DSM-5 drug use disorder: results from the national epidemiologic survey on alcohol and related conditions-III. *JAMA Psychiatry*. 2016;73(1):39–47.

15. Hartwell KJ, Prisciandaro JJ, Borckardt J, Li X, George MS, Brady KT. Real-time fMRI in the treatment of nicotine dependence: a conceptual review and pilot studies. *Psychol Addict Behav*. 2013;27(2):501–509.

16. Heilig M, Goldman D, Berrettini W, O'Brien CP. Pharmacogenetic approaches to the treatment of alcohol addiction. *Nat Rev Neurosci*. 2011;12(11):670–684.

17. Kerrigan AJ, Kaough JE, Wilson BL, Wilson JV, Bostick R. Vocational rehabilitation of participants with severe substance use disorders in a VA veterans industries program. *Subst Use Misuse*. 2004;39(13-14):2513–2523.

18. Klein JW. Pharmacotherapy for substance use disorders. *Med Clin North Am*. 2016;100(4):891–910.

19. Klostermann K, O'Farrell TJ. Treating substance abuse: partner and family approaches. *Soc Work Public Health*. 2013;28(3-4):234–247.

20. Koob GF, Mason BJ. Existing and future drugs for the treatment of the dark side of addiction. *Annu Rev Pharmacol Toxicol*. 2016;56:299–322.

21. Koob GF, Volkow ND. Neurobiology of addiction: a neurocircuitry analysis. *Lancet Psychiatry*. 2016;3(8):760–773.

22. Kosten T, Domingo C, Orson F, Kinsey B. Vaccines against stimulants: cocaine and MA. *Br J Clin Pharmacol*. 2014;77(2):368–374.

23. Kwako LE, Momenan R, Grodin EN, Litten RZ, Koob GF, Goldman D. Addictions Neuroclinical Assessment: a reverse translational approach. *Neuropharmacology*. 2017;122:254–264.

24. Kwako LE, Momenan R, Litten RZ, Koob GF, Goldman D. Addictions neuroclinical assessment: a neuroscience-based framework for addictive disorders. *Biol Psychiatry*. 2016;80(3):179–189.

25. MacKillop J. The Behavioral economics and neuroeconomics of alcohol use disorders. *Alcohol Clin Exp Res*. 2016;40(4):672–685.

26. Martins SS, Sarvet A, Santaella-Tenorio J, Saha T, Grant BF, Hasin DS. Changes in US lifetime heroin use and heroin use disorder: prevalence from the 2001-2002 to 2012-2013 national epidemiologic survey on alcohol and related conditions. *JAMA Psychiatry*. 2017;74(5):445–455.

27. McCrady BS, Wilson AD, Munoz RE, Fink BC, Fokas K, Borders A. Alcohol-focused behavioral couple therapy. *Fam Process*. 2016;55(3):443–459.

28. Medlock MM, Rosmarin DH, Connery HS, et al. Religious coping in patients with severe substance use disorders receiving acute inpatient detoxification. *Am J Addict*. 2017;26(7):744–750.

29. Muller Ewald VA, LaLumiere RT. Neural systems mediating the inhibition of cocaine-seeking behaviors. *Pharmacol Biochem Behav*. 2018;174:53–63.

30. Noormohammadi MR, Nikfarjam M, Deris F, Parvin N. Spiritual well-being and associated factors with relapse in opioid addicts. *J Clin Diagn Res*. 2017;11(3):VC07–VC10.

31. O'Brien CP. Review. Evidence-based treatments of addiction. *Philos Trans R Soc Lond B Biol Sci*. 2008;363(1507):3277–3286.

32. Pacher P, Steffens S, Hasko G, Schindler TH, Kunos G. Cardiovascular effects of marijuana and synthetic cannabinoids: the good, the bad, and the ugly. *Nat Rev Cardiol*. 2018;15:151–166.

33. Pierce RC, O'Brien CP, Kenny PJ, Vanderschuren LJ. Rational development of addiction pharmacotherapies: successes, failures, and prospects. *Cold Spring Harb Perspect Med*. 2012;2(6):a012880.

34. Reilly MT, Noronha A, Goldman D, Koob GFX. Genetic studies of alcohol dependence in the context of the addiction cycle. *Neuropharmacology*. 2012;122:3–21.

35. Rezapour T, DeVito EE, Sofuoglu M, Ekhtiari H. Perspectives on neurocognitive rehabilitation as an adjunct treatment for addictive disorders: from cognitive improvement to relapse prevention. *Prog Brain Res*. 2016;224:345–369.

36. Rojewski AM, Baldassarri S, Cooperman NA, et al. Exploring Issues of comorbid conditions in people who smoke. *Nicotine Tob Res*. 2016;18(8):1684–1696.

37. Salling MC, Martinez. Brain stimulation in addiction. *Neuropsychopharmacology*. 2016;41(12):2798–2809.

38. Schlossarek S, Kempkensteffen J, Reimer J, Verthein U. Psychosocial determinants of cannabis dependence: a systematic review of the literature. *Eur Addict Res*. 2016;22(3):131–144.

39. Sethuraman L, Subodh BN, Murthy P. Validation of vocational assessment tool for persons with substance use disorders. *Ind Psychiatry J*. 2016;25(1):59–64.

40. Silverman MJ. Effects of live and educational music therapy on working alliance and trust with patients on detoxification unit: a four-group cluster-randomized trial. *Subst Use Misuse*. 2016;51(13):1741–1750.

41. Siniscalchi A, Bonci A, Mercuri NB, et al. Cocaine dependence and stroke: pathogenesis and management. *Curr Neurovasc Res*. 2015;12(2):163–172.

42. Spagnolo PA, Goldman D. Neuromodulation interventions for addictive disorders: challenges, promise, and roadmap for future research. *Brain*. 2017;140(5):1183–1203.

43. Tracy K, Wallace SP. Benefits of peer support groups in the treatment of addiction. *Subst Abuse Rehabil*. 2016;7:143–154.

44. Volkow ND, Koob GF, McLellan AT. Neurobiologic Advances from the brain disease model of addiction. *N Engl J Med*. 2016;374(4):363–371.

45. Weinshenker D, Holmes PV. Regulation of neurological and neuropsychiatric phenotypes by locus coeruleus-derived galanin. *Brain Res*. 2016;1641(Pt B):320–337.

46. Wise RA, Koob GF. The development and maintenance of drug addiction. *Neuropsychopharmacology*. 2014;39(2):254–262.

47. Wong CC, Mill J, Fernandes C. Drugs and addiction: an introduction to epigenetics. *Addiction*. 2011;106(3):480–489.

14

Metabolomics in Drug Response and Addiction

RAIHAN K. UDDIN AND SHIVA M. SINGH

What Is Metabolomics?

Metabolomics is the newest addition to the "omics" science. An "omics" has been defined as a neologism referring to a holistic view on biologic macromolecules, such as in genomics or proteomics.[9] Genomics aims to understand the structure and function of the genome by studying all nucleotide sequences, including the structural genes, regulatory sequences, and noncoding DNA sequences in the chromosomes of any organism. It also examines the molecular mechanisms that maintain genomic integrity and allow its transmission and the expression including any interplay of genetic and environmental factors in disease. Proteomics involves the identification and study of the complete set of proteins in a species and the determination of their role in physiologic and pathophysiologic functions.[2,56] Together with these and other "omics" technologies, metabolomics contribute to the detailed understanding of the in vivo function of gene products, biochemical analysis, and regulatory networks. The metabolomics represents the collection of all low-molecular-weight molecules found in a given cell and can provide a snapshot of the physiology of a cell at a given time during development and differentiation including responses to food, drugs, and other challenges.[20]

Biochemists view metabolomics as metabolites profiling or the quantitative measurement of the dynamic multiparametric metabolic response of living systems to pathophysiological stimuli or genetic modification.[11] Biologists, particularly geneticists, on the other hand, view it as the science of a highly complex and organized biochemical network in which small molecules, such as metabolic substrates and products, lipids, small peptides, vitamins, amino acids, signaling molecules, and other protein cofactors, are interacting between them and with other biological macromolecules in the metabolome.[9] These small molecules are acting usually at very low concentrations in tissue-signaling functions.[18] Along with the understanding of the in vivo interaction of gene products, metabolomics also contributes a great deal to the mathematical description and simulation of the whole cell in the systems biology approach. Systems biology tries to integrate genomic, proteomic, transcriptomic, and metabolomic information to give a more complete picture of living organisms (Fig. 14.1). Here, the biological events in organisms are systematically interpreted through the combination of complex measurements from various methods resulting in high-throughput data. In this chapter, we discuss addiction as a problem of systems biology with emphasis on metabolomics.

Substance Abuse and Its Effect on Health and Economy

Substance use, abuse, and addiction that include but are not limited to alcohol,[41,61] nicotine,[17] opioids,[48] cocaine,[35] cannabinoids,[1] methamphetamine, and amphetamine,[33] continue to be a significant public health concern and pose tremendous cost to our society. In the United States alone, in 1998, the economic cost associated with illicit drug use was estimated to be US$280 billion, for nicotine US$158 billion,[7] and for alcohol abuse US$185 billion, with an average annual increase of 3.8% per year.[21] This brings the combined total estimated economic impact of substance abuse in the United States to over half a trillion dollars.[61] Recent data indicate that approximately 1.6 million people in the United States abuse or are dependent on prescription opioids.[48] In the United Kingdom, the cost associated with alcohol abuse

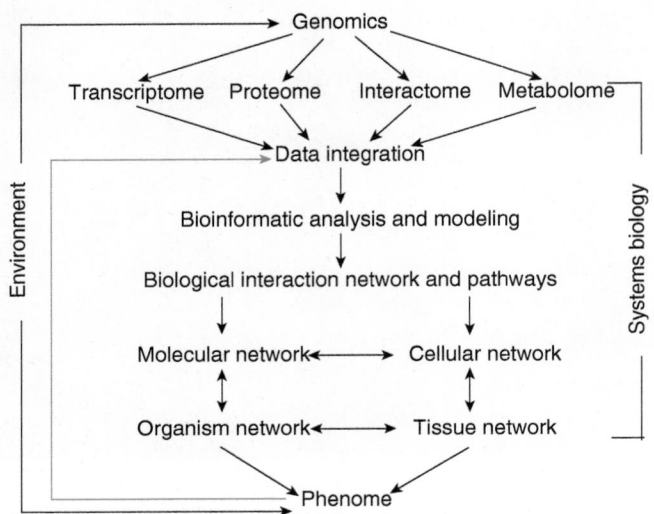

• **Fig. 14.1** Connection between "omics" sciences and systems biology. Functional genomics and other technologies are used to map the transcriptome (complete set of transcripts), proteome (complete set of proteins), interactome (complete set of interactions), metabolome (complete set of metabolites), and other "omics" knowledge bases. Bioinformatics analysis is done to model and infer network pathways from integrated data. Experimentally valid biological network of cells, tissues, and organs from particular organism are integrated with phenome (complete set of phenotypes) to obtain the complete picture about specific mechanism and disease.

is approximately $39 billion each year.[41] Drug and alcohol abuse is a major cause of morbidity and mortality both in the United States and worldwide. Alcohol use disorders including liver and heart diseases account for 4% of the global burden of disease and cause 1.8 million deaths.[41] The excessive burden of drug abuse on our health and economy makes it necessary for us to better understand how these drugs affect the metabolomics of our cellular systems, mechanisms of action in different parts of the body, and factors that determine the variability of addictive responses. A better insight into these mechanisms will offer a better understanding of the problem as well as identify effective treatment and preventative approaches to addiction, which remains insidious in most societies.

Substance Abuse Leads to Addiction

At the center of the problem of substance abuse is addiction to these substances. It has been long hypothesized that the combination of genetic and environmental factors following drug use and abuse alters cellular physiology. This alteration is expected to be cell and organ specific. In due course, it may follow physiological adaptation, leading to an urge for the drug response and the development of addiction.[27,37,61] Evidence for the involvement of genes in the drug addiction process comes from classical epidemiological and genetic studies. Data from both animal and humans support the relevance of genetic influences in substance abuse and dependence.[3,24,34,55] Twin studies, for example, have shown robust genetic components for alcohol, opiate, cocaine, and tobacco addictions.[5,28,54]

The major target of virtually all drugs in the human or animal body, either directly or indirectly, is the nervous system—specifically one or more pathways deep within the brain.[25,29,39,62] Drug-related, especially alcohol-related, brain damage and associated

neuropsychological changes have been well documented (see Oscar-Berman et al.[38,39]). There is increasing evidence that long-lasting changes in the brain result from the progression of casual user to addict.[37] Acute drug intoxication is accompanied by highly localized and dynamic patterns of brain activation and deactivation,[26,47] as well as complex cascades of transcriptional reprogramming.[63,64]

All compounds with abuse potential have the ability to disrupt information processing in the brain by subverting or affecting the expression of gene(s) involved in one or more of the common neurotransmitter systems (i.e., gamma-aminobutyric acid, glutamate, acetylcholine, dopamine, serotonin, and opioid peptides). However, an early increase in dopamine signaling has been one of the most consistent observations across studies of the reinforcing effects of drugs of abuse.[13,40,61] Although studies with various knockout mice have emphasized the role of specific gene products working in the brain (see Mayfield et al.,[34] such as Homer 2,[49] opioid receptors,[8] and alpha 4 nicotinic receptors[50] in conferring either protection from or increased risks of addiction). In addition it is apparent that the contribution of any single gene in the development of addition for any drug is only a small part of the picture. Like most familial behavioral phenotypes, drug and alcohol use disorders result from the complex interaction of multiple genes.[46] This complexity may account for ongoing challenges associated with the development of addiction and solutions to deal with them. Needless to say, multiple genes exert their effects in the context of genetic networks, which are typically under the influence of environmental factors. These early effects initiated by the gene product induced by drugs or alcohol most likely cascade through the signaling pathways and generate a domino effect.[59] To understand the complete molecular or gene expression changes that may occur in the brain due to drug and alcohol use it is important to capture those changes as a whole and perform a systematic analysis. One novel and effective approach that has been used in recent years to decipher and unravel this complex mystery is metabolomics.

Metabolomics: The Beginning

The completion of the human genome project has made it possible to investigate the whole genome using high-throughput technologies and analyze data via a systems approach (see Fig. 14.1). Derivation of molecular-based strategies, development of new computer application and technologies, and the application of bioinformatics are accelerating the elucidation of molecular underpinnings of human diseases as well as helping to effectively prevent, diagnose, and treat these diseases. These strategies can also be successfully applied in addiction-related disorders.

Since molecular biology's early years, biological questions have been successfully approached mainly by studying individual gene function(s) and gene products, one or a few at a time. Despite understanding the cause of many biological problems, however, many fundamental biological questions remain to be answered. This is mainly because the majority of gene products function together, interacting with other gene products and influencing multiple pathways. Therefore, biological processes should be considered as complex networks of interconnected components. In addition to studying the components individually, it is important to study the combined nature of these gene products in the metabolomic networks and pathways.

Metabolomics in Addiction Research: Current Approach

Selection of Technology to Capture Metabolomic Changes

Recent advances in the latest technologies allow profiling of all metabolic components in a biological system at any given time, investigating of dynamic changes in component quantity or quality in a system under external stimuli or perturbation, and finally, analyzing the changes of one component in relation to another. The goal here would be to generate protein-protein, protein-DNA, or other component-component mapping of the networking pathways involved. Gene expression microarray is one such high-throughput technology that allows detection of cellular changes at the transcript level and has been used extensively in research on alcohol and other drugs of abuse.[15,16,53] Gene expression profiling using microarray chips has proved to be the most successful genome-wide technology to capture the temporal-spatial expression pattern of a cell. Because the expression microarrays are an RNA-based method, they are highly effective in the simultaneous identification and measurement of virtually all transcripts that are differentially expressed between any two samples representing treatment (e.g., ethanol) and control. Transcript profiling using microarrays is the most widespread functional genomics technique because of its relative technical simplicity, low cost, and short turnaround time. In recent years, the development of high-density microarray chips has allowed us to present the entire transcriptome of more complex organisms such as human and mouse on a single chip. The availability of improved algorithms and easy to use software has made it possible to interpret and analyze the microarray data without much computer knowledge. Of all the addictions, such studies have been extensively used in alcoholism.

Over the last 5 years, studies on humans and animal models using microarray have contributed to our knowledge of the molecular effects of alcohol and identified a number of potential candidate genes of interest in the context of alcohol response alone. In addition, microarray experiments generate a large number of ethanol-responsive genes, some of which are repeatedly identified as such in multiple reports regardless of experimental paradigm. However, it would be extremely difficult and time consuming to investigate this large number of genes using a single or candidate gene approach. Because these genes belong to multiple biochemical pathways including stress response, gene regulation, apoptosis, cell growth, and cell signaling,[53,57] we need to analyze them altogether in the context of cell and tissue system.

Tissue and Organ of Interest

In order to investigate the effect on gene expression following drug or alcohol exposure, cells or tissues from participants and their matched controls are needed. In most cases brain and brain regions are viewed as most appropriate. However, matched samples of brains are not available for such studies. The next best option is to make use of brain bank samples. This too is not always practical. More importantly, matching participant and control brains is not an easy task, as they differ in a large number of parameters that may affect gene expression. We will not discuss this issue any further except to state that in the lack of human brain matched samples, and due to the problem of manipulative experiments on humans, most studies have relied on a number of animal models. Of course this approach has its own drawbacks. With

this realization, we focus this discussion on one of the favored animal model (e.g., mouse). This has a number of advantages. Established genetic strains of mice are available and widely used that differ in responses to various drugs, including preference to voluntary alcohol consumption. For example, strain C57BL/6 J consistently demonstrates high ethanol preference, which is about 60% in comparison to strains A/J (26%), BALB/CJ (30.4%), and DBA/2 J (11.8%), given the free choice of water and 10% ethanol over a 14-day period.[31] Once a suitable genetic animal model is selected and the drug preference phenotype is reconfirmed with an in-house study, the animal model can be used in necessary experimental treatment with the drug under study following appropriate methods. This allows collection of the desired organ following appropriate treatment along with strain/genotype-, age-, and sex-matched controls. The drug treatment may involve various modes and durations as appropriate. It is also possible to include various environmental manipulations including stresses before or after the exposure to the addictive drug being investigated. The tissue of interest (e.g., brain) is collected at the appropriate time and processed for studies on DNA, RNA, and protein including structural and developmental alterations that may be affected in any drug response including addiction. Although such studies in the past have concentrated on RNA and protein including cellular changes, it is important to point out that future studies may include DNA and protein changes, reflecting epigenetic modifications. In fact it is likely that the addiction to a drug that is acquired following repeated exposures may involve epigenetic changes (DNA methylation, histone modification including chromatin alterations), which has remained on the side line of such a research. We will not go into any detail except to point out that such changes will explain a variety of RNA and protein changes that have been reported in response to drugs and drug addictions. For mainstream research in the new genomic era, the tissues of interest are harvested from an experimental animal model and used for RNA isolation. The purified RNA is hybridized to a suitable expression array, which allows identification of genes that are affected as a result of drug exposures.

Generating a Gene List

The microarray is hybridized, scanned, and analyzed following the manufacturer's recommended method and software. Microarray experiments generate a large number of genes, which are analyzed further using bioinformatics tools and software. It is beneficial to develop a list of genes that show significant difference in expression between treatment, gender, and age, or any other selected parameters. This list can be further refined by primarily excluding genes for which no information is available in the public databases such as the National Center for Biotechnology Information (NCBI; http://www.ncbi.nlm.nih.gov/), Ensembl (http://www.ensembl.org/index.html), GO (http://www.geneontology.org/), UCSC (http://genome.ucsc.edu/), and so on (see Verstreken et al.[60]). These genes are used in the subsequent analysis as explained in Fig. 14.2.

Bioinformatics Tools and Analysis

It is apparent that in most cases a single gene may carry out several functions in the cell by interacting with other genes in the network. In this way, the action of one gene product dynamically affects the action of others in a cascading fashion in the cellular pathways, generating a complex global network.[22] In order to identify how a particular gene interacts in a subsystem, how all the subsystems coordinate into a particular pathway, and how the collective actions of multiple implicated pathways emerge into a global network in the metabolome, causing multifaceted alcohol or drug effect, the genes are analyzed using specialized software to predict biological association network. Currently many biological pathway analysis and visualization software programs are available. Some of the commercial and free software are listed in Table 14.1.

Genes from the list are used as input in pathway analysis software to study the neurometabolomics and to predict biological association (Fig. 14.3). These programs are generally connected with underlying database(s) and allow the user to query the database(s) for genes of interest. These databases for human, mouse, rat, yeast, or any other organisms are compiled by retrieving relevant published scientific information from public databases such as PubMed (http://www.ncbi.nlm.nih.gov/pubmed/) using automated natural language processing or other data mining techniques. The retrieved information is then curated and stored in the database, for example, in the form of cellular events such as regulation, interaction, and modifications among proteins, cell processes, and small cellular molecules. Upon query to the

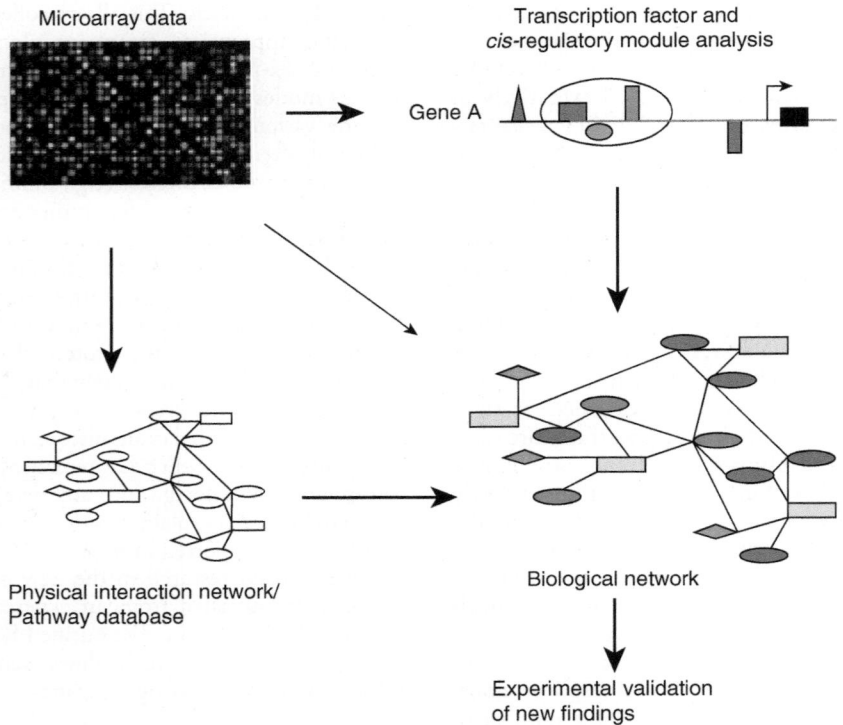

• **Fig. 14.2** Overall view of an integrated approach to constructing pathway or regulatory interaction network. Data generated from microarray experiment can be used to perform transcription regulatory network and/or biological interaction network.

TABLE 14.1	Useful Bioinformatics Software Tools and Databases for Protein-Protein Interaction and Transcription Regulatory Network Pathway Analysis.	
Type of Resource	**Web Address (URL)**
Pathway Databases	
EcoCyc	http://ecocyc.org/
KEGG	http://www.genome.jp/kegg/
MIPS	http://mips.gsf.de/genre/proj/yeast/
PathGuide	http://www.pathguide.org/
REACTOME	https://www.reactome.org/
SigPath	https://bioconductor.org/packages/release/bioc/html/sigPathway.html
Pathway Analysis, Visualization, and Prediction Tools	
Bibliosphere (commercial)	http://www.genomatix.de/products/BiblioSphere/
BioLayout *Express*3D (free)	https://www.ebi.ac.uk/about/news/service-news/BioLayoutExpress3D

Continued

TABLE 14.1   Useful Bioinformatics Software Tools and Databases for Protein-Protein Interaction and Transcription Regulatory Network Pathway Analysis.—cont'd

Type of Resource	Web Address (URL)
Cytoscape (open source, free)	https://cytoscape.org/
GENECENSUS	http://bioinfo.mbb.yale.edu/genome/
GenMAPP (free)	http://www.genmapp.org/introduction.html
GNA (Genetic Network Analyzer)	http://ralyx.inria.fr/2008/Raweb/ibis/uid16.html
Ingenuity Pathway Analysis (commercial)	http://www.ingenuity.com/products/pathways_analysis.html
Osprey (free)	http://biodata.mshri.on.ca/osprey/servlet/Index
Pathway Studio (commercial)	http://www.ariadnegenomics.com/products/pathway-studio/
VisANT	http://visant.bu.edu/
Transcription Regulatory Databases	
DBTSS	http://dbtss_old.hgc.jp/hg17/
EPD	https://epd.epfl.ch//index.php
JASPER	http://jaspar.cgb.ki.se/cgi-bin/jaspar_db.pl
PReMOD	http://genomequebec.mcgill.ca/PReMod/
Rvista	http://genome.lbl.gov/vista/index.shtml
TRANSFAC	http://www.gene-regulation.com/pub/databases.html
TRED	http://rulai.cshl.edu/cgi-bin/TRED/tred.cgi?process=home
TRRD	http://wwwmgs.bionet.nsc.ru/mgs/gnw/trrd/
Regulatory Network Analysis Tools	
GEMS Launcher (commercial)	http://www.genomatix.de
Gene Regulation Tools	http://zlab.bu.edu/zlab/gene.shtml
GeneExpress	http://wwwmgs.bionet.nsc.ru/mgs/systems/geneexpress/
RSAT	http://rsat.ulb.ac.be/rsat/
Toucan (open source, free)	http://homes.esat.kuleuven.be/~saerts/software/toucan.php
Protein Interaction Databases	
3DID	http://3did.irbbarcelona.org/
AfCS	http://www.signaling-gateway.org/
BIND	https://www.ebi.ac.uk/miriam/main/collections/MIR:00000001
DIMA	http://mips.gsf.de/genre/proj/dima2/
DIP	http://dip.doe-mbi.ucla.edu/
HPRD	http://www.hprd.org/
INTACT	http://www.ebi.ac.uk/intact/site/index.jsf
iPfam	http://ipfam.sanger.ac.uk/
MINT	http://mint.bio.uniroma2.it/mint/Welcome.do
PDZBase	http://icb.med.cornell.edu/services/pdz/start
PIBASE	http://modbase.compbio.ucsf.edu/pibase/queries.html
Prolinks	http://mysql5.mbi.ucla.edu/cgi-bin/functionator/pronav

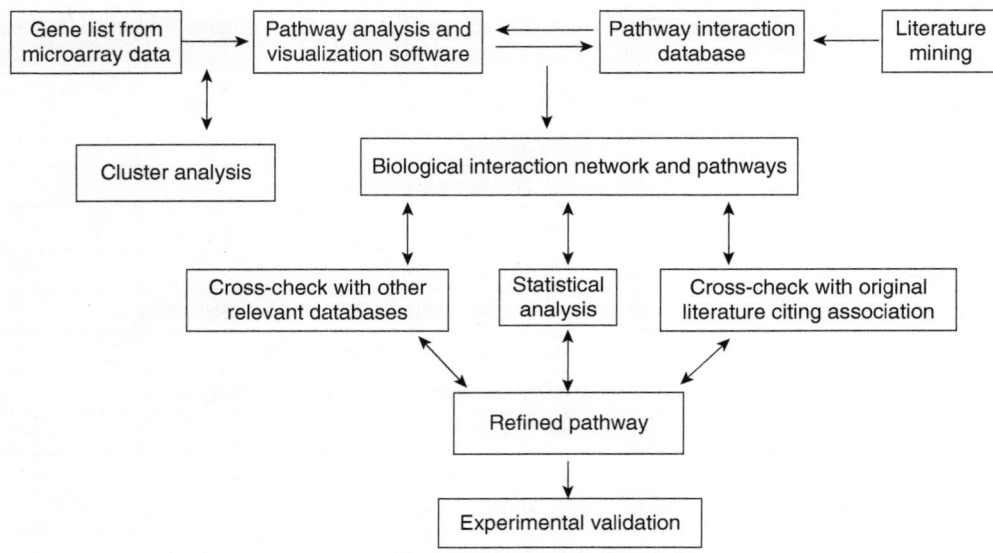

• **Fig. 14.3** Workflow of constructing meaningful biological interaction network and pathways from microarray data.

database, the software program will construct a biological interaction network and provide visualization in a graph format for further exploration, examination, and prediction. Some of the programs also have a built-in Gene Ontology search while others have additional features such as integrated transcription factor and *cis*-regulatory sequence analysis option (e.g., Bibliosphere). Commercial pathway analysis software is generally easy to use with available guides and tutorials, where the open source or free software requires an extra learning curve and customization based on user's need.

An initial output from such analysis may generate a network graph that may seem highly complex due to the presence of all possible associations among all matching gene products upon query to the database. Fig. 14.4 shows an example of a simplified view of one such initial outputs from PathwayStudio pathway analysis software. In this example, mouse Affymetrix chips were used to assess the relative expression of genes in the brain in response to acute ethanol treatment on two genetic strains of mice (DBA/2 J or D2 and C57BL/6 J or B6) that are known to differ with respect to their responses to alcohol.[53] The expression array results showed that the genes fall into two main categories: strain-specific and strain-specific ethanol-responsive genes. Only the ethanol-responsive gene data set, containing about 60 genes, was then used in cluster analysis to predict genes that tend to coexpress in response to ethanol treatment. The results revealed that eight of the genes show downregulation at the same level in both B6 and D2 mice in response to ethanol and nine demonstrate upregulation, which is higher in D2 mice than in B6 mice, while 24 of the genes show upregulation at the same magnitude in both B6 and D2 mice. This last cluster was further analyzed in the PathwayStudio software. The output was filtered to include only protein, cell complex, functional class, cell process, and cell object. All irrelevant interactions and associations were removed from the network and the result, as shown in Fig. 14.4, represents the most relevant biological associations among 24 ethanol-responsive genes. A network graph like this one is generally composed of nodes and lines. Nodes are shown by symbols of different shapes and sizes (e.g., circular, oval, triangle, rectangle, of different colors), which can

represent any biomolecule such as protein, enzyme, cell complex, cell process, treatment, DNA, RNA, and metabolite. Nodes are connected by lines (straight or curved) representing physical interaction, association, or relationship between nodes (e.g., protein-protein, protein-DNA, and protein-cell process). In addition, the lines can also be of different types to indicate the type of association such as binding, regulation, and expression. A positive or negative sign can be associated with each type to represent the specific nature of the interaction. Color code can be used to include metabolomic category of the genes being studied. In a transcription regulatory network, the nodes generally represent transcription factors, cofactors, and DNA *cis*-regulatory elements. Lines in a regulatory network would indicate physical interaction between transcription factors and *cis*-regulatory elements, that is, protein-DNA interactions.

Once the initial network is developed, each interaction between two nodes (e.g., cell processes, proteins, enzymes, cell complex, and treatment) should be verified individually by examining the cited curation and literature. Any irrelevant and indirect relationship should also be excluded from the network during final analysis. The result is also further cross-checked with other relevant database entries and can be statistically validated using an appropriate algorithm. This kind of rigorous exercise helps reveal significant and fruitful information generally hidden in the network. For example, an analysis similar to the one described in Fig. 14.4 starting with all 60 ethanol-responsive genes was narrowed down to only 7 genes that showed direct connection to ethanol in closely interacting pathways in the brain (Fig. 14.5). The result shows that ethanol affects multiple cellular events, which include synthesis and degradation, gene regulation, transcription, translation and expression, phosphorylation, molecular transport, biogenesis, and various enzymatic activities. Through this and other subsequent downstream events, ethanol contributes both positively and negatively to a large number of biochemical pathways. Although drugs of abuse act on different receptor systems, they activate common downstream sequences of events, which underlie characteristic behavioral phenotypes such as compulsive drug-taking, craving, and relapse.[42]

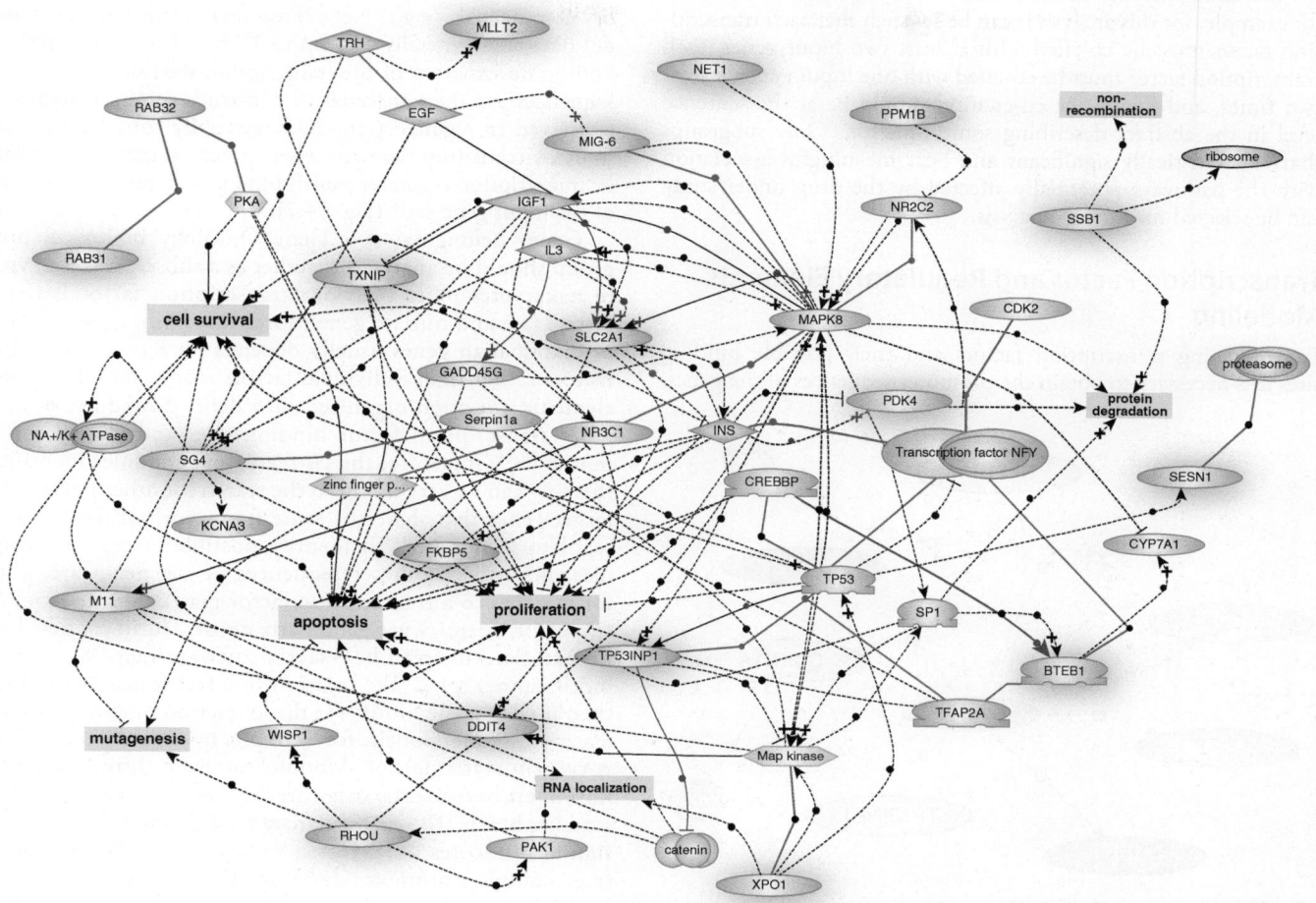

• **Fig. 14.4** Functional interactions of 24 ethanol-responsive gene products. Ethanol-responsive gene products (*orange ovals* shaded in *green*) are shown with other cellular objects such as protein (*orange ovals*), cell complex (e.g., transcription factor NFY, Na+/K+ ATPase), and cell process (*yellow rectangles*). These interactions could be of several different types: expression (e.g., *blue lines* connecting two cell objects), regulation (e.g., *gray lines*), and binding (e.g., *purple lines*). The interactions of these ethanol-responsive genes contribute directly or indirectly to a number of cell processes, specifically apoptosis, cell survival, and proliferation. (Reproduced from Uddin RK, Singh SM. Cis-Regulatory sequences of the genes involved in apoptosis, cell growth, and proliferation may provide a target for some of the effects of acute ethanol exposure. *Brain Res.* 2006;1088(1):31–44, with permission from Elsevier.)

Transcription Regulatory Network in Drug Metabolomics

As described in the preceding text, the action of ethanol and other drugs may be realized through the transcriptional control of gene expression, transcriptional regulators, or factors, and their combinatorial control on *cis*-regulatory elements play a critical role in the coexpression of these genes. This affects the interaction of genes in the metabolome and thus may affect signals that cascade through cellular pathways. There has been rapid progress in recent years in the development of a systems approach for identifying such transcriptional regulatory networks from high-throughput data generally generated from microarray experiments.[4,51,58] A summary of this powerful approach is outlined in Fig. 14.6.

Gene Selection and Literature Analysis

Because this approach can also use microarray technology, a list of genes showing significant difference between experimental and control cells or tissues can be developed using microarray experiments as described in the previous strategy or using similar comparable methods. Now we need to investigate all possible physical interactions between transcription factors and between transcription factors and *cis*-regulatory elements, for example, promoters, enhancers, and other *cis*-acting regulatory elements on the promoter regions involving these genes. Various free and commercial software packages are available for this purpose (Table 14.1) that offer a number of modeling tools integrated with statistical algorithms and curated literature and transcription factor databases. The strategy outlined below can be performed using either free software tools such as the TOUCAN package or commercial software such as the GEMS Launcher package (see Table 14.1).

Once the genes are selected, they are used in literature analysis to identify possible transcription factors that interact with their promoter sequences either manually or by using commercially available software such as Bibliosphere (http://www.genomatix.de). This analysis is performed to subgroup the initial gene set into overexpressed Gene Ontology groups based on the results from the literature analysis. The stringency level can be set by the user, for example, for this analysis it can be set such that each transcription factor must be co-cited with at least two input genes, each transcription factor must be co-cited with one input genes at least two times, and finally the co-citation should be at the sentence level in the abstract describing some function. Only subgroups that are statistically significant and bear meaningful association with the pathways potentially affected by the drug under study can be selected for further analysis.

Transcription Factor and Regulatory Elements Modeling

For modeling transcription factors and their possible binding sites it is necessary to obtain the promoter sequences of the genes.

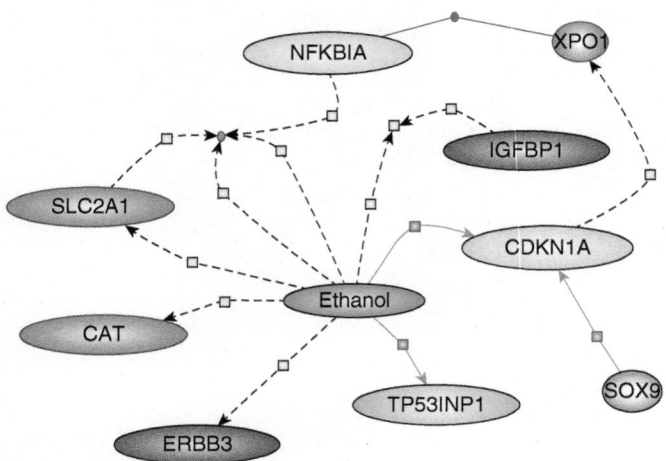

• **Fig. 14.5** An example of a final interaction network. A proposed pathway for ethanol's action on genes is shown where they directly interact with ethanol and other genes in the brain. This kind of small network showing the most relevant associations can be developed from an initial output of a pathway analysis software and can be used for further experimental validation. (Reprinted from Uddin RK, Treadwell JA, Singh SM. Towards unraveling ethanol-specific neuro-metabolomics based on ethanol responsive genes in vivo. *Neurochem Res.* 2005;30(9):1179–1190, with permission from Springer Science + Business Media.)

They can be retrieved from any public (e.g., NCBI and Ensembl) or commercial (e.g., Gene2Promoter http://www.genomatix.de) databases generally 500 bp to 1 kb upstream and 100 bp to 200 bp downstream of the transcription start site. The promoter sequences are then analyzed to construct common significantly conserved *cis*-regulatory modules, generally consisting of two or more *cis*-regulatory elements where potential transcription factors or transcription regulator motifs bind on the promoter sequences of the input gene set[58] (Fig. 14.7).

Genes belonging to a Gene Ontology biological process group should be analyzed together as a subset. It is known that in eukaryotes more than one transcription factor is required to regulate and initiate gene expression. Also, the coregulation of mammalian genes usually depends on sets of transcription factors rather than individual factors alone, and *cis*-regulatory elements are often organized into defined modules of two or more transcription factor binding sites and clusters of such motifs.[10,14] Therefore, the *cis*-regulatory modules identified in this way can be very useful in the search for other potential new target genes that share the same framework of the known *cis*-regulatory modules. To identify possible *cis*-regulatory modules, first, the promoter sequences of the genes are scanned for matches to a transcription factor matrix library (e.g., Mat-Inspector, http://www.genomatix.de or MotifScanner, http://homes.esat.kuleuven.be/~saerts/software/help/WebServices/motifscanner.htm). The transcription factor matches found are then used as basic motifs for the extraction of common *cis*-regulatory module models, for example, by FrameWorker (http://www.genomatix.de) or ModuleSearchers (http://homes.esat.kuleuven.be/~saerts/software/help/WebServices/modulesearcher.htm).. The *cis*-regulatory module models with the best significant scores are selected to scan other DNA sequences (e.g., complete promoter database of organism or animal under study) for matches to these models. This would also verify the specificity of the models generated by the modeling software used. The bioinformatics tools that can be used for this search are, for example, ModelInspector (http://www.genomatix.de) or MotifSampler (http://homes.esat.kuleuven.be/~saerts/software/tutorial1/TOUCAN_Tutorial_MotifSampler.html). This approach also can identify other potential target genes of *cis*-regulatory module models predicted above.

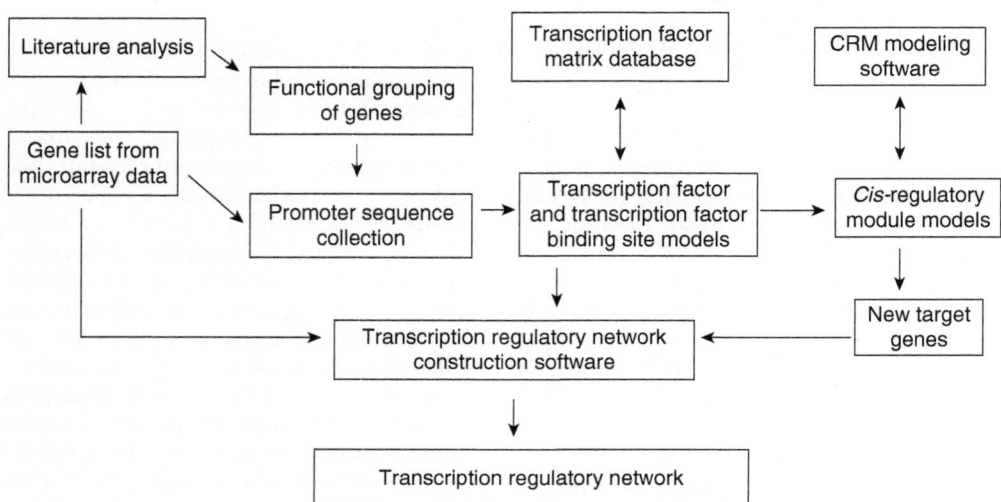

• **Fig. 14.6** Workflow of generating transcription regulatory network.

The use of this strategy in research on drugs of abuse has shown promising results. For example, one research involving alcohol has shown that the alcohol-responsive metallothionein genes[31,32] Mt1 and Mt2, are regulated by transcription factor cyclic AMP responsive element-binding protein and metal-activated transcription factor 1 and involved primarily in zinc ion homeostasis.[58] Cyclic AMP responsive element binding is known to control gene expression for a variety of functions in the central nervous system and thought to be associated with both anxiety and alcohol preference. Haplodeficiency of the cyclic AMP responsive element binding gene and ethanol-induced decreases in cyclic AMP responsive element binding function have been shown to be associated with increased alcohol drinking in mice.

The search in the modeling databases for genes that share the same cis-regulatory module as cyclic AMP responsive element binding has revealed new target genes Synj1 (synaptojanin 1) and Tph1 (tryptophan hydroxylase 1), potentially regulated by this module. Synj1 is known to be involved in the regulation of synaptic vesicle function and has been studied as a potential candidate gene for psychiatric disorders.[43,60] Of interest, the Tph1 gene product is known as a rate-limiting enzyme in the biosynthesis of serotonin and its activity is most abundant in the brain. Alteration in brain serotonin level has been implicated as an important contributing factor in many psychiatric disorders including alcoholism.[3] Altered arrangement of transcription factor binding sites in the module can direct the action of these and other target genes in intracellular signaling cascades, cell growth, and/or maintenance. In addition to cyclic AMP responsive element binding, other key transcription factors identified are EVI1 (ecotropic viral integration site-1) and SP1. These factors modulate the contribution of the target ethanol-responsive genes in cell cycle regulation and apoptosis or programmed cell death. Multiple lines of evidence indicate that different groups of ethanol-responsive genes are involved in different biological processes, and their coregulation most likely results from different sets of regulatory modules.

Construction of Transcription Regulatory Network

The new target genes identified are added to the original list and the newly compiled list of genes is used to construct a regulatory

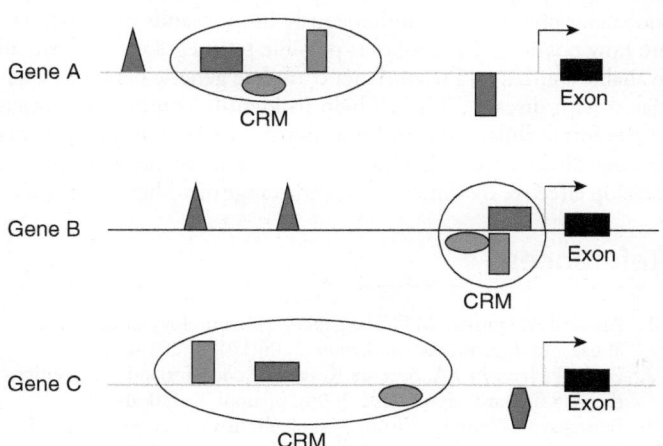

• Fig. 14.7 Transcription factor and regulatory elements modeling. The figure shows a common cis-regulatory module (CRM) consisting of three common transcription factors (shown as colored shapes) shared by genes A, B, and C.

network using the information available in the interaction databases. This way the microarray gene expression data profiles and transcription factor cis-regulatory module analysis data are integrated into protein-protein and protein-DNA interaction data available in the databases to obtain a broader systems view. Because gene expression and cis-regulatory module location data provide complementary information, integration of these data sources can emphasize the functional part of the network and thus make the inferred network more biologically relevant. There has been significant progress in the development of interaction databases (see Table 14.1). These databases are constructed by storing curated published protein-DNA or protein-protein interaction obtained from extensive literature mining where in the literature protein-DNA interaction was validated using ChIP-chip analysis and protein-protein interaction was measured by two-hybrid system, Co-IP and mass spectrometry experiments. Results from other high-throughput technologies, such as genome-wide location analysis and cap analysis of gene expression, that experimentally map many types of functional DNA elements on the genome are also used. Although the use of different databases in constructing the regulatory network may vary, the basic construction principle would be the same as constructing a pathway (see Fig. 14.2).

A refined regulatory network constructed from an integrated approach can provide novel biological insight into cellular interactions in response to drugs and alcohol. This may predict new genes that are contributing in a particular pathway or indicate up or downstream effects of other pathways. Now would be time to experimentally validate these findings with rigorous testing. However, before jumping into experiment one must consider that the predicted networks are time, space, and condition dependent, that is, different parts of the network will likely be active in different conditions. They have to be evaluated under the specific condition of interest.

A network established this way is termed as a static network. This kind of network can be generated for a given dose of drug or alcohol for each cell, tissue, or organ type for an animal system. A number of static networks can be connected and mapped together to generate a tissue- and drug-specific dynamic network (see Fig. 14.1), which would provide significant knowledge toward our understanding of the metabolomics of drugs of abuse.

Application of Metabolomics in Solving Addiction Disorders

The strategies presented have been successfully applied in studying tissue- and disease-specific regulatory networks for human diseases, including cancer,[44,52] cardiac hypoxia,[12] innate immunity,[19] and inflammation.[6] They were also used in the past to study the metabolomics of alcohol action.[57-59] Most recently,[30] a similar method was used to develop a common molecular network underlying addiction to different abusive substances. Using literature mining, a Knowledgebase of Addiction-Related Genes (KARG) was developed (http://opendata.pku.edu.cn/dataset.xhtml?persistentId=doi:10.18170/DVN/OZUJRU&language=en) that contains over 2000 items of evidence linking 1500 human genes to addiction. Sequences of nearly 400 human addiction-related genes were analyzed using bioinformatics tools, for example, KOBAS software,[45] and mapped to statistically significant, biologically meaningful, experimentally validated pathways in the Kyoto Encyclopedia of Genes and Genomes (KEGG) database.[23] Molecular pathways that

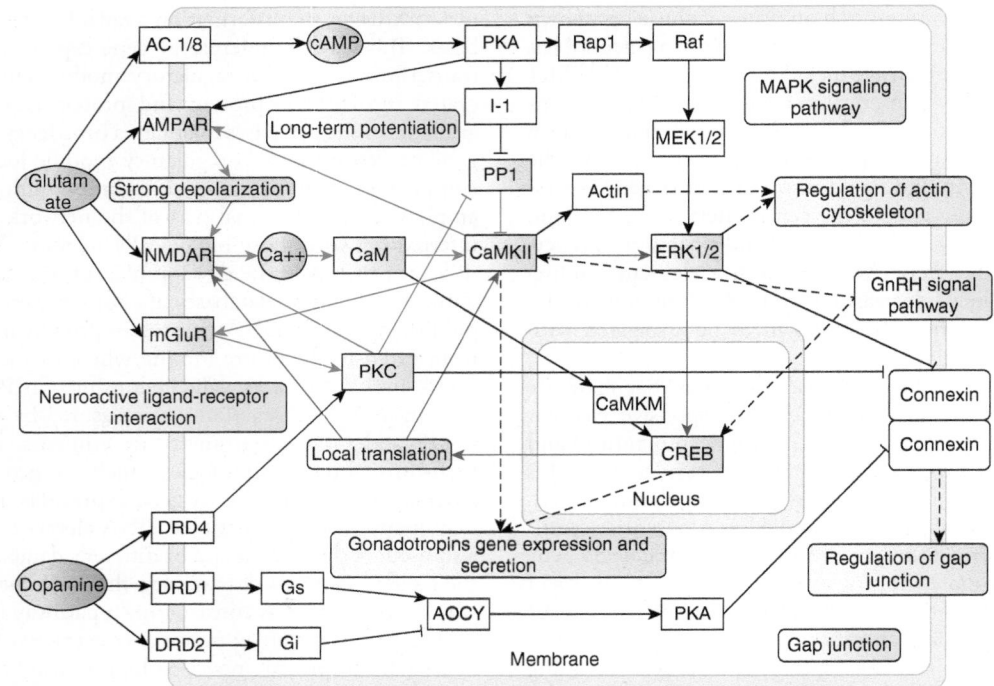

• **Fig. 14.8** Hypothetical common molecular network for drug addiction. The network was constructed manually based on the common pathways identified and protein interaction data. Addiction-related genes were represented as *white boxes* while neurotransmitters and secondary messengers were highlighted in *purple*. The common pathways are highlighted in *green boxes*. Related functional modules such as "regulation of cytoskeleton," "regulation of cell cycle," "regulation of gap junction," and "gene expression and secretion of gonadotropins" were highlighted in *carmine boxes*. Several positive feedback loops were identified in this network. Fast positive feedback loops were highlighted in *red lines* and slow ones were highlighted in *blue lines*. (Reprinted from Li CY, Mao X, Wei L. Genes and (common) pathways underlying drug addiction. *PLoS Comput Biol.* 2008;4(1):e2, with permission.)

were identified as significantly enriched for four drugs of abuse including cocaine, alcohol, opioids, and nicotine were selected as common pathways for drug addiction. This study found several pathways shared by all four addictive substances—long-term potentiation, mitogen-activated protein kinase (MAPK) signaling pathway, GnRH signaling pathway, and gap junction—and by connecting these pathways with additional protein-protein interaction data constructed a hypothetical common molecular network for drug addiction (Fig. 14.8). Of interest, cyclic AMP (cAMP) responsive element binding, an important transcription factor implicated in alcohol research,[58] has also been identified in this common pathway.

Integration of Systems Biology to Medication Discovery

Common human diseases are driven by complex networks of genes and a number of environmental factors. To understand this complexity in order to identify targets and develop medications against disease, a systematic approach is required to elucidate the genetic and environmental factors and interactions among and between these factors, and to establish how these factors induce changes in gene networks that in turn lead to disease.

The rapid progress in the development of large-scale high-throughput genetic screening technologies, and the availability

of super computing power of modern specialized software and instant high-speed web access to numerous genetic data repository have enabled researchers to take a more systems biology approach to study complex traits like disease. Genotyping of hundreds of thousands of DNA markers, scanning through millions of single nucleotide polymorphisms, and profiling tens of thousands of molecular phenotypes simultaneously in thousands of individuals are now possible. This makes it possible to integrate data from all available sources and reconstruct complete genetic networks associated with disease. This can help us identify common pathways in the intracellular signaling cascades shared by the causal factors driving disease, formulate clinical approach for prevention, and develop effective treatments for a wide range of addictive disorders.

References

1. Agrawal A, Lynskey MT. The genetic epidemiology of cannabis use, abuse and dependence. *Addiction.* 2006;101(6):801–812.
2. Baak JP, Janssen EA, Soreide K, et al. Genomics and proteomics – the way forward. *Ann Oncol.* 2005;16(suppl 2):ii30–ii44.
3. Banerjee N. Neurotransmitters in alcoholism: a review of neurobiological and genetic studies. *Indian J Hum Genet.* 2014;20(1):20–31.
4. Bansal M, Belcastro V, Ambesi-Impiombato A, et al. How to infer gene networks from expression profiles. *Mol Syst Biol.* 2007;3:78.
5. Beirut LJ. Genetic vulnerability and susceptibility to substance dependence. *Neuron.* 2011;69(4):618–627.

6. Calvano SE, Xiao W, Richards DR, et al. A network-based analysis of systemic inflammation in humans. *Nature.* 2005;437(7061):1032–1037.

7. CDC. *Targeting Tobacco Use: The Nation's Leading Cause of Death.* Atlanta, GA: National Center for Chronic Disease Prevention and Health Promotion, Centers for Disease Control and Prevention; 2005.

8. Chefer VI, Kieffer BL, Shippenberg TS. Contrasting effects of mu opioid receptor and delta opioid receptor deletion upon the behavioral and neurochemical effects of cocaine. *Neuroscience.* 2004;127(2):497–503.

9. Claudino WM, Quattrone A, Biganzoli L, et al. Metabolomics: available results, current research projects in breast cancer, and future applications. *J Clin Oncol.* 2007;25(19):2840–2846.

10. Elkon R, Linhart C, Sharan R, et al. Genome-wide in silico identification of transcriptional regulators controlling the cell cycle in human cells. *Genome Res.* 2003;13(5):773–780.

11. Faber JH, Malmodin D, Toft H, et al. Metabonomics in diabetes research. *J Diabetes Sci Technol.* 2007;1(4):549–557.

12. Feala JD, Coquin L, Paternostro G, et al. Integrating metabolomics and phenomics with systems models of cardiac hypoxia. *Prog Biophys Mol Biol.* 2008;96(1–3):209–225.

13. Feltenstein MW, See RE. The neurocircuitry of addiction: an overview. *Br J Pharmacol.* 2008;154(2):261–274.

14. Fessele S, Maier H, Zischek C, et al. Regulatory context is a crucial part of gene function. *Trends Genet.* 2002;18(2):60–63.

15. Flatscher-Bader T, van der Brug MP, Landis N, et al. Comparative gene expression in brain regions of human alcoholics. *Genes Brain Behav.* 2006;5(suppl 1):78–84.

16. Flatscher-Bader T, Zuvela N, Landis N, et al. Smoking and alcoholism target genes associated with plasticity and glutamate transmission in the human ventral tegmental area. *Hum Mol Genet.* 2008;17(1):38–51.

17. Gardner TJ, Kosten TR. Therapeutic options and challenges for substances of abuse. *Dialogues Clin Neurosci.* 2007;9(4):431–445.

18. German JB, Hammock BD, Watkins SM. Metabolomics: building on a century of biochemistry to guide human health. *Metabolomics.* 2005;1(1):3–9.

19. Gilchrist M, Thorsson V, Li B, et al. Systems biology approaches identify ATF3 as a negative regulator of Toll-like receptor 4. *Nature.* 2006;441(7090):173–178.

20. Gomase VS, Changbhale SS, Patil SA, et al. Metabolomics. *Curr Drug Metab.* 2008;9(1):89–98.

21. Harwood HJ, Fountain D, Fountain G. Economic cost of alcohol and drug abuse in the United States, 1992: a report. *Addiction.* 1999;94(5):631–635.

22. Huang S. Back to the biology in systems biology: what can we learn from biomolecular networks? *Brief Funct Genomic Proteomic.* 2004;2(4):279–297.

23. Kanehisa M, Goto S, Hattori M, et al. From genomics to chemical genomics: new developments in KEGG. *Nucleic Acids Res.* 2006;34(Database issue):D354–D357.

24. Kendler KS, Jacobson KC, Prescott CA, et al. Specificity of genetic and environmental risk factors for use and abuse/dependence of cannabis, cocaine, hallucinogens, sedatives, stimulants, and opiates in male twins. *Am J Psychiatry.* 2003;160(4):687–695.

25. Koob GF The neurobiology of addiction: a neuroadaptational view relevant for diagnosis. *Addiction.* 2006;101(suppl 1):23–30.

26. Koob GF, Vokow ND. Neurocircuitry of addiction. *Neuropsychopharmacology.* 2010;35(1):217–238.

27. Kreek MJ. Drug addictions. Molecular and cellular endpoints. *Ann NY Acad Sci.* 2001;937:27–49.

28. Kreek MJ, Nielsen DA, LaForge KS. Genes associated with addiction: alcoholism, opiate, and cocaine addiction. *Neuromolecular Med.* 2004;5(1):85–108.

29. Leshner AI. Addiction is a brain disease, and it matters. *Science.* 1997;278(5335):45–47.

30. Li CY, Mao X, Wei L. Genes and (common) pathways underlying drug addiction. *PLoS Comput Biol.* 2008;4(1):e2.

31. Loney KD, Uddin KR, Singh SM. Strain-specific brain metallothionein II (MT-II) gene expression, its ethanol responsiveness, and association with ethanol preference in mice. *Alcohol Clin Exp Res.* 2003;27(3):388–395.

32. Loney KD, Uddin RK, Singh SM. Analysis of metallothionein brain gene expression in relation to ethanol preference in mice using cosegregation and gene knockouts. *Alcohol Clin Exp Res.* 2006;30(1):15–25.

33. Maxwell JC, Rutkowski BA. The prevalence of methamphetamine and amphetamine abuse in North America: a review of the indicators, 1992–2007. *Drug Alcohol Rev.* 2008;27(3):229–235.

34. Mayfield RD, Harris RA, Schuckit MA. Genetic factors influencing alcohol dependence. *Br J Pharmacol.* 2008;154(2):275–287.

35. Minozzi S, Amato L, Davoli M, et al. Anticonvulsants for cocaine dependence. *Cochrane Database Syst Rev.* 2008;2:CD006754.

36. Reference deleted in review.

37. O'Brien CP. Research advances in the understanding and treatment of addiction. *Am J Addict.* 2003;12(suppl 2):S36–S47.

38. Reference deleted in review.

39. Oscar-Berman M, Shagrin B, Evert DL, et al. Impairments of brain and behavior: the neurological effects of alcohol. *Alcohol Health Res World.* 1997;21(1):65–75.

40. Oswald LM, Wand GS. Opioids and alcoholism. *Physiol Behav.* 2004;81(2):339–358.

41. Parker AJ, Marshall EJ, Ball DM. Diagnosis and management of alcohol use disorders. *BMJ.* 2008;336(7642):496–501.

42. Ron D, Jurd R. The "ups and downs" of signaling cascades in addiction. *Sci STKE.* 2005;2005(309):re14.

43. Saito T, Guan F, Papolos DF, et al. Mutation analysis of SYNJ1: a possible candidate gene for chromosome 21q22-linked bipolar disorder. *Mol Psychiatry.* 2001;6(4):387–395.

44. Segal E, Friedman N, Kaminski N, et al. From signatures to models: understanding cancer using microarrays. *Nat Genet.* 2005;37(suppl):S38–S45.

45. Shi YH, Zhu SW, Mao XZ, et al. Transcriptome profiling, molecular biological, and physiological studies reveal a major role for ethylene in cotton fiber cell elongation. *Plant Cell.* 2006;18(3):651–664.

46. Singh SM, Treadwell J, Kleiber ML, et al. Analysis of behavior using genetical genomics in mice as a model: from alcohol preferences to gene expression differences. *Genome.* 2007;50(10):877–897.

47. Stein EA, Pankiewicz J, Harsch HH, et al. Nicotine-induced limbic cortical activation in the human brain: a functional MRI study. *Am J Psychiatry.* 1998;155(8):1009–1015.

48. Sullivan LE, Fiellin DA. Narrative review: buprenorphine for opioid-dependent patients in office practice. *Ann Intern Med.* 2008;148(9):662–670.

49. Szumlinski KK, Dehoff MH, Kang SH, et al. Homer proteins regulate sensitivity to cocaine. *Neuron.* 2004;43(3):401–413.

50. Tapper AR, McKinney SL, Nashmi R, et al. Nicotine activation of alpha4* receptors: sufficient for reward, tolerance, and sensitization. *Science.* 2004;306(5698):1029–1032.

51. Tegner J, Bjorkegren J. Perturbations to uncover gene networks. *Trends Genet.* 2007;23(1):34–41.

52. Tomlins SA, Mehra R, Rhodes DR, et al. Integrative molecular concept modeling of prostate cancer progression. *Nat Genet.* 2007;39(1):41–51.

53. Treadwell JA, Singh SM. Microarray analysis of mouse brain gene expression following acute ethanol treatment. *Neurochem Res.* 2004;29(2):357–369.

54. True WR, Xian H, Scherrer JF, et al. Common genetic vulnerability for nicotine and alcohol dependence in men. *Arch Gen Psychiatry.* 1999;56(7):655–661.

55. Tsuang MT, Lyons MJ, Meyer JM, et al. Co-occurrence of abuse of different drugs in men: the role of drug-specific and shared vulnerabilities. *Arch Gen Psychiatry.* 1998;55(11):967–972.

56. Tyers M, Mann M. From genomics to proteomics. *Nature.* 2003;422(6928):193–197.

57. Uddin RK, Singh SM. Cis-Regulatory sequences of the genes involved in apoptosis, cell growth, and proliferation may provide a target for some of the effects of acute ethanol exposure. *Brain Res.* 2006;1088(1):31–44.

58. Uddin RK, Singh SM. Ethanol-responsive genes: identification of transcription factors and their role in metabolomics. *Pharmacogenomics J.* 2007;7(1):38–47.

59. Uddin RK, Treadwell JA, Singh SM. Towards unraveling ethanol-specific neuro-metabolomics based on ethanol responsive genes in vivo. *Neurochem Res.* 2005;30(9):1179–1190.

60. Verstreken P, Koh TW, Schulze KL, et al. Synaptojanin is recruited by endophilin to promote synaptic vesicle uncoating. *Neuron.* 2003;40(4):733–748.

61. Volkow ND, Li TK. Drugs and alcohol: treating and preventing abuse, addiction and their medical consequences. *Pharmacol Ther.* 2005;108(1):3–17.

62. Weil ZM, Norman GJ, DeVries AC, Nelson RJ. The injured nervous system: a Darwinian perspective. *Prog Neurobiol.* 2009;86(1):48–59.

63. Yuferov V, Kroslak T, Laforge KS, et al. Differential gene expression in the rat caudate putamen after "binge" cocaine administration: advantage of triplicate microarray analysis. *Synapse.* 2003;48(4):157–169.

64. Zhang D, Zhang L, Lou DW, et al. The dopamine D1 receptor is a critical mediator for cocaine-induced gene expression. *J Neurochem.* 2002;82(6):1453–1464.

15

Neuroimaging Findings in Substance Use Disorders

ASHLEY ACHESON

Introduction

A comprehensive understanding of the underlying neurobiology of alcohol and other drug use will likely prove essential in developing more effective prevention, early intervention, and treatment strategies. Ethical limitations prevent the use of many of the techniques developed to study brains in animal models of addiction; however, technical advancements in neuroimaging are increasingly allowing for more in-depth brain assessments in humans. This chapter reviews findings on brain structure and function in individuals with alcohol and other substance use disorders.

These insights into brain alterations associated with addictions are often limited by questions of causality. Most studies report cross-sectional comparisons between addicted individuals and healthy controls, and thus obscuring whether differences are due to substance use, preexisting differences that may have contributed to risk, or some combination of these two factors. To help address this, relevant studies examining at-risk individuals prior to the onset of substance use disorders are also discussed in this chapter.

Structural Alterations

Brain Volume

Differences in brain volume can be measured noninvasively through high-resolution structural magnetic resonance imaging (MRI) scans. Studies investigating differences in gray or white matter volume may manually trace regions of interest in high-resolution MRI scans and calculate volumes; however, automated analysis techniques like brain voxel-based morphometry are more common,[6] as they are less time consuming and easier for comparing multiple brain regions than manual tracing methods. Despite these advantages, automated methods can have problems with accuracy in regions with anatomical variations between subjects, such as folds in the cortex.[107]

Gray Matter Volume

Alcohol dependence is associated with reduced gray matter in the prefrontal cortex, insula, ventral striatum, amygdala, and hippocampus,[14,36,112] and gray matter deficits appear more pronounced in female than male patients,[41] suggesting that female patients may be more sensitive to the neurotoxic effects of alcohol. Similarly, a recent voxel-based meta-analysis of gray matter volume comparisons in heavy users of cocaine, methamphetamine, and amphetamine and healthy controls found that the most consistently reported findings were gray matter volume reductions in the insula, thalamus, middle and inferior frontal gyrus, and anterior cingulate.[26] Reduced insula, thalamus, and anterior cingulate volumes have also been correlated with greater methamphetamine cravings in users.[69] Reduced insula and striatal volumes have also been observed in chronic heroin users.[31,86] A recent meta-analysis on gray matter deficits in marijuana users reported somewhat mixed findings, although reduced hippocampal volumes do appear to be a consistent finding.[80] Finally, tobacco smokers show decreased insula, orbitofrontal, prefrontal, and cingulate cortex volumes.[30,76] Collectively these findings suggest that gray matter volume deficits are present across different classes of substance use disorders, with insula, prefrontal, and cingulate cortexes commonly affected.

It is unclear to what extent gray matter deficits associated with substance use disorders are a direct consequence of substance use. Prefrontal gray matter deficits were found to worsen over a 5-year period in people with chronic alcoholism,[78] and there is evidence that gray matter deficits are attenuated with extended alcohol abstinence.[112] Similarly, daily morphine administration in patients with chronic pain reduces volumes of orbitofrontal cortex and amygdala[55,111] providing further evidence that at least some gray matter deficits may be a consequence of chronic use. However, nonabusing individuals who have family histories of alcohol or other substance use disorders (FH+) have reduced amygdala volumes,[24,38] and although findings in other brain regions are somewhat mixed,[23] this does suggest that at least some gray matter deficits may predate excessive substance use.

White Matter Volume

Alcohol dependent patients have decreased frontal white matter volumes, and these deficits are more pronounced in patients with Wernicke encephalopathy.[14,36,112] Similar to sex differences in gray matter deficits, female patients with alcoholism show more pronounced white matter deficits than male patients.[41] There is mixed evidence for greater white matter volume deficits in alcoholic patients with comorbid cocaine dependence[10] and tentative evidence for frontal white matter deficits in cocaine-dependent patients without comorbid alcohol dependence.[53] Findings on white matter volumes in marijuana users are mixed,[80] but frontal white matter volume deficits have been observed in individuals who abused marijuana along with cocaine and or heroin but not alcohol.[84] Similarly, reduced white matter volumes were found in opioid-dependent patients[50] and long-term tobacco smokers.[76] Collectively these findings suggest that frontal white matter volume deficits are also broadly associated with different classes of substance use disorders, although they may be a marker for more extensive substance use than gray matter reductions.

White matter volume deficits appear to be a consequence of problem substance use, at least in the case of alcohol use disorders. White matter volume improvements during abstinence have been documented in alcohol-dependent patients,[14,112] although it is not clear that full recovery is possible. Unlike gray matter volume deficits, white matter volume deficits have not been reported in nonabusing FH+ individuals,[112] suggesting that these deficits are not present before the onset of problem substance use.

White Matter Microstructure

White matter microstructure can be assessed using diffusion tensor imaging to index fractional anisotropy (FA) of water diffusion in white matter tracts. FA describes the directional selectivity of the random diffusion of water molecules.[8,21,79,96] Higher FA values (maximum theoretical value is 1.0) are observed along heavily myelinated white matter tracts. The structure of the axonal cell membranes and myelin sheath hinders the diffusion of water molecules in all directions except along the fiber tract, thereby producing highly anisotropic water diffusion.[79] Thus decreased FA values in white matter tracts may indicate decreased myelin levels or damage to axons due to processes such as inflammation.[88,89]

Decreased frontal white matter FA values have been found in nearly all classes of substance use disorders. For instance, alcohol-dependent patients had reduced frontal white matter FA that was associated with higher self-reported impulsivity, longer duration of drinking,[59] and slower processing speeds on cognitive measures.[90] Frontal white matter FA deficits were also present in adolescent binge drinkers,[66] suggesting that relatively limited exposure to large alcohol doses may impair white matter integrity in youths, while frontal white matter FA increases in alcohol-dependent patients with extended abstinence.[77] Similarly, frontal white matter FA deficits have also been reported in cocaine-dependent patients,[53,63] and FA deficits in cocaine-dependent patients were also associated with greater impulsivity[81] and was more pronounced in individuals who abused additional substances.[48] Similarly, frontal white matter FA deficits have also been observed in individuals who abuse methamphetamine,[19,49] opioids,[57,97] marijuana,[34,35] and tobacco.[32,82] Collectively, these findings suggest that white matter FA deficits may be a common phenotype across multiple classes of substance use disorders.

Although there is evidence of improvement in frontal white matter FA during abstinence, there is also evidence that FA deficits are at least partially premorbid. Nonabusing FH+ adolescents and young adults have been found to have decreased frontal white matter FA values,[1,2,3,37] and these deficits have been shown to be proportional to the number of biological parents and grandparents with substance use disorders,[2,3] suggesting a possible hereditary influence. Of interest, similar FA deficits were not observed in FH+ youths with low levels of externalizing behaviors and other risk-related characteristics,[91] suggesting that frontal white matter FA deficits may be closely linked to the behavioral phenotype underlying risk in FH+, typically referred to as behavioral undercontrol[85] or neurobehavioral inhibition.[92]

Collectively, these findings indicate that white matter microstructure deficits are present in individuals with substance use disorders and appear to both partially predate substance use and worsen as a consequence of heavy substance use. Additional studies are needed to determine how frontal white matter FA deficits may contribute to risk of substance use disorder, as well as what specific underlying white matter dysfunctions the decreased FA values reflect.

Summary of Structural Brain Findings

Collectively, these studies indicate that, across different classes, substance use disorders are associated with structural brain alterations in both gray and white matter tissue, commonly involving the prefrontal and frontal brain regions. In several instances these alterations were related to increased impulsivity and other problem behaviors, suggesting a possible neural substrate for behavioral dysfunctions commonly associated with substance use disorders. Brain alterations found in substance users are often assumed to be a consequences of substance use, and there is evidence that substance use is directly associated with structural brain changes. However, given that tobacco use is both directly linked to frontal gray and white matter alterations and not controlled for in most studies, it is difficult to rule out a direct contribution of smoking to the findings described earlier. Finally there is evidence that some gray matter and white matter alterations may predate problem substance use.

Dopamine and Other Neurotransmitter Systems

It is possible to study neurotransmitter systems in humans using techniques such as positron emission tomography (PET), which involves administering radiolabeled ligands and thus exposing participants to low levels of radiation. Although these studies are generally quite safe, since radiation is involved they are generally restricted to adult populations and not children and adolescents. Thus, PET imaging studies are more readily used in adult populations with existing substance use disorders rather than in youth populations prior to the onset of substance use disorders or with limited substance use histories.

Dopamine

Dopamine (DA) has received extensive attention in the addiction field, due in no small part to the finding that nearly all drugs of abuse induce increased dopamine levels in the striatum, and the DA system has been studied extensively in addicted populations using PET imaging.[43,95] With PET imaging it is possible to study DA-receptor availability and distribution and stimulant-induced DA release using radiolabeled ligands for specific DA receptors (D2, D3, or D4) or DA transporters, and to monitor DA synthesis using radiolabeled levodopa (L-DOPA).

Decreased striatal D2 receptor availability has been observed across most drug addictions included alcohol, cocaine, methamphetamine, opiates, and tobacco (see Trifilieff et al.[95] for review), and these deficits appear to persist even with extended abstinence (e.g., Volkow et al.[100–103]). It appears that decreased striatal D2 receptor availability may be at least partially a consequence of heavy substance use, as prolonged exposure to drugs such as cocaine or methamphetamine decreases D2 receptor density in animal models.[68,94] Furthermore, striatal D2 receptor availability in FH+ adults with no substance use disorders has been reported to be increased relative to FH– controls[101] or no different from FH– controls.[17,71] However, other studies have also associated decreased D2 receptor availability with substance use disorder risk factors such as increased impulsivity in both individuals with substance use disorders and healthy controls as well as in animal models (see Trifilieff et al.[95]). Thus D2 receptor availability deficits also may at least partially predate substance use disorders and contribute to substance use disorder risk.

PET studies have also been used to index stimulant-induced striatal DA release by comparing DA receptor binding before and after administering drugs like amphetamine. Similar to findings on DA receptor availability, individuals with alcohol, cocaine, methamphetamine, opiates, and tobacco all show blunted DA release in this assay, and again similar findings are observed in animal models with prolonged exposure to drugs of abuse (see Trifilieff et al.[95] for review). Findings in FH+ adults are mixed, with one study reporting blunted DA release in this assay,[17] and another reporting no differences in DA release from FH– controls.[71] Blunted stimulant-induced striatal DA release has also been associated with increased impulsivity both in healthy normal adults[73] and individuals with substance use disorders (see Trifilieff et al.[95]). Thus as with D2 receptor availability deficits, decreased stimulant-induced DA release also may partially predate substance use disorders and contribute to substance use disorder risk.

In contrast with findings on D2 receptor availability and stimulant-induced DA release, findings on DA transporter levels in individuals with substance use disorders appear mixed, with some studies reporting decreases relative to controls and other studies reporting no differences (see Hou et al.[43] for reviews). Findings on presynaptic DA synthesis in individuals with substance use disorders are also divergent, with some studies reporting increases, decreases, and no differences, respectively (see Hou et al.[43] for

reviews). These findings suggest that DA transporter levels and presynaptic DA release are less consistently affected in individuals with substance use disorder, although additional studies with larger sample sizes may be necessary to clarify this.

Other Neurotransmitters Systems

PET imaging has been used to a lesser extent to study other neurotransmitter systems in addicted populations. During abstinence, μ-opioid receptor binding increases in cortical and striatal regions in heavy users of alcohol, cocaine, and opioids, and these increases appear to be related to cravings (see Jones et al.[45] and Volkow et al.[104] for reviews). Some studies report both increases and decreases in serotonin transporters in the mid- and hind-brains of heavy users of alcohol and other drugs.[56,104] Reduced γ-aminobutyric acid A (GABA$_A$) receptor binding in cortical and striatal regions has been observed in heavy users of alcohol and opiates.[58,104] Reduced metabotropic glutamate receptor binding in the prefrontal cortex has been observed in smokers but not cocaine users,[93] suggesting that this may be specific to nicotine dependence. Finally, there is reduction in cannabinoid-type 1 receptor binding in both heavy users of marijuana and alcohol, with both groups showing deficits in cortical regions and only alcohol users showing deficits in subcortical regions.[39]

Summary of Neurotransmitter Findings

Collectively these results indicate that substance use disorders are associated with widespread disruptions in the DA system along with other neurotransmitter systems. Decreased striatal D2 receptor availability and decreased striatal DA release appear to be clear addiction biomarkers and provide insight into how reward circuitry is altered in addictions. However, additional studies are needed to better understand how these DA and other neurotransmitter systems are synergistically affected in addicted individuals and how these systems affect chronic drug use. Restrictions on the use of PET in children and adolescents make studying these systems in nonabusing FH+ and other at risk populations prior to the onset of substance use more difficult, thereby making it harder to determine to what extent alterations may predate substance use.

Functional Imaging Findings

Functional brain activity is frequently measured using functional MRI (fMRI) to monitor changes in blood oxygenation level–dependent (BOLD) signaling. Increasing activity in a brain region is followed a few seconds later by an increase in BOLD signaling, reflecting an increase in oxygen carrying blood to that area. Thus BOLD levels are not a direct marker of neural activity, but rather a delayed indicator with a temporal resolution (changes over seconds) on a vastly different scale than the activity of neurons (changes over milliseconds). Despite these limitations, the combinations of spatial and temporal resolution possible with fMRI make it an extremely popular choice for studying human brain activity. This section reviews findings in addicted populations, focusing on brain activations associated with alcohol and other drug cues, nondrug rewards, delay discounting, response inhibition, and, finally, resting state connectivity.

Alcohol and Other Drug-Cue Reactivity

Exposure to alcohol and other drug-related cues consistently induced activations in reward circuitry in addicted populations.[18,22,45,52]

Alcohol and other drug cues (stimuli that have been associated with substance use through repeated pairings) can induce strong attentional biases and cravings in heavy users.[28] Imaging studies have most often compared activations to alcohol, cocaine, tobacco, or other drug cues relative to neutral cues in heavy users of those substances. The drug cues used typically involve viewing substance use–related words, images, and videos, hearing scripts about substance use; handling substance use paraphernalia; and/or smelling or tasting alcohol or drugs. Cues that involve more than one sensory modality appear to invoke neural activations with more robust relationships with craving and other clinical indicators of addiction severity.[110] Recent meta-analyses have found that drug cue–induced activations appear largely consistent across drug classes. For instance, heavy drinkers and patients with alcohol use disorders exposed to alcohol cues had increased activations in regions including the striatum, amygdala, anterior cingulate, middle frontal cortex, and orbitofrontal cortex.[52,83] Similarly, heavy cocaine users exposed to cocaine cues had increased activations in the striatum, amygdala, anterior and posterior cingulate, and insula, and heavy tobacco users exposed to tobacco cues had increased activity in the striatum, amygdala, and anterior cingulate cortex.[52]

Collectivity, these studies indicate that stimuli associated with substance use produce a generally common pattern of robust activations in reward-related circuitry across different classes of substance use disorders. These neural activations show significant promise as biomarkers for predicting treatment response and measuring treatment outcomes.[22]

Nondrug Reward Reactivity

Many studies have found that patients with substance use disorders have altered functioning of reward circuitry in response to nondrug rewards like money; however, the direction of these effects are varied.[42] For example, one of the most commonly used paradigms involving nondrug rewards has been the monetary incentive delay task, which examines neural responses to cues predicting monetary gains and losses as well as gain and loss outcomes.[7] Alcohol-dependent patients performing this task have been reported to have striatal activity that is reduced,[9,108] increased,[99] or not different from healthy controls.[11,12] Similarly, striatal activity in cocaine-dependent individuals performing this task has been reported to be reduced,[15] increased,[46] or similar to controls.[75] Likewise, marijuana users performing these tasks have also been reported to have striatal activity that is reduced,[98] increased,[72] or similar to controls.[29] A recent meta-analysis of studies of individuals with substance disorders performing fMRI tasks involving reward anticipation and delivery (including monetary incentive delay tasks) reported overall that individuals with substance use disorders have relatively reduced striatal activity during the anticipation of rewards and relatively increased striatal activity during the delivery of rewards, which the authors note to be difficult to interpret in the context of current neurobiological theories of addiction.[62]

Delay Discounting

Delay discounting has received extensive attention in the addiction field because discounting or devaluing of delayed rewards has been observed in nearly all classes of substance use disorders as well in nonabusing FH+ individuals.[33] However, relatively few functional imaging studies on delay discounting in addicted populations have been published, and findings are mixed. For instance, heavy alcohol users have been reported to have greater activations in prefrontal, frontal, and occipital cortical regions.[5,20] In contrast, heavy methamphetamine users performing delay-discounting tasks have been reported to have decreased activity in frontoparietal regions,[40,67] and smokers have been reported to have decreased activity in parietal and occipital cortical regions.[51]

The mixed results observed may be partially due to things like variations in tasks designs and analytical strategies, so caution is warranted in interpreting differences in delay-discounting associated neural activity across different substance use disorders. Furthermore, the limited published studies on delay discounting in addicted populations likely reflect inherent difficulties in adapting complex paradigms like delay discounting for imaging to compare different populations. Thus, despite clear behavioral evidence of increased delay discounting in addicted populations, it is less clear how neural activity underlying delay discounting may be altered in these individuals.

Response Inhibition

Response inhibition, or the ability to inhibit proponent responding, has also been found to be consistently impaired in individuals with substance use disorders as well as in nonabusing FH+ individuals, typically measured with stop signal or go/no go tasks.[25] These tasks activate a predominantly right-sided network of structures including the inferior frontal gyrus, anterior cingulate cortex, presupplementary motor area, and dorsolateral prefrontal cortex. Findings in individuals with substance use disorders are generally mixed, although it does appear somewhat more common for addicted individuals to have relative decreases in activity in these structures.[61] Thus similar to delay discounting, it is not entirely clear how neural activity is altered in addicted populations to account for their impairments in response inhibition.

Resting State Functional Connectivity

Resting state functional connectivity (rsFC) is emerging as a potentially powerful measure for studying psychiatric disorders.[87] Unlike fMRI tasks, where participants are shown images or required to perform tasks, resting state scanning procedures typically involve imaging subjects instructed to let their minds wander and not fixate on any particular topic. At rest, brain circuits such as the default mode network show correlated patterns of neural activity, and alterations in rsFC have been observed in psychiatric disorders such as depression, autism, and schizophrenia.[87]

Individuals with substance use disorders have been reported to have altered rsFC patterns; however, the directions of findings are mixed.[74] For instance, alcohol-dependent patients have been reported to have decreased rsFC between the ventral striatum and ventromedial prefrontal cortex, insula, and putamen,[16,70] with poorer connectivity predicting relapse in short-term abstinent alcoholics.[16] In contrast, although cocaine-dependent patients have been reported to show poorer rsFC between the putamen and insula and postcentral gyrus,[65] compulsive cocaine use has been associated with increased rsFC between the striatal and anterior prefrontal/orbital prefrontal cortex,[44] and relapse in cocaine-dependent patients has been predicted by increased rsFC between the posterior hippocampus and posterior cingulate.[4] Likewise, opioid-dependent patients have been reported to have decreased rsFC between both the ventral striatum and insula[97] and caudate and dorsolateral prefrontal cortex,[105] but have also been reported to have increased rsFC, both between the ventral striatum and prefrontal and orbitofrontal cortexes[64] and between the hippocampus and the caudate, putamen, insula, and posterior cingulate.[113] Increases and decreases in rsFC have also been observed for regular marijuana users[13,60,106] and tobacco smokers.[27,54,109] Collectively, these findings suggest that substance users have altered rsFC, although the direction of the findings may depend on both the drug class and specific circuits examined.

Functional Imaging Summary

The most reliable functional imaging findings in addicted populations appear to be increased reactivity in reward-related circuitry in response to alcohol and other drug cues, and this holds promise as a biomarker for predicting treatment outcomes and indexing therapeutic effects. Findings in other areas appear much more varied; however, several caveats are important to keep in mind. Functional imaging studies place greater demands on participants than structural imaging studies, and in some paradigms it can be difficult to measure how fully participants are complying with instructions and engaging with procedures. Many studies, particularly older ones, used fairly small samples, which may not only have resulted in some false-positive findings but also considerable heterogeneity across study samples in potential confounding variables such as comorbid psychiatric conditions and other substance use. Thus studies with enough participants to find significant group differences in a particular study may not have been large enough to find activation differences reliably associated with substance use disorders across studies. Finally, differences in analytical procedures may also have contributed to significant variability across studies.

Conclusion

Overall, the most consistent neuroimaging findings appear to be reduced gray and white matter volumes in frontal brain regions, impaired frontal white matter microstructure, decreased striatal D2 receptor availability and blunted striatal DA release, and increased activity in response to alcohol and other drug cues in reward-related circuitry. Many of these alterations appear to be at least partially present before the onset of substance use, associated with behavioral risk characteristics, worsening with continued substance use, and in some cases show recovery with extended abstinence. The extent of brain alterations present in addicted populations highlight the need for more multimodal neuroimaging studies, or least consideration in how functional imaging study results are interpreted (e.g., caution assuming increased frontal cortical activity on an fMRI task activity simply reflects increased cognitive effort). Large sample, longitudinal multimodal imaging studies, such as the current Adolescent Brain and Cognition Development (ABCD; https://addictionresearch.nih.gov/abcd-study) study offer significant promise for furthering our understanding of the neurobiological basis of addiction.

References

1. Acheson A, Tagamets MA, Winkler A, et al. Striatal activity and reduced white matter increase frontal activity in youths with family histories of alcohol and other substance-use disorders performing a go/no-go task. *Brain and Behavior*. 2015;5:e00352.
2. Acheson A, Wijtenburg SA, Rowland LM, et al. Combining diffusion tensor imaging and magnetic resonance spectroscopy to study reduced frontal white matter integrity in youths with family histories of substance use disorders. *Hum Brain Mapp*. 2014;35:5877–5887.
3. Acheson A, Wijtenburg SA, Rowland LM, et al. Assessment of whole brain white matter integrity in youths and young adults with a family history of substance-use disorders. *Hum Brain Mapp*. 2014;35:5401–5413.
4. Adinoff B, Gu H, Merrick C, McHugh M, et al. Basal hippocampal activity and its functional connectivity predicts cocaine relapse. *Biol Psychiatry*. 2015;78:496–504.
5. Amlung M, Sweet LH, Acker J, Brown CL, MacKillop J. Dissociable brain signatures of choice conflict and immediate reward preferences in alcohol use disorders. *Addict Biol*. 2014;19:743–753.
6. Ashburner J, Friston KJ. Voxel-based morphometry--the methods. *Neuroimage*. 2000;11:805–821.
7. Balodis IM, Potenza MN. Anticipatory reward processing in addicted populations: a focus on the monetary incentive delay task. *Biol Psychiatry*. 2015;77:434–444.
8. Basser PJ. Focal magnetic stimulation of an axon. *IEEE Transactions on Biomedical Engineering*. 1994;41:601–606.
9. Beck A, Schlagenhauf F, Wustenberg T, et al. Ventral striatal activation during reward anticipation correlates with impulsivity in alcoholics. *Biol Psychiatry*. 2009;66:734–742.
10. Bjork JM, Grant SJ, Hommer DW. Cross-sectional volumetric analysis of brain atrophy in alcohol dependence: effects of drinking history and comorbid substance use disorder. *Am J Psychiatry*. 2003;160:2038–2045.
11. Bjork JM, Smith AR, Chen G, Hommer DW. Mesolimbic recruitment by nondrug rewards in detoxified alcoholics: effort anticipation, reward anticipation, and reward delivery. *Hum Brain Mapp*. 2012;33:2174–2188.
12. Bjork JM, Smith AR, Hommer DW. Striatal sensitivity to reward deliveries and omissions in substance dependent patients. *Neuroimage*. 2008;42:1609–1621.
13. Blanco-Hinojo L, Pujol J, Harrison BJ, et al. Attenuated frontal and sensory inputs to the basal ganglia in cannabis users. *Addict Biol*. 2016.
14. Buhler M, Mann K. Alcohol and the human brain: a systematic review of different neuroimaging methods. *Alcohol Clin Exp Res*. 2011;35:1771–1793.
15. Bustamante JC, Barros-Loscertales A, Costumero V, et al. Abstinence duration modulates striatal functioning during monetary reward processing in cocaine patients. *Addict Biol*. 2014;19:885–894.
16. Camchong J, Stenger A, Fein G. Resting-state synchrony during early alcohol abstinence can predict subsequent relapse. *Cereb Cortex*. 2013;23:2086–2099.
17. Casey KF, Benkelfat C, Cherkasova MV, Baker GB, Dagher A, Leyton M. Reduced dopamine response to amphetamine in subjects at ultra-high risk for addiction. *Biol Psychiatry*. 2014;76:23–30.
18. Chase HW, Eickhoff SB, Laird AR, Hogarth L. The neural basis of drug stimulus processing and craving: an activation likelihood estimation meta-analysis. *Biol Psychiatry*. 2011;70:785–793.
19. Chung A, Lyoo IK, Kim SJ, et al. Decreased frontal white-matter integrity in abstinent methamphetamine abusers. *Int J Neuropsychopharmacol*. 2007;10:765–775.
20. Claus ED, Kiehl KA, Hutchison KE. Neural and behavioral mechanisms of impulsive choice in alcohol use disorder. *Alcohol Clin Exp Res*. 2011;35:1209–1219.
21. Conturo TE, McKinstry RC, Akbudak E, Robinson BH. Encoding of anisotropic diffusion with tetrahedral gradients: a general mathematical diffusion formalism and experimental results. *Magn Reson Med*. 1996;35:399–412.
22. Courtney KE, Schacht JP, Hutchison K, Roche DJ, Ray LA. Neural substrates of cue reactivity: association with treatment outcomes and relapse. *Addict Biol*. 2016;21:3–22.
23. Cservenka A. Neurobiological phenotypes associated with a family history of alcoholism. *Drug Alcohol Depend*. 2016;158:8–21.
24. Dager AD, McKay DR, Kent Jr JW, et al. Shared genetic factors influence amygdala volumes and risk for alcoholism. *Neuropsychopharmacology*. 2015;40:412–420.

25. Dalley JW, Robbins TW. Fractionating impulsivity: neuropsychiatric implications. *Nat Rev Neurosci.* 2017;18:158–171.

26. Ersche KD, Williams GB, Robbins TW, Bullmore ET. Meta-analysis of structural brain abnormalities associated with stimulant drug dependence and neuroimaging of addiction vulnerability and resilience. *Curr Opin Neurobiol.* 2013;23:615–624.

27. Fedota JR, Stein EA. Resting-state functional connectivity and nicotine addiction: prospects for biomarker development. *Ann N Y Acad Sci.* 2015;1349:64–82.

28. Field M, Cox WM. Attentional bias in addictive behaviors: a review of its development, causes, and consequences. *Drug Alcohol Depend.* 2008;97:1–20.

29. Filbey FM, Dunlop J, Myers US. Neural effects of positive and negative incentives during marijuana withdrawal. *PLoS One.* 2013;8:e61470.

30. Gallinat J, Meisenzahl E, Jacobsen LK, et al. Smoking and structural brain deficits: a volumetric MR investigation. *Eur J Neurosci.* 2006;24:1744–1750.

31. Gardini S, Venneri A. Reduced grey matter in the posterior insula as a structural vulnerability or diathesis to addiction. *Brain Res Bull.* 2012;87:205–211.

32. Gogliettino AR, Potenza MN, Yip SW. White matter development and tobacco smoking in young adults: a systematic review with recommendations for future research. *Drug Alcohol Depend.* 2016 ;162:26–33.

33. Gray JC, MacKillop J. Impulsive delayed reward discounting as a genetically-influenced target for drug abuse prevention: a critical evaluation. *Front Psychol.* 2015;6:1104.

34. Gruber SA, Dahlgren MK, Sagar KA, Gonenc A, Lukas SE. Worth the wait: effects of age of onset of marijuana use on white matter and impulsivity. *Psychopharmacology (Berl).* 2014;231:1455–1465.

35. Gruber SA, Silveri MM, Dahlgren MK, Yurgelun-Todd D. Why so impulsive? White matter alterations are associated with impulsivity in chronic marijuana smokers. *Exp Clin Psychopharmacol.* 2011;19:231–242.

36. Hashimoto E, Riederer PF, Hesselbrock VM, et al. Consensus paper of the WFSBP task force on biological markers: biological markers for alcoholism. *World J Biol Psychiatry.* 2013;14:549–564.

37. Herting MM, Schwartz D, Mitchell SH, Nagel BJ. Delay discounting behavior and white matter microstructure abnormalities in youth with a family history of alcoholism. *Alcohol Clin Exp Res.* 2010;34:1590–1602.

38. Hill SY, Wang S, Carter H, McDermott MD, Zezza N, Stiffler S. Amygdala volume in offspring from multiplex for alcohol dependence families: the moderating influence of childhood environment and 5-HTTLPR variation. *J Alcohol Drug Depend.* 2013;(suppl 1).

39. Hirvonen J. In vivo imaging of the cannabinoid CB1 receptor with positron emission tomography. *Clin Pharmacol Ther.* 2015;97:565–567.

40. Hoffman WF, Schwartz DL, Huckans MS, et al. Cortical activation during delay discounting in abstinent methamphetamine dependent individuals. *Psychopharmacology (Berl).* 2008;201:183–193.

41. Hommer D, Momenan R, Kaiser E, Rawlings R. Evidence for a gender-related effect of alcoholism on brain volumes. *Am J Psychiatry.* 2001;158:198–204.

42. Hommer DW, Bjork JM, Gilman JM. Imaging brain response to reward in addictive disorders. *Ann N Y Acad Sci.* 2011;1216:50–61.

43. Hou H, Wang C, Jia S, Hu S, Tian M. Brain dopaminergic system changes in drug addiction: a review of positron emission tomography findings. *Neurosci Bull.* 2014;30:765–776.

44. Hu Y, Salmeron BJ, Gu H, Stein EA, Yang Y. Impaired functional connectivity within and between frontostriatal circuits and its association with compulsive drug use and trait impulsivity in cocaine addiction. *JAMA Psychiatry.* 2015;72:584–592.

45. Jasinska AJ, Stein EA, Kaiser J, Naumer MJ, Yalachkov Y. Factors modulating neural reactivity to drug cues in addiction: a survey of human neuroimaging studies. *Neurosci Biobehav Rev.* 2014;38:1–16.

46. Jia Z, Worhunsky PD, Carroll KM, et al. An initial study of neural responses to monetary incentives as related to treatment outcome in cocaine dependence. *Biol Psychiatry.* 2011;70:553–560.

47. Jones T, Rabiner EA, Company PETRA. The development, past achievements, and future directions of brain PET. *J Cereb Blood Flow Metab.* 2012;32:1426–1454.

48. Kaag AM, van Wingen GA, Caan MW, Homberg JR, van den Brink W, Reneman L. White matter alterations in cocaine users are negatively related to the number of additionally (ab)used substances. *Addict Biol.* 2017;22(4):1048–1056.

49. Kim IS, Kim YT, Song HJ, et al. Reduced corpus callosum white matter microstructural integrity revealed by diffusion tensor eigenvalues in abstinent methamphetamine addicts. *Neurotoxicology.* 2009;30:209–213.

50. Kivisaari R, Rapeli P, Van Leemput K, et al. Cerebral measurements and their correlation with the onset age and the duration of opioid abuse. *J Opioid Manag.* 2010;6:423–429.

51. Kobiella A, Ripke S, Kroemer NB, et al. Acute and chronic nicotine effects on behaviour and brain activation during intertemporal decision making. *Addict Biol.* 2014;19:918–930.

52. Kuhn S, Gallinat J. Common biology of craving across legal and illegal drugs - a quantitative meta-analysis of cue-reactivity brain response. *Eur J Neurosci.* 2011;33:1318–1326.

53. Lim KO, Wozniak JR, Mueller BA, et al. Brain macrostructural and microstructural abnormalities in cocaine dependence. *Drug Alcohol Depend.* 2008;92:164–172.

54. Lin F, Wu G, Zhu L, Lei H. Altered brain functional networks in heavy smokers. *Addict Biol.* 2015a;20:809–819.

55. Lin JC, Chu LF, Stringer EA, et al. One month of oral morphine decreases gray matter volume in the right amygdala of individuals with low back pain: confirmation of previously reported magnetic resonance imaging results. *Pain Med.* 2015b.

56. Lin SH, Lee LT, Yang YK. Serotonin and mental disorders: a concise review on molecular neuroimaging evidence. *Clin Psychopharmacol Neurosci.* 2014;12:196–202.

57. Lin WC, Chou KH, Chen CC, et al. White matter abnormalities correlating with memory and depression in heroin users under methadone maintenance treatment. *PLoS One.* 2012;7:e33809.

58. Lingford-Hughes A, Myers J, Watson B, et al. Using [(11)C]Ro15 4513 PET to characterise GABA-benzodiazepine receptors in opiate addiction: similarities and differences with alcoholism. *Neuroimage.* 2016;132:1–7.

59. Liu IC, Chiu CH, Chen CJ, Kuo LW, Lo YC, Tseng WY. The microstructural integrity of the corpus callosum and associated impulsivity in alcohol dependence: a tractography-based segmentation study using diffusion spectrum imaging. *Psychiatry Res.* 2010;184:128–134.

60. Lopez-Larson MP, Rogowska J, Yurgelun-Todd D. Aberrant orbitofrontal connectivity in marijuana smoking adolescents. *Dev Cogn Neurosci.* 2015;16:54–62.

61. Luijten M, Machielsen MW, Veltman DJ, Hester R, de Haan L, Franken IH. Systematic review of ERP and fMRI studies investigating inhibitory control and error processing in people with substance dependence and behavioural addictions. *J Psychiatry Neurosci.* 2014;39:149–169.

62. Luijten M, Schellekens AF, Kuhn S, Machielse MW, Sescousse G. Disruption of reward processing in addiction: an image-based meta-analysis of functional magnetic resonance imaging studies. *JAMA Psychiatry.* 2017.

63. Ma L, Hasan KM, Steinberg JL, et al. Diffusion tensor imaging in cocaine dependence: regional effects of cocaine on corpus callosum and effect of cocaine administration route. *Drug Alcohol Depend.* 2009;104:262–267.

64. Ma N, Liu Y, Li N, Wang CX, et al. Addiction related alteration in resting-state brain connectivity. *Neuroimage.* 2010;49:738–744.

65. McHugh MJ, Demers CH, Braud J, Briggs R, Adinoff B, Stein EA. Striatal-insula circuits in cocaine addiction: implications for impulsivity and relapse risk. *Am J Drug Alcohol Abuse.* 2013;39:424–432.

66. McQueeny T, Schweinsburg BC, Schweinsburg AD, et al. Altered white matter integrity in adolescent binge drinkers. *Alcohol Clin Exp Res.* 2009;33:1278–1285.

67. Monterosso JR, Ainslie G, Xu J, Cordova X, Domier CP, London ED. Frontoparietal cortical activity of methamphetamine-dependent and comparison subjects performing a delay discounting task. *Hum Brain Mapp.* 2007;28:383–393.

68. Moore RJ, Vinsant SL, Nader MA, Porrino LJ, Friedman DP. Effect of cocaine self-administration on dopamine D2 receptors in rhesus monkeys. *Synapse.* 1998;30:88–96.

69. Morales AM, Kohno M, Robertson CL, Dean AC, Mandelkern MA, London ED. Gray-matter volume, midbrain dopamine D2/D3 receptors and drug craving in methamphetamine users. *Mol Psychiatry.* 2015;20:764–771.

70. Muller-Oehring EM, Jung YC, Pfefferbaum A, Sullivan EV, Schulte T. The resting brain of alcoholics. *Cereb Cortex.* 2015;25:4155–4168.

71. Munro CA, McCaul ME, Oswald LM, et al. Striatal dopamine release and family history of alcoholism. *Alcohol Clin Exp Res.* 2006;30:1143–1151.

72. Nestor L, Hester R, Garavan H. Increased ventral striatal BOLD activity during non-drug reward anticipation in cannabis users. *Neuroimage.* 2010;49:1133–1143.

73. Oswald LM, Wong DF, Zhou Y, et al. Impulsivity and chronic stress are associated with amphetamine-induced striatal dopamine release. *Neuroimage.* 2007;36:153–166.

74. Pariyadath V, Gowin JL, Stein EA. Resting state functional connectivity analysis for addiction medicine: from individual loci to complex networks. *Prog Brain Res.* 2016;224:155–173.

75. Patel KT, Stevens MC, Meda SA, et al. Robust changes in reward circuitry during reward loss in current and former cocaine users during performance of a monetary incentive delay task. *Biol Psychiatry.* 2013;74:529–537.

76. Peng P, Wang Z, Jiang T, Chu S, Wang S, Xiao D. Brain-volume changes in young and middle-aged smokers: a DARTEL-based voxel-based morphometry study. *Clin Respir J.* 2017;11(5):621–631.

77. Pfefferbaum A, Rosenbloom MJ, Chu W, et al. White matter microstructural recovery with abstinence and decline with relapse in alcohol dependence interacts with normal ageing: a controlled longitudinal DTI study. *Lancet Psychiatry.* 2014;1:202–212.

78. Pfefferbaum A, Sullivan EV, Rosenbloom MJ, Mathalon DH, Lim KO. A controlled study of cortical gray matter and ventricular changes in alcoholic men over a 5-year interval. *Arch Gen Psychiatry.* 1998;55:905–912.

79. Pierpaoli C, Basser PJ. Toward a quantitative assessment of diffusion anisotropy. *Magn Reson Med.* 1996;36:893–906.

80. Rocchetti M, Crescini A, Borgwardt S, et al. Is cannabis neurotoxic for the healthy brain? A meta-analytical review of structural brain alterations in non-psychotic users. *Psychiatry Clin Neurosci.* 2013;67:483–492.

81. Romero MJ, Asensio S, Palau C, Sanchez A, Romero FJ. Cocaine addiction: diffusion tensor imaging study of the inferior frontal and anterior cingulate white matter. *Psychiatry Res.* 2010;181:57–63.

82. Savjani RR, Velasquez KM, Thompson-Lake DG, et al. Characterizing white matter changes in cigarette smokers via diffusion tensor imaging. *Drug Alcohol Depend.* 2014;145:134–142.

83. Schacht JP, Anton RF, Myrick H. Functional neuroimaging studies of alcohol cue reactivity: a quantitative meta-analysis and systematic review. *Addict Biol.* 2013;18:121–133.

84. Schlaepfer TE, Lancaster E, Heidbreder R, et al. Decreased frontal white-matter volume in chronic substance abuse. *Int J Neuropsychopharmacol.* 2006;9:147–153.

85. Schuckit MA, Smith TL. The relationship of behavioural undercontrol to alcoholism in higher-functioning adults. *Drug Alcohol Rev.* 2006;25:393–402.

86. Seifert CL, Magon S, Sprenger T, et al. Reduced volume of the nucleus accumbens in heroin addiction. *Eur Arch Psychiatry Clin Neurosci.* 2015;265:637–645.

87. Shen HH. Core concept: resting-state connectivity. *Proc Natl Acad Sci U S A.* 2015;112:14115–14116.

88. Song SK, Sun SW, Ju WK, Lin SJ, Cross AH, Neufeld AH. Diffusion tensor imaging detects and differentiates axon and myelin degeneration in mouse optic nerve after retinal ischemia. *Neuroimage.* 2003;20:1714–1722.

89. Song SK, Yoshino J, Le TQ, et al. Demyelination increases radial diffusivity in corpus callosum of mouse brain. *Neuroimage.* 2005;26:132–140.

90. Sorg SF, Squeglia LM, Taylor MJ, Alhassoon OM, Delano-Wood LM, Grant I. Effects of aging on frontal white matter microstructure in alcohol use disorder and associations with processing speed. *J Stud Alcohol Drugs.* 2015;76:296–306.

91. Squeglia LM, Jacobus J, Brumback T, Meloy MJ, Tapert SF. White matter integrity in alcohol-naive youth with a family history of alcohol use disorders. *Psychol Med.* 2014;44:2775–2786.

92. Tarter RE, Kirisci L, Mezzich A, et al. Neurobehavioral disinhibition in childhood predicts early age at onset of substance use disorder. *Am J Psychiatry.* 2003;160:1078–1085.

93. Terbeck S, Akkus F, Chesterman LP, Hasler G. The role of metabotropic glutamate receptor 5 in the pathogenesis of mood disorders and addiction: combining preclinical evidence with human Positron Emission Tomography (PET) studies. *Front Neurosci.* 2015;9:86.

94. Thanos PK, Kim R, Delis F, Rocco MJ, Cho J, Volkow ND. Effects of chronic methamphetamine on psychomotor and cognitive functions and dopamine signaling in the brain. *Behav Brain Res.* 2017;320:282–290.

95. Trifilieff P, Ducrocq F, van der Veldt S, Martinez D. Blunted dopamine transmission in addiction: potential mechanisms and implications for behavior. *Semin Nucl Med.* 2017;47:64–74.

96. Ulug AM, Barker PB, van Zijl PC. Correction of motional artifacts in diffusion-weighted images using a reference phase map. *Magn Reson Med.* 1995;34:476–480.

97. Upadhyay J, Maleki N, Potter J, et al. Alterations in brain structure and functional connectivity in prescription opioid-dependent patients. *Brain.* 2010;133:2098–2114.

98. van Hell HH, Vink M, Ossewaarde L, Jager G, Kahn RS, Ramsey NF. Chronic effects of cannabis use on the human reward system: an fMRI study. *Eur Neuropsychopharmacol.* 2010;20:153–163.

99. van Holst RJ, Clark L, Veltman DJ, van den Brink W, Goudriaan AE. Enhanced striatal responses during expectancy coding in alcohol dependence. *Drug Alcohol Depend.* 2014;142:204–208.

100. Volkow ND, Fowler JS, Wang GJ, et al. Decreased dopamine D2 receptor availability is associated with reduced frontal metabolism in cocaine abusers. *Synapse.* 1993;14:169–177.

101. Volkow ND, Wang GJ, Begleiter H, et al. High levels of dopamine D2 receptors in unaffected members of alcoholic families: possible protective factors. *Arch Gen Psychiatry.* 2006;63:999–1008.

102. Volkow ND, Wang GJ, Maynard L, et al. Effects of alcohol detoxification on dopamine D2 receptors in alcoholics: a preliminary study. *Psychiatry Res.* 2002;116:163–172.

103. Volkow ND, Wang GJ, Smith L, et al. Recovery of dopamine transporters with methamphetamine detoxification is not linked to changes in dopamine release. *Neuroimage.* 2015;121:20–28.

104. Volkow ND, Wiers CE, Shokri-Kojori E, Tomasi D, Wang GJ, Baler R. Neurochemical and metabolic effects of acute and chronic alcohol in the human brain: studies with positron emission tomography. *Neuropharmacology.* 2017;122:175–188.

105. Wang Y, Zhu J, Li Q, et al. Altered fronto-striatal and fronto-cerebellar circuits in heroin-dependent individuals: a resting-state FMRI study. *PLoS One.* 2013;8:e58098.

106. Wetherill RR, Fang Z, Jagannathan K, Childress AR, Rao H, Franklin TR. Cannabis, cigarettes, and their co-occurring use: disentangling differences in default mode network functional connectivity. *Drug Alcohol Depend.* 2015;153:116–123.

107. Winkler AM, Kochunov P, Blangero J, et al. Cortical thickness or grey matter volume? The importance of selecting the phenotype for imaging genetics studies. *Neuroimage.* 2010;53:1135–1146.

108. Wrase J, Schlagenhauf F, Kienast T, et al. Dysfunction of reward processing correlates with alcohol craving in detoxified alcoholics. *Neuroimage.* 2007;35:787–794.

109. Wu G, Yang S, Zhu L, Lin F. Altered spontaneous brain activity in heavy smokers revealed by regional homogeneity. *Psychopharmacology (Berl).* 2015;232:2481–2489.

110. Yalachkov Y, Kaiser J, Naumer MJ. Functional neuroimaging studies in addiction: multisensory drug stimuli and neural cue reactivity. *Neurosci Biobehav Rev.* 2012;36:825–835.

111. Younger JW, Chu LF, D'Arcy NT, Trott KE, Jastrzab LE, Mackey SC. Prescription opioid analgesics rapidly change the human brain. *Pain.* 2011;152:1803–1810.

112. Zahr NM. Structural and microstructral imaging of the brain in alcohol use disorders. *Handb Clin Neurol.* 2014;125:275–290.

113. Zhai TY, Shao YC, Xie CM, et al. Altered intrinsic hippocampus declarative memory network and its association with impulsivity in abstinent heroin dependent subjects. *Behav Brain Res.* 2014;272:209–217.

16

Neurobiological Basis of Drug Reward and Reinforcement

DAVID M. LOVINGER

CHAPTER OUTLINE

Introduction

Drug use disorders involve a number of factors including genetic and environmentally influenced predispositions, the actions of the drugs themselves, the immediate environment, and the neurobiological mechanisms that promote and support drug actions and addiction. This chapter deals mostly with the latter aspect of drug use, abuse, and addiction, as we explore the ways in which the brain is built to adapt to environmental circumstances, and how these aspects of neural function can promote the continued use and abuse of certain drugs and ultimately promote disorders related to these drugs. We then consider the mechanisms through which drugs of abuse interact with the brain systems that promote maladaptive drug use and addiction.

Drug use disorders have been defined in several different ways, most of which stress the habitual or compulsive nature of addictive behavior; the physical, psychological, and social damage produced by the behavior; and the trauma associated with cessation of the behavior. Drug use disorders also share many features in common with disorders related to natural biological drives (e.g., sex and food consumption), physical activities (e.g., excessive exercise), and relatively benign drugs (e.g., caffeine) (discussed in Brunton et al.[24] and Koob and Le Moal[102]). Drugs of abuse with harmful effects are the main focus of the present discussion. In addition, excessive use of drugs may lead to health and psychological problems even in the absence of an agreed-upon definition of use disorders. Thus, it is important to understand the neural mechanisms that contribute to prolonged and maladaptive drug use.

The *Diagnostic and Statistical Manual of Mental Disorders*, Fifth Edition (DSM-5),[4] covers substance-related and addictive disorders. It should be noted that addiction per se is not a diagnosis recommended in the manual, as the term substance use disorder is preferred. Within this classification, the manual defines substance use disorder as a "…cluster of cognitive, behavioral, and physiological symptoms indicating that the individual continues using the substance despite significant substance-related problems." Common features of these disorders are cognitive, affective, sleep, and behavioral changes that center on use or cessation of use of the addictive substance or action (sometimes referred to as a habit). Central features of the use disorder are risky drug use, craving, social impairment, continued use despite negative consequences, and the possible negative consequences of cessation of drug use. All of these aspects of substance use and addictive disorders can be seen to relate to innate brain mechanisms underlying processes referred to as reinforcement and/or reward. In this context, it is important to discuss current ideas about the neural mechanisms of reinforcement and reward before discussing the impact of drugs of abuse on these processes.

Experimental Psychology Concepts of Reward and Reinforcement

An important aspect of the use and abuse of a wide range of drugs is their reinforcing properties. A reinforcer is defined in experimental psychology as a substance or stimulus presented following a behavior that increases the incidence of the behavior above baseline levels. As Skinner[180] wrote:

The operation of reinforcement is defined as the presentation of a certain kind of stimulus in a temporal relation with either a stimulus or a response. A reinforcing stimulus is defined as such by its power to produce the resulting change [in the response]. There is no circularity about this; some stimuli are found to produce the change, others not, and they are classified as reinforcing and nonreinforcing accordingly.

It is worth highlighting the dual use of the term stimulus by Skinner to refer to both the result of the action (the reinforcer), and a stimulus within the environment that can become associated with the response and the reinforcer. One definition of reinforcement, although not Skinner's position, is that it involves a strengthening of the ability of stimuli to elicit responses (the so-called stimulus-response model[81]), while a somewhat looser definition is a strengthening of the ability of the environment in general, including some neural activity within the animal itself and the animal's past history in that environmental context, to elicit the response.[48]

The concept of reinforcement is best known from the work of Konorski and Skinner on what is now called operant or instrumental conditioning.[9,180] However, the term reinforcement has also been used in the context of Pavlovian, or classical, conditioning. One use of this term is that presentation of an unconditioned stimulus subsequent to the conditioned stimulus reinforces the ability of the conditioned stimulus to elicit a conditioned response. This term has also been used to refer to the effects of stimuli that predict the value of a rewarding stimulus presented prior to presentation of food or another naturally desirable outcome.[155,175,176] For example, in the paradigm used by Schultz,[175,176] responding for food (licking) as well as neuronal activity related to stimulus presentation and responding can be measured. Dayan and Balleine provided a nice discussion of the distinctions between reinforcement in the context of Pavlovian and instrumental conditioning.[42]

Two forms of reinforcement, termed positive and negative, have also been postulated. Positive reinforcement refers to the process in which delivery of a desirable consequence increases the incidence of the behavior. This is easily understood in the context of the instrumental or operant conditioning paradigm in which delivery of palatable food will increase bar pressing by a rodent or key pecking by a pigeon.[180] Negative reinforcement occurs when the performance of an action results in omission or avoidance of an undesirable stimulus (e.g., foot shock), and the incidence of the behavior increases as a result of this learning process.[181] The initial phases of learning some skills, such as swimming, involve what might be termed negative reinforcement, as the skill helps to reduce the undesirable effects of the environment. Many investigators do not subscribe to the idea that positive and negative reinforcement are distinct processes, as both types of reinforcement basically refer to something that increases the incidence of a given behavior. However, negative reinforcement is a useful concept when measuring stimulus-behavior relationships, as it describes a condition in which increasing behavior leads to omission/avoidance of a stimulus. Learning in everyday life will often involve both positive and negative reinforcement.

Two other terms that have come to be used in the context of instrumental learning and addiction are punishment and reward. Consideration of the conditions that promote cessation of behavior led to the definition of the undesirable outcome as punishment,[8,196] although the role of punishment has been hotly debated.[182] The term reward was not so readily accepted by early behaviorists but has come into common use as a reference to the desirable outcome in an instrumental learning paradigm. The terms reward and positive reinforcement are often used interchangeably, but as we will discuss, these terms can be used to refer to different processes that control instrumental learning of actions, including drug self-administration.

Studies conducted over the last few decades have led to the refinement of the concepts of instrumental conditioning, reward, and reinforcement based on the role of the outcome produced by a particular behavior in conditioning paradigms. Dickinson, Balleine, and others have shown that responses developed under certain types of conditioning schedules will rapidly diminish if the value of the outcome is decreased or if receipt of the outcome is no longer contingent on making the response.[1,12,33] This learning of action-outcome contingencies is best achieved with training schedules where the outcome is easily predictable and the probability of obtaining the outcome is enhanced with increased rates of responding (e.g., fixed or random ratio schedules). In this case, the outcome has been termed to have a rewarding action, based on its intrinsic value to the organism at the time of testing and association with the instrumental action itself.

In contrast, training with schedules where predictability is poorer and increasing rates do not increase probability of successful outcomes (e.g., random interval schedules) produces responding that is insensitive to outcome devaluation or noncontingent presentation of the outcome.[12,45,78] This stimulus-response type of conditioning can also occur with extensive training using schedules with higher predictability (discussed in Yin and Knowlton[219]). In the case of stimulus-response learning, the association is made between antecedent environmental stimuli and the subsequent response, with the outcome serving as a reinforcer regardless of the immediate value of this outcome to the animal. As you can see, this is closer to the classical definitions of reinforcement favored by stimulus-response theorists, Donahoe, and perhaps Skinner.[48,180] It should also be noted that White[210] drew a similar distinction between reward and reinforcement, albeit with a more traditional behaviorist emphasis on the definitions of these terms. Other investigators have defined reward in terms of positive reinforcement in combination with positive hedonic value,[102] an idea that suggests more overlap between the two processes. Although the separate definitions of reward and reinforcement in this context may be debated, there is strong evidence for the two instrumental conditioning processes themselves. Thus the differentiation of the roles of stimuli/environment and outcome in the two different learning processes is important, and separate discussion of reward and reinforcement in these contexts is useful.

Before we consider how reward and reinforcement contribute to addiction it is worth discussing the adaptive purpose of these neural systems. Behaviors that lead to enhanced survival and/or reproduction are necessary for propagation of genes and species. Innate feeding, reproductive, and harm-avoidance behaviors exist in all animals, but learning about features of the environment is necessary to obtain the opportunity to express these innate behaviors. Pavlovian conditioning is one such learning process whereby performance of something approximating an innate or reflexive behavior can come to be elicited by stimuli that were originally neutral with respect to predicting a particular outcome (e.g., obtaining food or avoiding harm). Instrumental conditioning adds another layer of sophistication to this process. Animals with this capacity can learn to perform new actions and new sets of actions to obtain a positive consequence or avoid punishment. Both types of learning have obvious adaptive utility, as the animal can now integrate complex features of the world and new behavioral strategies into maintaining safety, as well as the quest for food and mating partners. The power of the neural mechanisms involved in reward and reinforcement likely derives from this relationship to survival and reproductive success.[126]

However, there is the possibility that reward and reinforcement mechanisms will not always be used for adaptive purposes. One such example is the phenomenon of self-starvation. Animals that are trained to perform an intracranial self-stimulation task, described later, will perform this task at the expense of sufficient eating if access to food is time-restricted.[166] Similar self-starvation is observed if animals are given the opportunity to run on a wheel when on a limited food access schedule.[18,165] This particular form of self-starvation has been considered as a model of human anorexia nervosa,[18] which itself is clearly an example of maladaptive behavior involving the brain systems we will consider. Stimuli that originally signal a positive outcome can change their predictive value (a certain location may contain food at one time and a predator at another). Furthermore, stimuli or substances that interact with the neural mechanisms involved in reinforcement may come to have reinforcing value even when they are not coupled to a favorable outcome, or even when they are associated with harmful results. Most drugs of abuse can act in this manner, and can lead to reinforcement of what we might call maladaptive behaviors. In the remainder of this chapter we will consider the brain circuitry and cellular and molecular mechanisms involved in reinforcement. Consideration of this topic will also entail some discussion of the experimental techniques used to uncover these mechanisms.

Neurotransmitters and Neural Circuitry: Involvement in Different Aspects of Reward, Reinforcement, and Addiction

Although the concept of instrumental learning had begun to crystallize by the early 1930s mainly due to the work of Konorski and Skinner,[98,180,222] little was known about the neural circuits involved in this behavior. Konorski and Divac both obtained evidence from studies involving lesions of the caudate nucleus implicating this part of the striatum in instrumental conditioning.[47,98] The discovery by Olds and Milner[136] of intracranial self-stimulation provided an important clue as to the importance of at least one pathway within the basal ganglia. In the original intracranial self-stimulation paradigm, the animal was implanted with an electrode that could stimulate fibers in the medial forebrain bundle. Investigator-initiated stimulation at this site led the animal to repeat the behaviors that were ongoing at the time when the stimulus was delivered. Thus activation of this neural pathway was in and of itself rewarding or reinforcing. It was later discovered that a key set of axons within the medial forebrain bundle supplied dopaminergic afferents to the forebrain regions known collectively as the striatum.[36,150,214] This finding stimulated work on the role of dopamine in brain mechanisms of reward and addiction that has continued to this day.

The dopaminergic pathways in the brain are now well known. The somata of the majority of neurons that use dopamine as a neurotransmitter are concentrated in contiguous ventral midbrain structures called the substantia nigra pars compacta (SNc), or A-9 nucleus, and the ventral tegmental area, or A-10 nucleus.[95] The neurons in these two regions project to different striatal subregions and other forebrain targets. Neurons from the substantia nigra pars compacta primarily innervate the dorsal striatum (the caudate and putamen nuclei in primates). In contrast, dopaminergic neurons from the ventral tegmental area (VTA) project strongly to the ventral portion of the striatum, particularly a striatal subregion

called the nucleus accumbens that sits in the ventromedial region of the striatum. Neurons within the VTA also send dopaminergic afferents to the prefrontal, orbitofrontal (insular), and cingulate cortices, with more minor projections to other cortical regions such as the limbic cortical subregions.[135]

The initial data suggesting that dopaminergic neuronal activity is crucial for intracranial self-stimulation was later supplemented by the finding that intracranial self-stimulation could be produced by stimulation within the ventral midbrain regions where the dopaminergic neurons reside. Intracranial self-stimulation is supported by stimulation in the VTA, as well as at subregions of the SNc.[36,132,156] These studies did not rule out the possibility that stimulation of fibers that originated elsewhere and passed through the ventral midbrain contributed to intracranial self-stimulation. Nonetheless, the combination of these findings with those findings that dopaminergic manipulations alter intracranial self-stimulation strongly implicated dopamine coming from ventral midbrain neurons in the mechanisms that underlie reward and reinforcement during this process.

The focus on dopamine in the context of reward and reinforcement often overshadows the role of other neurotransmitters. Indeed, dopamine is a modulatory neurotransmitter that in and of itself is not capable of strong excitation or inhibition of neurons within this circuitry. Furthermore, there is evidence indicating that dopaminergic transmission is not required for certain aspects of behavior that are thought to involve reward or reinforcement. For example, gene-targeted mice that lack dopamine are still able to learn the location of food, but appear to require dopamine to express the learned behavior.[160] This finding and similar data from other studies seems to indicate that dopamine is necessary for the motivational aspects of reward seeking[21,141] or incentive salience.[17] In addition, there is evidence that neurochemical lesions of the dopaminergic system do not eliminate self-administration of drugs of abuse such as heroin and ethanol[147,154] suggesting that dopaminergic transmission may not be necessary for all of the rewarding or reinforcing effects of drugs of abuse. Thus, we need to consider the role of other neurotransmitters in reward, reinforcement, and addiction. An exhaustive description of all the neurotransmitters involved in these processes is beyond the scope of the present chapter. Instead, the role of particular neurotransmitters with intriguing roles in the brain reward/reinforcement circuitry are discussed.

Within the central nervous system, the neurotransmitters glutamate and γ-aminobutyric acid (GABA) are responsible for the majority of fast synaptic transmission.[95] Glutamate directly excites neurons via the activation of ligand-gated cation channel-type receptors, whereas GABA activates anion-preferring channels and generally has an inhibitory action. Both of these neurotransmitters have been implicated in brain mechanisms of reward, reinforcement, and drug actions.[50,60,94]

One approach that has been used to examine the role of glutamate and GABA in reward, reinforcement, and addiction-related behaviors is blockade of receptors with specific antagonists, usually injected into a specific brain area.[39,41,179,186] These approaches have proven to be effective in altering behavior and have implicated certain subtypes of ionotropic glutamate receptors in reward and addiction-related behaviors. However, it is sometimes difficult to discern the specific behavioral role of glutamate and its receptors using antagonist blockade, as antagonists of ionotropic glutamate receptor will almost certainly decrease neuronal activity and disrupt circuit activity. Thus, the antagonist effect may not necessarily reflect a need for activation of the receptor so much as the necessity of activity of a particular set of neurons. The opposite case often exists for GABAergic activity, as blockade of GABA receptors, GABA$_A$ receptors in particular, tends to increase neuronal activity and may stimulate circuitry. For these reasons, much recent research on the roles of GABA and glutamate in reinforcement, reward, and addiction has focused on the role of particular glutamate receptor and GABA$_A$ receptor subunit proteins.

The ligand-gated ion channels that mediate fast excitatory and inhibitory synaptic transmission are multimeric proteins that can be formed by numerous subunits and subunit combinations. Chronic exposure to addictive drugs alters the expression of particular ionotropic GABA and glutamate receptor subunits.[27,89,105] Manipulating subunit expression can subtly alter receptor function without eliminating receptor activity. This has allowed investigators to explore the roles of these receptors in drug- and addiction-related behaviors without major disruption of the activity of neurons within the reward/reinforcement circuitry. This line of research has been boosted immensely by techniques for transgenic receptor expression and gene-targeted receptor modification and disruption (i.e., so-called knock in and knockout techniques). Transgenic and gene-targeting mice that express higher or lower amounts of a desired receptor subunit are quite useful, as are mice that express a slightly mutated version of a receptor. Viral-based gene overexpression, often involving microinjection of constructs into specific brain regions, is also being widely used to enhance protein function in neurons within reward/reinforcement circuitry. Development of new techniques to alter receptor expression or structure using the Talen and clusters of regularly interspaced short palindromic repeats (CRISPR) techniques has enhanced the rate at which gene-targeted mice and viruses can be developed and employed.[80,87,124] Altering expression of the GluR1 alpha-amino-3-hydroxy-5-methylisoxazole-4-propionic acid (AMPA) receptor subunit in gene-targeted mice alters instrumental learning[88,197] and reduces morphine dependence and sensitization.[204] Altered acute responses to drugs of abuse, as well as changes in ethanol tolerance and dependence, have been observed in mice in which GABA$_A$ receptors have been altered by gene targeting of alpha2, alpha5, and delta subunits.[110,121,203] However, one caveat that must be added to this discussion is that neuronal activity has not been measured in vivo in the animals used in these studies, and thus, the extent to which subunit loss alters circuit activity has yet to be determined in any of the aforementioned experimental models.

The neuromodulatory transmitter serotonin (or 5-hydroxytryptamine) can influence the brain reward and reinforcement circuitry, in part through actions on dopaminergic neurons.[60,79] Serotonin can also influence goal-directed and habitual behavior through its role in control of affect and in impulsivity. The likelihood of choosing new actions without strong outcome control has been linked to disorders of brain serotonergic systems. Impulsivity is responsive to some treatments aimed at the serotonergic system.[60,143] Because of the disregard for outcomes, impulsive responding may be a first step in the process leading to stimulus control of behavior and maladaptive habits. Measures of impulsivity in animal models have been suggested to predict a pattern of addiction-like drug taking in rodents.[15] Serotonin levels in several brain regions are elevated during administration of psychostimulant drugs such as amphetamine and cocaine, and there is evidence that excessive serotonergic transmission contributes to the addictive effects of these drugs, in addition to the well-characterized role of dopamine in these processes.[59,75,79,129,188]

Opioid neuropeptides are widely distributed in the brain, including in the action/reinforcement/reward circuitry discussed at present.[95] These peptides, enkephalins, and endorphins, in particular, are perhaps best known for their roles in analgesia. However, it is now well established that opioid peptide production and release is increased in response to stressful stimuli and other environmental challenges.[53,149] In addition, brain opioid systems have been implicated in mechanisms of reward, particularly in relation to food and drugs of abuse. Studies of food-related behaviors generally indicate that opioid peptides signal something about the hedonic value or desirability of the food, sometimes called "liking."[16,21,69,163] Opiate drugs that act as agonists at mu- and delta-type opiate receptors are self-administered in instrumental paradigms (reviewed in Gratton[63]), and opiate agonists produce decreases in the threshold for intracranial self-stimulation.[22,208] Opiate antagonists can also influence intracranial self-stimulation.[209] These findings indicate that activation of the brain opioid system has rewarding effects.

The brain endocannabinoid system has also begun to receive a great deal of attention as a mediator of instrumental learning and addiction. Endocannabinoids are lipid metabolites that act on the cannabinoid receptors, the receptors originally discovered as mediators of the psychoactive effects of drugs such as marijuana and hashish.[134] In the brain, endocannabinoid agonists act mainly through the cannabinoid-1 (CB1) receptor to produce short- and long-lasting synaptic plasticity.[109] The role of the brain endocannabinoid systems in responses to a variety of drugs of abuse is a fascinating topic that has received a great deal of attention in recent years, and this subject is discussed later in this chapter. Recent studies using instrumental conditioning techniques indicate that CB1 receptors play a role in the transition from action-outcome to stimulus-response (habit) learning.[58,64,72] Thus the endocannabinoid system may play an important role in reinforcement-based instrumental learning. It is not yet clear if alterations in dopaminergic transmission or effects on other neurotransmitter systems are involved in this habit-promoting effect of endocannabinoids. The CB1 receptor is highly expressed throughout the brain circuitry thought to mediate instrumental conditioning.[71,77] Within these circuits, CB1 receptors are expressed on axon terminals of glutamatergic and GABAergic neurons (reviewed in Lovinger[109]), and may well regulate release of other neurotransmitters including catecholamines.[192] Thus there are many possible sites where endocannabinoid-dependent synaptic plasticity may play a role in this type of learning and in addiction.

The foregoing discussion should make it clear that to better understand the neuronal mechanisms contributing to reward, reinforcement, and addiction we need to understand more fully the brain circuits involved in the control of actions and the instrumental learning of actions and association of actions with stimuli. We must also gain a better understanding of the roles of particular neurotransmitters and receptors in different parts of these circuits. The forebrain, in conjunction with the ventral midbrain, can be conceptualized as a series of parallel cortico-basal-ganglia-cortex circuits that can also be serially interconnected (see Yin and Knowlton[219] for review). The ultimate function of these circuits is to modify cortical and brainstem output to control the selection, initiation, and timing of actions to produce effective integrated behaviors. Neurons and synapses within these circuits can undergo plastic changes that are thought to contribute to learning of new actions and association of actions with conditioned stimuli.

In an admittedly simplistic scheme, this circuitry can be separated into at least three parallel circuits[219] (Fig. 16.1). (More circuits have been suggested,[3,220] and undoubtedly further subdivisions will emerge based on the complex afferent and efferent connectivity of the striatum.[73,82,185]) Each of the circuits consists of a cortical component, a striatal component, downstream basal ganglia components, and a thalamic component. The sensorimotor circuit comprises the primary and secondary sensory and motor cortices and the SNc, which project to the putamen (the dorsolateral striatum in rodents), which then projects to the motor regions of the globus pallidus, ultimately influencing the ventral thalamus and closing the loop back at the sensory and motor cortices (see Fig. 16.1A). The associative circuitry involves similar connections between associative areas of the cortex (including the prefrontal and parietal regions), the SNc, the caudate nucleus (the dorsomedial striatum in rodents), associative regions of the pallidum, and the mediodorsal and ventral thalamus (see Fig. 16.1B). The limbic circuitry involves the limbic cortices (including not only neocortical prefrontal and temporal areas, but also archicortical regions such as the hippocampus and basolateral amygdala), the VTA, the ventral striatum/accumbens, the ventral pallidum, and the mediodorsal thalamus (see Fig. 16.1C). One can even consider connections within the amygdala to have a similar organization, with the cortical component being the basolateral amygdala, the VTA projections providing the dopaminergic modulatory input, the striatal components being the central amygdala and bed nucleus of the stria terminals, and downstream targets leading ultimately to cortical outputs (see Fig. 16.1D). Evidence for interconnections among the circuits at the level of striatonigral-striatal projections can help to coordinate the different systems.[14,68,184,219] To fully understand reward and reinforcement-dependent learning and resultant behavioral output in the mammalian brain, it is necessary to consider all of the components in this circuitry.

Recent studies have begun to shed light on the role of these different forebrain circuits in instrumental and Pavlovian conditioning, and the ideas generated from these studies are now being applied to examination of drug actions.[12,49,57,219,220] Based on excitotoxic lesioning and local pharmacological manipulations, evidence has accumulated that the associative circuit involving the dorsomedial striatum and associated circuitry, including the basolateral amygdala,[139,140] has key roles in action-outcome learning. Afferent inputs from the prefrontal cortex to neurons in the dorsomedial striatum provide one source of input containing information relevant to action selection, and the cingulate cortex may provide input about discriminative stimuli.[12] The dopaminergic input from the substantia nigra may provide information about reward value. The contribution of action-outcome learning to drug taking is easy to conceptualize. Intrinsically rewarding effects of drugs likely control behavior even in recreational or social users seeking the euphoric effects of cocaine and amphetamine or the anxiety-reducing effects of alcohol. Indeed, studies in rat indicate that cocaine-seeking behavior, measured as an instrumental response normally associated with drug availability, is rapidly lost with devaluation under certain conditioning regimens.[137] It is not yet clear if action-outcome contingencies continue to drive drug seeking and self-administration after long-term drug use and in addicted individuals. It is tempting to speculate that addiction involves a shift in behavioral control from action-outcome/reward to stimulus-controlled/reinforcement mechanisms such as those described in the next few paragraphs. Of interest, Pelloux et al.[145] have shown that rats given limited experience with cocaine seeking and taking will readily suppress seeking responses when intermittent punishment is given, while prolonged exposure to this paradigm reveals a subgroup of rats that will not show this punishment-suppression effect. Furthermore, rats allowed to orally self-administer cocaine continued to show instrumental responses associated with the drug even after cocaine devaluation.[123] Thus evidence is developing that prolonged exposure to psychostimulants can lead to a shift from action-outcome to stimulus-driven behavior.

The sensorimotor circuit involving the dorsolateral striatum appears to play a prominent role in stimulus-response or habit learning. In this circuit the neocortical components and the dorsolateral striatum process information about the relationship between stimulus presentation and response performance, with the dopaminergic inputs from the substantia nigra (and the ventral tegmental area to some extent) providing a reinforcing signal to promote the stimulus-response association.[12] It has been suggested that the role of dopamine is required for the initial stages of this association, but that behaviors become ingrained and resistant to dopaminergic manipulations once the stimulus-response association is formed and habitual behavior is in place.[211] Ultimately, output from the motor cortex and thalamus is important for behavioral performance, and thus, this circuit can produce relatively straightforward throughput from sensory input to motor output. Habitual responding has been postulated to contribute to drug-taking behavior, such that when an individual is in the proper environment with the drug available, the actions involved in drug administration will be automatized and will often continue regardless of the specific outcome of drug usage. There is emerging evidence that this sort of responding may contribute to cocaine- and alcohol-related behaviors in rodents[46,122,145] (see also Sampson et al.[169]) However, to date the role of stimulus-response associations in drug administration and relapse has not yet been thoroughly examined and fully dissociated from the stimulus-dependent forms of learning thought to be mediated by the limbic circuit (described in subsequent text).

Among the roles of the limbic circuit is the integration of information for Pavlovian and instrumental conditioning in a type of learning called Pavlovian-instrumental transfer.[38,219,220] In this circuit, limbic neocortical areas such as the ventral prefrontal cortex provide information relevant to task outcomes to the nucleus accumbens. The basolateral amygdala provides input on reward and appetitive incentive value to the accumbens, where it is combined with the other cortical information. Dopaminergic inputs to the basolateral amygdala, limbic neocortex, and ventral tegmental area also provide information about reward value, while the orbitofrontal cortex may provide information important about the relationship of particular stimuli to task outcomes.[138] The role of the hippocampus and other limbic cortical regions that project to the nucleus accumbens is less clear. The net result is development of associations between environmental stimuli and task outcome (sometimes called stimulus-outcome learning), through which discrete stimuli gain control over particular instrumental responses. In this way the Pavlovian association of the stimulus transfers to the performance of the instrumental response. A role for this type of learning within the context of addiction is easy to postulate. It has long been thought that stimuli that are associated with, and predictive of, drug administration (e.g., needles, liquor bottles) can stimulate drug seeking and taking.[57,99,162] Indeed, there is experimental evidence that this sort of cue-induced relapse and drug craving can be induced in both humans and experimental animals.[19,30,31,99,162]

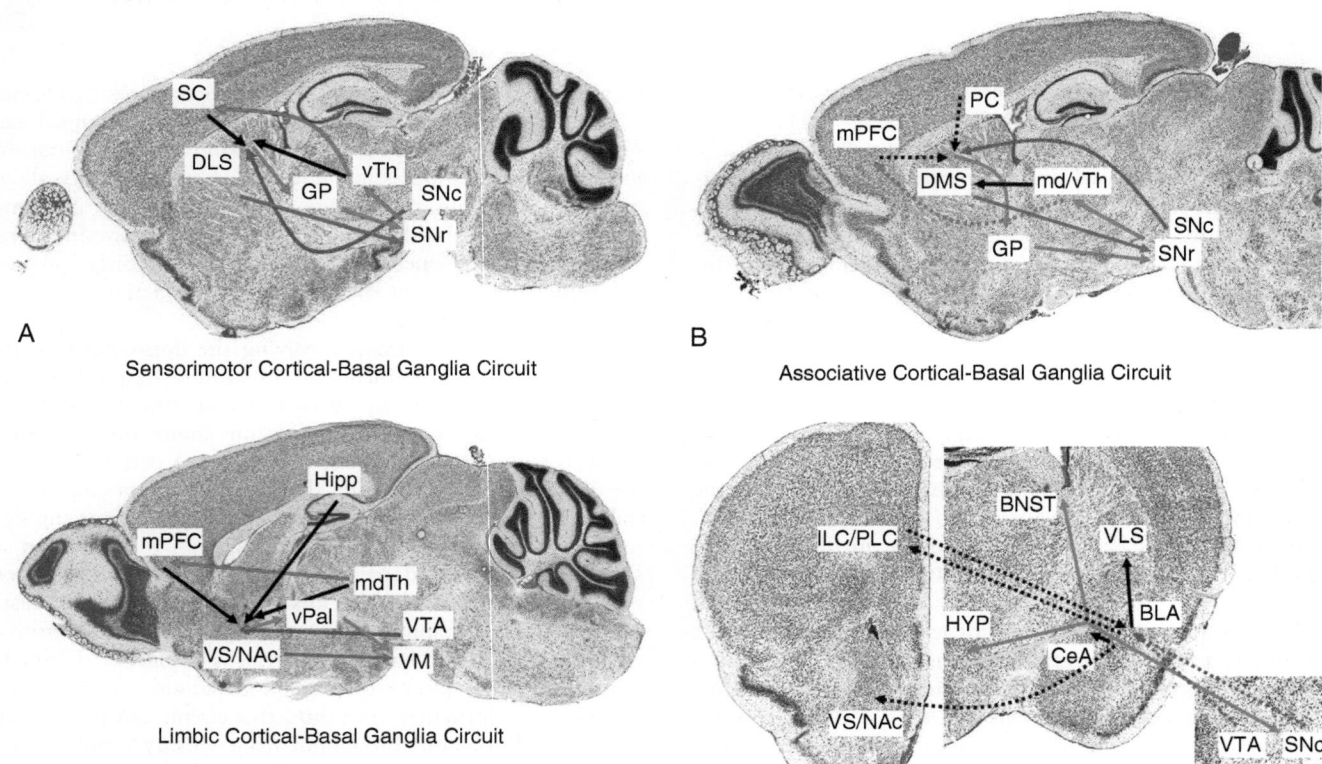

A

Sensorimotor Cortical-Basal Ganglia Circuit

B

Associative Cortical-Basal Ganglia Circuit

C

Limbic Cortical-Basal Ganglia Circuit

D

Amygdala-Basal Ganglia-Cortical Circuit

• **Fig. 16.1** Schematic diagram of the reward/reinforcement circuits in the rodent brain. (A) The sensorimotor circuit (shown in a parasagittal orientation) contains glutamatergic connections from the somatosensory and motor cortices and the thalamus to the dorsolateral striatum (putamen equivalent in rodents); γ-aminobutyric acid (GABA)ergic connections from the dorsolateral striatum to the substantia nigra pars reticulata and motor pallidum (the direct and indirect pathways, respectively); GABAergic connections from pallidum to nigra reticulata; GABAergic connections from the nigra reticulata to the thalamus; and glutamatergic thalamocortical projections back to the sensory and motor cortices. Dopaminergic inputs to the dorsolateral striatum come from the substantia nigra pars compacta. (B) The associative circuit contains glutamatergic connections from, for example, the medial prefrontal and parietal cortices, as well as thalamus, to the dorsomedial striatum (caudate equivalent in rodents); GABAergic connections from the dorsomedial striatum to the nigra reticulata and pallidum (direct and indirect pathways, respectively); GABAergic connections from pallidum to nigra reticulata; and glutamatergic thalamocortical projections back to the associative cortex. Dopaminergic inputs to the dorsomedial striatum come from the substantia nigra pars compacta. (C) The limbic circuit contains glutamatergic connections from the limbic cortical and limbic areas such as the prefrontal cortex, hippocampus, and basolateral amygdala, as well as from thalamus, to the ventral striatum/nucleus accumbens; GABAergic nucleus accumbens connections to the ventral mesencephalon and ventral pallidum (direct and indirect pathways); GABAergic connections from ventral pallidum to ventral mesencephalon; and glutamatergic thalamocortical connections back to the limbic cortex. Dopaminergic inputs to the nucleus accumbens come from the ventral tegmental area. (D) The basolateral and central amygdala connect to a variety of brain regions involved in motivation, reward, and reinforcement (shown here using separate brain sections). The basolateral amygdala receives dopaminergic input from the substantia nigra and ventral tegmental area, as well as glutamatergic input from the medial prefrontal cortex. Glutamatergic efferents from the basolateral amygdala innervate the medial prefrontal cortex, central amygdala, dorsal striatum, and nucleus accumbens. The central amygdala receives afferent input from the hypothalamus as well as glutamatergic input from the basolateral amygdala. GABAergic efferent output from the central amygdala innervates the hypothalamus, the bed nucleus of the stria terminalis, and several hindbrain areas including the interstitial nucleus of the posterior limb of the anterior commissure, the SNc, the periaqueductal gray area, the parabrachial nucleus the nucleus of the solitary tract, and the pedunculopontine nucleus (only SNc projections are shown in this figure). *Solid arrows* depict connections within the plane of the single brain section depicted, while *dashed lines* show connections that run out of the plane of the section. *Black arrows,* glutamatergic corticostriatal, thalamostriatal, and BLA projections; *green arrows,* GABAergic striatal and pallidal indirect pathway, and BLA projections; *blue arrows,* GABAergic striatal direct pathway afferents; *red arrows,* glutamatergic thalamocortical afferents; *brown arrows,* dopaminergic nigral and ventral tegmental afferents; *yellow arrow,* hypothalamic projection to CeA. *BLA,* Basolateral amygdala; *BNST,* bed nucleus of the stria terminalis; *CeA,* central amygdala; *DLS,* dorsolateral striatum; *DMS,* dorsomedial striatum; *GP,* globus pallidus; *Hipp,* hippocampus; *HYP,* hypothalamus; *ILC,* infralimbic prefrontal cortex; *mdTh,* mediodorsal thalamus; *md/vTh,* mediodorsal and ventral thalamus; *mPFC,* medial prefrontal cortex; *PC,* parietal cortex; *PLC,* prelimbic prefrontal cortex; *SC,* sensory cortex; *SNc,* substantia nigra pars compacta; *SNr,* substantia nigra pars reticulata; *VLS,* ventrolateral striatum; *VM,* ventral mesencephalon; *VS/NAc,* ventral striatum/nucleus accumbens; *vPal,* ventral pallidum; *VTA,* ventral tegmental area; *vTh,* ventral thalamus.

The characterization of the limbic circuit as the mediator of reward and/or reinforcement is an idea that has captured the imagination of neurobiologists and addiction researchers.[7,61,83,96] However, it is now becoming clear that the circuitry that includes the dorsal striatum has an equally important role in these processes (see Yin et al.[220] for review). In addition to the studies mentioned that implicated the associative and sensorimotor circuits in action-outcome and stimulus-response learning, there is also evidence that dopaminergic innervation of the dorsal striatum plays important roles in instrumental learning. Stimulation of dopaminergic neurons in the substantia nigra pars compacta supports intracranial self-stimulation, as mentioned earlier. Furthermore, activation of substantia nigra neurons with intracranial self-stimulation–inducing patterns enhances learning and striatal synaptic plasticity.[156] An elegant series of studies by the Palmiter laboratory indicate a key role for dorsal striatal dopamine in instrumental learning and performance. Using dopamine restored in the dorsal striatum of mice that have been engineered to lack the neurotransmitter, these investigators have shown that food-seeking and instrumental learning/performance were rescued.[159,161] Thus full neurochemical integration within the dorsal striatum is all that is needed for proper motivational signaling and instrumental performance. This is not to say that the limbic circuitry does not have reward-related functions, but rather that an intact limbic circuit may not be necessary for proper learning and performance of a purely instrumental task.

In recent years, researchers have also focused on the circuitry involved in generating undesirable effects that contribute to drug taking and relapse, and the effects of the drugs themselves on this circuitry (reviewed in Koob[100] and Koob and Le Moal[102]). There is evidence for reduction in the positive hedonic effects of drugs after sustained self-administration, and negative consequences of drug use and withdrawal increase with repeated use and withdrawal.[a] The amygdala and associated structures appear to have prominent roles in this scenario. The amygdala has generally been thought of as a brain region involved in the processing of information related to emotion, and the role of the amygdala in anxiety and responses to stress is widely known.[107] However, one can also view the role of the amygdala as providing a neural index of the incentive value of a particular stimulus or event.[12,168,200] In this context, the amygdala plays roles in both reward and reinforcement processes as defined earlier. Furthermore, it is now clear that the structure we call the amygdala can be subdivided based on cytoarchitecture and afferent/efferent connections. Two well-characterized amygdalar subregions are the basolateral and central nuclei. The basolateral amygdala is an archicortical structure containing mainly glutamatergic projection neurons and a small number of GABAergic interneurons. The basolateral amygdala innervates other structures within the amygdala, but also has connections with parts of the prefrontal cortex, and the dorsomedial and ventral regions of the striatum.[167] Input to the basolateral amygdala from areas such as the ventral tegmental area and the locus coeruleus provides information about arousal and motivational state[152]; thus, one possible role for this brain region is to integrate information necessary for a reward signal and relay that information to the associative circuit involved in action-outcome learning. The central amygdala is similar in cytoarchitecture to the striatum, having a large proportion of GABAergic projection neurons.[167] This structure receives excitatory input from the basolateral amygdala, neocortical, and paleocortical regions, as well as information about motivational

state via neuromodulatory regions such as the hypothalamus.[167] Output from the central amygdala is sent to the bed nucleus of the stria terminalis, hypothalamus, and other subcortical regions, as well as to the substantia nigra and ventral tegmental area, where it can influence the circuitry involved in stimulus-response and stimulus-outcome learning.[152,167] In addition, the amygdala has emerged as a brain region with important roles in conditioned responses related to the rewarding effects of drugs studied using the conditioned place preference task described in the following section.[23,65] The amygdala interconnections with the bed nucleus of the stria terminalis, a subcortical nucleus with a striatal-like organization (i.e., populated predominantly by GABAergic projection neurons), have generated a great deal of interest, as the bed nucleus of the stria terminalis has been implicated in the actions of drugs of abuse as well as in drug self-administration and relapse.[6,66,206]

Clearly, a better understanding of the brain regions in involved in learning and control of behavior involving reward and reinforcement is emerging. In addition, methodology is emerging that will help define the roles of brain circuitry and circuit physiology in behavior, and to refine our behavioral models based on neuroscientific findings. One of the challenges in addiction research in the coming years will be to determine how the function of these brain circuits contributes to responses to drugs of abuse, maladaptive use of the drugs, and addiction.

Models of Drug Use and Drug Addiction

Examination of the neural basis of drug actions, drug use, and addiction has relied to a great extent on development of laboratory animal models. A great deal of progress has been made with this approach. However, it has proven difficult to model all aspects of drug actions and addiction. For example, how does one assess euphoria or craving in an animal that is incapable of verbal self-report. Progress was slow at times for development of reasonable models of self-administration for drugs such as alcohol, cannabinoids, and nicotine.[111,170,183] Agreeing on a universal definition of addiction and developing an animal model thereof has also proven to be difficult. Nonetheless, several decades of research have led to the development of a variety of behavioral tests that assay various aspects of drug action, drug use, and addiction (Table 16.1). These techniques continue to be refined and combined with new techniques for neuroscientific investigation to provide more complete information about relevant neural mechanisms. The following discussion will describe some of these animal models, with an emphasis on models of drug reward, reinforcement, and addiction.

A seemingly direct way to measure the reinforcing effects of a substance is to determine whether delivery of the drug itself will support learning or continued performance of a particular action or set of actions. This so-called self-administration paradigm has been used to examine the reinforcing actions of many drugs of abuse in a variety of animal models, and in general all of these drugs have been found to support self-administration under at least one schedule of drug administration.[57] Comparisons of self-administration in humans and laboratory animals have indicated similarities that auger well for the experimental use of these procedures.[142] The general procedure is to train the animal to press a lever or nose-poke an object in order to receive the drug either by oral, intravenous, or intracranial routes of administration. Using the basic instrumental training schedule, animals can also be tested in a final short extinction session in which no drug is

TABLE 16.1	Models of Drug Reward and Reinforcement: Relation to Phenotypes of Human Drug Use, Dependence, and Addiction.

Model	Human Drug Use Phenotype
Simple operant self-administration	Hedonic value, liking/wanting
Devaluation	Goal-directed versus habitual responding
Intracranial self-stimulation threshold changes	Hedonic value, anhedonia
Conditioned place preference/aversion	Reinforcement, incentive sensitization, resistance to negative outcome
Progressive ratio breakpoint	Hedonic value, compulsivity
Behavioral cost	Hedonic value, compulsivity
Response persistence without drug	Compulsivity
Punished responding/ pairing with undesirable tastant	Compulsivity, resistance to negative outcome
Cue-induced reinstatement	Craving, incentive sensitization
Secondary reinforcement	Craving, habitual responding
Psychomotor stimulation/ sensitization	Incentive sensitization
Incubation	Craving, incentive sensitization

available to see if they perform the operant behavior. This helps to assess the drug-seeking behavior without any interference from neural actions of the drug itself (e.g., depressant effects that reduce rate of responding). Variations of this basic procedure include the use of secondary reinforcers (e.g., stimuli paired with the opportunity for drug self-administration that come to elicit behavior themselves),[15,49] and use of a progressive ratio schedule in which animals must increase their responses exponentially[157] with each trial in order to continue drug delivery. In this latter procedure, the investigator assesses the breakpoint, which is the response requirement beyond which the subject will no longer work for the drug. This procedure can be used to determine the relative reinforcing efficacy of a particular drug. This approach has the advantage of direct measurement of the animal's willingness to use the drug. However, there are some drawbacks to self-administration techniques. For example, self-administration leading to high levels of drug in the brain that impair subsequent performance of the actions needed for further drug taking (reviewed in Hemby et al.[70]). Oral self-administration of drugs such as ethanol brings into play factors such as taste that affect the willingness of certain animals to ingest the desired drug.[62] Use of instrumental self-administration procedures also necessitates consideration of separate neural control of drug seeking and drug taking.[15,162,170] Nonetheless, self-administration procedures are arguably the most direct measure of use and abuse, particularly given the variety of procedures that have been developed using instrumental paradigms. Self-administration procedures also allow investigators to examine the effects of treatments on drug use in preclinical assays.

In light of the previous discussion of reinforcement and reward, or action-outcome and habit learning, it seems important to evaluate which of these modes of behavior actually drives drug self-administration. As mentioned in the preceding text, investigators have found evidence that drugs of abuse promote habit learning[37,46,122,145] (see also Samson[169]). Another common variant of the drug self-administration procedure is cue-induced drug-related responding and reinstatement of this responding and/or drug taking. It has clearly been demonstrated that cues signaling the opportunity to respond instrumentally and obtain a drug can come to elicit responding in the absence of the drug, and especially robustly when the drug has been omitted for long periods.[19,93,177] This procedure involves a component of stimulus-outcome learning or Pavlovian-instrumental transfer with the cue serving as the Pavlovian conditioned stimulus. Indeed, this type of conditioning has become pretty much the standard in instrumental self-administration procedures, as some explicitly paired cue, most often a light, is included in most such studies. This may be one reason for the large number of studies implicating the aforementioned limbic circuitry in drug-seeking behavior, as this circuitry appears to have important roles in stimulus-outcome learning. There is certainly some heuristic value to such studies in the context of human addiction, as it is easy to imagine how environmental stimuli that signal drug availability might trigger drug seeking and relapse.

Other surrogate measures of the rewarding effects of drugs of abuse have been developed. Drawing on the intracranial self-stimulation paradigm discussed earlier, investigators have examined the ability of drugs of abuse to shift the threshold stimulus intensities needed to support self-stimulation. Several abused drugs produce a leftward shift in the stimulus-response curve or increase rates of responding, indicating that they enhance the reinforcing properties of intracranial self-stimulation (see Wise[215] for review). Drugs with this sort of action include those that are strongly self-administered such as cocaine and amphetamine, as well as other drugs of abuse, although studies of ethanol have yielded mixed results that might be explained by variables such as route of drug administration.[10,103,125] This technique can reveal indirectly the rewarding or reinforcing effects of drugs, but thus far the emphasis has mainly been on the effects of investigator-administered drugs and involvement of the limbic circuitry. It would be interesting to see this line of research extended to include more self-administration/intracranial self-stimulation studies and examination of different circuitry and component brain regions.

Recent studies have focused on identifying behaviors that might be indicative of an addictive phenotype in experimental animals. One approach has been to develop a battery of tests designed to measure continued drug seeking and taking under conditions where these behaviors become increasingly difficult and costly. Deroche-Gamonet et al.[44] have developed a three-test battery consisting of: (1) measuring the progressive ratio breakpoint mentioned earlier; (2) measuring the persistence of instrumental responding on a previously cocaine-associated manipulandum even when a signal indicates no drug availability; and (3) determining whether cocaine self-administration will continue even when associated with electric foot shock (a paradigm also used in Pelloux et al.[145] and Vanderschuren and Everitt[201]). Of interest, Wolffgramm and Heyne[217] and Petry and Heyman[146] have used a conceptually similar approach with alcohol. Wolffgramm and Heyne[217] provided the alcohol in a solution with a normally aversive tastant, and they found that this procedure decreased drinking in animals that had short-term alcohol drinking experience, while drinking was maintained at much higher levels in animals that had been drinking alcohol for a long period (at least 9 months). Petry and Heyman[146] steadily increased the behavioral cost necessary to obtain an alcohol-containing solution and found that rats with experience drinking alcohol maintained their drinking despite the increasing cost, while similar effects were not observed with palatable nutrient-containing solutions. These sorts of techniques are now being used to examine factors that predispose animals to uncontrolled/compulsive drug self-administration. Everitt and coworkers[15] have determined that what appears to be impulsive responding in a five-choice serial reaction time test is predictive of later abusive drug use in this paradigm. This paradigm has been used by investigators to identify subgroups of rats that are especially vulnerable to what might be termed addiction. It is interesting to note that only a relatively modest subgroup of rats given extensive self-administration experience show maintained responding in the second and third tests and also show high breakpoints in test 1.[44] It is hoped that this approach will provide a powerful tool for identifying genetic, neuronal, and circuit differences that contribute to enhanced susceptibility to drug addiction.

Although this approach has some face validity, it is not clear that a model of all aspects of addiction can be developed in rodents. Most rodent drug self-administration paradigms use operant responding for drug delivery, and often with intravenous drug administration directly contingent upon the operant action. The measurements in such experiments are generally number of lever presses and number of drug infusions. However, because infusion will occur following the prescribed number of lever presses there is no way to separate drug seeking (i.e., operant responding) from drug taking (infusion). Thus it is unclear if the different manipulations are altering the operant responses or the drug control of these responses. Investigators have tried to separate the seeking and taking aspects in operant self-administration (SA) procedures using second order schedules and oral drug taking (especially for ethanol). The two aspects can be controlled separately, indicating a confound in interpreting effects of experimental manipulations in operant SA studies. Another problem is the method of scoring in such studies. The protocol is designed to identify the top scorers in a particular test within a given cohort of a given rodent strain. This system generally ignores important genetic and cohort effects that influence behavior toward drugs of abuse. Indeed, C57Bl6J mice will more readily self-administer several drugs of abuse in comparison to other mouse strains, and the genes that regulate these differences are being characterized.[43,106,130] Thus, even the top scorers from these other strains may not reach the mean level achieved by mice from the more self-administration-prone strain. It is difficult to see how one can label mice as "addiction-prone" when there are large numbers of mice from another strain that show more severe drug-related behaviors. There are additional problems in the case of alcohol, where self-administration often involves oral intake. In general, it has been difficult to induce rodents to drink to the same blood alcohol levels and levels of intoxication achieved by humans.[13] New techniques have been developed for increasing rodent alcohol intake, and older techniques are being revisited.[13] However, it is important to consider other animals that show excessive alcohol intake, such as nonhuman primates.[11,86] Overall, development of a single rodent model that captures all aspects of addiction is an overly ambitious undertaking.

An alternative experimental approach is to examine key phenotypic behaviors associated with drug use disorders and attempt to determine the molecules, cells, and circuits that control these behaviors.[91] For example, phenotypes such as excessive drug intake following abstinence, cue-induced reinstatement of drug self-administration, incubation of increased lever-pressing, or outcome-resistant drug intake can all be coupled with neurophysiological measurements and manipulation of particular brain circuits to better understand the neural underpinnings of different facets of the response to drugs of abuse and drug-seeking/taking behaviors (see Table 16.1). The ultimate goal of this research is to develop therapies aimed at these brain components to reduce harmful aspects of drug use disorders.

One important phenotype is the rewarding effects of the drug itself. Investigators have long used Pavlovian conditioning to examine whether drug administration can be used to produce a conditioned place preference in an animal.[198] In this paradigm, the animal is given the drug paired with one of two or three chambers in an apparatus, and then tested later for location preference. In a final drug-free test, the animal is then free to choose a location in which to spend the trial. If more time is spent in a particular location, this is thought to indicate that the drug paired with this location has a preferred or rewarding effect. This technique has the advantage that the animals are not subjected to drug intoxication at the time of testing, so there is little chance of impairment of behavior by the drug itself. However, it must be stressed that the location is a conditioned stimulus and not a primary reward or reinforcer of any kind in this paradigm. Thus the technique does not measure these functions per se, that is, the animal does not have to repeat an action to obtain an outcome, and thus, it is at best a surrogate measure of the underlying construct and one that may be subject to influence by properties of the environment or drug that are not directly related to its reinforcing effects. Nonetheless, strong progress has been made in identifying the neural mechanisms underlying conditioned place preference,[22,64,74,178,179] and there is considerable overlap with mechanisms implicated in reward circuitry.

The psychomotor stimulant effects of drugs have also been proposed to provide a measure of drug reinforcement, reward, and addiction.[216] Administration of many drugs will produce forward locomotion and it has been theorized that this represents an operant approach response indicative of positive reinforcement by the drug.[216] That forward locomotion is elicited by stimulation of the medial forebrain bundle, the site where stimulation yields intracranial self-stimulation, was also advanced as evidence that the mechanisms underlying this locomotion are linked to positive reinforcement. However, it is possible that locomotor activation is merely an adjunct consequence of drug exposure and medial forebrain bundle stimulation. The circuitry that controls performance of voluntary actions overlaps extensively with that involved in reinforcement, reward, habit formation, and addiction. Thus, it is possible that drug actions produce separate effects that both influence locomotion and drug reward or drug seeking, but that these effects are separable. Indeed, elegant studies showed just such a separation for regions of the ventral tegmental area and nucleus accumbens implicated in cocaine- and opiate-induced locomotor stimulation and conditioned place preference or self-administration.[178,179] In addition, mice that lack dopamine show a nearly complete loss of morphine-stimulated locomotion but continue to show morphine-induced conditioned place preference.[74] Locomotor stimulation and reward/reinforcement can also be separated pharmacologically. In the case of alcohol, stimulation of forward locomotion is inconsistent in rats, and locomotor depressant effects are most often observed,[54,113] but rats clearly show other signs of ethanol reward and reinforcement (see Koob[99,100] for examples). Furthermore, Risinger et al.[158] and Sanchez et al.[172] found differences in genetic factors underlying ethanol-induced locomotor stimulation and conditioned place preference for ethanol. Thus, it is not clear that forward locomotion is a good proxy for the actual reinforcing effects of the drug.

The idea of sensitization, an increase in frequency and intensity of a behavior elicited by a stimulus or treatment, has also figured prominently in models of drug abuse and addiction. Repeated administration of certain drugs of abuse, psychostimulants in particular, elicits successively larger increases in locomotor activity in rodents. It has been speculated that this locomotor sensitization is a result of the underlying neuroadaptive processes that contribute to addiction following repeated drug exposure. However, it is still not clear that the locomotor-stimulating effects are related to reward or reinforcement per se, for the same reasons discussed in the preceding paragraphs. In one sense, however, drug seeking and self-administration must involve some form of sensitization, as these behaviors involve increases in responding elicited by the drug or drug-related environments or cues. One theory advanced to account for this aspect of drug-related behavior is the incentive-sensitization model.[162] This theory provides a reasonable explanation for the willingness of addicts to expend a great deal of energy and engage in new behaviors to obtain drugs, and also can explain the greater motivation of animals to work for previously used drugs in tasks such as the progressive ratio/breakpoint paradigm mentioned in the preceding text. Other behavioral measures in laboratory animals provide evidence for enhanced incentive to seek and use drugs. For example, conditioned place preference and cue-induced reinstatement of drug seeking indicate that the motivational value of previously neutral stimuli is enhanced when these stimuli are associated with drugs of abuse (reviewed in Robinson and Berridge[162]). Thus although simple locomotor sensitization may provide only limited information about drug effects on the brain reward/reinforcement system, the concept of sensitization is important within this context.

A role for negative reinforcement in addiction is also easily conceptualized, and experimental models based on this idea have been developed to provide information on important drug abuse-related phenotypes and neural mechanisms. Drugs such as benzodiazepines have known anxiolytic properties[23] and thus reduce an aversive state. The psychostimulants produce acute mood elevation that may provide temporary relief from negative affect (although these drugs are by no means effective antidepressants). Thus negative reinforcement may be a strong driving force for acute drug use.

Relief of the negative symptoms encountered during drug withdrawal can also be characterized as a negative reinforcing component of addiction. Withdrawal following chronic use of different drugs of abuse produces symptoms ranging from heightened anxiety and irritability (benzodiazepines, alcohol) and dysphoria and depression (psychostimulants) to severe physiological symptoms such as abdominal cramps (heroin).[23,118] Withdrawal from drugs is associated with higher thresholds for intracranial self-stimulation in experimental animals, indicating dysphoria associated with this state.[101,174] Relief from these symptoms has been postulated to drive relapse to drug use.[100,102] Indeed, animals made dependent on drugs will increase self-administration and drug-related instrumental responding following drug withdrawal (reviewed in Koob and Le Moal[102]). This sort of reinstatement

responding has also been observed in alcohol-dependent animals and is referred to as the "alcohol deprivation effect" (reviewed in Spanagel[189]). Animals that have undergone conditioned aversion in which withdrawal is rapidly induced and paired with previously neutral stimuli show reinstatement of heroin self-administration and elevation of intracranial self-stimulation thresholds, as if the aversive effects of withdrawal were reducing rewarding drug effects while driving relapse.[145] It is easy to imagine how this withdrawal-relief model can explain relapse after full-blown symptoms have begun. However, it is not so clear that this model can explain continuous drug use in the absence of withdrawal sufficient to produce symptoms. The ability of this model to explain relapse long after the cessation of withdrawal symptoms is also not as clear. Processes such as incubation, as lasting neuroadaptation that leads to greater drug seeking after prolonged abstinence, may more readily account for this type of relapse.[205] Several brain regions within the associative and limbic circuitry have been implicated in the incubation process.[25,148] In addition, lasting recruitment of drug effects on brain systems involved in stress responding has been suggested to underlie the long-term susceptibility to relapse.[102]

The concept of negative reinforcement is also built into addiction theories based on the Opponent-Process idea.[102,187] These theories essentially propose that net emotional state is the result of competition between emotions (e.g., elation vs. fear), and that changes in the competitive balance over time can lead to changes in net emotion and behavior. Within the context of addiction one can easily envision that the euphoric high achieved just after administration of a drug like cocaine can dissipate and be replaced by depression as the neurochemical effects of the drug wear off.[202] With repeated drug use, the euphoria becomes less pronounced as the depression is enhanced, and the user ends up taking the drug to relieve the depression, which could be termed a negative reinforcement model. This process has been modeled with cocaine and heroin self-administration, and it was found that both intracranial self-stimulation thresholds and cocaine or heroin self-administration escalated after several cycles of self-administration and withdrawal.[2,97] Koob, LeMoal, and coworkers have extended these ideas to include the concept of allostasis[117,213] in which the emotional set-point resulting from the new balance of opponent processes is altered toward a more depressed level with repeated drug use.[100,102] The addict ends up using the drug to maintain this new set-point, often relieving more adverse emotional symptoms. Experimental models such as withdrawal-induced excessive self-administration have been used in conjunction with neurochemical approaches to implicate the extended amygdala and associated brain regions in these allostatic changes and the accompanying negative reinforcement driving drug taking and relapse (reviewed in Koob[100] and Koob and Le Moal[102]). Brain systems for responding to environmental stress and internal anxiety may provide the aversive effects that interact with brain reward/reinforcement circuitry to drive drug use in these models.[101]

Actions of Addictive Drugs Within the Reinforcement and Reward Circuitry

The majority of abused substances act on specific molecular targets within the brain. These drug actions influence mechanisms thought to be involved in addiction, usually by producing a direct reinforcing or rewarding effect. Using the aforementioned addiction models combined with neurochemical and pharmacological techniques, investigators have discovered a number of molecular interactions produced by acute and chronic drug exposure that underlie the rewarding and reinforcing effects of drugs of abuse. The mechanisms that are easiest to appreciate are those triggered by the so-called psychostimulant drugs, such as cocaine and amphetamine. These compounds act directly on the protein known as the dopamine transporter to enhance the concentration of dopamine present in the synaptic cleft following release of the neurotransmitter.[104] Cocaine is a competitive inhibitor of dopamine transporter that reduces the reuptake of dopamine into neurons, while amphetamine can also increase release of dopamine directly through the dopamine transporter.[92] It is easy to see how these molecular actions have rewarding and reinforcing consequences, given that dopamine has an important role in both of these processes, and these drugs will enhance dopamine signaling.

Given that cocaine is thought to act primarily on the dopamine transporter, it is surprising that evidence has emerged for actions of drugs of abuse that could be construed as indicating reinforcing effects of cocaine even in the absence of the transporter.[164,188] However, it appears that blockade of serotonin reuptake indirectly mediates this effect. Even more surprising is the finding that serotonin mediates cocaine conditioned place preference in dopamine-deficient mice.[75] These mice show a conditioned place preference for morphine.[74] Thus, dopamine itself may not be necessary for this drug-related learning. However, evidence that manipulations that decrease the firing of dopaminergic neurons reduce conditioned place preference in these dopamine-deficient mice suggest that another factor released by these neurons may have important roles in drug-related reward.[75]

The actions of many other drugs of abuse have also been suggested to involve dopamine, but in a less-direct manner. For example, opiates, nicotine, and alcohol all increase dopamine levels in regions of the brain such as the ventral and dorsal striatum, and appear to do so by increasing the firing rate of the dopaminergic neurons themselves (reviewed in Pierce and Kumaresan[151]). Hypotheses about the mechanisms underlying the reinforcing effects of these drugs of abuse have generally centered on the idea that enhancement of dopaminergic transmission leads to reward or reinforcement, and that all drugs of abuse work through this mechanism in one way or another. However, this idea is undoubtedly too simplistic given the evidence discussed earlier that dopamine is not necessary for reward-related learning. Furthermore, dopamine does not appear to be necessary for self-administration and the reinforcing effects of all drugs of abuse, particularly for drugs with indirect effects on the dopaminergic system. Studies of the effects of dopaminergic lesions and dopamine receptor antagonists on ethanol self-administration have yielded mixed results in a variety of self-administration and operant paradigms. D2 receptor antagonists and D1 antagonists and knockout of D1 and D2 reduce self-administration in some paradigms, but alcohol intake is not abolished after lesions of the dopaminergic system or by other dopamine receptor antagonists.[151,154,171] The evidence for dopamine involvement in opiate self-administration and opiate-related reward/reinforcement is likewise mixed, including evidence for lack of effect of dopaminergic lesions.[147,151] Thus, it appears that dopaminergic transmission is not strictly necessary for alcohol and opiate intake. Dopamine is probably not the final common pathway for drug reward, reinforcement, and self-administration as was once imagined, and the focus has now shifted to the importance of the circuitry that is influenced by dopamine.

The primary targets of almost all drugs of abuse are cell surface proteins that regulate synaptic transmission. The role of neurotransmitter transporters as targets for psychostimulants has already been discussed. Drugs such as nicotine, benzodiazepines, barbiturates, and, to some extent, alcohol produce their actions by altering the neurotransmitter receptors known as ligand-gated ion channels.[24] These receptors mediate fast synaptic transmission in the brain and can directly influence the activity of neurons within the brain reward/reinforcement circuitry. An assortment of other psychoactive and addictive drugs, including opiates, cannabinoids, and hallucinogens, produce their actions via G protein–coupled receptors.[24] This class of receptors produces neuromodulatory actions of neurotransmitters by initiating or influencing intracellular molecular signaling pathways.[24,95] The subtle changes in neuronal activity and gene expression produced by drug actions at these receptors can have profound acute and long-lasting effects on the brain reward and reinforcement systems.

Opiate drugs produce their intoxicating and rewarding effects through activation of mu, and to a lesser extent delta and kappa, opiate receptors.[35,114] Opioid peptides and their receptors have also been implicated in the rewarding effects of drugs of abuse, including effects of nicotine, cannabinoids, and alcohol (reviewed in Contet et al.[35] and Gaveriaux-Ruff and Kieffer[55]). There is also considerable evidence that opiate receptor blockade reduces rewarding and reinforcing effects of a variety of drugs of abuse, as well as drug seeking and taking in animal models of addiction (see Boutrel[20] for review). The opiate receptor antagonist naltrexone can also produce lower sensitivity to intracranial self-stimulation, but this is seen mainly with stimulation in the ventral striatum and not with ventral tegmental area stimulation.[209] Thus, there is reason to believe that opioid peptides can mediate the reinforcing and rewarding effects of drugs of abuse, perhaps independent of the actions of dopamine.

As mentioned in the preceding text, the cannabinoid drugs produce their intoxicating actions mainly via brain CB1 receptors. Delta-9-tetrahydrocannabinol, the main psychoactive ingredient in cannabis-derived drugs, is a partial agonist of the CB1 receptor. Several synthetic delta-9-tetrahydrocannabinol analogs and other CB1 agonists also produce intoxicating effects. Emerging evidence indicates an important role for endocannabinoids and the CB1 receptor in drug self-administration. Antagonist blockade or gene-targeted knockout of CB1 receptors decreases self-administration of a variety of drugs of abuse in animal models.[112] Blockade of the receptor decreases intake and operant self-administration of ethanol.[32,207] Antagonists of the CB1 receptor also reduce increases in extracellular dopamine produced by several drugs of abuse,[29] and thus, endocannabinoids may alter the rewarding *or* reinforcing actions of drugs of abuse via this mechanism.

Chronic exposure to drugs of abuse is thought to bring about neuroadaptive changes that alter the brain reinforcement/reward circuitry. Recent studies have focused on changes in the efficacy of synaptic transmission and alterations in dendritic morphology in neurons within the ventral tegmental area and nucleus accumbens. Cocaine exposure has been demonstrated to produce changes in the ratio of excitatory synaptic responses mediated by AMPA and N-methyl-D-aspartate–type glutamate receptors, a change thought to reflect long-term plasticity of glutamatergic synapses.[5,195,199] This sort of synaptic plasticity has been observed in recordings from both nucleus accumbens medium spiny neurons and ventral tegmental area dopaminergic neurons.[195,199] Even a single dose of cocaine appears to produce this plastic change in excitatory transmission.[199] Other drugs of abuse, including ethanol, alter efficacy of both excitatory and inhibitory transmission in the ventral tegmental area.[119,190] Synaptic plasticity produced by drug exposure may condition synapses within the reinforcement/reward circuits to enhance responses to subsequent exposure to drugs or drug-related stimuli. This could occur at the expense of using this circuitry to learn other, more adaptive, responses to environmental stimuli.

Chronic drug exposure also alters long-term synaptic depression mediated by endocannabinoids and the CB1 receptor. Repeated exposure to delta-9-tetrahydrocannabinol for days eliminates this form of long-term synaptic depression in the dorsal striatum, hippocampus, and nucleus accumbens,[76,116,131] and this adaptation appears to involve decreases in the presynaptic actions of CB1 receptors. Even a single exposure to delta-9-tetrahydrocannabinol produces a similar action.[115] A single treatment with cocaine also eliminates endocannabinoid-dependent long-term synaptic depression,[52] and chronic ethanol exposure has been reported to have a similar action in the striatum.[218] Loss of endocannabinoid-dependent long-term depression (LTD) is associated with enhanced habit learning in mice.[131] Given the role of CB1 receptors in response to the drugs of abuse mentioned previously, it is possible that adaptations in endocannabinoid/CB1 function underlie neuroadaptations that lead to altered reinforcing and rewarding properties of many drugs of abuse.

Repeated exposure to cocaine, amphetamine, alcohol, and other such drugs of abuse changes the dendritic structure of the neurons in the prefrontal cortex, nucleus accumbens, and dorsal striatum.[40,85,128,163] Changes in spine density and dendritic branching are seen, with differential effects in different brain regions. These morphological changes are thought to lead to alterations in the ability of neurons within this circuitry to respond to normal levels of synaptic input. Ultimately, this dendritic rearrangement could lead to less plasticity within the circuitry and help to rigidify behaviors related to the addictive drug.

There are also a host of cellular and molecular changes within the reinforcement/reward circuitry that have been related to drugs of abuse (see Nestler[133] for review), and there is simply not space within this review to cover all of these changes. However, interesting information is emerging from examination of drug-induced changes in glutamatergic synaptic transmission within the circuitry of interest. Glutamate signaling through G protein–coupled receptors called metabotropic glutamate receptors is one system implicated in these drug-induced changes.[67,193] The metabotropic glutamate receptors come in a variety of subtypes.[34] The different metabotropic glutamate receptor subtypes produce diverse cellular actions including inhibition and stimulation of neurotransmitter release and activation of intracellular signaling pathways that contribute to changes in neuronal excitability and long-lasting plasticity of synaptic transmission.[34] Group I metabotropic glutamate receptors are implicated in neuroadaptations to abused drugs, as well as drug self-administration.[67,193] The expression and function of metabotropic glutamate receptor-5 is downregulated following chronic administration of cocaine and withdrawal, but upregulated by alcohol exposure (reviewed in Szumlinski et al.[193]). At the same time, expression of the Homer protein that interacts with this receptor and changes its signaling functions undergoes similar drug-related upregulation.[191,193,194] The group I metabotropic glutamate receptors are implicated in forms of synaptic plasticity throughout the brain reward/reinforcement circuitry, including endocannabinoid-dependent long-term synaptic depression.[67] Thus, cocaine-induced downregulation of metabotropic glutamate receptor-5 in brain regions such as the nucleus accumbens

following chronic drug exposure could underlie loss of metabotropic glutamate receptor–mediated synaptic plasticity.[52,67,173] In the case of alcohol, increased metabotropic glutamate receptor/Homer expression may be part of a general increase in glutamatergic signaling after repeated drug administration and withdrawal, contributing to plastic changes in the circuitry that ultimately foster increased drug seeking and self-administration.[185] This idea is consistent with the finding that a metabotropic glutamate receptor-5 antagonist decreases alcohol seeking and relapse in animals with self-administration experience.[9]

Roles in chronic drug actions and relapse for the presynaptically localized metabotropic glutamate receptor 2 (mGluR2) are emerging from recent research. Early studies by Kalivas and coworkers indicated that increased extracellular glutamate produced by changes in transporter function leads to mGluR2 activation following chronic cocaine exposure.[127] This feedback mechanism may help to limit hyperactivation of key cortical glutamatergic inputs that help drive drug seeking and taking. Indeed, recent studies support the idea that deficient mGluR2 activity contributes to increased seeking and taking of cocaine, ethanol, and nicotine.[26,90,120,221] A positive allosteric modulator of mGluR2 shows promise for reducing drug seeking after chronic exposure and abstinence in animal models.[26,90]

However, despite this wealth of knowledge, it is still not clear how the cellular and molecular changes brought about by drugs of abuse contribute to overall changes in circuit function that ultimately lead to addiction. Addressing this topic will require more sophisticated analysis of neuronal and circuit function in vivo, combined with continued work at the molecular, cellular, and behavioral levels. Clearly, this is a key direction for future research on the neural basis of drug reinforcement and reward.

What Drives Drug Use, Abuse, and Addiction: The Direction of Future Research

Ultimately, the goals of research on drugs and use disorders are to gain a better understanding of how drugs act on the brain, and to develop better approaches for minimizing and treating drug abuse-related problems. The neurobiological mechanisms discussed in this chapter indicate that brain mechanisms of reward and reinforcement are more complicated than most of us previously imagined in terms of both the circuitry involved and the underlying neurochemistry.

The interactions of drugs of abuse with these systems are likewise complex. It is likely that drugs engage multiple aspects of the different circuits during the initial phases of exposure. Drug actions on dopaminergic transmission and other aspects of the associative circuit will signal the positive hedonic value of the drug and establish the motivation to continue to take the drug. At the same time, drug-associated cues and environmental connections to drug availability will be signaled and learned through the limbic circuitry, likely contributing to the sensitized incentive described by Robinson and Berridge.[162] It is currently thought that the role of the sensorimotor circuitry in drug seeking and taking develops rather slowly during the course of experience with drugs.[49,57] However, effects on this circuitry of drugs such as ethanol occur with acute and short-term chronic exposure.[40,144,212] Furthermore, the rate of recruitment of this system may depend on the schedule and contingencies of drug availability, especially in relation to instrumental behaviors. Furthermore, engagement of the sensorimotor circuitry likely develops in parallel with activation of the other circuits, and there may be competition between the different circuits for control of behavior.[37] Ultimately the involvement of the systems will likely depend on the pattern of recruitment of different circuit elements. However, there is emerging evidence that reinforcing effects of drugs ultimately lead to involvement of the sensorimotor circuitry and establishment of drug-related habits.[14,49,57,219] One intriguing scenario is a shift from a purely stimulus-outcome–based mode of responding to one that also includes stimulus-response–based actions. Thus a drug user may initially come to associate certain cues with the rewarding effects of a drug, and this may initially drive drug seeking. With continued drug exposure, the stimulus-response circuitry becomes progressively more engaged as drugs reinforce the stimulus/environment control of drug seeking and use. Indeed, the work of Everitt and colleagues appears to support such a transition from limbic to sensorimotor circuit control of drug-related actions.[14,49] It remains to be seen how action-outcome–based learning plays a role in this scenario, but this form of learning will almost certainly play a role in drug use and abuse in humans. One possibility is that action-outcome–based learning may drive the acquisition of new behaviors that are designed to locate and obtain drugs of abuse, providing another mechanism through which incentive sensitization takes over brain function to promote drug seeking and use. Brain mechanisms involved in stress responsivity and production of aversive responses to drug withdrawal also become progressively more involved as drug use and abuse continue, and these circuits likely interact with mechanisms of reward and reinforcement to promote relapse to drug use (Fig. 16.1).

The effects of stress on the prefrontal cortex are of interest in this regard. Studies showing that exposure to acute or chronic stress and corticosterone treatment stunts the dendritic morphology of neurons in the medial prefrontal cortex,[28,84,153] suggesting that the circuitry involving this brain region is impaired during stress. These dendritic stunting effects have been postulated to impair executive decision-making capabilities.[162] One result of this neurotoxic stress effect may be to drive behavior away from goal-directed actions and toward habitual responding.[51] Thus stress may act on the reward/reinforcement circuitry at a number of levels to promote inflexible drug seeking and use. Ultimately, drug use and abuse are initiated and sustained by a number of intrinsic neural mechanisms including goal-directed behavior, environmentally stimulated instrumental behavior, habitization of drug-related responses, and negative reinforcement/allostasis that promotes a return to drug use.

Determining the relative roles of these different neural mechanisms and neural circuits in drug use, abuse, and addiction will require new avenues of research at the molecular, cellular, systems, and behavioral levels. Ultimately, an integrative approach that incorporates all of these levels of analysis is needed. Behavioral models of different phenotypes relevant to drug reward, reinforcement, seeking, and taking need to be used with an eye to determining the roles of the underlying changes in circuits, cells, and molecules. In using these models it will be necessary to bear in mind all of the possible processes that contribute to drug use, relapse, and addiction, including goal-directed behavior, cue-related conditioning, avoidance of aversive consequences, incubation, and development of habitual actions. The development of models that allow investigators to select animals that are highly sensitive to compulsive drug use should provide the opportunity to examine genetic, epigenetic, and environmental factors that have predispositional effects in these animals. However, the generality of these models to multiple drugs of abuse needs to be demonstrated, and it will be important to determine if the same factors play a role in the development of compulsive use of different drugs. It is very likely that no one model will be able to tell us all that we need to know to understand maladaptive drug use and addiction. Thus it is important to continue to cultivate useful models and develop new ones, always with an eye toward determining the underlying neurobiology.

In considering the role of neural circuitry in drug reward, reinforcement, and addiction, a more inclusive approach will likely be needed. Basic neuroscientific research is now revealing multiple parallel brain systems for control of different aspects of action production and action learning. Movement beyond the monolithic concept of a single neural reward/reinforcement system is necessary. It is likely that these systems will have similar roles in behavior directed toward drugs of abuse, and this must be considered in designing experiments aimed at determining the neural basis of drug seeking and use.

At the cellular and molecular levels, a number of changes brought about by drug exposure and related conditioning have been described. However, little is known about the role of most of these changes in the development of maladaptive drug use and/or addiction. Consideration of the wide variety of neurotransmitters and receptors that participate in normal and abnormal functioning of the relevant brain circuitry is especially important. Experimental approaches designed to manipulate particular molecules within given cell types and circuits (e.g., local drug application, disconnection analyses, opto- and chemogenetic techniques, and the use of sophisticated genetically manipulated mice) will play an ever-increasing role in our quest to determine which molecular and cellular changes are important and which are merely epiphenomena or secondary to the truly causal changes. The powerful tools for genetic and circuit manipulation, molecular analysis, examination of neurophysiology and neurochemistry at the in vitro and in vivo levels, and ever more sophisticated behavioral analysis in a variety of organisms should allow investigators to make rapid progress in this area in the coming years.

References

1. Adams CD, Dickinson A. Instrumental responding following reinforcer devaluation. *Q J Exp Psychol*. 1981;33B:109–121.
2. Ahmed SH, Kenny PJ, Koob GF, Markou A. Neurobiological evidence for hedonic allostasis associated with escalating cocaine use. *Nat Neurosci*. 2002;5:625–626.
3. Alexander GE, Delong MR, Strick PL. Parallel organization of segregated circuits linking basal ganglia and cortex. *Ann Rev Neurosci*. 1986;9:357–381.
4. American Psychiatric Association. *Diagnostic and Statistical Manual of Mental Disorders V: Substance-Related and Addictive Disorders*. 5th ed. Washington, DC: American Psychiatric Publishing; 2016.
5. Argilli E, Sibley DR, Malenka RC, England PM, Bonci A. Mechanism and time course of cocaine-induced long-term potentiation in the ventral tegmental area. *J Neurosci*. 2008;28(37):9092–1000.
6. Aston-Jones G, Harris GC. Brain substrates for increased drug seeking during protracted withdrawal. *Neuropharmacol*. 2004;47(suppl 1):167–179.
7. Atallah HE, Lopez-Paniagua D, Rudy JW, O'Reilly RC. Separate neural substrates for skill learning and performance in the ventral and dorsal striatum. *Nat Neurosci*. 2007;10(1):126–131.
8. Azrin NH, Holz WC. Punishment. In: Honig WK, ed. *Operant Behavior: Areas of Research and Application*. New York: Appleton-Century-Crofts; 1966:380–447.

9. Backstrom P, Bachteler D, Koch S, Hyytia P, Spanagel R. mGluR5 antagonist MPEP reduces ethanol-seeking and relapse behavior. *Neuropsychopharmacology.* 2004;29:921–928.

10. Bain GT, Kornetsky C. Ethanol oral self administration and rewarding brain stimulation. *Alcohol.* 1989;6(6):499–503.

11. Baker EJ, Farro J, Gonzales S, Helms C, Grant KA. Chronic alcohol self-administration in monkeys shows long-term quantity/frequency categorical stability. *Alcohol Clin Exp Res.* 2014;38(11):2835–284.

12. Balleine BW. Neural bases of food-seeking: affect, arousal and reward in corticostriatolimbic circuits. *Physiol Behav.* 2005;86(5):717–730.

13. Becker HC, Ron D. Animal models of excessive alcohol consumption: recent advances and future challenges. *Alcohol.* 2014;48(3):205–208.

14. Belin D, Everitt BJ. Cocaine seeking habits depend upon dopamine-dependent serial connectivity linking the ventral with the dorsal striatum. *Neuron.* 2008;57(3):432–441.

15. Belin D, Mar AC, Dalley JW, Robbins TW, Everitt BJ. High impulsivity predicts the switch to compulsive cocaine-taking. *Science.* 2008;320(5881):1352–1355.

16. Berridge KC. Food reward: brain substrates of wanting and liking. *Neurosci Biobehav Rev.* 1996;20:1–25.

17. Berridge KC, Robinson TE. What is the role of dopamine in reward: hedonic impact, reward learning, or incentive salience? *Brain Res Rev.* 1998;28(3):309–369.

18. Boakes RA. Self-starvation in the rat: running versus eating. *Span J Psychol.* 2007;10(2):251–257.

19. Bonson KR, Grant SJ, Contoreggi CS, et al. Neural systems and cue-induced cocaine craving. *Neuropsychopharmacology.* 2002;26:376–386.

20. Boutrel B. A neuropeptide-centric view of psychostimulant addiction. *Br J Pharmacol.* 2008;154(2):343–357.

21. Brabano MF, Cador M. Opioids for hedonic experience and dopamine to get ready for it. *Psychopharmacology (Berl).* 2007;191(3):497–506.

22. Broekkamp CLE, Phillips AG, Cools AR. Facilitation of self-stimulation behavior following intracerebral microinjections of opioids into the ventral tegmental area. *Pharmacol Biochem Behav.* 1979;11:289–295.

23. Brown EE, Fibiger HC. Differential effects of excitotoxic lesions of the amygdala on cocaine-induced conditioned locomotion and conditioned place preference. *Psychopharmacology (Berl).* 1993;113:123–130.

24. Brunton L, Lazo J, Parker K. *Goodman & Gilman's the Pharmacological Basis of Therapeutics.* New York: McGraw-Hill; 2005.

25. Caprioli D, Venniro M, Zhang M, Bossert JM, Warren BL, Hope BT, Shaham Y. Role of dorsomedial striatum neuronal ensembles in incubation of methamphetamine craving after voluntary abstinence. *J Neurosci.* 2017;37(4):1014–1027.

26. Caprioli D, Venniro M, Zeric T, et al. Effect of the novel positive allosteric modulator of metabotropic glutamate receptor 2 AZD8529 on incubation of methamphetamine craving after prolonged voluntary abstinence in a rat model. *Biol Pychiatry.* 2015;78(7):463–473.

27. Carlezon Jr WA, Nestler EJ. Elevated levels of GluR1 in the midbrain: a trigger for sensitization to drugs of abuse? *Trends Neurosci.* 2002;25:610–615.

28. Cerqueira JJ, Pêgo JM, Taipa R, Bessa JM, Almeida OF, Sousa N. Morphological correlates of corticosteroid-induced changes in prefrontal cortex-dependent behaviors. *J Neurosci.* 2005;25(34):7792–7800.

29. Cheer JF, Wassum KM, Sombers LA, et al. Phasic dopamine release evoked by abused substances requires cannabinoid receptor activation. *J Neurosci.* 2007;27(4):791–795.

30. Childress AR, Ehrman RN, Rohsenow D, Robbins SJ, O'Brien CP. Classically conditioned factors in drug dependence. In: Lowinson J, Ruiz P, Millman R, eds. *Comprehensive Textbook of Substance Abuse.* Baltimore: Williams & Wilkins; 1993:56–69.

31. Childress AR, Mozley PD, McELgin W, Fitzgerald J, Reivich M, O'Brien CP. Limbic activation during cue-induced cocaine craving. *Am J Psychiatry.* 1999;156:11–18.

32. Colombo G, Orrù A, Lai P, Cabras C, Maccioni P, Rubio M, Gessa GL, Carai MA. The cannabinoid CB1 receptor antagonist, rimonabant, as a promising pharmacotherapy for alcohol dependence: preclinical evidence. *Mol Neurobiol.* 2007;36(1):102–112.

33. Colwill RM, Rescorla RA. Effect of reinforcer devaluation on discriminative control of instrumental behavior. *J Exp Psychol Anim Behav Proc.* 1990;16(1):40–47.

34. Conn PJ, Pin JP. Pharmacology and functions of metabotropic glutamate receptors. *Ann Rev Pharmacol Toxicol.* 1997;37:205–237.

35. Contet C, Kieffer BL, Befort K. Mu opioid receptor: a gateway to drug addiction. *Curr Opin Neurobiol.* 2004;J14(3):370–378.

36. Corbett D, Wise RA. Intracranial self-stimulation in relation to the ascending dopaminergic systems of the midbrain: a moveable electrode mapping study. *Brain Res.* 1980;85(1):1–15.

37. Corbit LH, Janak PH. Habitual alcohol seeking: neural bases and possible relations to alcohol use disorders. *Alcohol Clin Exp Res.* 2016;40(7):1380–13837.

38. Corbit LH, Janak PH, Balleine BW. General and outcome-specific forms of Pavlovian-instrumental transfer: the effect of shifts in motivational state and inactivation of the ventral tegmental area. *Eur J Neurosci.* 2007;26(11):3141–3149.

39. Cornish J, Kalivas P. Glutamate transmission in the nucleus accumbens mediates relapse in cocaine addiction. *J Neurosci.* 2000;20(RC89):81–85.

40. Cuzon Carlson VC, Seabold GK, Helms CM, et al. Synaptic and morphological neuroadaptations in the putamen associated with long-term, relapsing alcohol drinking in primates. *Neuropsychopharm.* 2011;36(12):2513–2528.

41. Dalley JW, Laane K, Theobald DE, Armstrong HC, Corlett PR, Chudasama Y, Robbins TW. Time-limited modulation of appetitive Pavlovian memory by D1 and NMDA receptors in the nucleus accumbens. *Proc Natl Acad Sci USA.* 2005;102(17):6189–6194.

42. Dayan P, Balleine BW. Reward, motivation, and reinforcement learning. *Neuron.* 2002;36(2):285–298.

43. Deroche V, Caine SB, Heyser CJ, Polis I, Koob GF, Gold LH. Differences in the liability to self-administer intravenous cocaine between C57BL/6 x SJL and BALB/cByJ mice. *Pharmacol Biochem Behav.* 1997;57(3):429–440.

44. Deroche-Gamonet V, Belin D, Piazza PV. Evidence for addiction-like behavior in the rat. *Science.* 2004;305(5686):1014–1017.

45. Dickinson A, Nicholas DJ, Adams CD. The effect of the instrumental training contingency on susceptibility to reinforcer devaluation. *Q J Exp Psychol.* 1983;35B:35–51.

46. Dickinson A, Wood N, Smith JW. Alcohol seeking by rats: action or habit? *Q J Exp Psychol B.* 2002;55(4):331–348.

47. Divac I, Rosvold HE, Szwarcbart MK. Behavioral effects of selective ablation of the caudate nucleus. *J Comp Physiol Psychol.* 1967;63:184–190.

48. Donahoe J, Palmer D, Burgos J. The unit of selection: what do reinforcers reinforce? *J Exp Anal Behav.* 1997;67(2):259–273.

49. Everitt BJ, Robbins TW. Neural systems of reinforcement for drug addiction: from actions to habits to compulsion. *Nat Neurosci.* 2005;8(11):1481–1489.

50. Feltenstein MW, See RE. The neurocircuitry of addiction: an overview. *Br J Pharmacol.* 2008;154(2):261–274.

51. Ferreira ED, Sousa JC, Melo I, et al. Chronic stress causes frontostriatal reorganization and affects decision-making. *Science.* 2009;325(5940):621–625.

52. Fourgeaud L, Mato S, Bouchet D, Hémar A, Worley PF, Manzoni OJ. A single in vivo exposure to cocaine abolishes endocannabinoid-mediated long-term depression in the nucleus accumbens. *J Neurosci.* 2004;24(31):6939–6945.

53. Frederickson RC, Geary LE. Endogenous opioid peptides: review of physiological, pharmacological and clinical aspects. *Prog Neurobiol.* 1982;19(1–2):19–69.

54. Frye GD, Breese GR. An evaluation of the locomotor stimulating action of ethanol in rats and mice. *Psychopharmacology.* 1981;75:372–379.

55. Gaveriaux-Ruff C, Kieffer BL. Opioid receptor genes inactivated in mice: the highlights. *Neuropeptides.* 2002;36:62–71.

56. Gawin FH, Kleber HD. Abstinence symptomatology and psychiatric diagnosis in cocaine abusers: clinical observations. *Arch Gen Psychiatry.* 1986;43:107–113.

57. Gerdeman GL, Partridge JG, Lupica CR, Lovinger DM. It could be habit forming: drugs of abuse and striatal synaptic plasticity. *Trends Neurosci.* 2003;26(4):184–192.

58. Gerdeman GL, Schechter JB, French ED. Endocannabinoid signaling at striatal CB1 receptors is critical for the consolidation of stimulus-response memories. 2007 symposium on the cannabinoids. Burlington, Vermont: International Cannabinoid Research Society; 2007:123. www.cannabinoidsociety.org.

59. Giros B, Jaber M, Jones SR, Wightman RM, Caron MG. Hyperlocomotion and indifference to cocaine and amphetamine in mice lacking the dopamine transporter. *Nature.* 1996;379:606–612.

60. Goodman A. Neurobiology of addiction. An integrative review. *Biochem Pharmacol.* 2008;75(1):266–322.

61. Grace AA, Floresco SB, Goto Y, Lodge DJ. Regulation of firing of dopaminergic neurons and control of goal-directed behaviors. *Trends Neurosci.* 2007;30:220–227.

62. Grahame NJ, Cunningham CL. Intravenous ethanol self-administration in C57BL/6 J and DBA/2 J mice. *Alcohol Clin Exp Res.* 1997;21:56–62.

63. Gratton A. In vivo analysis of the role of dopamine in stimulant and opiate self-administration. *J Psychiatry Neurosci.* 1996;21(4):264–279.

64. Gremel CM, Chancey JH, Atwood BK, Luo G, Neve R, Ramakrishnan C, Deisseroth K, Lovinger DM, Costa RM. Endocannabinoid modulation of orbitostriatal circuits gates habit formation. *Neuron.* 2016;90(6):1312–1324.

65. Gremel CM, Cunningham CL. Roles of the nucleus accumbens and amygdala in the acquisition and expression of ethanol-conditioned behavior in mice. *J Neurosci.* 2008;28(5):1076–1084.

66. Grueter BA, McElligott ZA, Robison AJ, Mathews GC, Winder DG. In vivo metabotropic glutamate receptor 5 (mGluR5) antagonism prevents cocaine-induced disruption of postsynaptically maintained mGluR5-dependent long-term depression. *J Neurosci.* 2008;28(37):9261–9270.

67. Grueter BA, McElligott ZA, Winder DG. Group I mGluRs and long-term depression: potential roles in addiction? *Mol Neurobiol.* 2007;36(3):232–244.

68. Haber SN, Fudge JL, McFarland NR. Striatonigrostriatal pathways in primates form an ascending spiral from the shell to the dorsolateral striatum. *J Neurosci.* 2000;20:2369–2382.

69. Hayward MD, Pintar JE, Low MJ. Selective reward deficit in mice lacking beta-endorphin and enkephalin. *J Neurosci.* 2002;22(18):8251–8258.

70. Hemby SE, Johnson BA, Dworkin SI. Neurobiological basis of drug reinforcement. In: Johnson BA, Roache JD, eds. *Drug Addiction and Treatment, Nexus of Neuroscience and Behavior.* Philadelphia: Lippincott Raven; 1997:2–19.

71. Herkenham M, Lynn AB, Johnson MR, Melvin LS, de Costa BR, Rice KC. Characterization and localization of cannabinoid receptors in rat brain: a quantitative in vitro autoradiographic study. *J Neurosci.* 1991;11:563–583.

72. Hilário MRF, Clouse E, Yin HH, Costa RM. Endocannabinoid signaling is critical for habit formation. *Front Integr Neurosci.* 2007;1:1–12.

73. Hintiryan H, Foster NN, Bowman I, et al. The mouse corticostriatal projectome. *Nat Neurosci.* 2016;19:1100–1114.

74. Hnasko TS, Sotak BN, Palmiter RD. Morphine reward in dopamine-deficient mice. *Nature.* 2005;438:854–857.

75. Hnasko TS, Sotak BN, Palmiter RD. Cocaine-conditioned place preference by dopamine-deficient mice is mediated by serotonin. *J Neurosci.* 2007;27(46):12484–12488.

76. Hoffman AF, Oz M, Caulder T, Lupica CR. Functional tolerance and blockade of long-term depression at synapses in the nucleus accumbens after chronic cannabinoid exposure. *J Neurosci.* 2003;23(12):4815–4820.

77. Hohmann AG, Herkenham JM. Localization of cannabinoid CB1 receptor mRNA in neuronal subpopulations of rat striatum: a double-label in situ hybridization study. *Synapse.* 2000;37:71–80.

78. Holman EW. Some conditions for the dissociation of consummatory and instrumental behavior in rats. *Learn Motiv.* 1975;6:358–366.

79. Howell LL, Kimmel HL. Monoamine transporters and psychostimulant addiction. *Biochem Pharmacol.* 2008;75(1):196–217.

80. Hsu PD, Lander ES, Zhang F. Development and applications of CRISPR-Cas9 for genome engineering. *Cell.* 2014;157(6):1262–1278.

81. Hull CL. *Principles of Behavior.* New York: Appleton-Century-Crofts; 1943.

82. Hunnicutt BJ, Jongbloets BC, Birdsong WT, Gertz KJ, Zhong H, Mao T. A comprehensive excitatory input map of the striatum reveals novel functional organization. *Elife.* 2016;28:5.

83. Hyman SE, Malenka RC, Nestler EJ. Neural mechanisms of addiction: the role of reward-related learning and memory. *Annu Rev Neurosci.* 2006;29:565–598.

84. Izquierdo A, Wellman CL, Holmes A. Brief uncontrollable stress causes dendritic retraction in infralimbic cortex and resistance to fear extinction in mice. *J Neurosci.* 2006;26(21):5733–5738.

85. Jedynak JP, Uslaner JM, Esteban JA, Robinson TE. Methamphetamine-induced structural plasticity in the dorsal striatum. *Eur J Neurosci.* 2007;25(3):847–853.

86. Jimenez VA, Grant KA. Studies using macaque monkeys to address excessive alcohol drinking and stress interactions. *Neuropharmacology.* 2017;122:127–135.

87. Jinek M, Chylinski K, Fonfara I, Hauer M, Doudna JA, Charpentier E. A programmable dual-RNA-guided DNA endonuclease in adaptive bacterial immunity. *Science.* 2012;337(6096):816–821.

88. Johnson AW, Bannerman D, Rawlins N, Sprengel R, Good MA. Targeted deletion of the GluR-1 AMPA receptor in mice dissociates general and outcome-specific influences of appetitive rewards on learning. *Behav Neurosci.* 2007;121(6):1192–1202.

89. Jones S, Bonci A. Synaptic plasticity and drug addiction. *Curr Opin Pharmacol.* 2005;5(1):20–25.

90. Justinova Z, Panlilio LB, Secci ME, et al. The novel metabotropic glutamate receptor positive allosteric modulator, ASD8529, decreases nicotine self-administration and relapse in squirrel monkeys. *Biol Psychiatry.* 2015;78(7):452–462.

91. Kaffman A, Krystal JH. New frontiers in animals research of psychiatric illness. *Methods Mol Biol.* 2012;829:3–30.

92. Kahlig KM, Galli A. Regulation of dopamine transporter function and plasma membrane expression by dopamine, amphetamine, and cocaine. *Eur J Pharmacol.* 2003;479(1–3):153–158.

93. Kalivas PW, McFarland K. Brain circuitry and the reinstatement of cocaine-seeking behavior. *Psychopharmacology (Berl).* 2003;168(1–2):44–56.

94. Kalivas PW, O'Brien C. Drug addiction as a pathology of staged neuroplasticity. *Neuropsychopharmacology.* 2008;33(1):166–180.

95. Kandel ER, Schwartz JH, Jessell TM. *Principles of Neural Science.* New York: McGraw-Hill; 2000.

96. Kelley AE. Ventral striatal control of appetitive motivation: role in ingestive behavior and reward-related learning. *Neurosci Biobehav Rev.* 2004;27(8):765–776.

97. Kenny PJ, Chen SA, Kitamura O, Markou A, Koob GF. Conditioned withdrawal drives heroin consumption and decreases reward sensitivity. *J Neurosci.* 2006;26(22):5894–5900.

98. Konorski J. *Integrative Activity of the Brain.* Chicago: University of Chicago; 1967.

99. Koob G. The neurobiology of addiction: a neuroadaptational view relevant for diagnosis. *Addiction.* 2006;101(suppl 1):23–30.

100. Koob G. Neurobiological substrates for the dark side of compulsivity in addiction. *Neuropharmacology.* 2008;56(suppl 1):18–31.

101. Koob G, Kreek MJ. Stress, dysregulation of drug reward pathways, and the transition to drug dependence. *Am J Psychiatry.* 2007;164(8):1149–1159.

102. Koob G, Le Moal M. Addiction and the brain antireward system. *Annu Rev Psychol.* 2008;59:29–53.

103. Kornetsky C, Bain GT, Unterwald EM, Lewis MJ. Brain stimulation reward: effects of ethanol. *Alcohol Clin Exp Res.* 1988;12(5):609–616.

104. Kuhar MJ, Sanchez-Roa PM, Wong DF, et al. Dopamine transporter: biochemistry, pharmacology and imaging. *Eur Neurol Suppl.* 1990;1:15–20.

105. Kumar S, Fleming RL, Morrow AL. Ethanol regulation of gamma-aminobutyric acid A receptors: genomic and nongenomic mechanisms. *Pharmacol Ther.* 2004;101(3):211–226.

106. Kumar V, Kim K, Joseph C, et al. C57BL/6N mutation in the cytoplasmic FMRP interactions protein 2 regulates cocaine response. *Science.* 2013;342(6165):1508–1512.

107. LeDoux J. The amygdala. *Curr Biol.* 2007;17(20):R868–R874.

108. Leventhal AM, Kahler CW, Ray LA, Stone K, Young D, Chelminski I, Zimmerman M. Anhedonia and amotivation in psychiatric outpatients with fully remitted stimulant use disorder. *Am J Addict.* 2008;17(3):218–223.

109. Lovinger DM. Presynaptic modulation by endocannabinoids. *Handb Exp Pharmacol.* 2008;184:435–477.

110. Löw K, Crestani F, Keist R, et al. Molecular and neuronal substrate for the selective attenuation of anxiety. *Science.* 2000;290(5489):131–134.

111. Maldonado R. Study of cannabinoid dependence in animals. *Pharmacol Ther.* 2002;2:153–164.

112. Maldonado R, Valverde O, Berrendero F. Involvement of the endocannabinoid system in drug addiction. *Trends Neurosci.* 2006;29(4):225–232.

113. Masur J, Oliveira De Souza ML, Zwicker AP. The excitatory effect of ethanol: absence in rats, no tolerance and increased sensitivity in mice. *Pharmacol Biochem Behav.* 1986;24:1225–1228.

114. Matthes HWD, Maldonado R, Simonin F, et al. Loss of morphine-induced analgesia, reward effect and withdrawal symptoms in mice lacking the μ-opioid receptor gene. *Nature.* 1996;383:819–823.

115. Mato S, Chevaleyre V, Robbe D, Pazos A, Castillo PE, Manzoni OJ. A single in-vivo exposure to delta 9THC blocks endocannabinoid-mediated synaptic plasticity. *Nat Neurosci.* 2004;7(6):585–586.

116. Mato S, Robbe D, Puente N, Grandes P, Manzoni OJ. Presynaptic homeostatic plasticity rescues long-term depression after chronic Delta 9-tetrahydrocannabinol exposure. *J Neurosci.* 2005;25(50):11619–11627.

117. McEwen BS, Wingfield JD. The concept of allostasis in biology and biomedicine. *Horm Behav.* 2003;43(1):2–15.

118. McGregor CM, Srisurapanont M, Jittiwutikarn J, Laobhripatr S, Wongtan T, White JM. The nature, time course and severity of methamphetamine withdrawal. *Addiction.* 2005;100:1300–1329.

119. Melis M, Camarini R, Ungless MA, Bonci A. Long-lasting potentiation of GABAergic synapses in dopamine neurons after a single in vivo ethanol exposure. *J Neurosci.* 2002;22(6):2074–2082.

120. Meinhardt MW, Hansson AC, Perreau-Lenz S, et al. Rescue inhibition of infralimbic mGluR2 deficit restores control over drug-seeking behavior in alcohol dependence. *J Neurosci.* 2013;33(7):2794–2806.

121. Mihalek RM, Bowers BJ, Wehner JM, et al. GABA(A)-receptor delta subunit knockout mice have multiple defects in behavioral responses to ethanol. *Alcohol Clin Exp Res.* 2001;25:1708–1718.

122. Miles FJ, Everitt BJ, Dalley JW, Dickinson A. Conditioned activity and instrumental reinforcement following long-term oral consumption of cocaine by rats. *Behav Neurosci.* 2004;118(6):1331–1339.

123. Miles FJ, Everitt BJ, Dickinson A. Oral cocaine seeking by rats: action or habit? *Behav Neurosci.* 2003;117(5):927–938.

124. Mojica FJ, Montoliu L. On the origin of CRISPR-Cas technology: from prokaryotes to mammals. *Trends Microbiol.* 2016;24(10):811–820.

125. Moolten M, Kornetsky C. Oral self-administration of ethanol and not experimenter-administered ethanol facilitates rewarding electrical brain stimulation. *Alcohol.* 1990;7:221–225.

126. Moore BR. The evolution of learning. *Biol Rev.* 2004;79:301–335.

127. Moussawi K, Kalivas PW. Group II metabotropic glutamate receptors (mGlu2/3) in drug addiction. *Eur J Pharmacol.* 2010;639(1–3):115–122.

128. Mulholland PJ, Chandler LJ. The thorny side of addiction: adaptive plasticity and dendritic spines. *Sci World J.* 2007;7:9–21.

129. Müller CP, Carey RJ, Huston JP, De Souza Silva MA. Serotonin and psychostimulant addiction: focus on 5-HT1A-receptors. *Prog Neurobiol.* 2007;81(3):133–178.

130. Mulligan MK, Ponomarev I, Boehm 2nd SL, et al. Alcohol trait and transcriptional genomic analysis of C57BL/6 substrains. *Genes Brain Behav.* 2008;7(6):677–689.

131. Nazzaro C, Greco B, Cerovic M, et al. SK channel modulation rescues striatal plasticity and control over habit in cannabinoid tolerance. *Nat Neurosci.* 2012;15(2):284–293.

132. Nazzaro JM, Seeger TF, Gardner EL. Morphine differentially affects ventral tegmental and substantia nigra brain reward thresholds. *Pharmacol Biochem Behav.* 1981;14(3):325–331.

133. Nestler EJ. Molecular neurobiology of addiction. *Am J Addict.* 2001;10(3):201–217.

134. Nicoll RA, Alger BE. The brain's own marijuana. *Sci Am.* 2004;291(6):68–75.

135. Oades RD, Halliday GM. Ventral tegmental (A10) system: neurobiology. 1. Anatomy and connectivity. *Brain Res.* 1987;434(2):117–165.

136. Olds J, Milner P. Positive reinforcement produced by electrical stimulation of septal area and other regions of rat brain. *J Comp Physiol Psychol.* 1954;47(6):4194–4127.

137. Olmstead MC, Lafond MV, Everitt BJ, Dickinson A. Cocaine seeking by rats is a goal-directed action. *Behav Neurosci.* 2001;115(2):394–402.

138. Ostlund SB, Balleine BW. Orbitofrontal cortex mediates outcome encoding in Pavlovian but not instrumental conditioning. *J Neurosci.* 2007;27(18):4819–4825.

139. Ostlund SB, Balleine BW. Differential involvement of the basolateral amygdala and mediodorsal thalamus in instrumental action selection. *J Neurosci.* 2008;28(17):4398–4405.

140. Ostlund SB, Balleine BW. Theories of goal-directed behavior. In: Squire LR, ed. *Encyclopedia of Neuroscience.* Vol. 4. Oxford: Academic Press; 2009:943–949.

141. Palmiter RD. Dopamine signaling in the dorsal striatum is essential for motivated behaviors: lessons from dopamine-deficient mice. *Ann NY Acad Sci.* 2008;1129:35–46.

142. Panlilio LV, Goldberg SR. Self-administration of drugs in animals and humans as a model and an investigative tool. *Addiction.* 2007;102(12):1863–1870.

143. Pattij T, Vanderschuren LJ. The neuropharmacology of impulsive behaviour. *Trends Pharmacol Sci.* 2008;29(4):192–199.

144. Patton MH, Roberts BM, Lovinger DM, Mathur BN. Ethanol disinhibits dorsolateral striatal medium spiny neurons through activation of a presynaptic delta opioid receptor. *Neuropsychopharmacology.* 2016;41(7):1831–1840.

145. Pelloux Y, Everitt BJ, Dickinson A. Compulsive drug seeking by rats under punishment: effects of drug taking history. *Psychopharmacology (Berl).* 2007;194(1):127–137.

146. Petry NM, Heyman GM. Behavioral economics of concurrent ethanol-sucrose and sucrose reinforcement in the rat: effects of altering variable ratio requirements. *J Exper Anal Behav.* 1995;64:331–359.

147. Pettit HO, Ettenberg A, Bloom FE, Koob GF. Destruction of dopamine in the nucleus accumbens selectively attenuates cocaine but not heroin self-administration in rats. *Psychopharmacology.* 1984;84:167–173.

148. Pickens CL, Airavaara M, Theberge F, Fanous S, Hope BT, Shaham Y. Neurobiology of the incubation of drug craving. *Trends Neurosci.* 2011;34(8):411–420.

149. Pfaff DW, Kieffer BL, Swanson LW. Mechanisms for the regulation of state changes in the central nervous system: an introduction. *Ann NY Acad Sci.* 2008;1129:1–7.

150. Phillips AG, Fibiger HC. Dopaminergic and noradrenergic substrates of positive reinforcement: differential effects of d- and l-amphetamine. *Science.* 1973;179(73):575–577.

151. Pierce RC, Kumaresan V. The mesolimbic dopamine system: the final common pathway for the reinforcing effect of drugs of abuse? *Neurosci Biobehav Rev.* 2006;30(2):215–238.

152. Pitkänen A. Connectivity of the rat amygdaloid complex. In: Aggleton JP, ed. *The Amygdala: a Functional Analysis.* Oxford: University Press; 2000:31–115.

153. Radley JJ, Sisti HM, Hao J, Rocher AB, McCall T, Hof PR, McEwen BS, Morrison JH. Chronic behavioral stress induces apical dendritic reorganization in pyramidal neurons of the medial prefrontal cortex. *Neuroscience.* 2004;125:1–6.

154. Rassnick S, Stinus L, Koob GF. The effects of 6-hydroxydopamine lesions of the nucleus accumbens and the mesolimbic dopamine system on oral self-administration of ethanol in the rat. *Brain Res.* 1993;623:16–24.

155. Rescorla RA, Wagner AR. A theory of Pavlovian conditioning: variations in the effectiveness of reinforcement and nonreinforcement. In: Black AH, Prokasy WF, eds. *Classical Conditioning II: Current Research and Theory.* New York: Appleton-Century-Crofts; 1972:64–99.

156. Reynolds JN, Hyland BI, Wickens JR. A cellular mechanism of reward-related learning. *Nature.* 2001;413(6851):67–70.

157. Richardson NR, Roberts DC. Progressive ratio schedules in drug self-administration studies in rats: a method to evaluate reinforcing efficacy. *J Neurosci Methods.* 1996;66(1):1–11.

158. Risinger FO, Malott DH, Prather LK, Niehus DR, Cunningham CL. Motivational properties of ethanol in mice selectively bred for ethanol-induced locomotor differences. *Psychopharmacology (Berl).* 1994;116(2):207–216.

159. Robinson S, Rainwater AJ, Hnasko TS, Palmiter RD. Viral restoration of dopamine signaling to the dorsal striatum restores instrumental conditioning to dopamine-deficient mice. *Psychopharmacology (Berl).* 2007;191(3):567–578.

160. Robinson S, Sandstrom SM, Denenberg VH, Palmiter RD. Distinguishing whether dopamine regulates liking, wanting, and/or learning about rewards. *Behav Neurosci.* 2005;119:5–15.

161. Robinson S, Sotak BN, During MJ, Palmiter RD. Local dopamine production in the dorsal striatum restores goal-directed behavior in dopamine-deficient mice. *Behav Neurosci.* 2006;120(1):196–200.

162. Robinson TE, Berridge KC. Review. The incentive sensitization theory of addiction: some current issues. *Philos Trans R Soc Lond B Biol Sci.* 2008;363(1507):3137–3146.

163. Robinson TE, Kolb B. Structural plasticity associated with exposure to drugs of abuse. *Neuropharmacology.* 2004;47(suppl 1):33–46.

164. Rocha BA, Fumagalli F, Gainetdinov RR, et al. Cocaine self-administration in dopamine-transporter knockout mice. *Nat Neurosci.* 1998;1(2):132–137.

165. Routtenberg A, Kuznesof AW. Self-starvation of rats living in activity wheels on a restricted feeding schedule. *J Comp Physiol Psych.* 1967;64:414–421.

166. Routtenberg A, Lindy J. Effects of the availability of rewarding septal and hypothalamic stimulation on bar pressing for food under conditions of deprivation. *J Comp Physiol Psychol.* 1965;60:158–161.

167. Sah P, Faber ES, Lopez De Armentia M, Power J. The amygdaloid complex: anatomy and physiology. *Physiol Rev.* 2003;83(3):803–834.

168. Salinas JA, Parent MB, McGaugh JL. Ibotenic acid lesions of the amygdala basolateral complex or central nucleus differentially effect the response to reductions in reward. *Brain Res.* 1996;742:283–293.

169. Samson HH, Cunningham CL, Czachowski CL, Chappell A, Legg B, Shannon E. Devaluation of ethanol reinforcement. *Alcohol.* 2004;32(3):203–212.

170. Samson HH, Czachowski CL. Behavioral measures of alcohol self-administration and intake control: rodent models. *Int Rev Neurobiol.* 2003;54:107–143.

171. Samson HH, Tolliver GA, Haraguchi M, Hodge CW. Alcohol self-administration: role of mesolimbic dopamine. *Ann NY Acad Sci.* 1992;654:242–253.

172. Sanchez FP, Dickenson L, George FR. Ethanol self-administration is genetically independent of locomotor stimulation in fast and slow mice. *Alcohol.* 1996;13(1):79–84.

173. Scheyer AF, Wolf ME, Tseng KY. A protein synthesis-dependent mechanism sustaines calcium-permeable AMPA receptor transmission in nucleus accumbens synapses during withdrawal from cocaine self-administration. *J Neurosci.* 2014;34(8):3095–3100.

174. Schulteis G, Markou A, Cole M, Koob GF. Decreased brain reward produced by ethanol withdrawal. *Proc Natl Acad Sci USA.* 1995;92(13):5880–5884.

175. Schultz W. Predictive reward signal of dopamine neurons. *J Neurophysiol.* 1998;80:1–27.

176. Schultz W. Getting formal with dopamine and reward. *Neuron.* 2002;36:241–263.

177. See RE. Neural substrates of cocaine-cue associations that trigger relapse. *Eur J Pharmacol.* 2005;526(1–3):140–146.

178. Sellings LH, McQuade LE, Clarke PB. Evidence for multiple sites within rat ventral striatum mediating cocaine-conditioned place preference and locomotor activation. *J Pharmacol Exp Ther.* 2006;317(3):1178–1187.

179. Shabat-Simon M, Levy D, Amir A, Rehavi M, Zangen A. Dissociation between rewarding and psychomotor effects of opiates: differential roles for glutamate receptors within anterior and posterior portions of the ventral tegmental area. *J Neurosci.* 2008;28:8406–8416.

180. Skinner BF. *The Behavior of Organisms.* New York: Appleton-Century-Crofts; 1938.

181. Skinner BF. Are theories of learning necessary? *Psychol Rev.* 1950;57(4):193–216.

182. Skinner BF. *Science and Human Behavior.* New York: Macmillan; 1953.

183. Slifer BL. Schedule-induction of nicotine self-administration. *Pharmacol Biochem Behav.* 1983;19(6):1005–1009.

184. Smith AD, Bolam JP. The neural network of the basal ganglia as revealed by the study of synaptic connections of identified neurones. *Trends Neurosci.* 1990;13(7):259–265.

185. Smith JB, Klug JR, Howard CD, et al. Genetic-based dissection unveils the inputs and outputs of the striatal patch and matrix compartments. *Neuron.* 2016;91(5):1069–1084.

186. Smith-Roe SL, Kelley AE. Coincident activation of NMDA and dopamine D1 receptors within the nucleus accumbens core is required for appetitive instrumental learning. *J Neurosci.* 2000;20(20):7737–7742.

187. Solomon RL, Corbit JD. An opponent-process theory of motivation: 1 temporal dynamics of affect. *Psychol Rev.* 1974;81:119–145.

188. Sora I, Wichems C, Takahashi N, et al. Cocaine reward models: conditioned place preference can be established in dopamine- and in serotonin-transporter knockout mice. *Proc Natl Acad Sci USA.* 1998;95:7699–7704.

189. Spanagel R. Recent animal models of alcoholism. *Alcohol Res Health.* 2000;24(2):124–131.

190. Stuber GD, Hopf FW, Hahn J, Cho SL, Guillory A, Bonci A. Voluntary ethanol intake enhances excitatory synaptic strength in the ventral tegmental area. *Alcohol Clin Exp Res.* 2008;32(10):1714–1720.

191. Swanson C, Baker D, Carson D, Worley P, Kalivas P. Repeated cocaine administration attenuates group I metabotropic glutamate receptor-mediated glutamate release and behavioral activation: a potential role for Homer 1b/c. *J Neurosci.* 2001;21:9043–9052.

192. Szabo B, Schlicker E. Effects of cannabinoids on neurotransmission. *Handb Exp Pharmacol.* 2005;168:327–365.

193. Szumlinski KK, Ary AW, Lominac KD. Homers regulate drug-induced neuroplasticity: implications for addiction. *Biochem Pharmacol.* 2008;75(1):112–133.

194. Szumlinski KK, Lominac KD, Oleson EB, et al. Homer2 is necessary for EtOH-induced neuroplasticity. *J Neurosci.* 2005;25:7054–7061.

195. Thomas MJ, Beurrier C, Bonci A, Malenka RC. Long-term depression in the nucleus accumbens: a neural correlate of behavioral sensitization to cocaine. *Nat Neurosci.* 2001;4(12):1217–1223.

196. Thorndike CL. Reward and punishment in animal learning. *Comp Psychol Monogr.* 1932;8:29.

197. Todtenkopf MS, Parsegian A, Naydenov A, Neve RL, Konradi C, Carlezon Jr WA. Brain reward regulated by AMPA receptor subunits in nucleus accumbens shell. *J Neurosci.* 2006;26(45):11665–11669.

198. Tzschentke TM. Measuring reward with the conditioned place preference paradigm: a comprehensive review of drug effects, recent progress and new issues. *Prog Neurobiol.* 1998;56:613–672.

199. Ungless MA, Whistler JL, Malenka RC, Bonci A. Single cocaine exposure in vivo induces long-term potentiation in dopamine neurons. *Nature.* 2001;411(6837):583–587.

200. Uwano T, Nishijo H, Ono T, Tamura R. Neuronal responsiveness to various sensory stimuli, and associative learning in the rat amygdala. *Neuroscience.* 1995;68:339–361.

201. Vanderschuren LJ, Everitt BJ. Drug seeking becomes compulsive after prolonged cocaine self-administration. *Science.* 2004;305(5686):1017–1019.

202. Van Dyke C, Byck R. Cocaine. *Sci Am.* 1982;246:128–141.

203. van Rijnsoever C, Täuber M, Choulli MK, et al. Requirement of alpha5-GABAA receptors for the development of tolerance to the sedative action of diazepam in mice. *J Neurosci.* 2004;24(30):6785–6790.

204. Vekovischeva OY, Zamanillo D, Echenko O, et al. Morphine-induced dependence and sensitization are altered in mice deficient in AMPA-type glutamate receptor-A subunits. *J Neurosci.* 2001;21(12):4451–4459.

205. Venniro M, Caprioli D, Shaham Y. Animal models of drug relapse and craving: From drug priming-induced reinstatement to incubation of craving after voluntary abstinence. *Prog Brain Res.* 2016;224:25–52.

206. Walker JR, Ahmed SH, Gracy KN, Koob GF. Microinjections of an opiate receptor antagonist into the bed nucleus of the stria terminalis suppress heroin self-administration in dependent rats. *Brain Res.* 2000;854(1–2):85–92.

207. Wang L, Liu J, Harvey-White J, Zimmer A, Kunos G. Endocannabinoid signaling via cannabinoid receptor 1 is involved in ethanol preference and its age-dependent decline in mice. *Proc Natl Acad Sci USA.* 2003;100(3):1393–1398.

208. Weibel SL, Wolf HH. Opiate modification of intracranial self-stimulation in the rat. *Pharmacol Biochem Behav.* 1979;101:71–78.

209. West TE, Wise RA. Effects of naltrexone on nucleus accumbens, lateral hypothalamic and ventral tegmental self-stimulation rate-frequency functions. *Brain Res.* 1988;462(1):126–133.

210. White NM. Reward or reinforcement: what's the difference? *Neurosci Biobehav Rev.* 1989;13(2–3):181–186.

211. Wickens JR, Horvitz JC, Costa RM, Killcross S. Dopaminergic mechanisms in actions and habits. *J Neurosci.* 2007;27(31):8181–8183.

212. Wilcox MV, Cuzon Carlson VC, Sherazee N, et al. Repeated binge-like ethanol drinking alters ethanol drinking patterns and depresses striatal GABAergic transmission. *Neuropsychopharmacology.* 2014;39(3):579–594.

213. Wingfield JC. Anniversary essay: control of behavioural strategies for capricious environments. *Anim Behav.* 2003;66:807–816.

214. Wise RA. Catecholamine theories of reward: a critical review. *Brain Res.* 1978;152(2):215–247.

215. Wise RA. Addictive drugs and brain stimulation reward. *Annu Rev Neurosci.* 1996;19:319–340.

216. Wise RA, Bozarth MA. A psychomotor stimulant theory of addiction. *Psychol Rev.* 1987;94(4):469–492.

217. Wolffgramm J, Heyne A. From controlled drug intake to loss of control: the irreversible development of drug addiction in the rat. *Behav Brain Res.* 1995;70:77–94.

218. Xia JX, Li J, Zhou R, Zhang XH, Ge YB, RuYuan X. Alterations of rat corticostriatal synaptic plasticity after chronic ethanol exposure and withdrawal. *Alcohol Clin Exp Res.* 2006;30(5):819–824.

219. Yin HH, Knowlton B. The role of the basal ganglia in habit formation. *Nat Rev Neurosci.* 2006;7(6):464–476.

220. Yin HH, Ostlund SB, Balleine BW. Reward-guided learning beyond dopamine in the nucleus accumbens: the integrative functions of cortico-basal ganglia networks. *Eur J Neurosci.* 2008;28(8):1437–1448.

221. Zhou Z, Karlsson C, Liang T, et al. Loss of metabotropic glutamate receptor 2 escalates alcohol consumption. *Proc Natl Acad Sci USA.* 2013;110(42):16963–16968.

222. Zielinski K. Jerzy Konorski on brain associations. *Acta Neurobiol Exp (Wars).* 2006;66(1):75–84.

17

Neurobehavioral Toxicology of Substances of Abuse

MARTIN A. JAVORS, THOMAS S. KING, BRETT C. GINSBURG, GREGORY T. COLLINS, AND LISA R. GERAK

CHAPTER OUTLINE

Ethanol (Alcohol)

History

Ethanol is surely the oldest known substance of abuse. The details of the original discovery of fermented beverages have been lost to time because of the unavailability of the written word. Thus no one really knows exactly when humans started drinking fermented beverages. Animals such as birds, insects, and elephants have shown signs of drunkenness by purposefully eating ripened fruit in which yeast produced ethanol.[97] It is known that intentionally fermented beverages existed as early as 10,000 BCE.[226] Aristotle, the founding father of the scientific method, showed in the 3rd century BCE that boiled wine lost its intoxicating character, but he never took the next step of condensing the ethanol.[97] The distillation of ethanol from wine was discovered by a Muslim chemist in the 8th century. There are a myriad of accounts of the incorporation of alcoholic beverages into the daily life of every society. As with all substances of abuse, ethanol was probably not used abusively at first. For example, early versions of beer were used as food. Alcoholic beverages such as beer and wine were used in ritualistic religious exercises, and evidence of the use of beer and wine as medicinal remedies exist from at least 2000 BCE.

A recently published book describes in detail the cultural history of alcohol.[97] The use of alcoholic beverages in most societies is certainly evident. It has produced social and health benefits as well as significant detrimental forensic and health problems. For example, light to moderate alcohol intake may be associated with lower risk of cardiovascular mortality in hypertensive men.[183,198] On the other hand, excessive ethanol consumption is closely associated with abnormal elevation of blood pressure in normotensive and hypertensive individuals.[198] Despite its social and possible health benefits, excessive ethanol consumption is a major medical health problem. In 1995, it was reported that about 10 million Americans were considered to be alcoholic.[9]

Chemical Properties

Ethanol is a relatively simple molecule (C_2H_6O) with a molecular weight of 46 and density of 0.789 g/cm^3. At ambient temperatures, it is a clear, colorless liquid that is highly volatile, flammable, and miscible with water and many other organic solvents. Its lipid-to-water partition coefficient is 0.096, so the distribution of ethanol favors an aqueous versus a lipid phase.[217] In humans, this solubility ratio explains the distribution of ethanol in total body water.

Ethanol concentration is expressed in a variety of ways depending on the area of application. For example, a blood alcohol concentration of 0.1% (w/v) is the upper limit of the legal range while driving a car in many states. This concentration can also be expressed as 100 mg%, 100 mg/dL, 1 g/L, and 21.7 mM. The concentration of ethanol in commercially available forms of consumable, distilled alcoholic beverages is expressed in terms of proof, which is a number that is approximately double the percentage of ethanol (200 proof = 100% ethanol). Of interest, the term "proof" was used in the 19th century by English sailors who developed a test for the minimal concentration of ethanol in rum. If the sailor could successfully ignite gun powder soaked in the rum, it was proof that the rum was acceptably potent and had not been diluted with water. At least 50% (v/v) of ethanol is necessary to ignite gun powder. This simple test was important because the sailors were given rum as part of their pay.

Pharmacokinetics

Routes of Administration

Alcohol is one of the drugs of abuse that can be legally purchased, with age as the only restriction. Humans self-administer ethanol by the oral route exclusively. There are many forms of commercially available alcoholic beverages with widely varying percentages by volume, including beer (~5%), malt liquor (~7%), wine (~12%), sherry or port (~17%), cordials or liqueur (~24%), brandy (~40%), and distilled spirits (~40%–50%).

Absorption and Distribution

After oral administration, ethanol is rapidly absorbed into the blood principally from the small intestine, but also from the stomach and colon.[55,90,14] It is known that food, ethanol concentration, and liquid volume affect the gastric emptying rate and gastric absorption of ethanol, but once ethanol reaches the small intestine, its absorption is rapid and complete.[147,310] For example, when a nonintoxicating dose of ethanol (~0.5 g/kg) is ingested over a relatively short period of time (~30 minutes) on an empty stomach, ethanol reaches its maximal concentration in the blood within 15–30 minutes.[17] In fact, intravenous administration of ethanol combined with quantification of either breath or blood ethanol concentration has been used to estimate total body water.[217]

Metabolism

The metabolism of ethanol occurs mainly in the liver by oxidation of ethanol to acetaldehyde by alcohol dehydrogenase and conversion of nicotinamide adenine dinucleotide to nicotinamide adenine dinucleotide hydrate. A secondary pathway of oxidative ethanol metabolism occurs in liver microsomal tissue in the smooth endoplasmic reticulum.[172] Chronic consumption of ethanol increases the capacity of the liver microsomal ethanol oxidizing system, with an increase in several cytochrome P450s (CYPs), especially a nicotinamide adenine dinucleotide phosphate-requiring enzyme (CYP2E1). This system provides a higher rate of ethanol oxidation and is important to the development of tolerance to alcohol.[172] Both of these mechanisms produce acetaldehyde, which is then converted to acetate by the action of aldehyde dehydrogenase.

Elimination/Excretion

The disappearance of ethanol from the blood or breath was originally thought to be a linear, zero order function, that is, independent of the blood ethanol concentration and probably due to saturation of alcohol dehydrogenase.[191] However, it has been shown more recently that the elimination profile is more accurately described by Michaelis-Menten kinetics.[309] Nevertheless, at higher doses of ethanol, there is an apparent linear phase (15 mg%/hour) that starts at the completion of the absorption-distribution phases and extends to a blood ethanol concentration of about 20 mg%. Below this concentration, the elimination becomes curvilinear. The elimination half-life of ethanol is about 2–4 hours. Between 90% and 95% of ingested ethanol is converted to acetaldehyde and acetate and then eliminated in the urine. About 3%–5% of a dose of ethanol is eliminated unchanged in the urine, breath, or through the skin.[309] Less than 2% of ethanol is metabolized nonoxidatively to ethyl glucuronide, ethyl sulfate, phosphatidyl ethanol, and fatty acid methyl esters. Of interest, these direct metabolites of ethanol are measurable as markers for ethanol consumption.

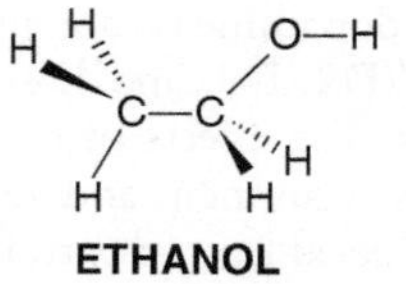

• **Fig. 17.1** Structure of ethanol.

Pharmacodynamics

The small size and simplicity of ethanol's structure (Fig. 17.1) is in contrast to its significant and complicated pharmacodynamic effects. When compared with most other drugs, very high concentrations of ethanol, in the millimolar range, are required to produce biological effects. Because of its simple chemical structure and the concentrations required for physiological effects, ethanol binding sites with high affinity (μM or nM range) most likely do not exist. It has been proposed that an ethanol binding site exists on γ-aminobutyric acid A ($GABA_A$) receptors that contain a combination of $\alpha 4$ (or $\alpha 6$), $\beta 3$, and δ subunits, making them sensitive to concentrations of ethanol as low as 3 mM.[114,301] Furthermore, relatively recent reports indicate that a certain domain of the enzyme adenylyl cyclase is responsible for sensitivity to ethanol.[114] Amino acid mutations of target proteins designed to modify ethanol's effects have suggested that specific groups of amino acid residues in transmembrane regions of proteins may be binding sites for ethanol.[196] The results of these relatively recent studies suggest that ethanol situates itself into tiny pockets in protein structures to produce significant changes in biochemical, physiological, and behavioral functions (see Fig. 17.1)

Neuropharmacological Effects

The neuropharmacological effects of ethanol have been identified and measured at biological levels from the molecular to the behavioral.

At the cellular/molecular level, it has been shown that acute, physiologically relevant concentrations of ethanol (5–50 mM) affect the function of numerous different receptor types.[292] Ethanol inhibits N-methyl-D-aspartate (NMDA) receptors[126,178] and L-type Ca^{2+} channels[302] and enhances the function of $GABA_A$ receptors,[8,63a] glycine receptors,[196] serotonin-3 receptors,[177] and neuronal nicotinic acetylcholine receptors.[6,209]

Effects of ethanol on the aforementioned receptor systems (e.g., a neurotransmitter receptor or ion channel) can often be demonstrated using electrophysiological techniques, thereby showing effects on neurons or neuronal systems. If ethanol affects the rate of neuronal firing, membrane potential, or other cellular parameters, the effects of ethanol on receptor systems and perhaps specific brain areas can sometimes be linked to certain behaviors.[64] Electrophysiological studies have shown that ethanol affects the firing rate of neurons in several brain areas, including the cerebellum, inferior olivary nucleus, locus coeruleus, ventral tegmental area, substantia nigra, hippocampus, and septal area.[64] Furthermore, these effects of ethanol on single cells are thought to modify neurotransmission in the mammalian central nervous system, especially in the hippocampus, locus coeruleus, cerebellum, spinal cord, and cortex via pre- and postsynaptic effects.[64]

From a behavioral perspective, acute low doses of ethanol are anxiolytic and can enhance mood and produce euphoric feelings in humans. In fact, the use of ethanol as a disinhibitor in social settings is well known and widespread throughout recorded history.[97] For individuals who have the ability to limit ethanol intake,

there appear to be social and health benefits. On the other hand, higher acute doses cause intoxication, sedation, sleep, and hangover, and very high acute doses can induce coma and possibly death as a result of respiratory depression. Studies with laboratory rodents showed effects of ethanol to produce hypothermia, analgesia, motor activation, and, at higher doses, motor incoordination. Chronic, heavy alcohol consumption produces a myriad of problems as discussed later in this chapter.

The behavioral consequences of acutely administered, lower doses (<30 mM) of ethanol may be linked to certain receptor systems. For example, intoxication, sedation, and motor incoordination are probably mediated via certain subunit configurations of the $GABA_A$ receptor.[64,301] In addition, there is thought to be differential sensitivity among presynaptic, postsynaptic, and extrasynaptic $GABA_A$ receptors, with the extrasynaptic types being the most sensitive.[82] Ethanol-induced hypothermia and analgesia are not thought to be mediated by $GABA_A$ receptors, but by inwardly rectifying G protein–gated K^+ channels.[20,136,156] The concentration of ethanol required to affect other receptors is very high (>50 mM), so the involvement of these receptors at physiological concentrations is not clear.

A discussion of the neuropharmacology of ethanol would not be complete without comments about acetaldehyde. Acetaldehyde is the first metabolic product of ethanol in vivo and is produced by the action of alcohol dehydrogenase. Acetaldehyde may be responsible for some of the effects of ethanol, probably mostly the unpleasant and chronic side effects.[64,301] The mechanism whereby these effects of acetaldehyde occur may be due to aldehyde-amine condensation products of amino acid side chains on proteins.[64] Humans who carry a certain inactive form of mitochondrial aldehyde dehydrogenase do not metabolize acetaldehyde and have an uncomfortable facial flushing reaction after drinking alcohol.[200] In addition, the hangover that occurs after a bout of heavy drinking is probably caused by high concentrations of acetaldehyde.[301]

Toxicology

Whether ethanol produces an acute, satisfying, possibly beneficial effect versus an acute or chronic, unhealthy toxic effect is related to the concentration of ethanol, the dose of ethanol, and the length of exposure to ethanol. From a medical perspective, ethanol consumption of less than two standard drinks per day (≤ ~30 g) by humans appears to decrease mortality[13] and the mechanism is probably related to a reduction of coronary heart disease.[56] Thus low or moderate levels of ethanol consumption are thought to be healthful. On the other hand, chronic heavy ethanol consumption of five standard drinks per day (~75 g) or more for men and four standard drinks per day (~60 g) or more for women, or frequent binging, can cause severe, detrimental health problems.[171] These health problems result from direct toxic effects of ethanol on the liver, heart, brain, kidneys, and stomach. Indirectly, the replacement of calories from food by calories from ethanol (malnutrition) can cause additional negative effects on these organ systems.[171] These serious effects of ethanol abuse can eventually result in alcoholism, a pathology that includes very serious medical and behavioral difficulties.

Cocaine

History

Cocaine is a derivative of the coca plant *Erythroxylon coca*, which is native to the mountains of South America. Traditionally, South

American natives have chewed coca leaves as a stimulant to fend off fatigue, especially at relatively hypoxic elevations of the Andes Mountains. In 1574, the Spanish physician Nicolas Bautista Alfaro (1493–1588) published a description of the plant, its use, and its effects.[38] In 1862, the German chemist Albert Neiman (Gottingen, Germany, 1834–1861) isolated the active component of the coca plant and called it cocaine. He was also the first to report the local anesthetic properties of cocaine, noting its numbing effects on his own tongue. In 1880, pharmacologist Basil Von Anrep of the University of Leipzig proposed use of cocaine as a surgical anesthetic in humans.[298] Canadian surgeon William S. Halsted became the first physician to use cocaine for a nerve block during surgery and subsequently became the first known physician to develop a cocaine addiction. In 1884, psychiatrist Sigmund Freud published a cocaine monograph entitled *Uber Coca* in which he advocated for the use of cocaine to treat a variety of conditions including asthma, wasting diseases, and syphilis.[92] Freud also eventually became addicted to cocaine. In the late 1800s, cocaine was added to a number of beverages including the "medicinal" wine Vin Mariani in France. In 1895, *The Lancet* published a report of six cocaine-associated deaths, underscoring the significant potential toxicity of this drug. Cocaine was an ingredient in the original version of John Pemberton's Coca Cola; cocaine was removed from the popular soft drink in 1906. With passage of the Harrison Narcotics Tax Act in 1914, nonprescription use of cocaine was made illegal. In 1970 cocaine was classified as a Schedule II drug (Comprehensive Drug Abuse Prevention and Control Act).

Pharmacodynamics

Cocaine is a tropane (aminoester) alkaloid with a pK_a of 8.6. Crack cocaine (free-base) is produced by combining cocaine HCl with an alkali. Crack cocaine is more heat-stable than is cocaine HCl and therefore can be smoked.[77]

Cocaine interacts primarily with these central nervous system biogenic amine systems. Cocaine blocks the in vitro reuptake of norepinephrine, dopamine, and serotonin.[139] Saturable, high-affinity Na^+-independent and Na^+-dependent [^3H]-cocaine binding has been associated with sites for serotonin and for dopamine reuptake, respectively, in the central nervous system.[238] With acute or low-dose administration of cocaine, this reuptake inhibition leads to increased aminergic concentrations within aminergic synapses and increased binding both to pre- and postsynaptic aminergic receptors. Chronic cocaine administration is generally believed to result in aminergic depletion for the duration of drug exposure.[139] However, unlike high doses of methamphetamine,[135] chronic cocaine does not produce dopamine nerve terminal degeneration, at least in the prefrontal and frontal cortex or dorsal raphe.[60]

Various addictive drugs such as cocaine that act as positive reinforcers increase synaptic dopaminergic concentrations in selected areas such as the nucleus accumbens. Homologous recombination targeting the dopamine transporter results in an absence of cocaine- or amphetamine-induced behavioral activation.[106] The ventral tegmental area, nucleus accumbens, and caudate nucleus, areas rich in the neurotransmitter dopamine, are collectively considered the reward pathway.[159,160] Cocaine antagonism of presynaptic dopamine transport results in elevated dopamine levels in mesolimbic synapses with resultant drug reinforcement. Maintenance of higher dopamine levels in reward pathway synapses leads to feelings of euphoria and a cocaine high. The increased

availability of synaptic dopamine is thought to act on D1-like (D1 and D5) and D2-like (D2, D3, and D4) receptors in the mesocorticolimbic synapses. The effects of cocaine acting on the D1 receptor in the nucleus accumbens and ventral tegmental area are thought to be responsible, at least in part, for the reinforcing properties associated with long-term exposure to this drug.[266]

Long-term cocaine use is associated with a selective decrease in D1 receptors in striatal reward areas both in rodents[35,36,39] and in nonhuman primates.[204] Dopamine depletion using the neurotoxin 6-hydroxydopamine infused into either the nucleus accumbens or the ventral tegmental area results in an attenuation of the reinforcing effects of cocaine self-administration. Similarly, dopamine D1 receptor knockout mice have demonstrated a lack of reinforcing effect of cocaine in contrast to wild-type controls.[37] D1 and D2 receptors have opposing intracellular and behavioral effects and thus may differentially affect drug-reinforcing behaviors. David Self and colleagues[266] demonstrated that cocaine self-administration behavior was mediated by dopamine D1 and not by dopamine D2 receptors and that this behavior progressively diminished in rats when cocaine was replaced with saline (extinction behavior).

Cocaine also blocks voltage-gated sodium channels and thus reversibly attenuates conduction of nerve impulses, which accounts for the local anesthetic properties of the drug.[238] Depending on the relative distribution of the drug, a relatively selective depression of inhibitory neurons can produce cerebral excitation at lower concentrations of the drug, and this in turn can lead to generalized convulsions. At high concentrations, cocaine could produce more profound depression of brain function and ultimately coma, cardiorespiratory arrest, and death.

Pharmacokinetics

Distribution

Cocaine is rapidly absorbed across nasal, tracheal, and laryngeal epithelial membranes within minutes of its administration. Peak plasma concentrations of 120–474 ng/mL are reached within 30–60 minutes of intranasal administration and remain detectable up to 6 hours after administration.[16,288] Cocaine may limit its own absorption due to its activity as a potent vasoconstrictor.[309] Bioavailability of intranasal cocaine (i.e., area under the plasma concentration-time curve) is approximately 5 times less than that for equivalent intravenous dosing (0.19–2.0 mg/kg). The biological half-life for cocaine is 0.5–1.5 hours with a volume of distribution of 2.0 L/kg and a systemic clearance of 2.0 L/minutes.[139]

Metabolism/Elimination

Cocaine metabolism is catalyzed by esterase activity, principally within plasma and liver. Liver esterase activity accounts for 30%–50% of the metabolism of cocaine to ecgonine methyl ester. Another 30%–40% of cocaine is nonenzymatically hydrolyzed into benzoylecgonine (Fig. 17.2). The elimination half-lives of these major metabolites of cocaine are 6 and 4 hours, respectively. These metabolites can be detected in urine samples up to 60 hours after cocaine administration. A small amount (1%–5%) of cocaine is excreted unchanged in urine within 8 hours of administration.[139] Individuals with liver dysfunction or malnutrition, or who are being treated with plasmapheresis, who are pregnant, or who have taken anticholinesterase medication (e.g., echothiophate eye drops, neostigmine) are relatively esterase-deficient, resulting in reduced capacity to degrade cocaine and thus elevated circulating levels of the drug with the potential for increased toxicity (see Fig. 17.2).

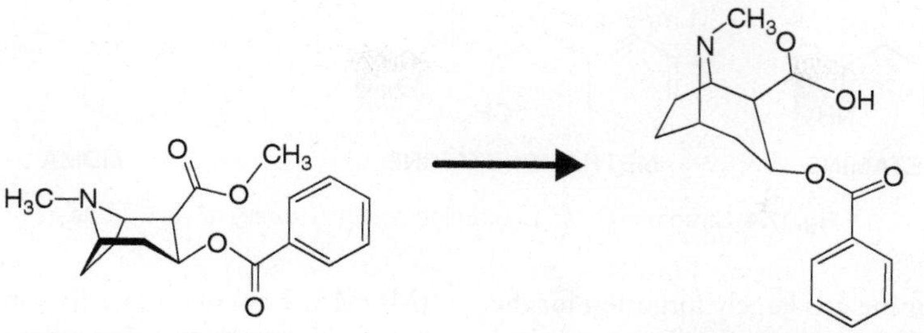

• **Fig. 17.2** Structures of cocaine and its metabolite benzoylecgonine.

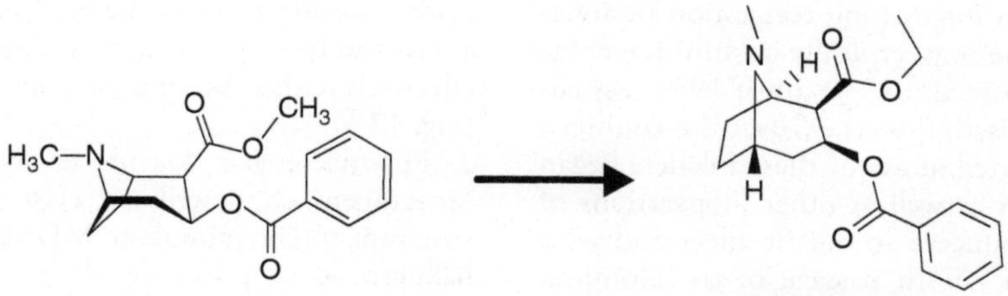

• **Fig. 17.3** Structures of cocaine and cocaethylene.

Cocaine metabolism demonstrates first-order kinetics over a wide range of doses. Within 4–5 hours, almost all of a dose of cocaine has been metabolized, with metabolites present in urine for 4–8 hours following intranasal dosing.[139] Measurable levels of the metabolite benzoylecgonine may be detected in urine as long up to 60 hours after a single dose of cocaine and for up to 3 weeks after heavy use of cocaine.

Less than 10% of cocaine is *N*-methylated into the active metabolite norcocaine. Liver *N*-methylation activity is increased by progesterone. *N*-methylation of cocaine into norcocaine is thus enhanced under conditions of elevated progesterone, for example, during pregnancy. This may account for the reported increased cocaine-associated cardiotoxicity during pregnancy.

Concurrent use of cocaine and alcohol results in the production of the active metabolite cocaethylene (ethylbenzoylecgonine) (Fig. 17.3).[268] Cocaethylene has a significantly longer elimination half-life than cocaine and may be more cardiotoxic than cocaine[247] (see Fig. 17.3).

Toxicology

Cocaine-induced antagonism of nigrostriatal dopamine activity may result in extrapyramidal motor dysfunction including bradykinesia, akinesia, akathisia, catalepsy and dystonic reactions.[91] In a study conducted between 1979 and 1990 by the medical examiner's office for Dade County, Florida, excited delirium was associated with approximately one in every six cocaine-related deaths. These victims were described as having experienced an immediate onset of bizarre and sometimes violent behavior, including extreme paranoia, ending in cardiorespiratory collapse and death.

In addition, cocaine abuse is associated with both acute and long-term cardiotoxicity.[245,284] Acutely, cocaine acts as a vasoconstrictor, reducing blood flow to myocardium with an increased risk for cardiac ischemia and infarction. Cocaine-inhibited reuptake of norepinephrine also leads to increased intracellular concentrations of calcium within cardiocytes, which through membrane depolarization can trigger sustained action potentials, extrasystolic

contractions, and tachycardia. Long-term effects of cocaine on cardiac function can include a depression in contractility, in part related to the activity of cocaine as a local anesthetic. Cardiomyopathy associated with long-term cocaine abuse may be a result of oxidative stress to the myocardium.[137] Systemic effects include peripheral vascular constriction with resultant ischemic compromise of various organs.

Long-term use of cocaine is also associated with elevated circulating levels of muscle enzymes such as creatine kinase, suggesting muscle degradation or rhabdomyolysis.[248] Thirty-three percent of the participants in a study of cocaine-induced rhabdomyolysis experienced acute renal failure, severe liver dysfunction, and disseminated intravascular coagulation; six of them died.

Cocaine has been shown repeatedly to adversely affect reproductive function in female rats,[83,84] male and female nonhuman primates,[192] and male[47] and female[27] humans. In the rat, cocaine administration produces loss of estrous cyclicity, which at higher doses of cocaine may become permanent.[152] Maternal cocaine use during gestation has also been associated with numerous adverse effects on the developing fetus, including growth retardation, dysmorphic features, seizures and strokes, and numerous postnatal behavioral abnormalities.[297] Because such fetuses are typically exposed to various confounding variables, such as a lack of prenatal care, poor maternal nutrition, and polydrug exposures, the idea of a specific cocaine teratophilia (or "cocaine baby") syndrome has been called into question.[158]

Amphetamine and Amphetamine-Analogs

History

The Chinese plant ma hung (*Ephedra vulgaris*) has been used traditionally to treat asthma. In the 1920s the active ingredient in extracts of this plant was identified as ephedrine. In 1887, the Romanian chemist Lazar Edeleanu (1861–1941) first synthesized alpha-methylphenethylamine,[76] now more commonly known as amphetamine (**alpha-methylphenethylamine**). Originally named

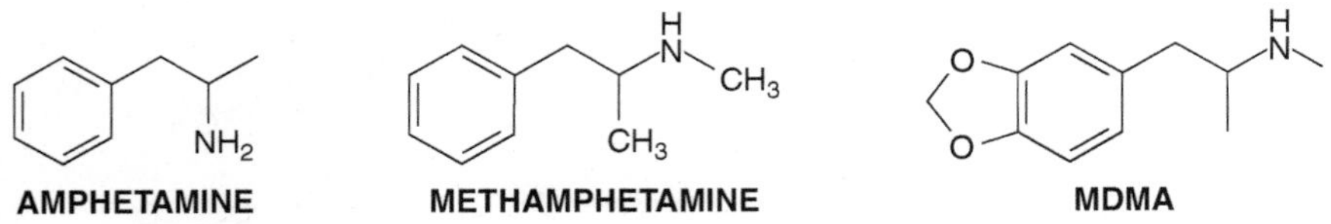

• **Fig. 17.4** Structures of amphetamine and structurally related drugs.

phenylisopropylamine, amphetamine was largely forgotten for the next four decades. In the late 1930s, amphetamine was prescribed for narcolepsy as well as hyperactivity syndromes. In 1932, the pharmaceutical company Smith, Kline & French marketed the racemic amphetamine (*dl*-amphetamine) mixture Benzedrine as an over-the-counter medication for treating congestion by inhalation of the drug. Benzedrine was typically administered via inhalers. From its introduction in the 1930s until 1954, ephedrine was available without prescription (i.e., over-the-counter). By the 1940s and 1950s, reported abuse of these inhalers began to emerge. Benzedrine inhalers as well as other preparations of the drug could be used to produce a stimulant effect and were sometimes abused as "bennies." With passage of the Comprehensive Drug Abuse Prevention and Control Act in 1970, methamphetamine and amphetamine became classified as Schedule II and III drugs, respectively. The following year, the classification of amphetamine was changed to Schedule II.

The term "amphetamines" also refers to a class of drugs derived from amphetamine, the substituted amphetamines. In recent years, the easily synthesized *N*-methylated form of amphetamine, methamphetamine (METH), has become readily available and one of the most commonly abused stimulants in the United States. But METH is not a recent addition to the list of amphetamine-related drugs. In 1885, the Japanese physician-chemist Nagayoshi Nagai (1844–1929) isolated ephedrine from the plant *E. vulgaris* and, in 1893, synthesized METH by reduction of ephedrine using red phosphorus and iodine.[174] In 1929, he was the first to synthesize and elucidate the structure of ephedrine. In 1919, the Japanese chemist Akira Ogata (1887–1978) synthesized crystallized METH. In the 1980s, METH became increasingly more popular as a street drug. In 1996, the Methamphetamine Control Act was enacted, to regulate the key ingredients (e.g., ephedrine, pseudoephedrine, phenylpropanolamine), in manufacturing METH and increasing criminal penalties for possession, distribution, and manufacturing of the drug. The price of methamphetamine is largely determined by the availability of ephedrine, a key ingredient. Regulation of ephedrine, and its resulting unavailability, has increased its wholesale price. As a result, drug traffickers have switched to a less regulated and more economical substitute, pseudoephedrine. However, the Combat Methamphetamine Epidemic Act of 2005, a part of HR 3199, was enacted regulating over-the-counter sales of cold medicines containing pseudoephedrine. Methamphetamine can be smoked, snorted, or injected and has significantly longer-lasting stimulant effects than cocaine and is generally much less expensive to purchase than cocaine.[193] Methamphetamine is considered highly addictive. Methamphetamine users typically develop tolerance to the drug that leads to higher and more frequent use.

Amphetamine is a homologue of phenethylamine and a weak base with a chemical structure very similar to that of dopamine and norepinephrine. Amphetamine is the parent compound for a class of similar psychoactive drugs including the *N*-methylated form of amphetamine, methamphetamine, and the methylenedioxy analog of methamphetamine, 3,4-methylenedioxy-*N*-methylamphetamine

(MDMA; Ecstasy). Typically formulated as a racemic mixture (*d*- and *l*-amphetamine), *d*-amphetamine is thought to act primarily on the dopaminergic systems, whereas *l*-amphetamine is comparatively norepinephrinergic (noradrenergic). Amphetamine and related drugs are lipid-soluble in nonionized form and as such are readily absorbed across the gastrointestinal tract lining as well as across the blood-brain barrier. Amphetamines can thus be taken effectively either by oral or parenteral routes of administration (Fig. 17.4).

Pharmacologist David E. Nichols formulated the term "enactogen" to describe a class of synthetic drugs similar in structure to the stimulant MDMA (Ecstasy) but which exhibit hallucinogenic properties.[214,215] The term "entactogen" is a combination of the roots "en" (Greek: *within*), "tactus" (Latin: *touch*), and "gen" (Greek: *produce*).[215] Enactogens are characterized by a substituted amphetamine core thus belonging to the phenethylamine class of psychoactive drugs. Enactogens include 3,4-methylenedioxyamphetamine (MDA or tenamfetamine), 4-methylenedioxy-*N*-ethylamphetamine, (MDEA), 3,4-methylenedioxy-alpha-ethyl-*N*-methylphenethylamine (MBDB; EDEN or Methyl-J), α-ethyltryptamine (etryptamine, α-ethyltryptamine, α-ET, or AET), and 4-bromo-2,5-dimethyphenethylamine (2C-B). MDMA is also often considered a member of the entactogen family.

4-Bromo-2,5-dimethyphenethylamine, or 2C-B, was first synthesized from 2,5-dimethoxybenzaldehyde by the Russian-American pharmacologist Alexander Shulgin in 1974. In the late 1970s, the German pharmaceutical company Drittewelle began manufacturing and marketing the drug as an aphrodisiac called Eros. Shortly after its introduction to clinical psychiatry, 2C-B made its way into the recreational drug scene. 2C-B remains popular within the rave subculture but is often confused with MDMA (Ecstasy). 2C-B and related entactogens are now classified as Schedule I drugs in the United States.

Based on the known mechanisms of action of MDMA, entactogens are thought to act by increasing synaptic levels of dopamine (DA), norepinephrine (NE), and serotonin (5-HT). However, there have been very few research studies to examine the pharmacology of entactogens in humans or experimental animal models.

Mechanism of Action

Amphetamines are CNS and sympathetic nervous system stimulants, acting on biogenic amine pathways.[193] Physical effects include reduced appetite, hyperactivity, restlessness and insomnia, tachycardia, and increased blood pressure and constipation. Behavioral effects include anxiety and generalized excitability, a perception of increased energy, repetitive actions, increased alertness, emotional lability and, with higher or long-term dosing, occasional psychosis. These effects are similar to those of other stimulates such as cocaine. The amount of releasable as well as previously released DA at dopaminergic nerve terminals is closely regulated by two selective membrane-bound transporters.[146,203,243,249] DA is moved via vesicular monoamine transporter-2 (VMAT-2) into synaptic vesicles for storage and eventual release. Without vesicular transport, DA remains within the cytoplasm where it is subject to degradation including oxidation and presynapse via the DA transporter (DAT). DAT inhibition or blockade results in increased levels of extracellular DA. Amphetamines induce presynaptic DA release, block DA reuptake, inhibit DA storage within presynaptic vesicles, and block enzyme-catalyzed DA metabolism. Shortly after amphetamine administration, reversal of the DAT results in nonvesicular DA efflux.[161,281] In addition, the movement of DA into synaptic vesicles is blocked by amphetamine, resulting in increased DA release into the synapse and the potential for DA oxidation and damaging free radical formation within the presynapse. Although also acting through similar mechanisms on NE and, to a lesser extent, 5HT terminals, amphetamine's reinforcing and behavioral-stimulant effects are associated with enhanced dopaminergic activity, primarily within the mesolimbic DA system.[65,203] The targeted effects of amphetamine on dopaminergic activity in caudate nucleus, nucleus accumbens, and ventral striatum correlate well with stereotypic onset of euphoria associated with this drug.[73,145] Amphetamine also acts to increase glutamate release in selected brain areas such as the nucleus accumbens, striatum, and prefrontal cortex.[65] These areas are implicated in reward pathways.

In similar fashion to the DA transporter (DAT), amphetamine can also induce reverse the direction of serotonin movement via the serotonin transporter (SERT).[282] Amphetamine interacts with the serotoninergic system in selected brain regions such as the mesocorticolimbic pathway.[123] Similar to amphetamine, methamphetamine induces release of 5HT, DA, and NE as well as blockade of 5HT, DA, and NE transporters within the CNS, leading to increased synaptic activities of these biogenic amines.

Formation of free radicals including oxygen and nitrogen species (ROS and RNS, respectively) is particularly characteristic of methamphetamine administration.[105,165,320] An amphetamine analog, methamphetamine, induces selective degeneration of DA neuron terminals without cell body loss. Methamphetamine-induced terminal degeneration may be mediated in part by excitatory amino acid (e.g., glutamate) activity.[59] Methamphetamine also induces rapid and reversible decreases in the rate-limiting enzyme for serotonin (5-hydroxytrypamine, 5-HT) synthesis, leading to reduced levels of this biogenic amine within various CNS areas.[14,130,228]

Amphetamine, MDMA, and other psychotropic agents may also interact with a relatively new class of receptors called the trace amine-associated receptors (TAARs).[24] TAARs represent a class of G protein–coupled binding sites for endogenous trace amines, metabolic products of the better-known biogenic amines such as NE, DA, 5HT, and histamine. Trace amines are normally present in very low (nanomolar) concentrations and include tyramine, octopamine, tryptamine and β-phenylethylamine. Trace amines such as β-phenylethylamine may function to modulate biogenic amine synaptic activities in select brain areas related to affective states and thus in maintaining levels of excitement and alertness.[281] Branchek and Blackburn[28] have hypothesized a role for trace amines in substance abuse, depression, attention-deficit/hyperactivity disorder, eating disorders, schizophrenia, and other neuropsychiatric diseases.

Pharmacokinetics

Metabolism and Elimination

Metabolism of amphetamine is almost exclusively hepatic. In the liver, amphetamine can be hydroxylated (phenyl ring), deaminated, or conjugated.[311] Methamphetamine is N-demethylated. In a study of human subjects given measured doses of amphetamine orally, 34% of the drug was excreted unchanged in urine.[227] Metabolites of the drug included benzoic acid and parahydroxy-amphetamine. These metabolites were themselves further converted into hippuric acid and parahydroxyephedrine, respectively.

Toxicology

The toxic effects of amphetamine and related drugs can be dangerous and potentially fatal.[66] Short-term effects of amphetamine include increased heart rate and blood pressure, decreased appetite, feelings of elation and self-assuredness, and reduced fatigue. Long-term, repetitive amphetamine use has been associated with insomnia and restlessness, significant weight loss, hallucinations, and paranoid psychosis. Amphetamine use can also include psychic dependence and tolerance as well as psychotic episodes in some individuals.[54] Continuous high-dose amphetamine use has been associated with a state of paranoid (amphetamine) psychosis closely resembling the symptoms of paranoid schizophrenia. Symptoms include hyperactivity, anxiety, paranoid delusions, and auditory-tactile hallucinations in a setting of clear consciousness with little if any disorientation.

Use of amphetamines and related stimulants is particularly dangerous in patients with a history of heart disease or underlying hypertension as well as patients with glaucoma.[66] Amphetamines and stimulants should also be avoided by anorexic individuals because of the appetite- suppressing properties of these drugs. In addition, amphetamines can cause life-threatening hypertensive crisis and possibly neurotoxic reactions when taken with monoamine oxidase (MAO) inhibitors for clinical depression. Amphetamine-associated death is considered to be a direct consequence of excessive sympathomimetic activity. Amphetamine toxicity includes hypertension, hyperpyrexia, delirium, convulsions, and severe tachycardia leading to cardiovascular collapse. Amphetamine also increases sympathetic tone, regulating smooth muscle contraction and thus can affect adversely the functions of the gastrointestinal tract, uterus, urinary bladder, and other organs dependent on smooth muscle activity.

MDMA has been associated with serotoninergic depletion and neuronal degeneration in rodent and nonhuman primate models.[118,239,240,273] These neurotoxic effects were more pronounced in nonhuman primates than in rodents.[273] Within 3 weeks of MDMA administration, profound serotoninergic neurodegeneration was seen in nonhuman primates in most brain areas.[241] Some CNS areas showed evidence of partial recovery, that is, hippocampus, caudate nucleus, and frontal cortex. However, the partial recoveries appeared to be short-term, with a return to the dramatic patterns of serotoninergic losses seen 2 weeks after drug exposure.

Colado and colleagues[48] reported that MDMA administration to pregnant rats does not produce damage to 5-HT nerve terminals in the brains of the fetuses, in contrast to the serotoninergic neurodegeneration seen in the CNS of the mothers. They hypothesized that this contrast in maternal versus fetal effects may be due to MDMA converted into free radical–associated metabolites in the adult brain but not in the immature brain. Alternatively, the developing CNS may have more effective or more active free radical scavenging mechanisms than the mature adult CNS.

Therapeutic administration of amphetamines is usually by the oral route. When used recreationally/illicitly, amphetamines are taken orally, snorted, smoked, or by intravenous injection.[78]

Methamphetamine's methyl group is lipid soluble and easily transported across the blood-brain barrier as well as relatively resistant to enzymatic degradation catalyzed by MAO activity. After an oral administration (4 x 10 mg), methamphetamine is initially detected in plasma samples within 15 minutes to 2 hours. Maximal plasma concentrations (14.5–33.8 μg/L) are achieved within 2–12 hours and the drug remains measurable for 36–72 hours after administration.[258] Methamphetamine has an elimination half-life of 9–15 hours primarily via urinary excretion. Methamphetamine elimination half-life varies with differences in urinary pH. One of the metabolites of methamphetamine is amphetamine.

Amphetamine and amphetamine-like derivatives are potent CNS stimulants affecting regulatory centers for heart rate, body temperature, blood pressure, appetite, attention, mood, and responses associated with alertness or alarm responses.[66] Physiological and psychological responses to amphetamines closely resemble the sympathetic nervous system–induced fight-or-flight responses, including increased heart rate and blood pressure, vasoconstriction, bronchodilation, and hyperglycemia. Users report increased ability to focus on tasks, an overall increase in mental alertness, avoidance of fatigue, and decrease in appetite.

Drug tolerance develops rapidly in amphetamine abuse.[169] Tolerance to the drug's effects results in increasing amounts of the drug needed to obtain similar rewarding effects. However, chronic amphetamine use can produce so-called reverse tolerance, or sensitization to some of the psychological effects of the drug. Amphetamine users will often take more of the drug during withdrawal periods and may use other drugs such as benzodiazepines, or less commonly, barbiturates to lessen the effects of withdrawal.[14,169]

Methamphetamine administration is associated with both dopaminergic and serotoninergic neurodegeneration. The generation of free radicals as a byproduct of increased DA and 5HT metabolism is postulated to play a key role in this neurodegeneration.[105,320] Blocking increases in METH-induced release of DA or 5HT reduce the neurodegeneration seen with administration of this drug. In addition, pretreating with multiple injections of escalating doses of methamphetamine produces tolerance to the long-term neurotoxic effects of methamphetamine on striatal DA neurons.[278] Although not yet well defined, the mechanism for this tolerance may be related to aberrant monoamine transporter-2 (VMAT-2) and dopamine transporter function in these neurons.

Cathinone and Synthetic Cathinone Derivatives

History

The leaves of the *Catha edulis* (khat) plant, which is native to the Horn of Africa and Arabian Peninsula, have been chewed for thousands of years, purportedly for their stimulant-like effects. In 1930, Wolfes identified the primary active constituent of khat to be cathine [(+) pseudonorephedrine]; cathinone [β-keto-amphetamine] was later identified to be a more potent contributor to the stimulant effects of khat[287] and for which cathine is a primary metabolite.[155]

Recent estimates suggest that khat is used daily by approximately 20 million people[88]; however, because its use is concentrated in the Arabian Peninsula and portions of Eastern Africa, it is not considered to a represent a major public health problem worldwide. Nevertheless, khat has received significant attention from international regulators, with its potential for abuse/dependence first discussed by the League of Nations in 1935, and again

by the United Nations and World Health Organization at the Single Convention on Narcotic Drugs in 1961. However, it was not until the Convention on Psychoactive Substances in 1971 that cathinone was placed on the international list of Schedule I drugs. Subsequently, the US Drug Enforcement Administration (DEA) added cathinone to its list of Schedule I drugs in 1993.

Because of its use as a precursor to the chemical synthesis of ephedrine and norephedrine, cathinone was first synthesized in 1915 by Eberhard.[75] With slight modifications to Eberhard's synthesis, Adams and colleagues[134] (Hyde et al., 1928) developed a method for synthesizing cathinone and several derivatives of cathinone that are still in use today. Driven in large part by chemical and pharmacological similarities among cathinone, ephedrine, and the amphetamines, numerous cathinone derivatives have been synthetized and patented by drug companies for their putative antidepressant and/or antiparkinsonian effects. For instance, methcathinone (α-methylamino-propiophenone) was first patented in Germany in 1936 (German Patent 639,126) as a chemical precursor for the synthesis of ephedrine (and ephedrine derivatives), later used in the Soviet Union for its antidepressant properties (1930s to 1940s), and subsequently patented by Parke Davis in 1957 (US Patent 2802865). Because of concern for abuse, methcathinone was listed as a Schedule I drug in 1994 by the International Convention on Psychotropic Substances, as well as the DEA.

Although recreational use of methcathinone in the 1970s provided early indications that synthetic cathinones possess high abuse potential, it was not until mephedrone (4-methylmethcathinone) and methylone (3,4-methylenedioxy-N-methylcathinone) emerged on the European club scene in around 2000 that these cathinone derivatives gained widespread popularity among drug abusers. Since that time, the recreational use of synthetic cathinones has increased dramatically around the world. They are widely available, marketed as "bath salts," "research chemicals," or "plant food," and can be easily purchased on the Internet and in local shops as "safe" and "legal highs." Indeed, anecdotal and survey data suggest that their effects are similar to those produced by cocaine and methamphetamine.[33,40,51,314] Coincident with the increasing popularity of these agents as recreational drugs, poison control centers and emergency departments around the world have seen dramatic increases in the number of patients presenting with cardiovascular and/or neuropsychiatric toxicities as well as overdose fatalities related to the use of synthetic cannabinoids and/or cathinones.[19,74] Because of the rapid increase in abuse and toxicity associated with the recreational use of these synthetic cathinone derivatives, in 2011 the DEA used its emergency scheduling authority to temporarily list three synthetic cathinones (mephedrone, methylone, and MDPV) as Schedule I. Although these regulations temporarily reduced the production/sale/use of these particular compounds, new derivatives with similar pharmacologic properties, and presumably high potential for abuse, quickly took their place in the market. In 2014, the list of synthetic cathinones placed under Schedule I was expanded to include 10 additional derivatives (4-MEC [4-methylethcathinone], 4-MePPP [4'-methyl-α-pyrrolidinopropiophenone], α-PVP [α-(pyrrolidin-1-yl)valerophenone], butylone [β-keto-N-methylbenzodioxolylbutanamine], pentedrone [α-methylamino-valerophenone], pentylone [β-keto-methylbenzodioxolylpentanamine], 4-FMC [flephedrone; 4-fluoromethcathinone], 3-FMC [3-fluoromethcathinone], naphyrone [naphthylpyrovalerone], and α-PBP [α-(pyrrolidinobuterophenone]), bringing the total number of synthetic cathinones listed as Schedule I drugs to 13 as of 2016.

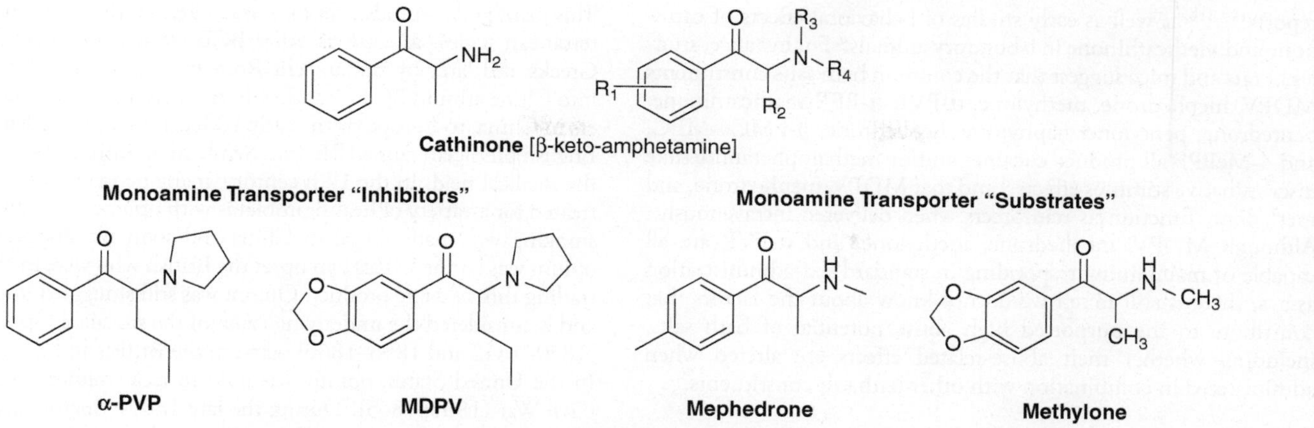

• **Fig. 17.5** Cathinone. Monoamine transporter "inhibitors" and monoamine transporter "substrates."

Chemical Properties

Similar to amphetamine, cathinone is a chemical derivative of phenethylamine; however, in addition to the alkyl group on the alpha carbon, cathinone also contains a ketone group on the beta carbon (i.e., β-keto-amphetamine). This core cathinone structure (phenethylamine with an alkyl group on the alpha carbon and a ketone group on the beta carbon) contains four locations for chemical modification (see Fig. 17.1), and is conserved across the more than 200 chemical derivatives of cathinone that have been described. Despite similarities among the chemical structures of the synthetic cathinones, the cathinone superfamily has a relatively heterogeneous pharmacology, with two main subfamilies of compounds defined by their capacity to inhibit the uptake monoamines by their transporters (i.e., inhibitors), or to both inhibit the uptake and stimulate the release of monoamines (i.e., substrates)[83,84,269,270] (Fig. 17.5).

Pharmacokinetics

Cathinone and its derivatives are readily absorbed and have high blood-brain barrier permeability,[269] with behavioral effects apparent within minutes after systemic administration in rodents.[a] Although the pharmacokinetic profiles of cathinone and several of the abused cathinone derivatives (e.g., MDPV, α-PVP, mephedrone, and methylone) have been examined, little is known about the pharmacokinetic properties of the majority of the synthetic cathinones. As with most amphetamine-like compounds, cathinone and its derivatives are metabolized primarily by liver enzymes. Although it is well known that cathinone is metabolized to pharmacologically active compounds (i.e., cathine and norephedrine), less is known about the pharmacologic activities of the metabolites of other cathinone derivatives. Of interest, whereas some of the synthetic cathinones (e.g., MDPV) exhibit linear pharmacokinetics,[10] other cathinone derivatives exhibit nonlinear pharmacokinetics. For example, whereas methylone is metabolized primarily by CYP2D6, it is also known to function as a mechanism-based inactivator of CYP2D6 function, effectively inhibiting its own metabolism in a time- and dose-dependent manner.[79,229]

Pharmacodynamics

Similar to other CNS and sympathetic nervous system stimulant drugs, cathinone and its synthetic derivatives increase extracellular levels of monoamines through their interactions with transporters for dopamine (DAT), norepinephrine (NET), and serotonin (SERT). As mentioned earlier in this chapter text, chemical diversity within the cathinone superfamily has resulted in subfamilies of compounds with slight, but important, differences in their primary mechanism of action. Similar to amphetamine, cathinone and some of its derivatives (e.g., substrates such as mephedrone, methylone, and 3-FMC) are known to both inhibit the uptake and stimulate the release of dopamine, norepinephrine, and serotonin, whereas other cathinone derivatives (e.g., inhibitors such as MDPV, α-PVP, naphyrone) are capable of inhibiting monoamine uptake without stimulating their release, a mechanism of action more similar to that of cocaine than amphetamine. In addition to differences in their effects at monoamine transporters (i.e., release and/or inhibition), a great deal of diversity exists among the synthetic cathinones with respect to the selectivity with which they act at dopamine, norepinephrine, and serotonin transporters, as well as other nontransporter sites.[83,84,269,270] For example, among inhibitors, some compounds (e.g., naphyrone, pentylone) inhibit the uptake of dopamine, norepinephrine, and serotonin at comparable doses, whereas other compounds, including MDPV, and α-PVP, are potent inhibitors of dopamine and norepinephrine uptake with low affinity for the serotonin transporter.[18,84,269] Similar differences are also apparent among substrates, with compounds such as cathinone being more potent at releasing dopamine than serotonin, whereas other cathinone derivatives, such as mephedrone, are equipotent at releasing dopamine and serotonin.[83,269,270]

Although relatively little is known about the effects of synthetic cathinones at sites other than the monoamine transporters, affinity for serotonin (1A, 2A, and/or 2C) and/or adrenergic (α1, α2a) receptors has been reported for some cathinones.[269,270] Similar binding profiles have been reported for other amphetamine-like compounds (e.g., amphetamine, methamphetamine, MDMA); however, it is worth noting that unlike many amphetamine-like compounds, beta-keto containing cathinones appear to be devoid of activity at TAARs.[269,270]

To date, the majority of preclinical studies on the behavioral effects of cathinones have focused on characterizing their acute locomotor effects.[b] Although the discriminative stimulus and reinforcing effects of cathinones have been described in much less detail, preliminary evidence is generally consistent with human

---

[a]References 18, 51, 86, 94–96, 186, 187.

[b]References 2, 94–96, 176, 187, 318.

reports[142,314] as well as early studies of behavioral effects of cathinone and methcathinone in laboratory animals.[c] For instance, studies in rats and mice suggest that the common bath salts constituents MDPV, mephedrone, methylone, α-PVP, α-PBP, methcathinone, pentedrone, pentylone, naphyrone, flephedrone, 3-FMC4-MEC, and 4-MePPP all produce cocaine- and/or methamphetamine-like discriminative stimulus effects,[d] and that MDPV, mephedrone, and methylone, function as reinforcers when delivered intravenously.[e] Although MDPV, mephedrone, methylone, and α-PVP are all capable of maintaining responding in standard self-administration assays, there is still much we do not know about the factors that contribute to the purported high abuse potential of bath salts, including whether their abuse-related effects are altered when administered in combination with other bath salt constituents.

Toxicology

Although national drug use surveys (e.g., Substance Abuse and Mental Health Services Administration [SAMSHA] National Survey on Drug Use and Health) have yet to be updated to include data on synthetic cathinone (i.e., bath salts) overdoses, the Drug Abuse Warning Network recorded over 20,000 emergency department visits involving bath salts in 2011 alone.[74] As with other stimulants, the most common symptoms associated with bath salts overdose are cardiovascular (e.g., tachycardia, hypertension, and chest pain) and/or neuropsychiatric complications (e.g., agitation, paranoia, and hallucination (see references 19, 199, and 237). Whereas acute myocardial infarction can seriously compromise the health of the user, case reports suggest that the paranoia and hallucinations produced by bath salts can precipitate self-destructive or violent behavior that can put users, their families, and medical staff at risk.[188,274] (Stimulants such as cocaine, methamphetamine, and MDMA have well-characterized cardiovascular effects in rats[122,259,290] and preliminary evidence suggests that mephedrone and MDPV produce similar, if not greater, increases in heart rate and mean arterial pressure.[18,157,261,289]) Given the overlap between the toxic effects of cathinones and other stimulants (e.g., cocaine, methamphetamine, MDMA), it is not surprising that current treatments for cathinone overdose parallel those used for cocaine, including the use of benzodiazepines to decrease cardiovascular effects and agitation. In some cases, haloperidol has been used to decrease the central stimulant effects of cathinones; however, as with cocaine, beta-blockers are contraindicated for the treatment of hypertension because they have been shown to result in further increases in blood pressure.

However, it should be noted that because bath salts preparations often contain multiple psychoactive compounds, with mixtures of two cathinones, and mixtures of a cathinone and caffeine being the most common,[f] it is difficult to say whether the toxicities observed in bath salts can be attributed to a single cathinone, or whether they result from interactions among the various bath salts constituents.

Opiates

History

Crude opium is a component of the opaque, milky-white sap obtained from the seedpods of the poppy plant (*Papaver somniferum*).[32]

[c]References 107, 141, 148, 256, 257, 317, 321.
[d]References 115, 122, 123, 128, 143.
[e]References 1, 2, 112, 206, 260, 303, 304.
[f]References 29, 42, 63, 264, 277, 324.

This plant and its product opium were likely cultivated in the Mediterranean region as early as 5000 BCE by ancient Egyptians and Greeks and later by the ancient Romans. Opium was introduced into China around BC 800 and, with the arrival of European explorers to China, to Europe by the early 18th century. In 1680, a famous English physician named Thomas Syndenham introduced opium to the medical field. In the 17th century, many people in Europe were treated for a variety of health problems with opium. In 1729, opium smoking was made illegal in China and soon the importation of opium was banned. This ban upset the British who were in charge of trading this valuable product. Opium was still smuggled into China and is considered the underlying cause of the so-called Opium Wars (1839–1842 and 1856–1860) between the British and the Chinese. In the United States, opium was used to treat soldiers during the Civil War (1861–1865). During the late 1800s, doctors prescribed "tonics" containing opiates for many conditions. Typically, these medicines failed to list opiates as one of the ingredients.

Opium represents a complex of sugars, proteins, fats, water, meconic acid, plant wax, latex, gums, ammonia, sulfuric and lactic acids, and numerous alkaloids. Alkaloids present in opium include morphine (10%–15%), codeine (1%–3%), papaverine (1%–3%), and thebaine (1%–2%). Noscapine, narceine, and approximately 25 other alkaloids are also present, but have essentially little to no effect on the CNS and are not usually considered to be opiates. Thebaine is considered highly toxic and thus not used therapeutically[4]; it acts as a potent stimulant rather than as a depressant, at higher concentrations, causing strychnine-like convulsions. Thebaine can be used to produce the semisynthetic morphine analogues oxycodone, dihydromorphinone, hydrocodone, and etorphine.

In 1805 the German pharmacist Frederick Serturner isolated morphine from opium. He named this newfound compound after Morpheus, the Greek god of dreams. Morphine-related analogues include the diphenylpropylamines (e.g., methadone), the 4-phenylpiperidines (e.g., meperidine), the morphinans (e.g., levorphanol), and 6,7-benzomorphans (e.g., metazocine), each of which has in common a piperidine ring or a key component of that ring structure. Heroin was first synthesized in 1874 by the British chemist C. Adler Wright. Heroin is synthesized from morphine. Heroin is the 3, 6-diacetyl ester of morphine, that is, diacetylmorphine (see Fig. 17.5). Heroin became widely accepted within the medical community in the early 1900s. The high risk for addiction was not initially recognized by physicians at that time. With a better understanding of its abuse potential, heroin was later regulated with passage of the Harrison Narcotics Tax Act of 1914. The drug is now classified as a Schedule I substance with significant abuse potential but no accepted medical use.

The term "opiate" refers to morphine-like alkaloids (e.g., morphine itself, heroin, codeine, thebaine, and papaverine) derived from opium as well as a number of semisynthetic and synthetic opiates. Opioid refers to endogenous substances with morphine-like activity. Endogenous opioids include dynorphins, enkephalins, endorphins, endomorphins, and nociceptin/orphanin FQ. The term "endorphin" was first used in the mid-1970s to describe any endogenous morphine-like substance, now classified as endogenous opioidergic peptides. We now recognize several classes of endogenous opioidergic peptides including enkephalins, endorphins, dynorphins, and endomorphins. Opiates such as morphine and heroin bind to and activate the same receptors used by endogenous opioidergic peptides, namely mu (μ), kappa (κ) and delta (δ) receptors.

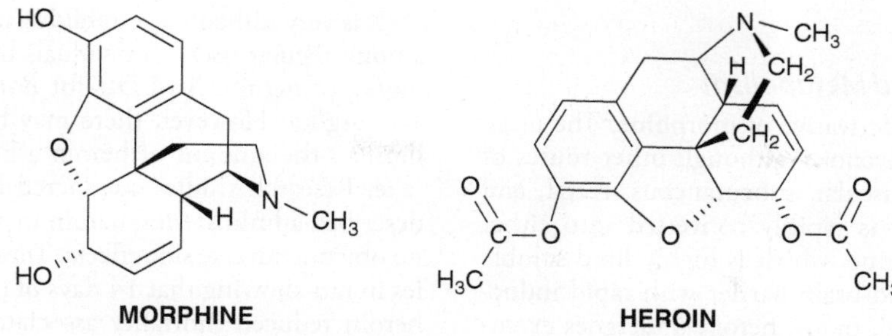

• **Fig. 17.6** Structures of morphine and heroin.

Opioidergic receptors are expressed only in the CNS, gastrointestinal tract, and vas deferens. Most opioid receptors are linked to an inhibitory G protein (G_i). Thus endogenous opioidergic peptide receptor binding is associated with inhibition of adenylate/cAMP second-messenger systems and inhibition of the target neuron.

Endogenous opioidergic peptides are generally involved with homeostasis or regulation of basic physiological functions including respiration, endocrine functions, and nociception (pain). Endogenous opioidergic peptides may also play important roles in mood and affect. The greatest density of opioidergic receptors is found in the limbic system (emotions and affect) and in the dorsal horn of the spinal cord (nociception). Thus it should not be surprising that endogenous opioidergic peptides are thought to integrate euphoric and emotional components of pain relief (Fig. 17.6).

According to the Department of Health and Human Services, the United States is currently in the midst of an opiate epidemic.[295] Prescription opiates are now the most commonly prescribed class of drugs in the United States,[296] and although they are effective and an important component of balanced pain management,[46] the increased clinical use is associated with increased risks. For example, abuse of prescription opiates has increased dramatically in the last two decades,[150] with more than 10 million people in the United States using prescription opiates nonmedically.[272] As a direct result of increased abuse, there has been a dramatic escalation in overdose deaths.[250,272] Nearly 500,000 people in the United States died from a drug overdose between 2000 and 2014, with more than 61% of those fatalities attributed to opiates.[250] Moreover, the death rate from opiate overdose has grown every year since 2000, and the rate of fatal overdose increased 14% from 2013 to 2014.[250] Prescription opiate abuse is also fueling an increase in heroin abuse, because heroin is often cheaper and more accessible than other opiates[53]; as a result, the death rate due to heroin overdose increased 26% from 2013 to 2014.[53] In addition to declaring that opiate overdose fatalities have reached epidemic levels, the US Department of Health and Human Services now advocates for greater access to treatment for opiate abusers.[295] In addition, the Centers for Disease Control and Prevention has issued new guidelines for prescribing opiates that includes 12 recommendations for clinicians who are treating patients with chronic pain.[72]

Mechanism of Action

Opiate agonists and antagonists bind to stereospecific, saturable receptors in the brain and other tissues. CNS opioidergic receptors are widely but unevenly distributed. These receptors were originally classified according to their affinity for binding agonists: mu (μ) receptors preferentially bind to morphine, kappa (κ) receptors to ketocyclazocine, and delta (δ) receptors to deltorphin II. Morphine also binds to both kappa and delta receptors, although with less affinity than to mu receptors. In 2000, these receptors were reclassified as OP_1 (delta), OP_2 (kappa), and OP_3 (μ) by a subcommittee of the International Union of Basic and Clinical Pharmacology.[138] Mu receptors are located widely throughout the CNS, especially in the limbic system (frontal and temporal cortex, amygdala, and hippocampus); thalamus; striatum; hypothalamus; and midbrain. Kappa receptors are located primarily in the spinal cord, periaqueductal gray area, and cerebral cortex. Delta receptors are located primarily in pontine nuclei, amygdala, olfactory bulbs, and deep cerebral cortex. Opiate receptors are G-protein-coupled and function as modulators, both positive and negative, of synaptic transmission. Most known opiates exhibit no ceiling effect for analgesia with the exception of codeine for which a ceiling effect is estimated as 7mg/kg. Mu receptor activation results in analgesia, euphoria, respiratory depression, miosis, decreased gastrointestinal motility, and physical dependence. Kappa-receptor stimulation also produces analgesia, miosis, respiratory depression, as well as dysphoria and some psychomimetic effects (i.e., disorientation and/or depersonalization). Delta receptor activation produces dysphoria, is hallucinogenic, and produces respiratory depression at high doses and cardiac stimulation. Opiates working primarily through mu receptors also suppress cough reflex. The antitussive effects of codeine are mediated through direct action on receptors in the cough center of the medulla.

Heroin is transported rapidly across the blood-brain barrier and metabolized into morphine and related compounds. It is generally assumed that heroin itself has only minor pharmacological effects. Most of the pharmacological effects associated with heroin are actually caused by morphine as well to some degree, the other two major metabolites 6-acetylmorphine (6-AM) and metabolites 6-acetylmorphine (M6G).[305] M6G possesses analgesic properties, although M3G does not seem to have any agonistic effect either in vivo or in cell cultures.[121]

Most opiates such as heroin and morphine produce a profound sense of euphoria in most users, although this effect diminishes with development of tolerance to the drug. Heroin and morphine share in common the ability to induce euphoria, relaxation, as well as, with time, drowsiness and sleepiness. Short-term studies among users suggested that heroin tolerance develops no more rapidly than tolerance to morphine.[285] This is perhaps not surprising given the physicochemical properties of heroin and morphine and the metabolism of heroin metabolism to morphine.

Pharmacokinetics

Routes of Administration and Metabolism

Heroin represents the diacetyl derivative of morphine. The usual route of administration is intravenous, although other routes of administration include intramuscular, subcutaneous, rectal, and intranasal. After absorption, it is rapidly converted into either morphine or monoacetylmorphine, which is highly lipid soluble and thus easily crosses the blood-brain barrier with rapid induction of euphoria.[216] When taken orally, heroin undergoes extensive first-pass metabolism via deacetylation into morphine in the liver. Thus heroin can be considered a prodrug.[254] In contrast, intravenous injection of the drug essentially bypasses first-pass metabolism with rapid distribution across the blood-brain barrier due to the presence of acetyl groups, which makes the drug more lipid soluble than morphine.[154] Within the brain, heroin is deacetylated into 3- and 6-monoacetylmorphine and into morphine, which binds to μ-opioid receptors. Most of the morphine is further converted to morphine-3-glucuronide (M3G; approximately 50%) and morphine-6-glucuronide (M6G; approximately 10%).[5] Recent studies have demonstrated that the brain, pancreas, and myocardium can also produce morphine.[22]

Morphine is metabolized primarily into morphine-3-glucuronide and morphine-6-glucuronide via glucuronidation catalyzed by the liver enzyme UDP glucuronosyl transferase 2B7 (UGT2B7).[151] Morphine is similarly metabolized in brain and kidneys. At least in studies using rodent models, morphine-6-glucuronide is far more potent an analgesic than morphine itself. However, this morphine metabolite crosses the blood-brain barrier poorly in contrast to morphine.

Toxicology

The psychological dependence associated with opioidergic addiction is both protracted and complex. Well beyond the recovery from the physical need for the drug, the opiate addict may obsess about use of the drug and feel an inability to deal with daily activities without use of the drug. These individuals are at high risk for relapse assuming neither the physical environment.

Opiate withdrawal symptoms in opiate users can be seen as early as 2–3 hours after the last dose of drug.[210] Major withdrawal signs peak between 48 to 72 hours after last dose and subside within 9 to 12 days. Initial signs of withdrawal include dilated pupils, profuse sweating, and anxiety. These individuals also experience progressively stronger drug craving, severe abdominal distress, diarrhea, nausea and vomiting, restlessness, muscle and bone pain, insomnia, cold flashes with goose bumps ("cold turkey") alternating with high temperature spiking ("hot flashes"), and kicking movements ("kicking the habit"). Severe depression is a common manifestation. Opiate withdrawal is rarely fatal, although sudden withdrawal by heavily dependent users in poor health may be fatal. Opiate withdrawal is considered less risky than alcohol, benzodiazepine, or barbiturate withdrawal.

Following intravenous infusion of heroin, the user experiences a surge of euphoria ("rush") along with dry mouth, a warm flushing of the skin, and a heaviness of the extremities.[185] The user then becomes alternately somnolent and alert ("on the nod"), shifting between wakeful and drowsy states. Mental functioning declines. Tolerance to the effects of the drug develop over time and regular use. In effect, the user must use more heroin to achieve the same intensity of effect. Eventually, drug-induced neural plasticity within reward pathways of the brain results in addiction to the drug.

It is very difficult to establish a lethal dose50 (LD_{50}) for heroin among regular users. Individuals have overdosed on as little as 1 mg/kg of heroin. An LD_{50} for nonaddicts has been suggested as 1–5 mg/kg. However, there may be no easily identifiable upper limit to the amount of heroin a heavily addicted individual can take. Research studies conducted in the 1920s in opiate addicts described administering heroin in doses of 1600 to 1800 mg with no obvious adverse side effects. These results are supported by studies in rats showing that 14 days of pretreatment with morphine or heroin reduced mortality associated with subsequent morphine administration.[280] Thus long-term opiate abuse is typically associated with development of highly significant drug tolerance.

Neurological complications associated with heroin use include peripheral neuropathies, nerve pressure palsies, hypoxic encephalopathy, seizures, rhabdomyolysis, and transverse myelopathies. Spongiform leukoencephalopathy is a relatively rare complication of heroin use, with only 70 reported cases from the first reported case in 1984 through 2004.[113] This complication is typically seen among users who inhale fumes generated by heating heroin, a practice called "chasing the dragon."[124] The typical lesions include abnormal white matter with patchy spongiform change and prominent reactive fibrous gliosis consisting of glial fibrillary acidic protein- (GFAP-)positive fibrous astrocytes. Symptoms vary according the brain regions involved but often include cognitive dysfunction, cerebellar ataxia, dysarthria, and motor restlessness with an estimated mortality rate of approximately 25%.

Heroin-related death has been associated with the phenomenon of place tolerance and overdose as a result of using the drug in an unaccustomed environment.[99] The mechanism for fatal overdosing in this situation was described as an overriding of conditioned or place tolerance. Because heroin use is such a highly ritualized behavior, long-time users exhibit increased tolerance to the drug in locations in which they have repeatedly administered heroin. When they used in a different location, this environment-conditioned tolerance does not occur, which produces enhanced effects of the drug. In response to this decrease in tolerance, the user increases the typical dose of the drug. If extreme in self-dosing, the result can be a fatal overdose.

Morphine also affects immune system function via interactions with dendritic cells.[195] Dendritic cells, a type of antigen-presenting cell, express opiate receptors. Dendritic cells exposed to morphine during their maturation produce increased levels of interleukin-12, a cytokine responsible for promoting the proliferation, growth, and differentiation of T lymphocytes, which are active in adaptive immune responses and less so, interleukin-10, a cytokine responsible for promoting B-lymphocyte responsiveness.

Hallucinogens

History

Hallucinogens comprise a class of drugs defined by their ability to induce changes in the user's perception of reality. Users describe seemingly real images, sounds, and sensations that do not in fact exist.[212] Traditionally, these drugs were derived from plant sources but are now synthetic with resultant greater purity of product (Drug Enforcement Administration, Drug Descriptions: Hallucinogens). Commonly used hallucinogens include lysergic acid diethylamide (LSD) and psilocybin (Fig. 17.7).

Lysergic acid is a component of ergot alkaloids found in the ergot fungus (*Claviceps purpurea*), which infects cereal grains including rye.[211] Ergot alkaloids are very potent compounds

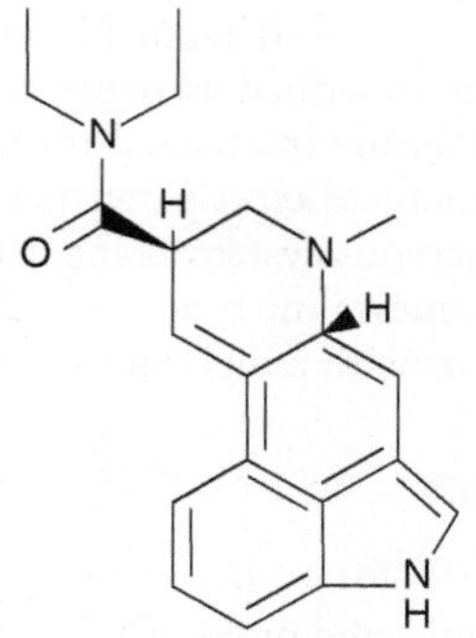

• **Fig. 17.7** Structure of LSD.

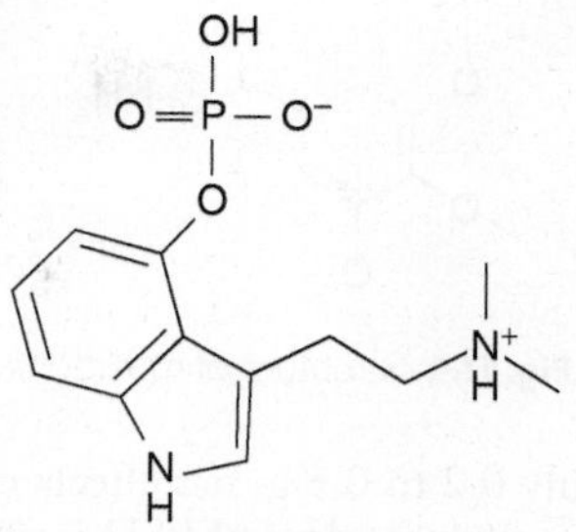

PSILOCYBIN

• **Fig. 17.8** Structure of psilocybin.

responsible for ergotism (also known as ergotoxicosis, ergot poisoning, and St. Anthony's Fire) characterized by convulsive and vasoconstrictive symptoms including gangrene and hallucinations, mania and psychoses.

Lysergic acid diethylamide (or LSD) was first synthesized in 1938 by Swiss chemist Albert Hofmann (1905–2008).[127] The hallucinogenic effects of LSD were not immediately recognized and the drug was ignored over the next several years. But in 1943, Hofmann accidentally absorbed a very small amount of LSD and experienced first-hand the psychogenic effects of the drug. He then followed up with an additional self-administration of LSD, later reporting the intensely psychedelic effects associated with the drug. The abbreviation LSD is derived from its early codename *LSD-25* (German "lysergsäure-diethylamid" followed by a sequential development number). LSD was initially marketed by Sandoz Laboratories as a therapeutic drug with numerous potentially useful psychiatric applications. However, the drug's entry into the illicit, recreational environment with ensuing political repercussions eventually precluded further interest in the drug among pharmaceutical companies and physicians. The substance was eventually banned for any use other than research as a DEA Schedule I substance.

For a time during the 1950s and early 1960s, intelligence agencies in the United States and other countries had an interest in use of LSD to facilitate interrogations and mind control.[286] The Central Intelligence Agency (CIA) conducted such studies through the Office of Scientific Intelligence largely in response to similar studies employed by the Soviet Union and China in the early 1950s. One such study involved the use of US soldiers dosed with LSD to study the effects of panic. By the late 1960s the CIA had ended these LSD studies, the results of which were considered too unpredictable.

The principal psychoactive component of so-called magic mushrooms is an indole related to tryptamine, psilocybin. Use of hallucinogenic mushrooms (Psilocybe cubensis and *P. semilanceata*) may go back as far as prehistoric humans, although conclusive evidence for this is lacking. Their early use was probably associated with religious communing, divination, and healing just as they are among some present-day Native Americans. Bernardino de Sahagún (1499–1590), a Franciscan missionary, described the ritualistic use of teonanácatl or "flesh of the gods" among the Central American Aztecs. In the 1960s, recreational use of hallucinogenic mushrooms was promoted by R. Gordon and Valentina Wasson, Timothy Leary, and others, which led to the popularization of a number of psychoactive *Psilocybe* species found in North America, Europe, and Asia.

In 1958, Hofmann had identified psilocin and psilocybin as the active compounds in psychoactive mushrooms. By the early 1970s, a number of psychoactive *Psilocybe* species were described, these variants being found in North America, Europe, and Asia. These mushrooms may also contain small amounts of other psychoactive tryptamines. Psilocybin and psilocin are listed as Schedule I drugs in the United States and many other countries (Fig. 17.8).

Mushroom concentrations of psilocybin and psilocin vary significantly among varieties of psychoactive mushrooms but averages 0.5%–2.0% of the dry weight of the average mushroom. The more common species *P. cubensis* contains approximately 10–25 mg psilocybin and psilocin. When psilocybin is ingested, it is broken down to produce psilocin, which is responsible for the hallucinogenic effects. Twenty-five milligrams to 50 mg of psilocybin and/or psilocin is generally thought to be a heavy psychoactive dose of these drugs.

Pharmacodynamics

Mechanisms of Action

The hallucinogenic effects of LSD and phenethylamine hallucinogens are thought to be mediated by the binding of these drugs to the $5HT_{2A}$ receptor.[184] LSD administered in so-called recreational doses has been shown to interact with $5-HT_{1A}$, $5-HT_{2A}$, $5-HT_{2C}$, $5-HT_{5A}$, $5-HT_{5B}$, and $5-HT_6$ receptors. More specifically, the hallucinogenic effects of LSD have been attributed to the drug's strong partial agonist effects at $5-HT_{2A}$ receptors[184]; selective $5-HT_{2A}$ specific antagonists block the psychotropic activity of LSD. With the exception of the ligand-gated ion channel $5-HT_3$ receptor, all other 5-HT receptors are G-protein-coupled seven transmembrane receptors that activate intracellular second messenger pathways. The exact sites and mechanisms of action and are not yet known. In addition to the drug's effects on $5HT_{2A}$ receptors, LSD has been shown to affect glutaminergic systems within the CNS. Systemic LSD (0.1 mg/kg, i.p.) or direct LSD infusion (10 μM) into prefrontal cortex has been associated with elevated levels of glutamate release in this brain region, an effect blocked by administration of the $5HT_{2A}$ antagonist M100907 (0.05 mg/kg, i.p.). Chronically, LSD may activate dopamine- and cyclic AMP-regulated phosphoprotein with molecular weight 32 kDa (DARPP-32)–related pathways, a mechanism of action shared by numerous other psychoactive drugs including cocaine, amphetamine, methamphetamine, nicotine, caffeine, LSD, PCP, ethanol, and morphine.

Typical doses of LSD are measured in microgram amounts rather than the more typical milligram amounts associated with other drugs of abuse. Hofmann determined that an active dose

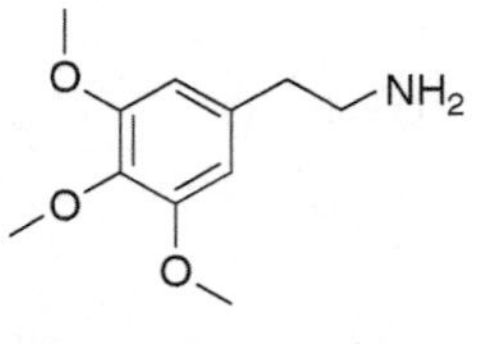

• **Fig. 17.9** Structure of mescaline.

of mescaline, roughly 0.2 to 0.5 g, has effects comparable to 100 µg or less of LSD.[127] A single dose of LSD is typically 100 to 500 µg; threshold psychotropic effects of the drug experienced with as little as 25 µg.[109] The LD_{50} for LSD has been estimated to range from 200 µg/kg to more than 1 mg/kg, although there are no known deaths attributed directly to the use of LSD. LSD users do not exhibit the typical features of drug addiction and dependence; however, tolerance to the drug can develop rapidly. Users demonstrate cross-tolerance between LSD and psilocybin. Attenuation of tolerance to LSD is thought to be related to drug-induced downregulation of $5HT_{2A}$ receptors in as yet undefined CNS areas.

Adverse reactions to LSD have been treated using fast-acting benzodiazepines such as diazepam or triazolam. These serve as anxiolytics, calming the patient but without directly blocking LSD binding at $5HT_{2A}$ sites. Theoretically, specific $5\text{-}HT_{2A}$ receptor antagonists, for example, the atypical antipsychotic quetiapine fumarate, would act to block LSD binding at these receptors, thus attenuating the psychoactive effects of LSD.

Mescaline (3,4,5-trimethoxyphenethylamine) is a naturally occurring hallucinogenic phenethylamine. Mescaline is one of several psychoactive alkaloids produced by several species of cactus including the peyote cactus (*Lophophora williamsii*), the San Pedro cactus (*Echinopsis pachanoi*), and the Peruvian Torch cactus (*Echinopsis peruviana*).[162] The peyote cacti are primarily subterranean, with underground roots and a relatively small above-ground crown consisting of several disk-shaped "buttons." These buttons are cut from the cactus and dried. Peyote includes a number of alkaloids including mescaline. Peyote has been used as a part of religious rites by Native American Indians of the arid northern Mexico and southwest United States for thousands of years. Peyote buttons with measurable levels of mescaline were found within prehistoric native Indian ruins and traced back to 3780–3660 BCE by radiocarbon dating.[80] Mescaline was first isolated and identified in 1897 by German chemist Arthur Heffter and first synthesized in 1919 by Ernst Späth (Fig. 17.9).

Mescaline is rapidly absorbed after oral ingestion by rats.[223] In human, the effective dose range is 300–500 mg of pure mescaline. The hallucinogenic effects of associated with ingestion of mescaline are seen in doses of 300–600 mg, the equivalent of 9–20 small peyote cactus tops. Mescaline is 1000–3000 times less potent than LSD, and 30 times less potent than psilocybin. The LD_{50} has been estimated as 212 mg/kg, i.p., for mice; 132 mg/kg, i.p., for rats; and 328 mg/kg, i.p., for guinea pigs. About half the initial dosage is excreted after 6 hours, but some studies suggest that it is not metabolized at all before excretion. The effects of mescaline can last up to 12 hours. Tolerance to mescaline increases with repeated administration. Mescaline may exhibit cross-tolerance with either LSD or psilocin. Equipotent doses of mescaline and LSD have been described as all but indistinguishable in psychoactivity.[263] A significant amount (20%–50%) of an ingested dose of mescaline is excreted in the urine unchanged in canine experimental models. Lesser amounts (7%) are excreted in urine by humans.

In contrast to LSD-induced hallucinations, those associated with mescaline use are described as being consistent with actual experiences but are typically intensified through visual and auditory inputs.[68,231] Mescaline elicits a pattern of sympathetic arousal, with the peripheral nervous system being a major target for this drug. Similar to LSD, mescaline binds to and activates brain serotonin $5\text{-}HT_{2A}$ receptors with a high nanomolar affinity.[202]

Pharmacokinetics

Routes of Administration

LSD is typically administered orally. Often absorbent paper, sugar cubes, or gelatin cubes are used as vehicles to deliver very small amounts of the drug. Unlike most other medicinal or illicit drugs dosed in milligram concentrations, psychoactive doses are measured in microgram concentrations. Liquid forms of the drug can be administered either intramuscularly or intravenously. Twenty micrograms to 30 µg is thought to be a threshold dose to experience psychoactive effects.[109] The psychoactive effects of a threshold dose (20–30 µg) of LSD typically last from 6–12 hours depending on tolerance, body weight, and age. These effects do not last longer than measurable blood levels of LSD as was once thought. Aghajanian and Bing[100] reported that LSD had an elimination half-life of 175 minutes. In a case study involving a single adult male, a 1 µg/kg dose of LSD orally had a plasma half-life of 5.1 hours, with a peak plasma concentration of 5 ng/mL 3 hours after drug administration. These investigators also reported a close correlation between measurable blood concentrations of LSD and the time course of the subject's difficulties with simple arithmetic problems. Recent research suggests that LSD binds to the $5\text{-}HT_{2A}$ receptor in such a way that locks it into the receptor binding site, preventing rapid dissociation of the molecule and potentially leading to prolonged action.[300] Following ingestion, psilocybin is rapidly absorbed and dephosphorylated to psilocin.[116] Similar to LSD, psilocin is a highly potent $5HT_{1A}$, $5\text{-}HT_{2A}$, and $5\text{-}HT_{2C}$ receptor agonist. The receptor binding potency of psilocin correlates strongly with its potency as a hallucinogen.[225] The psychoactive effects of psilocin can be highly variable among individuals. Effects reported by many individuals include strong visual and auditory components. Ingestion of psilocybin and/or psilocin is associated with an increase in the ability to concentrate on memories, feelings of time expansion, abstract and distractive thought patterns, as well as indecisiveness, phonetic experimentation (glossolalia), and epiphanies about life.[225,315]

Psilocybin has a reported onset of action of 15–30 minutes following ingestion, with psychoactive effects lasting 5–8 hours.[246] The duration of psychoactive effects correlates with dosage, itself a function of mushroom preparation and storage, and with variations in metabolism among users.

Toxicology

LSD has been shown to bind to and induce conformational changes in the structure of the DNA helix.[69] And although LSD has been reported to be mutagenic at higher doses in animal models, no detectable DNA damage or increased incidence of cancers has been seen with LSD use in humans.

In fact, most hallucinogens are not known to have long-term toxicities. However, an important caveat is the potential for MDMA to produce free radicals as a side reaction to the effects of this drug on biogenic amine systems in the CNS. These free radicals may induce neurodegeneration within various brain areas with resultant disease states.[49] Hallucinogen persisting perception disorder (HPPD; Fourth Edition of the *Diagnostic and Statistical Manual of Mental Disorders* [DSM-IV] diagnosis: diagnostic code 292.89) represents a condition in which the vision system-related effects of drug persist over a long period of time.[85] HPPD is distinctly different from so-called "flashbacks" in being persistent. The mechanism for this disorder has not been defined.

To date no significant toxicities have been associated with ingestion of psilocybin mushrooms. However, a lethal dose in humans has not been established. The oral LD_{50} in rats is 280 mg/kg.[225] Psilocybin represents approximately 1% of the dried weight of the *P. cubensis* mushroom. An adult weighing 60 kg would have to ingest 1.7 kg of dried mushrooms to reach a dosage equivalent to the oral LD_{50} in rats. Psilocybin and psilocin are not considered addictive, although both can induce short-term increases in tolerance of users.

Therapeutic Use

Recent research suggests that hallucinogens might be used therapeutically in some situations. Results of clinical trials have shown positive effects of MDMA in depression and posttraumatic stress disorder, and as an anxiolytic for terminally ill patients.[17,110,182,308] Recent pilot studies have even examined the potential of psilocybin to treat addiction to tobacco and alcohol.[23,71,143]

Cannabis

History

In 1378, the Emir of the Joneima in Arabia, Soudoun Sheikouni issued the first recorded edict prohibiting cannabis use.[170] He ordered all cannabis plants in the region destroyed and that those convicted of ingesting the plant have all of their teeth removed. Fewer than 20 years later, in 1393, use of cannabis in Arabia had increased.[170] And so it goes even today with the allure of this unique plant. Despite centuries of government edicts from all corners of the globe, cannabis remains the most popular psychoactive substance on the planet with the exception of caffeine, tobacco, and ethanol.

Cannabis has been used in China for over 5000 years.[189] Its use in the Middle East is probably similarly ancient. The translation of the ingredients of the holy oil used by Aaron and his sons to anoint the tabernacle of Moses consisted of myrrh, cinnamon, cassia (commonly used as cinnamon in North America), and calamus extracted into olive oil. However, in the original Hebrew text, the last ingredient is "kanah bosm," which some contend is actually the Sycthian etymological root of cannabis.[189] Indeed, the Greek historian Herodatus describes recreational use of cannabis among the Sycthians 2500–3000 years ago.

Cannabis is the genus name given to several strains of the plant commonly called hemp.[299] As early as 1855, it was recognized that hemp carefully cultivated in the gardens of the Near and Far East had vastly different properties when consumed than the hemp grown as a large scale crop in Europe, which was used in the production of fibers for rope, paper, and fabric.[299] For thousands of years in the Near and Far East, preparations of cannabis were smoked, eaten, or prepared in beverages. Thus although improvements in refining and distilling capabilities over the past 200 years have led to drastic increases in the potency and portability of drugs such as cocaine, morphine, and even ethanol, cannabis users continue to employ the same methods practiced by prehistoric peoples. However, modern methods of drug preparation, including extraction with carbon dioxide or solvents can produce a more concentrated product.[325] More recently, synthetic chemicals that mimic the effects of cannabis (synthetic cannabinoids) have gained popularity as recreational drugs. The first synthetic cannabinoids identified were developed by Roger Adams in the mid-20th century.[312] Over the next several decades, additional synthetic cannabinoids were developed; however, these molecules remained confined largely to research laboratories. In the mid-2000s, a team of chemists led by John Huffman synthesized a series of synthetic cannabinoids, with the goal of producing peripherally restricted cannabinoids with little or no psychoactive activity.[132] However, several of the molecules they synthesized had substantial psychoactive activity. The relatively simple synthesis and availability of precursors, combined with their legal status, resulted in large-scale production by international chemical laboratories. These chemicals continue to be incorporated into recreational drug products and sold worldwide as recreational drug products.[276]

These chemicals are derived from several different chemical classes, and are broadly described as synthetic cannabinoids. Because manufacturers are continuously altering the chemical structure, these drugs are often not detected using common drug test methods.[12] Emerging evidence indicates that these chemicals are more dangerous than phytocannabinoids produced by the cannabis plant, perhaps due to their greater pharmacological potency and efficacy.[12]

Chemical Properties

Raw cannabis contains 483 distinct chemical constituents, most of which are common to other plants.[81] However, the genus *Cannabis* alone produces the 66 known chemicals that constitute the cannabinoids.[81] Cannabinoids are terpenes joined to an alkyl-substituted resorcinol. Several of the cannabinoids are psychoactive, most notably Δ^9-tetrahydrocannabinol (THC; see Fig. 17.1). THC is regarded as the principal psychoactive constituent of cannabis, and can produce discriminative stimulus effects in experienced cannabis users. THC has a molecular weight of 314. It is insoluble in water, and experimental preparations commonly employ the use of an emulsifier such as vegetable oil to allow an injectable solution. The concentration of THC in cannabis depends upon the source, with levels ranging from 0.007% to almost 4.0%.[233] Although official reports released by the US Department of Justice assert that the concentration of THC in cannabis is increasing both in the United States and abroad, others, including the director of the Univ of Mississippi Marijuana Potency Monitoring Project Mohammed ElSohly, dispute this claim (http://www.slate.com/?id=2074151). Selective breeding techniques have undoubtedly resulted in enriched THC-containing strains, notably in Canada and The Netherlands; however, after several generations in the United States, the THC content of these strains recedes to levels common to American plants.[233] Climate, light, soil, humidity, and stress during the growing season all affect THC content.

Synthetic cannabinoids have been derived from at least five different chemical classes. These include classical cannabinoids, which share structural similarities with phytocannabinoids; nonclassical cannabinoids, which are similar to classical cannabinoids, but lack a third fused ring; aminoalkylindoles, which are structurally diverse and represent the most common synthetic cannabinoids used recreationally; eicosanoids, which are fatty acids that serve as endogenous cannabinoids in mammals; and others that are often chimeras from the other four classes.[323] Generally these compounds share the lipophilicity of phytocannabinoids. Thus preparation of these chemicals typically involves dissolving them in a solvent, and then applying the solution to nonpsychoactive plant material such as potpourri. Once the solvent evaporates, the synthetic cannabinoid-impregnated product is packaged and sold, to be smoked similar to cannabis by the consumer.[276] Although the raw material obtained from chemical suppliers is relatively pure,[140] this production results in widely variable concentrations, even within the same package. Furthermore, synthetic marijuana products often contain several different synthetic cannabinoid molecules. These factors make predicting the quality and intensity of the effect of these drugs highly unpredictable.

Pharmacokinetics

Routes of Administration

Marijuana is most commonly smoked. The plant material is macerated and rolled into cigarettes or loaded into a pipe. Some people utilize a water pipe in which the smoke is drawn through water, with the intent of removing toxic compounds resulting from pyrolysis. This method does appear to effectively reduce the ingestion of pyrolytic toxins.[230] However, a study funded by the Multidisciplinary Association for Psychedelic Studies (MAPS) and the California chapter of the National Organization to Reform Marijuana Laws (CaNORML) showed that while water pipes do filter out tar, the water also traps substantial amounts of THC, which leads the user to ingest more smoke, offsetting the benefits of water filtration.[101] An alternative to smoking that is growing in popularity is vaporization. This technique requires specialized equipment that heats the plant material up to 200°C, the vaporization temperature of THC[3] and related compounds, but not hot enough to result in combustion. This method has been shown to result in similar subjective effects (almost 90% of the vaporized substance is THC), yet almost completely eliminate combustion byproducts in the inhaled product.[49,102,120]

THC can also be eaten. Typically, fat-soluble cannabinoids are extracted into butter or some other oil, which is filtered and used to make foods. Although this method eliminates any byproducts of combustion, the onset of psychoactive effects is slower and more difficult for the user to titrate.[30,233] Alternatively, cannabinoids can be extracted from the plant material with ethanol. The ethanol can then be consumed or used as a tincture. Again, this method eliminates harmful byproducts resulting from combustion, but makes dose titration more difficult. Furthermore, impairment due to cannabis is enhanced by ethanol, possibly due to pharmacokinetic or pharmacodynamic interactions.[129,190] Oral and topical preparations were the most commonly used medicinal applications in the late 19th and early 20th centuries.

Another preparation, hashish, has been used for centuries in some regions. Hashish describes a preparation of the resin (which contains a high concentration of the psychoactive constituents in cannabis.[233] More recently, THC extract in a liquid or wax-based form has gained popularity. This can be accomplished by soaking raw cannabis in solvent (often butane) or exposing it to pressurized CO_2. The resulting product is a waxy substance with extremely high THC content.[325]

Synthetic cannabinoids can also be prepared in a liquid vehicle, often a propylene glycol/vegetable oil mixture, similar to the vehicle used in electronic cigarettes to deliver

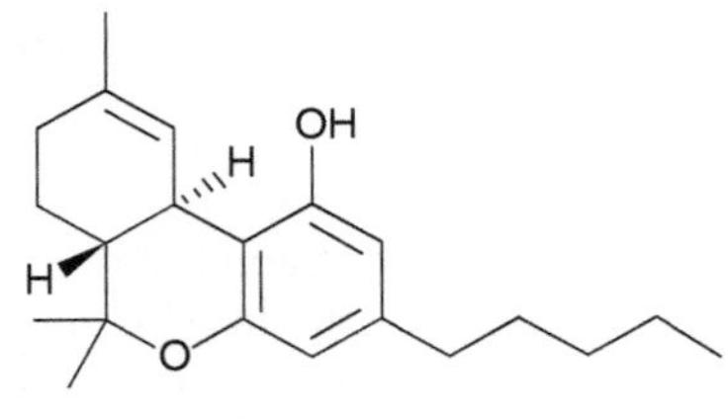

• **Fig. 17.10** Structure of Δ^9-tetrahydrocannabinol.

nicotine.[3,57,103] This preparation can be used in the same types of vaporizer pens used to consume liquid nicotine preparations (Fig. 17.10).

Δ^9-Tetrahydrocannabinol

Distribution and Bioavailability

Inhalation of THC results in rapid absorption, similar to other inhaled drugs. In addition, smoking and vaporization produce very similar pharmacokinetic profiles in the plasma of human volunteers.[292] Depending on the experience of the individual, 15% to 50% of the THC in the raw plant matter reaches the systemic circulation.[220] Oral consumption of cannabis leads to much slower and more variable absorption of THC, which may depend in part on the vehicle.

The volume of distribution for THC is about 10 L, and is primarily distributed to body fat, and internal organs with fatty compositions such as the liver, heart, mammary tissue, and brain. THC in plasma is almost entirely bound to lipoproteins, albumin, and red blood cells. Only about 3% of free THC is found in plasma.[220]

Pharmacokinetics of synthetic cannabinoids are less clear. This is largely because the particular molecules in recreational use are constantly changing and are often mixed with other synthetic cannabinoids or even other psychoactive chemicals.[12] In one case report, the synthetic cannabinoid MAB-CHMINACA was found in postmortem tissue at high concentrations in liver, pancreas, kidney, and other target organs, as well as in the blood (albeit at lower concentrations). Surprisingly, only low levels of the substance were found in adipose tissue.[115] Furthermore, levels of another synthetic cannabinoid found in the product the deceased consumed prior to death, 5-fluoro-ADB, were significantly lower than would be expected, based on the relative concentrations of each in the synthetic marijuana product.[115] This indicates that various synthetic cannabinoids might have unique pharmacokinetic profiles. Variable pharmacokinetics, in addition to the constantly changing molecules added to synthetic marijuana products, complicates detection of recent synthetic cannabinoid use, which is often reported as a reason for their use.[41]

Metabolism and Elimination

Metabolism of THC is primarily achieved by the liver, although other organs can metabolize THC. THC is hydroxylated into 11-OH-THC by mitochondrial cytochrome P450 (CYP), which maintains pharmacological activity.[220] Further metabolism by the same enzyme results in the inactive 11-nor-9-carboxy-THC.[220] One recent report determined the half-life of THC to be 1.4 hours, although this period is shorter than the results reported previously by others. Determination of the half-life of THC can be difficult, due to the slow development of equilibrium between plasma and fat-bound THC.

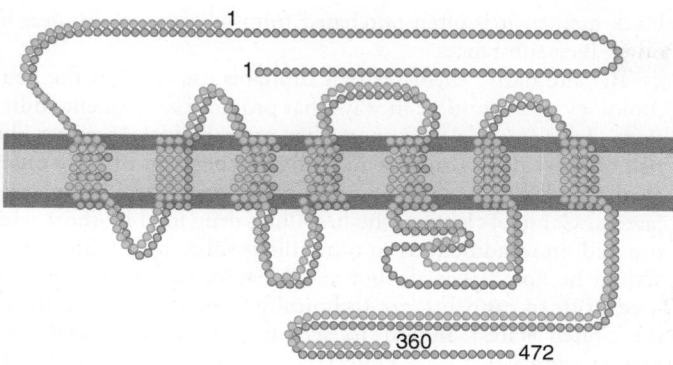

• **Fig. 17.11** Structure of CB1 (*blue*) and CB2 (*green*) receptors. Each receptor has a structure common to other seven transmembrane G-shaped protein receptors.

A recent study in pigs compared elimination of THC with that of the synthetic cannabinoids JWH-210 and RCS-4.[255] The authors found that a three-compartment model best fit all three cannabinoids, and central volumes of distribution were similar for THC and JWH-210, but about three times larger for RCS-4. Clearance rates were also similar for THC and JWH-210, but about twice as fast for RCS-4.

Pharmacodynamics

Pharmacology

There are two types of cannabinoid receptors that have been definitively identified. Both are G-protein-coupled receptors. CB1 receptors are widely expressed in the CNS, particularly in the hippocampus, cortex, cerebellum, and mesolimbic dopamine system. CB2 receptors were first identified on immune cells and thought to exist only in the periphery, but have recently been shown to be expressed by neurons and glial cells in the brain (Fig. 17.11).

Cellular Effects

Both CB1 and CB2 are G-protein-linked receptors with a homologous structure to other, similar receptor proteins (see Fig. 17.2). These receptors contain seven transmembrane-spanning domains with an extracellular head and intracellular tail.[235] Cannabinoid receptors are thought to associate primarily with the Gi/Go family of G-proteins, resulting in inhibition of adenylate cyclase and inhibition of calcium channels upon receptor activation.[219] However, more recent evidence suggests that at least the CB1 receptor may associate with alternative second messenger systems depending on the agonist or tissue preparation.

Tissue Effects

Due to the activated receptor complex coupling with inhibitory G-proteins, cannabinoid agonists tend to have inhibitory effects. CB1 receptors are enriched in brain and are generally thought to function as inhibitory feedback modulators of presynaptic neurons.[291] Stimulation of postsynaptic neurons results in liberation of membrane-bound endogenous cannabinoid agonists, which migrate back across the synapse to the presynaptic membrane. Stimulation of CB1 receptors then inhibits further production or release of neurotransmitter.[291]

Both CB1 and CB2 receptors appear to promote neurogenesis, particularly in the hippocampus.[140,274] However, the progenitor cells that result from the application of cannabinoid agonists remain undifferentiated, awaiting further signaling by other molecules. It remains unclear whether the levels of THC and other cannabinoid agonists ingested by cannabis users are able to produce these effects.

Immune Effects

Generally, cannabinoids consumed during moderate marijuana use have little effect on immune system function; however, immune function can be suppressed in cells directly exposed to smoke.[153] Consequences of heavy use on immune function remain unclear. Immune cells express CB2 receptors, with expression levels in B cells > natural killer cells > monocytes > neutrophils > T cells. Cannabinoid signaling is involved in migration of immune cells. Immune cells migrate up the concentration gradient toward the endogenous cannabinoid 2-AG. Agonists (including the partial agonist THC) interfere with this chemotaxis, and this inhibition of cell migration is antagonized by CB2 receptor antagonists.[197] Studies leading to this conclusion were performed in vitro with levels of cannabinoids unlikely to be found in recreational cannabis users. Indeed, recreational use of cannabis by immunocompromised individuals does not appear to result in increased HIV viral load or reduce the circulating T lymphocytes.[44,300]

Systemic Effects

CB1 receptors are highly enriched in the CNS, particularly in the hippocampus, cerebellum, cortex, and mesolimbic dopamine system.[235] CB1-specific agonists produce characteristic effects associated with cannabinoids, including hypothermia, antinociception, locomotor depression, and ataxia.[52] Cannabis intoxication in humans produces sedation, euphoria, time dilation, dry mouth, and perceptual disturbances.

Therapeutic Effects

Recently, Western medicine has rediscovered potential therapeutic uses for cannabis. Because THC simulates appetite and inhibits emesis, it has been used as a treatment for wasting due to chemotherapy in cancer patients as well as in HIV patients.[157,300] Because THC produces antinociception, it has been used as an adjunct to treat peripheral neuropathic pain in HIV and other patients.[232] The antispastic properties of cannabis have led to its use in patients with multiple sclerosis and its intraoptic pressure lowering properties have led to its use in glaucoma.[50,157] Clearly, the endogenous cannabinoid system is a rich target for therapeutic agents; however, promoting smoking as a delivery system is generally frowned upon. Thus other delivery systems have gained traction in recent years.[102,120,232]

Toxicology

Apoptosis

Application of THC to cultured hippocampal neurons can result in cell death due to apoptosis. Chan et al.[43] treated hippocampal slices from adult female rats with THC (0.2, 0.38, 0.5, 1, and 2 μM) daily and assessed cell viability over 10 days. THC concentrations of 0.5 μM and higher resulted in dose- and time-dependent decreases in cell viability over the first 6 days. The apoptotic effect of THC appears to be mediated by CB1 receptor–mediated activation of c-Jun N-terminal kinase (JNK), initiating the caspase-3 programmed cell death pathway. However, in aggregating brain cell cultures consisting primarily of neurons, glia, or a mixture of the two, repeated treatment with 1 and 2 μM did not result in cell death, although a marker for GABAergic, cholinergic, and astrocytic markers was reduced following treatment.[201]

It is important to note that these concentrations of THC are likely higher than those achieved in vivo. Postmortem brain samples in cannabis users revealed THC levels ranging from 3nM to 0.1 µM, well below concentrations used in studies in vitro.[207] Blood levels were lower than brain levels in every subject. Consumption of a marijuana cigarette (3.55% THC) resulted in THC levels up to 0.85 µM; however, peak levels were rapid in onset and dissipated rapidly.[131] Thus the relevance of apoptosis due to concentrations of THC at or above 0.5 µM remains unclear. Further studies designed to examine apoptosis following systemic THC administration would help clarify the impact of THC on neuronal cell death.

Lung Cancer

Because smoked cannabis delivers comparable or even higher levels of tar than tobacco cigarettes, there is some interest in the relative risk of developing cancer due to chronic use.[242,283,319] Such studies are difficult to undertake as many cannabis users also use other recreational substances, especially tobacco.[308] To date, studies have reported mixed results.[252,294] Recently, a pooled analysis of six case-controlled studies across the United States, Canada, the United Kingdom, and New Zealand found cannabis users were at no greater statistical risk than those who never used cannabis.[322a]

Head and Neck Cancer

Although heavy cannabis use may lead to the development of lung cancer, cannabis use is not linked to increased incidence of head and neck cancer.[308] Heavy use of cannabis (>8.3 cigarettes/day/year) resulted in a slight increase in the prevalence of head and neck cancers; however, this increase was nonsignificant. In contrast, alcohol or tobacco use significantly increased the risk of developing head and neck cancer in this study.

Mental Disorders-Psychosis

Perhaps the most controversial possible toxic effect of cannabis use at present is the possible link between cannabis use in adolescence and subsequent development of psychosis. Cannabis use can result in acute psychotic episodes.[173] More recent studies have suggested that prolonged cannabis use during adolescence can increase the likelihood of psychotic symptoms in young adulthood.[30]

Depression

Few studies have investigated links between cannabis use and major depressive disorder. Wilcox et al.[307] and Lynskey et al.[181] found that initiation of cannabis use during adolescence increased the risk of subsequent depressive disorder. However, these studies are not conclusive. Furthermore, basic research has demonstrated an antidepressive effect of indirect cannabinoid agonists.[25,108] Thus a causal link between cannabis use and depression has not been decisively established.

Drug Addiction

Perhaps the most contentious debate over possible psychiatric sequelae of cannabis use relates to the gateway theory. That is, that use of cannabis leads to an increased likelihood of subsequent addiction to other illicit substances.[208] Currently, the most widely held opinion is the Correlated Vulnerabilities Theory, which posits a predisposition toward illicit substance use. Thus those who use cannabis could have a more permissive attitude toward illicit substances in general and may be more willing to try other illicit substances. Furthermore, where cannabis is only available on the black market, it is often purchased from sellers who also deal in other illicit substances.

The alternative theory is that cannabis use changes the neurobiology of the initiate in ways that promote subsequent addictions. Lynskey et al.[181] report that cannabis use increases the risk of subsequent drug use in twins independent of early onset alcohol and tobacco use or other behavioral or environmental factors. Cannabis is often the first illicit drug used by those who proceed on to addictions to other illicit substances (although it should be noted that alcohol and tobacco, which are typically used prior to cannabis, are technically illegal for adolescents in the United States). Indeed, tobacco use appears to precede and predict cannabis use.[149] However, more recently, Patton et al. reported that cannabis use precedes and predicts tobacco use. Thus it does not appear that the gateway phenomenon is specific to cannabis, and these results support the correlated vulnerabilities theory.

Synthetic Cannabinoid Intoxication

For the most part, synthetic cannabinoids produce similar toxicity as phytocannabinoids, including delusions, lethargy, confusion, and dizziness. However, case reports are beginning to characterize a cluster of effects that appear unique to synthetic cannabinoid overdose. These effects include hyperemesis, agitation or psychotic-like behavior, seizures, extreme hypertension and chest pain, breathing difficulty, and acute kidney injury.[26] These adverse effects of overdose are alarming and appear to describe a cluster of adverse effects unique to synthetic cannabinoids, perhaps due to their higher potency or efficacy.[236]

Treatment of Cannabis and Synthetic Cannabinoid Addiction

No pharmacotherapy is presently approved for use in cannabinoid dependence. The development of CB1 receptor antagonists such as rimonabant has provided a potential candidate, although approval for clinical use of rimonabant in the United States was recently denied due to safety concerns.[167] At present, the only treatments shown to be effective for cannabinoid addiction or dependence are behavioral therapies, including cognitive behavioral therapy, motivational enhancement therapy, and contingency management, or some combination of these three.[34] Due to the controversy surrounding the clinical relevance of cannabis dependence and addiction, potential treatments for the disorder have not been as widely researched as for other substance use disorders such as alcohol or cocaine.

Nicotine

History

Tobacco is a plant native to the Americas. Before domestication, only one strain probably existed; however, propagation of tobacco use across the world under widely varying conditions has produced up to 40 unique species (1). Likely for thousands of years, tobacco was used by pre-Columbian Americans in religious ceremonies. Shamens used tobacco in combination with other substances to simulate near-death experiences.[299a]

Tobacco was introduced to Europe by Christopher Columbus's crew in the late 1400s after they returned from the Bahamas. The natives they encountered smoked cigars which they called *tabacos*. Tobacco was rolled into maize leaves and smoked. Natives of Hispanola burned tobacco over open coals and inhaled the smoke through the nose. The Aztecs smoked tobacco mixed with fragrant herbs and resins from clay pipes, but also insufflated dried, crushed leaves (snuff), and chewed leaves mixed with lime. However, pre-Colombian tobacco use appears to have been confined to North and Central America as the people of South America (with the notable exception of Peru) did not produce pipes or other smoking devices, nor was tobacco part of their folklore or culture before the arrival of Spaniards.[299a] In 1559, Jean Nicot was sent to Lisbon on a diplomatic mission for France. While there, he was introduced to the tobacco plant and snuff, which he brought back to France.[234] Very soon afterward, the use of snuff (kept in sufficiently impressive boxes) was widespread among the nobility of France. For introducing this plant to greater Europe, the genus of tobacco (*Nicotiana*) and its primary psychoactive constituent (nicotine) bear the name of Nicot.[234]

The United States was established, in part, to produce tobacco to meet the growing demand in Europe. From the 1600s on, tobacco use spread widely and quickly around the world. Only within the past 40 years, as the serious health concerns arising from tobacco use have become generally accepted, have smoking rates begun to decline. Since 1965, smoking prevalence among adults in the United States has declined from 40%–50% to 10%–20%.[212a] A recent advent that might alter this trajectory is the development of flavored nicotine solutions used in vaporizer pens.[195a] These products may increase the initiation of teenagers and young adults to nicotine dependence and ultimately could lead to higher levels of nicotine dependence in the coming decades.[195a] Other hazards of this form of consumption, such as serious lung disease, have also become apparent.[121a]

Chemical Properties

The primary active ingredient in tobacco is nicotine. The structure of nicotine is shown in Fig. 17.12. Nicotine has a molecular weight of 162.26 g/mol and is soluble in water. Indeed, nicotine extracted from tobacco in water has been used as an insecticide since 1746.[234]

Pharmacokinetics

Routes of Administration

Tobacco is most commonly rolled into cigarettes and smoked. This has not always been the case. Until the 20th century, tobacco was most commonly chewed, insufflated as snuff, or smoked in pipes.[217a,299a] The advent of cigarette rolling machines led to increased production capacity and ultimately increased consumption of cigarettes. During the 1900s, cigarette manufacturers expended enormous resources on developing improvements in the paper, filters, flavorings, and even the tobacco blends used in cigarettes to produce brand-specific cigarette qualities and to increase consumer desire and demand.[217a]

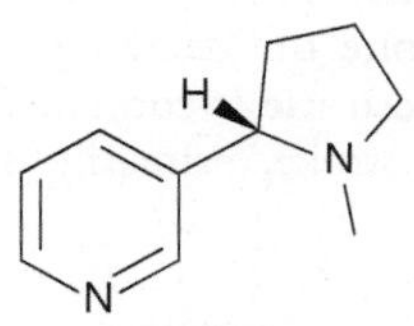

Nicotine

• **Fig. 17.12** Chemical structure of nicotine.

Inhalation of cigarette smoke results in a rapid transfer of nicotine from the lungs into the blood and then into the brain. Nicotine migration from inhaled smoke to lung to brain within 10 seconds has been linked to its high abuse and addiction liability,[121a] though this has recently been questioned.[60a] Because nicotine is a polar compound (weak base with pKa = 8), the use of ammonia during the production process results in a free-base form of the compound which speeds the transfer from lung to blood. Tobacco manufacturers insist that ammonia is used in the production of cigarettes to enhance the flavor of the product, rather than to enhance the psychopharmacological effects of nicotine. However, industry documents show that tobacco companies have known for several decades that the use of ammonia enhances nicotine delivery.[310a]

Tobacco can also be smoked loose in a pipe or rolled into tobacco leaves as a cigar. Many users perceive that such use is less harmful that smoking tobacco in cigarettes. Reasons for these beliefs include the notion that nicotine is an additive in cigarettes but is not present in cigar or pipe tobacco, that cigar or pipe tobacco is less processed or "more organic," and that cigar or pipe smoking behavior is typically more moderate than cigarette smoking.[282a] In fact, smoking tobacco in any formulation presents a similar health risk of developing lung, larnygeal, or oral cancers as well as other diseases that increase morbidity and mortality.[282a]

Smokeless tobacco includes snuff, which is insufflated; dip or chew, which is kept in the mouth in contact with the buccal lining; and several newer formulations, including snus, a Scandinavian snuff product which is held in the mouth inside a pouch. While these forms do not expose the user or bystanders to harmful smoke, smokeless tobacco contains known carcinogens. Exposure to nitrosoamines is extremely high in users of smokeless tobacco, and over a 20-year period of use, exposure levels can reach those known to produce tumors in rodents.[22a] Although results are mixed and at times difficult to interpret due to differences in socioeconomic status, diet, and genetic background, the use of smokeless tobacco generally increases the risk of developing cancer (especially oral, esophageal, and pancreatic cancers), though not as much as use of smoked tobacco.

More recently, electronic cigarettes and other novel nicotine delivery devices have been manufactured.[302a] These cigarettes contain no tobacco and do not burn. Rather, a battery powered atomizer heats a nicotine formulation contained in a disposable filter pack. Users puff on the device just as they would puff on a tobacco cigarette and the tip glows red to simulate the smoking experience. Because the user (and bystanders) are not exposed to smoke or tobacco, these products are touted as safer than other tobacco formulations. However, the cost is more prohibitive than tobacco products (though this may depend on local laws and fees and product packaging,[147a] and no long-term data on the potential health consequences or maintenance of use is yet available on these devices.

Distribution/Bioavailability

A dose of 60 mg of free-base nicotine is considered lethal in humans.[234] Even a dose as low as 4 mg can produce symptoms consistent with acetylcholinesterase inhibitor poisoning, including salivation, vomiting, muscle weakness, convulsions, and fibrillation. Smoke from modern cigarettes yields between 1 and 2 mg of nicotine per cigarette. Nicotine replacement gum is sold in 2- and 4-mg formulations, with the higher dose recommended for heavy (>25 cigarettes/day) smokers who presumably have developed tolerance to nicotine.

Metabolism/Elimination

In animals, only a small portion of administered nicotine is eliminated unchanged. Nicotine and its metabolic products are largely excreted in urine, with a single dose requiring 16 hours for complete elimination.[311a] Nicotine is metabolized to cotinine primarily by the liver, specifically by CYP2A6, CYP2B6, and CYP2E1.[18a] Cotinine has a longer half-life than nicotine (16 hours versus 2 hours, respectively), and thus is increasingly used as a clinical biomarker of recent (2–3 days) nicotine use.[18a]

Pharmacodynamics

Generally, nicotine has a biphasic dose-effect curve, with low doses producing tachycardia, hypertension, and general arousal and higher doses producing bradycardia, hypotension, and sedation.[18a] Still higher doses can produce salivation, emesis, and convulsions. All of these effects of nicotine are subject to rapid and dramatic tolerance upon continued use. Tolerance to central nervous system and cardiovascular effects can occur within a day of use (with a return to morning levels due to abstinence imposed by sleep).

Pharmacological Effects

Nicotine binds to nicotinic achetylcholine (nACh) receptors. These receptors are located in the central nervous system and distributed presynaptically, postsynaptically, and on the cell soma (15). The nicotinic receptors consist of pentomers composed of either five alpha ($\alpha2$–$\alpha10$) subunits or a combinations of alpha and beta ($\beta2$–$\beta4$) subunits.[18a,235a] The most abundant subunits are the $\alpha4$ and $\beta2$, and receptors comprised of these subunits may account for 90% of all nicotine binding sites in the brain.[18a] When acetylcholine or nicotine binds to the recognition site at the interface between an alpha subunit and an adjacent (alpha or beta) subunit, the conformation of the receptor changes, which opens a channel to allow sodium and calcium to enter the cell.[235a] This, in turn, facilitates the release of neurotransmitters—particularly dopamine in the midbrain region but also norepineprine, GABA, glutamate, and endorphins. Because midbrain dopamine appears to be a common pathway activated by drugs of abuse and other pleasurable events, it is believed that this action is central to the addictive nature of tobacco.[18a]

Tissue Effects

In brain, acute administration of nicotine leads to a complex pattern of effects. As noted above, nicotine has a direct effect on neurons, facilitating release of neurotransmitters, including norepiniephrine. The release of norepinephrine from the adrenal cortex and stimulation of the reticular formation results in increased arousal reflected by a decrease in alpha activity of an electroencephalogram.[113a] Respiration is increased due to direct stimulation of the medulla. Nicotine also stimulates the brain region responsible for emesis, leading to vomiting following high doses or in inexperienced users.[113a]

In the periphery, nicotine receptors are found primarily in the neuromuscular junction of voluntary muscles.[113a] Nicotinic stimulation of these receptors can lead to tremor. In the cardiovascular system, nicotine increases heart rate and constricts capillaries in the skin, which leads to increased blood pressure. Nicotine also inhibits stomach secretion and stimulates bowel activity.[113a]

Systemic Effects

Because nicotine produces rapid and profound tolerance, systemic effects of nicotine differ between smokers and nonsmokers.

In smokers, nicotine improves motor performance (in simulated driving tasks) and learning but impairs fine motor control due to the voluntary muscle tremor it produces.[113a] While nicotine administration results in heightened arousal, most smokers report that nicotine is relaxing. This paradoxical effect on mood has been widely studied and may owe more to the other trappings of smoking (holding the cigarette, lighting it, and stopping other activities to focus on the act of smoking) rather than due to a direct effect of nicotine.[113a] Clearly, though, nicotine is reinforcing and promotes subsequent seeking and consumption of the substance, as evidenced by the high rates of addiction to nicotine.[113a]

Toxicology

Acute

High doses of nicotine can lead to respiratory depression and increased secretion of saliva and mucus similar to the effects of a cholinesterase inhibitor. As previously noted, nicotine can increase blood pressure and induce vomiting.

Withdrawal

Tobacco use leads to profound tolerance.[18a] Abrupt cessation of nicotine leads to a wide array of withdrawal signs and syptoms including axiety, dizziness, nausea, constipation, inability to concentrate, weight gain, and sleep disturbances.[113a] The use of nicotine replacement or varenicline can minimize these problems.[169a]

Cardiopulmonary System

Toxic effects of tobacco use on the lungs are due to the inhalation of smoke rather than to direct effects of nicotine. Ash, tar, and products of pyrolysis are deposited in the lungs. The pyrolytic products in the smoke are especially harmful, particularly benz[a]pyrine, which is metabolized into a carcinogenic compound by P-450 enzymes in lung tissue.[234,265a] Nicotine inhibits the action of cilia in the lungs, which normally would move the tar up and out of the lungs and into the esophagus, leading to increased exposure to these toxic chemicals.[113a,152a] Ultimately, this repeated insult to the lining of the lungs can lead to emphysema and lung cancer.[225a,302a]

Tobacco use is clearly linked to an increased risk of heart disease. Direct effects of nicotine on the heart and vasculature are compounded by effects of carbon monoxide and other pyrolytic compounds derived for the accompanying smoke.[113a] Reduced systemic oxygen perfusion further taxes the heart and brain. Additionally, smoking contributes to the deposition of cholesterol on the vascular walls, causing athlerosclerosis.[113a] This also reduces blood perfusion and increases the circulatory pressure.

Stroke

Because smoking is clearly linked to vascular disease, one might assume that smoking could be causally linked to acute cerebral ischemic events (stroke). However, such a relationship has been difficult to demonstrate. In a literature review, Giroud and Dumas[106a] conclude that smoking increases the risk of stroke 1.7 to 5.7 times. Despite the relative lack of data demonstrating a causal link, tobacco use is contraindicated in those at risk of or recovering from stroke, primarily due to its hypertensive effects.[60a,88]

Cancer

While the link between some cancers and smoking is debated,[113a] the link between smoking and lung cancer is clear. By one estimate, 90% of all lung cancer is attributable to exposure to tobacco smoke.[302a] A major constituent of smoke produced by burning tobacco is benzo[a]pyrene, which is oxidized by the P-450 enzyme to trans-7, 8-diol-9, 10-epoxide—a potent carcinogen.[234] While the use of smokeless tobacco can certainly reduce the risk of lung cancer, smokeless tobacco may lead to an increase in oral, esophageal, and pancreatic cancer.[22a] Nitrosoamines that naturally occur in tobacco at extremely high levels are likely the causative element in these cancers, though carcinogenic effects of nicotine itself may also play a role by promoting the growth of cancer cells.[22a,41a]

Therapeutic Effects

Nicotine can improve cognitive function, especially in those afflicted with neurodegenerative disorders such as Alzheimer and Parkinson disease. The use of nicotinic agonists in such patients has recently been suggested.[47a] However, due to the known perils of smoking and even smokeless nicotine delivery, such therapeutic use awaits the development of novel nicotinic agonists and improved delivery methods.

Treatment for Cessation of Smoking

A vast array of drugs has been tested as pharmacotherapeutics for smoking cessation.[169a] Yet few of these studies have proven success over placebo. Presently, the best candidates for pharmacotherapy of smoking include buproprion and nicotine (delivered via gum or a transdermal patch formulation). Varenicline is an exciting new development currently approved as a smoking cessation therapy. Additionally, recent studies suggest that contingency management may be an effective means to reduce smoking in those who wish to stop, as well as in those who do not.

Buproprion appears to be effective in some patients.[308a] It works by blocking reuptake of synaptic dopamine and norepinephrine, which are thought to be important in the reinforcing and conditioned aspects of nicotine effects, respectively.[169a] Nicotine replacement therapy has been shown to be effective in some individuals. Nicotine is provided in chewing gum or on a transdermal patch. Smokers can use the gum as desired while the patch is applied and remains continuously affixed. Nicotine replacement reduces the urge to smoke by providing an alternative means of administration. However, due to potential teratogenic effects of nicotine, its use in pregnant and nursing mothers has been debated.[274a] Varenicline is a nicotinic receptor partial agonist. By occupying nicotine-binding sites, varenicline can blunt or block receptor activation by nicotine, but due to its low efficacy agonist effects, it provides a low level of nicotinic signalling on its own. This compound is approved for use, yet some questions remain over its long-term safety, particularly regarding the potential for development of depression, especially during smoking cessation.[131a,235b] Taken together, several promising pharmacotherapies (including buproprion, nicotine replacement, and varenicline) exist for treatment of tobacco addiction, each of which is more effective than placebo.[77]

In addition to pharmacotherapies, behavioral therapies for smoking have been shown to be effective.[163a] Most promising is contingency management. In this procedure, reducing tobacco use is reinforced, usually with a monetary payout contingent on reduced carbon monoxide or salivary cotinine levels. Even those not wishing to stop smoking reduce their consumption of cigarettes when subjected to contingency management.[163b]

Combining pharmacotherapy with behavioral therapy may be more effective than either alone, though this has yet to be definitively confirmed.[202a]

Inhalants

History

Probably the first wave of inhalant abuse was launched by the discovery of the euphoric properties of ether. During a short-lived prohibition on alcohol in Ireland during the late 19th century, the ethanol-like properties of ether made it an attractive alternative.[233] Volatile substance abuse was first described in 1951, and reports of "sudden sniffing deaths" began appearing in the 1960s.[175] It was at this time that amyl nitrate became widely available. After over-the-counter sales of amyl nitrate were curtailed, other related nitrates were substituted, as were nitrous oxide in the form of small canisters used as whipped cream propellant and solvents such as those found in fuels, paints, and other industrial products. The median age at first inhalant use is 13 years. The lifetime prevalence of use is similar in girls and boys.

Mechanism of Action

Inhalants are generally grouped into three categories. The most commonly used are volatile hydrocarbons, which include fuels such as gasoline and solvents such as toluene.[175] These are the most commonly abused compounds. Volatile alkyl nitrites have distinct pharmacological and behavioral effects and are considered a unique class of inhalant.[175] Finally, nitrous oxide is not a hydrocarbon, but is widely abused as an inhalant.

Historically, the Meyer-Overton hypothesis was invoked to explain inhalant action. Inhalants are highly lipophilic, and the Meyer-Overton hypothesis posits that anesthetic action is related to the disruption of the orientation of membrane-bound proteins by perturbing the lipid membrane, especially in the CNS. This hypothesis was also used for many years to explain the actions of ethanol. However, as with ethanol, more recent evidence suggests that specific alterations in proteins are responsible for neurotransmission, particularly glutamatergic, GABAergic, and opioidergic pathways. In particular, abused volatile solvents appear to share pharmacological effect with certain benzodiazepines, which act as positive allosteric modulators at GABA_A receptors, whereas nitrous oxide appears to share pharmacological effects with NMDA receptor antagonists such as phencyclidine or ketamine.[267]

Smooth Muscle Relaxation

Although other volatile hydrocarbon effects are apparent at specific proteins in the CNS, the alkyl nitrites have not been shown to specifically alter proteins involved in neurotransmission. Rather, these compounds are thought to produce smooth muscle relaxation, perhaps by liberating nitrous oxide.[175] Alternatively, effects due to these drugs could be indirect, resulting from biotransformation into other pharmacologically active chemicals, such as isobutyl alcohol.[175]

NMDA

The first evidence that inhalants could alter ion channel function specifically, rather than nonspecifically by inserting in the lipid bilayer came from Cruz et al.[58] In this study, toluene dose-dependently inhibited inward cationic currents through recombinant *Xenopus* NMDA receptors. The site of action appeared to be in the NR1/NR2B subunit combination, although other combinations were also affected to a lesser extent. Addition of glycine or NMDA did not alter the inhibitory effect of toluene, which would be expected if toluene was acting as an antagonist at the NMDA or glycine site. It is important to note that NMDA function was inhibited at concentrations well below those that altered the conductance of the membrane, indicating that the effects were not due to general disruption of the membrane. AMPA and kainate receptors were not similarly affected. Subsequently, Bale[15] replicated these findings in primary neuronal cultures. Additional evidence for specific action of inhalants at NMDA receptors is the upregulation of NMDA receptors following chronic exposure.[26] Like the volatile hydrocarbons, nitrous oxide also inhibits NMDA receptors.

GABA

Volatile hydrocarbons increase GABA$_A$ receptor function.[175] The site of action on GABA$_A$ receptors appears to be the α1β1 subunit.[166] One volatile convulsant solvent, flurothyl, inhibits recombinant GABA$_A$ receptor. Nitrous oxide does not influence GABAergic signaling. Taken together, volatile hydrocarbon inhalants (excepting alkyl nitrites) share similar pharmacological effects with ethanol, namely inhibition of NMDA receptors and enhancement of GABAergic signaling.

Dopamine

Based on the widespread abuse of inhalants, and the involvement of the dopaminergic system in reinforcing actions of many abused drugs, one might expect inhalants to enhance dopaminergic signaling. Indeed, brief exposure to toluene increases dopaminergic firing from the ventral tegmental area and increases extracellular dopamine in the nucleus accumbens.[166] Although this evidence is consistent with dopaminergic effects of other abused drugs, it is likely that these effects are due to indirect actions of solvents at GABA receptors, rather than to a direct effect on dopamine receptors.[166]

Other Receptors and Ion Channels

There is some evidence of opioidergic involvement in the effects of inhalants. The antinociceptive effects of nitrous oxide are antagonized by naloxone, although the anesthetic effects are not.[175] Acute toluene exposure increases μ-opioid receptor protein levels in the brainstem.[179] There is also evidence of volatile organic solvents affecting serotonin (5HT3) receptors, P2X receptors, and voltage-gated ion channels, although the relationship between these effects and behavioral effects remains murky.

Pharmacokinetics

Generally, inhalants are highly lipophilic, and are rapidly absorbed and eliminated. Inhalants are eliminated unchanged by respiration, are metabolized in the liver, or both.[175] Nitrous oxide is eliminated unchanged by respiration, whereas aromatic hydrocarbons are largely metabolized by hepatic mechanisms. Alkyl nitrites may be converted to alcohols as well as nitric oxide donors. Metabolism of aromatic hydrocarbons in the liver occurs via the CYP system. The CYP2E1 enzyme appears to be the primary enzyme recruited.[175] Extrahepatic metabolism of aromatic hydrocarbons occurs to a lesser extent and may result in organ-specific toxicity.

Pharmacodynamics

Toluene produces a biphasic effect on locomotion, similar to ethanol. Low doses result in hyperlocomotion, with higher doses progressing from sedation to motor impairment to anesthesia.[166] Inhalants can protect against seizures in animals, although convulsions have also been seen. In humans, inhalants rarely produce convulsions.[166] Toluene exerts anxiolytic effects in animal models, which might be expected due to activity at GABA$_A$ receptors. Rats exposed to toluene chronically show deficits in learning and memory as assessed by the Morris-water maze inhalant abusers.

Operant work with inhalants is sparse. One major impediment is producing consistent exposure conditions inside of the chamber typically used for such studies. However, operant responding for food is diminished by acute exposure to inhalants, regardless of the schedule of reinforcement employed.[166] Toluene and other solvents share discriminative stimulus effects with other classic CNS depressants such as ethanol. This is not surprising considering the effects on GABA$_A$ and NMDA receptors common to these drug classes. Although some have reported success at training rodents to self-administer solvents intravenously, establishing inhalant self-administration has yet to be reported.[166] Proper containment of the volatilized solvent and consistent delivery contingent upon an appropriate response will be required to perform such procedures.

Toxicology

Each class of inhalants presents its own unique toxicology. Chronic use of any inhalant can lead to neuropathy. Volatile organic solvents present the most overt and widespread toxicological effects, including cardio, renal, and hepatic toxicities. Amyl nitrites also produce direct toxic effects, whereas toxic effects of nitrous oxide are indirect.

Volatile organic solvent abuse leads to an array of toxic effects. Most common are neuropathies. Neurological damage is generally not dose related. However, there may be a relationship between neurological damage and duration of use.[179] Chronic abuse of n-hexane (found in glues and fuel) is associated with peripheral neuropathy, whereas toluene is associated with cerebellar disease.[179] Neuropathy related to volatile organic solvent use can present as euphoria and hallucinations, headache dizziness progressing to slurred speech, confusion, tremor, and weakness. Transient cranial nerve palsy can also occur. Heavy use of these agents leads to white matter degeneration and demyelination evidenced by perivascular macrophages containing coarse or laminar myelin debris.

Pulmonary effects are due to either direct damage to lung tissue or asphyxiation.[179] Hypoxia causes pulmonary toxicity and is usually due to the method of administration (mask/rebreathing) rather than overabundance of hydrocarbons.[175] Also inadvertent aspiration of liquid hydrocarbon can injure tissue.

Acute cardiotoxicity is usually the cause of sudden sniffing death. It is thought that the inhalant sensitizes the myocardium by blocking the potassium current, prolonging repolarization—a substrate for dysrhythmia.[175] Chronic use can result in chronic myocarditis with fibrosis, and present as palpitations, shortness of breath, syncope, and electrocardiographic abnormalities.[175] Renal disorders are especially associated with toluene abuse. In particular, chronic toluene exposure is considered causal for tubular acidosis, urinary calculi, glomerulonephritis, and renal failure. Distal renal tubular acidosis can result in hypokalemia and muscle weakness. Hepatic failure has also been observed, primarily following halogenated hydrocarbon use, such as carbon tetrachloride or refrigerants, probably due to a reactive metabolite withdrawal nsity in rod.

Volatile alkyl nitrite use is associated with methemoglobinemia.[175] This may be a result of the ability of these strong oxidants to change the charge on the ferrous ion from Fe^{2+} to Fe^{3+}.[175] The most prominent toxic effects of nitrous oxide are due to asphyxiation and auto accidents, rather than to a direct effect of the agent. Chronic abuse can lead to irreversible oxidation of cobalamin (vitamin B_{12}), which leads to aberrations in the myelin sheath.

Barbiturates

History

Among classes of abused drugs, barbiturates are relative newcomers, with a history of just over 100 years of use and abuse. The primary reason for this rather short history is that, unlike drugs from other pharmacological classes, barbiturates have not been found in nature and had to be developed in the laboratory. In 1864, Adolf von Baeyer synthesized the first barbiturate, malonylurea, which was later named barbituric acid.[176] With the perfection of the synthetic process by Edouard Grimaux in 1879, derivatives of barbituric acid could be widely developed, including diethyl-barbituric acid or barbital, which became the first barbiturate on the market in 1904.[176] The clinical success of barbiturates led to the synthesis of more than 2500 different compounds, with 50 of them available clinically.

Barbiturates were initially introduced as hypnotics, although other effects became evident with their continued development and clinical use. For example, the anticonvulsant effects were discovered in 1912, the same year that phenobarbital was first available commercially.[128,176] Systematic use of barbiturates in intravenous anesthesia did not occur until 1927, with pentobarbital introduced in anesthesia in 1930, and thiopental and methohexital introduced later (1936 and 1956, respectively). These therapeutic effects led to the huge popularity and widespread use of the barbiturates, which peaked during the 1930s and 1940s.[128] In addition to the therapeutic effects of barbiturates, adverse effects were also increasingly evident. One effect that took very little time to emerge was the development of dependence. Evidence that dependence developed with repeated barbiturate administration appeared in the literature in 1905, 1 year after the introduction of barbital.[176] Another problem associated with the use of barbiturates was fatal overdose. In fact, the two scientists who were responsible for the introduction of barbital in 1904, Josef von Mering and Emil Fischer, are thought to have been dependent on barbiturates and to have died of a possible overdose.[176] The abuse potential of these drugs was not reliably documented until the 1950s.[128] Together, these adverse effects led to the decline of the clinical use of barbiturates, which was further exacerbated by the introduction of the benzodiazepines in the 1960s. This new class of drugs produced similar therapeutic effects with a greater margin of safety. Today, barbiturates are used clinically for some indications, mostly for certain types of seizures and for induction of anesthesia.

Chemical Properties

Barbituric acid is 2,4,6-trioxohexahydropyrimidine (see Fig. 17.11). Clinically useful barbiturates are formed by the addition of alkyl or aryl groups at position 5.[125] Salts can result when the carbonyl group on position 2 takes on an acidic character, thereby improving solubility in water and increasing absorption.[125] Thus sodium salts are more amenable to intravenous administration and are the form of barbiturates used in anesthesia. Although barbiturates are highly lipid soluble, replacing the oxygen at C2

with sulfur decreases partition coefficients, resulting in drugs with shorter onsets and durations of action.[125] These barbiturates, which include thiopental, have been used extensively to induce anesthesia (Fig. 17.13).

Pharmacokinetics

Routes of Administration

Because mechanism of action does not vary among barbiturates, these drugs are generally classified according to their pharmacokinetics, specifically by their duration of action.[67] Differences in formulations, therapeutic use, and abuse of barbiturates are due to differences in their duration of action. For example, ultrashort-acting barbiturates, such as methohexital and thiopental, are available only for intravenous use and are used exclusively for induction of anesthesia. Short- to intermediate-acting barbiturates, such as pentobarbital, are available in capsules, suppositories, or in solution for intravenous or intramuscular administration. Long-acting barbiturates, such as phenobarbital, are available only for oral use.

Absorption and Distribution

After oral administration, barbiturates are rapidly and completely absorbed from the upper part of the small intestine. Long-acting barbiturates are absorbed more slowly than shorter-acting drugs.[313] Barbiturates are widely distributed, beginning with highly vascularized areas like the brain. For the highly lipid-soluble, ultra-short-acting drugs, these initially high concentrations of barbiturates in the CNS decline as the drug distributes to less vascularized areas like muscle and fat.[125] This redistribution of barbiturates from the brain to other tissues contributes to the very short duration of action of these drugs.

Metabolism and Excretion

Barbiturates are almost completely metabolized in the liver before renal excretion, and unchanged barbiturates infrequently appear in urine.[313] Microsomal enzymes oxidate the larger of the two substituent groups at position 5, forming alcohols, phenols, ketones, or carboxylic acids.[125] Repeated administration of barbiturates results in the induction of the hepatic enzymes responsible for their inactivation. This metabolic tolerance shortens the half-life of barbiturates as well as that of any other drugs metabolized through the same enzymes.

Pharmacodynamics

Mechanism of Action

Barbiturates act at $GABA_A$ receptors. The $GABA_A$ receptor complex is a transmembrane protein complex that is formed by five subunits with multiple binding sites on each $GABA_A$

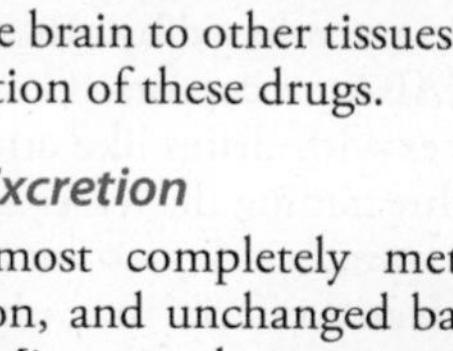

• **Fig. 17.13** Structure of barbituric acid. (From http://pubchem.ncbi.nlm.nih.gov.)

receptor. When GABA binds to its distinct sites on this protein complex, channels open and Cl⁻ enters the cell. Other sites on the GABA$_A$ receptor complex are modulatory sites, and drugs acting at these sites can alter the effects of GABA. Barbiturates act at distinct modulatory sites to facilitate the actions of GABA, thereby increasing Cl⁻ flux.[7] At large concentrations, barbiturates can activate channels even in the absence of GABA$_A$.[7,89,244]

Pharmacological Effects

The primary pharmacological effect of barbiturates is to decrease activity of the CNS. The most prominent effects of barbiturates are their sedative effects, which vary with dose from mild sedation to general anesthesia. These drugs decrease sleep latency and the number of awakenings and can also affect the stages of sleep by decreasing time spent in rapid-eye-movement and slow-wave sleep.[125] Barbiturates can also reduce anxiety, although sometimes this effect is difficult to dissociate from sedative effects. The ability of barbiturates to prevent and reverse convulsions continues to be exploited clinically.

Toxicology

In addition to these therapeutic effects, depression of the CNS also accounts for the most serious acute toxicological effect of barbiturates. When CNS activity is reduced, there is a concomitant decrease in ventilation. Barbiturates affect both respiratory drive and its rhythmic characteristics, and at large doses, these effects can be sufficiently severe to eliminate respiration. Thus acute barbiturate overdose can be fatal. The respiratory-depressant effects of barbiturates can also be exacerbated by other drugs, particularly those with actions at GABA$_A$ receptors. Combinations of sublethal doses of barbiturates with drugs like ethanol or benzodiazepines can result in life-threatening decreases in ventilation.

In addition to their respiratory-depressant effects, barbiturates produce several other adverse effects that ultimately led to the decline of their clinical use. Perhaps the most serious problems occur when the drugs are administered repeatedly. Chronic use or abuse of sedative doses of barbiturates can result in the development of tolerance or dependence. In addition to pharmacokinetic tolerance that occurs when hepatic microsomal enzymes are induced, pharmacodynamic tolerance can also develop, which likely involves changes in GABA$_A$ receptor structure or function. One change that occurs in GABA$_A$ receptors during chronic barbiturate treatment is a functional uncoupling of binding sites.[322] Regardless of the mechanism, the development of tolerance has multiple consequences. First, a larger dose or more frequent administration is needed to maintain the desired effect. Because pharmacokinetic tolerance shortens the duration of action of a drug without altering the amount of drug needed to produce an effect, use of larger doses could lead to overdose.[313] Even if overdose is avoided by increasing frequency rather than dose, the escalating intake is more likely to result in the development of dependence and the emergence of a more robust withdrawal syndrome.

A second important consequence of chronic barbiturate treatment is the development of dependence, which is evident when withdrawal signs emerge following abrupt discontinuation of treatment. Signs begin to appear 24 hours after the last dose of the barbiturate, peak within 2–3 days, and subside slowly over the next 10–14 days.[93,306] The withdrawal syndrome has been classified based on the severity of signs and symptoms. For example, mild signs include apprehension, muscle weakness, tremors, twitches, orthostatic hypotension, anorexia, insomnia, anxiety, and profuse sweating, whereas severe withdrawal includes tonic-clonic seizures and psychosis, which usually resembles delirium tremens that are observed when alcohol use is discontinued.[306] Increasing the dose, frequency, or duration of chronic barbiturate treatment will increase the severity of the withdrawal syndrome that emerges when treatment is terminated. Because the most serious signs of barbiturate withdrawal can be life-threatening, one approach that has been used to decrease barbiturate use while avoiding severe withdrawal signs has been to substitute an equivalent dose of a longer-acting barbiturate, such as phenobarbital, for the drug administered chronically.[275] The slow offset of the longer-acting drug results in the maintenance of more constant blood levels of the barbiturate, thereby preventing the emergence of severe withdrawal; the dose of phenobarbital can be decreased slowly over time until the individual can safely stop taking barbiturates altogether.

Although barbiturate abuse has declined over the last 40 years along with the decline of clinical use, barbiturates have been abused more frequently than other CNS depressants except for alcohol. Some people abuse barbiturates exclusively. Often, use of barbiturates began when they were prescribed for the treatment of some disorder. With continued use and possibly escalating intake due to the development of tolerance, dependence also developed, leading to the emergence of withdrawal when treatment was discontinued. These abusers continue to take barbiturates to avoid withdrawal, as opposed to taking the drug to treat the condition that prompted the initial use of barbiturates.[67] In contrast, other abusers take barbiturates in small doses, infrequently, or for short periods so that dependence does not develop. These abusers often use barbiturates in combination with other drugs of abuse, including ethanol, opioids, and psychoactive stimulants.

Benzodiazepines

History

The history of the benzodiazepines is even shorter than that of the barbiturates. In the 1930s, Dr. Leo Sternbach was working on a chemical group called heptoxdiazines, which did not seem to have biological activity.[163] He moved from Poland to the United States to work for Hoffmann-LaRoche where he resumed his study of these compounds. In 1957, pharmacological effects, including sedative effects, were observed for one of his compounds (Ro#5-0690); the chemists later found that the compound had undergone a molecular rearrangement to become a 1,4-benzodiazepine.[163] Initially, the compound was called methaminodiazepoxide, although the name was later changed to chlordiazepoxide. The clinical effectiveness of chlordiazepoxide was not immediately evident. In fact, chlordiazepoxide was nearly discarded because a large dose was given to geriatric patients, which resulted in ataxia.[163] Eventually, more appropriate doses were used and its clinical utility and safety were established. It was introduced in 1960 with the more successful benzodiazepine diazepam introduced in 1963. More than 3000 benzodiazepines have been synthesized, with as many as 35 in clinical use around the world. Because benzodiazepines have a larger margin of safety, as compared with the barbiturates, they quickly became the drugs of choice to reduce anxiety, promote sleep, and reverse convulsions.

Although benzodiazepines are still used widely today for some indications, their use is now being strongly discouraged in patients who are receiving opioids to treat pain or opioid abuse because it has become clear that the risk of fatal opioid overdose is increased by the concurrent use of benzodiazepines.[g] Most opioid abusers, including those in treatment programs, also abuse benzodiazepines. Moreover, benzodiazepines are often prescribed with opioids; concomitant prescribing of opioids and benzodiazepines increased 41% between 2002 and 2014,[133] and concurrent therapeutic use of opioids and benzodiazepines increased 53% between 2003 and 2011 among US veterans.[119] Clearly, people are using or abusing opioids and benzodiazepines together, and concurrent use of drugs from these two pharmacological classes is the factor most often associated with opioid overdose and death.[31,61,144,168] In addition, overdose is more likely in pain patients who are prescribed both opioids and benzodiazepines, as compared with patients receiving prescription opioids and not benzodiazepines.[224,262] Given the large body of evidence indicating the serious risks involved with combined use, the Centers for Disease Control and Prevention has recommended that clinicians avoid prescribing benzodiazepines with opioids[72] and the US Food and Drug Administration has added a boxed warning to all benzodiazepines and opioids marketed to treat pain or cough (a total of nearly 400 products) with information about the risks of concurrent use.[87]

Chemical Properties

Benzodiazepine refers to the chemical structure of the drug, which has a benzene ring fused to a seven-member diazepine ring; benzodiazepines that are used clinically have 1,4-diazepine rings.[125] Substituent groups at positions 1 and 3 can vary widely. Unlike diazepam (see Fig. 17.13), some benzodiazepines have triazolo (e.g., triazolam, alprazolam) or imidazolo (e.g., midazolam) rings fused at positions 1 and 2.[125] Another drug with a fused imidazolo ring at positions 1 and 2 also has a methyl group at position 4 and a keto group replacing the ring at position 5; these structural variations dramatically change the pharmacology, resulting in the benzodiazepine antagonist flumazenil.[125] Like barbiturates, benzodiazepines have high lipid-to-water distribution coefficients; unfortunately, benzodiazepines do not form salts as readily as barbiturates do. With exception of midazolam and chlordiazepoxide, which can form hydrochloride salts, benzodiazepines are insoluble in water (Fig. 17.14).

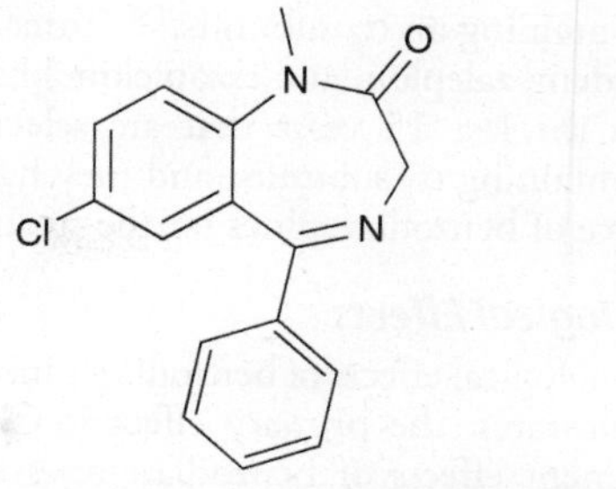

Pharmacokinetics

Routes of Administration

Another similarity between barbiturates and benzodiazepines is that within each class of compounds, the mechanism of action does not vary. Consequently, benzodiazepines are also generally classified according to their pharmacokinetics, specifically by their duration of action. Short-acting benzodiazepines generally have a half-life of minutes to a few hours; these drugs, which include midazolam, are primarily used for conscious sedation or the induction of anesthesia and are, therefore, available in commercially prepared solutions for intravenous administration. Intermediate-acting benzodiazepines, such as alprazolam or lorazepam, are used orally for anxiety and insomnia, although lorazepam is also available for

• **Fig. 17.14** Structure of diazepam. (From http://pub.chem.ncbi.nlm.nih.gov.)

parenteral administration, primarily to reverse convulsions. Long-acting drugs, such as diazepam, are generally used orally.

Absorption and Distribution

The benzodiazepines that are currently used clinically are completely absorbed after oral administration. Once in the systemic circulation, they bind to plasma proteins, with the extent of binding varying with lipid solubility from 70% for alprazolam to 99% for diazepam.[125] Redistribution can occur for drugs with the highest lipid solubility.

Metabolism and Excretion

Benzodiazepines are extensively metabolized by several hepatic microsomal systems. The most important aspect of the pharmacokinetics of benzodiazepines is the formation of active metabolites. Although a few benzodiazepines (e.g., lorazepam) are inactivated by the initial metabolic reaction, most are converted to metabolites that have the same mechanism of action as the parent compound. For some drugs, more than one biotransformation reaction is needed to inactivate the drug and often the subsequent reactions occur more slowly than the initial reaction. Consequently, the duration of action of most benzodiazepines has little to do with its half-life in plasma. The hepatic enzymes responsible for metabolism of benzodiazepines are not induced by chronic benzodiazepine treatment.

Pharmacodynamics

Mechanism of Action

Like barbiturates, benzodiazepines act at their own distinct sites on $GABA_A$ receptors, where they facilitate the actions of GABA.[218] One distinct difference between benzodiazepines and barbiturates is that benzodiazepines do not activate the channel directly and their actions are dependent on the presence of GABA.[117,271] $GABA_A$ receptors are formed by 5 protein subunits, which form the ion channel. Based on their amino acid sequence, several classes of subunits have been identified with multiple variants within each class.[180] The large number of subunits that can be combined to form $GABA_A$ receptor complexes indicates that many variations of this complex are possible. The subunit composition of $GABA_A$ receptors is clearly important in forming modulatory sites, particularly benzodiazepine sites. The $GABA_A$ receptor complex often includes 2α, 1β, and 2γ subunits. Benzodiazepine binding sites are formed when a γ_2 subunit is coexpressed with any α and any β,[180] with the subtype of the α subunit conferring selectivity to benzodiazepine ligands.[70] Generally, 1,4-benzodiazepines bind with high affinity to benzodiazepine receptors containing an α_1, α_2, α_3, or α_5 subunit and do not bind, or bind with very low affinity, to receptors containing an α_4 subunits.[180] Three nonbenzodiazepine drugs (zolpidem, zaleplon, and eszopiclone) have been introduced clinically in the last 15 years that are selective benzodiazepine receptors containing α_1 subunits, and they have been used extensively in place of benzodiazepines for the treatment of insomnia.

Pharmacological Effects

The pharmacological effects of benzodiazepines are similar to those of the barbiturates; the primary effect is CNS depression. The most prominent effects of benzodiazepines are their anxiolytic, sedative, and anticonvulsant effects, although other therapeutic uses include their use as muscle relaxants or to induce anesthesia. In terms of clinical utility, benzodiazepines are similar to barbiturates in many ways. For example, drugs from these pharmacological classes promote sleep by decreasing sleep latency, the number of awakenings, and the time spent in rapid-eye-movement and slow-wave sleep while increasing the time spent in stage 2 sleep.[125] One way in which drugs from these classes differ is their ability to relieve anxiety; the anxiolytic effects of benzodiazepines are evident at doses that do not produce sedation, whereas doses of barbiturates that produce anxiolytic effects also produce sedation.

Toxicology

Benzodiazepines are relatively safe drugs. Although CNS depression by benzodiazepines results in decreased ventilation, these respiratory-depressant effects are mild. Even when the dose of benzodiazepines is increased, the effects on respiration are not sufficiently severe to be life-threatening. From a clinical perspective, benzodiazepines are much safer than barbiturates because of differences in the severity of respiratory-depressant effects; this larger margin of safety of benzodiazepines has resulted in their widespread use and contributed to the decline of the clinical use of barbiturates. When administered alone, benzodiazepine overdose does not result in life-threatening respiratory depression; however, these effects can be exacerbated by other drugs. Ventilation can be dramatically decreased when benzodiazepines are administered in combination with ethanol, other positive $GABA_A$ modulators, or drugs with primary mechanisms of action at receptors other than gamma receptors, such as opioids.

Although overdose of benzodiazepines does not result in severe acute effects, their use is limited by other adverse effects, particularly by effects that occur during chronic treatment. For example, the use of sedative doses of benzodiazepines for 2 weeks can result in the development of tolerance. Escalating intake to maintain the therapeutic effect can exacerbate the development of dependence. To avoid both phenomena, physicians generally limit the duration of benzodiazepine use to less than 2 weeks. Because drugs selective for benzodiazepine receptors containing α_1 subunits have sedative effects and are less likely to produce tolerance, the introduction of these drugs has led to a decline in the use of benzodiazepines for insomnia. Tolerance is less problematic when benzodiazepines are used for other indications, such as anxiety, because smaller doses are needed to produce the therapeutic effect and tolerance is less likely to develop under those treatment conditions.

Another consequence of long-term use of benzodiazepines is the development of dependence, and the signs and symptoms that emerge when benzodiazepine treatment is discontinued are similar to those that are evident following termination of barbiturate treatment. Like barbiturate withdrawal, signs and symptoms of benzodiazepine withdrawal can be separated into categories based on their severity. Minor withdrawal symptoms include increased anxiety, involuntary muscle twitches, tremor, progressive weakness, dizziness, visual illusions, nausea, insomnia, weight loss, and orthostatic hypotension; major withdrawal symptoms include tonic-clonic seizures and psychosis resembling delirium tremens that occurs when alcohol use is discontinued.[221] More recently, the importance of other withdrawal symptoms, such as sleep disturbances, has been recognized.[205,236] Although the signs and symptoms of withdrawal are similar for benzodiazepines and barbiturates, the time course for the development of dependence and the emergence of withdrawal varies slightly between these classes of drugs. Benzodiazepine dependence becomes evident only after long periods of treatment, often requiring 3 months or longer.[313] Moreover, because of the long duration of action of benzodiazepines and the formation of active metabolites, withdrawal might not emerge until 3–7 days after discontinuation of treatment. The availability of benzodiazepines with long durations of action increases the feasibility of using a drug with a slow offset to maintain more constant blood levels of a benzodiazepine while slowly reducing the dose. In this manner, benzodiazepine use can be decreased while avoiding the emergence of robust withdrawal.

Like other drugs that act at $GABA_A$ receptors, benzodiazepines are abused, and benzodiazepine abuse appears to be increasing. From 2000 to 2014, there was a 1.5-fold increase in abuse of benzodiazepines alone.[38a] Despite these recent increases, the incidence of primary benzodiazepine abuse remains low in the general population; however, benzodiazepine abuse is high in some groups, particularly among people who abuse other drugs. For example, the incidence of benzodiazepine use is high among opioid abusers.[98,111] Dependence can develop during chronic benzodiazepine abuse, and the emergence of withdrawal can impact treatment outcome. Individuals sometimes prolong their drug use or abuse in order to avoid withdrawal, and relapse is common as they try to alleviate withdrawal symptoms.[11] For example, when treatment is discontinued in individuals using benzodiazepines for insomnia, the relapse rate is 43%.[205] Similarly, 50% of polydrug abusers experiencing withdrawal from large doses of benzodiazepines resume drug use within 2–3 days, with individuals describing extreme measures taken to avoid withdrawal.[265] Thus emergence of benzodiazepine withdrawal could have severe consequences in drug abusers, possibly leading to increased abuse of benzodiazepines and other drugs.

References

1. Aarde SM, Creehan KM, Vandewater SA, Dickerson TJ, Taffe MA. In vivo potency and efficacy of the novel cathinone α-pyrrolidinopentiophenone and 3,4-methylenedioxypyrovalerone: self-administration and locomotor stimulation in male rats. *Psychopharmacology (Berl)*. 2015;232:3045–3055.
2. Aarde SM, Huang PK, Creehan KM, Dickerson TJ, Taffe MA. The novel recreational drug 3,4-methylenedioxypyrovalerone (MDPV) is a potent psychomotor stimulant: self-administration and locomotor activity in rats. *Neuropharmacology*. 2013;71:130–140.
3. Abrams DI, et al. Vaporization as a smokeless cannabis delivery system: a pilot study. *Clin Pharmacol Ther*. 2007;82:572–578.
4. Aceto MD, Harris LS, Abood ME, et al. Stereoselective mu- and delta-opioid receptor-related antinociception and binding with (+)-thebaine. *Eur J Pharmacol*. 1999;365:143–147.
5. Aderjan RE, Skopp G. Formation and clearance of active and inactive metabolites of opiates in humans. *Ther Drug Monit*. 1998;20:561–569.

5a. Aghajanian GK, Bing OH. Persistence of lysergic acid diethyl-amidein the plasma of human subjects. *Clin Pharmacol Therap*. 1964;5:611–614.

6. Aistrup GL, Marszalec W, Narahashi T. Ethanol modulation of nicotinic acetylcholine receptor currents in cultured cortical neurons. *Mol Pharmacol*. 1999;55:39–49.

7. Allan AM, Harris RA. Anesthetic and convulsant barbiturates alter gamma-aminobutyric acid-stimulated chloride flux across brain membranes. *J Pharmacol Exp Ther*. 1986;238:763–768.

8. Allan AM, Harris RA. Acute and chronic ethanol treatments alter gaba receptor-operated chloride channels. *Pharmacol Biochem Behav*. 1987;27:665–670.

9. Angell M, Kassirer JP. Alcohol and other drugs - toward a more rational and consistent policy. *N Engl J Med*. 1994;331:537–539.

10. Anizan S, Concheiro M, Lehner KR, et al. Linear pharmacokinetics of 3,4-methylenedioxypyrovalerone (MDPV) and its metabolites in the rat: relationship to pharmacodynamic effects. *Addict Biol*. 2016;21:339–347.

11. Ashton H. The diagnosis and management of benzodiazepine dependence. *Curr Opin Psychiatry*. 2005;18:249–255.

12. Ashton JC. Synthetic cannabinoids as drugs of abuse. *Curr Drug Abuse Rev*. 2012;5:158–168.

13. Bagnardi C, Zambon A, Quatto P, et al. Flexible meeta-regression functions for modeling aggregate dose-response data, with an application to alcohol and mortality. *Am J Epidemiol*. 2004;159:1077–1086.

14. Bakhit C, Gibb JW. Methamphetamine-induced depression of tryptophan hydroxylase: recovery following acute treatment. *Eur J Pharmacol*. 1981;76:229–233.

15. Bale AS, Tu Y, Carpenter-Hyland EP, et al. Alterations in glutamatergic and gabaergic ion channel activity in hippocampal neurons following exposure to the abused inhalant toluene. *Neuroscience*. 2005;130:197–206.

16. Barnett G, Hawks R, Resnick R. Cocaine pharmacokinetics in humans. *J Ethnopharmacol*. 1981;3:353–366.

17. Barquin J, de Dios Luna J, Hernandez AF. A controlled study of the time-course of breath alcohol concentration after moderate ingestion of ethanol following a social drinking session. *Forensic Sci Int*. 2008;177:140–145.

18. Baumann MH, Partilla JS, Lehner KR, et al. Powerful cocaine-like actions of 3,4-methylenedioxypyrovalerone (MDPV), a principal constituent of psychoactive "bath salts" products. *Neuropsychopharmacology*. 2013;38:552–562.

18a. Benowitz NL. Neurobiology of nicotine addiction: implications for smoking cessation treatment. *Am J Med*. 2008;121(4 suppl 1):S3–S10.

19. Benzie F, Hekman K, Cameron L, et al. Emergency department visits after use of a drug sold as " bath salts " — Michigan, November 13, 2010-March 31, 2011. *Morbid Mortal Weekly Rep*. 2011;60:624–627.

20. Blednov YA, Stoffel M, Alva H, et al. A pervasive mechanism for analgesia: activation of GIRK2 channels. *Proc Natl Acad Sci USA*. 2003;100:277–282.

21. Bleich A, Gelkopf M, Schmidt V, Hayward R, Bodner G, Adelson M. Correlates of benzodiazepine abuse in methadone maintenance treatment. A 1 year prospective study in an Israeli clinic. *Addiction*. 1999;94:1533–1540.

22. Boettcher C, Fellermeier M, Boettcher C, et al. How human neuroblastoma cells make morphine. *Proc Natl Acad Sci USA*. 2005;102:8495–8500.

22a. Boffetta P, Hecht S, Gray N, Gupta P, Straif K. Smokeless tobacco and cancer. *Lancet Oncol*. 2008;9(7):667–675.

23. Bogenschutz MP, et al. Psilocybin-assisted treatment for alcohol dependence: a proof-of-concept study. *J Psychopharmacol Oxf Engl*. 2015;29:289–299.

24. Borowsky B, Adham N, Jones KA, et al. Trace amines: identification of a family of mammalian G protein-coupled receptors. *Proc Natl Acad Sci USA*. 2001;98:8966–8971.

25. Bortolato M, Mangieri RA, Fu J, et al. Antidepressant-like activity of the fatty acid amide hydrolase inhibitor URB597 in a rat model of chronic mild stress. *Biol Psychiatry*. 2007;62:1103–1110.

26. Bowen SE, Batis JC, Paez-Martinez N, et al. The last decade of solvent research in animal models of abuse: mechanistic and behavioral studies. *Neurotoxicol Teratol*. 2006;28:636–647.

27. Bracken MB, Eskenazi B, McSharry J-E, et al. Association of cocaine use with sperm concentration, motility, and morphology. *Fertil Steril*. 1990;53:315–322.

28. Branchek TA, Blackburn TP. Trace amine receptors as targets for novel therapeutics: legend, myth and fact. *Curr Opin Pharmacol*. 2003;3:90–97.

29. Brandt SD, Sumnall HR, Measham F, Cole J. Analyses of second-generation 'legal highs' in the UK: initial findings. *Drug Test Anal*. 2010;2:377–382.

30. Brenneisen R. Pharmacokinetics. In: Grotenhermen F, Russo E, eds. *Cannabis and Cannabinoids: Pharmacology, Toxicology, and Therapeutic Potential*. Binghamton, NY: Hayworth Integrative Healing; 2002:67–73.

31. Bretteville-Jensen AL, Lillehagen M, Gjersing L, Andreas JB. Illicit use of opioid substitution drugs: prevalence, user characteristics, and association with non-fatal overdoses. *Drug Alcohol Depend*. 2015;147:89–96.

32. Brownstein MJ. A brief history of opiates, opioid peptides, and opioid receptors. *Proc Natl Acad Sci USA*. 1993;90:5391–5393.

33. Brunt TM, Poortman A, Niesink RJ, van den Brink W. Instability of the ecstasy market and a new kid on the block: mephedrone. *J Psychopharmacol*. 2011;25:1543–1547.

34. Budney AJ, Roffman R, Stephens RS, et al. Marijuana dependence and its treatment. *Addict Sci Clin Pract*. 2007;4:4–16.

35. Caine SB, Heinrichs SC, Coffin VL, et al. Effects of the dopamine D-1 antagonist SCH 23390 microinjected into the accumbens, amygdala or striatum on cocaine self-administration in the rat. *Brain Res*. 1995;692:47–56.

36. Caine SB, Koob GF. Effects of dopamine D-1 and D-2 antagonists on cocaine self-administration under different schedules of reinforcement in the rat. *J Pharmacol Exp Ther*. 1994;270:209–218.

37. Caine SB, Thomsen M, Gabriel KI, et al. Lack of self-administration of cocaine in dopamine D1 receptor knock-out mice. *J Neurosci*. 2007;27:13140–13150.

38. Calatayud J, Gonzalez A. History of the development and evolution of local anesthesia since the coca leaf [see comment]. *Anesthesiology*. 2003;98:1503–1508.

38a. Calcaterra SL, Severtson SG, Bau GE, et al. Trends in intentional abuse or misuse of benzodiazepines and opioid analgesics and the associated mortality reported to poison centers across the United States from 2000 to 2014. *Clin Toxicol (Phila)*. 2018;56(11):1107–1114.

39. Callahan PM, De la GR, Cunningham KA. Discriminative stimulus properties of cocaine: modulation by dopamine D1 receptors in the nucleus accumbens. *Psychopharmacology*. 1994;115:110–114.

40. Carhart-Harris RL, King LA, Nutt DJ. A web-based survey on mephedrone. *Drug Alcohol Depend*. 2011;118:19–22.

41. Castaneto MS, et al. Synthetic cannabinoids: epidemiology, pharmacodynamics, and clinical implications. *Drug Alcohol Depend*. 2014. https://doi.org/10.1016/j.drugalcdep.2014.08.005.

41a. Catassi A, Servent D, Paleari L, Cesario A, Russo P. Multiple roles of nicotine on cell proliferation and inhibition of apoptosis: implications on lung carcinogenesis. *Mutat Res*. 2008;659(3):221–231.

42. Caudevilla-Gálligo F, Ventura M, Iciar BI, Ruiz I, Fornís I. Presence and composition of cathinone derivatives in drug samples taken from a Drug Test Service in Spain (2010–2012). *Hum Psychopharmacol*. 2013;28:341–344.

43. Chan GC, Hinds TR, Impey S, et al. Hippocampal neurotoxicity of Delta9- tetrahydrocannabinol. *J Neurosci*. 1998;18:5322–5332.

44. Chao C, Jacobson LP, Tashkin D, et al. Recreational drug use and T lymphocyte subpopulations in HIV-uninfected and HIV-infected men. *Drug Alcohol Depend*. 2008;94:165–171.

45. Reference deleted in review.
46. Cheatle MD. Prescription opioid misuse, abuse, morbidity, and mortality: balancing effective pain management and safety. *Pain Med*. 2015;16:S3–S8.
47. Cocores JA, Dackis CA, Gold MS. Sexual dysfunction secondary to cocaine abuse in two patients. *J Clin Psychiatry*. 1986;47:384–385.
47a. Cincotta SL, Yorek MS, Moschak TM, Lewis SR, Rodefer JS. Selective nicotinic acetylcholine receptor agonists: potential therapies for neuropsychiatric disorders with cognitive dysfunction. *Curr Opin Investig Drugs*. 2008;9(1):47–56.
48. Colado MI, O'Shea E, Granados R, et al. In vivo evidence for free radical involvement in the degeneration of rat brain 5-HT following administration of MDMA ('ecstasy') and p-chloroamphetamine but not the degeneration following fenfluramine. *Br J Pharmacol*. 1997;121:889–900.
49. Colado MI, O'SheaE GR, Murray TK, Green AR. In vivo evidence for free radical involvement in the degeneration of rat brain 5-HT following administration of MDMA ('ecstasy') and p-chloroamphetamine but not the degeneration following fenfluramine. *Br J Pharmacol*. 1997;21:889–900.
50. Colasanti BK, Craig CR, Allara RD. Intraocular pressure, ocular toxicity and neurotoxicity after administration of cannabinol or cannabigerol. *Exp Eye Res*. 1984;39:251–259.
51. Collins GT, Abbott M, Galindo K, Rush EL, Rice KC, France CP. Discriminative stimulus effects of binary drug mixtures: studies with cocaine, MDPV, and caffeine. *J Pharmacol Exp Ther*. 2016;359:1–10.
52. Compton DR, Bagley RB, Katzen JS, et al. (+)- and (-)-N-allyl-normetazocine binding sites in mouse brain: in vitro and in vivo characterization and regional distribution. *Life Sci*. 1987;40:2195–2206.
53. Compton WM, Jones CM, Baldwin GT. Relationship between nonmedical prescription-opioid use and heroin use. *N Engl J Med*. 2016;374:154–163.
54. Connell PH. The use and abuse of amphetamines. *Practitioner*. 1968;200:234–243.
55. Cooke AR, Birchall MB, Birchall A. Absorption of ethanol from the stomach. *Gastroenterology*. 1969;57:269–272.
56. Corrao G, Bagnardi C, Zambon A, et al. A meta-analysis of alcohol consumption and the risk of 15 diseases. *Preventive Med*. 2004;38:613–619.
57. Cranford JA, Bohnert KM, Perron BE, Bourque C, Ilgen M. Prevalence and correlates of 'Vaping' as a route of cannabis administration in medical cannabis patients. *Drug Alcohol Depend*. 2016;169:41–47.
58. Cruz SL, Mirshahi T, Thomas B, et al. Effects of the abused solvent toluene on recombinant N-methyl-D-aspartate and non-N-methyl-D-aspartate receptors expressed in Xenopus oocytes. *J Pharmacol Exp Ther*. 1998;286:334–340.
59. Cubells JF, Rayport S, Rajendran G, et al. Methamphetamine neurotoxicity involves vacuolation of endocytic organelles and dopamine-dependent intracellular oxidative stress. *J Neurosci*. 1994;14:2260–2271.
60. Cunningham ET, Paris JM, Goeders NE. Chronic cocaine enhances serotonin autoregulation and serotonin uptake binding. *Synapse*. 1992;11:112–123.
60a. Dalal PM. Ischaemic strokes: management in first six hours. *Neurol India*. 2001;49(2):104–115.
60b. Dar R, Frenk H. Reevaluating the nicotine delivery kinetics hypothesis. *Psychopharmacology (Berl)*. 2007;192(1):1–7.
61. Darke S, Marel C, Mills KL, et al. Patterns and correlates of non-fatal heroin overdose at 11-year follow-up: findings from the Australian Treatment Outcome Study. *Drug Alcohol Depend*. 2014;144:148–152.
62. Darke S, Ross J, Mills K, Teesson M, Williamson A, Havard A. Benzodiazepine use among heroin users: baseline use, current use and clinical outcome. *Drug Alcohol Rev*. 2010;29:250–255.
63. Davies S, Wood DM, Smith G, et al. Purchasing "legal highs" on the Internet--is there consistency in what you get? QJM. *Int J Med*. 2010;103:489–493.
63a. Davis WC, Ticku MK. Ethanol enhances [3H]diazepam binding at the benzodiazepine-gamma-aminobutyric acid receptor-ionophore complex. *Mol Pharmacol*. 1981;20:287–294.
64. Deitrich RA, Dunwiddie TV, Harris RA, et al. Mechanism of action of ethanol: initial central nervous system actions. *Pharmacol Rev*. 1989;41:489–537.
65. Del AA, Gonzalez-Mora JL, Armas VR, et al. Amphetamine increases the extracellular concentration of glutamate in striatum of the awake rat: involvement of high affinity transporter mechanisms. *Neuropharmacology*. 1999;38:943–954.
66. Derlet RW, Rice P, Horowitz BZ, et al. Amphetamine toxicity: experience with 127 cases. *J Emergency Med*. 1989;7:157–161.
67. Devenyi P, Wilson M. Barbiturate abuse and addiction and their relationship to alcohol and alcoholism. *Can Med Assoc J*. 1971;104:215–218.
68. Diaz J. *How Drugs Influence Behavior*. Englewood Cliffs, NJ: Prentice Hall; 1996.
69. Dishotsky NI, Loughman WD, Mogar RE, et al. LSD and genetic damage. *Science*. 1971;172:431–440.
70. Doble A, Martin IL. Multiple benzodiazepine receptors: no reason for anxiety. *Trends Pharmacol Sci*. 1992;13:76–81.
71. Dos Santos RG, et al. Antidepressive, anxiolytic, and antiaddictive effects of ayahuasca, psilocybin and lysergic acid diethylamide (LSD): a systematic review of clinical trials published in the last 25 years. *Ther Adv Psychopharmacol*. 2016;6:193–213.
72. Dowell D, HaegerichTM CR. CDC guidelines for prescribing opioids for chronic pain—United States, 2016. *JAMA*. 2016;315:1624–1645.
73. Drevets WC, Gautier C, Price JC, et al. 2001;Amphetamine-induced dopamine release in human ventral striatum correlates with euphoria. *Biol Psychiatry*. 2001;49:81–96.
74. Drug Abuse Warning Network. *The DAWN Report: "Bath Salts" Were Involved in Over 20,000 Drug-Related Emergency Department Visits in 2011*; 2013.
75. Eberhard A. Ueber die synthese des inaktiven ephedrine bez. *Pseudoephedrins. Archives die Pharmazie*. 1915;258:97–129.
76. Edeleanu L. Uber einige derivate der Phenylmethacrylsaure und der Phenylisobutter-saure. *Ber Deutsch Chem Ges*. 1887;20:616–622.
77. Eisenberg MJ, Filion KB, Yavin D, et al. Pharmacotherapies for smoking cessation: a meta-analysis of randomized controlled trials. *CMAJ*. 2008;179:135–144.
78. Ellison JM, Dobies DF. Methamphetamine abuse presenting as dysuria following urethral insertion of tablets. *Ann Emergency Med*. 1984;13:198–200.
79. Elmore JS, Dillon-Carter O, Partilla JS, et al. Pharmacokinetic profiles and pharmacodynamic effects for methylone and its metabolites in rats. *Neuropsychopharmacology*. 2017;42:649–660.
80. El-Seedi HR, DeSmet PA, Beck O, et al. Prehistoric peyote use: alkaloid analysis and radiocarbon dating of archeological specimens of Lophophora from Texas. *J Ethnopharmacol*. 2005;101:238–242.
81. ElSohly MA. Chemical contituents of cannabis. In: Grotenhermen F, Russo E, eds. *Cannabis and Cannabinoids*. Binghamton, NY: Hayworth Integrative Healing; 2002:27–37.
82. Enoch MA. Review: the role of GABAA receptors in the development of alcoholism. *Pharmacol Biochem Behav*. 2008;90:95–104.
83. Eshleman AJ, Wolfrum KM, Hatfield MG, Johnson RA, Murphy KV, Janowsky A. Substituted methcathinones differ in transporter and receptor interactions. *Biochem Pharmacol*. 2013;85:1803–1815.
84. Eshleman AJ, Wolfrum KM, Reed JF, et al. Structure-activity relationships of substituted cathinones, with transporter binding, uptake, and release. *J Pharmacol Exp Ther*. 2017;360:33–47.
85. Espiard ML, Lecardeur L, Abadie P, et al. Hallucinogen persisting perception disorder after psilocybin consumption: a case study. *Eur Psychiatry: J Assoc Eur Psychiatrists*. 2005;20:458–460.

86. Fantegrossi WE, Gannon BM, Zimmerman SM, Rice KC. In vivo effects of abused "bath salt" constituent 3,4-methylenedioxypyrovalerone (MDPV) in mice: drug discrimination, thermoregulation, and locomotor activity. *Neuropsychopharmacology*. 2013;38: 563–573.

87. FDA. FDA Drug Safety Communication: FDA warns about serious risks and death when combining opioid pain or cough medicines with benzodiazepines; requires its strongest warning. 2016. http://www.fda.gov/Drugs/DrugSafety/ucm518473.htm.

88. Flemming KD, Brown RD. Secondary prevention strategies in ischemic stroke: identification and optimal management of modifiable risk factors. *Mayo Clin Proc*. 2004;79(10):1330–1340.

89. French-Mullen JM, Barker JL, Rogawski MA. Calcium current block by (-)-pentobarbital, phenobarbital, and CHEB but not (+)-pentobarbital in acutely isolated hippocampal CA1 neurons: comparison with effects on GABA-activated Cl? current. *J Neurosci*. 1993;13:3211–3221.

90. Finch JE, Kendall MJ, Mitchard M. An assessment of gastric emptying by breathalyser. *Br J Clin Pharmacol*. 1974;1:233–236.

91. Fines RE, Brady WJ, DeBehnke DJ. Cocaine-associated dystonic reaction. *Am J Emergency Medi*. 1997;15:513–515.

92. Freud S. Centralblatt für die ges. *Therapie*. 1884;2:289–314.

93. Gardner AJ. Withdrawal fits in barbiturate addicts. *Lancet*. 1967;2:337–338.

94. Gatch MB, Dolan SB, Forster MJ. Comparative behavioral pharmacology of three pyrrolidine-containing synthetic cathinone derivatives. *J Pharmacol Exp Ther*. 2015;354:103–110.

95. Gatch MB, Rutledge MA, Forster MJ. Discriminative and locomotor effects of five synthetic cathinones in rats and mice. *Psychopharmacology (Berl)*. 2015;232:1197–1205.

96. Gatch MB, Taylor CM, Forster MJ. Locomotor stimulant and discriminative stimulus effects of 'bath salt' cathinones. *Behav Pharmacol*. 2013;24:437–447.

97. Gately I. *Drink: A Cultural History of Alcohol*. New York, NY: Gotham Books; 2008.

98. Gelkopf M, Bleich A, Hayward R, et al. Characteristics of benzodiazepine abuse in methadone maintenance treatment patients: a 1 year prospective study in an Israeli clinic. *Drug Alcohol Depend*. 1999;55:63–68.

99. Gerevich J, Bacskai E, Farkas L, et al. A case report: pavlovian conditioning as a risk factor in heroin 'overdose' death. *Harm Reduction J*. 2005;2:11–14.

100. Reference deleted in review.

101. Gieringer D. Marijuana research: waterpipe study. *MAPS Bulletin*. 1996;6(3). Multidisciplinary Association for Psychedelic Studies 9-10-2008.

102. Gieringer DS, Laurent J, Goodrich S. Cannabis vaporizer combines efficient delivery of THC with effective suppression of pyrolytic compounds. *J Cannabis Ther*. 2004;4:7–27.

103. Gieringer DH. Cannabis 'vaporization'. *J Cannabis Ther*. 2001;1:153–170.

104. Reference deleted in review.

105. Giovanni A, Liang LP, Hastings TG, et al. Estimating hydroxyl radical content in rat brain using systemic and intraventricular salicylate: impact of methamphetamine. *J Neurochem*. 1995;64:1819–1825.

106. Giros B, Jaber M, Jones SR, et al. Hyperlocomotion and indifference to cocaine and amphetamine in mice lacking the dopamine transporter. *Nature*. 1996;379:606–612.

106a. Giroud M, Dumas R. [Effect of smoking in cerebral vascular accidents]. *Presse Med*. 1994;23(22):1037–1039.

107. Glennon RA, Yousif M, Naiman N, Kalix P. Methcathinone: a new and potent amphetamine-like agent. *Pharmacol Biochem Behav*. 1987;26:547–551.

108. Gobbi G, Bambico FR, Mangieri R, et al. Antidepressant-like activity and modulation of brain monoaminergic transmission by blockade of anandamide hydrolysis. *Proc Natl Acad Sci USA*. 2005;102:18620–18625.

109. Greiner T, Burch NR, Edelberg R. Psychopathology and psychophysiology of minimal LSD-25 dosage; a preliminary dosage-response spectrum. *Arch Neurol Psychiatry*. 1958;79: 208–210.

110. Grob CS, et al. Pilot study of psilocybin treatment for anxiety in patients with advanced-stage cancer. *Arch Gen Psychiatry*. 2011;68:71–78.

111. Gutierrez-Cebollada J, de la TR, Ortuno J, et al. Psychotropic drug consumption and other factors associated with heroin overdose. *Drug Alcohol Depend*. 1994;35:169–174.

112. Hadlock GC, Webb KM, Mcfadden LM, et al. 4-Methylmethcathinone (Mephedrone): neuropharmacological effects of a designer stimulant of abuse. *J Pharmacol Exp Therap*. 2011;339:530–536.

113. Halloran O, Ifthikharuddin S, Samkoff L. Leukoencephalopathy from "chasing the dragon. *Neurology*. 2005;64:1755.

113a. Hancock S, McKim W. Drugs and Behavior: An Introduction to Behavioral Pharmacology, Books a la Carte (8th Edition) [Internet]. Pearson; [cited 2019 Sep 9]. Available at: https://www.biblio.com/book/drugs-behavior-introduction-behavioral-pharmacology-books/d/1246540701.

114. Harris RA, Trudell JR, Mihic SJ. Ethanol's molecular targets. *Sci Signaling*. 2008;1:e7.

115. Hasegawa K, et al. Postmortem distribution of MAB-CHMINACA in body fluids and solid tissues of a human cadaver. *Forensic Toxicol*. 2015;33:380–387.

116. Hasler F, Bourquin D, Brenneisen R, et al. Determination of psilocin and 4-hydroxyindole acetic acid in plasma by HPLC-ECD and pharmacokinetic profiles of oral and intravenous psilocybin in man. *Pharmacologica Acta Helvetica*. 1997;72:175–184.

117. Hattori K, Oomura Y, Akaike N. Diazepam action on gamma-aminobutyric acid-activated chloride currents in internally perfused frog sensory neurons. *Cell Mol Neurobiol*. 1986;6:307–323.

118. Hatzidimitriou G, McCann UD, Ricaurte GA. Altered serotonin innervation patterns in the forebrain of monkeys treated with (+/?)3,4-methylenedioxymethamphetamine seven years previously: factors influencing abnormal recovery. *J Neurosci*. 1999;19:5096–5107.

119. Hawkins EF, Malte CA, Grossbard JR, Saxon AJ. Prevalence and trends in concurrent opioid analgesic and benzodiazepine use among Veterans Affairs patients with post-traumatic stress disorder, 2003-2011. *Pain Med*. 2015;16:1943–1954.

120. Hazekamp A, Ruhaak R, Zuurman L, et al. Evaluation of a vaporizing device (Volcano) for the pulmonary administration of tetrahydrocannabinol. *J Pharm Sci*. 2006;95:1308–1317.

121. Hemstapat K, Smith SA, Monteith GR, et al. The neuroexcitatory morphine metabolite, morphine-3-glucuronide (M3G), is not neurotoxic in primary cultures of either hippocampal or cerebellar granule neurones. *Pharmacol Toxicol*. 2003;93:197–200.

121a. Henningfield JE, Keenan RM. Nicotine delivery kinetics and abuse liability. *J Consult Clin Psychol*. 1993;61(5):743–750.

121b. Henry TS, Kanne JP, Kligerman SJ. Imaging of Vaping-Associated Lung Disease. *N Engl J Med*. 2019. [Epub ahead of print].

122. Hicks AR, Ogden BA, Varner KJ. Cardiovascular responses elicited during binge administration of cocaine. *Physiol Behav*. 2003;80:115–122.

123. Hilber B, Scholze P, Dorostkar MM, et al. Serotonin-transporter mediated efflux: a pharmacological analysis of amphetamines and non-amphetamines. *Neuropharmacology*. 2005;49:811–819.

124. Hill MD, Cooper PW, Perry JR. Chasing the dragon - neurological toxicity associated with inhalation of heroin vapour: case report. *CMAJ Canadian Med Assoc J*. 2000;162:236–238.

125. Hobbs WR, Rall TW, Verdoorn TA. Hypnotics and sedatives; ethanol. In: Hardman JG, Limbird LE, eds. *Goodman & Gilman's the Pharmacological Basis of Therapeutics*. New York, NY: McGraw-Hill; 1996:361–396.

126. Hoffman PL, Rabe CS, Moses F, et al. N-Methyl-D-Aspartate receptors and ethanol - inhibition of calcium flux and cyclic-GMP production. *J Neurochem*. 1989;52:1937–1940.

127. Hofmann A. *LSD-my Problem Child.* New York, NY: McGraw-Hill; 1980.

128. Hollister LE. The pre-benzodiazepine era. *J Psychoactive Drugs.* 1983;15:9–13.

129. Hollister LE. Interactions of cannabis with other drugs in man. *NIDA Res Monogr.* 1986;68:110–116.

130. Hotchkiss AJ, Gibb JW. Long-term effects of multiple doses of methamphetamine on tryptophan hydroxylase and tyrosine hydroxylase activity in rat brain. *J Pharmacol Exp Ther.* 1980;214:257–262.

131. Huestis MA, Henningfield JE, Cone EJ. Blood cannabinoids I. Absorption of THC and formation of 11-OH-THC and THC-COOH during and after smoking marijuana. *J Anal Toxicol.* 1992;16:276–282.

131a. Hughes JR. Varenicline as a Cause of Suicidal Outcomes. *Nicotine Tob Res.* 2016;18(1):2–9.

132. Huffman JW, et al. Structure-activity relationships for 1-alkyl-3-(1-naphthoyl)indoles at the cannabinoid CB(1) and CB(2) receptors: steric and electronic effects of naphthoyl substituents. New highly selective CB(2) receptor agonists. *Bioorg Med Chem.* 2005;13:89–112.

133. Hwang CS, Kang EM, Kornegay CJ, Staffa JA, Jones CM, McAninch JK. Trends in the concomitant prescribing of opioids and benzodiazepines, 2002-2014. *Am J Prev Med.* 2016;51:151–160.

134. Hyde JF, Browning E, Adams R. Synthetic homologs of d,L'ephedrine. *J Am Chem Soc.* 1928;50:2287–2292.

135. Ikawa K, Watanabe A, Motohashi N, et al. The effect of repeated administration of methamphetamine on dopamine uptake sites in rat striatum. *Neurosci Lett.* 1994;167:37–40.

136. Ikeda K, Kobayashi T, Kumanishi T, et al. Molecular mechanisms of analgesia iduced by opioids and ethanol: is the GIRK channel one of the keys? *Neurosci Res.* 2002;44:121–131.

137. Isabelle M, Vergeade A, Moritz F, et al. NADPH oxidase inhibition prevents cocaine-induced up-regulation of xanthine oxidoreductase and cardiac dysfunction. *J Mol Cell Cardiol.* 2007;42:326–332.

138. *IUPHAR Compendium of Receptor Characterization and Classification.* 2nd ed. London: IUPHAR Media; 2000:321–333.

139. Jatlow PI. Drug of abuse profile: cocaine. *Clin Chem.* 1987;33:Suppl–71B.

140. Jiang W, Zhang Y, Xiao L, et al. Cannabinoids promote embryonic and adult hippocampus neurogenesis and produce anxiolytic- and antidepressant-like effects. *J Clin Invest.* 2005;115:3104–3116.

141. Johanson CE, Schuster CR. A comparison of the behavioral effects of l- and dl-cathinone and d-amphetamine. *J Pharmacol Exp Ther.* 1981;219:355–362.

142. Johnson PS, Johnson MW. Investigation of "bath salts" use patterns within an online sample of users in the United States. *J Psychoactive drugs.* 2014;46:369–378.

143. Johnson MW, Garcia-Romeu A, Cosimano MP, Griffiths RR. Pilot study of the 5-HT2AR agonist psilocybin in the treatment of tobacco addiction. *J Psychopharmacol Oxf Engl.* 2014;28:983–992.

144. Jones CM, Mack KA, Paulozzi LJ. Pharmaceutical overdose deaths, United States, 2010. *J Am Med Assoc.* 2013;309:657–659.

145. Jones S, Kornblum JL, Kauer JA. Amphetamine blocks long-term synaptic depression in the ventral tegmental area. *J Neurosci.* 2000;20:5575–5580.

146. Kahlig KM, Binda F, Khoshbouei H, et al. Amphetamine induces dopamine efflux through a dopamine transporter channel. *Proc Natl Acad Sci USA.* 2005;102:3495–3500.

147. Kalant H. Absorption, diffusion, distribution, and elimination of ethanol. In: Kissin B, Begleiter H, eds. *Effects on Biological Membranes in the Biology of Alcoholism.* New York, NY: Plenum; 1971:1–46.

147a. Kamerow D. Big Tobacco lights up e-cigarettes. *BMJ.* 2013;346: f3418.

148. Kaminski BJ, Griffiths RR. Intravenous self-injection of methcathinone in the baboon. *Pharmacol Biochem Behav.* 1994;47:981–983.

149. Kandel DB, Yamaguchi K, Chen K. Stages of progression in drug involvement from adolescence to adulthood: further evidence for the gateway theory. *J Stud Alcohol.* 1992;53:447–457.

150. Kanouse AB, Compton P. The epidemic of prescription opioid abuse, the subsequent rising prevalence of heroin use, and the federal response. *J Pain Palliat Care Pharmaco.* 2015;59:102–114.

151. Kilpatrick GJ, Smith TW. Morphine-6-glucuronide: actions and mechanisms. *Med Res Rev.* 2005;25:521–544.

152. King TS, Schenken RS, Kang IS, et al. Cocaine disrupts estrous cyclicity and alters the reproductive. *Neuroendocrinology.* 1990;51:15–22.

152a. Kitamura S. Effects of cigarette smoking on metabolic events in the lung. *Environ Health Perspect.* 1987;72:283–296.

153. Klein TW, Newton C, Larsen K, et al. The cannabinoid system and immune modulation. *J Leukoc Biol.* 2003;74:486–496.

154. Klous MG, Van den BW, Van Ree JM, et al. Development of pharmaceutical heroin preparations for medical co-prescription to opioid dependent patients. *Drug Alcohol Depend.* 2005;80: 283–295.

155. Knoll J. Studies on the central effects of (-)cathinone. *NIDA Res Monogr.* 1979;27:322–323.

156. Kobayashi T, Ikeda K, Kojima H, et al. Ethanol opens G-protein-activated inwardly rectifying K+ channels. *Nat Neurosci.* 1999;2:1091–1097.

157. Kogan NM, Mechoulam R. Cannabinoids in health and disease. *Dialogues Clin Neurosci.* 2007;9:413–430.

158. Konkol RJ. Is there a cocaine baby syndrome? *J Child Neurol.* 2008;9:225–226.

159. Koob GF. Drugs of abuse: anatomy, pharmacology and function of reward pathways. *Trends Pharmacol Sci.* 1992;13:177–184.

160. Koob GF. Neural mechanisms of drug reinforcement. *Ann NY Acad Sci.* 1992;654:171–191.

161. Kuczenski R, Segal D. Concomitant characterization of behavioral and striatal neurotransmitter response to amphetamine using in vivo microdialysis. *J Neurosci.* 1989;9:2051–2065.

162. LaBarre W. *The Peyote Cult.* Hamden, CT: Archon Books; 1975.

163. Lader M. History of benzodiazepine dependence. *J Subst Abuse Treat.* 1991;8:53–59.

163a. Lamb RJ, Kirby KC, Morral AR, Galbicka G, Iguchi MY. Improving contingency management programs for addiction. *Addict Behav.* 2004;29(3):507–523.

163b. Lamb RJ, Morral AR, Kirby KC, Javors MA, Galbicka G, Iguchi M. Contingencies for change in complacent smokers. *Exp Clin Psychopharmacol.* 2007;15(3):245–255.

164. Lavie E, Fatséas M, Denis C, Auriacombe M. Benzodiazepine use among opiate-dependent subjects in buprenorphine maintenance treatment: correlates of use, abuse and dependence. *Drug Alcohol Depend.* 2009;99:338–344.

165. LaVoie MJ, Hastings TG. Dopamine quinone formation and protein modification associated with the striatal neurotoxicity of methamphetamine: evidence against a role for extracellular dopamine. *J Neurosci.* 1999;19:1484–1491.

166. Law R, et al. Notes from the field: increase in reported adverse health effects related to synthetic cannabinoid use - United States, january-may 2015. *MMWR Morb Mortal Wkly Rep.* 2015;64:618–619.

167. Le Foll B, Goldberg SR. Cannabinoid CB1 receptor antagonists as promising new medications for drug dependence. *J Pharmacol Exp Ther.* 2005;312:875–883.

168. Leece P, Cavacuiti C, Macdonald EM, et al. Predictors of opioid-related death during methadone therapy. *J Subst Abuse Treat.* 2015;57:30–35.

169. Leith NJ, Kuczenski R. Chronic amphetamine: tolerance and reverse tolerance reflect different behavioral actions of the drug. *Pharmacol Biochem Behav.* 1981;15:399–404.

169a. Lerman C, LeSage MG, Perkins KA, et al. Translational research in medication development for nicotine dependence. *Nat Rev Drug Discov.* 2007;6(9):746–762.

170. Lewin L. *Indian Hemp: Cannabis Indica. Phantastica: A Classic Survey on the Use and Abuse of Mind-Altering Plants*. Rochester, VT: Park Street; 1998:89–102.

171. Lieber CS. Medical disorders of alcoholism. *NE J Med*. 1995;333:1058–1065.

172. Lieber CS. Microsomal ethanol-oxidizing system (MEOS): the first 30 years (1968-1998) - a review. *Alcohol Clin Exp Res*. 1999;23:991–1007.

173. Linszen D, van Amelsvoort T. Cannabis and psychosis: an update on course and biological plausible mechanisms. *Curr Opin Psychiatry*. 2007;20:116–120.

174. Lock M. *East Asian Medicine in Urban Japan: Varieties of Medical Experience*. Berkeley: University of California; 1984.

175. Long H. Inhalants. In: Flomenbaum NE, Goldfrank LR, Hoffman RS, Howland MA, Lewin NA, Nelson LS, eds. *Goldfrank's Toxicologic Emergencies*. New York, NY: McGraw-Hill; 2006.

176. López-Arnau R, Martínez-Clemente J, Pubill D, Escubedo E, Camarasa J. Comparative neuropharmacology of three psychostimulant cathinone derivatives: butylone, mephedrone and methylone. *Br J Pharmacol*. 2012;167:407–420.

177. Lovinger DM. Inhibition of 5-Ht3 receptor-mediated ion current by divalent metal-cations in NCB-20 neuroblastoma-cells. *J Neurophysiol*. 1991;66:1329–1337.

178. Lovinger DM, White G, Weight FF. Ethanol inhibits NMDA-activated ion current in hippocampal-neurons. *Science*. 1989;243:1721–1724.

179. Lubman DI, Yücel M, Lawrence AJ. Inhalant abuse among adolescents: neurobiological considerations. *Br J Pharmacol*. 2008;154:316–326.

180. Luddens H, Korpi ER, Seeburg PH. GABAA/benzodiazepine receptor heterogeneity: neurophysiological implications. *Neuropharmacology*. 1995;34:245–254.

181. Lynskey MT, Glowinski AL, Todorov AA, et al. Major depressive disorder, suicidal ideation, and suicide attempt in twins discordant for cannabis dependence and early-onset cannabis use. *Arch Gen Psychiatry*. 2004;61:1026–1032.

182. Mahapatra A, Gupta R. Role of psilocybin in the treatment of depression. *Ther Adv Psychopharmacol*. 2017;7:54–56.

183. Malinski MK, Sesso HD, Lopez-Jiminez F, et al. Alcohol consumption and cardiovascular disease mortality in hypertensive men. *Archiv Intern Med*. 2004;164:623–628.

184. Marek GJ, Aghajanian GK. LSD and the phenethylamine hallucinogen DOI are potent partial agonists at 5-HT2A receptors on interneurons in rat piriform cortex. *J Pharmacol Exp Ther*. 1996;278:1373–1382.

185. Martin WR, Fraser HF. A comparative study of physiological and subjective effects of heroin and morphine administered intravenously in postaddicts. *J Pharmacol Exp Ther*. 1961;133:388–399.

186. Marusich JA, Antonazzo KR, Wiley JL, Blough BE, Partilla JS, Baumann MH. Pharmacology of novel synthetic stimulants structurally related to the "bath salts" constituent 3,4-methylenedioxypyrovalerone (MDPV). *Neuropharmacology*. 2014;87:206–213.

187. Marusich JA, Grant KR, Blough BE, Wiley JL. Effects of synthetic cathinones contained in "bath salts" on motor behavior and a functional observational battery in mice. *Neurotoxicology*. 2012;33:1305–1313.

188. McGraw M, McGraw L. Bath salts: not as harmless as they sound. *J Emerg Nurs*. 2012;38:582–588.

189. McKim WA. *Cannabis. Drugs and Behavior: An Introduction to Behavioral Pharmacology*. Englewood Cliffs, NJ: Prentice-Hall; 1986:211–234.

190. Mechoulam R, Parker L. Cannabis and alcohol - a close friendship. *Trends Pharmacol Sci*. 2003;24:266–268.

191. Mellenby E. Alcohol: its absorption into and disappearance from the blood under different conditions. *Med Res Council Special Rep Service No*; 1919:31.

192. Mello NK, Sarnyai Z, Mendelson JH, et al. Acute effects of cocaine on anterior pituitary hormones in male and female rhesus monkeys. *J Pharmacol Exp Ther*. 1993;266:804–811.

193. Mendelson J, Uemura N, Harris D, et al. Human pharmacology of the methamphetamine stereoisomers. *Clin Pharmacol Ther*. 2006;80:403–420.

194. Reference deleted in review.

195. Messmer D, Hatsukari I, Hitosugi N, et al. Morphine reciprocally regulates IL-10 and IL-12 production by monocyte-derived human dendritic cells and enhances T cell activation. *Mol Med*. 2006;12:284–290.

195a. Miech R, Patrick ME, O'Malley PM, Johnston LD. What are kids vaping? Results from a national survey of US adolescents. *Tob Control*. 2017;26(4):386–391.

196. Mihic SJ, Ye Q, Wick MJ, et al. Sites of alcohol and volatile anaesthetic action on GABA(A) and glycine receptors. *Nature*. 1997;389:385–389.

197. Miller AM, Stella N. CB2 receptor-mediated migration of immune cells: it can go either way. *Br J Pharmacol*. 2008;153:299–308.

198. Miller PM, Anton RF, Egan BM, et al. Excessive alcohol consumption and hypertension: clinical implications of current research. *J Clin Hypertens*. 2005;7:346–351.

199. Reference deleted in review.

200. Mizoi Y, Ijiri I, Tatsuno Y, et al. Relationship between facial flushing and blood-acetaldehyde levels after alcohol intake. *Pharmacol Biochem Behav*. 1979;10:303–311.

201. Monnet-Tschudi F, Hazekamp A, Perret N, et al. Delta-9-tetrahydrocannabinol accumulation, metabolism and cell-type-specific adverse effects in aggregating brain cell cultures. *Toxicol Appl Pharmacol*. 2008;228:8–16.

202. Monte AP, Waldman SR, Marona-Lewicka D, et al. Dihydrobenzofuran analogues of hallucinogens. 4. Mescaline derivatives. *J Med Chem*. 1997;40:2997–3008.

202a. Mooney M, Babb D, Jensen J, Hatsukami D. Interventions to increase use of nicotine gum: a randomized, controlled, single-blind trial. *Nicotine Tob Res*. 2005;7(4):565–579.

203. Moore KE. The actions of amphetamine on neurotransmitters: a brief review. *Biol Psychiatry*. 1977;12:451–462.

204. Moore RJ, Vinsant SL, Nader MA, et al. Effect of cocaine self-administration on dopamine D2 receptors in rhesus monkeys. *Synapse*. 1998;30:88–96.

205. Morin CM, Belanger L, Bastien C, et al. Long-term outcome after discontinuation of benzodiazepines for insomnia: a survival analysis of relapse. *Behav Res Ther*. 2005;43:1–14.

206. Motbey CP, Clemens KJ, Apetz N, et al. High levels of intravenous mephedrone (4-methylmethcathinone) self-administration in rats: neural consequences and comparison with methamphetamine. *J Psychopharmacol*. 2013;27:823–836.

207. Mura P, Kintz P, Dumestre V, et al. THC can be detected in brain while absent in blood. *J Anal Toxicol*. 2005;29:842–843.

208. Murray RM, Morrison PD, Henquet C, et al. Cannabis, the mind and society: the hash realities. *Nat Rev Neurosci*. 2007;8:885–895.

209. Narahashi T, Aistrup GL, Lindstrom JM, et al. Ion channel modulation as the basis for general anesthesia. *Toxicol Lett*. 1998;101:185–191.

210. National Institute on Drug Abuse. *InfoFacts: Heroin*; 2006.

211. National Institute on Drug Abuse. *InfoFacts: LSD*; 2006.

212. National Institute on Drug Abuse. *Research Report: Hallucinogens and Dissociative Drugs*; 2001.

212a. National Institutes of Health/ National Cancer Institute. *Cancer Trends Progress Report*; 2018. Available at: http://progressreport.cancer.gov.

213. Reference deleted in review.

214. Nichols DE. Differences between the mechanism of action of MDMA, MBDB, and the classic hallucinogens. Identification of a new therapeutic class: entactogens. *J Psychoactive Drugs*. 1986;18:1305–1313.

215. Nichols DE, Hoffman AJ, Oberlender RA, et al. Derivatives of 1-(1,3-benzodioxol-5-yl)-2-butanamine: representatives of a novel therapeutic class. *J Med Chem.* 1986;29:2009–2015.

216. *NIDA Research Report - Heroin Abuse and Addiction: NIH Publication No. 05-4165*, Printed October 1997, Reprinted September, 2000, Revised May 2005.

217. Norberg A, Gabrielsson J, Jones AW, et al. Within- and between-subject variations in pharmacokinetic parameters of ethanol by analysis of breath, venous blood, and urine. *Br J Clin Pharmacol.* 2000;49:399–408.

217a. Norman V. The history of cigarettes. Changes of smoke chemistry of modern day cigarettes. Truth Tobacco Industry Documents. 1983. Available at: https://www.industrydocuments.ucsf.edu/tobacco/docs/#id=szcw0105.

218. Obata T, Morelli M, Concas A, Serra M, Yamamura HI. Modulation of GABA-stimulated chloride influx into membrane vesicles from rat cerebral cortex by benzodiazepines and nonbenzodiazepines. In: Biggio G, Costa E, eds. *Chloride Channels and Their Modulation by Neurotransmitters and Drugs.* New York, NY: Raven; 1988:175–187.

219. Onaivi ES, Chakrabarti A, Chaudhuri G. Cannabinoid receptor genes. *Prog Neurobiol.* 1996;48:275–305.

220. ONDCP Public Affairs. Study Finds Highest Levels of THC in U.S. Marijuana To Date. whitehousedrugpolicy.gov. 5-1-0007. *Office of National Drug Control Policy.* 2008;9-10.

221. Owen RT, Tyrer P. Benzodiazepine dependence. A review of the evidence. *Drugs.* 1983;25:385–398.

222. Reference deleted in review.

223. Palenicek T, Balikova M, Bubenikova-Valesovas V, et al. Mescaline effects on rat behavior and its time profile in serum and brain tissue after a single subcutaneous dose. *Psychopharmacology.* 2008;196:51–62.

224. Park TW, Saitz R, Ganoczy D, Ilgen MA, Bohnert AS. Benzodiazepine prescribing patterns and deaths from drug overdose among US veterans receiving opioid analgesics: case-cohort study. *BMJ.* 2015;350:h2698.

225. Passie T, Seifert J, Schneider U, et al. The pharmacology of psilocybin. *Addiction Biol.* 2002;7:357–364.

225a. Patel RR, Ryu JH, Vassallo R. Cigarette smoking and diffuse lung disease. *Drugs.* 2008;68(11):1511–1527.

226. Patrick CH. *Alcohol, Culture, and Society.* Durham, NC: Duke University; 1952.

227. Patrick RL. Amphetamine and cocaine: biological mechanisms. In: Barchas JD, Berger PA, Ciaranello RD, eds. *Psychopharmacology: From Theory to Practice.* New York, NY: Oxford University; 1977:331–340.

228. Peat MA, Warren PF, Bakhit C, et al. The acute effects of methamphetamine, amphetamine and p-chloroamphetamine on the cortical serotonergic system of the rat brain: evidence for differences in the effects of methamphetamine and amphetamine. *Eur J Pharmacol.* 1985;116:11–16.

229. Pedersen AJ, Petersen TH, Linnet K. In vitro metabolism and pharmacokinetic studies on methylone. *Drug Metab Dispos.* 2013;41:1247–1255.

230. Peles E, Schreiber S, Adelson M. Factors predicting retention in treatment: 10-year experience of a methadone maintenance treatment (MMT) clinic in Israel. *Drug Alcohol Depend.* 2006;82:211–217.

231. Pelner L. Peyote cult, mescaline hallucinations, and model psychosis. *NY State J Med.* 1967;67:2838–2843.

232. Perez J, Ribera MV. Managing neuropathic pain with Sativex: a review of its pros and cons. *Expert Opin Pharmacother.* 2008;9:1189–1195.

233. Perrine DM. *Dissociatives and Cannabinoids: PCP, THC, ETCs.* In: *The Chemistry of Mind-Altering Drugs: History, Pharmacology, and Cultural Context.* Washington, DC: American Chemical Society; 1996:333–394.

234. Perrine DM. Stimulants: nicotine, caffeine, cocaine, amphetamines. In: *The Chemistry of Mind-Altering Drugs: History, Pharmacology, and Cultural Context.* Washington, DC: American Chemical Society; 1996:171–218.

235. Pertwee RG. Pharmacology of cannabinoid CB1 and CB2 receptors. *Pharmacol Ther.* 1997;74:129–180.

235a. Picciotto MR, Addy NA, Mineur YS, Brunzell DH. It is not "either/or": activation and desensitization of nicotinic acetylcholine receptors both contribute to behaviors related to nicotine addiction and mood. *Prog Neurobiol.* 2008;84(4):329–342.

235b. Popkin MK. Exacerbation of recurrent depression as a result of treatment with varenicline. *Am J Psychiatry.* 2008;165(6):774.

236. Poyares D, Guilleminault C, Ohayon MM, et al. Chronic benzodiazepine usage and withdrawal in insomnia patients. *J Psychiatr Res.* 2004;38:327–334.

237. Reference deleted in review.

238. Reith ME. Cocaine receptors on monoamine transporters and sodium channels. *NIDA Res Monogr.* 1988;88:23–43.

239. Ricaurte GA, DeLanney LE, Irwin I, et al. Toxic effects of MDMA on central serotonergic neurons in the primate: importance of route and frequency of drug administration. *Brain Res.* 1988;446: 165–168.

240. Ricaurte GA, DeLanney LE, Wiener SG, et al. 5-Hydroxyindoleacetic acid in cerebrospinal fluid reflects serotonergic damage induced by 3,4-methylenedioxymethamphetamine in CNS of non-human primates. *Brain Res.* 1988;474:359–363.

241. Ricaurte GA, Martello AL, Katz JL, et al. Lasting effects of (±)-3,4-methyle-nedioxymethamphetamine (MDMA) on central serotonergic neurons in nonhuman primates: neurochemical observations. *J Pharmacol Exp The.* 1992;261:616–622.

242. Rickert WS, Robinson JC, Rogers B. A comparison of tar, carbon monoxide and pH levels in smoke from marihuana and tobacco cigarettes. *Can J Public Health.* 1982;73:386–391.

243. Riddle EL, Fleckenstein AE, Hanson GR. Mechanisms of methamphetamine-induced dopaminergic neurotoxicity. *AAPS J.* 2006;8: E413–E418.

244. Robertson B. Actions of anaesthetics and avermectin on GABAA chloride channels in mammalian dorsal root ganglion neurones. *Br J Pharmacol.* 1989;98:167–176.

245. Robledo-Carmona J, Ortega-Jimenez MV, Garcia-Pinilla JM, et al. Severe cardiomyopathy associated to cocaine abuse. *Int J Cardiol.* 2006;112:130–131.

246. Rold JF, Mushroom madness. Psychoactive fungi and the risk of fatal poisoning. *Postgraduate Med.* 1986;79:218–228.

247. Rose JS. Cocaethylene: a current understanding of the active metabolite of cocaine and ethanol. *Am J Emergency Med.* 1994;12: 489–490.

248. Roth D, Alarcon FJ, Fernandez JA, et al. Acute rhabdomyolysis associated with cocaine intoxication. *N Engl J Med.* 1988;319: 673–677.

249. Rothman RB, Baumann MH. Balance between dopamine and serotonin release modulates behavioral effects of amphetamine-type drugs. *Ann NY Acad Sci.* 2006;1074:245–260.

250. Rudd RA, Aleshire N, Zibbell JE, Gladden RM. Increases in drug and opioid overdose deaths—United States, 2000-2014. *MMWR Morb Mortal Wkly Rep.* 2016;64:1378–1382.

251. San L, Tato J, Torrens M, Castillo C, Farré M, Camí J. Flunitrazepam consumption among heroin addicts admitted for in-patient detoxification. *Drug Alcohol Depend.* 1993;32:281–286.

252. Sasco AJ, Merrill RM, Dari I, et al. A case-control study of lung cancer in Casablanca, Morocco. *Cancer Causes Control.* 2002;13: 609–616.

253. Reference deleted in review.

254. Sawynok J. The therapeutic use of heroin: a review of the pharmacological literature. *Can J Physiol Pharmacol.* 1986;64:1–6.

255. Schaefer N, et al. Distribution of synthetic cannabinoids JWH-210, RCS-4 and Δ 9-tetrahydrocannabinol after intravenous administration to pigs. *Curr Neuropharmacol.* 2016.

256. Schechter MD, Glennon RA. Cathinone, cocaine and methamphetamine: similarity of behavioral effects. *Pharmacol Biochem Behav.* 1985;22:913–916.

257. Schechter MD. Potentiation of cathinone by caffeine and nikethamide. *Pharmacol Biochem Behav.* 1989;33:299–301.

258. Schepers RJ, Oyler JM, Joseph Jr RE, et al. Methamphetamine and amphetamine pharmacokinetics in oral fluid and plasma after controlled oral methamphetamine administration to human volunteers. *Clin Chem.* 2003;49:121–132.

259. Schindler CW, Thorndike EB, Blough BE, Tella SR, Goldberg SR, Baumann MH. Effects of 3,4-methylenedioxymethamphetamine (MDMA) and its main metabolites on cardiovascular function in conscious rats. *Br J Pharmacol.* 2014;171:83–91.

260. Schindler CW, Thorndike EB, Goldberg SR, et al. Reinforcing and neurochemical effects of the "bath salts" constituents 3,4-methylenedioxypyrovalerone (MDPV) and 3,4-methylenedioxy-N-methylcathinone (methylone) in male rats. *Psychopharmacology (Berl).* 2016;233:1981–1990.

261. Schindler CW, Thorndike EB, Suzuki M, Rice KC, Baumann MH. Pharmacological mechanisms underlying the cardiovascular effects of the "bath salt" constituent 3,4-methylenedioxypyrovalerone (MDPV). *Br J Pharmacol.* 2016;173:3492–3501.

262. Schuman-Olivier Z, Hoeppner BB, Weiss RD, Borodovsky J, Shaffer HJ, Albanese MJ. Benzodiazepine use during buprenorphine treatment for opioid dependence: clinical and safety outcomes. *Drug Alcohol Depend.* 2013;132:580–586.

263. Schwartz RH. Mescaline: a survey. *Am Family Physician.* 1988;37:122–124.

264. Seely KA, Patton AL, Moran CL, et al. Forensic investigation of K2, Spice, and "bath salt" commercial preparations: a three-year study of new designer drug products containing synthetic cannabinoid, stimulant, and hallucinogenic compounds. *Foren Sci Int.* 2013;233:416–422.

265. Seivewright N, Dougal W. Withdrawal symptoms from high dose benzodiazepines in poly drug users. *Drug Alcohol Depend.* 1993;32:15–23.

265a. Seliskar M, Rozman D. Mammalian cytochromes P450--importance of tissue specificity. *Biochim Biophys Acta.* 2007;1770(3):458–466.

266. Self DW, Belluzzi JD, Kossuth S, et al. Self-administration of the D1 agonist SKF 82958 is mediated by D1, not D2, receptors. *Psychopharmacology.* 1996;123:303–306.

267. Shelton KL. Discriminative stimulus effects of abused inhalants. *Curr Top Behav Neurosci.* 2016. https://doi.org/10.1007/7854_2016_22.

268. Signs SA, Ckey-White HI, Vanek VW, et al. The formation of cocaethylene and clinical presentation of ED patients testing positive for the use of cocaine and ethanol. *Am J Emergency Med.* 1996;14:665–670.

269. Simmler LD, Buser TA, Donzelli M, et al. Pharmacological characterization of designer cathinones in vitro. *Br J Pharmacol.* 2013;168:458–470.

270. Simmler LD, Rickli A, Hoener MC, Liechti ME. Monoamine transporter and receptor interaction profiles of a new series of designer cathinones. *Neuropharmacology.* 2014;79:152–160.

271. Simmonds MA. Distinction between the effects of barbiturates, benzodiazepines and phenytoin on responses to gamma-aminobutyric acid receptor activation and antagonism by bicuculline and picrotoxin. *Br J Pharmacol.* 1981;73:739–747.

272. Skolnick P, Volkow ND. Re-energizing the development of pain therapeutics in light of the opioid epidemic. *Neuron.* 2016;92:294–297.

273. Slikker Jr W, Holson RR, Ali SF, et al. Behavioral and neurochemical effects of orally administered MDMA in the rodent and nonhuman primate. *Neurotoxicology.* 1989;10:529–542.

274. Slomski A. A trip on "bath salts" is cheaper than meth or cocaine but much more dangerous. *JAMA.* 2014;308:2445–2447.

274a. Slotkin TA. If nicotine is a developmental neurotoxicant in animal studies, dare we recommend nicotine replacement therapy in pregnant women and adolescents? *Neurotoxicol Teratol.* 2008;30(1):1–19.

275. Smith DE, Wesson DR. Phenobarbital technique for treatment of barbiturate dependence. *Arch Gen Psychiatry.* 1971;24:56–60.

276. Spaderna M, Addy PH, D'Souza DC. Spicing things up: synthetic cannabinoids. *Psychopharmacology (Berl.).* 2013;228:525–540.

277. Spiller HA, Ryan ML, Weston RG, Jansen J. Clinical experience with and analytical confirmation of "bath salts" and "legal highs" (synthetic cathinones) in the United States. *Clin Toxicol.* 2011;49:499–505.

278. Stephans S, Yamamoto B. Methamphetamines pretreatment and the vulnerability of the striatum to methamphetamine neurotoxicity. *Neuroscience.* 1996;72:593–600.

279. Stitzer ML, Griffiths RR, McLellan AT, Grabowski J, Hawthorne JW. Diazepam use among methadone maintenance patients: patterns and dosages. *Drug Alcohol Depend.* 1981;8:189–199.

280. Strandberg JJ, Kugelberg FC, Alkass K, et al. Toxicological analysis in rats subjected to heroin and morphine overdose. *Toxicol Lett.* 2006;166:11–18.

281. Sulzer D, Chen TK, Lau YY, et al. Amphetamine redistributes dopamine from synaptic vesicles to the cytosol and promotes reverse transport. *J Neurosci.* 1995;15:4102–4108.

282. Sulzer D, Sonders MS, Poulsen NW, et al. Mechanisms of neurotransmitter release by amphetamines: a review. *Prog Neurobiol.* 2005;75:406–433.

282a. Symm B, Morgan MV, Blackshear Y, Tinsley S. Cigar smoking: an ignored public health threat. *J Prim Prev.* 2005;26(4):363–375.

283. Tashkin DP, Gliederer F, Rose J, et al. Tar, CO and delta 9THC delivery from the 1st and 2nd halves of a marijuana cigarette. *Pharmacol Biochem Behav.* 1991;40:657–661.

284. Tazelaar HD, Karch SB, Stephens BG, et al. Cocaine and the heart. *Hum Pathol.* 1987;18:195–199.

285. Tschacher W, Haemmig R, Jacobshagen N. Time series modeling of heroin and morphine drug action. *Psychopharmacology.* 2003;165:188–193.

286. Congress US. *The select Committee to study governmental Operations with respect to intelligence activities, Foreign and Military intelligence [Church Committee report].* Washington, D.C.: GPO; 1976. Report no. 94-755, 94th Congress, 2d Session.

287. UN Document. *Studies on the Chemical Composition of Khat. Iii. Investigations on the Phenylalkylamine Fraction.* United Nations Laboratory document MNAR/11/75, GE; 1975:75–1264.

288. Van DC, Barash PG, Jatlow P, et al. Cocaine: plasma concentrations after intranasal application in man. *Science.* 1976;191:859–861.

289. Varner KJ, Daigle K, Weed PF, et al. Comparison of the behavioral and cardiovascular effects of mephedrone with other drugs of abuse in rats. *Psychopharmacology.* 2013;225:675–685.

290. Varner KJ, Ogden BA, Delcarpio J, Meleg-smith S. Cardiovascular responses elicited by the "binge" administration of methamphetamine. *J Pharmacol Exp Therap.* 2002;301:152–159.

291. Vaughan CW, Christie MJ. Retrograde signalling by endocannabinoids. *Handb Exp Pharmacol.* 2005;168:367–383.

292. Vengeliene V, Bilbao A, Molander A, et al. Neuropharmacology of alcohol addiction. *Br J Pharmacol.* 2008;154:299–315.

293. Reference deleted in review.

294. Voirin N, Berthiller J, Benhaïm-Luzon V, et al. Risk of lung cancer and past use of cannabis in Tunisia. *J Thorac Oncol.* 2006;1:577–579.

295. Volkow ND, Frieden TR, Hyde PS, Cha SS. Medication-assisted therapies--tackling the opioid overdose epidemic. *N Engl J Med.* 2014;370:2063–2066.

296. Volkow ND, McLellan AT. Opioid abuse in chronic pain—misconceptions and mitigation strategies. *N Engl J Med.* 2016;374:1253–1256.

297. Volpe FH. Effect of cocaine use on the fetus. *N Engl J Med.* 1992;327:399–407.

298. Von Anrep B. Ueber die physiologische Wirkung des Cocain. *E Pfluger Arch Ges Physiol.* 208;21:38–77.

299. Von Bibra BEF. *Hashish. Plant Intoxicants: A Classic Text on the Use of Mind-Altering Plants.* Rochester, VT: Healing Arts; 1995:147–165.

299a. von Bibra BE. *Plant Intoxicants: A Classic Text on the Use of Mind-Altering Plants.* Rochester, VT: Healing Arts Press; 1995.

300. Wacker D, et al. Crystal structure of an LSD-bound human serotonin receptor. *Cell.* 2017;168:377–389. e12.

301. Wallner M, Olsen RW. Physiology and pharmacology of alcohol: the imidazobenzodiazepine alcohol antagonist site on subtypes of GABAA receptors as an opportunity for drug development. *Br J Pharmacol*. 2008;154:288–298.

302. Wang XM, Wang G, Lemos JR, et al. Ethanol directly modulates gating of a dihydropyridine-sensitive Ca2+ channel in neurohypophyseal terminals. *J Neurosci*. 1994;14:5453–5460.

302a. Warner K. Will the next generation of "safer" cigarettes be safer? *J Pediatr Hematol Oncol*. 2005;27(10):543–550.

303. Watterson LR, Hood L, Sewalia K, et al. The reinforcing and rewarding effects of methylone, a synthetic cathinone commonly found in "bath salts. *J Addict Res Therap*. 2012;suppl 9:1–18.

304. Watterson LR, Kufahl PR, Nemirovsky NE, et al. Potent rewarding and reinforcing effects of the synthetic cathinone 3,4-methylenedioxypyrovalerone (MDPV). *Addict Biol*. 2014;19:165–174.

305. White JM, Irvine RJ. Future directions in opioid overdose. *Addiction*. 1999;94:978–980.

306. Wikler A. Diagnosis and treatment of drug dependence of the barbiturate type. *Am J Psychiatry*. 1968;125:758–765.

307. Wilcox HC, Anthony JC. The development of suicide ideation and attempts: an epidemiologic study of first graders followed into young adulthood. *Drug Alcohol Depend*. 2004;76(Suppl):S53–S67.

308. Wilcox JA. Psilocybin and obsessive compulsive disorder. *J Psychoactive Drugs*. 2014;46:393–395.

308a. Wilkes S. The use of bupropion SR in cigarette smoking cessation. *Int J Chron Obstruct Pulmon Dis*. 2008;3(1):45–53.

309. Wilkinson PK. Pharmacokinetics of ethanol: a review. *Alcoholism: Clin Exp Res*. 1980;4:6–21.

310. Wilkinson PK, Sedman AJ, Sakmar E, et al. Pharmacokinetics of ethanol after oral administration in the fasting state. *J Pharmacokinet Biopharm*. 1977;5:207–224.

310a. Willems EW, Rambali B, Vleeming W, Opperhuizen A, van Amsterdam JGC. Significance of ammonium compounds on nicotine exposure to cigarette smokers. *Food Chem Toxicol*. 2006;44(5):678–688.

311. Williams RT, Caldwell RJ, Dreng LG. Comparative metabolism of some amphetamines in various species. In: Schneider SH, Esdin E, eds. *Frontiers of Catecholamine Research*. Oxford; England: Pergamon; 1973:927–932.

311a. Williams RT. Detoxication mechanisms in man. *Clin Pharmacol Ther*. 1963;4(2):234–254.

312. Williams EG, Himmelsbach CK, Wikler A, Ruble DC, Lloyd BJ. Studies on marihuana and pyrahexyl compound. 1896-1970 61 *Public Health Rep*. 1946:1059–1083.

313. Winger G, Hofmann FG, Woods JH. *A Handbook on Drug and Alcohol Abuse*. New York, Oxford: University Press; 1992.

314. Winstock AR, Mitcheson LR, Deluca P, Davey Z, Corazza O, Schifano F. Mephedrone, new kid for the chop? *Addiction*. 2011;106:154–161.

315. Wittman M, Carter O, Hasler F, et al. Effects of psilocybin on time perception and temporal control of behavior in humans. *J Psychopharmacol*. 2007;21:50–64.

316. Woody GE, Mintz J, O'Hare K, O'Brien CP, Greenstein RA, Hargrove E. Diazepam use by patients in a methadone program—how serious a problem? *J Psychedelic Drugs*. 1975;7:373–379.

317. Woolverton WL, Johanson CE. Preference in rhesus monkeys given a choice between cocaine and dl-cathinone. *J Exp Analysis Behav*. 1984;41:35–43.

318. Wright MJ, Angrish D, Aarde SM, et al. Effect of ambient temperature on the thermoregulatory and locomotor stimulant effects of 4-methylmethcathinone in Wistar and Sprague-Dawley rats. *PLoS One*. 2012;7:e44652.

319. Wu TC, Tashkin DP, Rose JE, et al. Influence of marijuana potency and amount of cigarette consumed on marijuana smoking pattern. *J Psychoactive Drugs*. 1988;20:43–46.

320. Yamamoto BK, Zhu W. The effects of methamphetamine on the production of free radicals and oxidative stress. *J Pharmacol Exp Ther*. 1998;287:107–114.

321. Young R, Glennon RA. Discriminative stimulus effects of S(-)-methcathinone (CAT): a potent stimulant drug of abuse. *Psychopharmacology*. 1998;140:250–256.

322. Yu R, Ticku MK. Effects of chronic pentobarbital treatment on the GABAA receptor complex in mammalian cortical neurons. *J Pharmacol Exp Ther*. 1995;275:1442–1446.

322a. Zhang LR, Morgenstern H, Greenland S, et al. Cannabis smoking and lung cancer risk: Pooled analysis in the International Lung Cancer Consortium. *Int J Cancer*. 2015;136(4):894–903.

323. Znaleziona J, et al. Determination and identification of synthetic cannabinoids and their metabolites in different matrices by modern analytical techniques – a review. *Anal Chim Acta*. 2015;874: 11–25.

324. Żukiewicz-Sobczak W, Zwoliński J, Chmielewska-Badora J, et al. Analysis of psychoactive and intoxicating substances in legal highs. *Ann Agricul Environ Med*. 2012;19:309–314.

18

Animal Models of Substance Use Disorders: Motivational Perspective

GEORGE F. KOOB

Definitions Relevant to Animal Models

Drug addiction, also known as substance use disorder,[8] is a chronically relapsing disorder that is characterized by (1) compulsion to seek and take the drug, (2) loss of control in limiting intake, and as defined by the present author and others, (3) emergence of a negative emotional state (e.g., dysphoria, anxiety, irritability) when access to the drug is prevented.[87,152]

Drug addiction has been conceptualized as a disorder that involves elements of both impulsivity and compulsivity, in which impulsivity can be defined behaviorally as "a predisposition toward rapid, unplanned reactions to internal and external stimuli without regard for the negative consequences of these reactions to themselves or others."[116] Compulsivity can be defined as elements of behavior that result in perseveration in responding in the face of adverse consequences or perseveration in the face of incorrect responses in choice situations. The compulsivity element could be considered analogous to some of the symptoms of substance use disorder that is outlined by the American Psychiatric Association (i.e., continued substance use despite knowledge of having had a persistent or recurrent physical or psychological problem and a great deal of time spent in activities necessary to obtain the substance).[8]

Collapsing the cycles of impulsivity and compulsivity yields a composite addiction cycle that comprises three stages—binge/intoxication, withdrawal/negative affect, and preoccupation/anticipation (craving). Impulsivity often dominates at early stages, and compulsivity dominates at terminal stages. As an individual moves from impulsivity to compulsivity, a shift occurs from positive reinforcement that drives the motivated behavior to negative reinforcement that drives the motivated behavior[78] (Fig. 18.1). Negative reinforcement can be defined as the process by which the removal of an aversive stimulus (e.g., negative emotional state of drug withdrawal) increases the probability of a response (e.g., dependence-induced drug intake). These three stages are conceptualized as interacting with each other, becoming more intense, and ultimately leading to the pathological state known as addiction.[87] The present review focuses on the role of animal models of dependence that are associated with the negative emotional state of the withdrawal/negative affect stage of the addiction cycle (see Fig. 18.1).

The diagnostic criteria for addiction that are described by the Fifth Edition of the *Diagnostic and Statistical Manual of Mental Disorders* (DSM-5)[8] have evolved over the past 30 years, with a shift from an emphasis on and necessary criteria of tolerance and withdrawal to other criteria that are directed more at compulsive use, craving, and relapse. The number of criteria that are met by individuals who meet the criteria for addiction varies with the severity of addiction, the stage of the addiction process, and the drug in question, but the criteria are well represented by symptoms that coalesce around the withdrawal/negative affect and preoccupation/anticipation stages[29,33] (see Fig. 18.1).

Important for the present chapter is the distinction between physical or somatic signs of withdrawal and motivational signs of withdrawal. Both reflect dependence in the classic sense,[66] but only the motivational signs of withdrawal are argued herein to be relevant to the syndrome of addiction (see discussion of somatic vs. motivational withdrawal in subsequent text of this chapter). Thus, although historically the diagnostic criteria have focused on physical (somatic) signs of withdrawal, more motivational signs have been neglected, and the argument of the present treatise is that motivational signs of withdrawal remain a critical aspect of the addiction process.

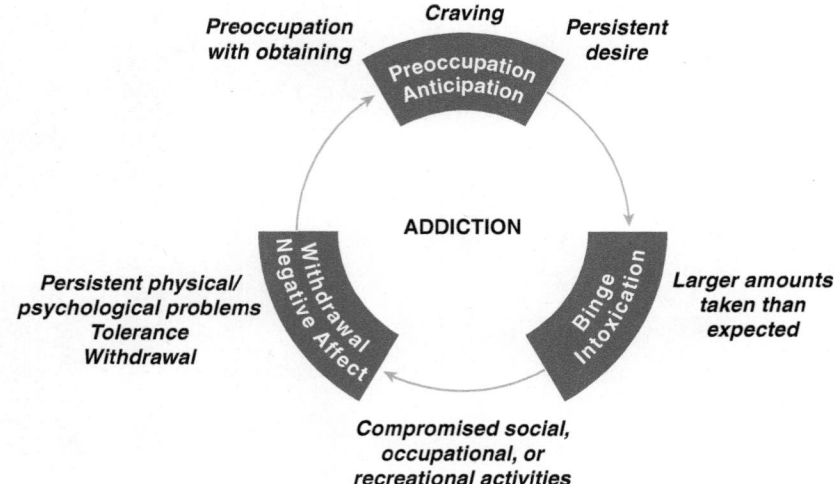

• **Fig. 18.1** Diagram describing the three stages of the addiction cycle—preoccupation/anticipation, binge/intoxication, and withdrawal/negative affect—from a psychiatric perspective with the different criteria for substance dependence incorporated from the DSM-5. Bolded symptoms from the DSM reflect changes during the three stages of the addiction cycle. (Reprinted with permission from Koob.[80])

Different drugs produce different patterns of addiction, with an emphasis on different components of the addiction cycle. The classic drugs of addiction are opioids. A pattern of intravenous or smoked drug taking evolves, including intense intoxication, the development of tolerance, escalation of intake, and profound dysphoria, physical discomfort, and somatic withdrawal signs during abstinence. Intense preoccupation with obtaining opioids (craving) develops that often precedes the somatic signs of withdrawal and is linked not only to stimuli that are associated with obtaining the drug but also to stimuli that are associated with withdrawal and internal and external states of stress. A pattern develops in which the drug must be taken to avoid the severe dysphoria and discomfort of abstinence. Other drugs of abuse follow a similar pattern but may involve more the binge/intoxication stage (e.g., psychostimulants and alcohol) or less binge/intoxication and more withdrawal/negative affect and preoccupation/anticipation stages (e.g., nicotine and cannabinoids).

Animal Models of Withdrawal

Somatic Signs

Two drugs, opioids and alcohol, provide classic examples of the somatic signs of withdrawal and have served as models for measures of withdrawal per se. Indeed, as discussed earlier, these somatic measures are basically a "red herring" for the more motivational measures of withdrawal from the perspective of negative reinforcement, drug seeking, and craving that are associated with acute and protracted abstinence. However, the somatic signs of withdrawal are an index of neuroadaptational changes that reflect sufficient drug intake to produce motivational measures, given that motivational measures occur at lower doses and earlier than somatic signs.[162]

For opioids, somatic withdrawal signs in humans are dramatic and dose-dependent and duration-of-abstinence-dependent and include a number of overt measurable signs, such as yawning,

lacrimation, rhinorrhea, perspiration, gooseflesh, tremor, dilated pupils, anorexia, nausea, emesis, diarrhea, weight loss, and elevations of temperature and blood pressure.[66] In animals (rodents), opioid withdrawal signs are well characterized when precipitated by the administration of a competitive opioid receptor antagonist, such as naloxone.[51,107] A weighted scale was developed and widely adopted that included graded signs of weight loss, diarrhea, escape attempts, wet dog shakes, abdominal constrictions, facial fasciculations/teeth chattering, salivation, ptosis, abnormal posture, penile grooming/erection/ejaculation, and irritability[51] (Table 18.1). When the somatic signs of opioid withdrawal are directly compared with more motivational measures, the motivational measures are more sensitive and show more efficacy in defining the withdrawal state.[162] Spontaneous withdrawal shows many of the same signs, but they are significantly less intense[131] (see Table 18.1).

For alcohol, the somatic signs of withdrawal in humans are equally dramatic but also life-threatening and are characterized by tremor, increases in heart rate, increases in blood pressure, increases in body temperature, anorexia, and convulsions. In its severest form, alcohol withdrawal can result in pronounced hyperthermia that can evolve into delirium tremens, a state of marked sympathetic hyperactivity, hyperthermia (which can be fatal), and hallucinations.[56] In animals (rodents), alcohol withdrawal signs are characterized by hyperactivity, tail tremors, tail stiffness, head tremors, general tremors, ventromedio-distal flexion, wet shakes, teeth chattering, akinesia, spastic rigidity, and induced and spontaneous convulsions[102] (see Table 18.1). With alcohol, the withdrawal is only spontaneous because no known competitive antagonist can precipitate withdrawal. Similar to opioids, withdrawal from alcohol is dose- and duration-of-abstinence-dependent, with peak withdrawal ranging from 10 to 16 hours with high-dose blood alcohol levels at the time of withdrawal (300–400 mg/dL).[102]

Motivational Signs

Animal models of the withdrawal/negative affect stage include increases in anxiety-like responses, measures of conditioned place

TABLE 18.1 Somatic withdrawal signs

OPIOID WITHDRAWAL	
Rats	Humans
Weight loss	Weight loss
Diarrhea	Diarrhea
Escape attempts	Yawning
Wet dog shakes	Lacrimation
Abdominal constrictions	Rhinorrhea
Facial fasciculations	Perspiration
Teeth chattering	Gooseflesh
Salivation	Tremor
Ptosis	Dilated pupils
Abnormal posture	Anorexia
Penile grooming	Nausea
Erection/ejaculation	Emesis
Irritability	Hyperthermia
	Increased blood pressure

ALCOHOL WITHDRAWAL	
Rats	Humans
Hyperactivity	Tremor
Tail tremors	Increased heart rate
Tail stiffness	Increased blood pressure
Akinesia	Increased body temperature
Spastic rigidity	Anorexia
Convulsions	Convulsions
	Hyperthermia
	Delirium tremens

TABLE 18.2 Animal Models Associated With the Different Stages of the Addiction Cycle

Stage of Addiction Cycle	Animal Model
Binge/intoxication	• Drug/alcohol self-administration • Conditioned place preference • Brain stimulation reward thresholds
Withdrawal/negative affect	• Anxiety-like responses • Conditioned place aversion • Brain stimulation reward • Escalation of drug self-administration with extended access or dependence
Preoccupation/anticipation	• Drug-induced reinstatement • Cue-induced reinstatement • Stress-induced reinstatement • Protracted abstinence

aversion (rather than preference), and elevations of brain stimulation reward thresholds in response to precipitated withdrawal or spontaneous withdrawal from chronic administration of a drug[a] (Table 18.2).

Anxiety-Like Symptoms

A common response to acute withdrawal and protracted abstinence from all major drugs of abuse is the manifestation of anxiety-like responses. Animal models have revealed anxiety-like responses to all major drugs of abuse during acute withdrawal, with the dependent variable often a passive response to a novel and/or aversive stimulus, such as the open field or elevated plus maze, or an active response to an aversive stimulus, such as defensive burying of an electrified metal probe. Withdrawal from repeated administration of cocaine produces an anxiogenic-like response in the elevated plus maze and defensive burying test, both of which are reversed by administration of corticotropin-releasing factor (CRF) antagonists[16,155] (Fig. 18.2). Precipitated withdrawal in opioid dependence and nicotine dependence also produces anxiety-like effects.[52,60,163] Spontaneous alcohol withdrawal produces anxiety-like behavior.[b]

Dysphoria-Like Symptoms

Place aversion has been used to measure the aversive stimulus effects of withdrawal, mostly in the context of opioids[59,179]

[a]References 43, 49, 104, 133, 161, 162.
[b]References 13, 23, 75, 129, 137, 183, 185.

(Fig. 18.3). In contrast to conditioned place preference, rats that are exposed to a particular environment while undergoing precipitated withdrawal from opioids spend less time in the withdrawal-paired environment when subsequently presented with a choice between that environment and an unpaired environment. Such an association continues to be manifested weeks after the animals are "detoxified" (e.g., after the morphine pellets are removed[12,178]) and can be measured from 24 hours to 16 weeks later.[59,178,179] Additionally a place aversion in opioid-dependent rats can be observed with doses of naloxone below which somatic signs of withdrawal are observed.[162] Although naloxone itself will produce a place aversion in nondependent rats, the threshold dose that is required to produce a place aversion decreases significantly in dependent rats.[59]

The place aversion to opioids does not require the maintenance of opioid dependence for its manifestation, and a variation of this approach is to explore the place aversion that is produced following a naloxone injection after a single acute injection of morphine. Acute opioid dependence has been defined as the precipitation of withdrawal-like signs by opioid receptor antagonists following a single opioid dose or short-term administration of an opioid receptor agonist.[106] Rats exhibit a reliable conditioned place aversion that is precipitated by a low dose of naloxone after a single morphine injection that reflects a motivational component of acute withdrawal.[11] Similar acute withdrawal-like effects have been observed using anxiety-like responses following bolus injections of alcohol.[207]

Reward Thresholds

Electrical brain stimulation reward or intracranial self-stimulation has a long history as a measure of activity of the brain reward system and of the acute reinforcing effects of drugs of abuse. All drugs of abuse, when administered acutely, lower brain reward thresholds.[93] Brain stimulation reward involves widespread neurocircuitry in the brain, but the most sensitive sites, defined by the lowest thresholds, involve the trajectory of the medial forebrain bundle that connects the ventral tegmental area with the basal forebrain.[126] Although much emphasis was placed initially on the role of the ascending monoamine systems in the medial forebrain bundle, other nondopaminergic, descending systems in the medial forebrain bundle clearly play a key role.[64]

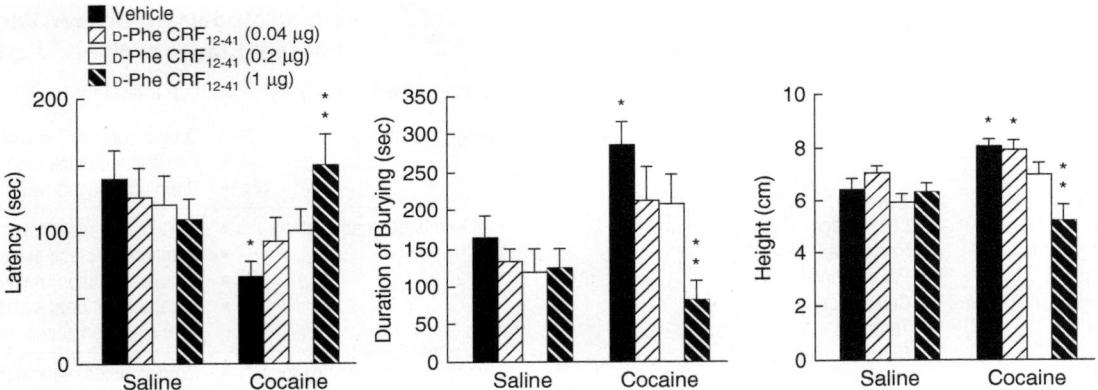

• **Fig. 18.2** Effect of intracerebroventricular administration of the corticotropin-releasing factor (CRF) antagonist D-Phe CRF$_{12-41}$ on anxiogenic-like effects in the defensive burying paradigm following chronic cocaine administration. Rats received chronic cocaine (20 mg/kg, i.p., for 14 days) or saline (1 ml/kg, i.p.). Animals were then tested in the defensive burying paradigm 48 h after the last injection. D-Phe CRF$_{12-41}$ (0, 0.04, 0.2, and 1.0 mg/5 mL) was administered immediately after the animal touched the electrified probe and received the shock and 5 min before the testing session. The data are expressed as mean ± standard error of the mean (SEM; n = 10–14/group). The left panel shows the latency to start burying in all experimental groups (*p < 0.05, compared with saline/vehicle group; **p < 0.01, compared with cocaine/vehicle group; Duncan post hoc test). The middle panel represents the total duration of burying behavior in all experimental groups (*p < 0.05, compared with chronically saline-treated groups; **p < 0.01, compared with cocaine/vehicle group; Duncan post hoc analysis). The right panel represents the height of bedding material at the junction between the probe and the wall of the testing cage (*p < 0.05, compared with saline/vehicle group; **p < 0.01, compared with other chronically cocaine-treated groups; Duncan post hoc analysis). (Reprinted with permission from Basso et al.[16] [Springer Science+Business Media].)

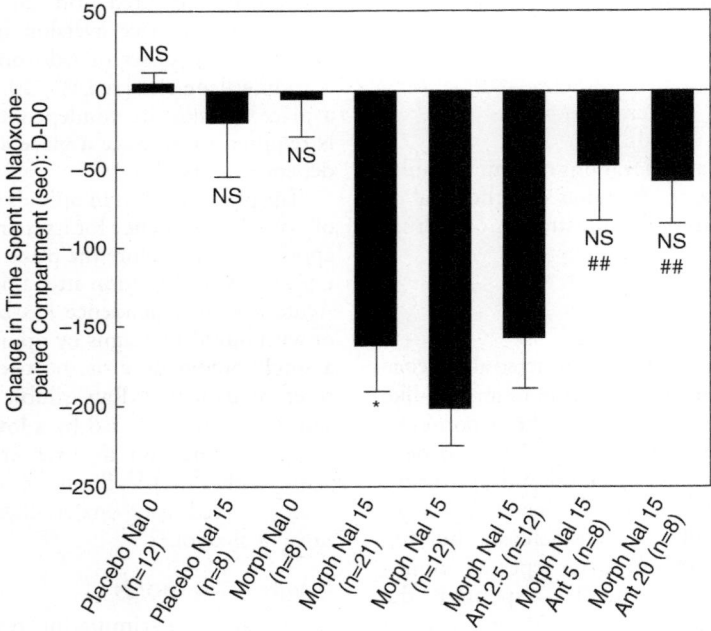

• **Fig. 18.3** The corticotropin-releasing factor-1 antagonist antalarmin (Ant) reduced naloxone (NAL)-precipitated place aversion conditioning in morphine (Morph)-dependent rats. Morphine dependence was induced by subcutaneous implantation of two slow-release, morphine-containing pellets, each containing 75 mg of morphine base. Placebo-pelleted rats received placebo morphine pellets that were implanted subcutaneously. Separate groups of morphine-dependent rats that received naloxone (15 μg/kg, subcutaneously) immediately prior to conditioning (Morph-Nal) were also injected 30 min before naloxone on days 6, 8, and 10 with antalarmin (2.5, 5, 10, or 20 mg/kg, intraperitoneally; n = 8–12/group). Although antalarmin at doses of 2.5 and 5 mg/kg was ineffective, doses of 10 and 20 mg/kg blocked the place aversion that was produced by naloxone in morphine-dependent rats and returned values to levels that were observed with naloxone in placebo-pelleted rats and in morphine-no naloxone (Morph-Nal 0) rats. *p < 0.05, within each dose group treatment (Wilcoxon signed-rank test). NS refers to no significant place preference or place aversion with the Wilcoxon signed-rank test. ##p < 0.01, compared with Morph-Nal 15 group (between-group comparisons, Mann-Whitney test [ΔD]). (Reprinted with permission from Stinus et al.[177])

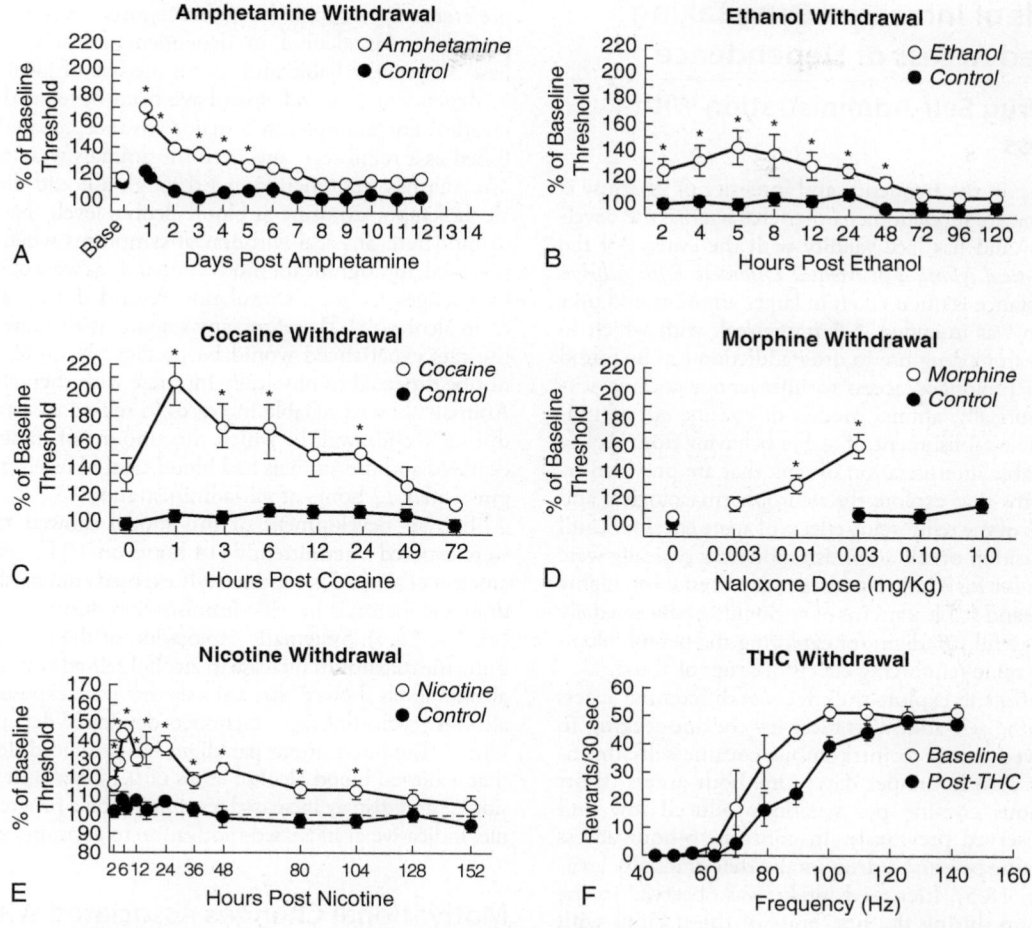

• **Fig. 18.4** (A) Mean intracranial self-stimulation reward thresholds (± SEM) in rats during amphetamine withdrawal (10 mg/kg/day for 6 days). Data are expressed as a percentage of the mean of the last five baseline values prior to drug treatment. *$p < 0.05$, compared with saline control group. (Reprinted with permission from Paterson et al.[133] [Springer Science+Business Media].) (B) Mean intracranial self-stimulation reward thresholds (± SEM) in rats during alcohol withdrawal (blood alcohol levels achieved: 197.29 mg%). Elevations of thresholds were time-dependent. *$p < 0.05$, compared with control group. (Reprinted with permission from Schulteis et al.[161]) (C) Mean intracranial self-stimulation thresholds (± SEM) in rats during cocaine withdrawal 24 h following the cessation of cocaine self-administration. *$p < 0.05$, compared with control group. (Reprinted with permission from Markou and Koob[104].) (D) Mean intracranial self-stimulation reward thresholds (± SEM) in rats during naloxone-precipitated morphine withdrawal. The minimum dose of naloxone that elevated intracranial self-stimulation reward thresholds in the morphine group was 0.01 mg/kg. *$p < 0.05$, compared with control group. (Reprinted with permission from Schulteis et al.[162]) (E) Mean intracranial self-stimulation reward thresholds (± SEM) in rats during spontaneous nicotine withdrawal following surgical removal of osmotic minipumps that delivered nicotine hydrogen tartrate (9 mg/kg/day) or saline. *$p < 0.05$, compared with control group. (Data adapted from Epping-Jordan et al.[43]) (F) Mean intracranial self-stimulation reward thresholds (± SEM) in rats during withdrawal from an acute 1.0 mg/kg dose of Δ^9-tetrahydrocannabinol (THC). Withdrawal significantly shifted the reward function to the right (indicating lower reward). (Reprinted with permission from Gardner and Vorel[49].) Note that because different equipment systems and threshold procedures were used in the collection of the above data, direct comparisons among the magnitude of effects that were induced by these drugs cannot be made.

Acute intravenous cocaine self-administration in animals lowers reward thresholds, consistent with the well-documented effects of drugs of abuse in lowering brain reward thresholds.[69] However, with more prolonged access to the drug, the lowering of reward thresholds (i.e., rewarding effects) are replaced with elevations of reward thresholds (i.e., anti-rewarding effects) after the initial lowering of reward thresholds, presumably reflecting an acute withdrawal or opponent process-like effect. Such elevations of reward thresholds begin rapidly,

can be observed within a single session of self-administration, and are greater with greater exposure to cocaine,[73] bearing a striking resemblance to human subjective reports.[24,186] Chronic administration or self-administration of all drugs of abuse produces elevations of reward thresholds during spontaneous or precipitated acute withdrawal (Fig. 18.4). These elevations of threshold can be short (minutes to hours) or can last for days, depending on dose, drug, time of exposure, and precipitant.

Animal Models of Increased Drug Taking With Prolonged Access or Dependence

Escalation of Drug Self-Administration With Extended Access

A progressive increase in the frequency and intensity of drug use is one of the major behavioral phenomena that characterize the development of addiction and has face validity with the criteria of the *Diagnostic and Statistical Manual of Mental Disorders Fifth Edition* (DSM-5): "The substance is often taken in larger amounts and over a longer period than was intended."[8] A framework with which to model the transition from drug use to drug addiction can be found in animal models of prolonged access to intravenous cocaine self-administration. Historically, animal models of cocaine self-administration involved the establishment of stable behavior from day to day to allow the reliable interpretation of data that are provided by within-subjects designs that explore the neuropharmacological and neurobiological bases of the reinforcing effects of acute cocaine. Until 1998, after the acquisition of self-administration, rats typically were allowed access to cocaine for 3 hours or less per day to establish highly stable levels of intake and stable patterns of responding between daily sessions. This was a useful paradigm for exploring the neurobiological substrates for the acute reinforcing effects of drugs of abuse.

However, in an effort to explore the effects of differential access to intravenous cocaine self-administration on cocaine-seeking in rats, rats were allowed access to intravenous cocaine self-administration for 1 hour or 6 hours per day.[4] One-hour access (short access) to intravenous cocaine per session produced low and stable intake, as observed previously. In contrast, 6-hour access (long access) to cocaine produced drug intake that gradually escalated over days (Fig. 18.5). Increased intake was observed in the extended-access group during the first hour of the session, with sustained intake over the entire session and an upward shift in the dose-effect function, suggesting an increase in hedonic set point. When animals were allowed access to different doses of cocaine, both the long- and short-access animals titrated their cocaine intake, but the long-access rats consistently self-administered almost twice as much cocaine at any dose tested, further suggesting an upward shift in the set point for cocaine reward in the escalated animals.[5,38,103] Such increased self-administration in dependent animals has now been observed with cocaine, methamphetamine, nicotine, heroin, and alcohol[4,6,32,42,74] (see Fig. 18.5). This model is a key element for evaluating the motivational significance of changes in the brain reward and stress systems in addiction that lead to compulsivity in addiction. Similar changes in the reinforcing and incentive effects of cocaine have been observed following extended access and include increased cocaine-induced reinstatement after extinction and decreased latency to goal time in a runway model for cocaine reward.[36] Altogether, these results suggest that drug taking with extended access changes the motivation to seek the drug. Whether this enhanced drug taking reflects the sensitization of reward or a reward deficit state remains under discussion,[189] but the brain reward and neuropharmacological studies that are outlined in subsequent text argue for a reward deficit state that drives the increased drug taking during extended access.

Withdrawal-Induced Drinking

Historically, animal models of negative reinforcement that is associated with alcohol dependence have proven difficult, especially with rodents. The induction of physical dependence could enhance the preference for alcohol,[c] but other reports did not support enhanced preference for alcohol in dependent animals.[20,118,205] Over the past 30 years, reliable and useful models of alcohol consumption in dependent rats and mice have been developed in several laboratories. For example, in a major advance, alcohol first was established as a reinforcer, and then the animals were made dependent. The animals were maintained through a liquid diet or continuous alcohol vapor exposure at blood alcohol levels that produced mild-to-moderate physical withdrawal symptoms when the alcohol was removed, but significant motivational signs were observed, measured by changes in brain stimulation reward during acute withdrawal from alcohol.[161] Therefore, any somatic withdrawal symptoms that the rats experienced would be predictably quite mild and would not be expected to physically interfere with their ability to respond. Animals showed reliable increases in self-administration of alcohol during withdrawal, in which the amount of intake approximately doubled and the animals had blood alcohol levels from 0.10 to 0.15 gm% after 12 hours of self-administration.[146]

Further development of this model showed that animals that were exposed intermittently (14 hours on/10 hours off) to the same amount of alcohol as continuously exposed animals showed even more dramatic increases in self-administration during acute withdrawal[125] (see Fig. 18.5). Systematic exploration of the parameters that determine the maximum increase in alcohol self-administration and blood alcohol levels showed that animals that were exposed to intermittent alcohol via alcohol vapor chambers developed dependence more rapidly.[125] The intermittent paradigm has produced dependent animals that achieved blood alcohol levels of 0.15 gm% in a 30-minute session[140] and display increased responding on a progressive-ratio schedule, indicative of increased motivation to consume alcohol.[193]

Motivational Changes Associated With Increased Drug Intake During Extended Access or Dependence

The hypothesis that compulsive drug use is accompanied by a chronic perturbation in brain reward homeostasis has been tested in an animal model of the escalation of drug intake with prolonged access combined with measures of brain stimulation reward thresholds. Animals that were implanted with intravenous catheters and allowed differential access to intravenous self-administration of cocaine or heroin showed increases in drug self-administration from day to day in the long-access group but not in the short-access group. The differential exposure to drug self-administration had dramatic effects on reward thresholds that progressively increased in long-access rats but not in short-access or control rats across successive self-administration sessions[2,72] (Fig. 18.6). Elevations of baseline reward thresholds temporally preceded and were highly correlated with the escalation of cocaine intake. Postsession elevations of reward thresholds failed to return to baseline levels before the onset of each subsequent self-administration session, thereby deviating progressively more from control levels. The progressive elevation of reward thresholds was associated with the dramatic escalation of cocaine consumption that was observed previously. After escalation had occurred, an acute cocaine challenge facilitated brain reward responsiveness to the same degree as before but resulted in higher absolute brain reward thresholds in long-access compared with short-access rats.[2] Similar results have been observed with extended access to heroin,[72] in which rats that were allowed 23-hour access to

---

[c]References 39, 40, 68, 146, 153, 160, 187, 206.

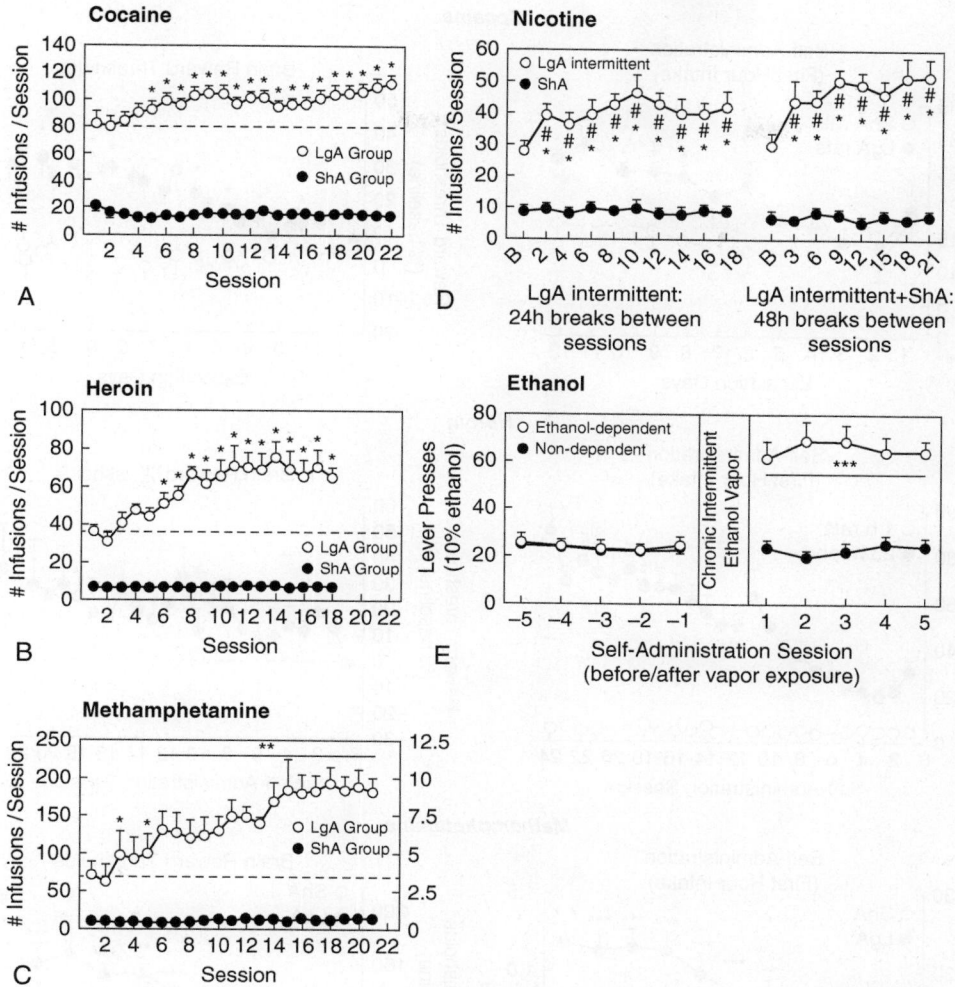

• **Fig. 18.5** Escalation of drug intake. (A) Effect of drug availability on cocaine intake (mean ± SEM). In long-access (LgA) rats ($n = 12$) but not short-access (ShA) rats ($n = 12$), the mean total cocaine intake started to increase significantly from session 5 ($p < 0.05$; sessions 5 to 22 compared with session 1) and continued to increase thereafter ($p < 0.05$; session 5 compared with sessions 8–10, 12, 13, and 17–22). (Reprinted with permission from Ahmed and Koob.[4]) (B) Effect of drug availability on total intravenous heroin self-infusions (mean ± SEM). During the escalation phase, rats had access to heroin (40 μg per infusion) for 1 h (ShA rats, $n = 5$-6) or 11 h per session (LgA rats, $n = 5$-6). Regular 1-h (ShA rats) or 11-h (LgA rats) sessions of heroin self-administration were performed 6 days per week. The dotted line indicates the mean ± SEM number of heroin self-infusions in LgA rats during the first 11-h session. *$p < 0.05$, different from the first session (paired t-test). (Reprinted with permission from Ahmed et al.[6]) (C) Effect of extended access to intravenous methamphetamine on self-administration as a function of daily sessions in rats trained to self-administer 0.05 mg/kg/infusion of intravenous methamphetamine during 6-h sessions. ShA, 1-h session ($n = 6$). LgA, 6-h session ($n = 4$). *$p < 0.05$, **$p < 0.01$, compared with day 1. (Reprinted with permission from Kitamura et al.[74]) (D) Nicotine intake (mean ± SEM) in rats that self-administered nicotine under a fixed-ratio (FR) 1 schedule in either 21-h (long access [LgA]) or 1-h (short access [ShA]) sessions. LgA rats increased their nicotine intake on an intermittent schedule with 24–48 h breaks between sessions, whereas LgA rats on a daily schedule did not. The left shows the total number of nicotine infusions per session when the intermittent schedule included 24-h breaks between sessions. The right shows the total number of nicotine infusions per session when the intermittent schedule included 48-h breaks between sessions. #$p < 0.05$, compared with baseline; *$p < 0.05$, compared with daily self-administration group. $n = 10$ per group. (Reprinted with permission from Cohen et al.[32]) (E) Ethanol self-administration in ethanol-dependent and nondependent animals. The induction of ethanol dependence and correlation of limited ethanol self-administration before and excessive drinking after dependence induction following chronic intermittent ethanol vapor exposure is shown. ***$p < 0.001$, significant group × test session interaction. With all drugs, escalation is defined as a significant increase in drug intake within-subjects in extended-access groups, with no significant changes within-subjects in limited-access groups. (Reprinted with permission from Edwards et al.[42])

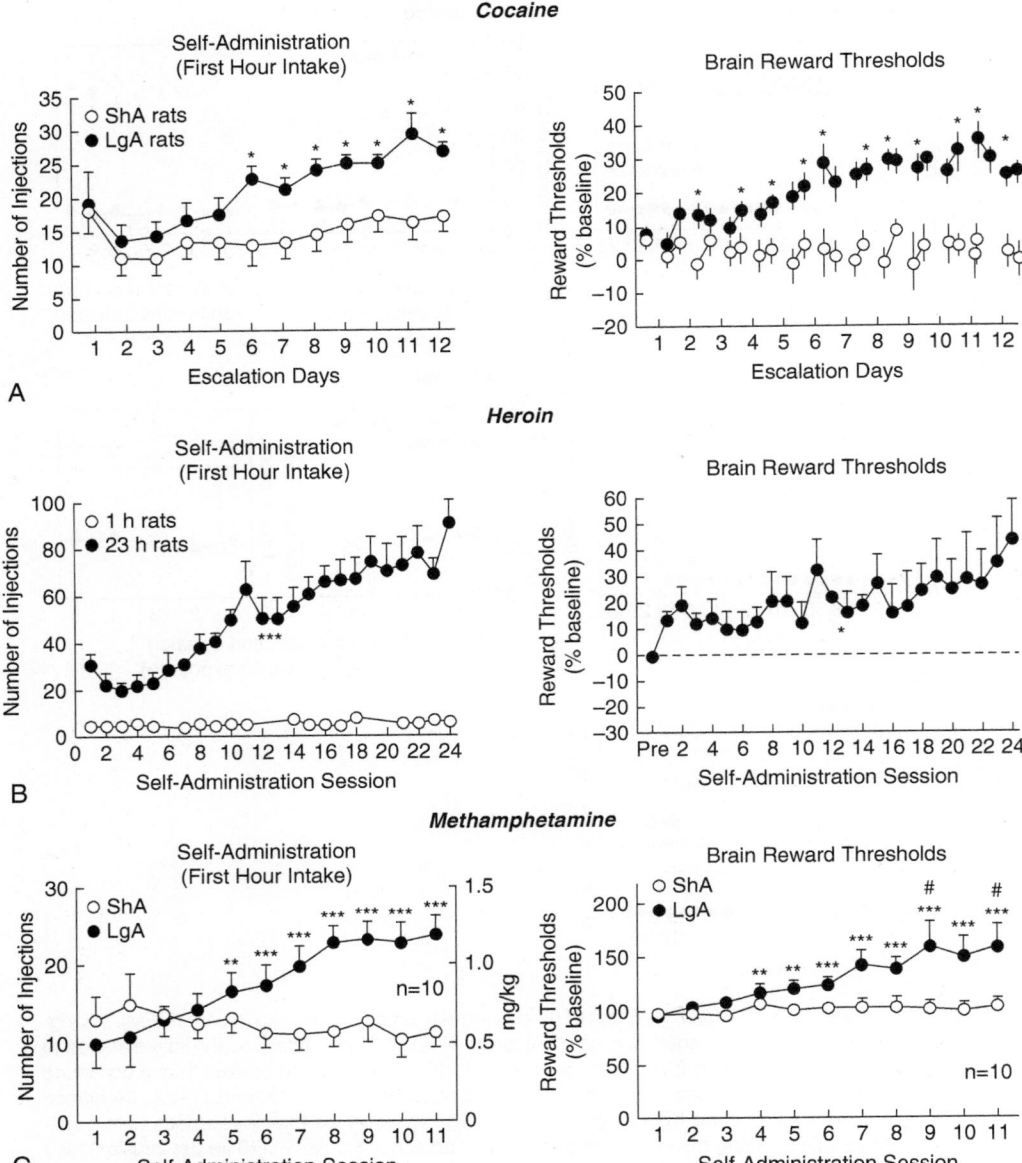

• **Fig. 18.6** (A) Relationship between elevation in of intracranial self-stimulation (ICSS) reward thresholds and cocaine intake escalation. (*Left*) Percent change from baseline response latencies (3 h and 17–22 h after each self-administration session; first data point indicates 1 h before the first session). (*Right*) Percent change from baseline ICSS thresholds. *$p < 0.05$, compared with drug-naive and/or ShA rats (tests for simple main effects). (Reprinted with permission from Ahmed et al.[2]) (B) Unlimited daily access to heroin escalated heroin intake and increased reward thresholds. (*Left*) Heroin intake (± SEM; 20 µg per infusion) in rats during limited (1 h) or unlimited (23 h) self-administration sessions. ***$p < 0.001$, main effect of access (1 or 23 h). (*Right*) Percent change from baseline ICSS thresholds (± SEM) in 23 h rats. Reward thresholds, assessed immediately after each daily 23 h self-administration session, became progressively more elevated as exposure to self-administered heroin increased across sessions. *$p < 0.05$, main effect of heroin on reward thresholds. (Reprinted with permission from Kenny et al.[72]) (C) Escalation of methamphetamine self-administration and ICSS in rats. Rats were daily allowed to receive ICSS in the lateral hypothalamus 1 h before and 3 h after intravenous methamphetamine self-administration with either 1- or 6-h access. (*Left*) Methamphetamine self-administration during the first hour of each session. (*Right*) ICSS measured 1 h before and 3 h after methamphetamine self-administration. *$p < 0.05$, **$p < 0.01$, ***$p < 0.001$, compared with session 1; #$p < 0.05$, compared with LgA 3 h after. (From Jang et al.[70])

heroin showed a time-dependent elevation of reward thresholds that paralleled the increases in heroin intake (see Fig. 18.6).

Another reflection of the change in motivation that is associated with dependence is a measure of reinforcement efficacy, measured by changes in progressive-ratio responding. In the progressive-ratio procedure, rats are first allowed to reach baseline responding

for cocaine under a fixed-ratio 1 schedule of reinforcement. For a progressive-ratio schedule, the response requirement (i.e., the number of lever responses that are required to receive a drug injection, or "ratio") increases using an exponential function, such as $5^{(0.2 \cdot \text{infusion number})} - 5$, yielding response requirements of 1, 2, 4, 6, 9, 12, 15, 20, 25, 32, 40, 50, 62, 77, 95, 118, 146, 178, 219, and

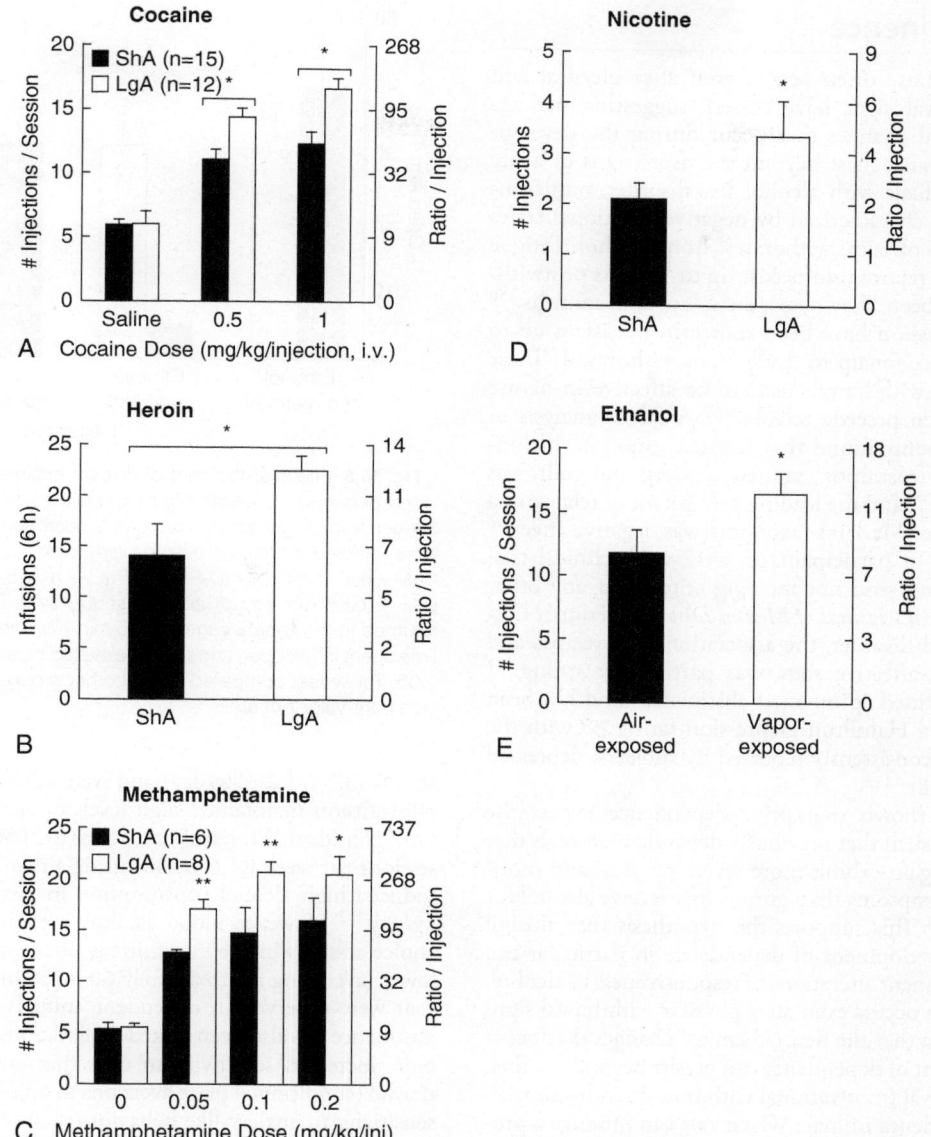

• **Fig. 18.7** (A) Dose-response function of cocaine self-administration in rats under a progressive-ratio schedule. Test sessions under a progressive-ratio schedule ended when rats did not achieve reinforcement within 1 h. The data are expressed as the number of injections per session on the left axis and ratio per injection on the right axis. *$p < 0.05$, compared with short-access (ShA) rats at each dose of cocaine. (Reprinted with permission from Wee et al.[197]) (B) Responding for heroin under a progressive-ratio schedule of reinforcement in ShA and long-access (LgA) rats. *$p < 0.05$, LgA significantly different from LgA. (Modified with permission from Barbier et al.[14]) (C) Dose-response for methamphetamine under a progressive-ratio schedule. Test sessions under a progressive-ratio schedule ended when rats did not achieve reinforcement within 1 h. *$p < 0.05$, **$p < 0.01$, LgA significantly different from ShA. (Modified with permission from Wee et al.[199]) (D) Breakpoints on a progressive-ratio schedule in LgA rats that self-administered nicotine with 48 h abstinence between sessions. LgA rats on an intermittent schedule reached significantly higher breakpoints than LgA rats that self-administered nicotine daily. The data are expressed as mean ± SEM. *$p < 0.05$. $n = 9$ rats per group. (Reprinted with permission from Cohen et al.[32]) (E) Mean (± SEM) breakpoints for alcohol while in nondependent and alcohol-dependent states. **$p < 0.01$, main effect of vapor exposure on alcohol self-administration. (Reprinted with permission from Walker and Koob.[193])

268, etc.[148] Sessions on this schedule are terminated when more than three times the animal's longest baseline interresponse time has elapsed since the last self-administered cocaine injection.[19] Animals normally respond for 11–15 injections of cocaine, and the breakpoint is defined as the highest completed ratio in a session. The dependent measure in progressive-ratio experiments is the total number of injections that are obtained per session and

the breakpoint. Extended access to drugs that results in escalated intake is also associated with an increase in breakpoint for cocaine on a progressive-ratio schedule, suggesting enhanced motivation to seek cocaine or the lower efficacy of cocaine reward.[132,197] Similar results have been observed with methamphetamine and withdrawal-induced drinking in rats that were made dependent with alcohol vapor[193] (Fig. 18.7).

Protracted Abstinence

Relapse to drugs of abuse often occurs even after physical and motivational withdrawal signs have ceased, suggesting perhaps that the neurochemical changes that occur during the development of dependence can persist beyond the overt signs of acute withdrawal. In individuals with alcohol use disorder, numerous symptoms that can be characterized by negative emotional states persist long after acute physical withdrawal from alcohol. Fatigue and tension have been reported to persist up to 5 weeks postwithdrawal.[7] Anxiety has been shown to persist up to 9 months,[150] and anxiety and depression have been shown to persist in up to 20%–25% of alcoholics for up to 2 years postwithdrawal. These symptoms, post-acute withdrawal, tend to be affective in nature and subacute and often precede relapse.[9,65] A factor analysis of Marlatt's relapse taxonomy found that negative emotion, including elements of anger, frustration, sadness, anxiety, and guilt, was a key factor in relapse,[208] and the leading precipitant of relapse in a large-scale replication of Marlatt's taxonomy was negative affect.[99] In secondary analyses of participants in a 12-week clinical trial with alcohol dependence and not meeting criteria for any other *Diagnostic and Statistical Manual of Mental Disorders*, Fourth Edition (DSM-IV), mood disorder, the association with relapse and a subclinical negative affective state was particularly strong.[111] This state has been termed "protracted abstinence" and has been defined in humans as a Hamilton Depression rating ≥8 with the following three items consistently reported by subjects: depressed mood, anxiety, and guilt.[111]

Animal work has shown that prior dependence lowers the dependence threshold such that previously dependent animals that are made dependent again exhibit more severe physical and motivational withdrawal symptoms than groups that receive alcohol for the first time.[17,18,21,23] This supports the hypothesis that alcohol experience and the development of dependence in particular can lead to relatively permanent alterations of responsiveness to alcohol. However, relapse often occurs even after physical withdrawal signs have ceased, suggesting that the neurochemical changes that occur during the development of dependence can persist beyond the final overt signs of withdrawal (motivational withdrawal syndrome).

A history of dependence in male Wistar rats can produce a prolonged elevation of alcohol self-administration in daily 30-minute sessions after acute withdrawal and detoxification.[142,143,147,174] This increase in self-administration of alcohol is accompanied by increases in blood alcohol levels and persists for up to 8 weeks postdetoxification. The increase in self-administration is also accompanied by increased behavioral responsivity to stressors and increased responsivity to antagonists of the brain CRF systems.[50,174,185] The persistent increase in alcohol self-administration has been hypothesized to involve an allostatic-like adjustment such that the set point for alcohol reward is elevated.[88,147] These persistent alterations of alcohol self-administration and residual sensitivity to stressors can be arbitrarily defined as a state of "protracted abstinence." Protracted abstinence, defined as such in the rat, spans a period after acute physical withdrawal has disappeared when elevations of alcohol intake over baseline and increased behavioral responsivity to stress persist (2–8 weeks postwithdrawal from chronic alcohol).

Significant self-administration of high amounts of alcohol that are similar to those that are observed in alcohol-preferring animals and during protracted abstinence has been observed using other methods. Here, the animals exhibited tolerance but no somatic withdrawal. Rats that received passive intragastric infusion of alcohol for 3–6 days at levels that are observed in alcohol-preferring

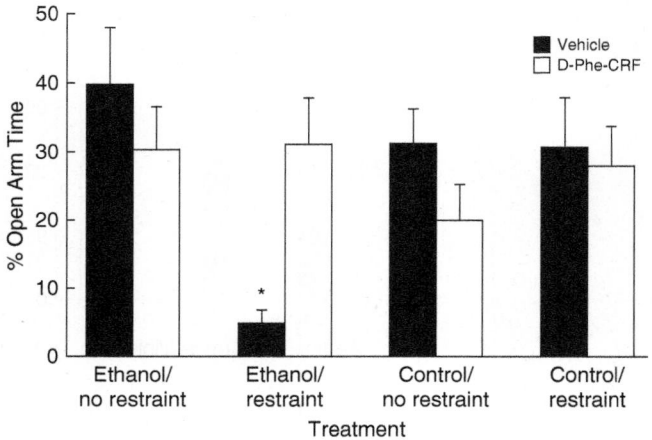

• **Fig. 18.8** Effect of restraint stress on exploratory behavior in the elevated plus maze 6 weeks after exposure to an alcohol liquid diet over a 3-week period. Control rats received a sucrose-containing liquid diet. Rats were injected intracerebroventricularly with 10 μg of [D-Phe^{12}, Nle^{21,38}, CαMeLeu^{37}]rCRF$_{12-41}$ (D-Phe-CRF$_{12-41}$; n = 8-11 per group) or vehicle (n = 7 or 8 per group) and subsequently placed in restraint tubes or returned to their home cages for 15 min. The mean (± SEM) percentage of time spent in the open arms of the elevated plus maze was measured. *p < 0.05, Tukey test compared with all other groups. (Reprinted with permission from Valdez et al.[185])

strains (3.3–12.2 g/kg/day) and were allowed access to intragastric self-infusion maintained high levels of alcohol self-administration (4–7 g/kg/day).[45] Intermittent access to 20% alcohol (three 24-hour sessions per week for 6 weeks) using a two-bottle choice procedure induced high alcohol consumption in rats to levels up to 5–6 g/kg/day.[172] However, blood alcohol levels in 30-minute two-bottle choice sessions in the intermittent 20% animals were significantly lower (averaging approximately 60 mg% in Wistar rats) than those that were observed in dependent animals (see above). Protracted abstinence has also been linked to elevations of brain reward thresholds, increased sensitivity to cues that are associated with withdrawal (conditioned place aversions to opioids), and increases in the sensitivity to anxiety-like behavior (alcohol) that have been shown to persist after acute withdrawal symptoms have subsided in animals with a history of dependence.[123,173,178,184,185]

Stress-induced reinstatement of drug-seeking and stress-induced reinstatement of anxiety-like states during protracted abstinence represent models of the persistent preoccupation/anticipation (craving) stage of the addiction cycle. Protracted abstinence, largely described in alcohol dependence models, appears to involve overactive glutamatergic and CRF systems.[34,184] Rats that were made dependent with chronic continuous exposure to alcohol exhibited anxiety-like behavior on the elevated plus maze at 4 weeks postwithdrawal.[184] CRF receptor antagonists that are injected intracerebroventricularly or systemically block the potentiated anxiety-like responses to stressors that are observed during protracted abstinence from chronic alcohol.[d] In one example, rats that were tested on the elevated plus maze 3–5 weeks postwithdrawal did not exhibit an anxiogenic-like response at baseline, but an anxiogenic-like response was provoked by mild restraint stress only in rats with a history of alcohol dependence (Fig. 18.8). This stress-induced anxiogenic-like response was reversed by a competitive CRF receptor antagonist[185] (see Fig. 18.8).

---

[d]References 22, 23, 67, 130, 185, 204.

In human studies, situations of stress are the most likely triggers for relapse to drug-taking.[25,105] In parallel, there is evidence of stress-induced reinstatement in animal studies. In animals that are made dependent, stressors have a greater impact. Animal models of stress-induced reinstatement show that stressors elicit strong recovery of extinguished drug-seeking behavior in the absence of further drug availability.[3,44,168] The delivery of acute intermittent footshock induced the reinstatement of cocaine-seeking behavior after prolonged extinction, and this was as effective as a priming injection of cocaine.[3,37,44] Such effects are also observed after a 4- to 6-week drug-free period[44] and appear to be drug-specific, in which food-seeking behavior was not reinstated.[3] Other stressors that have been shown to be effective in reinstating drug seeking include food deprivation, restraint stress, tail pinch stress, swim stress, conditioned fear, social defeat stress, and administration of the α_2-adrenergic receptor antagonist yohimbine (an activator of the sympathetic nervous system).[e] Stress-induced reinstatement is mediated by norepinephrine and CRF, with a focus on the bed nucleus of the stria terminalis (for review, see reference 166 and 167).

Neurobiological Bases of Increased Drug Taking During Extended Access or Dependence

In a within-system adaptation, repeated drug administration elicits an opposing reaction within the same system in which the drug elicits its primary reinforcing actions.[84] For example, if the synaptic availability of the neurotransmitter dopamine is responsible for the acute reinforcing actions of cocaine, then the within-system opponent process neuroadaptation would be a decrease in the synaptic availability of dopamine. In a between-system adaptation, repeated drug administration recruits a different neurochemical system, one that is not involved in the acute reinforcing effects of the drug but that when activated or engaged acts in opposition to the primary reinforcing effects of the drug. For example, chronic cocaine may activate the neuropeptide dynorphin, and dynorphin produces dysphoria-like effects that would be opposite to those of dopamine.

Within-System Changes: Dopamine

Within-system neuroadaptations to chronic drug exposure include decreases in function of the same neurotransmitter systems in the same neurocircuits that are implicated in the acute reinforcing effects of drugs of abuse during drug withdrawal in animal studies. Decreases in activity of the mesolimbic dopamine system and decreases in serotonergic neurotransmission in the nucleus accumbens are well documented.[114,151,201,202] Imaging studies in drug-addicted humans have consistently shown long-lasting decreases in the numbers of dopamine D_2 receptors in drug abusers compared with controls.[191] Additionally, cocaine abusers have lower dopamine release in response to a pharmacological challenge with a stimulant drug.[110,192] Decreases in the number of dopamine D_2 receptors, coupled with the decrease in dopaminergic activity, in cocaine, nicotine, and alcohol abusers results in the lower sensitivity of reward circuits to stimulation by natural reinforcers.[109,190] These findings suggest an overall reduction of the sensitivity of the dopamine component of reward circuitry to natural reinforcers and other drugs in drug-addicted individuals.

Psychostimulant withdrawal in humans is associated with fatigue, depressed mood, and psychomotor retardation and in animals is associated with lower motivation to work for natural rewards[15]

and a decrease in locomotor activity,[135] behavioral effects that may involve decreases in dopaminergic function. Animals during amphetamine withdrawal exhibited decreased responding on a progressive-ratio schedule for a sweet solution, and this decreased responding was reversed by the dopamine receptor partial agonist terguride,[15,128] suggesting that low dopamine tone contributes to the motivational deficits that are associated with psychostimulant withdrawal.

Under this conceptual framework, other within-system neuroadaptations would induce greater sensitivity of receptor transduction mechanisms in the nucleus accumbens. The activation of adenylate cyclase, protein kinase A, cyclic adenosine monophosphate response-element binding protein, and ΔFosB has been observed during drug withdrawal.[121,124,164,169] The ΔFosB response is hypothesized to represent a neuroadaptive change that extends long into protracted abstinence.[122]

Between-System Changes: Role of Corticotropin-Releasing Factor

A prominent role for the activation of brain stress systems and inhibition of anti-stress systems in acute withdrawal and protracted abstinence has been established.[79] The neurobiological systems in the brain that constitute the brain stress systems that are engaged by the addiction process include CRF, dynorphin, norepinephrine, hypocretin, vasopressin, glucocorticoids, and neuroinflammatory factors. Perhaps the most compelling data derive from studies of the extrahypothalamic CRF system. CRF controls hormonal and behavioral responses to stressors, but the extrahypothalamic CRF system is hypothesized to mediate behavioral responses to stressors.[62] In addiction, CRF plays a key role via both the hypothalamic-pituitary-adrenal axis and extrahypothalamic CRF stress system, with a common response of elevated adrenocorticotropic hormone, corticosterone, and amygdala CRF during acute withdrawal[f] (Fig. 18.9). Data that support the role of CRF in mediating the negative emotional responses that are associated with acute and protracted abstinence have largely been generated by preclinical studies with animal models. The negative emotional-like states that are associated with acute withdrawal and protracted abstinence from all major drugs of abuse in animal models can be reversed by CRF receptor antagonists.[82] The effects of CRF antagonists have been localized to the central nucleus of the amygdala.[137] Critically, activation of the hypothalamic-pituitary-adrenal axis may be an early dysregulation that is associated with excessive drug taking that ultimately produces a "kindling" or sensitization of the extrahypothalamic CRF systems.[86,188]

Using the conditioned place aversion paradigm, the opioid receptor partial agonist buprenorphine dose-dependently decreased place aversion that was produced by precipitated opioid withdrawal. Systemic administration of a CRF_1 receptor antagonist and direct intracerebral administration of a peptide CRF_1/CRF_2 antagonist also decreased opioid withdrawal–induced place aversions.[63,177] Functional noradrenergic receptor antagonists also blocked opioid withdrawal–induced place aversion.[35]

The ability of CRF antagonists to block the anxiogenic-like and aversive-like motivational effects of drug withdrawal would predict motivational effects of CRF antagonists in animal models of extended access to drugs (Table 18.3). CRF antagonists selectively blocked the increased self-administration of drugs that was associated with extended access to intravenous self-administration of cocaine,[175] nicotine,[52] and heroin.[57]

---

[e]References 94, 98, 100, 138, 139, 154, 168, 170.

[f]References 35, 81, 85, 115, 127, 136, 144, 145.

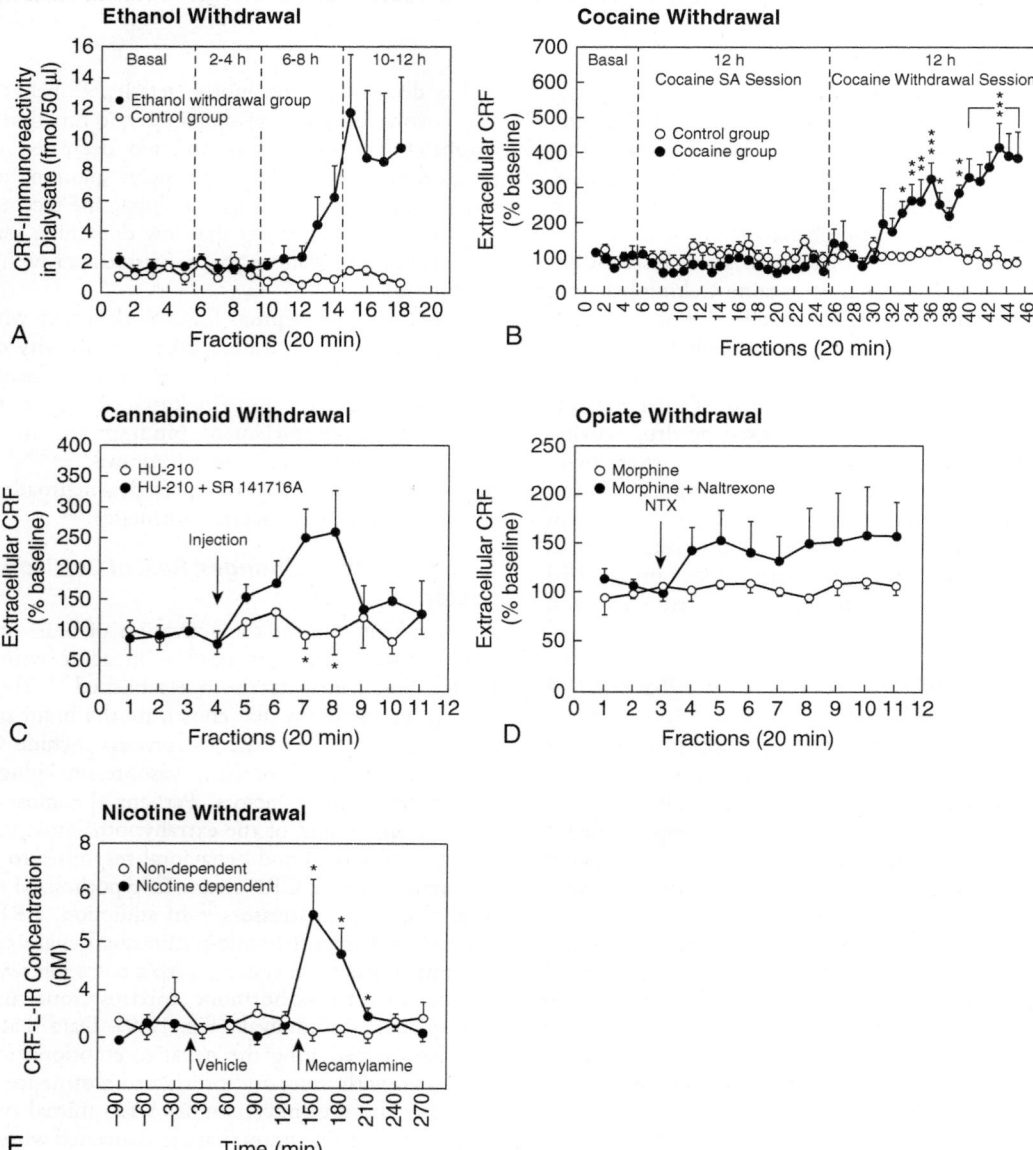

• **Fig. 18.9** (A) Effects of alcohol withdrawal on corticotropin-releasing factor (CRF)–like immunoreactivity in the rat amygdala, determined by microdialysis. Dialysate was collected over four 2-h periods that regularly alternated with nonsampling 2-h periods. The four sampling periods corresponded to the basal collection (before removal of alcohol), and 2–4 h, 6–8 h, and 10–12 h after withdrawal. Fractions were collected every 20 min. Data are represented as mean ± SEM ($n = 5$ per group). Analysis of variance confirmed significant differences between the two groups over time ($p < 0.05$). (Reprinted with permission from Merlo-Pich et al.[115]) (B) Mean (± SEM) dialysate CRF concentrations collected from the central nucleus of the amygdala in rats during baseline, 12 h cocaine self-administration (SA), and a subsequent 12-h withdrawal period (cocaine group, $n = 5$). The figure shows CRF levels in rats with the same history of cocaine self-administration training and drug exposure but not given access to cocaine on the test day (Control group, $n = 6$). The data are expressed as percentages of basal CRF concentrations. Dialysates were collected over 2-h periods that alternated with 1-h nonsampling periods, as shown by the timeline at the top. During cocaine self-administration, dialysate CRF concentrations in the cocaine group decreased by ~25% compared with control animals. In contrast, the termination of access to cocaine resulted in a significant increase in CRF release that began approximately 5 h postcocaine and reached 400% of presession baseline levels at the end of the withdrawal session. *$p < 0.05$, **$p < 0.01$, ***$p < 0.001$, simple effects after overall mixed-factorial analysis of variance. (Reprinted with permission from Richter and Weiss[141] [John Wiley & Sons, Inc.].) (C) Effects of cannabinoid CB_1 receptor antagonist SR 141716A (3 mg/kg) on CRF release from the central nucleus of the amygdala in rats that were pretreated for 14 days with the CB_1 receptor agonist HU-210 (100 mg/kg). Cannabinoid withdrawal that was induced by SR 141716A was associated with increased CRF release (*$p < 0.005$, $n = 5$–8). Vehicle injections did not alter CRF release ($n = 5$–7). Data were standardized by transforming dialysate CRF concentrations into percentages of baseline values based on averages of the first four fractions. (Reprinted with permission from Rodriguez de Fonseca et al[149] [American Association for the Advancement of Science].) (D) Effects of morphine withdrawal on CRF release in the central nucleus of the amygdala. Withdrawal was precipitated by administration of naltrexone (NTX; 0.1 mg/kg) in rats that were prepared with chronic morphine pellet implants. (Reprinted with permission from Weiss et al[200] [Wiley].) (E) Effect of mecamylamine (1.5 mg/kg, intraperitoneally)-precipitated nicotine withdrawal on CRF release in the central nucleus of the amygdala measured by in vivo microdialysis in chronic nicotine pump-treated (nicotine-dependent, $n = 7$) and chronic saline pump-treated (non-dependent, $n = 6$) rats. *$p < 0.05$, compared with nondependent. (Reprinted with permission from George et al.[52])

TABLE 18.3 | **Role of Corticotropin-Releasing Factor in Dependence**

Drug	Withdrawal-Induced Changes in Extracellular Corticotropin-Releasing Factor in CeA	CORTICOTROPIN-RELEASING FACTOR RECEPTOR ANTAGONIST EFFECTS			
		Withdrawal-Induced Anxiety-Like or Aversive Responses	Baseline Self-Administration or Place Preference	Dependence-Induced Increases in Self-Administration	Stress-Induced Reinstatement
Cocaine	↑	↓	—	↓	↓
Opioids	↑	↓	—	↓	↓
Alcohol	↑	↓	—	↓	↓
Nicotine	↑	↓	—	↓	↓
Δ⁹-THC	↑	↓			

—, no effect; blank entries indicate not tested. CeA, central nucleus of the amygdala. Δ^9-THC, Δ^9-tetrahydrocannabinol.
(Reprinted with permission from Koob.[79])

A particularly dramatic example of the motivational effects of CRF in dependence can be observed in animal models of alcohol self-administration in dependent animals. During alcohol withdrawal, extrahypothalamic CRF systems become hyperactive, with an increase in extracellular CRF in the central nucleus of the amygdala and bed nucleus of the stria terminalis in dependent rats[47,115,127] (see Fig. 18.9). The dysregulation of brain CRF systems is hypothesized to underlie the enhanced anxiety-like behaviors and the enhanced alcohol self-administration that are associated with alcohol withdrawal.

Supporting this hypothesis, exposure to repeated cycles of chronic alcohol vapor produced substantial increases in alcohol intake in rats both during acute withdrawal and during protracted abstinence (2 weeks post-acute withdrawal).[125,142] The subtype nonselective CRF receptor antagonists α-helical CRF$_{9-41}$ and D-Phe CRF$_{12-41}$ (intracerebroventricular administration) reduced alcohol self-administration in dependent and postdependent animals.[174,184] When administered directly into the central nucleus of the amygdala, a CRF$_1$/CRF$_2$ antagonist blocked alcohol self-administration in alcohol-dependent rats during withdrawal.[47] Systemic injections of small-molecule CRF$_1$ antagonists also blocked the increased alcohol intake and anxiety-like responses that were associated with acute withdrawal.[48,75,129] These data suggest an important role for CRF, primarily in the central nucleus of the amygdala, in mediating the increased self-administration that is associated with dependence (see Table 18.3).

As noted previously, exposure to repeated cycles of chronic alcohol vapor produced substantial increases in alcohol intake in rats during both acute withdrawal and protracted abstinence (2 weeks post-acute withdrawal).[125,142] Intracerebroventricular administration of a CRF$_1$/CRF$_2$ receptor antagonist blocked the dependence-induced increase in alcohol self-administration during both acute withdrawal and protracted abstinence.[184] Central nucleus of the amygdala administration of a CRF$_1$/CRF$_2$ antagonist[47] and systemic injections of small-molecule CRF$_1$ receptor antagonists blocked the increased alcohol intake that was associated with acute withdrawal.[48] Systemic administration of a small-molecule CRF$_1$ antagonist also blocked the increased alcohol intake in protracted abstinence,[50] and intracerebroventricular administration of a CRF$_1$/CRF$_2$ receptor antagonist blocked the increased anxiety-like responses that were provoked by a stressor during protracted abstinence (see Fig. 18.8). These results suggest that brain CRF systems remain hyperactive during protracted abstinence, and this hyperactivity has motivational significance for excessive alcohol drinking.

Between-System Changes: Role of Other Neuropharmacological Systems

Other modulatory brain neurotransmitter systems that have pro-stress actions converge on the extended amygdala and include norepinephrine, vasopressin, substance P, hypocretin (orexin), and dynorphin, all of which may contribute to negative emotional states that are associated with drug withdrawal or protracted abstinence.[79] κ-Opioid receptor agonists and dynorphins produce aversive-like effects in both animals and humans[117,134,171,196] and have been hypothesized to mediate negative emotional states that are associated with drug withdrawal.[g] High compulsive-like drug intake that is associated with extended access and dependence for methamphetamine, heroin, and alcohol is blocked by κ-opioid receptor antagonists.[158,194,198,203] Two sites for these actions are the shell of the nucleus accumbens and amygdala,[71,119,158] suggesting a κ-opioid receptor/dynorphin contribution within the extended amygdala to negative emotional states.[27] High compulsive-like drinking in dependent rats during withdrawal can also be blocked by a β-adrenergic receptor antagonist, α$_1$ adrenergic receptor antagonist, κ-opioid receptor antagonist, vasopressin 1b receptor antagonist, glucocorticoid receptor antagonist, and neuroimmune system antagonist.[79,83] High compulsive-like heroin intake in the model of extended-access self-administration was blocked by a substance P receptor antagonist and hypocretin-2 receptor antagonist[14,159] (see Fig. 18.5).

Neurotransmitter systems that are implicated in anti-stress actions include neuropeptide Y (NPY), nociceptin, and endocannabinoids. NPY has powerful orexigenic and anxiolytic effects and has been hypothesized to act in opposition to the actions of CRF in addiction.[61] The activation of NPY in the central nucleus of the amygdala has effects that are opposite to CRF, in which NPY blocks the increase in γ-aminobutyric acid (GABA) release in the central nucleus of the amygdala that is produced by alcohol, blocks high compulsive-like alcohol administration, and blocks the transition to excessive drinking with the development of dependence.[53,54,180,181,182] Nociceptin (also known as orphanin FQ) has anti stress-like effects in animals.[30,108] Nociceptin and synthetic nociceptin/orphanin FQ peptide (NOP) receptor agonists have effects on GABA synaptic activity in the central nucleus of the amygdala that are similar to NPY and can block high alcohol consumption in a genetically selected line of rats that is known to be hypersensitive to stressors.[41] Evidence also

[g]References 26, 76, 96, 97, 101, 112, 113, 138, 157.

implicates endocannabinoids in the regulation of affective states, in which reductions of cannabinoid CB_1 receptor signaling produce anxiogenic-like behavioral effects.[165] Blocking endocannabinoid clearance can also block some drug-seeking behaviors.[1,46,156] Thus, endocannabinoids play a protective role in preventing drug dependence by buffering the stress activation that is associated with withdrawal (see Fig. 18.5 and Fig. 18.9).

Homeostatic Versus Allostatic View of Dependence

The development of the aversive emotional state that drives the negative reinforcement source of motivation in addiction has been defined as the "dark side" of addiction[89,90] and is hypothesized to be the b-process of the hedonic dynamic that is known as opponent process when the a-process is euphoria. Two processes are hypothesized to form the neurobiological basis for the b-process: loss of function in the reward systems (within-system neuroadaptation) and recruitment of a negative emotional state via the brain stress or anti-reward systems (between-system neuroadaptation).[84,87] Anti-reward is a construct based on the hypothesis that brain systems are in place to limit reward.[90] As dependence and withdrawal develop, brain stress systems, such as CRF, norepinephrine, and dynorphin, are recruited, producing the negative emotional state.[10,77,120] At the same time, within the motivational circuits of the ventral striatum-dorsal striatum, reward function decreases. The combination of decreases in reward neurotransmitter function and the recruitment of anti-reward systems provides a powerful source of negative reinforcement that contributes to compulsive drug-seeking behavior and addiction.

An overall conceptual theme that is argued here is that drug addiction represents a break with homeostatic brain regulatory mechanisms that regulate the emotional state of the animal. However, the view that drug addiction represents a simple break with homeostasis is insufficient to explain a number of key elements of addiction. Drug addiction, similar to other chronic physiological disorders, such as high blood pressure, worsens over time, is subject to significant environmental influences, and leaves a residual neuroadaptive trace that allows rapid "re-addiction," even months and years after detoxification and abstinence. These characteristics of drug addiction imply more than simply a homeostatic dysregulation of hedonic function and executive function, but rather a dynamic break with homeostasis of these systems that has been termed "allostasis."

Allostasis, originally conceptualized to explain the persistent morbidity of arousal and autonomic function, is defined as "stability through change" and differs significantly from homeostasis.[176] Allostasis involves a feed-forward mechanism rather than the negative feedback mechanisms of homeostasis, with continuous reevaluation of need and continuous readjustment of all parameters toward new set points. Allostatic mechanisms have been hypothesized to be involved in maintaining a functioning brain reward system that has relevance for the pathology of addiction.[88] Repeated challenges, such as the case with drugs of abuse, lead to attempts of the brain via molecular, cellular, and neurocircuitry changes to maintain reward stability but at a cost. For the drug addiction framework elaborated here, the residual deviation from normal brain reward threshold regulation is termed an "allostatic state." This state represents a combination of chronic elevation of reward set point that is engaged by the motivational changes that involve decreased function of reward circuits and recruitment of anti-reward systems, and both may contribute to the compulsivity of drug seeking and drug taking. Determining how these systems are modulated by other known brain emotional systems that are

localized to the extended amygdala and how individuals differ at the molecular-genetic level of analysis to convey loading on these circuits remain challenges for future research.

Animal Models of Dependence: Validity and Relevance to Treatment

Face Validity

Animal models of motivational withdrawal have substantial face validity. The hypothetical constructs that are associated with models of motivational withdrawal—anxiety, dysphoria, and lower reward—all are hypothesized to reflect such symptoms in humans. However, the major limitation of face validity here is that arguing that a rat is truly experiencing "dysphoria" is virtually impossible because no verbal reports can be obtained from a rat. In contrast, from a behaviorist perspective, one could argue that a verbal report in a human is only one measure of dysphoria and that the human symptoms can also be measured in a place aversion situation. Clearly, the translation of animal models to the human condition has not reached such a level of sophistication but see reference 95. With regard to other symptoms of addiction that are associated with the withdrawal/negative affect stage, such as escalation with extended access or dependence-induced drinking, face validity is again limited. Animals in the conditions that are designed by the researcher are indeed self-administering intoxicating amounts of drugs. However, the social situations for animals versus humans are vastly different, and a requirement for true face validity would be restrictive and unproductive. Certainly, some new information would be obtained if one had a model of free-ranging rats drank alcohol in the context of burrow dominance hierarchy. Such studies can and have been done with success in nonhuman primates, in which the social impact has more construct validity for the human condition. Indeed, construct validity—not face validity—in animal models is critical for the heuristic study of biological processes in the human condition and more specifically the understanding of the neurobiology of addiction.

Construct Validity

The models of the compulsive-like drug seeking and taking that are associated with the withdrawal/negative affect stage have construct validity (i.e., they have explanatory power for the human condition or functional equivalence for the human condition). For example, ample evidence indicates impaired reward function in animals that exhibit the escalation of drug intake with extended access to intravenous drugs of abuse and in animals with withdrawal-induced excessive drinking. Similarly, evidence exists for impaired stress responsivity during drug withdrawal that is paralleled in the human condition.[55,86,140] Ample evidence suggests that the decrease in dopaminergic function in the mesocorticolimbic dopamine system in rats during acute withdrawal is robust in humans.[190]

Emphases on face validity[31] may be misplaced and can be argued to undermine progress in the field. For example, the method of induction of opioid dependence (e.g., pellets vs. self-administration) appears to matter little compared with the dose of opioid employed (Table 18.4). Clearly, high opioid doses over time produce dose-dependent somatic withdrawal symptoms and excessive drug seeking, measured by intake or reinforcement efficacy. Different patterns of administration of the drug (intermittent exposure to alcohol vs. continuous alcohol) may also

TABLE 18.4 Heroin Self-Administration as a Function of Opioid-Induction Procedure.

Method of Induction	Escalation Time	Total Heroin Intake*	Reference
Morphine pellets (2 × 75 mg, subcutaneously)	0–3 days	~1,200 µg/kg (8 h)	195
Heroin self-administration (12-h access; 60 µg/kg/infusion)	0–20 days	~2,400 µg/kg (12 h)	58
Heroin self-administration (23-h access; 60 µg/kg/infusion)	0–35 days	~3,000 µg/kg (23 h)	28

*Note that the total dose per day, extrapolated to 24 h, would be similar with all three methods of induction.

ultimately have motivational effects.[125] However, the unspoken view that to have a valid model of alcoholism "one must show that a rat can drink whiskey from a bottle in a paper bag on a street corner while smoking a cigarette" is misleading and counterproductive. A case in point is a historical comparison of a classic Southern European alcoholic (who never showed public intoxication but imbibed several bottles of wine per day and clearly met the criteria for somatic withdrawal when deprived of alcohol) to the binge alcoholic of Northern Europe. Would one argue that the biological bases of liver toxicity, frontal cortex dysfunction, or activation of the brain stress systems during motivational withdrawal that are sufficient to induce excessive drinking are different for such different phenotypes of alcoholism? There are numerous examples of the induction of a disease state (such as in cancer, diabetes, pain, and obesity), independent of the exact human pattern of disease induction, that has construct validity for understanding the underlying biology but not necessarily face validity. Thus, emphasis must be placed on construct validity and the reliability of animal models and not the red herring of face validity.

Relevance to Medications Development

The thesis of this chapter is that animal models of motivational dependence provide a heuristic framework for understanding a key and previously neglected source of reinforcement that is associated with addiction. An interactive, iterative process can be established whereby existing medications that interact with the withdrawal/negative affect stage of the addiction cycle would be used to validate and improve animal and human laboratory models and then predict viable candidates for novel medications.[81,91,92] Medications that are currently on the market for the treatment of addiction have provided not only a window on the opportunities for facilitating treatment but also a means by which to evaluate future medications development. A combination of excellent and validated animal models of addiction and an enormous surge in understanding through basic research of the neurocircuits and neuropharmacological mechanisms that are involved in the neuroadaptive changes that account for the transition to dependence and the vulnerability to relapse have provided numerous viable targets for future medications development. The development of human laboratory studies for these stages of the addiction cycle is critical and will allow

dynamic iterative feedback to and from the animal models that are key to identifying novel candidates for treatment.[91] Novel neurobiological targets will be derived from this basic research on addiction with a focus on the withdrawal/negative affect stage and protracted abstinence component of the preoccupation/anticipation stages of the addiction cycle. Indeed, some would argue that targets that restore homeostasis of reward function rather than block reward function will be significantly more valuable to the field.[90,91,92]

Acknowledgments

The author would like to thank Michael Arends for his assistance with manuscript preparation.

References

1. Adamczyk P, McCreary AC, Przegalinski E, et al. The effects of fatty acid amide hydrolase inhibitors on maintenance of cocaine and food self-administration and on reinstatement of cocaine-seeking and food-taking behavior in rats. *J Physiol Pharmacol.* 2009;60:119–125.
2. Ahmed SH, Kenny PJ, Koob GF, et al. Neurobiological evidence for hedonic allostasis associated with escalating cocaine use. *Nat Neurosci.* 2002;5:625–626.
3. Ahmed SH, Koob GF. Cocaine- but not food-seeking behavior is reinstated by stress after extinction. *Psychopharmacology.* 1997;132:289–295.
4. Ahmed SH, Koob GF. Transition from moderate to excessive drug intake: change in hedonic set point. *Science.* 1998;282:298–300.
5. Ahmed SH, Koob GF. Long-lasting increase in the set point for cocaine self-administration after escalation in rats. *Psychopharmacology.* 1999;146:303–312.
6. Ahmed SH, Walker JR, Koob GF. Persistent increase in the motivation to take heroin in rats with a history of drug escalation. *Neuropsychopharmacology.* 2000;22:413–421.
7. Alling C, Balldin J, Bokstrom K, et al. Studies on duration of a late recovery period after chronic abuse of ethanol: a cross-sectional study of biochemical and psychiatric indicators. *Acta Psychiatr Scand.* 1982;66:384–397.
8. American Psychiatric Association. *Diagnostic and Statistical Manual of Mental Disorders.* 5th ed. Washington DC: American Psychiatric Publishing; 2013.
9. Annis HM, Sklar SM, Moser AE. Gender in relation to relapse crisis situations, coping, and outcome among treated alcoholics. *Addict Behav.* 1998;23:127–131.
10. Aston-Jones G, Delfs JM, Druhan J, et al. The bed nucleus of the stria terminalis: a target site for noradrenergic actions in opiate withdrawal. In: McGinty JF, ed. *Advancing from the Ventral Striatum to the Extended Amygdala: Implications for Neuropsychiatry and Drug Abuse. Annals of the New York Academy of Sciences.* Vol. 877. New York: New York Academy of Sciences; 1999:486–498.
11. Azar MR, Jones BC, Schulteis G. Conditioned place aversion is a highly sensitive index of acute opioid dependence and withdrawal. *Psychopharmacology.* 2003;170:42–50.
12. Baldwin HA, Koob GF. Rapid induction of conditioned opiate withdrawal in the rat. *Neuropsychopharmacology.* 1993;8:15–21.
13. Baldwin HA, Rassnick S, Rivier J, et al. CRF antagonist reverses the "anxiogenic" response to ethanol withdrawal in the rat. *Psychopharmacology.* 1991;103:227–232.
14. Barbier E, Vendruscolo LF, Schlosburg JE, et al. The NK1 receptor antagonist L822429 reduces heroin reinforcement. *Neuropsychopharmacology.* 2013;38:976–984.
15. Barr AM, Phillips AG. Withdrawal following repeated exposure to d-amphetamine decreases responding for a sucrose solution as measured by a progressive ratio schedule of reinforcement. *Psychopharmacology.* 1999;141:99–106.

16. Basso AM, Spina M, Rivier J, et al. Corticotropin-releasing factor antagonist attenuates the "anxiogenic-like" effect in the defensive burying paradigm but not in the elevated plus-maze following chronic cocaine in rats. *Psychopharmacology*. 1999;145:21–30.

17. Becker HC. Positive relationship between the number of prior ethanol withdrawal episodes and the severity of subsequent withdrawal seizures. *Psychopharmacology*. 1994;116:26–32.

18. Becker HC, Hale RL. Ethanol-induced locomotor stimulation in C57BL/6 mice following RO15–4513 administration. *Psychopharmacology*. 1989;99:333–336.

19. Bedford JA, Bailey LP, Wilson MC. Cocaine reinforced progressive ratio performance in the rhesus monkey. *Pharmacol Biochem Behav*. 1978;9:631–638.

20. Begleiter H. Ethanol consumption subsequent to physical dependence. In: Gross MM, ed. *Alcohol Intoxication and Withdrawal: Experimental Studies II. Advances in Experimental Medicine and Biology*. Vol. 59. New York: Plenum; 1975:373–378.

21. Branchey M, Rauscher G, Kissin B. Modifications in the response to alcohol following the establishment of physical dependence. *Psychopharmacologia*. 1971;22:314–322.

22. Breese GR, Overstreet DH, Knapp DJ. Conceptual framework for the etiology of alcoholism: a "kindling"/stress hypothesis. *Psychopharmacology*. 2005a;178:367–380.

23. Breese GR, Overstreet DH, Knapp DJ, et al. Prior multiple ethanol withdrawals enhance stress-induced anxiety-like behavior: inhibition by CRF1- and benzodiazepine-receptor antagonists and a 5-HT1a-receptor agonist. *Neuropsychopharmacology*. 2005b;30:1662–1669.

24. Breiter HC, Gollub RL, Weisskoff RM, et al. Acute effects of cocaine on human brain activity and emotion. *Neuron*. 1997;19:591–611.

25. Brown SA, Vik PW, Patterson TL, et al. Stress, vulnerability and adult alcohol relapse. *J Stud Alcohol*. 1995;56:538–545.

26. Chartoff E, Sawyer A, Rachlin A, et al. Blockade of kappa opioid receptors attenuates the development of depressive-like behaviors induced by cocaine withdrawal in rats. *Neuropharmacology*. 2012;62:167–176.

27. Chavkin C, Koob GF. Dynorphin, dysphoria and dependence: the stress of addiction. *Neuropsychopharmacology*. 2016;41:373–374.

28. Chen SA, O'Dell L, Hoefer M, et al. Unlimited access to heroin self-administration: independent motivational markers of opiate dependence. *Neuropsychopharmacology*. 2006;31:2692–2707. [corrigedum: 31:2802].

29. Chung T, Martin CS. Classification and course of alcohol problems among adolescents in addictions treatment programs. *Alcohol Clin Exp Res*. 2001;25:1734–1742.

30. Ciccocioppo R, Economidou D, Fedeli A, et al. The nociceptin/orphanin FQ/NOP receptor system as a target for treatment of alcohol abuse: a review of recent work in alcohol-preferring rats. *Physiol Behav*. 2003;79:121–128.

31. Cicero TJ. A critique of animal analogs of alcoholism. In: Majchrowicz E, Noble EP, eds. *Biochemistry and Pharmacology of Ethanol*. Vol. 2. New York: Plenum; 1979:533–560.

32. Cohen A, Koob GF, George O. Robust escalation of nicotine intake with extended access to nicotine self-administration and intermittent periods of abstinence. *Neuropsychopharmacology*. 2012;37:2153–2160.

33. Crowley TJ, Macdonald MJ, Whitmore EA, et al. Cannabis dependence, withdrawal, and reinforcing effects among adolescents with conduct symptoms and substance use disorders. *Drug Alcohol Depend*. 1998;50:27–37.

34. de Witte P, Littleton J, Parot P, et al. Neuroprotective and abstinence-promoting effects of acamprosate: elucidating the mechanism of action. *CNS Drugs*. 2005;19:517–537.

35. Delfs JM, Zhu Y, Druhan JP, et al. Noradrenaline in the ventral forebrain is critical for opiate withdrawal-induced aversion. *Nature*. 2000;403:430–434.

36. Deroche V, Le Moal M, Piazza PV. Cocaine self-administration increases the incentive motivational properties of the drug in rats. *Eur J Neurosci*. 1999;11:2731–2736.

37. Deroche V, Marinelli M, Le Moal M, et al. Glucocorticoids and behavioral effects of psychostimulants: II. Cocaine intravenous self-administration and reinstatement depend on glucocorticoid levels. *J Pharmacol Exp Ther*. 1997;281:1401–1407.

38. Deroche-Gamonet V, Belin D, Piazza PV. Evidence for addiction-like behavior in the rat. *Science*. 2004;305:1014–1017.

39. Deutsch JA, Koopmans HS. Preference enhancement for alcohol by passive exposure. *Science*. 1973;179:1242–1243.

40. Deutsch JA, Walton NY. A rat alcoholism model in a free choice situation. *Behav Biol*. 1977;19:349–360.

41. Economidou D, Hansson AC, Weiss F, et al. Dysregulation of nociceptin/orphanin FQ activity in the amygdala is linked to excessive alcohol drinking in the rat. *Biol Psychiatry*. 2008;64:211–218.

42. Edwards S, Guerrero M, Ghoneim OM, Roberts E, Koob GF. Evidence that vasopressin V1b receptors mediate the transition to excessive drinking in ethanol-dependent rats. *Addict Biol*. 2011;17:76–85.

43. Epping-Jordan MP, Watkins SS, Koob GF, et al. Dramatic decreases in brain reward function during nicotine withdrawal. *Nature*. 1998;393:76–79.

44. Erb S, Shaham Y, Stewart J. Stress reinstates cocaine-seeking behavior after prolonged extinction and a drug-free period. *Psychopharmacology*. 1996;128:408–412.

45. Fidler TL, Clews TW, Cunningham CL. Reestablishing an intragastric ethanol self-infusion model in rats. *Alcohol Clin Exp Res*. 2006;30:414–428.

46. Forget B, Coen KM, Le Foll B. Inhibition of fatty acid amide hydrolase reduces reinstatement of nicotine seeking but not break point for nicotine self-administration: comparison with CB$_1$ receptor blockade. *Psychopharmacology*. 2009;205:613–624.

47. Funk CK, O'Dell LE, Crawford EF, et al. Corticotropin-releasing factor within the central nucleus of the amygdala mediates enhanced ethanol self-administration in withdrawn, ethanol-dependent rats. *J Neurosci*. 2006;26:11324–11332.

48. Funk CK, Zorrilla EP, Lee MJ, et al. Corticotropin-releasing factor 1 antagonists selectively reduce ethanol self-administration in ethanol-dependent rats. *Biol Psychiatry*. 2007;61:78–86.

49. Gardner EL, Vorel SR. Cannabinoid transmission and reward-related events. *Neurobiol Dis*. 1998;5:502–533.

50. Gehlert DR, Cippitelli A, Thorsell A, et al. 3-(4-Chloro-2-morpholin-4-yl-thiazol-5-yl)-8-(1-ethylpropyl)-2,6-dimethyl-imidazo[1,2-b]pyridazine: a novel brain-penetrant, orally available corticotropin-releasing factor receptor 1 antagonist with efficacy in animal models of alcoholism. *J Neurosci*. 2007;27:2718–2726.

51. Gellert VF, Holtzman SG. Development and maintenance of morphine tolerance and dependence in the rat by scheduled access to morphine drinking solutions. *J Pharmacol Exp Ther*. 1978;205:536–546.

52. George O, Ghozland S, Azar MR, et al. CRF-CRF1 system activation mediates withdrawal-induced increases in nicotine self-administration in nicotine-dependent rats. *Proc Natl Acad Sci USA*. 2007;104:17198–17203.

53. Gilpin NW, Misra K, Herman MA, et al. Neuropeptide Y opposes alcohol effects on gamma-aminobutyric acid release in amygdala and blocks the transition to alcohol dependence. *Biol Psychiatry*. 2011;69:1091–1099.

54. Gilpin NW, Stewart RB, Murphy JM, et al. Neuropeptide Y reduces oral ethanol intake in alcohol-preferring (P) rats following a period of imposed ethanol abstinence. *Alcohol Clin Exp Res*. 2003;27:787–794.

55. Goeders NE. Stress and cocaine addiction. *J Pharmacol Exp Ther*. 2002;301:785–789.

56. Goldstein DB. *Pharmacology of Alcohol*. New York: Oxford University; 1983.

57. Greenwell TN, Funk CK, Cottone P, et al. Corticotropin-releasing factor-1 receptor antagonists decrease heroin self-administration in long-, but not short-access rats. *Addict Biol*. 2009a;14:130–143.

58. Greenwell TN, Walker BM, Cottone P, et al. The α_1 adrenergic receptor antagonist prazosin reduces heroin self-administration in rats with extended access to heroin administration. *Pharmacol Biochem Behav*. 2009b;91:295–302.

59. Hand TH, Koob GF, Stinus L, et al. Aversive properties of opiate receptor blockade: evidence for exclusively central mediation in naive and morphine-dependent rats. *Brain Res.* 1988;474:364–368.

60. Harris GC, Aston-Jones G. β-Adrenergic antagonists attenuate withdrawal anxiety in cocaine- and morphine-dependent rats. *Psychopharmacology.* 1993;113:131–136.

61. Heilig M, Koob GF. A key role for corticotropin-releasing factor in alcohol dependence. *Trends Neurosci.* 2007;30:399–406.

62. Heinrichs SC, Koob GF. Corticotropin-releasing factor in brain: a role in activation, arousal, and affect regulation. *J Pharmacol Exp Ther.* 2004;311:427–440.

63. Heinrichs SC, Menzaghi F, Schulteis G, et al. Suppression of corticotropin-releasing factor in the amygdala attenuates aversive consequences of morphine withdrawal. *Behav Pharmacol.* 1995;6:74–80.

64. Hernandez G, Hamdani S, Rajabi H, et al. Prolonged rewarding stimulation of the rat medial forebrain bundle: neurochemical and behavioral consequences. *Behav Neurosci.* 2006;120:888–904.

65. Hershon HI. Alcohol withdrawal symptoms and drinking behavior. *J Stud Alcohol.* 1977;38:953–971.

66. Himmelsbach CK. Can the euphoric, analgetic, and physical dependence effects of drugs be separated? IV. With reference to physical dependence. *Fed Proc.* 1943;2:201–203.

67. Huang MM, Overstreet DH, Knapp DJ, et al. Corticotropin-releasing factor (CRF) sensitization of ethanol withdrawal-induced anxiety-like behavior is brain site specific and mediated by CRF-1 receptors: relation to stress-induced sensitization. *J Pharmacol Exp Ther.* 2010;332:298–307.

68. Hunter BE, Walker DW, Riley JN. Dissociation between physical dependence and volitional ethanol consumption: role of multiple withdrawal episodes. *Pharmacol Biochem Behav.* 1974;2:523–529.

69. Izenwasser S, Kornetsky C. Brain-stimulation reward: a method for assessing the neurochemical baes of drug-induced euphoria. In: Watson RR, ed. *Drugs of Abuse and Neurobiology.* Boca Raton, FL: CRC; 1992:1–21.

70. Jang CG, Whitfield T, Schulteis G, Koob GF, Wee S. A dysphoric-like state during early withdrawal from extended access to methamphetamine self-administration in rats. *Psychopharmacology.* 2013;225:753–763.

71. Kallupi M, Wee S, Edwards S, et al. Kappa opioid receptor-mediated dysregulation of GABAergic transmission in the central amygdala in cocaine addiction. *Biol Psychiatry.* 2013;74:520–528.

72. Kenny PJ, Chen SA, Kitamura O, et al. Conditioned withdrawal drives heroin consumption and decreases reward sensitivity. *J Neurosci.* 2006;26:5894–5900.

73. Kenny PJ, Polis I, Koob GF, et al. Low dose cocaine self-administration transiently increases but high dose cocaine persistently decreases brain reward function in rats. *Eur J Neurosci.* 2003;17:191–195.

74. Kitamura O, Wee S, Specio SE, et al. Escalation of methamphetamine self-administration in rats: a dose-effect function. *Psychopharmacology.* 2006;186:48–53.

75. Knapp DJ, Overstreet DH, Moy SS, et al. SB242084, flumazenil, and CRA1000 block ethanol withdrawal-induced anxiety in rats. *Alcohol.* 2004;32:101–111.

76. Knoll AT, Meloni EG, Thomas JB, et al. Anxiolytic-like effects of κ-opioid receptor antagonists in models of unlearned and learned fear in rats. *J Pharmacol Exp Ther.* 2007;323:838–845.

77. Koob GF. Neuroadaptive mechanisms of addiction: studies on the extended amygdala. *Eur Neuropsychopharmacol.* 2003;13:442–452.

78. Koob GF. Allostatic view of motivation: implications for psychopathology. In: Bevins RA, Bardo MT, eds. *Motivational Factors in the Etiology of Drug Abuse.* Vol. 50. Nebraska Symposium on Motivation. Lincoln NE: University of Nebraska; 2004:1–18.

79. Koob GF. A role for brain stress systems in addiction. *Neuron.* 2008a;59:11–34.

80. Koob GF. Neurobiology of addiction. In: Galanter M, Kleber HD, eds. *Textbook of Substance Abuse Treatment.* 4th ed. Washington, DC: American Psychiatric; 2008b:3–16.

81. Koob GF. New dimensions in human laboratory models of addiction. *Addict Biol.* 2009;14:1–8.

82. Koob GF. The dark side of emotion: the addiction perspective. *Eur J Pharmacol.* 2015;753:73–87.

83. Koob GF. *Antireward, Compulsivity, and Addiction: Seminal Contributions of Dr. Athina Markou to Motivational Dysregulation in Addiction.* Psychopharmacology: in press; 2017.

84. Koob GF, Bloom FE. Cellular and molecular mechanisms of drug dependence. *Science.* 1988;242:715–723.

85. Koob GF, Heinrichs SC, Menzaghi F, et al. Corticotropin releasing factor, stress and behavior. *Semin Neurosci.* 1994;6:221–229.

86. Koob GF, Kreek MJ. Stress, dysregulation of drug reward pathways, and the transition to drug dependence. *Am J Psychiatry.* 2007;164:1149–1159.

87. Koob GF, Le Moal M. Drug abuse: hedonic homeostatic dysregulation. *Science.* 1997;278:52–58.

88. Koob GF, Le Moal M. Drug addiction, dysregulation of reward, and allostasis. *Neuropsychopharmacology.* 2001;24:97–129.

89. Koob GF, Le Moal M. Plasticity of reward neurocircuitry and the 'dark side' of drug addiction. *Nat Neurosci.* 2005;8:1442–1444.

90. Koob GF, Le Moal M. Addiction and the brain antireward system. *Annu Rev Psychol.* 2008;59:29–53.

91. Koob GF, Lloyd GK, Mason BJ. Medications development for treatment of drug addiction: a Rosetta stone approach. *Nat Rev Drug Discov.* 2009;8:500–515.

92. Koob GF, Mason BJ. Existing and future drugs for the treatment of the dark side of addiction. *Annu Rev Pharmacol Toxicol.* 2016;56:299–322.

93. Kornetsky C, Esposito RU. Euphorigenic drugs: effects on the reward pathways of the brain. *Fed Proc.* 1979;38:2473–2476.

94. Kreibich AS, Blendy JA. cAMP response element-binding protein is required for stress but not cocaine-induced reinstatement. *J Neurosci.* 2004;24:6686–6692.

95. Kwako LE, Momenan R, Litten RZ, et al. Addictions neuroclinical assessment: a neuroscience-based framework for addictive disorders. *Biol Psychiatry.* 2016;80:179–189.

96. Land BB, Bruchas MR, Lemos JC, et al. The dysphoric component of stress is encoded by activation of the dynorphin κ-opioid system. *J Neurosci.* 2008;28:407–414.

97. Land BB, Bruchas MR, Schattauer S, et al. Activation of the kappa opioid receptor in the dorsal raphe nucleus mediates the aversive effects of stress and reinstates drug seeking. *Proc Natl Acad Sci U S A.* 2009;106:19168–19173.

98. Le AD, Harding S, Juzytsch W, et al. Role of alpha-2 adrenoceptors in stress-induced reinstatement of alcohol seeking and alcohol self-administration in rats. *Psychopharmacology.* 2005;179:366–373.

99. Lowman C, Allen J, Stout RL. Replication and extension of Marlatt's taxonomy of relapse precipitants: overview of procedures and results. *Addiction.* 1996;91(suppl):s51–s71.

100. Lu L, Shepard JD, Hall FS, et al. Effect of environmental stressors on opiate and psychostimulant reinforcement, reinstatement and discrimination in rats: a review. *Neurosci Biobehav Rev.* 2003;27:457–491.

101. Mague SD, Pliakas AM, Todtenkopf MS, et al. Antidepressant-like effects of κ-opioid receptor antagonists in the forced swim test in rats. *J Pharmacol Exp Ther.* 2003;305:323–330.

102. Majchrowicz E. Induction of physical dependence upon ethanol and the associated behavioral changes in rats. *Psychopharmacologia.* 1975;43:245–254.

103. Mantsch JR, Yuferov V, Mathieu-Kia AM, et al. Effects of extended access to high versus low cocaine doses on self-administration, cocaine-induced reinstatement and brain mRNA levels in rats. *Psychopharmacology.* 2004;175:26–36.

104. Markou A, Koob GF. Post-cocaine anhedonia: an animal model of cocaine withdrawal. *Neuropsychopharmacology.* 1991;4:17–26.

105. Marlatt G, Gordon J. Determinants of relapse: implications for the maintenance of behavioral change. In: Davidson P, Davidson S, eds. *BehavioralMedicine: Changing Health Lifestyles.* New York: Brunner/Mazel; 1980:410–452.

106. Martin WR, Eades CG. A comparison between acute and chronic physical dependence in the chronic spinal dog. *J Pharmacol Exp Ther.* 1964;146:385–394.

107. Martin WR, Wikler A, Eades CG, et al. Tolerance to and physical dependence on morphine in rats. *Psychopharmacologia.* 1963;4:247–260.

108. Martin-Fardon R, Zorrilla EP, Ciccocioppo R, et al. Role of innate and drug-induced dysregulation of brain stress and arousal systems in addiction: focus on corticotropin-releasing factor, nociceptin/orphanin FQ, and orexin/hypocretin. *Brain Res.* 2010;1314:145–161.

109. Martin-Solch C, Magyar S, Kunig G, et al. Changes in brain activation associated with reward processing in smokers and non-smokers: a positron emission tomography study. *Exp Brain Res.* 2001;139:278–286.

110. Martinez D, Narendran R, Foltin RW, et al. Amphetamine-induced dopamine release: markedly blunted in cocaine dependence and predictive of the choice to self-administer cocaine. *Am J Psychiatry.* 2007;164:622–629.

111. Mason BJ, Ritvo EC, Morgan RO, et al. A double-blind, placebo-controlled pilot study to evaluate the efficacy and safety of oral nalmefene HCl for alcohol dependence. *Alcohol Clin Exp Res.* 1994;18:1162–1167.

112. McLaughlin JP, Li S, Valdez J, et al. Social defeat stress-induced behavioral responses are mediated by the endogenous kappa opioid system. *Neuropsychopharmacology.* 2006;31:1241–1248.

113. McLaughlin JP, Marton-Popovici M, Chavkin C. κ Opioid receptor antagonism and prodynorphin gene disruption block stress-induced behavioral responses. *J Neurosci.* 2003;23:5674–5683.

114. Melis M, Spiga S, Diana M. The dopamine hypothesis of drug addiction: hypodopaminergic state. *Int Rev Neurobiol.* 2005;63:101–154.

115. Merlo-Pich E, Lorang M, Yeganeh M, et al. Increase of extracellular corticotropin-releasing factor-like immunoreactivity levels in the amygdala of awake rats during restraint stress and ethanol withdrawal as measured by microdialysis. *J Neurosci.* 1995;15:5439–5447.

116. Moeller FG, Barratt ES, Dougherty DM, et al. Psychiatric aspects of impulsivity. *Am J Psychiatry.* 2001;158:1783–1793.

117. Mucha RFHerz A. Motivational properties of kappa and mu opioid receptor agonists studied with place and taste preference conditioning. *Psychopharmacology.* 1985;86:274–280.

118. Myers RD, Stoltman WP, Martin GE. Effects of ethanol dependence induced artificially in the rhesus monkey on the subsequent preference for ethyl alcohol. *Physiol Behav.* 1972;9:43–48.

119. Nealey KA, Smith AW, Davis SM, et al. κ-opioid receptors are implicated in the increased potency of intra-accumbens nalmefene in ethanol-dependent rats. *Neuropharmacology.* 2011;61:35–42.

120. Nestler EJ. Molecular basis of long-term plasticity underlying addiction. *Nat Rev Neurosci.* 2001;2:119–128.

121. Nestler EJ. Historical review: molecular and cellular mechanisms of opiate and cocaine addiction. *Trends Pharmacol Sci.* 2004;25:210–218.

122. Nestler EJ, Malenka RC. The addicted brain. *Sci Am.* 2004;290:78–85.

123. Niikura K, Zhou Y, Ho A, et al. Proopiomelanocortin (POMC) expression and conditioned place aversion during protracted withdrawal from chronic intermittent escalating-dose heroin in POMC-EGFP promoter transgenic mice. *Neuroscience.* 2013;236:220–232.

124. Nye HE, Nestler EJ. Induction of chronic Fos-related antigens in rat brain by chronic morphine administration. *Mol Pharmacol.* 1996;49:636–645.

125. O'Dell LE, Roberts AJ, Smith RT, et al. Enhanced alcohol self-administration after intermittent versus continuous alcohol vapor exposure. *Alcohol Clin Exp Res.* 2004;28:1676–1682.

126. Olds JMilner P. Positive reinforcement produced by electrical stimulation of septal area and other regions of rat brain. *J Comp Physiol Psychol.* 1954;47:419–427.

127. Olive MF, Koenig HN, Nannini MA, et al. Elevated extracellular CRF levels in the bed nucleus of the stria terminalis during ethanol withdrawal and reduction by subsequent ethanol intake. *Pharmacol Biochem Behav.* 2002;72:213–220.

128. Orsini C, Koob GF, Pulvirenti L. Dopamine partial agonist reverses amphetamine withdrawal in rats. *Neuropsychopharmacology.* 2001;25:789–792.

129. Overstreet DH, Knapp DJ, Breese GR. Modulation of multiple ethanol withdrawal-induced anxiety-like behavior by CRF and CRF$_1$ receptors. *Pharmacol Biochem Behav.* 2004;77:405–413.

130. Overstreet DH, Knapp DJ, Breese GR. Drug challenges reveal differences in mediation of stress facilitation of voluntary alcohol drinking and withdrawal-induced anxiety in alcohol-preferring P rats. *Alcohol Clin Exp Res.* 2007;31:1473–1481.

131. Papaleo F, Contarino A. Gender- and morphine dose-linked expression of spontaneous somatic opiate withdrawal in mice. *Behav Brain Res.* 2006;170:110–118.

132. Paterson NE, Markou A. Increased motivation for self-administered cocaine after escalated cocaine intake. *Neuroreport.* 2003;14:2229–2232.

133. Paterson NE, Myers C, Markou A. Effects of repeated withdrawal from continuous amphetamine administration on brain reward function in rats. *Psychopharmacology.* 2000;152:440–446.

134. Pfeiffer A, Brantl V, Herz A, et al. Psychotomimesis mediated by κ opiate receptors. *Science.* 1986;233:774–776.

135. Pulvirenti LKoob GF. Lisuride reduces psychomotor retardation during withdrawal from chronic intravenous amphetamine self-administration in rats. *Neuropsychopharmacology.* 1993;8:213–218.

136. Rasmussen DD, Boldt BM, Bryant CA, et al. Chronic daily ethanol and withdrawal: 1. Long-term changes in the hypothalamo-pituitary-adrenal axis. *Alcohol Clin Exp Res.* 2000;24:1836–1849.

137. Rassnick S, Heinrichs SC, Britton KT, et al. Microinjection of a corticotropin-releasing factor antagonist into the central nucleus of the amygdala reverses anxiogenic-like effects of ethanol withdrawal. *Brain Res.* 1993;605:25–32.

138. Redila VA, Chavkin C. Stress-induced reinstatement of cocaine seeking is mediated by the kappa opioid system. *Psychopharmacology.* 2008;200:59–70.

139. Ribeiro Do Couto B, Aguilar MA, Manzanedo C, et al. Social stress is as effective as physical stress in reinstating morphine-induced place preference in mice. *Psychopharmacology.* 2006;185:459–470.

140. Richardson HN, Lee S, O'Dell LE, et al. Alcohol self-administration acutely stimulates the hypothalamic-pituitary-adrenal (HPA) axis but dependence leads to a dampened neuroendocrine state. *Eur J Neurosci.* 2008;28:1641–1653.

141. Richter RMWeiss F. In vivo CRF release in rat amygdala is increased during cocaine withdrawal in self-administering rats. *Synapse.* 1999;32:254–261.

142. Rimondini R, Arlinde C, Sommer W, et al. Long-lasting increase in voluntary ethanol consumption and transcriptional regulation in the rat brain after intermittent exposure to alcohol. *FASEB J.* 2002;16:27–35.

143. Rimondini R, Sommer WH, Dall'Olio R, et al. Long-lasting tolerance to alcohol following a history of dependence. *Addict Biol.* 2008;13:26–30.

144. Rivier J, Rivier C, Vale W. Synthetic competitive antagonists of corticotropin-releasing factor: effect on ACTH secretion in the rat. *Science.* 1984;224:889–891.

145. Roberto M, Cruz MT, Gilpin NW, et al. Corticotropin releasing factor-induced amygdala gamma-aminobutyric acid release plays a key role in alcohol dependence. *Biol Psychiatry.* 2010;67:831–839.

146. Roberts AJ, Cole M, Koob GF. Intra-amygdala muscimol decreases operant ethanol self-administration in dependent rats. *Alcohol Clin Exp Res.* 1996;20:1289–1298.

147. Roberts AJ, Heyser CJ, Cole M, et al. Excessive ethanol drinking following a history of dependence: animal model of allostasis. *Neuropsychopharmacology.* 2000;22:581–594.

CHAPTER 18 Animal Models of Substance Use Disorders: Motivational Perspective 263

148. Roberts DCS, Richardson NR. Self-administration of psychomotor stimulants using progressive ratio schedules of reinforcement. In: Boulton AA, Baker GB, Wu PH, eds. *Animal Models of Drug Addiction. Neuromethods.* Vol. 24. Totowa, NJ: Human; 1992:233–269.
149. Rodriguez de Fonseca F, Carrera MRA, Navarro M, et al. Activation of corticotropin-releasing factor in the limbic system during cannabinoid withdrawal. *Science.* 1997;276:2050–2054.
150. Roelofs SM. Hyperventilation, anxiety, craving for alcohol: a subacute alcohol withdrawal syndrome. *Alcohol.* 1985;2:501–505.
151. Rossetti ZL, Hmaidan Y, Gessa GL. Marked inhibition of mesolimbic dopamine release: a common feature of ethanol, morphine, cocaine and amphetamine abstinence in rats. *Eur J Pharmacol.* 1992;221:227–234.
152. Russell MAH. What is dependence? In: Edwards G, ed. *Drugs and Drug Dependence.* Lexington, MA: Lexington Books; 1976:182–187.
153. Samson HH, Falk JL. Alteration of fluid preference in ethanol-dependent animals. *J Pharmacol Exp Ther.* 1974;190:365–376.
154. Sanchez CJ, Sorg BA. Conditioned fear stimuli reinstate cocaine-induced conditioned place preference. *Brain Res.* 2001;908:86–92.
155. Sarnyai Z, Biro E, Gardi J, et al. Brain corticotropin-releasing factor mediates "anxiety-like" behavior induced by cocaine withdrawal in rats. *Brain Res.* 1995;675:89–97.
156. Scherma M, Panlilio LV, Fadda P, et al. Inhibition of anandamide hydrolysis by cyclohexyl carbamic acid 3'-carbamoyl-3-yl ester (URB597) reverses abuse-related behavioral and neurochemical effects of nicotine in rats. *J Pharmacol Exp Ther.* 2008;327:482–490.
157. Schindler AG, Li S, Chavkin C. Behavioral stress may increase the rewarding valence of cocaine-associated cues through a dynorphin/κ-opioid receptor-mediated mechanism without affecting associative learning or memory retrieval mechanisms. *Neuropsychopharmacology.* 2010;35:1932–1942.
158. Schlosburg JE, Whitfield Jr TW, Park PE, et al. Long-term antagonism of κ opioid receptors prevents escalation of and increased motivation for heroin intake. *J Neurosci.* 2013;33:19384–19392.
159. Schmeichel BE, Barbier E, Misra KK, et al. Hypocretin receptor 2 antagonism dose-dependently reduces escalated heroin self-administration in rats. *Neuropsychopharmacology.* 2015;40:1123–1129.
160. Schulteis G, Hyytia P, Heinrichs SC, et al. Effects of chronic ethanol exposure on oral self-administration of ethanol or saccharin by Wistar rats. *Alcohol Clin Exp Res.* 1996;20:164–171.
161. Schulteis G, Markou A, Cole M, et al. Decreased brain reward produced by ethanol withdrawal. *Proc Natl Acad Sci USA.* 1995;92:5880–5884.
162. Schulteis G, Markou A, Gold LH, et al. Relative sensitivity to naloxone of multiple indices of opiate withdrawal: a quantitative dose-response analysis. *J Pharmacol Exp Ther.* 1994;271:1391–1398.
163. Schulteis G, Stinus L, Risbrough VB, et al. Clonidine blocks acquisition but not expression of conditioned opiate withdrawal in rats. *Neuropsychopharmacology.* 1998;19:406–416.
164. Self DW, McClenahan AW, Beitner-Johnson D, et al. Biochemical adaptations in the mesolimbic dopamine system in response to heroin self-administration. *Synapse.* 1995;21:312–318.
165. Serrano AParsons LH. Endocannabinoid influence in drug reinforcement, dependence and addiction-related behaviors. *Pharmacol Ther.* 2011;132:215–241.
166. Shaham Y, Shalev U, Lu L, et al. The reinstatement model of drug relapse: history, methodology and major findings. *Psychopharmacology.* 2003;168:3–20.
167. Shalev U, Grimm JW, Shaham Y. Neurobiology of relapse to heroin and cocaine seeking: a review. *Pharmacol Rev.* 2002;54:1–42.
168. Shalev U, Highfield D, Yap J, et al. Stress and relapse to drug seeking in rats: studies on the generality of the effect. *Psychopharmacology.* 2000;150:337–346.
169. Shaw-Lutchman TZ, Barrot M, Wallace T, et al. Regional and cellular mapping of cAMP response element-mediated transcription during naltrexone-precipitated morphine withdrawal. *J Neurosci.* 2002;22:3663–3672.
170. Shepard JD, Bossert JM, Liu SY. The anxiogenic drug yohimbine reinstates methamphetamine seeking in a rat model of drug relapse. *Biol Psychiatry.* 2004;55:1082–1089.
171. Shippenberg TS, Zapata A, Chefer VI. Dynorphin and the pathophysiology of drug addiction. *Pharmacol Ther.* 2007;116:306–321.
172. Simms JA, Steensland P, Medina B, et al. Intermittent access to 20% ethanol induces high ethanol consumption in Long-Evans and Wistar rats. *Alcohol Clin Exp Res.* 2008;32:1816–1823.
173. Skjei KL, Markou A. Effects of repeated withdrawal episodes, nicotine dose, and duration of nicotine exposure on the severity and duration of nicotine withdrawal in rats. *Psychopharmacology.* 2003;168:280–292.
174. Sommer WH, Rimondini R, Hansson AC, et al. Upregulation of voluntary alcohol intake, behavioral sensitivity to stress, and amygdala *crhr1* expression following a history of dependence. *Biol Psychiatry.* 2008;63:139–145.
175. Specio SE, Wee S, O'Dell LE, et al. CRF₁ receptor antagonists attenuate escalated cocaine self-administration in rats. *Psychopharmacology.* 2008;196:473–482.
176. Sterling P, Eyer J. Allostasis: a new paradigm to explain arousal pathology. In: Fisher S, Reason J, eds. *Handbook of Life Stress, Cognition and Health.* Chichester: Wiley; 1988:629–649.
177. Stinus L, Cador M, Zorrilla EP, et al. Buprenorphine and a CRF1 antagonist block the acquisition of opiate withdrawal-induced conditioned place aversion in rats. *Neuropsychopharmacology.* 2005;30:90–98.
178. Stinus L, Caille S, Koob GF. Opiate withdrawal-induced place aversion lasts for up to 16 weeks. *Psychopharmacology.* 2000;149:115–120.
179. Stinus L, Le Moal M, Koob GF. Nucleus accumbens and amygdala are possible substrates for the aversive stimulus effects of opiate withdrawal. *Neuroscience.* 1990;37:767–773.
180. Thorsell A, Rapunte-Canonigo V, O'Dell L, et al. Viral vector-induced amygdala NPY overexpression reverses increased alcohol intake caused by repeated deprivations in Wistar rats. *Brain.* 2007;130:1330–1337.
181. Thorsell A, Slawecki CJ, Ehlers CL. Effects of neuropeptide Y and corticotropin-releasing factor on ethanol intake in Wistar rats: interaction with chronic ethanol exposure. *Behav Brain Res.* 2005a;161:133–140.
182. Thorsell A, Slawecki CJ, Ehlers CL. Effects of neuropeptide Y on appetitive and consummatory behaviors associated with alcohol drinking in wistar rats with a history of ethanol exposure. *Alcohol Clin Exp Res.* 2005b;29:584–590.
183. Tucci S, Cheeta S, Seth P, et al. Corticotropin releasing factor antagonist, α-helical CRF₉₋₄₁, reverses nicotine-induced conditioned, but not unconditioned, anxiety. *Psychopharmacology.* 2003;167:251–256.
184. Valdez GR, Roberts AJ, Chan K, et al. Increased ethanol self-administration and anxiety-like behavior during acute withdrawal and protracted abstinence: regulation by corticotropin-releasing factor. *Alcohol Clin Exp Res.* 2002;26:1494–1501.
185. Valdez GR, Zorrilla EP, Roberts AJ, et al. Antagonism of corticotropin-releasing factor attenuates the enhanced responsiveness to stress observed during protracted ethanol abstinence. *Alcohol.* 2003;29:55–60.
186. Van Dyke CByck R. Cocaine. *Sci Am.* 1982;246:128–141.
187. Veale WLMyers RD. Increased alcohol preference in rats following repeated exposures to alcohol. *Psychopharmacologia.* 1969;15:361–1372.
188. Vendruscolo LF, Barbier E, Schlosburg JE, et al. Corticosteroid-dependent plasticity mediates compulsive alcohol drinking in rats. *J Neurosci.* 2012;32:7563–7571.
189. Vezina P. Sensitization of midbrain dopamine neuron reactivity and the self-administration of psychomotor stimulant drugs. *Neurosci Biobehav Rev.* 2004;27:827–839.
190. Volkow ND, Fowler JS. Addiction, a disease of compulsion and drive: involvement of the orbitofrontal cortex. *Cerebr Cortex.* 2000;10:318–325.

191. Volkow ND, Fowler JS, Wang GJ. Role of dopamine in drug reinforcement and addiction in humans: results from imaging studies. *Behav Pharmacol.* 2002;13:355–366.

192. Volkow ND, Wang GJ, Fowler JS, et al. Decreased striatal dopaminergic responsiveness in detoxified cocaine-dependent subjects. *Nature.* 1997;386:830–833.

193. Walker BM, Koob GF. The γ-aminobutyric acid-B receptor agonist baclofen attenuates responding for ethanol in ethanol-dependent rats. *Alcohol Clin Exp Res.* 2007;31:11–18.

194. Walker BM, Zorrilla EP, Koob GF. Systemic κ-opioid receptor antagonism by nor-binaltorphimine reduces dependence-induced excessive alcohol self-administration in rats. *Addict Biol.* 2010;16:116–119.

195. Walker JR, Chen SA, Moffitt H, et al. Chronic opioid exposure produces increased heroin self-administration in rats. *Pharmacol Biochem Behav.* 2003;75:349–354.

196. Wee S, Koob GF. The role of the dynorphin-κ opioid system in the reinforcing effects of drugs of abuse. *Psychopharmacology.* 2010;210:121–135.

197. Wee S, Mandyam CD, Lekic DM, et al. α₁-Noradrenergic system role in increased motivation for cocaine intake in rats with prolonged access. *Eur Neuropsychopharmacol.* 2008;18:303–311.

198. Wee S, Orio L, Ghirmai S, et al. Inhibition of kappa opioid receptors attenuated increased cocaine intake in rats with extended access to cocaine. *Psychopharmacology.* 2009;205:565–575.

199. Wee S, Wang Z, Woolverton WL, Pulvirenti L, Koob GF. Effect of aripiprazole, a partial D2 receptor agonist, on increased rate of methamphetamine self-administration in rats with prolonged access. *Neuropsychopharmacology.* 2007;32:2238–2247.

200. Weiss F, Ciccocioppo R, Parsons LH, et al. Compulsive drug-seeking behavior and relapse: neuroadaptation, stress, and conditioning factors. In: Quinones-Jenab V, ed. *The Biological Basis of Cocaine Addiction. Annals of the New York Academy of Sciences.* Vol. 937. New York: New York Academy of Sciences; 2001:1–26.

201. Weiss F, Markou A, Lorang MT, et al. Basal extracellular dopamine levels in the nucleus accumbens are decreased during cocaine withdrawal after unlimited-access self-administration. *Brain Res.* 1992;593:314–318.

202. Weiss F, Parsons LH, Schulteis G, et al. Ethanol self-administration restores withdrawal-associated deficiencies in accumbal dopamine and 5-hydroxytryptamine release in dependent rats. *J Neurosci.* 1996;16:3474–3485.

203. Whitfield Jr TW, Schlosburg J, Wee S, et al. κ Opioid receptors in the nucleus accumbens shell mediate escalation of methamphetamine intake. *J Neurosci.* 2015;35:4296–4305.

204. Wills TA, Knapp DJ, Overstreet DH, et al. Sensitization, duration, and pharmacological blockade of anxiety-like behavior following repeated ethanol withdrawal in adolescent and adult rats. *Alcohol Clin Exp Res.* 2009;33:455–463.

205. Winger G. Effects of ethanol withdrawl on ethanol-reinforced responding in rhesus monkeys. *Drug Alcohol Depend.* 1988;22:235–240.

206. Wolffgramm JHeyne A. Social behavior, dominance, and social deprivation of rats determine drug choice. *Pharmacol Biochem Behav.* 1991;38:389–399.

207. Zhang Z, Morse AC, Koob GF, et al. Dose- and time-dependent expression of anxiety-like behavior in the elevated plus-maze during withdrawal from acute and repeated intermittent ethanol intoxication in rats. *Alcohol Clin Exp Res.* 2007;31:1811–1819.

208. Zywiak WH, Connors GJ, Maisto SA, et al. Relapse research and the Reasons for Drinking Questionnaire: a factor analysis of Marlatt's relapse taxonomy. *Addiction.* 1996;91(suppl):s121–s130.

19

Novel Methodologies: Proteomic Approaches in Substance Abuse Research

SCOTT E. HEMBY, WENDY LYNCH, AND NILESH S. TANNU

Introduction

The comprehensive sequencing of human and other important genomes has enhanced our understanding of the cellular organization and function in higher organisms. This has been largely accomplished by the innovations in large-scale analysis of messenger RNA (mRNA) expression (microarrays, serial-analysis of gene expression [SAGE], and differential display). Genomics-based approaches have led to unprecedented advances in our understanding of the biological basis of substance abuse; however, the next step in systems biology is the examination of coordinate expression of the entire complement of proteins, including modifications and protein-protein interactions—proteomics. The broad-scale analysis of proteins in health and disease is essential given that proteins are central components of cellular physiology carrying out the greater part of biological events in the cell, even though certain mRNAs can act as effector molecules. Furthermore, it is important to note that mRNA and protein analyses are not interchangeable, with each being governed by distinct spatial, temporal, and physiological processes that generally prevent correlation of mRNA and protein expression in neuronal systems.[1,21]

Proteomics involves the evaluation of the entire complement of proteins in a biological system with respect to structure, expression level, protein-protein interactions, posttranslational modifications (PTMs)—often referred to as structural, functional, and expression proteomics, respectively. The majority of early efforts in proteomics have been directed toward a comparison of differential protein expression and identification in disease and control tissues. However, changes in protein abundance do not define protein function exclusively, as many vital functions are brought about by PTMs, interactions among proteins, and differential distribution in subcellular components. Multiple proteomic strategies are needed to capture the involvement of regulatory mechanisms that affect protein abundance and function, such as protein-protein interactions and subcellular distribution.

The advent of proteomics can be attributed in part to the rapid development of mass spectrometry (MS), bioinformatics, and the current accessibility of vast protein databases from various organisms. These rapid advancements have improved our understanding of the cellular structure and function within the brain and the roles of various proteins and protein interactions in health and disease. However, the central nervous system poses unique challenges to proteomic inquiries, including the temporal and spatial expression characteristics of neurons and glia, the cellular heterogeneity of brain regions, the connectivity and communication between neurons, and the dynamic structural and functional alterations in neurons and glia that occur as a function of the interaction between the organism and the environment, development, learning and memory, and disease. These challenges can be overcome to some extent by combining specific isolation and fractionation procedures with high-throughput protein separation and analysis strategies to yield a more global view of the proteome in different physiological states than has been available previously. For example, before the advent of high-throughput proteomics technologies, our knowledge of protein alterations and the durations of those alterations induced by substance abuse was limited to fewer than 100 proteins—primarily expression levels of proteins assessed either individually or a few proteins at a time. With the development of proteomic technologies and strategies, it is now possible to evaluate significant portions of the neuroproteome (thousands of proteins) from crude homogenates to discrete cellular domains. Proteomic analysis strategies allow the simultaneous assessment of thousands of proteins of known and unknown function, thereby enabling a more comprehensive view of the protein orchestration in addictive disorders. Broad-scale evaluations of protein expression are well suited to the study of drug abuse, particularly in light of the complexity of the brain compared with other tissues, the multigenic nature of drug addiction, the vast representation of expressed proteins in the brain, and our relatively limited knowledge of the molecular pathology of this illness.

The development of innovative strategies has been ongoing in neuroproteomics, in particular for the study of PTMs, mapping of proteins from multiprotein complexes, and mapping of organelle proteomes.[14] An understanding of the proteins in neurons along with their expression levels, their PTMs, as well as the protein-protein interaction maps would revolutionize addiction biology and addiction medicine in that we would then be able to expand our knowledge of the biochemical alterations specifically associated with substance abuse. Such information would be used to identify new targets for medication development.

Technology and Methods for Expression Proteomics

Protein Fractionation

The biological samples subjected to proteomic analysis in neuroscience include tissue, distinct cell populations, and cerebrospinal fluid (CSF). Each type of sample is extremely complex, as the protein constituents vary in charge, molecular mass, hydrophobicity, PTM, as well as spatial and temporal expression. The number of coding genes for the CNS fluctuate between 25,000 and 30,000.[94] This added complexity of the neuroproteome will be overwhelming if we hypothesize that each protein on average has 10 splice variants, cleavage products, and PTMs, yielding approximately 250,000 to 300,000 protein isoforms to assess. Currently, there are no proteomic methods that have the capacity to separate and identify the entire proteome. One approach is to reduce the complexity of the proteome by subcellular fractionation procedures, thereby allowing a more thorough assessment of cellular domains (e.g., synapse, membrane, nucleus, and cytoplasm) while enriching low-abundance proteins that may not be detectable at the level of whole cell protein analysis.[101]

Protein stability and purity as well as prevention of protein degradation and modification are of critical importance throughout various stages of proteomic analysis. Rapid removal of brain tissue, dissection, and freezing are imperative for the maintenance of the proteome state in the sample. Protease and phosphatase inhibitors are used to help prevent degradation and dephosphorylation of proteins during protein preparation[67]; however, care should be taken that adducts and charge trains are not introduced by these inhibitors. Purification of proteins from other cellular substances is also necessary, for example, lipids, several proteins (e.g., albumin and immunoglobulin are particularly abundant in the brain), and nucleic acids should be eliminated from the protein sample. The most common methods of purification rely on selective precipitation including acetone and trichloroacetic acid, although a number of commercially available kits are available.[77]

Cerebrospinal Fluid

CSF is secreted by the choroid plexus in the lateral ventricles and is found in the cerebral ventricles and in the subarachnoid space flowing down the spinal canal as well as upward over the brain convexities. CSF, which an important determinant of the extracellular fluid (ECF) surrounding neurons and glia in the CNS, removes harmful brain metabolites, provides a mechanical cushion, and serves as a conduit for peptide hormones secreted by the hypothalamus. CSF is in steady state with the ECF and thus is considered to contain biochemical constituents that reflect neural activity.

Although proteomic studies of neuronal tissue have multiple challenges including the use of postmortem tissue and invasive biopsies from antemortem tissues, CSF proteomics is amenable to serial analysis by minimally invasive lumbar puncture. A change in the expression of CSF constituents may provide important insights into various CNS diseases by improving our understanding of the molecular basis of disease as well as providing disease biomarkers. Given the low protein concentration (~150–450 µg/mL) and the high salt concentration (>150 mmol/L) of CSF and the abundance of albumin (~60% of the total CSF protein) and immunoglobulin,[27] it is necessary to deplete these abundant proteins (e.g., affinity removal, solid phase extraction) and reduce the salt concentration (e.g., protein affinity columns, ultrafiltration, and dialysis) to improve protein recovery and allow better detection of low-abundance proteins. This limitation, the depletion of some of the proteins of interest, can be overcome by a separate analysis of the depleted abundant proteins to ensure the analysis of proteins interacting with the abundant proteins.

Cellular Domain

Several recent proteomics studies have employed fractionation methods that allow collection of multiple cellular components from one tissue source.[17,35,99] This allows a greater amount of each fraction to be used initially, thereby enabling analysis of low-abundance proteins. As the fractions are generated from the same samples, the experimental variability is reduced with the additional advantage of an additive increase in the whole proteome analyzed. The crucial drawback has been the overlap of the proteins between fractions.

Cytoplasm

Because the current proteomic strategies rely heavily on two-dimensional (2D) gel electrophoresis, which has been optimized for the analysis of soluble protein fractions, it is not surprising that most initial phases of proteomic analysis have focused on profiling of the cytoplasm. Most of the key regulators of the signaling pathways are housed in the cytoplasm, where, beside regulating the expression of receptors, they also channel important cytodynamic information between the nucleus and the membrane proteins. Some of the recent studies profiling the cytoplasm have revealed interesting new paradigms in our understanding of neurobiology.

Nucleus

The nucleus has a high degree of organization, consisting of structurally and functionally distinct compartments: nucleolus, nuclear speckles, nuclear pore complex, and nuclear envelope. The nucleus is a highly organized organelle consisting of domains that are fundamental for preserving the homeostasis of the cellular milieu. The profiling of the nuclear proteome in neuroscience has been the slowest of all subcellular fractions. However, there have been some good studies documenting the need to do so. In addition to the soluble fraction of nucleus, there has been an interest in other compartments of nucleus—nuclear envelope, nuclear pore complex, and nucleolus—although no studies to date have been published using such methods in addiction biology research.

Mitochondria

The mitochondria is a complex structure involved in fundamental processes, such as the tricarboxylic acid (TCA) cycle, β-oxidation of fatty acids, the urea cycle, electron transport, oxidative phosphorylation, apoptosis, and heme synthesis. Neuroproteomic analyses of the mitochondria have focused on the abundance in different brain regions.[51,117] Data sets from mitochondrial proteomes from different species and tissues have documented 400–700 mitochondrial-associated proteins, which will enable scientists to better understand the mitochondrial machinery in health and disease.[60,103]

Membrane

Membrane and the membrane-associated proteins constitute nearly a third of the cellular proteins and represent targets of approximately two-thirds of pharmaceutical agents.[95,113] These proteins are involved in various cellular processes including signal transduction, cell adhesion, exocytosis, and metabolism and ion transport. Because membrane proteins are amphipathic, their hydrophobic nature makes them difficult to study and necessitates different strategies for analysis as compared to cytosolic proteins, for example. Therefore, although great strides have been made toward the analysis of soluble cellular proteins, the analysis of membrane proteins reported in proteomic analyses has been underrepresented.[111] The traditional proteomic approach of two-dimensional gel electrophoresis (2DGE) has many limitations for analyzing membrane proteins[12]—including the insolubility of hydrophobic proteins in a nondetergent sample buffer and inadequate alkaline-protein resolution. To a large extent, these issues can be overcome using a variety of combinations of liquid chromatographic separation techniques.

Synaptosomes and Postsynaptic Density

Synapses can be fractionated into synaptosomes as well as distinct pre- and postsynaptic components. Synaptosomes constitute the entire presynaptic terminal (including mitochondria and synaptic vesicles) and portions of the postsynaptic terminal (including postsynaptic membrane and postsynaptic density [PSD]). The study of synaptic proteomes is an important starting point in neuroscience for understanding complex brain functions, critical for understanding neuroplasticity as well as the neuropathology associated with drugs of abuse.

Synaptosomes are subcellular membranous structures formed during mild disruption of brain tissue. The shearing forces cause the nerve endings to break off and subsequent resealing of the membranes form the synaptosomes. The synaptosomes have a complex structure equipped with components of signal transduction, metabolic pathways, and organelles as well as structural components required for vesicular transport. Synaptosomes can be isolated from brain homogenate by differential and density-gradient centrifugation.[86]

The postsynaptic density (or PSD) is a disk-like structure with a thickness of ~30–40 nm and width of ~100–200 nm. The most important structures associated with it are the cytoskeletal proteins, regulatory enzymes, and neurotransmitter receptors and associated proteins. These constitute a very highly structured framework with a definite association of the receptors and ion channels with the signaling molecules and the cytoskeletal elements to play an imperative role in signal transduction as well as synaptic plasticity. There are several available fractionation methods for isolation of the PSD.[70,105]

Separation

Gel-Based Methods

Expression proteomics refers to the determination of protein levels without regard to PTMs. Gel-based as well as chromatographic separation approaches have been integral in generating proteomic profiles in numerous tissues including brain; however, research into the neuroproteome to date has been predominantly gel based.

Two-Dimensional Gel Electrophoresis

The basic principles of 2DGE remain the same since its introduction, namely the separation of proteins by *isoelectric focusing* (IEF; first dimension) followed by sodium dodecyl sulfate polyacrylamide **gel** electrophoresis (SDS-PAGE; second dimension), which involves the separation of proteins by their molecular weight.[46,66] In standard 2DGE experiments, approximately 1000–2000 proteins spots are visualized on a gel representing the most abundant proteins, while other low-abundance proteins are largely obscured by the more abundant proteins. Subcellular fractionation can be used to enrich the representation of low-abundance proteins. Caveats of the 2DGE procedure include (1) the possibility of comigration of proteins (i.e., many proteins in a spot); (2) migration of proteins as multiple spots (i.e., due to charge trains, PTMs, isoforms, and so on); (3) intensive image analysis requiring manual removal of artifacts; (4) inability or difficulty of large and hydrophobic proteins to be isolated in first-dimension gels; and (5) poor representation of highly acidic and basic proteins (i.e., membrane-bound proteins). In general, 2DGE variability is approximately 20%–30% due to sample preparation, reagent sources, staining methods, image analysis software, and technical expertise and experience.[59]

Isoelectric Focusing. Following protein solubilization, the next step in 2DGE is isoelectric focusing (or IEF), which separates the proteins in the first dimension according to their isoelectric point (or pI). The pI of a protein is primarily a function of the amino acid side chains that are protonated or deprotonated, depending on the pH of the solution in which the protein is present. For IEF, protein samples are loaded onto strip gels consisting of a gradient of pH values, and electrophoresis leads protein migration depending on the net charge of each protein in the sample. At a specific pI, the protein will reach the point in the pH gradient where the net charge of the protein is zero and stop migrating.

SDS-PAGE. Next, the IEF gel or strip is equilibrated with sodium dodecyl sulfate (SDS) and placed on top of the SDS acrylamide gel. The equilibration step is necessary to allow the SDS molecules to complex with the proteins and produce anionic complexes with net negative charge roughly equivalent to the molecular weight of the protein. Proteins are electrophoresed migrating from the IEF gel and into the SDS gel, where they separate according to molecular weight (second dimension). Both conventional SDS-PAGE instruments, such as those used for western blotting, and special purpose apparatuses can be used for this step.

Gel Staining. Following electrophoresis, it is imperative to visualize gel spots for subsequent isolation and MS analysis. Coomassie Brilliant Blue (CBB), silver nitrate, and negative staining are common postelectrophoresis methods available for the

2D gel-based proteomics analysis. The sensitivity of these stains range from 100 ng (e.g., CBB) to 1 ng (e.g., silver nitrate) for individual protein spot detection.[65,85] In acidic medium, CBB binds to the amino acids by electrostatic and hydrophobic interactions; however, some of the proteins release the dye during the destaining procedure, which may cause problems with reproducibility and quantitative reliability. CBB is compatible with MS, as complete destaining of the gel can be achieved using bicarbonate. As a rule of thumb, proteins detected visually by CBB are sufficiently abundant for characterization by MS. Disadvantages of CBB staining include low sensitivity and a narrow dynamic range, which however is better than silver stain. Silver staining is widely used for quantitative analysis due to its high sensitivity. Despite its excellent sensitivity, silver staining lacks reproducibility, has a limited linear dynamic range, subjective judgment of the staining end-point, and interferes with the MS compatibility, resulting in a much lower sequence coverage compared to CBB.[61] Even though silver staining is still used currently, there has been an increasing trend to use the new-generation fluorescent stains.

Fluorescence-based detection methods are more sensitive than the absorbance-based methods given the difference in detected and incident wavelengths, which lead to lower background values.[110] SyproRuby dye (Molecular Probes, Eugene, OR), the first of the fluorescent stains, is part of a stable organic complex composed of ruthenium, which interacts noncovalently with basic amino acids in proteins.[6] The stain can be visualized using a wide range of excitation sources commonly used in the image analysis systems. It has a sensitivity that approximates silver staining with a linear dynamic range of three orders of magnitude. DeepPurple (GE Healthcare, Piscataway, NJ) possesses a broad dynamic detection range over four orders of magnitude with limited speckling and background staining,[55,91] appears to result in increased peptide recovery from in-gel digests compared to SyproRuby stain and improves matrix-assisted laser desorption/ionization time of flight (MALDI-ToF) MS-based identification of lower abundance protein spots by increasing sequence coverage.[102]

Two-Dimensional Difference in Gel Electrophoresis

Whereas 2DGE has been the workhorse of proteomics for several decades, the method has been plagued by issues of reproducibility and quantitation given that multiple gels have to be compared. Two-dimensional difference in gel electrophoresis (2D-DIGE)[106] allows the labeling of two to three samples with different dyes on the same 2D gel, thereby reducing spot-pattern variability and the number of gels in an experiment—with the result of making spot matching much more simple and accurate. The most popularized experimental design has been the use of a pooled internal standard (sample composed of equal aliquots of each sample in the experiment) labeled with the Cy2 dye and labeling control and experimental samples with Cy3 or Cy5 dyes swapped equally across the samples, respectively. Following first- and second-dimension electrophoresis, gels are sequentially scanned for Cy2-, Cy3-, and Cy5-labeled proteins by the following lasers/emission filters; 488-/520-, 532-/580-, and 633-nm/670-nm, respectively. The scanned images of the fluorescence-labeled proteins are sequentially analyzed by differential in-gel analysis (DIA; performs Cy5/Cy3: Cy2 normalization) followed by biological variation analysis (BVA; performs inter-gel statistical analysis to provide relative abundance in various groups). These log abundance ratios are then compared between the control and diseased/treatment samples from all the gels using statistical analysis (t test and analysis of variance [ANOVA]).

A modification of 2D-DIGE in which cyanine dyes that label all of the cysteine residues of proteins has been introduced with a detection limit for saturation labeling of 0.1 ng protein per spot thereby reducing the amount of protein sample required for analysis.[88] This procedure provides a very attractive alternative for performing quantitative 2D-DIGE when dealing with low sample amounts, typical in neuroscience, even though only two saturation dyes are currently available (Cy3 and Cy5).

Chromatographic Separation of Proteins

The coupling of efficient chromatographic and electrophoretic separation methods with high-performance MS holds great promise for qualitative and quantitative characterization of highly complex protein mixtures. The advances in chemical tagging and isotope-labeling techniques have enabled the quantitative analysis of proteomes. Multidimensional liquid chromatographic separation (also known as multidimensional protein identification technology; MudPIT[108]) is typically based on using two or more physical properties of peptides (size, charge, hydrophobicity, and affinity) to reduce the complexity of the proteome. Methods commonly used to separate peptides based on physical and chemical properties include ultracentrifugation (density), capillary electrophoresis (size and charge), isoelectric focusing (isoelectric point), size-exclusion chromatography (Stoke's radius), ion-exchange chromatography (charge), hydrophobic interaction chromatography (hydrophobicity), reverse-phase chromatography (hydrophobicity), and affinity chromatography (biomolecular interactions).

A major advantage of multidimensional approaches over 2DGE methods is the ability to isolate low-abundance proteins as well as the proteins with extreme pI, molecular weight, and hydrophobicity.[23,69,108] In most multidimensional separation approaches, proteins are digested into peptides prior to separation yielding complex peptide mixtures but with increased solubility due to the elimination of nonsoluble hydrophobic peptides—a critical caveat for the study of membrane proteins that are insoluble in aqueous buffers.

Several strategies have been developed for relative quantitation of protein expression between samples including (1) isotopic labeling of separate protein mixtures, (2) combined digestion of the labeled proteins followed by multidimensional liquid chromatographic separation, (3) automated tandem mass spectroscopy (MS/MS) of the separated peptides, and (4) automated database search to identify the peptide sequences and quantify the relative protein abundance based on the MS/MS.

Isotope-Coded Affinity Tags (ICAT and iTRAQ)

Isotope-coded affinity tags (ICAT) used to be is one of the most popular methods for quantitative proteome analysis before the inception of isobaric tags for relative and absolute quantitation (iTRAQ) multiplex quantitation strategy.[22] The ICAT reagent is composed of a cysteine-reactive group, a linker containing the heavy or light isotopes (d8/d0), and a biotin affinity tag. The labeling method involves in vitro derivatization of cysteine residues in a protein with d0 or d8 followed by enzymatic digestion of the combined sample. All cysteine biotin-tagged residues are selectively separated by avidin column followed by further separation using reverse-phase chromatography. The isotopically tagged peptides give quantitative mass spectrometry analysis based on the relative peak intensities/areas of d0 and d8 labeled peptides.[24] Another advantage is the ability to analyze peptides with molecular weight more than 3000 Da easily because the mass difference between the coded isoforms is sufficiently large.

A major limitation of ICAT is the exclusive analysis of cysteine containing peptides (10%–20% of the peptides). The resolution is greatest in the case of smaller peptides where the d8/d0 ratio is higher and with peptides that have multiple cysteine residues.[80] Another limitation is that the biotin affinity tag remains linked to the peptides throughout the analysis, causing shifts in chromatographic separation, shifts in the mass-to-charge ratio (m/z), and changes to MS/MS spectra relative to the unlabeled peptides complicating the manual or computer-assisted interpretation.[16,24] Most analyses of ICAT have utilized the combination of strong cation exchange (SCX) chromatography with reverse-phase microbore liquid chromatography coupled with on-line (RP-μLC) with MS and MS/MS.[24,50,108] Data-dependent software is used to select specific mass/charge (m/z) peptides for CID, alternating MS and MS/MS scans for collecting qualitative and quantitative data. Alternative strategies such as per-methyl esterification of carboxylic acid groups,[18] specific labeling of lysine residues,[71] and peptide N-termini[62] have also been used recently. Quantification software has been developed, which can assemble a composite ratio for a protein based on the calculated expression ratio from all the peptides from a single protein such as XPRESS (http://tools.proteomecenter.org/XPRESS.php) and ProICAT (Applied Biosystems, Foster City, CA) The data obtained from these applications can be analyzed collectively using INTERACT for multiple experiments.[28]

iTRAQ methodology is an extension of ICAT, which uses four isobaric reagents (114, 115, 116, and 117), allowing the multiplexing of four different samples in a single LC-MS/MS experiment. More recently, iTRAQ 8Plex, which has four more isobaric reagents (113, 118, 119, and 121) in addition to the traditional four iTRAQ reagents, expands the possibilities of using more experimental variables for comparison. A major advantage of this technique over the ICAT is the ability to label multiple peptides per protein; this increases the confidence of identification as well as quantitation. A recent study comparing 2 DGE and iTRAQ reported a confidence interval of 0.24 for isobaric tagging versus 0.31 for 2 DGE as well as a greater range of expression ratios.[11] A more recent study compared 2D-DIGE, ICAT, and iTRAQ and reported that iTRAQ was more sensitive than the ICAT, which was equisensitive to 2D-DIGE. The complementary nature of these techniques was confirmed by the limited overlap of the proteins characterized.[114]

Top-Down Proteomics

The aforementioned techniques (bottom-up proteomics) are based on consistent enzymatic conversion of proteins to peptides. It is customary to accurately make mass measurements by MS/MS of lower molecular-weight peptides rather than higher molecular-weight intact proteins; however, the bottom-up approach increases the sample complexity, and the entire sequence coverage for proteins is rarely achieved, thereby limiting site-specific PTM analysis of proteins. Such limitations have renewed interest in top-down proteome characterization strategies. Such techniques characterize individual proteins by MS *without* prior enzymatic cleavage. Capillary isoelectric focusing (CIEF) coupled with Fourier transform-ion cyclotron resonance (FTICR) MS is one such strategy for analyzing complex protein mixtures using a top-down approach.[39,107] One potential major limitation is that the level of information is not always sufficient for confident protein identification due to the possibilities of point mutations, PTMs,

and the presence of open reading frames having high-sequence homology. This problem can be overcome somewhat by incorporation of isotopically labeled amino acids into the cellular proteins of unicellular model organisms. The partial amino acid content information obtained combined with CIEF-FTICR, enables identification of proteins from genome databases without MS/MS information.[39,57] Other limitations include the large amount of sample required and the low-throughput that is not amenable to automation.

Mass Spectrometry

Mass spectrometers consist of three major units: the ion source, the mass analyzer, and the ion detection system. MS is based on the separation of ionized proteins or peptides according to the mass to charge ratio (m/z). Tandem mass spectrometry (or MS/MS), on the other hand, couples two mass spectrometers in time and space and has revolutionized the field of expression and functional proteomics.[92] MS/MS involves selection of peptides of a certain mass and the subsequent fragmentation and mass analysis (in two stages). In the first stage, the precursor ion produced by the ion source is selected for fragmentation. The fragmentation results in production of product ions to be analyzed in the second stage of mass analysis. The inconvertible link between the precursor ion and the product ions is responsible for the unique molecular specificity of MS/MS.

Ion Source

A number of ionization technologies exist including fast ion bombardment (FAB),[4] matrix-assisted laser desorption ionization (MALDI),[42] and electrospray ionization (ESI).[15] MALDI and ESI are the techniques of choice for most proteomic applications of neuroscience research. MALDI works by mixing the protein sample with a light-absorbing matrix that forms a crystal. This is usually done on some form of plate with multiple positions for different samples. When the plate is pulsed with a laser of a particular wavelength, the energy from the laser is absorbed by the crystal matrix and the proteins within the crystal are ionized and desorbed (ejected) from the plate into the mass analyzer.

In ESI (and nanospray ionization), ions are produced in a liquid phase. The protein sample, in a solvent solution, is ejected as a mist of droplets from a charged capillary tip. As the solvent in the droplets evaporates, the total charges of the proteins in the droplet remain but with a reduced surface area of the droplet. This continues to a point at which individual ions leave the droplet. Individual ions then pass on into the mass analyzer.

Mass Analyzers

Whichever method of ionization is used, once the ions are created they must be separated before being detected in such a way as to provide information on the m/z ratio. Mass analyzers do not actually detect the ions or measure ion mass; they are used only to separate ions according to their m/z ratio. A number of mass analyzer types exist: time-of-flight (ToF), quadrapole, ion trap, and Fourier transform ion cyclotron resonance (or FTICR).

ToF mass analyzers can be thought of as a tube. The ionized proteins enter the tube by passing through a high-voltage accelerator. The speed at which the ion travels is proportional to its mass (m). The number of ions are produced simultaneously and pass through the ToF tube and to a detector; the ions with a higher m/z ratio will travel faster and reach the detector first. Since the distance traveled and time are all known, the m/z ratio can be calculated and from that the mass.

Quadrapole mass analyzers also involve ions traveling down what can be thought of as a tube. In this case though, the tube consists of four parallel rods. The rods are two pairs of two that can be tuned to different currents and radio frequencies. The two pairs of rods have opposite currents and shifted radio frequencies allowing a form of tuning in which only ions of a particular m/z ratio pass though the tube. A range of m/z ratios can be scanned, generating an m/z profile of the sample. Quadrapole mass analyzers are often used with an ESI ion source.

Ion trap mass analyzers use the same principles as the quadrapole in that specific combinations of current and radio frequencies are used to select particular m/z ratios. The ion trap can be thought of as a small ball with one electrode around the equator and two more electrodes at the poles. Ions are introduced into the center of the ball and are kept in orbits within the trap. By changing current and radio frequency combinations, particular m/z ratio ions are ejected from the ion trap through a port to the detector. By scanning though these voltages and radio frequencies a complete m/z profile can made.

A number of hybrids of these separation strategies exist, all of which are generally designed to increase the accuracy of m/z measurements and sensitivity to low-abundance ions. ToF analyzers can be placed in series (ToF/ToF) with a reflectron or collision cell between them, quadrupoles and ToF can be placed in series (Q-ToF), and extremely powerful magnets and Fourier transform algorithms (FTICR) can be used to determine the m/z ratios of all ions within an ion trap. Detectors change the kinetic energy of the ions into an electrical current that can be measured and passed along to a computer. Although these detectors give information on the abundance of ions, quantitation of protein abundance differences between samples by MS is limited unless samples are linked to isotopes (see ICAT).

All of these MS techniques can be applied to complex protein samples, that is, a mixture of hundreds or thousands of proteins. It is important to separate the use of MS instruments to separate proteins from the MS used for protein identification, as will be described later. As described in subsequent text, quantitative analysis by MS is limited to techniques like ICAT. For researchers looking to profile the expression of proteins in a large number of samples, MS can be problematic and requires a great deal of time on expensive instruments.

Protein Identification

No matter the separation and quantitation methods used, at the end of the experiment the proteins must be identified. Most approaches use mass spectrometry. Peptide mass fingerprinting (PMF) and tandem mass spectrometry (or MS/MS) are the main methods for determining protein identities. PMF was developed by a number of research groups[36,56,68] and begins with digestion of a protein with an enzyme, typically trypsin. Trypsin cleaves proteins at very specific locations, resulting in a series of peptides. If this mixture of peptides is analyzed by MS, a series of peptide masses is created. These masses are searched against databases using one of a number of programs (e.g., ProFound and MASCOT). These programs take DNA sequence databases translated into protein sequences and calculate the resulting peptide masses if these protein sequences were digested with trypsin. The peptide masses generated from the MS of the digested protein of interest is then compared against these databases and

the protein can be identified. PMF of spots from 2DGE gels is one very common application. Gel plugs are either excised by hand or robot. These plugs contain the proteins of interest and the proteins are digested in the plugs with trypsin. With visual stains, the plug must often be destained, and some stains work better than others. Silver stains that use glutaraldehyde are not compatible with MS.

Even if MS instead of 2DGE was chosen as the method of protein separation, MS is also used for protein identification through a process called tandem mass spectrometry (or MS/MS). A number of different strategies exist for MS/MS; in general the process entails the selection of one ion/peptide generated during initial MS and then fragmenting this ion/peptide into smaller pieces and measuring the mass of the resulting ions. These secondary ions can be decoded into peptide sequence information that can be searched against protein sequence databases to identify the protein. Almost all of the ionization and mass analyzer types can all be used for MS/MS, provided that the instrument is appropriately configured. One MS/MS method that is particularly suited for proteome determination, but less so for quantitation, is multidimensional protein identification technology (or MudPIT).[108] In this method all the proteins in a sample are digested and loaded onto LC columns (see previous explanation). After fractionation of the peptides, the peptides are fed into an MS/MS instrument for protein identification. This method has identified thousands of proteins, can detect membrane proteins, and is similar in concept to shotgun sequencing of DNA.

Some of the more traditional methods for identifying proteins are still used for proteomic experiments. Edman protein sequencing can be performed on proteins or peptides extracted from gels or blotted from gels, although the method is limited by low throughput and requires a comparatively large amount of protein. Another technique is the far western blot, where a 2DGE gel is blotted and probed with an antibody against a specific protein. This approach does not offer much progress over conventional immunoblotting.

Protein Arrays

Protein arrays provide a means to characterize the function, interactions, and activities of a large number of target proteins. Protein arrays are generally divided into three categories: antibody (analytical protein) arrays, functional protein arrays, and reverse-phase protein arrays[96] Antibody arrays utilize either antibody capture of labeled proteins[25] or the sandwich-based immunoassay in which the protein of interest is captured by one antibody adhered to the array surface and a second antibody that is labeled for detection.[25,76] Antibody arrays are probably most applicable in addiction medicine as a means of quantifying protein levels in various tissues and fluids as well as a rapid assay for potential biomarkers. Functional protein arrays are useful for determining the biochemical properties of proteins including protein binding and enzyme-substrate interactions. Arrays are produced by adhering purified proteins to the array surface and probing with labeled proteins or substrates. This type of array is used to study the following types of functional protein interactions: protein/protein,[118] protein/peptide,[41] protein/DNA,[26] protein/RNA,[93] protein/lipid,[84] protein/small molecule,[118] and protein/glycan.[7]

Due to some of the limitations of electrophoresis and MS methods, selected research groups are attempting to create proteomic chips/arrays.[72,112] Antibodies or other affinity reagents (e.g., aptamers, peptides) are spotted onto some sort of matrix.

Hundreds to thousands of spots are on a single array. A labeled sample is then washed across the array and proteins bind to their specific antibody. The process can also be reversed whereby the protein samples of interest are spotted onto the matrix and then probed with different affinity reagents. Although these array or chip approaches have potential for greatly increasing the throughput of proteomic experiments, the use of affinity reagents as the separation method is a severely limiting factor and cannot be ignored. A high-quality antibody is needed for each protein of interest and each modification of that protein. To generate quantitative data from antibody arrays, and because association kinetics between different antibodies and antigens can vary tremendously, relative concentrations of each antibody and antigen have to optimized for each protein. Although there seem to be a number of pitfalls to proteomic chips/arrays as an open-screen technique, they do hold promise for routine examination of a small group of proteins. Well-known pathways or gene families could be easily examined by such an approach.

Implementation for Drug Abuse Studies

Proteomic Analysis of Cocaine

Whereas several studies have assessed gene and subsequent protein expression as a function of cocaine administration in humans and animal models, few studies to date have employed high-throughput proteomic technologies to examine the effects of psychomotor stimulant administration on protein expression patterns in discrete brain regions. Two examples of such approaches in this area include comparative analyses of proteomic alterations in the nucleus accumbens (NAc) of cocaine overdose victims and controls, and a complementary study in this region from rhesus monkeys self-administering cocaine for 18 months and controls.

The abuse liability of cocaine has been linked to the direct effects of the drug on dopamine uptake blockade yielding elevated extracellular dopamine concentrations that occur in discrete areas of the brain, specifically the NAc and the ventral tegmental area (VTA), prefrontal cortex—regions of the mesolimbic dopamine pathway that originate in the VTA and project to several forebrain regions, most notably the NAc. Numerous studies in rodent self-administration models have demonstrated definitively an important role for the NAc in the reinforcing effects of cocaine.[32–34,73,119] Recent imaging studies in humans have revealed cocaine-induced functional activation of the NAc following acute drug administration in cocaine-dependent subjects[8] and bilateral activation of the NAc following imagery-induced drug craving.[45] In addition to the acute neurochemical and neurophysiological changes that occur as a function of cocaine, continued administration exerts biochemical adaptations in reinforcement-relevant brain regions[48,63,109] that are apparent at the structural, genomic, and proteomic levels and likely provide the biochemical foundation for sensitization, craving, withdrawal, and relapse.[64] For example, studies in rodent models indicate that chronic cocaine administration leads to persistent or even permanent biochemical alterations in the cAMP pathway (e.g., Carlezon et al.,[10] Pliakas et al.,[75] Self et al.,[87] and Terwilliger et al.[104]), activator protein 1 family members (e.g., Hiroi et al.,[37] Hope et al.,[38] and Pich et al.[74]), glutamate, dopamine, γ-aminobutyric acid (GABA) and opiate receptors, growth factors, cytoskeletal elements, and circadian genes.[a]

Human

Whereas animal studies have advanced our understanding of the neurobiological basis of drug addiction, the evaluation of similar questions in human tissue are few yet are essential. Although there are many difficulties with postmortem brain studies, it is one of the most promising ways to view biochemical changes that are relevant to human drug abusers and to educate the public about the consequences of cocaine abuse. By assessing changes in defined biochemical pathways in human postmortem tissue, we can begin to ascertain the fundamental molecular and biochemical processes that are associated with long-term cocaine use. Furthermore, studies utilizing human postmortem tissue will reveal whether the regulatory adaptations that occur in rodents and monkeys are applicable to human brain and will reveal which changes are state or trait markers in human drug abusers.

To examine the neuropathological consequences of chronic cocaine abuse in the human brain, 2DIGE was used to compare protein alterations in the NAc between cocaine overdose victims (CODs) and controls.[100] The NAc was dissected from coronal blocks of frozen brain tissue that had been obtained previously from subjects that were matched on a number of demographic and pathological indices. Tissue was fractionated into membrane, nuclear, and cytoplasmic fractions as described previously,[35,98] with only cytosolic fractions used for this study. Following image normalization between gels, spots with significantly differential image intensities were identified, excised, and trypsin digested. Differentially expressed proteins were identified by MALDI-ToF/ToF MS. Mass lists were submitted to MASCOT using GPS Explorer to search against the NCBInr (National Centre for Biotechnology Information non-redundant) *primate* database for protein identification. The criterion for identification include a MASCOT confidence interval greater than 95%. Protein identification was confirmed by checking the protein mass and pI accuracy. A total of 1407 spots were found to be present in a minimum of five subjects per group and the intensity of 18 spots was found to be differentially abundant between the groups, leading to the eventual positive identification of 15 proteins by PMF. In addition, 32 spots that were constitutively expressed were positively identified by PMF. The identified proteins can be categorized as cell structure, synaptic plasticity/signal transduction, mitochondria, and metabolism and are representative of functional classes that are affected either directly or indirectly by cocaine administration. For example, previous studies in human COD have reported significant dysregulation of ionotropic glutamate receptors in mesolimbic brain areas (VTA and NAc)—an effect that likely has far-reaching implications in terms of the mechanisms that support increased expression as well as the physiological implications of this upregulation. For example, liprin α3 (upregulated over 2.5-fold in COD) belongs to a family of proteins whose postsynaptic expression is involved in the transport of N-methyl-D-aspartate (NMDA) receptor vesicles along microtubules. Along with increased beta tubulin (2.72-fold in COD), these results begin to provide a framework that could mediate the increased levels of inotropic glutamate receptor (iGluR) subunits at the membrane surface in COD.[35]

In addition to protein alterations that likely are involved in the maintenance of iGluR expression, the abundance of several metabolic proteins was altered in COD that may be related to the consequence of increased iGluR expression—such as increased calcium flux and resulting oxidative stress. For example, peroxiredoxin 2, a neuronal protein involved in redox regulation, was decreased in COD. Prior studies showed have reported that

---

[a] References 2, 3, 19, 31, 40, 52, 97, 115, 116.

cocaine administration increases lipid peroxidation,[47] alters antioxidant enzyme activity and elevates reactive oxygen species in dopaminergic projection areas.[13,54] The mitochondrial protein ATP synthase beta chain, a protein that produces ATP from ADP that is generated from electron transport complexes involved in mitochondrial respiration, was also decreased in COD. These data provide but two examples by which chronic cocaine exposure profoundly affects processes that are integral to normal neuronal function (i.e., decreased ability to reduce reactive oxygen species and improper functioning of energy metabolism). Such changes are likely reflected in changes in glucose metabolism and utilization following cocaine administration in rats,[78] monkeys,[53,79] and humans.[8,83] Understanding the coordinated involvement of multiple proteins in human brain as a function of cocaine abuse provides unique insight into the molecular basis of the disease, offers new targets for pharmacotherapeutic intervention for drug-abuse related disorders, and has the potential to reshape the debate on which biochemical indices are most relevant to the human condition.

Nonhuman Primate

Whereas studies in human brain are important for understanding the neuropathological consequences of chronic cocaine intake, factors such as agonal state, postmortem interval, variability in drug intake, and disease comorbidity may affect the stability of proteins as well as their posttranslational modification. The use of nonhuman primate models of cocaine self-administration provide a critical bridge between human studies and basic research whereby the aforementioned variables that may confound human postmortem studies are better controlled, allowing more precise correlation between drug intake and altered protein expression and function. Using a nonhuman primate model of cocaine self-administration with chronic access (18 months), the effects on protein abundance and phosphorylation were determined in the NAc of rhesus monkeys using 2D-DIGE and 2DGE, followed by gel staining with Pro-Q Diamond phospho-protein gel stain, respectively. As detailed for the aforementioned studies in human postmortem tissue, gel images were normalized for each set of experiments and spots with significantly differential image intensities ($P < 0.05$) were identified, excised and trypsin digested, and analyzed by MALDI-ToF/ToF MS. Eighteen positively identified were found to be differentially expressed in the accumbens between the groups—a significant number of which were either directly or indirectly related to the hyperglutamatergia identified in both COD and rhesus monkeys self-administering cocaine.[35,99] Of interest, the study identified several proteins that complement/supplement the results of the study in COD, including proteins involved in cell structure, synaptic plasticity/signal transduction, metabolism, and mitochondrial function. Specifically, glial fibrillary acidic protein (GFAP), syntaxin binding protein 3, protein kinase C isoform, adenylate kinase isoenzyme 5, and mitochondrial-related proteins were increased in monkeys self-administering cocaine while beta-soluble NSF attachment protein (β SNAP) and neural and nonneural enolase were decreased. In addition to determination of overall protein abundance, the study also explored the functional proteome of the accumbens, in this case by evaluating the expression of phosphorylated proteins. Of the identified spots on the gel, 15 phosphoproteins were positively identified including increased levels of GABA$_A$ receptor–associated protein 1, 14-3-3 gamma protein, glutathione S-transferase, and brain type aldolase, and decreased levels of beta-actin, Rab GDP dissociation inhibitor, guanine deaminase, peroxiredoxin 2 isoform b, and several mitochondrial proteins. Results from this study complement those previously obtained for cocaine-induced biochemical alterations in COD using an animal model that closely recapitulates the human condition. The findings suggest a coordinated dysregulation of proteins related to cell structure, signaling, metabolism, and mitochondrial function that likely indicates long-term compromised cellular function. The reversal or attenuation of these biochemical alterations are important targets for addressing the neuropathology associated with drug abuse.

Rodent

Rodent models of drug abuse provide an economically viable approach for studying the continuum of proteomic changes associated with cocaine addiction (initial use, chronic use and binging, withdrawal, and so on) as well as determining the functional significance of such changes. The majority of proteomic analyses of cocaine's effects in rodent brain have been undertaken following experimenter administration of acute or subchronic dosing regimens of cocaine. Although such studies provide insight into the initial pharmacological effects of cocaine on brain protein expression, changes may or may not be parallel changes associated with the reinforcing effects of the drug as modeled by the intravenous self-administration paradigm.

Proteomic studies using rodents have focused on four brain regions associated with the reinforcing and behavioral effects of drugs: striatum, nucleus accumbens, medial prefrontal cortex, and amygdala.[20,49,81,82,90] Shen and colleagues utilized a novel ion current–based approach in combination with LTQ Orbitrap MS/MS analysis to identify over 2000 proteins in the striatum following 1 and 22 days of withdrawal from noncontingent chronic cocaine administration. Thirteen of the 166 proteins differentially expressed between the two time points were expressed at both withdrawal time points. Of interest, the majority of proteins confirmed findings from previous studies.[89] Kalivas and colleagues queried the PSD fraction of the NAc proteome using iTRAQ labeling and multidimensional liquid chromatographic separation followed by MALDI-ToF/ToF analysis. Of the 42 proteins that were differentially expressed in the PSD accumbens fraction, AKAP79/150 was significantly increased. Injection of an AKAP peptide into this region reduced cocaine reinstatement, indicating a functional role for this protein in relapse vulnerability.[81] Lichti et al. queried the accumbens proteome to identify proteins mediating the addiction protective phenotype of environmental enrichment.[49] The effect of isolation versus environmental enrichment was assessed following 14 days of cocaine self-administration. Accumbens protein isolates were separated by the nanoLC chromatography system and analyzed using the LTQ-Orbitrap Velos MS/MS. The study quantified over 1900 proteins differentially expressed as a function of cocaine self-administration, environmental enrichment, and the interaction of cocaine and environmental enrichment. A thorough discussion of the findings is beyond the scope of the chapter; however, pooling accumbens from two subjects per group may not reflect the complexities and subtleties of differences between the groups.

A recent study brings together the power of the rodent self-administration behavioral approach with state of the art protein analysis to provide novel insights into the mechanisms underplaying memory extinction and reconsolidation of cocaine-related cues.[82] Rich and colleagues assessed the phosphoproteome of the basolateral amygdala in rats with a history of cocaine self-administration using titanium dioxide (TiO$_2$) spin columns to isolate multiply phosphorylated peptides, nano-LC separation, and LTQ Orbitrap MS/MS for peptide identification. Identified peptides were used to create a list for quantitative selected reaction monitoring analysis on the QTRAP 5500. Comparisons were made between groups to identify phosphopeptides regulated by cocaine-associated memory extinction and reconsolidation, leading to the discovery that the phosphorylation of calcium-calmodulin-dependent kinase II α at serine 331 was memory dependent. By pharmacological inhibition of this in the basolateral amygdala, the team was able to reduce cocaine reinstatement by improving memory extinction and attenuating cocaine-related memory reconsolidation.

Proteomic Analysis of Alcohol

Similar to cocaine, the majority of proteomic analyses for alcohol abuse have been conducted in human postmortem tissue and the research has been guided largely by previous studies detailing significant changes in brain morphology, such as cortical and subcortical atrophy. Alcohol-induced changes in cortical and subcortical structure volumes have been correlated with both white and gray matter damage; overall brain shrinkage in alcoholism is largely attributable to cortical white matter loss.[9,29] Thus, in one of the first published proteomic studies of the effects of alcohol in the human brain, Matsumato and colleagues compared the proteomic profile of white matter in the dorsolateral prefrontal cortex between controls, uncomplicated alcoholics (>80 g of ethanol/day, no postmortem evidence of cirrhosis or Wernicke-Korsakoff syndrome [WKS]), alcoholics complicated with hepatic cirrhosis (>80 g of ethanol consumed per day, postmortem confirmation of hepatic cirrhosis, and no postmortem evidence of WKS), reformed alcoholic (>120 g of beer/day for 10 years; abstained last 14 years, no postmortem evidence of cirrhosis or WKS). The elegant experimental design addresses multiple comparisons simultaneously, including the effects of alcoholism in the human brain (controls versus uncomplicated alcoholics), peripheral versus centrally mediated effects on protein alterations (uncomplicated alcoholics versus alcoholics complicated with hepatic cirrhosis), and the transient or permanent nature of alcoholism on brain protein changes (uncomplicated alcoholics versus reformed alcoholics). Following dissection of the dorsolateral prefrontal cortex (DLPFC), crude protein homogenate was isolated from each subject and separated using 2DGE followed by protein identification using MALDI-ToF MS. The study found 60 protein spots that were differentially expressed between controls and alcoholics, of which18 were positively identified representing 11 proteins including proteins involved in cell structure and metabolism, with the most interesting finding being that thiamine deficiency may be related to alcohol-induced brain damage to this region. Of interest, NADH2 dehydrogenase and fructose-biphosphate aldolase C were the only two proteins that were differentially expressed between the uncomplicated and complicated alcoholics.

Complementary proteomic analyses have also been conducted in the genu[43] and splenium[44] of the corpus callosum (CC)—a structure whose volume is decreased in alcoholics.[30] The CC is of particular interest, given that it is the major white matter structure connecting the total cerebral hemispheres, allowing exchange of sensory, motor, and cognitive information. Using similar cohorts and proteomic approaches, two regions of the CC were assessed—the genu and splenium. In the splenium, 43 proteins were found to be differentially expressed between alcoholics and controls, with 26 proteins present in the complicated alcoholic group that were involved in oxidative stress, lipid peroxidation, and apoptosis networks. The prevalence of protein alterations in the complicated alcoholic group suggests a potential relationship with liver dysfunction and cirrhosis. Similarly, 50 identified proteins were differentially expressed in alcoholics in the genu of the CC, with 7 proteins unique to the uncomplicated alcoholic group and 28 unique to the complicated alcoholic group. Differentially expressed proteins were categorized as cytoskeletal, metabolic, oxidative stress related, calcium regulation, and signaling proteins. Comparative analysis between the three studies indicated significant region-specific protein expression in different regions of white matter (CC genu, CC splenium, and DLPFC), suggesting that there are regional differences in their susceptibility to the effects of chronic alcohol.

In addition to determining potential protein correlates of regional white matter alterations induced by alcohol, separate studies have explored alcohol-induced alterations in the hippocampus of human postmortem tissue[58] and in the NAc and amygdala of a rodent model of chronic alcohol intake.[5] These regions are known to be sensitive to the effects of alcohol, with changes in the functional integrity that affect short-term and spatial memory and reward circuitry. Both studies utilized standard 2DGE approaches and MALDI-ToF MS analysis. In the human postmortem study, crude protein homogenates from the hippocampus were compared between uncomplicated alcoholics and controls. Seventeen proteins were identified that were differentially expressed between the groups—proteins involved in metabolism, signaling, and oxidative stress. Comparison with other data from this group emphasizes the regional specificity of alcohol-induced changes and provides a framework for determining the biochemical mechanisms of alcohol-induced neuropathology.

In addition to the use of human postmortem tissue to understand the effects of alcohol, the field has benefited by the use of well-characterized rodent models that exhibit varying degrees of alcohol consumption. Because the aforementioned studies in humans have provided exceptional insight into the pathology associated with chronic alcohol intake, the continuum of alcohol abuse and alcoholism includes biochemical changes in regions associated with the rewarding effects of alcohol—for example, the NAc and amygdala. Using the inbred alcohol-preferring rat line, Bell and colleagues compared the effects of alcohol access (continuous, multiple scheduled access, and ethanol naïve) on the expression of proteins obtained from crude protein homogenates. Data revealed proteins in the accumbens and amygdala that changed in the same direction in the continuous and multiple scheduled access groups suggesting that these proteins were altered as a function of alcohol consumption. In addition, numerous proteins were found to be differentially expressed based on brain region and on exposure to alcohol. The amygdala appeared to be more sensitive to the cellular stress–related effects of chronic alcohol, whereas protein identification in the accumbens reflected alterations in synaptic and cytoskeletal activity that led the authors to suggest increased neuronal function. Examination of the differentially expressed proteins identified in this study, in other behavioral models, and at various times along the alcohol exposure continuum is warranted.

Conclusion

The advent of proteomics technologies provides a unique opportunity to discover and explore biochemical substrates and consequences associated with abused substances. Results from rodent, nonhuman primate, and human postmortem studies indicate significant impairments in neuronal function and plasticity in several brain regions. To date the majority of studies have utilized rodents to model human cocaine intake; however, growing evidence indicates the need to refine rodent and nonhuman primate models to better recapitulate human drug intake and associated neuropathologies. As in other psychiatric and neurological illnesses, researchers should identify the molecular pathologies associated with cocaine addiction in humans and attempt to recapitulate such biological alterations in animal models.

Understanding the coordinated involvement of multiple proteins with chronic cocaine and alcohol addiction provides insight into the molecular basis of drug dependence in general and may offer novel targets for pharmacotherapeutic intervention. Although significant advances have been made in the identification of neurochemical and neurobiological substrates involved in the behavioral effects of abused drugs, the relationship between these effects and resultant alterations in protein expression remain in their infancy and the application of this information to the development of treatment strategies has not been fruitful for several reasons. One explanation is that research in the areas of neurobehavioral pharmacology and molecular biology has proceeded in relative isolation of each other. To date, there have been few published studies combining models of self-administration with proteomic approaches. Other possible explanations include (1) the inappropriate use of experimental models, (2) reliance on non-neuronal systems or neuronal tissue not directly involved in the reinforcing effects of the drug, and (3) the lack of definable neural substrates at the cellular or biochemical level. The combination of appropriate behavioral models of drug reinforcement, specific neurobiological systems, and state of the art molecular techniques will provide the most pertinent data for understanding the molecular basis of drug reinforcement and for potentially establishing novel targets for treatment.

A more detailed understanding of the molecular and biochemical cascades in specific neuronal populations and the interactions between well-defined neuronal populations within discrete brain regions could lead to a greater knowledge of the basic neurobiological processes involved in drug reinforcement. Future efforts investigating the biological basis of drug reinforcement should be directed at specific cellular targets in brain regions considered to be involved in drug reinforcement and should focus on cortical influence on behavior—structures that are best studied in human postmortem tissue and in nonhuman primate models. The integration of basic neuroscience and behavior offers the most productive avenue for delineating the complexity of the neurobiological underpinnings of drug reinforcement and the subsequent development of effective pharmacotherapies to treat addiction.

Acknowledgment

The writing of this chapter was supported in part by funding of the following NIH grants: DA012498, DA003628, and DA06634 (SEH).

References

1. Anderson L, Seilhamer J. A comparison of selected mRNA and protein abundances in human liver. *Electrophoresis*. 1997;18(3-4):533–537.
2. Backes E, Hemby SE. Discrete cell gene profiling of ventral tegmental dopamine neurons after acute and chronic cocaine self-administration. *J Pharmacol Exp Ther*. 2003;307(2):450–459.
3. Bahi A, Dreyer JL. Cocaine-induced expression changes of axon guidance molecules in the adult rat brain. *Mol Cell Neurosci*. 2005;28(2):275–291.
4. Barber M, et al. Fast atom bombardment mass spectrometry of bleomycin A2 and B2 and their metal complexes. *Biochem Biophys Res Commun*. 1981;101(2):632–638.
5. Bell RL, et al. Protein expression changes in the nucleus accumbens and amygdala of inbred alcohol-preferring rats given either continuous or scheduled access to ethanol. *Alcohol*. 2006;40(1):3–17.
6. Berggren K, et al. A luminescent ruthenium complex for ultrasensitive detection of proteins immobilized on membrane supports. *Anal Biochem*. 1999;276(2):129–143.
7. Blixt O, et al. Printed covalent glycan array for ligand profiling of diverse glycan binding proteins. *Proc Natl Acad Sci U S A*. 2004;101(49):17033–17038.
8. Breiter HC, et al. Acute effects of cocaine on human brain activity and emotion. *Neuron*. 1997;19(3):591–611.
9. Carlen PL, et al. Reversible cerebral atrophy in recently abstinent chronic alcoholics measured by computed tomography scans. *Science*. 1978;200(4345):1076–1078.
10. Carlezon Jr WA, et al. Regulation of cocaine reward by CREB. *Science*. 1998;282(5397):2272–2275.
11. Choe LH, et al. A comparison of the consistency of proteome quantitation using two-dimensional electrophoresis and shotgun isobaric tagging in Escherichia coli cells. *Electrophoresis*. 2005;26(12):2437–2449.
12. Churchward MA, et al. Enhanced detergent extraction for analysis of membrane proteomes by two-dimensional gel electrophoresis. *Proteome Sci*. 2005;3(1):5.
13. Dietrich JB, et al. Acute or repeated cocaine administration generates reactive oxygen species and induces antioxidant enzyme activity in dopaminergic rat brain structures. *Neuropharmacology*. 2005;48(7):965–974.
14. Dreger M. Subcellular proteomics. *Mass Spectrom Rev*. 2003;22(1):27–56.
15. Fenn JB, et al. Electrospray ionization for mass spectrometry of large biomolecules. *Science*. 1989;246(4926):64–71.
16. Ferguson PL, Smith RD. Proteome analysis by mass spectrometry. *Annu Rev Biophys Biomol Struct*. 2003;32:399–424.
17. Fountoulakis M. Application of proteomics technologies in the investigation of the brain. *Mass Spectrom Rev*. 2004;23(4):231–258.
18. Goodlett DR, et al. Differential stable isotope labeling of peptides for quantitation and de novo sequence derivation. *Rapid Commun Mass Spectrom*. 2001;15(14):1214–1221.
19. Graham DL, et al. Tropomyosin-related kinase B in the mesolimbic dopamine system: region-specific effects on cocaine reward. *Biol Psychiatry*. 2009;65:696–701.
20. Guan X, Guan Y. Proteomic profile of differentially expressed proteins in the medial prefrontal cortex after repeated cocaine exposure. *Neuroscience*. 2013;236:262–270.
21. Gygi SP, et al. Correlation between protein and mRNA abundance in yeast. *Mol Cell Biol*. 1999;19(3):1720–1730.
22. Gygi SP, et al. Quantitative analysis of complex protein mixtures using isotope-coded affinity tags. *Nat Biotechnol*. 1999;17(10):994–999.
23. Gygi SP, et al. Evaluation of two-dimensional gel electrophoresis-based proteome analysis technology. *Proc Natl Acad Sci U S A*. 2000;97(17):9390–9395.
24. Gygi SP, et al. Proteome analysis of low-abundance proteins using multidimensional chromatography and isotope-coded affinity tags. *J Proteome Res*. 2002;1(1):47–54.
25. Haab BB. Antibody arrays in cancer research. *Mol Cell Proteomics*. 2005;4(4):377–383.
26. Hall DA, et al. Regulation of gene expression by a metabolic enzyme. *Science*. 2004;306(5695):482–484.
27. Hammack BN, et al. Improved resolution of human cerebrospinal fluid proteins on two-dimensional gels. *Mult Scler*. 2003;9(5):472–475.
28. Han DK, et al. Quantitative profiling of differentiation-induced microsomal proteins using isotope-coded affinity tags and mass spectrometry. *Nat Biotechnol*. 2001;19(10):946–951.

29. Harper C, et al. Neuropathological alterations in alcoholic brains. Studies arising from the New South Wales Tissue Resource Centre. *Prog Neuropsychopharmacol Biol Psychiatry*. 2003;27(6):951–961.

30. Harper CG, Kril JJ. Corpus callosal thickness in alcoholics. *Br J Addict*. 1988;83(5):577–580.

31. Hemby SE, Horman B, Tang W. Differential regulation of ionotropic glutamate receptor subunits following cocaine self-administration. *Brain Res*. 2005;1064(1-2):75–82.

32. Hemby SE, Johnson BA, Dworkin SI. Neurobiological basis of drug reinforcement. In: Johnson BA, Roache JD, eds. *Drug Addiction and Its Treatment: Nexus of Neuroscience and Behavior*. Philadelphia: Lippincott-Raven Publishers; 1997:137–169.

33. Hemby SE, et al. Differences in extracellular dopamine concentrations in the nucleus accumbens during response-dependent and response-independent cocaine administration in the rat. *Psychopharmacology (Berl)*. 1997;133(1):7–16.

34. Hemby SE, et al. Synergistic elevations in nucleus accumbens extracellular dopamine concentrations during self-administration of cocaine/heroin combinations (Speedball) in rats. *J Pharmacol Exp Ther*. 1999;288(1):274–280.

35. Hemby SE, et al. Cocaine-induced alterations in nucleus accumbens ionotropic glutamate receptor subunits in human and nonhuman primates. *J Neurochem*. 2005;95(6):1785–1793.

36. Henzel WJ, et al. Identifying proteins from two-dimensional gels by molecular mass searching of peptide fragments in protein sequence databases. *Proc Natl Acad Sci U S A*. 1993;90(11):5011–5015.

37. Hiroi N, et al. FosB mutant mice: loss of chronic cocaine induction of Fos-related proteins and heightened sensitivity to cocaine's psychomotor and rewarding effects. *Proc Natl Acad Sci U S A*. 1997;94(19):10397–10402.

38. Hope B, et al. Regulation of immediate early gene expression and AP-1 binding in the rat nucleus accumbens by chronic cocaine. *Proc Natl Acad Sci U S A*. 1992;89(13):5764–5768.

39. Jensen PK, et al. Probing proteomes using capillary isoelectric focusing-electrospray ionization Fourier transform ion cyclotron resonance mass spectrometry. *Anal Chem*. 1999;71(11):2076–2084.

40. Jiang X, et al. Human BDNF isoforms are differentially expressed in cocaine addicts and are sorted to the regulated secretory pathway independent of the Met66 substitution. *Neuromolecular Med*. 2009;11:1–12.

41. Jones RB, et al. A quantitative protein interaction network for the ErbB receptors using protein microarrays. *Nature*. 2006;439(7073):168–174.

42. Karas M, Hillenkamp F. Laser desorption ionization of proteins with molecular masses exceeding 10,000 daltons. *Anal Chem*. 1988;60(20):2299–2301.

43. Kashem MA, Harper C, Matsumoto I. Differential protein expression in the corpus callosum (genu) of human alcoholics. *Neurochem Int*. 2008;53(1-2):1–11.

44. Kashem MA, et al. Differential protein expression in the corpus callosum (splenium) of human alcoholics: a proteomics study. *Neurochem Int*. 2007;50(2):450–459.

45. Kilts CD, et al. The neural correlates of cue-induced craving in cocaine-dependent women. *Am J Psychiatry*. 2004;161(2):233–241.

46. Klose J. Protein mapping by combined isoelectric focusing and electrophoresis of mouse tissues. A novel approach to testing for induced point mutations in mammals. *Humangenetik*. 1975;26(3):231–243.

47. Kloss MW, Rosen GM, Rauckman EJ. Biotransformation of norcocaine to norcocaine nitroxide by rat brain microsomes. *Psychopharmacology (Berl)*. 1984;84(2):221–224.

48. Koob GF, Le Moal M. Drug addiction, dysregulation of reward, and allostasis. *Neuropsychopharmacology*. 2001;24(2):97–129.

49. Lichti CF, et al. Environmental enrichment alters protein expression as well as the proteomic response to cocaine in rat nucleus accumbens. *Front Behav Neurosci*. 2014;8:246.

50. Link AJ, et al. Direct analysis of protein complexes using mass spectrometry. *Nat Biotechnol*. 1999;17(7):676–682.

51. Lovell MA, et al. Quantitative proteomic analysis of mitochondria from primary neuron cultures treated with amyloid beta peptide. *Neurochem Res*. 2005;30(1):113–122.

52. Lynch WJ, et al. Gene profiling the response to repeated cocaine self-administration in dorsal striatum: a focus on circadian genes. *Brain Res*. 2008;1213:166–177.

53. Lyons D, et al. Cocaine alters cerebral metabolism within the ventral striatum and limbic cortex of monkeys. *J Neurosci*. 1996;16(3):1230–1238.

54. Macedo DS, et al. Cocaine alters catalase activity in prefrontal cortex and striatum of mice. *Neurosci Lett*. 2005;387(1):53–56.

55. Mackintosh JA, et al. A fluorescent natural product for ultra sensitive detection of proteins in one-dimensional and two-dimensional gel electrophoresis. *Proteomics*. 2003;3(12):2273–2288.

56. Mann M, Hojrup Roepstorff. Use of mass spectrometric molecular weight information to identify proteins in sequence databases. *Biol Mass Spectrom*. 1993;22(6):338–345.

57. Martinovic S, et al. Selective incorporation of isotopically labeled amino acids for identification of intact proteins on a proteome-wide level. *J Mass Spectrom*. 2002;37(1):99–107.

58. Matsuda-Matsumoto H, et al. Differential protein expression profiles in the hippocampus of human alcoholics. *Neurochem Int*. 2007;51(6-7):370–376.

59. Molloy MP, et al. Overcoming technical variation and biological variation in quantitative proteomics. *Proteomics*. 2003;3(10):1912–1919.

60. Mootha VK, et al. Integrated analysis of protein composition, tissue diversity, and gene regulation in mouse mitochondria. *Cell*. 2003;115(5):629–640.

61. Mortz E, et al. Improved silver staining protocols for high sensitivity protein identification using matrix-assisted laser desorption/ionization-time of flight analysis. *Proteomics*. 2001;1(11):1359–1363.

62. Munchbach M, et al. Quantitation and facilitated de novo sequencing of proteins by isotopic N-terminal labeling of peptides with a fragmentation-directing moiety. *Anal Chem*. 2000;72(17):4047–4057.

63. Nestler EJ. Molecular basis of long-term plasticity underlying addiction. *Nat Rev Neurosci*. 2001;2(2):119–128.

64. Nestler EJ, Aghajanian GK. Molecular and cellular basis of addiction. *Science*. 1997;278(5335):58–63.

65. Neuhoff V, et al. Essential problems in quantification of proteins following colloidal staining with coomassie brilliant blue dyes in polyacrylamide gels, and their solution. *Electrophoresis*. 1990;11(2):101–117.

66. O'Farrell PH. High resolution two-dimensional electrophoresis of proteins. *J Biol Chem*. 1975;250(10):4007–4021.

67. Olivieri E, Herbert B, Righetti PG. The effect of protease inhibitors on the two-dimensional electrophoresis pattern of red blood cell membranes. *Electrophoresis*. 2001;22(3):560–565.

68. Pappin DJ. Peptide mass fingerprinting using MALDI-TOF mass spectrometry. *Methods Mol Biol*. 2003;211:211–219.

69. Peng J, et al. Evaluation of multidimensional chromatography coupled with tandem mass spectrometry (LC/LC-MS/MS) for large-scale protein analysis: the yeast proteome. *J Proteome Res*. 2003;2(1):43–50.

70. Peng J, et al. Semiquantitative proteomic analysis of rat forebrain postsynaptic density fractions by mass spectrometry. *J Biol Chem*. 2004;279(20):21003–21011.

71. Peters EC, et al. A novel multifunctional labeling reagent for enhanced protein characterization with mass spectrometry. *Rapid Commun Mass Spectrom*. 2001;15(24):2387–2392.

72. Petricoin EF, et al. Clinical proteomics: translating benchside promise into bedside reality. *Nat Rev Drug Discov*. 2002;1(9):683–695.

73. Pettit HO, et al. Destruction of dopamine in the nucleus accumbens selectively attenuates cocaine but not heroin self-administration in rats. *Psychopharmacology*. 1984;84(2):167–173.

74. Pich EM, et al. Common neural substrates for the addictive properties of nicotine and cocaine. *Science*. 1997;275(5296):83–86.

75. Pliakas AM, et al. Altered responsiveness to cocaine and increased immobility in the forced swim test associated with elevated cAMP response element-binding protein expression in nucleus accumbens. *J Neurosci*. 2001;21(18):7397–7403.

76. Poetz O, et al. Protein microarrays: catching the proteome. *Mech Ageing Dev*. 2005;126(1):161–170.

77. Polson C, et al. Optimization of protein precipitation based upon effectiveness of protein removal and ionization effect in liquid chromatography-tandem mass spectrometry. *J Chromatogr B Analyt Technol Biomed Life Sci*. 2003;785(2):263–275.

78. Porrino LJ. Functional consequences of acute cocaine treatment depend on route of administration. *Psychopharmacology (Berl)*. 1993;112(2-3):343–351.

79. Porrino LJ, et al. Cocaine self-administration produces a progressive involvement of limbic, association, and sensorimotor striatal domains. *J Neurosci*. 2004;24(14):3554–3562.

80. Regnier FE, et al. Comparative proteomics based on stable isotope labeling and affinity selection. *J Mass Spectrom*. 2002;37(2):133–145.

81. Reissner KJ, et al. AKAP signaling in reinstated cocaine seeking revealed by iTRAQ proteomic analysis. *J Neurosci*. 2011;31(15):5648–5658.

82. Rich MT, et al. Phosphoproteomic Analysis reveals a novel mechanism of camkiialpha regulation inversely induced by cocaine memory extinction versus reconsolidation. *J Neurosci*. 2016;36(29):7613–7627.

83. Risinger RC, et al. Neural correlates of high and craving during cocaine self-administration using BOLD fMRI. *Neuroimage*. 2005;26(4):1097–1108.

84. Saliba AE, et al. A quantitative liposome microarray to systematically characterize protein-lipid interactions. *Nat Methods*. 2014;11(1):47–50.

85. Scheler C, et al. Peptide mass fingerprint sequence coverage from differently stained proteins on two-dimensional electrophoresis patterns by matrix assisted laser desorption/ionization-mass spectrometry (MALDI-MS). *Electrophoresis*. 1998;19(6):918–927.

86. Schrimpf SP, et al. Proteomic analysis of synaptosomes using isotope-coded affinity tags and mass spectrometry. *Proteomics*. 2005;5(10):2531–2541.

87. Self DW, et al. Involvement of cAMP-dependent protein kinase in the nucleus accumbens in cocaine self-administration and relapse of cocaine-seeking behavior. *J Neurosci*. 1998;18(5):1848–1859.

88. Shaw J, et al. Evaluation of saturation labelling two-dimensional difference gel electrophoresis fluorescent dyes. *Proteomics*. 2003;3(7):1181–1195.

89. Shen S, et al. Ion-current-based temporal proteomic profiling of influenza-a-virus-infected mouse lungs revealed underlying mechanisms of altered integrity of the lung microvascular barrier. *J Proteome Res*. 2016;15(2):540–553.

90. Shen S, et al. Large-scale, ion-current-based proteomic investigation of the rat striatal proteome in a model of short- and long-term cocaine withdrawal. *J Proteome Res*. 2016;15(5):1702–1716.

91. Smejkal GB, Robinson MH, Lazarev A. Comparison of fluorescent stains: relative photostability and differential staining of proteins in two-dimensional gels. *Electrophoresis*. 2004;25(15):2511–2519.

92. Smith RD. Trends in mass spectrometry instrumentation for proteomics. *Trends Biotechnol*. 2002;20(suppl 12):S3–S7.

93. Song G, Neiswinger J, Zhu H. Characterization of RNA-binding proteins using protein microarrays. *Cold Spring Harb Protoc*. 2016;2016(10). https://doi.org/10.1101/pdb.prot087973.

94. Southan C. Has the yo-yo stopped? An assessment of human protein-coding gene number. *Proteomics*. 2004;4(6):1712–1726.

95. Stevens T, et al. Mechanisms regulating endothelial cell barrier function. *Am J Physiol Lung Cell Mol Physiol*. 2000;279(3):L419–L422.

96. Sutandy FX, et al. Overview of protein microarrays. *Curr Protoc Protein Sci*. 2013;Chapter 27:Unit 27.1.

97. Tang W, et al. Alterations in ionotropic glutamate receptor subunits during binge cocaine self-administration and withdrawal in rats. *J Neurochem*. 2004;89(4):1021–1033.

98. Tang W-X, et al. Molecular profiling of midbrain dopamine regions in cocaine overdose victims. *J Neurochem*. 2003;85:911–924.

99. Tang WX, et al. Molecular profiling of midbrain dopamine regions in cocaine overdose victims. *J Neurochem*. 2003;85(4):911–924.

100. Tannu N, Mash DC, Hemby SE. Cytosolic proteomic alterations in the nucleus accumbens of cocaine overdose victims. *Mol Psychiatry*. 2007;12(1):55–73.

101. Tannu NS, et al. Comparative proteomes of the proliferating C(2) C(12) myoblasts and fully differentiated myotubes reveal the complexity of the skeletal muscle differentiation program. *Mol Cell Proteomics*. 2004;3(11):1065–1082.

102. Tannu NS, et al. Effect of staining reagent on peptide mass fingerprinting from in-gel trypsin digestions: a comparison of SyproRuby and DeepPurple. *Electrophoresis*. 2006;27(15):3136–3143.

103. Taylor SW, et al. Characterization of the human heart mitochondrial proteome. *Nat Biotechnol*. 2003;21(3):281–286.

104. Terwilliger RZ, et al. A general role for adaptations in G-proteins and the cyclic AMP system in mediating the chronic actions of morphine and cocaine on neuronal function. *Brain Research*. 1991;548(1-2):100–110.

105. Trinidad JC, et al. Phosphorylation state of postsynaptic density proteins. *J Neurochem*. 2005;92(6):1306–1316.

106. Unlu M, Morgan ME, Minden JS. Difference gel electrophoresis: a single gel method for detecting changes in protein extracts. *Electrophoresis*. 1997;18(11):2071–2077.

107. Valaskovic GA, Kelleher NL. Miniaturized formats for efficient mass spectrometry-based proteomics and therapeutic development. *Curr Top Med Chem*. 2002;2(1):1–12.

108. Washburn MP, Wolters D, Yates 3rd JR. Large-scale analysis of the yeast proteome by multidimensional protein identification technology. *Nat Biotechnol*. 2001;19(3):242–247.

109. White FJ, Kalivas PW. Neuroadaptations involved in amphetamine and cocaine addiction. *Drug Alcohol Depend*. 1998;51(1-2):141–153.

110. White IR, et al. A statistical comparison of silver and SYPRO Ruby staining for proteomic analysis. *Electrophoresis*. 2004;25(17):3048–3054.

111. Wilkins MR, et al. Two-dimensional gel electrophoresis for proteome projects: the effects of protein hydrophobicity and copy number. *Electrophoresis*. 1998;19(8-9):1501–1505.

112. Wilson DS, Nock S. Recent developments in protein microarray technology. *Angew Chem Int Ed Engl*. 2003;42(5):494–500.

113. Wu CC, et al. A method for the comprehensive proteomic analysis of membrane proteins. *Nat Biotechnol*. 2003;21(5):532–538.

114. Wu WW, et al. Comparative study of three proteomic quantitative methods, DIGE, cICAT, and iTRAQ, using 2D gel- or LC-MALDI TOF/TOF. *J Proteome Res*. 2006;5(3):651–658.

115. Yuferov V, et al. Microarray studies of psychostimulant-induced changes in gene expression. *Addict Biol*. 2005;10(1):101–118.

116. Zhang D, et al. Repeated cocaine administration induces gene expression changes through the dopamine D1 receptors. *Neuropsychopharmacology*. 2005;30(8):1443–1454.

117. Zhang S, Fu J, Zhou Z. Changes in the brain mitochondrial proteome of male Sprague-Dawley rats treated with manganese chloride. *Toxicol Appl Pharmacol*. 2005;202(1):13–17.

118. Zhu H, Snyder M. Protein arrays and microarrays. *Curr Opin Chem Biol*. 2001;5(1):40–45.

119. Zito KA, Vickers G, Roberts DC. Disruption of cocaine and heroin self-administration following kainic acid lesions of the nucleus accumbens. *Pharmacol Biochem Behav*. 1985;23(6):1029–1036.

20

Neuroinflammatory Processes in Drug Addiction

LEON G. COLEMAN, JR., AND FULTON T. CREWS

Innate Immune Signaling in the Brain

Immune Cells of the Brain

Historically the brain has been considered an "immune privileged" organ, meaning it is protected from immune activation that occurs in the periphery. Currently, this is largely considered true; however, the brain has its own immune defenses. The resident immune defenses in the brain are known to be composed of innate immune responses. This allows for recognition and elimination of viral, bacterial, and fungal pathogens. Historically, immune function in the brain has primarily been considered the role of glial—microglia and astrocytes. Microglia are the resident macrophages of the brain and derive from mesodermal tissue-specific monocytes. Microglia transition from a resting state to various stages of activation in response to infections, stressors, and drugs of abuse such as alcohol and cocaine.[a] Stages of microglial activation have been traditionally classified as M1 (proinflammatory) and M2 (antiinflammatory). M1 activation is associated with the release of canonical proinflammatory cytokines such as tumor necrosis factor α (TNFα), interleukin 1β (IL-1β), and IL-6, as well as

[a]References 20, 45, 76, 79, 142, 154, 167.

generation of reactive oxygen species (ROS) through increased inducible nitric oxide synthase (iNOS) and nicotinamide adenine dinucleotide phosphate (NADPH)-oxidase expression. The M2 state is associated with the release of canonical antiinflammatory cytokines such as IL-10 and IL-4. Microglia also regulate physiological processes in the healthy brain, such as synaptic pruning, debris clearance, immune surveillance/defense, and neurogenesis.[96,97] Astrocytes are another important cell type in the neuroimmune system.[64] Astrocytes express immune receptors and cytokines in response to immune activation.[89] Astrocytes undergo an activation known as reactive gliosis to help limit tissue damage in different contexts.[141] Some suggest that astrocytes adopt proinflammatory and antiinflammatory states, similar to microglia.[87,111a] Astrocytes are also involved in numerous physiological processes, such as maintenance of fluid homeostasis, metabolic support of neurons, and modulation of synaptic transmission through uptake of glutamate.[98] Both alcohol and cocaine also cause astrocyte activation.[2,142,178] It is important to note that both microglia and astrocytes regulate synaptic plasticity. Thus their activation by drugs of abuse might result in synaptic changes and neuronal firing. Of interest, neurons have also been proposed to play a role in innate immune responses through modulation of glia and the induction of cytokines.[105,106] In addition, a variety of cytokine receptors, such as those for,[97a] suggesting that neurons respond to cytokines. Indeed, IL-1β, monocyte chemoattractant protein-1 (MCP-1) and other immune-signaling molecules alter neuronal firing and modulates γ-aminobutyric acid (GABA) transmission.[11,12,159] These studies indicate that in the brain, cytokines and other immune-signaling molecules modify synapses and neurocircuits similar to neurotransmitters.

Pattern Recognition Receptors and Their Ligands

The innate immune system functions to recognize foreign pathogens for their elimination. These pathogenic elements are detected by pattern recognition receptors (PRRs). These receptors recognize specific molecular signatures associated with bacteria and viruses, termed pathogen-associated molecular patterns (PAMPs). PRRs are promiscuous receptors that have also been

TABLE 20.1   Selected Toll-like Receptors (TLRs) implicated in Addiction and Neurological Diseases

TLR	Foreign Immunogen	Endogenous TLR Ligand	Neuropsychiatric Disease
2	Bacterial di- and tri-acylated polypeptides[37] Gram (+) lipoglyans[24]	α-Synuclein	Alcoholism Parkinson disease[99]
3	dsRNA	Stathmin, dsRNA	Alzheimer disease[85] Multiple sclerosis[36]
4	Bacterial endotoxin Peptidoglycans	HMGB1 HSPs 60, 70/72[176]	Alcoholism[50] Cocaine abuse Stroke, traumatic brain injury Chronic pain
7	ssRNA[109]	Let-7, miR-21	Alcoholism[45] Alzheimer disease[110] Chronic pain[136]

HMGB1. High-mobility group box.

found to recognize endogenous molecules associated with cell stress or trauma, known as damage-associated molecular patterns (DAMPs). This is considered "sterile" inflammation, when innate immune activation occurs without the presence of a foreign pathogen. The release of DAMPs has been implicated in the pathologies of numerous peripheral immunological diseases. DAMP release also occurs in the brain, which is normally a sterile environment. PRRs play critical roles in addiction pathology.[49] To date, five classes of PRRs have been identified including: Toll-like receptors (TLRs), C-type lectin receptors, nucleotide binding domain receptors (leucine-rich repeat containing or nucleotide-binding oligomerization domain [NOD]-like receptors), RIG-I-like receptors, and absent in melanoma 2 (AIM2)-like receptors[35]. TLRs are the most studied PRRs, and have been implicated in both cocaine and alcohol addiction.[8,130,143] To date, 10 TLRs have been identified in humans and 12 in mice.[35] TLR ligands include a variety of molecules from bacterial endotoxin to mammalian high-mobility group box 1 (HMGB1) and heat shock proteins[176] (Table 20.1). TLRs are characterized by an N-terminal extracellular leucine-rich repeat sequence and an intracellular Toll/IL-1 receptor/resistance motif (TIR).[170] TLR signaling operates through key adapter proteins that initiate the signaling cascade upon ligand recognition. All TLRs, except for TLR3, utilize the MyD88 adapter protein complex. TIRAP/MyD88 complex formation causes activation of the IL-1 receptor–associated kinases (IRAKs) and the TNF receptor–associated factor 6 (TRAF6) leading to IκB and MAPK activation. IκB and MAPK activation result in activation of the nuclear factor kappa-light-chain-enhancer of activated B cells (NF-κB) and activated protein-1 (AP-1) transcription factors, respectively. These transcription factors regulate the expression of proinflammatory cytokines that propagate and magnify the immune response. Because TLRs share common intracellular signaling with several cytokines, subsequent cytokine release leads to an amplification of immune responses. Activation of these transcription factors is involved in addiction (detailed below). TLR signaling was initially described in peripheral immune cells. Thus the precise signaling pathways for the TLRs in each brain cell type have yet to be delineated. Both microglia and astrocytes appear to show canonical TLR4 signaling in response to ethanol resulting in NF-κB activation. However, responses in neurons are poorly understood. There is debate on whether neurons are capable of

activating NF-κB. Some suggest that neurons do,not[118] while others find that NF-κB activation in glutamatergic and cultured neurons regulates plasticity, learning, and memory.[93,106] Furthermore, activated NF-κB subunit colocalizes with dorsal horn spinal neurons[10] and different neuronal cell lines exhibit NF-κB-dependent regulation of μ-opioid receptor expression.[31,185]

A key feature of TLR signaling is the induction of proinflammatory DAMP release. These DAMPs can subsequently further TLR activation by binding to their respective receptors. Because the brain is sterile, TLR activation in the brain in response to drugs of abuse likely involves DAMP-mediated signaling. One such DAMP that has been found to play a role in alcohol addiction in particular is the protein high-mobility group box 1 (or HMGB1), a nuclear chromatin binding protein that can be released during cellular stress, activation, or damage. Upon its release, HMGB1 acts as an immune mediator via TLR4 or RAGE receptors.[88,127] HMGB1 has been implicated in alcohol addiction pathology and might be involved in other drugs of abuse (detailed further later in this chapter). HMGB1 is also released prior to hyperexcitable states, such as seizures, and modulates glutamatergic signaling.[119a] Neuroimmune activation and neuronal signaling could be interconnected by DAMP release. Several cytokines have been found to regulate normal brain function and could be dysregulated by drugs of abuse. Thus DAMP and cytokine paracrine and autocrine signaling across glia through kinase cascades may represent brain plasticity mechanisms that could contribute to the development of addiction

Immune Signaling Molecules as Neuromodulators

In the brain, the neuroimmune system functions not only to address foreign pathogens, but also regulates normal brain function. Recently, numerous immune signaling molecules have also been found to be important for synaptic activity, learning, and memory. For example, the classic proinflammatory cytokine TNFα is required for development of long-term potentiation (LTP) in the visual cortex[168] and is critical for synaptic strength.[18] At higher concentrations, however, TNFα disrupts LTP.[171] This translates into behavioral alterations, as TNFα-overexpressing mice show decreased performance on spatial learning and memory tasks.[4]

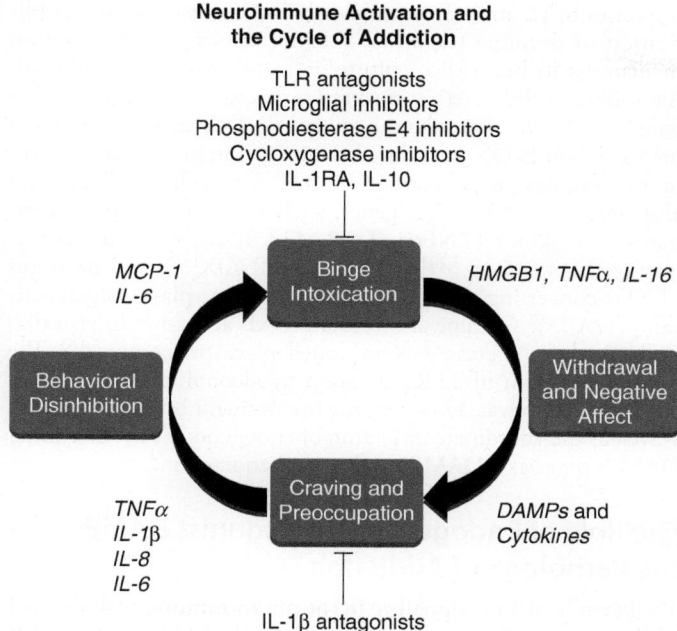

Neuroimmune Activation and the Cycle of Addiction

- Fig. 20.1 Neuroimmune contributions during the various stages of addiction.

The cytokine IL-1β also modulates LTP, promoting it at lower levels, but disrupting LTP at higher concentrations.[74,147,148] In addition, IL-1β modulates neuronal GABA transmission in the central amygdala.[11,12] The M2 (antiinflammatory) microglia-associated protein TGF-β1 promotes LTP and object recognition memory.[40] IL-4 and IL-13 knockout (KO) mice show learning and memory impairments.[34,62] The inflammatory chemokines MIP-1α and CX3CL1 also regulate synaptic plasticity and memory function.[22,119] CX3CL1 KO mice show impaired LTP, whereas exogenously added MIP-1α impairs LTP. These immune-associated molecules have multiple functions. Thus in the brain, immune signaling molecules seem to function as endogenous neuromodulators. Disruption of the expression or release of these molecules by drugs of abuse could alter synaptic activity and behavior.

Addiction as a Neuroimmune Disease

Neuroimmune Components of the Stages of Addiction

The neuroimmune contribution to the pathology of addiction has become the topic of recent numerous reviews.[b] Neuroimmune signaling has been identified in each of the stages of addiction. The pathology of addiction has been modeled by a three-stage process to identify different features that may be targeted by intervention.[58,183] Addicted individuals cycle through binge intoxication, withdrawal and negative affect, craving, and preoccupation, and back to binge intoxication[102] (Fig. 20.1). Much work remains to be done to better understand the impact of innate immune activation during the various stages; however, several inflammatory

mediators have been found to play important roles at various stages.

During the binge/intoxication stage, several immune-regulating interventions have been found to alter alcohol consumption. Immune activation by injection of the TLR4 agonist lipopolysaccharide (LPS) increases ethanol consumption in mice,[29] whereas local knockdown of TLR4 in the central amygdala also decreases ethanol self-administration.[114] MCP-1 increases alcohol self-administration after intracerebroventricular injection in rats.[177] Meanwhile, the antiinflammatory mediators IL-1 receptor antagonist and IL-10 each reduce alcohol self-administration when injected into the basolateral amygdala.[121,122] Blocking IL-1β signaling in the VTA also prevents cocaine-induced dopamine release in the nucleus accumbens.[130] Furthermore, ablation of certain key neuroimmune genes, such as IL-6, IL-1ra, Ccr2, Ccl2, and Ccl3, decreases ethanol consumption.[28,30] Compounds that inhibit microglia also reduce the binge/intoxication stage. Minocycline, a microglial inhibitor, reduces ethanol self-administration[1] and conditioned place preference to cocaine.[130] An analysis of genetically paired rodents found that high ethanol drinking animals show increased NF-κB and other proinflammatory gene expression.[128] These studies suggest that neuroimmune activation may play a role in the rewarding properties of drugs of abuse. However, care should be taken when extrapolating rodent studies to humans, as in addicted humans, the rewarding properties of drugs of abuse shift from the drug itself to cues associated with the drug.[102] The majority of rodent work to date has been done in nondependent animals and should be interpreted in that context.

Neuroimmune activation also occurs during the craving/preoccupation stage. In human alcoholics, increased plasma levels of multiple proinflammatory cytokines have been found such as TNFα[80] (which correlates with severity of alcoholism), and IL-1β, IL-6, and IL-8, which correlate with alcohol craving.[80,108] TNFα, IL-6, and IL-1β each cross the blood-brain barrier to exert their CNS effects.[16,17] Infusion of the opioid-insensitive TLR4 antagonist (+)-naltrexone during withdrawal reduces cue-induced heroine seeking.[173] More work needs to be done to discern the role of neuroimmune activation in the craving of drugs of abuse. However, these findings suggest a potential role and a possibility of immune therapeutics to prevent drug-associated craving.

Neuroimmune activation is also involved in the withdrawal/negative affect stage of addiction. A large body of literature does suggest that the development of negative affective states such as anxiety and dysphoria contribute to the maintenance of addiction.[101] The negative affect stage is often described as stress. It is thought that continued substance abuse is an attempt to alleviate these negative states. Alcohol withdrawal causes increased inflammatory cytokines in the brain.[101] In addition, intracerebroventricular injection of cytokines sensitizes anxiety-like behavior during alcohol withdrawal.[33] Thus, cytokine induction is thought to contribute to negative affect associated with withdrawal. Heightened activation of stress pathways during withdrawal also cause neuroinflammation. Stress causes sensitization of microglia to inflammation in an HMGB1-dependent manner.[191] TLR4 activation modulates serotonin transporter (SERT) function and increases depression-like behavior.[199] Furthermore, various types of acute and chronic stress causes microglia activation in multiple brain regions[175] and leads to depression-like behavior. The proinflammatory cytokines TNFα, IL-6, and IL-1β contribute to the pathologies of mood disorders.[20a,20b] Agents that inhibit microglial activation block the development of depression-like behavior.[69,103,175,194] Ethanol increases microglial markers such

[b]References 15, 49, 51, 52, 54, 56, 57, 86, 115, 123, 124, 126, 129, 156, 180.

as CD11b and Iba1,[66,149] consistent with microglial activation, and primes the microglial response to peripheral inflammation.[149] In addition, stress also causes NF-κB activation. Human psychosocial stress causes NF-κB activation in blood monocytes.[23] Restraint stress in rodents causes NF-κB activation with subsequent production of TNFα and proinflammatory prostaglandins.[23,117] Ethanol activates NF-κB in rat and mouse brain,[151,189] and human astrocytes.[60] Therefore, it is clear that both stress and alcohol can affect glia and lead to neuroimmune activation. The exact neuroimmune milieu associated with drug withdrawal–induced stress is not clear. However, stress pathways overlap with neuroimmune pathways associated with drug withdrawal and are clearly activated. Further work needs to be done to determine the exact contributions of neuroimmune activation to negative affect and stress associated with drug withdrawal.

Neuroimmune Signaling in Alcoholism

Alcohol use activates the neuroimmune system, contributing to the development of alcohol use disorders.[49,52,56,180] Findings from postmortem human alcoholic brain tissue, rodent studies, and cell culture work support this hypothesis. Postmortem human alcoholic brains show increased microglial[79,160] and astrocyte markers.[160] Postmortem human alcoholic brains show increased expression of neuroimmune molecules, such as MCP-1, TLR2, TLR3, TLR4, TLR7, and HMGB1.[50,79] Ethanol exposure studies in vivo also find increased expression of TLRs2–4 in cortex and cerebellum, with subsequent NF-κB activation and cytokine induction.[50,113] Binge alcohol treatment persistently increases neuroimmune molecules such as TLR3, TLR4, HMGB1, and RAGE. [179,181] Ethanol also sensitizes neuroimmune responses to TLR3 and TLR4 agonists.[149,154] Studies in vitro find that ethanol directly activates immune cells. Alcohol activates microglia in vitro, increasing expression of TNFα, IL-1β, iNOS, and NADPH oxidase.[66,149,155] In addition, alcohol activates astrocytes, with increases in GFAP.[3,71] These effects in vitro and in vivo involve TLR activation. TLR4 activation has been shown to play a pivotal role in alcohol-induced neuroimmune signaling.[3] TLR4 KOs and TLR4 KO glia are protected from much of neuroimmune activation by ethanol including glial cell activation, NF-κB activation, caspase-3 activation, anxiety-like behavior, and memory impairment.[c] Astrocytes treated in vitro with siRNA against TLR4 or MD-2 and CD14 (critical adaptor molecules for TLR4 signaling) are protected from ethanol-induced NF-κB induction.[25] In addition, ethanol increases the formation of TLR4/TLR2 heterodimers in microglia cell membrane, causing iNOS induction and MAPK activation.[65] Both TLR4 and TLR2 KOs were protected. In an alcohol-preferring rat strain (p-rats), increased expression of TLR4 in the VTA was found to correspond with binge ethanol responding,[92] with TLR4 expression being regulated by GABA(A)α2 receptor[114] and the stress-associated corticotropin-releasing factor (CRF).[92] TLR4 activation has also been implicated in cocaine and heroin abuse.[130,143,173] Furthermore, ethanol-induced innate immune activation caused impairment of short and long-term memory for object recognition in mice.[137] This was accompanied by a reduction of H3 and H4 histone acetylation as well as histone acetyltransferase activity in the frontal cortex, striatum, and hippocampus. TLR4 KO mice were protected from behavioral impairments and histone modifications. TLR7 has also been identified as important in neuroimmune activation by ethanol leading to hippocampal neurodegeneration, and should be investigated further.[45] Activation of TLRs is a central feature in the neuroimmune

responses to ethanol. This leads to NF-κB activation and amplification of immune responses. Ethanol causes NFκB activation in neurons in brain slice culture[45,200] and in vivo.[189] Although the unique cellular activation patterns need to be further elucidated, it is clear that ethanol activates NFκB in brain. Ethanol increases NFκB-DNA binding both in vivo in mice[47] and in vitro in rat hippocampal-entorhinal cortex slice culture.[200] Ethanol also induces NFκB target genes, such as MCP-1,[79] proinflammatory cytokines (TNFα, IL-1β, and IL-6),[152] proinflammatory oxidases (iNOS,[3,201] COX,[3,25] and NOX[155]), and proteases (TNFα-converting enzyme [TACE] and tissue plasminogen activator [tPA]).[201] Cocaine also causes NF-κB activation in vivo that is required for increased conditioned place preference.[5,161] The exact mechanism of TLR activation by alcohol and other drugs of abuse is not clear. However, the involvement of multiple TLRs as well as the coordinate induction of endogenous TLR-activating DAMPs suggests a DAMP-mediated phenomenon.

The Role of Endogenous TLR Agonist DAMPs in the Pathology of Addiction

The key role of TLR signaling in the neuroimmune pathology of addiction begs the question of—What is the mechanism of TLR activation? The brain is typically a sterile environment; however, TLRs are expressed and follow differential developmental expression patterns.[95] Certain TLRs have also been found to have nonimmune functions, such as TLR3 and TLR8, which regulate axonal and neurite outgrowth, respectively.[39,116] Thus TLR signaling occurs in brain function in the absence of infection, through the release of endogenous TLR agonists. This led to the hypothesis that TLR activation in addiction is mediated through the release of endogenous agonists. Indeed, induction of DAMPs has been found in the pathology of alcoholism. The endogenous TLR4 and RAGE agonist, HMGB1, in particular, has been identified as a critical neuroimmune mediator in alcoholism. HMGB1 is increased in postmortem human alcoholic brain in several brain regions and correlates with lifetime alcohol consumption.[45,50,179] Ethanol administration in vivo increases HMGB1 in cortex and cerebellum.[50,113] In addition, microglia secrete HMGB1 in response to ethanol as well as tobacco smoke extract.[42,45,50,106,203] Thus ethanol and other drugs of abuse can cause sterile inflammation by the release of HMGB1. Recently, ethanol has been found to cause TLR7 activation through the vesicular secretion of the miRNA let-7b DAMP.[45] Let-7b binds the single-stranded RNA sensing TLR7 leading to neuroimmune activation and neurodegeneration. HMGB1 is actually required for immune responses to TLRs 3, 7, and 9.[196] Therefore, HMGB1 may represent a critical modulator of multiple neuroimmune signals. Indeed, blocking HMGB1 release prevents cytokine induction by chronic ethanol.[193] Methamphetamine also induces HMGB1 in vivo and in vitro, with HMGB1 inhibition preventing neuroimmune activation by methamphetamine.[70]

Neuroimmune Activation and the Progression to Addiction

The progression from drug or alcohol abuse to addiction occurs over time (Fig. 20.2). This progression often begins during adolescence. Alcohol and drug abuse during adolescence are common.[107] Regarding alcoholism, the age at drinking onset is strongly related to the risk of developing an alcohol use disorder

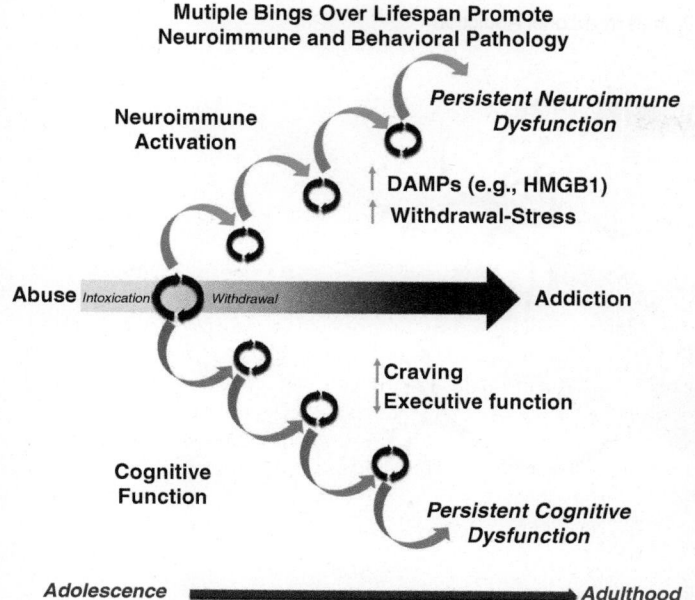

Mutiple Bings Over Lifespan Promote Neuroimmune and Behavioral Pathology

Neuroimmune Activation

Persistent Neuroimmune Dysfunction

↑ DAMPs (e.g., HMGB1)
↑ Withdrawal-Stress

Abuse Intoxication Withdrawal → Addiction

↑Craving
↓Executive function

Cognitive Function

Persistent Cognitive Dysfunction

Adolescence → Adulthood

• **Fig. 20.2** Multidrug exposures amplify neuroimmune signals and cognitive decline.

in adulthood.[61,75] Adolescence is a unique developmental period during which maturation of key structures that regulate cognitive function and decision-making occurs (for review see Crews et al.[54]). Binge drinking during this time has long-lasting effects including persistent neuroimmune activation, leading to prolonged cognitive dysfunction.[43,179] Indeed, neuroimmune markers in alcoholics correlate with lifetime alcohol consumption and age at drinking onset,[45,50,52,179,181] with some remaining elevated long after ethanol administration, during abstinent periods.[45,50,179] It is well known that repeated cycles of binge exposure and withdrawal amplify alcohol-induced pathology.[32,120] This is similar to the innate imune system, as autocrine and paracrine signaling by the release of DAMPS, such as HMGB1, amplify immune responses with each recurring exposure. This amplification might be similar to an LTP-type of phenomenon, and could represent neuroimmune plasticity. This is interesting, especially given the modulation of LTP systems in the brain by many proinflammatory cytokines. The recurrent and persistent NF-κB activation by repeated alcohol or drug intake might mimic a chronic inflammatory state. This is supported by the increased innate immune markers in the postmortem brains of human alcoholics,[45,50] as well as the upregulation of NF-κB target genes.[135] This persistent and chronic immune response has also been seen after one dose of systemic LPS, a TLR4 agonist. One administration of high-dose LPS (5 mg/kg) causes persistent microglial activation with ongoing ROS generation leading to dopaminergic neuron loss over a period of months.[152] Although seemingly on a lower scale, binge-ethanol causes similar pathophysiology.[13,154,201] The recurrent and prolonged amplification of neuroimmune responses causes TLR and NF-κB activation, leading to further increased TLR expression, cytokine production, and DAMP release. This involves the release of HMGB1 as well as miRNA-let-7b -containing microvesicles.[14,45,169] Let-7 isoforms are increased in postmortem human alcoholic brain and in rodent chronic ethanol models.[111,131] Furthermore, ethanol induces ROS generation that also activates NF-κB and leads to further cytokine release and

paracrine signaling.[144,151,172] Each progressive binge may increase the neuroimmune baseline, leading to further damage and pathology. This "smoldering" level of inflammation due to repeated drug binges, as is typical with alcoholism and drug abuse, might underpin the transition from abuse to addiction. Intervention of this feature of disease pathology might belay this transition.

Another important cognitive feature in the progression to addiction is a loss in frontal cortical mediated executive function. These functions include motivation, planning and goal setting, and behavioral flexibility. Frontal cortical dysfunction results in perseveration and repetition of previously learned behaviors due to failure to associate new information (e.g., negative consequences) into decision-making. Binge drinkers report more negative mood and perform worse on executive functioning tasks.[174,192] In alcoholics this is common[48] and manifests in impulsivity and behavioral inflexibility. Reversal learning—the ability to change previously learned behaviors—is an index of behavioral flexibility.[162,165] Both human alcoholics[68,91] and cocaine addicts[165] demonstrate reversal learning deficits. Rodents also show persistent deficits in reversal learning following binge ethanol[9,43,132] or cocaine.[38,163] Frontal cortical function is key in this circuitry that involves loops between the prefrontal cortex, striatum, and amygdala.[84] Frontal cortical regulation of mood and cognition occurs through reciprocal glutamatergic connections with multiple brain regions. A hyperglutamatergic state has also been demonstrated in both cocaine- and stimulant-addicted brains.[157] Astrocytes are key regulators of synaptic glutamate levels. Ethanol exposure induces NF-κB activation in astrocytes, leading to increased expression of proinflammatory genes[140,200,201] and impaired astrocyte glutamate transport.[202] Increased extracellular glutamate levels cause enhanced neuronal excitation, microglial activation, and excitotoxicity.[190,200] TLR4 KOs are protected from this ethanol induced-hyperglutamatergic state and its associated neurotoxicity.[3,100] Innate immune gene induction in the frontal cortex contributes to glutamatergic hyperexcitability and the impairment of executive function.[100,156] Thus, neuroimmune activation by ethanol may be a component of the progressive development of hyperexcitability and cognitive dysfunction seen in alcohol use disorders.

Neuroimmune Basis of Addiction—A Work in Progress

We have presented much of the work that shows that neuroimmune activation is a key feature in the pathology of addiction. However, much work remains to be done. Little research has been done regarding brain regional differences in neuroimmune responses to drugs of abuse. Each brain region has specific populations of neurons that may respond differently to alcohol and other drugs of abuse. Furthermore, the complex interactions between cell types—neurons, microglia, and astrocytes—need to be further elucidated. In Fig. 20.3, we summarize some of the cell-cell interactions between neurons and glia regarding HMGB1, let-7b, and TLRs 4 and 7. However, there remains much to be discovered regarding these interactions. In addition, the interaction between stress, psychiatric disorders, and drugs of abuse on the neuroimmune system is also likely very important in human populations. Stress is a key feature in the cycle of addiction; however, addiction-related stress needs to be better differentiated from other non–addiction-related stressors. A hypothesis is presented in this chapter of stress and drug-induced neuroimmune signaling that inactivates frontal cortex and sensitizes limbic circuitry. This leads to persistent increases in TLRs and DAMPs (e.g., HMGB1) amplified by

Glial-Neuronal Neuroimmune Signals in Alcohol Addiction

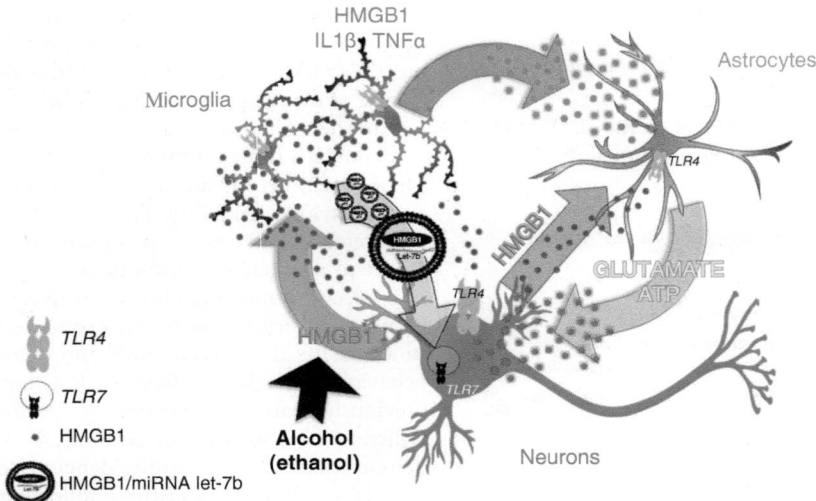

• **Fig. 20.3** Neuron-glia cell-cell interactions in neuroimmune responses to alcohol.

cycles of stress and intoxication. Innate immune signaling impacts cognitive and emotive function, leading to dysfunction.[59,77,134,197] These mechanisms might underlie the progressive and persistent nature of addiction. Currently, neuroimmune mechanisms have been most studied in the context of alcohol abuse and alcoholism. Considerable emerging evidence supports a role for HMGB1/TLR signaling, innate immune gene induction, and alterations in epigenetics and neurotransmission as culminating in the neurobiology of alcoholism.[54,58,180] Innate immune activation and TLR signaling seem to be essential for ethanol induction of pathology. Ethanol and other drugs of abuse promote innate immune gene induction,[52,79,155] which seems to be linked to changes in executive function, reinforcement-reward, and negative affect-craving-anxiety to promote addiction.[180] Although much of this work is convincing regarding the presence of a role of neuroimmune activation involvement in the pathology of addiction, there remain many gaps regarding the precise mechanism and the significance of immune activation. Nonetheless, significant findings exist to warrant the investigation of neuroimmune therapies for efficacy in the treatment or prevention of addiction.

Future Immune Therapies for Addiction

Toward Novel Addiction Treatment Strategies Based on Immune Pharmacology

Given the data presented, several potential neuroimmune therapies are given in Table 20.2. Some of these medications are currently being tested in clinical trials for alcohol use disorders. Due to the challenges to the human condition associated with translating animal models of alcohol and drug abuse, and gaps in knowledge, it is unclear whether these therapies would be of highest benefit for prevention or recovery from addiction. It is known that neuroimmune activation and addiction can cause neurodegeneration.[51,152,158,184,186] Although immune therapies would likely not be of benefit in brain regions where neurodegeneration has already occurred, there may still be a benefit for recovery of normal synaptic function and neuroplasticity. Microglia and cytokines can

alter synaptic signaling.[104] For example, IL-1β reduces eIPSCs in the central amygdala to modulate ethanol effects on GABA receptors.[11] Therefore, significant exploration of immune therapies in various models of alcohol abuse is warranted. Many US Food and Drug Administration (FDA)–approved drugs have also been found to have antiinflammatory actions in the CNS. Table 20.2 lists some candidate drugs that have been found to be beneficial in the context of addiction or other neuroimmune conditions. For example, minocycline is a tetracycline antibiotic and microglial inhibitor[146] that prevents ethanol induced–microglial activation and reduces alcohol self-administration.[1,149] A recent human study found that in a laboratory setting minocyline did not alter subjective responses to ethanol or ethanol-induced craving; however, alcohol self-administration has not yet been reported in humans.[143a] Phosphodiesterase 4 (PDE4) inhibitors reduce inflammation by increasing cAMP concentration, resulting in reduced NF-κB activation.[90] Recently, these agents have been found to reduce ethanol intake in rodents.[19,27,81] A recent phase 2 clinical trial using the PDE4 inhibitor ibudilast showed beneficial effects, including improvements in mood after stress and alcohol-cue exposures, and reduced levels of tonic craving.[155a] A different placebo-controlled trial found that ibudilast reduced some of the rewarding effects of methamphetamine.[195] PPARγ agonists might also be helpful in alcohol use disorders through their antiinflammatory activities. The PPARγ agonist pioglitazone is a microglial inhibitor[166] that reduces neurotoxicity in fetal alcohol spectrum disorder models[63,94] that could potentially play a beneficial role in alcoholism. Each of these drugs, and others with antiinflammatory actions, should be investigated for their potential efficacy in alcohol use disorders.

Acknowledgments

We thank the National Institute on Alcohol Abuse and Alcoholism for its support through the Neurobiology of Adolescent Drinking in Adulthood (NADIA) consortium (AA020024, AA020023), the Bowles Center for Alcohol Studies (AA011605), and the U54 collaborative partnership among NCCU, and UNC (AA019767), and K08-AA024829.

TABLE 20.2	Potential Neuroimmune Therapies for the Treatment of Addiction	
Drug	**Mechanism Primary Immune**	**CNS Activity**
Minocycline	Tetracycline antibiotic Microglial inhibitor	Reduces alcohol self-administration[1] Reduces ethanol microglia activation[149] Prevents reinstatement of morphine and amphetamine seeking[6,7]
Rapamycin	Macrolide antibiotic mTORC1 inhibitor	Reduces binge ethanol intake in male patients[46] Neuroprotection via autophagy promotion[41,145]
Azithromycin	Macrolide antibiotic Microglial inhibitor	Promotes antiinflammatory M2 microglial activation state[198]
Rifampin	Bacterial RNA polymerase inhibitor TLR4 inhibition	Inhibits microglia activation to TLR4[21,187]
Indomethacin	COX-2 inhibitor	Reduces alcohol self-administration[73] Reduces ethanol neurotoxicity[140]
Simvastatin	HMG-CoA Reductase inhibitor NF-κB inhibition	Reduces inflammation and neurotoxicity to ischemia and injury[112,164]
Glycyrrhizin	HMGB1 inhibition	Blocks ethanol-induced cytokine release[203] Reduces neuroinflammation after traumatic brain injury[133]
Pioglitazone, DHA	PPARγ agonists	Reduce toxicity and proinflammatory cytokines in fetal alcohol spectrum disorder model[63,94]
Ibudilast, mesopram, rolipram, CDP 840	Phosphodiesterase 4 inhibition	Reduce ethanol intake in C57BL/6J mice[27] Reduces ethanol self-administration in rats[19]
Naltrexone/naloxone and nalmefene	μ-Opioid antagonists TLR4 inhibition	Reduces alcohol self-administration Binds TLR4 adaptor protein MD2[82,188] Prevent neuroimmune activation by ethanol[125]
Etanercept	TNFα antagonist	Prevents REM sleep disruption in alcoholics[83]

CNS, Central nervous system; *HMGB1*. high-mobility group box; *NF-κB*, nuclear factor kappa B; *REM*, rapid eye movement; *TLR*, Toll-like receptor; *TNF*, tumor necrosis factor.

References

1. Agrawal RG, Hewetson A, George CM, Syapin PJ, Bergeson SE. Minocycline reduces ethanol drinking. *Brain, Behavior Immunity*. 2011;25(suppl 1):S165–S169. https://doi.org/10.1016/j.bbi.2011.03.002.

2. Alfonso-Loeches S, Pascual-Lucas M, Blanco AM, Sanchez-Vera I, Guerri C. Pivotal role of TLR4 receptors in alcohol-induced neuroinflammation and brain damage. *J Neurosci*. 2010;30:8285–8295. https://doi.org/10.1523/JNEUROSCI.0976-10.2010.

3. Alfonso-Loeches S, Pascual-Lucas M, Blanco AM, Sanchez-Vera I, Guerri C. Pivotal role of TLR4 receptors in alcohol-induced neuroinflammation and brain damage. *J Neurosci*. 2010;30:8285–8295. https://doi.org/10.1523/JNEUROSCI.0976-10.2010.

4. Aloe L, et al. Learning abilities, NGF and BDNF brain levels in two lines of TNF-alpha transgenic mice, one characterized by neurological disorders, the other phenotypically normal. *Brain Res*. 1999;840:125–137.

5. Ang E, et al. Induction of nuclear factor-kappaB in nucleus accumbens by chronic cocaine administration. *J Neurochem*. 2001;79:221–224.

6. Arezoomandan R, Haghparast A. Administration of the glial cell modulator, minocycline, in the nucleus accumbens attenuated the maintenance and reinstatement of morphine-seeking behavior. *Can J Physiol Pharmacol*. 2016;94:257–264. https://doi.org/10.1139/cjpp-2015-0209.

7. Attarzadeh-Yazdi G, Arezoomandan R, Haghparast A. Minocycline, an antibiotic with inhibitory effect on microglial activation, attenuates the maintenance and reinstatement of methamphetamine-seeking behavior in rat. *Prog Neuro-Psychopharm Bio Psychiatry*. 2014;53:142–148. https://doi.org/10.1016/j.pnpbp.2014.04.008.

8. Bachtell R, et al. Targeting the toll of drug abuse: the translational potential of toll-like receptor 4. *CNS Neurol Disord Drug Targets*. 2015;14:692–699.

9. Badanich KA, Becker HC, Woodward JJ. Effects of chronic intermittent ethanol exposure on orbitofrontal and medial prefrontal cortex-dependent behaviors in mice. *Behav Neurosci*. 2011;125:879–891. https://doi.org/10.1037/a0025922.

10. Bai L, et al. Toll-like receptor 4-mediated nuclear factor-kappaB activation in spinal cord contributes to chronic morphine-induced analgesic tolerance and hyperalgesia in rats. *Neurosci Bulletin*. 2014;30:936–948. https://doi.org/10.1007/s12264-014-1483-7.

11. Bajo M, et al. IL-1 interacts with ethanol effects on GABAergic transmission in the mouse central amygdala. *Front Pharm*. 2015;6:49. https://doi.org/10.3389/fphar.2015.00049.

12. Bajo M, et al. Role of the IL-1 receptor antagonist in ethanol-induced regulation of GABAergic transmission in the central amygdala. *Brain Behav Immun*. 2015;45:189–197. https://doi.org/10.1016/j.bbi.2014.11.011.

13. Bala S, Marcos M, Gattu A, Catalano D, Szabo G. Acute binge drinking increases serum endotoxin and bacterial DNA levels in healthy individuals. *Plos One*. 2014;9:e96864. https://doi.org/10.1371/journal.pone.0096864.

14. Bala S, et al. Up-regulation of microRNA-155 in macrophages contributes to increased tumor necrosis factor α (TNFα) production via increased mRNA half-life in alcoholic liver disease. *J Biol Chem*. 2011;286:1436–1444. https://doi.org/10.1074/jbc.M110.145870.

15. Ballester J, Valentine G, Sofuoglu M. Pharmacological treatments for methamphetamine addiction: current status and future directions. *Exp Rev Clin Pharm*. 2017;10:305–314. https://doi.org/10.1080/17512433.2017.1268916.

16. Banks WA, Kastin AJ, Broadwell RD. Passage of cytokines across the blood-brain barrier. *Neuroimmunomodulation*. 1995;2:241–248.

17. Banks WA, Kastin AJ, Gutierrez EG. Penetration of interleukin-6 across the murine blood-brain barrier. *Neurosci Lett*. 1994;179:53–56.

18. Beattie EC, et al. Control of synaptic strength by glial TNFalpha. *Science*. 2002;295:2282–2285. https://doi.org/10.1126/science.1067859.

19. Bell RL, et al. Ibudilast reduces alcohol drinking in multiple animal models of alcohol dependence. *Addict Biol*. 2015;20:38–42. https://doi.org/10.1111/adb.12106.

20. Beynon SB, Walker FR. Microglial activation in the injured and healthy brain: what are we really talking about? Practical and theoretical issues associated with the measurement of changes in microglial morphology. *Neuroscience*. 2012;225:162–171. https://doi.org/10.1016/j.neuroscience.2012.07.029.

20a. Bhattacharya A, Derecki NC, Lovenberg TW, Drevets WC. Role of neuro-immunological factors in the pathophysiology of mood disorders. *Psychopharmacology (Berl)*. 2016;233(9):1623–1636.

20b. Bhattacharya A, Drevets WC. Role of neuro-immunological factors in the pathophysiology of mood disorders: implications for novel therapeutics for treatment resistant depression. *Curr Top Behav Neurosci*. 2017;31:339–356.

21. Bi W, et al. Rifampicin inhibits microglial inflammation and improves neuron survival against inflammation. *Brain Res*. 2011;1395:12–20. https://doi.org/10.1016/j.brainres.2011.04.019.

22. Bian C, Zhao ZQ, Zhang YQ, Lu N. Involvement of CX3CL1/CX3CR1 signaling in spinal long term potentiation. *Plos One*. 2015;10:e0118842. https://doi.org/10.1371/journal.pone.0118842.

23. Bierhaus A, et al. A mechanism converting psychosocial stress into mononuclear cell activation. *Pro Nat Acad Sci U S A*. 2003;100:1920–1925. https://doi.org/10.1073/pnas.0438019100.

24. Blanc L, et al. Gram-positive bacterial lipoglycans based on a glycosylated diacylglycerol lipid anchor are microbe-associated molecular patterns recognized by TLR2. *Plos One*. 2013;8:e81593. https://doi.org/10.1371/journal.pone.0081593.

25. Blanco AM, Valles SL, Pascual M, Guerri C. Involvement of TLR4/type I IL-1 receptor signaling in the induction of inflammatory mediators and cell death induced by ethanol in cultured astrocytes. *J Immunol*. 2005;175:6893–6899.

26. Reference deleted in review.

27. Blednov YA, Benavidez JM, Black M, Harris RA. Inhibition of phosphodiesterase 4 reduces ethanol intake and preference in C57BL/6J mice. *Front Neurosci*. 2014;8:129. https://doi.org/10.3389/fnins.2014.00129.

28. Blednov YA, et al. Perturbation of chemokine networks by gene deletion alters the reinforcing actions of ethanol. *Behav Brain Res*. 2005;165:110–125. https://doi.org/10.1016/j.bbr.2005.06.026.

29. Blednov YA, et al. Activation of inflammatory signaling by lipopolysaccharide produces a prolonged increase of voluntary alcohol intake in mice. *Brain Behav Immun*. 2011;25(suppl 1):S92–S105. https://doi.org/10.1016/j.bbi.2011.01.008.

30. Blednov YA, et al. Neuroimmune regulation of alcohol consumption: behavioral validation of genes obtained from genomic studies. *Addict Biol*. 2012;17:108–120. https://doi.org/10.1111/j.1369-1600.2010.00284.x.

31. Borner C, Hollt V, Kraus J. Mechanisms of the inhibition of nuclear factor-kappaB by morphine in neuronal cells. *Mol Pharmacol*. 2012;81:587–597. https://doi.org/10.1124/mol.111.076620.

32. Breese GR, Overstreet DH, Knapp DJ. Conceptual framework for the etiology of alcoholism: a "kindling"/stress hypothesis. *Psychopharmacology*. 2005;178:367–380. https://doi.org/10.1007/s00213-004-2016-2.

33. Breese GR, et al. Repeated lipopolysaccharide (LPS) or cytokine treatments sensitize ethanol withdrawal-induced anxiety-like behavior. *Neuropsychopharmacology*. 2008;33:867–876. https://doi.org/10.1038/sj.npp.1301468.

34. Brombacher TM, et al. IL-13-mediated regulation of learning and memory. *J Immunol*. 2017;198:2681–2688. https://doi.org/10.4049/jimmunol.1601546.

35. Brubaker SW, Bonham KS, Zanoni I, Kagan JC. Innate immune pattern recognition: a cell biological perspective. *Ann Rev Immunol*. 2015;33:257–290. https://doi.org/10.1146/annurev-immunol-032414-112240.

36. Bsibsi M, et al. The microtubule regulator stathmin is an endogenous protein agonist for TLR3. *J Immunol*. 2010;184:6929–6937. https://doi.org/10.4049/jimmunol.0902419.

37. Buwitt-Beckmann U, et al. TLR1- and TLR6-independent recognition of bacterial lipopeptides. *J Bio Chem*. 2006;281:9049–9057. https://doi.org/10.1074/jbc.M512525200.

38. Calu DJ, Roesch MR, Stalnaker TA, Schoenbaum G. Associative encoding in posterior piriform cortex during odor discrimination and reversal learning. *Cerebral Cortex*. 2007;17:1342–1349. https://doi.org/10.1093/cercor/bhl045.

39. Cameron JS, et al. Toll-like receptor 3 is a potent negative regulator of axonal growth in mammals. *J neurosci*. 2007;27:13033–13041. https://doi.org/10.1523/JNEUROSCI.4290-06.2007.

40. Caraci F, et al. A key role for TGF-beta1 in hippocampal synaptic plasticity and memory. *Sci Rep*. 2015;5:11252. https://doi.org/10.1038/srep11252.

41. Chen G, et al. Autophagy is a protective response to ethanol neurotoxicity. *Autophagy*. 2012;8:1577–1589. https://doi.org/10.4161/auto.21376.

42. Chen Y, et al. Translocation of endogenous danger signal HMGB1 from nucleus to membrane microvesicles in macrophages. *J Cel Physiol*. 2016;231:2319–2326. https://doi.org/10.1002/jcp.25352.

43. Coleman Jr LG, He J, Lee J, Styner M, Crews FT. Adolescent binge drinking alters adult brain neurotransmitter gene expression, behavior, brain regional volumes, and neurochemistry in mice. *Alcohol Clin Exp Res*. 2011;35:671–688. https://doi.org/10.1111/j.1530-0277.2010.01385.x.

44. Reference deleted in review.

45. Coleman Jr LG, Zou J, Crews FT. Microglial-derived miRNA let-7 and HMGB1 contribute to ethanol-induced neurotoxicity via TLR7. *J Neuroinflam*. 2017;14:22. https://doi.org/10.1186/s12974-017-0799-4.

46. Cozzoli DK, et al. Functional regulation of PI3K-associated signaling in the accumbens by binge alcohol drinking in male but not female mice. *Neuropharmacology*. 2016;105:164–174. https://doi.org/10.1016/j.neuropharm.2016.01.010.

47. Crews F, et al. BHT blocks NF-kappaB activation and ethanol-induced brain damage. *Alcohol Clin Exp Res*. 2006;30:1938–1949. https://doi.org/10.1111/j.1530-0277.2006.00239.x.

48. Crews FT, Boettiger CA. Impulsivity, frontal lobes and risk for addiction. *Pharmacol Biochem Behavior*. 2009;93:237–247. https://doi.org/10.1016/j.pbb.2009.04.018.

49. Crews FT, Lawrimore CJ, Walter TJ, Coleman LG. The role of neuroimmune signaling in alcoholism. *Neuropharm*. 2017. https://doi.org/10.1016/j.neuropharm.2017.01.031.

50. Crews FT, Qin L, Sheedy D, Vetreno RP, Zou J. High mobility group box 1/Toll-like receptor danger signaling increases brain neuroimmune activation in alcohol dependence. *Biol Psychiatry*. 2013;73:602–612. https://doi.org/10.1016/j.biopsych.2012.09.030.

51. Reference deleted in review.

52. Crews FT, Vetreno RP. Neuroimmune basis of alcoholic brain damage. *Internat Rev Neurobiol*. 2014;118:315–357. https://doi.org/10.1016/B978-0-12-801284-0.00010-5.

53. Reference deleted in review.

54. Crews FT, Vetreno RP, Broadwater MA, Robinson DL. Adolescent alcohol exposure persistently impacts adult neurobiology and behavior. *Pharmacol Rev.* 2016;68:1074–1109. https://doi.org/10.1124/pr.115.012138.

55. Crews FT, Zou J, Qin L. Induction of innate immune genes in brain create the neurobiology of addiction. *Brain Behav Immun.* 2011;25(suppl 1):S4–S12. https://doi.org/10.1016/j.bbi.2011.03.003.

56. Crews FT, et al. Neuroimmune function and the consequences of alcohol exposure. *Alcohol Res.* 2015;37:331–341. 344–351.

57. Cui C, Shurtleff D, Harris RA. Neuroimmune mechanisms of alcohol and drug addiction. *Internat Rev Neurobiol.* 2014;118:1–12. https://doi.org/10.1016/B978-0-12-801284-0.00001-4.

58. Cui C, et al. Brain pathways to recovery from alcohol dependence. *Alcohol.* 2015;49:435–452. https://doi.org/10.1016/j.alcohol.2015.04.006.

59. Dantzer R, O'Connor JC, Freund GG, Johnson RW, Kelley KW. From inflammation to sickness and depression: when the immune system subjugates the brain. *Nat Rev Neurosci.* 2008;9:46–56. https://doi.org/10.1038/nrn2297.

60. Davis RL, Syapin PJ. Ethanol increases nuclear factor-kappa B activity in human astroglial cells. *Neurosci Letters.* 2004;371:128–132. https://doi.org/10.1016/j.neulet.2004.08.051.

61. Dawson DA, Goldstein RB, Chou SP, Ruan WJ, Grant BF. Age at first drink and the first incidence of adult-onset DSM-IV alcohol use disorders. *Alcohol Clin Exp Res.* 2008;32:2149–2160. https://doi.org/10.1111/j.1530-0277.2008.00806.x.

62. Derecki NC, et al. Regulation of learning and memory by meningeal immunity: a key role for IL-4. *J Exp Med.* 2010;207:1067–1080. https://doi.org/10.1084/jem.20091419.

63. Drew PD, Johnson JW, Douglas JC, Phelan KD, Kane CJ. Pioglitazone blocks ethanol induction of microglial activation and immune responses in the hippocampus, cerebellum, and cerebral cortex in a mouse model of fetal alcohol spectrum disorders. *Alcohol Clin Exp Res.* 2015;39:445–454. https://doi.org/10.1111/acer.12639.

64. Farina C, Aloisi F, Meinl E. Astrocytes are active players in cerebral innate immunity. *Trends Immunol.* 2007;28:138–145. https://doi.org/10.1016/j.it.2007.01.005.

65. Fernandez-Lizarbe S, Montesinos J, Guerri C. Ethanol induces TLR4/TLR2 association, triggering an inflammatory response in microglial cells. *J Neurochem.* 2013;126:261–273. https://doi.org/10.1111/jnc.12276.

66. Fernandez-Lizarbe S, Pascual M, Guerri C. Critical role of TLR4 response in the activation of microglia induced by ethanol. *J Immunol.* 2009;183:4733. https://doi.org/10.4049/jimmunol.0803590.4744.

67. Reference deleted in review.

68. Fortier CB, et al. Delay discrimination and reversal eyeblink classical conditioning in abstinent chronic alcoholics. *Neuropsychol.* 2008;22:196–208. https://doi.org/10.1037/0894-4105.22.2.196.

69. Frank MG, Baratta MV, Sprunger DB, Watkins LR, Maier SF. Microglia serve as a neuroimmune substrate for stress-induced potentiation of CNS pro-inflammatory cytokine responses. *Brain Behav Immun.* 2007;21:47–59.

70. Frank MG, et al. The danger-associated molecular pattern HMGB1 mediates the neuroinflammatory effects of methamphetamine. *Brain Behav Immun.* 2016;51:99–108. https://doi.org/10.1016/j.bbi.2015.08.001.

71. Franke H. Influence of chronic alcohol treatment on the GFAP-immunoreactivity in astrocytes of the hippocampus in rats. *Acta Histochem.* 1995;97:263–271. https://doi.org/10.1016/S0065-1281(11)80187-X.

72. Freeman K, et al. Temporal changes in innate immune signals in a rat model of alcohol withdrawal in emotional and cardiorespiratory homeostatic nuclei. *J Neuroinflammation.* 2012;9:97. https://doi.org/10.1186/1742-2094-9-97.

73. George FR. The role of arachidonic acid metabolites in mediating ethanol self-administration and intoxication. *Ann N Y acad sci.* 1989;559:382–391.

74. Goshen I, et al. A dual role for interleukin-1 in hippocampal-dependent memory processes. *Psychoneuroendocrinology.* 2007;32:1106–1115. https://doi.org/10.1016/j.psyneuen.2007.09.004.

75. Grant BF, Dawson DA. Age of onset of drug use and its association with DSM-IV drug abuse and dependence: results from the National Longitudinal Alcohol Epidemiologic Survey. *J Substance Abuse.* 1998;10:163–173.

76. Guo ML, et al. Cocaine-mediated microglial activation involves the ER stress-autophagy axis. *Autophagy.* 2015;11:995–1009. https://doi.org/10.1080/15548627.2015.1052205.

77. Hanke ML, Kielian T. Toll-like receptors in health and disease in the brain: mechanisms and therapeutic potential. *Clin Sci.* 2011;121:367–387. https://doi.org/10.1042/CS20110164.

78. Reference deleted in review.

79. He J, Crews FT. Increased MCP-1 and microglia in various regions of the human alcoholic brain. *Exp Neurol.* 2008;210:349–358. https://doi.org/10.1016/j.expneurol.2007.11.017.

80. Heberlein A, et al. TNF-alpha and IL-6 serum levels: neurobiological markers of alcohol consumption in alcohol-dependent patients? *Alcohol.* 2014;48:671–676. https://doi.org/10.1016/j.alcohol.2014.08.003.

81. Hu W, et al. Inhibition of phosphodiesterase-4 decreases ethanol intake in mice. *Psychopharmacology.* 2011;218:331–339. https://doi.org/10.1007/s00213-011-2290-8.

82. Hutchinson MR, et al. Evidence that opioids may have toll-like receptor 4 and MD-2 effects. *Brain Behav Immun.* 2010;24:83–95. https://doi.org/10.1016/j.bbi.2009.08.004.

83. Irwin MR, Olmstead R, Valladares EM, Breen EC, Ehlers CL. Tumor necrosis factor antagonism normalizes rapid eye movement sleep in alcohol dependence. *Bio Psychiatry.* 2009;66:191–195. https://doi.org/10.1016/j.biopsych.2008.12.004.

84. Izquierdo A, Brigman JL, Radke AK, Rudebeck PH, Holmes A. The neural basis of reversal learning: an updated perspective. *Neuroscience.* 2016. https://doi.org/10.1016/j.neuroscience.2016.03.021. [Epub ahead of print] https://doi.org/10.1016/j.neuroscience.2016.03.021.

85. Jackson AC, Rossiter JP, Lafon M. Expression of Toll-like receptor 3 in the human cerebellar cortex in rabies, herpes simplex encephalitis, and other neurological diseases. *J Neurovirol.* 2006;12:229–234. https://doi.org/10.1080/13550280600848399.

86. Jacobsen JH, Hutchinson MR, Mustafa S. Drug addiction: targeting dynamic neuroimmune receptor interactions as a potential therapeutic strategy. *Curr Opin Pharmacol.* 2016;26:131–137. https://doi.org/10.1016/j.coph.2015.10.010.

87. Jang E, et al. Phenotypic polarization of activated astrocytes: the critical role of lipocalin-2 in the classical inflammatory activation of astrocytes. *J Immunol.* 2013;191:5204–5219. https://doi.org/10.4049/jimmunol.1301637.

88. Janko C, et al. Redox modulation of HMGB1-related signaling. *Antioxid Redox Signal.* 2014;20:1075–1085. https://doi.org/10.1089/ars.2013.5179.

89. Jensen CJ, Massie A, De Keyser J. Immune players in the CNS: the astrocyte. *J Neuroimmune Pharmacol.* 2013;8:824–839. https://doi.org/10.1007/s11481-013-9480-6.

90. Jimenez JL, Punzon C, Navarro J, Munoz-Fernandez MA, Fresno M. Phosphodiesterase 4 inhibitors prevent cytokine secretion by T lymphocytes by inhibiting nuclear factor-kappaB and nuclear factor of activated T cells activation. *J Pharmacol Exp Therap.* 2001;299:753–759.

91. Jokisch D, Roser P, Juckel G, Daum I, Bellebaum C. Impairments in learning by monetary rewards and alcohol-associated rewards in detoxified alcoholic patients. *Alcohol Clin Exp Res.* 2014;38:1947–1954. https://doi.org/10.1111/acer.12460.

92. June HL, et al. CRF-amplified neuronal TLR4/MCP-1 signaling regulates alcohol self-administration. *Neuropsychopharmacology.* 2015;40:1549–1559. https://doi.org/10.1038/npp.2015.4.

93. Kaltschmidt B, Kaltschmidt C. NF-kappab in long-term memory and structural plasticity in the adult mammalian brain. *Front Mol Neurosci.* 2015;8:69. https://doi.org/10.3389/fnmol.2015.00069.

94. Kane CJ, et al. Protection of neurons and microglia against ethanol in a mouse model of fetal alcohol spectrum disorders by peroxisome proliferator-activated receptor-gamma agonists. *Brain Behav Immun.* 2011;25(suppl 1):S137–S145. https://doi.org/10.1016/j.bbi.2011.02.016.

95. Kaul D, et al. Expression of Toll-like receptors in the developing brain. *Plos One.* 2012;7:e37767. https://doi.org/10.1371/journal.pone.0037767.

96. Kettenmann H, Hanisch UK, Noda M, Verkhratsky A. Physiology of microglia. *Physiol Rev.* 2011;91:461–553. https://doi.org/10.1152/physrev.00011.2010.

97. Kettenmann H, Kirchhoff F, Verkhratsky A. Microglia: new roles for the synaptic stripper. *Neuron.* 2013;77:10–18. https://doi.org/10.1016/j.neuron.2012.12.023.

97a. Khairova RA, Machado-Vieira R, Du J, Manji HK. *Int J Neuropsychopharmacol.* 2009;12(4):561–578.

98. Khakh BS, Sofroniew MV. Diversity of astrocyte functions and phenotypes in neural circuits. *Nat Neurosci.* 2015;18:942–952. https://doi.org/10.1038/nn.4043.

99. Kim C, et al. Neuron-released oligomeric alpha-synuclein is an endogenous agonist of TLR2 for paracrine activation of microglia. *Nature Commun.* 2013;4:1562. https://doi.org/10.1038/ncomms2534.

100. Knapp DJ, Crews FT. Induction of cyclooxygenase-2 in brain during acute and chronic ethanol treatment and ethanol withdrawal. *Alcohol Clin Exp Res.* 1999;23:633–643.

101. Koob GF, Le Moal M. Plasticity of reward neurocircuitry and the 'dark side' of drug addiction. *Nat neurosci.* 2005;8:1442–1444. https://doi.org/10.1038/nn1105-1442.

102. Koob GF, Volkow ND. Neurocircuitry of addiction. *Neuropsychopharmacology.* 2010;35:217–238. https://doi.org/10.1038/npp.2009.110.

103. Kreisel T, et al. Dynamic microglial alterations underlie stress-induced depressive-like behavior and suppressed neurogenesis. *Molecular Psychiatry.* 2014;19:699–709. https://doi.org/10.1038/mp.2013.155.

104. Lacagnina MJ, Rivera PD, Bilbo SD. Glial and neuroimmune mechanisms as critical modulators of drug use and abuse. *Neuropsychopharmacol.* 2017;42:156–177. https://doi.org/10.1038/npp.2016.121.

105. Lawrimore C, Crews F. Neuron-like cell line SH-SY5Y displays different ethanol-induced immune signal molecule response and NFkB activation compared to microglia-like BV2. *Res Society Alcohol Ann Meeting Poster Abstract.* 2016.

106. Lawrimore C, Crews F. Ethanol, TLR3, and TLR4 agonists have unique innate immune responses in neuron-like SH-SY5Y and microglia-like BV2. *Alcohol Clin Exp Res.* 2017;41:939–954.

107. Johnston LD, Miech RA, O'Malley PM, et al. *Monitoring the Future: National Results on Adolescent Drug Use 2018.* Ann Arbor, MI: University of Michigan Institute for Social Research, June 2018. http://www.monitoringthefuture.org//pubs/monographs/mtf-overview2018.pdf.

108. Leclercq S, De Saeger C, Delzenne N, de Timary P, Starkel P. Role of inflammatory pathways, blood mononuclear cells, and gut-derived bacterial products in alcohol dependence. *Biol Psychiatry.* 2014;76:725–733. https://doi.org/10.1016/j.biopsych.2014.02.003.

109. Lehmann SM, et al. Extracellularly delivered single-stranded viral RNA causes neurodegeneration dependent on TLR7. *J Immunol.* 2012;189:1448–1458. https://doi.org/10.4049/jimmunol.1201078.

110. Lehmann SM, et al. An unconventional role for miRNA: let-7 activates Toll-like receptor 7 and causes neurodegeneration. *Nat Neurosci.* 2012;15:827–835. https://doi.org/10.1038/nn.3113.

111. Lewohl JM, et al. Up-regulation of microRNAs in brain of human alcoholics. *Alcohol Clin Exp Res.* 2011;35:1928–1937. https://doi.org/10.1111/j.1530-0277.2011.01544.x.

111a. Liddelow SA, Guttenplan KA, Clarke LE, et al. Neurotoxic reactive astrocytes are induced by activated microglia. *Nature.* 2017;541(7638):481–487.

112. Lim SW, et al. Simvastatin therapy in the acute stage of traumatic brain injury attenuates brain trauma-induced depression-like behavior in rats by reducing neuroinflammation in the hippocampus. *Neurocrit Care.* 2017;26(1):122–132. https://doi.org/10.1007/s12028-016-0290-6.

113. Lippai D, et al. Alcohol-induced IL-1beta in the brain is mediated by NLRP3/ASC inflammasome activation that amplifies neuroinflammation. *J Leukocyte Biol.* 2013;94:171–182. https://doi.org/10.1189/jlb.1212659.

114. Liu J, et al. Binge alcohol drinking is associated with GABAA alpha2-regulated Toll-like receptor 4 (TLR4) expression in the central amygdala. *Proc Natl Acad Sci U S A.* 2011;108:4465–4470. https://doi.org/10.1073/pnas.1019020108.

115. Loftis JM, Janowsky A. Neuroimmune basis of methamphetamine toxicity. *Internat Rev Neurobiol.* 2014;118:165–197. https://doi.org/10.1016/B978-0-12-801284-0.00007-5.

116. Ma Y, et al. Toll-like receptor 8 functions as a negative regulator of neurite outgrowth and inducer of neuronal apoptosis. *J Cell Bio.* 2006;175:209–215. https://doi.org/10.1083/jcb.200606016.

117. Madrigal JL, Moro MA, Lizasoain I, Lorenzo P, Leza JC. Stress-induced increase in extracellular sucrose space in rats is mediated by nitric oxide. *Brain Res.* 2002;938:87–91.

118. Mao XR, Moerman-Herzog AM, Chen Y, Barger SW. Unique aspects of transcriptional regulation in neurons--nuances in NFkappaB and Sp1-related factors. *J Neuroinflammation.* 2009;6:16. https://doi.org/10.1186/1742-2094-6-16.

119. Marciniak E, et al. The Chemokine MIP-1alpha/CCL3 impairs mouse hippocampal synaptic transmission, plasticity and memory. *Sci Rep.* 2015;5:15862. https://doi.org/10.1038/srep15862.

119a. Maroso M, Balosso S, Ravizza T, et al. Interleukin-1 type 1 receptor/Toll-like receptor signalling in epilepsy: the importance of IL-1beta and high-mobility group box 1. *J Intern Med.* 2011;270(4):319–326.

120. Marshall SA, Geil CR, Nixon K. Prior binge ethanol exposure potentiates the microglial response in a model of alcohol-induced neurodegeneration. *Brain Sci.* 2016;6:16. https://doi.org/10.3390/brainsci6020016.

121. Marshall SA, McKnight KH, Blose AK, Lysle DT, Thiele TE. Modulation of binge-like ethanol consumption by IL-10 signaling in the basolateral amygdala. *J Neuroimmune Pharmacol.* 2017;12:249–259. https://doi.org/10.1007/s11481-016-9709-2.

122. Marshall SA, et al. IL-1 receptor signaling in the basolateral amygdala modulates binge-like ethanol consumption in male C57BL/6J mice. *Brain Behav Immun.* 2016;51:258–267. https://doi.org/10.1016/j.bbi.2015.09.006.

123. Mayfield J, Ferguson L, Harris RA. Neuroimmune signaling: a key component of alcohol abuse. *Curr Opin Neurobiol.* 2013;23:513–520. https://doi.org/10.1016/j.conb.2013.01.024.

124. Montesinos J, Alfonso-Loeches S, Guerri C. Impact of the innate immune response in the actions of ethanol on the central nervous system. *Alcohol Clin Exp Res.* 2016;40:2260–2270. https://doi.org/10.1111/acer.13208.

125. Montesinos J, Gil A, Guerri C. Nalmefene prevents alcohol-induced neuroinflammation and alcohol drinking preference in adolescent female mice: role of TLR4. *Alcohol Clin Exp Res.* 2017;41:1257–1270. https://doi.org/10.1111/acer.13416.

126. Most D, Ferguson L, Harris RA. Molecular basis of alcoholism. *Handbook Clin Neurol.* 2014;125:89–111. https://doi.org/10.1016/B978-0-444-62619-6.00006-9.

127. Muller S, Ronfani L, Bianchi ME. Regulated expression and subcellular localization of HMGB1, a chromatin protein with a cytokine function. *J Internal Med.* 2004;255:332–343.

128. Mulligan MK, et al. Toward understanding the genetics of alcohol drinking through transcriptome meta-analysis. *Pro Nat Acad Sci U S A.* 2006;103:6368–6373. https://doi.org/10.1073/pnas.0510188103.

129. Neupane SP. Neuroimmune interface in the comorbidity between alcohol use disorder and major depression. *Front Immunol.* 2016;7:655. https://doi.org/10.3389/fimmu.2016.00655.

130. Northcutt AL, et al. DAT isn't all that: cocaine reward and reinforcement require Toll-like receptor 4 signaling. *Mol Psychiatry.* 2015;20:1525–1537. https://doi.org/10.1038/mp.2014.177.

131. Nunez YO, et al. Positively correlated miRNA-mRNA regulatory networks in mouse frontal cortex during early stages of alcohol dependence. *Bmc Genomics.* 2013;14:725. https://doi.org/10.1186/1471-2164-14-725.

132. Obernier JA, White AM, Swartzwelder HS, Crews FT. Cognitive deficits and CNS damage after a 4-day binge ethanol exposure in rats. *Pharmacol Biochem Behav.* 2002;72:521–532.

133. Okuma Y, et al. Glycyrrhizin inhibits traumatic brain injury by reducing HMGB1-RAGE interaction. *Neuropharmacology.* 2014;85:18–26. https://doi.org/10.1016/j.neuropharm.2014.05.007.

134. Okun E, et al. Toll-like receptor 3 inhibits memory retention and constrains adult hippocampal neurogenesis. *Proc Natl Acad Sci U S A.* 2010;107:15625–15630. https://doi.org/10.1073/pnas.1005807107.

135. Okvist A, et al. Neuroadaptations in human chronic alcoholics: dysregulation of the NF-kappaB system. *Plos One.* 2007;2:e930. https://doi.org/10.1371/journal.pone.0000930.

136. Park CK, et al. Extracellular microRNAs activate nociceptor neurons to elicit pain via TLR7 and TRPA1. *Neuron.* 2014;82:47–54. https://doi.org/10.1016/j.neuron.2014.02.011.

137. Pascual M, Balino P, Alfonso-Loeches S, Aragon CM, Guerri C. Impact of TLR4 on behavioral and cognitive dysfunctions associated with alcohol-induced neuroinflammatory damage. *Brain Behav Immun.* 2011;25(suppl 1):S80–91. https://doi.org/10.1016/j.bbi.2011.02.012.

138. Reference deleted in review.

139. Reference deleted in review.

140. Pascual M, Blanco AM, Cauli O, Minarro J, Guerri C. Intermittent ethanol exposure induces inflammatory brain damage and causes long-term behavioural alterations in adolescent rats. *Eur J Neurosci.* 2007;25:541–550. https://doi.org/10.1111/j.1460-9568.2006.05298.x.

141. Pekny M, Pekna M. Astrocyte reactivity and reactive astrogliosis: costs and benefits. *Physiol Rev.* 2014;94:1077–1098. https://doi.org/10.1152/physrev.00041.2013.

142. Periyasamy P, Guo ML, BuchS. Cocaine induces astrocytosis through ER stress-mediated activation of autophagy. *Autophagy.* 2016;12:1310–1329. https://doi.org/10.1080/15548627.2016.1183844.

143. Periyasamy P, et al. Cocaine-mediated downregulation of miR-124 activates microglia by targeting KLF4 and TLR4 signaling. *Mol Neurobiol.* 2018;55:3196–3210. https://doi.org/10.1007/s12035-017-0584-5.

143a. Petrakis IL, Ralevski E, Gueorguieva R, et al. Targeting neuroinflammation with minocycline in heavy drinkers. *Psychopharmacology (Berl).* 2019 Mar 27. https://doi.org/10.1007/s00213-019-05205-3. [Epub ahead of print]

144. Pietri M, et al. Reactive oxygen species-dependent TNF-alpha converting enzyme activation through stimulation of 5-HT2B and alpha1D autoreceptors in neuronal cells. *Faseb J.* 2005;19:1078–1087. https://doi.org/10.1096/fj.04-3631com.

145. Pla A, Pascual M, Guerri C. Autophagy constitutes a protective mechanism against ethanol toxicity in mouse astrocytes and neurons. *Plos One.* 2016;11:e0153097. https://doi.org/10.1371/journal.pone.0153097.

146. Plane JM, Shen Y, Pleasure DE, Deng W. Prospects for minocycline neuroprotection. *Arch Neurol.* 2010;67:1442–1448. https://doi.org/10.1001/archneurol.2010.191.

147. Prieto GA, Cotman CW. Cytokines and cytokine networks target neurons to modulate long-term potentiation. *Cytokine Growth Factor Rev.* 2017;34:27–33. https://doi.org/10.1016/j.cytogfr.2017.03.005.

148. Prieto GA, et al. Synapse-specific IL-1 receptor subunit reconfiguration augments vulnerability to IL-1beta in the aged hippocampus. *Proc Nat Acad Sci U S A.* 2015;112:E5078–E5087. https://doi.org/10.1073/pnas.1514486112.

149. Qin L, Crews FT. Chronic ethanol increases systemic TLR3 agonist-induced neuroinflammation and neurodegeneration. *J Neuroinflam.* 2012;9:130. https://doi.org/10.1186/1742-2094-9-130.

150. Reference deleted in review.

151. Qin L, Crews FT. NADPH oxidase and reactive oxygen species contribute to alcohol-induced microglial activation and neurodegeneration. *J Neuroinflam.* 2012;9:5. https://doi.org/10.1186/1742-2094-9-5.

152. Qin L, et al. Increased systemic and brain cytokine production and neuroinflammation by endotoxin following ethanol treatment. *J Neuroinflam.* 2008;5:10. https://doi.org/10.1186/1742-2094-5-10.

153. Reference deleted in review.

154. Qin L, et al. Systemic LPS causes chronic neuroinflammation and progressive neurodegeneration. *Glia.* 2007;55:453–462.

155. Qin L, Liu Y, Hong JS, Crews FT. NADPH oxidase and aging drive microglial activation, oxidative stress, and dopaminergic neurodegeneration following systemic LPS administration. *Glia.* 2013;61:855–868. https://doi.org/10.1002/glia.22479.

155a. Ray LA, Bujarski S, Shoptaw S, et al. Development of the neuroimmune modulator ibudilast for the treatment of alcoholism: a randomized, placebo-controlled, human laboratory trial. *Neuropsychopharmacology.* 2017;42(9):1776–1788.

156. Ray LA, Roche DJ, Heinzerling K, Shoptaw S. Opportunities for the development of neuroimmune therapies in addiction. *Internat Rev Neurobiol.* 2014;118:381–401. https://doi.org/10.1016/B978-0-12-801284-0.00012-9.

157. Reissner KJ, Kalivas PW. Using glutamate homeostasis as a target for treating addictive disorders. *Behav Pharmacol.* 2010;21:514–522. https://doi.org/10.1097/FBP.0b013e32833d41b2.

158. Rocha NP, de Miranda AS, Teixeira AL. Insights into neuroinflammation in parkinson's disease: from biomarkers to anti-inflammatory based therapies. *Biomed Res Internat.* 2015:628192. https://doi.org/10.1155/2015/628192. 2015.

159. Rostene W, Kitabgi P, Parsadaniantz SM. Chemokines: a new class of neuromodulator? *Nat rev Neurosci.* 2007;8:895–903. https://doi.org/10.1038/nrn2255.

160. Rubio-Araiz A, et al. Disruption of blood-brain barrier integrity in postmortem alcoholic brain: preclinical evidence of TLR4 involvement from a binge-like drinking model. *Addict Biol.* 2017;22:1103–1116. https://doi.org/10.1111/adb.12376.

161. Russo SJ, et al. Nuclear factor kappa B signaling regulates neuronal morphology and cocaine reward. *J Neurosci.* 2009;29:3529–3537. https://doi.org/10.1523/JNEUROSCI.6173-08.2009.

162. Schoenbaum G, Roesch MR, Stalnaker TA. Orbitofrontal cortex, decision-making and drug addiction. *Trend Neurosci.* 2006;2:116–124. https://doi.org/10.1016/j.tins.2005.12.006.

163. Schoenbaum G, Saddoris MP, Ramus SJ, Shaham Y, Setlow B. Cocaine-experienced rats exhibit learning deficits in a task sensitive to orbitofrontal cortex lesions. *Eur J Neurosci.* 2004;19:1997–2002. https://doi.org/10.1111/j.1460-9568.2004.03274.x.

164. Sironi L, et al. Activation of NF-kB and ERK1/2 after permanent focal ischemia is abolished by simvastatin treatment. *Neurobiol Dis.* 2006;22:445–451. https://doi.org/10.1016/j.nbd.2005.12.004.

165. Stalnaker TA, Takahashi Y, Roesch MR, Schoenbaum G. Neural substrates of cognitive inflexibility after chronic cocaine exposure. *Neuropharmacology.* 2009;56(suppl 1):63–72. https://doi.org/10.1016/j.neuropharm.2008.07.019.

166. Storer PD, Xu J, Chavis J, Drew PD. Peroxisome proliferator-activated receptor-gamma agonists inhibit the activation of microglia and astrocytes: implications for multiple sclerosis. *J Neuroimmunol.* 2005;161:113–122. https://doi.org/10.1016/j.jneuroim.2004.12.015.

167. Streit WJ. Microglia as neuroprotective, immunocompetent cells of the CNS. *Glia.* 2002;40:133–139. https://doi.org/10.1002/glia.10154.

168. Sugimura T, Yoshimura Y, Komatsu Y. TNFalpha is required for the production of T-type Ca(2+) channel-dependent long-term potentiation in visual cortex. *Neurosci Res.* 2015;96:37–44. https://doi.org/10.1016/j.neures.2015.02.005.

169. Szabo G, Lippai D. Converging actions of alcohol on liver and brain immune signaling. *Internat Rev Neurobio.* 2014;118:359–380. https://doi.org/10.1016/B978-0-12-801284-0.00011-7.

170. Takeuchi O, Akira S. Pattern recognition receptors and inflammation. *Cell.* 2010;140:805–820. https://doi.org/10.1016/j.cell.2010.01.022.

171. Tancredi V, et al. Tumor necrosis factor alters synaptic transmission in rat hippocampal slices. *Neurosci Lett.* 1992;146:176–178.

172. Thakur V, McMullen MR, Pritchard MT, Nagy LE. Regulation of macrophage activation in alcoholic liver disease. *J Gastroenterol Hepatol.* 2007;22(suppl 1):S53–56. https://doi.org/10.1111/j.1440-1746.2006.04650.x.

173. Theberge FR, et al. Effect of chronic delivery of the Toll-like receptor 4 antagonist (+)-naltrexone on incubation of heroin craving. *Biological Psychiatry.* 2013;73:729–737. https://doi.org/10.1016/j.biopsych.2012.12.019.

174. Townshend JM, Duka T. Mixed emotions: alcoholics' impairments in the recognition of specific emotional facial expressions. *Neuropsychologia.* 2003;41:773–782.

175. Tynan RJ, et al. Chronic stress alters the density and morphology of microglia in a subset of stress-responsive brain regions. *Brain Behav Immun.* 2010;24:1058–1068. https://doi.org/10.1016/j.bbi.2010.02.001.

176. Vabulas RM, et al. The endoplasmic reticulum-resident heat shock protein Gp96 activates dendritic cells via the Toll-like receptor 2/4 pathway. *J Biol Chem.* 2002;277:20847–20853. https://doi.org/10.1074/jbc.M200425200.

177. Valenta JP, Gonzales RA. Chronic intracerebroventricular infusion of monocyte chemoattractant protein-1 leads to a persistent increase in sweetened ethanol consumption during operant self-administration but does not influence sucrose consumption in long-evans rats. *Alcohol Clin Exp Res.* 2016;40:187–195. https://doi.org/10.1111/acer.12928.

178. Valles SL, Blanco AM, Pascual M, Guerri C. Chronic ethanol treatment enhances inflammatory mediators and cell death in the brain and in astrocytes. *Brain Pathol.* 2004;14:365–371.

179. Vetreno RP, Crews FT. Adolescent binge drinking increases expression of the danger signal receptor agonist HMGB1 and Toll-like receptors in the adult prefrontal cortex. *Neurosci.* 2012;226:475–488. https://doi.org/10.1016/j.neuroscience.2012.08.046.

180. Vetreno RP, Crews FT. Current hypotheses on the mechanisms of alcoholism. *Handb Clin Neurol.* 2014;125:477–497. https://doi.org/10.1016/B978-0-444-62619-6.00027-6.

181. Vetreno RP, Qin L, Crews FT. Increased receptor for advanced glycation end product expression in the human alcoholic prefrontal cortex is linked to adolescent drinking. *Neurobiol Dis.* 2013;59:52–62. https://doi.org/10.1016/j.nbd.2013.07.002.

182. Reference deleted in review.

183. Volkow ND, Koob GF, McLellan AT. Neurobiologic advances from the brain disease model of addiction. *N Eng J Med.* 2016;374:363–371. https://doi.org/10.1056/NEJMra1511480.

184. von Bernhardi R, Eugenin-von Bernhardi L, Eugenin J. Microglial cell dysregulation in brain aging and neurodegeneration. *Front Aging Neurosci.* 2015;7:124. https://doi.org/10.3389/fnagi.2015.00124.

185. Wagley Y, et al. Inhibition of c-Jun NH2-terminal kinase stimulates mu opioid receptor expression via p38 MAPK-mediated nuclear NF-kappaB activation in neuronal and non-neuronal cells. *Biochim Biophys Acta.* 2013;1833:1476–1488. https://doi.org/10.1016/j.bbamcr.2013.02.017.

186. Wang WY, Tan MS, Yu JT, Tan L. Role of pro-inflammatory cytokines released from microglia in Alzheimer's disease. *Ann Trans Med.* 2015;3:136. https://doi.org/10.3978/j.issn.2305-5839.2015.03.49.

187. Wang X, et al. Rifampin inhibits Toll-like receptor 4 signaling by targeting myeloid differentiation protein 2 and attenuates neuropathic pain. *Faseb J.* 2013;27:2713–2722. https://doi.org/10.1096/fj.12-222992.

188. Wang X, et al. Pharmacological characterization of the opioid inactive isomers (+)-naltrexone and (+)-naloxone as antagonists of toll-like receptor 4. *Br J Pharm.* 2016;173:856–869. https://doi.org/10.1111/bph.13394.

189. Ward RJ, et al. Identification of the nuclear transcription factor NFkappaB in rat after in vivo ethanol administration. *Febs Letters.* 1996;389:119–122.

190. Ward RJ, et al. Neuro-inflammation induced in the hippocampus of 'binge drinking' rats may be mediated by elevated extracellular glutamate content. *J Neurochem.* 2009;111:1119–1128. https://doi.org/10.1111/j.1471-4159.2009.06389.x.

191. Weber MD, Frank MG, Tracey KJ, Watkins LR, Maier SF. Stress induces the danger-associated molecular pattern HMGB-1 in the hippocampus of male Sprague Dawley rats: a priming stimulus of microglia and the NLRP3 inflammasome. *J Neurosci.* 2015;35:316–324. https://doi.org/10.1523/JNEUROSCI.3561-14.2015.

192. Weissenborn R, Duka T. Acute alcohol effects on cognitive function in social drinkers: their relationship to drinking habits. *Psychopharmacology.* 2003;165:306–312. https://doi.org/10.1007/s00213-002-1281-1.

193. Whitman BA, Knapp DJ, Werner DF, Crews FT, Breese GR. The cytokine mRNA increase induced by withdrawal from chronic ethanol in the sterile environment of brain is mediated by CRF and HMGB1 release. *Alcohol Clin Exp Res.* 2013;37:2086–2097. https://doi.org/10.1111/acer.12189.

194. Wohleb ES, et al. beta-Adrenergic receptor antagonism prevents anxiety-like behavior and microglial reactivity induced by repeated social defeat. *J Neurosci.* 2011;31:6277–6288. https://doi.org/10.1523/JNEUROSCI.0450-11.2011.

195. Worley MJ, Heinzerling KG, Roche DJ, Shoptaw S. Ibudilast attenuates subjective effects of methamphetamine in a placebo-controlled inpatient study. *Drug Alcohol Depend.* 2016;162:245–250. https://doi.org/10.1016/j.drugalcdep.2016.02.036.

196. Yanai H, et al. HMGB proteins function as universal sentinels for nucleic-acid-mediated innate immune responses. *Nature.* 2009;462:99–103. https://doi.org/10.1038/nature08512.

197. Yirmiya R, Goshen I. Immune modulation of learning, memory, neural plasticity and neurogenesis. *Brain Behav Immun.* 2011;25:181–213. https://doi.org/10.1016/j.bbi.2010.10.015.

198. Zhang B, et al. Azithromycin drives alternative macrophage activation and improves recovery and tissue sparing in contusion spinal cord injury. *J Neuroinflam.* 2015;12:218. https://doi.org/10.1186/s12974-015-0440-3.

199. Zhu CB, et al. Interleukin-1 receptor activation by systemic lipopolysaccharide induces behavioral despair linked to MAPK regulation of CNS serotonin transporters. *Neuropsychopharmacol.* 2010;35:2510–2520. https://doi.org/10.1038/npp.2010.116.

200. Zou J, Crews F. CREB and NF-kappaB transcription factors regulate sensitivity to excitotoxic and oxidative stress induced neuronal cell death. *Cel mol neurobio.* 2006;26:385–405. https://doi.org/10.1007/s10571-006-9045-9.

201. Zou J, Crews F. Induction of innate immune gene expression cascades in brain slice cultures by ethanol: key role of NF-kappaB and proinflammatory cytokines. *Alcohol Clin Exp Res.* 2010;34:777–789. https://doi.org/10.1111/j.1530-0277.2010.01150.x.

202. Zou JY, Crews FT. TNF alpha potentiates glutamate neurotoxicity by inhibiting glutamate uptake in organotypic brain slice cultures: neuroprotection by NF kappa B inhibition. *Brain Res.* 2005;1034:11–24. https://doi.org/10.1016/j.brainres.2004.11.014.

203. Zou JY, Crews FT. Release of neuronal HMGB1 by ethanol through decreased HDAC activity activates brain neuroimmune signaling. *Plos One.* 2014;9:e87915. https://doi.org/10.1371/journal.pone.0087915.

21

Alcohol: Clinical Aspects

BANKOLE A. JOHNSON, GABRIELLE MARZANI, DEREK BLEVINS, AND SURBHI KHANNA

CHAPTER OUTLINE

Introduction

Alcohol is one of the oldest and the most widely used psychoactive substances in the world, second only to caffeine. The use of alcohol is a part of most cultures worldwide, and it is recognized that there are both positive and negative aspects of alcohol consumption. Positive aspects might include the socialization, stimulation of appetite, more rapid onset of sleep, and reduction in the incidence of heart disease. The negative aspects include poor judgment, liver disease, hypertension, memory problems, and even death. Of course, as with all drugs, there is a risk of addiction to alcohol, which exacerbates the negative aspects of alcohol use and leads to its own sequelae of complications and disorders. The National Institute on Alcohol Abuse and Alcoholism notes that "men who drink 5 or more standard drinks in a day (or more than 14 per week) and women who drink 4 or more in a day (or more than 7 per week) are at increased risk for alcohol-related problems."[79]

The six levels of alcohol use are abstention, experimentation, social or recreational use, habituation, abuse, and, finally, addiction. Abstention is nonuse. Experimentation is the use of alcohol for curiosity and without any subsequent alcohol-seeking behavior. Social or recreational use of alcohol involves sporadic infrequent drinking without any real pattern. Habituation involves drinking with an established pattern, but without any major negative consequences. Abuse of alcohol is the continuation of drinking despite negative consequences. Finally, addiction involves a compulsion to drink, an inability to stop drinking, and the progression of major life dysfunction with continued use.[52] The fifth edition of the *Diagnostic and Statistical Manual of Mental Disorders* (DSM-5) has consolidated these last two levels of alcohol use to a diagnosis of alcohol use disorder (AUD), which is then rated by severity.[1]

In the United States, the per-capita consumption of alcohol from beer, wine, and spirits combined in 2013 was 2.34 gallons. This value was unchanged from 2012 but represents the highest per-capita consumption since before 1990. Essentially, after a steady decrease in the mid- to late 1990s, there has been a general increase in per-capita consumption of alcohol since 1999.[81]

Alcohol use is a significant cause of morbidity and mortality in the United States and worldwide. The World Health Organization reports that the deaths of 3.3 million men and women around the globe were attributable to alcohol consumption,[114] making alcohol use the leading risk factor for premature death and disability among persons ages 15 to 49.[66] In 2014, 16.3 million adults had a past year alcohol use disorder in the United States.[13] Mortality rates follow drinking levels. A European study of 25 countries found that a rise of 1 L per capita in alcohol intake was associated with a 1% rise in all causes of morbidity.[49] The global economic burden of alcohol was estimated to be in the range of $210–665 billion in 2002.[4] The Centers for Disease Control and Prevention (CDC) estimated this figure at $232.5 billion in 2006 in the United States alone.[14]

In the United States, more than 50% of adults have a close family member who is dependent on alcohol.[25] More than 25%

of youths younger than the age of 18 years are aware of a relative who is dependent on alcohol.[47] Alcohol dependence runs in families.[7,21,72]

The burden of the alcohol dependence disease is not equal across all regions. The disease impact of alcohol dependence is greatest in regions where the per-capita consumption is highest, such as Latin America, as compared with the Middle East. In addition, other factors, such as increasing economic growth, have raised the risk of alcohol dependence in Europe.[90]

Alcohol consumption increases the risk of harm or death in the context of the operation of heavy machinery, fires, falls, and water activities. In the United States, approximately 40% of all traffic fatalities are alcohol related.[19] Trauma and aggressive behavior are associated highly with alcohol consumption less than 6 hours before the event.

Alcohol-Related Disorders

Alcohol is associated with many physical and mental disorders. Perhaps the most well-documented physical disorder is alcohol-related liver disease. Alcohol-induced fatty liver disease and obesity are both associated with progression to cirrhosis.[18,26] In the United States, more than 600,000 individuals have cirrhosis; about 20%–25% of these cases are attributed to excessive alcohol consumption.[97,102] Typically, the development of cirrhosis requires the consumption of at least 30 grams of ethanol daily for women and 50 grams daily for men for at least 5 years.[5] In addition, the presence of hepatitis C virus in the context of alcohol dependence is associated with increased rates of cirrhosis.[94,98] Women have an increased incidence of liver cirrhosis compared to men with the same amount of alcohol consumption and their dose-dependent increase in risk is steeper.[5,18] Globally, esophageal cancers, head and neck cancers, and liver cancers are of great concern, and are associated with alcohol use disorders.[12]

Individuals with mental illness are susceptible to alcohol use disorders. This, in part, may be due to attempts to self-medicate underlying anxiety, depression, mania, or psychosis. However, drinking alcohol in excess tends to worsen underlying psychiatric illness. Excessive use of alcohol is associated with a poorer chance of recovery from anxiety and depressive disorders.[48] Bipolar disorders and other impulse control disorders are associated with high rates of alcohol dependence. Dually diagnosed individuals have a poorer prognosis than those with just one of these disorders.[27,105] Drinking more than 29 drinks per week can double the risk of a psychiatric disorder. Neurocognitive disorders such as Alzheimer's dementia or multiinfarct dementia, can be worsened or be caused by alcohol, and the relationship between the two can be difficult to determine.[96] Alcohol use disorders are common in individuals with schizophrenia and worsen symptoms of the disease.[34,38,64] Unfortunately, individuals with mental illness tend to underreport their use of alcohol[104] and remain untreated as a result.

Age at Onset of Drinking Behavior

The age at onset of drinking has a significant role in outcomes. An individual who starts drinking before the age of 15 years is approximately four times more likely to develop alcohol dependence, and this rate increases the earlier the onset of drinking.[29] Data collected from the 2015 National Survey on Drug Use and Health found that 8.7 million 12 to 20 year olds were past-month drinkers, of which 5.3 million reported binge drinking and 1.3

million reported heavy use.[13] Furthermore, according to the Monitoring the Future survey in 2015, 10% of 8th graders, 22% of 10th graders, and 35% of 12th graders reported past-month alcohol consumption.[57] The risk of developing alcohol dependence and a more relapsing illness is greater in adolescents than in adults.[50] Notably, between 20% and 30% of early alcohol drinkers progress to heavy drinking in adulthood.[36,41] Children who drink often have behavioral problems, especially conduct disorders.[32,55] Frequently, adolescents, much like adults, are self-medicating for anxiety and depression.[61,93]

Alcohol dependence is a heterogeneous disorder and consists of subtypes, each with "varying degrees of biological and psychosocial antecedents."[8,21,56,99] The relationship between biological vulnerability, the environment, and their interactions in the development of alcohol dependence is the subject of active research.[60] Current evidence suggests that alcoholism is 50%–60% determined genetically in both men and women.[31] The term "psychiatric pharmacogenetics" has now entered the alcohol literature. Its purpose is to use genetic testing to predict, on an individual level, which treatment will be efficacious.[45]

Contrary to conventional wisdom, there are a number of studies showing that alcohol dependence is not always a chronic and progressive disease. This assertion is based on longitudinal studies and national surveys. It appears that persons who develop alcohol dependence in middle age have the most stability in terms of the disease. In this population, alcoholism can be a chronic remitting disease.[41,42,109,111,112] In contrast, individuals who develop alcoholism after the age of 50 years will often decrease their drinking as they age. Of interest, alcohol dependence in persons over 65 years of age continues to increase in the United States.

The 2001–2002 National Epidemiologic Survey on Alcohol and Related Conditions analyzed recovery rates of alcohol-dependent adults over a 1-year period. This population tended to be middle-aged, white males who were well educated (60% college educated); thus the generalizability is limited. More than half of the 4422 adults had experienced the onset of alcohol dependence between the ages of 18 and 24, and only 25% had ever received any treatment for alcohol problems. At 1 year, 35.9% were fully recovered (17.7% low-risk drinkers plus 18.2% abstainers), 25% were still dependent, 27.3% were in partial remission, and 11.8% were asymptomatic drinkers. Only 25% of the group had ever received any type of treatment.[25]

Effects of Ethnicity, Gender, Place of Residence, and Religion on Alcohol Consumption

Ethnicity is a complex and multifaceted construct, and often the terms used by demographers do not reflect the different subgroups. For example, Korean Americans and Chinese Americans are both considered as Asian, but drinking patterns are quite distinct between these two groups. A study conducted in 2004 found a lower rate of alcohol dependence in Chinese-American college students (5%) as compared with Korean-American college students (13%).[33] First-generation Mexicans and native-born Mexicans behave differently in their drinking patterns.[17,39] Whites have the highest consumption levels, followed by Latinos and, then, Blacks. There is considerable ethnic disparity in the progression of drinking behavior. White men peak first (18–25 years), followed by Hispanic and Black men, with peak ages between 26 and 30 years. Although levels of drinking tend to be low among native-born Latinos, acculturation stress increases alcohol abuse and dependence with migration and first-generation populations.[11,17] Ethnicity and socioeconomic status are also tied to the level of drinking.[40]

Currently, women have nearly the same rates of alcohol dependence as men. This is in contrast with 1940, when men were more than twice as likely to be dependent on alcohol. Of interest, women often have a more severe disease course—perhaps due to reduced access to care, a greater time period before seeking treatment, or both.

Despite common misperceptions, the extent of drinking among Native Americans varies tremendously by tribe. The proportion of Native Americans who reported being current drinkers ranged from a low of 30% to a high of 84%. This wide range of reported drinking behavior is indicative of considerable variance between the alcohol use in Native American tribes. Furthermore, it has been reported that Northern reservations have a higher incidence of hospital admittance for an alcohol-related medical problem than Southern reservations (111/1000 versus 11/1000, respectively).[107] On some Native American reservations, high quantities of alcohol are consumed per episode, but the frequency of binge drinking is low.[84]

Location also matters. Urban and suburban dwellers have higher rates of dependence compared with their rural counterparts. Drinking styles also differ.

Religion appears to be an important determinant for drinking.[73] Jews, Episcopalians, and Baptists living in rural areas show low rates of alcohol dependence compared with the general population.

Clinical Picture

Alcoholism can present in a multitude of ways, and at times its clinical effects can be subtle. Although there is no typical clinical pattern for an individual's progression from excessive drinking to alcohol dependence, there are certain themes that prevail. These are based on the pathophysiology of alcohol.

An early manifestation of excessive drinking is intoxication. This can begin with one's peers or by the influence of an older individual or family member. Some individuals note stress, depressed mood, or negative affect as a driving force, although at times it is elation. For others, there is an urge to drink, or craving. Although the concept of craving appears simple, the craving literature has found it difficult to define with consensus. When alcohol consumption leads to repeated bouts of intoxication and becomes a fixed pattern of behavior, the likelihood of alcohol-related problems increases.

As the body adapts to excessive alcohol consumption, tolerance develops. With tolerance, an increasingly greater amount of alcohol consumption is needed to obtain the same physiological effects. This can manifest as worsening grades or sick days among college students and workers and, for both, an increase in stress within interpersonal relationships, often characterized by greater irritability and moodiness. Furthermore, driving while under the influence of alcohol becomes more likely, and can lead to legal complications as well as morbidity and mortality to drivers, passengers, and other bystanders.

Heavy drinking can lead to blackouts, a failure to recall the events around the intoxication, due to the brain's inability to process and lay down the memory in the hippocampus.

Hangovers, which are associated with headaches and nausea, can manifest the next morning after a bout of heavy drinking. Often, as duties and responsibilities lapse, attention to hygiene can wane, and the chronic drinker's demeanor and behavior change. Memory lapses or forgetfulness may become more evident. In addition, the chronic excessive drinker may report guilt, remorse, and self-loathing after consuming alcohol and might conceal his or her drinking in order to avoid dealing with others. Such individuals tend to minimize the severity of their drinking behavior and its impact on others.

When drinking is being concealed, social isolation tends to occur, and to block or dampen guilt and anxiety, "relief drinking" can happen. Relief drinking may serve not only to temper these feelings but also to transiently reduce the resulting insomnia. Relief drinking might also temporarily ameliorate withdrawal symptoms upon drinking cessation (often starting within a few hours), which are the consequence of sympathetic nervous system hyperactivity. These symptoms can include tremulousness and anxiety and can proceed to a spectrum of serious withdrawal patterns, including delirium tremens. Despite any painful consequences such as loss of relationships, employment, legal entanglements, and physical and psychological complications, drinking can become the individual's sole goal. The physical features of the disease are described below.

Signs and Symptoms

Cardiovascular System

Although it has been consistently shown that light-to-moderate drinking reduces the risk of coronary artery disease, there still remain severe risks to the cardiovascular system for people who are heavy alcohol drinkers.[62,68,88,91] Cardiovascular conditions that may result from heavy drinking include hypertension, cardiac arrhythmias, and dilated cardiomyopathy.

The relationship between hypertension and heavy alcohol use has been known for more than three decades. Although a mechanism has yet to be elucidated, several clinical studies have confirmed this relationship.[59,63,69] Clinicians in all fields of medicine should be aware that hypertension can be the result of heavy and chronic alcohol consumption.

The incidence of cardiac arrhythmias following excessive alcohol consumption is commonly known as "holiday heart phenomenon" following the observation that supraventricular arrhythmias in alcoholics most often occur on Mondays or between Christmas and New Year's Day.[35] Although the direct cause of arrhythmias following heavy drinking is not explicitly known, it has been suggested that it could be due to myocardial damage, vagal reflexes, electrolyte or metabolic effects, or changes in conduction and refractory periods. Regardless of the root cause, the incidence of cardiac arrhythmias doubles for heavy drinkers compared with light drinkers.[22]

Dilated cardiomyopathy is characterized by an enlarged heart with weakened contraction. Sustained heavy alcohol use is thought to be a major contributing factor to dilated cardiomyopathy.[58] Although the prevalence of alcohol-induced dilated cardiomyopathy is not fully known, it is estimated that up to 40% of dilated cardiomyopathy cases are a result of excessive alcohol consumption.[28,44] The clinical picture may initially involve nonspecific electrocardiographic findings and possible rhythm disturbances but may progress to congestive heart failure, chronic rhythm disturbances, and even death.[9,87]

Gastrointestinal System

Excessive alcohol consumption can cause gastroesophageal reflux disease, gastritis, or ulcers in the lining of the stomach. These can manifest as a burning in the throat or stomach or complaints of dark stools (i.e., melena). In individuals who present with a long history of gastroesophageal reflux disease, there is an increased incidence of Barrett's esophagus, a metaplastic conversion of the mucosa of the lower esophagus; it is a well-known precursor lesion for esophageal cancer.

Chronic excessive alcohol consumption can cause varices, both gastric and esophageal. When varices rupture, often during severe retching, the individual may present with bright red blood. Bleeding varices are life-threatening medical emergencies. Mallory-Weiss tears from esophageal varices often require monitoring in intensive care settings due to their risk for re-bleeding with a high rate of blood loss.

Hepatic System

Chronic excessive alcohol consumption is associated with an increased risk for the development of liver disease. In the United States, 2 million people have alcoholic liver disease, ranging in severity from fatty liver to alcoholic hepatitis and end-stage cirrhosis.[77]

Fatty liver is the accumulation of fatty acids in the liver. The pathogenesis of fatty liver is due to the overproduction of protonated nicotinamide adenine dinucleotide from alcohol dehydrogenase, which, in turn, leads to the inhibition of fatty acid oxidation, the citric acid cycle, and gluconeogenesis.[65] It is the inhibition of fatty acid oxidation, as well as an increased synthesis of triglycerides, followed by the inhibition of the secretion of lipoprotein from the liver, which all contribute to fatty liver.[100]

Alcoholic hepatitis causes inflammation of the liver along with areas of fibrosis and necrosis. In the United States, approximately 10%–35% of heavy drinkers develop alcoholic hepatitis. It can take months to years to develop this condition, and the only method to arrest its progress is through abstinence. Nevertheless, even with the cessation of alcohol consumption, the resulting scarring of the liver and any other collateral damage remain.[74] The mortality rate in individuals with alcoholic hepatitis is 15%–20%, and even despite abstinence, many cases progress to cirrhosis.[85]

Cirrhosis is characterized by progressive scarring of the liver due to the toxic effects of excessive alcohol use and alcohol's metabolites. Cirrhosis, the most advanced form of alcoholic liver disease, is the leading cause of death among alcoholics. In 2010, approximately 490,000 deaths occurred due to alcohol-related liver disease, which represented 0.9% of all global deaths.[89]

More than 15,000 Americans die each year from cirrhosis due to excessive alcohol use.[115] Individuals with a diagnosis of both alcoholic hepatitis and cirrhosis have a death rate of more than 60% over a 4-year period. Most individuals die within the first 12 months of receiving the diagnosis.[77] Although the progression of cirrhosis might be halted by abstinence, cirrhosis is very difficult to treat, and the damage to the liver cannot be reversed.

Endocrine System

Pancreatitis, both acute and chronic, is another complication of excessive alcohol use. Pancreatic insufficiency or malabsorption presents with gray, foul-smelling stools that float. Pancreatitis typically manifests with pain in the center of the abdomen that radiates to the back. Pancreatitis ranges from an uncomfortable but stable condition to a medical emergency, depending on the severity of the event. Individuals with chronic pancreatitis may have calcifications that can be seen on a plain radiographic film.

Diabetes, both type 1 and type 2, can be a consequence of excessive alcohol use. The development of type 1 diabetes is rare and is due to almost complete destruction of the pancreas. Type 2 diabetes is more common and due to weight gain from carbohydrate ingestion. Hypogonadism and osteoporosis are other complications. Thyroid disease also can be a sequela of excessive alcohol use, abuse, or dependence.

Rheumatic and Immune System

Chronic excessive alcohol consumption has been linked with an increase in illness and death from infectious diseases. Due to alcohol's immunosuppressive effects, there is an increased susceptibility to bacterial pneumonia, pulmonary tuberculosis, and hepatitis C. There is even some speculation that chronic excessive alcohol users are at increased risk for HIV infection due to lowered immune response, and that those with HIV may have a quicker progression from HIV to full-blown AIDS.[77]

Gout is a common complication of chronic excessive alcohol consumption. Podagra (gout in the big toe) is a typical complaint. Alcohol use appears to mitigate certain autoimmune conditions such as systemic lupus erythematosus and rheumatoid arthritis.

Hematological/Hematopoietic System

Anemias, both macrocytic and microcytic, are possible. Macrocytic anemia can be due to folate or vitamin B_{12} deficiency. An increased mean corpuscular volume can reflect macrocytic anemia. Of note, an increased mean corpuscular volume can also be a result of liver disease when the lipid bilayers that hold the red cell do not form correctly. When liver disease is severe, platelets can be destroyed or can sequester in an enlarged spleen. Microcytic anemias are related to active bleeding or blood loss and should prompt evaluation for a gastrointestinal disorder or lesion. Sideroblastic anemia can also occur.

Central Nervous System

The brain is sensitive to alcohol's toxic effects. Areas that are particularly sensitive include the hippocampus and the cerebellum, which can result in memory deficits and dementias as well as abnormal gait and intention tremors. Rarely, central pontine myelinolysis can occur. These central nervous system deficits are discussed in detail in subsequent text of this chapter.

Peripheral Neurological System

Changes in position and vibration sense occur after prolonged excessive alcohol use and are due to vitamin B_{12} or folate deficiencies, or both. Myopathy can be a rare manifestation of alcohol dependence.

Integumentary System (Skin)

Psoriasis vulgaris, acne rosacea, and erythropoietic protoporphyria are all common skin conditions associated with excessive alcohol use. With liver disease, spider nevi, telangiectasias, palmar erythema (reddened palms), spider angiomas, and hepatic porphyrias, particularly porphyria cutanea tarda (bullous erosions, blistering, crusting lesions, and scarred healing with hyperpigmentation or depigmentation on the face, the side of the neck, and the back of the hands), might be found.

Nutritional Status

Low levels of potassium, magnesium, and phosphorus are common in individuals with severe alcohol dependence. Hypophosphatemia and hypomagnesemia also can be complications of severe nutritional deficiency. A refeeding syndrome that can lead to diaphragmatic paralysis and respiratory failure can occur. On many blood chemistries, magnesium and phosphorus are not part of the panel. Therefore, it is prudent to check these electrolytes in an alcohol-dependent individual who appears nutritionally compromised. Low levels of potassium can cause additional medical complications (particularly cardiovascular) if not replaced; however, this can be difficult to achieve in the setting of low magnesium. Therefore, magnesium and potassium need to be replenished simultaneously. As noted previously, thiamine replacement is also often required.

Oncology

An increasing number of cancers are being associated with excessive alcohol use or dependence. Traditionally, alcohol-related cancers include oropharyngeal, esophageal, gastric, pancreatic, and rectal cancers. In women, alcohol abuse has been reported to contribute to the etiology of breast cancer.

Fetal Development

The consumption of alcohol during pregnancy has been linked with poor birth outcomes, the potential for long-term developmental disabilities, and the manifestation of fetal alcohol spectrum disorder, which includes fetal alcohol syndrome.[2] According to the CDC, 1 in 10 pregnant women reported consuming alcohol in the past 30 days and 1 in 33 reported binge drinking in 2011–2013. Whereas among nonpregnant women the prevalence rate of any alcohol use was 53.6%, pregnant women had a rate of 10.2%.[108]

It has been estimated that the annual cost of care for those diagnosed with fetal alcohol spectrum disorders is $3.6 billion and that the lifetime cost for a single individual is $2.9 million.[67] These numbers are staggering considering that maternal alcohol use during pregnancy is the leading cause of preventable birth defects and neurodevelopmental disabilities in the United States.[43,80] The health care community continues to emphasize prevention and stresses abstinence from alcohol for women who are pregnant or considering becoming pregnant. Research into the clinical management of persons diagnosed with fetal alcohol spectrum disorders is still emerging, but human studies using behavioral intervention are encouraging.

The clinical manifestations of fetal alcohol exposure fall under the classification of fetal alcohol spectrum disorders. Fetal alcohol spectrum disorders can be further subdivided into four categorical syndromes: (1) fetal alcohol syndrome; (2) partial fetal alcohol syndrome; (3) alcohol-related neurodevelopmental disorder; and (4) alcohol-related birth defects.[8] In a study of first grade children, the authors reported an estimated prevalence of fetal alcohol syndrome between 1 and 9 per 1000 and an estimated prevalence of combined fetal alcohol syndrome plus partial fetal alcohol syndrome to be much higher at 17–26 per 1000.[70] This rate is significantly higher when compared to CDC data, which estimates a prevalence of 0.3 per 1000 children.[15]

A clinical diagnosis of fetal alcohol syndrome requires alcohol exposure, a recognizable facial pattern that includes short palpebral fissures (<10th percentile), thin upper vermilion lip, and smooth philtrum, evidence of growth retardation or malformation, and evidence of neurocognitive defects. Newborns with fetal alcohol syndrome may exhibit irritability, tremors, hypotonia, and even withdrawal symptoms. Partial fetal alcohol syndrome is diagnosed when there is confirmation of alcohol consumption during pregnancy and, although not all the features of fetal alcohol syndrome are present, neurocognitive and some craniofacial features are present. Children diagnosed with alcohol-related neurodevelopmental disorder do not typically have the growth retardation or facial features characteristic of fetal alcohol syndrome, but the resulting neurocognitive defects are more pronounced. A diagnosis of alcohol-related birth defect requires some of the facial features characteristic of fetal alcohol syndrome, but it is the behavioral features or structural abnormalities that are more prominent.[75]

In addition to the physical impairments inflicted by alcohol, there is a spectrum of cognitive problems that children who are diagnosed with fetal alcohol spectrum disorders exhibit. These problems include difficulties with hyperactivity, sustained and focused attention, cognitive flexibility, learning and memory, and social understanding.[54] Aside from cognitive deficits, these children can also exhibit psychological and behavioral difficulties such as psychiatric problems, inappropriate sexual behavior, and alcohol and/or drug abuse.[106] In fact, 90% of children diagnosed with fetal alcohol spectrum disorders have some form of diagnosable psychiatric disorder, ranging from attention deficit disorder to depression to schizophrenia. Fifty percent have been confined in either a mental health or criminal justice institution.[67]

Although perinatal exposure to alcohol is known to be detrimental to fetal development, there is some debate as to whether it is ethanol or its metabolite acetaldehyde that causes the developmental abnormalities found in fetal alcohol syndrome. Acetaldehyde is 10 times more teratogenic than alcohol.[86] However, this differential in teratogenicity is, perhaps, countered by the fact that blood ethanol concentration is 10 times higher than acetaldehyde in the typical person.

Acetaldehyde levels in excess of 35 µg can cause damage to a fetus, but acetaldehyde is rapidly metabolized by the placenta, and, after the third month of pregnancy, no acetaldehyde is detectable in the fetus.[83] The placenta is, however, permeable to ethanol, and the fetus does not have ethanol dehydrogenase, the enzyme required to break down ethanol. It is, therefore, reasonable to propose that an hour or two following alcohol ingestion, the ethanol concentration in the mother's blood may be falling while the ethanol concentration of the fetus may be rising.[53] Although it is not clear whether it is alcohol itself or its metabolite acetaldehyde that is responsible for the developmental abnormalities found in fetal alcohol spectrum disorders, the physical findings in fetal alcohol syndrome do point to an interesting fact: it is not the disruption of developing tissues but rather the reduction in the number of cells and the subsequent cell migration abnormalities, particularly of the central nervous system, that causes the anomalies found in fetal alcohol syndrome.

Psychological and Psychiatric Complications of Alcohol

Individual differences in human physiology cause varying physical manifestations of the effects of both acute and long-term use of alcohol. Alcohol affects almost all organ systems through the natural progression of the disease. These are characterized as acute, chronic, and withdrawal effects.

Acute Effects

The acute effects of alcohol ingestion can be tracked progressively using the concentration of alcohol in a person's blood, or blood alcohol concentration. The unit of measurement for blood alcohol concentration is weight by volume, such as milligrams per deciliter, but it can also be expressed as a percentage, such as 5% alcohol by volume.[3] The acute effects of alcohol consumption follow the typical dose-response relationship characteristic of all drugs in that the bigger the dose, the bigger the effect.[77] The typical progressive effects of alcohol intoxication in relation to blood alcohol concentration are illustrated in Table 21.1[77,78] ;however, there is considerable personal variation.

The metabolism of alcohol occurs at a rate of about 1 ounce of pure alcohol (2 drinks) eliminated from the body every 3 hours. Following alcohol consumption, it takes about 15–20 minutes for alcohol to reach the brain and cause impairment. The maximum blood alcohol concentration is reached 30–90 minutes following the ingestion of alcohol.[76]

It is generally accepted that the consumption of a standard serving of alcohol (14 g, or 17.74 mL ethanol content) will increase the average person's blood alcohol concentration by 0.02%–0.05%. The average person's blood alcohol concentration decreases approximately 0.015% per hour following complete cessation of alcohol intake. A blood alcohol concentration of 0.20% represents very serious intoxication. A blood alcohol concentration ranging between 0.35% and 0.40% could be potentially fatal alcohol poisoning. The accepted LD_{50} for alcohol—that is, the dose that is lethal for 50% of the adult human population—is 0.40%.[78]

Besides the well-known acute effects of alcohol consumption such as lowered inhibitions, impaired ability to drive, slowed reaction time, slurred speech, and blackouts, some rare complications can occur. These include alcohol-induced psychotic disorder, central pontine myelinolysis, and acute alcoholic myopathy.

Alcohol-induced psychotic disorder or alcohol hallucinosis occurs most often in the context of drinking but can also occur in the presence of withdrawal. It is characterized by the acute onset of visual and auditory hallucinations and often includes delusions of a persecutory nature. These hallucinations and delusions usually resolve within 48 hours, although in some cases they can last much longer.

Central pontine myelinolysis is a rare disorder that is most often found in individuals who abuse alcohol. This disorder typically evolves over days to weeks, and the individual presents with mental confusion along with dysarthria, mutism, dysphagia, conjugate gaze palsies, and facial and neck weakness. Chronic hyponatremia seems to be a precipitating factor in the development of central pontine myelinolysis. Characteristic of the complication is bilaterally symmetrical focal destruction of white matter in the ventral pons. Approximately 10% of individuals display extrapontine lesions in the thalamus, basal ganglia, cerebellum, and

TABLE 21.1 The Progressive Effects of Alcohol.		
Blood Alcohol Concentration	**Changes in Behavior**	**Activity Impairment**
0.01–0.05	Relaxation Feeling of well-being Loss of shyness Loss of inhibitions Exaggerated behaviors	Impaired alertness Impaired judgment Minor impairment of memory Minor impairment of reasoning
0.06–0.10	Feeling of euphoria Feeling of pleasure Numbness of feelings Nausea and sleepiness	Impaired coordination Impaired balance Impaired speech Impaired vision Slow reaction time
0.11–0.20	Anger Mood swings Feeling of sadness Confusion Feeling of restlessness Nausea and vomiting Disorientation	Impaired reasoning Impaired depth perception Inappropriate social behavior Impairment of motor coordination Slurred speech Severely impaired judgment Severe memory impairment Blackouts
0.21–0.30	Aggression Depression Stupor Reduced sensations Nausea and vomiting	Loss of balance Loss of temperature regulation Loss of consciousness May be difficult to awaken
0.31–0.40	Unconsciousness Coma Death possible	Loss of bladder control Difficulty breathing Slowed heart rate
0.41 and greater	Death	

Adapted from tables in the National Institute on Alcohol Abuse and Alcoholism[77,78] as well as Inaba and Cohen.[52]

cerebral white matter. As the name of the disorder implies, these lesions are typified by a loss of myelin.[30] With proper support, individuals diagnosed with this condition typically regain some or all function after a few weeks.[16]

Acute alcoholic myopathy is a severe and life-threatening disorder that typically presents following several days of binge drinking.[46] Individuals typically present with pain, tenderness, cramps, proximal weakness, and swelling of the muscles, which can lead to cardiac arrhythmias. Further complications of acute alcoholic myopathy include hyperkalemia, renal failure, and even death. Following abstinence, recovery takes from a few days to weeks.

Chronic Effects

Although the physical effects of chronic alcohol abuse or dependence are well characterized, the psychological and psychiatric consequences are less familiar. Such chronic complications from chronic alcohol abuse or dependence include Wernicke encephalopathy, Korsakoff psychosis, alcoholic neuropathy, chronic alcoholic myopathy, and alcoholic dementia.

Wernicke's encephalopathy is caused by thiamin (vitamin B_1) deficiency and is usually diagnosed by a triad of symptoms: ataxia, oculomotor abnormalities, and global confusion.[92,113] Wernicke encephalopathy, however, is not just a condition of alcoholics but is found in people who are malnourished due to persistent vomiting, are experiencing starvation, or are undergoing renal dialysis. Gait ataxia is a prominent symptom, as are nystagmus and bilateral rectus palsies. The global confusion is characterized by sleepiness, disorientation, and inattention. Treatment (i.e., vitamin B_1 supplements) can correct most or all of the disturbances, but if left untreated, the mortality rate is 10%–20%. Individuals surviving Wernicke encephalopathy, however, tend to acquire Korsakoff psychosis.[6,67]

Korsakoff psychosis is a chronic amnesic disorder that can occur in individuals who have had Wernicke encephalopathy. Like Wernicke encephalopathy, Korsakoff psychosis is the result of thiamine deficiency. It is manifested by retrograde and anterograde amnesia, the latter caused by an inability to lay down new memories. Although immediate recall remains intact, short-term memory is impaired. Individuals are unaware of their memory deficits, and confabulation is common. The most probable cause of the memory deficits is lesions in the dorsal medial nuclei of the thalamus.[101] Although 20% of individuals recover completely over several months with vitamin B_1 supplements, approximately 25% never recover and subsequently require long-term care.[106]

Alcoholic neuropathy is the most commonly reported neurological complication in people addicted to alcohol. These individuals present with paresthesias, pain, and weakness; they may also have reduced pain and temperature sensations. Typically, there is axonal degeneration and demyelination, possibly due to a neurotoxic effect of ethanol on the peripheral nerves.[20,71] Although recovery is possible, it requires total abstinence and may take months.

The development of chronic alcoholic myopathy manifests as a painless syndrome wherein the individual has muscle weakness. The severity of the myopathy is directly related to the amount of alcohol consumed.[110] It is thought that chronic alcoholic myopathy is the result of the toxicity of ethanol and its metabolites, such as acetaldehyde, as opposed to nutritional deficiencies.[2,54,103] Individuals typically improve a few months after the discontinuation of alcohol.

The diagnostic criteria for alcoholic dementia remain controversial. There are currently no acceptable criteria available to diagnose definite alcohol-related dementia. There do exist, however, criteria for diagnosing probable alcohol-related dementia. These criteria include: (1) a clinical diagnosis of dementia at least 60 days after alcohol exposure and (2) significant alcohol use as defined by 35 or more standard drinks/week for men and 28 or more standard drinks/week for women for 5 years or longer. Furthermore, the onset of dementia must fall within a 3-year period of significant alcohol use.[51.] The neuropathic changes that usually accompany individuals diagnosed with alcoholic dementia include cortical atrophy, the loss of cortical neurons, and enlargement of the lateral ventricles.[24] The cognitive function of these individuals tends to improve after a few months of abstinence. Even the neuroimaging of these individuals reveals decreased ventricular dilation following a few months of abstinence.[76]

Conclusions

Alcohol-related disorders are an important global health problem. Not only is there a significant economic burden, but the negative personal effects of excessive alcohol consumption may be both physically and psychologically devastating. Many factors, including age at onset, ethnicity, gender, place of residence, and religion must all be considered in regard to the clinical picture of alcohol use and abuse. The clinical picture of alcohol is different for every individual but there are consistent themes, based on the pathophysiology of alcohol. Intoxication, blackouts, and hangovers are all typical clinical manifestations of excessive alcohol use. Although these manifestations may be readily apparent, other signs and symptoms may remain subtle, especially at the onset of excessive alcohol consumption. Many organ systems may be negatively affected by alcohol consumption. Alcohol-related liver disease, holiday heart phenomenon, gastroesophageal reflux disease, and anemia may all result from the prolonged use of alcohol, especially in excessive amounts. Furthermore, the excessive consumption of alcohol not only harms the individual who is drinking but may also have serious physical effects on the developing fetus. The psychological and psychiatric picture of alcohol consumption can be divided into acute and chronic effects. The acute effects of alcohol consumption, such as a loss of inhibitions and feelings of pleasure and euphoria, are well known, and these well-known effects entice individuals to consume alcoholic beverages. Finally, the continued excessive use of alcoholic beverages may result in severe chronic psychological and psychiatric effects such as Wernicke encephalopathy or Korsakoff psychosis.

Acknowledgments

We thank Catharine Helms and Robert H. Cormier, Jr., for their assistance with manuscript preparation.

References

1. American Psychiatric Association. *Diagnostic and Statistical Manual of Mental Disorders.* 5th ed. Arlington, VA: American Psychiatric Publishing; 2013.
2. Bailey BA, Sokol RJ. Pregnancy and alcohol use: evidence and recommendations for prenatal care. *Clin Obstet Gynecol.* 2008;51: 436–444.
3. Bailey WJ. Indiana prevention resource center factline on high potency alcoholic beverages [Online]; 1998. Available at: http://www.drugs.indiana.edu/publications/iprc/factline/high_potency.html. Accessed 16 Jan 2009.
4. Baumberg B. The global economic burden of alcohol: a review and some suggestions. *Drug Alcohol Rev.* 2006;25:537–551.
5. Becker U, Deis A, Sorensen TI, et al. Prediction of risk of liver disease by alcohol intake, sex, and age: a prospective population study. *Hepatology.* 1996;23:1025–1029. https://doi.org/10.1002/hep.510230513.
6. Bishai DM, Bozzetti LP. Current progress toward the prevention of the wernicke-korsakoff syndrome. *Alcohol Alcohol.* 1986;21: 315–323.
7. Bohman M, Sigvardsson S, et al. Maternal inheritance of alcohol abuse. Cross-fostering analysis of adopted women. *Arch Gen Psychiatry.* 1981;38:965–969.
8. Bucholz KK, Heath AC, et al. Can we subtype alcoholism? A latent class analysis of data from relatives of alcoholics in a multicenter family study of alcoholism. *Alcohol Clin Exp Res.* 1996;20: 1462–1471.

9. Burch GE, Phillips Jr JH, Ferrans VJ. Alcoholic cardiomyopathy. *Am J Med Sci.* 1966;252:123/189–138/104.

10. Reference deleted in review.

11. Caetano R, Ramisetty-Mikler S, et al. The Hispanic Americans baseline alcohol survey (HABLAS): DUI rates, birthplace, and acculturation across Hispanic national groups. *J Stud Alcohol Drugs.* 2008;69:259–265.

12. Carigulo T. Understanding the health impact of alcohol dependence. *Am J Health Syst Pharm.* 2007;64(5 suppl 3):S5–S11.

13. Center for Behavioral Health Statistics and Quality. *Behavioral health trends in the United States: Results from the 2014 National Survey on Drug Use and Health (HHS Publication No. SMA 15-4927, NSDUH Series H-50)*; 2015. Retrieved from http://www.samhsa.gov/ data.

14. Centers for Disease Control and Prevention. *Excessive drinking costs U.S. $223.5 billion*; 2014. Retrieved from http://www.cdc.gov/features/alcoholconsumption/.

15. Centers for Disease Control and Prevention. Fetal alcohol syndrome among children aged 7–9 years – Arizona, Colorado, and New York, 2010. *MMWR Morbidity and Mortality Weekly Report.* 2015;64(3):54–57.

16. Charness ME, Diamond I. Alcohol and the nervous system. *Curr Neurol.* 1984;5:383–422.

17. Cherpitel CJ, Robertson M, et al. Comorbidity for alcohol use disorders and drug use in Mexican-origin groups: comparison of data from national alcohol surveys in the U.S. and mexico. *Subst Use Misuse.* 2007;42:1685–1703.

18. Cholet F, Nousbaum JB, et al. Factors associated with liver steatosis and fibrosis in chronic hepatitis C patients. *Gastroenterol Clin Biol.* 2004;28:272–278.

19. Chou SP, Dawson DA, et al. The prevalence of drinking and driving in the United States, 2001–2002: results from the national epidemiological survey on alcohol and related conditions. *Drug Alcohol Depend.* 2004;83:137–146.

20. Claus D, Eggers R, Engelhardt A, Neundorfer B, Warecka K. Ethanol and polyneuropathy. *Acta Neurol Scand.* 1985;72:312–316.

21. Cloninger CR, Bohman M, Sigvardsson S. Inheritance of alcohol abuse. cross-fostering analysis of adopted men. *Arch Gen Psychiatry.* 1981;38:861–868.

22. Cohen EJ, Klatsky AL, Armstrong MA. Alcohol use and supraventricular arrhythmia. *Am J Cardiol.* 1988;62:971–973.

23. Reference deleted in review.

24. Courville CB, ed. *Effects of Alcohol on the Nervous System of Man.* Los Angeles, CA: San Lucas; 1955.

25. Dawson DA, Grant BF, et al. Recovery from DSM-IV alcohol dependence: United States: 2001–2002. *Addiction.* 2005;100:281–292.

26. Day CP. Who gets alcoholic liver disease: nature or nurture? *J R Coll Physicians Lond.* 2000;34:557–562.

27. DelBello MP, Strakowski SM, et al. Familial rates of affective and substance use disorders in patients with first-episode mania. *J Affect Disord.* 1999;56:55–60.

28. Demakis JG, Proskey A, Rahimtoola SH, et al. The natural course of alcoholic cardiomyopathy. *Ann Intern Med.* 1974;80:293–297.

29. DeWit DJ, Adlaf EM, et al. Age at first alcohol use: a risk factor for the development of alcohol disorders. *Am J Psychiatry.* 2000;157:745–750.

30. Diamond I, Messing RO. Neurologic effects of alcoholism. *West J Med.* 1994;161:279–287.

31. Dick DM, Bierut LJ. The genetics of alcohol dependence. *Curr Psychiatry Rep.* 2006;8:151–157.

32. Donovan JE, Jessor R, et al. Problem drinking in adolescence and young adulthood. a follow-up study. *J Stud Alcohol.* 1983;44:109–137.

33. Duranceaux NC, Schuckit MA, et al. Ethnic differences in level of response to alcohol between Chinese Americans and Korean Americans. *J Stud Alcohol Drugs.* 2008;69:227–234.

34. Eriksson A, Tengstrom A, et al. Typologies of alcohol use disorders among men with schizophrenic disorders. *Addict Behav.* 2007;32:1146–1163.

35. Ettinger PO, Wu CF, De La Cruz Jr C, Weisse AB, Ahmed SS, Regan TJ. Arrhythmias and the holiday heart: alcohol-associated cardiac rhythm disorders. *Am Heart J.* 1978;95:555–562.

36. Fillmore KM, Midanik L. Chronicity of drinking problems among men: a longitudinal study. *J Stud Alcohol.* 1984;45:228–236.

37. Reference deleted in review.

38. Gerding LB, Labbate LA, et al. Alcohol dependence and hospitalization in schizophrenia. *Schizophr Res.* 1999;38:71–75.

39. Gilder DA, Lau P, et al. A co-morbidity of alcohol dependence with other psychiatric disorders in young adult Mexican Americans. *J Addict Dis.* 2007;26:31–40.

40. Gilman SE, Breslau J, et al. Education and race-ethnicity differences in the lifetime risk of alcohol dependence. *J Epidemiol Community Health.* 2008;62:224–230.

41. Grant BF. Prevalence and correlates of alcohol use and DSM-IV alcohol dependence in the United States: results of the National longitudinal alcohol epidemiologic survey. *J Stud Alcohol.* 1997;58:464–473.

42. Grant BF, Dawson DA. Age of onset of drug use and its association with DSM-IV drug abuse and dependence: results from the national longitudinal alcohol epidemiologic survey. *J Subst Abuse.* 1998;10:163–173.

43. Grant T, Huggins J, Connor P, Pederson JY, Whitney N, Streissguth A. A pilot community intervention for young women with fetal alcohol spectrum disorders. *Community Mental Health J.* 2004;49:85–91.

44. Guzzo-Merello G, Cobo-Marcos M, Gallego-Delgado M, Garcia-Pavia P. Alcoholic cardiomyopathy. *World J Cardiol.* 2014;6(8):771–781.

45. Haile CN, Kosten TA, et al. Pharmacogenetic treatments for drug addiction: alcohol and opiates. *Am J Drug Alcohol Abuse.* 2008;34:355–381.

46. Haller RG, Knochel JP. Skeletal muscle disease in alcoholism. *Med Clin North Am.* 1984;68:91–103.

47. Harlem Brundtland G. *WHO European Ministerial Conference on Young People and Alcohol.* Sweden: World Health Organization; 2001.

48. Haynes JC, Farrell M, et al. Alcohol consumption as a risk factor for non-recovery from common mental disorder: results from the longitudinal follow-up of the national psychiatric morbidity survey. *Psychol Med.* 2008;38:451–455.

49. Her M, Rehm J. Alcohol and all-cause mortality in Europe 1982–1990: a pooled cross-section time-series analysis. *Addiction.* 1998;93:1335–1340.

50. Hingson RW, Heeren T, et al. Age at drinking onset and alcohol dependence: age at onset, duration, and severity. *Arch Pediatr Adolesc Med.* 2006;160:739–746.

51. Hulse GK, Lautenschlager NT, Tait RJ, Almeida OP. Dementia associated with alcohol and other drug use. *Int Psychogeriatrics.* 2005;17:S109–S127.

52. Inaba DS, Cohen WE. *Uppers, Downers, All Arounders: Physical and Mental Effects of Psychoactive Drugs.* 5th ed. Ashland OR. CNS Publications; 2004.

53. Itthagarun A, Nair RG, Epstein JB, King NM. Fetal alcohol syndrome: case report and review of the literature. *Oral Surg Oral Med Oral Pathol Oral Radiol Endod.* 2007;103:e20–e25.

54. Jacobson JL, Jacobson SW. Effects of prenatal alcohol exposure on child development. *Alcohol Res Health.* 2002;26:282–286.

55. Jessor R. Problem-behavior theory, psychosocial development, and adolescent problem drinking. *Br J Addict.* 1987;82:331–342.

56. Johnson BA, Cloninger CR, Roache JD, et al. Age of onset as a discriminator between alcoholic subtypes in a treatment-seeking outpatient population. *Am J Addict.* 2000;9:17–27.

57. Johnston LD, O'Malley PM, Miech RA, Bachman JG, Schulenberg JE. *Monitoring the Future National Survey Results on Drug Use, 1975-2015: Overview, Key Findings on Adolescent Drug use*. Ann Arbor: Institute for Social Research, The University of Michigan; 2016.

58. Kasper EK, Willem WRP, Hutchins GM, Deckers JW, Hare JM, Buaghman KL. The causes of dilated cardiomyopathy. Clinicopathologic review of 673 consecutive patients. *J Am Coll Cardiol*. 1994;23:586–590.

59. Keil U, Swales JD, Grobbee DE. Alcohol intake and its relation to hypertension. In: Verschuren PM, ed. *Health Issues Related to Alcohol Consumption*. Washington, DC: ILSI; 1993.

60. Kendler KS, Schmitt E, et al. Genetic and environmental influences on alcohol, caffeine, cannabis, and nicotine use from early adolescence to middle adulthood. *Arch Gen Psychiatry*. 2008;65:674–682.

61. Kessler RC, Crum RM, et al. Lifetime co-occurrence of DSM-III-R alcohol abuse and dependence with other psychiatric disorders in the National Comorbidity Survey. *Arch Gen Psychiatry*. 1997;54:313–321.

62. Klatsky AL. Epidemiology of coronary heart disease – influence of alcohol. *Alcohol Clin Exp Res*. 1994;18:88–96.

63. Klatsky AL. Blood pressure and alcohol intake. In: Laragh JH, Brenner BM, eds. *Hypertension: Pathophysiology, Diagnosis, and Management*. 2nd ed. New York: Raven; 1995.

64. Konarzewska B, Poplawska R, et al. Impact of alcohol dependence on the course and psychopathology of schizophrenia. *Psychiatr Pol*. 2007;41:715–726.

65. Lieber CS. Alcohol and the liver: 1994 update. *Gastroenterology*. 1994;106:1085.

66. Lim SS, Vos T, Flaxman AD. A comparative risk assessment of burden of disease and injury attributable to 67 risk factors and risk factor clusters in 21 regions, 1990–2010: a systematic analysis for the global burden of disease study 2010. *Lancet*. 2012;380(9859):2224–2260.

67. Lupton C, Burd L, Harwood R. The cost of fetal alcohol spectrum disorders. *Am J Med Genet C Sem Med Genet*. 2004;127C:42–50.

68. Maclure M. Demonstration of deductive meta-analysis: ethanol intake and risk of myocardial infarction. *Epidemiology Rev*. 1993;15:328–351.

69. MacMahon S. Alcohol consumption and hypertension. *Hypertension*. 1987;9:111–121.

70. May PA, Baete A, Russo J, et al. Prevalence and characteristics of fetal alcohol spectrum disorders. *Pediatrics*. 2014;134:855–888.

71. McLane JA. Decreased axonal transport in rat nerve following acute and chronic ethanol exposure. *Alcohol*. 1987;4:385–389.

72. Merikangas KR, Stolar M, et al. Familial transmission of substance use disorders. *Arch Gen Psychiatry*. 1998;55:973–979.

73. Michalak L, Trocki K, et al. Religion and alcohol in the U.S. National Alcohol Survey: how important is religion for abstention and drinking? *Drug Alcohol Depend*. 2007;87:268–280.

74. Moddrey WC. Alcoholic hepatitis: clinicopathologic features and therapy. *Sem Liver Dis*. 1988;8:91–102.

75. Mukherjee RAS, Hollins S, Turk J. Fetal alcohol spectrum disorder: an overview. *J R Soc Med*. 2006;99:298–302.

76. National Institute on Alcohol Abuse and Alcoholism. *Alcohol Metabolism*. Alcohol Alert No. 35; 1997. Retrieved from www.niaaa.nih.gov. Accessed 5 April 2016.

77. National Institute on Alcohol Abuse and Alcoholism. Medical consequences of alcohol abuse. *Alcohol Res Health*. 2000;24:27–31.

78. National Institute on Alcohol Abuse and Alcoholism. *Understanding Alcohol: Investigations into Biology and Behavior*; 2003.

79. National Institute on Alcohol Abuse and Alcoholism. *Helping Patients who Drink too Much: a Clinician's Guide*; 2007.

80. National Institute on Alcohol Abuse and Alcoholism. *Fetal Alcohol Exposure*; 2015. Retrieved from www.niaaa.nih.gov. Assessed 5 April 2016.

81. National Institute on Alcohol Abuse and Alcoholism. *Surveillance Report #102: Apparent per Capita Alcohol Consumption: National, State, and Regional Trends*; 2015:1977–2013.

82. Reference deleted in review.

83. Noble EP. A health caution: fetal alcohol syndrome. In: *National Institute on Alcohol Abuse and Alcoholism*. Washington, DC: U.S. Department of Health, Education and Welfare; 1977.

84. O'Connell J, Novins DK, et al. The relationship between patterns of alcohol use and mental and physical health disorders in two American Indian populations. *Addiction*. 2006;101:69–83.

85. Orrego H, Israel Y, Blake JE, et al. Assessment of prognostic factors in alcoholic liver disease: towards a global quantitative expression of severity. *Hepatology*. 1983;3:896.

86. Pratt OE. Introduction: what do we know of the mechanisms of alcohol damage in utero? *Ciba Found Symp*. 1984;105:1–7.

87. Regan TJ. Alcoholic cardiomyopathy. *Prog Cardiovasc Dis*. 1984;27:141–152.

88. Rehm JT, Bondy SJ, Sempos CT, Vuong CV. Alcohol consumption and coronary heart disease morbidity and mortality. *Am J Epidemiol*. 1997;146:495–501.

89. Rehm J, Samokhvalov AV, Shield KD. Global burden of alcoholic liver diseases. *J Hepatol*. 2013;59(1):160–168.

90. Rehm J, Sulkowska U, et al. Alcohol accounts for a high proportion of premature mortality in central and eastern Europe. *Int J Epidemiol*. 2007;36:458–467.

91. Renaud S, Criqui MH, Farchi G, Veenstra J. Alcohol drinking and coronary heart disease. In: Verschuren PM, ed. *Health Issues Related to Alcohol Consumption*. Washington, DC: ILSI; 1993.

92. Reuler JB, Girard GE, Conney TG. Wernicke's encephalopathy. *N Engl J Med*. 1985;312:1035–1038.

93. Rohde P, Lewinsohn PM, et al. Psychiatric comorbidity with problematic alcohol use in high school students. *J Am Acad Chil Adolesc Psychiatry*. 1996;35:101–109.

94. Safdar K, Schiff ER. Alcohol and hepatitis C. *Semin Liv Dis*. 2004;24:305–315.

95. Reference deleted in review.

96. Saxton J, Munro CA, et al. Alcohol, dementia, and Alzheimer's disease: comparison of neuropsychological profiles. *J Geriatr Psychiatry Neurol*. 2000;13:141–149.

97. Scaglione S, Kliethermes S, Shoham D, Durazo R, Luke A, Volk ML. The Epidemiology of cirrhosis in the United States: a population-based study. *J Clin Gastroenterol*. 2015;49(8):690–696. https://doi.org/10.1097/MCG.0000000000000208.

98. Schiff ER, Ozden N. Hepatitis C and alcohol. *Alcohol Res Health*. 2003;27:232–239.

99. Schuckit MA, Tipp JE, et al. An evaluation of type a and b alcoholics. *Addiction*. 1995;90:1189–1203.

100. Seitz HK, Sutter PM. Ethanol toxicity and nutritional status. In: Kotsonis FN, Mackey M, Hjelle J, eds. *Ethanol Toxicity and Nutritional Status*. New York: Raven; 1994.

101. Shimamura AP, Jernigan TL, Squire LR. Korsakoff's syndrome: radiological (CT) findings and neuropsychological correlates. *J Neurosci*. 1988;10:561–565.

102. Singal AK, Anand BS. Recent trends in the epidemiology of alcoholic liver disease. *Clinical Liver Disease*. 2013;2:53–56. https://doi.org/10.1002/cld.168.

103. Song SK, Rubin E. Ethanol produces muscle damage in human volunteers. *Science*. 1972;175:327–328.

104. Stasiewicz PR, Vincent PC, et al. Factors affecting agreement between severely mentally ill alcohol abusers' and collaterals' reports of alcohol and other substance abuse. *Psychol Addict Behav*. 2008;22:78–87.

105. Strakowski SM, DelBello MP, et al. Effects of co-occurring alcohol abuse on the course of bipolar disorder following a first hospitalization for mania. *Arch Gen Psychiatry*. 2005;62:851–858.

106. Streithguth AP, O'Malley K. Neuropsychiatric implications and long term consequences of fetal alcohol spectrum disorders. *Sem Clin Neuropsychiatry*. 2000;5:177–190.

107. Szlemko WJ, Wood JW, et al. Native Americans and alcohol: past, present, and future. *J Gen Psychol*. 2006;133:435–451.

108. Tan CH, Denny CH, Cheal NE, Sniezek JE, Kanny D. Alcohol use and binge drinking among women of childbearing age-united states, 2011-2013. *MMWR: Morbid Mortal Weekly Rep.* 2015;25(37):1042–1046.

109. Temple MT, Fillmore KM. The variability of drinking patterns and problems among young men, age 16–31: a longitudinal study. *Int J Addict.* 1985;20:1595–1620.

110. Urbano-Marquez A, Estruch R, Navarro-Lopez F, Grau JM, Mont L, Rubin E. The effects of alcoholism on skeletal and cardiac muscle. *N Engl J Med.* 1989;320:409–415.

111. Vaillant GE. Natural history of male psychological health: VIII. Antecedents of alcoholism and "orality." *Am J Psychiatry.* 1980;137:181–186.

112. Vaillant GE, Gale L, et al. Natural history of male alcoholism. II. The relationship between different diagnostic dimensions. *J Stud Alcohol.* 1982;43:216–232.

113. Victor M, Adams RD, Collins GH. *The Wernicke's-Korsakoff Syndrome and Related Neurologic Disorders due to Alcoholism and Malnutrition.* Philadelphia, PA: FA Davis; 1989.

114. World Health Organization. *Global Status Report on Alcohol and Health;* 2014. Retrieved from http://www.who.int/substance_abuse/publications/global_alcohol_report/msb_gsr_2014_1.pdf?ua=1.

115. Young-Hee Y, Chen CM, Hsiao-ye Yi. *Liver Cirrhosis Mortality in the United States: National, State, and Regional Trends: 2000-2011.* Surveillance Report #100. Bethesda, MD: National Institute on Alcohol Abuse and Alcoholism; 2014.

22
Cocaine

ROBERT BEECH AND RAJITA SINHA

CHAPTER OUTLINE

Introduction

The effects of cocaine on the nervous system have been studied for more than a hundred years. Early observers noted that among the symptoms produced by frequent cocaine use, one of the most prominent was cocaine craving.[54] In time, this craving for cocaine develops into a disorder termed cocaine dependence or addiction. Cocaine addiction is a chronic disorder characterized by compulsive drug seeking, frequent relapses, and continued drug use despite negative consequences.[31,41,58] On a personal level, the disease is associated with devastating consequences including loss of employment, disruption of marriage and family stability, risk of imprisonment, and associated health risks such as viral hepatitis and HIV.[26,52,139]

On a societal level, the costs associated with cocaine addiction include increases in violent crime, increased prevalence of blood-borne/sexually transmitted infections, and a soaring population of incarcerated addicts.[44] Data from 2014 indicate that there were 1.5 million current cocaine users 12 years of age or older in the United States.[141] Although this is decreased from previous years, it still represents a significant public health burden. Worldwide, rates of cocaine use remain high despite a decline in Europe and the United States, and access to treatment is extremely limited.[171] In this chapter we review the definitions and diagnostic criteria for the various cocaine-related disorders as well as the current understanding of the molecular biological basis for these disorders and current approaches to treatment.

Historical Aspects

Cocaine is a naturally occurring substance derived from the leaves of the *Erythroxylum coca* plant. Its use is thought to have originated more than 5000 years ago in religious ceremonies among the ancient civilizations of South America, but was greatly increased following the conquest of South America by the Spanish, who valued its effects in decreasing appetite and increasing stamina in the slaves who worked in the silver mines.[57,74,175] The first chemical purification of cocaine was achieved by Albert Niemann in 1860 and shortly thereafter it was incorporated into a variety of patent medicines and "tonics," including the original recipe for Coca-Cola, which was marketed as a temperance drink, "offering the virtues of coca, without the vices of alcohol."[57] Its use was promoted by several prominent figures of the time, perhaps most notably by Sigmund Freud.[57,74] Growing concern about the potential toxicity of cocaine helped lead to the passage of the Harrison Narcotics Tax Act in 1914. However, cocaine continued to be sold over the counter in the United States in a variety of forms until 1916.

Sex and Gender Differences

A variety of studies over the past decade have shown that the responses of men and women to cocaine differ markedly in several important aspects.[42,49,114] These differences extend to all phases of the addictive process including induction, maintenance, relapse, and response to treatment. Compared to men, women have been reported to initiate cocaine use at later ages, but progress more rapidly from first use to dependence, a phenomenon termed "telescoping."[180] Women have also been reported to experience decreased subjective effects of cocaine, including both positive ("feel high") and negative ("paranoid/suspicious," "heart racing/pounding") effects,[163] a phenomenon that may be partly explained by the lower peak blood levels of cocaine observed in women after administration of a the same dose of cocaine,[100] although other studies have reported an increase in negative nervousness effects among women.[89] Cocaine-dependent women have also been reported to differ from their male counterparts in their subjective[4] and physiological[47] response to stress, factors that may place them at increased risk for stress-induced relapse after an initial period of sobriety.[49] This is consistent with recent findings that severity of childhood trauma is predictive of cocaine-relapse outcomes in women but not men.[70] Cocaine-dependent women have also been reported to have a higher incidence of psychiatric, medical, social/family, and employment problems than men.[114] Moreover, cocaine-dependent men and women may have differential responses to treatment for cocaine dependence. A recent meta-analysis[33] found that compared with men, women had poorer treatment outcomes on multiple measures of cocaine use during treatment and at posttreatment follow-up. These differences may relate to the finding that disulfiram appears to be less effective in women than in men (see section below on treatment).

Animal studies have shown that estrogen and progesterone have opposing effects on cocaine-enhanced behavioral responses, with estrogen generally increasing sensitivity to the behavioral effects of cocaine while progesterone blunts those effects.[46] Recently, progesterone was found to reduce reinstatement of cocaine-seeking behavior in female rats, but not in male rats, while the combination of progesterone and the norepinephrine reuptake inhibitor, atomoxetine, was effective in both male and female rats.[168] Progesterone has been found to decrease the effects of smoked cocaine in women, but not in men.[38] Pregnancy is a condition during which levels of progesterone naturally rise by several-fold. Pregnancy is also a time when cocaine-dependent women often reduce their use of cocaine, with a resumption of cocaine use after delivery when progesterone levels fall. A recent pilot study found evidence that exogenous progesterone, given after delivery, could reduce the self-reported days of cocaine use during a 12-week trial compared to placebo, although there was no significant difference in the proportion of women with urine tests that are positive for cocaine.[185]

In addition, progesterone has differential effects on response to stress, with women but not men reporting lower rates of stress-induced negative emotion if they were treated with progesterone.[50] These effects may be mediated by the conversion of progesterone to the neuroactive steroid allopregnanolone (ALLO). A recent study in our lab found that exogenous progesterone increased levels of ALLO. This was associated with normalized basal and stress response levels of cortisol, decreased cocaine craving, and improvements in positive emotion and Stroop performance in response to stress and drug-cue exposures.[110] These findings highlight the need to consider individual factors including gender when discussing both the pathophysiology and approaches to treatment for cocaine dependence.

Pregnancy and Effects of Prenatal Exposure

The increasing prevalence in recent years of cocaine use among women of childbearing age has significance not only for the women themselves, but for the potential consequences to children exposed in utero. The pathophysiology of cocaine's effects on the developing nervous system has been conceptualized as occurring along three interrelated pathways.[93] The first of these is the direct neurochemical effects of cocaine on the developing nervous system, the second are sequelae related to the vasoconstrictive effects of cocaine on both the fetal and placental vessels. Finally, and perhaps most insidious are the epigenetic changes that may be induced by cocaine's effects on the developing brain, leading to long-term changes in both reward and stress-related circuits in the brain.[92,184] Studies using animal models of in utero cocaine exposure, suggest that there may be latent differences in neurocircuitry that are not revealed until the offspring are exposed to various stressors in adulthood.[20] Moreover, neuroimaging studies of adolescents who were exposed prenatally to cocaine confirm the presence of subtle differences in brain activation.[32] These differences in brain function may interact with various environmental factors to increase the risk for a variety of adverse outcomes including the development of cocaine dependence. An ongoing longitudinal study of a cohort of children who were exposed to cocaine in utero and followed from the fourth gestational month found that exposure to cocaine during the first trimester was associated with self-reported delinquent behavior; poorer problem solving and abstract reasoning; and reduced weight, height, and head circumference at 15 years of age.[134] Additional effects of cocaine during pregnancy and development are discussed in Chapter 71.

Youth

Data from the National Institute on Drug Abuse (NIDA) Monitoring the Future Study[125] show that cocaine use among youth has declined somewhat over the past four years. Lifetime use of cocaine among 8th graders decreased from 1.9% in 2012 to 1.6% in 2015. Among 10th graders it decreased from 3.3% to 2.7%, and among 12th graders from 4.9% to 4.0%. Furthermore, all of these numbers represent a substantial decrease from the peak levels seen in the late 1970s and early 1980s,[124] suggesting that efforts aimed at primary prevention are having some effect. However, given the devastating consequences associated with cocaine abuse and dependence, these numbers are certainly not cause for complacency.

Criminality

Studies conducted in the 1990s have suggested that the arrival of crack cocaine in urban centers in the United States and elsewhere was associated with a significant increase in the rates of a variety of types of crime.[8,60] Concerns about the relationship between cocaine use and criminality have resurfaced at the end of the first decade of the 21st century in connection with the drug wars taking place in Columbia and along Mexico's northern border.

Broadly speaking, the relationship between cocaine use and criminality can be considered in (at least) two complementary ways. The first is the relationship between cocaine use and criminality on the local level by users and small-scale dealers of cocaine (frequently these groups overlap). The second is the relationship between the illegal sale of cocaine and criminality on the national or international scale. On the individual level, cocaine use and dependence clearly increase the likelihood of engaging in other criminal activity including prostitution, theft, and violent crime.[26,71] Conversely, successful treatment of substance dependence is associated with decreased likelihood of re-offending among substance abusers in the criminal justice system.[126] On the national and international scale, the funds provided to international criminal organizations through the sale of illegal drugs and the violence perpetrated by these organizations can undermine the stability of entire nations and regions.[5] These findings highlight the need for new approaches to treatment for cocaine-abusing individuals in the criminal justice system, as well as improved national and international efforts to direct treatment to persons in need.

Cocaine Use Disorder

Definition/Diagnostic Criteria

Cocaine addiction or dependence can be conceptualized in a number of different ways. As defined by the *Diagnostic and Statistical Manual of Mental Disorders, Fifth Edition* (DSM-5),[1] the previous categories of "cocaine dependence" and "cocaine abuse" have been combined into a single category termed "cocaine use disorder," with modifiers for "mild," "moderate," or "severe," depending on the number of diagnostic criteria met by the individual. Diagnosis of stimulant use disorder is based on the same criteria used to diagnose substance use disorders involving other drugs of abuse. These include the presence of at least two of the following within the past year[1]:

1. Taking cocaine in larger amounts or over a longer period than was intended.
2. Persistent desire or unsuccessful efforts to cut down or control cocaine use.
3. Spending a great deal of time in activities necessary to obtain cocaine, use cocaine, or recover from its effects.
4. Craving, or a strong desire or urge to use cocaine.
5. Failure to fulfill major role obligations at work, school, or home as a result of recurrent cocaine use.

6. Continued cocaine use despite persistent or recurrent social or interpersonal problems caused or exacerbated by the effects of cocaine.
7. Giving up or reducing important social, occupational, or recreational activities because of cocaine use.
8. Repeatedly using cocaine in situations in which it is physically hazardous.
9. Continued cocaine use despite persistent or recurrent physical or psychological problems caused or exacerbated by cocaine.
10. Tolerance, as defined by either of the following:
    - Needing increased amounts of cocaine to achieve intoxication or desired effects.
    - Diminished effects with continued use of the same amount of cocaine.
11. Withdrawal, as manifested by either of the following:
    - The characteristic withdrawal syndrome for cocaine (see section on cocaine withdrawal, below).
    - Cocaine (or a closely related substance) is taken to relieve or avoid withdrawal symptoms.

Patients who meet two to three of these criteria are classified as a having a mild substance use disorder, those meeting four or five criteria would be classified as moderate, and those meeting six or more criteria would be classified as severe.

Note that this definition does not require the presence of physiological dependence, although the presence of physiological dependence may contribute to making the diagnosis (i.e., criteria 10 or 11 in the preceding text). Rather, as conceptualized in DSM-5, the diagnosis of Cocaine use disorder is made primarily based on the pattern of maladaptive behavior associated with its use. Moreover, when symptoms of tolerance and withdrawal are associated with appropriate medical treatment with prescribed medications (e.g., use of stimulants to treat attention-deficit/hyperactivity disorder [ADHD]), those symptoms are specifically NOT counted toward a diagnosis of a substance use disorder. However, since there are no US Food and Drug Administration (FDA)–approved indications for cocaine, symptoms of tolerance and withdrawal should be counted toward a diagnosis of cocaine use disorder.

Physiological dependence on cocaine is characterized by tolerance (criteria 10, above) and the occurrence of specific withdrawal symptoms when use is stopped. Symptoms of cocaine withdrawal include cocaine craving, depressed mood, sleep disturbance, appetite disturbance, and increased anxiety.[13,14,27,162] These symptoms have been incorporated into the current diagnostic criteria for cocaine withdrawal (discussed in subsequent text) and standardized instruments have been developed for rating the severity of these symptoms.[80]

Molecular/Biological Basis

Development of cocaine dependence is thought to be due to long-term consequences of repeated cocaine use in several areas of the brain, particularly those related to processing of reward-related information and executive control of behavior.[39,101,183] Molecular changes that occur following chronic administration of cocaine include changes in both dopaminergic[94] and glutamatergic[145] signaling pathways. Chronic administration of cocaine increases the expression of a number of important genes including tyrosine hydroxylase (TH), the rate-limiting enzymes in dopamine synthesis, glutamate receptor GluR1, and the transcription factor Δ FosB.[119] These effects are mediated, at least in part, by the transcription factor cyclic AMP (cAMP) response element binding protein (CREB).[117] More recent work has focused on the role of epigenetic mechanisms in maintaining the altered state of brain circuitry through long-lasting changes in gene expression.[81,120] These mechanisms include changes in DNA methylation and the expression and phosphorylation state of methyl CpG binding protein 2 (MeCP2)[3]; changes in histone acetylation and methylation[174]; changes in RNA-binding proteins[16]; and changes in the expression of noncoding RNAs (microRNAs) that regulate the half-life and expression of coding RNAs.[35]

Studies in animals show that the effects of cocaine use on the brain can be extremely long lasting, and in some cases can continue to increase during a period of abstinence such that the abstinent user, far from being back to normal after a brief or even a prolonged period of abstinence, may be even more sensitive to drug-related cues than someone who is actively using.[146,183] In addition to the changes in brain chemistry described earlier, long-term exposure to cocaine can also cause structural changes in the brain. In particular, long-term exposure to cocaine can increase the number of dendritic branches and the density of spines in a part of the brain called the nucleus accumbens,[136,145] part of the limbic system that regulates our response to natural rewards such as food or sex. Dendrites, and more specifically dendritic spines, are the specialized parts of brain cells that receive input from other cells and other brain regions. Changes in the number and structure of dendritic branches in the nucleus accumbens may account for some of the extremely long-lasting changes in brain function seen in cocaine addiction.[79,116,145] With this in mind, treatment strategies for cocaine dependence must focus on long-term treatment outcomes and developing strategies for preventing or minimizing the impact of relapses over the lifetime of the cocaine-dependent patient.

Treatment Approaches

Pharmacologic Treatments for Cocaine Dependence

Strategies for treating cocaine dependence include both pharmacologic treatments (discussed below) and nonpharmacologic treatments.[36] Several classes of medications have been investigated in clinical trials with patients with cocaine dependence. These include anticonvulsants,[112] antidepressants,[130] antipsychotics,[72,83] dopamine agonists,[111] and other psychostimulants,[104,167] and even cocaine vaccines.[88] Unfortunately, most of these trials have failed to demonstrate clinical meaningful results and none of these treatments is currently approved by the FDA for the treatment of cocaine dependence.[82] Additional details on two groups of medications, those targeting γ-aminobutyric acid (GABA)ergic and dopaminergic synapses, are provided below.

GABAergic Medications

GABAergic medications studied for the treatment of cocaine dependence include topiramate, baclofen, tiagabine, and vigabatrin. Topiramate is an anticonvulsant medication with activity at a variety of different ion channels and receptors including voltage-activated Na^+ channels, high voltage-activated Ca^{2+} channels, $GABA_A$ receptors, and α-amino-3-hydroxy-5-methyl-4-isoxazolepropionic acid (AMPA)/kainate receptors.[147] Topiramate is FDA approved for treatment and prophylaxis of migraine headache in adults and has been examined in a number of studies as a possible treatment for cocaine dependence. However, a recent meta-analysis[155] concluded that current evidence does not support the use of topiramate for cocaine-use disorder.

Baclofen is a $GABA_B$ agonist that is used primarily to treat muscle spasticity.[122] Animal studies have shown that baclofen inhibits cocaine-induced dopamine release in the nucleus accumbens.[40] In humans, initial open label trials indicated that baclofen might reduce cocaine craving.[96] However, results from two double-blind, placebo-controlled trials showed no significant overall difference between baclofen-treated and placebo-treated subjects.[76,149] Tiagabine inhibits the reuptake of GABA, and thus acts as an indirect GABA agonist.[91] It is FDA approved as an adjunct medication for the treatment of partial seizures. In a double-blind, placebo-controlled trial of methadone-maintained cocaine-dependent patients treated with tiagabine (24 mg/day; n = 25) versus gabapentin (n = 26) or placebo (n = 25), there was reduced cocaine use in the tiagabine compared to the other two groups.[59] However, in two other double-blind, placebo-controlled trials of tiagabine (20 mg/day) in cocaine-dependent subjects there was no difference between the tiagabine and the placebo groups.[181,182] Thus available evidence does not support the use of tiagabine to treat cocaine dependence.[112]

Vigabatrin is an irreversible inhibitor of GABA transaminase (GABA-T), the enzyme that breaks down GABA, and thus serves to increase GABAergic neurotransmission.[51] A series of open-label treatment studies[11,12,43] of vigabatrin in cocaine- and/or methamphetamine-abusing subjects suggested that vigabatrin might be helpful in reducing cocaine use. To date, there have been two double-blind, placebo-controlled trials of vigabatrin in subjects with cocaine dependence.[10,164] The first of these studies[10] was conducted with treatment-seeking Mexican parolees who were randomized to vigabatrin (n = 50) or placebo (n = 53) for 9 weeks with a 4-week follow-up assessment. The investigators found a greater rate of abstinence during the last 3 weeks of the trial in the vigabatrin group (28%, 14 subjects) compared to placebo (7.5%, 4 subjects). In addition, they found a higher rate of abstinence from alcohol among subjects who were initially using both substances in the vigabatrin group (43.4%, 10 subjects) compared to placebo (6.3%, 1 subject). The second study[164] was a 12-week trial with follow-up visits at weeks 13, 16, 20, and 24 conducted in 11 US sites, and included 186 subjects randomized to vigabatrin (n = 92) or placebo (n = 94). Unfortunately, this trial found no differences between vigabatrin and placebo in any of the primary or secondary outcomes. It is unclear if the differences between the two studies relate to the subjects studied (Mexican parolees versus general US population), length of trial, or other unknown variables. However, due to the negative outcome in the larger US study, a recent meta-analysis concluded that the available data do not support the use of vigabatrin (or any other anticonvulsant) for treatment of cocaine dependence.[112]

Dopaminergic Agents

Based on the successful use of replacement strategies for the treatment of opiate and nicotine dependence, a number of investigators have explored the possible use of agents that, like cocaine, lead to activation of dopamine receptors.[104,167] Dopaminergic agents evaluated for the treatment of cocaine dependence include bupropion, carbidopa/levodopa, amantadine, and a number of different stimulants used for the treatment of ADHD.

Bupropion, an atypical antidepressant that inhibits reuptake of both norepinephrine and dopamine, also acts as an antagonist at nicotinic acetylcholine receptors.[53] In a 12-week, placebo-controlled, randomized double-blind trial in methadone-maintained subjects[103] bupropion was not effective in reducing cocaine use. A later study by the same group that combined bupropion with contingency management (CM) found that bupropion (300 mg/d) potentiated the effect of CM in reducing cocaine use but had no effect in patients receiving noncontingent rewards.[132] A more recent study of bupropion in combination with cognitive behavioral therapy,[148] found no benefit of bupropion over placebo.

The combination of carbidopa and levodopa is a mainstay in the treatment of Parkinson disease.[127] Levodopa is the precursor of dopamine. Carbidopa is an inhibitor of dopa decarboxylase that does not cross the blood-brain barrier. By inhibiting the decarboxylation of levodopa in the circulation, the combination of levodopa and carbidopa allows higher concentrations of levodopa to reach the brain, and thus increases the amount of dopamine that is synthesized. In principle, this combination might act to decrease cravings for cocaine during withdrawal, and/or exacerbate the aversive effects of cocaine use in a manner similar to that proposed for disulfiram (see below). To date, there have been six randomized, double blind, placebo-controlled trials evaluating the combination of levodopa and carbidopa for the treatment of cocaine dependence. A recent meta-analysis based on these studies found no difference between carbidopa/levodopa for any of the outcome measures examined.[111]

Amantadine is a weak, noncompetitive N-methyl-D-aspartate (NMDA) receptor antagonist that both increases dopamine release and blocks dopamine reuptake.[6,86] It is used in the treatment of both Parkinson disease and influenza. To date there have been 10 studies that compared amantadine with placebo for the treatment of cocaine dependence, and an additional 5 studies that compared amantadine with an antidepressant (4 with desipramine and 1 with fluoxetine). Meta-analysis of these data showed no benefit of amantadine over either placebo or antidepressant treatment.[111]

Other stimulants evaluated for the treatment of cocaine dependence include bromocriptine cabergoline, mazindol, dextroamphetamine, methylphenidate, and modafinil. Like cocaine, all of these drugs inhibit the reuptake of dopamine or directly activate dopamine receptors, and thus can be considered as a form of replacement therapy, analogous to the well-known use of methadone in the treatment of opiate dependence. However, a recent meta-analyses[111] found no evidence of decreased cocaine use or improved retention, either for stimulants as a class of medications or for any individual medication in this class.

An alternative strategy involves the use of dopamine antagonists or partial agonists to block the reinforcing effects of cocaine-induced increases in dopaminergic signaling. Dopamine antagonists or partial agonists studied for the treatment of cocaine dependence include conventional, or typical, antipsychotic medications, which block signaling primarily at dopamine D_2 receptors, and newer, atypical antipsychotic medications, which in addition to D_2 receptors (among other receptors), also block signaling at serotonin $5HT_{2}A$ and $5HT_{2}C$ receptors, resulting in a different side-effect profile, and possibly differences in target symptoms in the treatment of schizophrenia.[166] Animal studies have suggested that treatment with typical antipsychotic medications can either decrease[133] or increase[87,135] self-administration of cocaine. A 2016 Cochrane Database Systematic Review[72] examined the evidence supporting the use of antipsychotic medications for cocaine dependence including risperidone, olanzapine, quetiapine, lamotrigine, aripiprazole, haloperidol, and reserpine, and concluded that the available evidence does not support the use of any antipsychotic medication in the treatment of cocaine dependence. One study reported that patients receiving quetiapine showed reductions in weekly cocaine use and craving; however, this outcome did not differ significantly from placebo.[169]

Medications Targeting Other Mechanisms: Dopamine-β-Hydroxylase

Disulfiram is an inhibitor of acetaldehyde dehydrogenase used in the treatment of alcohol dependence. Inhibition of acetaldehyde dehydrogenase leads to an accumulation of acetaldehyde, an intermediate in the metabolism of alcohol, and leads to symptoms similar to a severe hangover, including skin flushing, rapid heart rate, shortness of breath, nausea, vomiting, and throbbing headache. In severe cases it can cause visual disturbance, mental confusion, and even circulatory collapse. Disulfiram also inhibits dopamine-β-hydroxylase (DBH), one of the key enzymes involved in the catabolism of dopamine.[177] Elevated levels of dopamine may help to attenuate cocaine craving. On the other hand, in the presence of cocaine or other stimulants, inhibition of DBH may lead to a dramatic rise in synaptic dopamine levels, resulting in insomnia, paranoia, and, in extreme cases, stimulant psychosis.[61] A meta-analysis published in 2010 of data from seven trials of disulfiram for treatment of cocaine dependence (four compared to placebo and three compared to naloxone) found only "low evidence, at the present, supporting the clinical use of disulfiram for the treatment of cocaine dependence."[129] This was based in part on the authors' conclusions that available data showed "low quality of evidence, due to study design, small sample size and heterogeneity in terms of outcome operational definition." Moreover, gender analyses of these trials indicate that the positive effects reported for disulfiram in the treatment of cocaine dependence come largely from benefit in men and not women.[33,123]

More recent studies of disulfiram in the treatment of cocaine dependence have focused on the role of possible role of specific gene variants in explaining some of the observed heterogeneity in the response to disulfiram. Studied gene variants include DPH (the enzyme that catalyzes the conversion of dopamine to norepinephrine),[90] ANKK1 (ankyrin repeat and kinase domain containing 1, which regulates the synthesis of dopamine in the brain[121]), and the D_2 dopamine receptor[165] and the alpha1 adrenergic-receptor gene.[150] These results hold out the promise that the decision to treat (or not treat) cocaine dependence with disulfiram could be based on tests for specific gene variants that could influence treatment outcome. However, all of these findings are preliminary and have yet to be replicated in larger studies.

Nonpharmacologic Treatments for Cocaine Dependence

Nonpharmacologic treatments for cocaine dependence include a variety of individual psychotherapies,[28,138] group therapies,[176] and 12-step programs such as Narcotics Anonymous. Not surprisingly perhaps, the primary determinant of outcome for most such psychosocial treatments appears to be length of retention in treatment, with better outcomes generally reported by those treated 90 days or longer in both residential and outpatient settings.[154] These findings reinforce the need to focus on long-term outcomes and relapse prevention as the primary goal of treatments (both pharmacological and psychosocial) for cocaine dependence. Specific psychotherapeutic approaches to the treatment of cocaine dependence are discussed in more detail in the section on craving and relapse.

Intoxication

Definition/Diagnostic Criteria

Acute cocaine intoxication is typically characterized by a high feeling and stimulant effects including euphoria, increased pulse and blood pressure, and psychomotor activation. It can also include any of the following: alertness, anger, anxiety, belligerence, cognitive impairment, gregariousness, grandiosity, hyperactivity, hypervigilance, impaired judgment, impaired social and occupational functioning, interpersonal sensitivity, mood lability, restlessness, stereotyped and repetitive behavior, increased talkativeness, and tension. With chronic intoxication there can also be depressant effects such as social withdrawal, sadness, bradycardia, decreased blood pressure, and decreased psychomotor activity. Both acute and chronic intoxication are associated with impaired social and occupational function. Severe intoxication is associated with a number of medical complications including seizures, cardiac arrhythmias, hyperpyrexia, and vasoconstriction, leading to increased risk for myocardial infarction, stroke, and even death. Diagnostic criteria for cocaine intoxication include

A. Recent use of cocaine.
B. A clinically significant maladaptive behavioral or psychological changes (described above) that develops during or shortly after use of cocaine.
C. Two (or more) of the following physical symptoms:
   1. tachycardia or bradycardia
   2. papillary dilation
   3. altered blood pressure (elevated or lowered)
   4. chills or perspiration
   5. nausea or vomiting
   6. evidence of weight loss
   7. psychomotor agitation or retardation
   8. muscular weakness, respiratory depression, chest pain, or cardiac arrhythmias
   9. confusion, seizures, dyskinesias, dystonias, or coma
D. The symptoms observed are not due to a general medical condition or better accounted for by another mental disorder.[2]

Molecular/Biological Basis

Cocaine, administered by any of the commonly used routes including snorting, smoking, and intravenous injection, enters the bloodstream and rapidly crosses the blood-brain barrier. Although cocaine inhibits reuptake of all three monoamine neurotransmitters (dopamine, norepinephrine, and serotonin), both the acute effect of cocaine and the long-term changes responsible for the development of cocaine dependence are thought to be related primarily to its effects on dopamine signaling.[118] The neurotransmitter dopamine is synthesized in a small number of specialized dopamine-producing (dopaminergic) cells in the brain, and serves to regulate a number of important physiological processes. In particular, dopaminergic signaling in the so-called limbic system, including the ventral tegmental area (which produces dopamine) and the nucleus accumbens (one of the main sites of dopamine's actions), functions to signal the presence of naturally occurring rewards. Cocaine inhibits the reuptake of the neurotransmitter dopamine from the synaptic cleft and thus prolongs its actions in the brain. Increased dopamine activity in the nucleus accumbens is thought to produce the high felt after cocaine use.[69,118] In addition to its effects on the brain, cocaine can have direct effects on the circulatory system, leading to increased blood pressure and risk for myocardial infarction and stroke.[9,84,173]

Treatment Approaches

There are no specific treatments for cocaine intoxication, and in most cases acute cocaine intoxication can be managed with supportive care. Benzodiazepines are considered first-line treatment for agitation associated with acute cocaine intoxication. Typical antipsychotic medications (e.g., perphenazine and haloperidol) can be used for treatment of paranoia or psychosis associated with cocaine intoxication; however, these should be used with caution because of the possibility of acute hyperthermia syndromes associated with acute cocaine intoxication, which may be confused with neuroleptic malignant syndrome.[66] Cardiac or neurological symptoms associated with severe intoxication may require referral to an intensive care unit. Patients who are pregnant will require additional monitoring, since vasoconstriction associated with cocaine intoxication may lead to premature delivery.

Given the chronic, relapsing nature of cocaine abuse and dependence it is important to focus, as soon as possible, on planning for long-term treatment and relapse prevention. In most cases referral to residential or other long-term treatment modalities can be made, even prior to the resolution of the acute symptoms associated with cocaine intoxication.

Withdrawal

Definition/Diagnostic Criteria

Withdrawal from cocaine occurs after cessation or reduction of heavy and prolonged cocaine use and is characterized by dysphoric mood and two or more of the following:

A. fatigue
B. vivid, unpleasant dreams
C. insomnia or hypersomnia
D. increased appetite
E. psychomotor retardation or agitation.

These symptoms must also cause clinically significant distress or impairment in social, occupational, or other important areas of functioning in order to be diagnosed as cocaine withdrawal.[2] In some cases this is associated with a profound depression and suicidal ideation and actions can occur.

Molecular/Biological Basis

Cocaine withdrawal is thought to occur as the result of long-term adaptations in brain physiology and functioning caused by prolonged exposure to cocaine. Such adaptations are generally homeostatic in nature.[85] That is to say, they oppose the acute effects of cocaine and enable the brain to function as well as possible despite the massive barrage of dopamine signaling induced by cocaine. The synaptic architecture and signaling properties of a number of brain regions, including the limbic system, frontal cortex, and amygdala, is reconfigured such that functioning in the presence of cocaine becomes the new normal. The abrupt withdrawal or reduction of cocaine intake is perceived as a state of dopamine deficiency, and triggers the occurrence of the symptoms described earlier, as well as an intense desire to resume cocaine use in order to restore what is now perceived as a normal level of functioning. Molecular changes associated with the development of cocaine withdrawal include the accumulation of the transcription factor ΔFosB and increased cAMP-CREB signaling in the medium spiny neurons of the nucleus accumbens, increases in tyrosine hydroxylase (the rate limiting enzyme in dopamine synthesis), and increased neurotrophin and CREB signaling in the ventral tegmental area where the dopaminergic projections to the nucleus accumbens originate. These changes have the net effect of decreasing basal dopamine signaling, but increasing cocaine-stimulated release of dopamine, and thus reduce to body's ability to respond to rewards other than cocaine.[106,117,118] It is notable that although the acute phase of cocaine withdrawal typically resolves within several days, some of the neuroadaptations induced by prolonged exposure to cocaine may persist for months or even longer, resulting in a heightened sensitivity to both cocaine and cocaine-associated cues.[102,146] Thus resolution of acute withdrawal symptoms does not imply that the patient is no longer dependent on cocaine.

Treatment Approaches

There are no specific treatments for cocaine withdrawal, and in most cases acute cocaine withdrawal can be managed with supportive care. Mood changes including depression, irritability, anhedonia, emotional lability and disturbances in attention and concentration are common. In some instances, cocaine withdrawal can be associated with a profound depressive state, and suicidal ideation and actions are not infrequent. In these cases, hospitalization to prevent self-harm may be necessary. As noted above, resolution of acute withdrawal symptoms should not be construed as implying that the patient is no longer dependent on cocaine. Therefore, as soon as possible, the focus of treatment should shift to planning for long-term treatment. Ideally this should include referral to residential or other long-term treatment modalities with a focus on relapse prevention.

Craving and Relapse

Definition/Diagnostic Criteria

Cocaine craving and relapse are not specific diagnoses but are associated with all cocaine-related disorders. As discussed above, prolonged use of cocaine results in an intense desire to consume more cocaine. This effect has been noted for over 100 years[54] and is one reason that cocaine dependence is so difficult to treat. Relapse refers to the resumption of drug use after a period of abstinence. However, defining relapse in cocaine users is complex, since many users frequently engage in binge and other styles of periodic use, such that short intervals of abstinence are the rule even among current users.[62] Factors associated with increased risk for relapse include current levels of cocaine craving, exposure to stress or drug-related cues, and history of childhood abuse.[70,128,157]

Molecular/Biological Basis

As discussed in the preceding text, prolonged exposure to cocaine or other drugs of abuse produces homeostatic changes in the brain, such that it is no longer able to function normally in the absence of the abused drug.[85] Changes in glutamatergic signaling from the anterior cingulate and orbitofrontal cortex to the nucleus accumbens may be important in the transition from abuse to dependence (end-stage addiction).[78,79] Animal studies suggest roles for the basolateral amygdala in cue-primed reinstatement, the ventral tegmental area in drug-primed reinstatement, and adrenergic innervation of the extended amygdala in stress-primed reinstatement.[78] All three forms of priming may converge on the anterior cingulate cortex and have a final common output through the core of the nucleus accumbens. Neuroimaging studies also support a role for the projections from the anterior cingulate and orbitofrontal cortex to the nucleus accumbens in drug addiction.[22,58,79]

Parallel evidence from human laboratory and relapse outcome studies also substantiate preclinical evidence of neuroadaptations in brain stress and reward pathways that are associated with increased stress- and drug cue–induced drug craving, anxiety and dysfunctional physiological, and neuroendocrine responses in treatment-engaged cocaine-dependent individuals as compared to healthy social drinkers.[48,129,156] Stress- and cue-induced cocaine craving and neuroendocrine responses have been shown to predict cocaine relapse outcomes.[128,156] Brain imaging studies of stress- and drug cue–induced cocaine craving show specific positive association with the dorsal striatum regions,[158,159] whereas inhibitory control deficits show decreased activity in the prefrontal and anterior cingulated regions in cocaine-dependent individuals.[95]

Treatment Approaches

Treatments for cocaine craving and relapse are at the heart of all treatments for cocaine addiction. These include both pharmacologic and nonpharmacologic treatments. As discussed above, pharmacological approaches to the treatment of cocaine addiction include dopaminergic, GABAergic, and glutamatergic agents, although none are specifically approved by the FDA for this use.[36] Psychosocial approaches to the treatment of cocaine craving and relapse include contingency management, relapse prevention, general cognitive behavior therapy, and treatments combining cognitive behavior therapy and contingency management.[36] Contingency management interventions are based on principles of operant conditioning and offer monetary and/or nonmonetary rewards that are contingent on negative toxicology screens, indicating abstinence from drug use.[64] This approach has been evaluated in several controlled trials,[63,75,151-153] and has shown consistent, if modest, effects in reducing relapse (reviewed in Dutra et al.[36]). Potential barriers to more widespread use of this approach include costs associated with monetary incentives and frequent drug testing as well as social prohibitions against paying drug users for good behavior. However, some studies have found that contingency management approaches using prizes worth from $1 to $100 can achieve short-term abstinence with a lower per-patient cost.[131]

Relapse prevention is an alternative approach that focuses on identifying high-risk situations for relapse to drug use and avoiding or managing these situations by rehearsing alternative responses. Several studies have evaluated the effectiveness of relapse prevention techniques in cocaine-dependent subjects with mixed results. A 1991 study by Carroll et al.,[18] that compared relapse prevention therapy (RPT) to interpersonal psychotherapy (IPT) found no significant main effect for treatment. However, among the subgroup of more severe users, subjects who received RPT were significantly more likely to achieve abstinence (54% versus 9%) and be classified as recovered (54% versus 0%) than those who received IPT, while among the less severely addicted group there was no difference between the two treatments. A 1994 study by the same group comparing RPT to pharmacologic treatment with the antidepressant imipramine or a combination of RPT + desipramine found no significant effects in outcome for either RPT or medication. However, a 1-year follow-up study showed evidence of significant continuing improvement among the group who had received RPT.[19] Another study comparing RPT to 12-step programs in a group of 110 treatment-seeking subjects found no difference between the two treatments.[179] Thus the available evidence is limited and does not strongly support RPT over other approaches to treating cocaine craving and relapse.

Intoxication Delirium

Definition/Diagnostic Criteria

Cocaine intoxication-induced delirium refers to an acute disturbance in consciousness and cognition that occurs during cocaine intoxication, is in excess of the cognitive disturbances usually associated with cocaine intoxication, and when the symptoms are sufficiently severe to warrant independent clinical attention. Diagnostic criteria for cocaine intoxication-induced delirium are identical to those for other substance-induced deliriums and include:

A. Disturbance of consciousness (i.e., reduced clarity of awareness of the environment) with reduced ability to focus, sustain, or shift attention.
B. A change in cognition (such as memory deficit, disorientation, language disturbance) or the development of a perceptual disturbance that is not better accounted for by a preexisting, established, or evolving dementia.
C. The disturbance develops over a short period of time (usually hours to days) and tends to fluctuate during the course of the day.
D. Evidence from the history, physical examination, or laboratory findings that these symptoms (1) developed during the course of cocaine intoxication, and/or (2) cocaine use is etiologically related to the disturbance in consciousness.[2]

Molecular/Biological Basis

The precise molecular biological basis of cocaine intoxication-induced delirium is currently unknown. However, postmortem studies of patients with delirium or chronic cocaine abusers have shown reduced levels of the mRNA encoding the dopamine transporter (DAT)[21,97] and the transcription factor NURR1,[7] which regulates the expression of DAT. These changes would be expected to raise extracellular levels of dopamine in the brain, and thus interfere with the normal modulatory roles of dopamine on a variety of signaling mechanisms throughout the brain.

Treatment Approaches

There is no specific treatment of cocaine intoxication-induced delirium, and in most cases the delirium can be managed with supportive care. However, such patients will require more intensive monitoring than patients with typical cocaine intoxication, due to the elevated risk for cocaine-induced rhabdomyolysis.[140] Hyperthermia in patients with cocaine intoxication can be a sign of impending rhabdomyolysis. This condition must be recognized early to prevent secondary renal failure. Treatment of rhabdomyolysis focuses on ensuring adequate urine output and, possibly, alkalization of the urine. Dialysis may be necessary in extreme cases.[68] One study found that 24% of patients presenting to the emergency room for acute cocaine-related disorders had some degree of rhabdomyolysis, many of which were not apparent from the clinical history or physical examination making laboratory assessment, including measurement of serum creatinine phosphokinase and urinary myoglobin, an essential part of the evaluation and treatment of such patients.[178] Cardiac monitoring should also be considered given the risk of cocaine-induced arrhythmias, vasoconstriction, and myocardial infarction.[34]

Cocaine-Induced Psychotic Disorder

Definition/Diagnostic Criteria

Cocaine-induced psychotic disorder refers to the presence of psychotic symptoms in excess of those typically seen in patients with cocaine intoxication or withdrawal. These can include delusions or hallucinations or both. Delusions may be of any type but typically are paranoid and/or grandiose in nature. Diagnostic criteria for this disorder are the same as those used to diagnose other substance-induced psychotic disorders, and include:

A. Prominent hallucinations or delusions. Note: Do not include hallucinations if the person has insight that they are substance induced.
B. Evidence from the history, physical examination, or laboratory findings that these symptoms (1) developed during the course of cocaine intoxication or withdrawal, and/or (2) cocaine use is etiologically related to the development of psychotic symptoms.
C. The disturbance is not better accounted for by a psychotic disorder that is not substance induced. Evidence that the symptoms are better accounted for by a primary psychotic disorder that is not substance induced might include the following:
   • psychotic symptoms that precede the onset of cocaine use;
   • psychotic symptoms that persist for a substantial period of time (e.g., about a month) after the cessation of acute withdrawal or severe intoxication;
   • other evidence that suggests the existence of an independent non–substance-induced psychotic disorder (e.g., a history of recurrent non–substance-related episodes).
D. The disturbance does not occur exclusively during the course of a delirium.[2]

Subtypes

• With delusions: This subtype is used if delusions are the predominant symptom.
• With hallucinations: This subtype is used if hallucinations are the predominant symptom.

Molecular/Biological Basis

The precise molecular/biological basis of cocaine-induced psychotic disorder is currently unknown. However, there is evidence for a genetic vulnerability to the development of psychotic symptoms in individuals who abuse cocaine. In particular, genetic variants associated with low plasma levels of DBH, an enzyme that converts dopamine to norepinephrine and thus affects the balance between these two neurotransmitters in the brain have been associated with increased risk for cocaine-induced psychotic symptoms.[29,77] Individuals with lower levels of DBH would be expected to have a higher ratio of dopamine to norepinephrine, and thus be more sensitive to drugs such as cocaine that lead to unbalanced dopamine signaling in the brain.

Treatment Approaches

There is no specific treatment for cocaine-induced psychosis, and in most cases the psychotic symptoms will resolve within a few days after cessation of cocaine use. Benzodiazepines can be used for patients who are agitated. Care must taken in using neuroleptics to treat cocaine-induced psychosis because most antipsychotic medications will increase the QTc interval and may thus increase the risk for cocaine-associated cardiac arrhythmias.[186]

Cocaine-Induced Anxiety Disorder

Definition/Diagnostic Criteria

Cocaine-induced anxiety disorder can occur during either cocaine intoxication or cocaine withdrawal. Like other substance-induced anxiety disorders, cocaine-induced anxiety disorder is distinguished from a primary anxiety disorder by the fact that a substance is judged to be etiologically related to the symptoms. Diagnostic criteria for this disorder are the same as those for other substance-induced anxiety disorders and include:

A. The presence of prominent anxiety, panic attacks, or obsessions or compulsions.
B. Evidence from the history, physical examination, or laboratory findings that these symptoms (1) developed during the course of cocaine intoxication or withdrawal, and/or (2) cocaine use is etiologically related to the development of psychotic symptoms.
C. The disturbance is not better accounted for by an anxiety disorder that is not substance induced. Evidence that the symptoms are better accounted for by an anxiety disorder that is not substance induced might include:
   • anxiety symptoms that precede the onset of cocaine use;
   • anxiety symptoms that persist for a substantial period of time (e.g., about a month) after the cessation of acute withdrawal or severe intoxication;
   • other evidence that suggests the existence of an independent non–substance-induced anxiety disorder (e.g., a history of recurrent non–substance-related episodes).

Molecular/Biological Basis

While the precise molecular biological basis of cocaine-induced anxiety disorder is unknown, it has been suggested that the development of cocaine-induced anxiety or panic symptoms can be explained in terms of limbic-neuronal hyperexcitability induced by cocaine through a kindling mechanism.[98]

Treatment Approaches

There is no specific treatment of this disorder, and in some cases the psychotic symptoms will resolve within a few days after cessation of cocaine use. In cases where the symptoms do not resolve following cessation of cocaine use, treatment of is usually similar to treatment for a primary anxiety disorder such as generalized anxiety disorder, phobias, panic disorder, or obsessive-compulsive disorder. It has been suggested that clonazepam and/or carbamazepine may be more effective in the treatment of cocaine-induced panic symptoms than shorter-acting benzodiazepines such as alprazolam, possibly because of their greater anticonvulsant properties.[98] Of note, antidepressants, and particularly tricyclic antidepressants, have been reported to ineffective in the treatment of cocaine-induced panic symptoms. One study found that 60% of patients with cocaine-induced panic symptoms experienced a worsening of their symptoms when treated with tricyclic antidepressants.[99]

Cocaine-Induced Mood Disorder

Definition/Diagnostic Criteria

Cocaine-induced mood disorder refers to a prominent and persistent disturbance in mood that is judged to be due to the direct physiological effects of cocaine. Diagnostic criteria for this disorder are the same as for other substance-induced mood disorders and include:

A. A prominent and persistent disturbance in mood predominates in the clinical picture and is characterized by either (or both) of the following: (1) depressed mood or markedly diminished interest or pleasure in all, or almost all, activities, or (2) elevated, expansive, or irritable mood
B. Evidence from the history, physical examination, or laboratory findings that these symptoms (1) developed during the course of cocaine intoxication or withdrawal, and/or (2) cocaine use is etiologically related to the development of psychotic symptoms.
C. The disturbance is not better accounted for by a mood disorder that is not substance induced.
D. The disturbance does not occur exclusively during the course of a delirium.[2]

Molecular/Biological Basis

The neurobiological mechanisms underlying the development of cocaine dependence and mood disorders share a number of similarities.[15,105] These include a prolonged activation of the hypothalamic-pituitary-adrenal (HPA) axis and overexpression of the neuropeptide corticotropin-releasing factor (CRF).[56] There is abundant evidence from both animal[37,142] and human[157,160] studies showing that stress, and the associated increase in HPA activity, can trigger relapse to cocaine use. Conversely, prolonged elevation of HPA activity as a result of chronic cocaine use may result in a negative affective state provides a powerful motivational force for the continuation of drug self-administration [85]. Treatments that target this heightened HPA activity may thus represent important potential treatments for both mood[65,115] and cocaine-induced mood disorders.[143]

Treatment Approaches

Mood disorders that are directly attributable to cocaine can be difficult to distinguish from the frequent case of comorbid cocaine abuse or dependence with a primary mood disorder, either major depression or bipolar disorder. By definition, substance-induced mood disorders arise only in association with intoxication or withdrawal states, whereas primary Mood Disorders may precede the onset of substance use or may occur during times of sustained abstinence. However, in many cases both cocaine use and mood symptoms are longstanding, and it may be difficult to identify significant periods of time when either was absent. In addition, because the withdrawal state for cocaine can be relatively protracted, mood symptoms can persist in an intense form for several weeks after the cessation of cocaine use. Features that would suggest a primary mood disorder include (1) persistence of mood symptoms for a substantial period of time (i.e., a month or more) after cessation of cocaine use, (2) the development of mood symptoms that are substantially in excess of what would be expected given the amount or the duration of cocaine use; or (3) a history of prior recurrent primary episodes of mood disorder.[2]

Both cocaine-induced and primary mood disorders require clinical attention, especially when symptoms have been persistent and severe prior to treatment. The preponderance of evidence from both randomized clinical trials (RCTs) that prospectively targeted both depression and cocaine dependence and RCTs in which post hoc analyses demonstrated efficacy in the subgroup of cocaine abusers with comorbid depression, appears to support the use of antidepressant medication in patients with comorbid major depression and cocaine dependence (reviewed in Rounsaville et al.[137] and Torrens et al.[170]). In general selective serotonin reuptake inhibitors (SSRIs) appear to work poorly in dually diagnosed patients (e.g., Cornelius et al.[25] and Schmitz et al.[144]), whereas positive studies have used agents such as desipramine[17,55] or bupropion[103] that are more activating.

Cocaine-Induced Sexual Dysfunction

Definition/Diagnostic Criteria

Cocaine-induced sexual dysfunction refers to a clinically significant sexual dysfunction that results in marked distress or interpersonal difficulty that is judged to be fully explained by the direct physiological effects of cocaine. Subtypes may include: cocaine-induced sexual dysfunction (1) with impaired desire, (2) with impaired arousal, (3) with impaired orgasm, and (4) with sexual pain.[2]

Molecular/Biological Basis

Acute administration of cocaine is associated with an increase in sexual drive, an effect that may be due to increased section of luteinizing hormone.[30,108] However, chronic cocaine use induces a number of neuroendocrine abnormalities, including alterations in levels of prolactin secretion[24,107] (hypothesized to occur as a result of increased dopamine depletion in the tubuloinfundibular tract[23,30]). Elevated levels of prolactin would be expected to inhibit pituitary gonadotroph secretion,[109] which may contribute to the development of cocaine-induced sexual dysfunction in some patients.

Treatment Approaches

Since by definition cocaine-induced sexual dysfunction is fully explained by the direct physiological effects of cocaine, the primary focus of treatment should be on cessation of cocaine use. Expected improvements in sexual functioning may become a motivating factor to seek treatment for some cocaine-dependent subjects. If sexual function does not return to normal following a prolonged period of abstinence (i.e., 1 month or more), consideration should be given to the possibility that the patient has a primary sexual dysfunction. Contributing psychological factors such as possible comorbid major depression or anxiety disorders should also be taken into consideration. Phosphodiesterase-5 inhibitors (sildenafil, tadalafil, vardenafil) are commonly prescribed. However, some studies suggest that these drugs are more commonly taken to enhance sexual experience than to treat erectile dysfunction,[67] and may contribute to unsafe sex practices[45] and the consequent risk for infection among active cocaine users as well as the risk for adverse cardiac events.[73,161] Thus, it is important to take a careful sexual history and discuss openly the associated risks and benefits before prescribing these medications.

Cocaine-Induced Sleep Disorder

Definition/Diagnostic Criteria

Cocaine-induced sleep disorder refers to a prominent disturbance in sleep sufficiently severe to warrant independent clinical attention that is judged to be due to the direct physiological effects of cocaine and does not occur exclusively during the course of a delirium. Subtypes may include insomnia type, hypersomnia type, parasomnia type, which include a variety of sleep-related disorders, including confusional arousals, sleepwalking (somnambulism), and sleep terrors (night terrors) or mixed type (i.e., if more than one sleep disturbance is present and none predominates).[2] The onset of the sleep disorder can occur either during intoxication or during withdrawal. The diagnosis of cocaine-induced sleep disorder is made only when the symptoms cause clinically significant distress or impairment in social, occupational, or other important areas of functioning and the symptoms are in excess of those usually associated with cocaine intoxication or withdrawal. Typically, cocaine intoxication produces insomnia, whereas cocaine withdrawal is associated with hypersomnia.

Molecular/Biological Basis

In addition to changes in the total number of hours slept, chronic cocaine use is associated with significant changes in sleep architecture and deficits in sleep-related cognitive performance (e.g., sleep-dependent learning).[113,172] It has been suggested that this may be due to alterations in GABA signaling that are the result of adaptation to repeated overstimulation of monoaminergic pathways.[113] Of interest, although self-reports of sleep quality typically improve following cocaine abstinence, polysomnographic studies have shown that changes in sleep architecture and sleep-related cognitive performance do not improve, at least over the first three weeks of abstinence, suggesting that there may be long-lasting deficits in sleep quality that occur as a result of chronic cocaine use that are not necessarily appreciated by the patients themselves.

Treatment Approaches

Alterations in sleep architecture that occur during prolonged withdrawal from cocaine (reviewed in Morgan and Malison[113]) include an initial suppression of rapid eye movement (REM) sleep, followed after about 3 days by a rebound in REM sleep and an increase in total hours of sleep. After 2.5 weeks of abstinence from cocaine, users have sleep architecture similar to patients with chronic insomnia, that is, increased sleep latency, decreased sleep efficiency (% time spent asleep while in bed), and decreased total hours of sleep. As discussed in Morgan and Malison[113], this suggests that agents such as tiagabine that improve slow-wave sleep and possibly deficits in sleep-related cognitive performance may be more beneficial than benzodiazepines, which extend sleep by promoting stage 2 sleep. Several of the GABAergic medications discussed earlier that are being tested for treatment of cocaine dependence (topiramate, baclofen, tiagabine, and vigabatrin) may also be helpful in treating cocaine-induced sleep disorders.

References

1. APA. *Diagnostic and Statistical Manual of Mental Disorders (DSM-5)*. 5th ed. Arlington, VA: American Psychiatric Publishing; 2013.
2. APA. *Diagnostic and Statistical Manual of Mental Disorders, Fourth Edition, Text Revision (DSM-IV-TR)*. Washington, DC: American Psychiatric Association; 2000.

3. Ausio J. MeCP2 and the enigmatic organization of brain chromatin. Implications for depression and cocaine addiction. *Clinical Epigenetics.* 2016;8:58.

4. Back SE, Brady KT, Jackson JL, Salstrom S, ZinzowH. Gender differences in stress reactivity among cocaine-dependent individuals. *Psychopharmacology (Berl).* 2005;180:169–176.

5. Bagley B. *Drug Trafficking and Organized Crime in the Americas: Major Trends in the Twenty-First Century Woodrow Wilson Center Update on the Americas.* Washington, DC: Woodrow Wilson International Center For Scholars; 2012.

6. Bailey EV, Stone TW. The mechanism of action of amantadine in Parkinsonism: a review. *Arch Int Pharmacodyn Ther.* 1975;216:246–262.

7. Bannon MJ, Pruetz B, Manning-Bog AB, et al. Decreased expression of the transcription factor NURR1 in dopamine neurons of cocaine abusers. *Proc Natl Acad Sci U S A.* 2002;99:6382–6385.

8. Baumer E. Poverty, crack, and crime: a cross-city analysis. *J Res Crime Delinq.* 1994;31:311–327.

9. Benzaquen BS, Cohen V, Eisenberg MJ. Effects of cocaine on the coronary arteries. *Am Heart J.* 2001;142:402–410.

10. Brodie JD, Case BG, Figueroa E, et al. Randomized, double-blind, placebo-controlled trial of vigabatrin for the treatment of cocaine dependence in Mexican parolees. *Am J Psychiatry.* 2009;166:1269–1277.

11. Brodie JD, Figueroa E, Dewey SL. Treating cocaine addiction: from preclinical to clinical trial experience with gamma-vinyl GABA. *Synapse.* 2003;50:261–265.

12. Brodie JD, Figueroa E, Laska EM, Dewey SL. Safety and efficacy of gamma-vinyl GABA (GVG) for the treatment of methamphetamine and/or cocaine addiction. *Synapse.* 2005;55:122–125.

13. Brower KJ, Maddahian E, Blow FC, Beresford TP. A comparison of self-reported symptoms and DSM-III-R criteria for cocaine withdrawal. *Am J Drug Alcohol Abuse.* 1988;14:347–356.

14. Brower KJ, Paredes A. Cocaine withdrawal. *Arch Gen Psychiatry.* 1987;44:297–298.

15. Bruijnzeel AW, Repetto M, Gold MS. Neurobiological mechanisms in addictive and psychiatric disorders. *Psychiatr Clin North Am.* 2004;27:661–674.

16. Bryant CD, Yazdani N. RNA-binding proteins, neural development and the addictions. *Genes Brain Behav.* 2016;15:169–186.

17. Carroll KM, Nich C, Rounsaville BJ. Differential symptom reduction in depressed cocaine abusers treated with psychotherapy and pharmacotherapy. *J Nerv Ment Dis.* 1995;183:251–259.

18. Carroll KM, Rounsaville BJ, Gawin FH. A comparative trial of psychotherapies for ambulatory cocaine abusers: relapse prevention and interpersonal psychotherapy. *Am J Drug Alcohol Abuse.* 1991;17:229–247.

19. Carroll KM, Rounsaville BJ, Nich C, Gordon LT, Wirtz PW, Gawin F. One-year follow-up of psychotherapy and pharmacotherapy for cocaine dependence. Delayed emergence of psychotherapy effects. *Arch Gen Psychiatry.* 1994;51:989–997.

20. Chae SM, Covington CY. Biobehavioral outcomes in adolescents and young adults prenatally exposed to cocaine: evidence from animal models. *Biol Res Nurs.* 2009;10:318–330.

21. Chen L, Segal DM, Moraes CT, Mash DC. Dopamine transporter mRNA in autopsy studies of chronic cocaine users. *Brain Res Mol Brain Res.* 1999;73:181–185.

22. Childress A, Franklin T, Listerud J, Acton P, O'Brien C. Neuroimaging of cocaine craving states: cessation, stimulant administration, and drug cue pardigms. In: Davis K, Charney D, Coyle J, Nemeroff C, eds. *Neuropsychopharmacology: The Fifth Generation of Progress.* New York: Lippincott Williams & Wilkins; 2002:1575–1590.

23. Cocores JA, Miller NS, Pottash AC, Gold MS. Sexual dysfunction in abusers of cocaine and alcohol. *Am J Drug Alcohol Abuse.* 1988;14:169–173.

24. Contoreggi C, Herning RI, Koeppl B, et al. Treatment-seeking inpatient cocaine abusers show hypothalamic dysregulation of both basal prolactin and cortisol secretion. *Neuroendocrinology.* 2003;78:154–162.

25. Cornelius JR, Salloum IM, Thase ME. Fluoxetine versus placebo in depressed alcoholic cocaine abusers. *Psychopharmacol Bull.* 1998;34:117–121.

26. Cornish JW, O'Brien CP. Crack cocaine abuse: an epidemic with many public health consequences. *Annu Rev Public Health.* 1996;17:259–273.

27. Cottler LB, Shillington AM, Compton WM 3rd, Mager D, Spitznagel EL. Subjective reports of withdrawal among cocaine users: recommendations for DSM-IV. *Drug Alcohol Depend.* 1993;33:97–104.

28. Crits-Christoph P, Siqueland L, Blaine J, et al. Psychosocial treatments for cocaine dependence: National Institute on drug abuse collaborative cocaine treatment study. *Arch Gen Psychiatry.* 1999;56:493–502.

29. Cubells JF, Kranzler HR, McCance-Katz E, et al. A haplotype at the DBH locus, associated with low plasma dopamine beta-hydroxylase activity, also associates with cocaine-induced paranoia. *Mol Psychiatry.* 2000;5:56–63.

30. Dackis CA, Gold MS, Davies RK, Sweeney DR. Bromocriptine treatment for cocaine abuse: the dopamine depletion hypothesis. *Int J Psychiatry Med.* 1985;15:125–135.

31. Dackis CA, O'Brien CP. Cocaine dependence: a disease of the brain's reward centers. *J Subst Abuse Treat.* 2001;21:111–117.

32. Derauf C, Kekatpure M, Neyzi N, Lester B, Kosofsky B. Neuroimaging of children following prenatal drug exposure. *Semin Cell Dev Biol.* 2009;20:441–454.

33. DeVito EE, Babuscio TA, Nich C, Ball SA, Carroll KM. Gender differences in clinical outcomes for cocaine dependence: randomized clinical trials of behavioral therapy and disulfiram. *Drug Alcohol Depend.* 2014;145:156–167.

34. Devlin RJ, Henry JA. Clinical review: Major consequences of illicit drug consumption. *Crit Care.* 2008;12:202.

35. Doura MB, Unterwald EM. MicroRNAs modulate interactions between stress and risk for cocaine addiction. *Front Cell Neurosci.* 2016;10:125.

36. Dutra L, Stathopoulou G, Basden SL, Leyro TM, Powers MB, Otto MW. A meta-analytic review of psychosocial interventions for substance use disorders. *Am J Psychiatry.* 2008;165:179–187.

37. Erb S, Shaham Y, Stewart J. The role of corticotropin-releasing factor and corticosterone in stress- and cocaine-induced relapse to cocaine seeking in rats. *J Neurosci.* 1998;18:5529–5536.

38. Evans SM, Foltin RW. Exogenous progesterone attenuates the subjective effects of smoked cocaine in women, but not in men. *Neuropsychopharmacology.* 2006;31:659–674.

39. Everitt BJ. Neural and psychological mechanisms underlying compulsive drug seeking habits and drug memories--indications for novel treatments of addiction. *Eur J Neurosci.* 2014;40:2163–2182.

40. Fadda P, Scherma M, Fresu A, Collu M, Fratta W. Baclofen antagonizes nicotine-, cocaine-, and morphine-induced dopamine release in the nucleus accumbens of rat. *Synapse.* 2003;50:1–6.

41. Falck RS, Wang J, Carlson RG. Crack cocaine trajectories among users in a midwestern American city. *Addiction.* 2007;102:1421–1431.

42. Fattore L, Melis M, Fadda P, Fratta W. Sex differences in addictive disorders. *Front Neuroendocrinol.* 2014;35:272–284.

43. Fechtner RD, Khouri AS, Figueroa E, et al. Short-term treatment of cocaine and/or methamphetamine abuse with vigabatrin: ocular safety pilot results. *Arch Ophthalmol.* 2006;124:1257–1262.

44. Fischer B, Coghlan M. Crack use in North American cities: the neglected 'epidemic. *Addiction.* 2007;102:1340–1341.

45. Fisher DG, Malow R, Rosenberg R, Reynolds GL, Farrell N, Jaffe A. Recreational viagra use and sexual risk among drug abusing men. *Am J Infect Dis.* 2006;2:107–114.

46. Forray A, Sofuoglu M. Future pharmacological treatments for substance use disorders. *Br J Clin Pharmacol.* 2014;77:382–400.

47. Fox HC, Garcia M Jr, Kemp K, Milivojevic V, Kreek MJ, Sinha R. Gender differences in cardiovascular and corticoadrenal response to stress and drug cues in cocaine dependent individuals. *Psychopharmacology (Berl)*. 2006;185:348–357.

48. Fox HC, Hong KI, Siedlarz K, Sinha R. Enhanced sensitivity to stress and drug/alcohol craving in abstinent cocaine-dependent individuals compared to social drinkers. *Neuropsychopharmacology*. 2008:33796–33805.

49. Fox HC, Sinha R. Sex differences in drug-related stress-system changes: implications for treatment in substance-abusing women. *Harv Rev Psychiatry*. 2009;17:103–119.

50. Fox HC, Sofuoglu M, Morgan PT, Tuit KL, Sinha R. The effects of exogenous progesterone on drug craving and stress arousal in cocaine dependence: impact of gender and cue type. *Psychoneuroendocrinology*. 2013;38:1532–1544.

51. French JA. Vigabatrin. *Epilepsia*. 1999;40(suppl 5):S11–S16.

52. Friedman H, Pross S, Klein TW. Addictive drugs and their relationship with infectious diseases. *FEMS Immunol Med Microbiol*. 2006;47:330–342.

53. Fryer JD, Lukas RJ. Noncompetitive functional inhibition at diverse, human nicotinic acetylcholine receptor subtypes by bupropion, phencyclidine, and ibogaine. *J Pharmacol Exp Ther*. 1999;288:88–92.

54. Fullerton A. Toxic effects of cocaine and their treatment. *Lancet*. 1891;138:663–664.

55. Giannini AJ, Malone DA, Giannini MC, Price WA, Loiselle RH. Treatment of depression in chronic cocaine and phencyclidine abuse with desipramine. *J Clin Pharmacol*. 1986;26:211–214.

56. Goeders NE. A neuroendocrine role in cocaine reinforcement. *Psychoneuroendocrinology*. 1997;22:237–259.

57. Goldstein RA, DesLauriers C, Burda AM. Cocaine: history, social implications, and toxicity--a review. *Dis Mon*. 2009;55:6–38.

58. Goldstein RZ, Volkow ND. Drug addiction and its underlying neurobiological basis: neuroimaging evidence for the involvement of the frontal cortex. *Am J Psychiatry*. 2002;159:1642–1652.

59. Gonzalez G, Desai R, Sofuoglu M, et al. Clinical efficacy of gabapentin versus tiagabine for reducing cocaine use among cocaine dependent methadone-treated patients. *Drug Alcohol Depend*. 2007;87:1–9.

60. Grogger J, Willis M. The emergence of crack cocaine and the rise in urban crime rates. *Review of Economics and Statistics*. 2000;82:519–529.

61. Hameedi FA, Rosen MI, McCance-Katz EF, et al. Behavioral, physiological, and pharmacological interaction of cocaine and disulfiram in humans. *Biol Psychiatry*. 1995;37:560–563.

62. Havassy BE, Wasserman DA, Hall SM. Relapse to cocaine use: conceptual issues. *NIDA Res Monogr*. 1993;135:203–217.

63. Higgins ST, Budney AJ, Bickel WK, Hughes JR, Foerg F, Badger G. Achieving cocaine abstinence with a behavioral approach. *Am J Psychiatry*. 1993;150:763–769.

64. Higgins ST, Delaney DD, Budney AJ, et al. A behavioral approach to achieving initial cocaine abstinence. *Am J Psychiatry*. 1991;148:1218–1224.

65. Holsboer F. Corticotropin-releasing hormone modulators and depression. *Curr Opin Investig Drugs*. 2003;4:46–50.

66. Holstege C, Holstege L, Charlton N. *Cocaine-Related Psychiatric Disorders*. eMedicine, WebMD; 2008.

67. Horvath KJ, Calsyn DA, Terry C, Cotton A. Erectile dysfunction medication use among men seeking substance abuse treatment. *J Addict Dis*. 2007;26:7–13.

68. Huerta-Alardin A, Varon J, Marik P. Bench-to-bedside review: rhabdomyolysis - an overview for clinicians. *Critical Care*. 2005;9:158–169.

69. Hyman SE, Malenka RC. Addiction and the brain: the neurobiology of compulsion and its persistence. *Nat Rev Neurosci*. 2001;2:695–703.

70. Hyman SM, Paliwal P, Chaplin TM, Mazure CM, Rounsaville BJ, Sinha R. Severity of childhood trauma is predictive of cocaine relapse outcomes in women but not men. *Drug Alcohol Depend*. 2008;92:208–216.

71. Inciardi JA, Surratt HL. Drug use, street crime, and sex-trading among cocaine-dependent women: implications for public health and criminal justice policy. *J Psychoactive Drugs*. 2001;33:379–389.

72. Indave BI, Minozzi S, Pani PP, Amato L. Antipsychotic medications for cocaine dependence. *Cochrane Database Syst Rev*. 2016;3:Cd006306.

73. Jackson G. PDE 5 inhibitors and HIV risk: current concepts and controversies. *Int J Clin Pract*. 2005;59:1247–1248.

74. Johanson CE, Fischman MW. The pharmacology of cocaine related to its abuse. *Pharmacol Rev*. 1989;41:3–52.

75. Jones HE, Johnson RE, Bigelow GE, Silverman K, Mudric T, Strain EC. Safety and efficacy of L-tryptophan and behavioral incentives for treatment of cocaine dependence: a randomized clinical trial. *Am J Addict*. 2004;13:421–437.

76. Kahn R, Biswas K, Childress AR, et al. Multi-center trial of baclofen for abstinence initiation in severe cocaine-dependent individuals. *Drug Alcohol Depend*. 2009;103:59–64.

77. Kalayasiri R, Sughondhabirom A, Gueorguieva R, et al. Dopamine beta-hydroxylase gene (DbetaH) -1021C-->T influences self-reported paranoia during cocaine self-administration. *Biol Psychiatry*. 2007;61:1310–1313.

78. Kalivas PW, McFarland K. Brain circuitry and the reinstatement of cocaine-seeking behavior. *Psychopharmacology (Berl)*. 2003;168:44–56.

79. Kalivas PW, Volkow ND. The neural basis of addiction: a pathology of motivation and choice. *Am J Psychiatry*. 2005;162:1403–1413.

80. Kampman KM, Volpicelli JR, McGinnis DE, et al. Reliability and validity of the cocaine selective severity assessment. *Addict Behav*. 1998;23:449–461.

81. Kenny PJ. Epigenetics, microRNA, and addiction. *Dialogues Clin Neurosci*. 2014;16:335–344.

82. Kim JH, Lawrence AJ. Drugs currently in phase II clinical trials for cocaine addiction. *Expert Opin Investig Drugs*. 2014;23:1105–1122.

83. Kishi T, Matsuda Y, Iwata N, Correll CU. Antipsychotics for cocaine or psychostimulant dependence: systematic review and meta-analysis of randomized, placebo-controlled trials. *J Clin Psychiatry*. 2013;74:e1169–1180.

84. Konzen JP, Levine SR, Garcia JH. Vasospasm and thrombus formation as possible mechanisms of stroke related to alkaloidal cocaine. *Stroke*. 1995;26:1114–1118.

85. Koob GF, Le Moal M. Drug addiction, dysregulation of reward, and allostasis. *Neuropsychopharmacology*. 2001;24:97–129.

86. Kornhuber J, Weller M, Schoppmeyer K, Riederer P. Amantadine and memantine are NMDA receptor antagonists with neuroprotective properties. *J Neural Transm*. 1994;(suppl 43):91–104.

87. Kosten TA. Enhanced neurobehavioral effects of cocaine with chronic neuroleptic exposure in rats. *Schizophr Bull*. 1997;23:203–213.

88. Kosten TR, Domingo CB, Shorter D, et al. Vaccine for cocaine dependence: a randomized double-blind placebo-controlled efficacy trial. *Drug Alcohol Depend*. 2014;140:42–47.

89. Kosten TR, Kosten TA, McDougle CJ, et al. Gender differences in response to intranasal cocaine administration to humans. *Biol Psychiatry*. 1996;39:147–148.

90. Kosten TR, Wu G, Huang W, et al. Pharmacogenetic randomized trial for cocaine abuse: disulfiram and dopamine beta-hydroxylase. *Biol Psychiatry*. 2013;73:219–224.

91. Leach JP, Brodie MJ. Tiagabine. *Lancet*. 1998;351:203–207.

92. Lester BM, Conradt E, Marsit CJ. Are epigenetic changes in the intrauterine environment related to newborn neurobehavior? *Epigenomics*. 2014;6:175–178.

93. Lester BM, Padbury JF. Third pathophysiology of prenatal cocaine exposure. *Dev Neurosci*. 2009;31:23–35.

94. Levran O, Randesi M, da Rosa JC, et al. Overlapping dopaminergic pathway genetic susceptibility to heroin and cocaine addictions in African Americans. *Ann Hum Genet*. 2015;79:188–198.

95. Li CS, Huang C, Yan P, Bhagwagar Z, Milivojevic V, Sinha R. Neural correlates of impulse control during stop signal inhibition in cocaine-dependent men. *Neuropsychopharmacology.* 2008;33:1798–1806.

96. Ling W, Shoptaw S, Majewska D. Baclofen as a cocaine anti-craving medication: a preliminary clinical study. *Neuropsychopharmacology.* 1998;18:403–404.

97. Little KY, McLaughlin DP, Zhang L, et al. Brain dopamine transporter messenger RNA and binding sites in cocaine users: a post-mortem study. *Arch Gen Psychiatry.* 1998;55:793–799.

98. Louie AK, Lannon RA, Ketter TA. Treatment of cocaine-induced panic disorder. *Am J Psychiatry.* 1989;146:40–44.

99. Louie AK, Lannon RA, Rutzick EA, Browne D, Lewis TB, Jones R. Clinical features of cocaine-induced panic. *Biol Psychiatry.* 1996;40:938–940.

100. Lukas SE, Sholar M, Lundahl LH, et al. Sex differences in plasma cocaine levels and subjective effects after acute cocaine administration in human volunteers. *Psychopharmacology (Berl).* 1996;125:346–354.

101. Luscher C. The emergence of a circuit model for addiction. *Annu Rev Neurosci.* 2016;39:257–276.

102. Luscher C, Bellone C. Cocaine-evoked synaptic plasticity: a key to addiction? *Nat Neurosci.* 2008;11:737–738.

103. Margolin A, Kosten TR, Avants SK, et al. A multicenter trial of bupropion for cocaine dependence in methadone-maintained patients. *Drug Alcohol Depend.* 1995;40:125–131.

104. Mariani JJ, Levin FR. Psychostimulant treatment of cocaine dependence. *Psychiatr Clin North Am.* 2012;35:425–439.

105. Markou A, Kosten TR, Koob GF. Neurobiological similarities in depression and drug dependence: a self-medication hypothesis. *Neuropsychopharmacology.* 1998;18:135–174.

106. McClung CA, Nestler EJ. Regulation of gene expression and cocaine reward by CREB and DeltaFosB. *Nat Neurosci.* 2003;6:1208–1215. Epub 2003 Oct 1219.

107. Mendelson JH, Teoh SK, Lange U, et al. Anterior pituitary, adrenal, and gonadal hormones during cocaine withdrawal. *Am J Psychiatry.* 1988;145:1094–1098.

108. Mendelson JH, Teoh SK, Mello NK, Ellingboe J, Rhoades E. Acute effects of cocaine on plasma adrenocorticotropic hormone, luteinizing hormone and prolactin levels in cocaine-dependent men. *J Pharmacol Exp Ther.* 1992;263:505–509.

109. Meston CM, Frohlich PF. The neurobiology of sexual function. *Arch Gen Psychiatry.* 2000;57:1012–1030.

110. Milivojevic V, Fox HC, Sofuoglu M, Covault J, Sinha R. Effects of progesterone stimulated allopregnanolone on craving and stress response in cocaine dependent men and women. *Psychoneuroendocrinology.* 2016;65:44–53.

111. Minozzi S, Amato L, Pani PP, et al. Dopamine agonists for the treatment of cocaine dependence. *Cochrane Database Syst Rev.* 2015:Cd003352.

112. Minozzi S, Cinquini M, Amato L, et al. Anticonvulsants for cocaine dependence. *Cochrane Database Syst Rev.* 2015:Cd006754.

113. Morgan PT, Malison RT. Cocaine and sleep: early abstinence. *ScientificWorldJournal.* 2007;7:223–230.

114. Najavits LM, Lester KM. Gender differences in cocaine dependence. *Drug Alcohol Depend.* 2008;97:190–194.

115. Nemeroff CB. The corticotropin-releasing factor (CRF) hypothesis of depression: new findings and new directions. *Mol Psychiatry.* 1996;1:336–342.

116. Nestler EJ. Molecular basis of long-term plasticity underlying addiction. *Nat Rev Neurosci.* 2001;2:119–128.

117. Nestler EJ. Is there a common molecular pathway for addiction? *Nat Neurosci.* 2005;8:1445–1449.

118. Nestler EJ. The neurobiology of cocaine addiction. *Sci Pract Perspect.* 2005;3:4–10.

119. Nestler EJ. Review. Transcriptional mechanisms of addiction: role of DeltaFosB. *Philos Trans R Soc Lond B Biol Sci.* 2008;363:3245–3255.

120. Nestler EJ. Epigenetic mechanisms of drug addiction. *Neuropharmacology.* 2014;76 Pt B:259–268.

121. Neville MJ, Johnstone EC, Walton RT. Identification and characterization of ANKK1: a novel kinase gene closely linked to DRD2 on chromosome band 11q23.1. *Human Mutation.* 23:540–545.

122. Newberry NR, Nicoll RA. Direct hyperpolarizing action of baclofen on hippocampal pyramidal cells. *Nature.* 1984;308:450–452.

123. Nich C, McCance-Katz EF, Petrakis IL, Cubells JF, Rounsaville BJ, Carroll KM. Sex differences in cocaine-dependent individuals' response to disulfiram treatment. *Addict Behav.* 2004;29:1123–1128.

124. NIDA. The epidemiology of cocaine use and abuse. In: Schober S, Schade C, eds. *Research Monograph 110.* Vol. 110. Rockvile, MD: U.S. Department Of Health And Human Services; 1991.

125. NIDA. *Monitoring the Future: Trends in The Availability of Various Drugs (Revised June 2016).* In: U.S.D.O.H.A.H. SERVICES (Ed.). Betheda, MD: National Institutes of Health; 2016.

126. NIDA. *Principles of Drug Abuse Treatment for Criminal Justice Populations: A Research-Based Guide.* In: U.S.D.o.H.a.H. Services (Ed.). Bethesda, MD: National Institutes of Health.

127. Nutt JG, Wooten GF. Clinical practice. Diagnosis and initial management of Parkinson's disease. *N Engl J Med.* 2005;353:1021–1027.

128. Paliwal P, Hyman SM, Sinha R. Craving predicts time to cocaine relapse: further validation of the now and brief versions of the cocaine craving questionnaire. *Drug Alcohol Depend.* 2008;93:252–259.

129. Pani PP, Trogu E, Vacca R, Amato L, Vecchi S, Davoli M. Disulfiram for the treatment of cocaine dependence. *Cochrane Database Syst Rev.* 2010:Cd007024.

130. Pani PP, Trogu E, Vecchi S, Amato L. Antidepressants for cocaine dependence and problematic cocaine use. *Cochrane Database Syst Rev.* 2011:Cd002950.

131. Petry NM, Martin B. Low-cost contingency management for treating cocaine- and opioid-abusing methadone patients. *J Consult Clin Psychol.* 2002;70:398–405.

132. Poling J, Oliveto A, Petry N, et al. Six-month trial of bupropion with contingency management for cocaine dependence in a methadone-maintained population. *Arch Gen Psychiatry.* 2006;63:219–228.

133. Rasmussen TG, Sauerberg P, Nielsen EB, et al. Muscarinic receptor agonists decrease cocaine self-administration rates in drug-naive mice. *Eur J Pharmacol.* 2000;402:241–246.

134. Richardson GA, Goldschmidt L, Larkby C, Day NL. Effects of prenatal cocaine exposure on adolescent development. *Neurotoxicol Teratol.* 2015;49:41–48.

135. Roberts DC, Vickers G. The effect of haloperidol on cocaine self-administration is augmented with repeated administrations. *Psychopharmacology (Berl).* 1987;93:526–528.

136. Robinson TE, Kolb B. Alterations in the morphology of dendrites and dendritic spines in the nucleus accumbens and prefrontal cortex following repeated treatment with amphetamine or cocaine. *Eur J Neurosci.* 1999;11:1598–1604.

137. Rounsaville BJ. Treatment of cocaine dependence and depression. *Biol Psychiatry.* 2004;56:803–809.

138. Rounsaville BJ, Carroll KM. Back S. individual psychotherapy. In: Lowinson JH, Ruiz P, eds. *Substance Abuse: A Comprehensive Textbook.* Baltimore, MD: Williams and Wilkins; 2005:653–670.

139. Roy E, Arruda N, Bruneau J, Jutras-Aswad D. Epidemiology of injection drug use: new trends and prominent issues. *Can J Psychiatry.* 2016;61:136–144.

140. Ruttenber AJ, McAnally HB, Wetli CV. Cocaine-associated rhabdomyolysis and excited delirium: different stages of the same syndrome. *Am J Forensic Med Pathol.* 1999;20:120–127.

141. SAMHSA. Behavioral *Health Trends in the United States: Results from the 2014 National Survey on Drug Use and Health.* HHS Publication No. SMA 15-4927, NSDUH Series H-50. Rockville, MD: Center for Behavioral Health Statistics and Quality; 2015.

142. Sarnyai Z. Neurobiology of stress and cocaine addiction. Studies on corticotropin-releasing factor in rats, monkeys, and humans. *Ann N Y Acad Sci.* 1998;851:371–387.

143. Sarnyai Z, Shaham Y, Heinrichs SC. The role of corticotropin-releasing factor in drug addiction. *Pharmacol Rev*. 2001;53:209–243.

144. Schmitz JM, Averill P, Stotts AL, Moeller FG, Rhoades HM, Grabowski J. Fluoxetine treatment of cocaine-dependent patients with major depressive disorder. *Drug and Alcohol Dependence*. 2001;63:207–214.

145. Scofield MD, Heinsbroek JA, Gipson CD, et al. The nucleus accumbens: mechanisms of addiction across drug classes reflect the importance of glutamate homeostasis. *Pharmacol Rev*. 2016;68:816–871.

146. Shaham Y, Hope BT. The role of neuroadaptations in relapse to drug seeking. *Nat Neurosci*. 2005;8:1437–1439.

147. Shank RP, Gardocki JF, Streeter AJ, Maryanoff BE. An overview of the preclinical aspects of topiramate: pharmacology, pharmacokinetics, and mechanism of action. *Epilepsia*. 2000;41(suppl 1):S3–S9.

148. Shoptaw S, Heinzerling KG, Rotheram-Fuller E, et al. Bupropion hydrochloride versus placebo, in combination with cognitive behavioral therapy, for the treatment of cocaine abuse/dependence. *J Addict Dis*. 2008;27:13–23.

149. Shoptaw S, Yang X, Rotheram-Fuller EJ, et al. Randomized placebo-controlled trial of baclofen for cocaine dependence: preliminary effects for individuals with chronic patterns of cocaine use. *J Clin Psychiatry*. 2003;64:1440–1448.

150. Shorter D, Nielsen DA, Huang W, Harding MJ, Hamon SC, Kosten TR. Pharmacogenetic randomized trial for cocaine abuse: disulfiram and alpha1A-adrenoceptor gene variation. *Eur Neuropsychopharmacol*. 2013;23:1401–1407.

151. Sigmon SC, Correia CJ, Stitzer ML. Cocaine abstinence during methadone maintenance: effects of repeated brief exposure to voucher-based reinforcement. *Exp Clin Psychopharmacol*. 2004;12:269–275.

152. Silverman K, Higgins ST, Brooner RK, et al. Sustained cocaine abstinence in methadone maintenance patients through voucher-based reinforcement therapy. *Arch Gen Psychiatry*. 1996;53:409–415.

153. Silverman K, Robles E, Mudric T, Bigelow GE, Stitzer ML. A randomized trial of long-term reinforcement of cocaine abstinence in methadone-maintained patients who inject drugs. *J Consult Clin Psychol*. 2004;72:839–854.

154. Simpson DD, Joe GW, Fletcher BW, Hubbard RL, Anglin MD. A National evaluation of treatment outcomes for cocaine dependence. *Arch Gen Psychiatry*. 1999;56:507–514.

155. Singh M, Keer D, Klimas J, Wood E, Werb D. Topiramate for cocaine dependence: a systematic review and meta-analysis of randomized controlled trials. *Addiction*. 2016;111:1337–1346.

156. Sinha R. The role of stress in addiction relapse. *Curr Psychiatry Rep*. 2007;9:388–395.

157. Sinha R, Garcia M, Paliwal P, Kreek MJ, Rounsaville BJ. Stress-induced cocaine craving and hypothalamic-pituitary-adrenal responses are predictive of cocaine relapse outcomes. *Arch Gen Psychiatry*. 2006;63:324–331.

158. Sinha R, Lacadie C, Skudlarski P, et al. Neural activity associated with stress-induced cocaine craving: a functional magnetic resonance imaging study. *Psychopharmacology (Berl)*. 2005;183:171–180.

159. Sinha R, Li CS. Imaging stress- and cue-induced drug and alcohol craving: association with relapse and clinical implications. *Drug Alcohol Rev*. 2007;26:25–31.

160. Sinha R, Talih M, Malison R, Cooney N, Anderson GM, Kreek MJ. Hypothalamic-pituitary-adrenal axis and sympatho-adrenomedullary responses during stress-induced and drug cue-induced cocaine craving states. *Psychopharmacology (Berl)*. 2003;17062–72.

161. Smith KM, Romanelli F. Recreational use and misuse of phosphodiesterase 5 inhibitors. *J Am Pharm Assoc*. 2003;45(2005):63–72; quiz 73-65.

162. Sofuoglu M, Dudish-Poulsen S, Brown SB, Hatsukami DK. Association of cocaine withdrawal symptoms with more severe dependence and enhanced subjective response to cocaine. *Drug Alcohol Depend*. 2003;69:273–282.

163. Sofuoglu M, Dudish-Poulsen S, Nelson D, Pentel PR, Hatsukami DK. Sex and menstrual cycle differences in the subjective effects from smoked cocaine in humans. *Exp Clin Psychopharmacol*. 1999;7:274–283.

164. Somoza EC, Winship D, Gorodetzky CW, et al. A multisite, double-blind, placebo-controlled clinical trial to evaluate the safety and efficacy of vigabatrin for treating cocaine dependence. *JAMA Psychiatry*. 2013;70:630–637.

165. Spellicy CJ, Kosten TR, Hamon SC, Harding MJ, Nielsen DA. ANKK1 and DRD2 pharmacogenetics of disulfiram treatment for cocaine abuse. *Pharmacogenet Genomics*. 2013;23:333–340.

166. Stahl S. Describing an Atypical Antipsychotic: Receptor Binding and Its Role in Pathophysiology. *Primary Care Companion J Clin Psychiatry*. 2003;5:9–13.

167. Stoops WW, Rush CR. Agonist replacement for stimulant dependence: a review of clinical research. *Curr Pharm Des*. 2013;19:7026–7035.

168. SwalveN Smethells JR, Zlebnik NE, Carroll ME. Sex differences in reinstatement of cocaine-seeking with combination treatments of progesterone and atomoxetine. *Pharmacol Biochem Behav*. 2016;145:17–23.

169. Tapp A, Wood AE, Kennedy A, Sylvers P, Kilzieh N, Saxon AJ. Quetiapine for the treatment of cocaine use disorder. *Drug Alcohol Depend*. 2015;149:18–24.

170. Torrens M, Fonseca F, Mateu G, Farre M. Efficacy of antidepressants in substance use disorders with and without comorbid depression. A systematic review and meta-analysis. *Drug Alcohol Depend*. 2005;78:1–22.

171. UNODC. *World Drug Report*. New York: United Nations Office on Drugs and Crime; 2015.

172. Valladares EM, Irwin MR. Polysomnographic sleep dysregulation in cocaine dependence. *ScientificWorldJournal*. 2007;7:213–216.

173. Vasica G, Tennant CC. Cocaine use and cardiovascular complications. *Med J Aust*. 2002;177:260–262.

174. Walker DM, Cates HM, Heller EA, Nestler EJ. Regulation of chromatin states by drugs of abuse. *Curr Opin Neurobiol*. 2015;30:112–121.

175. Warner EA. Cocaine Abuse. *Ann Intern Med*. 1993;119:226–235.

176. Washton AM. Group therapy with outpatients. In: Lowinson JH, Ruiz P, eds. *Substance Abuse: A Comprehensive Textbook*. Baltimore, MD: Williams and Wilkins; 2003:671–680.

177. Weinshenker D, Schroeder JP. There and back again: a tale of norepinephrine and drug addiction. *Neuropsychopharmacology*. 2007;32:1433–1451.

178. Welch RD, Todd K, Krause GS. Incidence of cocaine-associated rhabdomyolysis. *Ann Emerg Med*. 1991;20:154–157.

179. Wells EA, Peterson PL, Gainey RR, Hawkins JD, Catalano RF. Outpatient treatment for cocaine abuse: a controlled comparison of relapse prevention and twelve-step approaches. *Am J Drug Alcohol Abuse*. 1994;20:1–17.

180. White KA, Brady KT, Sonne S. Gender differences in patterns of cocaine use. *Am J Addict*. 1996;5:259–261.

181. Winhusen T, Somoza E, Ciraulo DA, et al. A double-blind, placebo-controlled trial of tiagabine for the treatment of cocaine dependence. *Drug Alcohol Depend*. 2007;91:141–148.

182. Winhusen TM, Somoza EC, Harrer JM, et al. A placebo-controlled screening trial of tiagabine, sertraline and donepezil as cocaine dependence treatments. *Addiction*. 2005;100(suppl 1):68–77.

183. Wolf ME. Synaptic mechanisms underlying persistent cocaine craving. *Nat Rev Neurosci*. 2016;17:351–365.

184. Yohn NL, Bartolomei MS, Blendy JA. Multigenerational and transgenerational inheritance of drug exposure: the effects of alcohol, opiates, cocaine, marijuana, and nicotine. *Prog Biophys Mol Biol*. 2015;118:21–33.

185. Yonkers KA, Forray A, Nich C, et al. Progesterone for the reduction of cocaine use in post-partum women with a cocaine use disorder: a randomised, double-blind, placebo-controlled, pilot study. *The Lancet Psychiatry*. 2014;1:360–367.

186. Zemrak WR, Kenna GA. Association of antipsychotic and antidepressant drugs with Q-T interval prolongation. *Am J Health Syst Pharm*. 2008;65:1029–1038.

23
Nicotine

DAVID L. ATKINSON, JENNIFER MINNIX, PAUL M. CINCIRIPINI, AND
MAHER KARAM-HAGE

CHAPTER OUTLINE

Epidemiology

Cigarette smoking is the principal cause of premature death and disability in the United States. In 2016 about 480,000 deaths in the United States were caused by cigarette smoking.[312] According to the International Agency for Research on Cancer, tobacco smoking is causally linked to at least 13 different types of neoplastic disease.[152] However, despite education about the health hazards of smoking and other tobacco control efforts, many smokers continue to encounter extreme difficulty quitting and staying tobacco-free long-term.

With the advent of electronic cigarettes, nicotine addiction has now taken on a new form outside of the traditional route of cigarette smoking. E-cigarettes have been seen both as a public health benefit and a potential danger. E-cigarette use is now more common than combustible nicotine products among youth. This raises the interesting question of what harm does nicotine addiction do apart from the largely known risks of cancer, respiratory, and cardiovascular disease due to the smoke in combustible tobacco? The answer to this question affects millions of people in the United States and around the world. According to the Centers for Disease Control and Prevention (CDC), 16% of US adults have ever used e-cigarettes as of 2016 and about 4% are current users, the highest use is in the age 18–24 group; however, the relatively good news is that most of that age group seem to be using non-nicotine content e-cigarettes.[310]

The latest annual National Survey on Drug Use and Health (NSDUH) in 2017 covered ≈70,000 noninstitutionalized US residents 12 years of age or older and reported that tobacco use in past month has declined in recent years, from the highest rate of 42% in 1965 to the lowest reported rate of 23.5% in 2016.[266] Surveys with different methodologies and definitions of smoking have produced varying rates of smoking prevalence. The latest CDC report from 2017 estimates that 14% of the US population were current smokers (10.5% are daily smokers); it also reported that smoking is more prevalent in men (16.7%) than in women (13.6%), in those with less than a high school diploma (24.2%), and in those under the poverty level (26.1%). In another epidemiological study, the latest data from the 2012 National Health Interview Survey (NHIS) reported that 18% of the US population age 18 years or older were current smokers (21% of men and 16% of women). Smoking rates were substantially higher among individuals with less than a high school education. What is interesting is that, according to CDC, 55% of current smokers made at least one quit attempt of at least 24 hours in the previous year and 70% are interested in quitting.[322a]

The latest University of Michigan Monitoring the Future survey from 2018 found a continued decrease in lifetime prevalence of cigarette smoking to historic lows among 8th, 10th, and 12th graders with 9.4%, 15.9%, and 26.6%, respectively. This survey also reported a continuing decline in smoking in the last 30 days, with 1.9%, 5.0%, and 7.6%, respectively.[158a] Although the trend is downward, the above numbers highlight the magnitude of the problem with smoking and nicotine dependence, with past 30-day use trailing only cannabis and alcohol in terms of past 30-day prevalence. Adolescents from different background or life trajectories have very different smoking behaviors, 21.9% of those who do not plan to complete a 4-year college are smokers versus 8.9% of those who plan to do 4 years. Furthermore, 15% of Caucasians were smokers during the past 30 days, versus 6.9% of African Americans.

The evolving trend of e-cigarettes has shown rapid growth in recent years. Levels of nicotine vaping in the past year increased dramatically in 2018. In 10th and 12th grades, the annual increases are the largest ever recorded for any substance in the 44 years that MTF has tracked adolescent drug use. From 2017 to 2018 nicotine vaping increased by 3.4, 8.9, and 10.9 percentage points in 8th, 10th, and 12th grades. These increases resulted in yielded prevalence levels of 11%, 25%, and 30%, respectively. Although e-cigarettes have been touted as a potential smoking cessation tool, the evidence is that the majority of young e-cigarette users are not using them to quit, but are using them for motives such as novelty. The percent of 12th grade students who reported use of nicotine in the past 30 days significantly increased to 28.5% in 2018 from 23.7% in 2017. Nicotine use is indicated by any use of cigarettes, large cigars, flavored or regular small cigars, hookah, smokeless tobacco, or a vaping device with nicotine. This increase was driven entirely by vaping. Use of each of the other tobacco products was slightly down in 2018, although none of these decreases were statistically significant. Having flavors that are enjoyable and acceptable to young people is leading to greater youth acceptance. In 2018, of youth who use vaporized e-cigarettes, 13.5% did so because it looks cool, 22% use because of boredom, and 20.7% use to relieve tension and relax, whereas only 9.6% say they are using e-cigarettes to help them quit regular cigarettes. On the other hand, 53.6% say they vape because they want to experiment and 38.4% because they think e-cigarettes taste good.[215a]

In 2016, among baseline e-cigarette users, conversion to combustible tobacco smoking was much greater in a longitudinal school-based assessment study.[199] Whereas it is almost certain that much of this overlap represents correlated liabilities to both combustible and e-cigarette use, it shows that the e-cigarettes did not have much of a protective effect and that this group is at high-risk of conversion. New aspects of e-cigarette use are constantly being elucidated, and the practice of "dripping," where the liquid is dripped directly onto the heating element to increase flavor and throat-hit, has been reported recently.[184] The use of flavors in e-cigarettes continues to be a topic of controversy, and it could be associated with its own health consequences.[197]

Hookah, water pipe, shisha, or narghile' smoking is an increasingly prevalent method of using tobacco. Although it is commonly thought to be safer for the lungs, this is not borne-out by the scientific research.[132] In addition to the higher level of carbon monoxide (CO), the charcoal used to heat the tobacco discharges carbon nanoparticles that can impair the respiratory system,[227] and filtering through water is not effective to eliminate CO, carbon, or other particles and toxins. Furthermore, the hit of the tobacco from these devices can be substantial, and lead to a greater dose of nicotine with greater cardiac effects.[338] In youth, the hookah/water pipe may be associated with different gateway effects on the later use of other substances,[113] but this will need to be investigated further. The amount of tobacco consumed in the

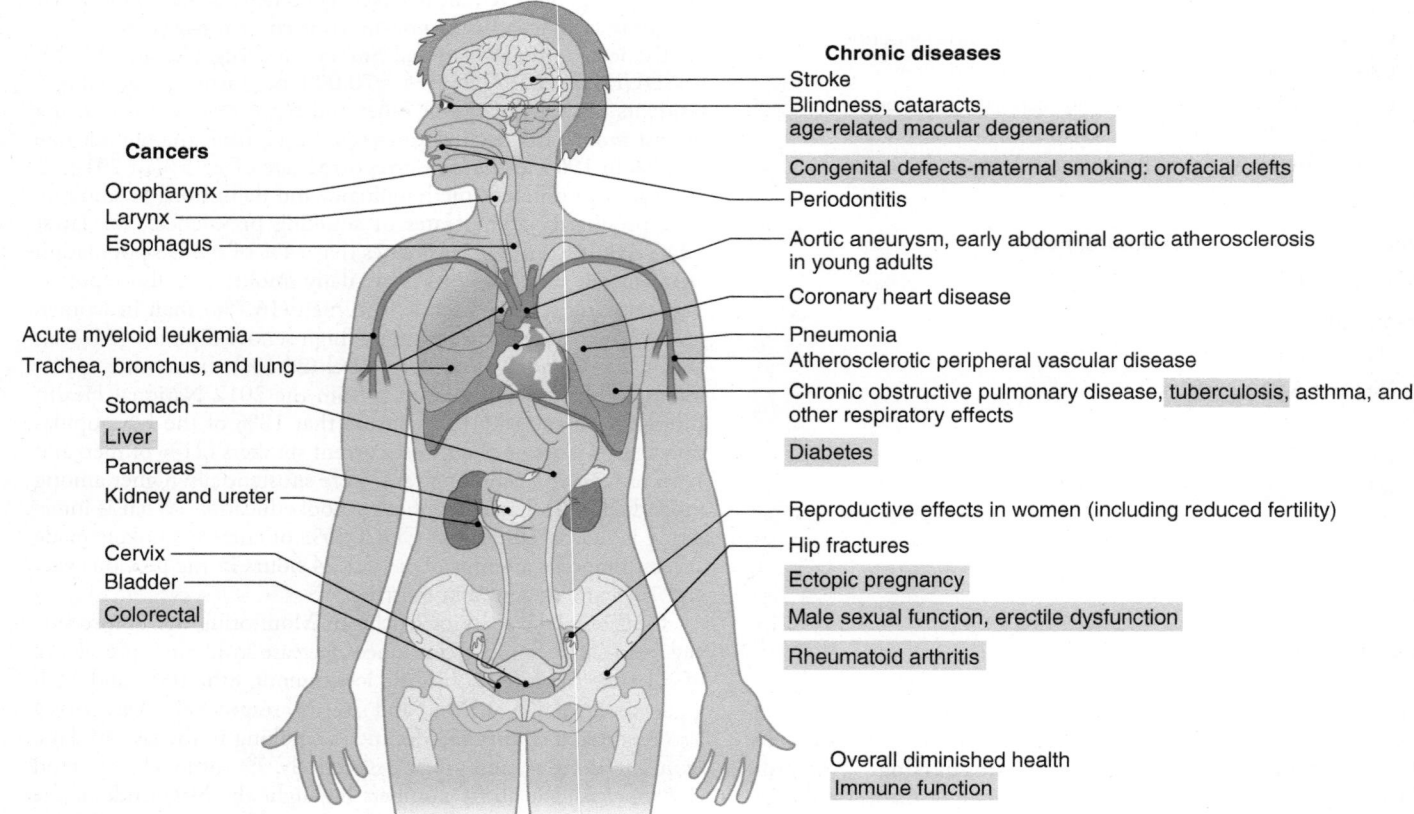

• **Fig. 23.1** Health consequences of smoking on body organs. Each condition shaded in red is a new disease causally linked to smoking in the 2014 Surgeon General's Report, *The Health Consequences of Smoking—50 Years of Progress.* (From the Centers for Disease Control and Prevention.)

session may be quite large, and water pipe smoking exposes people to risks of smoking not seen with other products, such as acute carbon monoxide poisoning.[98,168]

The number of young smokers needs to be closely watched because tobacco prevention is preferred over treatment due to the difficulty of treating an established nicotine dependence. The difficulty in overcoming nicotine dependence is illustrated by the poor success rates among smokers who try to quit. The majority of smokers (~70%) report an interest in quitting, and around 55% have attempted to quit in the previous year. However, only ~7% of smokers are abstinent at 1 month after their quit date and fewer than 2% are abstinent 1 year after quitting, including those who receive assistance in smoking cessation.[311] It is worth noting that the difficulty in maintaining abstinence is strongly related to affective and cognitive dysfunction, which may persist in some smokers for some time after the initial cessation, as well as postcessation cigarette cravings.[175] The health consequences associated with smoking tobacco are substantial and life-threatening (Fig. 23.1). Smoking is the primary causal factor for 30% of all cancer deaths and 80% of deaths related to chronic obstructive pulmonary disease.[308] According to the CDC,[308] cigarette smoking or exposure to tobacco smoke resulted in 443,000 premature deaths and 5.1 million years of potential life lost from 2000 to 2004. The three leading causes of smoking-attributable deaths were lung cancer, ischemic heart disease, and chronic obstructive pulmonary disease. In addition, an estimated 776 infant deaths attributed to smoking during pregnancy occurred annually from 2000 to 2004. Sadly, despite the fact that cigarette use has declined substantially since the 1960s, the number of smoking-related deaths has remained relatively unchanged.[309]

Biological, Behavioral, and Cognitive Aspects of Nicotine Dependence

The Reward Pathway

Among the more than 9000 components of tobacco smoke, about 70 are known carcinogens.[205] The most studied component of tobacco smoke is nicotine, which is the major psychoactive ingredient in tobacco smoke and the component most associated with tobacco dependence.[27] Like many drugs associated with abuse and dependence, nicotine ingestion stimulates a rapid increase in dopamine in the nucleus accumbens and the ventral tegmental area, typically within 10 seconds of smoking a cigarette.[231,235,246] Under normal circumstances, the nucleus accumbens and ventral tegmental area are activated by food, social affiliation, and sexual activity, all of which are linked to survival (Fig. 23.2A).

The key component of the reward pathway within the mesocorticolimbic system is the neurotransmitter dopamine, the pathways of which project from the nucleus accumbens and ventral tegmental area to the prefrontal cortex, the amygdala, and the olfactory tubercle[116] (Fig. 23.2B). At the same time that dopamine is released from the ventral tegmental area, a signal is sent to the amygdala, which stamps-in the positive associations of pleasure with the environmental cues that were presented at the time, as well as the delivery of the reinforcing dopamine in the accumbens shell.[163] This means that previously neutral stimuli, such as a brand of cigarette, a package, a vaporizing device, or even a painful burn on the throat (termed, "throat hit") are now associated with reinforcement. Repeat appearances of cues such as the cigarette, the logo, or even the locations in which one has smoked will trigger the craving and expectation of reward—and when the

anticipatory firing of dopamine is not met with actual delivery, it leads to frustration and continued or intensified craving.[321]

Although dopamine appears to be the final common neurotransmitter of this pathway, other neurotransmitter systems such as γ-aminobutyric acid, glutamate, cholinergics, and anticholinergic are believed to be involved in the activation of the reward pathway and the sustainability of substance sue.[206]

Nicotine affects the reward pathway by more than one mechanism; for example, in animal studies, dopamine antagonists or the destruction of dopaminergic neurons in the nucleus accumbens results in a decrease of nicotine self-administration in laboratory animals.[89] Nicotinic acetylcholine receptors (nAChRs) are a subtype of cholinergic receptors present throughout the central nervous system (CNS) and exert varying effects (excitatory, inhibitory, or modulatory) depending on their location in the brain. In turn, nAChRs have an impact on the activity of several neurotransmitters, including dopamine, norepinephrine, serotonin, glutamate, and γ-aminobutyric acid, and of endogenous opioid peptides.[6] Prior research has focused primarily on dopamine as a main determinant of nicotine and other drug addictions,[61,154,288] as well as the effect of nicotine on the nucleus accumbens and the similarity of that to other addictive drugs. However, the cholinergic mechanism is also obviously an important determinant[288] and the role of glutamate is ubiquitous to any CNS process[115] (Fig. 23. 2C).[6] The endogenous opioid, or endorphin, system is also involved in nicotine dependence, and naloxone can precipitate withdrawal in nicotine-dependent individuals.[179] Most recently the emphasis is shifting to include most if not all the other major neurotransmitter systems in the brain.[319] Finally, cannabinoid-1 (CB$_1$) receptors also seem to be involved in nicotine dependence and the activation of dopaminergic neurons in the mesocorticolimbic system,[75,187] highlighting once more the importance of broadening the horizon and scope of our research efforts to include other systems in addition to dopamine and the reward pathway, and other downstream effects of nicotine addiction.

Neuronal Adaptation

Most if not all substances of abuse and dependence initially produce desirable and pleasant effects. However, not everyone who uses these substances goes on to chronically use them, and not all long-term substance abusers become dependent or addicted to them. Genetic, environmental, and cultural factors may all interact to predispose some individuals to substance use and subsequent dependence/addiction.

The pleasurable sensation produced by reward pathway activation is associated with acute use of the substance, whereas repeated administration of nicotine over months or years is likely to lead to increased tolerance and withdrawal in the absence of nicotine. Tolerance and withdrawal are the physiological hallmarks of dependence, and they may be reflecting the neuroadaptive effects occurring within the brain.[28] Of interest, the chronic use of drugs appears to cause a generalized decrease in dopaminergic neurotransmission, likely in response to the intermittent yet repetitive increases in dopamine-inducing presynaptic downregulation of dopamine as a compensatory mechanism for supraphysiological levels of signaling[273,318] (Fig. 23.3). Using and withdrawing from drugs also increase the levels of corticotropin-releasing factor (CRF), which is associated with the activation of central stress pathways. In vivo animal studies utilizing microdialysis during withdrawal from ethanol, cocaine, nicotine, or tetrahydrocannabinol showed an increase in extracellular CRF.[182] Of interest, the direct injection of a CRF antagonist into the amygdala

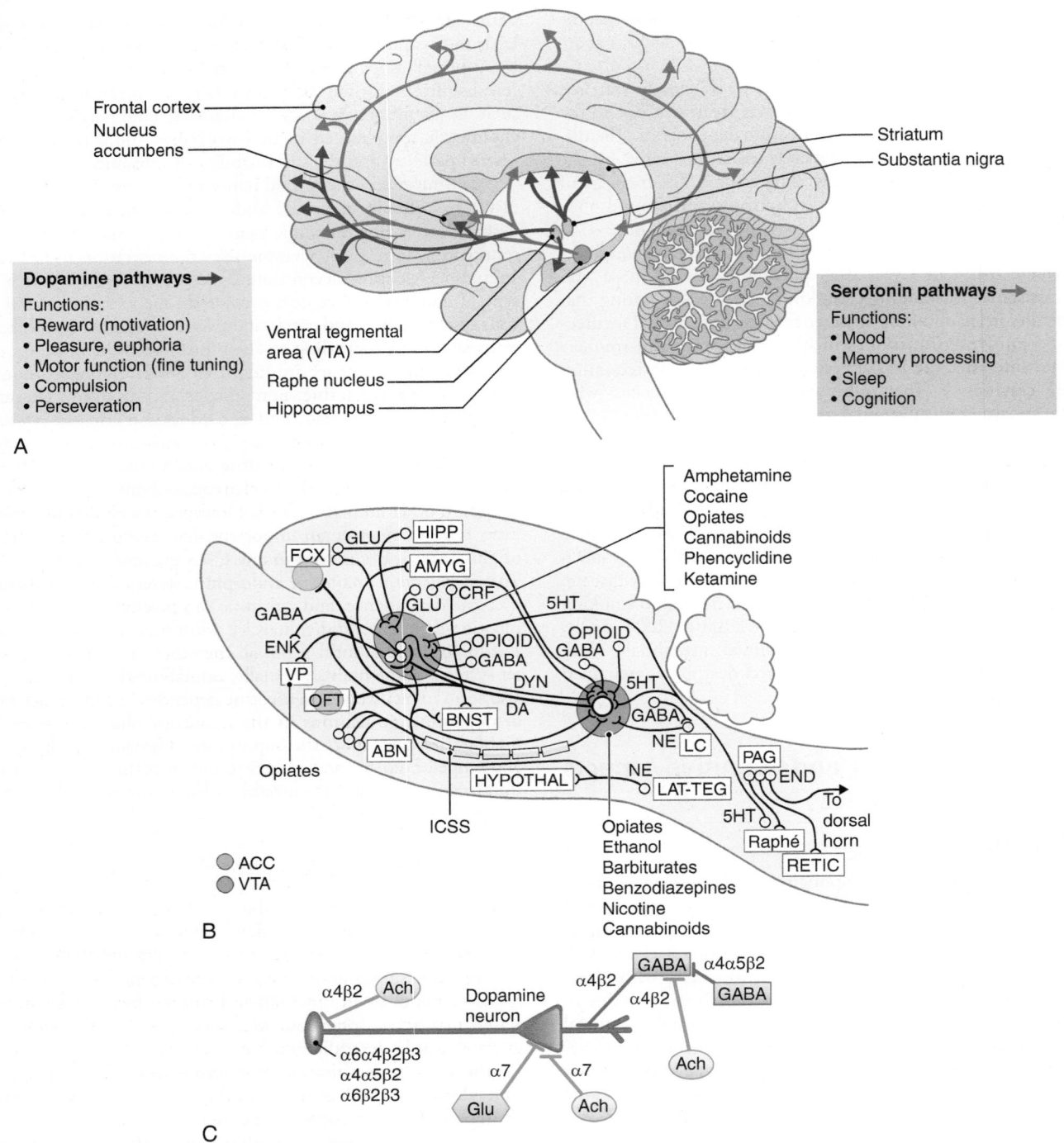

• **Fig. 23.2** (A) The reward pathway with projections to the frontal and prefrontal cortex. (B) Reward pathway interplay with other neuronal systems and the impact of different substances of use. (C) Diagram of the complex regulation of dopamine release by excitatory (glutamate [Glu]), inhibitory (gamma aminobutyric acid [GABA]), and cholinergic (acethylcoline [Ach]) neurons. (C, From Albuquerque EX, Pereira EFR, Alkondon M, Rogers SW. Mammalian nicotinic acetylcholine receptors: from structure to function. *Physiol Rev.* 2009;89[1]:73–120.)

reversed some of the symptoms of withdrawal (i.e., anxiogenic behaviors).[183,236,258,259,320]

Two neuroadaptive models have been used to explain how changes in reward function are associated with the development of substance dependence: sensitization and counter adaptation.

The sensitization model[259] postulates that there is an increased desire for the drug without a corresponding increase in pleasure, and often with a decrease in pleasure, following intermittent but administration of a drug. This is in contrast to the pharmacological tolerance to a substance, which occurs after continuous

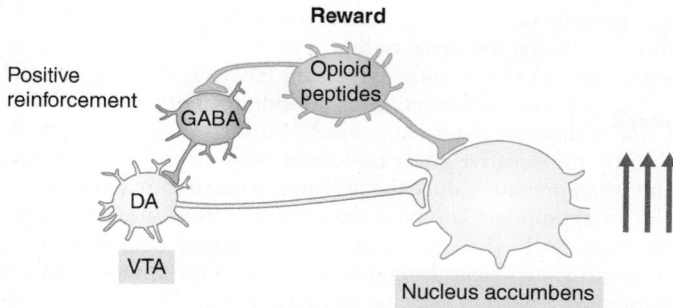

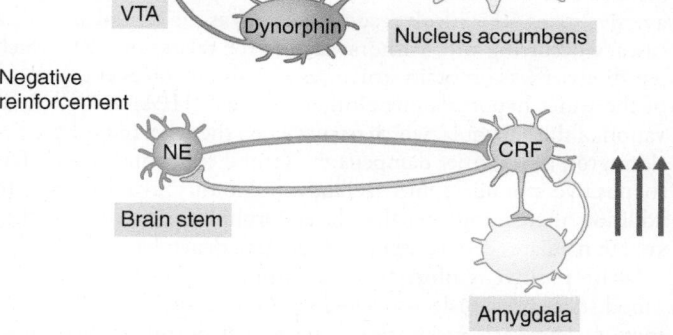

Reward

Positive reinforcement

Opioid peptides
GABA
DA
VTA
Nucleus accumbens

Within-system neuroadaptations

Positive reinforcement

Opioid peptides
GABA
DA
VTA
Nucleus accumbens

Between-system neuroadaptations

Positive reinforcement

Opioid peptides
GABA
DA
κ⊖
κ⊖
VTA
Dynorphin
Nucleus accumbens

Negative reinforcement

NE
CRF
Brain stem
Amygdala

• **Fig. 23.3** Negative reinforcement in drug addiction: the darkness within. *CRF*, •••; *DA*, •••; *NE*, •••; *VTA*, ventral tegmental area. (From Koob GF. Negative reinforcement in drug addiction: the darkness within. *Curr Opin Neurobiol.* 2013;23[4]:559–563.)

exposure to a drug. Sensitization can be thought of as the increase in wanting a drug after intermittent use and can facilitate the transition from occasional use to chronic use and tolerance.[258] This phenomenon is well described and summarized in a paper by Nora Volkow, titled: "Decreased Reward Sensitivity and Increased Expectation Sensitivity Conspire to Overwhelm the Brain's Control Circuit."[320]

The counteradaptation model postulates that the initial positive feelings of reward resulting from the use of a drug are followed by an opposing rather than synchronous development of tolerance that is manifested by the appearance of withdrawal associated with the lack of the substance.[304] The positive rewarding effects diminish gradually with sustained use, whereas tolerance for the

effect of a drug takes longer to dissipate after stopping the use; a cycle of escalating drug use may follow after each cessation and consequent withdrawal. When the neurotransmitter system of the reward pathway is overactivated through escalating drug use, the system may not be able to maintain an increasingly pleasurable response to the drug. The individual is motivated to escalate the amount of use, to compensate for not delivering the reward that was expected based-on previous experience. This is evidenced in microdialysis experiments that have documented decreases in dopaminergic and serotonergic transmission in the nucleus accumbens after chronic and escalating use.[298] Increase in CRF and concomitant decrease in neuropeptide Y during substance withdrawal (including nicotine) are associated with increases in anxiety. In turn, during substance withdrawal, activation of norepinephrine pathways stimulates additional CRF, possibly resulting in an amplification of arousal and stress, and even neurotoxic effects if this amplification of arousal and stress are long-lasting.[268]

Of course, the two previous models are not mutually exclusive. One aspect of withdrawal that expands the concept of negative reinforcement is the effects of withdrawal on the brain's prefrontal control circuit,[110] and the depletion of inhibitory capacity.[109,140] The state of withdrawal alters the ability of the individual to resist drug-related opportunities, and cigarettes are no exception.[219] The brain needs to have sufficient "energy" to inhibit drug cravings, and this has been a point of practical wisdom in mutual help groups, which warn that individuals who are tired are at greater risk of relapse.[109]

Other models of nicotine addiction have been proposed, based on mechanisms associated with cognitive control and reinforcement learning,[80] particularly the negative reinforcement associated with the reduction in negative affect that may follow smoking after a period of abstinence (withdrawal).[19] These models are discussed in detail later in this chapter.

Cognitive Impairment

Although much of the focus of previous research has been related to nicotine's effects on reward processes and mesolimbic dopamine neurotransmission,[61,154,231] a growing body of literature suggests that nicotine's noradrenergic and dopaminergic effects on attention, information processing, and affective regulation may be of considerable importance in understanding the maintenance of a nicotine use disorder. Neurological deficits common to attention and substance use disorders, such as impaired performance, lack of motivation, decreased working memory, and impaired executive function, have been well documented[329] in both children and adults who have these disorders.[21,26,97,270,291] Current lines of investigation suggest that overlapping interrelated brain areas are responsible for explaining the attentional and executive impairments common to the two disorders.[64,105] The involvement of two areas, in particular the prefrontal cortex and anterior cingulate cortex, highlights the commonalities between drug dependence and attentional disorders, including nicotine and neurophysiological deficits related to cognitive dysfunction. It also may be that nicotine causes a distinct problem with decision-making, as evidenced by smokers' performance on the Iowa Gambling Task.[51] Stopping smoking can partially reverse these deficits. Longitudinal studies will be needed to determine how much of the decision-making deficit was preexisting (and predisposed the individual to substance use), and how much was an effect of the drug. Likewise, it is important to see if group differences between current and former smokers are due to acute drug-effects, or represent a different set of neurobiological characteristics in those who have been able to quit and those who have not.

The prefrontal cortex regulates goal-directed behavior, thought, and affect by using working memory to provide representational knowledge about past or future events and integrating this information into a plan for action or to exercise inhibitory control over inappropriate actions or thoughts.[256] In attentional/cognitive disorders these processes are impaired and manifested in symptoms that involve poor attention, planning, impulse control, and monitoring of one's behavior. Disentangling the direct relationship of these processes to a substance use disorder is difficult, because these individuals also have neurochemical deficits in the mesolimbic dopamine system.[232] Studies indicate that the right prefrontal cortex in humans is particularly important in the inhibition of activity (i.e., Stop or Go-No Go tasks).[15] The orbital and ventral prefrontal cortex may also have a similar inhibitory effect in the affective domain, thus permitting appropriate social behaviors.[287,302] In attention-deficit/hyperactivity disorder (ADHD), for example, the anterior cingulate cortex has been implicated in the regulation of the motivational aspects of attention as well as in the regulation of response selection and inhibition.[329] Thus researchers have begun to characterize ADHD as a disorder with deficits in inhibitory processes involving frontal cortical structures.[21] Notably, there is a significant relationship between a history of ADHD and smoking.[180] If a person must mentally manipulate information and make a response, the anterior cingulate cortex (with its connections to the prefrontal cortex) becomes active.[230] This area become particularly active in tasks where inhibitory control or divided attention are necessary.[253]

The importance of the inhibitory role of these structures in drug dependence has also been highlighted by several researchers. Drug-addicted individuals, including smokers, continue to use drugs even when faced with negative consequences and diminished reward, suggesting an apparent loss of control.[258] The failure to regulate (i.e., inhibit) this drive points to a dysfunction within the prefrontal cortex[319] and related areas including the anterior cingulate and orbitofrontal cortices.[207] These prefrontal dysfunctions may themselves be caused by deficits in the limbic structures, or exacerbated by them.[91,232] As shown in Fig. 23.3, the resulting persistence of the behavior is not necessarily due to continued reinforcement by the drug (mesolimbic dopamine) but rather to the enhanced saliency of the drug and drug cues that have been firmly established (learned) in memory during the acquisition of dependence. During maintenance of substance use disorders, these super-salient drug-related cues, including the effects of priming doses from the first amount of administration, overcome the inhibitory control of the prefrontal cortex that might normally inhibit the response to take the drug due to perceived costs (consequences) with decreasing hedonistic properties. The expectation of reward is maintained by the brain as it releases significant dopamine when approaching an opportunity to use a substance, even if the actual hedonic enjoyment of that substance has decreased with the development of tolerance. This causes the individual to escalate their use, and sometimes attempt to recreate the level of stimulation that they have previously experienced, and will forever remember that state when presented with cues to use (often termed "euphoric recall"). The development of tolerance occurs over time and leads to the individual needing to consume an increasing amount of the drug, particularly because the effects of the first use of the drug remain the ones that are expected and predicted by the user.[63]

Preclinical studies suggest that the impairment in prefrontal cortex function may be related to significant dendritic branching and spine density resulting from repeated drug administration,[260] thus amplifying the signal of salient events. Moreover, abstinence from the drug significantly reduces the efficiency of the prefrontal cortex to process information in working memory, thereby interfering with its regulatory function.[337] Such effects might be mediated by the negative affect associated with nicotine withdrawal, and when present, reduce the probability that a smoker may exercise an appropriate coping response and increase the probability of relapse.[19,337] There is electroencephalography (EEG) evidence supporting persistent frontal lobe dysfunction among smokers using tasks related to working memory (P300). Neuhaus and colleagues[228] found a hypoactivation of the anterior cingulate, orbitofrontal, and prefrontal cortices among both current and former smokers compared to never smokers, suggesting that the dysfunctional activation patterns found in smokers may not completely remit after quitting; a fact that may increase their vulnerability to relapse. It remains to be seen whether this is an effect of smoking, or a preexisting risk factor that led these individuals to be more likely to smoke.

A model by Curtin, Baker, and colleagues[80] attempts to address the conditions under which cognitive control mechanisms affect the processing of motivationally relevant information (i.e., smoking cues) and the execution of situationally appropriate behavior. The model holds that once dependence is established, drug use motivation is frequently driven by implicit processes that are largely automatic and outside of the user's awareness (contextual cueing involving the hippocampus and amygdala, and discrete cueing involving the basolateral amygdala).[66,153] These implicit processes are developed and maintained by negative and positive reinforcement learning.

In the case of negative reinforcement, internal states associated with negative affect or drug withdrawal can engage motivational systems and drug use behavior in an attempt to ameliorate these aversive states. This involves such processes as the central amygdala cascade occurring with withdrawal, and the release of CRF, which has direct effects on brain structures and also involves engagement of the wider hypothalamus-pituitary-adrenal (HPA) axis.[271] Activation of the habenula, which occurs when there is a reward prediction error, also further dampens the ventral tegmental area (VTA) to positive stimuli[210] and facilitates inhibitory avoidance.[248] In addition, there is evidence that the endorphin (endogenous opioid) system mediates certain aspects of nicotine dependence.[155,179,305]

With positive reinforcement, environmental cues and positive mood states previously associated with rewarding drug effects can increase approach motivation. The model postulates that these learned associations trigger subcortical, "bottom-up" processes that can influence drug-seeking behavior implicitly by engaging appetitive or avoidance motivational systems. Thus the drug user may frequently engage in drug-use behaviors for reasons that are outside of conscious awareness, and each use will reinforce the strength of the circuit.

Although the model proposed by Curtin et al.[80] holds that drug sensitization is largely maintained by the implicit influence of learned associations on motivation, the authors also speculate about circumstances in which drug use comes under explicit or cognitive control. Cognitive control can be defined as the effortful application of attentional resources to meaningful information and tasks.[41] Cognitive control is crucial to learning as it is activated when an organism encounters unexpected outcomes, unfavorable outcomes, or response errors.[144] In this model, cognitive control is important because it is elicited during response conflict, which can occur when the user attempts to regulate the craving and drug-seeking behaviors that result from exposure to conditioned cues.

Ultimately, cognitive control is what allows a drug user to engage in less well-learned alternatives to drug-seeking behavior when drug craving and approach motivation is activated. However, it is during instances of response conflict and engagement of cognitive control mechanisms that drug craving will be most acutely experienced by the drug user. If there are clear processing deficits engendered in the management of response conflict (also pertinent to error monitoring in the anterior cingulate cortex), then behavioral resistance to the increased craving is also diminished.

Development of Nicotine Dependence Risk, and the Effect on Other Substance Use Disorders

Effect on Comorbid Substance Use

All substances use, share, and activate the same underlying neuronal pathways of reward and reinforcement; nicotine may be strengthening the circuits involved in the maintenance of all-drug taking behaviors. Such that these circuits are primed to carry-out addictive behaviors for substances that the nicotine users subsequently experiment with and use regularly, the brain effects of nicotine use mean that individuals are often craving when they are in withdrawal, which can begin within hours of cessation of use. It is unknown what effect this may have on alcohol consumption or other drug use, and traditionally clinical recommendations have often proceeded from the assumption that it will be too difficult for individuals to simultaneously quit nicotine and other substances of abuse as that might incur increased risk of relapse to the other substance. However, the data continue to accumulate against that concept. It seems that quitting smoking (tobacco use) while in treatment either has no impact or, in some studies, has a favorable impact on the ability to quit and stay quit from other substances.[295] Therefore it is important to systematically assess for tobacco use disorder while people come in for treatment of other substance use disorders and offer them assistance to quit.

Because nicotine is one of the earliest drugs to be used, it is important to assess whether use by youth has a gateway effect toward other substances of abuse. For "gateway effect," the order of the substance may not be as important, but rather that the use of one substance leads to greater vulnerability for the subsequent use and addiction to other substances. The tobacco gateway seems to open quickly for urban adolescent smokers, who demonstrate a very high rate of concomitant substance use in a recent study.[213] The uptake of cannabis seems to be much greater for youth with preexisting nicotine dependence,[137,314] with the route of administration being an important variable, as smoking had greater risks than chewing tobacco.[5] Furthermore, there is strong evidence that the relationship between cannabis and nicotine is bidirectional,[15] with cannabis use being one of the strongest predictors of the subsequent onset of daily nicotine use after controlling for other variables.[24]

The effects of nicotine cessation on other substances of abuse have been studied, even in high-risk groups like adolescents diagnosed with ADHD and substance use disorders. Still the cessation of nicotine did not increase the rate of relapse to other substances.[130,237] Furthermore, the addition of smoking cessation to an established cannabis intervention did not adversely affect quit rates.[188] In recent years there has seemed to be an increase in the number of adolescents and young adults who are moving away from tobacco and nicotine dependence to use other substances,[159]

which ultimately could make the costs to society even greater. Conversely, not ceasing the use of other substances does increase the uptake of nicotine use.[36]

Nicotine and Negative Affect

Relative to some other substances of abuse (e.g., cocaine), negative reinforcement plays a more powerful role in the maintenance of tobacco use disorders. Negative reinforcement is the process of strengthening a behavior by having an aversive state removed after the behavior is performed, such as the smoking of a cigarette to avoid nicotine withdrawal.[191] One of the most fundamental aspects of nicotine dependence involves its neuroregulatory function on mood. The negative emotions involve decreased experience of reward, increased perception of threat, increased activation of what Panskepp termed the "rage system," and increased sensations of tension (possibly with relative disinhibition of locomotor activity).[238] The experience of frustrated nonreward recruits more motivation and energy for reward seeking, and increases the probability of reward attainment. To resist this frustration, an individual would need to have a good level of inhibition and an ability to tolerate negative affect.

The relationship between negative affect and the ability to sustain cessation of smoking behavior plays a prominent role in theories of nicotine dependence.[19] It has been theorized that individuals addicted to a substance learn to detect internal cues that negative affect is approaching as drug levels fall within the body. To prevent the onset of these negative feelings, the addicted person self-administers the drug, although often this process proceeds without conscious awareness. The longer the individual is without the drug, the more likely these negative feelings are to enter conscious awareness, providing direct reinforcement that taking the drug relieves negative affect (Fig. 23.4). This relationship has driven the development of new pharmacological[68,133,150] and behavioral[54,134] approaches to treatment. The experience of negative affect is a significant contributor to the risk of relapse, and negative affect reduction is cited by many smokers as an important reason to smoke. This is, of course, a fool's errand, as the negative affect is not truly relieved, but simply postponed. Newer approaches such as the ecological momentary assessment are helpful tools for tobacco researchers to look at the day-to-day, moment-to-moment correlates of smoking that could lead to the targeting of specific moments and tailoring strategies to forestall the resumption of tobacco consumption.[218] Improving the understanding of the psychobiological and genetic mechanisms associated with the modulation of mood by nicotine will help us better understand the mechanisms of nicotine dependence and the relationship between these mechanisms and treatment success (see Fig. 23.4).[19]

The term "negative affect" refers to a composite index of many negative mood states, including feelings of depression, dysphoria, irritability, and nervousness, and is usually measured by Likert-type scales such as the Positive and Negative Affect Scale (PANAS),[323] Profile of Mood States (POMS),[214] or other similar adjective checklists.[272] Research on the relationship between negative affect and smoking behavior has included evaluation of the effects of a past history of major depression, which may serve as a marker for vulnerability to future depressed mood, and evaluation of the effects of precessation and postcessation negative affect.

Indeed, the presence of negative affect following cessation has been found to characterize over 50% of all smoking lapses, with 19% of all lapses occurring under conditions of extreme negative

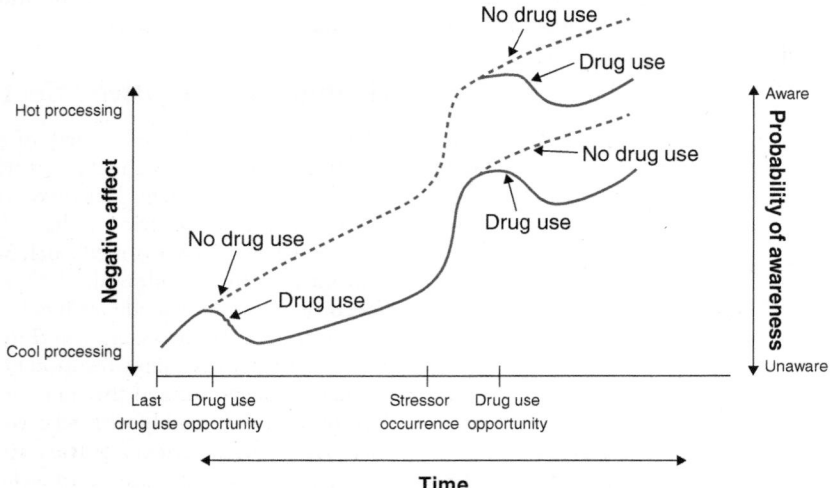

The role of affect and awareness in drug motivation

• **Fig. 23.4** Affective processing model of negative reinforcement in addiction. The *horizontal axis* represents time since last drug use, and the *vertical axis* represents intensity of the affective response. Affect increases in direct proportion to the amount of time since last drug use. As affect grows, the probability of the affect being consciously available grows as well. In addition, as the affect escalates, information processing begins to be dominated by the hot system rather than the cool system. If the drug is used optimally, nascent negative affect will be quelled before it becomes available to consciousness. If drug use is impeded at this point, however, affect may become conscious, and the addicted individual may be aware that negative affect decreases following renewed drug use. Negative affect spurred by exteroceptive stressors can become conscious as well and may be relieved by drug use. (Reprinted from Baker TB, Piper ME, McCarthy DE, Majeskie MR, Fiore MC. Addiction motivation reformulated: An affective processing model of negative reinforcement. *Psychol Rev.* 2004;111[1]:33–51)

mood.[272] Negative affect appears to be the component of nicotine withdrawal that most profoundly influences relapse and the trajectory of nicotine withdrawal symptoms.[175,242–244] The expectation that nicotine will produce desirable emotional consequences[326] has also been shown to inversely predict cessation success. In addition to postcessation negative affect, precessation levels of negative affect,[69,119,175,176,178] have been shown to predict cessation outcome. Negative affect following a quit attempt has been related to treatment failure and relapse across a variety of treatment modalities.[39,57,175]

When a smoker quits using tobacco, the above biological, cognitive, and behavioral aspects of dependence may increase the risk of relapse. However, many factors are associated with an increased risk for relapse after quitting smoking, including the availability of cigarettes, an increase in psychological stressors, and a triggering of conditioning factors (cues). Visual cues can be seeing people smoking or going to a location where one used to smoke or obtain cigarettes. Such factors may trigger the enduring adaptational changes that occurred in the brain during the period of nicotine consumption and subsequent addiction. The amygdala is very slow to forget, if it ever does, positively reinforced cues, in a term called incubation of drug craving.[203]

Genetics

Longitudinal twin studies have shown that the genetic risk for all substance use is shared[339] and there is substantial genetic contribution,[208,209] although there can be a substantial reduction in heritability in rural environments,[190] where the cultural factors are more important. There is some evidence of a specific genetic risk factor for nicotine dependence that does not significantly overlap with other substance use risk.[171] There is a noteworthy distinction between

the factors and processes leading to the initiation of a drug and the persistence of its use, and these factors are particularly important for a drug with as widespread exposure as nicotine. The persistence of nicotine dependence displays some difference in the genetics of initiation and persistence.[138] Genetic studies have been performed to take into consideration a very large number of single nucleotide polymorphisms (SNPs); we see that a substantial portion of variance in cigarette use can be explained by genetic effects that also mediate behavioral disinhibition.[322] Some of these genes could be involved in many different pathways, and it will take time to see if there are groups of genetic markers involved in similar or overlapping processes. Currently, there is no genetic test that can precisely determine an individual's risk of developing a tobacco use disorder.

Heritability

Recent family, twin, and molecular genetic studies provide compelling evidence of a role for genetic factors governing smoking initiation, continuation, and cessation, with estimated heritability rates ranging from 47%–76% for initiation and 62% for persistence.[a] The concordance rates for smoking, not smoking, and quitting are higher for monozygotic than for dizygotic twins, and the concordance rates for smoking in 108 pairs of identical twins reared apart (where 82 smoked) was 75.9%. Although monozygotic concordance rates for initiation and continuation of smoking were both above 80% in another study,[209] the weighted correlation in liability to lifetime regular smoking was 0.80 in monozygotic twins, and 0.53 in dizygotic twins, suggesting that the heritability of liability to regular smoking is likely 50% to 60%.[170] A meta-analysis of data from six studies revealed an

---

[a]References 60, 192, 194, 245, 264, 282.

estimated heritability rate of 0.6 for males and 0.48 for females for smoking persistence.[201] For the maintenance of dependent smoking behavior, the percent genetic contribution seems to be about 70%.[300] Three linkage studies of smoking behavior[31,93,286] suggest that alleles that influence smoking behavior occur in only a small proportion of families.

Genome-Wide Association Studies of Nicotine Dependence

Relatively recent genome-wide association studies related to nicotine dependence have been published. Uhl et al.[306] used 520,000 SNPs using a DNA pooling approach. They prepared pools of DNA from nicotine-dependent European-American smoking cessation trial participants and control individuals. Because in the DNA pooling technique individual genotypes are not available, they compared genotypes from the entire group of nicotine-dependent research participants to genotypes from European-American research volunteers free from any substantial lifetime use of any addictive substance. They performed analyses using smokers versus nonsmokers and successful versus nonsuccessful quitters and identified several genes of interest.

A study by Berrettini and colleagues[32] examined nicotine dependence using genome-wide association data from proprietary databases (GlaxoSmithKline) established to study cardiovascular and other common diseases. In this study, nicotine dependence was studied using a single indicator: cigarettes per day where cases were defined as smokers consuming >25 cigarettes per day and controls were noted as consuming <5 cigarettes per day. Their initial analysis identified a significant relationship ($P = .0006$) between a SNP in the cholinergic receptor nicotinic alpha 3 subunit (CHRNA3) region, rs6495308, although the P-value fell below the 10^{-7} expected for genome-wide analysis. Nevertheless in a replication sample, another SNP in this same region, rs1317286, did meet the expected P-value for a relationship with cigarettes per day.

Bierut et al.[34] performed a genome-wide association on 1050 nicotine-dependent cases and 879 nondependent smokers. This was a two-stage study in which DNA pooling was used in the first stage of analyses and 31,960 SNPs were selected and genotyped in the nicotine-dependent cases and nondependent controls. They identified 35 SNPs with P-values less than 10^{-6}; however, none of these SNPs maintained significance after correcting for multiple testing. However, this study did identify several candidate genes. In a follow-up study, Bierut[35] used data from The Collaborative Study on the Genetics of Alcoholism (COGA) and contrasted smokers who consumed over 20 cigarettes per day with those who smoked >100 cigarettes in their lifetime but never more than 10 cigarettes per day. The results showed the nonsynonymous coding SNP of the CHRNA5 gene, rs16969968 ($P = 0.007$), was associated with habitual smoking. Other SNPs in this region that were highly correlated with rs16969968 included rs2036527, rs17486278, rs1051730, and rs17487223 ($r^2 > 0.79$). A second independent finding noted by these authors in this gene cluster, was an association with rs578776, for which a low correlation with rs16969968 ($r^2 < 0.15$) was observed.

Three recent genome-wide association studies have identified gene variants in a region on the long arm of chromosome 15 (15q24/15q25.1) as significant contributors to the risk of lung cancer, as well as nicotine dependence. The region of interest encompasses the nicotinic acetylcholine receptor subunit genes CHRNA3, CHRNA5, and CHRNB4, and involves several SNPs in strong linkage disequilibrium with each other. These include rs10517309,145,294 and rs8034191.[9,145] In the case control study by Amos[9] and in a further analysis of these and other data by Spitz and colleagues,[281] a significant relationship was noted for gene variants in this region (the A variant for rs1051730 in this analysis) associated with lung cancer, nicotine dependence, and smoking quantity indices in cases and controls, as well as earlier age of smoking initiation and time to first cigarette in controls. A nonsignificant trend was also noted for an inverse relationship between the adverse allele and duration of cessation. Thorgeirsson and colleagues[294] also found a significant relationship between risk of lung cancer and peripheral artery disease and the T variant (TT TG GG) of rs1051730. A significant association was also found between the adverse allele likelihood of being a former smoker, and as with the previous study, associations were also noted between the minor allele and smoking quantity, Fagerström Test for Cigarette Dependence scores, and symptoms of nicotine dependence from the *Diagnostic and Statistical Manual of Mental Disorders, Fourth Edition, Text Revision* (DSM-IV TR). Of interest, the genome-wide association study by Hung and colleagues[149] also noted a significant risk of lung cancer and the variant alleles of rs1051730 and rs8034191, but unlike the other two genome-wide association studies for lung cancer, these authors did not note an association with nicotine dependence, a finding which is at variance with several recent studies of nicotine dependence not involving cancer patients. For example, the rs1051730 SNP is in strong linkage disequilibrium (correlated) with the CHRNA5 SNP, rs16969968, for which the A variant has been shown to increase the risk of nicotine dependence in the studies noted earlier.[35,265] This SNP also has an r^2 of .18 and .90 with rs6495308 and rs1317286, respectively, which are two SNPs in this CHRNA3-A5 region that have been shown to predict cigarettes per day in heavy smokers in the genome-wide association study by Berrettini and colleagues.[32] Furthermore, in the study of Thorgeirsson et al.,[294] the relationship of rs1051730 with FTCD scores or symptoms on the DSM-IV, was at a level similar to that observed in a candidate gene study using low frequency smokers as controls.[265]

Candidate Gene Studies for Nicotine Dependence

An examination of the literature in this area shows that over 60 unique genes have been noted in candidate gene studies of nicotine dependence. Several reviews have been published in this area,[b] with most concluding that small sample size and replicability pose significant issues in interpreting these results. In addition, the limited characterization of the phenotype (i.e., simple classification as a smoker or not) may further restrict the information that can be obtained from these studies. Most of the candidate genes studied to date fall into two categories: Nicotine metabolism and CNS receptor or neurotransmitter function. An example of the metabolism is the cytochrome P450 (CYP)2A polymorphisms have also been associated with different risks for tobacco use disorders.[226] The receptor and neurotransmitter studies have included all the major SNPs that have been researched in the smoking literature related to dopamine pathways and nicotinic receptors—for example dopamine receptor D2 (DRD2), dopamine (DOPA), ankyrin repeat and kinase domain containing 1 (ANKK1), dopamine transporter (DAT), catechol-O-methyltransferase (COMT), cholinergic receptor nicotinic alpha 4 subunit (CHRNA4), and cholinergic receptor nicotinic beta 2 subunit (CHRNB2) (see Blomqvist et al.,[37] Huang et al.,[145] Hutchison et al.,[151] Saccone et al.,[265] and Zhang et al.[341]).

---

[b]References 62, 198, 201, 202, 222–224.

Genome-Wide Studies Predicting Nicotine Cessation Treatment Outcome

Uhl and colleagues[307] recently[265] conducted a genome-wide association study examining successful versus unsuccessful quitters across three clinical trials: one used nicotine replacement therapy (NRT), and results from this sample were also previously published by this group[306]; and two used bupropion, in mixed racial samples. The combined sample for all three trials totaled 540 individuals, with individual trial samples 266 and 150 for the two bupropion trials and 124 in the NRT trials. This group of investigators used a DNA pooling strategy and Monte Carlo simulation analysis of gene frequencies to identify SNPs that differentiated abstainers and nonabstainers, as well as those that were specific to nicotine replacement therapy or bupropion. In total, they noted several thousand SNPs with nominal significance covering over 100 genes, involved in numerous biological processes ranging from cell adhesion, transcription regulation, intracellular signaling, cell structure, and unknown function. Although intriguing and suggestive of a pharmacogenetic effect, the results from this study are difficult to interpret given the sheer number of hits and the complex biological processes involved. Clearly, much more information is needed, taking a more traditional approach to genome-wide association techniques to examine both predictors of abstinence and pharmacogenetic effects of smoking cessation medications.

Candidate Gene Studies Predicting Treatment Outcome

A handful of candidate studies have examined genetic predictors of NRT and bupropion. Like the candidate gene studies on nicotine dependence, most of these studies have focused on markers in the dopamine pathway, given the importance of the dopaminergic neurotransmission in nicotine reinforcement. For example, several polymorphisms in the D2 receptor gene (DRD2), including the following variants: C957T, -141Cins/del and Taq1A (ANKK1), C32806T, and a variable-number-of-tandem-repeat (VNTR) in the DRD4 (C-521T) have been shown to predict cessation outcome to NRT.[84,160,193,340] Others have identified genes associated with opioid or serotonergic pathways.[85,196] With the exception of the study by David,[84] most have predicted only end of treatment success. Similarly, many of these same markers (Taq1A, --141Cins/del),[82,86,87,193,289] and others (COMT, cytochrome P450 2B6 [CYP 2B6], DAT)[33,83,195] have been associated with successful treatment by bupropion, as well as another antidepressant, venlafaxine.[68,70] One recent candidate gene study took a systems approach to identifying SNPs associated with smoking cessation using bupropion.[76] This study involved a population of 217 and 195 smokers receiving bupropion or placebo, respectively. Using a systems-based candidate gene approach this study identified polymorphisms (rs2072661 and rs2072660) within the β2nicotinic acetylcholine receptor (CHRNB2), which showed significant association with abstinence rates at end of treatment and at 6-month follow-up in a placebo-controlled trial of bupropion for smoking cessation. The association with the two SNPs was very high ($r^2 = 0.96$). These effects were independent of treatment but there was some indication that abstinence might be modulated by bupropion. For example, there was a substantial increase in relapse rates for those individuals carrying the minor allele after treatment was discontinued. Subsequent analyses of rs2072661 showed a significant relationship with time to relapse at the 6-month follow-up period and modulation of withdrawal symptoms at the target quit date.

TABLE 23.1   Items and Scoring for the Fagerström Test for Cigarette Dependence.

Questions	Answers	Points
1. How soon after you wake up do you smoke your first cigarette?	Within 5 min	3
	6–30 min	2
	31–60 min	1
	After 60 min	0
2. Do you find it difficult to refrain from smoking in places where it is forbidden, e.g., in church, at the library, in cinema, etc.?	Yes	1
	No	0
3. Which cigarette would you hate most to give up?	The first one in the morning	1
	All others	0
4. How many cigarettes/day do you smoke?	10 or less	0
	11–20	1
	21–30	2
	31 or more	3
5. Do you smoke more frequently during the first hours after waking than during the rest of the day?	Yes	1
	No	0
6. Do you smoke if you are so ill that you are in bed most of the day?	Yes	1
	No	0

Reprinted from Heatherton et al.[139] with permission: John Wiley & Sons, Inc.

Diagnosis

In 2013, the Fifth Edition of the *Diagnostic and Statistical Manual of Mental Disorders* (DSM-5) was published, and included several changes to the section now entitled: Substance Related and Addictive Disorders. Tobacco Use Disorder has replaced nicotine dependence and has the same general 11 symptoms like other substance use disorders. The new list of 11 symptoms was basically a combination of the DSM-IV-TR abuse and dependence symptoms with the removal of "legal consequences" from the list in exchange for "craving, or strong desire or urge to use." Although all seven of the prior dependence symptoms were retained, the newly added symptoms are "recurrent tobacco use in situations in which it is physically hazardous," continued use despite the social or interpersonal problems caused or exacerbated by tobacco, and recurrent tobacco use resulting in a failure to fulfill major role obligations at work, school, or home. Nicotine is reported to be among the most addictive of substances of use, especially when consumed through smoking tobacco. After prolonged smoking, the user develops nicotine tolerance and exhibits withdrawal symptoms when nicotine is absent; these are two physiological symptoms of dependence (addiction). Furthermore, nicotine may be responsible for other criteria for dependence: loss of control over smoking (e.g., not being able to reduce or stop smoking; or smoking more than intended), compulsive use (e.g., spending more time using the substance or giving up important events to use the substance), and continued smoking despite adverse consequences (e.g., heart attack, emphysema, or cancer). The presence of any two or more of those 11 criteria for at least a year satisfies the definition of tobacco use disorder, previously called dependence and classically known as addiction.[8]

A commonly used scale for assessing nicotine dependence is the Fagerström Test for Nicotine Dependence (or FTCD) (Table 23.1).[139] The FTCD measures physiological dependence (tolerance and withdrawal) reliably well, but does not reliably measure some of the other dimensions of nicotine dependence (especially the behavioral ones). Of particular importance is the first item of the scale (How soon after you wake up in the morning you smoke your first cigarette?), which has been validated recently as a proxy for nicotine dependence and called "heaviness of smoking index" (HIS).[20] Most research studies until now have used the total FTCD score of equal to or greater than 4, as a cutoff as synonymous to physiological dependence to nicotine.[239,250] The Wisconsin Inventory of Smoking Dependence Motives (WISDM-68)[247] and its shortened version (WISDM-37)[279] are more recently developed multidimensional scales of nicotine dependence. These are usually used in research as they are more comprehensive and detailed than the FTCD and include measures of cognitive enhancement, negative reinforcement, positive reinforcement, automaticity, affiliative attachment, loss of control, behavioral choice/amelioration, craving, cue exposure/associative processes, social/environmental goals, taste/sensory processes, weight control, and tolerance (see Table 23.1).

Smoking and Psychiatric Comorbidities

There is substantial evidence to suggest that smoking is closely linked with several psychiatric comorbidities, suggesting shared biological pathways between nicotine dependence and these psychiatric conditions. For example, current smoking rates among those with no mental illness, lifetime mental illness, and past-month mental illness has been reported as 22.5%, 34.8%, and 41.0%, respectively. Remarkably, smokers with a mental disorder in the past month reportedly consumed 44.3% of all cigarettes smoked in this nationally representative sample.[185] Several studies have demonstrated a strong relationship between alcohol, substance abuse, and other psychiatric disorders and smoking.[c] For example, the lifetime prevalence rate of alcohol dependence or drug abuse is estimated at 23%–30% among adult smokers,[23,43] and this number is higher among the young adult cohort.[290] Among nondependent and dependent current smokers, lifetime rates of mood and anxiety disorders have been reported as 12%–26.7%, and 33.5%–46.5%, respectively.[43] In addition, there is an elevated risk of first onset of major depression, panic disorder, and generalized anxiety disorder among smokers.[48,49,52,158,172] A significant shared familial risk of depression and smoking has been identified for heavy and nonheavy nicotine-dependent smokers,[157] and a history of major depression[7] has been associated with an increased prevalence of smoking,[45,47,121,173] nicotine dependence,[46] and greater nicotine withdrawal severity. Some studies have found an inverse relationship between major depression history and quitting success, but these findings have not been uniform.[50,119,142,221,229]

Some data have suggested that treatment with sequential fluoxetine, beginning 8 weeks before the target quit rate, is associated with enhancement of quit rate, and significantly reduced negative affect during the withdrawal state.[53] In addition, bipolar disorders have been shown to have a relationship to smoking, with rates nearly as high as those for schizophrenia. As with posttraumatic stress disorder (PTSD), which carries a very strong association with tobacco use.[164]

In the area of neurodevelopmental disorders, odds ratios comparing "ever" with "never" smokers were positively related to the number of ADHD symptoms. Among those reporting regular smoking over their lifetime, an inverse relationship between number of ADHD symptoms and age at onset, and a positive relationship between symptoms and number of cigarettes smoked, has also been observed.[180] The time to first use of cigarette in the morning, the number of cigarettes smoked in a day, and the likelihood of smoking when sick, have all been correlated with ADHD symptoms.[330] In addition, in longitudinal studies of individuals with ADHD, it has been revealed that hyperactive-impulsive symptoms were risk factors for multiple substance use disorder, and inattentive symptoms only predicted nicotine dependence[96]; the links persisted even after controlling for the presence of conduct disorder. The association with ADHD naturally raised the question of whether treatment with stimulants might affect nicotine dependence risk. In clinical laboratory studies, the acute administration of methylphenidate is associated with greater nicotine use in controls,[263] and in ADHD individuals,[317] but one study showed the effect of increasing cigarette intake to be curiously correlated with decreases in food intake.[316] Clinical trials using osmotic-released methylphenidate led to no clinical improvement or worsening of smoking for ADHD individuals,[335] but had some benefit for nonwhites,[78] and has generally been established to be relatively safe in a substance-using population.[334] A meta-analysis of several studies showed a relationship between treating ADHD symptoms with stimulants and reduced rates of smoking: "effect sizes were larger for studies that used clinical samples, included more women, measured smoking in adolescence rather than adulthood, conceptualized stimulant treatment as consistent over time, and accounted for comorbid conduct disorder."[269]

Conduct disorder (CD) has also been associated with smoking, "with a dose-dependent effect,"[212,255] as it has been associated with all other substances of abuse. The general lack of response to aversive information relative to healthy controls (CD individuals are relatively insensitive to punishment) is associated with substance use in this population,[107] and may require alteration in the common approaches to substance abuse treatment in this population.

Eating disorders are linked with tobacco, as the use of nicotine for weight reduction is an important factor in smoking, particularly for women.[177] A drive for thinness has been associated with smoking on a daily basis.[77] Smokers have a greater prevalence of eating pathology[77] and body shape concerns,[174] and among women, bulimia nervosa and binge-eating disorder are associated with higher rates of smoking.[280] Subtyping of the eating disorders appears important, because both the binge-purge types of anorexia and bulimia have been shown to have higher odds-ratios of smoking than the other subtypes.[13] There is concern that smoking cessation could lead to reemergence of anorexia symptoms in remitted anorexics, triggered by the rapid weight-gain with smoking cessation,[275] and caution certainly needs to be exercised in this population, with careful planning around triggers to relapse of both disorders. Smoking status affects the resting energy expenditure in patients with anorexia, and should be considered during refeeding.[315] In smokers, comorbid bulimia and binge-eating disorder have higher rates of depression and alcohol use,[267,327] and binge-eating and smoking carry an additional risk of panic disorder and PTSD.[327]

The impact of comorbid psychiatric symptoms on the ability to quit using tobacco varies according to the disorder. Certain comorbidities such as ADHD and social anxiety may strongly predict relapse rates[148] and provide opportunities for intervention to improve outcomes by treating the comorbid disorder.[56]

---

[c]References 22, 40, 44, 79, 121, 136, 185, 332.
[d]References 10, 42, 57, 121, 122, 325.

Prevention Science

Prevention science is suggesting that there are weak and inconsistent effects of school policies on tobacco use.[114,135] However, enforcing the laws regarding tobacco use and its sales to minors can affect the rate of its use.[90] In addition, there are studies showing the use of graphic warning labels that can induce brain responses that effectively change the individual's motivation to use a substance.[2,88,131,233,234] Early prevention and interactive education using audiovisual technologies such as the ASPIRE program seem to be successful in lowering the uptake of smoking from 6% to 2% among high school students who participated versus controls.[251] The Good Behavior Game showed decreased rates of regular smoking from ages 19 to 21,[169] and Unplugged[112] has been associated with decreased rates of smoking uptake and slower progression of increased rates of smoking. Unplugged uses a social influence model to decrease the normative perception of peers using tobacco, and increased the refusal skills for tobacco.[118] The Unplugged curriculum may have the critical difference of using teachers to deliver the evidence-based prevention of substance use. The relationship of the teachers to the students helps the message remain salient for the individual.

A public health campaign in the United States has shown some effect,[94,211] and it is partly responsible for the downtrend in American youth use of combustible tobacco. The decreased frequency of combustible tobacco use in the American population means that there have been demographic and psychological drifts in the makeup of the average smoker. Today's smokers have become increasingly concentrated among those with psychiatric diagnosis, less wealth, or living in rural areas. Demographic shifts are important to consider when designing prevention efforts. The targeting of peer-crowds (groups of adolescents or youth who share similarities across the nation, for example, alternative, hipster, hip-hop, and country) seems to be a promising way to tailor prevention messages using the cutting-edge techniques (and science) of marketing.[204] The tactic of tobacco prevention using messages tailored to specific peer crowds on social media is a promising intervention being used in the Commonwealth of Virginia.[189]

Increasingly a large proportion of individuals who smoke are diagnosed with a mental illness.[200] In addition to the seriously mentally ill (schizophrenia and bipolar disorder), of particular concern is the correlation of cigarette smoking with depressive symptoms,[120] due to the high prevalence of depression in the general population. This raises an ethical concern with the state and federal government filling tax coffers with the taxation of cigarettes, because the burden of that taxation is increasingly falling on the marginalized[71] and persons living with mental illness.[120,186] This is not to say that the taxation should not occur because increases in cost greatly decrease the prevalence of smoking,[156] but the shifting burden onto vulnerable users highlights a moral imperative that the funds garnered from the taxation of cigarettes should be reinvested into smoking cessation efforts, in particular for those who are marginalized and/or diagnosed with mental disorders.

For youth, living in a smoking home can be a risk factor independent of having smoking parents.[126] There is limited evidence that family-based interventions can affect the risk of smoking in youth unless they are intensive.[293] Two studies showed that these can be additive beyond the interventions at school, and one study showed that the effects on smoking were comparable to those of the Good Behavior Game.[293] Anti-tobacco mass-media campaigns are likely to be more effective when they are buttressed by the interventions being delivered in the classroom.[143]

Treatment

As smoking becomes less prevalent, treatment may become a more difficult task for individuals who continue to smoke, and especially residual smokers who have failed earlier treatments for nicotine dependence. The current smoker is more likely to be more dependent on nicotine and have low motivation to change, most likely due to prior failed attempts—what has been termed a "hardening effect"—whereby a greater proportion of those with high motivation to change have already ceased tobacco use, leaving a more difficult-to-treat cohort.[92] Other markers of continuing to smoke and unsuccessful quitting (hard core smoker) are lower education and lower socioeconomic status.[71,312] Newer, tailored, and perhaps more comprehensive approaches may be needed for the more recalcitrant and difficult to quit population.

The US Public Health Service along with the Department of Health and Human Services, and in concert with other public health agencies, has sponsored general guidelines for the treatment of tobacco use and dependence. The first guideline was initially published in 1996 (summarizing 3000 publications), updated in 2000 (adding 2000 publications), and further updated in 2008, when information was added from about 2700 newer publications and had 10 key recommendations[108] (Table 23.2). The latest review in 2015 done by the US preventative task force (a group of independent scientists focus on reviewing the literature for evidence in prevention) assigned the evidence for effectiveness of tobacco treatment as having the highest possible category A, with the standard of care being counseling plus medications.[276]

The chance for recovery from nicotine dependence is maximized when a comprehensive biological, psychological, and social (biopsychosocial) assessment is done. Such assessments, which should account for the smoker's motivation for change, can guide both psychosocial therapy and pharmacological treatment. Pharmacological treatments produce the best results when combined with psychosocial therapy by doubling the odds of quitting smoking of either alone.[276] However, medications are often used alone or with minimal support and they do alleviate some of the effects of nicotine withdrawal, decrease cravings for tobacco use, and decrease the risk of relapse.

Nicotine replacement therapies (or NRTs) and non–nicotine-based medications such as sustained-release bupropion-SR (Zyban or Wellbutrin-SR) and varenicline (Chantix) have been shown to reduce cravings and nicotine withdrawal symptoms when used as aids to quitting smoking. NRTs, Bupropion-SR, and varenicline are first-line therapies for tobacco dependence, whereas nortriptyline (Pamelor) and clonidine (Catapres) are considered second-line (Table 23.3). Although there have been reported mood alterations that occur with varenicline, bupropion and other medications while patients try to quit smoking, multiple studies concluded that the risk is fairly minimal and insignificant, even among people with current or past but stable psychiatric disorders.[11,65,252] As a result, in December 2016, the US Food and Drug Administration (FDA) revised the packet insert and removed the black box warning for both varenicline and bupropion, replacing it with an adverse effect precaution. A historic decision, as the FDA has never before removed a black box warning from any medication insert.

According to their mechanism of action, the FDA approved-pharmacological agents for nicotine dependence may be grouped into three categories: nicotine agonists (i.e., nicotine replacement therapies [or NRTs]), nicotine antagonist (bupropion), and nicotine partial agonist (varenicline).

TABLE 23.2 Ten-key Guideline Recommendations.

The overarching goal of these recommendations is that clinicians strongly recommend the use of effective tobacco dependence counseling and medication treatments to their patients who use tobacco, and that health systems, insurers, and purchasers assist clinicians in making such effective treatments available.

1. Tobacco dependence is a chronic disease that often requires repeated intervention and multiple attempts to quit. Effective treatments exist, however, that can significantly increase rates of long-term abstinence.

2. It is essential that clinicians and health care delivery systems consistently identify and document tobacco use status and treat every tobacco user seen in a health care setting.

3. Tobacco dependence treatments are effective across a broad range of populations. Clinicians should encourage every patient willing to make a quit attempt to use the counseling treatments and medications recommended in this Guideline.

4. Brief tobacco dependence treatment is effective. Clinicians should offer every patient who uses tobacco at least the brief treatments shown to be effective in this Guideline.

5. Individual, group, and telephone counseling are effective, and their effectiveness increases with treatment intensity. Two components of counseling are especially effective, and clinicians should use these when counseling patients making a quit attempt:
   - Practical counseling (problem solving/skills training)
   - Social support delivered as part of treatment

6. Numerous effective medications are available for tobacco dependence, and clinicians should encourage their use by all patients attempting to quit smoking—except when medically contraindicated or with specific populations for which there is insufficient evidence of effectiveness (i.e., pregnant women, smokeless tobacco users, light smokers, and adolescents).
   - Seven first-line medications (five nicotine and two non-nicotine) reliably increase long-term smoking abstinence rates:
   - Bupropion SR, Nicotine gum, Nicotine inhaler, Nicotine lozenge, Nicotine nasal spray, Nicotine patch, Varenicline
   - Clinicians also should consider the use of certain combinations of medications identified as effective in this Guideline.

7. Counseling and medication are effective when used by themselves for treating tobacco dependence. The combination of counseling and medication, however, is more effective than either alone. Thus, clinicians should encourage all individuals making a quit attempt to use both counseling and medication.

8. Telephone quitline counseling is effective with diverse populations and has broad reach. Therefore, both clinicians and health care delivery systems should ensure patient access to quitlines and promote quitline use.

9. If a tobacco user currently is unwilling to make a quit attempt, clinicians should use the motivational treatments shown in this Guideline to be effective in increasing future quit attempts.

10. Tobacco dependence treatments are both clinically effective and highly cost-effective relative to interventions for other clinical disorders. Providing coverage for these treatments increases quit rates. Insurers and purchasers should ensure that all insurance plans include the counseling and medication identified as effective in this Guideline as covered benefits.

Reprinted from Treating Tobacco use and Dependence 2008 Update,[108] US Department of Health and Human Services website.

TABLE 23.3 FDA-Approved Dosage and Rx Availability for Pharmacological Agents for Smoking Cessation.

Cessation Agent	Dosage	Label Indication and Use	Availability in United States	RR of Efficacy (95% CI)
Nicotine gum	2 mg and 4 mg	2 mg ≤25 cig/day and 4 mg ≥25 cig/day; one piece every 1–2 hours for weeks 1–6, one every 2–4 hours for weeks 7–9, and one every 4–8 hours for weeks 10–12	OTC; traditional, mint, and orange flavors, generic available	1.49 (1.40–1.60)[a]
Nicotine patch	21 mg, 14 mg, and 7 mg	≥10 cig/day: 21 mg for 6 weeks, then 14 mg for 2 weeks; then 7 mg for 2 weeks, ≤10 cig/day: 14 mg for 6 weeks, then 7 mg for 2 weeks	OTC; clear and skin color; generic available	1.64 (1.53–1.75)[a]
Nicotine nasal spray	10 mg/mL, 0.5 mg/squirt	2 squirts (one dose) per hour, minimum 8 doses/day, maximum 40 doses/day; recommended up to 3 months	Prescription only, 100 mg/bottle; no generic	2.02 (1.49–2.73)[a]
Nicotine oral inhaler	10 mg/cartridge, 4 mg delivered	6–16 cartridges/day up to 12 weeks, then gradual reduction for another 12 weeks; usually individualized	Prescription only, 168 cartridges/box; no generic	1.90 (1.36–2.67)[a]
Nicotine lozenges	2 mg and 4 mg	If first cig is ≤30 minutes after waking, use 4-mg lozenge; if ≥30 minutes, use 2-mg lozenge; use one every 1–2 hours for 6 weeks, then one every 2–4 hours for 3 weeks, then one every 4–8 hours for 3 weeks; minimum 8 lozenges/day, maximum 20 lozenges/day	OTC; mint and cherry flavors; no generic	1.52 (1.32–1.74)[a]
Bupropion-SR	100 mg and 150 mg	150 mg every morning for 3 days, then 150 mg twice daily; recommended for 3 months	Prescription available; generic available	1.94 (1.72–2.19)[b]
Varenicline	0.5 mg and 1 mg	0.5 mg every morning for 3 days, then 0.5 mg twice daily for 4 days, then 1 mg twice daily up to 3 months; if successful may extend another 3 months	Prescription only; no generic	2.24 (2.06–2.43)[c]

[a]RR/comparative efficacy for nicotine replacement therapies with control (placebo), as reviewed by Hartmann-Boyce et al.[135a]

[b]RR for overall bupropion-SR efficacy, as reviewed by Hughes et al.[146]

[c]RR for varenicline efficacy compared with placebo by Cahill et al.[58]

Cig, Cigarettes; *FDA*, US Food and Drug Administration; *OTC*, over the counter; *RR*, risk ratio.

Nicotine Agonists

NRTs were the first pharmacological treatments to be offered for smoking cessation. The quit rate among smokers who take an NRT is about double that of smokers who do not; some NRTs are available by prescription only (Rx), and some are available over the counter (OTC).[165] The FDA has approved the following NRTs for smoking cessation: polacrilex gum (OTC); patches (16- or 24-hour; Rx and OTC); nasal spray (Rx); buccal inhaler (Rx); flavored gum (OTC); and lozenges (OTC). Table 23.3 provides detailed information on NRTs.

In a 2018 analysis, Hartmann-Boyce et al.[135a] included 133 trials, with 64,640 participants. They reported that the overall risk ratio (RR) for abstinence with NRTs compared with control (placebo) was 1.55 (95% confidence interval [CI] 1.49–1.61). In addition, they reported that combinations of NRTs were more effective than a single NRT, and they confirmed the following conclusions in an earlier review by Silagy et al.[274]: (1) 8 weeks of patch therapy is as effective as longer courses of patch therapy, and there is no evidence that tapering therapy is better than abruptly ending therapy; (2) wearing a patch only during waking hours (16 hours/day) is as effective as wearing a patch for 24 hours/day; (3) gum may be offered on a fixed-dose or as-needed basis; (4) highly dependent smokers (e.g., those who need to smoke within 30 minutes of waking) and those who have been unable to quit with 2-mg gum can be offered 4-mg gum; and (5) the effectiveness of NRTs appears to be largely independent of the intensity of psychosocial therapeutic support provided to the smoker. Finally, the review stated that practitioners should give the patient brief advice on how to quit and an overview of ways to improve the effectiveness of treatment.

Two considerations in offering combined NRTs are the patient's previous success with an NRT and the extent of nicotine dependence. If someone has had prior success quitting on one type of NRT, it is recommended that the same product be used again, assuming that the patient is interested in NRTs rather than non–nicotine-based medications. Patient education and management of expectations are key aspects of the clinical visit before treatment begins. This is especially true for combination approaches, such as the simultaneous use of two NRTs or of bupropion and an NRT. Patients may hesitate to use such combinations because all NRT labels still have a warning against combining NRTs as well as against continuing to smoke after starting an NRT. To note, both the combination of NRTs and using NRTs with concurrent smoking have been deemed safe.[108] Results from several studies demonstrate the safety of combining NRTs[217]; other studies have explicitly used NRTs (gums, inhalers, or patches), even if patients continue to smoke. Using NRTs in this way has helped reduce the number of cigarettes smoked each day by up to 50% in participants who were not motivated to quit. Those studies pointed out a lack of significant nicotine toxicity or major adverse events if using NRTs while continuing to smoke.[38,101,324]

The dosing of nicotine replacement up to and exceeding 42 mg/day may be necessary to relieve symptoms of withdrawal.[285] Although this is not a standard strategy, improved outcomes are shown in many instances when these higher doses are used. To obtain an adequate dose of nicotine, it is important to estimate the amount of nicotine intake a person has; that is due to interindividual differences in pharmacokinetics, inhalation technique. Furthermore, with the combined use of nicotine vaporizers and cigarettes now more common, it is important to get quantification beyond the simple pack-year.[254] One can assess the levels of cotinine in the blood, saliva, or urine to determine the severity of nicotine dependence,[102,111] and there is also a rapid urine screen available to detect the presence or absence of the drug.[1] Expired breath carbon monoxide (CO) levels above 4 mmol/L are also used to detect nonabstinence from cigarettes.[29]

It is important to note that many smokers have used nicotine vaporizers as treatments for cigarette smoking,[3] but this is less commonly the motive in teens and young adults.[181] There are significant differences between nicotine vaporizers, and it is sufficient to say that they were not designed by health scientists with goal to diminish nicotine dependence. Some more recent vaporizing devices, Mark 10 and Vuse, were designed with the express goal of increasing nicotine delivery and allowing a comparable nicotine delivery device for cross-consumption with combustible nicotine products, which may sustain the dependence on nicotine. They are sold with cartridges specific for the device, and one brand actually has chemical additives designed to provide a marker signal to burn the throat.[100] Newer devices like JUUL offer many attractive flavors and unique features. They are small and sleek, have a much smaller vape cloud, and look like flash drives. All of this has made them easy to conceal from parents and teachers. By adding benzoic acid to nicotine salts, these devices achieve a higher absorption rate of nicotine, and therefore a lower heating temperature can induce absorption of nicotine into bloodstream at levels similar to those obtained from smoking a cigarette.[163a] In one study, cutting nicotine concentration in half over an 8-month period did not change the levels of cotinine in blood.[102] The individuals seemed to increase the amount of liquid used and may have auto-adjusted other parameters to maintain their levels of nicotine.

Older vaporizers delivered nicotine at a low rate and may have provided nicotine levels more comparable to a nicotine replacement dosing that would relieve withdrawal symptoms than to a high level obtained from smoked tobacco. Another important issue with nicotine vaporization is the idea that without total cessation of combustible nicotine, vaporization could sustain nicotine dependence, as the vaporizer would be used in situations such as breaks from work, where the use of combustible nicotine is not ideal or permitted.

In one study in e-cigarette-naive tobacco users in Belgium, there was a substantial decrease in the amount of cigarettes smoked per day in 44% of the e-cigarette users. The most striking result was that the 34% of e-cigarette users had stopped smoking combustible tobacco cigarettes versus 0% in the control group.[3] In another recent study in young, not-ready-to-quit smokers, e-cigarettes helped reduce number of smoked cigarettes by 50% at the end of treatment (3 weeks), another indication of the potential effect of e-cigarettes on smoking.[301]

Nicotine Antagonists

Bupropion

The FDA-approved bupropion-SR (amfebutamone) for the treatment of tobacco dependence in 1991 under the new trade name Zyban. Bupropion-SR therapy is typically started 1–2 weeks before the planned quit date at a dosage of 150 mg per day for 3–7 days. The dosage should then be increased to 300 mg/day (divided into two doses, or once daily if the XL formulation is used). Bupropion-SR was originally approved as an antidepressant; it is considered an atypical antidepressant because it does not have a clearly known mechanism of action. Its pharmacodynamic properties include inhibition of norepinephrine reuptake and a modest inhibition of dopamine reuptake.[16] These properties are thought to contribute to bupropion-SR's antidepressant and antismoking action. In addition, later studies[277] have suggested that bupropion-SR acts as a noncompetitive antagonist on high-affinity (a4b2) subnicotinic acetylcholine (nACh) receptors. One of bupropion-SR's metabolites, (2S, 3S)-hydroxybupropion, has been hypothesized to be an even more powerful antagonist at a4b2 nicotine receptors than bupropion-SR itself. Therefore, (2S,3S)-hydroxybupropion may also reduce nicotine reward, withdrawal symptoms, and cravings.[81]

Bupropion-SR is contraindicated in patients with a family history or personal history of seizure and in those who have ever had a significant head trauma that resulted in a loss of consciousness for more than 10 minutes. Patients who have anxiety, insomnia, dry mouth, or tremors may experience a worsening of these symptoms with bupropion-SR. In patients with elevated liver enzyme levels, bupropion-SR metabolites may accumulate and lead to toxicity.[241]

Hughes et al.[81,146] analyzed the efficacy data on bupropion-SR as the sole therapy in a recent meta-analysis of 44 clinical trials that included more than 13,728 smokers. The meta-analysis found that patients taking bupropion-SR were more likely than those taking a placebo to achieve long-term tobacco abstinence (relative risk [RR] 1.62; 95% CI 1.49–1.76). Bupropion-SR also has been shown to be effective in several special clinical populations such as schizophrenic patients,[103] depressed patients,[55] veterans,[25] and smokers with PTSD,[141] and in primary care settings.[225]

The addition of an NRT to bupropion-SR therapy is believed to produce immediate relief from nicotine withdrawal, at least in the immediate postcessation period. A large controlled trial showed that the combination of bupropion and one form of NRT (the patch), while more effective than the monotherapies at the end of treatment, was not more effective than bupropion-SR alone at the 1-year follow-up.[162] Bupropion-SR can offer unique advantages for smokers who also have depression or attention-deficit/hyperactivity disorder because it may alleviate some of the resulting comorbid symptoms. It may also be an advantageous treatment choice in individuals who are overweight or afraid of gaining weight after they quit smoking as it seems to help in attenuating the weight gain associated with smoking cessation.[220] Bupropion seems to have a subtle but important positive effect on sexual dysfunction that seems to occur with chronic smoking, especially when the dysfunction is also related to the use of selective serotonin reuptake inhibitors.[73]

Although other antidepressants and anxiolytics have not generally been found efficacious for smoking cessation,[146] bupropion's antidepressant actions may make it a particularly attractive choice for smokers vulnerable to negative affect or among those with some level of affective and/or cognitive impairment. For example, in one study relative to placebo, bupropion has been shown to be effective among smokers with a history of depression,[278] although absolute cessation rates among depression history positive and negative smokers may not differ.[146] Apart from smoking, bupropion has long been indicated for the treatment of depression, and recent studies have shown additional benefits including prevention of the recurrence and improved efficacy for depressed patients with concomitant anxiety,[72] as well as a favorable outcome for the treatment of cocaine addiction when combined with behavioral treatment.[249] In a study of bupropion with 497 depressed smokers, depression symptoms did not seem mediate the effect on smoking abstinence. Similarly, given concerns about bupropion's seizure potential during alcohol withdrawal, it has not been used directly in the treatment of smokers with current alcohol or other

substance use disorders. However, among those who are in full remission from alcohol and other substances it seems to have a favorable effect on smoking cessation outcome and on reduction in number of cigarettes per day.[166,167] Nortriptyline, a tricyclic antidepressant, has noradrenergic properties similar to those of bupropion and it is the only antidepressant that has shown similar efficacy in the treatment of smokers as well as smoker-alcoholics regardless of existence of depressive symptoms.[299] In addition, among those with elevated depressive symptoms treatment with sequential fluoxetine, beginning 8 weeks before the target quit rate was associated with higher quit rate, and significantly reduced negative affect during immediately after quitting.[53]

Mecamylamine

Mecamylamine, a nicotine receptor antagonist, is used as a second-line therapy for smoking cessation. The addition of mecamylamine was shown in preclinical and clinical studies to increase the efficacy of nicotine patch therapy from 27.5%–29% to 47.5%–58%. However, a later multisite-controlled study reported that the increase in efficacy was not statistically significant.[123]

Mecamylamine produces unpleasant side effects, such as postganglionic effects (e.g., orthostatic hypotension) and strong anticholinergic effects (e.g., dry mouth and constipation), which have limited its use to either clinical or laboratory research settings.

Nicotine Partial Agonists

Varenicline

Varenicline (Chantix in the United States and Champix internationally) is the first pharmaceutically designed compound with partial agonist effects at nicotine receptors to become available in the market. Varenicline is a selective partial agonist that stimulates the a4b2 nicotine cholinergic receptors and consequently stimulates dopamine release in the nucleus accumbens, although to a lesser extent (40%–60% less) than nicotine itself. Varenicline displays antagonistic properties as well; by binding to nicotine receptors with a relatively long half-life (24 hours), it prevents the full stimulation of the receptors that ensues when nicotine is coadministered.[74] Because of these properties, varenicline may provide relief from withdrawal symptoms (an agonist effect) while blocking the rewarding effects of nicotine (an antagonist effect).[296] In addition, animal studies have shown that varenicline acts as a full agonist of the alpha-7 nicotine cholinergic receptor. Although this property has no clear benefit for smoking cessation,[216] it may have benefits for patients with chronic mental disorders (e.g., schizophrenia).

Varenicline is highly effective, and it may have lower side-effects with comparable efficacy when given at lower doses.[58] In addition, it is a relatively safe medication among patients with psychiatric disorders as there are no confirmed associations between varenicline and suicidal behavior.[58] Danicline was another nicotinic partial agonist drug; it had low efficacy rates and as a result its development was halted.[58] Clinical trials have shown varenicline to be more effective than bupropion-SR or placebo for smoking cessation, with a resulting odds ratio of 3:1 compared to placebo (see Table 23.3). Two randomized double-blind clinical trials had compared varenicline (2 mg), bupropion (300 mg), and placebo and led to varenicline's approval as a smoking cessation treatment. One showed overall continuous abstinence rates from the end of treatment through 1 year of 21.9%, 16.1%, and 8.4%, respectively[124]; and the other, 23%, 14.6%, and 10.3%.[161] In all these comparisons, continuous abstinence rates were significantly higher for varenicline than for bupropion or placebo, even at 1-year follow-up with medication. In a combined analysis of the two trials, varenicline resulted in significantly higher continuous abstinence rates at 1 year than either placebo or bupropion (all *P* values < 0.05).[125] In this pooled analysis, varenicline nearly tripled the odds of quitting smoking compared with placebo, even when using continued abstinence as a measure during the last 4 weeks of medication treatment (odds ratio [OR] 3.09; 95% CI 1.95–4.91; $p < 0.001$). In an extension study, additional 12 weeks of varenicline therapy (a total of 24 weeks) was given to those who abstained from smoking at some point during the first 3 months of varenicline therapy, which significantly reduced the risk of relapse among smokers who were abstinent at the end of the first 12 weeks.[297] Compared with smokers who received a placebo in this double-blind continuation trial, those who received varenicline reported significantly less cravings and diminished withdrawal symptoms throughout the trial.[59]

The most common adverse effects of varenicline are nausea, which occurs in up to 30% of patients (approximately twice the rate of nausea among those taking a placebo), flatulence, and vivid/abnormal dreams (10%–15%). In 2008–2009, the FDA received a large amount of reports indicating increased depressive symptoms, occurrence or increase in suicidal ideation, and difficulty with coordination. Further analysis of existing data[292] and prospective studies were requested to clarify the relationship of the medication and the magnitude of such occurrences, in particular among those with psychiatric disorders. None of the studies done in depression,[12] bipolar disorder,[65] or schizophrenia[104,331] found correlation with using varenicline. It is recommended that patients stop the medication and advise their health care provider immediately if they develop changes in behavior or any of the above symptoms.[313] In December 2016, the FDA took the unprecedented action of the first time in removing a blackbox warning; this was regarding the risk of neuropsychiatric effects of varenicline.[106] This action was based on above-mentioned analysis and studies including the largest prospective controlled double-blind study on smoking cessation study to date EAGLES with 8000 subjects worldwide,[11] not showing an increased risk. Most recently, the EAGLES extension study to determine if there is an increase in serious cardiovascular events between the groups did not show any significant difference when comparing varenicline, bupropion, patch, and placebo.[30] For many patients, the prospect of using varenicline, a newer option, seem to motivate them to quit smoking, especially for those who have not succeeded with older smoking cessation medications. In addition, combining varenicline with bupropion-SR might provide better smoking cessation efficacy for those who are highly nicotine dependent,[95] in particular males,[261,262] whereas it does not seem to offer an advantage for those who are not heavily dependent on nicotine.[67]

Cytisine

Cytisine (also known as Tabex) is a nicotine-like alkaloid derived from the plant species *Laburnum anagyroides*. Little was known about cytisine in the United States until the fall of the Soviet Union in the 1990s. Most studies of cytisine for smoking cessation were open-label trials, and those that were controlled were not done so rigorously. Furthermore, most of the studies were from Bulgaria and none were published in the English-language literature, making it difficult for investigators in the United States to form a definitive scientific opinion on the efficacy of cytisine for smoking cessation.[303] Two trials of cytisine (937 people) found that more participants taking cytisine stopped smoking compared with placebo at longest follow-up, with a pooled risk ratio (RR) of 3.98 (95% CI 2.01–7.87; low-quality evidence). One recent trial comparing cytisine with NRT in 1310 people found a benefit for cytisine at 6 months (RR 1.43, 95% CI 1.13–1.80).[58]

Other Medications

Clonidine, a second-line pharmacotherapy, has exhibited modest efficacy in smoking-cessation trials. Clonidine increased the chances of quitting (RR 1.63; 95% CI 1.22–2.18), but this was offset by a dose-dependent rise in adverse events.[58a]

Several tricyclic antidepressants, which inhibit the reuptake of norepinephrine and serotonin, in particular nortriptyline, might facilitate smoking cessation either alone or in combination with behavioral treatment. Nortriptyline increased the chances of quitting compared to placebo (RR 2.03; 95% CI 1.48–2.78).[58a] However, tricyclic antidepressants have significant disadvantages, including anticholinergic burden, cardiac side effects, and potential for lethality in an overdose.

Other potentially useful medications that are not FDA approved at this time for smoking cessation include rimonabant (Acomplia), a cannabinoid receptor CB_1 blocker[117,257]; Quitpack, a combination of mecamylamine and bupropion-SR; and a nicotine vaccine as an active immunization to help the immune system recognize nicotine as a foreign and develop antibodies against it.[240] Establishing efficacy of these treatments will require further study.

Nonpharmacological Treatments

As noted earlier, recovery from nicotine dependence is maximized when treatment includes pharmacological and psychosocial approaches.[276] Research shows that providing cessation interventions is feasible and effective in substance use disorder samples.[14] Research in this area has been codified within clinical practice guidelines for tobacco cessation that recommend the use of both psychosocial (skills-based, problem-solving, and motivational enhancement approaches) and pharmacological interventions (bupropion, varenicline, nicotine replacement therapies) for all smokers, including those with complex comorbidities such as substance use and mental health disorders.[108] The best evidence for psychosocial interventions supports the use of behavioral and motivational approaches along with medications,[14,284] with evidence supporting their use in high smoking groups.[333] Behavioral interventions are especially useful for patients who are interested in tobacco cessation and can help patients develop new skills for addressing the stress in the lives, learn and practice strategies for coping with nicotine cravings, make environmental changes that support abstinence, and support patients' use of combination nicotine replacement therapy. As the population of smokers decreases and those who need to quit represent longer-term, more addicted smokers, those who come for treatment may have low readiness for or interest in quitting. For these smokers, motivational approaches can help patients identify personal reasons for quitting, reduce tobacco use as a start on the path toward cessation, and learn skills that can be used in future quit attempts.

Behavioral and motivational approaches can be delivered in different ways: brief intervention from a health care worker, telephone counseling, and self-help materials all promote cessation.[284] There is growing evidence to support web and mobile platforms for providing behavioral interventions,[128,328] and strong evidence supporting the use of state-funded tobacco quitlines that provide telephone counseling and nicotine replacement therapy for several weeks.[17,108,283] Many have been shown to help even smokers who are not willing to quit.[336] A widely used framework for assessing and intervening around tobacco use is called the 5 A's of tobacco cessation: (1) Ask patients if they smoke; (2) Advise them to quit; (3) Assess motivation for change; (4) Assist if they are willing to change; and (5) Arrange for follow-up. Research finds that use of the 5 A's framework is feasible in a range of health care settings and leads to increased rates of tobacco cessation.[4] Overall, there are range of behavioral and motivational options that can easily be delivered within medical, addiction, or mental health treatment settings by a range of treatment providers. Given the great harm from smoking and nicotine dependence, it is critical that all approaches be offered to and used with all smokers.

Summary

Long term tobacco use, usually resulting in nicotine dependence, is the leading cause of preventable disease and death in the United States and worldwide. Nicotine addiction activates the reward pathway, and consequently the prefrontal cortex, in a manner similar to that of other addictions. Familial traits and genetics are responsible for up to 60% of the variance for nicotine dependence; several SNPs and specific chromosomes have been implicated. Smoking cigarettes is a fast and effective tool for nicotine delivery, and nicotine dependence is a multifaceted syndrome consisting of biological, behavioral, and cognitive components. After a cessation attempt, the emerging negative affect (anxiety, depression, irritability, and so on) has been found to correlate with relapse to smoking. Therefore the treatment of nicotine dependence often requires an integrated approach that includes behavioral and motivational therapy in addition to medication. The diagnosis of nicotine dependence is usually made clinically; however, there are several scales that can be used to quantify the level of dependence, such as the FTCD and the WISDM. After more than two decades of research and development, health professionals can now turn to an arsenal of efficacious pharmacotherapies to treat smoking cessation. These agents often double the odds for quitting over placebo and in some cases almost triple those odds. Indeed, many smokers have benefited from these treatments and quit successfully. However, despite these advances, many smokers relapse, and unfortunately the long-term abstinence rates among smokers who are interested in quitting smoking remain low despite the best efforts and pharmacological treatment.[20]

References

1. Acosta M, Buchhalter A, Breland A, Hamilton D, Eissenberg T. Urine cotinine as an index of smoking status in smokers during 96-hr abstinence: comparison between gas chromatography/mass spectrometry and immunoassay test strips. *Nicotine Tob Res.* 2004;6(4):615–620. https://doi.org/10.1080/14622200410001727867.

2. Adebiyi AO, Uchendu OC, Bamgboye E, Ibitoye O, Omotola B. Perceived effectiveness of graphic health warnings as a deterrent for smoking initiation among adolescents in selected schools in southwest Nigeria. *Tob Induc Dis.* 2016;14:7. https://doi.org/10.1186/s12971-016-0074-y.

3. Adriaens K, van Gucht D, Declerck P, Baeyens F. Effectiveness of the electronic cigarette: an eight-week Flemish study with six-month follow-up on smoking reduction, craving and experienced benefits and complaints. *Int J Environ Res Public Health.* 2014;11(11):11220–11248. https://doi.org/10.3390/ijerph111111220.

4. Agency for Healthcare Research and Quality. Five Major Steps to Intervention (The "5 A's"): The five major steps to intervention are the "5 A's": Ask, Advise, Assess, Assist, and Arrange. http://www.ahrq.gov/professionals/clinicians-providers/guidelines-recommendations/tobacco/5steps.html. Updated Dec 2012. Accessed April 16, 2018.

5. Agrawal A, Lynskey MT. Tobacco and cannabis co-occurrence: does route of administration matter? *Drug Alcohol Depend.* 2009;99(1–3):240–247. https://doi.org/10.1016/j.drugalcdep.2008.08.007.

6. Albuquerque EX, Pereira EFR, Alkondon M, Rogers SW. Mammalian nicotinic acetylcholine receptors: from structure to function. *Physiol Rev.* 2009;89(1):73–120. https://doi.org/10.1152/physrev.00015.2008.

7. American Psychiatric Association. *Diagnostic and Statistical Manual of Mental Disorders.* 4th ed. Washington, DC: American Psychiatric Association; 1994.

8. American Psychiatric Association. *Diagnostic and Statistical Manual of Mental Disorders.* 5th ed. Arlington, VA: American Psychiatric Association; 2013.

9. Amos CI, Wu X, Broderick P, et al. Genome-wide association scan of tag SNPs identifies a susceptibility locus for lung cancer at 15q25.1. *Nat Genet.* 2008;40(5):616–622.

10. Anda RF, Williamson DF, Escobedo LG, Mast EE, Giovino GA, Remington PL. Depression and the dynamics of smoking: a national perspective. *J Am Med Assoc.* 1990;264(12):1541–1545.

11. Anthenelli RM, Benowitz NL, West R, et al. Neuropsychiatric safety and efficacy of varenicline, bupropion, and nicotine patch in smokers with and without psychiatric disorders (EAGLES): a double-blind, randomised, placebo-controlled clinical trial. *Lancet.* 2016;387(10037):2507–2520. https://doi.org/10.1016/S0140-6736(16)30272-0.

12. Anthenelli RM, Morris C, Ramey TS, et al. Effects of varenicline on smoking cessation in adults with stably treated current or past major depression: a randomized trial. *Ann Intern Med.* 2013;159(6):390–400. https://doi.org/10.7326/0003-4819-159-6-201309170-00005.

13. Anzengruber D, Klump KL, Thornton L, et al. Smoking in eating disorders. *Eat Behav.* 2006;7(4):291–299. https://doi.org/10.1016/j.eatbeh.2006.06.005.

14. Apollonio D, Philipps R, Bero L. Interventions for tobacco use cessation in people in treatment for or recovery from substance use disorders. *Cochrane Database Syst Rev.* 2016;11:CD010274. https://doi.org/10.1002/14651858.CD010274.pub2.

15. Aron AR, Robbins TW, Poldrack RA. Inhibition and the right inferior frontal cortex. *Trends Cogn Sci.* 2004;8(4):170–177.

16. Ascher JA, Cole JO, Colin JN, et al. Bupropion: a review of its mechanism of antidepressant activity. *J Clin Psychiatry.* 1995;56:395–401.

17. Babb S, Malarcher A, Schauer G, Asman K, Jamal A. Quitting smoking among adults - United States, 2000-2015. *MMWR Morb Mortal Wkly Rep.* 2017;65(52):1457–1464. https://doi.org/10.15585/mmwr.mm6552a1.

18. Badiani A, Boden JM, Pirro S de, Fergusson DM, Horwood LJ, Harold GT. Tobacco smoking and cannabis use in a longitudinal birth cohort: evidence of reciprocal causal relationships. *Drug Alcohol Depend.* 2015;150:69–76. https://doi.org/10.1016/j.drugalcdep.2015.02.015.

19. Baker TB, Piper ME, McCarthy DE, Majeskie MR, Fiore MC. Addiction motivation reformulated: an affective processing model of negative reinforcement. *Psychol Rev.* 2004;111(1):33–51. https://doi.org/10.1037/0033-295X.111.1.33.

20. Baker TB, Piper ME, McCarthy DE, et al. Time to first cigarette in the morning as an index of ability to quit smoking: implications for nicotine dependence. *Nicotine Tob Res.* 2007;9(suppl 4):S555–S570. https://doi.org/10.1080/14622200701673480.

21. Barkley RA. Behavioral inhibition, sustained attention, and executive functions: constructing a unifying theory of ADHD. *Psychol Bull.* 1997;121(1):65–94.

22. Barkley RA, Fischer M, Edelbrock CS, Smallish L. The adolescent outcome of hyperactive children diagnosed by research criteria: I. An 8-year prospective follow-up study. *J Am Acad Child Adolesc. Psychiatry.* 1990;29(4):546–557.

23. Batel P, Pessione F, Maitre C, Rueff B. Relationship between alcohol and tobacco dependencies among alcoholics who smoke. *Addiction.* 1995;90(7):977–980.

24. Becker J, Schaub MP, Gmel G, Haug S. Cannabis use and other predictors of the onset of daily cigarette use in young men: what matters most? Results from a longitudinal study. *BMC Public Health.* 2015;15:843. https://doi.org/10.1186/s12889-015-2194-3.

25. Beckham JC. Smoking and anxiety in combat veterans with chronic posttraumatic stress disorder: a review. *J Psychoactive Drugs.* 1999;31(2):103–110.

26. Beitchman JH, Douglas L, Wilson B, et al. Adolescent substance use disorders: findings from a 14-year follow-up of speech/language-impaired and control children. *J Clin Child Psychol.* 1999;28(3):312–321.

27. Benowitz NL. Pharmacology of nicotine: addiction and therapeutics. *Annu Rev Pharmacol Toxicol.* 1996;36:597–613.

28. Benowitz NL. Neurobiology of nicotine addiction: implications for smoking cessation treatment. *Am J Med.* 2008;121(4 suppl 1):S3–S10.

29. Benowitz NL, Ahijevych K, Hall S, et al. Biochemical verification of tobacco use and cessation. *Nicotine Tob Res.* 2002;4:149–159. https://doi.org/10.1080/14622200210123581.

30. Benowitz NL, Pipe A, West R, et al. Cardiovascular safety of varenicline, bupropion, and nicotine patch in smokers: a randomized clinical trial. *JAMA Intern Med.* 2018. https://doi.org/10.1001/jamainternmed.2018.0397.

31. Bergen AW, Korczak JF, Weissbecker KA, Goldstein AM. A genome-wide search for loci contributing to smoking and alcoholism. *Genet Epidemiol.* 1999;17(suppl 1):S55–S60.

32. Berrettini W, Yuan X, Tozzi F, et al. Alpha-5/alpha-3 nicotinic receptor subunit alleles increase risk for heavy smoking. *Mol Psychiatr.* 2008;13(4):368–373.

33. Berrettini WH, Wileyto EP, Epstein L, et al. Catechol-O-methyltransferase (COMT) gene variants predict response to bupropion therapy for tobacco dependence. *Biol Psychiatry.* 2007;61(1):111–118.

34. Bierut LJ, Madden PAF, Breslau N, et al. Novel genes identified in a high density genome wide association study for nicotine dependence. *Hum Mol Genet.* 2006;16:24–35.

35. Bierut LJ, Stitzel JA, Wang JC, et al. Variants in nicotinic receptors and risk for nicotine dependence. *Am J Psychiatry.* 2008;165(9):1163–1171. https://doi.org/10.1176/appi.ajp.2008.07111711.

36. Blanco C, Hasin DS, Wall MM, et al. Cannabis use and risk of psychiatric disorders: prospective evidence from a US national longitudinal study. *JAMA Psychiatry.* 2016;73(4):388–395. https://doi.org/10.1001/jamapsychiatry.2015.3229.

37. Blomqvist O, Gelernter J, Kranzler HR. Family-based study of DRD2 alleles in alcohol and drug dependence. *Am J Med Genet.* 2000;96(5):659–664.

38. Bolliger CT, Zellweger JP, Danielsson T, et al. Smoking reduction with oral nicotine inhalers: double blind, randomised clinical trial of efficacy and safety. *BMJ.* 2000;321(7257):329–333.

39. Borelli B, Niaura RS, Keuthen NJ, et al. Development of major depressive disorder during smoking-cessation treatment. *J Clin Psychiatry.* 1996;57(11):534–538.

40. Borland BL, Heckman HK. Hyperactive boys and their brothers. A 25-year follow-up study. *Arch Gen Psychiatry.* 1976;33(6):669–675.

41. Botvinick MM, Braver TS, Barch DM, Carter CS, Cohen JD. Conflict monitoring and cognitive control. *Psychol Rev.* 2001;108(3):624–652.

42. Brandon TH, Tiffany ST, Obremski KM, Baker TB. Postcessation cigarette use: the process of relapse. *Addict Behav.* 1990;15:105–114. https://doi.org/10.1016/0306-4603(90)90013-N.

43. Breslau N. Psychiatric comorbidity of smoking and nicotine dependence. *Behav Genet.* 1995;25(2):95–101.

44. Breslau N, Johnson EO, Hiripi E, Kessler R. Nicotine dependence in the United States: prevalence, trends, and smoking persistence. *Arch Gen Psychiatry.* 2001;58(9):810–816.

45. Breslau N, Kilbey M, Andreski P. Nicotine dependence, major depression, and anxiety in young adults. *Arch Gen Psychiatry.* 1991;48(12):1069–1074.

46. Breslau N, Kilbey MM, Andreski P. Nicotine dependence, major depression, and anxiety in young adults. *Arch Gen Psychiatry.* 1991;48:1069–1074.

47. Breslau N, Kilbey MM, Andreski P. Nicotine dependence and major depression: new evidence from a prospective investigation. *Arch Gen Psychiatry.* 1993;50:31–35.

48. Breslau N, Klein DF. Smoking and panic attacks: an epidemiologic investigation. *Arch Gen Psychiatry.* 1999;56(12):1141–1147.

49. Breslau N, Peterson EL, Schultz LR, Chilcoat HD, Andreski P. Major depression and stages of smoking: a longitudinal investigation. *Arch Gen Psychiatry.* 1998;55:161–166.

50. Breslau N, Peterson EL, Schultz LR, Chilcoat HD, Andreski P. Major depression and stages of smoking. A longitudinal investigation. *Arch Gen Psychiatry.* 1998;55(2):161–166.

51. Briggs Z, O'Connor M, Jollans EK, O'Halloran L, Dymond S, Whelan R. Flexible emotion-based decision-making behavior varies in current and former smokers. *Addict Behav.* 2015;45:269–275. https://doi.org/10.1016/j.addbeh.2015.02.011.

52. Brown DC. Smoking cessation in pregnancy. *Can Fam Physician.* 1996;42:102–105.

53. Brown RA, Abrantes AM, Strong DR, et al. Efficacy of sequential use of fluoxetine for smoking cessation in elevated depressive symptom smokers. *Nicotine Tob Res.* 2014;16(2):197–207. https://doi.org/10.1093/ntr/ntt134.

54. Brown RA, Kahler CW, Niaura RS, et al. Cognitive-behavioral treatment for depression in smoking cessation. *J Consult Clin Psychol.* 2001;69(3):471–480.

55. Brown RA, Niaura RS, Lloyd-Richardson EE, et al. Bupropion and cognitive-behavioral treatment for depression in smoking cessation. *Nicotine Tob Res.* 2007;9(7):721–730.

56. Buckner JD, Zvolensky MJ, Jeffries ER, Schmidt NB. Robust impact of social anxiety in relation to coping motives and expectancies, barriers to quitting, and cessation-related problems. *Exp Clin Psychopharmacol.* 2014;22(4):341–347. https://doi.org/10.1037/a0037206.

57. Burgess ES, Kahler CW, Niaura RS, Abrams DB, Goldstein MG, Miller IW. Patterns of change in depressive symptoms during smoking cessation: who's at risk for relapse? *J Consult Clin Psychol.* 2002;70(2):356–361.

58. Cahill K, Lindson-Hawley N, Thomas KH, Fanshawe TR, Lancaster T. Nicotine receptor partial agonists for smoking cessation. *Cochrane Database Syst Rev.* 2016;5:CD006103. https://doi.org/10.1002/14651858.CD006103.pub7.

58a. Cahill K, Stevens S, Perera R, Lancaster T. Pharmacological interventions for smoking cessation: an overview and network meta-analysis. *Cochrane Database Syst Rev.* 2013;5:CD009329.

59. Cappelleri JC, Baker CL, Bushmakin AG, Reeves K. *Effects of Varenicline on Craving and Withdrawal Symptoms;* 2006. Orlando, FL.

60. Carmelli D, Swan GE, Robinette D, Fabsitz R. Genetic influence on smoking--A study of male twins. *N Engl J Med.* 1992;327:829–833.

61. Carr LA, Basham JK, York BK, Rowell PP. Inihibition of uptake of 1-methyl-4-phenylpyridinium ion and dopamine in striatal synaptosomes by tobacco smoke components. *Eur J Pharmacol.* 1992;215:285–287.

62. Carter BL, Long TY, Cinciripini PM. A meta-analytic review of the CYP2A6 genotype and smoking behavior. *Nicotine Tob Res.* 2004;6(2):221–227.

63. Center for Substance Abuse Treatment. Treatment for Stimulant Use Disorders. *Chapter 4—Practical Application of Treatment Strategies:* Substance Abuse and Mental Health Services Administration (US). 1999. Treatment Improvement Protocol (TIP) Series, No. 33. https://www.ncbi.nlm.nih.gov/books/NBK64334/.

64. Chambers RA, Taylor JR, Potenza MN. Developmental neurocircuitry of motivation in adolescence: a critical period of addiction vulnerability. *Am J Psychiatry.* 2003;160(6):1041–1052.

65. Chengappa KN, Perkins KA, Brar JS, et al. Varenicline for smoking cessation in bipolar disorder: a randomized, double-blind, placebo-controlled study. *J Clin Psychiatry.* 2014;75(7):765–772.

66. Childress AR, Ehrman RN, Wang Z, et al. Prelude to passion: limbic activation by "unseen" drug and sexual cues. *PLoS One.* 2008;3(1):e1506.

67. Cinciripini PM, Minnix JA, Green CE, et al. An RCT with the combination of varenicline and bupropion for smoking cessation: clinical implications for front line use. *Addiction.* 2018;113(9):1673–1682. https://doi.org/10.1111/add.14250.

68. Cinciripini PM, Tsoh JT, Wetter DW, et al. Combined effects of venlafaxine, nicotine replacement & brief counseling on smoking cessation. *Exp Clin Psychopharmacol.* 2005;13(4):282–292. https://doi.org/10.1037/1064-1297.13.4.282.

69. Cinciripini PM, Wetter DW, Fouladi RT, et al. The effects of depressed mood on smoking cessation: mediation by post-cessation self-efficacy. *J Consult Clin Psychol.* 2003;71(2):292–301. https://doi.org/10.1037/0022-006X.71.2.292.

70. Cinciripini PM, Wetter DW, Tomlinson GE, et al. The effects of the DRD2 polymorphism on smoking cessation and negative affect: evidence for a pharmacogenetic effect on mood. *Nicotine Tob Res.* 2004;6(2):229–239.

71. Clare P, Bradford D, Courtney RJ, Martire K, Mattick RP. The relationship between socioeconomic status and 'hardcore' smoking over time--greater accumulation of hardened smokers in low-SES than high-SES smokers. *Tob Control.* 2014;23(e2):e133–e138. https://doi.org/10.1136/tobaccocontrol-2013-051436.

72. Clayton AH. Extended-release bupropion: an antidepressant with a broad spectrum of therapeutic activity? *Expert Opin Pharmacother.* 2007;8(4):457–466.

73. Clayton AH, Pradko JF, Croft HA, et al. Prevalence of sexual dysfunction among newer antidepressants. *J Clin Psychiatry.* 2002;63(4):357–366.

74. Coe JW, Brooks PR, Vetelino MG, et al. Varenicline: an alpha-4beta2 nicotinic receptor partial agonist for smoking cessation. *J Med Chem.* 2005;48(10):3474–3477. https://doi.org/10.1021/jm050069n.

75. Cohen C, Kodas E, Griebel G. CB1 receptor antagonists for the treatment of nicotine addiction. *Pharmacol Biochem Behav.* 2005;81(2):387–395.

76. Conti DV, Lee W, Li D, et al. Nicotinic acetylcholine receptor beta2 subunit gene implicated in a systems-based candidate gene study of smoking cessation. *Hum Mol Genet.* 2008;17(18):2834–2848.

77. Copeland AL, Spears CA, Baillie LE, McVay MA. Fear of fatness and drive for thinness in predicting smoking status in college women. *Addict Behav.* 2016;54:1–6. https://doi.org/10.1016/j.addbeh.2015.11.010.

78. Covey LS, Hu M-C, Winhusen T, Weissman J, Berlin I, Nunes EV. OROS-methylphenidate or placebo for adult smokers with attention deficit hyperactivity disorder: racial/ethnic differences. *Drug Alcohol Depend.* 2010;110(1–2):156–159. https://doi.org/10.1016/j.drugalcdep.2010.02.002.

79. Covey LS, Hughes DC, Glassman AH, Blazer DG, George LK. Ever-smoking, quitting, and psychiatric disorders: evidence from the Durham, North Carolina, epidemiologic catchment area. *Tob Control.* 1994;3:222–227.

80. Curtin JJ, McCarthy DE, Piper ME, Baker TB. Implicit and explicit drug motivational processes: a model of boundary conditions. In: Reinout R, Stacy A, eds. *Handbook of Implicit Cognition and Addiction.* Thousand Oaks, CA: SAGE Publications; 2006: 233–250.

81. Damaj MI, Carroll FI, Eaton JB, et al. Enantioselective effects of hydroxy metabolites of bupropion on behavior and on function of monoamine transporters and nicotinic receptors. *Mol Pharmacol.* 2004;66(3):675–682.

82. David SP, Brown RA, Papandonatos GD, et al. Pharmacogenetic clinical trial of sustained-release bupropion for smoking cessation. *Nicotine Tob Res.* 2007;9(8):821–833. https://doi.org/10.1080/14622200701382033.

83. David SP, Brown RA, Papandonatos GD, et al. Pharmacogenetic clinical trial of sustained-release bupropion for smoking cessation. *Nicotine Tob Res.* 2007;9(8):821–833.

84. David SP, Munafo MR, Murphy MF, Proctor M, Walton RT, Johnstone EC. Genetic variation in the dopamine D4 receptor (DRD4) gene and smoking cessation: follow-up of a randomised clinical trial of transdermal nicotine patch. *Pharmacogenomics J.* 2008;8(2):122–128.

85. David SP, Munafo MR, Murphy MF, Walton RT, Johnstone EC. The serotonin transporter 5-HTTLPR polymorphism and treatment response to nicotine patch: follow-up of a randomized controlled trial. *Nicotine Tob Res.* 2007;9(2):225–231.

86. David SP, Niaura RS, Papandonatos GD, et al. Does the DRD2-Taq1 A polymorphism influence treatment response to bupropion hydrochloride for reduction of the nicotine withdrawal syndrome? *Nicotine Tob Res.* 2003;5(6):935–942. https://doi.org/10.1080/14622200310001615295.

87. David SP, Strong DR, Munafo MR, et al. Bupropion efficacy for smoking cessation is influenced by the DRD2 Taq1A polymorphism: analysis of pooled data from two clinical trials. *Nicotine Tob Res.* 2007;9(12):1251–1257. https://doi.org/10.1080/14622200701705027.

88. Deeming tobacco products to be subject to the federal food, drug, and Cosmetic act, as amended by the family smoking prevention and tobacco control act; Restrictions on the sale and distribution of tobacco products and required warning statements for tobacco products. Final rule. *Fed Regist.* 2016;81(90):28973–29106.

89. Di Chiara G. Role of dopamine in the behavioural actions of nicotine related to addiction. *Eur J Pharmacol.* 2000;393:295–314.

90. DiFranza JR, Savageau JA, Fletcher KE. Enforcement of underage sales laws as a predictor of daily smoking among adolescents: a national study. *BMC Public Health.* 2009;9:107. https://doi.org/10.1186/1471-2458-9-107.

91. Dobrossy MD, Furlanetti LL, Coenen VA. Electrical stimulation of the medial forebrain bundle in pre-clinical studies of psychiatric disorders. *Neurosci Biobehav Rev.* 2015;49:32–42. https://doi.org/10.1016/j.neubiorev.2014.11.018.

92. Docherty G, McNeill A, Gartner C, Szatkowski L. Did hardening occur among smokers in England from 2000 to 2010? *Addiction.* 2014;109(1):147–154. https://doi.org/10.1111/add.12359.

93. Duggirala R, Almasy L, Blangero J. Smoking behavior is under the influence of a major quantitative trait locus on human chromosome 5q. *Genet Epidemiol.* 1999;17(suppl 1):S139–S144.

94. Duke JC, Davis KC, Alexander RL, et al. Impact of a U.S. anti-smoking national media campaign on beliefs, cognitions and quit intentions. *Health Educ Res.* 2015;30(3):466–483. https://doi.org/10.1093/her/cyv017.

95. Ebbert JO, Hatsukami DK, Croghan IT, et al. Combination varenicline and bupropion SR for tobacco-dependence treatment in cigarette smokers: a randomized trial. *J Am Med Assoc.* 2014;311(2):155–163.

96. Elkins IJ, McGue M, Iacono WG. Prospective effects of attention-deficit/hyperactivity disorder, conduct disorder, and sex on adolescent substance use and abuse. *Arch Gen Psychiatry*. 2007;64(10):1145–1152. https://doi.org/10.1001/archpsyc.64.10.1145.

97. Epstein JN, Conners CK, Erhardt D, March JS, Swanson JM. Asymmetrical hemispheric control of visual-spatial attention in adults with attention deficit hyperactivity disorder. *Neuropsychology*. 1997;11(4):467–473.

98. Etemadi A, Khademi H, Kamangar F, et al. Hazards of cigarettes, smokeless tobacco and waterpipe in a Middle Eastern population: a cohort study of 50 000 individuals from Iran. *Tob Control*. 2016. https://doi.org/10.1136/tobaccocontrol-2016-053245.

99. Etter JF. Cytisine for smoking cessation: a literature review and a meta-analysis. *Arch Intern Med*. 2006;166(15):1553–1559.

100. Etter J-F. Throat hit in users of the electronic cigarette: an exploratory study. *Psychol Addict Behav*. 2016;30(1):93–100. https://doi.org/10.1037/adb0000137.

101. Etter JF, Laszlo E, Zellweger JP, Perrot C, Perneger TV. Nicotine replacement to reduce cigarette consumption in smokers who are unwilling to quit: a randomized trial. *J Clin Psychopharmacol*. 2002;22(5):487–495.

102. Etter J-F. A longitudinal study of cotinine in long-term daily users of e-cigarettes. *Drug Alcohol Depend*. 2016;160:218–221. https://doi.org/10.1016/j.drugalcdep.2016.01.003.

103. Evins AE, Cather C, Deckersbach T, et al. A double-blind placebo-controlled trial of bupropion sustained-release for smoking cessation in schizophrenia. *J Clin Psychopharmacol*. 2005;25(3):218–225.

104. Evins AE, Cather C, Pratt SA, et al. Maintenance treatment with varenicline for smoking cessation in patients with schizophrenia and bipolar disorder: a randomized clinical trial. *J Am Med Assoc*. 2014;311(2):145–154. https://doi.org/10.1001/jama.2013.285113.

105. Faraone SV, Biederman J. Efficacy of Adderall for attention-deficit/hyperactivity disorder: a meta-analysis. *J Atten Disord*. 2002;6(2):69–75.

106. FDA Chantix Fact Sheet. 2016.

107. Finn PR, Mazas CA, Justus AN, Steinmetz J. Early-onset alcoholism with conduct disorder: go/no go learning deficits, working memory capacity, and personality. *Alcohol Clin Exp Res*. 2002;26(2):186–206.

108. Fiore MC, Jaen CR, Baker TB, et al. *Treating Tobacco Use and Dependence*: 2008 update, clinical practice guideline. PM:18807274. Updated March 4, 2015.

109. Freeman SM, Aron AR. Withholding a reward-driven action: studies of the Rise and fall of motor activation and the effect of cognitive depletion. *J Cogn Neurosci*. 2016;28(2):237–251. https://doi.org/10.1162/jocn_a_00893.

110. Froeliger B, McConnell PA, Stankeviciute N, McClure EA, Kalivas PW, Gray KM. The effects of N-Acetylcysteine on frontostriatal resting-state functional connectivity, withdrawal symptoms and smoking abstinence: a double-blind, placebo-controlled fMRI pilot study. *Drug Alcohol Depend*. 2015;156:234–242. https://doi.org/10.1016/j.drugalcdep.2015.09.021.

111. Fu M, Martinez-Sanchez JM, Agudo A, et al. Nicotine dependence and salivary cotinine concentration in daily smokers. *Eur J Cancer Prev*. 2012;21(1):96–102. https://doi.org/10.1097/CEJ.0b013e32834a7e59.

112. Gabrhelik R, Duncan A, Miovsky M, Furr-Holden CDM, Stastna L, Jurystova L. "Unplugged": a school-based randomized control trial to prevent and reduce adolescent substance use in the Czech Republic. *Drug Alcohol Depend*. 2012;124(1–2):79–87. https://doi.org/10.1016/j.drugalcdep.2011.12.010.

113. Galanti MR, Al-Adhami M. Use of a water pipe is not an alternative to other tobacco or substance use among adolescents: results from a national survey in Sweden. *Nicotine Tob Res*. 2015;17(1):74–80. https://doi.org/10.1093/ntr/ntu132.

114. Galanti MR, Coppo A, Jonsson E, Bremberg S, Faggiano F. Anti-tobacco policy in schools: upcoming preventive strategy or prevention myth? A review of 31 studies. *Tob Control*. 2014;23(4):295–301. https://doi.org/10.1136/tobaccocontrol-2012-050846.

115. Gao M, Jin Y, Yang K, Zhang D, Lukas RJ, Wu J. Mechanisms involved in systemic nicotine-induced glutamatergic synaptic plasticity on dopamine neurons in the ventral tegmental area. *J Neurosci*. 2010;30(41):13814–13825.

116. Gardner EL. Addiction and brain reward and antireward pathways. *Adv Psychosom Med*. 2011;30:22–60. https://doi.org/10.1159/000324065.

117. George TP, O'Malley SS. Current pharmacological treatments for nicotine dependence. *Trends Pharmacol Sci*. 2004;25(1):42–48.

118. Giannotta F, Vigna-Taglianti F, Rosaria Galanti M, Scatigna M, Faggiano F. Short-term mediating factors of a school-based intervention to prevent youth substance use in Europe. *J Adolesc Health*. 2014;54(5):565–573. https://doi.org/10.1016/j.jadohealth.2013.10.009.

119. Ginsberg D, Hall SM, Reus VI, Muñoz RF. Mood and depression diagnosis in smoking cessation. *Exp Clin Psychopharmacol*. 1995;3(4):389–395. https://doi.org/10.1037/1064-1297.3.4.389.

120. Glasheen C, Hedden SL, Forman-Hoffman VL, Colpe LJ. Cigarette smoking behaviors among adults with serious mental illness in a nationally representative sample. *Ann Epidemiol*. 2014;24(10):776–780.

121. Glassman AH, Helzer JE, Covey LS, et al. Smoking, smoking cessation, and major depression. *J Am Med Assoc*. 1990;264(12):1546–1549.

122. Glassman AH, Stetner F, Walsh BT, et al. Heavy smokers, smoking cessation, and clonidine: results of a double-blind, randomized trial. *J Am Med Assoc*. 1988;259:2863–2866.

123. Glover ED, Laflin MT, Schuh KJ, et al. A randomized, controlled trial to assess the efficacy and safety of a transdermal delivery system of nicotine/mecamylamine in cigarette smokers. *Addiction*. 2007;102(5):795–802.

124. Gonzales D, Rennard SI, Nides M, et al. Varenicline, an alpha-4beta2 nicotinic acetylcholine receptor partial agonist, vs sustained-release bupropion and placebo for smoking cessation: a randomized controlled trial. *J Am Med Assoc*. 2006;296(1):47–55. https://doi.org/10.1001/jama.296.1.47.

125. Gonzales DH, Rennard SI, Billing CB, Reeves K, Watsky E, Gong J. *A Pooled Analysis of Varenicline, an Alpha 4 Beta 2 Nicotinic Receptor Partial Agonist vs Bupropion, and Placebo for Smoking Cessation*; 2006. Orlando, FL.

126. Gorini G, Carreras G, Cortini B, et al. Smoke-free homes and youth smoking behavior in Italy: findings from the SIDRIAT longitudinal study. *Nicotine Tob Res*. 2016;18(11):2075–2082. https://doi.org/10.1093/ntr/ntw149.

127. Gourlay SG, Stead LF, Benowitz NL. Clonidine for smoking cessation. *Cochrane Database Syst Rev*. 2004;3:CD000058-CD000058.

128. Graham AL, Jacobs MA, Cohn AM, et al. Optimising text messaging to improve adherence to web-based smoking cessation treatment: a randomised control trial protocol. *BMJ Open*. 2016;6(3):e010687. https://doi.org/10.1136/bmjopen-2015-010687.

129. Grant BF, Hasin DS, Chou SP, Stinson FS, Dawson DA. Nicotine dependence and psychiatric disorders in the United States: results from the national epidemiologic survey on alcohol and related conditions. *Arch Gen Psychiatry*. 2004;61(11):1107–1115.

130. Gray KM, Riggs PD, Min S-J, Mikulich-Gilbertson SK, Bandyopadhyay D, Winhusen T. Cigarette and cannabis use trajectories among adolescents in treatment for attention-deficit/hyperactivity disorder and substance use disorders. *Drug Alcohol Depend*. 2011;117(2–3):242–247. https://doi.org/10.1016/j.drugalcdep.2011.02.005.

131. Green AE, Mays D, Falk EB, et al. Young adult smokers' neural response to graphic cigarette warning labels. *Addict Behav Rep*. 2016;3:28–32. https://doi.org/10.1016/j.abrep.2016.02.001.

132. Haddad L, Kelly DL, Weglicki LS, Barnett TE, Ferrell AV, Ghadban R. A systematic review of effects of waterpipe smoking on cardiovascular and respiratory health outcomes. *Tob Use Insights.* 2016;9:13–28. https://doi.org/10.4137/TUI.S39873.

133. Hall SM, Humfleet GL, Reus VI, Munoz RF, Hartz DT, Maude-Griffin R. Psychological intervention and antidepressant treatment in smoking cessation. *Arch Gen Psychiatry.* 2002;59: 930–936.

134. Hall SM, Sees KL, Munoz RF, et al. Mood management and nicotine gum in smoking treatment: a therapeutic contact and placebo-controlled study. *J Consult Clin Psychol.* 1996;64(5):1003–1009.

135. Hallingberg B, Fletcher A, Murphy S, et al. Do stronger school smoking policies make a difference? Analysis of the health behaviour in school-aged children survey. *Eur J Public Health.* 2016;26(6):964–968. https://doi.org/10.1093/eurpub/ckw093.

135a. Hartmann-Boyce J, Chepkin SC, Ye W, et al. Nicotine replacement therapy versus control for smoking cessation. *Cochrane Database Syst Rev.* 2018;5:CD000146.

136. Hartsough CS, Lambert NM. Pattern and progression of drug use among hyperactives and controls: a prospective short-term longitudinal study. *J Child Psychol.Psychiatry.* 1987;28(4):543–553.

137. Haug S, Nunez CL, Becker J, Gmel G, Schaub MP. Predictors of onset of cannabis and other drug use in male young adults: results from a longitudinal study. *BMC Public Health.* 2014;14:1202. https://doi.org/10.1186/1471-2458-14-1202.

138. Heath AC, Martin NG, Lynskey MT, Todorov AA, Madden PAF. Estimating two-stage models for genetic influences on alcohol, tobacco or drug use initiation and dependence vulnerability in twin and family data. *Twin Res.* 2002;5(02):113–124. https://doi.org/10.1375/twin.5.2.113.

139. Heatherton TF, Kozlowski LT, Frecker RC, Fagerström KO. The Fagerström test for nicotine dependence: a revision of the Fagerström tolerance questionnaire. *Br J Addiction.* 1991;86(9):1119–1127. https://doi.org/10.1111/j.1360-0443.1991.tb01879.x.

140. Heckman BW, Ditre JW, Brandon TH. The restorative effects of smoking upon self-control resources: a negative reinforcement pathway. *J Abnorm Psychol.* 2012;121(1):244–249. https://doi.org/10.1037/a0023032.

141. Hertzberg MA, Moore SD, Feldman ME, Beckham JC. A preliminary study of bupropion sustained-release for smoking cessation in patients with chronic posttraumatic stress disorder. *J Clin Psychopharmacol.* 2001;21(1):94–98.

142. Hitsman B, Borrelli B, McChargue DE, Spring B, Niaura RS. History of depression and smoking cessation outcome: a meta-analysis. *J Consult Clin Psychol.* 2003;71(4):657–663.

143. Hoffman SJ, Tan C. Overview of systematic reviews on the health-related effects of government tobacco control policies. *BMC Public Health.* 2015;15:744. https://doi.org/10.1186/s12889-015-2041-6.

144. Holroyd CB, Coles MGH. The neural basis of human error processing: reinforcement learning, dopamine, and the error-related negativity. *Psychol Rev.* 2002;109(4):679–709.

145. Huang W, Payne TJ, Ma JZ, et al. Significant association of ANKK1 and detection of a functional polymorphism with nicotine dependence in an African-American sample. *Neuropsychopharmacol.* 2009;34(2):319–330. https://doi.org/10.1038/npp.2008.37.

146. Hughes JR, Stead LF, Hartmann-Boyce J, Cahill K, Lancaster T. Antidepressants for smoking cessation. *Cochrane Database Syst Rev.* 2014;1:CD000031.

147. Hughes JR, Stead LF, Lancaster T. Nortriptyline for smoking cessation: a review. *Nicotine Tob Res.* 2005;7(4):491–499.

148. Humfleet GL, Prochaska JO, Mengis M, et al. Preliminary evidence of the association between the history of childhood attention-deficit/hyperactivity disorder and smoking treatment failure. *Nicotine Tob Res.* 2005;7(3):453–460.

149. Hung RJ, McKay JD, Gaborieau V, et al. A susceptibility locus for lung cancer maps to nicotinic acetylcholine receptor subunit genes on 15q25. *Nature.* 2008;452(7187):633–637.

150. Hurt RD, Sachs DP, Glover ED, et al. A comparison of sustained-release bupropion and placebo for smoking cessation. *N Engl J Med.* 1997;337(17):1195–1202.

151. Hutchison KE, Allen DL, Filbey FM, et al. CHRNA4 and tobacco dependence: from gene regulation to treatment outcome. *Arch Gen Psychiatry.* 2007;64(9):1078–1086.

152. IARC. *Tobacco smoke and involuntAry smoking.* Updated October 13, 2014.

153. Ito R, Robbins TW, McNaughton BL, Everitt BJ. Selective excitotoxic lesions of the hippocampus and basolateral amygdala have dissociable effects on appetitive cue and place conditioning based on path integration in a novel Y-maze procedure. *Eur J Neurosci.* 2006;23(11): 3071–3080. https://doi.org/10.1111/j.1460-9568.2006.04883.x.

154. Izenwasser S, Cox BM. Inhibition of dopamine uptake by cocaine and nicotine: tolerance to chronic treatments. *Brain Res.* 1992;573:119–125.

155. Jackson KJ, Muldoon PP, Biasi M de, Damaj MI. New mechanisms and perspectives in nicotine withdrawal. *Neuropharmacology.* 2015;96(Pt B):223–234. https://doi.org/10.1016/j.neuropharm.2014.11.009.

156. Jha P, Peto R. Global effects of smoking, of quitting, and of taxing tobacco. *N Engl J Med.* 2014;370(1):60–68. https://doi.org/10.1056/NEJMra1308383.

157. Johnson EO, Rhee SH, Chase GA, Breslau N. Comorbidity of depression with levels of smoking: an exploration of the shared familial risk hypothesis. *Nicotine Tob Res.* 2004;6(6):1029–1038.

158. Johnson RA, Hoffmann JP. Adolescent cigarette smoking in U.S. racial/ethnic subgroups: findings from the National Education Longitudinal Study. *J Health Soc Behav.* 2000;41(4):392–407.

158a. Johnston LD, Miech RA, O'Malley PM, et al. *Monitoring the Future National Survey Results on Drug Use 1975-2018: Overview, Key Findings on Adolescent Drug Use.* Ann Arbor, MI: Institute for Social Research, University of Michigan; 2019.

159. Johnston LD, O'Malley PM, Miech RA. *Monitoring the Future national survey results on drug use, 1975-2016: overview, key findings on adolescent drug use.* http://www.monitoringthefuture.org/pubs/monographs/mtf-overview2016.pdf; 2017. Accessed May 30, 2017.

160. Johnstone EC, Yudkin PL, Hey K, et al. Genetic variation in dopaminergic pathways and short-term effectiveness of the nicotine patch. *Pharmacogenetics.* 2004;14(2):83–90. https://doi.org/10.1097/01.fpc.0000054154.92680.6d.

161. Jorenby DE, Hays JT, Rigotti NA, et al. Efficacy of varenicline, an alpha4beta2 nicotinic acetylcholine receptor partial agonist, vs placebo or sustained-release bupropion for smoking cessation: a randomized controlled trial. *J Am Med Assoc.* 2006;296(1):56–63. https://doi.org/10.1001/jama.296.1.56.

162. Jorenby DE, Leischow SJ, Nides MA, et al. A controlled trial of sustained-release bupropion, a nicotine patch, or both for smoking cessation. *N Engl J Med.* 1999;340(9):685–691.

163. Juarez B, Han M-H. Diversity of dopaminergic neural circuits in response to drug exposure. *Neuropsychopharmacol.* 2016;41(10):2424–2446. https://doi.org/10.1038/npp.2016.32.

163a. JUUL Labs. *JUULpods Ingredients.* https://www.juul.com/learn/pods#juulpods-ingredients; 2019. Accessed October 15, 2019.

164. Kalman D, Morissette SB, George TP. Co-morbidity of smoking in patients with psychiatric and substance use disorders. *Am J Addict.* 2005;14(2):106–123. https://doi.org/10.1080/10550490590924728.

165. Karam-Hage M, Cinciripini PM. Pharmacotherapy for tobacco cessation: nicotine agonists, antagonists, and partial agonists. *Curr Oncol Rep.* 2007;9/6:509–516.

166. Karam-Hage M, Robinson JD, Brower KJ. Bupropion-SR for smoking reduction and cessation in alcohol-dependent outpatients: a naturalistic, open-label study. *Curr Clin Pharmacol.* 2014;9(2):123–129.

167. Karam-Hage M, Strobbe S, Robinson JD, Brower KJ. Bupropion-SR for smoking cessation in early recovery from alcohol dependence: a placebo-controlled, double-blind pilot study. *Am J Drug Alcohol Abuse.* 2011;37(6):487–490. https://doi.org/10.3109/00952990.2011.598591.

168. Katurji M, Daher N, Sheheitli H, Saleh R, Shihadeh A. Direct measurement of toxicants inhaled by water pipe users in the natural environment using a real-time in situ sampling technique. *Inhal Toxicol.* 2010;22(13):1101–1109. https://doi.org/10.3109/08958378.2010.524265.

169. Kellam SG, Mackenzie ACL, Brown CH, et al. The good behavior game and the future of prevention and treatment. *Addict Sci Clin Pract.* 2011;6(1):73–84.

170. Kendler KS. *The Genetic Epidemiology of Smoking: Section II: Nicotine-Individual Risk Factors for Initiation.* Bethesda, MD: Addicted to Nicotine: A National Research Forum; 1998.

171. Kendler KS, Myers J, Prescott CA. Specificity of genetic and environmental risk factors for symptoms of cannabis, cocaine, alcohol, caffeine, and nicotine dependence. *Arch Gen Psychiatry.* 2007;64(11):1313–1320. https://doi.org/10.1001/archpsyc.64.11.1313.

172. Kendler KS, Neale MC, MacLean CJ, Heath AC, Eaves LJ, Kessler RC. Smoking and major depression: a casual analysis. *Arch Gen Psychiatry.* 1993;50(1):36–43.

173. Kendler KS, Neale MC, MacLean CJ, Heath AC, Eaves LJ, Kessler RC. Smoking and major depression. A causal analysis. *Arch Gen Psychiatry.* 1993;50(1):36–43.

174. Kendzor DE, Adams CE, Stewart DW, Baillie LE, Copeland AL. Cigarette smoking is associated with body shape concerns and bulimia symptoms among young adult females. *Eat Behav.* 2009;10(1):56–58. https://doi.org/10.1016/j.eatbeh.2008.10.012.

175. Kenford SL, Smith SS, Wetter DW, Jorenby DE, Fiore MC, Baker TB. Predicting relapse back to smoking: Contrasting affective and physical models of dependence. *J Consult Clin Psychol.* 2002;70:216–227. https://doi.org/10.1037/0022-006X.70.1.216.

176. Killen JD, Fortmann SP, Kraemer HC, Varady AN, Davis L, Newman B. Interactive effects of depression symptoms, nicotine dependence, and weight change on late smoking relapse. *J Consult Clin Psychol.* 1996;64(5):1060–1067. https://doi.org/10.1037/0022-006X.64.5.1060.

177. King L, Saules KK, Irish J. Weight concerns and cognitive style: which carries more "weight" in the prediction of smoking among college women? *Nicotine Tob Res.* 2007;9(5):535–543. https://doi.org/10.1080/14622200701188935.

178. Kinnunen T, Doherty K, Militello FS, Garvey AJ. Depression and smoking cessation: characteristics of depressed smokers and effects of nicotine replacement. *J Consult Clin Psychol.* 1996;64:791–798. https://doi.org/10.1037/0022-006X.64.4.791.

179. Kishioka S, Kiguchi N, Kobayashi Y, Saika F. Nicotine effects and the endogenous opioid system. *J Pharmacol Sci.* 2014;125(2):117–124.

180. Kollins SH, McClernon FJ, Fuemmeler BF. Association between smoking and attention-deficit/hyperactivity disorder symptoms in a population-based sample of young adults. *Arch Gen Psychiatry.* 2005;62(10):1142–1147.

181. Kong G, Morean ME, Cavallo DA, Camenga DR, Krishnan-Sarin S. Reasons for electronic cigarette Experimentation and Discontinuation among adolescents and young adults. *Nicotine Tob Res.* 2015;17(7):847–854. https://doi.org/10.1093/ntr/ntu257.

182. Koob GF. Stress, corticotropin-releasing factor, and drug addiction. *Ann N Y Acad Sci.* 1999;897:27–45.

183. Koob GF. Negative reinforcement in drug addiction: the darkness within. *Curr Opin Neurobiol.* 2013;23(4):559–563. https://doi.org/10.1016/j.conb.2013.03.011.

184. Krishnan-Sarin S, Morean M, Kong G, et al. E-cigarettes and "dripping" among high-school youth. *Pediatrics.* 2017;139(3). https://doi.org/10.1542/peds.2016-3224.

185. Lasser K, Boyd JW, Woolhandler S, Himmelstein DU, McCormick D, Bor DH. Smoking and mental illness: a population-based prevalence study. *J Am Med Assoc.* 2000;284(20):2606–2610. https://doi.org/10.1001/jama.284.20.2606.

186. Lawrence D, Mitrou F, Zubrick SR. Smoking and mental illness: results from population surveys in Australia and the United States. *BMC Public Health.* 2009;9:285. https://doi.org/10.1186/1471-2458-9-285.

187. Le Foll B, Forget B, Aubin H-J, Goldberg SR. Blocking cannabinoid CB1 receptors for the treatment of nicotine dependence: insights from pre-clinical and clinical studies. *Addict Biol.* 2008;13(2):239–252. https://doi.org/10.1111/j.1369-1600.2008.00113.x.

188. Lee DC, Budney AJ, Brunette MF, Hughes JR, Etter J-F, Stanger C. Outcomes from a computer-assisted intervention simultaneously targeting cannabis and tobacco use. *Drug Alcohol Depend.* 2015;155:134–140. https://doi.org/10.1016/j.drugalcdep.2015.08.001.

189. Lee YO, Jordan JW, Djakaria M, Ling PM. Using peer crowds to segment Black youth for smoking intervention. *Health Promot Pract.* 2014;15(4):530–537. https://doi.org/10.1177/1524839913484470.

190. Legrand LN, Keyes M, McGue M, Iacono WG, Krueger RF. Rural environments reduce the genetic influence on adolescent substance use and rule-breaking behavior. *Psychol Med.* 2008;38(9):1341–1350. https://doi.org/10.1017/S0033291707001596.

191. Lerman C, Audrain-McGovern J. Reinforcing effects of smoking: more than a feeling. *Biol Psychiatry.* 2010;67(8):699–701. https://doi.org/10.1016/j.biopsych.2010.02.014.

192. Lerman C, Caporaso NE, Audrain J, et al. Evidence suggesting the role of specific genetic factors in cigarette smoking. *Health Psychol.* 1999;18(1):14–20.

193. Lerman C, Jepson C, Wileyto EP, et al. Role of functional genetic variation in the dopamine D2 receptor (DRD2) in response to bupropion and nicotine replacement therapy for tobacco dependence: results of two randomized clinical trials. *Neuropsychopharmacol.* 2006;31(1):231–242. https://doi.org/10.1038/sj.npp.1300861.

194. Lerman C, Shields PG, Audrain J, et al. The role of the serotinin transporter gene in cigarette smoking. *Cancer Epidem Biomar.* 1998;7:253–255.

195. Lerman C, Shields PG, Wileyto EP, et al. Effects of dopamine transporter and receptor polymorphisms on smoking cessation in a bupropion clinical trial. *Health Psychol.* 2003;22(5):541–548.

196. Lerman C, Wileyto EP, Patterson F. The funtional mu opioid receptor (OPRM1) Asn40Asp variant predicts short-term response to nicotine replacement therapy in a clinical trial. *Pharmacogenomics J.* 2004;4:184–192.

197. Lerner CA, Sundar IK, Yao H, et al. Vapors produced by electronic cigarettes and e-juices with flavorings induce toxicity, oxidative stress, and inflammatory response in lung epithelial cells and in mouse lung. *PLoS One.* 2015;10(2):e0116732. https://doi.org/10.1371/journal.pone.0116732.

198. Lessov-Schlaggar CN, Pergadia ML, Khroyan TV, Swan GE. Genetics of nicotine dependence and pharmacotherapy. *Biochem Pharmacol.* 2008;75(1):178–195.

199. Leventhal AM, Zvolensky MJ. Anxiety, depression, and cigarette smoking: a transdiagnostic vulnerability framework to understanding emotion-smoking comorbidity. *Psychol Bull.* 2015;141(1):176–212.

200. Leyro TM, Crew EE, Bryson SW, et al. Retrospective analysis of changing characteristics of treatment-seeking smokers: implications for further reducing smoking prevalence. *BMJ Open.* 2016;6(6):e010960. https://doi.org/10.1136/bmjopen-2015-010960.

201. Li MD. The genetics of smoking related behavior: a brief review. *Am J Med Sci.* 2003;326(4):168–173.

202. Li MD. Identifying susceptibility loci for nicotine dependence: 2008 update based on recent genome-wide linkage analyses. *Hum Genet.* 2008;123(2):119–131.

203. Li X, Caprioli D, Marchant NJ. Recent updates on incubation of drug craving: a mini-review. *Addict Biol.* 2015;20(5):872–876. https://doi.org/10.1111/adb.12205.

204. Lisha NE, Jordan JW, Ling PM. Peer crowd affiliation as a segmentation tool for young adult tobacco use. *Tob Control.* 2016;25(suppl 1):i83–i89. https://doi.org/10.1136/tobaccocontrol-2016-053086.

205. Loddenkemper R, Kreuter M, eds. *The Tobacco Epidemic.* 2nd, Revised and Extended Edition. Vol. 42. Basel, New York: Karger: Progress in respiratory research; 2015:1422–2140.

206. Lowinson JH, Ruiz P, Millman RB, Langrod JG. *Substance Abuse: A Comprehensive Textbook.* New York, NY: Lippincott Williams & Wilkins; 2005.

207. Lubman DI, Yucel M, Pantelis C. Addiction, a condition of compulsive behaviour? Neuroimaging and neuropsychological evidence of inhibitory dysregulation. *Addiction.* 2004;99(12):1491–1502.

208. Lynskey MT, Agrawal A, Heath AC. Genetically informative research on adolescent substance use: Methods, findings, and challenges. *J Am Acad Child Adolesc Psychiatry.* 2010;49(12):1202–1214. https://doi.org/10.1016/j.jaac.2010.09.004.

209. Maes HH, Woodard CE, Murrelle L, et al. Tobacco, alcohol and drug use in eight- to sixteen-year-old twins: the virginia twin study of adolescent behavioral development. *J Stud Alcohol.* 1999;60(3):293–305. https://doi.org/10.15288/jsa.1999.60.293.

210. Matsumoto M. Role of the lateral habenula and dopamine neurons in reward processing. *Brain Nerve.* 2009;61(4):389–396.

211. McAfee T, Davis KC, Alexander JR RL, Pechacek TF, Bunnell R. Effect of the first federally funded US antismoking national media campaign. *Lancet.* 2013;382(9909):2003–2011. https://doi.org/10.1016/S0140-6736(13)61686-4.

212. McCutcheon VV, Scherrer JF, Grant JD, et al. Parent, sibling and peer associations with subtypes of psychiatric and substance use disorder comorbidity in offspring. *Drug Alcohol Depend.* 2013;128(1–2):20–29. https://doi.org/10.1016/j.drugalcdep.2012.07.015.

213. McKelvey KL, Ramo DE, Delucchi K, Rubinstein ML. Polydrug use among urban adolescent cigarette smokers. *Addict Behav.* 2017;66:145–150. https://doi.org/10.1016/j.addbeh.2016.11.017.

214. McNair DM, Lorr M, Droppleman LF. *Profile of Mood States Manual.* San Diego, CA: Education and Industrial Testing Service; 1992.

215. Miech RA. Monitoring the Future: National Adolescent Drug Trends in 2017: Findings Released. http://www.monitoringthefuture.org.

215a. Miech R, Johnston L, O'Malley PM, et al. Adolescent vaping and nicotine use in 2017-2018 - U.S. national estimates. *N Engl J Med.* 2019;380(2):192–193.

216. Mihalak KB, Carroll FI, Luetje CW. Varenicline is a partial agonist at alpha4beta2 and a full agonist at alpha7 neuronal nicotinic receptors. *Mol Pharmacol.* 2006;70(3):801–805.

217. Mills EJ, Wu P, Lockhart I, Thorlund K, Puhan M, Ebbert JO. Comparisons of high-dose and combination nicotine replacement therapy, varenicline, and bupropion for smoking cessation: a systematic review and multiple treatment meta-analysis. *Ann Med.* 2012;44(6):588–597. https://doi.org/10.3109/07853890.2012.705016.

218. Minami H, Tran LT, McCarthy DE. Using ecological measures of smoking trigger exposure to predict smoking cessation milestones. *Psychol Addict Behav.* 2015;29(1):122–128. https://doi.org/10.1037/adb0000017.

219. Mitchell SH. Effects of short-term nicotine deprivation on decision-making: delay, uncertainty and effort discounting. *Nicotine Tob Res.* 2004;6(5):819–828. https://doi.org/10.1080/14622200412331296002.

220. Mooney ME, Sofuoglu M. Bupropion for the treatment of nicotine withdrawal and craving. *Expert Rev Neurother.* 2006;6(7):965–981. https://doi.org/10.1586/14737175.6.7.965.

221. Morris S, Mermelstein R. Depression and relapse: Antecedent or Consequence? Conference Name: SRNT Fifth Annual Conference; February; San Diego, CA, San Diego, CA.

222. Munafò M, Clark T, Johnstone E, Murphy M, Walton R. The genetic basis for smoking behavior: a systematic review and meta-analysis. *Nicotine Tob Res.* 2004;6(4):583–597.

223. Munafò MR, Flint J. Meta-analysis of genetic association studies. *Trends Genet.* 2004;20(9):439–444.

224. Munafo MR, Johnstone EC. Genes and cigarette smoking. *Addiction.* 2008;103(6):893–904.

225. Murray RL, Coleman T, Antoniak M, et al. The effect of proactively identifying smokers and offering smoking cessation support in primary care populations: a cluster-randomized trial. *Addiction.* 2008;103(6):998–1006.

226. Mwenifumbo JC, Tyndale RF. Genetic variability in CYP2A6 and the pharmacokinetics of nicotine. *Pharmacogenomics.* 2007;8(10):1385–1402. https://doi.org/10.2217/14622416.8.10.1385.

227. Nelson MD, Rezk-Hanna M, Rader F, et al. Acute effect of hookah smoking on the human Coronary Microcirculation. *Am J Cardiol.* 2016;117(11):1747–1754. https://doi.org/10.1016/j.amjcard.2016.03.007.

228. Neuhaus A, Bajbouj M, Kienast T, et al. Persistent dysfunctional frontal lobe activation in former smokers. *Psychopharmacology (Berl).* 2006;186(2):191–200.

229. Niaura RS, Britt DM, Borrelli B, Shadel WG, Abrams DB, Goldstein MG. History and symptoms of depression among smokers during a self-initiated quit attempt. *Nicotine Tob Res.* 1999;1(3):251–257.

230. Nielsen K, Petersen SE, Orntoft T. A comparison between stereological estimates of mean nuclear volume and DNA flow cytometry in bladder tumours. *APMIS.* 1989;97(10):949–956.

231. Nisell M, Marcus M, Nomikos GG, Svensson TH. Differential effects of acute and chronic nicotine on dopamine output in the core and shell of the rat nucleus accumbens. *J Neural Transm.* 1997;104:1–10.

232. Nisell M, Nomikos GG, Svensson TH. Nicotine dependence, midbrain dopamine systems and psychiatric disorders. *Pharmacol Toxicol.* 1995;76(3):157–162.

233. Noar SM, Francis DB, Bridges C, Sontag JM, Ribisl KM, Brewer NT. The impact of strengthening cigarette pack warnings: systematic review of longitudinal observational studies. *Soc Sci Med.* 2016;164:118–129. https://doi.org/10.1016/j.socscimed.2016.06.011.

234. Noar SM, Hall MG, Francis DB, Ribisl KM, Pepper JK, Brewer NT. Pictorial cigarette pack warnings: a meta-analysis of experimental studies. *Tob Control.* 2016;25(3):341–354. https://doi.org/10.1136/tobaccocontrol-2014-051978.

235. Nomikos GG, Damsma G, Wenkstern D, Fibiger HC. Acute effects of bupropion on extracellular dopamine concentrations in rat striatum and nucleus accumbens studied by in vivo microdialysis. *Neuropsychopharmacol.* 1989;2:273–279.

236. O'Connor PG, Fiellin DA. Pharmacologic treatment of heroin-dependent patients. *Ann Intern Med.* 2000;133(1):40–54.

237. Pagano ME, Delos-Reyes CM, Wasilow S, Svala KM, Kurtz SP. Smoking cessation and adolescent treatment response with comorbid ADHD. *J Subst Abuse Treat.* 2016;70:21–27. https://doi.org/10.1016/j.jsat.2016.07.008.

238. Panksepp J. Affective neuroscience of the emotional BrainMind: Evolutionary perspectives and implications for understanding depression. *Dialogues Clin Neurosci.* 2010;12(4):533–545.

239. Payne TJ, Smith PO, McCracken LM, McSherry WC, Antony MM. Assessing nicotine dependence: a comparison of the Fagerstrom Tolerance Questionnaire (FTQ) with the Fagerstrom Test for Nicotine Dependence (FTND) in a clinical sample. *Addict Behav.* 1994;19(3):307–317.

240. Pentel PR, LeSage MG. New directions in nicotine vaccine design and use. *Adv Pharmacol.* 2014;69:553–580. https://doi.org/10.1016/B978-0-12-420118-7.00014-7.

241. Physician Digital Reference. PDR 2017. http://www.pdr.net/drug-summary/Wellbutrin-SR-bupropion-hydrochloride-238.5891. Accessed June 2017.

242. Piasecki TM, Jorenby DE, Smith SS, Fiore MC, Baker TB. Smoking withdrawal dynamics: I. Abstinence distress in lapsers and abstainers. *J Abnorm Psychol.* 2003;112(1):3–13. https://doi.org/10.1037/0021-843X.112.1.3.

243. Piasecki TM, Jorenby DE, Smith SS, Fiore MC, Baker TB. Smoking withdrawal dynamics: II. Improved tests of withdrawal--relapse relations. *J Abnorm Psychol.* 2003;112(1):14–27. https://doi.org/10.1037/0021-843X.112.1.14.

244. Piasecki TM, Jorenby DE, Smith SS, Fiore MC, Baker TB. Smoking withdrawal dynamics: III. Correlates of withdrawal heterogeneity. *Exp Clin Psychopharmacol*. 2003;11:276–285. https://doi.org/10.1037/1064-1297.11.4.276.

245. Picciotto MR, Zoli M, Rimondini R, et al. Acetylcholine receptors containing the beta2 subunit are involved in the reinforcing properties of nicotine. *Nature*. 1998;391:173–177. https://doi.org/10.1038/34413.

246. Pidoplichko VL, DeBiasi M, Williams JT, Dani JA. Nicotine activates and desensitizes midbrain dopamine neurons. *Nature*. 1997;390(6658):401–404. https://doi.org/10.1038/37120.

247. Piper ME, Piasecki TM, Federman EB, et al. A multiple motives approach to tobacco dependence: the Wisconsin Inventory of Smoking Dependence Motives (WISDM-68). *J Consult Clin Psychol*. 2004;72(2):139–154. https://doi.org/10.1037/a0013298.

248. Pobbe RLH, Zangrossi JR H. Involvement of the lateral habenula in the regulation of generalized anxiety- and panic-related defensive responses in rats. *Life Sci*. 2008;82(25–26):1256–1261. https://doi.org/10.1016/j.lfs.2008.04.012.

249. Poling J, Oliveto A, Petry N, et al. Six-month trial of bupropion with Contingency management for cocaine dependence in a methadone-maintained population. *Arch Gen Psychiatry*. 2006;63(2):219–228.

250. Pomerleau CS, Pomerleau OF, Majchrzak MJ, Kloska DD, Malakuti R. Relationship between nicotine tolerance questionnaire scores and plasma cotinine. *Addict Behav*. 1990;15(1):73–80. https://doi.org/10.1016/0306-4603(90)90009-M.

251. Prokhorov AV, Kelder SH, Shegog R, et al. Impact of A Smoking Prevention Interactive Experience (ASPIRE), an interactive, multimedia smoking prevention and cessation curriculum for culturally diverse high-school students. *Nicotine Tob Res*. 2008;10(9):1477–1485. https://doi.org/10.1080/14622200802323183.

252. Raich A, Ballbe M, Nieva G, et al. Safety of varenicline for smoking cessation in psychiatric and Addicts patients. *Subst Use Misuse*. 2016;51(5):649–657. https://doi.org/10.3109/10826084.2015.1133646.

253. Raichle ME, Fiez JA, Videen TO, et al. Practice-related changes in human brain functional anatomy during nonmotor learning. *Cereb Cortex*. 1994;4(1):8–26.

254. Ramesh D, Schlosburg JE, Wiebelhaus JM, Lichtman AH. Marijuana dependence: not just smoke and mirrors. *ILAR J*. 2011;52(3):295–308. https://doi.org/10.1093/ilar.52.3.295.

255. Riala K, Ilomaki E, Hakko H, Rasanen P. Is the severity of adolescent conduct disorder associated with the level of nicotine dependence? *Eur Child Adolesc Psychiatry*. 2011;20(8):393–399. https://doi.org/10.1007/s00787-011-0189-x.

256. Ridderinkhof KR, Ullsperger M, Crone EA, Nieuwenhuis S. The role of the medial frontal cortex in cognitive control. *Science*. 2004;306(5695):443–447. https://doi.org/10.1126/science.1100301.

257. Robinson JD, Cinciripini PM, Karam-Hage M, et al. Pooled analysis of three randomized, double-blind, placebo controlled trials with rimonabant for smoking cessation. *Addict Biol*. 2017. https://doi.org/10.1111/adb.12508.

258. Robinson TE, Berridge KC. Incentive-sensitization and addiction. *Addiction*. 2001;96(1):103–114.

259. Robinson TE, Berridge KC. The incentive sensitization theory of addiction: some current issues. *Philos Trans R Soc Lond B Biol Sci*. 2008;363(1507):3137–3146.

260. Robinson TE, Gorny G, Mitton E, Kolb B. Cocaine self-administration alters the morphology of dendrites and dendritic spines in the nucleus accumbens and neocortex. *Synapse*. 2001;39(3):257–266.

261. Rose JE, Behm FM. Combination treatment with varenicline and bupropion in an adaptive smoking cessation paradigm. *Am J Psychiat*. 2014;171(11):1199–1205. https://doi.org/10.1176/appi.ajp.2014.13050595.

262. Rose JE, Behm FM. Combination varenicline/bupropion treatment benefits highly dependent smokers in an adaptive smoking cessation paradigm. *Nicotine Tob Res*. 2016:ntw283. https://doi.org/10.1093/ntr/ntw283.

263. Rush CR, Higgins ST, Vansickel AR, Stoops WW, Lile JA, Glaser PEA. Methylphenidate increases cigarette smoking. *Psychopharmacology (Berl)*. 2005;181(4):781–789. https://doi.org/10.1007/s00213-005-0021-8.

264. Sabol SZ, Nelson ML, Fisher C, et al. A genetic association for cigarette smoking behavior. *Health Psychol*. 1999;18(1):7–13.

265. Saccone SF, Hinrichs AL, Saccone NL, et al. Cholinergic nicotinic receptor genes implicated in a nicotine dependence association study targeting 348 candidate genes with 3,713 SNPs. *Hum Mol Genet*. 2007;16(1):36–49. https://doi.org/10.1093/hmg/ddl438.

266. SAMHSA. 2016 National Survey on Drug Use and Health: NSDUH.https://www.samhsa.gov/data/sites/default/files/NSDUH…/NSDUH-DetTabs-2016.pdf. Updated September 2017. Accessed April 16, 2018.

267. Sandager N, Peterson CB, Allen S, Henderson KE, Crow S, Thuras P. Tobacco use and comorbidity in bulimia nervosa. *Int J Eat Disord*. 2008;41(8):734–738. https://doi.org/10.1002/eat.20572.

268. Sarnyai Z. Neurobiology of stress and cocaine addiction. Studies on corticotropin-releasing factor in rats, monkeys, and humans. *Ann N Y Acad Sci*. 1998;851:371–387.

269. Schoenfelder EN, Faraone SV, Kollins SH. Stimulant treatment of ADHD and cigarette smoking: a meta-analysis. *Pediatrics*. 2014;133(6):1070–1080. https://doi.org/10.1542/peds.2014-0179.

270. Seidman LJ, Biederman J, Faraone SV, Weber W, Ouellette C. Toward defining a neuropsychology of attention deficit-hyperactivity disorder: performance of children and adolescents from a large clinically referred sample. *J Consult Clin Psychol*. 1997;65(1):150–160.

271. Semba J. Nicotine withdrawal induces subsensitivity of hypothalamic–pituitary–adrenal axis to stress in rats: implications for precipitation of depression during smoking cessation. *Psychoneuroendocrinology*. 2004;29(2):215–226. https://doi.org/10.1016/S0306-4530(03)00024-6.

272. Shiffman S, Paty J, Gnys M, Kassel J, Hickcox M. First lapses to smoking: within-subjects analysis of real-time reports. *J Consult Clin Psychol*. 1996;64(2):366–379. https://doi.org/10.1037/0022-006X.64.2.366.

273. Siciliano CA, Calipari ES, Ferris MJ, Jones SR. Adaptations of presynaptic dopamine terminals induced by psychostimulant self-administration. *ACS Chem Neurosci*. 2015;6(1):27–36. https://doi.org/10.1021/cn5002705.

274. Silagy C, Lancaster T, Stead L, Mant D, Fowler G. Nicotine replacement therapy for smoking cessation. *Cochrane Database Syst Rev*. 2004;3:CD000146-CD000146.

275. Simioni N, Cottencin O. Resurgence of anorexic symptoms during smoking cessation in patients with a history of anorexia nervosa: an unseen problem?--Report of two cases. *Int J Eat Disord*. 2015;48(6):798–801. https://doi.org/10.1002/eat.22428.

276. Siu AL. Behavioral and pharmacotherapy interventions for tobacco smoking cessation in adults, including pregnant women: U.S. Preventive Services Task Force Recommendation StatementUSPSTF recommendation Statement for interventions for tobacco smoking cessation. *Ann Intern Med*. 2015. N/A(N/A):N/A-N/A. https://doi.org/10.7326/M15-2023..

277. Slemmer JE, Martin BP, Damaj I. Bupropion is a nicotine antagonist. *J Pharmacol Exp Ther*. 2000;295:321–327.

278. Smith SS, Jorenby DE, Leischow SJ, et al. Targeting smokers at increased risk for relapse: treatming women and those with a history of depression. *Nicotine Tob Res*. 2003;5:99–109.

279. Smith SS, Piper ME, Bolt DM, et al. Development of the brief Wisconsin Inventory of smoking dependence motives. *Nicotine Tob Res*. 2010;12(5):489–499. https://doi.org/10.1093/ntr/ntq032.

280. Solmi M, Veronese N, Sergi G, et al. The association between smoking prevalence and eating disorders: a systematic review and meta-analysis. *Addiction*. 2016;111(11):1914–1922. https://doi.org/10.1111/add.13457.

281. Spitz MR, Amos CI, Dong Q, Lin J, Wu X. The CHRNA5-A3 region on chromosome 15q24-25.1 is a risk factor both for nicotine dependence and for lung cancer. *J Nat Cancer Inst.* 2008;100(21):1552–1556.

282. Spitz MR, Shi H, Hudmon KS, et al. A case-control study of the dopamine D2 receptor gene and smoking status in lung cancer. *J Natl Cancer Inst.* 1998;90(5):358–363.

283. Stead LF, Hartmann-Boyce J, Perera R, Lancaster T. Telephone counselling for smoking cessation. *Cochrane Database Syst Rev.* 2013;8:CD002850.

284. Stead LF, Koilpillai P, Lancaster T. Additional behavioural support as an adjunct to pharmacotherapy for smoking cessation. *Cochrane Database Syst Rev.* 2015;10:CD009670.

285. Stead LF, Perera R, Bullen C, et al. Nicotine replacement therapy for smoking cessation. *Cochrane Database Syst Rev.* 2012;11:CD000146-CD000146. https://doi.org/10.1002/14651858.CD000146.pub4.

286. Straub RE, al e. Susceptibility genes for nicotine dependence: a genome scan and followup in an independent sample suggest that regions on chromosomes 2, 4, 10, 16, 17, and 18 merit further study. *Mol Psychiatr.* 1999;4:129–144.

287. Stuss DT, Gow CA, Hetherington CR. "No longer Gage": frontal lobe dysfunction and emotional changes. *J Consult Clin Psychol.* 1992;60(3):349–359.

288. Subramaniyan M, Dani JA. Dopaminergic and cholinergic learning mechanisms in nicotine addiction. *Ann N Y Acad Sci.* 2015;1349:46–63. https://doi.org/10.1111/nyas.12871.

289. Swan GE, Jack LM, Valdes AM, et al. Joint effect of dopaminergic genes on likelihood of smoking following treatment with bupropion SR. *Health Psychol.* 2007;26(3):361–368.

290. Talati A, Wickramaratne PJ, Keyes KM, Hasin DS, Levin FR, Weissman MM. Smoking and psychopathology increasingly associated in recent birth cohorts. *Drug Alcohol Depend.* 2013;133(2):724–732. https://doi.org/10.1016/j.drugalcdep.2013.08.025.

291. Tapert SF, Baratta MV, Abrantes AM, Brown SA. Attention dysfunction predicts substance involvement in community youths. *J Am Acad Child Adolesc Psychiatry.* 2002;41(6):680–686.

292. Thomas KH, Martin RM, Davies NM, Metcalfe C, Windmeijer F, Gunnell D. Smoking cessation treatment and risk of depression, suicide, and self harm in the Clinical Practice Research Datalink: prospective cohort study. *BMJ.* 2013;347:f5704.

293. Thomas RE, Baker PRA, Thomas BC, Lorenzetti DL. Family-based programmes for preventing smoking by children and adolescents. *Cochrane Database Syst Rev.* 2015;(2):CD004493. https://doi.org/10.1002/14651858.CD004493.pub3.

294. Thorgeirsson TE, Geller F, Sulem P, et al. A variant associated with nicotine dependence, lung cancer and peripheral arterial disease. *Nature.* 2008;452(7187):638–642.

295. Thurgood SL, McNeill A, Clark-Carter D, Brose LS. A systematic review of smoking cessation interventions for adults in substance abuse treatment or recovery. *Nicotine Tob Res.* 2016;18(5):993–1001. https://doi.org/10.1093/ntr/ntv127.

296. Tonstad S, Hays JT, Jorenby DE, et al. Varenicline phase III Studies; November; Dallas, TX.

297. Tonstad S, Tonnesen P, Hajek P, Williams KE, Billing CB, Reeves KR. Effect of maintenance therapy with varenicline on smoking cessation: a randomized controlled trial. *J Am Med Assoc.* 2006;296(1):64–71.

298. Torregrossa MM, Kalivas PW. Microdialysis and the neurochemistry of addiction. *Pharmacol Biochem Behav.* 2008;90(2):261–272.

299. Torrens M, Fonseca F, Mateu G, Farre M. Efficacy of antidepressants in substance use disorders with and without comorbid depression. A systematic review and meta-analysis. *Drug Alcohol Depend.* 2005;78(1):1–22. https://doi.org/10.1016/j.drugalcdep.2004.09.004.

300. True WR, Heath AC, Scherrer JF, et al. Genetic and environmental contributions to smoking. *Addiction.* 1997;92(10):1277–1287.

301. Tseng T-Y, Ostroff JS, Campo A, et al. A randomized trial comparing the effect of nicotine versus placebo electronic cigarettes on smoking reduction among young adult smokers. *Nicotine Tob Res.* 2016;18(10):1937–1943. https://doi.org/10.1093/ntr/ntw017.

302. Tsoh JY, Cinciripini PM, Wetter D, et al. Depression history, negative affect, and stages of change in smoking cessation. *Ann Behav Med.* 1999;21(supplement):205.

303. Tutka P, Zatonski W. Cytisine for the treatment of nicotine addiction: from a molecule to therapeutic efficacy. *Pharmacol Rep.* 2006;58(6):777–798.

304. Ueda H. Anti-opioid systems in morphine tolerance and addiction-locus-specific involvement of nociceptin and the NMDA receptor. *Novartis Found Symp.* 2004;261:155–162.

305. Ueno K, Kiguchi N, Kobayashi Y, et al. Possible involvement of endogenous opioid system located downstream of alpha7 nicotinic acetylcholine receptor in mice with physical dependence on nicotine. *J Pharmacol Sci.* 2014;124(1):47–53.

306. Uhl GR, Liu QR, Drgon T, Johnson C, Walther D, Rose JE. Molecular genetics of nicotine dependence and abstinence: whole genome association using 520,000 SNPs. *BMC Genet.* 2007;8:10.

307. Uhl GR, Liu QR, Drgon T, et al. Molecular genetics of successful smoking cessation: convergent genome-wide association study results. *Arch Gen Psychiatry.* 2008;65(6):683–693.

308. US Centers for Disease Control and Prevention. Annual smoking-attributable mortality, years of potential life lost, and productivity losses - United States, 1997-2001. *MMWR Morb Mortal Wkly Rep.* 2005;54(25):625–628.

309. US Centers for Disease Control and Prevention. Smoking-attributable mortality, years of potential life lost, and productivity losses--United States, 2000-2004. *MMWR Morb Mortal Wkly Rep.* Updated March 4, 2015.

310. US Centers for Disease Control and Prevention. QuickStats: percentage of adults who ever used an E-cigarette and percentage who currently use E-cigarettes, by age group - national health interview survey, United States, 2016. *MMWR Morb Mortal Wkly Rep.* 2017;66(33):892. https://doi.org/10.15585/mmwr.mm6633a6.

311. US Department of Health and Human Services. *Reducing Tobacco use: A Report of the Surgeon General.* Atlanta, GA: US Department of Health and Human Services, Centers for Disease Control and Prevention, National Center for Chronic Disease Prevention and Health Promotion. Office on Smoking and Health; 2000.

312. US Department of Health and Human Services. *The Health Consequences of Smoking--50 Years of Progress: A Report of the Surgeon General.* Atlanta, GA: Surgeon General's Report; 2014.

313. US Food and Drug Administration. *Public Health Advisory, Important Information on Chantix (Varenicline).* Rockville: MD; 2008.

314. van Prince Leeuwen A, Creemers HE, Verhulst FC, et al. Legal substance use and the development of a DSM-IV cannabis use disorder during adolescence: the TRAILS study. *Addiction.* 2014;109(2):303–311. https://doi.org/10.1111/add.12346.

315. van Wymelbeke V, Brondel L, Marcel Brun J, Rigaud D. Factors associated with the increase in resting energy expenditure during refeeding in malnourished anorexia nervosa patients. *Am J Clin Nutr.* 2004;80(6):1469–1477.

316. Vansickel AR, Poole MM, Stoops WW, et al. Stimulant-induced changes in smoking and caloric intake: influence of rate of onset. *Pharmacol Biochem Behav.* 2009;92(4):597–602. https://doi.org/10.1016/j.pbb.2009.02.012.

317. Vansickel AR, Stoops WW, Glaser PEA, Poole MM, Rush CR. Methylphenidate increases cigarette smoking in participants with ADHD. *Psychopharmacology (Berl).* 2011;218(2):381–390. https://doi.org/10.1007/s00213-011-2328-y.

318. Volkow ND, Fowler J, Wang G-J. Role of dopamine in drug reinforcement and addiction in humans: results from imaging studies. *Behav Pharmacol.* 2002;13:355–366.

319. Volkow ND, Fowler JS, Wang GJ. The addicted human brain viewed in the light of imaging studies: brain circuits and treatment strategies. *Neuropharmacology.* 2004;47(suppl 1):3–13.

320. Volkow ND, Wang GJ, Fowler JS, Tomasi D, Telang F, Baler R. Addiction: decreased reward sensitivity and increased expectation sensitivity conspire to overwhelm the brain's control circuit. *Bioessays*. 2010;32(9):748–755. https://doi.org/10.1002/bies.201000042.

321. Volkow ND, Wang GJ, Telang F, et al. Cocaine cues and dopamine in dorsal striatum: mechanism of craving in cocaine addiction. *J Neurosci*. 2006;26(24):6583.

322. Vrieze SI, McGue M, Miller MB, Hicks BM, Iacono WG. Three mutually informative ways to understand the genetic relationships among behavioral disinhibition, alcohol use, drug use, nicotine use/dependence, and their co-occurrence: twin biometry, GCTA, and genome-wide scoring. *Behav Genet*. 2013;43(2):97–107. https://doi.org/10.1007/s10519-013-9584-z.

322a. Wang TW, Asman K, Gentzke AS, et al. Tobacco Product Use Among Adults - United States, 2017. *MMWR. Morb Mortal Wkly Rep*. 2018;67(44):1225–1232. https://doi.org/10.15585/mmwr.mm6744a2.

323. Watson D, Clark LA, Tellegen A. Development and validation of brief measures of positive and negative affect: the PANAS Scales. *J Pers Soc Psychol*. 1988;54:1063–1070. https://doi.org/10.1037/0022-3514.54.6.1063.

324. Wennike P, Danielsson T, Landfeldt B, Westin A, Tonnesen P. Smoking reduction promotes smoking cessation: results from a double blind, randomized, placebo-controlled trial of nicotine gum with 2-year follow-up. *Addiction*. 2003;98(10):1395–1402.

325. Wetter DW, Kenford SL, Smith SS, Fiore MC, Jorenby DE, Baker TB. Gender differences in smoking cessation. *J Consult Clin Psychol*. 1999;67(4):555–562. https://doi.org/10.1037/0022-006X.67.4.555.

326. Wetter DW, Smith SS, Kenford SL, et al. Smoking outcome expectancies: factor structure, predictive validity, and discriminant validity. *J Abnorm Psychol*. 1994;103:801–811.

327. White MA, Grilo CM. Psychiatric comorbidity in binge-eating disorder as a function of smoking history. *J Clin Psychiatry*. 2006;67(04):594–599. https://doi.org/10.4088/JCP.v67n0410.

328. Whittaker R, McRobbie H, Bullen C, Rodgers A, Gu Y. Mobile phone-based interventions for smoking cessation. *Cochrane Database Syst Rev*. 2016;4:CD006611. https://doi.org/10.1002/14651858.CD006611.pub4.

329. Wilens TE, Biederman J. Alcohol, drugs, and attention-deficit/hyperactivity disorder: a model for the study of addictions in youth. *J Psychopharmacol*. 2005.

330. Wilens TE, Vitulano M, Upadhyaya H, et al. Cigarette smoking associated with attention deficit hyperactivity disorder. *J Pediatr*. 2008;153(3):414–419. https://doi.org/10.1016/j.jpeds.2008.04.030.

331. Williams JM, Anthenelli RM, Morris CD, et al. A randomized, double-blind, placebo-controlled study evaluating the safety and efficacy of varenicline for smoking cessation in patients with schizophrenia or schizoaffective disorder. *J Clin Psychiatry*. 2012;73(5):654–660.

332. Williams JM, Ziedonis D. Addressing tobacco among individuals with a mental illness or an addiction. *Addict Behav*. 2004;29(6):1067–1083.

333. Wilson A, Guillaumier A, George J, Denham A, Bonevski B. A systematic narrative review of the effectiveness of behavioural smoking cessation interventions in selected disadvantaged groups (2010-2017). *Expert Rev Respir Med*. 2017;11(8):617–630. https://doi.org/10.1080/17476348.2017.1340836.

334. Winhusen TM, Lewis DF, Riggs PD, et al. Subjective effects, misuse, and adverse effects of osmotic-release methylphenidate treatment in adolescent substance abusers with attention-deficit/hyperactivity disorder. *J Child Adolesc Psychopharmacol*. 2011;21(5):455–463. https://doi.org/10.1089/cap.2011.0014.

335. Winhusen TM, Somoza EC, Brigham GS, et al. Impact of attention-deficit/hyperactivity disorder (ADHD) treatment on smoking cessation intervention in ADHD smokers: a randomized, double-blind, placebo-controlled trial. *J Clin Psychiatry*. 2010;71(12):1680–1688. https://doi.org/10.4088/JCP.09m05089gry.

336. Wu L, Sun S, He Y, Zeng J. Effect of smoking reduction therapy on smoking cessation for smokers without an Intention to quit: an updated systematic review and meta-analysis of randomized controlled. *Int J Environ Res Public Health*. 2015;12(9):10235–10253. https://doi.org/10.3390/ijerph120910235.

337. Xu J, Mendrek A, Cohen MS, et al. Brain activity in cigarette smokers performing a working memory task: effect of smoking abstinence. *Biol Psychiatry*. 2005;58(2):143–150.

338. Yildirim F, Cevik Y, Emektar E, Corbacioglu SK, Katirci Y. Evaluating ECG and carboxyhemoglobin changes due to smoking narghile. *Inhal Toxicol*. 2016;28(12):546–549. https://doi.org/10.1080/08958378.2016.1224957.

339. Young SE, Rhee SH, Stallings MC, Corley RP, Hewitt JK. Genetic and environmental vulnerabilities underlying adolescent substance use and problem use: general or specific? *Behav Genet*. 2006;36(4):603–615. https://doi.org/10.1007/s10519-006-9066-7.

340. Yudkin P, Munafo M, Hey K, et al. Effectiveness of nicotine patches in relation to genotype in women versus men: randomised controlled trial. *BMJ*. 2004;328(7446):989–990. https://doi.org/10.1136/bmj.38050.674826.

341. Zhang H, Ye Y, Wang X, Gelernter J, Ma JZ, Li MD. DOPA decarboxylase gene is associated with nicotine dependence. *Pharmacogenomics*. 2006;7(8):1159–1166.

24

Cannabis: An Overview of the Empirical Literature

MICHAEL J. ZVOLENSKY, SAMANTHA G. FARRIS, TERESA M. LEYRO, KIRSTEN J. LANGDON, AMIT BERNSTEIN, AND MARCEL O. BONN-MILLER

Introduction

Marijuana (also referred to as cannabis) is a drug that is derived from the flowers, stems, leaves, and seeds of the hemp plant (*Cannabis sativa*). Cannabis is the generic term that refers to the psychoactive substances derived from the plant, including cannabis-like substances (e.g., synthetic cannabinoid compounds). In this chapter, we utilize the term cannabis, but it should be noted marijuana is used as frequently in the literature. The need for public health awareness and evidence-based clinical care for cannabis use and its disorder remains a major health care priority in the United States and beyond. Indeed, cannabis has been the most widely used illicit substance in the United States for the past 30 consecutive years,[101] with approximately 12% of individuals 12 years of age or older having used cannabis in the past year.[148] An estimated 9% of persons who have ever used cannabis will become dependent,[117] with prevalence estimates of 17% among those who start using cannabis in adolescence and upwards of 50% among daily users.[75] These rates in the United States represent a significant public health concern considering that several well-documented negative consequences have been associated with daily or weekly drug use (e.g., disrupted cortical development, increased risk of severe medical and psychiatric disease, increased risk of motor-vehicle accidents, and impaired lifetime achievement).[184]

The overarching aim of the present chapter is to provide an overview of cannabis use and its disorder. The chapter is organized into seven sections. In the first section we describe the prevalence of cannabis use and cannabis use disorder. In the second section we clarify the nature of cannabis use in terms of its pharmacokinetics and acute intoxication features. The third section details the classification of cannabis use disorder using the current diagnostic nomenclature. The fourth section discusses the motivational bases for use of the drug. In the fifth section we provide a synopsis of some problems associated with cannabis use and disorder, including health problems, social problems, and psychological disturbances. The sixth section provides a summary of the scientific work focused on cannabis, the reasons for its use, and users' relative success in quitting. In the final section, we describe some practically oriented clinical issues for primary care medical practitioners to consider in terms of the recognition and treatment of cannabis use and its disorder.

Prevalence

Cannabis has been the most widely used illicit substance for 30 consecutive years in the United States, with approximately 12% of individuals (12 years of age or older) having endorsed cannabis use in the past year. Of those who have ever used cannabis, nearly 9% of individuals will become dependent. Among those who initiated cannabis use in adolescence, an estimated 17% will become dependent, while 50% of daily cannabis users will become dependent. Probability estimates of transitioning from cannabis use to dependence indicate that cannabis is associated with a high rate of dependence potential.[117] For example, the probability that cannabis users develop dependence is approximately 9%, half of whom develop dependence within 5 years after initial onset of cannabis use, which is faster than the transition of nicotine or alcohol dependence.[117] Furthermore, greater levels of use are related to an increased risk for dependence. Studies suggest that the rate of dependence is 20%–30% among those persons using cannabis on a regular (weekly) basis.[74] Cosubstance use with cannabis is common, and approximately 80% of cannabis users met criteria for an additional substance use disorder (e.g., alcohol, nicotine).[117] It is important to note that the current prevalence estimates are based on the *Diagnostic and Statistical Manual of Mental Disorders, Fourth Edition, Text Revision* (DSM-IV-TR),[4] which was revised in 2013 (*Diagnostic and Statistical Manual of Mental Disorders, Fifth Edition* [DSM-5][5]). This update resulted in changes to the classification of disordered cannabis use, which may affect the prevalence estimates.[5] However, to date, the bulk of the literature has naturally reported prevalence estimates prior to the update.

Of special relevance to clinical practitioners, many treatment and community studies have examined prevalence rates of cannabis use among different samples with a variety of medical and psychological problems. This is important given psychiatric comorbidity is associated with transition from cannabis use to dependence.[117] For example, 23% of individuals seeking treatment for psychosis report cannabis use, with about half of that group misusing the drug.[71] Cannabis use is associated with earlier first episode of psychosis, which is particularly evident in high-potency cannabis use.[60] These findings are consistent with a recent meta-analysis indicating cannabis abuse/dependence is associated with increased likelihood of transition to psychosis in ultra-high-risk individuals.[108] Another community-based study found that approximately 16% of patients with spinal cord injury used cannabis.[187] Among individuals with current and lifetime chronic pain, the prevalence of past-month cannabis use was 22.9% and 34.9%, respectively.[190] In addition, among HIV-infected individuals, past-month cannabis use is estimated to range from 23% to 65%.[91,141] Cannabis use disorder is also common among military veterans,[19] which may be underestimated due to underdiagnosis.[19] Other work found that cannabis use is common among recently homeless individuals (16%[179]). Moreover, data indicate that cannabis use accounts for as much as 25% of the primary drug problems of individuals seeking residential drug treatment.[62] Similarly, among adolescents seeking outpatient services for cannabis abuse or dependence, approximately 38% reported depression and 29% reported acute levels of anxiety.[61] These studies suggest that cannabis use: (1) may be overrepresented among certain vulnerable populations and (2) is a primary clinical concern.

Nature of Cannabis Use: Pharmacokinetics and Acute Intoxication Features

Pharmacokinetics

Cannabis can be consumed via smoking (e.g., hand-rolled cigarettes, water pipes, nonwater pipes, vaporizers), ingestion (e.g., mixed into foods or used in the process of brewing tea), transdermally, or rectally. Cannabis shares some qualities with tobacco in that it is composed principally of plant material, often is used via smoking routes (e.g., pipes, joints), and contains a myriad of chemical compounds. Unlike tobacco,

however, the active agents in cannabis are cannabinoids (unique to the marijuana plant). There are at least 100 different cannabinoids in marijuana, although the pharmacokinetics of most of these compounds is largely unknown.[7] Of these, the most abundant cannabinoid is tetrahydrocannabinol (THC),[172] which is considered responsible for the main psychotropic effects of cannabis. The THC content of plants from a range of sources and strains varies dramatically.[132] With a focus on improved plant breeding and improved growing techniques, the THC content of cannabis has increased dramatically in a short period of time. As one illustrative example, THC content from a typical cannabis cigarette (joint) in the 1960s was 10 mg, whereas estimates suggest that it currently is around 1 g (or 150–200 mg).[7] Cannabidiol (CBD) is another constituent in cannabis that lacks the same psychoactive effects as THC, and instead appears to act as an antagonist of some of the negative psychoactive effects of THC.[124,136,145] Data indicate that CBD has a range of therapeutic effects including anticonvulsant, antipsychotic, analgesic, and neuroprotective properties.[63,145] In addition, there is growing prevalence in the use of synthetic cannabis compounds, which include oral formulations (pill, capsules) of cannabis that are available for prescription (e.g., nabilone, dronabinol), and other nonmedical synthetic cannabinoids products (e.g., K2, spice).[150]

Since the discovery of a cannabinoid receptor within the brain in the late 1980s, researchers have been able to explicate the process by which THC acts on the brain. Currently, there is evidence of three potential cannabinoid receptors, only one of which is located within the brain (the cannabinoid-1 receptor).[172] When THC is inhaled into the body via cannabis smoking, it passes from the lungs into the bloodstream.[87] Once in the blood, THC attaches to cannabinoid receptors, such as the cannabinoid-1 receptor, adding to or reducing the naturally occurring endogenous ligands for these receptors (e.g., anandamide).[59] The cannabinoid-1 receptor, in particular, has been found to mediate both neurochemical and behavioral properties of these cannabinoids, including tolerance.[172] It also is noteworthy that THC and other cannabinoids move rapidly into fat and other bodily tissues but are released relatively slowly from these tissues back into the bloodstream.[96] Eventually, cannabinoids are cleared from the body via urine and fecal matter,[172] although elimination is relatively slow.[95] The detection window in urine depends upon various factors, including drug dose, form of administration, duration/frequency of use, and individual differences in absorption, metabolism, and excretion.[118] Specifically, urinary detection windows (via 11-nor-9-carboxy-THC [THCOOH] metabolite) ranges from several days in infrequent users to months in frequent users.[118]

Acute Intoxication Features

THC can produce a range of acute psychosensory experiences including perceptual distortions (e.g., hallucinogenic properties), relaxation, anxiety, acute paranoia, inhibition, and so on.[99] Periods of intoxication depend on use patterns and potency but tend to last for at least a few hours.[39,133,149] The acute effects of THC also impair executive functioning, including working memory, attentional and information processing, and impulsivity,[52] as well as psychomotor performance on complex, demanding tasks.[75,142,160] There is a dose-dependent relation between THC and psychomotor and cognitive impairment, with higher doses being associated with more impairment for

TABLE 24.1	Criteria for Cannabis Use Disorder.

A. A problematic pattern of cannabis use, leading to clinically significant impairment or distress, as manifested by at least two of the following, occurring within a 12-month period:

1. Cannabis is often taken in larger amounts or over a longer period than was intended.
2. There is a persistent desire or unsuccessful efforts to cut down or control cannabis use.
3. A great deal of time is spent in activities necessary to obtain cannabis, use cannabis, or recover from its effects.
4. Craving, or a strong desire or urge to use cannabis.
5. Recurrent cannabis use resulting in a failure to fulfill major role obligations at work, school, or home.
6. Continued cannabis use despite having persistent or recurrent social or interpersonal problems caused or exacerbated by the effects of cannabis.
7. Important social, occupational, or recreational activities are given up or reduced because of cannabis use.
8. Recurrent cannabis use in situations in which it is physically hazardous.
9. Cannabis use is continued despite knowledge of having a persistent or recurrent physical or psychological problem that is likely to have been caused or exacerbated by cannabis.
10. Tolerance, as defined by either of the following:
    (a) A need for markedly increased amounts of cannabis to achieve intoxication or desired effect
    (b) Markedly diminished effect with continued use of the same amount of cannabis
11. Withdrawal, as manifested by either of the following:
    (a) The characteristic withdrawal syndrome for the cannabis (*see A and B of the criteria set for cannabis withdrawal*, Table 24.2)
    (b) Cannabis (or closely related substance) is taken to relieve or avoid withdrawal symptoms

From APA. *Diagnostic and Statistical Manual of Mental Disorders*, Fifth Edition (DSM-5). Washington, DC: American Psychological Association; 2013.

TABLE 24.2	Cannabis Withdrawal (Criteria A and B).

A. Cessation of cannabis use that has been heavy or prolonged (i.e., usually daily or almost daily use over a period of at least a few months).
B. Three (or more) of the following signs and symptoms develop within approximately 1 week after Criterion A:
    1. Irritability, anger, or aggression
    2. Nervousness or anxiety
    3. Sleep difficulty (e.g., insomnia, disturbing dreams)
    4. Decreased appetite or weight loss
    5. Restlessness
    6. Depressed mood
    7. At least one of the following physical symptoms causing significant discomfort: abdominal pain, shakiness/tremors, sweating, fever, chills, or headache

Data from Budney AJ, Hughes JR, Moore BA, Vandrey R. Review of the validity and significance of cannabis withdrawal syndrome. *Am J Psychiatry*. 2004;161 (11):1967-1977; Levin KH, Copersino MI, Heishman SJ, Liu F, Kelly DL, Boggs DL, et al. Cannabis withdrawal symptoms in non-treatment-seeking adults cannabis smokers. *Drug Alcohol Depend*. 2010;111(1):120-127.

more demanding tasks.[7,75,142] Although cognitive impairment for hours after exposure to THC is a well-replicated phenomenon in laboratory studies,[160] there has been consistent debate about the permanent cognitive effects of THC.[7] Data are mixed as to whether there are long-term effects of THC on impulsivity; however, attention and working memory appear to be largely unaffected.[52] Although decision-making and risk-taking behavior are not consistently affected by acute intoxication, one study found that heavy cannabis users who abstained from cannabis use had impaired decision-making capacities and great risk-taking tendencies.[186] The observed deficits appear to be more clearly documented among chronic, heavy cannabis users, relative to occasional or light users.[52]

Classification of Cannabis Use Disorder

According to the DSM-5,[5] cannabis use disorder is used to classify problematic cannabis use (see Table 24.1 for the diagnostic criteria for cannabis use disorder). Cannabis use disorder is a pattern of problematic cannabis use despite significant problems from use that produce cognitive, behavioral, and physiological symptoms due to continued cannabis use. These symptoms broadly reflect impaired control (symptoms 1–4), social impairment (symptoms 5–7), risky use (symptoms 8–9), and pharmacological criteria (symptoms 10–11). Unique to the current diagnostic formulation is the unidimensional diagnostic classification, which reflects

a range of the disorders, from mild to severe in form. Specifically, three severity specifiers are used based on the number of symptoms present: mild (presence of 2–3 symptoms), moderate (presence of 4–5 symptoms), and severe (presence of 6 or more symptoms). This is in contrast to the prior diagnostic classification of cannabis use disorders in the DSM-IV-TR,[4] which included two disorders that were designed to reflect harmful consequences of frequent use (marijuana abuse) relative to more severe compulsive use (marijuana dependence).

This change to the diagnostic classification was based in part on the limited empirical data that supported the validity of distinguishing marijuana abuse and dependence,[11,44,121,176] and lack of scientific consensus for a marijuana dependence syndrome.[31] Data indicate that the five most commonly endorsed symptoms are: hazardous use (24.8%), persistent desire/attempts to stop or cut down (15.9%), craving (13.9%), continued use despite interpersonal problems (10.7%), and neglect of work/school/home responsibilities (10.4%).[43]

One additional change in the diagnostic classification of cannabis use disorder is the recognition of cannabis withdrawal syndrome (see Table 24.2 for list of common cannabis withdrawal symptoms[31,114]), which can contribute to difficulties in quitting cannabis.[34,70] Based on the DSM-5-defined cannabis withdrawal symptoms, one study found that 11.9% of cannabis users met criteria for cannabis withdrawal, male relatives of female users were significantly more likely to report withdrawal symptoms (16.4% vs. 9.0%), and withdrawal symptoms are moderately heritable.[183] Finally, the DSM-5 includes the addition of cannabis craving, or strong desire or urge to use cannabis.

Although limited research to date has examined the comparability of the previous and current diagnostic criteria, one study found considerable diagnostic agreement between DSM-IV and DSM-5 (92.9% agreement), although slightly higher prevalence estimates were observed in the DSM-5 definition relative to the DSM-IV (41.0% relative to 39.4%).[135] However, this pattern of results has not been observed consistently. For example, lower diagnostic correspondence has been observed for cannabis use disorder (kappa range .43–.79 depending on the number of symptoms endorsed), and is less concordant relative to other substance use disorders (alcohol, cocaine, and opioid).[43] Other data indicate that DSM-5 cannabis use disorder is less prevalent than DSM-IV abuse/dependence,[126] which has been observed only in European American cannabis users, but not African American users.[2] Diagnostic shifts have been deemed minimally related to the removal of the legal problems criterion or addition of the craving criterion.[135] Regarding severity thresholds, 67%-97.5% of marijuana dependent individuals per the DSM-IV-TR definition would meet criteria for a severe cannabis use disorder,[107,135] indicating relatively strong diagnostic concordance. However, greater discrepancies are observed among those with a marijuana abuse diagnosis: 56% received a diagnosis of mild cannabis use disorder, 21% received a moderate cannabis use disorder diagnosis, and 23% received no diagnosis. Indeed, interrater diagnostic reliability was lower for mild cannabis use disorder, relative to moderate or severe cannabis use disorder, although all DSM-5 cannabis use disorders showed greater reliability relative to DSM-IV abuse/dependence disorders.[57] More data are needed to estimate the prevalence of the DSM-5 cannabis use disorder, at varying severity levels.

To date, researchers have employed standardized interviews to index cannabis diagnoses in a manner identical to those for other types of substances (e.g., alcohol, tobacco). At the same time, in contrast to the diagnostic classification system, pattern of cannabis use (quantity/frequency of use) is not considered.[44] Despite this, it has been more common historically to denote cannabis use variability by asking respondents to indicate their level of use (e.g., frequency) over a specified period of time.[55] From this perspective, having participants specify the frequency, and perhaps quantity, of cannabis use also can be a common assessment method.[40] Collectively, then, deciding on whether nosological classification and/or a use-oriented assessment protocol (i.e., volume and frequency) is indicated may depend on the specific clinical need or research question being posed and the theoretical basis for it.

Motivational Bases of Cannabis Use

Researchers and clinicians also have increasingly found merit in applying motivational models to understand and clinically intervene with cannabis use and its disorder. This work has built from the motivational study of alcohol[46,51,169,170] and tobacco[97,137,144,191] use. At the most basic level, such an approach recognizes that there are a number of distinct motives for using cannabis that can vary both between and within individuals.[45] That is, two individuals may use cannabis for different reasons, and one individual may use for multiple types of reasons. Motivational models predict that distinct motives may theoretically be related to particular types of problems.[45] For example, specific motives may play unique roles in various aspects of use (e.g., addictive use, withdrawal symptoms, craving) or problems related to use (e.g., psychological disturbances, risk-taking behavior). Thus enhancing efforts to explicate cannabis use motives empirically will presumably facilitate the nature of cannabis use and its disorders as well as linkages between cannabis use and its clinically important correlates, as it has for alcohol and tobacco use.[45,137]

Recognizing the practical importance of theoretically delineating and empirically measuring cannabis use motives, Simons and colleagues developed the Marijuana Motives Measure.[157,158] Studies have evaluated the factor structure of the Marijuana Motives Measure among young adults in the United States (*n* = 161),[158] young adults and adolescents in France (*n* = 114),[38] young adult cannabis users in the United States (*n* = 227),[193] and young adult frequent cannabis users in the Netherlands (*n* = 600).[10] Using a combination of exploratory and confirmatory factor analytic approaches, the Marijuana Motives

Measure demonstrated a multidimensional measurement model across extant work—specifically, a five-factor solution denoting Enhancement, Conformity, Expansion, Coping, and Social motives for cannabis use, each with satisfactory levels of internal consistency,[10,38,158,193] and preliminary evidence for routine motives (i.e., using cannabis out of boredom, out of habit.)[10] The Comprehensive Marijuana Motives Questionnaire is another self-report assessment developed by Lee and colleagues[110,111] that taps 12 different motivational aspects of use: Enjoyment, Conformity, Coping, Experimentation, Boredom, Alcohol, Celebration, Altered Perceptions, Social Anxiety, Relative Low Risk, Sleep, and Availability. This measure was developed and validated among young adult college students (n = 346)[110] and suggests that this population may have several unique reasons for using cannabis. It is also worth noting that existing assessments of cannabis motives assume cross-situational consistency; however, motives may change within a person depending on situational characteristics.[154,155]

Existing motivation-oriented work on cannabis is important in terms of informing the understanding of how and why cannabis use may be related to certain patterns of substance use, problems related to use, and psychological problems. For example, using the Marijuana Motive Measures, greater levels of Coping, Enhancement, Social, and Expansion motives for cannabis use have each been found to be concurrently significantly associated with frequency of past 30-days of cannabis use.[21,38,157,158] These associations between motives for use and frequency of use do not appear to be attributable to other alternative factors such as amount of time being a cannabis user or other types of concurrent substance use.[21] Moreover, coping motives appear to be uniquely related to likelihood of having cannabis dependence, at least cross-sectionally.[10,35,65] Using the Comprehensive Marijuana Motives Questionnaire, coping and sleep/rest motives are uniquely related to cannabis-related problems.[110] However, the exact directional relation between cannabis motives and patterns of cannabis use remains underexplored. It is noteworthy that other work suggests that specific motives may be relevant to the understanding of psychological vulnerability. For example, coping motives for cannabis use, but not other motives, have been significantly predictive of negative affect, anxious arousal, and anhedonic depressive symptoms,[127] especially among more frequent users relative to less frequent/occasional users.[22] These types of findings may have important theoretical implications for a better understanding of previous research linking cannabis use to affect-based psychological vulnerability.

Negative Correlates of Cannabis Use and Its Disorders

Historically, cannabis has been viewed by some as a less severe, or "soft," drug,[163] and policy shifts toward medicalization and legalization of cannabis have been observed in recent years. Although significant variability presently exists in legality of cannabis across states in the United States,[12] there is increasing public support for the legalization of cannabis. Specifically, recent public opinion data from 2015 indicate that 53% of adults in the United States are in favor of legalizing cannabis, which is in contrast to 2006 data when 32% were in favor of legalization.[140] In contrast, scientific study has provided a corpus of empirical evidence that cannabis use and its disorders are associated with a number of clinically significant problems.[184] Indeed, there are several empirically documented negative consequences of frequent or problematic cannabis use (typically defined as weekly or daily use). These negative effects are evident in physical, social, interpersonal, and, more recently, psychological realms.[77] In this section of the chapter, we describe some examples of work pertaining to possible negative correlates of cannabis use.

Health-Related Problems

One of the foremost negative effects of cannabis use is long-term cognitive impairment.[161] A wealth of research indicates that long-term and heavy cannabis use may cause neuropsychological impairment,[64,98,125,161,162] which may last even after abstinence.[17,125,139] For example, one large study of 1037 individuals followed from birth until age 38 examined the longitudinal association between intelligent quotient (IQ) and cannabis use.[125] Data indicated that (a) individuals who persistently met criteria for regular cannabis use and/or cannabis dependence had significant declines in global IQ a loss of approximately 6 IQ points). These effects were significant after adjusting for other drug dependence, tobacco use, alcohol dependence, schizophrenia, and number of years of education. It is notable that early onset of cannabis use was linked to greater IQ decline (initiation of cannabis use in adolescence vs. adulthood). Persistent cannabis dependence was also associated with decreased likelihood of pursuing education after high school and greater attention/memory problems identified by a collateral informant. Moreover, the effects of cannabis cessation did not fully restore neuropsychological functioning among individuals who initiated cannabis use in adolescence.[125]

There have been a series of important large-scale prospective studies documenting the negative effects of cannabis over time on pulmonary functioning (e.g., Sherrill et al.[153] and Tashkin et al.[173,175]). Although the results across investigations are not fully consistent,[138,174] they converge on the observation that greater duration of cannabis use is related to increased bronchitis symptoms (e.g., coughing, wheezing).[173] Some data also indicate that the combination of smoking tobacco and cannabis relative to tobacco alone is associated with greater odds of respiratory symptoms[128] and increased odds of having chronic obstructive pulmonary disease if more than 50 cannabis cigarettes were used in lifetime.[171] Some data indicate that among certain subpopulations of users (e.g., those using cannabis more frequently), the negative medical effects of this drug are, perhaps, even more clinically noteworthy. For example, frequent cannabis use is associated with an increased risk of severe respiratory illnesses, especially chronic bronchitis[16]; however, pulmonary effects are not similarly observed among lighter/occasional lifetime users.[138] In addition, there are studies of the relation between cannabis use and cancer. Epidemiological data indicate that heavy cannabis use (smoking at least 50 cannabis cigarettes in lifetime) is associated with a twofold increased risk of developing lung cancer[36]; however, controlled studies of these cancer-related negative effects of cannabis use are underrepresented in the literature. Overall, more research is needed to understand the effects of inhaled cannabis on the effects of pulmonary health.[14]

It is also noteworthy that some research suggests that cannabis use may be related to poor cardiovascular health, especially following acute cannabis use and among those with coronary artery disease,[177] although the mechanism underlying this risk is not well understood. Cannabis use is also associated with impaired immune system functioning, but these investigations, again, have not been consistently replicated.[42,90,104] Upon close inspection of these studies, it becomes clear that some of the inconsistencies of these investigations may be related to problems in the measurement of cannabis use, individual differences in use, or confounded by other health risk behaviors (e.g., tobacco smoking). A similar set of issues is evident for linkages between cannabis use and impaired reproductive effects. Here, nonhuman research suggests that heavier cannabis use is related to impaired reproductive capacity,[76] but controlled evidence among humans is currently lacking.[37]

It should be noted that although most research has focused on elucidating putative negative health consequences or correlates of cannabis use, there has been scientific and clinical interest in possible health benefits of the drug.[102] Namely, cannabis use has been suggested to improve certain disease symptoms (e.g., by decreasing eye pressure, involuntary movement, and perceived pain) and stimulate appetite.[89,90] Although this body of work is complicated, the strongest evidence of possible health benefits for cannabis use appears to be focused on increasing appetite, decreasing nausea and vomiting, preventing systemic weight loss, and possibly improving pain tolerance.[9,88,90]

Social Problems

In addition to the potential risk of a number of negative physical consequences, adverse social consequences related to certain types of cannabis use have been reported (e.g., frequent users, such as those who use on a daily or weekly basis). Lynskey and Hall,[119] for example, reviewed evidence suggesting that cannabis use was a contributing factor to impaired educational attainment, and others have found that cannabis use leads to reduced workplace productivity,[112] as well as impaired judgment within hours after cannabis use (e.g., among airline pilots).[113] It is possible that (1) cannabis use causes poor educational attainment, (2) cannabis use is a consequence of poor educational attainment, (3) both are true, or (4) shared risk factors increase the likelihood of both cannabis use and poor educational performance (e.g., cognitive impairment, attention-deficit/hyperactivity disorder).[77] Although the direct patterning of effects is unknown, a consistent pattern emerges: the greater the amount of use (measured in frequency of use or severity of use), the greater the impairment. The specific mechanism(s) underlying these use-related effects are as yet theoretically and empirically unspecified.

As another example, cannabis use has been linked to fatal traffic accidents and general driving impairment. Cannabis is the most common illicit drug detected among drivers who were tested for drugs.[25,85] The prevalence of positive cannabis results among drivers who died in a motor vehicle crash have increased from 4.2% in 1999 to 12.2% in 2010[26]; this increase was not observed for positive alcohol results. Driving-simulation and on-road studies indicate that reaction time, road tracking, speed, divided attention, and visual processing speed are impaired by THC, although these results have not been consistently documented, perhaps due to variability in methodological approaches.[85] In addition, data convincingly indicate that performance is increasingly impaired as blood concentrations of THC increase, and that the risk associated with cannabis is incrementally increased when considered used with alcohol.[85]

Other work suggests that frequent or more severe cannabis use may lead to using more severe forms of other drugs (e.g., widely publicized, but sometimes controversial, gateway theories of the developmental nature of substance use patterns).[77,130,184] One overarching limitation to the vast majority of work linking certain types of cannabis use to social and interpersonal functioning, and even future use of other substances, is that there is a dearth of (controlled) prospective evaluations. Thus conclusions drawn from extant work should be viewed conservatively.

Psychological Problems

There have been a variety of psychological problems associated with cannabis use and its disorder. Perhaps the most well-known psychological problem(s) associated with cannabis use has been psychotic-spectrum disorders. There are numerous lines of empirical evidence that have provided robust evidence of an association between cannabis use and psychotic-spectrum disorders.[77] Indeed, case reports of cannabis use have documented that such drug use can precede the onset of certain psychotic-spectrum disorders such as schizophrenia at higher rates than expected by chance of psychosis among regular cannabis users.[23] Although the directional nature of the cannabis-psychotic-spectrum problem association has been the subject of consistent intellectual debate (e.g., Hambrecht et al.[78]), one position has been that the use of cannabis may actually increase the risk of psychotic-spectrum disorders.[23] Consistent with this cannabis-to-psychotic symptoms/disorders perspective, the acute effects of cannabis use have been found to contribute to the elicitation of psychotic episodes and exacerbations of such symptoms among previously afflicted persons (e.g., the recurrence of psychotic symptoms[122]). Other research has found that intravenous THC administered to antipsychotic-treated patients with schizophrenia and nonpsychiatric controls exacerbated positive schizophrenic symptoms in the patient sample and induced positive symptoms in controls.[54] Neuroimaging studies have also found similarities between neural networks impaired by cannabis use and those known to be implicated in the etiology of schizophrenia (see Loeber et al.[116] for a review). Finally, in a meta-analytic review of the existing empirical literature, Semple and colleagues[152] concluded that the early use of cannabis increased the risk of schizophrenia or a schizophrenia-like psychotic illness by approximately threefold. Although a model indicating that cannabis may lead to psychotic-spectrum disorders provides only one possible way in which these factors may be related, it documents the importance of understanding cannabis in the context of severe mental illness. It is worth noting that the scientific literature also indicates that cannabidiol (CBD) may attenuate the effects of THC on psychosis symptoms[156]; in turn CBD may[106] have beneficial antipsychotic effects. This area of study requires further attention.

In another area of research, scientific activity has been focused on addressing the relationship between cannabis and depressive symptoms or problems.[72] The interest in this line of inquiry appears to have been historically fueled by the clinical observation that regular (i.e., on a daily or weekly basis) cannabis users often reported a lack of motivation for completing day-to-day activities (e.g., going to school).[181] The depression-cannabis literature has sometimes identified statistically significant relations between cannabis use and depressive symptoms and disorders.[41] However, the most recent work in this domain has indicated that the strength of such cannabis-depressive associations may be relatively weak, and markedly attenuated, or even nonexistent, after adjusting for common variables such as gender.[56] As one illustrative example, Brook and colleagues[27] completed a study that involved a two-time (1- to 2-year interval) prospective study of Colombian adolescents (n = 2226; 48.2% female) who were 12- to 17-years-old. Findings indicated that cannabis use in early adolescence did not significantly predict later depressive symptoms (time 2) after controlling for distress and interpersonal functioning in earlier adolescence (time 1). However, among a large sample of Australian adolescents ages 14–15 (n = 1601) who were followed for 7 years, the prevalence of depression and anxiety increased as the frequency of cannabis use increased.[134] This effect was observed particularly in females, relative to males.[134] This work, when considered in the context of the psychotic-spectrum research, highlights that cannabis should not be considered to have the same types of linkages with all forms of mental illness.

Another area of research has begun to address the relations between cannabis use and anxiety symptoms and disorders. This work was initially stimulated by the observation that cannabis use may acutely promote heightened levels of anxiety symptoms and elicit panic attacks under certain conditions or in certain individuals.[89,178,181] For example, when a person is intoxicated from using cannabis, they may experience acute paranoia, escalating anxiety symptoms, and perhaps a panic attack. This type of experience makes intuitive sense in that cannabis can elicit a wide range of acute sensory-oriented experiences and distortions that may be perceived as out of the person's control and could be interpreted as threatening by some persons who are fearful of such internal stimuli and experiences. Some evidence appears consistent with this perspective. For example, Hathaway[86] found that among weekly users of cannabis (n = 104), approximately 40% reported having had at least one panic attack related to such use. These prevalence rates are noteworthy in light of lifetime rates of panic attacks among the general population of approximately 5%–8%.[105] Another study found that, after covarying cigarettes per day, alcohol use, and negative affectivity, the interaction between cannabis use and anxiety sensitivity (fear of anxiety and related internal sensations) is related to increased levels of anxiety symptoms among cannabis users who also use tobacco.[189] Thus, certain individual differences such as anxiety sensitivity may be important to consider in understanding the linkages between cannabis use and anxiety states and disorders.

Another study involving a representative sample (n = 4745) found that a lifetime history of marijuana dependence, but not use or abuse, was related to an increased risk of panic attacks after covarying the effects of polysubstance use, alcohol abuse, and demographic variables.[188] In a more recent investigation, Zvolensky and colleagues[192] prospectively evaluated marijuana use, abuse, and dependence in relation to the onset of panic attacks and panic disorder. Participants at the start of the study were adolescents (n = 1709) with a mean age of 16.6 years (SD = 1.2; time 1) and were reassessed 1 year later (time 2) and then again as young adults (time 3; mean age = 24.2 years, SD = 0.6). Results indicated that adolescent-onset marijuana use and dependence were significantly prospectively associated with increased odds for the development of panic attacks and panic disorder. However, marijuana use or dependence was not *incrementally* associated with the development of panic after controlling for daily cigarette smoking. There is also growing research in the area of cannabis and posttraumatic stress disorder (PTSD). For example, nationally representative data indicate that PTSD is associated with increased likelihood of using cannabis in the past year, which was significant after adjusting for cooccurring anxiety and depressive disorders.[50,106] In addition, among a sample of military veterans exposed to combat who were enrolled in a residential treatment program for PTSD, those who had a cannabis use disorder relative to those without had less change in PTSD symptom severity posttreatment.[18] Collectively, these recent findings underscore the importance of considering the role of cannabis use with regard to understanding anxiety vulnerability.

It is worth noting that the anxiety-cannabis link may be driven by the effects of THC relative to CBD.[145] Indeed, a review of preclinical and clinical studies indicated that CBD is associated with anxiolytic effects relevant to various psychological disorders (PTSD, generalized anxiety disorder, panic disorder, obsessive-compulsive disorder, social anxiety disorder).[15] This effect was consistently observed in 29 of 33 pretrials and 7 of 10 clinical trials.[15]

Cannabis: Motivation to Quit, Reasons for Quitting, and Success in Quitting

Although historically and presently presumed by some key segments of the general public to be relatively harmless,[6] cannabis has many cardinal features of addiction similar to more "hard drugs." Indeed, for many individuals who use cannabis, tolerance to the drug develops and, presumably, contributes to more frequent or heavier use patterns or dosing with more potent (more pure tetrahydrocannabinol) forms of the drug.[75] For example, nonhuman research and, human empirical data suggest that cannabis discontinuation among regular users produces an internally consistent withdrawal pattern (see Budney et al.[31] for a review), and cannabis withdrawal syndrome and symptoms are now recognized in the DSM-5.[5] Disrupted sleep, nightmares, nausea, anxiety, tension, and irritability are common withdrawal symptoms,[30-32,83] any of these symptoms appear early after drug discontinuation,[32] and some symptoms may last for weeks beyond the quit day (e.g., disrupted sleep).[31,32] This withdrawal profile can appear relatively quickly during the course of use (e.g., relative early in the cannabis using career,[29,48,164,166] and may have clinical importance in terms of predicting relapse.[33] With the recognition that cannabis use and its disorder are common addictive behaviors and can be related to life impairment and a variety of related negative consequences, it is natural to question how motivated users are to quit, what their reasons are for quitting, and what their relative degree of success is in doing so?

Motivation to Quit

Two bodies of empirical evidence indicate that a large number of individuals who use cannabis on a regular basis (e.g., monthly) and who meet a range of diagnostic criteria (from use through cannabis use disorder) are motivated to quit. The first research evaluated treatment-seeking behavior. Here, the Drug Abuse Reporting Program[151] and other reports[159] documented that a clinically significant number of individuals were seeking therapeutic services for problematic cannabis use. Other large-scale surveys independently replicated such findings.[67,92] Dennis and colleagues[58] reported that of "the 1.5 million adult admissions to the U.S. public treatment system in 1998, 35% were admitted for treatment of cannabis problems" (p. 9). Such rates are higher than those found for cocaine (32%), opioids (18%), stimulants (9%), and other psychoactive substances (12%).[58] Similarly, national survey data indicate that 1 million people age 12 or older received treatment for cannabis in the past year, which was higher than for any other illicit drug.[146] In addition, other reports involving national databases have found that the demand for treatment of cannabis use and its disorder was 21% higher in 2010 than in 2000 among individuals ages 12 or older.[147] It also is important to note that cannabis treatment outcome studies have documented that a large number of treatment-seeking cannabis users are *not*

current polysubstance abusers.[163,164] For example, Stephens and colleagues[166] found that 80% of a large, treatment-seeking marijuana-dependent sample (n = 309) did not report abuse of other substances in the past 90 days and 40% reported never abusing an illicit drug other than cannabis. Moreover, among military veterans, the prevalence of polysubstance use among individuals with a cannabis use disorder was found to be about 50%.[19] These data indicate that cannabis represents a significant clinical and public health problem in its own right and commonly prompts treatment-seeking behavior even in the absence of other drug use.

The second body of evidence related to motivation to quit suggests that, despite the notable rates of documented treatment-seeking behavior, most persons using or with a cannabis use disorder actually attempt to quit on their own.[49,53,185] For example, in 2010, approximately half of individuals age 12 or older who received treatment for alcohol or illicit drug use in the past year sought treatment at a self-help group.[146] Self-quit behavior is operationally defined as attempts to quit without professional assistance (i.e., enrolling in a formal treatment program that uses pharmacological, psychosocial, or combined therapeutic approaches).[49] Numerous studies have reported that by young adulthood, many individuals have made multiple cannabis quit attempts on their own. It also is noteworthy that rates of self-quit attempts from cannabis are generally similar to those observed for other substances (e.g., tobacco).[93] For example, studies of weekly cannabis users have indicated that by age 30, individuals have reported a range of three to seven quit attempts on their own (e.g., Copersino et al.[49] and Stephens et al.[166]). However, the rates of successful self-guided reduction or cessation is low among most users.[28] Although some of these unsuccessful quitters may ultimately seek professional treatment when they continue to fail in their quit efforts, it is not presently clear what percentage will ultimately do so and under what circumstances.

These data are noteworthy for two chief reasons. First, these data suggest that a large proportion of cannabis use disordered individuals are interested in and pursue quitting on their own. Second, there is little empirical knowledge about the phenomenology of these quit attempts (e.g., latency to lapse and relapse, withdrawal symptoms) or the mechanisms underlying success or failure in cessation attempts among self-quitters not seeking professional treatment. Such knowledge is essential for understanding malleable processes underlying cannabis lapse and relapse versus sustained abstinence and, therefore, will ultimately facilitate future translational efforts to develop innovative cannabis treatment strategies targeting those at high risk for relapse.

Reasons for Quitting

Current cannabis users, ranging from monthly users to those dependent on the drug, report multiple concurrent reasons for quitting.[69,120,166,185] Among adults, worry about physical and psychological effects of cannabis use is the most often cited factor for wanting to quit.[120,185] For example, Copersino et al.[49] reported that 60% of non–treatment-seeking adult weekly cannabis users reported worry about health problems (both real and perceived) as a motivating factor for quitting, and 63% desired to quit in order to gain more self-control over their lives. In another study, Reilly and colleagues[143] similarly found that anxiety or depressive symptoms were the most commonly reported negative effects of cannabis use and that the primary reason for quitting among weekly non–treatment-seeking cannabis users (n = 268). Others have reported similar findings among both nontreatment seekers[24] and treatment seekers[166]; such findings do not appear to vary as a function of the type of cannabis use problem.[24] Overall, these data suggest that cannabis users typically express multiple reasons for quitting, with the most common reasons pertaining to excessive negative emotional symptoms (e.g., anxiety and depression and worry about negative health effects of cannabis use) and impaired levels of personal self-control associated with regular cannabis use.

Success in Quitting

Individuals attempting to quit cannabis experience marked difficulty whether they make a quit attempt on their own or seek professional (formal) treatment. Numerous survey studies, for example, have documented that current, regular cannabis users (both those who are and are not dependent on the drug) who try to quit on their own report difficulty in maintaining abstinence, as indexed by numerous unsuccessful cessation attempts.[49,94,185]

Although self-quit attempts (without professional assistance) tend to be the most frequently employed cessation strategy,[24] it is striking that even among those who *do* seek professional treatment, relapse to use is a common experience. Indeed, in a critical review of the treatment outcome literature for marijuana dependence, McRae and colleagues[123] concluded: "studies suggest that many patients do not show a positive treatment response, indicating that marijuana dependence is not easily treated" (p. 369). For example, one large-scale controlled study (*n* = 291) found that 63% of adults receiving two of the best available intervention strategies—motivational individualized intervention or cognitive-behavioral therapy—relapsed to regular use within 4 months.[165] For comparison purposes, the delayed treatment (control) condition reported that 91% of individuals were not abstinent at the 4-month assessment.[165] At 16 months, relapse rates among the active treatment conditions rose to 71% and 72% for the motivational individualized intervention and cognitive-behavioral therapy, respectively.[165] Other studies have reported similar results.[48,163,167] In addition, Moore and Budney[84] reported that among marijuana-dependent adult outpatients receiving treatment (*n* = 152), 71% lapsed (defined as any cannabis use) within 6 months, 46% within 3 months, and 24% within 1 month. In the same study, 71% of lapsers ultimately experienced a full relapse (defined as 4 or more days of use per week).[129]

It also should be noted that there have been historically few pharmacotherapy options available for cannabis use disorders. In fact, currently, there are no medications approved by the US Food and Drug Administration (FDA) for cannabis use disorders, although a number of agents are currently being investigated. See Chapter 56 for further details. Several human laboratory–based investigations have tested the effect of several pharmacological interventions on cannabis withdrawal symptoms and relapse behavior (e.g., quetiapine, nabilone, baclofen, mirtazapine, lofexidine, Zolpidem, nabiximols).[3,47,79-82,182] These studies have generally found an effect for reducing certain withdrawal symptoms (e.g., improved sleep quality, decreased weight loss, decreased irritability and craving)[3,47,79,81,182]; however, minimal effects on reducing relapse with the exception of nabilone have been documented.[79]

Although cannabis relapse is now a well-documented, prevalent clinical problem, there has been relatively little scientific work focused on predictors of success or failure in attempts to quit using cannabis. The work that has been completed in this regard has been broadly guided by social learning,[8] stress and coping,[103] and behavioral economic[13] theories of substance use and relapse. These studies have thus far provided a number of initial and important

observations: (1) early lapses are predictive of later relapses, regardless of whether they receive formal treatment[1,84,109]; (2) personal stressors (e.g., family conflict) are related to relapse among individuals receiving outpatient treatment[68]; (3) other substance use and peers' substance use (alcohol and other drugs) are predictive of relapse to cannabis use among adolescent outpatients[109]; and (4) the level of self-efficacy (i.e., beliefs regarding one's ability to refrain from use) for abstaining from cannabis use among adults seeking treatment is predictive, albeit modestly in terms of effect size, of later relapse.[20,115,168]

Cannabis: Overview of Clinical Issues Relevant to Practitioners

Given that cannabis use and disorder are common and can be associated with a relatively wide variety of negative problems, clinicians such as primary care physicians who interact with patients in nonspecialty clinical settings ought to be knowledgeable of basic issues in clinical care for this drug problem. To facilitate this process, we now turn to a discussion of (1) barriers and facilitators of treatment and (2) some core clinical competencies by highlighting basic assessment and treatment strategies. This discussion is broadly relevant to clinical practitioners working in the medical, dental, and psychological sectors of the health care industry. The topics discussed in this domain are not intended to be exhaustive or indicative of the full range of possible clinically relevant issues. They are, however, intended to offer some initial insight into the basic skills and knowledge that may be required to interact effectively with the cannabis-using population.

Barriers to and Facilitators of Treatment

Provider knowledge of cannabis use treatment is important in order to facilitate appropriate treatment referral. Data indicate that general practitioners and nurses are not as a rule trained in how to handle cannabis-related issues, although it is generally acknowledged that effects psychological treatments exist for addressing cannabis use.[131] In addition, low confidence in knowledge about the treatment of cannabis use is common among providers,[131] as many feel as though it is not within their expertise to treat cannabis use and often recommend that patients seeking these services be referred to drug service specialists.[186a] Low confidence or knowledge in assessment and treatment of cannabis use may serve as a barrier to facilitating treatment in individuals who use cannabis.[131] Moreover, not viewing cannabis use as a problem is both a patient- and provider-level barrier to treatment seeking.[66]

Basic Competencies

The most basic level of competency of clinical relevance focuses on simply being aware of the scientifically developed knowledge on the prevalence and impact of cannabis and its disorders. Here, clinicians should initially strive to attain an overall awareness of cannabis use and behavior as it relates to their patient population(s). Specifically, it is important for clinicians to recognize that cannabis use is integrally related to a wide range of negative life problems (e.g., respiratory illness). By obtaining such knowledge of cannabis use and its disorder, the clinician is better equipped to offer patients accurate information about problems related to cannabis use. This information can include psychoeducational facts (e.g., how cannabis may impact cognitive processes), but also may involve strategies designated (through scientific evaluation) as helpful to quitting, such as brief motivational interventions.[166] To gain access to this information, practicing clinicians can consider both informal and formal methods of education. More specific goal-oriented targets can include, but are not limited to, being able to efficiently and capably (1) describe the prevalence of cannabis use and disorder, (2) describe regional cannabis use patterns, (3) describe the negative physical and psychological consequences of cannabis use and cannabis use disorder, (4) describe the importance and role of cannabis treatment, particularly those methods based on evidence-based resources, (5) maintain a general awareness of emerging research related to the treatment of cannabis use and disorder, (6) understand the criteria used for defining cannabis use and cannabis use disorder, and (7) communicate an interest and willingness to consult with other resources when cannabis knowledge may be limited. It is important to note that practicing clinicians should discuss the relative potential benefits of cannabis use as well as the harms associated with use.

A second basic competency skill domain pertains to developing counseling skills for effectively dealing with cannabis use and its disorder. This domain of competence naturally builds from the foregoing description of general knowledge and awareness. This area of work necessarily begins with developing a level of clinical comfort with cannabis use topics and being capable of engaging a patient in a discussion focused on this topic. For this reason, the basic competency element in this domain requires counseling skills that strengthen interpersonal connection (e.g., rapport, listening to patient concerns). From the counseling perspective, a variety of core skills are necessary. These include, but are not limited to (1) having the capacity to be an active listener and demonstrate an empathetic stance regarding clinical care involving cannabis-related issues, (2) being able to communicate the strengths and challenges to evidence-based care treatment approaches for cannabis use and its disorder in a nonthreatening manner, (3) being able to understand basic models of behavior change that pertain to cannabis use and meaningfully communicate levels of motivational stage and readiness to clients, and (4) being able to elicit motivational aspects of patients' cannabis use and communicating psychoeducation about the effects of cannabis related to reasons for individuals' use.

From an assessment perspective, basic competencies are needed to adequately understand how to evaluate cannabis use behavior and history. Without this level of proficiency, it will be challenging to document readiness to quit or success in doing so. In the assessment process, there are both historical and current factors to evaluate. The overarching goal is to learn to comprehensively document and obtain accurate information that can be used in a clinically meaningful manner. The assessment process can be usefully divided into two global phases: intake (or initial assessment) and ongoing assessment. For the intake assessment, key variables to assess include: the extent and nature of cannabis use from a lifetime and current perspective; documenting current interest and motivation in quitting; employing evidence-based technologies for documenting marijuana use disorder; identifying (with the client) barriers to quitting currently; identifying strengths in the client or the environment (e.g., social support) for quitting; documenting the nature of past quit history and the relative degree of success in such attempts; and personal as well as cultural variables that may impact cannabis use and decisions regarding use. The intake assessment process should also integrate information about the client's medical and psychological history (e.g., concurrent substance use) in order to understand how such factors may influence the ongoing cannabis use or attempts to quit.

Ongoing assessments require an understanding of each client and the specific variables that need to be regularly tracked in order to accurately and objectively document (and understand) the motivation to quit and cannabis use behavior. Here there will be differences across individuals, but in most instances, cannabis use behavior, ongoing life stressors, motivation for use, and current motivation to quit are possibly important targets. This information can be used to track and understand ongoing efforts to quit. For example, clinicians should take note of each client's specific thoughts related to cannabis use (e.g., belief that cannabis use functions as an effective method of stress management, attenuate physical symptoms), primary reason(s) for wanting to quit use (e.g., health, social stigma), and situations in which cannabis use is most likely to occur (e.g., when drinking alcohol). This information, in turn, can be applied to help educate clients about their specific cannabis use patterns and, ultimately, to help them formulate a plan for making a quit attempt that is individualized to their specific needs and life circumstances.

Aside from the individual level of commitment to professional development, it is a reality that most medical care occurs within a context that intersects with other health care professionals. When enlisted in an integrated manner, the systems involved in such clinical work may be a powerful resource for dealing with cannabis use and its disorder. The need for such systems-oriented care is particularly evident given that educational efforts focused solely on the individual have not always been met with large degrees of success in the substance use field (e.g., Thorndike et al.[180]). In addition, many individuals seek medical care in medical systems governed by managed care businesses or other third party payers. As a result, changes to a system of medical care can have a major impact in terms of the type and quality of care administered by practitioners working within that system.

Summary

Understanding and treating cannabis use is an important public health priority. The next decade promises to be an important time to marshal resources in order to bridge major knowledge gaps and translate such developments into promising prevention and treatment approaches.

References

1. Agosti V, Levin FR. Predictors of cannabis dependence recovery among epidemiological survey respondents in the United States. *Am J Drug Alcohol Abuse*. 2007;33(1):81–88.
2. Agrawal A, Lynskey MT, Bucholz KK, Kapoor M, Almasy L, Dick DM, et al. DSM-5 cannabis use disorder: a phenotypic and genomic perspective. *Drug Alcohol Depend*. 2014;134:362–369.
3. Allsop DJ, Copeland J, Lintzeris N, Dunlop AJ, Montebello M, Sadler C, et al. Nabiximols as an agonist replacement therapy during cannabis withdrawal: a randomized clinical trial. *JAMA Psychiatry*. 2014;71(3):281–291.
4. APA. *Diagnostic and Statistical Manual of Mental Disorders*. 4th ed. Washington, DC: American Psychological Association; 2000.
5. APA. *Diagnostic and Statistical Manual of Mental Disorders*, 5th ed (DSM-5). Washington, DC: American Psychological Association; 2013.
6. Ashton CH. Adverse effects of cannabis and cannabinoids. *Br J Anaesth*. 1999;83(4):637–649.
7. Ashton CH. Pharmacology and effects of cannabis: a brief review. *Br J Psychiatry*. 2001;178(2):101–106.

8. Bandura A. *Social-Cognitive Theory, Encyclopedia of Psychology*. Washington, DC: American Psychological Association; 2000:329–332.

9. Belendiuk KA, Baldini LL, Bonn-Miller MO. Narrative review of the safety and efficacy of marijuana for the treatment of commonly state-approved medical and psychiatric disorders. *Addict Sci Clin Pract*. 2015;10(1):1.

10. Benschop A, Liebregts N, van der Pol P, Schaap R, Buisman R, van Laar M, et al. Reliability and validity of the Marijuana motives measure among young adult frequent cannabis users and associations with cannabis dependence. *Addict Behav*. 2015;40:91–95.

11. Beseler CL, Hasin DS. Cannabis dimensionality: dependence, abuse and consumption. *Addict Behav*. 2010;35(11):961–969.

12. Bestrashniy J, Winters KC. Variability in medical marijuana laws in the United States. *Psychol Addict Behav*. 2015;29(3):639.

13. Bickel WK, Vuchinich RE. *Reframing Health Behavior Change with Behavioral Economics*. Psychology Press; 2000.

14. Biehl JR, Burnham EL. Cannabis smoking in 2015: a concern for lung health? *Chest J*. 2015;148(3):596–606.

15. Blessing EM, Steenkamp MM, Manzanares J, Marmar CR. Cannabidiol as a potential treatment for anxiety disorders. *Neurotherapeutics*. 2015;12(4):825–836.

16. Bloom JW, Kaltenborn WT, Paoletti P, Camilli A, Lebowitz MD. Respiratory effects of non-tobacco cigarettes. *Br Med J (Clin Res Ed)*. 1987;295(6612):1516–1518.

17. Bolla KI, Brown K, Eldreth D, Tate K, Cadet J. Dose-related neurocognitive effects of marijuana use. *Neurol*. 2002;59(9):1337–1343.

18. Bonn-Miller MO, Boden MT, Vujanovic AA, Drescher KD. Prospective investigation of the impact of cannabis use disorders on posttraumatic stress disorder symptoms among veterans in residential treatment. *Psychological Trauma*. 2013;5(2):193.

19. Bonn-Miller MO, Harris AH, Trafton JA. Prevalence of cannabis use disorder diagnoses among veterans in 2002, 2008, and 2009. *Psychological Services*. 2012;9(4):404.

20. Bonn-Miller MO, Moos RH, Boden MT, Long WR, Kimerling R, Trafton JA. The impact of posttraumatic stress disorder on cannabis quit success. *Am J Drug Alcohol Abuse*. 2015;41(4):339–344.

21. Bonn-Miller MO, Zvolensky MJ, Bernstein A. Marijuana use motives: Concurrent relations to frequency of past 30-day use and anxiety sensitivity among young adult marijuana smokers. *Addict Behav*. 2007;32(1):49–62.

22. Bonn-Miller MO, Zvolensky MJ, Bernstein A, Stickle TR. Marijuana coping motives interact with marijuana use frequency to predict anxious arousal, panic related catastrophic thinking, and worry among current marijuana users. *Depress Anxiety*. 2008;25(10):862–873.

23. Bowers Jr M, Boutros N, D'Souza DC, Madonick S. Substance abuse as a risk factor for schizophrenia and related disorders. *Int J Ment Health*. 2001;30(1):33–57.

24. Boyd SJ, Tashkin DP, Huestis MA, Heishman SJ, Dermand JC, Simmons MS, et al. Strategies for quitting among non-treatment-seeking marijuana smokers. *Am J Addict*. 2005;14(1):35–42.

25. Brady JE, Li G. Prevalence of alcohol and other drugs in fatally injured drivers. *Addict*. 2013;108(1):104–114.

26. Brady JE, Li G. Trends in alcohol and other drugs detected in fatally injured drivers in the United States, 1999–2010. *Am J Epidemiol*. 2014;179(6):692–699.

27. Brook JS. The effect of early marijuana use on later anxiety and depressive symptoms. *NYS Psychol*. 2001;13:35–40.

28. Buckner JD, Zvolensky MJ, Ecker AH. Cannabis use during a voluntary quit attempt: an analysis from ecological momentary assessment. *Drug Alcohol Depend*. 2013;132(3):610–616.

29. Budney AJ, Higgins ST, Radonovich KJ, Novy PL. Adding voucher-based incentives to coping skills and motivational enhancement improves outcomes during treatment for marijuana dependence. *J Consult Clin Psychol*. 2000;68(6):1051.

30. Budney AJ, Hughes JR, Moore BA, Novy PL. Marijuana abstinence effects in marijuana smokers maintained in their home environment. *Arch Gen Psychiatry*. 2001;58(10):917–924.

31. Budney AJ, Hughes JR, Moore BA, Vandrey R. Review of the validity and significance of cannabis withdrawal syndrome. *Am J Psychiatry*. 2004;161(11):1967–1977.

32. Budney AJ, Moore BA, Vandrey RG, Hughes JR. The time course and significance of cannabis withdrawal. *J Abnorm Psychol*. 2003;112(3):393.

33. Budney AJ, Novy PL, Hughes JR. Marijuana withdrawal among adults seeking treatment for marijuana dependence. *Addict*. 1999;94(9):1311–1322.

34. Budney AJ, Vandrey RG, Hughes JR, Thostenson JD, Bursac Z. Comparison of cannabis and tobacco withdrawal: severity and contribution to relapse. *J Subst Abuse Treat*. 2008;35(4):362–368.

35. Bujarski SJ, Norberg MM, Copeland J. The association between distress tolerance and cannabis use-related problems: the mediating and moderating roles of coping motives and gender. *Addict behav*. 2012;37(10):1181–1184.

36. Callaghan RC, Allebeck P, Sidorchuk A. Marijuana use and risk of lung cancer: a 40-year cohort study. *Cancer Causes Control*. 2013;24(10):1811–1820.

37. Caplan GA, Brigham BA. Marijuana smoking and carcinoma of the tongue. Is there an association? *Cancer*. 1990;66(5):1005–1006.

38. Chabrol H, Ducongé E, Casas C, Roura C, Carey KB. Relations between cannabis use and dependence, motives for cannabis use and anxious, depressive and borderline symptomatology. *Addict Behav*. 2005;30(4):829–840.

39. Chait L, Zacny JP. Reinforcing and subjective effects of oral Δ9-THC and smoked marijuana in humans. *Psychopharmacol*. 1992;107(2-3):255–262.

40. Chen K, Kandel DB, Davies M. Relationships between frequency and quantity of marijuana use and last year proxy dependence among adolescents and adults in the United States. *Drug Alcohol Depend*. 1997;46(1):53–67.

41. Chuan-Yu C, Wagner FA, Anthony JC. Marijuana use and the risk of Major Depressive Episode Epidemiological evidence from the United States National Comorbidity Survey. *Soc Psychiatry Psychiatr Epidemiol*. 2002;37(5):199.

42. Coates RA, Farewell VT, Raboound J, Read SE, Macfadden DK, Calzavara LM, et al. Cofactors of progression to acquired immunodeficiency syndrome in a cohort of male sexual contacts of men with human immunodeficiency virus disease. *Am J Epidemiol*. 1990;132(4):717–722.

43. Compton WM, Dawson DA, Goldstein RB, Grant BF. Crosswalk between DSM-IV dependence and DSM-5 substance use disorders for opioids, cannabis, cocaine and alcohol. *Drug Alcohol Depend*. 2013;132(1):387–390.

44. Compton WM, Saha TD, Conway KP, Grant BF. The role of cannabis use within a dimensional approach to cannabis use disorders. *Drug Alcohol Depend*. 2009;100(3):221–227.

45. Cooper ML. Motivations for alcohol use among adolescents: development and validation of a four-factor model. *Psychol Assess*. 1994;6(2):117.

46. Cooper ML, Frone MR, Russell M, Mudar P. Drinking to regulate positive and negative emotions: a motivational model of alcohol use. *J Pers Soc Psychol*. 1995;69(5):990.

47. Cooper ZD, Foltin RW, Hart CL, Vosburg SK, Comer SD, Haney M. A human laboratory study investigating the effects of quetiapine on marijuana withdrawal and relapse in daily marijuana smokers. *Addiction biology*. 2013;18(6):993–1002.

48. Copeland J, Swift W, Roffman R, Stephens R. A randomized controlled trial of brief cognitive-behavioral interventions for cannabis use disorder. *J Subst Abuse Treat*. 2001;21(2):55–64; discussion 65-56.

49. Copersino ML, Boyd SJ, Tashkin DP, Huestis MA, Heishman SJ, Dermand JC, et al. Quitting among non-treatment-seeking marijuana users: reasons and changes in other substance use. *Am J Addict*. 2006;15(4):297–302.

50. Cougle JR, Bonn-Miller MO, Vujanovic AA, Zvolensky MJ, Hawkins KA. Posttraumatic stress disorder and cannabis use in a nationally representative sample. *Psychol Addict Behav.* 2011;25(3):554.

51. Cox WM, Klinger E. A motivational model of alcohol use. *J Abnormal Psychol.* 1988;97(2):168.

52. Crean RD, Crane NA, Mason BJ. An evidence based review of acute and long-term effects of cannabis use on executive cognitive functions. *J Addict Med.* 2011;5(1):1.

53. Cunningham JA. Remissions from drug dependence: is treatment a prerequisite? *Drug Alcohol Depend.* 2000;59(3):211–213.

54. D'Souza DC, Abi-Saab WM, Madonick S, Forselius-Bielen K, Doersch A, Braley G, et al. Delta-9-tetrahydrocannabinol effects in schizophrenia: implications for cognition, psychosis, and addiction. *Biol Psychiatry.* 2005;57(6):594–608.

55. Day NL, Wagener DK, Taylor PM. Measurement of substance use during pregnancy: methodologic issues. *Current Research on the Consequences of Maternal Drug Abuse.* Rockville, MD: US Department of Health and Human Services; 1985:36–47.

56. Degenhardt L, Hall W, Lynskey M. Alcohol, cannabis and tobacco use among Australians: a comparison of their associations with other drug use and use disorders, affective and anxiety disorders, and psychosis. *Addict.* 2001;96(11):1603–1614.

57. Denis CM, Gelernter J, Hart AB, Kranzler HR. Inter-observer reliability of DSM-5 substance use disorders. *Drug Alcohol Depend.* 2015;153:229–235.

58. Dennis M, Babor TF, Roebuck MC, Donaldson J. Changing the focus: the case for recognizing and treating cannabis use disorders. *Addict.* 2002;97(s1):4–15.

59. Devane WA, Hanus L, Breuer A, Pertwee RG, Stevenson LA, Griffin G, et al. Isolation and structure of a brain constituent that binds to the cannabinoid receptor. *Science.* 1992;258(5090):1946–1949.

60. Di Forti M, Sallis H, Allegri F, Trotta A, Ferraro L, Stilo SA, et al. Daily use, especially of high-potency cannabis, drives the earlier onset of psychosis in cannabis users. *Schizophrenia Bulletin.* 2014;40(6):1509–1517.

61. Diamond G, Panichelli-Mindel SM, Shera D, Dennis M, Tims F, Ungemack J. Psychiatric syndromes in adolescents with marijuana abuse and dependency in outpatient treatment. *J Child Adoles Subst Abuse.* 2006;15(4):37–54.

62. Didcott P, Flaherty B, Muir C, Wales NS. *A Profile of Addicts in Residential Treatment in New South Wales.* Directorate of the Drug Offensive; 1988.

63. Fernández–Ruiz J, Sagredo O, Pazos MR, García C, Pertwee R, Mechoulam R, et al. Cannabidiol for neurodegenerative disorders: important new clinical applications for this phytocannabinoid? *Br J Clin Pharmacol.* 2013;75(2):323–333.

64. Fletcher JM, Page JB, Francis DJ, Copeland K, Naus MJ, Davis CM, et al. Cognitive correlates of long-term cannabis use in Costa Rican men. *Arch Gen Psychiatry.* 1996;53(11):1051–1057.

65. Fox CL, Towe SL, Stephens RS, Walker DD, Roffman RA. Motives for cannabis use in high-risk adolescent users. *Psychol Addict Behav.* 2011;25(3):492.

66. Gates P, Copeland J, Swift W, Martin G. Barriers and facilitators to cannabis treatment. *Drug and Alcohol Review.* 2012;31(3):311–319.

67. Gerstein DR, Johnson RA. Nonresponse and selection bias in treatment follow-up studies. *Substance Use Misuse.* 2000;35(6-8):971–1014.

68. Godley MD, Kahn JH, Dennis ML, Godley SH, Funk RR. The stability and impact of environmental factors on substance use and problems after adolescent outpatient treatment for cannabis abuse or dependence. *Psychol Addict Behav.* 2005;19(1):62.

69. Goodstadt MS, Sheppard MA, Chan GC. Non-use and cessation of cannabis use: neglected foci of drug education. *Addict behav.* 1984;9(1):21–31.

70. Gorelick DA, Levin KH, Copersino ML, Heishman SJ, Liu F, Boggs DL, et al. Diagnostic criteria for cannabis withdrawal syndrome. *Drug Alcohol Depend.* 2012;123(1):141–147.

71. Green B, Young R, Kavanagh D. Cannabis use and misuse prevalence among people with psychosis. *Br J Psychiatry.* 2005;187(4):306–313.

72. Green BE, Ritter C. Marijuana use and depression. *J Health Soc Behav.* 2000;41(1):40–49.

73. Hall W, Degenhardt L. Adverse health effects of non-medical cannabis use. *Lancet.* 2009;374(9698):1383–1391.

74. Hall W, Johnston L, Donnelly N. *Epidemiology of Cannabis use and its Consequences.* Toronto, Canada: Centre for Addiction and Metnal Health; 1999.

75. Hall W, Solowij N. Adverse effects of cannabis. *Lancet.* 1998;352(9140):1611–1616.

76. Hall W, Solowij N, Lemon J. *The Health and Psychological Consequences of Canna-bis Use.* Canberra, Australia: Australian Government Publishing Service; 1994.

77. Hall WD. Cannabis use and the mental health of young people. *Aust N Z J Psychiatry.* 2006;40(2):105–113.

78. Hambrecht M, Häfner H. Cannabis, vulnerability, and the onset of schizophrenia: an epidemiological perspective. *Aust N Z J Psychiatry.* 2000;34(3):468–475.

79. Haney M, Cooper ZD, Bedi G, Vosburg SK, Comer SD, Foltin RW. Nabilone decreases marijuana withdrawal and a laboratory measure of marijuana relapse. *Neuropsychopharmacology.* 2013;38(8):1557–1565.

80. Haney M, Hart CL, Vosburg SK, Comer SD, Reed SC, Cooper ZD, et al. Effects of baclofen and mirtazapine on a laboratory model of marijuana withdrawal and relapse. *Psychopharmacology.* 2010;211(2):233–244.

81. Haney M, Hart CL, Vosburg SK, Comer SD, Reed SC, Foltin RW. Effects of THC and lofexidine in a human laboratory model of marijuana withdrawal and relapse. *Psychopharmacology.* 2008;197(1):157–168.

82. Haney M, Hart CL, Vosburg SK, Nasser J, Bennett A, Zubaran C, et al. Marijuana withdrawal in humans: effects of oral THC or divalproex. *Neuropsychopharmacology.* 2004;29(1):158–170.

83. Haney M, Ward AS, Comer SD, Foltin RW, Fischman MW. Abstinence symptoms following smoked marijuana in humans. *Psychopharmacology.* 1999;141(4):395–404.

84. Harrison PA, Asche SE. Adolescent treatment for substance use disorders: outcomes and outcome predictors. *J Child Adolesc Subst Abuse.* 2001;11(2):1–17.

85. Hartman RL, Huestis MA. Cannabis effects on driving skills. *Clinical Chemistry.* 2013;59(3):478–492.

86. Hathaway AD. Cannabis effects and dependency concerns in long-term frequent users: a missing piece of the public health puzzle. *Addict Res Theory.* 2003;11(6):441–458.

87. Herkenham M, Lynn AB, Little MD, Johnson MR, Melvin LS, De Costa BR, et al. Cannabinoid receptor localization in brain. *Proc Natl Acad Sci U S A.* 1990;87(5):1932–1936.

88. Hill KP. Medical marijuana for treatment of chronic pain and other medical and psychiatric problems: a clinical review. *Jama.* 2015;313(24):2474–2483.

89. Hollister LE. Health aspects of cannabis. *Pharmacol Rev.* 1986;38(1):1–20.

90. Hollister LE. Marijuana and immunity. *J Psychoactive drug.* 1992;24(2):159–164.

91. Hosek SG, Harper GW, Domanico R. Predictors of medication adherence among HIV-infected youth. *Psychol Health Med.* 2005;10(2):166–179.

92. Hubbard RL, Collins JJ, Rachal JV, Cavanaugh ER. The criminal justice client in drug abuse treatment. *NIDA Res Monogr.* 1988;86:57–80.

93. Hughes JR. The future of smoking cessation therapy in the United States. *Addiction.* 1996;91(12):1797–1802.

94. Hughes JR, Peters EN, Callas PW, Budney AJ, Livingston AE. Attempts to stop or reduce marijuana use in non-treatment seekers. *Drug Alcohol Depend.* 2008;97(1):180–184.

95. Hunt CA, Jones RT. Tolerance and disposition of tetrahydrocannabinol in man. *J Pharmacol Exp Ther.* 1980;215(1):35–44.

96. Hunt CA, Jones RT, Herning RI, Bachman J. Evidence that cannabidiol does not significantly alter the pharmacokinetics of tetrahydrocannabinol in man. *J Pharmacokinet Biopharm.* 1981;9(3):245–260.

97. Ikard FF, Green DE, Horn D. A scale to differentiate between types of smoking as related to the management of affect. *Int J Addict.* 1969;4(4):649–659.

98. Jnr HP, Yurgelun-Todd D. The residual cognitive effects of heavy marijuana use in college students. *J Clin Forensic Med.* 1996;3(4):188.

99. Johns A. Psychiatric effects of cannabis. *Br J Psychiatry.* 2001;178(2):116–122.

100. Johnston L, O'Malley P, Bachman J. *Monitoring the Future: National Survey Results on Drug Use, 1975–2002.* Bethesda, MD: National Institute of Drug Abuse; 2003.

101. Johnston L, O'Malley P, Bachman J, Schulenberg J. *Monitoring the Future: National Survey Results on Drug Use, 1975–2003.* Institute for Social Research; 2004.

102. Joy JE, Watson Jr SJ, Benson Jr JA. *Marijuana and Medicine: Assessing the Science Base.* National Academies Press; 1999.

103. Kaplan HB. *Psychosocial Stress From the Perspective of Self Theory.* Academic Press; 1996.

104. Kaslow RA, Blackwelder WC, Ostrow DG, Yerg D, Palenicek J, Coulson AH, et al. No evidence for a role of alcohol or other psychoactive drugs in accelerating immunodeficiency in HIV-1—positive individuals: a report from the Multicenter AIDS Cohort Study. *JAMA.* 1989;261(23):3424–3429.

105. Katerndahl DA, Realini JP. Lifetime prevalence of panic states. *Am J Psychiatry.* 1993;150:246.

106. Kevorkian S, Bonn-Miller MO, Belendiuk K, Carney DM, Roberson-Nay R, Berenz EC. Associations among trauma, posttraumatic stress disorder, cannabis use, and cannabis use disorder in a nationally representative epidemiologic sample. *Psychol Addict Behav.* 2015;29(3):633.

107. Kopak AM, Proctor SL, Hoffmann NG. An assessment of the compatibility of DSM-IV and proposed DSM-5 criteria in the diagnosis of cannabis use disorders. *Subst Use Misuse.* 2012;47(12):1328–1338.

108. Kraan T, Velthorst E, Koenders L, Zwaart K, Ising H, van den Berg D, et al. Cannabis use and transition to psychosis in individuals at ultra-high risk: review and meta-analysis. *Psychol Med.* 2016;46(4):673–681.

109. Latimer WW, Winters KC, Stinchfield R, Traver RE. Demographic, individual, and interpersonal predictors of adolescent alcohol and marijuana use following treatment. *Psychol Addict Behav.* 2000;14(2):162.

110. Lee CM, Neighbors C, Hendershot CS, Grossbard JR. Development and preliminary validation of a comprehensive marijuana motives questionnaire. *J Stud Alcohol Drugs.* 2009;70(2):279–287.

111. Lee CM, Neighbors C, Woods BA. Marijuana motives: young adults' reasons for using marijuana. *Addict behav.* 2007;32(7):1384–1394.

112. Lehman WE, Simpson DD. Employee substance use and on-the-job behaviors. *J Appl Psychol.* 1992;77(3):309.

113. Leirer VO, Yesavage JA, Morrow DG. Marijuana carry-over effects on aircraft pilot performance. *Aviation, Space, and Environmental Medicine*; 1991.

114. Levin KH, Copersino ML, Heishman SJ, Liu F, Kelly DL, Boggs DL, et al. Cannabis withdrawal symptoms in non-treatment-seeking adult cannabis smokers. *Drug Alcohol Depend.* 2010;111(1):120–127.

115. Litt MD, Kadden RM, Stephens RS. Coping and self-efficacy in marijuana treatment: results from the marijuana treatment project. *J Consult Clin Psychol.* 2005;73(6):1015–1025.

116. Loeber RT, Yurgelun-Todd DA. Human neuroimaging of acute and chronic marijuana use: implications for frontocerebellar dysfunction. *Human Psychopharmacol.* 1999;14(5):291–304.

117. Lopez-Quintero C, De los Cobos JP, Hasin DS, Okuda M, Wang S, Grant BF, et al. Probability and predictors of transition from first use to dependence on nicotine, alcohol, cannabis, and cocaine: results of the National Epidemiologic Survey on Alcohol and Related Conditions (NESARC). *Drug Alcohol Depend.* 2011;115(1):120–130.

118. Lowe RH, Abraham TT, Darwin WD, Herning R, Cadet JL, Huestis MA. Extended urinary Δ9-tetrahydrocannabinol excretion in chronic cannabis users precludes use as a biomarker of new drug exposure. *Drug Alcohol Depend.* 2009;105(1):24–32.

119. Lynskey M, Hall W. The effects of adolescent cannabis use on educational attainment: a review. *Addiction.* 2000;95(11):1621–1630.

120. Martin CE, Duncan DF, Zunich EM. Students' motives for discontinuing illicit drug-taking. *Health Values.* 1983;7(5):8–11.

121. Martin CS, Chung T, Kirisci L, Langenbucher JW. Item response theory analysis of diagnostic criteria for alcohol and cannabis use disorders in adolescents: implications for DSM-V. *J Abnormal Psychol.* 2006;115(4):807.

122. Mathers D, Ghodse A. Cannabis and psychotic illness. *Br J Psychiatry.* 1992;161(5):648–653.

123. McRae AL, Budney AJ, Brady KT. Treatment of marijuana dependence: a review of the literature. *J Subst Abuse Treat.* 2003;24(4):369–376.

124. Mechoulam R, Parker LA, Gallily R. Cannabidiol: an overview of some pharmacological aspects. *Int J Basic Clin Pharmaco.* 2002;42(S1):11S–19S.

125. Meier MH, Caspi A, Ambler A, Harrington H, Houts R, Keefe RS, et al. Persistent cannabis users show neuropsychological decline from childhood to midlife. *Proc Natl Acad Sci U S A.* 2012;109(40):E2657–E2664.

126. Mewton L, Slade T, Teesson M. An evaluation of the proposed DSM-5 cannabis use disorder criteria using Australian national survey data. *J Stud Alcohol Drugs.* 2013;74(4):614–621.

127. Mitchell H, Zvolensky MJ, Marshall EC, Bonn-Miller MO, Vujanovic AA. Incremental validity of coping-oriented marijuana use motives in the prediction of affect-based psychological vulnerability. *J Psychopathol Behav Assess.* 2007;29(4):277–288.

128. Moore BA, Augustson EM, Moser RP, Budney AJ. Respiratory effects of marijuana and tobacco use in a US sample. *J Gen Intern Med.* 2005;20(1):33–37.

129. Moore BA, Budney AJ. Relapse in outpatient treatment for marijuana dependence. *J Subst Abus Treat.* 2003;25(2):85–89.

130. Newcomb MD, Bentler PM. *Consequences of Adolescent Drug Use: Impact on the Lives of Young Adults.* Sage Publications, Inc; 1988.

131. Norberg MM, Gates P, Dillon P, Kavanagh DJ, Manocha R, Copeland J. Screening and managing cannabis use: comparing GP's and nurses' knowledge, beliefs, and behavior. *Subst Abuse Treat Prev Policy.* 2012;7(1):1.

132. O'Dea PJ, Murphy B, Balzer C. Traffic and illegal production of drugs in rural America. *NIDA Res Monogr.* 1997;168:79–89.

133. Ohlsson A, Lindgren JE, Wahlen A, Agurell S, Hollister L, Gillespie H. Plasma delta-9-tetrahydrocannabinol concentrations and clinical effects after oral and intravenous administration and smoking. *Clin Pharmacol Ther.* 1980;28(3):409–416.

134. Patton GC, Coffey C, Carlin JB, Degenhardt L, Lynskey M, Hall W. Cannabis use and mental health in young people: cohort study. *BMJ.* 2002;325(7374):1195–1198.

135. Peer K, Rennert L, Lynch KG, Farrer L, Gelernter J, Kranzler HR. Prevalence of DSM-IV and DSM-5 alcohol, cocaine, opioid, and cannabis use disorders in a largely substance dependent sample. *Drug Alcohol Depend.* 2013;127(1):215–219.

136. Pertwee R. *The Pharmacology and Therapeutic Potential of Cannabidiol.* Dordrecht, Netherlands: Kluwer Academic Publishers; 2004.

137. Piper ME, Piasecki TM, Federman EB, Bolt DM, Smith SS, Fiore MC, et al. A multiple motives approach to tobacco dependence: the Wisconsin Inventory of Smoking Dependence Motives (WISDM-68). *J Consult Clin Psychol.* 2004;72(2):139.

138. Pletcher MJ, Vittinghoff E, Kalhan R, Richman J, Safford M, Sidney S, et al. Association between marijuana exposure and pulmonary function over 20 years. *JAMA.* 2012;307(2):173–181.

139. Pope HG, Gruber AJ, Hudson JI, Cohane G, Huestis MA, Yurgelun-Todd D. Early-onset cannabis use and cognitive deficits: what is the nature of the association? *Drug Alcohol Depend.* 2003;69(3):303–310.

140. PRC. *In Debate Over Legalizing Marijuana.* Disagreement Over Drug's Dangers; 2015.

141. Prentiss D, Power R, Balmas G, Tzuang G, Israelski DM. Patterns of marijuana use among patients with HIV/AIDS followed in a public health care setting. *JAIDS J Acquir Immune Defic Syndr.* 2004;35(1):38–45.

142. Ranganathan M, D'souza DC. The acute effects of cannabinoids on memory in humans: a review. *Psychopharmacology.* 2006;188(4):425–444.

143. Reilly D, Didcott P, Swift W, Hall W. Long-term cannabis use: characteristics of users in an Australian rural area. *Addiction.* 1998;93(6):837–846.

144. Russell M, Peto J, Patel U. The classification of smoking by factorial structure of motives. *J R Stat Soc Ser A Stat.* 1974:313–346.

145. Russo E, Guy GW. A tale of two cannabinoids: the therapeutic rationale for combining tetrahydrocannabinol and cannabidiol. *Medical Hypotheses.* 2006;66(2):234–246.

146. SAMHSA. *Results from the 2010 National Survey on Drug Use and Health: Summary of National Findings.* Rockville, MD: Substance Abuse and Mental Health ServicesAdministration; 2011.

147. SAMHSA. *Center for Behavioral Health Statistics and Quality. Treatment Episode Data Set (TEDS): 2000-2010.* Rockville, MD: Substance Abuse and Mental Health Services Administration; 2012.

148. SAMHSA. *National Survey on Drug Use and Health.* Rockville, MD: Substance Abuse & Mental Health Services Administration; 2013.

149. Schuckit MA. *Drug and Alcohol Abuse: a Clinical Guide to Diagnosis and Treatment.* Vol. 3. New York, NY, England: Plenum Medical Book Co/Plenum; 1989.

150. Seely KA, Prather PL, James LP, Moran JH. Marijuana-based drugs: Innovative therapeutics or designer drugs of abuse? *Molecular Interventions.* 2011;11(1):36.

151. Sells SB. The effectiveness of drug abuse treatment. I & II; 1974.

152. Semple DM, McIntosh AM, Lawrie SM. Cannabis as a risk factor for psychosis: systematic review. *J Psychopharmacol.* 2005;19(2):187–194.

153. Sherrill DL, Krzyzanowski M, Bloom JW, D'Lebowitz M. Respiratory effects of non-tobacco cigarettes: a longitudinal study in general population. *Int J Epidemiol.* 1991;20(1):132–137.

154. Shrier LA, Scherer EB. It depends on when you ask: motives for using marijuana assessed before versus after a marijuana use event. *Addict Behav.* 2014;39(12):1759–1765.

155. Shrier LA, Walls C, Rhoads A, Blood EA. Individual and contextual predictors of severity of marijuana use events among young frequent users. *Addict Behav.* 2013;38(1):1448–1456.

156. Silva TBG, Balbino CQ, Weiber AFM. The relationship between cannabidiol and psychosis: a review. *Annals Clin Psychiatry.* 2015;27(2):134–141.

157. Simons J, Correia CJ, Carey KB. A comparison of motives for marijuana and alcohol use among experienced users. *Addict Behav.* 2000;25(1):153–160.

158. Simons J, Correia CJ, Carey KB, Borsari BE. Validating a five-factor marijuana motives measure: relations with use, problems, and alcohol motives. *Consult Clin Psychol.* 1998;45(3):265.

159. Simpson DD. *Evaluation of Drug Abuse Treatments, Based on First Year Followup: National Followup Study of Admissions to Drug Abuse Treatments in the DARP During 1969-1972* (Vol. 2): US Department of Health, Education, and Welfare, Public Health Service, Alcohol, Drug Abuse, and Mental Health Administration. National Institute on Drug Abuse; 1978.

160. Solowij N. *Cannabis and Cognitive Functioning.* Cambridge University Press; 2006.

161. Solowij N, Battisti R. The chronic effects of cannabis on memory in humans: a review. *Current Drug Abuse Rev.* 2008;1(1):81–98.

162. Solowij N, Stephens RS, Roffman RA, Babor T, Kadden R, Miller M, et al. Cognitive functioning of long-term heavy cannabis users seeking treatment. *JAMA.* 2002;287(9):1123–1131.

163. Stephens R. Effects of brief and extended treatment on marijuana use and related problems. Paper presented at the T. Babor (Chair), Treatment of marijuana dependence. Symposium conducted at the meeting of the American Public Health Association, Chicago; 1999.

164. Stephens RS, Babor TF, Kadden R, Miller M. The Marijuana Treatment Project: rationale, design and participant characteristics. *Addiction.* 2002;97(s1):109–124.

165. Stephens RS, Roffman RA, Curtin L. Comparison of extended versus brief treatments for marijuana use. *J Consult Clin Psychol.* 2000;68(5):898.

166. Stephens RS, Roffman RA, Simpson EE. Adult marijuana users seeking treatment. *J Consult Clin Psychol.* 1993;61(6):1100.

167. Stephens RS, Roffman RA, Simpson EE. Treating adult marijuana dependence: a test of the relapse prevention model. *J Consult Clin Psychol.* 1994;62(1):92.

168. Stephens RS, Wertz JS, Roffman RA. Self-efficacy and marijuana cessation: a construct validity analysis. *J Consult Clin Psychol.* 1995;63(6):1022.

169. Stewart SH, Zeitlin SB, Samoluk SB. Examination of a three-dimensional drinking motives questionnaire in a young adult university student sample. *Behav Res Ther.* 1996;34(1):61–71.

170. Stewart SH, Zvolensky MJ, Eifert GH. Negative-reinforcement drinking motives mediate the relation between anxiety sensitivity and increased drinking behavior. *Pers Individ Dif.* 2001;31(2):157–171.

171. Tan WC, Lo C, Jong A, Xing L, FitzGerald MJ, Vollmer WM, et al. Marijuana and chronic obstructive lung disease: a population-based study. *Can Med Assoc J.* 2009;180(8):814–820.

172. Tanda G, Goldberg SR. Cannabinoids: reward, dependence, and underlying neurochemical mechanisms—a review of recent preclinical data. *Psychopharmacol.* 2003;169(2):115–134.

173. Tashkin D. Is frequent marijuana smoking harmful to health? *West J Med.* 1993;158(6):635.

174. Tashkin DP. Effects of marijuana smoking on the lung. *Ann Am Thorac Soc.* 2013;10(3):239–247.

175. Tashkin DP, Simmons MS, Sherrill DL, Coulson AH. Heavy habitual marijuana smoking does not cause an accelerated decline in FEV1 with age. *Am J Respir Crit Care Med.* 1997;155(1):141–148.

176. Teesson M, Lynskey M, Manor B, Baillie A. The structure of cannabis dependence in the community. *Drug Alcohol Depend.* 2002;68(3):255–262.

177. Thomas G, Kloner RA, Rezkalla S. Adverse cardiovascular, cerebrovascular, and peripheral vascular effects of marijuana inhalation: what cardiologists need to know. *Am J Cardiol.* 2014;113(1):187–190.

178. Thomas H. A community survey of adverse effects of cannabis use. *Drug Alcohol Depend.* 1996;42(3):201–207.

179. Thompson RG, Hasin DS. Cigarette, marijuana, and alcohol use and prior drug treatment among newly homeless young adults in New York City: relationship to a history of foster care. *Drug Alcohol Depend.* 2011;117(1):66–69.

180. Thorndike AN, Rigotti NA, Stafford RS, Singer DE. National patterns in the treatment of smokers by physicians. *JAMA.* 1998;279(8):604–608.

181. Tunving K. Psychiatric effects of cannabis use. *Acta Psychiatrica Scandinavica.* 1985;72(3):209–217.

182. Vandrey R, Smith MT, McCann UD, Budney AJ, Curran EM. Sleep disturbance and the effects of extended-release zolpidem during cannabis withdrawal. *Drug Alcohol Depend.* 2011;117(1):38–44.

183. Verweij K, Agrawal A, Nat N, Creemers H, Huizink A, Martin N, et al. A genetic perspective on the proposed inclusion of cannabis withdrawal in DSM-5. *Psychol Med.* 2013;43(08):1713–1722.

184. Volkow ND, Baler RD, Compton WM, Weiss SR. Adverse health effects of marijuana use. *N Engl J Med.* 2014;370(23):2219–2227.

185. Weiner MD, Sussman S, McCuller WJ, Lichtman K. Factors in marijuana cessation among high-risk youth. *J Alcohol Drug Educ.* 1999;29(4):337–357.

186. Whitlow CT, Liguori A, Livengood LB, Hart SL, Mussat-Whitlow BJ, Lamborn CM, et al. Long-term heavy marijuana users make costly decisions on a gambling task. *Drug Alcohol Depend.* 2004;76(1): 107–111.

186a. Wilson I, Whiting M, Scammell A. Addressing cannabis use in primary care: GPs' knowledge of cannabis-related harm and current practice. *Prim Health Care Res Dev.* 2007;8(3):216–225.

187. Young ME, Rintala DH, Rossi CD, Hart KA, Fuhrer MJ. Alcohol and marijuana use in a community-based sample of persons with spinal cord injury. *Arch Phys Med Rehabil.* 1995;76(6):525–532.

188. Zvolensky MJ, Bernstein A, Sachs-Ericsson N, Schmidt NB, Buckner JD, Bonn-Miller MO. Lifetime associations between cannabis, use, abuse, and dependence and panic attacks in a representative sample. *J Psychiatr Res.* 2006;40(6):477–486.

189. Zvolensky MJ, Bonn-Miller MO, Bernstein A, McLeish AC, Feldner MT, Leen-Feldner EW. Anxiety sensitivity interacts with marijuana use in the prediction of anxiety symptoms and panic-related catastrophic thinking among daily tobacco users. *Behav Res Ther.* 2006;44(7):907–924.

190. Zvolensky MJ, Cougle JR, Bonn–Miller MO, Norberg MM, Johnson K, Kosiba J, et al. Chronic pain and marijuana use among a nationally representative sample of adults. *Am J Addict.* 2011;20(6):538–542.

191. Zvolensky MJ, Feldner MT, Leen-Feldner E, Bonn-Miller MO, McLeish AC, Gregor K. Evaluating the role of anxiety sensitivity in smoking outcome expectancies among regular smokers. *Cognitive Therapy and Research.* 2004;28(4):473–486.

192. Zvolensky MJ, Lewinsohn P, Bernstein A, Schmidt NB, Buckner JD, Seeley J, et al. Prospective associations between cannabis use, abuse, and dependence and panic attacks and disorder. *J Psychiatr Res.* 2008;42(12):1017–1023.

193. Zvolensky MJ, Vujanovic AA, Bernstein A, Bonn-Miller MO, Marshall EC, Leyro TM. Marijuana use motives: a confirmatory test and evaluation among young adult marijuana users. *Addict Behav.* 2007;32(12):3122–3130.

25

Opiates and Prescription Drugs

JOHN A. RENNER AND JOJI SUZUKI

Classification

Medications derived from *Papaver somniferum*, the opium poppy, have played a central role in medical practice for well over 3500 years. Sumerian clay tablets, which include our oldest known medical texts, called the opium poppy "Hul Gil," the "Joy Plant." In the Greco-Roman era, poppies were cultivated for their pain-relieving, antidiarrheal, and sedative properties. Today, medications in this class are divided into two groups. Opiates are naturally occurring compounds derived from the active alkaloids of the opium poppy. This group includes morphine, codeine, and thebaine. Opioids, defined as compounds that bind to opioid receptors, are typically manufactured medications that are classified as either fully synthetic or semisynthetic. Medications in the synthetic opioid group include alfentanil (Alfenta, Rapifen), fentanyl, meperidine (Demerol), methadone (Dolophine), pentazocine (Talwin), propoxyphene (Darvon), and sufentanil (Sufenta). Included in the semisynthetic opioid group are buprenorphine (Bunavail, Buprenex, Probuphine, Suboxone, Subutex, and Zubsolv), hydrocodone (Hycodan), oxycodone (Percodan), and oxymorphone (Numorphan), all of which are derived from thebaine. Other semisynthetic compounds derived from the opium poppy are hydromorphone (Dilaudid) and heroin, which is metabolized to morphine. Both of these drugs are highly abusable. The human body also produces a number of endogenous opioids, such as endorphins, enkephalins, and dynorphins. Other opioids that exist in nature, but are not related to opiates, include salvinorin A (from *Salvia divinorum*) and mitragynine (from *Mitragyna speciosa*).

Etiology

There is no clearly defined etiology for opiate use disorder. Risk is determined by multiple factors including genetics, psychiatric comorbidity, and social and environmental factors, including drug exposure. Twin studies suggest that genetics alone accounts for 45%–50% of the risk for opioid dependence. Recent work has identified two sites on chromosome 17 that are associated with an increased risk for drug dependence; one of these sites is connected to severe symptoms of opioid dependence, but not to dependence on other drugs.[47] Further work is needed to identify the specific genes that are associated with the unique risk for opioid dependence.

Epidemiology

Patterns of Use

For most of the 21st century, heroin was the primary opiate abused in the United States. There were major epidemics after World War I, World War II, and the Vietnam War. Among the general population, it is estimated that 10%–30% of individuals who are exposed to licit and illicit opioids may develop symptoms of an opioid use disorder. These numbers may be significantly higher in individuals with co-occurring psychiatric disorders, particularly those exposed to sexual abuse or combat trauma. Although regular estimates of drug use in adults and adolescents have been available from the Monitoring the Future study and the National Survey on Drug Use and Health, information on drug use disorders has rarely been collected.[63,153] There was a 16-year gap between publication of the 1990–1992 National Comorbidity Survey data and the 2000 National Survey on Drug Use and Health, which collected 12-month prevalence data on drug use disorders.[153] Depending on the survey and the criteria used, estimates for the lifetime prevalence of any drug use disorders have ranged from 0.4% to 7.5%.[30,51,73,133]

For many years, it was assumed that the lifetime risk for heroin use disorder was relatively low and ranged from 0.4% to 0.7%. In 2006, the National Survey on Drug Use and Health reported that 3.79 million individuals used heroin at least once in their lifetime and 323,000 were classified with either dependence or abuse of heroin. In addition, it was estimated that there were 250,000 individuals in methadone maintenance treatment. From 1984 to 1994, new users of heroin each year ranged between 28,000 and 80,000. From 1995 to 2001, the number averaged over 100,000; in 2006, it dropped slightly to 91,000.[35] Heroin use began to increase gradually after 2006 and the number of new users reached 268,000 in 2014, representing almost a 100% increase in that time frame (Fig 4; NSDUH 2015, Figure 13). Even more concerning, the number of overdose deaths related to heroin increased by almost 300% during the same period.[65]

Incidence of Substance Use Disorders

The most recent national survey, the 2001–2002 National Epidemiologic Survey on Alcohol and Related Conditions, was designed to collect data on drug use disorders and, for the first time in a national survey, to collect separate data on both illicit drugs and prescribed medications. The National Epidemiologic Survey on Alcohol and Related Conditions surveyed 43,093 adults (18 years of age or older) in the United States, and captured data at the time when the United States' epidemic of prescription opioid abuse was at its peak. The National Comorbidity Survey and the Environmental Catchment Area Survey combined data on heroin and other opiates into a broad drug abuse category that also included other illicit drugs, thus making it impossible to get specific data on opiates, or to separate out information on heroin from data on prescribed opiates.[30,62] The National Epidemiologic Survey on Alcohol and Related Conditions reported the prevalence of 12-month and lifetime drug abuse as 1.4% and 7.7%, respectively, and the rates of drug dependence as 0.6% and 2.6%, respectively. Rates of abuse and dependence were significantly higher in men than in women and in Native Americans than in whites, blacks, and Hispanics.[30] The lifetime prevalence of nonmedical prescription opioid drug use was 4.7%. The lifetime prevalence of nonmedical opioid drug use disorders was 1.4%, indicating that approximately

30% of users were at risk for developing an opioid drug use disorder. Men were significantly more likely to progress from use to abuse to dependence than were women, as were Native Americans as compared with whites. The mean age at onset of opioid abuse or dependence was 22.8 years, and the mean age at first treatment was 26.2 years, a lag of 3.4 years. Approximately two-thirds of individuals with opioid use disorders never received treatment.[62] This prevalence of nonmedical opioid use disorders is two to three times higher than prior estimates of the prevalence of heroin use disorders.

Abuse of Opioid Analgesics

The abuse of opioid analgesics was traditionally thought to be a relatively small part of the drug problem in the United States. Although there were few data on the risk for dependence among individuals treated for chronic pain, the risk was assumed to be minimal.[125,129] During the 1960s, the introduction of pentazocine (Talwin) triggered a period of abuse after opiate addicts discovered that the injected combination of Talwin and amphetamines ("T's and Blues") produced a potent euphoric effect. After this problem was identified, the US Food and Drug Administration (FDA) required that the medication be reformulated as a combination tablet of Talwin and naltrexone (TalwinNX).[100] This formulation produced an antagonist reaction in addicted individuals if the tablets were crushed and injected, essentially eliminating significant misuse of this medication. The abuse of other opioid analgesics remained a minimal problem until the introduction of OxyContin in 1996. From 1970 to 1995, the National Survey on Drug Use and Health reported that the annual number of new nonmedical users of pain relievers ranged from 700,000 to 1,000,000.[153] In the 5 years following 1996, this number almost tripled to 2,500,000.[35] These numbers reflected a new epidemic of misuse of pain relievers in the United States (Fig. 25.1). The number of nonmedical users of pain relievers began to decline

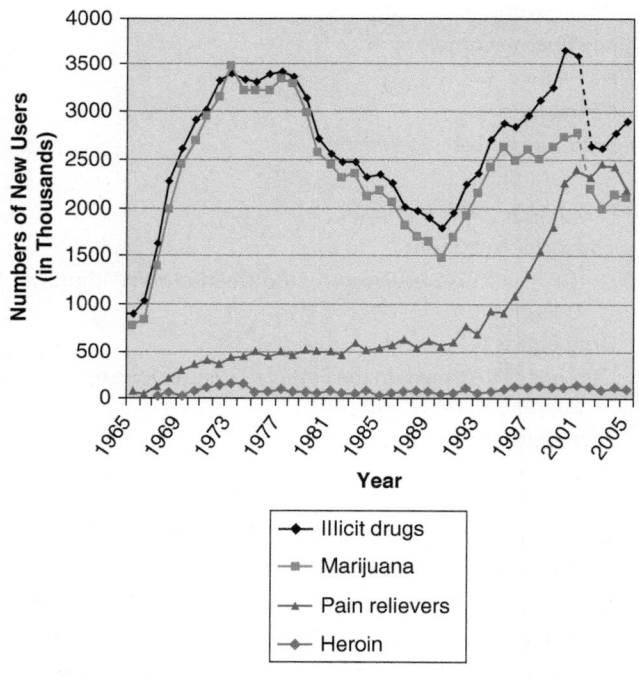

• **Fig. 25.1** New drug user patterns, 1965–2005.[35]

after 2006. In 2014 it was estimated at 10.34 million noninstitutionalized persons 12 years of age or older (see Fig. 25.4).[29]

As noted previously, prior to 2000, the National Survey on Drug Use and Health reported only drug use data, not data on drug use disorders.[30] In 2005, the National Survey on Drug Use and Health reported that 4.9% of 12- to 17-year-olds had used prescription pain relievers nonmedically in the past year. This was more than 24 times the reported use of heroin in this group (0.2% versus 4.9%). In this cohort, past-year dependence or abuse was 1.1% (275,000 individuals) for pain relievers versus 0.0% (fewer than 9000 individuals) for heroin dependence or abuse.[153] In 2006, the National Survey on Drug Use and Health reported that 33,422,000 Americans 12 years of age or older admitted to the nonmedical use of pain relievers at least once in their lives and that 12,649,000 had done so in the last year. The survey classified 1,635,000 individuals 12 years of age or older with dependence or abuse of pain relievers, as compared with 323,000 individuals classified with dependence or abuse of heroin. The 2006 National Survey on Drug Use and Health estimated that 7,800,000 adults in the United States (3.2% of the total population) were in need of treatment for some type of illicit drug problem; less than 20% of that group received any treatment in 2006. By 2015, there were more than 2.1 million new illicit users of pain relievers, making the misuse of pain relievers the second most common new drug of misuse, ahead of marijuana (2.6 million). In comparison, there were only 135,000 new initiates to heroin misuse in 2015 (Fig. 25.2). These data make it clear that the misuse of pharmaceutical analgesics has replaced heroin as the dominant opioid misuse problem in the United States.[35]

Risks Associated With the Use of Opioid Analgesics

For many years, pain management specialists had voiced concern about the undertreatment of pain. The pharmaceutical industry also identified a need for less abusable and more potent opioids for pain management. In the 1980s, the Bard Corporation developed a sustained-release technology suitable for morphine.

This led to the marketing of sustained-release morphine in England under the brand name of MST Continus; in 1984, the same medication was introduced in the United States by Purdue Pharma as MS-Contin. This formulation proved effective in preventing significant abuse, and the medication gained wide acceptance in the American market. The expanding use of opioids for the treatment of severe pain led to an interest in a medication with greater potency, longer duration of action, and low abuse potential. Oxycodone provided the desired potency, but it could not be successfully formulated with the sustained-release technology that had been effective with morphine. This problem was resolved in 1996 when Purdue introduced OxyContin, a time-release formulation of oxycodone with an acrylic coating that was designed to dissolve slowly and provide 12 h of pain control, permitting individuals with pain to sleep through the night. This formulation permitted delivery of doses ranging from 10 to 160 mg—doses far in excess of the 30-mg maximum dose previously available in oxycodone tablets. This was a major advance in the management of severe pain. Based on the experience with MS-Contin, both Purdue and the FDA assumed that this formulation would have low abuse potential, and Purdue was permitted to market the medication as a potent, long-acting narcotic with a lower abuse potential than other opioid analgesics. Consequently, Purdue marketed OxyContin as a first-line agent for the treatment of nonmalignant pain. At that time, there was a general presumption that iatrogenic addiction secondary to the treatment of legitimate pain was a rare event. This assumption was based on a series of articles published between 1977 and 1982, all of which reported a minimal risk of iatrogenic addiction in the treatment of acute pain.[99,125,129] This view was reinforced by Portenoy and Foley,[128] who found evidence of abuse problems in only 2 of 38 individuals chronically treated with opiates for nonmalignant pain. They concluded that opioid maintenance therapy was safe, except in individuals with a history of drug abuse. In 2000, Joranson et al. reviewed emergency room data from the Drug Abuse Warning Network and found no evidence of an increase in analgesic abuse, despite significant increases in the prescription of opioid analgesics.[66]

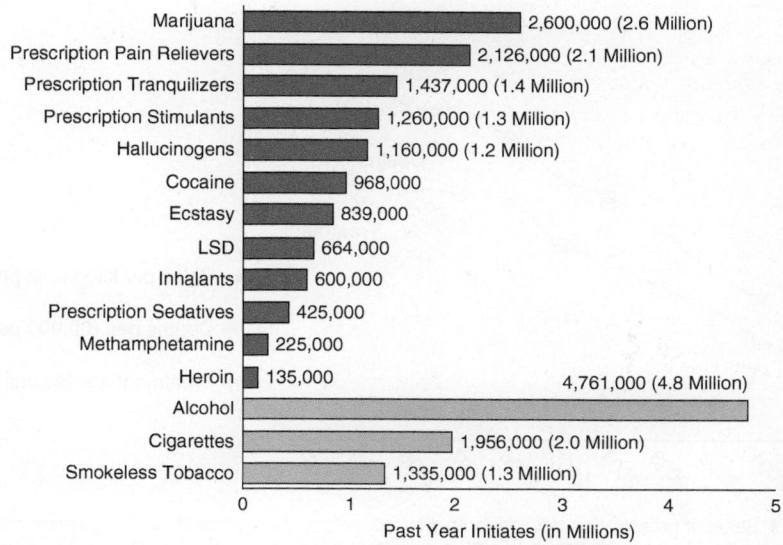

• **Fig. 25.2** Numbers of past year initiates of substances among people 12 years of age or older: 2015. *LSD,* Lysergic acid diethylamide. (From the National Survey on Drug Use and Health: 2015, Figure 10.[157])

In the late 1990s, clinicians in rural Virginia and northern Maine reported that young people were crushing OxyContin tablets and snorting or injecting the drug. This method of ingestion produced a highly euphoric and reinforcing experience; abusers were exposed to very high doses of oxycodone, and many quickly became addicted. There was also a corresponding spike in overdose deaths. Despite growing evidence of addiction and overdose deaths, Purdue executives remained convinced of the efficacy and safety of their medication. By 2000, sales of Oxy-Contin reached over $1 billion/year and the company was marketing it as a first-line agent for a wide variety of pain syndromes, with recommendations that it be used before lower scheduled narcotics, or even before Ultram (tramadol), a nonnarcotic.[100] In 2001, the FDA required a new label for OxyContin that dropped claims about a reduced risk of abuse. By this time it had become apparent that overdose deaths and reports of addictive behavior did not just involve individuals who were illicitly using the drug, but that some people being treated for legitimate pain problems were becoming addicted and finding it impossible to stop their use of the drug. In retrospect, clinicians realized that the bulk of the medical literature claiming a minimal risk of iatrogenic addiction primarily reported on experience using opioids to treat acute pain and that there were few data on the risk of addiction in individuals treated for chronic pain.[66] Similarly, there were no data on the addiction risks associated with the use of long-acting high-potency agents such as OxyContin for either acute or chronic pain. All of the published research on the abuse risk of chronic opioid treatment preceded the marketing of those medications.

As physicians became aware of the problems associated with OxyContin, many shifted to oral methadone as a safer alternative for the management of chronic pain. From 1998 to 2006, the number of methadone prescriptions for pain in the United States increased from 0.5 million to over 4 million. Unfortunately, there was a linear relationship between opioid-related overdose deaths and the increase in prescription of pain relievers (Fig. 25.3).[110]

Starting in the late 2000s, national surveys began to identify an increase in the number of individuals reporting the use of heroin[29] (Fig. 25.4). By 2014, even though the rate of non-medical use of prescription opioids had been steadily declining, the rate of heroin use had spiked considerably. Indeed, in 2014, there were 910,000 individuals who had used heroin during the previous year, which is almost double from a decade prior. Consequently, there has been a dramatic increase in the number of heroin-related overdoses during that same time period. In 2014, there was a 300% increase in the number heroin-related overdoses compared to 2010[29] (Fig.25.5). The number of treatment admissions for opioid use disorder remained fairly steady from 2011 to 2014 at slightly below 500,000 admissions per year, although the number related to the misuse of opioid analgesics dropped to 132,000, whereas the number related to heroin increased to over 357,000.[156]

Neurobiology

The functions of all the compounds in this class (opiates, synthetic opioids, and endogenous opioids) are mediated through a variety of receptors in the central and peripheral nervous systems. The mu, delta, and kappa opioid receptors are well defined, and genes encoding for these receptors have been cloned.[25,26,41,70] The mu receptor was named because of the affinity of morphine for this receptor. Full agonists at the mu receptor activate the receptor, are highly reinforcing, and include the most abused types of opioids. There are two primary subtypes of the mu receptor; subtype 1 (mu$_1$) apparently mediates analgesic effects, whereas subtype 2 (mu$_2$) is likely responsible for the symptoms associated with opioid overdose (including respiratory depression) and withdrawal. Agonists at the mu receptor include morphine, methadone, and beta-endorphin. These compounds also have agonist activity at the delta receptor (named because of their presence in the vas deferens). The primary agonists at the delta receptor are met-enkephalins and leu-enkephalins.

Another group of receptors were named kappa because of their affinity for the opioid agonist ketazocine. Kappa receptors bind endogenous dynorphin and are thought to mediate spinal cord analgesia. They are also involved in the

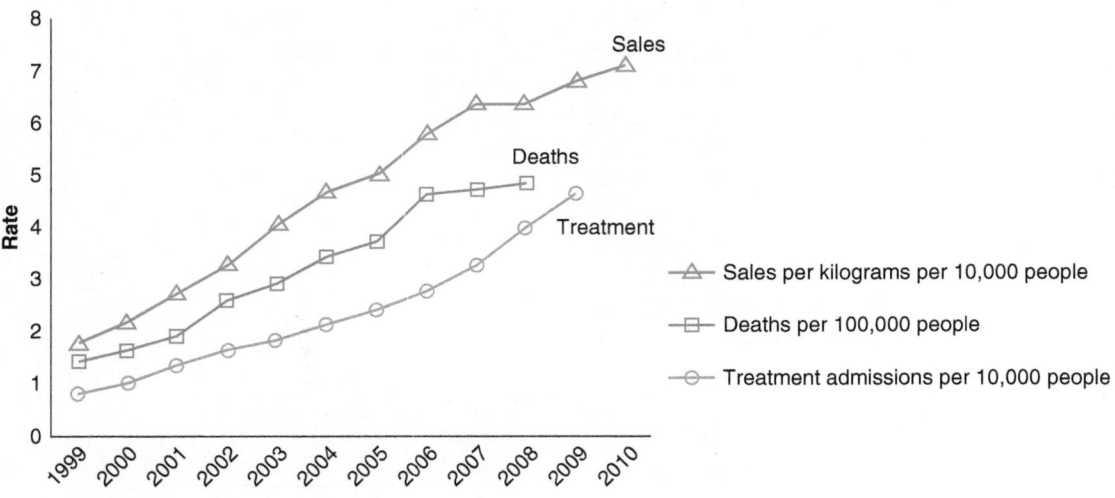

• **Fig. 25.3** Sales of prescription opioids, opioid overdose deaths, and treatment admission during 1999–2010. (From the National Vital Statistics System, 1999–2008; Automation of Reports and Consolidated Orders System [ARCOS] of the Drug Enforcement Administration [DEA], 1999–2010; Treatment Episode Data Set, 1999–2009.[110])

psychotomimetic and dysphoric effects seen in overdoses of pentazocine and other kappa-active synthetic opiates. Opioid antagonists (naloxone and naltrexone) are synthetic derivatives of oxymorphone and act primarily at the two mu receptor sites, although they also have some antagonist activity at the kappa receptor (Fig. 25.6).

There is another group of medications that have mixed agonist-antagonist properties. For example, pentazocine acts as a kappa agonist and as a weak mu antagonist. Butorphanol has mixed kappa and mu agonist properties and weak antagonist properties. Buprenorphine is classified as a partial opioid agonist at the mu and kappa receptors and an antagonist at the delta receptor.

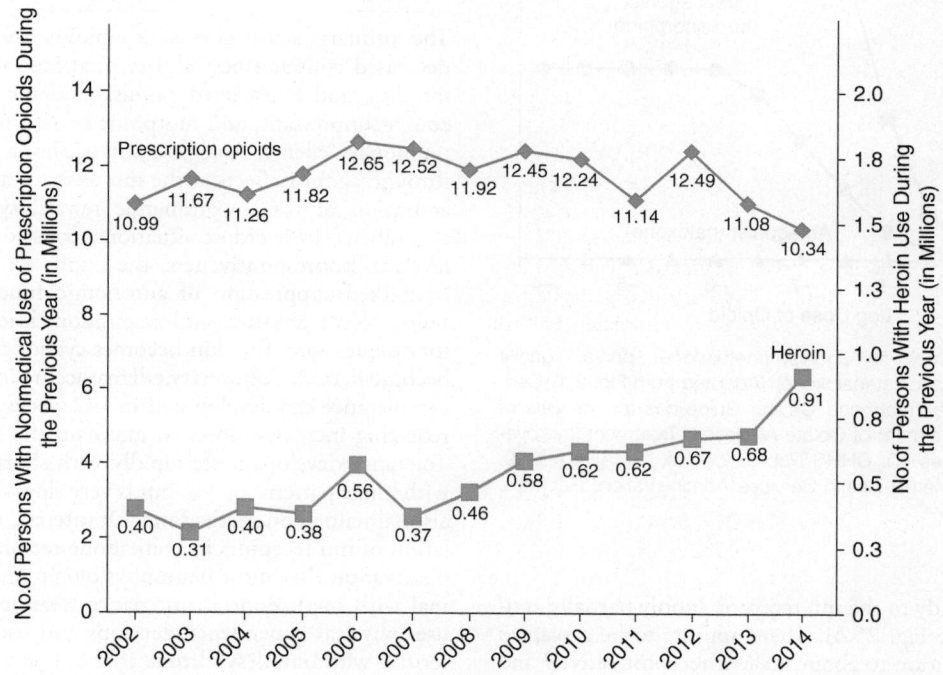

• **Fig. 25.4** Nonmedical use of prescription opioids and heroin during the previous year among noninstitutionalized persons 12 years of age or older, 2002–2014. (From Compton WM, Jones CM, Baldwin GT. Relationship between nonmedical prescription-opioid use and heroin use. *N Engl J Med*. 2016;374:154–163.)

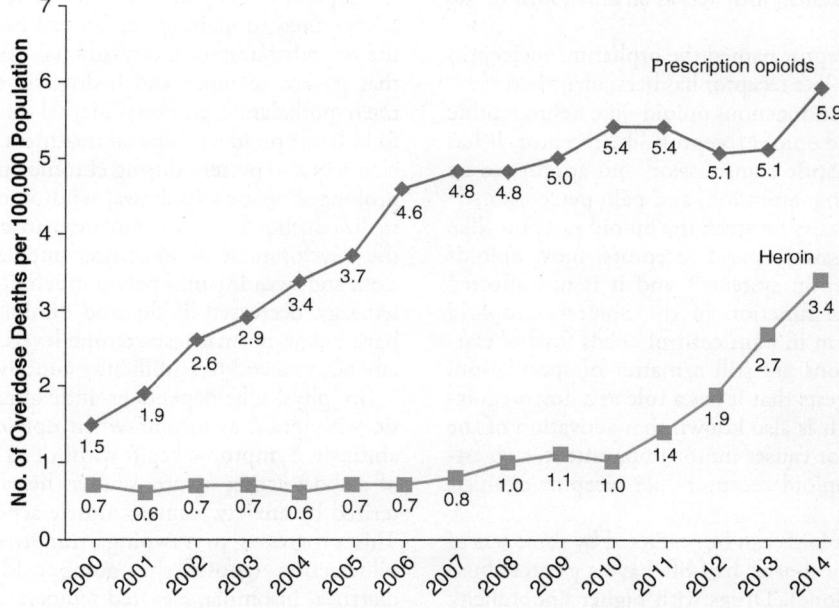

• **Fig. 25.5** Age-adjusted rates of death related to prescription opioids and heroin drug poisoning in the United States, 2000–2014. (From Compton WM, Jones CM, Baldwin GT. Relationship between nonmedical prescription-opioid use and heroin use. *N Engl J Med*. 2016;374:154–163.)

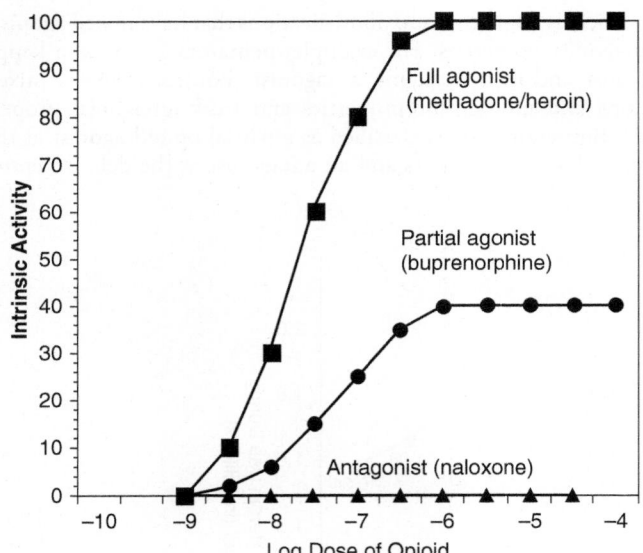

• **Fig. 25.6** Intrinsic activity: full agonist (methadone), partial agonist (buprenorphine), and antagonist (naloxone) (Adapted from Fig. 2.1, Center for Substance Abuse Treatment. Clinical Guidelines for the Use of Buprenorphine in the Treatment of Opiate Addiction. Treatment Improvement Protocol [TIP] Series 40. DHHS Publication No. [SMA] 40–3939. Substance Abuse and Mental Health Services Administration, Rockville, MD, 2004.)

Although it binds tightly to the mu receptor, it only partially activates the receptor (see Fig. 25.4). There appears to be a plateau effect that limits activation to about 50% of receptor activity and prevents the respiratory depression seen with full mu receptor agonists; of interest, the analgesic effect of buprenorphine does not seem to be limited by the plateau effect.[33] When a partial agonist is administered in the presence of a full agonist, the partial agonist either displaces the full agonist or prevents its binding to the receptor. As a result, the partial agonist acts as an antagonist to the full agonist.[167]

More recently, a new receptor named the orphanin/nociceptin receptor or opioid receptor–like receptor has been identified.[32,104] Orphanin/nociceptin is an endogenous opioid–like neuropeptide that acts as an agonist at the opioid receptor–like receptor. It has an inhibitory effect on synaptic transmission and appears to be involved in memory, learning, attention, and pain perception.[121] Despite the structural similarity between the opioid receptor–like receptor and the three classical opioid receptors, most opioids lack affinity for the nociceptin system,[59] and it is not affected by opioid antagonists. The function of the nociceptin/opioid receptor–like receptor system in pain control needs further clarification, and other functions are still a matter of speculation, although investigation suggests that it has a role as a downregulator of immune function.[45] It is also known that activation of the opioid receptor–like receptor causes motor impairment, suggesting that development of opioid receptor–like receptor agonists would be difficult.

The abuse potential of opioids can be predicted by three sets of characteristics. Drugs with a shorter half-life have a greater abuse potential (heroin > methadone). Drugs with higher lipophilicity cross the blood-brain barrier more rapidly and are more likely to be abused (heroin > morphine > methadone). Finally, those drugs with a faster route of administration have a higher abuse potential (intravenous injection > subcutaneous injection > oral ingestion). Heroin (di-acetyl-morphine) has two acetyl groups that render it very lipophilic, enabling it to cross the blood-brain barrier more rapidly than morphine, thereby making it a preferred drug for injecting opioid abusers.[123,146]

Biological Effects of Use

The primary acute effects of opioids are euphoria, analgesia, decreased consciousness and respirations, vomiting, reduced gut motility, and constricted pupils. Codeine is also effective as a cough suppressant, and morphine is used to treat cardiac-related pulmonary edema. Analgesia and euphoria are produced directly through agonist effects at the mu receptor and indirectly through activation of the dopaminergic reward system in the nucleus accumbens. In overdose situations, consciousness is depressed to levels of nonresponsiveness, the pupils are pin point, and there is marked suppression of autonomic functions with decreased pulse, blood pressure, and respiration, leading to lethal respiratory depression. The skin becomes cyanotic, and skeletal muscles become flaccid. Pulmonary edema occurs in 50% of cases. Physical tolerance can develop within 1–2 weeks with repeated dosing, requiring increased doses to maintain the original opioid effect. Tolerance develops more rapidly with shorter-acting opiates and with binge patterns of use, but is very slow to develop in individuals maintained on methadone. Of interest, there is no downregulation of mu receptors in methadone recipients,[76] supporting the observation that most neurophysiologic functions return to normal with methadone maintenance treatment.[82,84] With chronic use, physical dependence develops and users manifest a characteristic withdrawal syndrome if the dose is reduced or stopped. In some animal models, physical dependence has developed in the absence of tolerance, suggesting that these are dissociable phenomena.[131] Tolerance develops more quickly to opiate side effects than to the analgesic effect. Chronic opiate use leads to reduced dopaminergic tone and decreased binding capacity at the D_2 dopamine receptor.[8,83,162,163] Once tolerance develops, opiates are required to maintain an altered homeostatic set-point within the hypothalamic-pituitary-adrenal axis and within the pathways that govern memory and hedonistic desires.[81] Abnormalities in the hypothalamic-pituitary-adrenal axis may persist for over 1 year following opioid withdrawal treatment. A relative endorphin deficiency is also present during chronic opiate misuse and during the prolonged opiate withdrawal syndrome, but endorphin levels normalize during methadone maintenance treatment.[79,82,145] Despite the development of tolerance, pupillary constriction, constipation, and sweating may persist indefinitely. Long-term users report lethargy, decreased libido, and diminished sexual function; men have below-normal testosterone levels, and women may develop amenorrhea and have difficulty conceiving.

In physically dependent individuals, there is a characteristic withdrawal syndrome when opioids are reduced or stopped abruptly. Symptoms begin within 6–12 h following the last dose of a short-acting opiate, such as heroin. Early stages are characterized by anxiety, nausea, muscle aches, and abdominal cramps. This progresses to yawning, rhinorrhea, lacrimation, sweating, piloerection (gooseflesh, "going cold turkey"), dilated pupils, diarrhea, insomnia, elevated temperature, heart rate, blood pressure, and respirations. In the most severe stage, the syndrome includes severe craving, abdominal cramps, diarrhea, and painful

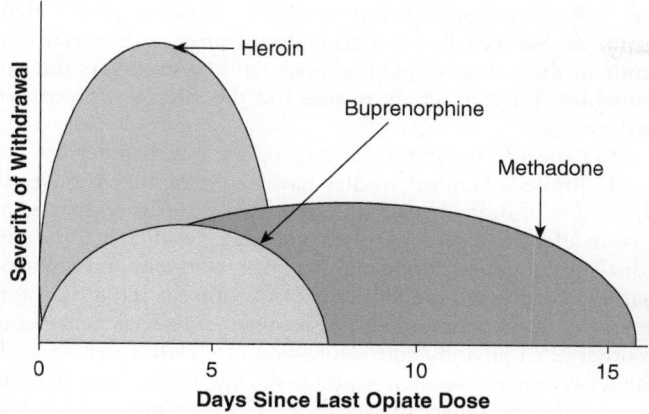

• **Fig. 25.7** Comparison of spontaneous withdrawals (Heroin > Buprenorphine > Methadone Withdrawal). The graph illustrates the severity of opioid-withdrawal symptoms after abrupt discontinuation of equivalent doses of heroin, buprenorphine, and methadone. (Copyright © 2004 Massachusetts Medical Society. All rights reserved.[80])

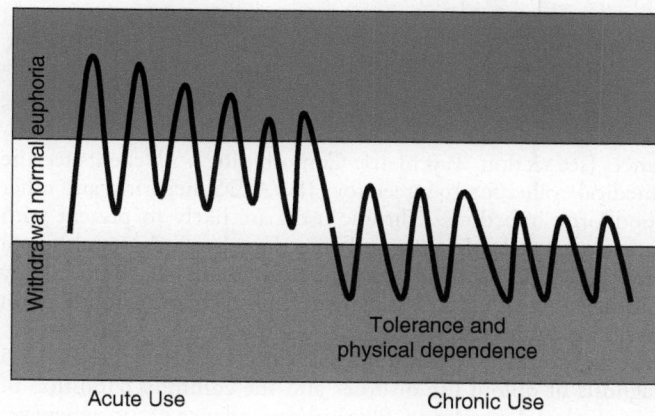

• **Fig. 25.8** Natural history of opioid dependence. (Courtesy Daniel P. Alford, MD.)

TABLE 25.1	Characteristics of Spontaneous Opioid Withdrawal.		
Drug	**Onset**	**Peak**	**Duration**
Heroin	6–12 h	~3 days	4–7 days
Buprenorphine	1–3 days	~4 days	5–7 days
Methadone	1–2 days	~7 days	12–14 days

cramps and muscle spasms ("kicking the habit"). Many of the acute symptoms of opiate withdrawal are driven by an overactive catecholaminergic system located in the locus coeruleus and by dopaminergic neurons located in the ventral tegmental area. The syndrome is most severe in individuals dependent on short-acting opiates such as heroin, but it clears in 4–7 days. Withdrawal from long-acting opioids, such as methadone, is less severe but can last for 14 days or more. Withdrawal symptoms from the partial agonist buprenorphine are slightly less severe than those caused by methadone and last 5–7 days, making it the preferred opioid for use in medically supervised withdrawal (Fig. 25.7 and Table 25.1). Following withdrawal, many addicts experience a prolonged state of dysphoria that may last for months. Indeed, the negative emotional states during withdrawal and periods of abstinence is a result of the adaptations in the fear circuitry, which includes the extended amygdala. The fear circuitry becomes overactive, and the addicted individual begins to seek drug use to find relief from these negative emotional states.[164]

Psychological Effects of Use

In nontolerant users, opioids produce sedation, analgesia, and, in some cases, euphoria and a profound sense of well-being. This is often described as being "high" or "on the nod." Many users also report an antidepressant effect from opioids. As use becomes more frequent, users cycle between states of euphoria and normality (Fig. 25.8).

Regular use eventually leads to physical tolerance, a state where progressively higher doses are required to produce the desired experience of euphoria. Eventually the individual becomes physically dependent and starts to experience withdrawal symptoms whenever the euphoria wears off. Drug craving becomes progressively more severe, and higher doses are required to prevent the development of withdrawal. In this later stage of dependency, users rarely feel normal and typically cycle between states of low-level intoxication and withdrawal (see Fig. 25.8). Large doses of opiates are needed to eliminate withdrawal symptoms, and it may be difficult for the addicted individual to achieve any state approaching normality, let alone euphoria. At this stage, individuals addicted to opioids are chronically irritable and depressed. Individuals maintained on stable doses of long-acting opioids such as methadone, levo-alpha acetyl methadol, or buprenorphine become tolerant to any sedative effects, and they generally report the absence of craving, euphoria, or withdrawal symptoms. They often feel more alert and energized following their daily dose. However, many individuals on maintenance treatment fail to develop tolerance to the side effects of constipation and sweating.

Diagnosis

The 2013 the fifth edition of the *Diagnostic and Statistical Manual of Mental Disorders* (DSM-5) brought substantial changes to the diagnostic criteria for substance use disorders.[4] The diagnoses of substance abuse and substance dependence were combined to create one diagnosis: substance use disorder. The decision to make this change was based on the weaknesses of the previous nosology, including the low reliability and validity of the substance abuse diagnosis, that the majority of substance abuse diagnoses were made with only one criterion (hazardous use criterion), and the incorrect assumption that substance abuse is a less severe or prodromal version of substance dependence.[58] In addition, one of the criteria from substance abuse—recurrent legal problems stemming from substance use—was dropped because the criteria was met very infrequently and because patients rarely endorse legal problems alone in the absence of other criteria. Finally, the decision was made to add a criterion for cravings because of empirical support from behavioral, neuroimaging, pharmacology, and genetic studies, as well as greater coherence with ICD-10, which already includes craving as a criteria.[4]

Clients may present with the typical symptoms of either opioid intoxication or withdrawal described in the sections that follow titled "Opioid Overdose" and "Opioid Withdrawal Syndromes." A urine toxicology examination should be obtained on all clients to confirm current use and to screen for the misuse of other substances (see section "Psychiatric Comorbidity"). All clients require a medical evaluation to screen for HIV/AIDS, hepatitis, and other bloodborne infections. Chronic users are likely to present with track marks and other signs of injection drug misuse, although some individuals addicted to pain relievers may have no history of intravenous drug use and may present no abnormal findings on physical examination.

Some confusion continues to exist between the DSM-5 diagnosis of opioid use disorder and the common condition of physiological dependence. Physical dependence occurs whenever there is ongoing use of opiates for medical treatment. Physically dependent individuals may manifest both tolerance and withdrawal symptoms, but they show no symptoms of craving or loss of control, and the majority are able to taper off opiates with little or no difficulty. A few individuals, particularly those treated with high-potency opioids, may experience prolonged and severe withdrawal symptoms and will require a much more gradual medication taper. For some clients (between 3% and 30%), long-term treatment with opiates may trigger an iatrogenic addiction. They may experience euphoria when initially treated, and then go on to develop craving and loss of control of their medication use, eventually meeting full DSM-5 criteria for opioid use disorder.[4] When evaluating these clients, it may be useful to look for the presence of the "4 Cs" commonly associated with addiction: Craving, Compulsive use, loss of Control, and Continued use despite apparent harm.[3] Clinical experience suggests that individuals at highest risk for misusing pain medications are those with a prior history of alcohol use disorder or other substance misuse, family history of substance use disorders, and with co-occurring psychiatric disorders, including antisocial personality disorder.

Psychiatric Comorbidity

Dependence on alcohol and other classes of drugs is common in the majority of individuals with opioid disorder and has a significant impact on the outcome of treatment. There is also a high rate of comorbidity between all of the drug use disorders and other psychiatric disorders. With few exceptions, the National Epidemiologic Survey on Alcohol and Related Conditions data showed positive and significant correlations between drug use disorders, alcohol use disorders, nicotine dependence, and antisocial personality disorder.[30] As Kessler noted in his reviews of the literature on the epidemiology of comorbidity of mental and substance use disorders, the available data have consistently shown that comorbid disorders are more chronic and have a significantly more persistent and severe course.[71,72,74] Unfortunately, methodologic limitations in the original National Comorbidity Survey, the Environmental Catchment Area Survey, and the National Comorbidity Survey Replication make it difficult to get specific comorbidity estimates regarding opioid use, misuse, and dependence.[57,62] Although the National Comorbidity Survey found an odds ratio of 2.4 for comorbidity between any lifetime alcohol or drug use disorder and any lifetime DSM-III revised mental disorder,[73] there were no drug-specific data available in that study. Responses on opiates, cocaine, cannabis, and hallucinogens were combined under a single category of drug use disorders.[5] Both the National Comorbidity Survey and the Environmental Catchment Area Survey relied on data collected prior to the recent epidemic of the misuse of pain relievers, and these surveys did not distinguish between heroin misuse and the misuse of prescribed medications.

Data specific to comorbidity in opiate use disorder are relatively limited. Clinical studies have reported that a range of 55%–74% of individuals with opioid use disorder in treatment have an affective disorder.[132] Brooner et al.[17] evaluated 716 individuals seeking methadone maintenance treatment and reported that 47% of the sample met criteria for other psychiatric disorders. The most common diagnoses were antisocial personality disorder (25.1%) and major depression (15.8%). Rosen and colleagues recently evaluated a group of 140 methadone maintenance participants over the age of 50. In this sample, 57.1% had at least one other psychiatric disorder in the previous year. The most prevalent disorders in this cohort were major depression (32.9%), posttraumatic stress disorder (27.8%), and generalized anxiety disorder (29.7%); women had higher levels of depression than men (43.8% vs. 27.2%) and had twice the prevalence rate of panic disorder and agoraphobia.[139] As indicated above, depression and anxiety disorders are common in this population and are associated with increased severity of substance use disorders and poorer treatment outcome.[17,135] Other substance use disorders are also common in individuals dependent on opiates. Brooner et al.[16] evaluated 68 methadone maintenance participants enrolled in an HIV education program. In this group, lifetime rates for abuse or dependence were as follows: cocaine 55.9%, sedative/hypnotics 53%, marijuana 47.1%, and alcohol 47.1%. Forty-eight percent of the sample met criteria for a nonsubstance use psychiatric disorder, the most common being antisocial personality disorder (29%) and major depression (19%). Individuals with other psychiatric disorders also had a greater number of substance use disorders and a more severe clinical course.

The association between heroin misuse and antisocial personality disorder reflects an overlap of genetic and psychological factors. Individuals willing to initiate heroin use are often impulsive, and typically see themselves as nonconformists, or risk takers, and in defiance of social convention. Their use of heroin is not surprising given the illegality of heroin and the commonly acknowledged social deviation associated with intravenous drug use. The National Epidemiologic Survey on Alcohol and Related Conditions study showed strong associations between drug use disorders, other substance use disorders, and antisocial personality disorder.[30] The authors suggested that this association is related to the unique genetic factors that underlie these groups of disorders.

As compared with earlier national epidemiologic surveys, the National Epidemiologic Survey on Alcohol and Related Conditions provided more specific information on opiate dependence and other co-occurring psychiatric and substance use disorders. Individuals identified in the National Epidemiologic Survey on Alcohol and Related Conditions who were dependent on one type of prescription medication were highly likely to have clinically significant drug use disorders for both illicit drugs and other classes of nonmedical prescription drugs. There was a high comorbidity for mood, anxiety, personality, and other substance use disorders, including nicotine and alcohol. The specific odds ratios for comorbidity between opioid use disorders and other conditions were other nonmedical prescription drug use disorder (80.1), other illicit drug use disorder (28.1), alcohol use disorder (11.4), nicotine dependence (6.7), any mood disorder (4.6), bipolar I disorder (4.9), any anxiety disorder (3.0), panic with agoraphobia (4.3), any personality disorder (4.9), and antisocial personality disorder (8.1). These conditions were all diagnosed according to the criteria of the DSM-IV, which required the criteria of clinical significance and ruled out conditions considered to be substance-induced.[62]

Co-occurring Psychiatric Disorders and the New Opioid-Dependent Population

Recent studies suggest that some features of psychiatric comorbidity and opioid use disorder have changed during the last decade. The availability of cheap, high-quality heroin has meant that most initiates begin by snorting the drug; some become addicted yet never progress to intravenous use. Members of this group minimize the risk of nonintravenous drug use. They see snorting heroin as relatively socially acceptable and do not see themselves as socially deviant (and indeed are probably less antisocial than earlier generations of heroin users). Similarly, misusers of pain relievers are even less likely to see their behavior as dangerous or antisocial (they naively assume that legal drugs are both safe and less likely to lead to addiction). Data from the 2015 National Survey on Drug Use and Health showed that more than 53.7% of the misusers of pain relievers were given the drug for free or bought or took the drug from friends or relatives; less than 4.9% purchase from drug dealers[158] (Fig. 25.9).

This type of distribution system reinforces the perception that the illicit use of these drugs is normative. It is only after these individuals become physically dependent and have escalating habits that they are forced to seek out illicit suppliers. At some point they may recognize that heroin is cheaper than opioid pharmaceuticals and they may then switch to snorting and/or intravenous heroin use. As the severity of their opioid dependence progresses, they are also likely to manifest symptoms of a substance-induced personality disorder, with both dependent and antisocial features. Such substance-induced antisocial traits typically resolve when these individuals become engaged in addiction treatment, but they may reappear during periods of relapse.

Iatrogenic Addiction

There is a growing and less well-defined group of individuals who may present with iatrogenic opioid use disorder. Since the mid-1990s, careless and overenthusiastic prescribing of highly potent opioid analgesics has placed many individuals at increased risk for addiction. Of particular concern are veterans returning from combat in Iraq and Afghanistan who may have both combat stress and physical injuries requiring treatment with potent opioids. Comparison of individuals who misuse prescription opioids and individuals who misuse heroin shows higher levels of chronic pain, depression, and benzodiazepine use among those who misuse prescription opioids.[13,105] They are also less likely to use illicit nonopioid drugs or to inject drugs.[147] As compared with individuals with heroin use disorder, this group is more likely to have had psychiatric treatment, yet they have fewer family problems, are more socially stable, and have fewer illegal sources of income.[13,28] They also tend to resist referrals for methadone maintenance and are likely better candidates for naltrexone treatment or office-based buprenorphine treatment.[43]

The misuse of other substances is also less common in this population as compared with individuals who misuse heroin.[147] Alcohol misuse has been a longstanding problem among individuals on methadone maintenance. Marijuana use is also very common, although clinicians have disagreed over the clinical significance of this behavior. During the 1980s, cocaine misuse became rampant among those who misuse opioids. Although this problem has declined in the general population, it remains epidemic in individuals with heroin use disorder. The concurrent misuse of all of these substances continues to be a problem among those on methadone maintenance; however, clinicians report less-frequent problems of this type in clients treated with buprenorphine in the office-based setting. Dobler-Mikola et al. reported on the first 6 months of methadone maintenance treatment for 103 participants and noted that 51% continued to use cocaine and 61% continued to use heroin.[38] In contrast, Mintzer et al. reported that 54% of Suboxone recipients at 6 months had no urine tests that were positive for illicit substances.[102] In a separate study, Fiellin et al. reported that the self-reported frequency of

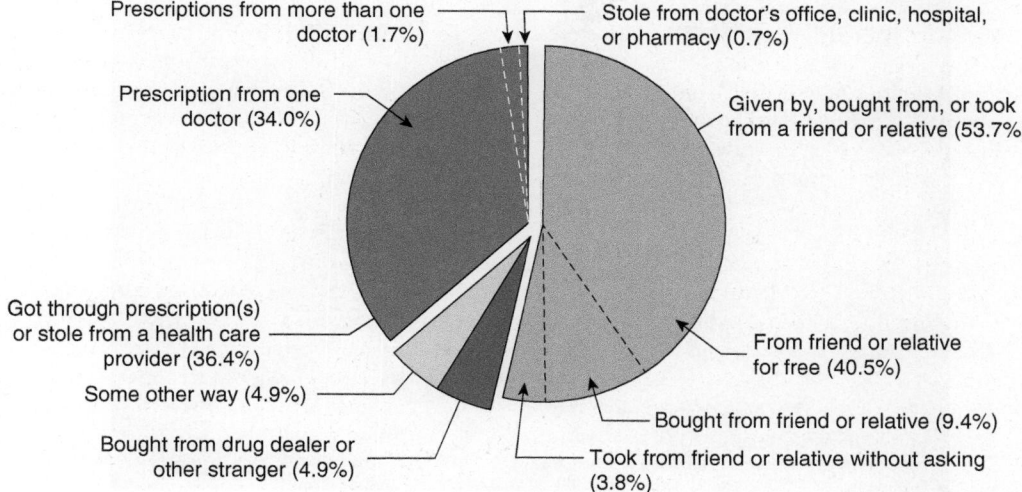

• **Fig. 25.9** Source where pain relievers were obtained for most recent misuse among people 12 years of age or older who misused prescription pain relievers in the past year: Percentages, 2015. (From the National Survey on Drug Use and Health, Figure 24.[158])

opiate use dropped from 5.3 days per week to 0.4 days per week during a 6-month buprenorphine maintenance trial; 50%–57% of the participants had at least one cocaine-positive urine test during the 6-month trial.[44]

The demographics of this new population with opioid use disorder are more apparent in individuals being treated with buprenorphine. The Substance Abuse and Mental Health Services Administration was required by the legislation (Drug Addiction Treatment Act of 2000) that authorized the office-based use of buprenorphine to complete a national survey reviewing demographic data on buprenorphine recipients who were being treated in that setting. As compared with individuals on methadone, this study indicated that buprenorphine recipients were younger, included higher percentages of whites and women, and were far more likely to be employed and have higher levels of education (Fig. 25.10).[158]

Clinicians have generally reported that these clients are less deteriorated, appear much less socially deviant, and are more typical of the general population. On average, addicted individuals enter buprenorphine maintenance treatment 5 years earlier than methadone maintenance clients enter treatment. They are significantly less likely to have used needles and consequently have a much lower incidence of hepatitis C and HIV disease.

Clinical Management

Opiate Overdose

Opiate overdose is a life-threatening emergency. Patients typically present with depressed consciousness, depressed respirations, and miotic pupils. With meperidine (Demerol) overdoses, the pupils may not be miotic. Similarly, with severe hypoxia or in overdoses with multiple classes of drugs, the pupils may be dilated. It is also common to see hypotension and diminished heart rate and occasionally pulmonary edema. The patient should be checked for venous sclerosis (track marks), but these may be missing in younger individuals who may be taking prescription medications orally or may be inhaling or smoking heroin. A drug overdose should be suspected in any comatose individual, and serum toxicology and blood glucose should be obtained immediately.

The primary goal of treatment is to sustain or restore vital functions and to immediately reverse the overdose with an opioid antagonist.

1. Immediately assess the adequacy of airway, breathing, and circulation (ABC). Initiate intubation and resuscitation, and support vital functions as needed. Signs of overdose include slow or shallow breathing, loud snoring or gasping for air, cyanotic skin, bradycardia, and unresponsiveness to sternal rub. If there is no evidence of respirations, and the individual is not in a medical setting, activate emergency medical services (EMS) by calling 911.
2. Establish an intravenous line and administer a 50% dextrose/water solution.
3. In cases of suspected recent oral drug ingestion, gastric lavage should be initiated. Care must be taken to avoid aspiration; patients should be intubated if there is evidence of respiratory depression.
4. Naloxone (Narcan) 0.2–0.4 mg intravenously will begin to reverse the effects of an opiate overdose within 1 minute. If there is no response to the initial dose, repeat doses may be administered every 2–3 minutes. If there is no response after a total dose of 10 mg naloxone, it can be assumed that the coma is not solely caused by an opiate. However, data from fentanyl overdoses appear to indicate that even higher doses of naloxone may be needed to reverse the overdose. Nevertheless, the patient should then be evaluated for other causes of coma, including the ingestion of other drugs, trauma, and diabetic coma. If not in a medical setting, naloxone rescue kits can also be used by lay people. Traditionally, naloxone kits required assembly by the person administering the dose, but more recently the FDA has approved both an intramuscular

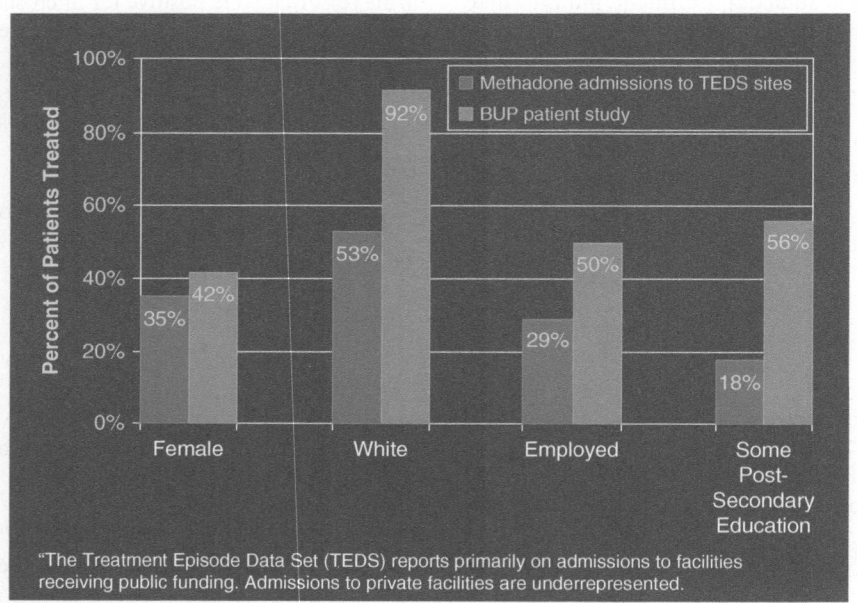

• **Fig. 25.10** Methadone recipients* and buprenorphine (BUP) recipients study sample: demographic differences.

injector (Evzio Auto-Injector) and a nasal spray (Narcan Nasal Spray). Neither of the new kits require any assembly, and both come with instructions for lay people.

5. All overdose patients should be hospitalized and monitored for a minimum of 24 h, particularly if an ingestion of multiple drugs is suspected.

6. Patients who have overdosed on long-acting opioids such as methadone or propoxyphene need to be monitored for 24–48 h. Since the antagonist effects of naloxone will last for only 30–90 minutes, such patients should be monitored in an intensive care unit and placed on an intravenous naloxone drip.

7. Patients who present with symptoms of interstitial pneumonia, pulmonary congestion, or edema should be treated with oxygen, and with intubation and assisted ventilation if required. In these circumstances, cardiac function is normal and there is no change in heart size. Treatment with diuretics and digitalis will be ineffective and should be avoided.

8. Any overdose patient should have a psychiatric evaluation and should be referred for treatment for a substance use disorder. Physicians need to stress the importance of further treatment and to strongly encourage attempts to curb or eliminate further drug use. Whenever possible, opiate overdose kits containing intranasal naloxone or the intramuscular injector and instructions for managing overdoses should be provided to all drug-abusing individuals and their friends and families.

Opiate Withdrawal Syndromes

The withdrawal syndrome for short-acting opiates (heroin or morphine) begins 6–12 h after the last use. Early symptoms include opiate craving, anorexia, anxiety, and irritability. These are coupled with clinical signs of increased respirations and blood pressure, sweating and yawning, lacrimation, rhinorrhea, piloerection (gooseflesh), tremor, and dilated pupils. After 48–72 h, the symptoms progress to include nausea, vomiting, diarrhea, insomnia, tachycardia, abdominal cramps, and involuntary muscle spasms and limb movements. Observable signs subside over 5–7 days, but a prolonged state of craving, depression, irritability, and dysphoria may persist for months.

The signs and symptoms associated with withdrawal from longacting opioids such as methadone or propoxyphene are similar to those described above, but they may not begin until 24–48 h after the last dose and may last for 3 weeks or more. Individuals tapering from methadone maintenance also complain of deep bone pain that may last for weeks. As with individuals who are withdrawing from short-acting opiates, there is a similar protracted withdrawal state. Buprenorphine has a withdrawal syndrome similar to other long-acting opioids, but it is usually less intense and of shorter duration (see Fig. 25.5).[80]

Opiate Withdrawal Treatment

Similar to the treatment of other withdrawal syndromes, the primary objective is to substitute the short-acting drug to which the patient is dependent with a longer-acting drug in the same class and gradually taper at a rate that prevents severe withdrawal and avoids intoxication or excessive sedation. The preferred medications for opiate withdrawal treatment are oral methadone and sublingual buprenorphine.[78,127] Clinical experience suggests that methadone is preferred for less-motivated individuals with larger opiate habits, or for individuals with histories of polydrug abuse

or significant psychiatric comorbidity. Buprenorphine is preferred for highly motivated individuals with smaller habits. In circumstances where opioids are not available, the alpha-adrenergic agonist clonidine may be substituted. Clonidine moderates autonomic withdrawal symptoms but does not control insomnia, restlessness, craving, or dysphoria. In combination with methadone, it may permit more rapid withdrawal treatment with lower doses of opioids. However, clonidine alone is not an adequate treatment for the withdrawal syndrome. Addicts rarely prefer clonidine, and relapse rates are higher than those seen with other medications.[49]

Before starting withdrawal medication, the client should have a thorough physical with urine toxicology and a complete drug and medical history. Except in those patients who are currently on medication-assisted treatment with either methadone or buprenorphine, it is almost impossible to accurately estimate the person's level of physical dependence. Clients' reports are often misleading, and it is highly dangerous to estimate the quality and quantity of street drugs. Even when clients are transferred from maintenance programs, the clinician must always contact program staff to verify the dose before starting treatment. The only safe way to avoid an inadvertent overdose is to document the presence of mild opiate withdrawal before initiating treatment. This is best done using a standard opiate withdrawal scale such as the Clinical Opiate Withdrawal Scale or the Objective Opiate Withdrawal Scale.[56,168] Once clients score in the mild to moderate withdrawal range on the Clinical Opiate Withdrawal Scale, they can be given an initial dose of 20 mg methadone orally or 4 mg buprenorphine sublingually.

For younger individuals with minimal habits, it is prudent to start with 10 mg methadone or 2 mg buprenorphine. Clients should be periodically monitored with a withdrawal scale and can be redosed in 2–4 h if withdrawal symptoms do not subside. If 10–20 mg methadone was effective as an initial dose, it may be repeated in 12 h if necessary. In no circumstance should the total 24-h dose exceed 40 mg methadone or 12 mg buprenorphine. If symptoms progress on the second treatment day, the total daily dose may be increased to 60 mg methadone or 16 mg buprenorphine, but doses in this range are rarely necessary in inpatient settings. Once symptoms are adequately controlled, the dose should be tapered at a rate that prevents further withdrawal and minimizes distress. Methadone can be decreased 5 mg/day or a maximum of a 20% dose reduction per day. Inpatient methadone withdrawal treatment can usually be completed in 5–7 days.[127] Buprenorphine can be decreased at the rate of a 50% dose reduction per day, although a more gradual reduction spread over 13 days has a better outcome and was significantly more effective than clonidine.[84] One review compared buprenorphine withdrawal treatment with clonidine and methadone.[49] Compared with clonidine, buprenorphine-treated clients stayed in treatment longer (particular in outpatient withdrawal treatment), had fewer withdrawal symptoms, and were more likely to complete treatment.[88] There was no significant difference in outcome comparing methadone to buprenorphine in severity of withdrawal or completion of treatment, but withdrawal symptoms resolved more quickly in buprenorphine-treated individuals.

Although withdrawal treatment can be accomplished on either an inpatient or an outpatient basis, the best results are seen with very prolonged outpatient tapers, or with a 1- to 2-week inpatient withdrawal treatment followed by long-term residential care. Brief (3- to 4-day) inpatient treatment has a very high relapse rate, averaging 90%–95% within 1 year. Better outcomes are seen with multiyear maintenance treatment followed by gradual outpatient medication taper. Yet, in the best of circumstances, there is an 80% relapse rate within 1 year.[7] Because the fatality rate for active opiate use disorder ranges from 8% to 20% per year, addicts need to understand the risks when withdrawal treatment is not followed by long-term residential treatment.

Other protocols for opiate withdrawal treatment have involved a rapid inpatient clonidine taper combined with a transition to narcotic antagonist treatment utilizing naltrexone or naloxone. Naltrexone is used to precipitate withdrawal, and then increasing doses of clonidine are used to suppress withdrawal symptoms as naltrexone is quickly increased to antagonist maintenance levels.[118,137] Although this approach provides a quick and cost-effective model for withdrawal treatment, there is no evidence that it produces higher levels of long-term abstinence as compared with other treatment approaches.[50] Ultra-rapid withdrawal treatment protocols have been proposed utilizing escalating doses of naltrexone given under general anesthesia or heavy sedation.[14] O'Connor and Kosten reviewed the existing literature on rapid and ultra-rapid withdrawal treatment and concluded that the studies are inadequate because of the small numbers of subjects included, variations in protocols utilized, lack of randomized design and/or control groups, and lack of long-term follow-up.[117] Well-designed, long-term studies are necessary to demonstrate that these procedures have greater efficacy over standard treatment protocols beyond the short-term treatment period.[148] In addition, deaths have been reported during the 16–40 h following ultra-rapid withdrawal treatment[69]; for this reason alone, ultra-rapid withdrawal treatment procedures cannot be recommended.

Other medications have been proposed for opiate withdrawal treatment, but none have been studied adequately. Proposed agents include N-methyl-D-aspartate (NMDA) receptor antagonists, such as dextromethorphan and memantine, and the serotonin type 1A receptor agonist buspirone. Buydens-Branchey et al. compared placebo with a methadone taper versus two dose levels of buspirone. There was no significant difference noted between the subjects treated with a methadone taper and those treated with either buspirone dose.[19]

Opiate Pharmacotherapy

Naltrexone

Naltrexone is a long-acting, competitive mu opioid receptor antagonist with an active metabolite (6-B-naltrexol). It displaces other opioids from the receptor and prevents further opioid binding for approximately 24 h (see Fig. 25.4). Oral naltrexone was approved for the treatment of opioid use disorder in 1984 but had minimal use because of patient compliance issues.[116] With the exception of some physicians in state monitoring programs, most clients would not comply with the medication unless daily administration was monitored by another individual.[141] Extended-release naltrexone (ER-NX) (Vivitrol) is the most recent medication given FDA approval for the treatment of opioid use disorder.[27] ER-NX is administered as a monthly 380 mg injection, thus resolving short-term compliance issues. Long-term blockade of the mu-receptor prevents the reinforcing effects of opioids and leads to gradual extinction of drug seeking and craving. It decreases drug-conditioned cues and minimizes the pathological responses contributing to relapse. Clients report an absence of urges to use opioids. Trials comparing the oral and ER formulations have demonstrated retention in treatment of 50%–70% at

6 months, with ER retention at twice the rate of the oral formulation and the majority of retained clients being abstinent from opioids. FDA approval for the treatment of opioid use disorder was granted in 2010 based on a single randomized, double-blind, placebo-controlled trial in a Russian population with no access to agonist therapy.[85] The relevance of these findings to US clients has been questioned.[31] For treatment with ER-NX to be initiated, clients must be opioid free for 5 to 7 days. Clients are initially given low doses of oral naltrexone to ensure an opioid-free state and to avoid the risk of inducing severe opioid withdrawal with the first injection. Sustaining a drug-free state during this lead-in period is a challenge for some clients and limits the utility of this treatment option. There are no published data comparing the efficacy of methadone to buprenorphine to ER-NX, thus making it difficult to identify the patients most likely to benefit from ER-NX. Clinicians generally recommend ER-NX for younger clients or individuals with shorter and less severe forms of opioid use disorder, clients unwilling to commit to maintenance, or those who have done poorly on methadone or buprenorphine. Some individuals who have been successful on maintenance may see ER-NX as a logical next step in their recovery program. It may also be a treatment option for very highly motivated individuals, professionals in formal monitoring programs, or individuals on parole or recently released from residential or controlled settings. Clinical challenges with ER-NX include difficulty maintaining abstinence during the lead-in phase, overdose risks in individuals who terminate treatment, and management of acute severe pain, which may require an inpatient admission to override the blockade.

Methadone

Methadone was developed as an analgesic during World War II. It is a full agonist at the mu and delta receptors (see Fig. 25.4) and acts as an NMDA antagonist.[54] In 1965, Dole and Nyswander reported its successful use as a maintenance medication for chronic opiate addiction. It is a highly lipophilic, long-acting, and orally effective medication that controls craving and opiate withdrawal with a single daily dose. In company with counseling and other supportive services, up to 70% of addicts are able to eliminate their opiate use.[7,39] Clients demonstrate no euphoria, mental dulling, or motor impairment. Long-term methadone dosing normalizes brain endocrine physiology and reestablishes normal activity along the hypothalamic-pituitary-adrenal axis.[81] Federal regulations limit maintenance treatment to highly regulated methadone clinics, and individuals must document a 1-year history of addiction and a current state of physiologic dependence to qualify for maintenance treatment. Successful treatment requires adequate dosing (60–120 mg daily), strong ancillary services delivered by professionally trained therapists, and long-term, if not indefinite, treatment.[7,20,97,151] Methadone has typical opiate side effects and does not appear to have significant hepatotoxicity.

Methadone should not be started in maintenance clients until opiate withdrawal has been documented, and the starting dose should not exceed 30 mg orally, with a maximum of 40 mg as the total first-day dose. In individuals with significant persistent withdrawal symptoms, the dose may be increased to 50 mg on the second day, but from that point forward, dose increases should be held to a maximum of 10 mg/week. Reports of prolonged QTc waves and torsade de pointes have raised concerns about the safety of methadone, particularly in individuals with histories of cardiac disease or those at doses over 100 mg. Deaths have been reported among individuals being treated for pain when doses were increased rapidly. Because of its long half-life, methadone may quickly accumulate to toxic levels if individuals are not given adequate time to develop tolerance to previous doses. Electrocardiograms should be obtained before starting treatment and should be repeated regularly in patients at risk for cardiac problems. Methadone is metabolized by the cytochrome P450 (CYP)4503A4 system. Drugs that induce that system, such as phenytoin, rifampin, or efavirenz, may reduce methadone levels and precipitate withdrawal. Similarly, drugs that inhibit the CYP4503A4 system, such as cimetidine or the macrolide antibiotics, will increase methadone levels.

Levo-Alpha Acetyl Methadol

Levo-alpha acetyl methadol is an orally effective, long-acting derivative of methadone that has been approved for maintenance treatment. Because of its long half-life, it can be dosed thrice weekly.[111] Despite clinical efficacy,[64] levo-alpha acetyl methadol was never widely accepted by methadone clinics or opiate addicts. It has particular utility in individuals who are rapid metabolizers of methadone and have traditionally been difficult to stabilize on methadone. After the FDA required a black-box warning because of the risk of death associated with prolonged QTc intervals and torsade de pointes, the manufacturer voluntarily withdrew levo-alpha acetyl methadol from the market.

Buprenorphine

Buprenorphine, a partial agonist at the mu-opiate receptor, was approved by the FDA in 2002 for the treatment of opiate dependence. Its effectiveness has been demonstrated in a number of double-blind, placebo-controlled trials.[65,67,90,152] Buprenorphine is available in a sublingual formulation, either alone (Subutex) or in a combination formulation with naloxone (Bunavail, Suboxone, and Zubsolv), and as 6 month implants (Probuphine). As a partial opiate agonist, it binds tightly to opiate receptors but does not fully activate the receptor. Because of this ceiling effect, there is no significant respiratory depression regardless of the dose of buprenorphine ingested (see Fig. 25.4). For this reason, it has been recognized as an unusually safe opioid. This property, coupled with a slow onset of action and the combination formulation with naloxone (to reduce the illicit intravenous use of the medication), was thought to limit the misuse potential of the medication. Both the FDA and the Drug Enforcement Administration approved its use in office-based settings, without the regulatory limitations placed on methadone maintenance treatment. The introduction of office-based buprenorphine treatment has been a major public health success.[158] As anticipated, the availability of maintenance treatment in private office settings has attracted a large population of addicted but higher-functioning individuals. There are currently over 600,000 individuals receiving office-based buprenorphine treatment in the United States, and an additional 12,500 receiving buprenorphine in opioid treatment programs, compared with 350,000 individuals on methadone maintenance. Individuals are attracted to the greater flexibility of office-based treatment and to the lesser intensity and shorter duration of withdrawal symptoms with buprenorphine as compared with methadone. It should be noted, however, that there is no evidence that buprenorphine withdrawal treatment is associated with any less of a long-term relapse rate than is seen with methadone. It is critical that all maintenance clients be engaged in individual or group counseling and/or 12-step programs. Pharmacotherapy without ancillary services is rarely effective.[53,97,107]

Federal regulations limit practitioners of office-based buprenorphine treatment to an initial limit of 30 active clients and require a waiver for a second Drug Enforcement Administration number based on American Board of Psychiatry and Neurology certification in addiction psychiatry, certification in addiction medicine by the American Society of Addiction Medicine or the American Osteopathic Association, or completion of an 8-h training course. After holding a waiver for 1 year, clinicians may apply for an increase to treat up to 100 clients. In 2016, the Substance Abuse and Mental Health Services Administration revised regulations to permit clinicians to apply for an increased waiver limit of 275 clients after 1 year at the 100 client limit. Nurse practitioners and physician assistants are now also permitted to apply for the waiver, but must complete 24 h of training. To qualify for treatment, clients must be at least 16 years old and must meet DSM-5 criteria for opiate use disorder, moderate or severe. In comparison with methadone, this permits the treatment of younger people with short addiction histories. These individuals are more likely to primarily misuse pain relievers, not heroin, and many have never misused intravenous drugs. As a group, they are less likely to be HIV positive, to have hepatitis C, or to have criminal records, and are more likely to be employed and to have had some college education. Clinicians have reported that most of their buprenorphine recipients are highly motivated and respond very positively to treatment.[107,157]

Treatment initiation with buprenorphine requires careful attention to its antagonist-like properties. Because of its high affinity for the opiate receptor, buprenorphine will displace most other agonists. However, as a partial agonist, it does not fully activate the receptor. The net result is that the addict experiences this action as an antagonist effect. Severe but relatively brief withdrawal may be precipitated whenever buprenorphine is taken in the presence of a full agonist. To initiate buprenorphine treatment successfully, the clinician must therefore determine that the client is currently opiate free. This is best done by counseling the client to abstain from opiates for at least 24 h and by documenting the presence of opiate withdrawal using withdrawal scales such as the Clinical Opiate Withdrawal Scale. Once the individual demonstrates mild to moderate withdrawal on the Clinical Opiate Withdrawal Scale, he or she may safely take the first buprenorphine dose. It is recommended that an initial dose of 4 mg sublingually be given under observation in the clinician's office and that the client be observed for an additional 2 h to ensure that there is no precipitated withdrawal. Supplemental doses can be given if withdrawal symptoms persist, with a maximum recommended first-day dose of 8 mg. The dose can be raised in 2- to 4-mg increments over the next 2–3 days to a dose that eliminates any further withdrawal symptoms and craving. The usual maintenance dose ranges between 12 and 16 mg sublingually daily. Urine samples should be monitored regularly. Higher doses should be considered if craving and opiate use do not cease within 1–3 weeks. Because of the ceiling effect, there is no pharmacological justification for daily doses over 32 mg. The implant formulation was approved in 2016 and is recommended only for patients who have previously established stable recovery on a sublingual buprenorphine/naloxone dose of 8 mg/2 mg.[89]

Novel Anticraving Medications

Although agonist replacement and antagonist treatments have demonstrated efficacy in reducing craving for opiates, other pharmacologic agents have also been investigated. Only a small number of studies have been conducted with these medications, and further studies are needed to determine their efficacy. A 12-week randomized, placebo-controlled trial showed that baclofen recipients remained in treatment longer, but baclofen did not reduce the rate of opioid-positive urine samples.[6] In a small trial, pentazocine-dependent individuals were given either naltrexone alone or gabapentin and naltrexone. Participants given gabapentin and naltrexone reported less craving during and shortly after withdrawal treatment than those given naltrexone alone.[86] In another small, 12-week trial, methadone maintenance participants who were given magnesium had fewer urine samples that tested positive for opiates than those given placebo.[95] Although topiramate has been investigated for its use in withdrawal treatment,[173,174] there are no trials to date that have tested its efficacy in reducing craving for opiates.

Psychosocial Treatment

A variety of psychosocial treatments have been used to treat substance use disorders. Although pharmacotherapy is an important component of treatment, nonpharmacological strategies remain crucial for the overall success of treatment. Although most of these treatments are not specific to opiate use disorder, this section will review the psychosocial treatments in common use.

Outpatient Drug-Free Programs (Postmedication Withdrawal Treatment)

A variety of individual and group psychotherapies may be very helpful in modifying clients' behaviors and lifestyles. Commonly used individual psychotherapies include cognitive behavioral therapy, contingency management, motivational enhancement therapy, and 12-step facilitation. In addition, various group therapies are also frequently utilized, including family therapy and intensive outpatient group treatment.

Relatively few randomized trials have been conducted to examine the effects of psychosocial treatments for opiate dependence in the outpatient drug-free postdetoxification setting. Nevertheless, a recent meta-analysis of controlled trials for psychosocial treatments concluded that contingency management and cognitive behavioral therapy for opiate dependence produced effect sizes that are low-moderate to high-moderate, comparable to the effect size of pharmacologic treatment for anxiety disorders.[40]

Cognitive behavioral treatments are among the most frequently employed interventions that are empirically tested across a broad range of substances, including opiates.[22] Cognitive behavioral therapy attempts to help clients learn the various feelings, thoughts, behaviors, and situations that raise the likelihood of drug use, and to help them cope more effectively with negative emotional states. Individuals are also taught to avoid triggers and situations that promote drug use. Typically, cognitive behavioral therapy approaches place an emphasis on functional analysis of drug use as well as skills training.[22] Several studies have reported positive results utilizing cognitive behavioral therapy, but not in a drug-free context.[9,87,132] A recent study also showed positive results with exposure therapy in a drug-free setting, a behavioral technique aimed at reducing cue reactivity by exposing abstinent individuals to drug-related cues while preventing their conditioned responses.[96] Community reinforcement approaches, also based on operant conditioning theory, have been shown to be helpful for clients on methadone maintenance treatment, who have been shown to reduce their use of illicit opiates if given alternate reinforcers—that is, take-home methadone.[1,150]

Contingency management is a generic behavioral intervention based on the principles of operant conditioning, using primarily positive reinforcements to promote abstinence.[60] A common strategy involves the use of a voucher that can be used to purchase retail items in the community if therapeutic goals are met—that is, negative urine toxicology results.[139] There are two randomized trials to date that have shown positive results when contingency management is used in conjunction with naltrexone.[23,24] One study examined voucher reinforcement for heroin and cocaine users in an outpatient drug-free program but did not show any significant difference with the no-voucher group.[68] This finding is consistent with those of other studies that have found an increased likelihood of negative results when treating individuals with polysubstance use disorder.[40] A meta-analysis examining all the studies that utilized voucher-based reinforcement therapy or related monetary-based incentives to treat substance use disorders concluded that overall voucher-based treatments were superior to control treatments.[92]

Motivational enhancement interventions include the various strategies that attempt to increase clients' motivation to change their drug use, reduce ambivalence, and increase commitment to abstinence.[37] This approach uses the stages of change model to help identify where clients are in the recovery process and to help them progress more rapidly. Motivational interviewing is the most frequently utilized interviewing style that attempts to increase motivation for change.[101] No studies have been conducted for opiate-dependent individuals in a drug-free setting. One study has been conducted with participants in a methadone program, but it did not contain all the components necessary to qualify as motivational enhancement therapy and did not show any reduction in opiate use as compared with controls.[143]

Twelve-step facilitation is a manualized, evidence-based treatment with a large research base that can be integrated with other therapies that the client is receiving.[136] It is a technique used to help clients engage in and maximize their response to 12-step meetings. Twelve-step facilitation was initially created for Project MATCH and was shown to be as effective in reducing alcohol use as was motivational enhancement therapy and cognitive behavioral therapy.[112] However, no studies have examined the efficacy of 12-step facilitation specifically for individuals with opioid use disorder in a drug-free setting. Gossop[48] reported that more frequent attenders at 12-step meetings were more likely to be abstinent from opiates and alcohol compared with nonattenders or less frequent attenders, but the study was not designed to determine whether attendance had a causal effect on abstinence or was simply a characteristic of more successful clients. A randomized trial of standard outpatient buprenorphine maintenance treatment compared to buprenorphine with intensive counseling services reported that 12-step attendance was associated with better 6-month treatment outcomes, but there was no added benefit if 12-step meeting attendance was a required condition of treatment.[106]

Group therapy is the most widely used psychosocial treatment for substance use disorders.[15] Because clients may be less likely to trust clinicians and others in a position of authority, group treatments utilizing family members, peers, and other clients can dilute the negative countertransferences that some clients experience. Groups can be offered in a wide variety of settings (inpatient, outpatient, and residential), target specific populations (such as gay men and lesbians, women with posttraumatic stress disorder, combat veterans, or individuals with bipolar disorder), and can have a variety of theoretical approaches (12-step, cognitive behavioral therapy, and interpersonal). Groups can provide relief from the tremendous shame and isolation that clients experience, as well as provide a safe environment for obtaining support, confirmation, and advice.[15] Furthermore, groups can correct disturbed interpersonal interactions by establishing a healthy and mutually supportive attachment to others.[46] Several studies have examined group therapy for individuals with opiate use disorder in the setting of agonist maintenance treatment (see the subsequent section "Outpatient Treatment in the Setting of Methadone and Buprenorphine Maintenance").

Family therapy includes treatments that involve family members of the client. It is designed to help the family manage and cope with the distress caused by the negative consequences of drug misuse.[120] A particularly well-studied family therapy is behavioral couples therapy, which is designed for married or cohabiting couples.[119] This treatment works to promote a cohesive relationship and better communication with family members, which in turn can lower the risk of relapse.

McLellan et al. have defined intensive outpatient programs as programs that offer at least 9 h/week of structured programming and partial hospital programs as programs that offer at least 20 h of services per week.[97] In one study, compared with individuals in traditional outpatient treatment, which offers no more than 4 h of programming per week, clients in intensive programs received more addiction-focused treatment but fewer medical and employment-focused services. At 6-month follow-up, both groups had notable improvements in substance misuse, health, and social functioning.[97] In another study, graduates from an intensive program were more likely to be abstinent from drugs at the 6-month follow-up and less likely to be incarcerated than those who did not complete the program.[165]

Drug Courts

Drug courts are being utilized increasingly to offer treatment in place of incarceration.[138] Standard features of drug courts include regular and close monitoring of progress by the judicial officer, urine drug testing, coordinated aftercare plans, and dismissal or reduction of charges upon successful completion of treatment.[138] Although not specific to individuals with an opioid use disorder, an extensive meta-analysis revealed that drug court participants had lower re-arrest and conviction rates than those who did not participate.[160]

Outpatient Treatment in the Setting of Methadone and Buprenorphine Maintenance

Individuals maintained on methadone or buprenorphine clearly benefit from additional psychosocial interventions. In a study by Woody and colleagues, methadone maintenance clients who received professional treatment (cognitive or supportive-expressive therapy) showed greater improvements than those individuals who received only drug counseling.[170] The greater benefit was found to be sustained at the 12-month follow-up, and similar results were replicated in a community sample.[171] A recent meta-analysis of psychosocial treatments combined with agonist maintenance treatment concluded that the addition of psychosocial support to standard methadone maintenance treatment significantly reduces the misuse of heroin during treatment.[2]

A number of studies have investigated the value of psychosocial treatment added to standard buprenorphine maintenance. One study specifically tested the benefit of cognitive behavioral therapy combined with buprenorphine maintenance treatment.[107] Although the participants were dually dependent on cocaine and opiates, those who attended more therapy sessions had significantly more negative urine toxicology results for opiates and cocaine. Although the study duration was only 70 days, the results appeared to support previous data that showed beneficial effects of buprenorphine and cognitive behavioral therapy for maintenance clients.[67] Kakko et al.[67] compared buprenorphine maintenance with placebo; all subjects received weekly group cognitive behavioral therapy and weekly individual counseling. One-year retention in treatment was 75% in the buprenorphine group and 0% in the placebo group. Although not the primary hypothesis of the study, these results suggest that 6 days of medication treatment followed by placebo coupled with cognitive behavioral therapy and individual counseling was a very ineffective treatment for chronic opioid dependence.[67] In another study, standard methadone maintenance treatment was compared with methadone maintenance plus weekly group therapy. At 6 months, the group therapy clients had significantly less drug use than the control group.[144]

Two randomized trials of buprenorphine treatment failed to show the benefit of cognitive behavioral therapy above and beyond medical management. In the study by Fiellin and colleagues, 141 opioid-dependent primary care patients receiving buprenorphine were randomized to physician management or physician management plus cognitive behavioral therapy. At 24 weeks, similar results in opioid outcomes were reported.[42] Similar to cognitive behavioral therapy, contingency management in conjunction with buprenorphine treatment has led to mixed results. In a study of 202 opioid-dependent patients receiving buprenorphine, patients were randomized to receive concurrent cognitive behavioral therapy, contingency management, both, or neither. No differences in opioid use was found among the four treatment groups.[91] At present, no conclusive evidence exists that adding either cognitive behavioral therapy or contingency management will improve opioid-use outcomes when added to buprenorphine provided with standard medical management. Finally, in a study of 653 patients with prescription opioid dependence treated with buprenorphine, those randomized to receiving medical management alone had opioid misuse outcomes similar to those randomized to receiving medical management and manualized drug counseling.[166] These findings highlight the importance of individualizing treatment with close physician monitoring and ensuring the availability of additional psychosocial interventions for patients who request them.

Therapeutic Communities

Therapeutic communities for substance use disorders are based both in the community and in prisons and include a variety of short- and long-term residential and ambulatory programs that provide medical, mental health, vocational, educational, family counseling, legal, and administrative services.[34] The general goal of therapeutic communities is to promote abstinence, change antisocial behaviors, and develop prosocial attitudes and skills by living together with others in a structured environment.[172] Features that differentiate therapeutic communities from other residential treatments are their coordination of a comprehensive range of treatment services in one setting, use of the community itself as the therapist and teacher, and a view that holds that the individual, not the drug, is the essence of the disorder.[34] Another element of therapeutic communities is the encounter, a variety of peer-led supportive/confrontational sessions aimed at giving members feedback from others on whether they are meeting community expectations of recovery.[34]

A recent meta-analysis examining the efficacy of therapeutic communities showed that there is little evidence that therapeutic communities offer significant benefits compared with other residential treatments, or that one type of therapeutic community is better than another.[149] However, the authors also acknowledged that the analysis may be biased and that firm conclusions cannot be drawn.

Therapeutic communities have been utilized frequently in correctional facilities.[169] One meta-analysis demonstrated that prisoners with substance use disorders treated in therapeutic community programs have lower recidivism rates compared with those without treatment.[124] Another study examined prison-based psychosocial treatments and reached a similar conclusion.[103] Optimal results were seen when inmates participated in prison-based therapeutic communities that were followed by community-based aftercare.[61,93]

Conclusions Regarding Psychosocial Treatment

Although relatively few studies have been conducted exclusively with individuals with opioid use disorders, the psychosocial therapies described have been shown to be effective in this population and are critical in the overall treatment of addiction. A wide variety of these treatments can be offered to suit the needs of individual clients. Although no one psychosocial intervention has been shown to be superior to another, the evidence taken as a whole favors incorporating psychosocial therapies, with or without pharmacologic treatments. In addition, the efficacy of pharmacologic therapies is clearly improved when combined with psychosocial treatments. Nonetheless, recent investigations of buprenorphine treatment also demonstrate the value of close physician monitoring.

Co-occurring Psychiatric Disorders

The Incidence of Co-occurring Psychiatric Disorders

The incidence of co-occurring psychiatric disorders in individuals with opioid use disorder ranges from 13% to 85% (Table 25.2).[142] The lifetime prevalence for any drug use disorder is 37.5% in individuals with bipolar I disorder.[51] There is also a high lifetime prevalence of posttraumatic stress disorder in patients with substance use disorder, although clients may initially deny a posttraumatic stress disorder history. Individuals with posttraumatic stress disorder may only be willing to discuss this problem after they have developed a more trusting relationship with their clinician. Villagomez et al. reported a lifetime posttraumatic stress disorder prevalence of 20% in women and 11% in men.[161] The prevalence is even higher in adolescents with substance use disorders, with a 24.3% incidence in boys and a 45.3% incidence in girls.[36] Similarly high rates of co-occurring disorders are reported in older methadone clients.[140] These findings indicate that all individuals with opioid use disorder should be screened for other psychiatric disorders on admission. Severe problems such as suicidal or

TABLE 25.2	Lifetime Prevalence in Opioid-Dependent Individuals.	
	Men (%)	Women (%)
Affective disorders	70.7	85.4
Anxiety disorders	13.2	25.4
Phobic disorder	8.2	13.9

Adapted from Rounsaville BJ, Weissman MM, Kleber HD, et al. Heterogeneity of psychiatric diagnosis in treated opiate addicts. *Arch Gen Psychiatry*. 1982;39:161–168.

homicidal ideation, or psychosis, require immediate assessment and consideration for hospitalization. Less severe symptoms of anxiety and depression are very common in individuals entering treatment; many of these symptoms are substance-induced and will clear once the client's substance use is under control. Appropriate diagnosis is difficult when clients are either intoxicated or in withdrawal. The first goal of treatment is, therefore, to stabilize the addiction.

Substance-Induced Disorders Versus Independent Disorders

Once the individual has achieved abstinence or has been stabilized on methadone or buprenorphine, a more comprehensive psychiatric evaluation should be done to determine whether there are any persistent psychiatric symptoms. The first step in this evaluation is to separate substance-induced psychiatric disorders from independent psychiatric disorders. The DSM-5 criteria for a substance-induced disorder require that symptoms occur during, or within 1 month of, intoxication, withdrawal, or taking a substance/medication, and that the substance is thought to be capable of producing the mental disorder. If symptoms persist 1 month beyond substance use, they are presumed to reflect an independent psychiatric disorder.[4] Independent psychiatric disorders are more likely if there is a family history of psychiatric disorders. These symptoms do not diminish with sobriety, and they typically continue with little change during prolonged periods of abstinence. The age at onset for most psychiatric disorders is in the early teens and typically precedes the development of any substance use disorder by 5–10 years. A careful longitudinal history will clarify the sequence of symptoms and will help to separate an independent psychiatric disorder from any substance-induced psychopathology. It is difficult to make this assessment in the presence of active substance use. Unless there is a clear history that confirms the presence of other psychiatric disorders, treatment should focus primarily on the addiction.

Managing Co-occurring Psychiatric Disorders

In the case of co-occurring psychiatric disorders, a more comprehensive treatment plan is required to address both conditions. Treatment is most effective if the psychiatric treatment is integrated into the addiction treatment program. All involved clinicians should work in close collaboration to ensure coordinated care. Treatment elements need to be integrated throughout the entire course of treatment, from assessment, to initial medication withdrawal treatment or maintenance/stabilization, and through aftercare.[18] Clients with a substance use disorder will respond to most standard evidence-based forms of psychiatric treatment, including psychotherapy and pharmacotherapy.[159] However, standard treatments for psychiatric disorders cannot be expected to treat the substance misuse problem. Sobriety from all substances of misuse must remain a primary treatment goal and will require active participation in addiction treatment. Structured psychotherapy approaches are most effective, particularly cognitive behavioral therapy. The seeking safety treatment model developed by Najavits for treating co-occurring posttraumatic stress disorder and substance use disorders is particularly useful for managing addicted individuals with a range of psychopathology.[108]

There are few published data on the treatment of co-occurring depressive disorders in individuals with opioid use disorder; most of the available data come from studies on methadone maintenance clients. In a placebo-controlled trial, Nunes et al. demonstrated efficacy for imipramine in the treatment of depressed methadone maintenance clients.[114] Results with selective serotonin reuptake inhibitors in this population have generally been negative,[126] although two studies reported improvement in depression in methadone recipients using sertraline.[21,55] Kosten et al. failed to demonstrate efficacy for desipramine in the treatment of depressed buprenorphine-maintained subjects, and warned against using this combination of medications.[77]

Although it is common practice to prescribe selective serotonin reuptake inhibitors and other antidepressants to treat anxiety disorders in individuals with substance use disorders,[122] including those maintained on methadone and buprenorphine, there are few data to demonstrate efficacy in this specific population. McRae et al. have demonstrated efficacy for buspirone in the treatment of anxiety disorders in methadone recipients.[98] Short-acting benzodiazepines are typically avoided in this population because of concerns about misuse and toxicity.[11] However, Bleich et al. demonstrated efficacy for the long-acting benzodiazepine, clonazepam, in the treatment of anxiety disorders in methadone recipients with a prior history of benzodiazepine misuse.[10] There has been particular concern about prescribing benzodiazepines for individuals maintained on buprenorphine, related to reports of overdose deaths in France secondary to the intravenous injection of combinations of buprenorphine and high-potency benzodiazepines.[12,75,115] Despite these concerns about the risks of benzodiazepine misuse in opioid addicts, a comprehensive review of the literature has shown efficacy for the treatment of generalized anxiety disorder, panic disorder, and agoraphobia and probable efficacy for social phobia, with little evidence of added risk for medication misuse or increased relapse[130] (also see Osser et al.[122]).

There are relatively few data on the treatment of schizophrenia and co-occurring opioid use disorder. The incidence of schizophrenia is thought to be relatively low in this population, although the Environmental Catchment Area Survey reported a 47% lifetime prevalence for any substance use disorder in this population.[133] Alcohol use disorders are the most common substance use disorders seen. Methadone clinics report a very low incidence of psychosis. In general, individuals with schizophrenia and co-occurring opioid dependence are poorly compliant with medication, do not respond well to typical antipsychotics, and show high rates of relapse and hospitalization. However, this population has responded positively to treatment with the atypical antipsychotics, particularly clozapine. It has been speculated that clozapine (a weak D_2 blocker, but a potent noradrenergic A_2 blocker) may normalize mesolimbic dopamine circuits and thus reduce craving for opiates and other illicit drugs.[52]

When considering pharmacotherapy for any psychiatric disorders, caution is required to avoid the use of abusable medications, especially short-acting benzodiazepines. Treatment should always begin with nonabusable medications with proven efficacy for the specific condition. Clients need to be monitored closely to ensure sobriety and compliance with treatment. Depressed clients can be treated with most of the standard antidepressants. When treating anxiety disorders, attention should be given to psychological therapies and coordinated pharmacotherapy. Benzodiazepines should be used with caution and should not be prescribed unless the individual has failed to respond to adequate trials of antidepressants or buspirone. If required, long-acting benzodiazepines are preferred to the more abusable shorter-acting drugs such as alprazolam. Atypical antipsychotic medications may be particularly effective in this population, although quetiapine should be used with caution because of its misuse potential. Any client who fails to respond to treatment should be monitored closely to ensure medication compliance and to rule out any relapse to substance misuse.

Primary Prevention

For many years, prevention activities in the United States have focused on interdiction and on public education with a primary abstinence message, Just say no. A gradual decline in the misuse of marijuana, cocaine, and heroin[35,63] suggested that this approach may have had a positive impact on the misuse of some illicit substances. However, the recent epidemic of the misuse of prescription pain relievers and a corresponding increase in opioid-related overdose deaths indicate the need to reassess prevention techniques. Young adults, in particular, seem to have interpreted the messages against illicit drugs to imply that licit drugs are safe and nonaddictive. The medical community also underestimated the addictive risks involved in the use of opioids to treat acute and chronic pain. There is clearly a need for a national education campaign to inform the public and physicians about the risks associated with prescription pain relievers and the availability of effective treatment.[30] Physicians have not been well trained in the management of pain or in the safe prescription of potent opioids with long half-lives. In 2008, the Center for Substance Abuse Treatment of the Substance Abuse and Mental Health Services Administration launched a major campaign to improve physician education in these areas. These have been reinforced by recent announcements by the Centers for Disease Control and Prevention and by the office the US Surgeon General. Other efforts are underway to improve medical school curricula and residency training to achieve a better understanding of the addictive disorders and to improve substance use disorder screening and the management of individuals at risk for substance use disorders.[94,109,134] FDA approval of a variety of alcohol anticraving medications and the availability of buprenorphine for the office-based treatment of opioid use disorders have opened a new era for the medical treatment of substance use disorders. Corresponding changes in physician education are necessary if these new treatment options are to achieve their full potential. Physicians and the public need education to destigmatize substance use disorders, and to improve general awareness of the effectiveness of addiction pharmacotherapy and manually guided therapies such as cognitive behavioral therapy, motivational enhancement therapy, and 12-step facilitation.

Epidemiologic evidence has consistently shown that primary psychiatric disorders strongly predict the later development of substance use disorders, with a range of 5–10 years between the onsets of the two conditions. This presents a clear opportunity for primary prevention. Kessler has estimated that the effective early treatment of psychiatric disorders would prevent as much as 50% of all substance use disorders.[72] Needle exchange programs provide another opportunity for the prevention of disease and outreach to opiate abusers. A large percentage of new cases of hepatitis C are a direct result of injection drug users sharing hypodermic needles. To prevent the spread of hepatitis C and HIV, needle exchange programs were developed to provide sterile needles and associated injection supplies at no cost. Sometimes the dirty needles must be exchanged for clean needles. These programs also typically offer a variety of other services, such as "bleach kits," naloxone rescue kits, HIV testing, condoms, and referrals to treatment.

Conclusion

As with other chronic relapsing medical disorders, physicians and other clinicians have important roles to play in long-term treatment approaches that integrate appropriate pharmacotherapy with psychotherapy and self-help interventions. Routine screening, particularly for adolescents and young adults, client education about the risks and benefits of potent pain relievers, conservative management of less severe pain syndromes, and early and aggressive treatment of depression and anxiety disorders all will play a role in reducing the incidence of opioid use disorders. Once patterns of opioid misuse are identified, referrals for treatment, including appropriate pharmacotherapy, and long-term management approaches hold the most promise for successful control and amelioration of the problems associated with opioid use disorder.

References

1. Abbott PJ, Weller SB, Delaney HD, et al. Community reinforcement approach in the treatment of opiate addicts. *Am J Drug Alcohol Abuse.* 1998;24:17–30.
2. Amato L, Minozzi S, Davoli M, et al. Psychosocial combined with agonist maintenance treatments versus agonist maintenance treatments alone for treatment of opioid dependence. *Cochrane Database Syst Rev.* 2004;18(4):CD004147.
3. American Academy of Pain Medicine, American Pain Society, American Society of Addiction Medicine. *Public Policy Statement on the Rights and Responsibilities of Healthcare Professionals in the Use of Opioids for the Treatment of Pain*; 2004. http://www.ampainsoc.org/advocacy/rights.htm.
4. American Psychiatric Association. *Diagnostic and Statistical Manual of Mental Disorders.* 5th ed. Arlington, VA: American Psychiatric Association; 2013.
5. Anthony JC, Warner LA, Kessler RC. Comparative epidemiology of dependence on tobacco, alcohol, controlled substances, and inhalents: basic findings from the national comorbidity survey. *Exp Clin Psychopharmacol.* 1994;3:224–268.
6. Assadi SM, Radgoodarzi R, Ahmed-Abhari SA. Baclofen for maintenance treatment of opioid dependence: a randomized double-blind placebo-controlled clinical trial. *BMC Psychiatry.* 2003;18(3):16.
7. Ball J, Ross A. *The Effectiveness of Methadone Maintenance Treatment.* New York: Springer; 1991.
8. Bart G, Borg L, Schluger JH, et al. Suppressed prolactin response to dynorphin A1–13 in methadone-maintained versus control subjects. *Pharmacol Exp Ther.* 2003;306(2):581–587.
9. Bickel WK, Amass L, Higgins ST, et al. Effects of adding behavioral treatment to opioid detoxification with buprenorphine. *J Consult Clin Psychol.* 1997;65:803–810.
10. Bleich A, Gelkopf M, Weizman T, et al. Benzodiazepine abuse in a methadone maintenance treatment clinic in Israel: characteristics and a pharmacotherapeutic approach. *Isl J Psychiatry Relat Sci.* 2002;39:104–112.
11. Borron SW, Monier C, Risede P, et al. Funitrazepam variably alters morphine, buprenorphine, and methadone lethality in the rat. *Hum Exp Toxicol.* 2002;21:599–605.
12. Boyd J, Randell T, Luurila H, Kuisma M. Serious overdoses involving buprenorphine in Helsinki. *Acta Anaesthesiol Scand.* 2003;47:1031–1033.
13. Brands B, Blake J, Sproule B, et al. Prescription opioid abuse in patients presenting for methadone maintenance treatment. *Drug Alcohol Depend.* 2004;73:199–207.
14. Brewer C. Ultra-rapid antagonist-precipitated opiate detoxification under general anaesthesia or sedation. *Addict Biol.* 1997;2:291–302.
15. Brook DW. Group therapy. In: Galanter M, Kleber HD, eds. *Textbook of Substance Abuse Treatment.* 4th ed. Washington, DC: American Psychiatric Publishing; 2008.
16. Brooner RK, Bigelow GE, Regier MW. Methadone maintenance: high rate of other substance use disorders and relationship to psychiatric comorbidity. *NIDA Res Monogr.* 1989;95:442.
17. Brooner RK, King VL, Kidorf M, et al. Psychiatric and substance use comorbidity among treatment-seeking opioid abusers. *Arch Gen Psychiatry.* 1997;54(1):71–80.
18. Brunette MF, Mueser KT. Psychosocial interventions for the long-term management of patients with severe mental illness and co-occurring substance use disorders. *J Clin Psychiatry.* 2006;67(suppl 7):10–17.
19. Buydens-Branchey L, Branchey M, Reel-Brander C. Efficacy of buspirone in the treatment of opioid withdrawal. *J Clin Psychopharmacol.* 2005;25:230–236.
20. Calsyn DA, Malcy JA, Saxon AJ. Slow tapering from methadone maintenance in a program encouraging indefinite maintenance. *J Subst Abuse Treat.* 2006;30:159–163.
21. Carpenter KM, Brooks AC, Vosburg SK, et al. The effect of sertraline and environmental context on treating depression and illicit substance use among methadone maintained opiate dependent patients: a controlled clinical trial. *Drug Alcohol Depend.* 2004;74:123–134.
22. Carroll KM. Cognitive-behavioral therapies. In: Galanter M, Kleber HD, eds. *Textbook of Substance Abuse Treatment.* 4th ed. Washington, DC: American Psychiatric Publishing; 2008.
23. Carroll KM, Ball SA, Nich C, et al. Targeting behavioral therapies to enhance naltrexone treatment of opioid dependence: efficacy of contingency management and significant other involvement. *Arch Gen Psychiatry.* 2001;58:755–761.
24. Carroll KM, Sinha R, Nich C, et al. Contingency management to enhance naltrexone treatment of opioid dependence: a randomized clinical trial of reinforcement. *Exper Clin Psychopharmacol.* 2002;10:54–63.
25. Chen Y, Mestek A, Liu J, et al. Molecular cloning and functional expression of a mu-opioid receptor from rat brain. *Mol Pharmacol.* 1993;44:8–12.
26. Chen Y, Mestek A, Liu J, et al. Molecular cloning of a rat kappa opioid receptor reveals sequence similarities to mu and delta opioid receptors. *Biochem J.* 1993;295:625–628.
27. Comer SD, Sullivan MA, Yu E, et al. Injectable, sustained-release naltrexone for the treatment of opioid dependence: a randomized, placebo-controlled trial. *Arch Gen Psychiatry.* 2006;63:210–218.
28. Compton WM, Denisco R. Prescription drug abuse. In: Galanter M, Kleber HD, eds. *Textbook of Substance Abuse Treatment.* 4th ed. Washington DC: American Psychiatric Publishing; 2008.
29. Compton WM, Jones CM, Baldwin GT. Relationship between nonmedical prescription-opioid use and heroin use. *N Engl J Med.* 2016;374:154–163.
30. Compton WM, Thomas YF, Stinson FS, et al. Prevalence, correlates, disability, and comorbiduty of DSM-IV drug abuse and dependence in the United States. Results from the national

epidmeiologic survey on alcohol and related conditions. *Arch Gen Psychiatry.* 2007;64:566–576.

31. Connery HS. Medication-assisted treatment of opioid use disorder: review of the evidence and future directions. *Har Rev Psychiatry.* 2015;23(2):63–75.

32. Corbett AD, Henderson G, McKnight AT, et al. 75 years of opioid research: the exciting but vain quest for the Holy Grail. *Br J Pharmacol.* 2006;147(suppl 1):S153–S162.

33. Cowan A. Buprenorphine: the basic pharmacology revisited. *J Addict Med.* 2007;1:68–72.

34. DeLeon G. Therapeutic communities. In: Glanater M, Kleber HD, eds. *Textbook of Substance Abuse Treatment.* 4th ed. Washington, DC: American Psychiatric Publishing; 2008.

35. Department of Health and Human Services, Substance Abuse and Mental Health Services Administration, Office of Applied Studies, Results from the 2006 National Survey on Drug Use and Health. http://oas.samhsa.gov/NSDUH/2k6NSHDUH/2k6results.cfm#Ch5. Accessed 29 June 2008.

36. Deykin EY, Buka SL. Prevalance and risk factors for posttraumatic stress disorder among chemically dependent adolescents. *Am J Psychiatry.* 1997;154(6):752–757.

37. DiClemente CC, Garay M, Gemmell L. Motivational enhancement. In: Galanter M, Kleber HD, eds. *Textbook of Substance Abuse Treatment.* 4th ed. Washington, DC: American Psychiatric Publishing; 2008.

38. Dobler-Mikola A, Hattenschwiler J, Meili D, et al. Patterns of heroin, cocaine, and alcohol abuse during long-term methadone maintenance treatment. *J Subst Abuse Treat.* 2005;29(4):259–265.

39. Dole VP, Nyswander M. A medical treatment for diacetylmorphine (heroin) addiction. A clinical trial with methadone hydrochloride. *JAMA.* 1965;193:646–650.

40. Dutra L, Stathopoulou G, Basden SL, et al. A meta-analytic review of psychosocial interventions for substance use disorders. *Am J Psychiatry.* 2008;165:179–187.

41. Evans CJ, Keith Jr DE, Morrison H, et al. Cloning of a delta-opioid receptor by functional expression. *Science.* 1992;258:1952–1955.

42. Fiellin DA, Barry DT, Sullivan LE, et al. A randomized trial of cognitive behavioral therapy in primary care-based buprenorphine. *Am J Med.* 2013;126(1):74. e11–7.

43. Fiellin DA. Buprenorphine: effective treatment of opioid addiction starts in the office. *Am Fam Physician.* 2006;73:1513–1514.

44. Fiellin DA, Pantalon MV, Chawarski MC, et al. Counseling plus buprenorphine–naloxone maintenance therapy for opioid dependence. *N Eng J Med.* 2006;355(4):365–374.

45. Finley MJ, Happel CM, Kaminsky DE, et al. Opioid and nocicpetin receptors regulate cytokine and cytokine receptor expression. *Cell Imunol.* 2008;252(1–2):146–154.

46. Flores PJ. *Addiction as an Attachment Disorder.* Jason. Lanham, MD: Aronson; 2004.

47. Gelernter J, Panhuysen C, Wilcox M, et al. Genomewide linkage scan for opioid dependence and related traits. *Am J Hum Genet.* 2006;78(5):759–769.

48. Gossop M, Stewart D, Marsden J. Attendance at Narcotics Anonymous and Alcoholics Anonymous meetings, frequency of attendance, substance use outcomes after residential treatment for drug dependence: a 5-year follow-up study. *Addiction.* 2007;103:119–125.

49. Gowing L, Ali R, White J. Buprenorphine for the management of opioid withdrawal (Cochrane review). *Cochrane Database Syst Rev.* 2006;2:CD002025.

50. Gowing L, Ali R, White J. Opioid antagonists with minimal sedation for opioid withdrawal (Cochrane review). *Cochrane Database Syst Rev.* 2006;1:CD002021.

51. Grant BF. Prevalence and correlates of drug use and DSM-IV drug dependence in the United States: results from the National Longitudinal Alcohol Epidemiologic Survey. *J Subst Abuse.* 1996;8:195–21.

52. Green AI, Noordsy DL, Brunette MF, et al. Substance abuse and schizophrenia: pharmacotherapeutic intervention. *J Subst Abuse Treat.* 2008;34(1):61–71.

53. Green MD, Renner JA. Buprenorphine for the management of opioid dependence, feature article. *Essential Psychopharmacol.* 2009;7(3):73–87.

54. Gutstein HB, Akil H. Opioid analgesics. In: Hardman JG, Limbird LL, eds. *Goodman and Gilman's the Pamacologicbasis of Terapetics.* New York: McGraw-Hill; 2001.

55. Hamilton SP, Nunes EV, Janal M, et al. The effect of sertraline on methadone plasma levels in methadone-maintained patients. *Am J Addict.* 2000;9(1):63–69.

56. Handelsman L, Cochrane KJ, Aronson MJ, et al. Two new rating scales for opiate withdrawal. *Am J Alcohol Abuse.* 1987;13:293–308.

57. Hasin DS, Hatzenbueler M, Smith S, et al. Co-occurring DSM-IV drug abuse in DSM-IV drug dependence: results from the national epidemiologic survey on alcohol and related conditions. *Drug Alcohol Depend.* 2005;80(1):117–123.

58. Hasin DS, O'Brien CP, Auriacombe M, et al. DSM-5 criteria for substance use disorders: recommendations and rationale. *Am J Psychiatry.* 2013;170(8):834–851.

59. Hawkinson JE, Acosta-Burruel M, Espita SA. Opioid activity profiles indicate similarities between the nociceptin/orphanin FQ and opioid receptors. *Eur J Pharmacol.* 2000;389(2–2):107–114.

60. Higgins ST, Silverman K. Contingency management. In: Galanter M, Kleber HD, eds. *Textbook of Substance Abuse Treatment.* 4th ed. Washington, DC: American Psychiatric Publishing; 2008.

61. Hiller ML, Knight K, Simpson DD. Prison-based substance abuse treatment, residential aftercare and recidivism. *Addiction.* 1999;94(6):833–842.

62. Huang B, Dawson DA, Stinson FS, et al. Prevalence, correlates, and comorbidty of nonmedical prescription drug use and drug use disorders in the United States: results of the national epidemiologic survey on alcohol and related conditions. *J Clin Psychiatry.* 2006;67:1062–1073.

63. Johnson LD, O'Malley PM, Bachman JG, et al. *Monitoring the Future: National Survey Results on Drug Use; 1975–2004.* Bethesda, MD: National Institute on Drug Abuse; 2005.

64. Johnson RE, Chutuape MA, Strain EC, et al. A comparison of levomethadyl acetate, buprenorphine, and methadone for opioid dependence. *N Eng J Med.* 2000;343:1290–1297.

65. Jones CM, Logan J, Gladden RM, et al. Vital signs: demographic and substance use trends among heroin users – United States, 2002-2013. *MMWR Morb Mortal Wkly Rep.* 2015;64(26):719–725.

66. Joranson DE, Ryan KM, Gilson AM, et al. Trends in medical use and abuse of opioid analgesics. *JAMA.* 2000;283:1710–1714.

67. Kakko J, Svanborg KD, Kreek MJ, et al. 1-year retention and social function after buprenorphine-assisted relapse prevention treatment for heroin dependence in Sweden: a randomized, placebo-controlled trial. *Lancet.* 2003;361(9358):662–668.

68. Katz EC, Chutuape MA, Jones HE, et al. Voucher reinforcement for heroin and cocaine abstinence in an outpatient drug-free program. *Drug Alcohol Depend.* 2002;10(2):136–143.

69. Kaye AD, Gervitz C, Bosscher HA, et al. Ultrarapid opiate detoxification: a review. *Can J Anaesth.* 2003;50:663–671.

70. Keiffer BL, Befort K, Gaveriaux-Ruff C, et al. The delta-opioid receptor: isolation of a cDNA by expression cloning and pharmacological characterization. *Proc Natl Acad Sci USA.* 1992;89:12048–12052. erratum in *Proc Natl Acad Sci USA.* 1994;91:1193.

71. Kessler RC. Epidemiology of psychiatric comorbidity. In: Tsuang MT, Tohen M, Zahner GEP, eds. *Textbook in Psychiatric Epidemiology.* New York: Wiley; 1995.

72. Kessler RC. The epidemiology of dual diagnosis: impact of substance abuse on the diagnosis, course, and treatment of mood disorders. *Biol Psychiatry.* 2004;56:730–737.

73. Kessler RC, McGonagle KA, Zhao S, et al. Lifetime and 12-month prevalence of DSM-III-R psychiatric disorders in the United States:

results from the national comorbidity survey. *Arch Gen Psychiatry.* 1994;51:8–19.

74. Kessler RC, Nelson CB, McGonagle KA, et al. The epidemiology of co-occurring addictive and mental disorders: implications for prevention and service utilization. *Am J Orthopsychiatry.* 1996;66:17–31.

75. Kintz P. A new series of 13 buprenorphine-related deaths. *Clin Biochem.* 2002;35:513–516.

76. Kling MA, Carson RE, Borg L, et al. Opioid receptor imaging with PET and [(18)F] cyclofoxy in long-term methadone-treated former heroin addicts. *J Pharmacol Exp Ther.* 2000;295:1070–1076.

77. Kosten T, Falcioni, Oliveto A, Feingold A. Depression predicts higher rates of heroin use on desipramine with buprenorphine than with methadone. *Am J Addict.* 2004;13:191–201.

78. Kosten TR, Kleber HD. Buprenorphine detoxification from opioid dependence: a pilot study. *Life Sci.* 1988;42:635–671.

79. Kosten TR, Morgan C, Kreek MJ. Beta endorphine levels during heroin, methadone, buprenorphine, and naloxone challenges: preliminary findings. *Biol Psychiatry.* 1992;32:523–528.

80. Kosten TR, O'Connor PG. Management of drug and alcohol withdrawal. *N Engl J Med.* 2003;348:1786–1795.

81. Kreek MJ. Neurobiology of opiates and opioids. In: Galanter M, Kleber HD, eds. *Textbook of Substance Abuse Treatment.* 4th ed. Washington, DC: American Psychiatric Publishing; 2008.

82. Kreek MJ, Ragunath J, Plevy S, et al. ACTH, cortical and beta-endorphin response to metyrapone testing during chronic methadone maintenance treatment in humans. *Neuropeptides.* 1984;5:277–278.

83. Kreek MJ, Schluger J, Borg L, et al. Dynorphin A1–13 causes elevation of serum levels of prolactin through an opioid receptor mechanism in humans: gender differences and implications for modulations of dopaminergic tone in the treatment of addictions. *J Pharmacol Exp Ther.* 1999;288:260–269.

84. Kreek MJ, Wardlaw SL, Hartman N, et al. Circadian rhythms and levels of beta-endorphin, ACTH, and cortisol during chronic methadone maintenance treatment in humans. *Life Sci.* 1983;33(suppl 1):409–411.

85. Krupitsky E, Nunes EV, Ling W, et al. Injectible extended-release naltrexone for opioid dependence: a double-blind, placebo-controlled, multicenter randomized trial. *Lancet.* 2011;377:1506–1513.

86. Kumar P, Jain MK. Gabapentin in the management of pentazocine dependence: a potent analgesic-anticraving agent. *J Assoc Physicians India.* 2003;51:673–676.

87. Linehan MM, Dimeff LA, Reynolds SK, et al. Dialectal behavior therapy versus comprehensive validation therapy plus 12-step for the treatment of opioid dependent women meeting criteria for borderline personality disorder. *Drug Alcohol Depend.* 2002;67:13–26.

88. Ling W, Amass L, Shoptaw S, et al. A multi-center randomized trial of buprenorphine-naloxone versus clonidine for opioid detoxification: findings from the national institute on drug abuse clinical trials network. *Addiction.* 2005;100(8):1090–1100.

89. Ling W, Casadonte P, Kampman KM, et al. Buprenorphine implants for treatment of opioid dependence: a randomized controlled trial. *JAMA.* 2010;304(4):1576–1583.

90. Ling W, Charuvastra C, Collins JF, et al. Buprenorphine maintenance treatment of opiate dependence: a multicenter, randomized clinical trial. *Addiction.* 1998;93:475–486.

91. Ling W, Hillhouse M, Ang A, et al. Comparison of behavioral treatment conditions in buoprenorphine maintenance. *Addiction.* 2013;108(10):1788–1798.

92. Lussier JP, Heil SH, Mongeon JA, et al. A meta-analysis of voucher-based reinforcement therapy for substance use disorders. *Addiction.* 2006;101(2):192–203.

93. MacKenzie DL. *What Works in Corrections: Reduciing the Criminal Activities of Offenders and Delinquents.* New York: Cambridge University; 2006.

94. Madras B. *Screening, Brief Intervention, Referral and Treatment (SBIRT) Abstract #164901. 5.* Washington, DC: American Public Health Association 135th Annual Meeting; 2007.

95. Margolin A, Kantak K, Copenhaver M, et al. A preliminary, controlled investigation of magnesium L-aspartate hydrochloride for illicit cocaine and opiate use in methadone-maintained patients. *J Addict Dis.* 2003;22(2):49–61.

96. Marissen MAE, Franken IH, Blanken P, et al. Cue exposure therapy for the treatment of opiate addiction: results of a randomized controlled clinical trial. *Psychother Psychosom.* 2007;76:97–105.

97. McLellan AT, Hagan TA, Meyers K, et al. "Intensive" outpatient substance abuse treatment: comparisons with "traditional" outpatient treatment. *J Addict Dis.* 1997;16(2):57–84.

98. McRae AL, Sonne SC, Brady KT, et al. A randomized, placebo-controlled trial of buspirone for the treatment of anxiety in opioid-dependent individuals. *Am J Addict.* 2004;13:53–63.

99. Medina JL, Diamond S. Drug dependency in patients with chronic headaches. *Headache.* 1997;17(1):12–14.

100. Meier B. *Pain killer.* New York: Rodale, St Martin's; 2003.

101. Miller WR, Rollnick S. *Motivational Interviewing: Preparing People for Change.* 2nd ed. New York: Guilford; 2002.

102. Mintzer IL, Eisenberg M, Terra M, et al. Treating opioid addiction with buprenorphine-naloxone in community-based primary care settings. *Ann Fam Med.* 2007;5(2):146–150.

103. Mitchell O, MacKenzie DL, Wilson DB. *The Effectiveness of Incarceration-Based Drug Treatment on Criminal Behavior.* Paper approved by the campbell collaboration, criminal justice review group; 2006. http://www.campbellcollaboration.org/doc-pdf/Incarceration-BasedDrugTxSept06final.pdf. Accessed 31 May 2010.

104. Mollereau C, Parmentier M, Mailleux P, et al. ORL1, a novel member of the opioid receptor family. Cloning, functional expression and localization. *FEBS Lett.* 1994;341(1):33–38.

105. Monga N, Rehm J, Fischer B, et al. Using latent class analysis (LCA) to analyze patterns of drug use in a population of illegal drug abusers. *Drug Alcohol Depend.* 2007;88:1–8.

106. Monico LB, Gryczynski J, Mitchell SG, et al. Buprenorphine treatment and 12-step meeting attendance: conflicts, compatibilities and patient outcomes. *J Subst Abuse Treat.* 2015;57:89–95.

107. Montoya ID, Schroeder JR, Preston KL, et al. Influence of psychotherapy attendance on buprenorphine treatment outcome. *J Subst Abuse Treat.* 2005;28(3):247–254.

108. Najavits LK. *Seeking Safety: A Treatment Manual for PTSD and Substance Abuse.* New York: Guilford; 2002.

109. National Institutes of Health, National Institute of Alcohol Abuse and Alcoholism. *Helping Patients Who Drink too Much: A Clinician's Guide*; 2005; updated 2005 edn.

110. National Vital Statistics System, 1999-2008; Automation of Reports and Consolidated Orders System (ARCOS) of the Drug Enforcement Administration (DEA) (1999-2010) Treatment Episode Data Set, 1999-2009.

111. Neff JA, Moody DE. Differential N-demethylation of L-a-acetyl-methadol (LAAM) and norLAAM by cytochrome P450 s 2B6, 2C18, and 3A4. *Biochem Biophys Res Commun.* 2001;284:751–756.

112. Nowinski J, Baker S, Carroll K. NIAAA project MATCH Monograph Series, Vol 1. *Twelve-Step Facilitation Therapy Manual: a Clinical Research Guide for Therapists Treating Individuals with Alcohol Abuse and Dependence.* Washington, DC: Government Printing Office; 1992.

113. Nunes EV, Quitkin FM, Donovan SJ, et al. Imipramine treatment of opiate-dependent patients with depressive disorders: a placebo-controlled trial. *Arch Gen Psychiatry.* 1998;55:153–160.

114. Nunes EV, Sullivan MA, Levin FR. Treatment of depression in patients with opiate dependence. *Biol Psychiatry.* 2004;56:793–802.

115. Obadia Y, Perrin V, Feroni I, et al. Injecting misuse of buprenorphine among French drug users. *Addiction.* 2001;96:267–272.

116. O'Brien C, Greenstein RA, Mintz J, et al. Clinical experience with naltrexone. *Am J Drug Alcohol Abuse*. 1975;2:365–377.
117. O'Connor PG, Kosten TR. Rapid and ultra-rapid opioid detoxification techniques. *JAMA*. 1998;297(3):229–234.
118. O'Connor PG, Waugh ME, Carroll KM, et al. Primary care-based ambulatory opioid detoxification: the results of a clinical trial. *J Gen Intern Med*. 1995;10:255–260.
119. O'Farrell TJ, Fals-Stewart W. *Behavioral Couples Therapy for Alcoholism and Drug Abuse*. New York: Guilford; 2006.
120. O'Farrell TJ, Fals-Stewart W. Family therapy. In: Galanter M, Kleber HD, eds. *Textbook of Substance Abuse Treatment*. 4th ed. Washington, DC: American Psychiatric Publishing; 2008.
121. Orsini MJ, Nesmelovai I, Young HC, et al. The nociceptin pharmacophore site for opioid receptor binding derived from the NMR structure and bioactivity relationships. *J Biol Chem*. 2005;280(9):8134–8142.
122. Osser DN, Renner JA, Bayog R. *Algorithm for the Pharmacotherapy of Anxiety in Chemical Abusers. Psychopharmacology Algorithm Project*. Harvard Medical School; 2006. http://mhc.com/algorithms/ver4/startAnx.html. Accessed 24 July 2008.
123. Pasternak GW. Opioid receptos. In: Meltzer H, ed. *Psychopharmacology: The Third Generation of Progress*. New York: Raven; 1987.
124. Pearson F, Lipton D. A meta-analytic review of the effectiveness of corrections-based treatments for drug abuse. *Prison J*. 1999;79:384–410.
125. Perry S, Heidrich G. Management of pain during debridement: a survey of U.S. burn units. *Pain*. 1982;13(3):267–280.
126. Petrakis I, Carrol KM, Nick C, et al. Fluoxetine treatment of depressive disorders in methadone-maintained opioid addicts. *Drug Alcohol Depend*. 1998;50:221–226.
127. Polydorou S, Kleber HD. Detoxification of opioids. In: Galanter M, Kleber HD, eds. *Textbook of Substance Abuse Treatment*. 4th ed. Washington, DC: American Psychiatric Publishing; 2008.
128. Portenoy RK, Foley KM. Chronic use of opioid analgesics in non-malignant pain: report of 38 cases. *Pain*. 1986;25(2):171–186.
129. Porter J, Jick H. Addiction rare in patients treated with narcotics. *N Eng J Med*. 1980;302(2):123.
130. Posternak MA, Mueller TI. Assessing the risks and benefits of benzodiazepines for anxiety disorders in patients with a history of substance abuse or dependence. *Am J Addict*. 2001;10(1):48–68.
131. Raehal KM, Bohn LM. Mu opioid receptor regulation and opioid responsiveness. *AAPS J*. 2005;7:E587–E591.
132. Rawson RA, McCann MJ, Shoptaw SJ, et al. Naltrexone for opioid dependence: evaluation of a manualized psychosocial protocol to enhance treatment response. *Drug Alcohol Res*. 2001;20:67–78.
133. Regier DA, Farmer ME, Rae DS, et al. Comorbidity of mental disorders with alcohol and other drug abuse: results from the epidemiologic catchment area (ECA) study. *JAMA*. 1990;264(19):2511–2518.
134. Renner JA. How to train residents to identify and treat dual diagnosis. *Biol Psychiatry*. 2004;56(10):810–816.
135. Renner JA, Baxter JD, Suzuki J, et al. Substance abuse and depression. In: Ciraulo DA, Shader RI, eds. *Pharmacology of Depression*. 2nd ed. Totowa, NJ: Humana; 2007.
136. Ries RK, Galante M, Tonigan JS. Twelve-step facilitation. In: Galanter M, Kleber HD, eds. *Textbook of Substance Abuse Treatment*. 4th ed. Washington, DC: American Psychiatric Publishing; 2008.
137. Riordan CE, Kleber HD. Rapid opiate detoxification with clonidine and naloxone (letter). *Lancet*. 1980;1:1079–1080.
138. Ritvo JI, Causey HL. Community-based treatment. In: Galanter M, Kleber HD, eds. *Textbook of Substance Abuse Treatment*. 4th ed. Washington DC: American Psychiatric Publishing; 2008.
139. Robles E, Stitzer MI, Strain EC, et al. Voucher-based reinforcement of opiate abstinence during methadone detoxification. *Drug Alcohol Depend*. 2002;65(92):179–189.
140. Rosen D, Smith ML, Reynolds CF. The prevalence of mental and physical health disorders among older methadone maintenance patients. *Am J Geriatric Psychiatry*. 2008;16(6):488–497.
141. Roth A, Hogan I, Farren C, et al. Naltrexone plus group therapy for the treatment of opiate-abusing health-care professionals. *J Subst Abuse Treat*. 1997;14:19–22.
142. Rounsaville BJ, Weissman MM, Kleber HD, et al. Heterogeneity of psychiatric diagnosis in treated opiate addicts. *Arch Gen Psychiatry*. 1982;39:161–168.
143. Saunders B, Wilkinson C, Phillips M. The impact of a brief motivational intervention with opiate users attending a methadone program. *Addiction*. 1995;90(3):415–424.
144. Scherbaum N, Kluwig J, Spicka M, et al. Group psychotherapy for opiate addicts in methadone maintenance treatment – a controlled trial. *Eur Addict Res*. 2005;11(4):163–171.
145. Schluger JH, Bart G, Green M, et al. Corticotropin-releasing factor testing reveals a dose-dependent difference in methadone maintained vs. Control subjects. *Neuropsychopharmacology*. 2003;28(5):985–994.
146. Shader RI, Renner JA. Opioid abuse and dependence: acute and chronic treatment. In Shader R, ed. *Manual of Psychiatric Therapeutics*. 4th ed. Baltimore, MD: Lippincott Williams & Wilkins.
147. Sigmon SC. Characterizing the emerging population of prescription opioid abusers. *Am J Addict*. 2006;15:208–212.
148. Singh J, Basu D. Ultra-rapid opioid detoxification: current status and controversies. *J Postgrad Med*. 2004;50:227–232.
149. Smith LA, Gates S, Foxcroft D. Therapeutic communities for substance related disorder. *Cochrane Database Syst Rev*. 2006;1:CD005338.
150. Stitzer ML, Iguchi MY, Kidorf M, et al. Contingency management in methadone treatment: the case for positive incentives. *NIDA Res Monogr*. 1993;137:19–36.
151. Strain EC, Bigelow GE, Liebson IA, et al. Moderate- vs. high-dose methadone in the treatment of opioid dependence: a randomized trial. *JAMA*. 1999;281:1000–1005.
152. Strain EC, Stitzer ML, Liebson IA, et al. Comparison of buprenorphine and methadone in the treatment of opioid dependence. *Am J Psychiatry*. 1994;151:1025–1030.
153. Substance Abuse and Mental Health Services Administration. *Office of Applied Studies Results From the 2004 National Survey on Drug Use and Health: National Findings*. Rockville, MD: Department of Health and Human Services, NSDUH Series H-28, DHHS publication SAM 05–4062; 2005.
154. Substance Abuse and Mental Health Services Administration, Center for Substance Abuse Treatment. *2007 SAMHSA evaluation of the impact of the DATA waiver program*; 2007. http://www.buprenorphine.samhsa.gov/evaluation.html. Accessed 4 Aug 2008.
155. Substance Abuse and Mental Health Services Administration. *Office of Applied Studies. Results from the 2013 National Survey on Drug Use and Health: Summary of National Findings, NSDUH Series H-48*. Rockville, MD: HHS Publication No. (SMA) 14-4863; 2014.
156. Substance Abuse and Mental Health Services Administration, Center for Behavioral Health Statistics and Quality. *Treatment Episode Data Set (TEDS): 2004-2014*. National Admissions to Substance Abuse Treatment Services
157. Substance Abuse and Mental Health Services Administration. Center for Behavioral Health Statistics and Quality. Risk and protective factors and estimates of substance use initiation: Results from the 2015 National Survey on Drug Use and Health. *NSDUH Data Review*; 2016. Retrieved from http://samhsa.gov/data/.
158. Subtance Abuse and Mental Health Services Administration, Center for Behavioral Health Statistics and Quality. *Prescription Drug Use and Misuse in the United States: Results From the 2015 National Survey on Drug Use and Health: HSDUH Data Review*; 2016. Retrieved from http://samhsa.gov/data/.
159. Tiet QQ, Mausbach B. Treatments for patients with dual diagnosis: a review. *Alcohol Clin Exp Res*. 2007;31(4):513–536.
160. United States Government Accountability Office. *Adult Drug Courts: Evidence Indicates Recidivism Reductions and Mixed Results for Other Outcomes (GAO-05–219)*. Washington, DC: US GAO; 2007.

161. Villagomez RE, Meyer TJ, Lin MM, et al. Post-traumatic stress disorder among inner city methadone maintenance patients. *Subst Abuse Treat*. 1995;12:253–257.

162. Volkow ND. Imaging the addicted brain: from molecules to behavior. *J Nucl Med*. 2004;45:13N–22N.

163. Volkow ND, Fowler JS, Wang GJ. The addicted human brain: insights from imaging studies. *J Clin Invest*. 2003;111:1444–1451.

164. Volkow ND, Koob GF, McLellan AT. Neurobiologic advances from the brain disease model of addiction. *N Engl J Med*. 2016;374(4):363–371.

165. Wallace AE, Weeks WB. Substance abuse intensive outpatient treatment: does program graduation matter? *J Subst Abuse Treat*. 2004;27(1):27–30.

166. Weiss ED, Potter JS, Fiellin DA, et al. Adjunctive counseling during brief and extended buprenorphine-naloxone treatment for prescription opioid dependence: a 2-phase randomized controlled trial. *Arch Gen Psychiatry*. 2011;68(12):1238–1246.

167. Welsh C, Sherman SG, Tobin KE. A case of heroin overdose reversed by sublingually administered buprenorphine/naloxone (Suboxone). *Addiction*. 2008;103(7):1226–1228.

168. Wesson D, Ling W. The clinical opiate withdrawal scale (COWS). *Psychoactive Drugs*. 2003;35(2):253–259.

169. Wexler HK. The success of therapeutic communities for substance abusers in American prisons. *J Psychoactive Drugs*. 1995;27(1):57–66.

170. Woody GE, Luborsky L, McLellan AT, et al. Psychotherapy for opiate addicts. Does it help? *Arch Gen Psychiatry*. 1983;40(6):639–645.

171. Woody GE, McLellan AT, Luborsky L, et al. Psychotherapy in community methadone programs: a validation study. *Am J Psychiatry*. 1995;152(9):1302–1308.

172. Yablonski L. *The Tunnel Back*. New York: Macmillan; 1965.

173. Zullino DF, Cottier A, Besson J. Case report: topiramate in opiate withdrawal. *Prog Neuro-Psychopharmacol Biol Psychiatry*. 2002;26(6):1221–12123.

174. Zullino DF, Krenz S, Zimmerman G, et al. topiranate in opiate withdrawal – comparison with clonidine and with carbamazepine/mianserin. *Subst Abuse*. 2004;25(4):27–33.

26

Clinical Aspects of Methamphetamine

NICOLE LEE

CHAPTER OUTLINE

Introduction

Methamphetamine, developed in 1893, is a synthetic stimulant that affects the central nervous system and other major organ systems. Until the 1950s, no prescription was necessary to obtain methamphetamine or other amphetamine-containing products. Prescriptions for variants of these drugs were freely dispensed in the 1960s. Different versions of methamphetamine became popular in the 1960s, and "ice," a smokable derivative, emerged in the late 1980s in Hawaii. The evolution of methamphetamine use since 1988 has varied. The early to mid-1990s witnessed escalating problems with methamphetamine throughout many parts of the world. In the United States the highest rates of use were in the Western region of the country, particularly in suburban and rural communities. Australia also saw increases in use and, in the same region, Southeast Asia also reported escalating prevalence. Relatively little use is reported in the United Kingdom and the rest of Europe.

One of the key enablers of the growth of methamphetamine use was the wide availability of pseudoephedrine, the primary precursor of methamphetamine, which was contained in many over-the-counter cold medications including Sudafed, Nyquil, and Claritin-D. Methamphetamine was manufactured and distributed by small homemade "kitchen chemists," as well as larger syndicates and drug cartels. Those exposed to active methamphetamine production sites, including children, can have serious health consequences from explosions, fires, and toxic gases and wastes. Consequently, methamphetamine use and methamphetamine use disorder have had a substantial impact on the treatment, health care, criminal justice, and social welfare systems. From 2003 to 2006, many jurisdictions around the world, including the United States, imposed strict precursor control laws that restrict the retail sales of medications that contain pseudoephedrine. These efforts have substantially reduced the availability of methamphetamine and increased its price in many areas of the United States.

In the United States, from the early 1990s through 2005, numerous indicators have shown steady increases in the use of methamphetamine. However, in the early to mid-2000s, many areas in the world have started to show a reduction in people who use the drug. In 2007 in the United States, 529,000 people 12 years of age or older were current users of methamphetamine, a reduction from 731,000 in 2006.[104] Similarly, the Community Epidemiology Work Group of the National Institute on Drug Abuse reported that methamphetamine indicators from law enforcement (arrests and seizures) and emergency room data from 20 of 22 metropolitan areas, showed either a stable or downward trend of methamphetamine use during 2006 and 2007.[68] Similarly, treatment admissions for methamphetamine, which increased dramatically from the 1990s to 2005, showed a decline in 2006.

In other parts of the world, similar declines have been reported. In Australia, for example, there has been a decreasing trend in reported methamphetamine use since 1998, and the 2016 National Drug Strategy Household Survey[2] shows methamphetamine at its lowest point since recording began. However, harm indicators have continued to increase, including ambulance callouts,[60] treatment presentations,[2] and drug-related deaths,[23] largely due to a change in reported preference for the more potent and pure crystal form (ice) over the powdered form (speed).

Neurobiological Impact of Methamphetamine Use

Some caution is required in interpreting neurocognitive studies, as most are cross-sectional and cannot confirm whether cognitive deficits are predrug or postdrug use. In addition, some longitudinal studies show that childhood deficits in executive function can predict adolescent drug use, suggesting that some of the cognitive problems could be premorbid.[106] Frequency, duration, and quantity of use does not appear to predict level of cognitive impairment, suggesting a vulnerability to the toxic effects of methamphetamine among some people who use it.[55] However, regular long-term methamphetamine use has been associated with significant impairment relative to age- and education-matched controls on a range of cognitive domains[96] and self-reported functional impairments correspond with neurocognitive deficits.

Methamphetamine has a significant impact on the structure and chemistry of the brain, largely through disruption of the dopamine system.[24] Methamphetamine releases stores of dopamine into the synapse, and then blocks its reuptake, resulting in significantly increased levels of dopamine in the synapse of neurons, particularly in the prefrontal cortex and the limbic regions of the brain. Among people who use methamphetamine occasionally, these changes to the dopamine system correct themselves after a few days, and dopamine stores return to preuse levels once the methamphetamine has been eliminated from the body. However, among people who use methamphetamine regularly, depleted dopamine stores do not have sufficient time to replenish. Methamphetamine also increases the cytoplasmic concentration of dopamine, which promotes oxidation products that are toxic to the nerve terminals,[85] and long-term use has been associated with a fourfold increase in risk of Parkinson disease.[22] The neurotoxicity of methamphetamine is further accentuated by its prolonged half-life and long duration of action.

After regular use, there is evidence of damage to the structures of the dopamine system, significantly affecting executive functioning, episodic memory, and motor functioning.[24,96] The magnitude of the impairments is significant[96] compared to other drugs such as cocaine[58] and cannabis.[40]

For regular and dependent methamphetamine users who enter treatment, attention, memory, and executive function seem to decline further in the first 2 weeks of abstinence potentially due to the deprivation of the acute benefits of methamphetamine on cognition, sleep disturbance, or neuropsychiatric sequelae. After 6 months of abstinence, cognitive test performance is worse than in people who had either relapsed or continued to use,[99] with little significant improvement in the first 12 months.[113] However, one study showed some improvement after an average of 13 months, with the range up to 42 months, on some domains (motor functioning and information processing speed but not learning, memory, and executive functioning).[55]

The level of dopamine depletion is a predictor of relapse risk.[112] People who use methamphetamine over a long period also demonstrate attentional bias for drug-related stimuli,[45] which has been shown to predict poorer treatment outcomes.[15] Cognitive impairment is generally associated with poorer treatment retention.[17]

Effects of Methamphetamine Use and Methamphetamine Use Disorder

Acute and Chronic Physical Effects of Methamphetamine Use

At low doses, euphoria, increased blood pressure, elevated body temperature, and rapid heart and breathing rates are commonly experienced acute effects of methamphetamine use. Other immediate clinical symptoms include reduced fatigue, reduced hunger, increased energy, increased sexual drive, and increased self-confidence.

At higher doses causing moderate intoxication, negative acute physiological effects can include intense stomach cramps, shaking, bruxism, disrupted menstrual cycles, formication (i.e., the sensation of insects creeping on the skin), and insomnia.[86]

Toxicity, or overdose, can manifest in cardiovascular, central nervous system, and respiratory problems. Death is relatively rare but can occur.[23] Cardiopulmonary consequences are among the more common health complications among people who use methamphetamine, with chest pain, hypertension, shortness of breath, tachycardia and acute coronary syndrome common in emergency room cases involving methamphetamine toxicity.[116] Turnipseed and colleagues[110] documented acute coronary syndrome in 25% of people who use methamphetamine regularly and admitted for chest pain, possibly resulting from myocardial ischemia and the risk of arrhythmias and cardiogenic shock.[115] Cardiomyopathy related to methamphetamine use may be reversible; if drug use ceases.[54] Pulmonary edema was found in over 70% of methamphetamine-related deaths.[59] Damage to small blood vessels in the brain can result in stroke, paralysis, and brain damage.[114] Central nervous system[7] manifestations of methamphetamine use include agitation, violent behavior, and self-harm; coma; seizure; movement disorders; confusion, psychosis, paranoia, hypersexuality, and hallucinations; and headache. Respiratory manifestations of methamphetamine use include dyspnea (shortness of breath), wheezing, and pneumothorax.[108] "Meth mouth" and other oral complications are common among people who use methamphetamine regularly.[97] Like many drugs, methamphetamine reduces saliva production, increasing risk of dental caries, enamel erosion, and gum disease.[41] Studies also suggest poor oral hygiene, teeth grinding, and jaw clenching (bruxism), and direct caustic effects of methamphetamine may also contribute to oral problems.[26]

Compulsive skin picking can occur among people who use methamphetamine regularly, resulting in sores and ulcers. This is commonly in response to sensations of bugs crawling below the skin (formication).[6] Formication is essentially a tactile hallucination accompanied by the delusion that insects are causing the sensation.[95] Methamphetamine also raises body temperature and increases perspiration, and restricts blood flow to the surface of the skin, which can contribute to both skin irritation, resulting in picking, and poor skin health. Cellulitis and abscesses resulting from injection of methamphetamine may also affect skin condition.

Many people who use methamphetamine have psychiatric comorbidity, particularly psychosis, depression, and suicidal ideation.[75,120] Nearly 25% of people who use methamphetamine at least monthly have experienced a clinically significant symptom of psychosis, with people who are dependent on methamphetamine three times more likely to have experienced symptoms of psychosis.[72] There is some evidence that methamphetamine increases risk of mental health problems, rather than merely co-occurring.[61]

Sexual Behavior and Communicable Diseases

Several surveys have shown high rates of methamphetamine use among men who have sex with men, estimated to be around 11%.[35] Men who have sex with men and who use methamphetamine are more likely to report a greater number of sex partners, greater likelihood of sex with an HIV-infected partner, and unprotected anal intercourse than men who have sex with men who do not use methamphetamine.[14,34] There is some evidence that methamphetamine use directly increases sexual risk behavior among men who have sex with men, rather than just co-occurring[47]

A study by Rawson and colleagues[87] found that both men and women who use methamphetamine tend to engage in frequent sexual activity, to have multiple, anonymous sexual partners, and to report low rates of condom use and high rates of unprotected anal and vaginal sex, increasing HIV risk.

Studies of people who use methamphetamine in general also show strong associations between methamphetamine use and communicable disease risk, including HIV; hepatitis A, B, C; and other sexually transmitted infections, due to risky sexual and drug use practices.[82] Risky drug use practices among people who use methamphetamine, including injection and drug-sharing behaviors (e.g., sharing water for needle or pipe preparations and/or to rinse syringes/pipes and cotton) have also significantly increased the risk of infectious diseases.[38,39,87,91,111]

Specific Populations

Youth

Methamphetamine use is low among teenagers,[57] but young people in their 20s have the highest rate of use.[3,105] However, there is a worldwide downward trend in use in this group. The literature on clinical risk factors associated with methamphetamine use among youth suggests that young people who use methamphetamine have a high rate of past history of physical and sexual abuse/trauma, family history of substance use problems, and current psychological problems, including affective emotional and conduct disorders.[80,81,90,118]

Women

Research indicates that women use methamphetamine at rates similar to those of men, and suggests that compared to men, women tend to begin use earlier, are more prone to dependence, experience greater psychological distress, but also have better treatment outcomes.[5,29] Almost half (46%) of national admissions to publicly funded treatment in the United States are adult women who use methamphetamine, compared with 31% of admissions for other drugs (i.e., heroin, alcohol, marijuana).[104] A large body of literature comparing drug-dependent women with drug-dependent men indicates that women are more likely than men to report extensive histories of trauma, neglect, and abuse.[79] Between 70% and 85% of women who develop methamphetamine dependence have reported a history of sexual and physical abuse.[8,78,86] Such histories have been linked to an increased likelihood of domestic violence in adult relationships, chronic addiction, criminal activity, homelessness, and psychiatric cooccurring illness.[76] Women offenders who are dependent on methamphetamine tend to have had significantly greater exposure to childhood abuse and household dysfunction than have methamphetamine-dependent men, and more often reported sexual abuse in adolescence and as an adult.[77]

Pregnant Women and Their Children

There is limited evidence on the impact of prenatal methamphetamine exposure on the developing fetus and most is complicated by the high level of polydrug use and poor social conditions to which women who are dependent on methamphetamine may be exposed. Studies that are available suggest higher rates of preterm birth, placental abruption, cardiac anomalies, smaller head circumference, fetal distress, and fetal growth restriction.[100] Women who use methamphetamine tend to have a lower body mass index, increasing risk of pregnancy complications, and more frequent and longer hospital stays.[27] Women who use methamphetamine risk intrauterine growth retardation and insufficient amount of oxygen to the fetus,[28,117] resulting in low birth weight, relatively small gestational size, and increased risk of neurodevelopmental problems.[1] Around 4% of babies born to women who use methamphetamine go through withdrawal.[51] There is some limited evidence of longer-term behavioral effects of children born to women who use methamphetamine.[117]

Criminal Offenders

The numbers of incarcerations and other problems within the criminal justice system among methamphetamine-dependent individuals have increased, which supports the strong association between methamphetamine use disorder and participation in illegal behaviors.[33] Since 2002, the criminal justice system has been the top referral source for methamphetamine treatment.[18] The latest national statistics indicate that a large proportion of admissions for primary methamphetamine/amphetamine use across the country was from the criminal justice system (49%), compared with 34% for other categories of drugs.[104] In California, more than half of offenders who used drugs and were diverted from the judicial system to treatment in lieu of incarceration primarily used methamphetamine.[32]

Offenders who are dependent on methamphetamine and who are seeking treatment may require different treatment options and plans tailored to their special characteristics.[18] It has been suggested that drug courts may be an effective tool for promoting successful treatment outcomes for methamphetamine-dependent offenders.[52] Drug courts are governed by a number of key components, including the integration of treatment with criminal case processing; early identification and prompt placement of eligible drug offenders into the program; provision of a continuum-of-services treatment plan; alcohol and drug testing; and ongoing judicial interaction.[109] One study examined the treatment response of methamphetamine-dependent individuals within a drug court setting and found that drug court participation was associated with better rates of engagement, retention, completion, and abstinence compared with people who use methamphetamine who did not participate in a drug court treatment setting.[67] Follow-up analyses revealed that participants who were enrolled in the drug court intervention used methamphetamine significantly less frequently compared with people who use methamphetamine without drug court supervision.

People With Co-occurring Disorders

Many people who are dependent on methamphetamine present for treatment with symptoms of psychiatric problems. Although distinguishing the degree to which these symptoms can be attributed to methamphetamine use versus a premorbid disorder is often difficult, the treatment is the same. Clinically, high rates of depression coupled with impulsivity put people who use methamphetamine regularly at higher risk of suicidal behavior. Some research has implicated methamphetamine-related intoxication, withdrawal, and psychiatric symptoms in elevating risk of depression and suicide.[64]

Reducing Harms Associated With Methamphetamine Use

By far the majority of people who use methamphetamine do so infrequently and irregularly, and for a short period in their lives. More than weekly use is associated with dependence and the dependence rate among people who currently use methamphetamine is around 10%–15%, with use of the crystal form resulting in higher rates of regular use and methamphetamine use disorder. Numerous harms can affect people who use methamphetamine, whether they are dependent or not, including high rates of polydrug use, mental health problems, and acute toxicity effects.

Around 10% of people inject the drug, with the majority smoking or using other routes of administration. Clean needle programs have been shown to be effective in reducing harms associated with injecting, such as bloodborne viruses, and can be an effective way to provide health information to people who use drugs, but with low rates of injecting among people who use methamphetamine, access to this group is more difficult. Our understanding of harm reduction strategies for this group is more limited than for other drugs.

Toxicity, or overdose, can happen to anybody, including people using for the first-time and those who use regularly. Useful harm reduction messages to reduce the risk of toxicity include using only a small amount in the first instance to test the strength of the methamphetamine; avoiding mixing of methamphetamine with alcohol or other drugs; avoiding lengthy binge sessions that put the body under extreme stress; taking as many breaks as possible from using methamphetamine; and understanding the actions and effects of methamphetamine and being vigilant for early warning signs of overdose. An ambulance should be called immediately if overdose is suspected. In the event of overdose, keep the person cool (e.g., moist towels) and reduce stimulation in the environment (e.g., lower the lights, turn off music, speak quietly and calmly, and reassure the person) until the ambulance arrives.

Methamphetamine use reduces the sedating effects of alcohol, and some people use methamphetamine so they can drink more. A lethal dose of alcohol is around 4 grams of alcohol per 100 mL of blood (i.e., a blood alcohol concentration [BAC] of ≥0.4) and this does not change in the presence of methamphetamine. However, methamphetamine may mask the effects of alcohol so people feel less drunk at the same BAC. People should be informed of the risk of alcohol poisoning and should be advised to monitor their drinking to reduce that risk.

Sharing equipment increases risk of bloodborne viruses, including HIV and hepatitis. Sharing pipes to smoke crystal meth also increases potential exposure to blood through cracked or cut lips. Methamphetamine use can reduce inhibitions and increase sexual desire and risk taking. Some use methamphetamine specifically to enhance sexual encounters; for others sex may be spontaneous. This effect of methamphetamine puts people who use methamphetamine at high risk of sexually transmitted infections. People who use methamphetamine should be encouraged to use their own equipment and be prepared at all times and have access to condoms, dental dams, and lubricant.

Methamphetamine affects sleep, nutrition, and dental hygiene. Because of the stimulating effects of methamphetamine, people often have trouble maintaining a healthy sleeping pattern. Methamphetamine can keep people who use it awake for long periods of time and also disrupt the timing of sleep. People who use methamphetamine should be encouraged to go to bed and get up at regular times, even if they cannot sleep, rest without sleep still allows the body some recovery time. Lack of appetite is typical among people who use methamphetamine and they may go for several days without eating. Eating something (healthy) like a banana or a healthy shake is beneficial even if appetite is poor. Regular exercise has been shown to reduce symptoms of depression and anxiety among people newly abstinent from methamphetamine.[88] Brushing and flossing of teeth, drinking a sufficient amount of water each day, and chewing sugar-free gum can help to reduce the risk of dental caries often associated with regular methamphetamine use.

Acute Management of Methamphetamine Problems

Managing Methamphetamine Intoxication

Acute agitation from methamphetamine intoxication is most often the condition that leads people who use methamphetamine to seek medical attention, and talking down the patient in a calm environment is a first course of action if possible. For mild agitation, administration of benzodiazepines can useful. For severe behavioral disturbances, droperidol[13,53] is the recommended agent; the addition of olanzapine may also be helpful in some cases.[107]

Managing Acute Methamphetamine Psychosis

Symptoms of methamphetamine-induced psychosis can be difficult to differentiate from those of other disorders that may predate drug use, and so a definitive diagnosis is required before commencing treatment. People who use methamphetamine regularly frequently report auditory hallucinations, which is more typical of schizophrenia, in addition to visual (flashing lights, peripheral artifacts), olfactory, and tactile sensations. Symptoms of methamphetamine psychosis include persecutory delusions, ideas of reference, hallucinations (visual and auditory, olfactory, tactile), relative clear sensorium, stereotypy and compulsive acts, anhedonia and depression, blunt affect, poverty of speech, and being prone to excited delirium and violence.

Methamphetamine-induced acute psychosis, which generally is transient, can require use of either a benzodiazepine or an antipsychotic, both of which may be halted when acute symptoms have resolved. Low-dose antipsychotics between psychotic episodes may be useful, but there is no empirical guidance on the efficacy or appropriateness of such treatment. Such agents are contraindicated for adolescents and young adults, in whom methamphetamine-induced psychosis has increased more than fivefold from 1993 to 2002.[19] Treatment of this population should follow the treatment described above for intoxication.

Managing Chronic Methamphetamine Psychosis

Symptoms of persistent or chronic methamphetamine psychosis are often so similar to those of schizophrenia that some clinicians may regard them as clinically equivalent conditions, and most likely in these cases methamphetamine has acted as the trigger for schizophrenia. Symptoms of schizophrenia and of persistent methamphetamine-related psychosis are not readily distinguishable, and the treatment for this condition remains basically the same as in recent practice.

Managing Methamphetamine Withdrawal

Methamphetamine withdrawal symptoms consist of severe fatigue, cognitive impairment, feelings of depression and anxiety, anergia, confusion, and paranoia. For the majority of individuals experiencing acute withdrawal/early phase abstinence, most symptoms resolve over 7–14 days.[71,119] Often the physical withdrawal symptoms are mild, and rest, exercise, and a healthy diet may be a suitable management approach for most people. Those with heightened agitation and sleep disturbance may respond to benzodiazepines, but acute depression and anhedonia associated with early abstinence generally resolve without intervention. Clinicians should be aware of possible dehydration and hyperthermia. Drug craving may be addressed via behavioral treatments or periods of residential care. No pharmacotherapy has been shown to be effective in other symptoms of methamphetamine withdrawal.

Certain groups of individuals present for treatment with special concerns, as detailed below:

- *Women who use methamphetamine*—higher rates of depression, often with histories of sexual and physical abuse; responsibilities for children.
- *People who inject methamphetamine*—very high rates of psychiatric symptoms; severe withdrawal syndromes; high rates of hepatitis.
- *Homeless, chronically mentally ill individuals*—high levels of psychiatric symptoms at admission and during treatment.
- *Individuals under the age of 21*—antipsychotic medications and other mediations should be avoided or used with caution.
- *Men who have sex with men*—at very high risk for HIV, hepatitis, and other sexually transmitted diseases.

Treatment for People Who Use Methamphetamine

A body of literature has been developed on treatment outcomes for methamphetamine use. Engagement in treatment, retention in treatment for at least 90 days, abstinence during treatment, and treatment completion have consistently been shown to successfully predict positive treatment outcomes with methamphetamine-dependent populations.[42,46] One study found that people who use methamphetamine have better treatment outcomes than people who use alcohol or other drugs,[65] demonstrating at least that treatment for this group is effective.

Risk factors for poor treatment outcomes have been identified as daily methamphetamine use, injection methamphetamine use, having less than a high school education, young age at treatment admission, having a disability,[9] polydrug use,[10] childhood trauma and abuse,[78] and having an underlying psychotic disorder[36] or major depression.[37] Treatment participation and active recovery efforts, including frequent 12-step program participation, have been associated with successful treatment outcomes.[48] Research has also shown that women and men respond to treatment similarly in terms of retention and completion, although women tend to have slightly better treatment outcomes, including more improved relationships with family and fewer medical problems as compared with men.[8,49]

Few studies to date have examined the longer-term impact of treatment, including patterns of use and psychosocial outcomes. Despite the success in treatment, McKetin et al.[73] showed that posttreatment relapse rates are high among people who use methamphetamine. Three months after residential treatment, for example, relapse rates were around 45%, after 1 year around 80%, and by 3 years after treatment rates of relapse were similar to those who did not enter treatment, at around 90%. In one longitudinal examination of outcomes over a 10-year period, Hser and colleagues[48] found that quitting was predicted by current treatment and self-help participation among people who use stimulants (including people who use methamphetamine and cocaine), and that cessation of drug use was less likely among people who use methamphetamine with an early drug-use onset relative to people who use cocaine or heroin. Lubman et al. also found that engagement with posttreatment support such as SMART Recovery or other mutual aid groups increased the likelihood of abstinence.[65]

The majority of studies investigating the effectiveness of treatment for stimulant addiction have focused on cocaine use and methamphetamine use disorder, with fewer studies on methamphetamine. Despite differences between the two stimulants in individual health, psychological, and cognitive effects, both groups tend to show comparable responses to psychosocial behavioral treatments.[20,50,66]

Evidence-based behavioral treatment for methamphetamine-dependent individuals *does* work, as documented by the authors and colleagues.[31,62,98] Treatment has profound effects, including reductions in methamphetamine use during treatment, increased treatment retention, decreased use of other drugs, decreased criminal involvement, and reduced high-risk sexual practices among gay and heterosexual people who use methamphetamine.[83,89]

Cognitive Behavioral Therapy

Cognitive behavioral therapy is a short-term, focused approach to help people who use alcohol and other drugs reduce use, become abstinent, or avoid relapse. The underlying assumption is that learning processes play an important role in the development and continuation of substance use. Key elements of cognitive behavioral therapy are:

- Functional analyses of substance use
- Individualized training in recognizing emotional states
- Exercises, such as thought stopping and managing thoughts about drug use
- Coping skills, problem-solving, planning for emergencies, and refusal skills
- Examination of the client's cognitive processes related to substance use
- Identification and debriefing of past and future high-risk situations
- Encouragement and review of extrasession implementation of skills
- Practice of skills within sessions.

Cognitive behavioral therapy promotes abstinence via skill training, including learning and practicing strategies for: (1) reducing availability and exposure to drugs and related cues, (2) fostering resolution to stop drug use by exploring positive and negative consequences of continued use, (3) self-monitoring to identify high-risk situations and to conduct functional analyses of substance use, (4) recognition of conditioned craving and development of strategies to cope with craving, (5) identification of seemingly irrelevant decisions that can culminate in high-risk situations, (6) preparing for emergencies and coping with relapse to substance use, (7) drug refusal skills, and (8) identifying and confronting thoughts about drugs. Several versions or packages of cognitive behavioral therapy–based interventions are available in manual form.

Cognitive behavioral therapy ranges from very brief to longer more intensive interventions, all within the same broad theoretical approach.

A brief therapy trialed in Australia[4] showed significant increases in abstinence rates among people who received only two sessions of motivational interviewing and cognitive behavioral therapy compared to a self-help booklet. People who received four sessions of motivational interviewing and cognitive behavioral therapy showed the same outcomes, and also significantly reduced symptoms of depression.

A comparison of the 4-session brief intervention of Baker et al. with 12 weeks of acceptance and commitment therapy (ACT), a form of cognitive behavioral therapy incorporating mindfulness strategies, showed no significant differences.[101] There was a high dropout in the ACT group and the average number of sessions attended was three.

Among intensive interventions, The Matrix Model offers a blended treatment approach that incorporates principles of cognitive behavioral therapy in individual and group settings, family education, motivational interviewing, and behavioral therapy; while not a pure cognitive behavioral therapy intervention, the Matrix Model employs cognitive behavioral therapy principles. This manualized therapy has been proven effective in reducing methamphetamine use during the 16-week application of the intervention, in comparison with a treatment as usual condition in a large Center for Substance Abuse Treatment–funded multisite trial.[91,92] The Matrix Model also has been evaluated as a stand-alone treatment for subgroups of people who use methamphetamine (e.g., gay and bisexual men and heterosexuals) and as the behavioral treatment platform in pharmacotherapy trials for methamphetamine use disorder.[30] The National Institute on Drug Abuse had also trialed a manualized cognitive behavioral therapy, based on coping skills therapy, of 12-sessions approach.[16]

Contingency Management

Also known as motivational incentives, contingency management is an intervention for drug use that employs immediate reinforcement for demonstration of desired behaviors (e.g., a drug-free urine test). Contingency management appears to produce the most robust reductions in methamphetamine use of any single technique. Roll and colleagues[94] conducted an early multisite clinical trial in which a contingency management protocol was evaluated as an addition to an outpatient methamphetamine treatment program. Participants in the contingency management condition demonstrated a superior clinical performance on multiple outcome measures (number of methamphetamine-negative urine samples, number of consecutive weeks of abstinence, percent that completed the trial with continual abstinence). A later trial by the same group to determine whether varying the duration of contingency management produced different rates of abstinence. Participants received standard psychosocial treatment or psychosocial treatment plus either 1-month, 2-month, or 4-month of contingency management. They found that participants were more likely to remain abstinent with longer contingency management duration.[93] Menza et al.[74] found that among men who have sex

with men and use methamphetamine, contingency management increased frequency of use, and the authors did not recommend the intervention for this group.

Medications for Treatment of Methamphetamine Use and Methamphetamine Use Disorder

Although multiple medications have been investigated for treating methamphetamine use disorder, none has shown to be sufficiently effective for widespread use. Brensilver and colleagues[11] concluded that although some medications have shown promising results (methylphenidate, naltrexone, bupropion, and mirtazapine), no pharmacotherapy has been found to be broadly effective.

Reviews by Stoops and Rush[102,103] of clinical and laboratory trials of agonist replacement medication and combination pharmacotherapies for stimulant use disorder identify potentially promising directions but no widely effective option.

A Cochrane Review of psychostimulant medications for amphetamine dependence[84] reviewed 11 studies of dexamphetamine, bupropion, methylphenidate, and modafinil. No significant differences were found between these medications and placebo in effect on reducing amphetamine use or craving, increasing length of abstinence; the retention in treatment studies was low and a similar proportion of adverse events prompting dropout was evident for both psychostimulants and placebo groups.

Since the publication of these reviews, 12 new clinical studies have been published.

Overall, among the medications that have been subject to controlled trials, only five have more than three published reports, offering more confidence in the results: dexamphetamine, modafinil, methylphenidate, naltrexone, and bupropion. All had some studies in support and some finding no difference to placebo. Dexamphetamine may reduce the severity of dependence but not use; only short-acting dexamphetamine has been evaluated in clinical studies, and longer-acting formulations may yield different results. Methylphenidate may reduce use and craving.[63] Modafinil may reduce use.[70] Naltrexone may also reduce use and craving and improve retention.[56] Bupropion may reduce use, and also has the benefit of reducing tobacco use.[69] Bupropion may have more benefit for people whose use is lighter.[31,43] Although all reported that these medications were safe and tolerable, studies tend to show a high dropout and low medication adherence.

Lower baseline amphetamine use is strongly related to benefit from treatment,[25] suggesting that earlier intervention, at least with bupropion, may yield better results. The complex action of methamphetamine in the brain[44,96] affects multiple systems, meaning a single medication may not be effective.

Future Directions in Research and Practice

There are many areas where knowledge about methamphetamine effects and actions is limited. Our understanding of the effects of methamphetamine on the brain is relatively limited and topics that are garnering increased attention include: (1) cellular mechanisms of action of methamphetamine and their relationship to neurotoxicity; (2) the interplay between the limbic brain circuitry underlying reward and the frontal brain that exercises control over the limbic brain, and (3) the disinhibition of the limbic brain resulting from functional or structural disconnection from the executive brain. As knowledge emerges about these complex interactions, researchers and clinicians face new challenges as well as new opportunities for the development and implementation of pharmacological and behavioral treatment strategies to address methamphetamine use disorder.

Although there are some evidence-based behavioral interventions for methamphetamine use disorder, they are relatively limited compared to treatments for other mental health disorders, and further research to broaden treatment options is needed.

Most people who use drugs do not need treatment, and even those that do have periods of use while they find the treatment that is most effective for them to assist in achieving abstinence. Most people who start using drugs use only occasionally and for a very short period in the lives. Many regions in the world have well-developed strategies to reduce harms from opioid use—such as clean needle programs and replacement pharmacotherapy—but these are less relevant to people who use methamphetamine, who tend to use routes of administration other than injecting. Given the paradoxical increase in harms despite the decrease in use in many parts of the world, research is needed that helps our understanding of ways to keep people safer in the short period they are experimenting with drugs, or before they get into treatment.

Regardless of the advances in scientific understanding of methamphetamine use and responses, utilization of such knowledge often occurs with much delay and sometimes never happens. The real world in which clinical researchers conduct investigations of new treatments and in which clinicians treat clients is not always receptive to findings from human laboratory studies or even phase III trials, and implementation of research-proven practices never occur in an optimally timely manner without first overcoming various obstacles.

The first part of any solution to the problems associated with methamphetamine use involves greater awareness by all those involved in pertinent disciplines, from basic scientists to primary care physicians. To accomplish at least part of that awareness raising, new curricula need to be developed and refined at all levels, in academic institutions at the undergraduate and postgraduate levels and in community practice settings, where clinicians may seek and find definitive training in the science and practice of addiction medicine.

References

1. American College of Obstetricians and Gynecologists. Committee opinion methamphetamine abuse in women of reproductive age. *Obstet Gynecol.* 2011;117(51–55).
2. Australian Institute of Health and Welfare. *Alcohol and Other Drug Treatment Services in Australia 2015-16.* Drug Treatment Series No. 29. Cat. No. Hse 187. Canberra: AIHW; 2017.
3. Australian Institute of Health and Welfare. *National Drug Strategy Household Survey 2016: Detailed Findings.* Drug Statistics Series No. 31. Cat. No. Phe 214. Canberra: AIHW; 2017.
4. Baker A, Lee NK, Claire M, Lewin TJ, Grant T, Pohlman S, et al. Brief cognitive behavioural interventions for regular amphetamine users: a step in the right direction. *Addiction.* 2005;100(3):367–378.
5. Boles SM, Joshi V, Grella C, Wellisch J. Childhood sexual abuse patterns, psychosocial correlates, and treatment outcomes among adults in drug abuse treatment. *J Sexual Abuse.* 2005;14(1):39–55.
6. Bostwick MJ, Lineberry TW. The 'meth' epidemic: managing acute psychosis, agitation, and suicide risk. *Current Psychiatry.* 2006;5(11):46–60.
7. Bowyer JF, Thomas M, Schmued LC, Ali SF. Brain region-specific neurodegenerative profiles showing the relative importance of amphetamine dose, hyperthermia, seizures, and the blood-brain barrier. *Ann N Y Acad Sci.* 2008;1139(1):127–139.
8. Brecht ML, Brien A, von Mayrhauser C, O' Anglin MD. Methamphetamine use behaviors and gender differences. *Addict Behav.* 2004;29(1):89–106.
9. Brecht ML, Greenwell L, Anglin MD. Methamphetamine treatment: trends and predictors of retention and completion in a large state treatment system (1992-2002). *J Subst Abuse Treat.* 2005;29(4):295–306.
10. Brecht ML, Huang D, Evans E, Hser YI. Polydrug use and implications for longitudinal research: ten-year trajectories for heroin, cocaine, and methamphetamine users. *Drug Alcohol Depend.* 2008;96(3):193–201.
11. Brensilver M, Heinzerling KG, Shoptaw S. Pharmacotherapy of amphetamine-type stimulant dependence: an update. *Drug Alcohol Rev.* 2013;32:449–460.
12. Reference deleted in review.
13. Calver L, Page CB, Downes MA, Chan B, Kinnear F, Wheatley L, et al. The safety and effectiveness of droperidol for sedation of acute behavioral disturbance in the emergency department. *Ann Emerg Med.* 2015;66(3):230–238.e1.
14. Carey JW, Mejia R, Bingham T, Ciesielski C, Gelaude D, Herbst JH, et al. Drug use, high-risk sex behaviors, and increased risk for recent HIV infection among men who have sex with men in Chicago and Los Angeles. *AIDS Behav.* 2009;13(6):1084–1096.
15. Carpenter KM, Schreiber E, Church S, McDowell D. Drug stroop performance: relationships with primary substance of use and treatment outcome in a drug-dependent outpatient sample. *Addict Behav.* 2005;31:174–181.
16. Carroll KM. *A Cognitive-Behavioral Approach: Treating Cocaine Addiction (NIH Publication No. 98-4308).* National Institute on Drug Abuse Rockville MD; 1998.
17. Carroll KM, Kiluk BD, Nich C, Babuscio TA. Cognitive function and treatment response in a randomized clinical trial of computer-based training in cognitive-behavioral therapy. *Subst Use Misuse.* 2011;46(1):23–34.
18. Center for Substance Abuse Research. Dramatic increase in national treatment admissions for methamphetamine coincides with increase in criminal justice referrals. *CESAR FAX.* 2006;15(22):1.
19. Cooper WO, Arbogast PG, Ding H, Hickson GB, Fuchs DC, Ray WA. Trends in prescribing of antipsychotic medications for us children. *Ambul Pediatr.* 2006;6(2):79–83.
20. Copeland AL, Sorensen JL. Differences between methamphetamine users and cocaine users in treatment. *Drug Alcohol Depend.* 2001;62(1):91–95.
21. Reference deleted in review.
22. Curtin K, Fleckenstein AE, Robison RJ, Crookston MJ, Smith KR, Hanson GR. Methamphetamine/amphetamine abuse and risk of parkinson's disease in Utah: a population-based assessment. *Drug Alcohol Depend.* 2014;146:30–38.
23. Darke S, Kaye S, Duflou J. Rates, characteristics and circumstances of methamphetamine-related death in Australia: a national 7-year study. *Addiction.* 2017;112:2191–2201.
24. Dean AC, Groman SM, Morales AM, London ED. An evaluation of the evidence that methamphetamine abuse causes cognitive decline in humans. *Neuropsychopharmacology.* 2013;38(2):259–274.
25. Dean AC, London ED, Sugar CA, Kitchen CM, Swanson A, Heinzerling KG, et al. Predicting adherence to treatment for methamphetamine dependence from neuropsychological and drug use variables. *Drug Alcohol Depend.* 2009;105(1):48–55.
26. De-Carolis C, Boyd GA, Mancinelli L, Pagano S, Eramo S. Methamphetamine abuse and "meth mouth" in Europe. *Med Oral Patol Oral Cir Bucal.* 2015;20(2):e205–e210.
27. Denison FC, Norwood P, Bhattacharya S, Duffy A, Mahmood T, Morris C, et al. Association between maternal body mass index during pregnancy, short–term morbidity, and increased health service costs: a population–based study. *BJOG Int J Obstetric Gynaecol.* 2014;121(1):72–82.

28. Derauf C, LaGasse LL, Smith LM, Grant P, Shah R, Arria A, et al. Demographic and psychosocial characteristics of mothers using methamphetamine during pregnancy: preliminary results of the infant development, environment, and lifestyle study (ideal). *Am J Drug Alcohol Abuse.* 2007;33(2):281–289.

29. Dluzen DE, Liu B. Gender differences in methamphetamine use and responses: a review. *Gend Med.* 2008;5(1):24–35.

30. Elkashef A, Rawson RA, Smith E, Pearce V, Flammino F, Campbell J, et al. The NIDA methamphetamine clinical trials group: a strategy to increase clinical trials research capacity. *Addiction.* 2007;102(suppl 1):107–113.

31. Elkashef AM, Rawson RA, Anderson AL, Li SH, Holmes T, Smith EV, et al. Bupropion for the treatment of methamphetamine dependence. *Neuropsychopharmacology.* 2008;33(5):1162–1170.

32. Evans E, Longshore D, Prendergast M, Urada D. Evaluation of the substance abuse and crime prevention act: client characteristics, treatment completion and re-offending three years after implementation. *J Psychoactive Drugs.* 2006;38(suppl 3):357–367.

33. Farabee D, Prendergast M, Cartier L. Methamphetamine use and HIV risk among substance-abusing offenders in California. *J Psychoactive Drugs.* 2002;34:295–300.

34. Forrest DW, Metsch LR, LaLota M, Cardenas G, Beck DW, Jeanty Y. Crystal methamphetamine use and sexual risk behaviors among HIV-positive and HIV-negative men who have sex with men in South Florida. *J Urban Health.* 2010;87(3):480–485.

35. Freeman P, Walker BC, Harris DR, Garofalo R, Willard N, Ellen JM, et al. Methamphetamine use and risk for HIV among young men who have sex with men in 8 US cities. *Arch Pediatr Adolesc Med.* 2011;165(8):736–740.

36. Glasner-Edwards S, Mooney LJ, Marinelli-Casey P, Hillhouse M, Ang A, Rawson RA. Risk factors for suicide attempts in methamphetamine dependent patients. *Am J Addict.* 2008;17(1):24–27.

37. Glasner-Edwards S, Mooney LJ, Marinelli-Casey P, Hillhouse M, Ang A, Rawson RA. Identifying methamphetamine users at risk for major depressive disorder: findings from the methamphetamine treatment project at 3-year follow-up. *Am J Addict.* 2008;17(2):99–102.

38. Gonzales R, Marinelli-Casey P, Hillhouse M, Hunter J, Ang A, Rawson RA, et al. Hepatitis A and B virus infection among methamphetamine dependent users. *J Subst Abuse Treat.* 2008;35(3):351–352.

39. Gonzales R, Marinelli-Casey P, Shoptaw S, Ang A, Rawson RA. Hepatitis C virus infection among methamphetamine-dependent individuals in outpatient treatment. *J Subst Abuse Treat.* 2006;31(2):195–202.

40. Grant I, Gonzalez R, Carey CL, Natarajan L, Wolfson T. Non-acute (residual) neurocognitive effects of cannabis use: a meta-analytic study. *Soc J Int Neuropsychol.* 2003;9(5):679–689.

41. Hamamoto D, Rhodus N. Methamphetamine abuse and dentistry. *Oral Disease.* 2008;15(1):27–37.

42. Hartz DT, Frederick-Osborne SL, Galloway GP. Craving predicts use during treatment for methamphetamine dependence: a prospective, repeated-measures, within-subject analysis. *Drug Alcohol Depend.* 2001;63(3):269–276.

43. Heinzerling KG, Swanson A, Hall TM, Yi Y, Wu Y, Shoptaw SJ. Randomized, placebo-controlled trial of bupropion in methamphetamine-dependent participants with less than daily methamphetamine use. *Addiction.* 2014;109(11):1878–1886.

44. Herin DV, Rush C. Grabowski J Agonist–like pharmacotherapy for stimulant dependence: preclinical, human laboratory, and clinical studies. *Ann N Y Acad Sci.* 2010;1187:76–100.

45. Hester R, Lee N, Pennay A, Nielsen S, Ferris J. The effects of modafinil treatment on neuropsychological and attentional bias performance during 7-day inpatient withdrawal from methamphetamine dependence. *Exp Clin Psychopharmacol.* 2010;18(6):489–497.

46. Hillhouse MP, Marinelli–Casey P, Gonzales R, Ang A, Rawson RA. Predicting in–treatment performance and post–treatment outcomes in methamphetamine users. *Addiction.* 2007;102(s1):84–95.

47. Hoenigl M, Chaillon A, Moore DJ, Morris SR, Smith DM, Little SJ. Clear links between starting methamphetamine and increasing sexual risk behavior: a cohort study among men who have sex with men. *J Acquir Immune Defic Syndr.* 2016;71(5):551–557.

48. Hser YI, Evans E, Huang D, Brecht ML, Li L. Comparing the dynamic course of heroin, cocaine, and methamphetamine use over 10 years. *Addict Behav.* 2008;33(12):1581–1589.

49. Hser YI, Evans E, Yu-Chuang H. Treatment outcomes among women and men methamphetamine abusers in california. *J Subst Abuse Treat.* 2005;28(1):77–85.

50. Huber A, Ling W, Shoptaw S, Gulati V, Brethen P, Rawson R. Integrating treatments for methamphetamine abuse: a psychosocial perspective. *J Addict Dis.* 1997;16(4):41–50.

51. Hudak ML, Tan RC, Frattarelli DA, Galinkin JL, Green TP, Neville KA, et al. Neonatal drug withdrawal. *Pediatrics.* 2012;129(2):e540–e560.

52. Huddleston CW. *Drug courts: An effective strategy for communities facing methamphetamine, in Bureau of Justice Assistance Bulletin May 2005.* U.S. Department of Justice, Office of Justice Programs; 2005:1–15.

53. Isbister GK, Calver LA, Page CB, Stokes B, Bryant JL, Downes MA. Randomized controlled trial of intramuscular droperidol versus midazolam for violence and acute behavioral disturbance: the DORM study. *Ann Emerg Med.* 2010;56(4):392–401.e1.

54. Islam MN, Kuroki H, Hongcheng B, Ogura Y, Kawaguchi N, Onishi S, et al. Cardiac lesions and their reversibility after long term administration of methamphetamine. *Forensic Sci Int.* 1995;75(1):29–43.

55. Iudicello JE, Woods SP, Vigil O, Scott JC, Cherner M, Heaton RK, et al. Longer term improvement in neurocognitive functioning and affective distress among methamphetamine users who achieve stable abstinence. *Exp Neuropsychol Au.* 2010;32(7):704–718.

56. Jayaram-Lindstrom N, Hammarberg A, Beck O, Franck J. Naltrexone for the treatment of amphetamine dependence: a randomized, placebo-controlled trial. *Am J Psychiatr.* 2008;165(11):1442–1448.

57. Johnston LD, O'Malley PM, Bachman JG, Schulenberg JE. *Monitoring te Future: National Results on Adolescent Drug Use: Overview of Key Findings, 2007.* Bethesda MD: National Institute on Drug Abuse; 2008.

58. Jovanovski D, Erb S, Zakzanis KK. Neurocognitive deficits in cocaine users: review of the evidence. *J Clin Exp Neuropsychol.* 2005;27:189–240.

59. Karch SB, Stephens BG, Ho CH. Methamphetamine-related deaths in San Francisco: demographic, pathologic, and toxicologic profiles. *J Forensic Sci.* 1999;44(2):359–368.

60. Killen J, Matthews S, BakSheev G, Lloyd S. *Ambo Project: Alcohol and Drug Related Ambulance Attendances - 2014-15 Summary Bulletin.* Melbourne: Turning Point.

61. Lee NK, Harney AM, Pennay AE. Examining the temporal relationship between methamphetamine use and mental health comorbidity. *Adv Dual Diagn.* 2012;5(1):23–31.

62. Lee NK, Rawson RA. systematic review of cognitive and behavioural therapies for methamphetamine dependence. *Drug Alcohol Rev.* 2008;27(3):309–317.

63. Ling W, Chang L, Hillhouse M, Ang A, Striebel J, Jenkins J, et al. Sustained–release methylphenidate in a randomized trial of treatment of methamphetamine use disorder. *Addiction.* 2014;109(9):1489–1500.

64. Ling W, Rawson R, Shoptaw S. Management of methamphetamine abuse and dependence. *Curr Psychiatry Rep.* 2006;8:345–354.

65. Lubman D, Manning V, Best D, et al. *A Study of Patient Pathways in Alcohol and Other Drug Treatment.* Turning Point Fitzroy; 2014.

66. Luchansky B, Krupski A, Stark K. Treatment response by primary drug of abuse: does methamphetamine make a difference? *Abuse treat. J Subst Abuse Treat.* 2007;32:89–96.

67. Marinelli-Casey P, Gonzales R, Hillhouse M, Ang A, Zweben J, Cohen J, et al. Drug court treatment for methamphetamine dependence: treatment response and posttreatment outcomes. *J Subst Abuse Treat.* 2008;34(2):242–248.

68. Maxwell JC, Rutkowski BA. The prevalence of methamphetamine and amphetamine abuse in North America: a review of the indicators, 1992-2007. *Drug Alcohol Rev.* 2008;27(3):229–235.

69. McCann DJ, Li SH. A novel, nonbinary evaluation of success and failure reveals bupropion efficacy versus methamphetamine dependence: reanalysis of a multisite trial. *CNS Neurosci Ther.* 2012;18(5):414–418.

70. McEihiney MC, Rabkin JG, Rabkin R, Nunes EV. Provigil (modafinil) plus cognitive behavioral therapy for methamphetamine use in HIV+ gay men: a pilot study. *Am J Drug Alcohol.* 2009;35:34–37.

71. McGregor C, Srisurapanont M, Jittiwutikarn J, Laobhripatr S, Wongtan T, White JM. The nature, time course and severity of methamphetamine withdrawal. *Addiction.* 2005;100(9):1320–1329.

72. McKetin R, McLaren J, Lubman DI, Hides L. The prevalence of psychotic symptoms among methamphetamine users. *Addiction.* 2006;101(10):1473–1478.

73. McKetin R, Najman JM, Baker AL, Lubman DI, Dawe S, Ali R, et al. Evaluating the impact of community–based treatment options on methamphetamine use: findings from the methamphetamine treatment evaluation study (mates). *Addiction.* 2012;107(11):1998–2008.

74. Menza TW, Jameson DR, Hughes JP, Colfax GN, Shoptaw S, Golden MR. Contingency management to reduce methamphetamine use and sexual risk among men who have sex with men: a randomized controlled trial. *BMC Public Health.* 2010;10(1):774.

75. Meredith CW, Jaffe C, Ang-Lee K, Saxon AJ. Implications of chronic methamphetamine use: a literature review. *Harvard Rev Psychiatry.* 2005;13(3):141–154.

76. Messina N, Grella C. Childhood trauma and women's health outcomes: a California prison population. *Am J Public Health.* 2006;96(10):1842–1848.

77. Messina N, Grella C, Burdon W, Prendergast M. Childhood adverse events and current traumatic distress: a comparison of men and women prisoners. *Criminal Justice Behav.* 2007;34(11):1385–1401.

78. Messina N, Marinelli-Casey P, Hillhouse M, Rawson R, Hunter J, Ang A. Childhood adverse events and methamphetamine use among men and women. *J Psychoactive Drugs Suppl.* 2008;5:399–409.

79. Messina NP, Burdon WM, Prendergast ML. Assessing the needs of women in institutional therapeutic communities. *J Offender Rehabil.* 2003;37(2):89–106.

80. Miura H, Fujiki M, Shibata A, Ishikawa K. Prevalence and profile of methamphetamine users in adolescents at a juvenile classification home. *Psychiatry Clin Neurosci.* 2006;60(3):352–357.

81. National Center on Addiction and Substance Abuse. *The Formative Years: Pathways to Substance Abuse Among Girls and Young Women Ages.* New York: CASA: Columbia University; 2003:8–22.

82. National Institute on Drug Abuse. *Methamphetamine abuse and addiction, in Research Report Series, NIH Publication No. 02-4210.* Bethesda MD: NIDA; 2002.

83. Peck JA, Reback CJ, Yang X, Rotheram-Fuller E, Shoptaw S. Sustained reductions in drug use and depression symptoms from treatment for drug abuse in methamphetamine-dependent gay and bisexual men. *J Urban Health.* 2005;82:i100–i108.

84. Perez-Mana C, Castells X, Torrens M, Capella D, Farre M. Efficacy of psychostimulant drugs for amphetamine abuse or dependence. *Cochrane Database Syst Rev.* 2013;9.

85. Pierce RC, Kumaresan V. The mesolimbic dopamine system: the final common pathway for the reinforcing effect of drugs of abuse? *Neurosci Biobehav Rev.* 2006;30(2):215–238.

86. Rawson R, Gonzales R, Ling W. Methamphetamine abuse and dependence: an update. *Directions in Psychiatry.* 2006;26(10):131–144.

87. Rawson R, Pearce V, Ang A, Marinelli-Casey P, Brummer J, Authors MTPC. Methamphetamine dependence and human immunodeficiency virus risk behavior. *J Subst Abuse Treat.* 2008;35(3):279–284.

88. Rawson RA, Chudzynski J, Gonzales R, Mooney L, Dickerson D, Ang A, et al. The impact of exercise on depression and anxiety symptoms among abstinent methamphetamine-dependent individuals in a residential treatment setting. *J Subst Abuse Treat.* 2015;57:36–40.

89. Rawson RA, Gonzales R, Marinelli–Casey P, Ang A. Methamphetamine dependence: a closer look at treatment response and clinical characteristics associated with route of administration in outpatient treatment. *Am J Addict.* 2007;16(4):291–299.

90. Rawson RA, Gonzales R, Obert JL, McCann MJ, Brethen P. Methamphetamine use among treatment-seeking adolescents in southern california: participant characteristics and treatment response. *J Subst Abuse Treat.* 2005;29(2):67–74.

91. Rawson RA, Marinelli–Casey P, Anglin MD, Dickow A, Frazier Y, Gallagher C, et al. A multi–site comparison of psychosocial approaches for the treatment of methamphetamine dependence. *Addiction.* 2004;99(6):708–717.

92. Rawson RA, McCann MJ, Flammino F, Shoptaw S, Miotto K, Reiber C, et al. A comparison of contingency management and cognitive-behavioral approaches for stimulant-dependent individuals. *Addiction.* 2006;101(2):267–274.

93. Roll JM, Chudzynski J, Cameron JM, Howell DN, McPherson S. Duration effects in contingency management treatment of methamphetamine disorders. *Addict Behav.* 2013;38(9):2455–2462.

94. Roll JM, Petry NM, Stitzer ML, Brecht ML, Peirce JM, McCann MJ, et al. Contingency management for the treatment of methamphetamine use disorders. *Am J Psychiatry.* 2006;163(11):1993–1999.

95. Rusyniak DE. Neurologic manifestations of chronic methamphetamine abuse. *Neurol Clin.* 2011;29(3):641–655.

96. Scott JC, Woods SP, Matt GE, Meyer RA, Heaton RK, Atkinson JH, et al. Neurocognitive effects of methamphetamine: a critical review and meta-analysis. *Neuropsychol Rev.* 2007;17(3):275–297.

97. Shetty V, Harrell L, Murphy DA, Vitero S, Gutierrez A, Belin TR, et al. Dental disease patterns in methamphetamine users: findings in a large urban sample. *J Am Dent Assoc.* 2015;146(12):875–885.

98. Shoptaw S, Reback CJ, Peck JA, Yang X, Rotheram-Fuller E, Larkins S, et al. Behavioral treatment approaches for methamphetamine dependence and HIV-related sexual risk behaviors among urban gay and bisexual men. *Drug Alcohol Depend.* 2005;78(2):125–134.

99. Simon SL, Dean AC, Cordova X, Monterosso JR, London ED. Methamphetamine dependence and neuropsychological functioning: evaluating change during early abstinence. *J Stud Alcohol Drugs.* 2010;71(3):335–344.

100. Smith LM, Diaz S, LaGasse LL, Wouldes T, Derauf C, Newman E, et al. Developmental and behavioral consequences of prenatal methamphetamine exposure: a review of the infant development, environment, and lifestyle (ideal) study. *Neurotoxicol Teratol.* 2015;51:35–44.

101. Smout MF, Longo M, Harrison S, Minniti R, Wickes W, White JM. Psychosocial treatment for methamphetamine use disorders: a preliminary randomized controlled trial of cognitive behavior therapy and acceptance and commitment therapy. *Subst Abus.* 2010;31:98–107.

102. Stoops WW, Rush CR. Agonist replacement for stimulant dependence: a review of clinical research. *Curr Pharm Des.* 2013;19:7026–7035.

103. Stoops WW, Rush CR. Combination pharmacotherapies for stimulant use disorder: a review of clinical findings and recommendations for future research. *Expert Rev Clin Pharmacol.* 2014;7:363–374.

104. Substance Abuse and Mental Health Services Administration. *Results From the 2007 National Survey on Drug Use and Health: National findings in Office of Applied Studies, NSDUH Series H-34, DHHS Publication No. SMA 08-4343.* Rockville, MD: SAMHSA; 2008:08–4343.

105. Substance Abuse and Mental Health Services Administration. *Results From the 2013 National Survey on Drug Use and Health: Summary of National Findings. in NSDUH Series H-48, HHS Publication No. (SMA) 14-4863.* Rockville MD: SAMHSA; 2014.

106. Tarter RE, Kirisci L, Habeych M, Reynolds M, Vanyukov M. Neurobehavior disinhibition in childhood predisposes boys to substance use disorder by young adulthood: direct and mediated etiologic pathways. *Drug Alcohol Depend.* 2004;73(2): 121–132.

107. Taylor DM, Yap CY, Knott JC, Taylor SE, Phillips GA, Karro J, et al. Midazolam-droperidol, droperidol, or olanzapine for acute agitation: A randomized clinical trial. *Ann Emerg Med.* 2017;69(3):318–326.e1.

108. Thompson CA J. Pulmonary arterial hypertension seen in methamphetamine abusers. *Am Syst Pharm.* 2008;65(12):1109–1110.

109. Turner S, Longshore D, Wenzel S, Deschenes E, Greenwood P, Fain T. A decade of drug treatment court research. *Subst Use Misuse.* 2002;37(12 and 13):1489–1527.

110. Turnipseed SD, Richards JR, Kirk JD, Diercks DB, Amsterdam EA. Frequency of acute coronary syndrome in patients presenting to the emergency department with chest pain after methamphetamine use. *J Emerg Med.* 2003;24:369–373.

111. Vogt TM, Perz JF, Van Houten CK, Harrington R, Hansuld T, Bialek SR. An outbreak of hepatitis b virus infection among methamphetamine injectors: the role of sharing injection drug equipment. *Addiction.* 2006;101(5):726–730.

112. Wang G, Smith L, Volkow N, Telang F, Logan J, Tomasi D, et al. Decreased dopamine activity predicts relapse in methamphetamine abusers. *Mol Psychiatry.* 2012;17(9):918–925.

113. Wang G, Volkow ND, Chang L, Miller E, Sedler M, Hitzemann R, et al. Partial recovery of brain metabolism in methamphetamine abusers after protracted abstinence. *Am J Psychiatry.* 2004;161(2):242–248.

114. Wang SJ, Ju T, Chen C, Liao K, Fuh J, Hu H. Stroke associated with methamphetamine inhalation. *Eur Neurol.* 1994;34(1):16–22.

115. Wijetunga M, Bhan R, Lindsay J, Karch S. Acute coronary syndrome and crystal methamphetamine use: a case series. *Hawaii Med J.* 2004;63:8–13.

116. Won S, Hong RA, Shohet RV, Seto TB, Parikh NI. Methamphetamine-associated cardiomyopathy. *Clin Cardiol.* 2013;36(12):737–742.

117. Wouldes T, LaGasse L, Sheridan J, Lester B, NZ. Maternal methamphetamine use during pregnancy and child outcome: what do we know. *NZ Med J.* 2004;117(1206):1–10.

118. Yen CF, Su YC. The associations of early-onset methamphetamine use with psychiatric morbidity among taiwanese adolescents. *Subst Use Misuse.* 2006;41:35–44.

119. Zorick T, Nestor L, Miotto K, Sugar C, Hellemann G, Scanlon G, et al. Withdrawal symptoms in abstinent methamphetamine-dependent subjects. *Addiction.* 2010;105:1809–1818.

120. Zweben JE, Cohen JB, Christian D, Galloway GP, Salinardi M, Parent D, et al. Psychiatric symptoms in methamphetamine users. *Am J Addict.* 2004;13(2):181–190.

27

Sedative-Hypnotics and Anxiolytics

BACHAAR ARNAOUT AND ISMENE L. PETRAKIS

Introduction

The sedative-hypnotics and anxiolytics are central nervous system depressants that also have muscle relaxant and anticonvulsant effects and are widely used in psychiatry, neurology, anesthesiology, and general medicine. The most common of these are the benzodiazepines and the new-generation nonbenzodiazepine hypnotics (i.e., zaleplon, zolpidem, and eszopiclone), which due to their better safety profiles have largely replaced the barbiturates and other older agents, particularly in the treatment of insomnia and anxiety. This group of medications also includes chloral hydrate, meprobamate, carisoprodol, glutethimide, and methaqualone. γ-Hydroxybutyrate, which has some properties associated with the sedative-hypnotics, is usually classified as a club drug.

Beyond their use in the treatment of anxiety disorders and insomnia, the benzodiazepines also are often used for the management of agitation, the treatment of seizures, as muscle relaxants, for premedication in anesthesiology, and as the mainstay of treatment for the management of medication detoxification from alcohol. The new-generation nonbenzodiazepine hypnotics are used primarily for the treatment of insomnia. The barbiturates are most commonly prescribed for the treatment of epilepsy and for anesthesia, and they can also be used for detoxification from alcohol. The older sedative-hypnotic and anxiolytic agents such as chloral hydrate, meprobamate, carisoprodol, glutethimide, and methaqualone are less commonly used nowadays.

These groups of medications have a similar mechanism of action in that they all enhance the activity of the brain's main inhibitory neurotransmitter, γ-aminobutyric acid (GABA), leading to the opening of chloride channels and cell membrane hyperpolarization. In a simplified but clinically useful model, the central nervous system maintains a balance between inhibitory signals mediated by GABA and signals mediated by the brain's primary excitatory neurotransmitter, glutamate.[27] When the balance sways toward glutamate-mediated excitatory transmission, the individual experiences arousal and anxiety; conversely, GABA-mediated inhibitory transmission results in tranquility and sedation. The benzodiazepines bind to GABA$_A$ receptors, where they enhance GABA activity.[62] The new-generation nonbenzodiazepine hypnotics have a similar mode of action but appear to have relative selectivity to certain subunits of the GABA$_A$ receptor, resulting in a prominent sedative-hypnotic effect and a relatively weaker anxiolytic effect.[22] In addition, the barbiturates potentiate GABA activity at the GABA$_A$ receptor, but may additionally exert a direct effect on opening the chloride channel.[48] Chloral hydrate, meprobamate, carisoprodol, glutethimide, and methaqualone also appear to exert their effects through GABAergic transmission. All of these medications can be used to reduce anxiety at lower doses and to induce sleep at higher doses. Commonly used sedative-hypnotics and anxiolytic drugs, along with their approximate dose equivalencies, are included in Table 27.1. Because all of these drugs have wide therapeutic applications and are among the most commonly used, the conceptualization of what constitutes inappropriate use of the sedative-hypnotics and anxiolytics is often difficult to determine. The use of these drugs in a fashion other than as prescribed (i.e., nonmedical use) has been defined as "misuse," and the terms "abuse" and "dependence" have been replaced by the term "substance use disorder" in the *Diagnostic and Statistical Manual of Mental Disorders, Fifth Edition* (DSM-5).[1]

Despite their most common appropriate therapeutic use, nonmedical use of the sedative-hypnotics and anxiolytics can be problematic and often occurs in individuals with other substance use disorders as well as those with general psychiatric disorders. In the 2014 National Survey on Drug Use and Health, with a sample of 67,901 respondents representative of the United States, 0.1% and 0.7% of people 12 years of age or older were current nonmedical users of sedatives or tranquilizers, respectively.[9] In the National Epidemiologic Survey on Alcohol and Related Conditions, conducted in 2001–2002 with a sample of 43,093 respondents representative of the United States, the lifetime prevalence of nonmedical use of sedatives and tranquilizers was 4.1% and 3.4%, respectively, and the lifetime prevalence of sedative and tranquilizer use disorder was 1.1% and 1.0%, respectively.[45] In the same survey, the 12-month prevalence rates were 0.16% for sedative

TABLE 27.1	List of Sedative-Hypnotics and Anxiolytics With Approximate Dose Equivalencies.	
Generic Name	Trade Name	Approximate Dose Equivalency (mg)
Benzodiazepines		
Alprazolam	Xanax	1
Chlordiazepoxide	Librium	25
Clonazepam	Klonopin	1
Clorazepate	Tranxene	15
Diazepam	Valium	10
Estazolam	ProSom	1
Flurazepam	Dalmane	20
Lorazepam	Ativan	2
Oxazepam	Serax	20
Quazepam	Doral	20
Temazepam	Restoril	20
Triazolam	Halcion	0.25
Non-Benzodiazepine Hypnotics		
Eszopiclone	Lunesta	3
Zaleplon	Sonata	10
Zolpidem	Ambien	10
Barbiturates		
Amobarbital	Amytal	100
Butabarbital	Butisol	100
Butalbital	Fiorinal	100
Pentobarbital	Nembutal	100
Phenobarbital	Luminal	30
Secobarbital	Seconal	100
Other Agents		
Chloral hydrate	Noctec	500
Glutethimide	Doriden	250
Meprobamate	Miltown	800
Methaqualone	Quaalude	300

use disorder and 0.13% for tranquilizer use disorder.[96] The survey reported high rates of lifetime comorbidity between sedative and tranquilizer use disorders and alcohol use disorders (odds ratios of 13.4 and 14.2, respectively), mood disorders (odds ratios of 4.9 and 4.8, respectively), anxiety disorders (odds ratios of 3.7 and 4.2, respectively), and personality disorders (odds ratios of 5.6 and 6.6, respectively).[94] Comorbidity is likely to be even higher in clinical populations. For example, in a sample of 427 treatment-seeking individuals with alcohol use disorders, the lifetime prevalence of anxiolytic use disorder was 20%[80]; and in a survey of 194 patients on methadone maintenance, 47% reported a history of benzodiazepine use, and 39.8% reported a history of nonmedical benzodiazepine use.[11] Conversely, in a sample of 30 consecutive

patients undergoing inpatient detoxification from benzodiazepines because of severe benzodiazepine dependence, 100% had another lifetime substance use disorder, 33% had lifetime major depression, and 30% had lifetime panic disorder.[8]

Intoxication and Overdose

As noted earlier, the benzodiazepines are most commonly used as anxiolytics and sedative-hypnotics. However, there are reports of their consumption for the purpose of intoxication, which is described as similar to alcohol intoxication,[84] leading to the saying, "benzodiazepines are the driest of martinis."[32] There are, however, some differences between intoxication from benzodiazepines and alcohol intoxication. For example, benzodiazepine users less commonly report the social disinhibition associated with alcohol use. Disinhibition and aggression related to benzodiazepine use is relatively rare and is more likely to occur in persons with high baseline levels of hostility as well as those with preexisting brain damage.[41] With dose escalation, pleasurable intoxication may progress to manifestations of more profound toxicity, such as impairment in attention or memory, slurred speech, incoordination, unsteady gait, nystagmus, stupor or coma, and eventually respiratory depression. The benzodiazepines have a fairly wide therapeutic index, and overdose rarely results in death in healthy individuals. However, although safer than the barbiturates,[88] the benzodiazepines have been associated with lethal overdoses when used alone,[23] and especially when combined with other central nervous system depressants, such as alcohol[49,88] and opioids, including buprenorphine.[47,99,108] Recent data are very concerning, as rates of both benzodiazepine prescriptions and benzodiazepine-related overdose deaths rose considerably in the first decade of the century,[5] and their use was involved in 30.6% of prescription drug-related overdose deaths in 2013.[10] In addition, a recent large retrospective cohort study found an association between anxiolytic and hypnotic use and an increased risk of mortality.[104]

The mechanism by which benzodiazepines manifest their rewarding potential is not well understood. Recent findings suggest that benzodiazepines share their reinforcing effects with other addictive drugs by activating the mesolimbic reward pathway.[97] Laboratory studies that have tried to evaluate the rewarding properties of the benzodiazepines have found that healthy individuals have no preference for the benzodiazepines over placebo—in fact, healthy subjects have demonstrated a preference for placebo over higher doses of the benzodiazepines.[110] However, individuals with a substance use disorder history, especially to sedatives, may be more likely to experience benzodiazepines as rewarding.[110] In addition, there is evidence that individuals with a history of moderate alcohol consumption, anxiety, and insomnia,[37] as well as children of alcoholics,[14,15] may be more likely to experience the reinforcing effects of the benzodiazepines. Of interest though, research on the use of the benzodiazepines for the treatment of anxiety disorders in individuals with a prior history of substance use disorder found little evidence for induction of relapse to substance use.[63,68] There is some evidence that benzodiazepines with a rapid onset of action such as diazepam[35,36] and those with a short half-life such as alprazolam,[3] may have a relatively more reinforcing effect, although these results are controversial.[82] Taking the drug intravenously also has been associated with increased reinforcing effects.[89]

When misused, the central nervous system depressants are often taken in combination with other drugs,[18,19] often leading to complex and dangerous interactions. For example, individuals may use the benzodiazepines to enhance intoxication with opioids or alcohol, or to self-medicate the anxiety associated with stimulant use as well as the discomfort associated with stimulant or opioid withdrawal.

The nonbenzodiazepine hypnotics are even less likely to be taken for intoxication; however, they carry a risk of misuse, especially among individuals with other substance use disorders and psychiatric comorbidity.[13,38] Although they are likely safer than the benzodiazepines, there have been reports of coma, respiratory depression, and fatal overdoses on high doses of zolpidem, especially when combined with other drugs.[17] The barbiturates have a narrower therapeutic window in comparison with the benzodiazepines and carry more risk of dangerous central nervous system depression and death on overdose. Fatal overdose also may occur with other older agents; however, both their medical and recreational use has declined since the introduction of the benzodiazepines.

Benzodiazepine intoxication is managed according to the level of severity. Mild intoxication can be managed with supportive care and medical monitoring, while overdose is managed in an intensive care setting. Flumazenil, a benzodiazepine receptor antagonist, can be used intravenously to reverse benzodiazepine overdose.[105] Flumazenil should be used with caution as its use may induce benzodiazepine withdrawal and increase the risk of grand mal seizures.[105] Flumazenil also has been used in overdose related to the new-generation nonbenzodiazepine hypnotics.[12,29,42] Because the barbiturates exert their activity independently of the benzodiazepine binding site, flumazenil does not block their effects and is not useful in barbiturate overdose.

Tolerance and Withdrawal

Physiological dependence requires the presence of tolerance or withdrawal. Tolerance is marked by the gradual need to use increased doses of the substance to achieve the same effect, or a diminished effect with the same dose. Tolerance to the sedative-hypnotics and anxiolytics occurs through central nervous system adaptation to the drug at the receptor level.[7] Depending on the agent used, its dose, and the duration of use, tolerance can develop in days to months. Tolerance to the benzodiazepines is more likely to develop to the sedative-hypnotic and motor impairment effects than to the anxiolytic and short-term memory impairment effects.[33,54] Tolerance can be minimized by using the medication for a short period, taking "drug holidays," and using the lowest effective dose. Cross-tolerance can occur between the benzodiazepines and other depressant drugs, including alcohol.[46]

Withdrawal is marked by the presence of a characteristic syndrome on cessation or reduction in the use of the substance and can be avoided or relieved by taking the same or closely related substance. Symptoms of withdrawal from the benzodiazepines resemble those of alcohol withdrawal, and are generally the result of central nervous system excitation, which is the opposite of the primary action of the drug. Withdrawal progresses from a syndrome of anxiety, insomnia, and tremor to nausea, vomiting, diaphoresis, tachycardia, hypertension, and rarely to grand mal seizures[58] and delirium in rare, severe cases.[53,112] Withdrawal usually develops after taking the benzodiazepines for months; however, milder withdrawal may emerge after days to weeks of use. Withdrawal severity correlates with the duration of use[72] and the potency and dose of the drug taken,[58] as well as individual susceptibility and general health status.

Syndromes that occur commonly after cessation of use of the benzodiazepines can be divided into:
- Acute withdrawal, characterized by relatively severe symptoms emerging several hours to days following dose reduction or cessation of use. Use of short-acting agents is associated with relatively more intense but shorter duration of acute withdrawal symptoms, peaking 2 days after discontinuation, whereas longer-acting agents result in milder but longer withdrawal, peaking in 4–7 days.[65,74]
- Protracted withdrawal, characterized by ongoing anxiety and depression, as well as mild sensory and motor disturbances that can linger for months.[4] More severe presentations such as psychotic depression also have been reported.[61]
- Symptom recurrence, which is the reemergence of preexisting symptoms, such as anxiety, that were previously masked by the benzodiazepine.[65] Although often difficult to distinguish, reemerging symptoms tend to be stable over time, unlike withdrawal symptoms, which tend to subside gradually.
- Symptom rebound, which is the exacerbation of preexisting symptoms after cessation of use, and is, therefore, a combination of genuine withdrawal and symptom reemergence.[25,65]

Of note, physiological dependence (i.e., tolerance or withdrawal) may occur even when the medications are adequately used at therapeutic doses and does not necessarily indicate that a substance use disorder has developed, as defined by the DSM-5. Nonetheless, the presence of physiological dependence should alert the clinician that the individual may have developed a substance use disorder, in which case the presence of tolerance and withdrawal is associated with greater severity of the disorder.[83] The term "addiction," although not an official diagnostic term in the DSM-5, is commonly used to refer to the more severe forms of substance use disorder.

Benzodiazepine withdrawal can be managed by supportive measures in mild cases. In more severe cases, pharmacological detoxification is often achieved by substituting the substance with a long-acting benzodiazepine such as clonazepam or chlordiazepoxide and gradually reducing the dose over several days in inpatient detoxification programs. Intermediate-acting benzodiazepines, such as lorazepam, also are effective, and a simple taper of the original medication can also be used. Although inpatient detoxification may be needed when concurrently detoxifying from several drugs such as alcohol and opiates, a more gradual taper also can be achieved over several weeks to months in the outpatient setting.[87] Evidence suggests that gradual detoxification is more effective than abrupt discontinuation, which is associated with a higher dropout rate.[21] It also is recommended that the taper be slower after reaching about 50% of the original dose.[75,87] An older method, using phenobarbital substitution,[92] is less common, but is used when detoxifying individuals from the barbiturates.[91] Because benzodiazepine or barbiturate withdrawal is associated with serious morbidity and the possibility of mortality, the clinician should evaluate individuals carefully and consider pharmacologic management of benzodiazepine withdrawal. Of other, non–sedative-hypnotic/anxiolytic medications studied for benzodiazepine detoxification, the anticonvulsant carbamazepine has the most promising data, suggesting its possible utility when used as an adjunct to the benzodiazepines,[86] and its use also may improve drug-free outcomes.[21] The adjunctive use of pregabalin may have a role in improving subjective sleep quality during benzodiazepine tapers.[81]

The literature on physiological dependence to the new-generation nonbenzodiazepine hypnotics has been scarce.

Tolerance and withdrawal from these drugs have been reported but appear to be relatively rare, as compared with the benzodiazepines,[38] possibly due to their relative selectivity at the $GABA_A$ receptor. Caution, however, is advised, as there have been reported cases of withdrawal seizures,[16] as well as withdrawal delirium and psychosis, after discontinuation of the use of the new-generation nonbenzodiazepine hypnotics.[98,100,109] A detoxification regimen similar to that used with the benzodiazepines and barbiturates has been suggested in managing withdrawal from these agents.[70]

Withdrawal from the barbiturates and other older agents is associated with a clinical picture comparable to that of the benzodiazepines and may lead to withdrawal seizures as well as delirium. Treatment includes detoxification with phenobarbital, a benzodiazepine, or by a gradual taper of the original substance.

Substance Use Disorder

The DSM-5[1] offers a clear definition of substance use disorder that applies to most classes of substances of abuse (the exception is drugs that do not haven an established withdrawal syndrome), including the sedative-hypnotics and anxiolytics.

Evaluating for sedative, hypnotic, and anxiolytic use disorder when a patient has been prescribed the medication by a physician is potentially difficult. For example, if an individual manifests psychosocial deterioration, it is often difficult to determine whether it is related to a substance use disorder or the result of an undertreated anxiety disorder. The trajectory of the patient's level of functioning may be a good clinical barometer—if their level of functioning improves with the use of a benzodiazepine, then it is likely that the prescribed substance is beneficial. Conversely, the patient's demand for increasing doses of the medications despite deteriorating psychosocial functioning is one indication that a substance use disorder may have developed. The patient's level of functioning can be evaluated by accessing previous records, as well as collateral information and involvement of significant others, after obtaining the patient's consent.

Other indicators of the presence of a substance use disorder are reports of loss of prescriptions, running out of the medication, obtaining the medication from several prescribers, and other signs of loss of control over use of the substance. Even when these signs are present, the physician should consider the possibility that the behavior could be related to the patient's efforts to obtain a medication that they need for a genuine disorder. In such instances, with adequate treatment of the underlying psychiatric disorder, this behavioral pattern should resolve. Naturally, there is no simple strategy to managing these complex clinical situations, and in all cases the clinician should clarify the reasons for the patient's use of these agents, evaluate the risk/benefit ratio of prescribing, and subsequently use clinical judgment to develop a reasonable treatment plan in collaboration with the patient.

A common clinical dilemma revolves around whether a physician should prescribe benzodiazepines to individuals with a history of other (nonbenzodiazepine) substance use disorders. Although their use is unquestionably of great value in detoxification from alcohol and other substances, their value as anxiolytics and sedative-hypnotics in this patient population is difficult to determine. The prudent course seems to be that although the benzodiazepines should not be absolutely contraindicated in patients with a history of substance use disorders, since some individuals may in fact benefit from treatment with benzodiazepines without misusing them, special care should be exercised and, if possible,

the benzodiazepines should not be the first line of treatment. When prescribed, their use should be monitored and the clinical course followed over time for signs of a substance use disorder.

Treatment of sedative-hypnotic and anxiolytic use disorder usually involves successful detoxification, followed by psychosocial interventions aimed at achieving long-term abstinence. People with sedative-hypnotic and anxiolytic use disorder often have other co-occurring substance use disorders and psychiatric disorders,[45] which should be screened for, adequately diagnosed, and concurrently treated. There are no agents approved by the US Food and Drug Administration (FDA) for the long-term treatment of benzodiazepine use disorder. However, pharmacologic strategies are being investigated to target achieving abstinence from the benzodiazepines. Agents that have shown promising potential include the benzodiazepine antagonist flumazenil[30,44] although further study is clearly needed, as its use may carry a high risk of precipitating seizures in patients with physiological dependence.[55] Other promising agents include the anticonvulsants carbamazepine[21] and valproate.[39,77] Although controversial, maintenance substitution treatment with a long-acting agent, such as clonazepam, also has been suggested.[106] Long-acting benzodiazepines may provide adequate relief from low-grade anxiety, which may be a trigger to relapse to other benzodiazepine and alcohol use. These strategies, although interesting and promising, are still in their investigational stages, and data supporting their safety and efficacy are limited.

Data on the new-generation nonbenzodiazepine hypnotics have been scarce; however, there is emerging evidence that they do carry a risk of substance use disorder, especially among individuals with other substance use disorders and psychiatric comorbidity.[13,38] Although use disorder related to these medications seems to be less likely than with the benzodiazepines, caution should nonetheless be exercised with their prolonged use. Since the introduction of the benzodiazepines, use of the barbiturates and other older agents has been declining, and use disorders related to these agents are relatively rare.

Mood and Anxiety Disorders

The benzodiazepines, unlike many other medications used in psychiatry, offer patients substantial and quick relief from anxiety and insomnia, which, whether primary or related to other disorders such as depression or psychosis, are among the most common symptoms in the practice of psychiatry. The benzodiazepines can be taken continuously or as needed and often lack many of the side effects common to psychiatric medications such as weight gain, liver toxicity, and sexual dysfunction. However, although often prescribed for the initial phases of anxiety disorders and depression, the controversy lies in their continued use beyond the acute phase. Some research suggests that they display continued efficacy for the long-term treatment of panic disorder, without the need for progressive dose escalation.[73,111] Many long-term benzodiazepine users actually decrease their dose and make attempts to stop use.[78] Other research, however, questions the long-term efficacy of the benzodiazepines for the treatment of anxiety and depression,[67] and suggests that their chronic use may be associated with depressive symptomatology,[90] although direct causation has not been clearly established. There is also concern that continued use may result in interdose rebound symptoms or simply mask withdrawal rather than treat an underlying anxiety disorder. Moreover, some research has demonstrated that anxiety levels may actually decrease after successful discontinuation of benzodiazepine use.[37]

In addition, there is evidence suggesting that both short-term and long-term use of the benzodiazepines may interfere with other effective treatments, such as cognitive behavioral therapy for panic disorder,[66,102] and that benzodiazepine use may be associated with poorer maintenance of gains after exposure therapy for posttraumatic stress disorder,[79] although direct causality is not possible to establish based on current data. As noted earlier, depression and psychotic depression have been described in protracted withdrawal from the benzodiazepines.[4,61] Additional precautions in prescribing these medications should be taken due to the frequent use of the benzodiazepines in suicide attempts[60] and accidental overdose.

It is recommended to use nonbenzodiazepine medications such as the selective serotonin reuptake inhibitors, as well as other antidepressants and buspirone, as first-line agents for mood and anxiety disorders, especially in individuals with a history of substance use disorder. Other strategies to manage acute anxiety include the use of anticonvulsants, antihistamines, and antipsychotics. Effective psychotherapies, such as cognitive behavioral therapy, also have been developed for specific disorders. The benzodiazepines are safest when reserved either as short-term adjuvants to other medications in the initial stages of treatment or as long-term treatment only in refractory cases. Moreover, they should be generally avoided in individuals with an active substance use disorder and cautiously in those with a remitted substance use disorder.

Many long-term benzodiazepine users can be gradually detoxified from these drugs on an outpatient basis. The difficulty often lies in patients' perception that the benzodiazepines are the only effective medications. With a good therapeutic alliance, a detoxification regimen often can be successfully negotiated and achieved. Patients should be reassured that there are numerous nonbenzodiazepine medications that are effective in managing insomnia and anxiety disorders. In treating these individuals, clinicians need to distinguish between protracted withdrawal and the reemergence of symptoms of a mood or an anxiety disorder (i.e., symptom relapse).

Cognitive Disorders

Acute use of the benzodiazepines is known to cause cognitive impairment, especially among the elderly and those with preexisting brain damage, and it is likely to resolve after tapering or discontinuing the medication. In more severe cases, this may progress to developing delirium.[28] As noted earlier, delirium also can be a sign of withdrawal from the benzodiazepines.

The extent of the effects of prolonged use of the benzodiazepines on cognition is difficult to determine. Research has demonstrated lack of tolerance to benzodiazepine-associated short-term memory impairment even after years of use.[33,54] After cessation of use, cognition is likely to gradually improve within weeks[76]; however, some cognitive deficit after prolonged use may linger even months after stopping the medication, and it is unclear whether this reflects permanent residual cognitive deficit.[6,95,103] A recent case-control study found an association between benzodiazepine use and the risk of dementia,[20] although causality is impossible to ascertain based on the presented data. Findings of a subsequent prospective cohort study did not support a causal relationship between benzodiazepine use and dementia.[34] In light of this evidence, caution should be taken with use of the benzodiazepines, especially in those prone to cognitive impairment, who are at an increased risk for confusion and falls.

Use of other GABAergic drugs, including the new-generation nonbenzodiazepine hypnotics, can cause cognitive impairment.[59] Delirium also may be associated with the use and withdrawal from the new-generation nonbenzodiazepine hypnotics,[98,109] as well as other GABAergic agents.

Psychotic Manifestations

Psychosis related to the use of the benzodiazepines is relatively rare. However, psychosis may be associated with benzodiazepine withdrawal delirium[40] and is an indication for medically supervised detoxification. When part of delirium, psychotic symptoms should be considered as part of the withdrawal picture and treated with appropriate, often very high doses of the benzodiazepines with close medical monitoring. Antipsychotic medications should be used with caution and only as adjuncts to the benzodiazepines. It remains unclear to what extent antipsychotics are beneficial in treating withdrawal delirium beyond their sedative effect, and although they may be useful in managing agitation, they may also inappropriately cover underlying withdrawal symptoms. Antipsychotic medications can also lower the seizure threshold and potentiate delirium due to anticholinergic activity. If antipsychotics need to be used in combination with the benzodiazepines to manage agitation in the context of benzodiazepine withdrawal, high-potency antipsychotics such as haloperidol should be considered. As noted earlier, psychotic depression also has been reported as a presentation of protracted benzodiazepine withdrawal.[61]

Psychosis, marked by hallucinations and delusions after weeks of benzodiazepine use at a therapeutic level, has been reported and may be related to underlying brain damage.[107] In this case, psychosis is likely to resolve with dose reduction or cessation of benzodiazepine use. Psychosis may also be associated with intoxication or withdrawal from the new-generation nonbenzodiazepine hypnotics[57,98,100] as well as other GABAergic sedative-hypnotics and anxiolytics.

Sleep Disorders

Short-term use of the benzodiazepines results in a decrease in sleep latency and the number of awakenings, an increase in total sleep time, and improvement in sleep quality.[43,64] Other effects of short-term use include daytime drowsiness,[43] as well as disruption of sleep architecture: stage 2 increases, slow-wave sleep decreases, and rapid-eye-movement sleep latency decreases.[69] Continued use of benzodiazepines can result in tolerance to their sedative action, which may occur after several days,[93] and can eventually lead to rebound insomnia when their use is stopped.[94] There also is concern that chronic use may be simply masking rebound insomnia rather than treating an underlying sleep problem.[37] Individuals who demand escalating doses of the benzodiazepines may be misinterpreting tolerance and rebound insomnia as a need for a dose increase.

As noted earlier, the new-generation nonbenzodiazepine hypnotics may be less likely to result in tolerance, especially when used at therapeutic doses. Eszopiclone and the extended-release form of zolpidem (Ambien CR) have been shown to be effective and safe in the long-term management of insomnia in a double-blind, placebo-controlled design,[50,51] and zolpidem and zaleplon have been shown to have long-term efficacy in open-label studies.[2,56] These data may encourage physicians to prescribe these medications more freely than the benzodiazepines. However, an assessment group from the National Institute for Health and Clinical

Excellence, an independent organization providing guidance on health-related issues in the United Kingdom, concluded that randomized controlled trials have not been able to demonstrate substantial consistent differences between zolpidem, zaleplon, zopiclone (of which eszopiclone is the (S)-isomer), and the benzodiazepines in terms of their efficacy or in treatment-emergent adverse events.[24] Overall, caution should be exercised with prolonged use of all GABAergic sedative-hypnotics, and other strategies such as cognitive behavioral therapy should be incorporated into treatment. Other pharmacologic strategies are also available, such as ramelteon (Rozerem), a melatonin receptor agonist with no known abuse potential.[71]

The barbiturates and other older agents share many characteristics of the benzodiazepines and the new-generation nonbenzodiazepine hypnotics but are less likely to be prescribed for the treatment of insomnia.

Sexual Dysfunction

Data on the effect of the benzodiazepines on sexual dysfunction are scarce, at times conflicting, and mostly based on prospective data with certain design limitations as well as on retrospective data and case reports. Benzodiazepine use has been associated with sexual dysfunction in both men and women, manifested as decreased sexual desire, erectile dysfunction, inhibited orgasm, and inhibited ejaculation.[26,31,101] These side effects seem to emerge after weeks of use and are likely to subside after dose reduction or cessation of use. There are few available data on sexual dysfunction related to the new-generation nonbenzodiazepine hypnotics, the barbiturates, chloral hydrate, meprobamate, carisoprodol, glutethimide, and methaqualone. A recent review concluded that there are insufficient data to clearly ascertain the effects of anxiolytic medications on sexual function.[52]

Although not a specific side effect of the medication, the dangers of sedative-hypnotic and anxiolytic misuse also include drug-facilitated sexual assaults (date rape), especially when potent fast-acting agents are added to alcoholic beverages, inducing passivity and amnesia. Flunitrazepam (Rohypnol), which is not approved by the FDA but is available illicitly, has been associated with drug-facilitated sexual assaults. Other drugs that have been associated with drug-facilitated sexual assaults include other benzodiazepines, zolpidem, chloral hydrate, meprobamate, and other agents.[85]

Summary

The benzodiazepines, the new-generation nonbenzodiazepine hypnotics, and the barbiturates, as well as other older agents, share a similar mode of action by enhancing GABAergic transmission in the central nervous system. Although all of these medications have legitimate medical uses, they also are associated with the risk of misuse and substance use disorder, particularly in individuals with other substance use disorders. They also are associated with psychiatric and medical complications. These medications are safest when they are prescribed for short periods and at the lowest effective dose, their use is monitored, and special precautions are taken when prescribing them for individuals with a substance use disorder history.

Acknowledgments

The authors would like to thank the National Institute on Alcohol Abuse and Alcoholism, the Center for the Translational Neuroscience of Alcoholism, and Diana Limoncelli for technical assistance.

References

1. American Psychiatric Association. *Diagnostic and Statistical Manual of Mental Disorders.* 5th ed. Arlington, VA: American Psychiatric Association; 2013.
2. Ancoli-Israel S, Richardson GS, Mangano RM, et al. Long-term use of sedative hypnotics in older patients with insomnia. *Sleep Med.* 2005;6:107–113.
3. Apelt S, Schmauss C, Emrich HM. Preference for alprazolam as opposed to diazepam in benzodiazepine-dependent psychiatric inpatients. *Pharmacopsychiatry.* 1990;23:70–75.
4. Ashton H. Protracted withdrawal syndromes from benzodiazepines. *J Subst Abuse Treat.* 1991;8:19–28.
5. Bachhuber MA, Hennessy S, Cunningham CO, Starrels JL. increasing benzodiazepine prescriptions and overdose mortality in the United States, 1996–2013. *Am J Public Health.* 2016;106(4):686–688.
6. Barker MJ, Greenwood KM, Jackson M, et al. Persistence of cognitive effects after withdrawal from long-term benzodiazepine use: a meta-analysis. *Arch Clin Neuropsychol.* 2004;19:437–454.
7. Barnes Jr EM. Use-dependent regulation of GABAA receptors. *Int Rev Neurobiol.* 1996;39:53–76.
8. Busto UE, Romach MK, Sellers EM. Multiple drug use and psychiatric comorbidity in patients admitted to the hospital with severe benzodiazepine dependence. *J Clin Psychopharmacol.* 1996;16:51–57.
9. Center for Behavioral Health Statistics and Quality. Behavioral health trends in the United States: Results from the 2014 National Survey on Drug Use andHealth (HHS Publication No. SMA 15-4927, NSDUHSeries H-50); 2015. Retrieved from http://www.samhsa.gov/data/.
10. Centers for Disease Control and Prevention. *National Vital Statistics System mortality data; 2015.* Retrieved from http://www.cdc.gov/nchs/deaths.htm.
11. Chen KW, Berger CC, Forde DP, D'Adamo C, Weintraub E, Gandhi D. Benzodiazepine use and misuse among patients in a methadone program. *BMC Psychiatry.* 2011;11(1):1.
12. Cienki JJ, Burkhart KK, Donovan JW. Zopiclone overdose responsive to flumazenil. *Clin Toxicol (Phila).* 2005;43:385–386.
13. Cimolai N. Zopiclone: is it a pharmacologic agent for abuse? *Can Fam Physician.* 2007;53:2124–2129.
14. Ciraulo DA, Barnhill JG, Ciraulo AM, et al. Parental alcoholism as a risk factor in benzodiazepine abuse: a pilot study. *Am J Psychiatry.* 1989;146:1333–1335.
15. Ciraulo DA, Sarid-Segal O, Knapp C, et al. Liability to alprazolam abuse in daughters of alcoholics. *Am J Psychiatry.* 1996;153:956–958.
16. Cubala WJ, Landowski J. Seizure following sudden zolpidem withdrawal. *Prog Neuropsychopharmacol Biol Psychiatry.* 2007;31:539–540.
17. Darcourt G, Pringuey D, Sallière D, et al. The safety and tolerability of zolpidem—an update. *J Psychopharmacol.* 1999;13:81–93.
18. Darke S, Ross J, Cohen J. The use of benzodiazepines among regular amphetamine users. *Addiction.* 1994;89:1683–1690.
19. Darke SG, Ross JE, Hall WD. Benzodiazepine use among injecting heroin users. *Med J Aust.* 1995;162:645–647.
20. de Gage SB, Moride Y, Ducruet T, Kurth T, Verdoux H, Tournier M, et al. Benzodiazepine use and risk of Alzheimer's disease: case-control study. *BMJ.* 2014;349:g5205.
21. Denis C, Fatséas M, Lavie E, et al. Pharmacological interventions for benzodiazepine mono-dependence management in outpatient settings. *Cochrane Database Syst Rev.* 2006;3:CD005194.
22. Drover DR. Comparative pharmacokinetics and pharmacodynamics of short-acting hypnosedatives: zaleplon, zolpidem and zopiclone. *Clin Pharmacokinet.* 2004;43:227–238.
23. Drummer OH, Ranson DL. Sudden death and benzodiazepines. *Am J Forensic Med Pathol.* 1996;17:336–342.

24. Dündar Y, Dodd S, Strobl J, et al. Comparative efficacy of newer hypnotic drugs for the short-term management of insomnia: a systematic review and meta-analysis. *Hum Psychopharmacol.* 2004;19:305–322.

25. Fontaine R, Chouinard G, Annable L. Rebound anxiety in anxious patients after abrupt withdrawal of benzodiazepine treatment. *Am J Psychiatry.* 1984;141:848–852.

26. Fossey MD, Hamner MB. Clonazepam-related sexual dysfunction in male veterans with PTSD. *Anxiety.* 1994;1:233–236.

27. Foster AC, Kemp JA. Glutamate- and GABA-based CNS therapeutics. *Curr Opin Pharmacol.* 2006;6:7–17.

28. Foy A, O'Connell D, Henry D, et al. Benzodiazepine use as a cause of cognitive impairment in elderly hospital inpatients. *J Gerontol A Biol Sci Med Sci.* 1995;50:M99–M106.

29. Garnier R, Guerault E, Muzard D, et al. Acute zolpidem poisoning--analysis of 344 cases. *J Toxicol Clin Toxicol.* 1994;32: 391–404.

30. Gerra G, Zaimovic A, Giusti F, et al. Intravenous flumazenil versus oxazepam tapering in the treatment of benzodiazepine withdrawal: a randomized, placebo-controlled study. *Addict Biol.* 2002;7: 385–395.

31. Ghadirian AM, Annable L, Belanger MC. Lithium, benzodiazepines, and sexual function in bipolar patients. *Am J Psychiatry.* 1992;149:801–805.

32. Gitlow S. *Substance use Disorders: A Practical Guide.* Lippincott Williams & Wilkins; 2007:86.

33. Gorenstein C, Bernik MA, Pompeia S. Differential acute psychomotor and cognitive effects of diazepam on long-term benzodiazepine users. *Int Clin Psychopharmacol.* 1994;9:145–153.

34. Gray SL, Dublin S, Yu O, et al. Benzodiazepine use and risk of incident dementia or cognitive decline: prospective population based study. *BMJ.* 2016;352:i90.

35. Griffiths RR, Johnson MW. Relative abuse liability of hypnotic drugs: a conceptual framework and algorithm for differentiating among compounds. *J Clin Psychiatry.* 2005;66(suppl 9):31–41.

36. Griffiths RR, Wolf B. Relative abuse liability of different benzodiazepines in drug abusers. *J Clin Psychopharmacol.* 1990;10: 237–243.

37. Griffiths RR, Weerts EM. Benzodiazepine self-administration in humans and laboratory animals—implications for problems of long-term use and abuse. *Psychopharmacology (Berl).* 1997;134: 1–37.

38. Hajak G, Müller WE, Wittchen HU, et al. Abuse and dependence potential for the non-benzodiazepine hypnotics zolpidem and zopiclone: a review of case reports and epidemiological data. *Addiction.* 2003;98:1371–1378.

39. Harris JT, Roache JD, Thornton JE. A role for valproate in the treatment of sedative-hypnotic withdrawal and for relapse prevention. *Alcohol Alcohol.* 2000;35:319–323.

40. Heritch AJ, Capwell R, Roy-Byrne PP. A case of psychosis and delirium following withdrawal from triazolam. *J Clin Psychiatry.* 1987;48:168–169.

41. Hoaken PN, Stewart SH. Drugs of abuse and the elicitation of human aggressive behavior. *Addict Behav.* 2003;28:1533–1554.

42. Hojer J, Salmonson H, Sundin P. Zaleplon-induced coma and bluish-green urine: possible antidotal effect by flumazenil. *J Toxicol Clin Toxicol.* 2002;40:571–572.

43. Holbrook AM, Crowther R, Lotter A, et al. Meta-analysis of benzodiazepine use in the treatment of insomnia. *CMAJ.* 2000;162:225–233.

44. Hood SD, Norman A, Hince DA, Melichar JK, Hulse GK. Benzodiazepine dependence and its treatment with low dose flumazenil. *Br J Clin Pharmacol.* 2014;77(2):285–294.

45. Huang B, Dawson DA, Stinson FS, et al. Prevalence, correlates, and comorbidity of nonmedical prescription drug use and drug use disorders in the United States: results of the national epidemiologic survey on alcohol and related conditions. *J Clin Psychiatry.* 2006;67:1062–1073.

46. Khanna JM, Kalant H, Weiner J, et al. Rapid tolerance and cross-tolerance as predictors of chronic tolerance and cross-tolerance. *Pharmacol Biochem Behav.* 1992;41:355–360.

47. Kintz P. Deaths involving buprenorphine: a compendium of French cases. *Forensic Sci Int.* 2001;121:65–69.

48. Koltchine VV, Ye Q, Finn SE, et al. Chimeric GABAA/glycine receptors: expression and barbiturate pharmacology. *Neuropharmacology.* 1996;35:1445–1456.

49. Koski A, Ojanpera I, Vuori E. Alcohol and benzodiazepines in fatal poisonings. *Alcohol Clin Exp Res.* 2002;26:956–959.

50. Krystal AD, Walsh JK, Laska E, et al. Sustained efficacy of eszopiclone over 6 months of nightly treatment: results of a randomized, double-blind, placebo-controlled study in adults with chronic insomnia. *Sleep.* 2003;26:793–799.

51. Krystal AD, Erman M, Zammit GK, et al. Long-term efficacy and safety of zolpidem extended-release 12.5 mg, administered 3 to 7 nights per week for 24 weeks, in patients with chronic primary insomnia: a 6-month, randomized, double-blind, placebo-controlled, parallel-group, multicenter study. *Sleep.* 2008;31:79–90.

52. La Torre A, Giupponi G, Duffy DM, et al. Sexual dysfunction related to psychotropic drugs: a critical review. Part III: mood stabilizers and anxiolytic drugs. *Pharmacopsychiatry.* 2014;47(1):1–6.

53. Levy AB. Delirium and seizures due to abrupt alprazolam withdrawal: case report. *J Clin Psychiatry.* 1984;45:38–39.

54. Lucki I, Rickels K, Geller AM. Chronic use of benzodiazepines and psychomotor and cognitive test performance. *Psychopharmacology (Berl).* 1986;88:426–433.

55. Lugoboni F, Faccini M, Quaglio GL, Albiero A, Casari R, Pajusco B. Intravenous flumazenil infusion to treat benzodiazepine dependence should be performed in the inpatient clinical setting for high risk of seizure. *J Psychopharmacol.* 2011;25(6): 848–849.

56. Maarek L, Cramer P, Attali P, et al. The safety and efficacy of zolpidem in insomniac patients: a long-term open study in general practice. *J Int Med Res.* 1992;20:162–170.

57. Markowitz JS, Brewerton TD. Zolpidem-induced psychosis. *Ann Clin Psychiatry.* 1996;8:89–91.

58. Martínez-Cano H, Vela-Bueno A, de Iceta M, et al. Benzodiazepine withdrawal syndrome seizures. *Pharmacopsychiatry.* 1995;28: 257–262.

59. Mattila MJ, Vanakoski J, Kalska H, et al. Effects of alcohol, zolpidem, and some other sedatives and hypnotics on human performance and memory. *Pharmacol Biochem Behav.* 1998;59:917–923.

60. Mendelson WB, Rich CL. Sedatives and suicide: the San Diego study. *Acta Psychiatr Scand.* 1993;88:337–341.

61. Modell JG. Protracted benzodiazepine withdrawal syndrome mimicking psychotic depression. *Psychosomatics.* 1997;38:160–161.

62. Mohler H, Fritschy JM, Rudolph U. A new benzodiazepine pharmacology. *J Pharmacol Exp Ther.* 2002;300:2–8.

63. Mueller TI, Pagano ME, Rodriguez BF, et al. Long-term use of benzodiazepines in participants with comorbid anxiety and alcohol use disorders. *Alcohol Clin Exp Res.* 2005;29:1411–1418.

64. Nowell PD, Mazumdar S, Buysse DJ, et al. Benzodiazepines and zolpidem for chronic insomnia: a meta-analysis of treatment efficacy. *JAMA.* 1997;278:2170–2177.

65. Noyes Jr R, Garvey MJ, Cook B, et al. Controlled discontinuation of benzodiazepine treatment for patients with panic disorder. *Am J Psychiatry.* 1991;148:517–523.

66. Otto MW, Bruce SE, Deckersbach T. Benzodiazepine use, cognitive impairment, and cognitive-behavioral therapy for anxiety disorders: issues in the treatment of a patient in need. *J Clin Psychiatry.* 2005;66(suppl 2):34–38.

67. Pélissolo A, Maniere F, Boutges B, et al. Anxiety and depressive disorders in 4,425 long term benzodiazepine users in general practice [French]. *Encephale.* 2007;33:32–38.

68. Posternak MA, Mueller TI. Assessing the risks and benefits of benzodiazepines for anxiety disorders in patients with a history of substance abuse or dependence. *Am J Addict.* 2001;10:48–68.

69. Poyares D, Guilleminault C, Ohayon MM, et al. Chronic benzodiazepine usage and withdrawal in insomnia patients. *J Psychiatr Res*. 2004;38:327–334.

70. Rappa LR, Larose-Pierre M, Payne DR, et al. Detoxification from high-dose zolpidem using diazepam. *Ann Pharmacother*. 2004;38:590–594.

71. Reynoldson JN, Elliott Sr E, Nelson LA. Ramelteon: a novel approach in the treatment of insomnia. *Ann Pharmacother*. 2008;42:1262–1271.

72. Rickels K, Case WG, Downing RW, et al. Long-term diazepam therapy and clinical outcome. *JAMA*. 1983;250:767–771.

73. Rickels K, Schweizer E. Panic disorder: long-term pharmacotherapy and discontinuation. *J Clin Psychopharmacol*. 1998;18(6 suppl 2):12S–18S.

74. Rickels K, Schweizer E, Case WG, et al. Long-term therapeutic use of benzodiazepines. I. Effects of abrupt discontinuation. *Arch Gen Psychiatry*. 1990;47:899–907.

75. Rickels K, DeMartinis N, Rynn M, et al. Pharmacologic strategies for discontinuing benzodiazepine treatment. *J Clin Psychopharmacol*. 1999;19(6 suppl 2):12S–16S.

76. Rickels K, Lucki I, Schweizer E, et al. Psychomotor performance of long-term benzodiazepine users before, during, and after benzodiazepine discontinuation. *J Clin Psychopharmacol*. 1999;19: 107–113.

77. Rickels K, Schweizer E, Espana FG, Case G, DeMartinis N, Greenblatt D. Trazodone and valproate in patients discontinuing long-term benzodiazepine therapy: effects on withdrawal symptoms and taper outcome. *Psychopharmacology*. 1999;141(1):1–5.

78. Romach M, Busto U, Somer G, et al. Clinical aspects of chronic use of alprazolam and lorazepam. *Am J Psychiatry*. 1995;152: 1161–1167.

79. Rosen CS, Greenbaum MA, Schnurr PP, Holmes TH, Brennan PL, Friedman MJ. Do benzodiazepines reduce the effectiveness of exposure therapy for posttraumatic stress disorder?[CME]. *J Clin Psychiatry*. 2013;74(12):1–478.

80. Ross HE. Benzodiazepine use and anxiolytic abuse and dependence in treated alcoholics. *Addiction*. 1993;88:209–218.

81. Rubio G, Bobes J, Cervera G, et al. Effects of pregabalin on subjective sleep disturbance symptoms during withdrawal from long-term benzodiazepine use. *European Addiction Research*. 2011;17(5): 262–270.

82. Rush CR, Higgins ST, Bickel WK, et al. Abuse liability of alprazolam relative to other commonly used benzodiazepines: a review. *Neurosci Biobehav Rev*. 1993;17:277–285.

83. Schuckit MA, Daeppen JB, Danko GP, et al. Clinical implications for four drugs of the DSM-IV distinction between substance dependence with and without a physiological component. *Am J Psychiatry*. 1999;156:41–49.

84. Schuckit MA, Greenblatt D, Irwin M, et al. Reactions to ethanol and diazepam in healthy young men. *J Stud Alcohol*. 1991;52: 180–187.

85. Schwartz RH, Milteer R, LeBeau MA. Drug-facilitated sexual assault ('date rape'). *South Med J*. 2000;93:558–561.

86. Schweizer E, Rickels K, Case WG, Greenblatt DJ. Carbamazepine treatment in patients discontinuing long-term benzodiazepine therapy: effects on withdrawal severity and outcome. *Arch Gen Psychiatry*. 1991;48(5):448–452.

87. Schweizer E, Rickels K, Case WG, et al. Long-term therapeutic use of benzodiazepines. II. Effects of gradual taper. *Arch Gen Psychiatry*. 1990;47:908–915.

88. Serfaty M, Masterton G. Fatal poisonings attributed to benzodiazepines in Britain during the 1980s. *Br J Psychiatry*. 1993;163:386–393.

89. Singh RK, Jain R, Ray R, et al. Abuse liability of diazepam through different routes. *Indian J Physiol Pharmacol*. 2001;45:181–190.

90. Smith BD, Salzman C. Do benzodiazepines cause depression? *Hosp Community Psychiatry*. 1991;42:1101–1102.

91. Smith DE, Wesson DR. Phenobarbital technique for treatment of barbiturate dependence. *Arch Gen Psychiatry*. 1971;24:56–60.

92. Smith DE, Wesson DR. Benzodiazepine dependency syndromes. *J Psychoactive Drugs*. 1983;15:85–95.

93. Smith RB, Kroboth PD. Influence of dosing regimen on alprazolam and metabolite serum concentrations and tolerance to sedative and psychomotor effects. *Psychopharmacology (Berl)*. 1987;93:105–112.

94. Soldatos CR, Dikeos DG, Whitehead A. Tolerance and rebound insomnia with rapidly eliminated hypnotics: a meta-analysis of sleep laboratory studies. *Int Clin Psychopharmacol*. 1999;14: 287–303.

95. Stewart SA. The effects of benzodiazepines on cognition. *J Clin Psychiatry*. 2005;66(suppl 2):9–13.

96. Stinson FS, Grant BF, Dawson DA, et al. Comorbidity between DSM-IV alcohol and specific drug use disorders in the United States: results from the national epidemiologic survey on alcohol and related conditions. *Drug Alcohol Depend*. 2005;80: 105–116.

97. Tan KR, Brown M, Labouèbe G, et al. Neural bases for addictive properties of benzodiazepines. *Nature*. 2010;463(7282):769–774.

98. Toner LC, Tsambiras BM, Catalano G, et al. Central nervous system side effects associated with zolpidem treatment. *Clin Neuro-Pharmacol*. 2000;23:54–58.

99. Tracqui A, Kintz P, Ludes B. Buprenorphine-related deaths among drug addicts in France: a report on 20 fatalities. *J Anal Toxicol*. 1998;22:430–434.

100. Tsai MJ, Huang YB, Wu PC. A novel clinical pattern of visual hallucination after zolpidem use. *J Toxicol Clin Toxicol*. 2003;41: 869–872.

101. Uhde TW, Tancer ME, Shea CA. Sexual dysfunction related to alprazolam treatment of social phobia. *Am J Psychiatry*. 1998;145:531–532.

102. van Balkom AJ, de Beurs E, Koele P, et al. Long-term benzodiazepine use is associated with smaller treatment gain in panic disorder with agoraphobia. *J Nerv Ment Dis*. 1996;184:133–135.

103. Verdoux H, Lagnaoui R, Begaud B. Is benzodiazepine use a risk factor for cognitive decline and dementia? A literature review of epidemiological studies. *Psychol Med*. 2005;35:307–315.

104. Weich S, Pearce HL, Croft P, et al. Effect of anxiolytic and hypnotic drug prescriptions on mortality hazards: retrospective cohort study. *BMJ*. 2014;348:g1996.

105. Weinbroum AA, Flaishon R, Sorkine P, et al. A risk-benefit assessment of flumazenil in the management of benzodiazepine overdose. *Drug Saf*. 1997;17:181–196.

106. Weizman T, Gelkopf M, Melamed Y, et al. Treatment of benzodiazepine dependence in methadone maintenance treatment patients: a comparison of two therapeutic modalities and the role of psychiatric comorbidity. *Aust N Z J Psychiatry*. 2003;37:458–463.

107. White MC, Silverman JJ, Harbison JW. Psychosis associated with clonazepam therapy for blepharospasm. *J Nerv Ment Dis*. 1982;170:117–119.

108. Wolf BC, Lavezzi WA, Sullivan LM, et al. Alprazolam-related deaths in palm beach county. *Am J Forensic Med Pathol*. 2005;26: 24–27.

109. Wong CP, Chiu PK, Chu LW. Zopiclone withdrawal: an unusual cause of delirium in the elderly. *Age Ageing*. 2005;34:526–527.

110. Woods JH, Katz JL, Winger G. Abuse liability of benzodiazepines. *Pharmacol Rev*. 1987;39:251–413.

111. Worthington 3rd JJ, Pollack MH, Otto MW, et al. Long-term experience with clonazepam in patients with a primary diagnosis of panic disorder. *Psychopharmacol Bull*. 1998;34:199–205.

112. Zalsman G, Hermesh H, Munitz H. Alprazolam withdrawal delirium: a case report. *Clin Neuropharmacol*. 1998;21:201–202.

28

Clinical Aspects of Inhalant Addiction

YU-CHIH SHEN AND SHIH-FEN CHEN

CHAPTER OUTLINE

Types of Inhalants Being Abused

Inhalants encompass a wide range of pharmacologically diverse substances that readily vaporize. Unlike most other substances of abuse, which are classified into groups that share a specific central nervous system (CNS) action or perceived psychoactive effect, inhalants are grouped by their common route of administration. Inhalants are classified into three groups on the basis of their currently known pharmacologic actions (Table 28.1).[25] Group I includes volatile solvents, fuels, and anesthetics that contain aliphatic, aromatic, or halogenated hydrocarbons. All of these ingredients are found in thousands of commonly used and readily available consumer products. Group II includes nitrous oxide. Group III includes volatile alkyl nitrites. The most commonly abused inhalants are found in Group I. Virtually any hydrocarbon can have mind-altering effects when inhaled in large enough doses. Nitrous oxide, or "laughing gas," is diverted from medical or dental anesthesia use and sold in balloons for inhalation or is simply inhaled from whipped cream aerosol cans. Alkyl nitrites, or "poppers," are also abused; typically, amyl nitrite ampoules intended to treat angina are "popped" open and inhaled. The fifth edition of the *Diagnostic and Statistical Manual of Mental Disorders* (DSM-5) excludes Group II and III inhalants from the inhalant-related disorders, which are classified as other (or unknown) substance-related disorder.[1]

Epidemiology

Inhalants are easily available, legal, and inexpensive, which contribute to the high use of inhalants among poor and young persons. According to the 2018 National Institute on Drug Abuse (NIDA) survey of the United States, the past year use of inhalants is at its lowest levels in the history of the survey among 10th and 12th graders (2.4% and 1.6%, respectively). Rates of inhalant use are traditionally highest among 8th graders. Past year use among this age group is at 4.6%, down from 12.8% at its peak rate in 1995. In another 2017 survey by the National Survey on Drug Use and Health (NSDUH), past year inhalant use among individuals 12 to 17, 18 to 25, and 26 years of age or older are 2.3, 1.6, and 0.3 percent, respectively.

According to the NIDA and NSDUH surveys, most inhalant users are male; however, 8th grade girls are more likely to try inhalants than are 8th grade boys. In terms of ethnicity, Hispanics have the highest rates of past year use among 8th and 10th graders, compared to both African Americans and Caucasians. Urban and rural settings see comparable rates of inhalant abuse. Inhalant abusers may be related to certain occupations where abusable solvents, propellants, or anesthetics are readily available. Inhalants are sometimes referred to as gateway drugs, which means they are among the first drugs people try before moving on to other substances, such as alcohol, marijuana, and cocaine. Inhalant use accounts for 1% of all substance-related death and around 0.5% of all substance-related emergency room visits. Twenty-two percent of inhalant users who die of sudden sniffing death syndrome (SSDS) have no history of previous inhalant abuse—they are first-time users.

Mechanisms of Action

The immediate effects of group I and II inhalants are similar to the early classic stages of anesthesia.[3] The abuser is initially stimulated and then disinhibited and prone to impulsive behaviors. Speech becomes slurred and gait is uneven. Euphoria, frequently with hallucinations, is followed by drowsiness and sleep, particularly after repeated inhalations. Coma is unusual because, as the user becomes drowsy, exposure to the inhalant is terminated before large enough doses are absorbed. The mechanisms of action of these inhalants have not been well defined. It is likely that inhalants act as a mix of N-methyl-D-aspartic acid (NMDA) antagonist and γ-aminobutyric acid (GABA) agonist to produce CNS depressant effects.[4]

Nitrites have pharmacologic effects that are significantly different from those of other inhalants. Instead of direct CNS effects, they primarily cause vasodilation and smooth muscle relaxation.[21] The sensations of floating and increased skin tactility as well as warmth and throbbing occur within 10s of inhalation and then diminish within 5 min. Abuse of nitrites may result in tachycardia, flushing, blurred vision, headache, lightheadedness, significant hypotension, syncope, and high enough levels of methemoglobinemia to cause cyanosis and lethargy. Other inhalants are used

TABLE 28.1	Pharmacologic Classification of Inhalants and Common Street Names.
Group	**Common Street Names**
Volatile solvents, fuels, and anesthetics	Air blast, discorama, hippie crack, medusa, moon gas, oz, poor man's pot
Nitrous oxide	Laughing gas, buzz bomb, shoot the breeze
Volatile alkyl nitrites	Poppers, snappers, boppers, pearls, amys, quicksilver

TABLE 28.2	*Diagnostic and Statistical Manual of Mental Disorders, Fifth Edition,* Inhalant-Related Disorders.
Inhalant use disorder	
Inhalant-induced disorders	
Inhalant intoxication	
Inhalant intoxication delirium	
Inhalant-induced persisting dementia	
Inhalant-induced psychotic disorder[a]	
Inhalant-induced anxiety disorder[a]	
Inhalant-induced mood disorder[a]	
Other inhalant-induced disorders	

[a]Specify if: with onset during intoxication.

to alter mood, but nitrites are inhaled to enhance sexual feelings, penile engorgement, and anal sphincter relaxation to intensify sexual experience.

Morbidity and Mortality

Inhalant abuse causes psychosocial as well as organic morbidity. Ongoing inhalant abuse is associated with failure in school, delinquency, and an inability to adjust to societal norms.[7] The chief organic morbidity is CNS damage, resulting in dementia and cerebellar dysfunction.[9,11,22] Typically, there is a loss of cognitive and other higher functions, gait disturbances, and loss of coordination. Imaging studies demonstrate a loss of brain mass[11] and white matter degeneration.[9,22] Other organic effects are related to specific chemicals found in some but not all products. The strength of the association ranges from definite to likely to speculative. Definite associations include peripheral neuropathy, deafness, and metabolic acidosis. Likely morbidities include embryopathy, neonatal withdrawal, and lung damage. Speculative morbidities include cardiomyopathy, toxic hepatitis, decreased visual acuity, aplastic anemia, and leukemia.[25]

Death due to inhalant abuse can occur by several mechanisms, including asphyxia, suffocation, risky behaviors, aspiration, and SSDS.[20] Asphyxia is probably of only theoretical concern because it requires the partial pressure of the inhalant to be so high that oxygen is displaced. Suffocation occurs when the mode of use involves inhalation through the nose and mouth from a plastic bag, which may occlude the airway if the user loses consciousness. Disinhibition while under the influence of inhalants may cause dangerous behaviors such as drowning, jumps or falls from heights, hypothermia, and fire-associated deaths (due to the flammability of most inhalants). The risk of death from aspiration is similar to that for alcohol or other depressants and is related to the combination of decreased level of consciousness and loss of protective airway reflexes. SSDS is usually associated with cardiac arrest. The inhalant causes the heart to beat rapidly and erratically, resulting in cardiac arrest.

Chronic nitrous oxide abuse causes short-term memory loss and peripheral neuropathy.[5] The peripheral neuropathy results when nitrous oxide inactivates vitamin B_{12} and mediates a pernicious anemia–type syndrome, which includes anemia, leukopenia, sensorimotor neuropathy, and posterior/lateral column spinal cord disease. Nitrites are abused mainly for their sensory and sexual effects, and use may promote higher-risk sexual practices, facilitate transmission of sexually transmitted infections, and result in pharmacologic interactions, such as with sildenafil (Viagra).[21] Chronic abuse of volatile alkyl nitrites has

documented hematologic and immune system effects without associated cognitive deficits.[21]

Psychiatric Disorders in Inhalant Users

The DSM-5 provides two categories of inhalant-related disorders (Table 28.2).[1] The first category is inhalant use disorders, which are characterized by a maladaptive pattern of inhalant use leading to clinically significant impairment or distress. The second category, inhalant-induced disorders (intoxication, intoxication delirium, persisting dementia, psychotic disorder, anxiety disorder, and mood disorder), results from the toxic effects of inhalants. Other inhalant-induced disorders is the DSM-5 recommended diagnosis for inhalant-related disorders that do not fit into one of the diagnostic categories discussed earlier. Conditions related to abuse of either anesthetic gases or nitrites are not listed under the DSM-5 categories for inhalant-related disorders. Instead, these are classified as other (or unknown) substance-related disorders. Some effects and disorders associated with those compounds are discussed briefly elsewhere in this chapter.

Inhalant Use Disorder

The cardinal feature of inhalant use disorder is repeated use of inhalants, resulting in combinations of social or physical consequences, loss of control, or development of tolerance, and so on. Despite the absence of an inhalant withdrawal diagnosis in the DSM-5, some people still complain about withdrawal symptoms, including sleep disturbances, irritability, sweating, tachycardia, nausea, shakiness, illusions, delusions, and hallucinations.[15]

Two differential diagnoses should be considered.[23] First, polysubstance dependence is common in adolescents. Abuse of other drugs can be traced through an individual's history, physical findings, and drug screens. Second, impulsive behaviors during chronic inhalant use might mimic or be comorbid with conduct disorder or antisocial personality disorder. Conduct or antisocial behaviors that appear before the onset of inhalant abuse or in periods of abstinence suggest the presence of these disorders.

No controlled studies guide the treatment of inhalant use disorder. Treatment usually takes a long time and involves enlisting the support of the person's family, changing the friendship network if the individual uses with others, teaching coping skills, and helping the individual increase his or her self-esteem.

In research with animal models of inhalant abuse, NMDA, GABA, glycine, nicotine, and 5-hydroxytryptamine type 3 (5-HT3) receptors appear to be important targets of action for several abused solvents. Emerging evidence suggests that other receptor subtypes and nerve membrane ion channels are also involved.[4] Evidence suggests that lamotrigine (Lamictal), a phenyltriazine anticonvulsant, might be effective for inhalant use disorder because it modulates release of glutamate, blocks 5-HT3 receptors, and inhibits dopamine uptake.[24] Baclofen (Lioresal), a selective GABA$_B$ receptor agonist, might be effective for inhalant use disorder because its agonistic action at GABA$_B$ receptors in the ventral tegmental area might control the activity of the mesolimbic dopamine pathway to reduce the reinforcing effects of inhalants.[14] Buspirone (BuSpar) and risperidone (Risperdal) have also been reported to be effective for treating inhalant use disorder.[18,19] Overall, the efficacy of these agents in inhalant use disorder requires additional investigation.

In addition to inhalant use disorder, most inhalant users have comorbid conduct disorder, attention-deficit/hyperactivity disorder (ADHD), major depressive disorder, dysthymic disorder, alcohol dependence, and psychosis.[16,23] Psychiatrists often prescribe bupropion (Wellbutrin) or atomoxetine (Strattera) for ADHD, antidepressants for depression, naltrexone (Revia) or acamprosate (Campral) for comorbid alcohol dependence, and antipsychotics for psychotic symptoms.[23] In addition to psychiatric management, appropriate medical care is also required for the disorder's medical sequelae.[17]

Inhalant-Induced Disorders

Inhalant Intoxication and Inhalant Intoxication Delirium

When too much of an inhalant is taken, the user becomes intoxicated. According to the DSM-5, the signs of inhalant intoxication include dizziness, nystagmus, incoordination, slurred speech, unsteady gait, lethargy, depressed reflexes, psychomotor retardation, tremor, generalized muscle weakness, blurred vision, diplopia, euphoria, stupor, or coma. Inhalant intoxication delirium is a state in which a person gets extremely intoxicated, with a disturbance of consciousness and a change in cognition.

Differentiation of the diagnosis of inhalant intoxication from that of other types of substance intoxication depends on an individual's history and the evidence of inhalant use such as perioral rash and the presence of inhalant odor and residue. Polysubstance dependence is common among inhalant users. Concomitant intoxication with other substances may be assessed by history and toxicologic examinations.[23] Intravenous injection of dextrose and naloxone (Narcan) will help rule out coma due to diabetes and coma of narcotic origin, respectively.[17] If the mood disturbance, anxiety, or psychosis appears prominently during inhalant intoxication and is sufficiently severe to warrant clinical attention, the diagnosis should be inhalant-induced mood, anxiety, or psychotic disorder, respectively. If delirium develops in the course of inhalant intoxication, the diagnosis is inhalant intoxication delirium rather than inhalant intoxication.[8]

Inhalants are rapidly metabolized and excreted. Inhalant intoxication usually lasts a few hours or less unless there are medical complications. Inhalant intoxication usually resolves spontaneously and requires no medical attention.[10] However, medical complications such as cardiac arrhythmias, trauma, bronchospasm,

or laryngospasm need treatment, and clinicians should note the client's vital signs and level of consciousness.[17] The treatment of inhalant intoxication delirium is similar to that used for inhalant intoxication, but the variations of levels of consciousness require special attention to the individual's safety. If the delirium results in severe behavioral disturbances or cognition changes, short-term treatment with a dopamine receptor antagonist may be helpful.[13] Sedative medications, including benzodiazepines, are contraindicated because they may enhance the inhalant's depression of the CNS.[4]

Inhalant-Induced Persisting Dementia

Inhalants are commonly used both in industry and by consumers as fat solvents. Thus because the brain is a lipid-rich organ, chronic solvent abuse is neurotoxic and can cause dementia.[9,11,22] Inhalant-induced dementia is typically associated with memory impairment and at least one of the following: aphasia, apraxia, agnosia, and executive function disturbance. These symptoms can be associated with delirium, which can persist beyond the usual duration of inhalant intoxication or withdrawal.[1]

There are, typically, two other differential diagnoses that should be considered among individuals who are suspected of having inhalant-induced persisting dementia. First, many inhalant abusers concomitantly abuse alcohol or other sedatives that can also produce dementia. Second, histories of head injury are common among those who are inhalant abusers.[17,23] Thus even among individuals with a documented course of inhalant-induced persisting dementia, other causes of dementia also need to be considered in the differential diagnosis.

Few inhalant abusers have been studied prospectively. Despite some reports of improvement after abstention from inhalants, most neurocognitive deficits persist and worsen.[26] In addition, as neurocognitive deficits progress to dementia, inhalant abusers gradually lose the cognitive capacity to avoid relapses, and each relapse may accelerate brain degeneration.

No controlled studies have been performed to guide the treatment of individuals with inhalant-induced persisting dementia. Correcting the reversible and slowing the progression of irreversible factors of inhalant-induced dementia are the primary approaches to treatment. Individuals may require extensive support within their families or in foster or domiciliary care.

Inhalant-Induced Psychotic Disorder

Clinical evidence suggests that tetraethyl lead can provoke psychotic symptoms.[6] The cardinal features of inhalant-induced psychotic disorder are prominent delusions or hallucinations (mostly visual) developing during or within 1 month of inhalant use. These psychotic symptoms can occur during intoxication, delirium, and even some time after the inhalant has been withdrawn, and they can complicate a preexisting psychotic disorder.[1]

The course of inhalant-induced psychotic disorder is typically brief, lasting a few hours to days beyond the intoxication. Treatment of medical complications, together with conservative management of inhalant intoxication, is appropriate.[17] Agitation, confusion, and psychosis may respond to the administration of antipsychotics such as haloperidol (Haldol).[13]

A thorough search of the literature revealed only one controlled study that investigated therapy among people with inhalant-induced psychotic disorder.[13] In this study, 40 male patients admitted to an acute psychiatric unit for treatment of inhalant-induced psychotic disorder were assigned to receive 5 weeks of treatment with carbamazepine (Tegretol) or haloperidol (Haldol), supplied in identical-appearing capsules. Individuals in both treatment groups improved significantly over time, but adverse effects were significantly more common and more severe in the haloperidol group. Carbamazepine appears to have comparable efficacy but fewer adverse effects than haloperidol for the treatment of inhalant-induced psychotic disorder. Nevertheless, because there was no placebo group in this study, these data cannot establish that medication was better than no medication.

Inhalant-Induced Anxiety Disorder

The essential features of inhalant-induced anxiety disorder are prominent anxiety, panic attacks, obsession, or compulsion developing during or within 1 month of inhalant intoxication or withdrawal. Inhalant use that is etiologically related to the disturbance causes clinically significant distress or impairment in social or occupational life, or disruptions in other important areas of functioning. The anxiety symptoms are not better accounted for by an anxiety disorder that is not inhalant induced, and the anxiety does not occur exclusively during the course of a delirium.[1]

The course and treatment of inhalant-induced anxiety disorders are like those of inhalant intoxication. Sedative medications, including benzodiazepines, are contraindicated because they may enhance the inhalant's depressant effects on the CNS, thereby precipitating inhalant-induced anxiety disorder.[4]

Inhalant-Induced Mood Disorder

The essential features of inhalant-induced mood disorder include prominent and persistent disturbance in mood with (1) depressed mood or markedly diminished interest or pleasure in daily life and activities and (2) elevated, expansive, or irritable mood developing during or within 1 month of substance intoxication or withdrawal. The depressed mood is not better accounted for by a mood disorder that is not inhalant induced, and the mood disturbance does not occur exclusively during the course of an episode of delirium.[1]

The course and treatment of inhalant-induced mood disorders are like those of inhalant intoxication. The course is brief, lasting a few hours to days beyond the intoxication. Although antidepressants or antimanic medications are seldom appropriate for these relatively brief disorders, the risk of suicide requires a carefully monitored psychosocial intervention. Suicidality has a very strong relationship with inhalant use disorder. Inhalant use disorder in incarcerated youth may signal elevated suicide risk.[12] Suicide risk assessments, therefore, should include questions about inhalant use.

Prevention and Management Considerations

As with other types of substance abuse, the most effective way to curtail use is through prevention.[2] There are many potentially preventive strategies; however, most of these have proved to be impractical. Restricting the availability of some of these products merely results in a shift to the use of other products. Limiting the availability of inhalants is impractical because they comprise a large group of products that are universally available and have legitimate uses. Reformulating a product by replacing the hydrocarbons with other chemicals is not practical because this usually results in a less-effective product. Adding a noxious chemical to the product to prevent misuse also is ineffective because there are multiple products that would require such adulterants. Warning labels on packages may be counterproductive because they allow children to identify sniffable substances more easily. Criminalization of the user is not a meaningful deterrent for the prevention of inhalant abuse, either for the experienced user or for the person who is experimenting for the first time. Criminalization of the vendor is ineffective, again because of the issue of dealing with multiple products that have legitimate uses.

Education is considered to be the most effective preventive strategy.[2] Progressive, school-based inhalant abuse prevention courses, taught beginning in kindergarten, with developmentally appropriate modules taught throughout elementary school, are seen as the most efficient strategy and should be implemented—particularly in areas where inhalant abuse is prevalent. Offering alternative activities in recreational facilities, for example, and promoting traditional cultural values encourage positive lifestyles, thereby reducing the risk for inhalant abuse and other destructive behaviors. Prevention workers are especially effective when they are from the local community. However, they must be appropriately trained and have access to ongoing support.

Psychiatrists are encouraged to be aware that inhalant abuse can occur in all client populations, including their own. They need to be knowledgeable about the epidemiology of inhalant abuse, particularly regarding local and regional trends, and about the serious health consequences of inhalant abuse. In particular, they need to know about unique clinical features such as CNS damage and SSDS. Finally, they need to help educate children, adolescents, parents, teachers, media representatives, and vendors of volatile substances about inhalant abuse prevention and the health risks of inhalant use. Psychiatrists can serve as a valuable community resource regarding inhalant use awareness, prevention, detection, and management.[25]

Treating inhalant users is difficult because of the many pharmacologic, clinical, and demographic factors that make this type of substance abuse unique. Treatment strategies are still being developed, and additional research is needed to identify effective strategies to help these individuals.

References

1. American Psychiatric Association. *Diagnostic and Statistical Manual of Mental Disorders.* 5th ed. Arlington, VA: American Psychiatric Publishing; 2013.
2. Anderson CE, Loomis GA. Recognition and prevention of inhalant abuse. *Am Fam Physician.* 2003;68:869–874.
3. Balster RL. Neural basis of inhalant abuse. *Drug Alcohol Depend.* 1998;51:207–214.
4. Bowen SE, Batis JC, Paez-Martinez N, et al. The last decade of solvent research in animal models of abuse: mechanistic and behavioral studies. *Neurotoxicol Teratol.* 2006;28:636–647.
5. Brouette T, Anton R. Clinical review of inhalants. *Am J Addict.* 2001;10:79–94.
6. Candura SM, Butera R, Gandini C, et al. Occupational poisoning with psychiatric manifestations. *G Ital Med Lav Ergon.* 2000;22:52–61; discussion 62–63.
7. Chadwick OF, Anderson HR. Neuro-psychological consequences of volatile substance abuse: a review. *Hum Toxicol.* 1989;8:307–312.
8. Evren C, Barut T, Saatcioglu O, et al. Axis I psychiatric comorbidity among adult inhalant dependents seeking treatment. *J Psychoactive Drugs.* 2006;38:57–64.
9. Filley CM, Heaton RK, Rosenberg NL. White matter dementia in chronic toluene abuse. *Neurology.* 1990;40:532–534.
10. Flanagan RJ, Ives RJ. Volatile substance abuse. *Bull Narc.* 1994;46:49–78.
11. Fornazzari L, Wilkinson DA, Kapur BM, et al. Cerebellar, cortical and functional impairment in toluene abusers. *Acta Neurol Scand.* 1983;67:319–329.

12. Freedenthal S, Vaughn MG, Jenson JM, et al. Inhalant use and suicidality among incarcerated youth. *Drug Alcohol Depend.* 2007;90:81–88.

13. Hernandez-Avila CA, Ortega-Soto HA, Jasso A, et al. Treatment of inhalant-induced psychotic disorder with carbamazepine versus haloperidol. *Psychiatr Serv.* 1998;49:812–815.

14. Kandasamy A, Jayaram N, Benegal V. Baclofen as an anti-craving agent for adolescent inhalant dependence syndrome. *Drug Alcohol Rev.* 2015;34:696–697.

15. Keriotis AA, Upadhyaya HP. Inhalant dependence and withdrawal symptoms. *J Am Acad Child Adolesc Psychiatry.* 2000;39:679–680.

16. Mackesy-Amiti ME, Fendrich M. Inhalant use and delinquent behavior among adolescents: a comparison of inhalant users and other drug users. *Addiction.* 1999;94:555–564.

17. Meadows R, Verghese A. Medical complications of glue sniffing. *South Med J.* 1996;89:455–462.

18. Misra LK, Kofoed L, Fuller W. Treatment of inhalant abuse with risperidone. *J Clin Psychiatry.* 1999;60:620.

19. Niederhofer H. Treating inhalant abuse with buspirone. *Am J Addict.* 2007;16:69.

20. Ramsey J, Anderson HR, Bloor K, et al. An introduction to the practice, prevalence and chemical toxicology of volatile substance abuse. *Hum Toxicol.* 1989;8:261–269.

21. Romanelli F, Smith KM, Thornton AC, et al. Poppers: epidemiology and clinical management of inhaled nitrite abuse. *Pharmacotherapy.* 2004;24:69–78.

22. Rosenberg NL, Spitz MC, Filley CM, et al. Central nervous system effects of chronic toluene abuse—clinical, brainstem evoked response and magnetic resonance imaging studies. *Neurotoxicol Teratol.* 1988;10:489–495.

23. Sakai JT, Hall SK, Mikulich-Gilbertson SK, et al. Inhalant use, abuse, and dependence among adolescent patients: commonly comorbid problems. *J Am Acad Child Adolesc Psychiatry.* 2004;43:1080–1088.

24. Shen YC. Treatment of inhalant dependence with lamotrigine. *Prog Neuropsychopharmacol Biol Psychiatry.* 2007;31:769–771.

25. Williams JF, Storck M. Inhalant abuse. *Pediatrics.* 2007;119:1009–1017.

26. Yamanouchi N, Okada S, Kodama K, et al. Effects of MRI abnormalities on WAIS-R performance in solvent abusers. *Acta Neurol Scand.* 1997;96:34–39.

29

Anabolic-Androgenic Steroids

KIRK J. BROWER

Introduction

Anabolic-androgenic steroids (AASs) refer to the male hormone, testosterone, and many of its natural and synthetic derivatives. All AASs have androgenic (masculinizing) and muscle-specific (anabolic) effects, but some are relatively more anabolic or androgenic than others. Oxandrolone, for example, has greater anabolic activity and less androgenic activity than testosterone.[108a] All AASs share a cholesterol-like and -derived chemical structure in common with other classes of steroid compounds, such as corticosteroids, mineralocorticoids, and estrogens. Synthetic selective androgen receptor modulators are nonsteroidal anabolic-androgenic drugs,[119] but little is known about the addiction potential of these premarketed substances.

Although AAS use is widely focused on the illicit uses to increase muscle growth and strength, several established medical uses exist for these substances. The US Food and Drug Administration (FDA)–approved medical uses of AASs include male hypogonadism (androgen deficiency),[5] hereditary angioedema (a dermatological disorder), treatment of weight loss associated with AIDS, burns, and other catabolic states,[108a] and relatively rare types of anemias including Fanconi and those related to bone marrow suppression (aplastic anemia).[94a,142] Other uses of AASs, including experimental ones, have included male contraception,[130] postmenopausal hormonal therapy, and treatment of depression[136a] and sexual disorders.[12a]

AASs are rarely used in isolation. Typical appearance and performance enhancing drug (APED) use involves several synthetic androgens and some combination of legal stimulants, illegal stimulants/thermogenic drugs, illicit nonsteroidal anabolics, and legal supplement use.[110a] Within the international sports community, APEDs are commonly referred to as "doping agents" and subject to detection by the World Anti-Doping Agency.[4,119] The use of APEDs by athletes to increase performance constitutes only a small subset of APED users,[111] and the secrecy of this form of drug use prevents any substantial literature on specific patterns of use among athletes. Unlike recreational users, fear of detection leads athletes to use a range of evasion strategies including use of masking agents, altered drug use schedules, and designer drug use.

AASs have some superficial similarities to so-called classical addictive drugs, such as alcohol, cocaine, nicotine, and opioids. A major difference is that AASs are not taken to induce euphoria and have little interoceptive detectability.[62a] Rather, APEDs are often taken in the context of a fitness-focused lifestyle that prohibits use of classical drugs of abuse.[90] Although not part of the motivating salience of APEDS, many of these substances have known psychoactive effects. For instance, the psychoactive influence of testosterone on mood has historically been a source of investigation in medicine that persists.[136a,137] Recent advances in the neurobiology of AASs have further increased overall attention to the neurobiology androgen effects on reward. There is now general consensus that AASs are reinforcing[139] and have important psychiatric effects,[107a] including the potential for addiction-like pattern of use.[139]

Epidemiology

AASs first entered the mainstream athletic spotlight with the 1956 World Games. The Russian team was discovered to be using AASs at the Vienna weightlifting championships, leading other teams to introduce this seemingly miraculous drug to their athletes. As elite sports athletes continued to misuse these substances, AASs became banned drugs by the International Olympic Committee in 1975. During the Montreal Olympic Games in 1976, eleven athletes were disqualified as a result of urine steroid screening tests that were instituted.[50]

Since then, AAS use has become more commonplace within the population. A meta-analysis of 271 studies[110] yielded a global lifetime prevalence rate of 3.3%, with males significantly more likely than females to have used (6.4% vs. 1.6%). The highest rates were found in "recreational sportspeople" (18.4%) and athletes (13.4%), followed by prisoners and arrestees (12.4%). In the United States., between 2.9 million and 4 million people have tried AAS.[104] In 1990, Congress passed the Anabolic Steroid Control Act, in an effort to reduce use, and anabolic steroids became a Schedule III controlled substance. Anabolic steroid use had spread from professional athletes and body builders to high school athletes and non-athletes striving to improve strength and physical appearance. According to the National Youth Risk Behavior Survey, the percentage of all high school students who ever took steroids without a doctor's prescription is 3.5. The prevalence of taking steroids without a prescription was higher among male (4.0%) than female (2.7%) students. According to the results from this survey, the prevalence of having ever taken steroids without a doctor's prescription increased from 1991 to 2001 (2.7%–5.0%) and then decreased somewhat from 2001 to 2015 (5.0%–3.5%).[65] In addition, the University of Michigan Monitoring the Future study, which conducts an annual survey on substance use among high school students, has collected data on steroid use in 8th, 10th, and 12th grade students since 1989. These data show a fairly stable rate of increase from 1991 to 1998 across these groups in overall annual prevalence rate and a gradual decline in use from 1999 to 2016. Lifetime prevalence of AAS use in 12th graders significantly decreased from 2.3% in 2015 to 1.6% in 2016. A consistent finding is that males outnumber females in prevalence of AAS use,[a] with onset commonly occurring in one's early 20s, and risk persisting into middle age.

Overall, men who train extensively by lifting weights for athletic or aesthetic purposes are at highest risk to use AASs.[3] Most studies also support a correlation with alcohol and other drug abuse,[110a] with some exceptions (e.g., Striegel et al.[123]). Conduct disorder during childhood and adolescence and adolescent body image and muscularity concerns are predictive of AAS use in male weightlifters.[105] Body dissatisfaction commonly co-occurs with AAS use,[11,64] but this finding is not consistent.[43] A severe form of body dissatisfaction among male AAS users has been called muscle dysmorphia (MD),[88a] although women may also have it.[37] Individuals with muscle dysmorphia exhibit a persistent belief that they are too weak or small and whose daily behavior is severely impacted by a preoccupation with increasing muscle mass. This syndrome has been compared to eating disorders—thus historically referred to as *reverse anorexia nervosa* or *bigorexia*.[22,62,89] Individuals with MD may share patterns of cognitive functioning that are similar to individuals

with eating and body image disturbances.[89a] Specifically, set-shifting difficulties and weak central coherence are positively associated with the drive for muscularity, a symptom of MD.[40] MD also has features of obsessive-compulsive disorder.[19,20]

Pharmacology

Chemical Structure

Derived from cholesterol, AASs have a 4-ring structure with 19 carbon atoms. Modifications at C-17 and other carbon atoms are responsible for much of the variety among synthetic AASs.[69] Alkylation at the C-17 atom in its alpha position results in most of the oral forms of AASs, because this structural modification confers resistance to first-pass liver metabolism. The C-17-alkyl-AASs may also be more likely to cause liver toxicity and cholesterol abnormalities. Esterification at the C-17 atom in its beta position results in the commonly injected testosterone esters (testosterone cypionate, testosterone enanthate, and testosterone propionate). Because testosterone is rapidly metabolized by the liver, the testosterone esters were designed as depot medications, and are released slowly from the muscles into which they are injected.

Pharmacokinetics

Most oral forms of AASs are relatively short-acting with half-lives of approximately 24 h, whereas injected AASs are relatively long-acting with half-lives of several days to weeks. Thus testosterone esters when injected for medically indicated replacement therapy are usually administered every 2–4 weeks, whereas oral forms are typically administered daily. Gel forms and transdermal forms of testosterone are applied topically to, and absorbed by, the skin for replacement therapy. Their pharmacokinetics also require daily administration. A buccal form of testosterone is available that is applied to the upper gingiva and requires dosing every 12 h. The topical forms of testosterone are not typically used illicitly, however, because they are difficult to administer in the supraphysiological doses preferred by illicit users.

Testosterone can be viewed as a "prohormone" for both dihydrotestosterone[28] and estradiol. When testosterone is aromatized by the enzyme, aromatase, estradiol is formed and acts on estrogen receptors. When reduced by the enzyme 5α-reductase, dihydrotestosterone is formed and acts on androgen receptors. Testosterone also acts directly on androgen receptors, but dihydrotestosterone is about 10 times more potent. Different organs are genetically programmed to express one enzyme or the other preferentially depending on its function. Thus, 5α-reductase predominates in the testes where spermatogenesis occurs, and aromatase predominates in the female breast causing enlargement. In the human brain, aromatase regulates the androgen-to-estrogen ratio in a tissue-specific manner.[6] Similarly, preferential gene expression may drive the synthesis of either estrogen or androgen receptors depending on the tissue site and function of the organ, in particular, the brain.

Urine Testing

Testing for AASs in the urine, although critical for athletic competitions at the elite level, is rarely performed in routine clinical practice, including addiction treatment settings. One reason is that AAS users are not frequently seen in addiction treatment

---

[a]References 54, 60, 85, 90, 94, 104, 110.

TABLE 29.1	Representative Anabolic-Androgenic Steroids Used by Weightlifters and Bodybuilders.

Injected testosterone esters
Testosterone cypionate
Testosterone propionate (Testoviron)
Testosterone enanthate (Delatestryl)
Testosterone ester mixture (Sustanon)
Injected veterinary forms
Boldenone undecylenate (Equipoise)
Stanozolol (Winstrol-V)
Trenbolone acetate (Finajet, Finaplex)
Other injected forms
Nandrolone decanoate (Deca-Durabolin)
Nandrolone phenpropionate (Durabolin)
Oral forms
Methandrostenolone (Dianabol), also known as methandienone
Methyltestosterone (Android, Testred)
Oxandrolone (Anavar)
Oxymetholone (Anadrol)
Stanozolol (Winstrol)

settings. Another reason is that testing is expensive and requires specialized laboratories that can perform mass spectrometry/gas chromatography across a large number of different AASs (Table 29.1). The detection of AASs in urine has recently been reviewed.[2]

Patterns of Illicit Use

Users often take AAS with the very specific goals of improving physical appearance and athletic abilities. Thus they tend to take these substances in strategic doses and combinations for varying durations. Multiple substances are often combined ("stacked") to maximize effects and to achieve supraphysiological dosages. These substances are self-administered during the drug cycles that typically last between 4 and 12 weeks.[29] AAS use is sometimes started at low doses and increased to a peak, and then gradually reduced, a pattern referred to as "pyramid" dosing. The polypharmacy of the APED cycle can be complex and relies on recipes passed via expert user circles of an individual trial and error knowledge based in self experimentation. Often ignored, APED users use specific exercise and dietary practices in conjunction with the cycle and postcycle recovery period. Many surveys suggest that AAS users are more likely than nonusers to misuse other addictive drugs. In this regard, it is of interest that AASs can increase sensitivity to alcohol,[58] amphetamine,[7,121] and opioids.[18] This sensitivity is likely part of a larger adaptation of the central nervous system to rewards of all types.

AASs are readily available through social networks associated with weightlifting gyms.[84] Although classified as Schedule III controlled substances in the Unites States, AASs are available on the Internet, although the real contents may be suspect.

Adverse Medical Effects

Adverse medical effects of AASs have been well reviewed.[49a,107a] Adverse medical effects may be transient, relatively reversible, and limited to periods of use and acute withdrawal; or long-term, relatively irreversible, and persistent during periods of sustained abstinence. The short-term effects generate less disagreement among experts than do the long-term effects, because good epidemiological studies of the latter are lacking. The major organ systems that are adversely affected by AASs are endocrine, hepatic, and cardiovascular.

Effects on the Endocrine System

Endocrine side effects result from having too high or too low concentrations of gonadotropins and sex steroids. Given that AAS use involves introducing exogenous androgens to the system, it results in a series of endocrinological events. Increased levels of free androgens through AAS use stimulate the secretion of aromatases, which break down the androgen molecules to be cleared from the system. This process, aromatization, causes circulating androgens to be converted to estradiol and other estrogens, leading to higher levels of estrogens in the system and resulting in unwanted physical feminization effects. For instance, gynecomastia or the development of breast tissue, female-pattern fat deposition, and water retention are common effects of aromatization that occur through AAS use. Gynecomastia, particularly when painful, may require surgical correction. In men, these effects also include testicular atrophy, abnormal and reduced spermatogenesis,[63,91] premature male pattern baldness, and loss of libido, although these physical effects are most often transient and reverse shortly upon ending AAS use. In addition, most users are aware of the common adverse effects and will often take ancillary drugs to combat these physical changes. In women, the endocrine side effects of AAS use include clitoral hypertrophy, decreased breast size, hirsutism including abnormal facial hair (such as mustache and beard growth), menstrual irregularities, reduction of breast size, infertility, and deepened voice. In females, some of these physical changes may be permanent and irreversible.[33,91] If taken during pregnancy, AASs can masculinize a female fetus.

Effects on the Hepatic System

Adverse effects on the liver—such as impaired excretion function, cholestasis, peliosis hepatis, and liver cancer—from AAS have been observed through animal studies, raising health concerns for individuals administering AAS in supraphysiological doses.[8,55,72] In addition, there have been a number of case studies that have reported the presence of liver disorders in young athletes using AAS.[14,25] However, it should be noted that these adverse effects have been observed only with the use of orally active 17-alpha alkylated AAS, such as methyltestosterone, oxymetholone, fluoxymesterone, norethandrolone, and methandienone. This type of AAS is less aromatizable and sought out by users who are attempting to avoid the androgenic effects that lead to excessive estrogen.[66,72] Systematic research has shown mild and reversible elevation of transaminase levels from the use of oral 17-alpha alkylated AAS, although this relationship has never been associated with the use of injectable steroids.[72]

Effects on the Circulatory System

Cardiovascular effects include hypertension, abnormal cholesterol levels, and cardiomyopathy as well as numerous case reports of myocardial infarction or stroke. Some effects may be confounded by strenuous exercise that accompanies AAS use. The lack of controlled trials of the cardiac effects of AAS since it is an illicit substance, combined with polypharmacy, also creates a problem when investigating whether AAS have a direct effect on the circulatory system. Nevertheless, a review of autopsy data from 1990 to 2012 revealed 19 fatalities in AAS users due to cardiac causes.[33a]

Although the American College of Sports Medicine concluded that there was a clear relationship between AAS use and hypertension in a position paper, this claim was based on the findings of a single study that has not been replicated.[86] Other studies have not found AAS use to have any effect on hypertension.[83,106] Possible effects that anabolic steroids may have on hypertension include their potential to increase blood pressure through observed effects on water retention in users, especially with use of oral anabolics. In addition, it is possible that some anabolic steroids with erythropoietic effects, such as boldenone undecylante, raise blood pressure when they increase blood volume to support the higher levels of red blood cells that accrue. This idea could explain symptoms that have been reported in AAS users, such as nosebleeds, which may be caused by the increased blood volume from oral anabolics and boldenone; however, this relationship has not yet been empirically proven, since these substances cannot be legally administered in the United States.[72]

Several studies have established a relationship between some forms of AAS use and decreased serum high-density lipoprotein (HDL) and an increase in low-density levels, which is an identified risk factor for heart disease.[1,52,106] Although these effects on serum cholesterol levels have been the most commonly cited negative effect of AAS use, studies have shown that serum cholesterol levels return to normal after stopping AAS use.[73,106] It is believed that the effects on HDL levels are not from testosterone, but rather the estrogen that it is converted to after aromatization. Thus, using low-aromatization AAS or using antiestrogenics in order to avoid the unwanted androgenic effects of AAS, puts users at a greater risk for lowered HDL.[72]

Other adverse effects include acne, peripheral edema due to water retention, polycythemia, exacerbation of tic disorders, sleep disorders,[136] and infections due to nonsterile injection practices. Taken by children, AASs can cause premature closure of epiphyseal growth plates in long bones, resulting in small stature.

Psychiatric Aspects and Effects

There is general consensus that AASs are psychoactive drugs that can contribute to and cause psychiatric effects in vulnerable individuals.[3,86a,99a,103,109] Many factors can influence the development of adverse psychiatric effects to drugs. Such factors include genetic vulnerability, social context, stress, personality characteristics, a past history of psychiatric problems, use of other substances, and expectancies. Case reports, retrospective studies, and psychiatric diagnostic studies of AASs users provide some clues regarding the range of adverse psychiatric effects observed, however, it can be difficult to prove that AASs, rather than coexisting factors (e.g., other drug use, predisposition, or environment) were responsible. Therefore, double-blind placebo-controlled trials that measure psychiatric effects of AASs are more conclusive (see below).

The most frequently described adverse psychiatric effects of AASs are extreme mood reactivity, marked aggression including homicidal thoughts and behavior (roid rage), grandiose and paranoid delusions, and addiction-like behavior.[77,103] Mania or hypomania, violent aggression, and delusions typically begin during a course of AAS use, whereas depressive episodes and suicide attempts are most likely to occur within 3 months of stopping AAS use, that is, during AAS withdrawal.[79] Fortunately, most psychiatric effects such as mood swings are reversible with medically monitored cessation of AAS use, but suicides and homicides are obviously irreversible. These data are not based on placebo-controlled studies and most recreational users report limited psychiatric complications during their use.

The true rate of adverse psychiatric effects among AAS users is unknown. Studies of illicit AAS users typically include small numbers of participants who may not be representative of all AAS users; and the studies rely on self-report of past events, which may not always be accurate.[92,97,106] One controlled study of 160 athletes reported that 23% of 88 AAS users were diagnosed with major mood disorders (i.e., mania, hypomania, or depression) in association with their AAS use, including 11% diagnosed with major depression.[106] That study also suggested that psychiatric effects are dose related: none of the AAS users taking low doses had major depression, whereas medium-dose and high-dose users had rates of 6 and 28%, respectively. Another study[79] found that rates of depression were higher during AAS withdrawal than when actively taking AASs (6.5% versus 1.3%). That study also found that 3.9% of 77 illicit AAS users had attempted suicide during the withdrawal period.[79] An autoptic study found that, compared to deceased amphetamine or heroin users, AAS users are more likely to die at a younger median age and violently, such as through suicide or homicide.[99] Rates of completed suicides, however, are especially hard to estimate. In a series of 34 forensically evaluated deaths among male AAS users, 11 users committed suicide, 9 were victims of homicide, 12 deaths were judged as accidental, and 2 were indeterminate.[129] Another study examined 24 cases of unnatural or unexpected deaths in AAS users and found that the majority (62.5%) were due to drug toxicity, 16.7% suicide, and 12.5% homicide.[27] This finding demonstrates the lack of clear causality in deaths of AAS users, since there is often comorbid polysubstance-related behaviors. Several studies have investigated the link between testosterone levels and suicide with conflicting findings. Some have found significantly low testosterone levels after suicide attempts,[81,134] which supports the link between AAS withdrawal and depression symptoms. Another study observed no association between testosterone levels and history of suicide attempt in male veterans with posttraumatic stress disorder.[13] Similarly, a comparison of testosterone levels in male suicide attempters and healthy controls found no difference between the two groups.[95] However, results from a study examining testosterone levels in suicide attempters with bipolar disorder found a positive correlation between testosterone and the number of manic episodes and suicide attempts.[118] Thus the precise pathophysiological relationship between testosterone and suicidal behavior remains unclear.

Adverse psychiatric effects appear to be dose related.[93] There are at least four double-blind, randomized placebo-controlled trials that employed relatively high doses of AASs.[107,124,133,144] Three of these studies indicate that some individuals will experience severe, adverse psychiatric effects after high doses of AASs are administered.[107,124,144] although one study found no evidence of psychiatric effects.[133] Averaging across studies, recent reviews have concluded that the incidence of prominent irritability or hypomania attributable to steroids during controlled trials is 5%.[107,114] These gold standard studies, however, are likely to underestimate the incidence and severity of psychiatric effects, because ethical considerations limit the maximum doses of AASs that can be administered to human subjects.[107] Illicit AAS users typically consume 10–100 times the therapeutic doses prescribed legitimately by physicians to restore testosterone levels in patients who cannot make their own. By contrast, the maximum doses administered in the cited controlled trials were 5–6 times the therapeutic dose.[107,124,133,144]

Neurobiology

The following structures have been implicated in the psychoactive properties of AASs: the midbrain,[35,59] nucleus accumbens,[34] amygdala,[23] hippocampus,[36,57,75] and prefrontal cortex.[35,56] Androgen receptors are prominent in the hippocampus, amygdala, and prefrontal cortex,[57] structures involved in learning and/or aggression. Synaptic density in the hippocampus is androgen-dependent.[75] The size of the medial amygdala is also AAS dependent.[23] More recent studies have examined structural brain imaging in human AAS users.[40b]

Neurotransmitter systems altered by AASs include γ-aminobutyric acid,[34,41,42] glutamate, which correlated with aggressive behavior,[31] dopamine,[34,70,71,115] opioids,[59,76,98] norepinephrine,[126] and serotonin.[26,74,108,126]

The mechanism of action of AASs can vary depending on the availability (in different brain regions) of specific enzymes such as 5α-reductase or aromatase, and receptors such as androgen or estrogen. This is because many of the metabolites of testosterone are active.[34,36] Thus the actions of AASs on the brain can be exceedingly complex. The inherent polypharmacy of AASs also complicates the basic understanding of its neurobiology. Stimulants are commonly used among AAS users and ultimately have less controversial and robust effects on mood and aggression, with known central nervous system effects.[112]

A modern theory of AAS misuse positions these substances as catalysts for allostatic response (i.e., homeostasis maintaining) to the musculoskeletal and stress systems. This adaptation involves increased endorphin/opioid response to exercise stress that produces an exercise high that is highly reinforcing. Over time, this model suggests that the natural allostatic responses in the hypothalamic-pituitary-gonadal axis and adrenal axis eventually reach a state of allostatic overload, where the AAS user would require constant AASs to achieve normal functioning within these respective systems.[48]

Addiction

The term "addiction" is used here synonymously with moderate to severe substance use disorders, as defined by the *Diagnostic and Statistical Manual of Mental Disorders, Fifth Edition* (DSM-5) criteria. The generally accepted abuse potential of AASs led to their classification in 1991 by the Drug Enforcement Administration as Schedule III Controlled Substances. Addiction to AAS was originally proposed in a peer-reviewed journal in 1989.[67] Repetitive, rigorous weight training activity might be reinforcing in itself, similar to exercise dependence, or psychosocially (if not monetarily) rewarding in terms of winning competitions, or having athletic prowess or a fit-appearing body. It remains true that AASs are not generally used nonmedically in the absence of regular and intense exercise, suggesting that exercise may be *essential* to any addictive syndrome that includes AASs.[44] Nevertheless, it is now generally accepted that AASs have a potential for addiction.[40a,62a]

Rodents will self-administer AASs and show clear evidence of mild reinforcing effects,[139] although self-administration is paradigm dependent.[32] The reinforcing effects appear larger for AASs have moderate aromatizing (i.e., metabolize into estrogens) effects suggesting an estrogenic mechanism is involved in AASs reinforcing properties.[138] The evidence of addiction to AASs from animal studies was a subject of comprehensive review,[140] and the evidence suggests that AASs somehow alter the opiate system.

Frequencies of withdrawal symptoms are shown in Table 29.2. Pope et al.[104] recently reviewed 10 studies of rates of AAS users who fit DSM-III-R or DSM-IV diagnostic criteria for substance dependence for AAS use. Three of the published studies[79,105,106] assessed for lifetime prevalence of AAS dependence, whereas six[12,24,39,53,88,96] assessed only for current AAS dependence. Both types of studies produced similar estimates of AAS dependence within users, however, with a mean (95% confidence interval) across studies of 32.5% (25.4%, 39.7%), with a median of 29.5%.

All reported instances of AAS dependence have occurred in nonmedical or illicit users who took AASs for weightlifting and bodybuilding. It is important to note that no cases of AAS dependence have been reported in patients legitimately taking medically prescribed AASs for clinical indications, which is primarily an issue of dose. Medical indications only require doses to restore normal physiologic function, whereas use for athletic performance or aesthetic appearance require supraphysiological doses of AASs. In contrast to prescription opioid dependence, therefore, the development of addiction to AASs does not appear to start with therapeutic doses that escalate over time as addiction emerges. Rather, dependence on AASs seems to require deliberate self-administration of supratherapeutic doses from the beginning and the co-occurrence of intense exercise. The lack of AAS dependence in individuals taking them for legitimate medical purposes has led to the erroneous conclusion that dependence does not develop without compulsive weightlifting activity, but this conclusion is confounded by the correlation between exercise and supratherapeutic doses.

Screening and Assessment

History

There is one published and validated structured interview for APED use: the Appearance and Performance Enhancing Drug Use Schedule (APEDUS).[46] The interview covers 10 core areas related to clinical concern among APED users. It categorizes APEDs according to licit and illicit substances and lists a broad range of symptoms and side effects of the complex polypharmacy found among users. In general, it is advised to identify the "recipe" of drug use for screening purposes. This accomplishes some key risk information and also establishes credibility to your screening approach. In addition, the interview contains questions regarding body image, exercise, and dietary practices. These sections are all designed to cover core pathology associated with problematic APED use. Finally, sections related to socialization and intentions for future drug use are included to contextualize the point in an individual trajectory of drug use.

Physical

Vital signs—hypertension. *Appearance*—muscle hypertrophy that is disproportionately larger in the upper torso than lower torso. *Skin*—acne, needle marks in large muscle groups, especially the gluteals, male pattern baldness or alopecia in men and abnormal facial hair in women, jaundice if severe liver disease. *Eyes*—jaundice if severe liver disease. *Chest*—gynecomastia and tender breasts in men or decreased breast size in women. *Abdomen*—right upper quadrant tenderness, enlarged liver if diseased. *Urogenital system*—prostatic hypertrophy and testicular atrophy in men and clitoral hypertrophy in women. *Extremities*—edema/water retention.

TABLE 29.2 Endorsed Anabolic-Androgenic Steroid Withdrawal Symptoms.

Symptom	Brower et al. [12] N = 49	Midgley et al. [88] N = 50	Copeland et al. [24] N = 100	*Hildebrandt et al. [45] N = 400
Anorexia	24%	–	33%	–
Acne				57.8%
Anxiety	–	–	12%	21%
Body image dissatisfaction	42%	–	38%	–
Decreased libido	20%	10%	1%	26.8%
Decreased size or weight	–	52%	–	–
Decreased strength	–	38%	–	–
Depressed mood	41%	–	31%	–
Depressed (due to size loss)	–	30%	–	–
Depression (unexplained)	–	6%	–	20.8%
Desire to take more steroids	52%	–	28%	–
Fatigue	43%	4%	24%	–
General loss of interest	–	–	23%	–
Headaches	20%	–	6%	–
Increased aggression	–	10%	–	33%
Insomnia	20%	–	–	47.3%
Nausea	–	–	2%	–
Nosebleeds	–	–	1%	–
Restlessness	29%	–	10%	–
Suicidal thoughts	4%	–	2%	–
Sweating	–	–	1%	–

Study reported self-reported side effects associated with AAS, not specific to withdrawal symptoms.

Mental Status

Large clothes may be worn to hide physical build if there is a body image disorder. Deepened voice and other masculine features may be observed in women. In terms of psychomotor behavior, speech, mood and affect, thought content, thought processes, and perception, the mental status exam can be consistent with depression, hypomania, or mania, with or without psychotic features. Suicidal and/or homicidal ideation must be assessed due to well-documented increases in aggression and impulsivity. Paranoid ideation or delusions with or without hallucinations are also important to assess.

Labs

The most common laboratory test to detect the use of AASs is an analysis of urine.[113] Although most clinical laboratories do not do these tests because they are specialized and expensive (most will eventually involve mass spectrometry/gas chromatography), clinicians should not hesitate to ask their local labs to send samples to where they can be analyzed. While waiting for the results, some common blood tests can be ordered as reviewed below.

Muscle enzymes can be elevated because of intensive weight training and intramuscular injections. Because alanine transaminase

and aspartate transaminase overlap with liver enzymes, creatinine phosphokinase should also be ordered. Cases of rhabdomyolysis have been reported.

Liver enzymes can be elevated because many of the oral AASs, especially the 17-alpha-alkylated ones, are metabolized there and can be toxic to the liver. Because alanine transaminase and aspartate transaminase overlap with muscle enzymes, bilirubin should also be ordered. Needle sharing, while not as common as among heroin addicts, can also infect the liver with hepatitis B or C.

A complete blood count may reveal elevations in hemoglobin, hematocrit, or red blood cell count, because AASs can stimulate erythropoiesis.

Chemically Activated LUciferase gene eXpression (CALUX) bioassays for androgen receptors (ARs) can accurately capture the androgen activity of plasma without direct knowledge of the cocktail of AASs taken.[51] This method achieves this goal by quantifying the degree of luciferase released upon activation of the specific receptor. The use of these assays overcomes the problem of drug heterogeneity caused by the common forms of polypharmacy encountered among AAS users.[45]

Levels of the hormones, luteinizing hormone and follicle-stimulating hormone, can be expected to be decreased, due to negative feedback of AASs on the hypothalamus and pituitary gland. Testosterone and estradiol will be elevated with use of testosterone esters, but endogenous output of these hormones will be minimal.

A cholesterol profile will likely show elevated low-density lipoprotein cholesterol and decreased high-density lipoprotein cholesterol. Because this profile is generally associated with cardiac disease, it is important to bring it to the attention of the user. Electrocardiography and echocardiography may reveal cardiac disease more directly if present. Left ventricular hypertrophy is typical in AAS users and sometimes other weightlifters, but diastolic dysfunction is more likely in AAS users, and may also extend to the right ventricle.[68]

A sperm analysis is not required but it will likely reveal either a decreased or zero sperm count, abnormal morphology, and reduced motility.

Treatment

AAS users are not commonly seen in addiction treatment settings, unless they are also dependent on or abusing other substances like alcohol, opioids, or stimulants.[21] They may present for psychiatric symptoms, but are most likely to be seen in primary care clinics or sports medicine clinics. It must be emphasized that no controlled studies of treating AAS-related disorders exist.[9,103] In the absence of a higher-level evidence base, the best we can do is borrow strategies shown to be effective for treating other substance-related disorders, while at the same time both respecting and targeting some unique features found among AAS users. As with dependence on other substances, the goals of treatment are abstinence from all addictive drugs, restoration of physical and mental health, and improved coping and psychosocial functioning. Whether maintenance with testosterone agonist therapy is a reasonable goal will be discussed below. The remaining part of this section will be organized by specific AAS-related disorders.

Anabolic-Androgenic Steroid Use Disorder

AAS abuse is defined as recurrent use that either causes adverse consequences or occurs in situations that are physically hazardous. Usually treatment is aimed first at motivating AAS users to stop their use via motivational interviewing, leveraging significant others affected by their use, or legal/medical consequences related to their use. and involvement of their social support network. The nature and severity of the adverse consequences require discussion in the context of the potential benefits of AASs that users perceive for themselves.

Anabolic-Androgenic Steroid Withdrawal

The degree of risk associated with acute cessation of AAS is not known, however, tapering off the substances under regular medical supervision is recommended. AAS users whose pattern of use included cycling and pyramid dosing, already know how to taper themselves from AASs and should be encouraged to do so. Those who are motivated to stop using but have difficulty doing it will likely have need pharmacological assistance in managing this withdrawal. There are neither controlled studies nor agreement about how to do it. Suggested techniques include testosterone substitution therapy followed by a taper at a rate that is tolerable and safe.[10] Prior to such treatment, blood work for follicle-stimulating hormone, luteinizing hormone, testosterone, and estrogen should be obtained. There are several cases described of persisting human

pituitary gonadotropin abnormalities weeks to months after tapering. Persisting human pituitary gonadotropin abnormalities may manifest clinically as sterility or depression, the latter of which should be treated as an AAS-induced mood disorder (see below). Whether these cases may possibly benefit from long-term testosterone supplementation, analogous to agonist therapy for opioid dependence, is unknown and regarded as experimental. In addition, testosterone supplementation would not correct sterility. Instead, medications that stimulate the human pituitary gonadotropin axis such as human chorionic gonadotropin,[87] luteinizing hormone, gonadotropin-releasing hormone,[135] and estrogen blockers,[117,127] may be required. These latter hormones are also used illicitly.[122] AAS withdrawal shares characteristics with other endocrine withdrawal syndromes.[49]

Severe Anabolic-Androgenic Steroid Use Disorder

Treatment of AAS dependence is subject to the same challenges as addiction therapy in general. Users often fail to appreciate the adverse consequences of their use and/or overvalue the perceived benefits of their use. Thus, they lack motivation to stop using. Motivational interviewing and motivational enhancement therapy may be indicated for these cases. For individuals whose dependence is associated with intolerable withdrawal symptoms that lead to relapse, agonist therapy with testosterone may be considered with an endocrine consult. Agonist therapy has the advantages of replacing illicit drugs of unknown contents with pharmaceutical-grade medication that is injected by a nurse or doctor every 2–4 weeks during an office visit. Unfortunately, there are no controlled trials of any of these approaches.

In approaching the psychological aspects of treatment, several differences from other drugs of abuse are important to consider. One difference between AAS-dependent individuals and many other addicts is that getting high is not the predominant goal of using AASs (even though AAS users may have used other substances to get high). Instead, the goals of using AASs are very culturally congruent with American values: to be bigger, better, competitive, and a winner. Reaching such goals requires hard work, discipline, and delayed gratification whether or not one uses AASs. Accordingly, AASs are used to align with, not escape from, mainstream societal values.

Another difference is that AAS users are more likely than other individuals with substance use disorders to be preoccupied with their bodies and physical attributes as a source of identity and self-esteem. Their goals, daily activities, and ways of coping with interpersonal conflicts will likely reflect their being a physical presence in the world. This is not to minimize anyone's intellectual abilities. Rather, it is to highlight that a reliance (or overreliance) on physical attributes, and anything which interferes with that, may be expected to emerge as a therapeutic issue. The livelihood and self-esteem of professional athletes, bodybuilders, male models, and so on, depend on it. Although this is a crucial difference, it has some similarity to what is expected of other addicted individuals—that they let go of a substance and sometimes a lifestyle on which they have come to depend and value highly.

Physical attributes can refer to appearance or athleticism. For individuals focused on appearance, Pope et al.[101] and others[15,47] have drawn deserved attention to the underlying body image distortion that can drive AAS use. The struggle to get bigger, no matter how big one already is, has been referred to as "reverse anorexia nervosa." Later, the term, "body dysmorphic disorder," was coined by Pope and colleagues[102] and is a preferred descriptive, because distorted body image, not disordered eating, is at the core of the disorder (even though AAS use has been linked to disordered eating[100]). Although using AASs for their myoactive effects is a crucial difference between AAS users and other substance users, it bears a resemblance to addicted individuals who use substances to overcome and self-medicate social anxiety, depression, and chronic pain as a step toward functioning better, not worse, in our society. As with other individuals, the original goals are important to understand and manage in other ways, but this only works well when the addiction itself is treated.

Anabolic-Androgenic Steroid-Induced Mood Disorder

AAS-induced mood disorder may resemble mania during episodes of use and depression during episodes of withdrawal. The cycling of mood states can resemble bipolar disorder, and parallel the cycling on and off the AASs. Acute mania is best treated with antipsychotic medication, but mood stabilizers are not necessary when individuals are willing to stop using AASs unless an independent mood disorder with bipolar features co-occurs. Whether a mood stabilizer would normalize bipolar-like symptoms for those who resist stopping AASs is not known.

For individuals diagnosed with major depression who have no history of manic or hypomanic episodes (whether or not AAS induced), antidepressant medication is indicated. For depressed individuals with a history of manic or hypomanic episodes that were only AAS induced, antidepressant therapy should be initiated cautiously and monitored closely. Whether AAS-induced mania or hypomania predicts antidepressant-induced mania or hypomania is unknown. There is anecdotal case-report data that AAS-induced depression can be treated successfully with selective serotonin reuptake inhibitors.[78] For individuals who do not respond to an adequate trial with selective serotonin reuptake inhibitors and who also have below-normal testosterone levels in the morning, consideration may be given to augmentation with testosterone gel.[101] Another approach involves short-term use of human growth hormone.[38] Suicides have been reported in AAS users, especially during withdrawal,[99] and safety must be prioritized, including hospitalization when needed.

Although medication can address the biological aspects of depression, AAS users may also feel depressed in response to losing momentum with their training activities. Individuals cannot be expected to achieve or maintain the peak physical progress they made on AASs with training and diet alone. Thus they may feel smaller and weaker from losing muscle size and strength, which can contribute to depression. Individuals may need guidance in setting realistic expectations for themselves and in balancing their lives with other enjoyable activities that do not depend on muscle size and strength. This may entail a similar kind of lifestyle change that other individuals with addiction need to make to stay clean and sober. Alternative social supports and sources of gratification is a common theme in addiction treatment. In addition to selective serotonin reuptake inhibitors, cognitive behavioral therapy that challenges body image distortions may also help to alleviate depression in individuals with muscle dysphoria.

Anabolic-Androgenic Steroid-Induced Psychotic Disorder

AAS-induced psychotic disorder may require hospitalization for safety reasons and to ensure abstinence. Treatment includes cessation of AAS use and the temporary use of antipsychotic medication. With proper treatment, psychosis can be expected to remit within a few weeks.

Conclusions

AASs, which consist of testosterone, selected metabolites, and synthetic derivatives with cholesterol-like chemical structures, have both anabolic (muscle-building) and androgenic (masculinizing) properties and legitimate medical uses. Their use is endemic among some groups of bodybuilders and male athletes, who take supratherapeutic doses (10–100 times therapeutic doses) primarily for their anabolic effects. By 1990, an estimated 1 million Americans had tried AASs. Nonmedical or illicit use is characterized by combining (stacking) multiple forms, including oral and intramuscularly injected preparations, as well as taking various other substances to augment their effects, ameliorate side effects, or escape detections. Use may occur in cycles, with drug-free intervals between cycles. A variety of adverse medical consequences are known, involving the endocrine, cardiovascular, hepatic, and central nervous systems. Psychiatric effects result from the neurobiological actions of AASs and include mood disorders, psychotic disorders, aggressive and impulsive behaviors with suicide and homicide as extreme outcomes, and addiction. Addiction treatment should account for both similarities and differences in taking AASs when compared with classical addictive drugs such as stimulants, opioids, and alcohol, but controlled trials are lacking to guide clinical practice.

References

1. Alén M, Rahkila P. Anabolic-androgenic steroid effects on endocrinology and lipid metabolism in athletes. *Sports Med.* 1988;6:327–332.
2. Anawalt BD. Detection of anabolic androgenic steroid use by elite athletes and by members of the general public. *Mol Cellular Endocrinol.* 2018;464:21–27.
3. Bahrke MS, Yesalis CE, Wright JE. Psychological and behavioural effects of endogenous testosterone and anabolic-androgenic steroids. *Sports Med.* 1996;22:367–390.
4. Barroso O, Mazzoni I, Rabin O. Hormone abuse in sports: the antidoping perspective. *Asian J Androl.* 2008;10:391–402.
5. Bhasin S, Cunningham GR, Hayes FJ, Matsumoto AM, Snyder PJ, Swerdloff RS, Montori VM. Testosterone therapy in men with androgen deficiency syndromes: an Endocrine Society clinical practice guideline. *J Clin Endocrinol Metab.* 2010;95:2536–2359.
6. Biegon A. In vivo visualization of aromatase in animals and humans. *Front Neuroendocrinol.* 2016;40:42–51.
7. Birgner C, Kindlundh-Högberg AM, Nyberg F, Bergström L. Altered extracellular levels of DOPAC and HVA in the rat nucleus accumbens shell in response to sub-chronic nandrolone administration and a subsequent amphetamine challenge. *Neurosci Lett.* 2007;412:168–172.
8. Bronson FH, Matherne CM. Exposure to anabolic-androgenic steroids shortens life span of male mice. *Med Sci Sports Exerc.* 1997;29:615–619.
9. Brower K. Assessment and treatment of anabolic steroid abuse, dependence, and withdrawal. *Anabolic Steroids in Sport and Exercise.* 2nd ed. Champaign, IL: Human Kinetics. 2000:305–332.
10. Brower K. Withdrawal from anabolic steroids. *Curr Ther Endocrinol Metab.* 1997;6:338.
11. Brower KJ, Blow FC, Hill EM. Risk factors for anabolic-androgenic steroid use in men. *J Psychiatr Res.* 1994;28:369–380.
12. Brower KJ, Blow FC, Young JP, Hill EM. Symptoms and correlates of anabolic–androgenic steroid dependence. *Addiction.* 1991;86:759–768.

12a. Buster JE. Managing female sexual dysfunction. *Fertil Steril.* 2013;100:905–915.

13. Butterfield MI, Stechuchak KM, Connor KM, et al. Neuroactive steroids and suicidality in posttraumatic stress disorder. *Am J Psychiatry.* 2005;162:380–382.

14. Cabasso A. Peliosis hepatis in a young adult bodybuilder. *Med Sci Sports Exerc.* 1994;26:2–4.

15. Cafri G, Thompson JK, Ricciardelli L, McCabe M, Smolak L, Yesalis C. Pursuit of the muscular ideal: physical and psychological consequences and putative risk factors. *Clin Psychol Rev.* 2005;25:215–239.

16. Reference deleted in review.

17. Reference deleted in review.

18. Célérier E, Yazdi MT, Castañé A, Ghozland S, Nyberg F, Maldonado R. Effects of nandrolone on acute morphine responses, tolerance and dependence in mice. *Eur J Pharmacol.* 2003;465:69–81.

19. Chandler CG, Grieve FG, Derryberry WP, Pegg PO. Are anxiety and obsessive-compulsive symptoms related to muscle dysmorphia? *Int J Men's Health.* 2009;8:143.

20. Chung B. Muscle dysmorphia: a critical review of the proposed criteria. *Perspect Biol Med.* 2001;44:565–574.

21. Clancy GP, Yates WR. Anabolic steroid use among substance abusers in treatment. *J Clin Psychiatry.* 1992;53(3):97–100.

22. Cole JC, Smith R, Halford JC, Wagstaff GF. A preliminary investigation into the relationship between anabolic-androgenic steroid use and the symptoms of reverse anorexia in both current and ex-users. *Psychopharmacology.* 2003;166:424–429.

23. Cooke B. Steroid-dependent plasticity in the medial amygdala. *Neuroscience.* 2006;138:997–1005.

24. Copeland J, Peters R, Dillon P. Anabolic-androgenic steroid use disorders among a sample of Australian competitive and recreational users. *Drug Alcohol Depend.* 2000;60:91–96.

25. Creagh T, Rubin A, Evans D. Hepatic tumours induced by anabolic steroids in an athlete. *J Clin Pathol.* 1988;41:441–443.

26. Daly RC, Su T-P, Schmidt PJ, Pickar D, Murphy DL, Rubinow DR. Cerebrospinal fluid and behavioral changes after methyltestosterone administration: preliminary findings. *Arch Gen Psychiatry.* 2001;58:172–177.

27. Darke S, Torok M, Duflou J. Sudden or unnatural deaths involving anabolic–androgenic steroids. *J Forensic Sci.* 2014;59:1025–1028.

28. Edinger KL, Frye CA. Intrahippocampal administration of an androgen receptor antagonist, flutamide, can increase anxiety-like behavior in intact and DHT-replaced male rats. *Horm Behav.* 2006;50:216–222.

29. Evans NA. Current concepts in anabolic-androgenic steroids. *Am J Sports Med.* 2004;32:534–542.

30. Fingerhood MI, Sullivan JT, Testa M, Jasinski DR. Abuse liability of testosterone. *J Psychopharmacol.* 1997;11:59–63.

31. Fischer SG, Ricci LA, Melloni RH. Repeated anabolic/androgenic steroid exposure during adolescence alters phosphate-activated glutaminase and glutamate receptor 1 (GluR1) subunit immunoreactivity in Hamster brain: correlation with offensive aggression. *Behav Brain Res.* 2007;180:77–85.

32. Foltin R. The importance of drug self–administration studies in the analysis of abuse liability. *Am J Addict.* 1992;1:139–149.

33. Franke WW, Berendonk B. Hormonal doping and androgenization of athletes: a secret program of the German Democratic Republic government. *Clin Chem.* 1997;43:1262–1279.

33a. Frati P, Busardo F, Cipolloni L, De Dominicis E, Fineschi V. Anabolic androgenic steroid (AAS) related deaths: autoptic, histopathological and toxicological findings. *Curr Neuropharmacol.* 2015;13:146–159.

34. Frye CA. Some rewarding effects of androgens may be mediated by actions of its 5α-reduced metabolite 3α-androstanediol. *Pharmacol Biochem Behav.* 2007;86:354–367.

35. Frye CA, Babson A, Walf AA. Self-administration of 3α-androstanediol increases locomotion and analgesia and decreases aggressive behavior of male hamsters. *Pharmacol Biochem Behav.* 2007;86:415–421.

36. Frye CA, Edinger KL. Testosterone's metabolism in the hippocampus may mediate its anti-anxiety effects in male rats. *Pharmacol Biochem Behav.* 2004;78:473–481.

37. Gonzalez-Marti I, Fernández-Bustos JG, Contreras Jordan OR, Sokolova M. Muscle dysmorphia: detection of the use-abuse of anabolic androgenic steroids in a Spanish sample. *Adicciones.* 2018;30:243–250.

38. Graham MR, Davies B, Kicman A, Cowan D, Hullin D, Baker JS. Recombinant human growth hormone in abstinent androgenic-anabolic steroid use: psychological, endocrine and trophic factor effects. *Curr Neurovasc Res.* 2007;4:9–18.

39. Gridley D, Hanrahan S. Anabolic-androgenic steroid use among male gymnasium participants: dependence, knowledge and motives. *Sport Health.* 1994;12. 11–11.

40. Griffiths S, Murray SB, Touyz S. Disordered eating and the muscular ideal. *J Eat Disord.* 2013;1:15.

40a. Grönbladh A, Nylander E, Hallberg M. The neurobiology and addiction potential of anabolic androgenic steroids and the effects of growth hormone. *Brain Res Bull.* 2016;126:127–137.

40b. Hauger LE, Westlye LT, Fjell AM, Walhovd KB, Bjørnebekk A. Structural brain characteristics of anabolic–androgenic steroid dependence in men. *Addiction.* 2019;114:1405–1415.

41. Henderson L, Penatti C, Jones B, Yang P, Clark A. Anabolic androgenic steroids and forebrain GABAergic transmission. *Neuroscience.* 2006;138:793–799.

42. Henderson LP. Steroid modulation of GABA A receptor-mediated transmission in the hypothalamus: effects on reproductive function. *Neuropharmacology.* 2007;52:1439–1453.

43. Hildebrandt T, Alfano L, Langenbucher JW. Body image disturbance in 1000 male appearance and performance enhancing drug users. *J Psychiatr Res.* 2010;44:841–846.

44. Hildebrandt T, Lai JK, Langenbucher JW, Schneider M, Yehuda R, Pfaff DW. The diagnostic dilemma of pathological appearance and performance enhancing drug use. *Drug Alcohol Depend.* 2011;114:1–11.

45. Hildebrandt T, Langenbucher JW, Carr SJ, Sanjuan P. Modeling population heterogeneity in appearance-and performance-enhancing drug (APED) use: applications of mixture modeling in 400 regular APED users. *J Abnorm Psychol.* 2007;116:717.

46. Hildebrandt T, Langenbucher JW, Lai JK, Loeb KL, Hollander E. Development and validation of the appearance and performance enhancing drug use schedule. *Addict Behav.* 2011;36:949–958.

47. Hildebrandt T, Schlundt D, Langenbucher J, Chung T. Presence of muscle dysmorphia symptomology among male weightlifters. *Compr Psychiatry.* 2006;47:127–135.

48. Hildebrandt T, Yehuda R, Alfano L. What can allostasis tell us about anabolic-androgenic steroid addiction? *Dev Psychopathol.* 2011;23:907–919.

49. Hochberg Ze, Pacak K, Chrousos GP. Endocrine withdrawal syndromes. *Endocr Rev.* 2003;24:523–538.

49a. Horwitz H, Andersen JT, Dalhoff KP. Health consequences of androgenic anabolic steroid use. *J Internal Med.* 2019;285:333–340.

50. Houlihan B. *Dying to Win: Doping in Sport and the Development of Anti-Doping Policy.* Council of Europe; 2002.

51. Houtman CJ, Sterk SS, Van de Heijning MP, et al. Detection of anabolic androgenic steroid abuse in doping control using mammalian reporter gene bioassays. *Analytica Chimica Acta.* 2009;637:247–258.

52. Hurley BF, Seals DR, Hagberg JM, et al. High-density—lipoprotein cholesterol in bodybuilders v powerlifters: negative effects of androgen use. *JAMA.* 1984;252:507–513.

53. Ip EJ, Lu DH, Barnett MJ, Tenerowicz MJ, Vo JC, Perry PJ. Psychological and physical impact of Anaboli–androgenic Steroid steroid dependence. *Pharmacotherapy: The Journal of Human Pharmacology and Drug Therapy.* 2012;32:910–919.

54. Irving LM, Wall M, Neumark-Sztainer D, Story M. Steroid use among adolescents: findings from Project EAT. *J Adolesc Health.* 2002;30:243–252.

55. Ishak KG. Hepatic lesions caused by anabolic and contraceptive steroids. In: *Seminars in Liver Disease.* © 1981 by Thieme Medical Publishers, Inc.; 1981:116–128.

56. Janowsky J. The role of androgens in cognition and brain aging in men. *Neuroscience.* 2006;138:1015–1020.

57. Janowsky JS. Thinking with your gonads: testosterone and cognition. *Trends Cogn Sci.* 2006;10:77–82.

58. Johansson P, Lindqvist A-S, Nyberg F, Fahlke C. Anabolic androgenic steroids affects alcohol intake, defensive behaviors and brain opioid peptides in the rat. *Pharmacol Biochem Behav.* 2000;67:271–279.

59. Johansson P, Ray A, Zhou Q, Huang W, Karlsson K, Nyberg F. Anabolic androgenic steroids increase β-endorphin levels in the ventral tegmental area in the male rat brain. *Neurosci Res.* 1997;27:185–189.

60. Johnston LD, O'Malley PM, Miech RA, Bachman JG, Schulenberg JE. *Monitoring the Future National Survey Results on Drug Use, 1975-2016: Overview, Key Findings on Adolescent Drug Use.* Ann Arbor: Institute for Social Research, The University of Michigan; 2017:113.

61. Kanayama G, Amiaz R, Seidman S, Pope Jr HG. Testosterone supplementation for depressed men: current research and suggested treatment guidelines. *Exp Clin Psychopharmacol.* 2007;15:529.

62. Kanayama G, Barry S, Hudson JI, Pope Jr M, Harrison G. Body image and attitudes toward male roles in anabolic-androgenic steroid users. *Am J Psychiatry.* 2006;163:697–703.

62a. Kanayama G, Brower KJ, Wood RI, Hudson JI, Pope Jr HG. Anabolic–androgenic steroid dependence: an emerging disorder. *Addiction.* 2009;104:1966–1978.

63. Kanayama G, Hudson JI, DeLuca J, Isaacs S, Baggish A, Weiner R, Bhasin S, Pope HG Jr. Prolonged hypogonadism in males following withdrawal from anabolic–androgenic steroids: an under-recognized problem. *Addiction.* 2015;110:823–831.

64. Kanayama G, Pope HG, Cohane G, Hudson JI. Risk factors for anabolic-androgenic steroid use among weightlifters: a case–control study. *Drug Alcohol Depend.* 2003;71:77–86.

65. Kann L. Youth risk behavior surveillance—United States, 2015. *MMWR Surveill Summ.* 2016:65.

66. Karasawa T, Shikata T, Smith RD. Report of nine cases. *Pathol Int.* 1979;29:457–469.

67. Kashkin KB, Kleber HD. Hooked on hormones?: an anabolic steroid addiction hypothesis. *JAMA.* 1989;262:3166–3170.

68. Kasikcioglu E, Oflaz H, Umman B, Bugra Z. Androgenic anabolic steroids also impair right ventricular function. *Int J Cardiol.* 2009;134:123–125.

69. Kicman A. Pharmacology of anabolic steroids. *Br J Pharmacol.* 2008;154:502–521.

70. Kindlundh A, Lindblom J, Bergström L, Wikberg JE, Nyberg F. The anabolic–androgenic steroid nandrolone decanoate affects the density of dopamine receptors in the male rat brain. *Eur J Neurosci.* 2001;13:291–296.

71. Kindlundh AM, Rahman S, Lindblom J, Nyberg F. Increased dopamine transporter density in the male rat brain following chronic nandrolone decanoate administration. *Neurosci Lett.* 2004;356:131–134.

72. Langenbucher J, Hildebrandt T, Carr SJ. Medical consequences of anabolic steroids. *Handbook of the Medical Consequences of Alcohol and Drug Abuse.* 2008:385–421.

73. Lenders J, Demacker P, Vos J, et al. Deleterious effects of anabolic steroids on serum lipoproteins, blood pressure, and liver function in amateur body builders. *Int J Sports Med.* 1988;9:19–23.

74. Lindqvist A-S, Johansson-Steensland P, Nyberg F, Fahlke C. Anabolic androgenic steroid affects competitive behaviour, behavioural response to ethanol and brain serotonin levels. *Behav Brain Res.* 2002;133:21–29.

75. MacLusky N, Hajszan T, Prange-Kiel J, Leranth C. Androgen modulation of hippocampal synaptic plasticity. *Neuroscience.* 2006;138:957–965.

76. Magnusson K, Hallberg M, Bergquist J, Nyberg F. Enzymatic conversion of dynorphin A in the rat brain is affected by administration of nandrolone decanoate. *Peptides.* 2007;28:851–858.

77. Majewska MD. Neuronal actions of dehydroepiandrosterone possible roles in brain development, aging, memory, and affect. *Ann N Y Acad Sci.* 1995;774:111–120.

78. Malone DA, Dimeff RJ. The use of fluoxetine in depression associated with anabolic steroid withdrawal: a case series. *J Clin Psychiatry.* 1992.

79. Malone Jr DA, Dimeff RJ, Lombardo JA, Sample RB. Psychiatric effects and psychoactive substance use in anabolic-androgenic steroid users. *Clin J Sport Med.* 1995;5:25–31.

80. Reference deleted in review.

81. Markianos M, Tripodianakis J, Istikoglou C, et al. Suicide attempt by jumping: a study of gonadal axis hormones in male suicide attempters versus men who fell by accident. *Psychiatry research.* 2009;170:82–85.

82. Matthiesson KL, McLachlan RI. Male hormonal contraception: concept proven, product in sight? *Hum Reprod Update.* 2006;12:463–482.

83. Mauss J, Börsch G, Bormacher K, Richter E, Leyendecker G, Nocke W. Effect of long-term testosterone oenanthate administration on male reproductive function: clinical evaluation, serum FSH, LH, testosterone, and seminal fluid analyses in normal men. *Acta Endocrinologica.* 1975;78:373–384.

84. Maycock BR, Howat P. Social capital: implications from an investigation of illegal anabolic steroid networks. *Health Educ Res.* 2007;22:854–863.

85. McCabe SE, Brower KJ, West BT, Nelson TF, Wechsler H. Trends in non-medical use of anabolic steroids by US college students: results from four national surveys. *Drug Alcohol Depend.* 2007;90:243–251.

86. Medicine ACoS. *Position Stand on the Use of Anabolic-Androgenic Steroids in Sports.* Lippincott Williams & Wilkins; 1987.

86a. Medras M, Brona A, Józków P. The central effects of androgenic-anabolic steroid use. *J Addict Med.* 2018;12:184–192.

87. Menon DK. Successful treatment of anabolic steroid–induced azoospermia with human chorionic gonadotropin and human menopausal gonadotropin. *Fertil Steril.* 2003;79:1659–1661.

88. Midgley SJ, Heather N, Davies JB. Dependence-producing potential of anabolic-androgenic steroids. *Addict Res.* 1999;7:539–550.

88a. Mitchell L, Murray SB, Cobley S, et al. Muscle dysmorphia symptomatology and associated psychological features in bodybuilders and non-bodybuilder resistance trainers: a systematic review and meta-analysis. *Sports Med.* 2017;47:233–259.

89. Mosley PE. Bigorexia: bodybuilding and muscle dysmorphia. *Eur Eat Disord Rev.* 2009;17:191–198.

89a. Murray SB, Rieger E, Touyz SW, García Dla G, Lic Y. Muscle dysmorphia and the DSM–V conundrum: where does it belong? A review paper. *Int J Eating Dis.* 2010;43:483–491.

90. Neumark-Sztainer D, Cafri G, Wall M. Steroid use among adolescents: longitudinal findings from Project EAT. *Pediatrics.* 2007;119:476–486.

91. Nieschlag E, Vorona E. Mechanisms in endocrinology: Medical consequences of doping with anabolic androgenic steroids: effects on reproductive functions. *Eur J Endocrinol.* 2015;173:R47–R58.

92. O'Sullivan AJ, Kennedy MC, Casey JH, Day RO, Corrigan B, Wodak AD. Anabolic-androgenic steroids: medical assessment of present, past and potential users. *Med J Aust.* 2000;173:323–327.

93. Pagonis TA, Angelopoulos NV, Koukoulis GN, Hadjichristodoulou CS. Psychiatric side effects induced by supraphysiological doses of combinations of anabolic steroids correlate to the severity of abuse. *Eur Psychiatry.* 2006;21:551–562.

94. Pallesen S, Jøsendal O, Johnsen B-H, Larsen S, Molde H. Anabolic steroid use in high school students. *Subst Use Misuse.* 2006;41:1705–1717.

94a. Paustian L, Chao MM, Hanenberg H, et al. Androgen therapy in Fanconi anemia: a retrospective analysis of 30 years in Germany. *Ped Hematol Oncol.* 2016;33:5–12.

95. Perez-Rodriguez MM, Lopez-Castroman J, Martinez-Vigo M, et al. Lack of association between testosterone and suicide attempts. *Neuropsychobiology.* 2010;63:125–130.

96. Perry PJ, Lund BC, Deninger MJ, Kutscher EC, Schneider J. Anabolic steroid use in weightlifters and bodybuilders: an internet survey of drug utilization. *Clin J Sport Med.* 2005;15:326–330.

97. Perry PJ, Yates WR, Andersen KH. Psychiatric symptoms associated with anabolic steroids: a controlled, retrospective study. *Ann Clin Psychiatry.* 1990;2:11–17.

98. Peters K, Wood R. Androgen dependence in hamsters: overdose, tolerance, and potential opioidergic mechanisms. *Neuroscience.* 2005;130:971–981.

99. Petersson A, Garle M, Holmgren P, Druid H, Krantz P, Thiblin I. Toxicological findings and manner of death in autopsied users of anabolic androgenic steroids. *Drug Alcohol Depend.* 2006;81:241–249.

99a. Piacentino D, Kotzalidis G, del Casale A, et al. Anabolic-androgenic steroid use and psychopathology in athletes. A systematic review. *Curr Neuropharmacol.* 2015;13:101–121.

100. Pisetsky EM, May Chao Y, Dierker LC, May AM, Striegel–Moore RH. Disordered eating and substance use in high–school students: results from the youth risk behavior surveillance system. *Int J Eat Disord.* 2008;41:464–470.

101. Pope Jr HG, Cohane GH, Kanayama G, Siegel AJ, Hudson JI. Testosterone gel supplementation for men with refractory depression: a randomized, placebo-controlled trial. *Am J Psychiatry.* 2003;160:105–111.

102. Pope HG, Gruber AJ, Choi P, Olivardia R, Phillips KA. Muscle dysmorphia: an underrecognized form of body dysmorphic disorder. *Psychosomatics.* 1997;38:548–557.

103. Pope Jr HG, Kanayama G. Treatment of anabolic-androgenic steroid related disorders. In: *Textbook of Addiction Treatment: International Perspectives.* Springer; 2015:621–636.

104. Pope HG, Kanayama G, Athey A, Ryan E, Hudson JI, Baggish A. The lifetime prevalence of anabolic–androgenic steroid use and dependence in Americans: current best estimates. *Am J Addict.* 2014;23:371–377.

105. Pope HG, Kanayama G, Hudson JI. Risk factors for illicit anabolic-androgenic steroid use in male weightlifters: a cross-sectional cohort study. *Biol Psychiatry.* 2012;71:254–261.

106. Pope HG, Katz DL. Psychiatric and medical effects of anabolic-androgenic steroid use: a controlled study of 160 athletes. *Arch Gen Psychiatry.* 1994;51:375–382.

107. Pope HG, Kouri EM, Hudson JI. Effects of supraphysiologic doses of testosterone on mood and aggression in normal men: a randomized controlled trial. *Arch Gen Psychiatry.* 2000;57:133–140.

107a. Pope Jr HG, Wood RI, Rogol A, Nyberg F, Bowers L, Bhasin S. Adverse health consequences of performance-enhancing drugs: an Endocrine Society scientific statement. *Endocr Rev.* 2013;35:341–375.

108. Ricci LA, Rasakham K, Grimes JM, Melloni RH. Serotonin-1A receptor activity and expression modulate adolescent anabolic/androgenic steroid-induced aggression in hamsters. *Pharmacol Biochem Behav.* 2006;85:1–11.

108a. Ring J, Heinelt M, Sharma S, Letourneau S, Jeschke MG. Oxandrolone in the treatment of burn injuries: a systematic review and meta-analysis. *J Burn Care Res.* 2019. [Epub ahead of print].

109. Rubinow DR, Schmidt PJ. Androgens, brain, and behavior. *Am J Psychiatry.* 1996;153:974.

110. Sagoe D, Andreassen CS, Molde H, Torsheim T, Pallesen S. Prevalence and correlates of anabolic–androgenic steroid use in a nationally representative sample of 17-Year-Old Norwegian adolescents. *Subst Use Misuse.* 2015;50:139–147.

110a. Sagoe D, McVeigh J, Bjørnebekk A, Essilfie MS, Andreassen CS, Pallesen S. Polypharmacy among anabolic-androgenic steroid users: a descriptive metasynthesis. *Subst Abuse Treat Prev Policy.* 2015;10:12.

111. Sagoe D, Molde H, Andreassen CS, Torsheim T, Pallesen S. The global epidemiology of anabolic-androgenic steroid use: a meta-analysis and meta-regression analysis. *Ann Epidemiol.* 2014;24:383–398.

112. Sanjuan PM, Langenbucher JL, Hildebrandt T. Mood symptoms in steroid users: the unexamined role of concurrent stimulant use. *J Subst Use.* 2016;21:395–399.

113. Saudan C, Baume N, Robinson N, Avois L, Mangin P, Saugy M. Testosterone and doping control. *Br J Sports Med.* 2006;40:i21–i24.

114. Schmidt PJ, Berlin KL, Danaceau MA, et al. The effects of pharmacologically induced hypogonadism on mood in healthymen. *Arch Gen Psychiatry.* 2004;61:997–1004.

115. Schroeder JP, Packard MG. Role of dopamine receptor subtypes in the acquisition of a testosterone conditioned place preference in rats. *Neurosci Lett.* 2000;282:17–20.

116. Reference deleted in review.

117. Shabsigh A, Kang Y, Shabsign R, et al. Clomiphene citrate effects on testosterone/estrogen ratio in male hypogonadism. *J Sex Med.* 2005;2:716–721.

118. Sher L, Grunebaum MF, Sullivan GM, Burke AK, Cooper TB, Mann JJ, Oquendo MA. Testosterone levels in suicide attempters with bipolar disorder. *J Psychiatr Res.* 2012;46:1267–1271.

119. Solomon ZJ, Mirabal JR, Mazur DJ, Kohn TP, Lipshultz LI, Pastuszak AW. Selective androgen receptor modulators: current knowledge and clinical applications. *Sexual Med Rev.* 2019;7(1):84–94.

120. Somboonporn W: *Testosterone Therapy for Postmenopausal Women: Efficacy and Safety. In Seminars in Reproductive Medicine.* Copyright© 2006 by Thieme Medical Publishers, Inc., 333 Seventh Avenue, New York, NY 10001, USA.; 2006: 115–124.

121. Steensland P, Hallberg M, Kindlundh A, Fahlke C, Nyberg F. Amphetamine-induced aggression is enhanced in rats pre-treated with the anabolic androgenic steroid nandrolone decanoate. *Steroids.* 2005;70:199–204.

122. Stenman UH, Hotakainen K, Alfthan H. Gonadotropins in doping: pharmacological basis and detection of illicit use. *Br J Pharmacol.* 2008;154:569–583.

123. Striegel H, Simon P, Frisch S, et al. Anabolic ergogenic substance users in fitness-sports: a distinct group supported by the health care system. *Drug Alcohol Depend.* 2006;81:11–19.

124. Su T-P, Pagliaro M, Schmidt PJ, Pickar D, Wolkowitz O, Rubinow DR. Neuropsychiatric effects of anabolic steroids in male normal volunteers. *JAMA.* 1993;269:2760–2764.

125. Reference deleted in review.

126. Tamaki T, Shiraishi T, Takeda H, Matsumiya T, Roy RR, Edgerton VR. Nandrolone decanoate enhances hypothalamic biogenic amines in rats. *Med Sci Sports Exerc.* 2003;35:32–38.

127. Tan RS, Vasudevan D. Use of clomiphene citrate to reverse premature andropause secondary to steroid abuse. *Fertil Steril.* 2003;79:203–205.

128. Thiblin I, Garmo H, Garle M, et al. Anabolic steroids and cardiovascular risk: a national population-based cohort study. *Drug Alcohol Depend.* 2015;152:87–92.

129. Thiblin I, Lindquist O, Rajs J. Cause and manner of death among users of anabolic androgenic steroids. *J Forensic Sci.* 2000;45:16–23.

130. Thirumalai A, Page ST. Recent developments in male contraception. *Drugs.* 2019;79:11–20.

131. Tracz MJ, Sideras K, Bolona ER, et al. Testosterone use in men and its effects on bone health. A systematic review and meta-analysis of randomized placebo-controlled trials. *J Clin Endocrinol Metab.* 2006;91:2011–2016.

132. Trenton AJ, Currier GW. Behavioural manifestations of anabolic steroid use. *CNS Drugs.* 2005;19:571–595.

133. Tricker R, Casaburi R, Storer T, et al. The effects of supraphysiological doses of testosterone on angry behavior in healthy eugonadal men--a clinical research center study. *J Clin Endocrinol Metab.* 1996;81:3754–3758.

134. Tripodianakis J, Markianos M, Rouvali O, Istikoglou C. Gonadal axis hormones in psychiatric male patients after a suicide attempt. *Eur Arch Psychiatry Clin Neurosci.* 2007;257:135–139.

135. Van Breda E, Keizer H, Kuipers H, Wolffenbuttel B. Androgenic anabolic steroid use and severe hypothalamic-pituitary dysfunction: a case study. *Int J Sports Med.* 2003;24:195–196.

136. Venâncio DP, Tufik S, Garbuio SA, da Nóbrega ACL, de Mello MT. Effects of anabolic androgenic steroids on sleep patterns of individuals practicing resistance exercise. *Eur J Appl Physiol.* 2008;102:555–560.

136a. Walther A, Breidenstein J, Miller R. Association of testosterone treatment with alleviation of depressive symptoms in men: a systematic review and meta-analysis. *JAMA Psychiatry.* 2019;76:31–40.

137. Werner AA. The male climacteric. *JAMA.* 1939;112:1441–1443.

138. Wood RI. Anabolic steroids: a fatal attraction? *J Neuroendocrinol.* 2006;18:227–228.

139. Wood RI. Anabolic-androgenic steroid dependence? Insights from animals and humans. *Front Neuroendocrinol.* 2008;29:490–506.

140. Wood RI. Anabolic–androgenic steroid dependence? Insights from animals and humans. *Front Neuroendocrinol.* 2008;29:490–506.

141. Yates WR, Perry PJ, MacIndoe J, Holman T, Ellingrod V. Psychosexual effects of three doses of testosterone cycling in normal men. *Biol Psychiatry.* 1999;45:254–260.

142. Young NS. Aplastic anemia. *N Engl J Med.* 2018;379:1643–1656.

30

Caffeine

JACK E. JAMES

CHAPTER OUTLINE

Introduction

Caffeine is the most widely consumed drug in history.[118] Indeed, caffeine is unusual among psychoactive compounds in being part of the daily diet of most people. With more than 80% of people worldwide consuming caffeine daily,[125] current usage transcends almost every social barrier, including age, gender, geography, and culture. No other psychoactive substance—including nicotine, alcohol, and the many illicit drugs—comes close to caffeine in popularity.

Caffeine occurs naturally in a number of plant species, where it serves as a protective toxin to defend against predation by insects and herbivores. A common but erroneous belief, sometimes implied in advertisements for caffeine products, is that caffeine has always been widely present in the human diet. In fact, it was not until after European colonization in the 17th and 18th centuries that caffeine products, previously unavailable to most people, became widely accessible. That is, the ubiquitous presence of caffeine in the human diet is a phenomenon of fairly recent origin.

The aim of this chapter is to provide an overview of caffeine and its use, with particular attention being given to consequences for health and well-being. In that context, the emphasis throughout is on dietary use, taking account of both acute and chronic effects. Following relevant background, including mention of the main sources of caffeine and prevailing patterns of use, attention is given to the pharmacology of caffeine, including the main mechanism of action and the key processes of physical dependence and tolerance. This is followed by a discussion of the psychopharmacology of caffeine, with particular attention being given to effects on psychomotor performance and mood, and the processes of withdrawal and withdrawal reversal.

The remainder of the chapter deals mostly with the health consequences of dietary caffeine, beginning with mental health and well-being. That section is followed by two separate sections dealing with physical health, the first of which is concerned with cardiovascular disease, and the second with cancer, maternal consumption, consumption among children and adolescents, and potential adverse interactions between caffeine and other drugs. Questions concerning caffeine "addiction" and whether there is a safe level of consumption are examined, followed by reviews of emerging interest in potential health benefits of caffeine beverages, including compounds other than caffeine, with particular reference to type 2 diabetes mellitus and Parkinson disease. The section thereafter considers processes that threaten the integrity of caffeine science, a topic that to date has received far less attention than it deserves. The section preceding the conclusions contains discussions of public policy and regulation of caffeine exposure, and strategies that have been found useful for reducing and quitting caffeine.

Main Sources of Caffeine and Patterns of Consumption

The main dietary sources of caffeine are tea and coffee beverages, and increasingly, soft drinks (e.g., colas) and so-called energy drinks. The tea plant is indigenous to regions of China, South Asia, and India. Written accounts in China of tea leaves being used to brew a beverage date to as early as 350 CE, and by about 600 CE tea had been introduced to Japan from China. It is unclear, however, to what extent tea was consumed by the general population of either country during these early periods. In the 17th century, the Dutch introduced tea to Europe and America, and today tea is cultivated commercially in about 30 countries. Coffee is indigenous to Ethiopia, from where it was transported for cultivation to Arabia in the 15th century. By the early 16th century, the practice had been established in the Islamic world of extracting caffeine by infusing ground roasted beans. The Dutch brought coffee plants to Europe in the early 17th century, and established plantations in the Dutch East Indies. Subsequent colonization by other European powers led to new and extensive plantations being established in the West Indies, Latin America, Africa, and India.

By the late 18th century, coffee replaced tea in popularity in the United States, and today coffee is the main source of caffeine globally. Tea continues to be consumed more widely, but qualifies as the second main source because its caffeine content is generally lower than that of coffee. Other common sources of caffeine include cocoa and chocolate (in both solid and beverage form), but the caffeine content of these is generally low and represents a negligible fraction of the total amount of caffeine consumed. In addition, although the daily intake of caffeine from sources specific to particular regions (e.g., maté in parts of South America) may be substantial for particular groups of consumers, the overall intake from such sources is small relative to total global consumption of the drug. Similarly, some medications, both prescribed and over-the-counter, contain as much as 200 mg (approximately 2–4 cups of coffee or tea) per tablet or capsule, and could be an important (even the main) source of caffeine for some individuals. For the general population, however, caffeine-containing medications are typically taken intermittently, or not at all, thereby contributing little to total population caffeine intake. Notwithstanding variations in per capita consumption between geographic regions, intake for the majority of consumers ranges from about 200 to 400 mg of caffeine per day (the approximate equivalent of 2–6 cups of coffee or tea per day).

Caffeine soft drinks are an increasingly important source of the drug, and often the main source for children. The more recently developed energy drinks are also increasing in importance as a source of caffeine for young people. Whereas the caffeine in sodas and energy drinks sometimes derives partly from plant products involved in manufacture (e.g., cacao, cola nut, guarana), most of the caffeine content of such drinks is added in refined form. That is, these products, which are targeted primarily at children and adolescents, are explicitly designed to be psychoactive. The seemingly inexorable growth in the consumption of caffeine by children has become a cause for concern in its own right (e.g., Heatherley et al.[98]) as well as giving rise to concerns that caffeine

in the form of sodas and energy drinks may serve as a gateway to increased use of other drugs.

The popularity of caffeine is often attributed to perceived consumer benefits. For example, participants in a recent survey of more than 1200 college students reported a host of effects including perceived improvements in wakefulness, concentration, physical energy, and mood.[190] However, as explained in more detail below, it is a mistake to assume that such reports reflect primary effects of the drug. Rather, it is known that physical dependence rapidly develops in response to repeated ingestion of caffeine, as is confirmed by feelings of sleepiness, poorer concentration, less physical energy, and negative mood following relatively brief periods of caffeine abstinence. As such, the benefit that consumers report is largely illusory. They are not due to the primary actions of the drug but to the reversal of abstinence-induced withdrawal effects. That is, notwithstanding perceptions, performance is merely restored to what would be normal for the individual were they not a caffeine consumer in the first place, leaving little or no net benefit attributable to caffeine.

Although consumption patterns relating to the various main sources of caffeine may change during the lifespan (e.g., an individual may switch from drinking sodas during childhood to coffee in adulthood), exposure to caffeine is essentially lifelong for the majority of people. Indeed, the first exposure for most people precedes birth. Caffeine crosses the placenta,[24,305] and because most women consume caffeine while pregnant, the majority of newborns show pharmacologically active levels of plasma caffeine.[51] Exposure typically continues during childhood, with patterns of use tending to consolidate during adolescence and early adulthood. Thereafter, usage tends to stabilize, generally undergoing little change for the remainder of life.[125] The unparalleled prevalence of caffeine use introduces multipliers in relation to the possible impact of the drug. At the individual level, lifelong use could lead to effects accumulating over the lifespan. Furthermore, considering the near-universal use of caffeine, individual effects, even if small, could have a substantial cumulative impact when assessed across entire populations.

Pharmacology of Caffeine

Caffeine belongs to a family of purine derivative methylated xanthines often referred to as methylxanthines or merely xanthines. At room temperature, caffeine is a white odorless powder with a bitter taste.[307] Caffeine was first isolated from green coffee beans in 1820 by Ferdinand Runge in Germany, and later was found to be present in a variety of other species (e.g., tea, maté, and cacao). Fig. 30.1 shows the structure of caffeine (1, 3, 7-trimethylxanthine) and the three dimethylxanthine primary metabolic products of caffeine in humans. Following oral ingestion, caffeine is rapidly absorbed into the bloodstream from the gastrointestinal tract.[10] Approximately 90% of the caffeine contained in a cup of coffee is cleared from the stomach within 20 min,[34] and peak plasma concentration is typically reached within about 40–60 min.[234]

Once ingested, caffeine is readily distributed throughout the body, and the concentrations attained in blood are highly correlated with those found in the brain, saliva, breast milk, semen, amniotic fluid, and fetal tissue.[125] The drug has an elimination half-life of about 5 h in adults,[228] and typical consumption patterns of 3–4 doses (e.g., cups) per day result in plasma concentrations that remain at pharmacologically active levels for most of the waking hours. In adults, caffeine is virtually completely

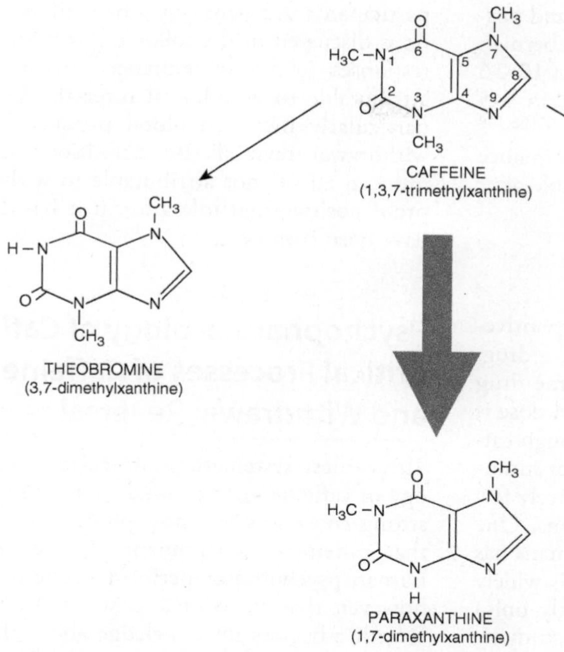

CAFFEINE
(1,3,7-trimethylxanthine)

THEOBROMINE
(3,7-dimethylxanthine)

THEOPHYLINE
(1,3-dimethylxanthine)

PARAXANTHINE
(1,7-dimethylxanthine)

• **Fig. 30.1** Caffeine and its dimethylated metabolites in humans (*arrow widths* indicate approximate relative proportions of the metabolites in plasma).

transformed by the liver, with less than 2% of the ingested compound being recoverable in urine.[278] Although the beverages and foods that contain caffeine may have other constituents (e.g., sugar, milk) that possess nutritional value, caffeine itself has no nutritional value.

Main Mechanism of Action

Caffeine exerts a variety of pharmacological actions at diverse sites, both centrally and peripherally, which are generally believed to be due mostly to competitive blockade of adenosine receptors.[52] Adenosine is a neuromodulator that acts on specific cell-surface receptors distributed throughout the body.[26,44,204,314] Due to similarities in the molecular structure of caffeine and adenosine, caffeine occupies adenosine receptor sites, with A_1 and A_{2A} receptors appearing to be the primary targets. Table 30.1 summarizes some of adenosine's main actions, which are generally to inhibit physiological activity. At typical dietary levels of intake, caffeine blocks adenosine receptors, producing effects broadly opposite to those summarized in Table 30.1.[18,27,73,185] It appears, also, that A_1 and A_{2A} receptors interact in functionally important ways with dopamine receptors.[63,83] In particular, A_{2A} receptors may be involved in the control of the dopaminergic signaling system essential to motor control.[65] In addition, caffeine has been reported to stimulate neuroendocrine activity, especially the catecholamine stress hormones of epinephrine and norepinephrine (e.g., Lane et al.[180]). Increases in serum cortisol and/or urinary cortisol metabolites have also been reported.[174,194,195,230,231] However, findings have not been entirely consistent in that some investigators have found cortisol levels to be unresponsive to caffeine.[171,222] The inconsistencies may be due to the typical challenge of about 250 mg (2–3 cups of coffee), being a borderline dose to which some people are unresponsive. For example, in one study, 250 mg of caffeine had no effect, whereas 500 mg increased plasma cortisol levels.[280]

TABLE 30.1	Some Acute Biological Effects of Adenosine.[a]
Biological System	**Effect**
Central nervous system	Decreased transmitter release, sedation
Cardiovascular	Dilated cerebral and coronary blood vessels
Renal	Antidiuresis
Respiratory	Bronchoconstriction
Gastrointestinal	Inhibition of acid secretion
Metabolic	Inhibition of lipolysis

[a]By blocking adenosine receptors, caffeine has effects broadly opposite to those summarized above.

Physical Dependence

Repeated use of caffeine, such as occurs in the context of dietary use, generally leads to the development of physical dependence, evidenced by the appearance of behavioral, physiological, and subjective withdrawal effects provoked by abrupt cessation of use.[153,179,283,313] Although incompletely understood, the mechanism responsible for caffeine physical dependence is believed to involve adenosine. Repeated exposure to caffeine, including dietary use, is thought to result in an increased number of adenosine receptors and/or enhanced affinity, resulting in hypersensitivity during abstinence.[18,225,311] Sleepiness, lethargy, and headache are common symptoms of caffeine withdrawal in humans,[a] and

[a]References 56, 79, 82, 92, 107, 127, 172, 177, 229, 282.

cessation of as little as 100 mg (1 cup of coffee) per day, and possibly considerably less, can produce symptoms (e.g., Lieberman et al.[191] and Smit et al.[271]). These may be felt within about 12–16 h, with a peak at around 24–48 h, generally abating within 3–5 days, and only infrequently extending for up to 1 week.[91,108,109] Notably, studies show that decreases in psychomotor performance (not necessarily discernible to the individual) are detectable after as little as 6–8 h since caffeine was last ingested.[99]

Tolerance

Drug tolerance refers to the progressive reduction in responsiveness that sometimes accompanies repeated exposure to a drug. It is evidenced by a decline in efficacy, whereby the same drug dose has less effect following repeated use or an increased dose is required to produce effects previously experienced. Although caffeine tolerance has been shown in relation to the locomotor stimulant effects of the drug in rats,[66,105] there have been relatively few empirical demonstrations of caffeine tolerance in humans. One focus of attention in relation to caffeine tolerance in humans has been the drug's cardiovascular effects,[47,120,121] which it is widely believed undergo tolerance. The most often (and frequently, only) cited source for the claim of hemodynamic tolerance is a study by Robertson and colleagues,[239] which is widely misquoted as having demonstrated complete hemodynamic tolerance to dietary caffeine. James[118] (pp. 111–113) has shown that the Robertson et al.[239] study did not demonstrate complete tolerance to caffeine, and that due to its many methodological limitations, the study could not have demonstrated complete tolerance. On the contrary, as discussed in more detail below, notwithstanding some contradictory findings, empirical evidence from diverse sources mostly converges to show that blood pressure remains reactive to the pressor action of caffeine despite repeated exposure such as that which occurs when caffeine is part of the daily diet (e.g., James[120,121,129]).

Overall, it appears unlikely that complete tolerance occurs in relation to most effects arising from typical patterns of caffeine consumption. It is important to note that the response magnitude to successive doses of the drug is generally inversely proportional to plasma caffeine level.[170,275] Specifically, whereas larger doses generally produce larger effects than smaller doses (dose-response relationship), the effect of successive doses of equivalent size is such that the difference in effect of each dose and the one before it diminishes (i.e., the difference in effect between the first and second dose is larger than the difference in effect between the second and third dose, and so on). It is also notable that overnight abstinence, which characterizes usual patterns of consumption, results in almost complete depletion of systemic caffeine by early morning.[189,228,265] Several lines of inquiry suggest that any tendency there might otherwise be toward the long-term development of tolerance is curbed by the pattern of diurnal depletion of systemic caffeine experienced by most consumers.

Indeed, the very fact that many hundreds of published experiments have reported significant caffeine-induced behavioral, physiological, and subjective effects provides strong evidence that the usual patterns of consumption do *not* produce complete tolerance. Most participants in such experiments have been typical caffeine consumers who arrive at the experimental laboratory following a brief period of abstinence. Notwithstanding the brevity of the typical period of abstinence (e.g., overnight) employed in experimental studies of the acute effects of caffeine,

participants are generally observed to be caffeine responsive. As is discussed in the following section, some caffeine-induced responses (especially enhanced performance and mood) are attributable to withdrawal reversal. However, other responses, particularly increased blood pressure, are not attributable to withdrawal reversal. By definition, any persistent caffeine-induced effects not attributable to withdrawal reversal provide proof positive that tolerance, if it has developed at all, cannot have been complete.

Psychopharmacology of Caffeine: The Critical Processes of Caffeine Withdrawal and Withdrawal Reversal

The earliest systematic examinations of the psychopharmacology of caffeine were conducted about a century ago.[103,104] The strong consensus for most of the intervening period has been that caffeine is a stimulant capable of enhancing aspects of human psychomotor performance and mood. In recent years, however, that traditional view has been essentially disproved. Recent advances in knowledge about the dynamics of caffeine withdrawal and withdrawal reversal have radically transformed our understanding of caffeine psychopharmacology. In a typical study, behavioral and psychological outcomes are measured in healthy volunteers before and after double-blind administration of caffeine and placebo, and (compared with baseline and placebo) changes have often been reported in postcaffeine outcomes. This has been particularly evident in studies of performance and mood, wherein it has often been concluded that caffeine has *enhancing* properties. However, a critical appraisal of the typical study design shows that the findings yielded by such studies are, at best, ambiguous.[119,133,147]

Paralleling the time-honored practice of placebo-controlled studies of medications, caffeine is typically withheld for a period prior to testing for effects, with the aim of ensuring all participants are equivalent in systemic drug levels at the time of testing. Such efforts to achieve experimental control are inadequate for assessing caffeine effects, because the drug is used daily by most people. Typically, caffeine is consumed in separate portions throughout the day, with fewer portions consumed later in the day, followed by overnight abstinence.[125] With the half-life of caffeine in healthy adults being approximately 5 h,[228] overnight abstinence usually leads to complete or near-complete elimination of systemic caffeine by early morning.[188,189] Consequently, when employing the placebo-controlled paradigm, caffeine researchers have frequently made use of naturally occurring overnight abstinence by asking participants to forgo their usual morning caffeine beverage prior to laboratory testing.

What was not fully appreciated in the past (and, alas, continues to be ignored by some today; see James[133,147] for an extended review) is that having avoided caffeine since the evening before, study participants are generally entering the early stages of caffeine withdrawal by the time they are tested in the laboratory (typically, at least 12–14 h since caffeine was last ingested) (see James[118] and James et al.[147]). As explained earlier, habitual use of caffeine produces physical dependence, evidenced by the appearance of readily measurable withdrawal symptoms following periods of abstinence (e.g., Juliano et al.[153]). Thus, there remains the crucial question (discussed in the section to follow): To what extent do effects (e.g., enhanced performance and mood) generally attributed to caffeine represent genuine net effects of the drug or reversal of withdrawal effects induced by short periods of abstinence[119]?

Performance and Mood

The fact that caffeine is consumed daily by most people as part of a normal diet presents formidable methodological obstacles when trying to accurately isolate the net effects of the drug. Although the problem had been ignored for decades, systematic attempts have tackled the key methodological challenges posed by caffeine withdrawal and withdrawal reversal. Approaches have varied, but generally fall into three broad categories, consisting of studies that compare consumers and low/nonconsumers, pretreatment and ad lib consumption studies, and long-term withdrawal studies.[125,147] The first two approaches (studies comparing consumers with low/nonconsumers and pretreatment/ad lib consumption studies) have been shown to involve substantial limitations (for a discussion see James[125,133] and James and Rogers[147]). In contrast, the third approach (long-term withdrawal) has proven successful. This has entailed taking the core features of the traditional drug-challenge paradigm, with its attendant strengths of double blinding and placebo control, and extending them to include alternating periods of daily caffeine use and nonuse (abstinence).

Table 30.2 summarizes the core design features of an experimental paradigm employed successfully by James and colleagues (e.g., see James[117,120,127] and Keane et al.[160]) to elucidate caffeine's net effects using long-term withdrawal. During caffeine phases of that paradigm, participants ingest the approximate equivalent of 1 cup of coffee three times daily, thereby simulating the typical population pattern of caffeine consumption. The protocol employs six consecutive days of placebo/caffeine intake to achieve stability of responding before challenging participants on the seventh day of each alternating 1-week period. The 1-week time frame was chosen on the grounds that studies of caffeine tolerance in humans have generally found that effects plateau within 3–5 days of continuous use.[47,120,121,238] In addition, there is a strong body of evidence showing that withdrawal effects generally abate within

a similar time frame of 3–5 days (e.g., Griffiths et al.[91] and Hughes et al.[108]). The full research design, as shown in Table 30.2, offers the substantial benefit of being able to examine and compare the separate acute and chronic effects of caffeine in the one experiment. An abridged version of the design has also been used, consisting of the "PP" and "CC" conditions outlined in Table 30.2 without the "PC" and "CP" conditions (e.g., James et al.[138-140]). While not elucidating the more detailed processes of withdrawal and tolerance, the abridged design allows key questions concerning caffeine's net effects to be addressed.

Long-term caffeine withdrawal studies have provided strong support for the withdrawal reversal hypothesis in relation to cognitive performance and mood.[133,147] That is, overnight caffeine abstinence has been found to be detrimental to performance and mood, with these adverse effects being removed when caffeine is reingested (restoration due to reversal of withdrawal effects). It is important to note that recent studies have yielded consistent evidence of caffeine having little or no net beneficial effect on cognitive performance and mood under conditions of sustained caffeine use versus sustained abstinence.[127,138,140] Several other studies, which may not all strictly qualify as long-term studies, have reported similar results in relation to performance and mood in adults[152,238,243,244] and children.[98] Unfortunately, the same level of rigor has yet to be applied in studies of physical performance. As such, there is little justification for oft-repeated claims about caffeine being an effective ergogenic aid.[130]

To repeat, the classic drug-challenge protocol, long considered the gold standard of drug research, is not a suitable design for revealing the effects of a drug that is consumed daily by most people and is subject to the development of physical dependence and associated symptoms of withdrawal.[133] Nevertheless, essentially uninterpretable studies continue to be published in which a standard drug-challenge design has been used to examine the effects of caffeine on performance, both cognitive (e.g., Borota et al.[22]) and physical (e.g., Lara et al.[182]). Evidently, there is need on the part of editors and reviewers to be better informed about the inherent ambiguity of results arising from such studies. Unfortunately, however, there is evidence that some journal editors may be resistant to

TABLE 30.2 Summary of a Double-Blind Placebo-Controlled Crossover Protocol Incorporating Alternating Periods of "Long-Term" Caffeine Exposure and Abstinence.[a]

Week	Run-in Days (Days 1–6)	"Challenge" (Day 7)	Condition (abbreviation)	Effects Revealed by Challenge
1	Placebo	Placebo	PP	Sustained abstinence (i.e., caffeine "wash out"). Serves as a caffeine-free baseline.
2	Placebo	Caffeine	PC	Acute challenge. When compared with PP and CC, reveals the presence of tolerance.
3	Caffeine	Placebo	CP	Acute abstinence. When compared with PP and CC, reveals the presence of withdrawal.
4	Caffeine	Caffeine	CC	Habitual use. When compared with PP, reveals the net effects of habitual consumption.

PP, Placebo ingested for 6 consecutive days followed by 1 day of placebo challenge; *PC*, 6 days of placebo followed by 1 day of caffeine challenge; *CP*, 6 days of caffeine followed by 1 day of placebo challenge; *CC*, 6 days of caffeine followed by 1 day of caffeine challenge.

[a]Design originally described by James and colleagues,[120,121,127] versions of which have been employed by the same authors in subsequent studies (e.g., James and Gregg,[138,139] James et al.,[140] Keane et al.[160]).

scientific challenges to cherished beliefs about caffeine having performance-enhancing stimulant-like effects.[134] It is misleading, however, to refer to caffeine as a stimulant, if that term is used to refer to enhanced or supranormal performance. Rather, the stimulant properties of caffeine, especially at higher dose levels, are in the form of psychomotor agitation, including feelings of jitteriness and restlessness.

Sleep and Wakefulness

Persistent beliefs about caffeine being capable of enhancing psychomotor performance and mood are matched by equally strong beliefs that caffeine is effective in reversing negative effects of sleep loss.[141] Until recently, however, studies of caffeine and sleep failed to take account of the processes of withdrawal and withdrawal reversal. Employing the abbreviated version of the experimental paradigm summarized in Table 30.2 (i.e., PP versus CC as defined in the table), James et al.[140] examined the effects of dietary caffeine in healthy volunteers who alternated weekly between placebo and caffeine and who were either rested or deprived of more than 50% of their usual nighttime sleep on the evening before testing. Confirming previous studies, caffeine was found to have no significant net enhancing effects for either performance or mood when participants were rested, while also having no net restorative effects when performance and mood were negatively affected by sleep restriction. Indeed, James and Gregg[138] found that caffeine exacerbated the marked adverse effects of sleep restriction on mood.

Similarly, after controlling for caffeine withdrawal effects, Rogers et al.[243] found that cognitive performance was unimproved by caffeine in participants who were sleep restricted. Acute (overnight) caffeine withdrawal was found to impair performance on tasks requiring sustained attention, and subsequent caffeine intake merely prevented further deterioration in performance (withdrawal reversal). In contrast, the significantly better levels of performance on the same tasks shown by long-term (3 weeks) withdrawn participants were not improved by caffeine. In addition, acute caffeine withdrawal had a variety of negative effects on mood. More recently, Keane et al.[160] examined the effects of caffeine on patterns of electroencephalographic activity in a rare example of a study of electroencephalography in which caffeine withdrawal and withdrawal reversal were controlled. While again finding little evidence of positive stimulant effects, Keane et al.[160] found some similarities in effects on brain activity following caffeine ingestion (challenge) and acute caffeine withdrawal. As such, these findings and others by the same investigators[159] are consistent with results from studies of performance and mood in which caffeine withdrawal and withdrawal reversal had been controlled. That is, rather than having positive stimulant effects, a change in drug state, whether in the form of acute caffeine challenge or acute caffeine withdrawal, may disrupt normal electrophysiological activity in the brain, which may in turn be the substrate for the observed negative effects on performance and mood.

The terms "sleep" and "wakeful" lack precise definition, and are sometimes used as if they were exact antonyms of one another. Possibly everyone, however, has had the experience of being both sleepy and wakeful (i.e., tired but unable to sleep, for example, during periods of acute worry). This should not be surprising, since it is unlikely that a single mechanism controls the processes of sleepiness and wakefulness. As such, caffeine may directly interfere with an aspect of sleep (e.g., block receptors in the adenosine mechanism) and thereby forestall sleep while only poorly benefiting alertness. At the same time, sleepiness is a reliable effect of even brief periods of caffeine abstinence.

One source of confusion concerning caffeine's putative antisoporific effects is the fact that withdrawal-induced sleepiness is reversible by ingesting caffeine, thereby creating the illusion that caffeine is effective in stimulating wakefulness and overcoming sleepiness. In reality, the overall effect of caffeine on the sleep cycle is primarily that of disruption, involving increased risk of caffeine-induced sleep delay and withdrawal-induced periods of sleepiness. The former, caffeine-induced sleep delay, is possibly largely avoided by the majority of consumers who typically do not ingest caffeine after early evening. In contrast, although sleepiness induced by caffeine withdrawal is possibly widely experienced, most people are probably unaware of it (i.e., unaware of caffeine withdrawal as a cause of daytime sleepiness). Indeed, there is a strong possibility, yet to be verified, that sleepiness induced by caffeine withdrawal is a common, although largely unrecognized, cause of fatigue-related traffic and industrial accidents.

Considering the overall evidence, there can be little confidence in the conclusions and recommendations promulgated by a Task Force established by the American Academy of Sleep Medicine to specifically examine the use of caffeine (and other "stimulants") for countering the effects of sleep loss.[21] The available evidence does not justify the Task Force's claim that caffeine is an effective sleep-loss prophylactic. A similarly disappointing view must be taken of a more recent analysis published under the auspices of the Cochrane Database of Systematic Reviews.[162] That review concluded that "there is no reason for healthy individuals who already use caffeine within recommended levels to improve their alertness to stop doing so." Unfortunately, the reviewers took no account of caffeine withdrawal and withdrawal reversal, which may account for them being led to a conclusion that is not merely misleading but also potentially dangerous. Whereas it is reasonable to advise current caffeine consumers to intermittently consume caffeine as a countermeasure to withdrawal-induced sleepiness when engaged in important real-life settings, such as long-distance driving and shift work, it is important to note, however, that withdrawal-induced sleepiness can be best avoided by not being a caffeine consumer, thereby obviating the need for intermittent caffeine ingestion to maintain wakefulness. Indeed, if there is benefit to be had from caffeine's antisoporific effects, that benefit is likely to be most effectively exploited by taking the drug only on infrequent occasions when sleepiness must be forestalled, but to otherwise abstain from the drug.

To summarize, a substantial research effort to elucidate the effects of caffeine on sleep and wakefulness, undertaken over a period spanning decades, has often been ambiguous and sometimes misleading due to failure to recognize that habitual use of caffeine, even at moderate levels, leads to physical dependence, evidenced by measurable behavioral and subjective effects in response to abstinence involving periods as short as 6–8 h. The few adequately controlled studies that have been done suggest that caffeine exacerbates, rather than benefits, performance and mood degraded by sleep loss. More studies are needed to better characterize sleep-related problems associated with caffeine withdrawal, and in particular to gauge the extent to which caffeine withdrawal may be a common, if largely unrecognized, cause of fatigue-related traffic and industrial accidents.

Mental Health and Well-Being

Major systems of medical and psychiatric diagnosis give formal recognition to disorders of psychological function arising from caffeine misuse. Notably, misuse in this context includes levels of use falling within the range seen in the general caffeine-consuming population. Because formal diagnoses can only be made after affected persons come to the attention of relevant professionals, it follows that a sizable proportion of the general public may be engaging in caffeine misuse even if a formal diagnosis has not been made. The 10th revision of the *International Statistical Classification of Diseases and Related Health Problems* (ICD-10)[320] has a specific diagnostic classification of mental and behavioral disorders due to use of *other stimulants*, including caffeine, with subcategories for acute intoxication, dependence syndrome, and withdrawal state. Similarly, under the label of caffeine-related disorders, within the broader rubric of substance-related disorders, the *Diagnostic and Statistical Manual of Mental Disorders, Fifth Edition* (DSM-5)[6] includes several caffeine-related diagnoses.

As with the ICD-10[320], the DSM-5[6] includes several caffeine-related diagnoses. Specifically, caffeine is listed as one of 10 separate classes of drugs in the diagnostic category of *Substance-related and Addictive Disorders*, which in turn is divided into two groups: *substance use disorders* and *substance-induced disorders*. In the *use* category, caffeine is a proposed clinical diagnosis that has yet to be formally accepted as disorder. In the *substance-induced* category, however, there are four specific caffeine-related disorders: *caffeine intoxication*, *caffeine withdrawal* (elevated from a proposed diagnosis in the previous edition of DSM[5,110]), *other caffeine-induced disorders*, and *unspecified caffeine-related disorder*. The diagnostic criteria for caffeine intoxication and caffeine withdrawal are shown in Tables 30.3 and 30.4, respectively. The rubric, *other caffeine-induced disorders*, includes *caffeine-induced anxiety disorder*, referring to "panic attacks or anxiety" believed to be precipitated by caffeine; and *caffeine-induced sleep disorder*, referring to a "prominent and severe disturbance in sleep" induced by caffeine.

The Epidemiology of Caffeine Disorders

Given the generally low level of awareness of caffeine-induced dysfunction in both lay and professional communities, it is likely that caffeine disorders remain substantially undiagnosed despite the existence of formal diagnostic protocols. Moreover, caffeine ingestion and withdrawal undoubtedly have undiagnosed biobehavioral outcomes that are not covered by current formal diagnostic categories but are nevertheless potentially serious. For example, as well as the likelihood that withdrawal-induced sleepiness sometimes contributes to fatigue-related accidents, evidence indicates that surgical patients commonly experience perioperative caffeine-withdrawal headache due to the requirement that they fast (and therefore do not receive their usual caffeine intake) prior to anesthesia.[57,59,79,218] Prophylactic administration of caffeine appears to provide a simple and effective remedy.[95,315] Indeed, the reversal of headache under such circumstances is further evidence of the role of caffeine withdrawal in the development of headache. In addition, in reference to medical operations, caffeine-induced hand tremor has been found to undermine surgical precision. In a double-blind placebo-controlled crossover study, Urso-Baiarda et al.[298] found that moderate amounts of caffeine had a detrimental effect on microsurgical ability due to the adverse effect of the drug on hand steadiness. That this should be of concern is all the more evident in light of evidence that surgeons often use caffeine (most often in the form of coffee) to maintain wakefulness during long working hours.[74] Varied findings such as these contribute to the impression that the population prevalence of caffeine-induced harm far exceeds that which would be implied by the frequency with which such problems are formally diagnosed in clinical settings.

Dietary Caffeine and Physical Health: Cardiovascular Disease

When considered in totality, the large and diverse body of relevant scientific literature is conclusive in pointing to adverse acute effects of caffeine on cardiovascular function, especially blood

---

TABLE 30.3	Diagnostic Criteria for Caffeine Intoxication.

A. Recent consumption of caffeine, usually in excess of 250 mg (e.g., more than 2–3 cups of brewed coffee).
B. Five (or more) of the following signs, developing during, or shortly after, caffeine use:
  (1) Restlessness
  (2) Nervousness
  (3) Excitement
  (4) Insomnia
  (5) Flushed face
  (6) Diuresis
  (7) Gastrointestinal disturbance
  (8) Muscle twitching
  (9) Rambling flow of thought and speech
  (10) Tachycardia or cardiac arrhythmia
  (11) Periods of inexhaustibility
  (12) Psychomotor agitation
C. The signs or symptoms in criterion B cause clinically significant distress or impairment in social, occupational, or other important areas of functioning.
D. The signs or symptoms are not attributable to another medical condition and are not better explained by another mental disorder, including intoxication with another substance.

Adapted from the American Psychiatric Association[6] [pp. 503–504].

TABLE 30.4	Diagnostic Criteria for Caffeine Withdrawal.

A. Prolonged daily use of caffeine.
B. Abrupt cessation of or reduction in caffeine use, followed within 24 hours by three (or more) of the following signs or symptoms:
  (1) Headache.
  (2) Marked fatigue or drowsiness
  (3) Dysphoric mood, depressed mood, or irritability.
  (4) Difficulty concentrating.
  (5) Flu-like symptoms (nausea, vomiting, or muscle pain/stiffness).
C. The signs or symptoms in criterion B cause clinically significant distress or impairment in social, occupational, or other important areas of functioning.
D. The signs or symptoms are not associated with the physiological effects of another medical condition (e.g., migraine, viral illness) and are not better explained by another mental disorder, including intoxication or withdrawal from another substance.

Adapted from the American Psychiatric Association[6] [p. 506].

pressure. Although evidence of chronic effects is less conclusive (for reasons outlined below), the available evidence nevertheless provides strong grounds for regarding dietary caffeine a significant factor in the development of cardiovascular disease. The extent of the evidence is such as to suggest the need for primary prevention at a population-wide level, including appeals to consumers to avoid caffeine in the interests of cardiovascular health. Such action, however, has been largely absent and it is important to examine reasons for that neglect. Accordingly, this section provides an overview of relevant experimental and epidemiological findings, and considers possible reasons as to why the relevant evidence has not attracted the level of serious attention that it deserves. Two main reasons for this neglect, considered below, appear to be: confusion regarding the epidemiology of caffeine and cardiovascular disease arising from exposure misclassification, confounders, and possible misunderstanding of putative threshold effects; and the ill-founded belief that habitual caffeine use leads to the development of tolerance to the cardiovascular effects of the drug.

Concerns for cardiovascular health in the context of dietary caffeine have a firm foundation in demographics. Cardiovascular disease is the leading worldwide cause of mortality and morbidity.[137] As well as being of high prevalence, cardiovascular diseases are generally of long latency, and have complex multifactorial causation implicating diverse aspects of lifestyle including diet. As discussed in preceding text, the prevalence of dietary caffeine is extremely high and essentially lifelong. In that context, it is noteworthy that adenosine has an important role in the regulation of cardiovascular function as well as being the main mechanism of action for caffeine, thereby providing strong biological plausibility for a possible link between the two. Blood pressure level is of particular concern, because it is the single most important predictor of population levels of cardiovascular disease,[240,241] and compared with several other key indices of cardiovascular function blood pressure is markedly more responsive to dietary caffeine.

Acute Effects of Caffeine on Blood Pressure

It has been shown conclusively that caffeine increases blood pressure acutely, with reports generally indicating increases in the range of 5–15 mg Hg systolic and 5–10 mg Hg diastolic. This acute pressor effect occurs across a wide age range, with effects lasting for up to several hours in healthy men and women (see James[125,129] for a discussion). In addition, the pressor effect of caffeine is additive to that of cigarette smoking,[76,146,274] is at least additive (e.g., France et al.,[72] Greenberg et al.,[89] James,[117,121] and Lane et al.[180]) and may be synergistic (e.g., al' Absi et al.[3] and Lane et al.[181]) to the pressor effect of psychosocial stress, and is evident in persons with hypertension as well as in normotensives (e.g., Hartley et al.[87] and Shepard et al.[264]). Furthermore, studies show that caffeine produces acute increases in aortic stiffness and enhances wave reflection, both of which contribute to increased blood pressure as well as being independent risk factors for cardiovascular disease.[158,202,308,309] Again, these effects have been observed in persons who are normotensive as well as those being treated for hypertension and appear to be synergistic to similar effects from cigarette smoking.[310] Increased consumption of caffeinated energy drinks has reawakened interest in the cardiovascular effects of caffeine, and recent studies of popular energy drinks such as Red Bull have confirmed earlier findings regarding the blood pressure–elevating effects of caffeine (e.g., Grasser et al.,[87] Kurtz et al.,[165] and Miles-Chan et al.[210]).

Epidemiology of Caffeine and Cardiovascular Disease

More than 100 large epidemiological studies in more than a dozen countries have reported data on the relationship between dietary caffeine and cardiovascular function, morbidity, and/or mortality. Although when taken as a whole the epidemiological findings suggest that dietary caffeine is harmful to cardiovascular health,[129] there has been a trend in more recent population surveys for coffee and caffeine to be reported as "protective." However, one feature of this large literature is the many inconsistencies in the reported findings. The response of some commentators and reviewers to this inconsistency has been to dismiss concerns about caffeine, a response that is neither logical nor consistent with overall findings. Dismissing concerns is particularly unjustified in light of the large and consistent body of evidence from experimental studies. By their nature, experimental studies afford a greater level of control than epidemiological approaches. Indeed, by integrating experimental and epidemiological findings, the former help to clarify inconsistencies in the latter. Considered comprehensively, the experimental and epidemiological findings raise concerns over the implications of dietary caffeine for population cardiovascular health. The assumption that clear consistency should have emerged in the epidemiological findings, if caffeine were having substantive population effects, fails to take account of the many methodological limitations in the epidemiological literature.

Misclassification

A major limitation of many studies is poor measurement of the key exposure variable, namely, caffeine consumption. Whereas this limitation has long been the subject of criticism (e.g., Gilbert,[85] James,[118] and Schreiber et al.[259]), there has been relatively little improvement or innovation to overcome the problem. Although dietary caffeine levels can be measured reliably using detailed self-report inventories,[144] many studies have employed poor self-report protocols and have shown little regard for the reliability of the measurements employed. Moreover, whereas many epidemiological studies of caffeine and cardiovascular health collected blood samples (mostly for the purpose of measuring serum lipid levels), there has been a failure to take the obvious next step of measuring systemic levels of caffeine or its metabolites.[128] As such, use has not been made of the fact that good estimates of dietary caffeine levels can be obtained by analyzing plasma and saliva caffeine (or paraxanthine, the major metabolite in humans) using high-performance liquid chromatography (e.g., Abu-Zeid et al.[1]) or enzyme immunoassay techniques.[139]

Confounding in Epidemiological Research

A frequent erroneous observation about the epidemiology of caffeine and cardiovascular health is that much of the research has ignored the influence of confounders. This confounder myth[118] asserts that reports of significant positive correlations between caffeine consumption and cardiovascular disease are the result of failure to control confounders, especially cigarette smoking. As well as being a cardiovascular risk factor, smoking has been found to be positively correlated with caffeine use (e.g., Klesges et al.,[163] Patton et al.,[224] and Trichopoulas et al.[293,295]). The myth, however, arises from the fact that, for the past three to four decades, epidemiological studies of caffeine have routinely controlled for cigarette smoking. Excepting one or two early studies, virtually all of the literature reporting a positive correlation between caffeine consumption and cardiovascular disease controlled for the influence of cigarette smoking.

In the context of population studies there is always a risk of unanticipated influence of an as-yet unidentified confounder. However, in epidemiological studies of dietary caffeine and health, the list of potential or presumed confounders that have been controlled for is very long, and includes: age, gender, cigarette smoking, alcohol consumption, body mass index, dietary factors, serum cholesterol, blood pressure, medical history, use of oral contraceptives, family history of heart disease, physical activity, personality, region of residence, education level, and religion.[118] Indeed, there has probably been a tendency toward overadjustment for confounders in epidemiological studies of caffeine (e.g., La Croix et al.[170] and Rosenberg et al.[249]). In particular, findings have frequently been adjusted for blood pressure and cholesterol, which may be caffeine-related and coffee-related causal pathways in their own right.

Some of the problems associated with statistical control of putative confounders are evident in a recent large study by Freedman et al.[75] of reputed health benefits and harms of habitual coffee/caffeine consumption. The study included over 400,000 participants between 50 and 71 years of age, who were free of major disease at baseline. During 14 years of follow-up, over 50,000 of the original study participants died. Notable, in analyses that were adjusted only for age (a standard adjustment in virtually all health-related population surveys), there was a dose-response association between coffee consumption and *increased* mortality, with a similar result being reported in another large and more recent similar study by Liu et al.[193] However, for Freedman et al.[75] but not Liu et al.,[193] that pattern was *reversed* after extensive multivariate adjustment for reputed confounders, including smoking, alcohol consumption, body mass index, and various demographic and health-related exposures (e.g., diet, physical activity). Only after such adjustment, did Freedman et al.[75] find coffee drinking to be beneficial to health.

In addition to reporting number of cups drunk per day, coffee drinkers in the Freedman et al.[75] study were also categorized according to whether the coffee they drank was caffeinated or decaffeinated "more than half the time." In analyses stratified by type of coffee predominantly consumed (caffeinated or decaffeinated), similar associations were observed for the two types of coffee, suggesting that compounds in coffee (e.g., antioxidants, including polyphenols) other than caffeine were responsible for the reputed health benefit. In that regard, the findings were consistent with other epidemiological studies that have also reported inverse (protective) associations between coffee consumption and cause-specific mortality including heart disease,[321] stroke,[183] and diabetes.[111]

Although the Freedman et al. study [75] supports an emerging consensus that coffee has health benefits, inconsistencies between observational findings such as theirs and findings from experimental studies suggest the need for caution. Well-controlled experimental studies have shown definitively that caffeine increases blood pressure acutely, and although it is sometimes asserted that tolerance develops to the pressor effects of caffeine, the empirical evidence shows that tolerance is partial and not complete.[58,120,121,129,196] Although long-term blood pressure increases caused by the caffeine in coffee are modest, a contribution to increased population levels of heart disease and stroke would be expected in view of the near-universal population exposure to caffeine.[126] It is possible that antioxidants or other compounds in coffee counter the pressor effects of caffeine; however, if that were so, long-term patterns of mortality would be different between consumers of caffeinated and decaffeinated beverages, with the latter displaying better

cardiovascular health. Yet, the Freedman et al. study[75] reported similar outcomes for caffeinated and decaffeinated coffee.

Threshold Effects

It is common in epidemiological studies of caffeine to stratify according to level of reported caffeine use. A proportion of studies adopting that approach have reported the existence of a threshold, whereby a positive association (i.e., higher level of disease) is observed in consumers reporting higher levels of intake (e.g., 6 or more cups of coffee per day) but not in consumers reporting lower levels of intake. Although such reports may be reassuring for average consumers, the notion of an actual threshold in this context is not persuasive. Experimental studies of caffeine have consistently found the acute hemodynamic effects of caffeine to be proportional to systemic caffeine level (e.g., Smits et al.[275,276]). In the absence of other intervening variables, this dose-response effect would be expected to result in a relatively continuous relationship between caffeine and cardiovascular disease outcomes rather than one marked by a threshold. Unreliability in the data, especially due to imprecise measurement of dietary exposure (as outlined above), is a more likely explanation of the threshold effects sometimes reported in epidemiological studies of caffeine and population cardiovascular disease.

Epidemiology of Caffeine and Blood Pressure

As part of the larger body of epidemiological research on caffeine and cardiovascular disease, James[129] identified 18 population studies that were specifically concerned with caffeine and blood pressure. Of these, five reported no association between dietary caffeine and blood pressure, six reported a significant positive association for systolic and/or diastolic pressure, and seven reported an inverse association for either systolic or diastolic pressure. The diverse findings are not explained by differences in the study populations, as these were similar in demographics and socioeconomics. Indeed, the level of inconsistency highlights the extent of the limitations that exist in the epidemiological findings, which contrast the largely consistent pattern of pressor effects reported in experimental studies (discussed in subsequent text). Of particular concern is that epidemiological studies have generally ignored issues related to the plasma caffeine concentration time course and associated pressor effects. The general pattern is shown in Fig. 30.2, which is a schematic representation of the estimated 24-h plasma caffeine concentration time course, assuming an elimination half-life of 5 h and ingestion of the approximate equivalent of 1 cup of coffee in the morning, mid-morning, and mid-afternoon.

Fig. 30.2 helps to show that the strength, and even the sign, of the correlation between dietary caffeine and blood pressure level depends on the timing of blood pressure measurement relative to when caffeine was last ingested.[129] Using 24-h ambulatory monitoring, James[120] found that overnight abstinence produced transient modest decreases in blood pressure. Thus, taking a cross-section of the population, recent caffeine consumption is likely to have a pressor effect (positive association), whereas brief caffeine abstinence (10–12 h) may have no effect, and longer periods of abstinence (12–24 h) may decrease blood pressure modestly (inverse association due to withdrawal). In view of this analysis, a noteworthy feature of several of the studies in which dietary caffeine was said to have been protective (i.e., inverse association between intake and blood pressure) is that participants were asked to fast before being examined.[129] Specifically, participants

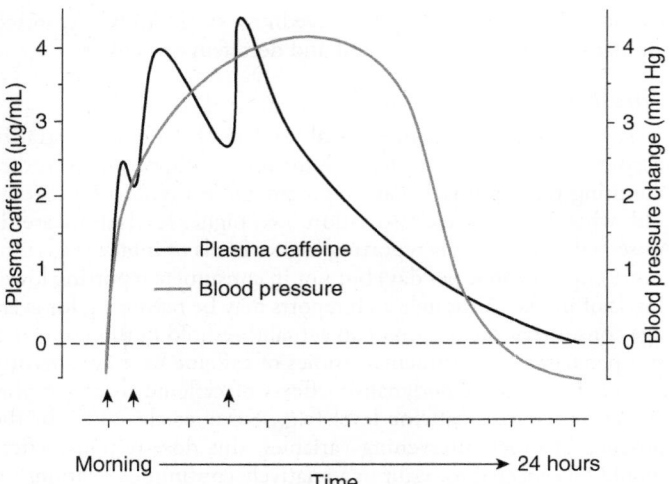

• **Fig. 30.2** Schematic representation of estimated 24-h plasma dietary caffeine concentration time course and associated change in blood pressure. Estimated plasma caffeine concentration assumes an elimination half-life of 5 h and ingestion of 1 cup of coffee after awakening and at two further time points (*arrows*) during the earlier part of the day (with evening and overnight abstinence). Associated blood pressure changes are relative to caffeine-free levels in long-term abstinent individuals.

in five of the seven relevant studies were reported to have fasted, while one reported nonfasting and one omitted to report whether participants fasted or not. Thus, in the majority of the studies involved, caffeine consumers' blood pressure readings were likely to have been transiently lower (due to withdrawal) than normal for themselves and potentially lower also than their nonconsuming counterparts.

Although interpretation of the findings of epidemiological studies of caffeine and blood pressure depends crucially on knowing when blood pressure was measured relative to when participants ingested caffeine, with one exception,[267] none of the relevant studies provides that level of detail. In the one exception, an overall analysis revealed no association between caffeine consumption and blood pressure level after adjustment for age, body mass, cigarette smoking, alcohol consumption, serum cholesterol, and family history of hypertension.[267] On closer examination, however, the authors reported that participants who had consumed caffeine during the 3 h prior to measurement had significantly elevated blood pressure compared with participants consuming no caffeine for the same period. It is notable that because the increases in blood pressure associated with recent ingestion of caffeine were independent of average daily intake (a measure of habitual use), the results also confirm experimental findings that habitual caffeine consumption does not lead to complete tolerance to the pressor action of the drug.

Chronic Effects of Dietary Caffeine on Blood Pressure

In early direct (i.e., experimental) examinations of the chronic hemodynamic effects of dietary caffeine, modest sustained decreases in blood pressure were reported when caffeine beverages were either removed from the diet[13] or replaced by decaffeinated alternatives.[303,304] Similar results were reported in a number of subsequent studies in which ambulatory monitoring was used to measure blood pressure level for extended time

periods.[88,120,150,233,285] Moreover, it is known that blood pressure responses of similar magnitude may be accompanied by different patterns of change in cardiac output and total peripheral resistance, and that these differences in hemodynamic profile may be implicated in cardiovascular pathology.[90] Speculation has existed as to whether caffeine-induced pressor effects are due to stimulation of contractility of heart muscle leading to increased cardiac output, or vasoconstriction leading to increased total peripheral resistance. Findings generally suggest that the blood pressure–elevating effect of caffeine is due primarily to increased vascular resistance.[40,78,96,139,273] Because greater risk has been attached to hemodynamic reactivity in which vascular, rather than myocardial, responses predominate,[153] findings of caffeine-induced vascular resistance add to concerns regarding the possible implications of dietary caffeine for cardiovascular health.

Dietary Caffeine and Population Blood Pressure Levels

If, as this review indicates, dietary caffeine contributes to statistically significant elevations in blood pressure, it should be noted that such increases are modest in absolute terms, amounting to possibly 2–4 mm Hg for most waking hours of the day. The question, therefore, that needs to be considered is whether such increases are likely to have an appreciable effect on population cardiovascular mortality and morbidity. It is sometimes presumed that increases of such magnitude are not meaningful, on the grounds that blood pressure level is inherently variable. However, it should be remembered that the effects of caffeine are at least additive, and possibly synergistic, to blood pressure increases due to a variety of other factors (e.g., smoking, hypertension, stress). In this sense, caffeine represents a preventable additional burden on the cardiovascular system.

The clearest insight into the contribution of blood pressure increases to cardiovascular disease is provided by population statistics describing the relationship between blood pressure level and cardiovascular mortality and morbidity. Because the association between the population distribution of blood pressure and cardiovascular disease is primarily linear, any contribution by caffeine to population blood pressure level may be expected to contribute to the overall incidence of cardiovascular mortality and morbidity.[200,201,232,241,302] It is important to remember that exposure to caffeine is generally long (essentially lifelong for most consumers), the prevalence of exposure is high (more than 80% in most countries), and the incidence of cardiovascular disease is high throughout the world. Although reduced blood pressure associated with reductions in dietary caffeine may be expected to be modest in absolute terms, even modest absolute changes in population levels of blood pressure translate to significant changes in the population burden of cardiovascular death and disease.

For example, it has been estimated that a downward shift of 2–3 mm Hg in the population distribution of blood pressure would produce life-saving benefits equal to the cumulative benefits achieved by antihypertensive treatment.[241,247] It has also been estimated that population-wide reductions of 2 mm Hg would avert 5% of deaths from coronary heart disease and 15% of stroke deaths.[240,241] More specifically, James[126] estimated that if caffeine consumption had the effect of elevating average population blood pressure by 2–4 mm Hg, a reasonable inference considering the relevant experimental data (e.g., James,[126,129] Jiang et al.,[151] and Takei et al.[286]), extrapolation based on epidemiological blood pressure data[200,201] suggests that population-wide cessation of caffeine use could lead to a reduction of 9%–14% of premature deaths from coronary heart disease and 17%–24% of premature deaths from stroke. If caffeine were removed from the diet in populations where coffee specifically is widely consumed, additional benefits might be achieved due to the adverse impact of that beverage on serum cholesterol and homocysteine.[129]

As an approach to scientific enquiry, the statistical control characteristic of epidemiological research is a poor substitute for the level of control offered by experimental science. Given the widespread consumption of coffee (and the near-universal consumption of caffeine beverages generally), substantial opportunities for enhancing health could be in the offing through discovery of whether and which components of coffee benefit or harm consumers, under what circumstances, and in relation to which outcomes. More and bigger observational studies are unlikely to give the certainty of knowledge that is needed for framing clinical advice for individual patients and general health advice for populations. In the end, the only sure method we have for teasing apart the undoubtedly complex cause-and-effect relationships between coffee/caffeine and health is experimental method.

Long-term clinical trials in which participants are assigned to respective caffeine and placebo groups (with verification of adherence via salivary or plasma bioassay) should be regarded a high priority by the research community including research funding agencies. In the meantime, observational findings should be regarded with caution, especially when they contradict predictions arising from experimental studies. Potentially helpful in suggesting lines of inquiry to be undertaken using randomized controlled trials, observational studies of caffeine and health should not be accepted as the last word.[131] Notably, a recent review of caffeine and cardiovascular effects, sponsored by the leading industry lobby (discussed below), makes no mention of caffeine's effects on blood pressure and takes no account of those effects as part of that article's broadly favorable assessment of caffeine and health.[50]

Dietary Caffeine and Physical Health: Noncardiovascular Disease

Cancer

Studies of cultured cells in vitro have reported both mutagenic and antimutagenic potential for caffeine/coffee,[19,29] and in vivo studies of intact nonhuman animals have suggested variously that caffeine is not a carcinogen, is carcinogenic under some conditions, and is antitumoric under other conditions.[125] Moreover, the relevance of the in vitro and in vivo findings to lifelong dietary use of caffeine in humans remains unclear. Currently, there is a strong consensus that the experimental evidence as a whole suggests that the drug is not a significant carcinogen in humans. In addition, there has been extensive epidemiological study of caffeine beverage consumption and cancer. Most of that research has been concerned primarily with coffee consumption, although over the past decade tea has also been a focus of attention. Because comparatively few studies have examined caffeine specifically, it is necessary to treat the findings for coffee and tea consumption as being only indirectly suggestive of the carcinogenic potential of caffeine.

All Cancers

Cancer is not a single disease, and therefore it is not surprising that most studies have been concerned with cancers located at one or a small number of specific sites rather than overall cancer rates. However, regarding overall rates, studies have tended to suggest

no adverse impact of caffeine on cancer mortality (e.g., LeGrady et al.[187] and Martin et al.[205]). On the other hand, studies of specific sites indicate more complex associations than those suggested by examination of the relationship between caffeine consumption and all-cancer incidence.

Lower Urinary Tract

Following an early report of a significant association between coffee consumption and cancer of the lower urinary tract (renal pelvis, bladder, and urethra),[39] there has been considerable epidemiological interest in coffee as a possible cause of bladder cancer. The substantial body of literature that has accumulated tends to suggest a positive but weak association.[112,118] However, although the association has been reported in different populations,[35,45,213,277] there is doubt as to whether the relationship is causal.

Pancreas

Early studies reported an association between caffeine beverages and pancreatic cancer,[199,283] one of the most rapidly fatal of human malignancies. Subsequent epidemiological studies, however, yielded mixed results. In a review of relevant research conducted before 1990, the International Agency for Research on Cancer[112] concluded that the evidence was suggestive of a weak relationship between high levels of coffee consumption and the occurrence of pancreatic cancer but cautioned that even this association could be due to bias or confounding. More recent studies have tended not to support the existence of even a modest positive correlation,[77,156,266,322,324] although in one meta-analysis it was concluded that small amounts of coffee may be protective while high intake increases disease risk.[219]

Breast

The epidemiology of caffeine and breast disease is somewhat mixed, especially among older studies, with some reporting a modest increased risk associated with caffeine consumption,[168,184,203,246] and others reporting no association.[197,248,255] More recent studies have tended increasingly to report no association,[67,208,272] and, more recently still, reports have appeared of an inverse association (i.e., protective effect) between caffeine consumption and breast cancer. Unfortunately, however, the pattern of findings has been inconsistent, with one study, for example, reporting an inverse association in premenopausal women and no association postmenopause,[14] and another study reporting a weak inverse association in postmenopausal women but no association for the cohort overall.[208]

Colon

Results of studies of caffeine consumption and cancer of the colon and/or rectum have also been highly varied. Some reported no association between coffee consumption and increased risk of disease,[186,209,220,223] whereas others reported an increased risk.[270,275,277] Still others, however, have reported a reduced risk.[b] Alleged reduced risk (i.e., potential protective effect) has led to speculation about possible mechanisms of action, including rates of bile acid secretion and colonic motility.[116,209,288]

Other Cancer Sites

Results for other cancer sites also tend to be mixed, with a pattern seeming to emerge of more recent studies reporting no association, or even a protective effect in some instances, thereby contradicting

[b]References 1, 15, 30, 114, 116, 166, 169, 269, 288.

earlier findings of adverse effects. For example, Armstrong and Doll[9] reported a positive correlation between coffee consumption and cancer of the kidney, whereas later studies, with the exception of Asal et al.,[11] have mostly failed to observe any relationship between coffee and/or tea consumption and kidney cancer. Similarly, whereas several earlier studies reported significantly increased risk of ovarian cancer in coffee consumers,[167,293,319] more recent studies have tended to report no association.[102,279,287]

Maternal Consumption of Caffeine

As mentioned in the preceding text, caffeine readily crosses the placenta during pregnancy. Thus at any time during the pregnancy of caffeine-consuming mothers-to-be, the developing fetus is exposed to concentrations of the drug equal to systemic levels in the mother. Naturally questions arise regarding the implications of this exposure, especially considering the known pharmacological actions of caffeine. In 1980, responding to reasonable suspicions and then-recent empirical findings, the US Food and Drug Administration (FDA) issued a warning advising pregnant women to restrict, or eliminate, coffee consumption. The focus of this warning was in relation to morphological (i.e., physical) abnormalities that had been observed in animal studies. However, the animal studies usually used dosing levels higher than those typical of human dietary use, and the consensus today is that dietary levels are unlikely to result in morphological abnormalities.[125]

Notwithstanding reassurance regarding gross defects, the question arises as to what represents an appropriate margin of safety for intrauterine exposure to caffeine in the human fetus. The usual safety standard employed by the FDA in relation to the human consumption of food additives is one-hundredth the maximum safe level of exposure in animals.[296] By that standard, virtually any pattern of regular caffeine consumption by a woman who is pregnant would put her unborn child at risk. That is, applying the FDA's usual standards, pregnant women should abstain from caffeine completely. Moreover, teratology (the scientific study of conditions caused by the interruption or alteration of normal development) includes not only the study of physical defects, but also the study of more subtle behavioral and emotional anomalies. Although a wide range of caffeine-induced developmental effects on behavior and neurochemistry have been demonstrated in animals, there have been very few reported studies in humans. The results that have been reported point to the need for further studies to examine caffeine as a potential behavioral teratogen.[125]

Pregnancy Outcomes

Several studies have reported a positive association between maternal caffeine use and spontaneous abortion,[38,49,84,235,317] whereas some others have found no association.[61,212] It has been suggested that positive findings could be due to confounding from pregnancy-induced nausea, which is less frequent in pregnancies that miscarry than those that go to term. It is plausible that women who experience nausea might respond by reducing their caffeine intake. Consequently, it could be this "loss of taste" for caffeine rather than reduced caffeine per se that might be the basis for the observed positive correlation between higher caffeine use and spontaneous abortion. However, the nausea hypothesis has not been supported by studies that took account of nausea experienced during pregnancy.[28,84]

In relation to findings for fetal growth, most studies have reported an inverse association (i.e., higher caffeine consumption is associated with lower birth weight),[60,155,214,254,281,306]

although some studies reported no association.[27,36,70,93,208,268] Notably, a recent Norwegian study of dietary caffeine and pregnancy outcomes involving almost 60,000 expectant mothers, the most comprehensive and thorough of its kind undertaken to date, found that caffeine intake was robustly associated with lower birth weight.[262] Indeed, notwithstanding inconsistencies in some of the earlier published findings, the current weight of evidence strongly points to harm from maternal caffeine consumption, with a number of meta-analyses concluding that caffeine consumption during pregnancy is a risk factor for lower birth weight.[33,62,251]

Taken as a whole, the relevant literature has led to increasingly unequivocal conclusions. An early systematic review concluded that there was tentative support for the conclusion that caffeine contributes to fetal growth restriction and lower birth weight.[145] That review highlighted various methodological limitations in the then extant literature and called for more research employing improved methods for measuring caffeine exposure and better controls against potential confounders, especially alcohol and tobacco use. An updated review published 6 years later concluded that the evidence had strengthened[118] and another review published 6 years after that concluded that the evidence had become strong.[125] Existence of a dose-response relation is an additional indicator of causation.[136] Studies published during the past decade provide no justification for continuing to ignore the now scientifically robust finding that maternal caffeine consumption contributes to lower birth weight.

The absence of a threshold effect is further indication of the urgent clinical need for action to counter the current widespread patterns of maternal caffeine consumption. Recommendations advising moderation (i.e., to limit consumption to low or moderate levels)[154] are without scientific foundation. Taking account of all the relevant science, the only justifiable recommendation that can be made at this time is for caffeine abstinence during pregnancy. In that context, caffeine abstinence refers specifically to avoidance of coffee, tea, cola, and other caffeine-containing beverages such as sodas and energy drinks. The low caffeine content of chocolate and chocolate confectionaries, chocolate cake, hot chocolate, and decaffeinated coffee and tea is such that those products probably need not form part of a maternal caffeine-abstinence regimen.

Children and Adolescents

From among the many caffeine products that have newly emerged, children and adolescents have been specifically targeted as consumers in the rapidly expanding market of energy drinks.[16,80,258] There has been simultaneous growth in awareness that caffeine consumption within that group is associated with negative behavior and other harmful outcomes. In particular, increased dietary caffeine among children and adolescents has been found to be associated with caffeine withdrawal symptoms,[8] poorer academic achievement,[142] increased daytime sleepiness[142] and reduced total sleep time,[8] increased somatic and social problems,[8] anger and violence,[143] and serious poisoning with fatal and near-fatal outcomes especially when ingested with alcohol.[94,132] In addition, there is speculation that adolescent dietary caffeine may function as a gateway to use of other substances, including alcohol, nicotine, and illicit drugs.[142,164,236,289,291]

Much attention has been given to the concomitant consumption of caffeine and alcohol, especially in relation to the now common practice among youth of mixing caffeine, particularly in the form of energy drinks, with alcohol. Consumption of the two substances combined has a pharmacological basis. As a nonselective adenosine receptor antagonist, caffeine counteracts the somnogenic effects of alcohol, and alcohol may in turn ameliorate the anxiogenic effects of caffeine.[261] By offsetting the sedating effects of alcohol, caffeine may reduce the sensation of intoxication. Any reduction in subjective intoxication is likely to impair judgments about risky behavior (e.g., drink-driving), and encourage higher consumption of alcohol, with further impairments to judgment and neurocognitive functioning.[64] This hypothetical sequence of events is supported by a substantial and growing body of evidence, which suggests that compared to alcohol alone, the concomitant consumption of caffeine increases the risk of assaultive and other violent behavior.[23,64,106,211,221]

Adverse Interactions Between Caffeine and Other Drugs

Taking into account the near-universal use of caffeine, it is inevitable that the taking of other drugs will often coincide with that of caffeine. Regarding recreational drugs, it is commonplace to see smokers light up when drinking a caffeine beverage, and indeed cigarette smokers consume more caffeine on average than nonsmokers. Similarly, alcohol is sometimes consumed in conjunction with caffeine, either as separate beverages or, as has become popular among some younger-age groups, in a single beverage containing both alcohol and caffeine. Caffeine is also sometimes used to "cut" illicit drugs such as heroin, cocaine, and amphetamine, with the users of those drugs sometimes consuming substantial amounts of caffeine even when not intending to so do. Particular concerns, however, arise in relation to pharmaceuticals with which caffeine may interact adversely or whose therapeutic efficacy may be undermined by caffeine (e.g., benzodiazepines and some antibiotics).[118,125]

Is Caffeine Addictive and Is There a Safe Level of Consumption?

The evidence reviewed in the preceding text indicates that dietary caffeine is a probable risk to cardiovascular health, poses a threat to fetal growth, interacts adversely with common therapeutic drugs, and produces dysphoric effects after brief abstinence. Therefore, taking account of its widespread and persistent use, should caffeine be considered a drug of addiction? Physical dependence is a prototypic characteristic of drugs widely regarded as addictive, and the relevant evidence pertaining to caffeine is conclusive. The occurrence of a characteristic syndrome of abstinence effects shows that repeated caffeine use leads to the development of physical dependence. Accordingly, it may reasonably be said that caffeine is a drug of addiction. On the other hand, the term "addiction" has wide currency and carries a variety of emotive connotations (e.g., illicit use, criminality, and violence) that have little relevance to dietary caffeine. Accordingly, it might be prudent not to be strident in labeling caffeine an addictive substance. That stance, however, should not distract us from the evidence that dietary caffeine is habit-forming as well as harmful.

Considering the evidence of harm, it is appropriate to ask: Is there a safe level of consumption? The inescapable (if unpopular) fact is that there is no daily level of intake that can be regarded as risk free.[125] The equivalent of as little as 1 cup of coffee produces a modest increase in blood pressure lasting 2–3 h, which if experienced daily over a lifetime probably contributes to increased cardiovascular disease; any level of habitual caffeine consumption

during pregnancy exposes the fetus to a dose equivalent to that received by the mother and evidently impedes fetal growth; caffeine interacts negatively with some therapeutic drugs; and dietary use produces physical dependence.

Does Caffeine Have Health Benefits?

There has long been interest in caffeine beverages as possible sources of benefit, and much of that interest has centered on the putative benefits of caffeine for psychomotor performance and mood. However, as discussed earlier, there is now a firm body of evidence showing that caffeine has little or no net benefits for performance or mood. Nevertheless, due at least partly to industry-sponsored efforts, there has been a substantial growth of interest in caffeine beverages as possible sources of benefit for physical health, especially in relation to diabetes and Parkinson disease.

Type 2 Diabetes Mellitus

Several epidemiological studies have reported significant dose-dependent reductions in the risk of developing type 2 diabetes mellitus in association with caffeine and coffee consumption.[c] Although findings have prompted some authors to claim that caffeine and coffee protect against type 2 diabetes, it is important to note that the studies in question were nonexperimental and shared many of the same potential confounder effects that have generally undermined interpretation of epidemiological studies of caffeine and health. More importantly, experimental studies have found the opposite pattern of results than would be expected from the population studies.

Double-blind placebo-controlled trials have consistently found that caffeine impairs glucose tolerance and decreases insulin sensitivity, and the findings have been reported for a wide range of participant groups, including persons with diabetes and those without.[d]). As such, it is difficult to reconcile how caffeine could offer protection against type 2 diabetes when experimental studies have shown that it compromises glucose metabolism both before and after development of the disease. Thus, although caffeine appears distinctly unlikely to confer any protection against the development of diabetes, one issue is whether there may be a compound other than caffeine in coffee that offers such benefit. If such a compound exists, to be of benefit, it would need to be sufficiently potent not only to negate, but to exceed, the negative effects of caffeine.

Considering the epidemiological and experimental evidence, it can be seen that a similar dilemma as that described above for cardiovascular disease also exists in relation to the possible involvement of caffeine in glucose metabolism and the development of type 2 diabetes. Although observational studies have tended to report that coffee provides protection against diabetes, experimental studies of healthy adults and patients alike provide strong evidence that caffeine impairs glucose homeostasis through transient increases in insulin resistance.[173] As with caffeine and blood pressure, if compounds in coffee other than caffeine protect against diabetes, this should be evident in long-term differences between consumers of caffeinated and decaffeinated coffee, but as with heart disease and stroke, such differences have generally not been reported (e.g., Freedman et al.[75]) in relation to diabetes. These inconsistencies raise doubts about the soundness of the observational findings from epidemiological studies. Apart from

---

[c]References 2, 75, 151, 250, 252, 300, 301.
[d]References 86, 161, 173, 175–178, 191, 227, 301.

causation not being able to be determined from observational studies, it is also the case that the statistical methods of control employed cannot guarantee adequate confounder adjustment or overadjustment.

Parkinson Disease and Age-Related Neurodegeneration

There is a substantial body of epidemiological evidence of an inverse association between caffeine consumption and the development of Parkinson disease (e.g., Ascherio et al.,[12] Costa et al.,[43] Hernan et al.,[100] and Ross et al.[251]). That finding has been widely assumed to be causal, and has contributed to speculation about the neuroprotective action of caffeine. In particular, attention has focused on interactions between the dopaminergic and adenosinergic systems and caffeine's putative ability to forestall dopaminergic neuron degeneration through its action on the A_{2A} adenosine receptor.[e] An earlier population study by Jarvis[149] is sometimes cited as support for the idea that caffeine has neuroprotective properties, not solely in relation to Parkinson disease but also other neurodegenerative diseases such as Alzheimer disease (e.g., Eskelinen et al.[54]). In a cross-section of the population, Jarvis reported that higher caffeine intake was positively related to better performance on certain psychomotor and cognitive tasks, and the effect was reported to have been larger in older participants. However, a more recent prospective study involving a larger population sample found little evidence of improved performance associated with caffeine consumption or of any protective action of caffeine on age-related cognitive decline.[299]

Moreover, Evans et al.[55] recently suggested that the inverse association between caffeine consumption and Parkinson disease, and the similar relationship that exists between cigarette smoking and Parkinson disease (which has fostered the belief that nicotine is neuroprotective), may be an epiphenomenon rather than a causal connection. Broadly, Evans et al.[55] argued that confounding due to individual differences in the personality disposition of impulsive sensation seeking may have led to misunderstanding of the findings. The authors cited evidence that sensation seeking is inversely associated with Parkinson's disease, with higher sensation seeking also being associated with higher caffeine consumption and smoking. Evans et al.[55] hypothesized that there are biological features characteristic of low sensation-seeking individuals that also predispose to Parkinson disease. Thus rather than indicating any neuroprotective capability, higher caffeine and nicotine intake may simply be two behavioral manifestations of a generalized personality disposition, namely, impulsive sensation-seeking, which itself is the expression of a biological substrate that confers a level of protection against the development of Parkinson disease.

Findings from the Lothian Birth Cohort 1936 Study, Scotland,[41] give further reason to doubt any direct neuroprotective role for caffeine or coffee.[131] The Lothian study is unique among studies of coffee and cognitive aging, because it derives from a large cohort of elderly participants (70+ years) whose IQ had been comprehensively measured at age 11 years. The study found that individuals with higher childhood IQ generally performed better on tests of cognitive performance in adulthood than individuals with lower childhood IQ. In addition, higher-IQ children consumed more coffee in adulthood than lower-IQ children; a lifestyle-related choice among persons possessing the higher social status that tends to accompany higher IQ. Analyses showed that coffee-related

superior cognitive ability in adulthood was not due to the protective effects of coffee but was the result of lifelong cognitive advantage stemming from superior cognitive ability in childhood.

The salutary lesson to be taken from the Lothian study[41] is that the opposite conclusion to the finding that coffee had no protective effect for cognitive function in older age would have been suggested had childhood IQ scores not been available. Consequently, doubt is cast over the findings of reputed benefits in all other studies of coffee and neurodegenerative disease, because none included measurements of childhood IQ. This is not to argue that the same specific variables of childhood IQ and associated socioeconomic status are necessarily key potential confounders in all observational studies of dietary coffee and health-related outcomes. Rather, the crucial point is that great caution is needed when interpreting findings from epidemiological studies, and such caution is possibly greater for studies of coffee consumption than almost any other health-related behavior. This is because of what Turkheimer[294] described the "etiological distance" between the putative causal variable (coffee in this instance) and outcomes of interest (the chronic diseases that occur in later life). The acute effects of coffee are generally modest, and the decades-long consumption characteristic of older-aged coffee consumers is but one of countless potential biobehavioral variables that might conceivably benefit or harm health. In such circumstances, it is essentially unknowable what variables to control for and what to ignore. Measuring every conceivable variable for inclusion in statistical models is not the answer, as so doing merely creates other problems including overadjustment bias (e.g., Schisterman et al.[257]).

Other Active Compounds in Caffeine Beverages

Notwithstanding the strength of the evidence that dietary caffeine poses a number of significant risks to health, an important caveat arises when other compounds in caffeine beverages are considered. Whereas caffeine is generally accepted as being the main biologically active ingredient of those beverages, the presence of other compounds also having biological effects has become a focus of interest. Of course, the other active compounds could have either positive or negative implications for health. An example of the latter is the presence of a cholesterol-raising factor in unfiltered brewed coffee.[253,297,312,318] However, influenced by many years of industry-sponsored research, there has been substantial investment in the search for beneficial effects from noncaffeine active compounds in coffee and tea. Accordingly, any assessment of the overall health implications of caffeine beverages must take into account the benefits, if any, of these other compounds present in caffeinated beverages.

In particular, it is claimed that polyphenols, especially chlorogenic acid, in coffee have potential cardiovascular benefits due to their antioxidant properties (e.g., Bonita et al.[20]). Similarly, theanine, a nonproteinic amino acid, has been posited as having a blood pressure-lowering effect (e.g., Rogers et al.[245]). Nevertheless, the importance of such findings is not immediately obvious. Antioxidants are present in many foods (e.g., fruits, vegetables, and nuts) and it is questionable whether beverages that contain potentially harmful caffeine should be recommended as good sources of dietary antioxidants. Alternatively, whenever such beverages are endorsed for their antioxidant content, it would seem self-evidently preferable to recommend decaffeinated varieties. However, it has long been recognized that consumers of decaffeinated

---

[e]References 28, 32, 157, 207, 260, 292.

beverages consume fewer cups per day than consumers of beverages containing caffeine,[37] a pattern that is consistent with what is known about caffeine's pharmacological properties. That is, taking into account the rapidity with which caffeine physical dependence develops, it is to be expected that caffeinated varieties encourage a higher level of intake than the same beverages without caffeine. Thus, any explicit recommendation to consume decaffeinated varieties of coffee and tea is tantamount to encouragement to consume less of such beverages, which in turn necessarily means smaller profits for manufacturers.

In that context, it should be acknowledged that the caffeine industry is extensively involved in research concerned with the purported benefits of caffeinated beverages. Industry involvement includes basic and applied animal and human studies, as well as sponsorship of articles in scientific outlets that are favorable to industry interests. The conflicts of interest inherent in industry-sponsored research raise serious questions about the integrity of caffeine science, especially in relation to the increasingly frequent "scientific" assertions about "benefits" from caffeine-beverage consumption.

Threats to the Integrity of Caffeine Science

It is important to acknowledge that the academic pursuit of research on caffeine is extensively linked to the trade in caffeine products. Each of the main sources of caffeine, namely, coffee, tea, soft drinks, and energy drinks, is a multinational, multibillion dollar enterprise. By their own account, these industries have sought to counter evidence that threatens their commercial interests [see 122 and 128]. Over several decades, industry has been engaged in extensive efforts to influence public and scientific opinion about caffeine and caffeine products by various means both direct and indirect, including sponsorship of meetings of "experts," collaboration with public institutions, dissemination of selected information, and funding for selected caffeine research.[122]

In the 20 years from 1962 to 1982, the average number of cups of coffee consumed per day in the United States declined 39%,[206] and it is evident from caffeine-industry publications that manufacturers attributed much of that decline to increased public awareness of scientific concern about possible caffeine-induced harmful effects.[122] Around 1990, there was an arrest in the downward trend, and thereafter a reversal evidenced by substantially increased sales of all categories of caffeine beverages. Manufacturers of caffeine products have been in no doubt about the reason for the improved commercial outlook for caffeine products. Industry representatives congratulated themselves on the success of their campaign to counter scientific findings that threatened their interests.[101,237] In that regard, there is a parallel between actions by the caffeine industry to use science to protect profits and similar activities by the tobacco, alcohol, food, pharmaceutical, and other industries.[137]

Industry Influences on Research

Actions of the International Life Sciences Institute (ILSI),[114] headquartered in Washington, DC, show that the parallel between caffeine-industry manipulation of science and similar action by other international corporate conglomerates is *not* coincidental. Established in 1978 in response to commercial concerns from threatened increases in public regulation of caffeine products, ILSI has evolved into a global network of "collaborative science [to improve] human and environmental health and safety worldwide"

(http://www.ilsi.org/Pages/Mission.aspx). Its governing board includes representatives from the agrochemical, beverage, food, and pharmaceutical industries, with the balance largely comprising individual university-based scientists. ILSI's caffeine-industry partners include familiar brand names such as Coca-Cola, Kraft Foods, Mars, Nestlé, Procter & Gamble, and Unilever. ILSI publicly disavows the term "industry lobby," preferring euphemisms such as "advocacy" and "promotion" to describe its efforts to use "evidence-based science as an aid" to decision-making that protects private profit at the potential cost of public health.

ILSI's general success as a third-part representative for industry[128] owes much to its history of successful lobbying on behalf of the caffeine industry (http://www.ilsi.org/Pages/Risk_Science_Toxicology.aspx). Following passage by the US Congress of laws on foods and drugs in 1958, a list was compiled of some hundreds of additives, including caffeine, that were generally recognized as safe (GRAS). Subsequent revisions of GRAS compounds were conducted by the FDA and by the time of ILSI's foundation in 1978, with funding from soda manufacturers,[226] caffeine was under direct threat of being removed from the GRAS list. In 1980, the FDA issued a warning cautioning pregnant women against the use of coffee. With caffeine's safe status in serious jeopardy, ILSI responded by initiating its own investigations.

A budget of US$1.2 million was allocated to the task and funds were distributed to a wide range of universities and institutes (http://www.ilsi.org/Pages/Risk_Science_Toxicology.aspx). Findings were submitted to the FDA in the form of extensive reports, which were subsequently published as collections of chapters in book form, edited by scholars affiliated with two of the funded institutions—Harvard Medical School[48] and the Mario Negri Institute (Italy).[81] The pattern established at that time has continued as a characteristic feature of ILSI's diverse sponsored workshops and publications (e.g., Doepker et al.[50] and Institute of Medicine[113]). Using a tactic that had previously been exploited by the tobacco industry,[217] erudite works describing basic science are juxtaposed alongside skewed accounts that dampen potential health concerns, such that the latter are given credibility by association with the former.[123,124,128] Adverse attention is typically diverted by creating the false impression of scientific consensus, while simultaneously calling for further research to address contested issues, which if acknowledged outright would threaten commercial interests.

ILSI's extensive success in infiltrating high-level public institutions has attracted sharp criticism. Its affiliations include the National Academy of Sciences and the Institute of Medicine in the United States,[113] the European Food Safety Authority, the United Nations Food and Agriculture Organization, and the World Health Organization (WHO). Although affiliation with industry does not itself constitute evidence of wrongdoing, ILSI has fostered collaborations with public institutions worldwide and wrongdoing has indeed been exposed.

A WHO Committee of Experts on Tobacco Industry Documents reported that for many years tobacco companies operated with the "purpose of subverting the efforts of the World Health Organization to address tobacco issues [and that the] attempted subversion was elaborate, well financed, sophisticated and usually invisible"[323] (p. 18). Subsequently, the Tobacco Free Initiative, a WHO project, identified ILSI as one such group.[198,215] In addition, in the scholarly literature, ILSI has been the subject of editorial criticism for failing to declare conflict of interest in relation to the publication of literature dealing with the science of alcohol and health,[53] during which the picture emerged of an institute presenting itself as dispassionate and independent while actually serving as a third party representative of interested corporations.[128] The skill with which ILSI infiltrates public institutions is further illustrated by the extensive public funding it has garnered in the form of research grants from the European Union and instances of previously hidden support such as that from the European Food Safety Authority, which ILSI has used to fund its information dissemination and lobbying activities.[42]

Concealment is a recurring feature of ILSI activities, as evidenced by a recent self-congratulatory article, published in a peer-reviewed journal, in which ILSI is extolled as a "global leader" in health research.[286] The author byline states no affiliation and the "competing interests" statement at the end of the article states, "The author has no conflict of interest directly relevant to the content of this article." Yet, the author, Ayako Takei (http://www.zoominfo.com/p/Ayako-Takei/1507069701), is an agrochemical specialist with close ties to the Health and Environment Sciences Institute, which operates as a nonprofit charity and global branch of ILSI.

It is important that ways are found for ensuring exposure of possible conflicts of interest where they are not freely declared. Where possible conflicts do exist, ways must be found to safeguard against resulting threats to scientific integrity.[128] The importance and urgency of steps by the scientific community to counter such threats is highlighted by extensive empirical evidence of bias in industry-sponsored biomedical research.[4,137] In the final analysis, assurances of integrity in caffeine science will almost certainly depend on the severing of entanglement between academic researchers and corporate sponsors, including third-party representatives such as ILSI, in the same way that such steps were found necessary in the field of tobacco-related research.

Conflict of Interest and the Self-Serving Bias

A conflict of interest exists when an ethical or professional interest clashes with a pecuniary self-interest. Although a necessary prerequisite for openness, the mere declaration of a conflict of interest is unlikely to foil outcome bias in industry-sponsored research. For one thing, a simple declaration provides no basis for consumers of scientific research, including scientists, policy makers, and the public, to judge the nature and extent of any consequential bias. Indeed, drawing on relevant experimental findings from social psychology, Dana and Loewenstein[46] have argued that declaring a conflict of interest can actually be counterproductive by exacerbating the declarer's bias. Dana and Loewenstein[46] explained that part of the difficulty in dealing with the problem is that it is usually assumed that bias founded on a conflict of interest is a matter of deliberate choice. This perspective contributes to the indignation that is sometimes expressed when the subject is raised. Unfortunately, however, the "deliberate choice" view of bias arising from conflicts of interest is inconsistent with empirical findings, which show that even when individuals try to be objective their judgments are subject to an unintentional self-serving bias.[46] In other words, self-serving bias is part of human nature. It is the role of the scientist to safeguard the integrity of research in the face of human limitations.

Indeed, unintentional self-serving bias might help to explain some apparent contradictions alluded to earlier. Weinstein[316] has shown that "behavioral performance tends to produce perceptions supportive of the behavior" (p. 2). If so, it is likely that caffeine consumers will be more readily accepting of conclusions consistent with their own extant caffeine-consuming behavior than findings that conflict with such behavior. Thus it is possible that a subtle inherent self-serving bias inclines consumers of caffeine products to be more influenced by neutral or positive findings concerning caffeine than is engendered by more objective assessments.

Despite the fact that epidemiological studies provide a shaky foundation for inferring causation, almost all of the evidence purporting to show that caffeine and coffee are health protective is derived from observational studies. To make matters worse, much of that which has been inferred about reputed health benefits from observational studies (for example, in relation to cardiovascular health, diabetes, and cognitive aging) contradicts that which is predicted from better controlled experimental studies. In normal science, experimental findings would generally be accorded greater plausibility over contradictory observational findings. In caffeine science, however, the opposite appears more often to be the case, with good news from observational findings, however, implausible, being preferred over cautionary findings from experimental studies.

Furthermore, because most people consume caffeine daily, it is likely that the large majority of researchers, reviewers, and editors of scientific literature are caffeine consumers. As such, the resulting impact of an inherent self-serving bias on the way scientific findings are promulgated could be pervasive. For example, experimental findings are ordinarily accepted as providing stronger evidence of causal relationships than epidemiological findings. Yet, the opposite view could be said to have been in operation in a number of important areas of caffeine research. In relation to cardiovascular disease and type 2 diabetes mellitus, in particular, there appears to have been a tendency to ignore experimental findings of likely harm in favor of accepting epidemiological findings of no harm or benefit. Unfortunately, however, there is relatively little published literature addressing the topic of self-serving bias in science, and therefore little systematic knowledge exists of this as a source of industry-based threats to integrity in caffeine science.

Public Policy and Regulation of Caffeine Exposure

As described earlier, the main sources of caffeine are those beverages in which it occurs naturally, namely coffee and tea, as well as the wide range of beverages, including sodas and energy drinks to which caffeine is added. Notwithstanding the ubiquity of those sources, the trend is for caffeine to be added to an ever-wider variety of products, including flavored milk, bottled water, confectionery, ice cream, chewing gum, yogurt, breakfast cereal, cookies, sunflower seeds, and beef jerky.[132,256] In addition, caffeine is present in prescribed and over-the-counter medications for weight loss, pain relief, colds and flu, and antisleep compounds. Miscellaneous products that contain caffeine include breath-freshener sprays and mints; caffeine powder and aerosol inhaler for "instant" delivery of psychoactive effects; skin lotions, cosmetics, soap, and shampoo; and caffeine-infused tights intended for weight loss. Furthermore, caffeine is frequently used as a diluent (cutting agent) in illicit drugs. Indeed, the ubiquity of caffeine is such that it has become a biologically significant contaminant of freshwater and marine systems due to disposal of unused caffeine into water systems (e.g., undrunk coffee down the kitchen sink).[242]

Largely in response to particular concerns about harm to children, some countries have undertaken tentative first steps toward regulation. Denmark, France, and Norway introduced sales restrictions on the energy drink, Red Bull. Canada requires labeling in relation to the same product, advising that it should not be mixed with alcohol. Labeling of "high caffeine content" exists on some products in some countries.[236] In Sweden, a reduction in the maximum quantity of caffeine tablets from 250 to 30 that can be obtained over the counter in a single purchase was introduced as a suicide-prevention intervention and appears to have been successful.[290] Overall, however, regulatory initiatives have been limited and there is no evidence of generalized reductions in population exposure to caffeine. Considering the extensive level of concern, both past and present, the current regulatory vacuum seems far from acceptable or prudent.

In 1911, acting on authority vested by the then recently enacted Food and Drug Act, agents in the United States seized quantities of Coca-Cola syrup because they considered the caffeine content to be a significant threat to public health.[263] Following lengthy legal proceedings, Coca-Cola agreed to decrease the caffeine content of the drink, and further legal action ceased. Armed with improved knowledge of caffeine toxicity and faced with extensive evidence of substantial harm to public health, today's authorities appear more perplexed and less decisive than their counterparts of more than a century earlier.[132] Since those initial actions in the early 20th century, attempts at regulation have been sporadic and fragmented, and have consistently fallen far short of addressing the totality of issues surrounding caffeine-related harm.

In particular, regulatory authorities might have been expected to show greater deference to the precautionary principle that ordinarily prevails in relation to concerns about public health, including when disagreement exists within the scientific community.[135] Broadly, the precautionary principle states that in the absence of scientific consensus regarding potential harm from a particular action, the burden of proof lies with those responsible for the action to demonstrate *absence* of harm. Responsibility for demonstrating absence of harm typically falls most strongly on purveyors of new products marketed to vulnerable groups such as expectant mothers, children, and adolescents. In light of evidence of widespread caffeine-related harm, including increased blood pressure, low birth weight, and physical dependence (as discussed throughout this chapter), absence of harm obviously has not been demonstrated. Thus persistent regulatory inaction represents a serious breach of the precautionary principle that underpins public health.

The outline of a broad policy framework for caffeine has been provided by James,[132] as follows:

- Labeling of caffeine products to indicate the caffeine content per stated serving size and the source of caffeine, stating in particular whether or not caffeine has been added to the product;
- restrictions on advertising, especially to children and adolescents, and inclusive of electronic and live media;
- pricing policies, including taxation and other financial measures of the kind found to be effective in curtailing consumption of cigarettes and alcohol[7,31]; and
- direct restrictions on sales, especially age restrictions.

Reducing and Quitting Caffeine

Despite long-standing concerns about high levels of dietary caffeine and abundant evidence of potential harm, few reports exist of systematic efforts to assist habitual consumers to reduce or cease their use of the drug. Indeed, following a brief rise in interest about two decades ago, reports of systematic attempts to manage caffeine intake appear to have all but disappeared from the literature. One early commentary on the subject more than a century ago advised that negative withdrawal effects could be avoided by

a gradual reduction of caffeine.[25] That advice has stood the test of time remarkably well. Using a single-subject experimental design, Foxx and Rubinoff [71] reported favorable results for three participants who received a program of behavioral intervention based on nicotine and cigarette "fading" methods that the same research group had developed for smokers.[69,70] Treatment consisted of a combination of self-monitoring and a series of predetermined step-wise reductions in daily caffeine consumption in the direction of a specified terminal goal of reduced daily intake. Subsequently, Foxx[68] obtained follow-up data from the three original participants, reporting that the reduced intake of all three was substantially maintained 40 months following the termination of treatment. Bernard et al.[17] employed similar procedures with a single subject, and again reported favorable results.

These generally promising initial findings were confirmed in a larger study by James et al.[148] in which 27 chronic heavy caffeine consumers were monitored before and during a 4-week treatment program and at 6- and 18-week follow-up. However, due to the results of this and all previous caffeine-reduction studies being expressed solely in terms of participant self-reports, the reliability of the findings could be open to question. Accordingly, James et al.[145] reported plasma concentrations of caffeine and its primary dimethylated metabolites (paraxanthine, theophylline, and theobromine) as well as self-reported caffeine intake during the course of a caffeine-fading regimen similar to that employed in a previous study by the same authors.[148] Results from 12 participants, each with a history of heavy caffeine consumption, again supported the general efficacy of the caffeine-fading approach. However, unlike all previous studies in which caffeine intake had been determined solely on the basis of self-report, follow-up plasma concentrations of caffeine and caffeine metabolites suggested that participants in the James et al.[145] study experienced partial relapse at 12 weeks of follow-up.

It has long been known that the accuracy of self-reports is enhanced when subjects are aware that their behavior may be independently checked (e.g., Lipinsky et al.[192] and Nelson et al.[216]). Hence, the independent measurement of plasma caffeine levels in the James et al.[145] study may have encouraged participants to be more accurate in reporting follow-up caffeine intake than their counterparts in previous studies. Nevertheless, despite the partial relapse suggested by the plasma concentration date of James et al.,[145] the overall (albeit limited) evidence indicates that motivated individuals wishing to reduce or quit their use of caffeine can so do without experiencing pronounced, if any, negative withdrawal effects, provided that consumption is reduced in a graduated (step-wise) fashion rather than abruptly. That broad conclusion was again confirmed in a recent study of caffeine consumers who had previously "tried unsuccessfully to quit using caffeine."[57] Marked reductions in caffeine consumption, maintained for up to 1 year of follow-up, were reported following brief therapist-guided manualized intervention that incorporated caffeine fading.

Conclusions

Claims that dietary caffeine is of little importance to health are ill founded. Short-term withdrawal of caffeine has negative effects on psychomotor performance and mood, and these effects may reoccur chronically in a substantial proportion of habitual consumers. In addition, caffeine produces modest increases in blood pressure that have long-term implications for cardiovascular health, caffeine interacts adversely with some medicines, there is suggestive evidence of increased risk of spontaneous abortion when caffeine is consumed during pregnancy and strong evidence of lower birth weight due to maternal caffeine consumption, and consistent evidence of associations between caffeine consumption and a host of behavioral and emotional problems in children and adolescents. There is little support for the frequent suggestion that caffeine harm is confined to groups characterized as heavy consumers. Conversely, most claims of benefits from dietary caffeine are derived from epidemiological studies that provide correlational rather than causal evidence that is vulnerable to confounding errors. Although urgent answers are needed in relation to many key questions, the health and well-being of caffeine consumers is further threatened due to concerns about the integrity of caffeine science arising from the widespread involvement of vested corporate interests in caffeine research. In the meantime, the precautionary principle indicates the need for a regulatory framework to limit caffeine harm.

References

1. Abu-Zeid HA, Choi NW, Hsu PH. Factors associated with risk of cancer of the colon and rectum. *Am J Epidemiol.* 1981;114:442.
2. Agardh EE, Carlsson S, Ahlbom A, Efendic S, Grill V, Hammar N, et al. Coffee consumption, type 2 diabetes and impaired glucose tolerance in Swedish men and women. *J Intern Med.* 2004;255:645–652.
3. al'Absi M, Lovallo WR, McKey B, Sung BH, Whitsett TL, Wilson MF. Hypothalamic-pituitary-adrenocortical responses to psychological stress and caffeine in men at high and low risk for hypertension. *Psychosom Med.* 1998;60:521–527.
4. Als-Nielsen B, Chen W, Gluud C, Kjaergard LL. Association of funding and conclusions in randomized drug trials: a reflection of treatment effect or adverse events? *J Am Med Assoc.* 2003;290:921–928.
5. American Psychiatric Association. *Diagnostic and Statistical Manual of Mental Disorders.* 4th ed, text revision. Washington, DC: Author; 2000.
6. American Psychiatric Association. *Diagnostic and Statistical Manual of Mental Disorders.* 5th ed. Washington, DC: Author; 2013.
7. Anderson P, Chisholm D, Fuhr DC. Alcohol and global health 2. Effectiveness and cost-effectiveness of policies and programmes to reduce the harm caused by alcohol. *Lancet.* 2009;373:2234–2246.
8. Anderson BL, Juliano LM. Behavior, sleep, and problematic caffeine consumption in a college-aged sample. *J Caffeine Res.* 2012;2:38–47.
9. Armstrong B, Doll R. Environmental factors and cancer incidence and mortality in different countries, with special reference to dietary practices. *Int J Cancer.* 1975;15:617–631.
10. Arnaud MJ. The pharmacology of caffeine. *Prog Drug Res.* 1987;31:273–313.
11. Asal NR, Geyer JR, Risser DR, Lee ET, Kadamani S, Cherng N. Risk factors in renal cell carcinoma. II. Medical history, occupation, multivariate analysis, and conclusions. *Cancer Detect Prev.* 1988;13:263–279.
12. Ascherio A, Zhang SM, Hernan MA, Kawachi I, Colditz GA, Speizer FE, et al. Prospective study of caffeine consumption and risk of Parkinson's disease in men and women. *Ann Neurol.* 2001;50:56–63.
13. Bak AA, Grobbee DE. A randomized study on coffee and blood pressure. *J Human Hypertens.* 1990;4:259–264.
14. Baker JA, Beehler GP, Sawant AC, Jayaprakash V, McCann SE, Moysich KB. Consumption of coffee, but not black tea, is associated with decreased risk of premenopausal breast cancer. *J Nutr.* 2006;136:166–171.
15. Baron JA, Gerhardsson-de-Verdier M, Ekbom A. Coffee, tea, tobacco, and cancer of the large bowel. *Cancer Epidemiol Biomarkers Prev.* 1994;3:565–570.
16. Batada A, Wootan MG. Nickelodeon markets nutrition-poor foods to children. *Am J Prev Med.* 2007;33:48–50.
17. Bernard ME, Dennehy S, Keefauver LW. Behavioural treatment of excessive coffee and tea drinking: a case study and partial replication. *Behav Ther.* 1981;12:543–548.
18. Biaggioni I, Paul S, Puckett A, Arzubiaga C. Caffeine and theophylline as adenosine receptor antagonists in humans. *J Pharmacol Exp Ther.* 1991;258:588–593.
19. Bichler J, Cavin C, Simic T, Chakraborty A, Ferk F, Hoelzl C, et al. Coffee consumption protects human lymphocytes against oxidative and 3-amino-1-methyl-5H-pyrido[4,3-b]indole acetate (Trp-P-2) induced DNA-damage: results of an experimental study with human volunteers. *Food Chem Toxicol.* 2007;45:1428–1436.
20. Bonita JS, Mandarano M, Shuta D, Vinson J. Coffee and cardiovascular disease: in vitro, cellular, animal, and human studies. *Pharmacol Res.* 2007;55:187–198.
21. Bonnet MH, Balkin TJ, Dinges DF, Roehrs T, Rogers NL, Wesensten NJ. The use of stimulants to modify performance during sleep loss: a review by the sleep deprivation and stimulant task force of the american academy of sleep medicine. *Sleep.* 2005;28:1163–1187.
22. Borota D, Murray E, Keceli G, Chang A, Watabe JM, Ly M, et al. Post-study caffeine administration enhances memory consolidation in humans. *Nature Neurosci.* 2014;17:201–203.
23. Brache K, Stockwell T. Drinking patterns and risk behaviors associated with combined alcohol and energy drink consumption in college drinkers. *Addict Behav.* 2011;36:1133–1140.
24. Brazier JL, Salle B. Conversion of theophylline to caffeine by the human fetus. *Seminars Perinatol.* 1981;5:315–320.
25. Bridge N. Coffee-drinking as a frequent cause of disease. *Trans Assoc Am Physicians.* 1893;8:281–288.
26. Bush A, Busst CM, Clarke B, Barnes PJ. Effect of infused adenosine on cardiac output and systemic resistance in normal subjects. *Br J Clin Pharmacol.* 1989;27:165–171.
27. Carter AJ, O'Connor WT, Carter MJ, Ungerstedt U. Caffeine enhances acetylcholine release in the hippocampus in vivo by a selective interaction with adenosine A1 receptors. *J Pharmacol Exp Ther.* 1995;273:637–642.
28. Cauli O, Morelli M. Caffeine and the dopaminergic system. *Behav Pharmacol.* 2005;16:63–77.
29. Cavin C, Holzhaeuser D, Scharf G, Constable A, Huber WW, Schilter B. Cafestol and kahweol, two coffee specific diterpenes with anticarcinogenic activity. *Food Chem Toxicol.* 2002;40:1155–1163.
30. Centonze S, Boeing H, Leoci C, Guerra V, Misciagna G. Dietary habits and colorectal cancer in a low-risk area: results from a population-based case-control study in southern Italy. *Nutr Cancer.* 1994;21:233–246.
31. Chaloupka FJ, Davidson PA. *Applying Tobacco control Lessons to Obesity: Taxes and Other Pricing Strategies to Reduce Consumption.* saint paul, MN: tobacco control legal consortium; 2010. Available at http://publichealthlawcenter.org/sites/default/files/resources/tclc-syn-obesity-2010.pdf. Accessed February 1, 2013.
32. Chen JF, Xu K, Petzer JP, Staal R, Xu YH. Beilstein M et al. Neuroprotection by caffeine and A(2A) adenosine receptor inactivation in a model of Parkinson's disease. *J Neurosci.* 2001;21:RC143.
33. Chen LW, Wu Y, Neelakantan N, et al. Maternal caffeine intake during pregnancy is associated with risk of low birth weight: a systematic review and dose response meta-analysis. *BMC Med.* 2014;12:174.
34. Chvasta TE, Cooke AR. Absorption and emptying of caffeine from the human stomach. *Gastroenterology.* 1971;61:838–843.
35. Chyou PH, Nomura AM, Stemmermann GN. A prospective study of diet, smoking, and lower urinary tract cancer. *Ann Epidemiol.* 1993;3:211–216.
36. Clausson B, Granath F, Ekbom A, Lundgren S, Nordmark A, Signorello LB, et al. Effect of caffeine exposure during pregnancy on birth weight and gestational age. *Am J Epidemiol.* 2002;155:429–436.

37. Clinton WP. The chemistry of coffee. In: MacMahon B, Sugimura T, eds. *Banbury Report 17: Coffee and Health*. New York: Cold Spring Harbor Laboratory; 1984:3–10.

38. Cnattingius S, Signorello LB, Anneren G, Clausson B, Ekbom A, Ljunger E, et al. Caffeine intake and the risk of first-trimester spontaneous abortion. *N Engl J Med*. 2000;343:1839–1845.

39. Cole P. Coffee drinking and cancer of the lower urinary tract. *Lancet*. 1971;2:1335.

40. Coney AM, Marshall JM. Role of adenosine and its receptors in the vasodilation induced in the cerbral cortex of the rat by systemic hypoxia. *J Physiol*. 1998;509:507–518.

41. Corley J, Jia X, Kyle JAM, et al. Caffeine consumption and cognitive function at age 70: the lothian birth cohort 1936 study. *Psychosom Med*. 2010;72:206–214.

42. Corporate Europe Observatory. *The International Life Sciences Institute (ILSI), a corporate lobby group: European parliament report on EFSA budget rightfully judges links to ILSI as conflicts of interest*; 2012. Available at http://corporateeurope.org/about-ceo. Accessed March 22, 2016.

43. Costa J, Lunet N, Santos C, Santos J, Vaz-Carneiro A. Caffeine exposure and the risk of Parkinson's disease: a systematic review and meta-analysis of observational studiess. *J Alzheimers Dis*. 2010;20(S1):221–238.

44. Cunha RA, Ferré S, Vaugeois J-M, Chen J-F. Potential therapeutic interest of adenosine A_{2A} receptors in psychiatric disorders. *Curr Pharm Des*. 2008;14:1512–1524.

45. D'Avanzo B, La-Vecchia C, Franceschi S, Negri E, Talamini R, Buttino I. Coffee consumption and bladder cancer risk. *Eur J Cancer*. 1992;28A:1480–1484.

46. Dana J, Loewenstein G. A social science perspective on gifts to physicians from industry. *JAMA*. 2003;290:252–255.

47. Denaro CP, Brown CR, Jacob PI, Benowitz NL. Effects of caffeine with repeated dosing. *Eur J Clin Pharmacol*. 1991;40:273–278.

48. Dews PB, ed. *Behavioral Effects of Caffeine*. Berlin: Springer-Verlag; 1984.

49. Dlugosz L, Belanger K, Hellenbrand K, Holford TR, Leaderer B, Bracken MB. Maternal caffeine consumption and spontaneous abortion: a prospective cohort study. *Epidemiol*. 1996;7:250–255.

50. Doepker C, Lieberman HR, Smith AP, Peck JD, El-Sohemy, Welsh BT A. Caffeine: friend or foe? *Annu Rev Food Sci Technol*. 2016;7:117–137.

51. Dumas M, Gouyon JB, Tenenbaum D, Michiels Y, Escousse A, Alison M. Systematic determination of caffeine plasma concentrations at birth in preterm and full-term infants. *Develop Pharmacol Ther*. 1982;4:182–186.

52. Dunwiddie TV, Masino SA. The role and regulation of adenosine in the central nervous system. *Annu Rev Neurosci*. 2001;24:31–55.

53. Edwards G, Savva S. ILSI Europe, the drinks industry, and a conflict of interest undeclared. *Addiction*. 2001;96:197–202.

54. Eskelinen MH, Kivipelto M. Caffeine as a protective factor in dementia and Alzheimer's disease. *J Alzheimers Dis*. 2010;20: S167–S174.

55. Evans AH, Lawrence AD, Potts J, MacGregor L, Katzenschlager R, Shaw K, et al. Relationship between impulsive sensation seeking traits, smoking, alcohol and caffeine intake, and Parkinson's disease. *J Neurol Neurosurg Psychiatry*. 2006;77:317–321.

56. Evans SM, Griffiths RR. Dose-related caffeine discrimination in normal volunteers: individual differences in subjective effects and self-reported cues. *Behav Pharmacol*. 1991;2:345–356.

57. Evatt DP, Juliano LM, Griffiths RR. A brief manualized treatment for problematic caffeine use: a randomized control trial. *J Consult Clin Psychol*. 2016;84:113–121.

58. Farag NH, Whitsett TL, McKey BS, et al. Caffeine and blood pressure response: sex, age, and hormonal status. *J Womens Health*. 2010;19:1171–1176.

59. Fennelly M, Galletly DC, Purdie GI. Is caffeine withdrawal the mechanism of postoperative headache? *Anesthesia Analgesia*. 1991;72:449–453.

60. Fenster L, Eskenazi B, Windham GC, Swan SH. Caffeine consumption during pregnancy and fetal growth. *Am J Public Health*. 1991;81:458–461.

61. Fenster L, Hubbard AE, Swan SH, Windham GC, Waller K, Hiatt RA, et al. Caffeinated beverages, decaffeinated coffee, and spontaneous abortion [see comment]. *Epidemiology*. 1997;8:515–523.

62. Fernandes O, Sabharwal M, Smiley T, Pastuszak A, Koren G, Einarson T. Moderate to heavy caffeine consumption during pregnancy and relationship to spontaneous abortion and abnormal fetal growth: a meta-analysis. *Reprod Toxicol*. 1998;12:435–444.

63. Ferré S. Mechanisms of the psychostimulant effects of caffeine: implications for substance use disorders. *Psychopharmacology*. 2016;233(10):1963–1979.

64. Ferré S, O'Brien MC. Alcohol and caffeine: the perfect storm. *J Caffeine Res*. 2011;1:153–162.

65. Ferré S, Schwarcz R, Li XM, Snaprud P, Ögren SO, Fuxe K. Chronic haloperidol treatment leads to an increase in the intramembrane interaction between adenosine A2 and dopamine D2 receptors in the neostriatum. *Psychopharmacology*. 1994;116: 279–284.

66. Finn IB, Holtzman SG. Pharmacologic specificity of tolerance to caffeine-induced stimulation of locomotor activity. *Psychopharmacology*. 1987;93:428–434.

67. Folsom AR, McKenzie DR, Bisgard KM, Kushi LH, Sellers TA. No association between caffeine intake and postmenopausal breast cancer incidence in the iowa women's health study. *Am J Epidemiol*. 1993;138:380–383.

68. Foxx RM. Behavioral treatment of caffeinism: a 40-month follow-up. *Behav Therapist*. 1982;5:23–24.

69. Foxx RM, Axelroth E. Nicotine fading, self-monitoring and cigarette fading to produce cigarette abstinence or controlled smoking. *Behav Res Ther*. 1983;21:17–27.

70. Foxx RM, Brown RA. Nicotine fading and self-monitoring for cigarette abstinence or controlled smoking. *J Appl Behav Anal*. 1979;2:111–125.

71. Foxx RM, Rubinoff A. Behavioral treatment of caffeinism: reducing excessive coffee drinking. *J Appl Behav Anal*. 1979;12: 344–355.

72. France C, Ditto B. Cardiovascular responses to the combination of caffeine and mental arithmetic, cold pressor, and static exercise stressors. *Psychophysiology*. 1992;29:272–282.

73. Franchetti P, Messini L, Cappellacci L, et al. 8-Azaxanthine derivatives as antagonists of adenosine receptors. *J Med Chem*. 1994;37:2970–2975.

74. Franke AG, Bagusat C, McFarlan C, Tassone-Steiger T, Kneist W, Lieb K. The use of caffeinated substances by surgeons for cognitive enhancement. *Ann Surg*. 2015;261:1091–1095.

75. Freedman ND, Park Y, Abne CC, et al. Association of coffee drinking with total and cause-specific mortality. *N Engl J Med*. 2012;366:1891–1904.

76. Freestone S, Yeo WW, Ramsay LE. Effect of coffee and cigarette smoking on the blood pressure of patients with accelerated (malignant) hypertension. *J Human Hypertens*. 1995;9:89–91.

77. Friedman GD, van den Eeden SK. Risk factors for pancreatic cancer: an exploratory study. *Int J Epidemiol*. 1993;22:30–37.

78. Fuller RW, Maxwell DL, Conradson T-BG, Dixon CMS, Barnes PJ. Circulatory and respiratory effects of infused adenosine in conscious man. *Br J Pharmacol*. 1987;24:309–317.

79. Galletly DC, Fennelly M, Whitwam JG. Does caffeine withdrawal contribute to postanaesthetic morbidity? *Lancet*. 1989;1:1335.

80. Gallimberti L, Buja A, Chindamo S, et al. Energy drink consumption in children and early adolescents. *Eur J Pediatr*. 2013;172:1335–1340.

81. Garattini S, ed. *Caffeine, Coffee, and Health*. New York, NY: Raven Press; 1993.

82. Garrett BE, Griffiths RR. Physical dependence increases the relative reinforcing effects of caffeine versus placebo. *Psychopharmacology*. 1998;139:195–202.

83. Garrett BE, Holtzman SG. Caffeine cross-tolerance to selective dopamine D1 and D2 receptor agonists but not to their synergistic interaction. *Eur J Pharmacol.* 1994;262:65–75.

84. Giannelli M, Doyle P, Roman E, Pelerin M, Hermon C. The effect of caffeine consumption and nausea on the risk of miscarriage. *Paediatr Perinatal Epidemiol.* 2003;17:316–323.

85. Gilbert RM. *Caffeine as a Drug of Abuse.* New York: Wiley; 1976.

86. Graham TE, Sathasivam P, Rowland M, Marko N, Greer F, Battram D. Caffeine ingestion elevates plasma insulin response in humans during an oral glucose tolerance test. *Can J Physiol Pharmacol.* 2001;79:559–565.

87. Grasser EK, Yepuri G, Dulloo AG, Montani JP. Cardio and cerebrovascular responses to the energy drink Red Bull in young adults: a randomized cross-over study. *Eur J Clin Nutr.* 2014;53:1561–1571.

88. Green PJ, Suls J. The effects of caffeine on ambulatory blood pressure, heart rate, and mood in coffee drinkers. *J Behav Med.* 1996;19:111–128.

89. Greenberg W, Shapiro D. The effects of caffeine and stress on blood pressure in individuals with and without a family history of hypertension. *Psychophysiology.* 1987;24:151–156.

90. Gregg ME, Matyas TA, James JE. A new model of individual differences in hemodynamic profile and blood pressure reactivity. *Psychophysiology.* 2002;39:64–72.

91. Griffiths RR, Bigelow GE, Liebson IA. Human coffee drinking: reinforcing and physical dependence producing effects of caffeine. *J Pharmacol Exp Ther.* 1986;239:416–425.

92. Griffiths RR, Evans SM, Heishman SJ, et al. Low-dose caffeine physical dependence in humans. *J Pharmacol Exp Ther.* 1990;255:1123–1132.

93. Grosso LM, Rosenberg KD, Belanger K, Saftlas AF, Leaderer B, Bracken MB. Maternal caffeine intake and intrauterine growth retardation. [Erratum appears in *Epidemiology* 2001;12(5):517.] *Epidemiology.* 2001;12:447–455.

94. Gunja N, Brown JA. Energy drinks: health risks and toxicity. *Med J Aust.* 2012;196:46–49.

95. Hampl KF, Schneider MC, Ruttimann U, Ummenhofer W, Drewe J. Perioperative administration of caffeine tablets for prevention of postoperative headaches. *Can J Anaesthesia.* 1995;42:789–792.

96. Hartley TR, Lovallo WR, Whitsett TL, Sung BH, Wilson MF. Caffeine and stress: implications for risk, assessment, and management of hypertension. *J Clin Hypertens.* 2001;3:354–361.

97. Hartley TR, Sung BH, Pincomb GA, Whitsett TL, Wilson MF, Lovallo WR. Hypertension risk status and effect of caffeine on blood pressure. *Hypertension.* 2000;36:137–1341.

98. Heatherley SV, Hancock KMF, Rogers PJ. Psychostimulant and other effects of caffeine in 9- to 11-year-old children. *J Child Psychol Psychiatry.* 2006;47:135–142.

99. Heatherley SV, Hayward RC, Seers HE, Rogers PJ. Cognitive and psychomotor performance, mood, and pressor effects of caffeine after 4, 6 and 8 h caffeine abstinence. *Psychopharmacology.* 2005;178:461–470.

100. Hernan MA, Takkouche B, Caamano-Isorna F, Gestal-Otero JJ. A meta-analysis of coffee drinking, cigarette smoking, and the risk of Parkinson's disease. *Ann Neurol.* 2002;52:276–284.

101. Heuman J. A look back on 1993. *Tea Coffee Trade J.* 1994;166:5–7.

102. Hirose K, Niwa Y, Wakai K, Matsuo K, Nakanishi T, Tajima K. Coffee consumption and the risk of endometrial cancer: evidence from a case-control study of female hormone-related cancers in Japan. *Cancer Sci.* 2007;98(3):411–415.

103. Hollingworth HL. The influence of caffeine on mental and motor efficiency. *Archiv Psychol.* 1912;22:1–166.

104. Hollingworth HL. The influence of caffeine on the speed and quality of performance in typewriting. *Psychol Rev.* 1912;19:66–73.

105. Holtzman SG, Finn IB. Tolerance to behavioral effects of caffeine in rats. *Pharmacol Biochem Behav.* 1988;29:411–418.

106. Howland J, Rohsenow DJ. Risks of energy drinks mixed with alcohol. *JAMA.* 2013;309:245–246.

107. Hughes JR, Higgins ST, Bickel WK, et al. Caffeine self-administration, withdrawal, and adverse effects among coffee drinkers. *Archiv Gen Psychiatry.* 1991;48:611–617.

108. Hughes JR, Oliveto AH, Bickel WK, Higgins ST, Badger GJ. Caffeine self-administration and withdrawal: incidence, individual differences and interrelationships. *Drug Alcohol Depend.* 1993;32:239–246.

109. Hughes JR, Oliveto AH, Helzer JE, Higgins ST, Bickel WK. Should caffeine abuse, dependence or withdrawal be added to DSM-IV and ICD-10? *Am J Psychiatry.* 1992;149:33–40.

110. Hughes JR, Oliveto AH, Liguori A, Carpenter J, Howard T. Endorsement of DSM-IV dependence criteria among caffeine users. *Drug Alcohol Depend.* 1998;52:99–107.

111. Huxley R, Lee CMY, Barzi F, et al. Coffee, decaffeinated coffee, and tea consumption in relation to incident type 2 diabetes mellitus: a systematic review with meta-analysis. *Arch Intern Med.* 2009;169:2053–2063.

112. IARC. Coffee, tea, mate, methylxanthines and methylglyoxal. *IARC Monograph Evaluating Carcinogenic Risks to Humans.* UK: WHO; 1991.

113. Institute of Medicine. *Caffeine in Food and Dietary Supplements: Examining Safety.* Washington, DC: The National Academies Press; 2014. Retrieved 10 March 2016 from http://www.nap.edu/catalog/18607/caffeine-in-food-and-dietary-supplements-examining-safety-workshop-summary.

114. International Life Sciences Institute. 2019. http://www.ilsi.org/. Accessed on 24 June 2019.

115. Jacobsen B, Bjelke E, Kvåle G, Heuch I. Coffee drinking, mortality, and cancer incidence: results from a Norwegian prospective study. *J Natl Cancer Inst.* 1986;76:823–831.

116. Jacobsen BK, Thelle DS. The Tromso heart study: is coffee drinking an indicator of a life style with high risk for ischemic heart disease? *Acta Med Scand.* 1987;222:215–221.

117. James JE. The influence of user status and anxious disposition on the hypertensive effects of caffeine. *Int J Psychophysiol.* 1990;10:171–179.

118. James JE. *Caffeine and Health.* London: Academic; 1991.

119. James JE. Does caffeine enhance or merely restore degraded psychomotor performance? *Neuropsychobiology.* 1994;30:124–125.

120. James JE. Chronic effects of habitual caffeine consumption on laboratory and ambulatory blood pressure levels. *J Cardiovasc Res.* 1994;1:159–164.

121. James JE. Psychophysiological effects of habitual caffeine consumption. *Int J Behav Med.* 1994;1:247–263.

122. James JE. Caffeine, health and commercial interests. *Addiction.* 1994;89:1595–1599.

123. James JE. Caffeine, psychomotor performance and commercial interests: reply to Smith. *Addiction.* 1995;90:1262–1265.

124. James JE. *Book Review of "Caffeine, Coffee, and Health" by S. Garattini (Ed.),* 1993, Raven Press, New York. Addiction. 1995;90, 137-138.

125. James JE. *Understanding Caffeine: A Biobehavioral Analysis.* Thousand Oaks, CA: Sage; 1997.

126. James JE. Caffeine and blood pressure: habitual use is a preventable cardiovascular risk factor. *Lancet.* 1997;349:279–281.

127. James JE. Acute and chronic effects of caffeine on performance, mood, headache, and sleep. *Neuropsychobiology.* 1998;38:32–41.

128. James JE. "Third party" threats to research integrity in public-private partnerships. *Addiction.* 2002;97:1251–1255.

129. James JE. A critical review of dietary caffeine and blood pressure: a relationship that should be taken more seriously. *Psychosom Med.* 2004;66:63–71.

130. James JE. Potential advances in knowledge from cross-fertilization between different fields of caffeine research. *J Caffeine Res.* 2012;2:1.

131. James JE. Coffee and mortality: urgent need for clinical trials to assess putative benefits and harms. *J Caffeine Res.* 2012;2:53–54.

132. James JE. Death by caffeine: how many caffeine-related fatalities and near-misses must there be before we regulate? *J Caffeine Res.* 2012;2:149–152.

133. James JE. Caffeine and cognitive performance: persistent methodological challenges in caffeine research. *Pharmacol Biochem Behav*. 2014;124:117–122.

134. James JE. Caffeine and cognitive performance: in search of balance in scientific opinion and debate. *J Caffeine Res*. 2014;4:107–108.

135. James JE. Dietary caffeine: "unnatural" exposure requiring precaution? *J Subst Use*. 2014;19:394–397.

136. James JE. Review: higher caffeine intake during pregnancy increases risk of low birth weight. *Evid Based Nurs*. 2015;18. 111-111.

137. James JE. *The Health of Populations: Beyond Medicine*. Oxford, UK: Elsevier-Academic Press; 2016.

138. James JE, Gregg ME. Effects of dietary caffeine on mood when rested and sleep restricted. *Human Psychopharmacol: Clin Exp*. 2004;19:333–341.

139. James JE, Gregg ME. Hemodynamic effects of dietary caffeine, sleep restriction, and laboratory stress. *Psychophysiology*. 2004;41:914–923.

140. James JE, Gregg ME, Kane M, Harte F. Dietary caffeine, performance and mood: enhancing and restorative effects after controlling for withdrawal relief. *Neuropsychobiology*. 2005;52:1–10.

141. James JE, Keane MA. Caffeine, sleep and wakefulness: implications of new understanding about withdrawal reversal. *Human Psychopharmacol: Clin Exp*. 2007;22:549–558.

142. James JE, Kristjansson AL, Sigfusdottir ID. Adolescent substance use, sleep, and academic achievement: evidence of harm due to caffeine. *J Adolescence*. 2011;34:665–673.

143. James JE, Kristjansson AL, Sigfusdottir ID. A gender-specific analysis of adolescent dietary caffeine, alcohol consumption, anger, and violent behavior. *Subst Use Misuse*. 2015;50:257–267.

144. James JE, Paull I. Caffeine and human reproduction. *Rev Environ Health*. 1985;7:151–167.

145. James JE, Paull I, Cameron-Traub E, Miners JO, Lelo A, Birkett DJ. Biochemical validation of self-reported caffeine consumption during caffeine fading. *J Behav Med*. 1988;11:15–30.

146. James JE, Richardson M. Pressor effects of caffeine and cigarette smoking. *Br J Clin Psychol*. 1991;30:276–278.

147. James JE, Rogers PJ. Effects of caffeine on performance and mood: withdrawal reversal is the most plausible explanation. *Psychopharmacology*. 2005;182:1–8.

148. James JE, Stirling KP, Hampton BAM. Caffeine fading: behavioral treatment of caffeine abuse. *Behav Ther*. 1985;16:15–27.

149. Jarvis MJ. Does caffeine intake enhance absolute levels of cognitive performance? *Psychopharmacology*. 1993;110:45–52.

150. Jeong D, Dimsdale JE. The effects of caffeine on blood pressure in the work environment. *Am J Hypertens*. 1990;3:749–753.

151. Jiang X, Zhang D, Jiang W. Coffee and caffeine intake and incidence of type 2 diabetes mellitus: a meta-analysis of prospective studies. *Eur J Nutr*. 2014;53:25–38.

152. Judelson DA, Armstrong LE, Sokmen B, Roti MW, Casa DJ, Kellogg MD. Effect of chronic caffeine intake on choice reaction time, mood, and visual vigilance. *Physiol Behav*. 2005;85:629–634.

153. Juliano LM, Griffiths RR. A critical review of caffeine withdrawal: empirical validation of symptoms and signs, incidence, severity, and associated features. *Psychopharmacology*. 2004;176:1–29.

154. Julius S. The blood pressure seeking properties of the central nervous system. *J Hypertens*. 1988;6:177–185.

155. Kaiser L, Allen LH, American Dietetic Association. Position of the American dietetic association: nutrition and lifestyle for a healthy pregnancy outcome. *J Am Dietetic Assoc*. 2008;108:553–561.

156. Kalapothaki V, Tzonou A, Hsieh CC, Toupadaki N, Karakatsani A, Trichopoulos D. Tobacco, ethanol, coffee, pancreatitis, diabetes mellitus, and cholelithiasis as risk factors for pancreatic carcinoma. *Cancer Causes Control*. 1993;4:375–382.

157. Kalda A, Yu L, Oztas E, Chen JF. Novel neuroprotection by caffeine and adenosine A(2A) receptor antagonists in animal models of Parkinson's disease. *J Neurol Sci*. 2006;248:9–15.

158. Karatzis E, Papaioannou TG, Aznaouridis K, Karatzi K, Stamatelopoulos K, Zampelas A, et al. Acute effects of caffeine on blood pressure and wave reflections in healthy subjects: should we consider monitoring central blood pressure? *Int J Cardiol*. 2005;98:425–430.

159. Keane MA, James JE. Effects of dietary caffeine on EEG, performance, and mood when rested and sleep restricted. *Human Psychopharmacol*. 2008;23:669–680.

160. Keane MA, James JE, Hogan MJ. Effects of dietary caffeine on topographic EEG after controlling for withdrawal and withdrawal reversal. *Neuropsychobiology*. 2007;56:197–207.

161. Keijzers GB, De Galan BE, Tack CJ, Smits P. Caffeine can decrease insulin sensitivity in humans. *Diabetes Care*. 2002;25:364–369.

162. Ker K, Edwards PJ, Felix LM, Blackhall K, Roberts I. Caffeine for the prevention of injuries and errors in shift workers. *Cochrane Database Syst Rev*. 2010;5:CD008508.

163. Klesges RC, Ray JW, Klesges LM. Caffeinated coffee and tea intake and its relationship to cigarette smoking: an analysis of the second national health and nutrition examination survey. *J Subst Abuse*. 1994;6:407–418.

164. Kristjansson AL, Sigfusdottir ID, Allegrante JP, James JE. Adolescent caffeine consumption, daytime sleepiness, and anger. *J Caffeine Res*. 2011;1:75–82.

165. Kurtz AM, Leong J, Anand M, Dargush AE, Shah SA. Effects of caffeinated versus decaffeinated energy shots on blood pressure and heart rate in healthy young volunteers. *Pharmacotherapy*. 2013;33:779–786.

166. La Vecchia C, Ferraroni M, Negri E, et al. Coffee consumption and digestive tract cancers. *Cancer Res*. 1989;49:1049–1051.

167. La Vecchia C, Franceschi S, Decarli A, et al. Coffee drinking and the risk of epithelial ovarian cancer. *Int J Cancer*. 1984;33:559–562.

168. La Vecchia C, Franceschi S, Decarli A, Parazzini F, Tognoni G. Coffee consumption and the risk of breast cancer. *Surgery*. 1986;100:477–481.

169. La Vecchia C, Negri E, Decarli A, et al. A case-control study of diet and colo-rectal cancer in northern Italy. *Int J Cancer*. 1988;41:492–498.

170. LaCroix AZ, Mead LA, Liang KY, Thomas CB, Pearson TA. Coffee consumption and coronary heart disease. *N Engl J Med*. 1987;316:947.

171. Lane JD. Neuroendocrine responses to caffeine in the work environment. *Psychosom Med*. 1994;546:267–270.

172. Lane JD. Effects of brief caffeine deprivation on mood, symptoms, and psychomotor performance. *Pharmacol Biochem Behav*. 1997;58:203–208.

173. Lane JD. Caffeine, glucose metabolism, and type 2 diabetes. *J Caffeine Res*. 2011;1:23–28.

174. Lane JD, Adcock RA, Williams RB, Kuhn CM. Caffeine effects on cardiovascular and neuroendocrine responses to acute psychosocial stress and their relationship to level of habitual caffeine consumption. *Psychosom Med*. 1990;52:320–336.

175. Lane JD, Barkauskas CE, Surwit RS, Feinglos MN. Caffeine impairs glucose metabolism in type 2 diabetes. *Diabetes Care*. 2004;27:2047–2048.

176. Lane JD, Feinglos MN, Surwit RS. Caffeine increases ambulatory glucose and postprandial responses in coffee drinkers with type 2 diabetes. *Diabetes Care*. 2008;31:221–222.

177. Lane JD, Hwang AL, Feinglos MN, Surwit RS. Exaggeration of postprandial hyperglycemia in patients with type 2 diabetes by administration of caffeine in coffee. *Endocrine Pract*. 2007;13:239–243.

178. Lane JD, Lane AJ, Surwit RS, Kuhn CM, Feinglos MN. Pilot study of caffeine abstinence for control of chronic glucose in type 2 diabetes. *J Caffeine Res*. 2012;2:45–47.

179. Lane JD, Phillips-Bute BG. Caffeine deprivation affects vigilance performance and mood. *Physiol Behav*. 1998;65:171–175.

180. Lane JD, Pieper CF, Phillips-Bute BG, Bryant JE, Kuhn CM. Caffeine affects cardiovascular and neuroendocrine activation at work and home. *Psychosom Med*. 2002;64:595–603.

181. Lane JD, Williams RB. Cardiovascular effects of caffeine and stress in regular coffee drinkers. *Psychophysiology.* 1987;24:157–164.

182. Lara B, Gonzalez-Millán C, Salinero JJ, Abian-Vicen J, Areces F, Barbero-Alvarez JC, et al. Caffeine-containing energy drink improves physical performance in female soccer players. *Amino Acids.* 2014;46:1385–1392.

183. Larsson SC, Orsini N. Coffee consumption and risk of stroke: a dose-response meta-analysis of prospective studies. *Am J Epidemiol.* 2011;174:993–1001.

184. Lawson DH, Jick H, Rothman KJ. Coffee and tea consumption and breast disease. *Surgery.* 1981;90:801–803.

185. LeBlanc J, Soucy J. Hormonal dose-response to an adenosine receptor agonist. *Can J Physiol Pharmacol.* 1994;72:113–116.

186. Lee S. Carcinogens and mutagens. *Tea Coffee Trade J.* 1993:5–6.

187. LeGrady D, Dyer AR, Shekelle RB, et al. Coffee consumption and mortality in the Chicago western electric company study. *Am J Epidemiol.* 1987;126:803–812.

188. Lelo A, Miners JO, Robson R, Birkett DJ. Assessment of caffeine exposure: caffeine content of beverages, caffeine intake, and plasma concentrations of methylxanthines. *Clin Pharmacol Ther.* 1986;39:54–59.

189. Lelo A, Miners JO, Robson RA, Birkett DJ. Quantitative assessment of caffeine partial clearances in man. *Br J Clin Pharmacol.* 1986;22:183–186.

190. Lieberman H, Marriott B, Judelson D, et al. Intake of caffeine from all sources including energy drinks and reasons for use in US college students. *FASEB J.* 2015;29(suppl 1):392–1.

191. Lieberman HR, Wurtman RJ, Emde GG, Roberts C, Coviella ILG. The effects of low doses of caffeine on human performance and mood. *Psychopharmacology.* 1987;92:308–312.

192. Lipinsky DP, Black JL, Nelson RO, Cimimero AR. The influence of motivational variables on the reactivity and reliability of self-recording. *J Consulting Clin Psychol.* 1975;43:637–646.

193. Liu J, Sui X, Lavie CJ, et al. Association of coffee consumption with all-cause and cardiovascular disease mortality. *Mayo Clin Proc.* 2013;88:1066–1074.

194. Lovallo WR, Farag NH, Vincent AS, Thomas TL, Wilson MF. Cortisol responses to mental stress, exercise, and meals following caffeine intake in men and women. *Pharmacol Biochem Behav.* 2006;83:441–447.

195. Lovallo WR, Pincomb GA, Sung BH, Passey RB, Suasen KP, Wilson MF. Caffeine may potentiate adrenocortical stress responses in hypertension-prone men. *Hypertension.* 1989;14:170–176.

196. Lovallo WR, Wilson MF, Vincent AS, et al. Blood pressure response to caffeine shows incomplete tolerance after short-term regular consumption. *Hypertension.* 2004;43:760–765.

197. Lubin JH, Burns PE, Blot WJ, Ziegler RG, Lees AW, Fraumeni JF. Dietary factors and breast cancer risk. *Int J Cancer.* 1981;28:685–689.

198. MacDonald R. WHO says tobacco industry "used" institute to undermine its policies. *Br Med J.* 2001;322:576.

199. MacMahon B, Yen S, Trichopoulos D, Warren K, Nardi G. Coffee and cancer of the pancreas. *N Engl J Med.* 1981;304:630–633.

200. MacMahon S. Blood pressure and the risk of cardiovascular disease. *N Engl J Med.* 2000;342:50–52.

201. MacMahon S, Peto R, Cutler J, et al. Blood pressure, stroke, and coronary heart disease. Part 1, prolonged differences in blood pressure: prospective observational studies corrected for the regression dilution bias. *Lancet.* 1990;335:765–774.

202. Mahmud A, Feely J. Acute effect of caffeine on arterial stiffness and aortic pressure waveform. *Hypertension.* 2001;38:227–231.

203. Mansel RE, Webster DJT, Burr M, Leger SS. Is there a relationship between coffee consumption and breast disease? *B J Surg.* 1982;69:295–296.

204. Marangos PJ, Boulenger JP. Basic and clinical aspects of adenosinergic neuromodulation. *Neurosci Biobehav Rev.* 1985;9:421–430.

205. Martin JB, Annegers JF, Curb JD, et al. Mortality patterns among hypertensives by reported level of caffeine consumption. *Prev Med.* 1988;17:310–320.

206. Masterson J. Trends in coffee consumption. *Tea Coffee Trade J.* 1983:24–25.

207. Menza M. The personality associated with Parkinson's disease. *Curr Psychiatry Rep.* 2000;2:421–426.

208. Michels KB, Holmberg L, Bergkvist L, Wolk A. Coffee, tea, and caffeine consumption and breast cancer incidence in a cohort of Swedish women. *Ann Epidemiol.* 2002;12:21–26.

209. Michels KB, Willett WC, Fuchs CS, Giovannucci E. Coffee, tea, and caffeine consumption and incidence of colon and rectal cancer. *J Natl Cancer Inst.* 2005;97:282–292.

210. Miles–Chan JL, Charrière N, Grasser EK, Montani JP, Dulloo AG. The blood pressure–elevating effect of Red Bull energy drink is mimicked by caffeine but through different hemodynamic pathways. *Physiol Rep.* 2015;3(2):e12290.

211. Miller KE. Energy drinks, race, and problem behaviors among college students. *J Adolesc Health.* 2008;43:490–497.

212. Mills JL, Holmes LB, Aarons JH, et al. Moderate caffeine use and the risk of spontaneous abortion and intrauterine growth retardation. *JAMA J Am Med Assoc.* 1993;269:593–597.

213. Momas I, Daures JP, Festy B, Bontoux J, Gremy F. Relative importance of risk factors in bladder carcinogenesis: some new results about Mediterranean habits. *Cancer Causes Control.* 1994;5:326–332.

214. Momoi N, Tinney JP, Liu LJ, Elshershari H, Hoffmann PJ, Ralphe JC, et al. Modest maternal caffeine exposure affects developing embryonic cardiovascular function and growth. *Am J Physiol – Heart Circulatory Physiol.* 2008;294:H2248–H2256.

215. Murphy P. ILSI responds to march 10 BMJ article. *Br Med J.* 2001;322:576.

216. Nelson RO, Lipinsky DP, Black JL. The effects of expectancy on the reactivity of self-recoding. *Behav Ther.* 1975;6:337–349.

217. Neuberger MB. *Smoke Screen: Tobacco and the Public Welfare.* Engelwood Cliffs, NJ: Prentice-Hall; 1963.

218. Nikolajsen L, Larsen KM, Kierkegaard O. Effect of previous frequency of headache, duration of fasting and caffeine abstinence on perioperative headache. *Br J Anaesthesia.* 1994;72:295–297.

219. Nishi M, Ohba S, Hirata K, Miyake H. Dose-response relationship between coffee and the risk of pancreas cancer. *Jpn J Clin Oncol.* 1996;26:42–48.

220. Nomura A, Heilbrun LK, Stemmermann GN. Prospective study of coffee consumption and the risk of cancer. *J Natl Cancer Inst.* 1986;76:587–590.

221. O'Brien MC, McCoy TP, Rhodes SD, et al. Caffeinated cocktails: energy drink consumption, high-risk drinking, and alcohol-related consequences among college students. *Acad Emerg Med.* 2008;15:453–460.

222. Oberman Z, Harell A, Herzberg M, Hoerer E, Jaskolka H, Laurian L. Changes in plasma cortisol, glucose and free fatty acids after caffeine ingestion in obese women. *Israel J Med Sci.* 1975;11:33–36.

223. Olsen J, Kronborg O. Coffee, tobacco and alcohol as risk factors for cancer and adenoma of the large intestine. *Int J Epidemiol.* 1993;22:398–402.

224. Patton GC, Hibbert M, Rosier MJ, Carlin JB, Caust J, Bowes G. Patterns of common drug use in teenagers. *Aust J Public Health.* 1995;19:393–399.

225. Paul S, Kurunwune B, Biaggioni I. Caffeine withdrawal: apparent heterologous sensitization to adenosine and prostacyclin actions in human platelets. *J Pharmacol Exp Ther.* 1993;267:838–843.

226. Pendergrast M. *Uncommon Grounds: the History of Coffee and How it Transformed our World.* New York, NY: Basic Books; 1999.

227. Petrie HJ, Chown SE, Belfie LM, Duncan AM, McLaren DH, Conquer JA, et al. Caffeine ingestion increases the insulin response to an oral-glucose-tolerance test in obese men before and after weight loss. *Am J Clin Nutr.* 2004;80:22–28.

228. Pfeifer RW, Notari RE. Predicting caffeine plasma concentrations resulting from consumption of food or beverages: a simple method and its origin. *Drug Intelligence Clin Pharm.* 1988;22: 953–959.

229. Phillips-Bute BG, Lane JD. Caffeine withdrawal symptoms following brief caffeine deprivation. *Physiol Behav.* 1998;63:35–39.

230. Pincomb GA, Lovallo WR, Passey RB, Brackett DJ, Wilson MF. Caffeine enhances the physiological response to occupational stress in medical students. *Health Psychol.* 1987;6:101–112.

231. Pincomb GA, Lovallo WR, Passey RB, Wilson MF. Effect of behavior state on caffeine's ability to alter blood pressure. *Am J Cardiol.* 1988;61:798–802.

232. Prospective Studies Collaboration. Age-specific relevance of usual blood pressure to vascular mortality: a meta-analysis of individual data for one million adults in 61 prospective studies. *Lancet.* 2002;360:1903–1913.

233. Rakic V, Burke V, Beilin LJ. Effects of coffee on ambulatory blood pressure in older men and women: a randomized controlled trial. *Hypertension.* 1999;33:869–873.

234. Rall TW. Drugs used in the treatment of asthma. The methylxanthines, cromolyn sodium, and other agents. In: Gilman AG, Rall TW, Nies AS, Taylor P, eds. *Goodman and Gilman's the Pharmacological Basis of Therapeutics.* New York: Pergamon; 1990:618–637.

235. Rasch V. Cigarette, alcohol, and caffeine consumption: risk factors for spontaneous abortion. *Acta Obstet Gynecol Scand.* 2003;82:182–188.

236. Reissig CJ, Strain EC, Griffiths RR. Caffeinated energy drinks: a growing problem. *Drug Alcohol Depend.* 2009;99:1–10.

237. Richards G. Tea in 1993. *Tea Coffee Trade J.* 1994;166:42–50.

238. Richardson NJ, Rogers PJ, Elliman NA, O'Dell RJ. Mood and performance effects of caffeine in relation to acute and chronic caffeine deprivation. *Pharmacol Biochem Behav.* 1995;52:313–320.

239. Robertson D, Wade D, Workman R, Woosley RL, Oates JA. Tolerance to the humoral and hemodynamic effects of caffeine in man. *J Clin Invest.* 1981;67:1111–1117.

240. Rodgers A, Lawes C, MacMahon S. Reducing the global burden of blood pressure-related cardiovascular disease. *J Hypertens.* 2000;18:S3–S6.

241. Rodgers A, MacMahon S. Blood pressure and the global burden of cardiovascular disease. *Clin Exp Hypertens.* 1999;21:543–552.

242. Rodriguez del Rey Z, Granek EF, Sylvester S. Occurrence and concentration of caffeine in Oregon coastal waters. *Mar Pollut Bull.* 2012;64:1417–1424.

243. Rogers PJ, Dernoncourt C. Regular caffeine consumption: a balance of adverse and beneficial effects for mood and psychomotor performance. *Pharmacol Biochem Behav.* 1998;59:1039–1045.

244. Rogers PJ, Heatherley SV, Hayward RC, Seers HE, Hill J, Kane M. Effects of caffeine and caffeine withdrawal on mood and cognitive performance degraded by sleep restriction. *Psychopharmacology.* 2005;179:742–752.

245. Rogers PJ, Smith JE, Heatherley SV, Pleydell-Pearce CW. Time for tea: mood, blood pressure and cognitive performance effects of caffeine and theanine administered alone and together. *Psychopharmacology.* 2008;195:569–577.

246. Rohan TE, McMichael AJ. Methylxanthines and breast cancer. *Int J Cancer.* 1988;41:390–393.

247. Rose J. Strategy of prevention: lessons from cardiovascular disease. *Br Med J.* 1981;282:1847–1851.

248. Rosenberg L, Miller DR, Helmrich SP, Kaufman DW, Schottenfeld D, Stolley PD, Shapiro S. Breast cancer and the consumption of coffee. *Am J Epidemiol.* 1985;122:391–399.

249. Rosenberg L, Palmer JR, Kelly JP, Kaufman DW, Shapiro S. Coffee drinking and nonfatal myocardial infarction in men under 55 years of age. *Am J Epidemiol.* 1988;128:570–578.

250. Rosengren A, Dotevall A, Wilhelmsen L, Thelle D, Johansson S. Coffee and incidence of diabetes in Swedish women: a prospective 18-year follow-up study. *J Intern Med.* 2004;255:89–95.

251. Ross GW, Abbott RD, Petrovitch H, Morens DM, Grandinetti A, Tung KH, et al. Association of coffee and caffeine intake with the risk of Parkinson disease. *JAMA.* 2000;283:2674–2679.

252. Salazar-Martinez E, Willett WC, Ascherio A, Manson JE, Leitzmann MF, Stampfer MJ, et al. Coffee consumption and risk for type 2 diabetes mellitus. *Ann Inter Med.* 2004;140:1–8.

253. Sanguigni V, Gallu M, Ruffini MP, Strano A. Effects of coffee on serum cholesterol and lipoproteins: the Italian brewing method. Italian group for the study of atherosclerosis and dismetabolic diseases, Rome II center. *Eur J Epidemiol.* 1995;11:75–78.

254. Santos IS, Victora CG, Huttly S, Morris S. Caffeine intake and pregnancy outcomes: a meta-analytic review. *Cad Saude Publica.* 1998;14(3):523–530.

255. Schairer C, Brinton LA, Hoover RN. Methylxanthines and breast cancer. *Int J Cancer.* 1987;40:469–473.

256. Schiffman SS, Warwick ZS. *Use of Flavor-Amplified Foods to Improve Nutritional Status in Elderly Persons.* New York Academy of Sciences; 1989.

257. Schisterman EF, Cole SR, Platt RW. Overadjustment bias and unnecessary adjustment in epidemiologic studies. *Epidemiol.* 2009;20:488–495.

258. Schneider MB, Benjamin HJ. Sports drinks and energy drinks for children and adolescents: are they appropriate? *Pediatrics.* 2011;127:1182–1189.

259. Schreiber GB, Robins M, Maffeo CE, Masters MN, Bond AP, Morganstein D. Confounders contributing to the reported associations of coffee or caffeine with disease. *Prev Med.* 1988;17: 295–309.

260. Schwarzschild MA, Xu K, Oztas E, Petzer JP, Castagnoli K, Castagnoli Jr N, et al. Neuroprotection by caffeine and more specific A2A receptor antagonists in animal models of Parkinson's disease. *Neurology.* 2003;61(suppl 6):S55–S61.

261. Seifert SM, Schaechter JL, Hershorin ER, Lipshultz SE. Health effects of energy drinks on children, adolescents, and young adults. *Pediatrics.* 2011;127:511–528.

262. Sengpiel V, Elind E, Bacelis J, Nilsson S, Grove J, Myhre R, et al. Maternal caffeine intake during pregnancy is associated with birth weight but not with gestational length: results from a large prospective observational cohort study. *BMC Med.* 2013;11:42. https://doi.org/10.1186/1741-7015-11-42.

263. Sepkowitz KA. Energy drinks and caffeine-related adverse effects. *JAMA.* 2013;309:243–244.

264. Shepard JD, al'Absi M, Whitsett TL, Passey RB, Lovallo WR. Additive pressor effects of caffeine and stress in male medical students at risk for hypertension. *Am J Hypertens.* 2000;13: 475–781.

265. Shi J, Benowitz NL, Denaro CP, Sheiner LB. Pharmacokinetic-pharmacodynamic modeling of caffeine: tolerance to pressor effects. *Clin Pharmacol Ther.* 1993;53:6–14.

266. Shibata A, Mack TM, Paganini-Hill A, Ross RK, Henderson BE. A prospective study of pancreatic cancer in the elderly. *Int J Cancer.* 1994;58:46–49.

267. Shirlow MJ, Berry G, Stokes G. Caffeine consumption and blood pressure: an epidemiologic study. *Int J Epidemiol.* 1988;17:90–97.

268. Shu XO, Hatch MC, Mills J, Clemens J, Susser M. Maternal smoking, alcohol drinking, caffeine consumption, and fetal growth: results from a prospective study. *Epidemiology.* 1995;6:115–120.

269. Slattery ML, Caan BJ, Anderson KE, Potter JD. Intake of fluids and methylxanthine-containing beverages: association with colon cancer. *Int J Cancer.* 1999;81:199–204.

270. Slattery ML, West DW, Robison LM, French TK, Ford MH, Schuman KL, Sorenson AW. Tobacco, alcohol, coffee, and caffeine as risk factors for colon cancer in a low-risk population. *Epidemiology.* 1990;1:141–145.

271. Smit HJ, Rogers PJ. Effects of caffeine on cognitive performance, mood and thirst in lower and higher caffeine consumers. *Psychopharmacology.* 2000;152:167–173.

272. Smith SJ, Deacon JM, Chilvers CE. Alcohol, smoking, passive smoking and caffeine in relation to breast cancer risk in young women. UK national case-control study group. *Br J Cancer.* 1994;70:112–119.
273. Smits P, Boekema P, de Abreu R, Thien T, van't Laar A. Evidence for an antagonism between caffeine and adenosine in the human cardiovascular system. *J Cardiovasc Pharmacol.* 1987;10:136–143.
274. Smits P, Temme L, Thien T. The cardiovascular interaction between caffeine and nicotine in humans. *Clin Pharmacol Ther.* 1993;54:194–204.
275. Smits P, Thien T, van't Laar A. Circulatory effects of coffee in relation to the pharmacokinetics of caffeine. *Am J Cardiol.* 1985;56:958–963.
276. Smits P, Thien T, van't Laar A. The cardiovascular effects of regular and decaffeinated coffee. *Br J Clin Pharmacol.* 1985;19:852–854.
277. Snowdon DA, Phillips RL. Coffee consumption and risk of fatal cancers. *Am J Public Health.* 1984;74:820–823.
278. Somani SM, Gupta P. Caffeine: a new look at an age-old drug. *Int J Clin Pharmacol Ther Toxicol.* 1988;26:521–533.
279. Song YJ, Kristal AR, Wicklund KG, Cushing-Haugen KL, Rossing MA. Coffee, tea, colas, and risk of epithelial ovarian cancer. *Cancer Epidemiol Biomarkers Prev.* 2008;17:712–716.
280. Spindel ER, Wurtman RJ, McCall A, et al. Neuroendocrine effects of caffeine in normal subjects. *Clin Pharmacol Ther.* 1984;36:402–407.
281. Spinillo A, Capuzzo E, Nicola SE, Colonna L, Egbe TO, Zara C. Factors potentiating the smoking-related risk of fetal growth retardation. *Br J Obstetrics Gynaecol.* 1994;101:954–958.
282. Stafford LD, Yeomans MR. Caffeine deprivation state modulates coffee consumption but not attentional bias for caffeine-related stimuli. *Behav Pharmacol.* 2005;16:559–571.
283. Stocks P. Cancer mortality in relation to national consumption of cigarettes, solid fuel, tea and coffee. *Br J Cancer.* 1970;24:215–225.
284. Streufert S, Pogash R, Miller J, et al. Effects of caffeine deprivation on complex human functioning. *Psychopharmacology.* 1995;118:377–384.
285. Superko HR, Myll J, DiRicco C, Williams PT, Bortz WM, Wood PD. Effects of cessation of caffeinated-coffee consumption on ambulatory and resting blood pressure in men. *Am J Cardiol.* 1994;73:780–784.
286. Takei A. ILSI Health and Environmental Sciences Institute (HESI), global leader in advancing translational science to create science-based solutions for a sustainable, healthier world. *Genes Environ.* 2015;37. https://doi.org/10.1186/s41021-015-0001-0.
287. Tavani A, Gallus S, Dal Maso L, Franceschi S, Montella M, Conti E, et al. Coffee and alcohol intake and risk of ovarian cancer: an Italian case-control study. *Nutr Cancer.* 2001;39:29–34.
288. Tavani A, La Vecchia C. Coffee, decaffeinated coffee, tea and cancer of the colon and rectum: a review of epidemiological studies, 1990-2003. *Cancer Causes Control.* 2004;15:743–757.
289. Temple JL. Caffeine use in children: what we know, what we have left to learn, and why we should worry. *Neurosci Biobehav Reviews.* 2009;33:793–806.
290. Thelander G, Jönsson AK, Personne M, et al. Caffeine fatalities—do sales restrictions prevent intentional intoxications? *Clin Toxicol.* 2010;48:354–358.
291. Thombs DL, O'Mara RJ, Tsukamoto M, et al. Event-level analyses of energy drink consumption and alcohol intoxication in bar patrons. *Addict Behav.* 2010;35:325–330.
292. Todes CJ, Lees AJ. The pre-morbid personality of patients with Parkinson's disease. *J Neurol Neurosurg Psychiatry.* 1985;48:97–100.
293. Trichopoulos D, Papapostolou M, Polychronopoulou A. Coffee and ovarian cancer. *Int J Cancer.* 1981;28:691–693.
294. Turkheimer E. Heritability and biological explanation. *Psychol Rev.* 1998;105:782–791.
295. Ungemack JA. Patterns of personal health practice: men and women in the United States. *Am J Prev Med.* 1994;10(1994):38–44.
296. United States Food and Drug Administration: Office of the Federal Register, National Archives and Records Administration. *Title 21, Code of Federal Regulations, 170.22. Safety factors to be considered. (Title 21, Code of Federal Regulations, Parts 170 to 1995).* Washington, DC: Office of the Federal Register US Government Printing Office; 1995.
297. Urgert R, van Vliet T, Zock PL, Katan MB. Heavy coffee consumption and plasma homocysteine: a randomized controlled trial in healthy volunteers. *Am J Clin Nutr.* 2000;72:1107–1110.
298. Urso-Baiarda F, Shurey S, Grobbelaar AO. Effect of caffeine on microsurgical technical performance. *Microsurgery.* 2007;27:84–87.
299. van Boxtel MP, Schmitt JA, Bosma H, Jolles J. The effects of habitual caffeine use on cognitive change: a longitudinal perspective. *Pharmacol Biochem Behav.* 2003;75:921–927.
300. van Dam RM, Feskens EJ. Coffee consumption and risk of type 2 diabetes mellitus. *Lancet.* 2002;360:1477–1478.
301. van Dam RM, Pasman WJ, Verhoef P. Effects of coffee consumption on fasting blood glucose and insulin concentrations: randomized controlled trials in healthy volunteers. *Diabetes Care.* 2004;27:2990–2992.
302. Van den Hoogen PC, Seidell JC, Menotti A, Kromhout D. Blood pressure and long-term coronary heart disease mortality in the Seven Countries study: implications for clinical practice and public health. *Eur Heart J.* 2000;21:1639–1642.
303. van Dusseldorp M, Katan MB. Headache caused by caffeine withdrawal among moderate coffee drinkers switched from ordinary to decaffeinated coffee: a 12 week double blind trial. *Br Med J.* 1990;300:1558–1559.
304. van Dusseldorp M, Smits P, Thien T, Katan MB. Effect of decaffeinated versus regular coffee on blood pressure. A 12-week, double-blind trial. *Hypertension.* 1989;14:563–569.
305. Van't Hoff W. Caffeine in pregnancy. *Lancet.* 1982;319(8279):1020.
306. Vik T, Bakketeig LS, Trygg KU, Lund-Larsen K, Jacobsen G. High caffeine consumption in the third trimester of pregnancy: gender-specific effects on fetal growth. *Paediatr Perinat Epidemiol.* 2003;17:324–331.
307. Vitzthum OG. Chemie und bearbeitung des kaffees. In: Eichler O, ed. *Kaffee Und Coffein.* 2nd ed. Berlin: Springer; 1976:3–64.
308. Vlachopoulos C, Hirata K, O'Rourke MF. Effect of caffeine on aortic elastic properties and wave reflection. *J Hypertens.* 2003;21:563–570.
309. Vlachopoulos C, Hirata K, Stefanadis C, Toutouzas P, O'Rourke MF. Caffeine increases aortic stiffness in hypertensive patients. *Am J Hypertens.* 2003;16:63–66.
310. Vlachopoulos C, Kosmopoulou F, Panagiotakos D, Ioakeimidis N, Alexopoulos N, Pitsavos C, et al. Smoking and caffeine have a synergistic detrimental effect on aortic stiffness and wave reflections. *J Am College Cardiol.* 2004;44:1911–1917.
311. von Borstel RW, Wurtman RJ. Caffeine withdrawal enhances sensitivity to physiologic level of adenosine in vivo. *Federation Proc.* 1982;41:1669.
312. Wahrburg U, Martin H, Schulte H, Walek T, Assmann G. Effects of two kinds of decaffeinated coffee on serum lipid profiles in healthy young adults. *Eur J Clin Nutr.* 1994;48:172–179.
313. Walters ER, Lesk VE. The effect of prior caffeine consumption on neuropsychological test performance: a placebo-controlled study. *Dement Geriatr Cogn Disord.* 2016;41:146–151.
314. Watt AH, Bayer A, Routledge PA, Swift CG. Adenosine-induced respiratory and heart rate changes in young and elderly adults. *Br J Clin Pharmacol.* 1989;27:265–267.
315. Weber JG, Ereth MH, Danielson DR. Perioperative ingestion of caffeine and postoperative headache. *Mayo Clinic Proc.* 1993;368:842–845.
316. Weinstein ND. Misleading tests of health behavior theories. [see comment]. *Ann Behav Med.* 2007;33(1):1–10.

317. Wen W, Shu XO, Jacobs Jr DR, Brown JE. The associations of maternal caffeine consumption and nausea with spontaneous abortion. *Epidemiology.* 2001;12:38–42.

318. Weusten-Van der Wouw MP, Katan MB, Viani R, et al. Identity of the cholesterol-raising factor from boiled coffee and its effects on liver function enzymes. *J Lipid Res.* 1994;35:721–733.

319. Whittemore AS, Wu ML, Paffenbarger Jr RS, et al. Personal and environmental characteristics related to epithelial ovarian cancer. II. Exposures to talcum powder, tobacco, alcohol, and coffee. *Am J Epidemiol.* 1988;128:1228–1240.

320. World Health Organization. *International Statistical Classification of Diseases and Related Health Problems. 10th Revision.* Geneva: WHO; 2007.

321. Wu J-N, Ho SC, Zhou C, et al. Coffee consumption and risk of coronary heart diseases: a meta-analysis of 21 prospective cohort studies. *Int J Card.* 2009;137:216–225.

322. Zatonski WA, Boyle P, Przewozniak K, Maisonneuve P, Drosik K, Walker AM. Cigarette smoking, alcohol, tea and coffee consumption and pancreas cancer risk: a case-control study from opole, poland. *Int J Cancer.* 1993;53:601–607.

323. Zeltner T, Kessler DA, Martiny A, Randera F. *Tobacco Company Strategies to Undermine Tobacco Control Activities at the World Health Organization.* Geneva: World Health Organization; 2000.

324. Zheng W, McLaughlin JK, Gridley G, et al. A cohort study of smoking, alcohol consumption, and dietary factors for pancreatic cancer (United States). *Cancer Causes Control.* 1993;4:477–482.

31

Serotonergic Hallucinogens

SHAUL LEV-RAN

Introduction

This chapter focuses on hallucinogens with psychoactive properties mediated through the serotonin system. Although commonly referred to as "hallucinogens," a lexigraphic disclaimer is warranted, as the experience elicited by these drugs commonly centers on distortion of perception, not true hallucinations. The most apt term is probably "psychedelic" from the Greek *psukhē*, meaning "mind" and *dēloun,* meaning "reveal" or "make visible." Although the enlightenment sought by recreational users may be an artifact of the psychoactive experience, researchers study these compounds hoping to gain insight into how the brain produces the mind. Nonetheless, in conforming to common usage, in this chapter these drugs will be referred to as hallucinogens.

History

Perceptions provide reassurance into our existence and the existence of the world around us. Thus it is not surprising that compounds capable of producing altered states of perception are regarded with mystical fascination and trepidation. The ritualistic consumption of plants, many of which derive their psychoactive properties through the serotonin system, has been an important part of religious and social ceremonies throughout human history.

Conceivably the oldest known ritualistic use of hallucinogens was in the Indus Valley during the second millennium BCE. A group of people known as Aryans worshiped a deity they named "Soma," which recent evidence suggests is the mushroom *Amanita muscaria* or Fly agaric.[159] These served as an inspiration to several later cultural sources: Aldous Huxley refers to soma as the "ideal pleasure drug" in his novel *Brave New World,* and the red and white spotted mushroom that is *A. muscaria* incidentally bears resemblance to the mushroom featured in the Mario Brothers video game worshiped by many adolescents in the second millennium CE.

Spiritual use of hallucinogens has been a part of various cultures throughout the world. In the 14th century CE, Aztecs and other Indians of Central America ingested psilocybin-containing mushrooms to bestow powers of clairvoyance during religious ceremonies. Contemporary South American and Caribbean peoples snorted a narcotic powder (Cohoba), which, reminiscent of modern club drugs, was used to promote friendliness during convulsive dance ceremonies. In Western cultures, hallucinogens may underlie mythos of witchcraft and sorcery. In his book *Hallucinogens and Shamanism*, Michael Harner[60] relates the symbol of a witch riding on a broomstick to the practice of medieval women achieving magical powers by anointing their mucous membranes with hallucinogenic substances. Linnda Caporael hypothesized that that the affliction of the girls sparking the Salem witch trials resulted from ergot (the natural substance from which lysergic acid diethylamine [LSD] is derived) poisoning caused by ingestion of rye grains contaminated with the fungus *Claviceps purpurea.*[27] More recently, a study conducted by Griffiths et al. found that when administered under supportive conditions psilocybin occasioned experiences similar to spontaneously occurring mystical experiences.[58]

The modern synthetic drug era began in the late 1960s with the legendary synthesis of LSD by the Swiss chemist, Albert Hoffman. While working at Sandoz Laboratories, Hoffman synthesized LSD as part of an effort to develop ergot derivatives capable of reducing postpartum bleeding. Not useful in this regard, the compound was shelved. Five years later, according to psychedelic lore, Hoffman was haunted by a "peculiar presentment" and repeated its synthesis. After accidentally absorbing a small amount he experienced its psychoactive effects while bicycling home. Psychedelic enthusiasts refer to this fateful day, April 16, 1943, as "Bicycle Day."

In the 1960s and 1970s, Timothy Leary brought LSD and other psychedelics to the forefront of pop culture. His introduction of psychedelic drugs to academic and therapeutic settings led to the research responsible for most of what is currently known about these drugs. However, his temerarious promotion of these drugs for individual enlightenment and the ensuing underground abuse precipitated strict government regulation, which for several decades halted substantial scientific research. In the 1980s, attention to hallucinogen use reemerged with the trend of all night dance parties known to as raves. These large gatherings featured electronic dance music and laser light shows. Attendees often used psychedelic drugs (most commonly 3,4-methylenedioxymethamphetamine—also known as MDMA or Ecstasy) to promote sociality and heighten the sensory stimuli of the music and lights. Despite the emergence of new hallucinogens, the use of LSD and the traditional psychedelics continued throughout recent decades.

Today, restrictions on research have loosened and there is a gradual increase in obtaining approval and carrying out research on psychedelic drugs. In recent years, emerging evidence is accumulating, indicating that serotonergic hallucinogens may be useful in a variety of clinical situations, such as treating cluster headaches,[138] anxiety associated with life-threatening diseases,[47] and substance use disorders.[23] Alongside the increased prevalence of hallucinogen use for individual enlightenment and therapeutic potential, concerns regarding potential adverse effects of these drugs increased as well. These include both physiological effects, which in some cases led to severe adverse effects (e.g., cases of seizures, cardiac arrhythmia, and death following ibogaine use[131]), as well as psychiatric adverse effects (e.g., include anxiety, flashbacks, psychosis following LSD use[4]). Accordingly, the use of hallucinogens for personal and spiritual growth was gradually met with concerns surrounding abuse of these substances, and particular concerns regarding their potential adverse effects.

Epidemiology

Hallucinogen use has declined since the 1970s, with the annual prevalence remaining below 10%.[76,109,111,148] The types of hallucinogens used have also changed. LSD, which was the most widely used hallucinogen, has been surpassed by newer synthetic club drugs. In 2014, the Substance Abuse and Mental Health Services Administration (SAMHSA) reported findings from the National Survey on Drug Use and Health (NSDUH),[7] indicating that use of hallucinogens has remained relatively steady since 2002. In 2014, 1.2 million people in the United States (0.4% of the population) reported using hallucinogens in the past month (use was higher among males compared to females: 748,000 vs. 426,000). In the same year, there were 936,000 people 12 years of age or older in the United States who had used hallucinogens for the first time within the past 12 months. According to the same report, the most common hallucinogen used was MDMA, with 609,000 people 12 years or older reporting use in the past month.

Classification

Serotonergic hallucinogens can be divided by chemical structure (Fig. 31.1). Indolealkylamines, which have more than one carbon ring and are structurally similar to serotonin, include LSD, ibogaine, psilocin, psilocybin, and N,N-dimethyltryptamine. The phenethylamines, that have only one carbon ring, more closely resemble amphetamine and the catecholamine neurotransmitters (dopamine, epinephrine, and norepinephrine). This class comprises mescaline, MDMA, 3,4-methylenedioxyamphetamine, and dimethoxymethylamphetamine. The psychopharmacology of all of the serotonergic hallucinogens (except for MDMA) is similar.

To avoid redundancy, this chapter begins with a general discussion of mechanism of action and then concentrates on representative indolealkylamines (LSD, psilocybin, and ibogaine) and phenethylamines (mescaline and MDMA), with LSD serving as a prototype for comparison.

Mechanism of Action

After nearly a half a century of research, it is currently understood that the psychoactive effects of both indolealkylamine and phenethylamine hallucinogens are mediated primarily through agonist activity at the 2A subtype of serotonergic receptors (as serotonin is also known as "5-hydroxytryptamine" [5HT], these are known as 5HT2A receptors). The structural resemblance of indolealkylamines to the serotonin neurotransmitter led researchers to suspect that their psychoactive effects were serotonergically mediated. Furthermore, the reported similarity of psychic experiences elicited by the phenethylamines and the indolealkylamines,[66] as well as cross-tolerance between the two classes,[18,160,161] suggest a shared mechanism of action, although distinct effects via distinct psychodynamic activity are yet to be understood.

Serotonin Receptor

The monoamine family of neurotransmitters comprises serotonin, epinephrine, norepinephrine, and dopamine. The serotonin receptor system is particularly complicated, with 14 distinct receptors belonging to 7 families (5HT1R–5HT7R) having been discovered so far. The system is made more complex by posttranslational receptor modifications, multiple G proteins, phenotypic switching, and crosstalk within and probably between receptor families.[70] All but one of the serotonin receptors are coupled to G proteins. The 5HT2A and 5HT2C receptors are similar and often referred to as the 5HT2A/2C receptor. There is a paucity of ligands with selectivity between these two subtypes, making it difficult to rule out an ancillary role of 5HT2C receptors in the psychoactive effects of hallucinogens.[44]

Indolealkylamine Hallucinogens

Lysergic Acid Diethylamide (LSD)
Street Information

Today, the majority of LSD is synthetic. However, it can be derived from two naturally occurring substances; the embryo of morning glory seeds (*Rivea corymbosa*) and *C. purpurea* (the parasitic fungus mentioned in the preceding text). Sunlight and chlorine—even at tap water concentrations—will inactivate LSD but it can be stored as a solid salt or dissolved in pure water as long as it is kept at low temperatures and protected from light and air.[140] Synthetic LSD is crystalline. It is crushed into a white odorless, tasteless powder that is dissolved and administered orally, sublingually, intramuscularly, or intravenously. Sublingual mediums include postage stamps, chewing gum, or sugar cubes often decorated with symbols (Fig. 31.2).

Street names for LSD, as for all of the serotonergic hallucinogens, are creative and include, but are not limited to, "acid," "blotter," "dots," and "Lucy." LSD is extremely potent and can even be absorbed subcutaneously. Doses of 20–30 µg produce psychoactive effects in humans,[57] and Hoffman estimated it to be 5000 to 10,000 times more potent than mescaline.[67] Although there is no standard dose for lysergic acid, the range of doses taken for

Indolealkylamine			
Serotinin	LSD (d-lysergic acid diethylamide)		Average dose: 30-300 µg Onset: 20-60 minutes Duration: 12 hours
	DMT (N,N-dimethyltryptamine)		Average dose: 60-100 mg smoked or intramuscular Onset: 3 minutes Duration: 30 minutes
	Ibogaine (12-methoxy-ibogamine)		Average dose: 2 to 5 grams Onset: 45 minutes Duration: up to 24 hours
	Psilocybin (O-phosphoryl-4-hydroxy-N,N-dimethyltryptamine)		Average dose: 10-30 mg Onset: 10-40 minutes Duration: 2-6 hours
	Psilocin (4-hydroxy-N,N-dimethyltryptamine)		(The active metabolite of psilocybin)
Amphetamine	Phenethylamine		
	Mescaline (3,4,5-trimethoxyphenethylamine)		Average dose: 300-500 mg Onset: 30 minutes Duration: 10-12 hours
	Ecstasy (MDMA; 3,4-methylenedioxy-methamphetamine)		Average dose: 80-160 mg Onset: 30-45 minutes Duration: 6 hours
	DOM (2,5-dimethoxy-4-methylamphetamine)		Average dose: 3-10 mg Onset: 30 minutes to 1 hour Duration: 14-20 hours
	MDA (3,4-methylene-dioxyamphetamine)		Average dose: 80-160 mg Onset: 1-1.5 hours Duration: 6-10 hours

• **Fig. 31.1** Chemical structures of indolealkylamine and phenethylamine hallucinogens.

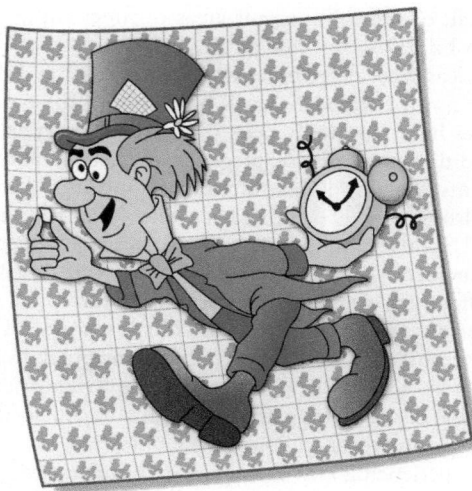

• **Fig. 31.2** Photograph of lysergic acid diethylamide (LSD) blotter sheet. (From the US Drug Enforcement Administration website.)

recreational purposes is generally between 50 and 400 µg, considerably lower than in the 1970s.[31,113,123] LSD is easily produced in great quantity. For example, 25 kg of ergotamine tartrate (a substrate for LSD) yields 5 kg of LSD or 100 million doses.

Physiological and Psychological Effects

LSD is hepatically metabolized and has no active metabolites. Maximal concentrations are reached between 0.5 and 4 hours after administration. Concentrations then decrease following first-order kinetics with a half-life of about 3.5 hours and slower elimination thereafter with a terminal half-life of close to 9 hours.[40] In a clinical study administering 200 µg to human subjects,[113,123] 1% of the orally administered LSD was eliminated in urine as LSD, and 13% was eliminated as 2-oxo-3-hydroxy-LSD within 24 hours. No sex differences were observed in the pharmacokinetic profiles of LSD. The acute subjective and sympathomimetic responses to LSD lasted up to 12 hours and were closely associated with the concentrations in plasma over time and exhibited no acute tolerance.[40] Users of LSD typically experience autonomic symptoms within several minutes and psychoactive effects approximately 10 minutes later. The autonomic symptoms are mainly sympathomimetic, that is, elevated blood pressure and pulse, diaphoresis, piloerection, nausea, uterine contractions, hyperreflexia, and tremor. Anisocoria (unequal pupils) and hippus (rhythmically dilating pupils) are not uncommon.[132]

Lysergic acid has several effects on psychological experience, including heightened mood, increased optimism, and trait-openness.[28] Additional reports of spiritual experiences and altered consciousness are common. Recent neuroimaging studies show increased global connectivity in high-level association cortices and the thalamus under the drug. The increase in global connectivity observed under LSD correlated with subjective reports of "ego dissolution."[149]

Not only does mood become amplified under the influence of LSD, but it can shift rapidly, and some users have reported experiencing multiple moods simultaneously. In addition, an increase in scores of psychotic-like symptoms are observed.[28] Sensory perceptions become enhanced and distorted.[78,90,110] Typical descriptions include vivid colorful geometric shapes, trails of actual objects, and seeing body parts separate from themselves. Dramatic complex disturbances may occur such as animation of inanimate objects or Satan's face appearing on someone's body.[135]

Auditory distortions are less common. At higher doses, synesthesia may occur (perceiving a sensation in different modality such as hearing colors). Distortions in the sense of time include time halting, stretching, repeating, and ceasing to exist.

When the overall experience is perceived as enlightening or emotionally stimulating, it is referred to as a "good trip." Other times the experience might be nightmarish, with fears of insanity or losing control. Such negative experiences are referred to "bad trips." While it has long been suggested that "set" (the individual's mindset) and "setting" (the physical and social environment) substantially affect psychedelic experience,[45a] it is unclear precisely what role they play in the cause of good trips versus bad trips. The clear association between the nature of a trip under the influence of LSD and subsequent experiences (good or bad) following ingestion is also unknown.

Hallucinogen Use Disorder

Tolerance to the psychological effects of LSD, but not the physiological effects, develops quickly.[22] In contrast to highly addictive drugs such as cocaine and heroin, with LSD there does not appear to be a withdrawal syndrome and users usually do not develop cravings or seek higher and higher doses. Although humans self-administer LSD, it does not serve as reinforcement in animal models. Nevertheless, because these physiological properties comprise only a couple of criteria for diagnosing a substance use disorder, other criteria (such as use in dangerous situations) are relevant and results from the National Epidemiologic Survey on Alcohol and Related Conditions (NESARC) indicate that the lifetime prevalence of hallucinogen use disorder is 0.6%.[138a]

Adverse Effects

Although LSD is considered relatively safe in terms of physical adverse effects when compared with other drugs of abuse, there are case reports of respiratory failure, hyperthermia, and coagulopathies associated with massive doses.[80] In general, there are three main reasons that people who use LSD come to clinical attention: the bad trip, hallucinogen persisting perceptual disorder (HPPD, also known as "flashbacks"), and psychosis.

The Bad Trip

Bad trips occur in about 1 in 10 LSD uses[39] and may lead to an emergency room visit. In addition to the psychological and physiological symptoms described earlier, patients usually have a clear sensorium without memory impairment and are able to provide a complete history. Furthermore, they often are accompanied by someone who was with them when they took the drug and who can confirm the suspected diagnosis.

In some cases a bad trip from LSD may be suspected but a confirmative history cannot be attained. For example, the individual may have unintentionally been exposed, may have been poisoned, or may simply be too agitated to provide a coherent history. Toxicology panels in most acute care settings do not routinely screen for LSD. In these cases, several additional etiologies should be considered such as intoxication with another hallucinogen, psychiatric illness, and delirium.

Differentiating LSD from other phenethylamine and indolealkylamine hallucinogens, for the most part, is academic, as they are treated similarly. It is, however, important to differentiate LSD from phencyclidine (PCP) intoxication because the pharmacological management differs. LSD is not smoked; therefore, if an individual reports having smoked the hallucinogen, PCP should be considered. In addition, individuals intoxicated on PCP are often brought in by authorities because of extremely disorganized, inappropriate, or combative behavior.

Acute LSD intoxication and the bad trip may superficially resemble psychiatric illnesses such as panic disorder, schizophrenia, or the mania of bipolar disorder. Sympathomimetic symptoms, ocular abnormalities (hippos and anisocoria) and visual perceptual disturbances suggest LSD intoxication but are not pathognomonic. Time is commonly the best way to differentiate LSD (substance-induced) psychosis from schizophrenia or mania. Generally, after several hours without pharmacological treatment, LSD intoxication wears off, whereas mania and schizophrenia do not. When substance-induced psychosis is suspected, this may remain a potential diagnosis for up to 4 weeks following last ingestion of the drug. Although feelings of being overwhelmed, scared, and afraid of losing control occur in panic attacks, LSD intoxication is further characterized by dramatic and persistent perceptual distortions. As with any altered mental state, the clinician should have a low threshold for suspecting delirium. Unlike delirium, there is generally no fluctuation in level consciousness with LSD intoxication.

The bad trip generally does not require inpatient hospitalization because of its time-limited course and quick recovery. The patient should be placed in a quiet, nonstimulating environment and provided continuous reassurance that his or her state of mind is drug induced and will not result in permanent brain damage.[146] Given that most emergency rooms are chaotic and understaffed, this may not be a realistic option. Furthermore, the patient may be too disorganized or combative to be talked down. When medications are needed, benzodiazepines are probably the best choice, so long as delirium has been ruled out. The use of neuroleptics should be reserved for instances in which none of the aforementioned efforts have succeeded. High-potency (less-anticholinergic) neuroleptics should be used because anticholinergic neuroleptics have been associated with paradoxical reactions,[137] hypotension, and anticholinergic crises.[91,142,143]

Hallucinogen Persisting Perceptual Disorder (HPPD)

Flashbacks are referred to as Hallucinogen Persisting Perception Disorder (HPPD) by the *Diagnostic and Statistical Manual of Mental Disorders, Fifth Edition* (DSM-5)[14] when they cause significant distress. They are defined as "the transient recurrence of disturbances in perception that are reminiscent of those experienced during one or more earlier hallucinogen intoxications."[44] The most common phenomena are visual distortions such as color confusion, geometric hallucinations, and trailing, but the content of the flashback may involve any of the senses.[69,139] It is not known what causes flashbacks. Theories include persisting damage to visual processing systems,[2,6] death of inhibitory cortical interneurons,[4,46] reverse tolerance,[144] and that they are an atypical dissociative state.[100]

Flashbacks may occur several days to several years after the antecedent use of LSD and have been reported with mescaline, PCP, and cannabinoids.[51,79,100] These recurrent visual disturbances, referred to as Hallucinogen Persistent Perceptual Disorder (or HPPD) are roughly divided into Flashback-Type (HPPD I) or HPPD-Type (HPPD II).[88] Flashback-Type visual disturbances are generally pleasant, short-term, reversible, nonintruding, nondistressing, nondisabling, and benign reoccurrences. whereas HPPD-Type visual disturbances are generally unpleasant, long-term, slowly reversible or irreversible, intruding, distressing, disabling, and pervasive reoccurrences.[86] Significant impairment in social, occupational, or other important areas of functioning is usually observed in HPPD II, but not HPPD I.[88]

It is unclear what determines who will experience HPPD and whether or not the experience will be pleasant. These perceptual disturbances have reportedly been induced by a myriad of situations including stress, exercise, pregnancy, sexual intercourse, dark environments, flashing lights, monotony, and use of other psychoactive drugs.[3,8,32,75,135] Individuals with HPPD II were found to initiate LSD use at an earlier age and report a higher number of overall incidents of use compared to those with HPPD I. Significant differences were found in the type of perceptual disorders between the two types of HPPD. Individuals with HPPD II more commonly report intentionally triggering perceptual disturbances and individuals with HPPD I more commonly report experiencing perceptual disorders triggered by sexual intercourse, dark environment, and looking at still or moving objects.

People experiencing HPPD may seek treatment with their general physician, ophthalmologists, neurologists, or psychiatrists with concerns about their vision, that they have a neurological disorder, or that they are losing their mind. There is no established pharmacological treatment,[83] but case reports suggest that such individuals may respond to typical antipsychotics,[16,85,101,107] clonidine,[84] benzodiazepines,[1,32,152] naltrexone,[87] or phenytoin.[151] The antipsychotic risperidone may exacerbate HPPD.[5,9,104] In addition, there have been reports of both exacerbation[95] and reduction[163] of HPPD following treatment with selective serotonin reuptake inhibitors. Despite their efficacy and minimal side effects, benzodiazepines may not be the first-line treatment for many individuals with HPPD because of abuse potential.

Psychosis

There have been a significant number of studies that have investigated LSD-induced psychosis and schizophrenia-like symptoms induced by LSD. In animal models, acute injection of the drug induced psychotic behaviors that were classified into positive symptoms, whereas chronic administration of LSD elicited positive symptoms as well as negative symptoms.[116] In humans, administration of LSD to healthy subjects results in an increase in positive schizophrenia-like symptoms.[28] On a population-based level, a study investigating emergency room visits following drug intoxication reported that among those patients referred to the emergency room following LSD ingestion, over 20% were found to have psychotic symptoms. Although this does not reflect the prevalence of psychosis among users of LSD, these rates are higher than those found for cannabinoids, amphetamine, and additional common substances.[155] Given accumulating evidence from preclinical, clinical, and population-based studies, LSD-induced psychosis is a serious concern, although specific data regarding rates of incidence among users are still lacking.

Psilocybin

Psilocybin, like LSD, is an indolealkylamine hallucinogen. Psilocybin can be derived from several genera of mushrooms—thus the street name "magic mushrooms." *Psilocybe cubensis* is the most common source of psilocybin. This mushroom grows on cow and horse manure in South America, Mexico, and most non-arid areas of the United States.[145] As with LSD, it was Albert Hoffman who isolated and then synthesized psilocybin. It was marketed by Sandoz laboratories under the trade name Indocybin as a potential tool for psychotherapy in the 1960s.

Psilocybin and its active metabolite psilocin are both Schedule I drugs. The spore prints, however, remain legal, presumably to provide mycologists the ability to grow pure psilocybin. Not surprisingly, several drug-oriented magazines advertise home cultivation kits that include live mycelia. The mushrooms can be eaten fresh, dried, or brewed. They are usually ingested orally but there is a case report of intravenous injection.[35] Psilocybin is metabolized into psilocin, which is responsible for the psychoactive effects.[89] Typical doses of psilocybin range from 4–20 mg (40 μg/kg) corresponding to 1–2 g of dried mushrooms.[145] Sympathomimetic symptoms occur at lower doses (3–5 mg), and psychological effects are elicited by doses above 8 mg.[124] Psychological effects begin within 30 minutes of ingestion, peak at 2–3 hours, and dissipate by 12 hours.[39]

Physiological changes are less pronounced than with LSD and are composed mainly of mydriasis and slight elevation in blood pressure and heart rate.[39] The psychological experience is similar to that with other indolealkylamine and phenethylamine hallucinogens, and cross-tolerance develops rapidly.[73,129] Some users report a more spiritual experience with psilocybin, but this may stem from its well-known use historically in spiritual ceremonies. Griffiths et al. conducted a double-blind controlled study in which hallucinogen-naïve subjects were given either psilocybin or amphetamine under conditions that would foster a spiritual experience. In this study, psilocybin occasioned sustained experiences similar to spontaneously occurring mystical experiences.[58]

In recent years there is a growing body of preclinical and clinical research into the physiological and psychological effects of psilocybin. An imaging study (on healthy humans receiving two doses of psilocybin—0.160 mg/kg and 0.215 mg/kg) showed increased perfusion in distinct right hemispheric frontal and temporal regions and bilaterally in the anterior insula, and decreased perfusion in left hemispheric parietal and temporal cortices and left subcortical regions.[88a] Potential therapeutic effects being explored include substance use disorders, depression, and anxiety.[75] Only one-third of magic mushrooms bought on the street actually contain psilocybin (many are simply store-bought mushrooms laced with PCP) and there are many wild poisonous mushrooms. Adulteration and misidentification seem to be a common cause of serious adverse outcomes.

Ibogaine

The indole alkaloid ibogaine is the most abundant hallucinogenic constituent present in the root bark of the West African rainforest shrub *Tabernanthe iboga*.[131] Extracts derived from this plant have a long history of traditional medicinal and ceremonial use by local people.[12,13] Ibogaine has been used as an experimental treatment for drug dependence since the 1960s,[10] particularly for cocaine and heroin dependence,[92,93] and recently clinical studies are emerging indicating that indeed it may be effective. The mechanism of action of ibogaine is unclear, and most probably includes several neurological receptors and transporters, including the sigma-2, kappa- and mu-opioid, serotonergic (5HT2 and 5HT3) receptors, α3β4 nicotinic receptors, and the *N*-methyl-D-aspartate (NMDA) ion channel.[50,93]

Despite evidence indicating the efficacy of ibogaine in treating substance use disorders, there are several concerns regarding its toxicity. Nausea and tremors have been reported following oral doses of ibogaine at 500, 600, and 800 mg.[96] In addition to these adverse effects, vomiting, and ataxia are common symptoms following

ibogaine ingestion.[131] Although these symptoms may resolve without further adverse effects, in other cases they herald the onset of more severe and, sometimes, life-threating clinical effects. These can include coma,[117] seizures,[24] respiratory difficulties,[11] cardiac arrhythmias,[126] and pulmonary aspiration.[11]

Because ibogaine is achieving widespread popularity for both recreational use as well as an alternate therapy for substance use disorders, there remains insufficient data regarding its efficacy and toxicity. Although a maximal oral dosage of 1 mg/kg has been suggested, using appropriate clinical trials to establish evidence of efficacy, and more importantly establish safe dose, are critical to prevent unnecessary deaths in individuals seeking treatment for substance use disorders.

Phenethylamine Hallucinogens

Mescaline

Mescaline (3,4,5-trimethoxyphenylethylamine), is a phenethylamine hallucinogen naturally found in several species of North and South American cacti. These cacti have been dubbed the "Divine Cacti" in reference to their several thousand year history of spiritual use by natives of Northern Mexico and the Southwestern United States. The North American peyote cactus, *Lophophora williamsii*, is a small, spineless cactus that grows in the Rio Grande and in parts of the Mexican plateau.

Mescaline was first isolated from peyote cacti in 1896 and was synthesized approximately 20 years later. It is extracted from the head (top) of the cactus, which must be carefully cut at ground level to allow regrowth. Improper harvesting will kill the plant.[94] Because of improper harvesting in Southern Texas, peyote is now listed as an endangered species. Peyote, like the other serotonergic hallucinogens is a Schedule I compound. However, many states allow "bona fide religious" use by members of the Native American Church.

Natural peyote has a bitter taste. It is dried and chewed, soaked in water, and drunk or injected. Mescaline is typically sold as disk-shaped "buttons" composed of either crushed peyote or synthetic mescaline. Genuine peyote is rare outside of the southwestern United States, with less than 17% of street samples actually containing mescaline.[134] The hallucinogenic dose is approximately 5 mg/kg (0.3–0.5 g). Each button contains about 50–100 mg of mescaline,[134] and users typically ingest 3–8 buttons.[81]

Mescaline is markedly less tolerable than the other serotonergic hallucinogens. Within the first 30 minutes, before the onset of psychological symptoms, users experience nausea, vomiting, restlessness, and headaches.[39,68] By 1–2 hours, however, these unpleasant physiological symptoms dissipate, and the psychic phase characterized by euphoria, sensory distortions, and feelings of confidence begins. The entire experience lasts up to 14 hours.[39,68] Treatment of acute intoxication and adverse consequences, as with LSD and psilocybin, involves reassurance (talking down) and use of benzodiazepines, if necessary.

3,4-Methylenedioxymethamphetamine (MDMA)

3,4-Methylenedioxymethamphetamine (MDMA/Ecstasy) is a synthetic drug that differs from traditional indolealkylamine and phenethylamine serotonergic hallucinogens in structure, pharmacology, and psychoactive properties, falling somewhere between amphetamine and mescaline. MDMA was first synthesized in

1912. It was patented as a precursor for a psychotherapeutic agent in 1914, as a cough suppressant in 1956, as a tranquilizer in 1960, and as an appetite suppressant in 1961, but it was never marketed.[30] In the early 1980s, MDMA was used in psychotherapy and was purported to improve self-esteem and therapeutic communication.[55] In 1985 the US Drug Enforcement Administration classified MDMA as a Schedule I drug. The United Nations Office on Drugs and Crime Report from 2015 indicates that up to 9,340,000 people globally reported use within the past year. Its use seems to be on the decline in the Americas, where MDMA seizures dropped by 81% between 2009 and 2012. The largest Ecstasy markets are currently East and Southeast Asia and Oceania.[153]

Pharmacology

Although MDMA promotes the release and inhibits the breakdown of all monoamine neurotransmitters (serotonin, dopamine, and norepinephrine), its most potent and probably most psychologically important interactions are with the serotonin system.[45,82] In addition to releasing serotonin and inhibiting its breakdown by monoamine oxidase, MDMA blocks serotonin reuptake by the serotonin transporter. In total, these actions lead to an acute increase of monoamines in the synaptic cleft followed by neuronal completion within 4–6 hours.[25,38,55,106] This depletion is exacerbated by its acute inhibition of tryptophan hydroxylase, the rate-limiting enzyme in the synthesis of serotonin.[21] The rank order of potency for stimulating monoamine release is norepinephrine = serotonin > dopamine.[122] It is hypothesized that the psychological effects result from MDMA's effects on the serotonin system, while its physiological effects are adrenergically mediated.[154]

In addition to these amphetamine-like effects, MDMA has affinity for 5HT2, M1-muscarinic, H1-histaminergic, and α2-adrenergic receptors, but the clinical significance of this receptor-binding profile is unclear. MDMA also indirectly raises blood levels of adrenocorticotropin-releasing hormone, antidiuretic hormone, cortisol, dehydroepiandrosterone, oxytocin, and prolactin.[38,150] Oxytocin and prolactin are naturally released following orgasm and childbirth and are thought to facilitate bonding. It has been hypothesized that MDMA-mediated release of these hormones results in the sense of intimacy central to the MDMA experience.[120,150]

MDMA is hepatically metabolized via the cytochrome P450 (CYP) system.[55] It has saturable kinetics, meaning that at higher doses metabolism is slower and toxicity is disproportionably more likely.[36,37,55] So far, identified metabolites include 3,4-methylenedioxyamphetamine, 4-hydroxy-3-methoxy-methamphetamine, 4-hydroxy-3-methoxyamphetamine, 3,4-dihydroxyamphetamine (also called alpha-methyldopamine), 3,4-methylenedioxyphenylacetone, and N-hydroxy-3,4-methylenedioxyamphetamine. The contribution of these metabolites to the psychoactive and toxic effects of MDMA is an area of active research.[157]

3,4-Methylenedioxyamphetamine is known to be psychoactive and like MDMA it causes release of serotonin and produces an empathogenic experience.[74,133] It also resembles the traditional serotonergic hallucinogens in that it has higher affinity for the 5HT2A receptor and produces more profound sensory disturbances. Much of the toxicity associated with MDMA has been attributed to this metabolite.[33] In addition to being a metabolite of MDMA, 3,4-methylenedioxyamphetamine has been synthesized and is used recreationally under the name MDA, or "Mellow Drug of America."

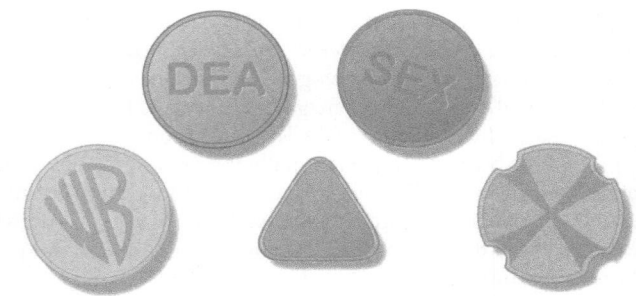

• **Fig. 31.3** Examples of 3,4-methylenedioxymethamphetamine. (MDMA; from the US Drug Enforcement Administration website.)

Street Information

MDMA is universally referred to as Ecstasy, but its street names include "XTC," "X," "E," "M," "Rolls," "Beans," "Disco Biscuit," "Adam," "Clarity," "Lovers speed," and "Hug Drug." The practices of combining MDMA with LSD or psilocybin to produce a more powerful psychological experience are referred to as "Candy Flipping" and "Hippie Flipping," respectively. Mentholated products such as cigarettes or vapor rub are often used to heighten the drug's effects.

MDMA is distributed as small single-dose tablets of various colors often decorated with icons or phrases (Fig. 31.3). These tablets usually contain 15–150 mg of MDMA. The tablet form lends a pharmaceutical appearance and a false impression that the contents are safe and uncontaminated. However, pure MDMA, as described below, is considerably less safe than perceived by most users, and often the contents are contaminated with acetaminophen, stimulants, or other hallucinogens.[20,53,136,162,164] Although MDMA is usually ingested orally, the tablets can be either crushed and snorted or dissolved and injected.[103,129]

MDMA is classified with other synthetic drugs such as gamma-hydroxy-butyrate, ketamine, and flunitrazepam as a club drug because of its popularity at dance parties, raves, and night clubs. In fact, it has been estimated that MDMA is present at 70% of raves, making it the most prevalent club drug.[77] Among 12th graders in the United States, 4.9% reported lifetime use of MDMA, and among individuals age 18–25 in the United States, 13.1% reported lifetime use.[29]

Physiological and Psychological Effects

MDMA is structurally similar to both amphetamine and mescaline; however, it seems less stimulating and addictive than amphetamine and produces less profound sensory distortions than mescaline and the other serotonergic hallucinogens.[26]

Physiological effects include sympathomimetic symptoms such as tachycardia, mydriasis, diaphoresis, tremor, and hypertension.[115] Urinary retention, esophoria (eyes turning inward), trismus, and bruxism, are also common.[72] MDMA users attempt to avoid the latter by sucking lollipops.[141] Of interest, with repeated administration these adverse effects become more pronounced and the sought-after psychological experiences diminish.[56]

The psychological experience begins 30–60 minutes following oral ingestion, peaks at 60–90 minutes, and last from 4 to 8 hours.[55,136] Users initially feel agitated, have decreased thirst and hunger, and experience a distorted sense of time. This is followed by increased energy with euphoria, enhanced sense of intimacy, and social tolerance.[42,59,105] Its effects on sociality have earned it the vernacular name "the luv drug" and the proposed pharmacological classification as an entactogen or empathogen.[112,156] Several days after ingestion of MDMA, users tend to experience depressive symptoms, referred to as "the midweek blues."[34,56,112,156,158]

In recent years there is increased interest regarding the therapeutic potential of MDMA in the treatment of posttraumatic stress disorder (PTSD). Initial clinical trials exploring the efficacy of MDMA-assisted psychotherapy (MDMA-AP) show significant improvements in treatment-resistant cases, and effect sizes are comparable with those of well-established therapies (such as prolonged exposure).[20a] Dropout rates for MDMA-AP were also reported to be lower than those cited in established psychotherapies for PTSD, indicating that this may be a promising treatment for this disorder. As of 2019, MDMA-AP psychotherapy for PTSD has entered the Phase 3 stage of drug development.

Adverse Effects

Untoward psychological experiences of MDMA include overarousal, sensory illusions, depersonalization, anxiety, and occasionally panic attacks.[125,158,164] As is the case with LSD-induced bad trip, benzodiazepines may be helpful.[99,118]

There is a growing body of evidence regarding potentially negative effects of MDMA on the brain. Deficits have been demonstrated in retrospective memory, prospective memory, higher cognition, complex visual processing, sleep architecture, sleep apnea, pain, neurohormonal activity, and psychiatric status. Neuroimaging studies have shown serotonergic deficits, which are associated with lifetime MDMA use, and a degree of neurocognitive impairment.[119] Despite this, much of this research includes heavy users and it is yet unclear what neurobiological long-term effects exist in casual, moderate users.[121]

MDMA use has been associated with severe life-threatening adverse consequences.[128] The risk of death for first-time users is estimated to be between 1 in 2000 and 1 in 50,000.[52] MDMA has received much of its notoriety for causing severe hyperpyrexia leading to rhabdomyolysis, disseminated intravascular coagulopathy, and multiorgan failure.[65] Via its effects on serotonin and dopamine, MDMA resets the body's internal thermostat. This is compounded by the hot, aerobically intensive dance party venues where it is often used[63] and by the frequent augmentation with diuretics such as alcohol and caffeine.

MDMA users are also susceptible to developing another hyperthermic condition—serotonin syndrome—particularly if they have ingested other serotonergic drugs. This is not unlikely given the multitude of drugs with effects on serotonin. Recreational drugs such as amphetamines or cocaine may intentionally be combined with MDMA. Inadvertent use of prescribed antidepressants as well as purposeful use of these drugs to boost the psychological effects of MDMA is also common. Unusual serotonin reuptake inhibitors such as phenylpiperidine opioids (methadone, meperidine, tramadol, propoxyphene) and monoamine oxidase inhibitors such as linezolid and isoniazid and ritonavir in combination with LSD might also precipitate a serotonin syndrome.[48,114] Serotonin syndrome is characterized by muscle rigidity, shivering, tremor, and increased deep tendon reflexes. The excessive muscle contraction leads to hyperthermia.[48] The associated mortality rate is 10%–15%.[59]

MDMA is associated with a host of other life-threatening consequences. It directly increases antidiuretic hormone release.[64] This combined with overhydration in response to the well-publicized concern of hyperthermia may induce dilutional hyponatremia and subsequent cerebral edema.[62,97] Symptoms include headache, delirium, irritability, nystagmus, and fatal cerebral herniation.[45] Perhaps because of its sympathomimetic properties,

there have been numerous case reports of an association with intracranial hemorrhage, venous sinus thrombosis,[49,61,71,130] and sudden death due to cardiac arrhythmias.[59,65,102,147] Of interest, there also appears to be an association, for unclear reasons, with pneumothoraces and pneumomediastinum.[16,19,98,127] Unrelated to hyperthermia-induced multiorgan failure, MDMA can cause liver failure that likely is mediated by a hypersensitivity reaction.[17,41,43] In individuals younger than 25-years-old, Ecstasy is a common cause of hepatic injury and should be suspected in any young person presenting with liver damage.[17]

Management of Acute Toxicity

Activated charcoal may be used in the acute management of MDMA toxicity in the unlikely scenario that the individual presents within 1 hour of ingestion. Otherwise, management involves fluid replacement in dehydrated patients with hypotension and tachycardia and use of labetalol for tachycardia and hypertension. Antihypertensive medications blocking both α- and β-adrenergic receptors are preferable. Unopposed β-receptor blockade may worsen hypertension due to loss of β-adrenergic–mediated vasodilation. Treatment of severe hyperthermia, whether due directly to MDMA or MDMA-induced serotonin syndrome, involves rapid cooling and supportive measures provided in an intensive care setting. Severe cases require sedation, intubation, and paralysis to decrease heat production from muscle contraction.[59] It is unclear at this point whether dantrolene is helpful.[59]

Conclusions

In conclusion, many serotonergic hallucinogens are naturally occurring compounds that have been used for thousands of years in spiritual practice and to induce perception-altering experiences. Fascination with these mind-altering drugs continues as clandestine chemists persist in synthesizing more varieties. Preclinical and clinical studies continue to shed light on the various neurobiological mechanisms involved in mediating the effects of serotonergic hallucinogens. Several physiological and psychological adverse effects of hallucinogen use have been repeatedly reported. Alongside these adverse effects warranting concern, there is growing interest and evidence regarding therapeutic effects of these substances in psychiatry and neurology.

References

1. Abraham H, Aldridge AM, Gogia P. The psychopharmacology of hallucinogens. *Neuropsychopharmacology*. 1996;14:285–298.
2. Abraham HD. A chronic impairment of colour vision in users of LSD. *Br J Psychiatry*. 1982;140:518–520.
3. Abraham HD. Visual phenomenology of the LSD flashback. *Arch Gen Psychiatry*. 1983;40:884–889.
4. Abraham HD, Aldridge AM. Adverse consequences of lysergic acid diethylamide. *Addiction*. 1993;88:1327–1334.
5. Abraham HD, Mamen A. LSD-like panic from risperidone in post-LSD visual disorder. *J Clin Psychopharmacol*. 1996;16:238–241.
6. Abraham HD, Wolf E. Visual function in past users of LSD: psychophysical findings. *J Abnorm Psychol*. 1988:443–447.
7. Administration Substance Abuse and Mental Health Services. *Results from the 2013 National Survey on Drug Use and Health: Summary of National Findings*. NSDUH Series H-48, HHS Publication No. (SMA) 14–4863. Rockville, MD: Author; 2014.
8. Alarcon RD, Dickinson WA, Dohn HH. Flashback phenomena. Clinical and diagnostic dilemmas. *J Nerv Ment Dis*. 1982;170:217–223.

9. Aldurra G, Crayton JW. Improvement of hallucinogen persisting perception disorder by treatment with a combination of fluoxetine and olanzapine: case report. *J Clin Psychopharmacol.* 2001;21. 343–324.

10. Alper KR, Beal D, Kaplan CD. A contemporary history of ibogaine in the United States and Europe. *Alkaloids Chem Biol.* 2001;56:249–281.

11. Alper KR, Lotsof HS, Geerte GMN, et al. Treatment of acute opioid withdrawal with ibogaine. *Am J Addict.* 1999;8:234–242.

12. Alper KR, Lotsof HS, Kaplan CD. The ibogaine medical subculture. *J Ethnopharmacol.* 2008;115:9–24.

13. Alper KR, Stajić M, Gill JR. Fatalities temporally associated with the ingestion of ibogaine. *J Forensic Sci.* 2012;57:398–412.

14. American Psychiatric Association. *Diagnostic and Statistical Manual of Mental Disorders.* 5th ed. Arlington; 2013.

15. Reference deleted in review.

16. Anderson WHO'Malley JE. Trifluoperazine for the trailing" phenomenon. *JAMA.* 1972;220:1244–1245.

17. Andreu V, Mas A, Bruguera M, et al. Ecstasy: a common cause of severe acute hepatotoxicity. *J Hepatol.* 1998;29:394–397.

18. Appel JB, Freedman DX. Tolerance and cross-tolerance among psychotomimetic drugs. *Psychopharmacologia.* 1968;13:267–274.

19. Badaoui R, El Kettani C, Fikri M, et al. Spontaneous cervical and mediastinal air emphysema after ecstasy abuse. *Anesth Analg.* 2002;95:1123.

20. Baggott M, Heifets B, Jones RT, et al. Chemical analysis of ecstasy pills. *JAMA.* 2000;284:2190.

20a. Bahji A, Forsyth A, Groll D, Hawken ER. Efficacy of 3,4-methylenedioxymethamphetamine (MDMA)-assisted psychotherapy for posttraumatic stress disorder: A systematic review and meta-analysis. *Prog Neuropsychopharmacol Biol Psychiatry.* 2019;96:109735.

21. Bengel D, Murphy DL, Andrews AM, et al. Altered brain serotonin homeostasis and locomotor insensitivity to 3, 4-methylenedioxymethamphetamine ("Ecstasy") in serotonin transporter-deficient mice. *Mol Pharmacol.* 1998;53:649–655.

22. Blaho K, Merigian K, Winbery S, et al. Clinical pharmacology of lysergic acid diethylamide: case reports and review of the treatment of intoxication. *Am J Ther.* 1997;4:211–221.

23. Bogenschutz MP, Forcehimes AA, Pommy JA, et al. Psilocybin-assisted treatment for alcohol dependence: a proof-of-concept study. *J Psychopharmacol.* 2015;29:289–299.

24. Breuer L, Kasper BS, Schwarze B, et al. "Herbal seizures" - atypical symptoms after ibogaine intoxication: a case report. *J Med Case Reports 2015.* 2015;91(58):1666–1672.

25. Brodkin J, Malyala A, Nash JF. Effect of acute monoamine depletion on 3,4-methylenedioxymethamphetamine-induced neurotoxicity. *Pharmacol Biochem Behav.* 1993;45:647–653.

26. Cami J, Farre M, Mas M, et al. Human pharmacology of 3,4-methylenedioxymeth-amphetamine ("ecstacy"): psychomotor performance and subjective effects. *J Clin Psychopharmacol.* 2000;20:455–466.

27. Caporael LR. Ergotism: the satan loosed in Salem? *Science.* 1976;192(80):21–26.

28. Carhart-Harris RL, Kaelen M, Bolstridge M, et al. The paradoxical psychological effects of lysergic acid diethylamide (LSD). *Psychol Med.* 2016;46:1379–1390.

29. Center for Behavioral Health Statistics and Quality. *2015 National Survey on Drug Use and Health.* Rockville, MD: Substance Abuse and Mental Health Services Administration; 2016.

30. Climko RP, Roehrich H, Sweeney DR, Al-Razi J. Ecstacy: a review of MDMA and MDA. *Int J Psychiatry Med.* 1987;16:359–372.

31. Cohen S. The hallucinogens and the inhalants. *Psychiatr Clin North Am.* 1984;7:681–688.

32. Reference deleted in review.

33. Colado MI, Williams JL, Green AR. The hyperthermic and neurotoxic effects of "Ecstasy" (MDMA) and 3,4 methylenedioxyamphetamine (MDA) in the Dark Agouti (DA) rat, a model of the CYP2D6 poor metabolizer phenotype. *Br J Pharmacol.* 1995;115:1281–1289.

34. Curran HV, Travill RA. Mood and cognitive effects of 3,4-methylenedioxymethamphetamine (MDMA, "ecstasy"): week-end "high" followed by mid-week low. *Addiction.* 1997;92:821–831.

35. Curry SCRose MC. Intravenous mushroom poisoning. *Ann Emerg Med.* 1985;14:900–902.

36. de la Torre R, Farré M, Ortuño J, et al. Non-linear pharmacokinetics of MDMA ('ecstasy') in humans. *Br J Clin Pharmacol.* 2000;49:104–109.

37. de la Torre R, Farré M, Roset PN, et al. Pharmacology of MDMA in humans. *Ann N Y Acad Sci.* 2000;914:225–237.

38. de la Torre R, Farré M, Roset PN, et al. Human pharmacology of MDMA: pharmacokinetics, metabolism, and disposition. *Ther Drug Monit.* 2004;26:137–144.

39. DiSclafani A, Hall RC, Gardner ER. Drug-induced psychosis: emergency diagnosis and management. *Psychosomatics.* 1981;22:845–855.

40. Dolder PC, Schmid Y, Haschke M, et al. Pharmacokinetics and concentration-effect relationship of oral LSD in humans. *Int J Neuropsychopharmacol.* 2016;19:1–7.

41. Ellis AJ, Wendon JA, Portmann B, Williams R. Acute liver damage and ecstasy ingestion. *Gut.* 1996;38:454–458.

42. European Monitoring Centre for Drugs and Drug Addiction. *Annual Report on the State of the Drugs Problem in the European Union and Norway.* Lisbon: EMCDDA; 2003.

43. Fidler H, Dhillon A, Gertner D, Burroughs A. Chronic ecstasy (3,4-methylenedioxymetamphetamine) abuse: a recurrent and unpredictable cause of severe acute hepatitis. *J Hepatol.* 1996;25:563–566.

44. Fiorella D, Helsley S, Lorrain DS, et al. The role of the 5-HT2A and 5-HT2C receptors in the stimulus effects of hallucinogenic drugs III: the mechanistic basis for supersensitivity to the LSD stimulus following serotonin depletion. *Psychopharmacology (Berl).* 1995;121:364–372.

45. Gahlinger PM. Club drugs: MDMA, gamma-hydroxybutyrate (GHB), rohypnol, and ketamine. *Am Fam Physician.* 2004;69:2619–2626.

45a. Garcia-Romeu A, Kersgaard B, Addy PH. Clinical applications of hallucinogens: a review. *Exp Clin Psychopharmacol.* 2016;24(4):229–268.

46. Garratt JC, Alreja M, Aghajanian GK. LSD has high efficacy relative to serotonin in enhancing the cationic current Ih: intracellular studies in rat facial motoneurons. *Synapse.* 1993;13:123–134.

47. Gasser P, Kirchner K, Passie T. LSD-assisted psychotherapy for anxiety associated with a life-threatening disease: a qualitative study of acute and sustained subjective effects. *J Psychopharmacol.* 2015;29:57–68.

48. Gillman PK. Monoamine oxidase inhibitors, opioid analgesics and serotonin toxicity. *Br J Anaesth.* 2005;95:434–441.

49. Gledhill JA, Moore DF, Bell D, Henry JA. Subarachnoid haemorrhage associated with MDMA abuse. *J Neurol Neurosurg Psychiatry.* 1993;56:1036–1037.

50. Glick SD, Maisonneuve IM, Kitchen BA, Fleck MW. Antagonism of α3β4 nicotinic receptors as a strategy to reduce opioid and stimulant self-administration. *Eur J Pharmacol.* 2002;438:99–105.

51. Goodman C, Bor O, Lev-Ran S. Synthetic cannabis substances (SPS) use and hallucinogen persisting perception disorder (HPPD): two case reports. *Isr J Psychiatry Relat Sci.* 2014;51:277–280.

52. Gore SM. Fatal uncertainty: death-rate from use of ecstasy or heroin. *Lancet.* 1999;354:1265–1266.

53. Graeme KA. New drugs of abuse. *Emerg Med Clin North Am.* 2000;18:625–636.

54. Reference deleted in review.

55. Green AR, Mechan AO, Elliott JM, et al. The pharmacology and clinical pharmacology of 3,4-methylenedioxymethamphetamine (MDMA, ecstasy"). *Pharmacol Rev.* 2003;55:463–508.

56. Greer GT, olbert R. Subjective reports of the effects of MDMA in a clinical setting. *J Psychoactive Drugs.* 1986;18:319–327.

57. Greiner T, Burch NR, Edelberg R. Psychopathology and psychophysiology of minimal LSD-25 dosage. *AMA Arch Neurol Psychiatry.* 1958;79:208–210.

58. Griffiths RR, Richards WA, McCann U, Jesse R. Psilocybin can occasion mystical-type experiences having substantial and sustained personal meaning and spiritual significance. *Psychopharmacology (Berl).* 2006;187:268–283.

59. Hall APHenry JA. Acute toxic effects of "Ecstasy" (MDMA) and related compounds: overview of pathophysiology and clinical management. *Br J Anaesth.* 2006;96:678–685.

60. Harner MM. *Hallucinogens and Shamanism.* London: Oxford University Press; 1973.

61. Harries DPDe Silva R. "Ecstasy" and intracerebral haemorrhage. *Scott Med J.* 1992;37:150–152.

62. Hartung TK, Schofield E, Short AI, et al. Hyponatraemic states following 3,4-methylenedioxymethamphetamine (MDMA, "ecstasy") ingestion. *QJM.* 2002;95:431–437.

63. Henry JA. Ecstasy and the dance of death. *BMJ.* 1992;305:5–6.

64. Henry JA, Fallon JK, Kicman AT, et al. Low-dose MDMA ("ecstasy") induces vasopressin secretion. *Lancet.* 1998;351:1784.

65. Henry JA, Jeffreys KJ, Dawling S. Toxicity and deaths from 3,4-methylenedioxymethamphetamine ("ecstasy"). *Lancet.* 1992;340:384–387.

66. Hoch PH, Cattell JP, Pennes HH. Effects of mescaline and lysergic acid (d-LSD-25). *Am J Psychiatry.* 1952;108:579–584.

67. Hofmann A. *LSD: My Problem Child.* New York: McGraw-Hill; 1980.

68. Hollister LE, Hartman AM. Mescaline, lysergic acid diethylamide and psilocybin: comparison of clinical syndromes, effects on color perception and biochemical measures. *Compr Psychiatry.* 1962;3:235–241.

69. Horowitz MJ. Flashbacks: recurrent intrusive images after the use of LSD. *Am J Psychiatry.* 1969;126:565–569.

70. Hoyer D, Hannon JP, Martin GR. Molecular, pharmacological and functional diversity of 5-HT receptors. *Pharmacol Biochem Behav.* 2002;71:533–554.

71. Hughes JC, McCabe M, Evans RJ. Intracranial haemorrhage associated with ingestion of "ecstasy". *Emerg Med J.* 1993;10:372–374.

72. Inman DS, Greene D. The agony and the ecstasy: acute urinary retention after MDMA abuse. *BJU Int.* 2003;91:123.

73. Isbell H, Wolbach AB, Wikler A, Miner EJ. Cross tolerance between LSD and psilocybin. *Psychopharmacologia.* 1961;2:147–159.

74. Johnson MP, Hoffman AJ, Nichols DE. Effects of the enantiomers of MDA, MDMA and related analogues on [3H]serotonin and [3H]dopamine release from superfused rat brain slices. *Eur J Pharmacol.* 1986;132:269–276.

75. Johnson MW, Griffiths RR. Potential therapeutic effects of psilocybin. *Neurotherapeutics.* 2017;14:734–740.

76. Johnston L, O'Malley P, Bachman J, Schulenberg JE. *Monitoring the Future National Results on Adolescent Drug Use: Overview of Key Findings, 2007* (NIH publication no. 08–6418). Bethesda, MD: National Institute on Drug Abuse; 2008.

77. Johnston LD, O'Malley PM, Bachman JG. *Monitoring the Future National Results on Adolescent Drug Use: Overview of Key Findings, 2002* (NIH publication no. 03–5374). Bethesda, MD: National Institute on Drug Abuse; 2003.

78. Katz MM, Waskow IE, Olsson J. Characterizing the psychological state produced by LSD. *J Abnorm Psychol.* 1968;73:1–14.

79. Keeler MH. Lysergic acid diethylamide. Adverse reactions and use in experimental therapy. *N C Med J.* 1967;28:323–327.

80. Klock JC, Boerner U, Becker CE. Coma, hyperthermia and bleeding associated with massive LSD overdose. A report of eight cases. *West J Med.* 1974;120:183–188.

81. Leikin JB, Krantz AJ, Zell-Kanter M, et al. Clinical features and management of intoxication due to hallucinogenic drugs. *Med Toxicol Adverse Drug Exp.* 1989;4:324–350.

82. Leonardi ETAzmitia EC. MDMA (ecstasy) inhibition of MAO type A and type B: comparisons with fenfluramine and fluoxetine (Prozac). *Neuropsychopharmacology.* 1994;10:231–238.

83. Lerner A, Gelkopf M, Skladman I. Flashback and hallucinogen persisting perception disorder: clinical aspects and pharmacological treatment approach. *Isr J Psychiatry Relat Sci.* 2002;39:92–99.

84. Lerner AG, Gelkopf M, Oyffe I, et al. LSD-induced hallucinogen persisting perception disorder treatment with clonidine: an open pilot study. *Int Clin Psychopharmacol.* 2000;8:35–37.

85. Lerner AG, Gelkopf M, Skladman I, et al. Clonazepam treatment of lysergic acid diethylamide-induced hallucinogen persisting perception disorder with anxiety features. *Int Clin Psychopharmacol.* 2003;18:101–105.

86. Lerner AG, Lev-Ran S. LSD-associated "Alice in Wonderland Syndrome" (AIWS): a hallucinogen persisting perception disorder (HPPD) case report. *Isr J Psychiatry Relat Sci.* 2015;52:67–68.

87. Lerner AG, Oyffe I, Isaacs G, Sigal M. Naltrexone treatment of hallucinogen persisting perception disorder. *Am J Psychiatry.* 1997;154:437.

88. Lerner AG, Rudinski D, Bor O, Goodman C. Flashbacks and HPPD: a clinical-oriented concise review. *Isr J Psychiatry Relat Sci.* 2014;51:296–301.

88a. Lewis CR, Preller KH, Kraehenmann R, et al. Two dose investigation of the 5-HT-agonist psilocybin on relative and global cerebral blood flow. *Neuroimage.* 2017;159:70–78.

89. Lindenblatt H, Krämer E, Holzmann-Erens P, et al. Quantitation of psilocin in human plasma by high-performance liquid chromatography and electrochemical detection: comparison of liquid–liquid extraction with automated on-line solid-phase extraction. *J Chromatogr B Biomed Sci Appl.* 1998;709:255–263.

90. Linton HB, Langs RJ. Subjective reactions to lysergic acid diethylamide (LSD-25). *Arch Gen Psychiatry.* 1962;6:352–368.

91. Lisansky J, Strassman RJ, Janowsky D, et al. *Transient Psychosis: Diagnosis, Management and Evaluation.* New York: Brunner/Mazel; 1984.

92. Lotsof HS, Alexander NE. Case studies of ibogaine treatment: implications for patient management strategies. *Alkaloids Chem Biol.* 2001;56:293–313.

93. Mačiulaitis R, Kontrimavičiūtė V, Bressolle F, Briedis V. Ibogaine, an anti-addictive drug: pharmacology and time to go further in development. A narrative review. *Hum Exp Toxicol.* 2008;27:181–194.

94. Mack RB. Marching to a different cactus: peyote (mescaline) intoxication. *N C Med J.* 1986;47:137–138.

95. Markel H, Lee A, Holmes RD, Domino EF. LSD flashback syndrome exacerbated by selective serotonin reuptake inhibitor antidepressants in adolescents. *J Pediatr.* 1994;125:817–819.

96. Mash DC, Kovera CA, Buck BE, et al. Medication development of ibogaine as a pharmacotherapy for drug dependence. *Ann N Y Acad Sci.* 1998;844:274–292.

97. Maxwell DL, Polkey MI, Henry JA. Hyponatraemia and catatonic stupor after taking ecstasy". *BMJ.* 1993;307:1993.

98. Mazur SHitchcock T. Spontaneous pneumomediastinum, pneumothorax and ecstasy abuse. *Emerg Med Australas.* 2001;13:121–123.

99. McCann UD, Ricaurte GA, Irwin I, Langston JW. MDMA ('ecstasy') and panic disorder: Induction by a single dose. *Biol Psychiatry.* 1992;32:950–953.

100. McGee R. Flashbacks and memory phenomena. A comment on "Flashback phenomena-clinical and diagnostic dilemmas". *J Nerv Ment Dis.* 1984;172:273–278.

101. Miller NS. *The principles and Practice of Addictions in Psychiatry.* Philadelphia: WB Saunders Company; 1997.

102. Milroy CM, Clark JC, Forrest AR. Pathology of deaths associated with ecstasy" and eve" misuse. *J Clin Pathol.* 1996;49:149–153.

103. Moore KA, Mozayani A, Fierro MF, Poklis A. Distribution of 3,4-methylenedioxymethamphetamine (MDMA) and 3,4-methylenedioxyamphetamine (MDA) stereoisomers in a fatal poisoning. *Forensic Sci Int.* 1996;83:111–119.

104. Morehead DB. Exacerbation of hallucinogen-persisting perception disorder with risperidone. *J Clin Psychopharmacol*. 1997;17:327–328.

105. Mørland J. Toxicity of drug abuse-amphetamine designer drugs (ecstasy): mental effects and consequences of single dose use. *Toxicol Lett*. 2000;112–113:147–152.

106. Morton J. Ecstasy. Pharmacology and neurotoxicity. *Curr Opin Pharmacol*. 2005;5:79–86.

107. Moskowitz D. Use of haloperidol to reduce LSD flashbacks. *Mil Med*. 1971;136:754–756.

108. Reference deleted in review.

109. National Drug Intelligence Center. *National Drug Threat Assessment 2006 (Product no. 2006-Q0317–001)*. Johnstown, PA: Author; 2006.

110. National Institute on Drug Abuse. *Research Report Series: Hallucinogens and Dissociative Drugs* (NIH publication no. 01–4209); 2001.

111. National Institute on Drug Abuse. *Epidemiologic trends in drug abuse: advance report (NIH publication no. . {x=[–]}. A)*. Bethesda, MD: Department of Health and Human Services, National Institutes of Health; 2006:06–5878.

112. Nichols DE. Differences between the mechanism of action of MDMA, MBDB, and the classic hallucinogens. Identification of a new therapeutic class: entactogens. *J Psychoactive Drugs*. 1986;18:305–313.

113. Nichols DE. Hallucinogens. *Pharmacol Ther*. 2004;101:131–181.

114. Oesterheld JR, Armstrong SC, Cozza KL. Ecstasy: pharmacodynamic and pharmacokinetic interactions. *Psychosomatics*. 2004;45:84–87.

115. Olson KR. *Poisoning & Drug Overdose*. 4th ed. Lange Medical New York: Books/McGraw-Hill; 2004.

116. Ouagazzal A, Grottick AJ, Moreau J, Higgins GA. Effect of LSD on prepulse inhibition and spontaneous behavior in the rat. A pharmacological analysis and comparison between two rat strains. *Neuropsychopharmacology*. 2001;25:565–575.

117. Paling FP, Andrews LM, Valk GD, Blom HJ. Life-threatening complications of ibogaine: three case reports. *Netherl J Med*. 2012;70:422–424.

118. Pallanti SMazzi D. MDMA (ecstasy) precipitation of panic disorder. *Biol Psychiatry*. 1992;32:91–95.

119. Parrott AC. Human psychobiology of MDMA or "Ecstasy": an overview of 25 years of empirical research. *Hum Psychopharmacol Clin Exp*. 2013;28:289–307.

120. Parrott AC, Buchanan T, Scholey AB, et al. Ecstasy/MDMA attributed problems reported by novice, moderate and heavy recreational users. *Hum Psychopharmacol Clin Exp*. 2002;17:309–312.

121. Parrott AC, Downey LA, Roberts CA, et al. Recreational 3,4-methylenedioxymethamphetamine or "ecstasy": current perspective and future research prospects. *J Psychopharmacol*. 2017;31:959–966.

122. Partilla JS, Dersch CM, Yu H, et al. Neurochemical neutralization of amphetamine-type stimulants in rat brain by the indatraline analog (-)-HY038. *Brain Res Bull*. 2000;53:821–826.

123. Passie T, Halpern JH, Stichtenoth DO, et al. The pharmacology of lysergic acid diethylamide: a review. *CNS Neurosci Ther*. 2008;14:295–314.

124. Passie T, Seifert J, Schneider U, Emrich HM. The pharmacology of psilocybin. *Addict Biol*. 2002;7:357–364.

125. Peroutka SJ, Newman H, Harris H. Subjective effects of 3,4-methylenedioxymethamphetamine in recreational users. *Neuropsychopharmacology*. 1988;1:273–277.

126. Pleskovic A, Gorjup V, Brvar M, Kozelj G. Ibogaine-associated ventricular tachyarrhythmias. *Clin Toxicol*. 2012;50:157.

127. Quin GI, McCarthy GM, Harries DK. Spontaneous pneumomediastinum and ecstasy abuse. *J Accid Emerg Med*. 1999;16:382.

128. Rejali D, Glen P, Odom N. Pneumomediastinum following ecstasy (methylenedioxymetamphetamine, MDMA) ingestion in two people at the same "rave". *J Laryngol Otol*. 2002;116:75–76.

129. Rohrig TP, Prouty RW. Tissue distribution of methylenedioxymethamphetamine. *J Anal Toxicol*. 1992;16:52–53.

130. Rothwell PM, Grant R. Cerebral venous sinus thrombosis induced by "ecstasy". *J Neurol Neurosurg Psychiatry*. 1993;56:1035.

131. Schep LJ, Slaughter RJ, Galea S, Newcombe D. Ibogaine for treating drug dependence. What is a safe dose. *Drug Alcohol Depend*. 2016;166:1–5.

132. Schiff PL. Ergot and its Alkaloids. *Am J Pharm Educ*. 2006;70:98. https://doi.org/10.5688/aj700598.

133. Schmidt CJ. Acute administration of methylenedioxymethamphetamine: comparison with the neurochemical effects of its N-desmethyl and N-ethyl analogs. *Eur J Pharmacol*. 1987;136:81–88.

134. Schwartz RH. Mescaline: a survey. *Am Fam Physician*. 1988;37:122–124.

135. Schwartz RH, Comerci GD, Meeks JE. LSD: patterns of use by chemically dependent adolescents. *J Pediatr*. 1987;111:936–938.

136. Schwartz RH, Miller NS. MDMA (ecstasy) and the rave: a review. *Pediatrics*. 1997;100:705–708.

137. Schwarz CJ. Paradoxical responses to chlorpromazine after LSD. *Psychosomatics*. 1967;8:210–211.

138. Sewell RA, Halpern JH, Pope HGJ. Response of cluster headache to psilocybin and LSD. *Neurology*. 2006;66:1920–1922.

138a. Shalit N, Rehm J, Lev-Ran S. Epidemiology of hallucinogen use in the U.S. results from the National Epidemiologic Survey on Alcohol and Related Conditions III. *Addict Behav*. 2019;89:35–43.

139. Shick JFE, Smith DE. Analysis of the LSD flashback. *J Psychedelic Drugs*. 1970;3:13–19.

140. Shulgin A, Shulgin A. *TIHKAL: The Continuation*; 1997.

141. Smith KM, Larive LL, Romanelli F. Club drugs: methylenedioxymethamphetamine, flunitrazepam, ketamine hydrochloride, and gamma-hydroxybutyrate. *Am J Heal Pharm*. 2002;59:1067–1076.

142. Solursh L. Emergency treatment of acute adverse reactions to hallucinogenic drugs. In: Bourne P, ed. *Acute Drug Emergencies*. New York: Academic Press; 1976:139–144.

143. Solursh LP, Clement WR. Use of diazepam in hallucinogenic drug crises. *JAMA J Am Med Assoc*. 1968;205:644–645.

144. Stahl S. Essential Psychopharmacology. *Neuroscientific Basis and Practical Applications*. Cambridge: University Press; 1996.

145. Stamets P. *Psilocybin Mushrooms of the World*. Berkeley: An Identification Guide; 1996.

146. Strassman RJ. Adverse reactions to psychedelic drugs. A review of the literature. *J Nerv Ment Dis*. 1984;172:577–595.

147. Suarez RV, Riemersma R. Ecstasy" and sudden cardiac death. *Am J Forensic Med Pathol*. 1988;9:339–341.

148. Substance Abuse and Mental Health Services Administration. *Results from the 2005 National Survey on Drug Use and Health: National findings (Office of Applied Studies, NSDUH Series H-30, DHHS publication no. SMA . –.)*. Rockville, MD: Author; 2006:06–4194.

149. Tagliazucchi E, Roseman L, Kaelen M, et al. Increased global functional connectivity correlates with LSD-induced ego dissolution. *Curr Biol*. 2016;26:1043–1050.

150. Thompson MR, Callaghan PD, Hunt GE, et al. A role for oxytocin and 5-HT1A receptors in the prosocial effects of 3,4 methylenedioxymethamphetamine ("ecstasy"). *Neuroscience*. 2007;146:509–514.

151. Thurlow HJ, Girvin JDP. Use of anti-epileptic medication in treating flashbacks" from hallucinogenic drugs. *Can Med Assoc J*. 1971;105:947–948.

152. Ungerleider JT, Frank IM. Management of acute panic reactions and drug flashbacks resulting from LSD ingestion. In: Bourne P, ed. *Acute Drug Emergencies*. New York: Academic Press; 1976:133–138.

153. United Nations Office on Drugs and Crime. *World Drug Report 2015 (United Nations publication, Sales No. E.15.XI.6)*. Vienna: Author; 2015.

154. Uys JNiesink R. Pharmacological aspects of the combined use of 3,4-methylenedioxymethamphetamine (MDMA, ecstasy) and gamma-hydroxybutyric acid (GHB): a review of the literature. *Drug Alcohol Rev.* 2005;24:359–368.
155. Vallersnes OM, Dines AM, Wood DM, et al. Psychosis associated with acute recreational drug toxicity: a European case series. *BMC Psychiatry.* 2016;16:293–301.
156. Velea D, Hautefeuille M, Vazeille G, Lantran-Davoux C. Nouvelles drogues synthetiques empathogenes [new synthesis empathogenic agents]. *Encephale.* 1999;25:508–514.
157. Verebey K, Alrazi J, Jaffe JH. The complications of "ecstasy" (MDMA). *JAMA.* 1988;259:1649–1650.
158. Vollenweider FX, Gamma A, Liechti M, Huber T. Psychological and cardiovascular effects and short-term sequelae of MDMA ("ecstasy") in MDMA-Naïve healthy volunteers. *Neuropsychopharmacology.* 1998;19:241–251.
159. Wasson RG. Soma of the Aryans: an Ancient Hallucinogen? *J Psychedelic Drugs.* 1971;3:40–46.
160. Winter JC. Tolerance to a behavioral effect of lysergic acid diethylamide and cross-tolerance to mescaline in the rat: absence of a metabolic component. *J Pharmacol Exp Ther.* 1971;178:625–630.
161. Wolbach AB, Isbell H, Miner EJ. Cross tolerance between mescaline and LSD-25 with a comparison of the mescaline and LSD reactions. *Psychopharmacologia.* 1962;3:1–14.
162. Wolff K, Hay AW, Sherlock K, Conner M. Contents of ecstasy. *Lancet.* 1995;346:1100–1101.
163. Young CR. Sertraline treatment of hallucinogen persisting perception disorder. *J Clin Psychiatry.* 1997;58:85.
164. Ziporyn T. A growing industry and menace: makeshift laboratory's designer drugs. *JAMA J Am Med Assoc.* 1986;256:3061–3063.

32

Ketamine and Phencyclidine

MICHAEL F. WEAVER AND SIDNEY H. SCHNOLL

CHAPTER OUTLINE

Introduction

Ketamine and phencyclidine are chemically related to each other and have psychotropic effects similar to those of other prototypical hallucinogens such as lysergic acid diethylamide. Phencyclidine was developed first as a dissociative anesthetic for animals and humans, but seizures, recreational abuse, and unpredictable effects have prevented its therapeutic use. Ketamine was developed after phencyclidine and has similar properties, although it is still used therapeutically as an anesthetic and analgesic in humans and animals and is currently being studied as a treatment for depression and suicidal ideation. Most ketamine used illicitly is diverted from veterinary supplies but is also relatively easy to synthesize. Both drugs have been abused since the 1970s and became popular again in the 2000s, especially among young adults who are active in the club scene.

Pharmacology

Mechanism of Action

Ketamine and phencyclidine are arylcyclohexylamines, which are dissociative anesthetics that produce perceptual distortions similar to those of hallucinogens, as well as other effects, so they are often classified as hallucinogens. Ketamine is a derivative of phencyclidine that is less potent and shorter-acting and is still used therapeutically in medical settings as an anesthetic and analgesic in humans,[8] especially in countries where opioids are not available. Ketamine and phencyclidine selectively reduce the excitatory actions of glutamate on central nervous system neurons mediated by the N-methyl-D-aspartate (NMDA) receptor complex.[4] These receptors mediate ion flux through channels permeable to sodium, potassium, and calcium, and are involved in synaptic transmission, long-term potentiation, and neuron plasticity. Pharmaco–magnetic resonance imaging (MRI) has confirmed that the subjective effects of ketamine are mediated by enhanced glutamate release.[14] In addition, phencyclidine affects mu opioid receptors,[18] blocks dopamine uptake,[5] and inhibits serotonin uptake.[51] Phencyclidine binds to specific receptors in the liver, kidney, lung, heart, and brain.[60] However, the exact mechanism of the effects of ketamine and phencyclidine has not been determined. Metabolism of ketamine and phencyclidine occurs in the liver by oxidation, hydroxylation, and then conjugation with glucuronic acid.[61]

Routes of Administration

Ketamine and phencyclidine can be taken orally, inhaled intranasally, smoked, or injected intramuscularly, subcutaneously, or intravenously. Ketamine is obtained primarily in powder form and taken by intranasal insufflation ("snorting") of lines,[28] which has a more rapid onset but a shorter duration of effects than when taken orally. Ketamine injection involves particular paraphernalia and high-risk practices.[31] Intramuscular injection is perceived as easier and less threatening than intravenous injection.[32]

Phencyclidine is taken as a tablet ("PeaCe Pill," or "PCP"), powder ("angel dust"), or liquid ("whack"). It is smoked alone or when added to tobacco cigarettes or marijuana joints, a combination known as "fry."[43] The onset of effects when smoked is almost immediate, similar to intravenous administration,[38] and is much more rapid than when taken orally (onset takes more than an hour).

Epidemiology

Ketamine

Ketamine was developed in the 1960s as a surgical anesthetic.[10] Recreational use began in the 1970s on the West Coast of the United States,[44] but it was not registered as a scheduled drug in the United States until 1997 or until 2006 in the United Kingdom. The prevalence of ketamine use appears to be stabilizing in the United States[29] but is rising in Europe and Asia.[28] There are

TABLE 32.1	Street Names.
Ketamine	**Phencyclidine**
Cat valium	Angel dust
K	Animal tranquilizer
Ket	Embalming fluid
Kit Kat	Fry
Special K	Hog
Super K	PCP
Vitamin K	PeaCe Pill
	Purple Haze
	Whack

many different street names for ketamine (Table 32.1). Nearly all ketamine users are polysubstance users, with 98% using drugs from three or more drug classes, such as inhalants and heroin.[63]

The National Institute on Drug Abuse (NIDA) has identified six drugs as club drugs, including ketamine. Club drugs are licit and illicit drugs from different classes that are used primarily by young adults in bars, clubs, concerts, and dance parties (or "raves"). These substances are used illicitly in those settings due to the perception that they enhance the sensory experience at dance parties where strobe lights, glow sticks, and techno music (wordless music with a driving beat) are part of the overall event.[58] More than 40% of individuals who use club drugs have tried ketamine.[35] Regular ketamine users are older (in their 20s as opposed to teens), employed, and better educated compared with most other club drug users.[15] Although ketamine use is very common among club goers—up to 66%—there is a very low prevalence of ketamine use among young people in the general population.[63]

Separate from clubs and raves, ketamine is also frequently used in other settings, such as at home or at a friend's house. In addition to club goers, it is used by young injection drug users,[31] health care workers,[40] and men who have sex with men.[9]

Phencyclidine

Phencyclidine was first synthesized in the 1950s as a dissociative anesthetic for therapeutic use and originally described as a drug of abuse in the 1960s. Phencyclidine at various times has achieved popularity as a street drug with many different street names (see Table 32.1), and is frequently sold in mixtures with other drugs.[49] Its use waxes and wanes because of its unpredictable effects. Its use increased in the 1970s and peaked in the 1980s but has experienced a resurgence in popularity since the late 1990s.[6] Although not classified as a club drug by NIDA, phencyclidine is used by young adults in settings similar to those of other club drugs.[6]

Trends in the popularity of specific drugs of abuse tend to be cyclic. Relatively large numbers of new users will experiment with a given drug or develop a pattern of recurrent use, often in combination with other substances. With more users, information about undesirable effects spreads among users, or public health concern prompts a response with dissemination of information about abuse and problems. Then the prevalence of abuse may subside for a while. Phencyclidine has gone through previous cycles of popularity because it is relatively easy to manufacture in clandestine laboratories. However, unpleasant effects of repeated use

(including propensity to violence and psychotic symptoms, as well as a high frequency of "bad trips") result in a drop in popularity. Phencyclidine use is on the rise again, along with the use of ketamine as part of the club drug scene.

Phencyclidine is often used in combination with other substances, primarily alcohol.[37] It may be added to tobacco cigarettes or marijuana joints, a combination known as "fry."[55] When added to tobacco, it is also called "Shermans" because it was first added to Sherman cigarettes, which are a private brand.

Use Disorders

Diagnostic and Statistical Manual of Mental Disorders Criteria

The criteria in the *Diagnostic and Statistical Manual of Mental Disorders, Fifth Edition* (DSM-5)[3] for use disorders for ketamine and phencyclidine do not differ significantly from the general criteria for substance use disorder (Table 32.2). Ketamine use disorder falls under the heading of phencyclidine-like substances in the DSM-5 and does not have a separate diagnosis or criteria set. A specific withdrawal syndrome has not been identified for these drugs, which is also the case for other hallucinogens. Therefore, criteria specific to withdrawal are not utilized to determine a diagnosis of use disorder for either ketamine or phencyclidine. There are no other unique criteria for ketamine or phencyclidine in the DSM-5.

Tolerance and Withdrawal

Tolerance develops rapidly to the desired effects,[30] resulting in reduced length of the subjective experience and requiring an increase in dose to maintain the expected effects. Users escalate the amount used to achieve the full hallucinogenic experience, up to seven times the original amount.[39] Use of higher recreational doses can result in more adverse effects, especially physiological side effects. Use of very high doses can result in onset of full anesthetic effects, which may result in an overdose situation for a recreational user. Continued use of ketamine or phencyclidine, despite experiencing these consequences, constitutes addiction.

A definitive physiological withdrawal syndrome does not appear to develop after stopping use of ketamine or phencyclidine. Phencyclidine users who smoked at least weekly and acknowledge psychological dependence reported no withdrawal symptoms upon stopping.[20]

Intoxication

Ketamine
Psychological Effects

Initial use of ketamine is based primarily on a desire for experimentation and openness to new experiences, and secondarily for pleasure.[39] Appealing effects described by users include visual hallucinations and out-of-body experiences; undesirable effects include memory loss and decreased sociability.[39] General central nervous system depressant effects include poor concentration and poor recollection similar to that associated with alcohol intoxication, which is not unexpected for an anesthetic drug.[45]

Ketamine effects include profound changes in consciousness and psychotomimetic effects such as changes in body image (feeling that the body is made of wood, plastic, or rubber) and possible

TABLE 32.2	**Use Disorder Criteria.**

A pattern of use leading to clinically significant impairment or distress, manifested by at least 2 of the following, occurring within a 12-month period:

1. Often taken in larger amounts or over a longer period than was intended.
2. Persistent desire or unsuccessful efforts to cut down or control use.
3. Great deal of time spent in activities necessary to obtain, use, or recover from its effects.
4. Craving, or a strong desire or urge to use.
5. Recurrent use resulting in failure to fulfill major role obligations at work (repeated absences or poor performance related to use), school (absences, suspensions, or expulsions), or home (neglect of children or household).
6. Continued use despite having persistent or recurrent social or interpersonal problems caused or exacerbated by the effects of the substance (arguments with a spouse about consequences of intoxication, physical fights).
7. Important social, occupational, or recreational activities are given up or reduced because of use.
8. Recurrent use in situations in which it is physically hazardous (driving an automobile or operating a machine when impaired).
9. Use is continued despite knowledge of having a persistent or recurrent physical or psychological problem that is likely to have been caused or exacerbated by the substance.
10. Tolerance, as defined by either:
    a. Need for markedly increased amounts to achieve intoxication or desired effect.
    b. Markedly diminished effect with continued use of the same amount.

Specify current severity:
1. Mild: presence of 2–3 symptoms.
2. Moderate: presence of 4–5 symptoms.
3. Severe: presence of 6 or more symptoms.

Specify if in remission:
1. Early: After full criteria were previously met, none of the criteria have been met for at least 3 months but for less than 12 months (with the exception of criterion #4, craving).
2. Sustained: After full criteria were previously met, none of the criteria have been met at any time during a period of 12 months or longer (with the exception of criterion #4, craving).

Specify if in a controlled environment: if the individual is in an environment where access to the substance is restricted (jail, therapeutic community, locked hospital unit).

---

feelings of spiritual separation from the body, including out-of-body experiences. At low doses, users describe mild dissociative effects, distortion of time and space, and hallucinations.[39] At large doses, users experience severe dissociation with intense detachment such that their perceptions seem to be located deep within their consciousness and reality is far off in the distance; this is called the "K-hole."[39]

The analgesic and dissociative effects may result in injury or even death in users.[39] The number of ketamine-related emergency department visits increased more than 500 percent between 2005 and 2011 (from 303 to 1550 visits).[53] Because of its lower potency and shorter duration of action, ketamine has less severe psychiatric issues than phencyclidine,[33] which may be why there are far fewer emergency department visits for ketamine than for phencyclidine. Cognitive impairments can occur even when a user is drug-free, and frequent users have greater impairment than infrequent users when drug-free.[12]

Several clinical trials have evaluated ketamine as a treatment for major depression that has been resistant to other medications and electroconvulsive therapy, and for depression associated with bipolar disorder.[1] Ketamine has been administered as an intravenous infusion in a medical setting with monitoring for 24 hours after. Response is rapid, with improvement rates of 25%–85% at 24 hours and 14%–70% at 72 hours, and side effects have been mild. Intranasal esketamine was recently approved for treatment-resistant depression. Phencyclidine has not shown such robust antidepressant effects.[33]

Physiological Effects

At low doses, ketamine causes stimulant effects with a temporary increase in blood pressure and heart rate, as well as diplopia and nystagmus.[23] Tachycardia and hypertension are the most common physical findings after illicit use.[59] Other findings of intoxication include pupil dilation and muscle rigidity. Rhabdomyolysis may result from muscle rigidity combined with exertion in severe agitation. Very large doses result in deep anesthesia with coma and respiratory depression.[47] Other physiologic effects of ketamine include severe epigastric pain known as "K-cramps," which may be due to smooth muscle relaxation in the biliary tract.[64]

Management

Management of ketamine intoxication is primarily supportive, and adverse effects typically resolve over several hours for mild to moderate intoxication. A thorough history and physical examination, along with toxicological screening for the presence of ketamine, establish the diagnosis. A quiet environment without bright light can help reduce the agitation and psychotic behaviors that are due to overstimulation.

Additional supportive care may be required for severe intoxication or overdose. Benzodiazepines such as lorazepam are helpful for more severe agitation, anxiety, and/or muscle rigidity.

Phencyclidine

Psychological Effects

A reason for initial use of phencyclidine has been described as a desire for enhancement of the user's everyday life.[16] Reasons for continuation of use include feelings of strength, power, and invulnerability, as well as psychic numbing to self-medicate anger and dysphoric symptoms.[20] The phencyclidine experience is regarded as pleasant only half the time and aversive the other half, but some users report that this unpredictability of effects is an attractive feature.[7]

Phencyclidine produces brief dissociative psychotic reactions, similar to schizophrenic psychoses. These reactions are characterized by changes in body image similar to those of ketamine as described in the preceding text. Moderate phencyclidine intake may lead to a catatonic-like presentation with the individual staring blankly and not responding to stimuli; the eyes remain open, even when the individual is in a comatose state. At higher doses, users have great difficulty differentiating between themselves and their surroundings. Some users have religious experiences while intoxicated, such as feelings of meeting God or knowledge of their own impending death.[19]

A dissociative phenomenon occurs occasionally, with phencyclidine abusers exhibiting dangerous or violent behaviors.[34] The individual also may appear psychotic. Previous psychiatric history is associated with a higher likelihood for assaultive behavior from phencyclidine use.[36] Levels of consciousness may fluctuate rapidly while the individual is recovering from the intoxication. The effects of phencyclidine can last for several days, since it is one of the longest-acting drugs of abuse.

The number of phencyclidine-related emergency department visits increased by more than 400% between 2005 and 2011 (from 14,825 to 75,538 visits), especially among young adults 25 to 34 years of age, and 69% of visits were by males; nearly half of visits were for phencyclidine in combination with other illicit drugs.[54] There is significant geographical variation among emergency department visits for phencyclidine use, with visits increasing in cities such as New York and Chicago, but remaining stable in other major metropolitan areas of the United States.

Physiological Effects

In low-dose intoxication, the individual presents with nystagmus, confusion, ataxia, and sensory impairment. This is the only drug of abuse that causes a characteristic vertical nystagmus (it can also cause horizontal or rotatory nystagmus), which helps to identify it as the cause when an individual presents with intoxication by an unknown drug. The DSM-5 provides a specific criteria set for phencyclidine intoxication[3] based primarily on physiological signs and behavioral changes (Table 32.3). Three stages of phencyclidine intoxication have been described,[46] and individuals may fluctuate between the first two stages for several hours; the third stage occurs when individuals take high doses (Table 32.4).

In high doses, the drug produces seizures and severe hypertension. The hypertension should be treated vigorously, since it may cause hypertensive encephalopathy or intracerebral bleeding. Phencyclidine can also cause life-threatening hyperthermia with temperatures over 106°F, which may occur many hours after use. Warning signs for hyperthermia include agitation, dry skin, and increased muscle tension.[56]

Management

The most effective treatment of phencyclidine intoxication is increasing its urinary excretion by acidifying the urine with ammonium chloride or ascorbic acid.[57] Urine acidification should be undertaken only after it is determined that the individual does not have myoglobinuria (indicating rhabdomyolysis) to prevent the development of acute renal failure. Some practitioners feel that the benefits of urine acidification are outweighed by the risks, especially in individuals with hepatic or renal impairment. If the individual is at low risk for hepatic or renal disease, acidification can be initiated. The urine pH should be monitored and kept at around 5.5, after which a diuretic can be administered to enhance excretion. The urine should be checked for the presence of phencyclidine to ensure that it is being excreted. Phencyclidine can be deposited in adipose tissue and released over time, which may

TABLE 32.3	*Diagnostic and Statistical Manual of Mental Disorders* (DSM-5) Criteria for Phencyclidine Intoxication.

A. Recent use of phencyclidine (or a related substance)
B. Clinically significant maladaptive behavioral changes that developed during or shortly after phencyclidine use. For example:
- Belligerence
- Assaultiveness
- Impulsiveness
- Unpredictability
- Psychomotor agitation
- Impaired judgment
- Impaired social or occupational functioning
C. Within an hour (less when smoked, "snorted", or used intravenously), 2 (or more) of the following signs:
- Vertical or horizontal nystagmus
- Hypertension or tachycardia
- Numbness or diminished responsiveness to pain
- Ataxia
- Dysarthria
- Muscle rigidity
- Seizures or coma
- Hyperacusis
D. The symptoms are not due to a general medical condition and are not better accounted for by another mental disorder.

result in a prolonged state of confusion that can last for weeks; urine acidification may be helpful to deplete the reserve drug.

In an individual who is hypertensive due to phencyclidine, intravenous antihypertensive medications should be administered to reduce blood pressure. Psychotic behavior can be treated with haloperidol. If the individual is severely agitated and poses a potential threat to self or others, haloperidol or lorazepam is effective to control agitation; barbiturates may be even more efficacious.[42] Hyperthermia requires rapid cooling measures such as ice packs or a cooling blanket.[56]

Phencyclidine Intoxication Delirium

Clinical Presentation

A psychiatric syndrome that brings phencyclidine users to medical attention is acute delirium. The duration and severity are dose-related, but the acute episode usually lasts 3–8 hours. Phencyclidine intoxication delirium is characterized by clouded consciousness that waxes and wanes (Table 32.5); this fluctuation may be due to periodic gastric secretion with intestinal reabsorption.[25] The individual's mental status fluctuates through paranoia, mania, rapid thought and speech, grandiosity, and emotional lability. All individuals initially experience distortion of body image (loss of body boundaries) and depersonalization (sense of unreality), followed by feelings of estrangement and loneliness; some individuals become catatonic and have dreamlike experiences. Clinically, individuals display insomnia, restlessness, hyperactivity, purposeless or bizarre behavior, perseveration, agitation, and aggression. Phencyclidine intoxication can be differentiated clinically from phencyclidine delirium because phencyclidine intoxication is accompanied by horizontal or vertical nystagmus, ataxia, or slurred speech, and occurs with a clear sensorium (similar to intoxication with other hallucinogens).

Phencyclidine delirium may persist much longer than the acute intoxication episode. There are three phases of phencyclidine

TABLE 32.4	Stages of Phencyclidine Intoxication.		
	Stage 1: Behavioral Toxicity	**Stage 2: Stupor**	**Stage 3: Coma**
Duration	1–2 h	1–2 h	1–4 days
Vital signs			
Blood pressure and heart rate	Mild elevation	Moderate elevation	Significant elevation
Body temperature	98–101°F	101–103°F	103–108°F (malignant hyperthermia)
Respiratory rate	Mild elevation	Moderate elevation	Periodic respirations, apnea
Visual			
Nystagmus	Horizontal, then vertical	Horizontal, vertical, rotary	Horizontal, vertical, rotary
Pupil response	Variable, often miotic	Reactive	Dilated
Gaze	Blank stare	Fixed stare or roving eyes	Disconjugate
Mental status	Poor concentration, repetitive movements, agitation	Catatonic (with eyes open)	Coma
Reflexes			
Deep tendon reflexes	Clonus	Crossed limb reflexes	Absent
Gag reflex	Increased	Repetitive swallowing	Absent
Corneal reflex	Normal	Absent	Absent
Response to pain	Reduced pinprick sensation	Response only to deep pain	No response to deep pain
Drooling	Mild	Moderate	Severe
Nausea	Mild	Moderate	Severe
Spasticity	Rigidity, spasms, ataxia, dysarthria, grimacing, bruxism	Rigidity, twitching, myoclonus, spasticity	Myoclonus, opisthotonos

delirium: agitated phase, mixed phase, and resolution phase. Each phase lasts around 5 days. The duration is influenced by the degree of exposure to phencyclidine, individual susceptibility, dosage of antipsychotic medication given, and whether urine acidification is undertaken.

Management

The hyperactivity, agitation, and aggression displayed by individuals with this condition result in intense physical exertion. Individuals with phencyclidine delirium are usually hospitalized in a closed psychiatric unit, but it is worthwhile to avoid use of physical restraints and to assure adequate hydration. Benzodiazepines and haloperidol may be helpful for phencyclidine delirium. Urine acidification facilitates excretion of phencyclidine and helps to ameliorate more rapidly the psychosis of this disorder. Urine acidification should continue for at least 3 days after the acute delirium has resolved, and individuals typically require 3–10 days of urine acidification. Electroconvulsive therapy is useful if individuals fail to respond to antipsychotic treatment after a week of inpatient treatment.[21,48]

Phencyclidine Organic Mental Disorder

Phencyclidine organic mental disorder is a mental impairment that may result from chronic phencyclidine use.[57] Characteristics include memory deficits, confusion or reduced intellectual function, assaultiveness, visual disturbances, and speech difficulty. The most common speech difficulty is blocking, which is the inability to retrieve the proper words. The course is variable, but the

confusional state may last 4–6 weeks. Urine acidification may shorten the course, although symptoms improve gradually with time if phencyclidine use does not recur.

Management involves protection from injury and helping to deal with disorientation. Excessive stimulation may result in agitation and violent behavior, so stimulation and sensory input should be minimized. A simple, structured, supportive approach works best in a nonthreatening environment with nonjudgmental staff.

Chronic Use

It can be difficult to differentiate whether specific long-term effects of chronic use of ketamine or phencyclidine are due solely to the ketamine or phencyclidine. Most users of ketamine or phencyclidine are polysubstance users, so attribution of chronic effects is complicated by use of multiple other substances that may produce their own adverse effects. The current generation of ketamine users is the first to have used it long-term. The chronic health effects of ketamine are not known. More research with studies of the effects of chronic ketamine and phencyclidine use on physical and mental health is necessary. This will help direct future prevention efforts.

Repeated use of ketamine or phencyclidine may result in long-term psychiatric consequences, such as anxiety, depression, or psychosis. The risk of a prolonged psychiatric reaction depends on the user's underlying predisposition to develop psychopathology, the amount of prior drug use, and the use of other drugs, as well as the dose and purity of the drug taken.[52] Individuals may present with

TABLE 32.5 *Diagnostic and Statistical Manual of Mental Disorders (DSM-5) Criteria for Phencyclidine Intoxication Delirium.*

Criteria	Specify If
A. Disturbance in attention (reduced ability to direct, focus, sustain, and shift attention) and awareness (reduced orientation to the environment).	1. Acute: lasting a few hours or days.
B. The disturbance develops over a short period of time (hours to a few days), represents a change from baseline attention and awareness, and tends to fluctuate in severity during the course of a day.	2. Persistent: lasting weeks or months.
C. An additional disturbance in cognition (memory deficit, disorientation, language, visuospatial ability, or perception).	
D. The disturbances in Criteria A and C are not better explained by another preexisting, established, or evolving neurocognitive disorder and do not occur in the context of a severely reduced level of arousal, such as coma.	1. Hyperactive: the individual has a hyperactive level of psychomotor activity that may be accompanied by mood lability, agitation, and/or refusal to cooperate with medical care.
E. Evidence from history, physical examination, or laboratory findings that the disturbance is a direct physiological consequence of substance intoxication.	2. Hypoactive: the individual has a hypoactive level of psychomotor activity that may be accompanied by sluggishness and lethargy that approaches stupor.
This diagnosis should be made instead of substance intoxication when the symptoms in Criteria A and C predominate in the clinical picture and when they are sufficiently severe to warrant clinical attention.	3. Mixed level of activity: the individual has a normal level of psychomotor activity even though attention and awareness are disturbed; also includes individuals whose activity level rapidly fluctuates.

TABLE 32.6 *Diagnostic and Statistical Manual of Mental Disorders (DSM-5) Criteria for Hallucinogen Persisting Perception Disorder.*

Criteria	Examples
A. Following cessation of use of phencyclidine or ketamine, the re-experiencing of one or more of the perceptual symptoms that were experienced while intoxicated.	1. Geometric hallucinations 2. False perceptions of movement in the peripheral visual fields 3. Flashes of color 4. Intensified colors 5. Trails of images of moving objects 6. Positive afterimages 7. Halos around objects 8. Macropsia (misperception of images as too large) 9. Micropsia (misperception of images as too small)
B. These symptoms cause clinically significant distress or impairment.	1. Social functioning 2. Occupational functioning 3. Other important areas of functioning
C. Symptoms are not attributable to another medical condition *and* are not better explained by another mental disorder *or* by another hypnopompic hallucinations.	1. Anatomical lesion of the brain 2. Infection of the brain 3. Migraine aura without headaches 4. Seizure disorders/visual epilepsies 1. Delirium 2. Major neurocognitive disorder 3. Schizophrenia 4. Other preexisting psychosis

apathy, hypomania, paranoia, delusions, hallucinations, formal thought disorder, or dissociative states. Treatment of prolonged anxiety, depression, or psychosis is the same as when these conditions are not associated with drug use.

Long-term adverse effects of the chronic use of ketamine include psychological problems such as dysphoria, apathy, or agitation, and impairment of short-term memory.[26] Chronic ketamine use results in impairment in semantic memory,[41] with greater impairment correlated with more frequent use; this improves with reduction in ketamine use. Impairment in episodic memory, attention deficit, and some schizotypal symptoms (dissociation, blunted affect, and cognitive disorganization) persists after 3 years despite cessation of ketamine use.[41] Long-term adverse effects of the chronic use of phencyclidine include intoxication delirium and organic mental disorder as described earlier.

The long-term consequence most commonly associated with the use of drugs such as ketamine and phencyclidine is Hallucinogen Persisting Perception Disorder (HPPD) [3], also known as "flashbacks." A flashback is an episode in which certain aspects of a previous psychedelic experience are unexpectedly reexperienced.[55] Triggers include stress, exercise, use of other drugs (especially marijuana), or entering a situation similar to the original drug experience; they may also occur spontaneously.[58] HPPD is thought to occur in a vulnerable subpopulation of users.[22] The DSM-5 provides a specific criteria set for HPPD (Table 32.6). The content varies widely and may include emotional or somatic components, but the perceptual distortions are most commonly reexperienced. This may consist of afterimages, trails behind moving objects, flashes of color, or lights in the peripheral visual fields. These episodes last several seconds to several minutes and are self-limited. The unpredictability of HPPD often provokes anxiety when episodes occur. However, they are fairly rare and tend over time to decrease in frequency, duration, and intensity, as long as no additional drug is taken.[52] Episodes are unlikely to occur more than 1 year after the original drug experience. Treatment of HPPD consists of supportive care, including reassurance that the episode will be brief; benzodiazepines help to reduce anxiety, but there are no randomized trials assessing the effectiveness of any pharmacotherapies.[22]

Chronic use of phencyclidine or ketamine may result in different physical health problems. Some health effects are related to the route of administration. Intranasal insufflation results in nasal problems according to studies of regular users.[39] Injection (whether subcutaneous, intramuscular, or intravenous) may result in exposure to blood-borne pathogens such as HIV or hepatitis C virus, subcutaneous abscesses, or bacterial endocarditis. The most common reason for ketamine users to seek medical attention due to ketamine use is from severe gastrointestinal cramping known as "K-cramps." Up to one-third of frequent ketamine users experience this,[39] but no treatment exists currently. One-fifth of users have reported bladder problems due to ulcerative cystitis,[50] which has a variable course, with one-third of cases resolving with stopping ketamine use, one-third with continuing symptoms, and one-third with worsening symptoms.[11] Another side effect of long-term ketamine use is headaches.

Addiction Treatment

Screening for ketamine and phencyclidine use by asking about drug use can be done in many settings, including by school counselors, nurses, primary care physicians, and others who interact with adolescents and young adults in high-risk setting for drug use such as the juvenile justice system and mental health services.[55] It is also important to ask about frequency of use, since those who have used weekly within the past year are much more likely to meet DSM-5 criteria for a diagnosis of a use disorder.[62]

The pattern of use of ketamine and phencyclidine is usually intermittent in social settings, so it may be perceived as less of a problem. This may limit willingness to consider addiction treatment by those who abuse these drugs. Adolescents and young adults are the primary users, so family members should be part of the treatment program. Treatment of abuse and dependence is often difficult due to the young age of most users and concurrent polysubstance use. Treatment involves components similar to that of other types of substance use disorders, including individual counseling, support groups, and 12-step self-help group attendance. Treatment settings focus on behavioral components such as individual and group counseling. Relapse prevention, a type of cognitive-behavioral therapy, has been recommended for ketamine use disorder.[27]

Individuals who chronically abuse phencyclidine display characteristics such as impulsiveness and poor interpersonal relationships.[57] This may make successful treatment more challenging, but a treatment environment with a supportive structure can be helpful. Due to the dissociative effects of ketamine and phencyclidine, those who abuse these drugs may have a sense of loss of contact with their bodies. Progressive relaxation techniques, yoga, and regular exercise may help individuals in treatment to focus and improve their concentration.[57] Chronic use of ketamine and phencyclidine may result in cognitive impairment, so a long-term treatment program must take this into consideration to be successful in maintaining abstinence. The treatment environment should provide a supportive structure,[57] recognition that initial engagement may be minimal, and utilization of routine and repetition. Treatment staff can improve the chances for a successful outcome by displaying patience and persistence with individuals.

There is no pharmacologic treatment available for phencyclidine or ketamine use.[2] Preclinical animal studies have shown that monoclonal antibodies against phencyclidine can be effective in treating overdose and intoxication, although human studies are necessary.[65] Single case reports have shown the potential utility of naltrexone[17] or lamotrigine[24] for treating cravings for ketamine in high-dose users, but further research into long-term pharmacotherapy is necessary.

References

1. Aan Het Rot M, Zarate Jr CA, Charney D, et al. Ketamine for depression: where do we go from here? *Biol Psychiatry*. 2012;72:537–547.
2. Abraham HD, Aldridge AM, Gogia P. The psychopharmacology of hallucinogens. *Neuro-Psychopharmacology*. 1996;14:285–298.
3. American Psychiatric Association. *Diagnostic and Statistical Manual of Mental Disorders*. 5th ed. Arlington, VA: American Psychiatric Publishing; 2013.
4. Anis NA, Berry SC, Burton N, et al. The dissociative anesthetics ketamine and phencyclidine selectively reduce excitation of central mammalian neurons by N-methyl-D-aspartate. *Br J Pharmacol*. 1983;79:565–575.
5. Bowyer JF, Spuhler KP, Weiner N. Effects of phencyclidine, amphetamine and related compounds on dopamine release from and uptake into striatal synaptosomes. *J Pharmacol Exp Ther*. 1984;229:671–680.
6. Bryant WK, Ompad DC, Ahern J, et al. Period and birth-cohort effects on age of first phencyclidine (PCP) use among drug users in New York City, 1960–2000. *Ann Epidemiol*. 2006;16:266–272.
7. Carroll ME. PCP, the dangerous angel. In: Snyder SH, ed. *Encyclopedia of Psychoactive Drugs*. New York: Chelsea House; 1985.
8. Chen G, Ensor CR, Russell D, et al. The pharmacology of 1-(1-phenylcyclohexyl) piperidine-HCl. *J Pharmacol Exp Ther*. 1959;127:241–250.
9. Clatts MC, Goldsamt L, Huso Y. Club drug use among young men who have sex with men in NYC: a preliminary epidemiological profile. *Subst Use Misuse*. 2005;40:1317–1330.
10. Corssen G, Domino EF. Dissociative anesthesia: further pharmacologic studies and first clinical experience with the phencyclidine derivative CI-581. *Anesth Analg Curr Res*. 1966;45:191–199.
11. Cottrell AM, Gillatt D. Consider ketamine misuse in patients with urinary symptoms. *Practitioner*. 2008;252:5.
12. Curran HV, Monaghan L. In and out of the K-hole: a comparison of the acute and residual effects of ketamine in frequent and infrequent ketamine users. *Addiction*. 2001;96:749–760.
13. Reference deleted in review.
14. Deakin JFW, Lees J, McKie S, et al. Glutamate and the neural basis of the subjective effects of ketamine: a pharmaco-magnetic resonance imaging study. *Arch Gen Psychiatry*. 2008;65:154–164.
15. Dillon P, Copeland J, Jansen K. Patterns of use and harm associated with non-medical ketamine use. *Drug Alcohol Depend*. 2003;69:23–28.
16. Feldman HW. *Angel Dust in Four American Cities: an Ethnographic Study of PCP Users*. Rockville, MD: U.S. Department of Health and Human Services; 1980.
17. Garg A, Sinha P, Kumar P, et al. Use of naltrexone in ketamine dependence. *Addictive Behaviors*. 2014;39:1215–1216.
18. Giannini AJ, Loiselle RH, Giannini MC, et al. Phencyclidine and the dissociatives. *Psychiatr Med*. 1984;3:197–217.
19. Gorelick DA, Wilkins JN, Wong C. Diagnosis and treatment of chronic phencyclidine (PCP) abuse. *NIDA Res Monogr*. 1986;64:218–228.
20. Gorelick DA, Wilkins JN, Wong C. Outpatient treatment of PCP abusers. *Am J Drug Alcohol Abuse*. 1989;15:367–375.
21. Grover D, Yeragani VK, Keshanan MS. Improvement of phencyclidine-associated psychosis with ECT. *J Clin Psychiatry*. 1986;47:477–478.
22. Halpern JH, Pope HG. Hallucinogen persisting perception disorder: What do we know after 50 years? *Drug Alcohol Depend*. 2003;69:109–119.
23. Harari MD, Netzer D. Genital examination under ketamine sedation in cases of suspected sexual abuse. *Arch Dis Child*. 1994;70:197–199.
24. Huang M-C, Chen L-Y, Chen C-K, et al. Potential benefit of lamotrigine in managing ketamine use disorder. *Medical Hypotheses*. 2016;87:97–100.

25. Hurlbut KM. Drug-induced psychoses. *Emerg Med Clin North Am.* 1991;9:31–52.
26. Jansen KLR. Ketamine—can chronic use impair memory? *Int J Addictions.* 1990;25:133–139.
27. Jansen KL, Darracot-Cankovic R. The non-medical use of ketamine, part two: a review of problem use and dependence. *J Psychoactive Drugs.* 2001;33:151–158.
28. Joe Laidler K. The rise of club drugs in a heroin society: the case of hong kong. *Subst Use Misuse.* 2005;40:1257–1278.
29. Johnston LD, O'Malley PM, Bachman JG, et al. *Monitoring the Future National Survey Results on Drug Use, 1975–2004, Secondary School Students.* Vol. 1. Bethesda, MD: National Institute on Drug Abuse; 2005.
30. Kamaya H, Krishna PR. Ketamine addiction. *Anaesthesiology.* 1987;67:861–862.
31. Lankenau SE, Clatts M. Drug injection practices among high-risk youths: the first shot of ketamine. *J Urban Health.* 2004;81:232–248.
32. Lankenau SE, Sanders B, Bloom JJ, et al. First injection of ketamine among young injection drug users (IDUs) in three U.S. cities. *Drug Alcohol Depend.* 2007;87:183–193.
33. Lodge D, Mercier MS. Ketamine and phencyclidine: the good, the bad and the unexpected. *Br J Pharmacol.* 2015;172:4254–4276.
34. Marrs-Simon PA, Weiler M, Santangelo MA, et al. Analysis of sexual disparity of violent behavior in PCP intoxication. *Vet Hum Toxicol.* 1988;30:53–55.
35. McCambridge J, Winstock A, Hunt N, et al. 5-year trends in use of hallucinogens and other adjunct drugs among UK dance drug users. *Eur Addict Res.* 2007;13:57–64.
36. McCardle L, Fishbein DH. The self-reported effects of PCP on human aggression. *Addict Behav.* 1989;14:465–472.
37. McCarron M, Schulze B, Thompson G, et al. Acute phencyclidine intoxication: clinical patterns, complications, and treatment. *Ann Emerg Med.* 1981;10:290–297.
38. Meng Y, Lichtman AH, Bridgen T, et al. Pharmacological potency and biodisposition of phencyclidine via inhalation exposure in mice. *Drug Alcohol Depend.* 1996;43:13–22.
39. Meutzelfeldt L, Kamboj SK, Rees H, et al. Journey through the K-hole: phenomenological aspects of ketamine use. *Drug Alcohol Depend.* 2008;95:219–229.
40. Moore NN, Bostwick JM. Ketamine dependence in anesthesia providers. *Psychosomatics.* 1999;40:356–359.
41. Morgan CJA, Monaghan L, Curran HV. Beyond the K-hole: a 3-year longitudinal investigation of the cognitive and subjective effects of ketamine in recreational users who have substantially reduced their use of the drug. *Addiction.* 2004;99:1450–1461.
42. Olney JW, Labruyere J, Wang G, et al. NMDA antagonist neurotoxicity: mechanism and prevention. *Science.* 1991;254:1515–1518.
43. Peters RJ, Kelder SH, Meshack A, et al. Beliefs and social norms about cigarettes or marijuana sticks laced with embalming fluid and phencyclidine (PCP): why youth use fry. *Subst Use Misuse.* 2005;40:563–571.
44. Petersen RC, Stillman RC. Phencyclidine (PCP) abuse: an appraisal. *NIDA Res Monogr.* 1978;21:1–17.
45. Pomarol-Clotet E, Honey GD, Murray GK, et al. Psychological effects of ketamine in healthy volunteers: phenomenological study. *Br J Psychiatry.* 2006;189:173–179.
46. Rappolt Sr RT, Gay GR, Farris RD. Phencyclidine (PCP) intoxication: diagnosis in stages and algorithms of treatment. *Clin Toxicol.* 1980;16:509–529.
47. Reich DL, Silvay G. Ketamine: an update on the first twenty-five years of clinical experience. *Can J Anaesth.* 1989;36:186–197.
48. Rosen AM, Mukherjee S, Shinbach K. The efficacy of ECT in phencyclidine-induced psychosis. *J Clin Psychiatry.* 1984;45:220–222.
49. Schnoll SH. Street PCP scene Issues on synthesis and contamination. *J Psychedelic Drugs.* 1980;12:229–233.
50. Shahani R, Streutker C, Dickson B, et al. Ketamine-associated ulcerative cystitis: a new clinical entity. *Urology.* 2007;69:810–812.
51. Smith RC, Melzer HY, Arora RC, et al. Effect of phencyclidine on 3H-catecholamine and 3H-serotonin uptake in synaptosomal preparations from rat brain. *Biochem Pharmacol.* 1977;26:1435–1439.
52. Strassman RJ. Adverse reactions to psychedelic drugs: a review of the literature. *J Nerv Ment Dis.* 1984;172:577–595.
53. Substance Abuse and Mental Health Services Administration, Drug Abuse Warning Network. *2011: National Estimates of Drug-Related Emergency Department Visits. HHS Publication No. (SMA) 13-4760, DAWN Series D-39.* Rockville, MD: Substance Abuse and Mental Health Services Administration; 2013.
54. Substance Abuse and Mental Health Services Administration, Center for Behavioral Health Statistics and Quality. *The DAWN Report: Emergency Department Visits Involving Phencyclidine (PCP).* Rockville, MD; November 12, 2013.
55. Weaver MF. Hallucinogens. In: Levesque RJ, ed. *Encyclopedia of Adolescence.* New York: Springer; 2012.
56. Weaver MF. Other drugs of abuse. In: McKean SC, Ross JJ, Dressler DD, et al., eds. *Principles and Practice of Hospital Medicine.* New York: McGraw-Hill; 2012.
57. Weaver MF, Schnoll SH. Phencyclidine and ketamine. In: Gabbard GO, ed. *Treatments of Psychiatric Disorders.* 4th ed. Washington, DC: American Psychiatric Publishing; 2007.
58. Weaver MF, Schnoll SH. Hallucinogens and club drugs. In: Galanter M, Kleber HD, eds. *Textbook of Substance Abuse Treatment.* 4th ed. Washington, DC: American Psychiatric Publishing; 2008.
59. Weiner AL, Vieira L, McKay CA, et al. Ketamine abusers presenting to the emergency department: a case series. *J Emerg Med.* 2000;18:447–451.
60. Weinstein H, Maayuni S, Glick S, et al. Integrated studies on the biochemical, behavioral and molecular pharmacology of phencyclidine: a progress report. In: Domino EF, ed. *Phencyclidine (PCP): Historical and Current Perspectives.* Ann Arbor, MI: NPP Books; 1981.
61. Wong LK, Biemann K. Metabolites of phencyclidine. *Clin Toxicol.* 1976;9:583–591.
62. Wu L-T, Ringwalt CL, Weiss RD, et al. Hallucinogen-related disorders in a national sample of adolescents: the influence of ecstasy/MDMA use. *Drug Alcohol Depend.* 2009;104:156–166.
63. Wu L-T, Schlenger WE, Galvin DM. Concurrent use of methamphetamine, MDMA, LSD, ketamine, GHB, and flunitrazepam among American youths. *Drug Alcohol Depend.* 2006;84:102–113.
64. Xu J, Lei H. Ketamine-an update on its clinical uses and abuses. *CNS NeuroScience & Therapeutics.* 2014;20:1015–1020.
65. Zalewska-Kaszubska J. Is immunotherapy an opportunity for effective treatment of drug addiction? *Vaccine.* 2015;33:6545–6551.

33

The Biology and Treatment of Gambling Disorder

IRIS M. BALODIS AND MARC N. POTENZA

CHAPTER OUTLINE

Introduction

Gambling has become increasingly accessible and socially acceptable over the past two decades, with an increasing number of venues and opportunities through casinos, video lottery terminals, sports betting venues, and online poker and other gambling sites. Although most people participate in gambling activities recreationally, some experience gambling problems, including the most severe form, gambling disorder.[107] Gambling disorder has been associated with significant financial debt, family tension, divorce, and criminal activity such as fraud and embezzlement.[77,88] Extreme cases have involved staged kidnappings and serious child neglect leading to death, murder, and suicide.[77]

Gambling disorder is defined as persistent and recurrent maladaptive gambling behavior that jeopardizes personal, occupational, or social functioning.[1] In the *Diagnostic and Statistical Manual of Mental Disorders, Fifth Edition* (DSM-5), gambling disorder is classified as the first non–substance-based disorder in a new addiction category.

The Psychiatric Nosology of Gambling Disorder

Gambling disorder has been conceptualized as a disorder falling within an obsessive-compulsive spectrum and as a "behavioral addiction."[9,92] Studies of impulse control disorders describe clinical elements including an urge to engage in a typically enjoyable yet, in the long term, counterproductive or harmful behavior, a mounting tension until the behavior is completed, a temporary abatement of tension following completion of the behavior, and a return of tension or appetitive urge following varying amounts of time.[67] Impulse control disorders have been described as having elements of impulsivity and compulsivity. Although the underlying motive of gambling disorder is initially pleasure, with increasing frequency individuals may feel out of control and their urges may become unpleasant or ego-dystonic.[67,73] Although some compulsive aspects to gambling are evident, the co-occurrence of obsessive compulsive disorder and gambling disorder is not that common, while comorbidity with substance dependence occurs frequently.[22,56,89] The diagnostic criteria of gambling disorder, listed in the DSM-5, share similarities with those for substance dependence. Individuals with gambling disorder can demonstrate tolerance and withdrawal symptoms as they gamble with increasing amounts of money in order to achieve the same hedonic experience, and they may become irritable or restless when attempting to cut down or quit their gambling.[1] Like individuals with drug addictions, those with gambling disorder demonstrate impaired control over their behavior and may hide the extent of their involvement from loved ones or commit forgery or fraud to sustain their gambling.[1] The term problem gambling has been at times used to describe less severe patterns of gambling than exhibited in gambling disorder. This category is conceptually similar to that of substance abuse, although no formal criteria exist for problem gambling.[118] In addition, the term has been used at times inclusive and at other times exclusive of gambling disorder. The most commonly used screening instrument for gambling disorder is the South Oaks Gambling Screen, and this screen queries the types and frequencies of gambling behaviors as well as gambling-related impact on life functioning, particularly with respect to borrowing money for gambling.[65] The South Oaks Gambling Screen is valid and reliable, and a score ≥5 signifies probable gambling disorder.[65]

Cognitive Distortions

A frequently acknowledged criterion of gambling disorder is the "chasing" of losses, whereby gamblers attempt to regain accumulated losses by returning to a gambling venue shortly following sustaining gambling losses. Nearly winning (e.g., receiving identical symbols on 2 of the 3 reels on an electronic gambling machine) has been suggested to contribute to gambling behaviors.[20] Individuals with gambling disorder, as well as recreational gamblers, may report other cognitive distortions, such as overestimating their chances of winning and their sense of control: "I know what it takes to win this game." In dice gambling and certain other forms, individuals may keep track of previous numbers in order to inform their subsequent bets with the thought that certain numbers will either appear more frequently because they have been observed previously ("hot numbers") or not ("numbers that are due"). Such a gambler's fallacy ignores laws of probability: that each role of the dice functions independently of the last. Superstitious behaviors ("I only play at nights") and attributional biases ("That dealer always makes me lose") are also expressed in gambling disorder as well as in recreational gambling groups.[121] Cognitive distortions may represent relevant considerations in the maintenance of gambling disorder, although their frequent occurrence in nonpathological gambling samples questions their centrality to the disorder.[74]

Prevalence Estimates and Characteristics

Precise gambling disorder prevalence estimates may be related to assessment measures and other factors. However, most studies report lifetime prevalence estimates ranging from 0.4% to 3% in the general population, representing approximately 2 to 3 million adults in the United States.[89,115,126] All types of gambling are also not equally represented in gambling disorder populations; one study suggests that pull-tabs, casino gambling, bingo, cards, lottery and sports betting, in descending order, are most strongly associated with gambling disorder,[130] and another study found the highest proportion of pathological gamblers at off-track compared with other venues.[77] Pathological gamblers may engage in multiple types of gambling.[130] Factors associated with gambling disorder include male sex, adolescent and young adult age, and presence of other psychiatric disorder(s).[107] In addition, minorities and persons with a lower socioeconomic status also appear more likely to gamble and may be at particular risk for gambling disorder.[130] Some studies have found that men and women with gambling disorder show similarities in demographic and clinical features, including time spent gambling, percentage of income lost through gambling, and gambling urge

severity.[40] Other studies have identified gender differences in manifestations of gambling behaviors that may have significant implications for prevention and treatment strategies. Although men constitute about two-thirds of the gambling disorder population and often show a longer duration of onset and begin gambling early in life (childhood/adolescence), women appear more likely to develop gambling disorder later in life and demonstrate a more rapid progression between onset and problematic engagement, a phenomenon observed in substance use behaviors and described as "telescoping."[40,117,129] Gender differences also exist in the types of gambling behavior and in gambling triggers. Women may report engaging in fewer forms of gambling, mostly bingo and slot machines, and often cite feeling prompted by negative mood states.[40] In contrast, men are more likely to gamble on cards or sporting events and report a greater saliency of sensory cues, such as sounds or advertisement, in their triggers for gambling.[40] In addition, women, as compared with men with gambling problems, may experience greater psychiatric comorbidity, particularly with mood and anxiety disorders.[26,27,89]

Gambling disorder frequently co-occurs with other psychiatric disorders.[93] Some studies estimate that up to three-fourths of individuals with gambling disorder report an alcohol use disorder, over 60% are daily tobacco smokers or nicotine dependent, and up to 40% report other drug abuse.[55,89] About half of individuals diagnosed with gambling disorder also experience a mood disorder, with a particularly high odds ratio of 8.6 for mania, and roughly 40% are also diagnosed with anxiety disorders.[89]

Estimates of personality disorders range from 29% to 93% in the gambling disorder population, with one study reporting an average of 4.6 personality disorders per person with gambling disorder.[11,80,89] Although borderline, histrionic, and antisocial personality disorders are most often cited, these may represent a component of an externalizing syndrome.[89] Personality and temperamental factors may play a role in the maintenance of gambling disorder, as pathological gamblers may show high levels of impulsiveness, novelty-seeking, rigidness, extravagance, and harm avoidance combined with low levels of self-directedness.[32,58,80] In particular, impulsivity has been investigated as a key underlying construct, and accordingly, in gambling disorder, severity of gambling behavior and psychological disturbances appear related to this measure.[112] Identification of co-occurring disorders is important as the disorders may guide treatment strategies and influence treatment outcome.[13]

The Biochemistry of Gambling Disorder

Serotonin

Pathological gambling shares similar biochemical features with substance dependence and other disorders characterized by impulsive features.[13] Low central levels of serotonin metabolites are observed in the cerebral spinal fluid samples of individuals with impaired impulse control including those with gambling disorder.[66,79,81,122,123] However, the precise nature of central serotonin function in gambling disorder is complicated by findings suggesting increased levels in gambling disorder.[81] Low endogenous levels of serotonin in gambling disorder are suggested by blunted prolactin responses following a pharmacological challenge.[75] Pharmacological challenges using the partial agonist metachlorophenylpiperazine produce a euphoric high in pathological gamblers, a response also observed in individuals with other impulsive disorders.[5,25,113] Together, these findings suggest a role for serotonin in gambling disorder, although the precise nature of its involvement requires further investigation.

Dopamine

Given a role for the mesocorticolimbic dopamine system in mediating the reinforcing properties of drugs,[60] dopamine has been hypothesized to be involved in gambling behaviors. The maturation of the mesocorticolimbic dopamine and other systems during adolescence may in part explain the high estimates of gambling problems evidenced during this period.[16] Some data suggest that dopamine levels may increase during gambling behaviors.[108] However, ligand-based imaging studies involving pathological gamblers have yet to be published in peer-reviewed journals. Like with serotonin, studies examining dopamine metabolites in gambling disorder populations have generated inconsistent findings. Although one study reported alterations in dopamine metabolites suggesting increased dopamine turnover in gambling disorder, this finding was largely mitigated when controlling for cerebrospinal fluid flow rates.[6,79]

During gambling activity, dopamine levels increase after longer playtimes in both recreational and pathological gamblers.[72,108] Consistent with the idea that gambling and stimulants generate similar effects, priming individuals with the prodopaminergic (and pronoradrenergic) drug amphetamine was associated with an increase in the desire to gamble and reduction in the confidence to resist gambling in pathological gamblers, and pleasurable and motivational responses were positively associated with problem gambling severity.[131] However, the dopamine D_2-like receptor antagonist haloperidol was also found to promote gambling thoughts and behaviors.[132] Hence, a precise role for dopamine in gambling disorder requires further investigation.

Individuals with Parkinson disease, a disorder characterized by dopamine system degeneration, have experienced gambling problems.[28,125,128] Dopamine agonists, such as pramipexole, ropinirole, and pergolide, have been associated with impulse control disorders such as gambling disorder in Parkinson disease.[99,124,127,128] Other factors, including levodopa dosage, age at Parkinson disease onset, marital status, family history of gambling problems, family or personal history of alcoholism, high levels of impulsivity, and presence of an impulse control disorder prior to Parkinson's disease onset have also been associated with impulse control disorders such as gambling disorder in Parkinson disease in systematic, cross-sectional studies.[99,127] As such, the extent to which gambling disorder in Parkinson disease reflects the pathophysiology of Parkinson disease, its treatment, a combination thereof, or other factors requires additional research.

Norepinephrine

Norepinephrine, implicated in sensation seeking and arousal, has also been investigated in the neurobiology of gambling disorder. Although healthy individuals demonstrate increased levels of norepinephrine prior to, as well as during, gambling sessions, pathological gamblers show particularly high levels of this neurochemical.[72,108] The desire to start or continue gambling positively correlated with norepinephrine levels in one study of pathological gamblers.[72] The report of altered catecholaminergic response patterns in gambling disorder subjects suggests that gambling may represent a compensatory behavior to heightened arousal levels.[72]

The Genetics of Gambling Disorder

An elevated frequency of gambling disorder in first-degree relatives of those with the disorder suggests a genetic component to the disorder.[8] Individuals who report gambling problems in their parents are themselves more likely to have higher scores on the South Oaks Gambling Screen; in addition, if their grandparents are also perceived as having gambling problems, these individuals may have a 12-fold higher odds of meeting criteria for gambling disorder.[33] The heritability estimate of a gambling disorder diagnosis from the Vietnam Era Twin registry is 46%, and lifetime prevalence estimates of gambling disorder in identical twins and fraternal twins are 22.6% and 9.8%, respectively.[29] A further analysis of this sample revealed that both identical and fraternal twins with subclinical gambling disorder symptoms were more likely to have a twin with full gambling disorder.[110] These results support a continuity model of gambling disorder, where subclinical gambling and gambling disorder are differentiated by the number rather than the type of contributing factors.[111] Genetic studies provide support for a familial co-aggregation of gambling disorder and other disorders, such as alcohol dependence, antisocial behaviors, and depression, with significant contributions stemming from shared genetic factors.[100,110,111]

Molecular genetics have inconsistently implicated allelic variants. In one early study of dopamine-related genes, a D_2 dopamine receptor gene variant associated with substance dependence[78] was found in 51% of pathological gamblers but only in 26% of controls.[19] Individuals with the most severe pathology and comorbid substance use were more likely to carry the D2A1 gene.[19] Altered distributions of other dopamine receptor gene variants (e.g., those encoding the D_1 and D_4 receptors) have been reported in pathological gamblers.[18] However, these early studies have been criticized on methodological grounds,[50] and a more recent study using a better controlled design and more thorough assessments did not replicate these findings.[23] As such, further research is needed to identify precise molecular genetic contributions to gambling disorder.

There are also suggestive data for serotonergic and noradrenergic genetic contributions to gambling disorder. One study found that men with gambling disorder are more likely to have a shorter variant of the gene coding for the serotonin transporter.[84] Other studies have also reported differential distributions of polymorphisms of monoamine oxidase-A–encoding genes in men with gambling disorder.[51,84] Larger, genome-wide studies are needed to identify more precisely genes implicated in gambling disorder and to investigate gene-by-environment and gene-by-gene interactions.

The Neuropsychology of Gambling Disorder

To date, few studies have examined neuropsychological functioning in pathological gamblers. Initial studies suggest deficits in executive functioning—not accounted for by intellectual differences, as assessed by standard intelligence quotient tests—in gambling disorder that are similar to those evidenced in substance-dependent populations.[32,35,37] Consistent with gambling disorder's classification as an impulse control disorder, pathological gamblers demonstrate impairments on response-inhibition tasks. The Stroop task assesses cognitive control involving attention, conflict monitoring, and response inhibition. Participants are required to name rapidly the ink color of matched (congruent) or mismatched (incongruent) color-word pairs. On congruent trials, the word "red" may be written in the color red while on incongruent trials the word "red" may be written in blue ink and, therefore, requires that the individual responds "blue." Not surprisingly, incongruent trials present greater difficulty as individuals are required to inhibit the prepotent reading response. Pathological gamblers show impairment on this task by producing more errors (i.e., reading the word, rather than naming the word's color) and in taking longer to respond.[32,101,105] Modified versions of this task, sometimes referred to as Emotional, Drug, or Gambling Stroop Tasks, use emotional, drug-related, or gambling-related words, respectively. Subjects are presented with neutral or theoretically disorder-valenced words in different-colored ink. In affected individuals as compared with healthy controls, the variant Stroop tasks tend to produce further delays and errors in processing. For example, in both recreational and pathological gamblers, when the words are theoretically more emotionally or motivationally salient rather than are neutral words (e.g., "dice" vs. "door"), a more pronounced Stroop effect is observed.[12,69] Such findings suggest not only an attentional bias for disorder-related stimuli, but also a certain level of automaticity in processing.[12]

The neuropsychological function of pathological gamblers, as compared with other subject groups, has been examined.[35–37] Four groups, consisting of individuals with gambling disorder, Tourette syndrome, alcohol dependence, or no psychiatric disorder, were compared on tasks assessing executive functioning.[35,37] On tasks involving response inhibition, including the Stroop Task, the three clinical groups performed significantly worse than did healthy controls, but did not differ from one another. This trend was also observed on the Wisconsin Card Sorting Task, a measure of cognitive flexibility. However, on tasks of planning and time estimation, pathological gamblers and alcohol-dependent individuals showed significantly poorer performance relative to healthy control subjects and those with Tourette syndrome.

The Iowa Gambling Task is a neurocognitive measure assessing risk/reward decision-making, where individuals can choose between different decks of cards with varying schedules of reward.[4] Two disadvantageous decks confer high rewards, but also present even higher penalties, thereby resulting in a net loss for players. Two advantageous decks provide low rewards, but even lower penalties. Therefore, consistent selections from these decks produce an overall gain in money. Pathological gamblers and alcohol-dependent subjects demonstrated disadvantageous performance compared with the healthy control group as well as the Tourette syndrome group. These findings are consistent with prior reports that pathological gamblers show disadvantageous performance on this task.[15,86] The performance profile of the gambling disorder group also showed that they responded faster, made fewer response shifts following losses, and demonstrated less conceptual knowledge about the task than did healthy controls.[35] These findings suggest an impulsive and perseverative response style, and this profile may relate to loss chasing or altered reward processing in the gambling disorder group. A separate study examining the psychophysiological correlates on the Iowa Gambling Task showed that, unlike healthy controls, pathological gamblers fail to show increases in skin conductance response or heart rate accelerations prior to making a disadvantageous choice.[36] These alterations in psychophysiological responses suggest an impairment in risk assessment related to disadvantageous risk-reward decision-making.[36]

Neurocognitive research findings in gambling disorder should be interpreted cautiously, as many studies do not control for comorbidity, medication status, gambling severity, or gambling type or provide comparison control groups.[35] Gambling motivations may also be important to consider when examining neurocognitive performance in pathological gamblers.[35] Whether individuals gamble in order to heighten arousal or relieve their dysphoric mood may relate to their performance and its underlying biobehavioral substrates. Impaired performance on some neurocognitive tasks assessing inhibition and decision-making may represent phenotypic markers in gambling disorder that have potential in predicting relapse.[38] More research is needed to identify intermediate phenotypic or endophenotypic markers that may be used in the diagnosis and treatment of gambling disorder.

Neuroimaging Studies

Neuroimaging studies suggest altered functioning in frontal, temporal, and limbic structures in pathological gamblers. The first published study using functional magnetic resonance imaging in gambling disorder utilized happy, sad, and gambling videotapes.[98] While viewing the videos, participants reported the onset of an emotional (e.g., feelings of sadness) or motivational (e.g., gambling urge) response by pressing a button. During the gambling scenarios (but not the happy or sad ones), pathological gamblers showed signal decreases in frontal and orbitofrontal cortical areas, thalamus, and basal ganglia. These brain changes occurred prior to conscious awareness of an emotional/motivational response, that is, preceding the button-press. This activation pattern contrasts with those from symptom provocation studies in obsessive compulsive disorder, in which increased activation of cortical-basal-ganglionic-thalamic circuitry is observed.[107]

During the viewing of the final portion of the gambling scenarios, when the most robust gambling stimuli were presented, pathological gamblers (relative to controls) showed less activation of the ventromedial prefrontal cortex. Subsequent studies using a functional magnetic resonance imaging Stroop task, a decision-making, and a simulated gambling task have also demonstrated relatively diminished activation of the ventromedial prefrontal cortex in association with gambling disorder.[96,102,116] The ventromedial prefrontal cortex has been implicated in mood regulation, decision-making, and impulsivity.[3,7,13,68] The ventral striatum, functionally connected to the ventromedial prefrontal cortex, has also been shown to activate less strongly in pathological gamblers.[94,102] Activation in the ventromedial prefrontal cortex and ventral striatum correlated inversely with gambling severity in pathological gamblers during simulated gambling, further suggesting the relevance of these regions to clinical aspects of gambling disorder.[102] Similar patterns of brain activations, including relatively diminished activation of ventral striatum, have been reported in cocaine-dependent subjects viewing cocaine tapes and gambling disorder subjects viewing gambling tapes, suggesting similar neural contributions to appetitive urge states across disorders.[94] These neurobiological findings support the conceptualization of gambling disorder as a behavioral or nonsubstance addiction.

Although to date fewer than 10 neuroimaging studies examining neural correlates in gambling disorder have been published, studies using healthy controls have investigated intertemporal choice, loss aversion, and other components influencing decision-making.[53,104,119] One functional magnetic resonance imaging study examining the neural correlates of loss-chasing behavior demonstrated increased ventromedial prefrontal cortex activation when healthy individuals tried to win back money lost on previous gambles.[14] Loss-chasing, therefore, appears linked to brain areas involved in reward processing[59] and raises the possibility that recreational gamblers may chase losses because they believe that winning is imminent.[14] The extent to which these findings relate to gambling disorder requires further, direct investigation.

Treatment

Few pharmacological and behavioral therapies targeting gambling disorder have been investigated with respect to their tolerabilities and efficacies. It is estimated that only 75%–12% of pathological gamblers seek formal treatment for gambling disorder.[61,109] These individuals may seek treatment for various reasons (e.g., threats of spousal divorce, suicide attempts), and thus treatment-seeking pathological gamblers may differ from pathological gamblers in the general population.[40]

Behavioral Treatments

Although Gamblers Anonymous is arguably the most widespread intervention for gambling disorder, questions exist regarding its effectiveness. One study reported that most individuals attend only one or two meetings and less than 10% remain in attendance after 1 year.[114] Cognitive therapies have shown promise in the treatment of gambling disorder. One cognitive therapy targets erroneous cognitions, such as illusions of control over random events, and was found to be helpful in an initial, small, wait-list–controlled study.[62] Following this treatment, approximately 86% of individuals no longer met gambling disorder criteria, and individuals reported greater self-efficacy and perception of control over their gambling problem. This type of therapy may also be effective in group format, and therapeutic gains appear to be maintained after 1 year.[63] Cognitive behavioral therapy for gambling disorder identifies gambling triggers and cognitive biases, reinforces nongambling behaviors, teaches coping skills, and addresses finance management and debt settlement.[87] Individuals receiving cognitive behavioral therapy showed greater reductions in gambling problems and time spent gambling than did those attending Gamblers Anonymous. However, both groups demonstrated improvements over time.

Other psychological interventions have been developed, including aversive therapy, imaginal desensitization, motivational enhancement, brief guided therapy, self-help workbooks, and eclectic therapies. The effectiveness of psychological interventions has been complicated by differences in assessments used to evaluate treatment outcome.[82] However, a review of behavioral therapy outcome studies showed that these interventions are associated with significant improvement both posttreatment and after long-term follow-up when compared with no treatment.[82] It should be noted, however, that drop-out rates in many studies approach 50%.[62] Future studies should examine the efficacy of combining different therapies that target different cognitive and motivational aspects of gambling disorder.

Pharmacological Treatments

Like in behavioral treatments, the evaluation of the efficacies of pharmacological therapies in gambling disorder is complicated by differences in sample sizes, trial durations, dosing strategies, trial designs, and outcome measures.

The findings of low serotonin levels in gambling disorder and blunted ventromedial prefrontal cortex to serotonergic drugs in impulse control disorders[103] suggest that selective serotonin reuptake inhibitors could be useful therapeutic agents for gambling disorder. Several studies have demonstrated that selective serotonin reuptake inhibitors such as fluvoxamine and paroxetine are associated with short-term improvement in pathological gamblers.[24,47,48,57] However, placebo-controlled trials of fluvoxamine and paroxetine have also yielded negative results.[10,39] Some variability in outcome may relate to heterogeneity of pathological gamblers, and guiding selection of therapies according to presence of co-occurring disorders (e.g., selective serotonin reuptake inhibitors for individuals with co-occurring gambling disorder and anxiety disorders) may help improve treatment outcomes.[43,93] Consistent with this notion, a study examining lithium in the treatment of individuals with co-occurring gambling disorder and bipolar-spectrum disorders found lithium to be superior to placebo in reducing symptoms of both gambling and mania.[49]

Three separate studies have found opioid antagonists (naltrexone and nalmefene) to be superior to placebo in the treatment of gambling disorder.[41,46,58] Individuals with a family history of alcoholism may be particularly responsive to treatment with an opiate antagonist.[42] Medications targeting dopamine receptors directly (e.g., the serotonin/dopamine antagonist olanzapine) have been shown in two placebo-controlled trials not to be superior to placebo in the treatment of gambling disorder.[31,70]

Natural Recovery

Like in drug addictions, untreated recovery appears to occur in gambling disorder Using cross-sectional data, it has been estimated that most pathological gamblers recover without any therapeutic intervention.[109] These findings suggest that gambling disorder in the community may represent an episodic rather than chronic disorder, and which factors influence its course require further investigation.[109,120]

Prevention Efforts

Few studies have investigated prevention efforts for gambling disorder. Primary prevention efforts for gambling might include more stringent regulation of gambling availability and advertisements and education initiatives on risks associated with gambling. The effectiveness of such interventions requires empirical testing. Given the exposure to nicotine and mutagens in some gambling environments, gambling may be associated with significant health risks.[54] Therefore, the amount of tobacco smoke exposure should be considered in discussions of healthy levels of gambling. A less-apparent health risk may be related to the significant increases in autonomic arousal associated with gambling[71,72]; approximately 83% of casino-related deaths may be attributable to sudden cardiac arrests.[52]

Identifying those individuals at greatest risk for developing gambling disorder may be important in developing effective prevention strategies. Many health care providers may not inquire about gambling disorder when assessing patients.[17] Like for substance abuse and dependence, screening tools for gambling disorder may be useful for medical practitioners, as associations between medical conditions and gambling disorder have been observed in community and medical clinic samples.[26,83,90,91,95] As discussed above, individuals with Parkinson disease should be monitored carefully during the course of their treatment to identify any changes in gambling behaviors.

Other prevention efforts include the use of gambling helplines and self-exclusion policies at casinos where individuals can voluntarily ask that they not be allowed on the gambling site premises.[61,97] The effectiveness of both of these prevention efforts has received relatively little study, although early analysis of self-exclusion programs suggest that they are associated with a 30% self-reported abstinence of gambling activities.[61,64] Self-exclusion programs may benefit from more extensive reinforcement through professional follow-up.[61]

Research Challenges and Future Directions

Over the last decade, several pharmacological and behavioral treatments of gambling disorder have received initial empirical support.[45,76] However, multiple questions and potentially confounding factors exist. For example, because relatively few pathological gamblers seek treatment, it is not clear whether those who do are representative of the larger gambling disorder population.[76] Individuals who seek help may demonstrate ambivalence toward treatment. For example, many individuals may still maintain positive feelings about gambling, and completion of even a short 6-week treatment study may be difficult to achieve.[120] The issue of monetary incentives for study participation may raise questions, as subjects may be motivated to participate by receipt of financial compensation rather than a genuine desire to stop gambling.[120] Moreover, the impetus for change in many pathological gamblers are financial crises that may not be resolved through psychological or pharmacological treatments.[120]

Many early treatment outcome studies have excluded individuals with co-occurring disorders. Given that many pathological gamblers have co-occurring disorders, questions are raised about the generalizability of such studies.[76] Initial studies suggest that co-occurring disorders influence treatment response.[93] Therefore, common co-occurring conditions should be identified and treatment outcome studies evaluated accordingly.[76] Furthermore, the use of a clinical control group in treatment studies, such as groups with other impulse control disorders or alcohol dependence, could be useful in identifying underlying biobehavioral factors and assessing similarities with other disorders.[34]

There are many unique populations affected by gambling disorder. However, to date, research, has included predominantly white males. Racial/ethnic differences have been observed with respect to gambling disorder in Asian,[85] Black,[2] Hispanic,[21] and Native American[30] groups. Differences in clinical characteristics of pathological gamblers have also been found to be associated with sexual orientation.[44] Individuals from minority populations may benefit preferentially from specific therapies. With respect to gender, although males and females with gambling disorder may both be willing to seek treatment, differences in clinical features may be important in guiding treatment.[40] For example, gambling triggers in females may be more strongly influenced by mood state, and thus therapy may preferentially target affective symptoms or mood regulation.[40]

Gambling disorder and substance dependence appear to involve similar patterns of dysregulation within ventral components of frontostriatal circuitry, neurocognitive impairments in inhibition and decision-making, and neurochemical and psychophysiological markers suggestive of arousal deficits. The frequent co-occurrence of gambling disorder and substance dependence disorders is consistent with the notion that similar mechanisms may underlie both disorders. Additional research may identify more specifically how gambling disorder relates to substance-based addictions and whether classification of gambling disorder as a nonsubstance addiction is appropriate.

The continued use of brain imaging techniques and the performance of large genetic studies should help advance the knowledge of the bio-behavioral basis of gambling disorder. The use of neuropsychological, neurochemical, neuroimaging, genetic, environmental, physiological, and self-report measures in treatment and community settings should facilitate integration of clinically relevant information.[34,40] An improved understanding of the relationship among these different facets should aid in establishing clinically relevant intermediary phenotypes for gambling disorder and advancing efforts in better characterization, diagnosis, and treatment of pathological gamblers.

References

1. American Psychiatric Association. *Diagnostic and Statistical Manual of Mental Disorders.* 5th ed. Washington, DC: American Psychiatric Association; 2013.
2. Barry DT, Steinberg MA, Wu R, Potenza MN. Characteristics of black and white callers to a gambling helpline. *Psychiatric Services.* 2008;59:1347–1350.
3. Bechara A. Risky business: emotion, decision-making, and addiction. *J Gambling Stud.* 2003;19:23–51.
4. Bechara A, Damasio H, Tranel D, Damasio AR. Deciding advantageously before knowing the advantageous strategy. *Science.* 1997;275:1293–1295.
5. Benkelfat C, Murphy DL, Hill JL, George DT, Nutt D, Linnoila M. Ethanollike properties of the serotonergic partial agonist m-chlorophenylpiperazine in chronic alcoholic patients. *Arch Gen Psychiatry.* 1991;48:383.
6. Bergh C, Eklund T, Sodersten P, Nordin C. Altered dopamine function in pathological gambling. *Psychol Med.* 1997;27:473–475.
7. Best M, Williams JM, Coccaro EF. Evidence for a dysfunctional prefrontal circuit in patients with an impulsive aggressive disorder. *Proc Natl Acad Sci USA.* 2002;99:8448–8453.
8. Black DW, Moyer T, Schlosser S. Quality of life and family history in pathological gambling. *J Nerv Ment Dis.* 2003;191:124–126.
9. Blanco C, Moreyra P, Nunes EV, Saiz-Ruiz J, Ibanez A. Pathological gambling: addiction or compulsion? *Semin Clin Neuropsychiatry.* 2001;6:167–176.
10. Blanco C, Petkova E, Ibanez A, Saiz-Ruiz J. A pilot placebo-controlled study of fluvoxamine for pathological gambling. *Ann Clin Psychiatry.* 2002;14:9–15.
11. Blaszczynski A, Steel Z. Personality disorders among pathological gamblers. *J Gambl Stud.* 1998;14:51–71.
12. Boyer M, Dickerson M. Attentional bias and addictive behaviour: automaticity in a gambling-specific modified Stroop task. *Addiction.* 2003;98:61–70.
13. Brewer JA, Potenza MN. The neurobiology and genetics of impulse control disorders: relationships to drug addictions. *Biochem Pharmacol.* 2008;75:63–75.
14. Campbell-Meiklejohn DK, Woolrich MW, Passingham RE, Rogers RD. Knowing when to stop: the brain mechanisms of chasing losses. *Biol Psychiatry.* 2008;63:293–300.
15. Cavedini P, Riboldi G, Keller R, D'Annucci A, Bellodi L. Frontal lobe dysfunction in pathological gambling. *Biol Psychiatry.* 2002;51:334–341.
16. Chambers RA, Potenza MN. Neurodevelopment, impulsivity and adolescent gambling. *J Gambling Stud.* 2003;19:53–84.

17. Christensen MH, Patsdaughter CA, Babington LM. Health care providers' experiences with problem gamblers. *J Gambl Stud.* 2001;17:71–79.

18. Comings DE, Gade-Andavolu R, Gonzalez N, et al. The additive effect of neurotransmitter genes in pathological gambling. *Clin Genet.* 2001;60:107–116.

19. Comings DE, Rosenthal RJ, Lesieur HR, et al. A study of the dopamine D2 receptor gene in pathological gambling. *Pharmacogenetics.* 1996;6:223–234.

20. Cote D, Caron A, Aubert J, Desrochers V, Ladouceur R. Near wins prolong gambling on a video lottery terminal. *J Gambl Stud.* 2003;19:433–438.

21. Cuadrado M. A comparison of Hispanic and Anglo calls to a gambling hotline. *J Gambling Stud.* 1999;15:71–82.

22. Cunningham-Williams RM, Cottler LB, Compton WM, Spitznagel EL. Taking chances: problem gamblers and mental health disorders – results from the St. Louis epidemiologic catchment area study. *Am J Public Health.* 1998;88:1093–1096.

23. da Silva Lobo DS, Vallada HP, Knight J, et al. Dopamine genes and pathological gambling in discordant sib-pairs. *J Gambl Stud.* 2007;23:421–433.

24. De La Gandara J, Sanz O, Gilaberte I. *Fluoxetine: Open-Trial in Pathological Gambling.* Washington, DC: American Psychiatric Association Annual Convention; 1999.

25. DeCaria CM, Begaz T, Hollander E. Serotonergic and noradrenergic function in pathological gambling. *CNS Spectr.* 1998;3:38–47.

26. Desai RA, Desai MM, Potenza MN. Gambling, health and age: data from the national epidemiologic survey on alcohol and related conditions. *Psychol Addict Behav.* 2007;21:431–440.

27. Desai RA, Potenza MN. Gender differences in the associations between past-year gambling problems and psychiatric disorders. *Soc Psychiatry Psychiatr Epidemiol.* 2008;43:173–183.

28. Dodd ML, Klos KJ, Bower JH, Geda YE, Josephs KA, Ahlskog JE. Pathological gambling caused by drugs used to treat Parkinson disease. *Arch Neurol.* 2005;62:1377–1381.

29. Eisen SA, Lin N, Lyons MJ, et al. Familial influences on gambling behavior: an analysis of 3359 twin pairs. *Addiction.* 1998;93:1375–1384.

30. Elia C, Jacobs DF. The incidence of pathological gambling among native Americans treated for alcohol dependence. *Int J Addictions.* 1993;28:659–666.

31. Fong T, Kalechstein A, Bernhard B, Rosenthal R, Rugle L. A double-blind, placebo-controlled trial of olanzapine for the treatment of video poker pathological gamblers. *Pharmacol Biochem Behav.* 2008;89:298–303.

32. Forbush KT, Shaw M, Graeber MA, et al. Neuropsychological characteristics and personality traits in pathological gambling. *CNS Spectr.* 2008;13:306–315.

33. Gambino B, Fitzgerald R, Shaffer H, Renner J, Courtnage P. Perceived family history of problem gambling and scores on SOGS. *Am J Psych.* 1993;9:169–184.

34. Goudriaan AE, Oosterlaan J, de Beurs E, van den Brink W. Pathological gambling: a comprehensive review of biobehavioral findings. *Neurosci Biobehav Rev.* 2004;28:123–141.

35. Goudriaan AE, Oosterlaan J, de Beurs E, van den Brink W. Decision making in pathological gambling: a comparison between pathological gamblers, alcohol dependents, persons with Tourette syndrome, and normal controls. *Brain Res Cogn Brain Res.* 2005;23:137–151.

36. Goudriaan AE, Oosterlaan J, de Beurs E, van den Brink W. Psychophysiological determinants and concomitants of deficient decision making in pathological gamblers. *Drug Alcohol Depend.* 2006;84:231–239.

37. Goudriaan AE, Oosterlaan J, de Beurs E, van den Brink W. Neurocognitive functions in pathological gambling: a comparison with alcohol dependence, Tourette syndrome and normal controls. *Addiction.* 2006;101:534–547.

38. Goudriaan AE, Oosterlaan J, De Beurs E, Van Den Brink W. The role of self-reported impulsivity and reward sensitivity versus neurocognitive measures of disinhibition and decision-making in the prediction of relapse in pathological gamblers. *Psychol Med.* 2008;38:41–50.

39. Grant J, Kim SW, Potenza MN, et al. Paroxetine treatment of pathological gambling: a multi-center randomized controlled trial. *Int Clin Psychopharmacol.* 2003;18:243–249.

40. Grant JE, Kim SW. Gender differences in pathological gamblers seeking medication treatment. *Compr Psychiatry.* 2002;43:56–62.

41. Grant JE, Kim SW, Hartman BK. A double-blind, placebo-controlled study of the opiate antagonist naltrexone in the treatment of pathological gambling urges. *J Clin Psychiatry.* 2008:e1–e7.

42. Grant JE, Kim SW, Hollander E, Potenza MN. Predicting response to opiate antagonists and placebo in the treatment of pathological gambling. *Psychopharmacology.* 2008;200:521–527.

43. Grant JE, Potenza MN. Escitalopram treatment of pathological gambling with co-occurring anxiety: an open-label pilot study with double-blind discontinuation. *Int Clin Psychopharmacol.* 2006;21:203–209.

44. Grant JE, Potenza MN. Sexual orientation of men with pathological gambling: prevalence and psychiatric comorbidity in a treatment-seeking sample. *Compr Psychiatry.* 2006;47:515–518.

45. Grant JE, Potenza MN. Treatments for pathological gambling and other impulse control disorders. In: Gorman J, Nathan P, eds. *A Guide to Treatments that Work.* Oxford, UK: University Press; 2007:561–577.

46. Grant JE, Potenza MN, Hollander E, et al. Multicenter investigation of the opioid antagonist nalmefene in the treatment of pathological gambling. *Am J Psychiatry.* 2006;163:303–312.

47. Hollander E, DeCaria C, Mari E, et al. Short-term single-blind fluvoxamine treatment of pathological gambling. *Am J Psych.* 1998;155:1781–1783.

48. Hollander E, DeCaria CM, Finkell JN, Begaz T, Wong CM, Cartwright C. A randomized double-blind fluvoxamine/placebo crossover trial in pathological gambling. *Biol Psychiatry.* 2000;47:813–817.

49. Hollander E, Pallanti S, Allen A, Sood E, Baldini Rossi N. Does sustained-release lithium reduce impulsive gambling and affective instability versus placebo in pathological gamblers with bipolar spectrum disorders? *Am J Psychiatry.* 2005;162:137–145.

50. Ibanez A, Blanco C, Perez de Castro I, Fernandez-Piqueras J, Saiz-Ruiz J. Genetics of pathological gambling. *J Gambl Stud.* 2003;19:11–22.

51. Ibanez A, de Castro IP, Fernandez-Piqueras J, Blanco C, Saiz-Ruiz J. Pathological gambling and DNA polymorphic markers at MAO-A and MAO-B genes. *Mol Psychiatry.* 2000;5:105–109.

52. Jason DR, Taff ML, Boglioli LR. Casino-related deaths in Atlantic city, New Jersey 1982–1986. *Am J Forensic Med Pathol.* 1990;11:112–123.

53. Kable JW, Glimcher PW. The neural correlates of subjective value during intertemporal choice. *Nat Neurosci.* 2007;10:1625–1633.

54. Kado NY, McCurdy SA, Tesluk SJ, et al. Measuring personal exposure to airborne mutagens and nicotine in environmental tobacco smoke. *Mutat Res.* 1991;261:75–82.

55. Kessler RC, Hwang I, Labrie R, et al. DSM-IV pathological gambling in the national comorbidity survey replication. *Psychol Med.* 2008;38:1351–1360.

56. Kessler RC, McGonagle KA, Zhao S, et al. Lifetime and 12-month prevalence of DSM-III-R psychiatric disorders in the United States. Results from the national comorbidity survey. *Arch Gen Psychiatry.* 1994;51:8–19.

57. Kim S, Grant JE, Adson DE, Shin YC, Zaninelli R. A double-blind, placebo-controlled study of the efficacy and safety of paroxetine in the treatment of pathological gambling disorder. *J Clin Psychiatry.* 2002;63:501–507.

58. Kim SW, Grant JE. Personality dimensions in pathological gambling disorder and obsessive-compulsive disorder. *Psychiatry Res.* 2001;104:205–212.

59. Knutson B, Fong GW, Bennett SM, Adams CM, Hommer D. A region of mesial prefrontal cortex tracks monetarily rewarding outcomes: characterization with rapid event-related fMRI. *Neuroimage.* 2003;18:263–272.

60. Koob GF, Nestler EJ. The neurobiology of drug addiction. *J Neuropsychiatry Clin Neurosci.* 1997;9:482–497.

61. Ladouceur R, Jacques C, Giroux I, Ferland F, Leblond J. Analysis of a casino's self-exclusion program. *J Gambl Stud.* 2000;16:453–460.

62. Ladouceur R, Sylvain C, Boutin C, et al. Cognitive treatment of pathological gambling. *J Nerv Ment Dis.* 2001;189:774–780.

63. Ladouceur R, Sylvain C, Boutin C, Lachance S, Doucet C, Leblond J. Group therapy for pathological gamblers: a cognitive approach. *Behav Res Ther.* 2003;41:587–596.

64. Ladouceur R, Sylvain C, Gosselin P. Self-exclusion program: a longitudinal evaluation study. *J Gambl Stud.* 2007;23:85–94.

65. Lesieur HR, Blume SB. The South Oaks Gambling Screen (SOGS): a new instrument for the identification of pathological gamblers. *Am J Psychiatry.* 1987;144:1184–1188.

66. Linnoila M, Virkkunen M, Scheinin M, Nuutila A, Rimon R, Goodwin FK. Low cerebrospinal fluid 5-hydroxyindoleacetic acid concentration differentiates impulsive from nonimpulsive violent behavior. *Life Sci.* 1983;33:2609–2614.

67. Marks I. Behavioural (non-chemical) addictions. *Br J Addict.* 1990;85:1389–1394.

68. Mayberg H, Liotti M, Brannan SK, et al. Reciprocal limbic-cortical function and negative mood: converging PET findings in depression and normal sadness. *Am J Psychiatry.* 1999;156:675–682.

69. McCusker CG, Gettings B. Automaticity of cognitive biases in addictive behaviours: further evidence with gamblers. *Br J Clin Psychol.* 1997;36(Pt 4):543–554.

70. McElroy SL, Nelson EB, Welge JA, Kaehler L, Keck Jr PE. Olanzapine in the treatment of pathological gambling: a negative randomized placebo-controlled trial. *J Clin Psychiatry.* 2008;69:433–440.

71. Meyer G, Hauffa BP, Schedlowski M, Pawlak C, Stadler MA, Exton MS. Casino gambling increases heart rate and salivary cortisol in regular gamblers. *Biol Psychiatry.* 2000;48:948–953.

72. Meyer G, Schwertfeger J, Exton MS, et al. Neuroendocrine response to casino gambling in problem gamblers. *Psychoneuroendocrinology.* 2004;29:1272–1280.

73. Miele GM, Tilly SM, First M, Frances A. The definition of dependence and behavioural addictions. *Br J Addict.* 1990;85:1421–1423; discussion 1429–1431.

74. Miller NV, Currie SR. A Canadian population level analysis of the roles of irrational gambling cognitions and risky gambling practices as correlates of gambling intensity and pathological gambling. *J Gambl Stud.* 2008;24:257–274.

75. Moreno I, Saiz-Ruiz J, Lopez-Ibor JJ. Serotonin and gambling dependence. *Human Psychopharmacol.* 1991;6:9–12.

76. Nathan PE. Methodological problems in research on treatments for pathological gambling. *J Gambl Stud.* 2005;21:109–116.

77. *National Gambling Impact Study Commission Final Report*; 1999.

78. Noble EP. Addiction and its reward process through polymorphisms of the D2 dopamine receptor gene: a review. *Eur Psychiatry.* 2000;15:79–89.

79. Nordin C, Eklundh T. Altered CSF 5-HIAA disposition in pathologic male gamblers. *CNS Spectr.* 1999;4:25–33.

80. Nordin C, Nylander PO. Temperament and character in pathological gambling. *J Gambl Stud.* 2007;23:113–120.

81. Nordin C, Sjodin I. CSF monoamine patterns in pathological gamblers and healthy controls. *J Psychiatr Res.* 2006;40:454–459.

82. Pallesen S, Mitsem M, Kvale G, Johnsen BH, Molde H. Outcome of psychological treatments of pathological gambling: a review and meta-analysis. *Addiction.* 2004;100:1412–1422.

83. Pasternak AV, Fleming MF. Prevalence of gambling disorders in a primary care setting. *Arch Fam Med.* 1999;8:515–520.

84. Perez de Castro I, Ibanez A, Saiz-Ruiz J, Fernandez-Piqueras J. Genetic contribution to pathological gambling: possible association between a functional DNA polymorphism at the serotonin transporter gene (5-HTT) and affected men. *Pharmacogenetics.* 1999;9:397–400.

85. Petry N. Gambling participation and problems among Southeast Asian refugees. *Psychiatric Services.* 2003;54:1142–1148.

86. Petry NM. Substance abuse, pathological gambling, and impulsiveness. *Drug Alcohol Depend.* 2001;63:29–38.

87. Petry NM, Ammerman Y, Bohl J, et al. Cognitive-behavioral therapy for pathological gamblers. *J Consult Clin Psychol.* 2006;74:555–567.

88. Petry NM, Kiluk BD. Suicidal ideation and suicide attempts in treatment-seeking pathological gamblers. *J Nerv Ment Dis.* 2002;190:462–469.

89. Petry NM, Stinson FS, Grant BF. Comorbidity of DSM-IV pathological gambling and other psychiatric disorders: results from the national epidemiologic survey on alcohol and related conditions. *J Clin Psychiatry.* 2005;66:564–574.

90. Pietrzak RH, Molina CA, Ladd GT, Kerins GJ, Petry NM. Health and psychosocial correlates of disordered gambling in older adults. *Am J Ger Psychiatry.* 2005;13:510–519.

91. Pietrzak RH, Morasco BJ, Blanco C, Grant BF, Petry NM. Gambling level and psychiatric and medical disorders in older adults: results from the national epidemiologic survey on alcohol and related conditions. *Am J Geriatr Psychiatry.* 2007;15:301–313.

92. Potenza MN. Should addictive disorders include non-substance-related conditions? *Addiction.* 2006;101:142–151.

93. Potenza MN. Impulse control disorders and co-occurring disorders: dual diagnosis considerations. *J Dual Diagn.* 2007;3:47–57.

94. Potenza MN. Review. The neurobiology of pathological gambling and drug addiction: an overview and new findings. *Philos Trans R Soc Lond B Biol Sci.* 2008;363:3181–3189.

95. Potenza MN, Fiellin DA, Heninger GR, Rounsaville BJ, Mazure CM. Gambling: an addictive behavior with health and primary care implications. *J Gen Intern Med.* 2002;17:721–732.

96. Potenza MN, Leung H-C, Blumberg HP, et al. An fMRI Stroop study of ventromedial prefrontal cortical function in pathological gamblers. *Am J Psychiatry.* 2003;160:1990–1994.

97. Potenza MN, Steinberg MA, McLaughlin SD, Wu R, Rounsaville BJ, O'Malley SS. Gender-related differences in the characteristics of problem gamblers using a gambling helpline. *Am J Psychiatry.* 2001;158:1500–1505.

98. Potenza MN, Steinberg MA, Skudlarski P, et al. Gambling urges in pathological gamblers: an fMRI study. *Arch Gen Psychiatry.* 2003;60:828–836.

99. Potenza MN, Voon V, Weintraub D. Drug Insight: impulse control disorders and dopamine therapies in Parkinson's disease. *Nat Clin Pract Neurol.* 2007;3:664–672.

100. Potenza MN, Xian H, Shah K, Scherrer JF, Eisen SA. Shared genetic contributions to pathological gambling and major depression in men. *Arch Gen Psychiatry.* 2005;62:1015–1021.

101. Regard M, Knoch D, Gutling E, Landis T. Brain damage and addictive behavior: a neuropsychological and electroencephalogram investigation with pathologic gamblers. *Cogn Behav Neurol.* 2003;16:47–53.

102. Reuter J, Raedler T, Rose M, Hand I, Glascher J, Buchel C. Pathological gambling is linked to reduced activation of the mesolimbic reward system. *Nat Neurosci.* 2005;8:147–148.

103. Rogers R, Everitt BJ, Baldacchino A, et al. Dissociable deficits in the decision-making cognition of chronic amphetamine abusers, opiate abusers, patients with focal damage to prefrontal cortex, and tryptophan-depleted normal volunteers: evidence for monaminergic mechanisms. *Neuropsychophamacology.* 1999;20:322–339.

104. Rogers RD, Ramnani N, Mackay C, et al. Distinct portions of anterior cingulate cortex and medial prefrontal cortex are activated by reward processing in separable phases of decision-making cognition. *Biol Psychiatry*. 2004;55:594–602.

105. Rugle L, Melamed L. Neuropsychological assessment of attention problems in pathological gamblers. *J Nerv Ment Dis*. 1993;181:107–112.

106. Reference deleted in review.

107. Shaffer HJ, Hall MN, Vander Bilt J. Estimating the prevalence of disordered gambling behavior in the United States and Canada: a research synthesis. *Am J Public Health*. 1999;89:1369–1376.

108. Shinohara K, Yanagisawa A, Kagota Y, et al. Physiological changes in Pachinko players; beta-endorphin, catecholamines, immune system substances and heart rate. *Appl Human Sci*. 1999;18:37–42.

109. Slutske WS. Natural recovery and treatment-seeking in pathological gambling: results of two U.S. national surveys. *Am J Psychiatry*. 2006;163:297–302.

110. Slutske WS, Eisen S, True WR, Lyons MJ, Goldberg J, Tsuang M. Common genetic vulnerability for pathological gambling and alcohol dependence in men. *Arch Gen Psychiatry*. 2000;57:666–673.

111. Slutske WS, Eisen S, Xian H, et al. A twin study of the association between pathological gambling and antisocial personality disorder. *J Abnorm Psychol*. 2001;110:297–308.

112. Steel Z, Blaszczynski A. Impulsivity, personality disorders and pathological gambling severity. *Addiction*. 1998;93:895–905.

113. Stein DJ, Hollander E, DeCaria CM, Simeon D, Cohen L, Aronowitz B. m-Chlorophenylpiperazine challenge in borderline personality disorder: relationship of neuroendocrine response, behavioral response, and clinical measures. *Biol Psychiatry*. 1996;40:508–513.

114. Stewart RM, Brown RI. An outcome study of gamblers anonymous. *Br J Psychiatry*. 1988;152:284–288.

115. Stucki S, Rihs-Middel M. Prevalence of adult problem and pathological gambling between 2000 and 2005: an Update. *J Gambl Stud*. 2007;23:245–257.

116. Tanabe J, Thompson L, Claus E, Dalwani M, Hutchison K, Banich MT. Prefrontal cortex activity is reduced in gambling and nongambling substance users during decision-making. *Hum Brain Mapp*. 2007;28:1276–1286.

117. Tavares H, Zilberman ML, Beites FJ, Gentil V. Gender differences in gambling progression. *J Gambl Stud*. 2001;17:151–159.

118. Toce-Gerstein M, Gerstein DR, Volberg RA. A hierarchy of gambling disorders in the community. *Addiction*. 2003;98:1661–1672.

119. Tom SM, Fox CR, Trepel C, Poldrack RA. The neural basis of loss aversion in decision-making under risk. *Science*. 2007;315:515–518.

120. Toneatto T. A perspective on problem gambling treatment: issues and challenges. *J Gambl Stud*. 2005;21:73–80.

121. Toneatto T, Blitz-Miller T, Calderwood K, Dragonetti R, Tsanos A. Cognitive distortions in heavy gambling. *J Gambl Stud*. 1997;13:253–266.

122. Virkkunen M, De Jong J, Bartko J, Goodwin FK, Linnoila M. Relationship of psychobiological variables to recidivism in violent offenders and impulsive fire setters. A follow-up study. *Arch Gen Psychiatry*. 1989;46:600–603.

123. Virkkunen M, Rawlings R, Tokola R, et al. CSF biochemistries, glucose metabolism, and diurnal activity rhythms in alcoholic, violent offenders, fire setters, and healthy volunteers. *Arch Gen Psychiatry*. 1994;51:20–27.

124. Voon V, Hassan K, Zurowski M, et al. Prevalence of repetitive and reward-seeking behaviors in Parkinson disease. *Neurology*. 2006;67:1254–1257.

125. Voon V, Potenza MN, Thomsen T. Medication-related impulse control and repetitive behaviors in Parkinson's disease. *Curr Opin Neurol*. 2007;20:484–492.

126. Weinstock J, Ledgerwood DM, Modesto-Lowe V, Petry NM. Ludomania: cross-cultural examinations of gambling and its treatment. *Rev Bras Psiquiatr*. 2008;(suppl 1):S3–S10.

127. Weintraub D, Koester J, Potenza MN, et al. *Dopaminergic Therapy and Impulse Control Disorders in Parkinson's Disease: A Cross-Sectional Study of Over 3,000 Patients*. Chicago, IL: Movement Disorders Society; 2008.

128. Weintraub D, Potenza MN. Impulse control disorders in Parkinson's disease. *Curr Neurol Neurosci Rep*. 2006;6:302–306.

129. Welte JW, Barnes GM, Tidwell MC, Hoffman JH. The prevalence of problem gambling among U.S. adolescents and young adults: results from a national survey. *J Gambl Stud*. 2008;24:119–133.

130. Welte JW, Barnes GM, Wieczorek WF, Tidwell MC, Parker JC. Risk factors for pathological gambling. *Addict Behav*. 2004;29:323–335.

131. Zack M, Poulos CX. Amphetamine primes motivation to gamble and gambling-related semantic networks in problem gamblers. *Neuropsychopharmacology*. 2004;29:195–207.

132. Zack M, Poulos CX. A D2 antagonist enhances the rewarding and priming effects of a gambling episode in pathological gamblers. *Neuropsychopharmacology*. 2007;32:1678–1686.

34

Implications of Food Addiction for Understanding and Treating Binge Eating Disorder

JACQUELINE C. CARTER, CAROLINE DAVIS, AND THERESE E. KENNY

Introduction

There has been considerable debate in the field about whether applying an addiction model could advance our understanding and treatment of compulsive overeating (e.g., Wilson[189]). Although we agree that an addiction model does not adequately address all of the core clinical features of eating disorders, we believe that this perspective may be useful in furthering our understanding of binge eating disorder (BED), in particular, and devising better treatments. BED is characterized by recurrent episodes of binge eating in the absence of the extreme weight control behaviors (e.g., fasting or self-induced vomiting) seen in anorexia nervosa and bulimia nervosa. Although acknowledging that BED and food addiction also have unique features that must be taken into consideration,[159] in this chapter, we argue that considering certain similarities between BED and substance use disorders would be useful in understanding the causes of compulsive overeating and in developing more effective treatments for BED. In presenting our case, we consider clinical and psychological parallels between binge eating and drug abuse. We also discuss the similarities in their psychobiological underpinnings

and the overlapping risk factors for their development. Finally, we consider the treatment implications of integrating an addiction model into empirically supported treatments for BED.

History and Background

Although people had written about the enslaving properties of opium and alcohol for centuries, it was not until the 1800s that the notion of drug abuse as a disease entity—rather than an issue of moral culpability—entered the general parlance of medical professionals.[111] Although the original (17th-century) use of the word *addicted* meant "to give over ... to someone or some practice," its first appearance with specific reference to narcotics was not until the early 20th century,[23] and for most of that time it was largely confined to the misuse of alcohol and the opiates. With the rise in popularity of psychiatry after World War II and the "rediscovery of addiction,"[22] other substances such as cocaine, amphetamine, and nicotine were added to the list of addictive drugs.

In recent years, there has been an interesting clinical and scientific shift in perspective, with many believing that addiction should encompass the compulsive engagement in activities such as gaming, Internet use, and shopping, in addition to its conventional relation with pharmacological rewards.[85,94,138,149] Current debate has even extended to the possibility that so-called behavioral addictions should include the abuse of *natural rewards*—that is, behaviors that are intrinsically necessary for our survival, and in which we freely engage with pleasure and without social sanction. Indeed, the *Diagnostic and Statistical Manual of Mental Disorders, Fifth Edition* (DSM-5) combines substance-related disorders and addictive disorders into a single category. Gambling disorder is the only currently recognized addictive disorder, with Internet gaming identified as a disorder requiring further study.

A few generations ago, it might have seemed heretical to suggest that food could be an addictive substance and that overeating could be an addictive behavior. As testament, we were able to find only six published references to such a viewpoint from 1950 to 1970, almost all of them written by T.G. Randolph,[150] the well-known founder of environmental medicine. However, an upsurge of change in perspective has occurred in the past few years, with a multitude of scientific journals publishing papers on food addiction, and the idea that certain foods, or food additives, have addictive properties has been accepted increasingly within the scientific community over the past decade.

Drugs as Food

Conventional evolutionary mismatch views of addiction propose that substance use is a relatively recent phenomenon in the history of our species and that it occurs largely because of the availability of purified and synthetic drugs and their direct routes of administration.[134,162] In other words, it is the ubiquity and concentrated doses of these substances that have contributed to widespread human drug abuse. By contrast, Sullivan and Hagen have pointed out that human beings shared a coevolutionary relationship with psychotropic plant substances in prehistory for millennia.[167] Indeed, they frequently ate them as food because their ingestion solved a recurrent problem faced by our ancestors.

The neurotransmitters that are essential for normal human functioning—and most implicated in substance use—are dopamine and serotonin, the precursors of which must be provisioned externally from high-quality nutrients such as protein. During most of our history, due to famines and seasonal food shortages, these precursors were nutritionally constrained and, consequently, people experienced neurotransmitter deficits with considerable regularity. Depletions of this sort tend to affect critical behaviors and emotions adversely, including motor activities, cognitive abilities, and mood.

In addition, it is generally believed that over our evolutionary history, certain plants developed chemical defenses against mammalian predators by producing neurotransmitter substitutes, which had toxic effects when ingested. Sullivan and Hagen argued that in response to this threat, "behaviourally sophisticated hominids" evolved to counterexploit the potential benefits of plant toxins.[167] For example, because these "neurotransmitter analogues" imparted energy, prevented fatigue, diminished appetite, and increased tolerance for hunger, they helped to avoid the maladaptive "behavioral sequelae of stress" in the absence of adequate food sources. In other words, plant substances served the dual purpose of substituting for more costly energy and buffering against the biological ravages of prolonged stress.

Thus, it seems reasonable and sensible to conclude that organic compounds in our environment can only be categorized as *beneficial* or *harmful* when we take account of dosage and the relevant characteristics of those who partake of them.[81]

Food as Drugs

This last point is particularly relevant when considering the typical macronutrient intake in current Western societies. Diets high in concentrated fats and sugars are not only dense in calories, but metabolically efficient because a large proportion of their energy is provided to the consumer. They also tend to elevate mood by releasing neuropeptides, which reinforce their selective preference.[101] Evolutionary biologists believe that cravings for sugar and fat evolved to enhance human energy intake in unpredictable nutritional environments, which were universally the norm until relatively recently.[81] However, in the quantities that many people ingest them today, they have an abuse potential rivaling that of popular addictive drugs.[96]

The food industry has become especially savvy in exploiting our natural human desire for sugar and fat by increasing manyfold their dose in much of our daily foods. For instance, there was a 42% per capita increase in the consumption of added fats and a 162% increase in cheese relative to only a 20% increase in fruits and vegetables between 1970 and 2000.[73] The sharply reduced cost of sugar and vegetable oils worldwide has greatly contributed to the production of highly palatable processed foods.[65] The incidence of snacking, especially in the form of carbohydrates, has also increased over the past 25 years, in tandem with the increase in daily energy intake.[160] Junk foods, which are the principal type of snack, have little nutritional value, but are highly appealing because of their high fat and sucrose content.

In the case of conventional drugs, greater potency tends to increase their addictive potential. Directly parallel to the notion of drug dosage is the size of the meals we are presently served. Wansink and Van Ittersum described the "portion-distorted embarrassment of food" in today's supermarkets and restaurants.[182] To illustrate, a fast-food restaurant meal—a burger, fries, soft drink, and dessert—can provide almost all of one's daily caloric requirements in a single serving. Moreover, the annual growth rate of fast food dining has increased threefold in the past generation compared with that of at-home consumption.[152] The sizes of plates, bowls, and glasses in our homes have also increased steadily over the years, and the serving size of some entrees has virtually doubled in recipe books since the 1930s.[182]

In summary, just as different drugs promote different degrees of dependence, foods also differ in their capacity to promote abuse.[178] Experts are now confident in claiming that the nutrients composing fast foods are inherently addictive because of their concentration and high volume of fats and sugars. In addition, like drugs of abuse, they have the ability to alter brain mechanisms in ways that contribute to their increasingly compulsive use (see Del Parigi et al.,[60] Grigson,[86] and Spring et al.[164]).

Clinical and Psychological Parallels

In making the argument for compulsive overeating as an addictive behavior, it is clearly not appropriate to include all cases of excessive food consumption in this taxon. Nor are we claiming that obesity and addiction are one and the same. However, we do believe that BED is a phenotype particularly well-suited to such a conceptualization, and that sound clinical and scientific evidence exists to support this viewpoint. Cassin and von Ranson[36] found, for example, that 94% of their adult BED sample described themselves as "food addicts" or "compulsive overeaters" and met the *Diagnostic and Statistical Manual of Mental Disorders, Fourth Edition* (DSM-IV) criteria for substance dependence disorder[5] when the term "substance" referred to "binge eating." When examined more objectively using the first edition of the *Yale Food Addiction Scale* (YFAS), food addiction symptoms also showed elevated overlap with BED, ranging from 42%–57%.[51,78,79] An updated version of the YFAS based on the DSM-5 diagnostic criteria for substance use disorder has recently been published.[77] Although there is not complete consensus among researchers on the defining features of all addictions, most would agree that there is a common set of defining characteristics. These include loss of control, tolerance and withdrawal, cravings, and repeated cycles of remission and relapse.

Loss of Control

Perhaps the most clear-cut feature of addiction is the increasingly compulsive use and abuse of the addictive substance or behavior, even in the face of detrimental consequences to health, safety, social relationships, and financial stability. In animal studies, for example, cocaine dependent[172] and binge-prone animals[139,140,174] will tolerate higher levels of foot shock to obtain cocaine and palatable food, respectively. Similarly, animals maintained on a palatable cafeteria diet will continue to consume food even when it has been laced with a bitter tasting substance.[93]

BED is characterized by recurrent episodes of binge eating without the regular use of compensatory behaviors such as purging, fasting, or excessive exercising. Feeling out of control of one's eating behavior is a defining feature of binge eating.[6] BED also appears to be a chronic and stable condition[148] with strong links to obesity.[61] Although initially believed to be a disorder of adulthood, there is growing evidence that BED also occurs in children and adolescents.[33] In addition to clinical research, there are good experimental paradigms whereby a subset of rats fed an intermittent diet of sugar have developed a pattern of copious consumption resembling human cases of BED (e.g., Avena et al.[12] and Colantuoni et al.[38]).

BED sufferers typically report distress and guilt about their eating habits, but they have great difficulty controlling these behaviors despite weight gain and ensuing medical problems such as diabetes and hypertension.[39,45] As a society, we are generally informed and knowledgeable about the negative consequences of poor nutrition and obesity and are sentient of dietary recommendations for good health, so we must conclude that binge eating—like drug addiction—exists despite an awareness of its poor health outcomes.

Tolerance and Withdrawal

In the most general sense, tolerance occurs when a stimulus of a particular magnitude elicits an increasingly diminished response with each repeated exposure and an increasingly higher dose is necessary to achieve the desired effect. This phenomenon is a key characteristic of all drug addictions—and one of the factors that fosters the escalation of intake. Animal studies have demonstrated that a sugar-enhanced diet is associated with increased daily food intake over time,[13] and decreased striatal dopamine response.[1] Individuals who report frequent ice-cream consumption also demonstrate decreases in striatal activation in response to an ice-cream–based milkshake,[34] suggesting similar neuroadaptations following prolonged exposure to highly palatable food in humans.

Direct evidence of tolerance in BED, however, arises primarily from clinical reports of individuals consuming more and more food in each binge as the disorder becomes more chronic. The finding that higher body weight correlates with the frequency and severity of binge eating episodes also provides indirect evidence of tolerance effects.[145] As well, a high proportion of adults with BED reported being overweight before the onset of their disordered eating, suggesting that over time, high-calorie diets prompt greater subsequent intake and may contribute to binge eating.[151]

The impact of tolerance on the progression of addictive behaviors is made more poignant by its synergy with the debilitating symptoms of withdrawal. Certain foods—particularly sugar—can cause pronounced withdrawal symptoms when removed from the diet, and these effects most clearly resemble the physical signs of distress seen in opiate withdrawal.[13] The most compelling evidence comes from animal research in which rats were initially maintained on a 25% glucose solution (e.g., Avena et al.[13] and Wideman et al.[188]) or high sucrose diet.[95] Following removal of the palatable diet, animals showed aggression, anxiety, a drop in body temperature, teeth chattering, forepaw tremor, head-shaking, and depressive-like behaviors—all symptoms associated with withdrawal from drugs such as heroin. Parallels have also been drawn between amphetamine and sugar withdrawal, both of which induce signs of increased impulsivity.[115,142] Although there is human evidence of sugar withdrawal, it comes mostly from clinical observation, self-help books, and Internet sites promoting weight-loss diets. They are, however, uniform in describing headaches, irritability, and flu-like symptoms among heavy sugar consumers who become abstinent.

Cravings and Relapse

One of the most distinguishing features of drug abuse is the pronounced sense of craving reported by addicts and their dismal and repeated failures at giving up the habit. Indeed, "craving" has been added to the list of diagnostic criteria for substance use disorder in the DSM-5. Addiction is rarely an acute illness. A decade ago, Leshner coined the term "chronic relapsing disorder" to describe addictive disorders because total and permanent abstinence seldom occurs after a single treatment episode.[106] For most individuals, there are repeated cycles of cessation and relapse. Human weight cycling is, almost by definition, a sign of repeated defeat in one's effort to curb overeating and is found to be a significant risk factor for the development of binge eating.[143]

The addict's powerful cravings that can be elicited from even a small dose—as well as from the many conditioned environmental cues—are thought to contribute to poor long-term treatment outcome. Studies have also demonstrated that food cravings are significantly higher in those who endorse food addiction symptoms[51,75,122] and in adults with binge eating disorder compared to their nonbingeing counterparts of comparable weight.[48,55,96,130,137] This meshes with other evidence that those with BED show enhanced preference for sweet and fatty foods compared with other obese individuals.[196] Craving in animals can only be inferred from their behavior and is typically defined as the enhanced motivation to procure an addictive drug by operant responding.[104] Such behavior has also been observed in rats who increased lever presses for glucose after a 4-week period of a sugar-enhanced diet relative to baseline,[13] and in animals maintained on a high sucrose diet compared to chow-fed controls.[174]

Neurobiological Parallels

Brain reward circuitry almost certainly evolved to foster our selective engagement in activities like eating, sex, and maternal behavior, which are the essence of our survival as a species. This otherwise highly adaptive neuroanatomical mechanism is also at the heart of all dependence disorders. Abused substances have psychomotor stimulant properties, which activate the same brain reward pathways as life's natural pleasures. In other words, there is a shared substrate for food and drug reward.[141] Due, however, to the potency of most addictive substances, and to their direct route of administration, the claim that drugs "hijack" the brain has become a popular idiom to describe the downwardly spiralling pattern of drug abuse.

Dopamine neurons in the ventral tegmental area send subcortical projections to striatal regions of the basal ganglia—importantly, the nucleus accumbens—and to various limbic structures such as the amygdala. Ventral tegmental area projections also extend to the prefrontal cortex. This mesocorticolimbic neural network is fundamentally complex and cleverly designed to regulate the many emotional, motivational, and cognitive processes involved in reward. For example, our engagement in these behaviors increases our sense of pleasure and well-being—events that galvanize our attention in preference to more neutral, and less essential, activities. Second, we have the desire to repeat these behaviors even in the face of distracting stimuli. They also nurture a strong positive memory, which increases their salience and enhances our appetitive motivation in their direction. Third, we quickly learn the cues in our environment that signal the approach or availability of these rewarding behaviors. Finally, we become resistant (temporarily) to their rewarding properties in order to move on to other activities.

Experts now generally agree that the reinforcing effects of addictive drugs and palatable foods are regulated, in large part, by the same dopamine pathways.[41,101,181] Although addictive drugs share with food the property of increasing dopamine in brain reward pathways, the former bypass the adaptive mechanisms of normal reward, such as the habituation that constrains the responsiveness of the brain to food reward.[63] Potent drugs abnormally facilitate Pavlovian incentive learning to drug-conditioned stimuli and sensitize the individual to cravings for the substance.[103] Drugs also cause a tolerance to their rewarding properties by the downregulation of dopamine receptors in the striatum[177] and a decrease in the function of the extended amygdala reward system, which produces the negative affect and anxiety associated with abstinence.[103] There is now compelling evidence that highly palatable foods eaten in abundance have the potential to cause these same neuroadaptations—alterations that increase compulsive use, foster strong cravings, contribute to the symptoms of withdrawal, and make abstinence increasingly difficult.[a]

Until relatively recently, the neurobiology of overeating was largely focused on the hypothalamus, while drug addiction research, by contrast, channelled its attention to the mesocorticolimbic pathways.[170] With the increasing sophistication of brain imaging techniques, we are now able to witness the activation of brain reward sites in response to palatable food.[15,161,180] Prefrontal systems also play a prominent role in eating and appetite. Opioid inhibition in the prefrontal cortex selectively decreases intake of palatable foods in animals demonstrating binge eating behavior.[24] Clinically, increased dysexecutive traits have been associated with binge eating and food cravings, just as they are with drug abuse.[163]

Some of the most compelling evidence for neurobiological parallels, especially those implicating dopaminergic systems, between drug addiction and binge eating comes from drug studies targeting dopamine receptors (e.g., Corwin et al.[42] and Grimm et al.[88]) A large body of research suggests that D_1 and D_2 receptor antagonism attenuates reinstatement of drug seeking for heroin,[29,198] nicotine,[109] ethanol,[110] and cocaine[3,8] in rats. Similarly, SCH 23390, a D_1 receptor antagonist, and raclopride, a D_2 receptor antagonist, decrease sugar consumption and seeking in rats who have had intermittent access to a sucrose solution and demonstrate binge-like behavior.[42,88] Research investigating D_3 receptor antagonism in binge eating has been less conclusive.[64,128,133] However, there is some evidence that D_3 receptors are involved in the motivational appeal of food in overweight and obese patients,[128] providing preliminary findings indicating parallels with the reinforcing properties of D_3 receptors in cocaine administration.[194,195]

Indirect support for dopaminergic parallels between drug addiction and binge eating comes from studies demonstrating that administration of GS 455534, an aldehyde dehydrogenase 2 (ALDH-2) inhibitor, decreases alcohol consumption and relapse rates,[10] reduces cocaine seeking,[197] and decreases consumption of palatable foods in animals who binge eat.[26] ALDH-2 is highly expressed in in the ventral tegmental area, predominantly in dopaminergic neurons,[119] and plays a role in dopamine metabolism, converting 3,4-dihydroxyphenylacetaldehyde (DOPAL) to 3,4-dihydroxyphenylacetic acid (DOPAC).[70] ALDH-2 inhibition by GS 455534 administration inhibits drug-induced dopamine increases in the nucleus accumbens without affecting basal levels of dopamine elsewhere in the brain,[10] providing a mechanism whereby GS 455534 may prevent drug/food seeking and consummatory behavior,[26] and pointing to the role of dopamine in addiction.

Other neurotransmitter systems such as γ-aminobutyric acid (GABA), the opioids, and serotonin are also integral to this process.[181] Drug-induced dopamine release is stimulated in the ventral tegmental area by opioid receptor activation via GABAergic inhibitory interneurons,[99] both of which have been implicated in animal studies of addiction (e.g., Cousins et al.[44] and Giuliano et al.[82]). Decreasing opioid receptor activation[62,82] or increasing GABA release[44,179] reduces drug administration in animals that are dependent on cocaine, heroin, nicotine, and alcohol. Moreover, combined administration of naltrexone (an opioid antagonist) and baclofen (a GABA agonist) suggests a potentiation of this effect in alcohol-dependent animals.[40,166] Naltrexone and baclofen exert similar effects in animals that demonstrate binge-like behavior, decreasing consumption of highly palatable (i.e., sweet or fatty) food when administered independently[21,24,32,42] or concurrently.[11] Although drugs acting on dopaminergic and opioid pathways exert similar effects in models of addiction and binge eating, with respect to food, dopamine release in the nucleus accumbens is generally associated with its reinforcing effects, while opioid signaling in this area regulates its palatability and hedonic properties.[43,66]

Recent research suggests there are many biological factors that contribute to individual differences in vulnerability to compulsive overeating (i.e., Davis[47] and Davis et al.[52]), factors that interact with environmental factors including the dramatic changes in our food environment (for review see Harris et al.[91]). In particular proneness to obesity seems to be associated with food addiction. Compared to obese-resistant animals, obese-prone animals demonstrate increased anxiety and craving following withdrawal from a high fat, high sugar diet,[144] alterations to dopaminergic and opioid receptors consistent with models of drug addiction,[4] and increased motivation for and decreased hedonic pleasure associated with highly palatable food.[153] Animals who attribute greater incentive salience to food cues, showing greater motivation for natural reinforcers, also demonstrate increased cocaine self-administration and dependence,[125,156] suggesting an unspecified predisposition toward addiction that develops uniquely given genetic (i.e., obesity proneness) and environmental factors (i.e., food marketing) acting on the organism. Due to the nature of these studies, however, we do not claim to know whether obese individuals are more susceptible to the reinforcing properties of food prior to the onset of obesity or if obesity leads to sensitization of the reinforcing effects of food. Rather we draw attention to this association to highlight the complex interaction between genetic and environmental factors in the development of compulsive overeating and possible parallels with other drugs of abuse.

Risk Factor Similarities

BED and drug addiction appear to share certain risk factors for their development. A recent study found significantly higher rates of psychopathology, including substance abuse, in first-degree relatives of women with BED compared with relatives of control women.[107] It is important to note, however, that all the disorders elevated in relatives with BED followed a pattern of independent transmission from BED, except for substance use disorder, the transmission pattern of which indicated a shared etiology. Although the vulnerability for both disorders has many social and cultural parallels, such as availability and cost contributing to their consumption, our review focuses only on common *psychobiological risks*.

---

[a]References 1, 34, 86, 89, 113, 141.

Impulsivity

High expression of impulsivity—a personality trait characterized by the diminished ability to inhibit behavior when restraint is the most advantageous and appropriate response in a particular situation—has strong links with both drug abuse[173, 176] and BED.[b] Neuroimaging studies have consistently demonstrated reduced lateral orbitofrontal cortical activation in individuals with BED during highly palatable food consumption, indicating decreased inhibitory control.[80] Davis (2013) found that obese individuals with BED who also met YFAS (1st edition) criteria for food addiction reported higher levels of impulsivity than those who did not.[48]

Impulsive individuals show pronounced weaknesses in learning appropriate associations between reward and punishment, which is essential to making advantageous choices.[72,184] Notably, research suggests that there are two underlying constructs of impulsivity that may predispose individuals to substance use and pathological eating behavior. Reward sensitivity increases preference for a substance (i.e., food or drug) and initiates ingestion, whereas rash spontaneous behavior impairs the ability to resist cravings.[59] Due to the challenges of doing prospective risk-factor research, it is not clear whether impulsive responding is a precursor to addiction disorders or whether it occurs only because of the brain alterations caused by excessive use. However, research examining nonclinical samples has provided some preliminary evidence addressing causality. Namely, correlations between overeating/binge eating and impulsivity[124] suggest that impulsive responding is not simply a consequence of brain alterations, but rather it can also precede the development of addictive disorders.

Reward Sensitivity

The sensitivity or reactivity of the common reward pathway is affected by several biological factors such as the density of dopamine receptors, the amount of dopamine released into the synapse, and the rapidity of its transport back into the cell by the reuptake protein. Individual differences in *reward sensitivity* have been strongly implicated in the risk for drug addiction[30,105,112,131] as well as compulsive overeating[52,57] and BED.[116,157] The research is divided, however, in terms of the causal direction of this association.

One argument favors the view that *hypo*-dopaminergic functioning—which has been called a "reward deficiency syndrome"—is a key factor in the development of addiction disorders.[25,98] The premise is that substances (such as addictive drugs and palatable food) are used as a form of self-medication to boost a sluggish dopamine system and increase hedonic capacity. Some studies have reported decreased striatal activation in individuals with BED compared to their weight-matched counterparts when presented with images of food[183] and gambling tasks,[14] although it must be noted that these individuals do not differ from normal-weight controls. The counterargument is that *hyper*-sensitivity to reward contributes to increased risk for addictive behaviors due to an enhanced motivation to engage in pleasurable activities. For instance, in several studies, heightened reward sensitivity was associated with emotional overeating, preference for high-fat food, binge eating, and food cravings, as well as with hazardous alcohol consumption.[56,71,112,158,180] One explanation for the apparent disagreement between the two bodies of research may be a *dual vulnerability* to addictions whereby both paths can confer risk, albeit in different individuals and perhaps with different levels of severity.

---

[b]References 9, 74, 92, 123, 124, 127, 165.

Impulsive Behavior and Decision-Making Deficits

Poor decision-making skills and difficulties with impulsivity are core symptoms of certain mental health problems but are perhaps most prominently seen in drug dependence.[17,19] Addicts tend to choose actions that bring immediate reward, even when this leads to a deleterious later outcome. The human ability to choose *present* options that favorably influence *future* outcomes depends crucially on an accumulated emotional memory of the consequences of our *past* interactions with similar events.[46] In other words, we form a probabilistic impression of how a particular action will turn out in the future from an emotionally biasing gut feeling, which was generated when that action caused either a positive or a negative reaction in the past. The orbitofrontal cortex, in particular, is critical for activating feelings or emotional states from thoughts about rewarding or punishing events that are not currently present in our environment.[16,18]

Much of the early research on decision making came from studying the social impairments of patients with ventromedial prefrontal cortical lesions and observing that their behavioral deficits are typically caused by an inability to assess future consequences advantageously.[7,155] In other words, they fail to weigh the pros and cons of their actions and to postpone immediate gratification, so their behavior is almost always guided by the negative or positive events present at the moment. A plethora of research using neuropsychological tests of decision-making ability has shown impairment in those dependent on a variety of addictive substances (e.g., Vassileva et al.[173] and Verdejo-Garcia et al.[176]). Similar impairments have been documented in individuals with BED,[114,116] bulimia nervosa, and in obese women.[27,31,54]

Negative Urgency and Emotion Regulation

Negative urgency is a facet of impulsivity that has been reliably associated with drug and alcohol addiction.[69,108,185,186,199] Whiteside and colleagues (2005, p. 561)[187] define negative urgency as the "tendency to engage in impulsive behaviors under conditions of negative affect, perhaps in order to alleviate negative emotions, despite the potentially harmful longer-term consequences." Negative urgency has also been shown to be associated with binge eating behavior[68,116,141] and symptoms of food addiction,[129,147] suggesting that it may be a shared risk factor for BED and addictive disorders.

Individuals who report high negative urgency tend to make rash behavioral decisions in response to negative emotional states,[183] pointing to the role of emotional-regulation deficits in addictive behaviors. Increased emotion-dysregulation scores have been associated with amphetamine[137] and marijuana[28] consumption. Such individuals endorse greater drug consumption following negative emotional states.[28,137] Similarly, in another study, increased depression scores predicted greater food consumption in individuals with BED,[132] and negative emotional states decreased in the 4 hours following an individual's first binge of the day.[20] Although the precise mechanisms by which consumption of an addictive substance relieves negative affective states are not known, animals who have been abstinent from sugar following prolonged access also tend to exhibit decreases in depressive-like behavior when they regain access to a high sucrose diet.[95] These findings suggest, at least in part, that the biological composition of addictive substances has mood-relieving properties, which may be enhanced by the inability to tolerate strong negative emotions and negative urgency.

Treatment of Binge Eating Disorder: Integrating an Addiction Perspective

Given the psychological and neurobiological overlaps between BED and substance use disorders, it may be useful for clinicians to integrate an addiction perspective into current treatments for BED.[49,50] There are presently no empirically supported guidelines for the treatment of food addiction, and we are not aware of any studies that have evaluated an addiction approach to the treatment of BED. There is however considerable empirical support for the efficacy of cognitive behavioral therapy (CBT) in the treatment of both BED and substance use disorders.[35,120,191,193] Indeed, the CBT approach for BED and the CBT approach for substance abuse share many strategies including psychoeducation, functional analysis, identifying triggers for problem behaviors, teaching coping skills for managing urges/cravings, cognitive restructuring techniques, and relapse prevention strategies.[67,117,121]

The following treatment considerations are intended to address features of food addiction among individuals presenting with BED, including food cravings, difficulties with inhibitory control, negative urgency, loss of control overeating, difficulties with emotion regulation, and emotionally driven overeating. They are not, however, intended for patients with bulimia nervosa (BN) or anorexia nervosa (AN). Although binge eating is a core feature of BN and occurs in about half of cases of AN, in the case of both of these eating disorders, the binge eating typically occurs in the context of extreme food restriction and normal or low body weight. This is in stark contrast to the usual clinical presentation of BED. Individuals with BED typically report experiencing a *general* lack of control over their eating outside binge eating episodes. Therefore, binge eating in BED typically occurs in the absence of extreme dietary restriction, and in the context of overweight or obesity.[117] As discussed by Wilson (2010), BN and AN therefore require a different treatment approach that has been well-described and empirically validated,[190] an approach that requires reduced dietary restriction.[146,192] Because individuals with BED typically do not report elevated dietary restriction between binge episodes, indeed they often report overeating between binge episodes, a different approach is needed. There is evidence, however, that many individuals with BED report elevated levels of dietary restraint—that is, they think they *should* restrict their food intake, but are typically not successful at doing so. Thus they often experience feelings of shame and guilt after eating, which may lead to further binge eating as a way of coping with these feelings. In addition, significantly more obese individuals with BED as compared to obese individuals without BED report overvaluation of shape and weight.[87] That is, not only are they dissatisfied with their shape and weight, but this dissatisfaction causes clinically significant distress and impairment. Effective treatments for BED must therefore also address these distinct core features of the psychopathology of BED.

As reviewed earlier in this chapter, there is growing evidence that certain types of highly processed foods or certain ingredients in these foods appear to hijack the brain of vulnerable individuals in a manner similar to that of addictive drugs.[76] Typically, it is these types of foods that are consumed during binge episodes among people with BED. We believe that controlled consumption, or even in some cases even abstinence from highly refined, processed foods among individuals with BED who also present with food addiction symptoms is recommended. Of course, not everyone with BED meets YFAS criteria for food addiction and not everyone who meets the YFAS criteria for food addiction

has BED. However, given the parallels between substance addiction and the excessive consumption of hyperpalatable, highly refined, processed foods during binge eating episodes, integrating an addiction perspective into current treatments for BED may improve outcomes.

Regarding the treatment of obesity, compulsive overeating is only one factor involved in the complex etiology of obesity. Approximately half of treatment-seeking obese people meet diagnostic criteria for BED and about half of these meet the YFAS criteria for food addiction.[78] Individuals who meet criteria for both BED and YFAS food addiction report more frequent binge eating, more intense cravings, more emotional eating, as well as greater depression symptoms than those with BED alone.[48] Gearhardt and colleagues (2012) have convincingly argued that the application of public health policies that have been successfully used to control the availability and use of addictive drugs should be applied to control addictive foods.[79] However, successful implementation of a public health approach to food addiction is likely to involve a lengthy process and, in the meantime, we require effective individual treatment strategies.

Because binge eating is a central feature of both BN and BED, most controlled treatment studies of BED to date have evaluated interventions with demonstrated efficacy for BN, particularly CBT and certain types of medications. The aim of psychological therapy is to interrupt cognitive, behavioral and emotional factors that are believed to perpetuate binge eating problems, whereas pharmacological interventions target mood regulation and the neurobiological basis of food intake regulation. Ideally, effective treatments for BED will eliminate the core behavior of binge eating, enhance healthy eating and exercise habits, reduce overvaluation of shape and weight, alleviate associated psychosocial problems, and produce clinically significant weight loss.

Psychoeducation

People with binge eating problems are often highly self-critical and report high levels of shame related to their disordered-eating behaviors.[84] Providing psychoeducation about the neurobiological and behavioral parallels between addiction disorders and compulsive overeating may be helpful. Understanding that they may be fighting a strong neurobiological drive to overeat in an environment that exploits these vulnerabilities could foster a therapeutic sense of self-compassion. It may also help them to accept that treatment is likely to involve enduring efforts to resist urges to overeat and to prevent relapse. Integrating compassion-focused interventions may be helpful for addressing the shame and guilt many individuals with BED experience with regard to their body image and eating behavior.[102]

Managing Food Cravings and Difficulties With Inhibitory Control

Craving is a core feature of both BED and addiction, and it has been added to the DSM-5 diagnostic criteria for addictive disorders.[6] Individuals with BED typically report intense food cravings in response to various conditioned environmental cues and strong corresponding urges to overeat that are experienced as difficult to resist despite typically being sufficiently nourished and, in most cases, overweight or obese.[58,135] Davis (2013) found that they also report intense food preoccupation even though they are typically not food deprived, and exhibit strong physiological responses to anticipatory food cues,[48] including thoughts or images of food.[80] This process is akin to the development of withdrawal symptoms in drug addiction. Certain vulnerable individuals seem more prone to experience the strong reinforcing properties of addictive foods or food ingredients. Thus in order to interrupt compulsive overeating symptoms, individuals with BED and food addiction symptoms need to develop strategies to increase their ability to tolerate food cravings and inhibit urges to overeat in response to triggers. A strategy adapted from Marlatt and Gordon's (1985) addiction treatment manual can be helpful in achieving this goal.[118] This strategy involves employing acceptance-oriented imagery to cope with urges—termed "urge-surfing"—in order to teach clients that food cravings will eventually subside if not acted upon. One study found evidence that a brief guided imagery intervention designed to interrupt elaboration of involuntary food thoughts was associated with reduced food cravings.[90] Similarly, mindfulness-skills training is recommended for developing a detached awareness of food cravings and urges to overeat.[37] In addition, distress-tolerance skills training—designed to help individuals tolerate the distress associated with food cravings and inhibit urges to overeat impulsively in response to food cravings—is likely to be of central importance in the treatment of food addiction.[37] Another potentially helpful strategy, adopted from substance-abuse treatment, is cue exposure with response prevention.[97] Treatment consists of repeated exposure to conditioned food cues (e.g., watching television), but eating (the response) is prevented. There is evidence from various small-scale studies that this approach results in reduced cravings and urges among binge eaters.[97]

Pharmacotherapy represents another possible avenue for the development of novel treatments for food addiction. There are a number of medications available for each of the major classes of addictive drugs which, in conjunction with psychosocial interventions, have been shown to be effective in reducing the likelihood of relapse by reducing urges and cravings.[136] An example of an anticraving medication is naltrexone, which works by blocking opiate receptors that regulate the release of dopamine in the reward pathways.[83] Although some researchers have suggested that naltrexone might be useful in the treatment of BED (e.g., deZwaan et al.[200]), there has been only one placebo-controlled, double-blind, randomized trial of naltrexone to date and it produced negative results.[2]

Dealing With Loss-of-Control

An inability to reduce or control consumption despite a strong desire to do so and despite negative consequences is a hallmark of both BED and substance addiction. In drug dependence, loss-of-control is indicated by the frequent consumption of a substance in larger quantities or over longer periods of time than intended.[6] In BED, loss-of-control is a central aspect of the definition of a binge and refers to a sense that one cannot control what or how much one is eating.[6] According to Volkow and Wise (2005), the consumption of hyperpalatable, highly processed foods is likely to have a priming effect that can trigger problematic overeating among vulnerable individuals.[177] Encouraging overweight individuals with BED who report symptoms of food addiction to limit or avoid consumption of hyperpalatable, highly processed foods may help reduce or eliminate the occurrence of this priming effect. Instead, patients should be encouraged to eat mainly unprocessed nutritious foods during their meals and snacks, which are more likely to satisfy their nutritional needs and reduce sensations of hunger and food cravings. Like drug abuse, binge eating is associated with impulsivity, including negative urgency, and impaired decision-making.[52,53,78] A strategy often used in the treatment of drug addiction, aimed at reducing impulsive responding and improving decision-making skills, is the use of guided imagery to

increase awareness of the likely negative consequences of problematic use.[120] This approach may also prove helpful in the treatment of compulsive overeating.

Addressing Emotionally-Driven Eating

Difficulties with emotion regulation are common to both BED and addictive disorders. People with BED and YFAS food addiction report higher levels of depression and emotion dysregulation than people with BED who do not meet criteria for YFAS food addiction.[78,147] They also report more binge eating, food cravings, emotionally driven eating, addictive personality traits, and impulsive behaviors, prompting the conclusion that comorbid food addiction reflects a more severe and more compulsive form of BED.[48] Negative affect may trigger cravings for hyperpalatable food that may be consumed as a maladaptive way to modulate negative emotional states or to increase pleasurable feelings or sensations.[20,100] For example, Udo, Grilo, and Brownell (2013) have shown that negative mood states in combination with food cravings reduced the ability of obese individuals to resist eating high calorie foods.[171] Therefore, the development of adaptive emotion-regulation skills, particularly distress tolerance skills, as discussed by Chen and Safer (2010) in their dialectical behavior therapy (DBT) approach,[37] is likely to play an important role in the effective treatment of BED and food addiction.

Enhancing Commitment to Change and Relapse Prevention

Another challenge common to the treatment of both substance use disorders and BED is enhancing motivation and commitment to change as well as preventing relapse. Motivational interviewing (MI) is a person-centered counseling style that grew out of the recognition that individuals with addictive disorders are often ambivalent about change and frequently drop out of treatment or relapse.[126] The goal of MI is to resolve ambivalence, enhance motivation and commitment for change, and improve treatment outcome. This approach has been applied to BED with promising results.[175] Anecdotally, individuals with binge eating problems commonly report that they find it difficult to remain committed to abstaining from overeating when they are in the midst of experiencing intense cravings. This is likely to be related to an interaction between the widespread neural changes associated with excessive consumption of hyperpalatable, highly processed foods as well as the challenges inherent in interrupting deeply ingrained learned habits.[169] Thus, motivational-enhancement strategies, designed to maintain abstinence from overeating during the moment-to-moment challenge of coping with intense cravings or urges to binge eat, is an important aspect of the treatment of food-addiction symptoms among individuals presenting with BED. Relatedly, it has been found that obese individuals who report food addiction symptoms, exhibit lower levels of perseverance; that is, persistence in the face of frustration.[129,168] This finding also reinforces the importance of distress tolerance and mindfulness skills training for BED.[154]

Summary and Conclusions

In summary, the compelling psychological and neurobiological parallels between BED and substance use disorders suggest that integrating an addiction perspective into current treatments for BED is likely to prove helpful. In this chapter, we reviewed the clinical, psychological, and neurobiological parallels between substance use disorder and BED. In addition, we discussed similarities in terms of the risk factor profiles of these two disorders.

Finally, we reviewed possible treatment strategies to address features of food addiction among individuals with BED including food cravings, difficulties with inhibitory control, negative urgency, loss-of-control overeating, emotionally driven eating, and maintaining motivation to change. In addition, we highlighted the importance of addressing the unique features of BED including overvaluation of shape and weight, as well as guilt and shame related to eating. As outlined in this chapter, we think that integrating an addiction perspective that considers the similarities between treating substance addiction and treating compulsive overeating may improve treatment outcomes for BED. Research evaluating the effectiveness of this approach is needed.

References

1. Ahmed S, Kashem MA, Sarker R, Ahmed EU, Hargreaves GA, McGregor IS. Neuroadaptations in the striatal proteome of the rat following prolonged excessive sucrose intake. *Neurochem Res.* 2014;39:815–824.
2. Alger SA, Schwalberg MD, Bigaouette JM, Michalek AV, Howard LJ. Effect of a tricyclic antidepressant and opiate antagonist on binge-eating behaviour in normal weight bulimic and obese binge-eating subjects. *Am J Clin Nutr.* 1991;53:865–871.
3. Alleweireldt AT, Hobbs RJ, Taylor AR, Neisewander JL. Effects of SCH-23390 infused into the amygdala or adjacent cortex and basal ganglia on cocaine seeking and self-administration in rats. *Neuropsychopharmacology.* 2006;31:363–374.
4. Alsio J, Olszewski PK, Norback AH, et al. Dopamine D1 receptor gene expression decreases in the nucleus accumbens upon long-term exposure to palatable food and differs depending on diet-induced obesity phenotype in rats. *Neuroscience.* 2010;171:779–787.
5. American Psychiatric Association. *Diagnostic and Statistical Manual of Mental Disorders.* 4th ed. Washington, DC: American Psychiatric Association Press; 1994.
6. American Psychological Association. *Diagnostic and Statistical Manual of mental Disorders.* 5th ed. Washington, DC: American Psychiatric Association Press; 2013.
7. Anderson SW, Bechara A, Tranel D, Damasio H, Damasio AR. Characterization of the decision-making defect of subjects with ventromedial frontal lobe damage. *Society for Neuroscience Abstracts.* 1994;24:1108.
8. Anderson SM, Schmidt HD, Pierce RC. Administration of the D2 dopamine receptor antagonist sulpiride into the shell, but not the core, of the nucleus accumbens attenuates cocaine priming-induced reinstatement of drug seeking. *Neuropsychopharmacology.* 2006;31:1452–1461.
9. Annagur B, Orhan O, Ozer A, Yalcin N, Tamam L. The effects of depression and impulsivity on obesity and binge eating disorder. *Bulletin of Clinical Psychopharmacology.* 2014;1:162–170.
10. Arolfo MP, Overstreet DH, Yao L, et al. Suppression of heavy drinking and alcohol seeking by a selective ALDH-2 inhibitor. *Alcohol Clin Exp Res.* 2009;33:1935–1944.
11. Avena NM, Bocarsly ME, Murray S, Gold MS. Effects of baclofen and naltrexone, alone and in combination, on the consumption of palatable food in male rats. *Exp Clin Psychopharmacol.* 2014;22:460–467. Refstyled.
12. Avena NM, Hoebel BG. A diet promoting sugar dependency causes behavioural cross-sensitization to a low dose of amphetamine. *Neuroscience.* 2003;122:17–20. Refstyled.
13. Avena NM, Rada P, Hoebel BG. Evidence for sugar addiction: behavioural and neurochemical effects of intermittent, excessive sugar intake. *Neurosci Biobehav Rev.* 2008;32:20–39.
14. Balodis IM, Kober H, Worhunsky PD, et al. Monetary reward processing in obese individuals with and without binge eating disorder. *Biol Psychiatry.* 2013;73:877–886.
15. Beaver JD, Lawrence AD, Van Ditzhuijzen J, Davis MH, Woods A, Calder AJ. Individual differences in reward drive predict neural responses to images of food. *J Neurosci.* 2006;26:5160–5166.
16. Bechara A. The role of emotion in decision-making: evidence from neurological patients with orbitofrontal damage. *Brain Cogn.* 2004;55:30–40.
17. Bechara A, Damasio H. Decision-making and addiction (part I): impaired activation of somatic states in substance dependent individuals when pondering decisions with negative future consequences. *Neuropsychologia.* 2002;40:1675–1689.
18. Bechara A, Damasio H, Damasio AR. Amygdala in brain function: basic and clinical approaches. *Ann N Y Acad Sci.* 2003;985:356–369.
19. Bechara A, Martin EM. Impaired decision making related to working memory deficits in individuals with substance abuse. *Neuropsychology.* 2004;18:152–162.
20. Berg KC, Crosby RD, Cao L, et al. Negative affect prior to and following overeating-only, loss of control eating-only, and binge eating episodes in obese adults. *Int J Eat Disord.* 2015;48:641–653.
21. Berner LA, Bocarsly ME, Hoebel BG, Avena NM. Baclofen suppresses binge eating of pure fat but not a sugar-rich or sweet-fat diet. *Behav Pharmacol.* 2009;20:631–634.
22. Berridge V. Two tales of addiction: opium and nicotine. *Hum Psychopharmacol Clin Exp.* 1997;12:S45–S52.
23. Berridge V, Mars S. History of addictions. *J Epidemiol Community Health.* 2004;58:747–750.
24. Blasio A, Steardo L, Sabino V, Cottone P. Opioid system in the medial prefrontal cortex mediates binge-like eating. *Addict Biol.* 2014;19:652–662.
25. Blum K, Braverman ER, Holder JM, et al. Reward deficiency syndrome: a biogenetic model for the diagnosis and treatment of impulsive, addictive, and compulsive behaviours. *J Psychoactive Drugs.* 2000;32(Suppl i-iv):1–112.
26. Bocarsly ME, Berner LA, Hoebel BG, Avena NM. Rats that binge eat fat-rich food do not show somatic signs or anxiety associated with opiate-like withdrawal: implications for nutrient-specific food addiction behaviours. *Physiol Behav.* 2011;104:865–872.
27. Boeka AG, Lokken KL. The Iowa gambling task as a measure of decision making in women with bulimia nervosa. *J Int Neuropsychol Soc.* 2006;12:741–745.
28. Bonn-Miller MO, Vujanovic AA, Zvolensky MJ. Emotional dysregulation: association with coping-oriented marijuana use motives among current marijuana users. *Subst Use Misuse.* 2008;43:1653–1665.
29. Bossert JM, Poles GC, Wihbey KA, Koya E, Shaham Y. Differential effects of blockade of dopamine D1-family receptors in nucleus accumbens core or shell on reinstatement of heroin seeking induced by contextual and discrete cues. *J Neurosci.* 2007;27:12655–12663.
30. Bowirrat A, Oscar-Berman M. Relationship between dopaminergic neurotransmission, alcoholism, and reward deficiency syndrome. *Am J Med Genet B Neuropsychiatr Genet.* 2005;132B:29–37.
31. Brand M, Franke-Sievert C, Jacoby GE, Markowitsch HJ, Tuschen-Caffier B. Neuropsychological correlates of decision making in patients with bulimia nervosa. *Neuropsychology.* 2007;21:742–750.
32. Buda-Levin A, Woknicki FHE, Corwin RL. Baclofen reduces fat intake under binge-type conditions. *Physiol Behav.* 2005;86:176–184.
33. Bulik CM, Brownley KA, Shapiro JR. Diagnosis and management of binge eating disorder. *World Psychiatry.* 2007;6:142–148.
34. Burger KS, Stice E. Frequent ice cream consumption is associated with reduced striatal response to receipt of an ice cream-based milkshake. *Am J Clin Nutr.* 2012;95:810–817.
35. Carroll KM, Onken LS. Behavioural therapies for drug abuse. *Am J Psychiatry.* 2005;162:1452–1460.
36. Cassin SE, von Ranson KM. Is binge eating experienced as an addiction? *Appetite.* 2007;49:687–690.

37. Chen EY, Safer DL. Dialectical behaviour therapy for bulimia nervosa and binge eating disorder. In: Grilo C, Mitchell J, eds. *The Treatment of Eating Disorders*. New York: Guilford Press; 2010.

38. Colantuoni C, Rada P, McCarthy J, et al. Evidence that intermittent, excessive sugar intake causes endogenous opioid dependence. *Obes Res*. 2002;10:478–488.

39. Colles SL, Dixon JB, O'Brien PE. Loss of control is central to psychological disturbance associated with binge eating disorder. *Obesity*. 2008;16:608–614.

40. Colombo G, Serra S, Vacca G, Carai MA, Gessa GL. Effect of the combination of naltrexone and baclofen, on acquisition of alcohol drinking behaviour in alcohol-preferring rats. *Drug Alcohol Depend*. 2005;77:87–91.

41. Corwin RL. Bingeing rats: a model of intermittent excessive behaviour? *Appetite*. 2006;46:11–15.

42. Corwin RL, Wojnicki FH. Baclofen, raclopride, and naltrexone differentially affect intake of fat and sucrose under limited access conditions. *Behav Pharmacol*. 2009;20:537–548.

43. Cota D, Tschop MH, Horwath TL, Levine AS. Cannabinoids, opioids and eating behaviour: the molecular face of hedonism? *Brain Res Rev*. 2006;51:85–107.

44. Cousins MS, Roberts DCS, de Wit H. GABAB receptor agonists for the treatment of drug addiction: a review of recent findings. *Drug Alcohol Depend*. 2002;65:209–220.

45. Curtis C, Davis C. A qualitative study of binge eating and obesity from an addiction perspective. *Eat Disord*. 2014;22:19–32.

46. Damasio AR. *Descartes' Error: Emotion, Reason, and the Human Brain*. New York: Grosset/Putnam; 1994.

47. Davis C. From passive overeating to "food addiction": a spectrum of compulsion and severity. *ISRN Obes*. 2013;2013:435027.

48. Davis C. Compulsive overeating as an addictive behaviour: overlap between food addiction and binge eating disorder. *Curr Obes Rep*. 2013;2:171–178.

49. Davis C, Carter JC. Compulsive overeating as an addiction disorder. A review of theory and evidence. *Appetite*. 2009;53:1–8.

50. Davis C, Carter JC. If certain foods are addictive, how might this change the treatment of compulsive overeating and obesity? *Curr Addict Rep*. 2014;1:89–95.

51. Davis C, Curtis C, Levitan RD, Carter JC, Kaplan AS, Kennedy JL. Evidence that 'food addiction' is a valid phenotype of obesity. *Appetite*. 2011;57:711–717.

52. Davis C, Levitan RD, Carter J, et al. Personality and eating behaviours: a case-control study of binge eating disorder. *Int J Eat Disord*. 2008;41(243):250.

53. Davis C, Levitan RD, Kaplan AS, et al. Reward sensitivity and the D2 dopamine receptor gene: a case-control study of binge eating disorder. *Prog Neuropsychopharmacol Biol Psychiatry*. 2008;32:620–628.

54. Davis C, Levitan RD, Muglia P, Bewell C, Kennedy J. 'Decision-making' deficits and overeating: a risk model for obesity. *Obes Res*. 2004;12:929–935.

55. Davis C, Patte K, Curtis C, Reid C. *Dopamine for Reward Motivation and Opioids for Pleasure: A Comparison of Binge Eating Disorder (BED) and Non-Bingeing Obese Adults*. Montreal: Paper presented at the annual meeting of the Eating Disorders Research Society; 2008.

56. Davis C, Patte K, Levitan RD, Reid C, Tweed S, Curtis C. From motivation to behaviour: a model of reward sensitivity, overeating, and food preferences in the risk profile for obesity. *Appetite*. 2007;48:12–19.

57. Davis C, Woodside DB. Sensitivity to the rewarding effects of food and exercise in the eating disorders. *Compr Psychiatry*. 2002;43:189–194.

58. Davis CA, Levitan RD, Reid C, et al. Dopamine for "wanting" and opioids for "liking": a comparison of obese adults with and without binge eating. *Obesity*. 2009;17:1220–1225.

59. Dawe S, Gullo MJ, Loxton NJ. Reward drive and rash impulsiveness as dimensions of impulsivity: implications for substance misuse. *Addict Behav*. 2004;29:1389–1405.

60. Del Parigi A, Chen KW, Salbe AD, Reimna EM, Tataranni PA. Are we addicted to food? *Obes Res*. 2003;11:493–495.

61. Devlin MJ. Is there a place for obesity in DSM-V? *Int J Eat Disord*. 2007;40:S83–S88.

62. Dhaher R, Toalston JE, Hauser SR, et al. Effects of naltrexone and LY255582 on ethanol maintenance, seeking, and relapse responding by alcohol-preferring (P) rats. *Alcohol*. 2012;46:17–27.

63. Di Chiara G, Bassareo V. Reward system and addiction: what dopamine does and doesn't do. *Curr Opin Pharmacol*. 2007;7:69–76.

64. Dodds CM, O'Neill B, Beaver J, et al. Effect of the dopamine D3 receptor antagonist GSK598809 on brain responses to rewarding food images in overweight and obese binge eaters. *Appetite*. 2012;59:27–33.

65. Drewnowski A. Nutrition transition and global dietary trends. *Nutrition*. 2000;16:486–487.

66. Esch T, Stefano GB. The neurobiology of pleasure, reward processes, addiction, and their health implications. *Neuro Endocrinol Lett*. 2004;25:235–251.

67. Fairburn CG, Marcus MD, Wilson GT. Cognitive-behavioural therapy for binge eating and bulimia nervosa: a comprehensive treatment manual. In: Fairburn C, Wilson TG, eds. *Binge eating: Nature, Assessment, and Treatment*. New York: Guilford Press; 1993:361–404.

68. Farstad SM, von Ranson KM, Hodgins DC, El-Guebaly N, Casey DM, Schopflocher DP. The influence of impulsiveness on binge eating and problem gambling: a prospective study of gender differences in Canadian adults. *Psychol Addict Behav*. 2015;29:805–812.

69. Fischer SSmith GT. Binge eating, problem drinking, and pathological gambling: linking behaviour to shared traits and social learning. *Pers Individ Dif*. 2008;44:789–800.

70. Florang VR, Rees JN, Brogden NK, Anderson DG, Hurley TD, Doorn JA. Inhibition of the oxidative metabolism of 3,4-dihydroxyphenylacetaldehyde, a reactive intermediate of dopamine metabolism, by 4-hydroxy-2-nonenal. *Neurotoxicology*. 2007;28:76–82.

71. Franken IHA, Muris P. Individual differences in reward sensitivity are related to food craving and relative body weight in healthy women. *Appetite*. 2005;45. 198–201.

72. Franken IHA, van Strien JW, Nijs I, Muris P. Impulsivity is associated with behavioural decision-making deficits. *Psychiatry Res*. 2008;158. 155–163.

73. Frazao E, Allshore J. Strategies for intervention: commentary and debate. *J Nutr*. 2003;133:844S–847S.

74. Galanti K, Gluck ME, Geliebter A. Test meal intake in obese binge eaters in relation to impulsivity and compulsivity. *Int J Eat Disord*. 2007;40:727–732.

75. Gearhardt AN, Boswell RG, White MA. The association of "food addiction" with disordered eating and body mass index. *Eat Behav*. 2014;15:427–433.

76. Gearhardt AN, Brownell KD. Can food and addiction change the game? *Biol Psychiatry*. 2013;73:802–803.

77. Gearhardt AN, Corbin WR, Brownell KD. Development of the yale food addiction scale version 2.0. *Psychol Addict Behav*. 2016;30:113–121.

78. Gearhardt AN, White MA, Masheb RM, Grilo CM. An examination of food addiction in a racially diverse sample of obese patients with binge eating disorder in primary care settings. *Compr Psychiatry*. 2013;54:500–505.

79. Gearhardt AN, White MA, Masheb RM, Morgan PT, Crosby RD, Grilo CM. An examination of the food addiction construct in obese patients with binge eating disorder. *Int J Eat Disord*. 2012;45:657–663.

80. Gearhardt AN, Yokum S, Orr PT, Stice E, Corbin WR, Brownell KD. Neural correlates of food addiction. *Arch Gen Psychiatry*. 2011;68:808–816.

81. Gerber LM, Williams GC, Gray SJ. The nutrient-toxin dosage continuum in human evolution and modern health. *Q Rev Biol.* 1999;74:273–289.

82. Giuliano C, Robbins TW, Wille DR, Bullmore ET, Everitt BJ. Attenuation of cocaine and heroin seeking by mu-opioid receptor antagonism. *Psychopharmacology.* 2013;227:137–147.

83. Gonzales RA, Weiss F. Suppression of ethanol-reinforced behaviour by naltrexone is associated with attenuation of the ethanol-induced increase in dialysate dopamine levels in the nucleus accumbens. *J Neurosci.* 1998;18:10663–10671.

84. Goss K, Allan S. Shame, pride and eating disorders. *Clin Psychol Psychother.* 2009;16:303–316.

85. Grant JE, Brewer JA, Potenza MN. The neurobiology of substance and behaviourial addictions. *CNS Spectr.* 2006;11:924–930.

86. Grigson PS. Like drugs for chocolate: separate rewards modulated by common mechanisms. *Physiol Behav.* 2002;76:389–395.

87. Grilo CM. Why no cognitive body image feature such as overvaluation of shape/weight in the binge eating disorder diagnosis? *Int J Eat Disord.* 2013;46:208–211.

88. Grimm JW, Harkness JH, Ratliff C, Barnes J, North K, Collins S. Effects of systemic or nucleus accumbens-directed dopamine D1 receptor antagonism on sucrose seeking in rats. *Psychopharmacology.* 2011;216:219–233.

89. Hajnal A, Margas WM, Covasa M. Altered dopamine D2 receptor function and binding in obese OLETF rat. *Brain Res Bull.* 2008;75:70–76.

90. Hamilton J, Fawson S, May J, Andrade J, Kavanagh DJ. Brief guided imagery and body scanning interventions reduce food cravings. *Appetite.* 2013;71:158–162.

91. Harris JL, Bargh JA, Brownell KD. Priming effects of television food advertising on eating behaviour. *Health Psychol.* 2009;28:404–413.

92. Hege MA, Stingl KT, Kullmann S, et al. Attentional impulsivity in binge eating disorder modulates response inhibition performance and frontal brain networks. *Int J Obes.* 2015;39:353–360.

93. Heyne A, Kiesselbach C, Sahun I, et al. An animal model of compulsive food-taking behaviour. *Addict Biol.* 2009;14:373–383.

94. Holden C. 'Behavioural' addictions: do they exist? *Science.* 2001;294. 980–982.

95. Iemolo A, Valenza M, Tozier L, et al. Withdrawal from chronic, intermittent access to a highly palatable food induces depressive-like behaviour in compulsive eating rats. *Behav Pharmacol.* 2012;23:593–602.

96. Innamorati M, Imperatori C, Balsamo M, et al. Food Cravings Questionnaire-Trait (FCQ-T) discriminates between obese and overweight patients with and without binge eating tendencies: the Italian version of the FCQ-T. *J Pers Assess.* 2014;96:632–639.

97. Jansen A. A learning model of binge eating: cue reactivity and cue exposure. *Behav Res Ther.* 1998;36:257–272.

98. Jimenez-Arriero MA, Ponce G, Rodriguez-Jimenez R, Aragues M, Galvan A, Rubio G. Taq1-A polymorphism linked to the DRD2 gene and P300 in alcoholic patients. *Eur J Psychiatry.* 2006;20:45–53.

99. Johnson SW, North RA. Opioids excite dopamine neurons by hyperpolarization of local interneurons. *J Neurosci.* 1992;12:483–488.

100. Joyner MA, Gearhardt AN, White MA. Food craving as a mediator between addictive-like eating and problematic eating outcomes. *Eat Behav.* 2015;19:98–101.

101. Kelley AE, Baldo BA, Pratt WE, Will MJ. Corticostriatal-hypothalamic circuitry and food motivation: integration of energy, action and reward. *Physiol Behav.* 2005;86:773–795.

102. Kelly AC, Carter JC. Self-compassion training for binge eating disorder: a pilot randomized controlled trial. *Psychol Psychother.* 2015;88:285–303.

103. Koob GF. The neurobiology of addiction: a neuroadaptational view relevant for diagnosis. *Addiction.* 2006;101(suppl 1):23–30.

104. Koob GF, Moal Le. Plasticity of reward neurocircuitry and the 'dark side' of drug addiction. *Nat Neurosci.* 2005;8:1442–1444.

105. Kreek MJ, Nielson DA, Butelman ER, LaForge KS. Genetic influences on impulsivity, risk taking, stress responsivity and vulnerability to drug abuse and addiction. *Nat Neurosci.* 2005;8:1450–1457.

106. Leshner AI. Addiction is a brain disease, and it matters. *Science.* 1997;278:45–47.

107. Lilenfeld LRR, Ringham R, Kalarchian MA, Marcus MD. A family history study of binge-eating disorder. *Compr Psychiatry.* 2008;49:247–254.

108. Littlefield AK, Sher KJ, Wood PK. Is "maturing out" of problematic alcohol involvement related to personality change? *J Abnorm Psychol.* 2009;118:360–374.

109. Liu X, Jernigen C, Gharib M, Booth S, Caggiula AR, Sved AF. Effects of dopamine antagonists on drug cue-induced reinstatement of nicotine-seeking behaviour in rats. *Behav Pharmacol.* 2010;21:153–160.

110. Liu X, Weiss F. Reversal of ethanol seeking behaviour by D1 and D2 antagonists in an animal model of relapse: differences in antagonist potency in previously ethanol-dependent versus nondependent rats. *J Pharmacol Exp Ther.* 2002;300:882–889.

111. London M. History of addiction: a UK perspective. *Am J Addict.* 2005;14:97–105.

112. Loxton NJ, Dawe S. Reward and punishment sensitivity in dysfunctional eating and hazardous drinking women: associations with family risk. *Appetite.* 2006;47:361–371.

113. Lu H, Zou Q, Chefer S, et al. Abstinence from cocaine and sucrose self-administration reveals altered mesocorticolimbic circuit connectivity by resting state MRI. *Brain Connect.* 2014;4:499–510.

114. Manasse SM, Forman EM, Ruocco AC, Butryn ML, Juarascio AS, Fitzpatrick KK. Do executive functioning deficits underpin binge eating disorder? A comparison of overweight women with and without binge eating pathology. *Int J Eat Disord.* 2015;48:677–683.

115. Mangabeira V, Garcia-Mijares M, Silva MT. Sugar withdrawal and differential reinforcement of low rate (DRL) performance in rats. *Physiol Behav.* 2015;139:468–473.

116. Manwaring JL, Green L, Myerson J, Strube MJ, Wilfley DE. Discounting of various types of rewards by women with and without binge eating disorder: evidence for general rather than specific differences. *Psychol Rec.* 2011;61:561–582.

117. Marcus MD. Adapting treatment for patients with binge-eating disorder. In: Garner DM, Garfinkel PE, eds. *Handbook of Treatment for Eating Disorders.* 2nd ed. New York: Guilford Press; 1997:484–493.

118. Marlatt GA, Gordon JR. *Relapse Prevention: Maintenance Strategies in the Treatment of Addictive Behavirors.* New York: Guilford Press; 1985.

119. McCaffery P, Drager UC. High levels of retinoic acid-generating dehydrogenase in the meso-telencephalic dopamine system. *Proc Natl Acad Sci.* 1994;91:7772–7776.

120. McGrady BS. Treatment of substance use disorders. In: Barlow DH, ed. *Handbook of Treatment of Psychological Disorders.* 5th ed. New York: Guilford Press; 2014:533–587.

121. McGrady BS, Merlo LJ. Psychological treatment for substance use disorders. In: Brownell KD, Gold MS, eds. *Food and Addiction: A Comprehensive Handbook.* Toronto, ON: Oxford University Press; 2012.

122. Meule A, Kubler A. Food cravings in food addiction: the distinct role of positive reinforcement. *Eat Behav.* 2012;13:252–255.

123. Meule A, Lutz A, Vogele C, Kubler A. Women with elevated food addiction symptoms show accelerated reactions, but no impaired inhibitory control, in response to pictures of high-calorie food-cues. *Eat Behav.* 2012;13:423–428.

124. Meule A, Platte P. Facets of impulsivity interactively predict body fat and binge eating in young women. *Appetite.* 2015;87:352–357.

125. Meyer PJ, Ma ST, Robinson TE. A cocaine cue is more preferred and evokes more frequency-modulated 50-kHz ultrasonic vocalizations in rats prone to attribute incentive salience to a food cue. *Psychopharmacology*. 2012;219:999–1009.

126. Miller WR, Rollnick S. *Motivational Interviewing: Preparing People for Change*. 2nd ed. New York: Guilford Press; 2002.

127. Mobbs O, Iglesias K, Golay A, Van der Linden M. Cognitive deficits in obese persons with and without binge eating disorder. Investigation using a mental flexibility task. *Appetite*. 2011;57:263–271.

128. Mogg K, Bradley BP, O'Neill B, et al. Effect of dopamine D(3) receptor antagonism on approach responses to food cues in overweight and obese individuals. *Behav Pharmacol*. 2012;23:603–608.

129. Murphy CM, Stojek MK, Mackillop J. Interrelationships among impulsive personality traits, food addiction, and body mass index. *Appetite*. 2013;73:45–50.

130. Mussell MP, Mitchellde Zwaan JE M, Crosby RD, Seim HC, Crow SJ. Clinical characteristics associated with binge eating in obese females: a descriptive study. *Int J Obes*. 1996;20:324–331.

131. Nader MA, Czoty PW. PET imaging of dopamine D2 receptors in monkey models of cocaine abuse: genetic predisposition versus environmental modulation. *Am J Psychiatry*. 2005;162:1473–1482.

132. Nasser JA, Bradley LE, Leitzsch JB, et al. Psychoactive effects of tasting chocolate and desire for more chocolate. *Physiol Behav*. 2011;104:117–121.

133. Nathan PJ, O'Neill BV, Mogg K, et al. The effects of the dopamine D(3) receptor antagonist GSK598809 on attentional bias to palatable food cues in overweight and obese subjects. *Int J Neuropsychopharmacol*. 2012;15:149–161.

134. Nesse RM. An evolutionary perspective on substance abuse. *Ethnology and Sociobiology*. 1994;15:339–348.

135. Ng L, Davis C. Cravings and food consumption in binge eating disorder. *Eat Behav*. 2013;14:472–475.

136. O'Brien CP. Anticraving medications for relapse prevention: a possible new class of psychoactive medications. *Am J Psychiatry*. 2005;162:1423–1431.

137. Okita K, Ghahremani DG, Payer DE, et al. Emotion dysregulation and amygdala dopamine D2-type receptor availability in methamphetamine users. *Drug Alcohol Depend*. 2016;161:163–170.

138. Orford J. *Excessive Appetites*. Chichester: John Wiley & Sons; 2001.

139. Oswald KD, Murdaugh DL, King VL, Boggiano MM. Motivation for palatable food despite consequences in an animal model of binge eating. *Int J Eat Disord*. 2011;44:203–211.

140. Pearson CM, Zapolski TC, Smith GT. A longitudinal test of impulsivity and depression pathways to early binge eating onset. *Int J Eat Disord*. 2015;48:230–237.

141. Pelchat ML. Of human bondage: Food cravings, obsession, compulsion, and addiction. *Physiol Behav*. 2002;76:347–352.

142. Peterson JD, Wolf ME, White FJ. Impaired DRL 30 performance during amphetamine withdrawal. *Behav Brain Res*. 2003;143:101–108.

143. Petroni ML, Villanova N, Avagnina S, et al. Psychological distress in morbid obesity in relation to weight history. *Obes Surg*. 2007;17:391–399.

144. Pickering C, Alsio J, Hulting AL, Schioth HB. Withdrawal from free-choice high-fat high-sugar diet induces craving only in obesity-prone animals. *Psychopharmacology*. 2009;204:431–443.

145. Picot AK, Lilenfeld LRR. The relationship among binge severity, personality psychopathology, and body mass index. *Int J Eat Disord*. 2003;34:98–107.

146. Pike KM, Carter JC, Olmsted MP. Cognitive Behaviour Therapy for Anorexia Nervosa. In: Grilos C, Mitchell J, eds. *Treatment of Eating Disorders*. New York: Guilford Press; 2010.

147. Pivarunas BConner BT. Impulsivity and emotion dysregulation as predictors of food addiction. *Eat Behav*. 2015;19:9–14.

148. Pope HG, Lalonde JK, Pindyck LJ, Walsh T, Bulik CM, Crow S. Binge eating disorder: a stable syndrome. *Am J Psychiatry*. 2006;163:2181–2183.

149. Potenza MN. Should addictive disorders include non-substance related conditions? *Addiction*. 2006;101(suppl 1):142–151.

150. Randolph TG. The descriptive features of "food addiction" – addictive eating and drinking. *Q J Stud Alcohol*. 1956;17:198–224.

151. Reas DL, Grilo CM. Timing and sequence of the onset of overweight, dieting, and binge eating in overweight patients with binge eating disorder. *Int J Eat Disord*. 2007;40:165–170.

152. Richards TJ, Patterson PM, Hamilton SF. Fast food, addiction, and market power. *J Agr Resour Econ*. 2007;32:425–447.

153. Robinson MJ, Burghardt PR, Patterson CM, et al. Individual differences in cue-induced motivation and striatal systems in rats susceptible to diet-induced obesity. *Neuropsychopharmacology*. 2015;40:2113–2123.

154. Safer DL, Robinson AH, Jo B. Outcome from a randomized controlled trial of group therapy for binge eating disorder: comparing dialectical behaviour therapy adapted for binge eating to an active comparison group therapy. *Behav Ther*. 2010;41:106–120.

155. Sanfey AG, Hastie R, Colvin MK, Grafman J. Phineas gauged: Decision-making and the human prefrontal cortex. *Neuropsychologia*. 2003;41:1218–1229.

156. Saunders BT, Robinson TE. A cocaine cue acts as an incentive stimulus in some but not others: implications for addiction. *Biol Psychiatry*. 2010;67:730–736.

157. Schag K, Teufel M, Junne F, et al. Impulsivity in binge eating disorder: food cues elicit increased reward responses and disinhibition. *PLoS One*. 2013;8:e76542.

158. Schienle A, Schafer A, Hermann A, Vaitl D. Binge-eating disorder: reward sensitivity and brain activation to images of food. *Biol Psychiatry*. 2009;65:654–661.

159. Schulte EM, Grilo CM, Gearhardt AN. Shared and unique mechanisms underlying binge eating disorder and addictive disorders. *Clin Psychol Rev*. 2016;44:125–139.

160. Sebastian RS, Cleveland LE, Goldman JD. Effect of snacking frequency on adolescents' dietary intakes and meeting national recommendations. *J Adolesc Health*. 2008;42:503–511.

161. Small DM, Zatore RJ, Dagher A, Evans AC, Jones-Gotman M. Changes in brain activity related to eating chocolate: from pleasure to aversion. *Brain*. 2001;124:1720–1733.

162. Smith TG, Tasnadi A. A theory of natural addiction. *Games and Economic Behaviour*. 2007;59:316–344.

163. Spinella M, Lyke J. Executive personality traits and eating disorders. *Int J Neurosci*. 2004;114:83–93.

164. Spring B, Schneider K, Smith M, et al. Abuse potential of carbohydrates for overweight carbohydrate cravers. *Psychopharmacology*. 2008;197:637–647.

165. Steiger H, Bruce KR. Phenotypes, endophenotypes, and genotypes in bulimia spectrum eating disorders. *Can J Psychiatry*. 2007;52:220–227.

166. Stromberg MF. The effect of baclofen alone and in combination with naltrexone on ethanol consumption in the rat. *Pharmacol Biochem Behav*. 2004;78:743–750.

167. Sullivan RJ, Hagen EH. Psychotropic substance-seeking: evolutionary pathology or adaptation? *Addiction*. 2002;97:389–400.

168. Sullivan S, Cloniger CR, Pryzbeck TR, Klein S. Personality characteristics in obesity and relationship with successful weight loss. *Int J Obes*. 2007;31:669–674.

169. Tomasi D, Volkow ND. Striatocortical pathway dysfunction in addiction and obesity: differences and similarities. *Crit Rev Biochem Mol Biol*. 2013;48:1–19.

170. Trinko R, Sears RM, Guarnieri DJ, DiLeone RJ. Neural mechanisms underlying obesity and drug addiction. *Physiol Behav*. 2007;91:499–505.

171. Udo T, Grilo CM, Brownell KD, Weinberger AH, Dileone RJ, McKee SA. Modeling the effects of positive and negative mood on the ability to resist eating in obese and non-obese individuals. *Eat Behav*. 2013;14:40–46.

172. Vanderschuren LJMJ, Everitt BJ. Drug seeking becomes compulsive after prolonged cocaine self-administration. *Science.* 2004;305:1017–1019.

173. Vassileva J, Petkova P, Georgiev S, et al. Impaired decision-making in psychopathic heroin addicts. *Drug Alcohol Depend.* 2007;86:287–289.

174. Velazquez-Sanchez C, Santos JW, Smith KL, Ferragud A, Sabino V, Cottone P. Seeking behaviour, place conditioning, and resistance to conditioned suppression of feeding in rats intermittently exposed to palatable food. *Behav Neurosci.* 2015;129:219–224.

175. Vella-Zarb RA, Mills JS, Westra HA, Carter JC, Keating L. A Randomized controlled trial of motivational interviewing + self-help versus psychoeducation + self-help for binge eating. *Int J Eat Disord.* 2015;48:328–332.

176. Verdejo-Garcia A, Benbrook A, Funderburk F, David P, Cadet J-L, Bolla KI. The differential relationship between cocaine use and marijuana use on decision-making performance over repeat testing with the Iowa Gambling Task. *Drug Alcohol Depend.* 2007;90: 2–11.

177. Volkow ND, Fowler JS, Wang G-J. Role of dopamine in drug reinforcement and addiction in humans: results from imaging studies. *Behav Pharmacol.* 2002;13:355–366.

178. Volkow ND, Wise RA. How can drug addiction help us understand obesity? *Nat Neurosci.* 2005;8:555–560.

179. Walker BM, Koob GF. The gamma-aminobutyric acid-B receptor agonist baclofen attenuates responding for ethanol in ethanol-dependent rats. *Alcohol Clin Exp Res.* 2007;31:11–18.

180. Wang GJ, Geliebter A, Volkow ND, et al. Enhanced striatal dopamine release during food stimulation in binge eating disorder. *Obesity.* 2011;19:1601–1608.

181. Wang G-J, Volkow ND, Thanos PK, Fowler JS. Similarity between obesity and drug addiction as assessed by neurofunctional imaging: a concept review. *J Addict Dis.* 2004;23:39–53.

182. Wansink B, Van Ittersum K. Portion size me: Downsizing our consumption norms. *J Am Diet Assoc.* 2007;107:1103–1106.

183. Weygandt M, Schaefer A, Schienle A, Haynes J-D. Diagnosing different binge-eating disorders based on reward-related brain activation pathways. *Hum Brain Mapp.* 2012;33:2135–2146.

184. Whiteside SP, Lynam DR. The five factor model and impulsivity: using a structural model of personality to understand impulsivity. *Pers Individ Dif.* 2001;30:669–689.

185. Whiteside SP, Lynam DR. Understanding the role of impulsivity and externalizing psychopathology in alcohol abuse: application of the UPPS impulsive behaviour scale. *Exp Clin Psychopharmacol.* 2003;11:210–217.

186. Whiteside SP, Lynam DR. Understanding the role of impulsivity and externalizing psychopathology in alcohol abuse: application of the UPPS impulsive behaviour scale. *Personality Disorders: Theory, Research & Treatment.* 2009;1:69–79.

187. Whiteside SP, Lynam DR, Miller JD, Reynolds SK. Validation of the UPPS impulsive behaviour scale: a four-factor model of impulsivity. *Eur J Pers.* 2005;19. 559–574.

188. Wideman CH, Nadzam GR, Murphy HM. Implications of an animal model of sugar addiction, withdrawal and relapse for human health. *Nutr Neurosci.* 2005;8. 269–276.

189. Wilson GT. The addiction model of eating disorders: a critical analysis. *Adv Behav Res Therapy.* 1991;13:27–72.

190. Wilson GT. Eating disorders, obesity and addiction. *Eur Eat Disord Rev.* 2010;18:341–351.

191. Wilson GT, Fairburn CG. Treatment for eating disorders. In: Nathan PE, Gorman JM, eds. *A Guide to Treatments that Work.* 3rd ed. New York: Oxford University Press; 2007:579–609.

192. Wilson GT, Fairburn CG, Agras WS. Cognitive-behavioural therapy for bulimia nervosa. In: Garner DM, Garfinkel PE, eds. *Handbook of Treatment for Eating Disorders.* 2nd ed. New York: Guilford Press; 1997:67–93.

193. Wilson GT, Wilfley DE, Agras S, Bryson SW. Psychological treatments of binge eating disorder. *Arch Gen Psychiatry.* 2010;67: 94–101.

194. Xi ZX, Gilbert JG, Pak AC, Ashby Jr CR, Heidbreder CA, Gardner EL. Selective dopamine D3 receptor antagonism by SB-277011A attenuates cocaine reinforcement as assessed by progressive-ratio and variable-cost-variable-payoff fixed-ratio cocaine self-administration in rats. *Eur J Neurosci.* 2005;21:3427–3438.

195. Xi ZX, Newman AH, Gilbert JG, et al. The novel dopamine D3 receptor antagonist NGB 2904 inhibits cocaine's rewarding effects and cocaine-induced reinstatement of drug-seeking behaviour in rats. *Neuropsychopharmacology.* 2006;31:1393–1405.

196. Yanovski SZ. Sugar and fat: cravings and aversions. *J Nutr.* 2003;133:835S–837S.

197. Yao L, Fan P, Arolfo M, et al. Inhibition of aldehyde dehydrogenase-2 suppresses cocaine seeking by generating THP, a cocaine use-dependent inhibitor of dopamine synthesis. *Nat Med.* 2010;16:1024–1028.

198. Yue K, Ma B, Chen L, et al. L-Stepholidine, a naturally occurring dopamine D1 receptor agonist and D2 receptor antagonist, attenuates heroin self-administration and cue-induced reinstatement in rats. *Neuroreport.* 2014;25:7–11.

199. Zapolski TC, Cyders MA, Smith GT. Positive urgency predicts illegal drug use and risky sexual behaviour. *Psychol Addict Behav.* 2009;23:348–354.

200. deZwaan M, Mitchell JE. Opiate antagonists and eating behaviour in humans: a review. *J Clin Pharmacol.* 1992;32:1060–1072.

35

Compulsive Buying

JOANNA M. MARINO, TROY W. ERTELT, JAMES E. MITCHELL, KATHY LANCASTER, AND JON E. GRANT

CHAPTER OUTLINE

Introduction

Kraepelin and Bleuler first identified oniomania, or the urge to buy, in the early 1900s.[7,39] Today, compulsive buying is likely a much different phenomenon from what it was when Kraepelin and Bleuler first conceptualized the disorder. In the United States, and likely in all industrialized nations, consumer spending takes place in both public places such as shopping centers, discount stores, or rummage sales and in private homes through the use of online shopping and television shopping networks. The set of symptoms known as compulsive buying, pathological buying, or buying disorder has recently received increased attention in both the consumer and mental health literatures, although data on the topic remain limited.

Diagnosis and Classification

Characteristics of compulsive buying include disinhibition or limited control over buying behavior.[6] Compulsive buying is not included in the *Diagnostic and Statistical Manual of Mental Disorders, Fourth Edition, Text Revision* (DSM-IV-TR); however, McElroy and colleagues[47] have outlined criteria that are consistent with the DSM-IV-TR format, and these have been widely adopted in defining and studying compulsive buying (Table 35.1).

Some have suggested that compulsive buying fits into the grouping of addictive and impulsive behaviors.[32] An individual with compulsive buying behavior may experience a cycle of urges and impulses, followed by pleasure or euphoria while shopping, and guilt after purchasing items, along with a drive to continue the behavior.[32,55] Impulse control disorders involve impulses or drives that the individual cannot resist, and these urges are harmful to oneself or another person.[55]

According to its current classification, compulsive buying is a "disorder of impulsive control-not otherwise specified" due, in part, to the limited research on this topic.[6] Some researchers have hypothesized that compulsive buying falls onto a spectrum, since the urge to buy may be variable in some individuals, or increasing and decreasing in certain situations, and the onset of compulsive buying behavior may be gradual.[14]

However, research has yet to determine whether compulsive buying fits better with obsessive-compulsive, addictive, or impulse control disorders. Black[5] conceptualized compulsive buying as obsessive thoughts followed by the compulsion to buy, and Frost and colleagues[26] found that compulsive buyers had higher scores on an obsessive-compulsive symptomatology scale when compared with controls. Christenson and colleagues[13] also suggested that compulsive buying might have features of both impulsive and compulsive disorders. Further research needs to delineate the relationship of compulsive buying to each of these theories.

Common factors among compulsive buying behavior are the desire, relief, and feeling of well-being that come from purchasing. Compulsive buyers may believe that their material possessions, not necessarily their personal characteristics, determine their identity. By purchasing, such individuals may feel that they are presenting a more desirable self to the world while hiding their shame over their debt and ongoing purchases. In addition, some research has suggested that a better conceptualization of compulsive buying may include compulsive acquisition, meaning that some individuals who exhibit compulsive buying behavior may feel the need to pick up or gather free items such as brochures or fliers.[26]

Individuals who exhibit compulsive buying behavior often appear to be upset over their own lying, such as hiding new packages from a spouse. For many compulsive buyers, the act of purchasing, rather than what they buy, is what leads to gratification.[14] Many who suffer from compulsive buying do not use the items that they purchase.[24] Some individuals may return or sell the item, although many keep the items.[13,29] This collection of items can lead to clutter or result in hoarding behavior. Some individuals with compulsive buying disorder spend their money on themselves, while others buy gifts.[24] Some have reported that their urge to shop has led them to seek out and rummage trash cans and dumpsters.

TABLE 35.1 **Diagnostic Criteria for Compulsive Buying.**

1. Maladaptive preoccupation with buying or shopping, or maladaptive buying or shopping impulses on behavior, as indicated by at least one of the following:

    a. Frequent preoccupation with buying or impulses to buy that is/are experienced as irresistible, intrusive and/or senseless.

    b. Frequent buying of more than can be afforded, frequent buying of items that are not needed, or shopping for longer periods of time than intended.

2. The buying preoccupations, impulses or behaviors cause marked distress, are time consuming, significantly interfere with social or occupational functioning, or result in financial problems (e.g., bankruptcy).

3. The excessive buying or shopping behavior does not occur exclusively during periods of hypomania or mania.

Adapted from McElroy SL, Keck PE Jr, Pope HG Jr. Compulsive buying: a report of 20 cases. *J Clin Psychiatry.* 1994;16:205–212.

Prevalence Rates and Subject Characteristics

The available data on prevalence rates of compulsive buying have proved to be variable. Koran and colleagues,[38] after conducting phone surveys, found a point prevalence of 5.8% in the United States, with female prevalence rates somewhat higher than males, at 6.0% and 5.5%, respectively. These numbers decreased to a 1.4% point prevalence when the Compulsive Buying Scale cutoff score was increased. Other studies have reported rates of compulsive buying of 1.9% among university students (n = 791) and 9.3% in psychiatric inpatients (n = 204).[28,59]

The age at onset for compulsive buying appears to typically be during late adolescence or early adulthood, although it may take several years to reach peak intensity.[7] Compulsive buying respondents tend to have incomes below $50,000, to be more likely to make minimum payments on credit cards, and to be within $500 of maximum credit limits.[38] Individuals with compulsive buying behavior also usually spend over $100 during compulsive buying episodes.[13] Christenson and colleagues[13] found that most individuals who exhibited compulsive buying behavior were experiencing indebtedness and that an average of almost half of the household's income went toward attempts to resolve debt caused by compulsive buying behavior. Differences in shopping tendencies between genders, among individuals of varying incomes, and during special events (e.g., holidays, birthdays, or anniversaries) are important considerations in studying compulsive buying behavior.[6]

One additional key feature of compulsive buying is the use of credit cards. O'Guinn and Faber[58] found that individuals who exhibited compulsive buying behavior, on average, tended to have more credit cards than general consumers and that more compulsive buyers' credit cards were within $100 of their limit. Access to credit cards is abundant in the United States, and cognitions associated with the use of credit cards (e.g., "I'm not paying for this right now," "I can afford this next month," or "I can pay off this credit card with another card") can often lead to the cycle of overspending. In addition, the desire for and value placed on the need to attain and have the most items possible are likely key aspects for many compulsive buyers. Others diagnosed with compulsive buying disorder may feel driven to purchase items because they have a collection of specific items. Still others feel the allure of the sense of saving when they see a sales rack, even when they spend money on an item that they do not need.

Economics and Consumerism

Economists have long studied the behavior of buyers. Some believe that it is best to conceptualize compulsive buying on a continuum with normal spending. However, compulsive buying is a disorder involving more than just indebtedness. Whereas individuals with compulsive buying behavior do have control over their spending, there are other factors influencing and sustaining the impulse to buy that make those with compulsive buying disorder feel that they can no longer control their buying.

External forces may have etiological importance in the development of compulsive buying. For example, in the United States, there appears to be a sense of importance attached to having higher end goods such as new, expensive cars and designer fashions. Others may feel pressures from the American culture's pursuit of youth. Individuals may experience a sense of psychological well-being when purchasing objects that fall into these categories and may think that these objects will make others perceive them as successful. Nevertheless, each individual may feel driven by a different factor or factors, and the concept of success may be different among individuals in different socioeconomic strata. Indeed, compulsive buying appears to affect individuals in varying socioeconomic categories.[14]

Shopping in the United States is a somewhat gender-specific leisure activity. Black[6] suggested that compulsive buying behavior and compulsive gambling behavior might be gender-specific variants of the same underlying pathology, with compulsive buying behavior manifesting itself in women and compulsive gambling behavior being more prevalent among men. Those with compulsive buying disorder often find themselves drawn to shopping for clothing, shoes, music CDs, jewelry, makeup, groceries, and décor for the home.[5,48] Larger items such as cars are also possible purchases, and for this reason, purchases differ depending on access to disposable income.

Etiology and Course

No one has extensively examined the possible etiologies of compulsive buying, although it will likely fit into a biopsychosocial etiological model.[21] The course for compulsive buying is probably chronic, with one study finding the mean age at onset in late adolescence.[13] Identification of buying as a problem tends to occur later, in one's late twenties or early thirties.[13] In many cases, the main thing that identifies compulsive buying is the large debt that subjects have accrued, followed by feedback from friends or family, legal problems, or guilt.[13]

Levels of materialism and youth are predictors of compulsive buying tendencies.[18] Women are more likely to be diagnosed with compulsive buying disorder, perhaps because women predominantly hold the shopping role in families.[13,46,63] Indeed, women are more likely to carry a diagnosis of compulsive buying. In addition, women have had higher scores on compulsive buying inventories, suggesting that compulsive buying may be more severe in females.[14] Compulsive buying is also related to low self-esteem and to problem credit-card use.[14,15,24,56,60]

Several variables may be important in determining etiological factors for compulsive buying behavior as well as differences in compulsive buying among younger individuals. Survey results of adolescents suggest a positive relationship between hours of television viewed per day and compulsive buying behavior. This may be due to the influence of materialism viewed on television.[15] There is also a significant correlation between compulsive buying behavior in adolescence and perceptions of parental compulsive buying behavior, possibly suggesting that compulsive buying is a learned behavior identified through modeling.[15] Adolescent girls appear to have higher compulsive buying scores than boys, which speaks to gender differences in diagnosis.[15] Predictive modeling of adolescent compulsive buying behavior suggests that gender, younger age, peer influence, parents' compulsive buying behavior, tangible family resources, family stressors, and lesser family communication may predict compulsive buying.[15,28] Others have found significant relationships between compulsive buying behavior and risk-taking behaviors such as smoking, alcohol and drug use, and unsafe sexual practices,[57] which may speak to the relationship between impulsivity and compulsive buying behavior.

Developmental learning may also affect the formation of compulsive buying. In examining retrospective recall of childhood buying behavior, d'Astous[14] found that the likelihood of compulsive buying increased in individuals who reported a history of being likely to spend money quickly after receiving it in childhood, as well as when they reported their parents buying "everything" they wanted.[14] In addition, susceptibility of influences from friends or social situations (e.g., feeling important when making a purchase, frustration when having fewer things than others do) was related to compulsive buying behavior.[14] Further research could better assess similarities in childhood experiences or modeling that may be precursors to compulsive buying.

There has been little research regarding the personal financial costs of compulsive buying. Miltenberger and colleagues[48] found that debt ranged from $0 to $30,000 in a small sample of individuals who exhibited compulsive buying behavior. Compulsive buying episodes can vary in duration from less than an hour to hours of shopping.[48]

A range of emotions can lead to compulsive buying episodes. Individuals with compulsive buying symptoms suggest that they often experience negative emotions before shopping, although some report elation, power, and joy beforehand.[13] Miltenberger and colleagues[48] also found that ratings of sadness or depressed mood were significantly higher before shopping when compared with mood during the shopping episode. Faber and Christenson[21] also reported that boredom, depressed mood, and anxiousness were moods experienced prior to shopping. Euphoria and excitement ratings were significantly higher during shopping episodes than afterwards.[48] These findings suggest that a negative mood state occurs before shopping and that shopping leads to a more positive change in an emotion. After shopping, a negative mood state is likely to emerge as individuals realize that they are unable to afford the purchased items. In most cases, negative emotion (e.g., tension/anxiousness, anger/irritation, self-criticalness, and boredom) scores were highest before shopping and decreased during and after the shopping episode.[48] This model of negative reinforcement may sustain compulsive buying behavior.[48]

Researchers have attempted to connect obsessive-compulsive spectrum disorders or impulse control disorder to compulsive buying, considering the possible role of serotonin in compulsive buying symptoms. In the only study directly examining this relationship, no differences emerged between compulsive buying participants and control participants in the rate of occurrence of two polymorphisms related to the serotonin transporter.[17]

Research on the pathophysiology of compulsive buying remains limited. In the one available study assessing the neurobiology of compulsive buying, functional magnetic resonance imaging (fMRI) assessments showed greater activation in the nucleus accumbens in participants with compulsive buying, compared to controls, when shown various products.[60] Consistent with these neurobiological findings, a study of neurocognition in compulsive buying found significant impairment in response inhibition, risk adjustment during decision making, and spatial working memory when compared to controls.[17]

Comorbidity

A number of studies have examined the relationship of compulsive buying with other psychiatric disorders. The most commonly reported comorbidities include mood disorders, anxiety disorders, substance use disorders, impulse control disorders, and eating disorders.[21,47,63] For example, when compared with control groups, it appears that persons with compulsive buying disorder are more likely to have a mood disorder or another psychiatric disorder than would be expected in the general population.[10] In individuals with compulsive buying disorder and their family members, depression and anxiety appear to be common.[10,24,26]

The relationship between compulsive buying and mood disorders is reasonably well established. In his examination of several case series, Black[6] identified comorbidity rates for compulsive buying disorder and mood disorders ranging from 28% to 95%. It is important to note that compulsive buying behavior is distinct from the symptoms of a manic or hypomanic episode. Additional research on how spending and buying differ in manic episodes compared with compulsive buying episodes would be useful in understanding the distinction.

Researchers have drawn a strong link between compulsive buying disorder and binge eating disorder.[22] Faber and colleagues[22] performed two studies to assess the link between these two disorders. In the first study, they examined compulsive buying in women diagnosed with binge eating disorder. The authors found that the women diagnosed with binge eating disorder had significantly more symptoms of compulsive buying than did matched controls. In the second study, the authors compared a group of participants (mostly women) with compulsive buying behavior with a group of participants whose buying behavior was normal. The authors found that those with compulsive buying behavior were significantly more likely to engage in behaviors characteristic of binge eating disorder. In addition, McElroy and colleagues[46] contributed a theoretical link between compulsive buying disorder and binge eating disorder, in that both disorders likely belong on the compulsive-impulsive behavior spectrum. Concerning other eating disorders, no one has shown a strong link between compulsive buying disorder and anorexia nervosa or bulimia nervosa.[50]

As mentioned previously, some have suggested that compulsive buying disorder is part of the obsessive-compulsive spectrum.[6] Interest in the obsessive-compulsive spectrum has increased over the last several years, and some have suggested that up to 10% of the population in the United States has an obsessive-compulsive spectrum problem that includes intrusive thoughts and/or repetitive behaviors.[33] However, the relationship of compulsive buying disorder to obsessive-compulsive disorder and obsessive-compulsive spectrum disorders is unclear. For example, Bienvenu and colleagues[4] examined a sample of individuals diagnosed with obsessive-compulsive disorder and their first-degree relatives. They identified only one case where compulsive buying disorder co-occurred with obsessive-compulsive disorder. In addition, Jaisoorya and colleagues[30] examined a large sample of individuals with obsessive-compulsive disorder and found only one individual with comorbid compulsive buying disorder. Although compulsive buying disorder symptoms seem to relate to the general symptoms of obsessive-compulsive disorder, it appears that the relationship between compulsive buying disorder and obsessive-compulsive disorder may be unremarkable.

Some have identified a relationship between compulsive buying disorder and kleptomania. McElroy and colleagues[46] presented a theoretical paper closely linking kleptomania and compulsive buying disorder. Lejoyeux and colleagues[44] identified a relative risk of comorbid kleptomania of 8.5% for those with compulsive buying disorder. It also seems possible that behaviors associated with kleptomania (e.g., shoplifting) may become more common in those with compulsive buying disorder as their financial situations deteriorate and they are unable to purchase the goods that they are compelled to obtain. Another disorder that some have speculated is closely related to compulsive buying disorder is pathological gambling. As noted above, Black[6] has conceptualized compulsive buying and pathological gambling as being gender-specific manifestations of a similar underlying psychopathology. In a sample of pathological gamblers, 23% had a lifetime history of compulsive buying disorder.[9] Christenson and colleagues.[13] found no difference between individuals who exhibited compulsive buying behavior and age-matched control subjects across trichotillomania, pyromania, kleptomania, intermittent explosive disorder, or pathological gambling. However, compulsive buying subjects were more likely to have any impulsive control disorder when compared with the age-matched control group.[13] Further research about the comorbidity among compulsive buying, kleptomania, and pathological gambling could help to explain the complex relationship observed among these disorders.

Schlosser and colleagues[65] reported on a sample of 46 individuals who met criteria for compulsive buying. Participants completed two assessments (Structured Interview for *Diagnostic and Statistical Manual of Mental Disorders, Third Edition*, Revised, Personality Disorders and Personality Diagnostic Questionnaire Revised), and the authors examined the extent to which the two instruments identified the same personality pathology. The most frequently identified personality disorder within the sample was obsessive-compulsive personality disorder. Twenty-two percent of the sample met the criteria for obsessive-compulsive personality disorder on both the Structured Interview for *Diagnostic and Statistical Manual of Mental Disorders, Third Edition*, Revised, Personality Disorders and Personality Diagnostic Questionnaire Revised. Avoidant personality disorder and borderline personality disorder were both present in 15% of the sample. Overall, 59% of the sample met criteria for a personality disorder on both the Structured Interview for *Diagnostic and Statistical Manual of Mental Disorders, Third Edition*, Revised, Personality Disorders and Personality Diagnostic Questionnaire Revised.[65]

The literature on hoarding is too large to review in this chapter; however, the literature regarding compulsive buying and hoarding is worth mentioning. Frost and Hartl[25] identified several important features of compulsive hoarding, including the acquisition of seemingly useless possessions and the inability to discard them, the negative effect of clutter created from compulsive hoarding on the activities of daily living, and the distress and impairment experienced because of compulsive hoarding. Others have suggested that those who compulsively hoard possessions attach sentimental meaning to items while others do not.[67] Hoarding behavior is more likely in those with compulsive buying disorder compared with a noncompulsive buying group.[26] No one thus far has proposed a diagnostic specifier for identifying hoarding behavior in compulsive buying; however, it may be that a hoarding specifier could help in differentiating compulsive buying disorder subtypes. That is, those with compulsive buying disorder who choose to give their items away may differ from those buyers who hoard items or see some sentimental value in the possession.[26] Indeed, Mueller and colleagues[52] suggested that compulsive buying behavior might be more severe in persons with compulsive buying who hoard compared with those who do not hoard items. Moreover, compulsive buying subjects with hoarding behavior are more likely to have an affective disorder, substance use disorder, eating disorder, or anxiety disorder than those subjects who only hoard, suggesting more comorbid psychopathology in those with both hoarding and compulsive buying behavior.[52] Further research is needed to identify whether those individuals with hoarding traits are different from those with compulsive buying without hoarding behavior and to determine how treatment may differ between these two groups.

Almost half of one compulsive buying sample had a substance abuse problem, with most subjects abusing or dependent on alcohol.[26] Researchers have shown that substance abuse is comorbid with compulsive buying behavior, although no research to the authors' knowledge has directly examined the relationship between the two disorders.

Cultural Considerations

Researchers have investigated compulsive buying in several countries, including the United States, Canada, Germany, Belgium, and the United Kingdom, with prevalence rates from 2% to 10% found in the United States, United Kingdom, and Germany.[56] Compulsive buying increased in Germany from 1991 to 2001.[56] Research in other countries has not yet determined whether compulsive buying behavior is on the rise.

Data comparing American and German samples suggest that the severity of compulsive buying in both samples is largely equivalent,[53] while German buyers were more likely to have a current or past psychiatric disorder and have a history of more psychiatric disorders, especially affective and anxiety disorders.[53] Substance abuse and binge eating were also highly comorbid disorders in the German sample.[53] Gwin and colleagues[29] have identified some significant predictors (e.g., gender, parents' compulsive buying, tangible family resources, communication style, and family stress) for compulsive buying tendencies in an adolescent sample from Mexico.

A study in South Korea comparing compulsive buying in American and South Korean college students revealed some similarities in their behavior.[42] However, different patterns emerged when the authors administered the Diagnostic Screener for Compulsive Buying, as developed by Faber and O'Guinn,[23] to samples from both the United States and South Korea. In the United States, the Diagnostic Screener for Compulsive Buying is unidimensional; however, in South Korea, the authors observed a bidimensional structure of the same measure.[41] The two dimensions suggested for the South Korean samples related to financial outcomes and unfettered spending.[41] The authors interpreted this difference in response to the Diagnostic Screener for Compulsive Buying as being indicative of culturally different manifestations of compulsive buying disorder.

In an analysis of Israeli consumers, Shoham and Brenčič[66] found that predictors of compulsive shopping behavior included unplanned purchasing, the tendency of consumers to buy items that were not on a list, and gender (i.e., females). The authors concluded that the in-store decision-making might lead to compulsive buying behavior.

Assessment

When assessing for compulsive buying, several factors are important to consider. First, the behavior cannot be better accounted for by another disorder such as mania or bulimia nervosa (in which individuals may buy large quantities of food to eat) or by an organic problem such as a brain injury.[6] Several instruments used in research and designed to characterize compulsive buying behavior (Table 35.2) also would be helpful in clinical populations.

TABLE 35.2	Instruments Useful in the Assessment of Compulsive Buying.

Addictive Buying Indicator[63]
Buying Cognitions Inventory[43]
Buying Impulsiveness Scale[61]
Compulsive Acquisition Scale[26]
Compulsive Buying Scale[23]
Compulsive Buying Scale[20]
Credit Card Use Scale[61]
Minnesota Impulsive Disorders Interview[59]
The Compulsive Buying Scale[68]
Yale-Brown Obsessive-Compulsive Scale-Shopping Version[51]

Treatment

Impulse control disorder treatment often involves problem solving, learning and employing alternative behaviors, cognitive restructuring, and relapse prevention interventions.[30] Compulsive buying has its own complexities, as buying behavior cannot ever be fully eliminated.[50] Randomized controlled trials of cognitive behavior therapy in a group format have shown promise.

Mitchell and colleagues[49] have created a self-help and group therapy manual that appears to be beneficial in the treatment of compulsive buying disorder. The following outline would typify a 10-week treatment plan:

- Week 1: Individuals are encouraged to calculate current debt, which is also essential in order for participants to determine a plan to resolve the debt that they have accrued. Many times, credit counselors are options for participants who are overwhelmed by their debt.
- Week 2: Like most cognitive-behavioral models, compulsive buying disorder treatment begins by encouraging individuals to identify their problem buying behaviors and the cues that lead to these behaviors (Fig. 35.1). Each week, subjects are required to complete a purchasing record to aid in the identification of problematic buying behavior.
- Week 3: Individuals who exhibit compulsive buying behavior are coached on how to avoid problematic situations, restrict their stimulus field (e.g., stopping only at specific, "low-risk" stores), and increase more desirable behaviors and activities. Delaying the response to buy by waiting at least 24 h can work to remedy impulse shopping.
- Week 4: Compulsive buying participants learn cash management techniques such as carrying small amounts of cash, paying off credit card debt, determining how much money they should place in a savings account each week, and balancing

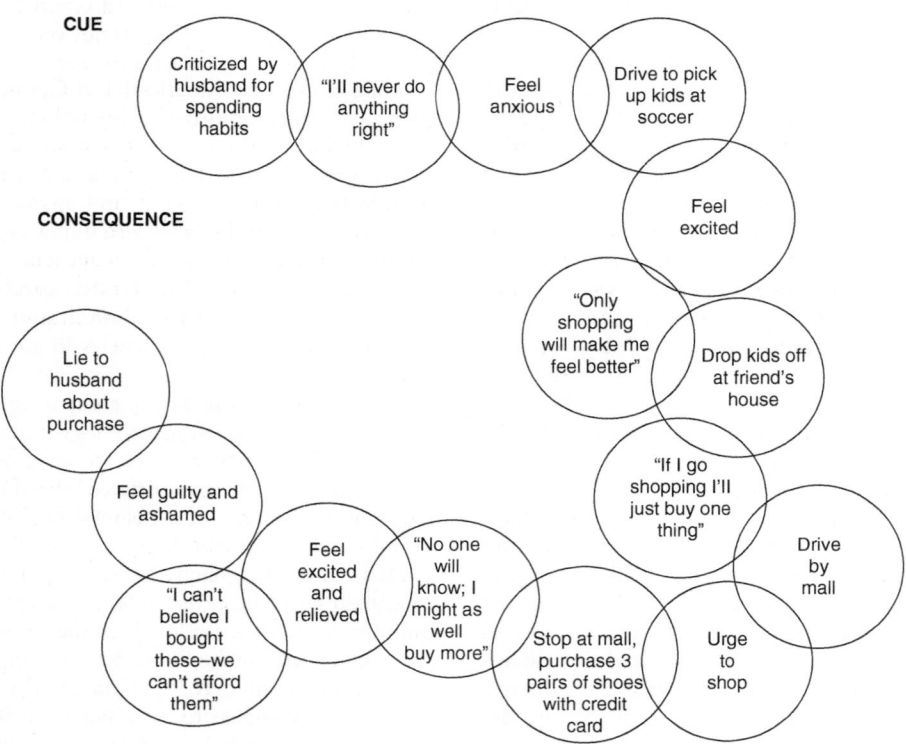

• **Fig. 35.1** Cue and consequence diagram.

a checkbook. Following an introduction to healthy buying behavior, participants begin to identify hoarding behavior as well as how to resolve this behavior.

- Week 5: There is a discussion of thoughts, feelings, and behaviors related to compulsive buying. Participants identify how cues lead to specific emotions, behaviors, and thoughts, and what consequences ensue.
- Week 6: There is a discussion of cognitive restructuring, especially challenging nonproductive thinking (e.g., "I can't live without my credit card" or "I have to go to the mall to feel better").
- Week 7: There is an examination of self-esteem, especially in relation to shopping and self-image.
- Weeks 8 and 9: In addressing exposure, stress managements, and problem solving skills, participants are encouraged to allow themselves into situations where they can identify and control their urge to buy and implement a new strategy for dealing with negative mood states.
- Week 10: In a discussion of relapse prevention plans, individuals learn to identify high-risk situations that may lead to lapses in compulsive buying behavior. They also identify how they can respond if a setback in buying occurs.

An examination of this cognitive-behavioral type therapy approach suggests positive results at the end of treatment and a 6-month follow-up, although the sample size in this pilot study was small.[49] Education about credit card use may be the key, as the use of cash and debit cards may have a very different impact on continued compulsive shopping, when compared with the continuing use of credit cards.[14,49] Posttreatment debts may be a concern in the resolution of mood symptoms.[49] Authors have also concluded that materialistic feelings and attitudes may be important predictors and subsequently important treatment factors in compulsive buying therapy.[18]

Randomized control trials have examined the CBT approach of Mitchell and colleagues.[49] Mueller and colleagues compared the 12-week program to a wait-list condition. Sixty participants were randomized to either group CBT or wait-list.[54] Those in the CBT condition showed improvement posttreatment and at 6-month follow-up. In a second study,[55] Müller and colleagues used a similar wait-list design and added a low-intensity guided self-help intervention as an additional active control. Participants randomized to the self-help spent time reading a manual and completing self-directed tasks and were also supported over the telephone at five time points during the 10-week period. Group CBT (n = 22) and self-help (n = 20) participants showed a marked improvement compared to wait-list, with equivalent symptom change. Finally, Benson and colleagues developed a program that integrated CBT, acceptance and commitment therapy, and psychodynamic principles.[3] Eleven participants were enrolled in a 12-week study comparing this program to wait-list. Those assigned to the treatment reported significantly greater reduction in compulsive buying symptoms.

In addition, a small case series (n = 4) of individuals with compulsive buying symptoms was treated with psychoanalysis.[40] The author suggested that internal emptiness is what created and maintained the compulsive buying behavior. There were no specific outcome data reported for this case series.

Support groups for treating addictions, such as Alcoholics Anonymous for alcoholism, have long been in use. Compulsive buying support groups have not become as common as other treatment groups, although Debtors Anonymous has been able to assist in debt management.[45] In addition, Brazer[12] outlined his method

for aiding individuals with money disorders, which includes the use of Debtors Anonymous in combination with psychoeducational group formats that discuss the disease model of addictions, educate individuals on debtors, deal with negative emotions such as anger and depression, improve self-esteem, and plan for the future. One major concern with using Debtors Anonymous is the group's limited number of locations. Black[5] also noted that several self-help books have been developed.[2,16,69]

Research on pharmacological treatment interventions has been mostly inconclusive, although researchers have studied several classes of medication. Case studies have suggested that naltrexone may be beneficial in the treatment of compulsive buying, since the medication specifically targets the urge to shop.[27]

Fluvoxamine has treated several psychological disorders including obsessive-compulsive disorder and depression. Black and colleagues[8] found similar and substantial improvement in a 9-week, double-blind comparison of fluvoxamine and placebo in compulsive buying subjects. Ninan and colleagues[57] found equivocal results between the control and fluvoxamine groups. However, in both studies, the authors suggested that psychoeducation related to compulsive buying symptoms and nonspecific therapeutic variables may have aided in the improvement of subjects.[8,57] These results suggest that self-help manuals or generalized therapeutic attention via more cost-effective support groups may be beneficial for individuals with compulsive buying disorder.

Koran and colleagues[35] investigated the use of escitalopram in conjunction with relapse prevention in compulsive buying and found that a similar number of both placebo and escitalopram subjects experienced relapses. Many of the subjects who relapsed in both groups appeared to have comorbid depression symptoms at the time of relapse or at baseline, suggesting the possibility of negative mood states as an etiological factor in compulsive buying.[35]

Koran and colleagues[36] also reported on open-label trials using citalopram for compulsive buying. The results appeared positive, as all subjects showed decreased scores on the Yale-Brown Obsessive-Compulsive Scale-shopping version and a depression scale.[36] Again, these authors suggested that the attention that individuals exhibiting compulsive buying behavior received in a clinical setting or the shopping logs that they completed might have had an important impact on the resolution of the compulsive buying systems, and that research with citalopram treatment alone is needed.[36] In a later study, Koran and colleagues[37] again found beneficial outcomes for all seven individuals randomized to the citalopram group in a double-blind study.

Aboujaoude and colleagues[1] conducted a 1-year follow-up with individuals who had exhibited compulsive buying behavior in the sample of Koran and colleagues.[36] At 3, 6, 9, and 12 months, over 70% of initial responders to citalopram were in remission.[1] The Yale-Brown Obsessive-Compulsive Scale-shopping version scores appeared to increase somewhat in persons who initially responded to citalopram, while total debt and shopping expenditures decreased.[1] Those who did not appear to respond to citalopram during the initial study showed poorer long-term outcomes.[1]

One clear problem with the pharmacological treatment studies thus far is small sample sizes. Further research clearly needs to determine how individuals will respond to varying selective serotonin reuptake inhibitors and other agents and what impact clinical attention has in these studies.

Future Research

Compulsive buying, while first identified nearly a century ago, has apparently become an increasingly common problem. This has led to increases in research in this area, but further study of the problem will need to determine which individuals on the compulsive buying spectrum will benefit from cognitive-behavioral therapy, behavioral therapy, or medication. Current literature on compulsive buying examines only cognitive-behavioral interventions; therefore, future research should likely examine other treatment interventions such as interpersonal therapy or behavioral therapy. In addition, compulsive buying treatment will likely need to address compulsive buying comorbidity. Finally, there needs to be further delineation of possible compulsive buying subtypes. The current chapter identified the state of research in this area, and further advances will help to identify and treat more appropriately those struggling with compulsive buying.

References

1. Aboujaoude E, Gamel N, Koran LM. A 1-year naturalistic follow-up of patients with compulsive shopping disorder. *J Clin Psychiatry*. 2003;64:946–950.
2. Arenson G. *Born to Spend: How to Overcome Compulsive Spending*. Blue Ridge Summit, PA: Tab Books; 1991.
3. Benson A, Eisenach D, Abrams L, van Stolk-Cooke K. Stopping overshopping: a preliminary randomized controlled trial of group therapy for compulsive buying disorder. *J Groups Addict Recovery*. 2014;9:97–125.
4. Bienvenu OJ, Samuels JF, Riddle MA, et al. The relationship of obsessive-compulsive disorder to possible spectrum disorders: results from a family study. *Biol Psychiatry*. 2000;48:287–283.
5. Black DW. Compulsive buying: a review. *J Clin Psychiatry*. 1996;57(suppl 8):50–55.
6. Black DW. Compulsive buying disorder: definition, assessment, epidemiology, and clinical management. *CNS Drugs*. 2001;15:17–27.
7. Black DW. Compulsive buying disorder: a review of the evidence. *CNS Spectr*. 2007;12:124–132.
8. Black DW, Gabel J, Hansen J, et al. A double-blind comparison of fluvoxamine versus placebo in the treatment of compulsive buying disorders. *Ann Clin Psychiatry*. 2000;12:205–211.
9. Black DW, Moyer T. Clinical features and psychiatric comorbidity of subjects with pathological gambling behaviors. *Psychiatr Serv*. 1998;49:1434–1439.
10. Black DW, Repertinger S, Gaffney GF, et al. Family history and psychiatric comorbidity in persons with compulsive buying: preliminary findings. *Am J Psychiatry*. 1998;155:960–963.
11. Reference deleted in review.
12. Brazer L. Psychoeducational group therapy for money disorders. In: Benson A, ed. *I Shop, Therefore I am – Compulsive Buying and the Search for Self*. New York: Jason Aronson; 2000.
13. Christenson GA, Faber RJ, de Zwaan M, et al. Compulsive buying: descriptive characteristics and psychiatric comorbidity. *J Clin Psychiatry*. 1994;55:5–11.
14. d'Astous A. An inquiry into the compulsive side of "normal" consumers. *J Consumer Res*. 1990;13:15–31.
15. d'Astous A, Maltais J, Roberge C. Compulsive buying tendencies of adolescent consumers. *Adv Consumer Res*. 1990;17:306–312.
16. Damon JE. *Shopaholics: Serious Help for Addicted Spenders*. Los Angeles: Price Stein Sloan; 1988.
17. Derbyshire KL, Chamberlain SR, Odlaug BL, Schreiber LR, Grant JE. Neurocognitive functioning in compulsive buying disorder. *Ann Clin Psychiatry*. 2014;26:57–63.
18. Devor EJ, Magee HJ, Dill-Devor RM, et al. Serotonin transporter gene (5-HTT) polymorphisms and compulsive buying. *Am J Med Genet B Neuropsychiatr Genet*. 1999;88:123–125.
19. Reference deleted in review.
20. Edwards EA. Development of a new scale for measuring compulsive buying behavior. *Financial Couns Plann*. 1993;4:67–84.
21. Faber RJ, Christenson GA. In the mood to buy: differences in the mood states experienced by compulsive buyers and other consumers. *Psychol Marketing*. 1993;13:803–819.
22. Faber RJ, Christenson GA, de Zwaan M, et al. Two forms of compulsive consumption: comorbidity of compulsive buying and binge eating. *J Consumer Res*. 1995;22:296–304.
23. Faber RJ, O'Guinn TC. A clinical screener for compulsive buying. *J Consumer Res*. 1992;19:459–469.
24. Faber RJ, O'Guinn TC, Krych R. Compulsive consumption. *Adv Consumer Res*. 1987;14:132–135.
25. Frost RO, Hartl TL. A cognitive-behavioral model of compulsive hoarding. *Behav Res Ther*. 1996;34:341–350.
26. Frost RO, Steketee G, Williams L. Compulsive buying, compulsive hoarding and obsessive-compulsive disorder. *Behav Ther*. 2002;33:201–214.
27. Grant J. Three cases of compulsive buying treated with naltrexone. *Int J Psychiatry Clin Pract*. 2003;7:223–225.
28. Grant JE, Levine L, Kim D, Potenza MN. Impulse control disorders in adult psychiatric inpatients. *Am J Psychiatry*. 2005;162(11):2184–2188.
29. Gwin C, Roberts J, Martinez CR. Does family matter: family influences on compulsive buying in Mexico. *Marketing Manag J*. 2003;14:45–62.
30. Hassay DN, Smith MC. Compulsive buying: an examination of the consumption motive. *Psychol Marketing*. 1996;13:741–753.
31. Reference deleted in review.
32. Hollander E, Allen A. Is compulsive buying a real disorder, and is it really compulsive? *Am J Psychiatry*. 2006;163:1670–1672.
33. Hollander E, Benzaquen SD. The obsessive-compulsive spectrum disorders. *Int Rev Psychiatry*. 1997;9:99–110.
34. Reference deleted in review.
35. Koran LM, Aboujaoude EN, Solvason B, et al. Escitalopram for compulsive buying disorder: a double-blind discontinuation study. *J Clin Psychopharmacol*. 2007;27:225–227.
36. Koran LM, Bullock KD, Hartston HJ. Citalopram treatment of compulsive shopping: an open-label study. *J Clin Psychiatry*. 2002;63:704–708.
37. Koran LM, Chuong HW, Bullock KD, et al. Citalopram for compulsive shopping disorder: an open-label study followed by double blind discontinuation. *J Clin Psychiatry*. 2003;64:7–10.
38. Koran LM, Faber RJ, Aboujaoude E. Estimated prevalence of compulsive buying behavior in the United States. *Am J Psychiatry*. 2006;163:1806–1812.
39. Kraepelin E. *Psychiatrie*. 8th ed. Leipzig: Verlag Von Johann Ambrosius Barth; 1915.
40. Krueger DW. On compulsive shopping and spending: a psychodynamic inquiry. *Am J Psychother*. 1988;42:574–584.
41. Kwak H, Zinkhan GM, Crask M. Diagnostic screener for compulsive buying: applications to the USA and South Korea. *J Consumer Affairs*. 2003;37:161–169.
42. Kwak H, Zinkhan GM, Lester Roushanzamir EP. Compulsive comorbidity and its psychological antecedents: a cross-cultural comparison between the US and South Korea. *J Consumer Market*. 2004;21:418–434.
43. Kyrios M, Frost RO, Steketee G. Cognitions in compulsive buying and acquisition. *Cogn Ther Res*. 2004;28:241–258.
44. Lejoyeux M, Tassain V, Soloman J, et al. Study of compulsive buying in depressed patients. *J Clin Psychiatry*. 1997;58:169–173.
45. Levine B, Kellen B. Debtors Anonymous and psychotherapy. In: Benson A, ed. *I Shop Therefore I Am—Compulsive Buying and the Search for Self*. New York: Jason Aronson; 2000.
46. McElroy SL, Keck PE, Phillips KA. Kleptomania, compulsive buying, and binge eating disorder. *J Clin Psychiatry*. 1995;56:14–26.
47. McElroy SL, Keck Jr PE, Pope Jr HG. Compulsive buying: a report of 20 cases. *J Clin Psychiatry*. 1994;16:205–212.

48. Miltenberger RG, Redlin J, Crosby RD, et al. Direct and retrospective assessment of factors contributing to compulsive buying. *J Behav Ther Exp Psychiatry.* 2003;34:1–9.
49. Mitchell JE, Burgard M, Farber R, et al. Cognitive behavioral therapy for compulsive buying disorder. *Behav Res Ther.* 2006;44:1859–1865.
50. Mitchell JE, Redlin J, Wonderlich SA, et al. The relationship between compulsive buying and eating disorders. *Int J Eat Disorder.* 2002;32:107–111.
51. Monahan P, Black DW, Gabel J. Reliability and validity of a scale to measure change in persons with compulsive buying. *Psychiatry Res.* 1995;64:59–67.
52. Mueller A, Mueller U, Albert P, et al. Hoarding in a compulsive buying sample. *Behav Res Ther.* 2007;45:2754–2763.
53. Mueller A, Mitchell JE, Mertens C, et al. Comparison of treatment seeking compulsive buyers in Germany and the United States. *Behav Res Ther.* 2007;45:1629–1638.
54. Mueller A, Mueller U, Silbermann A, et al. A randomized, controlled trial of group cognitive-behavioral therapy for compulsive buying disorder: posttreatment and 6-month follow-up results. *J Clin Psychiatry.* 2008;69:1131–1138.
55. Müller A, Arikian A, de Zwaan M, Mitchell J. Cognitive-behavioural group versus guided self-help for compulsive buying disorder: a preliminary study. *Clin Psychol Psychother.* 2013;20:28–35.
56. Neuner M, Raab G, Reisch LA. Compulsive buying in maturing consumer societies: an empirical re-inquiry. *J Econ Psychol.* 2005;26:509–522.
57. Ninan PT, McElroy SL, Kane CP, et al. Placebo-controlled study of fluvoxamine in the treatment of patients with compulsive buying. *J Clin Psychopharmacol.* 2000;20:362–366.
58. O'Guinn TC, Faber RJ. Compulsive buying: a phenomenological exploration. *J Consumer Res.* 1989;16:147–157.
59. Odlaug BL, Grant JE. Impulse-control disorders in a college sample: results from the self-administered Minnesota Impulse Disorders Interview (MIDI). Prim care companion. *J Clin Psychiatry.* 2010;12(2).
60. Raab G, Elger CE, Neuner M, Weber B. A neurological study of compulsive buying behavior. *J Consum Policy.* 2011;34:401–413.
61. Roberts JA, Jones E. Money attitudes, credit card use, and compulsive buying among American college students. *J Consumer Affairs.* 2001;35:213–240.
62. Reference deleted in review.
63. Rook DW, Fisher RJ. Normative influences on impulsive buying behavior. *J Consumer Res.* 1995;22:305–313.
64. Reference deleted in review.
65. Schlosser S, Black DW, Repertinger S, et al. Compulsive buying: demography, phenomenology, and comorbidity in 46 subjects. *Gen Hosp Psychiatry.* 1994;16:205–212.
66. Shoham A, Brenčič MM. Compulsive buying behavior. *J Consumer Marketing.* 2003;20:127–138.
67. Tolin DF, Frost RO, Steketee G. *Buried in Treasures: Help for Compulsive Acquiring, Saving, and Hoarding.* New York: Oxford University; 2007.
68. Valence G, d'Astrous A, Fortier L. Compulsive buying: concept and measurement. *J Consumer Policy.* 1988;11:419–433.
69. Wesson C. *Women Who Shop Too Much: Overcoming the Urge to Splurge.* New York: St. Martin's; 1990.

36

Sexual Behavior as an Addictive or Compulsive Phenomenon

KIMBERLY R. MCBRIDE, MICHAEL REECE, AND BRIAN DODGE

CHAPTER OUTLINE

Introduction

Due to the magnitude of the human immunodeficiency virus (HIV) and acquired immunodeficiency syndrome (AIDS) epidemic, and its profound impact on public health and social structures, an emphasis on the behavioral, social, and cultural factors associated with sexual risk and its relation to HIV transmission has been essential. However, an unanticipated artifact of disease-focused research is that much of the contemporary knowledge related to sexual behavior has been constructed in the context of HIV and other sexually transmitted infections. Recent sexual health research has made meaningful contributions to scientific understandings; however, scientists still know relatively little about sexuality in the general population in comparison with other aspects of health and human behavior.[41]

The void in scientific understanding has allowed sexual behaviors that are incongruent with dominant social norms to be constructed as pathologies despite a lack of empirical evidence to support proposed links between behavioral variations and negative outcomes.[42] A vivid example of this phenomenon can be seen in the social construction of sexual addiction, which proposes a threshold where sexual behavior becomes a clinical disorder. Although there has been substantial debate and controversy surrounding conceptualization of sexual behavior as an addictive phenomenon, the concept has been widely studied and measured in sexological, psychological, and public health research.[53] Numerous sexual scientists, clinicians, and support groups have increased awareness of, and treatments for, sexually compulsive behavior. However, studies of sexual compulsivity and its associations with sexual risk behavior have primarily assessed individuals who are already considered high risk for adverse sexual health outcomes due to other characteristics (e.g., substance use, higher number of sexual partners). Furthermore, systematic documentation of adverse outcomes associated with sexual compulsivity is lacking.

Recently, there has been a conceptual shift away from addiction models, and hypersexuality is now the dominant focus of the clinical and research literature. Variations in the definition of hypersexuality exist; however, the common theme is that sexual behavior, including thoughts or fantasies, is excessive. The most recent iteration of the *Diagnostic and Statistical Manual of Mental Disorders* (DSM-5) did not include hypersexuality as a diagnostic category despite some evidence to support the reliability and validity of proposed diagnostic criteria.[2,3,74] Currently, critical questions remain unanswered and controversy persists. Ongoing conceptual and methodological challenges make systematic research difficult. The scientific and clinical communities will need to address gaps in the literature through well-designed studies that test conceptual frameworks with rigorous methods and sound measures.

History of Sexual Addiction and Sexually Compulsive Behavior

The earliest descriptions of sexually compulsive behavior can be traced to Greek myths describing satyrs and the god Dionysius.[32,59] The term "nymphomania," historically used to describe female sexual excess, is also derived from Greek. The 19th century term "Don Juanism" was used in reference to male sexual excess.[32] In the late 19th century, Krafft-Ebing presented one of the first clinical case studies describing hypersexuality and its effects on life functioning.[52]

Sexual behavior viewed as an addictive or compulsive phenomenon is relatively recent.[38,51] During the mid-to-late 20th century, published case reports described similar clinical presentations of individuals reporting out-of-control sexual behaviors. However, there was inconsistency in the terms applied as well as conceptualizations of etiology.[a] Labels ranged from historical terms (e.g., nymphomania and Don Juanism) to moral reflections (e.g., perversions), to clinical terminology (e.g., paraphilias, compulsive sexual behavior, impulse control disorders, sexual addiction, and sexual compulsivity).

Currently, there is no universal agreement on terminology or a single accepted definition. The term hypersexuality dominates the contemporary literature but words such as sexual compulsivity, sexual impulsivity, and sexual addiction are still commonly used to reference sexual behavior that is beyond an individual's control, leading to impairment in life functioning and negative outcomes.[b] No single treatment strategy is widely accepted; rather, approaches range from individual cognitive and behavioral therapies, to the use of psychotropic medications, to group counseling..

Sex Outside the Norm

The idea that sexual behavior can exceed a threshold to become a clinical disorder has appeared in the scientific literature with increased frequency over the past 30 years. Prior to the emergence of HIV/AIDs in the late 1970s and early 1980s, interest in the phenomenon of out-of-control sexual behavior was limited primarily to researchers and clinicians from psychiatry, psychology, and medicine. In the early 1980s, the terms "sex addict" and "sexually compulsive" appeared in popular culture and were used to reference individuals whose sexual behaviors rested outside of accepted sociocultural norms. The emergence of HIV brought attention to sexual behaviors that increased the likelihood for transmission and sexual behavior perceived to be beyond an individual's control was identified as a risk factor.

In the decades following the initial HIV crisis, there has been a rapid proliferation of research examining the etiology, consequences, and approaches to treating out-of-control sexual behavior. Much of the literature has resulted from research focused on sexual risk-taking behaviors among gay men, pedophilic clinical samples, and self-identified sex addicts. Fewer studies have examined subclinical levels of out-of-control sexual behavior and nonclinical populations. Research has largely ignored women and populations at lower risk for HIV/sexually transmitted infection (STI). As a result, disease-focused models emphasizing the link between sexual behavior at the higher end of the behavioral continuum and adverse sexual health outcomes (e.g., HIV/STI) dominate the research literature. One consequence has been that variation in sexual behavior remains seated within a disease paradigm without sufficient acknowledgment of the methodological limitations and conceptual biases on which findings have been based.[83]

Although documentation linking out-of-control sexual behavior to adverse psychological and sexual health outcomes exists, the construct remains controversial within the scientific community. Scholars have argued that conceptualizations of normative sexual behavior are influenced by cultural and historical understandings that reflect sociocultural mores governing behavior.[35,51] Social and psychological theories are a reflection of existing norms that are

unique to time and place, and much of the debate surrounding sexual compulsivity centers on the ambiguities in the definition of "out-of-control." Historically, the universal standard for identification was behavioral frequency. In 2004, Bancroft and Vukadinovic wrote a critical review calling for scientific evidence that out of control sexual behavior is qualitatively different from normative sexual behavior that occurs at the high end of the continuum. In their critique, Bancroft and Vukadinovic maintained that it is negligent to assume that engaging in frequent sexual activity is inherently risky or problematic without documenting the occurrence of negative consequences.[9]

Other scientists have argued that perceptions of control over sexual behavior are social constructions, and that the importance and meaning of out-of-control models might reflect broader values related to self-control and self-consciousness that are unique to the American culture.[37,77] It has been suggested that diagnosis, and subsequent labeling, reflect attempts to pathologize and medicalize variations in sexual behavior.[37] Arguments in favor of this perspective often cite the fact that homosexuality was listed as a mental disorder in the *Diagnostic and Statistical Manual of Mental Disorders* of the American Psychiatric Association until the late 1970s. This point is central to understanding the lack of consensus in the scientific community given the rapidly emerging possibilities for the expression of sexuality and the diverse range of sexualities that exist in contemporary society. There remains a need for research that takes into account that sexual behaviors and norms vary among individuals and cultural groups. Indeed, what may be viewed as problematic for one individual, or within one culture, may be normative for another. The wide variation in contemporary sexual behavior, including behavioral frequency, makes it critical to systematically link behavior to adverse outcomes. Understanding the influence of sociocultural factors will allow scientists and clinicians to avoid errors in the diagnosis and treatment of problematic sexual behaviors.

Clinical Criteria

Despite some research linking out-of-control sexual behavior to adverse psychological and sexual health outcomes, the DSM-5 contains no specific diagnostic criteria or category for classification.[3] A categorization and diagnostic criteria for Hypersexual Disorder were proposed by Kafka in 2010.[44,45] Kafka characterized hypersexuality as a behavioral pattern involving repetitive and intense preoccupation with sexual fantasies, urges, and behaviors, leading to adverse consequences and clinically significant distress or impairment in social, occupational, or other important areas of functioning. Kafka also hypothesized that hypersexual individuals usually experience multiple unsuccessful attempts to control or reduce the amount of time spent engaging in sexual fantasies, urges, and behaviors in response to dysphoric mood states or stressful life events. Consistent with DSM criteria for other disorders, it was proposed that symptoms must be present for at least 6 months and occur independent of substance use, mania, or a medical condition in order for a diagnosis to be established.[1-3] Kafka recommended that an operational definition should be derived from large, nonclinical community samples where a range of normative sexual behaviors can be examined. He emphasized the need to consider demographic characteristics (e.g., age, gender, education, culture) when contextualizing sexual behaviors.

The results of a field trial designed to assess the reliability and validity of the diagnostic criteria proposed by Kafka reported high interrater reliability and stability of the criterion over time.[2,74,75]

---

[a] References 5, 23, 28, 30, 43, 61, 67, 79.
[b] References 11, 16, 17, 24, 33, 39, 49, 58, 72.

Sensitivity and specificity indices showed that criteria accurately reflected presenting problems and the diagnostic criteria demonstrated acceptable validity. Based on these findings, the Sexual and Gender Identity Disorders Working Group recommended the inclusion of hypersexual disorder as a diagnostic category; however, it was ultimately excluded from the final publication of the DSM-5.[3] Critics of the proposed category argued that the concept of hypersexuality resulted from moral norms and psychosocial values that should have no place diagnostic decision-making.[83]

Currently, diagnostic categorization lies in the hands of the practitioner. Options fall within one of three major categories: paraphilia, either one or more specifically identified or paraphilia not elsewhere classified; impulse control disorder not elsewhere classified; sexual disorder not elsewhere classified.

Despite the lack of specificity in diagnostic categorization, there is consensus among researchers regarding the relationship between hypersexuality and psychiatric comorbidity The literature reports consistent associations between out-of-control sexual behavior and psychological impairment and substance use disorders.[a] Scientists have begun to document comorbidities in nonclinical populations, community samples, and among groups at lower risk for HIV.

Raymond and colleagues reported that mood and anxiety disorders were the most consistent diagnoses among their community sample of 23 men and 2 women who self-identified as hypersexual, with 80% meeting the diagnostic criteria for an Axis I disorder at the time of data collection and 100% meeting the criteria across their lifetime.[68] Research has also established a link between hypersexuality and trait variables associated with psychological impairment. A study examining personality, psychological, and sexuality trait variables among 510 heterosexual, bisexual, and homosexual women and men who self-reported hypersexual behavior found that hypersexual behavior was related to depressed and anxious mood states and trait impulsivity.[87] Furthermore, higher neuroticism and lower agreeableness significantly predicted hypersexual behavior. Research examining sexual compulsivity in a sample of 235 women found that hypersexual behavior was predicted by psychoticism.[21] A similar study conducted among men ($N = 152$) reported finding that psychoticism, neuroticism, and agreeableness were significant predictors of hypersexual behavior.[65] Pachankas and colleagues (2014) established a relationship between maladaptive cognitions and hypersexuality among gay and bisexual men.[62]

A strong and consistent association between substance use and hypersexuality has been established. Grov et al. (2010) found that higher sexual compulsivity scores were associated with the use of ketamine, MDMA (ecstasy), gamma hydroxybutyrate (GBH), cocaine, and methamphetamines among a community-based sample of 1214 gay and bisexual men.[40] Kalichman and Cain found that higher levels of sexual compulsivity were linked to higher usage rates of alcohol, powder cocaine, crack cocaine, and inhalants.[46] Sutton et al. (2015) conducted chart reviews of patients referred for hypersexuality and found that there were more substance abuse disorders among those who were paraphilic when compared to other subtypes.[81]

The findings reported above are only a few examples of research documenting the association between psychiatric comorbidity and out-of-control sexual behavior. Numerous studies conducted over the past two decades have consistently found similar links. The observed associations between out-of-control sexual behavior and

psychiatric comorbidity have caused some scientists to question whether associations provide evidence that out-of-control sexual behavior is a unique psychiatric disorder, or whether it should be conceptualized as a behavioral symptom of an underlying condition. Although it is possible that out-of-control sexual behavior does warrant its own classification, it is also possible that individuals with other disturbances use sex as a means of self-medication to alleviate or temporarily escape discomfort caused by underlying distress. Research has shown that nonclinical negative mood states influence sexual interest among some individuals. The Dual Control Model (DCM) proposes that sexual arousal is influenced by two distinct psychophysiological systems: sexual excitation and sexual inhibition.[6-10] In this model, individuals with low inhibition and a high propensity for excitation may be more prone to problems of hypersexuality. Systematic investigation of the DCM as a possible explanation for hypersexuality in some individuals suggests that stress and dysphoric mood state may trigger hypersexual behavior.[76,78] These findings lend support to the hypothesis that some hypersexual behavior may represent attempts to escape psychological discomfort through sexual behavior.

Recent scientific attention has focused on examining psychological traits that may predispose individuals to hypersexuality. As interest in documenting the phenomenon among nonpatient populations has increased, there has been a shift toward understanding how structural dimensions of personality may influence hypersexual behavior. Prior research on the relationship between personality and addictive behavior has demonstrated positive associations among certain characteristics.[22,82,89] Studies examining hypersexuality and sexual risk-taking have also demonstrated significant associations between specific personality traits and out-of-control sexual behavior.[65,74] The Big Five model of personality developed by McCrea & Costa (1987) proposes five distinct structural dimensions of personality: Neuroticism, Extraversion, Openness to Experience, Agreeableness, and Conscientiousness.[57] Although there have been inconsistencies in the strength of relationships between personality traits and hypersexuality, studies have repeatedly found that higher levels of neuroticism and extraversion and lower levels of conscientiousness and agreeableness predict hypersexual behavior.[21,75,76]

When examining the evidence as a whole, there is support for the idea that there may be different types of sexual compulsivity that derive from different factors. Mood state might account for hypersexual behavior among some individuals, whereas others may be more prone to out-of-control behavior due to personality traits. A proportion of people may be using sexual behavior as a form of self-medication that allows them to alleviate negative emotions for some period of time. Observed comorbidities suggest that there may be some underlying mechanism causing dysregulation in both sexual behavior and mood. Additional research among diverse clinical and community samples will add specificity to our understandings of the mechanisms that cause and support hypersexual behavior. Debate about the construct is ongoing, with many scientists favoring the perspective that hypersexuality is a natural and harmless variation in sexual behavior, while others remain convinced that it is a psychiatric condition that warrants inclusion in the DSM.

Etiology

The ongoing debate regarding the construct of sexual compulsivity has resulted in varied perspectives on etiology. Many researchers have attempted to explain the development and maintenance of hypersexuality, which has resulted in several theoretical

---

[a] References 26, 46, 50, 69, 70, 86, 88.

representations of causation. Early theoretical explanations include Carnes' Addiction Model, Coleman's Compulsive Sexual Behavior Model, and Kalichman's Impulse Control Model.[19,26,50] More recent additions to the literature include Bancroft's Dual Control Model and Parson's Syndemic Model.[6-10,63] Parsons' model, which aims to explain hypersexuality in gay and bisexual men, is still in the early stages of testing and will not be reviewed here. However, preliminary evidence suggests that a three-group categorization of sexual compulsivity may be one systemic factor that explains HIV risk among gay and bisexual men. Each perspective suggests etiological explanations; however, overwhelming empirical evidence favoring any of these is markedly absent.

Carnes' Addiction Model

Carnes views sexual addiction as a chronic illness and has defined it as an extremely intense sex drive or obsession with sex.[19] From this perspective, sex becomes the most important need and drives the individual's behaviors.[20] Carnes operationally defined sex addiction as a pathological relationship with a mood-altering experience. According to Carnes, the hallmark of sexual addiction is the lack of ability to control sexual feelings, thoughts, and behaviors.[16,64] Rather than sex being a pleasurable act, Carnes asserts that for addicts, sex becomes a tool to ameliorate pain and relieve stress. He believes that the fear of abandonment and shame are at the core of sexual addiction.[19,20] Carnes likens the biological, neurological, and physiological responses that result from sexual stimulation to responses resulting from the consumption of alcohol and other drugs.[31,88]

Carnes advocates a 12-step treatment approach adapted from the Alcoholics Anonymous model. The underlying premise is that individuals are powerless over the amount or type of sexual behavior in which they engage.[19,59] Recovery is only possible when the individual has successfully progressed through the 12-Step process.

Coleman's Compulsive Sexual Behavior Model

Coleman first introduced the Compulsive Sexual Behavior (CSB) model of sexual compulsivity in 1990. Coleman theorized that CSB is a disorder characterized by intense sexually arousing fantasies, urges, and associated sexual behaviors that are intrusive, driven, and repetitive.[26] Individuals are described as lacking control over their sexual behavior, which they may perceive as excessive. Often these individuals experience serious comorbid symptoms and associated consequences including mood disorders, somatic complaints, substance abuse or dependency, HIV or other sexually transmitted infections, unwanted pregnancy, relationship problems, domestic violence, sexual dysfunction, or child abuse.[27] Furthermore, compulsive sexual behavior may lead to ethical, social, and legal problems, in addition to psychological distress.[27]

Coleman conceptualizes CSBs as fitting into one of two distinct categories, either paraphilic or nonparaphilic. Whereas paraphilic CSB comprises nonnormative sexual behavior that involves both distress and recurrent fantasies, nonparaphilic CSB involves the excessive and compulsive engagement in normative sexual behaviors.[19] The DSM-5 classifies eight paraphilic disorders: exhibitionistic disorder, fetishistic disorder, frotteuristic disorder, pedophilic disorder, sexual masochism disorder, sexual sadism disorder, transvestic disorder, and voyeuristic disorder.[3] Although there have been attempts to declassify many of these disorders, Coleman and colleagues rely on the criteria of distress and impaired functioning to distinguish

between varied sexual interests and actual psychiatric disorders.[3,27] According to Coleman, paraphilic behaviors inherently impair the ability to form reciprocal love relationships and achieve a sense of well-being, thus supporting underlying pathology.[27]

The term "nonparaphilic compulsive sexual behavior" has been used by Coleman to refer to typical sexual behavior occurring at the high end of the behavioral continuum. This conceptualization is most consistent with the phenomenon under exploration in this chapter. There is no clear diagnostic category for nonparaphilic CSB listed in the DSM-5.[3] Nonparaphilic CSB is thought to have at least seven subtypes: compulsive cruising and multiple partners, compulsive fixation on an unattainable partner, compulsive autoeroticism (masturbation), compulsive use of erotica, compulsive use of the Internet for sexual purposes, compulsive multiple love relationships, and compulsive sexuality within a relationship.[15,27] Nonparaphilic CSB is thought to be linked to a variety of adverse outcomes similar to those associated with paraphilic CSB.

Coleman and colleagues acknowledge that there is no clear division between subclinical symptoms and clinically significant conditions where diagnoses can be applied. Individuals may experience problematic sexual behaviors without meeting the clinical threshold for CSB.[27] Despite the lack of clear demarcation, Coleman et al. provide clinical criteria for making a CSB diagnosis.[27] According to the guidelines, criteria for CSB are met when the individual has recurrent and intense normophilic or paraphilic sexually arousing fantasies, sexual urges, and behaviors that cause clinically significant distress in social, occupational, or other areas of functioning; and these fantasies, sexual urges, and behaviors cannot be accounted for by another medical condition, substance use disorder, Axis I or II disorder, or developmental disorder. Furthermore, gender, sexual orientation, and sociocultural norms must be taken into account.

The etiology of CSB is described as complex and likely involves a variety of physiological and psychological factors.[27,69] Coleman has discussed links to both neuropsychiatric conditions such as temporal lobe lesions, epilepsy, and head trauma, as well as psychological disorders, particularly anxiety and depression. Coleman contends that neuropsychiatric causes should be considered when the onset of CSB is subsequent to a trauma, surgery, illness, or the use of a substance (prescribed or not). If neuropsychiatric causes are ruled out, it is important to consider psychological factors.[27,69]

The suggested treatment for CSB is a combination of pharmacotherapy and psychotherapy. According to Coleman's treatment paradigm, psychotherapy for CSB explores environmental and psychodynamic stressors that contribute to behavioral manifestations. Clients are taught coping mechanisms to manage stress, anxiety, and depression that might trigger problematic behavior. A group treatment approach is recommended; however, group treatments are not widely available. Because there are many types of CSB, Coleman suggests tailoring therapy to individuals within the group setting.[27] Couples and/or family therapy, in conjunction with individual or group treatment, may help facilitate healthy sexual and relational functioning. Favored pharmacological interventions include the use of selective serotonin reuptake inhibitors (SSRIs) or naltrexone. The body of evidence supporting the efficacy of SSRIs for treating compulsive sexual behavior comes from several small sample studies and case reports.[14,15,25,43] Likewise, there have been few studies examining the efficacy of naltrexone for treating compulsive sexual behavior.[69] Instead, much of the literature supporting the efficacy of naltrexone studied a variety of other disorders, including alcoholism, cocaine abuse, eating disorders, and pathological gambling.

Kalichman's Impulse Control Model

Kalichman's interest in out-of-control sexual behavior grew out of the desire to understand mediating factors associated with HIV risk and resistance to adopting risk-reduction strategies.[48] According to Kalichman, sexual compulsivity is a heterogeneous psychological construct that can include a preoccupation with sexual desires and behaviors to the degree that social, occupational, and daily life function are impaired.[46] Kalichman denotes that his conceptualization of sexual compulsivity is not synonymous with sex addiction, hypersexuality, or other clinically defined categories.[46] Kalichman defines sexual compulsivity as the propensity to experience sexual disinhibition and undercontrolled sexual impulses and behaviors as self-identified by the individual.[46] In addition, Kalichman believes that sexual compulsivity most likely has multiple forms and etiologies.

Because Kalichman's conceptualization of sexual compulsivity is nonclinical, the bulk of his work has focused on documenting the relationship between sexual compulsivity and HIV/STI risk, rather than trying to articulate theoretical underpinnings. Simply, he believes that individuals can only be identified as sexually compulsive when they self-report multiple markers of sexual preoccupation and undercontrolled sexual impulses, which are likely related to a lack of impulse control.[13,46]

Bancroft's Dual Control Model

Bancroft's Dual Control Model (DCM) was not specifically developed to explain hypersexuality but his conceptualizations and measures have been applied in research examining the phenomenon.[6-10] Bancroft believes that out-of-control sexual behavior is likely the result of multiple etiologies and a small proportion of cases may have features of obsessive-compulsive disorder.[6] However, he proposes that individual propensity toward excitation and inhibition may be applicable in many cases of hypersexuality.

The DCM hypothesizes that individual sexual arousal is dependent on responsiveness to two separate neurophysiological systems: sexual excitation and sexual inhibition.[6-10] These systems are thought to be mostly adaptive and functional, and individuals will vary in their propensity toward each. The balance between proneness toward excitation or inhibition will dictate the response.

The DMC has been used as a framework for understanding low (hypo) and high (hyper) sexual response in both men and women.[6-10] Those who are less responsive to inhibitory processes and more responsive to excitatory processes are thought to be the most likely to demonstrate hypersexual behavior. Although the link between higher sexual excitation and hypersexuality is consistently supported in the literature, the link between hypersexual behavior and sexual inhibition is less clear. Studies have found that higher levels of inhibition are associated with participation in risk behavior, which is counterintuitive to hypothesized relationships.[6] To account for the findings, researchers have suggested that individuals with high levels of inhibition may engage in behaviors associated with risk because they fear losing their sexual arousal. Bancroft notes that mood and personality traits may be important considerations when accounting for individual variation in patterns of response. For example, paradoxical patterns of high arousal in depressed individuals may lend support to the idea that some proportion of people are using sex as a form of self-medication.[6] He also recommends the use of SSRIs in cases where depression and/or anxiety are associated with hypersexuality because medications stabilize mood and may also inhibit sexual response.[6]

Measurement

A range of measures have been developed and used in research examining sexual compulsivity. The two most consistently cited measures are the Compulsive Sexual Behavior Inventory (CSBI) and the Sexual Compulsivity Scale (SCS).[26,49] The Cognitive and Behavioral Outcomes of Sexual Behavior Scale (CBOSBS) was developed in response to the lack of evidence linking sexual behaviors to negative outcomes. McBride and colleagues used outcomes proposed by the Society for the Advancement of Sexual Health in an attempt to create an outcomes-based measure that moved away from traditional focuses on behavioral frequency and sexual risk-taking.[55,56] Furthermore, they sought to develop a tool appropriate for use in community samples and one that would more accurately capture the experiences of women. A newer measure, The Hypersexual Disorder Screening Inventory (HDSI), was developed by the American Psychiatric Association's DSM-5 Workgroup committee as an instrument for screening hypersexuality during a field trial to test the reliability and validity of the diagnostic category.[2,64,74,75] The measure has not been widely used and initial validation was limited to patient populations. The HDSI requires additional testing before psychometric properties can be reported with confidence. Although we will not include further discussion on the HDSI in the section below, it is important for readers to be aware of this new tool.

Compulsive Sexual Behavior Inventory

The Compulsive Sexual Behavior Inventory (CSBI) was developed in response to the need for psychometrically sound measures to identify CSB.[26] The authors believed preexisting measures failed to incorporate all major components of the phenomenon. The CSBI was intended to create a standardized, reliable, and valid assessment tool for use in clinical and research settings. For validation purposes, it was hypothesized that no significant differences would be observed in scores obtained from those with paraphilic and nonparaphilic CSB but significant differences would be observed when the clinical group scores were compared to controls.

The preliminary study of reliability and validity included three groups: individuals diagnosed with paraphilic compulsive sexual behavior recruited from a sex-offender treatment program (N = 35); individuals with nonparaphilic compulsive sexual behavior recruited via advertisements (N = 15); control participants recruited via advertisements (N = 42). The initial inventory consisted of 42 items related to sexual control and various aspects of behavior associated with paraphilic and nonparaphilic CSB.[19] Participants rated their responses to items on a scale ranging from 1 = Very frequently to 5 = Never. A principal components factor analysis using varimax rotation was performed on the data and factor loadings that exceeded 0.60 after rotation were retained for the final scale. The reliability of the retained factors was tested using Cronbach's alpha and the data were tested using linear discriminant function analysis to determine the scale's ability to differentiate individuals with CSB from controls. In addition, three analyses of variance were conducted to explore mean differences for each group on identified subscales. A plot of data from the entire sample indicated that a three-factor solution, accounting for 58% of the variance, was the best fit. The first factor explained 42%, the second factor explained 10.1%, and the third factor accounted for 5.9% of the variance. The retention of items on each factor was determined by the magnitude of factor loading and subsequent assessments of face validity. A total of 28 items were retained, and the factors appeared to measure control, abuse, and violence.

Initial tests of validity were conducted using linear discriminant function analysis, testing the scale's ability to distinguish between groups believed to have CSB from those who did not. The classification matrix was reported to have correctly identified 92% of cases, with one normal control being incorrectly classified as compulsive and six compulsives being identified as normal. Further explorations of validity used the three subscales as independent variables in analyses of variance to explore group differences. The findings indicated significant effects for group on the control subscale. Pairwise comparisons demonstrated that pedophiles scored significantly lower on the subscale when compared with the other two groups. A significant main effect was found for the violence subscale, and subsequent pairwise comparisons showed that controls differed significantly from pedophiles. Table 36.1 reports the items contained in the CSBI.

Sexual Compulsivity Scale

Kalichman hypothesized that intrinsic factors (e.g., personality disposition) might play a role in HIV risk behaviors, and he was interested in exploring how Zuckerman's work on sensation seeking might apply within this context. Based on studies linking sensation seeking to high-risk sexual behaviors, Kalichman theorized that sensation seeking might be an important predictor of HIV risk and resistance to behavioral change.[34,48,60] Kalichman adapted the Sensation Seeking Scale to measure sensation seeking specific to sexual behavior and created a measure of sexual compulsivity.[90]

The Sexual Compulsivity Scale (SCS) was designed to measure two aspects of sexuality: hypersexuality and sexual preoccupation. The measure has been widely used in assessments of high-risk sexual behavior. Scale items were adapted from a 12-step self-help recovery manual for sex addicts[18,61] and the items were intended to capture "excessive preoccupation with sex acts and encounters."[49] The 10-item scale directs respondents to indicate the extent to which they agree with specific statements, and response options range from "not at all like me" to "very much like me."

Initial scale reliability and validity were tested in two samples; self-identified gay men (Sample 1) and inner-city men and women at high-risk for HIV (Sample 2). The majority of participants in sample 1 (N = 286) were white (63%) and reported an annual income over $20,000 (72%). Participants were recruited through fliers placed in bars and social organizations in Milwaukee, Wisconsin. Sample 2 was drawn from the community and consisted of 60 inner-city men and 98 women with characteristics that placed them at high-risk for HIV. Ninety-five percent of the sample identified as African American, and 94% reported an annual income of less than $20,000. Participants were recruited through local community agencies in Milwaukee, Wisconsin. Tests of reliability were performed by computing alpha coefficients. Internal consistency for Sample 1 was alpha = 0.86, and for Sample 2 alpha = 0.87. A 3-month retest was performed with both groups. For Sample 1 (N = 195) alpha = 0.64, and for Sample 2 (N = 52) alpha = 0.80. Construct validity was established by examining associations between scores on the SCS and reported engagement in risk behaviors. For Sample 1, positive associations were found between SCS scores, substance use, and sexual risk-taking behaviors. Inverse associations with self-esteem and the intention to reduce risk-taking behaviors were found. In Sample 2, positive associations between increased frequency of unprotected sex and higher number of sexual partners were reported, and these were also associated with pleasure activities. An inverse association

TABLE 36.1	Compulsive Sexual Behavior Inventory.

Please mark the response that best describes your behaviors or experiences[a]:

- How often have you had trouble controlling your sexual urges?
- Have you felt unable to control you sexual behavior?
- How often have you used sex to deal with worries or problems in your life?
- How often have you felt guilty or shameful about aspects of your sexual behavior?
- How often have you concealed or hidden your sexual behavior from others?
- How often have you been unable to control your sexual feelings?
- How often have you made pledges or promises to change or alter your sexual behavior?
- How often have your sexual thoughts or behaviors interfered with the formation of friendships?
- How often have you developed excuses and reasons to justify your sexual behavior?
- How often have you missed opportunities for productive and enhancing activities because of your sexual activity?
- How often have your sexual activities caused financial problems for you?
- How often have you felt emotionally distant when you were engaging in sex with others?
- How often have you had sex or masturbated more than you wanted to?
- Were you sexually abused as a child?
- Were you physically abused as a child?
- Other than parents or siblings, did you experience sexual activity as a child with someone more than 4–6 years older than you?
- Did you have sexual experiences with any of your siblings?
- Have you been forced to have sex with a stranger, casual acquaintance, or friend?
- How often have you been arrested or legally apprehended for your sexual behavior?
- Have you forced anyone against his or her will?
- Did you have sexual experiences with either of your parents?
- Have you ever hit, kicked, punched, thrown, chocked restrained, or beaten any of your sexual partners?
- Have you given others physical pain for sexual pleasure?
- In fighting, have you been hit, kicked, punched, slapped, thrown, chocked, restrained, or beaten by your current or most recent partner?
- Have you received physical pain for pleasure?
- Have you received money to have sex?
- Have you been forced to have sex with your husband, wife, or lover?
- Have you been watched masturbating or having sex without giving permission?

[a]Measured with a five-point response scale that includes *very frequently, often, occasionally, rarely,* and *never.*

Adapted from Coleman E, Miner M, Ohlerking F, et al. Compulsive sexual behavior inventory: a preliminary study of reliability and validity. *J Sex Marital Ther.* 2001;27:325-332.

between the intent to reduce risk was observed. Follow-up studies using the SCS have reported similar results.[12,13]

The SCS has received critique in the scientific literature. Since its initial publication, the scale has largely been used to assess sexual compulsivity and its relations to risky sexual behaviors among groups at high-risk for HIV infection (e.g., men who have sex with men, heavy substance abusers) and among samples with a positive HIV serostatus. Subsequent attempts to examine the scale's performance in general populations have found support for reliability and construct validity. For example, Dodge and colleagues

Please indicate the extent to which the following statements apply to you[a]:

- My sexual appetite has gotten in the way of my relationships.
- My sexual thoughts and behaviors are causing problems in my life.
- My desires to have sex have disrupted my daily life.
- I sometimes fail to meet my commitments and responsibilities because of my sexual behaviors.
- I sometimes get so horny I could lose control.
- I find myself thinking about sex while at work or in class.
- I feel that my sexual thoughts and feelings are stronger than I am.
- I have to struggle to control my sexual thoughts and behavior.
- I think about sex more than I would like to.
- It has been difficult for me to find sex partners who desire having sex as much as I want to.

[a]Measured with a four-point response scale that includes *never applies to me, sometimes applies to me, often applies to me,* and *always applies to me.*

Adapted from Kalichman and Rompa Frohlich P, Meston C. Sexual functioning and self-reported depressive symptoms among college women. *J Sex Res.* 2002;39:321–325.

examined the psychometric properties in a sample of nearly 900 heterosexual college students.[29] Significant relationships between sexual compulsivity and higher frequencies sexual behaviors (solo and partnered) and number of sexual partners were found and content validity was established. Higher sexual compulsivity scores were associated with higher frequencies of reported unprotected sexual behavior. Relationships between sexual compulsivity and solo, partnered, and unprotected sexual behaviors remained significant after controlling for demographic variables. Although the researchers found support for construct validity, they noted that it was not clear whether the scale distinctly measured sexual compulsivity or if it tapped into other constructs, such as sexual desire and sexual exploration. Table 36.2 lists the SCS items.

Cognitive and Behavioral Outcomes of Sexual Behavior Scale

The Society for the Advancement of Sexual Health (SASH) offered a list of outcomes that might indicate that behaviors (solo or partnered) are sexually compulsive. The outcomes outlined by SASH span six domains of life functioning: social, emotional, physical, legal, financial/occupational, and spiritual. Outcomes-based criteria suggests that behaviors are problematic when they lead to negative consequences in various areas of life functioning. For example, spending a great deal of time viewing sexually explicit material on the Internet may not necessarily be indicative of sexual compulsivity, but if that behavior results in the inability to relate to a romantic or relational partner, or creates other challenges such as loss of income, then it might indicate that the behavior has become problematic.[13]

Scales assessing cognitive and behavior outcomes of sexual behavior were developed by McBride and colleagues to assess both the extent to which an individual is concerned about negative outcomes resulting from their sexual behaviors, and the extent to which such outcomes were actually experienced by participants.[55,56] The scales were constructed based on the six domains articulated by SASH. The six domains assessed by the CBOSBS are: financial, legal, physical, psychological, spiritual, and social. The cognitive outcomes scale consists of 20 items and asks participants to rate the extent to which they worry that the things they

have done sexually may result in a specified outcome. Responses are measured on a four-point scale ranging from "never" to "always." Cognitive subscale scores were created from mean scores of the items making up each factor. The 16-item behavioral outcome scale assesses whether a participant has actually experienced an outcome. Responses are measured dichotomously as "yes" or "no." Behavioral outcome scores were the sum of the "yes" (1 point) versus "no" (0 points) answers to the items for each factor.

Tests of scale reliability and validity were conducted in a cross-sectional sample of 391 young adults, largely comprising women (70.3%, N = 274). The sample was chosen to explore whether negative cognitive and behavioral outcomes associated with sexual behavior could be detected in a nonclinical population at subclinical levels. The majority of participants were 21 years of age or younger (86.2%, N = 336) and overwhelming self-identified as heterosexual (95.4%, N = 372).

Analyses were conducted to assess the psychometric properties of the CBOSBS and the extent to which respondents reported experiencing negative outcomes resulting from sexual behaviors. Reliability of the CBOSBS was assessed using Cronbach's alpha for internal consistency reliability and separate analyses of the cognitive and behavioral items were conducted. Internal consistency for the 20-item cognitive scale was high (α = 0.89), with a slightly lower level of reliability (α = 0.75) for the 16-item behavioral scale. However, given that the response scale for the behavioral items was "yes" or "no," this level is quite acceptable.

Construct validity for the 20 cognitive outcomes items was tested using a principal component analysis with varimax rotation, specifying six factors because items were constructed to focus on the six outcome categories articulated by the SASH. The six-factor solution explained 74.8% of the total variance. The inter-item correlation matrix did not yield correlations high enough to suggest that the scale is unidimensional. Separate reliability estimates were calculated for each of the six factors (or subscales). Cronbach's alpha for internal consistency was found to be high for all of the factors, or subscales, indicating scale reliability in this sample. Table 36.3 contains the Cognitive and Behavioral Outcomes of Sexual Behavior Scale.

Implications for Clinical Practice

Research indicates that there is a threshold at which sexual behavior can lead to negative outcomes that include sexual risk-taking behavior and psychological distress.[55,56] These findings have important implications for HIV and STI prevention, as well as the prevention of adverse outcomes beyond risks to sexual health. Research has demonstrated that outcomes-focused assessment is appropriate for screening individuals with subclinical levels of hypersexuality and populations whose clinical presentations are different from those traditionally studied in research. For example, findings from the validation study of the CBOSBS indicate that women may be more likely to experience psychological, spiritual, and social distress related to their sexual behavior. Practitioners may need to reconceptualize approaches to both assessment and treatment based on this information,[55,56] whereas the same research indicates that men may primarily manifest sexual compulsivity in terms of physical sexual health outcomes, particularly those related to HIV/STI and unintended pregnancy in a female sexual partner. However, there is also evidence to suggest that young men experience disruptions in their social lives and other areas of functioning resulting from their sexual behavior. Therefore it may be appropriate to develop risk-reduction intervention

TABLE 36.3   Cognitive and Behavioral Outcomes of Sexual Behavior Scale.

Cognitive Outcomes

Below is a list of things that some people worry about as a result of their sexual activities (including things people do alone and those they do with others). Please indicate the extent to which the following apply to you. I am worried that the things I have done sexually[a]:

- Might have placed me or one of my sex partners at risk for pregnancy.
- Might have placed me or one of my sex partners at risk for a sexually transmitted infection (like herpes, gonorrhea, or crabs).
- Might have placed me or one of my sex partners at risk for HIV.
- Might have caused one of my sex partners to experience pain, injury, or other problems.
- Might have resulted in pain, injury, or other problems for myself.
- Might have presented the potential for serious physical injury or death.
- Might be leading to problems with my friends.
- Might be leading to problems with my family members.
- Might be leading to problems with my boyfriend/girlfriend/spouse.
- Might have placed me at risk of being arrested.
- Might have been against the law.
- Might have led to financial problems.
- Might have caused me to waste my money.
- Were interfering with my ability to complete tasks for work or school.
- Might have had presented the potential for me to lose my job.
- Could lead to school-related problems, such as probation, expulsion, or other sanctions.
- Were inconsistent with my spiritual beliefs.
- Were inconsistent with my religious values.
- Were making me feel guilty.
- Were making me ashamed of myself.

Behavioral Outcomes

Below is a list of things that sometimes happen to people as a result of their sexual activities (including those they do alone and those they do with others). Please indicate whether these things have happened to you during the last year as a result of your sexual activities. In the past year, as a result of the things you have done sexually, did the following happen to you[b]:

- I or my sexual partner (s) became pregnant.
- I contracted a sexually transmitted infection.
- I contracted HIV.
- I gave someone else a sexually transmitted infection.
- I gave someone else HIV.
- I caused pain, injury, or other physical problems for myself.
- I caused pain, injury, or other physical problems for a sex partner.
- My relationships with friends and/or family members were damaged.
- My relationships with a spouse or other relationship partner were damaged.
- I was arrested.
- I experienced financial problems.
- I experienced problems at school.
- I experienced problems at work.
- I experienced spiritual distress.
- I was embarrassed or ashamed of myself.
- I felt guilty.

[a]Measured with a four-point response scale that includes *never, sometimes, often,* and *always.*

[b]Measured with a dichotomous response scale that includes *yes* and *no.*

Adapted from McBride et al. Kalichman SC, Greenberg J, Abel GG. HIV-seropositive men who engage in high-risk sexual behavior: psychological characteristics and implications for prevention. *AIDS Care.* 1997;9:441–450.

strategies that address sexual-risk taking, while simultaneously providing other forms of treatment, including psychotherapy to address the psychological and social aspects of out-of-control sexual behavior.

Regardless of theoretical orientation, the majority of practitioners favor approaches that incorporate cognitive and behavioral dimensions related to developing and maintaining control. Research suggests that using the CBOSBS and measures that assess trait characteristics in conjunction with other screening tools allows clinicians to identify areas that direct the focus of treatment.[55,56] Observed gender differences in outcomes of hypersexuality suggests that clinicians may need to utilize different approaches in the assessment and treatment of sexual compulsivity based on the patient's gender. The literature consistently reports that women score lower on measures of hypersexuality and present for treatment less frequently than men. A possible explanation is that women are less likely to self-report problems related to out-of-control sexual behavior due to social and cultural stigma surrounding high sexual frequency or the behavioral expression of sexuality. Clinicians must take these issues into consideration to ensure that adequate assessments are performed.

Although preliminary research suggests that SSRIs and naltrexone may enhance the efficacy of treatment outcomes when used in conjunction with cognitive behavioral therapy, additional documentation is necessary due to the sampling limitations of the studies from which findings were drawn (i.e., small sample sizes and case study reports).[14,15,25,69]

Many clinicians have little or no training in the identification and treatment of hypersexuality. Because mental health professionals play a critical role in promoting health and well-being, it will be necessary to provide specialized training on the assessment and treatment of hypersexuality, particularly the identification of adverse outcomes resulting from sexual behavior. Providers need to be aware of the obvious risks to sexual and psychological health, as well as the potential for negative consequences across a variety of life domains.

Implications for Future Research

Historically, sexual compulsivity has been conceptualized as a phenomenon leading to sexual risk-taking with little focus on consequences beyond sexual health. More recent research suggests that qualitative differences exist. Research indicates that adverse outcomes resulting from sexual behavior may be indicative of subclinical levels of sexual compulsivity occurring in nonclinical populations. Longitudinal studies that link high scores on measures of sexual compulsivity to a progression in experiences of adverse cognitive and behavioral consequences is warranted. It may be that sexual compulsivity exists on a continuum in which individuals initially experience minor consequences, primarily limited to cognitive distress, and later progress to experiencing adverse behavioral consequences as the level of compulsivity increases. Studies that include clinical measures of psychological distress and the assessment of personality traits may provide additional insight into psychiatric comorbidities that have been linked to hypersexuality. If sexually compulsive behavior is, indeed, a mechanism of mood regulation (self-medication) for underlying psychiatric conditions, longitudinal studies might further our understanding of these associations.

Additional research is needed to determine the practical significance of sexual compulsivity in diverse populations.[29] Studies should aim to document actual adverse outcomes in individuals who score higher on measures of sexual compulsivity and who engage in more frequent sexual risk behaviors. The evidence provided would allow health professionals to develop and tailor HIV/STI education and intervention efforts to the unique needs of specific individuals and groups. Researchers should design, test, and refine potential therapeutic treatments for hypersexuality as its existence as a clinical condition becomes established through scientific inquiry.

Summary

Sexual behavior that goes beyond individual control has received a great deal of attention in the research literature, particularly as it relates to sexual risk-taking that presents the potential for HIV and STI transmission. Although many scientists support the existence of hypersexuality as a distinct psychiatric phenomenon, others have argued that no such phenomenon exists. Arguments against hypersexuality as a diagnostic category are rooted in the perspective that behaviors are merely normative sexual expression at the high end of the continuum and attempts to pathologize behavioral frequency reflect restrictive sociocultural norms that attempt to constrain behavior. The significant increase in opportunities for behavioral expression of individual sexuality through technological advances that present new avenues for sexual engagement (e.g. social media, Internet) add complexity. Shifting cultural and social norms have allowed for more open expressions of a range of sexualities and sexual behaviors, calling into question previous understandings of human sexuality and blurring the boundaries of normal.

Despite expanding possibilities and sociocultural shifts, there is scientific evidence to suggest that there is a point where sexual behavior becomes out-of-control, leading to adverse consequences. However, evidence documenting negative consequences beyond risks to sexual health has been sparse. Preliminary research suggests that a variety of negative consequences are associated with hypersexuality and may be important criteria for establishing the threshold at which behavior becomes out-of-control. Outcomes-based research is an important first step to improving understandings of the phenomenon and provides evidence to support construct validity. Outcomes-based research may contribute to improved understanding of etiologic mechanisms that contribute to the development and maintenance of sexual compulsivity.

An outcomes-focused approach may move science toward a more precise conceptual understanding of hypersexuality. Engaging in frequent sexual behavior is not inherently problematic, particularly if an individual is not experiencing impairment in functioning. Disease-focused explanations of out-of-control sexual behavior are limited to sexual compulsivity as it influences unprotected sex and the risk of disease. An outcomes-based understanding broadens the conceptualization and may help better explain instances when an individual is at low risk for disease but is experiencing impaired function in other areas of life. Consideration needs to be given to the role that personality traits play in the development and maintenance of hypersexuality. The value of diagnostic categorization remains in question because systematic evidence that unequivocally supports the construct is lacking. Priority should be given to well-designed studies that test conceptual frameworks with rigorous methods and sound measures.

References

1. American Psychiatric Association. *Diagnostic and Statistical Manual of Mental Disorders*. 4th ed. Washington, DC: American Psychiatric Association; 1994.
2. American Psychiatric Associations. *DSM-5 Workgroup on Sexual and Gender Identity Disorders*. Hypersexual Disorder Screening Inventory; 2010. http://www.dsm5.org/ProposedRevisions/Pages/proposedrevision.aspx?rid=415#. Accessed February 12, 2016.
3. American Psychiatric Association. *Diagnostic and Statistical Manual of Mental Disorders*. 5th ed. Washington, DC: American Psychiatric Association; 2013.
4. Reference deleted in review.
5. Auerback A. Satriasis and nymphomania. *Med Aspects Hum Sex*. 1968;2:39–45.
6. Bancroft J, Graham C, Janssen E, Sanders S. The dual control model: current status and future directions. *J Sex Res*. 2009;46:121–142.
7. Bancroft J, Janssen E. The dual control model of male sexual response: a theoretical approach to centrally mediated erectile dysfunction. *Neurosci Biobehav Rev*. 2000;24:571–579.
8. Bancroft J, Janssen E, Strong D, et al. The relation between mood and sexuality in heterosexual men. *Arch Sex Behav*. 2003;32:217–230.
9. Bancroft J, Janssen E, Strong D, et al. The relation between mood and sexuality in gay men. *Arch Sex Behav*. 2003;32:231–242.
10. Bancroft J, Vukadinovic Z. Sexual addiction, sexual compulsivity, sexual impulsivity, or what? Toward a theoretical model. *J Sex Res*. 2004;41:225–234.
11. Barth RJ, Kinder BN. The mislabeling of sexual impulsivity. *J Sex Martial Ther*. 1198;73:15–23.
12. Benotsch EG, Kalichman SC, Kelly JA. Sexual compulsivity and predictors of high-risk behaviors. *Addict Behav*. 1999;24:857–868.
13. Benotsch EG, Kalichman SC, Pinkerton SD. Sexual compulsivity in HIV-positive men and women: prevalence, predictors, and consequences of high-risk behaviors. *Sex Addict Compulsivity*. 2001;8:83–99.
14. Bourgeois JA, Klien M. Risperidone and fluoxetine in the treatment of pedophilia with comorbid dysthymia. *J Clin Psychopharm*. 1996;16:257–258.
15. Bradford JMW, Gratzer TG. A treatment for impulse control disorders and paraphilia: a case report. *Can J Psychiatry*. 1995;40:4–5.
16. Brandell JR, Nol J. Hypersexuality as a disorder of the self. *Psychotherapy Patient*. 1992;8:51–64.
17. Carnes P. *Out of the Shadows: Understanding Sexual Addiction*. Minneapolis, MN: Compcare; 1983.
18. Carnes P. *Sexual Dependency Inventory*. Minneapolis: MNGentle; 1988.
19. Carnes P. *Contrary to Love: Helping the Sexual Addict*. City Center, MN: Hazeldon; 1989.
20. Carnes P. *Out of the Shadows: Understanding Sexual Addiction*. 3rd edn. City Center, MN: Hazeldon; 2001.
21. Carvahlo J, Guerra L, Neves S, Norbre PJ. Psychopathological predictors characterizing sexual compulsivity in a nonclinical sample of women. *J Sex Marital Ther*. 2015;41(5):467–480.
22. Coëffec A. Les apports du modèle des cinq grands facteurs dans le domaine de l'alcoolodépendance [Big five factor contributions to addiction to alcohol]. *L'Encéphale*. 2011;37:75–82.
23. Coleman E. *Sexual Compulsivity: Definition, Etiology, and Treatment Considerations. Chemical Dependency and Intimacy Dysfunction*. New York: Haworth; 1988.
24. Coleman E. The obsessive-compulsive model for describing compulsive sexual behavior. *Am J Preven Psychiatry Neuro*. 1990;2:9–14.
25. Coleman E, Cesnick J, Moore A, et al. Exploratory study of the role of psychotropic medications in the psychological treatment of sex offenders. *J Offender Rehab*. 1992;44:75–88.

26. Coleman E, Miner M, Ohlerking F, et al. Compulsive sexual behavior inventory: a preliminary study of reliability and validity. *J Sex Marital Ther.* 2001;27:325–332.

27. Coleman E, Raymond N, McBean A. Assessment and treatment of compulsive sexual behavior. *Minnesota Med.* 2003;86:1–12.

28. Detre TP, Himmelhoch JM. Hyperlibido. *Med Aspects Hum Sex.* 1973;7:172–185.

29. Dodge B, Reece M, Cole S, et al. Sexual compulsivity among heterosexual college students. *J Sex Res.* 2004;41:343–350.

30. Eber M. Don juanism. *Bull Menninger Clin.* 1981;45:307–316.

31. Ferree MC. *No Stones: Women Redeemed from Sexual Shame.* Fairfax, VA: Xulon; 2002.

32. Finlayson AJR, Sealy J, Martin PR. The differential diagnosis of problematic hypersexuality. *Sex Addict Compulsivity.* 2001;8:241–251.

33. Fischer B. Sexual addiction revisited. *Addict Newslett.* 1995;2:27.

34. Fisher JD, Misovich SJ. Social influences and AIDS-preventive behavior. In: Edwards J, ed. *Social Influence Processes and Prevention.* New York: Plenum; 1990.

35. Foucault M. *The History of Sexuality: An Introduction.* New York: Random House; 1978.

36. Reference deleted in review.

37. Giugliano J. A sociohistorical perspective of sexual health: the clinician's role. *Sex Addict Compulsivity.* 2004;11:43–55.

38. Giugliano JR. A psychoanalytic overview of excessive sexual behavior and addiction. *Sex Addict Compulsivity.* 2003;10:275–290.

39. Goodman A. Sexual addiction. In: Lowinson JH, Ruiz P, Millman RB, Langrod JG, eds. *Substance Abuse: A Comprehensive Textbook.* 4th ed. Philadelphia: Williams & Wilkins; 2005.

40. Grov C, Parsons JT, Bimbi DS. Sexual compulsivity and sexual risk in gay and bisexual men. *Arch Sex Behav.* 2010;39(4):940–949.

41. Herbenick D, Reece M, Schick V, et al. Sexual behavior in the United States: results from a national probability sample of men and women ages 14–94. *J Sex Med.* 2010;7(s5):255–265.

42. Irvine J. *Disorders of Desire: Sexuality and Gender in Modern American Sexology.* Philadelphia: Temple University; 2005.

43. Kafka MP. Successful antidepressant treatment of nonparaphilic sexual addictions and paraphilias in men. *J Clin Psychiatry.* 1991;52:60–65.

44. Kafka MP. Hypersexual disorder: a proposed diagnosis for DSM-V. *Arch Sex Behav.* 2010;39:377–400.

45. Kafka MP. What happened to hypersexual disorder? *Arch Sex Behav.* 2014;43:1259–1261.

46. Kalichman SC, Cain D. The relationship between indicators of sexual compulsivity and high-risk sexual practices among men and women receiving services from a sexually transmitted infection clinic. *J Sex Res.* 2004;41:235–241.

47. Reference deleted in review.

48. Kalichman SC, Johnson JR, Adair V, et al. Sexual sensation seeking: scale development and predicting AIDS-risk behavior among homosexually active men. *J Pers Assess.* 1994;62:385–397.

49. Kalichman SC, Rompa D. Sexual sensation seeking and sexual compulsivity scales: reliability, validity, and predicting HIV risk behavior. *J Pers Assess.* 1995;65:586–601.

50. Kalichman SC, Rompa D. The sexual compulsivity scale: further development and use with HIV-positive persons. *J Pers Assess.* 2001;76:379–395.

51. Keane H. Disorders of desire: addiction and problems of intimacy. *J Med Humanit.* 2004;25:189–204.

52. Krafft-Ebing R. *Psychopathia Sexualis (trans: Rebman FJ).* New York: Paperback Library; 1965. 1886.

53. Levine MP, Troiden RR. The myth of sexual compulsivity. *J Sex Res.* 1988;25:347–363.

54. Reference deleted in review.

55. McBride K, Reece M, Sanders S. Predicting negative outcomes of sexual behavior using the compulsive sexual behavior inventory. *Int J Sex Health.* 2007;19:51–62.

56. McBride K, Reece M, Sanders S. Using the sexual compulsivity scale to predict outcomes of sexual behavior in young adults. *Sex Addict Compulsivity.* 2008;15:97–115.

57. McCrae RR, Costa T. Validation of the five-factor model of personality across instruments and observers. *J Pers Soc Psychol.* 1987;52:81–90.

58. Montaldi DF. Understanding hypersexuality with an axis II model. *J Psychol Human Sex.* 2002;14:1–22.

59. Myers WA. Addictive sexual behavior. *Am J Psychother.* 1995;49:473–483.

60. Newcomb MD, McGee L. Influence of sensation seeking on general deviance and specific problem behaviors from adolescence to young adulthood. *J Soc Pers Psychol.* 1991;61:614–628.

61. Orford J. Hypersexuality: implications for a theory of dependence. *B J Addict.* 1978;73:299–310.

62. Pachankis H, Redina J, Ventuneac A, Grov C, Parsons J. The role of maladaptive cognitions in hypersexuality among highly sexually active gay and bisexual men. *Arch Sex Behav.* 2014;43(4):669–683.

63. Parsons J, Redina J, Moody R, Ventuneac A, Grov C. Syndemic production and sexual compulsivity/hypersexuality in highly sexually active gay and bisexual men: further evidence for a three group conceptualization. *Arch Sex Behav.* 2015;44:1903–1913.

64. Parsons J, Redina J, Ventuneac A, et al. A psychometric investigation of the hypersexual disorder screening inventory among highly sexually active gay and bisexual men: an item response theory analysis. *J Sex Med.* 2013;10(12). https://doi.org/10.1111/jsm.12117.

65. Pinto J, Carvalho J, Nobre PJ. The relationship between the FFM personality traits, state psychopathology, and sexual compulsivity in a sample of male college students. *J Sex Med.* 2013;10(7):1773–1782.

66. Reference deleted in review.

67. Quadland MC, Shattls WD. AIDS, sexuality, and sexual control. *J Homosex.* 1987;4:277–298.

68. Raymond NC, Coleman E, Miner MH. Psychiatric comorbidity and compulsive/impulsive traits in compulsive sexual behavior. *Compr Psychiatry.* 2003;44. 370–338.

69. Raymond NC, Grant JE, Kim SW, et al. The treatment of compulsive sexual behaviour with naltrexone and serotonin reuptake inhibitors: two case studies. *Int Clin Psychopharm.* 2002;17:201–205.

70. Reece M. Sexual compulsivity and HIV serostatus disclosure among men who have sex with men. *Sex Addict Compulsivity.* 2003;10:1–11.

71. Reference deleted in review.

72. Reece M, Dodge BM, McBride K. Sexual compulsivity: issues and challenges. In: McAnulty RD, Burnette MM, eds. *Sex and Sexuality.* Westport, CT: Greenwood; 2006.

73. Reference deleted in review.

74. Reid RC, Carpenter BN, Hook JN, et al. Report of findings in a DSM-5 field trial for hypersexual disorder. *J Sex Med.* 2012;9(11):2868–2877.

75. Reid RC, Garos S, Carpenter BN. Reliability, validity, and psychometric development of the hypersexual behavior inventory in an outpatient sample of men. *Sex Addict Compulsivity.* 2011;18:30–51.

76. Rettenberger M, Klein V, Briken P. The relationship between hypersexual behavior, sexual excitation, sexuality inhibition, and personality traits. *Arch Sex Behav.* 2016;45:219–233.

77. Room R. Dependence and society. *B J Addict.* 1985;80:133–139.

78. Schultz K, Hook JN, Davis DE, et al. Non-paraphilic hypersexual behavior and depressive symptoms: a meta-analytic review of the literature. *J Sex Marital Ther.* 2014;40:477–487.

79. Schwartz MF, Brasted WS. Sexual addiction. *Med Aspects Hum Sex.* 1985;20:127–128.

80. Reference deleted in review.

81. Sutton KS, Stratton N, Pytyck J, et al. Patient characteristics by type of hypersexuality referral: a quantitative chart review of 115 consecutive male cases. *J Sex Marital Ther*. 2015;41(6):563–580.

82. Terracciano A, Costa PT. Smoking and the five factor model of personality. *Addiction*. 2004;99:472–481.

83. Toussaint I, Pitchot W. Hypersexuality will not be include in the DSM-V: a contextual analysis. *Rev Med Liege*. 2013;68(5-6): 348–353.

84. Reference deleted in review.

85. Reference deleted in review.

86. Wan M, Finlayson R, Rowles A. Sexual dependency treatment outcome study. *Sex Addict Compulsivity*. 2000;7:177–196.

87. Walton MT, Cantor JM, Lykins AD. An online assessment of personality, psychological, and sexuality trait variables associated with self-reported hypersexual behavior. *Arch Sex Behav*. 2016. https://doi.org/10.1007/s10508-015-0606-1.

88. Weiss D. The prevalence of depression in male sex addicts residing in the United States. *Sex Addict Compulsivity*. 2004;11:57–69.

89. Zagar Y, Ghaffari M. Simple and multiple relationships between big-five personality dimensions and addiction in university students. *Iran J Pub Health*. 2009;38:113–117.

90. Zuckerman M, Kolin EA, Price L, et al. Development of a sensation seeking scale. *J Consul Clinic Psychol*. 1964;28:477–482.

37

New Era of Internet Addiction Research in China

HANYUN HUANG AND LOUIS LEUNG

Introduction

In recent decades, one area of research on media effects has shed extensive light on problematic behavior in the use of media, particularly the overuse or the maladaptive use of the Internet, which is commonly known as Internet addiction (IA). Previous research supported the notion that the excessive use of technology could be problematic.[12] Young[54] posited that IA could be defined as an impulse-control disorder that does not involve an intoxicant. Recent research in IA has given rise to heated discussions and debates about the definition and assessment of IA and its related causes and consequences. Because the Internet has been widely adopted relatively recently in China, whether IA exists among Internet users as well as the symptoms and characteristics of addicts has become a focus of researchers in many disciplines (e.g., communication, psychiatry, psychology, sociology, public health, and education). Most scholars have agreed that IA research has significant implications for both theory and policy.

Despite the existing debate about the nature of IA, most researchers have considered previous definitions of addiction and integrated potential new symptoms. Hence, although different terminologies have been proposed (e.g., Internet dependency, problematic Internet use, and pathological Internet use), they include similar criteria for the assessment of the basic symptoms. Although certain aspects of this complex psychosocial process remain unclear, recent studies have reported important findings on diagnosing addictive symptoms, identifying predictors, and recommending preventive measures and treatments. However, because the previous IA research was conducted mainly in Western countries, little is known about the status of Internet addiction research in China. Thus, the aim of this chapter is to provide an overview of the work done in this emerging field in China, which has 731 million Internet users.[7]

Internet and Smartphone Penetration in China

With an internet penetration rate of 53.2%, the lives of Chinese are undergoing significant change. Among the new netizens in 2016, 80.7% used a mobile phone to go online. Moreover, research has shown a polarized trend in the age differences among netizens as increasing numbers of both youngsters and elders begin using the Internet.[7]

The number of mobile phone users reached 695 million at the end of 2016, and the percentage of people who used the telephone to go online increased from 90.1% in 2015 to 95.1% in 2016. Instant messaging (IM), search engine, and online news, as fundamental Internet services, showed steadily increasing usage at rates above 80%. On mobile phones, the most often used application was IM. The survey[7] revealed that up to 79.6% of netizens used WeChat the most often, followed by QQ (60%), Taobao, Baidu, and Alipay. In addition, Moments and Qzone, which are social services provided by WeChat and QQ, were also widely used at rates of 85.8% and 67.8%, respectively.[7] The 2016 China Social Media Influence Report released by Kantar[20] pointed out that over half of urban Chinese citizens were social media users. Moreover, compared with Americans, British, French, and Brazilian social media users, Chinese social media users ranked third in terms of activeness. Sixty-two percent of American interviewees reported using Facebook and/or Twitter, whereas 58% in Brazil and 56% in China (Weibo and/or WeChat) reported using these social media.

According to the report, there were 417 million online gamers in China, comprising 57% of the entire netizen population. There were 352 million mobile gamers, or 50.6% of all mobile phone users. The number of online shoppers reached 467 million, or 63.8% of all netizens. In particular, there were 441 million mobile-phone online shoppers, which was an annual increase of 29.8%.[7]

Live video streaming services increased throughout 2016 as capital poured into this newly developed industry, which is gaining popularity among Chinese netizens. At the end of 2016, the number of live streaming users had rocketed to 344 million, comprising 47.1% of all netizens. The usage rates of sports live, game live, and live chatting were 20.7%, 20%, and 19.8%, respectively.[7]

The 2015 Chinese Teenagers' Online Behavior Report, released by the China Internet Network Information Center (CNNIC)[7] revealed that at the end of 2015, there were 287 million teenage netizens in China, comprising 85.3% of the entire adolescent population, 90% of whom used mobile phone to access the Internet, whereas the percentages of personal computer and laptop users were 69% and 39.5%, respectively. The usage rates of IM, Weibo, and Bulletin Board System (BBS) were 92.4%, 37.6%, and 18%, respectively, all of which were higher than the average usage rate in China. At the end of 2015, the number of underage netizens reached 134 million, comprising 46.6% of all teenage netizens. It is worth noting that the usage rate of online gaming, which was 69.2%, was higher than that of the average rate of teenage netizens.

Theoretical Origin and Definition

Traditionally, the concept of addiction was based on a medical model that was specific to the bodily and psychological dependence on a physical substance. It was argued that the concept of addiction should be widened to cover a broader range of behaviors.[24,34,38] Griffiths proposed the concept of "technological addiction," which is nonchemical and behavioral, involving excessive human-machine interaction.[10] Derived from the substance-dependence criteria of the *Diagnostic and Statistical Manual of Mental Disorders, Fourth Edition* (DSM-IV),[1] Internet addiction disorder (IAD), the first listed Internet-related disorder, is defined as a behavioral addiction consisting of six core components: salience, mood modification, tolerance, withdrawal symptoms, conflict, and relapse.[11] Griffiths suggested that the source of this addiction could originate in one or more aspects of Internet use, including the process of typing, the medium of communication, the lack of face-to-face contact, Internet content, and online social activities. Young characterized IA as staying online for pleasure largely in chat rooms for an average of 38 hours or more per week, concluding that IA could shatter families, relationships, and careers. Utilizing an adapted version of the criteria for pathological gambling defined by the DSM-IV, Young developed eight criteria to provide a screening instrument for addictive Internet use. To be considered an addict, the individual must meet five of eight criteria for IA: (1) preoccupation with the Internet; (2) the need for greater amounts of time online; (3) repeated attempts to reduce Internet use; (4) mood modification by Internet use; (5) staying online longer than intended; (6) loss of a significant relationship, job, or educational, or career opportunity; (7) deception about the time spent online; (8) use of the Internet as a way of escaping from problems [5].

Recent Internet Addiction Research in China

In this chapter, a review of the literature is conducted to provide a broad account of the latest IA research in China. We performed an extensive search of the Social Science Citation Index and the Science Citation Index Expanded (SCI-E) of the ISI Web of the knowledge database of all published works related to IA research in China. A total of 101 relevant empirical studies, mostly journal articles spanning 2008 to 2016, were located. Among these

studies, the most relevant were selected for review. These studies were in communication, psychology, education psychology, sociology, information science, economics, business, and others.

The literature review is classified into six broad domains on IA research in China. The domains are national, regional, cross-cultural, mediating effects, Internet research in special groups, and studies using methods other than surveys.

National Internet Addiction Research in China

In 2009, a large-scale national survey of elementary and middle school students in 100 cities or towns in 31 provinces in China was conducted to investigate the prevalence of Internet addiction (IA).[30] The study was based on a probability sample of 24,013 respondents. The results showed that only 54.2% of the participants had access to the national Internet. The prevalence of IA was 6.3% in the total sample (N = 1523) and 11.7% among Internet users. Among the Internet users, males (14.8%) and rural students (12.1%) reported IA more often than females (7.0%) and urban students (10.6%). As the frequency of Internet use and time spent online per week increased, the percentage of IA increased. The study also reported that Internet cafés (18.1%) were the most typical location for surfing, and that playing Internet games (22.5%) was the most common purpose for Internet use. What is more, the most recent statistics on Internet penetration in China[7] shows that there might be 86 million Internet addicts in China. These indicate that IA has become an important social issue and has caught the attention of national policymakers.

In another national survey of Internet users, Jiang and Leung[19] posited that IA was a health risk and examined the effects of individual differences, awareness/knowledge, and acceptance of IA on the willingness of Chinese Internet users to change their Internet habits. In 2009, data were collected from an online survey of Internet users in urban China. The results showed that 12.3% of the participants were at high risk for having IAD.

As an increasing number of Chinese users connect to the Internet via their mobile devices; they use their smartphones or tablets to engage in various activities online. Therefore, this review of the literature in IA research included smartphone addiction studies. In a national online study, Bian and Leung[3] explored the roles of psychological attributes and smartphone usage patterns in predicting smartphone addiction symptoms and social capital. The results showed that those who scored higher in loneliness and shyness had a higher likelihood of being addicted to smartphone use. The results also indicated that loneliness was the most powerful predictor, inversely affecting both bonding and bridging social capital.

Regional Internet Addiction Research in China

In addition to national surveys, several IA studies were conducted in regional locations in China, especially economically well-developed urban areas. The literature review revealed that five major IA studies were conducted in Wuhan, which is a major city, that is, a first-tier city in China. The first study focused on the relationship between adolescent addictive Internet use (AIU) and drug abuse (DA).[10] The participants were from 15 secondary schools and one university. The prevalence rates of IA and drug use (DU) were 5% and 4%, respectively. The analysis, which used structural equation modeling, found that adolescent DU and DA were significantly predicted by AIU. The second study investigated the prevalence of problematic Internet use (PIU) among college students and the possible factors related to this disorder.[14] Students from eight universities completed a questionnaire survey. The results showed that 9.58% of the participants indicated PIU. Moreover, heavy Internet use habits, poor academic achievement, and lack of love from the family were found to be significantly related to PIU. The third study, which was also conducted in Wuhan, examined the prevalence and factors of IA among adolescents.[48] The results showed that a prevalence rate of IA at 13.5%. Internet addicts scored significantly lower in parental relationships and higher in hyperactivity-impulsivity than the non-Internet addicts did. Furthermore, better parental relationships were related to significantly decreased risk of IA in younger students than in older students. The fourth study investigated the clinical characteristics of IA by using a cross-sectional survey and a psychiatric interview.[43] A structured questionnaire was completed by students at two secondary schools. Subsequently, students with IAD were interviewed to confirm their diagnosis and evaluate their clinical characteristics. Among the respondents, 12.6% met the criteria for IAD. The results indicated that being male, in grades 7–9, having a poor relationship between parents, and higher self-reported depression scores were significantly related to the diagnosis of IAD. Finally, the last study examined the association between IA and stressful life events and psychological symptoms among a random sample of school students who were Internet users.[42] The findings indicated a high prevalence of IA among adolescent Chinese Internet users, indicating the importance of the stressors of interpersonal and school-related problems as risk factors for IA, which were mediated mostly through a negative coping style.

Three IA studies were conducted in Guangdong Province. One study examined the relationship between IA and self-injurious behavior (SIB) in adolescence.[23] The participants were high school students aged 13–18 years. The results showed that SIB was common among adolescence in this province. Addiction to the Internet was harmful to mental health and increased the risk of self-injury among adolescents. In a second study in the city of Guangzhou, Li and Wang[28] examined the role of cognitive distortion in online game addiction among Chinese adolescents. Adolescents from two middle schools completed a questionnaire survey. In addition, adolescents from a local mental hospital diagnosed with excessive online game play were randomly divided into to a cognitive behavior therapy group and a clinical control group to measure the severity of online game playing, anxiety, depression, and cognitive distortions according to a baseline after a 6-week intervention. The results showed that rumination and short-term thinking were the greatest predictors of online game addiction, and males were at a high risk of developing online game addiction. The third study was conducted in Guangzhou by Tan et al.[41] They explored the correlations between PIU, depression, and sleep disturbance. Their findings showed a high prevalence of PIU, depression, and sleep disturbance among the high school students, and PIU and depressive symptoms were strongly associated with sleep disturbance.

In a regional study of IA, the authors conducted an exploratory research on IM addiction among Chinese teenagers in Xiamen, Fujian.[14] The results showed that shyness and alienation from family, peers, and school had significant and positive correlations with levels of IM addiction. Both the level of IM use and the level of IM addiction were significantly related to decreases in academic

performance. In Wenzhou, Fujian Province, Jiang et al.[17] conducted a cross-sectional survey to assess the personality characteristics of college students with IA. The results showed that 6.9% of the sample had IA. Furthermore, there were significant differences in the personality characteristics, gender, ethnicity, and substance use patterns between students with and without IA.

Recently, Yang et al.[50] explored the dual effects of flow experience on high school students' IA and exploratory behavior. They also examined the effects of parental interventions on dual causal processes. The data were collected at eight high schools in a city in Hubei Province. The results revealed that flow experience had a positive influence on both high school students' IA and exploratory behavior. Moreover, parental support significantly reduced high school students' IA and increased their exploratory behavior on the Internet.

In a comparative study of two cities, Nanjing in the east and Urumqi in the west, Tao and Liu[44] explored the relationship between Internet dependence and eating disorders in a survey of secondary school and college students. The students were divided into Internet dependents and non-Internet dependents (control group). The results showed that the Internet dependents had significantly higher rates of symptoms of eating disorders than the control groups did. In a study of four cities in Guangdong Province (i.e., Shenzhen, Guangzhou, Zhanjiang, and Qingyuan), Wang et al.[46] investigated the prevalence of PIU and the potential risk factors for PIU among high school students. Among the participants, 12.2% met the criteria for PIU. The results showed that high study-related stress, having social friends, poor relations with teachers and students, and conflictive family relationships were risk factors for PIU. Similarly, a school-based study was also conducted in four cities (i.e., Shenyang, Guangzhou, Xinxiang, and Chongqing), which aimed to assess the correlations between PIU and physical and psychological symptoms among Chinese adolescents.[2] The results revealed that 11.7%, 24.9%, 19.8%, and 26.7% of the sample had PIU, physical symptoms, psychological symptoms, and poor sleep quality, respectively. Poor sleep quality was found to be an independent risk factor for both physical and psychological symptoms. The effects of PIU on physical and psychological symptoms were partially mediated by sleep quality.

In Hong Kong, Leung and Lee[26] examined the degrees to which demographics, addiction symptoms, information literacy, parenting styles, and Internet activities predicted Internet risk in a probability sample of 718 adolescents and teenagers aged 9–19 years. They conducted face-to-face interviews with the participants. The results showed that adolescents who were often targets of harassment tended to be older boys with a high family income. The findings indicated that they spent a significant amount of time on social networking sites (SNSs) and preferred the online setting. The adolescents who encountered the unwelcome solicitation of personal or private information online tended to be older girls. Regarding information literacy, they were generally very competent in using publishing tools, but they were not structurally literate (i.e., especially in understanding how information is socially situated and produced).

Using the same dataset, Leung and Lee[27] also examined the interrelationships among Internet literacy, IA symptoms, Internet activities, and academic performance. The regression results showed that the adolescent Internet addicts tended to be male, in low-income families, and lacking confidence in locating, browsing, and accessing information from multiple resources. However, they were technologically knowledgeable and frequent leisure users of SNSs and online games. Contrary to the hypothesis, Internet literacy, especially in publishing and technology, increased the likelihood of addiction to the Internet. As expected, Internet activities, especially SNSs and online games, were significantly and positively linked to IA as well as to all symptoms of IA. Furthermore, the higher the subjects scored on tool and social-structural literacy, the better their academic performance was. However, skills in technical literacy, such as publishing and technology literacy, were not significant predictors of academic performance.

Another study in Hong Kong was conducted to examine the correlations between heavy Internet use and various health risk behaviors and health-promoting behaviors in a university.[21] The results showed that 14.8% of the participants reported heavy Internet use, and that they had lower potential for health-promoting activities. Heavy Internet use was related to various risk behaviors, such as ignoring meals and sleeping late, as well as negative health outcomes, such as being overweight and hypersomnia.

Cross-Cultural Internet Addiction Research

In addition to large-scale national and regional research, IA research was also carried out in a number of comparative cross-cultural studies between China and the United States. One study that surveyed university students aimed to assess 10 IA symptoms. The findings revealed that the Chinese students in the sample showed a higher rate of IA than their US counterparts.[55] Another study explored the relationship between compulsive Internet use (CIU) and substance use in China and the United States.[40] The results found that CIU was related to substance use, but the relationship was not consistently positive.

Several studies were conducted in a range of countries and regions. Sariyska et al.[37] investigated the relationship between self-esteem, personality, and IA in Bulgaria, Germany, Spain, Colombia, China, Taiwan, and Sweden. The results showed that the personality dimension of self-directedness was negatively correlated with IA. However, no effect of the interaction between implicit and explicit self-esteem on IA was observed. Mak et al.[32] examined and compared the prevalence of Internet behaviors and addiction in adolescents in six Asian countries and regions (i.e., China, Hong Kong, Japan, South Korea, Malaysia, and the Philippines). The results showed that Hong Kong had the highest number of adolescents who reported daily Internet use. Moreover, Internet addictive behavior was common among adolescents in these Asian countries. Similarly, another study used structural equation modeling to explore the mediating role of IA in depression, social anxiety, and psychosocial well-being among adolescents in the same six Asian countries.[22] The results showed that IA mediated the relationship between social anxiety and poor psychosocial well-being in China, Hong Kong, and Malaysia.

Mediating Effects Studies in Internet Addiction Research

In addition to examining the linear, bivariate, and multivariate relationships, previous Internet addiction research also paid close attention to mediating effects. Yang et al. investigated the mediating role of life events in the relationship between IA and depression.[49] A school-based cross-sectional survey was conducted in junior and senior high schools in Hefei, China. The findings showed that life events fully mediated the relationship between IA and depression. Similarly, a survey of college students in five major cities in China was conducted to explore the effects of personality,

parental behaviors, and self-esteem on Internet addiction.[53] The results showed that psychoticism and neuroticism were both positively related to IA, and parental behaviors were also significantly linked to IA. Moreover, the study also found that the influence of emotional warmth from parents on IA was partially mediated by self-esteem.

A study was conducted in Xi'an, China, to examine whether father-child, mother-child, and peer attachment played mediating roles in parental marital conflict and IA.[51] The results indicated that mother-child and father-child attachments mediated the relationship between marital conflict and IA through peer attachment. Another study on PIU examined the unique roles of four dimensions of temperament (i.e., effortful control, sensation seeking, anger/frustration, and shyness) on adolescent PIU, as well as the mediating role of deviant peer affiliation (DPA) on these pathways.[29] The results showed that in all four temperament dimensions, DPA partially mediated the pathways to PIU.

Internet Addiction Research in Special Groups

In addition to adolescents and college students, the review revealed that previous IA research focused on many other special groups. In an experimental study, Zhong et al.[56] evaluated the effectiveness of a family-based intervention program for IA in Chinese adolescents The participants had been diagnosed as having IA by the Addiction Medical Treatment Center of the Beijing Military Zone General Hospital. The participants were divided randomly into an intervention group and a control group. The results showed that the family-based group intervention was more effective in reducing Internet use and enhancing family function. Another study examined the interrelationships between Internet connectedness, online gaming, Internet addiction symptoms, and academic performance decrement among young clients in one of the earliest and largest IA clinics in China.[18] The results showed that Internet café patrons and those who used the Internet with many goals or higher degrees of Internet adhesiveness exhibited a greater number of IA symptoms. As expected, the level of IA was significantly related to academic performance decrement. Other researchers proposed a model for understanding the contributors to and consequences of online gaming dependency.[35] A preliminary study surveyed 166 online gamers in China. The findings of the path analysis revealed that maladaptive cognitions, shyness, and depression were positively associated with online gaming addiction. Online gaming dependency was also positively related to different types of negative life consequences.

In addition to IA patients, migrant children (MC) and left-behind children (LBC) were evaluated for Internet addiction.[13] This study researched the associations between IA and depression in MC and LBC. LBC, MC, and non-left-behind rural children (RC) from 12 schools were surveyed using a cross-sectional design. LBC and RC were chosen from Henan and Shanxi Provinces, and MC was selected from the Shunyi and Changping districts of Beijing. The results showed that the prevalence of depression was 10.9%, 19.7%, and 14.3%, respectively, among RC, MCs, and LBC. The prevalence of IA was 3.7%, 6.4%, and 3.2% among RC, MC, and LBC, respectively. These findings suggested that IA might be related to the increased risk of depression in LBC, and migration was an important risk factor for depression in children.

Methodological Approaches in Internet Addiction Research

Most recent Chinese IA research employed the cross-sectional survey as the research method, and a few used other research tools. In 2010, one study on the prevalence of IA was conducted in Hong Kong using a two-wave panel household survey of 208 adolescents.[8] The participants self-reported their usage of the Internet, their symptoms of IA, and so on. Similarly, using a longitudinal panel survey design, in Time 1, Leung[25] collected data from 417 adolescents at two points. One year later, in Time 2, they examined the relationships between changes in Internet risk and social media gratifications-sought, IA symptoms, and social media use. By controlling for demographics and criterion variable scores in IA in Time 1, entertainment and IM use in Time 1 significantly predicted the increased IA measured in Time 2. The study also controlled for demographics and scores of criterion variables in Internet risk, including harassment, privacy exposure, and pornographic or violent content consumed in Time 1. Gratifications-sought (including status-gaining, expressing opinions, and identity experimentation), IA symptoms (including withdrawal and negative life consequences), and social media use (in particular, blogs and Facebook) significantly predicted the Internet risk changes in Time 2. These findings suggested that the predictors in Time 1 could be used to identify adolescents who are likely to develop IA symptoms and experience Internet risk based on their previous gratifications-sought, previous addiction symptoms, and their habits of social media use in Time 1.

Building on a framework developed from coding qualitative data, Rosenbaum and Wong[36] explored how IM services helped and hindered mental health among adolescents in China and the United States. The findings showed that young IM users in China and the United States received social support from their virtual relationships.

In addition to household and online surveys, Su et al. designed experiments to study the effects of intervention on online addiction in college students.[39] A pilot study of an intervention tool to help reduce Internet usage was conducted at the Healthy Online Self-Helping Center (HOSC). The participants were assigned randomly to four conditions in order to complete questionnaires at baseline and at 1-month follow-up. The results showed that under both natural and laboratory environments, HOSC effectively reduced the number of hours the participants spent online and their scores on Young's Diagnostic Questionnaire, as well as improving online satisfaction at 1-month follow-up. Wang et al.[47] used an event-related potential method to study the differences in the capacity for pain empathy in urban Internet-addicted LBC and nonaddicts. The participants took part in an event-related potential experiment that was conducted over 10 successive days. The results showed that IA influenced the capacity for pain empathy among urban LBC. In particular, it affected cognitive processing and assessment.

Yao et al.[52] conducted a retrospective nested case-control study to investigate mental health symptoms and levels of adaptation in Chinese college students in their freshman year as predictors of IA. The results revealed that freshman with characteristics of depression, learning maladaptation, and dissatisfaction could be an important intervention target to reduce IA.

The literature review also revealed that some research developed innovative tools for investigating IA. In recent years, microblogs have become more and more popular among college students. However, no published scale has been developed to assess the excessive use of microblogs. To develop their Microblog Excessive Use Scale (MEUS), Hou et al.[15] collected data from 3047 college students in China and compared their findings with the criteria used to assess IA. Another study examined the attraction of online games and their contribution to IA among college students in China.[45] This study tested the theoretical framework of online game attraction to develop the Online Game Attraction Inventory (OAI).

In 2009, the results of a bibliometric analysis of the scientific literature on Internet, video games, and cell phone addiction from 1996 to 2005 indicated that China had the second-highest rate of addiction.[4] Several IA studies were conducted in urban China. An empirical review examined 24 studies of IA treatment outcomes in China.[31] The review study used 15 attributes of the quality of evidence scores to evaluate these outcome studies. Based on the findings, it was recommended that further rigorously designed studies, accompanied by the transparent reporting of methods and findings, were needed to identify promising treatments for IA.

Conclusion

This chapter provided a broad overview of current IA research in China. The findings of this review showed that IA research has been conducted in different parts of China from different perspectives, and that many significant findings were obtained. Most of the existing research in China treated IA as a general phenomenon and reported different IA rates in a diverse range of samples. In recent years, many Chinese news reports and commentaries have begun to pay attention to specific types of IA addiction, such as online game addiction, online gambling addiction, pornography addiction, online shopping addiction, online chatting addiction, selfies addiction, photo-sharing addiction, and cybersex addiction. It is suggested that further social science research should be done to investigate particular types of IA addiction in China.

This review also revealed that most of Chinese IA research conducted in recent years employed the cross-sectional survey as the research method. Hence, qualitative research is needed to gain insights into the reasons for various kinds of IA addiction.

In China, the penetration of the Internet and smartphones increases rapidly every year. Many children and adolescents who use the Internet can become addicted to it. Lacking supervision, they can also encounter unhealthy and harmful information. Therefore, future research should go beyond examining the addiction rates to identifying the symptoms of IA addiction. Knowledge of these symptoms could help parents and educators detect and assess IA addiction in order to intervene appropriately at an early stage.

This review showed that the previous IA research in China has focused on adolescents and college students. Future IA studies should focus on groups such as white-collar workers, immigrant workers, and the middle-aged. Different groups may have specific characteristics, and they may be addicted to different functions of the Internet. Furthermore, as the rapidly developing technology of virtual reality (VR) and mobile/wearable devices becomes more ubiquitous and deeply affects our lives, addiction research into specific domain such as content addiction, applications addiction, and behavioral addiction will begin a new era in the advancement in Internet addiction research in China.

References

1. American Psychiatric Association. *Diagnostic and Statistical Manual for Mental Disorders*. 4th ed. Washington, DC: American Psychiatric Association; 1994.

2. An J, Sun Y, Wan YH, Chen J, Wang X, Tao FB. Associations between problematic internet use and adolescents' physical and psychological symptoms: possible role of sleep quality. *J Addict*. 2014;8(4):282–287.

3. Bian MW, Leung L. Linking loneliness, shyness, smartphone addiction symptoms, and patterns of smartphone use to social capital. *Soc Sci Comput Rev*. 2015;33(1):61–79.

4. Carbonell X, Guardiola E, Beranuy M, Belles A. A bibliometric analysis of the scientific literature on internet, video games, and cell phone addiction. *J Med Libr Assoc*. 2009;97(2):102–107.

5. CNNIC. *The Survey Report on Chinese Instant Message Market 2006*; 2006. http://www.cnnic.cn/html/Dir/2006/12/27/4367.htm. Accessed 25 June 2008.

6. CNNIC. *The 2015 Chinese Teenagers' online behavior report*; 2016. Accessed http://www.cnnic.net.cn/hlwfzyj/hlwxzbg/qsnbg/201608/P020160812393489128332.pdf.

7. CNNIC. *The 39th China Statistical Report on Internet Development*; 2017. http://www.cnnic.net.cn/hlwfzyj/hlwxzbg/hlwtjbg/201701/P020170123364672657408.pdf. Accessed 11 February 2017.

8. Fu K, Chan WSC, Wong PWC, Yip PSF. Internet addiction: prevalence discriminant validity and correlates among adolescents in Hong Kong. *Br J Psychiatry*. 2010;196(6):486–492.

9. Reference deleted in review.

10. Griffiths MD. Gambling on the internet: a brief note. *J Gambl Stud*. 1996;12:471–473.

11. Griffiths MD. Internet addiction: does it really exist? In: Gackenbach J, ed. *Psychology and The Internet: Intrapersonal, Interpersonal, and Transpersonal Applications*. New York: Academic; 1998.

12. Griffiths MD. Does internet and "addiction" exist? Some case study evidence. *Cyberpsychol Behav*. 2000;3:211–218.

13. Guo J, Chen L, Wang XH, et al. The relationship between internet addiction and depression among migrant children and left-behind children in China. *Cyberpsychol Behav Soc Netw*. 2012;15(11):585–590.

14. Huang HY, Leung L. Instant messaging addiction among teenagers in China: shyness, alienation, and academic performance decrement. *Cyberpsychol Behav*. 2009;12(6):675–679.

15. Hou J, Huang ZC, Li HX, et al. Is the excessive use of microblogs an internet addiction? Developing a scale for assessing the excessive use of microblogs in Chinese college students. *PLoS One*. 2014;9(11):e110960. https://doi.org/10.1371/journal.pone.0110960.

16. Reference deleted in review.

17. Jiang DG, Zhu S, Ye MJ, Lin CG. Cross-sectional survey of prevalence and personality characteristics of college students with internet addiction in Wenzhou, China. *Shanghai Arch Psychiatry*. 2012;24(2):99–107.

18. Jiang QL. Internet addiction among young people in China internet connectedness, online gaming, and academic performance decrement. *Internet Research*. 2014;24(1):2–20.

19. Jiang QL, Leung L. Effects of individual differences, awareness-knowledge, and acceptance of internet addiction as a health risk on willingness to change internet habits. *Soc Sci Comput Rev*. 2012;30(2):170–183.

20. Kantar. *China Social Media Influence Report, 2016*. 2016. http://www.cn.kantar.com/media/1190971/2016.pdf. Accessed 11 February 2017.

21. Kim JH, Lau CH, Cheuk K, Kan P, Hui HLC, Griffiths SM. Brief report: predictors of heavy internet use and associations with health-promoting and health risk behaviors among Hong Kong university students. *J Adolesc*. 2010;33(1):215–220.

22. Lai CM, Mak KK, Watanabe H, et al. The mediating role of internet addiction in depression, social anxiety, and psychosocial well-being among adolescents in six Asian countries: a structural equation modeling approach. *Public Health*. 2015;129(9):1224–1236.

23. Lam LT, Peng Z, Mai J, Jing J. The association between internet addiction and self-injurious behavior among adolescents. *Inj Prev*. 2009;15(6):403–408.

24. Lemon J. Can we call behaviors addictive? *Clin Psychol*. 2002;6:44–49.

25. Leung L. Predicting internet risks: a longitudinal panel study of gratifications-sought, internet addiction symptoms, and social media use among adolescents and children. *Health Psychol Behav Med*. 2014;2(1):424–439.

26. Leung L, Lee PSN. The influences of information literacy, internet addiction and parenting styles on internet risks. *New Media Soc*. 2012;14(1):115–134.

27. Leung L, Lee PSN. Impact of internet literacy, internet addiction symptoms, and internet activities on academic performance. *Soc Sci Comput Rev*. 2012;30(4):403–418.

28. Li HH, Wang S. The role of cognitive distortion in online game addiction among Chinese adolescents. *Child Youth Serv Rev*. 2013;35(9):1468–1475.

29. Li X, Newman J, Li DP, Zhang HY. Temperament and adolescent problematic internet use: the mediating role of deviant peer affiliation. *Comput Human Behav*. 2016;60:342–350.

30. Li YJ, Zhang XH, Lu FR, Zhang Q, Wang Y. Internet addiction among elementary and middle school students in China: a nationally representative sample study. *Cyberpsychol Behav Soc Netw*. 2014;17(2):111–116.

31. Liu C, Liao M, Smith DC. An empirical review of internet addiction outcome studies in China. *Res Soc Work Pract*. 2012;22(3):282–292.

32. Mak K, Lai M, Phil C, et al. Epidemiology of internet behaviors and addiction among adolescents in six Asian countries. *Cyberpsychol Behav Soc Netw*. 2014;17(11):720–728.

33. Reference deleted in review.

34. Orford J. *Excessive Appetites: A Psychological View of Addictions*. 2nd edn. Chichester, UK: Wiley; 2001.

35. Peng W, Liu M. Online gaming dependency: a preliminary study in China. *Cyberpsychol Behav Soc Netw*. 2010;13(3):329–333.

36. Rosenbaum MS, Wong IA. The effect of instant messaging services on society's mental health. *J Serv Mark*. 2012;26:124–135.

37. Sariyska R, Reuter M, Bey K, et al. Self-esteem, personality and internet addiction: a cross-cultural comparison study. *Pers Individ Dif*. 2014;X:28–33.

38. Shaffer HJ. Understanding the means and objects of addiction: technology, the internet and gambling. *J Gambl Stud*. 1996;12:461–469.

39. Su WL, Fang XY, Miller JK, Wang YY. Internet-based intervention for the treatment of online addiction for college students in China: a pilot study of the healthy online self-helping center. *Cyberpsychol Behav Soc Netw*. 2011;14(9):497–503.

40. Sun P, Johnson CA, Palmer P, et al. Concurrent and predictive relationships between compulsive internet use and substance use: findings from vocational high school students in China and the USA. *Int J Environ Res Public Health*. 2012;9(3):660–673.

41. Tan YF, Chen Y, Lu YG, Li LP. Exploring associations between problematic internet use, depressive symptoms and sleep disturbance among Southern Chinese adolescents. *Int J Environ Res Public Health*. 2016;13(3):313.

42. Tang J, Yu YZ, Du YK, Ma Y, Zhang DY, Wang JJ. Prevalence of internet addiction and its association with stressful life events and psychological symptoms among adolescent internet users. *Addict Behav*. 2014;39(3):744–747.

43. Tang J, Zhang Y, Li Y, et al. Clinical characteristics and diagnostic confirmation of internet addiction in secondary school students in Wuhan, China. *Psychiatry Clin Neurosci*. 2014;68(6):471–478.

44. Tao ZL, Liu Y. Is there a relationship between internet dependence and eating disorders? A comparison study of internet dependents and non-internet dependents. Eating and Weight Disorders Studies on Anorexia. *Bulimia and Obesity*. 2009;14(2-3):E77–E83.

45. Tone HJ, Zhao HR, Yan WS. The attraction of online games: an important factor for internet addiction. *Comput Hum Behav*. 2014;30:321–327.

46. Wang H, Zhou XL, Lu CY, Wu J, Deng XQ, Hong LY. Problematic internet use in high school students in Guangdong Province, China. *PLoS One.* 2011;6(5):e19660. https://doi.org/10.1371/journal.pone.0019660.

47. Wang T, Ge Y, Zhang JF, Liu J, Luo WB. The capacity for pain empathy among urban internet-addicted left-behind children in China: an event-related potential study. *Comput Hum Behav.* 2014;33:56–62.

48. Wu XH, Chen XG, Han J, et al. Prevalence and factors of addictive internet use among adolescents in Wuhan, China: interactions of parental relationship with age and hyperactivity-impulsivity. *PloS ONE.* 2013;8(4):e61782. https://doi.org/10.1371/journal.pone.0061782.

49. Yang LS, Sun L, Zhang ZH, Sun YH, Wu HY, Ye DQ. Internet addiction, adolescent depression, and the mediating role of life events: finding from a sample of Chinese adolescents. *Int J Psychol.* 2014;49(5):342–347.

50. Yang SQ, Lu YB, Wang B, Zhao L. The benefits and dangers of flow experience in high school students' internet usage: the role of parental support. *Comput Hum Behav.* 2014;41:504–513.

51. Yang XJ, Zhu L, Chen Q. Parent marital conflict and internet addiction among Chinese college students: the mediating role of father-child, mother-child, and peer attachment. *Comput Hum Behav.* 2016;59:221–229.

52. Yao B, Han W, Zeng LX, Guo X. Freshman year mental health symptoms and level of adaptation as predictors of internet addiction: a retrospective nested case-control study of male Chinese college students. *Psychiatry Research.* 2013;210(2):541–547.

53. Yao MZ, He J, Ko DM, Pang KC. The influence of personality, parental behaviors, and self-esteem on internet addiction: a study of Chinese college students. *Cyberpsychol Behav Soc Netw.* 2014;17(2):104–110.

54. Young KS. Internet addiction: the emergence of a new clinical disorder. *CyberPsychol Behav.* 1998;1:237–244.

55. Zhang L, Amos C, MacDowell WC. A comparative study of internet addiction. *Cyberpsychol Behav.* 2008;11(6):727–729.

56. Zhong X, Zu S, Sha S, et al. The effect of a family-based intervention model on internet-addiction Chinese adolescents. *Soc Behav Pers.* 2011;39(8):1021–1034.

38

Hoarding as a Behavioral Addiction

JESSICA R. GRISHAM, ALISHIA D. WILLIAMS, RAJA KADIB, AND PETER A. BALDWIN

Overview

Hoarding disorder (HD) is defined as the acquisition of—and inability to discard—a large number of possessions, to a degree that precludes intended use of living spaces and creates significant distress or impairment in functioning.[24,26] Hoarding can interfere with an individual's ability to work, interact with others, and perform basic activities, such as eating or sleeping. In severe cases, it may lead to dangerous, even life-threatening living conditions. Hoarding also is associated with a profound public health burden. In a survey of local health departments, 64% of health officers reported receiving hoarding complaints, some of which resulted in a significant cost to the community.[38] A large Internet survey of self-identified hoarding participants (N = 864) and family members (N = 655) revealed that compulsive hoarding is related to poor physical health, social service involvement, and significant occupational impairment.[102]

Hoarding has been linked previously to anxiety disorders, specifically obsessive-compulsive disorder (OCD); however, it is now defined in the *Diagnostic and Statistical Manual of Mental Disorders, Fifth Edition* (DSM-5) as a discrete disorder. Consistent with prominent models of anxiety disorders,[3a] individuals who hoard frequently report feelings of anxiety when they are asked to discard or organize their possessions. They also may demonstrate avoidance and safety behaviors connected to their hoarding-related beliefs and fears.[91] There is, however, a pleasurable or gratifying component associated with acquiring, collecting, and saving possessions that distinguishes hoarding from other anxiety-related problems.

This appetitive aspect of hoarding suggests that there are similarities between hoarding and behavioral addictions, which include several impulse control disorders (pathological gambling, pyromania, and kleptomania). In behavioral addictions, individuals experience pleasurable or gratifying feelings while engaging in the target behavior, followed by a decrease in arousal and feelings of guilt and remorse.[55] An individual who compulsively collects items from yard sales and thrift stores may similarly feel a rush of positive emotion upon finding an item that she feels is unique or valuable, followed by feelings of regret when she reflects upon how much the clutter is overtaking her home and negatively impacting her life. Although the anxiety-related aspects of hoarding have been the subject of several investigations,[26] the appetitive nature of this syndrome has been relatively understudied. Hoarding behavior is sometimes motivated by a desire to reduce anxiety; however, there are cases in which hoarding appears to be driven by anticipation of pleasure and impaired self-regulation.[46] There also may be cases in which both avoidance and approach behaviors play a role. From a clinical perspective, this underscores the importance of functional analysis in determining motivation for hoarding and, more specifically, acquisition behaviors.

Classification and Comorbidity

Hoarding was long considered a dimension or subtype of OCD.[94] Findings of moderate frequencies of hoarding behavior in OCD populations, ranging from 18% to 33%, supported this association.[29,83] Moreover, several studies found that individuals who hoard report more OCD symptoms than nonhoarding individuals do.[25,29] Frost and colleagues[37] compared individuals with OCD who hoarded versus those who did not, and found that the two groups did not differ on the number of OCD symptoms displayed, although they both reported more OCD symptoms than did anxious and nonclinical control participants.

Despite this association, mounting evidence began to suggest that hoarding was distinct from other OCD symptom dimensions. Most factor analyses of OCD symptoms found that hoarding constituted a separate factor from other obsessions and compulsions.[8,47,60,66,83] Furthermore, hoarding behavior has been reported in a variety of psychiatric disorders besides OCD, including schizophrenia,[64] organic mental disorders,[44] eating disorders,[24] brain injury,[17] and dementia.[20] Finally, hoarding is typically a poor predictor of treatment outcome in both psychological and pharmacological treatments for OCD,[9] although several recent studies have not confirmed this association.[16,85,90] In light of the conflicting evidence regarding the diagnostic status of hoarding, Wu and Watson[114] examined the relationship between OCD and hoarding in two large samples. They found that hoarding correlated only modestly with other OCD symptoms, which reliably correlated with each other. Furthermore, hoarding was not more strongly associated with OCD symptoms than other dimensions of psychopathology, such as depression. Subsequently, large epidemiological studies have demonstrated that hoarding difficulties are more prevalent than first thought, and are not definitively associated with one particular disorder.[50,82,97] Together, this research led to the development of criteria for hoarding disorder, which were included in the DSM-5.[2]

It is notable for the present discussion that not all individuals who hoard have comorbid symptoms reflective of typical OCD.[46] In addition, hoarding beliefs and behaviors do not always fit the OCD model. Steketee and Frost[91] noted that hoarding thoughts may not always impel the associated compulsive behaviors, may not be as intrusive as typical obsessions, and are not always viewed as ego-dystonic by the individual. In addition, many individuals who hoard lack insight into the severity of the consequences of their behaviors and can experience attenuated levels of distress compared with OCD clients.[91] The lack of insight and ego-syntonic nature of hoarding is similar to that observed in some addictive and impulse control disorders, suggesting some overlap in phenomenology between hoarding and many behavioral addictions.

Hoarding and Impulse Control Disorders

Most relevant to the current chapter is the association between hoarding and the spectrum of impulse control disorders. Impulse control disorders are positively reinforcing to the individual and are associated with a wide variety of emotional states, including pleasure or gratification. They are characterized by repetitive behaviors and impaired inhibition of these behaviors, and include pathological gambling, skin picking, and trichotillomania. Researchers have suggested that impulse control disorders may best be conceptualized as part of an obsessive compulsive spectrum,[54,71] as the urges and subsequent behavioral responses observed in impulse control disorders appear, at least superficially, similar to the excessive rituals observed in OCD.[6] Problems removing unwanted thoughts and deficits in decision making may also represent commonalities between OCD and impulse control disorders.

A key difference between impulse control disorders and OCD, however, is that an individual with an impulse control disorder experiences feelings of pleasure and gratification while engaging in the target behavior, in contrast to the anxiety experienced when individuals with OCD engage in a compulsion.[42] For example, the repetitive and often harmful rituals performed in OCD may appear similar to the wagering behaviors of compulsive gamblers. When significant monetary losses fuel chasing behavior, a compulsive gambler may feel compelled to gamble to avoid negative consequences in much the same way that rituals in OCD are performed in an effort to alleviate negative emotional states such as anxiety, shame, and guilt.[95] However, gambling behaviors are clearly pleasurable and reinforcing.[42] Individuals who hoard also derive a sense of pleasure and gratification from their acquisition behaviors, which may suggest that hoarding fits better among the impulse control disorders than its common conceptualization as a subtype of OCD.

Hoarding has been linked to poor impulse control in a variety of studies, suggesting the possibility of a common diathesis underlying both hoarding and certain impulse control disorders. Samuels et al.[83] reported a greater frequency of trichotillomania and skin picking among hoarding compared with nonhoarding individuals with OCD. Rasmussen et al.[77] found that hoarding individuals displayed poor response inhibition on standardized laboratory tasks relative to individuals with anxiety disorders, despite reporting similar levels of impulse control.

Frost et al.[30] found that pathological gamblers reported significantly more hoarding symptoms than light gamblers and speculated that both hoarding individuals and gamblers may share similar concerns about the loss of potential opportunities. Hoarding individuals believe that items may be needed for some future use and, therefore, fear discarding items as this would represent a lost opportunity for the item's use,[30] with some research suggesting that even the sight of a possession can trigger this fear.[32] Frost and colleagues[30] have suggested that pathological gamblers may have difficulty refraining from purchasing chances because of similar beliefs and fears about losing an opportunity to gain financial benefit. Although Grant et al.[41] found a low prevalence of impulse control disorders overall among individuals with OCD, OCD participants with a lifetime and current impulse control disorder were more likely to report hoarding symptoms. In addition, some research suggests that beliefs about possession and about buying are similar to the beliefs of those with compulsive hoarding.[58] The association between hoarding and impulse control disorders is consistent with McElroy and colleagues' conceptualization of a compulsive-impulsive spectrum[70] but requires further exploration.

Hoarding and Compulsive Acquisition

Compulsive acquisition is a central component of hoarding,[25,26] and is of particular significance when considering hoarding as a behavioral addiction. The compulsive acquisition component of hoarding consists, in part, of compulsive buying, which is classified as an impulse control disorder.[70] Compulsive buying has been defined as chronic, repetitive purchasing behavior in response to negative events and or/feelings that is difficult to stop and results in harmful consequences.[18] Similar to other impulse control disorders, compulsive buying is associated with a pattern of tension, pleasure, and subsequent feelings of guilt and remorse.[10] A high level of compulsive buying has been found among individuals who hoard,[28] and, conversely, a high level of hoarding symptoms have been found in compulsive buyers.[36] A study comparing compulsive buyers with noncompulsive buyers found that compulsive buyers scored higher on both OCD and hoarding symptoms, but the relationship between buying and OCD was mainly mediated by hoarding.[36] Of interest, this study found that while not all compulsive buyers suffer from compulsive hoarding, nearly all hoarding participants suffer from compulsive acquisition. Compulsive acquisition in hoarding, however, is not limited to buying, but includes collecting free things that are being given away or that have been discarded by others. However, Frost et al.[28] found that these behaviors were related; a measure of compulsive buying behavior was associated with a compulsive acquisition of free items.

The relationship between hoarding and compulsive buying may be accounted for by shared cognitive deficits and emotional dysregulation. Both hoarding and compulsive buying appear to be closely related to impaired mental control[28] and fears about decision making.[58] In addition, evidence suggests that similar cognitive biases about the meaning of possessions exist in both hoarding individuals and compulsive buyers.[58] Although O'Guinn and Faber[74] suggested that compulsive buyers may derive more emotional pleasure from the process of acquiring items, in contrast to hoarding individuals, who retain a sense of satisfaction from items even once ownership has been established, Kyrios et al.[58] found that compulsive buyers did hold beliefs about possession similar to those reported by hoarding participants. These beliefs included fears over lost opportunities to obtain objects, erroneous beliefs about the inherent value of possessions, and beliefs about personal responsibility for objects.[58] Research on hoarding has suggested that the sight of a possession activates the fear of losing an opportunity.[32]

Compulsive buying and hoarding also share problems with regulating emotions. Individuals who buy compulsively report difficulties accepting and coping with negative emotions,[110] similar to the difficulties in managing emotional distress that hoarding individuals report, both in response to their objects and in day-to-day life.[76,89] Compulsive buying and hoarding both appear to be driven by negative urgency—a tendency to react impulsively when experiencing negative emotion—which, in hoarding, intensifies emotional attachment to possessions.[76,110] Compulsive buying and hoarding difficulties are also related to low distress tolerance, in particular a low perceived ability to cope with distress, and the tendency to become absorbed or overwhelmed by the experience of distress.[96,99,110] Collectively, these findings suggest a diagnostic overlap between hoarding disorder and impulse control disorders.

Etiology/Biobehavioral Underpinnings of Hoarding

Over the past decade, much new evidence has emerged regarding the biological/neural underpinnings of hoarding. Several case reports have described cases of pathological collecting and saving that began after a brain injury, typically along with other changes in personality and social functioning.[17] These cases suggest that hoarding may be related to frontal lobe dysfunction. Other evidence for the biological correlates of hoarding has come from three domains of research: neuroimaging, electrophysiology, and genetics.

Neuroimaging

Numerous studies have investigated a possible neural basis of hoarding disorder.[45] Anderson et al.[119] conducted a study in which 13 of 86 individuals with focal lesions exhibited abnormal collecting behavior. All 13 of these individuals had damage to the mesial frontal region of the brain, including the anterior cingulate region. In addition, in the first study using positron emission tomography to examine compulsive hoarding, Saxena et al.[84] found that individuals with OCD who hoard had significantly lower glucose metabolism in the anterior and posterior regions of the cingulate gyrus when compared with individuals with OCD who did not hoard. The authors posited that lower activity in these regions may mediate the deficits in motivation, attention, memory, and decision-making that are associated with compulsive hoarding. Underactivity in these regions also has been observed in individuals who

misuse cocaine or alcohol regardless of whether they currently use these substances or have abstained for a lengthy period.[106-108]

Mataix-Cols et al.[67] conducted a functional magnetic resonance imaging (fMRI) study in which individuals with OCD were presented with pictures containing various types of OCD-related stimuli, including hoarding-related images (old newspapers, clothes, etc.). Participants were told to imagine that the items belonged to them and that they would have to discard them later. During this provocation, participants demonstrated greater activation than controls in the left precentral/superior frontal gyrus, left fusiform gyrus, and right orbitofrontal cortex.

Tolin et al.[105] engaged hoarding individuals in an in vivo acquiring and discarding task while undergoing fMRI. When discarding novel objects, hoarding individuals demonstrated reduced activation of the dorsal anterior cingulate cortex (ACC) and orbitofrontal cortex. When discarding their possessions, however, the same individuals demonstrated the reverse pattern. The ACC and insula became hyperactive relative to healthy individuals, with the greatest ACC activation observed on trials in which participants refused to discard. A similar pattern was observed in a subsequent trial of cognitive behavioral therapy (CBT) for hoarding[104]; however the ACC hyperactivity normalized after a treatment, in line with a reduction in hoarding severity. This finding led the authors to speculate that hoarding difficulties may be partially underpinned by an ACC-mediated error-monitoring system that is hypersensitive to possession.[104]

Electrophysiology

Several examinations of the error-related negativity (ERN) support the proposition that ACC-mediated error-monitoring systems are deficient in hoarding individuals. The ERN is an event-related potential component originating from the ACC that indexes error detection.[15,19,109] Mathews et al.[68] analyzed ERN data from several OCD samples and noted a trend for an enhanced ERN in hoarding OCD individuals compared to nonhoarding OCD individuals. Riesel, Kathmann, and Endrass[78] also examined the ERN in OCD individuals; however, these authors found an enhanced ERN in low hoarding relative to high hoarding OCD. Of interest, in the same sample, high-hoarding individuals displayed an enhanced ERN relative to healthy individuals. To begin to separate hoarding from OCD in examinations of disordered error monitoring processes, Mathews et al.[69] compared the ERN in HD individuals, OCD individuals, HD-and-OCD individuals, and healthy individuals. Individuals with an HD diagnosis exhibited a reduced ERN independent of the presence of OCD. Of interest, in this sample, HD-and-OCD participants demonstrated an ERN equivalent to that of the HD-only group. This differs from previous data[78], which found that the presence of hoarding symptoms in OCD differentiated the ERN from nonhoarding OCD individuals. Collectively, results of both neuroimaging and electrophysiology studies provide evidence that hoarding may reflect the dysregulation of several neural systems, in particular error-monitoring processes mediated by the ACC.

Genetics

Findings of several recent genetic studies also support the notion that hoarding represents a unique symptom subtype in OCD with a distinctive psychobiological profile. Lochner et al.[61] genotyped individuals with OCD and control participants of Afrikaner descent to investigate certain polymorphisms in genes hypothesized to be relevant to OCD. They reported that there may be a relationship between variation in the catechol-*O*-methyltransferase gene and compulsive hoarding. (Catechol-*O*-methyltransferase is an enzyme involved in the degradation of dopamine, a neurotransmitter with increased activity in OCD.) In another genetic study, Samuels et al.[81] treated compulsive hoarding as the phenotype of interest and stratified families with OCD into those with and without two or more relatives affected with compulsive hoarding. Results of the study suggested that a region on chromosome 14 was linked with compulsive hoarding behavior in families with OCD. Finally, Zhang et al.[115] conducted a genome scan of the hoarding phenotype on 77 sibling pairs who were concordant for a diagnosis of Gilles de la Tourette syndrome. Results of this study suggested joint effects for the hoarding phenotype of specific loci on 5q and 4q. Although the findings of these studies have not been conclusive, collectively they highlight possible regions of interest with respect to genetic correlates of compulsive hoarding.

Cognitive-Behavioral Theory and Evidence

Current cognitive-behavioral conceptualizations[26,94] specify a multidimensional model to explain the core manifestations of compulsive hoarding. Hoarding is posited to develop as a result of conditioned emotional responses associated with certain thoughts and beliefs concerning items or possessions. Acquisition and failure to discard possessions represent avoidance of the anxiety associated with discarding and decision making. In addition, similar to other behavioral addictions, excessive saving behavior is positively reinforced because the possessions attain a pleasurable or comforting quality. The prominent model of compulsive hoarding proposed by Steketee and Frost[94] consists of four main components: information-processing deficits, beliefs about and emotional attachments to possessions, and emotional distress and avoidance behaviors that develop as a result.

Information-Processing Deficits

The cognitive-behavioral model of hoarding suggests that individuals who hoard may possess information-processing deficits that result in confusion or misinterpretation about the value of possessions and difficulty organizing and discarding. Several neuropsychological studies of compulsive hoarding support the notion that there are cognitive deficits associated with this syndrome.

Grisham et al.[48] compared a compulsive hoarding group with a mixed clinical group and a community control group on a number of measures for attention, working memory, and verbal and nonverbal intelligence. They found that those in the hoarding group had intact verbal intelligence and working memory but were impaired on measures of attention and nonverbal intelligence. They also were slow to initiate responses and had difficulty inhibiting impulsive responses. Similarly, Hartl and colleagues[51] found that hoarding adults displayed symptoms consistent with attention-deficit/hyperactivity disorder on a self-report measure. Weaknesses in these neuropsychological domains of attention and nonverbal intelligence may, therefore, limit a hoarding individual's ability to sustain attention during a task (e.g., when deciding what possessions to save or discard) and to organize their possessions and reduce clutter. Other studies have found evidence for indecisiveness[31] and deficits in verbal and nonverbal memory.[53] Mackin et al.[65] compared 78 HD individuals to a healthy comparison group across multiple neuropsychological tests examining memory, reasoning, decision-making and speed-of-processing.

Relative to healthy participants, HD individuals displayed impairment in detecting, remembering, and categorizing visual information. However, when test-by-test comparisons were made within groups, HD displayed relative cognitive strengths in abstract reasoning using both verbal and visual information.

Hoarding behavior also appears to be associated with specific deficits in organizing and categorizing common objects.[63,111] Wincze et al.[111] compared the performance of hoarders with the performances of nonhoarders who had OCD and control participants on a sorting task. They found that participants in the hoarding group were underinclusive (i.e., they sorted the objects into a larger number of categories) compared with control participants. They also took a longer time than the controls to decide in what category the objects belonged, and they reported more distress during the sorting task. This was only true, however, when they were sorting personally relevant objects. These results suggest that the information-processing deficits due to an underinclusive categorization style are not global but are specific to relevant objects. Wincze at al.[111] suggested that a hoarding individual's difficulty categorizing objects may be due to the meaning attached to objects, which influences what features of the object are attended to during a sorting task. Luchian et al.[63] replicated this study with nonclinical hoarding and control participants and found similar results.

There are some inconsistencies in the research on hoarding and associated neuropsychological deficits. Although Grisham et al.[48] found that hoarding individuals displayed relatively intact decision making on a gambling task, Lawrence and colleagues[59] found that hoarding symptoms were associated with specific decision-making impairments on the same gambling task, in addition to poor set shifting on a sorting task. Lawrence et al.[59] suggested that hoarding individuals have difficulty deciding whether to save or discard a possession due to these difficulties in decision making. In addition, the risky behaviors exhibited by hoarding participants suggest that problems with impulse control may contribute to difficulties in decision making. Grisham et al.[48] did observe greater impulsivity in the hoarding group on measures of attention. The discrepancies between these studies are likely due to differences in the samples selected. In the Grisham et al.[48] study, the hoarding group consisted of participants who met the then proposed criteria for HD, regardless of whether they had OCD, while the hoarding group in Lawrence et al.[59] comprised individuals with OCD who also displayed hoarding behaviors.

The recent findings on specific neuropsychological characteristics associated with hoarding may elucidate the relationship between hoarding and addictions. Addictive disorders are characterized by repeated behaviors that are pleasurable to perform. Hoarding may similarly be associated with a pleasurable state upon acquisition of new items, but hoarding behaviors are also viewed as an attempt to avoid the emotional distress associated with discarding.[26] Although the motivations behind the behaviors (pleasure seeking versus distress avoiding) may vary, there is a degree of overlap that may be accounted for by similar neuropsychological deficits. Lubman et al.[62] argued that problematic drug use is associated with decreased inhibitory control, thus compromising decision-making ability. The poor inhibition and decision making are also evident in compulsive hoarding.[48] The deficits observed in hoarding participants on the gambling task[59] have also been found with drug-addicted individuals. Furthermore, these individuals show behavioral responses similar to the hoarding participants observed by Lawrence et al.[59] and individuals with lesions to the orbitofrontal cortex,[4] the same region implicated in positron emission tomographic studies of hoarding individuals. Drug-addicted individuals also show deficits in response inhibition[39] similar to those observed by Grisham et al.[48] with hoarding participants.

Emotional Attachment to Possessions

Maladaptive beliefs and excessive emotional attachment to possessions are also posited to play a central role in the maintenance of compulsive hoarding.[32,92] Research suggests that object-related beliefs cluster into four basic types: emotional attachment to possessions, memory-related concerns, responsibility for possessions, and control over possessions.[92] The beliefs and cognitions associated with excessive saving range from exaggerations of common beliefs, for example, "I need these sentimental possessions to remind me of important events in my life" to more idiosyncratic reasons for saving, for example, "These used Band-Aids are a part of me because they contain my blood." The individual's unrealistic beliefs about possessions are associated with excessive emotional attachment to objects, which leads to delaying or avoiding the process of making decisions and discarding.[25] Being particularly sensitive to anxiety or prone to rash decision-making appears to intensify beliefs about emotional attachment to possessions, which, in turn, exacerbates hoarding behavior.[76]

Excessive attachment to possessions can lead to a sense of grief and loss when individuals with compulsive hoarding are forced to discard items.[11] These reactions can even be comparable to the grief experienced due to the death of a loved one,[26] a finding that accords with a tendency for hoarding individuals to imbue their possessions with human qualities, thereby anthropomorphizing them.[43,98] As these reactions can inevitably provoke anxiety, avoidance of discarding is negatively reinforced because it prevents the experience of these emotions. Anxiety can also arise when others attempt to arrange or utilize a hoarding individual's possessions. Control over possessions appears to be partly related to a heightened sense of responsibility for keeping objects intact and to a sense of personal responsibility for being prepared in the event that an object is required at some point in the future.[27]

Assessment of Compulsive Hoarding

In early hoarding research, many studies used measures of OCD that included hoarding subscales, such as the Yale-Brown Obsessive Compulsive Scale,[40] the Obsessive Compulsive Inventory,[23] and the Obsessive Compulsive Inventory-Revised.[22] Some researchers raised concerns about using these items[91] due to questions about the definition of a hoarding obsession and the inability of these two items to assess many crucial aspects of hoarding behavior. One study of hoarding[75] used the Dimensional version of the Yale-Brown Obsessive Compulsive Scale.[80] This version was designed to assess OCD dimensions (contamination, cleaning, harm, hoarding, symmetry, sexual/religious, and miscellaneous obsessions and compulsions). The Dimensional version of the Yale-Brown Obsessive Compulsive Scale includes a series of clinician-administered scales that can be used to assess the presence and severity of each symptom dimension.

The Obsessive Compulsive Inventory and Obsessive Compulsive Inventory-Revised comprise several symptom subscales including Washing, Checking/Doubting, Obsessing, Mental Neutralizing, Ordering, and Hoarding. Both measures are somewhat better than the Yale-Brown Obsessive Compulsive Scale at assessing hoarding; however, the Hoarding subscales of both the original and revised Obsessive Compulsive Inventory can be problematic. This subscale failed to distinguish clinical from nonanxious controls adequately in the original Obsessive Compulsive Inventory,[23] and the revised inventory has demonstrated weak internal consistency.[49] In addition, Abramowitz and Deacon[1] found that the Obsessive Compulsive Inventory-Revised hoarding subscale correlated only weakly with the other Obsessive Compulsive Inventory-Revised subscales and did not correlate with the Yale-Brown Obsessive Compulsive Scale in a clinical sample of anxious participants. A recent adaption of the Obsessive Compulsive Inventory-Revised added three hoarding questions that better reflect the current DSM-5 criteria for HD, resulting in the OCI-HD. The OCI-HD demonstrated significantly greater diagnostic specificity than the original measure, correctly classifying 93% of clinically significant hoarding cases.[113] Although some concerns remain about the appropriateness of utilizing OCD measures to index hoarding thoughts and behaviors, the new OCI-HD instrument seems to provide a robust identifier of clinically significant hoarding in OCD samples.

Due to growing interest and research in hoarding, several measures have been developed to assess hoarding symptom severity and establish an HD diagnosis. The first systematic attempt to design a scale solely to measure hoarding symptoms was the Hoarding Scale,[25] a 22-item self-report questionnaire that assessed discarding behaviors, emotional reactions to discarding, problems with decisions regarding discarding, concerns over future use of discarded items, and sentimental attachment to possessions. The Hoarding Scale was found to be both reliable and valid in college, clinical, and community samples. In addition, it could discriminate between individuals who reported experiencing hoarding tendencies and community controls.[25] Although it possessed sound psychometric properties, the Hoarding Scale had inherent limitations, as subsequently identified by the primary author.[33] Given the limited information about hoarding behaviors at the time of its development, the Hoarding Scale did not assess all of the components that are now known to be important facets of hoarding, such as excessive acquisition. The scale also confounded beliefs about possessions with behavioral symptoms and included items about specific types of possessions that were not applicable to every individual with hoarding tendencies.[33] In addition, the Hoarding Scale did not adequately assess distress or impairment at the clinical/severe level.[91]

The recognition of the Hoarding Scale's limitations led to the development of a revised measure to address these concerns, the Saving Inventory-Revised[33]—a 23-item self-report questionnaire with three subscales assessing: (1) excessive acquisition of purchased and free items, (2) saving and discarding behaviors, and (3) excessive clutter as a result of these behaviors. The Saving Inventory-Revised has been shown to discriminate between identified hoarders and both nonhoarding controls and nonhoarding OCD cases.[33] The subscales have been shown to correlate with additional indices of hoarding interference, such as activity dysfunction and both self- and observer ratings of clutter in the home.[11,33,100]

There are several other self-report measures of hoarding. One commonly used measure, the Saving Cognitions Inventory,[92] is a 24-item self-report inventory that assesses beliefs and attitudes experienced when a person is trying to discard possessions. On a 7-point Likert scale, participants rate the extent to which a thought influences their decision about whether to discard a possession. The four subscales assess emotional attachment to objects, beliefs about objects as memory aids, responsibility for not wasting possessions, and the need for control over possessions, respectively.

In addition, a few studies have employed the Yale-Brown Obsessive Compulsive Scale: Acquisition and Saving Version,[93] a 10-item self-report measure that is modeled on the Yale-Brown Obsessive Compulsive Scale. The Acquisition and Saving Version indexes the severity of hoarding thoughts and behaviors and the subsequent interference and avoidance. Questions address time spent, distress, interference, and effort and success in resisting thoughts and hoarding behaviors. Finally, the Activities of Daily Living-Hoarding Subscale[94] is a 16-item inventory designed to assess interference in daily activities such as bathing, dressing, and preparing and cooking food due to clutter within the home. Items also assess general conditions within the home such as the presence of rotten food and associated safety/health issues (fire hazard, unsanitary conditions). The Activities of Daily Living-Hoarding Subscale is particularly useful when completed by two raters (e.g., by the hoarder and family member or clinician), as discrepancies between the two ratings can be indicative of poor insight.

Poor insight poses a problem for the assessment of hoarding when using measures that rely on self-disclosure of beliefs and behaviors. As noted previously, individuals with compulsive hoarding demonstrate limited recognition of the problem,[12,21,43,88] with up to 50% failing to recognize their behaviors as being problematic.[37,56] The validity of self-report inventories may, therefore, be compromised. In an effort to address this concern, Frost et al.[35] developed a pictorial measure to index the extent of clutter within the home. The Clutter Image Rating[35] includes nine pictures that vary in rating from 1 (no clutter) to 9 (severe clutter) for a kitchen, a living room, and a bedroom, with a mean composite score calculated across the three rooms (range 1–9). Respondents select the picture that most closely matches the amount of clutter in the corresponding room of their home.

In line with the development of criteria for HD,[2] researchers have developed two diagnostic interviews for HD. The Hoarding Rating Scale (HRS)[101] is a brief 5-item measure that can be administered in interview or questionnaire format. Individuals are asked to rate the severity of acquiring, clutter, difficulty discarding, emotional distress, and life impairment on a scale ranging from 0 (not difficult) to 8 (extremely difficult). The HRS demonstrates good convergent validity with DSM-5 criteria for HD. The Structured Interview for Hoarding Disorder[73] is a comprehensive diagnostic instrument that assesses the extent to which an individual meets each of the DSM-5 criteria and specifiers. The Structured Interview for Hoarding Disorder provides an algorithm for differentiating HD from hoarding related to neurological disease or lesion, OCD, or autism spectrum disorder (ASD), and also contains a risk assessment framework to help the assessor identify immediate threats to health and safety in the individual's home.

Treatment of Compulsive Hoarding

The presence of hoarding symptoms is often a negative predictor of treatment outcome for current treatments that are effective in treating OCD.[9] This is true for both pharmacological and psychological treatments.[5] It has been suggested that this is because those with hoarding problems often refuse treatment and/or are less motivated to engage due to poor insight. It is usually a family member or spouse that pressures the hoarder to seek treatment. Kozak and Foa[57] suggested that traditional treatments for OCD may be less effective because hoarding individuals often display perfectionistic thinking and magical ideas that interfere with the treatment components.

Biological Treatments

Most biological treatments have examined the effect of serotonergic medications on hoarding symptoms. In a study by Mataix-Cols et al.,[66] 150 individuals with OCD were treated with serotonergic reuptake inhibitors across six placebo-controlled medication trials. The authors examined whether different factor structures on the Yale-Brown Obsessive Compulsive Scale checklist predicted treatment response after controlling for baseline severity of symptoms. Only the hoarding dimension of the Yale-Brown Obsessive Compulsive Scale was associated with poorer outcomes on OCD symptom measures, suggesting that hoarding symptoms predict poor treatment outcome.

Winsberg et al.[112] investigated overall symptomatic improvement following treatment with serotonergic reuptake inhibitors in a sample of 20 hoarding individuals. Of the 18 participants who received an adequate trial, half showed an improvement by at least 25% on the Yale-Brown Obsessive Compulsive Scale, with one showing a marked response. It is unclear, however, whether these changes occurred in hoarding symptoms. All participants in the trials had other OCD symptoms, and the improvement in Yale-Brown Obsessive Compulsive Scale scores may have been due to changes in these symptoms. The nine individuals in the study who received CBT intervention for hoarding based on the treatment outline provided by Hartl and Frost[52] appeared to show somewhat greater improvements than those treated with medication alone. In another treatment study by Black et al.,[5] medication and cognitive behavioral treatments were compared with placebo. In a sample of 38 nondepressed individuals with OCD, approximately 18% of those who reported hoarding symptoms responded to treatment, compared with 40% of treatment responders in the nonhoarding group. These results are in accord with the suggestion that hoarding symptoms negatively predict treatment response. Other studies have found that early onset, poor insight, somatic obsessions,[16] sexual obsessions,[80a] and comorbidity[90] are predictors of poor treatment response to medications and not hoarding symptoms. One of these studies,[16] however, did find a statistical trend suggesting that hoarding may have been a negative predictor of treatment response.

Nevertheless, there is some promise for pharmacological and neuromodulatory treatments for hoarding. Recent pharmacotherapy studies[16,85] have found that hoarding individuals do respond, at least to some degree, to medication. Saxena et al.[85] found that hoarding OCD individuals responded as well to the serotonergic reuptake inhibitor medication paroxetine, as did nonhoarding OCD participants, although the treatment response of both groups was suboptimal. More recent trials of the serotonin and noradrenaline reuptake inhibitor venlafaxine-XR (Effexor-XR) have yielded reductions in hoarding symptoms comparable to that with CBT.[87] The inattention difficulties observed among some hoarding individuals[34,50] prompted a pilot trial of methylphenidate (Ritalin) pharmacotherapy. Despite some encouraging improvements in hoarding symptoms, participants found the drug's side effects difficult to tolerate.[79]

Most recently, researchers have examined the efficacy of repetitive transcranial magnetic stimulation (rTMS) protocols in hoarding similar to those that have proven fruitful in the treatment of depression.[13] In a single case study, 30 sessions of rTMS over the right dorsolateral prefrontal cortex led to moderate reductions in hoarding symptom severity, and the individual no longer met DSM-5 criteria for HD.[13] Taken together, recent research provides encouraging evidence that hoarding may respond to biological treatment regimens.

Psychological Treatments

CBT has had wider success in treating hoarding.[103] The current CBT approach is largely based on the model of compulsive hoarding described by Frost and Hartl.[26] Treatment may be in an individual or group format and usually involves therapists visiting clients' homes to complete exposure and discarding exercises.

CBT for hoarding covers five general themes: education about hoarding, improving decision-making capacity, development of an organizational system for possessions, graded exposure to avoidance behaviors, and cognitive restructuring around beliefs about possessions.[94] The exposure sessions are conducted both during sessions, with clients bringing in a selection of possessions, and within the home. Clients are expected to practice making decisions about the category to which possessions belong (i.e., discard, save, or retain for sorting later) and to follow through with these decisions. This exposes them to the emotional distress of discarding and challenges fears about making a mistake, missing information, and being responsible for discarded items. Therapists never touch clients' possessions without permission, so that the client is entirely responsible for the decision-making process. Clients are taught to challenge their beliefs about the emotional significance of their possessions, the cost of making a mistake, the need for perfectionism, and the importance of remembering/having access to information. In addition, they are required to create an organizational system and to categorize possessions that they decide to save based on this system in order to reduce clutter.

Growing evidence indicates that CBT for hoarding is effective but suboptimal in some respects. Hartl and Frost[52] conducted a multiple baseline experimental case study involving an individual with a longstanding hoarding problem. Therapy consisted of the strategies outlined earlier delivered in weekly 2-hour sessions combined with regular homework tasks. After 9 months, there was a reduction in hoarding symptoms, indecisiveness, and nonhoarding OCD symptoms. After 18 months, the targeted living spaces were almost completely free of clutter. Steketee et al.[93] conducted a larger-scale study for seven individuals over 20 weeks. Six of them attended group therapy and had individual home visits, while the seventh received individual home visits using a similar individual treatment applied by Hartl and Frost.[52] Scores on the Yale-Brown Obsessive Compulsive Scale showed some improvement after 15 sessions of treatment. Self-report ratings also improved on recognition of irrational reasons for saving, organization, and decision-making, although clutter was slow to improve. Scores on the Yale-Brown Obsessive Compulsive Scale and self-report measures improved further for participants who continued treatment every 2 weeks for a year.

Saxena et al.[86] reported similar improvement in a group of 20 hoarding individuals with OCD. A large group of individuals with nonhoarding OCD symptoms also received treatment. This included 6-week daily multimodal therapy involving cognitive behavioral therapy, selective serotonin reuptake inhibitor medications, and psychosocial rehabilitation. Scores on the Yale-Brown Obsessive Compulsive Scale following treatment showed improvement for both the hoarding and nonhoarding groups, although the improvement was less marked for the hoarding group. It is notable that improvements in mood and psychosocial functioning were similar for both groups.

Tolin et al.[103] conducted a meta-analysis of 12 treatment studies across individual and group formats, using both trained therapists and peer-support facilitators. CBT led to large reductions in difficulties with discarding, with more modest effects on clutter and excessive acquiring. The average number of sessions ranged from 13 to 35, and more than half of the studies included home visits in their treatment protocol. The number of sessions increased the effectiveness of CBT as did the number of home visits participants received, and studies with a greater proportion of individuals on pharmacotherapy yielded the largest reductions in difficulty discarding. Not all participants responded equally to CBT; younger age predicted a better response, and females benefited more than males. The authors concluded that although CBT for hoarding is effective, its effects are somewhat inconsistent across hoarding behaviors and cohorts.

Overall, research indicates that hoarding does respond to CBT, although improvements are not yet in line with gains observed in nonhoarders with OCD. There are a number of methodological limitations, however, that temper treatment research. First, there is a lack of properly controlled treatment studies that involve allocation to treatment (CBT or medication) and a placebo group. In addition, the focus on OCD-related hoarding measures used in earlier studies makes it difficult to determine whether improvements are due to changes in hoarding symptoms or other nonhoarding OCD symptoms. Up-to-date measures of hoarding symptoms should continue to be used to determine whether treatment is actually targeting hoarding.

Hoarding individuals may be responding relatively poorly to treatment due to a lack of insight and motivation to engage in treatment.[26] For this reason, more recent CBT manuals have incorporated motivational interviewing to increase individuals' insight into their hoarding problems.[94] Tolin et al.[100] reported that homework adherence was a positive predictor of treatment outcome, highlighting the importance of insight and motivation to overcome hoarding problems. Motivational interviewing[72] is often used in the treatment of addictions to resolve ambivalence about change and to help individuals identify the discrepancy between their current behavior and their goals for the future. A meta-analysis of randomized controlled trials examining the efficacy of motivational interviewing[7] found that this technique alone was as effective as other active treatments for problems involving drugs and alcohol, diet, and exercise.

Recent treatment research has directly addressed the cognitive deficits observed in some hoarding individuals. In a pilot study to assess treatment feasibility, DiMauro et al.[14] delivered computer-based cognitive attention training to 10 individuals with a primary HD diagnosis. The participants found the treatment acceptable and demonstrated improvements in visual attention, which generalized to other standardized tasks not targeted by the training. Ayers et al.[3] integrated cognitive remediation techniques into an existing CBT protocol for a group of older adults (mean age 66 years). Again, the cognitive remediation approach was acceptable to all participants, and response to treatment was double that of similar investigations that used only CBT. It appears that cognitive remediation represents an engaging and potentially fruitful addition to hoarding treatment.

Conclusions

In summary, it is useful to view hoarding from an addictions perspective in order to gain new insight into this complex phenomenon. First, this framework encourages us to shift our focus to the positively reinforcing aspects of hoarding behavior, rather than focusing solely on its anxiety-related features. Second, comparing hoarding with other types of behavioral addictions may shed light on some of the underlying neural mechanisms of hoarding, as well some of the cognitive and self-regulation deficits that may be associated with this disorder. Third, some of the challenges encountered in the treatment of hoarding, such as lack of insight or motivation, are common in substance abuse and behavioral addictions. We may be able to turn to this empirical literature for specific clinical strategies, such as motivational interviewing, that have been efficacious in treating addictive disorders.

References

1. Abramowitz JS, Deacon BJ. Psychometric properties and construct validity of the obsessive-compulsive inventory-revised: replication and extension with a clinical sample. 2006;20:1016–1035.
3a. Anderson SW, Damasio, H. Damasio AR. A neural basis for collecting behaviour in humans. *Brain.* 2005;128:201–212.
2. Association AP. *Diagnostic and Statistical Manual of Mental Disorders.* 5th ed. Arlington, VA: American Psychiatric Association; 2013.
3. Ayers CR, Saxena S, Espejo E, Twamley EW, Granholm E, Wetherell JL. Novel treatment for geriatric hoarding disorder: an open trial of cognitive rehabilitation paired with behavior therapy. *Am J Geriatric Psychiatry.* 2014;22:248–252.
3a. Barlow DH. *Anxiety and Its Disorders: The Nature and Treatment of Anxiety and Panic.* New York: Guilford Press, 2004.
4. Bechara A, Damasio H. Decision-making and addiction (part I): impaired activation of somatic states in substance dependent individuals when pondering decisions with negative future. *Neuropsychologia.* 2002;40:1675–1689.
5. Black DW, Monahan P, Gable J, Blum N. Hoarding and treatment response in 38 nondepressed subjects with obsessive-compulsive disorder. *J Clin Psychiatry.* 1998;59(8):420–425.
6. Blanco C, Moreyra P, Nunes EV, Saiz-Ruiz J, Ibanez A. Pathological gambling: addiction or compulsion? *Semin Clin Neuropsychiatry.* 2001;6:167–176.
7. Burke BL, Arkowicz H, Menchola M. The efficacy of motivational interviewing: a meta-analysis of controlled clinical trials. 2003;71:843–861.
8. Calamari JE, Wiegartz PS, Janeck AS. Obsessive–compulsive disorder subgroups: a symptom-based clustering approach. *Behav Res Ther.* 1999;37:113–125.
9. Christensen DD, Greist JH. The challenge of obsessive-compulsive disorder hoarding. *Prim Psychiatry.* 2001;8:79–86.
10. Christenson GA, Faber RJ, Mitchell JE. Compulsive buying: descriptive characteristics and psychiatric comorbidity. *J Clin Psychiatry.* 1994;55(1):5–11
11. Coles ME, Frost RO, Heimberg RG, Steketee G. Hoarding behaviors in a large college sample. *Behav Res Ther.* 2003;41:179–194. https://doi.org/10.1016/S0005-7967(01)00136-X.
12. Damecour CL, Charron M. Hoarding: a symptom, not a syndrome. *J Clin Psychiatry.* 1998;59:267–272.
13. Diefenbach GJ, Tolin DF, Hallion LS, et al. A case study of clinical and neuroimaging outcomes following repetitive transcranial magnetic stimulation for hoarding disorder. *Am J Psychiatry.* 2015;172:1160–1162. https://doi.org/10.1176/appi.ajp.2015.15060750.
14. DiMauro J, Genova M, Tolin DF, Kurtz MM. Cognitive remediation for neuropsychological impairment in hoarding disorder_ A pilot study. *J Obsessive Compuls Relat Disord.* 2014;3:132–138. https://doi.org/10.1016/j.jocrd.2014.03.006.
15. Doñamayor N, Heilbronner U, Münte TF. Coupling electrophysiological and hemodynamic responses to errors. *Hum Brain Mapp.* 2011;33:1621–1633. https://doi.org/10.1002/hbm.21305.
16. Erzegovesi S, Cavallini MC, Cavedini P, Diaferia G, Locatelli M, Bellodi L. Clinical predictors of drug response in obsessive-compulsive disorder. *J Clin Psychopharmacol.* 2001;21:488–492.
17. Eslinger PJ, Damasio AR. Severe disturbance of higher cognition after bilateral frontal lobe ablation Patient *EVR. Neurology.* 1985;35. 1731–1731.
18. Faber RJ, O'Guinn TC. A clinical screener for compulsive buying. *J Consum Res.* 2001;19:459–469.
19. Falkenstein M, Hoormann J, Christ S, Hohnsbein J. ERP components on reaction errors and their functional significance: a tutorial. *Biol Psychol.* 2000;51:87–107.
20. Finkel S, Costa G, Silva E, Cohen G, Miller S, Sartorius N. Behavioral and psychological signs and symptoms of dementia: a consensus statement on current knowledge and implications for research and treatment. *Int J Geriat Psychiatry.* 1997;12:1060–1061.
21. Fitzgerald PB. *The Bowerbird Symptom': A Case of Severe Hoarding of Possessions.* Vols. 1–4; 2007.
22. Foa EB, Huppert JD, Leiberg S, et al. The Obsessive-Compulsive Inventory: development and validation of a short version. *Psychol Assess.* 2002;14:485–496.
23. Foa EB, Kozak MJ, Salkovskis PM, Coles ME, Amir N. The validation of a new obsessive–compulsive disorder scale: the obsessive–compulsive inventory. *Psychol Assess.* 1998;10:206.
24. Frankenburg FR. Hoarding in anorexia nervosa. *Br J Med Psychol.* 1984;57:57–60.
25. Frost RO, Gross RC. The hoarding of possesions. *Behav Res Ther.* 1993;31:367–381.
26. Frost RO, Hartl TL. A cognitive behavioral model of compulsive hoarding. *Behav Res Ther.* 1996;34:341–350.
27. Frost RO, Hartl TL, Christian R, Williams N. The value of possessions in compulsive hoarding: patterns of use and attachment. *Behav Res Ther.* 1995;33:897–902.
28. Frost RO, Kim HJ, Morris C, Bloss C, Murray-Close M, Steketee G. Hoarding, compulsive buying and reasons for saving. *Behav Res Ther.* 1998;36:657–664. https://doi.org/10.1016/S0005-7967(98)00056-4.
29. Frost RO, Krause MS, Steketee G. Hoarding and obsessive-compulsive symptoms. *Behav Modif.* 1996;20:116–132.
30. Frost RO, Meagher BM, Riskind JH. Obsessive-compulsive features in pathological lottery and scratch-ticket gamblers. *J Gambl Stud.* 2001;17:5–19.
31. Frost RO, Shows DL. The nature and measurement of compulsive indecisiveness. *Behav Res Ther.* 1993;31:683–692.
32. Frost RO, Steketee G. Hoarding: clinical aspects and treatment strategies. *Obsessive-Compul Disord Pract Manag.* 1998.
33. Frost RO, Steketee G, Grisham J. Measurement of compulsive hoarding: saving inventory-revised. *Behav Res Ther.* 2004;42:1163–1182. https://doi.org/10.1016/j.brat.2003.07.006.
34. Frost RO, Steketee G, Tolin DF. Comorbidity in hoarding disorder. *Depress Anxiety.* 2011;28:876–884. https://doi.org/10.1002/da.20861.
35. Frost RO, Steketee G, Tolin DF, Renaud S. Development and validation of the clutter image rating. *J Psychopathol Behav Assess.* 2007;30:193–203. https://doi.org/10.1007/s10862-007-9068-7.
36. Frost RO, Steketee G, Williams L. Compulsive buying, compulsive hoarding, and obsessive-compulsive disorder. *Behav Ther.* 2002;33:201–214.
37. Frost RO, Steketee G, Williams LF, Warren R. Mood, personality disorder symptoms, and disability in obsessive-compulsive hoarders: a comparison with clinical and nonclinical controls. *Behav Res Ther.* 2000;38:1071–1081.
38. Frost RO, Steketee GS, Williams L. Hoarding: a community health problem. *Health Soc Care Community.* 2000;8:229–234.
39. Goldstein RZ, Volkow ND, Wang G-J, Fowler JS, Rajaram S. Addiction changes orbitofrontal gyrus function: involvement in response inhibition. *Neuroreport.* 2001;12:2595.
40. Goodman WK, Price LH, Rasmussen SA, et al. The yale-brown obsessive compulsive scale I. Development, use, and reliability. *Archiv Gen Psychiarty.* 1989;46:1006–1011.
41. Grant JE, Mancebo MC, Pinto A, Eisen JL, Rasmussen SA. Impulse control disorders in adults with obsessive compulsive disorder. *J Psychiatric Res.* 2006;40:494–501.
42. Grant JE, Potenza MN. Impulse control disorders: clinical characteristics and pharmacological management. *Annals Clin Psychiatry.* 2004;16:27–34.

43. Greenberg D. Compulsive hoarding. *Am J Psychother.* 1987;41:409–416.

44. Greenberg D, Witzum E, Levy A. Hoarding as a psychiatric syndrome. *J Clin Psychiatry.* 1990;51:417–421.

45. Grisham J, Baldwin P. Neuropsychological and neurophysiological insights into hoarding disorder. *NDT.* 2015;11:951–962. https://doi.org/10.2147/NDT.S62084.

46. Grisham JR, Brown TA, Liverant GI, Campbell-Sills L. The distinctiveness of compulsive hoarding from obsessive–compulsive disorder. *J Anxiety Disord.* 2005;19:767–779. https://doi.org/10.1016/j.janxdis.2004.09.003.

47. Grisham JR, Brown TA, Liverant GI, Campbell-Sills L. The distinctiveness of compulsive hoarding from obsessive–compulsive disorder. *J Anxiety Disord.* 2005;19:767–779. https://doi.org/10.1016/j.janxdis.2004.09.003.

48. Grisham JR, Brown TA, Savage CR, Steketee G, Barlow DH. Neuropsychological impairment associated with compulsive hoarding. *Behav Res Ther.* 2007;45:1471–1483. https://doi.org/10.1016/j.brat.2006.12.008.

49. Hajcak G, Huppert JD, Simons RF, Foa EB. Psychometric properties of the OCI-R in a college sample. *Behav Res Ther.* 2004;42:115–123.

50. Hall BJ, Tolin DF, Frost RO, Steketee G. An exploration of the comorbid symptoms and clinical correlates of clinically significant hoarding symptoms. *Depress Anxiety.* 2012;30:67–76. https://doi.org/10.1002/da.22015.

51. Hartl TL, Duffany S, Allen G, Steketee GS, Frost RO. Relationships among compulsive hoarding, trauma, and attention-deficit/hyperactivity disorder. *Behav Res Ther.* 2005;43:269–276. https://doi.org/10.1016/j.brat.2004.02.002.

52. Hartl TL, Frost RO. Cognitive-behavioral treatment of compulsive hoarding: a multiple baseline experimental case study. *Behav Res Ther.* 1999;37:451–461.

53. Hartl TL, Frost RO, Allen GJ, et al. Actual and perceived memory deficits in individuals with compulsive hoarding. *Depress Anxiety.* 2004;20:59–69. https://doi.org/10.1002/da.20010.

54. Hollander E. Obsessive-compulsive spectrum disorders: an overview. *Psychiatr Ann.* 1993;23:355–358.

55. Hollander E, Allen A. Is compulsive buying a real disorder, and is it really compulsive? *Am J Psychiatry.* 2006;163(10):1670–1672.

56. Kim H-J, Steketee G, Frost RO. Hoarding by elderly people. *Health Soc Work.* 2001;26:176–184.

57. Kozak MJ, Foa EB. *Mastery of Obsessive-Compulsive Disorder: A Cognitive-Behavioral Approach.* Oxford University Press; 2005.

58. Kyrios M, Frost RO, Steketee G. Cognitions in compulsive buying and acquisition. *Cognitive Therapy and Research.* 2004;28:241–258. https://doi.org/10.1023/b:cotr.0000021543.62799.32.

59. Lawrence NS, Wooderson S, Mataix-Cols D, David R, Speckens A, Phillips ML. Decision making and set shifting impairments are associated with distinct symptom dimensions in obsessive-compulsive disorder. *Neuropsychology.* 2006;20:409–419.

60. Leckman JF, Grice DE, Boardman J, et al. Symptoms of obsessive-compulsive disorder. *Am J Psychiatry.* 1997;154:911–917.

61. Lochner C, Kinnear CJ, Hemmings SM, et al. Hoarding in obsessive-compulsive disorder: clinical and genetic correlates. *J Clin Psychiatry.* 2005;66:1155–1160.

62. Lubman DI, Yücel M, Pantelis C. Addiction, a condition of compulsive behaviour? Neuroimaging and neuropsychological evidence of inhibitory dysregulation. *Addiction.* 2004;99:1491–1502.

63. Luchian S, McNally R, Hooley J. Cognitive aspects of nonclinical obsessive–compulsive hoarding☆. *Behav Res Ther.* 2007;45:1657–1662. https://doi.org/10.1016/j.brat.2006.08.014.

64. Luchins DJ, Goldman MB, Lieb M, Hanrahan P. Repetitive behaviors in chronically institutionalized schizophrenic patients. *Schizophrenia Res.* 1992;8:119–123.

65. Mackin RS, Vigil O, Insel P, et al. Patterns of clinically significant cognitive impairment in hoarding disorder. *Depress Anxiety.* 2016;33(3):211–218.

66. Mataix-Cols D, Matai RSL, Manzo PA, Jenike MA, Baer L. Use of factor-analyzed symptom dimensions to predict outcome with serotonin reuptake inhibitors and placebo in the treatment of obsessive-compulsive disorder. *Am J Psychiatry.* 1999;156:1409–1416.

67. Mataix-Cols D, Wooderson S, Lawrence N, Brammer MJ, Speckens A, Phillips ML. Distinct neural correlates of washing, checking, and hoarding symptom dimensionsin obsessive-compulsive disorder. *Archiv Gen Psychiarty.* 2004;61:564–576.

68. Mathews CA, Perez VB, Delucchi KL, Mathalon DH. Error-related negativity in individuals with obsessive–compulsive symptoms: toward an understanding of hoarding behaviors. *Biol Psychol.* 2012;89:487–494. https://doi.org/10.1016/j.biopsycho.2011.12.018.

69. Mathews CA, Perez VB, Roach BJ, et al. Error-related brain activity dissociates hoarding disorder from obsessive-compulsive disorder. *Psychol Med.* 2016;46(2):367–379.

70. McElroy SL, Keck PE, Phillips KA. Kleptomania, compulsive buying, and binge-eating disorder. *J Clin Psychiatry.* 1995;56:14–26.

71. McElroy SL, Keck PE Jr, Pope HG Jr, Smith JM, Strakowski SM. Compulsive buying: a report of 20 cases. 1994;55:242–248.

72. Miller WR, Rollnick S, Moyers TB. *Motivational Interviewing.* University of New Mexico; 1998.

73. Nordsletten AE, Fernandez De La Cruz L, Pertusa A, et al. *The Structured Interview for Hoarding Disorder (SIHD): Development, Further Validation, and Pragmatic Use*; 2013:1–10; Submitted for publication.

74. O'Guinn TC, Faber RJ. Compulsive buying: a phenomenological exploration. 198916:147–157.

75. Pertusa A, Fullana MA, Singh S, Alonso P, Menchon JM, Mataix-Cols D. Compulsive hoarding: OCD symptom, distinct clinical syndrome, or both? *Am J Psychiatry.* 2008;165:1289–1298. https://doi.org/10.1176/appi.ajp.2008.07111730.

76. Phung PJ, Moulding R, Taylor JK, Nedeljkovic M. Emotional regulation, attachment to possessions and hoarding symptoms. *Scand J Psychol.* 2015. https://doi.org/10.1111/sjop.12239.

77. Rasmussen JL, Brown TA, Steketee GS, Barlow DH. Impulsivity in hoarding. *J Obsessive Compuls Relat Disord.* 2013;2:183–191. https://doi.org/10.1016/j.jocrd.2013.02.004.

78. Riesel A, Kathmann N, Endrass T. Overactive performance monitoring in obsessive–compulsive disorder is independent of symptom expression. *Eur Arch Psychiatry Clin Neurosci.* 2014;264(8):707–717.

79. Rodriguez CI, Bender Jr J, Morrison S. Does extended release methylphenidate help adults with hoarding disorder? A case series. *J Clin Psychopharmacol.* 2013;33:444–447.

80. Rosario-Campos MC, Miguel EC, Quatrano S, et al. The dimensional yale–brown obsessive–compulsive scale (DY-BOCS): an instrument for assessing obsessive–compulsive symptom dimensions. *Mol Psychiatry.* 2006;11:495–504.

80a. Rufer M, Fricke S, Moritz, S, et al. Symptom dimensions in obsessive–compulsive disorder: prediction of cognitive-behavior therapy outcome. *Acta Psychiatrica Scandinavica.* 2006;13:440–446.

81. Samuels J, Shugart YY, Grados MA, et al. Significant linkage to compulsive hoarding on chromosome 14 in families with obsessive-compulsive disorder: results from the OCD collaborative genetics study. *Am J Psychiatry.* 2007;164(3):493–499.

82. Samuels JF, Bienvenu OJ, Grados MA, et al. Prevalence and correlates of hoarding behavior in a community-based sample. *Behav Res Ther.* 2008;46:836–844. https://doi.org/10.1016/j.brat.2008.04.004.

83. Samuels JF, Samue, Bienvenu III OJ, Riddle MA, et al. Hoarding in obsessive-compulsive disorder: results from a case-control study. *Behav Res Ther.* 2002;40:517–528.

84. Saxena S, Brody AL, Maidment KM. Cerebral glucose metabolism in obsessive-compulsive hoarding. *Am J Psychiatry.* 2004;161(6):1038–1048.

85. Saxena S, Brody AL, Maidment KM, Baxter Jr LR. Paroxetine treatment of compulsive hoarding. *J Psychiatric Res.* 2007;41:481–487. https://doi.org/10.1016/j.jpsychires.2006.05.001.

86. Saxena S, Maidment KM, Vapnik T, et al. Obsessive-compulsive hoarding: symptom severity and response to multimodal treatment. *J Clin Psychiatry*. 2002.

87. Saxena S, Sumner J. Venlafaxine extended-release treatment of hoarding disorder. *Int Clin Psychopharmacol*. 2014;29:266–273.

88. Shafran R, Tallis F. Obsessive-compulsive hoarding: a cognitive-behavioural approach. *Behav Cognit Psychother*. 1996;24:209–221.

89. Shaw AM, Timpano KR, Steketee G, Tolin DF, Frost RO. Hoarding and emotional reactivity: the link between negative emotional reactions and hoarding symptomatology. *J Psychiatric Res*. 2015;63:84–90. https://doi.org/10.1016/j.jpsychires.2015.02.009.

90. Shetti CN, Reddy YJ, Kandavel T, et al. Clinical predictors of drug nonresponse in obsessive-compulsive disorder. *J Clin Psychiatry*. 2005;66:1517–1523.

91. Steketee G, Frost R. Compulsive hoarding: current status of the research. *Clin Psychol Rev*. 2003;23:905–927. https://doi.org/10.1016/j.cpr.2003.08.002.

92. Steketee G, Frost RO, Kyrios M. Cognitive aspects of compulsive hoarding. *Cognit Ther Res*. 2003;27:463–479.

93. Steketee G, Frost RO, Wincze J, Greene KA, Douglass H. Group and individual treatment of compulsive hoarding: a pilot study. *Behav Cognit Psychother*. 2000;28:259–268.

94. Steketee GS, Frost RO. *Compulsive Hoarding and Acquiring: Therapist Guide*. USA: Oxford: University Press; 2006.

95. Tavares H, Gentil V. Pathological gambling and obsessive-compulsive disorder: towards a spectrum of disorders of volition. *Rev Brasil Psiquiatria*. 2007;29:107–117.

96. Timpano KR, Buckner JD, Richey JA, Murphy DL, Schmidt NB. Exploration of anxiety sensitivity and distress tolerance as vulnerability factors for hoarding behaviors. *Depress Anxiety*. 2009;26:343–353. https://doi.org/10.1002/da.20469.

97. Timpano KR, Exner C, Glaesmer H, et al. The Epidemiology of the proposed DSM-5 hoarding disorder. *J Clin Psychiatry*. 2011;72:780–786. https://doi.org/10.4088/JCP.10m06380.

98. Timpano KR, Shaw AM. Conferring humanness: the role of anthropomorphism in hoarding. *Pers Individ Dif*. 2013;54:383–388.

99. Timpano KR, Shaw AM, Cougle JR, Fitch KE. A multifaceted assessment of emotional tolerance and intensity in hoarding. *Behav Ther*. 2014;45:690–699. https://doi.org/10.1016/j.beth.2014.04.002.

100. Tolin DF, Frost RO, Steketee G. An open trial of cognitive-behavioral therapy for compulsive hoarding. *Behav Res Ther*. 2007;45:1461–1470. https://doi.org/10.1016/j.brat.2007.01.001.

101. Tolin DF, Frost RO, Steketee G. A brief interview for assessing compulsive hoarding: the hoarding rating scale-interview. *Psychiatry Res*. 2010;178:147–152. https://doi.org/10.1016/j.psychres.2009.05.001.

102. Tolin DF, Frost RO, Steketee G, Gray KD, Fitch KE. The economic and social burden of compulsive hoarding. *Psychiatry Res*. 2008;160:200–211. https://doi.org/10.1016/j.psychres.2007.08.008.

103. Tolin DF, Frost RO, Steketee G, Muroff J. Cognitive behavioral therapy for hoarding disorder: a meta-analysis. *Depress Anxiety*. 2015;32:158–166. https://doi.org/10.1002/da.22327.

104. Tolin DF, Stevens MC, Nave A, Villavicencio AL, Morrison S. Neural mechanisms of cognitive behavioral therapy response in hoarding disorder: a pilot study. *J Obsessive Compuls Relat Disord*. 2012;1:180–188. https://doi.org/10.1016/j.jocrd.2012.04.001.

105. Tolin DF, Stevens MC, Villavicencio AL, et al. Neural mechanisms of decision making in hoarding disorder. *Arch Gen Psychiatry*. 2012;69:832–841.

106. Volkow ND, Hitzemann R, Wang GJ, et al. Long-term frontal brain metabolic changes in cocaine abusers. 1992;11:184–190.

107. Volkow ND, Mullani N, Mull, Gould KL, Adler S, Krajewski K. Cerebral blood flow in chronic cocaine users: a study with positron emission tomography. *Br J Psychiatry*. 1988;152:641–648.

108. Volkow ND, Wang GJ, Fowler JS, et al. Decreased striatal dopaminergic responsiveness in detoxified cocaine-dependent subjects. *Nature*. 1997;386(6627):830–833.

109. Wessel JR. Error awareness and the error-related negativity: evaluating the frst decade of evidence. *Front Hum Neurosci*. 2012;6:88.

110. Williams AD, Grisham JR. Impulsivity, emotion regulation, and mindful attentional focus in compulsive buying. *Cognit Ther Res*. 2012;36:451–457. https://doi.org/10.1007/s10608-011-9384-9.

111. Wincze JP, Steketee G, Frost RO. Categorization in compulsive hoarding. *Behav Res Ther*. 2007;45:63–72. https://doi.org/10.1016/j.brat.2006.01.012.

112. Winsberg ME, Cassic KS, Koran LM. Hoarding in obsessive-compulsive disorder: a report of 20 cases. *J Clin Psychiatry*. 1999;60:591–597.

113. Wootton BM, Diefenbach GJ, Bragdon LB, Steketee G, Frost RO, Tolin DF. A contemporary psychometric evaluation of the obsessive compulsive inventory—revised (OCI-R). *Psychol Assess*. 2015;27:874–882. https://doi.org/10.1037/pas0000075.

114. Wu KD, Watson D. Hoarding and its relation to obsessive–compulsive disorder. *Behav Res Ther*. 2005;43:897–921. https://doi.org/10.1016/j.brat.2004.06.013.

115. Zhang H, Leckman JF, Pauls DL, et al. Genomewide scan of hoarding in sib pairs in which both sibs have Gilles de la Tourette syndrome. *Am J Hum Gen*. 2002;70:896–904.

39

Motivational Interviewing: Emerging Theory, Research, and Practice

KAREN S. INGERSOLL AND CHRISTOPHER C. WAGNER

CHAPTER OUTLINE

What Is Motivational Interviewing?

Motivational interviewing (MI) is a therapeutic approach used to explore and resolve ambivalence about behavior change. There is a strong evidence base to suggest that it reduces substance use problems and a growing evidence base for other problems. MI is an empathic therapeutic approach that explores and resolves lingering ambivalence about change. The clinician intentionally pursues the resolution of ambivalence and initiation of positive change as central goals, while maintaining focus on the client's concerns, perceptions, hopes, and goals rather than on those of the provider. MI communications are primarily reflections, open questions, and affirmations, avoiding an expert stance implied by a clinician-centered therapeutic agenda and heavy use of closed questions, information-provision, and advice. Thus while focusing on and eliciting the client's perceptions, the MI clinician explores areas of unresolved ambivalence and guides the client to resolve them to improve the client's life.

MI was first described as a way to work with people having problems with drinking.[49] From an MI perspective, addiction is viewed as "fundamentally a problem of motivation"[51] (p. 134). Cravings, urges, temptations, expectancies, problem recognition, perceived social norms and contingencies, perceived importance of and ability to change, and other addiction-related constructs all have significant motivational components. The development of addiction involves a process of diminishing volitional control of the addictive behaviors involved. As addiction intensifies, capacity for self-regulation diminishes—never below retrievable levels, but enough that it becomes ever more difficult for the person to consistently behave in consciously chosen ways.[50]

Along the pathway to addiction, people often have mixed feelings and thoughts about their drug and alcohol use. Although they may perceive some negative consequences of drinking or using, they also enjoy positive experiences such as intoxication, disinhibition, socialization, and pleasure. Alternatively, they may strongly want to change but feel unable. Whether mild or more extreme, these ambivalence conflicts often remain unresolved for years before significant changes are made. Understanding and resolving this ambivalence is a central goal of MI and is accomplished through elicitation rather than persuasion. Clinicians elicit the client's ideas and feelings about the current behavior, how the behavior fits in with their values, and what changes they might make to move toward a better future. The provider elicits the client's own motives and rationale for possible change, referred to in MI research as "change talk." In essence, MI is focused more on the *whether* and *why* to change than on the *how*.

Because MI is a therapy with a humanistic core, the basis of its conceptualization of addiction is that a person's process of natural growth and development is being blocked and that the person has become stuck. The process of helping the person is not one of curing a disorder or altering a learning history, but of enabling growth and development.[66] Like releasing a river that has become dammed, the process of helping may be as simple as opening up a channel to allow the flow to begin again; the river itself often takes care of the rest. Unresolved ambivalence makes up the core of the dam, slowing the river's momentum. Removing the barrier of unresolved ambivalence allows for a return to the natural flow toward health and well-being.

The counseling style used in MI is "quiet and eliciting" and the "therapeutic relationship is more like a partnership....than expert/recipient roles." [67] The spirit of MI may be more important than techniques, per se. The MI spirit is one of collaboration between two experts, the client having intimate knowledge of the self and the provider having skill in guiding conversations so that clarity of purpose emerges along with an increased sense of empowerment to take action. The spirit of MI is based on a respect and admiration for the client's autonomy, which is manifested as explicit support for the client's ability and authority to consider options, make choices, and take action. Finally, the spirit of MI is evocative. Clinicians explore and reflect the client's perceptions in such a way that a new understanding or commitment is evoked through the conversation. The provider explores the client's own concerns and elicits from the client a desire for change and a working plan to make it happen in a way that the client feels optimistic about it.

Although the clinician has a goal of facilitating the exploration and resolution of ambivalence, and may have ideas about promising directions, the provider is not attached to any single, specific outcome or pathway to get there. By remaining focused on the client's concerns and ideas about change, clinicians can assess the client's current readiness to change and tailor the strategies they use.

The relational stance in MI is one of respect and collaboration. MI clinicians believe that clients have expertise on themselves that can be used to make healthy changes. Using this approach, clinicians elicit more information than they provide. The client does more of the talking, explaining, exploring, and considering. Complementing the client's effort, the provider offers reflections, questions, and summaries, while affirming the client's work. Clinicians using the MI approach tend to ask rather than tell, and to listen rather than advise. MI clinicians show curiosity rather than content expertise, even when they have substantial expertise in the area of the client's concern. It is more important that the MI clinician focus on developing an understanding of the client's perspective rather than providing information, education, or persuasion, all of which may provoke resistance or reluctance.

MI practice builds upon this collaborative relationship with a basic communication style that is used throughout consultation or counseling sessions. The style is summarized with the acronym OARS—*O*pen questions that encourage further elaboration and consideration, *A*ffirmations that foster positive feelings in the consultation, *R*eflections that indicate that the provider has heard and accurately understood the client, and *S*ummaries that extend the basic reflections to include a sense of momentum or build interest in changing direction. These fundamental techniques are used to build rapport and gain understanding of a client's issues, to mend rifts in the treatment relationship, to redirect clients to more useful areas of consideration, and to solidify commitment to change in an established relationship where therapeutic alliance is strongly present.

In addition to the emphasis on using OARS as a basic communication style, MI clinicians use broader conversational strategies in the context of four general therapeutic processes: engaging, focusing, evoking, and planning.[55]

Engaging

MI is dependent on the development of a collaborative relationship between practitioner and client. Without this, the motivational influence of MI is likely to be quite limited. In MI, the engaging process involves two essential elements: (1) engaging them in a conversation that facilitates the process of self-exploration and disclosure; and (2) engaging them in a trusting, collaborative relationship focused on developing a shared understanding of the client's inner life as it relates to making positive changes. Good engagement brings clients to a place of openness and nondefensiveness. Clients let go of early questions they may have about the practitioner, the process of counseling, whether they will be looked down on or supported, how safe it is to reveal what they really think and do, and to what extent have they been telling themselves lies or half-truths about a stigmatized habit, pattern, or way of being. With these questions answered or at least made less prominent in clients' minds, they can more honestly and carefully consider their current situation and their options to move forward toward a better future.

Engagement is fostered through a skillful mix of open questions and reflections that highlight client experiences and perspectives. Engagement can be undermined when clinicians focus prematurely on issues that clients may feel defensive or vulnerable about before establishing a relatively strong therapeutic bond and a pattern of openness in discussion. Client engagement is also threatened when clinicians take an expert stance, in which the client's role is to simply report on problems, answer questions, provide information, and wait for the professional to sort out, solve, and render advice on how best to resolve the problems at hand. Beginning a clinical encounter with extensive assessment is especially risky as it combines both traps, pressing clients to discuss private and sensitive issues before a bond develops and putting them in the role of disempowered reporters who are simply to provide information to the expert on which to make a determination. When using MI, it may be best to delay any intensive assessment of clinical problems until after an initial conversation, and even then to sandwich the assessment between two brief MI-style conversations focusing more on the client's concerns, interests, and hopes.

Although we present engagement as the first process, following Miller and Rollnick,[55] it is important to highlight that it is not intended as a phase of treatment but as a therapeutic process that one may need to bring to the front at various points throughout treatment, when opening a new session or topic, when deepening the focus, and whenever clients are not fully engaged in an MI-style conversation and become defensive, detached, overwhelmed, or intellectualized. In these moments, returning to a focus on engaging can help reestablish the therapeutic bond and diminish whatever internal experience is threatening the client's sense of well-being and preventing them from engaging in an open, productive discussion.

Focusing

The second process, focusing, primarily involves the mutual discovery of the direction of client change and intended goals involved in making a change. Clients may initially present with a very clear direction and intended outcome. If so, the process of focusing is primarily about developing a shared understanding of what the client already knows. At other times, multiple change priorities may compete with one another, and focusing involves helping clients explore and sort those, as well as decide whether multiple discrete changes may be better bundled together in a broader program of change. Becoming more assertive is a broader theme that may be more readily addressed than focusing on each distinct situation in which the client feels unable to speak up, defend himself or herself, set limits, and so on. "Quitting use of all psychoactive substances" may be clearer and more attainable than "quitting smoking, reducing drinking, and moderating caffeine intake."

One strategy for focusing is *agenda mapping*. This is typically used when clients present with multiple competing issues. Agenda mapping involves having a metaconversation—stepping out of focusing on particular concerns or possibilities and instead having a discussion that attempts to sort out how to proceed forward. This involves first setting the stage to have the conversation, then developing a list of possible focus areas, then focusing on topics that could use fleshing out to establish a better understanding, then returning to a birds-eye view to examine how the topics fit together and to develop a plan for the journey ahead, deciding which topics/challenges to address first, second, at a later time, and so on. As the practitioner moves forward through the topics, he or she can wind the way back to the big picture to check if the priorities remain the same and adjust the plan as needed. Practitioners can also return to mapping if a topic of focus gets overly complex, seems unresolvable, or requires approaching in discrete steps with breaks in between, or if the topic is one that is emotionally intense.

Other clients may have no specific change goals or targets set, and only a vague sense of dissatisfaction, or a stronger sense of depression or anxiety, but these feelings seem disconnected from behavior. In these times, MI practitioners might shift from focusing on problems to focusing on possibilities, strengths, and successes. A given client may not be able to clearly define what the problem is for them or may have a clearly identified clinical issue such as maladaptive substance use, yet remain unable to perceive that to be a problem or not seem particularly ready to change it. Instead of engaging in guesswork regarding what problems might exist or risking ending up on opposing sides of ambivalence around clinical issues that clearly do exist, MI practitioners may shift the focus of conversation in a way that sidesteps the risk. For example, the client may be invited to *look back* and remember times that were better, or to recount some past successes about which he or she feels proud. The practitioner may invite the client to explore good things about his or her current situation, using that as a springboard for then inviting the client to identify what could be better. MI practitioners might also explore client-identified *strengths*, shifting the conversation toward more positive ground, and then eliciting ways in which clients could more intentionally utilize their strengths in their current situation. Or clients can be invited to look forward and *envision* a desired future, exploring imagined possibilities in order to make them seem more real and then utilizing the vision and emotional reactions to it as motivation to pull the client forward toward a better future. Alternatively, practitioners can broaden the conversation to have a more vague focus, a general sense of improvement, or happiness or satisfaction, and then narrow the conversation by inviting clients to begin to imagine what might lead them to greater fulfillment, thus returning to a clinical focus.

Finally, when practitioners and clients have different ideas about what to focus on or different opinions about which direction the client should pursue or how to go about it, the MI model cautions practitioners to monitor their "righting reflex," or their desires to fix things that are not going well in clients' lives. For example, clients may want to focus on specific circumstances that led to an arrest, while clinicians may think it more important to discuss the drinking and using patterns that led up to the event and that may lead to similar events in the future. Or a client may want to talk about apparent unfairness of cannabis laws or injustices in the criminal justice system, while the provider may want to focus on connections between the client's cannabis use and his or her inconsistent work history. Rather than fall into the righting reflex trap, practitioners may be better served by broadening the focus in a way that includes both concerns (e.g., the circumstances of the arrest as well as other circumstances in which no arrest occurred), finding subtle connections between the areas and then working forward by inviting the client to explore things in such a way that both focus areas become integrated into the discussion.

Regardless of which situation fits a specific client, the goal is to join them where they are and work together toward next steps.

Evoking

The third process is evoking, specifically evoking clients' motivation to change. For many clients with addiction problems, the benefits, drawbacks, and risks for continued substance use are generally well-known to them. There are genuinely few clients who are likely to be unaware of hazards and risks, and perhaps, unlike behavior change in other domains, there is generally little benefit in further provision of information about their situation, condition, or the possible future pathways available to them. Extrinsic motivation is simply not very motivating for people with substance use problems. Thus MI typically deemphasizes provision of general information or specific advice and emphasizes instead the process of eliciting clients' perspective and their own autonomous motivations to change. It does so by focusing attention on clients' values, preferences, hopes, and desires. Long-term change occurs when it is substantially motivated by these internal factors, independently chosen by the person, even though there may be external reinforcers involved (cf., self-determination theory; Markland et al.[47]).

The process of evoking is the core of motivational interviewing. Key tasks include *eliciting and responding to change talk* in order to build momentum toward making positive change, accepting and responding to sustain talk in ways that prevent either defensiveness or inertia, enhancing hope for success, and heightening clients' awareness of any discrepancies between their current choices and their goals or values in order to encourage greater convergence. Evidence (reviewed later) is accumulating that the counselor's therapeutic style and focus on eliciting and reinforcing change talk do in fact increase change talk, commitment to change, and subsequent action.

Two overarching strategies in the process of evoking client motivation in MI focus on increasing perceived *importance of making changes* and increased perceived *confidence about making changes.*

A number of simple strategies can be used to increase clients' sense of the importance of making changes. First, practitioners can explore the good and less good things about a current problematic habit like substance use. While exploring the status quo side of ambivalence (good things about staying the same, bad things about changing) may not be necessary and may be contraindicated for some clients, for others, particularly those who are defensive about their use, it can increase practitioners' understanding of client perspectives, help clients open up and bond with the practitioner, allow clients to vent so that they can then more productively consider change, and help identify potential obstacles that may arise later on in change attempts. Evocative questions focused on the subtypes of change talk related to importance (desire, reasons, needs) are simple strategies to help clients consider change. Such questions could include

- How would you like things to be different? (desire)
- What are some ways things could be better if you decided to quit drinking? (reasons)
- What would you say is the most important thing you could do now to prevent things from getting worse in the future? (need)

Practitioners can also do *importance scaling,* in which they ask the client to rate the importance of making a change on a scale from 0 to 10, and then follow-up by asking, "What makes your rating X instead of 0 (or another lower number)?" thus eliciting change talk (the client saying out loud what is important about making a change). *Looking back,* mentioned previously, can also be used to help clients remember how life was before problems developed (if relevant to their situation), thus eliciting motivation to regain what has been lost. *Envisioning* a better future can also increase clients' sense of importance of making a change. Finally, exploring client *values* can help identify discrepancies between their cherished values and the way they are actually living, or, in a less risky way, skipping the highlighting of discrepancy and just helping clients identify ways they could live in even greater congruence with their deeply held values.

Evoking greater client confidence about change is also motivating. Once again, practitioners can use evocative questions to elicit change talk (aimed at ability) in this regard, asking "What's something you'd feel pretty confident about trying now?" or "What would help you feel more confident about getting started?" and then reflecting and exploring client perspectives. Another parallel strategy is *confidence scaling,* using the same scaling approach as with importance, only this time focusing on confidence. An additional step with confidence scaling involves asking what would boost client's confidence by a couple of points, which can help when moving to the next process of planning. *Reviewing past successes* involves eliciting a discussion of previous accomplishments, how they prepared, what strategies they used, what barriers they faced, and how they worked around them. It can also help them reframe perceived failures as steps along the way to eventual change. Exploring *personal strengths* and available *supports* can also be motivating. Even if not directly applicable to the current change topic, building clients' sense that they are competent, worthwhile people with strengths and accomplishments, no matter how minor, can help them make difficult changes. A final confidence-building strategy involves *brainstorming hypothetical change.* People seem to find it easier to imagine what-if scenarios about change without the pressure of committing and therefore are less likely to get caught up in a crisis of confidence.

Planning

When people have mostly resolved their ambivalence and are interested in figuring out how to get started, MI practitioners use planning strategies to help them prepare for and initiate change. Clinicians can provide a *recapitulation,* or summary of the issues, focused on clients' perspectives on the importance of

making changes and their confidence, followed by a question such as "What now?" or "Where does this leave you?" The next step may include clarifying the goals of changing, and then exploring options for change with questions such as "What choices might you make?" or "Which options seem easier to try and more likely to succeed?" Clinicians now listen for *mobilizing change talk* and reflect and explore it. Mobilizing change talk relates to activation, or beginning to do something, and might sound like "I'm thinking about trying...," "I might...," or "I could...." Clinicians avoid pressing for firm commitment if clients are still tentative—and keep building momentum instead of risking turning clients away from change.

Another strategy to get started is to plan the steps toward change: What should happen and in what sequence? What supports can be rallied? When should various steps happen? What rewards can the client imagine will result? What might be some challenges that could interfere with the plan? Some clients like to develop a written change plan, while others prefer to make plans through conversation only.

As clients move into action, it can be helpful to continue to provide support and guidance, assisting them in self-monitoring their progress or finding a supportive mutual monitoring situation, such as a group or buddy. Part of moving into action may involve learning new skills, and it can be useful to bring in other therapies, classes, or practice opportunities at this point.

In addition to defining what MI includes, it is also useful to define what it does not include. For example, although occasional advice may be given to clients who are seeking it, unsolicited advice is not offered without first securing client permission. Similarly, clinicians do not confront or warn clients, engage in domineering or controlling interactions, or express their own concerns about clients or client choices (except in extenuating circumstances where clients may be in immediate danger). MI strategies or techniques are not simply added into interactions that are hierarchical in nature; rather, the MI style prescribes that the provider-client relationship is inherently nonhierarchical.

In summary, MI is a counseling approach in which clinicians use a client-centered stance paired with eliciting techniques to help clients explore and resolve their ambivalence about changing behaviors that are not optimally healthy. It is characterized by a collaborative, autonomy-supporting, and evocative style in which clinicians seek to understand clients' perspectives, while directing clients toward considering changing one or more behaviors by building a sense of discrepancy between the current and hoped-for self, avoiding confrontation, and supporting clients' optimism about the possibility and methods for change.

A Brief History of MI

Although it has strong roots in client-centered counseling, MI developed more out of practical experience than theoretical conviction and can be considered atheoretical or theoretically eclectic. Bill Miller's exploration with Norwegian colleagues of his intuitive practice guided him to elucidate the principles underpinning his approach, which integrated cognitive and behavioral elements into a broadly client-centered style. Miller's original principles were supplemented by collaborator Steve Rollnick's observation that ambivalence was a central aspect of change, and that MI specifically targeted ambivalence. Working together, Miller and Rollnick developed the clinical methods and described them in their 1991 book. They anchored their discussion of the rationale for elements of the clinical methods on discussion of the theories to which the elements were logically linked. The first related theory was Carl Rogers' theory of the necessary and sufficient conditions for therapeutic change, such as genuineness, congruence, and accurate empathy.[66] A second related theory was cognitive dissonance theory, in which Festinger posited that people would work to reduce thoughts that were strongly dissonant with their behaviors by altering either their attitudes/thoughts or their behaviors.[23] Although cognitive dissonance theory as a whole is no longer part of the model of MI, recent versions of MI have retained the idea of the related concept of discrepancy. A third related theory was Bem's self-perception theory, in which people observed themselves, their behaviors, and their statements, and inferred from those actions what they believed and valued.[10]

Although the scientific literature on MI helped to increase its popularity, a significant factor in its dissemination was the development of a network of skilled trainers who trained clinicians in MI across settings and in many countries across the globe. Rather than disseminating MI through writing only, Bill Miller and Steve Rollnick personally trained the first generation of MI Trainers. This group began meeting regularly at the time of the annual Training of New Trainers conducted by Miller and Rollnick and was initially a loose collaboration of volunteers. As new trainers were trained, the group outgrew its original small format and added online support for its growing community. With early technical assistance from the Mid-Atlantic Addiction Technology Transfer Center, the MI Network of Trainers grew into an active international community of many hundreds of trainers who interact via listservs, annual meetings, an online journal, and collaborative commercial and charitable training projects around the world. The MI Network of Trainers is now an independent entity that counts many of the most active MI researchers among its members, thus developing a strong communication loop between researchers, practitioners, and administrators in a wide variety of cultures and professional settings. MI researchers have had their own conference (International Conference on Motivational Interviewing) that has occurred biannually in Europe and the United States since 2008.

Theoretical Concepts and Emerging Models of MI

Although MI was derived from practice-based evidence, there are ongoing attempts to understand it theoretically. Currently, there is no comprehensive theory of MI that thoroughly explains its actions or drives its development, although there are several papers that hypothesize likely threads. In this section, we consider how an emerging model of MI might be woven from the threads of self-determination theory, the transtheoretical model of behavior change, emotions theory, interpersonal theory and psychotherapy, and data on MI and some of its potential mechanisms.

Defining MI

As practice evolves and new evidence about effectiveness and process-outcome relationships emerges, it is likely that definitions of MI will change. In some ways, this has already happened. There are at least four perspectives on defining MI. One is that MI *is a creation of and is defined by its original developers*. MI was described initially by Miller[49,52] and then by Miller and Rollnick,[53,54] and these founders of the approach may continually revise and update it as their own experiences and thoughts develop. Therefore

the principles, goals, techniques, strategies, and terms of MI follow from the founders' decisions, which may be influenced by data or practice or by exposure to other ideas. If the founders are the sole arbiters in defining MI, it is whatever they say it is, and elements may be added or deleted based on their preferences.

From the clinical research perspective, MI may be viewed instead as a set of attitudes, techniques, and strategies that can be described in a manual and can be evaluated with measures of treatment fidelity. This clinical research perspective focuses on sharp boundaries, specified timeframes, clearly defined strategies and techniques to address specific target behaviors, and attempts to isolate the unique elements of MI. The clinical research definition of MI results in a binary decision in that either MI is being done or MI is not being done. From this perspective, that MI is a specific definable intervention, a provider could be seen as doing MI in some sessions and not others, or possibly during some moments and not others.

Yet another perspective is the practitioner's angle. Practitioners might view MI as an overarching counseling style, a general way of working with clients. The practitioner using this style weaves whatever strands are most useful in the moment, no matter where those elements might have originated (in MI, in adaptations of MI, or in similar or complementary therapeutic approaches, disciplines, or experiences). From this perspective, practitioners may see themselves as doing MI even when a video sample of a discrete moment in therapy might show them to be providing a cognitive-behavioral therapy–derived intervention, albeit in an MI-consistent style. In such practice, a decision rule might be "can one smoothly transition in and out of elements borrowed from elsewhere?" The provider may be exploring ambivalence with a client and notice a bit of distorted thinking, slip unnoticed into working with the client on exploring the background of that thinking or its fit with reality or rationality, and then slip back out and back to exploring ambivalence. To the practitioner, this whole session may be thought of as MI if MI's spirit and techniques are present and if the client's responses indicate that the therapeutic alliance is steady.

A fourth perspective is that MI is a set of ideas or concepts that originated with Miller and Rollnick but are now independent from them. A conceptual perspective might define MI as a set of specific ideas that fit into a nomological net, a framework of logically coherent and connected constructs into which empirical and practice findings are placed and interrelated. A conceptual perspective on defining MI may be based less on either need for clear definition and fidelity to that definition, as in the clinical research perspective, or need for pragmatism and devotion to doing what works best in the moment, as in the practice perspective.

MI as an Activator of Autonomous Motivations and Growth

MI seeks to build internal motivation to change, even in the context of clients seeking to change due to some duress or external situation. Individuals with higher levels of internal motivation for change may be more likely to succeed in achieving and maintaining the desired change. MI seeks to elicit the person's healthy aspirations and propensity for positive growth. These aspirations and growth experiences are often internally motivating rather than resulting from external reinforcement alone. These goals of activating intrinsic motivations overlap somewhat with self-determination theory. Self-determination theory posits an alternative to some views of human motivation as originating in physiological needs, or as a drive state seeking to amend deficits. Instead, self-determination theory proposes that growth-oriented activity is the central source of motivation.[20] Self-determination theory states that people have innate needs for competence, relatedness, and autonomy, and that these needs can explain intrinsic motivation. Self-determination theory proposes that motivation becomes internalized naturally because humans are ready to internalize ambient values and regulations. Individuals come to grasp the importance of social values as children. Over time, they transform observed social mores into personal values and self-regulation. Self-determination theory proposes that internal motivation is most likely when a person has a sense of efficacy, control, or self-regulation with regard to the required behavior. Self-determination theory outlines a continuum of motivations ranging from externally regulated to truly intrinsic. Markland and colleagues propose that MI is not focused on truly intrinsic motivations (defined by self-determination theory as engaging in behaviors because they are inherently interesting or enjoyable).[47] Rather, MI focuses on a broader range of autonomous motivations regarding behaviors that lead toward desired outcomes for the person. These outcomes may involve extrinsic gain or increased coordination with one's values and self-identity.

MI as a Method to Move People Through Stages of Change

MI is a counseling style concerned with encouraging behavior change. The transtheoretical model[21,63] is a model of how people make deliberate changes, especially when it comes to eliminating problem behaviors and beginning new, healthier behaviors. The most well-known aspect of the transtheoretical model is the Stages of Change model, in which behavior change is seen as a process that progresses from low awareness and no intention to change through high awareness and active efforts to initiate or maintain change. The five stages of change are precontemplation, in which people may not recognize their behavior as problematic and are not planning to change; contemplation, in which people are considering change but remain ambivalent because there are also benefits resulting from their current behavior; preparation, in which people have decided to make a change and are making plans to change; action, in which people are actively taking steps to change, and maintenance, in which people are integrating the new behaviors into their ongoing lifestyle.

Although distinct, the transtheoretical model and model of stages of change and MI "grew up together" and complement one another.[22] Specifically, MI is a valuable approach to use when people are in the early stages of change, to build interest and motivation for change. The concept of stages may be better as a heuristic than as a reflection of reality. In clinical encounters, readiness for change can fluctuate within a single discussion about change. By maintaining a client-centered perspective and eliciting client readiness to change rather than attempting to use pressure to motivate change, the provider using MI can avoid evoking resistance that can inadvertently be elicited by getting ahead of the client.

MI as an Activator of Emotions and Openness

Most descriptions of MI and its work with ambivalence have focused on cognitive rather than emotional elements. The resolution of ambivalence is seen as a cognitive task, as in reaching a decision about which choice to make. MI techniques have been described in cognitive and behavioral terms, as means to positively resolve tension created by unresolved ambivalence about change. Wagner and Ingersoll presented an alternative conceptualization of MI.[79] Elicitation of negative emotions (e.g., by developing discrepancy) helps clients by narrowing their focus to areas in which they feel discontent, which leads toward them wanting to escape from the current unsatisfactory situation or avoid a future unsatisfactory situation. In contrast, the concept of positive reinforcement involves seeking positive states through behaviors that lead toward more satisfying conditions. From this perspective, motivation involves a desire to experience positive emotions. A positive emotions model encourages a view of motivation that emphasizes opening up to new experiences and actively seeking to build resources to support change and is consistent with the Broaden and Build model of positive emotions in motivation.[25,26] Elicitation of the positive emotion of interest may lead to greater openness to experiencing. When a client experiences interest (or related emotions such as wonder or curiosity), his or her cognitive focus broadens to consider options that previously had been overlooked or rejected. This increased flexibility in conceptualizing situations may then facilitate resolution of ambivalence and increased openness to engage in activities that lead toward change. As the person acts in the newly considered direction, he or she may improve certain skills and increase the likelihood of achieving a desired outcome. Movement in this positive direction may increase confidence, sense of accomplishment, self-esteem and mood, thus establishing these increased resources for the person to draw upon in service of even more profound changes. After analyzing common MI techniques and strategies through the lens of the broaden-and-build model, Wagner and Ingersoll concluded that MI elicits positive emotions of interest, hope, contentment, and inspiration by inviting clients to envision a better future, to remember past successes, and to gain confidence in their abilities to improve their lives.

MI as an Interpersonal Intervention

Interpersonal theory and research suggest that interpersonal interactions can be represented by two orthogonal (perpendicular) dimensions: control and affiliation.[39] The control dimension ranges from Dominance to Submission, whereas the affiliation dimension ranges from Warmth/Friendliness to Coldness/Hostility. When plotted, they form a circle that represents how controlling and affiliative a person is in interactions with others. Considerable evidence exists to support the idea that a friendly interpersonal style elicits reciprocal friendly responses from others and a hostile interpersonal style also elicits a reciprocal, hostile response.[38] Interpersonal theory also suggests that a dominant interpersonal style pulls for complementary submissive behavior, whereas submission pulls for complementary dominant behavior. However, although dominant behavior may pull for submissive behavior, it often elicits reciprocal dominant behavior as interactants struggle for the upper hand in a relationship.

Interpersonal theory has psychotherapeutic implications. Although submissive and friendly submissive clients may pull for and respond well to dominant and friendly dominant clinicians, clients having other baseline styles may not react as well to such a therapeutic stance. Clients presenting with hostile-dominance, who may be angry and lashing out, are unlikely to respond well to a provider who attempts to assert control or dominance over the interactions, even in a friendly dominant manner and even though this is a logical stance to take if the provider believes that the client's aggression must stop. Although being friendly and easygoing may be difficult to do in this situation, it is more likely to pull the client toward a friendly stance him or herself, which is likely to be more productive in moving forward. In contrast, with a client who is clinging and submissive, clinicians may be pulled to provide reassurance, structure, and direction, yet this is likely to reinforce the client's needy behavior. Instead, a provider may take an interpersonal stance that pulls for the client to become more assertive and assume greater ownership of his life, even though the client may be pulling for the provider to take a dominant stance. Fig. 39.1 shows an interpersonal circumplex with hypothetical MI-congruent provider behavior and client responsive behavior.

By definition, MI clinicians attempt to be both client-centered and directive. Regarding the client-centered aspect, it is useful to consider a continuum of provider-centered and client-centered responses. We first present the continuum in a linear fashion, with provider-centered behaviors that are hostile and controlling on the left and friendly but controlling to the right. Client-centered responses are in the center, ranging from deflecting on the hostile side to affirming on the warm side (Fig. 39.2).

On both ends of the continuum is the behavior "direct," because directing can be done in a hostile or warm manner. In our view, this behavior anchors the continuum up and around to the interpersonal circle to the top, which is dominance on the control dimension. Dominance is associated with being right, with being in authority, and with exerting authority or attempts to control others. These behaviors reflect the provider's perceptions and needs in a moment, and tend to indicate that the provider has moved away from being client-centered. Such provider-centered responses are more likely to elicit reactance, whether negative or positive, because they encroach upon the client's being by establishing a hierarchy in which the provider is above the client.

How might we classify particular provider statements to better understand how interpersonal interactions work in MI? A provider responding to a client's reduction in drinking may say, "I am proud of you." Upon first consideration, this appears to be a positive response, falling on the warm side of the affiliation dimension. However, this kind of statement is more likely to be perceived as approval, specifically praise, because it contains a dominant, judgmental element. Another example is "You worked really hard on that," which would be considered an affirmation, because it is an observation that notices the client's effort, rather than evaluating or praising the outcome. MI primarily uses the middle range of responses from deflection (occasionally, shifting focus) to affirmation. Responses near to these are also used in MI, but less often. In one demonstration video, Bill Miller agrees with a client angered by his previous treatment staff telling him that he must accept a label: "It doesn't make any sense to me! It's natural to push back when people push against you." Considering this continuum of possible provider statements, it appears that MI draws nearly exclusively from the client-centered range of responses.

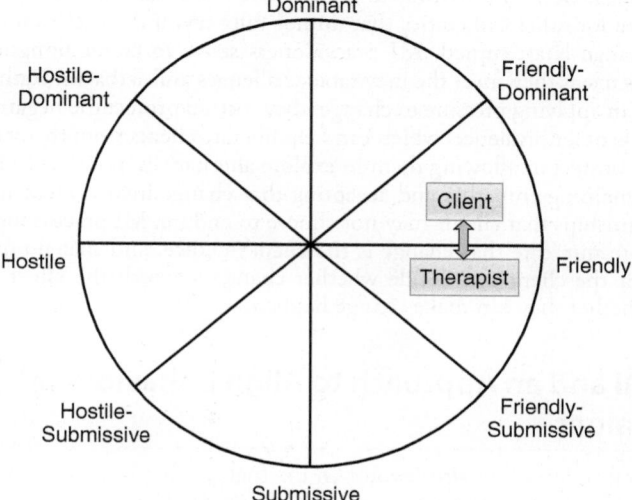

• **Fig. 39.1** Interpersonal circumplex with hypothesized MI–consistent provider characteristics and responsive client characteristics.

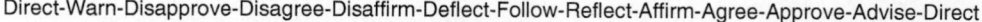

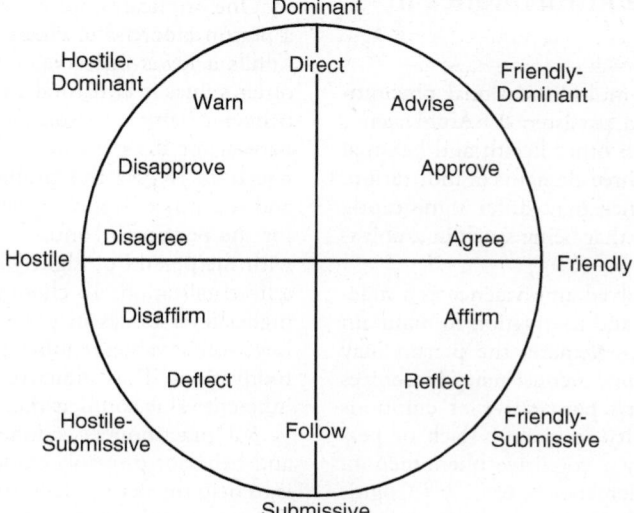

• **Fig. 39.2** Linear and circumplex depictions of provider-centered and client-centered provider behaviors in MI.

When considered in the context of the interpersonal circle model, the somewhat confusing left to right continuum becomes more meaningful (see Fig. 39.2). Approving and disapproving are not opposites of each other as they might at first seem, but both contain elements of dominance, although one is more hostile or cold and the other is more friendly or warm. Both, however, carry the risk of having the client feel as if he/she is being put in a submissive role and either accepting that, in which case the client is not in the best place for the kind of creative brainstorming that MI tries to bring out of people, or rejecting it and either withdrawing or fighting back against being dominated, even if only slightly. This key notion of reactance (reacting defensively to perception of being controlled) makes more sense when disapproval and approval are not seen as opposites but as partially opposite (one more hostile and the other more friendly) and partially similar (both taking a somewhat dominance or one-up stance).

Interpersonal theory has the potential to explain some mechanisms of action in MI. Interpersonally, MI clinicians tend to be friendly, which elicits a friendly, cooperative stance from most clients. Although MI has a directive component, in that the provider leads the client to explore and resolve ambivalence and initiate change, this directive process is not necessarily dominant interpersonally. For many people in a leadership role, it is natural to default to a more dominant style to lead, using either warm dominance by being outgoing, encouraging, praising, suggesting, and so on, or cold-dominance by directing, warning, confronting, or disapproving. Rather, the MI provider leads through affirmation, reflection, listening, and deflecting, all considered friendly to friendly-submissive behaviors. From the framework of interpersonal theory, these behaviors are less likely to elicit reactance, and are predicted instead to elicit reactions of more outgoing, spontaneous, confident, and self-reliant behaviors from clients. Thus clients take responsibility for deciding on and enacting steps toward change, increasing their self-efficacy for specific challenging behaviors, and building momentum and excitement about change. MI is thus almost entirely anchored in a friendly to friendly-submissive provider stance. This interpersonal stance in MI is paired with a leading/guiding/directing intent, and this unusual combination may contribute to the success of the MI approach.

MI as a Method to Resolve Ambivalence in the Direction of Change

Motivation can be understood as a multidimensional phenomenon including direction, effort, and persistence.[8] Ambivalence is highly prevalent in addiction, as in other health and habitual behaviors, and can interfere with all three elements of motivation. The targets or content of ambivalence may differ significantly among people, but the view in MI is that being stuck in ambivalence keeps people from changing.

The classic MI model casts unresolved ambivalence as a stalemate between motivation to change and motivation to maintain the status quo. In response to this stalemate, the person may experience inertia (lack of momentum), inconsistency in choices and behavior patterns as the person's perspective or emotions shift (lack of direction), or instability in change (lack of persistence). Ambivalence is not merely a cognitive phenomenon, but has emotional and behavioral elements as well.[79,80] Cognitively, ambivalence can pull people back and forth, from argument to counterargument about continuing to live as they are versus trying something new. Emotionally, people can experience

excitement, confidence, and determination about the possibilities in front of them, while also feeling dread, anger, or grief about the difficulties ahead and the comforts they may have to leave behind, along with disabling guilt or shame about the things they have done during their period of addiction. Behaviorally, some people make halting steps forward, unsure about moving at all, or backtrack at the first sign of potential failure. Others rush forward in a desire to change as quickly as possible, only to discover that they were not prepared for the challenges they face, possibly prompting a relapse.

Although MI practitioners tend not to focus their efforts on eliciting all sides of client ambivalence equally, putting more emphasis on change than the status quo, they also respectfully accept client hesitations, reservations, and defenses about change. Change is hard. It involves giving up valued parts of life and of oneself. New habits may feel awkward and may not pay off in the short term. Sometimes, unanticipated challenges or disadvantages appear along the pathway to change. Old habits may also compensate for other difficulties that do not fully reveal themselves until change is attempted. MI practitioners strive to come alongside clients as they meet the inevitable challenges and setbacks. Rather than applying pressure to change, they instead protect the negative side of ambivalence, which can help liberate clients from the need to protect it, allowing them to explore alternatives more freely. By remaining empathic and accepting that change involves loss and hardships that clients may not choose to endure, MI practitioners communicate that change is the client's choice, and that no one but the client can decide whether change is worth the effort or whether they can make change happen.

MI and an Approach to Align Behavior and Values

Ambivalence can also involve an internal conflict in personal values,[83] which can be seen as either behavioral ideals or preferences for experiences. As ideals, values provide judgments about what is good and not good. As preferences for experiences, values guide individuals toward seeking situations in which they may experience excitement, relaxation, novelty, competition, comfort, security, a sense of belonging, and so on.

One implication of Maslow's hierarchy of needs is that when a person is forced to choose between a behavior that exclusively fulfills a lower-order value and one that only fulfills a higher-order value, it is natural to choose the former. When addictive behavior helps a person escape pain or gain pleasure, then it is natural for the person to continue that behavior, despite social rejection. When the problem behavior meets both biological and social needs, such as belonging to a peer group, it is natural for the person to continue the behavior even when it interferes with the pursuit of higher-order strivings toward achievement or self-actualization. To choose a healthy behavior that meets these higher-level values in place of an addictive behavior that meets lower-order values requires a transcendence of the natural order of motivations. Thus addictive processes by their nature may contain inherent value conflicts that are difficult to resolve.

MI practitioners assume that a discrepancy between values and behavior probably exists, and therefore one therapeutic task is to help the person develop greater awareness of the discrepancy. Once some part of the behavior or its consequences becomes perceived as inconsistent with underlying values, the person is likely to become more motivated to change.

Summary: Emerging Relational and Technical Components in a Model or Theory of MI

In 2009, Miller and Rose summarized Miller's early work and proposed that two active components in combination lead to the efficacy of MI: a relational component that includes empathizing, collaborating, evoking client talk about their perspectives, and supporting client autonomy, and a technical component that includes evoking and reinforcing change talk.[56] Specifically, they hypothesized that MI would increase client change talk and reduce client resistance, that defense of the status quo by clients would relate negatively to change, and that change talk would relate positively to change. This model may provide a working model of MI in describing what happens; it is not an encompassing theory that attempts to explain why clients make changes after such interactions. An eventual model of MI would elucidate elements unique to MI and elements shared with other psychotherapies, and would demonstrate how the relational, technical, and interpersonal components work to produce client changes in beliefs, perspectives, emotions, and actions. However, of all the emerging theoretical elements, it has had the strongest influence over researchers examining the relationship between MI processes and outcomes, which we review in detail below.

Evidence About MI

Evidence About Efficacy

The evidence for the efficacy of MI is strong. Hundreds of randomized controlled trials (RCTs) of MI and its adaptations, such as Motivational Enhancement Therapy (MET), have been conducted. The literature amounts to so much evidence that there are now over 100 meta-analysis or synthesis studies of the impact of MI across a range of behaviors, topics, and disorders. Even the topics that are relatively less commonly studied have accrued some initial systematic reviews. In contrast, there are two areas, addiction and health care, with extensive and mature bodies of literature including systematic studies of the efficacy of MI. Across these studies of MI in addiction and health care, thousands of patients and study participants have contributed to a large set of diverse efficacy findings. It is perhaps inevitable that as that the evidence base has become more voluminous, it is sometimes contradictory or difficult to interpret. Given the large volume of evidence, here we review only those meta-analyses and systematic reviews published in peer-reviewed journals in the past 5 years (2012–2017) to examine what is now known about the use of MI to improve health behaviors and addictive behaviors.

Using MI in Medical Settings to Improve Health Behaviors

Of 15 systematic studies of trials in medical settings concerning health behaviors, five were published in the past 5 years. Taken together, they demonstrate a statistically significant, small to medium effect of MI that is robust across moderators such as setting, patient characteristics, and session length. For example, Lundahl et al.,[45] reviewed 48 randomized trials conducted across medical settings containing a wide range of patients and behavioral targets. They found that MI showed a significant ($P < .001$) overall effect across studies, associated with an odds ratio of 1.55 of better outcomes than various comparison interventions. Although effects were found for benefits of MI for HIV viral load, dental

outcomes, death rate, body weight, substance use, and sedentary behavior, MI was not effective with eating disorders and selected outcomes such as heart rate. Their overall conclusion was that MI can be used for many behavioral issues in health care. VanBuskirk and Wetherell[78] found significant small- to medium-sized effects of MI in a meta-analysis of 12 MI-specific primary care interventions, with strongest evidence for weight reduction (mean effect size [ES] = .47) and blood pressure (mean ES = .38), and more limited evidence for substance abuse (mean ES = –.22), adherence (mean ES = .19), and increases in physical activity (mean ES = .07). They also found that these effects can occur after as little as a single MI session and that the level of professional credentialing was a significant moderator of outcomes. Purath et al.[64] studied the impact of MI in primary care with older adults in a systematic review. They concluded that although MI shows promise to improve health behavior change among older adults, more study is needed due to wide variation in clinical implementation of MI and study flaws that limit confidence in findings. Morton et al.[58] reviewed the impact of MI in primary care settings by reviewing the components of MI in studies that sought to facilitate changes in activity, diet, and alcohol drinking. They found that over half of the 33 studies that met inclusion criteria demonstrated positive health behavior changes, yet concluded that clinical MI components and research methods and quality of studies varied so substantially that robust conclusions about the utility of MI in primary care could not be drawn. McKenzie et al.[48] conducted a systematic review of MI in health care to consider the potential relevance of MI to the increasing presence of multimorbidity among health care patients. Although they did not find controlled research specifically incorporating MI in relation to multimorbidity, they found small-to-medium effects across a range of behavioral targets relevant to multimorbidity such as diabetes, hypertension, HIV, and hyperlipidemia. Their findings pointed out the need for research into the effects of MI across multiple behavior change required to manage multimorbidity. Overall, these meta-analyses and systematic reviews indicate a consistent finding of a small-to-medium effect of MI on health behaviors that may be robust across settings. In addition, most investigators recommend improvements to study methodology and quality to allow for more confidence in these conclusions.

Using MI to Reduce or Prevent Addictive Behaviors

There are now 25 systematic reviews or meta-analyses in the area of substance use and addictive behaviors, with 16 of these studies published in the years 2012–2017. Earlier seminal systematic reviews such as the Mesa Grande study of the impact of various alcohol treatments[57] and a study of MI in health care that included alcohol behaviors[69] demonstrated consistent, significant effects of MI on alcohol intake and peak drinking; more recent studies reviewed below have assessed the impact of MI on drinking in specific populations, other drug use, and gambling.

Emergency Room MI for Heavy Drinking Youth

Kohler and Hoffmann[41] examined whether emergency room MI could reduce alcohol use in young people presenting with high levels of drinking following a precipitating event. Among studies of heavy drinkers, they found that MI (alone or in combination with normative resetting, skills training, or booster calls) decreased drinking frequency, drinking quantity, and alcohol-related consequences. There was significant variability across studies, however, in both quality and outcomes, leading the researchers to conduct best-case and worst-case scenarios. The best case scenario suggested that MI is at least as effective and possibly more effective than other brief interventions for reducing drinking among young people in the emergency context, and that it is more effective than educational materials, personal feedback, or referral to community services. The worst case scenario detected no differences.

In other reviews of specific applications of MI, meta-analyses and systematic reviews have shown evidence that MI increases near-term treatment adherence generally,[61] in chronic disease treatment,[86] in treatment of chronic pain,[2] HIV treatment,[33] in dentistry,[37] in smoking cessation,[44] in pediatric care,[11,31] and in regard to contraceptive use among women at high risk of unintended pregnancy.[84] Across all areas, investigators note the wide variability of quality and documentation in published studies, reflecting concerns expressed by the MI founders.[55a]

Brief Interventions for Drinking Adolescents and Young Adults

Tanner-Smith and Lipsey[76] found 185 studies of brief interventions for drinking among adolescents and young adults with varied levels of drinking problems and drinking severity. The greatest impact was found among interventions containing MI, decisional balancing, or goal setting. They found significant reductions in alcohol consumption and alcohol-related problems in both age groups. Modest effects were maintained over time, and interventions were low cost. In a subsequent meta-analysis, Tanner-Smith and Risser[77] found that significant alcohol reductions were reported following brief interventions, that the impact varied by measurement method, but that significant reductions were observed across measured. They concluded that even with modest effects, they were clinically significant and represented a reduction of overall risky drinking patterns among youth.

Prevention of Risky Drinking in College-Age Adults

Several studies examined the impact of MI when used as a prevention tool for risky drinkers in college students and other young adults. Samson and Tanner-Smith[70] studied single session alcohol interventions for heavy drinking college students. They found significant reductions in alcohol use, with larger effects of MI and MET and feedback interventions compared to CBT or psychoeducational interventions. They concluded that interventions for heavy drinking college students should include MI, MET, and feedback components. Huh et al.[35] examined studies of brief MI interventions for college drinking using advanced data modeling techniques. They found that overall effects on drinks per week and peak drinking were small, and that interventions combining individual MI with personalized feedback showed stronger results, but concluded that the efficacy and effect sizes of MI for college drinking prevention is weak. Similarly, Foxcroft et al.[24] conducted a Cochrane review of MI in preventing alcohol misuse in young adults and concluded that there is little evidence of the impact of MI as a preventive tool in this population, with no effects on important alcohol phenotype variables such as binge drinking, blood alcohol concentration, and alcohol-related risky behavior including driving.

Drug Use

Li et al.[43] examined MI to reduce drug use in adolescents. They found no effect of MI on drug use, and a significant publication bias. They concluded that MI has not been found to reduce adolescent illicit drug use. In contrast, a few studies examined the impact of MI on substance use across types of substances. Lenz et al.[42] conducted a meta-analysis of 25 studies of RCTs

of MET for reducing substance use among adults. They found a small to medium effect when compared to no treatment, and a small effect when compared to active treatments. Sayegh et al.[72] studied the impact of contingency management (CM) and MI on substance use among adults across types of drugs used. They found evidence for impact of each intervention, with CM producing medium-size effects that initially fade, while the small effects of MI lasted longer. Gates et al.[27] studied the impact of MI on cannabis use, examining a series of MI and CBT studies that used varied combinations of each treatment. Overall, they conclude that combining MI and CBT results in reductions in the frequency of use and severity of dependence at early treatment follow-ups, but that most results are no longer significant 9 months or later.

Alternate Modalities for Addictive Behaviors

Jiang et al[36] assessed the impact of MI on a range of addictive behaviors when delivered by telephone, Internet, or text messages rather than in face to face counseling, or in groups. Providing MI for drinking via telephone was effective in all included RCTs, as was Internet intervention and short message system (SMS) intervention for drinking. Results were mixed for targeting substance use other than alcohol and for group MI targeting alcohol and drug use cessation. The investigators concluded that there is strong evidence that telephone MI could supplement or replace face-to-face treatment, whereas there is not enough evidence yet for other modalities.

Problem Gambling

Cowlishaw et al.[16] focused on problem and pathological gambling, and found only four studies of MI, which tended to target problem rather than severely pathological gambling. The studies conducted so far demonstrated limited impact on financial loss and gambling frequency that is observed shortly after treatment, but with no impact on many other variables or at more distal follow-up points. They conclude that there is a need for more studies of the impact of MI, especially in the context of more severe gambling problems. Some studies evaluated the impact of MI as a preventive intervention, generally among young adults with minor harms from drinking behavior. A subsequent systematic review and meta-analysis of the efficacy of MI for disordered gambling found that MI was associated with significant reductions in gambling frequency across a full year and reduced dollars spent gambling in the short term.[85]

MI for Comorbid Alcohol and Depressive Disorders

Riper et al.[65] studied the impact of combining CBT and MI to target comorbid alcohol use disorders and major depressive disorder. They found a small and clinically significant impact in reducing alcohol consumption and symptoms of depression.

Similar to the literature on the efficacy of MI for health behaviors, these meta-analyses and systematic reviews indicate a very consistent, small to medium effect size of MI on a range of addictive behavior characteristics among adults. Results are more mixed for the efficacy of MI to reduce drinking and other addictive behaviors among adolescents and college students, with the most inconsistent findings for preventive rather than treatment uses of MI. MI is efficacious for reducing drinking among persons with harmful or disordered drinking, and shows promise in the treatment of other addictive disorders.

In conclusion, our review of this large set of meta-analytic and systematic studies of trials of the efficacy of MI has found that MI is efficacious for the improvement of health behaviors and in reducing substance use and related problems in people with unhealthy or disordered use. Its efficacy in prevention has not yet been established.

Evidence About MI Processes and Their Relationships With Outcomes

MI may be both blessed and cursed by its roots as a primarily atheoretical, clinically driven model of intervention. On the one hand, this aspect of MI has allowed it to be a dynamic method, shapeable as new ideas and evidence emerge. Accordingly, MI has undergone significant revision since its initial formulation, borrowing concepts from traditions as varied as cognitive dissonance theory, self-perception theory, and self-determination theory, and nearly as often, casting aside ideas that initially seemed to have promise but ultimately brought burdensome theoretical or philosophical accessories along with a core idea. Similarly, as an empirically based rather than theoretically derived model, the shape of MI has changed over time based on emerging evidence about the model as a whole as well as regarding which components appear to be effective in eliciting engagement and positive change in clients. Overall, it is yet to be determined just how flexible the MI model can be and just how closely its ongoing development will continue to reflect emerging empirical evidence. However, the intent to follow the data is there among MI's original developers and most current researchers.

On the other hand, this aspect of MI carries its own burden. Although an approach regularly updated to reflect emerging theoretical and empirical developments is dynamic, the cost is instability. With each new major update to the approach,[53-55] so many core and peripheral concepts are revised as to put earlier findings and conclusions in question, and with little in the way of core theoretical pillars to guide research, it is not entirely clear which elements researchers should include in studies and which should be focused on in published findings. This has led to an array of studies addressing related issues but constructed in ways that make them difficult to compare, which is a hindrance to establishing clear pathways for future development of the model.

As noted previously, Miller and Rose[56] contributed a model of the mechanisms of action in MI that contains core relational and technical components, the relational component including the core client-centered therapeutic stance, and the technical component primarily featuring the intentional evocation and reflection of client change talk (interest and hope in change) as well as avoidance of sustained exploration of client sustain talk (reluctance to change and defense of the status quo). This model has spurred nearly a decade of subsequent process-analysis studies that provide limited yet noteworthy support for the relational-technical model. As is often the case in model testing, however, answers to questions based on the relatively simple model provided by Miller and Rose have sometimes been less forthcoming than the emergence of more complex questions and conceptual possibilities. Although we cannot review all of the emerging pathways from this decade of exploration, in this section we review the primary findings. In addition, we note recent emerging evidence that does not appear to fit neatly into the relational-technical model of MI, harkening back to elements of the MI clinical model that have so far been underinvestigated in the mechanisms of action or process-outcome research based on the relational-technical model.

A review of 37 published research studies into various elements of the MI relational-technical model[68] identified substantial support for the core assertion that clinicians' MI-consistent behaviors are associated with in-session client change talk, which is in turn associated with subsequent positive external client change (across various behavioral domains). This is the core element of the technical aspect of the relational-technical model, and a 2014 meta-analysis of 12 primary studies reached a similar, if more tentative, conclusion (finding support for MI technical elements in influencing client reactions, but finding a positive, yet insignificant association between client change talk and positive outcome).[46] Expanding the focus to include therapist MI-inconsistent behaviors and sustain talk, an interesting pattern emerges. Although MI-inconsistent behaviors generally increase sustain talk and decrease change talk, and sustain talk predicts worse outcomes (all in line with the model), MI-consistent behaviors are associated with client change talk (as noted) but are also generally associated with increased client sustain talk. These studies have reflected both of these themes—that MI-inconsistent behaviors are associated with increased sustain talk and decreased change talk while MI-consistent behaviors are associated with increases in both types of talk, and that in-session sustain talk clearly predicts worse posttreatment outcomes while in-session change talk sometimes predicts better outcomes but other times predicts no change. Thus overall, it may be emerging that it is more important that clinicians avoid MI-inconsistent behaviors (e.g., confrontation, deficit focus) than that they actively engage in MI-prescribed behaviors (e.g., empathic reflections, focus on change talk).

These findings seem to partially contradict the technical hypothesis, but when expanding the scope of vision, they may reflect earlier, more comprehensive descriptions of MI that are geared more toward exploration and the resolution of ambivalence in the direction of change versus a narrower approach of simply evoking and reflecting change talk while ignoring sustain talk. The components of degree of engagement in the therapeutic process, the amount of exploration of ambivalence, and the depth of experiencing/processing are all current themes in MI process research. Looking more broadly at empathic speech, as well as more narrowly at prescribed MI micro-communications such as open questions, simple reflections (that reflect or paraphrase client statements), and complex reflections (that go beyond what clients have explicitly said), regular findings appear to be emerging that these MI-consistent communications foster client exploration of ambivalence as reflected in both change talk and sustain talk. One study found that of MI-consistent micro-communications, only affirmations served to differently elicit change talk versus sustain talk.[6] Furthermore, client self-exploration more generally predicts positive outcomes in instances when change talk does not.[8]

Attempts to unravel these seemingly contradictory findings have led to new, more complex developments in the understanding of MI processes and process-outcome relationships. A composite measure of change/sustain talk suggests that it may not be the amount of change talk that is important so much as the relative balance between change talk and sustain talk.[46] In other studies, neither the amount of sustain talk nor the overall balance was found to be as important in predicting outcome as the strength of change talk when it did emerge,[29,30] and yet another study found that a key element was the trend toward more change talk near the end of the intervention, a finding reflecting an earlier conceptualization by Amrhein et al.[3] that the most important element is the slope of change talk (trending upward, more positive). Additional studies found that simple measures of MI-consistent communications such as reflections or open questions were insufficient, and instead predictive power (in expected directions) was increased when these communications were coded in regard to their relative directionality toward change or status quo.[13] Finally, at least one as-yet unpublished study examines the context of discussion within which change talk emerges, and the subsequent association between this conversational context and postintervention outcomes. When MI sessions were divided into different conversational content focus areas (e.g., review of precipitating event, discussion of pros and cons, envisioning the future, and planning for change), change talk emerged differentially across topics; it was the change talk emerging during the "envisioning the future" segment that most reliably predicted change, whereas change talk during some of the other segments (e.g., change planning) was unrelated to postintervention change.[5]

Although most of the attention of process-outcome research in MI has focused on the technical arm of the relational-technical model, increasing interest is being given to the relational arm. Moyers[59] likens using MI without the requisite autonomy-supporting, empathic relationship to a "party trick" that "cannot be expected to lead to change" (p. 360). Yet as the technical aspect of MI has dominated consideration, relatively less is known about the contributing role of relationship in MI, either as a foundational aspect as Moyers describes, or as a direct contributor to positive change separate from the technical aspect. Furthermore, whereas the technical aspect of MI conduct has been largely reduced to the narrower and more behaviorally focused aspect of elicitation and reflection of change talk rather than the former broader concept of exploration and resolution of ambivalence about change, the role of relationship has perhaps been limited in more recent accountings of MI. As noted previously, however, some recent studies show that prescribed MI micro-communications evoke not only change talk but also sustain talk and that a greater degree of self-exploration sometimes predicts positive change outcomes even in the absence of signs of effectiveness of any MI-consistent therapist behaviors. Autonomy-restricting therapist behaviors, even in the absence of prescribed behavior, can lead to sustain talk, which can then lead to even greater degrees of autonomy-restrictive therapist behavior in a downward spiral.[40] In various other studies, relationship factors including acceptance, egalitarianism, warmth, genuineness, and empathy have predicted change talk[16,64] or reduced sustain talk.[9] Furthermore, the MI elements most predictive of outcome in some studies have included spirit (autonomy-support, evoking style, and collaboration).[12,15,28]

Overall, we conclude that there is positive support for aspects of both of the relational-technical components of MI. In addition, a careful review of the literature suggests that some recent descriptions of MI's technical element as elicitation and exploration of change talk, in the absence of exploration of sustain talk, may be too narrow. Instead, MI seems more effective when it includes a broader focus on exploration and the resolution of ambivalence. This approach may include strategic exploration of sustain talk when it deepens client self-experiencing. This may foster a deeper resolution of ambivalence than may be achieved through establishing momentum toward change through a focus on change talk alone. Increased attention to the purpose of therapist use of MI-consistent behaviors such as reflections and open questions will help to further elucidate the most effective ways of conducting MI, and attending to the context in which change talk emerges (in envisioning the future, toward the end of sessions/treatment) will help further hone MI practices. These assertions assume that MI development continues on a path of being guided by evidence rather than reverting to theoretical- or expert-driven development.

Other Developments in MI

MI Groups

MI was developed as an individual counseling approach. However, the adaptation of MI to groups is an emerging model for facilitating change.[81] Groups are a frequent treatment modality, useful both for their unique ability to tackle interpersonal and social difficulties directly and for cost-savings. MI groups are used increasingly as an alternative to dyadic MI to harness the power of a group of people who are in it together and who can provide support and encouragement to each other and learn from one another. These groups can be facilitated by practitioners with skills in MI and in group counseling and may vary considerably depending on how homogeneous or heterogeneous group members' presenting problems are. Some MI group leaders introduce topics and facilitate group discussion, while others facilitate the emergence of a group process that builds cohesion among members who navigate their way toward change with the support of the group.

Some aspects of fidelity can be measured with standard MI assessment instruments, while others require specialized measurement. Recently, MI groups have been defined and measured as including aspects of (1) group engagement (engaging, linking, openness, climate, cohesion, altruism), (2) client-centered foundation (framing in client perspective, autonomy, empathy, deepening focus, broadening focus, future focus), and (3) MI change focus (momentum, evoking motivation, narrowing focus, strengths, progress, hope).[82] As such, MI groups fit with the bulk of evidence-based group therapies, while retaining key MI features (and excluding features inconsistent with MI).

Evidence about MI groups is recent and still relatively minimal. To date, the strongest outcomes evidence is for the use of these groups for addiction-related issues[60] with some additional evidence in risk-reduction and disease coping.[81] With regard to process issues, MI groups can increase recognition of problems and ambivalence, increase perceived autonomy, self-efficacy, behavioral intentions, and readiness to change, and increase treatment engagement, attendance, and completion, as well as participation in aftercare. Recent process research on MI groups has also focused on change talk relatedness, in which the change talk of members appears to spur change talk in other members, establishing group momentum toward change.[74] Leader influences on group interactions appear strongest in the opening and closing segments of sessions, with change talk relatedness present in the middle of sessions.[34] Change talk can predict outcomes and can be influenced not only by differential responding by group leaders, but pooled change talk at the group level can predict individual member outcomes.[17] This last point reflects the theoretical proposition of implicit change talk,[81] that in group MI, members may benefit from simply listening to others speak positively toward change, without the requirement of the individual MI model that change is facilitated through explicit client change talk.

Given the recent development of MI in groups, certain aspects are still being explored for fit with the MI model, including such variations as that in group MI, clients often are not just talking about making changes outside of the session in their real life, as is typical in dyadic MI, but are actively making the changes within the group in interactions with other group members. While this aspect of group process is generally well-known, its fit with the MI model of in-session change talk leading to extrasession change is still being contemplated.

Preparing Clinicians to Use MI

Like any newer or emerging approach, much of the effort to train practitioners has been on-the-job or in the form of continuing education, rather than as a core element of preservice university training. Although this is changing as more university programs offer MI courses or sections, one-off workshops are still likely the most common exposure addiction services clinicians have to MI. However, these appear unlikely to be sufficient to bring most clinicians to competency using the approach. Several recent meta-analyses document the current state of MI training evaluations. Soderlund and colleagues[75] identified that the median length of training across identifiable studies was approximately 9 hours—addressing basic MI skills, spirit, identifying and reflecting change talk, and working with client resistance. Across meta-analyses, MI training appears to produce medium to large effect sizes in pre-post measured aspects of practice that were carried back into practice from training.[9,19,73,75] Unfortunately, gains in practice skills appear to be short-lived without follow-up training, coaching, and support[32,73] and are moderated by logistical parameters such as frequency, duration, and length of ongoing coaching. Another review found not only positive pre-post outcomes of training, but additionally that trained clinicians are significantly more proficient than a matched control group in MI skills.[19] However, in a review using a bar of basic competence to assess training outcomes, less than 15% of training studies reached a standard of at least 75% of trained clinicians demonstrating basic competence in MI skills.[32] The essential message is that single-event workshops appear useful to introduce MI and lay a foundation for basic skills. Although a few participants may be primed to reach competence in workshops, many do not achieve competency through this approach alone, and even fewer maintain skills on the job for more than a brief time. Ongoing feedback and coaching are the current standard approach for deepening and maintaining skills, and yet an array of logistical problems are reported on this approach, including attrition, lack of willingness to produce practice samples, time conflicts, and low availability of supervision. Some recent projects are focusing more on helping practitioners engage in self-development and on developing learning communities of interested clinicians to strengthen knowledge and skills outside of formal top-down implementation efforts.

Beyond training individual clinicians, current efforts are focused on system implementation of MI skills and practices, seen as the most promising approach for true integration of MI services into larger agencies or practice systems. This goal generally involves several steps, such as exploring provider and management perspectives about current services and competencies, broadening perspectives to build interest in adding skills to the clinicians' and agency's repertoires, and taking action to procure training, supervision, and organizational consultation. It is still relatively rare for an agency to take all of these steps, and to evaluate progress in a systematic way. How to train or produce MI-skillful organizations is a challenge already being addressed in some large scale projects, especially in the area of criminal justice. However, there is little current evidence about preferred methods in this area, and similarly, little evidence about best practices in training trainers.

Implementation science is currently being used to study the implementation and sustainability of MI interventions in community settings. The gap between research and practice settings is well-known and is a significant barrier to transferring knowledge and skills from controlled research settings to uncontrolled, variable and often chaotic environments of practice. Furthermore,

controlled efficacy studies simply cannot mirror the nature of clinical practice, which often simultaneously focuses on multiple conditions and target behaviors addressed across multiple (often rotating) clinicians. Establishing effective practice involves balancing fidelity with flexibility, attempting to provide adherent, competent practice of evidence-based approaches while adapting those approaches to idiosyncratic environments and developing program policies and practices, training and coaching practices, and fidelity monitoring that support not only adoption, but deep implementation and ongoing maintenance of those practices (Naar, personal communication, 2017). MI implementation science studies evaluate these variables while investigating how program development, training, supervision, and monitoring are conducted, with the aim of identifying effective and efficient ways to integrate MI into routine care.[1] Work in this complex area is ongoing, but it is too soon to draw generalized conclusions from published studies.

Summary

In summary, MI is an efficacious method to facilitate behavior change that has strong evidence for its positive impact on addictive and health behaviors. It may be practical, as it often achieves good outcomes with fewer sessions and less time than other substance abuse treatment methods. It has become a popular approach and is utilized around the world for the treatment of substance abuse and other behavior change challenges. Although the clinical methods have been detailed thoroughly, assessing practice and exploring process-outcome relationships are areas getting more attention recently, resulting in modest support for proposed mechanisms of action and suggesting that the actual process of change in MI is more complex than the simple models thus far proposed. As MI expands into new areas of application beyond its individual substance abuse counseling roots, there is a continued need to develop innovative methods of delivery and to provide effective training for providers, agencies, and trainers, all of which are being explored through various implementation science initiatives. Finally, the very definition of MI may be changing. It could become a clinical method that retains a distinct identity and is used in specific situations. Alternatively, it may become incorporated into broad practice and eventually lose its individual identity or become one of several specific approaches that focus on client motivation as a central component in fostering behavior change. Based on highly active research and training efforts globally, we are confident that MI will continue to evolve as knowledge about it expands.

References

1. Aarons G, Martino S, Naar S. Implementation science and motivational interviewing - researchers' brainstorming/planning *Forum. Forum Conducted at the International Conference on Motivational Interviewing (ICMI-5)*. Philadelphia, Pennsylvania; 2017.
2. Alperstein D, Sharpe L. The efficacy of motivational interviewing in adults with chronic pain: a meta-analysis and systematic review. *J Pain*. 2016;17(4):393–403.
3. Amrhein PC, Miller WR, Yahne CE, Palmer M, Fulcher L. Client commitment language during motivational interviewing predicts drug use outcomes. *J Consult Clin Psychol*. 2003;71:862–878.
4. Reference deleted in review.
5. Apodaca TR, Borsari B, Miller MB, Magill M, Jackson KM, Longabaugh R, et al. Do different MI components function differently in predicting change talk and outcomes? *Presented at the International Conference on Motivational Interviewing (ICMI-5)*. Philadelphia, Pennsylvania; 2017d.

6. Apodaca TR, Jackson KM, Borsari B, Magill M, Longabaugh R, Mastroleo NR, et al. Which individual therapist behaviors elicit client change talk and sustain talk in motivational interviewing? *J Subst Abuse Treat*. 2016;61:60–65.

7. Apodaca TR, Magill M, Longabaugh R, Jackson KM, Monti PM. Effect of a significant other on client change talk in motivational interviewing. *J Consult Clin Psychol*. 2013;81(1):35–46.

8. Arnold J, Randall R. *Work psychology: Understanding Human Behaviour in the Workplace*. Harlow, Essex: Pearson Education; 2010.

9. Barwick MA, Bennett LM, Johnson SNMJ, Moore JE. Training health and mental health professionals in motivational interviewing: a systematic review. *Child Youth Serv Rev*. 2012;34(9):1786–1795.

10. Bem DJ. Self-perception: an alternative interpretation of cognitive dissonance phenomena. *Psychol Rev*. 1967;74:183–200.

11. Borelli B, Tooley EM, Scott-Sheldon LAJ. Motivational interviewing for parent-child health interventions: a systematic review and meta-analysis. *Pediatric Dentistry*. 2015;37(3):254–265.

12. Borsari B, Apodaca TR, Jackson KM, Mastroleo N, Magill M, Barnett NP, et al. In-session processes of brief motivational interventions in two trials with mandated college students. *J Clin Psychol*. 2015;83(1):56–67.

13. Carcone AI, Naar S. Provider behaviors that predict change talk in HIV: A study of communication using the motivational interviewing framework. *Presented at the International Conference on Motivational Interviewing (ICMI-5)*. Philadelphia, Pennsylvania; 2017.

14. Catley D, Harris KJ, Mayo MS, Hall S, Okuyemi KS, Boardman T, et al. Adherence to principles of motivational interviewing and client within-session behavior. *Behav Cogn Psychother*. 2006;34:43–56.

15. Copeland L, McNamara R, Kelson M, Simpson S. Mechanisms of change within motivational interviewing in relation to health behaviors outcomes: a systematic review. *Patient Educ Couns*. 2015;98(4):401–411.

16. Cowlishaw S, Merkouris S, Dowling N, Anderson C, Jackson A, Thomas S. Psychological therapies for pathological and problem gambling. (11):CD008937.

17. D'Amico EJ, Houck JM, Hunter SB, Miles JNV, Osilla KC, Ewing BA. Group motivational interviewing for adolescents: change talk and alcohol and marijuana outcomes. *J Consult Clin Psychol*. 2015;83(1):68–80.

18. D'Amico EJ, Hunter SB, Miles JN, Ewing BA, Osilla KC. A randomized controlled trial of a group motivational interviewing intervention for adolescents with a first time alcohol or drug offense. *J Subst Abuse Treat*. 2013;45(5):400–408.

19. Reference deleted in review.

20. Deci EL, Ryan RM. *Intrinsic Motivation and Self-Determination in Human Behavior*. New York: Plenum Press; 1985.

21. DiClemente CC, Prochaska JO. Processes and stages of self-change: coping and competence in smoking behavior change. In: Shiffman S, Wills TA, eds. *Coping and Substance Use*. New York: Academic Press; 1985.

22. DiClemente CC, Velasquez M. Motivational interviewing and the stages of change. In: Miller WR, Rollnick S, eds. *Motivational interviewing*. 2nd ed. Preparing people for change. New York: Guilford; 2002.

23. Festinger L. *A Theory of Cognitve Dissonance*. Illinois: Row and Peterson; 1957.

24. Foxcroft DR, Coombes L, Wood S, Allen D, Almeida Santimano NM, Moreira MT. Motivational interviewing for the prevention of alcohol misuse in young adults.*Cochrane Database Syst Rev*. 2016;7:CD007025.

25. Fredrickson BL. Cultivating positive emotions to optimize health and well-being. *Prevent Treatment*. 2000;3(1).

26. Fredrickson BL. The value of positive emotions. *Am Scientist*. 2003;91(4):330–335.

27. Gates PJ, Sabioni P, Copeland J, Le Foll B, Gowing L. Psychosocial interventions for cannabis use disorder. (5).

28. Gaume J, Gmel G, Faouzi M, Daeppen JB. Counsellor behaviours and patient language during brief motivational interventions: a sequential analysis of speech. *Addiction*. 2008;103(11):1793–1800.

29. Gaume J, Longabaugh R, Magill M, Bertholet N, Gmel G, Daeppen JB. Under what conditions? therapist and client characteristics moderate the role of change talk in brief motivational intervention. *J Consult Clin Psychol*. 2016;84(3):211–220.

30. Gaume J, Magill M, Mastroleo NR, Longabaugh R, Bertholet N, Gmel G, et al. Change talk during brief motivational intervention with young adult males: strength matters. *J Subst Abuse Treat*. 2016;65:58–65.

31. Gayes LA, Steele RG. A meta-analysis of motivational interviewing interventions for pediatric health behavior change. *J Consult Clin Psychol*. 2014;82(3):521–535.

32. Reference deleted in review.

33. Hill S, Kavookjian J. Motivational interviewing as a behavioral intervention to increase HAART adherence in patients who are HIV-positive: a systematic review of the literature. *AIDS Care*. 2012;24(5):583–592.

34. Houck JM, Hunter SB, Benson JG, Cochrum LL, Rowell LN, D'Amico EJ. Temporal variation in facilitator and client behavior during group motivational interviewing sessions. *Psychol Addict Behav*. 2015;29(4):941–949.

35. Huh D, Mun EY, Larimer ME, White HR, Ray AE, Rhew IC, et al. Brief motivational interventions for college student drinking may not be as powerful as we think: an individual participant-level data meta-analysis. *Alcohol Clin Exp Res*. 2015;39(5):919–931.

36. Jiang S, Wu L, Gao X. Beyond face-to-face individual counseling: a systematic review on alternative modes of motivational interviewing in substance abuse treatment and prevention. *Addict Behav*. 2017;73:216–235.

37. Kay EJ, Vascott D, Hocking A, Nield H. Motivational interviewing in general dental practice: a review of the evidence. *Br Dent J*. 2016;221(12):785–791.

38. Kiesler DJ. The 1982 interpersonal circle: a taxonomy for complementarity in human transactions. *Psychol Rev*. 1983;90:185–214.

39. Kiesler DJ. *Contemporary Interpersonal Theory and Research: Personality, Psychopathology, and Psychotherapy*. New York: Wiley; 1996.

40. Klonek FE, Lehmann-Willenbrock N, Kauffeld S. Dynamics of resistance to change: a sequential analysis of change agents in action. *J Change Manag*. 2014;14(3):1–2.

41. Kohler S, Hofmann A. Can motivational interviewing in emergency care reduce alcohol consumption in young people? A systematic review and meta-analysis. *Alcohol Alcohol*. 2015;50(2):107–117.

42. Lenz AS, Rosenbaum L, Sheperis D. Meta-analysis of randomized controlled trials of motivational enhancement therapy for reducing substance use. *J Addict Offender Couns*. 2016;37(2):66–86.

43. Li L, Zhu S, Tse N, Tse S, Wong P. Effectiveness of motivational interieving to reduce illicit drug use in adolescents: a systematic review and meta-analysis. *Addiction*. 2016;111(5):795–805.

44. Lindson-Hawley N, Thompson TP, Begh R. Motivational interviewing for smoking cessation. 2015;(3):CD006936.

45. Lundahl B, Moleni T, Burke BL, Butters R, Tollefson D, Butler C, et al. Motivational interviewing in medical care settings: a systematic review and meta-analysis of randomized controlled trials. *Patient Edu Counsel*. 2013;93(2):157–168.

46. Magill M, GaumeApodaca J, Walthers TRJ, Mastroleo NR, Borsari B, Longabaugh R. The technical hypothesis of motivational interviewing: a meta-analysis of MI's key causal model. *J Consult Clin Psychol*. 2014;82(6):973–983.

47. Markland D, Ryan RM, Tobin V, Rollnick S. Motivational interviewing and self-determination theory. *J Soc Clin Psychol*. 2005;24:785–805.

48. McKenzie KJ, Pierce D, Gunn JM. A systematic review of motivational interviewing in healthcare: the potential of motivational interviewing to address the lifestyle factors relevant to multimorbidity. *J Comorbidity*. 2015;5(1):162–174.

49. Miller WR. Motivational interviewing with problem drinkers. *Behav Psycho-Therapy.* 1983;11:147–172.

50. Miller WR. Enhancing motivation for change. In: Miller WR, Heather N, eds. *Treating Addictive Behaviors: Processes of Change.* New York: Plenum Press; 1998:121.

51. Miller WR. Motivational factors in addictive behaviors. In: Miller WR, Carroll KM, eds. *Rethinking Substance Abuse: What Science Shows and What We Should Do About It.* New York: Guilford Press; 2006:134.

52. Miller WR, Gribskov CJ, Mortell RL. Effectiveness of a self-control manual for problem drinkers with and without therapist contact. *Int J Addictions.* 1981;16:1247–1254.

53. Miller WR, Rollnick S. *Motivational Interviewing: Preparing People to Change Addictive Behavior.* 1st ed. New York: Guilford Press; 1991.

54. Miller WR, Rollnick S. *Motivational Interviewing: Preparing People for Change.* 2nd ed. New York: Guilford Press; 2002.

55. Miller WR, Rollnick S. *Motivational Interviewing: Helping People Change.* 3rd ed. New York: Guilford Press; 2012.

55a. Miller WR, Rollnick S. The effectiveness and ineffectiveness of complex behavioral interventions: impact of treatment fidelity. *Contemp Clin Trials.* 2014;37(2):234–241.

56. Miller WR, Rose GS. Toward a theory of motivational interviewing. *Am Psychol.* 2009;64(6):527–537.

57. Miller WR, Wilbourne PL. Mesa grande: a methodological analysis of clinical trials of treatments for alcohol use disorders. *Addiction.* 2002;97(3):265–277.

58. Morton K, Beauchamp M, Prothero A, Joyce L, Saunders L, Spencer-Bowdage S, et al. The effectiveness of motivational interviewing for health behaviour change in primary care settings: a systematic review. *Health Psychol Rev.* 2015;9(2):205–223.

59. Moyers TB. The relationship in motivational interviewing. *Psychotherapy.* 2014;51:358–363.

60. Nyamathi AM, Sinha K, Greengold B, Marfisee M, Khalilifard F, Cohen A, et al. Effectiveness of intervention on improvement of drug use among methadone maintained adults. *J Addictiv Dis.* 2011;30(1):6–16.

61. Palacio A, Garay D, Langer B, Taylor J, Wood BA, Tamkariz L. Motivational interviewing improves medication adherence: a systematic review and meta-analysis. *J Gen Int Med.* 2016;31(8):929–940.

62. Reference deleted in review.

63. Prochaska JO, DiClemente CC. The transtheoretical approach. In: Norcross JC, Goldfried MR, eds. *Handbook of Psychotherapy Integration.* 2nd ed. New York: Oxford University; 2005:147–171.

64. Purath J, Keck A, Fitzgerald CE. Motivational interviewing for older adults in primary care: a systematic review. *Geriatric Nurs.* 2014;35(3):219–224.

65. Riper H, Andersson G, Hunter SB, de Wit J, Berking M, Cuijpers P. Treatment of comorbid alcohol use disorders and depression with cognitive-behavioural therapy and motivational interviewing: a meta-analysis. *Addiction.* 2014;109(3):394–406.

66. Rogers C. *On Becoming a Person: A Therapist's View of Psychotherapy.* London: Constable; 1961.

67. Rollnick S, Miller WR. What is motivational interviewing? *Behav Cognit Psychother.* 1995;23:325–334.

68. Romano M, Peters L. *Understanding the Process of Motivational Interviewing: A Review of the Relational and Technical Hypothesis.* Online first; 2014.

69. Rubak S, Sandbaek A, Lauritzen T, Christensen B. Motivational interviewing: a systematic review and meta-analysis. *Br J Gen Prac: J Royal College Gen Practitioners.* 2005;55(513):305–312.

70. Samson JE, Tanner-Smith EE. Single-session alcohol interventions for heavy drinking college students: a systematic review and meta-analysis. *J Studies Alcohol Drugs.* 2015;76(4):530–543.

71. Santa Ana EJ, Lamb K, Morgan-Lopez A, LaRowe S. Impact of group motivational interviewing (GMI) on dually diagnosed veterans with alcohol use disorders. *Drug Alcohol Depend.* 2014;140:e194.

72. Sayegh CS, Huey SJ, Zara EJ, Jhaveri K. Follow-up treatment effects of contingency management and motivational interviewing on substance use: a meta-analysis. *Psychol Addict Behav: J Soc Psychol Addict Behav.* 2017;31(4):403–414.

73. Schwalbe CS, Oh HY, Zweben A. Sustaining motivational interviewing: a meta-analysis of training studies. *Addiction.* 2014;109(8):1287–1294.

74. Shorey RC, Martino S, Lamb KE, LaRowe SD, Ana Santa EJ. Change talk and relatedness in group motivational interviewing: a pilot study. *J Subst Abuse Treat.* 2015;51:75–81.

75. Soderlund LL, Madson MB, Rubak S, Nilsen P. A systematic review of motivational interviewing training for general health care practitioners. *Patient Educ Couns.* 2011;84(1):16–26.

76. Tanner-Smith EE, Lipsey MW. Brief alcohol interventions for adolescents and young adults: a systematic review and meta-analysis. *J Subst Abuse Treat.* 2015;51:1–18.

77. Tanner-Smith EE, Risser MD. A meta-analysis of brief alcohol interventions for adolescents and young adults: variability in effects across alcohol measures. *Am J Drug Alcohol Abuse.* 2016;42(2):140–151.

78. VanBuskirk KA, Wetherell JL. Motivational interviewing with primary care populations: a systematic review and meta-analysis. *J Behav Med.* 2014;37(4):768–780.

79. Wagner CC, Ingersoll KS. Beyond cognition: broadening the emotional base of motivational interviewing. *J Psychother Integration.* 2008;18:191–206.

80. Wagner CC, Ingersoll KS. Beyond behavior: eliciting broader change with motivational interviewing. *J Clin Psychol.* 2009;65(11):1180–1194.

81. Wagner CC, Ingersoll KS. *Motivational Interviewing in Groups.* New York: Guilford Press; 2013.

82. Wagner CC, Ingersoll KS. Development and initial validation of the assessment of motivational interviewing groups – observer scales (AMIGOS). *Int J Group Psychother.* online first; 2017..

83. Wagner CC, Sanchez F. The role of values in motivational interviewing. In: Miller WR, Rollnick S, eds. *Motivational Interviewing: Preparing People to Change.* New York: Guilford Press; 2002:284.

84. Wilson A, Nirantharakumar K, Truchanowicz EG, Surenthirakumaran R, MacArthur C, Coomarasamy A. Motivational interviews to improve contraceptive use in populations at high risk of unintended pregnancy: a systematic review and meta-analysis. *Eur J Obstet Gynecol Reprod Biol.* 2015;191:72–79.

85. Yakovenko I, Quigley L, Hemmelgarn BR, Hodgins DC, Ronksley P. The efficacy of motivational interviewing for disordered gambling: systematic review and meta-analysis. *Addict Behav.* 2015;43:72–82.

86. Zomahoun HT, Guenette L, Gregoire JP, Lauzier S, Lawani AM, Ferdynus C, et al. Effectiveness of motivational interviewing interventions on medication adherence in adults with chronic diseases: a systematic review and meta-analysis. *Int J Epidemiol.* 2016;46(2):589–602.

40
Cognitive Behavioral Therapy for Addiction

MICHELLE VAUGHAN, SURBHI KHANNA, ELIZA BUELT, GABRIELA PACHANO, J. MORGAN PENBERTHY, AND J. KIM PENBERTHY

CHAPTER OUTLINE

Introduction

With the most recent revision (Fifth Edition) of the *Diagnostic and Statistical Manual of Mental Disorders* (DSM-5),[2] addictions are included in a larger category of Substance-Related and Addictive Disorders. Substance use disorders (SUDs) are now subcategorized into three levels of severity (mild, moderate, and severe). The specific criteria individuals must meet has remained similar, with recurrent legal problems no longer serving as a criterion, and craving/urge to use being added as an additional criterion.

Somewhat more stringent minimum criteria have been established for mild SUD (2–3 criteria vs. 1 or more for the old criteria of substance abuse), with 4–5 criteria needed for moderate SUD and 6 or more criteria for severe SUD. A withdrawal syndrome has also been added for cannabis within the newest version of the *International Classification of Diseases* (ICD-10).[88]

Cognitive behavioral therapy (CBT) has proven to be an effective psychotherapeutic treatment for psychiatric disorders such as mood and anxiety spectrum disorders, as well as SUDs. It is an individualized, collaborative approach to psychotherapy that emphasizes the importance of thoughts, feelings, and expectancies and also incorporates more traditional behavioral approaches that utilize counterconditioning and contingency management in addressing the problem of addiction.

CBT is based, in part, on social learning theory.[5] Thus an underlying assumption of cognitive and behavioral therapies[5,6] is that learning processes play an important role in the development and maintenance of SUDs. These same learning processes can be used to help individuals reduce their drug and alcohol use through modification and substitution of existing patterns. CBT is also based on stress and coping theories. These theories promote that life stressors are likely to trigger the use of avoidance or emotion-focused coping strategies such as substance use in individuals who have low self-efficacy and poor problem-solving coping skills in an attempt to avoid experiencing distress.[7] As such, CBT focuses on challenging individuals' positive expectancies about substance use, enhancing their self-confidence and self-efficacy to resist substance misuse, and improving their overall and specific skills for coping with life stress.

When applied to the addicted population, CBT helps a client change his or her drug or alcohol use as well as risky attitudes and beliefs.[7,44] CBT combines two very effective kinds of psychotherapy—cognitive therapy and behavioral therapy. CBT for SUDs focuses on helping clients in two major behavioral ways.[38] The first is to help reduce the intensity and frequency of their urges to use, by undermining their underlying beliefs or cognitions about using. The second is to teach the clients specific techniques for controlling or managing their urges to use or drink. In other words, the basic goals are to reduce the pressure to use and increase control. When a client's addiction is determined to be related to a co-occurring disorder, the psychiatric disorder also needs to be addressed by the mental health care provider.

Cognitive therapy focuses on how certain thinking patterns or beliefs cause symptoms.[6] Distorted or unproductive thoughts or cognitions can produce negative moods such as anxiety and depression, which can ultimately provoke more maladaptive thinking and/or behaviors that do not help facilitate positive change or affect. Cognitive therapy strategies focus on thought processes, recognizing that emotions and behaviors are best addressed by considering the faulty thought processes that precede such feelings and acts. Specifically, cognitive therapists collaborate with clients to define problems, explore beliefs, reexamine appraisals and thoughts about their use of substances, and modify these thoughts to promote more favorable and adaptive cognitions, which, in turn, impact positively both behaviors and mood. In addition, coping skills training expands this emphasis on thought processes by focusing clients on accepting stressors in their lives and constructively pursuing strategies to change their valence and tendency to pursue substances to escape and/or avoid situations. Although researchers/clinicians affirm the practicality of this approach as well, cognitive therapy cannot comprehensively address all aspects of SUDs without addressing the destructive behavioral inclinations common to substance users.

Behavioral therapy focuses on weakening the connections between troublesome situations and habitual behavioral reactions to them.[20] Strategies included in behavioral therapy include repeated behavioral practice of techniques such as distraction and relaxation and exploring consequences and reinforcement. A major goal of the behavioral component is to weaken the learned association between triggers such as the environment, situation, people, or moods, and the response of drug or alcohol use, and replace it with a more appropriate response. In time, the healthy response will become more familiar and replace the old response of using. Thus in many ways, the behavioral strategies employed are similar to those used for habit reversal or compulsive behaviors. These include teaching relaxation strategies such as deep breathing and progressive muscle relaxation, learning alternative responses such as drinking juice instead of alcohol, employing behavioral distraction, and avoiding triggers or risky situations. Two subtypes of this approach include contingency management (a positive-reinforcement treatment method in which clients are given rewards for constructive actions taken toward their recovery) and community reinforcement (a set of procedures that systematically reinforce treatment retention and substance reduction/abstinence). Clients may be rewarded for specific positive behaviors, such as producing drug-negative urine, returning to therapy, and specific lifestyle changes. These effective behavioral strategies frequently are incorporated into CBT for SUDs. CBT integrates both methods into a logical series of strategies that can identify maladaptive thoughts and resultant actions (via a decisional matrix and functional analysis), disrupt automatic patterns of functioning (through coping skills training and practice), reduce the impact of—and harmful response to—stress, and adopt more prosocial learning and interactions.

The goal of cognitive behavioral therapy can be either abstinence or moderate/controlled drinking or drug use (i.e., harm reduction), and is employed routinely for relapse prevention in abstinent individuals. CBT helps the client to identify his/her own unique high-risk situations for use. Then the client may develop plans and skills that are alternatives to using in these situations. CBT is designed to increase the client's confidence about his/her ability to resist using. Because SUDs have high rates of relapse, CBT includes effective relapse-prevention components of treatment.

Overview of Cognitive Behavioral Therapy

CBT combines two effective kinds of psychotherapy—cognitive therapy and behavioral therapy—to help clients change their drinking or drug use behavior and related risky attitudes and beliefs.[7] Cognitive therapy teaches individuals how certain thinking patterns contribute to their symptoms by giving them a distorted picture of events and interpersonal interactions in their lives, thus directly contributing to feelings of anxiety, depression, or anger that may provoke them into ill-chosen actions. Behavioral therapy helps individuals weaken the learned connections between troublesome situations and their habitual behavioral reactions to them.

Following the work of the more radical behaviorists (i.e., Skinner, Watson), Albert Ellis applied behavioral concepts to his work on human emotions in early work on addiction.[20] Ellis drew attention to the relationship between events (the "activating event"), personal beliefs, and resultant emotional responses. This model (a main component of rational emotive therapy) came to be known as ABC (A: activating event, B: beliefs, and C: emotional response), highlighting how a personal belief (B) about an activating event (A) could impact emotions (C). Ellis demonstrated that changing maladaptive beliefs (termed "irrational beliefs") regarding a client's perceptions of activating events to more rational and practical personal beliefs would lead to more desired emotional self-management. This model is used frequently in CBT and has been shown to be very effective in reducing substance use.[3]

Similarly, Aaron Beck extended Ellis' work to address irrational beliefs in primarily depressed clients. Because negative mood states have a high concordance rate with SUDs (13%–30%), Beck's strategies can be very helpful in addressing the myriad of irrational beliefs held by individuals with these disorders.[7] Specifically, Beck identified several common irrational beliefs held by these individuals that serve to reinforce their desires to use substances. These thought patterns include thoughts of helplessness, ideas that drugs improve their functioning, all-or-none thinking, self-criticism, assuming need for perfection, and mind reading. Failure to question the rationality of these thoughts relegates substance-using clients to repeat continuously the ABC cycle, with the addition of behaviorally acting on "C" in a way that further discourages the clients and reinforces the hopelessness that they feel through substance use. Through CBT, however, these irrational thoughts are explored extensively while supplanting drug behavior with healthy coping strategies. The goal of CBT can be to attain either no drinking/drug use (abstinence) or moderate/controlled drinking/use (i.e., harm reduction).

Beck found that underlying addictive beliefs result from dysfunctional core schemas in three areas: personal survival, autonomy, and freedom.[38] These addictive and dysfunctional thought patterns are experienced as taking over the individual's life, goals, and values, thereby leaving one's job and families as secondary priorities. The short-term gain of a high or a reduction of internal tension is followed by long-term negative consequences and problems.[38] To break this pattern, clients need to learn to cope directly with problems associated with SUDs, as well as to confront problems of everyday life in a more active and problem-solving manner.

The obstacle, unfortunately, in eliminating the substance use is the dysfunctional beliefs that the individual holds about the substance.[38] These beliefs range from the fear of the side effects of withdrawal to the belief that he/she cannot function without the substance. In addition, permission beliefs are common in addicted individuals. These are conceptualized as thoughts that allow or give permission to the individual to go ahead and use.

These thoughts include such self-statements as "Just one drink won't hurt anything. Go ahead and have one." Changing these schemas, maladaptive beliefs, thought patterns, and associations with common triggers is at the core of the cognitive approach. Thoughts must be altered to achieve long-term behavioral change.

When utilizing CBT, the client identifies his/her own unique high-risk situations for heavy drinking or drug use with the help of the therapist. Then, using CBT techniques, the therapist helps the client to develop plans and skills that are alternatives to using alcohol or drugs in these situations. Thus, using CBT also increases the client's confidence about his/her ability to resist using alcohol or drugs. Because people who are addicted typically demonstrate high rates of return to using, CBT also includes relapse-prevention training[55] and strategies to employ when lapses occur.

CBT has been used in both inpatient and outpatient settings. Therapists who provide CBT typically possess at least a master's-level degree plus specific training in this area, and more typically possess a Ph.D. in clinical or counseling psychology or an M.D. and advanced training in psychotherapy. Longabaugh and Morgenstern[50] recommended at least 12 sessions for clients with SUDs. In this way, CBT not only is clinically effective for substance treatment, but it is also efficient, time-limited, and cost-effective. Prior to initiating CBT, it is helpful for the therapist to assess the client across a number of functional areas in order to customize therapy to the client's specific needs. A thorough evaluation of readiness to change, mood, anxiety, and other emotional difficulties can be very helpful in defining the content of therapy. Information regarding the most recent negative consequences precipitated by substance use and the client's current stage of change[72] can be particularly helpful in determining how the therapist should interact with the client initially.

The transtheoretical model of Prochaska and Velicer[72] offers a useful conceptualization of a client's stage of change that can be used to motivate a client and better inform subsequent psychotherapy. The transtheoretical model of behavior change, or stages of change model, describes a series of six behavioral stages that an individual experiences in modifying a negative behavior in his/her life. These stages include denial, precontemplation, contemplation, preparation, action, and maintenance. Precontemplation is the first stage in this model and refers to individuals who do not consider their current behavior to be problematic and have not thought about stopping/changing their behavior within the past 6 months. If individuals begin to recognize the negative consequences of their behaviors, they find themselves in contemplation, where they begin to think about changing their behavior over the next 1–6 months and making plans for how to implement changes. In the action stage, individuals have made consistent behavior chances and have been able to sustain these changes for up to 6 months. In the maintenance stage, the individual has successfully changed his/her behavior and maintained these behavioral changes for 6 months or longer. By identifying a client's current stage of change, the cognitive behavioral therapist can better tailor the initial dialog of therapy to address related barriers to the client's desire to change and level of progress with respect to making changes.

Motivational interviewing[61] combines knowledge of individuals stage of change into a directive, collaborative process that builds self-efficacy through empathetic engagement with ambivalence. Often used in conjunction with CBT, these motivational enhancement strategies can reveal a client's maladaptive thought patterns that can be explored in more detail as the CBT sessions progress. Strategies such as using open-ended questions, affirming client thoughts, reflecting client statements, and summarizing client messages can be helpful in resolving clients' confusion and resistance to change. Clients in more advanced stages of change (action and maintenance) can begin CBT immediately. In such cases, motivational interviewing exercises such as the decisional matrix, which involves having the client list the pros and cons of using and not using substances, can be employed to clarify further any remaining ambivalence and reinforce motivation to change.

Cognitive Model of Addiction

Multiple interrelated cognitive models of addiction have been developed and evaluated since Bandura's classic presentations of social learning theory in the late 1960s and 1970s.[5] For example, Marlatt and Gordon[55] described four cognitive processes related to addictions that reflect the cognitive models: self-efficacy, outcome expectancies, attributions of causality, and decision-making processes. According to Beck et al.,[7] people try drugs initially to get pleasure, to experience the exhilaration of being high, and to share the excitement of using with others. In addition, often additional positive expectations are associated with use of the drug. For example, with cocaine, individuals expect greater energy, fluency, and creativity. They might desire reduced appetite that can lead to weight loss and greater productivity. For clients with alcohol use disorders, often the prime motivations for early use are greater sociability, reduced anxiety, and relief from boredom. These positive consequences often mask the negative consequences of drug use. Although these desired states may be based partly on real drug effects, substance users begin to distort the valence and importance of these effects over time. Cognitive distortions, in combination with life stressors (which ultimately increase as the person begins to neglect or avoid problems or responsibilities), lead to increased drug and alcohol use in pursuit of greater relief and/or pleasure, or a desire just to feel normal. Such problem-distracting behaviors have been described as self-medicating, whereby the person seeks to reduce the distress and problems associated with using through avoidance behavior and by increasing their use. This increased drug and alcohol use often leads to greater problems in the person's life and greater problem avoidance through greater and/or more frequent substance use.

In addition to the distorted thoughts that substances users hold regarding the positive effects of using, users have been found to have a significantly greater tendency to ruminate on irrational or automatic cognitive thoughts.[7] These thoughts include beliefs such as "I can't settle down without a few drinks," "I can't stand this feeling," and "people don't like me unless I am intoxicated." Such thoughts often relate to feelings of depression and anxiety, and the substance users seek the substance to reduce the distress of such thoughts. Drugs initially act as a distraction against these automatic and distressing thoughts and allow the person to forget the unpleasant ruminations. In this way, drugs appear to serve an adaptive function by allowing the person to turn off the ruminations temporarily. Unfortunately, this distraction is maladaptive over the long term, in that it prevents the individual from facing and dealing with problems in a healthy manner and creates more functional life problems. As the person becomes physiologically and psychologically dependent upon (or addicted to) the substance, the ability to change cognitive distortions without assistance becomes less and less likely. The goal of the cognitive therapist, then, becomes helping the client to recognize these distortions and to develop self-efficacy to actively address such thoughts in a more adaptive manner.

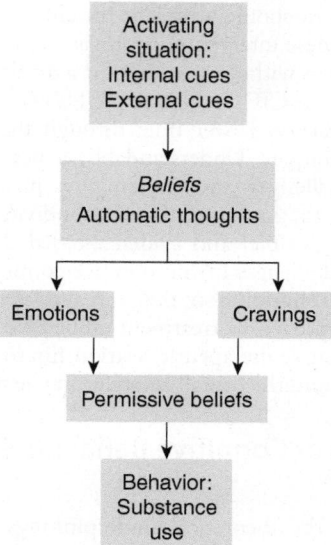

• **Fig. 40.1** Cognitive behavioral conceptualization of addiction.

In the context of development of and relapse from alcohol use disorder, Marlatt and Gordon[55] described the process of developing and relapsing from alcohol use disorders as a cognitive decision-making process. He proposed that substance use is a result of multiple decisions, which may or may not lead to further substance use and SUDs. He explained that although some decisions initially appear to be irrelevant to substance use, they nonetheless may result ultimately in an increased likelihood of relapse because of their incremental push toward higher-risk situations. To the extent that a person expects a greater positive versus negative outcome from drinking or using drugs (one's outcome expectancies), the person is likely to continue using the substance. Individuals' attributions of causality regarding substance use also play an important role in their continued use, as those who see their use as out of their own control or predestined (due to external factors) will likely maintain their use. Self-efficacy to cope with demanding or otherwise high-risk situations without the use of the substance are also crucial in the context of relapse, with rates of long-term abstinence likely to vary directly as a function of self-efficacy.[55]

From this perspective, the primary tasks of treatment are to identify and challenge the maladaptive cognitions/beliefs surrounding alcohol and drug use and replace them with more realistic and adaptive thoughts and beliefs in order to facilitate more adaptive behaviors of reduced use or abstinence. When more adaptive cognitive thinking has been restored, behavioral changes consistent with constructive thinking will follow. Fig. 40.1 portrays the cognitive behavioral conceptualization of addiction.

Behavioral Model of Addiction

From the perspective of cognitive behavioral theory, SUDs are viewed as learned behavior that is modeled, acquired, and reinforced through experience and learning.[55] If alcohol or drugs provide or are perceived to provide certain desired results (e.g., good feelings, reduced tension) on repeated occasions, the person may learn that the substance leads to the desired outcome. In other words, the substances and positive feelings become strongly associated with each other. People typically begin using drugs or alcohol as a positive reinforcement in their lives—to celebrate a

special occasion, as a reward, to reduce inhibitions, and/or to promote relaxation. In other words, initial use of drugs or alcohol is associated with its positive consequences, becoming the preferred way of achieving those results, particularly in the absence of other ways of meeting those desired ends. For some individuals, chronic use of drugs or alcohol can become a problem in cases where the substance is no longer used to feel good, but to avoid negative thoughts/feelings or to feel normal by reducing withdrawal symptoms. When this happens, substance use becomes a negative reinforcement instead of a positive one. From this perspective, the primary tasks of treatment are to (1) identify the specific needs that alcohol and drugs are being used to meet, and (2) develop skills that provide alternative ways of meeting those needs. In so doing, this breaks the learned associations between using drugs and alcohol and both the positive and negative reinforcements.

Persons with substance problems are highly vulnerable to high-risk stimuli for a variety of reasons.[55] Specifically, as people accommodate their drinking and drug habits, they begin to establish behavioral patterns in a variety of environmental contexts, which reinforce their intention to use as well as their experiential expectations. These environmental contexts become associated with the positive experiences of the drug over time and evolve into triggers that stimulate the user's desire for the drug. These triggers include both internal and external cues. Internal cues may include positive or negative emotions, pain, and/or frustration. External cues can include time of day (e.g., evening, night), place (e.g., at a friend's house, at a bar), or even other persons (e.g., friend, family). External cues also can include situations such as getting paid or working in an environment where alcohol is served (waitresses, bartenders). These triggers often activate clients' erroneous or irrational beliefs and lead them to make risky decisions that bring them closer to using. Such triggers must be identified and explored for underlying beliefs that shape physiological sensations linked to craving.

Case Conceptualization

As is the case in the treatment of other disorders, CBT for SUDs involves a unique case conceptualization for each individual. This forms the basis for a strong collaborative relationship between client and therapist, and effectively guides the content of the sessions. Through such collaboration, the client and therapist proceed to utilize specific, goal-oriented techniques tailored to the client's individualized needs and goals[50] while simultaneously enhancing the therapeutic alliance and collaborative nature of the work. Individuals are also taught to address and resolve naturally arising ambivalence about treatment to develop their motivation and progress toward their treatment goals. During therapy sessions, as well as through the use of self-help homework assignments, clients pursue solution-focused strategies that address the realities of recovery from addictive disorders. Psychotherapeutic innovations in relapse prevention often are implemented over the course of CBT for alcohol and other drug use disorders through identifying and reducing or learning to cope with high-risk use situations.

Case Example

Jonas is a 47-year-old man with a history of using alcohol since adolescence. He initially began using alcohol to reduce anxiety and facilitate dating experiences after he divorced his wife in his thirties. He began using alcohol as a way to enhance his ability to generate conversations in social situations. He works as an accountant and believes that others are very critical of him and see him as "stuffy" and "boring." He uses the alcohol mainly in the evenings

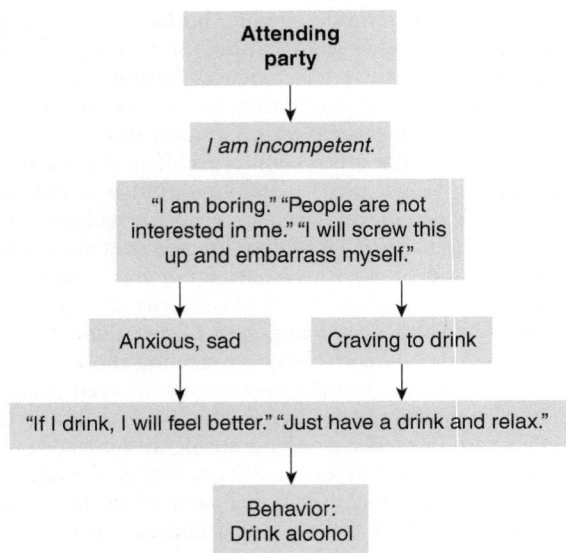

Attending party

↓

I am incompetent.

"I am boring." "People are not interested in me." "I will screw this up and embarrass myself."

↓ ↓

Anxious, sad   Craving to drink

↓ ↓

"If I drink, I will feel better." "Just have a drink and relax."

↓

Behavior: Drink alcohol

• **Fig. 40.2** Cognitive behavioral conceptualization of Jonas's case presentation.

when he goes out with business associates after work, although on weekends he has noticed that his drinking often starts early and continues all day long when he is visiting with friends or family.

When Jonas first divorced, he was quite anxious about becoming more social and going out with peers again. He started consuming a few alcoholic beverages as a way to reduce his anxiety and lower his inhibitions about making interesting conversation. In this way, Jonas's behavior was positively reinforced and he would later remember the situation as enjoyable and without anxiety. Over time, however, his tolerance for alcohol increased and he required more drinks to achieve his perceived degree of calmness required to make good conversation. He started feeling more anxious, and even depressed, if he could not consume alcohol, particularly when meeting with others.

Fig. 40.2 shows a cognitive behavioral case conceptualization of Jonas's alcohol use.

By understanding the relationships between Jonas's dysfunctional thoughts and behavioral patterns, insight regarding the nature of his alcohol problems can be gained and an individualized treatment program can be developed to address his unique needs. Since CBT has evidence-based techniques as its foundation, techniques such as recognizing and challenging maladaptive automatic thoughts, cue exposure, drug refusal training, and methods for coping with craving are used to help an individual break his/her pattern of addiction. Furthermore, because addictive disorders often involve deficits in areas such as social skills, management of emotions, and tolerance of difficult emotions, individuals often pursue progress in these areas within CBT. For example:

Jonas was encouraged to keep a diary of his thoughts and behaviors to help him understand and recognize the connection between his maladaptive thoughts and subsequent emotions and behaviors. With this information, Jonas and his therapist were able to challenge the veracity of his anxiety-provoking thoughts and substitute his critical interpretations with more rational views of his reality. In addition, Jonas was taught relaxation techniques (progressive muscle relaxation and imagery) to help manage his anxiety, as well as learning to tolerate some anxiety in his interactions with others. Finally, Jonas learned social skills regarding interactions with others, particularly in regard to his unrealistic

expectation that he should always be the entertainer in a conversation. Through these interventions, Jonas began to expose himself to social situations without reaching for a drink.

The rationale of CBT holds that SUDs are learned and, therefore, can be unlearned over time through the use of cognitive behavioral techniques. Understandably, a person with an SUD faces many challenges and, potentially, many serious consequences. However, through CBT, such individuals can take part in an effective, flexible, and evidence-based therapy specifically tailored to the challenges involved in overcoming SUDs and their individual needs. In doing so, they can avail themselves of a solution-focused approach to treatment embedded within a respectful and collaborative therapeutic relationship to facilitate recovery from addiction and the overall lifestyle change that they need.

Application of Cognitive Behavioral Therapy for Addiction

Understanding the theoretical underpinnings of cognitive and behavioral conceptualizations of addiction helps the therapist identify logical cognitive and behavioral targets for therapeutic intervention. This allows the therapist to individualize treatment for each client while remaining consistent with the general theoretical approach.

Therapy typically begins with an introduction to CBT and an opportunity for the client to disclose information about himself/herself. This is an important time for self-disclosure and building of the therapeutic alliance, as well as the beginning of the process of case conceptualization of the client and his/her presenting issues. During these early meetings, initial treatment goals are discussed. These goals are set collaboratively, with the client having the final say in the establishment of his/her goals. Abstinence is encouraged but may not be an absolute requirement. Treatment goals may involve substance use behaviors as well as other aspects of clients' lives, such as improved relationships, mood states, and level of functioning. Therapists work with clients to ensure that these goals are attainable (the client can produce them), realistic (the environment can produce them), and appropriate (they are related to the designated work to be done in therapy). Goals are revisited and revised as needed throughout treatment, based primarily upon the client's progress, which is assessed regularly.

The therapeutic process itself includes meeting regularly (usually for an hour weekly) for at least 3–6 months or longer if necessitated by continuation of symptoms or development of additional problems. Within each session, material is presented and reviewed regarding specific areas of concentration that relate to SUDs as well as more general issues related to emotional dysfunction. Session material may be presented orally and in writing (e.g., using written materials, flip charts, or a wipe-off board), and clients are encouraged to take notes, as visual learning significantly augments oral presentation of material and helps clients retain more information and stay involved in the session. There are issues that must be covered for the majority of clients receiving CBT, including: coping with cravings, thinking about using, problem solving, refusal skills, dealing with lapses, and relapse prevention. In addition, there often are additional issues that need to be addressed, such as assertiveness training, anger management, and recognizing and managing negative moods. These issues are addressed on an individual basis, but in a standardized cognitive behavioral conceptualization. Thus evidence-based treatment is tailored to the individual and provided in a consistent manner.

Weekly assignments or homework are assigned at each session and reviewed at the following session. The homework is a major part of CBT and ensures that clients are actively incorporating skills and techniques presented and reviewed in sessions in real life. Clients are encouraged to complete the homework, preferably in writing, and always through real-world practice. Research demonstrates that those clients who complete homework assignments more regularly consistently attain a better outcome from therapy, particularly those higher in readiness to change.[13,24,41] Therefore, homework completion is strongly encouraged. Compliance with homework can be increased in many ways: (1) through explaining the reasoning for the assignment and why and how it is theorized to help the client; (2) reviewing in session how to complete the homework; (3) assessing the client's motivation and ability to complete the homework by asking the client how likely he/she is to complete it and identifying any potential obstacles for completion, and then (4) clarifying ambivalence about homework and planning for obstacles, as well as (5) setting realistic expectations for the length of time and level of difficulty of the homework.

If a client is regularly noncompliant with homework, efforts are made to explore and change this therapy-interfering behavior. Specific techniques are employed to improve homework compliance, including making homework assignments specific and clear and explaining the rationale of the homework as well as the potential benefits of completing the assignment. As stated, setting realistic expectations for the homework is also important. Most assignments take less than 15 min to complete, and this needs to be made explicit to the client or else the client may overestimate the time needed to complete the assignment and may not even attempt it. Behavioral experiments need to be clearly defined and a rationale provided for their use, along with expected benefits. In addition, the client's level of motivation and commitment to completing the assignments can be assessed prior to the end of the session, so that realistic expectations are made regarding the homework. For instance, if a client understands the rationale of the homework and knows how to complete it and how long it will take, but still states that he/she does not want to do it and does not think that he/she is likely to complete it, then both the therapist and client understand that the homework will most likely not be completed unless the client's motivation changes. Some authors argue that homework non-compliance, to some degree, is an inevitable feature of CBT and, when effectively addressed, can yield some of the greatest opportunities for therapeutic change.[24] To that end, it is an expected and important component of CBT, and both clients and clinicians are wise to anticipate and prepare effectively for non-compliance issues.

General Components of Manualized Cognitive Behavioral Therapy for Addiction

CBT is commonly provided in a standard, manualized format for conceptualizing drinking and drug use problems and designing interventions that focus on developing healthier coping skills. It is often delivered in a collaborative motivational interviewing style, which facilitates the individual's progress through stages of change and therapeutic recovery. Manualized CBT is based on the early works of Beck et al.,[6] Ellis and Velten,[20] and the later works of Marlatt and Gordon.[55] These works eventually were condensed into the National Institute on Alcohol Abuse and Alcoholism's treatment protocol,[66] which has been broadly utilized in multi-site national addiction studies, including MATCH[73] and COMBINE.[71]

While there have been many variations and therapy subtypes that fall under the collective umbrella of CBT, this protocol specifically outlines standardized session themes and activities that have been shown to bring positive outcomes (reductions in drinking or drug use) and ensures systematic, effective, reliable, and replicable administration of treatment to individuals. The structure of CBT discussion topics and session activities for SUDs is designed to promote effective management of session time, focus on client thoughts, and development of more effective coping strategies.[36] It should be noted, however, that while this manualized approach has proven helpful and represents one of the most common cognitive behavioral frameworks for treating SUDs, therapists have considerable flexibility in matching unique client strengths and weaknesses to specific cognitive behavioral interventions within the weekly theme (such as role plays, review of take-home assignments, and construction of agenda). As such, the session is approached in a collaborative manner that tolerates modifications to planned activities as necessary. Yet, even with these potential changes and exploration of therapy-related themes, an overall commitment to therapeutic setting and following a set agenda is recommended to provide useful structure to the client problem-solving and coping resolution process.[36]

The following recommendations are based on results from the University of Virginia Center for Leading Edge Addiction Research (formerly the Center for Addiction Research and Education) clinic, which is part of the Department of Psychiatry and Neurobehavioral Sciences. Similar to the the National Institute on Alcohol Abuse and Alcoholism's CBT manual,[66] the clinic also administered CBT over 12 sessions in either group or individual format. There are seven core sessions, four elective sessions, and a termination session. Specific material is covered in each session as tolerated and has been designed and studied for optimum effectiveness.

Contraindications

There are some contraindications for use of CBT in populations with SUDs. First of all, this approach requires a minimum level of cognitive functioning. Specifically, abstract reasoning is deemed necessary for clients to understand and process session material and apply this knowledge to changing their behavior patterns and coping skills. Clients with serious psychopathology (such as manic episodes, psychosis, or acute intoxication) or low IQ/cognitive impairment may likely to have great difficulty understanding concepts such as cues or automatic thoughts and/or systematically adopting new coping skills. Furthermore, clients with a diffuse set of maladaptive thoughts and behaviors may require a greater number of sessions to achieve abstinence in comparison with those with specific, more circumscribed maladaptive symptoms. Finally, CBT is also directive in nature, with the therapist playing a major role in directing the focus and content of each session. As such, some clients may respond with resistance to this approach or demonstrate slow progress in therapy. Thus, it is important to be aware of the stage of change for your client and consider integrating a motivational interviewing style into your work if it is clear that the client is unwilling to admit that they have an addiction problem or if your client loses motivation at any time during treatment. If clients report that they do not wish to change their behavior, cognitive behavioral strategies, such as listing the pros and cons of using and quitting in the form of a decisional matrix (Box 40.1), clarifying values, examining consequences of use and challenging expectancy beliefs about use can successfully be utilized to clarify ambivalence and help refocus the therapeutic work on change.

Format/Length/Setting

Clients were seen either one-on-one or in a small group setting (2–5 individuals per group) in a private, confidential clinic for 12 sessions. Each individual session lasted approximately 60 min, and group sessions last approximately 90 min, although some sessions can be extended or reduced based on client needs. During the first session, the therapist devoted the time to develop a strong therapeutic alliance with the client, approaching the client in a friendly and neutral (i.e., not extremely dominant, not extremely submissive) interpersonal manner. In our clinic, clients were given a questionnaire every three sessions that assesses their interpersonal impression of the therapist and their working relationship. Research has shown that therapists who are able to maintain friendly and neutral interactions best facilitate client outcomes.[41] During each session, the therapist checks in with the client and reviews his/her progress over the preceding week. Then, the therapist reviewed the take-home assignment from the previous week, highlights achievements, and determines the cause of skill failures. Next, the therapist and the client create an agenda for the session duration that includes exploration of the weekly theme (see list of themes below). The remainder of the session explored new skill acquisition, and, together, the therapist and the client determined new practice activities and goals for the subsequent week.

Expectations of Therapist for Client

It is important for the therapist to discuss treatment expectations on the first day of therapy. Clients are expected to attend therapy regularly, on time, and sober. They are expected to report about their addiction honestly and to complete practice assignments before returning to therapy.

Functional Analysis

At the beginning, as well as throughout addiction treatment, clients and therapists should use monitoring records and functional analysis tools as a way to conceptualize clients' use and problems. In Table 40.1, clients are asked to notice and record the situations

in which they crave alcohol or drugs and record the severity of the craving and their subsequent behavior. By doing so, people increasingly become aware of the specific triggers in their environment and the variations in their cravings, as well as when they give in to their cravings. In Table 40.2, a functional analysis table, clients are asked to track the triggers (What set me up to use?), thoughts and feelings (What was I thinking and feeling?), behavior (What did I do?), and positive (What positive thing happened?) and negative (What negative thing happened?) consequences of their substance use. Clients should be instructed to write down every time they think about drinking or using a drug. It is important that clients record the time and day whenever they record an entry in this log to help with understanding behavioral patterns. In the "Triggers" column, clients should record who they are with, what they are doing, details about the situation, etc., to give a full picture of what was happening at the time a craving or urge to use or drink began. In the next column, they are to record specific thoughts and feelings that provoked the urge to use. In the middle "Behavior" column, clients should record how they were responding to the situations. Did they call a friend? Watch TV? Or pop open a can of beer? They should record all of this information here. In the last two columns, they should record the consequences, both positive and negative, of their behavior. Clients should bring this record with them to their next appointment for further review. These exercises should continue throughout treatment, particularly as clients become more skilled at choosing more adaptive coping strategies.

Skills Training

Clients also are taught pro-social adaptive coping skills to substitute maladaptive ways of coping. Specifically, clients are taught to set realistic self-goals, self-monitor thoughts and behaviors, challenge irrational thoughts, delay reacting to cravings, pursue distractions, confront problems directly, problem-solve actively, talk to others, avoid triggers, and reduce stress. These skills are assessed at baseline and tracked throughout treatment. Clients are taught to practice strategies between therapy sessions and to treat drinking opportunities as experiments for learning to implement new skills in the face of triggers to use.

Manualized Sessions—Sequence of Therapy Topics

Session 1: Introduction—Set goals, review therapy expectations and teach self-monitoring of triggers, thoughts, feelings, behaviors, and positive and negative consequences; also determine clients' drinking/using patterns. Clients are given a manual to reinforce weekly topics.

Session 2: Coping with Cravings—Explore a variety of active coping strategies to reduce cravings, such as: distraction, delaying use, pursuing social support, avoiding triggers, deep breathing/progressive muscle relaxation, imagery/urge surfing, and recalling negative consequences/planning ahead.

Session 3: Thinking about Using—Review thoughts common to persons with addiction problems, such as: nostalgia, disillu-

---

> **• BOX 40.1   Decisional Matrix or Advantages-Disadvantages Analysis**

Box 1: Good Things About Drinking

Box 2: Bad Things About Drinking

Box 4: Good Things About Changing My Drinking

Box 3: Bad Things About Changing My Drinking

TABLE 40.1   Self-Monitoring of Cravings.

Event/Situation	Intensity of cravings (0–100)	Behavior
Going to a party, feeling nervous	85%	Drink prior to going to party

---

TABLE 40.2   Functional Analysis: Self-Monitoring Record.

Triggers	Thoughts	Feelings	Behaviors	CONSEQUENCES Positive	Negative
3/9/16, 9 P.M. At home with girlfriend, arguing	I can't stand this; I need a drink	Angry 95%	Drank 4 beers	Calmed down	Girlfriend more mad; upset with myself

sionment, frustration, all-or-none thinking, self-doubt, feeling uncomfortable, helplessness, wanting to escape, crisis response, and testing control. Also consider how clients' expectations regarding how substance impacts thoughts/ feelings affect behavior.

Session 4: Problem Solving—Present a model for solving problems in an active way that considers generating a list of alternatives and evaluating pros and cons and the likelihood of positive outcomes, given the potential to resolve.

Session 5: Drink Refusal Skills—Consider ways to avoid giving in to requests by peers to use. Teach client to avoid these high-risk situations to the extent possible and, when unexpectedly exposed to triggers, to rely upon a predetermined plan to avoid use.

Session 6: Dealing with a Lapse—Describe how clients can lapse from time to time and how such lapses need not derail progress. Give strategies to help client return to recovery and refocus on treatment goals.

Session 7: Seemingly Irrelevant Decisions—Examine how small, seemingly irrelevant decisions that do not appear to affect drinking/use decisions can put a person at risk for relapse. Examine ways to prevent relapse through the deliberate choice of low-risk behavioral choices.

Last Session: Termination/Maintenance/Relapse Prevention—Review client progress over the course of therapy, re-examine client goals, review briefly all material, determine client skill achievements, recommend further practice with some skills, and make recommendations for follow-up.

Example of Skill Acquisition

Jonas completed a coping strategy questionnaire at baseline, indicating that he was relatively passive in dealing with his stress and anxiety and that he generally gave in to cravings when they developed. To collect more information about Jonas's coping skills and to help Jonas see a connection between his coping strategies and behaviors, he was assigned to complete a functional analysis diary. Jonas was initially reluctant to keep a diary regarding his daily drinking habits because he felt that he did not have any triggers and that he "just liked the taste" and "enjoyed a few drinks" with others. However, after reviewing his first week with his therapist and attempting to complete the diary retrospectively, Jonas became aware that much of his drinking related to feelings of inadequacy and loneliness. Jonas found that these feelings were reinforced each night with different people in that he was able to stop his feelings of anxiety by drinking "a few" beers. Unfortunately, the next day Jonas would always feel tired and disappointed by how many beers he had in fact drunk. He also worried about what he may have said in his "entertaining" conversations, as he often could not even remember much of the night beyond his second drink. In this way, the therapist was able to challenge his expectation that drinking made him entertaining and also help him to realize that drinking did not cure his anxiety over the long term; it only served to blunt temporarily all feelings. It also was determined by reviewing the diary that Jonas was going to nightly events that all involved opportunities to consume alcohol. With his therapist, he was able to recall healthier activities such as playing tennis or volunteering with a local charity. These activities helped to remove some of Jonas's temptation to drink, as well as distracting him for several hours in the evening, a time when his cravings were the most intense. Through the activities, Jonas learned how to cultivate a few new friendships without alcohol, which helped provide support for Jonas when he was

feeling stressed. Over time, Jonas was able to look forward to not going to the bars with his old friends; he then felt encouraged that he could tolerate some anxiety around others and developed pride that he did not need alcohol to endure his stress. Jonas continued to keep a journal of his thoughts and behaviors throughout therapy and became more aware of the great importance of monitoring his triggers, particularly when his problem seemed too overwhelming to overcome. Jonas completed a post-therapy coping skills questionnaire and was able to identify several strategies that he found to be helpful and effective for dealing with his cravings.

Research Support for Cognitive Behavioral Therapy in Addiction Literature

CBT has been demonstrated to facilitate effectively improvement for a number of mainstream SUDs. Across substances, more advanced stage of change/higher motivation to change at the start of treatment has generally been linked to improvements substance outcomes and/or treatment completion,[25,87] although not all studies have found such a relationship.[35] Consistent with the tenants of cognitive and behavioral therapies, client-reported self-efficacy[a] and outcome expectancies regarding substance use,[27,47] appear to play a critical role in the effectiveness of CBT for SUDs. However, empirical studies have failed to find a relationship between cognitive functioning and substance related outcomes with the use of CBT in SUD treatment,[26,42] indicating that cognitive functioning may not be as critical as hypothesized to the success of CBT in treatment for SUDs.

Treatment gains with respect to stimulant use have also been well established, with evidence that gains persist and grow over periods of 3–12 months.[b] The majority of this published empirical literature with respect to the effectiveness of CBT, however, has centered on the use of cocaine, methamphetamine, and/or nicotine.

Review of Cognitive Behavioral Therapy for Stimulant Drugs

Cocaine

Approximately 1.5 million adults use cocaine in the United States, often leading to problems in daily functioning and, ultimately, cocaine use disorders[15]. CBT has been demonstrated to be useful for managing and resolving the problems associated with SUDs. Marlatt and Gordon[55] introduced cognitive behavioral interventions as an effective approach that can alleviate psychological distress associated with repetitive physical and psychological habits arising from specific, reinforcing cognitive and behavioral patterns. Additional work by Carroll et al.[14] extended Marlatt and Gordon's work to include a specific, manualized protocol (see the National Institute on Drug Abuse–endorsed format for CBT sessions above) for treating cocaine disorders. Subsequent researchers studying the effectiveness of CBT protocols typically have adopted this manual.

A group of clients receiving CBT for cocaine use disorders was compared with a similar group receiving contingency management treatment (in which the client gets a reward contingent

[a] References 18, 23, 30, 35, 45, 47, 52, 80, 89.
[b] References 28, 33, 70, 75, 78, 79.

on reduced drug use).[75] Individuals in this study received three sessions of 90-min group CBT weekly, or three 2- to 5-min contingency management sessions (including receipt of voucher, if warranted), for a total of 16 weeks. Individuals demonstrated efficacious results 1 year after treatment was terminated, although these differences did not emerge until after treatment had ended. Although contingency management clients reported less use during the study, those who had received CBT did significantly better than contingency management clients at distant follow-up (6 months and 1 year later). In another comparison study of CBT versus interpersonal therapy and/or disulfiram administration, CBT was found to be at least as effective as these other therapies.[11]

Trujols and colleagues[85] undertook the painstaking task of evaluating specific CBT styles and techniques to determine the best practices within this model. These cognitive and/or behavioral therapy interventions included contingency management with vouchers, cue exposure treatment, relapse prevention therapy, and motivational interviewing. This review highlighted several strengths and weaknesses within these interventions. Contingency management interventions were found to present economic limitations, with questionable results regarding the maintenance of drug reduction outcomes. In contrast, cue exposure treatment (exposing individuals to cognitive cues that promoted drug use) resulted in definite treatment gains, including greater client retention and increased negative urine drug screens,[13] although Carroll et al.[13] noted that cravings initiated by cues outside the scope of clinical practice tended to perpetuate drug use. Researchers examined the role of at-home practice of cue exposure over 12 weeks of CBT and found that these reinforcing assignments resulted in higher program retention rates and thus kept clients committed to treatment.[13,24]

Schneider and Khantzian[81] further evaluated specific beneficial CBT mechanisms in an attempt to identify cocaine-dependent populations that could best benefit from CBT. They found that individuals' level of readiness for change differentiated treatment outcomes. They cautioned therapists to elicit and consider a client's stage of change prior to initiating any CBT technique, as some techniques can be contraindicated depending on where the client is in the cognitive process of making a change in his/her drug-use behavior.[53] Trujols and colleagues[85] concluded by noting that careful tailoring of CBT to the cocaine-dependent individual's needs in conjunction with other empirically derived biological approaches (i.e., pharmacotherapy) may ultimately equip these individuals with the best tools to overcome their addictive behaviors. The ability to choose appropriate homework tasks, therefore, may represent an important mechanism by which cocaine use disorders might be attenuated. Additionally, affective functioning (i.e., history of depression or anxiety) and deficits in abstract reasoning have been cited as important mediators in promoting superior CBT outcomes.[56] More recent work by Carroll and colleagues[12] has demonstrated the efficacy of cognitive behavioral therapies for cocaine use disorders provided via computer-biased training (CBT4CBT). In this study, individuals who received CBT4CBT along with methadone maintenance were more likely to be abstinent from cocaine for 3 or more consecutive weeks than those receiving methadone only, with effects persisting at 6 month follow up.

Knapp et al.[43] evaluated specific components of various therapies for SUDs to identify best-practice strategies in counseling substance-abusing or substance-dependent individuals. They identified five components as integral to the CBT process: (1) client-therapist collaboration, (2) case conceptualization, (3) structure, (4) socialization to the cognitive model, and (5) the use of cognitive and behavioral techniques. They also described a number of supplementary methods involved in cognitive behavioral approaches including Socratic questioning, analysis of advantages and disadvantages of use, monitoring of drug-related beliefs, activity monitoring and scheduling, behavioral experiments, and role playing. When 26 comparison studies (i.e., CBT vs. another psychosocial modality) were examined, mixed outcomes were reported. Although CBT emerged as a better therapy in approximately one-third of these studies, the loose conceptualizations and definitions used to characterize the CBT studies in this review likely obscured true differentiation of CBT versus other therapy effects. While additional research is warranted to understand better the precise mechanisms of action for effective CBT, available research to date confirms its potential value as an effective treatment approach for substance disorders.

Methamphetamines

In 2014, an estimated 1.6 million people aged 12 or older were current non-medical users of stimulants, and this included 569,000 (35.7%) people who were methamphetamine users.[15] Despite multiple efforts to reduce access and prevent experimentation, methamphetamine use disorders remain increasingly difficult to treat once an individual is introduced to this drug. While several psychosocial approaches have been explored and evaluated, CBT has emerged as a superior option in reducing or arresting drug consumption.[4]

Specifically, Rawson and colleagues[75] looked at several components of a Matrix model approach that was developed to impact the use of methamphetamines in dependent individuals. These components were derived from the CBT literature and included detailed information about the effects of stimulants, family education, 12-step program participation, and positive reinforcement for behavioral change and treatment compliance. Clients received 16 weeks (36 sessions) of CBT in a group format along with family education, social support, and individual counseling. While it is difficult to tease out the effect that additional therapies may have had on clients, these authors concluded that CBT techniques produced greater treatment adherence and greater abstinence than did various community treatment protocols.

In a randomized controlled trial of CBT for regular amphetamine users ($n = 32$), Baker and colleagues[3] reported on the feasibility of a brief (four-session) dose of CBT. They found that CBT was moderately effective among regular methamphetamine users in promoting abstinence, but cautioned that their results were preliminary and more research was needed. These initial findings were replicated in a larger study by the same authors in 2003.[4] In this more recent work, the authors found that ($n = 214$) there was a significant increase in the likelihood of abstinence from amphetamine use in those who received two or more treatment sessions. In addition, reductions in depression also were reported among CBT treatment groups. Given these findings, they recommended use of a stepped-care approach whereby the intervention starts with a structured assessment session and self-help material, followed by regular CBT sessions. The amount and dose of CBT is commensurate with the presentation of the clients' level of pathology (e.g., two sessions for regular users and additional sessions for those with moderate-to-severe levels of depression). Pharmacotherapy and/or longer-term CBT were recommended for non-responders.[4] Lee and Rawson,[46] however, emphasized the limited effectiveness of medications for methamphetamine users and acknowledged psychological interventions as the treatment of choice. These researchers reviewed randomized trials of CBT and found reductions in methamphetamine use, as well as other positive changes, even when treatment was limited to 2–4 sessions. The longevity of these effects, however, is not yet known. As such, CBT, even in its briefer adaptations, appears to be effective in reducing methamphetamine use.

In the context of a culturally-adapted version of CBT for gay and bisexual men abusing methaphetmine, Reback and Shoptaw[76] examined the effectiveness of a modified, gay-specific CBT (GCBT) with or without contingency management. They found that the GCBT alone was more effective in reducing methamphetamine use during treatment, these effects did not persist at 26-week follow-up.

Caffeine

Despite the widespread availability and cultural norm for caffeinated beverage consumption, little research exists examining the negative consequences of excessive and harmful caffeine consumption as well as consideration of potential interventions that might reduce these behaviors. Caffeine Use Disorder remains a condition for further study (vs. a formal diagnosis) in DSM-V,[1] and is included in the ICD-10 with other stimulant drugs. Ogawa and Ueki[68] advocated that caffeine manufacturers should clearly indicate caffeine content, specify a low-risk and safe amount of caffeine consumption, and state clearly that large quantities lead to long-term health risks. Through case studies, Ogawa and Ueki[68] revealed the nature of caffeine-related problems and requested further study for interventions that can impact the nature of these behaviors. As problems related to caffeine use resemble other psychostimulant addiction (although it is notably less risky), CBT represents a promising psychosocial approach by which to reduce excessive caffeine consumption. In an investigation of a single-session CBT intervention in 34 adults with symptoms of caffeine use disorder, Evatt, Juliano and Griffiths[22] found that individuals who received a 1 hour intervention and psychoeducational materials consumed less caffeine (verified by salivary caffeine tests) than a control group after treatment through 6 weeks post-treatment. However, these effects were not maintained at 6 month and 12 month follow up, leaving a need for future research in this area.

Nicotine

Tobacco use continues to be the leading cause of preventable death in the United States.[15] According to SAMHSA, an estimated 66.9 million people aged 12 or older were current users of a tobacco product including 55.2 million cigarette smokers in 2014.[15] CBT has been used to help smokers reduce or quit smoking with mixed success. In a study of outpatient smokers receiving CBT plus nicotine replacement therapy or placebo for 2 hours weekly for 5 weeks, 28% of those clients receiving CBT became abstinent from smoking and maintained that abstinence at 12 months.[77]

Hill and colleagues conducted a small-scale investigation of the effectiveness of a 10-week CBT intervention tailored to treat both nicotine and cannabis disorders along with nicotine replacement therapy. Significant reductions in tobacco use and indicators of severity of nicotine use disorders were found, demonstrating the feasibility and challenges of integrated treatment. In a group of cancer patients, although CBT reduced smoking behavior, it did no better than a basic health education condition in achieving smoking abstinence.[82] Sykes and Marks[83] developed a self-help

CBT program for disadvantaged smokers and reported abstinence or reduced consumption in clients who were provided with CBT tools.

Recent trends in CBT research and smoking have considered the role of depression in maintaining smoking abstinence. Hall and colleagues[29] randomized individuals in a 2 × 2 × 2 design whereby recently quitting smokers had a chance to receive CBT or no CBT and an antidepressant (nortriptyline or placebo). Analysis of the resultant data demonstrated that CBT was superior to other treatments for those reporting depressed mood but not for those with normal mood.[29] There was a non-significant trend favoring CBT in achieving abstinence, but CBT did not enhance smokers' compensatory coping skills. Discussion focuses currently on the need to examine a wide range of possible mediating variables in future research on CBT for smoking cessation.[84] Several clinical trials have tested whether CBT for smoking cessation would especially benefit depression-vulnerable smokers, with mixed results.[39]

Although data exists supporting the effectiveness of CBT for smoking cessation in African-Americans,[86] research on culturally-adapted CBT for individuals with nicotine use disorders has been rare. However, in a study of group-based culturally-specific or standard CBT with transdermal nicotine,[34] individuals who received culturally-specific CBT was more effective at one week into treatment, upon completion of treatment and at 3-month follow-up. These initial findings indicate that versions of CBT adapted to the unique social and cultural contexts of members of minority groups bear further consideration in future research.

Review of Treatment for Depressant Drugs

Alcohol

CBT for the treatment of alcohol use disorders likely represents one of the most studied treatments for the reduction or cessation of compulsive alcohol drinking. These CBT treatments have varied in length, modality (groups, individuals, or couples), content, treatment setting, and the addition of coping skills training.[62] Despite these differences, all CBT approaches focus on deficits in coping with stress and alcohol cues that maintain excessive drinking. Within these approaches, several strategies are explained: identification of situations likely to elicit inadequate coping, the use of instruction, therapist modeling, role playing, and behavioral rehearsal to enhance coping skills. Through repeated instruction and therapist support, clients begin to manage exposure to alcohol-related stimuli and handle stressful situations in more adaptive ways. Across 21 studies using CBT as a component of a larger treatment program, Longabaugh and Morgenstern[50] found that this treatment approach was more effective in reducing drinking than comparison treatment 71% of the time. Indeed, Miller and Wilbourne[62] documented significant and maintained improvements for alcohol-dependent individuals receiving CBT. Subsequent study replication by Kavanagh and colleagues[40] that compared additional cue exposure strategies with traditional CBT techniques (listed earlier), while demonstrating efficacy, did not further enhance the strength of these findings. In comparing cognitive behavioral strategies with other treatments with strong theoretical underpinnings, Longabaugh and Morgenstern[50] found equal effectiveness in 80% of cases.

More recent studies examining the effectiveness of CBT for disorders that often co-occur with alcohol use disorders have further bolstered the effectiveness of these therapies for comorbid disorders. Hien and colleagues[32] compared the effectiveness of

Seeking Safety, a present-focused CBT for Post Traumatic Stress Disorder (PTSD) and alcohol use disorder with and without a PTSD medication, sertraline. At the end of treatment as well as 6 months and 12 months post-treatment, both groups who received CBT demonstrated reductions in heavy drinking and drinks per drinking day and increases in abstinence, with no differences between groups. In a study comparing the effectiveness of treatments for anxiety use disorders and alcohol use disorders, Ciraulo and colleagues[16] utilized transdiagnostic CBT, an antidepressant (venlafaxine), and/or progressive muscle relaxation, CBT without medication had the greatest reduction in drinking during treatment above all other groups and was the only group superior to the control condition.

With respect to mood disorders and suicidality, Lydecker[51] utilized integrated group CBT for Major Depressive Disorder and SUDs (primarily alcohol) vs. twelve-step facilitation. Although twelve-step and ICBT groups both improved, the ICBT group showed more stability in reductions in use post-treatment. Esposito-Smythers[21] examined the effect of integrated, individual CBT for suicidality and alcohol use disorders in adolescence vs. treatment as usual within their randomized clinical trial. Results demonstrated significant reductions in both heavy drinking days and suicidal outcomes over the comparison group.

In a study of men who have sex with men who had alcohol use disorders and were also at risk for contracting HIV, Morgenstern and colleagues[63] compared the effectiveness of MI, MI with an culturally adapted version of CBT to a non-help-seeking group. Both treatment groups significantly reduced their drinking and other drug use during treatment, although MI only was superior to MI+CBT, contrary to the researchers' hypotheses. These reductions in use were sustained at 12 week and 12-month follow-up for both groups, demonstrating the overall effectiveness of a culturally-adapted version of CBT to sexual minority men.

In a more comprehensive review of behavioral and cognitive behavioral treatments for alcoholism, Kadden[38] explored several topics used within a CBT framework in an effort to identify inconsistencies in the literature and target research needs. In this paper, Kadden considered cue exposure, contingency management, community reinforcement, coping skills training, behavioral marital therapy, and client-treatment matching. Following an extensive review of the literature, he reported that coping skills training was ranked highest for effectiveness in treating alcoholism. The other approaches revealed mixed evidence in terms of efficacy and clear mechanism of action. Although coping skills training raised some concerns and limitations compared with other treatments, it increased consistently treatment effectiveness when used in conjunction with other CBT strategies. Kadden concluded by suggesting that treatment matching to individuals' characteristics may maximize the effectiveness of these interventions despite the lack of robust matching effects (in the absence of severe psychopathology) reported in previous publications of Project MATCH.[38,48]

In an attempt to understand better how mechanisms of action within CBT account for favorable outcomes, Long et al.[48] identified five promising variables in predicting treatment success: higher self-efficacy in positive social situations, greater treatment program involvement, a lower perception of staff control, a greater perception of treatment as helpful, and a reduction in psychological symptoms during treatment. As such, the authors suggested promoting clients' confidence and the perception of helpfulness in conjunction with skill-based relapse prevention strategies. Furthermore, social exchange models of intimate relationships also play a role in recovery, and therapy targeting the social functioning in an alcohol-dependent individual leads to improved relationship satisfaction, marital stability, and decreased domestic violence.[49] These CBT strategies promote better drinking outcomes associated with partner reinforcement of abstinence. Longabaugh and colleagues[50] cautioned, however, that more research is needed to confirm these preliminary findings.

In a more basic focus on social interactions, Meier and colleagues[59] considered the role of the therapeutic alliance in treating alcohol use disorders. The research thus far has indicated mixed results. While this set of authors found that early therapeutic alliance predicts engagement and retention in drug treatment, Dundon and colleagues[19] could only confirm these findings with non-CBT interventions. In this study, three groups were examined (a medication-only group, a medication plus medication-adherence focus group, and a medication plus CBT group); yet only the medication-only and medication plus adherence groups were associated with positive outcomes (number of sessions attended and/or days abstinent). It should be noted, however, that Dundon and colleagues[19] studied individuals interested in receiving pharmacotherapy, which may select for a different subject population from those who might benefit from the therapeutic alliance developed through psychotherapy alone. Also these researchers did not follow the role of changes in the therapeutic alliance over time, which can take time to develop and is likely to affect client behavior. More research is needed in this area to better inform CBT for alcohol use disorders.[78]

Benzodiazepines

Data regarding benzodiazepine use disorder and CBT is limited. Most patients abusing benzodiazepines suffer from underlying chronic anxiety or panic disorders. In a recent study, CBT was compared to benzodiazepine taper alone and taper plus relaxation condition among 47 patients with panic disorder seeking benzodiazepine taper. Results suggested that adjunct CBT facilitates discontinuation of benzodiazepine among those with panic disorder and prevents return of panic symptoms often seen with discontinuation.[8] Given the success of CBT with similar substances in this class, CBT would likely provide additional means by which to ameliorate benzodiazepine use disorders. Future research should consider how psychosocial interventions could enhance these efforts.

Barbiturates

The current state of barbiturate use disorders and CBT has not been studied. Most people with barbiturate problems are treated with pharmacotherapeutic dosing and medication strategies without psychosocial approaches. CBT would likely add benefits to these treatments.

Hypnotics

The long-term use of hypnotics for insomnia remains controversial. The management of hypnotic discontinuation following chronic use may be a challenge to both patients and providers.[83a] Further, recrudescence of insomnia symptoms after hypnotic discontinuation has been hypothesized to play a role in hypnotic-dependent insomnia.[64] In this way, clinicians may find it difficult to successfully taper these medications. CBT for insomnia (CBT-I) is often necessary to help hypnotic users to learn new skills to manage their sleep difficulties.[64] A study by Morin and colleagues[65] showed a greater proportion of drug free participants in the group who received a systematic hypnotic taper program combined with CBT compared to the group receiving taper alone (85% vs 48%).

Overall, research in the field of hypnotic use disorders and CBT is scarce and additional research is warranted in this area.

Cannabis

Marijuana use and related psychiatric comorbidities continues to be a growing concern in the U.S with an estimated 22.2 million aged 12 or older reporting use in the past month.[15] Despite the growing problem, treatment with pharmacotherapies continues to be an early stage and other psychosocial interventions are needed as augmenting strategies. CBT, motivational enhancement therapy and contingency management therapies have each been demonstrated to be efficacious for marijuana use disorders in a small number of studies to date.[58] For example, Copeland et al conducted a randomized control trial wherein 229 patients were randomly assigned to either a 6-session CBT or single session CBT) or delayed control treatment group (DTC).[17] Results showed that those in the the CBT groups were more likely to report abstinence, were significantly less concerned about their control over cannabis use, and reported fewer cannabis related problems compared to DTC group.

Berry and colleagues[9] examined the role of the alliance in predicting psychosis and substance-related outcomes in the context of a randomized controlled trial of motivational interviewing and CBT (MICBT) in individuals with recent onset psychosis and problematic cannabis use. They found alliance predicted levels of symptom and cannabis use during therapy and predicted symptoms and functioning (although not use) at follow-up. However, alliance failed to predict levels of substance misuse during therapy or at any of the follow-up points, casting additional doubt on the relationship between the alliance and substance-use outcomes long-term. Again, this is a potential area of research in the future and more studies are needed to demonstrate the effectiveness of CBT in cannabis use disorders.

Opioids

Amato and colleagues recently performed a systematic review of literature on opioid use disorders looking at various psychosocial interventions along with medications for opioid use disorders.[1] They concluded that the only benefit of adding psychosocial treatment was to increase the number of people remaining abstinent at follow up. It is worth noting that this review failed to compare different types of interventions like CBT, contingency management, biofeedback, and their separate roles are have not been systematically studied.

Despite the rising problem of opioid use disorders in the U.S, studies focusing on psychosocial interventions like CBT are scarce and more research is needed in this area.

Future Directions

In our clinic, our primary goals are to keep our clients safe and to keep them returning for therapy. If these goals cannot be met, no other goals can be achieved. As such, there are times when a CBT protocol must be adapted to meet these specific goals. Anecdotally, we have found that some sessions must run longer

or shorter than stated in the protocol to maintain these goals. In addition, there are times when one session must be reviewed a second time, or when a scheduled session's content must be truncated to address other issues that are more pressing in the client's life. Further research that tracks these CBT modifications and how they impact clients' outcomes is needed.

Additionally, future research needs to focus on the development of an effective working alliance between therapist and client. While past research has considered the working alliance at the first session, more information is needed regarding how the therapist/client relationship changes over time, how to augment these changes, and how best to achieve an effective relationship that promotes changes in clients' substance use.

Another area of research potential is treating substance-abusing individuals with co-occurring disorders (depression, anxiety, etc.). Thus far, CBT emerges as an effective adjunct for reducing addictive behaviors in depressed individuals when depression is targeted; yet additional research is needed to apply best these findings to the diverse populations who suffer from SUDs. To begin with, additional research is needed to determine the specific mechanisms of action at play in CBT that best promote the reduction of drug-seeking and drug-using behaviors. With the finding that individuals with SUDs also report high rates of depression, CBT strategies that specifically identify and target the unique thought patterns and behaviors of these individuals hold much promise. In fact, research that considers and targets all *Diagnostic and Statistical Manual of Mental Disorders*, 5th edition,[2] disorders in substance-abusing individuals should be examined using CBT as a potential therapeutic tool that can likely address both disorders in a way that medications and/or educational sessions cannot. Research that considers matching specific CBT strategies with specific disorders will likely prove very promising in addressing the unique experiences of substance use and comorbid disorders.

Another area of promising research considers the role of computers and electronic devices in promoting reduced addictive behaviors and/or reinforcing abstinence. Multiple websites have emerged that provide education and a chance to network with other addicts or specialists who can provide help during non-work hours when cravings and high-risk behaviors are more likely to take place. Carroll et al.[10] recently explored the use of a computer-assisted delivery of CBT for addiction and noted this agent to be an effective adjunct to standardized outpatient treatment for SUDs. More research is needed to expand on this likely successful variation of traditional CBT. Through exploration of these potential adjuncts to traditional CBT, treatment of SUDs will continue to improve and impact the lives of those who struggle with these conditions.

Despite the demonstrated effectiveness of CBT for the treatment of SUDs, there is still much about this therapy that remains unknown. Researchers continue to try to define specific dose-effect relationships by condensing treatment durations and identifying clients who are most suitable to benefit from fewer sessions. Research efforts need to compare directly the standard CBT with these briefer truncated cognitive behavioral interventions. In addition, the specific therapeutic mechanism(s) of change or action for CBT must still be identified.[72] Greater understanding of the impact of therapist variables on identified mechanism(s) of change also may be helpful in facilitating the development of efficacious, condensed forms of CBT.[31]

Kadden[37] has suggested that the study of CBT for relapse prevention may be advanced by identifying the most efficacious approaches to CBT, exploration of mediating factors, and identifying clients who are most likely to benefit from specific CBT strategies. Important elements of CBT selected for further investigation include cue exposure (i.e., factors that mediate or moderate cue reactivity), contingency management (i.e., optimal schedules for reinforcing abstinence and other supportive behaviors), community reinforcement (i.e., elements that are critical to maintaining outcomes), coping skills training (i.e., relative effectiveness of the various skills-training components, optimal combinations of them for different types of clients, and the optimal number and duration of treatment), the role of personality, interpersonal and environmental factors, and a re-examination of client-treatment matching. McKee and colleagues[57] have questioned further how future treatment might better motivate clients for successful CBT. Through greater understanding of the components of CBT and the interactions among client, therapist, and intervention factors in substance treatment, best-practice strategies can be developed to provide briefer, more effective CBT to clients with limited resources and/or need, for more immediate outcomes.

References

1. Amato L, Minozzi S, Davoli M, Vecci S. Psychosocial combined with agonist maintenance treatments versus agonist maintenance treatments alone for treatment of opioid dependence. *Cochrane Database Syst Rev*. 2008;4:CD004147.87.
2. American Psychiatric Association. *Diagnostic and Statistical Manual of Mental Disorders*. 5th ed. Arlington: VA: American Psychiatric Publishing; 2013.
3. Baker A, Boggs TG, Lewin TJ. Randomized controlled trial of brief cognitive-behavioural interventions among regular users of amphetamine. *Addiction*. 2001;96:1279–1287.
4. Baker A, Lee NK, Claire M, et al. Brief cognitive behavioural interventions for regular amphetamine users: a step in the right direction. *Addiction*. 2005;100(3):367–378.
5. Bandura A. Self-efficacy: toward a unifying theory of behavioral change. *Psychol Rev*. 1977;84:191–215.
6. Beck AT, Rush AJ, Shaw BF, Emery G. *Cognitive Therapy of Depression*. New York: Guilford; 1979.
7. Beck AT, Wright FD, Newman CF, Liese BS. *Cognitive Therapy of Substance Abuse*. New York: Guilford; 1993.
8. Bélanger L, Belleville G, Morin CM. Management of hypnotic discontinuation in chronic insomnia. *Sleep Med Clin*. 2009;4(4):583–592.
9. Berry K, Gregg L, Lobban F, Barrowclough C. Therapeutic alliance in psychological therapy for people with recent onset psychosis who use cannabis. *Compr Psychiatry*. 2016;67:73–80.
10. Carroll KM, Ball SA, Martino S, et al. Computer-assisted delivery of cognitive-behavioral therapy for addiction: a randomized trial of CBT4CBT. *Am J Psychiatry*. 2008;165:881–888.
11. Carroll KM, Fenton LR, Ball SA, et al. Efficacy of disulfiram and cognitive behavior therapy in cocaine-dependent outpatients: a randomized placebo-controlled trial. *Arch Gen Psychiatr*. 2004;61:264–272.
12. Carroll KM, Kiluk BD, Nich C, et al. Computer-assisted delivery of cognitive-behavioral therapy: efficacy and durability of CBT4CBT among cocaine-dependent individuals maintained on methadone. *Am J Psychiatr*. 2014;171:436–444.
13. Carroll KM, Nich C, Ball SA. Practice makes progress? Homework assignments and outcome in treatment of cocaine dependence. *J Consult Clin Psychol*. 2005;73:749–755.
14. Carroll KM, Rounsaville BJ, Gordon LT, et al. Psychotherapy and pharmacotherapy for ambulatory cocaine abusers. *Arch Gen Psychiatr*. 1994;51:177–187.
15. Center for Behavioral Health Statistics and Quality. Behavioral Health Trends in the United States: Results from the 2014 National Health Survey on Drug Use and Health. (HHS Publication no. SMA 15-4927, NSDUH Series H-50). 2015; Retrieved from http://www.samhsa.gov/data/.
16. Ciraulo DA, Barlow DH, Guillver SB, et al. The effects of venlafaxine and cognitive behavioral therapy alone and combined in the treatment of co-morbid alcohol use-anxiety disorders. *Behavior Res Ther*. 2013;51:729–735.
17. Copeland J, Swift W, Roffman R, Stephens R. A randomized controlled trial of brief cognitive–behavioral interventions for cannabis use disorder. *J Subst Abuse Treat*. 2001;21:55–64.
18. Davis AK, Osborn LA, Rosenberg H, et al. Psychometric evaluation of the marijuana reduction strategies self-efficacy scale with young recreational marijuana users. *Addict Behav*. 2014;39:1750–1754.
19. Dundon WD, Pettinati HM, Lynch KG, et al. The therapeutic alliance in medical-based interventions impacts outcome in treating alcohol dependence. *Drug Alcohol Depend*. 2008;95:230–236.
20. Ellis A, Velten E. *When AA Doesn't Work for You: Rational Steps to Quitting Alcohol*. Fort Lee, NJ: Barricade Books; 1992.
21. Esposito-Smythers C, Kahler CW, Spirito A, Kahler CW, Hunt J, Monti P. Treatment of co-occurring substance and suicidality among adolescents: a randomized trial. *J Consult Psych*. 2011;79:728–739.
22. Evatt DP, Juliano LM, Griffiths RR. A brief manualized treatment for problematic caffeine use: a randomized control trial. *J Consult Cl Psych*. 2016;84:113–121.
23. Glaser-Edwards S, Tate SR, McQuaid JR, et al. Mechanisms of action in integrated cognitive-behavioral treatment versus twelve-step facilitation for substance-dependent adults with comorbid major depression. *J Stud Alcohol Drugs*. 2007;68:663–672.
24. Gonzalez VM, Schmitz JM, DeLaune KA. The role of homework in cognitive-behavioral therapy for cocaine dependence. *J Consult Clin Psychol*. 2006;74:633–637.
25. Gouse H, Magidson JF, Burnhams W, et al. Implementation of cognitive-behavioral substance abuse treatment in Sub-Saharan Africa: treatment engagement and abstinence at treatment exit. *PLoS One*. 2016;11:1–19.
26. Granholm E, Tate SR, Link PC, et al. Neuropsychological functioning and outcomes of treatment for co-occurring depression and substance use disorders. *Am J Drug Alcohol Abuse*. 2011;37:240–249.
27. Gullo MJ, Matveeva M, Feeney GF, Young RM, Connor JP. Social cognitive predictors of treatment outcome in cannabis dependence. *Drug Alcohol Depend*. 2017;170:74–81.
28. Hall SM, Humfleet GL, Muñoz RF, et al. Using extended cognitive behavioral treatment and medication to treat dependent smokers. *Am J Pub Health*. 2011;101:2349–2356.
29. Hall SM, Reus VI, Muñoz RF. Nortriptyline and cognitive-behavioral therapy in the treatment of cigarette smoking. *Arch Gen Psychiatry*. 1998;55:683–690.
30. Hartzler B, Witkiewitz K, Villarroel N, Donovan D. Self-efficacy change as a mediator of associations between therapeutic bond and one-year outcomes in treatments for alcohol dependence. *Psych Addict Behav*. 2011;25:269–278.
31. Hazlett-Stevens H, Craske MG. Brief cognitive-behavioral therapy: definition and scientific foundations. In: Bond FW, Dryden W, eds. *Handbook of Brief Cognitive Behaviour Therapy*. New York: Wiley; 2002.
32. Hien DA, Levin FR, Ruglass LM, et al. Combining seeking safety with sertraline for PTSD and alcohol use disorders: a randomized controlled trial. *J Consul Clin Psych*. 2015;83:359–369.
33. Hooper MW, Antoni MH, Okuyemi K, Dietz NA, Resnicow K. Randomized controlled trial of group-based culturally specific cognitive behavioral therapy among African American smokers. *Nicotine Tob Res*. 2017;19:333–341.
34. Hooper MW, Antoni MH, Okuyemi K, Dietz NA, Resnicow K. Randomized controlled trial of group-based culturally specific cognitive behavioral therapy among African American smokers. *Nicotine Tob Res*. 2017;19:333–341.
35. Hunter-Reel D, McCrady BS, Hildebrandt T, Epstein EE. Indirect effect of social support for drinking on drinking outcomes: the role of motivation. *J Studies Alc Drugs*. 2010;71:930–937.
36. Kadden R, Kranzler H. Alcohol and drug abuse treatment at the University of Connecticut health center. *Br J Addict*. 1992;87:521–526.

37. Kadden RM. Behavioral and cognitive-behavioral treatments for alcoholism: research opportunities. *Recent Dev Alcohol.* 2003;16:165–182.

38. Kadden RM, Cooney NL, Litt GH. Matching alcoholics to coping skills or interactional therapies: Posttreatment results. *J Consult Clin Psychol.* 1989;57:698–704.

39. Kapson HS, Leddy MA, Haaga DAF. Specificity of effects of cognitive behavior therapy on coping, acceptance, and distress tolerance in a randomized controlled trial for smoking cessation. *J Clinical Psych.* 2012;68:1231–1240.

40. Kavanagh DJ, Sitharthan G, Young RM, et al. Addition of cue exposure to cognitive-behaviour therapy for alcohol misuse: a randomized trial with dysphoric drinkers. *Addiction.* 2006;101:1106–1116.

41. Kazantzis N, Deane FP, Ronan KR, L'Abate L., eds. *Using Homework Assignments in Cognitive Behavior Therapy.* New York: Routledge; 2005.

42. Kiluk BD, Nich C, Carroll KM. Relationship of cognitive function and the acquisition of coping skills in computer assisted treatment for substance use disorders. *Drug Alcohol Depend.* 2011;114:169–176.

43. Knapp WP, Soares BG, Farrel M, Lima MS. Psychosocial interventions for cocaine and psychostimulant amphetamines related disorders. *Cochrane Database Syst Rev.* 2007;3:CD003023.

44. Lazarus RS, Folkman S. *Stress, Appraisal, and Coping.* New York: Springer; 1984.

45. Lee M, Miller SM, Wen K, Hui SK, Roussi P, Hernandez E. Cognitive-behavioral intervention to promote smoking cessation for pregnant and postpartum inner city women. *J Behav Med.* 2015;38:932–943.

46. Lee NK, Rawson RA. A systematic review of cognitive and behavioural therapies for methamphetamine dependence. *Drug Alcohol Rev.* 2008;27:309–317.

47. Litt MD, Kadden RM, Kabila-Cormier E, Petry NM. Coping skills training and contingency management treatments for marijuana dependence: exploring mechanisms of behavior change. *Addiction.* 2008;103:638–648.

48. Long CG, Williams M, Midgley M, Hollin CR. Within-program factors as predictors of drinking outcome following cognitive-behavioral treatment. *Addict Behav.* 2000;25:573–578.

49. Longabaugh R, Donovan DM, Karno MP, McCrady BS, Morgenstern J, Tonigan JS. Active ingredients: how and why evidence-based alcohol behavioral treatment interventions work. *Alcohol Clin Exp Res.* 2005;29:235–247.

50. Longabaugh R, Morgenstern J. Cognitive-behavioral coping-skills therapy for alcohol dependence: current status and future directions. *Alcohol Res Health.* 1999;23:78–85.

51. Lydecker KP, Cummins KM, McQuaid J, Granholm E, Brown SA. Clinical outcomes of an integrated treatment for depression and substance use disorders. *Psych Addict Beh.* 2010;24:453–464.

52. Maisto SA, Roos CR, O'Sickey AJ, et al. The indirect effect of the therapeutic alliance and alcohol abstinence self–efficacy on alcohol use and alcohol–related problems in Project MATCH. *Alcohol Clin Exp Res.* 2015;39:504–513.

53. Margolin A, Avants SK, Kosten TR. Cue-elicited cocaine craving and autogenic relaxation. Association with treatment outcome. *J Subst Abuse Treat.* 1994;11:549–552.

54. Reference deleted in review.

55. Marlatt GA, Gordon JR. *Relapse Prevention: Maintenance Strategies in the Treatment of Addictive Behaviors.* New York: Guilford; 1985.

56. Maude-Griffin PM, Hohenstein JM, Humfleet GL, Reilly PM, Tusel DJ, Hall SM. Superior efficacy of cognitive-behavioral therapy for urban crack cocaine abusers: main and matching effects. *J Consult Clin Psychol.* 1998;66:832–837.

57. McKee SA, Carroll KM, Sinha R. Enhancing brief cognitive-behavioral therapy with motivational enhancement techniques in cocaine users. *Drug Alcohol Depend.* 2007;91:97–101.

58. McRae AL, Budney AJ, Brady KT. Treatment of marijuana dependence: a review of the literature. *J Subst Abuse Treat.* 2003;24:369–376.

59. Meier PS, Donmall MC, Barrowclough C, McElduff P, Heller RF. Predicting the early therapeutic alliance in the treatment of drug misuse. *Addiction.* 2005;100:500–511.

60. Reference deleted in review.

61. Miller MR. Motivational interviewing with problem drinkers. *Behav Psychother.* 1983;11:147–172.

62. Miller WR, Wilbourne PL. Mesa Grande: a methodological analysis of clinical trials of treatments for alcohol use disorders. *Addiction.* 2002;97:265–277.

63. Morgenstern J, Irwin TW, Weinberg ML, et al. A randomized controlled trial of goal choice interventions for alcohol use disorders among men who have sex with men. *J Consult Clin Psychol.* 2007;75:72–84.

64. Morin CM. *Insomnia: Psychological Assessment and Management.* New York: Guilford Press; 1993.

65. Morin CM, Bastien C, Guay B, Radouco-Thomas M, Leblanc J, Vallières A. Randomized clinical trial of supervised tapering and cognitive behavior therapy to facilitate benzodiazepine discontinuation in older adults with chronic insomnia. *Am J Psych.* 2004;161:332–342.

66. National Institute on Alcohol Abuse and Alcoholism. *Cognitive-Behavioral Coping Skills Therapy Skills;* 2003 (NIH Publication no. 94-3724). Retrieved from: https://pubs.niaaa.nih.gov/publications/projectmatch/match03.pdf.

67. O'Farrell TJ, Fals-Stewart W. *Behavioral Couples Therapy for Alcoholism and Drug Abuse.* New York: Guilford; 2000.

68. Ogawa N, Ueki H. Clinical importance of caffeine dependence and abuse. *Psychiatry Clin Neurosci.* 2007;61:263–268.

69. Otto MW, McHugh RK, Simon NM, Farach FJ, Worthingon JJ, Pollack MH. Efficacy of CBT for benzodiazepine discontinuation in patients with panic disorder: further evaluation. *Behav Res Ther.* 2010;48(8):720–727.

70. Peterson AV, Marek PM, Kealey KA, Bricker JB, Ludman EJ, Heffner JL. Does effectiveness of adolescent smoking-cessation intervention endure into young adulthood? 7-year follow-up results from a group-randomized trial. *PLoS One.* 2016;11(2).

71. Pettanati HM, Anton RF, Willenbring ML. The COMBINE Study—an overview of the largest pharmacotherapy study to date for treating alcohol dependence. *Psychiatr Times.* 2006;3:36–39.

72. Prochaska JO, Velicer WF. The transtheoretical model of health behavior change. *Am J Health Promot.* 1997;12:38–48.

73. Project MATCH Research Group. Project MATCH: rationale and methods for a multisite clinical trial matching patients to alcoholism treatment. *Alcohol Clin Exp Res.* 1993;17:1130–1145.

74. Project MATCH Research Group. Project MATCH secondary a priori hypotheses. *Addiction.* 1997;92:1671–1698.

75. Rawson RA, Huber A, McCann M, et al. A comparison of contingency management and cognitive-behavioral approaches during methadone maintenance treatment for cocaine dependence. *Arch Gen Psychiatr.* 2002;59:817–824.

76. Repack CJ, Shoptaw S. Development of an evidence-based, gay-specific cognitive behavioral therapy intervention for methamphetamine-abusing gay and bisexual men. *Addict Beh.* 2014;39:1286–1291.

77. Richmond RL, Kehoe L, de Ameida NAC. Three year continuous abstinence in a smoking cessation study using the nicotine transdermal patch. *Heart.* 1997;78:617–618.

78. Rodrigues NCP, Andrade MKD, O'Dwyer G, et al. Long-term effects of smoking cessation support in primary care: results of a two-year longitudinal study in Brazil. *J Bras Psiquiatr.* 2016;65:174–178.

79. Ruther T, Kiss A, Eberhardt K, Linhardt A, Kroger C, Pogarell O. Evaluation of the cognitive behavioral smoking reduction program 'Smoke_less': a randomized controlled trial. *Eur Arch Psychiatry Clin Neurosci.* 2018;268:269–277.

80. Sandahl C, Gerge A, Herlitz K. Does treatment focus on self-efficacy result in better coping? paradoxical findings from Psychodynamic and cognitive-behavioral group treatment of moderately alcohol-dependent patients. *Psychother Res.* 2004;14:388–397.

81. Schneider RJ, Khantzian EJ. Psychotherapy and patient needs in the treatment of alcohol and cocaine abuse. *Recent Dev Alcohol.* 1992;10:165–178.

82. Schnoll RA, Rothman RL, Wielt DB, et al. A randomized pilot study of cognitive-behavioral therapy versus basic health education for smoking cessation among cancer patients. *Ann Behav Med.* 2005;30:1–11.

83. Sykes CM, Marks DF. Effectiveness of a cognitive behaviour therapy self-help programme for smokers in London, UK. *Health Promot Int.* 2001;16:255–260.

83a. Santos C, Olmedo RE. Sedative-hypnotic drug withdrawal syndrome: Recognition and Treatment. *Emerg Med Pract.* 2017;19(3):1–20.

84. Thorndike FP, Friedman-Wheeler DG, Haaga DA. Effect of cognitive behavior therapy on smokers' compensatory coping skills. *Addict Behav.* 2006;31:1705–1710.

85. Trujols J, Luquero E, Siñol N, et al. Cognitive-behavioral therapy for the treatment of cocaine dependence [Spanish]. *Actas Esp Psiquiatr.* 2007;35:190–198.

86. Webb MS, de Ybarra DR, Baker EA, Reis IM, Carey MP. Cognitive–behavioral therapy to promote smoking cessation among African American smokers: a randomized clinical trial. *J Consult Clin Psychol.* 2010;78:24–33.

87. Weinstein A, Yemini Z, Greif J. Motivational and behavioral factors predicting success in cigarette smoking-cessation treatment combining group therapy with bupropion. *J Groups Addict Recovery.* 2008;3:79–92.

88. World Health Association. *The ICD-10 Classification of Mental and Behavioural Disorders: Clinical Descriptions and Diagnostic Guidelines.* Geneva: World Health Association; 1992.

89. Young RM, Connor JP, Feeney GFX. Alcohol expectancy changes over a 12-week cognitive–behavioral therapy program are predictive of treatment success. *J Subst Abuse Treat.* 2011;40:18–25.

41

Community Reinforcement Approach and Contingency Management Therapies

DANIELLE BARRY AND †NANCY M. PETRY

Introduction

This chapter describes the rationale behind and evidence in support of the efficacy of two reinforcement-based therapies: community reinforcement approach therapy and contingency management. The first section of the chapter reviews the evidence for the community reinforcement approach and recent studies extending the approach to adolescents with substance use disorders. The second section of this chapter details the theoretical basis and evidence of efficacy for contingency management interventions. The chapter concludes by discussing issues related to the cost-effectiveness of these interventions and their adoption in practice settings.

Community Reinforcement Approach Therapy

Community reinforcement approach therapy was first developed more than 40 years ago by Hunt and Azrin.[26] They described the

†Deceased.

community reinforcement approach as a comprehensive biopsychosocial treatment for alcohol dependence. It is based on the theoretical view that individuals use substances for their positive, reinforcing effects and that the relative lack of alternative, nondrug reinforcers maintains dependence. The development of alternative reinforcing activities that are incompatible with drug use is central to the community reinforcement approach.

The community reinforcement approach begins with a detailed functional analysis concerning the triggers and consequences of drug use behaviors. An example of a functional analysis is presented in Table 41.1. The treatment package itself includes a number of aspects: sobriety sampling, monitored disulfiram consumption (when appropriate), behavioral skills training, social and recreational counseling, behavioral marital therapy, problem solving, and drink refusal skills. Thus some of the components of the community reinforcement approach are similar to those of cognitive behavioral therapy (see Chapter 40).

The difference between the two types of therapies is that the community reinforcement approach is more directive, community based, and behavioral than cognitive behavioral therapy. In the community reinforcement approach, the therapist places a great deal of emphasis on changing environmental contingencies in the client's life. Employment, recreation, and family systems are all addressed to promote a lifestyle that is more reinforcing than substance use. Rather than being entirely office-based, the community reinforcement approach is typically performed, at least in part, in the community. If clients do not attend treatment or do not follow through with an employment or recreational goal, the therapist may go to their homes, take them to job interviews, or help them try a new recreational activity. The purpose of expanding the treatment beyond the office setting is to increase the positive reinforcing effects of non–substance-using activities by direct exposure.

Initial reports of the efficacy of the community reinforcement approach for the treatment of alcohol dependence were promising. Hunt and Azrin[26] and Azrin[3] described two early studies in which 16 and 18 alcohol-dependent individuals, respectively, were randomized to usual psychosocial therapy plus disulfiram or to the community reinforcement approach plus disulfiram. In both studies, the community reinforcement approach–treated individuals spent significantly fewer days drinking than did individuals

TABLE 41.1   Sample Functional Analysis Form for Use in Community Reinforcement Approach Therapy.

Day/Time	Situation	Thoughts/ Feelings	Substance Use? What and How Much?	Positive Consequences	Negative Consequences
Mon p.m.	Argument with neighbor	Angry!	Alcohol 9–10 beers	Forgot about neighbor for a while	Neighbor called cops because of noise.
Tues p.m.	Friend offered me a hit.	Terrible craving, really wanted to use.	Cocaine 1/2 g	Fun to be with old friend. Felt good.	Went home and drank more that night, even though I wasn't planning on drinking. Felt guilty next day.

Adapted from Budney AJ, Higgins ST. *A Community Reinforcement Approach: Treating Cocaine Addiction.* Vol 2. National Institute on Drug Abuse; 1998.

receiving usual care. The latter study had a long-term follow-up, which found that 90% of clients who had received the community reinforcement approach remained abstinent up to 2 years later.

Additional studies in alcohol-dependent individuals have found the community reinforcement approach to be of therapeutic benefit. For example, Azrin and colleagues[4] noted a therapeutic benefit of the community reinforcement approach, and Smith et al.[65] also reported that this approach led to greater abstinence during treatment than did usual care plus disulfiram treatment. Miller et al.[35,36] examined the various components of the community reinforcement approach and likewise found that this approach improved the treatment outcomes of individuals who received concomitant disulfiram treatment.

Several independent reviews and meta-analyses have concluded that the community reinforcement approach is an important, established, and effective treatment for alcohol use disorders.[14,24,25,37] Furthermore, in a systematic review of the community reinforcement approach's effectiveness, Roozen et al.[59] concluded that the community reinforcement approach, alone or with disulfiram, is efficacious for the treatment of alcohol dependence. The use of the community reinforcement approach in the treatment of other substance use disorders has not been examined as extensively.

Much recent research focuses on an adaptation of the community reinforcement approach for adolescents (A-CRA)[15] or combined with family training (CRAFT) to involve significant others in the treatment process and teach them how to maintain alternative reinforcements to substance use.[34] Randomized controlled trials of A-CRA demonstrate its efficacy in reducing cannabis use in adolescents.[15] So far, most clinics implementing A-CRA have done so in the context of grant-funded research studies,[28] and studies are underway to identify factors that facilitate sustained use of A-CRA after study funding ends.[27] A recent review of four studies suggests that CRAFT was associated with increased patient engagement and reduced depression symptoms relative to comparison treatments.[60]

Many studies have examined the community reinforcement approach in combination with another behavioral therapy, contingency management.

Contingency Management Interventions

Similar to the community reinforcement approach, contingency management is based on the principles of behavioral therapy. The primary difference between the two interventions is that contingency management provides *tangible* reinforcers for achieving target behaviors to increase the likelihood of those behaviors reoccurring, whereas the community reinforcement approach exposes clients to reinforcing activities and experiences. Typically, contingency management interventions identify an appropriate target

behavior (e.g., abstinence as verified by a negative urine toxicology test) and provide tangible reinforcers each time the target behavior occurs. The reinforcers are most often monetary-based vouchers exchangeable for retail goods and services and the chance to win prizes of varying magnitudes. If the target behavior does not occur, the reinforcers are removed.[18,41]

Contingency management is generally not provided as a standalone treatment for substance use disorders but instead is added to another treatment to improve outcomes. Contingency management is often combined with the community reinforcement approach in attempts to improve further the efficacy of the community reinforcement approach alone. An early study of voucher-based contingency management by Higgins et al.[20] offered the community reinforcement approach along with contingency management to 13 consecutively admitted cocaine-dependent outpatients and offered 12-step–based drug counseling to the next 15 consecutively admitted cocaine-dependent outpatients. In the contingency management condition, vouchers worth a specific amount of money were provided whenever individuals submitted cocaine-negative urine samples. Significant group differences emerged in the percentage of participants who remained in treatment for 12 weeks, with 85% in the community reinforcement approach plus contingency management group and 42% in the 12-step group remaining in treatment for the entire period. Participants in the community reinforcement approach plus contingency management group also achieved significantly longer periods of objectively verified continuous cocaine abstinence, with 77% versus 25%, respectively, achieving a month or more of continuous abstinence.

Higgins et al.[19] next conducted a 24-week randomized study comparing the same two treatments in a sample of 38 individuals, with half of them assigned to community reinforcement approach plus contingency management and the other half assigned to drug abuse counseling based on the 12-step model. Fifty-eight percent of the participants in the community reinforcement approach plus contingency management group completed treatment versus 11% of those in 12-step counseling. The groups also differed significantly on rates of continuous abstinence. Sixty-eight percent of participants receiving community reinforcement approach plus contingency management achieved 8 weeks of continuous abstinence compared with 11% in the 12-step counseling group. Group differences remained at 6-, 9-, and 12-month follow-up interviews.[17] Participants who received community reinforcement approach plus contingency management were more likely to self-report cocaine abstinence over the past 30 days and to submit cocaine-negative urine samples compared with those who received 12-step counseling.

To isolate the specific contribution of contingency management to these beneficial outcomes, Higgins and colleagues[18] next randomized 40 cocaine-dependent individuals to the community reinforcement approach alone or community reinforcement approach plus contingency management. Significantly more participants in the combined condition remained engaged in treatment for 24 weeks (75%) than in the community reinforcement approach-alone condition (40%). The longest duration of continuous abstinence differed between groups as well. Participants in the community reinforcement approach plus contingency management condition achieved an average of 11.7 (± 2.0) weeks of continuous abstinence from cocaine, whereas participants in the community reinforcement approach-alone condition achieved an average of 6.0 (± 1.5) weeks. These studies demonstrate that the community reinforcement approach plus contingency management is more effective than the community reinforcement approach alone for increasing the duration of abstinence. Furthermore, the benefits of community reinforcement approach plus contingency management persist up to a year beyond the end of the period during which vouchers are available.[16,23]

Although contingency management adds to the benefits of the community reinforcement approach, the converse is also true: including the community reinforcement approach improves the benefits associated with contingency management alone. Higgins et al.[22] assigned 100 cocaine-dependent individuals in a random fashion to either the combination of contingency management plus the community reinforcement approach or to contingency management alone. Participants who received the combined treatment remained in therapy longer, used cocaine less frequently during treatment, and reported a lower frequency of drinking to intoxication than did participants who received contingency management alone. Individuals treated with community reinforcement approach plus contingency management also evidenced improvements on other domains relative to individuals who received contingency management only. These included more days of employment, reduced depressive symptoms, and fewer hospitalizations and legal problems. Thus contingency management is an efficacious intervention for cocaine dependence, but it is most effective when administered in conjunction with the community reinforcement approach in this population.

Other studies have extended these benefits of community reinforcement approach plus contingency management to other substance-abusing populations. Bickel et al.[6] randomized 39 opioid-dependent individuals to a usual-care condition or community reinforcement approach plus contingency management. During treatment, abstinence rates were significantly higher among individuals who received contingency management. Using a nonrandomized design, Schottenfeld et al.[61] compared 117 opioid-maintained, cocaine- and opioid-dependent individuals who received either drug counseling or community reinforcement approach plus contingency management. Although retention and drug use did not differ between individuals receiving different forms of therapy in this report, engagement in community activities unrelated to drug use (e.g., parenting activities, employment, or planned recreational activities) was significantly associated with abstinence.

In the treatment of other drug use disorders such as nicotine, marijuana, or benzodiazepines, contingency management is typically applied as an adjunct to usual-care psychotherapies, rather than in conjunction with the community reinforcement approach. A variety of studies demonstrate that contingency management improves the treatment outcomes of marijuana-dependent individuals when added to motivational enhancement therapy or cognitive behavioral therapy.[8,9,30] Contingency management is also efficacious in the treatment of nicotine dependence[a] and benzodiazepine use.[68]

Two meta-analyses have demonstrated the therapeutic efficacy of contingency management in treating different substance use disorders.[33,54] Across 30 studies comparing treatments with and without the addition of voucher-based contingency management, Lussier et al.[33] found medium-sized group differences in length of abstinence from cocaine, opiates, tobacco, alcohol, and marijuana, with no significant difference in outcomes across specific drugs. More immediate delivery of reinforcement and higher reinforcement magnitude were associated with greater therapeutic benefit.[33] In an independent analysis of 47 contingency management trials that used vouchers as well as other forms of reinforcement (e.g., cash and privileges such as take-home methadone doses), Prendergast et al.[54] found that contingency management was most effective in reducing cocaine and opiate use. Smaller effects were noted with respect to reducing tobacco and polydrug abuse. Although both of these meta-analyses found benefits of contingency management, they included many studies that did not incorporate appropriate behavioral principles in the design of the reinforcement structure, such as frequent monitoring and reinforcement and escalating reinforcers with sustained behavioral change.[41] The benefits of contingency management are greater in studies that utilize appropriate behavioral principles.

Issues Hindering the Implementation of the Community Reinforcement Approach in Practice

Despite the strong research evidence that supports the efficacy of community reinforcement approach and contingency management in substance-abusing populations, these interventions are rarely implemented in clinical practice, although their use is growing. The primary reason for lack of use relates to costs. The community reinforcement approach is labor intensive and difficult to employ in practice settings, most of which are understaffed and underfunded. In its traditional sense, the community reinforcement approach is individually based and quite labor intensive in nature. Typically, one therapist will manage a small caseload of 10 or fewer clients.

To make the community reinforcement approach less labor intensive for therapists and more practical to implement in busy clinical practice settings, some studies have examined a modification of the approach by providing contingency management for completing goal-related activities. Rather than the therapist going out into the community with the client to ensure exposure to non–drug-related activities, the therapist will contract with the client each week to complete up to three goal-related activities. If the client engages in the activities and provides objective verification of completion, the client will earn tangible reinforcers such as vouchers. Table 41.2 provides an example of a typical activity contract.

This approach has been studied in several clinical trials. In a sample of polydrug-using individuals on methadone, Iguchi et al.[29] found that an intervention that provided tangible reinforcers for completion of goal-related activities resulted in lower drug use both during the treatment period and throughout the follow-up period than a usual contingency management approach that

---

[a]References 2, 13, 21, 57, 58, 63.

TABLE 41.2 **Sample Activity Contract.**

Specific Activity	Goal Area	Projected Date/Time of Completion	Things That Could Go Wrong	Problem Solve	Verification	Completed and Verified?
1. Complete draft of resume	Employment	Wed p.m.	Don't feel like it, No blank paper in house	Do on Thurs if not Wed, Bring blank paper from clinic	Bring in draft	
2. Go to 3 AA meetings	Sobriety	Wed p.m., Fri p.m., and Sat afternoon	Don't feel like going, car won't start	Make plans with Sally to go together and for coffee after meeting, ask Sally to drive	Signed attendance slip and coffee receipts	
3. Go to church	Recreation/ spirituality	Sunday 10 a.m.	Oversleep, no transportation	Set alarm Sat night, make plans to go with John	Bring back dated bulletin	

Adapted from Petry NM, Tedford J, Martin B. Reinforcing compliance with non-drug-related activities. *J Subst Abuse Treat.* 2001;20:33–44.

only reinforced drug abstinence. However, a subsequent study with cocaine-abusing individuals from psychosocial (nonmethadone) clinics failed to show a significant benefit of the contingency management for activity condition relative to usual care.[44] In that study, contingency management for submission of negative urine samples did significantly improve outcomes relative to standard care. Thus there is inconsistent evidence that this modified contingency management approach is sufficient to improve drug use outcomes in clinical settings.

It is important to note that contingent activity contracting is important for engaging individuals in drug-free recreational and other activities. If activity-contracting procedures are employed without contingent reinforcement, these activities are completed less than one-third of the time.[50] In contrast, when tangible reinforcers are provided in a contingent manner, these activities are completed about two-thirds of the time.[50,53] Furthermore, completion of these activities was typically associated with a reduction in drug use and improvements in psychosocial functioning. Individuals who completed family activities compared with those who did not reported a greater reduction in drug use as well as improvements in family functioning.[32] In sum, the reinforcement of salient non–drug-related activities through the use of tangible reinforcers has appeared to be an important method for decreasing drug use and should be more cost-effective than having therapists attend community events with their clients. Lower cost delivery systems, such as web-based programs, have also shown promise in improving outcomes for illicit drug users in outpatient addiction treatment.[10]

Issues Associated With Implementation of Contingency Management in Practice

Although contingency management can be used to reinforce engagement in non–drug-related activities, it is most often applied to encourage abstinence from using substances. Irrespective of the target behavior reinforced, contingency management has been criticized for being costly to implement, especially the voucher-based version.

An important component of contingency management is that the value of vouchers earned increases with each consecutive instance of a desired behavior. Thus the first negative specimen (or

activity completed) may result in a $2.50 voucher, the second a $3.25 voucher, the third a $4 voucher, and so on.[56,57] Thus by the end of a 12-week treatment period, individuals may be earning in excess of $40 for each negative sample or activity completed, and most effective voucher-based contingency management programs arrange for about $1000 in vouchers over the course of a 12-week treatment period Table 41.3). Hence, the costs of voucher-based contingency management are prohibitive for most community-based settings.

Studies that have attempted to reduce the amounts of vouchers available show that the procedure is less effective in decreasing drug use. Stitzer and Bigelow[66,67] found that nicotine abstinence increased as a function of the magnitude of the reinforcer, ranging from $0 to $12 per day. Dallery et al.[12] noted a direct relationship between voucher amounts and abstinence in another study of individuals receiving methadone maintenance treatment. These studies all suggest that the larger the magnitude of the reinforcer, the greater the improvement in treatment outcomes. Hence, reducing the value of the vouchers decreases their efficacy in promoting abstinence from substances.

Prize-Based Contingency Management

To address the issue of cost in contingency management interventions, Petry et al.[49] developed a prize-based contingency management intervention that provided tangible reinforcement on a variable ratio schedule. Individuals who provided objective evidence of abstinence or other target behaviors earned the opportunity to draw slips of paper that could be redeemed as prizes. The number of draws earned, similar to the voucher-based approach, increased with each consecutive negative sample, such that the first negative sample or completed activity resulted in one draw, the second in two draws, and so forth. Typically, the drawing of prizes was capped (e.g., at a maximum of eight draws per activity completed or negative sample submitted) after about 1 month of sustained behavioral change Table 41.4).

In most prize-based contingency management programs, clients draw from a bowl containing 500 slips of paper. Half the slips have encouraging messages but do not result in prizes, and half the slips result in a prize. There are typically three prize magnitudes, small (worth about $1), large (worth about $20), and jumbo (worth about $100). The majority of the slips (e.g., 209)

TABLE 41.3 Sample Voucher-Based Contingency Management Schedule.

Week	Sample	Points	Dollars	Bonus	Cumulative Earnings
1	Mon	10	$2.50		$2.50
	Wed	15	$3.75		$6.25
	Fri	20	$5.00	$10.00	$21.25
2	Mon	25	$6.25		$27.50
	Wed	30	$7.50		$35.00
	Fri	35	$8.75	$10.00	$53.75
3	Mon	40	$10.00		$63.75
	Wed	45	$11.25		$75.00
	Fri	50	$12.50	$10.00	$97.50
4	Mon	55	$13.75		$111.25
	Wed	60	$15.00		$126.25
	Fri	65	$16.25	$10.00	$152.50
5	Mon	70	$17.50		$170.00
	Wed	75	$18.75		$188.75
	Fri	80	$20.00	$10.00	$218.75
6	Mon	85	$21.25		$240.00
	Wed	90	$22.50		$262.50
	Fri	95	$23.75	$10.00	$296.25
7	Mon	100	$25.00		$321.25
	Wed	105	$26.25		$347.50
	Fri	110	$27.50	$10.00	$385.00
8	Mon	115	$28.75		$413.75
	Wed	120	$30.00		$443.75
	Fri	125	$31.25	$10.00	$485.00
9	Mon	130	$32.50		$517.50
	Wed	135	$33.75		$551.25
	Fri	140	$35.00	$10.00	$596.25
10	Mon	145	$36.25		$632.50
	Wed	150	$37.50		$670.00
	Fri	155	$38.75	$10.00	$718.75
11	Mon	160	$40.00		$758.75
	Wed	165	$41.25		$800.00
	Fri	170	$42.50	$10.00	$852.50
12	Mon	175	$43.75		$896.25
	Wed	180	$45.00		$941.25
	Fri	185	$46.25	$10.00	$997.50

Adapted from Budney AJ, Higgins ST. *A Community Reinforcement Approach: Treating Cocaine Addiction*. Vol 2. National Institute on Drug Abuse; 1998.

TABLE 41.4 Sample Drawing Schedule for Prize-Based Contingency Management.

Week	Sample	Draws
1	Mon	1
	Fri	2
2	Mon	3
	Fri	4
3	Mon	5
	Fri	6
4	Mon	7
	Fri	8
5	Mon	8
	Fri	8
6	Mon	8
	Fri	8
7	Mon	8
	Fri	8
8	Mon	8
	Fri	8
9	Mon	8
	Fri	8
10	Mon	8
	Fri	8
11	Mon	8
	Fri	8
12	Mon	8
	Fri	8
Total		164

Adapted from Petry NM, Alessi SM, Hanson T, Sierra S. Randomized trial of contingent prizes versus vouchers in cocaine-using methadone patients. *J Consult Clin Psychol*. 2007;75:983–991.

are associated with small prizes, and when clients draw a small slip, they select from items such as bus tokens, fast food gift certificates, food items, and toiletries. Fewer slips (e.g., 40) are exchangeable for large prizes such as portable CD players, telephones, telephone minutes, pot and pan sets, and $20 gift cards to stores and restaurants. One slip corresponds to a jumbo prize such a DVD player, stereo, or television. With this system, there is always an opportunity to earn something of high value, but overall earnings are expected to be relatively modest. On average, the maximal arranged reinforcement for a 12-week treatment period is about $250 to $400, and typically clients earn about half the programmed reinforcement.

Prize-based contingency management was first evaluated in a sample of 42 alcohol-dependent men participating in a Veterans Affairs outpatient substance abuse treatment program.[49] Twenty-three participants were assigned to standard care, a 4-week intensive outpatient program that included 12-step meetings, relapse prevention, coping skills training, and AIDS education, followed by 4 weeks of less-intensive aftercare. Nineteen individuals received the same standard care plus contingency management for abstinence and for compliance with treatment goals (a modification of the community reinforcement approach). All participants submitted Breathalyzer samples at each daily visit to the treatment program, and participants in the contingency management group who tested negative for alcohol earned the opportunity to draw for prizes. Contingency management participants also earned additional draws for completing activities related to their treatment goals, such as attending an Alcoholics Anonymous meeting, filling out a job application, or participating in planned recreational activities with non–drug-using family members. Individuals who received contingency management in addition to standard care were significantly more likely than individuals receiving standard care alone to remain in treatment for the 8 weeks of the study (84% vs. 22%) and to remain abstinent from alcohol for the duration of the study (69% vs. 39%). Individuals who received contingency management compared with individuals who received standard care were less likely to relapse to heavy alcohol use by the end of the study (26% vs. 61%). The average value of prizes earned by each participant in the contingency management condition was $200.

A direct comparison of voucher- and prize-based contingency management interventions for cocaine-abusing individuals entering a community-based, outpatient, drug-free treatment program found both approaches to contingency management to be more effective than standard care alone.[46] Both contingency management interventions compared with standard care increased retention in treatment and the duration of continuous abstinence from drugs significantly. Individuals in standard care, voucher-based contingency management, and prize-based contingency management remained in the program for 5.5 (± 3.6) weeks, 8.2 (± 3.8) weeks, and 9.3 (± 3.7) weeks, respectively. Although there was no statistically significant difference between the two contingency management groups, the trend toward longer retention in treatment in the prize-based contingency management group was notable. Individuals who received standard care achieved 4.6 (± 3.4) weeks of continuous abstinence compared with 7.0 (± 4.2) weeks in voucher-based contingency management and 7.8 (± 4.2) weeks in prize-based contingency management.

Petry and colleagues did a follow-up study to examine the relative efficacy of two contingency management approaches plus standard care versus standard care alone among cocaine-dependent individuals who were receiving methadone.[45] Participants were assigned in a random fashion to standard care, standard care plus prize-based contingency management, or standard care plus voucher-based contingency management. The amount of arranged reinforcement was twice as high in the voucher-based versus the prize-based contingency management condition. Both contingency management conditions increased the duration of abstinence and the proportion of cocaine-negative samples submitted; hence even the prize-based contingency management approach of lower cost was efficacious.

Because the low-cost prize-based contingency management approach had therapeutic benefit similar to that of the voucher-based contingency management program, the extent to which prize values could be reduced and still reduce drug use was examined in another study of cocaine-abusing outpatients.[52] In that study, one group received standard care at community-based drug-free clinics, and two groups received prize-based contingency management plus standard care. One contingency management group offered the opportunity to earn up to an average of $240 in prizes, whereas the other offered the chance to earn up to an average of $80 in prizes. Both contingency management conditions offered a similar number of opportunities to draw for prizes; however, compared with the $240 group, the prizes available in the $80 group were less valuable. Although contingency management with $240 available for prizes was significantly more efficacious than standard care, there was no difference between standard care and contingency management with $80 available for prizes. Therefore, although the prize-based version of contingency management does offer some cost advantage over its voucher-based counterpart, even within the prize-based version there appeared to be a lower bound or threshold in monetary value for it to be of greater therapeutic benefit than standard care.

Because the previous study suggests an association between prize magnitude and efficacy of contingency management, it would be worthwhile to determine whether and how much efficacy could be improved by increasing prize magnitude. A recent study compared higher and lower magnitude prize contingency management to voucher contingency management and usual care in a sample of cocaine-dependent methadone patients.[43] Patients assigned to voucher contingency management could earn up to $900 in vouchers over 12 weeks for providing cocaine-free urine specimens and alcohol-free breath samples. Patients assigned to the prize contingency management conditions could earn up to $900 in prizes on average in the high-magnitude condition and up to $300 on average in prizes in the low-magnitude condition. All three contingency management conditions yielded outcomes superior to those of usual care. In the usual care group, 36% of samples were negative for cocaine and alcohol over 12 weeks. In the contingency management groups, 55.5% of samples were negative in the low-magnitude contingency management group, 55.1% of samples were negative in the high-magnitude contingency management group, and 59.1% of samples were negative in the voucher group. Differences among the three contingency management groups were not significant. The mean longest duration of abstinence from cocaine and alcohol in the usual care group was 1.7 weeks. The mean longest duration of abstinence in the contingency management conditions were 3.1 weeks (low-magnitude prize contingency management), 3.7 weeks (high-magnitude prize contingency management), and 3.4 weeks (voucher contingency management). Contingency management was associated with longer duration of abstinence than usual treatment, and the three contingency management conditions did not differ from one another. This study suggests that a relatively low-cost contingency management procedure can reduce cocaine and alcohol use in patients receiving methadone maintenance with no significant benefit gained by increasing prize magnitude.

Prize-based contingency management was selected by the National Institute on Drug Abuse Clinical Trials Network for more extensive evaluation in community treatment settings[51] based on the encouraging results from controlled clinical studies. The goal of the Clinical Trials Network is to evaluate the effectiveness of treatments found to be efficacious in controlled studies done at specialized research centers in community-based clinical settings, where most individuals receive treatment for substance use disorders. In the largest studies of contingency management to date,[40,51] more than 800 stimulant (cocaine, methamphetamine, or amphetamine) abusers were recruited from community clinics throughout the United States. About half of the participants were recruited from psychosocial (drug-free) clinics ($N = 415$)[51] and half from methadone clinics (N = 388).[40] The clinics were located primarily in urban settings, but suburban and rural settings were represented as well. The duration of the combined studies was 12 weeks. As in other contingency management studies, participants were assigned to one of two groups, standard care or standard care plus prize-based contingency management using a system of escalating draws for consecutive stimulant-free urine samples. The maximum number of draws available was 204, with average maximal expected earnings of about $400 in prizes. In the psychosocial programs,[51] individuals who received contingency management plus standard care were significantly more likely than those receiving standard care alone to remain in treatment for the entire 12 weeks of the study (49% vs. 35%). Contingency management participants also attended more counseling sessions during the study period (19.2 ± 16.8) than did those receiving standard care (15.7 ± 14.4). The longest duration of continuous verified abstinence from stimulants was significantly greater in the contingency management group compared with the standard care group (8.6 ± 9.2 weeks vs. 5.2 ± 6.9 weeks), and contingency management participants were more likely than participants who were receiving standard care to achieve 4 (40% vs. 21%), 8 (26% vs. 12%), or 12 (19% vs. 5%) weeks of continuous abstinence from stimulants. Similar results were noted for participants maintained on methadone who abused stimulants.[40] Individuals who were assigned in a random fashion to the contingency management condition were significantly more likely to achieve long durations of abstinence and to submit higher proportions of stimulant-negative urine samples. The average amount of reinforcement earned in the methadone programs was $120 per individual, and in the psychosocial programs it was $203 per individual. Thus the costs of reinforcers in prize-based contingency management are relatively low, and the procedure is widely efficacious across settings and substance-abusing populations.

A meta-analysis of prize-based contingency management studies published between 2000 and 2013 indicates that prize contingency management increases abstinence from target substances during the implementation period with moderate effect sizes.[5] Significant effects were unfortunately not maintained 6 months after the prize-based interventions ended. Although the follow-up finding is consistent with outcomes for most substance use disorder treatments, including both behavior and pharmacological treatments, it suggests the need for further research on strategies for extending the beneficial effects of contingency management.

Cost-Effectiveness

Investigators have begun to examine the cost-effectiveness of contingency management. Using data from the Clinical Trials Network studies, Olmstead et al.[39] estimated resource utilization (treatment services including counseling sessions attended, urine and Breathalyzer tests, counselors' time associated with drawings, and value of prizes won) of individuals receiving standard care or standard care with contingency management at community-based outpatient psychosocial drug abuse treatment clinics. Unit costs of services were estimated via surveys administered at the eight participating clinics. Participant outcomes (primarily duration of continuous abstinence) were also obtained from the trials. The incremental cost to lengthen abstinence by 1 week was $258 (95% confidence interval, $191–$401) in psychosocial clinics.[39] In a follow-up analysis of the same data, Olmstead et al.[38] sought to determine by how much the cost-effectiveness of contingency management varied across the eight psychosocial clinics in the Clinical

Trials Network trial. Incremental costs, incremental outcomes, and incremental cost-effectiveness ratios of contingency management versus standard care were calculated for each clinic. The incremental cost of contingency management ranged across the clinics from an additional $306 to an additional $582 per individual. The effect of contingency management on abstinence ranged from an additional 0.5 weeks to an additional 4 weeks across the clinics. Incremental cost-effectiveness ratios for abstinence ranged from $145 to $666 per individual across the clinics. Thus the cost-effectiveness of contingency management did vary widely among clinics in the Clinical Trials Network trial, and future work is needed to focus on identifying sources of this variation, perhaps by identifying clinic-level best practices or identifying subgroups of individuals who respond the most cost-effectively, with the ultimate goal of improving the cost-effectiveness of contingency management overall.

Sindelar et al.[64] evaluated the incremental cost-effectiveness of contingency management in a study in which different magnitudes of the prize in the prize-based contingency management were compared. They found that the $240 prize-based contingency management condition produced outcomes at a lower per-unit cost than the $80 contingency management condition. This finding suggests that sometimes increasing up-front costs is more cost-effective overall. These results may be particularly relevant for substance-abusing populations who utilize high-cost resources such as inpatient medical and criminal justice services.

A systematic review of the published cost-effectiveness studies of contingency management suggests that existing studies have limited generalizability due to different treatment populations and different outcome measures across studies.[62] Further investigation is therefore needed, perhaps with collaboration among investigators to identify appropriate outcome measures and measures of treatment costs.

Challenges to Dissemination

Although the efficacy of the community reinforcement approach and contingency management for the treatment of substance use disorders in controlled settings is established, the adoption of these procedures by treatment providers in clinical practice has been limited. As noted earlier, the costs of the reinforcers and of staff time for administration of the procedures are some obstacles to implementation.

The costs associated with contingency management can be decreased by providing contingency management in a group context. Although typically implemented individually, prize-based contingency management can also be administered in a group format,[1,31,50] perhaps facilitating its adoption, as group therapy predominates in practice. Witnessing others winning prizes appears to lead to a camaraderie among clients, and group- and prize-based contingency management has been implemented at a fairly low cost (e.g., $15–$20 per week in direct costs).[31]

Cost is not the only barrier to implementation of these evidence-based practices. Implementation also depends on familiarity with and proficiency in techniques and principles of behavior modification. These include behavioral therapy and behavioral contracting and—in the case of contingency management—consistently applying contingencies, frequently monitoring and reinforcing behaviors, integrating escalating or bonus reinforcers, and providing adequate reinforcement magnitude.[41] Developing comprehensive training procedures for the community reinforcement approach and contingency management for community-based treatment staff is a large undertaking, but efforts toward dissemination are underway. Budney and Higgins[7] provided a treatment manual for the combination of the community reinforcement approach and voucher-based contingency management, and a training manual for prize-based contingency management is available at https://health.uconn.edu/contingency-management/training/training-related-links/.

Despite the barriers to adoption, the growing body of evidence for contingency management's efficacy has led to its being adopted by the US Department of Veterans Affairs and the UK National Health Service.[11,47] These large health care systems are committed to providing evidence-based treatments to their patient populations and have the resources to provide the required staff training and reinforcement systems to ensure that contingency management is delivered correctly. Studies of VA training programs indicate that they were effective in correcting misconceptions about contingency management and increasing willingness to implement it in practice.[55]

Other implementation concerns relate explicitly to prize-based contingency management. Because this procedure contains an element of chance, concerns have arisen that it might promote pathological gambling. However, gambling by definition involves risking something of value, which is not the case with contingency management. Examination of gambling behaviors among 803 individuals participating in the Clinical Trials Network prize-based contingency management studies found no evidence of increases in gambling behavior over time.[48] A retrospective analysis of three clinical trials suggested that participation in prize contingency management was actually associated with reductions in gambling among participants who had gambled in the month prior to treatment.[42] These studies suggest that prize-based contingency management is likely a safe intervention, even for substance users who gamble.

The ability of treatment systems that are under tight fiscal restraints and understaffed to absorb the additional costs of community reinforcement approach and contingency management is understandably met with skepticism. In the case of contingency management explicitly, reducing reinforcement magnitudes to under $240 for prize-based contingency management will compromise efficacy,[52] but it may be possible to offset costs in part or in full via fundraising or other strategies including the use of clinic privileges for some prizes. Moreover, the immediate costs of contingency management and the community reinforcement approach may pale in comparison to the societal and individual costs of continued drug abuse. Comprehensive cost-effectiveness analyses are needed to evaluate more clearly contingency management and the community reinforcement approach, when delivered either alone or together, relative to other modalities for treating substance abuse.

Conclusion

The community reinforcement approach and contingency management are efficacious interventions for the treatment of substance use disorders. The community reinforcement approach addresses the multiple biopsychosocial factors that contribute to substance abuse and provides intensive intervention to help individuals develop alternative forms of reinforcement to compete with substance use. Contingency management enhances the outcomes of the community reinforcement approach by providing tangible reinforcers for drug abstinence and other positive behaviors as clients learn self-reinforcement strategies, engage in new adaptive behaviors, and adopt a drug-free lifestyle. Numerous studies demonstrate the efficacy of these interventions as treatments for alcohol, cocaine, opiate, and marijuana use disorders.

Despite their efficacy, implementation of community reinforcement approach and contingency management has been slow in community settings. Many factors contribute to the implementation and sustainability of treatments, including the soundness of forged research-treatment partnerships, the readiness of communities to accept an innovation, and financial resources for training and implementation. Future adoption of these interventions for perhaps the most seriously impaired substance abusers may ultimately prove to be efficacious and cost-effective. Recent innovations such as using contingency management to reinforce community reinforcement approach activities (reducing the burden on counselors) and administering contingency management in group settings may facilitate wider adoption of these empirically validated treatments in practice. Adoption by large health care systems committed to providing evidence-based treatments can also accelerate adoption of these treatments in the broader community.

References

1. Alessi SM, Hanson T, Wieners M, Petry NM. Low-cost contingency management in community clinics: delivering incentives partially in group therapy. *Exp Clin Psychopharmacol.* 2007;15:293–300.
2. Alessi SM, Petry NM. Smoking reductions and increased self-efficacy in a randomized controlled trial of smoking abstinence-contingent incentives in residential substance abuse treatment patients. *Nicotine Tob Res.* 2014;16:1436–1445.
3. Azrin NH. Improvements in the community-reinforcement approach to alcoholism. *Behav Res Ther.* 1976;14:339–348.
4. Azrin NH, Sisson RW, Meyers R, Godley M. Alcoholism treatment by disulfiram and community reinforcement therapy. *J Behav Ther Exp Psychiatry.* 1982;13:105–112.
5. Benishek LA, Dugosh KL, Kirby KC, et al. Prize-based contingency management for the treatment of substance abusers: a meta-analysis. *Addiction.* 2014;109:1426–1436.
6. Bickel WK, Amass L, Higgins ST, Badger GJ, Esch RA. Effects of adding behavioral treatment to opioid detoxification with buprenorphine. *J Consult Clin Psychol.* 1997;65:803–810.
7. Budney AJ, Higgins ST. *A Community Reinforcement Approach: Treating Cocaine Addiction.* Vol. 2. National Institute on Drug Abuse; 1998.
8. Budney AJ, Higgins ST, Radonovich KJ, Novy PL. Adding voucher-based incentives to coping skills and motivational enhancement improves outcomes during treatment for marijuana dependence. *J Consult Clin Psychol.* 2000;68:1051–1061.
9. Budney AJ, Moore BA, Rocha HL, Higgins ST. Clinical trial of abstinence-based vouchers and cognitive-behavioral therapy for cannabis dependence. *J Consult Clin Psychol.* 2006;74:307–316.
10. Campbell AN, Nunes EV, Matthews AG, et al. Internet-delivered treatment for substance abuse: a multisite randomized controlled trial. *Am J Psychiatry.* 2014;17:683–690.
11. Carroll KM. Lost in translation? Moving contingency management and cognitive behavioral therapy into clinical practice. *Ann NY Acad Sci.* 2014;1327:94–111.
12. Dallery J, Silverman K, Chutuape MA, Bigelow GE, Stitzer ML. Voucher-based reinforcement of opiate plus cocaine abstinence in treatment-resistant methadone patients: effects of reinforcer magnitude. *Exp Clin Psychopharmacol.* 2001;9:317–325.
13. Donatelle R, Hudson D, Dobie S, Goodall A, Hunsberger M, Oswald K. Incentives in smoking cessation: status of the field and implications for research and practice with pregnant smokers. *Nicotine Tob Res.* 2004;6(suppl 2):S163–S179.
14. Finney JW, Monahan SC. The cost-effectiveness of treatment for alcoholism: a second approximation. *J Stud Alcohol.* 1996;57:229–243.

15. Godley SH, Meyers RJ, Smith JE, et al. The adolescent community reinforcement approach for adolescent cannabis users. *Cannabis Youth Treatment Series.* Vol. 4. MD: Silver Spring; 2002.

16. Higgins ST, Badger GJ, Budney AJ. Initial abstinence and success in achieving longer term cocaine abstinence. *Exp Clin Psychopharmacol.* 2000;8:377–386.

17. Higgins ST, Budney AJ, Bickel WK, Badger GJ, Foerg FE, Ogden D. Outpatient behavioral treatment for cocaine dependence: one-year outcome. *Exp Clin Psychopharmacol.* 1995;3:205–212.

18. Higgins ST, Budney AJ, Bickel WK, Foerg FE, Donham R, Badger GJ. Incentives improve outcome in outpatient behavioral treatment of cocaine dependence. *Arch Gen Psychiatry.* 1994;51:568–576.

19. Higgins ST, Budney AJ, Bickel WK, Hughes JR, Foerg F, Badger G. Achieving cocaine abstinence with a behavioral approach. *Am J Psychiatry.* 1993;150:763–769.

20. Higgins ST, Delaney DD, Budney AJ, et al. A behavioral approach to achieving initial cocaine abstinence. *Am J Psychiatry.* 1991;148:1218–1224.

21. Higgins ST, Heil SH, Solomon LJ, et al. A pilot study on voucher-based incentives to promote abstinence from cigarette smoking during pregnancy and postpartum. *Nicotine Tob Res.* 2004;6:1015–1020.

22. Higgins ST, Sigmon SC, Wong CJ, et al. Community reinforcement therapy for cocaine-dependent outpatients. *Arch Gen Psychiatry.* 2003;60:1043–1052.

23. Higgins ST, Wong CJ, Badger GJ, Ogden DE, Dantona RL. Contingent reinforcement increases cocaine abstinence during outpatient treatment and 1 year of follow-up. *J Consult Clin Psychol.* 2000;68:64–72.

24. Holder H, Longabaugh R, Miller WR, Rubonis AV. The cost effectiveness of treatment for alcoholism: a first approximation. *J Stud Alcohol.* 1991;52:517–540.

25. Holder HD, Blose JO. Typical patterns and cost of alcoholism treatment across a variety of populations and providers. *Alcohol Clin Exp Res.* 1991;15:190–195.

26. Hunt GM, Azrin NH. A community-reinforcement approach to alcoholism. *Behav Res Ther.* 1973;11:91–104.

27. Hunter SB, Ayer L, Han B, Garner BR, Godley SH. Examining the sustainment of the adolescent-community reinforcement approach in community addiction treatment settings: protocol for a longitudinal mixed method study. *Implement Sci.* 2014;9:104.

28. Hunter SB, Han B, Slaughter ME, Goldey SH, Garner BR. Associations between implementation characteristics and evidence-based practice sustainment: a study of the adolescent community reinforcement approach. *Implement Sci.* 2015;10:173.

29. Iguchi MY, Belding MA, Morral AR, Lamb RJ, Husband SD. Reinforcing operants other than abstinence in drug abuse treatment: an effective alternative for reducing drug use. *J Consult Clin Psychol.* 1997;65:421–428.

30. Kadden RM, Litt MD, Kabela-Cormier E, Petry NM. Abstinence rates following behavioral treatments for marijuana dependence. *Addict Behav.* 2007;32:1220–1236.

31. Ledgerwood DM, Alessi SM, Hanson T, Godley MD, Petry NM. Contingency management for attendance to group substance abuse treatment. *J Appl Behav Anal.* 2008;41:517–526.

32. Lewis MW, Petry NM. Contingency management treatments that reinforce completion of goal-related activities: participation in family activities and its association with outcomes. *Drug Alcohol Depend.* 2005;79:267–271.

33. Lussier JP, Heil SH, Mongeon JA, Badger GJ, Higgins ST. A meta-analysis of voucher-based reinforcement therapy for substance use disorders. *Addiction.* 2006;10:192–203.

34. Manuel JK, Austin JL, Miller WR, et al. Community reinforcement and family training: a pilot comparison of group and self-directed delivery. *J Subst Abuse Treat.* 2012;43:129–136.

35. Miller WR, Meyers RJ, Tonigan JS. A comparison of CRA and traditional approaches. In: Meyers RJ, Miller WR, eds. *A Community Reinforcement Approach to Addiction Treatment.* Cambridge: University Press; 2001.

36. Miller WR, Meyers RJ, Tonigan JS, Grant KA. Community reinforcement and traditional approaches: findings of a controlled trial. In: Meyers RJ, Miller WR, eds. *A Community Reinforcement Approach to Addiction Treatment.* Cambridge: University Press; 2001.

37. Miller WR, Wilbourne PL. Mesa grande: a methodological analysis of clinical trials of treatments for alcohol use disorders. *Addiction.* 2002;97:265–277.

38. Olmstead TA, Sindelar JL, Petry NM. Clinic variation in the cost-effectiveness of contingency management. *Am J Addict.* 2007;16:457–460.

39. Olmstead TA, Sindelar JL, Petry NM. Cost-effectiveness of prize-based incentives for stimulant abusers in outpatient psychosocial treatment programs. *Drug Alcohol Depend.* 2007;87:175–182.

40. Peirce JM, Petry NM, Stitzer ML, et al. Effects of lower-cost incentives on stimulant abstinence in methadone maintenance treatment: a national drug abuse treatment clinical trials network study. *Arch Gen Psychiatry.* 2006;63:201–208.

41. Petry NM. A comprehensive guide to the application of contingency management procedures in clinical settings. *Drug Alcohol Depend.* 2000;58:9–25.

42. Petry NM, Alessi SM. Prize-based contingency management is efficacious in cocaine-abusing patients with and without recent gambling participation. *J Subst Abuse Treat.* 2010;39:282–288.

43. Petry NM, Alessi SM, Barry DB, Carroll KM. Standard magnitude prize reinforcers can be as efficacious as larger magnitude reinforcers in cocaine-dependent methadone patients. *J Consult Clin Psychol.* 2015;83:464–472.

44. Petry NM, Alessi SM, Carroll KM, et al. Contingency management treatments: reinforcing abstinence versus adherence with goal-related activities. *J Consult Clin Psychol.* 2006;74:592–601.

45. Petry NM, Alessi SM, Hanson T, Sierra S. Randomized trial of contingent prizes versus vouchers in cocaine-using methadone patients. *J Consult Clin Psychol.* 2007;75:983–991.

46. Petry NM, Alessi SM, Marx J, Austin M, Tardif M. Vouchers versus prizes: contingency management treatment of substance abusers in community settings. *J Consult Clin Psychol.* 2005;73:1005–1014.

47. Petry NM, DePhilippis D, Rash CJ, Drapkin M, McKay JR. Nationwide dissemination of contingency management: the Veterans Administration initiative. *Am J Addict.* 2014;23:205–210.

48. Petry NM, Kolodner KB, Li R, et al. Prize-based contingency management does not increase gambling. *Drug Alcohol Depend.* 2006;83:269–273.

49. Petry NM, Martin B, Cooney JL, Kranzler HR. Give them prizes, and they will come: contingency management for treatment of alcohol dependence. *J Consult Clin Psychol.* 2000;68:250–257.

50. Petry NM, Martin B, Finocche C. Contingency management in group treatment: a demonstration project in an HIV drop-in center. *J Subst Abuse Treat.* 2001;21:89–96.

51. Petry NM, Peirce JM, Stitzer ML, et al. Effect of prize-based incentives on outcomes in stimulant abusers in outpatient psychosocial treatment programs: a national drug abuse treatment clinical trials network study. *Arch Gen Psychiatry.* 2005;62:1148–1156.

52. Petry NM, Tedford J, Austin M, Nich C, Carroll KM, Rounsaville BJ. Prize reinforcement contingency management for treating cocaine users: how low can we go, and with whom? *Addiction.* 2004;99:349–360.

53. Petry NM, Tedford J, Martin B. Reinforcing compliance with non-drug-related activities. *J Subst Abuse Treat.* 2001;20:33–44.

54. Prendergast M, Podus D, Finney J, Greenwell L, Roll J. Contingency management for treatment of substance use disorders: a meta-analysis. *Addiction.* 2006;101:1546–1560.

55. Rash CJ, DePhilippis D, McKay JR, Drapkin M, Petry NM. Training workshops positively impact beliefs about contingency management in a nationwide dissemination effort. *J Subst Abuse Treat.* 2013;45:306–312.

56. Roll JM, Higgins ST. A within-subject comparison of three different schedules of reinforcement of drug abstinence using cigarette smoking as an exemplar. *Drug Alcohol Depend.* 2000;58:103–109.

57. Roll JM, Higgins ST, Badger GJ. An experimental comparison of three different schedules of reinforcement of drug abstinence using cigarette smoking as an exemplar. *J Appl Behav Anal.* 1996;29:495–505.

58. Roll JM, Higgins ST, Steingard S, McGinley M. Use of monetary reinforcement to reduce the cigarette smoking of persons with schizophrenia: a feasibility study. *Exp Clin Psychopharmacol.* 1998;6:157–161.

59. Roozen HG, Boulogne JJ, van Tulder MW, van den Brink W, De Jong CA, Kerkhof AJ. A systematic review of the effectiveness of the community reinforcement approach in alcohol, cocaine and opioid addiction. *Drug Alcohol Depend.* 2004;74:1–13.

60. Roozen HG, de Waart R, van der Kroft P. Community reinforcement and family training: an effective option to engage treatment-resistant substance-abusing individuals in treatment. *Addiction.* 2010;105:1729–1738.

61. Schottenfeld RS, Pantalon MV, Chawarski MC, Pakes J. Community reinforcement approach for combined opioid and cocaine dependence. Patterns of engagement in alternate activities. *J Subst Abuse Treat.* 2000;18:255–261.

62. Shearer J, Tie H, Byford S. Economic evaluations of contingency management in illicit drug misuse programmes: a systematic review. *Drug Alcohol Rev.* 2015;34:289–298.

63. Sigmon SC, Miller ME, Meyer AC, et al. Financial incentives to promote extended smoking abstinence in opioid-maintained patients: a randomized trial. *Addiction.* [in press].

64. Sindelar J, Elbel B, Petry NM. What do we get for our money? Cost-effectiveness of adding contingency management. *Addiction.* 2007;102:309–316.

65. Smith JE, Meyers RJ, Delaney HD. The community reinforcement approach with homeless alcohol-dependent individuals. *J Consult Clin Psychol.* 1998;66:541–548.

66. Stitzer ML, Bigelow GE. Contingent reinforcement for reduced carbon monoxide levels in cigarette smokers. *Addict Behav.* 1982;7:403–412.

67. Stitzer ML, Bigelow GE. Contingent reinforcement for carbon monoxide reduction: within-subject effects of pay amount. *J Appl Behav Anal.* 1984;17:477–483.

68. Stitzer ML, Bigelow GE, Liebson IA, Hawthorne JW. Contingent reinforcement for benzodiazepine-free urines: evaluation of a drug abuse treatment intervention. *J Appl Behav Anal.* 1982;15:493–503.

42

Relapse Prevention and Recycling in Addiction

CARLO C. DICLEMENTE, MEREDITH A. HOLMGREN, DANIEL ROUNSAVILLE, CATHERINE CORNO, MEAGAN GRAYDON, DANIEL KNOBLACH, AND ALICIA WIPROVNICK

CHAPTER OUTLINE

Introduction

In the struggle to be free from addiction, for most individuals, repeated attempts are required to stop the addictive behavior. Multiple attempts to change and multiple treatment events are the norm rather than the exception in recovery from addiction.[46] There seems to be a predictable cycle in the path to recovery. Once addicted individuals become convinced that they need to change problematic addictive behaviors (illegal or nonprescription drug use, excessive alcohol consumption, tobacco use, or gambling), they will attempt either to quit completely or to significantly

modify these behaviors (e.g., cutting down or using methadone or buprenorphine instead of heroin). The majority of these individuals who make an attempt to change, however, are unsuccessful. In any cohort of individuals who enter treatment and make a bona fide attempt to change, the majority, between 60% and 80%, return to the problematic behavior after some period of success.[14,46] This event, although defined in various ways, has been labeled a "relapse."

Understanding the Concept of Relapse and Its Role in Recovery

The definition of what constitutes a relapse varies depending on the definition of success and failure in changing an addictive behavior. The most stringent definitions define success as complete abstinence from the behavior and identify relapse as any engagement in the addictive behavior (any consumption of alcohol, use of cocaine, and so on).[86] Other clinicians and researchers make a distinction between a slip or lapse and a full-blown relapse.[59] Slips and lapses have been defined variably as a single use, a single period of use, minimal amounts of use, or use without any consequences. Relapse is then a more significant engagement in the behavior than a single event or a brief period of use. Lapses could indicate that there are some vestiges of the behavior present that may create problems for sustained abstinence or lead to a relapse. Making a distinction between a lapse and a relapse can be clinically useful because the very strict definition of complete abstinence or failure can have unintended consequences, as described later. It is important first to note some common misconceptions about the phenomenon of relapse. Relapse is often viewed as a unique problem of substance abusers by practitioners and the public. However, relapse and lapsing back to unhealthy behaviors occur in all types of health behavioral change and is not limited to addictions. Many health behaviors, such as dietary change, diabetes management, regular physical activity, and medication adherence have a similar course, with large numbers of individuals lapsing and relapsing.[14,62] Relapse is not merely a function of physiological addiction, it is a function of the process of behavioral change when individuals attempt to change difficult-to-modify patterns of behavior.[31,63]

Another misconception is that relapse is often viewed as failure, since the desired behavioral change is not sustained. However, although it does not represent complete success, relapse is an integral part of learning during the recovery process. Individuals do not become addicted or recover from an addiction with a single learning event.[31] Within the stages of change model, relapse represents an event that not only involves a return to a problematic behavior but also signifies a return to an earlier stage of change for that behavior.[18,95] After relapsing, individuals can return to any of the pre-Action or even to Action stages; Precontemplation (not considering change in the near term), Contemplation (considering and decision making), Preparation (building commitment and planning), or Action (initial change lasting for 3–6 months). Individuals returning to the Precontemplation stage after relapse likely believe they cannot change or they are no longer interested in changing the addictive behavior. Relapsers who reconsider the pros and the cons of the addiction, try to resolve the associated ambivalence and make a new decision to quit have returned to the Contemplation stage. Those who determine what went wrong during the last quit attempt and are poised to make another attempt return to the Preparation stage. Relapsers who quickly make another attempt move back into the Action stage of change. The return to earlier stages of change after relapsing from the Action or Maintenance stage is called "recycling" back through the stages and often leads to another attempt that is successful.[32,51,98] The cyclical movement through the stages of change represents the learning process of successive approximations whereby an individual learns gradually through trial and error how to avoid the problems from past attempts and make a successful change in behavior.

Relapse, considered from this perspective, is not so much a failure as an opportunity to learn what went wrong and what was missing in the unsuccessful process of change. Most individuals who enter stable recovery do so only after multiple attempts to change. This pattern is true of individuals who have changed the addictive behavior without the aid of formal treatment as well as those who have been successful after a particular course of treatment.[33,67,72] In any case, understanding relapse and recycling is critical to understanding successful recovery. Helping individuals avoid relapse and/or to learn how to profit from the experience and become more successful is the goal of relapse prevention and of successful recycling. This chapter examines relapse prevention models, highlights critical components of relapse prevention, identifies key clinical strategies that can be used in the service of preventing relapse, and discusses how to promote successful recycling for those who were unable to change their behavior at any one point in time.

Relapse Prevention

As the field of addiction moved from a moral explanation of addiction to a focus on habit and disease, the challenge of maintaining change and avoiding relapse became a focus of research and theory.[14,56,59,93] Interest and research activity expanded to understand what precipitates relapse and the possible interventions that would reduce the relapse rate and increase the potential for recovery from a slip or a relapse. There were several dominant theories that were developed during the 20th century, not all of which were compatible with one another.

Models for Relapse Prevention

The two partially compatible models for understanding relapse came from different explanatory frameworks. The Medical Model

countered the prevailing perspective at the beginning of the 20th century that alcoholism and other addictions were moral problems that could be overcome with willpower and by observing moral standards. The view of addiction as a disease was intended to change the conversation about addiction, remove some of the stigma, and make it a medical condition that was treatable. This model was not only adopted by medical professionals but also by the influential founders of Alcoholics Anonymous and the Twelve-Step model for recovery.[86] At the same time in the academic community, the social and behavioral learning perspectives described addictions as overlearned behaviors that were supported by contextual forces. More recently, addiction has also been described as a reward deficit disorder in which an individual progresses from impulsivity to compulsivity and from positive reinforcement to negative reinforcement in the development of their addiction.[52] This model focuses more on how substances affect brain functioning, emotion regulation, and stress management, creating behaviors that are difficult to stop and maintain cessation. Of interest, all models arrived at some similar relapse-prevention strategies.

Medical and Mutual Help Model

In the Medical Model, addiction is viewed in terms of the changes that are made in the neurochemistry of the addicted individual, which causes physiological dependence. The perspective is that the addiction acts as a disease and changes biological processes which, in turn, pose significant barriers for change for the addicted individual. The physiological changes that result from prolonged substance abuse manifest themselves in craving, which continually pushes the addicted individual to return to the addictive behavior.[77] For the addicted individual, their normal biological state is inherently resistant to behavior change.[21,53] Medical Model–oriented interventions to prevent relapse include periods of hospitalization that focus on breaking the physiological and psychological connections to addiction as well as using medications that decrease cravings.

In the Medical/Mutual Help or Twelve-Step Model, addiction is also described as an illness or disease that addicted individuals are powerless to control.[78] One analogy for the disease is an allergy such that the individual cannot have contact with the substance without a loss of control. This perspective supports the view of relapse as any contact with addictive substance or behavior. The addicted individual is seen as someone who has a defect such that willpower cannot be the solution for recovery. Preventing relapse must include an admission of powerlessness and a reliance on a higher power, whether that is seen as a spiritual power or the power of the mutual help network that is created by associating with Alcoholics Anonymous and working the 12 steps of recovery. The program includes a number of strategies (e.g., approach recovery, one day at a time, you are always an alcoholic and must always be vigilant, meeting attendance) and support systems (e.g., sponsors, fellowship of Alcoholics Anonymous) for the prevention of relapse.

Reward Deficit Model

Addiction, particularly a severe alcohol use disorder, has been conceptualized as a reward deficit disorder. It is a chronically relapsing disorder that, like in the medical model, is defined by a loss of control in limiting one's intake. It is also characterized by a compulsion to use the substance driven also by the negative affectivity in the form of dysphoria, anxiety, or irritability occurring as a result of withdrawal from the substance. When an individual initiates substance use, impulsivity, a predisposition to quick unplanned actions without considering negative consequences, is the dominant precipitant to substance use. Later in the addiction cycle, once negative affectivity and withdrawal has begun, substance use becomes compulsive, meaning one continues to use the substance in the face of negative consequences. When substance use is more of an impulsive behavior, it is positively reinforced by the pleasurable effects of the drug. Use becomes compulsive as the motivational force changes to negative reinforcement and use becomes necessary to relieve a negative affective state. This model asserts that it is the reward deficit caused by neurobiological changes in the brain that is the chief vulnerability for relapse.[52] Interventions based on this model often include use of a pharmacological agent to assist in breaking the addiction cycle and in supporting behavioral strategies that will enable abstinence and avoidance of relapse.

Cognitive-Behavioral Models

In 1980, G. Alan Marlatt and Judith Gordon developed the Relapse Prevention Model, an extensive, empirically focused conceptual model that we use as the basis of our discussion of relapse in this chapter. Their cognitive-behavioral model of the relapse process[39] is based on social cognitive and learning models of behavior and posits that addiction stems from maladaptive habit patterns. Relapse is conceptualized as resulting from a series of predictable cognitive and behavioral events that lead to a return to substance use. This relapse prevention model hypothesizes that common cognitive, behavioral, and affective mechanisms underlie the process of relapse for a variety of problem behaviors. This view of recovery is based on learning theory and differs from the disease model in many ways, although it does share some theoretical precipitants of relapse.

The model assumes that a complex array of determinants is involved in the development of an addiction and the ability to successfully change addictive behaviors. Some influential factors include genetics, environmental/situational factors, family history of addiction, peer influence, early use of substances, and expectancies of the effects of the substance. During periods of abstinence, individuals must engage in cognitive and behavioral coping activities that lead to successful behavior change. Along the way, they are likely to face situations that put them at risk for relapse. High risk situations that become triggers for relapse are at the center of the cognitive-behavioral model of relapse.

The most recent refinement to this model emphasizes that relapse processes are interactive, dynamic, and nonlinear. They also define two sets of processes that contribute to relapse. More stable (called tonic) processes encompass risks for relapse that include background factors like genetics, social support, and dependence; cognitive processes include global self-efficacy, outcome expectancies, craving and motivation; as well as physical withdrawal. More immediate processes (called phasic) processes include the individual's affective states and coping behaviors (including cognitive/behavioral strategies and self-regulation). The more stable tonic processes determine one's vulnerability for relapse, but the more immediate phasic responses determine how and when that happens.[45]

Research has elucidated several experiences that lead to relapse, which have been incorporated into the cognitive-behavioral relapse model. Cummings et al.[27] found that the most frequently reported precipitants of relapse included negative emotional state (35% of relapses), social pressure (20%), interpersonal conflict (16%), and urges and temptations (9%). Factor analysis of the

Reason for Drinking Questionnaire[104] revealed three major factors that differentiated the types of relapses people experienced: (1) negative emotions, (2) social pressure and positive emotions with others, and (3) temptation and craving.

According to the cognitive-behavioral relapse model,[59] individuals who use effective coping responses and have high self-efficacy are less likely to relapse. Moreover, successful use of this coping behavior increases self-efficacy,[7,8] which should reduce the probability of subsequent relapse in similar high-risk situations. If an individual fails to use effective coping behaviors, the lure of the substances will increase while self-efficacy to abstain decreases, thereby escalating the likelihood that the individual will use the substance in that particular situation. Guilt and low self-esteem can occur if the substance is used during this period of abstinence. These feelings can propel an individual from the initial use of alcohol, often termed a "lapse," into a full-blown relapse.

Marlatt and Gordon[59,60] describe the onset of guilt and lowered self-efficacy as a possible effect of a lapse from an initial goal of abstinence. They label this reaction the Abstinence Violation Effect. This reaction is related to the individual's causal attribution for the slip. For example, when drinkers attribute the lapse to their own personal failure, they tend to experience guilt and negative emotions that can lead to increased drinking in an attempt to avoid or escape those feelings. When people attribute the lapse to stable, global factors that are beyond their control, they are more likely to avoid a full-blown relapse. A subsequent relapse is more likely for persons who attribute the lapse to a personal inability to cope with high-risk situations.[59] It is the individuals who are able to learn from the mistake and avoid future relapses that are better able to develop effective coping skills to deal with triggers.[55] Of interest, research has found that contrary to the proposed inevitable loss of control that occurs after a lapse, some people are able to slip or engage in a first use and then regain control.[36] If an individual is able to reinstate abstinence after a slip, they have achieved a *prolapse* or positive lapse experience.[45]

Review of Relapse Prevention and Substance Abuse Studies

Since the advent of a focus on relapse and maintenance and, in particular, the response to the detailed, conceptual perspective of the Relapse Prevention Model, interventions designed to prevent relapse have been developed as clinical applications of Marlatt and Gordon's model.[59] The conceptual foundations of this model and a review of its applications have been updated by Marlatt and Donovan[58] and Hendershot and colleagues.[45] These interventions are designed to enhance the maintenance stage tasks of sustaining and integrating change into the person's lifestyle and emphasize self-management and coping skills in order to withstand the challenges presented by relapse precipitants.[58] The goals of relapse prevention are twofold: to prevent an initial lapse and to provide lapse management to prevent a complete relapse if a lapse does occur. Most controlled studies that administered relapse prevention treatment measured outcome success based on the goal of abstinence, although treatment goals based on harm reduction and decreasing substance use have also been attempted.[19,48]

The effectiveness of relapse prevention as an intervention has been reviewed for different substances and compared to a number of alternative interventions. Relapse prevention programs have been designed specifically for smoking, alcohol, marijuana, cocaine, and other drug use. Although early reviews concluded that there was little evidence for differential effectiveness of relapse prevention across classes of substance abuse,[19] later reviews found some support for the greater effectiveness of relapse prevention when applied to alcohol or polydrug use disorders in combination with medication treatment.[48]

In terms of comparative efficacy, relapse prevention has been found to be superior to no-treatment control groups, and equally as effective as other treatments, such as supportive therapy, social support groups, and interpersonal psychotherapy.[19] Another review[48] found that relapse prevention has a greater impact on improving psychosocial functioning than on reducing substance use. In addition, relapse prevention was more effective when combined with the use of prescribed medication. Although results were based on a small number of studies and should be interpreted with caution, Irvin et al.[48] concluded that individual, group, and marital modalities were equally effective in preventing relapse in cohorts of substance abusers. What follows is a brief review of the literature on the efficacy and use of relapse- prevention strategies with different types of addictive behaviors. A detailed presentation of the standard elements is included in the section entitled "Strategies for Relapse Prevention."

Effectiveness Studies Across Addictive Behaviors

More research has been conducted on the effectiveness of relapse prevention for alcoholism and nicotine addiction than for any other addictive behaviors. The second edition of *Relapse Prevention* by Marlatt and Donovan[58] provides a detailed chapter on relapse prevention for each of the addictive behaviors. For most drugs of abuse, relapse prevention constructs and strategies have been applied in clinical settings. However, there is limited literature on specific relapse prevention treatments separate from more generic cognitive-behavioral approaches, and the research consists mainly of trials focusing on the Abstinence Violation Effect or other dimensions of the model. It is disappointing that more studies of the entire model and specifically its efficacy in preventing relapse across multiple behaviors have not been conducted. However, because cognitive-behavioral therapy approaches have incorporated many aspects of the relapse-prevention strategies, and evaluations of these approaches in addictions have been favorable in terms of effectiveness and efficacy in trials,[19] there is empirical support for many of the constructs and the strategies that are described later in this chapter.

Relapse prevention has been found to be most effective in treating alcohol and polysubstance use compared with other substances alone (cocaine, marijuana, cigarettes, and so on) or abusive behaviors.[48] Reviews of alcohol and drug treatment studies generally report a broad, multidimensional range of outcomes that include reductions in use, increased time before relapse, and improvement in functioning.[19]

In addition to the more commonly used cognitive-behavioral interventions, new theoretical approaches to relapse prevention are gaining popularity and being researched, including Mindfulness-Based Relapse Prevention (MBRP), which is discussed in more detail later in the chapter. A study that compared the effectiveness of MBRP, a standard cognitive-behavioral relapse-prevention protocol, and treatment as usual (TAU) among substance users who completed initial substance use treatment[12] found that there were no group differences at 3 months after treatment, yet at the 6-month follow-up, both MBRP and relapse prevention fared better than TAU in reducing the risk of relapse to heavy drinking and/or drug use. Of interest, relapse prevention performed better than MBRP in time to first drug use, while participants who received

MBRP had significantly fewer days of drug use and a lower probability of engaging in heavy drinking at the 12-month follow-up. This study is one of the first comparing these relapse prevention approaches and strongly supports the notion that continued intervention after initial treatment, particularly over extended periods, promotes relapse prevention among alcohol and drug users.

A recent comprehensive review of smoking cessation relapse prevention interventions found that self-help materials can promote relapse prevention among previously unaided quitters and that pharmacotherapies (i.e., varenicline, nicotine replacement therapy [NRT], and bupropion) can be effective in preventing relapse after initial treatment or a period of abstinence.[2] However, comprehensive reviews for smoking cessation conducted by the Cochrane Collaborative in 2009[43] and Agboola and colleagues[2] found insufficient evidence to support the use of behavioral approaches to prevent smoking relapse in individuals who already successfully quit— these interventions were aimed at teaching patients skills to identify and cope with triggering situations via face-to-face, telephone, or worksheet formats. However, the methodological soundness of these studies overall was low. Nevertheless, many relapse prevention strategies have been included in standard tobacco dependence treatment (knowing personal and environmental cues for smoking, delaying and urge management, relaxation, rewards, and so on) and are incorporated into self-help and Internet-assisted programs.[87] Thus relapse prevention has become a core component of intervention for smoking cessation, rather than a separate and independent intervention specifically designed to prevent relapse.

Critical Mechanisms for Relapse Prevention

An increasing number of studies indicate that the prevention of relapse or promotion of successful maintenance of change involves several key overarching constructs: motivation, coping, and self-efficacy. These three elements are critical to the long-term success of recovery and are important components to address in any program attempting to prolong abstinence and prevent relapse.

Motivation

Motivation plays an important role in relapse prevention. There is ample evidence that motivation for change as well as treatment outcome expectancy and client goals of abstinence are related to successful treatment outcomes.[1,64,81,82] Motivation at the beginning of treatment and the attitudes and intentions that individuals bring into treatment are related to early cessation of drinking and drug use as well as to long-term success.[68] Individuals who enter treatment after making a decision to change and taking steps toward change have a better prognosis compared with those who enter treatment and have not yet made a decision or taken steps.[49] Overall, motivation is one of the most consistent predictors of long-term outcomes.[9,44] In addition, studies have found that increase in motivation during pharmacobehavioral treatment predicted drinking outcomes posttreatment,[79] and relapse prevention is less effective for individuals who have low initial readiness.[37]

How motivation and expectancies affect successful change and prevent relapse are not completely understood. Motivation is clearly multidimensional and involves different mechanisms of change.[33] Motivation has been conceptualized as having multiple components: problem recognition and endorsement of taking steps toward changing. Problem recognition is necessary but not sufficient for change in substance use behavior; it is only when problem recognition is followed with commitment and endorsement of taking steps that there is a documented long-term change in substance use behavior.[3,17] Relapse prevention is less effective for individuals who have low initial readiness[37]; enhancing problem recognition should precede relapse prevention efforts

If motivation is viewed as a series of tasks outlined by the stages of change, there are multiple elements that are necessary for the success of recovery and the prevention of relapse. For example, to avoid relapse, addicted individuals need to have some continuing, compelling reasons to abstain, a firm decision based on realistic expectations, commitment to follow through despite difficulties, an effective set of strategies and plans on how to manage triggers, and the ability to problem solve effectively when the plan is not working. These tasks outlined in the five stages of change have to be accomplished adequately to be able to sustain change and overcome the difficult challenges presented to anyone stopping or modifying an addictive behavior.[31] As individuals begin to have some success at changing the addictive behavior, their motivation to make an attempt to change has to shift to motivation to sustain the change over time in the face of the multiple personal and environmental barriers that could undermine the decision, the commitment, the determination, and the plan. Triggers have to be met successfully and the centrifugal forces that bring one back to the addictive behavior, be they physiological, behavioral, or social/environmental, must be countered.

One way to understand the function of relapse in recovery is to see it as a sign that the motivational tasks involved in the stages have not been adequately addressed or successfully mastered. So relapse serves to indicate that the process of change has not been done well enough to support success. Recycling through the stages then serves to help the addicted individual adequately accomplish these tasks to a degree that enables change to be maintained and relapse to be avoided. Much of the work of relapse prevention has focused on the cues and triggers that precipitate relapse. Although those precipitants are important, they do not explain relapse.[87] Looking more broadly at the entire process of change and successful completion of multiple tasks of the stages can help clinicians explore a range of challenges and topics that span the entire motivational process instead of focusing only on the moment of the slip, lapse, or relapse.

Coping

Strong support also has been found for the relationship between coping and relapse prevention.[74] Individuals who fail to use any coping response in a crisis have been found to be more likely to relapse.[28] There are two main theoretical aspects of coping responses: (1) the focus of coping and (2) the methods of coping.[74] In both of these areas, there is an important distinction between active coping and avoidant coping. In terms of focus, active coping strategies are those which are oriented toward the problem, whereas avoidant coping strategies rely on avoidance of the problem. Active strategies are most appropriate when an individual has some control over the situation, whereas avoidant coping may be more useful when dealing with situations or events in which there is little or no control.[71] Methods of coping involve strategies and coping activities that involve both cognitive and behavioral strategies.

An individual's inability to utilize an effective coping behavior when he or she is experiencing a high-risk situation results in decreased self-efficacy and increased use of a substance as a coping mechanism.[59] However, differential effects have not been found for cognitive coping skills versus behavioral coping skills. Rather, actively engaging either type of coping skill seems to facilitate positive outcomes.[14,28,35] In summary, it appears that in preventing

relapse there is an important role for the addicted individual's response to any threats to abstinence or recovery. However, it is not only the actual effectiveness of the response that helps to prevent relapse but also the sense of confidence that the individuals have in their ability to perform the behaviors critical to recovery and needed to sustain change.

Self-Efficacy

Confidence in one's ability to perform behaviors seems to be a critical mechanism in intentional behavior change. Bandura[7] defined self-efficacy as the degree to which an individual feels confident and capable of performing a certain behavior in specific situations. The self-evaluation of one's confidence to remain abstinent has been associated with lower rates of relapse for both men and women, in inpatient and outpatient settings, and for both short-term and long-term follow-up.[15,39,81]

Deficits in abstinence self-efficacy have been found to be a significant predictor of relapse in a number of studies.[47,97] Ecological momentary assessment, or repeated sampling of research participants' experiences, has made possible the investigation of the dynamic nature of self-efficacy and other relapse predictors; a recent study of 305 recently abstinent smokers demonstrated that daily reports of lower abstinence self-efficacy and positive smoking outcome expectancies predicted the occurrence of a first lapse and that downward shifts in abstinence self-efficacy predicted onset of relapse.[42] Moreover, the longer an individual stays abstinent, the stronger their self-efficacy and sense of personal control becomes. Higher levels of self-efficacy have been found to be predictive of improved alcohol treatment and tobacco use outcomes in a variety of contexts[1,4,41,81]

In a study that investigated abstinence self-efficacy of inpatient alcoholics in predicting their ability to remain abstinent after treatment, the level of abstinence self-efficacy measured at discharge from the residential center was the strongest predictor of abstinence at 1-year follow-up.[47] A meta-analysis of self-efficacy and smoking cessation revealed that self-efficacy measured postquit has a stronger relation to future smoking behavior than when self-efficacy is measured prior to a quit attempt.[41] Additional support has been found for the predictive power of abstinence self-efficacy using the Alcohol Confidence Questionnaire.[97] Higher levels of confidence to resist the urge to drink in high-risk situations were associated with greater likelihood to maintain abstinence 6 months after treatment. In addition, lower levels of confidence in situations related to urges and testing control were found to predict relapse to heavy drinking during a 12-week treatment period.[10] Greenfield and colleagues[39] found that individuals who relapsed to alcohol the year after hospitalization had lower overall confidence scores than individuals who did not relapse. This later relapse onset for the group with higher self-efficacy indicates a relation between efficacy to abstain and duration of abstinent behavior following treatment.

A large clinical treatment trial for matching participants to optimal alcohol treatments based on a number of client characteristics, Project MATCH, considered abstinence self-efficacy to be an important variable for determining appropriate treatment. Levels of abstinence self-efficacy were measured at the start of the study (baseline) and at the end of treatment (posttreatment). For the outpatient arm of the study, baseline abstinence self-efficacy was predictive of drinking outcomes during treatment, throughout the 1-year follow-up, and at a 3-year follow-up.[34,82] However, for aftercare clients, baseline self-assessment of abstinence self-efficacy did not predict posttreatment drinking, suggesting that efficacy was a more powerful predictor for those individuals who were just beginning therapy compared with those who were continuing treatment and may have already experienced changes to their levels of abstinence self-efficacy or who evaluated their self-efficacy in a residential setting.

Strategies for Relapse Prevention

The challenge of preventing relapse is one of trying to find strategies that can support and increase motivation, can teach or implement appropriate coping activities when internal or external cues trigger a desire or temptation to drink or use drugs, and can encourage and strengthen the self-efficacy of the addicted individual. Proper motivation, coping and efficacy would then support recovery and prevent relapse. Most programs and models of treatment and mutual help provide activities and support that target these variables. Alcoholics Anonymous, for example, encourages continued self-reevaluation (e.g., moral inventories, reading supportive literature), active coping both in avoiding high-risk situations and turning to meetings and a sponsor to support sobriety, and supports efficacy with a focus on one day at a time and messages of empowerment based on support from a higher power. However, the most extensive discussion of relapse prevention strategies comes from the social learning and relapse prevention models.

Relapse prevention is best used with clients who have finished an initial detoxification round of treatment and/or may be coming to the end of initial phases of treatment, since these are the clients who have been able to achieve some measure of abstinence or change. In addition, rates of relapse are highest in the initial phases of the action stage and once initial treatment has been completed. Relapse prevention would also be appropriate for individuals who have experienced a slip after a period of sustained abstinence and as a follow-up treatment for individuals in the maintenance stage of change.[62]

Relapse prevention treatment strategies have been divided into five specific categories of activities: (1) assessment, (2) increasing insight/awareness, (3) skills trainings, (4) cognitive strategies, and (5) lifestyle interventions. Each of these activities will be described in detail below. The activities are interconnected and there is a logical flow beginning with the initial strategy of behavioral assessment, which often starts with self-monitoring by the client. The goal of this behavioral assessment is to get a clear and complete picture of the circumstances surrounding potential substance use and the client's reactions to each of those situations or cues. If the client is still actively using substances, it is critical to obtain accurate information about the amount, the environment surrounding the use, and the events that preceded and followed the use. The next step is to identify high-risk situations, coping skills, and the effectiveness of both cognitive and behavioral coping strategies being used to address the cues.[50,101]

Once key skill deficits are identified, coping skills training can be conducted using either group or individual sessions. An advantage of the group format is that peers are natural partners for role plays and can provide examples of coping or scenarios for group brainstorming. Including significant others in sessions can also potentially assist in cue reduction and coping training and have a comprehensive impact on a client's recovery.[50] Finally, the focus turns to the lifestyle of the individual to see how overall patterns of life activities can help or hinder continued recovery and the maintenance of change. We review each of these components in greater detail and then discuss two newer strategies that have been added to the relapse prevention tool box: mindfulness strategies and medications.

Assessment

Behavioral assessments can be conducted using direct observation by a therapist (when cues are available or presented), role play, interviews with family members or peers, self-report questionnaires (Alcohol or Drug Abstinence Self-Efficacy; Alcohol Confidence Questionnaire, Situational Confidence Questionnaire), and self-monitoring.[55,96,99] In fact, self-monitoring serves not only as a means of gathering information but also as an intervention. In a recent review, prompting self-monitoring and secondarily seeking commitment were found to be associated with better drinking outcomes in the use of brief interventions for excessive alcohol consumption.[66] Although clients may initially be resistant to self-monitoring as a homework assignment, frequently after completing it, they report that it is a positive experience. In addition to the insight gained though the self-assessment, monitoring often acts as a catalyst for behavioral change and leads to a reduction of the monitored behavior.[56] In addition, self-monitoring can be an effective tool to combat denial, challenge cognitive distortions, and identify substance-related automatic processes and negative thoughts that promote an automatic sequence of behaviors that lead to using.[99]

If the individual is still engaging in the addictive behavior, then using self-monitoring to assess the factors surrounding use is important. If the client has been able to achieve abstinence, a self-assessment of cravings is appropriate to identify their personal high-risk situations. A frequently used type of self-assessment is assigning a drinking diary or craving diary to identify habit patterns; potential triggers; high-risk situations; consequences of use to themselves as well as others; and the physical, emotional, and financial costs of using. It is important for the individual to understand the social, situational, emotional, cognitive, and physiological precipitants of relapse that make up a high-risk situation.[99] Technologies like telephone-based Interactive Voice Responding (IVR) and ecological momentary assessment (periodic daily assessment prompts) can be used for repeated self-monitoring.[23] More recently, this method of self-monitoring is being used in clinical settings to provide clients and clinicians with real-time information.[88]

High-risk situations are any situation that threatens an individual's abstinence self-efficacy and poses a strong potential for relapse back to the addictive behavior. High-risk situations include both intrapersonal determinants as well as interpersonal determinants. The intrapersonal determinants include both positive and negative emotional states as potential risk factors. Negative emotional states such as anger, depression, anxiety, boredom, and frustration can be triggering, particularly if substances were used as a way of dealing with the emotional states. Clients may need additional treatment such as anger management or therapy for depression in addition to drug counseling to give them the coping skills to deal with such negative emotions.[50] Positive emotional states such as feeling good, confident, or celebrating can bolster overconfidence in being able to handle "just one" use of the substance.[55] Interpersonal determinants include conflicts with friends, spouses, family members, and coworkers. Another interpersonal determinant is social pressure that can either be overt encouragement to use or covert pressure to conform in a situation where everyone else may be smoking, drinking, or drugging.[99]

Once the self-assessment has been completed, this information can be used to create a decisional balance sheet that helps to concretely lay out the pros and cons of using in particular situations.

Such a worksheet can clarify the specific reasons for maintaining abstinence and increase motivation, particularly for individuals who are not fully committed to treatment or recovery. Assessments not only identify high-risk situations but also examine the commitment, self-efficacy, and coping skills that the individual may use to address challenging situations.

Insight and Awareness

Increasing insight and awareness assists clients in understanding the processes that trigger a relapse, including social pressure, physiological mechanisms, and emotion management. Understanding these mechanisms is an important part of preparing for high-risk situations and unexpected triggers and urges. This can be made more concrete by creating an ongoing road map to relapse by which clients identify upcoming high-risk situations, as well as potential unexpected risks and emergency situations. They can also identify early warning signs that predict a high-risk situation.[38] The road map can also identify ways they can refrain from using with an effective coping strategy for a particular situation.[55] The next challenge is to make sure that clients have access to the types of skills and self-management strategies that would be needed to effectively address their risk situations that could provoke a return to the substance use or addictive behavior.

Behavioral Coping Skills

The behavioral skills training component involves training in a number of skills and strategies in different life domains to assist clients in resisting relapse. Skills training is designed to develop specific skills needed to cope with situations and to increase the client's sense of self-efficacy to sustain recovery and overcome risks for relapse. For example, relaxation training can be particularly helpful with clients who used substances to alleviate anxiety or to cope with stressful situations. Progressive relaxation training or mindfulness meditation can assist in decreasing anxiety in a high-risk situation sufficiently so that an alternative coping strategy can then be employed.[103] Assertiveness training, including practicing refusal skills, can assist clients with poor social skills in navigating interpersonal pressures to use and is associated with improved drinking outcomes, assisted by improved self-efficacy. Encouraging the use of social support has also led to continued abstinence, and perceived general social support is also associated with abstinence self-efficacy.[91] Practicing ways to refuse substances, deal with criticism, and appropriately express feelings of frustration, anger, or anxiety can assist clients in building their repertoire of coping skills.[99]

Cue exposure is another cognitive behavioral technique that is used to build up client's abstinence self-efficacy through gradually exposing them to substance-related cues. It is a counterconditioning procedure in which clients are progressively desensitized to the stimuli associated with the addictive behavior in controlled conditions. Clients practice using coping skills as they are gradually exposed to different high-risk situations. To avoid iatrogenic effects from putting clients in potentially very unsettling conditions, exposure should always end with adequate processing of the experience and debriefing, such as a relaxation exercise or meditation.[5,103] Clients who were encouraged to practice cue exposure with careful guidance from their therapist achieved significant improvement in drinking outcomes over time.[70]

There are numerous skills that can be developed and there are manuals for various types of addictive behaviors that contain modules for specific skills training in effective communication, anger management, coping with negative emotions, depression, assertiveness, handling rejection, meditation, and managing family members who use substances. These modules can be used depending on the types of situations that are identified by the addicted individual so that the relapse prevention strategies can be personalized to the types of situations and cues that are most salient for that individual.[69]

Cognitive Strategies

In addition to behavioral skills, there are also a number of cognitive strategies that can be taught and used to combat relapse. Often, relapse is precipitated not just by the external cues but by the interpretations and self-statements from within the individual when confronted with a high-risk situation. Cognitive strategies are designed to challenge and change ways that individuals process information and problematic self-statements that undermine coping and efficacy. These cognitive strategies include cognitive restructuring, relapse rehearsal, labeling and detachment, and coping imagery. Cognitive restructuring is the process of correcting addiction-related cognitive distortions and frequent patterns of thinking such as seemingly irrelevant decisions and the abstinence violation effect. Seemingly irrelevant decisions are decisions that are not inherently related to the actual substance use but can put the client in a high-risk situation. An example would be a client getting his car fixed at a mechanic one block from his favorite bar (alcohol-associated cues). Doing so could prompt him to go in to see if any friends (interpersonal pressure) were around as a way to alleviate the boredom (negative emotion) of waiting for his car to be fixed.[55] The goal of cognitive interventions is to help individuals examine and prevent such seemingly irrelevant decisions that put individuals in harm's way and can lead to relapse.

As was noted previously, the abstinence violation effect is a potential reaction to initial use or reengagement in the addictive behavior. If after a lapse, clients feel they have failed and experience a significant decrease in abstinence self-efficacy, they are more likely to go back to using as much as they used rather than attempt to regain abstinence. It is important to put a lapse into proper perspective so that clients can return to the recovery process rather than returning to their prior habits. Recovery from a slip seems to require an interpretation and attribution of the lapse as caused by external or environmental factors, a continuing commitment to the change goal, a confidence in the ability to recover from a lapse, and a reactivation of active coping to avoid or manage the triggering situations or cues.[55]

Relapse rehearsal and relapse fantasies are a means of associating the coping skills learned in treatment with a crisis situation. By imagining a high-risk situation and imagining oneself using an effective coping skill to avoid substance use, the client is able to prepare for a variety of high-risk situations and evaluate the expected effectiveness of different coping strategies. Coping imagery is another cognitive technique that can assist with combating high-risk situations. Making use of guided fantasy, the therapist and client can use personally relevant imagery that can bolster the client's self-efficacy to avoid relapse.[99]

Labeling and detachment are coping strategies aimed at helping clients experience urges and cravings without succumbing to them. This strategy reframes cravings as temporary sensations of desire as opposed to unending compulsions that dictate a client's behavior. Helping clients view cravings as coming from environmental cues, and not coming from within themselves, can assist in decreasing the subjective strength of the cravings.[66]

Cognitive coping strategies can be considered useful in two different contexts, both as *urge-specific coping strategies* and *general lifestyle change strategies*.[35] The former can best be used when cravings come on strong with little notice. If the client can practice these specific skills when exposed to threatening cues with their therapist, they will be more prepared to handle real-world high-risk situations outside of treatment. Lifestyle cognitive skills can be used at any time and are thought to prevent relapse independent of specific triggers. Numerous cognitive strategies have been found to be effectively used in either category, and include (1) identifying positive consequences of staying sober and negative consequences of returning to drinking, (2) using mastery/strength messages, (3) challenging thoughts, (4) thinking through a behavior chain from past consequences, (5) encouraging oneself to wait it out, (6) reminding oneself they are a sober person, and (7) leaving the situation.

Seeking support for abstinence and recovery from a slip involves both cognitive and behavioral strategies. Individuals that have social networks filled with drinking or drug use that they cannot leave are more prone to relapse and need to recognize the need to change the composition of the network and build another one that is supportive of recovery.[57] Mutual help groups like Alcoholics Anonymous and Smart Recovery provide opportunities to listen and understand the perspectives and experiences of others and offer both cognitive and behavioral coping activities for the addicted individual.[78]

Lifestyle Interventions

The final stage of the process of change is to integrate the new behavior into the lifestyle of the individual.[31] Replacing dependence with abstinence or excess with moderation generally involves a change not only in one behavior but in the addicted individual's overall way of life. Lifestyle interventions for relapse prevention include lifestyle balance, substitute indulgences, positive addictions, and stimulus control techniques. Lifestyle balance is a global strategy used to ameliorate stressful situations, promote appropriate coping, improve problem solving, and increase pleasurable activities such as hobbies or spending time with friends and family that were replaced by substance use. It is also important for clients to understand that their desires not to be depressed or to be social, which can lead to high-risk situations, are reasonable desires. However, they need to find alternative ways of fulfilling these needs without using substances or turning to other problematic, addictive behaviors.[55] In treatments that have encouraged clients to integrate new activities into their daily schedules, individuals with substance use disorders have reported experiencing decreased negative emotional states such as depression and anxiety.[29] Mutual help groups and activities can play an important role in offering a venue and a series of activities that can support the lifestyle changes.

Substitute indulgences are activities that are immediately gratifying and can serve as a substitute for the addictive behavior when a client experiences an urge or craving. One example is to take a hot shower or bubble bath instead of going to a bar to relax after a difficult day at work. It is important, however, that the pleasurable activities are not harmful in the long term. Positive addictions have a similar function in that they replace the activity of substance use, but have more long-term rewards and value, rather than immediate gratification. Examples of positive addiction include taking up a sport, regular exercise, or a new hobby. In general, increased engagement in substance-free behaviors is

associated with decreases in substance use in the general population.[26] In addition, individuals who identify future goals that are meaningful to them are less likely to have alcohol-related problems and heavy drinking episodes.[76] It is important that positive and enjoyable activities be practical and something that the client is able to perform and sustain on their own.[55]

Stimulus control techniques attempt to address the physical cues for relapse. A frequent example is the strong association of drinking and smoking, either of which could serve as a cue for the other. While experiencing some cues is inevitable, it is an important step for a client to eliminate the cues under their control by changing their routine as much as possible. An example for a client who is quitting smoking would be to throw out all cigarettes, ashtrays, and lighters, rearrange the furniture so that a favorite smoking area is not present, and change the morning routine so that it does not revolve around the first cigarette of the day.[55]

New Approaches for Relapse Prevention

Recently, another set of strategies has been added to relapse prevention treatment called Mindfulness-Based Relapse Prevention (or MBRP). The basic structure and goals of relapse prevention remain the same but there is an emphasis on the use of mindfulness techniques throughout the intervention process. Mindfulness meditation is a metacognitive skill learned through the practice of meditation that allows the individual to achieve perspective, patience, and inner peacefulness that can reduce relapse cues and create lifestyle changes to promote recovery.[11]

Mindfulness is a state of detached awareness of emotions, cognitions, and physical sensations. It is a state of attentional focus that can be used to change client's attitudes toward their thoughts, feelings, and sensations. MBRP uses development of the mindfulness state to disrupt maladaptive cognitions by heightening awareness of cravings without identifying with, judging, or reacting to them. The mindfulness state interrupts the chain of cognitions and emotions that follow an urge or craving, thus decreasing the likelihood of an action based on them.[103] A theorized mechanism on how MBRP works is that meditation improves higher-order executive control and loosens the strength of the learned reactions to the experienced cravings. As the number of automated reactions decrease, eventually the number of self-reported cravings also decreases.[102] Mindfulness appears to work differently than thought suppression, which prior studies have found to be an ineffective coping technique.[11] Researchers believe its long-term effects can be explained by an individual's improved ability to recognize and tolerate discomfort associated with craving or negative affect.[13]

Although much of the current research on relapse prevention strategies has assessed these approaches in the context of in-person therapy, there has been an effort to make these approaches available to the general public through technology. With the accessibility of the Internet and smart phones, researchers have begun to capitalize on these venues for treating addictions and preventing relapse. Given the novelty of these approaches, there are relatively few (and inconsistent) findings for relapse prevention. A review of text messaging–based interventions for smoking cessation and relapse prevention stated that all studies included demonstrated reduced smoking and prevention of relapse.[85] Furthermore, participants responded well to the application and its flexibility.[85, 89] One recent study investigated a mobile application that was used as a supplement to aftercare from residential treatment for alcohol abuse. This app included a component in which participants identified high-risk locations (i.e., bars they used to frequent), and the app would deliver just-in-time support to help participants cope with the high-risk situation. This app also included a panic button that participants could activate when they felt they might relapse. This feature provided automated support messages, computer generated alerts to key support people, and tools for addressing cravings. Participants who used the app and attended treatment had fewer risky (binge) drinking days at 4 and 12 months and were more likely to be abstinent at 8 and 12 months compared to a control group that received treatment as usual.[40] Alternatively, another study using a computer-delivered relapse prevention treatment for smoking showed no benefit compared with the assessment-only group.[100] Therefore it is clear that further research on these approaches is warranted, but initial findings suggest that the flexibility and accessibility of technology-based approaches are appealing to consumers and may add benefit to in-person treatment.

Medications for Relapse Prevention

Medications have also been found to be a useful adjunct to promote change and prevent relapse in treatments for nicotine, alcohol, and opiate addiction. Since the 1990s, both naltrexone and acamprosate (Campral), have been added to disulfiram (Antabuse) as approved medications in the United States to be prescribed for alcoholism treatment.[90] More recently on the market is an extended-release alternative form of naltrexone, under the trade name Vivitrol, requiring once monthly injections. Use of disulfiram causes a flushing or sick reaction when alcohol is ingested, which results in extremely low compliance, and as a result has not been found to be superior to placebo. Comprehensive reviews of acamprosate and naltrexone, conducted by the Cochrane Collaborative, revealed that both are effective in improving outcomes.[83,84] Acamprosate significantly reduced drinking risk, while also increasing days abstinent.[83] Alternatively, naltrexone was associated with 83% reduction in risk of heavy drink and a 4% decrease in drinking days.[84] Secondary outcomes for naltrexone were also significant, including reduction in the amount of alcohol consumed and fewer heavy drinking days. Therefore acamprosate may be more effective in promoting complete abstinence, while naltrexone may be more effective when the treatment goal is reduced drinking.

Methadone, buprenorphine, levo-alpha-acetylmethadol, and naltrexone have been used to treat heroin addiction. Opiate maintenance using methadone, buprenorphine, or levo-alpha-acetylmethadol assist in decreasing the extremely high rates of relapse in treatment of opiate addiction, although the medications themselves can be addictive at high doses, have negative side effects, and naltrexone specifically can have low compliance.[94] More recently, an injectable form of long-acting naltrexone has been approved to treat heroin dependence.[54] A comprehensive review showed promising results—the long-acting naltrexone was well tolerated by participants, had improved compliance, and was more effective for relapse prevention than the daily, oral tablets.

Medications for nicotine cessation include a variety of nicotine replacement products (i.e., NRT), varenicline tartrate (Chantix), and the antidepressant bupropion (Zyban). In a comprehensive review, the Cochrane Collaborative found that use of NRT, bupropion, or varenicline nearly doubles the likelihood of quitting compared with placebo. They also found that varenicline outperformed single forms of NRT but not combination NRT (e.g., patch plus gum). In addition, the effectiveness of medications are substantially increased when added to behavioral interventions.[16]

Although there have been studies of medications to treat cocaine addiction, they have not resulted in improved treatment outcomes with any consistency and there is currently no FDA-approved medication for treating cocaine addiction.[22] It is generally recommended that medications be administered in addition to a psychosocial intervention such as relapse prevention for opiate and nicotine treatment,[16] although investigations of combined therapy and medication have showed mixed results compared with either alone for treating alcoholism.[6,83,84]

When Relapse Prevention Fails

All of the above strategies are designed to help the addicted individual achieve and maintain change once initiated. However, as many of the studies demonstrated, these strategies are helpful to some but not others.[14,46] Even individuals who have been taught coping strategies and acknowledge the critical cues or triggers that make them vulnerable to relapse have not been successful in preventing relapse. This is when successful recycling has to be substituted for relapse prevention. Clinicians and researchers working in addictions have to take a life course perspective; abandon the single attempt, linear model of success; and see the process of successful change as better represented by a cyclical process that in the long run yields successful change.[80] We will discuss the life course perspective and the cyclical model below.

A Life Course Perspective on Recovery

Alcoholism and drug addictions are chronic conditions that can span decades and numerous periods of treatment, remission from drinking or drug use, relapse to uncontrolled drinking, and treatment re-entry. Treatment providers have a comparatively small amount of contact with clients in their overall treatment and recovery careers. It is important to understand the factors and context outside of treatment that are related to clients' entry into treatment and that precipitate relapse episodes. Taking the life course perspective of recovery is an important step for researchers to truly appreciate the full context in which a particular treatment episode succeeds or fails.[32]

Some individuals with less severe dependence are able to avoid the cycle of relapse and maintain either continued abstinence or a lower level of nonharmful substance use.[61] However, the recovery process of many addicted individuals is marked by multiple transitions in their treatment career. In long-term follow-up studies spanning up to 16 years, researchers have consistently found that individuals who received treatment sooner and spent more time in treatment had longer periods of remission from alcohol dependence. Greater use of alcohol was predicted by less self-efficacy, greater use of avoidance coping, and less of a perception that drinking was a significant problem.[72,73]

Successive Approximations, Recycling, and Learning From the Past

As described earlier, learning how to overcome an addiction and avoid relapse is essentially a process of successive approximations whereby addicted individuals try to modify the addictive behavior, fail to complete the change, and then try again until they are successful or until death, disability, or prison intervenes. There is no guarantee of success, even after multiple attempts because the learning may not be complete or the physiological or environmental barriers are too great for this individual to overcome. However, large numbers of individuals who have been classified as dependent on a substance have been successful in significantly changing addictive behaviors after multiple attempts. Half of the "ever smokers" in the United State have quit smoking successfully, and we have more than 40 million of these success stories.[20] An epidemiological study by Dawson and colleagues[30] examined more than 4000 individuals who had had a lifetime diagnosis of alcohol dependence. Based on past year drinking, they estimated that approximately 47% could be considered in full remission and were classified as either abstinent (18.2%), low-risk drinker (17.7%), or asymptomatic risk drinker (11.8%), with only 25% meeting the criteria for being dependent during the past year. This study highlights once again that the definition of relapse determines whether you consider someone in recovery or relapsed. Nevertheless, recovery does happen for many addicted individuals, demonstrating that over time there is significant change and successful self-management of addictive behaviors.

Relapse represents a problem in the preparation, planning, or implementation of the action plan. As such, it highlights some deficit or barrier that needs remediation or a different solution. Relapse then, should be viewed from a pragmatic and learning perspective. Trial and error are an integral part of psychological principles and medical practice. If one strategy or medication does not seem to help the individual completely manage the problem or begins to cause more problems than it solves (e.g., side effects), practitioners would quickly try another strategy or medication. However, often with addictions the inability to succeed has been viewed as a deficit of motivation, will, or character. A learning perspective that views the relapse as an opportunity to learn from the past and do something differently accurately reflects longitudinal research and is critical to creating effective relapse prevention activities that reflect the reality of recycling.

Promoting recycling represents a valid relapse prevention strategy that accepts the occurrence of relapse. Recycling engages individuals who have relapsed in a review of past success and failure with a view of finding what went right or wrong and when or where it occurred so that the deficits in motivation, coping, or self-efficacy can be remediated and the types of barriers that led to the relapse surmounted. In longitudinal studies, many individuals get stuck in the process of change and remain in precontemplation or contemplation for months or years.[18,95] The goal of recycling is to help individuals make another more successful attempt to change the addictive behavior more quickly and effectively. Policies and practices that limit access to services after a relapse or interpret relapse as a failure of the treatment undermine the recycling process.

Although relapse prevention is the focus of this chapter, there has been a recent shift in the field of addiction to understanding recovery as holistic, including but not exclusively defined by abstinence. The Substance Abuse Mental Health Services Administration (SAMSHA) recently developed a working definition of recovery: "a process of change through which individuals improve their health and wellness, live a self-directed life, and strive to reach their full potential." The four major dimensions of this definition include health (abstinence and health- wellness-promoting behaviors), home (stable and safe living situation), purpose (meaningful daily activities), and community (supportive social networks). From this perspective, holistic recovery constitutes the end goal of addiction treatment and recovery and is an important component of sustained change and long-term prevention of relapse.

Treatment Recommendations

There are several important considerations that summarize this review of relapse prevention and recycling in the addictions. Each of these considerations has important implications for treatment and research. Here we highlight the key considerations and implications:

1. Relapse is part of the process of successful behavioral change. Partial success and outright failure offer opportunities for learning that are critical for long-term successful recovery. As in other areas of life, the important reality is not that you have fallen down, but that you get back up and try again, ideally having learned important lessons about how to achieve the goal without falling down again. Relapse prevention begins at the start of the change process and should be an integral part of all treatment programs. However, addicted individuals may not be able to avoid and practitioners may not be able to prevent all relapse. In their efforts to promote maintenance and prevent relapse, treatments and treatment providers should concentrate on helping individuals manage motivation, engage in critical coping activities, and support and increase their self-efficacy to perform the behaviors needed to achieve abstinence and recovery. In addition, special attempts should be made to engage or reengage individuals who relapse in a conversation and collaboration to promote recycling to remedy the problems in the process of change that contributed to the relapse.

2. Maintaining change is the goal of relapse prevention. A number of elements have been identified as important maintenance enhancers that also act to prevent relapse. Commitment fueled by solid decision-making leading to adequate planning, skills acquisition and implementation, and a long-term goal and perspective seem to be critical to sustaining significant modification of addictive behaviors. A comprehensive perspective on the process of change and a life course perspective appear to be essential when addressing and comprehending relapse.

3. Support sustains success. Support from family, friends, and peers seems to play an important role in relapse prevention. Individuals who seek support and engage in mutual help groups have better outcomes.[92] Creating or supporting existing support groups and helping individuals to access and utilize the support can assist in relapse prevention. Integrating the relapse prevention model perspective with the mutual help perspective offers social interactions and support that can enhance personal coping, motivation, and self-efficacy.

4. Multiple problems complicate maintenance of change. Paying attention to complicating life problems—be they financial, family, social, medical, legal, or psychiatric in origin—can have an impact on successful recovery from addictions.[65] Psychiatric illness and emotional distress are risk factors for becoming addicted and act as barriers to beginning and remaining in recovery. Integration of treatment efforts across multiple problems seems to offer the best potential for successful change of the addiction as well as the other problems.

5. Stigma stifles success. Viewing relapse as a failure and relapsers as defective people who cannot change promotes failure identity and the stigmatization of addictions in general, and relapsers in particular. Relapse is a problem of behavior change and not a unique problem of addictions. Addressing and managing relapse is part and parcel of all efforts to change established patterns of behavior and to manage chronic illnesses from diabetes to addictions.

References

1. Adamson S, Sellman J, Frampton C. Patient predictors of alcohol treatment outcome: a systematic review. *J Subst Abuse Treat.* 2009;36(1):75–86.

2. Agboola S, McNeill A, Coleman T, Leonardi Bee J. A systematic review of the effectiveness of smoking relapse prevention interventions for abstinent smokers. *Addiction.* 2010;105(8):1362–1380.

3. Amrhein PC, Miller WR, Yahne CE, Palmer M, Fulcher L. Client commitment language during motivational interviewing predicts drug use outcomes. *J Consult Clin Psych.* 2003;71(5):862–878.

4. Annis HM, Davis CS. Self-efficacy and the prevention of alcoholic relapse: initial findings from a treatment trial. In: Baker TB, Cannon DS, eds. *Assessment and Treatment of Addictive Disorders.* New York: Praeger; 1988:88–112.

5. Annis HM, Schober R, Kelly E. Matching addiction outpatient counseling to client readiness for change: the role of structured relapse prevention counseling. *Exp Clin Psychopharmacol.* 1996;4(1):37–45.

6. Anton RF, et al. Combined pharmacotherapies and behavioral interventions for alcohol dependence: the combine study: a randomized controlled trial. *JAMA: J Am Med Assoc.* 2006;295(17):2003–2017.

7. Bandura A. Self-efficacy: toward a unifying theory of behavior change. *Psychol Rev.* 1977;84:191–215.

8. Bandura A. *Self-Efficacy: The Exercise of Control.* New York, NY: WH Freeman/Times Books/Henry Holt & Co; 1997P:ix, 604.

9. Reference deleted in review.

10. Blomquist O, Hernandez-Avila CA, Berleson JA, Ashraf A, Kranzler HR. Self-efficacy as a predictor of relapse during treatment for alcohol dependence. *Addict Disorders Treat.* 2003;2:135–145.

11. Bowen S, et al. The role of thought suppression in the relationship between mindfulness meditation and alcohol use. *Addict Behav.* 2007;32(10):2324–2328.

12. Bowen S, et al. Relative efficacy of mindfulness-based relapse prevention, standard relapse prevention, and treatment as usual for substance use disorders: a randomized clinical trial. *JAMA Psychiatry.* 2014;71(5):547–556.

13. Brewer J, Pbert L. Mindfulness: an emerging treatment for smoking and other addictions. *J Fam Med.* 2015;2(4):1035.

14. Brownell KD, et al. Understanding and preventing relapse. *Am Psychologist.* 1986;41(7):765–782.

15. Burling TA, et al. Self-efficacy and relapse among inpatient drug and alcohol abusers: a predictor of outcome. *J Studies Alcohol.* 1989;50(4):354–360.

16. Cahill K, Stevens S, Perera R, Lancaster T. Pharmacological interventions for smoking cessation: an overview and network meta-analysis. *Cochrane Db Syst Rev.* 2013;5(5).

17. Campbell S, Adamson S, Carter J. Client language during motivational enhancement therapy and alcohol use outcome. *Behav Cogn Psychoth.* 2010;38(4):399–415.

18. Carbonari JP, DiClemente CC, Sewell KB. Stage transitions and the transtheoretical 'stages of change' model of smoking cessation. *Swiss J Psychol/Schweizerische Zeitschrift für Psychologie/Revue Suisse de Psychologie.* 1999;58(2):134–144.

19. Carroll KM. Relapse prevention as a psychosocial treatment: a review of controlled clinical trials. *Exp Clin Psychol.* 1996;4(1):46–54.

20. CDC. Cigarette smoking among adults – United States, 2006. *MMWR 2006.* 2007;56:1157–1161.

21. Childress AR, Miller WR, Carroll KM. What can human brain imaging tell us about vulnerability to addiction and to relapse? In: *Rethinking Substance Abuse: What the Science Shows, and What We Should Do About It.* New York, NY: Guilford; 2006:46–60.

22. Ciccarone D. Stimulant abuse: pharmacology, cocaine, methamphetamine, treatment, attempts at pharmacotherapy. *Prim Care.* 2011;38(1):41–58.

23. Collins LR, Kashdan TB, Gollnisch G. The feasibility of cellular phones to collect ecological momentary assessment data:

24. Reference deleted in review.

25. Reference deleted in review.

26. Correia CJ, Benson T, Carey KB. Decreased substance use following increases in alternative behaviors: a preliminary investigation. *Addict Bheav.* 2005;30:19–27.

27. Cummings C, Gordon JR, Marlatt GA. Relapse: prevention and prediction. In: Miller WR, ed. *Addictive Behaviors.* New York: Pergamon; 1980:291–321.

28. Curry SG, Marlatt GA. Unaided quitters' strategies for coping with temptations to smoke. In: Wills TA, Shiffman S, eds. *Coping and Substance Use.* Orlando, FL: Academic Press; 1985:243–265.

29. Daughters SB, et al. Effectiveness of a brief behavioral treatment for inner-city illicit drug users with elevated depressive symptoms: the life enhancement treatment for substance use (LETS Act!). *J Clin Psychiat.* 2008;(1):122.

30. Dawson DA, et al. Recovery from DSM-IV alcohol dependence: United States, 2001–2002. *Alcohol Res Health.* 2006;29(2):131–142.

31. DiClemente CC. *Addiction and Change: How Addictions Develop and Addicted People Recover. Guilford Substance Abuse Series.* New York, NY: Guilford; 2003:317, xviii.

32. DiClemente CC. Natural change and the troublesome use of substances: a life-course perspective. In: Miller WR, Carroll KM, eds. *Rethinking Substance Abuse: What the Science Shows, and What We Should Do About It.* New York, NY: Guilford; 2006:81–96.

33. DiClemente CC. Mechanisms, determinants and process of change in the modification of drinking behavior. *Alcohol: Clin Exp Res.* 2007;31(S3):8.

34. DiClemente CC, Daniels JW, Carbonari JP. Determinants of alcohol abstinence self-efficacy: a test of Bandura's model. *Poster at Association for Advancement of Behavior Therapy.* 1997.

35. Dolan SL, Rohsenow DJ, Martin RA, Monti PM. Urge-specific and lifestyle coping strategies of alcoholics: relationships of specific strategies to treatment outcome. *Drug Alcohol Depen.* 2013;128:8–14.

36. Donovan D, Witkiewitz K. Relapse prevention: from radical idea to common practice. *Addict Res Theory.* 2012;20(3):204–217.

37. Gonzalez VM, Schmitz JM, DeLaune KA. The role of homework in cognitive-behavioral therapy for cocaine dependence. *J Consult Clin Psychol.* 2006;74(3):633–637.

38. Gorski TT. Relapse prevention: a state of the art overview. *Addiction Recovery.* 1993;13(2):25.

39. Greenfield S, Hufford M, Vagge L, Muenz L, Costello M, Weiss R. The relationship of self-efficacy expectancies to relapse among alcohol dependent men and women: a prospective study. *J Studies Alcohol.* 2000;61:345–351.

40. Gustafson DH, et al. A smartphone application to support recovery from alcoholism: a randomized clinical trial. *JAMA psychiatry.* 2014;71(5):566–572.

41. Gwaltney C, Metrik J, Kahler C, Shiffman S. Self-efficacy and smoking cessation: a meta-analysis. *Psychol Addict Behav.* 2009;23(1):56–66.

42. Gwaltney CJ, Shiffman S, Balabanis MH, Paty JA. Dynamic self-efficacy and outcome expectancies: prediction of smoking lapse and relapse. *J Abnorm Psychol.* 2005;114(4):661–675.

43. Hajek P, et al. Relapse prevention interventions for smoking cessation. *Cochrane Db Syst Rev.* 2013;8.

44. Heather N, McCambridge J. Post-treatment stage of change predicts 12-month outcome of treatment for alcohol problems. *Alcohol Alcohol.* 2013;48(3):329–336.

45. Hendershot CS, Witkiewitz K, George WH, Marlatt GA. Relapse prevention for addictive behaviors. *Subst Abuse Treat PR.* 2011;6(1):1.

46. Hunt WA, Barnett LW, Branch LG. Relapse rates in addiction programs. *J Clin Psychol.* 1971;27:455–456.

47. Ilgen M, McKellar J, Tiet Q. Abstinence self-efficacy and abstinence 1 year after substance use disorder treatment. *J Consult Clin Psychol.* 2005;73(6):1175–1180.

application to alcohol consumption. *Exp Clin Psychopharm.* 2003;11(1):73–78.

48. Irvin JE, Bowers CA, Dunn ME, Wang MC. Efficacy of relapse prevention: a meta-analytic review. *J Consult Clin Psychol.* 1999;67(4):563–570.

49. Isenhart C. Pretreatment readiness for change in male alcohol dependent subjects: predictors of one-year follow-up status. *J Studies Alcohol.* 1997;58:351–357.

50. Kadden RM, Cooney NL. Treating alcohol problems. In: Marlatt GAD, Dennis M, eds. *Relapse Prevention: Maintenance Strategies in the Treatment of Addictive Behaviors.* 2nd ed. New York, NY: Guilford; 2005:65–91.

51. Kirchner TR, Shiffman S, Wileyto EP. Relapse dynamics during smoking cessation: Recurrent abstinence violation effects and lapse-relapse progression. *J Abnorm Psychol.* 2012;121(1):187–197.

52. Koob GF. Theoretical frameworks and mechanistic aspects of alcohol addiction: alcohol addiction as a reward deficit disorder. In: *Behavioral Neurobiology of Alcohol Addiction.* Berlin Heidelberg: Springer; 2013:3–30.

53. Koob GF, et al. Neurobiology of addiction: a neuroadaptational view relevant for diagnosis. *Diagnostic Issues in Substance Use Disorders: Refining the Research Agenda for DSM-V.* Washington, DC: American Psychiatric Association; 2007:31–43.

54. Krupitsky EM, Blokhina EA. Long-acting depot formulations of naltrexone for heroin dependence: a review. *Curr Opin Psychiatr.* 2010;23(3):210–214.

55. Larimer ME, Palmer RS, Marlatt GA. Relapse prevention: an overview of Marlatt's cognitive-behavioral model. *Alcohol Res Health.* 1999;23(2):151–160.

56. Lichtenstein E, Danaher BG. Modification of smoking behavior: a critical analysis of theory, research and practice. In: *Advances in Behavior Modification.* New York: Academic Press; 1976:79–132.

57. Longabaugh R, et al. The effect of social investment on treatment outcome. *J Studies Alcohol.* 1993;54:465–478.

58. Marlatt GA, Donovan DM. *Relapse Prevention: Maintenance Strategies in the Treatment of Addictive Behaviors.* 2nd ed. New York: Guilford; 2005:416.

59. Marlatt GA, Gordon JR. *Relapse Prevention: Maintenance Strategies in the Treatment of Addictive Behaviors.* New York: Guilford; 1985.

60. Marlatt GA, Gordon JR. Determinants of relapse: implications for the maintenance of behavior change. In: Davidson PODSM, ed. *Behavior Medicine: Chaning Health Lifestyles.* New York: Brunner/Mazel; 1980.

61. Marlatt GA, Witkiewitz K. Harm reduction approaches to alcohol use: health promotion, prevention, and treatment. *Addict Behav.* 2002;27(6):867.

62. Marlatt GA, Witkiewitz K. Relapse prevention for alcohol and drug problems. In: Marlatt GA, Donovan DM, eds. *Relapse Prevention: Maintenance Strategies in the Treatment of Addictive Behaviors.* 2nd edn. New York, NY: Guilford; 2005:1–44.

63. McClelland DC. *Human Motivation.* New York: Cambridge University; 1987.

64. McKee S, O'Malley S, Salovey P, Krishnan-Sarin S, Mazure C. Perceived risks and benefits of smoking cessation: gender-specific predictors of motivation and treatment outcome. *Addict Behav.* 2005;30(3):423–435.

65. McLellan AT, et al. Predicting response to alcohol and drug abuse treatment. *Arch Gen Psychiatry.* 1983;40:620–625.

66. Michie S, et al. Identification of behaviour change techniques to reduce excessive alcohol consumption. *Addiction.* 2012;107(8):1431–1440.

67. Miller WR, Carroll KM. *Rethinking Substance Abuse: What the Science Shows, and What We Should Do About It.* New York, NY: Guilford; 2006:320, xvi.

68. Miller WR, Westerberg VS, Harris RJ, Tonigan JS. What predicts relapse? Prospective testing of antecedent models. *Addiction.* 1996;91(suppl):S155–S171.

69. Monti PM, et al. *Treating Alcohol Dependence: a Coping Skills Training Guide.* New York: Guilford; 1989.

70. Monti PM, et al. Naltrexone and cue exposure with coping and communication skills training for alcoholics: treatment process and 1–year outcomes. *Alcohol Clin Exp Res.* 2001;25(11):1634–1647.

71. Moos RH. *Coping Responses Inventory.* Odessa, FL: Psychological Assessment Resources; 1993.

72. Moos RH, Moos BS. Treated and untreated individuals with alcohol use disorders: rates and predictors of remission and relapse. *Int J Clin Health Psychol.* 2006;6(3):513–526.

73. Moos RH, Moos BS. Treated and untreated alcohol-use disorders: course and predictors of remission and relapse. *Evaluation Rev.* 2007;31(6):564–584.

74. Moser AE, Annis HM. The role of coping in relapse crisis outcome: a prospective study of treated alcholics. *Addiction.* 1996;91(8):1101–1113.

75. Reference deleted in review.

76. Murphy JG, Dennhardt AA, Skidmore JR, et al. A randomized controlled trial of a behavioral economic supplement to brief motivational interventions for college drinking. *J Consult Clin Psych.* 2012;80(5):876.

77. Niaura R. Cognitive social learning and related perspective on drug craving. *Addiction.* 2000;95(suppl 2):S155–S163.

78. Nowinski J, Baker S, Carroll K. *Twelve Step Facilitation Therapy Manual: A Clinical Research Guide for Therapists Treating Indivduals With Alcohol Abuse and Dependence.* Rockville, MD: NIAAA; 1992.

79. Penberthy JK, et al. Impact of motivational changes on drinking outcomes in pharmacobehavioral treatment for alcohol dependence. *Alcohol Clin Exp Res.* 2011;35(9):1694–1704.

80. Prochaska JO, DiClemente CC, Norcross JC. In search of how people change: applications to addictive behaviors. *Am Psychol.* 1992;47(9):1102–1114.

81. Project MATCH Research Group. Matching alcoholism treatments to client heterogeneity: project MATCH Posttreatment drinking outcomes. *J Studies Alcohol Drugs.* 1997;58(1):7–29.

82. Project MATCH Research Group. Matching alcoholism treatments to client heterogeneity: project MATCH three-year drinking outcomes. *Alcoholism: Clin Exp Res.* 1998;22(6):1300–1311.

83. Rösner S, et al. Acamprosate for alcohol dependence. *Cochrane Db Syst Rev.* 2010;9(9).

84. Rösner S, et al. Opioid antagonists for alcohol dependence. *Cochrane Db Syst Rev.* 2010;12.

85. Sampson A, Bhochhibhoya A, Digeralamo D, Branscum P. The use of text messaging for smoking cessation and relapse prevention: a systematic review of evidence. *J Smok Cessat.* 2015;10(01):50–58.

86. Sheehan T, Owen P. The disease model. In: Epstein BSMEE, ed. *Addictions: A Comprehensive Guidebook.* New York: Oxford University; 1999:268–286.

87. Shiffman S. Relapse prevention for smoking. In: Gordon GAMJ, ed. *Relapse Prevention: Maintenance Strategies in the Treatment of Addictive Behaviors.* New York: Guilford; 2005.

88. Simpson TL, Kivlahan DR, Bush KR, McFall ME. Telephone self-monitoring among alcohol use disorder patients in early recovery: a randomized study of feasibility and measurement reactivity. *Drug Alcohol Depen.* 2005;79(2):241–250.

89. Snuggs S, et al. Using text messaging to prevent relapse to smoking: intervention development, practicability and client reactions. *Addiction.* 2012;107(S2):39–44.

90. Spanagel R, Vengeliene V. New pharmacological treatment strategies for relapse prevention. In: *Behavioral Neurobiology of Alcohol Addiction.* Berlin Heidelberg: Springer; 2012:583–609.

91. Stevens E, Jason LA, Ram D, Light J. Investigating social support and network relationships in substance use disorder recovery. *Subst Abuse.* 2015;36(4):396–399.

92. Tonigan JS, Connors G, Miller WR. The alcoholics anonymous involvement scale (AAI): reliability and norms. *Psych Addict Behav.* 1996;10:75–80.

93. Vaillant GE. *The Natural History of Alcoholism: Causes, Patterns, and Paths to Recovery.* Cambridge, MA: Harvard University; 1983.

94. Veilleux JC, et al. A review of opioid dependence treatment: pharmacological and psychosocial interventions to treat opioid addiction. *Clin Psychol Rev.* 2010;30(2):155–166.

95. Velicer W, et al. Patterns of change: dynamic typology applied to smoking cessation. *Multivariate Behav Res.* 1990;25:587–611.

96. Velicer WF, et al. Relapse situations and self-efficacy: an integrative model. *Addict Behav.* 1990;15(3):271–283.

97. Vielva I, Iraurgi I. Cognitive and behavioural factors as predictors of abstinence following treatment for alcohol dependence. *Addiction.* 2001;96(2):297–303.

98. Wang SJ, et al. Short of complete abstinence: an analysis exploration of multiple drinking episodes in alcoholism treatment trials. *Alcohol Clin Exp Res.* 2002;26(12):1803–1809.

99. Wanigaratne S, Wallace W, Pullin J, Keaney F. *Relapse Prevention for Addictive Behaviors: A Manual for Therapists.* Chicago: Mosby; 1990.

100. Wetter DW, et al. A randomized clinical trial of a palmtop computer-delivered treatment for smoking relapse prevention among women. *Psychol Addict Behav.* 2011;25(2):365.

101. Witkiewitz K, Donovan DM, Hartzler B. Drink refusal training as part of a combined behavioral intervention: effectiveness and mechanisms of change. *J Consul Clin Psych.* 2012;80(3):440.

102. Witkiewitz K, Lustyk MK, Bowen S. Retraining the addicted brain: a review of hypothesized neurobiological mechanisms of mindfulness-based relapse prevention. *Psychol Addict Behav.* 2013;27(2):351–365.

103. Witkiewitz K, Marlatt GA, Walker D. Mindfulness-based relapse prevention for alcohol and substance use disorders. *J Cogn Psychother.* 2005;19(3):211–228. Special Issue: State-of-the-Art in Behavioral Interventions for Substance Use Disorders.

104. Zywiak WH, Connors GJ, Maisto SA, Westerberg VS. Relapse research and the reasons for drinking questionnaire: a factor analysis of Marlatt's relapse taxonomy. *Addiction.* 1996;91(suppl):S121–S130.

43

Brief and e-Health Interventions for the Treatment of Alcohol or Other Drug Addiction

ROBERT J. TAIT AND GARY K. HULSE

CHAPTER OUTLINE

Drug Use and Problems

A broad range of treatment approaches are available and necessary for the management of persons with problem drug and/or alcohol use. Individuals with problem substance use can present anywhere along a continuum, from early stage problems associated with acute, recreational, or binge use to severe dependence with major physical and psychosocial problems. This latter group commonly has multiple health problems with poor or negligible non–drug-using social support and requires intensive intervention, often with the objective of achieving abstinence. Traditionally, most therapeutic resources were directed at the management of this group. These interventions have generally been intensive in nature and costly to deliver and have failed to reach the majority of individuals using these substances.[85]

Although the impact of drug and alcohol dependence on health and society is widely recognized, the effects of nondependent excessive drug use are often underestimated by the community and the health care system. For example, the number of nondependent heavy drinkers far outweighs the number of dependent people.[87] Most alcohol-related problems result from people drinking below levels that cause major physical dependence. Nevertheless, the societal, family, and health impacts of nondependent drinking have a greater influence than dependent drinking on the community's burden of alcohol problems: the so-called prevention paradox.[56]

A report by the Institute of Medicine recommended that given the number of people with mild or moderate alcohol problems, a range of therapeutic approaches needed to be developed to cover the full gamut of alcohol use problems.[47] Similar conclusions could be drawn concerning clinical and subclinical use of other types of substances. Table 43.1 summarizes key definitions for problematic use of alcohol or other substances.

Drug Treatment in Primary Care and Nonspecialist Settings

People who consume hazardous levels of alcohol (use that will probably lead to harmful consequences for the user if it continues) rarely seek treatment.[87] Indeed, less than 30% of individuals with alcohol use disorders are likely to have sought professional care in the previous year,[98] and only 14% of those with other substance use disorders seek professional help.[6] People with early stage problem drug use commonly present to general practitioners or community health services for reasons that are not drug-related. Health workers in hospital emergency departments typically encounter a greater proportion of cases, such as acute trauma presentations, accident, injury, and overdose that are common consequences of drug use.[21]

The nondependent population, unlike their dependent counterparts, typically have an intact psychosocial fabric and, therefore, do not require the intensive interventions directed at dependent individuals.[72] The identification and effective management of these individuals before the development of more significant use, dependence, and associated major physical and/or psychosocial problems is clearly desirable. Individuals who have early problem

TABLE 43.1	Categories of Substance Use Disorders and Problems.
Category	**Description**
Dependence: DSM-5 (APA 2013)[5]	"…a cluster of cognitive, behavioral, and physiological symptoms indicating that the individual continues using the substance despite significant substance-related problems" (p. 483). Symptoms are grouped as relating to *impaired control* (e.g., inability to reduce use), *social impairment* (e.g., extensive time spent obtaining, using, and recovering from use), *risky use* (e.g., use in a situation that is physically hazardous, such as driving), and *pharmacological issues* (e.g., craving). Severity is categorized as mild (2–3 symptoms), moderate (4–5), or severe (6 or more symptoms).
Dependence: ICD-10 (WHO 2016)[109]	A syndrome of behavioral, cognitive, and physiological symptoms subsequent to repeated use of a substance. The criteria cover impaired control, withdrawal, tolerance, and preoccupation with use of the substance and persistent use despite evidence of the harmful consequences.
Harmful: ICD-10 (WHO 2016)[109]	Clear evidence of physical or psychological harm, including impaired judgment or dysfunctional behavior from substance use.
Additional ICD-10 diagnoses (WHO 2016)[109]	The ICD-10 diagnostic categories also include *Acute Intoxication, Withdrawal State, Withdrawal State with Delirium, Amnesic Syndrome, Psychotic Disorder,* and *Residual and Late Onset Psychotic Disorder.*
Hazardous[9]	Used by the WHO but not a diagnosis. Use of a drug that will probably lead to harmful consequences for the user if it continues at the same level.
Risky[45]	Those who drink/use other substances in a way that creates a risk of harm to themselves or others.

Current US alcohol guidelines recommend no more than two drinks (12 fluid ounces of regular beer, 5 fluid ounces of wine, or 1.5 fluid ounces of 80-proof distilled spirits) per day for men and one for women, with zero drinks being the only safe option in some cases (e.g., pregnancy, while operating machinery, or with some medications). US Department of Health & Human Services 2016.

Data from DSM-5, *Diagnostic and Statistical Manual of Mental Disorders, Fifth Edition*; ICD-10, International Statistical Classification of Diseases and Related Health Problems, 10th Revision; WHO, World Health Organization.

substance use but who are not dependent are a major target group for early identification. The importance of this approach has resulted in screening, brief intervention, and referral to treatment (SBIRT) being mandated in the United States for level 1 and 2 trauma centers.[3]

This approach has a sound rationale. Screening clients to identify at-risk users combined with brief interventions provides an efficient way of reaching a larger portion of clients with alcohol or other drug problems than provided by traditional intensive interventions, and may be especially suited to clients with less severe diagnoses.[69] By using opportunistic screening, brief interventions may reach a proportion of individuals who would not normally present at specialist treatment facilities.[15,103] Moreover, screening in primary care for subclinical alcohol consumption or other drug use to identify at-risk individuals allows preventive measures or treatment to be initiated before clinical-level disorders and the associated health and social problems develop.

A large number of short screening tests are available to aid in the systematic identification of alcohol or other drug use problems in primary care.[13] Two of the most commonly used tests are the Drug Abuse Screening Test[90] and the 10-item Alcohol Use Disorders Identification Test (AUDIT). The latter was developed by the World Health Organization and validated in numerous countries and populations.[85,86] It is also available in three shortened versions and has been used widely.[75] The Drug Abuse Screening Test is available as a 28-item form[90] or a 10-item short form[40] and screens for general drug abuse rather than a specific class of drug. The brevity of these instruments and their ease of use make them suitable for a range of general medical settings. Biological screening tests (e.g., breath, hair, urine, saliva, laboratory markers) would appear to offer a more robust assessment, but to date, these are of limited use in primary care, where results are needed quickly, must be inexpensive, and must show more than just recent use.[1,13,48] Therefore, biological assays may be more appropriate in specialist settings, clinical trials, or where they are required to comply with legal requirements.

What Is Screening and Brief Intervention?

Screening and brief intervention (SBI) is generally used as part of a consultation in a primary care setting—for instance, general practice or a community health service. However, as is explored in more detail below, some brief interventions may be initiated at a teachable moment such as in general hospital emergency, medical, or surgical departments, when individuals may be highly motivated to change their behavior.

Brief interventions are sometimes described as minimal interventions due to the less-intensive nature of the intervention required to effect changes toward more positive substance use patterns in nondependent individuals, or as early interventions because they are directed at individuals who have not progressed to more serious drug use patterns. However, even at the extreme end of the spectrum, SBI has a role in identifying people with dependence and enhancing referral for treatment.

There is no universally accepted definition of what constitutes a brief intervention. Babor provided a convenient heuristic where a single client contact with a professional constitutes a minimal intervention, 1–3 sessions constitute a brief intervention, 5–7 sessions a moderate intervention, and 8 or more an intensive intervention.[10] Miller and Wilbourne suggested that 1 or 2 sessions of treatment constitute a brief intervention,[66] whereas Moyer and colleagues used a threshold of 4 sessions to define brief interventions.[69] In the first section of this chapter, the focus is on interventions that can be delivered in 4 or fewer sessions. In the second section, the focus is on brief interventions to increase compliance with pharmacotherapies used in the treatment of problem alcohol or other drug use, which often extend over 12 or more sessions.

Notably, none of these definitions delineate the length or content of the intervention. Interventions are typically of 30- to 45-minute duration; however, within a community/primary care setting, interventions can be incorporated within a 5- to 10-minute physician consultation.[36] Five key elements have been identified for inclusion in an intervention. First, the clinician assesses the quantity and frequency of alcohol or other drug use and provides direct feedback to the client regarding health or psychosocial morbidity relevant to his or her level of use. Second, goals for alcohol or other drug use are established that are acceptable to both provider and client.

These goals may be a reduction in consumption, such as using alcohol in a low-risk fashion, or complete cessation, as is commonly employed with tobacco use. Third, the provider uses behavioral modification techniques—for example, to help the client identify high-risk situations and develop strategies to deal with these. Fourth, the clinician should supply support material on problems associated with substance use plus self-help techniques. Fifth, the provider should offer ongoing support.[36] Others have summarized the content under the acronym FRAMES[15]—that is, *F*eedback on personal risk, personal *R*esponsibility for the problem, *A*dvice that is clear and explicit, a *M*enu of options on how to change, an *E*mpathic style of counseling to avoid coercion or authoritarianism, and enhancement of the client's *S*elf-efficacy.[15]

Babor and colleagues provided a thorough discussion of the psychological principles and behavioral change strategies thought to underlie early or brief intervention programs; these incorporate principles from social, cognitive, and behavioral psychology to increase motivation and commitment to change.[12] For example, a health care professional can be seen as having social power, and, as a credible source of relevant health information, the provision of normative information allows social comparison and support networks to use social influence to modify behavior.[12]

A concept that often arises in the screening and brief intervention literature is that of the teachable moment when a person is particularly likely to be open to changing his or her behavior—for example, when a major health event or hospitalization related to substance use occurs.[41] McBride and colleagues suggested a model to help determine whether a given event, such as hospitalization for a substance-related morbidity, will cue the client to reduce his or her substance use.[65] First, does the event (e.g., hospitalization or ill health) serve to increase perceived risk from the client's use of the drug and the potential for positive outcomes to occur if the use is reduced or ceased? Second, does the event provoke a strong emotional response? Third, does it lead to redefining the person's self-concept? For instance, a child being diagnosed with asthma may be associated with smoking by a parent, leading to the parent reevaluating his or her role as a protective caregiver. Even in the presence of all these factors, preexisting individual factors may override the impact of the event. Nevertheless, delivering interventions at a teachable moment is likely to amplify greatly the impact of the intervention—for example, increasing cessation of smoking by up to 70% compared with a background quit rate of about 5%.[65]

Some have contended that the stress associated with a hospital presentation and the often chaotic environment in hospital emergency departments may mean that this is not a conducive setting in which to deliver an intervention. However, it may still be appropriate to use the opportunity to arrange a follow-up intervention,[61] and there is the possibility of using motivational techniques to encourage people to attend treatment rather than attempting to deliver treatment under these difficult conditions.

Screening and Brief Intervention—Effectiveness and Delivery

Alcohol

Of all the strategies and pharmacotherapies for treating alcohol use problems, there is more evidence, particularly from studies of high methodological quality, to support the use of SBI than any other type of intervention. Brief interventions are also the highest ranked intervention in clinical populations, although this form of intervention is most effective when individuals with more severe disorders are excluded.[69] The focus on clients with less-severe alcohol use problems means that low-risk use of alcohol can be the goal of the intervention rather than complete abstinence, which has been the traditional goal of more intensive interventions.

Although there is robust and extensive literature on the use of SBI for alcohol use problems,[15,69,106] a criticism has been raised that these conclusions were based on select populations and from tightly controlled clinical trials.[52] From a health care perspective, a critical concern is whether this type of intervention can be translated into the clinical setting of primary care. A meta-analysis of trials conducted in primary care using interventions that would be suitable for inclusion in clinical practice (i.e., physician interventions of 5–15 min or nurse interventions of 20–30 min) identified 28 trials, including 5 that used the motivational interviewing approaches.[52] Overall, brief interventions reduced alcohol consumption by 41 g/week at 1 year. Brief interventions also seem to be effective at reducing binge drinking and heavy drinking, albeit these conclusions are based on a limited number of studies and that the studies used different definitions to categorize heavy use of alcohol (criteria ranged from 20 to 35 drinks/week for men and 13 to 35 for women).[52] The main caveat identified by the research was the lack of a significant reduction in alcohol use by women, but this may be related to lack of statistical power, with only 499 of 7286 female participants included in the review.[52] This is a potentially important limitation, as women are more likely than men to seek help from primary care providers.[98] On the other hand, a recent meta-analysis did not find gender differences in the effectiveness of SBI,[69] suggesting that lack of statistical power may indeed be the explanation.

e-Health interventions cover a range of approaches that are mediated by electronic technology. At its most basic, this can be telephone support, but more frequently, interventions are provided via stand-alone computers, the Internet, smart phone applications, or text messages. Therefore, SBI can now be delivered by computers or remotely over the Internet (e-SBI) and can be accessed by nearly the entire population. e-SBI typically uses the same therapeutic approaches as a face-to-face intervention. Thus components may include a screening questionnaire, normative information, motivational enhancement, skills building, and relapse prevention. Although most data have been collected from tertiary student populations,[105] benefits have also been demonstrated in the general adult population,[78] with outcomes of a magnitude similar to those achieved by face-to-face brief interventions. e-SBI has also been evaluated in hospital emergency departments to address youth alcohol consumption and violence.[27]

Brief interventions including e-SBI also have a sound health economics rationale, with a positive cost-benefit ratio, with significant savings through reduced health costs as well as reduced costs to society—for instance, in reducing vehicle accidents.[30] The magnitude of this effect has been estimated at 5.6:1 at 12 months and 4.3:1 at 48 months when considering reduced health system costs alone.[37,38] Thus an intervention that cost $205 per individual to deliver resulted in an average benefit of $1151.[41] Including savings to the wider community, the total benefit was $7985 per intervention.[38]

There is some concern over the long-term effectiveness of e-SBI. In their meta-analysis, Donahue et al.[31] found a significant reduction in alcohol consumption between 3 and less than 12 months, but at 12 months and longer there was no significant difference between e-SBI and control groups. Similar findings were reported by Dedert et al.,[29] who reported that low-intensity e-interventions produced small reductions in alcohol consumption at 6 months, but there was little evidence for longer-term, clinically significant effects. Harris and Knight[43] conducted an extensive review of the use of e-SBI for alcohol use in medical settings, and found that although it was feasible and accepted by both staff and patients, the highly variable quality of data did not allow conclusions to be drawn regarding efficacy.

Tobacco

All forms of intervention to encourage the cessation of tobacco use are cost-effective in terms of cost per life-year saved,[102] with the cost of these interventions comparing favorably with virtually any other health care program.[99,102] Although improved rates of cessation accrue from more intensive interventions, these improvements do not keep pace with increased costs. However, this should not be used as a reason for not delivering more intensive interventions, which may be particularly efficacious in those with more severe problems, for whom brief interventions are typically less effective.[102]

Guidelines are available for primary care practitioners, such as physicians, nurses, and dentists, to aid in the development of screening procedures and the delivery of appropriate interventions for users of tobacco.[35,104] The United States guidelines evaluate a range of different psychosocial and pharmacological interventions as well as the management strategies for identifying and treating smokers in different primary care settings. The guidelines emphasize the importance of screening all patients for tobacco use and recommend strategies for approaching those willing to quit, those unwilling to quit, and those who have recently quit.[35] However, it also has been suggested that repeated advice to asymptomatic smokers may be counterproductive,[88] contrary to the guideline recommendation that smokers should be asked about their use of tobacco on every visit. Potentially, the importance of this guideline may be derived from the development of systems that help to ensure that cessation of tobacco use is thoroughly integrated into clinical practice rather than through increased benefits to an individual.

The initial approach recommended is a brief intervention that can be delivered in approximately 3 minutes, summarized under the mnemonic the 5 A's (Ask, Advise, Assess, Assist, and Arrange). These guide the practitioner to ask every client about tobacco use at each visit, to advise them clearly and in a personalized manner to quit tobacco use, to assess their current willingness to quit, to assist them in forming a cessation plan, to provide them with access to counseling and appropriate pharmacotherapies, and, finally, to arrange a follow-up appointment, if possible within a week of the agreed-upon quit date.[35]

If the client is not willing to quit, a further brief intervention can be delivered that focuses on increasing the motivation to quit (see Chapter 39 for detailed information on motivational interviewing). This brief intervention is formulated under the mnemonic the 5 R's (Relevance, Risks, Rewards, Roadblocks, and Repetition). Thus the intervention should focus on aspects that are personally relevant, such as current health problems, and should encourage the smoker to identify the risks of tobacco use and the rewards that will accrue with cessation. Any potential roadblocks to cessation should be addressed and solutions generated. Finally, the intervention should be repeated on each occasion that the client is seen.

Given the chronic relapsing nature of nicotine dependence and other addictive disorders, it is important also to plan and deliver relapse prevention interventions, especially in the first 3 months after a person has quit smoking. This typically involves the use of open-ended questions to encourage discussion of benefits, successes, and problems encountered as well as providing encouragement and help with significant problems, such as depression, weight gain, or withdrawal symptoms.

A meta-analysis of randomized trials with at least 6 months follow-up of brief interventions by physicians found that a single session lasting up to 20 minutes, plus up to one follow-up session, increased the rate of cessation by 1%–3% over the background rate of cessation (2%–3%).[91] The rate of mortality and morbidity due to smoking means that even small improvements in cessation result in noticeable benefits. However, the effectiveness of this approach is derived from screening all participants and intervening with those who are smokers. The main drawback identified was the difficulty of persuading physicians to incorporate systematic screening and intervention into regular practice. The development of online or smart phone cessation applications means that clinicians can easily advise clients to access additional supports or incorporate them with a face-to-face intervention.[20]

Brief interventions by nursing staff are also effective at producing small but significant increases in successful quitting. However, the authors of the analysis stress that statistical heterogeneity indicates that this finding may not generalize to all patient groups or clinical settings equally.[76] Nevertheless, the US guidelines recommend that interventions by all nonphysician clinicians (i.e., nurses, psychologists, and dentists) can be justified empirically compared with no treatment or self-help.[35] As with alcohol, there are now effective online smoking cessation programs, plus other electronic interventions such as text messages or smart phone applications.[20] These interventions yield small but important improvements in cessation.

Smoking cessation interventions delivered in a hospital would appear to be an ideal opportunity, particularly with the expansion of smoke-free hospital policies in many developed countries. However, a meta-analysis concluded that high-intensity behavioral interventions initiated in a hospital that included at least 1 month of postdischarge support were effective, but that lower-intensity and shorter-duration interventions were not found to be effective.[77] A more recent meta-analysis of trials that sought to reduce tobacco smoke exposure among hospitalized children found significant effects only in trials that measured maternal postpartum smoking relapse prevention.[28]

Illicit Drugs

The weight of evidence supporting the utility of brief interventions in treating alcohol use or cigarette smoking is in striking contrast with the limited studies on the use of these techniques for illicit substance use problems.[82] Two Cochrane reviews of psychosocial treatments for opiate use and of psychosocial and pharmacological treatment for opioid detoxification did not identify any studies that used brief interventions for the psychosocial component.[2] Similarly, a Cochrane review of psychosocial interventions to treat cocaine and other psychostimulant disorders failed to identify any brief interventions that matched the inclusion criteria.[55] A third Cochrane review of interventions to reduce drug use by young people conducted outside the school setting[39] and an earlier review of interventions for adolescent alcohol, tobacco, and other drug use[94] identified one brief intervention with adolescent substance users.[71]

In 2007, the National Institute on Drug Abuse concluded that there were too few data to support the use of screening, brief intervention, referral, and treatment (SBIRT) for illicit drug use and no research to support this with respect to prescription drug use.[23] Subsequently, a major trial was initiated with 459,599 people screened across a range of settings, including emergency departments, hospitals, community clinics, and schools.[63] Nearly 23% screened positive for heavy alcohol and or illicit drug use. By 6 months there were significant declines in use across all major categories (alcohol, cannabis, methamphetamine, and heroin).[63]

It is estimated that 15 million Americans misused prescription drugs in 2014.[19] The misuse of prescription and over-the-counter medications resulting in emergency department visits and other adverse outcomes, is a cause of concern that has resulted in calls for research funds to be directed to this area, including the evaluation of SBIRT programs to identify and intervene with the users of these licit substances.[22] The study by Madras and colleagues[63] reported reductions in other drug use, which included prescription medications, but further work focused on this category is required.

More recently, a number of studies have found SBI in illicit drug using populations to be both ineffective[80,83] and costly.[80,109] Roy-Byrne et al.[80] found no effect of a one-time brief intervention on illicit drug use among patients in a safety-net (low income) primary care setting. Another large and significant trial conducted among licit and illicit drug users in a primary care setting found no effect of SBI on any outcome measure. The authors concluded that SBI is not effective for this patient group.[83] Of interest, investigators examining the effect of access to an e-SBI site for illicit drug users, found no significant effects at 3- and 6-month follow-up, but did find a significant reduction in alcohol use in the intervention group at 12 months.[89] A review of online interventions for cannabis use or prevention of cannabis initiation identified 10 studies,[97] of which one was a single-session brief intervention[51] and one a face-to-face brief intervention plus online cognitive behavioral therapy.[54] Neither study achieved significant effects. It is important to note that although SBI is seemingly not effective in this patient group, the screening component should not be abandoned as an integral component of clinical assessment for at-risk groups.

An alternative approach is to use the screening and referral approach to encourage people to attend external agencies for treatment. This method has been used with adolescents presenting to emergency departments with alcohol or other drug problems. The authors reported that this type of intervention could be successfully delivered in emergency departments but noted that the yield (proportion of adolescents attending treatment), although significant compared with usual care, was low.[95,96] Further work is required to determine the best referral processes for specialist treatment for individuals who do not respond to brief interventions.[13]

Conclusions—Screening and Brief Interventions

Brief interventions including e-SBI are a well-recognized and empirically validated approach to the treatment of alcohol and nicotine disorders, particularly in the primary care setting. However, the key aspect is initiating procedures so that all clients are regularly asked about their alcohol or tobacco use and appropriate actions are taken. Nevertheless, some key shortcomings have been identified. First, there are few data to support the use of SBI

with illicit substances or the misuse of licit substances. Second, the effectiveness of SBI with women, at least for alcohol use problems, has yet to be definitively established. Given the greater use of primary care by women, this potential deficit is of concern. However, online alcohol interventions attract a greater proportion of women than traditional programs, which may provide a means of engaging with this group.[105] Third, the effectiveness of nonclinician screening and brief intervention programs for tobacco use needs further clarification.[35]

Improving Compliance/Adherence to Therapies

The first section of this chapter assessed brief interventions that aimed directly to address problem use of alcohol or other drugs. However, brief interventions also can be used to increase compliance with other treatment including pharmacotherapies. Used in this manner, they can have a role outside the specialist addiction treatment setting in addressing alcohol or other drug dependence. The following section reviews two models that have been used under this rubric.

Brief Behavioral Compliance Enhancement Treatment

Brief behavioral compliance enhancement treatment (BBCET) provides a standardized manual[50] that aims to improve the outcomes associated with pharmacotherapy, rather than constituting an independent intervention. It does this by enhancing behavioral compliance with a pharmacotherapy, in particular by increasing expectations of the effectiveness of that therapy. BBCET was developed from the clinical management used in the National Institute of Mental Health collaborative trial on depression.[34] The original trial included clinical management that aimed to maximize the effectiveness of the pharmacotherapy through improved compliance and, simultaneously, to minimize loss to follow-up to maintain the validity of the trial. It should, however, be emphasized that the clinical management used in the National Institute of Mental Health collaborative study did not include any elements that can be considered psychotherapy and that its content was not based on any validated data but rather on clinical experience.[34]

A manual-driven and standardized version of BBCET has been developed for clinical trials in the addictions, especially in the alcoholism field, and has now been used in several multisite studies. The BBCET is spread over 13, 10- to 20-minute sessions and is usually provided as weekly sessions.[50] An advantage of the BBCET over other brief interventions is that it is customized to suit the delivery of different types of medication. As part of this customization, the BBCET can be adapted to treatment protocols that target either abstinence or a reduction in hazardous drinking as the clinical endpoint. BBCET encourages compliance not only with pharmacotherapy but also with general treatment adherence. Indeed, providing encouragement to the patient, even for small treatment gains, is an important aspect of brief behavioral compliance enhancement treatment. Generally, the BBCET program consists of three phases covering initiation, maintenance, and termination of treatment. The initiation phase is critically important and seeks to engage the client in a positive and trusting relationship that fosters adherence with the treatment regimen and educates the patient with regard to the harmful effects of alcohol and the potential side effects of the medication. The clinician performing

BBCET emphasizes the importance of medication use, develops simple behavioral repertoires to enhance medication compliance, and builds a realistic expectation of success, but also discusses how potential side effects can be managed. Indeed, a flexible and naturalistic clinical feature of BBCET is that it can be administered by a trained provider within the scheduled format for the collection and discussion of side effects. In addition, from the first session, the clinician providing BBCET establishes a platform for ascertaining progress with changing drinking. Notably, a unique aspect of BBCET over other brief interventions is that the patient sets a weekly target drinking goal. The second phase aims to maintain compliance and, particularly, to avoid early termination of pharmacotherapy. The clinician explores the gains made by the client and addresses any medication side effects that have appeared. The final phase examines how medication use can be terminated while still maintaining improvement in drinking outcomes and how these gains can be maintained without assistance.[50] BBCET has also been incorporated into medication trials for other addictive disorders.[33] However, initial enthusiasm for the benefits of this approach need to be tempered by more recent data. In the best-designed randomized trials, few show improvements in adherence and clinical outcome measures.[70]

e-Health Interventions to Enhance Compliance to Therapies

As noted above, e-health interventions can be used as discrete screening and brief intervention programs. However, just as brief intervention techniques have been extended to cover multiple sessions in BBCET, e-health interventions can provide therapeutic support over many sessions. Carroll et al.[18] added computerized cognitive behavior therapy (CBT) to standard therapy, which included individual and group sessions based on CBT, and found significant reductions in drug use at 6 months. In addition, e-health interventions have been used successfully to replace some of the face-to-face therapy delivered to individuals on methadone programs.[64] In both these studies, the e-health components were provided in a clinical setting, rather than allowing participants remote access. This approach negates one of the principal advantages of Internet-based programs, the potential to reach many thousands of people, including those who may not access conventional treatment services. As an addition to other types of therapy, the most notable advantage of e-health interventions is their ability to ensure treatment fidelity and consistency across recipients.

Recent systematic reviews of the use of e-health interventions to improve medication adherence for persons with chronic diseases (e.g., asthma, diabetes, HIV) found that although results were generally supportive, the reviews noted that weak study designs and a reliance of self-report measures were a concern.[68] With respect to substance use, a recent study evaluated a mobile phone intervention to improve oral naltrexone adherence for individuals with alcohol dependence.[92] The small scale (n = 76) of the study means that the nonsignificant outcomes on the primary measure were unsurprising, but the study did find improvements on some measures of adherence with an increased period of adherence over the first month (19 vs. 3 days).

Conclusions—Compliance Enhancement

Brief interventions provide primary care health workers with a framework to deliver interventions to any client presenting with substance use disorders. Brief behavioral compliance enhancement treatment provides an extension to brief interventions if clients are interested in receiving pharmacotherapies to aid in cessation. Some elements of these pharmacotherapy compliance approaches appear simply to be good clinical practice, such as advising clients on how medications should be taken and warning of potential side effects. However, by providing these treatments as a structured manual-driven framework, they enable the clinician to approach with confidence a group of clients who are often regarded as difficult to treat in a variety of settings.

e-Health interventions have shown promise as adjuncts to standard clinical treatments in individuals with illicit drug disorders. However, although intuitively appealing as a means of improving medication adherence, further robust evaluation is required to support its use with antagonist medications like naltrexone.

Future Research

There is a growing literature on methods of improving adherence (now generally used instead of compliance due to its less-pejorative connotations) to psychotropic medications, especially among individuals with severe mental illness, such as those with schizophrenia.[17] It is estimated that about 76% of individuals with physical health problems are compliant with medications, compared with 65% of individuals prescribed antidepressants and 58% of individuals prescribed antipsychotic medications.[26] However, the high prevalence of comorbid alcohol or other drug problems and other mental health disorders, with an elevated level of associated mortality and morbidity[58,107] combined with the low rates of successful cessation in this population[42,79] illustrates the urgent need for the development of cessation programs for this group. The existing literature on adherence to psychotropic medication and the compliance enhancement programs for pharmacotherapies in treating alcohol or other drug problems suggests that it should be possible to design effective programs for this highly disadvantaged group.

Compliance enhancement interventions may also prove beneficial in supporting the use of pharmacotherapies with other addictive disorders. For instance, oral naltrexone has been approved for the management of heroin dependence, but poor compliance means that it is not generally regarded as an effective treatment.[67] However, in highly motivated individuals or with daily supervision, the effectiveness is increased.[46] Therefore, a trial using BBCET with oral naltrexone in a general heroin-using population appears to be warranted, with initial work having been initiated among individuals with alcohol dependence.[92]

Current research on SBI reveals some surprising findings. Although the approach is successful, albeit with small effects, on alcohol and tobacco use, the evidence of the approach translating to illicit drug users is more sporadic. Of particular concern is the lack of support in well-designed studies, that achieved high rates of retention and used biochemical confirmation of drug use.[81] This may reflect fundamental differences between individuals who use illicit rather than licit substances. Alternatively, many studies have included participants who use different drugs rather than addressing a specific type of drug. Where effects are likely to be small, generic interventions for a range of substances may not be appropriate.

Resources

Resources on alcohol use problems for professionals, clients, and families: http://www.niaaa.nih.gov
SAMHSA–HRSA Center for Integrated Health Solutions Screening, Brief Intervention and Referral for Treatment: http://integration.samhsa.gov/clinical-practice/SBIRT

Surgeon General Tobacco Use and Dependence Guidelines: http://www.ncbi.nlm.nih.gov/books/NBK63952/

Treatment Improvement Protocol 34: Brief Interventions and Brief Therapies for Substance Abuse: http://www.ncbi.nlm. nih.gov/books/NBK64947/pdf/Bookshelf_NBK64947.pdf

References

1. Aertgeerts B, Buntinx F, Ansoms S, Fevery J. Screening properties of questionnaires and laboratory tests for the detection of alcohol abuse or dependence in a general practice population. *Br J Gen Pract*. 2001;51:315–316.
2. Amato L, Minozzi S, Davoli M, Vecchi S Ferri M, Mayet S. Psychosocial and pharmacological treatments versus pharmacological treatments for opioid detoxification. *Cochrane Database Syst Rev*. 2011;9.
3. American College of Surgeons Committee on Trauma. *Resources for Optimal Care of the Injured Patient*. Chicago, IL: American College of Surgeons; 2014.
4. American Psychiatric Association. *Diagnostic and Statistical Manual of Mental Disorders*. 4th ed. Washington: APA; 1994.
5. American Psychiatric Association. *Diagnostic and Statistical Manual of Mental Disorders*. 5th ed. Washington, DC: APA; 2013.
6. Andrews G, Hall W, Teesson M, Henderson S. *The Mental Health of Australians. Canberra: Mental Health Branch*. Commonwealth Department of Health and Aged Care; 1999.
7. Reference deleted in review.
8. Reference deleted in review.
9. Babor T, Campbell R, Room R. *Lexicon of Alcohol and Drug Terms*. Geneva: World Health Organization; 1994.
10. Babor TF. Avoiding the horrid and beastly sin of drunkenness: does dissuasion make a difference? *J Consult Clin Psychol*. 1994;62:1127–1140.
11. Reference deleted in review.
12. Babor TF, Korner P, Wilber C, Good SP. Screening and early intervention strategies for harmful drinkers: initial lessons from the Amethyst project. *Aust Drug Alcohol Rev*. 1987;6:325–339.
13. Babor TF, McRee BG, Kassebaum PA, Grimaldi PL, Ahmed K, Bray J. Screening, brief intervention, and referral to treatment (SBIRT): toward a public health approach to the management of substance abuse. *Subst Abus*. 2007;39:7–30.
14. Reference deleted in review.
15. Bien TH, Miller WR, Tonigan JS. Brief interventions for alcohol problems: a review. *Addiction*. 1993;88:315–335.
16. Reference deleted in review.
17. Calhoun PS, Butterfield MI. Treatment adherence among individuals with serve mental illness. In: Bosworth HB, Oddone EZ, Weinberger M, eds. *Patient Treatment Adherence Concepts, Interventions, and Measurement*. Mahwah, NJ: Lawrence Erlbaum; 2006:307–328.
18. Carroll KM, Ball SA, Martino S, Nich C, Babuscio TA, Rounsaville BJ. Enduring effects of a computer-assisted training program for cognitive behavioral therapy: a 6-month follow-up of CBT4CBT. *Drug Alcohol Depend*. 2009;100:178–181.
19. Center for Behavioral Health Statistics and Quality. *Behavioral Health Trends in the United States: Results from the 2014 National Survey on Drug Use and Health*. NSDUH Series H-50. Rockville, MD: SAMHSA; 2015.
20. Chen Y, Madan J, Welton N, Yahaya I, Aveyard P. Effectiveness and cost-effectiveness of computer and other electronic aids for smoking cessation: a systematic review and network meta-analysis. *Health Technol Assess*. 2012;16:205.
21. Cherpitel CJ. Emergency room and primary care services utilization and associated alcohol and drug use in the United States general population. *Alcohol Alcohol*. 1999;34:581–589.
22. Clark HW. *The use and utility of prescription drug monitoring programs*. House energy and commerce oversight and investigations. 2007. Available from http://www.hhs.gov/asl/testify/2007/10/t20071024b.html. Accessed 7 Aug 2008.
23. Compton WM. How does SBIRT fit into the NIDA research program? *SBRIT Grantee Spring Meeting*; 2007. Available from http://www.mayatech.com/cti/sbirtgsm07/doc/day1_1030_Wilson-Compton_CabinetJudiciaryRoom.pdf. Accessed 31 July 2008.
24. Reference deleted in review.
25. Reference deleted in review.
26. Cramer JA, Rosenheck RA. Compliance with medication regimens for mental and physical disorders. *Psychiatr Serv*. 1998;49:196–201.
27. Cunningham RM, Chermack ST, Zimmerman MA, et al. Brief motivational interviewing intervention for peer violence and alcohol use in teens: one-year follow-up. *Pediatrics*. 2012;129:1083–1090.
28. Daly JB, Mackenzie LJ, Freund M, Wolfenden L, Roseby R, Wiggers JH. Interventions by health care professionals who provide routine child health care to reduce tobacco smoke exposure in children: a review and meta-analysis. *JAMA Pediatr*. 2015;170:1–10.
29. Dedert EA, McDuffie JR, Stein R, et al. Electronic interventions for alcohol misuse and alcohol use disorders: a systematic review. *Ann Intern Med*. 2015;163:205–214.
30. Donker T, Blankers M, Hedman E, Ljótsson B, Petrie K, Christensen H. Economic evaluations of Internet interventions for mental health: a systematic review. *Psychol Med*. 2015;45(16):3357–3376.
31. Donoghue K, Patton R, Phillips T, Deluca P, Drummond C. The effectiveness of electronic screening and brief intervention for reducing levels of alcohol consumption: a systematic review and meta-analysis. *J Med Internet Res*. 2014;16:e142.
32. Reference deleted in review.
33. Elkashef A, Kahn R, Yu E, et al. Topiramate for the treatment of methamphetamine addiction: a multi-center placebo-controlled trial. *Addiction*. 2012;107:1297–1306.
34. Fawcett J, Epstein P, Fiester SJ, Elkin I, Autry JH. Clinical management—imipramine/placebo administration manual: NIMH treatment of depression collaborative research program. *Psychopharmacol Bull*. 1987;23:309–324.
35. Fiore MC, Jaen CR, Baker TB, Bailey WC, Benowitz NL, Curry SJ, et al. *Treating Tobacco Use and Dependence: 2008 Update*. Rockville, MD: US Department of Health and Human Services; 2008.
36. Fleming M, Manwell LB. Brief intervention in primary care settings – a primary treatment method for at-risk, problem, and dependent drinkers. *Alcohol Res Health*. 1999;23:128–137.
37. Fleming MF, Mundt MP, French MT, Manwell LB, Stauffacher EA, Barry KL. Benefit-cost analysis of brief physician advice with problem drinkers in primary care settings. *Med Care*. 2000;38:7–18.
38. Fleming MF, Mundt MP, French MT, Manwell LB, Stauffacher EA, Barry KL. Brief physician advice for problem drinkers: long-term efficacy and benefit-cost analysis. *Alcohol Clin Exp Res*. 2002;26:36–43.
39. Gates S, McCambridge J, Smith LA, Foxcroft DR. Interventions for prevention of drug use by young people delivered in non-school settings. *Cochrane Database Syst Rev*. 2007. https://doi.org/10.1002/14651858.CD005030.pub2.
40. Gavin DR, Ross HE, Skinner HA. Diagnostic validity of the drug abuse screening test in the assessment of DSM-III drug disorders. *Br J Addiction*. 1989;84:301–307.
41. Gentilello LM, Duggan P, Drummond D, Tonnesen A, Degner EE, Fischer RP, et al. Major injury as a unique opportunity to initiate treatment in the alcoholic. *Am J Surg*. 1988;156:558–561.
42. Hagman BT, Delnevo CD, Hrywna M, Williams JM. Tobacco use among those with serious psychological distress: results from the national survey of drug use and health, 2002. *Addict Behav*. 2008;33:582–592.
43. Harris SK, Knight JR. Putting the screen in screening: technology-based alcohol screening and brief interventions in medical settings. *Alcohol Res: Curr Rev*. 2014;36:63–79.

44. Reference deleted in review.

45. Higgins-Biddle J, Babor T, Mullahy J, Daniels J, McRee B. Alcohol screening and brief intervention: where research meets practice. *Conn Med.* 1997;61:565–575.

46. Hulse GK, Basso MR. The association between naltrexone compliance and daily supervision. *Drug Alcohol Rev.* 2000;19:41–48.

47. Institute of Medicine. *Broadening the Base of Treatment for Alcohol Problems.* Washington, DC: National Academy; 1990.

48. Jaffee WB, Trucco E, Levy S, Weiss RD. Is this urine really negative? A systematic review of tampering methods in urine drug screening and testing. *J Subst Abuse Treat.* 2007;33:33–43.

49. Reference deleted in review.

50. Johnson BA, DiClemente CC, Ait-Daoud N, Stoks SM. (2003) Brief behavioral compliance enhancement treatment (BBCET) manual. In: Johnson BA, Ruiz P, Galanter M, eds. *Handbook of Clinical Alcoholism Treatment.* Baltimore: Lippincott Williams & Wilkins; 2003:282–301.

51. Jonas B, Tossmann P, Tensil M, Leuschner F, Struber E. Efficacy of a single-session online-intervention on problematic substance use [German]. *Sucht.* 2012;58:173–182.

52. Kaner EFS, Beyer F, Dickinson HO, Pienaar E, Campbell F, Schlesinger C, et al. Effectiveness of brief alcohol interventions in primary care populations. *Cochrane Database Syst Rev.* 2007. https://doi.org/10.1002/14651858.CD004148.pub3.

53. Karhuvaara S, Simojoki K, Virta A, Rosberg M, Löyttyniemi E, Nurminen T, et al. Targeted Nalmefene with simple medical management in the treatment of heavy drinkers: a randomized double-blind placebo-controlled multicenter study. *Alcohol Clin Exp Res.* 2007;31:1179–1187.

54. Kay-Lambkin FJ, Baker AL, Kelly B, Lewin TJ. Clinician-assisted computerised versus therapist-delivered treatment for depressive and addictive disorders: a randomised controlled trial. *Med J Aust.* 2011;195:S44–S50.

55. Knapp WP, Soares B, Farrel M, Lima MS. Psychosocial interventions for cocaine and psychostimulant amphetamines related disorders. *Cochrane Database Syst Rev.* 2007. https://doi.org/10.1002/14651858.CD003023.pub2.

56. Kreitman N. Alcohol consumption and the prevention paradox. *Br J Addiction.* 1986;81:353–363.

57. Reference deleted in review.

58. Lawrence D, Holman CD, Jablenski A, Hobbs MS. Death rate from ischaemic heart disease in Western Australian psychiatric patients 1980–1998. *Br J Psychiatry.* 2003;182:31–36.

59. Reference deleted in review.

60. Reference deleted in review.

61. Longabaugh R, Woolard RF, Nirenberg TD, Minugh AP, Becker B, Clifford PR, et al. Evaluating the effects of a brief motivational intervention for injured drinkers in the emergency department. *J Stud Alcohol.* 2001;62:806–816.

62. Reference deleted in review.

63. Madras BK, Compton WM, Avula D, Stegbauer T, Stein JB, Clark HW. Screening, brief interventions, referral to treatment (SBIRT) for illicit drug and alcohol use at multiple healthcare sites: comparison at intake and six months. *Drug Alcohol Depend.* 2009;99:280–295.

64. Marsch LA, Guarino H, Acosta M, et al. Web-based behavioral treatment for substance use disorders as a partial replacement of standard methadone maintenance treatment. *J Subst Abuse Treat.* 2014;46:43–51.

65. McBride CM, Emmons KM, Lipkus IM. Understanding the potential of teachable moments: the case of smoking cessation. *Health Educ Res.* 2003;18:156–170.

66. Miller WR, Wilbourne PL. Mesa Grande: a methodological analysis of clinical trials of treatments for alcohol use disorders. *Addiction.* 2002;97:265–277.

67. Minozzi S, Amato L, Vecchi S, Davoli M, Kirchmayer U, Verster A. Oral naltrexone maintenance treatment for opioid dependence. *Cochrane Database Syst Rev.* 2006. https://doi.org/10.1002/14651858.CD001333.pub2.

68. Mistry N, Keepanasseril A, Wilczynski NL, Nieuwlaat R, Ravall M, Haynes RB. Technology-mediated interventions for enhancing medication adherence. *J Am Med Inform Assoc.* 2015;22(e1): e177–e193.

69. Moyer A, Finney JW, Swearingen CE, Vergun P. Brief interventions for alcohol problems: a meta-analytic review of controlled investigations in treatment-seeking and non-treatment-seeking populations. *Addiction.* 2002;97:279–292.

70. Nieuwlaat R, Wilczynski N, Navarro T, Hobson N, Jeffery R, Keepanasseril A, et al. Interventions for enhancing medication adherence. *Cochrane Database Syst Rev.* 2014;11.

71. Oliansky DM, Wildenhaus KJ, Manlove K, Arnold T, Schoener EP. Effectiveness of brief interventions in reducing substance use among at-risk primary care patients in three community-based clinics. *Subst Abus.* 1997;18:95–103.

72. Orford J, Oppenheimer E, Edwards G. Abstinence or control: the outcome for excessive drinkers two years after consultation. *Behav Res Ther.* 1976;14:409–418.

73. Reference deleted in review.

74. Reference deleted in review.

75. Reinert DF, Allen JP. The alcohol use disorders identification test (AUDIT): a review of recent research. *Alcohol Clin Exp Res.* 2002;26:272–279.

76. Rice V, Stead L. Nursing interventions for smoking cessation. *Cochrane Database Syst Rev.* 2004. https://doi.org/10.1002/14651858.CD001188.pub2.

77. Rigotti NA, Munafo M, Stead LF. Interventions for smoking cessation in hospitalised patients. *Cochrane Database Syst Rev.* 2007. https://doi.org/10.1002/14651858.CD001837.pub2.

78. Riper H, Spek V, Boon B, Conijn B, Kramer J, Martin-Abello K, et al. Effectiveness of e-self-help interventions for curbing adult problem drinking: a meta-analysis. *J Med Internet Res.* 2011;13(2):e42.

79. Roick C, Fritz-Wieacker A, Matschinger H, Heider D, Schindler J, Riedel-Heller S, et al. Health habits of patients with schizophrenia. *Soc Psychiatry Psychiatr Epidemiol.* 2007;42:268–276.

80. Roy-Byrne P, Bumgardner K, Krupski A, et al. Brief intervention for problem drug use in safety-net primary care settings: a randomized clinical trial. *JAMA.* 2014;312:492–501.

81. Saitz R. Screening and brief intervention for unhealthy drug use: little or no efficacy. *Front Psychiatr.* 2014a;5:e1.

82. Saitz R, Alford DP, Bernstein J, Cheng DM, Samet J, Palfai T. Screening and brief intervention for unhealthy drug use in primary care settings: randomized clinical trials are needed. *J Addict Med.* 2010;4:123.

83. Saitz R, Palfai TP, Cheng DM, et al. Screening and brief intervention for drug use in primary care: the ASPIRE randomized clinical trial. *JAMA.* 2014;312:502–513.

84. Reference deleted in review.

85. Saunders JB, Aasland OG, Amundsen A, Grant M. Alcohol consumption and related problems among primary health care patients: WHO collaborative project on early detection of persons with harmful alcohol consumption – I. *Addiction.* 1993;88:349–362.

86. Saunders JB, Aasland OG, Babor TF, de la Fuente JR, Grant M. Development of the alcohol use disorders identification test (audit): who collaborative project on early detection of persons with harmful alcohol consumption – ii. *Addiction.* 1993;88:791–804.

87. Saunders JB, Lee NK. Hazardous alcohol use: its delineation as a subthreshold disorder, and approaches to its diagnosis and management. *Compr Psychiatr.* 2000;41:95–103.

88. Senore C, Battista RN, Shapiro SH, Segnan N, Ponti A, Rosso S, et al. Predictors of smoking cessation following physician' counseling. *Prev Med.* 1998;27:412–421.

89. Sinadinovic K, Wennberg P, Berman AH. Internet-based screening and brief intervention for illicit drug users: a randomized controlled trial with 12-month follow-up. *J Stud Alcohol Drugs.* 2014;75:313–318.

90. Skinner HA. The drug abuse screening test. *Addict Behav.* 1982;7:363–371.

91. Stead LF, Bergson G, Lancaster T. Physician advice for smoking cessation. *Cochrane Database Syst Rev.* 2008. https://doi.org/10.1002/14651858.CD000165.pub3.

92. Stoner SA, Hendershot CS. A randomized trial evaluating an mHealth system to monitor and enhance adherence to pharmacotherapy for alcohol use disorders. *Addict Sci Clin Pract.* 2012;7:9.

93. Reference deleted in review.

94. Tait RJ, Hulse GK. A systematic review of the effectiveness of brief interventions with substance using adolescents by type of drug. *Drug Alcohol Rev.* 2003;22:337–346.

95. Tait RJ, Hulse GK, Robertson SI. Effectiveness of a brief-intervention and continuity of care in enhancing attendance for treatment by adolescent substance users. *Drug Alcohol Depend.* 2004;74:289–296.

96. Tait RJ, Hulse GK, Robertson SI, Sprivulis P. Emergency department based intervention with adolescent substance users: 12-month outcomes. *Drug Alcohol Depend.* 2005;79:359–363.

97. Tait RJ, Spijkerman R, Riper H. Internet and computer based interventions for cannabis use: a meta-analysis. *Drug Alcohol Depend.* 2013;133:295.

98. Teesson M, Hall W, Lynskey M, Degenhardt L. Alcohol- and drug-use disorders in Australia: implications of the national survey of mental health and wellbeing. *Aust NZ J Psychiatry.* 2000;34:206–213.

99. Tengs TO, Adams ME, Pliskin JS, Safran DG, Siegel JE, Weinstein MC, et al. Five-hundred life-saving interventions and their cost-effectiveness. *Risk Anal.* 1995;15:369–390.

100. Reference deleted in review.

101. Reference deleted in review.

102. Warner KE. Cost effectiveness of smoking-cessation therapies. *Pharmacoeconomics.* 1995;11:538–549.

103. Werner MJ. Principles of brief intervention for adolescent alcohol, tobacco, and other drug use. *Pediatr Clin North Am.* 1995;42:335–349.

104. West R, McNeill A, Raw M. Smoking cessation guidelines for health professionals: an update. *Thorax.* 2000;55:987–999.

105. White A, Kavanagh DJ, Stallman H, Klein B, Kay-Lambkin F, Proudfoot J, et al. Online alcohol interventions: a systematic review. *J Med Internet Res.* 2010;12(5):e62.

106. Wilk AI, Jensen NM, Havighurst TC. Meta-analysis of randomized control trials addressing brief interventions in heavy alcohol drinkers. *J Gen Intern Med.* 1997;12:274–283.

107. Williams JM, Ziedonis D. Addressing tobacco among individuals with a mental illness or an addiction. *Addict Behav.* 2004;29:1067–1083.

108. World Health Organization. *International Statistical Classification of Diseases and Related Health Problems 10th Revision*; 2016. http://apps.who.int/classifications/icd10/browse/2016/en. Accessed on Jan 18 2016.

109. Zarkin G, Bray J, Hinde J, Saitz R. Costs of screening and brief intervention for illicit drug use in primary care settings. *J Stud Alcohol Drugs.* 2015;76:222–228.

44

Self-Help Approaches for Addictions

CHELSIE M. YOUNG, M. CHRISTINA HOVE, SHAUNA FULLER,
AND CLAYTON NEIGHBORS

Defining Self-Help

Help from without is often enfeebling in its effects, but help from within invariably invigorates.[190]

Self-help approaches to addiction encompass those strategies designed to reduce or eliminate substance use and/or associated negative consequences. As a construct, the boundaries that define self-help are potentially blurred. Virtually all successful and lasting change involves some degree of self-help and some measure of support by others. For the purposes of this chapter, we suggest two concrete boundary conditions that distinguish self-help strategies from other strategies: (1) the strategies are self-initiated and self-maintained and (2) the strategies do not involve enduring relationships with professional care providers, professional supervision or authority, or illicitly obtained prescription drugs. Under this umbrella fall techniques such as nonprescription substance replacement, bibliotherapy, helplines, spirituality and mindfulness, and Internet resources, as well as a variety of self-help groups. Interventions range in cost, intensity, accessibility, and efficacy, depending on the nature of the substance use.

This chapter begins with a brief review of relevant literature related to self-help in addiction, including reviews of natural recovery[103] and natural processes of change described in the Transtheoretical Model of Change.[168] Following a description of this literature, with the exception of self-help groups, this chapter reviews several self-help approaches and their applicability to the problematic use of specific substances.

Why Use Self-Help?

There are several reasons that an individual may opt for self-help methods as an alternative to professional care to manage substance use, including barriers in accessing treatment. In a national telephone survey of 14,985 residents from 60 randomly selected US communities, of those who reported that they needed help for substance abuse, well over one-third received no professional treatment, less treatment than they needed, or delays in treatment.[205] A commonly cited barrier to pursuing formal services for addiction concerns the high cost of treatment, which can lead some individuals who want help, but do not believe they can afford it, to manage their own care. Stigma and the associated negative attitudes that practitioners, medical staff, and other health professionals may convey toward the person seeking treatment often deter people from seeking professional rehabilitation services.[146] Feelings of shame, embarrassment, and failure only act to further embed fears of stigma. In these instances, self-help methods can provide an affordable, easily accessible, and anonymous point of entry into the recovery process.

Is Self-Help Good for Everyone?

Addictive behaviors can be and often are identified, modified, and resolved through self-initiated processes.[113,168] As reviewed later in this chapter, individuals who were once dependent on addictive substances have demonstrated the ability to change those maladaptive behaviors, often through means of self-help alone. Notwithstanding this, isolative and self-administered recovery, particularly in advanced cases of substance use disorders, may be ill-advised. With the exception of natural recovery (see subsequent text of this chapter), individuals fully entrenched in profound and active addiction are unlikely to manage successful and enduring recovery by relying exclusively on their own resources. In those cases, self-help interventions may best be understood as an initial stage in a multifaceted intervention approach, helping to facilitate a greater appreciation of the nature, symptoms, consequences, and resources available to combat substance use disorders.

Self-Help as Empowering

Although there are risks associated with self-administered treatment, there are also benefits in addition to alterations in substance use, which occur on an idiosyncratic level. Lacking professional intervention or guidance, individuals pursuing self-help interventions run the risk of potentially acquiring inadequate or ineffective information. However, self-help has the advantage of enabling individuals to achieve the internal resources necessary to feel a greater sense of autonomy and mastery over their behavior and their environment. This cultivated sense of power can have positive effects on self-esteem, self-efficacy, and personal responsibility.[16,17] These personal tools can breed the confidence and internal fortitude necessary to sustain recovery and prevent or recover from relapse.[168] Such changes in coping and identity may be instrumental and necessary for individuals to seek professional help in the process of recovery.[104]

Can Individuals Help Themselves?

At least two somewhat overlapping and extensive bodies of research literature have directly addressed the extent to which people can and do transition from problematic substance use, abuse, or dependence to less problematic use, moderate use, or abstinence without treatment or attendance in self-help groups such as 12-step or fellowship programs. These bodies of literature roughly correspond to the topics of *natural recovery* and the *Transtheoretical Model of Change*.

Natural Recovery

Natural recovery refers to the process by which many individuals who experience considerable difficulties related to their substance use successfully implement change without any formal assistance. Some individuals appear to simply "mature out," whereas others change in response to a specific event or set of circumstances. Sobell et al.[192] seminal examination of natural recovery from problematic alcohol and/or drug use (excluding tobacco) considered 40 samples of participants in 38 studies published between 1960 and 1997. Carballo and colleagues[36]

subsequently examined 22 studies published between 1999 and 2005 but used a more liberal time period in designation of substance use problem resolution.[103] Although the majority of studies of natural recovery have focused on alcohol, earlier studies also included heroin. In recent years, there has been a substantial surge in studies examining natural recovery from problematic cannabis use. These studies of natural recovery have largely relied on retrospective reports of participants' reasons for changing. These narrative accounts raise questions regarding potential memory distortions, self-serving biases, and/or inaccurate attributions of the effectiveness of specific factors leading to change. Nevertheless, they provide potentially important insights into successful self-help strategies. Combining the 40 studies from 1960 to 1997 reviewed by Sobell and colleagues[192] with the 22 studies from 1999 to 2005 examined by Carballo and colleagues,[36] we found that the most frequently reported reasons for reducing or eliminating substance use by successful self-changers were health-related (45%), financial (37%), negative personal reasons (e.g., shame and guilt, 35%), family-related (34%), significant other (32%), and religious reasons (31%). Factors most strongly associated with successful maintenance of change were social support (40%), family/significant other (34%), avoidance of substance use situations (24%), religion (23%), and developing non–substance-related interests (23%).

Maturation Effects

Related to the idea of natural recovery is the process of maturing out. Epidemiological literature and studies of natural history indicate that the highest rates of alcohol and other substance use occur during late adolescence and early adulthood.[12,103,132,182,226] Increasingly referred to as "emerging adulthood," the period corresponding from about high school graduation through the early 20s is associated with increased risk behaviors and experimentation across a range of high-risk behaviors, including substances of abuse. The majority of young adults who use substances during this developmental stage, even at problematic levels, reduce or eliminate use as they assume career and family responsibilities.[103] Individuals who experience substance use later in life and who reduce use without formal help tend to be in their mid-40s and report their heaviest use to be in their mid-to-late 20s,[177] further suggesting that, for many, natural recovery may be a maturational process.

With respect to research related to natural recovery, the majority of the literature has focused on alcohol. Other specific substances have also been examined in the context of natural recovery, including nicotine, marijuana, cocaine, and heroin, with relatively similar findings across substances. Natural recovery from nicotine, alcohol, and marijuana is reviewed below.

Nicotine

The vast majority (>80%) of individuals who quit smoking do so without treatment.[129,192] Narrative accounts of individuals who are successful with smoking cessation versus temporary cessation or current smokers suggest that the former who are successful report more severe consequences, more focused reasons for cessation, and more negative affect in describing reasons for quitting.[88,91] Successful quitters are also more likely to have and/or take advantage of good social support for cessation, to change their environment, and to feel less ambivalent about changes associated with the cessation process.

Alcohol

To date, the literature on natural recovery from substance use disorders has focused predominantly on alcohol. Consistent evidence now suggests that a large proportion of individuals who experience problems with alcohol are able to transition to moderate use or abstinence without formal help.[113,177,191] Heavy drinking is common in young adulthood but diminishes for most individuals as they take on traditional adult responsibilities (marriage, family, careers, and so on).[103] Beyond the developmental period of emerging adulthood, alcohol use disorders have continued to be viewed by many as resistant or impossible to change without assistance. These sentiments are a foundation underlying 12-step programs such as Alcoholics Anonymous (AA), where the fundamental premise stipulates that an individual is powerless over addiction and although it is not possible to be fully cured, continuous abstinence and therein remission is achievable by adhering to the program outlined in the 12 steps.[52,53] Within this framework, recovery is possible, whereas being cured or returned to a nonpathological use characterized by moderation, maturational effects, and natural recovery is not.

Individuals who successfully maintain natural recovery from problematic alcohol use often report initial motivation related to fear or anticipation of unacceptable life changes resulting from drinking, concern for the influence of one's drinking on his or her children, and religious inspiration.[35] Successful self-changers are more likely to have positive social support networks, be married, have higher self-esteem, and report less drug use and lower frequencies of intoxication.[177]

Marijuana

Relatively little research has examined natural recovery in the context of problematic cannabis use.[192] One 25-year follow-up of Vietnam Veterans found that 82.5% of cannabis cessation attempts occurred without treatment and that of those, 88.3% were successful.[167] Consistent with findings from the alcohol literature, successful self-help in cannabis use was most often initiated in response to changing views of personal use (cognitive evaluation) as well as negative consequences associated with continued use.[44,65] Strategies associated with successful change included modifications in lifestyle and the development of interests unrelated to cannabis use.

Processes of Change

Directly related to natural recovery, *processes of change* have been described as part of the Transtheoretical Model of Change (or Stages of Change Model).[60,168] The Transtheoretical Model of Change, which has been applied extensively to the field of substance use disorders and beyond, began with interviews of former smokers regarding their experiences with change. The model describes a sequence of stages in which individuals who are not initially aware of a need to change and are not in any way considering modification (precontemplation) over time begin to consider the possibility of making alterations (contemplation) and subsequently prepare for (preparation) and implement change (action). In the absence of relapse or regression to previous stages, individuals are ideally able to maintain change successfully (maintenance) over time. In the context of developing their model, Prochaska and DiClemente defined a number of processes that individuals identified as being important in their efforts to change. The processes of change include substitution, seeking information, cognitive evaluation, seeking support from others, self-rewards for change, affirmation of commitment, and restructuring one's environment. The Transtheoretical Model of Change and associated processes has provided a useful framework for considering how people identify, approach, and resolve problematic behavior. But it is also clear that original formulations of the model were overly simplistic.[59]

Self-Help Drug Replacement

Substance substitution or drug replacement therapy represents a potentially valuable self-help strategy for drug addictions. Substance substitution involves the practice of replacing specific substances to assist with the withdrawal or cessation of another drug or substance, the latter usually possessed of more significant, immediate, or well-known negative consequences. This method of intervention is also employed in some instances solely during the detox period, in order to facilitate fewer extreme withdrawal symptoms. There is some controversy around drug replacement therapy based on objections regarding the replacement of one addictive substance for another; however, it is a contemporarily well-accepted method of achieving harm reduction or abstinence from various substances. This is typically achieved by providing a lower dose of the same substance, varying the route of administration, or alternative substance replacement. Whether the goal is to provide a more predictable and manageable decline in substance dependence or to facilitate rapid removal, drug replacement therapy typically acts to reduce or mitigate the withdrawal symptoms commonly associated with physical dependence. To a lesser extent, it can also act as a means to replace, shift, or decrease the psychological correlates of addiction associated through habit, socialization, peer pressure, stress relief, and celebration. Although there are many pharmacological options available to manage withdrawal and cravings, this section focuses on nonmedically monitored options for drug replacement.

Replacement and Caffeine

Caffeine is a plant alkaloid found in numerous species, which acts as a central nervous system and metabolic stimulant. Estimates have indicated that upwards of 90% of American adults consume caffeine on a daily basis[123]; it is also believed to be one of the most widely used psychoactive substances in the world.[69] Caffeine is typically consumed to overcome lethargy, to promote vigilance and alertness, and to elevate mood. The major source of caffeine is coffee beans, but it is also commonly found in chocolate, tea, and soft drinks, as well as energy drinks and over-the-counter medications for headaches, pain relief, and appetite control. Although caffeine remains unscheduled and recognized by the US Food and Drug Administration (FDA) as a "safe food substance," it is an addictive substance that can lead to withdrawal symptoms after cessation of consistent use.[216] Caffeine may be commonly overlooked as a drug of abuse, in part due to its nearly universal legal status, prevalence as a normative food staple, and absence of commonly associated negative consequences. Furthermore, people may be unaware of or may underestimate their daily caffeine consumption, as the drug is associated mainly in connection with coffee. As a result, consumers may not be aware of the amount of regular consumption, impact on their daily functioning, or degree of physiologic and psychologic dependence.

The fifth edition of the American Psychiatric Association's *Diagnostic and Statistical Manual of Mental Disorders* (DSM-5) identifies Caffeine-Related Disorders to include Caffeine

Intoxication and Caffeine Withdrawal.[5] Currently, caffeine use cannot be diagnosed as a formal substance use disorder; however, Caffeine Use Disorder was identified as a condition for further study. The symptoms of acute caffeine intoxication may include restlessness, nervousness, hyperexcitability, insomnia, gastrointestinal disturbance, muscle twitching, rambling, tachycardia, and agitation. Very rarely, high doses of caffeine (>10 g) may produce respiratory failure or seizures. Regular users commonly develop tolerance to caffeine and may experience intense cravings after discontinuation. Withdrawal symptoms include headaches, flu-like symptoms, feelings of lethargy and reduced motivation, and dysphoric or irritable mood.

Individuals seeking to reduce or abstain from caffeine may find that the cravings can be managed by substance replacement. Because caffeine is less addictive than are other socially acceptable substances (e.g., alcohol, nicotine), replacement in social settings may be more easily achieved, providing a particularly effective way to reduce caffeine and mitigate adverse health consequences. The most popular replacement for caffeine is decaffeinated coffee, which contains between 2–15 mg of caffeine per 8-ounce cup compared to between 80–100 mg of caffeine in an 8-ounce cup of caffeinated drip coffee. International standards require that decaffeinated coffee beans are 97% free of caffeine, while the European Union standard requires that coffee beans are 99% caffeine-free by mass. This small amount of the active substance may help attenuate withdrawal symptoms including headaches, nausea, vomiting, muscle pain, and stiffness. Decaffeinated and herbal teas offer another option for caffeine replacement. Those individuals who are interested in reducing their caffeine intake from soft drinks have a variety of brand options offering caffeine-free drinks. There remains scant literature concerning the effectiveness of decaffeinated substitution for caffeine use; however, replacement in this manner can be a helpful harm reduction approach to significantly reduce one's intake of the drug (in the case of decaffeinated coffee) or to eliminate intake altogether.

Replacement and Nicotine

Both anecdotal evidence and scientific data speak to the highly addictive nature of nicotine, and more specifically, of nicotine found in tobacco products. Researchers regard nicotine as one of the most addictive recreational substances in use.[92,93] Similarly, the American Heart Association considers nicotine to be one of the hardest addictions to break. Nicotine, a central nervous system stimulant, is a plant alkaloid found most abundantly in tobacco leaves and is thought to be the main factor responsible for the dependence-forming properties of tobacco smoke. Although inhalation of tobacco smoke is the most common route of nicotine administration, tobacco may also be insufflated or chewed. Tobacco smoke contains carbon monoxide, as well as a mixture of particulate substances generated by the combustion process that make up tobacco tar.[69] Inhalation of carbon monoxide and tar is primarily responsible for the various diseases resulting from long-term use. Physiological and psychological dependence on nicotine generally develops quite rapidly, reflecting nicotine's pharmacokinetic properties, which are characterized by rapid distribution of nicotine to the brain that reaches peak levels within 10 seconds of administration. However, the acute effects of nicotine dissipate rapidly, as do the associated feelings of reward, promoting re-administration in order to maintain the drug's pleasurable effects and prevent withdrawal. This characteristic pattern of administration/reward and withdrawal/punishment is instrumental in maintaining nicotine use despite its negative consequences.

Rapid decreases in cigarette use can result in a variety of uncomfortable withdrawal effects including restlessness, increases in appetite, difficulty concentrating, irritability, constipation, and sleep disruption. Given the myriad of injurious and life-threatening implications of regular, heavy tobacco use, there have been massive public health initiatives to address this problem. Consistent and strong positive associations exist between cessation of use and maintaining a tobacco-free lifestyle. The US Department of Health and Human Services underscores that early tobacco use relapse is associated with difficulty coping with withdrawal symptoms.[215] In order to increase cessation success rates, nicotine replacement strategies were introduced to mitigate the early intense withdrawal symptoms linked with relapse,[165] and thereby improve successful cessation maintenance.

Nicotine Replacement Options

Perhaps the most widely known drug replacement approach is through the use of nicotine products. Nicotine replacement therapy is consistently found to be an efficacious front-line intervention designed to deliver nicotine with the intent to significantly reduce the severity and intensity of withdrawal symptoms. The FDA approved nicotine gum in the early 1980s, and by the mid-1990s nicotine patches were available without a prescription. The Tobacco Use and Dependence Guideline Panel reviewed and distilled more than 8700 research articles to establish clinical practice procedures in the treatment of tobacco use and dependence. Nicotine replacement was found to be so effective as a front-line treatment in tobacco dependence that it is included in five of the seven first-line medications identified as reliably curbing dependence and promoting long-term abstinence.[210] Over time, research has demonstrated that smoking cessation can be improved by approximately 50% when coupled with nicotine replacement therapy.[165] Nicotine replacement therapy is a recommended add-on for all smokers interested in quitting, with the exception of pregnant women, smokeless tobacco users, light smokers, and adolescents. Nicotine replacement products are available in various routes of administration such as gum, inhalers, patches, tablets, lozenges, and sprays. They are readily available over the counter in most pharmacies, drug stores, and grocery stores. Route of administration does not appear to impact outcomes.

More recently, electronic nicotine delivery systems (ENDS), such as electronic- or e-cigarettes, have become readily available and a popular alternative to tobacco cigarettes. ENDS are battery-powered instruments often manufactured to look like conventional cigarettes, cigars, or pipes, and referred to as vaporizers, vape pens, hookah pens, e-pipes, and e-cigarettes that deliver vaporized liquid nicotine. No smoke, tobacco, or combustion is part of its mechanism of action. ENDS work by heating liquid composed of propylene glycol, glycerin, flavoring, and nicotine until it vaporizes. They were developed in 2003, and by 2007 were marketed in the United States and Europe as a method to safely quit smoking. There are estimates that more than 250 different ENDS brands are currently available.

Although e-cigarettes have received a great deal of attention as a replacement for tobacco cigarettes, little is known about their addictive nature and potential harmful effects. Given that these products were not regulated by the FDA at their introduction, they were readily accessible to adolescents, and by 2012 use among this group doubled.[40] Despite their appeal to adolescents, ostensibly new nicotine users, research suggests that most users of e-cigarettes are current or former tobacco cigarette smokers.[181] In May 2016, the FDA extended federal authority to regulate e-cigarettes, thus prohibiting the sale of e-cigarettes to individuals under the age of 18.

Prior to that, *The New England Journal of Medicine*[105] reported that some e-cigarettes contain and release formaldehyde, further calling into question the possible carcinogenic effects and associated hazards, which remain largely unknown. The e-cigarette industry, which has until 2016 been essentially unregulated, also augments the vaporized liquid with supplementary additives and flavorings that have questionable safety implications.

ENDS have continued to gain momentum and popularity in recent years as a lifestyle product for smokers interested in mitigating the well-established risks associated with traditional cigarette smoking; their popularity continues to grow as they simulate the behavioral and sensory elements of smoking while being perceived as healthier.[162] They have been noted as playing a role in smoking cessation or tobacco harm reduction techniques.[128,169] A randomized controlled trial examined the efficacy of e-cigarettes compared with nicotine replacement therapy for smoking cessation and discovered moderate effectiveness in helping smokers quit with limited side effects.[34] Reviews of research focused on the effectiveness of e-cigarettes in the reduction or cessation of tobacco demonstrate positive, although weak, associations. However, little substantive information was gleaned from a current review of the literature due to a lack of longitudinal research and consistent limitations in study designs, suggesting that more research in this domain is sorely needed.[128]

Replacement and Alcohol

Alcohol use is common and prevalent, with estimates suggesting that three of four adults consume alcohol on at least a periodic or social basis. Low-level intoxication generally produces feelings of euphoria and relaxation and has been associated with pain relief. Higher levels of intoxication result in motor impairment, mood lability, memory loss, confusion, and toxicity. Consistent with standards established in the DSM-5, an Alcohol Use Disorder involves a repetitive pattern of use resulting in alcohol cravings, tolerance, withdrawal symptoms, and difficulty limiting or eliminating use despite overt negative consequences.[5] Treatment of Alcohol Use Disorders often involves both mitigating and ameliorating withdrawal effects, which when left untreated tend to perpetuate drinking cycles, while concurrently improving emotional regulation and functional coping skills.

Alcohol produces one of the more severe abstinence syndromes associated with withdrawal, which has the potential to result in delirium tremens (DTs); these are characterized by severe disorientation, confusion, hallucinations, blood pressure spikes, seizures, and in some cases death. Individuals who are most likely to experience withdrawal effects are those who have maintained a high blood alcohol content (BAC) level for several days in a row, have become intoxicated every evening for at least a month, and have histories of alcohol withdrawal symptoms. In short, the heavier the consumption and longer the time period, the more likely one is to experience withdrawal effects. Mild to moderate withdrawal symptoms include sleep difficulties/fragmentation, anxiety, sweating, increased blood pressure/pulse, tremors, and gastrointestinal upset. More severe withdrawal symptoms include DTs, which typically set in 48 hours or more after decline in alcohol consumption. It should be noted that generally mild to moderate withdrawal symptoms are not dangerous, although they can be for individuals with high blood pressure who have an additional risk of heart attack or stroke. Withdrawal symptoms generally remit after 24 hours following the last drink consumed.

Consequently, medically driven and supervised withdrawal is generally recommended, especially for individuals with chronic and heavy alcohol use histories. Despite this recommendation and the constellation of medical risks upon which it is based, many individuals prefer to step down their alcohol use through tapering procedures, thereby attenuating the effects of withdrawal. And although medical detox is safer, often more comfortable, and imposes structure that increases success, issues of geographic barriers, financial limitations, and psychiatric stigma remain instrumental in determining alcohol-related withdrawal preferences. Medical facilities increasingly prohibit patients from using nicotine products, while at the same time neglecting or refusing to provide nicotine replacement therapy, contributing to an already overwhelming process of withdrawal and discomfort, and which may act to dissuade an ambivalent patient from medically supervised detox. In addition, medical detox is most commonly accompanied with a diagnosis of Alcohol Use Disorder,[5] a historically stigmatizing label that can have an impact on contemporary and future medical treatment, health insurance, and vocational/academic opportunities. As a function of these and additional issues, many individuals make the decision to pursue self-managed tapering in order to decrease alcohol consumption while minimizing withdrawal effects.

Self-directed, nonmedical taper programs are available through online resources. Harm reduction, Abstinence and Moderation Support (HAMS) or the Harm Reduction for Alcohol network (hamsnetwork.org) publishes online resources regarding harm reduction approaches to alcohol use, which includes detailed instructions on a tapering program. The entirety of the program will not be repeated here; it can be accessed online through the HAMS network. Briefly, the approach involves moving alcohol consumption to beer and then drinking only a small amount to minimize or mitigate withdrawal effects. Critical to this plan is developing a personalized titration schedule in order to maximize program adherence. Although this can be a successful approach when followed appropriately, there are clearly a host of risks involved in self-managed titration of an addictive substance, including but not limited to infidelity to the program standards. If the taper schedule is self-monitored, there are no external checks in place to provide external supervision. In addition, the plan advocates the administration of a mind-altering substance that has a direct influence on frontal lobe functioning including disinhibition and impulsivity, depressant impact on motor cortex involving coordination, and additional physiological symptoms, all of which are well-established as negatively impacting decision-making. Disinhibition and impulsivity associated with alcohol may provide the user a feeling of license to deviate from the plan in a manner that is interpreted as acceptable at the time but potentially decreases the chances for successful implementation. In addition, any abrupt alteration of entrenched, heavy alcohol use including self-help taper programs increases the probability of an acute medical situation, which would occur in the absence of medical support and assistance.

Another commonly employed approach to alcohol replacement involves the consumption of nonalcoholic beer or wine in substitution of alcoholic beverages. This approach can be especially helpful in social settings, where the addition of normative peer pressure regarding alcohol consumption is relatively greater. In addition to issues of physiological dependence, the psychological facets of alcohol dependence can be overwhelming, in part because alcohol may serve an important social role in one's life. Low-alcohol substitutes approximate beer and wine without the alcohol content. These substitutes typically contain 0.5% or less of ethanol by volume, which is the maximum content that a beverage may contain to be legally called nonalcoholic in the United States. Thus the use of nonalcoholic beverages may help in the maintenance of abstinence by allowing an individual to continue to engage in social situations.

Drug substitution for alcohol may also be achieved with the use of herbal substances. Kudzu and kudzu extract have received attention recently as a potentially viable herbal supplement to attenuate the anxiogenic effects of withdrawal and perhaps even reduce cravings and urges to use alcohol. It is thought to reduce the intoxicating effects of alcohol and therefore to have potential in assisting users in moderating or reducing consumption.[124,187] Due to the paucity of research in this area, very little can be gleaned from the current literature; furthermore, this remains an untapped area for controlled studies.

Bibliotherapy

Perspectives in Bibliotherapy

Bibliotherapy, the belief that psychological and behavioral change can be affected by the content of written materials, has been a consistent method of self-help throughout history.[175] Religious materials such as the Bible, Sutras, Talmud, Quran, and the Vedas serve as enduring examples of self-directed tools for growth and change. Consistent with this, many psychiatric hospitals in the United States had established libraries by the middle of the 19th century.[178] Bibliotherapy remains a resource- and cost-effective intervention that is widely available, self-paced, and lacks the stigma associated with other interventions, which often deter individuals from seeking assistance.

Although there are clear benefits to bibliotherapy including availability, accessibility, and approachability, its efficacy in promoting change is less clear. As noted by Scogin,[183] many self-help books are not based on relevant theory or evidence-based treatments and therefore have predictable limitations in utility. Some research suggests that maladaptive habituated behavioral disruptions (i.e., alcohol consumption, smoking, nail-biting, and overeating) in general may not be as amenable to bibliotherapeutic interventions relative to other psychiatric conditions such as mood disorders.[88,184] In addition, individuals who benefit most from bibliotherapy tend to be self-referred,[9] thus the currently reported success rates might underestimate its effectiveness. Finally, variability in objective definition acts to diffuse the outcome of those investigations that do exist.

The concept of bibliotherapy is widely variable, such that references may describe a spectrum of behaviors and resources: from an individual reading a self-help manual to a professional care provider prescribing a relevant book chapter. For the purposes of this chapter, and consistent with a number of published studies,[9,122] the term bibliotherapy will refer to any self-directed therapeutic intervention presented in a written format that is designed to motivate and guide the process of change behavior. Those empirical investigations employing congruent definitions of bibliotherapy related to substance abuse were restricted to the reduction of nicotine, alcohol, and marijuana. A review of the literature did not find empirical research evaluating the efficacy of bibliotherapy for cocaine, opiates, or opioids.

Bibliotherapy for Nicotine

Smoking remains the leading annual cause of preventable premature morbidity and mortality annually in the United States.[141] Despite the fact that 40% of smokers attempt to quit each year (Centers for Disease Control and Prevention),[39] only about 5% are successful in maintaining abstinence for one year.[38,101] Various methods of assistance for smoking cessation, including counseling,[119,196,198] nicotine replacement therapy (NRT),[99,180,197] and pharmacotherapy such as buproprion[102,106] have been demonstrated to improve success rates.[239] Despite this, the majority of smokers who try to quit do so without seeking assistance or intervention.[71,163,188,239] Those smokers who employ interventions may represent the more nicotine-dependent proportion of the population,[71,188] who are at proportionally greater risk of relapse. Relapses, especially recurrent relapses, are generally detrimental to perseverance and successful cessation,[32,163,195,218,223] underscoring the importance of efficacious treatment interventions.

A vast array of bibliotherapeutic materials designed to promote smoking cessation exist,[81] from brief motivational pamphlets[3] to comprehensive manuals addressing initial cessation through relapse prevention.[4] These manuals are often based on cognitive behavioral models (e.g., social learning, transtheoretical model, relapse prevention) and designed as translations of therapist-administered multicomponent cessation programs. Despite the assortment of literature available, the evidence regarding the efficacy of bibliotherapeutic tools and, particularly, as applied in isolation is less compelling.

Although there appears to be preference for self-administered treatments such as bibliotherapy among individuals seeking to quit smoking,[71,188] research has not consistently demonstrated the ability of such materials to increase cessation and maintenance rates. Rather, only marginal benefits are associated with generic self-help materials (e.g., pamphlets, booklets) relative to no intervention.[76,119] Alternate treatment options including natural recovery,[72] telephone counseling,[57,153] and NRT[112] have demonstrated greater efficacy than generic bibliotherapy. Although research does not generally support the efficacy of generic bibliotherapeutic materials in isolation, there is evidence of increased cessation and maintenance rates when they are integrated with other treatments.

Tailoring written materials to specific individuals and populations whether in-person or via technology appears to increase the effectiveness of bibliotherapy. Self-help materials that are tailored to individual smokers appear marginally more effective than generic materials.[86,203] Meta-analytic studies have found that tailored materials have demonstrated greater efficacy for smoking cessation beyond no intervention[86,119] and relative to generic manuals (N = 20,414; odds ratio [OR] 1.42, 95% confidence interval [CI] 1.26 to 1.61).[119] Bibliotherapeutic materials were found to be efficacious in cessation and maintenance within intensive group programs when individuals participated in the prescribed activities associated with the reading.[54] This may be due to compliance with the program, inasmuch as individuals who are able to utilize and integrate self-help materials successfully are better able to adapt programmatic change into long-term lifestyle changes.[56] Although attempts to tailor self-help material to firefighters by employing language common to the fire service did not produce benefits beyond the American Lung Association's generic guide,[152] the combination of tailored smoking outcome and self-efficacy–enhancing information produced a significant effect on smoking cessation.[61] Thus the most promising effects for bibliotherapeutic interventions appear to be found in combinations of personalized adjuncts, such as written feedback in conjunction with outreach telephone counseling[57,153] or web-based, personalized feedback.[64] In sum, bibliotherapeutic interventions for smoking cessation appear most likely to be effective when tailored to specific population characteristics and include empirically based enhancements.

Bibliotherapy for Alcohol

Bibliotherapeutic materials designed to reduce maladaptive alcohol use are conceptually similar to smoking cessation publications in that they are often based on cognitive behavioral models, which are intended as easily digestible translations of multicomponent, professionally administered programs. The evidence regarding these resources is mixed but appears promising, particularly with the addition of technologically driven enhancements and when construed as the initial intervention in a stepped-care approach to alcohol treatment.[126,193]

Meta-analytic reviews of self-help programs designed to address problematic alcohol use have revealed differentially effective rates, somewhat dependent on the nature and severity of the treatment target. Research has not consistently revealed significant gains associated with bibliotherapy.[9,15] Greater efficacy has been associated with interpersonal intervention compared to bibliotherapy among at-risk users and those with severe alcohol use disorders. At-risk drinkers participating in individual or group alcohol skills training programs demonstrated greater preference, perceived assistance, and enduring change in alcohol use relative to those provided with bibliotherapeutic intervention only.[15] Among heavy drinkers, bibliotherapy alone was not found to be as effective as bibliotherapy in conjunction with brief advice or counseling.[233]

Despite this, other studies offer support for the efficacy of bibliotherapeutic interventions, particularly for early stage intervention. Bibliotherapeutic interventions appear better suited to address at-risk or mild cases of alcohol use disorders.[126] Apodaca and Miller's[9] meta-analysis revealed a small to medium effect size for bibliotherapy versus no intervention, and moderate support for bibliotherapy to reduce at-risk alcohol use. Consistent with these findings, a self-help manual in conjunction with limited professional contact (10 minutes) was found to be effective beyond treatment as usual in promoting alcohol cessation among pregnant women with mild alcohol abuse.[171] In a series of studies involving only limited professional contact (i.e., brief telephone contact and one 1-hour session), Miller and colleagues found reductions in alcohol consumption associated with a self-help manual that matched reductions associated with more involved treatment options,[136,139,140] which were found to be enduring.[135,138] Thus, there is mixed evidence regarding bibliotherapeutic efficacy. Based on this information, it appears likely that bibliotherapy is at least marginally more effective than no intervention, and may be more influential in early intervention than in later stages of addiction.

The most promising innovations in written interventions for alcohol use disorders appear to be within self-guided, technologically delivered interventions. It is important to note that these web-based interventions include significant professional contributions in development and thus may not be considered strictly bibliotherapeutic self-help; however, as noted earlier, the most effective print interventions are also the product of substantial professional contributions. Based on this, web-based interventions that were self-administered and self-directed were included in the current review. Self-help information presented within a technologically enhanced platform (e.g., web-based programming) appears to afford greater usability, and has demonstrated

efficacy across the range of alcohol use disorders. Interactivity and personalization appear to be essential features of successful web-based self-help interventions. For example, Riper and colleagues[173] found greater reductions in alcohol use among at-risk drinkers participating in a web-based, interactive, self-administered alcohol intervention relative to a web-based, generic, self-administered brochure. Similar web-based, personalized, self-administered programs have demonstrated efficacy in altering the motives that promote maladaptive alcohol use while also reducing contemporary alcohol consumption,[149] with demonstrated persistence in positive change.[147] These programs were also effective in reducing event-specific binge-drinking among at-risk drinkers (e.g., 21st birthday).[148] These findings extend to heavy drinkers, an area that bibliotherapeutic techniques have historically not been robustly effective. Reductions in alcohol consumption were found among heavy drinkers following participation in a web-based, self-administered intervention with gains persisting at 3 months.[51,117] Some research suggests that the addition of traditional bibliotherapeutic self-help materials to web-based interventions may produce additive benefits.[50] Furthermore, independent meta-analysis and reviews support the efficacy of technology-assisted self-help treatments,[151] although some professional contact may be optimal for sustained reductions in addictive behaviors.[111]

All told, although the research regarding bibliotherapeutic interventions for maladaptive alcohol use and web-based, personalized interventions appear promising, several caveats exist. Traditional and contemporary bibliotherapeutic interventions have the benefit of being nonintrusive, inexpensive, and, based on existing research, are perhaps best framed as an initial intervention in a stepped-care approach for mild or moderate alcohol abuse.[122] Bibliotherapeutic interventions that utilize interactive, fluid, web-based platforms demonstrate promising efficacy across a range of alcohol use disorders but perhaps particularly among at-risk drinkers. It is likely that continued development and adaptation in this area will contribute significantly to prevention and treatment in the future. These advances are most likely to be effective among groups with less access to traditional alcohol-related services such as women, younger individuals, and at-risk users.[224] In summary, when determining whether self-help is an appropriate treatment modality, individual characteristics, familiarity with web-based computer resources, access to professional care, and the severity of the substance use disorder should all be taken into consideration.[126]

Bibliotherapy for Marijuana

Based on a review of the literature to date, it is difficult to come to any conclusions regarding the utility of bibliotherapy as an intervention for marijuana use, particularly as a stand-alone intervention. A Canadian mental health study revealed that individuals acknowledging weekly cannabis use were more interested in receiving a self-help book or a computerized normative use summary than telephone counseling or individual psychotherapy.[48] Cannabis users may be well-suited to minimally intrusive interventions, since the majority, including those who meet criteria for dependence, will never seek treatment.[47] However, further research is required to elucidate the appropriateness and enduring benefits of bibliotherapy within this population.

Expressive Writing

Expressive writing is the practice of reflecting upon and ultimately writing down one's deepest thoughts and feelings, often regarding a specific topic. Expressive writing was first introduced by Pennebaker and Beall[159] as a means of examining whether writing about one's deepest thoughts and feelings about a traumatic event would improve one's health. Thirty years later, hundreds of research investigations have harnessed the power of writing to improve individuals' health and well-being and to decrease negative health behaviors (see references 160 and 161 for reviews). Expressive writing is thought to exert its effects by allowing individuals to disclose emotions that they may have been afraid to express previously, cognitively restructure and find meaning in their experiences, and learn how to better regulate themselves and their emotions. Since its creation, the expressive writing paradigm has been modified and applied more broadly as a health and well-being promoting intervention. Recent research has begun to explore the use of expressive writing as a self-help intervention for individuals engaging in substance use behaviors. The basic premise of expressive writing is that writing and reflecting on one's substance use behavior may result in a better understanding of one's feelings toward his/her substance use behavior and the impact that drug use has on his or her life and the lives of those close to them. This process of self-reflection may then motivate individuals to change their behavior and formulate plans for how to enact change in their lives.

Expressive Writing and Nicotine

The first study to implement an expressive writing paradigm to promote smoking cessation among young adult smokers found that adding a four-session expressive writing component to an existing counseling intervention did not improve intervention efficacy 6-months postbaseline.[6] The authors proposed that effects may not have been found because of the short follow-up period, so they conducted a second trial extending the follow-up period to 52 weeks and adding an additional writing session.[7] After 8 weeks of treatment, the expressive writing plus counseling group had significantly higher abstinence rates compared to the counseling only group; however, abstinence did not differ between treatment groups at 24- and 52-week follow-ups.[7] Although the research is limited, these studies do provide some support for adding an expressive writing component to an existing empirically supported intervention to potentially boost its efficacy. Furthermore, they suggest that using longer follow-ups and more frequent expressive writing sessions may be more likely to result in smoking abstinence, which can inform future expressive writing interventions to reduce smoking and promote change for other health behaviors.

Expressive Writing and Alcohol

To date, three studies have examined whether expressive writing leads to reductions in intentions for future drinking as well as reductions in actual drinking behavior. One study found that writing about a recent job loss reduced alcohol use at 6-week follow-up.[194] More recently, the expressive writing paradigm has been adapted to ask individuals to write about a negative heavy drinking episode. Results from two studies found that expressive writing about a negative heavy drinking occasion was associated with increased readiness to change one's drinking behavior,[174] and decreased intentions for engaging in future drinking.[234] Although expressive writing is itself not a new paradigm, adapting this approach for individuals to help them reduce their substance use is novel and largely unexplored. More investigations are needed to examine the efficacy of expressive writing as a brief intervention to reduce substance use behavior.

Helplines

A helpline is a telephone-based service that provides information, support, and advice to callers with a wide range of problems or concerns. This section focuses more specifically on quitlines/helplines through telephone intervention alone, since a separate section of this chapter is devoted to self-help through the use of web-based technology. Burgeoning web-based and phone applications have emerged as a means for providing accessible intervention in curbing the use of drugs and alcohol. More recently, in an effort to become increasingly accessible, some helplines are also offered in tandem with web-based programming.[145] A thorough review of the current literature did not reveal significant new contributions since the previous edition of this text. It is suspected that as technology has advanced, movement/interest has shifted away from telephone helplines and toward smart-phone and web-based applications. This section remains included, as quitlines remain a cost-effective, accessible, and viable option for specific groups, including older, lower income, rural, and minority populations.

Helplines offer a variety of distinct advantages unique to other forms of self-help, which may make them more accessible or appealing than seeking face-to-face counseling or professional treatment. Helplines provide an efficient means for delivering treatment to populations across wide geographic areas by eliminating barriers of access (e.g., transportation, child care, or scheduling conflicts). Many helplines are government funded and free of charge to callers, which enables them to reach more underserved populations (e.g., under/uninsured, low socioeconomic status).[8,22,154] Indeed, research has suggested that lower income, less educated, nonwhite, and older individuals tend to utilize telephone-based helplines (versus helplines coupled with Internet), suggesting that this remains a viable source of help for some populations.[145] Finally, helplines provide immediate treatment and support while preserving the caller's anonymity, a feature that may attract drug users who are already battling with stigma associated with their drug use.[100]

Helplines for Nicotine

The majority of published research on substance-abuse helplines has focused primarily on nicotine dependence, often referred to as "quitlines." Although quitlines are generally regarded as effective in helping smokers quit,[214] less in known about the effectiveness of helplines to treat other drug or alcohol use.[77] Therefore the majority of this section has been devoted to the evidence-based literature regarding quitlines. In the 1980s, television antismoking campaigns began in Australia and public service messages about the risks of smoking were introduced in the United States via 1-800-4-Cancer, which was launched as a call-in center to receive advice on smoking risks/cessation. Both programs demonstrated effectiveness in increasing motivation to quit, and as a result, quitlines gained both popularity and momentum.[165] Quitlines have since spread throughout North America, Europe, parts of South America, Asia, Australia, and South Africa.[8] Although many smokers are aware of quitlines as an adjunct support to smoking cessation, generally less than 5% of smokers actually access them.[179]

Nicotine Helpline Services

At a minimum, the majority of quitlines offer free self-help resources and other bibliotherapeutic information to callers. This is the most ubiquitous and standard service provided by quitlines.

Another common feature includes reactive smoking cessation counseling—reactive in the sense that the call is initiated by the smoker, who is able to speak with a counselor. Other services may include proactive counseling (counselor calls the client), replacement or cessation medication, chat rooms, referrals to other cessation resources, and recorded messages.[22,41,109,155]

Characteristics of Nicotine Helpline Callers and Specific Protocols

In general, smokers are four times more likely to use quitlines than face-to-face clinics.[109,238] Studies examining the characteristics of callers to a national reactive telephone quitline found an overrepresentation of disadvantaged (i.e., African-American, women, poorer, urban, less educated, older) and heavier smokers compared with the general population.[73,237] Due to the wide range of consumers, many quitlines have adopted specialized protocols to address the unique concerns of specific populations. Common specialized protocols exist for pregnant women, older adults, adolescents, ethnic minorities, smokeless tobacco users, and callers with multiple addictions.[46,209,236]

Nicotine Helplines and the Transtheoretical Model of Change

Although individuals committed to smoking cessation appear to benefit most from quitline support, research suggests that quitlines may be efficacious for individuals across a wide range of readiness to change. Previous research suggests that many first-time callers to smoking quitlines have already made plans to quit, and that these individuals tend to benefit most from the quitline intervention.[90,213] Helgason and colleagues[90] found that 22% of first-time callers were in the action stage (had quit for 6 months or less), 76% were in the preparation (planning to quit within the next 4 weeks) or the contemplation (interested in trying to quit within the next 6 months) stage, whereas only 2% were in the precontemplation stage (not interested in trying to quit within the next 6 months). Although callers who were smoke free (action/maintenance) at the start of the intervention had the highest likelihood of being abstinent at the end of the study, there were also positive outcomes for callers in the other three stages. Half of the first-time callers in the precontemplation stage advanced to either the contemplation or the action/maintenance stage by the end of the quitline intervention. Similarly, for callers in the contemplation stage at baseline, half progressed to either the preparation stage or the action/maintenance stage, whereas only 10% regressed to an earlier stage.[90] Of interest, although this research suggests that quitlines can help move callers from one stage of change to the next (e.g., from contemplation to action),[90,154] many quitlines in the United States restrict services to callers who are planning to quit.[46]

Helplines for Alcohol and Illicit Drugs

In a controlled experiment based in Wisconsin,[33] researchers recruited nearly 900 patients from clinic waiting rooms who were not necessarily seeking help for their drinking problems. Half of the participants received pamphlets about healthy living, while the remaining participants received telephone counseling in which counselors assisted in setting drinking goals and overcoming barriers to behavioral change. Telephone counseling reduced alcohol consumption by 17.3% for men and 13.9% for women, compared with 12.9% and 11%, respectively, for pamphlet-only conditions.[33]

The most promising research on alcohol helplines has been conducted on the UK telephone-based service known as "Drinkline." Established in 1993, Drinkline receives about 6000 calls a month, the majority of which are problem drinkers seeking help for themselves. Callers are given information about safe drinking levels, advice about how to control drinking or avoid alcohol, and suggestions for how to overcome any related problems. A survey of callers showed that 81% received the information that they needed and 91% intended to carry out a plan of action after calling Drinkline.[225] An extensive search failed to identify any comparable literature for alcohol helplines in the United States.

Despite the abundance of alcohol helplines, there remains a dearth of research on their protocol, services, and effectiveness. In a recent review of the effectiveness of alcohol and illicit drug use helplines, only 36 publications were identified. In total, 29 articles investigating or reporting on 19 different drug or alcohol helplines, (located in the United States, Europe, Australia, Asia, and Canada) were reported, further illustrating the paucity of research available in this domain.[77] A thorough review of the literature suggests that, for the most part, helplines focus primarily on alcohol and nicotine use.[198] Unfortunately an exhaustive review of the literature did not reveal any new investigations on helplines for alcohol.

Helplines for Anabolic-Androgenic Steroids

One of the most advanced, established, and researched helplines that specializes in steroid use remains the Anti-Doping Hot-Line founded by the Swedish health authorities with the support of the Swedish National Institute of Health.[63] This helpline provides information about side effects and risks associated with anabolic-androgenic steroids, as well as facilitating contact between users and health care agents. The telephone service not only reaches out to anabolic-androgenic steroid users and concerned family and friends but also informs health professionals and organizations (e.g., public schools) about doping issues. In fact, the majority of callers to the Anti-Doping Hot-Line are nonabusers.[63] Since the implementation and subsequent success of this Sweden-based helpline in 1993, Japan, France, Denmark, and other nations with high rates of anabolic-androgenic steroid abuse have followed suit with their own steroid helplines (primarily targeting athletes and adolescents).[18,21,209]

Helplines for Cocaine, Methamphetamines, and Opiates

Due to the highly addictive and harmful nature of drugs like cocaine, methamphetamines, and opiates, strictly outpatient and self-help methods of recovery, such as helplines, are less common. It is telling that there is nominal research on the topic. However, 24-hour, 7-days-a-week phone services remain available (e.g., Moderation Management, National Meth Helpline, Cocaine Addiction Helpline, and Heroin Addiction Helpline) that offer no-cost assessments and dispense advice on how to stop, how to help a loved one quit, interventions, information, and hallmark signs of addiction.

In recent years, prescription drug abuse has surged as a very serious public health concern. In an effort to address the rapid increase in prescriptive drug overdoses and deaths, the West Virginia Prescription Drug Abuse Quitline (WVPDAQ) was developed. The primary mission of the WVPDAQ is to provide support, information, and viable referral sources for individuals addicted to prescription medication. It was the first remotely operated quitline to provide telephone assistance for prescription drug addiction.[227] Only one investigation has been conducted on the WVPDAQ. Results indicated that between 2008 and 2010, there were 1056 calls received and self-report measures indicated that among callers, daily drug use declined.[240]

Helplines as Self-Help

Helplines ride a fine line between self-help and assisted interventions. On the one hand, many first-time callers to drug abuse helplines have taken proactive and self-initiated measures to make the call. From there, it is often up to the caller to decide the extent or breadth of services that he/she desires. Staying within the definition of self-help, callers can have a few questions answered or request that some information be sent to their homes. Helplines start to cross over into the zone of assisted, professional help when multiple counseling sessions are involved, the individual is referred to the helpline by a hospital or medical professional, or the caller enters proactive counseling with multiple phone sessions initiated by the counselor.

Religion, Spirituality, and Meditation

A long tradition of spirituality and religion exists in the contextualization and treatment of substance use disorders. In an open letter to Alcoholics Anonymous (AA)[1] founder William G. Wilson (Bill W), Carl Jung identified spiritual bankruptcy as an instrumental facet of addiction. "His craving for alcohol was the equivalent on a low level of the spiritual thirst of our being for wholeness … the union with God."[107] In contemporary practice, AA and similar 12-step Fellowships (e.g., Cocaine Anonymous [CA], Narcotics Anonymous [NA], Nicotine Anonymous [NicA]) remain a spiritual discipline, although they are not formally aligned with any religion.

Religion and spirituality are innately internal endeavors, albeit ones that often include corresponding external activities and, to varying extents, enduring relationships with professional providers and larger communities. A review of the literature did not produce research evaluating the role of religion or spirituality in recovery from addiction in a traditional, empirical fashion. The absence of such literature makes intuitive sense as it would be challenging to assign a random sample to a religious or spiritual condition or the absence thereof. However, given the emergence of significant research regarding these constructs in addiction, it is important to include a discussion of relevant findings. Thus this section includes a brief review of the literature on religion and spirituality in the sense that these constructs are self-initiated and self-maintained and are not externally imposed by scientists, physicians, or secular care providers. In addition, this section addresses empirical research involving meditation, which has received more recent attention as an intervention for substance use disorders.[27,184]

Religion and spirituality are conceptually distinct constructs, although they share some common features. For the purposes of this chapter, definitions of religion and spirituality will be based on those in the Handbook of Religion and Health[115] and consistent with existing literature.[78] Religion is defined as an organized system of beliefs, practices, rituals, and symbols designed to facilitate a relationship with the transcendent or sacred as well as with the greater community. Spirituality is defined as a less formal and more personal quest for meaning, designed to address questions about life and one's relationship with the transcendent

or sacred. Throughout this review, where no distinction has been made by contributing authors, the term r/s will be used to denote the phrase religion and spirituality.

Religion, Spirituality, and Nicotine

Previous research has found that both religion and spirituality (r/s) act as protective factors for nicotine addiction.[76,83,134] Both internal (e.g., religious importance, affiliation, personal devotion) and external (e.g., attendance, bible study) facets of religion have been significantly and inversely associated with tobacco initiation among children,[229] adolescents,[87,219] young adults,[211,228] and adults.[31] Consistently, older adults with a strong religious commitment were less likely to have ever smoked and, among those who did smoke, consumed fewer cigarettes.[115] Thus religion appears to act as a protective factor against the onset of nicotine use, thereby preventing the constellation of negative health consequences associated with nicotine addiction.

Although religion appears to act protectively against smoking onset, the impact of r/s on self-directed recovery from nicotine addiction is less clear. Despite the prevalence of r/s resources in the treatment of other substance use disorders, they have historically and inexplicably been absent from the treatment of nicotine addiction. Emerging research suggests this may reflect an area of potential growth in nicotine cessation interventions. A pilot study assessing interest in spiritual interventions for smoking cessation was well-received among current smokers with a history of spirituality, and particularly among older individuals (31–50+), females, and heavy smokers.[82] A culturally and religiously specific smoking cessation intervention designed to be conveyed through local churches for rural African Americans promoted greater positive movement in readiness to change than a tailored, minimal self-help intervention.[217] Consistent with these findings, smokers who reported the self-directed use of prayer for health and/or mind/body (m/b) therapies (e.g., biofeedback, meditation, hypnosis, yoga) were significantly more likely to have made attempts at quitting over the course of 12 months relative to those who did neither.[79] Of interest, however, Gillum and colleagues[79] did not find that this translated into greater success with smoking cessation; those reporting employing r/s and/or m/b were no more likely to report quitting. Thus current literature suggests some efficacy associated with r/s in the promotion of smoking cessation contemplation, if not overt attempts at change.

Based on the currently available information, r/s appears to be best understood as a motivational tool promoting interest in nicotine cessation rather than an independent intervention. There is no shortage of testimony of the positive health benefits of r/s; rather, there appears to be a paucity of well-controlled, sound investigations empirically corroborating those benefits,[20,189,212] such that the utility of r/s as an intervention, and particularly a self-administered intervention, remains unclear. In summary, although r/s has been well-received in the treatment of other substance use disorders, and recent studies appear intriguing, there is a dearth of well-controlled, empirically valid studies that lend support to the unqualified endorsement of r/s as a standalone intervention for smoking cessation.

Religion, Spirituality, and Alcohol

A substantial body of research delineates the protective role that religion[75,110,115] and spirituality[135] play in resilience against alcohol use disorders. Among adolescents, personal importance of religion was inversely associated with contemporary degree of alcohol and substance use.[68,137,170] Among college students, Stewart[202] found that those who rated spiritual beliefs highly drank less than those who rated spirituality as less important, although this protective effect diminished as the students aged. Similarly among college students, Leigh and colleagues[121] found alcohol use to be negatively correlated with scores on a spirituality scale. As spirituality scores increased, the use of alcohol decreased. Among adults, lower rates of alcohol use disorders have been associated with private practices of prayer and scripture reading.[114] Consistently, research has demonstrated that alcohol-related negative consequences and alcohol use disorders among the highest-risk religious group, drinking members of conservative Protestant denominations,[114,127] is still only 40% of that for drinkers with no religious affiliation.[98]

Furthermore, the absence of r/s may be a risk factor for developing maladaptive patterns of alcohol use. Individuals with alcohol and drug problems generally report lower religious commitment and involvement relative to the general population.[120,103,220] Consistent with these findings, descriptive studies suggest that individuals with alcohol and drug problems believe that receiving spiritually focused treatment would be helpful to their recovery.[13,58]

A number of sources suggest that religious or spiritual growth is an influential element in lasting recovery. Alcoholics Anonymous[1] frames addiction as a physical, mental, and spiritual disease requiring treatment in all three domains, the latter of which is an identified treatment stage (i.e., spiritual affiliation and growth) in their model of healthy and stable recovery. Previous research has found that the spirituality of AA members is positively associated with life satisfaction,[45] purpose in life, and duration of sobriety.[37,166] Similarly, a study of individuals in recovery found that higher levels of religious faith and spirituality were associated with a more optimistic life orientation, greater perceived social support, higher resiliency to stress, and lower levels of anxiety.[156] Some speculate that inasmuch as r/s is protective against addiction, the adoption of religious or spiritual beliefs may facilitate the process of recovery.[144]

Religion, Spirituality, and Other Substances

Consistent with the alcohol literature, r/s appears to have a protective influence against the onset of illicit drug use among adolescents[137,170] and adults.[76,83,134] Also analogous to the alcohol literature, a lack of religious commitment may be a risk factor for illicit drug use.[115] Stewart[202] found that 41% of college students who rated spirituality of low importance used marijuana, versus 15% of those rating spirituality of high importance.

Previous research suggests that religious and spiritual involvement exerts a positive influence in the treatment of substance use disorders. A recent study examining spiritual activities among heroin- and cocaine-dependent individuals revealed a weak but positive ($r = 0.16$, $p < .04$) association between spirituality and treatment outcome.[89] Individuals in this study who reported that they frequently spent time on religious or spiritual activities demonstrated significantly better outcomes in terms of subsequent drug use and treatment retention. Similarly, spirituality has also been associated with reduced severity of relapses[142] and treatment responsiveness.[164] In a study examining the effectiveness of coping techniques to reduce cocaine use after treatment, spirituality was one of a number of techniques associated with less cocaine use at 6-month follow-up.[175] Although these studies are promising, they do not address the role of r/s independent of formal treatment. As such, questions remain about the utility of r/s as an independent, self-administered mechanism of change for addictive disorders. Thus the current literature regarding r/s and recovery from illicit drug abuse and addiction appears to be at a stage of development where positive indications have been found, but these associations have not yet been fully elucidated.

Meditation and Mindfulness-Based Approaches

Meditation has been a spiritual and healing practice in some parts of the world for more than 5000 years. It has also become an increasingly common practice in Western cultures within the last 50 years. In the recent past, meditation and mindfulness-based approaches to substance use disorders have received a resurgence of attention in the empirical literature and popular press. Consistent with existing literature and a division of the National Institutes of Health, meditation will be referred to as techniques or practices intended to control or focus attention on emotions, thoughts, and sensations occurring in the present moment.[108,144] Analogous to the r/s findings, research has revealed support for this technique,[28,127] although a number of important questions remain.

Previous research suggests that meditation and mindfulness-based approaches to substance use disorders hold promise as a protective mechanism, intervention technique, relapse prevention tool, and a self-help approach. Transcendental meditation has demonstrated protective effects against alcohol use disorders.[14,183] Furthermore, transcendental meditation may be an effective coping technique for individuals at risk for developing alcohol use disorders. In a study evaluating various forms of relaxation techniques (transcendental-esque meditation, deep muscle relaxation, or quiet recreation) on patterns of heavy alcohol use among college students, Marlatt and colleagues[130] found that each technique produced reductions, but that meditation demonstrated the most consistent and reliable reductions over a 6-week intervention period, with an approximate 50% reduction in daily consumption. Similarly, among an incarcerated population, significant reductions in alcohol, marijuana, and crack cocaine use were found postincarceration for individuals who had participated in a Vipassana meditation course in conjunction with standard alcohol and drug classes.[27] Thus meditative practices appear to hold promise as a method of building resilience against maladaptive and clinically significant substance use disorders.

Among those with established substance use disorders, successful recovery is often related to an individual's ability to develop and employ a repertoire of coping behaviors to forestall or recover from relapse. Rates of relapse following substance abuse treatment are notoriously high, in excess of 60%,[131] which makes findings that meditation may be an effective skills-based coping tool that can extend the duration of treatment effects by countering relapse particularly powerful.[27,28,231,232] Mindfulness-Based Relapse Prevention (MBRP),[24] an integration of mindfulness meditative practice with established relapse prevention techniques, and administered professionally in conjunction with intensive substance use treatment, has demonstrated efficacy in lowering rates of relapse and reducing cravings at 4 months among individuals with alcohol use disorders,[23] and at 12 months with alcohol and substance use disorders.[26] Similar research has found reduced alcohol consumption or rates of relapse as well as additional psychiatric benefits including reduced subjective stress,[235] objective stress responding,[30] dysphoric symptom profile posttreatment,[230] and cravings[231] (see Bowen et al.[25] for review) associated with mindfulness-based interventions when administered as an adjunctive to formal therapy. These studies support MBRP interventions in formal treatment and may suggest the viability of benefits associated with self-administered practice.

However, not all research has demonstrated significant gains associated with meditative interventions. Individuals at a substance-abuse recovery house trained in mindfulness meditation did not demonstrate significant gains in duration of sobriety, life problems, or measures of psychological health compared to those who participated in traditional treatment.[2] Similarly, although Brewer and colleagues[30] found reductions in objective stress responding, there were no significant differences in treatment outcomes between those treated with traditional versus mindfulness-based therapeutic interventions. In addition to these concerns, vital questions remain about the mechanisms promoting change associated with meditation.[232]

In sum, existing research appears to support the positive influence of r/s and meditation in a multidimensional approach to protect against and in recovery from substance use disorders. In general, r/s and meditation appear to increase resiliency against substance abuse and dependence. More specifically, r/s is associated with increased personal satisfaction and resilience in recovery from alcohol use disorders, and r/s and meditation are associated with decreased use following treatment among other substance use disorders. MBRP is well-established as an efficacious intervention for reducing cravings, a significant trigger to relapse and continued addiction, and more generally, in promoting sustained recovery. Thus it seems practical to consider the positive impact of r/s and meditation in self-initiated endeavors to address substance use disorders. However, further research is required to elucidate the influence of these constructs distinct from formal treatment, and to evaluate their efficacy as self-administered interventions. Although r/s and meditation may play a positive and potentially significant role in recovery, it is not yet understood how and in what ways r/s[135,156] or meditation act to promote positive change[11,232] and whether those effects will extend to self-initiated and maintained treatment.

Internet Resources

Recent years have witnessed an ever-increasing reliance on the Internet and smartphones for accessing all types of health-related information. Estimates from the PEW research center found that Internet search for health information was the third most popular online activity, with 80% of adult Internet users reporting using the Internet to search for health information.[74] Accordingly, research evaluating Internet self-help websites and brief interventions has greatly expanded in recent years. The bulk of the research in this area has demonstrated that the Internet is a feasible and potentially efficacious source for self-help. Relatedly, a meta-analysis evaluating 85 computer-based interventions revealed that Internet interventions were associated with small but significant effects on health behaviors (d = .16).[222] More specifically, the review found that Internet-based interventions that heavily incorporate the theory of planned behavior tended to be significantly more effective (d = .360).[222] Furthermore, research on the efficacy of online interventions has found that the most successful web-based interventions tend to be interactive and tailored.[42,125,186]

A number of advantages of web-based self-help resources have been identified, including, most notably, convenience, low/no cost, availability, and anonymity. In addition, online self-help resources for additions are perceived positively by users,[53] online

communities can be helpful in providing users with social support, and such resources have been found to increase motivation to change.[97] The number of websites relevant to self-help for addictions is overwhelming in comparison with the relatively small burgeoning literature on Internet self-help. A quick Google search (June 28, 2016) on the phrase "quitting smoking" revealed over 2.7 million hits, with similar searches for alcohol (677,000) and marijuana (494,000) revealing smaller but still impressive numbers. Not surprisingly, a major challenge in using the Internet as a self-help tool is sorting wheat from chaff in identifying accurate and helpful information. Webliographies can help in this process and typically include descriptions of the content and purpose of a relatively small number of websites that are directly relevant and informative. In addition, self-help resources that have been empirically supported often have links to published manuscripts supporting their efficacy.

Internet Resources for Nicotine

Currently there are hundreds of commercial and free smoking cessation websites available, many of which have similar content, functions, and suggestions.[67] Typical content and functions focus on setting a quit date; finding alternative activities; recruiting social support; choosing a medication; information regarding risks and benefits; chat applications, and automated e-mails. Although limited research has evaluated these kinds of self-help resources, recent trials have shown significant but small effects on short-term abstinence ranging from 7 days up to 6 months.[a] A recent systematic review found that tailored, interactive online interventions were more effective than bibliotherapy for smoking cessation [42], further suggesting the potential of internet interventions in this area.

Internet Resources for Alcohol

A large number of websites are available that offer suggestions and tools for reducing or eliminating alcohol use. Self-help websites related to drinking often include the following: a short questionnaire followed by feedback regarding responses, including how the respondent's drinking compares with population norms for same-age, same-sex individuals; assessment of risk based on a screening measure; information about alcohol's effects on the body; tools for calculating blood alcohol content; and contact information for professional help or self-help groups.[49,70] Specifically, the Harm reduction, Abstinence, and Moderation Support (HAMS) website (www.HAMSnetwork.org) offers links to useful information, books, support groups, and online self-help websites such as the Drinker's Checkup[96,97] and Moderation Management.[95,94] The National Institute on Alcohol Abuse and Alcoholism (NIAAA) has a website called Rethinking Drinking (rethinkingdrinking.niaaa.nih.gov) that allows users to check their drinking patterns against recommended daily and weekly limits for safe drinking to assess their level of risk. The NIAAA website also provides tools for changing one's drinking including listing the pros and cons of drinking at their current level (i.e., decisional balance), encouraging the use of protective behavioral strategies such as alternating alcoholic and nonalcoholic beverages, and instructions on how to build drink refusal skills. Controlled trials of Internet-based self-help programs have generally demonstrated efficacy, with effect sizes in the small-to-medium range (e.g., references Cunningham et al.,[50] Kypri et al.,[118] Riper et al.,[172] Riper et al.,[173] White et al.[224]).

---

[a] References 42, 66, 67, 122, 158, 204, 206.

Internet Resources for Other Substances

Self-help options for substances other than nicotine and alcohol available through the Internet are relatively sparse. Although there are undoubtedly numerous websites that are relevant to self-help for substances other than nicotine and alcohol, the related research literature is scant, with the exception of a few feasibility studies (e.g., Ruggiero et al.[176]). However, a recent meta-analysis found that 10 randomized controlled trial online interventions (including guided and unguided) targeting marijuana use tended to have small but significant effects on reducing marijuana use.[208] Thus research is needed to examine the potential efficacy of online self-help interventions for substances other than alcohol and nicotine, as this medium is easily accessible to a wide audience, is cost-effective, and does not carry the stigma of being labeled with a substance abuse diagnosis.

Next Steps

Some important next steps in utilizing the Internet as a self-help resource for addictions include the use of social media websites such as Facebook and Twitter and smartphone applications. Although there are currently smartphone applications for substance use, most of the currently available applications allow individuals to track their substance use but do not necessarily contain evidence-based strategies for reducing substance use.[43] A meta-analysis of 24 smartphone health intervention studies found that this is a feasible medium and that users found smartphone-delivered interventions highly acceptable.[157] A valuable next step that is currently underway in several trials is the use of evidence-based intervention techniques for substance use transmitted via social media and smartphone applications. Feasibility information and initial results for these interventions is becoming available and is promising (e.g., Pechmann et al.[158]). The coming years will illuminate whether such self-help interventions can be successfully delivered via this technological medium.

Conclusions

Many individuals utilize self-help strategies in their efforts to overcome substance dependence and addiction. Existing research literature suggests that self-change (i.e., natural recovery) is in fact the most common route through which substance use changes occur. Self-help strategies seem to be less effective for individuals with more severe dependence. From a public health perspective, self-help strategies represent ideal mechanisms for reducing substance use–related problems because they are almost invariably low-cost relative to formal treatment, and because they can be disseminated widely (e.g., bibliotherapy, helplines, and the Internet). Moreover, the existing literature on self-help strategies is relatively promising, suggesting that in addition to being lower cost and widely available, self-help is also relatively effective.

The quantity and quality of the literature provide an important caveat for the rosy prospectus on self-help approaches. In comparison with the treatment literature, the literature on specific self-help strategies is considerably smaller and with fewer controlled studies. To some extent, this may be due to the inherent nature of self-help, the typical focus of health professionals on more formal treatment approaches, and perspectives on addiction that are incompatible with self-help as a viable option. By their nature, self-help strategies are less likely to draw attention from health care professionals or researchers in addiction. Thus the prevalence of self-help strategies has remained under the radar until recently. Although there is reasonably strong literature related to certain self-help approaches for some behaviors (e.g., replacement, bibliotherapy, and helplines) and substances (tobacco and alcohol), the literature related to other strategies (e.g., Internet resources and meditation) and other substances (e.g., steroids, cocaine, and heroin) is sparse. In some cases, this presents a quality control issue given the wide availability of Internet sites or self-help books with limited or no evidence that the specific suggestions proposed will be of benefit to the individual seeking change.

A number of deeper and broader issues underlie the consideration of self-help for addictions. To the extent that addiction is defined by one's inability to control use, self-help is somewhat of an oxymoron (i.e., if a person can stop, were they really addicted?). On the other hand, even formal treatment approaches require that individuals help themselves—whether practicing thought exercises or driving themselves to an appointment with a therapist. Regardless of how either self-help or addiction is defined, it seems clear that a desire to change is fundamental in determining the success of change efforts. For many, experiencing negative consequences related to substance use is enough to initiate a self-correction process, although the form of that process may vary by individual and by substance. This chapter represents an attempt to provide a broad overview of self-help approaches for addiction, with specific examples for specific substances. Based on the available evidence, self-help strategies appear to work well for many, especially those on the less severe end of the continuum, but more nuanced questions, such as which ones work for whom under what conditions and for what substances, are in need of critical and systematic investigation.

References

1. Alcoholics Anonymous. *Alcoholics Anonymous*. 3rd ed. New York; 1976.
2. Alterman ARI, Koppenhaver JM, Mulholland E, Ladden LJ, Baime MJ. Pilot trial of effectiveness of mindfulness meditation for substance abuse patients. *J Sub Use*. 2009;9:259–268.
3. American Cancer Society. *The Fifty Most Often Asked Questions About Smoking and Health and the Answers*. Atlanta, GA; 1982.
4. American Lung Association. *Freedom From Smoking Self-Help Manual*. New York; 1999.
5. American Psychological Association. *Diagnostic and Statistical Manual of Mental Disorders: DSM-5*. Washington, DC: American Psychiatric Association; 2013.
6. Ames SC, Patten CA, Offord KP, et al. Expressive writing intervention for young adult cigarette smokers. *J ClinPsychol*. 2005;61(12):1555–1570.
7. Ames SC, Patten CA, Werch CE, et al. Expressive writing as a smoking cessation treatment adjunct for young adult smokers. *Nicotine Tob Res*. 2007;9(2):185–194.
8. Anderson CMZhu SH. Tobacco quitlines: looking back and looking ahead. *Tob Control*. 2007;16:81–86.
9. Apodaca TR, Miller WR. A meta-analysis of the effectiveness of bibliotherapy for alcohol problems. *J Clin Psychol*. 2003;59:289–304.
10. Reference deleted in review.
11. Appel JKim-Appel D. Mindfulness: implications for substance abuse and addiction. *Int J Ment Health Addiction*. 2009;7:506–512.
12. Arnett JJ. The developmental context of substance use in emerging adulthood. *J Drug Issues*. 2005;35(2):235–254.
13. Arnold RM, Avants SK, Margolin A, Marcotte D. Patient attitudes concerning the inclusion of spirituality into addiction treatment. *J Subst Abuse Treat*. 2002;23:319–326.

14. Aron A, Aron EN. The transcendental meditation program's effect on addictive behaviors. *Addict Behav.* 1980;5:3–12.

15. Baer JS, Marlatt GA, Kivlahan DR, Fromme K, Larimer ME, Williams E. An experimental test of three methods of alcohol risk reduction with young adults. *J Consult Clin Psych.* 1992;60:974–979.

16. Bandura A. *Self-Efficacy: The Exercise of Control.* New York, NY: W H Freeman/Times Books/ Henry Holt & Co; 1997.

17. Bandura A. A sociocognitive analysis of substance abuse: an agentic perspective. *Psychol Sci.* 1999;10(3):214–217.

18. Bilard J, Ninot G, Hauw D. Motives for illicit use of doping substances among athletes calling a national antidoping phone-help service: an exploratory study. *Subst Use Misuse.* 2011;46:359–367.

19. Reference deleted in review.

20. Blumenthal JA, Babyak MA, Ironson G, et al. *Psychosom Med.* 2007;69:501–508.

21. Bojsen-Moller J, Christiansen AV. Use of performance- and image-enhancing substances among recreational athletes: a quantitative analysis of inquiries submitted to the Danish anti-doping authorities. *Scand J Med Sci Spor.* 2010;20:861–867.

22. Borland R, Segan CJ. The potential of quitlines to increase smoking cessation. *Drug Alcohol Rev.* 2006;25:73–78.

23. Bowen S, Chawla N, Collins SE, et al. Mindfulness-based relapse prevention for substance use disorders: a pilot efficacy trail. *Subst Abus.* 2009;30:295–305.

24. Bowen S, Chawla N, Marlatt GA. *Mindfulness-Based Relapse Prevention for the Treatment of Substance Use Disorders: A Clinician's Guide.* New York, NY: Guilford Press; 2010.

25. Bowen S, Witkiewitz K, Chawla N, Grow J. Integrating mindfulness and cognitive behavioral traditions for the long-term treatment of addictive behaviors. *J Clin Outcome Manag.* 2011;18:473–479.

26. Bowen S, Witkiewitz K, Clifasefi SL, et al. Relative efficacy of mindfulness-based relapse prevention, standard relapse prevention and treatment as usual for substance use disorders: a randomized clinical trial. *JAMA Psychiatry.* 2014;71:547–556.

27. Bowen S, Witkiewitz K, Dillworth TM, Chawla N, Simpson TL, Ostafin BD, et al. Mindfulness meditation and substance use in an incarcerated population. *Psychol Addict Behav.* 2006;20:343–347.

28. Bowen S, Witkiewitz K, Dillworth TM, Marlatt GA. The role of thought suppression in the relationship between mindfulness meditation and alcohol use. *Addict Behav.* 2007;32:2324–2328.

29. Reference deleted in review.

30. Brewer JA, Sinha R, Chen JA, et al. Mindfulness training and stress reactivity in substance abuse: results from a randomized, controlled stage I pilot study. *Subst Abuse.* 2009;30:306–317.

31. Brown QL, Linton SL, Harrell PT, et al. The influence of religious attendance on smoking. *Subst Use Misuse.* 2014;14:1392–1399.

32. Brown RA, Lejuez CW, Kahler CW, Strong DR. Distress tolerance and duration of past smoking cessation attempts. *J Abnorm Pschol.* 2002;111:180–183.

33. Brown RL, Saunders LA, Bobula JA, Mundt MP, Koch PE. Randomized-controlled trial of a telephone and mail intervention for alcohol use disorders: three-month drinking outcomes. *Alcohol Clin Exp Res.* 2007;31:1372–1379.

34. Bullen C, Howe C, Laugesen M, et al. Electronic cigarettes for smoking cessation: a randomized controlled trial. *Lancet.* 2013;382:1629–1637.

35. Burman S. The challenge of sobriety: natural recovery without treatment and self-help groups. *J Subst Abuse.* 1997;9:41–61.

36. Carballo JL, Fernández-Hermida JR, Secades-Villa R, Sobell LC, Dum M, García-Rodríguez O. Natural recovery from alcohol and drug problems: a methodological review of the literature from 1999 through 2005. In: Klingemann H, Sobell L, eds. *Promoting Self-Change From Addictive Behaviors: Practical Implications for Policy, Prevention, and Treatment.* New York: Springer; 87–101.

37. Carroll S. Spirituality and purpose in life in alcoholism recovery. *J Stud Alcohol.* 1991;54:297–301.

38. Centers for Disease Control and Prevention. Annual smoking-attributable mortality, years of potential life lost, and productivity losses -- United States, 1997-2001. *Morb Mortal Wkly Rep.* 2005;54:625–628.

39. Centers for Disease Control and Prevention. Tobacco use among adults -- United States, 2005. *Morb Mortal Wkly Rep.* 2006;55:1145–1148.

40. Centers for Disease Control and Prevention. Notes from the field: electronic cigarette use among middle and high school students-United States, 2011-2012. *MMWR. Morbidity and Mortality Weekly Report.* 2013;62(35):729.

41. Centers for Disease Control and Prevention. *Frequently asked questions about 1-800-QUIT-NOW and the national network of tobacco cessation quitlines.* Accessed on-line.

42. Civljak M, Stead LF, Hartmann–Boyce J, Sheikh A, Car J. *Internet–Based Interventions for Smoking Cessation.* The Cochrane Library; 2013.

43. Cohn A, Hunter-Reel D, Hagman BT, Mitchell J. Promoting behavior change from alcohol use through mobile technology: the future of ecological momentary assessment. *Alcohol Clin Exp Res.* 2011;35(12):2209–2215.

44. Copersino ML, Boyd SJ, Tashkin DP, et al. Gorelick Dermand JC, DA. Quitting among non-treatment-seeking marijuana users: reasons and changes in other substance use. *Am J Addiction.* 2006;15:297–302.

45. Corrington JC. Spirituality and recovery: relationships between levels of spirituality, contentment, and stress during recovery from alcoholism in AA. *Alcohol Treat Q.* 1989;6:151–165.

46. Cummins SE, Bailey L, Campbell S, Koon-Kirby C, Zhu SH. Tobacco cessation quitlines in North America: a descriptive study. *Tob Control.* 2007;16(suppl I):i9–i15.

47. Cunningham JA. Remissions from drug dependence: is treatment a prerequisite? *Drug Alcohol Depend.* 2000;59:211–213.

48. Cunningham JA. Is level of interest among cannabis users in self-help materials and other services aimed at reducing problem use? *Addiction.* 2005;100:561–562.

49. Cunningham JA. Internet-based interventions for alcohol, tobacco, and other substances of abuse. In: Miller PM, Kavanagh D, eds. *Translation of Addictions Science Into Practice.* New York; 2007.

50. Cunningham JA, Humphreys K, Koski-Jannes A, Cordingley J. Internet and paper self-help materials for problem drinking: is there an additive effect? *Addict Behav.* 2005;30:1517–1523.

51. Cunningham JA, Humpphreys K, Kypri K, van Mierlo T. Formative evaluation and three-month follow-up of an online personalized assessment feedback intervention for problem drinkers. *J Med Internet Res.* 2006;8:e5.

52. Cunningham JA, Sobell LC, Sobell MB. Awareness of self-change as a pathway to recovery for alcohol abusers: results from five different groups. *Addict Behav.* 1998;23:399–404.

53. Cunningham JA, Sobell LC, Sobell MB. Changing perceptions about self-change and moderate-drinking recoveries from alcohol problems: what can and should be done? *J Appl Soc Psychol.* 1999;29:291–299.

54. Curry SJ. Self-help interventions for smoking cessation. *J Consult Clin Psychol.* 1993;61:790–803.

55. Reference deleted in review.

56. Curry SJ, Marlatt GA, Gordon J, Baer JS. A comparison of alternative theoretical approaches to smoking cessation and relapse. *Health Psychol.* 1988;7:545–556.

57. Curry SJ, McBride C, Grothaus LC, Louie D, Wagner EH. A randomized trial of self-help materials, personalized feedback, and telephone counseling with nonvolunteer smokers. *J Consult Clin Psychol.* 1995;63:1005–1014.

58. Dermatis H, Guschwan MT, Galanter M, Bunt G. Orientation toward spirituality and self-help approaches in the therapeutic community. *J Addict Dis.* 2004;23:39–54.

59. DiClemente CC. Change is a process not a product: reflections on pieces to the puzzle. *Subst Use Misuse.* 2015;50(8–9):1225–1228.

60. DiClemente CC, Prochaska JO. Toward a comprehensive, trans-theoretical model of change. In: Miller WR, Heather N, eds. *Treating Addictive Behaviors*. New York; 1998.

61. Dijkstra A, De Vries H, Roijackers J. Long-term effectiveness of computer-generated tailored feedback in smoking cessation. *Health Educ Res*. 1998;13:207–214.

62. Reference deleted in review.

63. Eklöf AC, Thurelius AM, Garle M, Rane A, Sjöqvist F. The anti-doping hot-line, a means to capture the abuse of doping agents in the Swedish society and a new service function in clinical pharmacology. *Eur J Clin Pharmaco*. 2003;59:571–577.

64. Escoffery C, McCormick L, Bateman K. Development and process evaluation of web-based smoking cessation program for college smokers: innovative tool for education. *Patient Educ Couns*. 2004;53:217–225.

65. Ellingstad TP, Sobell LC, Sobell MB, Eickleberry L, Golden CJ. Self-change: a pathway to cannabis abuse resolution. *Addict Behav*. 2006;31:519–530.

66. Etter JF. Comparing the efficacy of two Internet-based, computer-tailored smoking cessation programs: a randomized trial. *J Med Internet Res*. 2005;7:e2.

67. Etter JF. Internet-based smoking cessation programs. *Int J Med Inform*. 2006;75:110–116.

68. Faulkner KK, Alcorn JD, Garvin RB. Prediction of alcohol consumption among fraternity pledges. *J Alcohol Drug Educ*. 1989;34:12–20.

69. Feldman RS, Myer JS, Quenzer LF. *Principles of Neuropsychopharmacology*. Sunderland, MA; 1997.

70. Finfgeld-Connet D. Web-based treatment for problem drinking. *J Psychosoc Nurs Ment Health Serv*. 2006;44:20–27.

71. Fiore MC, Novotny TE, Pierce JP, Giovino G, Hatziandreu EJ. Methods used to quit smoking in the United States. Do cessation programs help? *J Am Med Assoc*. 1990;263:2760–2765.

72. Fiore MC. US Public Health Services clinical practice guideline: treating tobacco use and dependence. *Respir Care*. 2000;45:1200–1262.

73. Firth A, Emmison M, Baker C. Calling for help: an introduction. In: Baker CD, Emmison M, Firth A, eds. *Calling for Help*. Philadelphia, PA; 2005.

74. Fox S. *Health Topics: 80% of Users Look for Health Information Online*. Washington, DC: Pew Internet & American Life Project; 2011. Retrieved from http://www.pewinternet.org/Reports/2011/HealthTopics.aspx.

75. Foxcroft DR, Lowe G. Adolescents drinking, smoking, and other substance use involvement: links with perceived family life. *J Adolesc*. 1995;18:159–177.

76. Gartner J, Larson DB, Allen GD. Religious commitment and mental health: a review of the empirical literature. *J Psychol Theol*. 1991;19:6–25.

77. Gates P. The effectiveness of helplines for the treatment of alcohol and illicit substance use. *J Telemed Telecare*. 2015;21:18–28.

78. Geppert C, Bogenschutz MP, Miller WR. Development of a bibliography on religion, spirituality and addictions. *Drug Alcohol Rev*. 2007;26:389–395.

79. Gillum FR, Bennett G, Santibantez S, Donahue M. Associations of prayer, mind-body therapy, and smoking cessation in a national survey. *Psychol Rep*. 2009;105:593–604.

80. Reference deleted in review.

81. Glynn TJ, Boyd GM, Gruman JC. *Self-Guided Strategies for Smoking Cessation: a Program Planner's Guide (NIH Publication No. 91-3104)*. Washington, DC: National Cancer Institute, Smoking and Tobacco Control Program.

82. Gonzales D, Redtomahawk D, Pizacani B, et al. Support for spirituality in smoking cessation: results of pilot survey. *Nicotine Tob Res*. 2007;9:299–303.

83. Gould RAClum GA. A meta-analysis of self-help treatment approaches. *Clin Psychol Rev*. 1993;13:169–186.

84. Reference deleted in review.

85. Reference deleted in review.

86. Hartmann-Boyce J, Lancaster T, Stead LF. Print-based self-help interventions for smoking cessation. *Cochran Database Syst Rev*. 2014;6. http://www.ncbi.nlm.nih.gov/pubmed/12137618.

87. Heath AC, Madden PAF, Grant JD, McLaughlin TL, Todorov AA, Bucholz KK. Resiliency factors protecting against teenage alcohol use and smoking: influences of religion, religious involvement and values, and ethnicity in the missouri adolescent female twin study. *Twin Res Hum Genet*. 1999;2:145–155.

88. Heatherton TF, Nichols PA. Personal accounts of successful versus failed attempts at life change. *Pers Soc Psychol Bull*. 1994;20:664–675.

89. Heinz A, Epstein DH, Preston KL. Spiritual/religious experiences and in-treatment outcome in an outcome in an inner-city program for heroin and cocaine dependence. *J Psychoactive Drugs*. 2007;39:41–49.

90. Helgason ÁR Tomson T, Lund KE, Galanti R, Ashnve S, Gilljam H. Factors related to abstinence in a telephone helpline for smoking cessation. *Eur J Public Health*. 2004;14:306–310.

91. Helvig TM, Sobell LC, Sobell MB, Simco ER. Smokers' narrative accounts of quit attempts: aids and impediments to success. *Psychol Addict Behav*. 2006;20:219–224.

92. Henningfield JE. Nicotine medications for smoking cessation. *N Engl J Med*. 1995;333:1196–1203.

93. Henningfield JE, Cohen C, Slade JD. Is nicotine more addictive than cocaine? *Br J Addict*. 1991;86:565–569.

94. Hester RK, Delaney HD, Campbell W, Handmaker N. A web application for moderation training: initial results of a randomized clinical trial. *J Subst Abuse Treat*. 2009;37:266–276.

95. Hester RK, Delaney HD, Campbell W. Moderatedrinking.com and moderation management: outcomes of a randomized clinical trial with non-dependent problem drinkers. *J Consult Clin Psych*. 2011;79:215–224.

96. Hester RK, Delaney HD, Campbell W. The college drinker's check-up: outcomes of two randomized clinical trials of a computer-delivered intervention. *Psychol Addict Behav*. 2012;26(1):1–12.

97. Hester RK, Squires DD, Delaney HD. The drinker's check-up: 12-month outcomes of a controlled clinical trial of a stand-alone software program for problem drinkers. *J Subst Abuse Treat*. 2005;28(2):159–169.

98. Hilton ME. The demographic distribution of drinking problems in 1984. In: Clark WB, Hilton ME, eds. *Alcohol in America: Drinking Practices and Problems*. Albany, NY; 1991.

99. Hjalmarson AI. Effect of nicotine chewing gum in smoking cessation: a randomized, placebo-controlled, double-blind study. *J Am Med Assoc*. 1984;252:2835–2838.

100. Hughes JR, Riggs RL, Carpenter MJ. How helpful are drug abuse helplines? *Drug Alcohol Depend*. 2001;62:191–194.

101. Hughes JR, Stead LF, Lancaster T. Shape of the relapse curve and long-term abstinence among untreated smokers. *Addiction*. 2004;99:29–38.

102. Hurt RD, Saches DPL, Glover ED, et al. A comparison of sustained-release buproprion and placebo for smoking cessation. *N Engl J Med*. 1997;337:1195–1202.

103. Jackson KM, Sartor CE, Sher K. The natural course of substance use and dependence. the oxford handbook of substance use and substance use disorders. *Two-Volume Set*. 2016;26(29):67–131.

104. Jackson R, Wernicke R, Haaga DAF. Hope as a predictor of entering substance abuse treatment. *Addict Behav*. 2003;28:13–28.

105. Jensen RP, Luo W, Pankow JF, Strongin RM, Peyton DH. Hidden formaldehyde in e-cigarette aerosols. *New Engl J Med*. 2015;372(4):392–394.

106. Jorenby DE, Leischow SJ, Nides MA, et al. A controlled trial of sustained-release bupropion, a nicotine patch, or both for smoking cessation. *N Engl J Med*. 1999;340:685–691.

107. Jung C. *Dr Carl Jung's Letter to Bill W., Jan 30, 1961*. 1961. Retrieved on 06/21/2016, from: http://www.silkworth.net/aahistory/carljung_billw013061.html.

108. Kabat-Zinn J. *Full Catastrophe Living: Using the Wisdom of your Body and Mind to Face Stress, Pain and Illness*. New York: Delta; 1990.

109. Keller PA, Bailey LA, Koss KJ, Baker TB, Fiore MC. Organization, financing, promotion, and cost of US quitlines, 2004. *Am J Prev Med.* 2007;32:32–37.

110. Kendler KS, Gardner CO, Prescott CA. Religion, psychopathology, and substance use and abuse: a multimeasure genetic-epidemiologic study. *Am J Psychiatry.* 1997;154:322–329.

111. Khadjesari Z, Murray E, Hewitt C, Hartley S, Godfrey C. Can stand-alone computer-based interventions reduce alcohol consumption? A systematic review. *Addiction.* 2011;106:267–282.

112. Killen JD, Fortmann SP, Newman B, Varady A. Evaluation of a treatment approach combining nicotine gum with self-guided behavioral treatments for smoking relapse prevention. *J Consul Clin Psychol.* 1990;58:85–92.

113. Klingemann H, Sobell LC. *Promoting Self-Change From Addictive Behaviors.* Springer; 2007.

114. Koenig HG, George LK, Meador KG, Blazer DG, Ford SM. Religious practices and alcoholism in a southern adult population. *Hosp Community Psychiatry.* 1994;45:225–231.

115. Koenig HG, Larson DB. Religion and mental health: evidence for association. *Int Rev Psychiatry.* 2001;13:67–78.

116. Reference deleted in review.

117. Koski-Jannes A, Cunningham JA, Tolonen K, Bothas H. Internet-based self-assessment of drinking 3-month follow up data. *Addict Behav.* 2007;32:533–542.

118. Kypri K, Saunders JB, Williams SM, McGee RO, Langley JD, Cashell Smith ML, et al. Web based screening and brief intervention for hazardous drinking: a double-blind randomized controlled trial. *Addiction.* 2004;99:1410–1417.

119. Lancaster T, Stead LF. Self-help interventions for smoking cessation. *Cochran Database Syst Rev.* 2005;3. http://www.ncbi.nlm.nih.gov/pubmed/12137618.

120. Larson DBWilson WP. Religious life of alcoholics. *South Med J.* 1980;73:723–727.

121. Leigh J, Bowen S, Marlatt GA. Spirituality, mindfulness and substance abuse. *Addict Behav.* 2005;30:1335–1341.

122. Lenert L, Muñoz RF, Perez JE, Bansod A. Automated email messaging as a tool for improving quit rates in an Internet smoking cessation intervention. *J Am Med Inform Assoc.* 2004;4:235–240.

123. Lovett R. Coffee: the demon drink? new scientist. *Feature.* 2005;21.

124. Lukes SE, Penetar D, Su Z, et al. A standardized kudzu extract (NPI-031) reduces alcohol consumption in nontreatment-seeking male heavy drinkers. *Psychopharmacology.* 2013;226:65–73.

125. Lustria MLA, Noar SM, Cortese J, Van Stee SK, Glueckauf RL, Lee J. A meta-analysis of web-delivered tailored health behavior change interventions. *J Health Commun.* 2013;18(9):1039–1069.

126. Mains JAScogin FR. The effectiveness of self-administered treatments: a practice-friendly review of the research. *J Clin Psychol.* 2003;59:237–346.

127. Mäkelä K. Consumption level and cultural drinking patterns as determinants of alcohol problems. *J Drug Iss.* 1975;5:344–357.

128. Malas M, Jan can der T, Schwartz R, et al. Electronic cigarettes for smoking cessation: a systematic review. *Nicotine Tob Res.* 2016;10:1093.

129. Marlatt GA, Curry S, Gordon JR. A longitudinal analysis of unaided smoking cessation. *J Consult Clin Psychol.* 1988;56:715–720.

130. Marlatt GA, Pagano RR, Rose RM, Marques JK. Effects of meditation and relaxation training upon alcohol use in male social drinkers. In: Shapiro DH, Walsh RN, eds. *Meditation: Classic and Contemporary Perspectives.* New York; 1984.

131. McLellan AT, Lewis DC, O'Brien CP, Kleber HD. Drug dependence, a chronic mental illness: implications for treatment, insurance, and outcome evaluations. *JAMA.* 2000;284:1689–1695.

132. Merrill JECarey KB. Drinking over the lifespan: focus on college ages. *Alcohol Res: Curr Rev.* 2016;38(1):103–114.

133. Reference deleted in review.

134. Michalak L, Trocki K, Bond J. Religion and alcohol in the US National Alcohol Survey: how important is religion for abstention and drinking? *Drug Alcohol Depend.* 2006;87:268–280.

135. Miller WR. Researching the spiritual dimensions of alcohol and other drug problems. *Addiction.* 1998;93:979–990.

136. Miller WR, Baca LM. Two-year follow-up of bibliotherapy and therapist-directed controlled drinking training for problem drinkers. *Behav Ther.* 1983;14:441–448.

137. Miller L, Davies M, Greenwald SM. Religiosity and substance use and abuse among adolescents in the. *National Comorbidity Survey J Am Acad Child Adolesc Psychiatry.* 2000;39:1190–1197.

138. Miller WR, Gribskov CJ, Mortell RL. Effectiveness of a self-control manual for problem drinkers with and without therapist contact. *Subst Use Misuse.* 1981;7:1247–1254.

139. Miller WR, Taylor CA. Relative effectiveness of bibliotherapy: individual and group self-control training in the treatment of problem drinkers. *Addict Behav.* 1980;5:13–24.

140. Miller WR, Taylor CA, West JC. Focused versus broad spectrum behavior therapy for problem drinkers. *J Consult Clin Psychol.* 1980;48:590–601.

141. Mokdad AH, Marks JS, Stroup DF, Gerberding JL. Actual causes of death in the United States, 2000. *JAMA.* 2004;291:1238–1245.

142. Morgenstern J, Frey RM, McCrady BS, Labouvie E, Neighbors C. Examining mediators of change in traditional chemical dependency treatment. *J Stud Alcohol.* 1996;57:53–64.

143. Reference deleted in review.

144. Muffler J, Langrod J, Larson D. "There is a balm in Gilead": religion and substance abuse treatment. In: Lowinson JH, Ruiz P, Millman RB, Langrod JG, eds. *Substance Abuse: A Comprehensive Textbook.* 2nd ed. Baltimore, MD; 1995.

145. Nash CM, Vickerman KA, Kellogg ES, Zbikowski SM. Utilization of a Web-based vs integrated phone/Web cessation program among 140,000 tobacco users: an evaluation across 10 free state quitlines. *J Med Internet Res.* 2015;17(2):e36.

146. Neale J, Tompkins C, Sheard L. Barriers to accessing generic health and social care services: a qualitative study of injecting drug users. *Health Soc Care Community.* 2008;16:147–154.

147. Neighbors C, Larimer ME, Lewis MA. Targeting misperceptions of descriptive drinking norms: efficacy of a computer-delivered personalized normative feedback intervention. *J Consult Clin.* 2004;72:434–447.

148. Neighbors C, Lee CM, Lewis MA, Fossos N, Walter T. Internet-based personalized feedback to reduce 21st birthday drinking: a randomized controlled trial of an event-specific prevention intervention. *J Consult Clin.* 2009;77:51–63.

149. Neighbors C, Lewis MA, Bergstrom RL, Larimer ME. Being controlled by normative influences: self-determination as a moderator of a normative feedback alcohol intervention. *J Health Psychol.* 2006;25:571–579.

150. Reference deleted in review.

151. Newman MG, Szkodny LE, Llera SJ, Przeworski A. A review of technology-assisted self-help and minimal contact therapies for drug and alcohol abuse and smoking addiction: is human contact necessary for therapeutic efficacy? *Clin Psychol Rev.* 2011;31:178–186.

152. O'Hara PO, Gerace TA, Elliot LL. Effectiveness of self-help smoking cessation guides for firefighters. *J Occup Med.* 1993;35:795–799.

153. Orleans CT, Schoenbach BJ, Wagner EH, Quade D, Salmon MA, Pearson DC, et al. Self-help quit interventions: effects of self-help materials, social support instructions, and telephone counseling. *J Consult Clin Psychol.* 1991;59:439–448.

154. Ossip-Klein DJ, Giovino GA, Meahed N, Black PM, Emont SL, Stiggins J, et al. Effects of a smokers' hotline: results of a 10-county self-help trial. *J Consult Clin Psychol.* 1993;59:325–332.

155. Ossip-Klein DJ, McIntosh S. Quitlines in North America: evidence base and applications. *Am J Med Sci.* 2003;326:201–205.

156. Pardini DA, Plante TG, Sherman A, Stump JE. Religious faith and spirituality in substance abuse recovery: determining the mental health benefits. *J Subst Abuse Treat.* 2000;19:347–354.

157. Payne HE, Lister C, West JH, Bernhardt JM. Behavioral functionality of mobile apps in health interventions: a systematic review of the literature. *JMIR Mhealth Uhealth.* 2015;3(1):e20.

158. Pechmann C, Pan L, Delucchi K, Lakon CM, Prochaska JJ. Development of a Twitter-based intervention for smoking cessation that encourages high-quality social media interactions via automessages. *J med Internet Res.* 2015;17(2):e50.

159. Pennebaker JW, Beall SK. Confronting a traumatic event. Toward an understanding of inhibition and disease. *J Abnorm Psychol.* 1986;95:274–281.

160. Pennebaker JW, Chung CK. Expressive writing, emotional upheavals, and health. *Handbook of Health Psychology.* 2007:263–284.

161. Pennebaker JW, Smyth JM. *Opening Up by Writing It Down: How Expressive Writing Improves Health and Eases Emotional Pain.* Guilford Publications; 2016.

162. Pepper JK, Brewer NT. Electronic nicotine delivery system (electronic cigarette) awareness, use, reactions and beliefs: a systematic review. *Tob Control.* 2014;23:375–384.

163. Piasecki TM. Relapse to smoking. *Clin Psychol Rev.* 2006;26:196–215.

164. Piedmont RL. Spiritual transcendence as a predictor of psychosocial outcome from an outpatient substance abuse program. *Psychol Addict Behav.* 2004;18:213–222.

165. Pierce JP, Cummins SE, White MM, Humphrey A, Messer K. Quitlines and nicotine replacement for smoking cessation: do we need to change policy? *AnnuRev Publ Health.* 2012;33:341–356.

166. Poage ED, Ketzenberger KE, Olson J. Spirituality, contentment, and stress in recovering alcoholics. *Addict Behav.* 2004;29:1857–1862.

167. Price RK, Risk NK, Spitznagel EL. Remission from drug abuse over a 25-year period: patterns of remission and treatment use. *Am J Pub Health.* 2001;91:1107–1113.

168. Prochaska JO, DiClemente CC. Norcross. In search of how people change: applications to addictive behavior. *Am Psychol.* 1992;47:1102–1114.

169. Rahman MA, Hann N, Wilson A, Mnatzaganian G, Worral-Carter L. E-cigarettes and smoking cessation: evidence from a systematic review and meta-analysis. *PLoS One.* 2015;10:e122544.

170. Rasic D, Kisely S, Langille DB. Protective associations of importance of religion and frequency of service attendance with depression risk, suicidal behaviours, and substance use in adolescents in Nova Scotia, Canada. *J Affect Disorders.* 2011;132:389–395.

171. Reynolds KD, Coombs DW, Lowe JB, Peterson PL, Gayoso E. Evaluation of a self-help program to reduce alcohol consumption among pregnant women. *Int J Addict.* 1995;30:427–443.

172. Riper H, Blankers M, Hadiwijaya H, et al. Effectiveness of guided and unguided low-intensity internet interventions for adult alcohol misuse: a meta-analysis. *PLoS One.* 2014;9(6):e99912.

173. Riper H, Kramer J, Smit F, Conjin B, Schippers G, Cuijpers P. Web-based self-help for problem-drinkers: a pragmatic randomized trial. *Addiction.* 2008;103:218–227.

174. Rodriguez LM, Young CM, Neighbors C, Campbell MT, Lu Q. Evaluating shame and guilt in an expressive writing alcohol intervention. *Alcohol.* 2015;49:491–498.

175. Rohsenow DJ, Martin RA, Monti PA. Urge-specific and lifestyle coping strategies of cocaine abusers: relationships to treatment outcomes. *Drug Alcohol Depend.* 2005;78:211–219.

176. Ruggiero KJ, Resnick HS, Acierno R, Carpenter MJ, Kilpatrick DG, Coffey SF, et al. Internet-based intervention for mental health and substance use problems in disaster-affected populations: a pilot feasibility study. *Behav Ther.* 2006;37:190–205.

177. Russell M, Peirce RS, Chan AWK, Wieczorek WF, Moscato BS, Nochajski TH. Natural recovery in a community-based sample of alcoholics: study design and descriptive data. *Subst Use Misuse.* 2001;36:1417–1441.

178. Salup BJ, Salup A. *Bibliotherapy: An Historical Overview;* 1978.

179. Schauer GL, Malarcher AM, Zhang L, Engstrom MC, Zhu S. Prevalence and correlates of quitline awareness and utilization in the United States: an update from the 2009-2010 national adult tobacco survey. *Nicotine Tob Res.* 2013;10:1093.

180. Schneider NG, Jarvik ME, Forsythe AB, Read LL, Elliot ML, Schweiger A. Nicotine gum in smoking cessation: a placebo-controlled, double-blind trial. *Addict Behav.* 1983;8:253–261.

181. Schoenborn CA, Gindi RM. Electronic cigarette use among adults: United States, 2014. *NCHS Data Brief.* no. 217, October 2015, 2014.

182. Schulenberg J, O'Malley PM, Bachman JG, Wadsworth KN, Johnston LD. Getting drunk and growing up: trajectories of frequent binge drinking during the transition to young adulthood. *J Stud Alcohol.* 1996;57(3):289–304.

183. Scogin FR. Introduction: integrating self-help into psychotherapy. *J Clin Psychol.* 2003;59:175–176. https://doi.org/10.1002/jclp.10139.

184. Scogin FR, Bynum J, Stephens G, Calhoon S. Efficacy of self-administered treatment programs: meta-analytic review. *Prof Psychol Res Pr.* 1990;21:42–47.

185. Reference deleted in review.

186. Shahab LM, cEwen A. Online support for smoking cessation: a systematic review of the literature. *Addiction.* 2009;104(11):1792–1804.

187. Shebek J, Rindone JP. A pilot study exploring the effect of kudzu root on the drinking habits of patients with chronic alcoholism. *J Altern Complemen Med.* 2000;6(1):45–48.

188. Shiffman S, Brockwell SE, Pillitteri JL, Gitchell JG. Use of smoking-cessation treatments in the United States. *Am J Prev Med.* 2008;34:102–111.

189. Sloan RP, Bagiella E, Powell T. Religion, spirituality and medicine. *Lancet.* 1999;353:664–667.

190. Smiles S. *Self-Help with Illustrations of Conduct and Perseverance.* London; 1905.

191. Sobell LC, Cunningham JA, Sobell MB. Recovery from alcohol problems with andwithout treatment: prevalence in two population surveys. *Am J Pub Health.* 1996;86:966–972.

192. Sobell LC, Ellingstad TP, Sobell MB. Natural recovery from alcohol and drug problems: methodological review of the research with suggestions for future directions. *Addiction.* 2000;95:749–764.

193. Sobell MB, Sobell LC. Stepped care as a heuristic approach to the treatment of alcohol problems. *J Consult Clin Psychol.* 2000;68:573–579.

194. Spera SP, Buhrfeind ED, Pennebaker JW. Expressive writing and coping with job loss. *Acad Manage J.* 1994;37(3):722–733.

195. Stapleton JA, Russell MA, Feyerabend C, et al. Dose effects and predictors of outcome in a randomized trial of transdermal nicotine patches in general practice. *Addiction.* 1995;90:31–42.

196. Stead LF, Lancaster T. Group behavior therapy programmes for smoking cessation. *Cochrane Database Syst Rev.* 2005;2. https://doi.org/10.1002/14651858.CD001007.pub2.

197. Stead LF, Perera R, Bullen C, Mant D, Lancaster T. Nicotine replacement therapy for smoking cessation. *Cochrane Database Syst Rev.* 2008. https://doi.org/10.1002/14651858.CD000146.

198. Stead LF, Perear R, Lancaster T. Telephone counseling for smoking cessation. *Cochrane Database Syst Rev.* 2006;3:1–86.

199. Reference deleted in review.

200. Reference deleted in review.

201. Reference deleted in review.

202. Stewart C. The influence of spirituality on substance use of college students. *J Drug Educ.* 2001;41:343–351.

203. Strecher VJ, Marcus A, Bishop K, et al. A randomized controlled trial of multiple tailored messages for smoking cessation among callers to the cancer information service. *J Health Commun.* 2005;10(S1):105–118.

204. Strecher VJ, Shiffman S, West R. Randomized controlled trial of a Web-based computer-tailored smoking cessation program as a supplement to nicotine patch therapy. *Addiction*. 2005;100:682–688.

205. Sturm R, Sherbourne CD. Are barriers to mental health and substance abuse care still rising? *J Behav Health Serv Res*. 2001;28:81–88.

206. Swartz LHG, Noell JW, Schroeder SW, Ary DV. A randomised control study of a fully automated Internet based smoking cessation programme. *Tob Control*. 2006;15:7–12.

207. Reference deleted in review.

208. Tait RJ, Spijkerman R, Riper H. Internet and computer based interventions for cannabis use: a meta-analysis. *Drug Alcohol Depen*. 2013;133(2):295–304.

209. Takahashi M, Tatsugi Y, Kohno T. Telephone counseling of athletes abusing anabolic-androgenic steroids. *J Sports Med Phy Fitness*. 2007;47:356–360.

210. The clinical practice guideline treating tobacco use and dependence 2008 update panel, liaisons, and staff. *Am J Prev Med*. 2008;35(2):158–176.

211. Timberlake DS, Rhee SH, Haberstick BC, et al. the moderating effects of religiosity on the genetic and environmental determinants of smoking initiation. *Nicotine Tob Res*. 2006;8:123–133.

212. Thoresen CE, Harris AHS. Spirituality and health: what's the evidence and what's needed? *Ann Behav Med*. 2002:3–13.

213. Tzelepis F, Paul CL, Walsh RA, McElduff P, Knight J. Proactive telephone counseling for smoking cessation: meta-analyses by recruitment channel and methodological quality. *J Natl Cancer I*. 2011;103(12):922–941.

214. Tzelepis F, Paul CL, Walsh RA, Wiggers J, Duncan SL, Knight J. Predictors of abstinence among smokers recruited actively to quitline support. *Addiction*. 2013;108:181–185.

215. U.S. Department of Health and Human Services. *The Health Consequences of Smoking: Nicotine & Addiction: A Report of The Surgeon General*. Rockville, MD: Center Disease Control, Center Health Promotion Education. Off. Smoke, Health; 1988:122.

215a. US Food and Drug Administration. Spilling the Beans: How Much Caffeine is Too Much? 2018. https://www.fda.gov/consumers/consumer-updates/spilling-beans-how-much-caffeine-too-much. Accessed June 21, 2019.

216. US Food and Drug Administration. *Code of Federal Regulations, Title 21, Volume 3*. Food for Human Consumption. the US Government Printing Office; 2016. https://www.accessdata.fda.gov/scripts/cdrh/cfdocs/cfcfr/cfrsearch.cfm. Accessed June 14, 2016.

217. Voorhees CC, Stillman FA, Swank RT, Heagerty PJ, Levine DM, Becker DM. Heart, body, and soul: impact of church-based smoking cessation interventions on readiness to quit. *Prev Med*. 1996;25:277–285.

218. Wagner EH, Schoenbach VJ, Orleans CT, Grothaus LC, Saunders KW, Curry SJ, et al. Participation in a smoking cessation program: a population-based perspective. *Am J Prev Med*. 1990;6:258–266.

219. Wallace Jr JM, Brown TN, Bachman JG, Laveist TA. The influence of race and religion on abstinence from alcohol cigarettes and marijuana among adolescents. *J Stud Alcohol*. 2003;64:843–848.

220. Walters OS. The religious background of 50 alcoholics. *Q J Stud Alcohol*. 1957;18:405–413.

221. Reference deleted in review.

222. Webb T, Joseph J, Yardley L, Michie S. Using the internet to promote health behavior change: a systematic review and meta-analysis of the impact of theoretical basis, use of behavior change techniques, and mode of delivery on efficacy. *J Med Internet Res*. 2010;12(1):e4.

223. Westman EC, Behm FM, Simel DL, Rose JE. Smoking behavior on the first day of a quit attempt predicts long-term abstinence. *Arch Intern Med*. 1997;157:335–340.

224. White A, Kavanagh E, Stallman H, et al. Online alcohol interventions: a systematic review. *J Med Internet Res*. 2010;12:e62.

225. White C, Ritchie J, Crisp D. *Help on Call: Callers' Evaluation of Drinkline, the National Alcohol Helpline*. London: Social and community planning research; 1996.

226. White HR, McMorris BJ, Catalano RF, Fleming CB, Haggerty KP, Abbott RD. Increases in alcohol and marijuana use during the transition out of high school into emerging adulthood: the effects of leaving home, going to college, and high school protective factors. *J Stud Alcohol*. 2006;67(6):810–822.

227. White RJ, Zullig KJ, Lander L, Shockley C, Pack R, Sullivan C. The West Virginia prescription drug abuse quitline. Challenges and lessons learned from running a remote quitline. *Health Promot Pract*. 2012;13:81–89.

228. Whooley MA, Boyd Al, Gardin JM, Williams DR. Religious involvement and cigarette smoking in young adults: the CARDIA study. *Arch Intern Med*. 2002;162:1604–1610.

229. Wills TA, Yaeger AM, Sandy JM. Buffering effect of religiosity for adolescent substance use. *Psychol Addict Behav*. 2003;17:24–31.

230. Witkiewitz K, Bowen S. Depression, craving, and substance use following a randomized trial of mindfulness-based relapse prevention. *J Consult Clin Psych*. 2010;78:362–374.

231. Witkiewitz K, Bowen S, Douglas H, Hsu SH. Mindfulness-based relapse prevention for substance craving. *Addict Behav*. 2013;38:1563–1571.

232. Witkiewitz K, Marlatt GA, Walker D. Mindfulness-based relapse prevention for alcohol and substance use disorders. *J Cogn Psychother Int Q*. 2005;19:211–228.

233. World Health Organization Brief Intervention Study Group. A randomized cross-national clinical trial of brief interventions with heavy drinkers. *Am J Pub Health*. 1996;86:948–955.

234. Young CM, Rodriguez LM, Neighbors C. Expressive writing as a brief intervention for reducing drinking intentions. *Addict Behav*. 2013;38:2913–2917.

235. Zgierska A, Rabago D, Zuelsdorff M, Coe C, Miller M, Fleming M. Mindfulness meditatioin for alcohol relapse preventions: a feasibility pilot study. *J Addict Med*. 2008;2:165–173.

236. Zhu S, Cummins SE, Wong S, Garmst AC, Tedeschi GJ, Reyes-Nocon J. The effects of a multilingual telephone quitline for Asian smokers: a randomized controlled trial. *J Natl Cancer Inst*. 2012;104:299–310.

237. Zhu S, Gardiner P, Cummins S, et al. Quitline utilization rates of African-American and White smokers: the California experience. *Am J Health Promot*. 2011;25:S51–S58.

238. Zhu SH, Anderson CM, Tedeschi GJ, Rosbrook B, Johnson CE, Byrd M, et al. Evidence of real-world effectiveness of a telephone quitline for smokers. *N Eng J Med*. 2002;347:1087–1093.

239. Zhu SH, Melcer T, Sun J, Rosbrook B, Pierce JP. Smoking cessation with and without assistance: a population-based analysis. *Am J Prev Med*. 2000;18:305–311.

240. Zullig KJ, Lander L, White RJ, Sullican C, Shockley C, Dong L. Preliminary evaluation of the WV prescription drug abuse quitline. *W VA Med J*. 2010;106:38–46.

45

Community Clinics

DOROTHY O. JACKSON

Introduction

The first section of this chapter traces the history of community clinic treatment for substance use disorders. Next, the chapter reviews various venues for community treatment and the effectiveness of approaches used where this is known. The definition of substance use disorders has been taken from the American Psychiatric Association's *Diagnostic and Statistical Manual of Mental Disorders, Fifth Edition* (DSM-5). There, "substance-related and addictive disorders" is defined and diagnostic criteria provided with the following specifiers: in early or sustained remission; in a controlled environment; and/or with perceptual disturbances. The disorders discussed in this chapter refer to substance-related and addictive disorders as described in the DSM-5. Where reviewed publications do not use these definitions, other terms used by the primary source are reported.

Although alcohol and nicotine abuse and dependence are listed in the DSM-5, coverage of community treatment is limited to exclude community interventions for these disorders. Community clinic is defined as an intervention that occurs in nonhospital settings and is affiliated with individual health practitioners, or community organizations.

Literature Review Methods

Several forms of literature search software were used to conduct this review. The primary sources have been PubMed and PsycINFO also included Google Scholar as a backup supplement. Key words used were: community clinic treatment for drug dependence (abuse, addiction, substance use disorder); community treatment for drug dependence (abuse, addiction, and so on); history of community clinic treatment for drug dependence (abuse, addiction, and so on); history of community treatment for drug dependence (abuse, addiction, and so on); substance-related disorders, psychotherapy, group, community health services, and adult. In addition, where particular authors or groups of authors have published widely, sources were searched by author names. Thus by definition other forms of addictive phenomena such as alcohol dependence, gambling, compulsive eating, sexual behavior, and other behaviors sharing similarities with the DSM-5-defined substance use disorders were excluded.

History of Community Substance Abuse Treatment

There is no obvious historical marker for when group treatment or community clinic treatment for substance use disorders began. It is likely that the first community treatment for substance use disorders in America originated in pharmacies when opium and laudanum were sold over the counter in community pharmacies. These drugs were widely available in the 1800s and much earlier before that in China, Great Britain, and other countries involved in trade with Asian sources of opium.[49] Historical sources document extensive morphine dependence as both a result of the US Civil War treatment of wounded soldiers and sales of over-the-counter potions and tonics laced with opium and cocaine. The residual addiction among Civil War veterans was called "army disease," and was treated extensively by physicians and community pharmacists with morphine or laudanum maintenance (our term), before the scientific discovery of the cause of addiction.[52] Likewise, dependence upon cocaine-laced tonics and potions was treated by community pharmacists in the same way by making maintenance or restorative doses of "Mrs. Winslow's Soothing Syrup," "Godfrey's Cordial," and other available over-the-counter tonics for those having the as-yet-to-be-identified withdrawal syndrome, and the modest fees to purchase them. Godfrey's Cordial was a mixture of opium sweetened by molasses and flavored with sassafras.[6] It appears that these early community treatments were individual ones rather than group interventions.

When the Harrison Act was passed in 1914, it required registration with the Internal Revenue Service by those involved in any phase of the opium or coca industry, and careful record keeping. The US government made an effort to establish some 40 community clinics to treat individuals who were addicted to morphine, and other opioids, and for whom the new law restricted and cut off their supply.[52] However, these clinics became the source of much controversy and were soon abandoned when the Internal Revenue Service declared them illegal and forced their closing. Persons still addicted faced the challenge of obtaining illegal supplies and risked arrest and incarceration for their opioid addiction. Some physicians continued to treat opioid addiction with prescription opioids, including morphine, even after the Harrison Act. However, in 1919 the Supreme Court ruled physicians could no longer prescribe narcotics for the purpose of treating addiction.[39] By making this community-based treatment illegal, the ruling curtailed this humane medical practice, driving addicted individuals to sources of illegal drugs, to immediate withdrawal, or attempts at detoxification.

The period between the Harrison Act in 1914 and 1935 marked a period where there were strong cultural beliefs and community emphasis on legal and moral sanctions against all narcotic addiction. This social context, including court rulings and Internal Revenue Service actions, proscribed a more humanitarian approach to addiction. Thus during this period there appears to be little, if any, available community clinic or group intervention for substance abuse disorders. However, 1935 marked a significant change in the US government's approach to addictive disorders.

A New Era Begins

In 1935 the US Public Health Service opened large institutions to treat narcotic addiction, first in Lexington, Kentucky, and 3 years later in Fort Worth, Texas. These programs were large federal facilities drawing clients from across the United States, mostly incarcerated addicts convicted of crimes. Although not community clinics, these institutions marked a new and growing attitude toward addictive disorders. These facilities set a precedent for subsequent development of local community clinics, group treatment, and other resources to treat addicted persons. The opening of these two federal treatment facilities that used a civil commitment approach to treat addiction was the beginning of a new era. Addiction became increasingly accepted by society as a disorder in need of special intervention, including medical intervention by community physicians and nonmedical individual and group intervention in various community agencies and programs. These were added to, but did not replace, the predominant community model and legal-based sanctions. Thus more-humane intervention for addictive disorders slowly developed and was accepted, if not widely supported, in subsequent years. Noteworthy is that research conducted at Lexington and Fort Worth greatly established a scientific understanding of the pharmacology and psychopharmacology of addiction, and many scientific behavioral principles that support and maintain addictive behavior, such as the function of drugs as behavioral reinforcers. These facilities also provided a platform for psychosocial assessment, individual and group treatment intervention and follow-up, and epidemiological methods that gradually spread to American urban areas where addictive disorders were prevalent.

Impact of the Community Mental Health Movement

In response to federal court rulings, the community mental health movement spread across the country during the 1960s, providing outpatient treatment for mental disorders. Many clinics developed group interventions for substance abuse and dependence. Most of these embedded substance use disorder clinics focused on alcohol dependence, which was the most prevalent disorder. However, forms of drug dependence were treated in community clinics, most using the Alcoholics Anonymous model prevalent at the time. In addition, during this period, religiously affiliated clinics developed to provide spiritually guided individual and group intervention for substance use disorders. Several of these are described in Milby,[52] but rarely, if ever, did reports of their work or evaluations of their effectiveness reach the professional health and addiction literature.

The Alcoholics Anonymous model can be conceptualized as a spiritually guided intervention that uses a manual. The manual, called the "Big Book," describes 12 steps guiding recovery from alcoholism. The recovery process is guided for each individual by a recovering sober sponsor. A key component of this intervention was the use of ubiquitous Alcoholics Anonymous community groups. As the Alcoholics Anonymous movement grew, the model provided widespread community intervention for alcoholism and gradually came to accept persons with other substance use disorders into their network of community Alcoholics Anonymous groups. Increased acceptance of individuals with substance use disorders was aided by the fact that most substance abusers also abused or were dependent on alcohol. The expansion of Alcoholics Anonymous peer-led community group meetings to Narcotics Anonymous helped gather and focus those with substance use disorders to participate in aftercare and continued rehabilitation and recovery efforts. Many persons entered these community-based groups after formal medical or psychosocial-based community treatment. However, despite the fact that Alcoholics Anonymous was one of the most widely utilized community interventions to treat substance use disorders, it was rarely scientifically evaluated. Only over the last 20 years have the Alcoholics Anonymous interventions been scrutinized with rigorous scientific methodology to study its efficacy and effectiveness.[65] A problem for individuals with co-occurring mental disorders and alcohol/drug dependence who utilized the Alcoholics Anonymous model treatment, especially peer-run aftercare groups, was the cultural bias against using a medication to treat a co-occurring disorder. Individuals with dual diagnoses sometimes found a lack of peer support for their medication treatment.

As community group interventions expanded, two predominant models emerged across American communities. One was the Alcoholics Anonymous movement, which focused initially on alcohol treatment and was especially influential as an aftercare intervention for the other, a medical model intervention. The medical model conceptualized addiction as a drug-induced disorder or disease maintained by an artificially induced biological drive from chronic addictive drug use.[21,35] Intervention required inpatient hospitalization for detoxification and restoration of abstinence and normalizing of natural biological drives devoid of addiction side effects and biological disruptions. Various psychosocial models were usually added to this medical approach, especially group rehabilitation and recovery procedures to support a drug-free lifestyle. As medical detoxification was studied, outcomes defined as return to abstinence after medical detoxification were considered successful, especially for inpatient detoxification. But outcomes defined as sustained abstinence at follow-ups were recognized as a dismal failure.[a] Such accumulating evidence provided the impetus for greater emphasis on developing psychosocial intervention to support behavioral lifestyle change, both during medical treatment but especially following hospitalization and in outpatient clinic group intervention and aftercare.

Community mental health interventions for substance abuse disorders and co-occurring mental and substance use disorders predominantly used a rehabilitation model for intervention, as distinguished from pharmacological and other somatic interventions.[24] Initial efforts to treat co-occurring disorders involved separate clinicians working for separate treatment agencies. These initial efforts met with failure, mainly due to problems in coordinating care and accessing needed services.[69]

The development of second-generation neuroleptic medication for serious mental illness was concurrent with refinement of psychosocial treatments, including group interventions, which, within community mental health clinics, served as a floor intervention. These emphasized development of a trusting relationship to help clients cope with a chronic mental illness. Within this relationship, clinician and client establish goals to maximize self-control over symptoms and minimize interference from the illness. This intervention is collaborative, utilizing psychosocial education, especially about the illness, and cognitive behavioral therapy. The intervention often involves peer groups to supplement individual counseling, psychotherapy, and medication monitoring. The recent decade has seen increasing emphases on involving families and use of evidence-based family interventions, and psychoeducation.[24] Drake and colleagues have contended that since the 1990s psychiatric rehabilitation became the dominant method employed in most community mental health clinics.

In the 1990s, specific approaches for treating co-occurring mental and substance use disorders began to be developed and tested.[7,62,87] However, as Drake et al. noted,[25] although controlled research has provided support for effectiveness of these integrated approaches, they are yet to be widely adopted in community clinics.

Effectiveness of Community Clinic Approaches 1935–1980

Community methadone maintenance treatment was initiated in New York City by Vincent Dole in 1965.[20] Based on a disease model of addiction, methadone, as a long-acting synthetic opiate, is given orally to opioid-addicted individuals as a treatment medication. It both alleviates withdrawal symptoms and blocks the effects of illicit opioid use. Methadone is a federally regulated, commercially pure medication, devoid of often dangerous adulterants (drug cutting/mixing agents), and administered in once daily doses in a medically supervised clinic. After initial assessment, many clients are administered take-home doses, which require less than daily attendance. As originally developed, psychosocial counseling and access to other community rehabilitation services provided additional therapeutic leverage for a changed lifestyle and sustained abstinence. The outcome studies of Dole and colleagues showed excellent treatment success as measured by the ability of addicts to reduce criminal activity, obtain or return to jobs or training programs, and otherwise make lifestyle changes to support abstinence.[20,22,23] The success of this early work soon led to a proliferation of methadone maintenance treatment across the nation and was supported by government grants to establish and maintain them with community matching funds. Although not as successful as original efforts by Dole and Nyswander, subsequent research from other communities generally found successful outcomes defined as treatment retention, reduced illicit drug use, criminal activity, and increased employment and other measured lifestyle changes.[4,52,55] However, when outcomes were considered as successful detoxification from methadone and sustained abstinence at follow-up, results were much less impressive.[43,53] Detoxification success was complicated by the discovery of a detoxification phobia, which hampered about 20%–30% of addicts in methadone maintenance from even attempting detoxification despite their goal to eventually do so.[33,55] Although it seems likely that some group psychosocial intervention was utilized in community methadone maintenance during this era, its use was not described in the studies cited here.

Much of the treatments predominantly oriented toward opioid dependence and most other polydrug abuse and dependence disorders were not treated in methadone maintenance programs. Rather, they were treated by other interventions. Many of these are reviewed later. Hospital-based inpatient treatment usually utilized medical procedures for detoxification, but these were embedded within a floor psychosocial recovery and rehabilitation intervention. When they first evolved, hospital stays of 1–2 months were common. However, these long stays succumbed to economic pressures from health insurance companies and gradually evolved to 28-day interventions.

Therapeutic community intervention usually involved the longest stays in a controlled access institutional environment, of up to 6 months or more, and many utilized psychosocial intervention conceptualized as community as the treatment intervention.[18] The community-as-intervention utilized peer group review and confrontation for antisocial and other nonadaptive behaviors that the community evaluated as nonadaptive for a drug-free lifestyle.

---

[a]References 13, 30, 32, 38, 43, 44, 52, 53, 75, 85.

These were usually staffed by few professional health personnel and relied heavily on recovering persons as peer mentors and group leaders. Finally, by far the widest used community intervention was drug-free clinics, where a variety of psychosocial and religious-spiritual intervention models were employed. Up until 1981 there was little scientifically sound clinical research on the effectiveness of any of these approaches (see Milby[52]; Chapters 9 and 10 for a review of these). Where outcome data were published, because of flawed research methods, occasional reported successful outcomes were interpreted with much skepticism.

Community Responses to the 1980s Cocaine Epidemic

During the 1980s, cocaine abuse and dependence increased dramatically in the United States with the availability of less-expensive free base crack cocaine crystals, which could be smoked instead of snorted or injected. This caused a great influx of clients to existing substance abuse community treatment programs at a time where there was no scientifically based effective treatment (medication or psychosocial intervention) available. University and community clinics treated this influx of new clients with their usual care, namely through medical or Alcoholics Anonymous models. However, the few studies that assessed clinical outcomes showed very disappointing results of high treatment dropouts and high relapse rates after treatment established abstinence.[28,29,40,82,83]

In response to this frustrating failure to provide a scientifically supported effective treatment for cocaine dependence, several empirically supported innovative interventions emerged in the 1990s. Two effective outpatient interventions emerged from university clinics and utilized either a group treatment model or a more individualized contingency management behavior therapy program.[12,34] Soon after that, Milby and colleagues[57] described a sufficiently effective community-based intervention for cocaine-dependent homeless persons that utilized contingency-managed access to abstinence-contingent housing and paid work/training along with a group-based behavioral day treatment. This effective community intervention has been improved and systemically replicated in three subsequent randomized trials[56,58,60] and found to be cost-effective.[73] However, to date there have been few efforts to transfer and systematically replicate this evidence-based intervention in other communities. In addition, during this period, other researchers developed community-based, empirically supported, effective group psychosocial interventions for cocaine dependence.[16,48,57,67,76]

Since initial studies by Higgins et al.[34] and Carroll et al.,[12] there has been steady development of effective psychotherapeutic interventions for cocaine dependence from randomized controlled trials employing both different study populations and interventions.[b] All of these, except perhaps Higgins et al. (who utilized an individual-focused intervention), utilized group interventions, which included psychoeducational group psychotherapeutic approaches, sometimes including couple or family interventions.[27,68] It is important to note that some of these recent studies have shown sustained abstinence at follow-up after initial treatment. This increased availability of research-based efficacious psychosocial interventions for cocaine dependence has led Carroll[9] to argue persuasively that manual-guided psychosocial

treatment should be used as a therapeutic platform to evaluate the efficacy of new pharmacotherapies.

Categories of Community Clinics

Rodgers and Barnett[70] examined types of community treatment programs and defined two main types: public and privately funded programs. These were further divided into four main types: public nonfederal programs (i.e., state-run or local programs), public federal programs, private nonprofit programs, and private for-profit programs. Data were derived from the 1991 National Drug and Alcoholism Treatment Unit Survey, and included a final total of 8865 programs. Some of these programs were inpatient hospital facilities, which are outside the scope of this chapter, but this study provides an introduction to different categories of substance abuse programs, as well as information about the differences among them. Overall, the largest number of programs were private nonprofit, followed by private for-profit, public nonfederal, and public federal programs. Thus the majority of programs were private programs comprising approximately 82.7% of the sample.

A key issue examined in comparisons among categories was staffing. Rodgers and Barnett[70] found that public nonfederal programs had the highest number of staff, followed by private nonprofit and private for-profit programs. Although public federal programs had the fewest number of staff, they were the most likely to employ doctoral level staff, followed closely by private for-profit programs. When examining the size of residential programs, federal programs were the largest, and private for-profit programs were the smallest. Public drug-free outpatient programs were also larger than the private drug-free outpatient programs. For-profit programs were the smallest. For methadone maintenance programs, private for-profit programs were the largest, with the rest of the categories lagging far behind.

The study of Rodgers and Barnett[70] also provided information on specific services offered by the different categories of substance abuse programs. Both public federal programs and private for-profit programs were most likely to offer aftercare and follow-up. Public federal programs were the most likely to offer medical care. All programs were equally likely to offer individual therapy; private nonprofit programs were slightly more likely than for-profit programs to offer group therapy, and private programs were more likely to offer family therapy. Their survey of services for special populations (discussed in more detail later), showed that public nonfederal programs were more likely to offer special services for pregnant individuals and youth. Private for-profit programs were more likely to offer services specialized for cocaine users.

There were also differences in funding sources for the categories of substance abuse treatment. Both private nonprofit and public nonfederal programs were more likely to receive Medicaid funding, although private for-profit programs that did receive Medicaid funding received more money than did public nonfederal programs. In addition, private for-profit programs were more likely to receive funding from both private insurance and client fees, and they also received the most from these funding sources, followed by nonprofit programs. Public federal programs received the least funding from these sources.

Overall, Rodgers and Barnett[70] found that private for-profit programs were smaller (with the exception of methadone maintenance programs), more specialized, and had less staff, but had staff with a higher level of training. These programs were also more likely to receive funding from private insurance and client fees, as opposed to Medicaid.

---

[b]References 10, 16, 27, 48, 56, 63, 68.

Types of Community Clinics

Therapeutic Communities

Therapeutic communities are one of the more common treatment methods present in community programs and have been included in large-scale studies such as the Drug Abuse Reporting Program.[78] Therapeutic communities are long-term, residential programs that utilize a social treatment approach. Therapeutic communities view drug abuse as a disorder of the person and the recovery process as development and integration of both psychological and social goals.[80] The community as a group aspect of treatment is seen as the major impetus toward growth and change. The community is made up of the social environment, peers, and staff, many of whom are successfully recovered addicts themselves.[18]

Both behavioral and social learning principles are utilized in therapeutic communities, and some techniques include efficacy training, social role training, and vicarious learning.[80] Physical addiction is seen as a symptom and is secondary in importance to the behavioral and psychological aspects of the individual's drug abuse. Maintaining a drug-free lifestyle is the main goal of therapeutic communities, which also utilize a present-oriented approach that emphasizes personal responsibility as well as the development of positive values such as honesty, good work ethic, and community involvement.[80] Although each individual is responsible for their own recovery process, the role each person plays in the recovery of others is also emphasized. Some of the daily activities of therapeutic communities include work, group sessions, and recreation. Individuals in the group serve as mediators and role models. They also confront misbehavior, rule violations, and share with one another during group sessions. Attitude and behavior change in relationships developed in the therapeutic communities serve an important function by helping maintain recovery after the individual leaves treatment.[80]

Condelli and Hubbard[15] provide a comprehensive chapter that discusses client outcomes for therapeutic communities from admission to posttreatment. These outcomes were not derived from scientifically controlled studies using rigorous randomized control methods. However, they do reflect what happens to clients admitted to therapeutic communities in community settings. This chapter examines outcomes from a large-scale series of studies derived from the Drug Abuse Reporting Program. Clients in these studies showed a decline in drug use, including opioid use as well as nonopioid use, and also showed a decrease in arrest and incarceration rates. One of the most important and consistent predictors of the success of individuals was the amount of time they spent in therapeutic communities, although the length of time necessary to see positive outcomes varied from study to study. In a Drug Abuse Reporting Program follow-up study, therapeutic communities showed more favorable outcomes than outpatient detoxification and intake-only; they did not differ significantly from methadone maintenance or outpatient drug-free counseling.[78]

In addition to the various categories of community clinics, there are also a variety of treatment approaches utilized. Although the list of various specific approaches is very long, there are a handful of approaches that were most commonly seen. What follows is a list of some of the most commonly used approaches, along with a description of some of the techniques and results of research studies, when available. Approaches discussed are contingency management, where group methods are employed; cognitive behavioral treatment (including relapse prevention); integrated group therapy for co-occurring bipolar and substance use disorders; 12-step facilitation; pharmacotherapeutic approaches (including methadone maintenance, buprenorphine, and so on), where group psychosocial or educational methods are used; and faith-based approaches.

Prize-Based Contingency Management

Prize-based contingency management is a viable option for community clinics and utilizes "an intermittent reinforcement contingency management approach" usually in the context of behavioral group therapy.[64] This differs from a voucher program in that prizes are not continuous, thus decreasing program costs. Many programs that utilize this approach offer draws from a container of chips that have different reward values marked on them, ranging from Good Job (no value) to Jumbo (gets to pick from prizes worth about $80–$100).[1,46,64] These draws can be made contingent on negative urine samples, participation in planned activities, or any other behaviors that the clinicians wish to reinforce. Another option is to set the program up with prize drawings every week. In this approach, clients are allowed to place their names into a bowl for each session that they attend, and then names are drawn each day to receive prizes.[1] These techniques can be utilized independently from each other or combined.

Petry et al.[64] utilized several programs from the Clinical Trials Network to look at the efficacy of prize-based contingency management in stimulant abusers. These programs all utilized the approach where clients earned draws from the container for chips with various reward values. The prize-based contingency management programs were compared with usual care, which was mostly group counseling. Participants in the prize-based contingency management programs showed more negative urine samples, as well as longer periods of abstinence. Other studies, which looked at both cocaine- and opioid-dependent individuals, showed similar results, each showing that participants in the prize-based contingency management program demonstrated longer periods of abstinence compared with those receiving standard treatment,[46] although the Alessi et al.[1] study failed to show an impact of contingency management prizes on attendance when prizes were awarded during group.

Day Treatment With Abstinence Contingencies and Vouchers

Day treatment with abstinence contingencies and vouchers[56,58,59,74] is an intensive program that focuses on substance abuse rehabilitation of homeless crack-cocaine abusers. Clients participate for 5.5 hours each day in the program for the first 2 months, during which time they are provided with lunch and transportation to and from the treatment center. Treatment services include: individual assessment and goal setting, individual and group counseling, and multiple psychoeducational groups. During weekly goal review groups, clients review contract goals and provide support and encouragement to each other and receive vouchers for goal attainment that may be applied toward renting low-cost, drug-free housing. Participants may also earn vouchers by engaging in proabstinence social and recreational activities. After 2 months, participants enter a 4-month vocational phase that includes both paid work and program-provided housing, which are abstinence contingent.

This day treatment approach has been shown to be effective compared with a treatment-as-usual individual and group counseling based on an Alcoholics Anonymous model, where clients

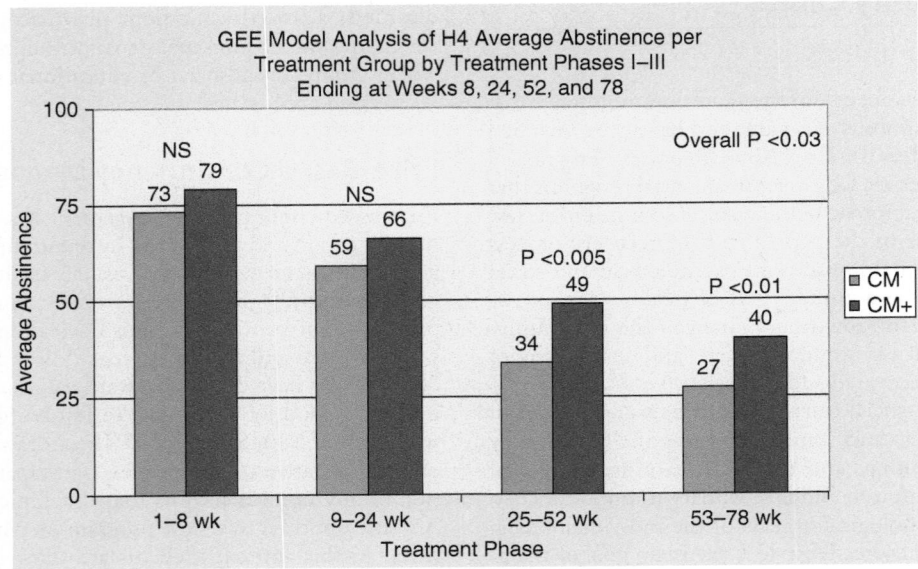

• **Fig. 45.1** H4 abstinence per group across phases: average abstinence per group across four phases of treatment as measured by observed urine collection and testing multiple times per week up to 24 weeks, and randomly thereafter through week 78 (18 months follow-up). *CM,* Contingency management; *GEE,* generalized estimating equations; *H4,* the study by Milby et al.[58]; *NS,* not significant. (From Milby JB, Schumacher JE, Vuchinich RE, Freedman MJ, Kertesz S, Wallace D. Toward cost-effective initial care for substance-abusing homeless. *J Subst Abuse Treat.* 2008;34(2):180–191.)

were referred to community resources for housing and work. Subsequent studies have utilized a dismantling design strategy where investigators systematically replicated the original behavioral day treatment,[57] while examining the contribution of key components.[56,58,74]

Results from the most recent study of Milby et al.[58] are shown in Fig. 45.1. In this study, designated H4, abstinence outcomes were compared between the two treatment groups to which participants were randomly assigned. The "CM" group received contingency-managed abstinence-contingent housing, work training, and paid work. The "CM+" group received the same contingency-managed components as the CM group, but in addition received a manualized effective cognitive behavioral day treatment used in previous studies. As Fig. 45.1 shows, abstinence levels for both groups during active treatment (weeks 1–24) are moderately high, ranging from 59% to 79%, with no differences between groups. However, at posttreatment follow-up, at 12 and 18 months, the CM+ group receiving additional cognitive behavioral intervention showed a delayed treatment effect of superior sustained long-term abstinence, which was measured rigorously using urine toxicologies. In a meta-analysis of treatment components, Schumacher et al.[74] found contingency-managed components to be those associated with greatest abstinence. All of these studies have shown modest improvements in both reduced homelessness and increased employment for all treatment groups from admission to long-term follow-up.

Cognitive Behavioral Treatment

According to McCarty et al.,[50] about one-third of treatment programs in the Clinical Trials Network utilized National Institute on Alcohol Abuse and Alcoholism treatment manuals, and 28% of those utilized cognitive behavioral treatment. In addition, approximately 26% of programs that utilized National Institute on Drug Abuse treatment manuals used *A Cognitive Behavioral Approach: Treating Cocaine Addiction.* The National Institute on Drug Abuse[63] provided a general description of cognitive behavioral therapy for substance use disorders as well as some information regarding its efficacy. Cognitive behavioral treatment is based on social learning theory and can be applied in a group or individual setting. Some of the foci are on increasing self-efficacy and reducing positive expectations about substance use, as well as teaching coping skills, especially in relapse situations. He reports that there are several studies that provide evidence for the efficacy of cognitive behavioral therapy in treating substance use disorders. In addition, a study by Maude-Griffin et al.[48] of crack-cocaine abusers showed that clients in cognitive behavioral treatment were more likely than clients in a 12-step facilitation program to achieve consecutive abstinence for one month. Clients in cognitive behavioral treatment also showed significantly better abstinence results at each of the follow-ups (weeks 4, 8, 12, and 26).

Rawson et al.[68] completed a study comparing cognitive behavioral treatment, contingency management, contingency management + cognitive behavioral therapy, and standard methadone treatment in a community clinic affiliated with the University of California Los Angeles. All of these treatments utilized group methods. During treatment and at week 17 follow-up, clients in the cognitive behavioral therapy did not show significantly more positive abstinence results than the standard methadone treatment, while both of the other two treatment conditions did. However, at the week 26 and week 52 follow-ups, the clients in the cognitive behavioral therapy showed the most positive abstinence results of all the treatment groups.

Relapse Prevention

Relapse prevention is a cognitive behavioral approach that strives for eventual abstinence by emphasizing reducing the risk of relapse. It is based on the theory that substance use disorders involve learned maladaptive behavior, and clients have the potential to reestablish previously adaptive non–drug use behaviors and develop new behaviors. Clients are taught to identify problem behavior and replace unhealthy behaviors with healthier substitutes. The cognitive behavioral treatment techniques are employed to identify risks and coping strategies to deal with those risks. Specific techniques utilized include (1) identifying disadvantages of continuing drug abuse; (2) self-monitoring drug use behavior to help identify situations that trigger maladaptive behaviors; and (3) developing effective coping strategies to curb craving and reduce stress. Although relapse prevention methods can be utilized in individual or group therapy, most community programs utilize groups.

Studies indicate that relapse prevention helps recovering drug addicts maintain abstinence longer by reducing the risk of relapse.[8,47] This method has also been found to reduce the impact of relapse if it should occur by preparing clients ahead of time with knowledge and tools to cope during distressing situations. The interested reader will find an excellent review by Carroll and Onken[11] of behavioral and cognitive behavioral therapies, some of which were conducted in group format or combined individual and group behavioral interventions. The review included studies with families and couples.

Integrated Group Therapy

Integrated group therapy is a manualized 20-session, 1-hour weekly group intervention that addresses substance use disorder simultaneously with co-occurring bipolar disorder. It emphasizes interaction between the disorders by examining similarities in cognitive and behavioral patterns involved in recovery from both.[84] Adverse effects of each disorder on the other are emphasized. For example, one session is "Dealing with Depression Without Using Alcohol or Drugs." Sessions involve a check-in, where clients report on substance use, moods, medication adherence, and the risky and stressful situations confronted. The check-in is followed by a planned psychoeducational topic and discussion. Their randomized controlled trial compared 20 weekly sessions of integrated group therapy with group drug counseling focused on the substance use disorder. Group drug counseling was an adaptation of the treatment delivered in the National Institute on Drug Abuse's Drug Abuse Collaborative Cocaine Treatment Study,[16] designed to approximate treatment in community substance use disorder programs. Group drug counseling also involved 20 weekly group sessions, each focused on a specific topic. Sixty-two participants with bipolar disorder and current substance dependence were treated with mood-stabilizing medications for 2 weeks or more and randomized to $N = 31$ in each group. Main outcomes were number of days of substance use and number of weeks ill with a mood disorder.

Results showed fewer days of substance use for integrated group therapy. Groups were similar for number of weeks ill with bipolar disorder during both treatment and follow-up; however, integrated group therapy had more depressive and manic symptoms. This study is notable for two reasons. First, the intervention was designed to be comparable to what many community clinics already do. That the integrated group therapy group showed better substance abuse outcomes, but not superior reductions in number of weeks ill with mood disorder, was a surprising finding. Integrated group therapy needs replication with larger N values and replication attempts in community clinic settings. If

integrated group therapy is shown effective in community clinics, its manualized format and straightforward procedures could yield significant impact on the treatment of co-occurring mental and substance use disorders in community substance abuse treatment programs, which rely heavily on group interventions. Integrated group therapy's potential impact on weekly mood disorder symptoms is troubling and could be a function of its weekly review of mood and medication compliance, which could increase participant's sensitivity to their bipolar symptoms. This impact is another reason for further study and replication before extensive community adoption is encouraged.

12-Step Facilitation

According to McCarty et al.,[50] of programs in the Clinical Trials Network that utilized National Institute on Alcohol Abuse and Alcoholism treatment manuals, 20% of those utilized 12-step facilitation. Although literature searches did not identify many studies on the efficacy of this approach specifically in community clinics, except as a comparison or control group, some more general information about it has been included.

Moos[61] provides a general description of 12-step facilitation for substance use disorders as well as some information on its efficacy. Twelve-step facilitation is based on the ideology of Alcoholics Anonymous and the disease model of addiction. Some of the main foci of this approach are on getting clients to admit that they have a problem, and that they are an alcoholic or addict. The emphasis is on abstinence, without accepting controlled drinking as an option. Clients are directed to develop and maintain strong relationships with positive individuals who support their sobriety, such as their family and other sober networks. They are also encouraged to turn themselves over to a Higher Power. Coping skills are taught, and self-efficacy is enhanced. Twelve-step facilitation is an all-encompassing approach, in that clients are asked to attend 12-step meetings, get a sponsor, read the literature, and regularly attend 12-step meetings. Moos reports that there are several studies that provide evidence that 12-step facilitation is effective for several different types of substance use disorders.

Faith-Based and Religiously Affiliated Programs

The faith-based and religious approach to substance use disorders is fairly common in community clinics.[52,77] However, there is little to no research on the efficacy of these approaches. In addition, there is little to no information regarding standard practice or techniques of these programs, other than that which is available on individual program websites. Twelve-step facilitation is spiritual in its approach, although it is not affiliated with a specific religious organization.

An article by Cnaan and Boddie[14] discusses a section of the Personal Responsibility and Work Opportunity Reconciliation Act of 1996 called Charitable Choice. This section encourages the participation of faith-based organizations in federally funded welfare services, including health services such and drug and alcohol treatment. In addition, since 1996, there have been other acts passed to further encourage the involvement of faith-based and religious organizations in social services. Furthermore, there is more protection for religious-based programs to maintain their themes and religious methods by being able to keep all religious symbols, literature, and so on, as well as protecting their ability to only hire employees who share or practice their religious beliefs and to fire those who do not.

Cnaan and Boddie[14] also discuss those studies that are focused on the effects of Charitable Choice. However, these studies only look at the awareness of Charitable Choice and an "assessment of the scope and nature of contracting relationships between faith-based organizations and the public sector." They also state that there are no studies on the effectiveness of the services provided by faith-based organizations.

Interventions for Specific Populations

The Substance Abuse and Mental Health Services Administration at the National Institutes of Health conducted the 2006 National Survey of Substance Abuse Treatment Services.[19] Data were collected on treatment facilities in the 50 states, the District Columbia, and US territories. The survey included information about programs tailored to treat specific populations. Specialized treatments include the treatment of adolescents, older adults, individuals with co-occurring mental/substance abuse disorders, gays/lesbians, driving under the influence/driving while intoxicated offenders, other substance-related criminal offenders, adult men, adult women, pregnant/postpartum women, and individuals with HIV.

It seems likely that clinics servicing large numbers of individuals are more likely to have a sufficient number of clients in more of these subgroups to enable the provision of specialized services. Thirty-two percent of facilities offer programs specifically for adult women and 25% for adult men. Services directed at treating pregnant or postpartum women are offered by 14% of facilities. Thirty-two percent of institutions also offer services designed for adolescents and 7% for older adults. Adolescent and senior services are offered most frequently by facilities operated by tribal governments (52 and 12%, respectively).

Women are often a minority in substance abuse treatment programs. Women have unique needs and problems associated with their gender, like child care and custody, and abuse by their partner, which may not be revealed or get much attention in male-dominated, mixed-gender group sessions. Thus many clinics have developed women's recovery groups. An example of such a specialty program for women is that of Greenfield and colleagues[31] in Boston. They have developed and completed an initial study of a manualized 12-session Women's Recovery Group. Women were randomized to either Women's Recovery Group or mixed-gender Group Drug Counseling. No differences in substance use were found during the 12-week treatment. However, at 6 months follow-up, Women's Recovery Group, but not Group Drug Counseling women, showed continued reductions in substance use. In addition, Women's Recovery Group women with alcohol dependence showed greater reductions in drinking. It is important to note that these results were associated with greater satisfaction among women treated in the Women's Recovery Group. Although this specialty group is early in its development and needs replication, both by the authors and those in another setting, it does suggest that such specialty groups can be supportive of longer-term clinical outcomes for women with substance use disorders.

Thirty-one percent of facilities offered special programs to driving under the influence/driving while intoxicated offenders. The majority of facilities offering offender services are private for-profit facilities (46%). Tribal government facilities offered 38% of substance abuse treatment specifically for persons with driving under the influence/driving while intoxicated charges. For other types of substance-related criminal offender populations, 28% of facilities offered tailored treatment. It is important to note that most, if not all, state and federal correctional facilities offer group interventions for inmates with substance use disorders, and some include within the correctional facility a residential therapeutic community where inmates are usually separated from the regular prison population.

Fewer facilities report offering services specifically designed for specialty populations, such as individuals with HIV/AIDS, older adults, and gays/lesbians. Only 10% of facilities report offering services for people with HIV/AIDS. Only 10% of federal government-operated facilities report offering services for older adults; however, this was greater than most other facilities. For the gay/lesbian client population, only 6% of facilities report offering specifically designed services. The percentage increases slightly (8%) for private, for-profit institutions who offer targeted treatment interventions for homosexuals. The literature that was reviewed did not mention whether these varieties of services are group services. However, it is likely that many of these categories are conducted in group intervention formats, especially therapy or psychoeducational groups.

Use of Evidence-Based Services in Community Clinic Substance Abuse Treatment

Treatment services operate with limited money and resources. Community substance abuse treatment services strive to be cost neutral for their planned budget expenditures. For-profit/private clinics aim to make a profit so the program can sustain, if not expand, its services. Thus a cost-effective program may come at the expense of maximizing treatment gains. Clinics using interventions that lack empirical evidence or have been deemed less beneficial than alternative methods, may prove in the long run to cost more to operate because of the need for longer treatment or increased risk of relapse. Thus it appears to be in the best long-term interest of facilities to find the most effective treatment that also results in long-term abstinence or maintenance of risk reduction, relapse prevention, shorter treatment time, and less manpower required for implementation. Overall, a treatment program that is both effective and efficient may be most beneficial for most treatment centers and clientele. Realistically, however, few community clinics have the resources to collect valid treatment outcome data to inform administrative decisions about what interventions are most effective or most cost-effective.

Community clinics that specialize in treatment of substance abuse or comorbid substance abuse and mental health disorders face an even greater need to maximize treatment gains in treating substance abuse because funding is often contingent upon these services. The 2005 American Psychological Association Statement defines effectiveness as treatment methods that are "… the integration of the best available research with clinical expertise in the context of patient characteristics, culture, and preferences."[3]

Treatment quality and effectiveness can be graded according to specific criteria. The Agency for Healthcare Research and Quality, US Department of Health and Human Services reported 40 systems of "grading the strength of a body of evidence." The National Guideline Clearinghouse, for example, requires developers to submit treatment guidelines based on quality of evidence criteria.

Standardization is important in promoting effectiveness of treatment by (1) comparing outcomes of one treatment to another, and thereby holding facilities accountable to reach expected outcomes and (2) training employees to administer treatment to clients while maintaining consistency of practice. Use of treatment guides and manuals can help employees check their actual treatment methods and behavior compared with what is specified and described in manuals or guidelines for high quality and/or effective treatment. In this way, treatment delivery fidelity may be more likely to result in positive outcomes obtained in clinical research using these same treatment manuals and methods. Standardization also helps to identify client variables that may contribute to good or poor treatment response by controlling for treatment methods. This form of standardization may facilitate practitioners to meet more needs of the clients.

Treatment guidelines are also published by agencies such as the National Institute of Drug Abuse.[63] Effective manualized interventions selected by or developed for the National Institute on Drug Abuse's National Drug Abuse Treatment Clinical Trials Network are available in the published clinical literature and posted on their website for use by community clinics outside of the network where original effectiveness research has been completed.

The Substance Abuse and Mental Health Services Administration has published and continues to provide an expanding library of treatment improvement manuals that are evidence-based and written for community substance abuse treatment program adoption. There appears to be a slowly growing trend among the more stably supported community substance abuse treatment programs, most of which utilize group interventions extensively, to adopt evidence-based interventions. However, it also seems that the diffusion of these evidence-based interventions is slow, and that the majority of community clinics have not yet fully embraced evidence-based services for their clients with substance use disorders.

The National Institute on Drug Abuse has produced a comprehensive handbook of evidence-based substance abuse treatments entitled *Principles of Drug Addiction Treatment: A Research-Based Guide.*[63] The guide outlines principles of effective treatment available in the United States and scientifically based approaches to drug addiction treatment as well as a list of resources and answers to some frequently asked questions for individuals and families seeking treatment. The document briefly describes studies supported by the National Institute on Drug Abuse that investigated interventions for substance use disorders, which were found to be efficacious and/or effective. Group treatment programs include long-term residential treatment, short-term residential programs, and outpatient drug-free treatment utilizing group intervention formats. The National Institute on Drug Abuse guide also describes agonist maintenance treatment (e.g., methadone treatment programs), narcotic antagonist treatment using naltrexone, and medical detoxification.

The National Institute on Drug Abuse's National Drug Abuse Treatment Clinical Trials Network

The mission of the Clinical Trials Network is to improve interventions available to persons with substance use disorders by studying the effectiveness of evidence-based treatment services in collaboration with community treatment agencies. Effectiveness research is conducted at collaborating community programs. The Clinical Trials Network aspires to replicate efficacious and effective treatment in clinical trials of substance abuse research by publishing findings from multiple community clinics and by allowing studies funded by other agencies to utilize Clinical Trials Network protocols. In addition, the Clinical Trials Network provides capabilities for access to Clinical Trials Network Node facilities (community clinics), new investigations, and Clinical Trials Network Nodes to serve as National Institutes of Health Training Centers.

The Clinical Trials Network consists of (1) 17 Nodes (Regional Research and Training Centers, all associated with five or more Community-Based Treatment Programs), (2) a Clinical Coordinating Center, and (3) a Data and Statistical Center. The network of multisites allows researchers to test the effectiveness of treatment on a large array of populations across the United States. The Clinical Trials Network also allows for new evidence-based practices to be diffused to and implemented by community clinics.

Virginia, Maryland, and Washington, DC, for example, are regions overseen by the Mid-Atlantic Node. This Clinical Trials Network Node is operated out of Johns Hopkins University (a Regional Research and Training Center) and is linked to seven Community-Based Treatment Programs such as the Chesterfield (Virginia) CSB Substance Abuse Service and the REACH Mobile Health Services in Catonsville, Maryland. The Mid-Atlantic Node, alone, has been involved in the implementation of nine substance abuse treatment protocols throughout this Node's affiliated community clinics.

Analogous to the network of National Institutes of Health–supported national cancer centers, but on a smaller scale, it is possible that the Clinical Trials Network could have a similar impact on community intervention for substance use disorders. Before national cancer centers were developed, effective treatments for cancers developed in academic medical centers were not transferred to local communities. Thus best practices remained relatively nonimplemented by local physicians. Treatment for substance use disorders is in a similar situation. Although there is an array of effective substance use disorder treatments, most studies at academic treatment centers have not yet been diffused to community clinics and programs. It is hoped that the Clinical Trials Network will increase the slow rate of diffusion of effective treatment and also accelerate discovery of the most effective of the efficacious interventions it studies.

Drug Abuse Reporting Program Studies

The Drug Abuse Reporting Program yielded a series of major large-scale studies that examined community-based drug abuse treatment agencies and their short- and long-term outcomes. The Drug Abuse Reporting Program was initiated in 1969 by the Institute of Behavioral Research at Texas Christian University. An article by Simpson and Sells[78] describes both the studies and the outcome measures. The Drug Abuse Reporting Program originally started with six treatment agencies, and expanded to include 52 in the United States and Puerto Rico, totaling 43,943 clients. It utilized client intake records, bimonthly treatment status records, and follow-up samples. Follow-up research began in 1974, after client intake records stopped being collected. Surveys lasted, on average, 5–7 years after admission, and 4 years after the end of treatment. The emphasis in the Drug Abuse Reporting Program was on community services and outcomes, not experimental interventions. Clinics included in the Drug Abuse Reporting Program continued with their normal procedures to collect data on client outcomes.

Follow-up outcome data were collected through a sample of reimbursed, face-to-face interviews. Interviews used retrospective self-reports on employment, drug and alcohol use, and return to treatment. The follow-up sample included 4627 clients from 34 Drug Abuse Reporting Programs. Five different types of community intervention in the follow-up sample included methadone maintenance, therapeutic communities, outpatient drug-free treatments, outpatient detoxification clinics, and the comparison group, which was intake only. The clients were also separated based on their addiction status and divided into three categories: active addicts (those who used opioids daily for 2 months before the Drug Abuse Reporting Program), former addicts (who had a history of daily opioid use, but not during the 2 months before the Drug Abuse Reporting Program), and nonaddicts (who had no history of daily opioid use). Outcomes examined at follow-up were illicit drug use, criminality indicators, alcohol use, return to treatment, and employment. The main outcome measures were illicit drug use and criminality

indicators. Highly favorable outcomes were defined as having no drug use and no arrests or incarcerations. Twenty-seven percent of clients in methadone maintenance met these standards, along with 28% in therapeutic communities, 24% in outpatient drug-free treatments, 15% in outpatient detoxification, and 14% in intake-only. Moderately favorable outcomes were defined as no daily drug use and no major criminality indicators, which were further defined as no crimes against persons or crimes of profit and no more than 30 days in jail or prison. Forty-one percent of clients from methadone maintenance met these standards, along with 40% in therapeutic communities, 33% in outpatient drug-free treatments, 25% in outpatient detoxification, and 27% in intake-only. More detailed results are found in Table 45.1.

Posttreatment data are for the first year after treatment, and persons included are black and white male opioid addicts.

The Drug Abuse Reporting Program follow-up results suggested that overall those clients in methadone maintenance, therapeutic communities, and outpatient drug-free treatments had better outcomes than those in the outpatient detoxification and intake-only groups. Long-term follow-up outcomes (i.e., those interviews conducted about 4 years after the Drug Abuse Reporting Program ended) continued with the same trend. Outcomes for clients in methadone maintenance, therapeutic communities, and drug-free treatments were more

TABLE 45.1	Pretreatment and Posttreatment Outcomes for the Drug Abuse Reporting Program Group Treatments.					
	THERAPEUTIC COMMUNITY (%)		OUTPATIENT DRUG FREE (%)		INTAKE ONLY (%)	
Outcome Measures	Pre-trx	Post-trx	Pre-trx	Post-trx	Pre-trx	Post-trx
Opioid Drugs						
Any use	100	58	100	64	100	70
Daily use	100	39	100	44	100	53
Marijuana						
Any use	56	62	52	69	49	67
Daily use	17	23	20	30	14	27
Other Nonopioid Drugs						
Any use	60	40	54	45	48	50
Daily use	10	10	11	10	7	11
Drug Abuse Treatment						
In 1+ months	53	32	48	33	50	43
Alcohol Use (80-proof)						
Over 4 oz per day	20	38	21	38	19	31
Over 8 oz per day	12	21	14	23	12	18
Employment						
Any employment	63	72	60	65	65	54
Employed 6+ months	20	61	24	52	21	44
Criminality						
Arrested 1+ times	95	33	87	34	86	39
Any jail or prison	83	33	66	34	68	41
Number of persons	582		256		152	

Adapted from data in Simpson DD, Sells SB. Effectiveness of treatment for drug abuse: an overview of the DARP research program. *Adv Alcohol Subst Abuse.* 1982;2(1):7–29.

positive, with an increased length of stay, with main results appearing between 90 days and 2 years. The outcomes for those who stayed only short term (less than 90 days) in these categories showed no significant difference between these clients and those who were in the outpatient detoxification and intake-only groups. Inspection of the follow-up records for 990 opioid addicts showed that 61% of that sample achieved opioid abstinence after the Drug Abuse Reporting Program treatment occurred. Throughout most of the Drug Abuse Reporting Program studies, the most important predictor variable was criminal history (arrests and incarcerations before entry into the Drug Abuse Reporting Program).

The Drug Abuse Reporting Program is still considered to be one of the great sources of information regarding client outcomes in community clinics. Some of the limitations of the Drug Abuse Reporting Program studies include the fact that they were not controlled studies. There was no randomization of clients into the different treatments. This meant that equality among the groups for gender, age, or any other variables was not controlled. However, this could also be considered a strength, because the studies allowed a real look into how clients actually arrive into various treatments. Another limitation was the fact that outcome data relied mostly on retrospective self-report, although some of the variables, such as criminality indicators, could be verified through records. The findings from this study utilized pre- and posttreatment data, with no rigorous experimental controls, so these methods prevent firm conclusions regarding treatment efficacy and effectiveness. For example, one major limitation of pre/post treatment studies is that in a recurring disorder like substance use disorder, abstinence and other functional indicators of treatment success naturally fluctuate in their usual course. Individuals seek treatment when they are at their worst and thus may show improvement or success as the natural course of their chronic disorder continues, rather than as a direct causal result of treatment.

A major strength of the Drug Abuse Reporting Program studies was the huge breadth of the research. Treatment agencies that were included in the Drug Abuse Reporting Program were very diverse, both in location and treatment philosophy. The studies were very consistent and provided similar results throughout the course of the program. One of the interesting findings of the Drug Abuse Reporting Program was that there were not any significant outcome differences between individual agencies or types of agencies. This could be considered a positive finding, showing more consistency than was necessarily expected. Overall, major Drug Abuse Reporting Program findings demonstrated positive outcomes for methadone maintenance, therapeutic community, and outpatient drug-free treatments among daily opioid users who remained in treatment for more than 90 days.

Additional Treatment Models

Some group methods investigated through the National Institute on Drug Abuse's support include Relapse Prevention (some have utilized individual therapy), the Matrix Model, Community Reinforcement Approach Plus Vouchers, and Day Treatment with Abstinence Contingencies and Vouchers. All are reviewed in the National Institute on Drug Abuse's *Principles of Drug Addiction Treatment*,[51] but this is not an exhaustive list of empirically based treatments. Numerous other substance abuse treatments not listed include an eclectic mixture of methods, theoretically driven techniques, or variations of other treatment procedures. Some evidence-based group treatments have not been evaluated extensively or have been found to be insufficiently efficacious or ineffective when rigorously evaluated in clinical settings. Still other substance use disorder treatments being utilized have been determined to be less effective than alternative evidence-based comparative treatments (e.g., Schumacher et al.[74]).

The Matrix Model

The Matrix Model[66,76] is a multifaceted manualized approach aimed at helping stimulant abusers obtain abstinence. Group treatment incorporates educating clients and their family members about addiction and relapse as well as self-help techniques. Abstinence is monitored by regular urine testing. A therapist acts as a mentor by educating, guiding, and supporting clients during recovery. Treatment focus is on positively reinforcing progression toward abstinence. The relationship between the therapist and client is positive, promoting an open and honest dialog between the two, avoiding authoritative and confrontational interactions. The matrix emphasis is on building clients' self-worth and confidence, helping clients resist temptations for using, and increasing the importance of the self, while reducing potential harm that may ensue through using drugs.

Treatment procedures incorporate effective elements of other empirically supported treatments.[67] As summarized by the National Institute on Drug Abuse's *Principles of Drug Addiction Treatment*,[63] specific techniques utilized in the Matrix Model include work sheets for individual sessions; group intervention components include family educational groups, early recovery skills groups, relapse prevention groups, conjoint sessions, 12-step programs, relapse analysis, and social support groups.

The Matrix Model has been shown in many studies to be effective at treating both drug and alcohol abuse as well as improving quality of life and reducing risky behaviors that may increase the risk of acquiring HIV.[76] Matrix treatment has been found to be equally effective for methamphetamine and cocaine abusers as well as enhancing the effectiveness of naltrexone treatment of opiate abusers.[36] Recently the Matrix Model has incorporated abstinence contingency management based on the voucher approach of Higgins et al.[34]

Challenges to Community-Based Clinics

In the previous section a number of empirically supported community treatments utilizing group interventions for substance use disorder have been described. These interventions have been carefully designed and rigorously tested. However, substance use disorder is still a major national problem. For example, despite some reduction in the prevalence of cocaine use since its peak in the 1980s, the prevalence of heavy cocaine use has not diminished.[72] In rural communities, methamphetamine has come to replace cocaine use in recent surveys.[81] These alarming substance abuse trends have been observed despite a wealth of evidence documenting the detrimental cognitive and physical effects of these substances.

A recent review of substance use disorder community treatment programs revealed a 15% closure rate within the first year of operation. Among those programs that survive the first year, up to 25% undergo a major shift in organization.[51] Most are taken over by a different administrative structure. The vast majority of programs report collecting more administrative data than clinically relevant information. Only 54% of programs perform on-site physical examinations at admission. A startling 28% of programs report no electronic information system, email, or even voice mail capabilities, whereas only 30% (largely housed under hospital and university settings) had full access to advanced information technology. The remaining 40% only had an information system available for administrative duties (i.e., budgeting, payroll, and billing), but the technology was not available to staff members that interact face-to-face with clients.[51]

It appears we are facing a paradox in the national effort to reduce substance use disorders. Health professionals have an increasing variety of effective interventions to treat persons with chemical dependencies, yet treatment programs in the community are struggling to remain open, let alone to address the rising population of persons with substance use disorders. Why is this? There are a number of barriers to the dissemination and maintenance of community addictions treatment programs. Most of these barriers can be categorized into one of three categories: (1) funding, (2) staffing, and (3) client-centered barriers.

Funding

Substance use disorder treatment programs have a myriad of funding sources to navigate. Each source has different eligibility requirements and payment mechanisms. The funding categories include: single state agencies, federal grants, local government, third-party reimbursements (e.g., private insurance and health maintenance organizations [HMOs]), private grants, client fees, and fundraising.[86] Community substance abuse treatment funding sources can be categorized as either the public or private sector. Funding sources, regardless of source, pose a number of barriers to substance use disorder treatment service delivery. The majority (more than 80%) of the nation's substance use disorder treatment programs are specialty care programs. Specialty care programs are small—typically treating fewer than 300 clients per year, community-based, outpatient, nonprofit organizations. Most utilized group interventions of various types with mostly unknown effectiveness. They are rarely affiliated with large medical care facilities. As freestanding entities, specialty care substance use disorder programs operate outside the realm of the mainstream health care system. The majority of their funding is government mandated (e.g., Medicaid and Veterans Administration) or provided by state and/or local criminal justice systems.[41] In most cases, these resources are limited, and the documentation and procedural requirements can be very time consuming. This is despite the fact that cost-benefit analyses overwhelmingly support a move toward increased government support of substance use disorder treatment programs.[79]

A few suggestions have been proposed to address the funding challenge facing substance use disorder treatment programs. A basic concern regarding program funding difficulties is the lack of information about available sources utilized by struggling agencies. This can be addressed by compiling a comprehensive list of available funding resources, such as the 1995 review by Zarkin and colleagues. In addition, it may prove beneficial to provide program directors and administrative staff with basic budget and resource allocation training. The use or expansion of self-funding may help some substance use disorder treatment programs. Self-funding programs can operate by placing fees for specific products to fund services that address the detrimental effects of its consumption, like cigarette taxes being used to fund cancer research.[79] In the case of illicit drug use, which, unlike alcohol and tobacco is not commercially marketed, restitution payments from those convicted of drug charges could be used to fund rehabilitation centers. The idea of self-funding programs is still relatively new, but if it proves to be a viable option for mitigating the pubic harm caused by alcohol and nicotine, it may be useful to consider for substance use treatment.

Staffing

A number of staffing difficulties face substance use disorder treatment programs. Some of these issues include: clinical staff training, caseloads, and staff retention/stability. McClellan and colleagues'[51] sample of community treatment programs found that 15% of program directors had no college degree, 58% had a bachelor's degree, and 20% had a master's degree. Nearly 72% of the directors for these programs worked full-time. Although 71% of the directors had worked within their program, most in a clinical position for more than a year, over half (54%) had been in the director position for less than a year. These statistics imply there is a problem of instability at the top administrative level of these programs.

If we look further at staff credentials, we find differences between private and public sector programs. The main difference is typically based on the program's funding source. Programs that receive at least 50% of their funding through public grants and/or contracts can be considered public sector programs. By this definition, private sector programs receive the majority of their funding from affiliated institutions, direct client payments, and third-party reimbursements.[71] One very notable distinction in staffing is that private sector programs, partially due to their hospital affiliations, are more likely to have a physician and master's level counselors available. This may have implications for these programs' viability, treatment quality, and success. Having higher educated staff allows more private sector programs to offer more innovative approaches, such as pharmacotherapy and other evidence-based psychosocial interventions—particularly those that require supervised training for implementation.[45]

Staff caseloads often present challenges for these programs. A number of treatment programs have been described as "choking on data collection requirements."[51] Administrative data reporting requirements are often time-consuming and cumbersome. This is particularly true for programs that hold contracts with multiple state agencies and managed care organizations. Each of these entities, for example, employment organizations, welfare departments, and criminal justice agencies, has unique requirements for record-keeping and billing. Caseworkers at many community programs report devoting 2–4 hours to collecting administrative data alone for each admission. This time and effort appears not to contribute to actual clinical assessment or treatment planning. Nevertheless, staff members in most treatment facilities find themselves busy completing a sizeable amount of paperwork and still left with the task of providing client care, in many cases without access to computers, email, fax, or even voicemail capabilities.

The most salient staff-related barrier to community treatment vitality is staff retention. Data from the National Treatment Center Study reveal an average turnover rate of 18.5% among addiction counselors.[45] This is much greater than national annual rates for other occupations that traditionally have high turnovers, such as teachers (13%) and nurses (12%).[37] Retention difficulties create numerous problems. In addition to recruiting costs, hiring, and training new counselors, high turnover rates compromise consistency of treatment and service delivery.[45] These staffing problems can have a variety of negative effects for clients such as increasing treatment drop-outs and exposing clients to rapidly changing staff—who may not be competent in delivering evidence-based, effective clinical interventions for their substance use disorders and other common comorbid mental disorders.

What can be done to address staff concerns? A survey of counselors and administrators in attendance at a 2003 training workshop yielded the following suggestions to address staff-related barriers to substance use disorder treatment programs: provide more relevant training, increase program support of staff, provide lighter workloads, and less redundancy in staff duties.[5] There is also a need to offer meaningful incentives to recruit physicians, nurses, psychologists, and counselors.[51] For instance, national educational loan forgiveness could help recruit health care professionals and make clinical careers in addiction treatment more valuable and rewarding if it were more accessible to community treatment programs. There is also a need to incorporate relevant continuing training opportunities, along with training for administrators in personnel management, accounting, budgeting, and other cornerstones of the small business industry. Administrators should streamline the amount of non-clinical data collection that is required.[51] Perhaps, by combining the administrative data with clinically pertinent information from admission, progress notes, and discharge assessments, the burden associated with required documentation can be partially alleviated.

Client-Centered Barriers

There are a number of barriers to substance use disorder program viability that are related to client-issues. One of the primary client-centered problems is motivation/treatment engagement. Client motivation has been shown to be a considerable predictor of treatment success.[42] This is even more evident when examining clients who do not enter treatment under criminal justice supervision. Surveys of substance use disorder programs have shown that clients are more likely to engage and remain motivated if they feel the staff has a vested interest in their recovery. This is especially true when clients feel a connection with their counselor. Good client-counselor rapport has been shown to be related to client engagement and subsequent success. A survey by Kirk and Amaranth[42] revealed a majority of clients preferred counselors with their own stories of recovery who are of the same gender, same cohort group, and with sensitivity to their client's culture.

In addition to client motivation/treatment engagement, many clients face practical obstacles that prevent their individual success, and when taken as a whole, become detrimental to the substance use disorder treatment program. Some of these challenges include transportation, child-care, and missed work. To address these issues, programs could offer incentives (e.g., meal and travel vouchers), daycare services, and vocational training to mitigate challenges, while maximizing the benefits of program attendance.

Opportunities to Expand Evidence-Based Substance Use Disorder Interventions

A great opportunity to expand program interventions is through university-affiliated translational research. Translational research emphasizes evaluations of treatments and interventions in clinically relevant settings. Continuing to increase knowledge about the efficacy and real-world implications of substance use disorder interventions is the first step toward increasing their availability. An additional way to improve substance use disorder program availability and effectiveness is with integrated mental health services. Despite barriers to prevent its occurrence, there remains a strong consensus to integrate mental health services with substance abuse treatment.[17] This is particularly important given that people with mental illness are 4–5 times as likely to develop a substance abuse disorder as the general population. Dual diagnosis significantly complicates treatment outcomes.[26] Drake and colleagues[25] concluded that "treatment in parallel and separate mental health and substance abuse treatment systems is remarkably ineffective." An integrated approach would make recovery the focus of treatment and would address parallel challenges associated with addiction and mental illness. Davidson and White[17] provided a thoughtful conceptualization of integrated treatment. Their table (adapted here as Table 45.2) details the key components of their integrated substance abuse and mental health treatment approach and illustrates how an integrated substance use disorder and mental health treatment approach might be structured.

Note suggestions for how substance use disorder and mental health treatment can be structured to impact both disorders.

TABLE 45.2   Key Components of Davidson and White Integrated Substance Abuse and Mental Health Treatment Approach.

Domain	Mental Illness	Addiction
Goals of care	Assist people in reducing the interference, impairment, disability, and discrimination associated with the condition(s) Support person's own efforts to manage his or her condition(s) while pursuing a dignified and gratifying life in the community	
Role of the person with the condition	Take ownership of his or her own recovery process Active involvement, including daily decision-making, for initiating and sustaining recovery Individual/family involvement, from policy development through service delivery and evaluation	
Underlying values	Sustained health care partnership model (vs. expert model) Hope-based Person- and family-centered Culturally competent Choice philosophy Promotes growth Builds on strengths and interests Focuses on overall life, including wellness, health, and spirituality Recovery-focused outcome measures	
Guiding principles	Recovery has multiple pathways and styles Recovery flourishes in supportive communities Recovery is enhanced by person–environment fit Recovery is voluntary Recovery outcomes vary across a heterogeneous population Recovery is a longitudinal, developmental process and a continuum Recovery is nonlinear Family involvement in recovery is helpful Peer support in recovery may be crucial Spirituality may be a critical component of recovery	
Strategies to facilitate recovery	Identify and engage early Carry and instill hope; offer role modeling Increase motivation for change (recovery priming) Offer information and education about the condition(s), recovery, available resources, and ways to self-manage the condition(s) Provide interventions effective in resolving crises, reducing or eliminating symptoms and/or impairments associated with condition(s), and improving health Provide opportunities, rehabilitation, and supports for persons to gain needed skills for occupying valued roles (e.g., student, spouse) Assertively connect person to other people in recovery, mutual support, recovery advocacy organizations, and indigenous recovery communities Provide posttreatment monitoring (recovery checkups) and support; active recovery coaching (stage-appropriate recovery education and advice); and, when necessary, early reintervention Offer community supports to enable person to lead a self-determined and meaningful life in the communities of his or her choice (e.g., supported housing, supported employment, supported education) Legal advocacy to counter stigma and discrimination, ensure the person's rights, and enable the person to regain the status of being a contributing member of society	
Essential ingredients of recovery-oriented systems	Motivation-based outreach and engagement interventions Basic (material and instrumental) support Pretreatment, in-treatment, and posttreatment recovery coaching/mentoring Assessment processes that are global, continual, and strengths-based Respite for people in recovery and families Rehabilitation and ongoing provision of community supports Peer support Family education and support Legal aid/advocacy Intensive clinical services, including crisis prevention and response, pharmacological and psychosocial treatments, and...	
	Acute inpatient care Illness management and recovery Assertive community treatment	Detox Contingency management Motivational interviewing

Adapted from an article by Davidson L, White W. The concept of recovery as an organizing principle for integrating mental health and addiction services. *J Behav Health Services Res.* 2007;34:109–122.

References

1. Alessi SM, Hanson T, Wieners M, Petry NM. Low-cost contingency management in community clinics: delivering incentives partially in group therapy. *Exp Clin Psychopharmacol.* 2007;15(3):293–300.
2. American Psychiatric Association. *Diagnostic and Statistical Manual of Mental Disorders.* 4th ed. Washington, DC: text revision; 2000.
3. American Psychological Association Statement. *Policy Statement on Evidence-Based Practice in Psychology.* Washington, DC: American Psychological Association; 2005.
4. Ball JD, Ross A. *The Effectiveness of Methadone Maintenance Treatment.* New York: Springer; 1991.
5. Bartholomew NG, Joe GW, Rowan-Szal GA, Simpson DD. Counselor assessments of training and adoption barriers. *J Subst Abuse Treat.* 2007;33(2):193–199.
6. Brecher EM. *Licit and Illicit Drugs.* Boston: Little Brown; 1972.
7. Carey KB. Substance use reduction in the context of outpatient psychiatric treatment: a collaborative, motivational, harm reduction approach. *Community Mental Health J.* 1996;32:291–306.
8. Carroll K, Rounsaville B, Keller D. Relapse prevention strategies for the treatment of cocaine abuse. *Am J Drug Alcohol Abuse.* 1991;17(3):249–265.
9. Carroll KM. Manual-guided psychosocial treatment. A new virtual requirement for pharmacotherapy trials? *Arch Gen Psychiatry.* 1997;54(10):923–928.
10. Carroll KM, Fenton LR, Ball SA, et al. Efficacy of disulfiram and cognitive behavior therapy in cocaine-dependent outpatients. *Archiv Gen Psychiatry.* 2004;61:264–272.
11. Carroll KM, Onken LS. Behavioral therapies for drug abuse. *Am J Psychiatry.* 2005;162(8):1452–1460.
12. Carroll KM, Rounsaville BJ, Nich C, Gordon LT, Wirtz PW, Gawin F. One year follow-up of psychotherapy and pharmacotherapy for cocaine dependence: delayed emergence of psychotherapy effects. *Archiv Gen Psychiatry.* 1994;51:989–997.
13. Chambers CD. The detoxification of narcotic addicts in outpatient clinics. In: Brill L, Lieberman L, eds. *Major Modalities in the Treatment of Drug Abuse.* New York: Behavioral Publications; 1972.
14. Cnaan RA, Boddie SC. Charitable choice and faith-based welfare: a call for social work. *Social Work.* 2002;47(3):224–235.
15. Condelli WS, Hubbard RL. Client outcomes from therapeutic communities. In: Tims FM, De Leon G, Jainchill N, eds. *Therapeutic Community: Advances in Research and Application.* (NIH Publication No. 94-3633). Rockville, MD: NIDA Research Monograph; 1994;144:80–98.
16. Crits-Christoph P, Siqueland L, Blaine J, Frank A, Luborsky L, Onken LS, et al. Psychosocial treatments for cocaine dependence: national institute on drug abuse collaborative cocaine treatment study. *Archiv Gen Psychiatry.* 1999;56:493–502.
17. Davidson L, White W. The concept of recovery as an organizing principle for integrating mental health and addiction services. *J Behav Health Services Res.* 2007;34:109–122.
18. De Leon G. The therapeutic community: toward a general theory and model. In: Tims FM, De Leon G, Jainchill N, eds. *Therapeutic Community: Advances in Research and Application.* (NIH Publication No. 94-3633). Rockville, MD: NIDA Research Monograph; 1994;144:16–52.
19. DHHS. *National Survey of Substance Abuse Treatment Services (N-SSATS): 2006, Data on Substance Abuse Treatment Facilities.* Rockville, MD: Substance Abuse and Mental Health Services Administration, Office of Applied Studies; 2006.
20. Dole VP, Nyswander ME. A medical treatment for diacetylmorphine (heroin) addiction: a clinical trial with methadone hydrochloride. *J Am Med Assoc.* 1965;193(8):80–84.
21. Dole VP, Nyswander ME. Heroin addiction – a metabolic disease. *Archiv Intern Med.* 1967;120:19–24.
22. Dole VP, Nyswander ME, Warner A. Successful treatment of 750 criminal addicts. *J Am Med Assoc.* 1968;206:2708–2711.
23. Dole VP, Robinson W, Orraca J, Towns E, Searcy P, Caine E. Methadone treatment of randomly selected criminal addicts. *N Engl J Med.* 1969;280(25):1372–1375.
24. Drake RE, Green AL, Mueser KT, Boldman HH. The history of community mental health treatment and rehabilitation for persons with severe mental illness. *Community Mental Health J.* 2003;39(5):427–440.
25. Drake RE, Mueser KT, Brunette MF. A review of treatments for people with severe mental illnesses and co-occurring substance use disorders. *Psychiatric Rehabil J.* 2004;27:360–374.
26. Epstein J, Barker P, Vorburger M, Murtha C. *Serious Mental Illness and Its Co-Occurrence With Substance Use Disorders.* Rockville, MD: Substance Abuse and Mental Health Services Administration, Office of Applied Studies; 2002.
27. Fals-Stewart WO, O'Farrell TJ, Birchler GR. Behavioral couples therapy for male methadone maintenance patients: effects on drug-using behavior and relationship adjustment. *Behav Therapy.* 2001;32:391–411.
28. Gawin FH, Kleber HD. Cocaine abuse treatment: an open pilot trial with lithium carbonate and desipramine. *Archiv Gen Psychiatry.* 1984;41:903–910.
29. Gawin FH, Kleber HD. Abstinence symptomatology and psychiatric diagnosis in cocaine abusers: clinical observations. *Archiv Gen Psychiatry.* 1986;47:861–868.
30. Gay G, Matzger A, Bathurst W, Smith D. Short-term heroin detoxification on an outpatient basis. *Int J Addictions.* 1971;6:259–260.
31. Greenfield SF, Trucco EM, McHugh RK, Lincoln M, Gallop RJ. The women's recovery group study: a stage I trial of women-focused group therapy for substance use disorders versus mixed-gender group drug counseling. *Drug Alcohol Depend.* 2007;1(6):39–47.
32. Guess LL, Tuchfeld BS. *Manual for Drug Abuse Treatment Program Self-Evaluation Supplement II: CODAP Tables.* Washington, DC: U.S. Government Printing Office; 1977.
33. Hall SM, Loeb PC, Kushner M. Methadone dose decreases and anxiety reduction. *Addict Behav.* 1984;9:11–19.
34. Higgins ST, Delaney DD, Budney AJ, Bickel WK, Hughes JR, Foerg F, et al. A behavioral approach to achieving initial cocaine abstinence. *Am J Psychiatry.* 1991;148(9):1218–1224.
35. Himmelsbach CK. Clinical studies of drug addiction: physical dependence, withdrawal, and recovery. *Archiv Intern Med.* 1942;69:766.
36. Huber A, Ling W, Shoptaw S, Gulati V, Brethen P, Rawson R. Integrating treatments for methamphetamine abuse: a psychosocial perspective. *J Addictive Dis.* 1997;16:41–50.
37. Ingersoll R. Teacher turnover and teacher shortages: an organizational analysis. *Am Educ Res J.* 2001;38:499–534.
38. Joe GW, Simpson DD. Research on Patient Retention in Treatment. *Paper presented at the American Psychological Association, New Orleans*; 1974.
39. Jones H. Addiction and pregnancy. In: Henningfield JE, Santora PB, Bickel WK, eds. *Addiction Treatment: Science and Policy for the Twenty-First Century.* Baltimore: Johns Hopkins University; 2007.
40. Kang SY, Kleinman PH, Woody GE, et al. Outcomes for cocaine abusers after once-a-week psychosocial therapy. *Am J Psychiatry.* 1991;148(5):630–635.
41. Kimberly J, McLellan T. The business of addiction treatment: a research agenda. *J Subst Abuse Treat.* 2006;31(3):213–219.
42. Kirk C, Amaranth K. Staffing issues in work with women at risk for and in recovery from substance abuse. *Women's Health Issues.* 1998;8(4):261–266.
43. Kleber HD. Detoxification from methadone maintenance: the state of the art. *Int J Addictions.* 1977;12(7):807–820.
44. Kleber HD, Riordan CE. The treatment of narcotic withdrawal: a historical review. *J Clin Psychiatry.* 1982;43(6.2):30–34.
45. Knudsen HK, Johnson A, Roman PM. Retaining counseling staff at substance abuse treatment centers: effects of management practices. *J Subst Abuse Treat.* 2003;24(2):129–135.

46. Ledgerwood DM, Petry NM. Does contingency management affect motivation to change substance use? *Drug Alcohol Depend.* 2006;83:65–72.

47. Marlatt GA, Gordon JR. *Relapse Prevention: Maintenance Strategies in the Treatment of Addictive Behaviors.* New York: Guilford; 1985.

48. Maude-Griffin PM, Hohenstein JM, Humfleet GL, Reilly PM, Tusel DJ, Hall SM. Superior efficacy of cognitive-behavioral therapy for crack cocaine abusers: main and matching effects. *J Consult Clin Psychol.* 1998;66:832–837.

49. Maurer DW, Vogel VH. *Narcotics and Narcotic Addiction.* 4th ed. Springfield, IL: Charles C. Thomas; 1973.

50. McCarty D, Fuller B, Kaskutas LA, et al. Treatment programs in the national drug abuse treatment clinical trials network. *Drug Alcohol Depend.* 2008;92:200–207.

51. McLellan AT, Carise D, Kleber HD. Can the national addiction treatment infrastructure support the public's demand for quality care? *J Subst Abuse Treat.* 2003;25(2):117–121.

52. Milby JB. *Addictive Behavior and its Treatment.* New York: Springer; 1981.

53. Milby JB. Methadone maintenance to abstinence: how many make it? *J Nervous Mental Dis.* 1988;176(7):409–422.

54. Milby JB, Garrett C, Meredith R. Iatrogenic phobic disorder in methadone maintenance treated patients. *Int J Addictions.* 1980;15(5):747–757.

55. Milby JB, Hohmann AA, Gentile M, et al. Methadone maintenance outcome as a function of detoxification phobia. *Am J Psychiatry.* 1994;151(7):1031–1037.

56. Milby JB, Schumacher JE, McNamara C, et al. Initiating abstinence in cocaine abusing dually diagnosed homeless persons. *Drug Alcohol Depend.* 2000;60(1):55–67.

57. Milby JB, Schumacher JE, Raczynski JM, et al. Sufficient conditions for effective treatment of substance abusing homeless persons. *Drug Alcohol Depend.* 1996;43(1–2):39–47.

58. Milby JB, Schumacher JE, Vuchinich RE, Freedman MJ, Kertesz S, Wallace D. Toward cost-effective initial care for substance-abusing homeless. *J Subst Abuse Treat.* 2008;34(2):180–191.

59. Milby JB, Schumacher JE, Vuchinich RE, et al. Transitions during effective treatment for cocaine-abusing homeless persons: establishing abstinence, lapse, and relapse, and reestablishing abstinence. *Psychol Addict Behav.* 2004;18(3):250–256.

60. Milby JB, Schumacher JE, Wallace D, Freedman MJ, Vuchinich RE. To house or not to house: the effects of providing housing to homeless substance abusers in treatment. *Am J Public Health.* 2005;95(7):1259–1265.

61. Moos RH. Theory based active ingredients of effective treatments for substance use disorders. *Drug Alcohol Depend.* 2007;88(2–3):109–121.

62. Mueser KT, Noorday DL, Drake RE, Fox L. *Integrated Treatment for Dual Disorders: A Guide to Effective Practice.* New York: Guilford; 2003.

63. National Institute on Drug Abuse. *Principles of Drug Addiction Treatment: a Research-Based Guide.* Washington, DC: NIH Publication No. 99-4180; 1999.

64. Petry NM, Peirce JM, Stitzer ML, et al. Effect of Prize-based Incentives on outcomes in stimulant abusers in outpatient psychosocial treatment programs. *Archiv Gen Psychiatry.* 2005;62:1148–1156.

65. Project MATCH Research Groups. Matching alcoholism treatments to client heterogeneity: project MATCH posttreatment drinking outcomes. *J Studies Alcohol.* 1997;58(1):7–29.

66. Rawson R, Obert JL, McCann MJ, Ling W. Psychological approaches for the treatment of cocaine dependence—a neurobehavioral approach. *J Addictive Dis.* 1991;11(2):97–120.

67. Rawson R, Shoptaw S, Obert JL, et al. An intensive outpatient approach for cocaine abuse: the matrix model. *J Subst Abuse Treat.* 1995;12(2):117–127.

68. Rawson RA, Huber A, McCann M, Shoptaw S, Farabee D, Ling W. A comparison of contingency management and cognitive-behavioral approaches during methadone maintenance treatment for cocaine dependence. *Archiv Gen Psychiatry.* 2002;59:593–600.

69. Ridgely MS, Goldman HH, Willenbring M. Barriers to the care of persons with dual diagnoses: organizational and financing issues. *Schizophr Bull.* 1990;16:123–132.

70. Rodgers JH, Barnett PG. Two separate tracks? A national multivariate analysis of differences between public and private substance abuse treatment programs. *Am J Drug Alcohol Abuse.* 2000;26(3):429–442.

71. Roman R, Ducharme L, Knudsen H. Patterns of organization and management in private and public substance abuse treatment programs. *J Subst Abuse Treat.* 2006;31(3):235–243.

72. SAMHSA. *National Survey on Drug Use & Health. Substance Abuse and Mental Health Services Administration,* Office of Applied Studies, Rockville, MD; 2004, 2004.

73. Schumacher JE, Mennemeyer ST, Milby JB, Wallace D, Nolan K. Costs and effectiveness of substance abuse treatments for homeless persons. *J Mental Health Policy Econ.* 2002;5(1):33–42.

74. Schumacher JE, Milby JB, Wallace D, et al. Meta-analysis of day treatment and contingency-management dismantling research: Birmingham homeless cocaine studies (1990–2006). *J Consult Clin Psychol.* 2007;75(5):823–828.

75. Sheffet A, Quinones M, Lavenhar MA, Doyle K, Prager H. An evaluation of detoxification as an initial step in the treatment of heroin addiction. *Am J Psychiatry.* 1976;133(3):337–339.

76. Shoptaw S, Rawson RA, McCann MJ, Obert JL. The matrix model of outpatient stimulant abuse treatment: evidence of efficacy. *J Addict Dis.* 1994;13(4):129–141.

77. Siegler M, Osmond H. Models of drug addiction. *Int J Addict.* 1968;3:3–24.

78. Simpson DD, Sells SB. Effectiveness of treatment for drug abuse: an overview of the DARP research program. *Adv Alcohol Subst Abuse.* 1982;2(1):7–29.

79. Tellez M. Isn't an alcohol- or drug-addicted adolescent worth a penny? Self-funding programs can make a difference. *J Emerg Nursing.* 2004;30(3):284–286.

80. Tims F, Jainchill N, De Leon G. Therapeutic communities and treatment research. In: Tims FM, DeLeon G, Jainchill N, eds. *Therapeutic Community: Advances in Research and Application.* Rockville, MD: NIDA Research Monograph 144 (NIH Publication No. 94-3633); 1994:1–15.

81. Volkow ND. The reality of co-morbidity: depression and drug abuse. *Biol Psychiatry.* 2004;56:714–717.

82. Wallace BC. Crack cocaine: what constitutes state of the art treatment? *J Addiction Dis.* 1991;11(2):79–95.

83. Washton AM, Stone-Washton N. Abstinence and relapse in outpatient cocaine addicts. *J Psychoactive Drugs.* 1990;22(2):135–147.

84. Weiss RD, Griffin ML, Kolodziej ME, et al. A randomized trial of integrated group therapy versus group drug counseling for patients with bipolar disorder and substance dependence. *Am J Psychiatry.* 2007;164(1):100–107.

85. Wilson BD, Elms RR, Thompson CP. Outpatient versus hospital methadone detoxification: an experimental comparison. *Int J Addictions.* 1975;10:13–21.

86. Zarkin G, Galinis D, French M, Fountain D, Ingram P, Guyett J. Financing strategies for drug abuse treatment programs. *J Subst Abuse Treat.* 1995;12(6):385–399.

87. Ziedonis DM, Fisher W. Motivation-based assessment and treatment of substance abuse in patients with schizophrenia. *Directions Psychiatry.* 1996;16:1–7.

46

Unhealthy Alcohol and Other Drug Use in Primary Care

MICHAEL F. BIERER AND RICHARD SAITZ

Introduction

The Health and Medicine Division, National Academies of Sciences, Engineering and Medicine has provided a working definition of primary care:

Primary care is the provision of integrated, accessible health care services by clinicians who are accountable for addressing a large majority of personal health care needs, developing a sustained partnership with patients, and practicing in the context of family and community.[47]

This definition emphasizes several aspects of care that impact individuals who use alcohol, tobacco, and other drugs.
1. Continuity of care over a "sustained" time period
2. Responsibility for addressing the majority of health care needs, including behavioral or psychological conditions
3. Coordination of "integrated" care that may include multiple consultants and groups
4. Inclusion of community and family issues that may challenge or promote health
5. Being "accountable" for care, implying some regard for efficiency and cost effectiveness, and for long-term outcomes across multiple conditions
6. Care is provided by clinical teams that might include physicians, nurses, counselors, physician's assistants, and others who are key to effective care.

They go on to describe core functions of primary care relevant to people who use substances.
1. Universal, selective, and indicated prevention, including screening for modifiable risk factors before consequences develop
2. Education of patients to help them live healthfully and to self-manage their health conditions and risks
3. Initial evaluation and treatment of health consequences as they emerge.

Primary care may be practiced by many medical professionals. Most readers will be familiar with general internists, family practitioners, or pediatricians in this role, but gynecologists, and other subspecialists, such as those in infectious disease, nephrology, or endocrinology, often provide primary care. In the United States, about half of the approximately one trillion doctor visits made in 2004 were to primary care clinicians (internal medicine, family medicine, and pediatrics).[3]

Given primary care's ubiquity and the multiplicity of functions (particularly the "ownership" in the long run of a patient's care), primary care providers are poised optimally to help patients with chronic behavioral health conditions, especially those that manifest with physical or emotional troubles that may cause someone to seek medical attention. Indeed, the setting for which the literature best supports the efficacy of brief interventions for alcohol is primary care practice. Conditions that are accompanied by shame and secrecy may need a trusted relationship with a professional to catalyze healthy change. The primary care clinician may be the only person in a patient's life who can fill that bill. Tobacco smoking, unhealthy alcohol and other drug use, and other drug and alcohol-related conditions are common among patients seeing primary care practitioners. About one in five adults visiting primary care clinicians drink above recommended limits or have consequences related to alcohol. Studies of primary care practices have demonstrated the success of care provided to people with unhealthy substance use, but also the large gap between its prevalence and the rates of screening, detection, and treatment.

This chapter addresses those gaps. Primary care clinicians are optimally positioned to identify, assess, manage, treat, and refer to specialty care as needed for unhealthy alcohol and other drug use as well as psychiatric and medical conditions that accompany or are caused by the substance use. The challenge to primary care in this arena is great; so too is the opportunity to make a profound difference in the lives of patients and their families.[46]

Screening

Unhealthy alcohol and other drug use is highly prevalent in the community and among primary care patients. It can result in physical and social deterioration and in increased use of costly medical resources. The primary care clinician can detect preclinical at-risk use or use with consequences and intervene effectively prior to the development of a substance use disorder. This paradigm is best studied and supported for alcohol and tobacco; whether detection and intervention for other drug use are effective remains controversial. It is for conditions for which we know that early versus later intervention can delay or diminish disease severity, morbidity, or mortality that a strong argument can be made for universal screening. Screening and screening tools can also be useful for identifying use, essential knowledge for diagnosis of medical symptoms, and for safe medication prescribing. The following sections review various screening strategies highlighting single-item tests that have the attractive attributes of convenience and good performance characteristics.

Screening for Alcohol Use

Surveys have found that screening is far from universal, and that only 13% of primary care clinicians use a validated instrument or tool to do so. When unhealthy use is identified, most primary care clinicians recommend self-help groups, but about a fifth of primary care clinicians offer no formal therapeutic intervention at all.[38] In a review of thousands of records, McGlynn et al. found that about one-half of recommended health services were provided to adult patients. Services for the *Diagnostic and Statistical Manual of Mental Disorders, Fourth Edition* (DSM-IV) alcohol dependence were at the lowest level: only 10% of patients with

alcohol dependence documented in the medical record had it addressed in any way.[63]

The US Preventive Services Task Force recommends screening and brief intervention for unhealthy alcohol use for adults and pregnant women. The US Preventive Services Task Force found that screening and brief intervention improves important health outcomes and that benefits outweigh any risks. The recommendation is as strong as that for screening mammography for women 40–50 years of age, osteoporosis screening for women 65 years or older, or cholesterol screening in young adults with other risk factors for coronary artery disease. One clear difference between screening and brief intervention for alcohol use and the other preventive services listed is that screening and brief intervention is a more time-consuming interaction with a patient than is ordering a radiological or blood test. In a revenue-driven health care environment, test ordering may add revenue to an institution. Prevention and reduction of alcohol use consequences, in contrast, may slow down the primary care clinician, decreasing volume-based-revenue, even with the prospect of downstream cost-savings. (This scenario may be mitigated in part by the existence of a billing code for screening and brief-intervention for substance use.) Indeed, screening and brief intervention may be cost-effective and even cost-saving, at least from a societal perspective, if the benefits of self-reported use translate into reduced health consequences and care utilization.[76] Based on randomized trials and simulation modeling, screening and brief intervention for alcohol ranks in the top five of preventive services in terms of cost-effectiveness.[59a,85]

Unhealthy Alcohol Use: Definitions

In the United States, about 70% of men and 60% of women 18 years of age or older drink alcohol.[27] Although there is evidence that low-level consumption is relatively low risk (although it does increase the risk for cancers, such as breast cancer),[95] higher amounts clearly risk numerous health consequences. Thus one dimension of screening for unhealthy alcohol use is solely based on quantity and frequency of intake. The other dimension that screening can address is alcohol consequences.

The National Institute on Alcohol Abuse and Alcoholism has defined cutoffs for unhealthy use that are empirically based in epidemiological literature. Risky drinking amounts are those above these cutoffs. For men, this level is greater than 14 drinks per week or >4 drinks on an occasion; for women this cutoff is >7 drinks/week or >3 drinks on an occasion. For individuals over 65 years of age, the cutoff is the same as that for women. A "drink" is defined, in the United States, as 12–14 g of ethanol (12 oz of beer, 5–6 oz of wine, or 1.5 oz of 80 proof spirits) (Table 46.1). Drinking risky amounts without associated consequences is risky drinking. If there are consequences, patients may have an alcohol use disorder (as defined in the *Diagnostic and Statistical Manual of Mental Disorders, Fifth Edition* [DSM-5]).[5] An important exception to using consumption to define unhealthy use is when even low-level use risks consequences. Aside from alcohol being a carcinogen, other examples include women intending pregnancy, pregnant women, people taking medications that interact with alcohol, and people with health conditions worsened by even small amounts (e.g., hepatitis C virus infection). The key distinction among individuals with unhealthy alcohol use is whether a moderate to severe alcohol use disorder (AUD) is present. Identifying such is important because the best advice and management are different, as discussed later in this chapter.

TABLE 46.1	Alcohol Use Definitions.	
	Quantity	**Alcohol-Related Consequences**
Lower risk use[a]	Below NIAAA-recommended limits	None
Unhealthy use		
Risky use	Above NIAAA-recommended limits	None
Use with consequences but no disorder	Not part of definition	Present but not meeting criteria for DSM-5 AUD
Mild AUD	Not part of definition	Meets 2-3 DSM-5 AUD criteria
Moderate/severe AUD	Not part of definition	Meets 4 or more DSM-5 Criteria

[a]The possible exceptions to the "lower risk" category are conditions in which any drinking may pose health risks. These include alcohol use disorder (e.g., past), family history of alcohol use disorder, intended pregnancy, pregnancy, use of medications that interact with alcohol, and disorders or symptoms usually made worse by alcohol (e.g., psychiatric symptoms or medical disorders such as hepatitis, peptic ulcer disease, or epilepsy).

Adapted from Akbik H, Butler SF, Budman SH, Fernandez K, et al. Validation and clinical application of the screener and opioid assessment for patients with pain (SOAPP). *J Pain Symptom Manage*. 2006;32:287–293; Cuijpers P, Riper H, Lemmers L. The effects on mortality of brief intervention for problem drinking: a metaanalysis. *Addiction*. 2004;99:829–845; O'Connor PG, Schottenfeld RS. Patients with alcohol problems. *New Eng J Med*. 1998;338:592–602.

What is the best way to screen for unhealthy alcohol use? Although we usually think about face-to-face discussions or questions in the clinical setting, screening runs the gamut from these to telephone or web-based instruments.[57] These approaches should be considered and adapted as appropriate, with an eye to optimal efficiency and effectiveness, for system-based approaches.

Any interaction between the primary care clinician and patient should serve to build the therapeutic relationship. Therefore history-taking should be conducted in an empathic, nonjudgmental way. Embedding questions about alcohol use among other routine medical history questions may serve to decrease resistance and improve both the tenor of the discussion and the quality of information generated. That said, screening is best done with interview questions that should be asked verbatim, as validated.

The first order of business is to ascertain whether the patient drinks at all. The clearest question is: "Do you sometimes drink beer, wine, or other alcoholic beverages?" If the patient does not drink at all, inquiring into the patient's rationale for abstaining may reveal that the patient has prior use with consequences. If the patient drinks at all, then quantity and frequency of drinking should be evaluated.

One wants to further characterize alcohol intake. It is important to assess the average number of drinks in a week and whether there are any heavy drinking episodes (i.e., drinking in excess of the single-occasion cut-offs delineated by the National Institute on Alcohol Abuse and Alcoholism). This brief screen can be done with three questions.[68]

1. On average, how many days per week do you have an alcoholic drink?
2. On a typical drinking day, how many drinks do you have?
3. What is the maximum number of drinks you had on any given occasion during the past month?

With the first two responses, the number of drinks per week can be calculated, and if weekly cutoffs are exceeded, then there is risky drinking. Similarly, if limits per episode are exceeded, the patient is drinking at a risky level.

The National Institute on Alcohol Abuse and Alcoholism Clinician's Guide recommends a *single* question to screen people who drink for unhealthy alcohol use[68]:

"How many times in the past year have you had X or more drinks in a day?" where X = 5 for men and 4 for women. A response >1 is considered positive.

This single item is both sensitive and specific for detecting unhealthy alcohol use, memorizable, requires no scoring, and is thus appropriate for most practices.[91] Single-question instruments are brief, valid, and efficient.

The Alcohol Use Disorders Identification Test (Table 46.2) is a 10-item instrument developed by the World Health Organization with good performance characteristics for identifying unhealthy alcohol use. It is scored from 0 to 40 with a score of 8 classically, but more recently scores of 5 (for men) and 4 (for women and those older than 60 years of age) have been considered positive. It requires scoring so may be better suited to a pen-and-paper or automated process than to verbal interview. The main advantage of the longer tool is that it provides more information for discussion and can suggest the presence of a disorder with a score of 15–20 or more.

A briefer validated screening tool is the Alcohol Use Disorders Identification Test-C. It comprises three consumption questions from the Alcohol Use Disorders Identification Test (the first three questions) and also requires scoring.[21,82] Using a score threshold (or cut-point) of 4 for males and 3 for females will identify unhealthy alcohol use, while a score of 7 or more suggests moderate to severe alcohol use disorder. This test is in wide use and is good for practices with workflows that permit scoring.

If a patient is NOT drinking above recommended cutoffs and has no absolute contraindication to any drinking, then the patient should be congratulated on the healthy pattern, educated about the risks and benefits of "moderate" (low amounts of) drinking (the best evidence for the former being for an increased risk for breast cancer and for the latter, possible decreased cardiovascular risk) and educated about optimal limits. If the screening is "positive," however, then further *assessment* is recommended for confirmation and to determine severity.

Screening for Tobacco Use

Evaluating the use of tobacco is by-and-large a simpler process than that for use of alcohol. The healthiest level of tobacco intake is none. Because efforts to make smoking a "vital sign," smoking status is now frequently recorded routinely at contacts with clinicians. A single question, such as "In the past year have you smoked cigarettes or used any other tobacco product?" should be asked of all patients. Caution should be taken with patients who define smoking as regular or current use; they may report they are

TABLE 46.2 | **AUDIT: The Alcohol Use Disorders Identification Test.**

FOR EACH QUESTION, CIRCLE THE ANSWER THAT BEST DESCRIBES YOUR EXPERIENCE.

Questions	0	1	2	3	4
1. How often do you have a drink containing alcohol?	Never	Monthly or less	2–4 times a month	2–3 times a week	4 or more times a week
2. How many drinks containing alcohol do you have on a typical day when you are drinking?	1 or 2	3 or 4	5 or 6	7 to 9	10 or more
3. How often do you have 5 or more drinks on one occasion?	Never	Less than monthly	Monthly	Weekly	Daily or almost daily
4. How often during the last year have you found that you were not able to stop drinking once you had started?	Never	Less than monthly	Monthly	Weekly	Daily or almost daily
5. How often during the last year have you failed to do what was normally expected of you because of drinking?	Never	Less than monthly	Monthly	Weekly	Daily or almost daily
6. How often during the last year have you needed a first drink in the morning to get yourself going after a heavy drinking session?	Never	Less than monthly	Monthly	Weekly	Daily or almost daily
7. How often during the last year have you had a feeling of guilt or remorse after drinking?	Never	Less than monthly	Monthly	Weekly	Daily or almost daily
8. How often during the last year have you been unable to remember what happened the night before because of your drinking?	Never	Less than monthly	Monthly	Weekly	Daily or almost daily
9. Have you or someone else been injured because of your drinking	No		Yes, but not in the last year		Yes, during the last year
10. Has a relative, friend, doctor, or other health care worker been concerned about your drinking or suggested you cut down?	No		Yes, but not in the last year		Yes, during the last year

Note: This questionnaire (the AUDIT) is reprinted with permission from the World Health Organization. To reflect standard drink sizes in the United States, the number of drinks in question 3 was changed from 6 to 5. A free AUDIT manual with guidelines for use in primary care settings is available online at www.who.org.

From National Institute on Alcohol Abuse and Alcoholism. *Helping Patients Who Drink Too Much: A Clinician's Guide.* 2005 ed. NIH Publication No. 07-3769. Bethesda, MD; NIH; 2007.

nonsmokers despite sporadic or recent but not current regular use. Finally, the presence of past or current smoking may itself raise concern for concomitant unhealthy alcohol or other drug use.[64]

Screening for Other Drug Use

The DAST-10 is a screening questionnaire that asks about drug use and consequences. A score of 3 or more is positive. The length of the questionnaire, and particularly the lack of validation studies in primary care settings, limits its utility.[90] The 10 questions probe for physical and social consequences (e.g., blackouts, withdrawal, relationship problems) and loss of control over use and do not identify the drug used.

The Alcohol Smoking and Substance Involvement Screening Test (ASSIST) is a complex instrument of 80 items yielding independent scores for each of multiple substances. A "positive" screening test can be defined as a score of 2 or greater (indicating any drug or alcohol use in the past 3 months), although the cutoff of 4 or greater is probably more clinically useful (indicating either weekly use or less-frequent recent use accompanied by consequences of use). ASSIST has been validated internationally. Although there are 80 items, if no use of a specific substance is reported, only 10 items need to be answered. If the patient reports any use of a substance, then a series of questions are asked about that substance. Its complexity, length, and need for scoring limit its utility in routine clinical primary care practice, although where computers are integrated into clinical or research settings, the test may be usable. The ASSIST is available online from the National Institute of Drug Abuse. Another major limitation of the ASSIST is that the results do not directly identify use of risky alcohol amounts per se, a critical target of screening in primary care settings because of the prevalence and proven value of brief intervention for such patients.[108]

The best approach to drug use screening in primary care is to ask one or two validated questions. The following single question test has been validated[65]: How many times in the past year have you used an illegal drug or used a prescription medication for non-medical reasons—for example, because of the experience or feeling it caused?[92]

Any nonzero response is considered positive. This has good sensitivity (>70% and specificity (>94%) and is appropriate for primary care settings. Because marijuana is becoming legal in many states, it can also be useful to simply ask about the frequency of any marijuana (cannabis) use and then determine if it is medicinal or whether there are any consequences of use in a further assessment.

Assessment

For any patient with unhealthy alcohol or other drug use, further assessment should delineate the role of the substance use in the patient's life. This runs the gamut among physical, emotional, interpersonal, and social/vocational functioning. Ultimately, ruling-in or ruling-out the diagnosis of moderate or severe substance use disorder is desirable, because management differs.

If the patient screens positive for drinking above recommended limits, there are several next steps: The primary objective of the evaluation is to determine if there is moderate to severe AUD. If there is only mild AUD, then brief counseling can have efficacy and is indicated. If there is severe AUD, then the effectiveness of brief intervention is less certain, but brief counseling with a goal of further care by the primary care clinician or via referral is desirable.[86] Moderate to severe AUD (per DSM-5) warrants an offer of pharmacotherapy, mutual help, and counseling. This can be provided by the primary care clinician if they have the skills, and if time permits, and/or by referral to specialty care, generally the favored approach if available and the patient is willing to go; more and more clinicians with behavioral health expertise are embedded and available in primary care settings, which is ideal as they are more accessible and familiar to patients in those settings. The other important objective of assessment here, irrespective of whether AUD is diagnosed, is to gather information about the impact of alcohol on the patient's life, both positive and negative, so that the patient can be counseled appropriately. Such insight into the personal impact of drinking may be at the core of effective motivational interviewing to assist with behavior change.[66]

One approach to assessment is oriented toward ruling in or out a diagnosis of AUD (recommended by the National Institute on Alcohol Abuse and Alcoholism Clinician's Guide).[68] The cardinal elements of AUD are loss of control, use despite negative consequences, and significant negative impact of use. A patient meets criteria for the diagnosis of AUD per DSM-5 if two or more of the following are present in a year, *accompanied by significant impairment or distress:*

1. Tolerance
2. Withdrawal
3. Spending substantial time getting, using, and recovering from use
4. Giving up important activities
5. Use despite known negative consequences
6. Inability to stop or cut down
7. Using more or more often than intended
8. Repeated use despite negative social consequences
9. Repeated use in hazardous situations
10. Craving
11. Use repeatedly resulting in failure to fulfill roles or functions.

AUD is rated as mild if 2–3 criteria are met, as moderate if 4–5 are met, and severe if 6–11 are met. Further assessment for psychiatric comorbidity is indicated when an alcohol use disorder is identified because it is common and needs to be addressed.

Some screening tests provide information regarding the presence of alcohol use disorders. Although a detailed interview is recommended for assessment, primary care providers often will not have such time available, particularly at the same visit in which a patient screens positive. As such, screening tests that provide information about consequences can help suggest the presence of more severe AUD.

Although not designed as an assessment tool, the 4-item CAGE questionnaire at a score of 2 or greater indicates a high likelihood of lifetime AUD. The four questions with which many primary care clinicians are already familiar are:

1. Have you ever felt you should *Cut down* on your drinking?
2. Have people *Annoyed* you by criticizing your drinking?
3. Have you ever felt bad or *Guilty* about your drinking?
4. Have you ever taken a drink first thing in the morning (*Eye-opener*) to steady your nerves or get rid of a hangover?

A positive answer is worth one point, and a score of 1 is 85% sensitive and 78% specific for an alcohol use disorder; a score of 2 is 71% sensitive and 91% specific.[2,25] The CAGE can serve as a starting point for a more detailed diagnostic assessment. The CAGE provides a natural segue to questions about the criteria for AUD that permit precise diagnosis.

Similarly for assessment and diagnosis of other drug use disorders, we recommend the ASSIST with a cutoff of 27 yielding high likelihood of a specific drug use disorder. Alternatively, the familiar CAGE questionnaire has been adapted to apply to drug use. The CAGE-AID is identical to the CAGE, one of the earliest validated alcohol screening questionnaires, with the exception that the clause "…or drug use" is appended to each of the four questions.[24] For example, the C question is: "Have you ever felt you should cut down on your drinking *or drug use*?" One affirmative response is a positive test. The CAGE-AID, like its source the CAGE, is limited in its focus on consequences, being less useful for identifying risky use. Again, the CAGE-AID, like the CAGE, is a jumping-off point for more detailed questions about consequences, leading to assessment of diagnostic criteria.

Management of Unhealthy Alcohol and Other Drug Use

Brief Intervention

Brief intervention is an essential part of the primary care clinician's management of patients with unhealthy behaviors in general, and unhealthy alcohol and other drug use in particular. It is covered in detail in the Chapter 43. Brief intervention is a brief, patient-centered counseling, a conversation of no more than 45 but usually 10–15 minutes. Informed by motivational interviewing, the primary care clinician provides feedback to the patient (after asking for permission to do so) about their substance use, use-related risks, and any consequences of importance to the patient (e.g., social, occupational, legal, medical, psychological consequences), and sometimes how their use compares to norms (Table 46.3). Along with the assessment should come clear and nonconfrontational advice about change, again after asking for permission to do so. The patient's desires and understanding about relevant behavior change should be elicited, as should their ability and readiness to change. Then with the patient's agreement, a menu of options for courses of action should be discussed. Their commitment, including an agreement about the next step and (long- and short-term) goals should be agreed upon and recorded. Finally, arrangement for follow-up should be made. The approach must be empathic and supportive of the patient's self-efficacy.

| TABLE 46.3 | Alcohol Epidemiology: Drinking Levels by Age and Sex of Community-Dwelling Adults in the United States. |

CUMULATIVE PERCENTILE OF DRINKS PER WEEK BY AGE AND GENDER

Age (yr)	0	1	2–3	4–5	6–8	9–12	13–19	20–29	30–39	40+
Men										
18–20	32	65	71	76	80	84	87	90	93	100
21–25	20	49	59	65	73	79	85	90	93	100
26–29	19	53	63	71	78	84	91	94	97	100
30–34	21	57	68	76	82	88	93	96	97	100
35–39	25	57	67	73	80	86	91	95	97	100
40–44	26	60	68	74	80	86	91	94	95	100
45–49	27	59	69	75	81	86	91	94	96	100
50–54	28	61	70	75	81	86	92	95	96	100
55–59	32	65	72	78	84	89	94	97	98	100
60–64	36	68	74	77	83	88	93	96	97	100
65+	45	73	78	82	87	91	95	98	99	100
Total	29	61	69	75	81	86	91	95	96	100
Women										
18–20	40	81	86	90	92	94	96	97	98	100
21–25	27	72	81	85	90	93	96	98	99	100
26–29	30	80	88	91	94	97	98	99	99	100
30–34	32	80	87	92	94	97	98	99	99	100
35–39	32	78	86	90	93	96	98	99	99	100
40–44	35	80	86	91	94	96	98	99	100	100
45–49	36	79	86	89	93	95	97	99	99	100
50–54	42	82	87	90	94	96	98	99	99	100
55–59	43	82	88	91	93	96	98	99	99	100
60–64	50	85	90	93	95	98	99	100	100	100
65+	63	89	92	94	96	98	99	100	100	100
Total	41	81	87	91	94	96	98	99	99	100

This table may be useful for helping patients understand how their level of drinking objectively compares to that of Americans of the same age and gender. For example, a 50-year-old woman who drinks two drinks every day can be provided advised that she drinks more than 98% of American women her age. Reprinted from Buchsbaum DG, Buchanan RG, Centor RM, et al. Screening for alcohol abuse using CAGE scores and likelihood ratios. *Annals Intern Med.* 1991;115(10):774–777, with permission from Elsevier.

More specifically, the clinician should determine the patient's perception of their use and need for change (e.g., "Do you think your drug use is a problem?").[86] For patients who are not ready to change, the goals are to increase problem awareness, express concern, and agree to disagree. Sometimes a trial of abstinence or cutting down can be useful. For patients considering change, the goal is to tip the balance toward change by eliciting positive and negative aspects of drinking and not drinking, to demonstrate discrepancies between patients' values and actions. Once the patient has decided to change, reviewing options for the next steps is recommended. The patient will need support and encouragement, and a reminder that the therapeutic relationship will continue regardless of continued unhealthy use or success in cutting down.

Management of Risky Alcohol and Drug Use

Brief intervention has been demonstrated to significantly improve self-reported drinking outcomes when delivered in many clinical settings and by varied clinical personnel, although the best controlled trial evidence is for screening and brief intervention in primary care settings by primary care clinicians.[17,34,35] Although they are less well-studied, brief interventions can also be written, phone, or computer/web-based, and can be single or multiple contacts.[57] The best evidence for efficacy is for multicontact interventions in people without a moderate to severe disorder. Implementation depends on the particular practice setting. The evidence for efficacy on health outcomes and utilization is inconclusive, although some individual studies are suggestive of benefit.

Fleming and colleagues demonstrated in a randomized controlled trial of a multicontact brief intervention, that significant effects on self-reported drinking and on health care utilization and expenditures can be detected for up to 4 years.[36] One meta-analysis demonstrated that brief intervention for alcohol decreases mortality.[29] Meta-analyses predict that on average alcohol intake will decline by 38 g per week (a 15% decrease)[16] and that the proportion of people drinking risky amounts decreases to 57% in brief intervention groups and 69% in controls.[14]

The evidence supporting brief intervention for drugs other than alcohol and tobacco is more limited. There are many high-quality randomized controlled studies demonstrating no significant effect of brief intervention on nonalcohol drug use. However, a small but growing number of controlled trials have successfully tested brief intervention for drugs after screening in outpatient settings. Bernstein and colleagues studied patients who used cocaine and or heroin who presented for care in outpatient (not primary care) settings. A single motivational brief intervention delivered by a trained health promotion advocate reduced cocaine and heroin use at 6 months more than written advice alone.[15] For example, more cocaine users who received brief intervention were abstinent than were controls (22% vs. 17%). The World Health Organization Alcohol Smoking and Substance Involvement Screening Test phase 3 trial found that brief intervention had efficacy with respect to intermediate outcomes, but there is doubt that the outcomes are clinically significant.[108] Blow and colleagues conducted a randomized controlled trial of brief intervention in urban emergency departments and found that certain methods (e.g., delivery by a trained therapist or by computer) resulted in significant decreases in drug use up to 12 months later.[18]

Brief interventions can decrease substance use, but even under the best circumstances (e.g., the evidence for alcohol brief intervention in primary care) many people continue to have unhealthy use. The effectiveness of repeated brief interventions is unknown, but primary care settings do provide the opportunity to assess alcohol use and consequences over time, and to address behavior change. Over time, with repeated conversations, the case for change can build in breadth and depth. As the clinician learns more about the patient and their substance use, the advice and rationale may become more personally salient and effective. The key for clinicians delivering longitudinal care is to maintain an empathic alliance and continue to address substance use. Drinking despite known negative consequences is a DSM-5 criterion for a disorder, so clinicians should remain alert to any consequences, and be clear in the education of the patient about the connection of the drinking and the consequence. Continued drinking in this case likely signals greater severity of the AUD.

If there is an important person in the patient's life, it may be effective to bring this person into the discussion, with the patient's consent. This person should be invited to a face-to-face visit with the patient. They may offer an important perspective, for instance by furnishing information about consequences of drinking or by assisting in the process of change. It may also be necessary for the behavior change to be a goal shared by the two people for success to take hold.

Once a patient has been able to reduce drinking to healthier levels, the clinician should recognize and affirm this success and monitor for any recurrence.

This discussion of management of drinking may be applied to use of other drugs. It should be noted that in many cases in the United States, the illegal activities involved in procuring illicit drugs is an obvious risk that can be used in motivational brief interventions, although it is becoming less an issue for cannabis/marijuana. Several drugs, depending on route of administration, induce physiological dependence at high rates, so controlled use will be rare; for instance, smoking freebase or crack cocaine is rarely a casual behavior over which there is robust control.

Management of Alcohol Use Disorder

Several approaches to moderate to severe alcohol use disorder (AUD) can be effective in primary care settings, namely, pharmacotherapy and counseling. Referrals to specialist care can also be helpful. Bear in mind that it is unlikely that a brief intervention alone will result in significant decrease in drinking of people with moderate to severe AUD.[104]

Pharmacotherapy

For the management of moderate to severe AUD alcohol dependence, acamprosate, naltrexone, and disulfiram have proven efficacy (see Chapter 51). A technical note: most such efficacy studies were in people with DSM-IV alcohol dependence, which is by and large similar to moderate to severe AUD. These medications, to be most effective, should be given along with counseling, which can be done in primary care settings and should *not* be withheld if the patient is not interested in formal psychotherapy visits.[78] Medications for alcohol use disorder are not "magic bullets" and should be considered as one of several effective approaches. Even with pharmacologic support, many patients find initiating and maintaining change to be challenging. We emphasize the importance of continued motivational counseling, mutual-help, and peer support in the community and attention to relapse prevention with or without medication use, based in large part on patient preferences and response to care. But no single approach is 100% effective for this chronic and serious condition so all known effective interventions should be considered. As such, offering and discussing medications with patients should be routine and realistic, addressing efficacy without falsely raising hopes. Because medication adherence is one of the most difficult challenges to overcome in primary care for all chronic diseases, let alone for behavioral conditions, minimizing and managing any side effects are critically important. Counseling designed to enhance medication adherence is also recommended.

Acamprosate has been approved for use in Europe since 1989 and in the United States since 2004. It has generally been studied in patients abstaining from alcohol for at least 5 days. If, however, abstinence cannot be achieved, initiating pharmacotherapy for AUD should be considered as clinical circumstances dictate. Acamprosate is an oral medication that is taken three times a day (two capsules each time for a total of six capsules daily). A congener of homotaurine, it is active at the γ-aminobutyric acid receptor and thought to modulate glutamatergic activity at the N-methyl-D-aspartate receptor. Its use is associated with an improvement in abstinence rates (15% in placebo vs. 23% for acamprosate-treated patients at 12 months) time to first drink, and days of cumulative abstinence, with a number needed to treat of 7.5 to achieve a 13% absolute risk reduction in relapse at 12 months.[19,60] In one study, it was effective when administered for a full year, and also reduced relapse for an additional year of follow-up. It is relatively well tolerated, reflected by low drop-out rates in clinical trials. The main side-effect is diarrhea, which improves with continued use of the medication. Renal insufficiency is a relative contraindication (dictates a dose reduction).[41,74,75]

Oral naltrexone has been approved to treat alcohol dependence (e.g., moderate to severe disorder) in the United States since 1994 and long-acting injectable naltrexone (monthly) since 2006. Naltrexone is a mu opioid receptor antagonist that is considered to block central endorphins and to decrease levels of dopamine released in the nucleus accumbens, a key event in euphoria and reward. Naltrexone has also generally been studied in abstinent patients,[97] and again, if impractical, starting the drug before a patient has achieved abstinence is acceptable practice. Orally it is taken daily usually at a dose of 50 mg, although starting with a dose of 25 mg a day for the first several days may increase tolerability. Most published studies are limited to a few months duration, but there is support for its use up to 6 months,[8] and in practice all of these medications should be continued as long as they continue to provide benefit and until the risk for relapse is low. Over weeks of ongoing treatment, measures of "craving" for alcohol diminish with time.[89] It may diminish craving and preoccupation with alcohol more than acamprosate.[52] There is good support for its role in decreasing rates of relapse to heavy drinking from 48% in controls to 37% in individuals taking naltrexone. Its effectiveness may be enhanced with cognitive behavioral therapy,[7] but it has also been effective in protocols with minimal counseling components,[72] making it well suited to the primary care setting. Other secondary outcomes are improved, including density of drinking and number of days without drinking, and abstinence. Medical outcomes, such as liver enzyme levels, improve with treatment as well.[12] It cannot be used in patients who require the use of opioids and should be withheld prior to elective procedures requiring opioid analgesia. Management of patients taking naltrexone with unanticipated need for opioid agonists, for example, trauma victims, may be complex, requiring high opioid doses and careful monitoring. It can be associated with gastrointestinal side effects, but these are generally self-limited and minor.[20,74] Naltrexone has reemerged in practice because of its significant superiority in a head-to-head trial versus acamprosate.[6,8] The long-acting form may help address the challenge of medication adherence, requiring but one injection every 4 weeks.[39]

Disulfiram is an inhibitor of aldehyde dehydrogenase, a step in the metabolism of alcohol. This causes the accumulation of acetaldehyde that in turn causes a range of reactions from an uncomfortable flushing reaction and nausea, to more severe problems such as vomiting, dehydration, and death. It is used as an "aversive" treatment to heighten the negative consequences of drinking. In placebo-controlled trials it fails to show efficacy, but this may make sense because its mechanism of action involves awareness that one is taking it. In more structured settings, such as when a family member may supervise and witness administration of the medication, it appears to be more efficacious. Several trials confirm that supervised administration is more effective than unsupervised dosing.[87] Because it has a high risk-to-benefit ratio, even in optimal settings, we do not typically choose this medication first. When it is prescribed, written informed consent should be obtained, reinforcing the supervisor's role as well as the possibly fatal consequences of coadministration with alcohol. Hepatitis is a feared side effect.[31]

Counseling in Primary Care

Even within the time constraints of primary care practice, there are models of counseling that can be adopted and adapted as feasible. Motivational interviewing is adapted as motivational enhancement therapy. Four sessions of motivational enhancement therapy was as effective as 12 sessions of cognitive behavioral therapy or 12-step facilitation in one large randomized trial. Motivational enhancement therapy, although more extensive, has many parallels to motivational brief interventions done in primary care settings.

One model of adherence enhancing counseling with the acronym BRENDA has been tested with oral and injectable naltrexone. The elements of the model, described in subsequent text, are individually or in combination supported by literature on depression and substance use management.[78]

The acronym indicates that the model begins with a *Biopsychosocial* evaluation, emphasizing there is more to AUD than physiological dependence. Providing feedback to the patient with a *Report* on this assessment is akin to brief intervention. *Empathic* understanding of the patient's situation as opposed to a confrontational style is a key element of interactions that fosters a strong therapeutic alliance. Rather than recommending one treatment to all patients, it is recommended that support and therapeutic interventions reflect the *Needs* collaboratively identified by the patient and the treatment provider. The many treatment types that have been demonstrated to improve drinking outcome with little evidence or clear superiority of any one, argue for acknowledgement of patient preferences. These first four BRENDA steps create a patient-centered, empathic alliance; they set the stage for and are recommended to precede the giving of *Direct* advice to the patient on how to meet the identified needs. Soliciting the patient's reaction to the advice and checking in as to the relevance and feasibility of the plan is key. This last step, to *Assess* reaction of the patient to advise and adjust as necessary for best care, permits the clinician and patient to arrive at a mutual plan. The patient role here may enhance self-efficacy (confidence to change), motivation, and ultimately behavior change.

An approach dubbed "medical management," tested in the "COMBINE" study, calls for an initial discussion lasting 45 minutes and eight follow-up sessions of approximately 20 minutes over the ensuing 4 months, on average every 2 to 3 weeks. The sessions covered a review of drinking and consequences, medication use and effects, and global functioning.[65] In the COMBINE study, medical management as described here proved more efficacious in increasing the number of days of abstinence than a more intensive behavioral counseling intervention. Although perhaps not a generalizable finding, this does reinforce the message of effectiveness of counseling that could be administered in the primary care setting.[7] Even if physician time is too limited for such counseling, health behavior change counselors in these settings could deliver it.

Primary care clinicians should adopt a proactive stance to supporting recovery activities. The counseling techniques described here are consistent with that general stance. It may be beneficial to discuss patient's participation in mutual-help groups in the community as a routine part of every visit. Exploring resistance to and benefits from meetings, suggesting active versus passive participation (e.g., working on "steps" or getting a sponsor), and recommending persistent and methodical attendance all promote engagement.[40,57]

Management of Tobacco Use

Brief interventions have been demonstrated to reduce smoking significantly. For patients who do not respond to brief counseling, the primary care clinician should be familiar with medication and counseling approaches to tobacco cessation.[11,43,49] Chapter 23 contains a detailed guide to the use of nicotine replacement therapies, bupropion, and varenicline for the treatment of tobacco use disorder. The essential approach described for AUD is applicable to tobacco: focus on the patient's distress, maintain an empathic connection, support medication use by monitoring side effects and responses, and continue to work toward sustaining all positive behavior changes.

Management of Opioid Use Disorder: Pharmacotherapy

Rates of relapse to opioids are high when patients do not receive opioid agonist treatment (OAT). A small minority of patients with OUD will be abstinent at 1 year if not receiving it. From 30% to 60% of patients provided OAT with methadone or buprenorphine are not using illicit drugs at 6 months. And at 4 years, up to 50% of patients no longer meet criteria for OUD.[106] Under the federal Drug Abuse Treatment Act of 2000,[103] specially qualified physicians may prescribe buprenorphine for sublingual administration for a limited number of patients with OUD . With the passage of new legislation in 2016, now nurse practitioners and physician assistants may qualify for prescriptive authority. The treatment of OUD with OAT, formerly legal only in methadone maintenance programs, has now begun to shift to outpatient clinicians outside of specialty settings and into the hands of primary care clinicans.[100] Qualifications for prescribing buprenorphine under the Drug Abuse Treatment Act of 2000 and the Comprehensive Addiction and Recovery Act (CARA) of 2016 are listed in Table 46.4. With documentation of qualifications, application is made to the US Food and Drug Administration (FDA) for a special Drug Enforcement Administration number to use when prescribing buprenorphine. In the first year, qualified prescribers can have 30 patients with active prescriptions at any one time. After a year of practice, application may be made to expand the allowed number of patients to 100. With new rules as of 2016, after a

TABLE 46.4	Provider Qualifications for Prescribing Buprenorphine for Opiate Use Disorder.

Valid license (MD, DO, NP, or PA)
Ability to refer to or provide appropriate psychosocial treatments
Must meet one or more of following:
- Subspecialty board certification in addiction psychiatry from the American Board of Medical specialties
- Subspecialty board certified in addiction medicine from the American Osteopathic Association (AOA)
- Addiction certification by the American Society of Addiction Medicine, ABAM, ABPM
- Successful completion of a qualifying 8-h (for MD or DO) or 24-h (for NP or PA) educational offering by the American Academy of Addiction Psychiatry, American Medical Association, AOA, American Society of Addiction Medicine, or any Department of Health and Human Services–approved organization
- Physician is an investigator in a clinical trial that led to approval of buprenorphine
- Training or experience as determined by a state licensing board

From the U.S. Department of Health and Human Services, Substance Abuse and Mental Health Services, Administration Center for Substance Abuse Treatment. Clinical Guidelines for the use of buprenorphine in the treatment of opioid addiction. Treatment Improvement Protocol (TIP) 40. Publication No. (SMA) 04-3939, 2004. From US Congress. *S524-Comprehensive Addiction and Recovery Act of 2016*; 2016.

year of having the waivered limit at 100, providers may apply to raise the patient number to 275. Expert credentialing as outlined below may permit accelerated increase of the patient number. As of 2016, there are some new stipulations about practice characteristics that may come to bear. Such stipulations include practice aspects such as the use of health information technology, use of statewide prescription-monitoring programs, having a drug "diversion control" plan, and acceptance of third-party coverage.

Buprenorphine is a mu-receptor partial agonist, meaning that it is active at the same receptor as morphine (and heroin, oxycodone, and other opioids) but with only partial activation. It therefore produces a weaker drug effect than the "pure" agonists, with less euphoria, less fatigue, and fewer side effects such as respiratory depression or constipation (i.e., it has a ceiling with respect to these effects). It is more tightly bound to the receptor; therefore agonists with stronger activity but weaker binding cannot occupy and activate the receptor. In fact it precipitates withdrawal from such substances by displacing them. The only medication approved thus far for use under the Drug Addiction Treatment Act of 2000 is buprenorphine. It is available alone or in combination with naloxone, the opioid antagonist that is usually administered intravenously. The buprenorphine and the buprenorphine/naloxone tablets or films are administered sublingually; via this route a negligible dose of naloxone is absorbed. The purpose of the addition of naloxone to the tablet is to decrease the desirability of diversion of the medication to parenteral use: when the combination is injected, the naloxone is fully active and blocks the effects of any opioid at the mu receptor, causing an abrupt withdrawal in patients who have circulating or bound mu opioid agonists. Buprenorphine is also now FDA approved and available as a depot-pellet that is surgically inserted subdermally and is active for 6 months. Its use is appropriate in certain situations and for patients who have been stable on low-dose sublingual buprenorphine or buprenorphine/naloxone. Special training and testing are required to permit prescribing or insertion of subdermal buprenorphine pellets.[24]

Patients meeting criteria for current moderate to severe DSM-5 OUD (or in some cases those in remission but at high risk of relapse) may be managed with the use of buprenorphine (or buprenorphine/naloxone). Detoxification or maintenance is possible, although relapse (and mortality) rates have been high after detoxification, and short-term outcomes of maintenance are superior.[50]

Patients optimally suited for OAT with buprenorphine should not require more structure than is likely in the primary care provider's office, should be able to adhere to office procedures and protocols, and should have no major comorbid psychiatric disorder and no dependence on a variety of other substances, for example, benzodiazepines. Occasionally, office-based buprenorphine treatment is the best option for a patient, even in the face of challenging comorbid issues; in these cases the clinician should offer OAT, balancing particular risks and benefits, understanding that patients can be referred for other modalities (e.g., methadone programs) should the treatment fail. The initial dosing of buprenorphine, evaluation, and follow-up require assiduous attention and can be complicated. Clinicians who have qualified and have obtained their special Drug Enforcement Administration "x-number" may receive ongoing advice and support through a Center for Substance Abuse Treatment–sponsored mentorship program, the Physician Clinical Support System (http://www.pcssmentor.org).[101]

The mu opioid antagonist naltrexone is approved for the treatment of OUD. Recent evidence has demonstrated improved 6-month relapse rates for people with heroin use disorder treated with injectable intramuscular extended-release naltrexone.[55,58]

A caveat with this medication is the accelerated loss of tolerance, and the theoretical increase in the risk of overdose with resumption of opioid use; this may be true for any OUD treatment that does not involve an agonist. Initiating full-dose mu antagonists requires that the patient have no agonist circulating so that withdrawal is not precipitated. This can be a barrier to outpatient initiation.

Referral to Specialty Care

For patients whose drinking or drug use meets the definition of substance use disorder (or SUD), the primary care clinician may refer to and collaborate with specialty care clinicians and should be familiar with available resources. Physicians should be familiar with local mutual help programs and how patients may join them. Primary care clinicians should be aware of resources listing local meetings and may consider attending meetings to be familiar with where they are sending patients. Many groups have representatives willing to come to physician offices or to meet patients to make referrals easier.

Primary care clinicians should also be familiar with local counseling resources, knowing what treatments are offered, and how, if, and which patients can access them. For patients with OUD, referral for methadone (or buprenorphine) should be considered. Finally, the primary care clinician should become aware of all local resources for referral of patients who exceed the clinician's capabilities or available time for appropriate management. Such specialized referrals are particularly important and useful for patients with serious psychiatric comorbidity, and for patients with substantial social service needs who may require intensive outpatient, residential, or inpatient care initially.

Patients in Remission

Primary care clinicians will care for many patients in remission from SUD.[38] Primary care clinicians who screen all patients and ask about lifetime use will be aware of such personal history. Supportive discussions about recovery should be part of every routine visit. When situations that may increase risk for relapse are encountered, or anticipated, problem-solving and recovery enhancement discussions should ensue. Patients should be advised to call for help. Any significant change in routine can signal risk. If patients change housing, relationships, or jobs, discussing relapse potential may be prudent. If the patient or a relative is experiencing significant medical illness or is diagnosed with a life-changing disease, the possibility of relapse should be discussed. If a patient with an active recovery routine supporting remission from SUD, for example, with regular participation in 12-step meetings, interrupts this practice, reasons should be explored, as such a change may herald relapse. And finally, when abstinent patients begin to experiment with "controlled" use of the problematic substance, empathic, clear concern should be expressed. If the patient is resistant to the notion that such use is itself problematic, it is good to discuss what warning signs would concern the patient. Discussing such hypothetical problems may be more palatable than facing imminent risk. The sound of the patient's own voice describing such problematic scenarios is sometimes enough to clarify the risk and catalyze improvement. Of note, in general, the safest and best recommendation for those with disorder is abstinence. Some may be able to continue low level use without consequences, but it is not possible to predict which patients will succeed with such an approach and it is not the majority.

Patients newly achieving abstinence or remission from SUD often feel shame and regret. This may extend to the sense of having mistreated their own bodies. Frequently, patients worry about the state of the liver, heart, brain, immune system, or kidneys after a prolonged time using alcohol or other drugs. This worry is often inaccurate or unrealistic. The primary care clinician can support abstinence by attending to such patients' concerns without being dismissive, but without augmenting the sense of urgency, absent significant physical or laboratory findings. It is normal for patients in early remission to feel malaise or fatigue; these are probably not symptoms of underlying disease. Changing sleep patterns and appetite are part of recovery as well. It is acceptable practice to monitor patients closely over time rather than sending off batteries of tests. Among exceptions to this approach of using the "test of time" would be for common infectious diseases that respond to treatment. Therefore repeated testing, for example, for exposure to HIV or hepatitis C virus would not be misplaced effort.

Treatment of Psychiatric Comorbidity

The details of the evaluation and management of comorbid psychiatric conditions are touched upon in various chapters throughout this book. There are higher rates of affective disorders among individuals who use alcohol, tobacco, and other drugs. Several core principles inform our practice and bear repeating for the primary care clinician. First, the primary care clinician should arrive at a mutual understanding with the patient about which symptoms are to be followed and evaluated as markers of the mental health condition. These may or may not be the most troubling for the patient. Those symptoms with higher frequency will be more sensitive bench marks than infrequent ones. Target symptoms should be clearly documented (e.g., sleep quality or quantity for people with depression; or numbers of episodes of tearfulness or guilty feelings). Second, patients should not titrate medications without speaking with the clinician. In part, substance use disorders may be thought of as pathologic self-pharmacotherapy. As such, it may be counterproductive to ask the patient to focus on and respond with self-medication to perceived internal distress.

It can be useful to try to ascertain whether there is a psychiatric diagnosis independent of the substance use condition. It is helpful to elicit a history of psychiatric disorders or mental health symptoms during periods of protracted abstinence, when they are less likely to have been due solely to the substance use. Still, the diagnosis is usually tentative rather than definitive. Management of symptoms or treatment of possible diagnoses with medications does not establish an independent diagnosis but can be helpful both with the substance use and with helping the patient feel and function better. The patient may have substance-related symptoms or syndromes that respond to treatment but do not meet criteria for a diagnosis. Nonetheless, it is important to treat these symptoms, as the approach will help management of the substance use disorder.

Consideration of withdrawal of the psychiatric medication when the patient is stable reduces the probability that patients without primary psychiatric problems will erroneously carry such a diagnosis long term. It is also important to remain vigilant about the emergence of new psychiatric problems. Abstinence may have disparate effects on psychiatric symptoms. Although, in general, recovery is associated with mitigation of psychologic distress and diminution of unpleasant psychiatric symptoms, abstinence may conversely elicit recrudescence or emergence of serious psychiatric distress, occasionally after months of seeming stability. Patients often discover persistence of guilt, poor sleep, or anxiety. Symptoms of posttraumatic stress disorder or mania may emerge in recovery. Moreover, there are well-described prolonged abstinence syndromes, such as the depression-like anergia and anhedonia of protracted cocaine abstinence that not only create a high relapse risk, but may benefit from pharmacotherapy.[40] Finally, medications that themselves can be misused or induce an SUD should generally be avoided. The risk of SUD development higher among individuals in early remission or with current or past SUD.[4] Such medications are almost never to be the first choice, and it is a rare situation that demands the use of risky medications at all. Benzodiazepines and psychostimulants are examples of drug classes of concern.

When treating depression or depressive symptoms in the setting of drug or alcohol use disorder, the primary care clinician needs to have a sense of how severe the symptoms are and how well the patient can safely and effectively engage in outpatient treatment in the primary care setting. When there is doubt, bringing in expert consultation of a psychiatric clinician versed in addiction is warranted. When the patient or others are at risk of imminent harm, emergency referral for safety is warranted.

For patients within the primary care clinician's expertise and comfort zone, management can be straightforward. The mainstays are psychotherapy and medication. Sometimes patients are resistant to a trial of medication for a variety of reasons, and their rationale should be discussed openly, although studies of depression management in primary care suggest that patients are generally more willing to accept medication than counseling.[105] Often, the notion that depression, like addiction, is a chemical disorder of the brain can be what enables an individual to accept pharmacotherapy. The primary care provider may allay fears of developing an SUD that involves a new medication or of stigmatization in abstinence-oriented therapy that mistakenly interprets use of medication as no different from an illicit drug. In addition, the evidence that treatment of depression in this setting has positive effects on addiction outcome should be reviewed.[70] Serotonin reuptake inhibitors such as citalopram or fluoxetine have demonstrated this dual efficacy in managing depression symptoms. Tricyclic antidepressants such as desipramine have been studied and supported in this setting as well, but may have a less favorable side effect profile.

Among the most distressing symptoms of early abstinence are disturbances of sleep. Hypersomnolence may be part of the "crash" from withdrawal from psychostimulants or the body's need to restore and heal after metabolic derangements associated with many drugs. It may also be one of several cardinal symptoms of depression. Other than treating depression if the diagnosis seems likely, we recommend no specific pharmacologic intervention here, other than to maintain good sleep hygiene and to avoid activities (e.g., driving) where significant fatigue poses a hazard. Insomnia is also frequent. Although patients often cite insomnia as a primary reason for relapse and persistence may be quite debilitating, randomized trials have not demonstrated an effect of insomnia treatment on abstinence rates. Nonetheless, many practitioners would use trazodone or a sedating antidepressant at least when depressive symptoms coexist. As with hypersomnolence, insomnia can be a symptom of affective disorders, which should remain in the differential diagnoses, as they would guide pharmacotherapy. In the absence of affective disorder, the physician

should review good sleep hygiene practices with the patient.[67] Among the mainstays of good sleep hygiene are minimal or no caffeine; 30 minutes of sunshine in the morning; exercise early in the day; a light meal in the evening; using the bed for sleep only; avoidance of media on back-lit screens; relaxation before bed; and maintaining a regular schedule.

As with depression, anxiety is associated with SUDs, and for some the anxiety disorder is primary. For others, periods of relative or complete alcohol or other substance abstinence, associated with adrenergic drive, causes or exacerbates anxiety symptoms, complicating early recovery and risking relapse due to self-medication. Patients may struggle with intolerable symptoms that threaten sobriety. If the history is clear that anxiety symptoms abate during abstinence, supportive counseling and cognitive therapy may suffice. However, diagnosis can be challenging. Symptoms may be part of generalized anxiety disorder, specific phobias, or posttraumatic stress disorder. Primary management in all cases should include nonpharmacological care. Support groups, cognitive therapy, and exposure-based therapies (for desensitization and coping strategies) are all possibilities. Posttraumatic stress disorder presents a challenge as to timing of therapy, with experts advising delay of intensive therapy to periods of stability. Pharmacotherapy for generalized anxiety disorder or posttraumatic stress disorder should involve a selective serotonin reuptake inhibitor as the gold standard. Treatment with buspirone can also be effective for anxiety symptoms and may have beneficial effects on alcohol consumption.[22,54] Benzodiazepines should generally be avoided for this indication in the primary care setting, carrying as they do the risk of incident benzodiazepine use disorder. For some patients, however, with close monitoring, they can be considered second- or third-line agents.[76]

It may be challenging to tease apart whether anxiety is a manifestation of mania or bipolar disorder, in which case an antidepressant as a sole agent may be contraindicated. When in doubt here, a mood stabilizer or sedating antipsychotic, such as quetiapine, may be preferable. Mood-stabilizing agents (such as valproic acid and carbamazepine) may become more common in such situations as we witness the possible emergence of topiramate, an anticonvulsant and a second-line mood-stabilizing agent, for use as a primary pharmacotherapy in AUD (controlled trials have demonstrated efficacy for alcohol dependence, but it is not currently approved for this indication by the FDA).[48] In this line, interest in the use of gabapentin for AUD is emerging, but clinical acceptance may be slowed by its misuse liability, especially among patients with OUD.[61]

Management of Withdrawal From Alcohol and Other Drugs

What follows is a general overview of considerations relevant to the primary care setting. More alcohol- and drug-specific recommendations follow in the next sections of this chapter.

"Withdrawal syndrome" refers to the physiological and behavioral response to sudden cessation or abrupt decrease in the intake of a drug to which physiological dependence has developed. In pharmacological dependence, the brain becomes adapted to the presence of the drug and develops compensatory mechanisms to function. When the drug is withdrawn, those compensatory changes are no longer opposed by the drug, and the result is the withdrawal syndrome. A simple analogy would be driving an automobile with the handbrake partially engaged. To maintain speed, supranormal acceleration is applied. If the brake is disengaged, the car will surge forward until a new balance is achieved.

Different drugs are associated with different withdrawal syndromes. Some are outwardly noticeable, as with the tremor of alcohol withdrawal or the dilated pupils of opioid withdrawal, and others may be invisible, as with the mental slowing and depression of cocaine withdrawal. The rate of decrease in drug dosage, as well as conditions of the patient, will affect the severity and manifestations of withdrawal.

It is critical to be familiar with withdrawal syndromes and their management. In particular, there are situations where the likelihood of complicated or dangerous withdrawal necessitates admission to an inpatient service. For frail or elderly patients, or those with unstable medical conditions, such as recent myocardial infarction, the risk of outpatient management is too great, and referral for admission should be made.

Even in otherwise healthy people, barbiturate and benzodiazepine withdrawal can be dangerous, as can severe alcohol withdrawal. Opioid withdrawal can lead to dehydration and metabolic abnormalities, but in healthy young people is usually tolerated. Psychostimulant, nicotine, and cannabis withdrawal are not typically dangerous, although they may be associated with subjective suffering that is real and significant. The management of withdrawal is termed "detoxification" and simply means supervised or medically treated withdrawal. Detoxification is not treatment of addiction per se; rather it is merely the process of ridding the body of the drug safely or with mitigated discomfort. As such, referral for detoxification should not be confused with addressing addiction treatment needs. In fact, in the United States, detoxification is most commonly not followed by effective addiction treatment. For OUD, OAT should typically be discussed.

Being aware of the withdrawal syndrome and attending to it are necessary to establish trust and to permit reasonable interactions with patients. It is inadvisable to engage in a long or complicated evaluation with a patient experiencing significant discomfort or craving because of withdrawal. Acknowledging and attending to a patient's comfort continuously to the extent possible is necessary. ("When did you last use? When will you need to again? Can we speak now?" are questions that may appropriately inaugurate all interactions with physiologically dependent patients seeking help).

There are other, nonmedical features that will make admission advisable. If the patient does not have a safe place to go where temptation or access to the substance is limited, then outpatient management is less likely to succeed, and offering inpatient admission is indicated. If there is no one to support the patient or to provide safe transportation, inpatient observation may be preferable. The American Society of Addiction Medicine has specific patient placement criteria that can help with such triage decisions.[10] Your office capabilities are also important in the decision to admit. Can you or staff see and evaluate the patient at sufficient frequency for safety? For moderate alcohol withdrawal, for example, evaluation daily with easy telephone availability throughout the first few days may be necessary.

In general, outpatient withdrawal can be achieved with reliable and motivated patients by advising them of safe symptom-driven and self-tapering schedules. Many patients will explain that they have done this on their own many times. Patients who are at low risk, or using low-dosages, or using a low-risk drug may try this safely. Depending on the level of physiological dependence, a typical recipe for self-tapering for short-acting opioids, benzodiazepines, and alcohol is to reduce the dose of the drug by 10%–20% per day, achieving abstinence in about a week or two. An exception is for long-acting drugs and for patients long histories

of benzodiazepine use disorder. In these cases, tapering schedules may be better tolerated over the course of weeks to months.[94]

We caution, again, that early relapse is common in severe OUD treated without continued OAT in the absence of a structured, supportive treatment program.

Many clinicians are reluctant to advise that a patient use the offending substance, even if it is part of a program to forestall withdrawal symptoms and to achieve abstinence. In this case, other medications can be prescribed. In principle, medications that are active at the same receptor or produce similar effects as the offending drug (i.e., cross-tolerance), have been demonstrated to help. Finally, patients may experience withdrawal from many substances simultaneously. It is often advisable to obtain objective identification of recently ingested drugs if possible, for instance with a urine, blood, or oral fluid toxicology panel or by confirming history with a trusted companion of the patient.

Alcohol Withdrawal

The primary care clinician should be familiar with inpatient detoxification, and can adapt protocols to the outpatient setting.[59] We address this section to the clinician interested in providing ambulatory detoxification because it is a complicated and intensive process requiring a high level of commitment personally and programmatically. For instance, face-to-face evaluation every 24 to 48 hours must be feasible on the part of both the patient and clinician. (Even when a trusted companion of the patient can assist remotely, hands-on care by the clinician should be possible for unexpected clinical events.) Alcohol withdrawal can be fatal or result in prolonged and complex hospitalization. Therefore the reflex may be to advise inpatient evaluation and management as a default. Most alcohol withdrawal, however, never comes to clinical attention and is not significant. Distinguishing cases that can be managed safely in the ambulatory arena from cases requiring inpatient management can be challenging and may make the difference between life and death. Some patients will not be willing for myriad reasons to consider inpatient detoxification, so distinguishing those cases where admission is elective can be critically important.[44]

In general, the severity of withdrawal can be predicted based on the severity of prior episodes. There is a loose relationship between intensity of drinking or blood alcohol level and severity of symptoms. But regardless, older patients, those with a history of head trauma or concomitant sedative use, and those with comorbid acute medical, surgical, or psychiatric illness, are at risk for more severe withdrawal. Outpatient management is generally safe in individuals who report their last drink over 36 hours prior (since more significant symptoms are unlikely to develop subsequently), have no other risk factors for severe withdrawal, and have a responsible other to accompany and monitor them. Inpatient detoxification should be considered when there is a history of seizure, other drug use, an anxiety disorder, multiple detoxifications, and/or a blood alcohol level over 150 mg/dL (the latter a sign of great tolerance and a risk for more severe withdrawal symptoms). Inpatient management is advisable for patients over age 60, those who have concurrent acute illness, seizure, or moderate to severe symptoms (because of the risks for delirium) as measured by an objective assessment scale such as the revised Clinical Institute Withdrawal Assessment for Alcohol scale.[99]

Patients whose conditions are uncomplicated may be advised to taper alcohol on their own at home. If instead, medications are to be used, several medications may be efficacious, including anticonvulsants. Despite the potential advantages of anticonvulsants that have fewer effects on cognition and alertness, we favor benzodiazepines because they are the only medications proven to decrease the severe and fatal complications of withdrawal in placebo-controlled trials.[62] Chlordiazepoxide and diazepam are convenient, rapidly absorbed orally, have long half-lives of elimination, and are inexpensive. Chlordiazepoxide is associated with less-intense initial euphoria, so may be preferable to diazepam for outpatient detoxification. The half-life of diazepam is 33 hours and that of desmethyl diazepam, its active metabolite, is 50 hours. Chlordiazepoxide is metabolized to nordiazepam, desmethyl diazepam, and oxazepam; the half-life is similarly prolonged. For patients with significant liver impairment (hypoalbuminemia or coagulopathy but not the more common mild transaminase elevation), benzodiazepines that are not hepatically metabolized are preferred. Oxazepam and lorazepam are frequent choices, having renal excretion. An objective measure of withdrawal should be used to monitor severity and response to treatment. For patients with moderate to moderate-severe withdrawal, that is, a revised Clinical Institute Withdrawal Assessment for Alcohol scale score of 8–20, diazepam 20 mg (or chlordiazepoxide 50 mg) orally may be given, and the patient reassessed after 2 hours. If the revised Clinical Institute Withdrawal Assessment for Alcohol scale score has increased, then inpatient admission should be considered. If the score remains above 8–12 (i.e., severity is more than "mild,") another dose of diazepam of 10 or 20 mg (or chlordiazepoxide 30-50 mg) should be given. If after 2 more hours, the revised Clinical Institute Withdrawal Assessment for Alcohol scale score has not decreased by 2 or more and/or remains above 15, admission should be advised. The median number of doses of diazepam required for patients with moderate to severe uncomplicated withdrawal is three.[88]

If the revised Clinical Institute Withdrawal Assessment for Alcohol scale score has decreased, the patient should be advised to take the same dose of benzodiazepine every 6–8 hours for three to four doses and be reevaluated within 48 hours, preferably the next day. Patients may need additional doses between these scheduled doses to treat reemergent symptoms. The revised Clinical Institute Withdrawal Assessment for Alcohol scale is administered at every clinical evaluation, although patients and their significant others should be told which symptoms to follow themselves (e.g., tremor, anxiety, agitation). The tapering of benzodiazepine can be advised over 3 to 5 days with clear follow-up and instructions to call for indications of over- or underdosing. When withdrawal is ablated after only a few doses of a long acting benzodiazepine have been administered, tapering may not be necessary, as the decrease in concentration is gradual.

Opioid Withdrawal

Like alcohol withdrawal, the intensity of opioid withdrawal syndromes is quite variable. Decisions about the choice between in- and outpatient detoxification, as with alcohol, depend on factors of social stability, comorbid illness, and the ability to resist illicit drug use as an outpatient. Unlike alcohol withdrawal, however, opioid withdrawal is less-often life-threatening in the absence of underlying disease. The most effective class of drugs for relieving withdrawal symptoms are opioids themselves, and many inpatient detoxification programs use long-acting oral medication such as methadone or sublingual medications such as buprenorphine for this purpose. In the absence of a special license (such as that under the Drug Addiction Treatment Act of 2000 permitting use of buprenorphine), however, it is currently illegal in the outpatient setting to prescribe opioids for the treatment of OUD or detoxification. (An exception is for patients with physiological dependence but without OUD; in this case, tapering doses of opioids may be prescribed to attenuate withdrawal symptoms. An example would be a patient on chronic opioids for sciatica who undergoes successful surgery and may taper off the analgesic.) Specially qualified physicians may prescribe buprenorphine and no other opioid for this purpose. Anyone with prescriptive authority may treat opioid withdrawal with non-opioids, however.

In general, all medications used for opioid withdrawal aim to attenuate the symptoms of withdrawal. Prominent symptoms or signs and the medications used to treat them are:

- Anxiety—benzodiazepines, buspirone, sedating antipsychotics
- Diarrhea or indigestion—hyoscyamine
- Insomnia—trazodone
- Muscle and bone aches—nonsteroidal anti-inflammatory drugs such as ibuprofen.
- Tachycardia, tremor—central alpha agonist clonidine either orally or transdermally.

Severity of withdrawal should be assessed using an objective scoring system such as the Clinical Opiate Withdrawal Scale or the Clinical Institute Narcotic Assessment Scale for Withdrawal Symptoms.[103] Treatment should match the pace of withdrawal. Therefore short-acting opioids that result in withdrawal syndromes that are themselves short will likely lead to a commensurately brief course of medication for withdrawal symptoms. Heroin withdrawal may gather intensity over 24–48 hours, so the dose of medication may need to be higher on the second day of withdrawal than the first.[53] Similarly, protracted withdrawal from, for example, methadone, may require several days or weeks of treatment. The severity of withdrawal symptoms is most effectively reduced by opioid replacement (e.g., methadone or buprenorphine). But the outcome of short-term detoxification alone, beyond symptom relief, is dismal with respect to relapse, unless the patient remains in a structured setting. As such, methadone or buprenorphine maintenance therapy is indicated. This is best begun by referral for opioid agonist treatment of withdrawal followed by continuation as treatment.

Medical Management (Including Preventive Care) of People With Unhealthy Alcohol and Other Drug Use

Regardless of whether or not substance use continues, the primary care clinician should attend to a number of other health issues. If use continues, driving habits should be assessed and clear advice given to abstain from driving when using alcohol or other drugs. For persons who continue to use opioids by injection, safer sterile injection techniques should be discussed (e.g., use of new syringes, avoidance of sharing, bleach cleaning of needles, never using without a partner or chaperone, taking a small test dose of a new batch of drug, and accessing needle exchange programs or supervised injection or observation sites). For individuals with continued opioid dependence, overdose prevention is paramount: provision of naloxone to the patient, contacts, and family, for use in the event of overdose can be lifesaving.

Preventive Care

Patients with unhealthy alcohol or other drug use often do not receive routine preventive health care. They may not have a primary care physician or health insurance, and they may not seek this care, in part as a result of substance use and related priorities and disorganization.[46] Furthermore, the physician-patient relationship may be less than optimal for people with SUDs, leading to lower quality of care received. Thus regardless of the status of the substance use, clinicians should make sure to offer such patients routine age- and sex-specific preventive care, as is indicated for all adults (e.g., colon and cervical cancer screening, vaccines, cholesterol testing), and facilitate its receipt to the extent possible. In addition, clinicians should be alert for signs of interpersonal violence and should ask about and recommend receipt of dental health care. On physical examination, cardiac auscultation is important for people who use injected drugs and who may have had endocarditis. Vaccination against hepatitis B should be considered in this high-risk population (particularly for those with a history of drug injection or risky sexual practices, or simply youth). Hepatitis A and/or B vaccination series are recommended when a patient is demonstrated to lack hepatitis antibodies and be and at-risk (e.g., injection drug use, unsafe sex). Patients who are sharing needles need to be reminded about the risk of transmission of HIV. Seronegative patients should be counseled about the availability of preexposure prophylaxis (PReP) with daily antiretroviral medications to reduce the risk of HIV infection. Patients who use injection drugs in high-risk situations (for instance, sharing needles with strangers or with people known to be infected with HIV) may consider PReP.[28a]

Pneumococcal vaccination is indicated for people with AUD. Risky sexual behavior is common in drug- and alcohol-using populations, so education and advice about risk, ensuring access to condoms, and screening for sexually transmitted diseases, especially HIV (now recommended universally for all adults by the Centers for Disease Control and Prevention), are prudent. Cervical cancer screening, also routine for adult sexually active women, is of particularly importance in smokers and those with risky sex practices, who are at higher risk for the disease. Similarly, breast cancer screening should be done, particularly in women with unhealthy alcohol use who are at greater risk. Osteoporosis screening (bone mineral density testing) is indicated for older women with risk factors, particularly smoking and heavy alcohol use. Consideration should also be given to screening for vitamin D deficiency because of poor diets and possible lack of sun exposure. Empirical recommendation of a multivitamin is another approach. Folate should be recommended for women of childbearing age. Other routine tests for individuals with alcohol and other drug use include the serum creatinine, tuberculosis skin testing, and liver enzymes and tests of synthetic function. Patients maintained on methadone, as with any medication that may alter cardiac conduction, should have periodic electrocardiograms as indicated. Lung cancer screening using low-dose computerized tomography (CT) scanning has been recommended by the United States Preventive Services Task Force (USPSTF) for people 55–80 years of age with a 30-pack year history who currently smoke or have been abstinent less than 15 years.

Managing Medical Consequences in the Face of Ongoing Substance Use

When patients are bothered enough by symptoms to bring them to the primary care clinician's attention, an opportunity often arises to link the unhealthy substance use to the symptom. This link, when pointed out by the physician nonjudgmentally and recognized by the patient, can serve as a "discrepancy" (between the goal of health/longevity and the current behavior) that motivates the patient to change.

A recurrent practical dilemma will arise for which there is no strong evidence to assist the primary care clinician in management. When a symptom or condition is likely related to the use of substances but can be treated with medication, primary care clinicians may be tempted to withhold medication, emphasizing instead the patient's responsibility to address the behavioral component (i.e., substance use). A common and representative scenario is hypertension related to excessive drinking of alcohol. An economical and healthy alternative to medication use is reduction of alcohol intake. The challenge to the primary care clinician is to decide with the patient what the best course of action will be. The use of medication in this case may be the best option, especially if the hypertension is severe. First, the reduction in the risk due to hypertension may be achieved more quickly with medication. Second, the significance of the risk may be made more salient by the physician's prescription of a medication. The behavioral component of the problem may thus be helped more than if medications were withheld. Clearly neither response precludes the other, so pursuing both courses is often the best option. If and when the drinking improves, pharmacological management may no longer be necessary. There are no hard and fast rules, here, however, and full and honest shared decision-making with the patient, while minimizing risk, is the optimal course. Prescription of known effective treatments, even in the face of a behavioral etiology of or contributor to disease, seems to be generally well accepted (e.g., medication for hypercholesterolemia in patients with poor diets; and asthma inhalers and even cardiac surgery for people who smoke cigarettes).

The vast number of signs, symptoms, and illnesses related to the entire spectrum of alcohol, tobacco, and other drug use precludes detailing them here. But several highlights most relevant to primary care clinicians follow.

Because tobacco smoking is a well-established risk factor for certain cancers and atherosclerotic disease, the primary care clinician will interpret symptoms with this risk in mind. Whereas pain in the arm in someone who does not smoke cigarettes may represent benign conditions, a Pancoast tumor or coronary insufficiency should be included in the differential diagnosis for someone who does. Shortness of breath and fatigue, among the most common symptoms brought to the primary care clinician's attention, may have serious causes in someone who smokes.

Heavy drinking is associated with disturbed sleep, gastroesophageal reflux disease symptoms, hypertension, peripheral neuropathy, hepatitis, coagulopathies, and cognitive problems. It is sometimes not clear when and how intensively to investigate causes other than alcohol of a particular medical condition. When the condition does not improve with abstinence or moderation, further testing is indicated, especially when these problems may be treatable or may represent important underlying conditions. Even when drinking is ongoing, however, it is prudent to rule out common, treatable problems and not simply attribute a sign, symptom, or condition to alcohol use. In the case of hepatitis, it is prudent to test for viral hepatitis or iron excess. If hypertension is refractory or severe, one may screen for secondary causes. Chronic esophagitis symptoms, refractory to proton pump inhibitors, may be an indication for endoscopy, even if drinking is ongoing. Cytopenias may represent a primary marrow dyscrasia. Neuropathy may be caused by a paraprotein (e.g., in multiple myeloma), diabetes, toxins, or other primary problems. Fatigue, tremor, and insomnia may all be attributable to thyroid dysfunction. Cognitive decline, coordination problems, seizures, or confusion may represent a subdural hematoma, cerebrovascular accident, or other central process. Vitamin B_{12} deficiency is not uncommon and may present with many signs or symptoms of chronic alcohol use, such as macrocytosis, anemia, neuropathy, or cognitive changes. Repletion of vitamin B_{12} can be straightforward and curative.

Hypertension or cardiac ischemia may be an acute presentation of cocaine use. If there are electrocardiographic changes consistent with ischemia, the patient needs to be admitted and observed, possibly to a cardiac care unit. In the presence of enhanced beta- and alpha-adrenergic tone that results from cocaine use, there is a risk that beta-blockers may cause unopposed alpha-adrenergic effects, such as vasoconstriction and hypertension. This risk has not been borne out in some retrospective clinical studies. Beta-blockade remains controversial, however, in the acute care of cocaine-related cardiac ischemia.[79] Anxiolytics, aspirin, and calcium channel blockers remain standard treatments.

Patients using parenteral drugs often present with skin problems caused by the needle use. Abscesses, ulcers, and cellulitis are common. Some ulcers are ischemic rather than infectious, typically when cocaine or other vasoconstrictive agents are injected subcutaneously or into muscle (e.g., when "skin-popping," the preferred route when veins become sclerosed and unusable after chronic intravenous administration). Needle use is also a risk for systemic infection. Viral infections include HIV and hepatitis. Fever in a person who injects drugs should always raise the possibility of systemic viral or bacterial infection. The venous system or right side is more likely affected than the arterial or left side, thus endocarditis is more often of the pulmonic or tricuspid valve. Pulmonary infiltrates or empyema may represent embolization of bacteria to the lung. Because persistence of the foramen ovale is common, patients may present with systemic embolization due to right-to-left shunting and passage of infected material (or bland particulate contaminants). So acute stroke, splenic infarcts, and limb ischemia due to emboli are possible presentations of injection drug use.

Viral hepatitis is common in people who inject drugs. Hepatitis C usually leads to chronic infection, and in a minority leads to cirrhosis, liver failure, or hepatocellular carcinoma. Effective treatments can result in permanent viral suppression. Current treatment is typically well tolerated, may be as short as 2 months, and depending on the genotype of the virus, is curative. Given the high prevalence of the infection in our patients, the qualitative improvement in treatment has been revolutionary.

Pain Management

Among the most challenging problems for people with established SUD is that of pain management. Perhaps because of the riskier lifestyles of people who use drugs and alcohol, trauma and pain are common. And pain thresholds are altered as either a cause or consequence of drug use. Use of opioids for analgesia or other drugs as muscle relaxants can lead to relapse.[81] There is a higher incidence of problems among chronic pain patients who have SUD than among those without.[107] But pain can also be a trigger for relapse, and when necessary, opioids may be prescribed. The key to navigating the difficult course here is to engage the patient in honest collaborative planning with the dual goal of minimizing both pain and the risk for relapse.

Clear enunciation of the risk of relapse may help the patient embrace, along with the primary care clinician, protocols that minimize such risk. Primary care clinicians might be wise to adopt some of these processes as "universal precautions" irrespective of a patient's prior history of addiction. Medications should

be prescribed in small amounts, for example, for days or weeks at a time, rather than for longer periods. Face-to-face visits should be frequent (especially for management of new pain); initially, prescriptions should be refilled only at visits. While ensuring adequate analgesia, clinicians should prescribe alternatives that have a lower street value, less abrupt onset of action, and longer half-life; such choices reduce the likelihood of misuse of prescribed drugs. It may be the case, paradoxically, that more aggressive pharmacological management to ablate pain may spare the patient the stress of discomfort and thus lower the likelihood of relapse, so long as the clinician and patient both keep the specter of relapse on the discussion agenda, and mutually agree to maintain tight control over drug quantities.

Discussion about perception of the drug effect may reveal that the patient is experiencing a high or euphoria or that the drug entrains preoccupation with the next dose or illicit drugs. Conversely, withdrawal may be experienced as pain. It may be impossible to distinguish the two; patient trust in the expertise and benevolence of the primary care clinician in these cases may permit trials of changes in medication or dose. For patients with chronic pain, whatever the cause, it is useful to identify measures other than the perceived severity of pain to monitor as the benchmarks for successful analgesia. It may be difficult for some patients to distinguish drug-hunger from somatic pain. Thus objective measures, such as duration of performance of an activity or distance walked, or questionnaires that assess physical function, are preferable to severity of pain.

Two commonly adopted protocols for the management of chronic pain with opioids in patients with addiction are contracts (i.e., written care agreements) and toxicology testing. Neither is well supported in objective literature, so the primary care clinician needs to think through the risks, benefits, and costs of either.[9] Many contracts specify expectations and the consequences of failing to meet them. Many of the behaviors that contracts seek to minimize are those that often accompany the development of moderate to severe SUD. Requests for early refills, lost medication, requests for brand name medications, and other behaviors may represent inadequate pain control. Diversion of medication for use in ways not prescribed (e.g., chewing, injecting, or snorting rather than swallowing oral medications), buying illicit drugs, or clandestinely obtaining medication from many prescribers, however, are clearer signs of SUD, although none of these is itself a reliable indicator. It is the pattern, intensity, and persistence of these behaviors that ought to raise suspicion of problems. As soon as the use of or desire for the drug on the patient's part becomes highly preoccupying, the strategy ought to change. The existence of a clear contract may make changes in management easier.

Contracts may present certain risks as well. If they are not utilized universally, they may stigmatize one group more than another and raise fairness or discrimination issues. They may undermine trust. There may be risks as well to the clinician: If not adhered to by the clinician, they appear to point out poor-quality care, as the primary care clinician is failing to adhere to a self-professed and written standard. This internal contradiction could raise the risk of litigation.

Written agreements might outline routines for monitoring toxicology tests,[26] expectations about nonpharmacological therapy (e.g., physical therapy), the prescribing clinician(s), designation of a single pharmacy, provisions for replacement medication for lost prescriptions or medication, the frequency of face-to-face visits, and the option of random call-in for pill counts and/or toxicologic screening.[10,33] Sample contracts can be reviewed online.[61]

Office protocols for coverage and shared responsibility should also be established to facilitate good continuity and communication. The checking of toxicology tests for the presence of illicit drugs (or the absence of prescribed drugs), although a common element of patient management, is complex, yielding false positives and false negatives. It has not been demonstrated to improve outcomes of management of pain.[52] Nonetheless, it can be useful in certain situations (e.g., to confirm that the patient is taking any of a prescribed controlled substance).

Because alcohol and other drug use disorders have both genetic and environmental causes, one should expect that family members of patients with SUD history are at risk themselves. Thus it is wise to discuss openly the risk of diversion of medications that may not be securely stored. Clear explanation of the patient's responsibility to protect medications and close monitoring of the rate of medication use are advisable. Primary care clinicians should know that some seemingly innocuous medications have addiction liability or a street value, either because of their direct euphorigenic effects or their role as adjunctive medications to augment euphoria. A partial list of such adjuncts includes quetiapine, gabapentin, carisoprodol, cyclobenzaprine, clonidine, baclofen, hydroxyzine, and promethazine.[12,66]

Other Challenging Medical Situations

Situations likely to be encountered by primary care physicians in the care of patients with alcohol or other drug use disorders include problems related to medications and medical procedures. For example, some patients report that opioids and anxiolytics prescribed for procedures, such as for colonoscopy, may lead to craving for illicit drugs. Similarly, use of needles for phlebotomy or medication injection may trigger craving. Anticipating this problem may prevent a relapse. Discussing it with the patient, having plans of patient action in place and for an increased intensity of supportive services may be indicated.

Confidentiality

The primary care clinician may not be familiar with laws concerning medical records and confidentiality of patients with SUDs. Patients may be ashamed of their use of alcohol or other drugs, and explaining the confidential nature of discussions can be reassuring. Indeed, such assurance may be necessary for good communication, although the assurance may not be enough as patients are often concerned that those with legal access to medical records (e.g., health insurers, employers, others to whom patients often must release information), will find out about their substance use (as is also true for cancer, diabetes, and other health conditions). The sharing of general medical records and information broadly comes under the Health Insurance Portability and Accountability Act of 1996.[102] According to this federal law, providers who share the care of a patient may communicate with one another about the patient. Such communication is critical for high-quality patient care and safety. This does not, however, apply to certain types of information or treatment settings. Notably, information about psychiatric and substance use disorders *sometimes* comes under a *more stringent* set of Federal regulations (42 CFR Part 2 revised in 1987 and again in 2017).[102] Recent revisions in these rules have been promulgated by the Substance Abuse and Mental Health Services Administration (SAMHSA) (https://www.federalregister.gov/documents/2017/01/18/2017-00719/confidentiality-of-substance-use-disorder-patient-records), responding to ongoing changes in the health care delivery

system, and seeking better coordination of care. Prior to the 2017 revisions, patients with SUDs could be systematically denied access to the benefits of information sharing. Under these new statutes, as before, protected information can be released to institutions, health care providers, or others *only with express and detailed written permission from the patient*. What is new is the ability of the patient to consent to general release of protected information to, for instance, "my treating providers" (rather than to specified individuals) permitting better integration of health information, while still protecting patients' privacy. Patients may specify what types of SUD information may be shared. It is stipulated that patients have the right to request the list of parties to whom information has been released, and that patients must be informed of that right at the time of consent. Information covered under CFR 42 Part 2 is highly protected and patients can be reassured it will not be released without their permission barring a court order (although patients can be required to sign such releases for various purposes, and insurers have access).

There are, however, a few important *exceptions* to the inviolability of this privacy. In a *medical emergency*, all relevant information should be shared. Many states have *mandatory reporting laws* with which primary care providers should be familiar. States vary, but in general, primary care providers are required to report to the relevant state authority certain high-risk situations when reason to suspect harm or risk of harm is substantial. Among these situations is suspected abuse or neglect of an elder or child, or specific intent to harm another person. Under some state mandatory reporting laws, it is illegal *not* to breach confidentiality and report the suspected risk to the mandated authority.

Primary care providers need to know these laws so as to be clear with patients about the bounds of confidentiality. It may be helpful to let patients know that, barring an emergency, the primary care provider will inform the patient *before* reporting a dangerous situation. In general, the situations requiring reporting are ones from which patients themselves would want to be protected, and knowing that the primary care provider will intercede, with warning, may be welcome.

Because many have misconceptions about alcohol and drug use health information privacy laws, the most important information for primary care providers to know about CFR 42 Part 2 is when it does *not* apply. In general it does *not* apply to primary care settings. CFR 42 Part 2 applies only to federally assisted individuals, entities, or identified units in medical facilities who *hold themselves out* as providing, and provide, alcohol, or drug use disorder diagnosis, treatment, or referral for treatment, or to health care personnel whose primary function is to do this and who are identified as such. Primary care settings and providers generally do not fall under this definition, although there may be exceptions. Merely prescribing medication for SUD does not trigger CFR 42 Part 2, if the prescriber is in a general medical facility and does not hold himself or herself out as primarily providing SUD care.

Summary and Conclusions

The primary care clinician is ideally positioned to identify patients with unhealthy alcohol or other drug use. The primary care clinician should be able to assess the severity of the substance use, to identify SUD, and perform brief interventions, if appropriate. While identifying and managing comorbid conditions, be they medical or psychiatric, incorporating the assistance of consultants and SUD specialists when needed can augment the quality of care. In addition to treating and referring, primary care clinicians have a critical role for patients with addictions who often need medical, mental health, and addictions services, as they coordinate and integrate care across these disparate and sometimes poorly connected systems. Primary care clinicians can prescribe pharmacotherapy or refer to specialists who can prescribe, for alcohol and opioid use disorders, and be the source of primary or adjunctive counseling. They can also treat comorbid psychiatric symptoms and syndromes. Care and coordination of care will be enhanced with judicious sharing of clinical information while protecting privacy and educating patients about the limits of confidentiality and the limits of disclosure. Finally, primary care providers should be familiar with treating medical problems, managing pain, and delivering preventive care to patients with substance-related diagnoses. With this knowledge and skill, primary care clinicians can make a difference for patients with substance use conditions by doing the right thing at the right time. Such practice is among the most rewarding activities in primary care settings.

References

1. Reference deleted in review.
2. Aertgeerts B, Buntinx F, Kester A. The value of CAGE in screening for alcohol abuse and alcohol dependence in general clinical populations. *J Clin Epidem.* 2004;57:30–39.
3. Agency for Healthcare Quality and Research. *Primary Care Doctors Account for Nearly Half of Physician Visits but Less Than one-Third of Expenses*; 2007. http://www.ahrq.gov/news/nn/nn042507.htm.
4. Akbik H, Butler SF, Budman SH, Fernandez K, et al. Validation and clinical application of the screener and opioid assessment for patients with pain (SOAPP). *J Pain Symptom Manage.* 2006;32:287–293.
5. American Psychiatric Association (APA). In: *Diagnostic and Statistical Manual of Mental Disorders.* 5th ed. *DSM-5 Revision.* Washington DC: American Psychiatric Association; 2013.
6. Anton RF. Naltrexone for the management of alcohol dependence. *NEJM.* 2008;359:715–721.
7. Anton RF, Moak DH, Latham P, et al. Naltrexone combined with either cognitive behavioral or motivational enhancement therapy for alcohol dependence. *J Clin Psychopharmacol.* 2005;25:349–357.
8. Anton RF, O'Malley S, Ciraulo DA, et al. Combined pharmacotherapies and behavioral interventions for alcohol dependence. The COMBINE study: a randomized controlled trial. *JAMA.* 2006;295(17):2003–3017.
9. Arnold RM, Han PKJ, Seltzer D. Opioid contracts in chronic nonmalignant pain management: objective and uncertainties. *Am J Med.* 2006;119:292–296.
10. ASAM (American Society of Addiction Medicine). *Patient Placement Criteria for the Treatment of Substance-Related Disorders (PPC-2R).* 2nd ed. Chevy Chase, MD: American Society of Addiction Medicine; 2001.
11. Aubin H-J, Bobak A, Britton JR, et al. Varenicline versus transdermal nicotine patch for smoking cessation: results from a randomized open-label trial. *Thorax.* 2008;63:717–724.
12. Balldin J, Berglund M, Borg S, et al. A 6 month controlled naltrexone study: combine effect with cognitive behavioral therapy in outpatient treatment of alcohol dependence. *Alc Clin Exp Res.* 2003;27:1142–1149.
13. Banta-Green C, Jackson TR, Hanrahan N, et al. Recent drug abuse trends in the Seattle-King County area. *Proc Community Epid Working Group.* 2004;2:1–23.
14. Beich A, Thorsen T, Rollnick S. Screening in brief interventions trials targeting excessive drinkers in general practice: systemic review and meta-analysis. *BMJ.* 2003;327:536.
15. Bernstein J, Bernstein E, Tassiopoulos K, et al. Brief motivational intervention at a clinic visit reduces cocaine and heroin use. *Drug Alcohol Depend.* 2005;77(1):49–59.
16. Bertholet N, Daeppen J-B, Wietlisbach V. Reduction of alcohol consumption by brief alcohol intervention in primary care. *Arch Intern Med.* 2005;165:986–995.
17. Bien TH, Miller WR, Tonigan JS. Brief interventions for alcohol problems: a review. *Addiction.* 1993;88:315–336.
18. Blow FC, Walton MA, Bohnert, et al. A randomized controlled trial of brief interventions to reduce drug use among adults in a low-income urban emergency department: the HealthiER You study. *Addiction.* 2017. https://doi.org/10.1111/add.13773.
19. Reference deleted in review.
20. Bouza C, Angeles M, Ana M, et al. The efficacy and safety of naltrexone and acamprosate in the treatment of alcohol dependence: a systematic review. *Addiction.* 2004;99:811–828.
21. Bradley KA, DeBenedetti AF, Volk RJ, et al. AUDIT-C as a brief screen for alcohol misuse in primary care. *Alcohol Clin Exp Res.* 2007;31:1209–1217.
22. Brady KT, Tolliver BK, Berduin ML. Alcohol use and anxiety: diagnostic and management issues. *Am J Psychiatry.* 2007;164:217–221.
23. Brown RL, Leonard T, Saunders LA, et al. Two-item conjoint screen for alcohol and other drug problems. *J Am Board Fam Pract.* 2001;14:95–106.
24. Brown RL, Rounds LA. Conjoint screening questionnaires for alcohol and other drug abuse: criterion validity in a primary care practice. *Wisconsin Med J.* 1995;94:135–140.
25. Buchsbaum DG, Buchanan RG, Centor RM, et al. Screening for alcohol abuse using CAGE scores and likelihood ratios. *Annals Intern Med.* 1991;115(10):774–777.
26. California Academy of Family Physicians. *Urine Drug Testing in Clinical Practice*; 2006. http://www.familydocs.org/monographs.php.
27. Canagasaby A, Vinson DC. Screening for hazardous or harmful drinking using one or two quantity-frequency questions. *Alcohol Alcohol.* 2005;40:208–213.
28. Chan KK, Neighbors C, Gilson M, et al. Epidemiologic trends in drinking by age and gender: providing normative feedback to adults. *Addict Behav.* 2007;32:967–976.
28a. Chou R, Evans C, Hoverman A, et al. Peexposure prophylaxis for the prevention of HIV infection. Evidence report and systematic review for the US Preventive Services Task Force. *JAMA.* 2019;321:2214–2230.
29. Cuijpers P, Riper H, Lemmers L. The effects on mortality of brief intervention for problem drinking: a metaanalysis. *Addiction.* 2004;99:829–845.
30. Micheli De, Fisberg M, Formigoni ML. Study on the effectiveness of brief intervention for alcohol and other drug use directed to adolescents in a primary health care unit. *Rev Assoc Med Bras.* 2004;50:305–313.
31. DeSousa A, Desousa A. An open randomized study comparing disulfiram and acamprosate in the treatment of alcohol dependence. *Alcohol Alcohol.* 2005;40(6):545–548.
32. Fiellin DA, Reid C, O'Connor PG. Outpatient management of patients with alcohol problems. *Ann Intern Med.* 2000;133:815–827.
33. Fishman SM, Kreis PG. The opioid contract. *Clin J Pain.* 2002;18(4):S70–S75.
34. Fleming MF, Barry KL, Manwell LB, et al. Brief physician advice for problem alcohol drinkers: a randomized controlled trial in community-based primary care practices. *JAMA.* 1997;277:1039–1045.
35. Fleming MF, Mundt MP, French MT, et al. Benefit-cost analysis of brief physician advice with problem drinkers in primary care settings. *Medical Care.* 2000;38:7–18.
36. Fleming MF, Mundt MP, French MT, et al. Brief physician advice for problem drinkers: long-term efficacy and benefit-cost analysis. *Alcohol Clin Exp Res.* 2002;26:36–43.
37. Friedmann PD, McCollough D, Chin MH, et al. Screening and intervention for alcohol problems. *J Gen Intern Med.* 2000;15:84–91.

38. Friedmann PD, Saitz R, Samet JH. Management of adults recovering from alcohol or other drug problems: relapse prevention in primary care. *JAMA*. 1998;279:1227–1231.

39. Garbutt JC, Kranzler HR, O'Malley SS, et al. Efficacy and tolerability of injectable naltrexone for alcohol dependence: a randomized controlled trial. *JAMA*. 2005;293:1617–1625.

40. Gawin FH, Ellinwood EH. Cocaine and other stimulants. Actions, abuse, and treatment. *N Engl J Med*. 1988;318:1173–1182.

41. Goh ET, Morgan MY. Review article: pharmacotherapy for alcohol dependence-the why, the what , and the wherefore. *Aliment Pharmacol Ther*. 2017;45(7):865–882.

42. Reference deleted in review.

43. Gonzales D, Rennard SI, Nides M, et al. Varenicline, an alph4beta2 nicotinic acetylcholine receptor partial agonist, vs sustained-release bupropion or placebo for smoking cessation. *JAMA*. 2006;296:47–55.

44. Hayashida M. An overview of outpatient and inpatient detoxification. *Alcohol Health Res World*. 1998;22:44–46.

45. Humphreys K. Professional interventions that facilitate 12 step self-help group involvement. *Alcohol Res Health*. 1999;23:93–98.

46. Institute of Medicine. *Improving the Quality of Health Care for Mental and Substance-use Conditions*. Washington, DC: National Academies; 2006.

47. Institute of Medicine. *Defining Primary Care: An Interim Report*; 1994. http://books.nap.edu/openbook.php?record_id=9153&page=15.

48. Johnson BA, Rosenthal N, Capece JA, et al. Topiramate for treating alcohol dependence: a randomized controlled trial. *JAMA*. 2007;298:1641–1651.

49. Jorenby DE, Hayes JT, Rigotti NA, et al. Efficacy of varenicline, an alph4beta2 nicotinic acetylcholine receptor partial agonist, vs placebo or sustained-release bupropion for smoking cessation. *JAMA*. 2006;296:56–63.

50. Kakko J, Svanborg KD, Kreek MJ, et al. *1-Year Retention and Social Function After Buprenorphine-Assisted Relapse Prevention Treatment for Heroin Dependence in Sweden: a Randomised*. Placebo-Controlled Trial; 2003.

51. Katz N, Fanciullo GJ. Role of urine toxicology testing in the management of chronic opioid therapy. *Clin J Pain*. 2002;18(4):S76–S82.

52. Kiefer F, Holger J, Tarnaske T, et al. Comparing and combining naltrexone and acamprosate in relapse prevention of alcoholism. *Arch Gen Psychiatry*. 2003;60:92–99.

53. Kosten TR, O'Connor PG. Management of drug and alcohol withdrawal. *New Engl J Med*. 2003;348:1786–1795.

54. Kranzler HR, Burleson JA, Del Boca FK, et al. Buspirone treatment of anxious alcoholics: a placebo-controlled trial. *Arch Gen Psychiatry*. 1994;51:720–731.

55. Krupitzky E, Nunes EV, Ling W, et al. Injectable extended-release naltrexone for opioid dependence: a double-blind, placebo-controlled, multicentre randomised trial. 2011;377(9776):1506–1513.

56. Reference deleted in review.

57. Kypri K, Saunders JB, Williams SM, et al. Web-based screening and brief intervention for hazardous drinking: a double-blind randomized controlled trial. *Addiction*. 2004;99:1410–1417.

58. Lee JD, Friedmann PD, Kinlock TW, et al. Extended-release naltrexone to prevent opioid relapse in criminal justice offenders. *N Engl J Med*. 2015;374:1232–1242.

59. Ling W, Casadonte P, Bigelow M, et al. Buprenophrine implants for treatment of opiate dependence A randomized controlded trial. *JAMA*. 2010;304:1576–1583.

59a Maciosek MV, LaFrance AB, Debmer SP, et al. Updated priorities among effective clinical preventive services. *Ann Fam Med*. 2017;15:14–22.

60. Mann K, Lehert P, Morgan MY. The efficacy of acamprosate in the maintenance of abstinence in alcohol-dependent individuals: results of a meta-analysis. *Alc Clin Exp Res*. 2004;28:51–63.

61. Mason BJ, Quello S, Goodell V, et al. Gabapentin treatment for alcohol dependence: a randomized clinical trial. *JAMA Intern Med*. 2014;174(1):70–77.

62. Mayo-Smith MF, et al. Pharmacological management of alcohol withdrawal. A meta-analysis and evidence based practice guideline. american society of addiction medicine working group on pharmacologic management of alcohol withdrawal. *JAMA*. 1997;278:144–151.

63. McGlynn EA, Asch SM, Adams J, et al. The quality of health care delivered to adults in the United States. *New Engl J Med*. 2003;348:2635–2645.

64. McKee SA, Falba T, O'Malley SS, et al. Smoking status as a clinical indicator for alcohol misuse in US adults. *Arch Intern Med*. 2007;167:716–721.

65. McNeely J, Cleland CM, Strauss SM, et al. Validation of self-administered single-item screening questions (SISQs) for unhealthy alcohol and drug use in primary care patients. *J Gen Intern Med*. 2015;301(12):1757–1764.

66. Miller WR, Rollnick S. *Motivational Interviewing: Preparing People to Change Addictive Behavior*. 2nd ed. New York: Guilford; 1991.

67. National Heart Lung and Blood Institute. *Your Guide to Healthy Sleep*. DHHS Publication No. 06-5271 http://www.nhlbi.nih.gov/health/public/sleep/healthy_sleep.pdf. Accessed 14 June 2008

68. National Institute on Alcohol Abuse and Alcoholism. *Helping Patients Who Drink Too Much: A Clinician's Guide*. 2005 ed. NIH Publication No. 07-3769. Bethesda, MD: NIH; 2007.

69. Nowinski J, Baker S, Carroll K. *Project MATCH Twelve Step Facilitation Therapy Manual. A Clinical Research Guide for Therapists Treating Individuals With Alcohol Abuse and Dependence*. Rockville: USDHHS; 1995.

70. Nunes EV, Levin FR. Treatment of depression in patients with alcohol or other drug dependence. *JAMA*. 2004;291:1887–1896.

71. O'Connor PG, Schottenfeld RS. Patients with alcohol problems. *New Eng J Med*. 1998;338:592–602.

72. O'Malley SS, Rounsaville BJ, Farren C, et al. Initial and maintenance naltrexone treatment for alcohol dependence using primary care versus specialty care. A nested sequence of 3 randomized trials. *Arch Intern Med*. 2003;163:1695–1704.

73. Oregon Health Sciences University (OHSU). *Chronic Pain Management*; 2008. http://www.ohsu.edu/ahec/pain/form.html. Accessed 28 Aug 2008.

74. Overman GP, Teter CJ, Guthrie SK. Acamprosate for the adjunctive treatment of alcohol dependence. *Ann Pharmacother*. 2003;37:1090–1099.

75. Paille FM, Guelfi JD, Perkins AC, et al. Double-blind randomized multicentre trial of acamprosate in maintaining abstinence from alcohol. *Alcohol Alcohol*. 1995;30:239–247.

76. Park TW. Debate: are benzodiazepines appropriate treatments for patients with substance use disorders? yes. *Addiction Med*. 2017;11(2):87–89.

77. Pettinati HM, O'Brien CP, Rabinowitz AR, et al. The status of naltrexone in the treatment of alcohol dependence; specific effects on heavy drinking. *J Clin Pharmacol*. 2006;26:610–625.

78. Pettinati HM, Weiss RD, Dundon W, et al. A structured approach to medical management: a psychosocial intervention to support pharmacotherapy in the treatment of alcohol dependence. *J Stud Alcohol*. 2005;suppl(15):179–187.

79. Rangel C, Shu RG, Lazar LD, et al. Beta blockers for chest pain associated with recent cocaine use. *JAMA*. 2010;170(10):874–879.

80. Reeves RR, Carter OS, Pinkofsky HB, et al. Carisoprodol (soma): abuse potential and physician unawareness. *J Addict Dis*. 1999;18:51–56.

81. Reid MC, Engles-Horton LL, Weber MB, et al. Use of opioid medications for chronic noncancer pain syndromes in primary care. *J Gen Intern Med*. 2002;17(3):173–179.

82. Reinert DF, Allen JP. The alcohol use disorders identification test (AUDIT): a review of recent research. *Alcohol Clin Exp Res*. 2002;26(2):272–279.

83. Rosenthal RN, Lofwall MR, Kim S, et al. Effect of buprenorphine implants on illicit opioid use among absinent adults with opioid dependence treated with sublingual buprenorphine: a randomized controlled trial. *JAMA*. 2016;316:282–290.

84. Saitz R. Unhealthy alcohol use. *New Engl J Med*. 2005;352:596–607.

85. Saitz R. Alcohol screening and brief intervention in primary care: absence of evidence for efficacy in people with dependence or very heavy drinking. *Drug Alchol Rev*. 2010;29(6):631–640.

86. Samet JH, Rollnick S, Barnes H. Beyond CAGE: a brief clinical approach after detection of substance abuse. *Arch Intern Med*. 1996;156:2287–2289.

87. Sass H, Soyka M, Mann K, et al. Relapse prevention by acamprosate: results from a placebo-controlled study on alcohol dependence. *Arch Gen Psychiatry*. 1996;53:673–680.

88. Sellars EM, Naranjo CA, Harrison M, et al. Diazepam loading: simplified treatment of alcohol withdrawal. *Clin Pharmacol Ther*. 1983;34:822–826.

89. Sinclair JD. Evidence about the use of naltrexone and for different ways of using it in the treatment of alcoholism. *Alcohol Alcohol*. 2001;36(1):2–10.

90. Skinner HA. The drug abuse screening test. *Addict Behav*. 1982;7(4):363–371.

91. Smith PC, Schmidt SM, Allensworth-Davies D, et al. Primary care validation of a single-question alcohol screening test. *J Gen Intern Med* 2009;24:783–788. [Erratum: (2010) *J Gen Intern Med*. 25(4):375.]

92. Smith PC, Schmidt SM, Allensworth-Davies D, et al. A Single-question screening test for drug use in primary care. *Arch Intern Med*. 2010;170(13):1155–1160.

93. Solberg LI, Maciosek MV, Edwards NM. Primary care intervention to reduce alcohol misuse: ranking its health impact and cost effectiveness. *Am J Prev Med*. 2008;34(2):143–152.

94. Soyka M. Treatmenet of benzodiazepine dependence. *N Engl J Med*. 2017;376:1147–1157.

95. Standridge JB, Zylstra RG, Adams SM. Alcohol consumption: an overview of benefits and risks. *So J Med*. 2004;97:664–672.

96. Starosta AN, Leeman RF, Volpicelli JR. The BRENDA model: integrating psychosocial treatment and pharmacotherapy for the treatment of alcohol use disorders. *J Psychiatric Pract*. 2006;12:80–89.

97. Streeton C, Whelan G. Naltrexone, a relapse prevention maintenance treatment of alcohol dependence: a meta-analysis of randomized controlled trials. *Alcohol Alcohol*. 2001;36:544–552.

98. Sullivan E, Fleming M. *A Guide to Substance Abuse Services for Primary Care Clinicians. Treatment Improvement Protocol (TIP) 24*. Department Health and Human Services Pub No. SMA 97–3139; 1997.

99. Sullivan JT, Sykora K, Schneiderman J, et al. Assessment of alcohol withdrawal: the revised clinical institute withdrawal instrument for alcohol scale (CIWA-Ar). *Br J Addiction*. 1989;84:1353–1357.

100. Sullivan LE, Fiellin DA. Narrative review: buprenorphine for opioid-dependent patients in office practice. *Ann Intern Med*. 2008;148:662–670.

101. US Congress. *S524-Comprehensive Addiction and Recovery Act of 2016*; 2016.

102. US Department of Health and Human Services. *The Confidentiality of Alcohol and Drug Abuse Patient Records Regulation and the HIPAA Privacy Rule: Implications for Alcohol and Substance Abuse Programs*; 2004. http://www.hipaa.samhsa.gov/download2/SAMHSA'sPart2–HIPAAComparisonClearedWordVersion.doc.

103. US Department of Health and Human Services. *Clinical Guidelines for the Use of Buprenorphine in the Treatment of Opioid Addiction. Treatment Improvement Protocol (TIP) 40*. DHHS Publication No. (SMA) 04-3939; 2004.

104. U.S. Preventive Services Task Force. Screening and behavioral counseling interventions in primary care to reduce alcohol misuse: recommendation statement. *Ann Intern Med*. 2004;140(554–556):557–568.

105. Unutzer J, Katon W, Callahan CM, et al. Collaborative care management of late-life depression in the primary care setting: a randomized controlled trial. *JAMA*. 2002;288:2836–2845.

106. Weiss RD, Potter JS, Griffin ML, et al. Long-term outcomes from the national drug abuse treatment clinical trials network prescription opioid addiction treatment study. *Drug Alc Depend*. 2015;150:112–119.

107. Wilson JF. Strategies to reduce opiate abuse. *Ann Intern Med*. 2007;146:887–890.

108. World Health Organization (WHO). *The Effectiveness of Brief Interventions for Illicit Drugs Linked to Alcohol, Smoking and Substance Involvement Screening Test (ASSIST) in Primary Health Care Settings: A Technical Report of Phase III Findings of the WHO ASSIST Randomized Controlled Trial*; 2008. http://www.who.int/substance_abuse/activities/assist_technicalreport_phase3_final.pdf. Accessed 28 Aug 2008.

47

Criminal Justice System and Addiction Treatment

KAREN L. CROPSEY, SAMANTHA P. SCHIAVON, FAYE S. TAXMAN, AND GLORIA D. ELDRIDGE

CHAPTER OUTLINE

Introduction

Compared with other nations, the United States incarcerates the largest percentage of its citizens, with close to 7 million adults[41b] and 650,000 youth under some form of criminal justice supervision, including prison, jail, and probation or parole supervision in the community.[71,81] Incarceration in the United States costs nearly $1.2 trillion each year in incarceration and societal costs,[52a] and 40%–60% of prison intakes result from failures in community supervision related to drug relapse.[30,46,62] Research consistently demonstrates the close connection between drug use and criminal justice involvement, with over 70% of offenders involved with drugs or alcohol at some point in their lifetimes.[78] About 36% of violent crimes involve alcohol and 40% of criminal offenders reported using alcohol at the time of their offense.[34] Many offenders are caught in a cycle of drug use, crime, arrest, and reincarceration.[4,31,75] Drug charges account for about one-third of re-arrests following release from prison or jail. Over half of all offenders are re-arrested within 12 months of release and over two-thirds are re-arrested within 3 years of release.[24a,79] Numerous studies have shown that involvement in community alcohol and drug treatment services delays re-arrest and reincarceration. The purpose of this chapter is to provide an overview of the drug and alcohol treatment needs of offenders and the mechanisms available in the criminal justice system to address these needs.

Prevalence of Substance Abuse and Dependence

Substance abuse is four times greater in the offender population than in the general population; 37% of offenders are estimated to have a substance abuse disorder, compared with 9% of the general population.[63] Over 80% of state prisoners reported a lifetime history of drug use[54] and about half of state prison inmates met *Diagnostic and Statistical Manual of Mental Disorders, Third Edition, Revised* (DSM-III-R) criteria for a substance use disorder.[44]

Compared with the nonoffender populations, offenders are more likely to abuse illicit and prescribed substances.[26] For example, about 11.3% of male and 20.8% of female prisoners reported daily opioid use in the 6 months preceding incarceration; 10% had a history of lifetime opioid dependence and 8% met criteria for current opioid dependence.[8] Abuse of prescribed opiates is a recent phenomenon and, according to the 2015 National Survey on Drug Use and Health, an estimated 3.8 million Americans 12 years of age or older used prescription opiates nonmedically in the past month, which represents three-fifths of all misusers of psychotherapeutic drugs. Among individuals who are 18 years of age or older who were arrested between 2002 and 2004, almost 30% had used prescription drugs nonmedically in the past year.[63] A recent study of prescription drug abuse among a large sample of prisoners found that 34% of male prisoners and 62% of female prisoners reported nonmedical use of prescription opiates.[92] Individuals who abused prescription opiates were more likely to have been involved in criminal activity and reported more drug charges, shoplifting, forgery, disorderly conduct, charges resulting in convictions, number of convictions, months incarcerated, and days incarcerated within the last month than individuals who had never abused prescription opiates.[92]

A recent study concluded that 64.5% of the inmate population in the United States met criteria for a substance use disorder,[8a] suggesting a large need for substance abuse services in facilities that are not equipped to offer such services. Because almost all arrestees are initially housed in jails while awaiting trial or sentencing, it is left to the jail facilities to treat the acute effects of drug use and withdrawal. For example, one-fourth (25%) of inmates reported withdrawal symptoms from active drug or alcohol use upon entering jail, but only 16% reported receiving medication for relief of withdrawal symptoms.[8]

Substance Abuse Comorbidities

Smoking

Smoking is the leading preventable cause of death in the United States, resulting in over 480,000 premature deaths each year and is implicated as a causal agent in an increasing range of cancers.[77] Prisoners, as a class, are especially vulnerable to the negative health consequences of smoking. Smoking rates are 3–4 times higher among prisoners than among individuals in the general population, and smoking is normative and nonstigmatized within the correctional environment.[17–19] Among male prisoners, smoking prevalence is 70%–80%.[13,14,17,18] Smoking rates among incarcerated women range from 42% to 91%—2–4 times greater than among women in the general population.[16,17]

Ninety percent of prisons prohibit smoking in medical, chapel, and vocational and educational areas; however, about 40% allow unrestricted smoking in common areas, housing units and cells, or in prison yards.[42,84] Due to a 2006 policy, cigarettes and other tobacco products are readily available in prison and tobacco products were banned from being sold in prison commissaries. In 2012, 30 states prohibited the use of tobacco inside state correctional facilities to reduce secondhand smoke.[14a] Due to the increase in smoke-free policies in prisons and jails, there has been an increase in tobacco contraband sold among prisoners.[47] Tobacco products are bartered among prisoners and employees and function as a form of prison currency.[47,56]

In an attempt to return nicotine products for sale in commissaries, electronic cigarettes have recently been developed specifically for use in correctional facilities.[94] If successful, electronic cigarettes will be sold in prisons across all 50 states, with calculated sales of nearly $330,000 per 100 inmates annually.[94] However, because of the high cost of cigarettes in prison, many prisoners purchase loose tobacco that they roll into nonfiltered cigarettes.[16,17] Thus smoking inside a correctional environment may present a higher risk for tobacco-related diseases than smoking in the community.

In contrast to the enormous literature focusing on smoking prevalence, prevention, cessation, and policies in other populations, smoking among prisoners remains virtually ignored, despite the enormous human, health, and economic costs.[2,16] Only five published studies have examined smoking interventions for prisoners.[17,20b,24a,25,58] All five suggest that prisoners are interested in smoking cessation and able to achieve smoking abstinence, despite pressures within the correctional environment to continue smoking. In the largest study to date of smoking cessation in a correctional setting, Cropsey and colleagues conducted a randomized controlled trial of a combined nicotine replacement and 10-week group smoking cessation intervention for female prisoners. Sustained cessation rates were comparable to cessation rates following smoking cessation interventions in the community.[17]

Psychiatric Disorders

According to a recent Report to Congress by the National Commission on Correctional Healthcare and National Institute on Justice on the health status of soon-to-be released inmates, rates of psychiatric disorders in US prisons and jails dramatically exceed general population rates.[55] A meta-analysis of 62 studies from 12 Western countries estimated that one in seven prisoners has a psychotic or major depressive disorder.[27] Prevalence estimates for psychiatric disorders among state *prison* inmates are schizophrenia (2%–4%), major depression (13%–19%), bipolar disorder (2%–5%), dysthymia (8%–14%), anxiety disorder (22%–30%), and posttraumatic stress disorder (6%–12%). Prevalence estimates for psychiatric disorders among *jail* inmates are similar: schizophrenia (1%), major depression (8%–15%), bipolar disorder (1%–3%), dysthymia (2%–5%), anxiety disorder (14%–20%), and posttraumatic stress disorder (4%–9%).[86] Approximately 50% of female inmates have mental illness.[22] A national study estimated rates of mental illness ranging from 3% to 23% for probationers and 1%–11% for parolees.[7] Finally, 6% of male and 15% of female jail inmates have acute psychiatric symptoms in need of treatment at the time of initial booking.[72,73]

Inmates with comorbid substance use and mental health problems report more numerous and serious past year and lifetime medical conditions and consume more medical services during incarceration and in the community[38]—underscoring the importance of psychiatric treatment in correctional settings. With the number of prisoners with serious psychiatric disorders exceeding the number of patients in psychiatric hospitals, jails and prisons have become "America's new mental hospitals" (p. 1612).[74] For many individuals with severe mental illness, most psychiatric care is provided in jails and prisons.[45] The high prevalence of psychiatric disorders in correctional populations is due, in part, to the deinstitutionalization of mentally ill persons, lack of access to community mental health services[50] and the criminalization of the mentally ill.[45] Unfortunately, most prisoners with psychiatric and substance use disorders do not receive adequate care during incarceration and are expected to serve 4 months longer than prisoners without a mental health problem.[27,41a] Although data are limited, most prisons and jails fail to conform to community standards for screening and treatment of mental disorders.[55,85] For example, 83% of jails offer screening, 60% offer mental health evaluations, 42% provide psychiatric medications, 43% offer crisis intervention, and 72% offer access to inpatient psychiatric treatment.[61] Jails and prisons differ in the type and range of mental health services; jails may provide management of acute symptoms and suicide prevention, whereas prisons may offer a range of services including long-term support and treatment. After incarceration, 34% of state prisoners received treatment, followed by 24% of federal prisoners and 17% of jail inmates.[41a] Medical and psychiatric treatment in criminal justice systems varies from state to state; some contract with independent companies to provide psychiatric and medical services for their populations. Often facilities offer specialized services such psychiatric or sex offender treatment units,[87] although little is known about the types and effectiveness of treatment programs offered.

HIV/AIDS and Sexually Transmitted Infections

The HIV/AIDS epidemic in the United States coincided with a sharp rise in incarceration related to the war on drugs, mandatory minimum sentencing, and truth in sentencing legislation in the

1980s and 1990s. As a result, many substance-abusing individuals at high risk for HIV/AIDS are also at high risk for criminal justice involvement. In 1997, 16% of individuals with AIDS and 22%–31% of individuals with HIV passed through a US correctional facility.[35] Between 1989 and 1999, 32.9% of positive HIV tests in Rhode Island came from the state correctional institution.[21] Between 1995 and 2004, the percentage of known HIV+ prisoners decreased from 2.3% to 1.9% of the prison population. AIDS-related deaths among state and federal prisoners declined from 2001 to 2010 by 16%.[51a] Despite that decline, the rate of confirmed AIDS in state and federal prisons was 3 times higher than in the overall US population—0.49% for prisoners and 0.14% for the US population.[79] In 2010, more than 20,000 inmates had HIV/AIDS, with the majority (91%) occurring in male inmates.[51a]

Offenders have histories of high-risk sexual behavior and high rates of sexually transmitted infections.[39,40] High-risk sexual behavior includes inconsistent condom use with multiple sexual partners, history of sexually transmitted infections, exchanging sex for money or drugs, and engaging in sexual intercourse with an injection drug user or under the influence of drugs or alcohol.[15,52] Rates of chlamydia and gonorrhea are 18–50 times higher in adult prisoners compared with adults in the general population.[9] Left untreated, chlamydia and gonorrhea may result in infertility, pelvic inflammatory disease, cervicitis, and ectopic pregnancy.[9] Rates of syphilis are also high in correctional populations; with 8% of male inmates and 5% of female inmates testing positive for syphilis,[12a] compared with less than 0.0001% of adults in the general population.[12a] High rates of untreated sexually transmitted infections enhance risk for HIV transmission or infection,[9]—suggesting the importance of addressing high-risk sexual behavior in the context of drug and alcohol abuse among criminal justice populations.

Other Infectious Diseases

Active or latent tuberculosis infections are higher among correctional populations than in the general population, with 20%–25% of prisoners testing positive for tuberculosis compared with 0.0048% of the general population.[3,10,11] Multidrug-resistant tuberculosis has become epidemic in prison institutions around the world, where high rates of HIV facilitate transmission of multidrug-resistant tuberculosis.[89] About one-third of prisoners test positive for hepatitis C, compared with general population rates of 2%.[12] The convergence of high rates of sexually transmitted infections, hepatitis C, HIV/AIDS, and tuberculosis among prisoners is not a coincidence; these diseases act synergistically in their infection rates and disease progression, making them more challenging to treat[89] and highlighting the importance of addressing them in the context of alcohol and drug abuse among correctional populations.

Pharmacotherapies for Substance Use

A review of the literature shows a dearth of research on pharmacological treatments for substance abuse among criminal justice populations, particularly in the United States.[20,27a] Providing effective treatment for opioid dependence decreases relapse to active substance use upon release from prison and prevents recidivism.[23] Despite this, very few correctional facilities provide methadone or other detoxification or maintenance for opioid-dependent prisoners.[5a,19,27a,43,49] A recent study demonstrated that initiating methadone maintenance therapy for prisoners with histories of opioid dependence prior to release facilitated entry into community treatment.[43] However, a primary disadvantage of methadone maintenance therapy is that the individual has to be treated at a methadone maintenance clinic after release from prison and waiting lists for such treatments in the community are long,[49] providing the opportunity for a recently released offender to fall between the cracks and miss the opportunity for immediate entry into methadone maintenance therapy upon release from prison.

An alternative treatment, oral naltrexone, an opiate antagonist, has been available for 20 years but has not been widely used, primarily due to problems with medication compliance. One review noted that less than 20% of recipients continued to take oral naltrexone 4 months after treatment was initiated.[57] Depot naltrexone has recently received US Food and Drug Administration (FDA) approval for use in treating alcohol dependence but does not have an indication for treating opioid dependence and is unlikely to be adopted by criminal justice authorities until FDA approval is obtained. However, studies are under way to investigate the use of depot naltrexone with individuals in community corrections, which may provide another option for pharmacotherapy for individuals under criminal justice supervision in the community.

Buprenorphine, a thebaine derivative, is a mu opioid partial agonist with a pharmacological profile that makes it attractive as a pharmacotherapy for the treatment of opioid dependence. Buprenorphine, like other full mu agonists, produces opioid-associated subjective and physiological effects, but its maximal effects are less than those of a full agonist such as morphine.[6] This property contributes to its utility in the treatment of opioid dependence in that buprenorphine is effective in preventing the onset of the opioid abstinence syndrome in opioid-dependent individuals. With escalating doses, buprenorphine produces less effect than full mu agonists and exhibits a ceiling effect at which further dose increases produce no additional effects.[88] In addition, buprenorphine has high affinity for the mu receptor, a property that produces blockade of the effects of full mu agonists, should these be administered during buprenorphine maintenance.

The safety of buprenorphine in nontolerant individuals (such as those exiting a controlled environment) was demonstrated by Walsh and colleagues,[88] where a plateau on subjective and respiratory dose effects resulted in sublingual doses up to 32 mg (2–4 times the recommended treatment dose) being well tolerated. Thus the ceiling effect associated with buprenorphine administration provides a wide margin of safety. Buprenorphine has fewer restrictions on its use for treatment of opioid addiction and provides an attractive alternative to methadone. In comparison with methadone and oral naltrexone, buprenorphine treatment demonstrated lower overall mortality related to its use.[29] Thus buprenorphine appears to have advantages over other opioid therapies, including better acceptance and compliance, a favorable safety profile, and the ability to deliver the medication by prescription in a general clinic practice after release from prison. A recent review concluded that the efficacy of buprenorphine has been firmly established for treatment of opioid dependence.[48] A cost-effectiveness study embedded in a randomized controlled trial of buprenorphine versus methadone concluded that buprenorphine is no more expensive than methadone maintenance therapy.[24] Buprenorphine has not been widely investigated with a corrections population, and adoption of this medication by criminal justice administrators has been nonexistent, despite the well-demonstrated efficacy of buprenorphine in noncriminal justice populations. One study

TABLE 47.1 **Substance Abuse Treatment Services in Community Supervision Agencies.**

Type of Service	% With Service	Estimated # of Offenders	SPECIALIZED FACILITIES % of ADP (Median)	% of Programs >90 Days	GENERIC PRISONS % of ADP (Median)	% of Programs >90 Days
Drug/alcohol education	53.1	190,906	7.7	78	8.6	56.9
Substance abuse group counseling: up to 4 h/week	47.1	141,263	4.8	90.9	3.3	62.8
Substance abuse group counseling: 5–25 h/week	21.2	37,090	1	87.9	2.7	92.9
Substance abuse group counseling: 26+ h/week	1.5	2,449	<1	71.8	1.1	24.2
Therapeutic community—segregated	3.7	17,579	27	24.3	2.6	77.2
Therapeutic community—non-segregated	3.4	9,815	100	0	6.6	86.8
Relapse prevention groups	34.3	43,740	<1	91.5	1.3	57.4
Case management	7.1	93,088	1.9	100	18	88.4

Note: % with service refers to the percentage of facilities that indicated that they offer the service. Estimated # of offenders is a national estimate of the sum of the number of offenders in the service on an average day. % of ADP refers to the percentage of the facility's population that is involved in the service on an average day.

Reprinted from Taxman FS, Perdoni ML, Harrison LD. Drug treatment services for adult offenders: the state of the state. *J Subst Abuse Treat.* 2007;32:239–254.

found that providing buprenorphine to women prior to release from the criminal justice system, reduced opiate use as they transitioned back into the community.[20a]

Community Corrections

The community corrections population has quadrupled over the past 25 years (1.12 million in 1980 to 6 million in 2006)[71, 81] and comprises the largest segment of the criminal justice population. The increase in criminal justice sanctions has been attributed to a change in US policy in the 1980s to "get tough on crime" and led to the war on drugs that continues today, with drug-related arrests skyrocketing over the past 35 years (322,300 drug arrests in 1970 to 1.65 million in 2005)[81]; driving under the influence continues to be the largest arrest category in the United States, with over 1.8 million arrests a year.[81]

Probation and Parole

At the end of 2006, there were over 6 million offenders on probation or parole in the United States (about 5,237,000 on probation and 798,200 on parole). Over half of these offenders have orders for substance abuse treatment services in the community, and providing care to these offenders is a challenge given the dearth of treatment services available in the community. For example, a recent survey of correctional agencies in the United States found that less than 10% of the offender population can participate in treatment services on a daily basis, due to the size of the population and the lack of availability of treatment services for offenders.[68] The majority of treatment services available to offenders are drug and alcohol education (53.1%), group counseling for less than 4 hours a week (47.1%), substance abuse counseling for 5 or more hours a week (21.2%), and therapeutic community or residential services (3.7%) (see Table 47.1). Even more revealing is that the most commonly offered services do not incorporate evidence-based treatment strategies such as

cognitive behavioral therapy, motivational interviewing, and therapeutic communities.[68]

Over the last three decades, different strategies have been used to address the large percentage of offenders that need treatment services. Most community correctional agencies use referrals to existing programs and services in the community to provide treatment for offenders. The referral process, generally referred to as the brokerage model, relies on the probation/parole officer giving a referral to the offender for a public health clinic(s) or a specific program. The success of the model relies on the offender obtaining services. Other variations to bridge the correctional and drug treatment systems have evolved over the past two decades to provide more direct access to treatment services by offenders. These variations include the Treatment Alternatives to Street Crime (now called Treatment Accountability for Safer Communities), drug treatment courts, "break the cycle" or seamless systems of care, or on-site treatment services.[1,65,70,91] Studies vary considerably on these different mechanisms, but generally research demonstrates that more offenders have access to treatment services and increased participation in treatment services when these options are available[65,66]

Another model is to train the probation/parole officer in a new role, which involves engaging the offender in the change process[65] by utilizing clinical skills such as motivational interviewing and addressing the offender's ambivalence toward involvement in treatment services. Studies of this approach have demonstrated that the altered role of the probation officer reduces technical violations compared with traditional intensive supervision programs where the parole officer's focus is solely on monitoring the offender after release.[28,65]

Drug Court

The drug court, a postadjudication sentencing program, was first established in 1989 and designed to reduce criminal involvement among drug-addicted offenders. By 2007 there were over 890 drug courts operating in the United States.[82] The theory that led to the formation of drug courts is that many drug-addicted offenders engage in criminal behavior as a means to acquire drugs; therefore, to reduce crime among drug-addicted offenders, the addiction must be treated.[32] The basic components of most drug courts include assessment of substance abuse disorder, assimilation of substance abuse treatment and criminal justice supervision through case management and weekly status hearings with judicial oversight, a continuum of care in which offenders have access to multiple services, frequent drug and alcohol screening, and continuous interactions between the offender and the criminal justice system (e.g., judges, case managers, and so on).[91] Drug treatment courts have revolutionized treatment for the criminal justice offender in that they provide a mechanism to ensure that monitoring, supervision, and treatment are intertwined. However, only about 3% of substance-abusing offenders have access to drug treatment courts.[68]

A number of studies have been conducted to determine the effectiveness of drug courts; findings are generally positive but mixed. Several studies have shown that participants in drug courts show diminished drug use and criminal activity and higher treatment retention rates compared with offenders in traditional treatment settings.[32,33,68,91] Belenko[5] reviewed evaluations of 37 drug courts nationwide and found that 47% of participants graduated successfully and that drug use and recidivism were low while clients were enrolled in drug court. However, most studies did not include long-term follow-up data, making postprogram outcomes unclear.[5] An empirical study of drug treatment courts found that treatment participation (29%–88%) and program graduation rates (29%–50%) varied considerably.[64]

A recent meta-analysis by Wilson et al. revealed that although individuals graduating from drug court have significantly lower arrest rates than nonparticipants, most drug court participants did not attend the minimum number of required treatment sessions and more than half were not given the minimum number of drug tests.[91] Taxman and colleagues report that treatment participation varied from 35% to 80% across drug courts.[64] In addition, none of the programs reviewed by Wilson and colleagues was based on a formal theory of the causes of addiction and most were using a mixed bag of therapeutic approaches without focusing on any one treatment method.[66,80] For example, some programs used 12-step approaches, which require addicts to turn over their addiction to a higher power in conjunction with cognitive-behavioral therapy, which focuses on thoughts and feelings and emphasizes learning new skills to change addictive behaviors. Unfortunately these two therapeutic approaches are incompatible in their views on the origins of addiction. In addition, although cognitive-behavioral therapy is widely considered one of the best approaches for treating substance abuse, it was used in only about 22% of therapy sessions.[64]

There also appears to be a dearth of family involvement and minority or culture-specific treatment in drug courts, all of which are important treatment components.[80] Many researchers have suggested that the lack of evidence- and theory-based practices in substance abuse treatment contributes significantly to rates of relapse and recidivism among offenders receiving treatment through drug courts.[80] Overall, it appears that the longer an offender is in treatment, the greater their chances are of succeeding in a drug court program—a finding consistent with research on all substance abuse treatment programs.[59,68]

Treatment Accountability for Safer Communities

Treatment Accountability for Safer Communities was developed in 1972 as a strategy to provide case management to bridge the gap between the criminal justice system and community substance abuse treatment. Treatment Accountability for Safer Communities models operate under the assumptions that drug addiction is prevalent among offenders; that there is a cycle of crime, incarceration, release, and relapse among drug-dependent individuals; and that this cycle provides frequent opportunities for treatment interventions.[41] Most Treatment Accountability for Safer Communities programs provide screening for program eligibility, assessment of treatment needs, referrals for treatment outside of Treatment Accountability for Safer Communities, and client-centered case management. Many programs emphasize a continuum of care and provide regular drug screens and correspondence with the criminal justice system regarding the client's progress. Treatment Accountability for Safer Communities currently operates in almost 40 states, and about 100 organizations use the Treatment Accountability for Safer Communities model.

Anglin and colleagues assessed Treatment Accountability for Safer Communities programs at five sites in the United States across three domains: service delivery, drug use, and recidivism. Compared with individuals receiving the standard strategy of referral to community treatment services, offenders participating in Treatment Accountability for Safer Communities had access to significantly more services at four of the five sites (drug counseling, urinalysis, and/or AIDS/HIV education). At three of the five sites, drug use decreased for Treatment Accountability for Safer Communities participants. However, there were no significant differences in recidivism (as assessed by re-arrest rates) among control and Treatment Accountability for Safer Communities groups. In fact, at two of the sites there were indications that Treatment Accountability for Safer Communities participants were more likely to be re-arrested than control group participants. More positive findings occurred at sites where the Treatment Accountability for Safer Communities services included group counseling and offenders did not have to go to another agency to acquire the needed clinical services treatment. Similar findings for intensive supervision programs (i.e., the probation officer monitors the offender through more frequent contact) suggest that increased monitoring leads to easier detection of criminal behavior among participants. Thus the increase in arrests among Treatment Accountability for Safer Communities participants can be seen as a success from a viewpoint of community safety, even though it increases technical violations and reincarcerations.[1] Other researchers have postulated that the case management approach taken by Treatment Accountability for Safer Communities programs does not decrease recidivism because it does not lead to increased participation in substance abuse treatment, treatment is usually of a short duration, and there are often no provisions in place for noncompliance (e.g., positive drug tests or missed treatment sessions).[67]

A more recent study revealed that jurisdictions with Treatment Accountability for Safer Communities had increased use of motivational interviewing, continuum of care policies, and services for offenders with cooccurring disorders.[93] In addition, the survey found that Treatment Accountability for Safer Communities administrators were stronger supporters of training initiatives likely to enhance cooperation among criminal justice organizations. A general survey of treatment services offered in correctional settings found that innovations tended to be clustered. Treatment

TABLE 47.2	Prevalence of Substance Abuse Services in Prisons.					
			SPECIALIZED FACILITIES		GENERIC PRISONS	
Type of Service	% With Service	Estimated # of Offenders	% of ADP (Median)	% of Programs >90 Days	% of ADP (Median)	% of Programs >90 Days
Drug/alcohol education	74.1	75,543	8.8	92.1	9	65.3
Substance abuse group counseling: up to 4 h/week	54.6	34,509	76.9	73.9	10	58
Substance abuse group counseling: 5–25 h/week	46	52,293	8.8	92.9	8	72.9
Substance abuse group counseling: 26+ h/week	11.2	12,182	11.3	78.9	18.6	24.3
Therapeutic community—segregated	19.5	34,776	8.8	84.3	15.5	74.8
Therapeutic community—non-segregated	9.2	10,710	5.7	91.6	14.4	66
Relapse prevention groups	44.5	39,493	13	74.3	3.8	62
Case management	6.9	10,761	100	91.1	9.1	40.7

Note: % with service refers to the percentage of facilities that indicated that they offer the service. Estimated # of offenders is a national estimate of the sum of the number of offenders in the service on an average day. % of ADP refers to the percentage of the facility's population that is involved in the service on an average day.

Reprinted from Taxman FS, Perdoni ML, Harrison LD. Drug treatment services for adult offenders: the state of the state. *J Subst Abuse Treat*. 2007;32:239–254.

Accountability for Safer Communities organizations are more likely than program and parole agencies to offer this clustering of innovative practices.[37] This finding allows a better understanding of implementation issues based on how organizations such as Treatment Accountability for Safer Communities, jails, and community correctional agencies affect the treatment delivery system. Overall, the survey findings suggest that communities that have organizations like Treatment Accountability for Safer Communities or Treatment Accountability for Safer Communities have made greater gains in improving service delivery for offenders in measurable ways, but that there is also considerable room for improvement in access to services and treatment and supervision outcomes.

Institutional Corrections

The availability of substance abuse treatment in correctional environments has decreased in the past two decades. In 1991, one-third of inmates who reported using drugs in the month prior to arrest received substance abuse treatment; in 1997, only 15% received treatment.[54] A recent survey of drug treatment services in the correctional setting found that less than 10% of the eligible inmate population receive drug treatment services in prison and that offenders in specialized treatment programs such as segregated therapeutic communities are more likely to be offered treatment services that are consistent with evidence-based practices.[68] Substance abuse treatment programs for inmates during and after incarceration are effective in reducing drug use and subsequent recidivism.[4,31,60] About one-fourth of inmates who participated in therapeutic community substance abuse treatment in prison and after release returned to prison, compared with 75% of prisoners who did not receive treatment or who received treatment in prison but no treatment after release.[51,60] The Washington State Institute for Public Policy noted that drug treatment in prison yields a benefit between $1.91 and $2.69 for every dollar invested in treatment. Drug treatment outside prison yielded a benefit of $8.87 for every dollar spent on treatment.[83] Thus substance abuse

treatment programs in and out of prison are successful in reducing substance abuse and recidivism and are cost effective.[36]

Prisons and Jails

Despite the potential benefits associated with delivery of drug treatment in correctional facilities, drug treatment is increasingly unavailable for drug-dependent offenders during incarceration, and the services provided are often not of sufficient duration or intensity and do not incorporate evidence-based practices. The National Criminal Justice Treatment Practices survey provided data on the availability of different types and intensities of drug treatment services offered in prisons and jails in the United States (Tables 47.2 and 47.3).[69] Substance abuse education and awareness is offered in 74% of prisons and 61% of jails and, as such, is the most prevalent form of drug treatment service provided. Group substance abuse counseling (≤4 h/week) is available in 55% of prisons and 60% of jails; group counseling 5–25 h/week is available in 46% of prisons and 23% of jails; and group counseling ≥26 h/week is available in 11% of prisons and 1% of jails. Counseling programs within prisons and jails incorporate various combinations of 12-step work, cognitive-behavioral skills training, life skills training, and drug education,[53] although less than 20% of sessions use cognitive or cognitive behavioral therapies.[69] Segregated therapeutic communities are available in 20% of prisons and 26% of jails; 45% of prisons and 51% of jails provide access to relapse-prevention groups.[69]

Although therapeutic communities are available in only a minority of prisons and jails in the United States, the aim of therapeutic communities goes beyond abstinence from drugs to complete lifestyle change for individuals involved in the therapeutic community, including development of prosocial attitudes and values and elimination of antisocial behaviors and attitudes. Therapeutic community members live with one another, ideally segregated from the general correctional population, and take responsibility for recovery through individual and group counseling, peer pressure, confrontation, and incentives and sanctions.[53,90]

TABLE 47.3	**Substance Abuse Services in Jails.**			
Type of Service	% With Service	Estimated # of Offenders in Service	% of ADP (Median) for General Facilities	% of Programs >90 Days for General Facilities
Drug/alcohol education	61.3	47,237	4.5	19.9
Substance abuse group counseling: up to 4 h/week	59.8	39,943	7.4	48.1
Substance abuse group counseling: 5–25 h/week	23.1	16,471	10.8	8.9
Substance abuse group Counseling: 26+ h/week	1.1	1,185	3.4	92.3
Therapeutic community—segregated	26.2	11,889	3	97.9
Therapeutic community—non-segregated	<1	282	4.3	75.4
Relapse prevention groups	50.7	20,173	3	93.6
Case management or treatment accountability for safer communities	22.8	15,235	7.7	89.8

Note: % with service refers to the percentage of facilities that indicated that they offer the service. Estimated # of offenders in service is a national estimate of the sum of the number of offenders in the service on an average day. % of ADP refers to the percentage of the facilities' population that is involved in the service on an average day.

Reprinted from Taxman FS, Perdoni ML, Harrison LD. Drug treatment services for adult offenders: the state of the state. *J Subst Abuse Treat.* 2007;32:239–254.

Despite the apparent availability of drug treatment services in prisons and jails, less than 10% of prison and jail inmates have daily access to drug treatment services.[69] One way of assessing the quality and appropriateness of services offered is to examine the proportion of prisons and jails that use evidence-based practices in their drug treatment programs. Less than 60% of available evidence-based practices were used in treatment programs for drug-involved adult offenders, suggesting that services available for drug-involved offenders in prisons and jails may be far from optimal.[28] Of interest, clusters of evidence-based practices tend to occur together, suggesting that some facilities may have overcome resource and philosophical barriers to the adoption of evidence-based practices—once one evidence-based practice is adopted, others may be adopted in the same setting with less difficulty.[37]

The effectiveness of drug treatment programs offered in prisons and jails can be evaluated in terms of reductions in postrelease drug use and in postrelease reoffending. A meta-analysis of 66 published and unpublished evaluations of incarceration-based drug treatment programs[53] provided support for the effectiveness of therapeutic communities in reducing postrelease drug use and reoffending. In contrast, other incarceration-based residential substance abuse treatment programs and group counseling programs reduced reoffending but were less effective in reducing drug use after release.

Conclusion

Research reviewed for this chapter documents the relationship between drug and alcohol abuse and dependence and criminal justice involvement, the relationship between drug and alcohol relapse and re-arrest and recidivism, the need for greater availability of drug and alcohol treatment within the criminal justice system, the need for strengthening treatment services by the inclusion of evidence-based practices and alternative forms of service delivery (such as drug courts and Treatment Accountability for

Safer Communities or Treatment Accountability for Safer Communities–like programs), the need for a coordinated system of care that bridges the gap between incarceration and return to the community, the need to introduce pharmacotherapy for addictions into drug treatment for criminal justice populations, and the urgent need for research into effective models of service delivery.

On the one hand, it is possible to look with horror at the system of drug treatment available for individuals under criminal justice supervision in the United States: as rates of incarceration and recidivism increase and comorbid conditions such as psychiatric disorders and infectious diseases become more prevalent, resources available to provide drug treatment become increasingly scarce. On the other hand, the association between criminal behavior and drug and alcohol abuse suggests a way out of the repeating cycle of drug abuse, criminal activity, incarceration, release, relapse, and re-arrest. Drug treatment reduces drug use and relapse and may reduce reoffense and re-arrest. Research is urgently needed to improve both access to and quality of drug treatment services for individuals under criminal justice supervision.

References

1. Anglin MD, Longshore D, Turner S. Treatment alternatives to street crime: an evaluation of five programs. *Criminal Justice Behav.* 1999;26:168–195.
2. Awofeso N. Implementing smoking cessation programs in prison settings. *Addiction Res Theory.* 2003;11(2):119–130.
3. Baillargeon J, Black SA, Pulvino J, Dunn K. The disease profile of Texas prison inmates. *Ann Epidemiol.* 2000;10:74–80.
4. Barton A. Breaking the crime/drugs cycle: the birth of a new approach? *Howard J Criminal Justice.* 2002;38:144–157.
5. Belenko S. *Research On Drug Courts: a Critical Review 2001 Update.* The National Center on Addiction and Substance Abuse (CASA) at Columbia University; 2001.
5a. Belenko S, Hiller M, Hamilton L. Treating substance use disorders in the criminal justice system. *Curr Psychiatry Rep.* 2013;15(11):414.

6. Bickel WK, Amass L. Buprenorphine treatment of opioid dependence: a review. *Exp Clin Psychopharm.* 1995;3:477–489.

7. Boone HB. Mental illness in probation and parole populations: results from a national survey. *Perspectives.* 1995;19:14–26.

8. Brooke D, Taylor C, Gunn J, Maden A. Substance misusers remanded to prison—a treatment opportunity? *Addiction.* 1998;93:1851–1856.

8a. Califano JA. *Behind Bars II: Substance Abuse and America's Prison Population.* New York, The National Center on Addiction and Substance Abuse at Columbia University (CASA); 2010, NCJ: 230327.

9. Center for Disease Control and Prevention. *Sexually Transmitted Disease Surveillance 2005 Supplement, 2005.* Atlanta, GA: U.S. Department of Health and Human Services, CDC; 2006.

10. Center for Disease Control and Prevention. *Reported Tuberculosis in the United States, 2005.* Atlanta, GA: U.S. Department of Health and Human Services, CDC; 2006.

11. Center for Disease Control and Prevention. *Reported Tuberculosis in the United States, 2007.* Atlanta, GA: U.S. Department of Health and Human Services, CDC; 2007.

12. Centers for Disease Control and Prevention. *Hepatitis C Fact Sheet, 2008.* Atlanta, GA: U.S. Department of Health and Human Services, CDC; 2008.

12a. Centers for Disease Control and Prevention. *Sexually Transmitted Disease Surveillance 2008.* Atlanta, GA: U.S. Department of Health and Human Services, CDC; 2009.

13. Colsher PL, Wallace RB, Loeffelholz PL, Sales M. Health status of older male prisoners: a comprehensive survey. *Am J Public Health.* 1992;82:881–884.

14. Conklin TJ, Lincoln T, Tuthill RW. Self-reported health and prior health behaviors of newly admitted correctional inmates. *Am J Public Health.* 2000;90:1939–1941.

14a. Cork K, Public Health Law Center. *Tobacco Behind Bars: Policy Options for the Adult Correctional Population (Appendix A).* St. Paul, MN: Public Health Law Center; 2012.

15. Cotton-Oldenburg NU, Jordan K, Martin SL, Kupper ML. Women inmates' risky sex and drug behaviors: are they related? *Am J Drug Alcohol Abuse.* 1999;25:129–130.

16. Cropsey K, Eldridge G, Ladner T. Smoking among female prisoners: an ignored public health epidemic. *Addict Behav.* 2004;29:425–431.

17. Cropsey K, Eldridge G, Weaver M, Villalobos G, Stitzer M, Best A. Smoking cessation intervention for female prisoners: addressing an urgent public health need. *Am J Public Health.* 2008;98:1894–1901.

17a. Cropsey KL, Jackson DO, Hale GJ, Carpenter MJ, Stitzer ML. Impact of self-initiated pre-quit smoking reduction on cessation rates: results of a clinical trial of smoking cessation among female prisoners. *Addict Behav.* 2011;36(1):73–78.

18. Cropsey KL, Kristeller JL. Motivational factors related to quitting smoking among prisoners during a smoking ban. *Addict Behav.* 2003;28:1081–1093.

19. Cropsey KL, Kristeller JL. The effects of a prison smoking ban on smoking behavior and withdrawal symptoms. *Addict Behav.* 2005;30:589–594.

20a. Cropsey KL, Lane PS, Hale GJ, et al. (2011). Results of a pilot randomized controlled trial of buprenorphine for opioid dependent women in the criminal justice system. *Drug Alcohol Depend.* 2011;119(3):172–178.

20b. Cropsey KL, McClure LA, Jackson DO, Villalobos GC, Weaver MF, Stitzer ML. The impact of quitting smoking on weight among women prisoners participating in a smoking cessation intervention. *Am J Public Health.* 2010;100(8):1442–1448.

20. Cropsey KL, Villalobos GC, St Clair CL. Pharmacotherapy treatment in substance dependent correctional populations: a review. *Substance Use Misuse.* 2006;40:1983–1999.

21. Desai AA, Latta ET, Spaulding A, Rich JD, Flanigan TP. The importance of routine HIV testing in the incarcerated population: the Rhode island experience. *AIDS Educ Prevent.* 2002;14(suppl B):45–52.

22. Ditton PM. *Mental Health and Treatment of Inmates and Probationers.* Washington, DC: Bureau of Justice Statistics Special Report: U.S. Department of Justice; 1999.

23. Dolan K, Hall W, Wodak A. The provisions of methadone within prison settings. In: Ward J, Mattick R, eds. *Methadone Maintenance Treatment and Other Opioid Replacement Therapies.* Amsterdam: Harwood Academic Publishers; 1998:379–396.

24. Doran CM, Shanahan M, Mattick RP, Aki R, White J, Bell J. Buprenorphine versus methadone maintenance: a cost-effectiveness analysis. *Drug Alcohol Depend.* 2003;71:295–302.

24a. Durose MR, Cooper AD, Snyder HN. *Recidivism of Prisoners Released in 30 States in 2005: Patterns from 2005 to 2010.* Bureau of Justice Statistics Special Report; 2014, NCJ 244205.

25. Edinger JD, Nelson WM, Davidson KM, Wallace J. Modification of smoking behaviors in a correctional institution. *J Clin Psychol.* 1978;34:991–998.

26. Farrell M, Boys A, Bebbington P, et al. Psychosis and drug dependence: results from a national survey of prisoners. *Br J Psychiatry.* 2002;181:393–398.

27. Fazel S, Danesh J. Serious mental disorder in 23000 prisoners: a systematic review of 62 surveys. *Lancet.* 2002;359:545–550.

27a. Friedmann PD, Hoskinson R, Gordon M, et al. Medication-assisted treatment in criminal justice agencies affiliated with the criminal justice-drug abuse treatment studies (CJ-DATS): availability, barriers, and intentions. *Subst Abus.* 2012;33(1):9–18.

28. Friedmann PD, Taxman FS, Henderson CE. Evidence-based treatment practices for drug-involved adults in the criminal justice system. *J Subst Abuse Treat.* 2007;32:267–277.

29. Gibson A, Degenhardt L. Mortality related to pharmacotherapies for opioid dependence: a comparative analysis of coronial records. *Drug Alcohol Rev.* 2007;26:405–410.

30. Glaze LE, Palla S. *Probation and Parole in the United States, 2004.* Bureau of Justice Statistics U.S. Department of Justice; 2005. NCJ 210676.

31. Gossop M, Marsden J, Stewart D, Rolfe A. Reductions in acquisitive crime and drug use after treatment of addiction problems: 1-year follow-up outcomes. *Drug Alcohol Depend.* 2000;58:65–72.

32. Gottfredson DC, Exum ML. The Baltimore city drug treatment court: one-year results from a randomized study. *J Res Crime Delinquency.* 2002;39:337–356.

33. Gottfredson DC, Najaka SS, Kearley BW. Effectiveness of drug treatment courts: evidence from a randomized trial. *Criminol Public Policy.* 2003;2:171–196.

34. Greenfeld LA. *Alcohol and Crime: An Analysis of National Data On the Prevalence of Alcohol Involvement in Crime.* U.S. Department of Justice, Bureau of Justice Statistics; 1998. NCJ 168632.

35. Hammett TM, Harmon P, Rhodes W. *The Burden of Infectious Disease Among Inmates and Releases from Correctional Facilities.* Chicago, IL: Prepared for National Commission on Correctional Health Care, National Institute of Justice; 1999.

36. Harwood HJ, Fountain D, Livermore G. *The Economic Cost of Alcohol and Drug Abuse in the United States, 1992.* Rockville, MD: National Institute on Drug Abuse and National Institute on Alcohol Abuse and Alcoholism; 1998.

37. Henderson CE, Taxman FS, Young DW. A Rasch model analysis of evidence-based treatment practices used in the criminal justice system. *Drug Alcohol Depend.* 2008;93:163–175.

38. Hiller ML, Webster JM, Garrity TF, Leukefeld C, Narevic E, Staton M. Prisoners with substance abuse and mental health problems: use of health and health services. *Am J Drug Alcohol Abuse.* 2005;31:1–20.

39. Hogben M, St Lawrence J, Eldridge G. Sexual risk behavior, drug use, and STD rates among incarcerated women. *Women Health.* 2001;34:63–78.

40. Hogben M, St Lawrence J, Hennessy MH, Eldridge G. Using the theory of planned behavior to understand the STD risk behaviors of incarcerated women. *Criminal Justice Behav.* 2003;30:187–209.

41. Inciardi JA, McBride DC. *Treatment Alternatives to Street Crime: History, Experiences and Issues.* Rockville, MD: National Institute of Drug Abuse; 1991.

41a. James DJ, Glaze LE. *Mental Health Problems of Prison and Jail Inmates* NCJ 213600 U.S. Department of Justice; 2006. http://www.bjs.gov/index.cfm?ty=pbdetail&iid=789.

41b. Kaeble D, Glaze LE. *Correctional Population in the United States, 2015* NCJ 250374. Washington, DC: Bureau of Justice Statistics; 2016.

42. Kauffman RM, Ferketice AK, Wewers ME. Tobacco policy in American prisons, 2007. *Tobacco Control.* 2008;17:357–360.

43. Kinlock TW, Gordon MS, Schwartz RP, O'Grady K, Fitzgerald TT, Wilson M. A randomized clinical trial of methadone maintenance for prisoners: results at 1-month post-release. *Drug Alcohol Depend.* 2007;91:220–227.

44. Kouri EM, Pope Jr HG, Powell KF, Olivia PS, Campbell C. Drug use history and criminal behavior among 133 incarcerated men. *Am J Drug Alcohol Abuse.* 1997;23:413–419.

45. Lamb HR, Weinberger LE. The shift of psychiatric inpatient care from hospitals to jails and prisons. *J Am Acad Psychiatry Law.* 2005;33:529–534.

46. Langan PA, Levin DJ. *Recidivism of Prisoners Released in 1994.* Bureau of Justice Statistics U.S. Department of Justice; 2002. NCJ 193427.

47. Lankanau SE. Smoke 'em if you got 'em: cigarette black markets in U.S. prisons and jails. *Prison J.* 2001;81:142–161.

48. Ling W, Wesson DR. Clinical efficacy of buprenorphine: comparisons to methadone and placebo. *Drug Alcohol Depend.* 2003;70:S49–S57.

49. Magura S, Rosenblum A, Lewis C, Joseph H. The effectiveness of in jail methadone maintenance. *J Drug Issues.* 1993;23:75–99.

50. Markowitz FE. Psychiatric hospital capacity, homelessness, and crime and arrest rates. *Criminology.* 2006;44:45–72.

51. Martin SS, Butzin CA, Saum CA, Inciardi JA. Three-year outcomes of therapeutic community treatment for drug-involved offenders in Delaware: from prison to work release to aftercare. *Prison J.* 1999;79:294–320.

51a. Maruschak LM. HIV in prisons, 2001-2010. US Department of Justice Bureau of Justice Statistics. 2015. https://www.bjs.gov/content/pub/pdf/hivp10.pdf.

52. McGowan RJ, Margolis A, Gaiter J, et al. Predictors of risky sex of young men after release from prison. *Int J STD AIDS.* 2003;14:519–523.

52a. McLaughlin M, Pettus-Davis C, Brown D, Veeh C, Renn T. The economic burden of incarceration in the U.S., institute for advancing justice research and innovation. Working Paper #AJI072016; 2016. https://joinnia.com/wp-content/uploads/2017/02/The-Economic-Burden-of-Incarceration-in-the-US-2016.pdf.

53. Mitchell O, Wilson DB, MacKenzie DL. Does incarceration-based drug treatment reduce recidivism? A meta-analytic synthesis of the research. *J Exp Criminol.* 2007;3:353–375.

54. Mumola CJ. *Substance Abuse and Treatment, State and Federal Prisoners.* Washington, DC: Office of Justice Programs; 1999:1–16.

55. National Commission on Correctional Health Care. *The Health Status of Soon-to-be-Released Inmates: A Report to Congress*; 2002. http://www.ncchc.org/pubs/pubs_stbr.html. Accessed 22 July 2005.

56. Patrick S, Marsh R. Current tobacco policies in U.S. adult male prisons. *Soc Sci J.* 2001;38:27–37.

57. Rabinowitz J, Cohen H, Tarrasch R, Kotler M. Compliance to naltrexone treatment after ultra-rapid opiate detoxification: an open label naturalistic study. *Drug Alcohol Depend.* 1997;47(2):77–86.

58. Richmond RL, Buler T, Belcher JM, Wodak A, Wilhelm KA, Baxter E. Promoting smoking cessation among prisoners: feasibility of a multi-component intervention. *Australian N Z J Public Health.* 2006;30:474–478.

59. Simpson DD, Joe GW, Broome KM, Hiller ML, Knight K, Rowan-Szal GA. Program diversity and treatment retention rates in the drug abuse treatment outcome study (DATOS). *Psychol Addict Behav.* 1997;11(4):279–293.

60. Simpson DD, Joe GW, Fletcher BW, Hubbard RL, Anglin MD. A national evaluation of treatment outcomes for cocaine dependence. *Archiv Gen Psychiatry.* 1999;56:507–514.

61. Steadman HJ, Veysey BM. *Providing Services for Jail Inmates with Mental Disorders.* Washington, DC: U.S. Department of Justice, NCJ 162207; 1997.

62. Stephan JJ. *State prison Expenditures, 2001.* Bureau of Justice Statistics U.S. Department of Justice, NCJ 202949; 2004.

63. Substance Abuse and Mental Health Services Administration. *Results From the 2006 National Survey on Drug Use and Health: National Findings.* Rockville, MD: Office of Applied Studies, NSDUH Series H-32, DHHS Publication No. SMA 07-4293; 2007.

64. Taxman FS, Bouffard J. Explaining drug treatment completion in drug court courts. *J Offender Rehabil.* 2005;42:23–50.

65. Taxman FS, Cropsey KL, Melnick G, Perdoni ML. COD services in community correctional settings: an examination of organizational factors that affect service delivery. *Behav Sci Law.* 2008;26:435–455.

66. Taxman FS, Cropsey KL, O'Boyle E, Gallant A (unpublished data). With limited room at the Inn: Examining the models for drug involved offenders.

67. Taxman FS, Cropsey KL, Young D, Wexler H. Screening, assessment and referral practices in adult correctional settings: a national perspective. *Criminal Justice Behav.* 2007;34:1216–1235.

68. Taxman FS, Pedroni ML, Harrison LD. Drug treatment services for adult offenders: the state of the state. *J Subst Abuse Treat.* 2007;32:239–254.

69. Taxman FS, Perdoni ML, Harrison LD. Drug treatment services for adult offenders: the state of the state. *J Subst Abuse Treat.* 2007;32:239–254.

70. Taxman FS, Thanner M. Risk, need, and responsivity (RNR): it all depends. *CrimeDelinquency.* 2006;52:28–51.

71. Taxman FS, Young DW, Wiersema B, Rhodes A, Mitchell S. The national criminal justice treatment practices survey: multilevel survey methods and procedures. *J Subst Abuse Treat.* 2007;32:225–238.

72. Teplin LA. Psychiatric and substance abuse disorders among male urban jail detainees. *Am J Public Health.* 1994;84:290–293.

73. Teplin LA, Abram KM, McClelland GM. Prevalence of psychiatric disorders among incarcerated women: pretrial jail detainees. *Archiv Gen Psychiatry.* 1996;53:505–512.

74. Torrey EF. Jails and prisons—America's new mental hospitals. *Am J Public Health.* 1995;85:1611–1613.

75. U.S. Department of Corrections. *Florida Department of Corrections Recidivism Report: Inmates Released from Florida Prisons July 1995 to June 2001*; 2003.

76. Reference deleted in review.

77. U.S. Department of Health and Human Services. *The Health Consequences of Smoking—50 Years of Progress: A Report of the Surgeon General.* Atlanta, GA: U.S. Department of Health and Human Services, Centers for Disease Control and Prevention, National Center for Chronic Disease Prevention and Health Promotion, Office on Smoking and Health; 2014.

78. U.S. Department of Justice. *Bureau of Justice Statistics Fiscal Year 1998: at a Glance.* Bureau of Justice Statistics Bulletin NCJ 169285; 1998.

79. U.S. Department of Justice. *HIV in Prison, 2001.* Bureau of Justice Statistics Bulletin NCJ 202293; 2004.

80. U.S. Department of Justice. Drug Courts. *The Second Decade. Office of Justice Programs.* National Institute of Justice; 2006.

81. U.S. Department of Justice. *Key Crime and Justice Facts at a Glance.* Bureau of Justice Statistics Bulletin; 2008. http://www.ojp.usdoj.gov/bjs/glance.htm. Accessed June 10, 2009.

82. U.S. Department of Justice. *Painting the Current Picture: A National Report Card on Drug Courts and Other Problem-Solving Court Programs in the United States. Office of Justice Programs.* National Institute of Justice; 2008.

83. U.S. Department of Justice. *Substance Abuse Treatment and Public Safety.* Justice Policy Institute, National Institute of Justice; 2008.

84. Vaughn MS, Del Carmen RV. Research note: a national survey of correctional administrators in the United States. *Crime Delinquency.* 1993;39(2):225–239.

85. Veysey BM, Bichler-Robertson G. *Providing Psychiatric Services in Correctional Settings. The Health Status of Soon-to-be-Released Inmates: a Report to Congress, 2, 157–165.* Chicago: National Commission on Correctional Health Care; 2002.

86. Veysey BM, Bichler-Robertson G. *Prevalence Estimates of Psychiatric Disorders in Correctional Settings*; 2002a. http://www/ncchc.org/pubs/pubs_stbr.html. Accessed 22 July 2005.

87. Veysey BM, Bichler-Robertson G. *Providing Psychiatric Services in Correctional Settings*; 2002b. http://www/ncchc.org/pubs/pubs_stbr.html. Accessed 22 July 2005.

88. Walsh SL, Preston KL, Stitzer ML, Cone EJ, Bigelow GE. Clinical pharmacology of buprenorphine: ceiling effects at high doses. *Clin Pharmacol Ther.* 1994;55:569–580.

89. Wells CD, Cegielski JP, Nelson LJ, et al. HIV infection and multidrug-resistant tuberculosis: the perfect storm. *J Infectious Dis.* 2007;196(suppl 1):S86–S107.

90. Welsh WN, Zajac G. A census of prison-based drug treatment programs: implications for programming, policy, and evaluation. *Crime Delinquency.* 2004;50:108–133.

91. Wilson DB, Mitchell O, Mackenzie DL. A systematic review of drug court effects on recidivism. *J Exp Criminol.* 2006;2:459–487.

92. Wunsch MJ, Nakamoto K, Goswami A, Schnoll SH. Prescription drug abuse among prisoners in rural Southwestern Virginia. *J Addict Disorders.* 2007;26:15–22.

93. Young DW, Taxman FS, Perdoni M, Melnick G. *TASC's Impact on Evidence-Based Practices in Corrections: Results From a National Survey.* Denver, CO: National TASC Association Meeting; 2007.

94. Young-Wolff KC, Karan LD, Prochaska JJ. (2015). Electronic cigarettes in jails: a panacea or public health problem? *JAMA Psychiatry.* 2015;72(2):103–104.

48

Adolescent Neurocognitive Development and School-Based Drug Abuse Prevention and Treatment

PALLAV POKHREL, DAVID S. BLACK, ADNIN ZAMAN, NATHANIEL R. RIGGS, AND STEVE SUSSMAN

CHAPTER OUTLINE

Introduction

Schools are an efficient and convenient choice of setting for intervention programs targeting adolescents. Schools provide access to a large number of adolescents in a learning environment in which adolescents are more likely to be receptive toward instructions involved in an intervention. Moreover, monitoring the fidelity of program implementation and assessing program effectiveness in a school setting are relatively easy.[76] In addition, the typical 4-year structure of school systems is conducive to tracking down students in order to obtain long-term follow-up data.

Prevention programming attempts to reach adolescents prior to the expected occurrence of certain problematic behavior such as drug abuse. The central focus of prevention is on the antecedents of problem behavior. Program participants are taught how to anticipate the impacts of these antecedents (e.g., such as desiring to feel good, cognitive exposure to drug-related cues, social influence, or cultural norms) and to counteract their potential impacts

with instruction of protective cognitions, behaviors, or access to protective social units (e.g., drug-free communities). Among these strategies are selective or indicated approaches that attempt to prevent individuals who are either currently at-risk for drug use behavior, by virtue of their membership in certain segments of the population, or who are already demonstrating early signs of drug use behavior, from developing clinically diagnosed drug use disorders.[51] Some researchers tend to refer to both indicated and selective programs as targeted programs.[79]

Cessation (treatment) programs are designed to assist in stopping drug use, given that youth were either not exposed or did not respond to prevention efforts. Cessation programs provide participants with strategies to cope with psychological dependence (emotional reliance) on and physiological withdrawal from a drug (e.g., what types of withdrawal symptoms to expect, how long one will experience these symptoms, and how to cope with these symptoms without relapsing). Cessation programs focus on stopping a current behavior from continuing to arrest ongoing consequences and permit recovery of health. The goal may also involve teaching one how to live with permanent changes (e.g., drug-related injury).

In the school setting, prevention efforts are generally delivered school-wide (i.e., universal prevention), whereas cessation programs are usually delivered outside of the classroom (e.g., with student assistance programs, in clinics, or perhaps involving the school nurse, possibly involving self-help support groups, which meet during lunchtime or after school). Exposure to early prevention programming could provide proactive interference against later drug-facilitative–type information, resulting in protection against drug misuse. These prevention efforts may inhibit, delay, or halt addiction, which is what makes cessation so difficult. For older adolescents who are caught up in cycles of drug misuse or abuse, prevention programming could help minimize the time spent in a using cycle.

A recent focus of adolescent school-based drug abuse prevention and cessation programming involves applying models of neurobiology/neuropsychology as potential influences on program outcomes. This chapter provides a brief overview of the application of neuroscience to adolescent development, indicates current school-based prevention and cessation strategies that may impact neuroscience-relevant adolescent functioning, and suggests new directions for the development and implementation of drug use prevention and cessation programs.

Brief Overview: Neuroscience and Adolescents

Adolescent vulnerability to substance use has been associated with the protracted morphological development of the neural systems responsible for self-control and regulation, in conjunction with a heightened tendency to seek novel experiences (e.g., Steinberg[9] and Chambers et al.[75]). The regions of the human brain linked to self-control and self-regulation are not fully developed until late adolescence. However, an increase in novelty-seeking behavior is evident when children transition into early adolescence. Thus increases in risk-taking and sensation-seeking tendencies among adolescents seem to precede the development of self-regulatory competencies.[75]

Several animal as well as human studies suggest that novelty-seeking behavior increases rapidly during adolescence[9]; this has been attributed to the changes that occur in the pro-motivational dopamine systems during this stage of ontological development.[9] The level of dopamine turnover among adolescents is likely to be higher than among children and adults.[9,73] Dopamine in the ventral striatum, which includes the nucleus accumbens, is believed to modulate the conversion of thoughts and emotions into motivated actions.[35] Dopamine release in the nucleus accumbens appears to filter and gate the motivational signals received from the cortical and limbic systems that are to be processed by the downstream motor systems.[9,35]

Several motivational stimuli have been associated with dopamine stimulation in the nucleus accumbens, including the drugs of misuse and agents of natural reward (e.g., food, sex). Furthermore, novel experiences tend to cause higher levels of dopamine stimulation compared with previously learned behaviors that have expected outcomes.[9] Hence, the same mesolimbic dopamine systems appear to mediate both drug- and novelty-seeking behaviors.[3] Conversely, concentrations of inhibitory motivation neurotransmitters such as serotonin appear to be lower in adolescent cerebrospinal fluid, which has been associated with higher impulsivity.[9] A greater tendency to act along with decreased inhibitory tendencies for self-destructive action could contribute to drug use experimentation.

Adolescents' vulnerability to drug use due to developmental changes in the dopaminergic system is further exacerbated by the relatively underdeveloped prefrontal cortex. Brain structure and function undergo significant changes throughout adolescence, notably in the forebrain regions, which comprise the prefrontal cortex. The prefrontal cortex is one of the last cortical structures to reach full ontogenetic development and may not achieve complete maturation until the third decade of a person's life.[19] This region of the brain is responsible for the spatiotemporal organization of goal-directed actions, which involve the carrying out of relevant actions in response to internal (e.g., memory) or external (e.g., environmental context) cues.[19,34] In other words, the principal function of the prefrontal cortex is to perform executive function. Executive function represents a complex set of interrelated functions that make the temporal organization of goal-directed behavior, language, and reasoning possible.[19] Methodologically, brain researchers find it difficult to separate the interrelated components of the executive system into discrete units (e.g., attention,

working memory, decision-making) and localize them to specific areas of the prefrontal cortex.[19] For example, the functional contribution of a specific prefrontal cortex area is difficult to measure after a discrete lesion, for such a lesion is likely to functionally affect the entire executive system.[19] Nonetheless, researchers have linked deficiencies in executive function to abnormalities related to attention, working memory, long-term memory retrieval, planning, temporal integration of memory and goal, decision-making, monitoring, and inhibitory control.[19]

Ability to exert sustained attention or manipulate the focus of one's attention is necessary to formulate a goal-directed thought or bring an action to completion. In turn, one needs to control distracting or interfering urges, both internal (e.g., thoughts, memory, instinctual) and external (e.g., environmental), in order to maintain sustained attention.[19] Working memory refers to the ability to retain information and utilize the information to execute a related action. Like most executive functions, working memory and sustained attention are interrelated and are essential for task perseverance. Furthermore, execution of actions involves foresight and planning. Planning represents the ability to utilize information obtained from selective retrieval of long-term memory, such as memory of past actions, for the anticipation of future events. Planning provides a conceptual scheme for the execution of a goal-directed behavior, and based on the anticipation of consequences, lays out the order of prospective actions. Individuals often have to choose among competing actions. The executive function of decision-making involves choosing an action after rationally evaluating the potential risks and rewards associated with its outcomes. Successful execution of goal-directed behaviors also depends largely on the ability to self-monitor. Monitoring enables one to assess the discrepancies between one's actions and one's goals, thus creating feedback which allows one to correct subsequent actions.

Inhibitory control involves controlling an impulse by inhibiting a response. According to Barkley,[4] response inhibition involves three processes: (1) inhibition of the prepotent response (i.e., a response linked in associational memory to immediate reinforcement), (2) stopping of an ongoing response in order to delay the final decision to respond, and (3) protecting this decision-making time interval from being interfered with by other competing stimuli and responses (i.e., interference control). Primary response inhibition partially aids the functioning of working memory, regulation of motivation, verbal internalization, and behavioral analyses.

Hence executive functions make the self-regulation of thoughts, emotion, and behavior possible. Conversely, deficiencies in executive function may result in poor impulse control, poor judgment, and disinhibited behavior.[4] Among adolescents, poor executive functioning has been consistently associated with higher rates of drug use (e.g., Grekin and Sher,[26] Mezzich et al.,[44] Tarter et al.,[82] and Xiao et al.[93]). Furthermore, early adolescent deficiencies in executive function have been found to predict later drug use disorders.[21,80] For example, Habeych et al.[28] found that attenuated amplitude of the P300 wave, an indicator of executive cognitive function, in late childhood predicted substance use disorders in late adolescent males.

Research suggests that executive function develops in sophistication at the same rate as the structural maturation of the prefrontal cortex; and age-related social and cognitive maturation during adolescence may be attributed to the concomitant structural changes in the brain.[19,75] For example, improvements in planning and decision-making have been linked with the structural developments in the dorsolateral and ventrolateral prefrontal cortex, respectively.[75] Most notable developmental changes in the forebrain region have been observed as changes in gray and white matter volumes. Recent neuroimaging studies suggest that there is a continuous increase in the brain white matter volume during adolescence.[23,55] For example, a significant growth is noticed in the posterior corpus callosum, the collection of over 200 million nerve fibers that allow communication between right and left hemispheres of the brain.[23,55] In addition, the gray matter volume, which increases substantially during childhood, appears to decrease during adolescence in certain cortical structures (e.g., the prefrontal cortex[22]).

Reduction in cortical gray matter volume might occur due to increased intracortical myelination and/or due to synaptic pruning.[55] Increased myelination of neurons results in a more efficient propagation of action potentials. Synaptic pruning involves selective removal of synapses that "do not efficiently transmit information pertaining to accumulating experience."[9] Synaptic pruning appears to serve a number of functions that facilitate cognitive development. For example, the process appears to stabilize the firing patterns of cortical neurons, which in turn is thought to enhance working memory performance.[9] In general, both myelination and synaptic pruning are believed to enhance the efficiency of cortical information processing as well as the connectivity between cortical and subcortical regions.[9,55,73,75]

Thus because adolescent prefrontal cortex is not yet fully developed, the associated executive functions are expected to be inadequately developed. As a result, adolescents tend to have lower regulatory competence, which makes them highly susceptible to drug use risk factors such as rash impulsiveness and poor decision-making.[81] For example, adolescents tend to be poor judges of the harmful consequences of drug use, yield easily to peer pressure, and seek immediate gratification.[81] Therefore it is not surprising that most adult drug users are likely to have initiated drug use in the period between early to mid-adolescence, before the brain regions associated with self-regulation are optimally developed.[81]

In summary, evidence suggests that the developmental upsurge in novelty seeking coupled with suboptimal brain development makes adolescents vulnerable to drug use. Thus to some extent, adolescent experimentation with drugs appears to be a normative behavior.[81] However, it should be noted that individual differences exist among adolescents with respect to both novelty seeking and executive functioning; some adolescents are always at a higher risk for developing substance use disorders than others.[3,81]

Negative Consequences of Drug Use on Teen Cognitive Function

Early onset of drug use, escalation of use, and possible dependence might subject adolescents to the risks of developing mental health disorders and experiencing social, academic, and legal consequences. The developing adolescent brain appears to be highly vulnerable to the neurotoxic effects of drugs, including those of licit drugs such as tobacco and alcohol and the so-called soft drugs such as marijuana. Prolonged exposure to drugs during adolescence may result in neuropsychological deficiencies and structural brain damage, especially in areas associated with memory and executive function.[37,38] Brown et al.[8] have reported that compared with a matched group of healthy youth, alcohol-dependent young adolescents (in the third week of abstinence) were found to perform poorly on verbal and visuospatial tasks, suggesting that protracted exposure to alcohol might have enduring adverse effects on the brain's functional ability involving memory and information

processing. In fact, magnetic resonance imaging results indicate that youth with alcohol use disorders tend to show smaller hippocampal and white matter volumes[10,11,49] and smaller prefrontal cortices.[12] De Bellis et al.[10] further found that the total hippocampal volume among adolescents with alcohol use disorder increased with the age at onset and decreased with the duration of disorder.

Although, taken together, the relatively limited extant neuroimaging studies fail to conclude whether chronic marijuana use is related to structural abnormalities in the brain (for review, see Quickfall and Crockford[61]), some of the findings (e.g., Wilson et al.[91]) suggest a relationship between age at first onset and decreased total brain volume. Furthermore, it appears that early marijuana use initiators (e.g., before the age of 17) tend to show significant later cognitive deficits (e.g., indicated by verbal IQ; visual scanning tasks) in comparison with nonusers and late-onset users.[14,59] Nicotine-dependent adolescents have been suggested to perform normally on working memory tasks following nicotine intake but poorly during withdrawal.[29,30] One neuroimaging study indicated that despite poor task performance, nicotine-dependent adolescents on withdrawal exhibited increased activities in the prefrontal cortex regions (e.g., dorsolateral prefrontal cortex) associated with working memory.[30] Because an optimal level of dopamine action is essential for normal working memory functioning, the adverse effects of tobacco use cessation on working memory suggest that regular nicotine use causes abnormal adaptations of the dopaminergic circuitries.[30] In fact, research on rodents has shown that the normal development of catecholaminergic systems during adolescence might be disrupted by protracted exposure to nicotine.[83–85] These studies have linked adolescent nicotine exposure with hippocampal damage and impairments in the midbrain catecholaminergic systems that play important roles in mood regulation and addiction development.[83–85]

By adversely affecting the normal development of the cortical and limbic brain structures associated with risk and reward calibration, decision-making, and inhibitory control, drug use not only exacerbates the loss-of-control due to incentive-sensitization[64] but also undermines the cognitive ability to stop using drugs voluntarily.[94] Evidence suggests that drug addiction might be related to impairments in ventromedial prefrontal and anterior cingulate cortices, brain regions associated with decision-making and inhibitory control.[94] Furthermore, acute withdrawal of drug use seems to affect the anterior cingulate cortex, consequently weakening inhibitory control.[94]

However, it should be noted that most of the research linking adolescent drug use, drug use withdrawal, and neuropsychological deficiencies has been cross-sectional, which makes any conclusion on their causal relationships open for debate.[94] Nonetheless, it seems that deficient neuropsychological functioning and adolescent drug use share a reciprocal relationship. For example, neuropsychological deficiencies in preteen years tend to predict drug use disorders (e.g., Tarter et al.[82]), and, similarly, early drug use onset or abuse also seems to predict neuropsychological deficiencies.[94] Such bidirectional relationships imply that adolescents with impaired neuropsychological functioning face the additional risk of drug use–mediated further neuropsychological deterioration.[94]

Thus there appear to be at least three important reasons that prevention or treatment targeting adolescent drug misuse should address motivation, decision-making, and inhibitory control. First, adolescents normally tend to show suboptimal development of regulatory competence.[11,75] Second, this regulatory competence is likely to be markedly lower among drug-misusing adolescents due to possible impairments in certain brain regions such as the prefrontal cortex, anterior cingulate cortex, and hippocampus.[10,12,94] Poor regulatory competence may not only make it difficult for these high-risk adolescents to stop using drugs but may also cause them to relapse easily in case of temporary successful cessation.[85] Third, adolescents at high risk for using drugs or developing drug use disorders are already likely to rank low on neurobehavioral inhibition,[82] which might additionally indicate that their executive functions have trait-based deficiencies.[4] Thus drug-abusing adolescents and adolescents at risk for developing drug dependence would benefit greatly from supplemental programming that promotes adaptive coping, impulse control, problem solving, and self-monitoring.

Brain Development and School-Based Drug Use Prevention and Treatment

It has become increasingly important for prevention researchers to take into account the findings made in neuroscience to guide their approach in designing drug use prevention programs for youth. In particular, researchers are interested in knowing whether developmental neurobiological and neurocognitive variables moderate and/or mediate prevention effects.[24,62] Currently, the research attempting to answer these questions seems to be at a preliminary stage.[24] For example, there is some evidence that adolescents' neurocognitive skills moderate their response to preventive intervention materials. In a study dealing with social competency skills training, adolescents with poor executive cognitive abilities were less likely to respond positively to the prevention curriculum.[17,18] Hence not all youth may be equally able to process prevention messages and instructions, and program materials may need to be individualized to address differential neurocognitive skills.

Alternatively, prevention or treatment programs may aim to enhance adolescent neurocognitive skills in order to counteract drug use behavior. Recent evidence suggests that practice in tasks requiring regulatory skills may enhance one's executive functioning, and this alteration appears to correspond to practice-induced structural changes in the brain (e.g., Kabat-Zinn[31] and Quickfall and Crockford[61]). Hence one might argue that repeated practice of skills and tasks demanding the use of executive functions (e.g., attention control, working memory) during childhood and adolescence, when cortical structures are likely to be most malleable, may assist the age-related development of executive functions, and in turn protect adolescents from engaging in risky behaviors.

Need for Tailoring Prevention and Treatment Programs

To promote program efficacy, prevention and treatment programming may need to be tailored to participants' personality characteristics. For example, outcomes may be enhanced a great deal if programs are designed to permit maximum processing of information by sensation-seeking recipients with neurocognitive processing that prefers presentations of rapidly changing stimuli.[57] As noted by Bardo et al.,[3] novelty exposure tends to activate the same neural substrates that mediate the rewarding effects of drugs of abuse. The reinforcing effects of drugs play a key role in promoting continued drug use behavior, especially among individuals who are more susceptible to drug effects (e.g., sensation-seeking or novelty-seeking individuals). Initial positive or neutral physical responses to drugs may encourage subsequent use, whereas initial aversive physical reactions may discourage subsequent use

behavior. One suggestion for prevention is to consider that at-risk youth (e.g., sensation-seeking youth) may process information differently than lower risk youth, and therefore prevention materials should be tailored accordingly.

Given the evidence that individuals higher in sensation seeking may have a neurobiologically based need for stimulation, it seems reasonable to assume that they need drug abuse prevention messages that are novel and exciting enough to grab their attention and pique their curiosity (e.g., see Pentz et al.[57]). In fact, Palmgreen et al.[54] found that high-sensation-seeking value-type public service announcements may have influenced higher sensation seekers' drug intake for several months following a media campaign. Fast-paced, novel, and stimulating media-type programs that grab or increase adolescents' attention and learning may more effectively influence sensation-seeking individuals with lower baseline dopamine turnover.[54]

Staiger et al.[74] have recently stated the need for tailoring drug abuse treatment programs with respect to three specific personality-based drug use risk factors, namely, reward sensitivity, behavior disinhibition (or rash impulsivity), and anxiety proneness. For example, contingency management could be used as a possible tactic for someone with high levels of reward sensitivity, as to replace drug-related reward with a prosocial alternative.[74] Similarly, treatment strategies such as meditation and mindfulness-based practices could be used to promote attention control and relaxation in order to address impulsiveness and anxiety proneness, respectively.[74]

Current School-Based Prevention Practices and Executive Functions

School-based programs designed for young children often focus on improving social-emotional competence (e.g., Greenberg et al.,[25] Shure,[70] and Shure[71]). Temperament characteristics such as emotionality predict adolescent problem behavior, including drug use behavior.[89] Wills and colleagues[88,90] argue that a person's childhood temperament characteristics and socialization affect his or her ability to self-regulate during adolescence, and in turn, his or her drug use behavior.[88,90] Promoting Alternative Thinking Strategies is a school-based prevention program that attempts to assist young children in social and emotional learning through the teaching and practice of executive function skills.[25] The Promoting Alternative Thinking Strategies curriculum is based on the affective-behavioral-cognitive-dynamic model of development.[24,25] The assumption underlying the affective-behavioral-cognitive-dynamic model is that due to delayed development of the neurocircuitry connecting cortical and limbic structures, children's cognitive and linguistic development tends to be inadequate when required to regulate complex emotional experiences. Thus children appear to have difficulty verbally internalizing emotional experience and managing related behavioral response. The Promoting Alternative Thinking Strategies curriculum uses the concepts of vertical control and horizontal communication to assist children's age-related neurocognitive development. Vertical control refers to the exertion of control by higher-order cognitive processes on the lower-order limbic impulses, and horizontal communication refers to mediated communication between the two hemispheres of the brain, a process integral to the internal verbalization of affect.[24,62]

Results demonstrate that Promoting Alternative Thinking Strategies can improve vertical control and horizontal communication. Vertical control is addressed though the combined use of curriculum lessons and the Control Signals Poster, which teach strategies for self-control, such as self-talk, that facilitate inhibitory control and planning.[24] The control signals poster uses a traffic-signal to guide goal-directed behaviors (e.g., red light signaling to stop and calm down, yellow light to slow down and think, and green light to try out the plan[62]). Horizontal communication is addressed through the identification and labeling of emotions and feelings through the combined use of curricular lessons and Feeling Face cards, which include color-coded facial images of affective states.[62]

A Promoting Alternative Thinking Strategies trial involving 7- to 9-year-olds recently found that the curriculum was effective in reducing externalizing and internalizing behaviors at 1-year follow-up, that Promoting Alternative Thinking Strategies had significant positive effects on verbal fluency and inhibitory control nine month posttest, that both inhibitory control and verbal fluency partially mediated internalizing behaviors, and that inhibitory control partially mediated the program effects on externalizing behaviors.[62]

Another example of a program for young children that focuses on social and emotional learning is the I Can Problem Solve program.[70,71] This program has been implemented on preschoolers through sixth graders and provides children with language and critical thinking skills that help them successfully resolve interpersonal problems with peers and adults through effective decision-making. The program is recommended to be implemented as a daily 20-minute classroom session for 15 months. All sessions are designed to foster interpersonal cognitive problem solving through dialogues, games, and group discussions that involve the use of words, pictures, puppets, and role playing. For example, students are taught to identify words that are precursors to understanding behavioral consequences and problem solving, and teacher-initiated interpersonal cognitive problem-solving dialogue is used to solve actual interpersonal problems among children. The program has been successful in reducing impulsivity and social inhibition (e.g., fear and timidity of others), which are related to the development of drug use and mental health disorders.[71]

Although it is common for prevention programs to include cognitive-behavioral skills training as a major component (e.g., life skills training),[6,7] executive function variables are not often directly measured as mediators of program effects.[62] However, in essence, such studies attempt to enhance the rate and quality of age-related cortical development. Several developmentally tailored life skills training trials have been successfully implemented in elementary, middle, and high schools to develop social and personal skills among youth.[65] The skills-building component of the program focuses on developing regulatory competence among youth necessary to counteract the social influences of drug use through training on, for example, coping and anxiety management (e.g., vertical control), and effective communication and assertiveness (e.g., horizontal communication).[65]

Recently, mindfulness-based interventions have emerged as having promising implications for executive function enhancement, with the potential to be applied to school-based drug use prevention.[56] Mindfulness refers to attaining a mental state in which attention is sustainably focused on the nonjudgmental awareness of thoughts and sensations passing through one at the given moment. Mindfulness interventions train participants to control their attention and emotions so as to focus on the present moment.[31] Essentially, mindfulness interventions provide training in self-regulation. Typically, mindfulness-based interventions use a simple sitting technique that teaches participants to focus on the breath, image, or mantra for as little as 10 minutes per session.[1] Since 2005, a number of studies have demonstrated that mindfulness training provided to children and adolescents may result in improved working memory, attention, and emotional regulation.[42,68] For example, researchers[16,50,68] have used task performance–based measures of executive function to show the effects of mindfulness-based interventions on improved working memory, attention-control, and cognitive flexibility among elementary school students.

The majority of mindfulness-based intervention studies involving adolescents have been school-based.[42] A recent systematic review by Felver et al.[15] identified 28 empirical studies that evaluated school-based mindfulness interventions for adolescents. Sixteen of the 28 studies involved a control group. In general, the studies tended to show that mindfulness intervention was associated with decreased externalizing and internalizing behaviors and mental health symptomology including anxiety, depression, and suicidal ideation. Although none of the studies assessed substance use as an outcome, the findings that mindfulness can modulate executive functions and reduce the more proximal risk factors of adolescent drug use such as externalizing behavior are very promising in regard to the successful application of mindfulness in school-based drug use prevention. Preliminary research on adolescent mindfulness and adolescent drug use is promising. For example, Pentz et al.[58] found trait mindfulness to buffer the effects of risk factors on adolescent drug use. Another study[2] showed that higher trait mindfulness was associated with reduced adolescent drug use through lower negative affect and lower perceived stress.

Clearly, more research is needed to better understand the potential protective effects of mindfulness-based interventions on executive functions and adolescent drug use. Even though a few studies have examined the effects of mindfulness on adolescents' executive functions as assessed with performance tasks, most school-based research still rely on self-reported measures as outcomes of mindfulness-based interventions.[15] Despite their merits, self-report measures may not be ideal to assess changes at the neurocognitive level. In addition, more research is needed to test hypothesis related to neurocognitive mechanisms that underlie the relationship between mindfulness and adolescent drug use.[32]

It appears that prevention programming would benefit additionally from the inclusion of a motivation component. Sussman et al.[79] evaluated 29 evidence-based, targeted drug abuse prevention programs for their effects on drug use or other problem behavior among high-risk youth. Eighteen of these programs involved school as a setting in some way. Of the 18 programs, 12 involved some motivation aspect, generally motivation enhancement, but sometimes they included extrinsic reinforcement strategies (i.e., reinforcement by manipulating environmental consequences of behavior such as by being paid contingent on performance). Sixteen of the 18 programs provided skills training, and 11 programs provided instruction in decision-making.

Taken together, these programs appear to define a type of programming referred to as the Motivation-Skills-Decision-making Model.[79] According to this model, targeted programming needs to: (1) motivate the at-risk recipients, who might have higher reward sensitivity,[74] to not desire to misuse drugs; (2) teach skills to enhance regulatory competence (e.g., self-control strategies[43]) and form prosocial bonds; and (3) facilitate decision-making and goal-directed behaviors. The Motivation-Skills-Decision-making Model tends to appear in a majority of the 18 programs; however, all three components were included together in only 5 of the programs.

The Reconnecting Youth program was one of the five programs and was implemented to youth at risk for school dropout.[13] The program involved 90 sessions within a comprehensive high school class, delivered generally over one semester, with small student groups and highly trained teachers. Instruction included use of group support and providing life skills training (norm setting, self-esteem enhancement, mood management, communication skills, self-monitoring, monitoring goals, school bonding, and social activities), with feedback to parents. Program goals were achieved through use of a quasi-experimental design, showing effects for school performance (18% improvement in grades), drug use (54% decrease in hard drug use), and suicide risk (32% decline in perceived stress). This program involved all three components of the Motivation-Skills-Decision-making Model, except that motivation was provided through peer group support, not through provision in motivational enhancement strategies. In essence, these targeted programs for high-risk populations could be interpreted as modifying phenotypical expressions of suboptimal neurobiological development. However, future integrative research will be needed to examine the reality of this speculation.

Schools as a Modality for Implementation of Cessation Programming

School-based interventions have been recognized as one of the most effective community-based means of delivering drug use treatment services to adolescents.[86] Empirical evidence indicates that most school-based drug use treatment programs tend to yield treatment outcomes that are, in terms of success, similar to outcomes of programs targeting adults.[86] Treatment services in schools can be delivered through school clinics (i.e., clinics located within schools), classroom-level interventions, or a combination of both.[77,86]

Traditionally, treatment services have been delivered to youth drug users by trained health professions in clinics located outside schools, such as in hospitals and universities.[86] With regard to adolescents, school-based treatment delivery options seem to have clear advantages over the traditional modes of service delivery, in terms of both identifying the need for and access to treatment.[86] Adolescents are not only less likely to recognize their own drug use problems but also less likely to make an effort to seek treatment services voluntarily.[86] Hence unless concerned adults guide them to treatment facilities, which is less likely to happen if the problems have not yet become serious, most adolescents requiring treatment might not receive any treatment at all. Moreover, visiting clinics situated in institutions other than schools might exact potentially deterring efforts from adults and adolescents alike, such as spending money and one's free time, and making appointments.[86] Ethnic minorities and individuals of lower socioeconomic status in particular might fail to take advantage of treatment opportunities offered outside schools.[86]

In a review of 66 adolescent tobacco use cessation programs, Sussman[77] found that 28 (i.e., 43% of the studies) of the programs used school-based clinics to deliver services and 9 programs used classroom-based programming, while the remaining involved systemwide efforts (e.g., mass-media campaigns, policy, or state wide), computer-based self-help, medical or recovery clinics, and family-based interventions. The review suggested that a school clinic is located within school premises and generally delivers services to students in nonclassroom sessions that usually address groups of 5 to 15 students during school hours.[77] On the other hand, classroom-based programs make use of course curricula to deliver services in classroom settings.[77] These programs often combine prevention and cessation components together.[77] Although school clinics are supposed to address subjects' individual needs and thus be more effective, among the studies reviewed by Sussman,[77] classroom-based programs showed higher quit rates (17%) compared with school clinics (12%). In fact, classroom-based programs showed the highest rates of cessation among all channels of program delivery.[77]

However, it seems unclear whether school clinics and classroom-based treatment programs function similarly for alcohol or illicit drug use problems. Most of the Motivation-Skills-Decision-making Model–based classroom programs that combine prevention and treatment objectives seem to target all drug use.[77] However, school-based interventions that target only alcohol or illicit drug use disorders seem to rely more on problem identification, referral (e.g., referring problem users or suspected users to outside facilities for treatment or screening), or group counseling (e.g., Student Assistance Programs).[86] Moreover, the efficaciousness of these interventions has not been rigorously researched.[87]

Treatment Strategies and Executive Function Skills

As with prevention programming, treatment programming for adolescent drug users is likely to benefit a great deal from motivational enhancement and skills training. Preparedness to change one's drug-using behavior (e.g., motivation) and drug use outcome expectancies is considered to be an important cognitive mediator of drug abuse treatment.[92] Treatment efforts are successful when drug abusers are receptive toward treatment, understand the risks of abusing drugs, and identify the benefits of stopping.[92] In other words, treatment efforts are more likely to be successful when subjects are adequately motivated to change their behaviors.

However, compared with adult drug abusers, adolescent abusers might be less motivated to change their behaviors and less likely to accept that they have drug abuse problems.[72] For example, a study on high school alcohol users found 49% of the sample at the precontemplation stage[60] of behavior change.[45] Hence treatment programs targeting adolescents need to be able to motivate them to seek treatment and comply by treatment protocol.[52] A large number of adolescents with less serious problems miss treatment opportunities because of lack of motivation.[52] In other words, motivation is a prerequisite for the success of other treatment strategies, such as cognitive-behavioral skills training, which includes self-control, planning, self-monitoring, and decision-making treatment strategies.

Smith and Anderson[72] argue that much of adolescent alcohol-related problem behaviors can be explained in terms of an interplay between personality factors such as behavioral disinhibition and learned or acquired pro-alcohol outcome expectancies. According to their model, over time, disinhibited adolescents learn to yield more readily to positive outcome expectancies of alcohol than negative.[72] Teaching adolescents cognitive skills such as self-instruction[41] to allocate attention on negative consequences of drug use rather than positive ones would be one way to treat biased outcome expectancies.[72] For example, an intervention could train adolescent drug users on mentally reviewing and countering the positive consequences of drug use with negative ones.[72] Another treatment strategy that Smith and Anderson[72] recommend deals with restructuring memory associations, such as replacing incentives associated with drug use in memory with deterrents. For example, metamemory techniques can be used to train adolescents on selectively retrieving negative experiences of past drug use episodes when confronted with a new drug use situation.[39,72] Treatment components should also include additional cognitive-behavioral strategies, particularly those dealing with self-control, stress management, and coping, which are especially important in helping individuals sustain through recovery. For example, meditation and mindfulness techniques, which are not commonly used in adolescent drug use treatment, can be implemented to improve attention and stress management[31] and reduce withdrawal-related symptoms.

Interventions based on motivational interviewing combine motivational enhancement with cognitive-behavioral therapy.[52] Brief motivational interviewing interventions have been found to be effective in reducing drug use among adults and young adults. Sussman's[77] review of youth tobacco use cessation programs found that most school-related programs tend to use cognitive-behavioral strategies compared with very few that use motivational enhancement, even though programs that use motivational enhancement tend to have higher quit rates.

Motivation Enhancement and Motivational Interviewing

Motivation enhancement techniques serve to clarify desire for and reduce ambivalence toward change. This may include, but is not restricted to, a specific strategy such as motivational interviewing.[46] Motivation enhancement helps participants to clarify their direction of change and increases their willingness to change. Motivation enhancement may also include use of response-contingent reinforcement, which reinforces quit behavior with the chance for extrinsic rewards such as money or prizes.[77] In one of the largest controlled field trials of a school-based teen smoking cessation program that uses various motivating activities (e.g., games, talk shows), Sussman et al.[78] found that 17% of adolescents who received the treatment stopped smoking at 3-month follow-up compared with 8% of the control adolescents. The clinic curriculum of Project EX consisted of eight sessions spread over 6 weeks.[78] The motivation component in the first session was represented by a talk show where family and friends confront smokers about their habits. In session three, adolescent smokers were involved in a game that intended to teach them about the negative effects on one's body of the harmful substances in tobacco.[78]

Motivational interviewing is a type of brief intervention (i.e., comprising one to five sessions), based on the theoretical principles of stages of change model (the transtheoretical model),[60] client-centered therapy,[65] and cognitive behavioral therapy. As advocated by client-centered therapy, motivational-interviewing attempts to motivate individuals to change their health risk behaviors through a nonjudgmental and nonconfrontational form of counseling.[46] In order to assist individuals to take action and maintain the behavior change, motivational interviewing programs usually intend to help individuals toward building self-regulatory skills that are essential in coping with stress and solving personal as well as interpersonal problems.[52]

As a treatment and harm-reduction technique, motivational interviewing has a relatively long history of effectiveness among alcohol-dependent adults.[52] More recently, researchers have begun to apply the technique on adolescent drug users too (e.g., Monti et al.[47]). In a systematic review of motivation interviewing trials on adolescents and emerging adults, Grenard et al.[27] located 17 treatment studies that dealt with alcohol use, tobacco use, multiple drug use, and injury-related outcomes. These interventions,

TABLE 48.1	Potential Intervention Strategies to Improve Adolescent Executive Function Skills.
Executive Functions	**Strategies**
Attention	Attentional control skills instruction (e.g., self-instruction strategies to help shift attention), mindfulness training
Memory	Training on metamemory (e.g., selective memory retrieval)
Working memory	Task practice (e.g., backward digit span task), mindfulness training
Inhibitory control	Self-control skills instruction (e.g., practice control signals poster, self-instruction, delay of gratification strategies)
Planning	Self-regulation skills instruction (e.g., making action plans; practice control signals poster), motivational interviewing
Decision making	Social and emotional problem-solving skills instruction (e.g., dialoguing, internal verbalization of speech), motivational interviewing
Monitoring	Self-regulation skills instruction (e.g., practice behavioral and emotional analyses, Feeling Face cards, life skills training)

five of which reported successful outcomes, were set in hospital outpatient clinics and emergency rooms (e.g., a youth visiting an emergency room after a drinking-related incident), colleges and universities, psychiatric hospitals, and other outpatient clinics. Evidently, most interventions tended to target adolescents with relatively serious drug use problems and none of them were school-based. Furthermore, the majority of the studies (i.e., 9 of 17) dealt with alcohol use only.[27]

Providing one-to-one motivational interviewing sessions in school-based settings might be a daunting effort, but it is certainly not impossible. Methods used by alcohol abuse interventions among young adults in college settings (e.g., Marlatt[40]) could be applied to adolescents in high schools. For example, drug-using adolescents could be screened and referred to school clinics, where they would be assisted by trained motivational interviewers.[48] Another possible way of utilizing motivational interviewing in school-based prevention or treatment practices is to combine it with a longer intervention. In an ongoing school-based intervention study, Sussman and colleagues are testing the effects of adding a telephone-based motivational interviewing component to an existing teen drug abuse prevention curriculum. Motivational interviewing has a prospect of proving effective in treating adolescent drug abuse in a school setting.

Conclusions and Future Directions

Table 48.1 lists examples of strategies that could be used to alter the executive functioning of children or adolescents with the aim of preventing or treating drug abuse. Novel techniques that might help assist age-related development of executive functioning are being increasingly tested (e.g., Klingberg et al.[33] and Olesen et al.[53]) and seem to have relevance to school-based prevention and cessation programming.

To implement these strategies, school-based drug use prevention and cessation programming should consider important findings from the field of neuroscience. First, programs should be tailored to meet the appropriate developmental stage of youth, considering both age and the special needs of certain subgroups (e.g., students raised in poverty or exposed to abuse). Treatments that require a certain level of emotional and cognitive processing should ensure that the psychophysiological skills have been developed by participants. Second, the neurocognitive mediators acting between the intervention and drug outcome need to be carefully measured. Third, the social environment must be considered, since resources, support systems, and messages delivered in the intervention may not be available in the general community (i.e., lack of community or family support not to use drugs, lack of financial resources to quit smoking such as the nicotine replacement patch). Thus it is important to assist youth to develop executive functioning skills to plan and obtain resources from their environment (identify treatment centers, plan transportation, consider options of treatment centers). Finally, much more research is needed to substantiate and improve the application of neuropsychological models to school-based drug use prevention and research.

Acknowledgment

This paper was supported by grants from the National Institute on Drug Abuse (No. DA13814, DA016090, DA020138, and P50 DA16094).

References

1. Black DS, Milam J, Sussman S. Sitting-meditation interventions among youth: a review of treatment efficacy. *Pediatrics*. 2009;124(3):532–541.
2. Black DS, Milam J, Sussman S, Johnson CA. Testing the indirect effect of trait mindfulness on adolescent cigarette smoking through negative affect and perceived stress mediators. *J Subst use*. 2012;17:417–429.
3. Bardo MT, Donohew RL, Harrington NG. Psychobiology of novelty seeking and drug seeking behavior. *Behav Brain Res*. 1996;77(1–2):23–43.
4. Barkley RA. Behavioral inhibition, sustained attention, and executive functions: constructing a unifying theory of ADHD. *Psychol Bull*. 1997;121(1):65–94.
5. Beauchemin J, Hutchins TL, Patterson F. Mindfulness meditation may lessen anxiety, promote social skills, and improve academic performance among adolescents with learning disabilities. *Complementary Health Pract Rev*. 2008;13(1):34–45.
6. Botvin G, Baker E, Dusenbury L, Tortu S, Botvin E. Preventing adolescent drug abuse through a multimodal cognitive-behavioral approach: results of three studies. *J Consult Clin Psychol*. 1990;58:437–446.
7. Botvin G, Schinke S, Epstein J, Diaz T. Effectiveness of culturally focused and generic skills training approaches to alcohol and drug abuse prevention among minority youths. *Psychol Addict Behav*. 1994;8:116–127.
8. Brown SA, Tapert SF, Granholm E, Delis DC. Neurocognitive functioning of adolescents: effects of protracted alcohol use. *Alcohol Clin Exp Res*. 2000;24(2):164–171.
9. Chambers RA, Taylor JR, Ponteza MN. Developmental neurocircuitry of motivation in adolescence: a critical period of addiction vulnerability. *Am J Psychiatry*. 2003;160:1041–1052.
10. De Bellis MD, Clark DB, Beers SR, Soloff P, Boring AM, Hall J. Hippocampal volume in adolescent onset alcohol use disorders. *Am J Psychiatry*. 2000;157:737–744.
11. De Bellis MD, Keshavan MS, Beers SR, Hall J, Frustaci K, Masalehdan A. Sex differences in brain maturation during childhood and adolescence. *Cereb Cortex*. 2001;11:552–557.
12. De Bellis MD, Narasimhan A, Thatcher DL, Keshavan MS, Soloff P, Clark DB. Prefrontal cortex, thalamus, and cerebellar volumes in adolescents and young adults with adolescent-onset alcohol use disorders and comorbid mental disorders. *Alcohol Clin Exp Res*. 2005;29(9):1590–1600.
13. Eggert LL, Thompson EA, Herting JR, Nicholas LJ, Dicker BG. Preventing adolescent drug abuse and high school dropout through an intensive school-based social network development program. *Am J Health Promotion*. 1994;8:202–215.
14. Ehrenreich H, Rinn T, Kunert HJ, Moeller MR, Poser W, Schilling L, et al. Specific attentional dysfunction in adults following early start of cannabis use. *Psychopharmacology*. 1999;142:295–301.
15. Felver JC, Celis-de Hoyos CE, Tezanos K, Singh NN. A systematic review of mindfulness-based interventions for youth in school settings. *Mindfulness*. 2016;7:34–45.
16. Felver JC, Tipsord JM, Morris MJ, Racer KH, Dishion TJ. The effects of mindfulness interventions on children's attention regulation. *J Atten Disord*. 2014. https://doi.org/10.1177/1087054714548032. Advanced online publication.
17. Fishbein DH. The importance of neurobiological research to the prevention of psychopathology. *Prevent Sci*. 2000;1(2):89–106.
18. Fishbein DH, Hydeb C, Eldreth D, Paschall MJ, Hubal R, Das A, et al. Neurocognitive skills moderate urban male adolescents' responses to preventive intervention materials. *Drug Alcohol Depend*. 2006;82:47–60.
19. Fuster JM. *The Prefrontal Cortex*. London: Elsevier; 2008.
20. Garrison Institute Report. *Contemplation and Education: A Survey of Programs Using Contemplative Techniques in K-12 Educational Settings a Mapping Report*. 2005. Retrieved October 12, 2008, from http://www.garrisoninstitute.org/programs/Mapping_Report.pdf. Accessed October 12, 2008.
21. Giancola PR, Tarter RE. Executive cognitive functioning and risk for substance abuse. *Psychol Sci*. 1999;10:203–205.
22. Giedd JN. Structural magnetic resonance imaging of the adolescent brain. *Ann NY Acad Sci*. 2004;1021:77–85.
23. Giedd JN, Blumenthal J, Jeffries NO, Castellanos FX, Liu H, Zijdenbos J, et al. Brain development during childhood and adolescence: a longitudinal MRI study. *Nat Neurosci*. 1999;2:861–863.
24. Greenberg MT. Promoting resilience in children and youth: preventive interventions and their interface with neuroscience. *Ann NY Acad Sci*. 2006;1094:139–150.
25. Greenberg MT, Kusché CA, Riggs N. The PATHS curriculum: theory and research on neurocognitive development and school success. In: Zins J, Weissberg R, Walber H, eds. *Building School Success on Social and Emotional Learning*. New York: Teachers College; 2004.
26. Grekin ER, Sher KJ. Alcohol dependence symptoms among college freshmen: prevalence, stability, and person-environment interactions. *Exp Clin Psychopharmacol*. 2006;14(3):329–338.
27. Grenard JL, Ames SL, Pentz MA, Sussman S. Motivational interviewing with adolescents and young adults for drug-related problems. *Int J Adolesc Med Health*. 2006;18(1):53–67.
28. Habeych ME, Sclabassi RJ, Charles PJ, Kirisci L, Tarter RE. Association among parental substance use disorder, p300 amplitude, and neurobehavioral disinhibition in preteen boys at high risk for substance use disorder. *Psychol Addict Behav*. 2005;19(2):123–130.
29. Jacobsen LK, Krystal JH, Mencl WE, Westerveld M, Frost SJ, Pugh KR. Effects of smoking and smoking abstinence on cognition in adolescent tobacco smokers. *Biol Psychiatry*. 2005;57(1):56–66.
30. Jacobsen LK, Mencl WE, Constable RT, Westerveld M, Pugh KR. Impact of smoking abstinence on working memory neurocircuitry in adolescent daily tobacco smokers. *Psychopharmacology*. 2007;193(4):557–566.
31. Kabat-Zinn J. *Full Catastrophe Living: Using the Wisdom of your Body and Mind to Face Stress, Pain, and Illness*. New York: Delacorte; 1990.

32. Kaunhoven RJ, Dorjee D. How does mindfulness modulate self-regulation in pre-adolescent children? An integrative neurocognitive review. *Neurosci Biobehav Rev.* 2017;74:163–184.

33. Klingberg T, Fernell E, Olesen PJ, Johnson M, Gustafsson P, Dahlström K, et al. Computerized training of working memory in children with ADHD – a randomized, controlled trial. *J Am Acad Child Adolesc Psychiatry.* 2005;44(2):177–186.

34. Kolb B, Wishaw IQ. *An Introduction to Brain and Behavior.* 2nd ed. New York: Worth Publisher; 2005.

35. Koob GF. Neural mechanisms of drug reinforcement. *Ann NY Acad Sci.* 1992;654:171–191.

36. Lee J, Semple RJ, Rosa D, Miller L. Mindfulness-based cognitive therapy for children: results of a pilot study. *J Cogn Psychotherapy.* 2008;22(1):15–28.

37. Lubman DI, Yucel M. Drugs, mental health and the adolescent brain: implications for early intervention. *Early Interv Psychiatry.* 2008;2:63–66.

38. Lubman DI, Yucel M, Hall WD. Substance use and the adolescent brain: a toxic combination? *J Psychopharmacol.* 2007;21(8):792–794.

39. Lyon GR, Krasnegor NA. *Attention, Memory, and Executive Functioning.* Baltimore: Paul H. Brookes; 1999.

40. Marlatt GA. Basic principles and strategies of harm reduction. In: Marlatt GA, ed. *Harm Reduction: Pragmatic Strategies for Managing High-Risk Behaviors.* New York: Guilford; 49–66.

41. Meichenbaum D. *Cognitive Behavior Modification: An Integrative Approach.* New York, NY: Plenum; 1977.

42. Meiklejohn J, Phillips C, Freedman ML, et al. Integrating mindfulness training into K-12 education: fostering the resilience of teachers and students. *Mindfulness.* 2012;3(4):291–307.

43. Metcalfe J, Mischel W. A hot/cool-system analysis of delay of gratification: dynamics of willpower. *Psychol Bull.* 1999;106(1):3–19.

44. Mezzich AC, Tarter RE, Giancola PR, Lu S, Kirisci L, Parks S. Substance use and risk sexual behavior in female adolescents. *Drug Alcohol Depend.* 1997;44:157–166.

45. Migneault JP, Pallonen UE, Velicer WF. Decisional balance and stage of change for adolescent drinking. *Addict Behav.* 1997;22(3):339–351.

46. Miller WR, Rollnick S. *Motivational Interviewing: Preparing People to Change Addictive Behavior.* New York: Guilford; 1991.

47. Monti PM, Barnett NP, O'Leary TA, Colby SM. Motivational enhancement for alcohol-involved adolescents. In: Monti PM, Colby SM, O'Leary TA, eds. *Adolescents, Alcohol, and Substance Abuse.* New York: Guilford; 2001.

48. Myers M, Brown SA, Tate S, Abrantes A, Tomlinson K. Toward brief interventions for adolescents with substance use and comorbid psychiatric problems. In: Monti PM, Colby SM, O'Leary TA, eds. *Adolescents, Alcohol, and Substance Abuse.* New York: Guilford; 2001.

49. Nagel BJ, Schweinsburg AD, Phan V, Tapert SF. Reduced hippocampal volume among adolescents with alcohol use disorders without psychiatric comorbidity. *Psychiatry Res.* 2005;139(3):181–190.

50. Napoli M, Krech P, Holley L. Mindfulness practice training for elementary school students. *J Appl School Psychol.* 2005;21:99–125.

51. National Institute on Drug Abuse. *Drug Abuse Prevention: What Works.* Bethesda, MD: National Institute on Drug Abuse; 1997.

52. O'Leary Tevyaw T, Monti PM. Motivational enhancement and other brief interventions for adolescent substance abuse: foundations, applications and evaluations. *Addiction.* 2004;99(2):63–75.

53. Olesen PJ, Westerberg H, Klingberg T. Increased prefrontal and parietal activity after training of working memory. *Nat Neurosci.* 2003;7:75–79.

54. Palmgreen P, Lorch EP, Stephenson MT, Hoyle RH, Donohew L. Effects of the office of national drug control policy's Marijuana initiative campaign on high-sensation-seeking adolescents. *Am J Public Health.* 2001;97(9):1644–1649.

55. Paus T. Mapping brain maturation and cognitive development during adolescence. *Trends Cogn Sci.* 2005;9(2):60–68.

56. Pentz MA. Integrating mindfulness into school-based substance use and other prevention programs. *Subst Use Misuse.* 2014;49:617–619.

57. Pentz MA, Jasuja GK, Rohrbach LA, Sussman S, Bardo MT. Translation in tobacco and drug abuse prevention research. *Evaluation Health Professions.* 1006;29(2):246–271.

58. Pentz MA, Riggs NR, Warren CM. Improving substance use prevention efforts with executive function training. *Drug Alcohol Depend.* 2014;163:S54–S59.

59. Pope HG, Gruber AJ, Hudson JI, Cohane G, Huestis MA, Yurgelun-Todd D. Early-onset cannabis use and cognitive deficits: what is the nature of the association? *Drug Alcohol Depend.* 2003;69:303–310.

60. Prochaska JO, DiClemente CC. Stages and processes of self-change of smoking: toward an integrative model of change. *J Consult Clin Psychol.* 1983;51(3):390–395.

61. Quickfall J, Crockford D. Brain neuroimaging in cannabis use: a review. *J Neuropsychiatry Clin Neurosci.* 2006;18(3):318–332.

62. Riggs NR, Greenberg MT. The role of neurocognitive models in prevention research. In: Fishbein D, ed. *The Science, Treatment, and Prevention of Antisocial Behaviors: Evidence-Based Practice.* Vol. II. Kingston, NJ: Civic Research Institute; 2004:8-1–8-20.

63. Riggs NR, Jahromi LB, Razza RP, Dilworth JE, Mueller U. Executive function and the promotion of social-emotional competence. *J Appl Develop Psychol.* 2006;27:300–309.

64. Robinson TE, Berridge KC. Incentive-sensitization and addiction. *Addiction.* 2001;96(1):103–114.

65. Rogers CR. The necessary and sufficient conditions of therapeutic personality change. *J Consult Psychol.* 1957;21(2):95–103.

66. Rones M, Hoagwood K. School-based mental health services: a research review. *Clin Child Family Psychol Rev.* 2000;3(4):223–241.

67. Saltzman A. *Mindfulness in the Classroom: Park Day School August 9th–10th 2008.* Research summary; 2008. Retrieved 1 September 2008 from http://www.stillquietplace.com.

68. Schonert-Reichl KA, Oberle E, Lawlor MS, et al. Enhancing cognitive and social-emotional development through a simple-to-administer mindfulness-based school program for elementary school children: a randomized controlled trial. *Dev Psychol.* 2015;51:52–66.

69. Semple RJ, Reid EFG, Miller L. Treating anxiety with mindfulness: an open trial of mindfulness training for anxious children. *J Cogn Psychotherapy.* 2005;19(4):379–392.

70. Shure MB. *I Can Problem Solve: An Interpersonal Cognitive Problem-Solving Program. Intermediate Elementary Grades.* Champaign, IL: Research; 1992.

71. Shure MB. *Raising a Thinking Preteen: The I Can Problem Solve Program for Eight-to-Twelve-Year-Olds.* New York: Owl/Holt; 2001.

72. Smith GT, Anderson KG. Personality and learning factors combine to create risk for adolescent problem drinking: a model and suggestions for intervention. In: Monti PM, Colby SM, O'Leary TA, eds. *Adolescents, Alcohol, and Substance Abuse.* New York: Guilford; 2001.

73. Spear L. The adolescent brain and age-related behavioral manifestations. *Neurosci Biobehav Rev.* 2000;24:417–446.

74. Staiger P, Kambouropoulos N, Dawe S. Should personality traits be considered when refining substance misuse treatment programs? *Drug Alcohol Rev.* 2007;26:17–23.

75. Steinberg L. Cognitive and affective development in adolescence. *Trends Cogn Sci.* 2005;9(2):69–74.

76. Sussman S. Development of a school-based drug abuse prevention curriculum for high-risk youths. *J Psychoactive Drugs.* 1996;28(2):169–182.

77. Sussman S. Effects of sixty-six adolescent tobacco use cessation trials and seventeen prospective studies of self-initiated quitting. *Tobacco Induced Dis.* 2002;1(1):35–81.

78. Sussman S, Dent CW, Lichtman KL. Project EX: outcomes of a teen smoking cessation program. *Addict Behav.* 2001;26(3):425–438.

79. Sussman S, Earleywine M, Wills T, et al. The motivation, skills, and decision-making model of drug abuse prevention. *Subst Use Misuse.* 2004;39(10–12):1971–2016.

80. Tarter R. Neurobehavior disinhibition in childhood predisposes boys to substance use disorder by young adulthood: direct and mediated etiologic pathways. *Drug Alcohol Depend.* 2004;73(2):121–132.

81. Tarter RE. Etiology of adolescent substance abuse: a developmental perspective. *Am J Addictions.* 2002;11(3):171–191.

82. Tarter RE, Kirisci L, Mezzich A, et al. Neurobehavioral disinhibition in childhood predicts early age at onset of substance use disorder. *Am J Psychiatry.* 2003;160:1078–1085.

83. Trauth JA, Seidler FJ, Ali SF, Slotkin TA. Adolescent nicotine exposure produces immediate and long-term changes in CNS noradrenergic and dopaminergic function. *Brain Res.* 2001;892(2):269–280.

84. Trauth JA, Seidler FJ, McCook EC, Slotkin TA. Adolescent nicotine exposure causes persistent upregulation of nicotinic cholinergic receptors in rat brain regions. *Brain Res.* 1999;851(1–2):9–19.

85. Trauth JA, Seidler FJ, Slotkin TA. An animal model of adolescent nicotine exposure: effects on gene expression and macromolecular constituents in rat brain regions. *Brain Res.* 2000;867(1–2):29–39.

86. Wagner EF, Tubman JG, Gil AG. Implementing school-based substance abuse interventions: methodological dilemmas and recommended solutions. *Addiction.* 2004;99(2):106–119.

87. Williams RJ, Chang SY. A comprehensive and comparative review of adolescent substance abuse treatment outcome. *Clin Psychol: Sci Pract.* 2000;7(2):138–166.

88. Wills TA, Dishion TJ. Temperament and adolescent substance use: a transactional analysis of emerging self-control [see comment]. *J Clin Child Adolesc Psychol.* 2004;33(1):69–81.

89. Wills TA, DuHamel K, Vaccaro D. Activity and mood temperament as predictors of adolescent substance use: test of a self-regulation mediational model. *J Pers Soc Psychol.* 1995;68(5):901–916.

90. Wills TA, Sandy JM, Yaeger A. Temperament and adolescent substance use: an epigenetic approach to risk and protection. *J Pers.* 2000;68(6):1127–1151.

91. Wilson W, Roy M, Turkington T, Hawk T, Coleman RE, Provenzale J. Brain morphological changes and early Marijuana use: a magnetic resonance and positron emission tomography study. *J Addict Dis.* 2000;19(1):1–22.

92. Winters KC. Assessing adolescent substance use problems and other areas of functioning: state of the art. In: Monti PM, Colby SM, O'Leary TA, eds. *Adolescents, Alcohol, and Substance Abuse.* New York: Guilford; 2001.

93. Xiao L, Bechara A, Cen S, Grenard JL, Stacy AW, Gallaher P, et al. Affective decision-making deficits, linked to a dysfunctional ventromedial prefrontal cortex, revealed in 10th-grade Chinese adolescent smokers. *Nicotine Tobacco Res.* 2008;10(6):1085–1097.

94. Yücel M, Lubman DI. Neurocognitive and neuroimaging evidence of behavioural dysregulation in human drug addiction: implications for diagnosis, treatment and prevention. *Drug Alcohol Rev.* 2007;26(1):33–39.

49

The Therapeutic Community for Drug Abuse Treatment: A Journey Yet Unfolding in the Recovery Movement

DAVID A. DEITCH AND LILIANE DRAGO

CHAPTER OUTLINE

Introduction

Since we finished this chapter in 2012, there has been a notable gap in therapeutic community outcome research. Although systematic reviews of the research in recent years on the therapeutic community conclude that therapeutic communities produce positive outcomes on substance use, employment, criminality and psychological health,[47,65] both interest and financial resources in support of this model have atrophied. Chief among the likely causes of this wane in interest in the therapeutic community model are funding sources that are increasingly limiting treatment duration and intensity, and the overarching concerns with promoting treatments whose effectiveness can be demonstrated in randomized controlled trials (RCTs). The random assignment of clients to treatment is ethically and practically challenging, as is the reduction of a purposefully multifaceted intervention such as the therapeutic community to a single controlled independent variable.

What studies that are marginally present seem to end by 2012 and those were of the therapeutic community in correctional settings. Even in this limited scope (i.e., prison-based treatment of substance use disorders) the therapeutic community model has given way to the pervasive dominance of evidence-based treatment practices, particularly cognitive behavioral therapy (CBT). Although many studies have supported the CBT outcomes, particularly in the management of depression and anxiety, which have had years of positive outcomes, these approaches have shown declines in effectiveness in the past few years.[36] The looming suspicions for this reversal are the fidelity of implementation, a problem associated with all of the RCT-supported treatment practices, most of which demonstrate their outcomes under conditions that are difficult to replicate with the resource limitations with which most substance use disorder treatment programs operate.

As with the limits imposed on substance use disorder treatment in the greater community, the longer-term therapeutic community approaches in corrections have been curtailed by housing and population control measures aimed at moving inmates out as soon as they are perceived to be safe to the greater civilian community.

Is this the beginning of the end for the therapeutic community model, once heralded as a breakthrough treatment, showing ambitious and meaningful outcomes on abstinence, employment, criminality, and psychological improvement?

Origins

It is wrong to assume that there has always been a specific and widely accepted understanding of what is meant by a therapeutic community. The designation has an ancient pedigree and a historic association with diseases of appetite and the concept of mutual help. By the late 20th century, it had come to identify a specific mode of treatment for substance misuse, addiction, and other behavioral disorders based on the power of the treatment community to change attitudes and behavior through mutual help and a regimen of structured activities and expectations. This is a regimen designed to promote compassion and responsibility, foster self-awareness, enable social learning, and make possible the acquisition of social capital.

At the dawn of the Christian era, in 25 BCE, Philo Judaeus wrote,

"They are called communitae therapeutrides ... because they profess an art ... more excellent than in general use ... for medicine only heals the bodies but [these] heal the souls which are under the mastery of terrible ... incurable diseases of pleasures and appetites."[29]

(Curiously, the term "appetitive" became a neurobehavioral declaration regarding addictive behavior in the late 20th and early 21st centuries—as supported by neuroimaging techniques that became available in the late 20th century.) Thus it appears that the struggle with uncontrolled appetite behavior was a challenge then, as it is now, and the ancients embraced an approach not unlike the therapeutic communities of today.[18]

We can presume that Philo, writing in Alexandria early in the 1st century, was describing the early Essene communities, where according to the Qumran Community rules of order and duty, life was meant to conform to the following principles: concern for the state of our soul and our physical survival; search for meaning (transcending truths); challenge and admonish with love; be invasive—accountable to the community; public disclosure of acts, fears, hopes, guilt; public expiation for wrongs done; banishment is possible—done with concern for survival; and leadership by elders—by models.

These same principles have been present in mutual help communities from early monastic splinter groups to the much later Methodist congregations that espoused a "return to first principles" and morphed into the early Oxford movement.[68] It may well be that combining two sets of rules—one imposing rigid moral and behavioral standards and the other promoting humanizing compassion and forgiveness—is why these principles have so often and so successfully been brought to bear on delinquent or deviant behavior, problems of social maladaptation, and finally on addictive behavior and other problems of appetite.

This can be seen in the spread of religiously based mutual help societies in Western Europe during the 17th and 18th centuries. Responding to the widespread overuse of alcohol, they launched temperance efforts in Europe, which spread to America. Many of these early attempts at appetite control included temporary residential support and pledges of abstinence.[68] Key principles embraced by these mutual help groups included disclosure (confession), admonition, commitment, and conversion of others. By the 1800s, the spread of these principles had influenced the development of the Washingtonian and numerous other small groups.

Before World War II, however, the term "therapeutic community" occurs only once, when it was applied to the care of orphans in 18th century Russia. It was next revived in wartime England at Northfield Hospital, a facility dedicated to the treatment of traumatized British troops. There, two psychiatric innovators, Maxwell Jones and Tom Maine, sought to reapportion authority and decision-making between staff and patients.[3,11]

They began referring to the democratic therapy that they introduced at Northfield Hospital as a therapeutic community, designed to reverse the dynamics of the traditional psychiatric hospital, which many had come to believe infantilized patients, exacerbating their disability and rendering them incapable of functioning outside the hospital environment. Patients in Northfield psychiatric units became the active decision makers, taking on increasing responsibility for ward management. Early discussions among these pioneers resulted in five basic assumptions: two-way communication at all levels; decision-making at all levels; shared leadership; consensus in decision-making, and social learning by social interaction with emphasis on the here and now.[37]

The horizontal, open system of communication, based on those five principles, was itself assumed to result in healing. It did, in fact, produce marked improvement among community members, and such success made the need for individualized treatment plans seem unnecessary (a notion that would later become doctrine in American drug treatment therapeutic communities). Maxwell Jones went on to become a teacher of this method in Europe and the United States throughout the 1950s and 1960s, influencing younger psychiatrists, particularly at state psychiatric hospitals in Washington, Oregon, New Mexico, and other Southwestern states.[38] However, not until the late 1970s did Jones become aware of and engage with the American drug treatment therapeutic community movement.[53]

The drug treatment therapeutic community was not introduced by any of the nurses or psychiatrists who, inspired by Jones, sought to develop similar treatment models. Its origin is attributed to a group that emerged in Venice Beach, California, in 1958, when an Alcoholics Anonymous member, Charles E. (Chuck) Dederich, started an organization he called Synanon, embodying mutual help principles of Alcoholics Anonymous and characterized by hierarchical structure, a semi-open communication system, and small group interactions focusing on behavioral change.

Not unlike other charismatic and gifted figures, Dederich brought his own background—corporate, Midwestern, and Depression-influenced—to the organization he founded. As is often the case when strong leading theoreticians mount efforts designed to alter human behavior, the organization took on the personality of its founder. Imitation of the leader—in dress, language, and general demeanor—became a defining characteristic of Synanon and an influence on subsequent therapeutic communities.

Dederich launched Synanon by breaking away from the Alcoholics Anonymous group he had been attending. Within the tradition of Alcoholics Anonymous, anyone can pick up the *Big Book* and start his own meeting. When Dederich and the few members who followed him started their meeting in Venice Beach in 1958, the community was loaded with "alkies," "pill-heads," and a few "junkies." These people, living on the edge of society in the pleasant, hospitable, Southern California beach community, were sleeping on the beach, begging for money, making drug deals, and essentially staying intoxicated with the drug of their choice or whatever else they could get. It was a setting ripe for an evangelical salvation-oriented mission.

With the help of a dedicated few, Dederich and his followers obtained funds to open a club and, in a tradition easily traced back 200 years, encouraged folks to drop in for conversation in hopes of gaining sobriety. Dederich began holding long meetings in which his innate verbal talents and wide range of interests—from corporate structures to Zen and Transcendental philosophies—drew growing audiences and proved a powerful magnet for membership.

Hearing of these meetings, the availability of food and rumors of easy sex, a few heroin users recently released from the California prison system dropped in. Contrary to their expectations, they were immediately confronted by a loud, bombastic host, who assured them they were welcome, but only if they were willing to help out. "There's no free lunch," Dederich told them, and this proved an attractive challenge to some, since it was such a departure from the traditional social work style they anticipated.[7]

A nascent community came into being made up of Dederich's Alcoholics Anonymous cadre, former prisoners, quasi-homeless addicts from the beach, and an upscale contingent of musicians and other artists. Core members from outside the area began moving in, renting the readily available small cabin rooms along Venice Beach. Later in that first year, the group acquired an armory on the beach in Santa Monica, which gave members a chance to live together, pool their funds, share meals, and begin to seek financial support in the community, soliciting donations of cash, foodstuffs, and other living supplies. It also challenged Dederich to organize, preside over, and control community life.

A large man, highly verbose and partially deaf, Dederich spoke at length and high volume. He loved to argue and debate, inspiring heated confrontation among members. These confrontations became a common style of interaction within the group, valued for the relief that many members claimed such abrasive exchanges brought them. Soon formalized, this mechanism was first called "The Synanon" after the name of their organization. By 1964 the Synanon began to be referred to as the "game."

It is from the Synanon game that the therapeutic community encounter evolved. What Dederich added to the fundamental Alcoholics Anonymous mechanism of self-disclosure was the muscle of confrontation. Alcoholics Anonymous rejects both invasiveness and cross-talking. Although no one at an Alcoholics Anonymous meeting interrupts, questions, or challenges a speaker, the game encouraged this kind of spirited exchange.

As the game developed, so did the ethical demands of mutual responsibility. Although no drug use was an early requirement of the group, many members continued to use. Troubling questions arose: What then is the responsibility of others in the group? Are they obliged to expose their drug-using fellow members?

The issue came to a head at what later became known as the "Night of the Big Cop-Out," when a number of drug users were "outed" and others "copped to" their use. At this point, the role of the community as monitor was established along with the principle of expulsion from the group for drug use.[7]

As a daily schedule took shape, work tasks necessary to operation of the community were assigned and a schedule of daily seminars established to broaden the intellectual horizon and knowledge base of members. A distinct corporate-like hierarchy was formed, with a top-down structure based on coercion ("our way or the highway") and leadership determined and rewarded by Dederich. The early rewards included special living quarters, special food, access to vehicles, and the ability to acquire girlfriends or boyfriends and sleep with them. (The euphemisms were "courting" and "steady dating.")

Early on, Synanon began organizing the process of drug treatment into a series of phases. Phase One was live in and work in; Phase Two, work out and live in; and Phase Three, live out, work out, and maintain membership. But very soon, by 1960, Phase One had grown from 2 to 6 months in response to relapse among members in Phases Two and Three.[28] By 1962, during a period of rapid membership growth, Phase One was extended to at least 1 year. Nevertheless, relapse continued to occur in Phases Two and Three. As a result, the work out and live out phases were entirely eliminated in 1964, with Dederich rationalizing that "Our members remain healthy and drug free while with us—so that we are obviously a healthier community than is the greater society."[21] At this point, the effort once labeled by *Life* magazine as a "Miracle on the Beach" began its drift into increasingly wilder utopian community fantasies and ultimately into a cult capable of criminal behavior (pleading no contest to charges of soliciting an assault and conspiracy to murder).

Early Expansion

Not surprisingly, and consistent with the experience of other psychosocial movements, there were breakaways from Synanon by 1964. These breakaways, while troubled by the Synanon's flaws, still took with them a deep belief in the essential elements of a treatment model that had made it possible for them to achieve and sustain abstinence. They also, however, carried with them a vision of treatment as redemption and the Synanon belief that they had the only right answer. Theirs was a point of view that perceived addiction, if not as a moral weakness and sin, then as a disorder of character.[7] Thus they were not only entitled to, but charged with, correcting such flaws by whatever means necessary within the limits of the law.

It was at this moment that new opportunities were created by growing demand for a response to the seemingly intractable problem of addiction to heroin and other illicit drugs. By the early 1960s, heroin use was expanding, particularly in urban America. The accompanying increase in crime brought to the surface public frustration with the failure of stern anti-addiction measures to effect change. Longer and longer minimum mandatory sentences for drug law offenses and civil commitment of addicts for treatment with lengthy stays in federal hospitals did not produce abstinence outcomes.

The notion that abstinence might not be a rational expectation had surfaced back in the early 1950s when Victor Vogel, MD, who then oversaw addiction treatment at the United States Public Health Hospital at Lexington, Kentucky, wrote that "If treatment results are compared with those in other chronic or recurrent diseases such as TB… arthritis… hypertension … diabetes … or cancer—results in this field (drug treatment) are good."[49] But this early glimpse of addiction as a chronic disease was ignored. Both the public and the afflicted either hoped for or wanted an answer called "cure." Synanon had promised such a miracle and so did the first spin-off, Daytop Lodge in New York.

Daytop Lodge was a research project based on Synanon. It was supervised by Brooklyn's Chief of Probation Joseph Shelly and his lead psychologist Alex Bassin. The acronym stood for Drug Addicts Treated on Probation. The population consisted of 35 male felons who accepted treatment at Daytop under probation supervision rather than prison sentences.[60] This marked a serious departure from the mutual help members involved in volitional recovery. Money in the past was begged or provided as charity. Now it was underwritten by government and administered by a criminal justice agency. It should be noted that this was the first step in what came to be known as therapeutic community institutionalization, and a new term, "ex-addict," came into use. The project had a shaky start with a rapid turnover of leadership. In October 1964, under a new and more experienced leadership team and with increased financial support from New York City, the program was reorganized, and Daytop Lodge morphed into Daytop Village.

Probation was no longer a requirement for admission, and the program now accepted women. A board of directors was formed, chaired by co-founder Monsignor William B. O'Brien, a Bronx priest with strong ties to the New York archdiocese.[56] Alex Bassin joined the board. Daniel Casriel, M.D., a psychiatrist who had written the first book about Synanon, *So Fair a House*, was now psychiatric director and David Deitch was clinical and program leader.[9] Soon, a growing number of candidates sought admission, and by the end of 1965, there were 100 members/residents in a larger facility.[19]

In 1966, New York City's mayor, John V. Lindsay, recruited Efren Ramirez, MD, a psychiatrist from San Juan, Puerto Rico, to coordinate the city's narcotic treatment programs as commissioner of the city's new Addiction Services Agency. Dr. Ramirez had already developed systems of community engagement, protracted client induction processes, and treatment approaches similar to those of Daytop Village ("Daytop"). Ramirez developed a close working relationship with the program, and Daytop staff became a resource for him as he set out to expand the city's response to a growing heroin epidemic. It was Ramirez, trained in the Max Jones model, who persuaded Daytop, which had been calling itself a "humanizing community," to adopt the term "therapeutic community" to better describe its approach.

Dr. Ramirez was soon joined by Mitchell S. Rosenthal, MD, a psychiatrist who had developed an alcohol and drug treatment hospital unit at the Oak Knoll Naval Hospital in Oakland, California. There, he had introduced many of structural and group characteristics he had observed at a Synanon facility in San Francisco. Ultimately, Ramirez made him deputy commissioner for rehabilitation.

Commissioner Ramirez was also reaching out to other young psychiatrists in hopes of expanding addiction treatment. He created a weekly get-together of Deitch, Rosenthal, and a young psychiatrist still in residency training, Judy Densen-Gerber Baden. These meetings provided the impetus for an explosive growth of the model in New York City. Rosenthal developed Phoenix House, and Judy Densen-Gerber created Odyssey House.[25] Daytop lent staff to each of these projects, and help also came from other former Synanon members.[56]

In short order, these projects spun off other new starts: Samaritan Village and Project Return in New York City; Gaudenzia in Philadelphia; Village South in Miami; and Gateway in Chicago. All of them shared many similar beliefs, hierarchical structures, group activities, and goals.

There was also a significant role in the expansion of the therapeutic community played by the young psychiatrists who finished their training and served in the US Public Health Service. The earliest concentrations of addiction treatment were located at the US Narcotic Farm in Lexington, Kentucky, run jointly by the Public Health Service and the US Prison Service, and a similar facility in Fort Worth, Texas. These facilities accepted voluntary admissions as well as addicts convicted in federal territories or found guilty of federal offenses.[5]

Three of these psychiatrists emerged as leaders in addiction research and treatment. Jerry Jaffe, who was to become the first White House director of the Special Action Office for Drug Abuse Prevention, currently referred to as the Office of National Drug Control Policy, became familiar with therapeutic community methods at Daytop while at Albert Einstein Hospital in at New York City. Recruited by the Department of Psychiatry at the University of Chicago to serve as the director of drug abuse treatment programs for the State of Illinois, he subsequently recruited two Daytop staff members who helped him to further develop Illinois' first therapeutic community, Gateway Foundation. In order to secure a facility for Gateway, Jaffe took a lien against his own home so that the therapeutic community model would be part of the broad array of programs, from outpatient detoxification through methadone maintenance, he created in Chicago.

A second US Public Health Service psychiatrist, Herbert D. Kleber, had his introduction to addictions at the Lexington Hospital and went on to the Department of Psychiatry at Yale's medical school. There, he recruited Daytop staff to develop a separate Daytop Connecticut in New Haven. Kleber was subsequently tapped to become the Office of National Drug Control Policy's first deputy director for demand reduction. Another US Public Health Service Hospital psychiatrist, Fred Glaser, helped bring the therapeutic community program Gaudenzia to Philadelphia while teaching at Temple University.

This rapid spread of therapeutic communities was made possible by program members seeking a cure and communities in search of new and better ways to confront addiction. Unlike the Alcoholics Anonymous movement, which holds that "members are in recovery not recovered," the therapeutic communities believed that cure was possible.[19] This belief was reinforced when peers were seen to succeed. Use of the term "ex-addict" grew, and the expansion of the therapeutic community was now fueled not only by former Synanon members, but by graduates of these new and exciting programs.

Proliferation of the therapeutic community was carried on a wave of optimism characteristic of the era—a period of seemingly infinite possibilities, before the war in Vietnam clouded the political landscape. The climate of the times made possible the spread of therapeutic community doctrine by outsiders, for here was a treatment model with no academic provenance or research history that essentially invented itself. Pioneering psychiatrists who embraced the model did not come from the medical or mental health mainstream, and few of those first-generation program leaders had any professional credentials at all. What they did have was an ideology. The concept of giving to get—the notion of helping others to facilitate one's own recovery—was a philosophical cornerstone, as was the belief that healing was possible only when one was part of something greater and more important than oneself. The men and women who staffed the early therapeutic communities strived to submerge their separate identities. To them, the golden word was "we." Many of these early staffers—formerly gone astray, isolated and addicted themselves—needed that merged identity to heal themselves before they could help others heal.

As Deitch wrote many years later,[72]

> These outsiders ... created humanizing communities that espoused dignity of all people, equality between races and sexes, nonviolence and peace, heightened consciousness and spirituality, and action as the road to personal and social change. These first-generation ideologists committed themselves to a way of life that provided health, safety, caring, and honesty—sometimes brutal honesty. They censured deception, cheating, and gain at others' expense. The original version of these early crusaders—a vision that still holds true today—was a commitment to live and act as agents of positive social transformation. We believed that what goes around comes around.

The Formative Years

Admissions

The mindset of first-generation US therapeutic communities was shaped by the realities of the heroin epidemics of the 1950s and 1960s and the lack of much in the way of alternative treatment resources. Candidates for admission were not then greeted with open arms—admission, it was felt, had to be earned. One had to prove oneself ready for treatment. In some programs this meant demonstrating that one had hit bottom.

Therapeutic community membership was then, as it is now, deemed to be voluntary. But few candidates at any time have sought admission without some form of persuasion, generally from family, employers, or the legal system. The pressure on addicts to seek therapeutic community treatment was particularly strong in the 1960s, when there was great threat of arrest or civil commitment, particularly in New York, which held the greatest concentration of first-generation therapeutic communities.

Admission to most therapeutic community programs then generally involved heavy doses of dissonance. These ranged from the demand that applicants demonstrate commitment by daily telephone calls to the program and long waits in the interviewee chair. Interviews could be conducted by three or four program members who would challenge the applicants' candor, belittle their claims of sincerity, and demand they drop their drug user's street facade and adopt new language and behavior.[70] Clearly, this type of challenge and the levels of dissonance discouraged many applicants and prompted others to leave soon after admission, feeling both angry and confused or compromised. For those who stayed, however, many would subsequently claim that the dissonance experience left them more invested in the process that followed.

The Role of Family

Then as now, the pressure that brought many applicants to treatment came from their families. This posed something of a problem for the therapeutic communities, which wanted to keep families engaged but distant. They needed families to understand that they were vulnerable to manipulation and exploitation and must to learn to resist pleas for help from their addicted children—particularly for money.

A favored practice for dealing with families that remained committed to their addicted children was bringing a group of families together to discuss their concerns and answer their questions. These sessions led to the creation of an education program that dealt not only with therapeutic community goals, structure, and methods but also with the stages and nature of addiction. This practice was, in many ways, an innovation that was adapted by other groups to help family members deal with such other disorders as mental illness, autism, and alcoholism.

Families were taught, as were their loved ones in the program, the notion that when you care about someone, you must set limits on their behavior, which may, at times, mean denying them money, shelter, and other benefits that might enable addicts to keep using without facing the natural consequences of their behavior. This later evolved into the tough love philosophy, one that would become a central theme to a self-help movement for parents and others intimately involved with addicts and others with problem behavior.

Eventually, many therapeutic communities formed small groups for family members, where the staff would lead discussions about their attitudes, behaviors, and values. This was considered a way to explore conflicts that potentially abetted their loved one's drug use. The preferred means of encouraging frank discussion was the encounter group that aimed at revealing differences between stated goals or needs and actual behavior. The intensity of interaction at these family groups, however, did not rise to the level practiced in the treatment community, and there was little acceptance or use of harsh confrontation.[29]

The Hierarchy of Roles

Once admitted to the residential setting, the new member was introduced to the community's elaborate and hierarchical structure, much of which remains as a cornerstone in the American therapeutic communities to this day. Rank and status were based on work assignment, and newcomers were assigned to what was considered a bottom function, such as cleaning the toilets or washing dishes. These jobs were meant to make clear to the client his position at the bottom in status, and the need to do the job well in order to gain status and move up in the hierarchy (which was often called "growing up"). But work was only one element on which moving up was based. Attitude, change, and commitment to the treatment community were also considered. The theme constantly reinforced by leaders to those beneath them was, You can have my job and you can be in charge, but you must earn it!

Each of these work assignments was real and necessary to the actual functioning of the community. Facilities needed to be cleaned; food prepared and cooked; cars oiled, gassed, and repaired; walls painted; and rooms renovated. Household needs had to be met, and effort was made to solicit contributions of everything from milk to gasoline from the greater community.

All donations were accepted: used clothing, slightly stale bread, fruit and vegetables, old dishes, and cookware. It was all needed. There were also cash gifts and, by incorporating as nonprofit organizations, therapeutic communities were able to add the inducement of a tax deduction to the selling points of personal recovery and self-reliance.

Much also had to be done to run what was, in reality, a small business—write the letters; answer the phones; make agendas; ensure positive behavior, coordinate between departments, and represent the therapeutic community in the outside world. Each task was the responsibility of a specific department. Each department had its place within the hierarchy, and one's status depended on one's role within the department and the department's place within the community. One gained status first by moving up within a department and then by moving on to a department with a more complex or demanding function.

Over time, each member, depending on his investment in treatment (judged to be doing well by peers and elders) was promoted upward. The promotions were done with drama and praise and were part of the reward system. Each promotion was discussed internally and was used as an example to guests and visitors to show how the therapeutic community structure rewarded one with increasing amounts of responsibility for areas of work, productiveness, and oversight of others.

During this time, youth and adults were mixed together, as were genders. All were treated with the same methods, expectations, and accountability demands. There was then no consciousness of a need for formal education for this predominantly adult population, and vocational training was done on the job, in the classic apprenticeship tradition. The need for supervision and oversight within the departments and within the community created an interesting tension between trust and scrutiny.

The Interactive Healing Life

Group processes were then and still are the lifeblood of the therapeutic community. Every day, every member, staff, or client, and even steady visitors and friends, became involved in one group process or another.[19]

The community began the day with a morning community meeting where concerns were expressed and problems were solved. These meetings always began with a prayer or a statement of the program philosophy. Each therapeutic community group strove to be unique, creating its own language and terms to describe shared activities common to all other therapeutic community groups. Program philosophies became a critical means of identification and morale building. Many were created by the members themselves and reflect the spirit of the times and the intense need for affiliation, membership, and family. Indeed, the greeting, "Good morning, family," permeated most American therapeutic communities and (at least until the mid-1970s) most therapeutic communities outside the United States.

During these early formative years, the problems that came up at morning meetings often dealt with issues of survival, such as getting food for the table. Others were more mundane, like dealing with laundry, announcing visitors that day, or welcoming new members. Some were personal disclosures, making the community aware of some member's personal distress. These morning meeting public disclosures were greeted with "reach-outs," expressions of concern and support from others. There were "pull-ups" for tasks left undone and also "push-ups," applause and recognition for tasks accomplished. These activities generated positive feelings—laughter and energy to start the day. The meetings usually ended with mutual hugs.

Intellectual Exchange

There was usually a break in the workday in mid-afternoon for lunch followed by the "daily seminar." Participation was mandatory for all, including the leadership. The goal of the seminar was to broaden the intellectual vista of community members. It was an opportunity to make them familiar with ideas and concepts that they had perhaps never heard of before. Everyone became a tutor or mentor, reading up on subjects so it could be brought to the group. There, members were encouraged, cajoled, and sometimes coerced into taking part in discussion of matters that ranged across vast subject areas. Philosophy was discussed, along with science and literature. Sessions might focus on the works of Nietzsche or Freud or the writing of Hemingway or Faulkner. The seminar was an important part of daily life, not only for its content, but as a means of helping members learn to conceptualize and verbalize.

Small Group Interventions

Generally, every evening was reserved for small group process. These sessions were at first called "encounters," although some used the language of Synanon and called them the "game." One dimension of the encounter was its formation, for the makeup of each group was usually decided by elders in the program drawing on information they had received from various members. No less than twice weekly, when the call went out "encounter-time," every member experienced a moment of tension and anxiety. One never knew until that moment who might be in their group and how they might be perceived or challenged about their behavior, attitude, or social contribution to learning to live drug free. Encounters involved challenge, and often exaggerated elaboration of a person's behavior would be used to elicit truth, the admission of error, and acceptance of corrective action.[10]

In 1968, the psychologist O. Horbart Mowrer, who visited Daytop frequently and was certainly in the behavioral therapy camp, made a unique contribution to the encounter group by adding a new aspect—promise-making. Members would now make a commitment to another (or many others) in the group to change or adapt some specific behavior. One did not necessarily have to believe in the need for or use of this behavior, one merely had to practice it. Subsequently, such phrases as "act as if" or "go through a motion" became a commonplace part of early therapeutic community life.

Also in 1964, Deitch and Casriel began experimenting with groups lasting 18–30 hours. This was not a physically impractical notion at a time when all community members, including the directors, paid staff, and program elders, all lived either in the same facility or one close by. Therapy was an ongoing process, 24 hours a day, and interactive dialogues were primary aspects of community life.[10]

These long-lasting groups became known as marathons, and a set of methods and procedures slowly evolved. The staff who selected marathon participants would consider how the process could be the most useful for the member. However, common to all was the expectation of going deep toward the past, toward unresolved guilt and unrevealed strengths to discover, in the process, that one could be vulnerable in the face of fears and, by doing so, gain strength. The format began with autobiography, particularly aimed at early feelings of fear, shame, and defenses that became self-defeating.[10]

As hours passed and intimacy grew, an atmosphere of caring emerged with expressions of compassion, and attempts at resolution became key. This experience was heightened by the combination of sleep deprivation, limited external stimuli, and selected stimuli to provoke moods (usually music, mirrors, drawing supplies, and occasional props such as photographs). Usually, by 24 hours, all had experienced a sense of catharsis and acceptance by the others over conflicts, guilt, and regrets.

This marathon session would be followed by a break during which each participant was asked to be alone and reflect on the experience. They were usually escorted by a nonparticipating member who had experience with the process to a quiet, private space to sleep, eat, and think. After this 6-hour break, participants reconvened for feedback. This process became very carefully regulated after the first few years, with the participants asking for feedback being given a scribe to record those portions of the feedback they requested. After feedback, the members would talk about their commitments to the group.

Considering the regressive possibilities of this type of group, there was a safety net provided by the fact that they all lived together in a larger community of others equally committed to being there for each other. Most often, this experience resulted in peaks of love and compassion and group bonding. At this point a follow-up plan could be developed to monitor the keeping of commitments made during the marathon.[10]

These marathons and shorter versions, with fixed targets of inquiry known as probes, ultimately morphed into a static group that met weekly and where the emphasis was on maintaining the intimacy created by the marathon or probe for further deep work. By 1979, static groups were created for members regardless of marathon participation.

The General Meeting: A Response to Crisis and Bad Behaviors

Unlike the daily morning meeting, when one heard the announcement of a general meeting, therapeutic community members immediately headed for the meeting space knowing something big or bad had happened. Here, unlike at traditional meetings, the chairs were not arranged in a circle, but rather in a classroom format, with the front reserved for standing elders who had a message to deliver. These meetings did not occur often. When they did occur, it had to do with a serious threat (usually by a member's behavior) to the community's two principal taboos—no violence or even the threat of violence, and no drugs or alcohol. (Cigarettes were used by all members, and smoking was considered normative.) Such violations usually called for banishment of the offender. The meeting was to bring focus to the event, generate anger toward the offender, challenge the offender's right to remain, and vent fury at the threat to the community. The decision about whether an offender stayed or was banished was made as a result of the group's assessment of the offender's display of regret, seeking of forgiveness, and pleas to stay. Such a visible display and catharsis for the entire community was considered necessary for safety and the community's drug-free goals.[8]

Public acts of contrition also permeated normal daily life. Signs were hung around member's necks describing their failures to be honest, their propensity for manipulation, or some other set of behaviors requiring a high level of focus and embarrassment to the person. These signs were often quite creative and developed for a specific individual and the particular offense. Other signs for more common offenses were used routinely and could be kept in a closet until needed.[19]

Treatment Duration

All of the New York therapeutic communities and many others maintained a phase system with an average prescribed length of stay, in order to complete all phases, of 2 to 2.5 years. The early therapeutic communities believed in a full character makeover and the creation of a new prosocial role in society. Indeed, such roles were made possible by becoming change agents and taking on careerist roles of therapeutic community staff, which were in high demand.[18]

Understandably, considering the length of the prescribed stay, the problem of sexual needs and interaction was always present. Many attempts were made to resolve this dilemma. At first, permission to have sex was given if the heterosexual couple was behaving well in their community life, presented as stable in courting, and had been in treatment long enough to presume greater stability. This approach varied from program to program and often within the same programs.

The tradition at that time was to insist on couples' education groups, followed by encounter groups for couples meant to explore feelings and conflicts. When such couples demonstrated that the relationship was not compromising their positive treatment engagement, they were permitted a designated space and privacy for a given time period. This ranged from 2 hours for beginners to an overnight visit for residents who had been in treatment for a considerable time.

By the early 1970s, the controversy and complexity of permitting, condoning, monitoring safety, public relations, and couples' conflict resolution soon gave way to exhaustion and brought about an official end to this era. Henceforth, sexual identity and romance could be discussed, but sanctioned sexual interactions were no longer permitted. The admonishment—You are here to get better; those other aspects are off the table and impede your personal recovery—eliminated the conversation but not the problem. However, sexual interactions between staff and clients continue to plague the recovery and mental health communities to this day.

The Therapeutic Community's Coming of Age

Therapeutic community treatment spread throughout country as well as to Europe and the Philippines (where there were new heroin epidemics). Expansion to Europe followed the visits of medical and psychiatric professionals to New York, then a hub of heroin use and treatment. Daytop (and later Phoenix House and Odyssey House) had a tradition of welcoming overseas visitors and enjoyed displaying their accomplishments. By 1970, this exposure had led Dr. Griffith Edwards, a leading addiction specialist in Britain, to sponsor Phoenix House London. Daytop sent staff to Sweden (1972) and Canada (1973). In 1972, Community Emiliehoefe in The Netherlands began shifting from a democratic (Jones) therapeutic community model to a US model therapeutic community. In 1976, the first world federation conference of therapeutic communities took place in Sweden. There was to be continued growth in Europe, where expansion, which had initially involved the American therapeutic communities, was soon undertaken by the Europeans themselves.[43]

In the United States, a national conference was organized by the National Institute on Drug Abuse and a very newly formed Therapeutic Communities of America in January 1976. Prominent among participants were the New York City therapeutic communities, but also represented were therapeutic communities from Florida, Canada, Pennsylvania, New Jersey, Washington, DC, Illinois, Washington, California, Ohio, Arizona, Rhode Island, Maryland, and Wisconsin.[53]

However, the majority of the incorporators of the Therapeutic Communities of America remained in steady stable roles as chief executive officers, and their organizations grew in numbers of people treated and locations throughout the United States.

A key finding of the 1976 conference was that "… the therapeutic community is now determined to succeed in the public arena. In part this choice is a reflex to survive, but the therapeutic community is aware that it is an evolving institution!" Certainly there was prescient truth of what continues to this day. In 1974 there were 15,000 people in therapeutic community treatment … and major new drug-taking trends of type, method, and user populations.[53]

The proceedings of the 1976 conference were sensitive to vulnerabilities of the past, noting that "the communities are still dependent upon the emergent sanctioned leader. Despite an ostensible peer dynamic, individual therapeutic communities and the therapeutic community movement as a whole are very hierarchical in their internal process particularly in the selection, cultivation, and acceptance of their leaders…."[53] This, however, proved no bar to expansion. Although the majority of the incorporators of the Therapeutic Communities of America remained in steady stable roles as chief executive officers, their organizations thrived, growing in size and spreading to new locations throughout the country.

Therapeutic Community Research

The 1976 conference proceedings also called for more research on both process and outcomes. Three researchers—George DeLeon hired by Phoenix House,[22] followed a few years later by Vincent Biase, hired by Daytop and Sherry Holland hired by Gateway—began to publish a set of promising outcome studies attesting to efficacy of the therapeutic community model.

The most prolific outcome spokesman for the therapeutic community movement was George DeLeon, who completed a series of 5-year follow-ups that revealed an important term for the entire drug abuse field. Time in program showed that any dose of drug treatment—regardless of type—of less than 3 months' duration did not appear helpful.

By 1984, DeLeon had published five papers, first describing the sociodemographics of New York Phoenix House therapeutic community members, then the signs or types of pathology and differences between men and women at Phoenix House. But it was the 1984 paper on a study of effectiveness that found that therapeutic community graduates had significant improvements in areas of drug use, criminality, and employment, which became the rallying point used by all therapeutic communities. These positive outcomes, with observable effect beginning after 90 days of treatment, were found to increase with the amount of time spent in treatment. The success rate at 2 years' posttreatment was approximately 90% for graduates (members who both completed residential care and achieved 6 months or more of aftercare in good status), 50% for completers, and 25% for dropouts who remain more than 6 months and less than 1 year.[23] The relationship between time in program and posttreatment success was found by other researchers as well.[32,62]

Although there were critics then as even now, all of DeLeon's publications gave the entire field a sense of accomplishment and a right to brag (sometimes boast) that this was a model that produced drug-free cures, and regardless of cure, helped reclaim lives.

Early Therapeutic Community Studies

Outcome research by De Leon and others continued to demonstrate the value of therapeutic community treatment. In 1988, in another study at Phoenix House, DeLeon found that over 75% of Phoenix House graduates were both drug and crime free 5–7 years after completing treatment. In contrast, dropouts in DeLeon's sample were 31% drug and crime free, and only 25% of individuals who received less than 1 year of treatment were drug and crime free.

Following the Drug Abuse Reporting Program studies,[62] a series of national studies in the 1990s with large samples of clients continued to demonstrate the efficacy of therapeutic community treatment. In the Treatment Outcomes Prospective Study, it was found that the longer clients spent in therapeutic communities, the less likely they were to use heroin, cocaine, marijuana, and psychotherapeutic drugs, and the more likely they were to be employed full-time and to have committed no predatory crimes during the follow-up year.[12]

In four large-scale follow-up studies interviewing samples of more than 1000 clients—the California Drug and Alcohol Treatment Assessment,[27] the Services Research Outcomes Study, the National Treatment Improvement Evaluation Study, and the Drug Abuse Treatment Outcomes Study[59]—long-term therapeutic community treatment was found to produce greater reductions in marijuana, cocaine, and crack use 1 year after treatment than any other modality. Heroin use was reduced nearly as much as by methadone maintenance. Similar effects were shown for reductions in arrests and in drug selling. The Drug Abuse Treatment Outcomes Study also reported that full-time employment following long-term residential treatment was more than 250% greater than for any other modality. The National Treatment Improvement Evaluation Study found employment among former participants in long-term residential treatment nearly 200% the rate for any other treatment modality.

Dropout rates early in therapeutic community treatment are high, but similar to those across all substance abuse treatment modalities.[23,32,62] In his early studies, DeLeon reported completion rates from 10% to 20%, and 1-year retention was from 15% to 30%, with the highest dropout within the first 30 days. In the mid-1980s, DeLeon and psychologist Steven Schwartz reported 12-month retention rates ranging from 4% to 21% at seven therapeutic communities, with the dropout rate highest in the first 14 days and declining thereafter.

The Treatment of Adolescents and Findings

The Drug Abuse Reporting Program and Treatment Outcomes Prospective studies of the effectiveness of the therapeutic community when adolescents were treated with adults in the same programs yielded mixed but disappointing results on the reduction of substance abuse, particularly alcohol and marijuana. Positive outcomes were found on employment and criminal involvement. Retention of adolescents was similar to that found for adults, as was the time-in-program correlation with posttreatment improvement.

However, as the 1970s witnessed an explosion in adolescent drug use and a significant decrease in the average age at onset of drug dependency, calls were being made to treat adolescents separately from adults. Therapeutic communities developed adolescent day and outpatient programs, as well as residential therapeutic communities for teens only.[20] The regimens of these programs were designed to be responsive to the developmental tasks of adolescents.

Many of the programs incorporated educational programs. In the case of some of the larger residential therapeutic communities, these were at times annexes of local high schools that offered a full range of academic courses and services.

School attendance and homework took the traditional place of job functions in the therapeutic community regimen for adolescents, with job assignments relegated to after-school hours and weekends, similar to the balance of work and school responsibilities of most adolescents in the community at large.[24]

Recreation was also more prominent in the therapeutic community regimens of adolescent facilities compared to those for adults, predicated on the notion that teens needed a physical outlet for their energies that otherwise would be channeled into misbehavior, and that they needed to find ways of amusing themselves that did not involve the use of intoxicants.

Work with the adolescent population also necessitated working with their families. At Phoenix House, the use of multifamily therapy was pioneered with adolescent clients and their families.[39] This treatment approach capitalized on the strengths of group therapy, helping parents and other family members reduce their sense of shame and guilt with the help of similar peers, and built on the merits of the therapeutic community by creating a sense of belonging, social support, and collective identification. Subsequently, multiple studies have demonstrated improved outcomes for clients whose families are included in the treatment process and have demonstrated support for the use group approaches for families.[39]

In a RAND study by Andrew Morral et al., teens randomly assigned to a therapeutic community residential program and other types of residential settings were compared.[51] The adolescents who were in the therapeutic community program had superior outcomes on measures of drug use, criminal activity, and measures of psychological dysfunction. These findings were substantiated in a study of adolescents in six different therapeutic communities, whose members were found to have significant reductions in alcohol, marijuana, and other illicit drug use, as well as criminal and other deviant behavior.[35]

The holistic therapeutic community approach for adolescents proved especially useful, with its emphasis on the broader range of developmental tasks instead of exclusive focus on drug taking, given that some drug and alcohol use and risk-taking behavior is normative for young people in their late teens and early twenties. If abstinence is achieved in the months they are in the treatment setting, and gains are made in educational achievement and psychosocial development and functioning, adolescents may well reap significant and valuable therapeutic benefit, avoiding the high likelihood of intransigent addiction known to be the trajectory for youngsters who initiate substance abuse in early adolescence.[24]

To the 21st Century

Responding to two decades of remarkable advances in our understanding of the addicted brain, therapeutic communities slowly modified the early treatment methods that were predicated on a view of addicts as they presented in the 1950s. As is true for most diseases, it was the grossest manifestations of addiction that first came to the attention of therapeutic community workers. This reflected more than the severity of their drug involvement. Because of the illegal nature of heroin (opiate) abuse, most addicts of the 1950s were stereotyped, marginalized, and imprisoned with all kinds of other criminals. As a result, they developed the competencies necessary to survive as outsiders. They may have wished they wanted to quit, but they continued to use because they had very little, if any, other identity.

The heroin epidemic continued through the 1960s, but with the 1970s came widespread misuse of such other drugs as amphetamines, hallucinogens, and cocaine, and a new and more diverse population of drug users. They came from all social strata and had a broader range of education and economic resources.

The image of the addict as an end-stage user with concomitant social and psychological disorders began to change with the emergence of the 1970s users, predominantly white and middle class, and included numbers of college age users of hallucinogens.

While the 1960s had seen an expansion of methadone maintenance and therapeutic community treatment for heroin addiction, a new model of treatment, neither residential nor pharmacological, was developed for the drug abusers of the 1970s. The introduction of ambulatory care, labeled "outpatient drug-free,"[59] swelled the ranks of behavioral health care professionals engaged in the treatment of drug misuse. They were quite unlike the men and women who provided most Alcoholics Anonymous and therapeutic community–based treatments, whose role was as much a commitment as a calling and who themselves suffered from the disorder, learned the lore of the model that had helped them, and presented the same with zeal and deep belief.

The outpatient drug-free community drew psychologists, social workers, and others from the helping professions. This new work force brought with it standards of practice based on the delivery of care during set hours and in discreet units of either individual counseling or group therapy. This was quite different from what was being practiced in the therapeutic community and 12-step world of full-time recovery engagement and constant involvement (albeit with sloppy boundaries). It was, however, this professional model that soon came to influence all of drug treatment, particularly that which was funded directly or indirectly by government.

Changing Therapeutic Community Practices

As federal and state substance abuse agencies were created in 1969 in response to President Nixon's War on Drugs, the influence of new regulatory demands and the increased demand for practices that closely resembled hospital and medical clinics markedly changed therapeutic community practices.

Basic to the therapeutic community was the concept of clients and staff belonging to a single community in which therapy was an ongoing process, interactive dialogues were a primary aspect of community life, and counselors were fully engaged in this process, regardless of the time it took. Imposition of a strict 40-hour work week in which at least 10 hours was needed for paperwork (case notes, group notes, counseling notes, treatment plans, and revisions) played havoc with this concept.

Regulation and credentialization raised therapeutic community costs. The early therapeutic communities, built upon adult care paradigms, utilized a client (resident) workforce to perform all the many tasks necessary to maintain the community—food services, cleaning and repairs, auto maintenance, escort service, and administrative chores. Residents, as they rose in the hierarchy, also undertook supervisory functions. Moreover, the early therapeutic community was also predicated on a long-term care model, which gave the population a substantial group of more mature members who were actualizing recovery skills in their daily lives. Regulations now barred residents from certain tasks. Because counselors now spent substantially less time with clients and there were fewer senior residents (the elders of the early years) to serve as role models and monitors, staff needs increased. Whereas once a ratio of one counselor for 20 or even 30 residents was sufficient, regulations now called for ratios closer to 1:15.

Funding sources responded to increased costs with demands for shorter lengths of stay, and therapeutic community programs attempted to control expenditures by creating economies of scale, developing treatment settings capable of housing a client population in excess of—often far in excess of—150 residents. Although these settings were often able to reduce fixed costs for food and building supplies, they created issues of clinical management that also limited the time and quality of client interactions. One must consider Bill White's admonition regarding threats to viability: "The twin threats of professionalism (preoccupation with power or status) and commercialism (preoccupation with money or property) have often proved fatal to advocacy movements."[69]

The nature of therapeutic community treatment also reflected a changing treatment population. This was due, in part, to the criminal justice system's widespread acceptance of treatment as an alternative to incarceration for most nonviolent drug law offenders. The courts, probation, and parole authorities became, for most therapeutic community programs in the United States, a major if not the sole source of referrals.

The therapeutic community client base had, over the decades, come to display a rising level of pathology as seen in multigenerational use of drugs, with new court referrals often reflecting three or four generations of family use. These clients were quite different from addicts of the 1950s, who were most often adults, usually the first in their families to use drugs, and who accepted the view that something was wrong with them because of their drug use. This view eroded in the 1980s as a growing number of addicts came to reject the social view of drug-taking as deviant. They considered their drug-taking normative and the laws as deviant and blindly prejudiced against them. Unlike the burned-out residents of the past, who arrived exhausted by their jail experiences and addiction lifestyle, these court referrals arrived resenting their mandated treatment. Rather than viewing treatment staff as helpers who cared deeply about them, they tended to view program staff as "jailers."

Added to the forces reshaping therapeutic community treatment was the competition for clients. The days when therapeutic communities were the only option available and clients needed to demonstrate their commitment to be admitted were long gone. Because few addicts were now eager to submit to the therapeutic community's demanding regimen, the programs became increasingly reliant on court referrals, who lacked any real choice.

At this point a further challenge emerged from academics and federal researchers who challenged therapeutic community claims of effectiveness. The landmark, long-term, follow-up studies of George DeLeon and others that had demonstrated the pivotal role of time in program were faulted for lacking random assignment and the control groups that make up the gold standard of experimental design. These critical voices reinforced a jaundiced view of therapeutic communities taken by a number of academically trained professionals entering the field, who not only challenged the utility of the therapeutic community, but raised as an issue the potential harmfulness of therapeutic community practices.[50] This came at a time when many researchers, particularly those studying the treatment of other life-threatening disorders, were adopting new and more rigorous experimental design.[54] The call for more credible studies and more evidence-supported practices extended throughout the field of medicine and behavioral health.

Buffeted by these forces, therapeutic community credibility began to wane. Some therapeutic communities faced these doubts by digging in their heels and becoming more rigid and orthodox. Others began to modify methods and incorporate new clinical practices into the therapeutic community regimen. However, the stereotype of shame-based, attack therapy that humiliated its members, screamed and yelled at them, and broke them down to build them back up was kept alive by those who questioned the validity of the therapeutic communities. Although the overwhelming majority of therapeutic communities had long ago abandoned such primitive practices, the field was demoralized in the late 1980s by its failure to shake off the stereotypes.

In 1992, however, a new and more favorable light was cast on therapeutic communities with the publication of studies that documented the effectiveness of therapeutic communities in prison settings to reduce recidivism and/or increase the length of time between release and reincarceration. New York's Stay'n Out program led the way.[67] Then, the prison therapeutic community was tried in Delaware with similar promising outcomes. Evaluations of the Key/Crest program found that significantly more of the clients who completed the in-prison program and the transitional aftercare program remained arrest free during the follow-up (55%) than an untreated comparison group (29%).[48] Those who also received outpatient aftercare following the transitional residential treatment had the best outcomes, with 69% being arrest free after 3 years. Results for relapse to drug use were similar, reported for 17% of those who completed the in-prison therapeutic community only, 27% who had both the in-prison treatment and transitional residential treatment, and 35% who also had outpatient aftercare remaining drug free during the follow-up, compared to only 5% of the comparison group.[48] Five-year outcomes were similar.[34] Recidivism rates were significantly lower for those who went through both Key and Crest or through Crest. Participation

in the in-prison therapeutic community treatment alone did not appear to significantly improve 5-year outcomes, although it was associated with higher rates of aftercare use.

The federal government's Substance Abuse and Mental Health Services Administration subsequently sponsored a treatment project in two of California's prisons, and, by 1992, Texas had adopted prison therapeutic communities as the state's primary means of halting an ever-growing demand for prison construction.[42] California followed Texas and, by 2000, close to 8500 therapeutic community treatment slots existed in California's prisons. In each state, outcome data supported the financial investment in prison-based therapeutic community as a means of reducing rates of recidivism and extending the length of time former inmates remained out of prison.[41]

In the Amity program at the R.J. Donovan prison in California, follow-up studies found that 3 years post-parole only 27% of individuals who received both in-prison and aftercare treatment were reincarcerated during the follow-up interval, compared to 75% in the comparison group, 79% who completed only the in-prison treatment, and 82% who were in-prison treatment dropouts.[66]

Evaluation of the Kyle/New Vision program in Texas demonstrated that completion of 3 months of residential aftercare in a transitional therapeutic community followed by up to another year of supervised outpatient aftercare was the strongest predictor of remaining arrest free for 2 years following release from prison, and aftercare completion was strongly associated with parolee satisfaction with these programs.[31] Three-year follow-up studies showed that in-prison treatment followed by aftercare was most effective for high-risk, high-need offenders.[46]

The research showed that positive outcomes would be sustained only if prison therapeutic community treatment was followed by transitional care in the community. Therapeutic communities have been shown to be effective within a prison environment and significantly reduce recidivism. Positive outcomes improve significantly when in-custody treatment is followed by community-based treatment.[42,48,66]

Also gaining traction in the 1990s were drug courts,[14] offering coerced and highly monitored treatment in the community in lieu of prison or jail. As the nation increasingly came to realize that the treatment of addicted offenders—whether in prison or mandated by the courts—was reducing the social cost of crime and promoting health,[46] the therapeutic community approach was reevaluated and its reputation was substantially restored.[64]

Further studies of prison therapeutic communities, showing substantial variations in outcome, highlighted the need for therapeutic community clinicians to better understand aspects of criminality.[44] Most treatment providers had then presumed that criminal acts were a result of addiction, although, for 30%–50% of this population, criminal activity preceded drug misuse. What was becoming clear was the need to recognize and respond to individual client differences.[40]

This perception was widespread—and not only in prison therapeutic communities. Programs throughout the country recognized the need for differentiated care and turned to a variety of validated assessment instruments as the basis for differential diagnoses and individual treatment plans. Disorders were becoming more recognized, particularly depression and anxiety, and in women, the presence of trauma and posttraumatic stress disorder. Such data demonstrated even further the need for a mix of methods, approaches, intensities, and time in treatment.[71] Increasingly therapeutic communities both in prison and in the community have come to recognize the need for and benefit of adopting other evidence-based approaches, although the resulting changes have been met with varying degrees of enthusiasm, readiness, and workforce willingness.

The therapeutic community has undergone an extraordinary evolution over the years. Yet some troubling issues are being resolved only now, in this first decade of the 21st century. Many have long been aware that the therapeutic community treatment model was, in large measure, based on male paradigms. But only with today's greater gender sensitivities have those in the field finally come to realize that, because of the staggering amount of trauma visited upon women; some traditional therapeutic community practices (particularly the mixed gender encounter groups)[50] can have profound iatrogenic effects on women.[15]

What the therapeutic community has proven during its evolution is that a system once rigid and orthodox is capable of extraordinary flexibility and adaptability. This can be seen in the use of medications, lengths of stay, settings (residential or outpatient), transdisciplinary staffs, and the adaptation of evidence-based practices and validated assessment instruments. But what makes the therapeutic community unique is not simply the power of the community as a treatment force but the uses to which this force is put.

When therapeutic community practitioners speak of treating the whole person, they have in mind all the dimensions of the individual—the emotional and psychological, the physical, the social and vocational, as well as the intellectual, ethical, and spiritual. For each of these dimensions, there are discrete goals and means of employing the elements of mutual help to identify strengths, remedy deficits, build competencies, and foster the capacity for continued growth.

The Future of Therapeutic Communities for the Treatment of Substance Use Disorders

Although the failure of traditional medical approaches to address this complex disorder spurred the evolution of the therapeutic community, the medical model is now poised to again dominate the paradigm of substance use disorder treatment. The Affordable Care Act entails several provisions to expand coverage for substance use disorder treatment and to shift the way services are paid for, from public monies to expanded, yet typically limited, coverage under Medicaid and private insurance. The expectation has been that the care will delivered in a more "ambulatory-based, medically oriented, and physician-directed system" and to "to make greater use of pharmacological treatment and services delivered by health professionals."[4] This seems to represent a reversal to the biological reductionism of the past, when the approach to addiction focused more on the physical causes and correlates of addiction and less on the psychological, social, environmental, behavioral, and cultural in which it is often grounded and perpetuated by. This model of care and the continuous shortening of treatment that has been imposed by managed care does not support the therapeutic community model of treatment at best and undermines its survival at worst.

People with moderate to severe substance use disorders often have a multitude of interrelated mental health, social, functional, and behavioral issues that will undermine either single or fragmented approaches. As addiction has flourished over many decades, the impact of multiple generations of drug misuse have left a terrible shadow of psychic and physical health complications on the current generation of substance users. Sizable percentages of clients with substance use disorders have histories of psychological trauma and psychiatric disorders, further pointing to the need for a robust regimen of treatment. Many observers have noted that substance use disorders are overdetermined[17,45] in regard to the multiplicity of causative and correlating problems. Others have pointed to the difficulty in treating the multiple-problem client.[26]

Many drug-use disordered individuals with lengthy histories of drug use have lived many years within the drug culture, failing to develop prosocial reward activities, work skills and attitudes, or a social support network. There is a large population with needs for more rigorous construction or reconstruction of prosocial resources, cognitions, behavior, and attitudes. If outcomes-driven, this requires a more-suitable duration of time than the usual, at best, 1-week limitation on residential care. Because all models of care have been shifted under the rubric of medical management, what we see is funding influencing form not function.

What is well documented in the research on substance use disorder treatment is the linear relationship between time in treatment and posttreatment outcomes, with 90 days being the minimum needed for improvement across treatment modalities, and the need for continuing care after treatment in the community.[13,16,33,61] To continuously reduce the treatment duration and intensity flies in the face of years of empirical evidence.

The following are distinctive features of therapeutic community treatment that make it especially effective for individuals with moderate to severe substance use disorders.

Effective Elements of Therapeutic Community Treatment

1. Holistic Treatment—The conceptualization of moderate to severe substance use disorders being ones of the whole person requiring multiple interventions is appropriate. The milieu of the therapeutic community allows for the incorporation of individual counseling, a multitude of various types of group counseling, including many cognitive behavioral therapies, behavior therapy, family therapy, psychoeducation, job skills training, and medical and mental health services, with the amount or frequency of each to be tailored to each individual's needs.

2. Community Separateness/Community Environment—The separation of the individual from the environment in which he or she uses drugs is key for individuals with moderate to severe substance use disorders. The immersion of the individual in an environment that resembles the greater society to which he or she will eventually return can facilitate the development of skills, cognitions, and behavior, which will result in successful adaptation to the demands of a lifestyle of recovery. The use of job functions and school for both adolescents and adults facilitates the acquisition of vital life skills that clients will need upon return to the community. This prorecovery environment provides an alternate culture to which members belong, with the goal of replacing the drug, street, and criminal subcultures to which most individuals with more severe substance use disorders belong.

3. Structured Day—The order and structure of the therapeutic community environment has a schedule of therapeutic activities throughout the day, consisting of the appropriate delegation of time for personal hygiene and self-care, work, education, counseling, social activities, and recreation, and so on provides a routine that is both habilitative and rehabilitative.

4. Self-Help and Mutual Self-Help—The use of self-help and mutual self-help empowers therapeutic community members, teaching them to rely on themselves and peers, as opposed to professional staff, as much as possible. Community members are encouraged to serve as role models and peer helpers, and to use social support as a coping mechanism. This provides an induction into the culture of recovery, which is essential for the maintenance of recovery in the community following treatment.

Current Practices That Enhance the Therapeutic Community Approach

1. Motivational Strategies in the Induction Phase to Engage Clients and Reduce Drop Out—As indicated earlier, the high attrition of clients in the first 30 days of treatment, common in all forms of treatment, can be improved with motivational interviewing, provided during the assessment and in individual and group counseling.[6,30,58]

2. Trauma-Informed Practices/Trauma Specific Treatment—The high prevalence of trauma in clients with substance use disorders, suggests that any type of treatment incorporate principles of trauma-informed care and provide either treatment of trauma or referral for care. Trauma-informed care necessitates the elimination of any vestiges of a character-disorder orientation, the use of harsh confrontation, and disciplinary practices that are overly punitive. Instead assurance is made to promote physical and emotional safety, choice, empowerment, and collaboration. *Seeking Safety*, an evidence-based manualized cognitive behavioral treatment, a first-stage trauma treatment developed specifically for those with substance use disorders, is especially appropriate as it is designed for stabilization and can be used in the earliest phases of treatment.[52]

3. Co-Occurring Disorder Capabilities—Many therapeutic communities are already providing integrated care for co-occurring psychiatric disorders, and this needs to continue and expand. This entails having appropriate staffing, medication monitoring, and appropriate psychoeducation and counseling, and to address co-occurring mental and substance-related disorders in policies and procedures, assessment, treatment planning, program content, and discharge planning.[1,57]

4. Motivational Incentives/Contingency Management—The use of behavioral contingencies has long been used in the therapeutic community; however, there has often been an overreliance on negative contingencies. Positive reinforcement, such as status changes and privileges, has typically been used for more complex behavioral change, which has made it largely unavailable to newer clients. Programs that use motivational incentives effectively will increase the ratio of positive to negative consequences, incorporating more tangible and social reinforcement, especially in the early phase of treatment, for small steps toward the target behavior, and in close temporal proximity to the target behavior.[63]

5. Person-Centered Practices—Many therapeutic communities are adopting more person-centered practices, and this needs to continue. This includes the collaboration of the client and his or her family in all aspects of treatment; attention to the strengths, needs, abilities and preferences of each client in individualized treatment plans; differential points of emphasis in the therapeutic community regimen of services and activities, and counseling practices such as motivational interviewing, which respects each client's autonomy and their right and responsibility to make choices that will affect their lives.

6. Medication-Assisted Treatment—Most therapeutic communities have moved away from the bias against medication-assisted treatment and incorporate the use of addiction medication. This has been a positive move and offers much potential for the appropriate combination of medication and other therapies.[4]

Conclusion

There are a few organizations remaining with most of the characteristics we have described in the body of the chapter, except one. They refuse public funding and rely instead on social enterprise, that is, finding ways through commerce to self-support their enterprises. Although such approaches may have separate issues of coercion, misuse, or exploitation, they regardless may be very much like the early monastic churches that withdrew from an expanding church with their diluted practices, and instead tried and often succeeded at building models more associated with the original purpose of survival of soul and life.

Although we welcome the definition of substance use disorders as a health problem, rather than a moral or criminal one, our hope is that we will resist its oversimplification and short-sighted evaluations of the cost-benefit of appropriate treatment. Research and history has taught us that we need a range of treatments and approaches to the treatment of substance use disorders, that no treatment is right for everyone, and that support for recovery has to be long term and extended into the communities in which recovering people will live.

It seems that a variety of funding mechanisms may be necessary to continue to provide treatment like the therapeutic community, which does not fall neatly into the medical, acute care, or fee-for-service models. Such mechanisms have been recently developed in New York State and some others, where therapeutic communities have advocated for and succeeded in maintaining funding through the state administered block grant and other public monies, public assistance funds for congregate housing, and Medicaid dollars for clinical services with a Centers for Medicare & Medicaid Services (CMS) waiver. Reimbursement through commercial insurance is not always possible, although some therapeutic community organizations have negotiated rates for extended coverage, given the modest cost of this treatment compared to hospital-based inpatient programs. Organizations in other states are still struggling to find ways of financing care in the therapeutic community.[2,55]

We may also be well served to consider adopting research designs and methods beyond those that demand the reduction of complex processes into a single variable. We believe that the therapeutic community has much to offer in the continuum of care for substance use disorders, albeit with a continuous focus on empirically based enhancements, and that its distinctive and considerable merits warrant its preservation.

References

1. American Society of Addiction Medicine. *Patient Placement Criteria for the Treatment of Substance-Related Disorders: ASAM PPC-2R*. 2nd ed. Chevy Chase, MD: American Society of Addiction Medicine; 2001.
2. Bloom SL. *The Sanctuary Model*; 2011. Retrieved October 18, 2011, from http://www.sanctuaryweb.com/trauma-informedsystems.php.
3. Bridger H. *The Therapeutic Community Today: Proceedings of the First World Institute of Therapeutic Communities*. Rome, Italy: Center Italiano di Solidarieta; 1984.
4. Buck JA. The looming expansion and transformation of public substance abuse treatment under the Affordable Care Act. *Health Affairs*. 2011;30(8):1402–1410.
5. Campbell N, et al. *The Narcotic Farm*. New York, UK: Abrams Books; 2008:59–61.
6. Carroll, Kathleen M, et al. Motivational interviewing to improve treatment engagement and outcome in individuals seeking treatment for substance abuse: a multisite effectiveness study. *Drug Alcohol Depend*. 81(3):301–312.

7. Casriel D. *So Fair a House.* Englewood Cliff, NJ: Prentice Hall; 1963.
8. Casriel D, Amen G. *Daytop: Three Addicts and Their Cure.* New York: Hill and Wang; 1971.
9. Casriel D, Deitch D. *New Success in the Cure of Narcotic Addicts.* Physicians' Panorama; 1968.
10. Casriel D, Deitch D. The marathon: the time extended group therapy. *Curr Psychiatric Therapies.* 1968;8. Grune and Stratton.
11. Clark D. *The Therapeutic Community Over 40 Years: Some Personal Reflections in Proceedings of the First World Institute of Therapeutic Communities.* Rome, Italy: Center Italiano di Solidarieta; 1984.
12. Condelli W, Hubbard R. Client outcomes from therapeutic communities. In: Tims F, DeLeon G, Jainchill N (eds). *Therapeutic Community: Advances in Research and Application.* NIDA Research Monograph 144 (National Institute on Drug Abuse, NIH Publication No. 94-3633). Rockville, MD: National Institute on Drug Abuse; 1994:80–98.
13. Condelli WS, Hubbard RL. Relationship between time spent in treatment and client outcomes from therapeutic communities. *J Subst Abuse Treat.* 1994;11(1):25–33.
14. Cooper C. The characteristics of American drug court programs, Chap 9. In: Knight K, Farabee D, eds. *Treating Addicted Offenders – A Continuum of Effective Practices.* Kingston, NJ: Civic Research Institute; 2004:1–11.
15. Covington S. Helping women recover: creating gender-responsive treatment. In: Straussner L, Brown S, eds. *Handbook of Women's Addictions Treatment.* San Francisco: Jossey-Bass; 2002.
16. De Leon G. Is the therapeutic community an evidence-based treatment? What the evidence says. *Therapeutic Communities.* 2010;31:104–128.
17. De Leon, George. Therapeutic Communities for substance abuse: Overview of approach and effectiveness. *Psychol Addict Behav.* 1989;3(3):140–147.
18. Deitch D. Treatment of drug abuse in the TC historical influences, current considerations and future outlook. In: *National Commission on Marijuana & Drug Abuse: Report to Congress and the President.* vol. 5. Washington, DC: US Government Printing Office; 1973.
19. Deitch D, Casriel D. *The Role of the Ex-Addict in the Treatment of Addiction.* Federal Probation; 1967.
20. Deitch D, Zweben J. The impact of social change on treating adolescents in therapeutic communities. *J Psychoactive Drugs.* 1976;8:3.
21. Deitch D, Zweben J. *Synanon: A Pioneering Effort in the Treatment of Drug Abuse and a Signal for Caution. Clinical Issues in Drug Abuse.* Baltimore, MD: Williams and Wilkins; 1981:289–302.
22. DeLeon G. *Psychologic and Socio-Demographic Profiles of Addicts in the Therapeutic Community.* New York: National Institute of Drug Abuse Grant No. DA-00831. Author; 1976.
23. DeLeon G. *The Therapeutic Community: Study of Effectiveness. National Institute on Drug Abuse Treatment Research Monograph Series (ADM 84-1286). Superintendent of Documents.* U.S. Washington, DC: Government Printing Office; 1984.
24. DeLeon G, Deitch D. Treatment of the adolescent substance abuser in a therapeutic community. In: Friedman S, Beschner G, eds. *Treatment Services for Adolescent Substance Abusers* (DHHS Publication No. [ADM] 85-1342, pp 216–230). Rockville, MD: National Institute of Drug Abuse; 1985.
25. Densen-Gerber J. *We Mainline Dreams: The Story of Odyssey House.* Garden City, New York: Doubleday; 1973.
26. Evans K, Sullivan JM. *Dual Diagnosis: Counseling the Mentally Ill Substance Abuser.* New York: Guilford Press; 1991.
27. Gerstein D, Harwood H, eds. *(Institute of Medicine) Treating Drug Problems. A study of the Evaluation, Effectiveness, and Financing of Public and Private Drug Treatment Systems.* Vol. A. Washington, DC: National Academy; 1990.
28. Gerstel D. *Paradise Incorporated: Presidio.* Novato, CA: Synanon; 1982.
29. Glaser F. Some historical and theoretical background of a self-help addiction treatment program. *Am J Drug Alcohol Abuse.* 1974;1:37–52.
30. Hettema J, Steele J, Miller WR. Motivational interviewing. *Annu Rev Clin Psychol.* 2005;1:91–111.
31. Hiller M, Knight K, Simpson D. Prison-based substance abuse treatment, residential aftercare, and recidivism. *Addiction.* 1999;94(6):833–842.
32. Hubbard R, Marsden M, Rachal J, Harwood H. *Drug Abuse Treatment: A National Study of Effectiveness.* Chapel Hill: University of North Carolina; 1989.
33. Hubbard RL, Craddock MS, Anderson MS. Overview of 5-year followup outcomes in the drug abuse treatment outcome studies (DATOS). *J Subst Abuse Treat.* 2003;25(3):125–134.
34. Inciardi J, Martin S, Butzin C, Hooper R, Harrison L. An effective model of prison-based treatment for drug-involved offenders. *J Drug Issues.* 1997;27(2):261–278.
35. Jainchill N. Therapeutic communities for adolescents: the same and not the same. In: Deleon G, ed. *Community as Method: Therapeutic Communities for Special Populations and Special Settings.* Westport, CT: Greenwood Publishing Group; 1997.
36. Johnson TJ, Friborg O. The effects of cognitive behavioral therapy as an anti-depressive treatment is failing: a meta-analysis. *Psychol Bull.* 2015. American Psychological Association.
37. Jones M. *The Therapeutic Community: A New Treatment Method in Psychiatry.* New York: Basic Books; 1953.
38. Jones M. *Social Psychiatry in Practice.* Harmondsworth: Penguin; 1968.
39. Kaufman E, Kaufman P. *Family Therapy of Drug and Alcohol Abuse.* Needham Heights, MA: Allyn and Bacon; 1992.
40. Knight K, Farabee D. Should in-prison drug treatment be mandated? Offender Substance Abuse Report. 3(6):81–84.
41. Knight K, Hiller M, Simpson D. Evaluating corrections-based treatment for the drug-abusing criminal offender. *J Psychoactive Drugs.* 1999;31(3):299–304.
42. Knight K, Simpson D, Hiller M. Three year re-incarceration outcomes for in-prison therapeutic community treatment in texas. *Prison J.* 1999;79(3):337–351.
43. Kooyman M. The history of therapeutic communities – a view from europe. In: Rawling B, Yates R, eds. *Therapeutic Communities for the Treatment of Drug Users.* UK: Jessica Kingsley; 2001.
44. LaTessa E, Holsinger A. The importance of evaluating corrections programs: assessing out come and quality. *Corrections Manage Q.* 1998;2(4):22–29.
45. Levin JD, Weiss RH. *The Dynamics and Treatment of Alcoholism: Essential Papers.* Jason Aronson; 1994.
46. Lowel L, Wexler H. *The R.J. Donnavan in-Prison and Community Substance Abuse Program – Three Year Return to Custody Data.* New York: National Development and Research Institute; 1998.
47. Malivert M, Fatséas M, Denis C, Langlois E, Auriacombe M. Effectiveness of therapeutic communities: a systematic review. *Eur Addict Res.* 2012;18(1):1–11.
48. Martin S, Butzin C, Saum C, Inciardi J. Three year outcomes of therapeutic communities treatment for drug involved offenders in delaware. *Prison J.* 1999;79(3):294–320.
49. Maurer D, Vogel V. *Narcotics and Narcotic Addiction.* Springfield, IL: Charles C Thomas; 1954.
50. Miller W, Hester R. *Treating Addictive Behaviors Process of Change.* New York: Plenum; 1986:135.
51. Morral A, McCaffrey D, Ridgeway G. Effectiveness of community-based treatment for substance-abusing adolescents: 12-month outcomes of youths entering Phoenix academy or alternative probation dispositions. *Psychol Addict Behav.* 2004;18(3):257–268.
52. Najavits LM. *Seeking Safety: A Treatment Manual for PTSD and Substance Abuse.* Guilford Press; 2002.
53. National Institute on Drug Abuse. DeLeon G, Beschner G (eds). *Proceedings of the Therapeutic Community of America Planning Conference;* January 29–30, 1976, National Institute on Drug Abuse Services Research Report, US Department of H.E.W, Public Health Service Alcohol Drug Abuse and Mental Health Administration, DHEW Publication No. (ADM); 1976:77–464.

54. National Institute on Drug Abuse. *New Directions in Therapeutic Communities Research: Building a Partnership Between Research and Practice.* San Francisco, CA: Conference Overview; 2000:7.

55. Norwig Debye-Saxinger, personal communications, February 28, 2017.

56. O'Brien W, Henican E. *You Can't Do it Alone: The Daytop Way to Make Your Child Drug Free.* New York: Simon & Schuster; 1993.

57. Perfas FB, Spross S. Why the concept-based therapeutic community can no longer be called drug-free. *J Psychoactive Drugs.* 2007;39:69–79.

58. Secades-Villa R, Ramón Fernánde-Hermida J, Arnáez-Montaraz C. Motivational interviewing and treatment retention among drug user patients: a pilot study. *Substance Use Misuse.* 2004;39(9):1369–1378.

59. Sells S, Demaree R, Simpson D, Joe G, Gorsuch R. Issues in the evaluation of drug abuse treatment. *Professional Psychology.* 1977;8(4):609–640.

60. Shelly J, Bassin A. Daytop lodge – a new treatment approach for drug addicts. *Corrective Psychiatry.* 1965;2(4):186–195.

61. Simpson D, Joe GW, Brown BS. Treatment retention and follow up outcomes in the Drug Abuse Treatment Outcome Study (DATOS). *Psychol Addict Behav.* 1997;11(4):294–330.

62. Simpson D, Sells S. Effectiveness of treatment for drug abuse: an overview of the DARP research program. *Adv Alcohol Subst Abuse.* 1982;2(1):7–29.

63. Stitzer ML, Petry NM, Peirce J. Motivational incentives research in the national drug abuse treatment clinical trials network. *J Subst Abuse Treat.* 2010;38:S61–S69.

64. Tims F, Inciardi J, Fletcher B, MacNeil Horton A. *The Effectiveness of Innovative Approaches in the Treatment of Drug Abuse. Contributions in Criminology and Penology* Chapter 5. New York: Greenwood; 1997.

65. Vanderplasschen W, Colpaert K, Autrique M, et al. *Therapeutic Communities for Addictions: A Review of Their Effectiveness From a Recovery Perspective.* The Scientific World Journal; 2013. Article ID 427817.

66. Wexler H, Melnick G, Lowe L, Peters J. Three-year re-incarceration outcomes for Amity in-prison therapeutic community and aftercare in california. *Prison J.* 1999;79(3):321–336.

67. Wexler H, Williams R. The stay'n out therapeutic community: prison treatment for substance abusers. *J Psychoactive Drugs.* 1989;18:221–230.

68. White W. *Slaying the Dragon the History of Addiction Treatment and Recovery in America,* 1, 5–11. Chestnut Health Systems/Light House Institute; 1998.

69. White W. *Lets Go Make Some History: Chronicles of the New Addiction Recovery Advocacy Movement.* Washington, DC: Johnson Institute; 2008.

70. Yablonsky L. *The Tunnel Back: Synanon.* New York, NY: Macmillan; 1965.

72. Zweben J. Special issues in treatment: women. In: Ries RK, Fiellin D, Miller S, Saitz R, eds. *Principles of Addiction Medicine.* 4th ed. Chevy Chase, MD: American Society of Addiction Medicine; 2007.

71. Special focus section: pioneering treatment and recovery models. Zweben J, Deitch D, eds. *J Psychoactive Drugs.* 1997;29(2):127–163.

50

Substance Use–Focused Mutual-Help Groups: Processes and Outcomes

CHRISTINE TIMKO, L. BRENDAN YOUNG, AND RUDOLF H. MOOS

CHAPTER OUTLINE

Introduction

Twelve-step mutual-help groups, often also called self-help or support groups, are an important component of the system of care for individuals with substance use disorders. Individuals make more visits to mutual-help groups for help with their own or family members' substance use and psychiatric problems than to all mental health professionals combined. About 9% of adults in the United States have been to an Alcoholics Anonymous meeting at some time in their life, and almost 80% of adults who seek help for alcohol use disorders participate in Alcoholics Anonymous.[18] Moreover, many substance use disorder treatment providers have adopted 12-step principles in treatment, and the majority of them refer clients to mutual-help groups.

Mutual-help groups offer a forum wherein members can express their feelings in a safe, structured setting, improve communication and interpersonal skills, better understand the reasons for their unhealthy substance use, learn self-control, and identify new activities and life goals. Accordingly, the American Psychiatric Association[1] and several other professional and health care organizations recommend referrals to mutual-help groups as an adjunct to the treatment of individuals with substance use disorders.

Major Types of Substance Use-Focused Mutual-Help Groups

The majority of the literature on mutual-help groups that address substance use focuses on traditional 12-step groups for individuals using alcohol and drugs or for their family members and friends. The most prevalent traditional 12-step groups are Alcoholics Anonymous, Narcotics Anonymous, Cocaine Anonymous, and Al-Anon Family Groups; other important substance-use–focused mutual-help groups include Secular Organizations for Sobriety, SMART Recovery (Self-Management and Recovery Training), Moderation Management, and LifeRing. These groups are briefly described next. Women for Sobriety, Double Trouble in Recovery, and Dual Recovery Anonymous are described in the sections on women and individuals with substance use and psychiatric disorders.

Alcoholics Anonymous

Alcoholics Anonymous is a fellowship with the primary purpose of helping individuals with alcohol-related problems maintain sobriety. It is structured around the 12 Steps (e.g., admission of powerlessness over alcohol, belief in a higher power) and 12 Traditions (e.g., an emphasis on the common welfare and recognition that personal recovery depends on Alcoholics Anonymous unity). (See www.aa.org/pdf/products/p-42_abriefguidetoaa.pdf for the Twelve Steps and Twelve Traditions.) Other key aspects of Alcoholics Anonymous involve open and closed group meetings and literature that describes Alcoholics Anonymous, shares its tenets, and provides guidance to recovering individuals. Estimated Alcoholics Anonymous membership is about 1,300,000 members and 60,000 groups in the United States, and about 2,041,000 members and 115,000 groups worldwide; about 38% of the members are women (see www.aa.org).

Narcotics Anonymous and Cocaine Anonymous

Narcotics Anonymous is a fellowship of recovering individuals with drug use disorders. It grew out of and is similar to Alcoholics Anonymous in that it provides a structured support network in which members share information about overcoming addiction and living productive, drug-free lives through adherence to the 12 Steps and 12 Traditions. Narcotics Anonymous encourages complete abstinence from all drugs, including alcohol, but, like Alcoholics Anonymous, accepts the use of prescribed medications for psychiatric and medical disorders. Narcotics Anonymous has about 63,000 weekly meetings in more than 130 countries worldwide; about 76% of the members are Caucasian and 43% are women (see www.na.org).

Cocaine Anonymous is a fellowship open to individuals who want to stop using cocaine, including crack cocaine and other mind-altering substances. Its program of recovery was adapted from Alcoholics Anonymous and uses the 12-step recovery approach. There are an estimated 30,000 members and more than 2000 groups (see www.ca.org).

Al-Anon and Nar-Anon

The purpose of Al-Anon Family Groups, a mutual-help organization more commonly known as Al-Anon, is to support people who are affected by another person's drinking and/or drug use. The history of Al-Anon is intertwined with that of Alcoholics Anonymous. Alateen is the affiliate of Al-Anon for young people (mainly adolescents) who are affected by another's substance use. Al-Anon is the most widely used form of help for concerned family members and friends in the United States.[23] Currently, there are more than 28,000 Al-Anon groups and over 24,000 Alateen groups in 130 countries (see www.al-anon.org). Of Al-Anon members in the United States and Canada, 83% are women and 93% are white; on average, members are 56 years old. Nar-Anon Family Groups (Nar-Anon) was begun to help with another's addiction to drugs other than alcohol. It is a worldwide fellowship adapted from Narcotics Anonymous.

Secular Organizations for Sobriety

Secular Organizations for Sobriety provides support for individuals who seek to achieve and maintain sobriety, a forum to express thoughts and feelings about recovery, and a nonreligious or secular approach that does not depend on the 12 Steps or 12 Traditions.

Members are expected to acknowledge their addiction and take responsibility for achieving and maintaining sobriety. Members tend to be well-educated individuals who have been in professional treatment and have attended and continue to attend Alcoholics Anonymous. The majority of the members are men (see www.secularsobriety.org).

SMART Recovery

SMART Recovery (or Self-Management and Recovery Training) espouses a rational treatment orientation and focuses on teaching individuals new coping skills and more logical ways of thinking and acting. Using trained facilitators in about 2000 groups, it emphasizes practical methods of changing maladaptive behavior rather than a 12-step or spiritual approach. SMART Recovery's 4-point program includes: (1) building and maintaining motivation to abstain; (2) learning how to cope with urges; (3) managing thoughts, feelings, and behavior; and (4) balancing momentary and enduring satisfactions (see www.smartrecovery.org). A comparison of three groups of SMART Recovery participants—those only attending meetings in person, those using only a web application of the program, and those attending meetings and employing the web application—found that these interventions were equally effective. That is, participants in all three groups were significantly more likely at follow-up to be abstinent and to have fewer drinking- and substance-related problems.[29]

Moderation Management

Moderation Management construes problem drinking as a habit that can be controlled by applying principles of cognitive-behavioral therapy in the context of a network of supportive peers. It provides an alternative to the spiritually oriented disease model of traditional 12-step mutual-help groups and to an abstinence goal; it allows members a choice of abstinence or moderate drinking goals. Moderation Management members tend to emphasize the value of self-control, insight, personal responsibility and choice, and rationality. Most Moderation Management members are Caucasian; they tend to be married, college educated, and employed, and more than half are women (see www.moderation.com).

LifeRing

LifeRing Secular Recovery is an organization of people who share practical experiences and sobriety support, embracing what works for each individual. LifeRing believes that each individual has the desire to find lasting sobriety, thought of as the Sober Self. With addiction, the Sober Self has been submerged, but still exists. People also have an Addict Self that tries to control decision-making and leads to substance use. LifeRing supports efforts to strengthen the Sober Self and weaken the Addict Self by sharing advice, understanding, and encouragement. It is thought to work by positive social reinforcement. The membership is primarily male (57%), white (96%), college educated (91%), and not religious (56%) (www.lifering.org).

Participation in Mutual-Help Groups and Substance Use Outcomes

Individuals with substance use disorders who participate in 12-step mutual-help groups, especially Alcoholics Anonymous and Narcotics Anonymous, tend to experience better alcohol and drug use outcomes than do individuals who do not participate in these groups. The most common index of participation has been attendance at group meetings; however, attention has also focused on aspects of involvement, such as reading 12-step literature, working the steps, obtaining a sponsor, and doing service work.

Attendance and Substance Use Outcomes

People who attend Alcoholics Anonymous in the first few weeks or months after treatment tend to experience good short-term substance use outcomes. For example, Project MATCH was a large clinical trial that compared 12-step facilitation, cognitive-behavioral, and motivational enhancement treatment for individuals with alcohol use disorders. Participants who attended Alcoholics Anonymous more often in each of the 3-month intervals after treatment were more likely to maintain abstinence from alcohol in that interval. In addition, more frequent Alcoholics Anonymous attendance in the first 3 months after treatment was related to a higher likelihood of abstinence and fewer alcohol-related consequences in the subsequent 3 months; these findings held for participants in each of the three types of treatment.[89]

Comparable findings were obtained in two projects conducted among individuals with substance use disorders who were treated in residential programs. Among individuals in hospital-based programs, those who participated in 12-step mutual-help groups in the 3 months before 1-year follow-up were more likely to be abstinent, in remission, and free of dependence symptoms. Clients who attended more group meetings experienced better outcomes than did clients who attended fewer meetings.[66] Among individuals in community-based programs, those who attended more 12-step mutual-help group meetings in the 3 months prior to a 1-year follow-up were more likely to be abstinent at follow-up.[60]

Individuals who continue to attend mutual-help groups for a longer interval are more likely to maintain abstinence than are individuals who stop attending. In a 9-year follow-up of individuals with substance use disorders who entered treatment, Witbrodt et al.[95] found that 12-step meeting attendance trajectories were aligned with abstinence patterns. Individuals who had continuing high attendance rates were more likely to be abstinent. Individuals who initially had high attendance rates were likely to be abstinent, but as their attendance declined by year 5, so did their likelihood of abstinence. Individuals who initially had high attendance and abstinence rates but no attendance after year 1 had a sharply declining rate of abstinence. Individuals who initially had low attendance, but then increased their attendance, also increased their abstinence rates. As expected, individuals who reported low or no attendance had the lowest abstinence rates. In a companion study, Witbrodt et al.[96] tested causal relationships between posttreatment 12-step group attendance and abstinence over 9 years. More 12-step attendance during years 1 and 5 was causally related to past-30-day abstinence at years 5 and 7, respectively, suggesting that 12-step attendance leads to abstinence well into the posttreatment period.

Another prospective study of individuals with alcohol use disorders showed that a longer duration of attendance in Alcoholics Anonymous in the first year after help-seeking was associated with a higher likelihood of 1-, 8-, and 16-year abstinence. These findings were based on better outcomes for individuals who attended Alcoholics Anonymous for 17 weeks or more. Individuals who attended Alcoholics Anonymous for only 1–16 weeks had no better outcomes than nonattendees did. Moreover, after controlling for the duration of Alcoholics Anonymous attendance in year 1, the duration of attendance in years 2–3 and 4–8 was related to a higher likelihood of 16-year abstinence.[57,59]

Despite findings that more 12-step group attendance is associated with better outcomes, it is possible that self-selection bias (i.e., individuals who attend meetings are more motivated to change) inflates estimates of the benefits of attendance. Humphreys et al.[30] employed instrumental variables models with six data sets to derive an estimate free of selection bias of the impact of Alcoholics Anonymous attendance. Increased attendance that could not be attributed to self-selection was associated with higher rates of abstinence.

Another question is the extent to which Alcoholics Anonymous is helpful to individuals using substances other than alcohol. Individuals with drug use problems are most likely to attend Alcoholics Anonymous, which has many easily accessible groups, even though the less easily accessible Narcotics Anonymous was created to enhance recovery from drug addiction. A study of young adults found that patients with drug use problems who attended more Alcoholics Anonymous than Narcotics Anonymous meetings were as likely to be abstinent as those who attended mainly Narcotics Anonymous meetings.[42] These findings suggest that patients with drug use problems may obtain as much benefit from participation in Alcoholics Anonymous relative to Narcotics Anonymous, boosting clinical confidence in making Alcoholics Anonymous referrals for these individuals when Narcotics Anonymous is less available.

Although many in the addiction field see 12-step group participation and medication-assisted treatment for substance addiction as compatible, individuals using such treatment who attend 12-step meetings may experience conflicts or pressures to discontinue medications. Despite such concerns, one study found improved long-term outcomes (between 18 months and 4 years) for patients using medication-assisted treatment who also attended 12-step groups.[69] Similarly, Monico and colleagues[55] found that more 12-step meeting attendance during the first 6 months of medication-assisted treatment did not precipitate treatment discontinuation and was associated with superior abstinence outcomes. Even so, treatment providers may need to help patients navigate using both medications and 12-step groups to achieve recovery; for example, patients may be encouraged to seek groups that are more accepting of medication treatments.

Involvement and Substance Use Outcomes

Attendance is an important indicator of mutual-help participation, but it may not adequately reflect an individual's level of group involvement, as shown by such indices as acceptance of 12-step ideology, having a spiritual awakening, giving Alcoholics Anonymous talks, socializing with Alcoholics Anonymous members, becoming a sponsor, and self-identification as a group member. These aspects of group involvement may be associated with substance use outcomes independent of the duration and frequency of attendance per se.

In support of this idea, individuals who held stronger beliefs in 12-step ideology were more likely to be abstinent independent of their 12-step group attendance.[26] In the National Institute on Drug Abuse Collaborative Cocaine Treatment Study, individuals who increased their 12-step involvement in the first 3 months of treatment had better cocaine and other drug use outcomes in the next 3 months. Individuals who regularly engaged in 12-step activities but attended meetings inconsistently had better drug use outcomes than did individuals who attended consistently but did not regularly engage in 12-step activities.[93]

Caldwell and Cutter[11] identified a group of individuals who showed substantial attendance at meetings but mixed involvement in Alcoholics Anonymous practices. These individuals were less enthusiastic about the concept of a higher power and Alcoholics Anonymous literature and were less involved with other Alcoholics Anonymous members. They also had high relapse rates. Individuals who attend mutual-help groups but are unable to embrace key aspects of the program appear to be less likely to benefit from it.

Participation and Outcomes Other Than Substance Use

Participation in mutual-help groups is associated primarily with better substance use outcomes; however, it has also been linked with more self-efficacy and spirituality and less distress, better social support and functioning, and enhanced coping skills and community participation.

Participation in mutual-help groups has been associated with stronger self-efficacy for abstinence, less distress and depression, and fewer psychiatric symptoms.[57,59,60,66] Compared with individuals who had not worked all 12 steps, those who had worked all 12 steps had more self-esteem and social confidence and were more optimistic and trusting.[78] In addition, some studies have shown an association between participation in mutual-help groups and higher levels of spirituality and perceived meaning of life.[48]

There is a relatively robust relationship between mutual-help group involvement and better social support and functioning. For example, individuals with alcohol use disorders who attended more Alcoholics Anonymous meetings over a 3-year interval had more friend-related support; individuals who attended Alcoholics Anonymous longer over 1-year and 8-year intervals also reported more support from friends.[81] Similarly, individuals who attended Narcotics Anonymous once a week or more had more friends than did individuals who did not attend Narcotics Anonymous or attended infrequently.[17]

In a review of this area, Groh and colleagues[27] concluded that more involvement in Alcoholics Anonymous was associated with larger friendship networks, primarily due to acquiring an Alcoholics Anonymous sponsor and the development of new 12-step friends. Involvement in Alcoholics Anonymous was also linked to more specific support for abstinence from friends and to higher quality friendships and more general support. It is important to note that the strength of affiliation among Alcoholics Anonymous members may be comparable to or even stronger than feelings for close friends and family members.

Affiliation with 12-step mutual-help groups tends to promote more reliance on approach coping and behaviorally oriented substance use coping processes. For example, Snow and colleagues[76] found that individuals who were more involved in Alcoholics Anonymous were more likely to rely on coping responses aimed toward reducing substance use, such as spending time with non-drinking friends, talking to someone about their drinking problems, rewarding themselves for trying to stop drinking, and becoming more aware of social efforts to help people stop drinking. In addition, individuals who attend Alcoholics Anonymous for longer intervals tend to rely more on approach coping and less on avoidance coping.[81]

There has been speculation that the admonition against public self-identification as a member of Alcoholics Anonymous or Narcotics Anonymous may discourage participation in community activities. However, many long-term Alcoholics Anonymous and Narcotics Anonymous members are active in established neighborhood organizations and civic groups, such as homeless coalitions and parent-teacher associations.[48] Similarly, Alcoholics Anonymous participation has been associated with community helping activities, such as mentoring youngsters or doing volunteer work among alcoholic individuals in recovery.[99]

Al-Anon Participation and Outcomes

Empirical studies of Al-Anon, some of which were conducted in the 1980s and 1990s, reported that more attendance was associated with better outcomes. Al-Anon members reported improvements in understanding alcoholism, and in depression, assertiveness, self-acceptance, and relationships.[16] Several studies have involved family members (known as Concerned Others) concerned about individuals with alcohol use disorders who were resistant to treatment. Compared to wait-list controls, Concerned Others who were referred to therapy based on Al-Anon concepts or to Al-Anon reported reduced personal problems and emotional distress (depression, anxiety, anger), and increased self-esteem, coping behaviors, and relationship happiness.[6,19,54,64,72]

At a 6-month follow-up of newcomers to Al-Anon, both those who sustained attendance and those who stopped attending reported gains from Al-Anon. However, sustained attendees were more likely than those who stopped attending to report benefits in a number of domains, including learning how to handle problems due to the drinker, general well-being, functioning, and psychological symptoms.[83] Attendees were also more likely than those who stopped attending to report increases in daily, in-person contact with the drinker. The main issues that prompted Concerned Others to initiate Al-Anon attendance were problems with overall quality of life, the drinker, stress, and anger; Al-Anon helps Concerned Others with these main concerns. Longer-term members were more likely than newcomers to report better functioning in these domains. A recent study in Iran also found that women attending Al-Anon for 6 months or longer were better off than women attending their first Al-Anon meeting on measures of problem solving and quality of life.[22]

Connections Between Mutual-Help Groups and Treatment

Many individuals who enter professional treatment also participate in mutual-help groups; in fact, 50%–80% of individuals in substance use disorder treatment also participate in mutual-help groups, and 60%–80% of Alcoholics Anonymous members have participated in treatment.[51] These two sources of help could contribute independently to better outcomes, or they could either bolster or detract from each other.

Participation in Treatment and Mutual-Help Groups

In general, individuals who enter treatment are more likely to participate in mutual-help groups than are individuals who do not enter treatment. Compared with help-seeking individuals who entered only Alcoholics Anonymous, individuals who entered both treatment and Alcoholics Anonymous participated as much or more in Alcoholics Anonymous in the subsequent 15 years. Individuals who stayed in treatment longer in the first year after seeking help subsequently showed more sustained participation in Alcoholics Anonymous. More extended treatment later in individuals' help-seeking careers was not associated with subsequent participation in Alcoholics Anonymous, which suggests that treatment providers' referrals to Alcoholics Anonymous have more influence in the context of an initial treatment episode.[58]

Moreover, individuals who participate in mutual-help groups are more likely to enter and complete treatment. Clients with drug use disorders who attended mutual-help groups weekly before treatment stayed in treatment longer and were more likely to complete treatment. In turn, clients who stayed in treatment longer subsequently were more likely to attend Alcoholics Anonymous at least weekly.[25] In a study of individuals with alcohol use disorders, those who participated in both treatment and Alcoholics Anonymous attended more treatment sessions and more Alcoholics Anonymous meetings than did those who participated only in treatment or only in Alcoholics Anonymous.[87]

Several studies have shown a more specific link, in that individuals who participate in 12-step treatment, which introduces clients to 12-step philosophy and encourages them to join a group, are more likely to affiliate with mutual-help groups than are individuals who participate in treatment that is not oriented toward 12-step principles. In Project MATCH, participants in 12-step facilitation treatment were more likely to attend and affiliate with Alcoholics Anonymous than were those in cognitive-behavioral treatment or motivational enhancement treatment.[89] Similarly, in another multisite study, participants in 12-step facilitation programs affiliated more with 12-step mutual-help groups after treatment than did persons who were treated in cognitive-behavioral treatment programs.[31]

Twelve-step facilitation treatment may enhance the effectiveness of 12-step mutual-help groups. Humphreys and colleagues[31] identified a stronger relationship between 12-step mutual-help group participation and better substance use outcomes among clients from 12-step facilitation treatment programs than among those from cognitive-behavioral treatment or eclectic programs. Posttreatment mutual-help group involvement partially explained the higher rates of abstinence among individuals from 12-step programs than among those from cognitive-behavioral treatment programs.

A supportive and spiritually oriented treatment environment can enhance participation in 12-step activities. Clients in more supportive treatment environments increased more in 12-step involvement during treatment; that is, they were more likely to acquire a sponsor and 12-step friends and to read 12-step literature. Moreover, when clients who had a high risk of discontinuing attendance at mutual-help groups after treatment were treated in a more supportive environment, their risk of discontinuing declined.[40]

These findings suggest that referral and alliance processes contribute to an association between participation in treatment and subsequent participation in mutual-help groups. A positive treatment alliance may enhance clients' motivation for recovery and underlie the impact of counselors' recommendations to attend mutual-help groups. Treatment that highlights the value of 12-step mutual-help groups in recovery encourages more mutual-help group involvement than treatment that does not highlight this value.

Participation in mutual-help groups may reduce the need for some costly treatment services. A 3-year prospective study of individuals with alcohol use disorders found that those who chose to attend only Alcoholics Anonymous had treatment costs that were 45% lower than costs for people who chose to attend outpatient treatment; outcomes were similar for both groups.[32]

A multisite study found that patients who received cognitive behavioral therapy made more use of treatment, whereas patients who received 12-step–oriented treatment attended more Alcoholics Anonymous meetings. Accordingly, at 1-year and 2-year follow-ups, annual treatment costs for the patients who had received 12-step–oriented treatment were 64% lower, and they had higher abstinence rates.[33,34] A 7-year follow-up of adolescents treated for substance use disorders found that each additional 12-step meeting attended was associated with an incremental medical cost reduction of 4.7% ($145 per year in 2010 US dollars). The medical cost offset was largely due to reductions in hospital inpatient days, psychiatric visits, and addiction treatment.[63]

Treatment, Mutual-Help Groups, and Substance Use Outcomes

Participation in treatment and participation in mutual-help groups have independent effects on substance use outcomes that tend to augment each other. Individuals who participated more intensively in mutual-help groups after treatment experienced better substance use outcomes, even after controlling for the effects of treatment completion and continuing care.[24] This finding was also obtained in follow-ups of individuals discharged from residential care.[60,67]

More importantly, participation in each of these two modalities of help can independently contribute to better outcomes. In a nationwide sample of alcohol-dependent individuals, persons who participated in 12-step mutual-help groups in addition to treatment were more than twice as likely to achieve an abstinent recovery as were individuals who participated in treatment alone.[18] Similarly, among clients with drug use disorders, longer episodes of treatment and weekly or more frequent mutual-help group attendance during and after treatment were each independently associated with 6-month abstinence.[25]

Participation in mutual-help groups may compensate for the lack of services provided in treatment. Among dually diagnosed participants in residential programs, the benefits of 12-step mutual-help group attendance depended on the intensity of treatment services. More 12-step mutual-help group attendance during treatment was associated with better alcohol and drug outcomes at discharge, only among individuals treated in low-service-intensity programs. More 12-step mutual-help group attendance after discharge from treatment was associated with better mental health and family/social functioning at 1 year, only among individuals receiving low-service-intensity care.[85]

Interventions to Enhance 12-Step Group Participation

Due in part to the convincing evidence that mutual-help group attendance and involvement are related to better substance use disorder outcomes, evidence-based interventions to facilitate 12-step group participation are now available. Twelve-step facilitation therapy, used in Project MATCH and now offered in both individual and group approaches, focuses on the first three of the 12 steps. Its goals are to facilitate patients' acceptance of having lost control over their substance use and the goal of abstinence, as well as patients' hope for recovery, faith in a Higher Power, and acknowledgment of the 12-step fellowship as instrumental in recovery. Project MATCH found that patients in Twelve-Step Facilitation, compared to those in motivational enhancement or cognitive behavioral therapy, attended more meetings and had better outcomes.[89]

Building on an earlier facilitation approach to connect 12-step volunteers with individuals with alcohol use disorders,[75] Timko et al.[80] found support for Intensive Referral, a brief facilitation intervention. Consisting of three sessions, Intensive Referral provides information about 12-step approaches, discusses patients' views of them, and links patients with 12-step volunteers to attend meetings together. Treatment providers or peer specialists follow up to reinforce attendance and involvement, including obtaining a sponsor. Patients who were assigned to Intensive Referral rather than standard referral had more 12-step group participation and less substance use at a 1-year postintervention follow-up.[79] Intensive Referral was adapted and empirically supported in a study of patients with co-occurring substance use and mental health disorders.[86]

Making AA Easier (MAAEZ) is designed to familiarize individuals with the culture of 12-Step meetings and help them anticipate and deal with concerns that could deter participation.[37] It is a manualized intervention consisting of six, 90-minute group sessions led by a counselor who is in recovery and has extensive personal experience with 12-step programs. Compared to patients in usual care only, patients in usual care plus MAAEZ were more likely to be abstinent at 1-year follow-up.[37]

Finally, Stimulant Abuser Groups to Engage in 12-Step (STAGE-12) was developed for individuals who use cocaine and amphetamines. It is composed of eight individual and group sessions that combine 12-step facilitation and intensive referral, in that they incorporate linkage with a 12-step volunteer and a focus on the first three of the 12 steps. During the 8-week intervention period, individuals who used stimulants receiving STAGE-12 as part of outpatient treatment were more likely to abstain from stimulants than were those who received usual care. The STAGE-12 group also reduced their drug use severity more at a 3-month follow-up.[20] Among patients receiving STAGE-12, those with more exposure to the intervention were more likely to be abstinent.[94]

Personal Factors, Participation, and Mutual-Help Group Outcomes

In an attempt to identify individuals who may be especially well-suited for participation in mutual-help groups, researchers have considered a range of personal factors, including severity and impairment related to substance use, and disease model beliefs and religious and spiritual orientation. In addition, studies have examined the suitability of mutual-help groups for individuals with substance use and psychiatric disorders, women, older adults, adolescents and emerging adults, and members of racial and ethnic minority groups.

Severity and Impairment

In general, individuals who use substances more heavily are more dependent on substances, have more substance-related problems, and lack control over substance use are more likely to affiliate with mutual-help groups. Clients with more impairment are more likely to continue mutual-help group attendance and less likely to drop out after treatment.[14] Among individuals with alcohol use disorders, compared with type A individuals in 12-step treatment, type B individuals, who have more severe alcohol-related problems, were more likely to attend Alcoholics Anonymous in the 12 months after treatment. Moreover, the type A individuals were

more than twice as likely to stop attending Alcoholics Anonymous after treatment.[88]

Compared with individuals with less severe substance use problems, those with more severe problems may benefit more from mutual-help group involvement. Morgenstern and colleagues[61] found that individuals with more severe substance use and psychosocial problems who had high levels of mutual-help group affiliation had better 6-month substance use outcomes; outcomes were poor when group affiliation was low. For individuals with less-severe problems, levels of mutual-help group affiliation were not related to outcomes.

In Project MATCH, among less impaired patients, adaptive social network changes and increases in social abstinence self-efficacy primarily explained the effect of Alcoholics Anonymous attendance on better alcohol outcomes. Among more impaired patients, in addition to these explanatory mediators, increased spirituality and reduced negative affect led to better outcomes of Alcoholics Anonymous attendance. For more severe patients, attending Alcoholics Anonymous reduces drinking by simultaneously reducing depression symptoms and increasing confidence in individuals' ability to resist alcohol when experiencing negative affect.[43]

Disease Model Beliefs and Religious and Spiritual Orientation

Individuals whose beliefs are more consonant with the 12-step orientation are more likely to affiliate with 12-step mutual-help groups. More specifically, people who believe in the disease model of substance use, have an abstinence goal, and see themselves as alcoholics or addicts tend to become more involved in mutual-help groups after discharge from acute treatment and are less likely to stop attending.[40]

Many individuals see a positive role for an emphasis on spirituality in mutual-help groups and focus on spirituality as a source of: (1) personal strength and self-protection (e.g., help in maintaining abstinence, reducing craving, and facing mortality) and (b) altruism and protection of others (e.g., not sharing drug paraphernalia or engaging in unsafe sexual practices).[2] Individuals with stronger religious beliefs are more likely to attend and become involved in 12-step mutual-help groups during and after treatment. In contrast, less religious individuals, including those who profess atheistic and agnostic beliefs, are less likely to attend and more likely to drop out of 12-step mutual-help groups. Nevertheless, when they do become involved in mutual-help groups, less religious individuals appear to obtain as much or more benefit from them as more religious individuals do.[38,40]

More generally, individuals whose religious and spiritual beliefs better match those of their primary mutual-help group tend to participate more in that group. More religious individuals are more likely to participate in 12-step than in other types of mutual-help groups; in contrast, religiosity does not seem to be associated with participation in SMART Recovery but is associated with less participation in Secular Organizations for Sobriety. Matching an individual's spiritual and religious beliefs to those of a mutual-help group may increase the individual's participation in the group and perhaps indirectly increase the likelihood of continued sobriety.[5]

Individuals who profess a stronger religious and spiritual orientation may be better able to accept their craving and, therefore, become more involved in 12-step mutual-help groups. Consistent with this view, clients who professed stronger spiritual and religious beliefs at intake to treatment improved more in acceptance-based responding between baseline and a 1-year follow-up. These individuals became more aware of and able to acknowledge internal experiences, such as cravings and distress, and were able to rely more on adaptive coping responses to confront and manage these experiences. In turn, enhanced acceptance-based responding at a 1-year follow-up predicted increased subsequent mutual-help group involvement. Thus together with treatment, spirituality and religiosity may promote self-regulation skills that contribute to 12-step mutual-help group affiliation.[12]

Whereas Alcoholics Anonymous and Narcotics Anonymous are spiritual 12-step groups, many religious congregations are now offering 12-step groups that incorporate a defined concept of higher power. For example, Saddleback Church in Southern California developed the faith-based Celebrate Recovery program using the 12 steps and adding "8 Recovery Principles" based on the Bible to define a Christian interpretation of higher power. These groups appeal to people who desire a specialized definition of higher power during 12-step participation. Celebrate Recovery reports over 500,000 participants and 10,000 participating churches worldwide from various Christian denominations (see www.celebraterecovery.com). A study of Celebrate Recovery participants found that spirituality was a significant component of their confidence to resist substance use.[10]

Individuals With Substance Use and Psychiatric Disorders

A high proportion of individuals with substance use disorders have co-occurring psychiatric disorders. With the exception of clients with psychotic disorders, these dually diagnosed individuals are as likely to attend 12-step mutual-help groups as are those with only substance use disorders. In general, individuals with dual diagnoses appear to benefit from substance-use–focused 12-step mutual-help groups as much as do those with only substance use disorders.[60,66]

A few studies have focused on participants with specific psychiatric disorders, especially posttraumatic stress disorder and major depression. Individuals with substance use disorders and posttraumatic stress disorder participated as much in 12-step mutual-help groups after treatment as did those with only substance use disorders. The dually diagnosed individuals who participated more in mutual-help groups were more likely to be abstinent and experienced less distress; they also were more likely to maintain stable remission over a 2-year follow-up.[67]

The situation may be different for clients who have substance use disorders and co-occurring major depression. Compared with individuals with only substance use disorders, those who also had major depression were less likely to become involved in 12-step mutual-help groups after treatment. At a 2-year follow-up, the association between mutual-help group involvement and abstinence was stronger for clients who had only substance use disorders than for those who also had major depression. These participants did not benefit as much from contact with a sponsor, 12-step friends, reading 12-step literature, and working the steps. Depressed individuals may have interpersonal problems that make it harder to develop friendships and to acquire and relate to a sponsor; thus they may need more support and guidance to become involved in and benefit from 12-step mutual-help groups.[40]

Traditional 12-step mutual-help groups may have some limitations for dually diagnosed individuals, who may be less able to bond with other members who do not share the experiences associated with psychiatric problems. Some group members may have ambivalent or negative attitudes about the use of medications to prevent relapse or alter mood. In addition, some dually diagnosed individuals may be alienated by 12-step philosophy, the emphasis on denial, and an apparent lack of empathy for individuals with psychiatric problems.

Given these issues, some dually diagnosed individuals may do better in dual-focused 12-step self-help groups, such as Double Trouble in Recovery. Double Trouble in Recovery is a 12-step fellowship adapted from the 12-step method of Alcoholics Anonymous; it is designed to meet the needs of individuals who have both substance use and psychiatric disorders. Double Trouble in Recovery specifically addresses the problems and benefits associated with psychiatric medications. It has amended steps 1 and 12 of the 12 steps to include mental health disorders so that, for example, step 1 is: "We admitted we were powerless over mental disorders and substance abuse—that our lives had become unmanageable" (see www.doubletroubleinrecovery.org).

Individuals who experience more psychiatric symptoms and more severe consequences of drug use are more likely to maintain attendance in Double Trouble in Recovery. As found in a study of Dual Diagnosis Anonymous, also a peer-support program for people with co-occurring disorders, this may be because group members feel accepted by others in the group, learn about how each disorder affects the other, feel comfortable having open discussions, and experience a focus on hope and recovery for both their substance use and mental health disorders.[71] With respect to outcomes, Double Trouble in Recovery members who engaged more in reciprocal learning and assuming a helping role were more likely to be abstinent at a 1-year follow-up. A 2-year follow-up showed that individuals who affiliated more strongly with Double Trouble in Recovery improved more in self-efficacy for recovery, leisure time activities, feelings of well-being, and social relationships.[52]

In a subsequent study, a cohort of dually diagnosed individuals who did not have Double Trouble in Recovery available during treatment was compared with a cohort exposed to it after Double Trouble in Recovery meetings were instituted in the treatment program. Compared with the pre–Double Trouble in Recovery cohort, the post–Double Trouble in Recovery cohort had significantly fewer days of alcohol and drug use, more frequently attended traditional 12-step group meetings outside the program, and better adherence to their psychiatric medications at a 6-month follow-up.[53]

In a randomized trial, Bogenschutz et al.[7] found that dually diagnosed patients who received 12-step facilitation Therapy in addition to usual care in a dual diagnosis program participated more in 12-step groups than patients in usual care. More participation in 12-step groups was associated with better drinking outcomes. In another randomized trial, dually diagnosed patients assigned to Double Trouble in Recovery used alcohol and other substances less at a 6-month follow-up than did waitlist control patients.[70] Twelve-step facilitation for dually diagnosed individuals is now a manualized treatment to help patients engage in Double Trouble in Recovery.[28]

Women

Women with alcohol or drug use disorders are at least as likely as men to attend and affiliate with mutual-help groups. Compared with men, women may be more likely to read Alcoholics Anonymous literature, call an Alcoholics Anonymous member for help, and experience a spiritual awakening. In a study of individuals with alcohol use disorders, women were more likely than men to attend Alcoholics Anonymous and went to more Alcoholics Anonymous meetings in the first year after initiating help-seeking. More extended participation in Alcoholics Anonymous was associated with a higher likelihood of 1-year remission for both women and men; however, the positive association between a longer duration of Alcoholics Anonymous attendance and stable remission was stronger for women.[60,84]

Compared with men, women may be more in tune with 12-step philosophy, which involves acceptance of powerlessness over the used substance and reliance on a higher power to attain sobriety. Mutual-help groups are nonhierarchical and nonauthoritarian and foster recovery in a relational, mutually enhancing, and safe context, which may especially appeal to women. In addition, compared with men, women may be more comfortable in mutual-help groups such as Alcoholics Anonymous because they are more interdependent with other people, more likely to gain self-esteem from developing and maintaining close relationships, and more at ease with emotional self-disclosure.[74]

Even though many women attend and benefit from Alcoholics Anonymous or Narcotics Anonymous, the emphasis in these groups on powerlessness, humility, and surrender alienates some women, who express discomfort with face-to-face self-disclosure in group meetings populated mostly by men. Alcoholics Anonymous may be especially problematic for women who drink for reasons associated with sexuality and gender roles. Many women report feeling that they do not fit in at Alcoholics Anonymous, and that they find it to be too negative, dislike the primary focus on the past, and feel that interchanges in Alcoholics Anonymous are dominated primarily by men.

These issues led to the development of Women for Sobriety, which provides an alternative for women who prefer an emphasis on improving self-esteem, independence, and personal responsibility rather than powerlessness, humility, and surrender. Women for Sobriety shares Alcoholics Anonymous' focus on meditation and spirituality but espouses the idea that sobriety is dependent on taking personal responsibility for one's behavior rather than on a higher power. Women for Sobriety seems to be especially attractive to well-educated, middle-aged, and middle- and upper-class women, many of whom, nevertheless, continue to attend Alcoholics Anonymous (see www.womenforsobriety.org).

In contrast to Alcoholics Anonymous, Women for Sobriety is based on the idea that women need a positive program that reinforces optimistic thinking about their abilities and independence, reduces their guilt, and enhances their coping skills. Many women report that they attend Women for Sobriety for support and nurturance, a safe environment, sharing about women's issues, and the positive emphasis on self-esteem. In this respect, there is an association between longer membership in Women for Sobriety and higher self-esteem.[35]

Adolescents and Emerging Adults

Only 12% and 13% of Alcoholics Anonymous and Narcotics Anonymous members, respectively, are younger than age 30, and only about 1% in both groups are younger than age 21 (www.aa.org; www.na.org). In addition, many youth may stop attending, possibly because they have difficulty accepting lifelong abstinence, relating to adults' concerns (e.g., jobs, marriage, children), and accessing meetings (lack of transportation). Even so, youth and emerging adults who attend more 12-step groups have better substance use outcomes.[41,46]

One study using data from the Drug Abuse Treatment Outcomes Studies for Adolescents (DATOS-A) found that, among adolescents with both drug and mental health disorders, participation in 12-step groups was positively associated with posttreatment abstinence.[77] In another study, dually diagnosed adolescents participated in 12-step groups at comparable or higher levels than adolescents with only substance use disorders, over 7 years. For both groups, participation was associated with abstinence at follow-ups.[13]

Older Adults

Late middle-aged and older adults participate in and benefit from 12-step mutual-help groups. In two studies, older clients (55+ years of age) with substance use disorders were matched with younger (aged 21–39) and middle-aged (aged 40–55) clients on the basis of race, education, marital status, and dual diagnosis status. These three groups of participants attended a comparable number of mutual-help group meetings during residential treatment and were equally likely to attend mutual-help groups in the first 2 years after treatment and to have a sponsor. Overall, individuals who attended more group meetings and those who obtained a sponsor in the first year experienced better 1-year alcohol and psychological distress outcomes. Participants who attended more meetings and had a sponsor in the second year reported less alcohol consumption at a 5-year follow-up. The three age groups did not differ in the associations between 12-step mutual-help group attendance and these outcomes.[49]

In a similar study of clients in community residential care, the three age-matched groups showed comparable mutual-help group attendance during treatment and in the year after entering treatment. A comparable percentage had a sponsor. Overall, clients who attended more mutual-help group meetings and those who had a sponsor a year after entering treatment had better alcohol-related and psychological distress outcomes at 1-year and 4-year follow-ups. Again, the three age groups did not differ in the associations between 12-step mutual-help group involvement and these outcomes.[50]

Race and Ethnicity

Compared with Caucasian clients, African American clients may be more likely to attend mutual-help groups as part of treatment and to increase their affiliation during treatment; in addition, they appear to be less likely to stop attending mutual-help groups after treatment.[47] Certain characteristics of 12-step mutual-help groups may especially appeal to African American clients, including the fact that meetings are widely available and open to anyone, and have a strong social and spiritual component. African American clients seem to be more likely to identify as Alcoholics Anonymous members, experience a spiritual awakening in Alcoholics Anonymous, and perform service at Alcoholics Anonymous meetings. In contrast, Caucasian clients are more likely to read 12-step literature and have a sponsor.[39,61]

In order to meet their unique recovery needs, African Americans appear to integrate cultural factors and a unique language and perspective in the process of affiliation with Alcoholics Anonymous. According to Durant,[21] African Americans are more likely to associate their problems with racism and economic disadvantage than with unhealthy alcohol use; they are less likely to accept the disease concept of alcoholism. Nevertheless, they are able to contrast the negative aspects of drinking with the positive aspects of abstinence, to respond to modeling and support from mentors and sponsors, to modify the moral aspects of Alcoholics Anonymous to meet their spiritual needs, and to adapt the Alcoholics Anonymous worldview to better fit their racial and cultural background.

Compared with non-Hispanic white individuals, Hispanic individuals may be less likely to attend Alcoholics Anonymous after treatment, perhaps because they tend to turn to their existing support system. However, attendance at Alcoholics Anonymous appears to be similarly associated with decreased alcohol consumption among both Hispanics and non-Hispanic whites.[3]

In Project MATCH, Hispanic individuals attended Alcoholics Anonymous less often after 12-step treatment than non-Hispanic white participants did. Nevertheless, as judged by self-identification as an Alcoholics Anonymous member, having an Alcoholics Anonymous sponsor, experiencing a spiritual awakening, and celebrating an Alcoholics Anonymous birthday, they were as committed to Alcoholics Anonymous as were non-Hispanic whites. Thus Hispanics' lower Alcoholics Anonymous attendance does not necessarily mean that they are less favorably inclined toward Alcoholics Anonymous. However, Hispanic clients who were more involved in specific Alcoholics Anonymous practices were not more likely to achieve abstinence.[4]

A comparison of urban Native American and non-Hispanic white attendees of Alcoholics Anonymous found that meeting attendance trajectories over a 9-month follow-up did not differ between the groups. American Indian participants discontinued attendance less often. For both groups, more attendance predicted abstinence.[90]

Active Ingredients of Mutual-Help Groups

The effectiveness of mutual-help groups in curtailing substance use is based largely on four key ingredients: (1) abstinence-specific and general support that emphasizes the value of identification with abstinence-oriented role models and strong bonds with family, friends, work, and religion; (2) the goal direction and structure of a consistent belief system that espouses a substance-free lifestyle; (3) involvement in rewarding activities that do not involve substance use; and (4) an emphasis on bolstering members' self-efficacy and coping skills and helping others overcome substance use problems.[56]

These critical factors appear to be common change factors that underlie long-term recovery from unhealthy substance use. A survey of mutual-help groups, including traditional 12-step groups, SMART Recovery, Secular Organizations for Sobriety, and Women for Sobriety, supported the idea of common change factors. It showed that active involvement in a support group was associated with a higher likelihood of long-term remission irrespective of the particular group to which the individual belonged.[5] Furthermore, the same active ingredients appear to be operative in Al-Anon as in other 12-step groups focused on substance use.[82] Specifically, bonding, goal direction, and access to peers in recovery and rewarding pursuits help to explain associations between sustained Al-Anon participation and improvements on key concerns of Al-Anon attendees.

Abstinence-Specific and General Support

Mutual-help groups are an important source of abstinence-specific and general support, and may be especially effective in counteracting the influence of people who use substances in a social network. Mutual-help groups provide modeling of substance use refusal skills, ideas about how to avoid relapse-inducing situations, practical advice for staying sober, and helpful hints about how to address the panoply of everyday life problems. Individuals who continue to attend Alcoholics Anonymous more regularly after treatment are more likely to have social network members who support cutting down or quitting substance use than are individuals who attend Alcoholics Anonymous less regularly. In fact, the increase in friends' abstinence-oriented and general support associated with involvement in mutual-help groups explains part of their positive influence on remission.[31,92] The rated quality of social interactions in 12-step groups increased over time among relatively new attendees, and higher-rated quality predicted increased 12-step–related behaviors and decreased alcohol use.[73]

According to Bond, Kaskutas, and Weisner,[9] individuals who have fewer individuals with unhealthy alcohol use in their social network and more people who encourage the reduction of drinking, as well as more Alcoholics Anonymous–based support for reducing drinking, are more likely to initiate and maintain abstinence; the number of Alcoholics Anonymous–based social network members who support reduced drinking explains part of Alcoholics Anonymous' effect on abstinence. In addition, involvement in Alcoholics Anonymous may protect individuals from the potential negative influence of a pro-drinking social network.[36] In support of these findings, analyses of Project MATCH data found that Alcoholics Anonymous attendance exerted its salutary effect on abstinence through reductions in pro-drinking network ties and, to a lesser degree, through increases in pro-abstinent social ties.[44]

Goal Direction and Structure

Mutual-help groups provide a context of goal direction and structure in the form of a shared ideology that enhances individuals' immersion into the group. The shared ideology, which is reinforced by explaining group beliefs in understandable terms, specifying changes needed to maintain sobriety, and providing the 12 steps as a guide for change, helps members to negotiate the recovery process. Alcoholics Anonymous norms appear to result in more personal and intimate self-disclosures and less conflict in Alcoholics Anonymous groups than in other support groups.[91,97]

In addition, there is a system of taking turns in Alcoholics Anonymous that exemplifies its egalitarian nature, nondifferentiated roles of members, and low levels of conflict. In this vein, members acknowledge and identify with previous speakers' contributions and do not openly confront or challenge them, thereby maintaining solidarity, communicating acceptance, and reducing the potential for conflict. Alcoholics Anonymous members tell life stories aligned with Alcoholics Anonymous principles, which supports the development of shared identities characterized by reliance on Alcoholics Anonymous and relevance to the 12 steps.[65]

The emphasis on spirituality is a key aspect of the goal direction in 12-step mutual-help groups. In this sense, Alcoholics Anonymous can be seen as a spiritual recovery movement that rewards compliance with its norms by engaging individuals in a social system that promotes new meaning in their lives. Among individuals in day hospital or residential treatment, increases in 12-step involvement from baseline to a 1-year follow-up predicted a higher likelihood of abstinence at follow-up. This relationship was explained partially by an increase in religious practices and spirituality. Thus spiritual change may contribute to recovery within the context of mutual-help group involvement.[98] According to

Project MATCH, attending Alcoholics Anonymous was associated with increases in spiritual practices, especially among individuals initially low on spirituality. Increases in spirituality partially mediated the association between meeting attendance and better subsequent alcohol outcomes.[45]

Involvement in Rewarding Activities

Another active ingredient of mutual-help groups involves their role in engaging members in rewarding substance-free social pursuits, such as home groups, parties, and community activities. Members who are more involved in group meetings and related activities, such as doing service and becoming a sponsor, are more likely to achieve and maintain abstinence.[36] Involvement in community groups predicted 1-year abstinence among drug-dependent individuals independent of attendance at Alcoholics Anonymous and Narcotics Anonymous and being a sponsor. By helping their members become more socially integrated, mutual-help groups increase the likelihood of sustained abstinence.[15]

Mutual-help groups also provide members with an opportunity to help other individuals in need, which tends to increase the helper's sense of purpose and personal responsibility, rewards for remaining sober, and commitment to recovery.[99] In a prospective study based on data from Project MATCH, recovering individuals who became sponsors or were otherwise engaged in helping others were less likely to relapse.[68] Similarly, compared with Double Trouble in Recovery members who were less involved in sharing at meetings and helping other members, those who were more involved in these activities were more likely to be abstinent at a 1-year follow-up.[52]

Sponsors provide other members with support and direction, 12-step instruction, tips to help promote abstinence and improve relationships, and crisis intervention. Engaging in these helping activities can improve the sponsor's self-esteem and social standing, strengthen the sponsor's social network, and provide a model of successful commitment to live a sober lifestyle. Accordingly, mutual-help group members who become sponsors are more likely to maintain abstinence than those who do not.[15]

Self-Efficacy and Coping

Affiliation with Alcoholics Anonymous tends to be associated with increases in members' self-efficacy and motivation for abstinence. For example, an analysis of data from Project MATCH showed that participation in Alcoholics Anonymous was positively related to self-efficacy to avoid drinking. Self-efficacy predicted a higher likelihood of abstinence and explained part of the association between participation in Alcoholics Anonymous and abstinence. In addition, Alcoholics Anonymous attendance at 6 months posttreatment predicted self-efficacy at 9 months, which predicted abstinence at 15 months. Self-efficacy to avoid drinking explained part of the effect of Alcoholics Anonymous attendance on abstinence for both less severe (type A) and more severe (type B) individuals with alcohol use disorders.[8,14]

A study that assessed individuals in 12-step treatment during treatment and at 1- and 6-month follow-ups focused on several common change factors, including self-efficacy, commitment to abstinence, appraisal of harm due to substance use, and active cognitive and behavioral coping. More affiliation with Alcoholics Anonymous in the month after treatment was associated with increases in these change factors and with better 1- and 6-month substance use outcomes. In addition, these common change

factors appeared to explain all of the effect of Alcoholics Anonymous affiliation on 6-month substance use outcomes.[62]

Affiliation with 12-step mutual-help groups promotes more reliance on coping responses directed toward reducing substance use. Individuals who are more involved in Alcoholics Anonymous are more likely to rely on coping skills directed toward controlling substance use, such as spending time with nondrinking friends, seeking advice about how to resolve their drinking problems, and rewarding themselves for trying to stop drinking.[76] The active ingredients of mutual-help groups that foster improvement in coping skills likely include modeling of substance use refusal skills, ideas about how to manage relapse-inducing situations, and practical advice for coping with craving.

Participation in mutual-help groups is also associated with improvements in general coping skills, that is, increases in approach coping and declines in avoidance coping.[62] Individuals who are more involved in 12-step groups tend to rely more on approach and less on avoidance coping; approach coping responses explained part of the effect of involvement in these groups on the reduction of substance use.[31]

Conclusions

The active ingredients of mutual-help groups tend to enhance motivation for recovery, self-efficacy to resist substance use, and effective coping skills. In this vein, increases in common change factors such as support, goal direction and structure, and involvement in rewarding activities are likely to result in increased motivation for recovery, self-efficacy to resist using alcohol and drugs, and approach coping.

Most generally, the finding that a longer duration of participation in mutual-help groups predicts better substance use outcomes indicates that mutual-help groups are most beneficial when they become a long-term supportive aspect of individuals' lives. Extended 12-step group engagement may initiate and maintain the personal and social changes needed to solidify recovery, especially abstinence-specific and general support, goal direction and structure, involvement in rewarding substance-free activities, and enhanced self-efficacy and coping skills. Mutual-help groups represent an important and complementary part of the array of effective interventions that can change the enduring aspects of individuals' life contexts and increase the likelihood of a long-term course of recovery.

Acknowledgments

Department of Veterans Affairs Health Services Research and Development Service funds (RCS 00-001) supported preparation of the manuscript. The views expressed here are those of the author.

References

1. American Psychiatric Association. *Practice guidelines for the treatment of patients with substance use disorders. Practice Guidelines for the Treatment of Psychiatric Disorders Compendium.* Washington, DC: American Psychiatric Association; 2010.
2. Arnold RM, Avants SK, Margolin A, Marcotte D. Patient attitudes concerning the inclusion of spirituality into addiction treatment. *J Subst Abuse Treat.* 2002;23:319–326.
3. Arroyo JA, Miller WR, Tonigan JS. The influence of Hispanic ethnicity on long-term outcome in three alcohol treatment modalities. *J Stud Alcohol.* 2003;64:98–104.

4. Arroyo JA, Westerberg VS, Tonigan JS. Comparison of treatment utilization and outcome for hispanics and non-hispanic whites. *J Stud Alcohol.* 1998;59:286–291.

5. Atkins RG, Hawdon JE. Religiosity and participation in mutual aid support groups for addiction. *J Subst Abuse Treat.* 2007;33:321–331.

6. Barber JG, Gilbertson R. An experimental study of brief unilateral intervention for the partners of heavy drinkers. *Res Soc Work Pract.* 1996;6:325–336.

7. Bogenschutz MP, Rice SL, Tonigan JS, et al. 12-step facilitation for the dually diagnosed: a randomized clinical trial. *J Subst Abuse Treat.* 2014;46:403–411.

8. Bogenschutz MP, Tonigan JS, Miller WR. Examining the effects of alcoholism typology and AA attendance on self-efficacy as a mechanism of change. *J Stud Alcohol.* 2006;67:562–567.

9. Bond J, Kaskutas LA, Weisner C. The persistent influence of social networks and alcoholics anonymous on abstinence. *J Stud Alcohol.* 2003;64:579–588.

10. Brown AE, Tonigan JS, Pavlik VN, Kosten TR, Volk RJ. Spirituality and confidence to resist substance use among celebrate recovery participants. *J Relig Health.* 2013;52:107–113.

11. Caldwell PE, Cutter HSG. Alcoholics anonymous affiliation during early recovery. *J Subst Abuse Treat.* 1998;15:221–228.

12. Carrico AW, Gifford EV, Moos R. Spirituality/religiosity promotes acceptance-based responding and twelve-step involvement. *Drug Alcohol Depend.* 2007;89:66–73.

13. Chi FW, Sterling S, Campbell CI, Weisner C. 12-step participation and outcomes over 7 years among adolescent substance use patients with and without psychiatric comorbidity. *Subst Abuse.* 2013;34:33–42.

14. Connors GJ, Tonigan JS, Miller WR. A longitudinal model of intake symptomatology, AA participation and outcome: retrospective study of the project MATCH outpatient and aftercare samples. *J Stud Alcohol.* 2001;62:817–825.

15. Crape BL, Latkin CA, Laris AS, Knowlton AR. The effects of sponsorship in 12-step treatment of injection drug users. *Drug Alcohol Depend.* 2002;65:291–301.

16. Cutter CG, Cutter HS. Experience and change in Al-Anon family groups: Adult children of alcoholics. *J Stud Alcohol Drugs.* 1987;48:29–32.

17. Davey-Rothwell MA, Kuramoto SJ, Latkin CA. Social networks, norms, and 12-step group participation. *Am J Drug Alcohol Abuse.* 2008;34:185–193.

18. Dawson DA, Grant BF, Stinson FS, Chou PS. Estimating the effect of help-seeking on achieving recovery from alcohol dependence. *Addiction.* 2006;101:824–834.

19. Dittrich JE, Trapold MA. A treatment program for wives of alcoholics: an evaluation. *Addict Behav.* 1984;3:91–102.

20. Donovan DM, Daley DC, Brigham GS, et al. Stimulant abuser groups to engage in 12-step (Stage-12): a multisite trial in the NIDA clinical trials network. *J Subst Abuse Treat.* 2013;44:103–114.

21. Durant A. African-American alcoholics: an interpretive/constructivist model of affiliation with alcoholics (AA). *J Ethnicity Subst Abuse.* 2005;4:5–21.

22. Etemadi A, Zarebahramabadi M, Mirkazemi R. Effect of Al-Anon attendance on family function and quality of life in women in Mashhad, Iran. *Am J Drug Alcohol Abuse.* 2015;41:442–448.

23. Fernandez AC, Begley EA, Marlatt GA. Family and peer interventions for adults: past approaches and future direction. *Psychol Addict Behav.* 2006;20:207–213.

24. Fiorentine R. After drug treatment: are 12-step programs effective in maintaining abstinence? *Am J Drug Alcohol Abuse.* 1999;25: 93–116.

25. Fiorentine R, Hillhouse MP. Drug treatment and 12-step program participation: the additive effects of integrated recovery activities. *J Subst Abuse Treat.* 2000;18:65–74.

26. Fiorentine R, Hillhouse MP. Exploring the additive effects of drug misuse treatment and twelve-step involvement: does twelve-step ideology matter? *Subst Use Misuse.* 2000;35:367–397.

27. Groh DR, Jason LA, Keys CB. Social network variables in alcoholics anonymous: a literature review. *Clin Psychol Rev.* 2008;28:430–450.

28. Hagler KJ, Rice SL, Muñoz RE, Salvador JF, Forcehimes AA, Bogenshultz MP. "It might actually work this time": benefits and barriers to adapted 12-step facilitation therapy and mutual-help group attendance from the perspective of dually diagnosed individuals. *J Addict Nurs.* 2015;26:120–128.

29. Hester RK, Lenberg KL, Campbell W, Delaney HD. Overcoming addictions, a web-based application, and SMART Recovery, an online and in-person mutual help group for problem drinkers, part 1: three-month outcomes of a randomized controlled trial. *J Med Internet Res.* 2013;15:134.

30. Humphreys K, Blodgett JC, Wagner TH. Estimating the efficacy of Alcoholics Anonymous without self-selection bias: an instrumental variables re-analysis of randomized clinical trials. *Alcohol Clin Exp Res.* 2014;38:2688–2694.

31. Humphreys K, Huebsch P, Finney J, Moos R. A comparative evaluation of substance abuse treatment: V. Substance abuse treatment can enhance the effectiveness of self-help groups. *Alcohol Clin Exp Res.* 1999;23:558–563.

32. Humphreys K, Moos R. Reduced substance-abuse-related health care costs among voluntary participants in Alcoholics Anonymous. *Psychiatr Serv.* 1996;47:709–713.

33. Humphreys K, Moos R. Can encouraging substance abuse patients to participate in self-help groups reduce demand for health care? A quasi-experimental study. *Alcohol Clin Exp Res.* 2001;25:711–716.

34. Humphreys K, Moos R. Encouraging posttreatment self-help group involvement to reduce demand for continuing care services: two-year clinical and utilization outcomes. *Alcohol Clin Exp Res.* 2007;31: 64–68.

35. Kaskutas LA. Predictors of self esteem among members of women for sobriety. *Addiction Res.* 1996;4:273–281.

36. Kaskutas LA, Ammon L, Delucchi K, Room R, Bond J, Weisner C. Alcoholics anonymous careers: patterns of AA involvement five years after treatment entry. Alcohol. *Clin Exp Res.* 2005;29: 1983–1990.

37. Kaskutas LA, Subbaraman MS, Witbrdot J, Zemore SE. Effectiveness of making alcoholics anonymous easier: a group format 12-step facilitation approach. *J Subst Abuse Treat.* 2009;37:228–239.

38. Kaskutas LA, Turk N, Bond J, Weisner C. The role of religion, spirituality, and alcoholics anonymous in sustained sobriety. *Alcohol Treat.* 2003;Q21:1–16.

39. Kaskutas LA, Weisner C, Lee M, Humphreys K. Alcoholics anonymous affiliation at treatment intake among white and black Americans. *J Stud Alcohol.* 1999;60:810–816.

40. Kelly J, Moos R. Dropout from 12-step self-help groups: prevalence, predictors, and counteracting treatment-related effects. *J Subst Abuse Treat.* 2003;24:241–250.

41. Kelly JF, Dow SJ, Yeterian JD, Kahler CW. Can 12-step group participation strengthen and extend the benefits of adolescent addiction treatment? A prospective analysis. *Drug Alcohol Depend.* 2010;110:117–125.

42. Kelly JF, Greene MC, Bergman BG. Do drug-dependent patients attending alcoholics anonymous rather than narcotics anonymous do as well? A prospective, lagged, matching analysis. *Alcohol Alcohol.* 2014;49:645–653.

43. Kelly JF, Hoeppner B, Stout RL, Pagano M. Determining the relative importance of the mechanisms of behavior change with Alcoholics Anonymous: a multiple mediator analysis. *Addiction.* 2012;107:289–299.

44. Kelly JF, Stout RL, Magill M, Tonigan JS. The role of Alcoholics Anonymous in mobilizing adaptive social network changes: a prospective lagged mediational analysis. *Drug Alcohol Depend.* 2011;114:119–126.

45. Kelly JF, Stout RL, Magill M, Tonigan JS, Pagano ME. Spirituality in recovery: a lagged mediational analysis of alcoholics anonymous' principal theoretical mechanism of behavior change. *Alcohol Clin Exp Res.* 2011;35:454–463.

46. Kelly JF, Stout RL, Slaymaker V. Emerging adults' treatment outcomes in relation to 12-step mutual-help attendance and involvement. *Drug Alcohol Depend.* 2013;129:151–157.

47. Kingree JB, Sullivan BF. Participation in alcoholics anonymous among African-Americans. *Alcohol Treat.* 2002;Q20:175–186.

48. Kurtz LF, Fisher M. Participation in community life by AA and NA members. *Contemp Drug Prob.* 2003;30:873–904.

49. Lemke S, Moos R. Treatment outcomes at 1-year and 5-years for older patients with alcohol use disorders. *J Subst Abuse Treat.* 2003;24:43–50.

50. Lemke S, Moos R. Treatment and outcomes of older patients with alcohol use disorders in community residential programs. *J Stud Alcohol.* 2003;64:219–226.

51. Magura S. The relationship between substance user treatment and 12-step fellowships: current knowledge and research questions. *Subst Use Misuse.* 2007;42:343–360.

52. Magura S, Laudet AB, Mahmood D, Rosenblum A, Vogel HS, Knight EL. Role of self-help processes in achieving abstinence among dually diagnosed persons. *Addict Behav.* 2003;28:399–413.

53. Magura S, Rosenblum A, Villano CL, Vogel HS, Fong C, Betzler T. Dual-focus mutual aid for co-occurring disorders: a quasi-experimental outcome evaluation study. *Am J Drug Alcohol Abuse.* 2008;34:61–71.

54. Miller RM, Meyers RJ, Tonigan JS. Engaging the unmotivated in treatment for alcohol problems: a comparison of three strategies for intervention through family members. *J Consult Clin Psychol.* 1999;67:688–697.

55. Monico LB, Gryczynski J, Schwartz RP, O'Grady K, Olsen YK, Jaffe JH. Buprenorphine treatment and 12-step meeting attendance: conflicts, compatibilities, and patient outcomes. *J Subst Abuse Treat.* 2015;57:89–95.

56. Moos R. Active ingredients of substance use focused self-help groups. *Addiction.* 2008;103:387–396.

57. Moos R, Moos B. Long-term influence of duration and frequency of participation in alcoholics anonymous on individuals with alcohol use disorders. *J Consult Clin Psychol.* 2004;72:81–90.

58. Moos R, Moos B. Paths of entry into Alcoholics Anonymous: effects on participation, perceived benefit, and outcome. *Alcohol Clin Exp Res.* 2005;29:1858–1868.

59. Moos R, Moos B. Participation in treatment and alcoholics anonymous: a 16-year follow-up of initially untreated individuals. *J Clin Psychol.* 2006;62:735–750.

60. Moos R, Schaefer J, Andrassy J, Moos B. Outpatient mental health care, self-help groups, and patients' 1-year treatment outcomes. *J Clin Psychol.* 2001;57:273–287.

61. Morgenstern J, Bux DA. Examining the effects of sex and ethnicity on substance abuse treatment and mediational pathways. *Alcohol Clin Exp Res.* 2003;27:1330–1332.

62. Morgenstern J, Labouvie E, McCrady BS, Kahler CW, Frey RM. Affiliation with Alcoholics Anonymous after treatment: a study of its therapeutic effects and mechanisms of action. *J Consult Clin Psychol.* 1997;65:768–777.

63. Mundt MP, Parthasarathy S, Chi FW, Sterling S, Campbell CI. 12-step participation reduces medical use costs among adolescents with a history of alcohol and other drug treatment. *Drug Alcohol Depend.* 2012;126:124–130.

64. Nowinski J. Self-help groups for addictions. In: McCrady BS, Epstein EE, eds. *Addictions: A Comprehensive Guidebook.* New York, NY, US: Oxford University Press; 1999:328–346.

65. O'Halloran S. Symmetry in interaction in meetings of alcoholics anonymous: the management of conflict. *Discourse Soc.* 2005;16:535–560.

66. Ouimette PC, Moos R, Finney J. Influence of outpatient treatment and 12-step group involvement on one-year substance abuse treatment outcomes. *J Stud Alcohol.* 1998;59:513–522.

67. Ouimette PC, Moos R, Finney J. Two-year mental health service use and course of remission in patients with substance use and posttraumatic stress disorders. *J Stud Alcohol.* 2000;61:247–253.

68. Pagano ME, Friend KB, Tonigan JS, Stout RL. Helping other alcoholics in alcoholics anonymous and drinking outcomes: findings from project MATCH. *J Stud Alcohol.* 2004;65:766–773.

69. Parran TV, Adelman CA, Merkin B, et al. Long-term outcomes of office-based buprenorphine/naloxone maintenance therapy. *Drug Alcohol Depend.* 2010;106:56–60.

70. Rosenblum A, Matusow H, Fong C, et al. Efficacy of dual focus mutual aid for persons with mental illness and substance misuse. *Drug Alcohol Depend.* 2014;135:78–87.

71. Roush S, Monica C, Carpenter-Song E, Drake RE. First-person perspectives on dual diagnosis anonymous (DDA): a qualitative study. *J Dual Diag.* 2015;11:136–141.

72. Rychtarik RG, McGillicuddy NB. Coping skills training and 12-step facilitation for women whose partner has alcoholism: effects on depression, the partner's drinking, and partner physical violence. *J Consult Clin Psychol.* 2005;73:249–261.

73. Rynes KN, Tonigan JS, Rice SL. Interpersonal climate of 12-step groups predicts reductions in alcohol use. *Alcohol Treat.* 2013;Q31:167–185.

74. Sanders JM. Women and the twelve steps of alcoholics anonymous: a gendered narrative. *Alcohol Treat.* 2016;Q24:3–29.

75. Sisson RW, Mallams JH. The use of systematic encouragement and community access procedures to increase attendance at Alcoholic Anonymous and Al-Anon meetings. *Am J Drug Alcohol Abuse.* 1981;8:371–376.

76. Snow MG, Prochaska JO, Rossi JS. Processes of change in alcoholics anonymous: maintenance factors in long-term sobriety. *J Stud Alcohol.* 1994;55:362–371.

77. Sterling S, Kohn CS, Lu Y, Weisner C. Pathways to chemical dependency treatment for adolescents in an HMO. *J Psychoactive Drugs.* 2004;36:439–453.

78. Suire JG, Bothwell RK. The psychosocial benefits of alcoholics anonymous. *Am J Addiction.* 2006;15:252–255.

79. Timko C, DeBenedetti A. A randomized controlled trial of intensive referral to 12-step self-help groups: one-year outcomes. *Drug Alcohol Depend.* 2007;90:270–279.

80. Timko C, DeBenedetti A, Billow R. Intensive referral to 12-Step self-help groups and 6-month substance use disorder outcomes. *Addiction.* 2006;101:678–688.

81. Timko C, Finney J, Moos R. The 8-year course of alcohol abuse: gender differences in social context and coping. *Alcohol Clin Exp Res.* 2005;29:612–621.

82. Timko C, Halvorson M, Kong C, Moos RH. Social processes explaining the benefits of Al-Anon participation. *Psychol Addict Behav.* 2015;29:856–863.

83. Timko C, Laudet A, Moos RH. Al-Anon newcomers: benefits of continuing attendance for six months. *Am J Drug Alcohol Abuse.* (in press).

84. Timko C, Moos R, Finney J, Connell E. Gender differences in help-utilization and the 8-year course of alcohol abuse. *Addiction.* 2002;97:877–889.

85. Timko C, Sempel JM. Intensity of acute services, self-help attendance, and one-year outcomes among dual diagnosis patients. *J Stud Alcohol.* 2004;65:274–282.

86. Timko C, Sutkowi A, Cronkite RC, Markin-Byrd K, Moos RH. Intensive referral to 12-step dual-focused mutual-help groups. *Drug Alcohol Depend.* 2011;118:194–201.

87. Tomasson K, Vaglum P. Psychiatric comorbidity and aftercare among alcoholics: a prospective study of a nationwide representative sample. *Addiction.* 1998;93:423–431.

88. Tonigan JS, Bogenschutz MP, Miller WR. Is alcoholism typology a predictor of both alcoholics anonymous affiliation and disaffiliation after treatment? *J Subst Abuse Treat.* 2006;30:323–330.

89. Tonigan JS, Connors GJ, Miller WR. Participation and Involvement in alcoholics anonymous. In: Babor TF, Del Boca FK, eds. *Matching Alcoholism Treatments to Client Heterogeneity: The Results of Project MATCH.* New York: Cambridge University; 2003:184–204.

90. Tonigan JS, Martinez-Papponi B, Hagler KJ, Greenfield BL, Venner KL. Longitudinal study of urban American Indian 12-step attendance, attrition, and outcome. *J Stud Alcohol Drugs*. 2013;74:514–520.

91. VanLear CA, Sheehan M, Withers LA, Walker RA. AA online: the enactment of supportive computer mediated communication. *West J Commun*. 2005;69:5–26.

92. Weisner C, DeLucchi K, Matzger H, Schmidt L. The role of community services and informal support on five-year drinking trajectories of alcohol dependent and problem drinkers. *J Stud Alcohol*. 2003;64:862–873.

93. Weiss RD, Griffin ML, Gallop RJ, et al. The effect of 12-step self-help group attendance and participation on drug use outcomes among cocaine-dependent patients. *Drug Alcohol Depend*. 2005;77:177–184.

94. Wells EA, Donovan DM, Daley DC, et al. Is level of exposure to a 12-step facilitation therapy associated with treatment outcome? *J Subst Abuse Treat*. 2014;47:265–274.

95. Witbrodt J, Mertens J, Kaskutas LA, Bond J, Chi F, Weisner C. Do 12-step meeting attendance trajectories over 9 years predict abstinence? *J Subst Abuse Treat*. 2012;43:30–43.

96. Witbrodt J, Ye Y, Bond J, Chi F, Weisner C, Mertens J. Alcohol and drug treatment involvement, 12-step attendance and abstinence: 9-year cross-lagged analysis of adults in an integrated health plan. *J Subst Abuse Treat*. 2014;46:412–419.

97. Wright KB. Shared ideology in alcoholics anonymous: a grounded theory approach. *J Health Commun*. 1997;2:83–99.

98. Zemore SE. A role for spiritual change in the benefits of 12-step involvement. *Alcohol Clin Exp*. 2007;Res 31(S3):76S–79S.

99. Zemore SE, Kaskutas LA, Ammon LN. 12-Step groups, helping helps the helper. *Addiction*. 2004;99:1015–1023.

51

Pharmacotherapy for Alcoholism and Some Related Psychiatric and Addictive Disorders: Scientific Basis and Clinical Findings

NASSIMA AIT DAOUD TIOURIRINE AND BANKOLE A. JOHNSON

CHAPTER OUTLINE

Introduction

In May 2013, the American Psychiatric Association issued the Fifth Edition of the *Diagnostic and Statistical Manual of Mental Disorders* (DSM-5) integrating the two DSM-IV disorders, alcohol abuse and alcohol dependence, into one single disorder called alcohol use disorder, with three levels of severity—mild, moderate, and severe. One of the goals in revising the DSM-IV-TR was to improve the scientific basis for psychiatric diagnosis and classification. Craving was introduced as a criterion for the diagnosis of alcohol use disorder given that some data that suggested a positive correlation with drinking severity and is the eighth most frequently reported symptom of the 12 symptoms that define the diagnosis of alcohol use disorder.[234]

Globally and in the United States, alcohol dependence is analogous to alcohol use disorder of moderate to severe rank, and rates as fifth and third, respectively, on the list of preventable causes of morbidity and mortality. From 2006 to 2010 in the United States, an average of 87,798 (27.9/100,000 population) deaths per year were attributed to alcohol, with 2.5 million (831.6/100,000) years of potential life lost to alcohol)[312a] and an overall estimated cost to the nation of about $249 billion.[280b] Results from the National Epidemiologic Survey on Alcohol and Related Conditions III collecting data on the new DSM-5 classification reported that the 12-month and lifetime prevalences of were 13.9% and 29.1%, respectively, with a prevalence that was highest for men (17.6% and 36.0%, respectively), whites (14.0% and 32.6%, respectively), and

Native Americans (19.2% and 43.4%, respectively).[110] Significant associations were found between 12-month and lifetime alcohol use disorder and other substance use disorders, major depressive, bipolar I disorders, and personality disorders across all levels of severity, with odds ratios (ORs) ranging from 1.2 (95% confidence interval [CI] 1.08–1.36) to 6.4 (95% CI 5.76–7.22). Associations between alcohol use disorder and panic disorder, specific phobia, and generalized anxiety disorder were modest; ORs ranged from 1.2 (95% CI 1.01–1.43) to 1.4 (95% CI 1.13–1.67) across most levels of severity.[110] Alcohol use disorder increases the risk of depression up to fourfold.[163,271] Depression in individuals with alcohol use disorder increases the degree of morbidity[256,257] and risk for suicide.[88,230] Individuals with bipolar disorder have a high prevalence of 46% to develop an alcohol-related disorder; indeed, the odds of a bipolar disorder if a person has an alcohol-related disorder are 5.1 times greater than in an individual without an alcohol-related disorder.[271] Individuals with comorbid bipolar and alcohol use disorder are at increased risk of violent behavior,[285] treatment nonadherence, high rates of hospitalization,[307] and mortality. Anxiety-related disorders also occur frequently among alcohol-dependent individuals (with a prevalence rate of 19.4%), especially general anxiety disorder, social phobia, and posttraumatic stress disorder.[271] Up to 90% of individuals with alcohol use disorders are smokers, and the heaviest drinkers tend to smoke the most.[15] In a sample size ranging from 80 to 1142, surveys of individuals with a diagnosis of moderate to severe alcohol use disorder from inpatient and outpatient treatment facilities showed an 86%–97% smoking rate among males and an 82%–90% rate among females.[39,74,171,331] Smoking increases the health risks and associated morbidity and mortality of alcohol use disorder greatly, and vice versa. Comorbid psychiatric disorder or smoking complicates the treatment of alcohol use disorder and increases the level of public health concern.

Alcohol use disorder is a chronic relapsing medical disorder.[226] Notwithstanding its psychological and social ramifications, once established, alcohol use disorder is essentially a brain disorder that bears many of the characteristics of other medical relapsing disorders such as diabetes and hypertension. Indeed, without a pharmacological adjunct to psychosocial therapy, the clinical outcome is poor, with up to 70% of clients resuming drinking within 1 year.[87,316] Comorbid psychiatric or smoking-related behavior with alcohol dependence would be expected to increase these rates of relapse.

Alcohol use disorder is a treatable disorder when efficacious medications are added to enhance the effects of psychosocial treatment. Advances in the neurosciences have facilitated the development of medications that target neurotransmitter systems, which modulate activity in the cortico-mesolimbic dopamine pathway, the primary circuit by which alcohol's reinforcing effects associated with its abuse liability are expressed. In addition, neuronal circuits in the extended amygdala modulate the expression of alcohol reinforcement in the cortico-mesolimbic dopamine pathway and increase the propensity for conditioned behaviors to trigger relapse.[169] It is now well accepted that some individuals with alcohol use disorder may possess a biological predisposition to the disease. These biologically vulnerable individuals with alcohol use disorder can be expected to benefit from specific adjunctive medications targeted toward correcting or ameliorating their underlying neurobiological abnormalities. Furthermore, we are now better at controlling the "dose" of adjunctive psychosocial treatments, thereby optimizing the therapeutic response of the candidate medicines. Targeting medicinal treatments toward psychiatric or smoking-related disorders that are comorbid with alcohol use disorder

is complex because the neuronal targets are broadened, and the implications of altering their function are less well understood.

Recently, the treatment of alcohol use disorder has been advanced by development of new models as well as broader therapeutic objectives. An important model is that with appropriate pharmacotherapy it is possible to initiate treatment while the individual is still drinking heavily and at the point of maximum crisis and help-seeking behavior.[153] To broaden access to treatment, effective but brief and standardized behavioral treatment has been developed to accompany medication delivery; thus these medications can now be provided more readily in the general practice setting.[152,263] Finally, it is now better recognized that although abstinence might be the ultimate goal in treating individuals with alcohol use disorder; reducing the frequency of heavy drinking has the major impact of decreasing alcohol-related consequences and improving quality of life.[153]

In this review, we focus on the development of those medications for which there is clinical information and that have been designed to reduce the desire to drink, to promote abstinence, or both. Basically, of the numerous neurotransmitter systems that have been identified for the development of new medicines, the most promising compounds appear to be those that modulate the function of opioids, glutamate with or without γ-aminobutyric acid (GABA), and serotonin. Other putative therapeutic medications including direct modulators of dopamine function, enzyme inhibitors, and neuroinflammatory pathways are also discussed. Each subsection of this chapter provides an overview of the basic science, clinical studies, and future directions for the development of specific promising medications from these neurobiological systems. Emphasis is made in places where the development of a particular medications has advanced the development of a new treatment model or broadened therapeutic objectives. As appropriate, subsections are expanded or added where there is the discussion of a medication that has been tested for the treatment of alcohol use disorder with a comorbid psychiatric disorder or smoking pertinent to this review. We conclude the chapter with remarks pertaining to current barriers to treatment and how they might be overcome.

Opioids: Mu Receptor Antagonist—Naltrexone

Basic Science and Human Laboratory Studies

The endogenous opioid system, particularly through its interactions with the cortico-mesolimbic dopamine system, is involved in the expression of alcohol's reinforcing effects[a] (Fig. 51.1). Obviously, opioid receptors also have interactions with other neurotransmitters, including those in the glutamate,[185] GABA,[89] serotonin,[218] cannabinoid,[208] and perhaps glycine[272] systems, that contribute to its effects on ethanol intake.

Although naltrexone has some affinity for the kappa-opioid receptor,[270] its principal pharmacological effect on alcohol consumption is through blockade of the mu-opioid receptor, as mice that lack the mu-opioid receptor do not self-administer alcohol.[275] Furthermore, alcohol intake increases beta-endorphin release in brain regions such as the nucleus accumbens,[209,250,268] an effect that is blocked by naltrexone.[343] Mu receptor antagonists such as naltrexone and naloxone also suppress ethanol intake across a

[a]References 102, 116, 130, 143, 159, 191, 219.

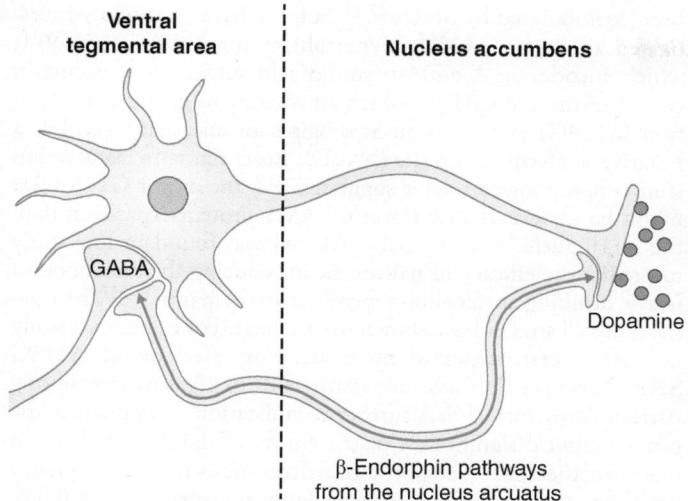

Ventral tegmental area

Nucleus accumbens

GABA

Dopamine

β-Endorphin pathways
from the nucleus arcuatus

• **Fig. 51.1** Schematic representation of opioid interactions with the cortico-mesolimbic dopamine reward pathway. Functional activity of beta-endorphin pathways primarily originating from the nucleus arcuatus can lead to increased dopamine release in the nucleus accumbens via two mechanisms. First, beta-endorphins can disinhibit the tonic inhibition of γ-aminobutyric acid (GABA) neurons on dopamine cells in the ventral tegmental area.[116,159,219] Second, beta-endorphins can stimulate dopamine cells in the nucleus accumbens directly. Both mechanisms may be important for alcohol reward. Alcohol stimulates beta-endorphin release in both the nucleus accumbens and ventral tegmental area.[297] Mu receptor antagonists such as naloxone and naltrexone block these central effects of beta-endorphins.[297,348] Embellished from Gianoulakis.[102] (Reprinted from Johnson and Ait-Daoud,[143] with kind permission from Springer Science+Business Media.)

wide range of animal paradigms[b] (cf. Berman et al.,[18] Juarez and Eliana,[160] and Ross et al.[278]). More recently, there also has been interest in elucidating the role of the hypothalamic-pituitary-adrenocortical axis in stress-induced ethanol consumption and sensitivity and how this might be influenced by naltrexone treatment.[164,337]

Ethanol has complex neurobiological interactions that affect the production, secretion, and binding of opioids to their receptors,[132] thereby hinting at a fundamental mechanistic process linking the two. This relationship does, however, remain imperfectly understood. For example, animals bred for high ethanol preference exhibit an exaggerated reactive rise in beta-endorphin level following ethanol intake.[103] Yet, naltrexone's ability to suppress ethanol-associated increases in beta-endorphin level appears greater in animals bred for low rather than high preference for alcohol.[343] Indeed, from a group of animals in the beta-endorphin–deficient mutant mouse line—C57BL/6-Pomc1(tm1Low)—the highest ethanol consumption occurred in the heterozygotes (50% beta-endorphin deficient) and not the homozygotes (no beta-endorphin) or control group of sibling wild-type mice from the same strain.[111] These findings do suggest, however, that molecular genetic differences that alter beta-endorphin expression, not simply its plasma levels, modulate the level of response to naltrexone. Nevertheless, there is growing evidence in humans that differences in the *OPRM1* mu-opioid receptor gene are associated with differential therapeutic response to naltrexone—a theme that is explored in detail later in this review.

Human laboratory studies that have evaluated naltrexone's effects on alcohol-induced positive subjective mood and craving

have yielded mixed results. Although it has been shown that naltrexone can reduce alcohol-induced positive subjective mood, albeit with increased sedation,[318] and increase the latency to consume alcohol among social drinkers,[65] others have reported no effect.[72] It does appear, however, that a positive familial loading for alcoholism might predict the potential anti-drinking and anti-craving effects of naltrexone in human laboratory studies. For example, King et al.[167] showed that social drinkers with a familial loading for alcoholism were more likely than those without it to exhibit a decrease in the stimulant effects of alcohol following naltrexone treatment. Nevertheless, they also reported concomitant negative mood exemplified by increased tension, fatigue, and confusion and decreased vigor, as well as notable adverse events such as nausea and vomiting following naltrexone. More recently, Krishnan-Sarin et al.[183] have shown that individuals with a family history of alcoholism, compared with their family history–negative counterparts, consumed less alcohol in a laboratory paradigm. Obviously, these results would lead to the speculation that there could be a genetic explanation for differential response to naltrexone's effects on craving and alcohol consumption among individuals with alcohol use disorder, which can be studied in the human laboratory. Nevertheless, even here, what has been demonstrated is that naltrexone increases the urge to drink among alcohol-dependent individuals who are aspartate (Asp) carriers of the *OPRM1* gene but has no effect on their homozygote, that is, asparagine-carrying, counterparts in a cue-reactivity laboratory paradigm.[223] Despite the dissimilarities between studies, including the subject's motivation toward seeking treatment, experimental set, setting, expectations, and paradigm, these results do appear to be in contrast with the report that naltrexone preferentially protected against relapse in Asp-carrying alcohol-dependent individuals.[257] The implications of these findings are discussed in the clinical subsection below.

In sum, basic science studies support the finding that naltrexone can reduce ethanol drinking and related behaviors in animals. Naltrexone appears most effective in suppressing the expected ethanol-induced increase in beta-endorphin level among animals that exhibit an exaggerated beta-endorphin response. The pharmacogenetic construct for understanding preferential response to naltrexone is not well understood and is even contrary to expectations. Generally, human laboratory studies provide some support for naltrexone as a medication that can reduce craving for alcohol as well as its consumption; however, these effects appear to be more readily demonstrable among individuals with high familial loading for alcoholism. An initial pharmacogenetic exploration did not demonstrate that naltrexone's anti-drinking effect is greatest among non–treatment-seeking, alcohol-dependent individuals who carry the Asp variant of the *OPRM1* gene.

Clinical Studies With Oral Naltrexone

In 1994, the US Food and Drug Administration (FDA) approved naltrexone for the treatment of alcohol dependence based on data from two relatively small (total *N* = 167) studies.[252,328] In those studies, recently abstinent, alcohol-dependent individuals who received naltrexone (50 mg/day), compared with their counterparts who got placebo, were less likely to relapse during the treatment period of 12 weeks. Nevertheless, 5 months after treatment, the relapse rates for the naltrexone and placebo groups were similar. The anti-alcohol-craving effects that were ascribed to naltrexone were based on three findings. First, individuals with the highest level of baseline craving appeared to benefit the most from

[b]References 7, 69, 90–92, 133, 162, 188, 282, 324, 327.

naltrexone.[135] Second, abstinent individuals who had received naltrexone had less of an impulse to initiate drinking.[253] Third, even among those who sampled alcohol, less pleasure was derived from the beverage.[329] These earlier studies were limited by the fact that only male veterans were tested in one of the studies,[328] and either there was no biomarker used to corroborate the self-reported data[251] or when the liver enzyme γ-glutamyl transferase was used as a biomarker the results were not contributory[328]—presumably due to the relative insensitivity of this measure to capture transient drinking patterns.

Notably, in two large meta-analyses,[32,312] naltrexone has been demonstrated to be efficacious at reducing the risk of relapse among recently abstinent, alcohol-dependent individuals. What has emerged from an examination of these studies was that naltrexone's effect size was small, with a corresponding number needed to treat (i.e., the number of individuals who need to be treated to prevent relapse in a single individual) of seven. An important threat to demonstrating efficacy for naltrexone is not having quite high enough levels of medication compliance. Indeed, in a 3-month follow-up and systematic replication of their study, Volpicelli et al.[330] found only a significant effect of naltrexone treatment compared with placebo recipients if the pill-taking rate exceeded 90%; even here, the difference in the percentage of drinking days between the naltrexone and placebo groups was small—3% and 11%, respectively.

Perhaps because of this small effect size, some studies have failed to demonstrate naltrexone's efficacy in treating alcohol dependence. For instance, in the United Kingdom collaborative trial led by Chick et al.,[46] no overall difference was found between the naltrexone 50 mg/day and placebo groups on any of the end-point measures; however, when individuals with less than 80% pill-taking compliance were excluded from the analysis, naltrexone was associated with a lower percentage of days drinking compared with placebo—12% versus 20%, respectively.[196,197] With naltrexone treatment, reduced pill-taking compliance is typically the result of adverse events such as nausea that can be reported as significant in up to 15% of trial participants.[60] Therefore, new technologies that aim to improve compliance by delivering naltrexone in depot form might possess a therapeutic advantage to the oral formulation. These technologies are discussed later in this section.

It is important to note that the landmark COMBINE study (N = 1383) has served to underscore that naltrexone (100 mg/day) plus medication management to enhance compliance compared with placebo reduced the risk of a heavy drinking day (hazard ratio [HR] 0.72, 97.5% CI 0.53–0.98; P = 0.02).[10] Uniquely, this study used a higher naltrexone dose (i.e., 100 mg/day vs. 50 mg/day), and the high compliance rate of pill taking—85.4%—improved clinical outcome.

Recently, it has been proposed that individuals with the Asp variant of the *OPRM1* gene exhibited preferentially higher relapse prevention rates when receiving naltrexone treatment.[257] As described previously, a similar response to naltrexone treatment on cue-elicited craving was not observed among non–treatment-seeking, alcohol-dependent individuals in a human laboratory study.[223] Furthermore, a recent clinical trial did not find a preferential effect of naltrexone treatment on any of the variants of the *OPRM1* gene.[97] Notably, the functional importance of variation in the *OPRM1* gene is still being elucidated. Although earlier studies in transfected cells suggested that the OPRM1-Asp[250] variant had a threefold higher affinity for beta-endorphin than OPRM1-Asn,[250] which would suggest enhanced function,[31] this has not

been corroborated by others.[17,19] In humans, a commonly investigated single-nucleotide polymorphism (or SNP), rs1799971, which encodes an Asn40Asp amino acid substitution, occurs in exon 1 of the OPRM1, in which an adenine to guanine substitution (A118G) exchanges an asparagine for an aspartic acid at a putative *N*-glycosylation site (N40D). Recent in vitro transfection studies have, however, have suggested that the minor G118 allele might be associated with lower OPRM1 protein expression than the A118 allele.[346] In humans, A118G was found in one study to predict the efficacy of naltrexone in reducing the likelihood of heavy drinking in alcohol-dependent participants.[11,257] In contrast, not all studies have shown these effects. For example, a study in male veterans reported no moderating effect of the A118G SNP[256] and the SNP did not improve drinking outcome among African Americans.[11,45] A further complication to estimating the general clinical significance of the effects of the Asp[250] allele on pharmacotherapeutic response to naltrexone is that its frequency can vary considerably between populations—from as low as 0.047 in African Americans to 0.154 in European Americans, and as high as 0.485 among those of Asian descent.[96,344] More genetic studies are, therefore, needed to elucidate fully the mechanistic effects of the Asp[250] allele, and to establish whether or not naltrexone response varies by variation at the *OPRM1* gene.

Certain clinical characteristics have been associated, however, with good clinical response to naltrexone, and these include a family history of alcohol dependence[135,231] or strong cravings or urges for alcohol.[231]

Naltrexone's utility compared with placebo as an add-on treatment in individuals with alcohol use disorder and comorbid bipolar I or II disorder was investigated recently.[291] All individuals received their concomitant medications prescribed for bipolar disorder prior to study entry, along with standardized cognitive behavioral therapy designed for the treatment of bipolar disorder and substance use at scheduled intervals during treatment.[284] Naltrexone showed trends (P < 0.10) toward a greater decrease in drinking days and alcohol craving but did not differ statistically from placebo on any outcome measure of drinking.

Naltrexone's utility compared with placebo as a treatment for alcohol dependence and smoking cessation also has been studied recently.[166] In that placebo-controlled study, there was no overall effect of naltrexone on either the consumption of alcohol or smoking. In a subsequent subset analysis confined to heavy drinkers (defined as those with at least one heavy drinking episode during the 2-week pre-enrollment baseline period), there was an effect of naltrexone to reduce heavy drinking; however, again there was no effect on smoking. Of interest, there was a significant negative association between quitting smoking and decreasing alcohol consumption, whereby greater success in stopping smoking was correlated with increased amounts of heavy drinking. These results do not provide strong support for the use of naltrexone as a medication for the simultaneous reduction or cessation of alcohol consumption and smoking among individuals comorbid for these conditions.

Although the use of naltrexone in the treatment of alcohol use disorder is supported by the scientific evidence and accepted by many regulatory agencies, most studies have looked at the target variable of naltrexone's propensity to prevent relapse. It is, therefore, not surprising that most studies have found that opioid antagonists reduce relapse to heavy drinking. It is notable that there also is some evidence that naltrexone may be more efficacious when prescribed to individuals who are actively drinking. This appears consistent with naltrexone's known effect on the endogenous opioid system, particularly through its interactions with the cortico-mesolimbic dopamine system. Alcohol stimulates beta-endorphin release in both the nucleus accumbens and ventral tegmental area, and opioid antagonists such as naltrexone block these central effects of beta-endorphins with the overall gain of a reduction in the reinforcing effect of alcohol. If there is no alcohol, then there is no alcohol-induced release of endogenous opioids for an opioid antagonist to block. In most clinical trials, no significant benefit from naltrexone was found while participants were abstinent, the primary effect of naltrexone was seen in participants who drank any alcohol while being enrolled in the trial. This work has been promoted by David Sinclair and his team in Finland. They provided evidence that opioid antagonists such as naloxone, nalmefene, or naltrexone had to be given in conjunction with alcohol drinking to produce positive results in animals. Furthermore, their results indicated that giving naltrexone, naloxone, or nalmefene during abstinence was not useful, as the major benefit from an opioid antagonist is produced by the mechanism of extinction.[297,299,300,302] Clinical trials from David Sinclair and his group showed that alcohol craving and drinking slowly diminished over many weeks in the form of an extinction curve.[c] Data from other clinical trials also showed that targeted prescription of naltrexone reduces heavy drinking when combined with some type of skill building intervention.[123,172,178]

Prescribing naltrexone to abstinent detoxified alcoholics is hypothesized to affect conditioned cue craving as the release of endorphins become conditioned to cues present around alcohol drinking. Naltrexone during abstinence could extinguish the ability of these cues to cause craving; however, it is possible that without the interaction of alcohol to allow for extinction of the behavior, the overall effect may be limited.

In sum, the majority of the data confirm that naltrexone is an efficacious medication for treating alcohol dependence. The therapeutic treatment effect size is, however, small, and poor pill-taking compliance can be associated with poor clinical outcome. Naltrexone can be used safely in individuals with alcohol use disorder without prior detoxification and could be effective even if it is taken only when drinking is expected, although more research evaluating the targeted approach to naltrexone treatment is needed. As a caution, it must be remembered that the FDA does have a black box warning that naltrexone administration could complicate or exacerbate liver damage among individuals with alcohol use disorder. There remains a dearth of published studies on the effects of different doses of naltrexone on drinking outcome. Further research is needed to establish whether naltrexone's therapeutic efficacy in treating alcohol use disorder differs among individuals who have variants of the *OPRM1* gene. Individuals with alcohol use disorder that have a positive family history or strong cravings for alcohol might benefit the most from naltrexone treatment. Naltrexone does not appear to be a promising medication for the contemporaneous reduction or cessation of alcohol consumption and smoking.

Clinical Studies With Depot Naltrexone

Three extended-release formulations of naltrexone for deep intramuscular injection have been developed—Vivitrol (Alkermes, Inc., Cambridge, MA, USA), Naltrel (Drug Abuse Sciences, Inc., Paris, France), and Depotrex (Biotek, Inc., Woburn, MA, USA). The premise for developing these depot formulations of

naltrexone is threefold. First, a well-formulated depot preparation can maintain relatively constant plasma levels by producing a slow but regular release of naltrexone. Individuals who take oral naltrexone and have notable adverse events such as nausea that can lead to study discontinuation probably experience this phenomenon due to the rapid rise in plasma levels following initial doses of oral naltrexone. Hence, a depot formulation might be expected to decrease these initial adverse events if it provided a more gradual rise in naltrexone plasma levels. Second, by providing a monthly depot preparation, compliance with receiving the medication is optimized and should be greater than reliance on remembering to take tablets. Third, because plasma levels should remain relatively constant throughout the month following the administration of a depot preparation, there should be relatively greater exposure to the therapeutic dose, thereby facilitating good clinical outcome. Information pertaining to the three depot preparations of naltrexone that are being tested is provided below.

Vivitrex or Vivitrol

Vivitrex, or Vivitrol as it is known now, is naltrexone formulated into poly-(lactide-co-glycolide),[293] small-diameter (<100 μm), injectable microspheres that contain other proprietary active moieties, which lead to its extended-release properties lasting for several weeks.[192] In 2004, Johnson et al.[149] published the initial safety, tolerability, and efficacy trial of Vivitrex for treating alcohol dependence. The design of the study was a 16-week randomized, placebo-controlled, double-blind clinical trial. Of the 25 alcohol-dependent individuals who participated in the trial, five received placebo and the remainder ($N = 20$) received 400 mg of Vivitrex. Results of that trial showed the safety of Vivitrex, with the most common adverse events being nonspecific abdominal pain, nausea, pain at the injection site, and headaches. None of the placebo recipients dropped out due to adverse events; in contrast, two of those who got Vivitrex discontinued for that reason. Due to the unbalanced design and small subject numbers, any inferences regarding efficacy had to be viewed quite cautiously. Nevertheless, there was a trend for those on Vivitrex, compared with placebo, to have a lower percentage of heavy drinking days—11.7% vs. 25.3%. Later, in a large placebo-controlled, double-blind, randomized, multisite, 24-week clinical trial, Garbutt et al.[95] showed that high-dose Vivitrex (380 mg) recipients had a significantly lower percentage of heavy drinking days than those who got placebo (HR 0.75, 95% CI 0.60–0.94; $P = 0.02$). Recipients of low-dose Vivitrex (190 mg) had outcomes similar to those who got placebo. The treatment response signal in the high-dose Vivitrex recipients came from the male participants, as the effect of both Vivitrex doses was no different from that in women who took placebo (HR 1.23, 95% CI 0.85–1.78; $P = 0.28$). The lack of efficacy for Vivitrol in women has been ascribed to greater subclinical affective symptoms, less of a family history of alcoholism (which is meant to be associated with good clinical outcomes to naltrexone), more responsiveness to placebo, and more clinical heterogeneity in the sample. In contrast with the premise for developing depot preparations, the dropout rate of 14.1% in the high-dose Vivitrex group was similar to that reported in studies with oral naltrexone. The chosen objective biomarker to corroborate the self-reported data—γ-glutamyl transferase—did not show a difference between any of the Vivitrex doses and the placebo group. The common reasons for study discontinuation were injection site reactions, headaches, and nausea. Serious adverse events were reported in two participants taking active medication that resulted in an interstitial pneumonia and an allergic-type eosinophilic pneumonia, both of which resolved after medical treatment. Thus the evidence remains that Vivitrol appears to be efficacious in preventing heavy drinking in men; however, it was approved by the FDA for treatment of both men and women based on the extant literature on naltrexone as a treatment for alcohol dependence. The expected advantage of Vivitrol for increasing compliance did not materialize quickly, although this might become more manifest in generic treatment settings rather than in a closely monitored clinical trial. The potential for hypersensitivity reactions to Vivitrol, although small, does require postmarketing evaluation by the FDA.

Naltrel

Naltrel consists of naltrexone incorporated into microspheres of poly-(DL-lactide) polymer. These microspheres, stored in single-dose vials, are suspended in a diluent that contains carboxymethylcellulose, mannitol, polysorbate 80, and water for injection. The polylactide polymer is metabolized to water and carbon dioxide. Then, as the microspheres degrade, naltrexone is released. In 2004, Kranzler et al.[179] studied the safety and efficacy of Naltrel in treating male and female alcohol-dependent individuals receiving monthly motivation enhancement-based therapy in a double-blind, placebo-controlled, 3-month randomized controlled trial ($N = 157$). The initial dose of Naltrel (150 mg) was delivered as a deep intramuscular injection into each buttock, and subsequent monthly doses were just 150 mg. Placebo injections were provided at the same frequency and constitution but lacked the active compound. Adverse events reported significantly more frequently in those who received Naltrel compared with those how received placebo included injection site reactions, chest pain, and upper abdominal pain. Placebo recipients were, however, more likely to report irritability than those who got Naltrel. Although 6 (3.8%) of the placebo recipients dropped out, 13 (8.2%) who got Naltrel discontinued treatment. Naltrel* was superior to placebo at increasing the mean number of cumulative abstinent days (52.8 days, 95% CI 48.5–57.2 days, vs. 45.6 days, 95% CI 41.1–50.0 days, respectively; $P = 0.018$) and having a longer median time to first drink (5 days, 95% CI 3–9 days, vs. 3 days, 95% CI 2–4 days, respectively; $P = 0.003$). The effects of gender on treatment outcome were not examined.

Somewhat in contrast, a single-site, 6-week trial of 16 alcohol-dependent individuals who received one intramuscular dose of Naltrel (300 mg)[344] suggested low tolerability, with 198 adverse events being reported. Of these, 17 were considered to be severe and included fatigue, gastrointestinal pain, irritability, nausea, somnolence (two reports), headache (four reports from three subjects), injection site pain, injection site mass, lethargy, depression, increased level of γ-glutamyl transferase (an index of heavy drinking[57]), back pain, and flatulence. No serious adverse events were reported. Drinking outcomes showed an improving trend over the duration of the trial.

Nevertheless, further studies on the safety and efficacy of the Naltrel formulation are warranted. Additional data are needed to determine whether, as with Vivitrol, there is a differential response on drinking outcomes between men and women who receive Naltrel.

Depotrex

Rather little public information is available on the Depotrex depot formulation. Like the other depot formulations, Depotrex appears to provide steady increases in plasma naltrexone levels[174] and is an effective mu-opioid receptor antagonist.[6,126] Pharmacokinetic data from 12 heroin-dependent individuals who received low and high doses of Depotrex—192 mg and 384 mg, respectively—showed that both doses maintained plasma naltrexone levels above 1 ng/mL for up to 4 weeks.[56] Average peak levels for the low and high doses of Depotrex were 3.8 ng/mL and 8.9 ng/mL, respectively. Plasma beta-naltrexol, the major metabolite of naltrexone, was greater proportionally but could not be detected 5 weeks following Depotrex administration. Both doses of Depotrex antagonized the positive subjective effects of heroin. Reported adverse events were minimal and included mild discomfort at the injection site, with no irritation or erythema. The promising earlier study by Kranzler et al.[174] of Depotrex (206 mg) in the treatment of alcohol dependence needs to be followed up.

In sum, depot formulations of naltrexone may offer some advantages such as increased compliance over the oral formulations. This advantage has, however, been difficult to demonstrate in randomized controlled trials but might become more apparent when these depot formulations are used in generic practices. Depot formulations do not appear to be more efficacious than the oral formulations, and with one of these—Vivitrol—no therapeutic effect in women has been demonstrated. The adverse event profiles of depot formulations of naltrexone that have been reported in randomized controlled trials appear similar in frequency and intensity to those observed for the oral formulation. The different depot formulations do appear to be similar in characteristics and profile, and more clinical information about which one to select to treat a particular alcohol-dependent individual, if all are approved by the FDA, shall be needed.

Nalmefene

Nalmefene is an opioid antagonist with the reported advantage over naltrexone being a longer half-life, greater oral bioavailability, and no evidence of liver toxicity. Also unlike naltrexone, which is principally an antagonist at mu and delta opioid receptors, nalmefene is a partial agonist at the kappa receptor. Of interest, it has been speculated that this effect of nalmefene on the kappa receptor would render it likely to be more effective than naltrexone. Specifically, notwithstanding its effects to modulate endogenous dopamine function by antagonism at the mu opioid receptor,[44,292] it also has been hypothesized that nalmefene may modulate the hypothesized overactivity of the dynorphin/kappa receptor by acting as a functional antagonist to decrease alcohol self-administration more markedly in alcohol-dependent compared with nondependent rats.[168,248] Nevertheless, even though it would be tempting to extend this hypothesis to humans, the relationship between dynorphin/kappa receptor and alcohol consumption remains complex and not well understood.[259]

In a small placebo-control, double-blind, randomized study of 21 individuals with alcohol-dependence, nalmefene 10 mg/day appeared to decrease significantly the number of drinks/drinking day but not any other measure of alcohol consumption.[210] In a second study by the same, 105 alcohol-dependent individuals were given a dosage of nalmefene 20 mg/day and 80 mg/day, and there was no significant difference among them, although more individuals relapsed to placebo (OR 2.4, 95% CI 1.05–5.59).[212] Nevertheless in a much larger controlled study of 270 alcohol-dependent individuals taking nalmefene at a dose of 5 mg/day, 20 mg/day, or 40 mg/day, there was no significant effect compared with placebo for any of the nalmefene doses.[9]

Nalmefene was, however, approved for the treatment of alcohol use disorder in Europe based on the results of three large-scale studies.[113,205,323] In the first 24-week, controlled study ($n = 604$), nalmefene 18 mg/day compared with placebo was associated with a significantly greater reduction in the number of heavy drinking days per month (–2.3 days, 95% CI –3.8 to –0.8). In addition, when the subjects consumed alcohol, they drank less significantly while on nalmefene compared with placebo (–11 g/day, 95% CI –16.8 to –5.1). In the second study (ESENSE 2; n = 718), which was 24 weeks in length, nalmefene (18 mg/day) also was given on an as-needed basis compared with placebo. Nalmefene compared with placebo was associated with a significantly greater reduction in the number of heavy drinking days per month (–1.7 days per month, 95% CI –3.1 to –0.4; $P = 0.012$) but not total alcohol consumption (–4.9 g/day; 95% CI –10.6 to 0.7; $P = 0.088$). Sub-population analysis from ESENSE 1 and 2 appeared to strengthen the data, whereby for the 667 individuals who met World Health Organization high-risk drinking level criteria (>60 g/day and >40 g/day, for men and women, respectively), the effect of nalmefene compared with placebo appeared to be more striking than that of the combined study population (n = 1.322) (–3.2 heavy drinking days, 95% CI –4.8 to –1.6; $P < 0.0001$ versus –2.0 heavy drinking days, 95% CI –3.0 to –1.0; $P < 0.0001$, respectively), and in alcohol consumption (–14.3 g/day, 95% CI –20.8 to –7.8; $P < 0.0001$ versus –7.6 g/day, 95% CI –11.6 to –3.5; $P < 0.0003$, respectively). For all the studies, the adverse event profile was mild to moderate, with the most common reactions being nausea, dizziness, insomnia, and headache. Confusion, and rarely, hallucinations and dissociations were reported.[259] Adverse events typically occurred early in treatment and were of relatively short duration. In sum, nalmefene under the brand name Selincro was approved in Europe in February 2013 for the treatment of alcohol use disorder, with the effect of reducing heavy drinking among those deemed not to be in need of detoxification.[308] Nalmefene appears to be well tolerated, although it remains unproven that it is any more efficacious than naltrexone despite the pharmacological expectations.

Glutamate

Metabotropic Glutamate Receptor-5 Modulator and N-Methyl-D-Aspartate Antagonist—Acamprosate

Acamprosate's principal neurochemical effects have been attributed to antagonism of N-methyl-D-aspartate glutamate receptors,[66,348] which restore the balance between excitatory and inhibitory neurotransmission that is dysregulated following chronic alcohol consumption.[67] Recently, however, it also has been proposed that acamprosate modulates glutamate neurotransmission at metabotropic-5 glutamate receptors.[118] Evidence that acamprosate modulates a novel site of action at metabotropic-5 glutamate receptors comes from the finding that it inhibits the binding and neurotoxic effects of (±)-1-aminocyclopentane-trans-1,3-dicarboxylic acid.[118] Acamprosate has been shown to decrease: (1) ethanol consumption in rodents,[29,61,189] but this effect may not be specific in food-deprived C57BL/6 J mice as both ethanol and water were reduced in a schedule-induced polydipsia task[81]; (2) dopamine hyperexcitability in the nucleus accumbens during alcohol withdrawal[62,279]; (3) general neuronal hyperexcitability[101,311]; (4) glutamatergic neurotransmission in alcohol-dependent rats[30,63];

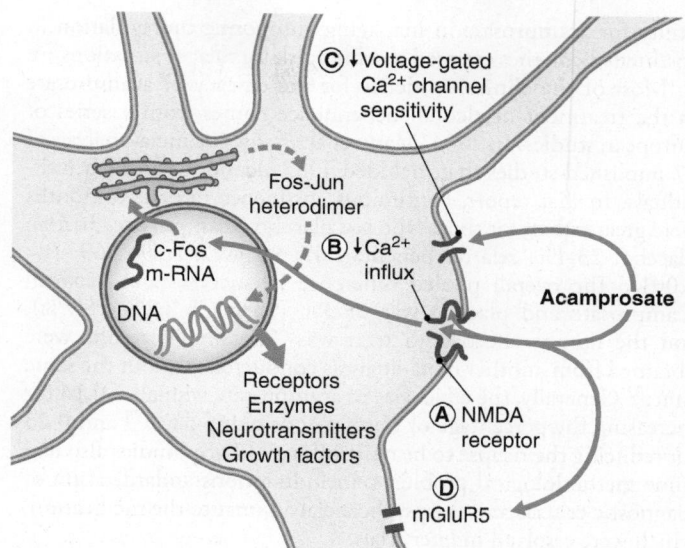

• **Fig. 51.2** Schematic representation of acamprosate's effects. Acamprosate has four principal effects: A, reducing postsynaptic excitatory amino acid neurotransmission at N-methyl-D-aspartate (NMDA); B, diminishing Ca^{2+} influx into the cell, which interferes with expression of the immediate early gene c-fos; C, decreasing the sensitivity of voltage-gated calcium channels; and D, modulating metabotropic-5 glutamate receptors (mGluR5s). mGluR5s are postsynaptic and are coupled to their associated ion channels by a second messenger cascade system (not shown). Also shown in this representation is synthesis of c-fos and c-jun in the endoplasmic reticulum, which can bind with DNA to alter the transcription of late effector genes. Late effector genes regulate long-term changes in cellular activity such as the function of receptors, enzymes, growth factors, and the production of neurotransmitters. (Adapted from Johnson and Ait-Daoud,[143] with kind permission from Springer Science+Business Media—adapted version reprinted from Johnson,[140] with permission from Elsevier—and from Spanagel and Zieglgansberger.[310])

(5) voltage-gated calcium channel activity, and (6) the expression of brain c-fos, an immediate early gene associated with alcohol withdrawal.[199,265] Nevertheless, it is acamprosate's ability to suppress alcohol-induced glutamate receptor sensitivity,[185] as well as conditioned cue responses to ethanol in previously dependent animals even after prolonged abstinence,[301,309,311,340] that has been linked with its therapeutic effect in humans—dampening negative affect and craving postabstinence[143,310] (Fig. 51.2).

Of interest, there has been a paucity of human laboratory studies that have examined the potential effects of acamprosate on alcohol-related behaviors associated with its abuse liability. Evidence from a human magnetic resonance imaging (MRI) study does, however, support acamprosate's ability to modulate glutamate neurotransmission as it decreases activity in brain regions rich in N-acetylaspartate and glutamate.[159] Human laboratory studies in both volunteers[213] and alcohol-dependent individuals[151] also have shown that acamprosate—that is, calcium acetyl homotaurinate—is relatively safe, with the most important adverse events being diarrhea, nervousness, and fatigue, especially at a relatively high dose (3 g/day). Because acamprosate is excreted unchanged in the kidneys, there is no risk of hepatotoxicity, but it should be used with caution in those with renal impairment.[151,217] Acamprosate has no significant clinical interaction with alcohol. Recently, it was shown that acamprosate can reduce heart rate response but not the increase in cortisol or subjective craving following the presentation of alcohol cues—a finding that suggests utility for acamprosate in managing autonomic dysregulation in abstinent alcoholics exposed to a high risk for relapse situations.[254]

Most of the clinical evidence for the efficacy of acamprosate in the treatment of alcohol dependence comes from a series of European studies. In 2004, Mann et al.[206] wrote a meta-analysis of 17 published studies that included 4087 alcohol-dependent individuals. In that report, continuous abstinence rates at 6 months were greater than for those who got placebo (acamprosate, 36.1%; placebo, 23.4%; relative benefit, 1.47; 95% CI 1.29–1.69; $P <$ 0.001). The overall pooled difference in success rates between acamprosate and placebo was 13.3% (95% CI 7.8%–18.7%), and the number needed to treat was 7.5. Similar results were obtained from another meta-analysis conducted at about the same time.[32] Generally, the effect size of acamprosate is small—0.14 for increasing the percentage of nonheavy drinking days[175] and 0.23 for reducing the relapse to heavy drinking.[47] Early studies also had some methodological problems, including nonstandardization of diagnostic criteria and the psychosocial adjunct to the medication, which were resolved in later trials.

Despite approval by the FDA on July 29, 2004, for the use of acamprosate in the treatment of alcohol dependence, largely based on the data from European studies, the results of studies in the United States have been disappointing. In the United States multisite trial by Lipha Pharmaceuticals, Inc., there was no overall clinical evidence that acamprosate was superior to placebo among a heterogeneous cohort of alcohol-dependent individuals; however, post hoc analysis suggested that a subgroup of alcoholics with a treatment goal of abstinence might derive benefit.[214] Furthermore, in 2006, the multi-site COMBINE study also failed to find any therapeutic benefit of acamprosate compared with placebo on any drinking outcome measures.[10] Obviously, the findings of these US studies have reduced the enthusiasm for using it by addiction specialists in the United States. From a scientific perspective, these findings do raise the question as to what type of alcohol-dependent individual benefits the most from acamprosate and why there is an important discrepancy between the results of US and European studies.

From the European studies, acamprosate appears to benefit alcohol-dependent individuals with increased levels of anxiety, physiological dependence, negative family history, late age at onset, and female gender.[326]

There are at least four possible explanations for the discrepancy between US and European studies. First, the populations sampled differ, with European, compared with US, studies having alcohol-dependent individuals with more prolonged drinking histories and alcohol-related neurological and psychosocial impairments. Thus it is tempting to speculate that European studies might have included individuals with greater neuroplasticity and, therefore, higher response to the ameliorating effects of anti-glutamatergic agents such as acamprosate. Second, US, compared with European, studies have tended to have higher levels of standardized psychosocial intervention as an adjunct to acamprosate, thereby masking the effect of the medication. Third, the therapeutic effect of acamprosate is small; hence, by chance, some trials can be expected to fail, especially those conducted in a multisite rather than a single-site environment due to the greater heterogeneity and variability of the cohort and research settings. Fourth, it is possible that future research might uncover other important differences between US and European cohorts to explain the discrepant findings such as potential differences in participants' subtype, stage of the alcoholism disease, or biomolecular constitution.

In sum, European studies have clearly demonstrated efficacy for acamprosate as a treatment for alcohol dependence. Acamprosate was FDA approved in the United States largely based on the results of the European studies. Acamprosate's therapeutic effect is small, but it is well tolerated, with the most prominent adverse events being diarrhea, nervousness, and fatigue, especially at a relatively high dose (3 g/day). In contrast, studies in the United States have, to date, been unable to find efficacy for acamprosate among a heterogeneous group of alcohol-dependent individuals. The reason for this discrepancy between the results of US and European studies has not been established. Perhaps, however, this discrepant finding might be due to differences in participants' selection, subtype, stage of the alcoholism disease, or biomolecular constitution that are yet to be determined. Intriguingly, preliminary results presented for the recently completed multisite collaborative European Study—Project Predict—also did not find an effect for acamprosate in the treatment of alcohol dependence.[207] Future studies are needed to delineate more clearly what type of alcohol-dependent individual can benefit from acamprosate treatment.

Other *N*-Methyl-D-Aspartate Receptor Antagonists

Other *N*-methyl-D-aspartate receptor antagonists such as memantine and neramexane are being studied for the treatment of alcohol dependence. Both compounds have been shown in animal models to suppress ethanol-induced *N*-methyl-D-aspartate receptor upregulation, thereby reducing ethanol sensitization and the propensity for subsequent drug use (for a review, see Nagy[240] and Kotlinska et al.[170]). In a human laboratory study, memantine reduced alcohol craving prior to but not after the experimental administration of alcohol. This would suggest that memantine might have the effect of reducing postcessation craving for alcohol.[21] This finding is supported by a later report that memantine might have effects comparable to diazepam at ameliorating alcohol withdrawal symptoms.[184] Nevertheless, despite the early preliminary findings, a recent pilot clinical trial comparing memantine with placebo for the treatment of alcohol dependence reported that the greater therapeutic effect at reducing the percentage of heavy drinking days and increasing the percentage of days abstinent[82] occurred among the placebo group. Although this pilot study did not provide support for memantine as an efficacious treatment for alcohol dependence, further studies are needed to make a final determination of memantine's therapeutic potential for this indication. Recently, it was reported that memantine was as effective as escitalopram (the S-enantiomer of citalopram, a selective serotonin reuptake inhibitor) for the treatment of alcohol dependence in individuals with comorbid major depressive disorder.[233] That study, however, lacked a placebo treatment arm; therefore, it has not been established that memantine is an efficacious treatment for alcohol dependence with comorbid major depression. No human study on the therapeutic effects of neramexane in treating alcohol dependence has been published.

Alpha-Amino-3-Hydroxy-5-Methylisoxazole-4-Propionic Acid and Kainate Glutamate Receptor Antagonist—Topiramate

Topiramate, a sulfamate-substituted fructopyranose derivative, has six important mechanisms of action. In addition to its ability to antagonize alpha-amino-3-hydroxy-5-methylisoxazole-4-propionic acid receptors and kainate glutamate receptors,[104,112,303] topiramate facilitates inhibitory $GABA_A$-mediated currents at nonbenzodiazepine sites on the $GABA_A$ receptor,[334,335] inhibits L-type calcium channels and limits calcium-dependent second messenger systems,[345] reduces activity-dependent depolarization and excitability of voltage-dependent sodium channels,[319] activates potassium conductance,[131] and is a weak inhibitor of carbonic anhydrase isoenzymes, CA-II and CA-IV,[183] which are found in both neuronal and peripheral tissues. In renal tubules, carbonic anhydrase isoenzyme inhibition reduces hydrogen ion secretion and increases secretion of Na^+, K^+, HCO_3^-, and water, thereby enhancing the likelihood of acidosis and renal stone formation.[70,290]

Johnson[137,138] has proposed a neuropharmacological model by which topiramate can decrease alcohol reinforcement and the propensity to drink (Fig. 51.3). Nevertheless, few studies on the effects of topiramate on ethanol consumption in animals have been published. An initial animal study had shown complex effects of topiramate on ethanol drinking in C57BL/6 mice. In that study, high-dose (50 mg/kg) but not low-dose (1, 5, and 10 mg/kg) topiramate suppressed ethanol intake 2 hours after it was injected into the animal. Topiramate also decreased saccharin preference, but its ability to suppress ethanol preference was associated with some increase in water intake.[94] Notably, in an elegant, recent animal study, Nguyen et al.[249] demonstrated that topiramate can suppress ethanol drinking in C57BL/6 mice; in addition, in contrast with the effects of naltrexone and tiagabine in the same animals, the mice treated with topiramate did not develop any tolerance to its anti-drinking effects. Furthermore, topiramate has been shown to suppress ethanol drinking persistently in alcohol-preferring (P) but not Wistar rats.[37] In addition to its ethanol-suppressing effects, there is evidence that topiramate can reduce alcohol- withdrawal symptoms in a model of handling-induced convulsions.[85] Hence, the preponderance of the animal literature does support topiramate as a promising medication for the treatment of alcohol dependence. Nevertheless, the effect of topiramate on ethanol drinking in animals appears to be less striking than that on drinking outcomes in humans, which are presented below. This challenges the notion that animal models can directly predict treatment response in humans, especially when a variety of models have not been used or been available to characterize or "fingerprint" response.[154] The results of additional animal experiments examining topiramate's mechanistic effects on ethanol consumption or related behaviors in animals are, therefore, awaited eagerly.

Recently, Johnson et al.[148,153] and Ma et al.[203] showed in a double-blind, randomized clinical trial that topiramate (up to 300 mg/day), compared with placebo, improved all drinking outcomes, decreased craving, and improved the quality of life of alcohol-dependent individuals who received 12 weeks of weekly brief behavioral compliance enhancement treatment.[152] The improvements in self-reported drinking outcomes were confirmed by plasma γ-glutamyl transferase, an objective biochemical measure of alcohol consumption.[57] The therapeutic effect size for the primary efficacy variable—percentage of heavy drinking days—was 0.63.

In a 6-week experimental study of 76 heavy drinkers who were not seeking treatment, Miranda et al.[229] showed that low-and high-dose topiramate—200 mg/day and 300 mg/day, respectively—were significantly better than placebo at decreasing the percentage of heavy drinking days.

Furthermore, in a subsequent 17-site (N = 371) US trial, topiramate (up to 300 mg/day) was again superior to placebo at

improving all self-reported drinking outcomes, γ-glutamyl transferase level, and some measures of quality of life among alcohol-dependent individuals who received 14 weeks of weekly brief behavioral compliance enhancement treatment.[155,157] Topiramate's therapeutic effect size for the reduction in percentage of heavy drinking days was 0.52, and the number needed to treat was 3.4.[147]

Topiramate's effects on glutamate receptors appear to be more potent and selective for those containing the GluK1 and GluK2 subunits encoded by GRIK1 and GRIK2, respectively. One SNP, rs2832407, a C-to-A noncoding substitution, has been found to be associated with alcohol use disorder, with the C allele being more common in subjects with the disorder.[181] The same allele was found to be related to significantly fewer adverse medications when participants were treated with topiramate.[269]

In a 12-week randomized placebo-controlled clinical trial of 138 individuals with alcohol use disorder, treatment with 200 mg of topiramate significantly reduced heavy drinking days and increased abstinent days as compared to placebo. In a subset of the population, mainly the European American subsample (N = 122), topiramate's effect on heavy drinking days was significantly influenced by the rs2832407 C-allele, with homozygotes having a more favorable response.[182]

Taken together, these clinical studies provide strong evidence that topiramate is a promising medication for the treatment of alcohol use disorder. Encouragingly, topiramate's therapeutic effect size is in the moderate range, and the clinical effects appear to increase with greater length of time on the medication.

Generally, topiramate has a favorable adverse event profile, with most reported symptoms being classified as mild to moderate.[138] The most common adverse events are paresthesia, anorexia, difficulty with memory or concentration, and taste perversion. Slow titration to the ceiling dose (up to 300 mg/day) for 8 weeks is critical to minimizing adverse events and improving tolerability (Table 51.1); however, about 10% of individuals taking topiramate may experience some cognitive difficulty, irrespective of the dose titration schedule.[22] Topiramate use has been linked with acute but rare visual adverse events. As of January 2005, there had been 371 spontaneous reports of myopia, angle-closure glaucoma, or increased intraocular pressure, for a rate of 12.7 reports per 100,000 patient-years exposure.[140] Usually, the syndrome of acute bilateral myopia associated with secondary angle-closure glaucoma presents as the acute onset of visual blurring, ocular pain, or both. Associated bilateral ophthalmologic findings can include myopia, shallowing of the anterior chamber, conjunctival hyperemia, and raised intraocular pressure. This syndrome resolves within a few days of discontinuing topiramate administration.[138]

Although topiramate has not shown efficacy in the treatment of bipolar disorder,[325] there is an ongoing National Institutes of Health–funded study of its efficacy in the treatment of individuals with comorbid alcohol use disorder and bipolar disorder. It is presumed that among individuals whose bipolar disorder is stabilized by concurrent medication prior to the trial, topiramate would have an added effect to improve drinking outcomes. Results of this study are awaited eagerly. Another anticonvulsant, valproic acid, is promising, as it has been shown to decrease heavy drinking in alcohol-dependent individuals with bipolar disorder.[281]

As a subgroup analysis of a 12-week double-blind, randomized, controlled trial, the effect of topiramate versus placebo among alcohol-dependent smokers was evaluated.[142] Topiramate recipients were significantly more likely than placebo recipients to become abstinent from smoking (OR 4.46, 95% CI 1.08–18.39;

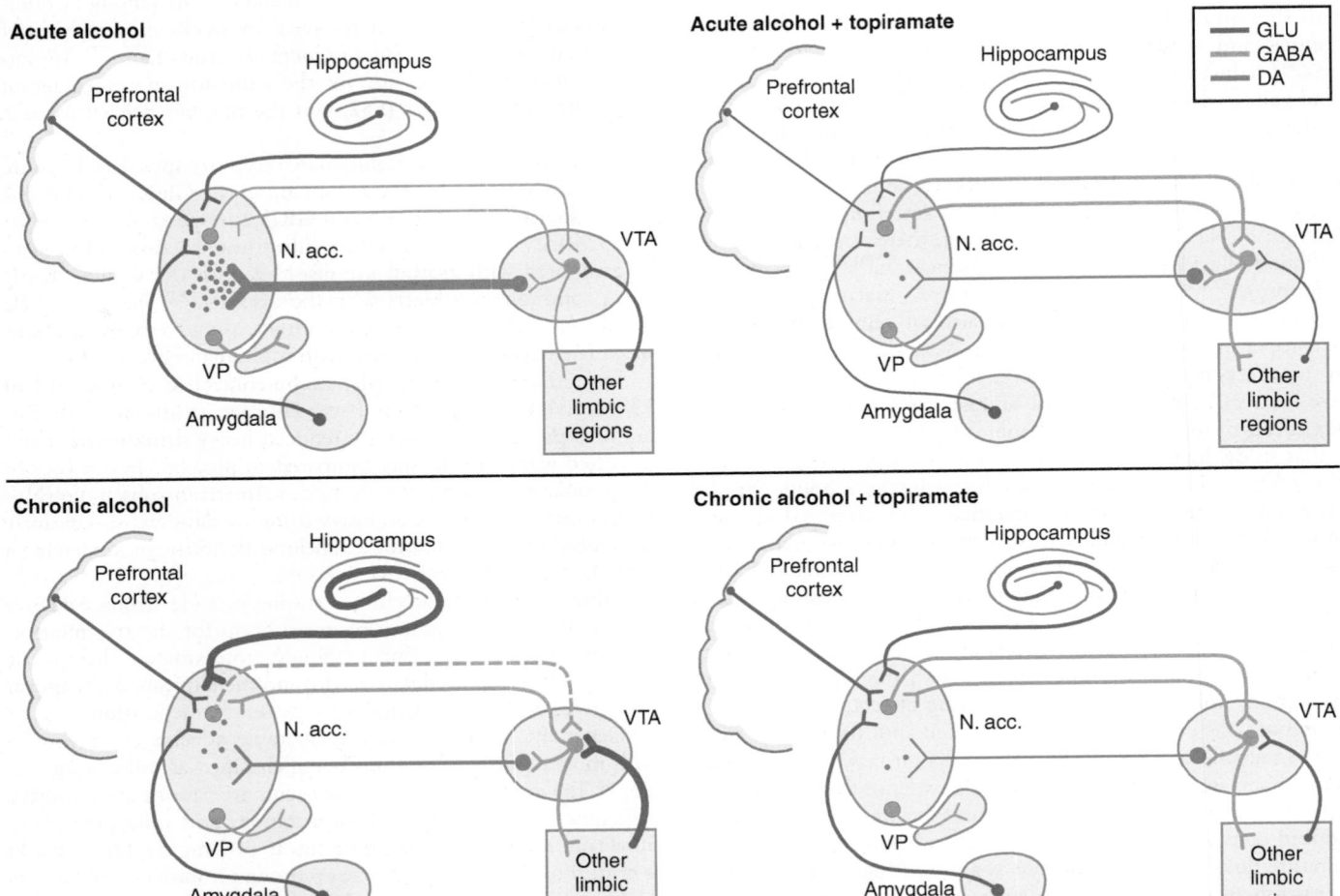

Acute alcohol

Prefrontal cortex

Hippocampus

N. acc.

VP

Amygdala

VTA

Other limbic regions

Acute alcohol + topiramate

Prefrontal cortex

Hippocampus

N. acc.

VP

Amygdala

VTA

Other limbic regions

GLU
GABA
DA

Chronic alcohol

Prefrontal cortex

Hippocampus

N. acc.

VP

Amygdala

VTA

Other limbic regions

Chronic alcohol + topiramate

Prefrontal cortex

Hippocampus

N. acc.

VP

Amygdala

VTA

Other limbic regions

• **Fig. 51.3** Schematic illustration of the hypothesized effects of acute and chronic alcohol, both with and without topiramate, on the cortico-mesolimbic dopamine (*DA*) reward circuit.[137] (*Upper left*) Acute alcohol suppresses the firing rate of ventral tegmental area (*VTA*) γ-aminobutyric acid (*GABA*) neurons, which leads to less suppression of VTA DA neuronal activity. This disinhibition leads to VTA DA neuronal firing and DA release in the nucleus accumbens (*N Acc*).[137] (*Lower left*) With chronic drinking, VTA GABA neurons are hyperexcitable, mainly because of increased glutamatergic input, less GABA tone from the N Acc, and rebound firing of GABA neurons because of their long-term suppression from repeated alcohol ingestion. This leads to VTA DA hypofunction and decreased release (compared with the acute condition) of DA in the N Acc.[137] (*Upper right*) During acute drinking, the GABAergic influence of topiramate probably predominates, particularly in the N Acc. This leads to greater inhibition of N Acc DA neurons, and greater GABA tone from the N Acc to the VTA suppresses VTA DA cell firing. Topiramate concomitantly inhibits the excitatory effects of glutamatergic neurons on DA neurons in the VTA and N Acc. These combined actions of topiramate should lead to profound suppression of DA neuronal activity and DA release in the N Acc. Hence, topiramate reduces the DA-mediated reinforcing effects of acute alcohol.[62] (*Lower right*) During chronic drinking, the predominant neuronal activity resides with the hyperexcitable state of VTA GABA neurons. Because of GABA-mediated inhibition and glutamatergic blockade of these neurons, topiramate "normalizes" VTA GABA neuronal activity. Although this would, at first, suggest that DA release in the N Acc would be enhanced, this does not occur, and DA release in the N Acc is most likely reduced because these N Acc terminals are contemporaneously inhibited by GABA inhibition and blockade of glutamate (*GLU*). In the chronic drinker, the anti-glutamatergic and L-type calcium channel effects of topiramate to block sensitization might predominate. Hence, topiramate would make it easier for a chronic alcoholic to withdraw from alcohol because rebound DA release would not occur (if drinking were ceased abruptly), and topiramate would aid in relapse prevention because alcohol's reinforcing effects would be decreased.[137] *Line weights* represent relative strengths of neuronal activity (heavy, medium, and light). The *broken line* represents decreased tone. *VP,* Ventral pallidum. (Reprinted from Johnson,[137] courtesy of Blackwell Publishing, Inc.)

TABLE 51.1   Topiramate Dose-Escalation Schedule.

Week	AM Dose	PM Dose	Total Daily Dose (mg)
1	0 mg	1 25-mg tablet	25
2	0 mg	2 25-mg tablets	50
3	1 25-mg tablet	2 25-mg tablets	75
4	2 25-mg tablets	2 25-mg tablets	100
5	2 25-mg tablets	1 100-mg tablet	150
6	1 100-mg tablet	1 100-mg tablet	200
7	1 100-mg tablet	1 100-mg tablet and 2 25-mg tablets	250
8	1 100-mg tablet and 2 25-mg tablets	1 100-mg tablet and 2 25-mg tablets	300

$P = 0.04$). Using a serum cotinine level of ≤ 28 ng/mL to segregate nonsmokers from smokers, the topiramate group had 4.97 times the odds of being nonsmokers (95% CI 1.1–23.4; $P = 0.04$). The strength of these results showing topiramate's treatment efficacy is bolstered by the fact that smoking cessation was not a goal of the study, and no specific measures, advice or counseling, or therapeutic targets were provided to help the participants quit smoking; thus the improvements in smoking rate represent a naturalistic change in behavior. Of interest, cigarette consumption and serum cotinine levels lessened as individuals became more abstinent in the topiramate group. In contrast, increasing abstinence from alcohol was associated with greater consumption of cigarettes and higher serum cotinine levels for the placebo group. These findings provide initial support for the proposal that topiramate may be an efficacious medicine for the simultaneous treatment of alcohol use disorder and smoking.

In sum, predicated upon a neuropharmacological conceptual model, there now is strong clinical support for topiramate as a promising medication for the treatment of alcohol use disorder. Topiramate's therapeutic effects appear to be robust, with a medium effect size, thereby potentially ushering in a new era of a reliably efficacious medicine for the treatment of alcohol use disorder with or without smoking. The moderator effect of rs2832407, if validated, would facilitate the identification of heavy drinkers who are likely to respond well to topiramate treatment with the best safety profile and provide an important personalized treatment option. Intriguingly, although the animal data also provide neuropharmacological support for topiramate's anti-drinking effects, more research is needed to characterize fully or fingerprint the pattern of response. Such preclinical studies should enable us to elucidate more clearly the basic mechanistic processes that underlie topiramate's efficacy as a treatment for alcohol use disorder. Although it is not yet known whether topiramate will be useful in treating alcohol-dependent individuals with bipolar disorder, another anticonvulsant (i.e., valproic acid) has shown some promise.

GABA Synthesis and Glutamate Synthesis Modulator—Gabapentin

Gabapentin is FDA approved for the treatment of epileptic seizures and neuropathic pain. The cellular and molecular targets of the actions of gabapentin are still not fully elucidated. Most studies would agree that gabapentin alters the metabolism or concentrations of glutamate, glutamine, and GABA in brain tissues. Gabapentin crosses the brain-blood barrier. It increases the concentration and probably the rate of synthesis of GABA and blocks a specific alpha-2d subunit of the voltage-gated Ca^{2+} channels at selective presynaptic sites. Gabapentin prevents neuronal death in several models, presumably by inhibition of glutamate synthesis by branched-chain amino acid aminotransferase (BCAA-t).[79]

Preclinical studies indicate that gabapentin may normalize stress-induced GABA activation in the amygdala that is associated with alcohol use disorder.[273] A human laboratory study found that gabapentin reduced alcohol cue craving and improved sleep quality in individuals with alcohol use disorder.[215] In a large outpatient clinical trial, gabapentin, particularly the 1800 mg dose, was found to significantly improve the rates of alcohol abstinence and reduce heavy drinking episodes in recently abstinent (3 days) individuals with alcohol use disorder. It was also found to be effective in treating symptoms of insomnia, dysphoria, and craving. Gabapentin was well tolerated, with the most common side effects including headache, fatigue, and insomnia. No significant difference in rate or severity was found between the adverse profile of placebo and active medication.[216] Gabapentin offers the advantage that it may be more readily adopted by primary care physicians for the treatment of alcohol use disorder as it is already commonly prescribed by them for other indications. Larger multisite studies are needed to replicate and extend these findings, and also to understand if there is a sustained posttreatment effect on drinking outcome.

Serotonin

For almost three decades, there has been intense interest in the effects of serotonergic agents in the treatment of alcohol use disorder. Encouraged by increased knowledge about the various serotonin receptor subtypes, researchers have examined the effects of various medications that bind to specific receptor sites. Here, we provide a synopsis of the preclinical and clinical studies that have been done on these serotonin function–altering medications in the treatment of alcohol use disorder.

Selective Serotonin Reuptake Inhibitors

For decades, it has been known that pharmacological manipulations that deplete the brain of serotonin decrease the preference for ethanol.[238,239] Using preference paradigms, pharmacological agents that inhibit serotonin reuptake from the synapse reduce the voluntary consumption of ethanol solutions using the preference paradigm.[d] Knockout mice at the serotonin transporter do, however, exhibit a general decrease in ethanol preference and consumption.[33] Thus there is ample preclinical support for the notion that selective serotonin reuptake inhibitors suppress ethanol consumption in animals.

Although these preclinical studies have shown that selective serotonin reuptake inhibitors can reduce ethanol consumption, the selectivity of this effect on reinforcement as opposed to general consummatory behaviors has been questioned.[26,27,220]

The inhibition of serotonin reuptake function has complicated the effects on food intake and fluid consumption.[105] Selective serotonin reuptake inhibitors do suppress food intake[109,295]

---

[d]References 64, 98, 106, 107, 222, 343.

and fluid consumption[105] and decrease palatability.[190] Yet, motivational factors exert some control on the expression of these behaviors.[314] For instance, selective serotonin reuptake inhibitors enhance satiety[26] but selectively reduce preference for certain macronutrients (i.e., sweet items and carbohydrates)[193,341,342] (cf. Heisler et al.[127] and Heisler et al.[128]) that increase the palatability and rewarding effects of food.[84,305,339] Hence, selective serotonin reuptake inhibitors might decrease ethanol consumption via the suppression of nonspecific general consummatory behaviors and specific anti-reinforcing effects.

Studies conducted using operant techniques have also supported a role for selective serotonin reuptake inhibitors in the suppression of ethanol consumption. Haraguchi et al.[117] showed that same-day pretreatments with fluoxetine dose-dependently reduced ethanol responding. Nevertheless, whereas the chronic administration of selective serotonin reuptake inhibitors to C57BL/6 J male mice produced an initial suppression of lever pressing for ethanol, there was a later rebound to baseline levels of responding for ethanol and ethanol consumption.[115] These results are somewhat similar to those of Murphy et al.,[235] who observed that fluoxetine administered to rats in a single daily infusion produced a significant reduction in ethanol-reinforced responding that started on the first day of treatment and increased on subsequent days of the 7-day treatment regimen. Responding for ethanol returned to pretreatment levels following cessation of fluoxetine treatment. Food intake, although somewhat suppressed initially, appeared to return to baseline levels on subsequent treatment days. Again, these results demonstrate that the suppression of ethanol intake by selective serotonin reuptake inhibitors follows a pattern of initial suppression of consummatory behavior followed by a reduction in reinforcement; thus when the selective serotonin reuptake inhibitors are discontinued, there is an extinction-like pattern of a return to the baseline behavior.

Despite the promise of these preclinical results, there is, at present, little support for the proposal that selective serotonin reuptake inhibitors are an efficacious treatment for a heterogeneous group of alcohol-dependent individuals. Initial studies of small sample size reported that selective serotonin reuptake inhibitors can produce short-term (1–4 week) decreases in alcohol consumption among problem drinkers.[242–247] Nevertheless, these studies were limited by at least three factors. First, most of the studies were conducted in men, thereby limiting the generalizability of the results to the general population.[243,245,246] Second, the adjunctive psychosocial treatment, which can decrease the apparent efficacy of the putative therapeutic medication because this too can have an important effect on drinking outcomes, was not standardized. Third, the treatment periods were short; thus it was not possible to determine whether these initial effects, which could be due to nonspecific factors, would be sustained. Indeed, the problem with studies of short duration that focus on a chronic relapsing disorder such as alcohol use disorder was highlighted in a later study by Gorelick and Paredes,[108] who found that there also was an effect for fluoxetine, compared with placebo, to decrease alcohol consumption by about 15% in the first 4 weeks of the trial but not over the entire length of the trial. In addition, Naranjo et al.[241] did not demonstrate that citalopram (40 mg/day) was superior to placebo in a 12-week treatment trial. Further, neither Kabel and Petty[161] nor Kranzler et al.[176] in two separate 12-week studies found fluoxetine (60 mg/day) to be superior to placebo for the treatment of alcohol use disorder.

There has been renewed understanding about how the administration of functionally different serotonergic agents can lead to different drinking outcomes among various subtypes of alcoholic

(for a review, see Johnson[136]). Adapted from Cloninger's classification scheme[50], two methods for subtyping alcoholics have been used in these pharmacotherapy studies. Basically, a particular type of alcoholic (i.e., Type A-like or late onset) characterized by a later age of onset of problem drinking (typically over the age of 25 years), a preponderance of psychosocial morbidity, and low familial loading can experience improved drinking outcomes after selective serotonin reuptake inhibitor treatment.

Although early human laboratory studies showed that Type B-like or early onset alcoholics, characterized by an early age of problem drinking onset (i.e., before the age of 25 years), high familial loading for alcohol use disorder, and a range of impulsive or antisocial traits, might be centrally deficient in the major metabolite of serotonin, 5-hydroxyindoleacetic acid,[40,194,195] the implications of this finding were, perhaps, oversimplified. At a cursory glance, it would appear that a selective serotonin reuptake inhibitor, by increasing serotonin turnover, would compensate for this dysfunction; thus these Type B-like or early onset alcoholics would then be expected to experience improved drinking outcomes following selective serotonin reuptake inhibitor treatment. Remarkably, the literature has demonstrated quite the opposite. For instance, Kranzler et al.[173] observed that fluoxetine treatment appeared to worsen the clinical benefit of the adjunctive cognitive behavioral treatment and that there was no difference from placebo. Actually, Type A-like or late-onset alcoholics, with presumably more normative serotonin function, have been observed to experience improved drinking outcomes from sertraline both during active treatment[240] and at 6-month follow-up.[75] In addition, Chick et al.[48] have shown that early onset or Type B-like alcoholics were more likely to relapse than their late-onset or Type A-like counterparts following fluvoxamine treatment.

Obviously, the relationship between serotonergic dysfunction and Type B-like or early onset alcoholism is not the simple result of a deficiency state. Indeed, Johnson[136] has hypothesized that an explanation for this effect might be allelic variation at the serotonin transporter, which leads to the differential expression of serotonin function. Of course, other biomolecular explanations are possible, and further research is needed to elucidate this important area of research.

Fluoxetine has been reported to be beneficial for the treatment of alcohol-dependent individuals with suicidal tendencies and severe comorbid depression.[58] A recent study did not find that sertraline treatment was more beneficial than placebo in treating depressed men and women with alcohol use disorder irrespective of the severity of the depression.[180] In another trial, sertraline was again found not to be beneficial in both men and women for the treatment of comorbid alcohol use disorder and depression, although women did have a very slight but not clinically meaningful improvement in depressive symptoms.[9] Notably, it has not been shown that the reduction in dysphoria in depressed alcoholics is associated with concomitant decreases in alcohol consumption.[211,224] Hence, the only conclusion that can be drawn at present is that except for a subtype of depressed alcoholic with suicidal tendencies or, perhaps, in women, there is not much evidence to recommend selective serotonin reuptake inhibitors over placebo for the treatment of depressed alcoholics.

Sertraline might have some utility in the treatment of alcohol-dependent individuals whose comorbid posttraumatic stress disorder is associated with early trauma,[36] thereby suggesting that different subtypes might vary in treatment response. In addition, there is promise that paroxetine might prove useful in treating alcohol-dependent individuals with social phobia.[267] There is no specific treatment, apart from symptomatic management, for the treatment of alcohol-dependent individuals with comorbid generalized anxiety disorder.[35]

In sum, despite strong animal data that would support the use of selective serotonin reuptake inhibitors as a promising treatment for alcohol use disorder, there is no evidence that they are of therapeutic benefit to a heterogeneous group of alcohol-dependent individuals. Notably, however, there is growing confirmation that selective serotonin reuptake inhibitors can improve the drinking outcomes of Type A-like or late-onset alcoholics. Rather than being a cause for discouragement, this finding might (a) open up the possibility of identifying important biogenetic or pharmacological mechanisms that underlie the alcoholism disease and (b) improve understanding about which type of alcohol-dependent individual can benefit the most from specific serotonergic treatment. Furthermore, there is no current evidence that providing a selective serotonin reuptake inhibitor to a depressed alcoholic without severe depressive symptoms and suicidal tendencies is of therapeutic benefit. Hence, what is clear is that clinicians should be cautious in prescribing selective serotonin reuptake inhibitors to alcohol-dependent individuals for the treatment of minor depressive or affective symptoms. Not only is this strategy unlikely to be a therapeutic benefit over placebo, and perhaps appropriate psychosocial management, but drinking outcomes can actually be worsened, especially if the alcohol-dependent individual is Type A-like or of late onset. There is some evidence that selective serotonin reuptake inhibitors might be useful in treating a cohort of alcohol-dependent individuals whose posttraumatic stress disorder is associated with early trauma, and in treating alcoholics with social phobia.

Serotonin-1 Partial Receptor Agonist

Preclinical studies have suggested that the serotonin-1A partial agonist, buspirone, may be effective at reducing ethanol consumption. Buspirone decreased volitional alcohol consumption from 60% to 30% in macaque monkeys, but there was considerable interindividual variation.[51] In Sprague-Dawley rats, buspirone significantly reduced ethanol intake in animals induced to drink by repeated brainstem injection of tetrahydropapaveroline. In a group of medium alcohol-preferring rats, buspirone (0.0025–0.63 mg/kg) reduced, while buspirone (>2.5 mg/kg) increased, alcohol consumption without affecting water consumption.[227] Although buspirone is a partial serotonin-1A agonist, the net effect of its repeated administration is to enhance serotonin function via facilitation of the postsynaptic receptor, which is more sensitive than the autoreceptor, and downregulation of autoreceptor function.[23] Nevertheless, this preclinical evidence would have been strengthened by operant studies examining the dose-response characteristics of buspirone as a function of ethanol concentration.

Buspirone has not been demonstrated to be an efficacious medication for the treatment of alcohol-dependent individuals without comorbidity. In a review of five published trials, buspirone was without a convincing effect in noncomorbid alcoholics; however, alcoholics with comorbid anxiety experienced some benefit.[38,204] Hence, buspirone's anxiolytic effects might translate to those who also are dependent on alcohol.

In summation, there is no current evidence that would suggest a role for buspirone in the treatment of alcohol use disorder without comorbid anxiety disorder.

Serotonin-2 Receptor Antagonist

Preclinical studies have suggested that the serotonin-2 receptor antagonist, ritanserin, can reduce ethanol consumption in animals[227, 236] (cf. Svensson et al.[315]). In addition, the serotonin-2 antagonists, amperozide[20,237,258] and FG5974,[187,274] significantly suppress ethanol intake without affecting water consumption. The exact mechanism by which serotonin-2 receptor antagonists might reduce ethanol consumption is unknown. It has been suggested, however, that they might exert their effects by acutely substituting for alcohol's pharmacobehavioral effects by facilitating burst firing in cortico-mesolimbic dopamine neurons,[322] or by the suppression of dopamine neurotransmission following their chronic administration.

In the clinical setting, ritanserin is not an efficacious treatment for alcohol use disorder. In a rigorously conducted, 12-week, multicenter clinical trial ($N = 423$) of ritanserin (2.5 or 5 mg/day) versus placebo as an adjunct to weekly cognitive behavioral therapy, none of the ritanserin doses was superior to placebo.[309] In a later study using similar methodology, ritanserin (2.5, 5.0, or 10.0 mg/day) was not superior to placebo at improving drinking outcomes.[336] Although higher doses of ritanserin might be of therapeutic benefit, testing these doses is precluded by ritanserin's potential to cause dose-dependent prolongation of the QTc interval on electrocardiography, thereby increasing the potential for life-threatening cardiac arrhythmias.

In summation, there is no clinical evidence that would support the use of ritanserin as a treatment for alcohol use disorder.

Serotonin-3 Receptor Antagonists

Preclinical studies provide strong support for the role of the serotonin-3 receptor in mediating alcohol's important neurochemical effects, and for serotonin-3 receptor antagonists to be promising treatment for alcohol use disorder.

In neurophysiological experiments, ethanol potentiates serotonin-3 receptor-mediated ion currents in NCB-20 neuroblastoma cells[202,347] and in human embryonic kidney 293 cells (or HEK 239, a specific cell line originally derived from human embryonic kidney cells) transfected with serotonin-3 receptor antagonist complementary DNA.[106] Serotonin-3 receptor antagonists block these effects.[201] Thus the serotonin-3 receptor is a site of action for ethanol in the brain.[200,202]

Pharmacobehavioral studies show that many of alcohol's reinforcing effects are mediated by serotonin-3 and dopamine interactions in the cortico-mesolimbic system.[13,129,145,169]

Serotonin-3 receptor antagonists have three principal effects that demonstrate their ability to modulate ethanol consumption and related behaviors. First, serotonin-3 receptor antagonists suppress hyperlocomotion in the rat induced by dopamine or ethanol injection into the nucleus accumbens[34]. Second, serotonin-3 receptor antagonists inhibit DiMe-C7 (a neurokinin)-induced hyperlocomotion, which also is reduced by the dopamine antagonist, fluphenazine.[95,312] Third, serotonin-3 receptor antagonists reduce ethanol consumption in several animal models and across different species[e] (cf. Beardsley et al.[16]).

Human laboratory studies have generally supported a role for the serotonin-3 antagonist ondansetron in reducing preference and craving for alcohol. In two distinct experiments, Johnson and Cowen[145] and Johnson et al.[150] showed that ondansetron

---

[e]References 13, 59, 72, 76, 134, 150, 221, 277, 288, 320.

pretreatment attenuated low-dose alcohol-induced positive subjective effects (including the desire to drink). Swift et al.,[317] using much higher alcohol and ondansetron doses, also discovered that ondansetron compared with placebo pretreatment reduced alcohol preference; however, a mixture of both stimulant and sedative interactions between ondansetron and alcohol also was observed. Whereas Doty et al.[73] did not find an effect of ondansetron on alcohol-induced mood, their experimental model of using a group rather than individual experimental setting could have decreased the sensitivity of their assessments.

Three clinical studies have provided evidence that ondansetron is a promising treatment for alcohol-dependent individuals, particularly those with an early onset or Type B-like subtype.

First, in a 6-week, double-blind, placebo-controlled study of 71 nonseverely alcohol-dependent males, Sellers et al.[287] observed that the 0.5-mg dose but not the 4-mg dose of ondansetron was associated with a nonsignificant trend ($P = 0.06$) toward a reduction in alcohol consumption. Post hoc analysis that eliminated 11 subjects who consumed less than 10 drinks/drinking day rendered the difference in drinking outcomes between the ondansetron 0.5 mg and placebo groups to be significant statistically ($P = 0.001$). Despite the limitations of this initial trial, which included a relatively short treatment period, the inclusion of just males, and the small number of subjects, the results of this study provided general support for ondansetron's promise in treating alcohol use disorder. In addition, these results showed that ondansetron may exhibit a nonlinear dose-response effect in the treatment of alcohol use disorder.

Second, in a large-scale ($N = 321$), 12-week, randomized, double-blind clinical trial in which alcohol-dependent individuals received weekly cognitive behavioral therapy, Johnson et al.[146] showed that ondansetron (1, 4, and 16 μg/kg, b.i.d.) was superior to placebo at improving drinking outcomes of those of the early onset or Type B-like subtype but not the late onset or Type A-like subtype. The self-reported decreases in alcohol consumption were corroborated by the concomitant reduction in carbohydrate-deficient transferrin level—a biomarker of transient alcohol consumption.

Third, Kranzler et al.[177] provided replication of the results by Johnson et al.[146] by showing that early onset (Type B-like) alcoholics had a significantly greater improvement in drinking outcomes compared with their late-onset (Type A-like) counterparts following 8 weeks of ondansetron (4 μg/kg, b.i.d.) treatment.

Intriguingly, these results demonstrate a differential effect of ondansetron treatment by subtype of alcohol-dependent individual. Indeed, the contrast is striking when compared with the effects of selective serotonin reuptake inhibitors on different subtypes of alcohol-dependent individuals as described earlier. Basically, early onset or Type B-like alcoholics with apparent serotonergic deficiency respond best to a medication that blocks the serotonin-3 receptor, whereas late-onset or Type A-like alcoholics with apparently normal serotonergic function derive the most benefit from a medication that can increase serotonin turnover and function. One potential disadvantage of subtyping by psychosocial variables is that they might not be stable across all populations (i.e., differences by ethnicity and regions could occur due to different exposure levels to alcohol), and the more complex algorithms for subtyping (e.g., into Type A or B) cannot be carried out prospectively or applied directly to a single individual. Arguably, more stable and generalizable dichotomization of different populations of alcoholics responsive to ondansetron might be achievable using pertinent and specific biomolecular variables.

As mentioned earlier, Johnson[136] has proposed a biomolecular explanation for these effects; however, other plausible possibilities might exist. A detailed elaboration of this concept is beyond the scope of this review. Nevertheless, the key feature is that polymorphic variation(s) at the serotonin transporter gene might result in a relative intrasynaptic hyposerotonergic state with consequent upregulation of postsynaptic serotonin receptors. Alcohol-dependent individuals with these polymorphic types may be prone to a heavier and more chronic pattern of drinking,[156, 207,277,289] perhaps through a counterregulatory mechanism to increase serotonin turnover. Because this attempted counterregulation through increased alcohol consumption can only be partially effective, as further drinking reduces the expression of the serotonin transporter gene further,[156] a vicious cycle is set up. Johnson[63] has proposed that ondansetron treatment may ameliorate heavy or severe drinking in such alcohol-dependent individuals, presumably by blockade of upregulated postsynaptic serotonin receptors. Indeed, preliminary statistical analysis of a recent clinical trial does suggest that ondansetron may have an effect to decrease severe drinking among individuals with specific polymorphisms of the serotonin transporter gene.

In a landmark controlled trial (n = 283), Johnson et al.[157a] showed that individuals with the LL genotype who received ondansetron had a lower mean number of drinks per drinking day (−1.62) and a higher percentage of days abstinent (11.27%) than those who received placebo. Among ondansetron recipients, the number of drinks per drinking day was lower (−1.53) and the percentage of days abstinent higher (9.73%) in LL compared with LS/SS individuals. LL individuals in the ondansetron group also had a lower number of drinks per drinking day (−1.45) and a higher percentage of days abstinent (9.65%) than all other genotype and treatment groups combined. For both number of drinks per drinking day and percentage of days abstinent, 5'-HTTLPR and rs1042173 variants interacted significantly. LL/TT individuals in the ondansetron group had a lower number of drinks per drinking day (−2.63) and a higher percentage of days abstinent (16.99%) than all other genotype and treatment groups combined. These results provided the proof of concept to show the efficacy of pharmacogenetic treatment of alcohol use disorder using ondansetron. In an extended evaluation of that study, Johnson et al.[158] also showed that individuals carrying one or more of genotypes rs1150226-AG and rs1176713-GG in HTR3A and rs17614942-AC in HTR3B showed a significant overall mean difference between ondansetron and placebo in drinks per drinking day (22.50; effect size = 0.867), percentage of heavy drinking days (220.58%; effect size = 0.780), and percentage of days abstinent (18.18%; effect size = 0.683). Combining these HTR3A/HTR3B and SLC6A4-LL/TT genotypes increased the target cohort from approaching 20% (identified in the previous study) to 34%. These added results present compelling evidence that a combined five-marker genotype panel can be used to predict the outcome of treatment of alcohol dependence with ondansetron. Thus certain subtypes of individuals with alcohol use disorder exist, whereby pharmacogenetic treatment using ondansetron can be targeted effectively toward a specific genetically defined cohort. Furthermore, these results open up the possibility of developing associated messenger RNA (mRNA) biomarkers to track treatment response with ondansetron.[158] It is intriguing that ondansetron also has shown efficacy in treating alcohol-dependent individuals with social phobia, presumably because of its anxiolytic effects.[304] The results of this study do, however, need to be validated by a larger clinical trial.

Acetylcholine: Cholinergic Receptor Antagonist—Varenicline

Varenicline is an agent that binds with high affinity to alpha-4/beta-2 nicotinic acetylcholine receptors to release dopamine in the cortico-mesolimbic dopamine system.[162] Hence it might mimic the effect of alcohol to excite central nicotinic acetylcholine receptors and cause cortico-mesolimbic dopamine activation.[24,25,78,306] Varenicline might, therefore, act as a substitute for the stimulating effects of alcohol. Animal studies have not, however, shown an effect of varenicline on self-administration[286] or conditioned place preference, although there was some attenuation of ethanol-induced locomotor effects.[114] Extrapolating these results to humans would suggest speculatively that varenicline might impair continued drinking once alcohol consumption has been initiated by reducing its stimulating effects. Some support for this was seen by Schacht et al.[283] in the human laboratory, where varenicline enhanced control over alcohol-related thoughts and cue-elicited activation in the orbitofrontal cortex; however, there was no effect on heavy drinking. Furthermore, the findings of Schacht et al.[283] do have some correlation but not complete agreement with an earlier human laboratory where varenicline attenuated alcohol-induced craving and positive subjective mood and decreased alcohol self-administration.[225] Roberts et al.[276] also showed that those receiving varenicline compared with placebo showed a smaller increase in alcohol craving in a human laboratory paradigm. Taken together, these animal and human laboratory studies point to a complex neuropharmacological effect of varenicline of alcohol craving, and cue-elicited response and subsequent drinking behavior, which might depend on conditioning, setting, neurobiological state, and environment. Nevertheless, clinical trials appeared to be warranted to test the potential efficacy of varenicline for the treatment of alcohol use disorder, given the high comorbidity of smoking behavior in this population, and because the FDA had approved varenicline as an aid to smoking cessation.[139]

Litten et al.[198] in a double-blind, placebo-controlled trial (n = 200) showed that varenicline 2 mg/day compared with placebo had significantly lower weekly percent heavy drinking days (primary outcome) (adjusted mean difference = 10.4), drinks per day, drinks per drinking day, and alcohol craving ($P < 0.05$). Nevertheless, in contrast, a subsequent double-blind, controlled clinical trial (n = 160), did not find an effect for varenicline compared with placebo to reduce heavy drinking.[68] Although there have been additional studies done,[80] the overall evidence for varenicline as a treatment for alcohol use disorder is not particularly compelling, and there seems to be no added effect to reduce nicotine intake among those who also smoke.

Dopamine

Dopamine Receptor Antagonists

Cortico-mesolimbic dopamine neurons have been implicated as the principal pathway by which alcohol and most other abused drugs express their reinforcing effects associated with abuse liability.[129,169,338] Yet it has been difficult to show evidence that direct dopamine receptor antagonists have a role in the treatment of alcohol use disorder. Presumably, direct opposition of dopamine pathways is associated with neuroadaptive changes that tend to reverse the initial effects of the blockade.[138] No traditional dopamine receptor blocker has been demonstrated to be an efficacious treatment for alcohol dependence. With the advent of atypical neuroleptics, there

has been renewed interest in testing these medications as potential treatment for alcohol dependence. Indeed, medications such as aripiprazole and quetiapine are currently in clinical testing, and the results are awaited eagerly. Other medications that are selective for dopamine-3 receptor antagonism also are under development.

Dopamine Receptor Agonists

At low doses, dopamine-2/dopamine-3 agonists such as bromocriptine and 7-OH-DPAT can reduce ethanol consumption in animals.[217,280,333] Although this might appear paradoxical to the dopamine theory of reinforcement for most abused drugs, it is possible that low-dose dopamine agonists preferentially augment autoreceptor function, thereby decreasing dopamine turnover.

An earlier report proposed that bromocriptine can decrease alcohol craving; however, subsequent studies have found no effect on alcohol drinking or related behaviors.[71,242,264] Nevertheless, perhaps due to the high addictive potential of dopamine agonists, this research approach has largely been abandoned in the clinical setting. Currently, dopamine receptor agonists do not hold promise as a treatment for alcohol dependence.

Gamma-Aminobutyric Acid-B Receptor Agonist—Baclofen

Animal studies have demonstrated that the $GABA_B$ receptor agonist, baclofen [beta-(4-chlorophenyl)-gamma-aminobutyric acid], causes decreases in voluntary ethanol intake,[52] the ethanol-deprivation effect,[53,266] and morphine-induced stimulation of ethanol consumption.[54]

Clinical trials have bolstered the findings of animal studies that suggest a role for baclofen in treating alcohol dependence. In an open-label, 4-week study, nine alcohol-dependent men were given baclofen (up to 30 mg/day). Seven of the nine men achieved abstinence, whereas the other two improved their drinking outcomes during the study period, according to self-reports corroborated by family members. Several objective biological markers of alcohol intake also showed significant reductions between the beginning and end of the study. Furthermore, craving, as measured by median Alcohol Craving Scale scores, decreased in the first study week and remained stable thereafter.[52]

In a 4-week, randomized, placebo-controlled, double-blind clinical trial with 39 alcohol-dependent individuals, 14 (70%) of 20 participants treated with baclofen (up to 30 mg/day) achieved abstinence, compared with 4 (21.1%) of 19 in the placebo group ($P < 0.005$). Baclofen treatment significantly improved drinking outcomes, state anxiety scores, and craving measures. Baclofen generally was well tolerated and had no apparent abuse liability. Adverse events, none of which were serious, consisted of nausea, vertigo, transient sleepiness, and abdominal pain.[2]

Recently, Addolorato and colleagues[1] reported in a randomized double-blind clinical trial that baclofen was more efficacious than placebo at promoting abstinence in alcohol-dependent individuals with liver cirrhosis. Because baclofen is primarily excreted unchanged in the urine and feces, it might be uniquely suitable for treating alcoholics with compromised hepatic function. Baclofen was well tolerated in this study, with few adverse events.

These findings indicate that baclofen is a promising medication for the treatment of alcohol dependence, particularly among those with compromised hepatic function. Additional studies of larger sample size and longer duration are awaited to establish the efficacy of baclofen for this indication.

Alcohol Metabolism Disruptor: Disulfiram

Disulfiram is an FDA-approved medication that has been used for treating alcoholism since the 1940s and is perhaps still the most widely used such medication in the United States today. Its principal mode of action is as an aversive agent. Disulfiram inhibits aldehyde dehydrogenase and prevents the metabolism of alcohol's primary metabolite, acetaldehyde. In turn, the accumulation of acetaldehyde in the blood causes unpleasant effects to occur if alcohol is ingested; these include sweating, headache, dyspnea, lowered blood pressure, flushing, sympathetic overactivity, palpitations, nausea, and vomiting. The association of these symptoms with drinking discourages further consumption of alcohol.[3] Serious side effects also have been reported, including hepatitis, hepatotoxicity, depression, and psychotic reactions.[255,294] Disulfiram also has been shown to reduce norepinephrine synthesis by inhibiting dopamine beta-hydroxylase,[262] a mode of action that has been proposed to support early reports of its potential efficacy as a treatment for cocaine dependence. For further details on the pharmacological effects of disulfiram, see also Johnson.[141] Although a review of disulfiram's potential effects on cocaine taking are outside the scope of this review, the reader is referred to recent studies by Petrakis et al.,[262] Carroll et al.,[43] and Baker et al.[12]

A 52-week, multisite, randomized, controlled trial with 605 alcohol-dependent men found that disulfiram might help prevent relapse in compliant individuals yet be ineffective at promoting continuous abstinence or a delay in the resumption of drinking.[93]

Disulfiram has no significant effect on craving for alcohol. Hence, individuals must be highly motivated to maintain disulfiram treatment, whereas those who wish to drink can simply stop taking the medication. The efficacy of disulfiram generally is limited to those who are highly compliant or who receive their medication under supervision—that is, the type of alcohol-dependent individuals who might be likely to abstain on their own, without adjunctive pharmacotherapy. Including a supportive spouse or partner in a disulfiram treatment plan helps to improve outcome.[3,8]

Disulfiram has been combined with naltrexone as a potential treatment for alcohol dependence with comorbid depression.[261] Although the combination appeared to be well tolerated, there was no significant advantage of the combination over either of the medications alone or placebo. These results do not support the use of the combination of disulfiram and naltrexone as a treatment for comorbid alcohol use disorder and depression.

Potential Treatments on the Horizon

Cannabinoid-1 Receptor Antagonists

Endocannabinoid receptors are found ubiquitously in the central nervous system, particularly in the cortex, hippocampus, basal ganglia, and cerebellum. Endogenous cannabinoids include anandamide and 2-arachidonylglycerol, which are metabolized by fatty acid amide hydrolase.[120]

In C57BL/6 J mice, cannabinoid-1 receptor blockade reduced ethanol consumption to the amounts ingested by cannabinoid-1 receptor null mutant mice.[332] Endocannabinoids may be involved in the neurochemical expression of susceptibility to the effects of ethanol. For instance, ethanol exposure can increase levels of brain 2-arachidonylglycerol and anandamide and downregulate cannabinoid-1 receptors.[14,41] In pharmacobehavioral studies, cannabinoid-1 receptor antagonists suppress ethanol intake in rats with a chronic history of alcohol administration,[186,277] reduce ethanol drinking in alcohol-preferring sP rats,[55,100] and decrease operant responding and cue-induced reinstatement of ethanol consumption.[49,77] It is plausible, however, that an important method by which cannabinoid-1 receptors influence ethanol taking is via their extensive connections to modulate other neuronal systems including monoamine pathways and their metabolism.[232,313,321] Fig. 51.4 shows the interactions between cannabinoid-1 and other neuronal systems.[139]

In Europe, initial human studies of the effects of cannabinoid receptor blockade on the drinking outcomes of alcohol-dependent individuals have been completed, and the results are awaited eagerly. Nevertheless, the recent finding that the cannabinoid-1 receptor antagonist (rimonabant) can increase mood disturbance and suicidality in smokers, which precluded the FDA from granting approval for that indication, might also impact the development of similar compounds for the treatment of alcohol use disorder.

Other Neurochemicals and Small Molecules

Presently, there are a host of other neurochemicals with potential benefit in treating alcohol use disorder. At this stage, testing remains within the animal literature and other preclinical models, and it would, therefore, be beyond the scope of this review to discuss them in detail. These compounds include antagonists at metabotropic-5 glutamate receptors, metabotropic-2/3 glutamate receptor agonists, stress-related neuropeptides such as corticotropin-releasing factor antagonists and modulators of neuropeptide Y, and nociceptin (for a review, see Heilig and Egli[120]). Recently, data from a combination of preclinical and human laboratory experiments were unveiled, showing that the neurokinin-1 antagonist LY686017 might be a promising medication for the treatment of alcohol use disorder.[99] These early results are being followed up by phase II clinical efficacy trials. Of interest, there has been renewed interest in γ-hydroxybutyrate as a treatment for alcohol use disorder; however, its successful use would require the development of a formulation that has very low addictive potential. For reviews, see Caputo and colleagues[42] and Addolorato and coworkers.[1] More recently, ABT-436, a vasopressin-1b receptor antagonist, compared with placebo, has shown promise at improving some measures of alcohol consumption, including increasing the percentage of days abstinent (51.2 vs 41.6,; p=0.037; d=0.31, respectively), an effect that was associated with a small but concomitant significant decrease in cigarette smoking.[280a] Presumably, the potential neuropharmacological effect of ABT-436 might be to decrease negative affective states associated with chronic alcohol consumption. Further studies are needed, however, to confirm this initial impression, and to determine whether certain types of individual with alcohol use disorder (e.g., those with associated mood or stress-related disorders) might derive particular benefit.

Combination Treatments

Combination treatments offer the promise of augmenting the effects of single medications by engaging multiple neuronal networks associated with the expression of alcohol's reinforcing effects associated with its abuse liability. Although this idea is alluring, medication combinations do create the potential for reduced compliance (due to the need to take additional tablets), heightened or new treatment emergent adverse events, or even inefficacy if the medications counteract one another.

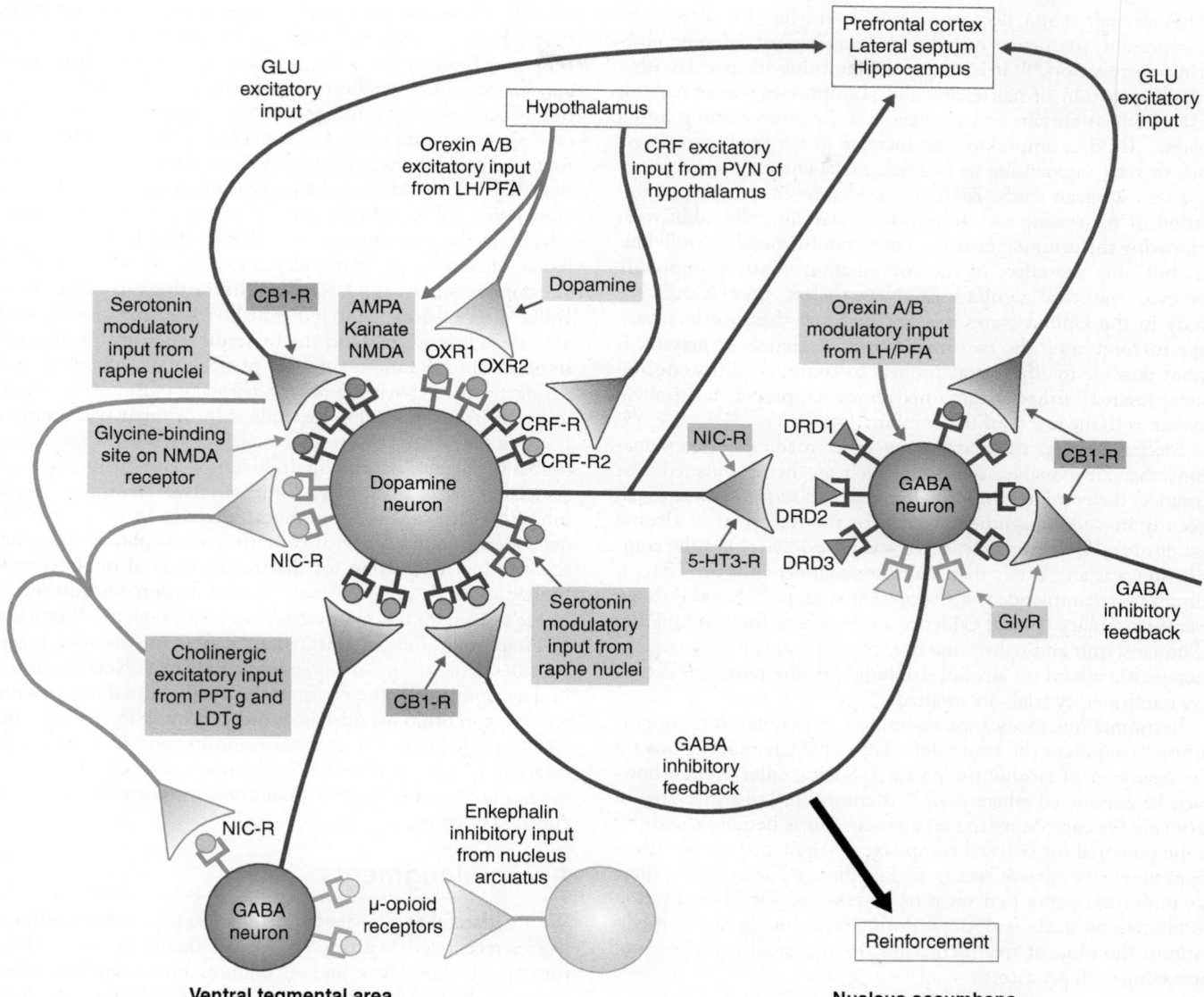

• **Fig. 51.4** Neuronal pathways involved with the reinforcing effects of alcohol, nicotine, and other abused drugs. Cholinergic inputs that arise the pedunculopontine tegmental nucleus (*PPTg*) and laterodorsal tegmental nucleus (*LDTg*) can stimulate ventral tegmental area (VTA) dopamine (DA) neurons. The VTA DA neuron projection to the nucleus accumbens (nACC) and cortex, the critical substrate for the reinforcing effects of abused drugs (including alcohol), is modulated by a variety of inhibitory (γ-aminobutyric acid [GABA] and opioid) and excitatory (nicotinic [*NIC-R*], glutamate [*GLU*], and cannabinoid-1 receptor [*CB1-R*]) inputs. The GLU pathways include those that express alpha-amino-3-hydroxy-5-methylisoxazole-4-propionic acid (*AMPA*), kainate, and *N*-methyl-D-aspartate (*NMDA*) receptors. Serotonin-3 receptors (*5-HT3-R*) also modulate DA release in the nACC. The glycine system, orexins, and cortico-trophin-releasing factor also are shown. *CRF-R1* and *CRF-R2*, Corticotropin-releasing factor receptors 1 and 2, respectively; *DRD1, DRD2,* and *DRD3,* DA receptors D1, D2, and D3, respectively; *GlyR,* glycine receptor; *LH/PFA,* periformical region of the lateral hypothalamus; *OXR1* and *OXR2,* orexin receptor types 1 and 2, respectively; *PVN,* paraventricular nucleus. (Adapted from Johnson[139]; copyright 2006, American Medical Association; all rights reserved and reprinted with permission from Johnson: *Am J Psych* [2010] 2010;167:630–639 [copyright 2010, American Psychiatric Association].)

Perhaps the best-studied medication combination so far has been that of naltrexone and acamprosate. This combination has been proposed to be of potential added therapeutic benefit for three reasons. First, naltrexone, by its action on endogenous opioids, modulates cortico-mesolimbic dopamine activity, thereby reducing the reinforcing effects of alcohol.[130,169] Acamprosate modulates alcohol withdrawal-induced increases in extracellular glutamate in the cortico-mesolimbic system.[62,63] Thus the combined effect of both naltrexone and acamprosate may be to modulate both the neurochemical effects responsible for triggering drinking and those associated with conditioned responses to drink, even after a prolonged period of abstinence. Second, although naltrexone decreases positive craving for alcohol,[329] acamprosate attenuates negative or conditioned craving post-drinking cessation.[310] It is, therefore, tempting to speculate that the combination of naltrexone and acamprosate would make it easier both to abstain and to prevent a slip from turning into a relapse. Third, acamprosate can increase blood levels of naltrexone, thereby augmenting its neurochemical effects.[151,213]

In a European study, Kiefer et al.[165] showed that the combination of naltrexone and acamprosate was clinically additive at improving the drinking outcomes of alcohol-dependent individuals, but only the effect of the combination versus acamprosate achieved statistical significance. Nevertheless, the COMBINE study in the United States did not find any therapeutic advantage to combining the two medications.[10] Hence, at present, it is not possible to advise practitioners to combine naltrexone and acamprosate. Further research may, however, provide a definitive answer as to the utility of the combination.

Mechanistically, there are many other medication combinations that are possible, some of which are being pursued. For instance, the combination of naltrexone and sertraline was tested recently in a pharmacotherapy trial for the treatment of alcohol use disorder. Unfortunately, there was no evidence that the combination was any better than naltrexone alone, and, therefore, it cannot be recommended as a treatment strategy.[86] Notably, however, preliminary clinical evidence suggests that the combination of ondansetron and naltrexone may result in added or synergistic therapeutic effects on alcohol drinking[4,144]; the results of definitive confirmatory trials are awaited.

In summation, medication combinations may afford the opportunity to augment the treatment effects of single medications for the treatment of alcohol use disorder. Such studies should, however, be conducted where there is a compelling pharmacological rationale for combining the medicines. This is because there also is the potential for reduced compliance, heightened or new treatment emergent adverse events, and inefficacy. Furthermore, there are important issues that must be determined for all medication combinations, such as optimal dosing, sequencing of the medications, duration of treatment, and the increased complexity of managing such protocols.

Conclusions

Recently, there has been renewed interest in developing efficacious medicines for the treatment of alcohol use disorder. Naltrexone and its depot formulations have demonstrated utility, but their therapeutic effect size is small. Despite FDA approval of acamprosate based on the positive results of European studies, there has, as yet, not been a clear demonstration of its efficacy in US studies. Even in the European studies, the therapeutic effect size of acamprosate is small. These discrepant findings might be the result of different populations of alcohol-dependent individuals, selection criteria, chronicity of the alcoholism disease, biomolecular differences, different methodologies between US and European studies, or sampling error due to the small effect size. For both naltrexone and acamprosate, research is ongoing to determine what type of alcohol-dependent individual benefits from using either medication. There also is the possibility that a pharmacogenetic approach may make it possible to improve the therapeutic outcome for those who receive naltrexone.. Topiramate is a promising medication for the treatment of alcohol use disorder with or without comorbid smoking. Based on two

studies, its therapeutic effect size appears to be in the medium range. Future research is needed to extend these results to other subpopulations of alcohol-dependent individuals. Gabapentin is another promising medication with encouraging results in reduction of alcohol relapse and relapse-associated symptoms involving craving, mood, and sleep, and had a favorable safety profile. Serotonergic medications need to be administered with care to ensure that they are provided to the subtype of alcohol-dependent individual who will benefit the most from such treatment. Although selective serotonin reuptake inhibitors benefit late-onset or Type A-like alcohol-dependent individuals, the serotonin-3 receptor antagonist ondansetron has efficacy in treating early onset or Type B-like alcohol-dependent individuals. Molecular genetic studies are ongoing to understand the underpinnings of this differential response among various subtypes of alcoholic to different serotonergic agents. Selective serotonin reuptake inhibitors might have utility in treating alcohol-dependent individuals with comorbid posttraumatic stress disorder associated with early trauma and, probably, alcohol-dependent individuals with major depression associated with suicidality. Both selective serotonin reuptake inhibitors and ondansetron appear effective in treating alcohol-dependent individuals with comorbid social phobia. Baclofen is a promising medication for the treatment of alcohol-dependent individuals with compromised hepatic function, but further studies are needed for this to be established. Although disulfiram is also FDA-approved for the treatment of alcohol use disorder, it is perhaps best utilized under supervised conditions. New medications in development for the treatment of alcohol use disorder with or without comorbid psychiatric disorder or smoking include varenicline, cannabinoid-1 receptor antagonists, and the neurokinin-1 receptor antagonist LY686017. Neuroscientific effort to uncover medication combinations with additive or synergistic therapeutic effects is ongoing.

Acknowledgments

We are grateful to Elsevier for permission to reproduce some text from a recent review article.[311] We also thank the National Institute on Alcohol Abuse and Alcoholism for its support through grants 5 R01 AA010522–14, 5 R01 AA012964–06, 5 R01 AA014628–04, and 5 R01 AA013964–05; the National Institutes of Health for its support through University of Virginia General Clinical Research Center Grant M01 RR00847, and Robert H. Cormier, Jr., Ann Richards, and Dr. Chamindi Seneviratne for their assistance with manuscript preparation.

References

1. LLFA Addolorato G, et al. Effectiveness and safety of baclofen for maintenance of alcohol abstinence in alcohol-dependent patients with liver cirrhosis: randomised, double-blind controlled study. *Lancet.* 2007;370(9603):1915–1922.
2. Addolorato G, et al. Baclofen efficacy in reducing alcohol craving and intake: a preliminary double-blind randomized controlled study. *Alcohol.* 2002;37:504–508.
3. Ait-Daoud N, Johnson BA. Medications for the treatment of alcoholism. In: Johnson BA, Ruiz P, Galanter M, eds. *Handbook of Clinical Alcoholism Treatment.* Baltimore, MD: Lippincott Williams & Wilkins; 2003:119–130.
4. Ait-Daoud N, et al. Combining ondansetron and naltrexone reduces craving among biologically predisposed alcoholics: preliminary clinical evidence. *Psychopharmacology.* 2001;154:23–27.

5. Alho H, Heinälä P, Kiianmaa K, Sinclair JD. Naltrexone for alcohol dependence: double-blind placebo-controlled Finnish trial. *Alcohol Clin Exp Res.* 1999;23:46A.

6. Alim TN, et al. Tolerability study of a depot form of naltrexone substance abusers [abstract]. In: Harris LS, ed. *Problems of Drug Dependence 1994: Proceedings of the 56th Annual Scientific Meeting, the College on Problems of Drug Dependence, Inc.,* Vol. II. NIDA Res Monogr. 1995; 153:253.

7. Altshuler HL, Phillips PE, Feinhandler DA. Alteration of ethanol self-administration by naltrexone. *Life Sci.* 1980;26:679–688.

8. Anton RF. Pharmacologic approaches to the management of alcoholism. *J Clin Psychiatry.* 2001;62(suppl 20 Review):11–17.

9. Anton RF, Pettinati H, et al. A multi-site dose ranging study of nalmefene in the treatment of alcohol dependence. *J Clin Psychopharmacol.* 2004;24(4):421–428.

10. Anton RF, et al. Combined pharmacotherapies and behavioral interventions for alcohol dependence – the COMBINE Study: a randomized controlled trial. *J Am Med Assoc.* 2006;295:2003–2017.

11. Anton RF, et al. An evaluation of mu-opioid receptor (OPRM1) as a predictor of naltrexone response in the treatment of alcohol dependence: results from the Combined Pharmacotherapies and Behavioral Interventions for Alcohol Dependence (COMBINE) study. *Arch Gen Psychiatry.* 2008;65:135–144.

12. Baker JR, Jatlow P, McCance-Katz EF. Disulfiram effects on responses to intravenous cocaine administration. *Drug Alcohol Depend.* 2007;87:202–209.

13. Barnes NM, Sharp T. A review of central 5-HT receptors and their function. *Neuropharmacology.* 1999;38:1083–1152.

14. Basavarajappa BS, Hungund BL. Chronic ethanol increases the cannabinoid receptor agonist anandamide and its precursor N-arachidonoylphosphatidylethanolamine in SK-N-SH cells. *J Neurochem.* 1999;72:522–528.

15. Batel P, et al. Relationship between alcohol and tobacco dependencies among alcoholics who smoke. *Addiction.* 1995;90:977–980.

16. Beardsley PM, et al. Serotonin 5-HT3 antagonists fail to affect ethanol self-administration of rats. *Alcohol.* 1994;11:389–395.

17. Befort K, et al. A single nucleotide polymorphic mutation in the human mu-opioid receptor severely impairs receptor signaling. *J Biol Chem.* 2001;276:3130–3137.

18. Berman RF, et al. Effects of naloxone on ethanol dependence in rats. *Drug Alcohol Depend.* 1984;13:245–254.

19. Beyer A, et al. Effect of the A118G polymorphism on binding affinity, potency and agonist-mediated endocytosis, desensitization, and resensitization of the human mu-opioid receptor. *J Neurochem.* 2004;89:553–560.

20. Biggs TA, Myers RD. Naltrexone and amperozide modify chocolate and saccharin drinking in high alcohol-preferring P rats. *Pharmacol Biochem Behav.* 1998;60(2):407–413.

21. Bisaga A, Evans SM. Acute effects of memantine in combination with alcohol in moderate drinkers. *Psychopharmacology.* 2004;172:16–24.

22. Biton V, et al. Topiramate titration and tolerability. *Ann Pharmacother.* 2001;35:173–179.

23. Blier P, de Montigny C. Modification of 5-HT neuron properties by sustained administration of the 5-HT1A agonist gepirone: electrophysiological studies in the rat brain. *Synapse.* 1987;1: 470–480.

24. Blomqvist O, et al. The mesolimbic dopamine-activating properties of ethanol are antagonized by mecamylamine. *Eur J Pharmacol.* 1993;249:207–213.

25. Blomqvist O, et al. Voluntary ethanol intake in the rat: effects of nicotinic acetylcholine receptor blockade or subchronic nicotine treatment. *Eur J Pharmacol.* 1996;314:257–267.

26. Blundell JE. Serotonin and appetite. *Neuropharmacology.* 1984;23:1537–1551.

27. Blundell JE, Latham CJ. In: Drugs, Appetite ST, eds. *Behavioural Pharmacology of Feeding.* London: Academic Press; 1982:41–80.

28. Bohn MJ, et al. Naltrexone and brief counseling to reduce heavy drinking. *Am J Addictions.* 1994;3(2):91–99.

29. Boismare F, et al. A homotaurine derivative reduces the voluntary intake of ethanol by rats: are cerebral GABA receptors involved? *Pharmacol Biochem Behav.* 1984;21:787–789.

30. Bolo N, et al. Central effects of acamprosate: part 2. Acamprosate modifies the brain in-vivo proton magnetic resonance spectrum in healthy young male volunteers. *Psychiatry Res.* 1998;82:115–127.

31. Bond C, et al. Single-nucleotide polymorphism in the human mu opioid receptor gene alters beta-endorphin binding and activity: possible implications for opiate addiction. *Proc Natl Acad Sci U S A.* 1998;95:9608–9613.

32. Bouza C, et al. Efficacy and safety of naltrexone and acamprosate in the treatment of alcohol dependence: a systematic review. *Addiction.* 2004;99:811–828.

33. Boyce-Rustay JM, et al. Ethanol-related behaviors in serotonin transporter knockout mice. *Alcohol Clin Exp Res.* 2006;30:1957–1965.

34. Bradbury AJ, et al. Laterality of dopamine function and neuroleptic action in the amygdala in the rat. 24Using Smart Source Parsing Dec. *Neuropharmacology.* 1985:1163–1170.

35. Brady KT. Evidence-based pharmacotherapy for mood and anxiety disorders with concurrent alcoholism. *CNS Spectr.* 2008;13(4 suppl 6):7–9.

36. Brady KT, et al. Sertraline in the treatment of co-occurring alcohol dependence and posttraumatic stress disorder. *Alcohol Clin Exp Res.* 2005;29:395–401.

37. Breslin FJ, Johnson BA, Lynch WJ. Effect of topiramate treatment on ethanol consumption in rats. *Psychopharmacology.* 2010;207:529–534.

38. Bruno F. Buspirone in the treatment of alcoholic patients. *Psychopathology.* 1989;22(suppl 1Using Smart Source Parsing):49–59.

39. Burling TA, Ziff DC. Tobacco smoking: a comparison between alcohol and drug abuse inpatients. *Addict Behav.* 1988;13:185–190.

40. Buydens-Branchey L, Branchey MH, Noumair D. Age of alcoholism onset. I. Relationship to psychopathology. *Arch Gen Psychiatry.* 1989;46:225–230.

41. Caille S, et al. Specific alterations of extracellular endocannabinoid levels in the nucleus accumbens by ethanol, heroin, and cocaine self-administration. *J Neurosci.* 2007;27:3695–3702.

42. Caputo F, et al. Gamma hydroxybutyric acid (GHB) for the treatment of alcohol dependence: a review. *Int J Environ Res Public Health.* 2009;6:1917–1929.

43. Carroll K, FLRBSA, et al. Efficacy of disulfiram and cognitive behavior therapy in cocaine-dependent outpatients: a randomized placebo-controlled trial. *Arch Gen Psychiatry.* 2004;61(3):264–272.

44. Chefer VI, et al. Ednogenous kappa-opioid receptor systems regulate mesoaccumbal dopamine dynamics ad vulnerability to cocaine. *J Neurosci.* 2005;25(20):304–318.

45. Chen AC, Morgenstern J, Davis CM, Kuerbis AN, Covault J, Kranzler HR. Variation in mu-opioid receptor gene (OPRM1) as a moderator of naltrexone treatment to reduce heavy drinking in a high functioning cohort. *J Alcohol Drug Depend.* 2013;1(1).

46. Chick J, et al. A multicentre, randomized, double-blind, placebo-controlled trial of naltrexone in the treatment of alcohol dependence or abuse. *Alcohol Alcohol.* 2000;35:587–593.

47. Chick J, et al. Does acamprosate improve reduction of drinking as well as aiding abstinence? *J Psychopharmacol.* 2003;17:397–402.

48. Chick J, et al. Efficacy of fluvoxamine in preventing relapse in alcohol dependence: a one-year, double-blind, placebo-controlled multicentre study with analysis by typology. *Drug Alcohol Depend.* 2004;74:61–70.

49. Cippitelli A, et al. Cannabinoid CB1 receptor antagonism reduces conditioned reinstatement of ethanol-seeking behavior in rats. *Eur J Neurosci.* 2005;21:2243–2251.

50. Cloninger CR. Neurogenetic adaptive mechanisms in alcoholism. *Science.* 1987;236:410–416.

51. Collins DM, Myers RD. Buspirone attenuates volitional alcohol intake in the chronically drinking monkey. *Alcohol*. 1987;4:49–56.

52. Colombo G, et al. Ability of baclofen in reducing alcohol intake and withdrawal severity: I—preclinical evidence. *Alcohol Clin Exp Res*. 2000;24:58–66.

53. Colombo G, et al. Suppression by baclofen of alcohol deprivation effect in Sardinian alcohol-preferring (sP) rats. *Drug Alcohol Depend*. 2003;70:105–108.

54. Colombo G, et al. Suppressing effect of the cannabinoid CB1 receptor antagonist, SR 141716, on alcohol's motivational properties in alcohol-preferring rats. *Eur J Pharmacol*. 2004;498:119–123.

55. Colombo G, et al. Suppression by baclofen of the stimulation of alcohol intake induced by morphine and WIN 55,212-2 in alcohol-preferring rats. *Eur J Pharmacol*. 2004;492:189–193.

56. Comer SD, et al. Depot naltrexone: long-lasting antagonism of the effects of heroin in humans. *Psychopharmacology*. 2002;159:351–360.

57. Conigrave KM, et al. CDT, GGT, and AST as markers of alcohol use: the WHO/ISBRA collaborative project. *Alcohol Clin Exp Res*. 2002;26:332–339.

58. Cornelius JR, et al. Fluoxetine in depressed alcoholics: a double-blind, placebo-controlled trial. *Arch Gen Psychiatry*. 1997;54:700–705.

59. Costall B, et al. Effects of the 5-HT3 receptor antagonist, GR38032F, on raised dopaminergic activity in the mesolimbic system of the rat and marmoset brain. *Br J Pharmacol*. 1987;92:881–894.

60. Croop RS, Faulkner EB, Labriola DF. The safety profile of naltrexone in the treatment of alcoholism. Results from a multicenter usage study. The Naltrexone Usage Study Group. *Arch Gen Psychiatry*. 1997;54:1130–1135.

61. Czachowski CL, Legg BH, Samson HH. Effects of acamprosate on ethanol-seeking and self-administration in the rat. *Alcohol Clin Exp Res*. 2001;25:344–350.

62. Dahchour A, De Witte P. Effects of acamprosate on excitatory amino acids during multiple ethanol withdrawal periods. *Alcohol Clin Exp Res*. 2003;27:465–470.

63. Dahchour A, et al. Central effects of acamprosate: part 1. Acamprosate blocks the glutamate increase in the nucleus accumbens microdialysate in ethanol withdrawn rats. *Psychiatry Res*. 1998;82:107–114.

64. Daoust M, et al. Isolation and striatal (3H) serotonin uptake: role in the voluntary intake of ethanol by rats. *Pharmacol Biochem Behav*. 1985;22:205–208.

65. Davidson D, Swift R, Fitz E. Naltrexone increases the latency to drink alcohol in social drinkers. *Alcohol Clin Exp Res*. 1996;20:732–739.

66. De Witte P, Bachteler D, Spanagel R. Acamprosate: preclinical data. In: Spanagel R, Mann KF, eds. *Drugs for Relapse Prevention of Alcoholism*. Basel, Switzerland: Birkhäuser Verlagp; 2005:73–83.

67. De Witte P, et al. Neuroprotective and abstinence-promoting effects of acamprosate: elucidating the mechanism of action. *CNS Drugs*. 2005;19:517–537.

68. deBejczy A, Lof E, Walther L, et al. Varenicline for treatment of alcohol dependence: a randomized, placebo-controlled trial. *Alcohol Clin Exp Res*. 2015;39(11):2189–2199.

69. DeWitte P. Naloxone reduces alcohol intake in a free-choice procedure even when both drinking bottles contain saccharin sodium or quinine substances. *Neuropsychobiology*. 1984;12:73–77.

70. Dodgson SJ, Shank RP, Maryanoff BE. Topiramate as an inhibitor of carbonic anhydrase isoenzymes. *Epilepsia*. 2000;41(suppl 1):S35–S39.

71. Dongier M, Vachon L, Schwartz G. Bromocriptine in the treatment of alcohol dependence. 15Using Smart Source Parsing Dec. *Alcohol Clin Exp Res*. 1991:970–977.

72. Doty P, de Wit H. Effect of setting on the reinforcing and subjective effects of ethanol in social drinkers. *Psychopharmacology*. 1995;118(1):19–27.

73. Doty P, Zacny JP, de Wit H. Effects of ondansetron pretreatment on acute responses to ethanol in social drinkers. *Behav Pharmacol*. 1994;5:461–469.

74. Dreher KF, Fraser JG. Smoking habits of alcoholic out-patients. *I Int J Addict*. 1967;2:259–270.

75. Dundon W, et al. Treatment outcomes in type A and B alcohol dependence 6 months after serotonergic pharmacotherapy. *Alcohol Clin Exp Res*. 2004;28:1065–1073.

76. Dyr W, Kostowski W. Evidence that the amygdala is involved in the inhibitory effects of 5-HT3 receptor antagonists on alcohol drinking in rats. *Alcohol*. 1995;12:387–391.

77. Economidou D, et al. Effect of the cannabinoid CB1 receptor antagonist SR-141716A on ethanol self-administration and ethanol-seeking behaviour in rats. *Psychopharmacology*. 2006;183:394–403.

78. Ericson M, et al. Voluntary ethanol intake in the rat and the associated accumbal dopamine overflow are blocked by ventral tegmental mecamylamine. *Eur J Pharmacol*. 1998;358:189–196.

79. Errante LD, Petroff OA. Acute effects of gabapentin and pregabalin on rat forebrain cellular GABA, glutamate, and glutamine concentrations. *Seizure*. 2003;12(5):300–306.

80. Erwin BLSlaton RM. Varenicline in the treatment of alcohol use disorders. *Ann Pharmacother*. 2014;48(11):1445–1455.

81. Escher T, Mittleman G. Schedule-induced alcohol drinking: non-selective effects of acamprosate and naltrexone. *Addict Biol*. 2006;11:55–63.

82. Evans SM, et al. A pilot double-blind treatment trial of memantine for alcohol dependence. *Alcohol Clin Exp Res*. 2007;31:775–782.

83. Fadda F, et al. MDL 72222, a selective 5-HT3 receptor antagonist, suppresses voluntary ethanol consumption in alcohol-preferring rats. *Alcohol Alcohol*. 1991;26:107–110.

84. Fantino M. Role of sensory input in the control of food intake. *J Auton Nerv Syst*. 1984;10:347–358.

85. Farook JM, et al. Topiramate (Topamax) reduces conditioned abstinence behaviours and handling-induced convulsions (HIC) after chronic administration of alcohol in Swiss-Webster mice. *Alcohol Alcohol*. 2007;42:296–300.

86. Farren CK, et al. A double-blind, placebo-controlled study of sertraline with naltrexone for alcohol dependence. *Drug Alcohol Depend*. 2009;99:317–321.

87. Finney JW, Hahn AC, Moos RH. The effectiveness of inpatient and outpatient treatment for alcohol abuse: the need to focus on mediators and moderators of setting effects. *Addiction*. 1996;91:1773–1796.

88. Flensborg-Madsen T, et al. Alcohol use disorders increase the risk of completed suicide–irrespective of other psychiatric disorders. A longitudinal cohort study. *Psychiatry Res*. 2009;167:123–130.

89. Foster KL, et al. GABA(A) and opioid receptors of the central nucleus of the amygdala selectively regulate ethanol-maintained behaviors. *Neuropsychopharmacology*. 2004;29:269–284.

90. Froehlich JC, et al. Naloxone attenuation of voluntary alcohol consumption. *Alcohol Alcohol*. 1987;(suppl 1):333–337.

91. Froehlich JC, et al. Naloxone attenuates voluntary ethanol intake in rats selectively bred for high ethanol preference. *Pharmacol Biochem Behav*. 1990;35:385–390.

92. Froehlich JC, et al. Importance of delta opioid receptors in maintaining high alcohol drinking. *Psychopharmacology*. 1991;103:467–472.

93. Fuller RK, et al. Disulfiram treatment of alcoholism. A Veterans Administration cooperative study. *J Am Med Assoc*. 1986;256:1449–1455.

94. Gabriel KI, Cunningham CL. Effects of topiramate on ethanol and saccharin consumption and preferences in C57BL/6J mice. *Alcohol Clin Exp Res*. 2005;29:75–80.

95. Garbutt JC, et al. Efficacy and tolerability of long-acting injectable naltrexone for alcohol dependence: a randomized controlled trial. *J Am Med Assoc*. 2005;293:1617–1625.

96. Gelernter J, Kranzler H, Cubells J. Genetics of two mu opioid receptor gene (OPRM1) exon I polymorphisms: population studies, and allele frequencies in alcohol- and drug-dependent subjects. *Mol Psychiatry*. 1999;4:476–483.

97. Gelernter J, et al. Opioid receptor gene (OPRM1, OPRK1, and OPRD1) variants and response to naltrexone treatment for alcohol dependence: results from the VA Cooperative Study. *Alcohol Clin Exp Res*. 2007;31:555–563.

98. Geller I. Effects of para-chlorophenylalanine and 5-hydroxytryptophan on alcohol intake in the rat. *Pharmacol Biochem Behav*. 1973;1:361–365.

99. George DT, et al. Neurokinin 1 receptor antagonism as a possible therapy for alcoholism. *Science*. 2008;319:1536–1539.

100. Gessa GL, et al. Suppressing effect of the cannabinoid CB1 receptor antagonist, SR147778, on alcohol intake and motivational properties of alcohol in alcohol-preferring sP rats. *Alcohol Alcohol*. 2005;40:46–53.

101. Gewiss M, et al. Acamprosate and diazepam differentially modulate alcohol-induced behavioral and cortical alterations in rats following chronic inhalation of ethanol vapor. *Alcohol Alcohol*. 1991;26:129–137.

102. Gianoulakis C. Alcohol-seeking behavior. The roles of the hypothalamic-pituitary-adrenal axis and the endogenous opioid system. *Alcohol Health Res World*. 1998;22:202–210.

103. Gianoulakis C, de Waele JP, Thavundayil J. Implication of the endogenous opioid system in excessive ethanol consumption. *Alcohol*. 1996;13:19–23.

104. Gibbs JW, et al. Cellular actions of topiramate: blockade of kainate-evoked inward currents in cultured hippocampal neurons. *Epilepsia*. 2000;41(suppl 1):S10–S16.

105. Gill K, Amit Z. Serotonin uptake blockers and voluntary alcohol consumption. A review of recent studies. *Recent Dev Alcohol*. 1989;7:225–248.

106. Gill K, Amit Z, Koe BK. Treatment with sertraline, a new serotonin uptake inhibitor, reduces voluntary ethanol consumption in rats. *Alcohol*. 1988;5:349–354.

107. Gill K, Filion Y, Amit Z. A further examination of the effects of sertraline on voluntary ethanol consumption. *Alcohol*. 1988;5:355–358.

108. Gorelick DA, Paredes A. Effect of fluoxetine on alcohol consumption in male alcoholics. *Alcohol Clin Exp Res*. 1992;16:261–265.

109. Gottfries CG. Influence of depression and antidepressants on weight. *Acta Psychiatr Scand Suppl*. 1981;290:353–356.

110. Grant BF, et al. Epidemiology of DSM-5 alcohol use disorder: results from the national Epidemiologic survey on alcohol and related conditions III. *JAMA psychiatry*. 2015;72(8):757–766.

111. Grisel JE, et al. Ethanol oral self-administration is increased in mutant mice with decreased beta-endorphin expression. *Brain Res*. 1999;835:62–67.

112. Gryder DS, Rogawski MA. Selective antagonism of GluR5 kainate-receptor-mediated synaptic currents by topiramate in rat basolateral amygdala neurons. *J Neurosci*. 2003;23:7069–7074.

113. Gual A, He Y, Torup L, et al. A randomized, double-blind, placebo-controlled, efficacy study of nalmefene, as-needed use, in patients with alcohol dependence. *Eur Neuropsychopharmacol*. 2013;23(11):1432–1442.

114. Gubner NR, McKinnon CS, Phillips TJ. Effects of varenicline on ethanol-induced conditioned place preference, locomotor stimulation, and sensitization. *Alcohol Clin Exp Res*. 2014;38(12):3033–3042.

115. Gulley JM, et al. Selective serotonin reuptake inhibitors: effects of chronic treatment on ethanol-reinforced behavior in mice. *Alcohol*. 1995;12:177–181.

116. Gysling K, Wang RY. Morphine-induced activation of A10 dopamine neurons in the rat. *Brain Res*. 1983;277:119–127.

117. Haraguchi M, Samson HH, Tolliver GA. Reduction in oral ethanol self-administration in the rat by the 5-HT uptake blocker fluoxetine. *Pharmacol Biochem Behav*. 1990;35:259–262.

118. Harris BR, et al. Acamprosate inhibits the binding and neurotoxic effects of trans-ACPD, suggesting a novel site of action at metabotropic glutamate receptors. *Alcohol Clin Exp Res*. 2002;26:1779–1793.

119. Reference deleted in review.

120. Heilig M, Egli M. Pharmacological treatment of alcohol dependence: target symptoms and target mechanisms. *Pharmacol Ther*. 2006;111:855–876.

121. Heinälä P, Alho H, Kuoppasalmi K, et al. Naltrexone in alcoholism treatment: Patient efficacy and compliance. In: *New Research. Program and Abstracts*. Washington, DC: American Psychiatric Association Annual Meeting; 1999. May 15–20, 1999.

122. Heinälä P, Alho H, Kuoppasalmi K, et al. (1999b) Use of naltrexone in the treatment of alcohol dependence — a double-blind placebo-controlled Finnish trial. *Alcohol Alcohol*. 1999;34:433.

123. Heinala PAH, Kiianmaa K, et al. Targeted use of naltrexone without prior detoxification in the treatment of alcohol dependence: a factorial double-blind, placebo-controlled trial. *J Clin Psychopharmacol*. 2001;21:287–292.

124. Heinälä P, et al. Naltrexone in alcoholism treatment: patient efficacy and compliance. In: *New Research. Program and Abstracts*. Washington, DC: American Psychiatric Association 1999 Annual Meeting; 1999.

125. Heinälä P, et al. Use of naltrexone in the treatment of alcohol dependence—a double-blind placebo-controlled Finnish trial. *Alcohol Alcohol*. 1999;34:433.

126. Heishman SJ, et al. Safety and pharmacokinetics of a new formulation of depot naltrexone [abstract]. In: Harris LS, ed. *Problems of Drug Dependence, 1993: Proceedings of the 55th Annual Scientific Meeting, the College on Problems of Drug Dependence, Inc.*, Vol II. NIDA Res Monogr. 1994; 141:82.

127. Heisler LK, Kanarek RB, Gerstein A. Fluoxetine decreases fat and protein intakes but not carbohydrate intake in male rats. *Pharmacol Biochem Behav*. 1997;58:767–773.

128. Heisler LK, Kanarek RB, Homoleski B. Reduction of fat and protein intakes but not carbohydrate intake following acute and chronic fluoxetine in female rats. *Pharmacol Biochem Behav*. 1999;63:377–385.

129. Hemby SE, Johnson BA, Dworkin SI. Neurobiological basis of drug reinforcement. In: Johnson BA, Roache JD, eds. *Drug Addiction and its Treatment: Nexus of Neuroscience and Behavior*. Philadelphia: Lippincott-Raven; 1997:137–169.

130. Hemby SE, et al. Differences in extracellular dopamine concentrations in the nucleus accumbens during response-dependent and response-independent cocaine administration in the rat. *Psychopharmacology*. 1997;133:7–16.

131. Herrero AI, et al. Two new actions of topiramate: inhibition of depolarizing GABA(A)-mediated responses and activation of a potassium conductance. *Neuropharmacology*. 2002;42:210–220.

132. Herz A. Endogenous opioid systems and alcohol addiction. *Psychopharmacology*. 1997;129:99–111.

133. Heyser CJ, Moc K, Koob GF. Effects of naltrexone alone and in combination with acamprosate on the alcohol deprivation effect in rats. *Neuropsychopharmacology*. 2003;28:1463–1471.

134. Hodge CW, et al. Specific decreases in ethanol- but not water-reinforced responding produced by the 5-HT3 antagonist ICS 205-930. *Alcohol*. 1993;10:191–196.

135. Jaffe AJ, et al. Naltrexone, relapse prevention, and supportive therapy with alcoholics: an analysis of patient treatment matching. *J Consult Clin Psychol*. 1996;64:1044–1053.

136. Johnson BA. Serotonergic agents and alcoholism treatment: rebirth of the subtype concept - an hypothesis. *Alcohol Clin Exp Res*. 2000;24:1597–1601.

137. Johnson BA. Progress in the development of topiramate for treating alcohol dependence: from a hypothesis to a proof-of-concept study. *Alcohol Clin Exp Res*. 2004;28:1137–1144.

138. Johnson BA. Recent advances in the development of treatments for alcohol and cocaine dependence: focus on topiramate and other modulators of GABA or glutamate function. *CNS Drugs.* 2005;19:873–896.

139. Johnson BA. New weapon to curb smoking: no more excuses to delay treatment. *Arch Intern Med.* 2006;166:1547–1550.

140. Johnson BA. Update on neuropharmacological treatments for alcoholism: scientific basis and clinical findings. *Biochem Pharmacol.* 2008;75(1):34–56.

141. Johnson BA. Disulfiram. In: Stolerman IP, ed. *Encyclopedia of Psychopharmacology.* Berlin: Springer-Verlag; 2010:413–416.

142. Johnson BA, et al. Use of oral topiramate to promote smoking abstinence among alcohol-dependent smokers: a randomized controlled trial. *Arch Intern Med.* 2005;165(14):1600–1605.

143. Johnson BA, Ait-Daoud N. Neuropharmacological treatments for alcoholism: scientific basis and clinical findings. *Psychopharmacology.* 2000;149:327–344.

144. Johnson BA, Ait-Daoud N, Prihoda TJ. Combining ondansetron and naltrexone effectively treats biologically predisposed alcoholics: from hypotheses to preliminary clinical evidence. *Alcohol Clin Exp Res.* 2000;24:737–742.

145. Johnson BA, Cowen PJ. Alcohol-induced reinforcement: dopamine and 5-HT3 receptor interactions in animals and humans. *Drug Dev Res.* 1993;30:153–169.

146. Johnson BA, et al. Ondansetron for reduction of drinking among biologically predisposed alcoholic patients: a randomized controlled trial. *J Am Med Assoc.* 2000;284:963–971.

147. Johnson BA, et al. Topiramate for treating alcohol dependence: a randomized controlled trial. *J Am Med Assoc.* 2007;298(14):1641–1651.

148. Johnson BA, et al. Oral topiramate for treatment of alcohol dependence: a randomised controlled trial. *Lancet.* 2003;361:1677–1685.

149. Johnson BA, et al. A pilot evaluation of the safety and tolerability of repeat dose administration of long-acting injectable naltrexone (Vivitrex®) in patients with alcohol dependence. *Alcohol Clin Exp Res.* 2004;28:1356–1361.

150. Johnson BA, et al. Attenuation of some alcohol-induced mood changes and the desire to drink by 5-HT3 receptor blockade: a preliminary study in healthy male volunteers. *Psychopharmacology.* 1993;112:142–144.

151. Johnson BA, et al. Dose-ranging kinetics and behavioral pharmacology of naltrexone and acamprosate, both alone and combined, in alcohol-dependent subjects. *J Clin Psychopharmacol.* 2003;23:281–293.

152. Johnson BA, et al. Brief behavioral compliance enhancement treatment (BBCET) manual. In: Johnson BA, Ruiz P, Galanter M, eds. *Handbook of Clinical Alcoholism Treatment.* Baltimore, MD: Lippincott Williams & Wilkins; 2003:282–301.

153. Johnson BA, et al. Oral topiramate reduces the consequences of drinking and improves the quality of life of alcohol-dependent individuals. *Arch Gen Psychiatry.* 2004;61:905–912.

154. Johnson BA, et al. Challenges and opportunities for medications development in alcoholism: an international perspective on collaborations between academia and industry. *Alcohol Clin Exp Res.* 2005;29:1528–1540.

155. Johnson BA, et al. Topiramate for treating alcohol dependence: a randomized controlled trial. *J Am Med Assoc.* 2007;298:1641–1651.

156. Johnson BA, et al. Can serotonin transporter genotype predict serotonergic function, chronicity, and severity of drinking? *Prog Neuropsychopharmacol Biol Psychiatry.* 2008;32:209–216.

157. Johnson BA, et al. Improvement of physical health and quality of life of alcohol-dependent individuals with topiramate treatment. *Arch Intern Med.* 2008;168(11):1188–1199.

157a. Johnson BA, et al. Pharmacogenetic approach at the serotonin transporter gene as a method of reducing the severity of alcohol drinking. *Am J Psychiatry.* 2011;168(3):265–275.

158. Johnson BA, Seneviratne C, Wang XQ, et al. Determination of genotype combinations that can predict the outcome of the treatment of alcohol dependence using the 5-HT(3) antagonist ondansetron. *Am J Psychiatry.* 2013;170(9):1020–1031.

159. Johnson SW, North RA. Opioids excite dopamine neurons by hyperpolarization of local interneurons. *J Neurosci.* 1992;12:483–488.

160. Juarez J, Eliana Bde T. Alcohol consumption is enhanced after naltrexone treatment. *Alcohol Clin Exp Res.* 2007;31:260–264.

161. Kabel DI, Petty F. A placebo-controlled, double-blind study of fluoxetine in severe alcohol dependence: adjunctive pharmacotherapy during and after inpatient treatment. *Alcohol Clin Exp Res.* 1996;20:780–784.

162. Kamdar NK, et al. Acute effects of naltrexone and GBR 12909 on ethanol drinking-in-the-dark in C57BL/6J mice. *Psychopharmacology.* 2007;192:207–217.

163. Kessler RC, et al. Lifetime co-occurrence of DSM-III-R alcohol abuse and dependence with other psychiatric disorders in the National Comorbidity Survey. *Arch Gen Psychiatry.* 1997;54(4):313–321.

164. Kiefer F, et al. Alcohol self-administration, craving and HPA-axis activity: an intriguing relationship. *Psychopharmacology.* 2002;164:239–240.

165. Kiefer F, et al. Comparing and combining naltrexone and acamprosate in relapse prevention of alcoholism: a double-blind, placebo-controlled study. *Arch Gen Psychiatry.* 2003;60:92–99.

166. King A, et al. Naltrexone decreases heavy drinking rates in smoking cessation treatment: an exploratory study. *Alcohol Clin Exp Res.* 2009;33:1044–1050.

167. King AC, et al. Effect of naltrexone on subjective alcohol response in subjects at high and low risk for future alcohol dependence. *Psychopharmacology.* 1997;129:15–22.

168. Kissler JL, et al. The one-two punch of alcoholism: role of central amygdala dynorphins/kappa-opioid receptors. *Biol Psychiatry.* 2014;75(10):774–782.

169. Koob GF. Neural mechanisms of drug reinforcement. *Ann N Y Acad Sci.* 1992;654:171–191. Review.

170. Kotlinska J, Bochenski M, Danysz W. N-methyl-D-aspartate and group I metabotropic glutamate receptors are involved in the expression of ethanol-induced sensitization in mice. *Behav Pharmacol.* 2006;17:1–8.

171. Kozlowski LT, Jelinek LC, Pope MA. Cigarette smoking among alcohol abusers: a continuing and neglected problem. *Can J Public Health.* 1986;77:205–207.

172. Kranzler HR. Treatment of alcohol dependence. *Liver Transplant Surg.* 1997;3(3):311–321.

173. Kranzler HR, et al. Fluoxetine treatment seems to reduce the beneficial effects of cognitive-behavioral therapy in type B alcoholics. *Alcohol Clin Exp Res.* 1996;20(9):1534–1541.

174. Kranzler HR, Modesto-Lowe V, Nuwayser ES. Sustained-release naltrexone for alcoholism treatment: a preliminary study. *Alcohol Clin Exp Res.* 1998;22:1074–1079.

175. Kranzler HR, Van Kirk J. Efficacy of naltrexone and acamprosate for alcoholism treatment: a meta-analysis. *Alcohol Clin Exp Res.* 2001;25:1335–1341.

176. Kranzler HR, et al. Placebo-controlled trial of fluoxetine as an adjunct to relapse prevention in alcoholics. *Am J Psychiatry.* 1995;152:391–397.

177. Kranzler HR, et al. Effects of ondansetron in early- versus late-onset alcoholics: a prospective, open-label study. *Alcohol Clin Exp Res.* 2003;27:1150–1155.

178. Kranzler HR, et al. Targeted naltrexone for early problem drinkers. *J Clin Psychopharmacol.* 2003;23:294–304.

179. Kranzler HR, et al. Naltrexone depot for treatment of alcohol dependence: a multicenter, randomized, placebo-controlled clinical trial. *Alcohol Clin Exp Res.* 2004;28:1051–1059.

180. Kranzler HR, et al. Sertraline treatment of co-occurring alcohol dependence and major depression. *J Clin Psychopharmacol.* 2006;26:13–20.

181. Kranzler HR, et al. Association of markers in the 3′ region of the GluR5 kainate receptor subunit gene to alcohol dependence. *Alcohol Clin Exp Res.* 2009;33(5):925–930.

182. Kranzler HR, et al. Topiramate treatment for heavy drinkers: moderation by a GRIK1 polymorphism. *Am J Psychiatry.* 2014;171(4):445–452.

183. Krishnan-Sarin S, et al. Family history of alcoholism influences naltrexone-induced reduction in alcohol drinking. *Biol Psychiatry.* 2007;62:694–697.

184. Krupitsky EM, et al. Effect of memantine on cue-induced alcohol craving in recovering alcohol-dependent patients. *Am J Psychiatry.* 2007;164:519–523.

185. Krystal JH, et al. Potentiation of low dose ketamine effects by naltrexone: potential implications for the pharmacotherapy of alcoholism. *Neuropsychopharmacology.* 2006;31:1793–1800.

186. Lallemand F, De Witte P. SR147778 a CB1 cannabinoid receptor antagonist, suppresses ethanol preference in chronically alcoholized Wistar rats. *Alcohol.* 2006;39:125–134.

187. Lankford MF, Bjork AK, Myers RD. Differential efficacy of serotonergic drugs FG5974, FG5893, and amperozide in reducing alcohol drinking in P rats. 13Using Smart Source Parsing Jul-Aug. *Alcohol.* 1996:399–404.

188. Le AD, et al. The effects of selective blockade of delta and mu opiate receptors on ethanol consumption by C57B1/6 mice in a restricted access paradigm. *Brain Res.* 1993;630:330–332.

189. Le Magnen J, Tran G, Durlach J. Lack of effects of Ca-acetyl homotaurinate on chronic and acute toxicities of ethanol in rats. *Alcohol.* 1987;4:103–108.

190. Leander JD. Fluoxetine suppresses palatability-induced ingestion. *Psychopharmacology.* 1987;91:285–287.

191. Lee YK, et al. Effects of naltrexone on the ethanol-induced changes in the rat central dopaminergic system. *Alcohol Alcohol.* 2005;40:297–301.

192. Lewis DH. Controlled release of bioactive agents from lactide/glycolide polymers. In: Chasin M, Langer R, eds. *Biodegradable Polymers as Drug Delivery Systems.* New York: Marcel Dekker; 1990:1–41.

193. Li ET, Anderson GH. 5-Hydroxytryptamine control of meal to meal composition chosen by rats. *Fed Proc.* 1983;42:542–548.

194. Linnoila M, De Jong J, Virkkunen M. Family history of alcoholism in violent offenders and impulsive fire setters. *Arch Gen Psychiatry.* 1989;46:613–616.

195. Linnoila M, VirkkunenM. Biologic correlates of suicidal risk and aggressive behavioral traits. *J Clin Psychopharmacol.* 1992;12(2 Suppl):19S–20S. Using Smart Source Parsing Apr.

196. Litten RZ, Allen J, Fertig J. Pharmacotherapies for alcohol problems: a review of research with focus on developments since 1991. *Alcohol Clin Exp Res.* 1996;20:859–876.

197. Litten RZ, Allen JP. Advances in development of medications for alcoholism treatment. *Psychopharmacology.* 1998;139:20–33.

198. Litten RZ, Ryan ML, Fertig JB, et al. A double-blind, placebo-controlled trial assessing the efficacy of varenicline tartrate for alcohol dependence. *J Addict Med.* 2013;7(4):277–286.

199. Littleton J. Acamprosate in alcohol dependence: how does it work? *Addiction.* 1995;90:1179–1188.

200. Lovinger DM. 5-HT3 receptors and the neural actions of alcohols: an increasingly exciting topic. *Neurochem Int.* 1999;35:125–130.

201. Lovinger DM. Inhibition of 5-HT3 receptor-mediated ion current by divalent metal cations in NCB-20 neuroblastoma cells. *J Neurophysiol.* 1991;66:1329–1337.

202. Lovinger DM, White G. Ethanol potentiation of 5-hydroxytryptamine3 receptor-mediated ion current in neuroblastoma cells and isolated adult mammalian neurons. *Mol Pharmacol.* 1991;40:263–270.

203. Ma JZ, Ait-Daoud N, Johnson BA. Topiramate reduces the harm of excessive drinking: implications for public health and primary care. *Addiction.* 2006;101:1561–1568.

204. Malec TS, Malec EA, Dongier M. Efficacy of buspirone in alcohol dependence: a review. *Alcohol Clin Exp Res.* 1996;20:853–858.

205. Mann K, Bladstrom A, et al. Extending the treatment options in alcohol dependence: a randomized controlled study of as-needed nalmefene. *Biol Psychiatry.* 2013;73(8):706–713.

206. Mann K, Lehert P, Morgan MY. The efficacy of acamprosate in the maintenance of abstinence in alcohol-dependent individuals: results of a meta-analysis. *Alcohol Clin Exp Res.* 2004;28:51–63.

207. Mann KF, Anton RF. Towards an individualized treatment in alcohol dependence: results from the US-combine study and German PREDICT study — in honor of past work of Dr. Jack Mendelson. Symposium presented at the 2008 Joint scientific Meeting of the research Society on Alcoholism and the international Society for Biomedical Research on alcoholism, June 29, 2008, Washington, DC. Alcohol Clin Exp Res, 2008. 32(s1):281A.

208. Manzanares J, et al. Interactions between cannabinoid and opioid receptor systems in the mediation of ethanol effects. *Alcohol Alcohol.* 2005;40:25–34.

209. Marinelli PW, Quirion R, Gianoulakis C. An in vivo profile of beta-endorphin release in the arcuate nucleus and nucleus accumbens following exposure to stress or alcohol. *Neuroscience.* 2004;127:777–784.

210. Mason BJ, et al. A double-blind, placebo-controlled pilot study to evaluate the efficacy and safety of oral nalmefene HCl for alcohol dependence. *Alcohol Clin Exp Res.* 1994;18(5):1162–1167.

211. Mason BJ, et al. A double-blind, placebo-controlled trial of desipramine for primary alcohol dependence stratified on the presence or absence of major depression. *J Am Med Assoc.* 1996;275:761–767.

212. Mason BJ, et al. A double-blind, placebo-controlled study of oral nalmefene for alcohol dependence. *Arch Gen Psychiatry.* 1999;56(8):719–724.

213. Mason BJ, et al. A pharmacokinetic and pharmacodynamic drug interaction study of acamprosate and naltrexone. *Neuropsychopharmacology.* 2002;27:596–606.

214. Mason BJ, et al. Effect of oral acamprosate on abstinence in patients with alcohol dependence in a double-blind, placebo-controlled trial: the role of patient motivation. *J Psychiatr Res.* 2006;40:383–393.

215. Mason BJ, et al. Proof-of-concept human laboratory study for protracted abstinence in alcohol dependence: effects of gabapentin. *Addict Biol.* 2009;14(1):73–83.

216. Mason BJ, et al. Gabapentin treatment for alcohol dependence: a randomized clinical trial. *JAMA Int Med.* 2014;174(1):70–77.

217. Mason GA, et al. The subchronic effects of the TRH analog TA-0910 and bromocriptine on alcohol preference in alcohol-preferring rats: development of tolerance and cross-tolerance. *Alcohol Clin Exp Res.* 1994;18:1196–1201.

218. Matsuzawa S, et al. Roles of 5-HT3 and opioid receptors in the ethanol-induced place preference in rats exposed to conditioned fear stress. *Life Sci.* 1999;64:PL241–PL249.

219. Matthews RT, German DC. Electrophysiological evidence for excitation of rat ventral tegmental area dopamine neurons by morphine. *Neuroscience.* 1984;11:617–625.

220. Maurel S, De Vry J, Schreiber R. Comparison of the effects of the selective serotonin-reuptake inhibitors fluoxetine, paroxetine, citalopram and fluvoxamine in alcohol-preferring cAA rats. *Alcohol.* 1999;17:195–201.

221. McBride WJ, Li TK. Animal models of alcoholism: neurobiology of high alcohol-drinking behavior in rodents. *Crit Rev Neurobiol.* 1998;12:339–369.

222. McBride WJ, et al. Serotonin and ethanol preference. *Recent Dev Alcohol.* 1989;7:187–209.

223. McGeary JE, et al. Genetic moderators of naltrexone's effects on alcohol cue reactivity. *Alcohol Clin Exp Res.* 2006;30:1288–1296.

224. McGrath PJ, et al. Imipramine treatment of alcoholics with primary depression: a placebo-controlled clinical trial. *Arch Gen Psychiatry.* 1996;53:232–240.

225. McKee SA, et al. Varenicline reduces alcohol self-administration in heavy-drinking smokers. *Biol Psychiatry*. 2009;66:185–190.

226. McLellan AT, et al. Drug dependence, a chronic medical illness: implications for treatment, insurance, and outcomes evaluation. *J Am Med Assoc*. 2000;284:1689–1695.

227. Meert TF. Effects of various serotonergic agents on alcohol intake and alcohol preference in Wistar rats selected at two different levels of alcohol preference. *Alcohol Alcohol*. 1993;28:157–170.

228. Meert TF, Janssen PA. Ritanserin, a new therapeutic approach for drug abuse. Part 1: effects on alcohol. *Drug Dev Res*. 1991;24:235–249.

229. Miranda R, et al. Effects of topiramate on urge to drink and the subjective effects of alcohol: a preliminary laboratory study. *Alcohol Clin Exp Res*. 2008;32(3):489–497.

230. Moak DH, et al. Sertraline and cognitive behavioral therapy for depressed alcoholics: results of a placebo-controlled trial. *J Clin Psychopharmacol*. 2003;23:553–562.

231. Monterosso JR, et al. Predicting treatment response to naltrexone: the influence of craving and family history. *Am J Addict*. 2001;10:258–268.

232. Moranta D, Esteban S, Garcia-Sevilla JA. Differential effects of acute cannabinoid drug treatment, mediated by CB1 receptors, on the in vivo activity of tyrosine and tryptophan hydroxylase in the rat brain. *Naunyn Schmiedebergs Arch Pharmacol*. 2004;369:516–524.

233. Muhonen LH, et al. Treatment of alcohol dependence in patients with co-morbid major depressive disorder — predictors for the outcomes with memantine and escitalopram medication. *Subst Abuse Treat Prev Policy*. 2008;3:1–7.

234. Murphy CM, et al. Craving as an alcohol use disorder symptom in DSM-5: an empirical examination in a treatment-seeking sample. *Exp Clin Psychopharmacol*. 2014;22(1):43–49.

235. Murphy JM, et al. Effects of fluoxetine on the intragastric self-administration of ethanol in the alcohol preferring P line of rats. *Alcohol*. 1988;5:283–286.

236. Myers RD, Lankford M, Bjork A. Selective reduction by the 5-HT antagonist amperozide of alcohol preference induced in rats by systemic cyanamide. *Pharmacol Biochem Behav*. 1992;43:661–667.

237. Myers RD, Lankford MF. Suppression of alcohol preference in high alcohol drinking rats: efficacy of amperozide versus naltrexone. 14Using Smart Source Parsing Feb. *Neuropsychopharmacology*. 1996:139–149.

238. Myers RD, Veale WL. Alcohol preference in the rat: reduction following depletion of brain serotonin. *Science*. 1968;160:1469–1471.

239. Nachman M, Lester D, Le Magnen J. Alcohol aversion in the rat: behavioral assessment of noxious drug effects. *Science*. 1970;168:1244–1246.

240. Nagy J. Renaissance of NMDA receptor antagonists: do they have a role in the pharmacotherapy for alcoholism? *Idrugs*. 2004;7:339–350.

241. Naranjo CA, Bremner KE, Lanctot KL. Effects of citalopram and a brief psycho-social intervention on alcohol intake, dependence and problems. *Addiction*. 1995;90:87–99.

242. Naranjo CA, George SR, Bremner KE. Novel neuropharmacological treatments of alcohol dependence. *Clin Neuropharmacol*. 1992;15(suppl 1 Pt A):74A–75A.

243. Naranjo CA, Sellers EM. Serotonin uptake inhibitors attenuate ethanol intake in problem drinkers. *Recent Dev Alcohol*. 1989;7:255–266.

244. Naranjo CA, et al. Zimelidine-induced variations in alcohol intake by nondepressed heavy drinkers. *Clin Pharmacol Ther*. 1984;35:374–381.

245. Naranjo CA, et al. The serotonin uptake inhibitor citalopram attenuates ethanol intake. *Clin Pharmacol Ther*. 1987;41:266–274.

246. Naranjo CA, et al. Fluoxetine differentially alters alcohol intake and other consummatory behaviors in problem drinkers. *Clin Pharmacol Ther*. 1990;47:490–498.

247. Naranjo CA, et al. Citalopram decreases desirability, liking, and consumption of alcohol in alcohol-dependent drinkers. *Clin Pharmacol Ther*. 1992;51:729–739.

248. Nealy KA, Smith AW, et al. K-opioid receptors are implicated in the increased potency of intra-accumbens nalmefene in ethanol-dependent rats. *Neuropharmacology*. 2011;61(1–2):35–42.

249. Nguyen SA, Malcolm R, Middaugh LD. Topiramate reduces ethanol consumption by C57BL/6 mice. *Synapse*. 2007;61:150–156.

250. Olive MF, et al. Stimulation of endorphin neurotransmission in the nucleus accumbens by ethanol, cocaine, and amphetamine. *J Neurosci*. 2001;21(RC184):1–5.

251. O'Malley SS, et al. 49Using Smart Source Parsing Nov. Naltrexone and coping skills therapy for alcohol dependence: a controlled study. *Arch Gen Psychiatry*. 1992:881–887.

252. O'Malley SS, et al. Naltrexone and coping skills therapy for alcohol dependence: a controlled study. *Arch Gen Psychiatry*. 1992;49:881–887.

253. O'Malley SS, et al. Experience of a "slip" among alcoholics treated with naltrexone or placebo. *Am J Psychiatry*. 1996;153:281–283.

254. Ooteman W, et al. The effect of naltrexone and acamprosate on cue-induced craving, autonomic nervous system and neuroendocrine reactions to alcohol-related cues in alcoholics. *Eur Neuropsychopharmacol*. 2007;17:558–566.

255. O'Shea B. Disulfiram revisited. *Hosp Med*. 2000;61:849–851.

256. Oslin DW, O'Brien CP, Katz IR. The disabling nature of comorbid depression among older DUI recipients. *Am J Addict*. 1999;8:128–135.

257. Oslin DW, et al. A functional polymorphism of the mu-opioid receptor gene is associated with naltrexone response in alcohol-dependent patients. *Neuropsychopharmacology*. 2003;28:1546–1552.

258. Overstreet DH, et al. Selective inhibition of alcohol intake in diverse alcohol-preferring rat strains by the 5-HT2A antagonists amperozide and FG 5974. 21Using Smart Source Parsing Nov. *Alcohol Clin Exp Res*. 1997:1448–1454.

259. Paille F, Martini H. Nalmefene: a new approach to the treatment of alcohol dependence. *Subst Abuse Rehabil*. 2014;5:87–94.

260. Reference deleted in review.

261. Petrakis I, et al. Naltrexone and disulfiram in patients with alcohol dependence and current depression. *J Clin Psychopharmacol*. 2007;27:160–165.

262. Petrakis IL, et al. Disulfiram treatment for cocaine dependence in methadone-maintained opioid addicts. *Addiction*. 2000;95:219–228.

263. Pettinati HM. et al. Medical management treatment manual: a clinical research guide for medically trained clinicians providing pharmacotherapy as part of the treatment for alcohol dependence. COMBINE Monograph Series, Vol. 2 (DHHS Publication No. 04–5289). Bethesda, MD: National Institute on Alcohol Abuse and Alcoholism. 2004.

264. Powell BJ, et al. A double-blind, placebo-controlled study of nortriptyline and bromocriptine in male alcoholics subtyped by comorbid psychiatric disorders. *Alcohol Clin Exp Res*. 1995;19:462–468.

265. Putzke J, et al. The anti-craving drug acamprosate reduces c-fos expression in rats undergoing ethanol withdrawal. *Eur J Pharmacol*. 1996;317(1):39–48.

266. Quintanilla ME, Perez E, Tampier L. Baclofen reduces ethanol intake in high-alcohol-drinking University of Chile bibulous rats. *Addict Biol*. 2008;13:326–336.

267. Randall CL, et al. Paroxetine for social anxiety and alcohol use in dual-diagnosed patients. *Depress Anxiety*. 2001;14:255–262.

268. Rawson RA, et al. A multi-site comparison of psychosocial approaches for the treatment of methamphetamine dependence. *Addiction*. 2004;99:708–717.

269. Ray LA, et al. A preliminary pharmacogenetic investigation of adverse events from topiramate in heavy drinkers. *Exp Clin Psychopharmacol*. 2009;17(2):122.

270. Raynor K, et al. Pharmacological characterization of the cloned kappa-, delta-, and mu-opioid receptors. *Mol Pharmacol.* 1994;45:330–334.

271. Regier DA, et al. Comorbidity of mental disorders with alcohol and other drug abuse. Results from the Epidemiologic Catchment Area (ECA) Study. *J Am Med Assoc.* 1990;264:2511–2518.

272. Resch GE, et al. Glycyl-glutamine in nucleus accumbens reduces ethanol intake in alcohol preferring (P) rats. *Brain Res.* 2005;1058:73–81.

273. Roberto M, et al. Cellular and behavioral interactions of gabapentin with alcohol dependence. *J Neurosci.* 2008;28(22):5762–5771.

274. Roberts AJ, et al. Effects of amperozide, 8-OH-DPAT, and FG 5974 on operant responding for ethanol. *Psychopharmacology.* 1998;137:25–32.

275. Roberts AJ, et al. Mu-opioid receptor knockout mice do not self-administer alcohol. *J Pharmacol Exp Ther.* 2000;293:1002–1008.

276. Roberts W, Harrison ELR, McKee S. Effects of varenicline on alcohol cue reactivity in heavy drinkers. *Psychopharmacology (Berl).* 2017;234(18):2737–2745.

277. Rodd-Henricks ZA, et al. Intracranial self-administration of ethanol into the posterior VTA of Wistar rats is mediated by 5-HT3 receptors [abstract]. *Alcohol Clin Exp Res.* 1999;23(suppl 5):49A.

278. Ross D, Hartmann RJ, Geller I. Ethanol preference in the hamster: effects of morphine sulfate and naltrexone, a long-acting morphine antagonist. *Proc West Pharmacol Soc.* 1976;19:326–330.

279. Rossetti ZL, Carboni S. Ethanol withdrawal is associated with increased extracellular glutamate in the rat striatum. *Eur J Pharmacol.* 1995;283:177–183.

280. Russell RN, et al. Apomorphine and 7-OH DPAT reduce ethanol intake of P and HAD rats. *Alcohol.* 1996;13:515–519.

280a. Ryan ML, Falk DE, Fertig JB, et al. A phase 2, double-blind, placebo-controlled randomized trial assessing the efficacy of ABT-436, a novel V1b receptor antagonist, for alcohol dependence. *Neuropsychopharmacology.* 2017;42(5):1012–1023.

280b. Sacks JJ, Gonzales KR, Bouchery EE, et al. 2010 national and state costs of excessive alcohol consumption. *Am J Prev Med.* 2015;49(5):e73–e79.

281. Salloum IM, et al. Efficacy of valproate maintenance in patients with bipolar disorder and alcoholism: a double-blind placebo-controlled study. *Arch Gen Psychiatry.* 2005;62:37–45.

282. Samson HH, Doyle TF. Oral ethanol self-administration in the rat: effect of naloxone. *Pharmacol Biochem Behav.* 1985;22:91–99.

283. Schacht JP, Anton RF, Randall PK, et al. Varenicline effects on drinking, craving and neural reward processing among non-treatment seeking alcohol-dependent individuals. *Psychopharmacology (Berl).* 2014;231(18):3799–3807.

284. Schmitz JM, et al. Cognitive-behavioral treatment of bipolar disorder and substance abuse: a preliminary randomized study. *Addict Disord Their Treat.* 2002;1:17–24.

285. Scott H, et al. Substance misuse and risk of aggression and offending among the severely mentally ill. *Br J Psychiatry.* 1998;172:345–350.

286. Scuppa G, Cippitelli A, Toll L, Ciccocioppo R, Ubaldi M. Varenicline decreases nicotine but not alcohol self-administration in genetically selected Marchigian Sardinian alcohol-preferring (msP) rats. *Drug Alcohol Depend.* 2015;1(156):126–132.

287. Sellers EM, et al. Clinical efficacy of the 5-HT3 antagonist ondansetron in alcohol abuse and dependence. *Alcohol Clin Exp Res.* 1994;18:879–885.

288. Sellers EM, et al. Serotonin and alcohol drinking. *NIDA Res Monogr.* 1992;119:141–145.

289. Seneviratne C, et al. Characterization of a functional polymorphism in the 3' UTR of SLC6A4 and its association with drinking intensity. *Alcohol Clin Exp Res.* 2009;33:332–339.

290. Shank RP, et al. An overview of the preclinical aspects of topiramate: pharmacology, pharmacokinetics, and mechanism of action. *Epilepsia.* 2000;41(suppl 1):S3–S9.

291. Sherwood Brown E, et al. A randomized, double-blind, placebo-controlled pilot study of naltrexone in outpatients with bipolar disorder and alcohol dependence. *Alcohol Clin Exp Res.* 2009;33:1863–1869.

292. Shippenberg TS, et al. Dynorphin and the pathophysiology of drug addiction. *Pharmacol Ther.* 2007;116(2):306–321.

293. Shive MS, Anderson JM. Biodegradation and biocompatibility of PLA and PLGA microspheres. *Adv Drug Deliv Rev.* 1997;28:5–24.

294. Sidmak Laboratories I. *Antabuse [package Insert].* East Hanover, NJ: Sidmak Laboratories, Inc.; 2001.

295. Simpson RJ, et al. Effect of zimelidine, a new antidepressant, on appetite and body weight. *Br J Clin Pharmacol.* 1981;11:96–98.

296. Sinclair D. Development in Finland of the extinction treatment for alcoholism with naltrexone. *Psychiatr Fenn.* 1997:76–97.

297. Sinclair J, Jääskeläinen IP. Continued efficacy after naloxone-induced suppression of alcohol drinking: dependence upon relative timing. *Alcohol Clin Exp Res.* 1995;19:13A.

298. Sinclair J, et al. Treatment of alcohol dependence with naltrexone utilizing an extinction protocol. In: *Abstracts: 38th Annual Meeting, National Institute of Mental Health (NIMH)-sponsored New Clinical Drug Evaluation Unit (NCDEU) Program.* Boca Raton, FL; 1998.

299. Sinclair JD. *Method for Treating Alcohol-Drinking Response.* Google Patents; 1989.

300. Sinclair JD. Drugs to decrease alcohol drinking. *Annals Med.* 1990;22(5):357–362.

301. Sinclair JD, Li TK. Long and short alcohol deprivation: effects on AA and P alcohol-preferring rats. *Alcohol.* 1989;6:505–509.

302. Sinclair JD, Scheinin H, Lammintausta R. *Method for Treating Alcoholism with Nalmefene.* Google Patents; 1992.

303. Skradski S, White HS. Topiramate blocks kainate-evoked cobalt influx into cultured neurons. *Epilepsia.* 2000;41(suppl 1):S45–S47.

304. Sloan TB, Roache JD, Johnson BA. The role of anxiety in predicting drinking behaviour. *Alcohol Alcohol.* 2003;38:360–363.

305. Smith GP. The physiology of the meal. In: Silverstone T, ed. *Drugs and Appetite.* London: Academic Press; 1982.

306. Söderpalm B, et al. Nicotinic mechanisms involved in the dopamine activating and reinforcing properties of ethanol. *Behav Brain Res.* 2000;113:85–96.

307. Sonne SC, Brady KT, Morton WA. Substance abuse and bipolar affective disorder. *J Nerv Ment Dis.* 1994;182:349–352.

308. Soyka MMuller CA. Pharmacotherapy of alcoholism – an update on approved and off-label medications. *Expert Opin Pharmacother.* 2017;18(12):1187–1199.

309. Spanagel R, Herz A, Shippenberg TS. Opposing tonically active endogenous opioid systems modulate the mesolimbic dopaminergic pathway. *Proc Natl Acad Sci U S A.* 1992;89:2046–2050.

310. Spanagel R, Zieglgansberger W. Anti-craving compounds for ethanol: new pharmacological tools to study addictive processes. *Trends Pharmacol Sci.* 1997;18:54–59.

311. Spanagel R, et al. Acamprosate and alcohol: I. Effects on alcohol intake following alcohol deprivation in the rat. *Eur J Pharmacol.* 1996;305:39–44.

312. Srisurapanont M, Jarusuraisin N. Opioid antagonists for alcohol dependence. *Cochrane Database Syst Rev.* 2005;1:CD001867.

312a. Stahre M, Roeber J, Kanny D, et al. *Contribution of Excessive Alcohol Consumption to Deaths and Years of Potential Life Lost in the United States.* 2014. https://www.cdc.gov/pcd/issues/2014/13_0293.htm.

313. Steffens M, Feuerstein TJ. Receptor-independent depression of DA and 5-HT uptake by cannabinoids in rat neocortex—involvement of Na(+)/K(+)-ATPase. *Neurochem Int.* 2004;44:529–538.

314. Stellar JR, Stellar E. *The Neurobiology of Motivation and Reward.* New York: Springer-Verlag; 1985.

315. Svensson L, et al. Involvement of the serotonergic system in ethanol intake in the rat. *Alcohol.* 1993;10:219–224.

316. Swift RM. Drug therapy for alcohol dependence. *N Engl J Med.* 1999;340:1482–1490.

317. Swift RM, et al. Ondansetron alters human alcohol intoxication. *Biol Psychiatry.* 1996;40:514–521.

318. Swift RM, et al. Naltrexone-induced alterations in human ethanol intoxication. *Am J Psychiatry.* 1994;151:1463–1467.

319. Taverna S, et al. Inhibition of transient and persistent Na+ current fractions by the new anticonvulsant topiramate. *J Pharmacol Exp Ther.* 1999;288:960–968.

320. Tomkins DM, Le AD, Sellers EM. Effect of the 5-HT3 antagonist ondansetron on voluntary ethanol intake in rats and mice maintained on a limited access procedure. *Psychopharmacology.* 1995;117:479–485.

321. Tzavara ET, et al. The cannabinoid CB(1) receptor antagonist SR141716A increases norepinephrine outflow in the rat anterior hypothalamus. *Eur J Pharmacol.* 2001;426:R3–R4.

322. Ugedo L, Grenhoff J, Svensson TH. Ritanserin, a 5-HT2 receptor antagonist, activates midbrain dopamine neurons by blocking serotonergic inhibition. *Psychopharmacology.* 1989;98:45–50.

323. Van den Brink W, Aubin HJ, Bladstrom A, et al. Efficacy of as-needed nalmefene in alcohol-dependent patients with at least a high drinking risk level: results from a subgroup analysis of two randomized controlled 6-month studies. *Alcohol Alcohol.* 2013;48(6):570–578.

324. van Ree JM, Kornet M, Goosen C. Neuropeptides and alcohol addiction in monkeys. *EXS.* 1994;71:165–174.

325. Vasudev K, et al. Topiramate for acute affective episodes in bipolar disorder. *Cochrane Database Syst Rev.* 2006;1:CD003384.

326. Verheul R, et al. Predictors of acamprosate efficacy: results from a pooled analysis of seven European trials including 1485 alcohol-dependent patients. *Psychopharmacology.* 2005;178:167–173.

327. Volpicelli JR, Davis MA, Olgin JE. Naltrexone blocks the post-shock increase of ethanol consumption. *Life Sci.* 1986;38:841–847.

328. Volpicelli JR, et al. Naltrexone in the treatment of alcohol dependence. *Arch Gen Psychiatry.* 1992;49:876–880.

329. Volpicelli JR, et al. Effect of naltrexone on alcohol "high" in alcoholics. *Am J Psychiatry.* 1995;152:613–615.

330. Volpicelli JR, et al. Naltrexone and alcohol dependence. Role of subject compliance. *Arch Gen Psychiatry.* 1997;54:737–742.

331. Walton RG. Smoking and alcoholism: a brief report. *Am J Psychiatry.* 1972;128:1455–1456.

332. Wang L, et al. Endocannabinoid signaling via cannabinoid receptor 1 is involved in ethanol preference and its age-dependent decline in mice. *Proc Natl Acad Sci U S A.* 2003;100:1393–1398.

333. Weiss F, et al. Free-choice responding for ethanol versus water in alcohol preferring (P) and unselected Wistar rats is differentially modified by naloxone, bromocriptine, and methysergide. *Psychopharmacology.* 1990;101:178–186.

334. White HS, et al. Topiramate enhances GABA-mediated chloride flux and GABA-evoked chloride currents in murine brain neurons and increases seizure threshold. *Epilepsy Res.* 1997;28:167–179.

335. White HS, et al. Topiramate modulates GABA-evoked currents in murine cortical neurons by a nonbenzodiazepine mechanism. *Epilepsia.* 2000;41(suppl 1):S17–S20.

336. Wiesbeck GA, et al. Ritanserin in relapse prevention in abstinent alcoholics: results from a placebo-controlled double-blind international multicenter trial. Ritanserin in Alcoholism Work Group. *Alcohol Clin Exp Res.* 1999;23:230–235.

337. Williams KL, Broadbear JH, Woods JH. Noncontingent and response-contingent intravenous ethanol attenuates the effect of naltrexone on hypothalamic-pituitary-adrenal activity in rhesus monkeys. *Alcohol Clin Exp Res.* 2004;28:566–571.

338. Wise RA, Bozarth MA. A psychomotor stimulant theory of addiction. *Psychol Rev.* 1987;94:469–492.

339. Wise RA, Raptis L. Effects of pre-feeding on food-approach latency and food consumption speed in food deprived rats. *Physiol Behav.* 1985;35:961–963.

340. Wolffgramm J, Heyne A. From controlled drug intake to loss of control: the irreversible development of drug addiction in the rat. *Behav Brain Res.* 1995;70(1):77–94.

341. Wurtman JJ, Wurtman RJ. Fenfluramine and fluoxetine spare protein consumption while suppressing caloric intake by rats. *Science.* 1977;198:1178–1180.

342. Wurtman JJ, Wurtman RJ. Drugs that enhance central serotoninergic transmission diminish elective carbohydrate consumption by rats. *Life Sci.* 1979;24:895–903.

343. Zalewska-Kaszubska J, et al. Effect of acute administration of ethanol on beta-endorphin plasma level in ethanol preferring and non-preferring rats chronically treated with naltrexone. *Pharmacol Biochem Behav.* 2006;85:155–159.

344. Zhang H, et al. Association between two mu-opioid receptor gene (OPRM1) haplotype blocks and drug or alcohol dependence. *Hum Mol Genet.* 2006;15:807–819.

345. Zhang X, et al. Modulation of high-voltage-activated calcium channels in dentate granule cells by topiramate. *Epilepsia.* 2000;41(suppl 1):S52–S60.

346. Zhang Y, et al. Allelic expression imbalance of human mu opioid receptor (OPRM1) caused by variant A118G. *J Biol Chem.* 2005;280:32618–32624.

347. Zhou Q, Lovinger DM. Pharmacologic characteristics of potentiation of 5-HT3 receptors by alcohols and diethyl ether in NCB-20 neuroblastoma cells. *J Pharmacol Exp Ther.* 1996;278:732–740.

348. Zieglgansberger W, et al. Actions of acamprosate on neurons of the central nervous system. In: Soyka M, ed. *Acamprosate in Relapse Prevention of Alcoholism.* Berlin: Springer; 1996:65–70.

52

Alcohol Withdrawal: Treatment and Application

NASSIMA AIT DAOUD TIOURIRINE, DEREK BLEVINS, AND ROBERT MALCOLM

CHAPTER OUTLINE

Introduction

Alcohol was used in Egypt since the time of the pharaohs, when wine played an important part in ceremonial life.[17] Egyptian texts more than 8000-years-old made reference to alcohol abuse and its consequences. The ancient Greeks were also experienced with alcohol use disorders. They first drank as part of a religious ritual to please their gods and forget their worries.[33,60] but soon realized that it caused seizures. In around 400 BCE, Hippocrates described seizures related to alcohol misuse and withdrawal, and the Romans used the term "morbius convivialis" to describe alcohol-related seizures.[23] European physicians in the late 18th and early 19th centuries gave detailed clinical descriptions of delirium tremens and noted a 50% mortality rate. Although delirium tremens was described as early as 1787, its relationship to acute alcohol withdrawal was not firmly established until the 21st century.[24,61]

Victor and Adams[74] described a series of alcohol-dependent patients admitted to a specialist unit in the United States. They identified the now well-recognized spectrum of symptoms—including tremor, nausea, anxiety, tinnitus, muscle cramps, diaphoresis, seizures, hallucinations, and delirium tremens—that constitute the alcohol withdrawal syndrome. Severe alcohol withdrawal has a mortality rate of up to 35% if untreated; if treated early, death rates range from 5% to 15%.[13]

Alcohol withdrawal is defined as a maladaptive behavioral change, with accompanying physiological and cognitive symptoms, that occurs in an individual whose blood- or tissue-alcohol concentrations decline following prolonged heavy use of alcohol.[1]

Withdrawal symptoms can occur when an individual who has consumed excessive alcohol daily stops drinking suddenly or reduces the quantity of alcohol. The likelihood of withdrawal symptoms increases with both the chronicity and quantity of drinking, the number of previous withdrawals, and the presence of complicating comorbid conditions.[5] Symptoms associated with the withdrawal syndrome include anxiety, psychomotor agitation, sweating, nausea, vomiting, insomnia, tremor, and rapid heart rate. In severe cases, delirium tremens, hallucinations, grand mal seizures, and disturbances in consciousness can occur.[1]

The goals of treatment for alcohol withdrawal include treating the immediate symptoms, preventing complications, and initiating long-term preventative therapy. The current agents of choice for the treatment of mild-to-moderate alcohol withdrawal in the outpatient setting are benzodiazepines.[48] Although the use of benzodiazepines is supported by an extensive body of literature, their use is limited by their potential for misuse, psychomotor sedation, and cognitive impairment. Benzodiazepines may also increase alcohol craving and early relapse to alcohol use[57] (Poulos and Zack, 2004) and increase the risk of misusing other substances in individuals with genetic predisposition to alcoholism or comorbid anxiety or personality disorder.[35,38] Furthermore, benzodiazepines have significant interactions with alcohol, opioids, and other CNS depressants. If taken together, they can increase the risk for respiratory depression and cognitive impairment. Some studies have suggested that benzodiazepine use itself may be associated with the development of delirium.[21]

Furthermore, although benzodiazepines are the standard of care for alcohol withdrawal, in clinical settings, the actual implementation varies dramatically. Some providers prefer a symptom-triggered approach, relying on elevated scores of the Clinical Institute of Withdrawal Assessment, revised (CIWA-Ar)[64] before administering any benzodiazepine, and others prefer a standard taper of preferably longer-acting benzodiazepines for a period of 3–5 days. The former strategy runs the risk of variability in CIWA-Ar scoring, and either under- or overestimating the need for benzodiazepines, whereas the latter may prolong inpatient hospitalizations for patients with less likelihood of experiencing alcohol withdrawal for various reasons, or conversely underdosing patients with larger degrees of alcohol tolerance. Many providers use a combination of these strategies by having a standard taper supplemented with as-needed benzodiazepines for "breakthrough" withdrawal symptoms. Overall, there is poor consensus regarding the most appropriate method, and this is likely largely due to variability in patients and systematic approaches to the treatment of substance withdrawal in hospital systems.

In light of the limitations associated with benzodiazepine use, there has been a growing interest in alternative treatment options for the alcohol withdrawal syndrome. A number of recent studies suggest that anticonvulsants might provide safe and effective alternatives to benzodiazepines, especially among those with moderate to severe alcohol withdrawal symptoms. These agents have demonstrated mood-stabilizing or anxiolytic effects, or both, in addition to their anticonvulsant activity, and are widely used in psychiatric practice.

Although their mechanism of action is not completely understood, the efficacy of anticonvulsants in the alcohol withdrawal syndrome is thought to be related to their ability to reduce "kindling" and facilitate γ-aminobutyric acid (GABA) inhibitory neurotransmission.[35] The kindling hypothesis proposes that long-term moderate to severe alcohol use disorder combined with repeated withdrawal episodes induces long-lasting neuronal and neurochemical changes in the brain. As a result of these neurobiological changes, the individual's response to alcohol is affected, resulting in increasingly severe episodes of withdrawal. An agent that ameliorates the kindling response might therefore prevent the summative effects of repeated drinking and withdrawal.[50]

Polycarpou et al.[56] published a 2005 *Cochrane Database* review of 48 studies with 3610 participants on the utility of anticonvulsants for treating alcohol withdrawal. Compared with placebo, there was a trend for anticonvulsants to improve the participants' global assessment of efficacy, and there was added protection against the development of seizures. Protection from seizures occurred whether anticonvulsants were given alone or in combination with other medications. In addition, anticonvulsants appeared to be superior to non-anticonvulsants at reducing the frequency of hallucinations, sweating, gastrointestinal symptoms, and sleep disorders. Furthermore, data from a subset of 12 of these studies (*N* = 960) that used anticonvulsants as antiwithdrawal agents—and in which mortality was reported as an outcome—showed that no participants died. Individuals who received anticonvulsants during detoxification from alcoholism, compared with those who received either placebo or benzodiazepines, were less likely to discontinue treatment due to adverse effects. The data from which the researchers could draw any conclusions to compare the efficacy of various anticonvulsants, especially the newer agents, against one another were too limited. Nevertheless, the authors of the *Cochrane Database* review exercised caution with the interpretation of their results because most studies were of small sample size, outcome measures were generally heterogeneous (a recommendation was made for the CIWA-Ar scale[72] to be used as the standard), and there was little consistency between studies on the methods and parameters for randomizing participants to treatment groups.

Anticonvulsants were found to be relatively safe and efficacious medications for treating alcohol withdrawal. Carbamazepine, the most studied medication compared with benzodiazepines, appears to confer added advantages such as fewer adverse events, no demonstrated abuse potential, and the lack of potentiation of alcohol's psychomotor and cognitive effects. Other anticonvulsants appear to share these properties, as well as being useful for reducing the frequency of a range of other withdrawal symptoms, including hallucinations, sweating, gastrointestinal disturbance, and sleep disorders. Although the *Cochrane Database* review did not provide any specific recommendations based on the statistical analysis,

clinical experience suggests that anticonvulsants should be considered the medication of choice among those with the potential to experience moderate to severe alcohol withdrawal symptoms and who can tolerate an oral route of administration. Adding benzodiazepines to an anticonvulsant regimen might confer some benefit patients with delirium tremens or severe agitation. This conclusion is further supported by a more recent *Cochrane Database* review that included 64 studies (n = 4309), evaluating benzodiazepines against placebos and other medications including anticonvulsants, and revealed that the only statistically significant finding was that benzodiazepines were more effective than placebo for preventing withdrawal seizures, but not statistically superior to anticonvulsants.[67]

Anticonvulsants in the Treatment of Alcohol Withdrawal

New insights into the pathophysiology of alcoholism have paved the way for studies of novel pharmacological tools for treating the behavioral, cognitive, and physiological symptoms associated with alcohol use disorder. Among anticonvulsant agents evaluated for efficacy in alcohol use disorder, some studies have found that carbamazepine treatment might reduce drinks per drinking day and time to first drink after withdrawal.[38,50] Small studies of valproate in alcohol-dependent individuals suggest that it might reduce relapse to heavy drinking and promote abstinence.[11,35] Of interest, in a recent placebo-controlled trial among alcoholics with comorbid bipolar disorder, valproate treatment was associated with a significant reduction of heavy drinking, and with better outcomes for those with higher serum valproate levels.[65]

Sodium Valproate

Sodium valproate is an antiepileptic compound with an unknown mechanism of action, although it is suggested that its antiepileptic action may be attributed to increased GABA levels in the brain.

Sodium valproate has been used for over 30 years for the treatment and prevention of alcohol withdrawal. A number of anecdotal and open-label studies indicate that the efficacy and safety of the anticonvulsant valproate (divalproex sodium) are similar to the effects of the anticonvulsant phenobarbital and the benzodiazepine lorazepam in reducing symptoms of alcohol withdrawal.[18] For example, Reoux et al.,[58] in a study of individuals with moderate alcohol withdrawal characterized as a score of ≥10 on the revised CIWA-Ar scale,[72] showed that sodium valproate treatment was well tolerated, reduced the need for benzodiazepine treatment, and led to a decreased likelihood of progression in severity of withdrawal symptoms compared with placebo.

An unblinded pilot study by Longo et al.[35] used stringent inclusion and exclusion criteria to compare the safety and efficacy of valproate with those of standard benzodiazepines for detoxification in a small (*N* = 16) inpatient population of individuals with mildly to moderately severe alcohol dependence and moderate alcohol withdrawal. Subjects received standard benzodiazepine detoxification (with lorazepam or chlordiazepoxide), 5-day detoxification with valproate, or detoxification with valproate plus 6-week maintenance. Valproate was administered using a loading-dose strategy (20 mg/kg/day in two doses 6–8 hours apart on day 1, then twice daily for 4 days or 6 weeks). Although the differences were not significant, perhaps due to small sample size, alcohol withdrawal symptom reduction tended to be more rapid in the valproate treatment group than in the benzodiazepine control group at 12- and 24-hour intervals. Four of five subjects (80%) in the valproate maintenance group were completely abstinent at the 6-week follow-up, compared with 5 of 11 (45%) in the combined detoxification-only groups. Furthermore, the participants receiving valproate showed lower liver transaminase levels than at baseline and no other hematological abnormalities at the 6-week follow-up.[35] This study demonstrated the importance of using a loading dose to achieve rapid therapeutic anticonvulsant blood levels. Despite the small sample size of this pilot study, the finding of higher abstinence rates at the 6-week follow-up in the valproate group supports further investigation of anticonvulsants as post-detoxification relapse prevention agents. A more recent retrospective chart review of 827 patients compared carbamazepine and valproate as adjunctive agents to the sedative-hypnotic clomethiazole and clonidine for inpatient detoxification and showed benefits of valproate over carbamazepine, including shorter pharmacological treatment, fewer transfers to the intensive care unit (ICU), fewer side effects, and a trend toward better effectiveness for preventing withdrawal seizures.[18] However, unlike the earlier pilot study, no comparator group was receiving an anticonvulsant agent without the sedative-hypnotic clomethiazole, thereby limiting generalizability of the utility of either carbamazepine or valproate.

Notably, most trials have been open-label; seizure rates were reported by only a few authors, and standardized multidimensional alcohol rating scales were seldom included. A notable limitation to the use of valproate for the prevention and treatment of alcohol withdrawal symptoms was its disadvantageous adverse events profile. Fatalities due to hepatic failure, life-threatening pancreatitis, and thrombocytopenia have all been reported among individuals who had received valproate or its derivatives. Its use is contraindicated in pregnancy due to teratogenic effects, and thus women of childbearing potential require a pregnancy test prior to initiation of valproate. Furthermore, because nonspecific gastrointestinal symptoms also have been reported following the ingestion of valproate, its clinical utility as an antiwithdrawal agent has been limited. In sum, however, it appears that it is at least as effective as benzodiazepines for treating alcohol withdrawal and has other advantages as a longer-term treatment for alcohol use disorders, particularly in individuals with comorbid bipolar disorder.

Carbamazepine and Oxcarbazepine

Placebo-controlled studies since the 1970s have supported the use of the potent anticonvulsant carbamazepine as a pharmacological agent for the treatment of acute alcohol withdrawal. Carbamazepine exerts its primary effects by blockade of voltage-sensitive sodium channels, as well as GABAergic and glutamatergic modulatory effects. Several double-blind studies have demonstrated that carbamazepine has efficacy at reducing alcohol withdrawal symptoms equal or superior to that of lorazepam, oxazepam, clomethiazole, tiapride, and placebo.[36,39] It also has been reported that carbamazepine can reduce effectively some measures of alcohol consumption (drinks per drinking day, number of heavy drinking days, and time to the first drinking day) during the postwithdrawal phase.[39,50]

Malcolm et al.[39] examined the efficacy of carbamazepine versus lorazepam for the treatment of alcohol withdrawal symptoms as well as drinking behavior in the 7 days immediately following the treatment period. They hypothesized that although both carbamazepine and lorazepam would suppress alcohol withdrawal,

carbamazepine would show the greater efficacy at ameliorating symptoms and reducing posttreatment drinking among those with a history of multiple episodes of previously treated alcohol withdrawal. In that double-blind trial ($N = 136$), carbamazepine 600–800 mg on day 1, tapered to 200 mg on day 5, was compared with lorazepam 6–8 mg on day 1, reduced to 2 mg on day 5, in a group of individuals experiencing moderate alcohol withdrawal. Participants were randomized to receive the carbamazepine or lorazepam fixed-dose taper across two levels of detoxification histories (0–1 or ≥2 prior medicated detoxifications). In addition, participants were administered the 10-item CIWA-Ar scale,[40] an aggregate measure of the severity of alcohol withdrawal that assessed individual symptoms such as nausea, tremor, sweating, anxiety, and agitation prior to medication treatment, daily for 5 days during the treatment phase, and on days 7 and 12 of the posttreatment period. The authors reported that carbamazepine and lorazepam were equally effective at decreasing the acute symptoms of alcohol withdrawal. There were no significant differences by treatment group in CIWA-Ar scale scores when all 12 study days were considered. There was, however, a significant treatment-group effect on posttreatment drinking. Participants who had zero or one previous detoxification episode showed no differences in posttreatment drinks per day based on treatment group. Among participants with multiple detoxifications, those who received carbamazepine drank an average of less than one drink/day compared with about five drinks/day among the lorazepam group ($P = 0.004$). Furthermore, the relative risk of having a first drink during the posttreatment period was three times higher for the lorazepam-treated group than for the carbamazepine group. Potential limitations of the study were the reliance on subjects' reports of previous medically treated withdrawal episodes, the fairly homogeneous demographic profile, and the low level of concomitant substance abuse by the participants. Nonetheless, the results of the study showed that carbamazepine was as efficacious as lorazepam at treating acute alcohol withdrawal, and had greater efficacy than lorazepam in preventing posttreatment relapse to drinking in participants with a history of multiple alcohol detoxifications.[39]

Psychosocial domains such as anxiety, depression, sleep quality, and the ability to return to work might be equally important in mediating outcomes of outpatient treatment but are often given only limited attention in the outpatient setting. Malcolm et al.,[37] therefore, extended their findings by comparing the effects of previous withdrawal history and treatment with carbamazepine or lorazepam on psychosocial outcome measures. In that study, designed as a 2 × 2 factorial (carbamazepine vs. lorazepam, 0–1 vs. ≥2 prior detoxifications), subjects completed a variety of self-rated measures of psychosocial function during the study period. The authors reported a statistically significant effect for scores to be lower for carbamazepine compared with lorazepam on the Zung anxiety scale[79] (34.8 vs. 38.9, respectively; $P = 0.01$) but to be higher on the visual analog scale of sleep quality (i.e., 62.1 vs. 51.2, respectively; $P = 0.02$). Neither the treatment group nor the number of previous withdrawals significantly affected the depression scores. Neither the carbamazepine or the lorazepam treatment groups produced a statistically significant effect on the ability to return to work.

The finding that carbamazepine was more efficacious than lorazepam at reducing anxiety and improving sleep is clinically important because the treatment of these psychiatric symptoms during acute detoxification could result in less distress and improved sleep during withdrawal—both of which could reduce the likelihood of relapse. Furthermore, these results have important implications for the subtle withdrawal symptoms, known as "protracted withdrawal syndrome," which can persist for weeks to months following the 5- to 7-day acute detoxification.[37] The symptoms that occur during the protracted withdrawal syndrome include anxiety, sleep disturbances, and mood instability. During the protracted withdrawal period, there is an increased risk of relapse to drinking. Thus the effective treatment of the symptoms of protracted withdrawal with carbamazepine during the acute detoxification period might improve long-term drinking outcomes. Although benzodiazepines have an indication for the 5- to 7-day acute detoxification period, they are not indicated for protracted withdrawal due to their addictive potential, synergistic effects with alcohol if patients relapse, and their own inherent potential to result in a protracted withdrawal syndrome similar to that of alcohol with long-term use.[2]

Oxcarbazepine, an analog of carbamazepine, has also shown efficacy in alcohol withdrawal, with the advantage of causing less induction of the cytochrome P450 (CYP) system and lower risk of neurological side effects, hormonal effects, and blood dyscrasias. In addition to blockade of voltage-sensitive sodium channels, like its antecedent, it also reduces glutamatergic transmission via reduction of high voltage-activated calcium currents.[77] A small (N = 29), randomized, single-blinded comparison of oxcarbazepine and carbamazepine showed similar effectiveness for alcohol withdrawal and no difference in side effects between the groups, but significantly less alcohol cravings in the oxcarbazepine group.[68] However, a larger (N = 50), double-blind, placebo-controlled study showed no differences in the need for rescue sedative-hypnotic medications (clothemiazole), withdrawal symptoms, or cravings, which the authors concluded may have been attributable to study design.[29]Although information could reasonably be extrapolated from the numerous studies of carbamazepine, and the newer analog has a favorable side effect profile, more research is needed to evaluate the efficacy of oxcarbazepine for alcohol withdrawal.

In sum, carbamazepine appears to be at least as effective as benzodiazepines in reducing the symptoms of mild-to-moderate alcohol withdrawal in relatively healthy individuals, although more evidence is needed for the newer oxcarbazepine. The doses given in these studies were generally lower than those that are used when the goal is to achieve anticonvulsant effects in patients with seizure disorders. In addition, carbamazepine appears to have efficacy that is superior or at least equal to that of other agents such as clomethiazole and tiapride in reducing withdrawal symptoms.[36] Systematic reviews have further verified carbamazepine's safety, tolerability, and effectiveness for the treatment of alcohol withdrawal in comparison to both placebo and benzodiazepines.[4,49] Despite the potential advantages of carbamazepine, its use can be associated with hepatotoxicity. Therefore the use of carbamazepine is contraindicated for the treatment of alcohol withdrawal among those with clinically significant hepatic disease. Because carbamazepine can cause blood dyscrasias, it should not be prescribed to individuals with either a propensity toward or a preexisting hematological disorder. And like valproate, it too can cause fetal neural tube defects, and is thus contraindicated for use in pregnant women.

Gabapentin

Gabapentin has a structural relationship similar to that of GABA,[47] and its mechanisms of action, although understood imperfectly, include the blockade of L-type calcium channels as well as facilitation of GABA synthesis.[47,55] Preclinical studies show that gabapentin decreases ethanol withdrawal–induced hyperexcitability in isolated slices of hippocampus[3] as well as convulsions and anxiety in alcohol-withdrawn mice.[76] In addition to these pharmacological properties, gabapentin's suitability as a promising candidate medication for treating alcohol withdrawal symptoms is aided by the fact that it does not induce hepatic enzymes and it is excreted unmetabolized in the urine. Hence, gabapentin will not exacerbate the hepatotoxic effects of alcohol.

Preliminary evidence supporting the potential of gabapentin to reduce alcohol withdrawal symptoms came from a case report[1] and a few case series that investigated the open-label use of the medication.[7,10,27,52,75] In a double-blind trial (N = 101), gabapentin was more efficacious than lorazepam at reducing insomnia during alcohol withdrawal[40] In addition, it has been proposed from a case series that gabapentin could be useful for a particular facet of a severe alcohol withdrawal syndrome—the reduction of tonic-clonic seizures.[63]

In a controlled study by Bonnet et al.[8] of gabapentin (400 mg four times daily) versus placebo for treating alcohol withdrawal symptoms in an inpatient setting, there was no significant difference between the two groups in the frequency and severity of their withdrawal symptoms or in the frequency with which the "rescue medication," clomethiazole, was used in the first 24 hours. However, the author followed this trial with an open trial of gabapentin for alcohol withdrawal using a loading protocol.[9] The protocol design effectively screened subjects to determine an early response, defined as symptom score reduction within 2 hours of administration of an 800 mg loading dose of gabapentin, and this group was treated for 2 days with gabapentin 600 mg, four times daily and then tapered. They treated 73% (N = 27) of the population as early responders and reclassified three participants as nonresponders due to worsening withdrawal in the following 36 hours—two participants of whom developed an epileptic seizure. The authors concluded that the gabapentin loading protocol was only helpful in less severe and less complicated acute alcohol withdrawal syndrome. Another open-label inpatient study by Mariani et al.[44] randomized participants (N = 27) to either a standard phenobarbital taper or gabapentin (1200 mg loading dose, with 2400 mg total in the first 24 hours, followed by a 3-day taper). The proportion of completers and of participants requiring rescue phenobarbital was not statistically significant between the groups. They did, however, find that those receiving gabapentin who required rescue phenobarbital had higher baseline CIWA-Ar scores. The same was true of the phenobarbital group, but this did not show statistical significance, whereas the gabapentin group did. Similar to the aforementioned study, the authors hypothesized that either gabapentin was underdosed for those in more severe withdrawal, or that gabapentin is ineffective for more severe manifestations of alcohol withdrawal.

Two outpatient studies further supported the utility of gabapentin in milder withdrawal syndromes. In a double-blind trial of gabapentin versus lorazepam, Myrick et al.[51] showed statistical superiority for higher-dose gabapentin (1200 mg tapering to 800 mg) in reduction of CIWA-Ar scores.[51] The lorazepam group was also more likely to drink on the first day of dose decrease, the second day off medication, and in the follow-up posttreatment period. A similar study comparing gabapentin to chlordiazepoxide for outpatient detoxification in a veteran population by Stock et al.[71] The gabapentin group started at 1200 mg for 3 days and then tapered down by 300 mg per day over the next 4 days, and showed a greater reduction in sedation (P = 0.04) and a trend to reducing alcohol cravings (P = 0.08), but no differences in reduction of CIWA-Ar scores.

Although large-scale controlled studies are needed to determine whether gabapentin can be useful in treating more severe manifestations of alcohol withdrawal, including tonic-clonic seizures, its utility may go well beyond its use in the acute withdrawal phase. Two smaller ($N = 21$ and $N = 60$), randomized double-blind trials[12,19] showed statistically significant improvements in various alcohol consumption measures in participants not in acute withdrawal. These results were followed by a larger ($N = 150$), randomized, double-blind trial by Mason et al.[46] that demonstrated a significant linear-dose effect for rates of abstinence and no heavy drinking, with the 1800 mg/day gabapentin group outperforming the 900 mg/day gabapentin and placebo groups. There were also significant benefits for sleep, mood, and cravings in the higher-dosed gabapentin group.

Thus the utility of gabapentin may extend well beyond acute alcohol withdrawal phase and potentially serve as a maintenance treatment for alcoholism, particularly in those who tolerate the medication well during acute withdrawal, but larger trials are needed in both acute withdrawal and long-term maintenance to fully evaluate its effectiveness. Although, unlike valproate and carbamazepine, the side effect profile is much more favorable due to the fact that it is renally excreted—the dose can be adjusted for renal impairment—and that it carries no black box warning.

Topiramate

Topiramate, a sulfamate-substituted derivative of fructopyranose, was identified originally as a potential antidiabetic agent.[70] Due to its structural similarity to known anticonvulsants, it was tested and found to have activity in several animal-seizure models. The compound was subsequently developed as an anticonvulsant based on its potency, duration of action, and neuroprotective effect.[70] The anticonvulsant effects of topiramate have been validated in the traditional rodent maximal-electroshock seizure test, as well as in several animal models of epilepsy. In the rat and mouse maximal-electroshock seizure test, topiramate showed potency similar to that of phenytoin and carbamazepine and greater than that of valproate.[70]

Recent studies of topiramate suggest that its pharmacokinetic properties provide several advantages over other antiepileptic agents. These advantages include its rapid and complete absorption, minimal metabolism, and minimal interaction with other medications, such as oral contraceptives. Similar to most marketed anticonvulsant agents, topiramate exerts its anticonvulsant effects through blockade of voltage-dependent sodium and L-type high voltage-gated calcium channels and facilitation of GABAergic neurotransmission via $GABA_A$. In addition, topiramate inhibits the activity of the alpha-amino-3-hydroxy-5-methylisoxazole-4-propionic acid (AMPA) and kainate subtypes of glutamate receptors, rather than the more traditional action at the N-methyl-D-aspartate (NMDA) subtype, and selectively inhibits carbonic anhydrase-II and carbonic anhydrase-IV.[70] Topiramate also has been reported to activate potassium conductance due to its ability to inhibit carbonic anhydrase.[38]

Titrating topiramate (over a range of 200–800 mg/day) produces a dose-proportional increase in its plasma concentration; both the maximal plasma concentration (C_{max}) and the area under the plasma concentration-time curve are linear and increase in proportion to the dose of topiramate at doses from 200 to 800 mg/day.[20,53] Due to its low binding to plasma proteins (9%–17%), topiramate is unlikely to be displaced by highly protein-bound medications, thus limiting the likelihood for its interaction

with other agents.[20] Furthermore, because topiramate is eliminated predominantly in the urine, with an elimination half-life of approximately 21 hours,[20,53,70] and is not metabolized extensively in humans (~20%),[20] topiramate will not exacerbate the hepatic-enzyme–inducing effects of alcohol.

The pharmacokinetic properties of topiramate might be altered in some special populations. Although no specific age-related changes in topiramate clearance or elimination half-life have been reported, a decline in renal function might occur with normal aging. Thus renal function should be evaluated in all elderly individuals receiving topiramate, since decreased renal function can alter the pharmacokinetics of medications eliminated by the kidneys, and adjustments of topiramate dose might be necessary in individuals with impaired renal function as well as in those undergoing hemodialysis.[20, 54]

Topiramate's pharmacodynamic profile would appear to make it an ideal treatment for alcohol withdrawal. Topiramate might reduce the overactivity of the sympathetic nervous system and neuronal hyperexcitability commonly seen in the early phase of alcohol withdrawal, through suppression of glutaminergic input, facilitation of $GABA_A$-mediated inhibitory impulse, blockade of sodium and calcium channels, and facilitation of potassium conductance.

Indeed, an open-label inpatient study by Choi et al.[14] found that topiramate 50 mg/day ($N = 25$) was as efficacious as lorazepam up to 4 mg/day ($N = 27$) at treating alcohol withdrawal, while allowing the individual to transition into outpatient care on the same regimen without the potential for abuse or the increased risk of relapse commonly seen in alcoholics treated with benzodiazepines. Previously, Rustembegovic et al.,[62] in a pilot open-label study ($N = 12$), found topiramate (50 mg twice daily) to be efficacious in the treatment of tonic-clonic seizures associated with alcohol withdrawal, with no side effects. Furthermore, Krupitsky and colleagues,[31] in a placebo-controlled, randomized single-blind study comparing the safety and efficacy of three antiglutamatergic agents—including topiramate (25 mg four times daily), memantine (10 mg three times daily), and lamotrigine (25 mg four times daily) versus diazepam (10 mg three times daily) for the treatment of alcohol withdrawal and detoxification in moderately severe alcoholic male patients ($N = 127$)—found that all active medications significantly reduced observer-rated and self-rated withdrawal severity, dysphoric mood, and supplementary use of diazepam compared with placebo. All medications were well tolerated. This study also provided suggestive evidence of subtle advantages of lamotrigine over memantine and topiramate in reducing observer-rated (CIWA-Ar[72]) and self-reported withdrawal severity. However, this study compared only single doses of each drug; the dose used for topiramate is not the one shown to be efficacious in outpatient trials, thereby rendering it difficult to extrapolate such conclusions from this study.

Because topiramate can be initiated while an individual with alcohol use disorder is still drinking, and has been shown to improve drinking outcomes in such individuals,[25,26] it is reasonable to hypothesize that topiramate treatment might be a strategy that can be used to decrease alcohol withdrawal as well as initiate and maintain abstinence from alcohol. Although its utility as monotherapy in the treatment of alcohol use disorder is more clearly delineated, more randomized trials are needed to determine its effectiveness in alcohol withdrawal syndrome, compared to benzodiazepines or barbiturates. Furthermore, individuals who receive topiramate treatment do need to be monitored closely during dose escalation to avoid adverse events such as sedation, paresthesia, anorexia, and cognitive impairment, and at all times for the rarer adverse events of glaucoma, transient blindness, nephrolithiasis, depression, and suicidal ideation.

Other Anticonvulsant Agents

Although other modulators of GABA function such as tiagabine and vigabatrin—anticonvulsants that inhibit GABA transport and metabolism,[66] respectively—have been proposed as potential treatment agents for alcohol withdrawal symptoms[41], there is at present no empirical support for their utility. Pregabalin, a drug that is structurally similar to gabapentin, which binds to an auxiliary subunit of voltage-dependent calcium channels[73] and thus reduces neuronal excitability, also showed promise for alcohol withdrawal in a single-blind comparison trial against tiapride and lorazepam.[45] The gabapentin-like drug was similar to comparators in most measures, including CIWA-Ar reduction, obsessive-compulsive drinking scales, and cravings, and outperformed on items regarding headache and orientation. However, a Swedish national register review revealed a signal for an association between pregabalin and misuse liability,[69] which may be related to its relatively greater potency and faster absorption compared to gabapentin, and raises concern for its utility in this population. Lamotrigine, a glutamate release inhibitor via blockade of sodium and calcium channels, was evaluated in the aforementioned randomized trial,[31] comparing three antiglutamatergic drugs (lamotrigine, topiramate, and memantine) to diazepam and placebo, and found significant reductions with all antiglutamatergic drugs, and suggested subtle advantages of lamotrigine over the other two antiglutamatergic agents, specifically for observe-rated CIWA-Ar scores. Finally, levetiracetam, an anticonvulsant with a poorly understood mechanism of action, showed positive results for alcohol withdrawal in an open-label trial ($N = 15$)[30]; a larger ($N = 106$), randomized, placebo-controlled trial did not support an addiction effect on the reduction of alcohol wihdrawal symptoms.[59] The utility of levetiracetam is also limited, particularly in this population, due to its known propensity to cause or worsen mood or behavioral problems.

Alpha-2 Adrenergic Agonists

In addition to glutamate and GABA, norepinephrine also plays a critical role in the alcohol withdrawal syndrome. Increases in norepinephrine explain certain alcohol withdrawal symptoms, and are positively correlated with the severity of withdrawal symptoms.[34] Thus the potential utility of agonists of the prejunctional, negative feedback, alpha-2 receptor is evident in the hyperadrenergic state of alcohol withdrawal. These agents specifically target the autonomic hyperactivity (i.e., increased blood pressure and heart rate) of the alcohol withdrawal syndrome but may also attenuate glutamate release by regulation of potassium and calcium currents[32] and thus also protect from alcohol withdrawal seizures. The pharmacodynamic and pharmacokinetic properties of the various alpha-2 agonists—including clonidine, dexmedetomidine, lofexidine, and guanfacine—may explain their effectiveness and clinical utility for alcohol withdrawal. Clonidine, the oldest of these agents, is also the most studied for alcohol withdrawal, with a 1975 double-blind trial ($N = 60$) comparing clonidine to placebo as an adjunctive agent during withdrawal showing faster improvements in tremor, systolic blood pressure, and less need for additional medication in the clonidine group.[6] A more recent randomized, controlled, double-blind trial compared 0.15 mg of

intrathecal and oral clonidine to a 10 mg dose of diazepam or placebo, in combination with intrathecal lidocaine, preoperatively in 45 alcohol-dependent men undergoing transurethral prostatectomy. Postoperatively, they observed significant differences in the CIWA-Ar scores of the clonidine groups (CIWA-Ar score = 1) compared to the diazepam group (CIWA-Ar score = 12), as well as a slightly decreased mean arterial blood pressure in the clonidine groups.[16] Although the study was limited by its sample size ($N = 45$) with four study arms, and the dose of diazepam was below what is typically needed in clinical practice when treating alcohol withdrawal, the CIWA-Ar score reduction in the clonidine groups was marked.

Dexmedetomidine is an intravenous alpha-2 adrenergic agonist used for ICU or procedural sedation that has the benefit of mild to moderate sedation without respiratory depression, and thus avoids the necessity of intubation. A review by Wong et al.[78] of 13 studies using dexmedetomidine for treatment of alcohol withdrawal in the ICU setting concluded that it was well tolerated, and decreased blood pressure and heart rate, but seizures occurred despite its use with or without benzodiazepines. More randomized, controlled, clinical trials are needed to elucidate the utility of dexmedetomidine as an adjunctive medication for the treatment of alcohol withdrawal in the ICU setting, but there is hope that it may reduce the amount of required benzodiazepines and limit the length of stay.

Lofexidine is an oral alpha-2 adrenergic agent similar to clonidine, but with less effect on blood pressure is approved in the United Kingdom for use in opioid withdrawal.[22] A 1985 placebo-controlled trial ($N = 63$) showed superiority of lofexidine over placebo for managing alcohol withdrawal, with six placebo patients and only one lofexidine patient requiring transition to benzodiazepine treatment,[15] whereas a 2001 double-blind, randomized, placebo-controlled trial ($N = 72$) actually showed that lofexidine as an adjunctive agent to chlordiazepoxide resulted in more severe withdrawal symptoms, more problems with hypotension, more adverse effects, and no improvement in retention rates.[28] Thus its utility remains unclear, and because it is not yet approved by the US Food and Drug Administration (FDA) in the United States, retrospective data that exists for its analogs, particularly clonidine, are lacking for lofexidine.

In summary, the potential utility of alpha-2 adrenergic agents in the treatment of alcohol withdrawal is evident due to their ability to reduce noradrenergic output that is a known phenomenon in the withdrawal state. In addition, they may play a role in reducing glutamatergic output in the CNMS, but perhaps not to the extent required to create equilibrium between glutamate and GABA in the brain. Maldonado et al.[42] have proposed a benzodiazepine-sparing algorithm for the treatment of alcohol withdrawal syndrome, utilizing the Prediction of Alcohol Withdrawal Severity Scale (PAWSS)[43] and combining anticonvulsant drugs with alpha-2 adrenergic agents. The algorithm is supported by data aforementioned in this chapter, but there are currently no clinical trial data suggesting superiority of this novel pharmacotherapeutic combination over benzodiazepines.

Summary and Conclusions

The use of anticonvulsant medications in treating individuals with alcohol use disorder proffers the novel approach of an antiwithdrawal agent, an antidrinking medication, or both. Anticonvulsants appear to be more effective than benzodiazepines against a larger range of withdrawal symptoms, with certain drugs being especially useful among individuals with moderate to severe withdrawal symptoms. In addition, anticonvulsants such as sodium valproate, gabapentin, and topiramate might have a further advantage over benzodiazepines in that they appear useful both for treating the acute withdrawal symptoms and, once abstinence has been achieved, for preventing relapse by modulating postcessation craving and affective disturbance. Obviously, this is an attractive pharmacological prospect, as the use of a single medication that is efficacious at the various stages of treatment reduces the need for polypharmacy, facilitates the buildup of dosing levels early in treatment, and minimizes the potential for unexpected adverse events and alcohol/medication interactions. Research specifically designed to determine the utility and feasibility of such an approach is needed.

Because of the potential utility of certain anticonvulsants, like valproate and gabapentin, in treating other psychiatric disorders such as bipolar disorder and anxiety, respectively, it is possible that their utility might also be extended to treating alcohol use disorders with a comorbid psychiatric condition.

Notably, the adverse events profiles of anticonvulsants have limited their use for treating the alcohol withdrawal syndrome. These limitations have highlighted the need for newer pharmacological agents that suppress withdrawal rapidly and have fewer adverse events, limited interaction with alcohol and other medications, and low potential for abuse. These agents should also be well tolerated in individuals with alcohol use disorder who also have comorbid psychiatric conditions.

Finally, the combination of anticonvulsants with other therapeutic agents that reduce autonomic hyperactivity, such as the alpha-2 agonists, warrants more clinical research to evaluate the safety and effectiveness of such novel detoxification regimens that could limit or entirely eliminate the need for benzodiazepines, given their misuse liability and other related adverse events.

References

1. American Psychiatric A. Substance-related disorders. In: *Diagnostic and Statistical Manual of Mental Disorders. DSM-IV-TR*. 4th ed. Text revision. Washington, D.C: American Psychiatric Association; 2000:191–223.
2. Ashton H. Protracted withdrawal syndromes from benzodiazepines. *J Subst Abuse Treat*. 1991;8(1):19–28.
3. Bailey C, Molleman A, Little H. Comparison of the effects of drugs on hyperexcitability induced in hippocampal slices by withdrawal from chronic ethanol consumption. *Br J Pharmacol*. 1998;123(2):215–222.
4. Barrons R, Roberts N. The role of carbamazepine and oxcarbazepine in alcohol withdrawal syndrome. *J Clin Pharm Ther*. 2010;35(2):153–167.
5. Becker HC. Alcohol withdrawal: neuroadaptation and sensitization. *CNS Spectr*. 1999;4(1):57–65. 38–40.
6. Björkqvist S. Clonidine in alcohol withdrawal. *Acta Psychiatr Scand*. 1975;52(4):256–263.
7. Bonnet U, et al. Treatment of alcohol withdrawal syndrome with gabapentin. *Pharmacopsychiatry*. 1999;32(03):107–109.
8. Bonnet U, et al. Treatment of acute alcohol withdrawal with gabapentin: results from a controlled two-center trial. *J Clin Psychopharmacol*. 2003;23:514–519.
9. Bonnet U, et al. An open trial of gabapentin in acute alcohol withdrawal using an oral loading protocol. *Alcohol Alcohol*. 2009;45(2):143–145.
10. Bozikas V, et al. Treatment of alcohol withdrawal with gabapentin. *Prog Neuropsychopharmacol Biol Psychiatry*. 2002;26:197–199.
11. Brady KT, et al. The use of divalproex in alcohol relapse prevention: a pilot study. *Drug Alcohol Depend*. 2002;67:323–330.
12. Brower KJ, et al. A randomized double-blind pilot trial of gabapentin versus placebo to treat alcohol dependence and comorbid insomnia. *Alcohol Clin Exp Res*. 2008;32:1429–1438.
13. Burns M, Price J, Lekawa M. *Delirium Tremens*. Emedicine from WebMD; 2008.
14. Choi EA, et al. The efficacy and safety of topiramate in the treatment of alcohol withdrawal. *J Korean Neuropsychiatr Assoc*. 2005;44:328–333.
15. Cushman P, et al. Alcohol withdrawal syndromes: clinical management with lofexidine. *Alcohol Clin Exp Res*. 1985;9(2):103–108.
16. Dobrydnjov I, et al. Intrathecal and oral clonidine as prophylaxis for postoperative alcohol withdrawal syndrome: a randomized double-blinded study. *Anesth Analg*. 2004;98(3):738–744.
17. El-Guebaly N, El-Guebaly A. Alcohol abuse in ancient Egypt: the recorded evidence. *Int J Addict*. 1981;16(7):1207–1221.
18. Eyer F, et al. Carbamazepine and valproate as adjuncts in the treatment of alcohol withdrawal syndrome: a retrospective cohort study. *Alcohol Alcohol*. 2011;46(2):177–184.
19. Furieri FA, Nakamura-Palacios EM. Gabapentin reduces alcohol consumption and craving: a randomized, double-blind, placebo-controlled trial. *J Clin Psychiatry*. 2007;68(11):1691–1700.
20. Garnett WR. Clinical pharmacology of topiramate: a review. *Epilepsia*. 2000;41(suppl 1):S61–S65.
21. Girard TD, Pandharipande PP, Ely EW. Delirium in the intensive care unit. *Crit Care*. 2008;12(3):S3.
22. Gowing L, et al. Alpha2-adrenergic agonists for the management of opioid withdrawal. *Cochrane Database Syst Rev*. 2016;(5).
23. Hauser A. Epidemiology of alcohol use and of epilepsy: the magnitude of the problem. In: Porter RJ, Mattson RH, Cramer JA, Diamond I, Schoenberg DG, eds. *Alcohol and Seizures–Basic Mechanisms and Clinical Concepts*. 1990:18.
24. Isbell H, et al. An experimental study of the etiology of "rum fits" and delirium tremens. *Q J Stud Alcohol A*. 1955.
25. Johnson BA, et al. Oral topiramate for treatment of alcohol dependence: a randomised controlled trial. *Lancet*. 2003;361:1677–1685.
26. Johnson BA, et al. Topiramate for treating alcohol dependence: a randomized controlled trial. *J Am Med Assoc*. 2007;298:1641–1651.
27. Karam-Hage M, Brower KJ. Gabapentin treatment for insomnia associated with alcohol dependence. *Am J Psychiatry*. 2000;157:151.
28. Keaney F, et al. A double-blind randomized placebo-controlled trial of lofexidine in alcohol withdrawal: lofexidine is not a useful adjunct to chlordiazepoxide. *Alcohol Alcohol*. 2001;36(5):426–430.
29. Koethe D, et al. Oxcarbazepine—efficacy and tolerability during treatment of alcohol withdrawal: a double–blind, randomized, placebo–controlled multicenter pilot study. *Alcohol Clin Exp Res*. 2007;31(7):1188–1194.
30. Krebs M, et al. Levetiracetam for the treatment of alcohol withdrawal syndrome: an open-label pilot trial. *J Clin Psychopharmacol*. 2006;26:347–349.
31. Krupitsky EM, et al. Antiglutamatergic strategies for ethanol detoxification: comparison with placebo and diazepam. *Alcohol Clin Exp Res*. 2007;31:604–611.
32. Lakhlani PP, Lovinger DM, Limbird LE. Genetic evidence for involvement of multiple effector systems in alpha 2A-adrenergic receptor inhibition of stimulus-secretion coupling. *Mol Pharmacol*. 1996;50(1):96–103.
33. Leibowitz J. Studies in the history of alcoholism—II. Acute alcoholism in ancient Greek and roman medicine. *Addiction*. 1967;62(1–2):83–86.
34. Linnoila M, et al. Alcohol withdrawal and noradrenergic function. *Ann Intern Med*. 1987;107(6):875–889.
35. Longo LP, Campbell T, Hubatch S. Divalproex sodium (Depakote) for alcohol withdrawal and relapse prevention. *J Addict Dis*. 2002;21:55–64.
36. Malcolm R, et al. Update on anticonvulsants for the treatment of alcohol withdrawal. *Am J Addict*. 2001;10 (suppl) Review:16–23.

37. Malcolm R, et al. The differential effects of medication on mood, sleep disturbance, and work ability in outpatient alcohol detoxification. *Am J Addict.* 2002;11:141–150.

38. Malcolm R, et al. The effects of carbamazepine and lorazepam on single versus multiple previous alcohol withdrawals in an outpatient randomized trial. *J Gen Intern Med.* 2002;17:349–355.

39. Malcolm R, et al. The effects of carbamazepine and lorazepam on single versus multiple previous alcohol withdrawals in an outpatient randomized trial. *J Gen Intern Med.* 2002;17(5):349–355.

40. Malcolm R, et al. Self-reported sleep, sleepiness, and repeated alcohol withdrawals: a randomized, double blind, controlled comparison of lorazepam vs gabapentin. *J Clin Sleep Med.* 2007;3(1):24–32.

41. Malcolm RJ. GABA systems, benzodiazepines, and substance dependence. *J Clin Psychiatry.* 2003;64(suppl 3):36–40.

42. Maldonado JR. Novel algorithms for the prophylaxis and management of alcohol withdrawal syndromes–beyond benzodiazepines. *Crit Care Clin.* 2017;33(3):559–599.

43. Maldonado JR, et al. The "Prediction of Alcohol Withdrawal Severity Scale" (Pawss): systematic literature review and pilot study of a new scale for the prediction of complicated alcohol withdrawal syndrome. *Alcohol.* 2014;48(4):375–390.

44. Mariani JJ, et al. A randomized, open-label, controlled trial of gabapentin and phenobarbital in the treatment of alcohol withdrawal. *Am J Addict.* 2006;15(1):76–84.

45. Martinotti G, et al. Pregabalin, tiapride and lorazepam in alcohol withdrawal syndrome: a multi–centre, randomized, single–blind comparison trial. *Addiction.* 2010;105(2):288–299.

46. Mason BJ, et al. Gabapentin treatment for alcohol dependence: a randomized clinical trial. *JAMA Int Med.* 2014;174(1):70–77.

47. McLean MJ. Gabapentin in the management of convulsive disorders. *Epilepsia.* 1999;40(suppl 6):S39–S50.

48. Miller MS, KS. *Detoxification and Substance Abuse Treatment.* Rockville, MD: Center for Substance Abuse Treatment; 2006.

49. Minozzi S, et al. *Anticonvulsants for Alcohol Withdrawal.* The Cochrane Library; 2010.

50. Mueller TI, et al. A double-blind, placebo-controlled pilot study of carbamazepine for the treatment of alcohol dependence. *Alcohol Clin Exp Res.* 1997;21:86–92.

51. Myrick H, et al. A double–blind trial of gabapentin versus lorazepam in the treatment of alcohol withdrawal. *Alcohol Clin Exp Res.* 2009;33(9):1582–1588.

52. Myrick H, Malcolm R, Brady KT. Gabapentin treatment of alcohol withdrawal. *Am J Psychiatry.* 1998;155:1632.

53. *Ortho-McNeil Pharmaceutical, I.* NJ: Raritan; 2003.

54. Ortho-McNeil Pharmaceutical I. *Topamax® [package Insert].* Raritan, NJ: Ortho-McNeil Pharmaceutical, Inc; 2008.

55. Petroff OA, et al. Effects of gabapentin on brain GABA, homocarnosine, and pyrrolidinone in epilepsy patients. *Epilepsia.* 2000;41:675–680.

56. Polycarpou A, et al. Anticonvulsants for alcohol withdrawal. *Cochrane Database Syst Rev.* 2005;3:CD005064.

57. Poulos C, Zack M. Low-dose diazepam primes motivation for alcohol and alcohol-related semantic networks in problem drinkers. *Behav Pharmacol.* 2004;15(7):503–512.

58. Reoux JP, et al. Divalproex sodium in alcohol withdrawal: a randomized double-blind placebo-controlled clinical trial. *Alcohol Clin Exp Res.* 2001;25:1324–1329.

59. Richter C, et al. Levetiracetam for the treatment of alcohol withdrawal syndrome: a multicenter, prospective, randomized, placebo-controlled trial. *J Clin Psychopharm.* 2010;30(6):720–725.

60. Rollbston J. Alcoholism in classical antiquity. *Addiction.* 1927;24(3):101–120.

61. Romano J. Early contributions to the study of delirium tremens. *Ann Med.* 1941;3(128):39.

62. Rustembegovic A, Sofic E, Kroyer G. A pilot study of topiramate (Topamax) in the treatment of tonic-clonic seizures of alcohol withdrawal syndromes. *Med Ar.* 2002;56:211–212.

63. Rustembegovic A, et al. A study of gabapentin in the treatment of tonic-clonic seizures of alcohol withdrawal syndrome. *Med Arh.* 2004;58:5–6.

64. Saitz R, et al. Individualized treatment for alcohol withdrawal: a randomized double-blind controlled trial. *JAMA.* 1994;272(7):519–523.

65. Salloum IM, et al. Efficacy of valproate maintenance in patients with bipolar disorder and alcoholism: a double-blind placebo-controlled study. *Arch Gen Psychiatry.* 2005;62:37–45.

66. Sarup A, Larsson OM, Schousboe A. GABA transporters and GABA-transaminase as drug targets. *Curr Drug Targets - CNS Neurol Disord.* 2003;2:269–277.

67. Schaefer TJ, Hafner JW. Are benzodiazepines effective for alcohol withdrawal? *Ann Emerg Med.* 2013;62(1):34–35.

68. Schik G, et al. Oxcarbazepine versus carbamazepine in the treatment of alcohol withdrawal. *Addiction Biol.* 2005;10(3):283–288.

69. Schwan S, et al. A signal for an abuse liability for pregabalin—results from the Swedish spontaneous adverse drug reaction reporting system. *Eur J Clin Pharmacol.* 2010;66(9):947–953.

70. Shank RP, et al. An overview of the preclinical aspects of topiramate: pharmacology, pharmacokinetics, and mechanism of action. *Epilepsia.* 2000;41(suppl 1):S3–S9.

71. Stock CJ, et al. Gabapentin versus chlordiazepoxide for outpatient alcohol detoxification treatment. *Ann Pharmacother.* 2013;47(7–8):961–969.

72. Sullivan JT, et al. Assessment of alcohol withdrawal: the revised clinical institute withdrawal assessment for alcohol scale (CIWA-Ar). *Br J Addict.* 1989;84:1353–1357.

73. Taylor CP, Angelotti T, Fauman E. Pharmacology and mechanism of action of pregabalin: the calcium channel α 2–δ (alpha 2–delta) subunit as a target for antiepileptic drug discovery. *Epilepsy Res.* 2007;73(2):137–150.

74. Victor M, Adams RD. The effect of alcohol on the nervous system. *Res Publ Assoc Res Nerv Ment Dis.* 1953;32:526.

75. Voris J, et al. Gabapentin for the treatment of ethanol withdrawal. *Subst Abus.* 2003;24:129–132.

76. Watson W, Robinson E, Little H. The novel anticonvulsant, gabapentin, protects against both convulsant and anxiogenic aspects of the ethanol withdrawal syndrome. *Neuropharmacology.* 1997;36(10):1369–1375.

77. Wellington K, Goa KL. Oxcarbazepine. *CNS Drugs.* 2001;15(2):137–163.

78. Wong A, Smithburger PL, Kane-Gill SL. Review of adjunctive dexmedetomidine in the management of severe acute alcohol withdrawal syndrome. *Am J Drug Alcohol Abuse.* 2015;41(5):382–391.

79. Zung W. A rating instrument for anxiety disorders. *Psychosomatics.* 1971;12:371–379.

53

Pharmacotherapy of Cocaine Addiction

†AHMED ELKASHEF AND FRANK VOCCI

Strategies for Selecting Candidate Medications for Testing

Bottom–Up Approach: Modulation of Appetitive Drives

Preclinical animal models of cocaine addiction, self-administration, reinstatement, and cue reactivity are commonly used to screen compounds for their potential as medications for treating cocaine dependence. These models, although helpful in selecting compounds, have very limited predictive validity. This issue is a critical one and will not be resolved fully until an effective medication is found that can be tested in animals for model validation. Until then, these limitations need to be factored in any go-no-go decision for advancing compounds for further development.

Preclinical Data

The role of corticotropin-releasing factor in drug addiction is very important, especially for relapse (which has been reviewed extensively.[72,112,125] Corticotropin-releasing factor appears to be a mediator of stress-induced reinstatement in rodent models. This effect was found not to be unique to cocaine in the rat models of stress-induced relapse[43,119] but also has been shown in heroin[119,120] and alcohol.[77] These data support the well-known notion that stress is a major precipitator of relapse in abstaining individuals. Modulating the stress circuitry will be beneficial not only for cocaine

but also for other substances. Multiple corticotropin-releasing factor-1 antagonists are currently in development for the treatment of depression and anxiety. One that is being developed in collaboration between the National Institute on Drug Abuse and the National Institute of Mental Health will be tested for addiction as well.

Dopamine D3 receptors, cloned in 1990,[1] are located mainly in the accumbens. This dopamine receptor subtype was found to be upregulated in postmortem brains of individuals with cocaine addiction who died of cocaine overdose.[123] D3 receptor levels, measured by the positron emission tomography (PET) ligand [11C]-+-PHNO, have been reported to be elevated in cocaine users by two independent groups.[86,102] D3 agonists exhibit cocaine-like effects in rodents and primates[1,123] and increased cocaine's subjective effects in human subjects[96]; see Table 53.1. D3 partial agonists have been shown to block cue-induced cocaine reinstatement,[40,106] cocaine-primed cocaine seeking,[40,49] and footshock-induced reinstatement of cocaine self-administration in rats,[132] suggesting overall a potential role for D3 antagonists in preventing the three triggers of relapse. However, the D3 antagonist GSK598809 increased blood pressure in dogs,[6] suggesting caution in advancing novel D3 antagonists to clinical studies.

Buspirone has recently emerged as a potential D3/D4 antagonist medication candidate. In self-administration studies in rhesus monkeys, the D3/D4 dopamine antagonist buspirone (intramuscular) reduced intravenous cocaine self-administration[11] and intravenous buspirone reduced intravenous cocaine self-administration in dominant rhesus monkeys, whereas it was ineffective in subordinate monkeys.[34] Buspirone (0.032 – 0.056 mg/kg/administered intravenously 20 minutes per hour for 23 hours) also reduced self-administration of the combination of cocaine and nicotine in rhesus monkeys.[88] PET studies in rhesus monkeys showed that buspirone, at intramuscular doses of 0.19 and 0.5 mg/kg and oral dose of 3 mg/kg, was extensively bound to D3 receptors in globus pallidus and midbrain.[71] These researchers also suggested that higher doses, approximately three times the 60 mg dose limit used to treat anxiety, would be needed to provide >80% sustained receptor occupancy. This has implications for the study reported by Winhusen et al.[131] as this trial may have used insufficient doses of buspirone (see Table 53.1).

The cannabinoid-1 receptor (CB-1) antagonists have been shown in different animal models to have potential to treat multiple addictions.[9,78] CB-1 antagonists act either by blocking the subjective/rewarding effects of drugs such as tetrahydrocannabinol or by blocking the ability of conditioned cues to promote

†Deceased.

TABLE 53.1	**Summary of Data on Published Medication Trials for Cocaine Dependence.**		
	Study	Outcome	Results
Dackis et al., 2005[36]	A double-blind, placebo-controlled trial of modafinil for cocaine dependence. 62 randomized subjects received a single morning dose of modafinil (400 mg) or matched placebo.	The primary efficacy measure was cocaine abstinence based on urine BE levels. Secondary measures were craving, cocaine withdrawal, retention and adverse events.	Subjects treated with modafinil provided significantly more cocaine-negative urine samples when compared with that of the placebo group.
Kaleschstein et al., 2013[62]	**Modafinil, but not escitalopram, improves working memory and sustained attention in long term-term, high-dose cocaine users.** 61 subjects were randomized to placebo ($n = 14$), escitalopram ($n = 16$), modafinil (200 mg, $n = 16$) or modafinil (200 mg) plus escitalopram ($n = 15$).	Measures included attention/information processing, episodic memory, working memory run at baseline and after 5 days of dosing.	Subjects treated with modafinil showed improved performance on two measures of working memory (mean n-back span, max n-back span), and trends toward improvement in visual working memory and sustained attention. Escitalopram did not improve cognitive measures.
Verrico et al., 2014[127]	Treatment with modafinil and escitalopram, alone or in combination, on cocaine-induced effects: a randomized, double-blind, placebo-controlled study. 64 subjects randomized to placebo ($n = 16$), modafinil (200 mg, $n = 16$), escitalopram, and modafinil (200 mg) plus escitalopram ($n = 15$).	Study participants were given a choice of cocaine or keeping money after 5 days of dosing. Participants rated the subjective effects of cocaine.	Modafinil attenuated many of the positive effects of cocaine. Escitalopram did not alter cocaine's subjective effects nor intensify the inhibitory effect of modafinil.
Anderson et al., 2009[5]	**Modafinil for the treatment of cocaine dependence.** Multicenter ($n = 6$) trial of 210 subjects randomized to placebo ($n = 72$), modafinil (200 mg, $n = 69$), or modafinil (400 mg, $n = 69$) and treated for 12 weeks.	Primary outcome measure was the weekly percentage of cocaine nonuse days. Secondary measure included maximum consecutive nonuse days and craving.	No significant difference was noted in the primary outcome measure, although the 200-mg modafinil group showed significant effects on the maximum number of nonuse days ($P = 0.02$) and craving ($P = 0.04$). Modafinil increased the weekly percentage of nonuse days in subjects without a history of alcohol dependence.
Dackis et al., 2012[37]	A double-blind, placebo-controlled trial of modafinil for cocaine dependence. 210 subjects were randomized to placebo, 200 mg, or 400 mg of modafinil and treated for 8 weeks.	Primary outcome measure was cocaine abstinence. Secondary measures included craving, cocaine withdrawal, retention, and tolerability.	No significant differences were seen on any measures although male subjects in the 400-mg group tended to be more abstinent than the placebo group ($P = 0.06$).
Kampman et al., 2015[65]	A double-blind, placebo-controlled trial of modafinil for the treatment of cocaine dependence without comorbid alcohol dependence. 94 cocaine-dependent men and women were evenly randomized to modafinil (300 mg) or placebo for 8 weeks.	Primary outcome measure was cocaine use by self-report, verified by twice-weekly urinalysis of benzoylecgonine. Secondary measures included cocaine craving (BSCS) and global improvement (CGI scale).	OR favored abstinence in the modafinil group (2.54; $P = 0.03$). Modafinil-treated subjects were more likely to be abstinent the last 3 weeks of the trial (23 vs 9 %, $P < 0.05$) and more likely to report low levels of craving intensity ($P = 0.03$) and duration ($P = 0.03$). Modafinil-treated subjects also were more likely to rate themselves much improved on the CGI ($P = 0.03$)
Nuijten et al., 2015[99]	Modafinil in the treatment of crack cocaine dependence in The Netherlands: Results of an open-label randomized controlled feasibility study. 65 crack-cocaine–dependent outpatients were randomized to receive either 12 weeks of CBT alone or CBT plus modafinil (400 mg/day) for 12 weeks.	The primary outcome measure was CBT retention. Secondary measure included modafinil adherence, tolerability, and safety; use of cocaine and other substances; cocaine craving/ health; social functioning; and patient satisfaction.	Modafinil had no effect on treatment retention, although adherence was low (10% completers). Post hoc exploratory analyses showed greater reduction in baseline use among highly adherent modafinil-treated subjects.
Morgan et al., 2016[94]	**Modafinil and sleep architecture in an inpatient-outpatient treatment study of cocaine dependence.** 57 cocaine-dependent subjects received either modafinil (400 mg) or placebo as inpatients followed by 6 weeks of outpatient treatment.	Primary outcome measure was the percentage of urine toxicology screens that were negative for cocaine. Polysomnographic sleep recordings were made prior to and after starting modafinil.	Modafinil was associated with a higher percentage of cocaine-free urine specimens (52% vs 26%, $P = 0.02$), an increase in N3 (stage 3) sleep time, more consecutive days abstinent and greater survival of abstinence.

TABLE 53.1	Summary of Data on Published Medication Trials for Cocaine Dependence.—cont'd		
Karila et al., 2016[69]	Dopamine transporter correlates and occupancy by modafinil in cocaine-dependent patients: A controlled study with high-resolution PET and [11C] - PE2I. 29 cocaine-dependent male subjects were randomized to modafinil or placebo. Modafinil was given as 400 mg/day for 26 days, 300 mg/day for 30 days, and 200 mg/day for 31 days. Dopamine transporter availability was measured with [11C]- PE2I prior to and after modafinil dosing.	Primary outcome measure was cocaine abstinence. Secondary measures included dopamine transporter occupancy, craving, depression, and decision making.	There were more therapeutic failures in the modafinil group. The dopamine transporter occupancy was reduced by 65.6% in patients receiving modafinil for 2 weeks.
Kampman et al., 2001[68]	Effectiveness of propranolol for cocaine-dependence treatment may depend on cocaine withdrawal symptom severity. 108 randomized subjects received 100 mg propranolol or matched placebo.	Quantitative urinary BE levels was the primary outcome measure. Secondary included treatment retention, ASI results, cocaine craving, mood and anxiety symptoms, cocaine withdrawal symptoms, and adverse events.	No comparison overall between the two groups with the exception of cocaine withdrawal symptoms in the propranolol subjects. However, propranolol-treated subjects with more severe cocaine withdrawal symptoms responded better than their placebo counterparts.
Kampman et al., 2006[63]	A double-blind, placebo-controlled trial of amantadine, propranolol, and their combination for the treatment of cocaine dependence in patients with severe cocaine withdrawal symptoms. 199 randomized patients received 300 mg/day of amantadine, 100 mg/day of propranolol, a combination of 300 mg/day or matching placebo.	Cocaine abstinence was the primary outcome measure.	The odds of cocaine abstinence improved significantly over time in propranolol-treated subjects who were highly adherent to study medication but not in placebo-treated subjects.
Brodie et al., 2003[16]	Treating cocaine addiction: from preclinical to clinical trial experience with gamma-vinyl GABA (GVG). 20 randomized subjects with a titration dose (1, 1.5, 2 g) of GVG.	Measuring 28 consecutive days clean (negative for cocaine).	Eight subjects successfully completed the program and were drug-free for periods ranging from 46–58 days.
Brodie et al., 2005[17]	Safety and efficacy of gamma-vinyl GABA (GVG) for the treatment of methamphetamine and/or cocaine addiction. 30 randomized.	Designed to include extensive visual field monitoring as well as outcome measures of therapeutic efficacy.	Sixteen of 18 subjects who completed the trial tested negative for methamphetamine and cocaine during the last 6 weeks of the trial. GVG did not produce any visual field defects or alterations in visual acuity.
Brodie et al., 2009[15]	Randomized, double-blind, placebo-controlled trial of vigabatrin for the treatment of cocaine dependence in Mexican parolees. Participants were randomly assigned to vigabatrin (n = 50) or placebo (n = 53) for 9 weeks. Maximum vigabatrin dose was 3000 mg/day and then the dose was tapered.	Cocaine use was measured twice weekly in urine samples. Primary outcome variable was 3 weeks of abstinence at the end of the trial. Secondary endpoints included alcohol use, craving, and CGI scores.	The vigabatrin group had a 28% abstinence rate vs 7.5% for placebo (P = 0.01). Retention was 62% in the vigabatrin group vs 41.5% for the placebo group. The alcohol abstinence rate was 43.5% vs. 6.3% in the placebo group.
Somoza et al., 2013[122]	A multisite, double-blind, placebo-controlled clinical trial to evaluate the safety and efficacy of vigabatrin for treating cocaine dependence. 186 subjects were randomized to vigabatrin (3000 mg/day) or placebo and dosed for 12 weeks.	The primary outcome variable was the proportion of participants with 2- week abstinence during the last 2 weeks of the trial.	No significant differences in the primary or secondary variables were observed across the groups. The vigabatrin group's adherence was marginal; urine measurement of vigabatrin suggested that 40% to 60% of the subjects may not have been dose adherent.
Kampman et al., 2004[66]	A pilot trial of topiramate for the treatment of cocaine dependence. 40 randomized titrating up to 200 mg/day of topiramate.	Cocaine abstinence was the primary outcome measure verified by twice weekly urine BE.	The topiramate-treated subjects were more likely to be abstinent from cocaine compared with placebo-treated subjects.
Kampman et al., 2013[67]	A double-blind, placebo-controlled trial of topiramate for the treatment of comorbid cocaine and alcohol dependence. 170 cocaine- and alcohol-dependent subjects were randomized to 300 mg topiramate or placebo for 13 weeks.	Primary outcome measures were self-reported cocaine and alcohol use with thrice weekly urine screens. Secondary measures included craving, Addiction Severity Index, cocaine withdrawal, and CGI improvement.	No significant difference on the primary outcome measure or in reducing alcohol use. Topiramate-treated subjects were more likely to be abstinent for the last 3 weeks of the trial. Subjects with more severe cocaine withdrawal symptoms fared better on topiramate.

Continued

TABLE 53.1   Summary of Data on Published Medication Trials for Cocaine Dependence.—cont'd

Johnson et al., 2013[59]	**Topiramate for the treatment of cocaine addiction: a randomized clinical trial.** 142 subjects were randomized to topiramate (300 mg/day maximum dose in weeks 6–12) or placebo.	Primary outcome measure was the weekly difference from baseline in the proportion of cocaine nonuse days. Secondary measures included urinary cocaine-free weeks, craving, and CGI improvement.	Topiramate was associated with an increased number of cocaine nonuse days relative to placebo ($P = 0.02$) and increased the likelihood of cocaine-free weeks (OR 3.21; $P = 0.02$).
Umbricht et al., 2014[126]	**Topiramate for cocaine dependence during methadone maintenance treatment: a randomized controlled trial.** 171 patients were randomized to topiramate (max dose 300 mg/day for weeks 8–15) or placebo and contingent or noncontingent vouchers for drug abstinence in a 2 × 2 design.	Primary outcome measures were cocaine abstinence measured by thrice weekly urinalysis, and retention. Voucher incentives were provided over 12 weeks. The analyses were conducted for the 12-week period in which vouchers were provided.	No significant differences emerged across the groups in terms of cocaine use or retention in the trial.
Nuijten et al., 2014[98]	Treatment of crack cocaine dependence with topiramate; a randomized-controlled feasibility trial in The Netherlands. 74 patients were randomized to receive CBT or topiramate (200 mg per day) plus CBT for 12 weeks.	Primary outcome measure was retention. Secondary outcome measures were medication adherence, safety, other substance use, health, social functioning, and patient satisfaction.	No differences were seen in retention or cocaine use, although adherence to topiramate was low. A post hoc analysis revealed a reduction in cocaine use only in patients with comorbid opioid dependence.
Gonzalez et al., 2003[50]	Tiagabine increases cocaine-free urines in cocaine-dependent methadone-treated patients: results of a randomized pilot study. 45 randomized to 12 or 24 mg of tiagabine or matched placebo.	Reduction of use as measured by cocaine-free urines.	In weeks 9 and 10, cocaine-free urine samples increased from baseline by 33% in subjects taking 24 mg/day and by 14% in those taking 12 mg/day and decreased by 10% with placebo-treated subjects.
Carroll et al., 1998[22]	Treatment of cocaine and alcohol dependence with psychotherapy and disulfiram. 122 randomized with 250–500 mg of disulfiram vs psychotherapy control (1 of 5 treatments).	Duration of continuous abstinence from cocaine or alcohol; frequency and quantity of cocaine and alcohol use by week, verified by urine toxicology and breathalyzer screens.	Disulfiram treatment was associated with better retention in treatment as well as longer duration of abstinence from alcohol and cocaine use. Two active psychotherapies (CBT and 12-step facilitation [TSF]) reduced cocaine use over time compared with the supportive treatment (clinical management).
George et al., 2000[48]	Disulfiram vs placebo for cocaine dependence in buprenorphine-maintained subjects: a preliminary trial. 20 randomized to 250 mg of disulfiram vs matched placebo.	Duration of abstinence from cocaine verified by urine test.	The total number of weeks abstinent from cocaine was higher in the disulfiram group versus placebo-treated subjects.
Petrakis et al., 2000[104]	Disulfiram treatment for cocaine dependence in methadone-maintained opioid addicts. 67 randomized to 250 mg disulfiram vs matched placebo.	Weekly assessments of the frequency and quantity of drug and alcohol use, weekly urine toxicology screens and breathalyzer readings.	Cocaine use was significantly decreased in quantity and frequency in subjects treated with disulfiram as compared with placebo-treated subjects.
Carroll et al., 2004[21]	Efficacy of disulfiram and cognitive behavior therapy in cocaine-dependent outpatients: a randomized placebo-controlled trial. 121 randomized to 250 mg/day of disulfiram or matched placebo.	Random regression analyses of self-reported frequency of cocaine use and results of urine toxicology screens.	Disulfiram-treated subjects reduced their cocaine use more than placebo-treated subjects.
Oliveto et al., 2011[101]	Randomized, double-blind, placebo-controlled trial of disulfiram for the treatment of cocaine dependence in methadone-stabilized patients. 161 cocaine- and opioid-dependent patients were randomized to 0, 62.5, 125, and 250 mg of disulfiram for weeks 3–14 of the trial.	The primary outcome measures were thrice weekly urine samples and weekly self-reported drug use.	Cocaine-positive urines increased in the 62.5 and 125-mg groups and decreased in the placebo and 250-mg dose groups ($P = 0.0001$). Self-reported cocaine use increased in the 125-mg group relative to the other dose groups ($P = 0.04$).
Carroll et al., 2012[24]	Efficacy of disulfiram and 12-step facilitation in cocaine-dependent individuals maintained on methadone: a randomized placebo-controlled trial. 112 study participants received either disulfiram (250 mg/day) or placebo and 12-step facilitation (TSF) or standard counseling in a 2 x 2 factorial design.	Primary outcome measure was urine benzoylecgonine levels.	The TSF group has fewer cocaine-positive urines throughout the trial. Disulfiram did not reduce cocaine use relative to placebo assignment, although a subgroup of disulfiram subjects without an alcohol use disorder showed greater reductions in cocaine use over time.

TABLE 53.1	Summary of Data on Published Medication Trials for Cocaine Dependence.—cont'd		
Kosten et al., 2013[75]	**Pharmacogenetic randomized trial for cocaine abuse: disulfiram and dopamine β-hydroxylase.** 74 cocaine- and opioid-dependent subjects received disulfiram (250 mg/day) or placebo and followed for 10 weeks.	Primary outcome measure was cocaine-positive urines. Participants were genotyped for the DβH gene polymorphism (rs1611115).	Disulfiram treatment reduced cocaine-positive urines relative to placebo (80% to 62%, respectively, $P = 0.001$). When stratified by DβH genotype, those subjects with the normal variant (CC) reduced their cocaine-positive urines from 84% to 56% ($P = 0.001$).
Schottenfeld et al., 2014[115]	**Randomized clinical trial of disulfiram for cocaine dependence or abuse during buprenorphine treatment.** 177 buprenorphine-treated subjects with cocaine dependence or abuse were randomized to disulfiram ($n = 91$, 250 mg/day) or placebo ($n = 86$).	Primary outcomes included days per week of cocaine use, number of cocaine-negative tests, and maximum consecutive weeks of cocaine abstinence. Participants were genotyped for the DβH gene polymorphism (84 CC homozygous, 71 CT or TT) and medication by genotype results were analyzed.	Self-reported use of cocaine was lowest in the CT or TT carriers, although there were no significant differences across the four groups in terms of cocaine-negative urine tests or consecutive weeks of cocaine abstinence.
Carroll et al., 2016[23]	A randomized factorial trial of disulfiram and contingency management to enhance cognitive behavioral therapy for cocaine dependence. 99 cocaine-dependent outpatients receiving CBT were assigned to disulfiram (250 mg/day) or placebo and contingency management (CM) or no CM in a 2 x 2 factorial design.	Primary outcome was percent days abstinent by self-report. Secondary outcome was cocaine use measured by three times weekly urinalysis.	There was no effect of disulfiram to reduce cocaine use. The order of effect in achieving self-reported 3 weeks continuous abstinence was CM + placebo > disulfiram with or without CM > placebo without CM.
Martell et al., 2005[84]	Vaccine pharmacotherapy for the treatment of cocaine dependence. 18 total randomized (10 received TA-DC 400 μg and 8 received 2000 μg) vs matched placebo.	Cocaine abstinence as verified by urine test.	The likelihood of using cocaine decreased in subjects who received the more intense vaccination schedule.
Martell et al., 2009[85]	Cocaine vaccine for the treatment of cocaine dependence in methadone-maintained patients: a randomized, double-blind, placebo-controlled efficacy trial. 115 patients were randomized to vaccine or placebo and followed for 12 weeks (weeks 8–20 of the trial).	The primary outcome measure was urinary benzoylecgonine measured three times weekly. Serum IgG levels of anti-cocaine antibodies were measured. Trials results were compared in those attaining a serum level of IgG anti-cocaine antibodies greater or less than 43 μg/mL.	Patients who had a serum level >43 μg/mL used less cocaine than those with levels <43 μg/mL. A higher proportion of patients with a serum level >43 μg/mL achieved a 50% reduction in cocaine use vs. those with a lower antibody level ($P = 0.048$).
Kosten et al., 2014[73]	Vaccine for cocaine dependence: a randomized double-blind placebo-controlled efficacy trial. 300 cocaine smokers were randomized to vaccine or placebo in this 16-week trial.	Primary outcome measure was urinary benzoylecgonine, collected thrice weekly. Analyses were conducted in the vaccine group dichotomized for serum IgG anti cocaine antibody levels ≥42 μg/mL and placebo group.	After week 8, more vaccinated than placebo-treated subjects had 2 weeks abstinence and the vaccine subgroup with IgG levels ≥42 μg/mL had the most cocaine-free urines for the last 2 weeks of the trial (OR = 3.02)
Kosten et al., 2003[74]	Desipramine and contingency management for cocaine and opiate dependence in buprenorphine-maintained patients. 160 randomized to 150 mg/day or matched placebo (with and without contingency management).	Cocaine abstinence as verified by urine test.	Cocaine-free and combined opiate and cocaine-free urines increased over time in those treated with either desipramine or contingency management and those receiving both had more drug-free urines (50%).
Poling et al., 2006[109]	Six-month trial of bupropion with contingency management for cocaine dependence in a methadone-maintained population. 106 randomized to 300 mg/day of bupropion or matched placebo (with and without voucher control and contingency management).	Reduction of cocaine use as tested by thrice-weekly urine toxicologic test results for cocaine and heroin.	Overall, voucher-based control and bupropion had fewer cocaine-positive urine drug screens than the other groups.
Ciraulo et al., 2005[28]	Nefazodone treatment of cocaine dependence with comorbid depressive symptoms. 69 randomized to 200 mg (bid) of nefazodone or matching placebo.	Cocaine use measured by urine BE and self-report.	Median weekly BE declined in the nefazodone group and scores for strength of cocaine craving decreased compared with placebo.

Continued

TABLE 53.1	Summary of Data on Published Medication Trials for Cocaine Dependence.—cont'd		
Winhusen et al., 2007[130]	A double-blind, placebo-controlled trial of reserpine for the treatment of cocaine dependence. 119 randomized to 0.5 mg/day of reserpine or matching placebo.	Cocaine use as determined by self-report confirmed with urine BE, cocaine craving, ASI and CGI scores.	No significant differences between reserpine and placebo.
Winhusen et al., 2007[129]	A double-blind, placebo-controlled trial of tiagabine for the treatment of cocaine dependence. 140 randomized to 20 mg/day of tiagabine or matching placebo.	Cocaine use as determined by self-report confirmed with urine BE, qualitative and quantitative urine toxicology measures.	Qualitative urine toxicology results suggest a possible weak signal for tiagabine in reducing cocaine use.
Kahn et al., 2009[61]	Multicenter trial of baclofen for abstinence initiation for severe cocaine dependence. 160 randomized to 60 mg of baclofen (max dose).	Cocaine use as determined by self-report confirmed by urine BE.	No significant effect between baclofen over placebo-treated subjects.
Elkashef A et al., 2006[42]	Double-blind, placebo-controlled trial of selegiline transdermal system (STS) for the treatment of cocaine dependence. 300 subjects to 20 mg of selegiline or placebo.	Self-reported cocaine use substantiated by urine BE.	There was no effect of selegiline over placebo-treated subjects.
Moeller et al., 2007[91]	Citalopram combined with behavioral therapy reduces cocaine use: a double-blind, placebo-controlled trial. 76 randomized to 20 mg/day of citalopram or matched placebo (with cognitive management and cognitive behavioral therapy).	Reduction in cocaine positive urines.	Cocaine treated subjects showed a significant reduction in positive urines during treatment as compared with placebo-treated subjects.
Johnson et al., 2006[60]	A preliminary randomized double-blind placebo-controlled study of the safety and efficacy of ondansetron in the treatment of cocaine dependence. 63 cocaine-dependent men and women were randomized to 0, 0.5, 2, and 8 mg/day of ondansetron and followed for 10 weeks.	Cocaine use by urine BE.	The 8 mg/day group had the lowest drop out and greater rate of negative urine BE ($P = 0.02$) compared with placebo. Ondansetron was well tolerated with no serious adverse events.
Mariani et al., 2012[83]	**Extended-release mixed amphetamine salts and topiramate for cocaine dependence: a randomized controlled trial.** 81 cocaine-dependent adult patients were randomized to mixed amphetamine salts plus topiramate or matching placebos.	The primary outcome measure was the proportion of subjects per group who achieved self-reported 3 weeks consecutive abstinence that was confirmed by self-report.	Participants in the mixed amphetamine salts plus topiramate group had a 33 % abstinence rate vs 16.7 % for placebo. There was a moderating effect of baseline cocaine use, suggesting the medication combination was more effective in those with high baseline cocaine use ($P = 0.05$).
Levin et al., 2015[79]	Extended-release mixed amphetamine salts vs placebo for comorbid adult attention deficit/hyperactivity disorder and cocaine use disorder: A randomized clinical trial. 126 adults diagnosed with comorbid adult attention deficit/hyperactivity disorder and cocaine use disorder were randomized to mixed amphetamine salts (60 or 80 mg) or placebo for 13 weeks.	ADHD symptomatology was measured by the Adult ADHD Investigator Symptom Rating Scale. Cocaine use was measured by self-report and weekly urine screens. The percentage of participants achieving three weeks abstinence was determined.	Seventy five percent of those in the 60 mg group ($P < 0.001$) and 58 % ($P = 0.07$) in the 80-mg group achieved a 30 % reduction in ADHD symptoms compared with 39.5 % in the placebo group. Rates of continuous abstinence for the last three weeks of the trial were 30.2 % in the 80-mg group ($P = 0.004$), 17.5 % in the 60 mg group ($P = 0.04$) vs a 7% rate for placebo.
Mooney et al., 2015[93]	**Pilot study of effects of lisdexamfetamine in cocaine use: A randomized, double-blind, placebo-controlled trial.** 43 cocaine-dependent participants were randomized to lisdexamfetamine ($n = 22$, 70 mg/day) or placebo ($n = 21$) and followed for 14 weeks.	Primary outcome measure was cocaine use, determined by twice weekly urinalysis.	No difference in cocaine use was noted between the two groups. Craving was lower in the lisdexamfetamine group.
Kampman et al., 2011[64]	**A double-blind, placebo-controlled pilot trial of acamprosate for the treatment of cocaine dependence.** 66 cocaine-dependent patients were enrolled in a 9-week trial where they received acamprosate (666 mg tid) or placebo for 8 weeks.	Primary outcome measure was cocaine use detected by twice weekly urinalysis.	The percent cocaine positive urines did not differ between the drug and placebo groups.

TABLE 53.1 | **Summary of Data on Published Medication Trials for Cocaine Dependence.—cont'd**

LaRowe et al., 2013[76]	A double-blind placebo-controlled trial of N-acetylcysteine in the treatment of cocaine dependence. 111 cocaine-dependent participants were randomized to N-acetylcysteine or placebo for 8 weeks.	Primary outcome measure was cocaine use, determined by thrice weekly urine collections.	No difference in cocaine use was noted between the N-acetylcysteine and placebo groups although N-acetylcysteine participants abstinent at randomization were less likely to relapse.
Pettinati et al., 2014[105]	**A pilot trial of injectable, extended-release naltrexone for the treatment of co-occurring cocaine and alcohol dependence.** 80 cocaine- and alcohol-dependent participants were randomized to two monthly injections of extended-release naltrexone or placebo injections.	Cocaine and alcohol use	No differences in either cocaine or alcohol use were seen in this pilot study.
Plebani et al., 2012[107]	Results of an initial trial of varenicline for the treatment of cocaine dependence. 37 cocaine-dependent participants were administered varenicline (1 mg bid) or placebo for 9 weeks.	Primary outcome measure was cocaine use, determined by thrice weekly urinalysis. Cocaine rewards was measured by the multiple-choice procedure (MCP).	Varenicline was associated with less cocaine use than placebo (OR = 2.02, $P = 0.08$). Varenicline deceased cocaine reward as measured in the MCP ($P = 0.02$).
Fox and Sinha, 2014[47]	The role of guanfacine as a therapeutic agent to address stress-related pathophysiology in cocaine-dependent individuals.	Laboratory challenge studies of stress and stress and cocaine cues.	Guanfacine, in doses of up to 3 mg/day, reduces cocaine craving, alcohol craving, anxiety, and negative emotion in women compared with women administered placebo.
Mooney et al., 2009[92]	Effects of oral methamphetamine on cocaine use: A randomized, double-blind, placebo-controlled trial. 82 cocaine-dependent participants were randomized to three medication treatment conditions 30-mg immediate-release methamphetamine, 30-mg sustained-release methamphetamine or matched placebo.	Cocaine use measured by urine BE; Medical adherence measured by pill count, urine riboflavin, methamphetamine and medication event monitoring system; craving by visual analogue scale, mood measured by BDI; adverse events and vital signs.	Participants who received sustained-release methamphetamines showed lower rates of cocaine positive urine samples (29%, $P < 0.0001$) and a greater reduction in craving ($P < 0.05$). BDI scores declined over the course of the trial. Similar retention rates between both forms of methamphetamines.
Schmitz et al., 2012[113]	Combination of modafinil and d-amphetamine for the treatment of cocaine dependence: a preliminary investigation. 73 participants were randomized to 400 mg modafinil, 60 mg d-amphetamine, 200 mg modafinil plus 30 mg d-amphetamine or matched placebo.	Primary outcome variables were retention and cocaine use by self-report and urine BE	No difference in retention rates between groups; Participants who received modafinil and d-amphetamine showed an increase in cocaine use over time with a low Bayesian probability of benefit (33%). Reduction in cocaine positive results in placebo and d-amphetamine only group.

ADHD, Attention-deficit/hyperactivity disorder; *ASI,* Addiction Severity Index; *BSCS,* Brief Substance Craving Scale; *BDI,* Beck Depression Inventory; *BE,* benzylecgonine; *CBT,* cognitive behavioral therapy; *CGI,* Clinical Global Impression; *OR,* odds ratio.

reinstatement of drug-seeking behavior in animals, presumably through the endocannabinoid system. Taken together, results suggest a role for the cannabinoid system for polysubstance addiction. However, the failure to gain marketing approval for rimonabant due to adverse events must be seen as a caution for advancing other CB-1 antagonists to clinical studies.

Vigabatrin is a γ-aminobutyric acid (GABA) transaminase inhibitor, which leads to marked elevation of GABA levels in the brain. It has been shown to be very effective in animal models to block cocaine self-administration, and to block dopamine release in a primate PET imaging study.[39] Early open-label pilot data in cocaine- and methamphetamine-addicted individuals showed promising results in facilitating abstinence.[17] Vigabatrin has been reported to cause visual field defects following prolonged use. In a 12-week study of vigabatrin (3000 mg/day) in cocaine users, no changes in visual acuity or peripheral field changes were noted (see Table 53.1).[10]

Dopamine β-hydroxylase (DβH) inhibitors have been studied in preclinical studies, clinical pharmacology studies, and clinical trials. Both disulfiram and nepicastat, another DβH inhibitor, were reported to attenuate cocaine-primed reinstatement in a rodent model,[116] but neither medication altered cocaine priming in the squirrel monkey.[29] In a placebo-controlled clinical pharmacology study, disulfiram dose was negatively correlated with cocaine choices.[53] In a second clinical pharmacology study with disulfiram, cocaine, and ethanol, disulfiram (0, 250, and 500 mg) doses were tested. Disulfiram (250 mg dose) did not enhance the cardiovascular effects of cocaine and may have reduced the subjective effects of cocaine. A disulfiram-ethanol response was seen with alcohol administration in disulfiram-treated participants. Cocaine did not exacerbate the response; in fact, it may have counteracted the hypotension but it increased tachycardia in two of seven participants. Clinical trial results with disulfiram are reported in Table 53.1. Nepicastat was reported to reduce the breakpoint in a progressive ratio model and attenuated cue-, cocaine prime-, footshock-, and yohimbine-induced reinstatement of cocaine-seeking behavior in the rodent.[117] In a clinical pharmacology study, nepicastat reduced the subjective effects of cocaine in non–treatment-seeking volunteers with cocaine use disorder.[35] A multicenter trial of nepicastat (120 mg per day or placebo) in cocaine-dependent study participants has been completed. The primary outcome measure is 2 weeks of abstinence at weeks 11 and 12 of the trial. Results are expected within the year.

Other compounds with interesting preclinical data include metabotropic glutamate receptor 5,[25] alpha-amino-3-hydroxy-5-methylisoxazole-4-propionic acid (AMPA) receptor antagonists,[7,31] orexin-A receptor antagonists,[14,54] opioid receptor-like 1 agonists,[26,27] N-acetylated-alpha-linked-acidic dipeptidase inhibitors,[121] and muscarinic M5 receptor ligands.[8,45] The partial mGluR5-negative allosteric modulators (NAMs) 5MPEP and Br-5MPEPy as well as MTEP, the full mGluR5 NAM, dose-dependently reduced cocaine self-administration and attenuated the discriminative stimulus properties of cocaine.[51] The mGluR5 NAM fenobam, which has been administered to human subjects in clinical trials, reduced intravenous cocaine self-administration, and cue-induced and cocaine-primed reinstatement behavior in rats.[70] Thus an mGluR5 compound could be tested in clinical studies in patients with cocaine use disorder.

Bottom–Up Approach: Pharmacotherapy of Reversal Learning/Cognitive Targets

Another pharmacotherapy target that has been discovered by basic neuroscience researchers is cocaine-induced deficits in reversal learning. Reversal learning, a test of cognitive flexibility, involves an organism's ability to determine that reward contingencies have changed and act accordingly. Cocaine has been shown to produce reversal learning deficits in an odor-discriminating task in rats trained to self-administer cocaine.[20] Lesions of the orbitofrontal cortex in rats also have been shown to cause reversal learning deficits in the odor discrimination model[114] and a serial discrimination reversal learning model.[13] Cocaine administered for 14 days can cause a failure to signal adverse outcomes in rats that also fail to reverse their cue selectivity, suggesting a failure of plasticity mechanisms in this brain region caused by the drug.[124] Cocaine administered to vervet monkeys for 14 days produced a reversal learning deficit of learned object discrimination.[58] Chronic cocaine users, but not amphetamine users, demonstrated reversal learning deficits in a probabilistic reversal learning task.[44]

Pharmacological modulation of reversal learning is in the early stages of testing. The serotonin-6 receptor antagonist Ro 04-6790 improved reversal learning in isolation-reared rats in the Morris water maze spatial discrimination task.[81] Several serotonin-6 receptor antagonists are in clinical testing,[55] suggesting that medications with this mechanism could be tested in chronic cocaine users in the probabilistic reversal learning task. The noradrenergic medications atomoxetine, desipramine, and methylphenidate improved reversal learning in a four-position discrimination task in rats and a three-choice visual discrimination task in Vervet monkeys,[118] whereas the dopamine transporter inhibitor GBR-12909 did not alter reversal learning. The authors noted that methylphenidate impaired retention in both rats and monkeys. Because it has been demonstrated that cocaine can produce reversal learning deficits, the obvious next studies that should be performed would be to test serotonin-6 receptor antagonists and norepinephrine transporter inhibitors in cocaine-affected animals. Positive results would provide a rationale for testing these medications in human subjects in the probabilistic reversal learning task mentioned above.

Prefrontal cortex (PFC) modulation of dopamine is largely influenced by serotonin (5-HT) in the frontal cortex.[57] Serotonin receptor 2A (5-HT$_{2A}$R) receptors are found in their highest density on layer V cortical pyramidal glutamatergic cells that project to subcortical structures.[30,89] Serotonin 2C (5-HT$_{2C}$R) receptors are located mainly on GABA interneurons with the prefrontal cortex[80] as well as dopaminergic and GABAergic neurons in the ventral tegmental area (VTA).[18] Elevation of 5-HT$_{2A}$R receptors in the VTA following injection of a plasmid containing the gene for 5-HT$_{2A}$R produced an enhanced response to cocaine-induced locomotor activity and rearing, suggesting a role for the 5-HT$_{2A}$R system in response to cocaine.[56] M100907, a 5-HT$_{2A}$R antagonist, administered intraperitoneally[97] or within the ventral medial PFC,[108] significantly attenuated cocaine cue-induced reinstatement behavior in rats. M100907 also attenuated cocaine-induced impulsivity in the differential reinforcement of low rate task and the one-choice serial reaction time task.[3] M100907 attenuated both cue- and cocaine-induced reinstatement behavior in rhesus monkeys, although cocaine self-administration was unaffected.[95] The 5-HT$_{2C}$R agonist Ro 60-0175 has been reported to attenuate cocaine-induced locomotor activity[52] and cocaine self-administration in rats.[46] The dose of the 5-HT$_{2C}$R agonist WAY 163909 needed to suppress the reinforcing efficacy of cocaine and cocaine-associated cues was 5–12-fold lower than that needed to suppress horizontal locomotor activity, suggesting a differential sensitivity to modulation of incentive salience of cocaine.[33] The 5-HT$_{2C}$R agonist MK 212 has been reported to attenuate the discriminative stimulus effects of cocaine.[19] Infusions of MK212 into the medial PFC attenuated the cue-induced and cocaine-prime induced reinstatement of self-administration behavior in rats.[103] In squirrel monkeys, the 5-HT$_{2C}$R agonist Ro 60-0175 was reported to attenuate the stimulant, reinforcing, and cocaine-priming effect on reinstatement of self-administration behavior.[82] The 5-HT$_{2C}$R system has also been studied for its effects on impulsivity and cocaine cue reactivity. Experiments in rats that had their 5-HT$_{2C}$R receptor population knocked down had an increase in impulsivity and reactivity to cocaine cues, suggesting that the 5-HT$_{2C}$R system modulates both of these behaviors.[4] Parallel studies in cocaine-dependent subjects with a single nucleotide polymorphism in the HTR2C gene noted that males with the Ser23 variant had greater attentional bias to cocaine cues in the Stroop test.[2] The recently approved 5-HT$_{2C}$R agonist lorcaserin will allow assessment of the possible efficacy of 5-HT$_{2C}$R agonism in the treatment of cocaine dependence.

Top–Down Approach

Marketed medications have been evaluated in different paradigms for efficacy in treating cocaine addiction. These medications were chosen based on different scientific rationales related to a known mechanism of action as a cocaine agonist or antagonist, and through modulating dopamine functions and the reward system. Some of these medications are direct dopamine agonists or antagonists, serotonin modulators, GABA agonists (both A and B), and glutamate modulators.

Our understanding of the addictive processes and neurobiology has greatly improved in the last two decades, thereby helping us to fine-tune our approach to pharmacological treatment.

Data are emerging from preclinical and clinical studies that suggest a selective role for specific medications in the addictive process. This would suggest that certain medications could be targeted at a specific phase of treatment or at a specific function involved in the addictive process—for example: (1) withdrawal phase (e.g., propranolol, amantadine); (2) active use phase (e.g., modafinil); (3) abstinence maintenance and relapse prevention (e.g., topiramate, other GABA agonists), stress modulators (e.g., corticotropin-releasing factor antagonists, lofexidine), cue-induced relapse (e.g., D3 antagonists, D-cycloserine), and priming (e.g., CB-1 antagonists, DβH inhibitors); (4) improvement of cognition (e.g., nootropic agents, D1 agonists); (5) modulation of frontal inhibitory mechanisms, such as strategic thinking and impulse control (e.g., modafinil, 5-HT$_{2A}$R antagonists, 5-HT$_{2C}$R agonists); and (6) modulation of reversal learning deficits (e.g., serotonin-6 antagonists, atomoxetine).

Clinical Trials in Cocaine Addiction

Table 53.1 summarizes clinical pharmacology studies and most of the conducted double-blind controlled trials in the last 20 years for treatment of cocaine dependence.

Multiple clinical trials of disulfiram, modafinil, topiramate, amphetamines, and vigabatrin have been conducted. The efficacy of disulfiram appears to be marginal and may be dependent on the level of DβH, although the Kosten et al.[75] and the Schottenfeld et al.[115] publications appear to be in conflict as to whether disulfiram is more efficacious in the normal variant or the variant that produces low DβH activity, respectively. It should be noted that the more recent clinical trials with disulfiram were conducted in populations that were codependent on opioids, with the exception of the study reported by Carroll et al.[75] Furthermore, contingency management was superior to disulfiram alone and disulfiram plus contingency management.[23] Disulfiram was also found to inhibit the plasma esterase that metabolizes cocaine to benzoylecgonine and leads to an increase in cocaine blood levels when coadministered with cocaine.[87] Clinicians need to caution patients and watch for increase in heart rate and blood pressure if patients continue to use cocaine while taking disulfiram. Overall disulfiram, approved in 1949, is prescribed less and less for alcohol-dependent patients because of its multiple side effects, risk of psychosis, and the fact that clinicians have better available medications. The field needs to move on to newer entities or develop better compounds with fewer side effects. One of these compounds is the selective DβH inhibitor, nepicastat, currently in trials for cocaine addiction.

The results of the trials with modafinil are somewhat more encouraging. Both the Anderson et al.[5] and the Kampman et al.[65] studies reported that modafinil significantly reduced cocaine use in participants without a history of alcohol dependence. The efficacy outcome variable, 3 weeks abstinence at the end of the study period, in the Kampman et al.[65] study, suggests that modafinil should be pursued further in patients with cocaine use disorder without a history of or current alcohol use disorder. The recent study by Morgan et al.,[94] in which modafinil was administered initially to cocaine-dependent inpatients (without a history of alcohol dependence) and then continued as outpatients, corroborated the findings of Anderson et al. and Kampman et al. Modafinil-treated patients in the study of Morgan et al. had reduced use of cocaine and a lesser propensity to return to cocaine use. The mechanism of efficacy in this case may be dopamine transporter occupancy, as modafinil has been reported to occupy 65.6% of dopamine transporters in cocaine-dependent subjects.[69]

The results for topiramate are mixed. Kampman et al.[67] reported that topiramate-treated patients were more likely to be abstinent for the last 3 weeks of the study, and Johnson et al.[59] reported that topiramate increased the number of cocaine non-use days and increased the likelihood of cocaine-free weeks. These preliminary results of efficacy were in contrast to those reported by Umbricht et al.[126]; in a methadone maintained, cocaine-dependent population, topiramate did not affect cocaine use relative to the topiramate placebo dose group. Given the reported efficacy of topiramate with treating alcohol dependence, further work with topiramate should be considered in cocaine- and alcohol-dependent populations. Unfortunately the trial for cocaine and alcohol dually dependent patients did not show effect[67]; however, it was conducted in an actively using population. Other anticonvulsant GABA agonists trials, for example, carbamazepine, gabapentin, lamotrigine, tiagabine, and vigabatrin were reviewed (Cochrane database systematic review) and found to have no evidence or low quality of evidence for cocaine use. Moderate quality evidence was reported for reducing dropout rate.[90] Further trials with topiramate and other GABA agonists should employ a relapse prevention design in abstinent patients that may be more promising than to initiate abstinence.

Amphetamines and their derivatives were tested in two clinical studies[92,93] with positive effects in lowering cocaine use and craving. The combination of mixed amphetamine salts and topiramate doubled the proportion of study participants abstinent from cocaine for the last 3 weeks of the trial relative to the placebo group.[83] This group followed up with a trial comparing extended-release mixed amphetamine salts for comorbid attention-deficit/hyperactivity disorder (ADHD) and cocaine use disorder.[79] The 60 and 80 mg doses of the amphetamine salts, dosed for 13 weeks, reduced ADHD symptoms to a greater extent than the reduction in the placebo group (60 mg $P < 0.001$; 80 mg $P = 0.07$). There was a dose-related increase in the proportion of participants abstinent from cocaine in the last 3 weeks of the trial. The percent abstinence rate for the placebo, 60 mg, and 80 mg groups was 7, 17.5 ($P = 0.04$), and 30.2 ($P = 0.004$), respectively. These robust findings should be followed up in a 6-month trial with abstinence for the last 2 months of the trial as the primary endpoint (see reference 128).

Two clinical trials of vigabatrin for the treatment of cocaine dependence have been reported in the last 10 years. One hundred and three cocaine-dependent parolees were randomly assigned to vigabatrin or placebo.[15] The 3-week abstinence rate of the vigabatrin group (28%) at the end of the study was almost four times higher than the rate seen in the placebo group (7.5%; $P = 0.01$). The results corroborated the initial study reported by Brodie et al.[16] in which 16 of 18 study participants who completed the study tested negative for cocaine and methamphetamine in the last 6 weeks of the trial. A multisite study was then performed by Somoza et al.[122] in which 186 study participants were randomized to vigabatrin (3000 mg/day) or placebo for 12 weeks. There was no difference in the abstinence rate between the two groups in the last 2 weeks of the trial. The adherence of the vigabatrin-treated subjects was considered marginal, as urine measurements of vigabatrin levels suggested that 40% to 60% of the participants may not have been medication adherent. As a result of the trial, the development of vigabatrin has been halted.

Cocaine Withdrawal

Most researchers do not assess symptoms of cocaine withdrawal or include it as an outcome except for the trials published by Kampman et al. Amantadine and propranolol have shown efficacy in helping individuals with severe withdrawal symptoms, as assessed by the Cocaine Symptom Severity Assessment scale devised by Kampman et al.[68] In a follow-up placebo-controlled study of either medication alone or in combination, only propranolol showed efficacy in the medication-adherent group analysis and not the intent-to-treat analysis. The combination did not prove to be superior to either medication alone.[67]

Comorbid Populations

Comorbid mental illness is more common than not in the addicted population. Prevalence rates range from 20% for attention-deficit disorders to 60% for bipolar disorders.[110] This adds another layer of complexity to the treatment approach and to participant selection criteria in clinical trials. This population has been ignored either intentionally or passively by mental health and addiction medication studies. Considering how common these conditions are, it is more sensible to face this issue head on and be more inclusive of this population with a priori hypotheses to test for variations in response or in biology, based on the underlying condition. A recent meta-analysis[100] showed that treating the underlying depression or anxiety was associated with some reduction in drug use; however, complete abstinence was hard to achieve. One study[79] tested the effect of mixed salt amphetamines in a dual diagnosis population of cocaine addiction and ADD, with significantly positive effects for both conditions.

Participant Heterogeneity

Participant demographics and clinical characteristics including patterns of use seem to be an important factor in predicting outcome. Baseline use always has been deemed one of the strongest predictors of outcome; this was very obvious in the data from the study of topiramate for cocaine dependence and the study of bupropion for methamphetamine dependence, where bupropion was found to be efficacious only in the group with low-to-moderate use at baseline. More recently, data from alcohol and nicotine studies highlight the role of pharmacogenomics as a very promising tool in predicting outcome.[38,111]

Genetic and clinical biomarkers predicting outcome could only improve our results and are being incorporated in many ongoing addiction trials to help elucidate subgroup response. This is a major step forward; we reviewed the data on biomarkers years ago[41] emphasizing the incorporation of some state and trait biomarkers to improve outcome. A more recent review of the topic[12] also emphasized the need for research to identify and validated these markers similar to in the cancer field.

Polysubstance Abuse

Although most patients with a substance use disorder would cite one drug of choice, most use more than one drug. This could be good or bad news. Having a polysubstance dependence could lead to treatment resistance, as in the case of the recently completed modafinil study for cocaine addiction, where the alcohol/cocaine dually dependent group showed no response to modafinil.

On the other hand, the good news is that medications that address common mechanisms in addiction could help polysubstance-addicted individuals; for example, topiramate seems to be promising for alcohol, stimulants, nicotine, and food addiction. Naltrexone has shown efficacy in alcohol, opiate, and stimulant addiction. These two medications should be tested in combination for relapse prevention in patients with polysubstance disorders. New molecular entities, for example, corticotropin-releasing factor, CB-1, and D3 antagonists—are all promising for polysubstance addiction as well. Further studies will tell.

Pharmacotherapy and Behavioral Therapy Combinations

Data from two cocaine studies suggest that the effect of the medication could be synergized when combined with contingency management. One using bupropion and the second using desipramine, in opiate-dependent, cocaine-abusing populations showed an enhanced effect of the medication and contingency management combination compared with each treatment arm alone.[74,115]

Summary

In general, it is sad to say that we are still nowhere close to finding a medication that is nearing approval or consistently showing an effect in cocaine trials. The three most studied marketed medicines so far are disulfiram, amphetamines, and modafinil. The rest of the 25 or so medications were all tested in one or two trials.

To follow the examples of currently approved medications for addiction treatment, for example, methadone and buprenorphine for opiate addiction or nicotine replacement therapy (NRT) products and varenicline for smoking, the cocaine field needs to find a powerful full agonist that mimics cocaine effects almost to the fullest. This is a very difficult task as cocaine affects almost all the neurotransmitters in the brain, either directly or indirectly, in contrast to opiates or nicotine. This is a task for medicinal chemistry, and it is indeed a tough one. Until a full cocaine agonist is found/synthesized, a combination of different medications with varying mechanisms may be needed to mimic cocaine's multiple effects. This approach is in practice clinically where polypharmacy and layering medications to achieve maximum response is the rule in treating many medical conditions, for example, hypertension, diabetes, and seizure disorders.

Relapse prevention approaches similar to naltrexone and nalmefene for alcohol and opiate relapse prevention, could include naltrexone, topiramate, GABA agonists, stress modulators (e.g., guanfacine, lofexidine), cue-induced relapse modulators (e.g., D3 antagonists, D-cycloserine), and priming modulators (e.g., CB-1 antagonists). This approach is hardly utilized in cocaine published studies. One study used buspirone for relapse prevention with no effect, possible because of inadequate dosing. More studies are needed with combinations of medications like naltrexone and topiramate along with contingency management.

Other therapeutic approaches target **improvement of cognition** (e.g., nootropic agents such as omega-3, and the D1 agonists), modulation of frontal inhibitory mechanisms (e.g., strategic thinking and impulse control) and modulation of reversal learning deficits (e.g., serotonin-6 antagonists).

As far as outcomes, a 3-week abstinence at the end of the trial period was proposed recently by the US Food and Drug Administration (FDA) as a meaningful clinical outcome; however, this benchmark is still hard to achieve as most cocaine trials report either no effect or reduction of cocaine use. The question becomes, is reduction of cocaine use a meaningful clinical outcome and what degree of reduction is considered clinically meaningful, especially if reduction of use is to be associated with improvement in other psychosocial outcomes (e.g., for general health, family, legal, psychiatric, or vocational, could this be a good outcome clinically?).

The field and the FDA need to agree on meaningful and reachable outcomes. Sensitive measures of psychosocial and health improvement during the relatively short duration of a clinical trial and follow-up period need to be developed. One study[32] investigated these issues in the National Institute on Drug Abuse

(NIDA) cocaine collaborative treatment study and reported that abstinence measures showed the highest correlation with abstinence at 1-year follow-up; however, the percentage of patients who achieved total abstinence in the study and during follow-up was very small (7.9%, 17/215). The authors also report very small or nonsignificant correlations between reduction of use and measures of functioning using the Addiction Severity Index at 12 months of follow-up. The study highlights the complexity of measuring cocaine outcomes and stresses the need to find more sensitive measures of change in functioning.

As a public health issue and a priority for NIDA, regular advisory meetings need to be reinstated with the FDA to discuss the current situation of pharmacotherapy, to review data, and to reach a consensus on achievable outcomes that will also help industry join in.

Trial designs that target subpopulations of patients with cocaine use disorder employing pharmacogenomics and biomarkers are being increasingly published, which will improve the yield of our trials and help us to better understand how to use medications for our heterogeneous population.

Industry partners need to be educated on the marketability of addiction medications and incentivized to participate in this field. Patent extension and exclusivity for marketed medications with expired patents for addiction indication may be a way. Partnership with NIDA for funding opportunities and experts' consultation, and academic institutions with experience in running trials for addiction will be a win-win situation for industry, especially small- to mid-sized companies that are hoping to create a niche in the market.

We hope that when it is time to revise this chapter a few years from now, we will have FDA-approved medication/s for cocaine addiction.

References

1. Acri JB, Carter SR, Alling K, et al. Assessment of cocaine-like discriminative stimulus effects of dopamine D3 receptor ligands. *Eur J Pharmacol*. 1995;281:R7–R9.
2. Anastasio NC, Liu S, Maili SE, et al. Variation within the serotonin (5-HT) 5-HT2C receptor system aligns with vulnerability to cocaine cue reactivity. *Transl Psychiatry*. 2014b;4:1–9.
3. Anastasio NC, Stoffel EC, Fox RG, et al. Serotonin (5-hydroxytryptamine) 5-HT (2A) receptor: association with inherent and cocaine-evoked behavioral disinhibition in rats. *Behav Pharmacol*. 2011;22(3):248–261.
4. Anastasio NC, Stutz SJ, Fox RG, et al. Functional status of the serotonin 5-HT2C receptor (5-HT2C R) drives interlocked phenotypes that precipitate relapse-like behaviors in cocaine dependence. *Neuropsychopharmacology*. 2014a;39:360–372.
5. Anderson AL, Reid MS, Li SH, et al. Modafinil for the treatment of cocaine dependence. *Drug Alcohol Depend*. 2009;104(1–2):133–139.
6. Appel NM, Li SH, Holmes TH, Acri JB. Dopamine D3 receptor antagonist (GSK598809) potentiates the hypertensive effect of cocaine in conscious, freely moving dogs. *J Pharmacol Exp Ther*. 2015;354(3):484–492.
7. Backstrom P, Hyytia P. Ionotropic glutamate receptor antagonists modulate cue-induced reinstatement of ethanol-seeking behavior. *Alcohol Clin Exp Res*. 2004;28:558–565.
8. Basile AS, Fedorova I, Zapata A, et al. Deletion of the M5 muscarinic acetylcholine receptor attenuates morphine reinforcement and withdrawal but not morphine analgesia. *Proc Natl Acad Sci USA*. 2002;99:11452–11457.
9. Beardsley PM, Thomas BF. Current evidence supporting a role of cannabinoid CB1 receptor (CB1R) antagonists as potential pharmacotherapies for drug abuse disorders. *Behav Pharmacol*. 2005;16:275–296.
10. Berezina T, Khouri AS, Winship MD, Fechtner ED. Visual field and ocular safety during short-term vigabatrin treatment in cocaine abusers. *Am J Ophthalmol*. 2012;154(2):326–332.
11. Bergman J, Roof RA, Furman CA, et al. Modification of cocaine self-administration by buspirone (buspar®): potential involvement of D3 and D4 dopamine receptors. *Int J Neuropsychopharmacol*. 2013;16(2):445–458.
12. Bough KJ, Amur S, Lao G, et al. Biomarkers for the development of new medications for cocaine dependence. *Neuropsychopharmacology*. 2014;39(1):202–219.
13. Boulougouris V, Dalley JW, Robbins TW. Effects of orbitofrontal, infralimbic, and prelimbic cortical lesions on serial spatial reversal learning in the rat. *Behav Brain Res*. 2007;179:219–228.
14. Boutrel B, Kenny PJ, Specio SE, et al. Role of hypocretin in mediating stress-induced reinstatement of cocaine-seeking behavior. *Proc Natl Acad Sci USA*. 2005;102:19168–19173.
15. Brodie JD, Case BG, Figueroa E, et al. Randomized, double-blind, placebo-controlled trial of vigabatrin for the treatment of cocaine dependence in Mexican parolees. *Am J Psychiatry*. 2009;166(11):1269–1277.
16. Brodie JD, Figueroa E, Dewey SL. Treating cocaine addiction: from preclinical to clinical trial experience with gamma-vinyl GABA. *Synapse*. 2003;50:261–265.
17. Brodie JD, Figueroa E, Laska EM, et al. Safety and efficacy of gamma-vinyl GABA (GVG) for the treatment of methamphetamine and/or cocaine addiction. *Synapse*. 2005;55:122–125.
18. Bubar MJ, Cunningham KA. Distribution of serotonin 5-HT2C receptors in the ventral tegmental area. *Neuroscience*. 2007;146:286–297.
19. Callahan PM, Cunningham KA. Modulation of the discriminative stimulus properties of cocaine by 5-HT1B and 5-HT 2C receptors. *J Pharmacol Exp Ther*. 1995;274:1414–1424.
20. Calu DJ, Stalnaker TA, Franz TM, et al. Withdrawal from cocaine self-administration produces long-lasting deficits in orbitofrontal-dependent reversal learning in rats. *Learn Mem*. 2007;14:325–328.
21. Carroll KM, Fenton LR, Ball SA, et al. Efficacy of disulfiram and cognitive behavior therapy in cocaine-dependent outpatients: a randomized placebo-controlled trial. *Arch Gen Psychiatry*. 2004;61:264–272.
22. Carroll KM, Nich C, Ball SA, et al. Treatment of cocaine and alcohol dependence with psychotherapy disulfiram. *Addiction*. 1998;93:713–727.
23. Carroll KM, Nich C, Petry NM, et al. A randomized factorial trial of disulfiram and contingency management to enhance cognitive behavioral therapy for cocaine dependence. *Drug Alcohol Depend*. 2016;160:135–142.
24. Carroll KM, Nich C, Shi JM, et al. Efficacy of disulfiram and Twelve Step Facilitation in cocaine dependent individuals maintained on methadone: a randomized placebo-controlled trial. *Drug Alcohol Depend*. 2012:224–231. 12691-2.
25. Chiamulera C, Epping-Jordan MP, Zocchi A, et al. Reinforcing and locomotor stimulant effects of cocaine are absent in mGluR5 null mutant mice. *Nat Neurosci*. 2001;4:873–874.
26. Ciccocioppo R, Economidou D, Fedeli A, et al. The nociceptin/orphanin FQ/NOP receptor system as a target for treatment of alcohol abuse: a review of recent work in alcohol-preferring rats. *Physiol Behav*. 2003;79:121–128.
27. Ciccocioppo R, Economidou D, Fedeli A, et al. Attenuation of ethanol self-administration and of conditioned reinstatement of alcohol-seeking behaviour by the antiopioid peptide nociceptin/orphanin FQ in alcohol-preferring rats. *Psychopharmacology*. 2004;172:170–178.

28. Ciraulo DA, Knapp C, Rotrosen J, et al. Nefazodone treatment of cocaine dependence with comorbid depressive symptoms. *Addiction*. 2005;100(suppl 1):23–31.

29. Cooper DA, Kimmel HL, Manvich DF, et al. Effects of pharmacological dopamine β-hydroxylase inhibition on cocaine-induced reinstatement and dopamine neurochemistry in squirrel monkeys. *J Pharmacol Exp Ther*. 2014;350(1):144–152.

30. Cornea-Hebert V, Riad M, Wu C, et al. Cellular and subcellular distribution of the serotonin 5- HT2A receptor in the central nervous system of adult rat. *J Comp Neurol*. 1999;409:187–209.

31. Cornish JL, Kalivas PW. Glutamate transmission in the nucleus accumbens mediates relapse in cocaine addiction. *J Neurosci*. 2000;20:RC89.

32. Crits-Christoph P, Gallop R, Gibbons MB, et al. Measuring outcome in the treatment of cocaine dependence. *J Alcohol Drug Depend*. 2013;1(2).

33. Cunningham KA, Fox RG, Anastasio NC, et al. Selective serotonin 5-HT (2C) receptor activation suppresses the reinforcing efficacy of cocaine and sucrose but differentially affects the incentive-salience value of cocaine- vs. sucrose-associated cues. *Neuropharmacology*. 2011;61(3):513–523.

34. Czoty PWNader MA. Effects of oral and intravenous administration of buspirone on food-cocaine choice in socially housed male cynomolgus monkeys. *Neuropsychopharmacology*. 2015;40(5):1072–1083.

35. De La Garza 2nd R, Bubar MJ, Carbone CL, et al. Evaluation of the dopamine β-hydroxylase (DβH) inhibitor nepicastat in participants who meet criteria for cocaine use disorder. *Prog Neuropsychopharmacol Biol Psychiatry*. 2015;59:40–48.

36. Dackis CA, Kampman KM, Lynch KG, et al. A double-blind, placebo-controlled trial of modafinil for cocaine dependence. *Neuropsychopharmacology*. 2005;30:205–211.

37. Dackis CA, Kampman KM, Lynch KG, et al. A double-blind, placebo-controlled trial of modafinil for cocaine dependence. *J Subst Abuse Treat*. Oct. 2012;43(3):303–312.

38. David SP, Munafo MR, Murphy MFG, et al. Genetic variation in the dopamine D4 receptor (DRD4) gene and smoking cessation: follow-up of a randomized clinical trial of transdermal nicotine patch. *Pharmacogenomics J*. 2008;8:122–128.

39. Dewey SL, Chaurasia CS, Chen CE, et al. GABAergic attenuation of cocaine-induced dopamine release and locomotor activity. *Synapse*. 1997;25:393–398.

40. Di Ciano P, Underwood RJ, Hagan JJ, et al. Attenuation of cue-controlled cocaine-seeking by a selective D3 dopamine receptor antagonist SB-277011-A. *Neuropsychopharmacology*. 2003;28:329–338.

41. Elkashef A, Biswas J, Acri JB, et al. Biotechnology and the treatment of addictive disorders. *BioDrugs*. 2007;21:259–267.

42. Elkashef A, Fudala PJ, Gorgon L, et al. Double-blind, placebo-controlled trial of selegiline transdermal system (STS) for the treatment of cocaine dependence. *Drug Alcohol Depend*. 2006;85:191–197.

43. Erb S, Shaham Y, Stewart J. The role of corticotropin-releasing factor and corticosterone in stress- and cocaine-induced relapse to cocaine seeking in rats. *J Neurosci*. 1998;18:5529–5536.

44. Ersche KD, Roiser JJP, Robbins TW, et al. Chronic cocaine but not chronic amphetamine use is associated with perseverative responding in humans. *Psychopharmacology*. 2008;197:421–431.

45. Fink-Jensen A, Fedorova I, Wortwein G, et al. Role for M5 muscarinic acetylcholine receptors in cocaine addiction. *J Neurosci Res*. 2003;74:91–96.

46. Fletcher PJ, Rizos Z, Sinyard J, et al. The 5-HT2C receptor agonist Ro-60-0175 reduces cocaine self-administration and reinstatement induced by the stressor yohimbine and contextual cues. *Neuropsychopharmacology*. 2008;33:1402–1412.

47. Fox H, Sinha R. The role of guanfacine as a therapeutic agent to address stress-related pathophysiology in cocaine-dependent individuals. *Adv Pharmacol*. 2014;69:217–265.

48. George TP, Chawarski MC, Pakes J, et al. Disulfiram versus placebo for cocaine dependence in buprenorphine-maintained subjects: a preliminary trial. *Biol Psychiatry*. 2000;47:1080–1086.

49. Gilbert JG, Newman AH, Gardner EL, et al. Acute administration of SB-277011A, NGB 2904, or BP 897 inhibits cocaine cue-induced reinstatement of drug-seeking behavior in rats: role of dopamine D3 receptors. *Synapse*. 2005;57:17–28.

50. Gonzalez G, Sevarion K, Sofuoglu M, et al. Tiagabine increases cocaine-free urines in cocaine-dependent methadone-treated patients: results of a randomized pilot study. *Addiction*. 2003;98:1625–1632.

51. Gould RW, Amato RJ, Bubser M, et al. Partial mGluR5 negative allosteric modulators attenuate cocaine-mediated behaviors and lack psychotomimetic- like effects. *Neuropsychopharmacology*. 2016;41:1166–1178.

52. Grottick AJ, Fletcher PJ, Higgins GA. Studies to investigate the role of 5-HT(2C) receptors on cocaine and food-maintained behavior. *J Pharmacol Exp Ther*. 2000;295:1183–1191.

53. Haile CN, De La Garza R, Mahoney JJ, et al. The impact of disulfiram treatment on the reinforcing effects of cocaine: a randomized clinical trial. *PLoS One*. 2012;7(11):e47702.

54. Harris GC, Wimmer M, Aston-Jones G. A role for lateral hypothalamic orexin neurons in reward seeking. *Nature*. 2005;437:556–559.

55. Heal DJ, Smith SL, Fisas A, et al. Selective 5-HT6 receptor ligands: progress in the development of a novel pharmacological approach to the treatment of obesity and related metabolic disorders. *Pharmacol Ther*. 2008;117:207–231.

56. Herin DV, Bubar MJ, Seitz PK, et al. Elevated expression of serotonin 5-HT2A receptors in the rat ventral tegmental area enhances vulnerability to the behavioral effects of cocaine. *Front Psychiatry*. 2013;4(2):1–12.

57. Howell LLCunningham KA. Serotonin 5-HT2 receptor interactions with dopamine function: implications for therapeutics in cocaine use disorder. *Pharmacol Rev*. 2015;67:176–197.

58. Jentsch JD, Olausson P, De La Garza 2nd R, et al. Impairments of reversal learning and response perseveration after repeated, intermittent cocaine administrations to monkeys. *Neuropsychopharmacology*. 2002;26:183–190.

59. Johnson BA, Ait-Daoud N, Wang XQ, et al. Topiramate for the treatment of cocaine addiction: a randomized clinical trial. *JAMA Psychiatry*. 2013;70(12):1338–1346.

60. Johnson BA, Roache JD, Ait-Daoud N, et al. A preliminary randomized, double-blind, placebo-controlled study of the safety and efficacy of ondansetron in the treatment of cocaine dependence. *Drug Alcohol Depend*. 2006;84:256–263.

61. Kahn R, Biswas K, Childress A, et al. Multi-center trial of baclofen for abstinence initiation for severe cocaine dependence. *Drug Alcohol Depend*. 2009;103:59–64.

62. Kalechstein AD, Mahoney JJ, Yoon JH, et al. Modafinil, but not escitalopram, improves working memory and sustained attention in long-term, high-dose cocaine users. *Neuropharmacology*. 2013;64:472–478.

63. Kampman KM, Dackis C, Lynch KG, et al. A double-blind, placebo-controlled trial of amantadine, propranolol, and their combination for the treatment of cocaine dependence in patients with severe cocaine withdrawal symptoms. *Drug Alcohol Depend*. 2006;85:129–137.

64. Kampman KM, Dackis C, Pettinati HM, et al. A double-blind, placebo-controlled pilot trial of acamprosate for the treatment of cocaine dependence. *Addict Behav*. Mar. 2011;36(3):217–221.

65. Kampman KM, Lynch KG, Pettinati HM, et al. A double-blind, placebo-controlled trial of modafinil for the treatment of cocaine dependence without co-morbid alcohol dependence. *Drug Alcohol Depend*. 2015;155:105–110.

66. Kampman KM, Pettinati HM, Lynch KG, et al. A pilot trial of topiramate for the treatment of cocaine dependence. *Drug Alcohol Depend*. 2004;75:233–240.

67. Kampman KM, Pettinati HM, Lynch KG, et al. A double-blind, placebo-controlled trial of topiramate for the treatment of comorbid cocaine and alcohol dependence. *Drug Alcohol Depend.Nov.* 2013;133(1):94–99.
68. Kampman KM, Volpicelli JR, Mulvaney F, et al. Effectiveness of propranolol for cocaine dependence treatment may depend on cocaine withdrawal symptom severity. *Drug Alcohol Depend.* 2001;63:69–78.
69. Karila L, Leroy C, Dubol M, et al. Dopamine transporter correlates and occupancy by modafinil in cocaine dependent patients: a controlled study with high-resolution PET and [11C]-PE2I. *Neuropsychopharmacol.* 2016.
70. Keck T, Yang HJ, Bi GH, et al. Fenobam sulfate inhibits cocaine-taking and cocaine- seeking behavior in rats: implications for addiction treatment in humans. *Psychopharmacology (Berl).* 2013;229(2):253–265.
71. Kim SW, Fowler JS, Skolnick P, et al. Therapeutic doses of buspirone block D3 receptors in the living primate brain. *In J Neuropsychopharmacol.* 2014;17(8):1257–1267.
72. Koob GF. Stress, corticotrophin-releasing factor, and drug addiction. *Ann N Y Acad Sci.* 1999;897:27–45.
73. Kosten TR, Domingo CB, Shorter D, et al. Vaccine for cocaine dependence: a randomized double-blind placebo-controlled efficacy trial. *Drug Alcohol Depend.* 2014;140:42–47.
74. Kosten T, Oliveto A, Feingold A, et al. Desipramine and contingency management for cocaine and opiate dependence in buprenorphine-maintained patients. *Drug Alcohol Depend.* 2003;70:P315–P325.
75. Kosten TR, Wu G, Huang W, et al. Pharmacogenetic randomized trial for cocaine abuse: disulfiram and dopamine β-hydroxylase. *Biol Psychiatry.* 2013;1(73):219–224 (3).
76. LaRowe SD, Kailvas PW, Nicholas JS, et al. A double-blind placebo-controlled trial of N-acetylcysteine in the treatment of cocaine dependence. *Am J Addict.* 2013;22(5). 443–352.
77. Le AD, Harding S, Juzytsch W, et al. The role of corticotrophin-releasing factor in stress-induced relapse to alcohol-seeking behavior in rats. *Psychopharmacology.* 2000;150:317–324.
78. Le Foll B, Goldberg SR. Cannabinoid CB1 receptor antagonists as promising new medications for drug dependence. *J Pharmacol Exp Ther.* 2005;312:875–883.
79. Levin FR, Mariani JJ, Specker S, et al. Extended-Release mixed amphetamine salts vs placebo for comorbid adult Attention-Deficit/Hyperactivity Disorder and cocaine use disorder: a randomized clinical trial. *JAMA Psychiatry.* 2015;72(6):593–602.
80. Liu S, Bubar MJ, Lanfracno MF, et al. Serotonin 2C receptor localization in GABA neurons of the rat medial prefrontal cortex: implications for understanding the neurobiology of addiction. *Neuroscience.* 2007;146:1677–1688.
81. Mann R, Lee V, Porkess MV, et al. Isolation rearing impairs recognition memory and reversal learning in rat. *J Psychopharmacol.* 2005;19:A39.
82. Manvich DF, Kimmel HL, Howell LL. Effects of serotonin receptor 2C agonists on the behavioral and neurochemical effects of cocaine in squirrel monkeys. *J Pharmacol Exp Ther.* 2012;341:424–434.
83. Mariani JJ, Pavlicova M, Bisaga A, et al. Extended-release mixed amphetamine salts and topiramate for cocaine dependence: a randomized controlled trial. *Biol Psychiatry.* 2012;72(1):950–956.
84. Martell BA, Mitchell E, Poling J, et al. Vaccine pharmacotherapy for the treatment of cocaine dependence. *Biol Psychiatry.* 2005;58:158–164.
85. Martell BA, Orson FM, Poling J, et al. Cocaine vaccine for the treatment of cocaine dependence in methadone-maintained patients: a randomized, double-blind, placebo-controlled efficacy trial. *Arch Gen Psychiatry.* 2009;66:1116–1123.
86. Matuskey D, Gallezot JD, Pittman B, et al. Dopamine D3 receptor alteration in cocaine-dependent humans imaged with [11C](+-) PHNO. *Drug Alcohol Depend.* 2014;139:100–105.
87. McCance-Katz EF, Kosten TR, Jatlow P. Disulfiram effects on acute cocaine administration. *Drug Alcohol Depend.* 1998;52:27–39.
88. Mello NK, Fivel PA, Kohut SJ. Effects of chronic buspirone treatment on nicotine and concurrent nicotine+ cocaine self-administration. *Neuropsychopharmacology.* 2013;38(7):1265–1275.
89. Miner LA, Backstrom JR, Sanders-bush E, Sesack SR. Ultrastructural localization of serotonin 2A receptors in the middle layers of the rat prelimbic prefrontal cortex. *Neuroscience.* 2003;116:107–117.
90. Minozzi S, Cinquini M, Amato L, et al. Anticonvulsants for cocaine dependence. *Cochrane Database Syst Rev.* 2015;17:4.
91. Moeller FG, Schmitz JM, Steinbert JL, et al. Citalopram combined with behavioral treatment reduces cocaine use: a double-blind, placebo-controlled trial. *Am J Drug Alcohol Abuse.* 2007;33:367–378.
92. Mooney ME, Herin DV, Schmitz JM, et al. Effects of oral methamphetamine on cocaine use: a randomized, double-blind, placebo-controlled trial. *Drug Alcohol Depend.* 2009;1(101):34–41 (1-2).
93. Mooney ME, Herin DV, Specker S, et al. Pilot study of the effects of lisdexamfetamine on cocaine use: a randomized, double-blind, placebo-controlled trial. *Drug Alcohol Depend.* 2015;153:94–103.
94. Morgan PT, Angarita GA, Canavan S, et al. Modafinil and sleep architecture in an inpatient-outpatients treatment study of cocaine dependence. *Drug Alcohol Depend.* 2016;160:49–56.
95. Murnane KS, Winschel J, Schmidt KT, et al. Serotonin 2A receptors differentially contribute to abuse-related effects of cocaine and cocaine-induced nigrostriatal and mesolimbic dopamine overflow in non-human primates. *J Neurosci.* 2013;33:13367–13374.
96. Newton TF, Haile CN, Mahoney JJ, et al. Dopamine D3 receptor –preferring agonists enhance the subjective effects of cocaine in humans. *Psychiatry Res.* 2015;230(1):44–49.
97. Nic Dhonnchadha BA, Dox RG, Stutz S, et al. Blockade of the serotonin 5-HT2A receptor suppresses cue-evoked reinstatement of cocaine-seeking behavior in a rat self-administration model. *Behav Neuosci.* 2009;123(2). 382–296.
98. Nuijten M, Blanken P, van den Brink W, Hendriks V. Treatment of crack-cocaine dependence with topiramate: a randomized controlled feasibility trial in The Netherlands. *Drug Alcohol Depend.* 2014;138:177–184.
99. Nuijten M, Blanken P, van den Brink W, Hendriks V. Modafinil I the treatment of crack cocaine dependence in The Netherlands: results of an open-label randomized controlled feasibility study. *J Psychopharmacol.* 2015;29(6):678–687.
100. Nunes EV, Levin ER. Treatment of depression in patients with alcohol or other drug dependence: a meta-analysis. *J Am Med Assoc.* 2004;291:1887–1896.
101. Oliveto A, Poling J, Mancino MJ, et al. Randomized, double-blind, placebo-controlled trial of disulfiram for the treatment of cocaine dependence in methadone-stabilized patients. *Drug Alcohol Depend.* 2011;113(2–3):184–191.
102. Payer DE, Behzadi A, Kish SJ, et al. Heightened D3 dopamine receptor levels in cocaine dependence and contribution to addiction behavioral phenotype: a positron emission tomography study with 11C]-+-PHNO. *Neuropsychopharmacology.* 2014;39(2):311–318.
103. Pentkowski NS, Duke FD, Weber SM, et al. Stimulation of medial prefrontal cortex serotonin 2C (5-HT (2C)) receptors attenuates cocaine-seeking behavior. *Neuropsychopharmacology.* 2010;35(10):2037–2048.
104. Petrakis IL, Carroll KM, Nich C, et al. Disulfiram treatment for cocaine dependence in methadone-maintained opioid addicts. *Addiction.* 2000;95:219–228.
105. Pettinati HM, Kampman KM, Lynch KG, et al. A pilot trial of injectable, extended-release naltrexone for the treatment of co-occurring cocaine and alcohol dependence. *Am J Addict.* 2014;23(6):591–597.

106. Pilla M, Perachon S, Sautel F, et al. Selective inhibition of cocaine-seeking behaviour by a partial dopamine D3 receptor agonist. *Nature*. 1999;400:371–375.

107. Plebani JG, Lynch KG, Yu Q, et al. Results of an initial clinical trial of varenicline for the treatment of cocaine dependence. *Drug Alcohol Depend*. 2012;1121 (1-2):163–166.

108. Pockros LA, Pentkowski NS, Swinford SE, Neiswander JL. Blockade of 5-HT2A receptors in the medial prefrontal cortex attenuates reinstatement of cue-elicited cocaine-seeking behavior in rats. *Psychopharmacology (Berl)*. 2011;213(2–3):307–320.

109. Poling J, Oliveto A, Petry N, et al. Six-month trial of bupropion with contingency management for cocaine dependence in a methadone-maintained population. *Arch Gen Psychiatry*. 2006;63:219–228.

110. Riggs P, Levin F, Green AI, et al. Comorbid psychiatric and substance abuse disorders: recent treatment research. *Subst Abuse*. 2008;29:51–63.

111. Rutter JL. Symbiotic relationship of pharmacogenetics and drugs of abuse. *AAPS J*. 2006;8:174–184.

112. Sarnyai Z, Shaham Y, Heinrichs SC. The role of corticotropin-releasing factor in drug addiction. *Phamacol Rev*. 2001;53:209–243.

113. Schmitz JM, Rathnayaka N, Green CE, et al. Combination of modafinil and d-amphetamine for the treatment of cocaine dependence: a preliminary investigation. *Front Psychiatry*. 2012;30(3):77.

114. Schoenbaum G, Nugent SL, Saddoris MP, et al. Orbitofrontal lesions in rats impair reversal but not acquisition of go, no go odor discriminations. *Neuroreport*. 2002;13:885–890.

115. Schottenfeld RS, Chawarski MC, Cubells JF, et al. Randomized clinical trial of disulfiram for cocaine dependence or abuse during buprenorphine treatment. *Drug Alcohol Depend*. 2014;136:36–42.

116. Schroeder JP, Cooper DA, Schank JR, et al. Disulfiram attenuates drug-primed reinstatement of cocaine seeking via inhibition of dopamine β-hydroxylase. *Neuropsychopharmacology*. 2010;35(12):2440–2449.

117. Schroeder JP, Epps SA, Grice TW, Weinshenker D. The selective dopamine β-hydroxylase inhibitor nepicastat attenuates multiple aspects of cocaine-seeking behavior. *Neuropsychopharmacology*. 2013;38:1032–1038.

118. Seu E, Lang A, Rivera RJ, et al. Inhibition of the norepinephrine transporter improves behavioral flexibility in rats and monkeys. *Psychopharmacology*. 2009;202:505–519.

119. Shaham Y, Erb S, Leung S, et al. CP-154–526, a selective, nonpeptide antagonist of the corticotropin-releasing factor1 receptor attenuates stress-induced relapse to drug seeking in cocaine- and heroin-trained rats. *Psychopharmacology*. 1998;137:184–190.

120. Shaham Y, Funk D, Erb S, et al. Corticotropin-releasing factor, but not corticosterone, is involved in stress-induced relapse to heroin-seeking in rats. *J Neurosci*. 1997;17:2605–2614.

121. Slusher BS, Thomas A, Paul M, et al. Expression and acquisition of the conditioned place preference response to cocaine in rats is blocked by selective inhibitors of the enzyme N-acetylated-alpha-linked-acidic dipeptidase (NAALADASE). *Synapse*. 2001;41:22–28.

122. Somoza EC, Winship D, Gorodetzky CW, et al. A multisite, double-blind, placebo-controlled clinical trial to evaluate the safety and efficacy of vigabatrin for treating cocaine dependence. *JAMA Psychiatry*. 2013;70(6):630–637.

123. Spealman RD. Dopamine D3 receptor agonists partially reproduce the discriminative stimulus effects of cocaine in squirrel monkeys. *J Pharmacol Exp Ther*. 1996;278:1128–1137.

124. Stalnaker TA, Roesch MR, Franz TM, et al. Abnormal associative encoding in orbitofrontal neurons in cocaine-experienced rats during decision-making. *Eur J Neurosci*. 2006;24:2643–2653.

125. Stewart J. Pathways to relapse: the neurobiology of drug- and stress-induced relapse to drug-taking. *J Psychiatry Neurosci*. 2000;25:125–136.

126. Umbricht A, DeFulio A, Winstanley EL, et al. Topiramate for cocaine dependence during methadone maintenance treatment: a randomized controlled trial. *Drug Alcohol Depend*. 2014;140:92–100.

127. Verrico CD, Haile CN, Mahoney JJ, et al. Treatment with modafinil and escitalopram, alone and in combination, on cocaine-induced effects: a randomized, double-blind, placebo-controlled trial. *Drug Alcohol Depend*. 2014;141:72–78.

128. Winchell C, Rappaport BA, Roca R, Rosebaugh CJ. Reanalysis of methamphetamine dependence treatment trial. *CNS Neurosci Ther*. 2012;18:367–368.

129. Winhusen T, Somoza E, Ciraulo D, et al. A double-blind, placebo-controlled trial of tiagabine for the treatment of cocaine dependence. *Drug Alcohol Depend*. 2007;91:141–148.

130. Winhusen T, Somoza E, Sarid-Segal O, et al. A double-blind, placebo-controlled trial of reserpine for the treatment of cocaine dependence. *Drug Alcohol Depend*. 2007;91:205–212.

131. Winhusen TM, Kropp F, Lindblad R, et al. Multisite, randomized, double-blind, placebo-controlled pilot clinical trial to evaluate the efficacy of buspirone as a relapse prevention treatment for cocaine dependence. *J Clin Psychiatry*. 2014;75(7):757–764.

132. Xi ZX, Gilbert J, Campos AC, et al. Blockade of mesolimbic dopamine D3 receptors inhibits stress-induced reinstatement of cocaine-seeking rats. *Psychopharmacology*. 2004;176:57–65.

54

Opioid Overdose

CHRISTOPHER WELSH AND JOY CHANG

History

Opiates have been used for thousands of years, with evidence of opium poppy (known as Hul Gil, "joy plant") cultivation more than 5000 years ago among the Sumerians in the area of Mesopotamia, near modern day Iraq. Its use for rituals and mystical purposes is evidenced by poppy seed capsules discovered in burial sites in Neuchatel, Switzerland and the *Cueva de los Murciélagos*, Spain, which have been carbon-14 dated to 4200 BCE.[449] As use spread throughout the Mediterranean, opium's medicinal properties were recognized.

The Greek physician Galen may have been the first to record an opium overdose in around 140 CE, during which he reportedly treated the patient with an emetic made of sweet wine.[398] In 1656, Christopher Wren experimented with intravenous administration (using animal bladders and goose quills) of opium to dogs and described overdose,[381] and several years later, German scientists J.D. Major and J.S. Elsholtz performed similar experiments on humans with reported toxicity.[25,91] A century and a half later, Friedrich Sertürner, the German pharmacist who isolated morphine from opium in the early 1800s, reported that he experimented with the alkaloid by administering it to himself, three boys, three dogs, and a mouse. One of the dogs reportedly died, and he described the effect that morphine had on himself and his three young "volunteers" as "near fatal."[321,345] The first recorded human fatality from a morphine overdose appears to be from the 1850s when Scottish physician Alexander Wood, one of the first to use and perfect the hypodermic needle and syringe, reportedly performed one of the first injections of morphine on his wife who subsequently died from respiratory depression,[66] although others claim that this story is not true.[183] Overdose is also discussed with regards to laudanum, a mixture of opium and alcohol, associated with overdose in mid-19th century. The *Brooklyn* (New York) *Daily Eagle*, January 10, 1861, reported two unrelated instances in a single day. Elizabeth Siddal an artist and wife of Dante Gabriel Rosetti, took laudanum for various illnesses and died of an overdose in February 1862.

Definitions

The term "overdose" is used variably by the lay public, health professionals, and in the medical literature and generally refers to an "excessive amount" of a substance (the noun) or the act of taking such an amount (the verb). This excessive amount is dependent on an individual's tolerance to the specific substance. Associated signs generally include the "opioid overdose triad" of constricted ("pinpoint") pupils, altered level of consciousness, and respiratory depression (both rate and effort). Additional signs may include blue or ashen skin, nails and lips; gurgling or snore-like sounds ("death rattle"); decreased blood pressure and heart rate; and pulmonary edema (Box 54.1).

There are no consistent guidelines or cutoffs to distinguish overdose from intoxication or being under the influence. Some consider an overdose only if the individual has lost consciousness and is unarousable by external stimulation. Number of breaths per minute used to define overdose range from less than 12 per minute to less than 8 per minute. The term "opioid-induced respiratory depression" is sometimes used to describe the side effect of opioid used medically in an attempt to distinguish this effect from the term "overdose" with the associated negative connotation. Another term used to address the complexities of tolerance, co-ingestion, medical comorbidities, and environmental context is "opioid-related overdose."

• **BOX 54.1** **Signs of Opioid Overdose**

"Overdose Triad"
    Constricted ("pinpoint") pupils
    Altered level of consciousness
    Respiratory depression (both rate and effort)
Blue or ashen skin, nails, and lips
Gurgling or snore-like sounds ("death rattle")
Decreased blood pressure and heart rate
"Froth" from mouth (from pulmonary edema)

The term "overdose" is not recognized in standard medical diagnostic nomenclature such as the *International Classification of Diseases and Related Health Problems, Tenth Revision, Clinical Modification* (ICD-10-CM) and the *Diagnostic and Statistical Manual of Mental Disorders, Fifth Edition* (DSM-5). What is commonly thought of as "overdose" can fall under one of two areas: "Poisoning" in the "Injury, Poisoning and Certain Other Consequences of External Causes" section or "Intoxication" in the "Mental, Behavioral and Neurodevelopmental Disorders" section.

International Statistical Classification of Diseases and Related Health Problems, Tenth Revision, Clinical Modification (ICD-10-CM)[716]

Injury, Poisoning, and Certain Other Consequences of External Causes

"Poisoning by, adverse effect of & under-dosing of drugs, medications & biological substances" (T26-50).

This category includes adverse effect of correct substance properly administered, poisoning by overdose of substance, poisoning by wrong substance given or taken in error, and under-dosing by taking less substance than prescribed or instructed. The determination of poisoning versus adverse effect is based on how the substance was used. If the correct substance was administered as prescribed, the condition is classified as an adverse effect. Using the prescribed medication less frequently than prescribed, in smaller amounts, or not using the medication as instructed by the manufacturer is not coded as poisoning but as underdosing. When the condition is a poisoning, the poisoning code is sequenced first, followed by additional codes for all manifestations. If there is also a diagnosis of abuse or dependence on the substance, the abuse or dependence is also coded. The poisoning code is also used when a condition results from interaction of a therapeutic drug used correctly with a nonprescription drug and/or alcohol. All involved substances should be coded separately.

Poisoning by opioids is designated by the code T40. There are specific codes (first decimal place) for heroin (T40.1), other opioids (T40.2), methadone (T40.3), and other synthetic narcotics (T40.4). In addition, a determination is to be made (third decimal place) as to whether the poisoning was unintentional (.XX1), intentional self-harm (.XX2), assault (.XX3), or undetermined (.XX4). Additional codes specify initial encounter, subsequent encounter, and sequela (fourth decimal place) (Box 54.2).

Mental, Behavioral and Neurodevelopmental Disorders: Mental and Behavioral Disorders Due to Psychoactive Substance Use

The diagnostic categories listed here are meant to designate the behavioral disorders of substance abuse and dependence.

• **BOX 54.2** **ICD-10 Multiple Cause-of-Death Codes for Poisoning**

T40.1 Poisoning by and adverse effect of HEROIN
T40.1X1 Poisoning by heroin, accidental (unintentional)
T40.1X2 Poisoning by heroin, intentional self-harm
T40.1X3 Poisoning by heroin, assault
T40.1X4 Poisoning by heroin, undetermined
T40.2 Poisoning by, adverse effect of OTHER OPIOIDS (natural and semisynthetic)
T40.2X1 Poisoning by other opioids, accidental (unintentional)
T40.2X2 Poisoning by other opioids, intentional self-harm
T40.2X3 Poisoning by other opioids, assault
T40.2X4 Poisoning by other opioids, undetermined
T40.2X5 Adverse effect of other opioids
T40.3 Poisoning by, adverse effect of METHADONE
T40.3X1 Poisoning by methadone, accidental (unintentional)
T40.3X2 Poisoning by methadone, intentional self-harm
T40.3X3 Poisoning by methadone, assault
T40.3X4 Poisoning by methadone, undetermined
T40.3X5 Adverse effect of methadone
T40.4 Poisoning by, adverse effect of OTHER SYNTHETIC NARCOTICS (other than methadone)
T40.4X1 Poisoning by other synthetic narcotics, accidental (unintentional)
T40.4X2 Poisoning by other synthetic narcotics, intentional self-harm
T40.4X3 Poisoning by other synthetic narcotics, assault
T40.4X4 Poisoning by other synthetic narcotics, undetermined
T40.4X5 Adverse effect of other synthetic narcotics

Although not meant to specifically designate the phenomenon of overdose, they are sometimes used interchangeably in studies, reports, and so on. They include Opioid use (F11.92), abuse (F11.12), or dependence (F11.22) with intoxication. Specifiers include uncomplicated (.XX0), with delirium (.XX1), with perceptual disturbance (.XX2), and unspecified (.XX9). There are not separate codes for the different types of opioid but the clinician is encouraged to add the name of the specific opioid (i.e., heroin, oxycodone, methadone) in addition to the numeric code.

Diagnostic and Statistical Manual of Mental Disorders, Fifth Edition (DSM-5)

The other major diagnostic coding system used for behavioral disorders in the United States is the *Diagnostic and Statistical Manual of Mental Disorders, Fifth Edition* (DSM-5).[11] Substance-Related and Addictive Disorders with Intoxication falls under the "Substance-Induced Disorder" category. With regard to Substance Use Disorders, the DSM-5 is similar to ICD-10-CM except it uses the term Opioid Use Disorder with the severity specifiers of Mild, Moderate, or Severe, whereas ICD-10-CM uses Abuse and Dependence codes (similar to the fourth edition [text revision] of the DSM [DSM-IV-TR]). With the DSM-5, a severity specifier of mild is the equivalent of ICD-10-CM abuse, whereas a severity specifier of moderate or severe is equivalent to ICD-10-CM dependence. The DSM-5 does not have a "Use" diagnostic category, although it does have an intoxication code for "Opioid Intoxication with no comorbid opioid use disorder." There are four criteria for Opioid Intoxication:

A. Recent use of an opioid.
B. Clinically significant problematic behavioral or psychological changes (e.g., initial euphoria followed by apathy, dysphoria, psychomotor agitation or retardation, impaired judgment) that developed during, or shortly after, opioid use.

C. Pupillary constriction (or pupillary dilation due to anoxia from severe overdose) and one (or more) of the following signs or symptoms developing during, or shortly after, opioid use: (1) drowsiness or coma, (2) slurred speech, (3) impairment in attention or memory.

D. The signs or symptoms are not attributable to another medical condition and are not better explained by another mental disorder, including intoxication with another substance.

The clinician can add a specifier "with or without perceptual disturbance."

Unlike DSM-IV-TR, where the intoxication and use disorder (abuse or dependence) were listed individually, DSM-5 uses a code that combines the use disorder and intoxication (in order to distinguish it from intoxication in an individual who does not have a history of a use disorder).

Defining Fatal Overdose

Historically, there has been a great deal of inconsistency in the way that "poisoning" or intoxication-related deaths have been categorized. Because some states have a system based on a centralized medical examiner, whereas others use jurisdictional coroners, there is often a great deal of variability within and between states. Because the numbers reported have significant implications for public health surveillance and resultant prevention strategies, it is extremely important that these deaths be reported in a manner that is consistent as possible. The National Association of Medical Examiners along with American College of Medical Toxicology released guidelines for the investigation, diagnosis, and certification of deaths related to opioid drugs.[190,191] These recommendations included a complete autopsy, a complete scene investigation (including reconciliation of prescription information and pill counts),[670] and comprehensive toxicological testing (of blood, urine, and vitreous humor) to include opioid and benzodiazepine analytes as well as other depressants, stimulants, and antidepressants. All of these are to be used in conjunction with medical history to determine four key components of the death certificate: Cause of Death, Other Significant Conditions Contributing to Death, Manner of Death, and How Injury Occurred. For Cause of Death, all substances believed to have been responsible for the death, and present in sufficient concentrations, are listed (as opposed to vague statements such as "mixed drug intoxication"). The Other Significant Conditions section lists conditions that might have predisposed a person to death (such as sleep apnea) but were neither necessary nor sufficient to cause the death. The Manner of Death is classified as either accident, suicide, homicide, or undetermined. The recommendations encouraged the use of "accident" for all cases of misuse or abuse without any apparent intent of self-harm and stressed that the "undetermined" designation should be reserved only for those cases for which the evidence exists to support more than one possible determination (as opposed to the more common use when the manner is not absolutely certain). Finally, the How Injury Occurred section should include the information about medical history, route of administration, drug formulation (long-acting, extended release, or immediate-release), and source of drug (prescription, illicit, diverted).

The Substance Abuse and Mental Health Services Administration (SAMHSA)[295] convened a consensus panel that addressed many of the same issues and added some additional case definitions: Drug-Caused Death, which refers to deaths that resulted from exposure to a substance regardless of the intent (accident, suicide, homicide) of the individual; and Drug-Detected Death, which refers to a death in which a drug is detected regardless of the drug's role in causing the death. A subcategory of Drug-Caused Death is Drug Poisoning Death, which refers specifically to deaths caused by acute exposure. The US National Center for Health Statistics (NCHS), which releases the annual National Vital Statistics Report *Deaths, Final Data*,[481] has also developed similar categories for drug-induced deaths; however, that classification also includes deaths involving adverse effects of drugs for therapeutic use.[480]

The Centers for Disease Control and Prevention (CDC), based on the external-cause-of-injury matrix, recommends defining an overdose when the first-listed E-code is "drug poisoning" and the principal diagnosis is "injury."[483,648] Consensus recommendations from the Safe States Alliance's Injury Surveillance Workgroup on Poisoning (ISW7)[326,346] recommends two alternative case definitions: one in which an overdose is defined when either the first-listed E-code or principal diagnosis indicates drug poisoning" and the second when an overdose is defined when any E-code or diagnosis lists drug poisoning. One study looking at data from Kentucky found a 50% increase in overdose cases identified when using the second ISW7 definition as compared to the CDC recommended definition.[606] In addition, in 1999, the ICD-10 replaced the previous revision of the ICD (ICD-9) as the classification system used by medical examiners in the determination of cause of death.

Epidemiology

Worldwide

Fatal Overdose

Reliable data on the epidemiology of the fatal overdose are variable and limited by the lack of consistency in case identification, coding, and reporting. The determination of the cause of death varies from country to country, within a given country and, often, within local jurisdictions. Toxicological verification is often not available, extremely limited, or imprecise. Many countries report on drug-related fatalities with some, in addition to drug overdoses, also including deaths due to HIV acquired through injecting drug use, suicide, and unintentional deaths and trauma due to illicit drug use. All of this makes comparisons between countries and regions difficult.[142] With this understanding, the World Health Organization (WHO) estimates that there were 187,100 drug-related deaths in 2013,[662] corresponding to a mortality rate of 40.8 drug-related deaths per million people 15–64 of age. By region, the estimated rates per million are: Africa, 61.9; North America, 136.8; Latin America and the Caribbean, 18.4; Asia, 28.2; West and Central Europe, 22.5; Eastern and Southeastern Europe, 41.5; and Oceania, 82.3. Although most countries report that opioids are the main drugs involved in these deaths, reliable numbers are not available for many countries. Other studies have looked at population-based crude and adjusted mortality rates in various areas and found a range of 0.04 to 46.6 per 100,000 person-years[243,244,436,652,653,696] and 0.11–253.8 per 100,000 person-years,[436,458] respectively. In addition, the largest systematic review of global deaths in people who inject drugs found that overdose is the leading cause in all areas of the world.[438]

The European Monitoring Centre for Drugs and Drug Addiction (EMCDDA) monitors drug-use patterns in the European Union (EU) as well as Norway and Turkey. Despite large variability in case definition and reporting, the EMCDDA represents the best estimate of drug-related morbidity and mortality in Europe. According to their data, most EU countries have seen increases in overdose deaths from 2003 to 2009, at which time there was a leveling or decline for several years in some countries.[246] Increases have been seen in a number of EU countries since 2012, with highest increases in Sweden, Spain, and Turkey as well as Ireland, Lithuania, and the United Kingdom (which saw a doubling of heroin-related overdoses between 2013 and 2015, the highest rates since the early 1990s). For most countries, between 2006 and 2014, overdose rates have increased in older adults and decreased in younger adults. Drug overdoses are estimated to account for 3.5% of all deaths among Europeans 15–39 years of age.[246] In 2014, there were approximately 6800 overdose deaths reported in the EU, 82% of which involved an opioid and 78% in males. The overall rate for the EU is approximately 19.2 overdose fatalities per million population 15–64 years of age (18.3 in the EU plus Turkey and Norway), with individual national rates ranging from 2.4 per million in Romania to 113 per million in Estonia. Other countries with rates over 40 per million include Denmark, Finland, Ireland, Lithuania, Norway, Sweden, and the United Kingdom. Heroin or its metabolites were found in the majority of fatal overdoses, although other substances were often found in combination. Prescription opioids most commonly mentioned in toxicology reports are methadone, fentanyl, tramadol, and buprenorphine. Starting in around 2013, parts of Europe also began to see increases in overdoses related to illicitly manufactured fentanyl and other designer fentanyl analogs.[22,246,326,334] Various areas of Canada have also seen substantial increases in overdose fatalities involving illicitly manufactured opioids.[83,325]

Nonfatal Overdose

Although fatalities related to opioid use are clearly tragic, nonfatal overdose is more common and exerts a huge cost, both economically and personally. Data on nonfatal overdoses are even more unreliable than data for fatal overdoses due to variability of definition, diagnosis, case identification, coding, and reporting. A number of studies from various parts of the world looking at individuals with histories of opioid misuse suggest that 16%–80% of those interviewed had experienced an overdose in their drug-using career, many of whom had experienced overdoses in the previous 6–12 months.[a] Other studies have estimated that 4%–5% of all overdose cases are fatal, with a cumulative risk of death increasing with each successive overdose.[133,169,242,653]

United States

Fatal Overdose

Although not as variable as the majority of other countries, data on overdose within the United States do exhibit a fair amount of variability from state to state. On average, about 81% of all death certificates list the specific drug(s) contributing to the death, with some states reporting the specific drug(s) in less than 50% of their death certificates. In addition, there are issues with the manner in which coded diagnosis are used in gathering data: some are based on the external-cause-of-injury code (E-code) and others are based on the principal diagnosis.

The United States reports one of the highest drug-related mortality rates worldwide (at 4.6 times the global average) and accounts for approximately 20% of drug-related deaths globally. The higher mortality rate in North America likely, in part, reflects better monitoring and reporting.[662,663] The relative contribution

of opioids to all overdose deaths has risen from about 38% in 2004 to more than 63% in 2013.[219,484] Prescription opioids account for approximately 75% of all prescription drug-related deaths.[522]

Given that data before and after 1999 are not entirely comparable, it still appears that fatalities related to drug overdose have increased steadily since the early 1970s. In 1980, there were an estimated 6100 drug poisoning deaths, a rate of 4.8 per 100,000.[690] During this period, the categorization of drug poisoning deaths did not allow easy distinction between deaths caused by prescription drugs and deaths caused by illicit drugs. Because the category of "opiates" did not distinguish between heroin and prescription opiates, it is difficult to determine how much of the change in opiate-related deaths was attributed to heroin and how much to prescription opioid analgesics.

Beginning in 1999, a new coding protocol was introduced that allowed researchers to better determine which drugs were involved in fatalities by allowing disaggregation of the "narcotics" category into the three largest components: heroin, cocaine, and opioid analgesics. Between 1999 and 2004, the number of annual deaths related to unintentional drug poisoning continued to rise to more than 20,000 in 2004. During this period, the gradual increase in cocaine-related mortality continued, whereas the number of deaths involving heroin stabilized. In contrast, the number of deaths involving prescription opioid analgesics increased from roughly 2900 in 1999 to 7500 in 2004, an increase of 160% in 5 years.[520,521,522] By 2004, opioid painkiller deaths numbered more than the total of deaths involving heroin and cocaine combined. Overdose deaths involving prescription opioids quadrupled between 1999 and 2014, from a rate of 1.5 deaths per 100,000 persons to 5.9 deaths per 100,000 persons (more than 165,000 deaths over that period).[109,112] The group with the highest risk for fatal prescription opioid–related poisoning was white, middle-aged men. As compared to the early 1990s, when overdose rates were lowest in the rural states, the highest mortality rates by 2004 were in New England, the Appalachian states, and the Southwest. In 2015, the four states with the highest drug overdose death rates per 100,000 population were West Virginia (41.5), New Hampshire (34.3), Kentucky (29.9), and Ohio (29.9).[333]

In addition, there was a correlation between state drug poisoning rates and state sales of prescription opioids, with a nearly fourfold difference among states in their use of opioid analgesics.[b] The number of prescriptions for opioids written in the United States (which prescribes an estimated 80% of all opioids prescribed in the world) more than tripled between 1991 (76 million prescriptions) and 2012 (259 million prescriptions).[98,99] The amount of opioid prescribed in the United States has been estimated to be the equivalent of 96 mg of morphine per person in 1997, 700 mg per person in 2007, 782 mg of morphine per person in 2010 (the peak), and decreasing gradually to 640 mg of morphine per person in 2015.[106,314] Despite the decline between 2010 and 2015, the amount in 2015 is still three times as high as the 1999 number. In addition, there is a great deal of variability across the country, with significantly higher rates in counties with a larger percentage of non-Hispanic whites, higher rates of unemployment and Medicaid enrollment, higher prevalence of diabetes and arthritis, and micropolitan (10,000 to 50,000 population) status.[20]

About 80% of individuals prescribed opioids receive less than 100 mg morphine equivalent per day from a single practitioner with another 10% receiving more than 100 mg morphine equivalents per day from a single provider. The remaining 10%

---

[a]References 43, 46, 68, 140, 160, 178, 184, 261, 262, 299, 363, 436, 544, 589, 723.

[b]References 97, 98, 436, 493, 521, 521, 666.

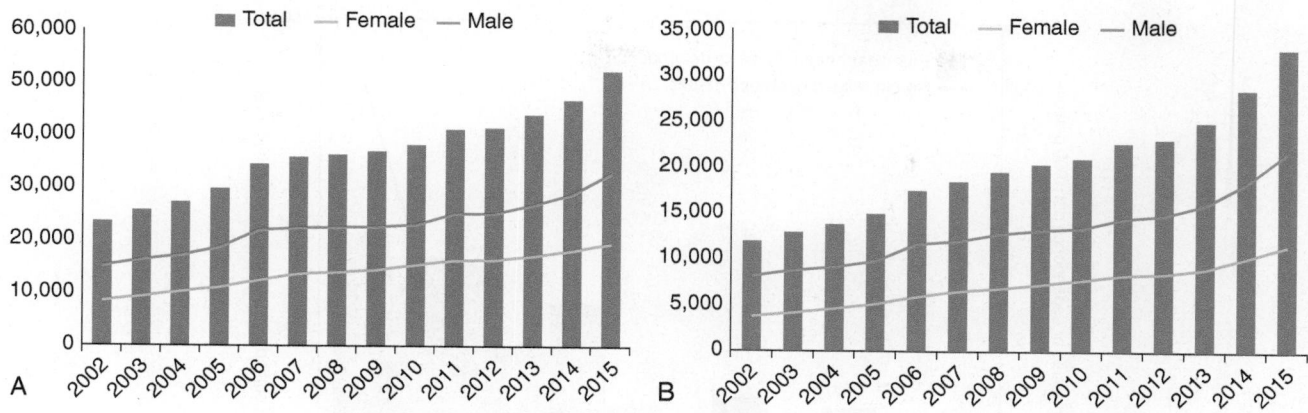

• **Fig. 54.1** Age-adjusted rate of drug overdose deaths (A) and drug overdose deaths involving opioids (B)—United States, 2002–2015. Age-adjusted death rates were calculated by applying age-specific death rates to the 2002 US standard population age distribution. Drug overdose deaths involving opioids are identified using the *International Statistical Classification of Diseases and Related Health Problems, Tenth Revision* (ICD-10) underlying cause-of-death codes X40–X44, X60–X64, X85, and Y10–Y14 with a multiple cause code of T40.0, T40.1, T40.2, T40.3, T40.4, or T40.6. Approximately one-fifth of drug overdose deaths lack information on the specific drugs involved. Some of these deaths might involve opioids. (From National Institute on Drug Abuse: https://www.drugabuse.gov/related-topics/trends-statistics/overdose-death-rates.)

of opioid prescription recipients tend to get higher doses (greater than 100 mg morphine equivalents per day) from multiple prescribers.[c]

Since 2004, overall rates of fatal overdose have continued to rise, reaching a high of 52,404 in 2015. Of this total, 33,091 fatalities were associated with any opioid, 63% of the total drug overdose deaths in 2015. This represented a 6.5% increase from the age-adjusted rate of 13.8 per 100,000 in 2013 to 16.3 per 100,000 in 2015[333,562,563] (Fig. 54.1). Rates of fatal overdose among non-Hispanic white persons has increased from 6.2 per 100,000 in 1999 to 21.1 per 100,000 in 2015. Increases for Hispanic and non-Hispanic black individuals have been much less dramatic.[333] From 2010 to 2015, 30 states and the District of Columbia saw increased fatality rates.[563]

The misuse of prescription opioids has continued to be a major public health problem, with an estimated 91.8 million persons 18 years of age or older (97.5 million including those 12 years of age or older) having used an opioid and 11.5 million (12.5 million including those 12 years of age or older; 4.7% of the US population over the age of 12) reporting nonmedical use in the past year. Of these, 59.9% reported using them without a prescription, with 40.8% reporting that they had obtained them from friends or relatives for free. Of those with a prescription, 22.2% used them in greater amounts than directed on their prescription, 14.6% used them more often than directed, and 13.1% used them longer than directed. Rates were higher in adults who were unemployed, uninsured, and with other behavioral health problems.[96,323,340] Although troublingly high, these numbers represent a decrease from a high of 12.65 million in 2006, and a slight increase from 2014, which had seen the lowest number since 2002. Despite this, there were 22,598 fatalities involving opioid analgesics in 2015, up from a previous peak of 16,917 in 2011, and following declines in 2012 and 2013.[333] The correlation between increased opioid prescribing and fatal overdose continued to be especially prevalent in rural areas including New England, Appalachia, and the southwest (Fig. 54.2).[d]

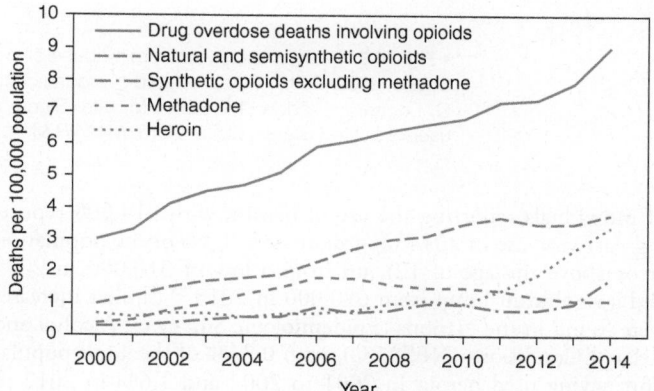

• **Fig. 54.2** Drug overdose deaths involving opioids by type of opioid—United States, 2000–2014. Age-adjusted death rates were calculated by applying age-specific death rates to the 2000 US standard population age distribution. Drug overdose deaths involving opioids are identified using the *International Statistical Classification of Diseases and Related Health Problems, Tenth Revision* (ICD-10) underlying cause-of-death codes X40–X44, X60–X64, X85, and Y10–Y14 with a multiple cause code of T40.0, T40.1, T40.2, T40.3, T40.4, or T40.6. (From Rudd R, Aleshire N, Zibbell J, Gladden R. Increases in drug and opioid overdose deaths-United States, 2000–2014. *MMWR Morb Mortal Wkly Rep.* 2016;64[50]: 1378–1382.)

Another study of substance abuse treatment–seeking individuals found that, of individuals who had developed an opioid use disorder and reported that they were first exposed to an opioid through a legitimate opioid prescription, approximately 95% reported that they had used another psychoactive substance (including alcohol, 93%; nicotine, 90%; and marijuana, 87%) prior to or coincident with the initial opioid use. In addition, 78% had used licit or illicit stimulants and 60% had used benzodiazepines with respondents reporting an average of four to five different substances used prior to the initial opioid.[131]

Unfortunately, the relative leveling off in prescription opioid misuse has been accompanied by a steady increase in the number

---

[c]References 60, 98, 99, 229, 233, 320, 321, 340.
[d]References 97, 98, 420, 459, 460, 562.

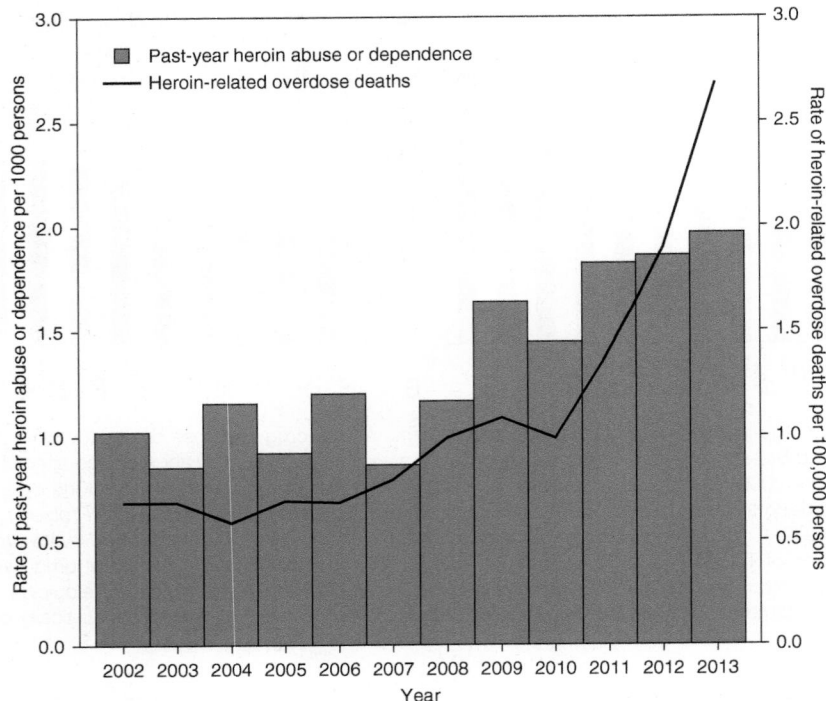

• **Fig. 54.3** Rates of past-year heroin abuse or dependence and heroin-related overdose deaths—United States, 2002–2013. Heroin-related overdose deaths increased by 286% from 2002 to 2013. (From Jones C, Logan J, Gladden M, Bohm M. Vital Signs: demographic and substance use trends among heroin users—United States, 2002–2013. *MMWR Morb Mortal Wkly Rep.* 2015;64[26];719–725.)

of individuals reporting the use of heroin, with 914,000 reporting past year use in 2014 (approximately 0.3% of the population at or above the age of 12), up from a low of 310,000 in 2003 and a significant jump from 680,000 in 2013.[88] Similar increases were found in the National Epidemiologic Survey on Alcohol and Related Conditions (NESARC), with 0.33% of the adult population having used heroin in 2001 to 2002 and 1.6% in 2012 to 2013.[435] The current heroin user tends to be slightly older, less urban, more often white, with a more even gender distribution than the typical heroin user of previous decades. The majority of the newer heroin users report being introduced to opioids through medical and nonmedical use of prescription opioids.[130,474] This increase in heroin use has been accompanied by a fivefold increase in heroin-related fatal overdoses between 2000 (1842 deaths) and 2014 (10,574 deaths)[109,355,482,484] (Figs. 54.3 and 54.4) and an increase of 20.6% just between 2014 and 2015 (12,989 deaths).[563]

Compared to other causes of unintentional injury deaths, poisoning has continued to increase over the past 15 years. In 2014, unintentional poisoning ranked in the top 10 causes of injury death in all age groups beginning at age 9, and was the leading cause for the age groups between 25- and 65-years-old.[483] Further evidence of the huge impact of overdose (primarily opioid but alcohol and other substances as well) comes from an analysis of all-cause mortality in the United States from 1993 to 2013.[90] The study found that, despite decades of steady decreases in mortality rates (by about 2% per year between 1978 and 1998) for all other age and demographic groups, there was an increase in overall mortality rates (by about 0.5% per year) in white non-Hispanics between 45- and 55-years-old. The majority of this increase was due to poisoning, although deaths from suicide and chronic liver disease also increased. This effect was sufficiently

significant to lower the life expectancy for this age group of white non-Hispanics by 0.1 years between 2013 and 2014.[156] A similar rise in mortality rates was not seen in other industrialized countries, including France, Germany, the United Kingdom, Canada, Australia, and Sweden.

Another indication of the growth of the problem related to poisoning fatalities can be seen in the comparison to fatalities related to car crashes. Once the leading cause of accidental fatalities, automobile crash fatalities have gradually declined since the 1970s. As overdose fatalities gradually increased, the numbers of related deaths intersected in 2008, at approximately 38,000 deaths, and have continued to move in opposite directions ever since[690] (Fig. 54.5). Complicating these statistics, however, a six-state study of fatally injured car drivers found that the prevalence of prescription opioids detected in postmortem toxicological testing increased from 1% in 1995 to 7.2% in 2015.[125]

Several specific situations deserve special attention. Overdose involving methadone has had a unique epidemiology, which has been fairly closely tied to the use of methadone for the treatment of pain. Methadone-related overdose deaths increased 22.1% per year between 2002 and 2006, and then declined approximately 6.5% per year between 2007 and 2014 (39% total decline).[107,255,354] The percentage of drug overdose deaths involving methadone also decreased from 12% in 2010 to 6% in 2015.[333] This closely paralleled the amount of methadone prescribed, which increased by 25.1% per year between 2002 and 2006 and declined 3.2% per year from 2006 to 2013 (Figs. 54.2 and 54.6). These rates peaked between 2005 and 2007 in all age groups younger than 55 years, but continued to increase in 55- to 64-year-olds. The declines were seen in all racial/ethnic groups and in males and females, although the rate of decline was slower among females.

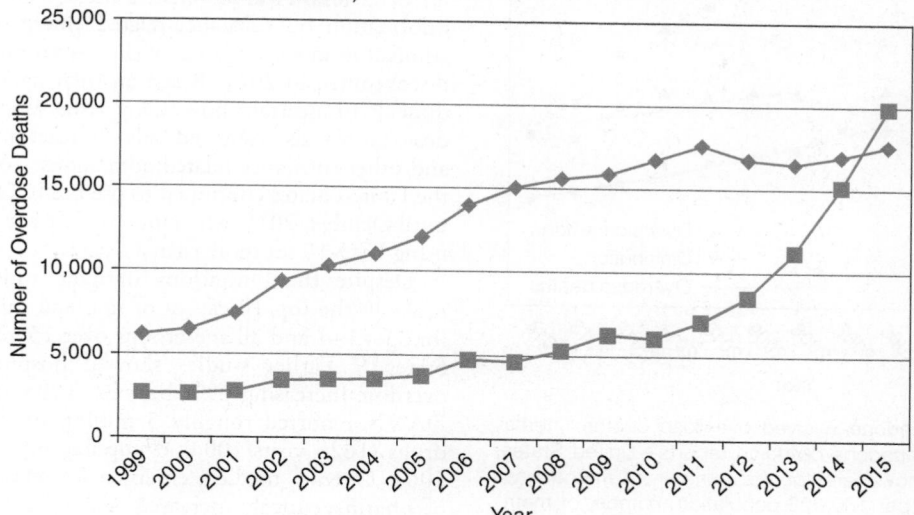

• **Fig. 54.4** Number of overdose deaths from prescription and illicit opioids in the United States, 1999–2015. Although it is sometimes difficult to distinguish illicitly manufactured versus pharmaceutical fentanyl, the numbers generally represent illicitly manufactured fentanyl, fentanyl analogues, and other nonpharmaceutical opioids as well as heroin. (From National Center on Health Statistics [NCHS] [2016]. National overdose deaths from select prescription and illicit drugs. https://www.drugabuse.gov/related-topics/trends-statistics/overdose-death-rates. Accessed July 26, 2017.)

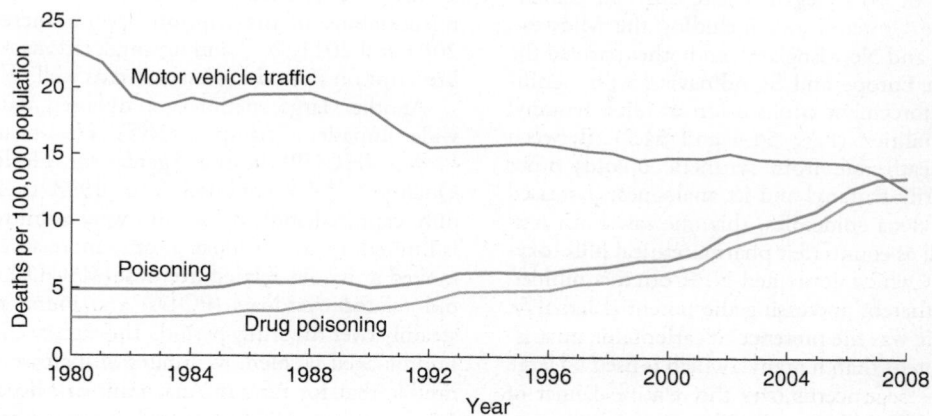

• **Fig. 54.5** Motor vehicle traffic and drug poisoning death rates—United States, 1980–2008. "Poisoning" also includes intentional poisonings (suicide). (From Warner M, Chen L, Makuc D, Anderson R, Miniño A. *Drug Poisoning Deaths in the United States, 1980–2008.* NCHS data brief, no 81. Hyattsville, MD: National Center for Health Statistics; 2011.)

The decline was also seen despite the fact that more than 100,000 individuals initiated methadone for the treatment of opioid use disorder during that period.

Another unique situation involves illicitly manufactured fentanyl (IMF), also known as nonpharmaceutical fentanyl (NPF), or its analogs (acetyl fentanyl, alpha-methylfentanyl, carfentanil, 3-methylfentanyl, and others) sold as heroin (often branded as more pure heroin under such names as China White, Tango & Cash, and TNT). Earlier epidemics were generally constrained to smaller areas starting in the late 1970s, with an outbreak (primarily in California) with at least 112 related deaths.[336] Over the next decade, sporadic clusters of fentanyl-associated fatalities were encountered in the mid-Atlantic region, with 16 deaths associated with the use of heroin contaminated with 3-methylfentanyl, in Pittsburgh 1986–1988[257,336,337,433] and 20 deaths associated with illicit fentanyl use in Baltimore in 1992.[607] From 2005 to 2007, a larger outbreak (more than 1000 fatalities) occurred over multiple metropolitan areas (Baltimore, Camden, Chicago, Detroit, Philadelphia, St. Louis, and Wilmington) as well as suburban and rural areas of Delaware, Illinois, Kentucky, Maine, Maryland, Massachusetts, Michigan, New Jersey, New Hampshire, Ohio, Pennsylvania, and Virginia.[4,57,97,646,712] When the source of that NPF was traced to a single lab in Mexico, which was dismantled, the outbreak came to an end.

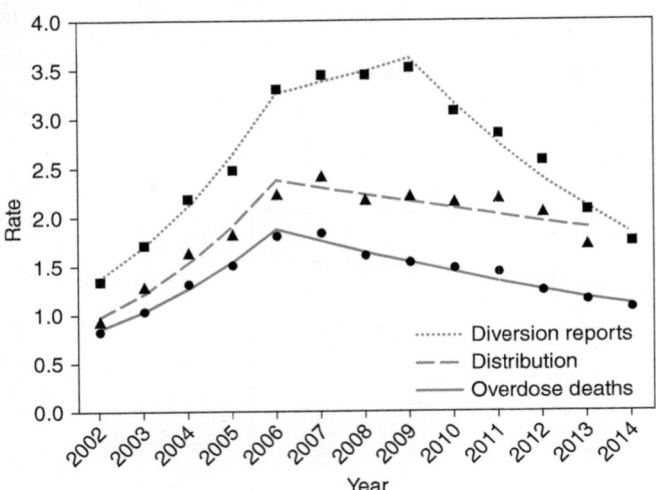

• **Fig. 54.6** Rates of methadone-involved overdose deaths, methadone distribution, and methadone diversion reports—United States, 2002–2014. The rates shown are for the number of methadone-involved overdose deaths per 100,000 population, number of methadone diversion reports per 100,000 population, and number of grams of methadone distributed per 100 population. (From Jones C, Baldwin G, Manocchio T, White J, Mack K. Trends in methadone distribution for pain treatment, methadone diversion, and overdose deaths—United States, 2002–2014. *MMWR Morb Mortal Wkly Rep.* 2016;65:667–671.)

The largest epidemic of NPF began in late 2013 in Canada and various parts of the United States including the Midwest, Southeast, mid-Atlantic, and New England, and other parts of the world including Eastern Europe and Scandinavia,[e] with significant increases in law enforcement confiscation of illicit fentanyl and related overdose fatalities[f] (Figs. 54.4 and 54.7). Between 2014 and 2015, the death rate from synthetic opioids other than methadone (primarily fentanyl and its analogues) increased 72%.[563] Unlike the previous epidemics, this one saw both fentanyl-laced heroin as well as counterfeit pharmaceutical pills (oxycodone, Xanax, Norco),[g] which contained NPF, often combined with a benzodiazepine, thereby increasing the potential lethality. Also new in this epidemic was the presence of carfentanil, an analogue 100 times more potent than fentanyl, which is used by large animal veterinarians.[161,502] Concerns over the relative danger of these analogues have lead the US Drug Enforcement Administration (DEA) and many local jurisdictions to implement enhanced precautions for first responders interacting with individuals and crime scenes that may have been exposed to fentanyl analogues.[226] In addition, this epidemic also saw the emergence of some novel opioids (AH-7921, MT-45, U-47700, and others) related to overdose fatalities in Canada, the United States, and Europe.[h]

Nonfatal Overdose

Numbers for nonfatal overdose are less reliable than those for fatalities. There is much more room for variability in coding. A heroin overdose may be coded as "respiratory depression" or "altered mental status" and "Heroin Use Disorder" and not detected as

a "poisoning." In addition, various databases may capture different components of the issue. The Drug Abuse Warning Network (DAWN), most recently overseen by SAMHSA and the Center for Behavioral Health Statistics and Quality (CBHSQ), collected information on substance-related emergency department (ED) admissions in various areas of the country from 1972, until it was discontinued in 2011. Based on their data, it can sometimes be difficult to ascertain how many visits were actually for an overdose, as they also captured "adverse reaction to a pharmaceutical" and other substance-related admissions. To add to the difficulty, the United States continued to use the ICD-9 for medical coding until October, 2015, when much of the rest of the world had been using ICD-10 for more than a decade.

Despite the limitations in data, unintentional poisoning ranks in the top 10 causes of nonfatal injury treated in an ED for ages 1–4 and all age groups over 15 years old in the United States.[483] Earlier studies showed hospitalizations for heroin overdose increasing 69% between 1993 and 2006.[658] In 2011, DAWN reported roughly 5 million total ED visits related to drugs (1626 visits/100,000 population) a 100% increase since 2004. Overall, medical emergencies related to nonmedical use of pharmaceuticals increased 132% in the period from 2004 to 2011 (1.2 million visits in 2011), with prescription opiate/opioid involvement rising 183% (approximately 348,000 visits in 2011). The specific drugs with the highest number of visits were oxycodone, hydrocodone, and methadone with 151,218, 82,480, and 66,870 visits, respectively. There were 258,482 visits related to heroin use, which constituted 83 visits/100,000 population, not a statistically significant rise from 2004.[626] Studies using other data sources similarly found ED visits involving misuse/abuse of prescription opioids increased 153% between 2004 and 2011,[95,358] and hospitalizations related to overdose on prescription opioid use increased as well.[137]

Another large, national study used data from the Nationwide Inpatient Sample (NIS) Healthcare Cost Utilization Project (HCUP) in the Agency for Healthcare Research and Quality[330,331,658] collected from 1993 to 2009. As these data only captured individuals who were admitted to the hospital, it is limited, in that it looks at only more severe cases. The authors looked at heroin-related overdoses (HODs) and prescription opioid–related overdoses (PODs) and found that PODs increased steadily over the study period. The highest increases were in white, middle-aged women, with rates of increase for whites more than double that for African Americans or Hispanics. Overall HODs increased from 1993 to 1999 but leveled off and decreased until they began to increase again around 2007. Since 1995, rates for African Americans and Hispanics decreased (with the exception of an uptick in 2009), whereas those for whites showed a gradual increase through most of the period with a significant increase beginning in 2007, surpassing African Americans for the first time in 2008. Yet another study using HCUP data found that the rate of hospital stays involving opioid overuse (which included treatment for opioid abuse and dependence in addition to overdose) among adults increased more than 150% between 1993 and 2012 when there were 709,500 opioid-related hospital stays representing a rate of 295.6 stays per 100,000 population.[513]

Looking at hospitalizations related to prescription opioids versus heroin using the NIS between 2000 and 2014, one study found significant geographic variation with PODs highest in the South and lowest in the Northeast and heroin-related overdoses highest in the Northeast and Midwest. Between 2012 and 2014, POD hospitalizations decreased in all areas of the United States

---

[e]References 22, 113, 220, 334, 608, 668.
[f]References 226, 276, 293, 484, 530, 608.
[g]References 222, 223, 265, 569, 631, 678.
[h]References 17, 34, 209, 225, 236, 359, 374, 463, 472, 561.

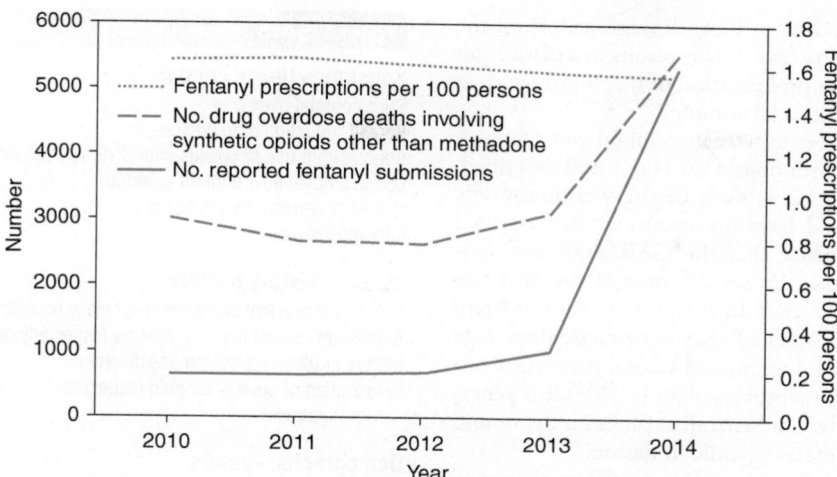

• **Fig. 54.7** Trends in number of drug overdose deaths involving synthetic opioids other than methadone,* number of reported fentanyl submissions to law enforcement,† and rate of fentanyl prescriptions§—United States, 2010–2014. (From Gladden RM, Martinez P, Seth P. Fentanyl law enforcement submissions and increases in synthetic opioid–involved overdose deaths—27 states, 2013–2014. *MMWR Morb Mortal Wkly Rep.* 2016;65:837–843.)

*Synthetic opioid–involved (other than methadone) overdose deaths are deaths with an ICD-10, underlying cause-of-death of X40–44 (unintentional), X60–64 (suicide), X85 (homicide), or Y10–Y14 (undetermined intent) and a multiple cause-of-death of T40.4 (poisoning by narcotics and psychodysleptics [hallucinogens]: other synthetic narcotics).
†Drug products obtained by law enforcement that tested positive for fentanyl are referred to as fentanyl submissions. Reports were supplied by the Drug Enforcement Administration's National Forensic Laboratory Information System and downloaded July 1, 2016.
§National estimates supplied by IMS National Prescription Audit and include short- and long-acting fentanyl prescriptions.

except New England, whereas heroin-related hospitalizations increased in all areas of the country.[660]

The preponderance of ED substance-related visits for children 5 years of age or younger involve accidental ingestions (which were recorded separately by DAWN). On average, more than 3200 children younger than 5 years of age are seen in the ED each year due to accidental opioid overdose.[77] In 2011, of a total of 113,634 visits, over 77,000 involved children in this age range. Pain relievers (including acetaminophen, aspirin, and nonsteroidal anti-inflammatories) were the most common class of drugs involved in accidental ingestion among children 5 years of age or younger, with 6.7% of visits related to opioids. Although overall visits for accidental ingestion by patients 5 years of age or younger were stable from 2004 to 2011, visits involving narcotic pain relievers increased 225% (from 1596 to 5187 per year).

Pathophysiology

As mentioned above, the hallmark of opioid overdose is constricted ("pinpoint") pupils, altered level of consciousness, and respiratory depression. This triad has been found to have 92% sensitivity and 76% specificity for heroin overdose.[614] The amount of a given opioid needed to produce these effects is dependent on tolerance, which is a complex interaction of single-cell and neuronal network-level alterations. Tolerance develops at different rates and to varied degrees to various clinical aspects of opioid intoxication, with that to respiratory depression developing slower and to a less complete extent than some other effects. Tolerance is also affected by nonpharmacological factors such as the environment in which the opioid is used. Animal studies and epidemiological data support the finding that fatal overdose is more likely when the opioid

is used in a novel setting as compared to a setting in which the drug has previously been used.[599,600-603]

The pupillary constriction, miosis, appears to be caused by parasympathetic excitation. This may not occur with overdose on meperidine, propoxyphene, and pentazocine.[376,377,703] Altered mental status may vary from mild sedation to stupor and coma. Gag reflex may also be suppressed. In addition to the typical, centrally mediated respiratory depression (discussed below), severe opioid overdose can also produce noncardiogenic pulmonary edema (NCPE) and bronchospasm. This typically presents with frothy, pink secretions and rales. In nontolerant individuals, opioid use can also cause nausea and vomiting. Rarely, overdose may also produce a centrally mediated muscle rigidity of the chest and abdominal wall. Rhabdomyolysis may be seen as a result of prolonged motionlessness and compression of muscle, typically in the context of coma. Hypotension, acidosis and dehydration may further increase the risk of this. There are also reports of rhabdomyolysis occurring in the absence of coma suggesting that it may, rarely, be a direct toxic effect or allergic reaction to heroin or an adulterant.[157]

Respiratory depression (decreased respiratory rate and effort, hypoxia, and hypercarbia) is the main cause of death due to opioid overdose, although cardiac arrest and arrhythmia induced by anoxia can also occur.[24,290,703] The mechanisms through which μ-opioid agonists suppress respiration are complex and not yet fully understood in humans. Opioid receptors are found in various central and peripheral areas including the pons and ventrolateral medulla in the brainstem; the insula, thalamus, and anterior cingulate cortex higher in the brain; the carotid bodies and vagus nerve; as well as in the epithelial, submucosal, and muscular layers of the airways themselves. It appears that the strongest effect on respiration by μ-opioid receptor agonists is mediated through a decrease in ventilatory response to CO_2 through action on the respiratory centers in the brainstem.[519] This results in a disruption of the respiratory pattern with prolongation of inspiration and, at higher opioid doses, changes in tidal volume.[390,391]

The mechanism by which benzodiazepines might worsen respiratory depression associated with opioid use is not well described. Benzodiazepines bind to the γ2 subunit of the γ-aminobutyric acid A receptor ($GABA_A$) and have no activity at the μ-opioid receptor. There is some evidence that the GABAergic and opioidergic systems are coexpressed in several areas of the rat brain and that there is anatomical overlap in receptors in various brain regions.[216,362] It has been postulated that benzodiazepines may also have effects on signal transduction and second messenger systems involved with μ-opioid receptor regulation.[535,536] It is generally felt that any potential effect of benzodiazepines on the opioid system is not primarily pharmacodynamic in nature.

Certain opioids have specific physiological effects that may contribute to the clinical picture in overdoses. Methadone and the related L-alpha-acetylmethadol (LAAM; not currently commercially available) are fairly unique among opioids in their potential to cause QTc prolongation and resultant torsade de pointes. The true prevalence of this QTc prolongation and torsade de pointes associated with methadone and the implication for methadone-related overdose are not clear.

Seizures have rarely been reported with morphine, fentanyl, sufentanil, alfentanil, and meperidine. Most of these have been reported only in conjunction with general anesthesia and were not confirmed with simultaneous electroencephalography (EEG) readings. It is possible that, what appears to be seizure activity may actually be rigidity, myoclonic jerks, and other nonepileptic movements.[i] Meperidine, however, has been associated with seizures, primarily due to the metabolite normeperidine. The risk of this is increased in the presence of renal impairment (which reduces the clearance of normeperidine) or concomitant use of medications that induce microsomal liver enzymes (through increased conversion of meperidine to normeperidine).[j]

Fentanyl and its analogs (e.g., acetylfentanyl, alfentanil, sufentanil) appear to be able to cause skeletal muscle rigidity (especially chest wall, sometimes referred to as "wooden chest"). It appears to be more common with rapid intravenous administration, although it is not dose dependent. Onset may be rapid and produce an inability to ventilate. It may be related to noradrenergic activation of spinal tracts associated with the locus coeruleus. Because the chest wall rigidity is not discernible after death, the role of this phenomenon in fatal overdose is not clear.[78]

Buprenorphine, a partial μ-opioid agonist that has been associated with a significantly lower risk of overdose, needs special consideration when discussing opioid-induced respiratory effects. At lower doses, buprenorphine produces CNS and respiratory depression in a dose-dependent manner. However, as the dose is increased, a plateau is reached at which these effects no longer continue to increase, making respiratory depression less likely than with other opioids. The ceiling effect on respiratory depression may be more evident in habitual users than in opioid naïve individuals, in whom respiratory depression may occur before reaching the ceiling.[k] Although the exact mechanism for this is not entirely clear, it appears that buprenorphine alone generally leads to mild decreases in PaO_2 with minimal increases in $PaCO_2$ as

---

[i]References 63, 89, 392, 462, 549, 570, 644.
[j]References 294, 318, 338, 361, 437, 636.
[k]References 155, 164, 311, 445, 720, 721.

• BOX 54.3 **Risk Factors for Opioid Overdose**

Substance Usage Factors
Prior nonfatal overdose
Recent reduction of tolerance
Concomitant use of opioids with CNS depressant substances
Use in a novel environment or alone
Higher or variable heroin purity
Intravenous use

Medical History Factors
Significant medical problems (especially hepatic and respiratory)
Significant mental health problems (especially depression and anxiety)
History of other substance use disorder
Prescription of opioids for pain (especially higher doses and longer-acting formulations)

Demographic Factors
Male
Middle-aged
Economically disadvantaged
Undereducated
Race (variable)

---

compared to the significant increase in $PaCO_2$ generally observed with full opioid agonists.[121,579]

Increased respiratory depression associated with the combination of buprenorphine and benzodiazepines has been reported in the anesthesia and animal literature since the mid-1980s.[251,273,312,447,535] This effect is generally found to be most pronounced for flunitrazepam, as compared to other benzodiazepines, with a relatively more pronounced effect on respiratory depression being observed when flunitrazepam is combined with buprenorphine as compared to some other opioids.[64] In addition, buprenorphine's main active N-dealkylated metabolite, norbuprenorphine, appears to produce considerably more potent respiratory depression than buprenorphine,[503,504] and buprenorphine itself may act as a protectant against norbuprenorphine's effects in rodents.[446]

Risk Factors

Over the past several decades, multiple studies have attempted to determine risk factors for overdose, both nonfatal and fatal.[l] Although there is some variation over time and across different areas of the world, there is a fair amount of consistency in many of these factors (Box 54.3).

Risk Related to Substance Use Factors

A *history of prior overdose*[m] is one of the strongest predictors of subsequent overdose. In addition, the risk of fatality appears to increase with each prior nonfatal overdose.[175,177,242,653]

A history of opioid dependence with *reduced tolerance* following medical detoxification,[n] release from incarceration (especially in

---

[l]References 24, 171, 174, 175, 178, 179, 566, 731.
[m]References 46, 59, 93, 139, 145, 174, 177, 178, 253, 254, 261, 375, 594, 619, 723.
[n]References 323, 422, 423, 450, 506, 541, 550, 584, 623, 637, 704, 707, 724, 731.

the first 1–2 weeks),[o] cessation of treatment (especially in the first month),[p] or self-imposed abstinence is also a very strong predictor of overdose. One study found that a total of 36 of 276 patients died after discharge from residential substance abuse treatment during the 8-year study period. Two-thirds of these deaths were classified as opiate overdose deaths, with six of these occurring within the first 4 weeks following discharge from the program, yielding an unadjusted excess mortality of 15.7 (rate ratio) in this period. There was no significant association between time in treatment and mortality after discharge, and no baseline characteristics correlated significantly with elevated mortality shortly after discharge.[550] Another study looking at more than 32,000 patients in California seeking methadone maintenance treatment over a 5-year period, found that the highest mortality risk occurred during the 2 weeks immediately following discontinuation of treatment, with a rate approximately 30 times that expected in the general population.[248] Yet another study found that victims of fatal overdose had significantly lower concentrations of morphine in hair samples compared to active heroin users, although their morphine levels were not significantly different than those in former heroin users who had been abstaining for several months prior to the study.[637]

Another highly correlated factor is the *concomitant use of opioids with CNS depressant substances*, especially alcohol, benzodiazepines, and barbiturates.[q] The relationship with alcohol use is not entirely straight forward, with some studies of fatalities showing higher alcohol levels correlated with lower morphine and 6-monoacetylmorphine (6-MAM) blood levels[175,172,281] but others finding no significant correlation.[459] One study actually found that complete abstinence from alcohol was a risk factor for opioid overdose fatality, possibly because individuals in that study who were not using alcohol tended to have higher rates of daily heroin use.[643] Studies looking at blood levels of sedatives and opioids in fatal overdoses have not demonstrated a clear relationship.[281,459,711]

Another important factor is *use in a novel* environment,[r] likely related to a decrease in tolerance, which appears to be classically conditioned through environmental cues.[494,599,603] This has also been reported in non–substance-abusing individuals who use opioids.[602] Related to this, being homeless[237] and *using alone* in secluded areas, often abandoned buildings, increases the risk of overdose and fatal overdose.[58] At least part of the increased risk can be explained by the lack of others to directly administer or seek medical assistance. Possibly related, several studies have shown that rushing the use of heroin, because of fear of being caught, may also raise the risk for overdose.[33]

Higher or variable heroin purity or "cut" is another important risk factor.[165,168,305,327,560] Darke et al.[167,168] measured the range and average heroin purity over a 2-year period and found that both were independent predictors of fatal overdoses and accounted for approximately 40% of the total variance.[167,168] Related to the purity of heroin, the cost of a gram of pure heroin (which, in the United States has decreased from $2690 in 1982 to $1237 in 1992, and to $552 in 2002 and $465 in 2012) has also been shown to be correlated with overdose, with a 2.9% increase in the

number of hospitalizations for overdose for every $100 decrease in the per gram price.[499,500,501,659,660] In addition, heroin *adulterated/substituted with other opioids*, especially fentanyl (or its analogs: acetyl fentanyl, alpha-methylfentanyl, carfentanil, 3-methylfentanyl, and others) also appears to raise the risk for nonfatal and fatal overdose.[s]

Some studies have shown a higher risk for overdose with *intravenous route of administration* of opioids,[33,193,194] whereas others have not found a significant correlation.[173,643,645]

Risk Related to Medical History Factors

The presence of other *significant medical conditions* (HIV, liver, or lung disease)[t] appears to increase the risk for overdose and fatality. Respiratory compromise related to conditions such as sleep apnea may convey a particularly increased risk[327].

Opioid users with *other psychiatric conditions* (especially depression and anxiety)[u] appear to be at higher risk for accidental overdose. Prior suicide attempts[68,436] have also been associated with accidental overdose in some but not all studies.[707] One study found that benzodiazepine users who did not initially use opioids were more likely than nonusers of benzodiazepines to later use opioids.[605]

A history of *other substance use disorder* is generally associated with prescription opioid overdose deaths—as is *poor compliance with or difficulty entering substance abuse treatment*,[v] although in a 5-year study of 155,434 patients treated with opioids in the United States by the Veterans Health Administration (VA), 60% of opioid-induced fatalities occurred in patients who did not have a history of a diagnosis of a substance use disorder.[60]

People who are *prescribed prescription opioids for pain*, in particular those on higher doses, on long-acting preparations, and with higher reports of pain, appear to have an increased risk for overdose.[w] The study by Dunn et al. found that, as prescription opioid dose escalates, the risk of prescription opioid overdose increases. Compared to persons taking opioid doses from 1–19 mg morphine-equivalent daily dose (MEDD), those persons taking 20–49 MEDD, 50–99 MEDD, and >100 MEDD had a 1.2-, 3-, and 11-fold increased risk of prescription opioid overdose, respectively. However, various studies have also found that many individuals who overdose are not chronic, daily opioid users[60,282,522] and are not on higher doses (more than 100 mg morphine equivalents/day).[60,228,229] Another study found that 10%–20% of people prescribed opioids received less than 100 mg MEDD from a single provider, 40% received more than 100 mg MEDD from a single provider, and 40% received more than 100 mg MEDD from multiple providers, but that 60% of all overdose fatalities from prescription opioids occurred in the 90% of the population who obtained their opioids from a single provider who was prescribing within guidelines.[99]

Risk Related to Demographic Factors

Certain demographic factors have been associated with overdose, although these factors vary in different parts of the world and

---

[o]References 15, 49, 50, 53, 52, 54, 139, 196, 252, 253, 302, 350, 364, 384, 450, 464, 559, 586, 597, 617, 714.

[p]References 136, 151, 152, 154, 176, 192, 197, 248, 300, 301.

[q]References 15, 33, 52, 53,116, 117, 118, 139, 149, 228, 305, 320, 322, 327, 329, 358, 422, 424, 490, 526, 565, 614, 653, 688, 690, 691, 692, 711, 731, 728, 734.

[r]References 172, 178, 289, 313, 329, 600, 602, 603.

[s]References 4, 57, 111, 113, 220, 257, 336, 385, 561, 562, 712.

[t]References 305, 307, 641, 675, 685, 690, 691, 731, 734.

[u]References 29, 82, 120, 229, 422, 604, 605, 630, 651, 690, 691, 693, 707, 726.

[v]References 168, 169, 171, 179, 248, 690, 691, 730.

[w]References 60, 61, 229, 228, 282, 357, 393, 455, 527, 552, 707, 709.

over time. Males have higher rates of overdose in most studies,[x] although there is evidence that rates in women have been increasing at a relatively faster rate.[19,101] Although all age groups beginning in adolescence are significantly impacted, higher rates have been reported in middle-age (variously defined but generally 35–54 years of age).[y] Lower levels of education are also associated with overdose with higher rates in individuals who did not graduate high school.[61,119,237,393]

Racial/ethnic characteristics appear to vary considerably over time and geography and are related to local heroin and prescription opioid use patterns in a given area. In the United States, through the 1980s and 1990s, heroin use tended to be concentrated in inner city neighborhoods with minority populations. During this period, overdose deaths were more common among African Americans and other minority groups. Various studies have reported increased risk in minorities: aboriginal individuals in Australia[364]; First Nations individuals in Canada[458]; non-Hispanic blacks and Hispanics in New York City[285]; and American Indian/Alaska Natives in the United States.[521,521,523] However, non-Hispanic whites have consistently had higher rates of overdose from prescription opioids and, as misuse of prescription opioids ,began to rise in the mid- to late-1990s, the proportion of opioid-related overdoses in non-Hispanic whites also rose. Beginning around 2010, as rates of heroin use began to increase in areas previously associated with prescription opioid use, the rates of heroin-related overdose began to rise significantly in non-Hispanic whites.[101,616]

Although heroin use and related overdose has been traditionally associated with urban settings,[130,195,204] increasingly, rural areas in the United States (especially the Appalachian region, Great Lakes, Southwest and New England) and other countries have seen a marked increase in overdose, initially related to an increase in prescription opioid use from the late 1999s to around 2010, with a switch to increased overdose related to heroin.[z] Whether urban or rural overdose rates, a common finding is an association of poverty with increased overdose rates. In a study of fatal overdose in New York City in 1996, deaths were more likely to occur in neighborhoods in the top decile of income inequality than in more equitable neighborhoods. This relationship seemed to be partially explained by the level of disorder in the environment.[476] Another study in New York City found that, compared with other unintentional, nonoverdose deaths, prescription opioid overdose deaths were more likely to occur in lower-income and fragmented neighborhoods, but when compared with heroin fatalities, they were more likely to occur in higher-income, less-fragmented neighborhoods.[116,117] Similarly, in rural Kentucky, fatality rates from prescription opioid overdose increased with the amount of poverty in the decedent's county of residence.[75] A similar pattern has been seen in other countries as well.[283]

Other risk factors for overdose that have been reported but with lower levels of support in the literature include: household members with a prescription for opioids, higher levels of dependence,[174,178] witnessing a family member overdose,[604] nicotine use,[355] and presence of tattoos.[88]

There have also been a few studies that have looked at the A118G single nucleotide polymorphism (SNP) of the mu-opioid receptor gene (*OPRM1*), which is found in about 5%–30% of the general population[638] and is associated with variability in nociception and opioid sensitivity.[48,62,124,259,378] It appears that this allele is associated with worse clinical severity in overdose.[427]

Risk Factors for Iatrogenic Overdose

Although opioid-induced respiratory depression is uncommon in the typical perioperative patient, there are several patient groups that are at higher risk: patients with sleep apnea, the morbidly obese, premature babies, the elderly, and the otherwise very ill.[91,162,163] There may also be some increased risk with patient-controlled analgesia (PCA), where studies have shown significant respiratory depression in 0.5%–2% of patients.[239,264,580,590,598,701] The use of very high-potency opioids such as remifentanil may also increase this risk.[65,122] A study looking at adverse events related to opioids in the ED setting found that errors included lack of attention to chronic health conditions that could predispose an individual to an opioid-related adverse event, failure to adjust opioid dosing in the elderly and for hepatic or renal impairment, concurrent use of multiple doses and routes of administration of opioids, coadministration of opioids with other sedating medications, and systems-based problems with patient handoffs and pharmacy oversight.[36]

Other data from MEDMARX (a national medication error reporting database) found that medical provider mistakes contributed significantly to opioid overdoses within the hospital. These overdoses occurred most often with hydromorphone, meperidine, fentanyl, and oxycodone. These errors include the interchanging of oral or intramuscular and intravenous formulations, interchanging of immediate release and extended release formulations, the incorrect administration time for intravenous drips (daily morphine dose being administered over 1 hour instead of 24 hours), and error in PCA settings.[231,239,635] Other studies have shown significant adverse events related to improper use of opioid conversion tables, limitations in these tables themselves and prescription guidelines that are not consistent on opioid rotation procedures.[389,425,693]

Methadone prescribed for pain has been found to be particularly associated with fatal overdose.[266,627,690,692,706,710] In addition to patient behaviors (such as concomitant use of sedative-hypnotics or nonmedical use of the prescribed drug), practitioner errors can contribute to this. These errors include overreliance on published equianalgesic conversion tables when converting from another opioid to methadone, initiation of methadone at too high a dose, titration of dose too rapidly, unfamiliarity with the unique pharmacokinetics and pharmacodynamics of methadone, inadequate identification and monitoring of patients at risk for substance misuse, failure to appreciate the incomplete tolerance to respiratory depression associated with chronic use of other opioids, and lack of education related to risk of QT interval prolongation and sleep apnea.[aa]

Methadone dispensed for the treatment of opioid use disorder has also been associated with nonfatal and fatal overdose,[bb] with many of the deaths occurring in the first 1–4 weeks of treatment.[cc] Although many of these involve the use of concomitant substances, it also appears that a good number of the deaths are related to the methadone dose being escalated too rapidly, typically as a result of an underappreciation of methadone's long elimination half-life,

[x]References 24,130, 357, 521, 521, 562, 690.
[y]References 237, 282, 521, 521, 562, 658.
[z]References 76, 130, 234, 237, 320, 322, 327, 436, 460, 523, 560, 616, 718.

[aa]References 14, 16, 266, 280, 377, 415, 692, 700.
[bb]References 32, 85–87, 136, 232, 369, 461, 529, 613, 729, 730.
[cc]References 151, 152, 154, 192, 197, 248, 369.

extensive bioavailability, tendency to accumulate with continuous dosing, and reduced elimination, as well as the role of underlying sleep apnea, QT-prolongation, and other substance use.[dd] One Australian study of patients on methadone maintenance treatment (MMT) found that 238 patients died between 1990 and 1995, 21% in the first week of treatment. Eighty-eight percent of these patients had other substances in their system. Only 10% of the patients who died in the first week of MMT tested positive for methadone alone.[730] There is also evidence that this may vary by setting, with lower rates in certain settings such as Norway, where all induction is done in specialty clinics,[13,14,136] as compared to higher overdose rates in the United Kingdom and Australia, where induction is often done in the primary care setting.[151,152,197]

Induction of patients onto buprenorphine or buprenorphine/naloxone appears to be much safer with significantly reduced risk for overdose compared to methadone.[42,369,416,430,432,534] One study of more than 19 million prescriptions over a 6-year period in the United Kingdom determined that buprenorphine is six times safer than methadone in terms of overdose risk.[432]

Prevention

As with many public health issues, prevention of overdose can be thought of in terms of (1) *Primary prevention*, focused on the reduction of use or misuse of opioids; (2) *Secondary prevention*, focused on the reduction of overdose; and (3) *Tertiary prevention*, focused on the reduction of deaths from overdose. Across these categories, there are efforts focused both on the individual patient and entire populations.

Primary Prevention

There is significant evidence that increased availability of prescription opioids has led to increased misuse and resultant overdose.[60,98,99,229,460] In addition, a relatively small number of patients appear to account for a disproportionate share of prescriptions.[419,420] Similarly, some research shows that a relatively small number of physicians are responsible for disproportionate numbers of opioid prescriptions.[203,634] As a result of these factors, a number of efforts have focused on reducing the prescribing, obtaining, use, and misuse of these medications. Although some efforts have been in existence for decades, there has been a significant increase in local, state, and federal efforts since the early to mid-2000s, with even further increase in 2014–2016.[ee] In 2011, The Office of National Drug Control Policy released *Epidemic: Responding To America's Prescription Drug Abuse Crisis*, which outlined a plan to reduce nonmedical use through: (1) Education, (2) Tracking and Monitoring, (3) Proper Medication Disposal, and (4) Enforcement.[497] Despite these various efforts, it is difficult to attribute any observed benefits to a given intervention as, in many cases, multiple interventions were in effect simultaneously.[ff] Reductions in overdose deaths related to methadone provide an example of the impact of multiple prevention efforts[354] (Box 54.4; see Fig. 54.6)

It is also important to point out that the success of many primary prevention initiatives in reducing the availability and misuse of prescription opioids may have played a role in the increased use of heroin and related overdose seen in the United States beginning

[dd]References 85, 86, 151, 152, 613, 711.
[ee]References 18, 200, 279, 485, 486, 497, 499, 669.
[ff]References 108, 110, 211, 212, 279, 349, 352, 406, 631.

• BOX 54.4 Prevention Strategies and Decreased Methadone-Related Overdose

- 2005—SAMHSA released Treatment Improvement Protocol (TIP) 43 "Medication-Assisted Treatment for Opioid Addiction in Opioid Treatment Programs."[115] Provided guidance on the safe use of methadone for the treatment of opioid use disorder
- 2006—FDA alert – "Methadone Use for Pain Control May Result in Death and Life-Threatening Changes in Breathing and Heart Beat." Warned about the risks of death, overdose, and cardiac arrhythmias when prescribing methadone for pain; revised the recommended dosing interval from every 3–4 hours to every 8–12 hours[267]
- 2007—SAMHSA released "Guidelines for the Accreditation of Opioid Treatment Programs."[625] Provided further recommendations for ensuring safe use of methadone in treatment programs mid-2000s (ongoing). Physician/Practitioner Clinical Support System (PCSS), funded by SAMHSA; coordinated by AAAP, AOAAM, APA, and ASAM, provided mentoring and continuing medical education focused on the use of medication-assisted treatment (initially buprenorphine but later including methadone) and the use of opioids in the management of pain (with a strong focus on methadone)
- Late 2000s (ongoing)—Opioid Treatment Program Clinical Staff Education, funded by SAMHSA, provided in-person trainings across the country on the safe use of methadone through best practices; provided technical assistance to programs providing methadone treatment
- 2008—Restriction of 40 mg methadone formulation to opioid use disorder treatment programs; coordinated effort of DEA and methadone manufacturers, attempted to better determine the source of diverted methadone, and attempted to control the availability and diversion of higher dosage form
- 2009—Recommendations for substantial reduction of the calculated dose on conventional equianalgesic conversion tables when switching from another opioid to methadone.[16,260,379]
- 2011—SAMHSA issued a document requesting that OTPs check prescription drug monitoring databases; increased importance because federal confidentiality law 42-CFR Part 2 prohibits the recording of methadone dispensed from an OTP into a state's PDMP
- 2012—REMS for methadone required by FDA
- 2013—States began removing methadone from preferred drug list for treatment of pain[531]; approximately one-third had done so by late 2016
- 2013—ASAM released a consensus statement on safe methadone induction and stabilization[32]
- 2014—APS issued a clinical practice guideline on the use of methadone for pain[123]
- 2014—AAPM recommended against methadone as a preferred analgesic[8,493]
- 2015—SAMHSA released a revision of their "Federal Guidelines for Opioid Treatment Programs"; provided further recommendations on improving safety when dispensing methadone[628]
- 2016—CDC published "CDC Guideline for Prescribing Opioids for Chronic Pain"[211,212]; recommended that methadone not be the first choice for a long-acting opioid and recommended that only clinicians who are familiar with methadone's unique risk profile and are prepared to educate and closely monitor their patients consider prescribing methadone for pain
- 2016—CMS issued recommendations on best practices for addressing prescription opioid addiction and overdose[114]; focused on steps insurers can take to reduce harms associated with methadone use for pain

AAAP, *American Academy of Addiction Psychiatry*; AAPM, *American Academy of Pain Medicine*; AOAAM, *American Osteopathic Academy of Addiction Medicine*; APA, *American Psychiatric Association*; APS, *American Pain Society*; ASAM, *American Society of Addiction Medicine*; CDC, *Centers for Disease Control and Prevention*; CMS, *Centers for Medicare & Medicaid Services*; FDA, *US Food and Drug Administration*; OTP, *Opioid Treatment Program*; REMS, *Risk Evaluation and Mitigation Strategies*; SAMHSA, *Substance Abuse and Mental Health Services Administration*.

around 2010,[gg] although this is far from a universally held belief.[hh] Similarly, it is not clear how many chronic pain patients are negatively affected by these same efforts as they have increased difficulty accessing opioids for appropriate use.[357]

Provider Education

Various initiatives to educate physicians and other health care providers have focused on education about evidence-based pain management, prescribing of controlled substances, and identification of substance misuse and use disorders.[492] Although generally believed to be effective at increasing knowledge, the evidence as to whether or not there are actual improvements in pain treatment or prescribing practices with provider education is limited.[ii] Some states require such education as part of the medical license renewal process, and there have been recommendations to include such education as a part of DEA registration renewal.[268,269]

Providers across the spectrum of medical practice continue to endorse insufficient education in pain or pain management.[326,332] The Office of National Drug Control Policy[497] recognized the need for evidence-based education for providers to identify, prevent, and treat substance use disorders and safe prescribing for pain. Partnered with National Institute on Drug Abuse (NIDA), the federal government released NIDAMED continuing medical education (CME) modules on opioid use disorders and pain management in 2012. In the 2 years after its debut, more than 90,000 providers had accessed and completed these modules.[663] At the state level as of 2017, 23 states and D.C. have developed requirements by statute, regulation, or board guidelines mandating continuing education in prescribing controlled substances, pain management, and identifying substance use disorders.[479] The 2011 Prescription Drug Abuse Prevention plan called for congressional amendment of federal law to require prescribers requesting DEA registration to participate in mandatory training on responsible opioid prescribing practices as a precondition to receiving a DEA number[663] but, as of 2017, participation in continuing education remains voluntary.

In 2009, the Food and Drug Administration (FDA) announced a Risk Evaluation and Mitigation Strategy (REMS) for extended-release (ER) and long-acting (LA) opioid medications.[268] This action required the producers of opioid medications to self-fund CME programming to prescribers at little or no cost based on a predetermined educational blueprint developed by the FDA[271] (Box 54.5).

Education about pain management in American medical schools has traditionally been very limited, with an average of less than 10 hours dedicated to the topic.[453] In 2016, the Association of American Medical Colleges (AAMC) released a statement committing to continued curriculum development and research efforts to elucidate addiction, pain, the brain, and behavior. More than 70 medical schools signed this statement in solidarity.

In March of 2016, the CDC released official guidelines for prescribing opioids for chronic pain,[211,212] targeting primary care providers in the outpatient setting who treat patients with chronic, noncancer pain. Existing guidelines developed by various professional associations and federal agencies shared common components such as dosing thresholds and risk mitigation strategies.[492] The guidelines were designed to assist with (1) determining when to initiate or continue opioids for chronic pain outside of active

---

[gg]References 127, 130, 146, 147, 149, 180, 407.
[hh]References 92, 146, 147, 211, 212, 326, 353, 357.
[ii]References 153, 158, 235, 317, 360, 413, 417, 656, 664, 727.

• BOX 54.5   FDA REMS for ER/LA Opioids: Content of Required Training for Prescribers

1. General information for safe opioid prescribing
   a. Patient selection and assessment
      i. Determine goal of therapy
      ii. Assessment of the risk of abuse, including history of substance abuse and serious mental illness
      iii. When relevant, determining if patient is opioid tolerant
   b. Considerations when prescribing opioids
      i. Pharmacokinetics and potential for overdose
      ii. Addiction, abuse, and misuse
      iii. Intentional abuse by patient or household contacts
      iv. Interactions with other medications/substances
   c. Managing patients taking opioids
      i. Establishing goals for treatment and evaluating pain control
      ii. Use of Patient Provider Agreements (PPAs)
      iii. Adherence to a treatment plan
      iv. Recognizing aberrant behavior
      v. Managing adverse events
   d. Initiating and modifying dosing of opioids for chronic pain
      i. As first opioid
      ii. Converting from one opioid to another
      iii. Converting from immediate-release to extended-release and long-acting products
      iv. Converting from one extended-release and long-acting product to another
      v. To effect/tolerability
      vi. How to deal with missed doses
   e. Maintenance
      i. Reassessment over time
      ii. Tolerance
   f. Monitoring patients for misuse and abuse
      i. Utilization of prescription monitoring programs to identify potential abuse
      ii. Understanding the role of drug testing
      iii. Screening and referral for substance abuse treatment
   g. How to discontinue opioid therapy when it is not needed any longer
2. Product-specific information
3. Patient counseling
   a. Information about prescribed opioid
   b. How to take opioid properly
      i. Adherence to dosing regimen
      ii. Risk from breaking, chewing, crushing certain products
      iii. Symptoms of overdose
   c. Reporting adverse effects
   d. Concomitant use of other CNS depressants, alcohol, or illegal drugs
   e. Discontinuation of opioid
   f. Risks associated with sharing, i.e., overdose prevention
   g. Proper storage in the household
      i. Avoiding accidental exposure
   h. Avoiding unsafe exposure by preventing theft and proper disposal
      i. Purpose and content of PPA

ER/LA, Extended-release and long-acting; FDA, US Food and Drug Administration; REMS, Risk Evaluation and Mitigation Strategy.
Excerpted from FDA Extended-Release (ER) and Long-Acting (LA) Opioid Analgesics Risk Evaluation and Mitigation Strategy (REMS); http://www.fda.gov/Drugs/DrugSafety/InformationbyDrugClass/ucm163647.htm.

---

cancer treatment, palliative care, and end-of-life care; (2) opioid selection, dosage, duration, follow-up, and discontinuation; and (3) assessment of risk and addressing harms of opioid use.

In the summer of 2016, as a part of his "Turn The TideRx" initiative, the Surgeon General mailed a letter to over 2.3 million health care professionals urging them to pledge to (1) educate themselves on how to treat pain safely and effectively, (2) screen their patients for opioid use disorders (and refer for evidence-based treatment if present), and (3) talk about and treat addiction as a chronic illness, not a moral failing. A companion website was created with various resources: http://turnthetiderx.org/

Prescription Guidelines

Implementation of prescribing guidelines is another means by which inappropriate prescribing of opioids can be reduced. National medical specialty organizations (such as the American College of Emergency Physicians and American Pain Society), large health care systems (such as the Veterans Administration/Department of Defense), health insurance companies, local and state health care agencies (New York City; Washington State) and hospitals have all issued clinical practice guidelines to improve quality of care and reduce negative outcomes through use of evidence-based practices. This has been done for specific drugs as well as for the prescribing of all opioids. Prescribing guidelines typically include limits on medications and formulations, initiation and titration of dose, maximum dose, drug switching, screening tools to assess risk for misuse, written treatment agreements, urine drug testing, and pill counts.[493]

Evidence that these recommendations can impact prescribing patterns is somewhat limited,[37,153,308,418,676] but some studies have shown reductions in number of patients managed with high-dose opioids, reductions in daily doses of prescribed opioids, increased percentages of providers reporting that they avoid using long-acting opioids for acute pain or in combination with benzodiazepines, and increases in use of drug screening by physicians.[jj] Effects on actual overdoses are difficult to determine but several studies have reported decreased deaths related to the use of prescribing guidelines.[138,275,277]

Prescription Drug Monitoring Programs

A prescription drug monitoring program (PDMP) is a state-run, statewide electronic database that collects information on prescribed/dispensed controlled substances (and, in a few cases, other drugs of concern) and makes that information available to authorized users. Similar programs exist in Canada,[612] Australia, and other European countries. California was the first state to establish such a (nonelectronic) monitoring program in 1939. In 2005, Congress passed the National All Schedules Prescription Electronic Reporting (NASPER) Act, authorizing federal funding and support for PDMPs. As of 2015, 49 states had active PDMPs in place.[478] Specifics of these programs vary considerably from state to state, with some focused more on improved clinical care and others focused more on law enforcement and diversion prevention. Programs differ as to whether they proactively report prescribing patterns to licensing boards, law enforcement, or insurance providers; whether prescribers/dispensers are required to register; whether clinicians must check the PDMP before prescribing; and if the PDMP is integrated with electronic health records. Twenty-nine states have mandatory access provisions in which regulation requires prescribers to query the PDMP for certain circumstances, such as in worker's compensation cases or prior to prescribing in a pain management clinic. The DEA does not play a role in the management of PDMPs.

These programs are generally believed to be helpful in identifying major sources of "doctor shopping" and prescription drug

diversion as well as improper prescribing and dispensing.[kk] Clinician acceptability, use, and actual impact on prescribing practices are variable.[256,309,348,366] A multicenter survey of emergency room physicians revealed that only 59% of respondents were registered for access to their respective state PDMP.[539] In a pre- and postevaluation of the implementation of Florida's PDMP and "pill mill laws," there was a small decrease in opioid prescriptions and morphine milligram equivalents prescribed. This was limited to prescribers and patients with the highest baseline opioid prescribing and use.[564] Another study of medical providers in Ohio emergency departments found that 41% of those given PDMP data altered their prescribing for patients found to be receiving multiple simultaneous controlled substance prescriptions.[23]

The state of Wyoming found that, when physicians and pharmacists received unsolicited PDMP reports concerning likely doctor shoppers, the number of patients meeting the criterion for doctor shopping dropped markedly, suggesting that PDMP reports prompted prescribers to reduce the availability of controlled substances to patients appearing to engage in doctor shopping.[546-548] In British Columbia, within 6 months of the inception of their PDMP, medically inappropriate prescriptions for opioids fell by 33% and for benzodiazepines by 49%.[210] Another study from Canada, however, found no difference in opioid prescribing between provinces with and without a PDMP.[261] Another study looking at disabled patients in the United States receiving Medicare found no correlation of PDMPs with reductions in opioid prescribing.[442] A study in France found a significant decrease in doctor shopping for buprenorphine with no effect on availability of the medication for treatment.[545]

Fewer studies have attempted to correlate the presence of a PDMP with reductions in overdose. One study in Florida found a 25% decrease in oxycodone-caused deaths after implementation of that state's PDMP in 2011.[199] Another study found no difference in the incidence of opioid overdose mortality between states with and without PDMPs,[523] whereas another study looking at states with PDMPs as of 2008 found wide variability across the United States, with some states recording increases in overdose fatalities and others, decreases.[409] A more recent study looked at 35 states that implemented a PDMP between 1999 and 2013 and found that a state's implementation of a program was associated with an average reduction of 1.12 opioid-related overdose deaths per 100,000 population in the year after implementation and that programs with more robust characteristics (such as monitoring for a greater numbers of drugs and weekly updating of data) had greater reductions in deaths, compared with states whose programs did not have these characteristics.[515]

Insurance Company Monitoring, Pill Limits, and Care Coordination

Insurance companies and pharmacy benefit managers (PBMs) have access to medical and pharmacy claims data that can be used to identify inappropriate prescribing practices and potential misuse of controlled substances by patients.[365,568] Various programs such as Patient Review and Restriction (PRR) programs (which limit "high utilizers" to single prescribers/pharmacies) and Drug Utilization Review (DUR) programs (which notify prescribers of patients with potential problematic use based on claims data) may help reduce misuse/diversion of controlled substances. Similarly, requirements for prior authorization and limits on medication quantity may also reduce misuse and diversion.[1,104]

[jj]References 138, 275, 277, 278, 342, 382, 468, 471, 493, 540, 587.

[kk]References 56, 306, 308, 317, 388, 470, 554, 655, 686, 717.

Although these interventions certainly make sense as useful interventions to decrease misuse and diversion of controlled substance, actual studies to support this are fairly limited.[317] Studies from individual state Medicaid and commercial insurance programs have found decreases in individual patient medication utilization as well as overall numbers of controlled substance prescriptions when PRR and DUR programs are used[ll] but some have not found a difference.[442] Similarly, studies looking at prior authorization requirements and quantity limits and patient care coordination have found reductions in amount of controlled substances prescribed and patient-level reductions in use.[287,469,489,508,509,681] One study found that the inclusion of methadone on the preferred drug lists (PDLs) of two states was associated with higher rates of fatal and nonfatal methadone overdose compared to a nearby state that did not include methadone on their PDL.[255]

FDA Changes in Scheduling and Postmarketing Surveillance of Opioids

Once the most widely prescribed medication in the United States (with over 137 million prescriptions per year), hydrocodone was moved from Schedule III to Schedule II by the DEA in 2014. One study found that the rescheduling resulted in an overall reduction of 26.3 million hydrocodone prescriptions (22% decrease form the year before the change), and 1.1 billion fewer hydrocodone tablets dispensed (16% decrease in the 12 months after rescheduling).[356] The study was not able to analyze the actual impact on overdoses.

In early 2016, the FDA also revised the requirements for extended-release and long-acting (or ER/LA) opioids to include additional postmarketing observational studies and clinical trials to assess the known serious risks of misuse, abuse, addiction, overdose, and death.[272]

Prescription Drug Identification Laws

Twenty-five states have laws either mandating or allowing pharmacists to request identification before dispensing prescription drugs. Most of the mandatory identification laws require a dispensing pharmacist to ask for identification if the person picking up the prescription is unknown to him or her. Five states have discretionary identification laws that allow the dispenser to demand patient identification rather than mandating that he or she do so.[105,477]

Electronic Prescriptions for Controlled Substances (EPCS)

Another attempt to reduce the diversion of controlled substances (as well as potential dosing mistakes due to illegible handwriting) is through the use of electronic prescribing. In 2010, the DEA published *Interim Final Rule for Electronic Prescriptions for Controlled Substances*, which allowed for Schedule II, III, and IV medications to be prescribed through electronic means as long as the prescriber uses a software application that conforms to regulatory standards and two-factor authentication.[17] The use of EPCS can also increase the likelihood that prescribers will check the PDMP prior to prescribing. Several states have passed legislation mandating the use of EPCS for controlled substances. No studies have yet demonstrated an impact on availability or misuse of controlled substances.

Laws Against Pill Mills and Doctor Shopping

In the first decade of the 21st century, a growing amount of attention was directed to the role of medical providers in the availability of misused opioids. Political and public concern over this issue led to, in early 2016, for the first time in the United States, a physician being convicted of murder for inappropriately prescribing opioids to patients who subsequently died of overdose. As a result of such concerns, various states have attempted to strengthen laws to decrease the ability of physicians to inappropriately prescribe opioids through underregulated facilities (pill mill laws) and identify/report patients who appear to be obtaining opioids inappropriately from multiple providers (doctor shopping laws; multiple provider laws). Pill mill laws typically require that a pain clinic be owned by a physician, that it not dispense opioids directly from the clinic, that it be registered with the DEA, that it agree to inspection, and that all prescriptions be reported to a state agency. Doctor shopping laws typically grant legal immunity to prescribers for reporting patients suspected of inappropriate prescription seeking. About one-fourth of US states have specific pill mill laws and about one-third have doctor shopping laws.[317]

Some studies have shown a decrease in actual numbers of clinics and opioid prescriptions[201,274,632] as well as overdoses[353] related to these laws. DEA and state law enforcement raids of pill mills (through Operation Pill Nation and Operation Oxy Alley) also contributed to the 27% decline in opioid deaths in Florida between 2010 and 2012.[108] In addition, in July of 2011, Florida instituted a law prohibiting physicians from dispensing Schedule II and III medications from their offices. Overdose deaths in the state attributed to hydrocodone product decrease from 315 in the year prior to the change to 245 in the year following the change (a 22.2% decline), whereas the prescribing rate of hydrocodone products per 100,000 population declined 9.7%. During the same period, overdose deaths attributed to oxycodone products declined 51.5% (from 1516 to 735), and the prescribing rate of oxycodone per 100,000 population declined 24%.[353]

Screening Pain Patients for Substance Misuse Risk

Universal screening of potential opioid recipients for risk of opioid misuse is another important measure in reducing opioid misuse. Various screening tools have been validated for this purpose including the Opioid Risk Tool (ORT); the Diagnosis, Intractability, Risk, and Efficacy inventory (DIRE); and the Screener and Opioid Assessment for Patients With Pain (SOAPP).[27,466,517,694] Similarly, once opioid treatment has been initiated, patients can be monitored on an ongoing basis with tools like the Current Opioid Misuse Measure.[80] For patients with a history of opioid or other substance use disorder, further assessment is necessary and increased care should be taken to reduce the risk of opioid misuse if the use of an opioid is determined to be necessary for pain management. Potential measures include enlistment of family members to monitor medication at home, increased "call-backs" and "pill counts," and prescriptions for smaller amounts of medication with more frequent follow-up visits. The impact of such measures on overdose has not been studied.

Public Awareness/Education

Public education has been a mainstay of prevention efforts to reduce substance use and misuse for many decades. From the Partnership For A Drug-Free America's 1987 "This Is Your Brain On Drugs" public service announcement (and its 1997 and 2016 updates) to their "Mind Your Meds" campaign (launched in 2013 and continuing through 2016), multi-media messages, often aimed at adolescents, have attempted to portray the risks of substance use and decrease the social acceptability of use. Although often felt to be helpful (or, at least, not harmful), it is generally

---

[ll]References 104, 182, 297, 339, 640, 733.

difficult to truly measure effects on actual substance use/misuse. However, examples of randomized trials of educational interventions (Iowa Strengthening Families Program; PROSPER) aimed at youth and/or families have shown effects on reducing prescription and illicit drug use in young adulthood.[250,577,611]

In another attempt to educate the general public about addiction as a whole, in November 2016, the US Surgeon General released the office's first ever report on the topic, *Facing Addiction in America: The Surgeon General's Report on Alcohol, Drugs, and Health*.[665] Another source of public education around the safe use, storage, and disposal of ER/LA opioids is through the REMS program (mentioned previously), which also requires drug manufacturers to produce medication guides and patient counseling documents for distribution by prescribers and pharmacies (Box 54.6; see Box 54.5).

Efforts focused on educating the public about safe storage and disposal of controlled substances have shown promise.[352,417,498] One example is the "Use Only as Directed" campaign in Utah targeted at adults through television and radio public service announcements, posters, patient information cards, bookmarks, and a website. This campaign promoted storage of **medications** in a safe place and disposal of unused or expired medications. In follow-up, 18% of **respondents** reported that they disposed of controlled substances as a result of the campaign and that they were also less likely to take a prescription medication that was not prescribed to them by a physician after the campaign.[352] The actual impact of such initiatives on overdose is not clear.

Prescription Medication Disposal and "Take-Back"

Another way to help reduce misuse of prescription opioids is to provide a safe means by which individuals can dispose of unused/expired medications in an environmentally safe manner. The Office of National Drug Control Policy (ONDCP) and FDA published guidelines on the safe disposal of unused medications, and in 2010, The Secure and Responsible Drug Disposal Act was passed to amend the Controlled Substances Act to allow a patient to deliver controlled substances to an entity that is authorized by federal law to dispose of them. DEA-sponsored National Prescription Drug Take-Back Day began in 2010 and has been held one or two times per year since then. The DEA has reported that the program has been successful, having collected almost 6.5 million pounds over the first 11 events, although it does not differentiate controlled substances from others.[221,224,303] As of 2014, the DEA also permitted manufacturers, distributors, law enforcement officials, treatment programs, pharmacies, and health care facilities to become authorized collectors of prescription medications.[218] Many jurisdictions have installed permanent drug drop boxes in law enforcement and health care facilities. Although these local efforts have been reported to be successful in removing controlled substances from the community,[304] the impact of these efforts on overdose is difficult to determine.

A related program called the fentanyl "Patch 4 Patch" Return program has been implemented in a number of jurisdictions in Canada beginning in 2013.[403,507] In it, a patient who is prescribed fentanyl patches for pain management must return the used patches in order to get new ones. Several of the jurisdictions have seen significant decreases in fentanyl-related overdoses since implementing the program.[518]

Abuse-Deterrent Formulations

Many individuals who misuse prescription opioids for nontherapeutic or recreational reasons often do so by chewing the pill to release the drug quickly, crushing it for increased ease of insufflation, or solubilizing it for intravenous injection. The goal of most abuse-deterrent formulations (ADFs) is to impose mechanical or chemical (such as gelling agents) barriers that make crushing or chewing the pill difficult.[3,467,558] Other strategies include combination of an opioid antagonist with an agonist (used with Suboxone) that largely blocks the μ-opioid effects when the medication is injected[269,270]; the addition of a substance which would

---

• BOX 54.6 REMS Patient Counseling Document

Patient Counseling Document on Extended-Release/Long-Acting Opioid Analgesics
Patient Name:
The DOs and DON'Ts of Extended-Release/Long-Acting Opioid Analgesics
DO:
- Read the Medication Guide
- Take your medicine exactly as prescribed
- Store your medicine away from children and in a safe place
- Flush unused medicine down the toilet
- Call your health care provider for medical advice about side effects. You may report side effects to FDA at 1-800-FDA-1088.
- Call 911 or your local emergency service right away if:
  - You take too much medicine
  - You have trouble breathing or shortness of breath
  - A child has taken this medicine by accident
- Talk to your health care provider:
  - If the dose you are taking does not control your pain
  - About any side effects you may be having
  - About all the medicines you take, including over-the-counter medicines, vitamins, and dietary supplements

DON'T:
- Give your medicine to others
- Take medicine unless it was prescribed for you
- Stop taking your medicine without talking to your health care provider
- Cut, break, chew, crush, dissolve, snort, or inject your medicine. If you cannot swallow your medicine whole, talk to your health care provider.
- Drink alcohol while taking this medicine

*For additional information on your medicine go to **dailymed.nlm.nih.gov***

Patient Counseling Document on Extended-Release/Long-Acting Opioid Analgesics
Patient Name:
Patient Specific Information:
_____
_____
_____
_____

Take this card with you every time you see your health care provider and tell him/her:
- Your complete medical and family history, including any history of substance abuse or mental illness
- If you are pregnant or are planning to become pregnant
- The cause, severity, and nature of your pain
- Your treatment goals
- All the medicines you take, including over-the-counter (nonprescription) medicines, vitamins, and dietary supplements
- Any side effects you may be having

Take your opioid pain medicine exactly as prescribed by your health care provider.

From FDA Risk Evaluation and Mitigation Strategy (REMS) for Extended-Release and Long-Acting Opioids. https://www.fda.gov/media/86281/download.

cause aversion if the formulation is altered (such as a nasal mucosa irritant); delivery systems that are difficult to manipulate (such as depot injections or subcutaneous implants); and prodrugs that require enzymatic activation in the body.[255] A novel form of abuse deterrence currently under development, known as XpiRx (pronounced "expire"), uses technology that "deactivates" the opioid in a tablet after a certain amount of time.

Abuse-deterrent formulations FDA-approved in the United States include OxyContin, an ER oxycodone tablet formulated to be more difficult to crush, break, or dissolve, and when dissolved, forms a viscous gel that is difficult to inject; Embeda, an ER morphine capsule formulated from pellets that contain a sequestered core of naltrexone (if the pellets are crushed, chewed, or dissolved, naltrexone is released, blocking morphine-induced euphoria); Hysingla, an ER hydrocodone tablet formulation that, when dissolved, forms a viscous gel that is difficult to inject through a hypodermic needle; Xtampza, an ER oxycodone capsule that contains microspheres formulated in such a way that is difficult to manipulate; Arymo, an ER morphine product tablet formulated with a polymer matrix that, when dissolved, forms a viscous gel that is difficult to inject through a hypodermic needle; Zohydro, an ER hydrocodone capsule formulation that incorporates excipients that form a viscous gel when the capsules are crushed and dissolved; and Targiniq, an opioid agonist/antagonist combination containing ER oxycodone and naloxone.

A number of studies have shown that the reformulation of Oxycontin has led to a significant reduction in misuse and related overdose.[mm] A study of opioid users entering substance abuse treatment found a significant reduction in self-reported misuse of reformulated Oxycontin following its release in 2010, although one-third of those who had used the pre- and post-reformulation products reported that they had successfully defeated the ADF mechanism and continued to inhale or inject the Oxycontin, and another significant number continued to misuse it orally.[128] In addition, that study found a significant rise in the initial use of heroin following the introduction of reformulated Oxycontin, although the authors stress that causality is difficult to establish. Another study found an increase in heroin and immediate-release oxycodone misuse associated with the decreased Oxycontin use.[150] Yet another study using national opioid prescription insurance claims found that the estimated prescription opioid overdose rate was 20% lower 2 years after introduction of the new formulation, but the estimated heroin overdose rate increased by 23%.[397] Other studies, however, have not found an increase in heroin use associated with a decrease in Oxycontin misuse.[92,328] More research is needed to better understand the true impact of these products on opioid use and overdose as a whole.[38,402]

Nonreinforcing Opioids

Medication development efforts continue attempts to develop opioid medications that provide the same amount of analgesia as typical opioid agonists without reinforcement or respiratory depression. One example is BU08028, a novel opioid compound that acts as an agonist at mixed μ-opioid peptide (MOP)/nociceptin-orphanin FQ peptide (NOP) receptors, and appears to have no tolerance, addiction potential, or respiratory depression.[205,410]

Possibly related to this, there are several studies that have shown an association between states with medical marijuana laws

and decreased urine positivity for opioids in individuals involved in fatal car crashes[346] and decreases in treatment admissions for opioid use disorder[543] and opioid-related overdose deaths.[31,543] The authors hypothesize that individuals in these areas are more likely to use marijuana for pain management. It is not possible to determine any causal relationship from these studies.

Increased Law Enforcement Interdiction

For decades, law enforcement interdiction, primarily focused on illicit drugs such as cocaine and heroin, had been a major component of the US War on Drugs. The High Intensity Drug Trafficking Areas (HIDTA) program was created as part of the Anti-Drug Abuse Act of 1988 with the purpose of providing assistance to federal, state, local, and tribal law enforcement agencies operating in areas determined to be critical drug-trafficking regions of the United States. The 28 HIDTAs, located in 48 states, Puerto Rico, the US Virgin Islands, and the District of Columbia cover approximately 17.6% of all counties in the United States and 63.5% of the US population.[501] A program known as the Drug Market Intervention (DMI) began in 2004 as an effort to bring together drug dealers, their families, law enforcement officials, drug treatment and other social service providers, and community leaders to help eliminate "open-air" drug markets.[487]

Beginning in the late 1990s, more focus was placed on diversion of controlled prescription medications. Since 2008, the DEA has partnered with various federal, state, and local law enforcement agencies to increase the number of Tactical Diversion Squads (TDS) targeting prescription opioid diversion. The DEA has also increased surveillance of DEA registrants with more diversion investigators.[574] Operation Pill Nation and Operation Oxy Alley (mentioned above) are examples of initiatives of the Organized Crime Drug Enforcement Task Force (OCDETF) targeting the illicit distribution of prescription opioids. Prescription Drug Monitoring Programs (or PDMPs) are also used in some states by law enforcement to look for providers who are overprescribing. The actual effect of law enforcement interdiction on medication misuse and overdose is not clear.

Secondary Prevention

Over the past 15–20 years, a growing amount of effort has been put into reducing/preventing opioid overdose and increasing help for those already addicted to opioids. Many of these interventions can be thought of as being both secondary and tertiary prevention, focused on reducing overdose and reducing related fatalities.

Prescriber Education

In addition to education aimed at reducing misuse and diversion of controlled substances mentioned earlier, some prescriber education has focused specifically on measures to reduce overdose. The risk evaluation and mitigation strategy (or REMS) for extended-release (ER) and long-acting (LA) opioid drugs specifically addresses the issue of minimizing risk for overdose. Consensus recommendations on the use of methadone for pain have also encouraged substantial reduction in calculated equianalgesic doses when converting from other opioids to methadone.[260,379] Another effort to increase prescriber awareness of the risk of combining opioids and benzodiazepines occurred in the fall of 2016 when the FDA added a Black Box Warning to all opioids and benzodiazepines highlighting the increased risk for overdose if taken in combination. As with primary prevention efforts, actual impact on overdose is difficult to determine.

[mm]References 81, 92, 129, 150, 328, 591, 592, 593.

Public/Opioid User Awareness/Education

Along with general information about substance misuse/abuse/use disorders, a growing amount of effort has been put into educating drug users and the general public about measures that can specifically help prevent overdose. Often provided through syringe exchange and other outreach programs, this messaging includes encouragement of practices such as "never use alone," "make an overdose prevention plan with your partner," "don't combine opioids with sedatives or alcohol," and "use a much lower amount if you have not used opioids for a while." Other efforts such as REMS (mentioned above) have specific messaging focused on preventing overdose (see Boxes 54.1 and 54.5). The actual impact of these efforts on overdose is difficult to determine.

Local Overdose Fatality Review Teams

Fatality review teams began in the late 1970s as a way to attempt to reduce future pediatric deaths by reviewing child fatality cases using a multidisciplinary team.[230] Overdose Fatality Review Teams (OFRT) use the same concept by gathering representatives from various agencies such as medical examiner's office, emergency medical services, drug treatment, social services, law enforcement, medical treatment, mental health treatment, and public health to review fatality cases to determine if there were things that might have helped prevent the death. The information is then used to inform policy and programmatic changes that might help prevent future overdoses. Although there have been no studies that have looked at the specific impact of these programs on overdose rates, the feeling that they help increase interagency communication and collaboration and resultant prevention efforts has been reported.[553]

Increased Drug Treatment

A great deal of evidence shows that proper treatment of opioid use disorders helps reduce opioid misuse and reduces opioid-related overdose.[5,6,192,193,196,440] Medication-assisted treatment (MAT), opioid maintenance treatment (OMT), or opioid substitution therapy are common terms used to refer to the use of methadone or buprenorphine for ongoing treatment. Although their use has been hampered by various federal and local policies/regulations,[134] as well as negative attitudes held by the general public, patients, medical providers, and many clinicians who work in the substance abuse treatment field,[380,680] the support of various government agencies (CDC, ONDCP)[497] and reforms in insurance coverage (Affordable Care Act; state Medicaid expansion) appear to be helping increase their availability.

Various studies in multiple countries have looked at reduced nonfatal and fatal overdose in patients receiving treatment,[nn] whereas others have looked at decreased rates across a larger population as treatment is introduced or expanded.[20,372,406,582] A large prospective cohort study of 10,545 heroin users entering treatment in Italy looked at standardized mortality ratio (SMR) estimates of excess mortality risk for heroin users in and out of treatment compared to the general population. It found that retention in any treatment was associated with decreased overdose compared to out of treatment (hazard ratio 0.09) with 10 overdose deaths in patients while in treatment versus 31 while out of treatment.[192] Another study followed a cohort of 296 Australian heroin users admitted to methadone maintenance over 15 years and found that patients were one-fourth as likely to die (included

overdose and suicide) while receiving methadone maintenance as those not in treatment.[86] Another Australian study, however, found that fatal overdose rates were higher in the first 28 days in patients receiving methadone versus buprenorphine or naltrexone implant and that, after 28 days, buprenorphine seemed to be the most protective against nonfatal overdose.[369] A meta-analysis of 19 treatment cohorts (including 122,885 individuals treated with methadone and 15,831 treated with buprenorphine) found that all cause rates of mortality were 11.3 per 1000 person years for those in methadone treatment versus 36.1 per 1000 person years for those out of treatment. Similarly, all-cause mortality was 4.3 per 1000 person years for those in buprenorphine treatment and 9.5 per 1000 person years for those out of treatment. Overdose mortality was similarly affected, with rates of 2.6 and 12.7 per 1000 person years for those in and out of methadone treatment, respectively, and 1.4 and 4.6 per 1000 person years for those in and out of buprenorphine treatment.[609]

In France, methadone maintenance was expanded and buprenorphine treatment introduced in 1995. In parallel with these actions, the number of lethal overdoses fell from 564 in 1994 to 393 in 1996 and 143 in 1998 (a 74.6% decrease in 4 years).[20,406] Another study in Baltimore, Maryland found a reduction in fatal heroin overdoses (from a high of 312 in 1999 to a low of 106 in 2008) related to the city's expansion of publicly funded methadone (in 2000) and buprenorphine (in 2003 and 2006) treatment. Both studies caution that it is difficult to rule out other social and public health factors from contributing to some of these results.[20,596]

Oral naltrexone, monthly ER injectable naltrexone (Vivitrol) and subcutaneous naltrexone implants (available in Russia and other countries) are also used. In addition, there are reports of increased overdose rates in patients taking oral naltrexone[291] related to the total loss of tolerance that occurs when taking a μ-opioid agonist. Outcome studies on Vivitrol/naltrexone implant are limited but have not shown increased rates of overdose so far[368,369,386,387,629] and one study with Vivitrol reported no overdoses compared to seven in the treatment as usual group after 18 months.[400] Another study from Australia found decreased rates of overdose in patients who had received a sustained release naltrexone implant,[341] with significantly less overdoses compared to patients receiving the oral naltrexone.[368]

Although difficult to substantiate, there are some who have raised the possibility that diverted maintenance medications (primarily buprenorphine) are largely used for self-management of opioid withdrawal and may help reduce overdose in those individuals using the medication illicitly.[315,465,581]

Safe Injection Facilities

Safe injection facilities (SIFs; variously referred to as Supervised Injecting/Consumption Centers/Rooms/Facilities, Drug Consumption Rooms, or Supervised Injection Services) are legally sanctioned facilities where individuals who use intravenous drugs can inject drugs under medical supervision (although a growing number of facilities target drug use via other routes of administration such as smoking). Such programs began more than three decades ago in Europe. As of 2016, more than 100 such facilities existed in 66 cities in Canada, Australia, and seven European countries (Switzerland, Germany, The Netherlands, Norway, Luxembourg, Spain, and Denmark). SIFs are designed to reduce the health and societal problems associated with injection drug use. Various studies have reported a reduction in opioid overdoses

---

nnReferences 72, 86, 135, 136, 152, 170, 176, 193, 208, 292, 395, 609, 643, 689.

related to SIFs.[oo] One study examined population-based overdose mortality rates for the several-year period before and after Sept 21, 2003, when the Vancouver SIF opened. The fatal overdose rate in the area 500 meters surrounding the SIF decreased by 35% after the opening of the SIF, from 253 to 165 deaths per 100,000 person-years ($P = 0.048$). By contrast, during the same period, the fatal overdose rate in the rest of the city decreased by only 9%, from 7.6 to 6.9 deaths per 100,000 person-years ($P = 0.490$).[431] It has been estimated that the facility has helped avert between 2 and 12 fatal overdoses per year.[456]

A few studies have not found a significant reduction in overdoses attributable to safe consumption facilities, and one found that overdoses, though none fatal, increased significantly within the facility.[185,227,443] As with many of the other prevention initiatives covered, it is very difficult to attribute any reductions in overdose to one intervention as it is often the case that multiple interventions are instituted at roughly the same time.[207]

Heroin Maintenance

Heroin-Assisted Treatment (HAT) [also referred to as poly-morphone-(or diamorphine or diacetylmorphine) Assisted Treatment or Supervised Injectable Heroin (SIH)] has been used in various countries at different times for over a century (including the United States in the early 1900s). It is currently part of standard medical practice for treatment-refractory heroin dependence in Canada, Switzerland, Germany, The Netherlands, and Denmark (as well as the United Kingdom where it can also be used for the treatment of pain). It is also approved in Belgium and Spain for use under research protocols. Several studies have reported a modest reduction in overdose correlated with the introduction of HAT.[pp]

A related clinical trial in Vancouver compared intravenous diacetylmorphine to hydromorphone and found lower overdoses (11 vs. 3, respectively) during the 6-month period of the study.[512] Reports on slow-release morphine, used as an alternative maintenance treatment in several European countries, have not reported on impact on overdose.[351]

Drug Testing

Drug testing/checking has been used for several decades primarily in settings where designer drugs such as 3,4-methylenedioxymethamphetamin (MDMA) are commonly used. More recently, such programs have emerged in Europe and Canada to test samples for the presence of synthetic opioids including fentanyl and some of its analogues.[73,94] The hope is that, if an individual knows that his/her drugs may contain a more potent, illicitly manufactured opioid, that individual might choose not to use the drug or to use a much smaller amount or use in a safe space like a safe consumption facility. Preliminary data from the Insite program in Vancouver, Canada have shown that the testing does influence the choices that the opioid user makes.[708] Further research is needed to determine the actual impact on overdose.

Tertiary Prevention

As mentioned earlier, many initiatives focus on prevention of both overdose and fatalities due to overdose. Most studies or evaluation efforts are unable to distinguish the relative effects of the two.

Public Education/Awareness

As the number of opioid-related overdoses began to increase in the early 2000s, public awareness campaigns began to increase in the affected areas of the United States. As was mentioned under secondary prevention, many of the education efforts were focused on both preventing overdose and preventing fatalities. Many of the education efforts were also combined with the provision of naloxone (see below) so the relative benefit of one versus the other is difficult to determine. One study of intravenous drug users found that they had improved knowledge of recognizing and responding to an overdose after viewing posters and leaflets displayed in an addiction treatment program.[69] A large event, International Overdose Awareness Day (August 31), originated in 2001with the aims "... to raise awareness of overdose and reduce the stigma of a drug-related death. It also acknowledges the grief felt by families and friends remembering those who have met death or permanent injury as a result of drug overdose."[347]

Naloxone Distribution to Illicit Opioid Users

Because one of the main risk factors for fatal opioid overdose is having experienced a prior nonfatal overdose and because many overdoses occur in settings where other opioid users are present, there is a strong argument for making naloxone widely available to illicit opioid users. Surveys of current or former illicit drug users have found that most are willing to administer naloxone to an individual who has overdosed.[qq]

The provision of naloxone to heroin users was first discussed in the mid-1990s[166,405,621] with small programs beginning distribution in around 1996.[100] By 2010, approximately 188 overdose education and naloxone distribution (OEND) programs existed in the United States (in 15 states and the District of Columbia) with many more added in the following 6 years. Multiple professional societies and government agencies have also made naloxone distribution a key component to their recommendations for battling the opioid overdose epidemic, including the American Academy of Addiction Psychiatry,[7] the American Heart Association (as part of the updated guidelines for cardiopulmonary resuscitation,[399] the American Medical Association,[9] the American Society of Addiction Medicine,[12] the American Pharmacists Association,[10] the American Psychiatric Association,[7] the Centers for Disease Control and Prevention,[213] the Office of National Drug Control Policy,[499] the Substance Abuse and Mental Health Services Administration,[627] the World Health Organization,[715] and the United Nations Office on Drugs and Crime.[647,661] Although naloxone is not classified as an over-the-counter medication by the FDA in the United States, a number of states have passed legislation for it to be distributed directly from a pharmacy under a blanket standing order.[249,620] Programs also exist in more than 15 other countries in Europe, Asia, and Australia,[rr] with more programs being added as the World Health Organization has encouraged the use of naloxone.

A survey of the 188 programs in the United States in 2010 found that they had distributed naloxone to over 50,000 individuals and had received reports of over 10,000 administrations of naloxone.[100] By 2014, these numbers had increased dramatically, with over 150,000 laypersons having received training and naloxone and program participants reporting reversal of more than 26,000 overdoses.[702] Various other studies have

---

[oo]References 198, 240, 241, 245, 431, 456, 457, 541, 542, 572, 576, 588, 618, 671.
[pp]References 258, 316, 429, 511, 528, 672, 673.

[qq]References 21, 370, 394, 533, 583, 624, 682.
[rr]References 202, 319, 324, 404, 439, 622, 657.

now shown that distribution of naloxone to opioid users can be done fairly easily and that a significant number of recipients use the naloxone to reverse an overdose.[ss] Although the majority of these studies are based on participant self-report of individuals trained in a single program, several have prospectively followed patient cohorts and found positive results.[202,286,288,622] A systematic review of 17 more rigorous studies found that 20 deaths occurred versus 2336 episodes of naloxone administration, or approximately one death per 123 administrations.[421] In some of the deaths, it is not clear if the victim was still alive when the naloxone was administered.[238]

Several studies have attempted to look at outcomes at a larger, population level. Following the implementation of OEND in various areas of Massachusetts in 2007, an analysis looked at areas with no OEND implementation versus those with low implementation (1–100 people trained per 100,000 population) and high implementation (greater than 100 people trained per 100,000 population). After adjusting for community level demographic and substance use factors, they found 27% and 46% reductions in opioid overdose mortality rates, respectively.[684] Naloxone distribution was also believed to play a major role in the dramatic reduction in heroin overdoses seen in San Francisco (from approximately 180 per year in the late 1990s to 10–11 per year from 2010–2012).[677] Another randomized controlled trial of naloxone distribution to opioid users upon release from prisons (16 prisons; 1685 prisoners) in Scotland showed a significant reduction in overdose fatalities during the period in which naloxone was supplied, although the trial was terminated early because only one-third of the reported naloxone administrations was to the ex-prisoners.[55,516]

One concern is the steadily rising cost of naloxone in the United States over the past 10–15 years. This is partially offset by the growing numbers of commercial and state Medicaid programs that cover the medication. Several studies have shown that OEND programs are cost effective, even if the full cost of the naloxone is absorbed by the program.[143,144]

Naloxone Distribution to Third Parties

Because opioid overdose often occurs when the victim is at home or with friends, family members and other acquaintances are often the best situated to act to administer naloxone. However, unlike the instances of prescribing to illicit opioid users or co-prescribing to individuals taking prescribed opioids chronically, in this case, the person to whom the naloxone is dispensed/prescribed is not the ultimate intended recipient of the medication, thus it does not neatly fall under the typical practice of medicine.[79] To address this, most states have created or amended laws to allow for the legitimate prescription to a third party (as well as some immunity from prosecution for the prescriber). Since 2001 when New Mexico first enacted such legislation, all 50 states and the District of Columbia have passed some type of law intended to increase prescribing and/or provide immunity to medical professionals who prescribe or dispense naloxone. The majority of these laws were passed between 2010 and 2015 and promote the use of naloxone in addition to training and education on recognizing and preventing overdoses.[186,189,488]

There are fewer publications available looking specifically at naloxone distribution to nonopioid using third parties, but available evidence suggests that the programs are easy to implement

and that trainees retain information even 12 months following the training,[132,408] and that these programs also contribute to a reduction in overdose fatalities.[215,684]

Naloxone Co-Prescribing to Patients Taking Opioids

Although not traditionally done by most prescribers and not always accepted by some,[51] the co-prescribing of naloxone with opioids (prescribed/dispensed either for pain or the treatment of opioid use disorder) has been encouraged increasingly through various initiatives including guidelines from the US Department of Veterans Affairs and the CDC.[211,212,505,683] Along with this are recommendations for opioid prescribers to assess all patients for risk of misuse and risk of overdose, and to educate patients and significant others about factors that can increase the risk of overdose (such as concurrent alcohol or sedative use) as well as safe storage of opioids.[40,181] Several studies have shown that this practice is feasible, generally well-accepted by patients, and associated with clinical benefits.[39] The NOSE (Naloxone for Opioid Safety Evaluation) study found that, in a chronic pain population, patients who had been prescribed naloxone had fewer opioid-related emergency department visits than those who were not prescribed naloxone.[141]

Naloxone With Law Enforcement and Other First Responders

In many areas, law enforcement personnel are likely to arrive at an overdose scene prior to emergency medical personnel. Traditionally, officers might be taught cardiopulmonary resuscitation but would not carry or administer any medications. As many areas have initiated and expanded distribution and prescribing of naloxone to opioid users and third parties, efforts have also been put in place to train law enforcement officers in recognizing and responding to overdose, including the use of naloxone. Studies have shown that law enforcement officers are generally in favor of naloxone distribution.[187,551] The ONDCP and the Department of Justice (DOJ) have urged police departments to have officers carry naloxone and the DOJ released a Naloxone Toolkit to help facilitate the increased use of naloxone by law enforcement officers.[667] As of late 2016, thousands of local and state police departments had implemented such programs.

Good Samaritan Laws

Related to the expansion of availability of naloxone to third parties is the issue of encouraging individuals to seek further medical assistance in the event of an overdose. Fear of arrest, either for drug possession, outstanding warrants, or for a possible bad outcome related to the overdose, has often been reported by bystanders as the main reason they do not call 911 in such an event.[tt] In an effort to address this, many states have enacted or expanded existing Good Samaritan laws (sometimes known as "medical amnesty laws") to provide legal protection to the overdose victim and/or the individual administering assistance.[186,188,189] Between 2007 (when New Mexico became the first state) and 2016, over two-thirds of states and the District of Columbia had enacted such legislation. Although this clearly can help increase the likelihood that bystanders will intervene and seek further medical assistance, there is also evidence that law enforcement is not always aware of the laws.[26]

There is also concern by some prescribers about legal consequences of prescribing naloxone.[41] As of 2016, a total of 32 states

---

[ss]References 2, 44, 45, 132, 206, 238, 335, 396, 401, 441, 473, 532, 533, 585, 650, 657, 725.

[tt]References 21, 184, 394, 538, 595, 649, 654.

had enacted specific legislation to provide full or partial civil immunity to medical professionals who prescribe naloxone as permitted by the law in their state.

Outreach Programs

States and local jurisdictions are increasingly looking for novel programs to enhance the tertiary prevention strategies mentioned here. Vancouver has instituted a Mobile Medical Unit in areas with high overdose rates in order to help provide additional rapid response medical capability to the already overwhelmed emergency medical system. States such as Rhode Island, Massachusetts, and Maryland have implemented outreach teams to try to engage overdose survivors and their social networks in order to offer prevention, education, treatment referrals and other social services.[249,573] The Boston Healthcare for the Homeless program has established a Supportive Place for Observation and Treatment (SPOT) where an individual who has recently used a substance can come to be monitored by medical staff while acutely intoxicated. The staff are able to provide supportive medical care and naloxone, should the intoxication progress to overdose.[249,283] Though these types of programs should be effective in reducing overdose fatalities, very little data exists in their effectiveness.

Use of Technology

Mobile and on-line technologies have also been used to help reduce overdose fatalities. Websites such as subreddit/r/opiates/wiki have been used to facilitate communication between drug users who post cautions such as areas where suspected fentanyl-laced heroin is being sold. A mobile phone app, Remote Egg Timer, allows an opioid user to program an emergency contact's number and then set a timer (for 10 minutes or so) prior to injecting. If the user does not push a stop button when the timer goes off, a text message is automatically sent to the emergency contact. Although it can be customized, the default message reads: "This is an automated request for help. Unresponsive after using. Would you mind checking up on me?" In order that the emergency contact can send help, the message can be made to send the user's GPS coordinates. Other mobile-phone apps (Trek Medics and OD Help) help connect potential opioid overdose victims with a crowd-sourced network of individuals who possess naloxone.[35,264]

Vaccines

Although early in development, a vaccine has been developed which appears to attenuate some of the psychoactive effects and respiratory depression of fentanyl and many of its analogues.[70] Similar vaccines have been developed which have demonstrated an attenuation of heroin's effects.[71,411,578]

Management

Opioid overdose is typically a true medical emergency and is best managed as such in a medical setting. This management should include establishment of an adequate airway with intubation, if necessary; support of adequate cardiac function; prevention of aspiration through intubation; replacement of fluids and electrolytes, if necessary; management of pulmonary edema with positive pressure oxygen; frequent monitoring of respiratory status and vital signs; and administration of naloxone (see below). Throughout, attention should be paid to potential co-occurring acute (such as rhabdomyolysis) and chronic (such as HIV, chronic obstructive pulmonary disease [COPD], or hepatic compromise)

medical problems.[120,448,495] Once the patients is stable, efforts should also be made to assess the patient's willingness to consider treatment for an opioid use disorder and/or to educate the patient to help reduce risk of a subsequent overdose. In one study, 26% of overdose victims sought treatment within 30 days of an overdose but most (57%–87%, depending on the setting) said that they had not received any information about resources from the treating medical staff.[537]

Naloxone (n-allyl noroxymorphone) is a pure, competitive antagonist at the μ, κ, and σ opioid receptors.[434] It is chemically similar to morphine with an =O group substituted for an -OH group to form oxymorphone and a subsequent methyl group substituted by an allyl group to form naloxone. It was synthesized in 1960 and first patented in 1961. It was approved by the FDA for the management of opioid overdose in 1971 and was placed on the World Health Organization's List of Essential Medicines in 1984.[713] Over the past four decades, multiple studies have shown that naloxone reverses respiratory depression caused by full opioid agonists.[298,414,444]

Naloxone reaches the brain very rapidly,[491,695] although the onset of action varies by route of administration: intravenous, 1–2 minutes; subcutaneous, 5–6 minutes; intranasal, 3–4 minutes; intramuscular, 2–6 minutes; intralingual, 30 seconds; and inhalational (nebulized), 5 minutes.[214,367,475,610,688] The duration of action is 30–90 minutes and depends on the dose, route of administration, and rate of elimination of both the agonist and naloxone.[47,247,674] It is metabolized by the liver into the inactive conjugate naloxone-3-glucuronide and has an elimination half-life of 30–90 minutes in adults,[721] and longer in neonates. It is significantly more potent at the μ-opioid receptor but will exert effects on the κ and σ receptors at higher doses.

There is no single, agreed-upon standard for dosing.[148] The duration and extent of naloxone-induced reversal of opioid-induced respiratory depression is highly variable and related to many factors, including the specific opioid used, the opioid dose, the route of administration, concurrent substances, other medical conditions, pain, genetic make-up of the patient, and exogenous stimulatory factors.[674] One milligram of naloxone given intravenously reverses the effects of 25 mg of diamorphine (heroin). In a study of healthy volunteers with no pain, the respiratory depression induced by the intravenous administration of 0.15 mg/kg of morphine was completely reversed by 0.4 mg of intravenous naloxone.[575]

In general, the goal is to give the lowest dose necessary to reverse the respiratory depression without precipitating withdrawal. The higher the dose, the higher the likelihood of precipitating withdrawal in a physically dependent individual. In the hospital setting, it is generally administered intravenously, although there is evidence that intramuscular and subcutaneous administration are just as effective but with a slightly longer time to onset of response.[688] A common protocol recommends giving 0.2 to 0.4 mg and repeating in 2 to 5 minutes if there is no initial effect. Another protocol recommends starting with a smaller dose with individuals who are known to be physically dependent: 0.04 mg and then increasing to 0.4 mg, 2 mg, and 10 mg if there is inadequate response at the lower doses.[67] Because the duration of action of naloxone is shorter than that of most opioids, it is recommended that an individual be monitored for several hours after he/she responds to naloxone. One recommended protocol found less negative outcomes if patients were kept until they could mobilize as usual, oxygenate on room air to greater than 92%, have a respiratory rate between 10 and

20 breaths/minute, have a temperature between 35.0°C and 37.5°C, have a heart rate between 50 and 100 beats/minute, and have a Glasgow Coma Scale score of 15.[126,137]

If a long-acting opioid such as methadone has been ingested, it will likely be necessary to repeat naloxone administration multiple times or place the patient on a continuous naloxone infusion ("drip"). One suggested protocol for this involves calculating two-thirds of the initial naloxone dose required for overdose reversal and giving that intravenously on an hourly basis.[296] This can be increased or decreased depending on the patient's clinical response. It is recommended that those individuals be monitored for 24 hours following response to naloxone. It is also important to remember that frequent monitoring of respiratory status is crucial even though the patient is on continuous infusion. An overdose on more potent opioids such as fentanyl or its analogues may require higher doses of naloxone.[uu] Overdose on buprenorphine may also require higher doses because of its high binding affinity for the μ-opioid receptor.[674,721]

Naloxone is generally felt to be extremely safe, with minimal, if any, side effects, even with higher doses of 10 mg.[vv] Agitation or aggression is sometimes seen, especially if a higher dose of naloxone is given and the victim is "pushed" into withdrawal.[43,74,367,371] Opioid withdrawal precipitated by naloxone administration generally occurs in less than 10% of cases and tends to dissipate in 30–60 minutes.[214,491] When side effects such as headache or confusion are reported, it is generally in more severe cases of overdose and it is difficult to ascertain whether the effects are due to the naloxone or to the hypoxia resulting from the overdose.[74,84] However, earlier reports from the 1970s with postoperative patients have suggested that naloxone use may, rarely, under certain specific circumstances, cause serious and possibly life-threatening side effects, such as pulmonary edema, cardiac arrhythmias, hypertension, and cardiac arrest.[263,454,514,639,642] High-dose and/or rapidly infused naloxone given to a patient who is hypotensive, hypovolemic, or previously in severe pain or stress, may, rarely, cause catecholamine-mediated cardiac arrhythmias and vasoconstriction, which might lead to a fluid shift from the systemic circulation to the pulmonary vascular bed, resulting in pulmonary edema.[263] Rarely, such serious events have been reported in overdose victims receiving naloxone from emergency medical services. In one study, of 453 patients treated with naloxone, 6 (1.3%) had complications such as cardiac arrest, pulmonary edema, and epileptic seizures, with the primary cause of cardiorespiratory complications from naloxone being a massive release of catecholamines.[510]

There are currently several commercially available formulations of naloxone in the United States: (1) a 0.4 mg/mL formulation approved for parenteral administration available in single-dose 1 mL vials and multidose 10 mL vials; (2) a 1 mg/mL formulation supplied in a single-dose 2 mg vial with a luer-lock syringe barrel (although approved for parenteral use, this formulation is often used off-label with a mucosal atomizer device [MAD] via the intranasal route, with half of the medication in the vial sprayed in each nostril); (3) an auto-injector that includes visual and voice instructions (via an imbedded speaker) that talks the user through the administration procedure and delivers 2 mg of naloxone (in 0.4 mL) per dose, intramuscularly or subcutaneously (this was specifically FDA approved for administration by lay persons); (4) a ready-to-use single-dose nasal spray in 2 mg/0.1 mL and 4 mg/0.1 mL also approved for administration by lay persons.[383]

Although intramuscular, subcutaneous, and intranasal routes of administration produce less-predictable absorption and a slower onset of action than intravenous administration, the actual efficacy is generally felt to be comparable because of the delay required in obtaining intravenous access.[30,367,567] Uncertainty exists as to the relative effectiveness of intranasally administered naloxone to individuals with nasal congestion/bleeding or with naloxone administered by any route to an individual in asystole without the concomitant use of cardiac compressions.

There are also reports of using buprenorphine/naloxone products to successfully reverse an opioid overdose.[697,698,732]

More recent research has looked at the role of the serotonin system in opioid-induced respiratory depression. The 5HT1A, 5HT4A, and 5HT7 receptor subtypes appear to be involved with modulation of respiratory centers in the brainstem.[ww] Preliminary animal studies with agonists at these serotonin receptor subtypes have demonstrated some positive results as far as reversal of respiratory depression due to opioids.[310,428,452,496,571,602] Other research looking at the role of the N-methyl-D-aspartate (NMDA) glutamate system, particularly modulators (ampakines) of the α-amino-3-hydroxy-5-methyl-4-isoxazole-proprionic acid (AMPA) receptors has also been promising.[555,556] Yet another line of research has looked at minocycline, a tetracycline antibiotic, with apparent neuroprotective and antiinflammatory properties possibly related to inhibition of glial activation. Studies in rats have demonstrated its potential for reversal and prevention of opioid-induced respiratory depression with simultaneous enhancement of opioid-induced analgesia.[159,343,344] Yet another line of research has been with inhibitors of the sodium/proton exchanger type 3 (NHE3) that appear to have a stimulatory effect on breathing due to an action within central respiratory pathways.[376,705] Research is also being conducted on devices that can monitor for physiological signals of overdose and call for help or automatically inject naloxone should an overdose occur.[249,679] Phrenic nerve stimulation devices have also been tested.[249,679]

Supports Following an Overdose

The effect of a fatal overdose on the friends, family, and other acquaintance of the victim can be devastating. Often, these significant others feel a great deal of guilt as they, usually unrealistically, believe that they could have done more to save their loved one. In addition, there is typically a great amount of shame, especially if the details of the death are made public. A number of organizations have arisen to assist the loved ones of victims of overdose.

- Grief Recovery After a Substance Passing (GRASP)—An expansion of "Jenny's Journey," an awareness program that was started in California in 1996 by a couple following the death of their daughter to a heroin overdose. It gradually grew to include support, and it has expanded to include more than 100 groups in over 30 states and Canada as well as a substantial support component through Facebook.
- Broken No More—Formed by families and friends of individuals with a drug disorder (addiction). The group's primary goals are to provide support, knowledge, and an information base for persons who have lost a loved one through the disorder of addiction.
- The Courage To Speak Foundation—Founded in 1996 by parents who lost their son to a heroin and diazepam overdose. Members provide presentations on drug prevention as well as

uuReferences 102, 103, 249, 412, 608, 633.
vvReferences 43, 67, 74, 284, 367, 371, 674, 699, 722.

wwReferences 28, 391, 557, 679, 687, 719.

full curricula for elementary, middle, and high school students and parents. The website contains resources and testimonials.

- Learn2Cope—A nonprofit support network that offers education, resources, peer support, and hope for parents and family members coping with a loved one who is addicted to opiates or other drugs. Founded by Joanne Peterson in 2004, the organization has grown to include over 7000 members as of August 2015, and has become a nationally recognized model for peer support and prevention programming.
- Let It Out—A support group started in Massachusetts that incorporates boxing with support for family members dealing with a loved one with addiction or the grief of a loved one lost to overdose.

Various memoirs have also been written by survivors of overdose victims, with the intent of providing support to others who have lost a loved-one.

- *When a Child Dies From Drugs* (2004) by Patricia and Russ Wittberger
- *I Am Your Disease* (2006) by Sheryl Letzgus McGinnis with Heiko Ganzer
- *Sunny's Story: How to Save a Young Life From Drugs* (2008) by Ginger Katz
- *Griefland: An Intimate Portrait of Love, Loss, and Unlikely Friendship* (2012) by Armen Bacon and Nancy Miller
- *Her: A Memoir* (2013) by Christa Parravani
- *Lord Fear: A Memoir* (2015) by Lucas Mann
- *Heroin Is Killing Our Children* (2016) by Missy H. Owen

Conclusion

Overdose from opioids has become a significant public health problem in the United States and other parts of the world. Despite various prevention efforts that have been implemented to try to reduce the misuse of opioids, increase treatment for persons with opioid use disorders, and reduce the likelihood of overdose and death from overdose, rates of overdose have continued to rise in many areas. Some of the increase appears to also be related to heroin cut with illicitly manufactured fentanyl analogues and other potent opioids. Efforts at international, national, and local levels continue to seek innovative approaches to address the problem.

References

1. Academy of Managed Care Pharmacy, Shoemaker S, Pozniak A, Subramanian R, et al. Effect of six managed care pharmacy tools: a review of the literature. *J Manag Care Pharm.* 2010;16(suppl 6):S3–S20.
2. Albert S, Brason F, Sanford C. Project Lazarus: community-based overdose prevention in rural North Carolina. *Pain Med.* 2011;12:S77–S85.
3. Alexander L, Mannion R, Weingarten B, et al. Development and impact of prescription opioid abusedeterrent formulation technologies. *Drug Alcohol Depend.* 2014;138:1–6.
4. Algren D, Monteilh C, Punja M, et al. Fentanyl-associated fatalities among illicit drug users in Wayne County, Michigan (July 2005-May 2006). *J Med Toxicol.* 2013;9(1):106–115.
5. Amato L, Davoli M, Perucci C, et al. An overview of systematic reviews of the effectiveness of opiate maintenance therapies: available evidence to inform clinical practice and research. *J Subst Abuse Treat.* 2005;28:321–329.
6. Amato L, Minozzi S, Davoli M, et al. Psychosocial and pharmacological treatments versus pharmacological treatments for opioid detoxification. *Cochrane Database Syst Rev.* 2011;(9):CD005031.
7. American Academy of Addiction Psychiatry. *Joint Position Statement of American Psychiatric Association and American Academy of Addiction Psychiatry: Opioid Overdose Education and Naloxone Distribution*; 2016. http://www.aaap.org/wp-content/uploads/2016/01/APA-AAAP-Stmt-on-Overdose-EducationBOT-Approved2.pdf.
8. American Academy of Pain Medicine. *The Evidence against Methadone as a "Preferred" Analgesic.* Chicago, IL: American Academy of Pain Medicine; 2014. http://www.painmed.org/files/the-evidence-againstmethadone-as-a-preferred-analgesic.pdf.
9. American Medical Association. *It's about Saving Lives: Increasing Access to Naloxone*; 2015. http://www.amaassn.org/ama/ama-wire/post/itssaving-lives-increasing-access-naloxone.
10. American Pharmacists' Association. *APhA Policy: Controlled Substances and Other Medications with Thepotential for Abuse and Use of Opioid Reversal Agents*; 2014. http://www.pharmacist.com/policy/controlled-substances-and-other-medications-potential-abuse-and-use-opioid-reversalagents-2.
11. American Psychiatric Association. *Diagnostic and Statistical Manual of Mental Disorders.* 5th ed. Arlington, VA: American Psychiatric Publishing; 2013.
12. American Society of Addiction Medicine. *Public Policy Statement on the Use of Naloxone for Theprevention of Drug Overdose Deaths*; 2014. Chevy Chase, MD. http://www.asam.org/docs/default-source/publicpolicystatements/1naloxone-rev-8-14.pdf.
13. Anchersen K, Clausen T, Gossop M, et al. Prevalence and clinical relevance of corrected QT intervalprolongation during methadone and buprenorphine treatment: a mortality assessmentstudy. *Addiction.* 2009;104:993–999.
14. Andrews C, Krantz M, Wedam E, et al. Methadone-induced mortality in the treatment of chronic pain:role of QT prolongation. *Cardiol J.* 2009;16(3):210–217.
15. Andrews J, Kinner S. Understanding drug-related mortality in released prisoners: a review of nationalcoronial records. *BMC Public Health.* 2012;12:270.
16. Argoff C. Clinical implications of opioid pharmacogenetics. *Clin J Pain.* 2010;26(suppl 10):S16–S20.
17. Armenian P, Olson A, Anaya A, et al. Fentanyl and a novel synthetic opioid U-47700 masquerading asstreet "Norco" in Central California: a case report. *Ann Emerg Med.* 2016;20. (Epub ahead of print).
18. Association of State and Territorial Health Officials. *ASTHO Prescription Drug Misuse and Abusestrategic Map: 2013-2015*; 2015. http://www.astho.org/Rx/Strategic-Map-2013-2015.
19. Astone N, Martin S, Aron L. *Death Rates for U.S. Women Ages 15 to 54; Some Unexpected Trends.* Washington, D.C: Urban Institute; 2015.
20. Auriacombe M, Fatséas M, Dubernet J, et al. French field experience with buprenorphine. *Am J Addict.* 2004;13(suppl 1):S17–S28.
21. Baca CGrant K. What heroin users tell us about overdose. *J Addict Dis.* 2007;26(4):63–68.
22. Bäckberg M, Beck O, Jonsson KH, et al. Opioid intoxications involving butyrfentanyl, 4 fluorobutyrfentanyl, and fentanyl from the Swedish STRIDA project. *Clin Toxicol.* 2015;53:609–617.
23. Baehren D, Marco C, Droz D, et al. A statewide prescription monitoring program affects emergency department prescribing behaviors. *Ann Emerg Med.* 2010;56:19–23.
24. Baldacchino A, Tolomeo S, Khan F, et al. Acute risk factors in fatal opioid overdoses as a result of hypoxia and cardiotoxicity. A systematic review and critical appraisal. *Heroin Addict Relat Clin Probl.* 2016;18(4):33–42.
25. Ball C. The early development of intravenous apparatus. *Anaesth Intensive Care.* 2006;34(suppl 1):22–26.
26. Banta-Green C, Beletsky L, Schoeppe J. Police officers' and paramedics' experiences with overdose and their knowledge and opinions of Washington State's drug overdose-naloxone-Good Samaritan law. *J Urban Health.* 2013;90(6):1102–1111.
27. Barclay J, Owens J, Blackhall L. Screening for substance abuse risk in cancer patients using the Opioid Risk Tool and urine drug screen. *Support Care Cancer.* 2014;22:1883–1888.

28. Barnes N, Sharp T. A review of central 5HT receptors and their function. *Neuropharmacology.* 1999;38:1083–1152.

29. Bartoli F, Carrà G, Brambilla G, et al. Association between depression and non-fatal overdoses among drug users: a systematic review and meta-analysis. *Drug Alcohol Depend.* 2014;134:12–21.

30. Barton ED, Colwell CB, Wolfe T, et al. Efficacy of intranasal naloxone as a needleless alternative for treatment of opioid overdose in the prehospital setting. *J Emer Med.* 2005;29:265–271.

31. Bachhuber M, Saloner B, Cunningham C, et al. Medical cannabis laws and opioid analgesic overdose mortality in the United States, 1999–2010. *JAMA Intern Med.* 2014;174(10):1668–1673.

32. Baxter L, Campbell A, Deshields M, et al. Safe methadone induction and stabilization: report of anexpert panel. *J Addict Med.* 2013;7:377–386.

33. Bazazi A, Zelenev A, Fu J, et al. High prevalence of non-fatal overdose among people who inject drugs in Malaysia: correlates of overdose and implications for overdose prevention from a cross-sectional study. *Int J Drug Policy.* 2015;26(7):675–681.

34. B.C. Coroners Service. *Fentanyl-Detected Illicit Drug Overdose Deaths January 1, 2012 to February 28, 2017.* http://www2.gov.bc.ca/assets/gov/public-safety-and-emergency-services/death-investigation/statistical/fentanyl-detected-overdose.pdf. Accessed August 6, 2017.

35. Beacon Dispatch. Community-based overdose response. *Trek Medics International.* 2017. https://www.trekmedics.org/beacon/overdose/.

36. Beaudoin F, Merchant R, Janicki A, et al. Preventing iatrogenic overdose: a review of in–emergency department opioid-related adverse drug events and medication errors. *Annals Emergency Med.* 2015;65(4):423–431.

37. Beaudoin F, Banerjee G, Mello M. State-level and system-level opioid prescribing policies: the impacton provider practices and overdose deaths, a systematic review. *J Opioid Manag.* 2016;12(2):109–118.

38. Becker WC, Fiellin DA. Abuse-deterrent opioid formulations — Putting the potential benefits into perspective. *N Engl J Med.* 2017;376:2103–2105.

39. Behar E, Rowe C, Santos G. Primary care patient experience with naloxone prescription. *Annals FamMed.* 2016;14(5):431–436.

41. Beletsky L, Rich J, Walley A. Prevention of fatal opioid overdose. *J Am Med Assoc.* 2012;308(18):1863–1864.

40. Beletsky L, Ruthazer R, Macalino G, et al. Physicians' knowledge of and willingness to prescribenaloxone to reverse accidental opiate overdose: challenges and opportunities. *J Urban Health.* 2007;84:126–136.

42. Bell J, Butler B, Lawrance A, et al. Comparing overdose mortality associated with methadone andbuprenorphine treatment. *Drug Alcohol Depend.* 2009;104:73–77.

43. Belz D, Lieb J, Rea T, et al. Naloxone use in a tiered-response emergency medical services system. *Prehosp Emerg Care.* 2006;10(4):468–471.

44. Bennett A, Bell A, Tomedi L, et al. Characteristics of an overdose prevention, response, and naloxone distribution program in Pittsburgh and Allegheny County, Pennsylvania. *J Urban Health.* 2011;88(6):1020–1030.

45. Bennett T, Holloway K. The impact of take-home naloxone distribution and training on opiate overdose knowledge and response: an evaluation of the project in wales. *Drugs-Education Prevention and Policy.* 2012;19(4):320–328.

46. Bergenstrom A, Quan VM, Van Nam L, et al. A cross-sectional study on prevalence of non-fatal drug overdose and associated risk characteristics among out-of-treatment injecting drug users in North Vietnam. *Subst Use Misuse.* 2008;43(1):77–84.

47. Berkowitz BA. The relationship of pharmacokinetics to pharmacological activity: morphine, methadone, and naloxone. *Clin Pharmacokinet.* 1976;1:219–230.

48. Beyer A, Koch T, Schroeder H, et al. Effects of the A118G polymorphis on binding affinity, potency, and agonist-meiated endocytosis, desensitization, and resensitization of the human mu-opioid receptor. *J Neurochem.* 2004;89:553–560.

49. Binswanger I, Blatchford P, Mueller S, et al. Mortality after prison release: opioid overdose and other causes of death, risk factors, and time trends from 1999 to 2009. *Annals Int Med.* 2013;159(9):592–600.

50. Binswanger I, Blatchford P, Yamashita, et al. Trends in overdose deaths after release from state prison,1999–2009. *Drug Alc Depend.* 2014;140:e14.

51. Binswanger I, Koester S, Mueller S, et al. Overdose education and naloxone for patients prescribed opioids in primary care: a qualitative study of primary care staff. *J Gen Intern Med.* 2015;30:1837–1844.

52. Binswanger I, Nowels C, Corsi K, et al. Return to drug use and overdose after release from prison: a qualitative study of risk and protective factors. *Addict Sci Clin Pract.* 2012;7(1):3.

53. Binswanger I, Stern M, Deyo R, et al. Release from prison- a high risk of death for former inmates. *N Engl J Med.* 2007;356(2):157–165.

54. Bird S, Hutchinson S. Male drugs-related deaths in the fortnight after release from prison: Scotland, 1996–99. *Addiction.* 2003;98:185–190.

55. Bird S, McAuley A, Perry S, et al. Effectiveness of Scotland's National Naloxone Programme for reducing opioid–related deaths: a before (2006–10) versus after (2011–13). *Comparison Addiction.* 2016;111(5):883891.

56. Blumenschein K, Fink J, Freeman P, et al. *Review of Prescription Drug Monitoring Programs in the United States: Independent Evaluation of the KASPER Program.* Lexington, Kentucky: University of Kentucky; 2010.

57. Boddiger D. Fentanyl-laced street drugs "kill hundreds." *Lancet.* 2006;368(9535):569–570.

58. Bohnert A, Nandi A, Tracy M, et al. Policing and risk of overdose mortality in urban neighborhoods. *Drug Alcohol Depend.* 2011;113(1):62–68.

59. Bohnert A, Tracy M, Galea S. Characteristics of drug users who witness many overdoses: implications for overdose prevention. *Drug Alcohol Depend.* 2012;120(1–3):168–173.

60. Bohnert A, Valenstein M, Bair MJ, et al. Association between opioid prescribing patterns and opioid overdose-related deaths. *J Am Med Assoc.* 2011;305(13):1315–1321.

61. Bonar E, Ilgen M, Walton M, et al. Associations among pain, non-medical prescription opioid use, and drug overdose history. *Am J Addict.* 2014;23:41–47.

62. Bond C, LaForge KS, Tian M, et al. Single nucleotide polymorphism in the human mu opioid receptorgene alters beta-endorphin binding and activity: possible implications for opiate addiction. *Proc Natl Acad Sci.* 1998;95:9608–9613.

63. Borgeat A, Biollaz J, Depierraz B, et al. Grand mal seizures after extradural morphine analgesia. *Br J Anaesth.* 1988;60:733–735.

64. Borron W, Monier C, Risède P, et al. Flunitrazepam variably alters morphine, buprenorphine and methadone lethality in the rat. *Hum Exp Toxicol.* 2002;21:599–605.

65. Bouillon T, Bruhn J, Radu-Radulescu L, et al. A model of the ventilatory depressant potency of remfentanil in the non-steady state. *Anesthesiology.* 2003;99:779–787.

66. Bovill J. Opium: a drug ancient and modern. In: Dahan A, van Kleef JW, eds. *Advances in Anesthesia and Analgesia: 22 Years of Research in Anesthesiology at Leiden University and LUMC.* Leiden: Department of Anesthesiology (LUMC); 2007:13–27.

67. Boyer EW. Management of opioid analgesic overdose. *N Eng J Med.* 2012;367:146–155.

68. Brådvik L, Frank A, Hulenvik P, et al. Heroin addicts reporting previous heroin overdoses also report suicide attempts. *Suicide Life Threat Behav.* 2007;37(4):475–481.

69. Branagan OGrogan L. Providing health education on accidental drug over-dose. *Nurs Times.* 2006;102:32–33.

70. Bremer P, Kimishima A, Schlosburg J, et al. Combatting synthetic designer opioids: a Conjugate Vaccine Ablates lethal doses of fentanyl class drugs. *Angew Chem Int Ed Engl.* 2016;55(11):3772–3775.

71. Bremer PT, Schlosburg JE, Banks ML, et al. Development of a clinically viable heroin vaccine. *J Am Chem Society*. 2017;139(25):8601–8611.

72. Brugal M, Domingo-Salvany A, Puig R, et al. Evaluating the impact of methadone maintenance programmes on mortality due to overdose and aids in a cohort of heroin users in Spain. *Addiction*. 2005;100(7):981989.

73. Brunt TM, Nagy C, Bücheli A, et al. Drug testing in europe: monitoring results of the Trans European Drug information (TEDI) project. *Drug Test Anal*. 2017;9:188–198.

74. Buajordet I, Naess A, Jacobsen D, et al. Adverse events after naloxone treatment of episodes of suspected acute opioid overdose. *Eur J Emerg*. 2004;11(1):19–23.

75. Buchanich JM, Balmert LC, Pringle JL, et al. Patterns and trends in accidental poisoning death rates in the US, 1979-2014. *Preventive Med*. 2016;89:317–323.

76. Bunn T, Yu L, Spiller H, et al. Surveillance of methadone-related poisonings in Kentucky using multiple data sources. *Pharmacoepidemiol Drug Saf*. 2010;19:124–131.

77. Burghardt LC, Ayers JW, Brownstein JS, et al. Adult prescription drug use and pediatric medication exposures and poisonings. *Pediatrics*. 2013;132(1):18–27.

78. Burns G, DeRienz R, Baker D, et al. Could chest wall rigidity be a factor in rapid death from illicit fentanyl abuse? *Clini Toxicol*. 2016;54(5):420–423.

79. Burris S, Beletsky L, Castagna C, et al. Stopping an invisible epidemic: legal issues in the provision of naloxone to prevent opioid overdose. *Drexel L Rev*. 2009;1:273.

80. Butler S, Budman S, Fanciullo G, et al. Cross validation of the current opioid misuse measure tomonitor chronic pain patients on opioid therapy. *Clin J Pain*. 2010;26:770–776.

81. Butler S, Cassidy T, Chilcoat H, et al. Abuse rates and routes of administration of reformulated extended-release oxycodone: initial findings from a sentinel surveillance sample of individuals assessed for substance abuse treatment. *J Pain*. 2013;14(4):351–358.

82. Cacioppo J, Hughts M, Waite L, et al. Loneliness as a specific risk factor for depressive symptoms: cross-sectional and longitudinal analyses. *Psychol Aging*. 2006;21:140–151.

83. Canadian Community Epidemiology Network on Drug Use. Deaths Involving Fentanyl in Canada 2009-2014. *CCENDU Bulletin Canadian Centre on Substance Abuse; 2015*. 2015.

84. Cantwell K, Dietze P, Flander L. The relationship between naloxone dose and key patient variables in the treatment of non-fatal heroin overdose in the prehospital setting. *Resuscitation*. 2005;65(3):315–319.

85. Caplehorn J. Deaths in the first two weeks of maintenance treatment in NSW in 1994: identifying cases of iatrogenic methadone toxicity. *Drug Alcohol Rev*. 1998;17(1):9–17.

86. Caplehorn J, Dalton M, Haldar F, et al. Methadone maintenance and addicts' risk of fatal heroin overdose. *Subst Use Misuse*. 1996;31(2):177–196.

87. Caplehorn J, Drummer O. Fatal methadone toxicity: signs and circumstances, and the role of benzodiazepines. *Aust N Z J Public Health*. 2002;26(4):358–362.

88. Carson H. The medium, not the message: how tattoos correlate with early mortality disclosures. *Am J Clin Pathol*. 2014;142(1):99–103.

89. Cascino GD, So EL, Sharbrough FW, et al. Alfentanil-induced epileptiform activity in patients with partial epilepsy. *J Clin Neurophysiol*. 1993;10:520–525.

90. Case A, Deaton A. Rising morbidity and mortality in midlife among white non-hispanic Americans in the 21st century. *Pro Nat Acad Sci*. 2015;112(49):15078–15083.

91. Cashman J, Dolins S. Respiratory and haemodynamic effects of acute postoperative pain management: evidence from published data. *Br J Anaesth*. 2004;93:212–223.

92. Cassidy T, Das Mahapatra P, Black R, et al. Changes in prevalence of prescription opioid abuse after introduction of an abuse-deterrent opioid formulation. *Pain Med*. 2014;15(3):440–451.

93. Caudarella A, Dong H, Milloy M, et al. Non-fatal overdose as a risk factor for subsequent fatal overdose among people who inject drugs. *Drug Alcohol Depend*. 2016;162:51–55.

94. Caudevilla F, Ventura M, Fornís I, et al. Results of an international drug testing service for cryptomarket users. *Int J Drug Policy*. 2016;35:38–41.

95. Center for Behavioral Health Statistics and Quality. *The DAWN Report: Highlights of the 2011 Drug Abuse Warning Network (DAWN) Findings on Drug-Related Emergency Department Visits*. Rockville, Md: Substance Abuse and Mental Health Services Administration; 2013.

96. Center for Behavioral Health Statistics and Quality. *2014 National Survey on Drug Use and Health: Detailed Tables*. Rockville, Md: Substance Abuse and Mental Health Services Administration; 2015.

97. Centers for Disease Control and Prevention. *Nonpharmaceutical Fentanyl-Related Deaths-Multiple States*, April 2005--March 2007. 2008; 57(29): 793–796.

98. Centers for Disease Control and Prevention. Vital signs: overdoses of prescription opioid pain relieversUnited States, 1998–2008. *MMWR (Morb Mortal Wkly Rep)*. 2011;60(43):1487–1492.

99. Centers for Disease Control and Prevention. CDC Grand Rounds: prescription drug overdoses- a U.S. epidemic. *MMWR (Morb Mortal Wkly Rep)*. 2012;61(01):10–13.

100. Centers for Disease Control and Prevention, Wheeler E, Davidson P, Jones T, Irwin K. Community-based opioid overdose prevention programs providing naloxone - United States, 2010. *MMWR (Morb Mortal Wkly Rep)*. 2012;61(6):101–105.

101. Centers for Disease Control and Prevention. *Vital Signs: Prescription Painkiller Overdoses: A Growingepidemic, Especially Among Women*; 2013. http://www.cdc.gov/vitalsigns/PrescriptionPainkillerOverdoses/index.html.

102. Centers for Disease Control and Prevention. Notes from the field: acetyl fentanyl overdose fatalities –Rhode Island, March-May 2013. *MMWR (Morb Mortal Wkly Rep)*. 2013;62(34):703–704.

103. Centers for Disease Control and Prevention. Recommendations for laboratory testing for acetyl fentanyl and patient evaluation and treatment for overdose for synthetic opioids. *HAN Health Advisory*. 2013. http://stacks.cdc.gov/view/cdc/25259.

104. Centers for Disease Control and Prevention. *Patient Review and Restriction Programs: Lessons Learned From State Medicaid Programs*. Atlanta, GA: CDC; 2013.

105. Centers for Disease Control and Prevention. *Public Health Law Program in the Office for State, Tribal, Local and Territorial Support & Division of Unintentional Injury Prevention*. Menu of State Prescription Drug Identification Laws; 2013. https://www.cdc.gov/phlp/menu-pdil.pdf.

106. Reference deleted in review.

107. Centers for Disease Control and Prevention. *(2014) WONDER [Database]*. Atlanta, GA: US Department of Health and Human Services, CDC; 2014. http://wonder.cdc.gov.

108. Centers for Disease Control and Prevention. Decline in drug overdose deaths after state policy changes – Florida, 2010–2012. *MMWR (Morb Mortal Wkly Rep)*. 2014;63:569–574.

109. Centers for Disease Control and Prevention. *Wide-ranging Online Data for Epidemiologic Research (WONDER); Multiple-Cause-of-Death File, 2000-2014*; 2015. http://wonder.cdc.gov/mcd-icd10.html.

110. Centers for Disease Control and Prevention. Decrease in rate of opioid analgesic overdose deaths — Staten Island, New York City, 2011–2013. *MMWR (Morb Mortal Wkly Rep)*. 2015;64:491–494.

111. Centers for Disease Control and Prevention. *Increases in Fentanyl Drug Confiscation and Fentanyl-Related Overdose Fatalities*; 2015. http://emergency.cdc.gov/han/han00384.asp.

112. Center for Disease Control and Prevention. *Wide-ranging Online Data for Epidemiologic Research (WONDER)*. Atlanta, GA: CDC, National Center for Health Statistics; 2016. Available at: http://wonder.cdc.gov.

113. Center for Disease Control and Prevention. Influx of fentanyl-laced counterfeit pills and toxic fentanyl related compounds further increases risk of fentanyl-related overdose and fatalities. *Health Alert Network*. 2016;25:1016.

114. Centers for Medicare & Medicaid Services. *CMCS Informational Bulletin: Best Practices for Addressing Prescription Opioid Overdoses, Misuse, and Addiction.* Baltimore, MD: US Department of Health and Human Services, Centers for Medicare & Medicaid Services; 2016. *www.medicaid.gov/federal-policy guidance/downloads/cib-02-02-16.pdf.*

115. Center for Substance Abuse Treatment. Medication-Assisted Treatment for Opioid Addiction in Opioid Treatment Programs. *Treatment Improvement Protocol (TIP) Series 43. HHS Publication No. (SMA) 12 4214.* Rockville, MD: Substance Abuse and Mental Health Services Administration; 2005.

116. Cerdá M, Ransome Y, Keyes K, et al. Prescription opioid mortality trends in New York City, 1990 2006: examining the emergence of an epidemic. *Drug Alcohol Depend.* 2013;132(1–2):53–62.

117. Cerdá M, Ransome Y, Keyes K, et al. Revisiting the role of the urban environment in substance use: the case of analgesic overdose fatalities. *Am J Public Health.* 2013;103(12):2252–2260.

118. Chan G, Stajic M, Marker E, et al. Testing positive for methadone and either a tricyclic antidepressant or a benzodiazepine is associated with an accidental overdose death: analysis of medical examiner data. *Acad Emerg Med.* 2006;13(5):543–547.

119. Cheng M, Sauer B, Johnson E, et al. Comparison of opioid-related deaths by work related injury. *Am J Ind Med.* 2013;56(3):308–316.

120. Cherubin CE, Sapira JD. The medical complications of drug addiction and the medical assessment of the intravenous drug user: 25 years later. *Ann Intern Med.* 1993;119(10):1017–1028.

121. Chevillard L, Mégarbane B, Risède P, et al. Characteristics and comparative severity of respiratory response to toxic doses of fentanyl, methadone, morphine and buprenorphine in rats. *Toxicol Lett.* 2009;191(23):327–340.

122. Choi S, Koo B-N, Nam S, et al. Comparison of remifentanil and fentanyl for postoperative pain control after abdominal hysterectomy. *Yonsei Med J.* 2008;49:204–210.

123. Chou R, Cruciani R, Fiellin D, et al. American Pain Society; Heart Rhythm Society. Methadone safety: a clinical practice guideline from the American pain society and College on problems of drug dependence, in collaboration with the Heart Rhythm society. *J Pain.* 2014;15:321–337.

124. Chou WY, Yang LC, Lu H, et al. Association of mu-opioid receptor gene polymorphism (A118G) with variation in morphine consumption for analgesia after total knee arthroplasty. *Acta Anaesthesiol Scand.* 2006;50:787–792.

125. Chihuri S, Li G. Trends in Prescription Opioids Detected in Fatally Injured Drivers in 6 U.S. States: 1995 2015. *Am J Public Health.* 2017;107(9):1487–1492.

126. Christenson J, Etherington J, Grafstein E, et al. Early discharge of patients with presumed opioid overdose; development of a clinical prediction rule. *Acad Emerg Med.* 2000;7(10):1110–1118.

127. Ciccarone D. Fentanyl in the US heroin supply: a rapidly changing risk environment. *Int J Drug Policy.* 2017;46:107–111.

128. Cicero T, Ellis M. Abuse-deterrent formulations and the prescription opioid abuse epidemic in the United States: lessons learned from OxyContin. *JAMA Psychiatry.* 2015;72(5):424–430.

129. Cicero T, Ellis M, Surratt H. Effect of abuse-deterrent formulation of OxyContin. *N Engl J Med.* 2012;367:187–189.

130. Cicero T, Ellis MS, Surratt HL, et al. The changing face of heroin use in the United States: a retrospective analysis of the past 50 years. *JAMA Psychiatry.* 2014;71(7):821–826.

131. Cicero TJ, Ellis MS, Kasper ZA. Psychoactive substance use prior to the development of iatrogenic opioid abuse: a descriptive analysis of treatment-seeking opioid abusers. *Addict Behav.* 2017;65:242–244.

132. Clark A, Wilder C, Winstanley E. A systematic review of community opioid overdose prevention and naloxone distribution programs. *J Addict Med.* 2014;8(3):153–163.

133. Clark M, Bates A. Nonfatal heroin overdoses in Queensland, Australia: an analysis of ambulance data. *J Urban Health.* 2003;80(2):238–247.

134. Clark R, Baxter J. Responses of state Medicaid programs to buprenorphine diversion: doing more harm than good? *JAMA Intern Med.* 2013;173:1571–1572.

135. Clausen T. Mortality is reduced while on opiate maintenance treatment, but there is a temporary increase in mortality immediately after starting and stopping treatment, a finding that may vary by setting. *Evid Based Med.* 2011;16:94–95.

136. Clausen T, Anchersen K, Waal H. Mortality prior to, during and after opioid maintenance treatment (OMT): a national prospective cross-registry study. *Drug Alcohol Depend.* 2008;94:151–157.

137. Coben J, Davis S, Furbee P, et al. Hospitalizations for poisoning by prescription opioids, sedatives, and tranquilizers. *Am J Preven Med.* 2010;38(5):517–524.

138. Cochella S, Bateman K. Provider detailing: an intervention to decrease prescription opioid deaths in Utah. *Pain Med.* 2011;12:S73–S76.

139. Coffey C, Wolfe R, Lovett A, et al. Predicting death in young offenders: a retrospective cohort study. *Med J Aust.* 2004;181(9):473–477.

140. Coffin P. *Overdose: a Major Cause of Preventable Death in Central and Eastern Europe and in Central Asia Recommendations and Overview of the Situation in Latvia, Kyrgyzstan, Romania, Russia and Tajikistan.* Vilnius, Lithuania: Eurasian Harm Reduction Network; 2008.

141. Coffin P, Behar E, Rowe C, et al. Nonrandomized intervention study of naloxone co-prescription for primary care patients receiving long-term opioid therapy for pain. *Ann Intern Med.* 2016;165:245–252.

142. Coffin P, Sherman S, Curtis M. Underestimated and overlooked: a global review of drug overdose and overdose prevention. In: Cook C, ed. *Global State of Harm Reduction 2010: Key Issues for Broadening the Response.* London: International Harm Reduction Association; 2010:2010.

143. Coffin P, Sullivan S. Cost-effectiveness of distributing naloxone to heroin users for lay overdose reversal. *Ann Intern Med.* 2013;158(1):1–9.

144. Coffin P, Sullivan S. Cost-effectiveness of distributing naloxone to heroin users for lay overdose reversal in Russian cities. *J Med Econ.* 2013;16(8):1051–1060.

145. Coffin P, Tracy M, Bucciarelli A, et al. Identifying injection drug users at risk of nonfatal overdose. *Acad Emerg Med.* 2007;14(7):616–623.

146. Compton W, Boyle M, Wargo E. Prescription opioid abuse: problems and responses. *Preven Med.* 2015;80:5–9.

147. Compton W, Jones C, Baldwin G. Relationship between nonmedical prescription-opioid use and heroin use. *N Engl J Med.* 2016;374(2):154–163.

148. Connors NJ, Nelson LS. The evolution of recommended naloxone dosing for opioid overdose by medical specialty. *J Med Toxicol.* 2016;12(3):276–281.

149. Cook S, Moeschler O, Michaud K, et al. Acute opiate overdose: characteristics of 190 consecutive cases. *Addiction.* 1998;93(10):1559–1565.

150. Coplan P, Kale H, Sandstrom L, et al. Changes in oxycodone and heroin exposures in the National Poison Data System after introduction of extended-release oxycodone with abuse-deterrent characteristics. *Pharmacoepidemiol Drug Saf.* 2013;22(12):1274–1282.

151. Corkery J, Schifano F, Ghodse A, et al. The effects of methadone and its role in fatalities. *Hum Psychopharmacol.* 2004;19(8):565–576.

152. Cornish R, Macleod J, Strang J, et al. Risk of death during and after opiate substitution treatment in primary care: prospective observational study in UK General Practice Research Database. *BMJ.* 2010;341.

153. Corson K, Doak M, Denneson L. Primary care clinician adherence to guidelines for the management of chronic musculoskeletal pain: results from the study of the effectiveness of a collaborative approach to pain. *Pain Med.* 2011;12:1490–1501.

154. Cousins G, Teljeur C, Motterlini N, et al. Risk of drug-related mortality during periods of transition in methadone maintenance treatment: a cohort study. *J Subst Abuse Treat.* 2011;41:252–260.

155. Cowan A, Doxey JC, Harry EJ. The animal pharmacology of buprenorphine, an oripavine analgesic agent. *Br J Pharmacol.* 1977;60:547–554.

156. Crimmins E, Zhang Y, Saito Y. Trends over four decades in disability-free life expectancy in the United States. *Amr Jrnl Pub Health.* epub April 14, 2016.

157. Crowe AV, Howse M, Bell GM, et al. Substance abuse and the kidney. *Q J Med.* 2009;93:147–152.

158. Crozier M, Mcmillan S, Hudson S, et al. The eastern North Carolina opioid prescribers project: a model continuing medical education workshop. *J Opioid Manag.* 2010;6(5):359–364.

159. Cui Y, Liao X, Liu W, et al. A novel role of minocycline: attenuating morphine antinociceptive tolerance by inhibition of p38 MAPK in the activated spinal microglia. *Brain Behav Immun.* 2008;22:114–123.

160. Cullen W, Bury G, Langton D. Experience of heroin overdose among drug users attending general practice. *Br J Gen Pract.* 2000;50(456):546–549.

161. Cuyahoga County Medical Examiner. *Medical Examiner Public Health Warning: Deadly Carfentanil Has Been Detected in Cuyahoga County*; 2016. http://executive.cuyahogacounty.us/en-US/ME Public-Health-Warning.aspx.

162. Dahan A, Aarts L, Smith T. Incidence, reversal, and prevention of opioid-induced respiratory depression. *Anesthesiology.* 2010;112(1):226–238.

163. Dahan A, Teppema L. Influence of anaesthesia and analgesia on the control of breathing. *Br J Anaesth.* 2003;91:40–49.

164. Dahan A, Yassen A, Romberg R, et al. Buprenorphine induces ceiling in respiratory depression but not in analgesia. *Br J Anaesth.* 2006;96(5):627–632.

165. Darke S, Duflou J, Torok M. A reduction in blood morphine concentrations amongst heroin overdose fatalities associated with a sustained reduction in street heroin purity. *Forensic Sci Int.* 2010;198(1–3):118–120.

166. Darke S, Hall W. The distribution of naloxone to heroin users. *Addiction.* 1997;92(9):1195–1199.

167. Darke S, Hall W, Kaye S, et al. Hair morphine concentrations of fatal heroin overdose cases and living heroin users. *Addiction.* 2002;97:977–984.

168. Darke S, Hall W, Weatherburn D, et al. Fluctuations in heroin purity and the incidence of fatal heroin overdose. *Drug Alcohol Depend.* 1999;54:155–161.

169. Darke S, Mattick RP, Degenhardt L. The ratio of non-fatal to fatal overdose. *Addiction.* 2003;98(8):1169–1170.

170. Darke S, Mills K, Ross J. Rates and correlates of mortality amongst heroin users: findings from the Australian Treatment Outcome Study (ATOS), 2001–2009. *Drug Alcohol Depend.* 2011;115:190–195.

171. Darke S, Ross J. Overdose risk perceptions and behaviours among heroin users in Sydney, Australia. *Eur Addict Res.* 1997;3:87–92.

172. Darke S, Ross J. Heroin-related deaths in south western Sydney Australia, 1992–1996. *Drug Alcohol Rev.* 1999;18:39–46.

173. Darke S, Ross J. Fatal heroin overdoses resulting from non-injecting routes of administration, NSW, Australia, 1992-1996. *Addiction.* 2000;95:569–573.

174. Darke S, Ross J, Hall W. Overdose among heroin users in Sydney, Australia: I. Prevalence and correlates of non-fatal overdose. *Addiction.* 1996;91(3):405–411.

175. Darke S, Sunjic S, Zador D, et al. A comparison of blood toxicology of heroin-related deaths and current heroin users in Sydney, Australia. *Drug Alcohol Depend.* 1997;47(1):45–53.

176. Darke S, Williamson A, Ross J, et al. Non-fatal heroin overdose, treatment exposure and client characteristics: findings from the Australian treatment outcome study (ATOS). *Drug Alcohol Rev.* 2005;24(5):425–432.

177. Darke S, Williamson A, Ross J, et al. Patterns of nonfatal heroin overdose over a 3-year period: findings from the Australian Treatment Outcome Study. *J Urban Health.* 2007;84(2):283–291.

178. Darke S, Zador D. Fatal heroin overdose: a review. *Addiction.* 1996;91:1765–1772.

179. Darke S, et al. Heroin-related deaths in south-western Sydney. *Med J Aus.* 1997;167:107.

180. Dart R, Surratt H, Cicero T, et al. Trends in opioid analgesic abuse and mortality in the United States. *N Engl J Med.* 2015;372:241–248.

181. Dasgupta N, Sanford C, Albert S, et al. Opioid drug overdoses: a prescription for harm and potential for prevention. *Am J Lifestyle Med.* 2010;4(1):32–37.

182. Daubresse M, Gleason P, Peng Y, et al. Impact of a drug utilization review program on high-risk use of prescription controlled substances. *Pharmacoepidemiol Drug Saf.* 2014;23:419–427.

183. Davenport-Hines R. *The Pursuit of Oblivion: A Global History of Narcotics.* W.W. Norton; 2003:68.

184. Davidson P, Ochoa K, Han J, et al. Witnessing heroin-related overdoses: the experiences of young injectors in San Francisco. *Addiction.* 2002;97(12):1511–1516.

185. Davies G. A critical evaluation of the effects of safe injection facilities. *J Global Drug Policy Pract.* 2007;1(3):9–19.

186. Davis C, Carr D. Legal changes to increase access to naloxone for opioid overdose reversal in the United States. *Drug Alcohol Depend.* 2015;157:112–120.

187. Davis C, Carr D, Southwell J, et al. Engaging law enforcement in overdose reversal initiatives: authorization and liability for naloxone administration. *Am J Public Health.* 2015;105(8):1530–1537.

188. Davis C, Chang S. *Legal Interventions to Reduce Overdose Mortality: Naloxone Access and Overdose Good Samaritan Laws.* The Network for Public Health Law: Robert Wood Johnson Foundation; 2014.

189. Davis C, Webb D, Burris S. Changing law from barrier to facilitator of opioid overdose prevention. *J Law Med Ethics.* 2013;41:33–36.

190. Davis G, et al. National Association of Medical Examiners position paper: recommendations for the investigation, diagnosis, and certification of deaths related to opioid drugs. *Acad Forensic Pathol.* 2013;3(1):77–83.

191. Davis G, et al. Complete Republication: national Association of Medical Examiners position paper: recommendations for the investigation, diagnosis, and certification of deaths related to opioid drugs. *J Med Toxicol.* 2014;10:100–106.

192. Davoli M, Bargagli A, Perucci C, et al. Risk of fatal overdose during and after specialist drug treatment: the VEdeTTE study, a national multi-site prospective cohort study. *Addiction.* 2007;102(12):1954–1959.

193. Degenhardt L, Bucello C, Mathers B, et al. Mortality among regular or dependent users of heroin and other opioids: a systematic review and meta-analysis of cohort studies. *Addiction.* 2011;106:32–51.

194. Reference deleted in review.

195. Degenhardt L, Hall W, Adelstein B. Ambulance calls to suspected overdoses: New South Wales patterns July 1997 to June 1999. *Aust N Z J Public Health.* 2001;25(5):447–450.

196. Degenhardt L, Larney S, Kimber J, et al. The impact of opioid substitution therapy on mortality post release from prison: retrospective data linkage study. *Addiction.* 2014;109:1306–1317.

197. Degenhardt L, Randall D, Hall W, et al. Mortality among clients of a state-wide opioid pharmacotherapy program over 20 years: risk factors and lives saved. *Drug Alcohol Depend.* 2009;105:9–15.

198. de Jong W, Weber U. The professional acceptance of drug use: a closer look at drug consumption rooms in The Netherlands, Germany and Switzerland. *Int J Drug Policy.* 1999;10:99–108.

199. Delcher C, Wagenaar A, Goldberger B, et al. Abrupt decline in oxycodone caused mortality after of Florida's Prescription Drug Monitoring Program. *Drug Alcohol Depend.* 2015;150:63–68.

200. Department of Health and Human Services. *Addressing Prescription Drug Abuse in the United States: Current Activities and Future Opportunities.* Washington, DC: Behavioral Health Coordinating Committee Prescription Drug Abuse Subcommittee; 2013. http://www.cdc.gov/drugoverdose/pdf/hhs_prescription_drug_abuse_report_09.2013.pdf.

201. DeRosier J. *Pain Clinic Legislation in Louisiana. Promising Legal Responses to the Epidemic of Prescription Drug Overdoses in the United States*. Atlanta, GA: CDC; 2008.

202. Dettmer K, Saunders B, Strang J. Take home naloxone and the prevention of deaths from opiate overdose: two pilot schemes. *BMJ*. 2001;322(7291):895–896.

203. Dhalla I, Mamdani MGT, et al. Clustering of opioid prescribing and opioid-related mortality among family physicians in Ontario. *Can Fam Physician*. 2011;57(3):e92–e96.

204. Dietze P, Jolley D, Cvetkovski S. Patterns and characteristics of ambulance attendance at heroin overdose at a local-area level in Melbourne, Australia: implications for service provision. *J Urban Health*. 2003;80(2):248–260.

205. Dinga H, Czotya P, Kiguchia N. A novel orvinol analog, BU08028, as a safe opioid analgesic without abuse liability in primates. 113(37):e5511–e5518.

206. Doe-Simkins M, Walley A, Epstein A, et al. Saved by the nose: Bystander-administered intranasal naloxone hydrochloride for opioid overdose. *Am J Public Health*. 2009;99(5):788–791.

207. Dolan K, Kimber J, Fry C, et al. Drug consumption facilities in Europe and the establishment of supervised injecting centres in Australia. *Drug Alcohol Rev*. 2000;19:337–346.

208. Dolan K, Shearer J, White B, et al. Four-year follow-up of imprisoned male heroin users and methadone treatment: mortality, re-incarceration and hepatitis C infection. *Addiction*. 2005;100(6):820–828.

209. Domanski K, Kleinschmidt K, Schulte J, et al. Two cases of intoxication with new synthetic opioid, U 47700. *Clin Toxicol*. 2017;55:46–50.

210. Dormuth C, Miller T, Huang A, et al. Effect of a centralized prescription network on inappropriate prescriptions for opioid analgesics and benzodiazepines. *CMAJ (Can Med Assoc J)*. 2012;184(16):e852–e856.

211. Dowell D, Haegerich T, Chou R. CDC guideline for prescribing opioids for chronic pain—United States, 2016. *MMWR Recomm Rep (Morb Mortal Wkly Rep)*. 2016;65(No. RR-1):1–49.

212. Dowell D, Haegerich T, Chou R. CDC guideline for prescribing opioids for chronic pain—United States, 2016. *J Am Med Assoc*. 2016;315:1624–1645.

213. Dowell D, Zhang K, Noonan R, et al. Mandatory provider review and pain clinic laws reduce the amounts of opioids prescribed and overdose death rates. *Health Aff*. 2016;35(10):1–9.

214. Dowling J, Isbister GK, Kirkpatrick CM, et al. Population pharmacokinetics of intravenous, intramuscular and intranasal naloxone in human volunteers. *Drug Moni*. 2008;30:490–496.

215. Doyon S, Benton C, Anderson B, et al. Incorporation of poison center services in a state-wide overdose education and naloxone distribution program. *Am J Addict*. 2016;25(4):301–306.

216. Drake CT, Milner TA. Mu-opioid receptors are in somatodendritic and axonal compartments of GABAergic neurons in rat hippocampal formation. *Brain Res*. 1999;849:203–215.

217. Drug Enforcement Administration. *Electronic Prescriptions for Controlled Substances*; 2014. https://www.deadiversion.usdoj.gov/fed_regs/rules/2010/fr0331.htm.

218. Drug Enforcement Administration. *Final Rule on Disposal of Controlled Substances*; 2014. https://www.federalregister.gov/articles/2014/09/09/2014-20926/disposal-of-controlled-substances.

219. Drug Enforcement Administration. *National Drug Threat Assessment Summary*; 2015. http://www.dea.gov/docs/2015%20NDTA%20Report.pdf.

220. Drug Enforcement Administration. *DEA Issues Nationwide Alert on Fentanyl as Threat to Health and Public Safety*; 2015. http://www.deadiversion.usdoj.gov/drug_chem_info/fentanyl.pdf.

221. Drug Enforcement Administration. *DEA'S Prescription Drug Take-Back Effort-- A Big Success*; 2015. https://www.dea.gov/divisions/hq/2015/hq100115.shtml.

222. Drug Enforcement Administration. *Counterfeit Pills Fueling U.S. Fentanyl and Opioid Crisis*; 2016. https://www.dea.gov/divisions/hq/2016/hq072216.shtml.

223. Drug Enforcement Administration. *DEA Intelligence Brief: Counterfeit Prescription Pills Containing Fentanyls: A Global Threat. DEA-DCT-DIB-021-16*; 2016. https://www.dea.gov/docs/Counterfeit%20Prescription%20Pills.pdf. Accessed September 19, 2016.

224. Drug Enforcement Administration. *DEA Collects Record-Setting Amount of Meds at Latest National Rx Take-Back Day*; 2016. https://www.dea.gov/divisions/hq/2016/hq050616.shtml.

225. Drug Enforcement Administration. Proposed rule: Schedules of controlled substances: temporary Placement of U-47700 into schedule I; 2016. www.federalregister.gov/documents/2016/09/07/2016-21477/schedules-of-controlled-substances-temporary-placement-of-u-47700-into-schedule-i.

226. Drug Enforcement Administration. *Fentanyl: A Briefing Guide for First Responders*; 2017. https://www.dea.gov/druginfo/Fentanyl_BriefingGuideforFirstResponders_June2017.pdf.

227. Drug Free Australia. *Analysis of KPMG Evaluation of the Sydney Medically Supervised Injecting centre*; 2010. www.drugfree.org.au/images/13Books FP/.../DFA_Analysis_Injecting_Room_2010.pdf.

228. Dunn K, Barrett F, Fingerhood M, et al. Opioid overdose history, risk behaviors, and knowledge in patients taking prescribed opioids for chronic pain. *Pain Med*. 2017;18(8):1505–1515.

229. Dunn K, Saunders K, Rutter C, et al. Opioid prescriptions for chronic pain and overdose: a cohort study. *Ann Intern Med*. 2010;152(2):85–92.

230. Durfee M, Parra J, Alexander R. Child fatality review teams. *Pediatr Clini Nor Am*. 2009;56(2):379–387.

231. Dy S, Shore A, Hicks R, et al. Medication errors with opioids: results from a national reporting system. *J Opioid Manag*. 2007;3:189–194.

232. Eap C, Buclin T, Baumann P. Interindividual variability of the clinical pharmacokinetics of methadone: implications for the treatment of opioid dependence. *Clin Pharmacokinet*. 2002;41(14):1153–1193.

233. Edlund M, Martin B, Fan M, et al. An analysis of heavy utilizers of opioids for chronic noncancer pain in the TROUP Study. *J Pain Symptom Manage*. 2010;40:279–289.

234. Edwards E, Searles J, Shapiro S. Deaths involving drugs in Vermont, 2004 through 2010. *Arch Intern Med*. 2011;171(18):1676–1678.

235. Elhwairis H, Reznich C. An educational strategy for treating chronic, non-cancer pain with opioids: a pilot test. *J Pain*. 2010;11:1368–1375.

236. Elliott S, Brandt S, Smith C. The first reported fatality associated with the synthetic opioid 3,4-dichloro N-[2-(dimethylamino)cyclohexyl]-N-methylbenzamide (U-47700) and implications for forensic analysis. *Drug Test Anal*. 2016;8(8):875–879.

237. Elzey M, Barden S, Edwards E. Patient characteristics and outcomes in unintentional, non-fatal prescription opioid overdoses: a systematic review. *Pain Physician*. 2016;19:215–228.

238. Enteen L, Bauer J, McLean R, et al. Overdose prevention and naloxone prescription for opioid users in San Francisco. *J Urban Health*. 2010;87(6):931–941.

239. Etches R. Respiratory depression associated with patient-controlled analgesia: a review of eight cases. *Can J Anaesth*. 1994;41:125–132.

240. European Monitoring Centre for Drugs and Drug Addiction. *European Report on Drug Consumption Rooms*. Lisbon, Portugal: Publications Office of the European Union; 2004.

241. European Monitoring Centre for Drugs and Drug Addiction. *Drug Consumption Facilities in Europe and beyond in: Harm Reduction: Evidence, Impacts and Challenges*. Lisbon, Portugal: Publications Office of the European Union; 2010.

242. European Monitoring Centre for Drugs and Drug Addiction. *European Drug Report 2010: Trends and Developments*. Luxembourg: Publications Office of the European Union; 2010.

243. European Monitoring Centre for Drugs and Drug Addiction. *2012 Annual Report on the State of the Drugs Problem in Europe*. Lisbon, Portugal; 2012.

244. European Monitoring Centre for Drugs and Drug Addiction. *European Drug Report 2014: Trends and Developments.* Luxembourg: Publications Office of the European Union; 2014.

245. European Monitoring Centre for Drugs and Drug Addiction. Drug consumption rooms: an overview of provision and evidence. http://www.emcdda.europa.eu/topics/pods/drug-consumption-rooms; 2015.

246. European Monitoring Centre for Drugs and Drug Addiction. *European Drug Report 2016: Trends and Developments.* Luxembourg: Publications Office of the European Union; 2016.

247. Evans J, Hogg M, Lunn J, et al. Degree and duration of reversal by naloxone of effects of morphine in conscious subjects. *Br Medical Jrnl.* 1974;2:589–591.

248. Evans E, Li L, Min J, et al. Mortality among individuals accessing pharmacological treatment for opioid dependence in California, 2006–10. *Addiction.* 2015;110:996–1005.

249. Fairbairn N, Coffin PO, Walley AY. Naloxone for heroin, prescription opioid, and illicitly made fentanyl overdoses: challenges and innovations responding to a dynamic epidemic. *Int J Drug Policy.* 2017;46:172–179.

250. Fang L, Schinke S. Two-year outcomes of a randomized, family-based substance use prevention trial for Asian American adolescent girls. *J Soc Psychol Addict Behav.* 2013;27(3):788–798.

251. Faroqui MH, Cole M, Curran J. Buprenorphine, benzodiazepines and respiratory depression. *Anaesthesia.* 1983;38(10):1002–1003.

252. Farrell M, Marsden J. *Drug-related Mortality Among Newly Released Offenders 1998 to 2000. Home Office Online Report.* London, UK: Home Office; 2005. Report No. 40/05.

253. Farrell M, Marsden J. Acute risk of drug-related death among newly released prisoners in England and Wales. *Addiction.* 2008;103:251–255.

254. Fathelrahman A, Ab Rahman A, Zain Z. Factors associated with adult poisoning in northern Malaysia: a case-control study. *Hum Exper Toxicol.* 2006;25:167–173.

255. Faul M, Bohm M, Alexander C. Methadone prescribing and overdose and the association with Medicaid preferred drug list policies- United States, 2007–2014. *MMWR (Morb Mortal Wkly Rep).* 2017;66:320–323.

256. Feldman L, Williams K, Coates J. Influencing controlled substance prescribing: attending and resident physician use of a state prescription monitoring program. *Pain Med.* 2012;13:908–914.

257. Fernando D. Fentanyl-laced heroin. *J Am Med Assoc.* 1991;12(22):2962.

258. Ferri M, Davoli M, Perucci C. Heroin maintenance for chronic heroin-dependent individuals. *Cochrane Database Syst Rev.* 2011;12 Art. No.: CD003410. https://doi.org/10.1002/14651858.CD003410.pub4.

259. Fillingim RB, Kaplan L, Staud R, et al. The A118G single nucleotide polymorphism of the mu-opioid receptor gene (OPRM1) is associated with pressure pain sensitivity in humans. *J Pain.* 2005;6:159–167.

260. Fine P, Portenoy R. Establishing "best practices" for opioid rotation: Conclusions of an expert panel. *J Pain Symptom Manage.* 2009;38(3):418–425.

261. Fischer B, Brissette S, Brochu S, et al. Determinants of overdose incidents among illicit opioid users in 5 Canadian cities. *Can Med Assoc J.* 2004;171(3):235–239.

262. Fischer B, Jones W, Krahn M, et al. Differences and over-time changes in levels of prescription opioid analgesic dispensing from retail pharmacies in Canada, 2005–2010. *Pharmacoepidemiol Drug Saf.* 2011;20(12):1269–1277.

263. Flacke J, Facke W, Williams G. Acute pulmonary edema following naloxone reversal of high-dose morphine anesthesia. *Anesthesiology.* 1977;47:376–378.

264. Fleming B, Coombes D. A survey of complications documented in a quality-control analysis of patient controlled analgesia in the postoperative patient. *J Pain Symptom Manage.* 1992;7:463–469.

265. Florida Department of Law Enforcement. *Buyer Beware - Deadly Super Pill Found in Central Florida*; 2016. http://www.fdle.state.fl.us/cms/News/2016/April/Buyer-Beware-%E2%80%93-deadly-super-pill-found-in Central.aspx.

266. Food and Drug Administration. *Public Health Advisory: Methadone Use for Pain Control Might Result in Death and Life-Threatening Changes in Breathing and Heartbeat.* Rockville, MD: Food and Drug Administration; 2006. http://www.fda.gov/Drugs/DrugSafety/PostmarketDrugSafetyInformationforPatientsandProviders/ucm124346.htm.

267. Food and Drug Administration Public Health Advisory. *Methadone use for pain control may result in death and life-threatening changes in breathing and heart beat;* 2006. Available at: http://www.fda.gov/ForConsumers/ConsumerUpdates/ucm124346.htm.

268. Food and Drug Administration. *Guidance for Industry-Format and Content of Proposed Risk Evaluation and Mitigation Strategies (REMS), REMS Assessments, and Proposed REMS Modifications;* 2009.

269. Food and Drug Administration. *FDA's efforts to address the misuse and abuse of opioids;* 2013. Available at: http://www.fda.gov/Drugs/DrugSafety/InformationbyDrugClass/ucm337852.htm.

270. Food and Drug Administration. *Guidance for Industry: Abuse-Deterrent Opioids Evaluation and Labeling;* 2015. http://www.fda.gov/downloads/Drugs/GuidanceComplianceRegulatoryInformation/Guidances/UCM334743.pdf.

271. Food and Drug Administration. *Introduction for the FDA Blueprint for Prescriber Education for Extended-Release and Long-Acting Opioid Analgesics.* Silver Spring, MD: Food and Drug Administration; 2016.

272. Food and Drug Administration. *Updated ER/LA Opioid Analgesic Postmarketing Requirements;* 2016. http://www.fda.gov/Drugs/DrugSafety/InformationbyDrugClass/ucm363722.htm.

273. Forrest A. Buprenorphine and lorazepam. *Anaesthesia.* 1983;38:598.

274. Forrester M. Ingestions of hydrocodone, carisoprodol, and alprazolam in combination reported to Texas poison centers. *J Addict Dis.* 2011;30:110–115.

275. Fox T, Li J, Stevens S, et al. A performance improvement prescribing guideline reduces opioid prescriptions for emergency department dental pain patients. *Ann Emerg Med.* 2013;62:237–240.

276. Frank RG, Pollack HA. Addressing the fentanyl threat to public health. *N Engl J Med.* 2017;376:605–607.

277. Franklin G, Fulton-Kehoe D, Turner J, et al. Changes in opioid prescribing for chronic pain in Washington state. *J Am Board Fam Med.* 2013;26:394–400.

278. Franklin G, Mai J, Turner J, et al. Bending the prescription opioid dosing and mortality curves: impact of the Washington state opioid dosing guideline. *Am J Ind Med.* 2013;55:325–331.

279. Franklin G, Sabel J, Jones CM, et al. A comprehensive approach to address the prescription opioid epidemic in Washington State: milestones and lessons learned. *Am J Public Health.* 2015;105:463–469.

280. Fredheim O, Moksnes K, Borchgrevink P, et al. Clinical pharmacology of methadone for pain. *Acta Anaesthesiol Scand.* 2008;52(7):879–889.

281. Fugelstad A, Ahlner J, Brandt L, et al. Use of morphine and 6-monoacetylmorphine in blood for the evaluation of possible risk factors for sudden death in 192 heroin users. *Addiction.* 2003;98(4):463–470.

282. Fulton-Kehoe D, Garg R, Turner J, et al. Opioid poisonings and opioid adverse effects in workers in Washington state. *Am J Ind Med.* 2013;56:1452–1462.

283. Gaeta J, Bock B, Takach M. Providing a safe space and medical monitoring to prevent overdose deaths. *Health Affairs Blog.* 2016. August 31, 2016. http://healthaffairs.org/blog/2016/08/31/providing-a-safe-space-and-medical-monitoring-to-prevent-overdose-deaths/.

284. Gal T. Naloxone reversal of bupreorphine-induced respiratory depression. *Clin Pharmacol Ther.* 1989;45:66–71.

285. Galea S, Ahern J, Tardiff K, et al. Racial/ethnic disparities in overdose mortality trends in New York City, 1990-1998. *J Urban Health*. 2003;80(2):201–211.

286. Galea S, Worthington N, Piper T, et al. Provision of naloxone to injection drug users as an overdose prevention strategy: early evidence from a pilot study in New York City. *Addict Behav*. 2006;31(5):907–912.

287. García M, Dodek A, Kowalski T, et al. Declines in opioid prescribing after a private insurer policy change — Massachusetts, 2011–2015. *MMWR (Morb Mortal Wkly Rep)*. 2016;65:1125–1131.

288. Gaston R, Best D, Manning V, et al. Can we prevent drug related deaths by training opioid users to recognize and manage overdoses? *Harm Reduct J*. 2009;6:26.

289. Gerevich J, Bácskai E, Farkas L, et al. A case report: Pavlovian conditioning as a risk factor of heroin 'overdose' death. *Harm Reduct J*. 2005;2:11.

290. Ghuran A, Nolan J. Recreational drug misuse: issues for the cardiologist. *Heart*. 2000;83(6):627–633.

291. Gibson A, Degenhardt L. Mortality related to pharmacotherapies for opioid dependence: a comparative analysis of coronial records. *Drug Alcohol Rev*. 2007;26:405–410.

292. Gibson A, Degenhardt L, Mattick R, et al. Exposure to opioid maintenance treatment reduces long-term mortality. *Addiction*. 2008;103:462–468.

293. Gladden RM, Martinez P, Seth P. Fentanyl law enforcement submissions and increases in synthetic opioid–involved overdose deaths — 27 States, 2013–2014. *MMWR (Morb Mortal Wkly Rep)*. 2016;65:837–843.

294. Goetting MG, Thirmam MJ. Neurotoxicity of meperidine. *Ann Emerg Med*. 1985;14:1007–1009.

295. Golberger BA, Maxwell JC, Campbell AC, et al. Uniform standards and case definitions for classifying opioid-related deaths: recommendations by a SAMHSA consensus panel. *J Addict Diseases*. 2013;32:231–243.

296. Goldfrank L, Weisman RS, Errick JK, et al. A dosing nomogram for continuous infusion intravenous naloxone. *Ann Emerg Med*. 1986;15:566–570.

297. Gonzalez A, Kolbasovsky A. Impact of a managed controlled-opioid prescription monitoring program on care coordination. *Am J Manag Care*. 2012;18:512–516.

298. Goodman A, Le Bourdonnec B, Dolle R. Mu opioid receptor antagonists: recent developments. *ChemMedChem*. 2007;2:1552–1570.

299. Gossop M, Griffiths P, Powis B, et al. Frequency of non-fatal heroin overdose: survey of heroin users recruited in non-clinical settings. *BMJ*. 1996;313(7054):402.

300. Gossop M, Stewart D, Tracy S, et al. A prospective study of mortality among drug misusers during a 4 year period after seeking treatment. *Addiction*. 2002;97:39–47.

301. Reference deleted in review.

302. Graham A. Post-prison mortality: Unnatural death among people released from Victorian prisons between January 1990 and December 1999. *Aust New Zeal J Criminol*. 2003;36(1):94–108.

303. Gray J, Hagemeier N. Prescription drug abuse and DEA-sanctioned drug take-back events: characteristics and outcomes in rural Appalachia. *Arch Intern Med*. 2012;172:1186–1187.

304. Gray J, Hagemeier N, Brooks B, et al. Prescription disposal practices: a 2-year ecological study of drug drop box donations in Appalachia. *Am J Public Health*. 2015;105(9):e89–e94.

305. Green T, Grau L, Carver H, et al. Epidemiologic trends and geographic patterns of fatal opioid intoxications in Connecticut, USA: 1997–2007. *Drug Alcohol Depend*. 2011;115(3):221–228.

306. Green T, Mann M, Bowman S. How does use of a prescription monitoring program change medical practice? *Pain Med*. 2012;13(10):1314–1323.

307. Green T, McGowan S, Yokell M, et al. HIV infection and risk of overdose: a systematic review and meta-analysis. *AIDS (London, England)*. 2012;26(4):403–417.

308. Green T, Zaller N, Rich J, et al. Revisiting Paulozzi et al.'s "prescription drug monitoring programs and death rates from drug overdose". *Pain Med*. 2011;12(6):982–985.

309. Griggs CA, Weiner SG, Feldman JA. Prescription drug monitoring programs: examining limitations and future approaches. *Western J Emerg Med*. 2015;16(1):67–70.

310. Guenther U, Manzke T, Wrigge H, et al. The counteraction of opioid-induced ventilatory depression by the serotonin 1A-agonist 8-OH-DPAT does not antagonize antinociception in rats in situ and in vivo. *Anesth Analg*. 2009;108:1169–1176.

311. Gueye P, Borron SW, Risède P, et al. Lack of effect of single high doses of buprenorphine on arterial blood gases in the rat. *Toxicol Sci*. 2001;62:148–154.

312. Gueye P, Borron SW, Risede P, et al. Buprenorphine and midazolam act in combination to depress respiration in rats. *Toxicol Sci*. 2002;65:107–114.

313. Gutiérrez-Cebollada J, de la Torre R, Ortuño J, et al. Psychotropic drug consumption and other factors associated with heroin overdose. *Drug Alcohol Depend*. 1994;35(2):169–174.

314. Guy GP, Zhang K, Bohm MK, et al. Vital signs: changes in opioid prescribing in the United States, 2006–2015. *MMWR (Morb Mortal Wkly Rep)*. 2017;66:697–704.

315. Gwin M, Kelly S, Brown B, et al. Uses of diverted methadone and buprenorphine by opioid addicted individuals in Baltimore, Maryland. *Am J Addict*. 2009;18(5):346–355.

316. Haasen C, Verthein U, Degwitz P, et al. Heroin-assisted treatment for opioid dependence: randomised controlled trial. *Br J Psychiatr*. 2007;191:55–62.

317. Haegerich T, Paulozzi L, Manns B, et al. What we know, and don't know, about the impact of state policy and systems-level interventions on prescription drug overdose. *Drug Alcohol Depend*. 2014;145:34–47.

318. Hagmeyer KO, Mauro LS, Mauro VF. Meperidine-related seizures associated with patient controlled analgesia pumps. *Ann Pharmacother*. 1993;27:29–32.

319. Håkansson A, Vedin A, Wallin C. Distribution of naloxone to prevent death from heroin overdose. Study of opioid dependent patients' attitudes to be part of the antidote program. *Lakartidningen*. 2013;110(29–31):1340–1342.

320. Hall AJ, Logan JE, Toblin RL, et al. Patterns of abuse among unintentional pharmaceutical overdose fatalities. *J Am Med Assoc*. 2008;300:2613–2620.

321. Hall W, Degenhardt L. Regulating opioid prescribing to provide access to effective treatment while minimizing diversion: an overdue topic for research. *Addiction*. 2007;102(11):1685–1688.

322. Hammersley R, Cassidy M, Oliver J. Drugs associated with drug-related deaths in Edinburgh and Glasgow, November 1990 to October 1992. *Addiction*. 1995;90(7):959–965.

323. Han B, Compton WM, Blanco C, et al. Prescription opioid use, misuse, and use disorders in U.S. adults: 2015 National Survey on Drug Use and Health. *Ann Intern Med*. 2017;167(5):293–301.

324. Hansen A. Norway tries naloxone in spray form to prevent deaths from drug overdose. *BMJ*. 2014;348:g1686.

325. Harm Reduction International, UK. *The Global State of Harm Reduction 2016*. London, UK: Harm Reduction International; 2017.

326. Harmon KJ, Proescholdbell S, Waller A, et al. *A Response to the Safe States Injury Surveillance Workgroup (ISW)-7 ICD-9-CM Poisoning Matrix*. Chapel Hill, North Carolina: Carolina Center for Health Informatics and the Injury Prevention Research Center (ICRC); The University of North Carolina; 2013.

327. Hasegawa K, Brown D, Tsugawa Y, et al. Epidemiology of emergency department visits for opioid overdose: a population-based study. *Mayo Clin Proc*. 2014;89(4):462–471.

328. Havens J, Leukefeld C, DeVeaugh-Geiss A, et al. The impact of a reformulation of extended-release oxycodone designed to deter abuse in a sample of prescription opioid abusers. *Drug Alcohol Depend*. 2014;139:9–17.

329. Havens J, Walker R, Leukefeld C. Prevalence of opioid analgesic injection among rural nonmedical opioid analgesic users. *Drug Alcohol Depend*. 2007;87:98–102.

330. HCUP. *Nationwide Inpatient Sample (NIS). Healthcare Cost and Utilization Project (HCUP)*. Agency for Healthcare Research and Quality; 1993-2009.

331. HCUP. *Nationwide Inpatient Sample Trends (NIS-Trends). Healthcare Cost and Utilization Project (HCUP)*. Agency for Healthcare Research and Quality; 1993-2009.

332. Heavner J. Teaching pain management to medical students. *Pain Pract*. 2009;9:85.

333. Hedegaard H, Warner M, Miniño AM. *Drug Overdose Deaths in the United States, 1999–2015. NCHS Data Brief, No 273*. Hyattsville, MD: National Center for Health Statistics; 2017.

334. Helander A, Bäckberg M, Signell P, Beck O. Intoxications involving acrylfentanyl and other novel designer fentanyls – results from the Swedish STRIDA project. *Clin Toxicol*. 2017;55(6):589–599.

335. Heller D, Stancliff S. Providing naloxone to substance users for secondary administration to reduce overdose mortality in New York City. *Public Health Rep*. 2007;122(3):393–397.

336. Henderson G. Fentanyl-related deaths: demographics, circumstances and toxicology of 112 cases. *J Forensic Sci*. 1991;36(2):422–433.

337. Hibbs J, Perper J, Winek C. An outbreak of designer drug-related deaths in Pennsylvania. *J Am Med Assoc*. 1991;265:1011–1013.

338. Hochman M. Meperidine associated myoclonus and seizures in long term hemodialysis patients. *Ann Neurol*. 1983;14:593.

339. Hoffman L, Enders J, Pippins J, et al. Reducing claims for prescription drugs with a high potential for abuse. *Am J Health Syst Pharm*. 2003;60:371–374.

340. Hughes A, Williams MR, Lipari RN, et al. *Prescription Drug Use and Misuse in the United States: Results from the 2015 National Survey on Drug Use and Health*. NSDUH Data Review; 2016. http://www.samhsa.gov/data/.

341. Hulse G, Tait R, Comer S, et al. Reducing hospital presentations for opioid overdose in patients treated with sustained release naltrexone implants. *Drug Alcohol Depend*. 2005;79(3):351–357.

342. Humphries C, Counsell D, Pediani R, et al. Audit of opioid prescribing: the effect of hospital guidelines. *Anaesthesia*. 1997;52:745–749.

343. Hutchinson M, Bland S, Johnson K, et al. Opioid-induced glial activation: mechanisms of activation and implications for opioid analgesia, dependence and reward. *Sci World J*. 2007;7:98–111.

344. Hutchinson M, Northcutt A, Chao L, et al. Minocycline suppresses morphine-induced respiratory depression, suppresses morphine-induced reward, and enhances systemic morphine-induced analgesia. *Brain Behav Immun*. 2008;22:1248–1256.

345. Huxtable R, Schwarz S. The isolation of morphine. *Mol Interv*. 2001;1:189–191.

346. Injury Surveillance Workgroup 7. *Consensus Recommendations for National and State Poisoning Surveillance*. Atlanta, GA: The Safe States Alliance; 2012.

347. International overdose awareness day. http://www.overdoseday.com/.

348. Islam M, McRae I. An inevitable wave of prescription drug monitoring programs in the context of prescription opioids: pros, cons and tensions. *BMC Pharmacol Toxicol*. 2014;15(46).

349. Jamison R, Sheehan K, Scanlan E, Matthews M, Ross E. Beliefs and attitudes about opioid prescribing and chronic pain management: survey of primary care providers. *J Opioid Manag*. 2014;10(6):375–382.

350. Jann M, Kennedy W, Lopez G. Benzodiazepines: a major component in unintentional prescription drug overdoses with opioid analgesics. *J Pharm Pract*. 2014;27:5–16.

351. Jegu J, Gallini A, Soler P, et al. Slow-release oral morphine for opioid maintenance treatment: a systematic review. *Br J Clin Pharmacol*. 2011;71(6):832–843.

352. Johnson E, Porucznik C, Anderson J, et al. State-level strategies for reducing prescription drug overdose deaths: Utah's prescription safety program. *Pain Med*. 2011;12(suppl 2):S66–S72.

353. Johnson H, Paulozzi L, Porucznik C, et al. Decline in drug overdose deaths after state policy changes – Florida, 2010-2012. *MMWR (Morb Mortal Wkly Rep)*. 2014;63(26):569–574.

354. Jones C, Baldwin G, Manocchio T, et al. Trends in methadone distribution for pain treatment, methadone diversion, and overdose deaths -United States, 2002–2014. *MMWR (Morb Mortal Wkly Rep)*. 2016;65:667–671.

355. Jones C, Gladden M, Bohm K. Vital signs: demographic and substance use trends among heroin users – 2002–2013. *MMWR (Morb Mortal Wkly Rep)*. 2015;64(26):719–725.

356. Jones C, Lurie P, Throckmorton D. Effect of US Drug Enforcement Administration's rescheduling of hydrocodone combination analgesic products on opioid analgesic prescribing. *JAMA Intern Med*. 2016;176(3):399–402.

357. Jones C, Lurie P, Woodcock J. Addressing prescription opioid overdose: data support a comprehensive policy approach. *J Am Med Assoc*. 2014;312:1733–1734.

358. Jones C, McAninch J. Emergency department visits and overdose deaths from combined use of opioids and benzodiazepines. *Am J Prev Med*. 2015;49(4):493–501.

359. Jones M, Hernandez B, Janis G, et al. A case of U-47700 overdose with laboratory confirmation and metabolite identification. *Clin Toxicol Aug*. 2016;23:1–5 (Epub ahead of print).

360. Kahan M, Gomes T, Juurlink D, et al. Effect of a course-based intervention and effect of medical regulation on physicians' opioid prescribing. *Can Fam Physician*. 2013;59(5):e231–e239.

361. Kaiko RF, Foley KM, Grabinsky PY. Central nervous system excitatory effects of meperidine in cancer patients. *Ann Neurol*. 1983;13:180–185.

362. Kalyuzhny AE, Dooyema J, Wessendorf MW. Opioid- and GABAA- receptors are co-expressed by neurons in rat brain. *Neuroreport*. 2000;11:2625–2628.

363. Karbakhsh M, Salehian Zandi N. Acute opiate overdose in Tehran: the forgotten role of opium. *Addict Behav*. 2007;32(9):1835–1842.

364. Kariminia A, Butler T, Corben S, et al. Extreme cause specific mortality in a cohort of adult prisoners 1998 to 2002: a data-linkage study. *Int J Epidemiol*. 2007;36(2):310–318.

365. Katz N, Birnhaum H, Brennan M, et al. Prescription opioid abuse: challenges and opportunities for payers. *J Manag Care*. 2013;19:295–302.

366. Reference deleted in review.

367. Kelly A, Kerr D, Dietze P, et al. Randomized trial of intranasal versus intramuscular naloxone in prehospital treatment for suspected opioid overdose. *Med J Aust*. 2005;182:24–27.

368. Kelty E, Hulse G. Examination of mortality rates in a retrospective cohort of patients treated with oral or implant naltrexone for problematic opiate use. *Addiction*. 2012;107(10):1817–1824.

369. Kelty E, Hulse G. Fatal and non-fatal opioid overdose in opioid dependent patients treated with methadone, buprenorphine or implant naltrexone. *Int J Drug Policy*. 2017;46:54–60.

370. Kerr D, Dietze P, Kelly A, et al. Attitudes of Australian heroin users to peer distribution of naloxone for heroin overdose: perspectives on intranasal administration. *J Urban Health*. 2008;85(3):352–360.

371. Kerr D, Kelly AM, Dietze P, et al. Randomized controlled trial comparing the effectiveness and safety of intranasal and intramuscular naloxone for the treatment of suspected heroin overdose. *Addiction*. 2009;104(12):2067–2074.

372. Kerr T, Fairbairn N, Tyndall M, et al. Predictors of non-fatal overdose among a cohort of polysubstance using injection drug users. *Drug Alcohol Depend*. 2007;87(1):9–45.

373. Kim J, Santaella-Tenorio J, Mauro C, et al. State medical marijuana laws and the prevalence of opioids detected among fatally injured drivers. *Am J Public Health*. 2016;106(11):2032–2037.

374. Kimergård, Breindahl T, Hindersson P, et al. Tampering of opioid analgesics: a serious challenge for public health? *Addiction.* 2016;111(10):1701–1702.

375. Kinner S, Milloy M-J, Wood E, et al. Incidence and risk factors for non-fatal overdose among a cohort of recently incarcerated illicit drug users. *Addict Behav.* 2012;37:691–696.

376. Kiwull-Schöne H, Kiwull P, Frede S, et al. Role of brainstem sodium/proton exchanger 3 for breathing control during chronic acid-base imbalance. *Am J Respir Crit Care Med.* 2007;176:513–519.

377. Kleinschmidt K, Wainscott M, Ford M. Opioids. In: Ford MD, Delaney KA, Ling LJ, et al., eds. *Ford: Clinical Toxicology.* 1st ed. Philadelphia, Pa: WB Saunders; 2001:627–639.

378. Klepstad P, Rakvag T, Kaasa S, et al. The 118 AG polymorphism in the human micro-opioid receptor gene may increase morphine requirements in patients with pain caused by malignant disease. *Acta Anaesthesiol Scand.* 2004;48:1232–1239.

379. Knotkova H, Fine P, Portenoy R. Opioid rotation: the science and limitations of the equianalgesic dose table. *J Pain Symptom Manage.* 2009;38(3):426–439.

380. Knudsen H, Abraham A, Roman P. Adoption and implementation of medications in addiction treatment programs. *J Addict Med.* 2011;5:21–27.

381. Kotwal A. Innovation, diffusion and safety of a medical technology: a review of the literature on injection practice. *Social Sci Med.* 2005;60(5):1133–1147.

382. Krebs E, Ramsey D, Miloshoff J, et al. Primary care monitoring of long-term opioid therapy among veterans with chronic pain. *Pain Med.* 2011;12:740–746.

383. Krieter P, Chiang N, Gyaw S, et al. Pharmacokinetic properties and human use characteristics of an fda approved intranasal naloxone product for the treatment of opioid overdose. *J Clin Pharmacol.* 2016;56(10):1243–1253.

384. Krinsky C, Lathrop S, Brown P, Nolte K. Drugs, detention, and death: a study of the mortality of recently released prisoners. *Am J Forensic Med Pathol.* 2009;30(1):6–9.

385. Krinsky C, Lathrop S, Crossey M, et al. A toxicology-based review of fentanyl-related deaths in New Mexico (1986–2007). *Am J Forensic Med Pathol.* 2011;32(4):347–351.

386. Krupitsky E, Nunes E, Ling W. Injectable extended-release naltrexone (XR-NTX) for opioid dependence: long-term safety and effectiveness. *Addiction.* 2013;108(9):1628–1637.

387. Krupitsky E, Zvartau E, Woody G. Use of Naltrexone to treat opioid addiction in a country in which methadone and buprenorphine are not available. *Curr Psychiatry Rep.* 2010;12(5):448–453.

388. Kuehn B. Major disparities in opioid prescribing among states: some states crack down on excess prescribing. *J Am Med Assoc.* 2014;312:684–686.

389. Kunins H, Farley T, Dowell D. Guidelines for opioid prescription: Why emergency physicians need support. *Ann Intern Med.* 2013;158:841–842.

390. Lalley P. Mu-opioid receptor agonist effects on medullary respiratory neurons in the cat: evidence for involvement in certain types of ventilatory disturbances. *Am J Physiol Regul Integr Comp Physiol.* 2003;285:R1287–R1304.

391. Lalley P, Bischoff A, Richter D. 5HT-1A receptor mediated modulation of medullary expiratory neurons in the cat. *J Physiol.* 1994;476:117–130.

392. Landow L. An apparent seizure following inadvertent intrathecal morphine. *Anaesthesiology.* 1985;62:545–562.

393. Lanier W, Johnson E, Rolfs R, et al. Risk factors for prescription opioid-related death, Utah, 2008-2009. *Pain Med.* 2012;13(12):1580–1589.

394. Lagu T, Anderson B, Stein M. Overdoses among friends: drug users are willing to administer naloxone to others. *J Subst Abuse Treat.* 2006;30(2):129–133.

395. Langendam M, van Brussel G, Coutinho R, et al. The impact of harm reduction-based methadone treatment on mortality among heroin users. *Am J Public Health.* 2001;91:774–780.

396. Lankenau S, Wagner K, Silva K, et al. Injection drug users trained by overdose prevention programs: responses to witnessed overdoses. *J Community Health.* 2013;38(1):133–141.

397. Larochelle M, Zhang F, Ross-Degnan D, et al. Rates of opioid dispensing and overdose after introduction of abuse-deterrent extended-release oxycodone and withdrawal of propoxyphene. *JAMA Intern Med.* 2015;175(6):978–987.

398. Latimer D, Goldberg J. *Flowers in the Blood: The Story of Opium.* New York: Franklin Watts; 1981.

399. Lavonas E, Drennan I, Gabrielli A, et al. Part 10: special circumstances of resuscitation: 2015 American heart association guidelines update for cardiopulmonary resuscitation and emergency Cardiovascular care. *Circulation.* 2015;132(18 suppl 2):S501–S518.

400. Lee J, Friedmann P, Kinlock T. Extended-release naltrexone to prevent opioid relapse in criminal justice offenders. *N Engl J Med.* 2016;374:1232–1242.

401. Leece P, Hopkins S, Marshall C, et al. Development and implementation of an opioid overdose prevention and response program in Toronto, Ontario. *Can J Public Health.* 2013;104(3):e200–e204.

402. Leece P, Orkin A, Kahan M. Tamper-resistant drugs cannot solve the opioid crisis. *CanMed Assoc J.* 2015;187:717–718.

403. Legislative Assembly of Ontario. *Bill 33: Safeguarding Our Communities Act (Patch for Patch Return Policy) Patch4Patch in Ontario;* 2015. http://www.ontla.on.ca/web/bills/bills%5fdetail.do%3flocale%3den&BillID%3d3059&isCurrent%3d&BillStagePrintId%3d6615&btnSubmit%3dgo.

404. Lenton S, Dietze P, Olsen A, et al. Working together: Expanding the availability of naloxone for peer administration to prevent opioid overdose deaths in the Australian Capital Territory and beyond. *Drug Alcohol Rev.* 2015;34(4):404–411.

405. Lenton S, Hargreaves K. Should we conduct a trial of distributing naloxone to heroin users for peer administration to prevent fatal overdose? *Med J Aust.* 2000;173(5):260–263.

406. Lepère B, Gourarier L, Sanchez M, et al. Reduction in the number of lethal heroin overdoses in France since 1994. Focus on substitution treatments. *Ann Med Interne.* 2001;152(suppl 3):IS5–IS12.

407. Levy B, Paulozzi L, Mack K, et al. Trends in opioid analgesic-prescribing rates by specialty, U.S., 2007–2012. *Am J Prev Med.* 2015;49(3):409–413.

408. Lewis D, Park J, Vail L, et al. Evaluation of the overdose education and naloxone distribution program of the Baltimore student harm reduction Coalition. *Am J Public Health.* 2016;106(7):1243–1246.

409. Li G, Brady J, Lang B, et al. Prescription drug monitoring and drug overdose mortality. *Injury Epidemiol.* 2014;1(9):1–8.

410. Li J. Buprenorphine analogue BU08028 is one step closer to the Holy Grail of opioid research. *Proc Natl Acad Sci U S A.* 113(37):10225–10227.

411. Li Q, Luo Y, Sun C, et al. A morphine/heroin vaccine with new hapten design attenuates behavioral effects in rats. *J Neurochem.* 2011;119(6):1271–1281.

412. Lofwall M, Martin J, Tierney M, et al. Buprenorphine diversion and misuse in outpatient practice. *J Addict Med.* 2014;8(5):327–332.

413. Lofwall M, Wunsch M, Nuzzo P, et al. Efficacy of continuing medical education to reduce the risk of buprenorphine diversion. *J Subst Abuse Treat.* 2011;41:321–329.

414. Longnecker D, Grazis P, Eggars G. Naloxone for antagonism of morphine-induced respiratory depression. *Anesth Analg.* 1973;52:447–453.

415. LoVecchio F, Pizon A, Riley B, et al. Onset of symptoms after methadone overdose. *Am J Emerg Med.* 2007;25(1):57–59.

416. Luty J, O'Gara C, Sessay M. Is methadone too dangerous for opiate addiction? *BMJ.* 2005;331:1352–1353.

417. McCauley J, Back S, Brady KT. Pilot of a brief, web-based educational intervention targeting safe storage and disposal of prescription opioids. *Addict Behav.* 2013;38:2230–2235.

418. McCracken L, Boichat C, Eccleston D. Training for general practitioners in opioid prescribing for chronic pain based on practice guidelines: a randomized pilot and feasibility trial. *J Pain.* 2012;13:32–40.

419. McDonald D, Carlson K. Estimating the prevalence of opioid diversion by "doctor shoppers" in the United States. *PLoS One.* 2013;8(7):e69241.

420. McDonald D, Carlson K, Izrael D. Geographic variation in opioid prescribing in the U.S. *J Pain.* 2012;13(10):988–996.

421. McDonald R, Strang J. Are take-home naloxone programmes effective? Systematic review utilizing application of the Bradford Hill criteria. *Addiction.* 2016;111(7):1177–1187.

422. McGregor C, Ali R, Lokan R, et al. Accidental fatalities among heroin users in South Australia, 1994 1997: toxicological findings and circumstances of death. *Addiction Res Theor.* 2002;10(4):335–346.

423. McGregor C, Darke S, Ali R, Christie P. Experience of non-fatal overdose among heroin users in Adelaide, Australia: circumstances and risk perceptions. *Addiction.* 1998;93:701–711.

424. Reference deleted in review.

425. Manchikanti L, Abdi S, Atluri S, et al. American Society of Interventional Pain Physicians (ASIPP) guidelines for responsible opioid prescribing in chronic non-cancer pain: Part I- evidence assessment. *Pain Physician.* 2012;15:S1–S65.

426. Man L-H, Best D, Gossop M, et al. Relationship between prescribing and risk of opiate overdose among drug users in and out of maintenance treatment. *Eur Addict Res.* 2004;10:35–40.

427. Manini AF, Jacobs MM, Vlahov D, et al. Opioid receptor polymorphism !118G associated with clinical severity in a drug overdose population. *J Med Toxicol.* 2013;9:148–154.

428. Manzke T, Guenther U, Ponimaskin E, et al. 5-HT4(a) receptors avert opioid-induced breathing depression without loss of analgesia. *Science.* 2003;301:226–229.

429. March J, Oviedo-Joekes E, Perea-Milla E, et al. Controlled trial of prescribed heroin in the treatment of opioid addiction. *J Substance Abuse Treat.* 2006;31(2):203–211.

430. Maremmani I, Gerra G. Buprenorphine-based regimens and methadone for the medical management of opioid dependence: selecting the appropriate drug for treatment. *Am J Addict.* 2010;19:557–568.

431. Marshall B, Milloy M, Wood E, et al. Reduction in overdose mortality after the opening of North America's first medically supervised safer injecting facility: a retrospective population-based study. *Lancet.* 2011;377(9775):1429–1437.

432. Marteau D, McDonald R, Patel K. The relative risk of fatal poisoning by methadone or buprenorphine within the wider population of England and Wales. *BMJ Open.* 2015;5:e007629.

433. Martin M, Hecker J, Clark R, et al. China White epidemic: an eastern United States emergency department experience. *Ann Emerg Med.* 1991;20(2):158–164.

434. Martin W. Naloxone. *Arch Int Med.* 1976;85:765–768.

435. Martine SS, Sarvet A, Santella-Tenorio J, et al. Changes in us lifetime heroin use and heroin use disorder prevalence from the 2001-2002 to 2012-2013 National Epidemiologic Survey on Alcohol and Related Conditions. *JAMA Psychiatry.* 2017;74(5):445–455.

436. Martins S, Sampson L, Cerda M, et al. Worldwide prevalence and trends in unintentional drug overdose: a systematic review of the literature. *Am J Public Health.* 2015;105(11):e29–e49.

437. Mather L, Tucker G. Systemic availability of orally administered meperidine. *Clin Pharmacol Ther.* 1976;120:535–540.

438. Mathers B, Degenhardt L, Bucello C, et al. Mortality among people who inject drugs: a systematic review and meta-analysis. *Bull World Health Organ.* 2013;91:102–123.

439. Matheson C, Pflanz-Sinclair C, Aucott L, et al. Reducing drug related deaths: a pre-implementation assessment of knowledge, barriers and enablers for naloxone distribution through general practice. *BMC Fam Pract.* 2014;15(1):12–21.

440. Mattick R, Breen C, Kimber J, et al. Buprenorphine maintenance versus placebo or methadone maintenance for opioid dependence. *Cochrane Database Syst Rev.* 2014;2:CD002207.

441. Maxwell S, Bigg D, Stanczykiewicz K, et al. Prescribing naloxone to actively injecting heroin users: a program to reduce heroin overdose deaths. *J Addict Dis.* 2006;25(3):89–96.

442. Meara E, Horwitz J, Powell W, et al. State legal restrictions and prescription-opioid use among disabled adults. *NEJM.* 2016;375(1):44–53.

443. Medically Supervised Injecting Centre [MISC] Evaluation Committee. *Final Report of the Evaluation of the Sydney Medically Supervised Injecting Centre*; 2003. http://www.indro-online.de/sydneyfinalreport.pdf.

444. Mégarbane B, Declèves X, Bloch V, et al. Case report: Quantification of methadone induced respiratory depression using toxicokinetic/toxicodynamic relationships. *Crit Care.* 2007;11:R5.

445. Mégarbane B, Hreiche R, Pirnay S, et al. Does high-dose buprenorphine cause respiratory depression? Possible mechanism and therapeutic consequences. *Toxicol Rev.* 2006;225(2):79–85.

446. Megarbane B, Marie N, Pirnay S. Buprenorphine is protective against the depressive effects of norbuprenorphine on ventilation. *Toxicol Appl Pharmacol.* 2006;212:256–267.

447. Megarbane B, Pirnay S, Borron S, et al. Flunitrazepam does not alter cerebral distribution of buprenorphine in the rat. *Toxicol Lett.* 2005;157(3):211–219.

448. Melandri R, Re G, Lanzarini C, et al. Myocardial damage and rhabdomyolysis associated with prolonged hypoxic coma following opiate overdose. *J Toxicol Clin Toxicol.* 1996;34(2):199–203.

449. Merlin M. *On the Trail of the Ancient Opium Poppy.* Cranbury, New Jersey: Farleigh Dickinson University Press; 1984.

450. Merrall E, Bird S, Hutchinson S. A record linkage study of drug-related death and suicide after hospital discharge among drug–treatment clients in Scotland, 1996–2006. *Addiction.* 2013;108:377–384.

451. Merrall E, Kariminia A, Binswanger I, et al. Meta-analysis of drug-related deaths soon after release from prison. *Addiction.* 2010;105(9):1545–1554.

452. Meyer L, Fuller A, Mitchell D. Zacopride and 8-OH-DPAT reverse opioid-induced respiratory depression and hypoxia but not catatonic immobilization in goats. *Am J Physiol Regul Integr Comp Physiol.* 2006;290:R405–R413.

453. Mezei L, Murinson B, Johns Hopkins Pain Curriculum Development Team. Pain education in North American medical schools. *J Pain.* 2011;12(12):1199–1208.

454. Michaelis L, Hickey P, Clark T. Ventricular irritability associated with the use of naloxone. *Ann Thoracic Surg.* 1974;18:608–614.

455. Miller M, Barber C, Leatherman S, et al. Prescription opioid duration of action and the risk of unintentional overdose among patients receiving opioid therapy. *JAMA Intern Med.* 2015;175(4):608–615.

456. Milloy M, Kerr t, Tyndall M, et al. Estimated drug overdose deaths averted by North America's first medically-supervised safer injection facility. *PLoS One.* 2008;3:e3351.

457. Milloy M, Wood E. Emerging role of supervised injecting facilities in human immunodeficiency virus prevention. *Addiction.* 2009;104(4):620–621.

458. Milloy M, Wood E, Reading C, et al. Elevated overdose mortality rates among First Nations individuals in a Canadian setting: a population-based analysis. *Addiction.* 2010;105(11):1962–1970.

459. Minett W, Moore T, Juhascik M, et al. Concentrations of opiates and psychotropic agents in polydrug overdoses: a surprising correlation between morphine and antidepressants. *J Forensic Sci.* 2010;55(5):1319–1325.

460. Modarai F, Mack K, Hicks P, et al. Relationship of opioid prescription sales and overdoses, North Carolina. *Drug Alcohol Depend.* 2013;132(1–2):81–86.

461. Modesto-Lowe V, Brooks D, Petry N. Methadone deaths: risk factors in pain and addicted populations. *J Gen Intern Med.* 2010;25(4):305–309.

462. Modica P, Tempelhoff R, White P. Pro- and anti-convulsant effects of anesthetics (part I and II). *Anesth Analg.* 1990;70:433–444.

463. Mohr A, Friscia M, Papsun D, et al. Analysis of novel synthetic opioids U-47700, U-50488 and Furanyl Fentanyl by LC-MS/MS in postmortem casework. *J Anal Toxicol.* 2016;40(9):709–717.

464. Moller L, Matic S, van den Bergh B, et al. Acute drug-related mortality of people recently released from prisons. *Publ Health*. 2010;124:637–639.

465. Monte A, Mandell T, Wilford B, et al. Diversion of buprenorphine/naloxone coformulated tablets in a region with high prescribing prevalence. *J Addict Dis*. 2009;28(3):226–231.

466. Moore T, Jones T, Bowder J, et al. A comparison of common screening methods for predicting aberrant drug-related behavior among patients receiving opioids for chronic pain management. *Pain Med*. 2009;10(8):1426–1433.

467. Moorman-Li R, Motycka C, Inge L, et al. A review of abuse-deterrent opioids for chronic nonmalignant pain. *PT*. 2012;37(7):412–418.

468. Morasco B, Duckart J, Dobscha S. Adherence to clinical guidelines for opioid therapy for chronic pain in patients with substance use disorder. *J Gen Intern Med*. 2011;26:965–971.

469. Morden N, Zerzan J, Rue T, et al. Medicaid prior authorization and controlled-release oxy-codone. *Med Care*. 2008;46:573–580.

470. Morgan L, Weaver M, Sayeed Z, Orr R. The use of prescription monitoring programs to reduce opioid diversion and improve patient safety. *J Pain Palliat Care Pharmacother*. 2013;27(1):4–9.

471. Morse J, Stockbridge H, Egan K, et al. Primary care survey of the value and effectiveness of the Washington state opioid dosing guideline. *J Opioid Manag*. 2012;7:427–433.

472. Mounteney J, Giraudon I, Denissov G, et al. Fentanyls: are we missing the signs? Highly potent and on the rise in Europe. *Int J Drug Policy*. 2015;26(7):626–631.

473. Mueller S, Walley A, Calcaterra S, et al. A review of opioid overdose prevention and naloxone prescribing: implications for translating community programming into clinical practice. *Subst Abuse*. 2015;36(2):240–253.

474. Muhuri P, Gfroerer J, Davies M. *Associations of Nonmedical Pain Reliever Use and Initiation of Heroin Use in the United States*. Rockville, Md: CBHSQ (Center for Behavioral Health Statistics and Quality) Data Review. SAMHSA; 2013. http://www.samhsa.gov/data/sites/default/files/DR006/nonmedical-pain-reliever use-2013.htm.

475. Mycyk M. Nebulized Naloxone gently and effectively reverses methadone intoxication. *J Emer Med*. 2003;24:185–187.

476. Nandi A, Galea S, Ahern J, et al. What explains the association between neighborhood-level income inequality and the risk of fatal overdose in New York City? *Soc Sci Med*. 2006;63(3):662–674.

477. National Alliance for Model State Drug Laws. *States that Require an ID From a Recipient Prior to Dispensing Prescriptions for Controlled Substances*; 2013. www.namsdl.org/library/B86EEA4F-1372-636C DD9DC3EC15AA9959/ +&cd=2&hl=en&ct= clnk&gl=us.

478. National Alliance for Model State Drug Laws. *Annual Review of Prescription Monitoring Programs*. Charlottesville, VA: National Alliance for Model State Drug Laws; 2015.

479. National Alliance for Model State Drug Laws. *Overview of State Pain Management and Prescribing Policies*. Charlottesville, VA: National Alliance for Model State Drug Laws; 2016.

480. National Center for Health Statistics (NCHS). *Vital Statistics: Instructions for Classifying Multiple Causes of Death. NCHS Instruction Manual, Part 2b*. Hyattsville, Md: NCHS; Department of Health and Human Services; 2009.

481. National Center for Health Statistics (NCHS). *Deaths; Final Data for 2010*. Hyattsville, Md: NCHS; Department of Health and Human Services; 2013.

482. National Center for Health Statistics (NCHS). *ICD–10: external cause of injury mortality matrix [online]*. Available from: https://www.cdc.gov/nchs/injury/injury_matrices.htm (Accessed November 27, 2016).

483. National Center for Health Statistics (NCHS). *Center for Disease Control and Prevention*. National Center for Injury Prevention and Control; 2015. http://www.cdc.gov/injury/images/lccharts/leading_causes_of_injury_deaths_unintentional_injury_2014_ 1040w740h.gif.

484. National Center on Health Statistics (NCHS). *National Overdose Deaths from Select Prescription and Illicit Drugs*; 2016. https://www.drugabuse.gov/related-topics/trends-statistics/overdose-death-rates.

485. National Conference of State Legislatures. *Prevention of Prescription Drug Overdose and Abuse*. Washington, DC; 2014. http://www.ncsl.org/research/health/prevention-of prescriptiondrug-ovrdose and-abuse.aspx.

486. National Governors Association. *Six strategies for reducing prescription drug abuse*; 2012. http://www.nga.org/files/live/sites/NGA/files/pdf/1209ReducingRxDrugsBrief.pdf.

487. National Network for Safe Communities. *Drug Market Intervention: An Implementation Guide*. Washington, DC: Office of Community Oriented Policing Services; 2015. ISBN: 978-1-935676-56 0. http://nnscommunities.org/our-work/strategy/drug-market-intervention.

488. Network for Public Health Law. *Legal Interventions to Reduce Overdose Mortality: Naloxone Access and Overdose Good Samaritan Laws*; 2016. https://www.networkforphl.org/_asset/qz5pvn/network-naloxone-10-4.pdf.

489. Neven D, Paulozzi L, Howell D, et al. A randomized controlled trial of a citywide emergency department care coordination program to reduce prescription opioid related emergency department visits. *J Emerg Med*. 2016;51(5):498–507.

490. New York City Department of Health and Mental Hygiene. Illicit drug use in New York City. *NYC Vital Signs*. 2010;9(1):1–4.

491. Ngai S, Berkowitz B, Yang J, et al. Pharmacokinetics of naloxone in rats and in man: basis for its potency and short duration of action. *Anesthesiology*. 1976;44(5):398–401.

492. Norn S, Kruse P, Kruse E. On the history of injection. *Dan Medicinhist Arbog*. 2006;34:104–111.

493. Nuckols T, Anderson L, Popescu I, et al. Opioid prescribing: a systematic review and critical appraisal of guidelines for chronic pain. *Annal Int Med*. 2014;160(1):38–47.

494. O'Brien C, Childress A, McLellan A, et al. A learning model of addiction. In: O'Brien C, Jaffe J, eds. *Addictive States*. New York: Raven Press; 1992:157–177.

495. O'Conner P, Selwyn P, Schottenfield R. Medical care for injection-drug users with human immunodeficiency virus infection. *N Engl J Med*. 1994;331(7):450–459.

496. Reference deleted in review.

497. Office of National Control Policy. *(2011) Epidemic: Responding to America's Prescription Drug Abuse*. Washington, DC; 2009. www.whitehouse.gov/sites/default/files/ondcp/issues content/prescriptiondrugs/rx_abuse_plan_0.pdf.

498. Office of National Drug Control Policy. *Proper Disposal of Prescription Drugs*. Washington D.C.

499. Office of National Drug Control Policy Executive. *National Drug Control Strategy: Data Supplement 2014*. Washington, DC: Office of the President of the United States; 2014; 2014. .

500. Office of National Drug Control Policy. *Fact Sheet: Opioid Abuse in the United States*; 2014. https://www.whitehouse.gov/sites/default/files/ondcp/Fact_Sheets/opioids_fact_sheet.pdf.

501. Office of National Drug Control Policy. High Intensity Drug Trafficking Areas (HIDTA) Program. https://www.whitehouse.gov/ondcp/high-intensity-drug-trafficking-areas-program (Accessed November 12, 2016).

502. Ohio Hamilton County Heroin Coalition. Heroin adulterant creating deadly combination; 2016. http://www.hamiltoncountyhealth.org/files/files/Press%20Releases/Carfentanil_7_15_2016.pdf.

503. Ohtani M, Kotaki H, Sawada Y, et al. Comparative analysis of buprenorphine- and norbuprenorphine induced analgesic effects based on pharmacokinetic-pharmacodynamic modeling. *J Pharmacol Exp Ther*. 1995;272:505–510.

504. Ohtani M, Kotaki H, Uchino K, et al. Pharmacokinetic analysis of enterohepatic circulation of buprenorphine and its active metabolite, norbuprenorphine, in rats. *Drug Metab Dispos*. 1994;22:2–7.

505. Oliva E, Nevedal A, Lewis E, et al. Patient perspectives on an opioid overdose education and naloxone distribution program in the U.S. Department of Veterans Affairs. *Subst Abus*. 2016;37:118–126.

506. Oliver P, Horspool M, Rowse G, et al. *A Psychological Autopsy Study of Non-deliberate Fatal Opiate Related Overdose*. London: National Treatment Agency for Substance Misuse; 2007.

507. Ontario Injury Prevention Resource Center. *Fentanyl Patch 4 Patch (P4P) Return Program Guidelines.* http://www.oninjuryresources.ca/downloads/news/P4P_Return_Program_Guidelines.pdf. Accessed (August 6, 2017).

508. Oregon State University. *Carisoprodol Quantity Limit Policy Impact Analysis.* Salem: OR: Oregon State University; 2004.

509. Oregon State University. *Drug Use Evaluation: Long-Acting Opioids (LAO).* Salem, OR: Oregon State University; 2012.

510. Osterwalder J. Naloxone for intoxications with intravenous heroin and heroin mixtures—Harmless or hazardous? *J Toxicol Clin Toxicol.* 1996;34:409–416.

511. Oviedo-Joekes E, Brissette S, Marsh D, et al. Diacetylmorphine versus methadone for the treatment of opioid addiction. *NEJM.* 2009;361(8):777–786.

512. Oviedo-Joekes E, Guh D, Brissette S, et al. Hydromorphone compared with diacetylmorphine for long term opioid dependence: a randomized clinical trial. *JAMA Psychiatry.* 2016;73(5):447–455.

513. Owens P, Barrett M, Weiss A, et al. *Hospital Inpatient Utilization Related to Opioid Overuse Among Adults, 1993-2012. HCUP Statistical Brief #177.* Rockville, MD: Agency for Healthcare Research and Quality; 2014. http://www.hcup-us.ahrq.gov/reports/statbriefs/sb177-Hospitalizations-for-Opioid-Overuse.pdf.

514. Partridge B, Ward C. Pulmonary edema following low-dose naloxone administration. *Anesthesiology.* 1986;65:709–710.

515. Patrick S, Fry C, Jones T, Buntin M. Implementation of prescription drug monitoring programs associated with reductions in opioid-related death rates. *Health Aff.* 2016;35(7):1–9.

516. Parmar MKB, Strang J, Choo L, et al. Randomized controlled pilot trial of naloxone-on-release to prevent post-prison opioid overdose deaths. *Addiction.* 2016;112:502–515.

517. Passik S, Kirsh K, Casper D. Addiction-related assessment tools and pain management: instruments for screening, treatment planning, and monitoring compliance. *Pain Med.* 2008;9(suppl S2):S145–S166.

518. Patch4Patch. *Patch 4 Patch Saves Lives*; 2017. http://patch4patch.ca/.

519. Pattinson K. Opioids and the control of respiration. *Br J Anaesth.* 2008;100(6):747–758.

520. Paulozzi L, Annest J. Unintentional poisoning deaths-United States, 1999-2004. *MMWR (Morb Mortal Wkly Rep).* 2007;56(5):93–96.

521. Paulozzi L, Budnitz D, Xi Y. Increasing deaths from opioid analgesics in the United States. *Pharmacoepidemiol Drug Saf.* 2006;15:618–627.

522. Paulozzi L, Jones C, Mack K. Vital signs: overdoses of prescription opioid pain relievers United States, 1999-2008. *MMWR (Morb Mortal Wkly Rep).* 2011;60(43):1487–1492.

523. Paulozzi L, Kilbourne E, Desai H. Prescription drug monitoring programs and death rates from drug overdose. *Pain Med.* 2011;12(5):747–754.

524. Paulozzi L, Ryan G. Opioid analgesics and the rates of fatal drug poisoning in the United States. *Am J Prev Med.* 2006;31:506–511.

525. Paulozzi L, Weisler R, Patkar A. A national epidemic of unintentional prescription opioid overdose deaths: how physicians can help control it. *J Clin Psychiatr.* 2011;72(5):589–592.

526. Paulozzi L, Xi Y. Recent changes in drug poisoning mortality in the United States by urban–rural status and by drug type. *Pharmacoepidemiol Drug Saf.* 2008;17(10):997–1005.

527. Paulozzi L, Zhang K, Jones C, et al. Risk of adverse health outcomes with increasing duration and regularity of opioid therapy. *J Am Board Fam Med.* 2014;27:329–338.

528. Perea-Milla E, Ayçaguer L, Cerdà J, et al. Efficacy of prescribed injectable diacetylmorphine in the Andalusian trial: Bayesian analysis of responders and non-responders according to a multi domain outcome.index. *Trials.* 2009;10:70.

529. Perret G, Déglon JJ, Kreek M, et al. Lethal methadone intoxications in Geneva, Switzerland, from 1994 to 1998. *Addiction.* 2000;95(11):1647–1653.

530. Peterson AB, Gladden RM, Delcher C, et al. Increases in fentanyl-related overdose deaths — Florida and Ohio, 2013–2015. *MMWR (Morb Mortal Wkly Rep).* 2016;65:844–849.

531. Pew Charitable Trusts. *Most States List Deadly Drug Methadone as a "Preferred Drug."* Philadelphia, PA: The Pew Charitable Trusts; 2015. 2015. http://www.pewtrusts.org/en/research-andanalysis/blogs/stateline/2015/4/23/ most-states-list-deadly-methadone-as-a-preferred-drug.

532. Piper T, Rudenstine S, Stancliff S, et al. Overdose prevention for injection drug users: lessons learned from naloxone training and distribution programs in New York City. *Harm Reduct J.* 2007;4:3.

533. Piper T, Stancliff S, Rudenstine S, et al. Evaluation of a naloxone distribution and administration program in New York City. *Subst Use Misuse.* 2008;43(7):858–870.

534. Reference deleted in review.

535. Pirnay S, Mégarbane B, Borron S, et al. Effects of various combinations of benzodiazepines with buprenorphine on arterial blood gases in rats. *Basic Clin Pharmacol Toxicol.* 2008;103(3):228–239.

536. Poisnel G, Dhilly M, Le Boisselier R, et al. Comparison of five benzodiazepine receptor agonists on buprenorphine-induced μ-opioid receptor regulation. *J Pharmacol Sci.* 2009;110:36–46.

537. Pollini R, McCall L, Mehta S, et al. Non-fatal overdose and subsequent drug treatment among injection drug users. *Drug Alcohol Depend.* 2006;83(2):104–110.

538. Pollini R, McCall L, Mehta S, et al. Response to overdose among injection drug users *American. J Prev Med.* 2006;31(3):261–264.

539. Pomerleau A, Nelson L, Hoppe J, et al. The impact of prescription drug monitoring programs and prescribing guidelines on emergency department opioid prescribing: a multi-center survey. *Pain Med.* 2016. Epublished March 19, 2016.

540. Porucznik C, Johnson E, Rolfs R, et al. Opioid prescribing knowledge and practices: provider survey following promulgation of guidelines—Utah, 2011. *J Opioid Manag.* 2013;9:217–224.

541. Poschadel S, Höger L, Schnitzler J, et al. *Evaluation der Arbeit der Drogenkonsumräume in der Bundesrepublik Deutschland', Nr 149, Schriftenreihe des Bundesministeriums für Gesundheit und Soziale Sicherheit.* Baden-Baden; 2003.

542. Potier C Laprévote V, Dubois-Arber F, et al. Supervised injection services: what has been demonstrated? A systematic literature review. *Drug Alcohol Depend.* 2014;145:48–68.

543. Powell D, Pacula R, Jacobson M. *Do Medical Marijuana Laws Reduce Addiction and Deaths Related to Pain Killers?* Cambridge, MA: National Bureau of Economic Research; 2015. Working Paper No. 21345.

544. Powis B, Strang J, Griffiths P, et al. Self-reported overdose among injecting drug users in London: extent and nature of the problem. *Addiction.* 1999;94(4):471–478.

545. Pradel V, Frauger E, Thirion X, et al. Impact of a prescription monitoring program on doctor-shopping for high dosage buprenorphine. *Pharmacoepidemiol Drug Safety.* 2009;18(1):36–43.

546. Prescription Drug Monitoring Program Center of Excellence. *Trends in Wyoming PMP prescription history reporting: evidence for a decrease in doctor shopping?* 2010. http://www.pdmpexcellence.org/sites/all/pdfs/NFF_ wyoming_rev_11_16_10.pdf 23.

547. Prescription Drug Monitoring Program Center of Excellence. *Nevada's Proactive PMP: The Impact of Unsolicited Reports, October, 2011;* 2011. http://www.pdmpexcellence.org/sites/all/pdfs/nevada_nff_10_26_11.pdf.

548. *Prescription Drug Monitoring Program (PDMP) Center of Excellence: Briefing on PDMP.* Waltham, Mass: Brandeis University; 2013.

549. Rao TLK, Mummaneni N, El-Etr AA. Convulsions: an unusual response to intravenous fentanyl administration [Letter]. *Anesth Analg.* 1982;61:1020–1021.

550. Ravndal E, Amundsen E. Mortality among drug users after discharge from inpatient treatment: an 8-year prospective study. *Drug Alcohol Depend.* 2010;108(1–2):65–69.

551. Ray B, O'Donnell D, Kahre K. Police officer attitudes towards intranasal naloxone training. *Drug Alcohol Depend.* 2015;146:107–110.

552. Ray W, Chung C, Murray K, et al. Prescription of long-acting opioids and mortality in patients with chronic noncancer pain. *J Am Med Assoc.* 2016;315(22):2415–2423.

553. Rebbert-Franklin K, Haas E, Singal P, et al. Development of Maryland local overdose fatality review teams: a localized, interdisciplinary approach to combat the growing problem of drug overdose deaths. *Health Promot Pract.* 2016;4:596–600.

554. Reifler L, Droz D, Bailey J, et al. Do prescription monitoring programs impact state trends in opioid abuse/misuse? *Pain Med.* 2012;13(3):434–442.

555. Ren J, Ding X, Funk G, et al. Ampakine CX717 protects against fentanyl-induced respiratory depression and lethal apnea in rats. *Anesthesiology.* 2009;110:1364–1370.

556. Ren J, Poon B, Tang Y, et al. Ampakines alleviate respiratory depression in rats. *Am J Respir Crit Care Med.* 2006;174:1384–1391.

557. Richter D, Manzke T, Wilken B, et al. Serotonin receptors: Guardians of stable breathing. *Trends Mol Med.* 2003;9:542–548.

558. Romach M, Schoedel K, Sellers E. Update on tamper-resistant drug formulations. *Drug Alcohol Depend1.* 2013;30(1–3):13–23.

559. Rosen D, Schoenbach V, Wohl D. All-cause and cause-specific mortality among men released from state prison, 1980–2005. *Am J Public Health.* 2008;98(12):2278–2284.

560. Rossen L, Khan D, Warner M. Trends and geographic patterns in drug-poisoning death rates in the U.S., 1999-2009. *Am J Prev Med.* 2013;45(6):e19–e25.

561. Ruan X, Chiravuri S, Kay A. Comparing fatal cases involving U-47700. *Forensic Sci Med Pathol.* 2016;12(3):369–371.

562. Rudd R, Aleshire N, Zibbell J, et al. Increases in drug and opioid overdose deaths-United States, 2000–2014. *MMWR (Morb Mortal Wkly Rep).* 2016;64(50):1378–1382.

563. Rudd RA, Seth P, David F, Scholl L. Increases in drug and opioid-involved overdose deaths — United States, 2010–2015. *MMWR (Morb Mortal Wkly Rep).* 2016;65:1445–1452.

564. Rutkow L, Chang H, Daubresse M, et al. Effect of Florida's prescription drug monitoring program and pill mill laws on opioid prescribing and use. *JAMA Int Med.* 2015;175(10):1642–1649.

565. Ruttenber A, Kalter H, Santinga P. The role of ethanol abuse in the etiology of heroin-related death. *J Forensic Sci.* 1990;35(4):891–900.

566. Ruttenber A, Luke J. Heroin-related deaths: new epidemiologic insights. *Science.* 1984;226(4670):14–20.

567. Sabzghabaee A, Eizadi-Mood N, Yaraghi A, et al. Naloxone therapy in opioid overdose patients: intranasal or intravenous? A randomized clinical trial. *Arch Med Sci.* 2014;10:309–314.

568. Sacciccio L. *Costs of prescription drug abuse in the Medicare part D program. Testimony before the US Senate Committee on Homeland Security and Govern-Mental Affairs Subcommittee on Federal Financial Management.* Government Information, Federal Services, and International Security; 2011.

569. Sacramento County Health and Human Services Department. *Drug Overdose Health Alert. Counterfeit Norco Containing Fentanyl;* 2016. http://www.dhhs.saccounty.net/PUB/Documents/AZ-Health-Info/ME Fentanyl+Alert_20160401.pdf.

570. Safwat AM, Daniel D. Grand mal seizure after fentanyl administration [Letter]. *Anesthesiology.* 1983;59:78.

571. Sahibzada N, Ferreira M, Wasserman A, et al. Reversal of morphine-induced apnea in the anesthetized rat by drugs that activate 5-hydroxytrptamine1A receptors. *J Pharmacol Exp Ther.* 2000;292:704–713.

572. Salmon A, Van Beek I, Amin J, et al. The impact of a supervised injecting facility on ambulance call outs in Sydney, Australia. *Addiction.* 2010;105:676–683.

573. Samuels E. Emergency department naloxone distribution: a Rhode Island department of health, recovery community, and emergency department partnership to reduce opioid overdose deaths. *Rhode Island Med J.* 2014;97(10):38–39.

574. Santos A. *Combating Pharmaceutical Diversion: Targeting 'rogue Pain Clinics' and 'Pill Mills';* 2013. http://www.deadiversion.usdoj.gov/mtgs/pharm_awareness/conf_2013/may_2013/santosII pdf.

575. Sarton E, Teppema L, Dahan A. Naloxone reversal of opioid-induced respiratory depression with special emphasis on the partial agonist/antagonist buprenorphine. *Adv Exp Med Biol.* 2008;605:486–491.

576. Schatz E, Nougier M. Drug consumption rooms: evidence and practice. *International Drug Policy Consortium.* 2012. 2012. http://idpc.net/publications/2012/06/idpc-briefing-paper-drug-consumption-rooms-evidence-and-practice.

577. Schinke S, Fang L, Cole K. Computer-delivered, parent-involvement intervention to prevent substance use among adolescent girls. *Prev Med.* 2009;49(5):429–435.

578. Schlosburg J, Vendruscoloa L, Bremer P, et al. Dynamic vaccine blocks relapse to compulsive intake of heroin. *Proc Nat Acad Sci.* 2013;110(22):9036–9041.

579. Schroeder CA, Smith LJ. Respiratory rates and arterial blood-gas tensions in healthy rabbits given buprenorphine, butorphanol, midazolam, or their combinations. *J Am Assoc Lab Anim Sci.* 2011;5(2):205–211.

580. Schug S, Torrie J. Safety assessment of postoperative pain management by an acute pain service. *Pain.* 1993;55:387–391.

581. Schuman-Olivier Z, Albanese M, Nelson S, et al. Self-treatment: illicit buprenorphine use by opioid dependent treatment seekers. *J Subst Abuse Treat.* 2010;39(1):41–50.

582. Schwartz R, Gryczynski J, O'Grady K, et al. Opioid agonist treatments and heroin overdose deaths in Baltimore, Maryland, 1995-2009. *Am J Public Health.* 2013;103(5):917–922.

583. Seal K, Downing M, Kral A, et al. Attitudes about prescribing take-home naloxone to injection drug users for the management of heroin overdose: a survey of street-recruited injectors in the San Francisco Bay area. *J Urban Health.* 2003;80(2):291–301.

584. Seal K, Kral A, Gee L, Moore L, et al. Predictors and prevention of nonfatal overdose among street recruited injection heroin users in the San Francisco Bay Area, 1998–1999. *Am J Public Health.* 2001;91(11):1842–1846.

585. Seal K, Thawley R, Gee L, et al. Naloxone distribution and cardio-pulmonary resuscitation training for injection drug users to prevent heroin overdose death: a pilot intervention study. *J Urban Health.* 2005;82(2):303–311.

586. Seaman S, Brettle R, Gore S. Mortality from overdose among injecting drug users recently released from prison: database linkage study. *BMJ.* 1998;316:426–428.

587. Sekhon R, Aminjavahery N, Davis C, et al. Compliance with opioid treatment guidelines for chronic non-cancer pain (CNCP) in primary care at a Veterans Affairs Medical Center (VAMC). *Pain Med.* 2013;14:1548–1556.

588. Semaan S, Fleming P, Worrell C, et al. Potential role of safer injection facilities in reducing HIV and hepatitis C infections and overdose mortality in the United States. *Drug Alcohol Depend.* 2011;118(2–3):100–110.

589. Sergeev B, Karpets A, Sarang A, Tikhonov M. Prevalence and circumstances of opiate overdose among injection drug users in the Russian Federation. *J Urban Health.* 2003;80(2):212–219.

590. Sertürner F. Uber das Morphium, eine neue salzfähige Grundlage, und die Mekonsäure, als Hauptbestandtheile des Opiums. *Ann Phys.* 1817;5:56–75.

591. Sessler N, Downing J, Kale H, et al. Reductions in reported deaths following the introduction of extended-release oxycodone (Oxy-Contin) with an abuse-deterrent formulation. *Pharmacoepidemiol Drug Saf.* 2014;23(12):1238–1246.

592. Severtson S, Bartelson B, Davis J, et al. Reduced abuse, therapeutic errors, and diversion following reformulation of extended-release oxycodone in 2010. *J Pain.* 2013;14(10):1122–1130.

593. Severtson S, Ellis M, Kurtz S, et al. Sustained reduction of diversion and abuse after introduction of an abuse deterrent formulation of extended release oxycodone. *Drug Alcohol Depend.* 2016;168:219–229.

594. Sherman S, Cheng Y, Kral A. Prevalence and correlates of opiate overdose among young injection drug users in a large U.S. city. *Drug Alcohol Depend.* 2007;88:182–187.

595. Sherman S, Gann D, Scott G, et al. A qualitative study of overdose responses among Chicago IDUs. *Harm Reduct J*. 2008;5:2.

596. Sherman S, Han J, Welsh C, et al. Efforts to reduce overdose deaths. *Am J Public Health*. 2013;103(8):e1–e2.

597. Shewan D, Hammersley R, Oliver J, et al. Fatal drug overdose after liberation from prison: a retrospective study of female ex-prisoners from Strathclyde region (Scotland). *Addiction Res*. 2000;8(3):267–278.

598. Sidebotham D, Dijkhuizen R, Schug S. The safety and utilization of patient-controlled analgesia. *J Pain Symptom Manage*. 1997;14:202–209.

599. Siegel S. Pavlovian conditioning analysis of morphine tolerance. *NIDA Res Monogr*. 1978;18:27–53.

600. Siegel S. Pavlovian conditioning and heroin overdose: reports from overdose victims. *Bull Psychonomic Soc*. 1984;22:428–430.

601. Siegel S. Pavlovian conditioning and drug overdose: when tolerance fails. *Addict Res Theory*. 2001;9(5):503–513.

602. Siegel S, Ellsworth D. Pavlovian conditioning and death from apparent overdose of medically prescribed morphine: a case report. *Bull Psychonomic Soc*. 1986;24(4):278–280.

603. Siegel S, Hinson R, Krank M, et al. Heroin "overdose" death: contribution of drug-associated environmental cues. *Science*. 1982;23:436–437.

604. Silva K, Schrager S, Kecojevic A, et al. Factors associated with history of non-fatal overdose among young nonmedical users of prescription drugs. *Drug Alcohol Depend*. 2013;128(1–2):104–110.

605. Skurtveit S, Furu K, Bramness J, et al. Benzodiazepines predict use of opioids—a follow-up study of 17,074 men and women. *Pain Med*. 2010;11(6):805–814.

606. Slavova S, Bunn TL, Talbert J. Drug overdose surveillance using hospital discharge data. *Publ Health Rep*. 2014;129:437–445.

607. Smialek J, Levine B, Chin L, et al. A fentanyl epidemic in Maryland 1992. *J Forensic Sci*. 1994;39:159–164.

608. Somerville NJ, O'Donnell J, Gladden RM, et al. Characteristics of fentanyl overdose — Massachusetts, 2014–2016. *MMWR (Morb Mortal Wkly Rep)*. 2017;66:382–386.

609. Sordo L, Barrio G, Bravo MJ, et al. Mortality risk during and after opioid substitution treatment: systematic review and meta-analysis of cohort studies. *BMJ*. 2017;357:1–14.

610. Reference deleted in review.

611. Spoth R, Trudeau L, Shin C, et al. Longitudinal effects of universal preventive intervention on prescription drug misuse: three RCTs with late adolescents and young adults. *Am J Public Health*. 2013;103(4):665–672.

612. Sproule B. *Prescription Monitoring Programs in Canada: Best Practice and Program Review*. Ottawa, ON: Canadian Centre on Substance Abuse; 2015.

613. Srivastava A, Kahan M. Methadone induction doses: are our current practices safe? *J Addict Dis*. 2006;25(3):5–13.

614. Steentoft A, Worm K, Christensen H. Morphine concentrations in autopsy material from fatal cases after intake of morphine and/or heroin. *J Forensic Sci Soc*. 1988;28(2):87–94.

615. Stewart D, Gossop M, Marsden J. Reductions in non-fatal overdose after drug misuse treatment: results from the National Treatment Outcome Research Study (NTORS). *J Subst Abuse Treat*. 2002;22(1):1–9.

616. Stewart K, Cao Y, Hsu M, et al. Geospatial analysis of drug poisoning deaths involving heroin in the USA, 2000–2014. *J Urban Health*. 2017;94(4):572–586.

617. Stewart L, Henderson C, Hobbs M, et al. Risk of death in prisoners after release from jail. *Aust N Z J Public Health*. 2004;28(1):32–36.

618. Stoltz J, Wood E, Small W, et al. Changes in injecting practices associated with the use of a medically supervised safer injection facility'. *J Public Health*. 2007;29(1):35–39.

619. Stoove M, Dietze P, Jolley D. Overdose deaths following previous non-fatal heroin overdose: record linkage of ambulance attendance and death registry data. *Drug Alcohol Rev*. 2009;28:347–352.

620. Stopka TJ, Donahue A, Hutcheson M, Green T. Nonprescription naloxone and syringe sales in the midst of opioid overdose and hepatitis C virus epidemics: Massachusetts, 2015. *J Am Pharm Assoc*. 2017;57(2)S:S34–S44.

621. Strang J, Darke S, Hall W, et al. Heroin overdose: the case for take-home naloxone. *Brit Med J*. 1996;312(7044):14351436.

622. Strang J, Kelleher M, Best D, et al. Emergency naloxone for heroin overdose. *BMJ*. 2006;333(7569):614–615.

623. Strang J, McCambridge J, Best D, et al. Loss of tolerance and overdose mortality after inpatient opiate detoxification: follow up study. *Br Med J*. 2003;326(7396):959–961.

624. Strang J, Powis B, Best D, et al. Preventing opiate overdose fatalities with take-home naloxone: pre launch study of possible impact and acceptability. *Addiction*. 1999;94(2):199–204.

625. Substance Abuse and Mental Health Services Administration. *Guidelines for the Accreditation of Opioid Treatment Programs: Revised July 20, 2007*. Rockville, MD: Substance Abuse and Mental Health Services Administration; 2007.

626. Substance Abuse and Mental Health Services Administration. *Drug Abuse Warning Network, 2011: National Estimates of Drug-Related Emergency Department Visits*. Rockville, MD: HHS Publication No. (SMA) 13-4760, DAWN Series D-39; 2013.

627. Substance Abuse and Mental Health Services Administration. *SAMHSA Opioid Overdose Prevention Toolkit*. Rockville MD: HHS publication no. (SMA) 13–4742; 2013.

628. Substance Abuse and Mental Health Services Administration. *Federal Guidelines for Opioid Treatment Programs. HHS Publication No. (SMA) PEP15-FEDGUIDEOTP*. Rockville, MD: Substance Abuse and Mental Health Services Administration; 2015.

629. Sullivan M, Bisaga A, Mariani J, et al. Naltrexone treatment for opioid dependence: does its effectiveness depend on testing the blockade? *Drug Alcohol Depend*. 2013;133:80–85.

630. Sullivan M, Edlund M, Zhang L, et al. Association between mental health disorders, problem drug use, and regular prescription opioid use. *Arch Intern Med*. 2006;166(19):2087–2093.

631. Sundwall D, Rolfs R. *Prescription Medication Deaths in Utah: Summary of Findings*. Utah Department of Health, Workgroup Meeting, October 24–25, 2005; 2005. Available at: http://health.utah.gov/prescription/pdf/Prescription_medication_deaths_in_utah.pdf.

632. Surratt H, O'Grady C, Kurtz S, et al. Reductions in prescription opioid diversion following recent legislative interventions in Florida. *Pharmacoepidemiol Drug Saf*. 2014;23:314–320.

633. Sutter M, Gerona R, Davis M, et al. Fatal fentanyl: one pill can kill. *Acad Emerg Med*. 2017;24(1):106–113.

634. Swedlow A, Ireland J, Johnson G. *Prescribing Patterns of Schedule II Opioids in California Workers' Compensation*. Oakland, CA: California Workers' Compensation Institute; 2011. http://www.cwci.org/document.php?file=1438.pdf.

635. Syed S, Paul J, Hueftlein M, et al. Morphine overdose from error propagation on an acute pain service. *Can J Anesth*. 2006;53:586–590.

636. Szeto HH, Inturrisi CE, Houde R, et al. Accumulation of normeperidine, an active metabolite of meperidine in patients with renal failure and cancer. *Ann Intern Med*. 1977;86:738–741.

637. Tagliaro F, Battisti Z de, Smith F, et al. Death from heroin overdose: findings from hair analysis. *Lancet*. 1998;351(9120):1923–1925.

638. Tan EC, Tan CH, Karupathivan U, et al. Mu opioid receptor gene polymorphism and heroin dependence in Asian populations. *Neurreport*. 2003;14(4):569–572.

639. Tanaka G. Hypertensive reaction to naloxone. *J Am Med Assoc*. 1974;228:25–26.

640. Tanenbaum S, Dyer J. The dynamics of prescription drug abuse and its correctives in one state Medicaid program. In: Wilford BB, ed. *Balancing the Response to Prescription Drug Abuse*. Chicago: American Medical Association; 1990:229–238.

641. Tardiff K, Marzuk P, Leon A, et al. HIV infection among victims of accidental fatal drug overdoses in New York City. *Addiction*. 1997;92:1017–1022.

642. Taff R. Pulmonary edema following naloxone administration in a patient without heart disease. *Anesthesiology.* 1983;59:576–577.

643. Teesson M, Marel C, Darke S, et al. Long-term mortality, remission, criminality and psychiatric comorbidity of heroin dependence: 11-year findings from the Australian Treatment Outcome Study. *Addiction.* 2015;110:986–993.

644. Templehoff R, Modica PA, Bernardo KL, et al. Fentanyl-induced electrographic seizures in patients with complex partial epilepsy. *J Neurosurg.* 1992;77:201–208.

645. Thiblin I, Eksborg S, Petersson A, et al. Fatal intoxication as a consequence of intranasal administration (snorting) or pulmonary inhalation (smoking) of heroin. *Forensic Sci Int.* 2004;139(2):241–247.

646. Thompson J, Baker A, Bracey A, et al. Fentanyl concentrations in 23 postmortem cases from the Hennepin county medical Examiner's office. *J Forensic Sci.* 2007;52:978–981.

647. Throckmorton D, Compton W, Lurie P. Management of opioid analgesic overdose. *NEJM.* 2012;367(14):1371.

648. Thomas KE, Johnson RL. *State Injury Indicators Report: Instructions for Preparing 2011 Data.* Atlanta: Centers for Disease Control and Prevention; National Center for Injury Prevention and Control; 2013.

649. Tobin K, Davey M, Latkin C, et al. Calling emergency medical services during drug overdose: an examination of individual, social and setting correlates. *Addiction.* 2005;100(3):397–404.

650. Tobin K, Sherman S, Beilenson P, et al. Evaluation of the Staying Alive programme: training injection drug users to properly administer naloxone and save lives. *Int J Drug Policy.* 2009;20:131–136.

651. Toblin R, Paulozzi L, Logan J, et al. Mental illness and psychotropic drug use among prescription drug overdose deaths: a medical examiner chart review. *J Clin Psychiatry.* 2010;71(4):491–496.

652. Tokar A, Andreeva T. Estimate of the extent of opiate overdose in Ukraine. *Tobac Contr Publ Health E Eur.* 2012;2(3):s57–s58.

653. Torralba L, Brugal MT, Villalbi JR, et al. Mortality due to acute adverse drug reactions: opiates and cocaine in Barcelona, 1989-93. *Addiction.* 1996;91(3):419–426.

654. Tracy M, Piper T, Ompad D, et al. Circumstances of witnessed drug overdose in New York City: implications for intervention. *Drug Alcohol Depend.* 2005;79(2):181–190.

655. Trust for America's Health. *Prescription Drug Abuse: Strategies to Stop the Epidemic;* 2013. http://healthyamericans.org/reports/drugabuse2013/TFAH2013RxDrugAbuseRpt12_no_embargo.pdf.

656. Turk D, Brody M, Okifuji E. Physicians' attitudes and practices regarding the long-term prescribing of opioids for non-cancer pain. *Pain.* 1994;59(2):201–208.

657. Tzemis D, Al-Qutub D, Amlani A, et al. A quantitative and qualitative evaluation of the British Columbia take home naloxone program. *CMAJ Open.* 2014;2(3):E153–E161.

658. Unick G, Rosenblum D, Mars S, et al. Intertwined epidemics: national demographic trends in hospitalizations for heroin- and opioid-related overdoses, 1993-2009. *PLoS One.* 2013;8(2):1–8.

659. Unick G, Rosenblum D, Mars S, et al. The relationship between US heroin market dynamics and heroin-related overdose, 1992–2008. *Addiction.* 2014;109:1889–1898.

660. Unick GJ, Ciccarone D. US regional and demographic differences in prescription opioid and heroin related overdose hospitalizations. *Int J Drug Policy.* 2017;46:112–119.

661. United Nations. *Office on Drugs and Crime World Drug Report.* Vienna, Austria; 2014. http://www.unodc.org/documents/wdr2014/World_-Drug_Report_2014_web.pdf.

662. United Nations Office on Drugs and Crime. *World Drug Report.* United Nations publication. Sales No. E.15.XI.6. 2015.

663. United States 2015, National Drug Control Strategy. *Office of National Drug Control Policy,* Executive Office of the President, Washington, D. C.

664. Ury W, Rahn M, Tolentino V, et al. Can a pain management and palliative care curriculum improve the opioid prescribing practices of medical residents? *J Gen Intern Med.* 2002;17:625–631.

665. U.S. Department Of Health and Human Services (HHS). *Office of the Surgeon General, Facing Addiction in America: The Surgeon General's Report on Alcohol, Drugs, and Health.* Washington, DC: HHS; 2016.

666. U.S. Department of Justice, Drug enforcement administration. *Automation of Reports and Consolidated Orders System (ARCOS).* Available at: http://www.deadiversion.usdoj.gov/arcos /index.html.

667. U.S. Department of Justice. *Law Enforcement Naloxone Toolkit;* 2015. https://www.bjatraining.org/tools/naloxone/.

668. U.S. Department of Justice. *Drug Enforcement Administration. DEA Investigative Reporting;* 2015. 2015.

669. U.S. Department of Justice. *Department of Justice Releases Strategy Memo to Address Prescription Opioid and Heroin Epidemic.* September 24, 2016. 2016 www.justice.gov/opa/pr/department-justice-releases strategy-memo-address-prescription-opioid-and-heroin-epidemic (Accessed October 9, 2016).

670. U.S. National Institute of Justice. *Office of Justice Programs (updated June, 2011): A guide to death scene investigation.* http://www.nij.gov/topics/law-enforcement/investigations/crime-scene/guides/death investigation/pages/welcome.aspx. (Accessed November 25, 2016).

671. Van Beek I, Kimber J, Dakin A, et al. The Sydney medically supervised injecting centre: reducing harm associated with heroin overdose. *Crit Public Health.* 2004;14:391–406.

672. Van den Brink W, Hendriks V, Blanken P, et al. *Medical Co-Prescription of Heroin. Two Trials.* The Hague: Central Committee on the Treatment Of Heroin Addicts; 2002.

673. Van den Brink W, Hendriks V, Blanken P, et al. Medical prescription of heroin to treatment resistant heroin addicts: two randomized controlled trials. *BMJ.* 2003;327:310–316.

674. Van Dorp E, Yassen A, Sarton E, et al. Naloxone reversal of buprenorphine-induced respiratory depression. *Anesthesiology.* 2006;105:51–57.

675. Van Haastrecht H, Mientjes G, van den Hoek A, et al. Death from suicide and overdose among drug injectors after disclosure of first HIV test result. *AIDS.* 1994;8:1721–1725.

676. Victor T, Alvarez N, Gould E. Opioid prescribing practices in chronic pain management: guidelines do not sufficiently influence clinical practice. *J Pain.* 2009;10:1051–1057.

677. Visconti AJ, Santos G, Lemos NP, et al. Opioid overdose deaths in the city and county of San Francisco: prevalence, distribution, and disparities. *J Urban Health Bull New York Acad Med.* 2015;92(4):758–772.

678. Vo K, van Wijk X, Lynch K, et al. Counterfeit Norco poisoning outbreak - san francisco Bay area, California, March 25-April 5, 2016. *MMWR (Morb Mortal Wkly Rep).* 2016;65:420–423.

679. Volkow N, Collins F. The role of science in addressing the opioid crisis. *NEJM.* 2017;377(4):391–394.

680. Volkow N, Frieden T, Hyde P, et al. Medication-assisted therapies- tackling the opioid-overdose epidemic. *NEJM.* 2014;370(22):2063–2066.

681. Von Korff M, Dublin S, Walker R, et al. The impact of opioid risk reduction initiatives on high-dose opioid prescribing for patients on chronic opioid therapy. *J Pain.* 2016;17:101–110.

682. Wakeman S, Bowman S, McKenzie M, et al. Preventing death among the recently incarcerated: an argument for naloxone prescription before release. *J Addict Dis.* 2009;28(2):124–129.

683. Reference deleted in review.

684. Walley A, Xuan Z, Hackman H, et al. Opioid overdose rates and implementation of overdose education and nasal naloxone distribution in Massachusetts: interrupted time series analysis. *BMJ.* 2013;346:f174.

685. Wang C, Vlahov D, Galai N, et al. The effect of HIV infection on overdose mortality. *AIDS.* 2005;19:935–942.

686. Wang J, Christo P. The influence of prescription monitoring programs on chronic pain management. *Pain Physician.* 2009;12(3):507–515.

687. Wang X, Dergacheva O, Kamendi H, et al. 5-hydroxytryp-tamine 1A/7 and 4α receptors differentially prevent opioid-induced inhibition of brain stem cardiorespiratory function. *Hypertension*. 2007;50:368–376.

688. Wanger K, Brough L, Macmillan I, et al. Intravenous vs subcutaneous naloxone for out-of-hospital management of presumed opioid overdose. *Acad Emerg Med*. 1998;5(4):293–299.

689. Ward J, Hall W, Mattick R. Role of maintenance treatment in opioid dependence. *Lancet*. 1999;353(9148):221–226.

690. Warner M, Chen LH, Makuc DM, et al. *Drug Poisoning Deaths in the United States, 1980–2008. NCHS Data Brief, No 81*. Hyattsville, MD: National Center for Health Statistics; 2011.

691. Warner-Smith M, Darke S, Lynskey M, et al. Heroin overdose: causes and consequences. *Addiction*. 2001;96(8):1113–1125.

692. Webster L, Cochella S, Dasgupta N, et al. An analysis of the root causes for opioid-related overdose deaths in the United States. *Pain Med*. 2011;12:S26–S35.

693. Webster L, Fine P. Review and critique of opioid rotation practices and associated risks of toxicity. *Pain Med*. 2012;13:562–570.

694. Webster L, Webster R. Predicting aberrant behaviors in opioid-treated patients: preliminary validation of the Opioid Risk Tool. *Pain Med*. 2005;6:432–442.

695. Weinstein S, Pfeiffer M, Schor J. Metabolism and pharmacokinetics of naloxone. *Psychopharmacol*. 1973;8:525–535.

696. Wells C. Deaths related to drug poisoning in England and Wales, 2008. *Health Stat Q*. 2009;43:48–55.

697. Welsh C, Doyon S. A case of heroin overdose reversed by sublingually-administered buprenorphine/naloxone film (Suboxone). *Clin Toxicol*. 2014;52(4):377–378.

698. Welsh C, Sherman S, Tobin K. A case of heroin overdose reversed by sublingually administered buprenorphine/naloxone (Suboxone®). *Addiction*. 2008;103(7):1226–1228.

699. Wermeling D. Review of naloxone safety for opioid overdose: practical considerations for new technology and expanded public access. *Ther Adv Drug Saf*. 2015;6(1):20–31.

700. Weschules D, Bain K. A systematic review of opioid conversion ratios used with methadone for the treatment of pain. *Pain Med*. 2008;9(5):595–612.

701. Wheatley R, Madej T, Jackson I, et al. The first year's experience of an acute pain service. *Br J Anaesth*. 1991;67:353–359.

702. Wheeler E, Jones S, Gilbert M, et al. Opioid overdose prevention programs providing naloxone to laypersons – United States, 2014. *MMWR (Morb Mortal Wkly Rep)*. 2015;64(23):631–635.

703. White M, Irvine J. Mechanisms of fatal opioid overdose. *Addiction*. 1999;94:961–972.

704. White S, Bird S, Merrall E, et al. Drugs-related death soon after hospital-discharge among drug treatment clients in Scotland: record linkage, validation, and investigation of risk-factors. *PLoS One*. 2015;10(11):e0141073.

705. Wiemann M, Piechatzek L, Göpelt K, et al. The NHE3 inhibitor AVE1599 stimulates phrenic nerve activity in the rat. *J Physiol Pharmacol*. 2008;59:27–36.

706. Williamson PA, Foreman KJ, White JM, et al. Methadone-related overdose deaths in South Australia, 1984-1994. How safe is methadone prescribing? *Med J Aust*. 1997;166(6):302–305.

707. Wines J, Saitz R, Horton N, et al. Overdose after detoxification: a prospective study. *Drug Alcohol Depend*. 2007;10(2–3):161–169. 89.

708. Winipeg Free Press. Drug tests at B.C. supervised injection site found 80% contained fentanyl. *Presentation at the 25th International Harm Reduction Conference*, Montreal, Canada; 2017. 2017. www.winnipegfreepress.com/arts-and-life/life/health/drug-checks-at-bc-supervised-injection-site found-80-contained-fentanyl-422316043.html.

709. Wisniewski AM, Purdy CH, Blondell RD. The epidemiologic association between opioid prescribing, non-medical use, and emergency department visits. *J Addict Dis*. 2008;27:1–11.

710. Wolf B, Lavezzi W, Sullivan L, et al. Methadone-related deaths in Palm Beach county. *J Forensic Sci*. 2004;49(2):375–378.

711. Wolf K. Characterization of methadone overdose: clinical considerations and the scientific evidence. *Ther Drug Monit*. 2002;24: 457–470.

712. Wong S, Mundy L, Drake R, et al. The prevalence of fentanyl in drug-related deaths in Philadelphia 2004-2006. *J Med Toxicol*. 2010;6(1):9–11.

713. World Health Organization. *Expert Committee on the Selection and Use of Essential Medicines (Including the Model List of Essential Medicines) 4th List*. Geneva, Switzerland: World Health Organization; 1984.

714. World Health Organization. *Prevention of Acute Drug-Related Mortality in Prison Populations during the Immediate post-release Period*. Geneva, Switzerland: World Health Organization; 2010.

715. World Health Organization. *Community Management of Opioid Overdose*. Geneva, Switzerland: World Health Organization; 2014.

716. World Health Organization. *International Statistical Classification of Diseases and Related Health Problems (10th Revision)*. Geneva, Switzerland: World Health Organization; 2016.

717. Worley J. Prescription drug monitoring programs, a response to doctor shopping: purpose, effectiveness, and directions for future research. *Issues Ment Health Nurs*. 2012;33:319–328.

718. Wunsch M, Nakamoto K, Behonick G, et al. Opioid deaths in rural Virginia: a description of the high prevalence of accidental fatalities involving prescribed medications. *Am J Addict*. 2009;18(1):5–14.

719. Yamauchi M, Dostal J, Kimura H, et al. Effects of buspirone on posthypoxic ventilatory behavior in the C57BL/6J and A/J mouse strains. *J Appl Physiol*. 2008;105:518–526.

720. Yassen A, Olofsen E, Romberg R, et al. Mechanism-based PK/PD modeling of the respiratory depressant effect of buprenorphine and fentanyl in healthy volunteers. *Clin Pharmacol Ther*. 2007;81(1):50–58.

721. Yassen A, Olofsen E, van Dorp E, et al. Mechanism-based pharmacokinetic-pharmacodynamic modelling of the reversal of buprenorphine-induced respiratory depression by naloxone: a study in healthy volunteers. *Clin Pharmacokinet*. 2007;46:965–980.

722. Yealy D, Paris P, Kaplan R, et al. The safety of prehospital naloxone administration by paramedics. *Ann Emerg Med*. 1990;19: 902–905.

723. Yin L, Gin G, Ruan Y, et al. Nonfatal overdose among heroin uses in southwestern China. *Am J Drug Alcohol Abuse*. 2007;33(4): 505–516.

724. Yokell M, Delgado M, Zaller N, et al. Presentation of prescription and nonprescription opioid overdoses to US emergency departments. *JAMA Intern Med*. 2014;174:2034–2037.

725. Yokell M, Green T, Bowman S, et al. Opioid overdose prevention and naloxone distribution in Rhode Island. *Med Health R I*. 2011;94(8):240–242.

726. Yoon YH, Chen C, Yi HY. Unintentional alcohol and drug poisoning in association with substance use disorders and mood and anxiety disorders: results from the 2010 Nationwide Inpatient Sample. *Inj Prev*. 2014;20:21–28.

727. Young A, Alfred K, Davignon P, et al. Physician survey examining the impact of an educational tool for responsible opioid prescribing. *J Opioid Manag*. 2012;8:81–87.

728. Zador D, Rome A, Hutchinson S, et al. Differences between injectors and non-injectors, and a high prevalence of benzodiazepines among drug related deaths in Scotland 2003. *Addict Res Theory*. 2007;15(6):651–662.

729. Zador D, Sunjic S. Methadone-related deaths and mortality rate during induction into methadone maintenance, New South Wales. *Drug Alcohol Rev*. 1996;21(2):131–136.

730. Zador D, Sunjic S. Deaths in methadone maintenance treatment in new south wales, Australia 1990–1995. *Addiction*. 2000;95(1): 77–84.

731. Zador D, Sunjic S, Darke S. Heroin-related deaths in New South Wales, 1992: toxicological findings and circumstances. *Med J Aust.* 1996;164:204–220.

732. Zamani N, Hassanian-Moghaddam H, Bayat A, et al. Reversal of opioid overdose syndrome in morphine-dependent rats using buprenorphine. *Toxicol Lett.* 2015;232(3):590–594.

733. Zarowitz B, Stebelsky L, Muma B, et al. Reduction of high-risk polypharmacy drug combinations in patients in a managed care setting. *Pharmacotherapy.* 2005;25:1636–1645.

734. Zedler B, Xie L, Wang L, et al. Risk factors for serious prescription opioid related toxicity or overdose among Veterans Health Administration patients. *Pain Med.* 2014;15:1911–1929.

55

Methamphetamine

LINDA P. DWOSKIN, EMILY R. HANKOSKY, PAUL E.A. GLASER, AND MICHAEL T. BARDO

Mechanism of Action

Methamphetamine is an indirect monoamine agonist that increases intracellular and extracellular levels of the monoamine neurotransmitters, dopamine, serotonin, and norepinephrine.[29,48] Methamphetamine gains entry into neurons either as a substrate at plasmalemmal neurotransmitter transporters or via diffusion across the plasmalemmal membrane as a result of its high lipophilicity. Once inside the presynaptic nerve terminal, methamphetamine inhibits neurotransmitter uptake at the vesicular monoamine transporter-2 located on synaptic vesicles and promotes neurotransmitter release from the vesicles, the result of which is to increase cytosolic neurotransmitter levels. In addition, methamphetamine inhibits monoamine oxidase, preventing a major route of intracellular metabolism of cytosolic neurotransmitter. The increased concentrations of cytosolic monoamines are available for reverse transport by the perisynaptic plasmalemmal neurotransmitter transporter. As neurotransmitter is transported from the cytosol to the extracellular space by the plasmalemmal transporter, methamphetamine is transported from the extracellular space into the cytosol. The outcome is that neurotransmitter concentration increases in the extracellular space. Finally, methamphetamine inhibits neurotransmitter uptake by the plasmalemmal monoamine transporters, contributing to the increased extracellular neurotransmitter concentrations.

Clinical Use of Methamphetamine

Methamphetamine is available on the market as a controlled substance, manufactured under the brand name Desoxyn (Ovation

Pharmaceuticals, Deerfield, IL). Methamphetamine has the same schedule II designation as other psychostimulant medications, such as amphetamine and methylphenidate, indicating both its therapeutic uses and high potential for misuse.[106,105] According to the package insert and labeling, methamphetamine can be used for the treatment of attention-deficit/hyperactivity disorder in children over the age of 6, short-term weight loss in obese individuals, and narcolepsy. The parameters for US Food and Drug Administration (FDA) approval in treating exogenous obesity include only short-term (i.e., a few weeks) usage in the context of a weight reduction plan including a structured diet with exercise, and only for patients in whom obesity has been refractory to other medications. In addition, methamphetamine use in obesity is discouraged if the patient is younger than age 12. Of interest, methamphetamine is not listed as a recommended therapy for the treatment of attention-deficit/hyperactivity disorder according to the current treatment guidelines from the American Academy of Pediatrics and the American Academy of Child and Adolescent Psychiatry.[3,111] Not surprisingly, it is rare for practicing physicians to prescribe methamphetamine for this indication.

The dosage recommendation by the package insert for attention-deficit/hyperactivity disorder starts with 5 mg given in the morning, and proceeds with weekly 5-mg increases until optimal clinical response has been achieved.[106] The usual dosing for childhood attention-deficit/hyperactivity disorder is 20–25 mg given as a once- or twice-daily dose. The recommended dosage in short-term obesity treatment is 5 mg taken 30 minutes before meals. Desoxyn is available only in 5-mg tablets, and no generic manufacturer currently exists. Abbott Pharmaceuticals produced Desoxyn since its introduction in 1942 and sold its rights to Ovation Pharmaceuticals in 2002, although Abbott maintains the facilities that manufacture the product. In addition, Abbott produced a sustained-release form of methamphetamine named Desoxyn Gradumet, utilizing a plastic matrix for gradual release of the methamphetamine. This product was available in 5-, 10-, and 15-mg doses. Manufacturing of the Desoxyn Gradumet was discontinued in 1999 due to "manufacturing difficulties."

No clinical trials are available by PubMed search for the use of methamphetamine in attention-deficit/hyperactivity disorder or obesity. However, methamphetamine and amphetamine are major metabolites of L-deprenyl (selegiline).[59] L-Deprenyl is commonly prescribed for Parkinson disease and has been evaluated in clinical trials for the treatment of attention-deficit/hyperactivity disorder. Results suggest that selegiline may be an efficacious medication for children with this disorder,[1,97] particularly children presenting with the inattentive subtype.[122] Although methamphetamine has not received official FDA approval for use in narcolepsy, this appears to be the main use for which it is prescribed in North America.[98] Methamphetamine is used along with other stimulants and L-deprenyl to treat the excessive sleepiness symptom of narcolepsy. The last trial evaluating methamphetamine in the treatment of narcolepsy was reported in 1993 and found that daytime sleepiness was treated successfully in adults with doses of 40–60 mg/day.[96]

Although methamphetamine may have proven efficacy and safety in the treatment of childhood attention-deficit/hyperactivity disorder and obesity, the risks of misuse and diversion along with its current negative stigma among health care workers and the public as an abused drug make it unlikely that many physicians will endorse its clinical use for these indications.

Diagnosis of Methamphetamine Use Disorder

With the transition to fifth edition of the *Diagnostic and Statistical Manual of Mental Disorders* (DSM-5), the term "use disorder" replaced "abuse" and "dependence" to describe what had been referred to as addiction. The basis of a substance use disorder is a cluster of symptoms, which indicate that an "individual continues using the substance despite significant substance-related problems."[4,5] The diagnosis is restricted to cases in which two or more symptoms have been present in the past 12 months. The symptoms incorporate four general categories including impaired control, social impairment, risky use, and pharmacological criteria (e.g., tolerance, withdrawal). Methamphetamine use disorder is classified under the broader category of stimulant use disorders. The severity of the disorder is specified based on the number of symptoms present: mild (2–3), moderate (4–5), and severe (6+). In addition to presenting as a primary disorder, methamphetamine use disorder also can be associated secondarily with the induction of psychotic disorders,[83] intoxication delirium, mood disorders, anxiety disorders, sleep disorders, and/or sexual dysfunction. Further notable changes to the symptom checklist between editions of the *Diagnostic and Statistical Manual of Mental Disorders* were the removal of legal problems and the addition of craving.[20]

Escalation of Methamphetamine Use

As is the case with other drugs of abuse, methamphetamine is often used in binge-like patterns that are characterized by periods of high intake, followed by "crashes" after the drug supply is depleted. Individuals often exhibit a developmental trajectory from experimentation with low doses, followed by escalation to higher binge intake, although the various patterns of intake that capture methamphetamine use across different individuals are difficult to characterize fully due to the clandestine nature of use within the population.[12,92] Interviews with chronic methamphetamine abusers suggest that most individuals initiate methamphetamine use by self-administering the drug at long intervals, a so-called recreational pattern.[22] Many individuals subsequently progress into dose escalation, with shorter intervals between successive self-administrations, thus manifesting as a binge-and-crash pattern. The escalation into higher dose intake may reflect, at least in part, tolerance to many of the peripheral and central effects of methamphetamine.[27,47]

Animal models have characterized the nature of escalation in methamphetamine use with repeated administration. Escalation

of methamphetamine use occurs when rats are given extended access to intravenous methamphetamine in an operant conditioning chamber.[74] With this procedure, rats are first trained to press a lever to intravenously self-infuse methamphetamine during daily 1-hour sessions. When subsequently shifted to 6-hour daily sessions, rats will escalate their intake pattern across sessions. This escalation is typically noted when comparing the intake of methamphetamine within rats across 6-hour sessions, as well as when comparing the intake of methamphetamine during the first hour of the 6-hour session with the intake of rats maintained on daily 1-hour sessions. Escalation of methamphetamine use enhances the ability of methamphetamine to prime reinstatement of extinguished lever-pressing,[118] suggesting that the development of an escalating pattern of intake may exacerbate the rate of relapse in abstinent humans.

Emerging research on age and sex differences in escalation has revealed that adolescents and females self-administer more methamphetamine during extended access conditions, compared to adults and males, respectively.[8,115] In an attempt to more closely model human binge patterns of intake, a recent study provided male and female rats with 96-hour access to intravenous methamphetamine over a 5-week period.[28] A crash was defined as no lever pressing for ≥6 hours and binges constituted all lever pressing in the 24+ hours prior to the crash. Using this model, duration of binge episodes increased from ~20 hours during week 1 to more than 50 hours by week 5. Furthermore, self-administration during normal sleep cycles and short interinfusions intervals (<1 minute) increased from week 1 to week 5. As such, this model of methamphetamine self-administration appears to closely parallel human patterns of binge exposure and may yield new mechanistic insights into the consequences of such exposure.

Attempts to attenuate escalation of methamphetamine self-administration using animal models of extended access have revealed promising effects of pharmacological and behavioral interventions. The group II metabotropic glutamate receptor agonist, LY379268, selectively and dose-dependently decreased methamphetamine self-administration under progressive ratio schedules of reinforcement both before and after extended access conditions.[32] Acute administration of the selective kappa opioid receptor antagonist, norbinaltorphimine (30 mg/kg, i.p.), blocked escalation of methamphetamine self-administration assessed for 11 days, as well as decreased responding on a progressive ratio schedule of reinforcement.[145] Attenuation of methamphetamine seeking was observed also following a single infusion of norbinaltorphimine (4 µg/0.5 µL) administered bilaterally and directly into nucleus accumbens shell. Assessments of behavioral interventions have supported a role for physical exercise in reducing methamphetamine seeking. Specifically, access to wheel running in the home cage attenuated escalation of methamphetamine self-administration relative to sedentary rats and rats with prior access to wheel running.[45] In another study, 30 days of wheel running during withdrawal from 22 days of extended access to methamphetamine reduced extinction responding as well as context- and cue-induced reinstatement.[129]

Escalation of methamphetamine use has a number of deleterious neurobehavioral effects. Compared with nonescalating use, escalating use of methamphetamine impairs performance on the novel object recognition test in rats,[115,118] which parallels neurocognitive impairments observed in abstinent methamphetamine abusers.[92] Furthermore, extended access to methamphetamine increases thresholds for intracranial self-stimulation of the medial forebrain bundle and other depressive-like behaviors.[67] In the prefrontal cortex, microRNAs associated with apoptosis and synaptic plasticity are increased following 14 days of extended access methamphetamine self-administration.[40] Escalation of methamphetamine use in rats also promotes cell death and decreases the genesis of neurons and glia (astrocytes and oligodendrocytes) in the medial prefrontal cortex.[82] The medial prefrontal cortex is a component of a complex frontal neurocircuitry involved in response inhibition and self-control.[72] Damage to the medial prefrontal cortex and related frontal structures may disinhibit behavior, thereby yielding a compulsive escalation of methamphetamine intake. In addition, because the medial prefrontal cortex is involved in the processing of stimulant reward,[54] it may be that damage to this region reduces the rewarding effect of methamphetamine, leading to a compensatory escalation of intake.

With extremely high doses of methamphetamine, profound hyperthermia and neurotoxicity are observed. In rats, neurotoxic effects can be observed following 1 day of high-dose methamphetamine treatment (10 mg/kg; 4 injections at 2-h intervals), an effect characterized by marked depletion of monoamine levels across various cortical and subcortical structures.[19,50,143] This neurotoxicity parallels the reductions in dopamine markers measured with positron emission tomography or with postmortem sampling in human methamphetamine abusers.[21,86,141,147] However, interpretation of results from studies using rats and the 1-day binge treatment protocol is limited, since human methamphetamine abusers do not typically reach high doses until long-term use leads to escalation of intake. In particular, a recent study by O'Neil et al.[104] demonstrated that the neurotoxic effects of a methamphetamine 1-day binge noted earlier in rats was blunted substantially when an escalating dose procedure was used. This decrease in neurotoxicity is not related to altered pharmacokinetics, as no changes in brain or plasma methamphetamine concentrations were observed following a methamphetamine binge in rats treated previously with escalating doses of methamphetamine.

Pharmacokinetics of Methamphetamine

Although methamphetamine is used clinically as an oral formulation, illicit use of methamphetamine more typically involves self-administration via the inhalation, intranasal, or intravenous routes. Unfortunately, information about the precise pharmacokinetics of methamphetamine use via these latter routes is sparse. Bioavailability via the intravenous route is 100%, whereas bioavailability via the intranasal route is 79% and via the inhalation route is 67%.[55] Although there is little opportunity to obtain blood samples from methamphetamine users during a binge, one study reported on blood concentrations taken from individuals arrested for suspicious behavior.[90] Among individuals in which methamphetamine was detected, the blood levels were found to range between ~0.5 and 10 μM. In controlled laboratory studies, the plasma half-life of methamphetamine was found to be approximately 10 hours in humans, which is considerably longer than the plasma half-life of 70 minutes found in rats.[55] In rats, the plasma concentration of methamphetamine reaches a maximum level faster following intraperitoneal administration (5–10 minutes) than following subcutaneous administration (20–30 minutes); however, ~42% of methamphetamine administered via intraperitoneal injection is subject to significant first-pass metabolism, which reduces bioavailability to ~52%.[51]

The major inactive metabolite of methamphetamine is p-hydroxymethamphetamine, which can be detected readily in the urine of methamphetamine abusers.[58] Methamphetamine is p-hydroxylated to p-hydroxymethamphetamine in liver microsomes. Of interest, in both rats and humans, a significant portion of methamphetamine is N-demethylated into amphetamine[17]. Amphetamine is also a potent psychostimulant that is p-hydroxylated to the inactive metabolite p-hydroxyamphetamine.[65] Because the conversion of methamphetamine to amphetamine is faster than the elimination of amphetamine from the blood, the concentration of amphetamine can actually exceed the level of methamphetamine when sampled at a long interval following a single bolus injection of intravenous methamphetamine.[22] In humans, the plasma half-life is slightly longer for L-methamphetamine than for D-methamphetamine (~14 hours vs. 10 hours).[91]

Mechanisms of Methamphetamine Reward

In addition to clear evidence of abuse, methamphetamine is a potent reinforcer in humans tested under highly controlled laboratory conditions. Methamphetamine reward is manifest both as a subjective report of liking and as a behavioral choice of methamphetamine self-administration over placebo. (We use the term "reward" to refer to both subjective and behavioral effects, whereas "reinforcement" is a more specific term that refers to operant behavior.) The response to oral methamphetamine (5 or 10 mg) or placebo was evaluated in healthy research participants in a residential laboratory facility.[57] Over an 8-day choice procedure, participants had the opportunity to self-administer the dose of methamphetamine that they most recently sampled or to receive a $1 voucher. As expected, methamphetamine was chosen more than placebo, and methamphetamine (10 mg) increased subjective ratings indicative of drug liking, demonstrating that oral methamphetamine is rewarding in humans. In another residential laboratory study, effects of repeated oral methamphetamine or placebo administration in humans were evaluated.[26] Relative to placebo, tolerance developed to the positive subjective effects of methamphetamine across repeated administration, which may be a factor leading to escalating use among at-risk individuals. Another study assessed the impact of an alternate reinforcer (money) on oral methamphetamine self-administration and employed individuals with a past-year history of methamphetamine use.[14] Choice of oral methamphetamine (8 or 16 mg) versus money ($0.25, up to $2) differed as a function of the response cost associated with the alternate reinforcer, such that methamphetamine was chosen more frequently when the response requirement for money was high. In any case, the majority of choices were for methamphetamine regardless of the response cost for money, demonstrating that the choice of methamphetamine was relatively resistant to changes in the cost for the alternate reinforcer.

Methamphetamine reward may be dependent to some extent on the pharmacokinetics of the drug. Drug reward is enhanced when there is a rapid onset of effect, which may explain why methamphetamine abusers tend to prefer the inhalation and intravenous routes of delivery over the oral route.[77] In addition, the rate of self-administration may be determined by the offset (elimination half-life) of the drug effect, with longer offset durations leading to less frequent self-administrations. These general principles may be important points to consider in attempts to develop effective pharmacotherapies for methamphetamine abuse. In particular, therapeutic agents designed to substitute for or block the rewarding effect of methamphetamine should ideally have a slow onset of action and a prolonged duration of action in order to minimize their potential for abuse. Nonetheless, it may be desirable for pharmacotherapeutic agents to have some rewarding effect because this will enhance patient compliance.

To better understand the neurobiological basis of methamphetamine reward and to develop new potential pharmacotherapies, a number of laboratory animal models have been developed. One widely used model is drug self-administration, which is based on fundamental principles of operant conditioning. In this model, rodents or nonhuman primates are trained to make an operant response (e.g., lever press) to receive a drug infusion. Responding is reinforced typically on a fixed ratio schedule in which a fixed number of responses lead to an infusion. Alternatively, a progressive ratio schedule can be used in which the number of responses required to earn an infusion increases incrementally after each infusion until a break point (cessation of responding) is achieved; the progressive ratio schedule is thought to estimate the relative effectiveness of the drug to serve as a reinforcer. A modification to the classic drug self-administration paradigm involves applying principles from behavioral economics.[64] A demand curve can be generated by increasing the fixed ratio requirement (i.e., up to fixed ratio 240) over several days and plotting the number of reinforcements earned (consumption) as a function of response requirement (price). Unit price defined as the response requirement per unit of reinforcer is useful for comparing reinforcers and minimizing the impact of a drug's pharmacological effects on drug seeking.[15] As expected based on human literature, both rats and nonhuman primates self-administer methamphetamine avidly and in a dose-dependent manner.[9,56,113]

Relapse is modeled in laboratory animals using a variety of reinstatement procedures that can be primed by exposure to the drug, drug-associated cues, or stress. For these assessments, rats are trained to self-administer the drug as described earlier and then undergo several days of extinction, during which the drug is no longer available and operant responding is extinguished. Thereafter, rats are primed to reinitiate drug-seeking through exposure to the drug, reintroduction of cues previously associated with delivery of the drug, or exposure to a stressor. It is important to note that tests of reinstatement are performed under extinction conditions. Increases in operant responding relative to extinction levels are interpreted as evidence of reinstatement of drug seeking.

Another model for measuring methamphetamine reward in rodents is the conditioned place preference preparation. This is a Pavlovian procedure in which the drug is paired with one distinct context and placebo is paired with a different context. When allowed to choose between the two different contexts in a drug-free state, rats show a preference for the drug-paired context. This preference is thought to reflect a secondary rewarding effect of the context due to its association with the drug, and it is a model of contextual control of drug seeking rather than a direct measure of the primary reinforcing effect of the drug per se.[11] Similar to self-administration, methamphetamine-conditioned place preference has been demonstrated in both rats and mice.[50,53,73]

Another animal model for evaluating methamphetamine reward is the brain stimulation reward preparation. In this model, a bipolar stimulating electrode is implanted chronically into the lateral hypothalamus, a region through which courses the medial forebrain bundle. The medial forebrain bundle connects dopaminergic cell bodies in the ventral tegmental area to the limbic terminal fields of the nucleus accumbens and prefrontal cortex, and stimulation of this pathway is highly reinforcing. Rats are first evaluated for brain stimulation reward threshold by adjusting the frequency of stimulation pulses in a series of ascending and descending increments. When a drug of abuse is subsequently administered, the brain stimulation threshold is lowered, thus providing an index of rewarding strength. Corroborating the findings

with self-administration and conditioned place preference, methamphetamine has been shown to decrease the threshold for brain stimulation reward.[130]

Animal models, coupled with neuroimaging technologies in humans, have uncovered some of the basic neural mechanisms that underlie methamphetamine reward. Although the reward circuitry is complex, involving multiple circuits and neurochemical systems,[71] dopaminergic neurotransmission in the mesocorticolimbic dopamine pathway undoubtedly plays a critical role in the psychostimulant effects of methamphetamine.[66,108,125] Methamphetamine reward results from increased dopamine release in limbic terminal fields, which is regulated by the vesicular monoamine transporter.[137] Methamphetamine increases extracellular dopamine concentrations by inhibiting the action of the vesicular monoamine transporter, which sequesters dopamine into vesicular stores, as well as by inhibiting monoamine oxidase, which diminishes dopamine metabolism, thereby making cytosolic dopamine more available for methamphetamine-induced reversal of the plasmalemmal dopamine transporter.[41,135] In addition to these dopamine-regulating cellular targets in the dopaminergic terminal fields, a number of other systems impinge on reward-relevant dopamine neurons, including γ-aminobutyric acid (GABA), glutamatergic, and nicotinic acetylcholine receptors localized within the midbrain ventral tegmental area region.[35] In addition, prefrontal cortical regions provide descending input into both the dopaminergic cell body and terminal regions.[71] Functional magnetic resonance imaging analyses in humans demonstrate that, in addition to increasing neural activity in the nucleus accumbens, methamphetamine increases activity in the orbitofrontal and anterior cingulate cortices.[142] Furthermore, using functional magnetic resonance and positron emission tomography imaging, abnormalities in brain structure and chemistry are observed in individuals using methamphetamine, including reductions in the density of dopamine transporters, dopamine D2 receptors, serotonin transporters, and vesicular monoamine transporters, particularly in striatum.[21]

A greater understanding of the neurocircuitry involved in methamphetamine reward has provided new targets for the development of medications to treat methamphetamine use disorder.[140] As mentioned previously, the dopamine transport inhibitor bupropion was found to be effective in a double-blind, placebo-controlled clinical trial.[44] However, because bupropion is also a nicotinic acetylcholine receptor antagonist,[95,128] it is not clear whether its efficacy is due to blockade of the dopamine transporter, blockade of nicotinic receptors, or blockade of both mechanisms concomitantly. Preclinical studies also have provided evidence that blockade of the vesicular monoamine transporter with lobeline or related synthetic analogs may be a beneficial approach.[a] Moreover, although direct blockade of dopamine D2 receptors is not a likely approach to treat methamphetamine abuse due to the induction of extrapyramidal side effects, effort has focused on atypical antipsychotics, such as sertindole or SB-277011A, which act at either serotonin-2 receptors[136] or dopamine D3 receptors,[130] respectively.

In addition to the direct effects of medications on the vesicular dopamine transporters, plasmalemmal transporters, and dopamine receptors, an alternative approach is to target systems that modulate mesocorticolimbic dopamine neurons. For example, preclinical work has indicated that medications that enhance GABA transmission by blocking the metabolic enzyme GABA

---

[a]References 2, 13, 41, 56, 103, 146.

transaminase may be useful for treating methamphetamine use disorders.[52] At least one study has shown that the GABA acid transaminase inhibitor, γ-vinyl GABA, is safe in human abusers, even among those who continue to use methamphetamine.[16] GABA receptor selective agonists are also under investigation,[53,113] as are glutamate receptor antagonists.[70]

Several other novel approaches for treating methamphetamine use disorder are in the pipeline. For example, novel congeners of the iboga plant alkaloid, ibogaine, may be useful,[107] although the potential utility of these alkaloids awaits characterization of their neuropharmacological mechanisms of action. In addition, a recent study indicates that medications that suppress the endogenous opioid peptide, nociceptin, may attenuate methamphetamine reward.[124] There is also accumulating preclinical evidence that oxytocin, the endogenous neuropeptide that is classically implicated in pair-bonding, decreases methamphetamine seeking and may have therapeutic potential.[10,30,31,46,63] Additional therapeutics gaining attention as potential treatments for methamphetamine use disorder are sigma receptor ligands[23,123] and N-acetylcysteine, the precursor to cysteine, with antioxidant properties.[89] Regardless of the mechanism, however, any pharmacotherapeutic approach for treating methamphetamine use disorder should be considered an adjunct to behavioral therapies. As mentioned earlier, the utility of contingency management and cognitive behavioral therapy to maintain abstinence rates among methamphetamine abusers has been demonstrated,[18,76,119,120] and further work is needed to determine whether the combination of pharmacotherapy and psychosocial interventions has a synergistic effect.

Human Studies in the Treatment of Methamphetamine Use Disorder

In response to a sharp increase in illicit use of methamphetamine in the mid- to late 1990s, the US government implemented supply-side interventions, including the Combat Methamphetamine Epidemic Act, to curtail illicit synthesis of methamphetamine by regulating the sale of its precursors (e.g., pseudoephedrine). These interventions resulted in short-term reductions in methamphetamine use.[38] As a consequence, methamphetamine has been supplied to users in the United States through its southern border. Illicit methamphetamine sales are estimated at $13 billion per year in the United States.[138] Methamphetamine smuggled into the United States is of high purity and low cost, leading to increased rates of methamphetamine overdose deaths, which more than doubled between 2010 and 2014.[144] Globally, methamphetamine is the most commonly seized amphetamine-type stimulant. In 2014, 108 tons of methamphetamine were seized worldwide, which was an increase of more than 300% since 2009.[138] Despite efforts to disrupt the supply, misuse of methamphetamine remains a global health problem.[84,112] Although many scientists and practitioners seem to assume that the more extensive experience and literature on the treatment of cocaine misuse can be extrapolated to methamphetamine, the mechanisms of action between cocaine and methamphetamine are sufficiently different, along with differences in the surrounding drug culture, to warrant independent trials and the unique treatment of people who misuse methamphetamine and wish to quit.[114]

A wide range of neuropharmacological strategies are being pursued in the search for an efficacious pharmacotherapy for methamphetamine use disorder. Recent evidence can be found through a search of registered clinical trials (clinicaltrials.gov), which is now

required for all institutional review board–approved clinical trials. A search of "methamphetamine" to capture both new and older terminologies (i.e., use disorder, dependence, abuse) yielded 271 listed studies, which is a sixfold increase in the number of clinical trials since the first edition of this chapter was published in 2011. Previously, few double-blind, randomized, placebo-controlled trials of pharmacotherapy for methamphetamine were available in the literature, but the National Institute on Drug Abuse Methamphetamine Clinical Trials Group clearly has contributed to the substantial increase in trials during the past 6 years.[42] These human and laboratory studies generally use one of two approaches for the treatment of methamphetamine use disorder. The more common approach has been medication repurposing, whereby medications with an existing approved indication (e.g., antidepressants) are evaluated for efficacy in treating methamphetamine use disorder. The second approach is to determine the safety and efficacy of novel candidate compounds as therapeutics for methamphetamine use disorder (e.g., Nickell et al.[103]).

For some users, the initial stage of treatment of methamphetamine use disorder is the medical management of withdrawal, particularly if the user is a binge or heavy user. This phase is characterized by increased sleep, eating, depressive symptoms, anxiety, poor concentration, and craving-related symptoms.[87] The other common scenario for withdrawal is when the user is incarcerated and unable to obtain methamphetamine.[7] A randomized, double-blind, placebo-controlled trial of the antidepressant mirtazapine in 31 outpatients undergoing treatment for methamphetamine withdrawal showed no benefit in terms of withdrawal symptoms or retention.[33] Mirtazapine, which acts as an antagonist or inverse agonist at 5-HT$_2$ receptors, improved time of sleep in the 2-week period during which it was evaluated. Mirtazapine was then assessed in conjunction with modafinil, a dopamine reuptake inhibitor used to treat narcolepsy and sleep apnea. An open-label comparison of modafinil (400 mg/day; $n = 14$) and mirtazapine (60 mg/day; $n = 13$) with treatment as usual with periciazine (2.5–10 mg/day) demonstrated less withdrawal severity with modafinil and mirtazapine[88]; however, these results must be interpreted with caution because this study lacked a placebo-controlled, double-blind design. A subsequent randomized, double-blind, placebo-controlled study revealed that mirtazapine (15 mg initial dose up to 30 mg/day at bedtime) administered to methamphetamine-using men who have sex with men, decreased methamphetamine use and decreased risky sexual behavior, suggesting that mirtazapine may be efficacious in a subset of methamphetamine users.[25]

Early clinical studies have identified the potential pharmacotherapeutic benefit of bupropion, a norepinephrine and dopamine reuptake inhibitor used as an antidepressant as well as for smoking cessation, in treating aspects of methamphetamine use disorder including memory function.[79] Initial safety studies indicated that methamphetamine administration during bupropion treatment was safe[101] and that bupropion reduced acute methamphetamine subjective effects and cue-induced craving for methamphetamine, supporting the evaluation of bupropion as a therapeutic.[102] Subsequently, a relatively large placebo-controlled trial evaluated the use of bupropion for the treatment of methamphetamine use disorder.[44,126] Twelve weeks of treatment with sustained-release bupropion (150 mg twice daily) versus placebo followed by a 30-day follow-up in five outpatient treatment facilities ($n = 152$ participants) showed some benefit when combined with behavioral interventions. In this study, bupropion treatment increased the number of weeks abstinent, although only the male subgroup that was ranked as low-to-moderate for methamphetamine usage showed significant improvement over placebo. Subsequent studies have confirmed findings from this original study suggesting that bupropion is not efficacious for maintaining abstinence,[6,148] except in a subset of individuals who adhered tightly to the medication regimen.[62] However, in a study including adolescents, bupropion was found in contrast to decrease the number of methamphetamine-free urine samples.[60] Taken together, bupropion may not be an effective candidate to treat methamphetamine use disorder, and in some populations, it appears to worsen outcomes.

An open-label study evaluated a sequential dosing algorithm consisting of hydroxyzine, flumazenil, and gabapentin to treat methamphetamine use disorder.[139] Hydroxyzine is a sedating antihistamine acting as an inverse agonist at histamine receptors that can be used to treat anxiety or allergies. Flumazenil is a benzodiazepine antagonist that is used to treat drowsiness. Gabapentin is an anticonvulsant that increases GABA neurotransmission and is used in the treatment of seizure disorders. In that study, 50 adults using methamphetamine were administered hydroxyzine (50 mg), followed 1 hour later by flumazenil (0.1–0.3 mg intravenously over 30 minutes) and gabapentin (initial dose 300 mg/day up to 1500 mg/day) for 4 weeks, and were followed for 8 weeks. A 47% reduction in methamphetamine use for the entire treatment group was found, with a 65% reduction specifically for the 36 participants who completed the 8-week evaluation, suggesting efficacy of the sequential medication regimen.[139] Caution is needed with respect to interpretation, however, due to the open-label design and lack of inclusion of a placebo comparison in the study design. In contrast, a randomized double-blind, placebo-controlled study evaluating 16 weeks of treatment with either gabapentin (800 mg twice daily; $n = 26$), baclofen (a muscle relaxant acting as a $GABA_B$ receptor agonist; 20 mg 3 times daily; $n = 25$), or placebo ($n = 37$) showed that neither medication was superior to placebo, revealing a lack of efficacy for methamphetamine use disorder.[61] A more recent study assessing hydroxyzine (50 mg), flumazenil (2 mg), and gabapentin (initial dose 300 mg up to 1200 mg/day) confirmed that the medication combination, termed PROMETA was no better than placebo in treating methamphetamine use disorder.[80]

A placebo-controlled, cross-over study investigating topiramate, an anticonvulsant used for seizures and migraines, showed that acute administration (up to 200 mg) enhanced, rather than attenuating, the positive subjective effects of methamphetamine.[69] A phase II double-blind, placebo-controlled, proof-of-concept study determined the safety and efficacy of chronic topiramate for the treatment of methamphetamine use disorder.[43] Participants ($n = 140$) meeting the DSM-IV criteria for methamphetamine dependence were randomized to receive topiramate at 25 mg escalating to 200 mg or placebo daily during weeks 1–5, and then topiramate 200 mg daily during weeks 6–12. The primary outcome measure was abstinence from methamphetamine during weeks 6–12. Generally, topiramate was well-tolerated and safe; however, no significant topiramate treatment effect was found. Exploratory data analyses indicated that participants ($n = 35$) whose baseline methamphetamine use was less than 18 days out of the previous 30, or who had negative urine prior to randomization ($n = 26$), experienced a topiramate treatment effect ($p = 0.03$ and 0.02, respectively). Thus despite the failure of the primary outcome variable, a subset of light methamphetamine users was identified as positive responders to treatment. In a subsequent study of 57 participants with methamphetamine use disorder, topiramate (50 mg initial dose up to 200 mg daily) significantly reduced positive urine screens at 6 weeks relative to placebo; however, no group

differences were found at any other time point, including at the conclusion of the 10-week study.[117] In addition, there were no differences between topiramate and placebo in retention or percent completion of the trial. Collectively, topiramate does not appear to be promising as a therapeutic for methamphetamine use disorder.

A small open-label study of 11 methamphetamine-dependent veterans showed decreased use with the atypical antipsychotic risperidone (average dose, 3.6 mg/day) over a 4-week treatment period.[93] A randomized, double-blind trial evaluating 80 participants with concurrent DSM-IV-defined bipolar I or II and methamphetamine or cocaine dependence showed that both quetiapine and risperidone, both serotonin-2 and dopamine D2 receptor antagonists used to treat psychiatric disorders including schizophrenia and bipolar disorder, reduced drug craving and improved manic, mixed, and depressive symptoms; however, limitations in interpretation are noted due to the lack of a placebo control group.[99]

Ondansetron (0.25, 1, or 4 mg twice daily) versus placebo was evaluated along with cognitive behavioral therapy in a small, randomized, double-blind, placebo-controlled trial in individuals seeking treatment for methamphetamine dependence.[68] Ondansetron is a serotonin-3 receptor antagonist used to treat nausea and vomiting. This 8-week trial found no benefit of ondansetron on any measured markers of methamphetamine use, withdrawal, or craving. Another trial evaluating sertraline (50 mg twice daily), a serotonin transporter inhibitor, which is used for the treatment of depression, anxiety, posttraumatic stress disorder, and obsessive-compulsive disorder, was found to worsen some outcome measures of methamphetamine use compared to placebo.[127]

Aripiprazole, a partial agonist at dopamine D2 receptors and approved by the FDA for the treatment of schizophrenia, was evaluated in human laboratory studies in which participants discriminated the interoceptive effects of 15 mg of D-amphetamine from placebo.[133] Aripiprazole (20 mg, but not at 10 mg) attenuated the discriminative stimulus effects of D-amphetamine; however, the high dose of aripiprazole alone produced performance decrements. The low dose of aripiprazole attenuated some of the subject-rated effects of D-amphetamine and did not impair performance, suggesting that aripiprazole may have therapeutic benefit.[133] In a subsequent double-blind inpatient study employing 16 methamphetamine-dependent participants, treatment with aripiprazole (15 mg orally) resulted in higher ratings on the Addiction Research Center Inventory subscales, reflecting euphoria and amphetamine-like effects following administration of methamphetamine (15 and 30 mg intravenously).[100] Furthermore, aripiprazole had no effect on abstinence-induced and cue-induced craving over the time course of treatment. In a study of seven non–treatment-seeking methamphetamine users, aripiprazole (15 mg) acutely decreased oral methamphetamine self-administration on a progressive ratio schedule of reinforcement and reduced some of the positive subjective effects of oral methamphetamine (4 and 8 mg) administration.[132] However, at the highest dose of methamphetamine (16 mg), aripiprazole augmented some of the positive subjective effects. Subsequent double-blind, placebo-controlled clinical trials found no differences between aripiprazole and placebo on methamphetamine abstinence,[24,134] although aripiprazole increased retention in one study.[134] Thus this dopamine D2 receptor partial agonist does not appear to be an effective treatment for methamphetamine use disorder.

A double-blind, placebo-controlled, between-group human laboratory study evaluated rivastigmine as a treatment for methamphetamine use disorder.[36] Rivastigmine is an acetylcholinesterase inhibitor used for the treatment of dementia. Initially, methamphetamine (30 mg) or placebo was self-administered intravenously in the controlled laboratory setting. Subsequently, participants chose either to self-administer a 3 mg dose of methamphetamine or placebo or to receive a monetary alternative ($0.05–$16). The number of choices for methamphetamine infusion was greater than for placebo, and the number of money choices was greater when placebo was available than when methamphetamine was available. Rivastigmine (1.5 or 3 mg; $n = 6$–9) did not alter the total number of methamphetamine infusions compared with placebo; however, the higher dose of rivastigmine reduced the positive subjective effects of self-administered methamphetamine. These findings were confirmed in a follow-up study, in which rivastigmine (6 mg) failed to reduce methamphetamine self-administration in participants with methamphetamine use disorder, but decreased "likely to use methamphetamine" at the lowest methamphetamine dose (15 mg, but not 30 mg) relative to placebo.[37] Thus a reduction in methamphetamine-induced subjective effects does not predict a decrease in self-administration.

Substitution therapies have proven beneficial in the treatment of nicotine and opioid use disorders, and recently, a similar approach has been evaluated for treatment of methamphetamine use disorder. D-Amphetamine is an indirect monoamine agonist used in the treatment of attention-deficit/hyperactivity disorder and narcolepsy. In a human laboratory setting, D-amphetamine (40 mg) was found to attenuate physiological and some subjective effects of intranasal methamphetamine, but failed to reduce intranasal methamphetamine (10, 20, 30 mg) self-administration.[110] A randomized, double-blind, placebo-controlled clinical trial found that D-amphetamine (60 mg/day) was no different from placebo on measures of methamphetamine use, but reduced symptoms of withdrawal and craving.[49] A study using a higher dose of D-amphetamine (110 mg/day), found that compared to placebo, D-amphetamine increased retention and modestly decreased psychometric measures of dependence, but there were no differences in self-report or physiological measures of methamphetamine use.[81]

Methylphenidate is an inhibitor at norepinephrine and dopamine transporters that is used also to treat attention-deficit/hyperactivity disorder and narcolepsy. Methylphenidate has been assessed in clinical trials for methamphetamine use disorder. In one randomized, double-blind, placebo-controlled, 22-week study, methylphenidate (up to 54 mg daily) increased participant retention in the study, but was no different from placebo on the number of methamphetamine positive urine screens.[94] In contrast, two subsequent randomized, double-blind, placebo-controlled studies found that treatment with methylphenidate (up to 54 mg daily) decreased methamphetamine use relative to placebo.[78,116] A consideration regarding the use of substitution therapies is the risk for misuse or diversion of the medications that are intended to treat the drug use disorder.[39] Coupled with the indeterminate nature of the clinical findings, substitution therapies for treating methamphetamine use disorder may not be the best approach.

Immunotherapies are emerging as potential treatments for methamphetamine use disorder.[109] An anti-methamphetamine monoclonal antibody, ch-mAb7F9, has been developed to reduce methamphetamine distribution to brain.[131] The antibody binds the methamphetamine in the peripheral compartment, and the antibody bound complex is too large to cross the blood-brain barrier, thereby preventing its pharmacological action in brain.[75] Recently, a phase I clinical trial followed 47 healthy volunteers for 147 days and determined that ch-mAb7F9 was safe and well-tolerated.[131]

Pharmacokinetic analyses revealed that pharmacologically relevant concentrations of ch-mAb7F9 were maintained for ~5 weeks following the highest dose (20 mg/kg) of antibody administered. An advantage of this approach is the long-time interval between administration of the therapy, which theoretically, could improve medication compliance. Some notable limitations of this approach include that active immunization is not tenable in immunocompromised individuals (e.g., HIV) and that beneficial effects can require several weeks needed for the appropriate immunological response to be realized, although passive immunization can circumvent some of these issues.[75] Ultimately, this approach may be most appropriate for highly motivated individuals as a prevention of relapse and likely will be most efficacious when paired with other pharmacotherapies and/or psychosocial interventions.

Medication nonadherence and enrollment of professional subjects recently have been identified as factors that may contribute to high rates of negative findings in clinical trials.[85] Medication nonadherence refers to participants not taking their study medication as instructed. Professional subjects refer to participants that feign or exaggerate symptoms of the disorder under study to enroll in the clinical trial for financial gain. Unwitting enrollment of professional subjects may artificially inflate the efficacy of placebo. Medication nonadherence has been reported to be as high as 39% in a recent review of eight clinical trials, and may obfuscate the therapeutic benefits of study medications.[85] Thus medication nonadherence and enrollment of professional subjects may culminate in a misrepresentation or underestimation of the efficacy of the pharmacotherapies being evaluated.[34] One approach to address this unanticipated problem may be to reevaluate potential therapeutics for methamphetamine use disorder that showed efficacy in human laboratory studies but not in clinical trials.

Finally, it is important to draw attention to the general consensus that any medication for methamphetamine abuse will be most effective in the context of concomitantly delivered behavioral therapies, much like other drugs of abuse.[121] Behavioral therapies have included cognitive behavioral therapy, contingency management, or both.[76] Outcome-based studies on cognitive behavioral therapy have shown reductions in methamphetamine abuse and relapse of abuse.[18] Contingency management procedures, although effective when individuals are actively in drug treatment, have not been shown to have long-term benefit once the individuals are on their own.[119]

Conclusions

Regulatory supply-side interventions to curtail illicit synthesis of methamphetamine provided short-term reductions in drug availability and the associated consequences, but methamphetamine misuse remains a global health crisis. Currently, no medications have been approved by the FDA for the treatment of methamphetamine use disorder. Recent advances in the understanding of the neurocircuitry involved in methamphetamine reward have provided new opportunities and rational targets that can be exploited for the development of pharmacotherapies to treat methamphetamine addiction. The efficacy and safety of these candidate pharmacotherapies require evaluation in adequately powered, double-blind, placebo-controlled trials; however, controlled human laboratory studies have the potential to evaluate more efficiently candidate treatments and provide information about whether the more expensive clinical trials are warranted. Currently, a wide range of neuropharmacological strategies are being pursued in the search for an efficacious pharmacotherapy for methamphetamine use disorder.

References

1. Akhondzadeh S, Tavakolian R, Davari-Ashtiani R, et al. Selegiline in the treatment of attention deficit hyperactivity disorder in children: a double blind and randomized trial. *Prog Neuropsychopharmacol Biol Psychiatry*. 2003;27:841–845.

2. Alvers KM, Beckmann JS, Zheng G, et al. The effect of VMAT2 inhibitor GZ-793A on reinstatement of methamphetamine-seeking in rats. *Psychopharmacol*. 2012;224:255–262.

3. American Academy of Pediatrics: Subcommittee on Attention-Deficit/Hyperactivity Disorder and Committee on Quality Improvement (AAP: SoADHDCoQI). Clinical practice guideline: treatment of the school-aged child with attention-deficit/hyperactivity disorder. *Pediatrics*. 2001;108:1033–1044.

4. American Psychiatric Association. *Diagnostic and Statistical Manual of Mental Disorders*. 5th ed. Arlington, VA: American Psychiatric Association; 2013.

5. American Psychiatric Association. *Highlights of Changes From DSM-IV-TR to DSM-5*. Arlington, VA: American Psychiatric Association; 2013.

6. Anderson AL, Li S, Markova D, et al. Bupropion for the treatment of methamphetamine dependence in non-daily users: a randomized, double-blind, placebo-controlled trial. *Drug Alcohol Depend*. 2015;150:170–174.

7. Anglin MD, Urada D, Brecht ML, et al. Criminal justice treatment admissions for methamphetamine use in California: a focus on Proposition 36. *J Psychoactive Drugs*. 2007;4 suppl:367–381.

8. Anker JJ, Baron TR, Zlebnik NE, et al. Escalation of methamphetamine self-administration in adolescent and adult rats. *Drug Alcohol Depend*. 2012;124:149–153.

9. Balster RL, Schuster CR. A comparison of d-amphetamine, l-amphetamine, and methamphetamine self-administration in rhesus monkeys. *Pharmacol Biochem Behav*. 1973;1:67–71.

10. Baracz SJ, Everett NA, McGregor IS. Oxytocin in the nucleus accumbens core reduces reinstatement of methamphetamine-seeking behaviour in rats. *Addict Biol*. 2014;21:316–325.

11. Bardo MT, Bevins RA. Conditioned place preference: what does it add to our preclinical understanding of drug reward? *Psychopharmacology (Berl)*. 2000;153:31–43.

12. Barr AM, Panenka WJ, MacEwan GW, et al. The need for speed: an update on methamphetamine addiction. *J Psychiatry Neurosci*. 2006;31:301–313.

13. Beckmann JS, Denehy ED, Zheng G, et al. The effect of a novel VMAT2 inhibitor, GZ-793A, on methamphetamine reward in rats. *Psychopharmacol*. 2012;220:395–403.

14. Bennett JA, Stoops WW, Rush CR. Alternate reinforcer response cost impacts methamphetamine choice in humans. *Pharmacol Biochem Behav*. 2013;103:481–486.

15. Bickel WK, DeGrandpre RJ, Higgins ST. Behavioral economics of drug self-administration: functional equivalence of response requirement and drug dose. *Life Sci*. 1990;47:1501–1510.

16. Brodie JD, Figueroa E, Laska EM, et al. Safety and efficacy of gamma-vinyl GABA (GVG) for the treatment of methamphetamine and/or cocaine addiction. *Synapse*. 2005;55:122–125.

17. Caldwell J, Dring LG, Williams RT. Metabolism of (14 C)methamphetamine in man, the Guinea pig and the rat. *Biochem J*. 1972;129:11–22.

18. Callaghan R, Taylor L, Victor JC, et al. A case-matched comparison of readmission patterns between primary methamphetamine-using and primary cocaine-using adolescents engaged in inpatient substance-abuse treatment. *Addict Behav*. 2007;32:3101–3106.

19. Cass WA. Decreases in evoked overflow of dopamine in rat striatum after neurotoxic doses of methamphetamine. *J Pharmacol Exp Ther*. 1997;280:105–113.

20. Center for Behavioral Health Statistics and Quality. *Impact of the DSM-IV to DSM-5 Changes on the National Survey on Drug Use and Health*. Rockville, MD: Substance Abuse and Mental Health Services Administration; 2016.

21. Chang L, Alicata D, Ernst T, et al. Structural and metabolic brain changes in the striatum associated with methamphetamine abuse. *Addiction*. 2007;102(suppl 1):16–32.

22. Cho AK, Melega WP, Kuczenski R, et al. Relevance of pharmacokinetic parameters in animal models of methamphetamine abuse. *Synapse*. 2001;39:161–166.

23. Cobos EJ, Entrena JM, Nieto FR. Pharmacology and therapeutic potential of sigma$_1$ receptor ligands. *Curr Neuropharmacol*. 2008;6:344–366.

24. Coffin PO, Santos G, Das M, et al. Aripiprazole for the treatment of methamphetamine dependence: a randomized, double-blind, placebo-controlled trial. *Addiction*. 2013;108:751–761.

25. Colfax GN, Santos G, Das M, et al. Mirtazapine to reduce methamphetamine use. *Arch Gen Psychiatry*. 2011;68:1168–1175.

26. Comer SD, Hart CL, Ward AS, et al. Effects of repeated oral methamphetamine administration in humans. *Psychopharmacology (Berl)*. 2001;155:397–404.

27. Cook CE, Jeffcoat AR, Sadler BM, et al. Pharmacokinetics of oral methamphetamine and effects of repeated daily dosing in humans. *Drug Metab Dispos*. 1992;20:856–862.

28. Cornett EM, Goeders NE. 96-hour methamphetamine self-administration in male and female rats: a novel model of human methamphetamine addiction. *Pharmacol Biochem Behav*. 2013;111:51–57.

29. Courtney KE, Ray LA. Methamphetamine: an update on epidemiology, pharmacology, clinical phenomenology, and treatment literature. *Drug Alcohol Depend*. 2014;143:11–21.

30. Cox BM, Bentzley BS, Regen-Tuero H, et al. Oxytocin acts in the nucleus accumbens to attenuate methamphetamine seeking and demand. *Biol Psych*. 2017;81:949–958.

31. Cox BM, Young AB, See RE. Sex differences in methamphetamine seeking in rats: impact of oxytocin. *Psychoneuroendocrinol*. 2013;38:2343–2353.

32. Crawford JT, Roberts DCS, Beveridge TJR. The group II metabotropic glutamate receptor agonist, LY379268, decreases methamphetamine self-administration in rats. *Drug Alcohol Depend*. 2013;132:414–419.

33. Cruickshank CC, Montebello ME, Dyer KR, et al. A placebo-controlled trial of mirtazapine for the management of methamphetamine withdrawal. *Drug Alcohol Rev*. 2008;27:326–333.

34. Czobor P, Skolnick P. The secrets of a successful clinical trial: compliance, compliance, compliance. *Mol Interv*. 2011;11:107–110.

35. Dani JA, Bertrand D. Nicotinic acetylcholine receptors and nicotinic cholinergic mechanisms of the central nervous system. *Annu Rev Pharmacol Toxicol*. 2007;47:699–729.

36. De La Garza R, Mahoney JJ, Culbertson C, et al. The acetylcholinesterase inhibitor rivastigmine does not alter total choices for methamphetamine, but may reduce positive subjective effects, in a laboratory model of intravenous self-administration in human volunteers. *Pharmacol Biochem Behav*. 2008;89:200–208.

37. De La Garza II R, Newton TF, Haile CN, et al. Rivastigmine reduces "likely to use methamphetamine" in methamphetamine-dependent volunteers. *Prog Neuropsychopharmacol Biol Psychiatry*. 2012;37:141–146.

38. Dobkin C, Nicosia N. The war on drugs: methamphetamine, public health, and crime. *Am Econ Rev*. 2009;99:324–349.

39. Dobry YSher L. Stimulant substitution in methamphetamine dependence. *Aust N Z J Psychiatry*. 2012;46:1201–1202.

40. Du H, Cao D, Ying C, et al. Alterations of prefrontal cortical microRNAs in methamphetamine self-administering rats: from controlled intake to escalated drug intake. *Neurosci Lett*. 2016;611.27–27.

41. Dwoskin LP, Crooks PA. A novel mechanism of action and potential use for lobeline as a treatment for psychostimulant abuse. *Biochem Pharmacol*. 2002;63:89–98.

42. Elkashef A, Rawson RA, Smith E, et al. The NIDA Methamphetamine Clinical Trials Group: a strategy to increase clinical trials research capacity. *Addiction*. 2007;102(suppl 1):107–113.

43. Elkashef AM, Kahn R, Yu E, et al. Topiramate for the treatment of methamphetamine addiction: a multi-center placebo-controlled trial. *Addiction*. 2011;107:1297–1306.

44. Elkashef AM, Rawson RA, Anderson AL, et al. Bupropion for the treatment of methamphetamine dependence. *Neuropsychopharmacology*. 2008;33:1162–1170.

45. Engelmann AJ, Aparicio MB, Kim A, et al. Chronic wheel running reduces maladaptive patterns of methamphetamine intake: regulation by attenuation of methamphetamine-induced neuronal nitric oxide synthase. *Brain Strut Funct*. 2014;219:657–672.

46. Ferland CL, Reichel CM, McGinty JF. Effects of oxytocin on methamphetamine-seeking exacerbated by predator odor pre-exposure in rats. *Psychopharmacol*. 2016;233:1015–1024.

47. Fischman MWSchuster CR. Tolerance development to chronic methamphetamine intoxication in the rhesus monkey. *Pharmacol Biochem Behav*. 1974;2:503–508.

48. Fleckenstein AE, Volz TJ, Riddle EL, et al. New insights into the mechanism of action of amphetamines. *Annu Rev Pharmacol Toxicol*. 2007;47:681–698.

49. Galloway GP, Buscemi R, Coyle JR, et al. A randomized, placebo-controlled trial of sustained-release dextroamphetamine for treatment of methamphetamine addiction. *Clin Pharmacol Ther*. 2011;89:276–282.

50. Gehrke BJ, Harrod SB, Cass WA, et al. The effect of neurotoxic doses of methamphetamine on methamphetamine-conditioned place preference in rats. *Psychopharmacology (Berl)*. 2003;166:249–257.

51. Gentry WB, Ghafoor AU, Wessinger WD, et al. (+)-Methamphetamine-induced spontaneous behavior in rats depends on route of (+)METH administration. *Pharmacol Biochem Behav*. 2004;79:751–760.

52. Gerasimov MR, Ashby Jr CR, Gardner EL, et al. Gamma-vinyl GABA inhibits methamphetamine, heroin, or ethanol-induced increases in nucleus accumbens dopamine. *Synapse*. 1999;34:11–19.

53. Goeders JE, Goeders NE. Effects of oxazepam on methamphetamine-induced conditioned place preference. *Pharmacol Biochem Behav*. 2004;78:185–188.

54. Goeders NE, Smith JE. Intracranial cocaine self-administration into the medial prefrontal cortex increases dopamine turnover in the nucleus accumbens. *J Pharmacol Exp Ther*. 1993;265:592–600.

55. Harris DS, Boxenbaum H, Everhart ET, et al. The bioavailability of intranasal and smoked methamphetamine. *Clin Pharmacol Ther*. 2003;74:475–486.

56. Harrod SB, Dwoskin LP, Crooks PA, et al. Lobeline attenuates d-methamphetamine self-administration in rats. *J Pharmacol Exp Ther*. 2001;298:172–179.

57. Hart CL, Ward AS, Haney M, et al. Methamphetamine self-administration by humans. *Psychopharmacology (Berl)*. 2001;157:75–81.

58. Hayakawa K, Miyoshi Y, Kurimoto H, et al. Simultaneous determination of methamphetamine and its metabolites in the urine samples of abusers by high performance liquid chromatography with chemiluminescence detection. *Biol Pharm Bull*. 1993;16:817–821.

59. Heinonen EH, Anttila MI, Lammintausta RA. Pharmacokinetic aspects of l-deprenyl (selegiline) and its metabolites. *Clin Pharmacol Ther*. 1994;56:742–749.

60. Heinzerling KG, Gadzhyan J, van Oudheusden, et al. Pilot randomized trial of bupropion for adolescent methamphetamine abuse/dependence. *J Adolesc Health*. 2013;52:502–505.

61. Heinzerling KG, Shoptaw S, Peck JA, et al. Randomized, placebo-controlled trial of baclofen and gabapentin for the treatment of methamphetamine dependence. *Drug Alcohol Depend*. 2006;85:177–184.

62. Heinzerling KG, Swanson A, Hall TM, et al. Randomized, placebo-controlled trial of bupropion in methamphetamine-dependent participants with less than daily methamphetamine use. *Addiction*. 2014;109:1878–1886.

63. Hicks C, Cornish JL, Baracz SJ. Adolescent pre-treatment with oxytocin protects against adult methamphetamine-seeking behavior in female rats. *Addict Biol*. 2014;21:304–315.

64. Hursh SR. Behavioral economics of drug self-administration and drug abuse policy. *J Exp Anal Behav*. 1991;56:377–393.

65. Hutchaleelaha AMayersohn M. Influence of activated charcoal on the disposition kinetics of methamphetamine enantiomers in the rat following intravenous dosing. *J Pharm Sci*. 1996;85:541–545.

66. Izawa J, Yamanashi K, Asakura T, et al. Differential effects of methamphetamine and cocaine on behavior and extracellular levels of dopamine and 3,4-dihydroxyphenylalanine in the nucleus accumbens of conscious rats. *Eur J Pharmacol*. 2006;549:84–90.

67. Jang C, Whitfield T, Schulteis G, et al. A dysphoric-like state during early withdrawal from extended access to methamphetamine self-administration in rats. *Psychopharmacol*. 2013;225:753–763.

68. Johnson BA, Ait-Daoud N, Elkashef AM, et al. A preliminary randomized, double-blind, placebo-controlled study of the safety and efficacy of ondansetron in the treatment of methamphetamine dependence. *Int J Neuropsychopharmacol*. 2008;11:1–14.

69. Johnson BA, Roache JD, Ait-Daoud N, et al. Effects of acute topiramate dosing on methamphetamine-induced subjective mood. *Int J Neuropsychopharmacol*. 2007;10:85–98.

70. Jun JH, Schindler CW. Dextromethorphan alters methamphetamine self-administration in the rat. *Pharmacol Biochem Behav*. 2000;67:405–409.

71. Kalivas PW, Peters J, Knackstedt L. Animal models and brain circuits in drug addiction. *Mol Interv*. 2006;6:339–344.

72. Kalivas PW, Volkow ND. The neural basis of addiction: a pathology of motivation and choice. *Am J Psychiatry*. 2005;162:1403–1413.

73. Kim HS, Jang CG. MK-801 inhibits methamphetamine-induced conditioned place preference and behavioral sensitization to apomorphine in mice. *Brain Res Bull*. 1997;44:221–227.

74. Kitamura O, Wee S, Specio SE, et al. Escalation of methamphetamine self-administration in rats: a dose-effect function. *Psychopharmacology (Berl)*. 2006;186:48–53.

75. Kosten T, Owens SM. Immunotherapy for the treatment of drug abuse. *Pharmacol Ther*. 2005;108:76–85.

76. Lee NK, Rawson RA. A systematic review of cognitive and behavioural therapies for methamphetamine dependence. *Drug Alcohol Rev*. 2008;27:309–317.

77. Lile JA. Pharmacological determinants of the reinforcing effects of psychostimulants: relation to agonist substitution treatment. *Exp Clin Psychopharmacol*. 2006;14:20–33.

78. Ling W, Chang L, Hillhouse M, et al. Sustained-release methylphenidate in a randomized trial of treatment of methamphetamine use disorder. *Addiction*. 2014;109:1489–1500.

79. Ling W, Rawson R, Shoptaw S. Management of methamphetamine abuse and dependence. *Curr Psychiatry Rep*. 2006;8:345–354.

80. Ling W, Shoptaw D, Hillhouse M. Double-blind placebo-controlled evaluation of the PROMETA protocol for methamphetamine dependence. *Addiction*. 2011;107:361–369.

81. Longo M, Wickes W, Smout M, et al. Randomized controlled trial of dexamphetamine maintenance for the treatment of methamphetamine dependence. *Addiction*. 2009;105:146–154.

82. Mandyam CD, Wee S, Eisch AJ. Methamphetamine self-administration and voluntary exercise have opposing effects on medial prefrontal cortex. *J Neurosci*. 2007;27:11442–11450.

83. Mathias S, Lubman DI, Hides L. Substance-induced psychosis: a diagnostic conundrum. *J Clin Psychiatry*. 2008;69:358–367.

84. Maxwell JC, Rutkowski BA. The prevalence of methamphetamine and amphetamine abuse in North America: a review of the indicators, 1992–2007. *Drug Alcohol Rev*. 2008;27:229–235.

85. McCann DJ, Petry NM, Bresell A. Medication nonadherence, "professional subjects," and apparent placebo responders. *J Clin Psychopharmacol*. 2015;35:566–573.

86. McCann UD, Wong DF, Yokoi F, et al. Reduced striatal dopamine transporter density in abstinent methamphetamine and methcathinone users: evidence from positron emission tomography studies with [11C]WIN-35,428. *J Neurosci.* 1998;18:8417–8422.

87. McGregor C, Srisurapanont M, Jittiwutikarn J, et al. The nature, time course and severity of methamphetamine withdrawal. *Addiction.* 2005;100:1320–1329.

88. McGregor C, Srisurapanont M, Mitchell A, et al. Symptoms and sleep patterns during inpatient treatment of methamphetamine withdrawal: a comparison of mirtazapine and modafinil with treatment as usual. *J Subst Abuse Treat.* 2008;35:334–342.

89. McKetin R, Dean OM, Baker AL. A potential role for N-acetylcysteine in the management of methamphetamine dependence. *Drug Alc Rev.* 2017;36:153–159.

90. Melega WP, Cho AK, Harvey D, et al. Methamphetamine blood concentrations in human abusers: application to pharmacokinetic modeling. *Synapse.* 2007;61:216–220.

91. Mendelson J, Uemura N, Harris D, et al. Human pharmacology of the methamphetamine stereoisomers. *Clin Pharmacol Ther.* 2006;80:403–420.

92. Meredith CW, Jaffe C, Ang-Lee K, et al. Implications of chronic methamphetamine use: a literature review. *Harv Rev Psychiatry.* 2005;13:141–154.

93. Meredith CW, Jaffe C, Yanasak E, et al. An open-label pilot study of risperidone in the treatment of methamphetamine dependence. *J Psychoactive Drugs.* 2007;39:167–172.

94. Miles SW, Sheridan J, Russel B, et al. Extended-release methylphenidate for treatment of amphetamine/methamphetamine dependence: a randomized, double-blind, placebo-controlled trial. *Addiction.* 2013;108:1279–1286.

95. Miller DK, Sumithran SP, Dwoskin LP. Bupropion inhibits nicotine-evoked [^{3}H]overflow from superfused rat striatal slices preloaded with [^{3}H]dopamine and from hippocampal slices preloaded with [^{3}H]norepinephrine. *J Pharmacol Exp Ther.* 2002;302:1113–1122.

96. Mitler MM, Hajdukovic R, Erman MK. Treatment of narcolepsy with methamphetamine. *Sleep.* 1993;16:306–317.

97. Mohammadi MR, Ghanizadeh A, Alaghband-Rad J, et al. Selegiline in comparison with methylphenidate in attention deficit hyperactivity disorder children and adolescents in a double-blind, randomized clinical trial. *J Child Adolesc Psychopharmacol.* 2004;14:418–425.

98. Morgenthaler TI, Kapur VK, Brown T, et al. Practice parameters for the treatment of narcolepsy and other hypersomnias of central origin. *Sleep.* 2007;30:1705–1711.

99. Nejtek VA, Avila M, Chen LA, et al. Do atypical antipsychotics effectively treat co-occurring bipolar disorder and stimulant dependence? A randomized, double-blind trial. *J Clin Psychiatry.* 2008;69:1257–1266.

100. Newton TF, Reid MS, De La Garza R, et al. Evaluation of subjective effects of aripiprazole and methamphetamine in methamphetamine-dependent volunteers. *Int J Neuropsychopharmacol.* 2008;11:1037–1045.

101. Newton TF, Roache JD, De La Garza R, et al. Safety of intravenous methamphetamine administration during treatment with bupropion. *Psychopharmacology.* 2005;182:426–435.

102. Newton TF, Raoache JD, De La Garza R, et al. Bupropion reduces methamphetamine-induced subjective effects and cue-induced craving. *Neurpsychopharmacology.* 2006;31:1537–1544.

103. Nickell JR, Siripurapu KB, Vartak A, et al. The vesicular monoamine transporter-2: an important pharmacological target for the Discovery of novel therapeutics to treat methamphetamine abuse. *Adv Pharmacol.* 2014;69:71–106.

104. O'Neil ML, Kuczenski R, Segal DS, et al. Escalating dose pretreatment induces pharmacodynamic and not pharmacokinetic tolerance to a subsequent high-dose methamphetamine binge. *Synapse.* 2006;60:465–473.

105. Ovation PI. *DESOXYN Methamphetamine Hydrochloride Tablets.* USP. Ovation Pharmaceuticals, Inc; 2007. http://www.ovationpharma.com/pdfs/products/product_1.pdf.

106. Ovation PI. *DESOXYN Medication Guide.* Ovation Pharmaceuticals, Inc; 2008. http://www.ovationpharma.com/pdfs/desoxyn.pdf.

107. Pace CJ, Glick SD, Maisonneuve IM, et al. Novel iboga alkaloid congeners block nicotinic receptors and reduce drug self-administration. *Eur J Pharmacol.* 2004;492:159–167.

108. Pereira FC, Lourenco E, Milhazes N, et al. Methamphetamine, morphine, and their combination: acute changes in striatal dopaminergic transmission evaluated by microdialysis in awake rats. *Ann N Y Acad Sci.* 2006;1074:160–173.

109. Peterson E, Laurenzana EM, Atchley WT, et al. Development and preclinical testing of a high-affinity single-chain antibody against (+)-methamphetamine. *J Pharmacol Exp Ther.* 2008;325:124–133.

110. Pike E, Stoops WW, Hays LR, et al. Methamphetamine self-administration in humans during d-amphetamine maintenance. *J Clin Psychopharmacol.* 2014;34:675–681.

111. Pliszka S. Practice parameter for the assessment and treatment of children and adolescents with attention-deficit/hyperactivity disorder. *J Am Acad Child Adolesc Psychiatry.* 2007;46:894–921.

112. Pluddemann A, Myers BJ, Parry CD. Surge in treatment admissions related to methamphetamine use in Cape Town, South Africa: implications for public health. *Drug Alcohol Rev.* 2008;27:185–189.

113. Ranaldi RPoeggel K. Baclofen decreases methamphetamine self-administration in rats. *Neuroreport.* 2002;13:1107–1110.

114. Rawson RA, Gonzales R, Marinelli-Casey P, et al. Methamphetamine dependence: a closer look at treatment response and clinical characteristics associated with route of administration in outpatient treatment. *Am J Addict.* 2007;16:291–299.

115. Reichel CM, Chan CH, Ghee SM, et al. Sex differences in escalation of methamphetamine self-administration: cognitive and motivational consequences. *Psychopharmacol.* 2012;223:371–380.

116. Rezaei F, Emami M, Zahed S, et al. Sustained-release methylphenidate in methamphetamine dependence treatment: a double-blind and placebo-controlled trial. *J Pharm Sci.* 2015;23:1–8.

117. Rezaei F, Ghaderi E, Mardani R, et al. Topiramate for the management of methamphetamine dependence: a pilot randomized, double-blind, placebo-controlled trial. *Fundam Clin Pharmacol.* 2016;30:282–289.

118. Rogers JL, De Santis S, See RE. Extended methamphetamine self-administration enhances reinstatement of drug seeking and impairs novel object recognition in rats. *Psychopharmacology (Berl).* 2008;199:615–624.

119. Roll JM. Contingency management: an evidence-based component of methamphetamine use disorder treatments. *Addiction.* 2007;102(suppl 1):114–120.

120. Roll JM, Petry NM, Stitzer ML, et al. Contingency management for the treatment of methamphetamine use disorders. *Am J Psychiatry.* 2006;163:1993–1999.

121. Rose ME, Grant JE. Pharmacotherapy for methamphetamine dependence: a review of the pathophysiology of methamphetamine addiction and the theoretical basis and efficacy of pharmacotherapeutic interventions. *Ann Clin Psychiat.* 2008;20:145–155.

122. Rubenstein S, Malone MA, Roberts W, et al. Placebo-controlled study examining effects of selegiline in children with attention-deficit/hyperactivity disorder. *J Child Adolesc Psychopharmacol.* 2006;16:404–415.

123. Sabino V, Hicks C, Cottone P. Sigma receptors and substance use disorders. *Adv Exp Med Biol.* 2017;964:177–199.

124. Sakoori K, Murphy NP. Endogenous nociceptin (orphanin FQ) suppresses basal hedonic state and acute reward responses to methamphetamine and ethanol, but facilitates chronic responses. *Neuropsychopharmacology.* 2008;33:877–891.

125. Shoblock JR, Maisonneuve IM, Glick SD. Differences between d-methamphetamine and d-amphetamine in rats: working memory, tolerance, and extinction. *Psychopharmacology (Berl).* 2003;170:150–156.

126. Shoptaw S, Heinzerling KG, Rotheram-Fuller E, et al. Randomized, placebo-controlled trial of bupropion for the treatment of methamphetamine dependence. *Drug Alcohol Depend*. 2008;96:222–232.

127. Shoptaw S, Huber A, Peck J, et al. Randomized, placebo-controlled trial of sertraline and contingency management for the treatment of methamphetamine dependence. *Drug Alcohol Depend*. 2006;85: 8–12.

128. Slemmer JE, Martin BR, Damaj MI. Bupropion is a nicotinic antagonist. *J Pharmacol Exp Ther*. 2000;295:321–327.

129. Sobieraj JC, Kim A, Fannon MJ, et al. Chronic wheel running-induced reduction of extinction and reinstatement of methamphetamine seeking in methamphetamine dependent rats is associated with reduced number of periaqueductal gray dopamine neurons. *Brain Struct Funct*. 2016;221:261–276.

130. Spiller K, Xi ZX, Peng XQ, et al. The selective dopamine D3 receptor antagonists SB-277011A and NGB 2904 and the putative partial D3 receptor agonist BP-897 attenuate methamphetamine-enhanced brain stimulation reward in rats. *Psychopharmacology (Berl)*. 2008;196:533–542.

131. Stevens MW, Henry RL, Owens MS, et al. First human study of a chimeric anti-methamphetamine monoclonal antibody in healthy volunteers. *mAbs*. 2014;6:1649–1656.

132. Stoops WW, Bennett JA, Lile JA, et al. Influence of aripiprazole pretreatment on the reinforcing effects of methamphetamine in humans. *Prog Neuropsychopharmacol Biol Psychiatry*. 2013;47:111–117.

133. Stoops WW, Lile JA, Glaser PE, et al. A low dose of aripiprazole attenuates the subjective-rated effects of d-amphetamine. *Drug Alcohol Depend*. 2006;84:206–209.

134. Sulaiman AH, Gill JS, Said MA, et al. A randomized, placebo-controlled trial of aripiprazole for the treatment of methamphetamine dependence and associated psychosis. *Int J Psychiatry Clin Pract*. 2013;17:131–138.

135. Suzuki O, Hattori H, Asano M, et al. Inhibition of monoamine oxidase by d-methamphetamine. *Biochem Pharmacol*. 1980;29:2071–2073.

136. Suzuki T, Misawa M. Sertindole antagonizes morphine-, cocaine-, and methamphetamine-induced place preference in the rat. *Life Sci*. 1995;57:1277–1284.

137. Takahashi N, Miner LL, Sora I, et al. VMAT2 knockout mice: heterozygotes display reduced amphetamine-conditioned reward, enhanced amphetamine locomotion, and enhanced MPTP toxicity. *Proc Natl Acad Sci USA*. 1997;94:9938–9943.

138. United Nations Office on Drugs and Crime, World Drug Report 2016 (United Nations publication, Sales No. E.16.XI.7).

139. Urschel HC, Hanselka LL, Gromov I, et al. Open-label study of a proprietary treatment program targeting type A γ-aminobutyric acid receptor dysregulation in methamphetamine dependence. *Mayo Clin Proc*. 2007;82:1170–1178.

140. Vocci FJAppel NM. Approaches to the development of medications for the treatment of methamphetamine dependence. *Addiction*. 2007;102(suppl 1):96–106.

141. Volkow ND, Chang L, Wang GJ, et al. Association of dopamine transporter reduction with psychomotor impairment in methamphetamine abusers. *Am J Psychiatry*. 2001;158:377–382.

142. Vollm BA, de Araujo IE, Cowen PJ, et al. Methamphetamine activates reward circuitry in drug naive human subjects. *Neuropsychopharmacology*. 2004;29:1715–1722.

143. Wallace TL, Gudelsky GA, Vorhees CV. Methamphetamine-induced neurotoxicity alters locomotor activity, stereotypic behavior, and stimulated dopamine release in the rat. *J Neurosci*. 1999;19:9141–9148.

144. Warner M, Trinidad JP, Bastian BA. *Drugs Most Frequently Involved in Drug Overdose Deaths: United States, 2010–2014*; 2016.

145. Whitfield TW, Schlosburg JE, Wee S, et al. K opioid receptors in the nucleus accumbens shell mediate escalation of methamphetamine intake. *J Neurosci*. 2015;35:4296–4305.

146. Wilmouth CE, Zheng G, Crooks PA, et al. Oral administration of GZ-793A, a VMAT2 inhibitor, decreases methamphetamine self-administration in rats. *Pharmacol Biochem Behav*. 2013;112:29–33.

147. Wilson JM, Kalasinsky KS, Levey AI, et al. Striatal dopamine nerve terminal markers in human, chronic methamphetamine users. *Nat Med*. 1996;2:699–703.

148. Winhusen TM, Brigham GS, Kropp F, et al. A randomized trial of concurrent smoking-cessation and substance use disorder treatment in stimulant-dependent smokers. *J Clin Psychiatry*. 2014;75: 336–343.

56

Potential Pharmacotherapies for Cannabis Dependence

MARC GRIFELL AND CARL L. HART

Introduction

Cannabis, which comprises Δ^9-tetrahydrocannabinol-containing products including marijuana and hashish, is the most widely used illicit drug in the world, with 183 million people reporting annual use in 2015.[123] During 2015, in the United States alone, an estimated 22.2 million (8.3%) individuals report current marijuana use, defined as use within the past 30 days.[22] Most users of cannabis consume the drug infrequently and without apparent negative consequences. There is, however, a small proportion of users who experience problems related to frequent cannabis use. It has been estimated that the cumulative probability of transitioning from use to dependence is 8.9% for cannabis users.[85] Although this number is low compared with dependence rates for nicotine users (67.5% of tobacco users will become dependent), rates of cannabis dependence in several countries have increased substantially over the past decade[9,22] as well as the number of individuals seeking treatment for cannabis-related problems.[3,22] The terms "dependence" and "dependent" encompass the *Diagnostic and Statistical Manual of Mental Disorders, Fourth Edition, Text Revision* (DSM-IV-TR) and the 10th revision of the *International Statistical Classification of Diseases and Related Health Problems.*

Although the total number of cannabis-dependent individuals who seek treatment is higher than the number of individuals who seek treatment for other illicit drugs, the relative proportion of those seeking treatment for cannabis dependence is low. For example, in the United States, the percentage of regular drug users who received treatment for a cannabis use disorder (includes cannabis abuse and dependence) in 2015 was around 5%, whereas this number was nearly 20% for cocaine users.[22] Several possible explanations for the relatively low percentage of cannabis treatment seekers include the fact that many individuals perceive cannabis as a relatively innocuous drug.[4] However, several investigators have reported that heavy, daily cannabis use is associated with an abstinence syndrome upon cessation of the drug (for review, see Budney[13]). Although cannabis withdrawal is not life-threatening, the accompanying symptoms such as irritability, anxiety, sleep disruptions, aches, and pains can be quite unpleasant. In addition, many individuals seeking treatment for cannabis dependence reported that these symptoms made it more difficult to maintain abstinence.[17]

In addition, heavy cannabis use has been reported to be associated with poor cognitive performance.[48,130,105,111] For example, Bolla and colleagues[10] reported that heavy use of cannabis was associated with poorer cognitive performance on a wide range of tasks (e.g., memory and executive functioning) and that decreased performance persisted as long as 28 days of abstinence. Lifetime exposure to cannabis alone higher than 7 joint-years is also possibly associated with pulmonary dysfunction.[104] The concept of joint-years indicates the cumulative dose of cannabis ingested in lifetime, being, for example, in the case of 7 joint-years either one joint every day during 7 years or seven joints every day during 1 year. Regarding the controverted relationship between cannabis and psychosis, Ksir and colleagues[77] published a recent review. In their study, they concluded that both early use of cannabis and heavy use of cannabis were more likely in individuals with a vulnerability to a variety of problems, such as early or heavy use of cigarettes or alcohol, use of other illicit drugs, and poor school performance. In some individuals, the same vulnerability also resulted in increased risk for psychosis or some other mental disorder.

Some investigators have speculated that the low percentage of individuals seeking treatment for cannabis dependence may be related to the fact that there are relatively few specific treatments for cannabis dependence,[113] although this issue does not appear to deter treatment-seeking cocaine abusers. Regular cannabis users may also be reluctant to participate in treatment programs dominated by alcohol-, cocaine-, and opioid-dependent individuals. Preference to quit without treatment and fear of stigma seem to be among the main barriers to seeking treatment.[40] There are data indicating that some cannabis dependence–specific therapies are successful in decreasing drug use and many associated negative consequences.[28,87] Other data, however, show that cannabis-dependent individuals exhibit high rates of relapse, similar to those found with other substances of abuse.[94] To date, the majority of treatment studies have investigated behavioral/psychosocial therapies. The development of pharmacotherapy presents another option that would be available to cannabis-dependent individuals who have a high relapse rate. Pharmacotherapies may be used alone, in combination with behavioral/psychosocial therapies, or in a staged manner following inadequate response to behavioral/psychosocial therapies. In general, the problem in treating substance-dependent individuals has been less that of treating withdrawal and more of preventing relapse. However, treating withdrawal symptoms continues to be an important first step in eventual success and one that clinicians often need to begin this therapeutic endeavor. The treatment of cannabis dependence in this regard is similar to efforts underway for decades for opioids, cocaine, and alcohol dependence.

Since the original review in 2005,[59] there have been several reviews addressing pharmacotherapies for cannabis dependence. This chapter incorporates most recent reviews and extends them by including the most recent studies. The chapter reviews findings from recent research on cannabinoids (a group of compounds related to Δ^9-tetrahydrocannabinol, the primary psychopharmacologically active constituent of marijuana smoke) that may be relevant for the development of pharmacotherapies for cannabis dependence. Data from studies that assessed the ability of medications to attenuate cannabinoid-related abstinence symptoms in laboratory animals and in humans will be reviewed. In addition, results from studies that have investigated the effects of pharmacological agents on response to cannabinoids are reviewed because these data may prove useful in informing the development of cannabis relapse prevention medications. The review begins with a brief overview of the different phases of the dependence cycle that cannabis pharmacotherapies might target as well as cannabinoid relevant neuropharmacology.

Detoxification and Relapse Prevention or Maintenance Phase

Medications are typically initiated at two different phases of the dependence cycle: during detoxification and prevention of relapse. Detoxification is usually an *initial and immediate goal* during which medications are administered to assuage unpleasant abstinence symptoms that may appear following abrupt cessation of drug use, for example, the administration of a benzodiazepine during alcohol withdrawal. Medications used in the detoxification phase are also sometimes used in the relapse prevention or maintenance phase, for example, nicotine replacement medications. Thus the distinction between a detoxification medication and a relapse prevention medication is sometimes less clear. It is also important for us to note that although we recognize that the goal of this chapter is to review pharmacotherapies that may have some utility in decreasing cannabis withdrawal symptoms, we want to be careful not to overstate the problem of cannabis withdrawal because such symptoms may play a limited role in the addictive process when compared with other important psychosocial factors.[60]

Maintenance medications can be viewed as a *longer-term strategy* used to help the dependent individual avoid relapsing to the abused drug. There are at least three major maintenance strategies. First, agonist or substitution therapy is used to induce cross-tolerance to the abused drug. For example, methadone (a long-acting μ-opioid agonist) and nicotine replacement medications have been used for opioid dependence and tobacco dependence, respectively, as agonist maintenance treatments to prevent relapse and cravings in individuals attempting to maintain abstinence. Agonist maintenance agents typically have safer routes of administration and diminished psychoactive effects relative to the abused drug. Second, antagonist therapy is used to produce extinction by preventing the user from experiencing the reinforcing effects of the abused drug. For example, the naltrexone blocks opioid mu receptors and agonists' associated effects and is therefore used as an antagonist therapy for opioid dependence. Finally, punishment therapy produces an aversive reaction following ingestion of the abused drug. For example, disulfiram (Antabuse) is used in the treatment of alcohol dependence. Disulfiram inhibits aldehyde dehydrogenase, a major enzyme involved in alcohol metabolism, thereby preventing the complete breakdown of alcohol, and the resultant accumulation of aldehyde produces unpleasant symptoms including headache, vomiting, and breathing difficulties.

Cannabinoid Neuropharmacology

Over the past two decades, data from basic research have contributed to an increased understanding of neuronal mechanisms involved in the effects of cannabinoids. Although a comprehensive review of cannabinoid neuropharmacology is beyond the scope of the current manuscript and such reviews have already been published,[37,73,132] a brief overview might be informative for the rationale regarding some of the medications presented in this review. Cannabinoids bind to two types of receptors: cannabinoid receptor 1 and cannabinoid receptor 2 (CB1 and CB2). These receptors are much more abundant than opioid receptors[109] suggesting that the potential actions of cannabinoids are widespread. CB2 receptors are found mainly outside of the brain in immune cells, suggesting that cannabinoids may play a role in the modulation of the immune response. CB1 receptors are found throughout the body, but primarily in the central nervous system. The regions in which central nervous system CB1 receptors reside may provide some clues about their functions. For example, the highest density of CB1 receptors has been found in cells of the basal ganglia, the primary components of which include the caudate nucleus, putamen, and globus pallidus (for review, see Pertwee and Ross[102] and Pertwee[101]). Cells of the basal ganglia are involved in coordinating body movements. Other regions that also contain a larger number of CB1 receptors include: the *cerebellum*, which coordinates fine body movements; the *hippocampus*, which is involved in aspects of memory storage; the *cerebral cortex*, which regulates the integration of higher cognitive functions; and the *nucleus accumbens*, which is involved in drug reinforcement. This suggests that endogenous cannabinoid activity modulates a broad range of behaviors.

Data from microdialysis studies have revealed that dopaminergic transmission is increased in the nucleus accumbens following acute administration of cannabinoid agonists[39,115] and this effect is blocked by the CB1 antagonist rimonabant (SR 141716A). Although it is possible that cannabinoid-induced dopamine elevations are a result of direct stimulation of dopamine neurons, accumulating evidence suggests a more likely mechanism of action is via disinhibition of dopamine-containing neurons that are under tonic γ-aminobutyric acid (GABA)ergic inhibition.[114] Consistent

TABLE 56.1 Published Studies That Have Employed Laboratory Animals to Evaluate Medication Effects on Precipitated Cannabinoid Withdrawal Symptoms.

Investigators	Species	Medication (dose)	Precipitant (dose)	Outcome
Verberne et al. 1981[129]	Rat	Δ^9-THC (6 mg/kg, i.v.)	Clomipramine (15 mg/kg, i.p.)	Δ^9-THC reduced withdrawal symptoms.
Lichtman et al. 2001[83]	Mouse	Δ^9-THC (30 mg/kg, i.v.)	Rimonabant (10 mg/kg, i.p.)	Δ^9-THC reversed withdrawal-related paw tremors.
Lichtman et al. 2001[83]	Mouse	Clonidine (0.125–1 mg/kg, i.p.)	Rimonabant (10 mg/kg, i.p.)	Clonidine reversed withdrawal-related paw tremors and head shakes.
Anggadiredja et al. 2003[2]	Mouse	Prostaglandin E_2 (1, 3.2 μg, i.c.v.)	Rimonabant (10 mg/kg, i.p.)	Prostaglandin E_2 lessened withdrawal symptoms.
Cui et al. 2001[30]	Rat	Lithium (4, 8, 16 mEq/kg)	AM281 (3 mg/kg, i.p.)	Lithium blocked withdrawal symptoms.

Δ^9-THC, Δ^9-tetrahydrocannabinol; i.v., intravenously; i.p., intraperitoneally; i.c.v., intracerebroventricularly.

neurochemical correlates during withdrawal from cannabinoids include reduced dopaminergic activity along the ventral tegmental area-nucleus accumbens pathway[32,117] and upregulated expression and release of corticotropin-releasing hormone in the central nucleus of the amygdala.[19,108] This growing body of knowledge, coupled with increasing numbers of individuals seeking treatment for cannabis dependence, has prompted research on the effects of cannabinoid antagonism on cannabis-associated reinforcement and research on the effects of cannabinoid agonists, as well as medications that decrease the stress response, on cannabis withdrawal.

Abstinence Symptoms Treatment Medications

Studies on Laboratory Animals

Prior to the availability of a cannabinoid antagonist, findings from investigations of cannabinoid-related withdrawal symptoms in laboratory animals were inconsistent. Some researchers found evidence of withdrawal symptoms upon abrupt cessation of drug administration,[6,71] whereas others failed to observe signs of withdrawal when drug administration was terminated.[31,57] Administration of the cannabinoid antagonist rimonabant, however, produces a reliable withdrawal syndrome in laboratory animals undergoing chronic cannabinoid treatment.[7] Behaviorally, this syndrome is most consistently characterized in rodents by wet-dog shakes, paw tremors, piloerection, and increased grooming.

The fact that cannabinoid-related withdrawal symptoms are reliably produced in laboratory animals not only provided evidence for physiological cannabinoid dependence, but it also provided an opportunity to examine systematically pharmacological agents for effectiveness in attenuating these symptoms. Table 56.1 summarizes selected studies that have employed laboratory animals to evaluate medication effects on precipitated cannabinoid withdrawal symptoms. Although the number of studies conducted evaluating potential cannabinoid treatment medications continues to grow, compared with medications development research for other drugs of abuse, this number is conspicuously low. In one earlier study, Verberne et al.[129]

administered intravenous Δ^9-tetrahydrocannabinol in escalating doses for five consecutive days to rats; on day 6, an acute dose of Δ^9-tetrahydrocannabinol or placebo was given 30 minutes prior to an intraperitoneal injection of clomipramine, a selective serotonin reuptake inhibitor (SSRI). The investigators reasoned that clomipramine would precipitate withdrawal in animals chronically exposed to Δ^9-tetrahydrocannabinol because fluoxetine, another SSRI, precipitated withdrawal in animals treated with a similar Δ^9-tetrahydrocannabinol dosing regimen.[128] Although clomipramine precipitated withdrawal symptoms in rats that received acute placebo, there were significantly fewer withdrawal symptoms observed in rats that received the acute dose of Δ^9-tetrahydrocannabinol. These findings, together with data from the report showing that fluoxetine also induces behavioral signs of withdrawal in rats chronically administered Δ^9-tetrahydrocannabinol,[128] suggest that increased serotonergic activity following abrupt discontinuation of repeated cannabinoid agonist treatment may be an important component in the behavioral expression of cannabinoid withdrawal. More recently, however, Touriño et al.[121] reported that the serotonin agonist 3,4-methylenedioxymethamphetamine dose-dependently attenuated rimonabant-precipitated Δ^9-tetrahydrocannabinol withdrawal symptoms in mice. The reasons for these apparent incongruent findings are unclear, but might be related to the fact that the tested medications have multiple sites of action. Some of these actions may overlap, whereas others may not. It is also important to note that there have been no published reports of clomipramine- or fluoxetine-precipitated cannabis withdrawal in humans, so it is not known whether precipitated withdrawal has not occurred. Thus the impact of increased serotonin activity on cannabinoid-related withdrawal is unclear.

Lichtman and colleagues demonstrated that Δ^9-tetrahydrocannabinol as well as clonidine, an α_2-receptor agonist, lessened rimonabant-precipitated withdrawal symptoms in mice.[83] In that study, mice were administered two daily subcutaneous injections of either Δ^9-tetrahydrocannabinol or vehicle for 2 days; on the third day, animals were given one injection of their respective treatment, followed 4 hours later with an intraperitoneal injection of rimonabant or vehicle. Five minutes after the rimonabant challenge dose, mice were administered either an intravenous injection of Δ^9-tetrahydrocannabinol (or placebo) or an intraperitoneal injection of clonidine (or placebo). Both Δ^9-tetrahydrocannabinol and clonidine reversed rimonabant-precipitated paw tremors, and this effect was independent of any generalized effects on movement. Although the finding that Δ^9-tetrahydrocannabinol reversed precipitated cannabinoid withdrawal is consistent with previous data,[129] these were the first published data to demonstrate that an α_2-receptor agonist was effective in alleviating symptoms of cannabinoid withdrawal. Clonidine has been shown to attenuate some withdrawal symptoms associated with alcohol[5,99] and opioid dependence[38,42,122] in humans and laboratory animals, suggesting that some features of withdrawal syndromes associated with drugs of abuse may share common underlying pathophysiological mechanisms. For instance, it is possible that withdrawal symptoms, at least in part, may be mediated by noradrenergic hyperactivity. This view is consistent with the observation that many humans experiencing withdrawal from commonly abused drugs, including alcohol, opioids, and cannabis, often report increased anxiety. One exception to this speculation, however, is the efficacy of bupropion in the treatment of nicotine dependence (see below).

Another interesting line of research aimed at understanding mechanisms underlying cannabinoid withdrawal is the examination of the role of the arachidonic acid cascade. Anggadiredja et al.[2] rendered mice Δ^9-tetrahydrocannabinol-dependent by administering two daily intraperitoneal injections of Δ^9-tetrahydrocannabinol for 5 days. On the sixth day, mice received one injection of Δ^9-tetrahydrocannabinol, followed 4 hours later with an intraperitoneal injection of rimonabant to precipitate withdrawal. Mice in an additional treatment group were given an intraventricular injection of prostaglandin E_2, an end-product of the arachidonic acid cascade, immediately before the rimonabant challenge dose. Prostaglandin E_2 dose-dependently attenuated rimonabant-precipitated withdrawal symptoms including forepaw tremors, forepaw licking, and facial preening. Although the exact mechanism(s) through which prostaglandin E_2 lessened withdrawal symptoms remains to be elucidated, it has been proposed that prostaglandin E_2 reduced symptoms of withdrawal via noradrenergic mechanisms.[2]

Convergent evidence supports this hypothesis. In an in vitro study of the effects of prostaglandin E_2 on electrically evoked tritiated norepinephrine overflow, Exner and Schlicker[36] found that prostaglandin E_2 inhibited the electrically evoked norepinephrine tritium overflow from mouse and rat brain cortex slices. Data from an earlier, similarly designed study[64] were consistent with those obtained by Exner and Schlicker.[36] In addition, as mentioned earlier, clonidine, administered 5 minutes after rimonabant in Δ^9-tetrahydrocannabinol-dependent mice, reversed the precipitated withdrawal,[83] providing further evidence for the role of noradrenergic processes in cannabinoid withdrawal.

The effects of lithium, a commonly used mood-stabilizing medication for the treatment of bipolar disorder, have also been assessed on cannabinoid withdrawal symptoms. Examination of lithium was based on the clinical observation that increased irritability, anxiety and depression often accompanies cannabis withdrawal; lithium effectively decreases these symptoms. Cui et al.[30] administered two daily injections of HU210, a synthetic cannabinoid agonist, to rats on 5 days; on the sixth day, animals were given one injection of their respective treatment, followed 4 hours later with an injection of AM281, a cannabinoid antagonist. The effects of lithium were examined by administering varying doses 15 minutes before the AM281 challenge dose. Lithium dose-dependently prevented symptoms of cannabinoid withdrawal. The investigators speculated that their findings were mediated via lithium-enhancing effects on central nervous system oxytocin

activity and were not related to lithium-associated mood-stabilizing effects. This hypothesis was based on the following observations: (1) oxytocin administration mimicked the effects of lithium on cannabinoid withdrawal; (2) pretreatment with an oxytocin receptor antagonist blocked lithium-related effects on cannabinoid withdrawal; (3) pretreatment with an oxytocin receptor antagonist alone enhanced AM281-precipitated cannabinoid withdrawal[30]; and (4) divalproex, another mood stabilizer used in the treatment of mania, failed to attenuate AM281-precipitated cannabinoid withdrawal (unpublished observations from the same group of researchers). The fact that animals exhibit a stress-like response (e.g., increased grooming behaviors and increased release of corticotropin-releasing hormone) during cannabinoid withdrawal, however, suggests that the mechanisms involved in the stress response may also play a role in the cannabinoid withdrawal syndrome. Given that increased oxytocinergic transmission markedly diminishes the stress response,[21,97,98] it seems plausible that oxytocin plays an integral role in lithium-related effects on cannabinoid withdrawal symptoms. Nevertheless, the exact mechanism responsible for lithium-associated ameliorating effects on cannabinoid withdrawal is an issue that can only be resolved with further research.

One important factor that might limit the generality of the above results is that cannabinoid drugs were administered to animals noncontingently; that is, they were not self-administered but were administered by the experimenter. Data from studies comparing noncontingent and contingent drug administration indicate that substantial differences (e.g., mortality rate and neurochemical) exist that are related to context of drug presentation.[34,63] Future studies should assess the utility of medications to alleviate cannabinoid withdrawal symptoms in animals undergoing abrupt discontinuation of self-administered cannabinoids.

Despite this potential limitation, the above results suggest that the administration of oral Δ^9-tetrahydrocannabinol might be a useful strategy to treat cannabis withdrawal. In addition, the data showing that clonidine mitigates cannabinoid withdrawal are encouraging and suggest that pharmacological agents that decrease noradrenergic output are excellent candidate medications to test in humans undergoing cannabis withdrawal. Although side effects, such as hypotension and sedation associated with clonidine may limit its clinical use for cannabis dependence, other α_2-receptor agonists such as lofexidine, which has a more favorable side effect profile, may hold promise in treating cannabis withdrawal. Indeed, this strategy was investigated in a recent study employing human marijuana abusers (see below). Data indicating that lithium, as well as oxytocin, prevented cannabinoid withdrawal provide potentially novel treatment strategies, although the clinical use of systemic oxytocin for anti-cannabinoid withdrawal effects might be limited because high doses may be required, which increase the likelihood of unpleasant peripheral side effects. Because oxytocin has been shown to produce effects similar to those of benzodiazepines,[124] an alternative approach might be to evaluate the effects of a benzodiazepine on cannabinoid withdrawal symptoms. Clinicians may be wary, however, about the potential for abuse associated with the use of some benzodiazepines, for example, alprazolam, particularly in sedative abusing populations,[18,82,135] thus others such as clonazepam or oxazepam may be more likely candidates. Finally, the data regarding the role of serotonergic activity in cannabinoid withdrawal are less clear: findings from two studies indicate that medications that augment serotonin activity may precipitate or worsen withdrawal, whereas results from another suggest that increased serotonin activity dampens withdrawal.

TABLE 56.2 Published Studies That Have Employed Human Research Participants to Evaluate Medication Effects on Marijuana Withdrawal Symptoms.

Investigators	Medication (dose, p.o.)	Outcome
Haney et al. 2001[54]	Bupropion (0, 300 mg/d)	Bupropion worsened symptoms during withdrawal.
Haney et al. 2003[51]	Nefazodone (0, 50 mg/d)	Nefazodone decreased some withdrawal symptoms, but it had no effect on most symptoms.
Haney et al. 2004[55]	Divalproex (0, 1500 mg/d)	Divalproex worsened mood and psychomotor performance during marijuana consumption and during marijuana withdrawal.
Haney et al. 2004[55]	Δ^9-THC (0, 50 mg/d)	Δ^9-THC reduced marijuana withdrawal symptoms and reversed the withdrawal-associated psychomotor performance decrements and weight loss associated with marijuana withdrawal.
Budney et al. 2007[16]	Δ^9-THC (0, 30, 90 mg/d)	Δ^9-THC dose-dependently attenuated marijuana withdrawal symptoms.

Δ^9-THC, Δ^9-tetrahydrocannabinol; *p.o.*, by mouth.

Studies on Human Research Participants

Although the majority of cannabis users may not experience symptoms of withdrawal, data from a variety of human laboratory and clinical studies demonstrate that an abstinence syndrome can be observed following abrupt cessation of heavy, near-daily use of smoked cannabis[14,58,75,94] or oral Δ^9-tetrahydrocannabinol.[53] Cannabinoid withdrawal syndrome in humans may include a variety of symptoms including increased negative mood states (e.g., increased anxiety, restlessness, depression, and irritability), disrupted sleep, decreased food intake, and in some cases, aggressive behavior.[15,76] These symptoms have been reported to begin 1 day after cannabinoid cessation, peak effects are observed on days 2–6, and most effects persist from 4 to 14 days, depending on an individual's level of cannabis dependence.[94] Because cannabis withdrawal may be one factor maintaining continued cannabis use (i.e., frequent marijuana smokers may continue their use not only for marijuana-related intoxicating effects, but also to avoid undergoing withdrawal symptoms), medications that would alleviate cannabis withdrawal symptoms could be useful.

Table 56.2 summarizes the studies that have employed human research participants to evaluate the potential of medications to alleviate marijuana withdrawal symptoms. As can be seen, the majority of the published research in this area has been conducted in our laboratory. Our group at Columbia University/New York State Psychiatric Institute has conducted a series of carefully controlled, within-participant design, residential laboratory studies. During these studies, nontreatment seekers, frequent marijuana smokers smoked active marijuana cigarettes on several consecutive days, five times per day, followed by several days of marijuana abstinence. During abstinence, placebo marijuana cigarettes were smoked and the effectiveness of potential treatment medications to attenuate marijuana withdrawal symptoms was examined. The first medication tested in these studies was bupropion 0, 300 mg/day, a US Food and Drug Administration (FDA)–approved tobacco smoking cessation aid and antidepressant.[54] Three hundred mg of bupropion were tested against a 0-mg control group. The rationale for the use of this medication was related to the observation that bupropion had been shown to maintain tobacco smoking abstinence, in part, because of its ability to decrease negative mood symptoms (e.g., increased anxiety, depression, and irritability) associated with nicotine withdrawal. Given that similar negative mood symptoms are also associated with marijuana withdrawal, bupropion was expected to improve symptoms of marijuana withdrawal. The data, however, indicated otherwise: bupropion worsened several ratings of mood, including irritability, restlessness and depression, and self-reported

sleep quality. The mechanism(s) mediating bupropion-worsening effects on marijuana withdrawal is unclear, but the mechanism of action most commonly attributed to bupropion is inhibition of dopamine reuptake and, to a lesser extent, norepinephrine reuptake inhibition.[35,78,112] Thus bupropion-associated effects on marijuana withdrawal symptoms could be related to enhanced norepinephrine activity. This suggestion is consistent with the above-cited data showing that clonidine, a medication that decreases noradrenergic activity, lessened precipitated Δ^9-tetrahydrocannabinol withdrawal symptoms[83] as well as the withdrawal symptoms associated with alcohol and opioid dependence.[74]

Another study conducted by our team investigated the effects of **nefazodone** 0, 450 mg/day on symptoms of marijuana withdrawal.[51] Participants were either administered 450 mg of nefazodone daily in the treatment group or 0 mg in the placebo control group. Nefazodone, an atypical antidepressant, is thought to exert its major therapeutic effects via antagonistic actions at the serotonin-2a receptor,[107,119] although it has also been shown to produce relatively weak inhibition of norepinephrine and serotonin uptake sites in vitro. A major reason for investigating nefazodone-related effects on marijuana withdrawal symptoms was that it had been demonstrated to effectively treat depression, agitation, and anxiety (symptoms also associated with marijuana withdrawal) in clinical populations.[136] Data from the study by Haney et al.[51] revealed that nefazodone decreased a few symptoms associated with marijuana withdrawal (i.e., ratings of "Anxious" and "Muscle Pain"), but it had no effect on most symptoms (e.g., ratings of "Irritable" and "Trouble Sleeping"). Because nefazodone did relieve some discomfort associated with marijuana withdrawal without worsening other symptoms and because only one active dose was tested, further study of this agent, using a broader dosing range, in the treatment of marijuana withdrawal could be warranted but may not occur because of the black box warning (i.e., the highlighted portion of the package insert) about hepatoxicity.

Divalproex 0, 1500 mg/day, approved for the treatment of epilepsy, mood disorders, and migraine headaches, was evaluated for effectiveness in decreasing marijuana withdrawal symptoms.[55] Study participants received either 1500 mg daily in the treatment group or 0 mg in the placebo control group. Divalproex's precise neurochemical mechanism of action remains unknown, although some divalproex-related therapeutic effects have been attributed to its ability to dampen sustained repetitive neuronal firing via modulation of Na$^+$ channel activity.[90] Other therapeutic effects might be related to its ability to increase central nervous system GABA activity.[23,103] The rationale for testing the effects of divalproex on marijuana withdrawal symptoms was not based on a proposed neurochemical mechanism of action, but instead was based on clinical evidence indicating that the medication had been used successfully to treat some symptoms commonly associated with marijuana withdrawal (e.g., irritability and mood lability[33]). Unfortunately, divalproex did not reduce marijuana withdrawal symptoms. In fact, many withdrawal symptoms, including anxiety and irritability, were significantly increased when participants were maintained on divalproex compared to when they were maintained on placebo.[55] Divalproex not only worsened marijuana withdrawal-associated mood, but it also produced psychomotor performance disruptions during marijuana consumption and during marijuana abstinence. The results are in agreement with data from the aforementioned unpublished study using rodents, which showed that divalproex had no effect on AM281-precipitated withdrawal. In short, these data do not support the use of divalproex as a marijuana treatment medication.

Two other groups of researchers have examined **lithium** carbonate, another mood stabilizer, for effectiveness in decreasing cannabis withdrawal symptoms. The rationale for testing lithium carbonate was based on encouraging data collected using laboratory animals in which the medication decreased cannabinoid-associated withdrawal symptoms.[30] Bowen et al.[30] and Winstock et al.[134] conducted open-label trials of the effects of lithium carbonate (500–900 mg/day) on cannabis withdrawal. In general, the researchers reported that the medication reduced withdrawal severity for most study participants, but both studies contained important limitations that decrease the generality of the findings. For example, the noncontrolled nature of these experiments may have increased expectancy effects; that is, the researchers' and the participants' knowledge that participants were receiving an active treatment medication influenced participants reported cannabis withdrawal intensity.

Another strategy tested for efficacy in attenuating human marijuana withdrawal is the administration of **oral Δ^9-tetrahydrocannabinol**. In a recently reported study, Haney and coworkers[55] investigated the effects of oral Δ^9-tetrahydrocannabinol (THC) 0, 10 mg administered five times per day, on marijuana withdrawal symptoms. Participants received either five capsules containing 0 mg of THC in the placebo control group or five capsules of 10 mg of THC each in the treatment group. The primary reason for evaluating the effects of oral Δ^9-tetrahydrocannabinol on marijuana withdrawal was based on the idea of substituting a longer-acting pharmacologically equivalent drug for the abused substance, stabilizing the individual on that drug, and then gradually withdrawing the substituted drug. In this way, the likelihood of precipitating abstinence symptoms is decreased. Nicotine replacement therapies have been used extensively in this capacity for the treatment of tobacco-related withdrawal, as has methadone for opioid withdrawal. Haney et al.[55] found that oral Δ^9-tetrahydrocannabinol markedly reduced symptoms associated with marijuana abstinence including self-reported ratings of marijuana craving, anxiety, misery, and sleep disturbance. The medication also reversed the withdrawal-associated psychomotor performance decrements as well as the anorexia and weight loss associated with marijuana withdrawal. It is important to note, too, that these effects occurred at an oral Δ^9-tetrahydrocannabinol dose indistinguishable from placebo (i.e., like placebo, active Δ^9-tetrahydrocannabinol produced no apparent subjective effects), highlighting the pharmacological specificity of marijuana withdrawal. Budney and colleagues[16] replicated and extended these findings by demonstrating that oral Δ^9-tetrahydrocannabinol (30 and 90 mg/day) dose-dependently suppressed cannabis withdrawal

in an outpatient environment. Together, these results are consistent with findings that showed that acute Δ^9-tetrahydrocannabinol administration substantially assuaged precipitated cannabinoid withdrawal in laboratory animals[83,129]; more importantly, they indicate that oral Δ^9-tetrahydrocannabinol might be beneficial in the treatment of marijuana dependence.

Several limitations of the above studies should be noted. First, most of the studies employed only one active dose of the treatment medication. Perhaps more cannabis-related withdrawal symptoms would have been alleviated if a wider range of medication doses were examined. This point is particularly relevant for the study that examined nefazodone because the tested active dose (450 mg/day), which was lower than doses regularly used clinically to treat anxiety and depression, showed a trend toward improved withdrawal symptomatology. Second, most study participants were seeking treatment to abstain from cannabis use. Because the study of cannabis-related effects in humans requires the administration of carefully controlled doses of smoked marijuana, ethical considerations dictate that research volunteers not only have current cannabis use histories, but that they are also not seeking treatment for their cannabis use.[44,52,] Thus it is possible that the above results may not generalize to persons who are requesting treatment for cannabis dependence. A related limitation is that although adolescents are more likely than adults to exhibit clinical features of cannabis dependence and experience difficulties abstaining from cannabis use,[24] none of the above studies included participants younger than 21 years of age. This was done because the studies involved the administration of smoked marijuana (a drug of abuse); thus it was believed inappropriate to expose children to smoked marijuana in the laboratory, even if the potential participant had reported previous use. Nonetheless, in light of the fact that a large proportion of cannabis-dependent persons under the age of 21 report using cannabis to alleviate withdrawal symptoms,[25] it may be important study the effects of potential treatment medications in older adolescents.

There are at least two issues of potential concern related to treating cannabis-dependent adolescents with medications such as oral Δ^9-tetrahydrocannabinol: (1) administration of a psychoactive drug to individuals whose brains are still developing can potentially hamper development, especially in areas like the prefrontal cortex, which is slower to develop than other cortical regions[125]; and (2) replacement of one psychoactive drug with abuse potential with another drug that has abuse potential. Although these concerns deserve serious consideration, it is important to note that the route of administration is a critical determinant of neurochemical consequences associated with drug administration, in part because neurochemical effects depend on the rate of rise of drug concentrations and the maximum drug concentrations achieved.[41] Thus administration of Δ^9-tetrahydrocannabinol via the oral route would be expected to produce less deleterious neuronal consequences than smoked marijuana. Regarding concerns about the abuse potential of oral Δ^9-tetrahydrocannabinol, data from a recent study completed in our laboratory showed that the drug produced low rates of self-administration in a sample of marijuana smokers, suggesting that the abuse potential of oral Δ^9-tetrahydrocannabinol is limited.[61] Note also that oral Δ^9-tetrahydrocannabinol, unlike smoked marijuana, is not associated with an increased risk of lung toxicity. Hence, from a risk-benefit perspective, oral Δ^9-tetrahydrocannabinol appears to be a safer therapeutic option. It should be noted that Gray et al.[45] recently assessed oral Δ^9-tetrahydrocannabinol (0, 2.5, 5, 10 mg/day) for tolerability in older adolescents (ages 16–21 years). They found that the drug produced dose-related increases in euphoria without producing significant

TABLE 56.3	Published Randomized Controlled and Quasi-Controlled Trials Evaluating Medications to Reduce Symptoms and Signs of Cannabis Withdrawal or Promote Cessation in Treatment-Seeking Cannabis-Dependent Subjects Without Comorbidity.	
Investigators	**Medication (dose)**	**Outcome**
Allsop et al. 2014[1]	Oral nabiximols (Sativex) 86.4 mg THC	Nabiximols significantly reduced the overall severity of cannabis withdrawal and increased treatment retention
Carpenter et al. 2009[20]	Oral nefazodone, 150 mg/day; to maximum 600 mg/day	Nefazodone not superior to placebo
Cornelius 2010[29]	Fluoxetine, 10 mg increasing to 20 mg/day after 2 weeks	Fluoxetine not superior to placebo
Gray et al. 2012[46]	N-acetylcysteine, 1200 mg twice daily	N-acetylcysteine increased THC-negative urines relative to placebo
Levin et al. 2004[79]	Oral divalproex sodium commenced at 500 mg/day, increasing to maximum of 2 g/day, depending on response	Divalproex sodium decreased self-reported marijuana use
Levin et al. 2011[80]	Oral dronabinol, commenced at 10 mg/day, titrated to 20 mg twice a day or the maximum tolerated	Dronabinol decreased withdrawal symptoms and increased treatment retention
Levin et al. 2013[81]	Venlafaxine-extended release, up to 375 mg on a fixed-flexible schedule	Venlafaxine not superior to placebo
Mason et al. 2013[89]	Oral gabapentin 300 mg, increasing to 1200 mg/day	Gabapentin decreased withdrawal symptoms and cannabis use
McRae-Clark et al. 2009[92]	Oral buspirone, initiated at 5 mg twice a day, increased to maximum 60 mg per day	Buspirone not superior to placebo but produced more adverse events
McRae-Clark et al. 2010[93]	Oral atomoxetine started at 25 mg, with further increase to 100 mg/day in week 4 if required	Atomoxetine not superior to placebo but produced more adverse events
Penetar et al. 2012[100]	Oral bupropion-SR (sustained release), 150 mg/day for days 1 to 3; then 150 mg twice a day	Bupropion decreased withdrawal symptoms and craving but produced more adverse events
Weinstein et al. 2014[133]	Escitalopram, 10 mg/day	Escitalopram not superior to placebo but was associated with higher drop-out rates

effects on cardiovascular measures, psychomotor performance, or negative subjective-effect ratings. Another limitation worth noting is that the same group of researchers has collected most of the published data in this research area, which highlights the need for replication of previous results and additional data.

The above limitations notwithstanding, the data obtained in human research participants demonstrate that while a growing number of medications have been tested, few show promise as potential treatment strategies for the amelioration of cannabinoid withdrawal symptoms. Findings from studies of bupropion and divalproex were discouraging, as these medications failed to assuage many marijuana withdrawal symptoms. In some cases, symptoms were worsened by the medication. Of the agents tested, clearly, oral Δ^9-tetrahydrocannabinol produced the most promising results. In addition, the limited results obtained in adolescents indicate that oral Δ^9-tetrahydrocannabinol is well tolerated and suggest further study of this medication in adolescent marijuana abusers. Although **no study has investigated the effects of benzodiazepines on human cannabis withdrawal symptoms**, data obtained in laboratory animals suggest that future studies should examine the ability of agents such as clonazepam or oxazepam to lessen severity of the withdrawal syndrome.

Randomized Controlled Trials

Table 56.3 shows results from clinical trials that have assessed pharmacotherapies for treating cannabis dependence. As is stated in a recent Cochrane review,[87] the evidence remains inconclusive, but there is moderate evidence indicating that oral THC increases the likelihood that participants will complete the trial. In addition, treatment with preparations containing THC reduces cannabis withdrawal symptoms and craving.

Relapse Prevention Medications

Drug self-administration procedures provide a reliable method for evaluating the reinforcing effects of psychoactive agents. Under these procedures, laboratory animals are provided an opportunity to self-administer intravenously doses of a drug contingent upon an operant response (e.g., lever pressing). These procedures have been used extensively not only to assess drug-related abuse liability, but also to evaluate the usefulness of potential pharmacotherapies in treating substance use disorders. If a potential treatment medication, for example, decreases self-administration of the abused drug in laboratory animals, then perhaps the treatment medication would be effective in curtailing human abuse of the drug. Although data from the majority of earlier studies showed that cannabinoids did not reliably maintain self-administration behavior in laboratory animals tested (e.g., Harris et al.[57] and Mansback et al.[85]; for review, see also Tanda et al.[118]), findings from recent studies clearly demonstrate that cannabinoids produce dose-related reinforcing effects in rats and squirrel monkeys.[68,88,118] The success of recent attempts to obtain reliable self-administration in laboratory animals has been attributed to the employment of lower Δ^9-tetrahydrocannabinol doses that were injected more rapidly than those previously investigated.

Because of the demonstration that Δ^9-tetrahydrocannabinol reliably serves as a reinforcer, Goldberg and colleagues have begun testing the ability of potential marijuana treatment medications to alter marijuana self-administration in squirrel monkeys. In the first study, monkeys were given an opportunity to self-administer Δ^9-tetrahydrocannabinol (2, 4 µg/kg) during sessions.[118] Both doses robustly maintained self-administration; when active Δ^9-tetrahydrocannabinol was substituted with vehicle, responding significantly decreased. Following the demonstration of Δ^9-tetrahydrocannabinol self-administration, the researchers then assessed the effects of the cannabinoid antagonist rimonabant, administered 1 hour before experimental sessions, on Δ^9-tetrahydrocannabinol as well as cocaine self-administration. The administration of rimonabant markedly reduced Δ^9-tetrahydrocannabinol self-administration, but had no effect on cocaine self-administration, indicating the selective involvement of the cannabinoid system in Δ^9-tetrahydrocannabinol reinforcing effects. These findings were recently extended when this group of investigators demonstrated that rimonabant blocked cue- and Δ^9-tetrahydrocannabinol–induced reinstatement of Δ^9-tetrahydrocannabinol self-administration by squirrel monkeys.[69] The finding that rimonabant suppressed Δ^9-tetrahydrocannabinol self-administration is an important one with respect to cannabis treatment medication development efforts. It suggests that cannabinoid antagonism might be a useful strategy for decreasing cannabis dependence in humans. In fact, Huestis et al.[65] reported that rimonabant (90 mg, by mouth) blocked the acute subjective and cardiovascular effects of smoked marijuana in human research volunteers. An important caveat to the above findings is that an acute rimonabant dosing regimen was employed in those studies. Because individuals undergoing treatment for cannabis dependence may require repeated administration of pharmacological agents, the clinical utility of rimonabant is unclear. In addition, although rimonabant-like medications may present an alternative option for individuals who do not want to be maintained on cannabinoid agonists, it is important to note that lack of compliance has been a major problem with antagonist therapy used in treating other substance use disorders (e.g., naltrexone for opioid dependence). Despite these concerns, the above data suggest that further study of rimonabant-like medications in the treatment of marijuana dependence is warranted.

In another study by this group of researchers, Justinova et al.,[67] using similar procedures, evaluated the effects of naltrexone, an opioid antagonist, on Δ^9-tetrahydrocannabinol self-administration behavior in monkeys. The rationale for the use of naltrexone stemmed from accumulating evidence obtained in laboratory animals, which suggests a reciprocal functional interaction between CNS cannabinoid and opioid systems.[86] Opioid antagonists, for example, have been demonstrated to precipitate withdrawal symptoms in rats dependent on cannabinoids.[72,95] Moreover, pretreatment with the opioid antagonist naloxone has been shown to decrease self-administration behavior maintained by cannabinoid agonists in rodents.[11,12,96] Justinova et al.[67] replicated and extended the self-administration data by demonstrating that Δ^9-tetrahydrocannabinol self-administration behavior in monkeys was significantly decreased in the presence of naltrexone. The dampening effect of naltrexone on Δ^9-tetrahydrocannabinol self-administration behavior was not as robust as those produced by the cannabinoid antagonist (described earlier). Although these data are congruent with the hypothesis that the endogenous opioid system modulates CNS cannabinoid effects and are suggestive of the idea that naltrexone might be useful in preventing relapse to marijuana use, data obtained using human research participants indicate that naltrexone does not alter marijuana-associated antinociceptive or subjective effects.[47,131] Indeed, Haney et al.[50] reported that naltrexone pretreatment (50 mg, oral) significantly increased positive subjective effects (e.g. ratings of "Good Drug Effect") of oral Δ^9-tetrahydrocannabinol (30 mg). Naltrexone also produced a moderate increase in choice to self-administer Δ^9-tetrahydrocannabinol, although this effect was not significant. More recently, Haney[49] investigated the effects of a lower, more selective dose of naltrexone (12 mg, oral) on response to oral Δ^9-tetrahydrocannabinol (0–40 mg) in nonmarijuana and marijuana smokers. Naltrexone-related effects varied as a function of marijuana use history: in nonmarijuana smokers, Δ^9-tetrahydrocannabinol–associated intoxicating effects (2.5 mg) were enhanced and Δ^9-tetrahydrocannabinol–associated anxiety (10 mg) was decreased, whereas, in marijuana smokers, Δ^9-tetrahydrocannabinol–associated intoxicating effects (20 mg) were reduced and Δ^9-tetrahydrocannabinol–associated anxiety (40 mg) was increased. The apparent lack of correspondence between data obtained using laboratory animals and those obtained with human research participants emphasizes the importance of not only testing potential marijuana pharmacotherapeutic agents in laboratory animals, but also evaluating the utility of these medications in human research participants.

In contrast to the large database describing the effects of relapse prevention medications in treating human alcohol and cocaine dependence (for review, see Karila et al.[70]), research evaluating potential cannabis pharmacotherapies is scarce. Of the few studies that have been published, most have focused primarily on the ability of the test medication to alter physiological and subjective effects of marijuana. Cone et al.,[27] for instance, showed that clonidine pretreatment reduced marijuana-related increase in heart rate, but had no effect on marijuana-related subjective effects, and as mentioned earlier, Huestis et al.[66] found that rimonabant pretreatment attenuated both the increased heart rate and intoxicating effects associated with smoked marijuana. Maintenance on a cannabinoid agonist has also been reported to decrease the intoxicating effects and increase heart rate following smoked marijuana.[66] These data indicate that some of marijuana-associated effects can be altered by various medications.

Although modification of subjective and cardiovascular effects produced by marijuana provides important information, the behavior of major interest in lab studies for the treatment of cannabis dependence is drug-taking. To date, only a few published studies have measured cannabis-taking behavior by human research volunteers while being maintained on a potential pharmacotherapeutic agent. The first study was a within-participant design, residential laboratory study during which the influence of oral Δ^9-tetrahydrocannabinol maintenance (0, 10, 20 mg, four times daily, each dose administered for three consecutive days) on choice to self-administer smoked marijuana was evaluated.[62] Hart et al.[62] reasoned that because Δ^9-tetrahydrocannabinol had been demonstrated to play an integral role in the behavioral effects of smoked marijuana[58] and because agonist therapies have been demonstrated to be effective in decreasing self-administration of other drugs of abuse,[8,26] marijuana-related reinforcing and subjective effects could be significantly attenuated during oral Δ^9-tetrahydrocannabinol maintenance. Yet, the choice to self-administer marijuana was not significantly altered by either of the two active Δ^9-tetrahydrocannabinol maintenance conditions, although some marijuana-associated positive subjective effect ratings (e.g., "Good Drug Effect") were reduced when participants were maintained on oral Δ^9-tetrahydrocannabinol. There exist several possible reasons that oral Δ^9-tetrahydrocannabinol maintenance did not alter marijuana self-administration, but two are of particular importance. First, the Δ^9-tetrahydrocannabinol maintenance regimen involved only three consecutive days of active treatment, which may have been an insufficient time frame to reduce marijuana self-administration by frequent marijuana users (prior to study enrollment, participants reported smoking an average of seven marijuana cigarettes per day). Second, none of the study participants were seeking treatment to abstain from marijuana use, further decreasing the likelihood of observing alterations in marijuana self-administration behavior. Given these observations, as well as the fact that some of marijuana's subjective effects decreased, the effect of longer oral Δ^9-tetrahydrocannabinol maintenance on self-administration of marijuana by different populations of marijuana-dependent individuals warrants further investigation.

In another laboratory study, Haney et al.[56] determined the effects of oral Δ^9-tetrahydrocannabinol (60 mg/day), lofexidine (2.4 mg/day), and the combination on symptoms of marijuana withdrawal and relapse, defined as a return to marijuana use after a period of abstinence. Oral Δ^9-tetrahydrocannabinol decreased most withdrawal symptoms, which replicates previous findings[23,55] but did not decrease marijuana relapse. Lofexidine was sedating and did not lessen withdrawal, but improved sleep and decreased marijuana relapse. The Δ^9-tetrahydrocannabinol–lofexidine combination most robustly improved sleep and attenuated marijuana withdrawal, craving, and relapse. These findings argue that the Δ^9-tetrahydrocannabinol–lofexidine combination should be examined further for its potential as a marijuana dependence treatment medication.

In a pilot outpatient trial, Levin et al.[79] tested divalproex as a marijuana abuse relapse prevention medication. This 12-week study utilized a double-blind placebo-controlled, crossover design, during which 25 individuals were initially randomized to either divalproex (average dose: 1673 mg/day) or placebo. Self-reported marijuana use and quantitative Δ^9-tetrahydrocannabinol urine levels were the primary outcome measures. Divalproex was not found to be more efficacious at curtailing marijuana use than placebo. In addition, divalproex, at doses tested, did not appear to be well tolerated, as compliance on the medication was poor. Together with the finding that divalproex was ineffective at decreasing symptoms of marijuana withdrawal,[55] these results suggest that divalproex is not a viable therapeutic option for marijuana dependence.

McRae et al.[91] used an open-label design to test buspirone (10–60 mg/day) as a potential marijuana dependence treatment medication. The rationale for testing buspirone was based on its ability to decrease anxiety, a symptom sometimes associated with cannabis withdrawal. This 12-week study enrolled 11 participants, but only two completed. The researchers reported that buspirone produced moderate reductions in self-reported marijuana craving and irritability and urine samples positive for marijuana metabolites. A major limitation associated with this study is that it was conducted under nonblinded conditions. As a result, the generality of the findings is limited.

In another open-label trial, the attention-deficit/hyperactivity disorder medication atomoxetine was investigated.[120] Tirado et al.[120] reasoned that atomoxetine would be an excellent candidate medication because impairments in attention, memory, executive function, and response inhibition seen in marijuana smokers resemble deficits seen in individuals with attention-deficit/hyperactivity disorder. During this 11-week trial, 13 cannabis-dependent treatment seekers were administered a flexible dose of atomoxetine (from 25 to 80 mg/day) depending upon individual tolerability, and self-reported cannabis use and use verified via urine toxicology were assessed. Self-reported cannabis use was decreased during medication treatment, but this was not confirmed by urine toxicology, as the number of tetrahydrocannabinol-positive urine screens did not vary as a function of treatment condition. In addition, atomoxetine was associated with significant adverse gastrointestinal symptoms (nausea, vomiting, dyspepsia, and diarrhea).

A growing number of clinical laboratory studies have demonstrated that the physiological and subjective effects of cannabis can be reduced by different classes of medications. Cannabis-related effects on heart rate are attenuated by the α_2-receptor agonist clonidine and by the cannabinoid antagonist rimonabant; cannabis-related intoxicating effects are dampened by rimonabant and by the cannabinoid agonist Δ^9-tetrahydrocannabinol. Such findings are encouraging, but clearly more research is needed to determine the clinical utility of these medications for cannabis dependence. Of the limited number of studies evaluating the effects of relapse prevention medications on cannabis-taking behavior by humans, one has shown a medication to decrease marijuana relapse; the Δ^9-tetrahydrocannabinol–lofexidine combination seems to be the most encouraging. The finding might ultimately prove beneficial in decreasing relapse to cannabis use in a treatment-seeking population of cannabis-dependent individuals, but further studies using different doses are needed to confirm data from the single available study.

Future Directions in Medication Development for Cannabis Dependence

Since 2000, there has been an increase in the popularity of smoking "blunts," marijuana wrapped in tobacco paper from inexpensive cigars such as Phillies Blunts or Dutch Masters.[43] Anecdotally, blunt smokers report that the combination of nicotine, derived from the tobacco wrapping, and tobacco enhances the psychoactive pleasurable effects of marijuana. Although there is currently a lack of scientific evidence substantiating this claim in humans, Valjent et al.[126] found that Δ^9-tetrahydrocannabinol–induced hypothermia, antinociception, and hypolocomotion were markedly facilitated by nicotine in mice. Consistent with these results, Solinas et al.[110] demonstrated that selective alpha7 nicotinic acetylcholine receptor antagonists disrupted the discriminative stimulus and reinforcing effects of cannabinoid receptor 1 agonists. They also found that selective alpha7 nicotinic acetylcholine receptor antagonists decreased Δ^9-tetrahydrocannabinol–induced dopamine elevations in the shell of the nucleus accumbens. In general, the preceding results are in line with a recent report indicating that symptoms of cannabis dependence are worsened by the combination of tobacco and marijuana smoking.[106] Together, these findings suggest that endocannabinoid and acetylcholinergic activity may produce synergetic effects and should be target for future medication development efforts for cannabis dependence.

Several new nicotinic acetylcholine receptor agonists are now in human clinical development for a variety of cognitive disorders and smoking cessation. Recently, varenicline, a nicotinic acetylcholine receptor partial agonist, was approved for smoking cessation with efficacy superior to nicotine replacement therapies and bupropion. Because of the overlap between nicotine and cannabis in terms of dependence and similarity in withdrawal symptoms,[17,127] pharmacotherapies, like varenicline and transdermal nicotine, may reduce the withdrawal effects associated with cannabis, particularly if the cannabis-dependent individuals are also dependent on tobacco.

In summary, research investigating the use of pharmacotherapies for cannabis use disorders continues to be refined. A growing number of medications have been shown to alleviate cannabinoid withdrawal symptoms in laboratory animals and may provide clues to the underlying neuronal mechanisms of cannabinoid dependence. In laboratory animals, only rimonabant has been shown to be particularly promising; in humans, a small number of medications have been demonstrated to decrease physiological and subjective effects of cannabis (clonidine, oral Δ^9-tetrahydrocannabinol, and rimonabant), and the Δ^9-tetrahydrocannabinol–lofexidine combination has been demonstrated to most effectively reduce relapse to cannabis use.

Acknowledgments

This research was supported by the National Institute on Drug Abuse grant #DA-03746. We gratefully acknowledge the efforts of Michaela Bamdad and Catalina Saldaña, who read an earlier version of the manuscript and made helpful suggestions. MG thanks the Instituto de Salud Carlos III for making his contribution possible through a Rio Hortega grant (CM18/00168)ISCIII/FSE

References

1. Allsop DJ, et al. Nabiximols as an agonist replacement therapy during cannabis withdrawal. *JAMA Psychiatry.* 2014;71:281.
2. Anggadiredja K, et al. Prostaglandin E2attenuates SR141716A-precipitated withdrawal in tetrahydrocannabinol-dependent mice. *Brain Res.* 2003;966:47–53.
3. Anthony JC, Warner LA, Kessler RC. Comparative epidemiology of dependence on tobacco, alcohol, controlled substances, and inhalants: basic findings from the national comorbidity survey. *Exp Clin Psychopharmacol.* 1994;2:244–268.
4. Apostolidis T, Fieulaine N, Simonin L, Rolland G. Cannabis use, time perspective and risk perception: evidence of a moderating effect. *Psychol Heal.* 2006;21:571–592.
5. Baumgartner GR, Rowen RC. Clonidine vs chlordiazepoxide in the management of acute alcohol withdrawal syndrome. *Arch Intern Med.* 1987;147:1223.
6. Beardsley PM, Balster RL, Harris LS. Dependence on tetrahydrocannabinol in rhesus monkeys. *J Pharmacol Exp Ther.* 1986;239.
7. Beardsley PM, Martin BR. Effects of the cannabinoid CB(1) receptor antagonist, SR141716A, after Delta(9)-tetrahydrocannabinol withdrawal. *Eur J Pharmacol.* 2000;387:47–53.
8. Benowitz NL, Zevin S, Jacob P. Suppression of nicotine intake during ad libitum cigarette smoking by high-dose transdermal nicotine. *J Pharmacol Exp Ther.* 1998;287:958–962.
9. Bhana A, et al. The South African Community epidemiology Network on drug Use (SACENDU) project, phases 1-8–cannabis and Mandrax. *S Afr Med J.* 2002;92:542–547.
10. Bolla KI, Brown K, Eldreth D, Tate K, Cadet JL. Dose-related neurocognitive effects of marijuana use. *Neurol.* 2002;2002(59):1337–1343.
11. Braida D, Pozzi M, Cavallini R, Sala M. Conditioned place preference induced by the cannabinoid agonist CP 55,940: interaction with the opioid system. *Neuroscience.* 2001;104:923–926.
12. Braida D, Pozzi M, Parolaro D, Sala M. Intracerebral self-administration of the cannabinoid receptor agonist CP 55,940 in the rat: interaction with the opioid system. *Eur J Pharmacol.* 2001;413:227–234.
13. Budney AJ. Review of the validity and significance of cannabis withdrawal syndrome. *Am J Psychiatry.* 2004;161:1967–1977.
14. Budney aJ, Hughes JR, Moore B, Novy PL. Marijuana abstinence effects in marijuana smokers maintained in their home environment. *Arch Gen Psychiatry.* 2001;58:917–924.
15. Budney AJ, Hughes JR. The cannabis withdrawal syndrome. *Curr Opin Psychiatry.* 2006;19:233–238.
16. Budney AJ, Vandrey RG, Hughes JR, Moore BA, Bahrenburg B. Oral delta-9-tetrahydrocannabinol suppresses cannabis withdrawal symptoms. *Drug Alcohol Depend.* 2007;86:22–29.
17. Budney AJ, Vandrey RG, Hughes JR, Thostenson JD, Bursac Z. Comparison of cannabis and tobacco withdrawal: severity and contribution to relapse. *J Subst Abuse Treat.* 2008;35:362–368.
18. Busto U, et al. Patterns of benzodiazepine abuse and dependence. *Br J Addict.* 1986;81:87–94.
19. Caberlotto L, Rimondini R, Hansson A, Eriksson S, Heilig M. Corticotropin-releasing hormone (CRH) mRNA expression in rat central amygdala in cannabinoid tolerance and withdrawal: evidence for an allostatic shift? *Neuropsychopharmacology.* 2004;29:15–22.
20. Carpenter KM, McDowell D, Brooks DJ, Cheng WY, Levin FR. A preliminary trial: double-blind comparison of nefazodone, bupropion-SR, and placebo in the treatment of cannabis dependence. *Am J Addict.* 2009;18:53–64.
21. Carter CS, Altemus M. Integrative fuctions of lactational hormones in social behavior and stress management. *Ann New York Acad Sci.* 1997;807:164–175.
22. Center for Behavioral Health Statistics and Quality. *Results from the 2015 National Survey on Drug Use and Health: Detailed Tables Prevalence Estimates*; 2016.
23. Chapman AG, Riley K, Evans MC, Meldrum BS. Acute effects of sodium valproate and gamma-vinyl GABA on regional amino acid metabolism in the rat brain: incorporation of 2-[14C]glucose into amino acids. *Neurochem Res.* 1982;7:1089–1105.
24. Chen CY, Anthony JC. Possible age-associated bias in reporting of clinical features of drug dependence: epidemiological evidence on adolescent-onset marijuana use. *Addiction.* 2003;98:71–82.
25. Coffey C, et al. Cannabis dependence in young adults: an Australian population study. *Addiction.* 2002;97:187–194.
26. Comer SD, Collins ED, Fischman MW. Buprenorphine sublingual tablets: effects on IV heroin self-administration by humans. *Psychopharmacology (Berl).* 2001;154:28–37.
27. Cone EJ, Welch P, Robert Lange W. Clonidine partially blocks the physiologic effects but not the subjective effects produced by smoking marijuana in male human subjects. *Pharmacol Biochem Behav.* 1988;29:649–652.
28. Copeland J, Clement N, Swift W. Cannabis use, harms and the management of cannabis use disorder. *Neuropsychiatry (London).* 2014;4:55–63.
29. Cornelius JR, et al. Double-blind fluoxetine trial in comorbid MDD-CUD youth and young adults. *Drug Alcohol Depend.* 2010;112:39–45.
30. Cui SS, et al. Prevention of cannabinoid withdrawal syndrome by lithium: involvement of oxytocinergic neuronal activation. *J Neurosci.* 2001;21:9867–9876.
31. Dewey WL, Harris LS, Kennedy JS. Some pharmacological and toxicological effects of 1-trans-8 and 1-trans-9-tetrahydrocannabinol in laboratory rodents. *Arch Int Pharmacodyn Ther.* 1972;196:133–145.
32. Diana M, Melis M, Gessa GL. Increase in meso-prefrontal dopaminergic activity after stimulation of CB1 receptors by cannabinoids. *Eur J Neurosci.* 1998;10:2825–2830.
33. Donovan SJ, et al. Divalproex treatment for youth with explosive temper and mood lability: a double-blind, placebo-controlled crossover design. *Am J Psychiatry.* 2000;157:818–820.
34. Dworkin SI, Mirkis S, Smith JE. Response-dependent versus response-independent presentation of cocaine: differences in the lethal effects of the drug. *Psychopharmacology (Berl).* 1995;117:262–266.
35. Dwoskin LP, Rauhut AS, King-Pospisil KA, Bardo MT. Review of the pharmacology and clinical profile of bupropion, an antidepressant and tobacco use cessation agent. *CNS Drug Rev.* 2006;12:178–207.
36. Exner H, Schlicker E. Prostanoid receptors of the EP3 subtype mediate the inhibitory effect of prostaglandin E2 on noradrenaline

release in the mouse brain cortex. *Naunyn Schmiedebergs Arch Pharmacol.* 1995;351:46–52.

37. Fattore L, Fadda P, Spano MS, Pistis M, Fratta W. Neurobiological mechanisms of cannabinoid addiction. *Mol Cell Endocrinol.* 2008;286.

38. Fielding S, et al. A comparison of clonidine with morphine for antinociceptive and antiwithdrawal actions. *J Pharmacol Exp Ther.* 1978;207:899–905.

39. Gardner EL. Addictive potential of cannabinoids: the underlying neurobiology. *Chem Phys Lipids.* 2002;121:267–290.

40. Gates P, Copeland J. *Barriers to treatment seeking for cannabis dependence (chapter 105). Handbook of Cannabis and Related Pathologies.* Elsevier Inc.; 2017. https://doi.org/10.1016/B978-0-12-800756-3/00123-X.

41. Gerasimov MR, et al. Comparison between intraperitoneal and oral methylphenidate administration: a microdialysis and locomotor activity study. *J Pharmacol Exp Ther.* 2000;295:51–57.

42. Gold MS, Redmond DE, Kleber HD. Clonidine blocks acute apiate-withdrawal symptoms. *Lancet.* 1978:599–602.

43. Golub A, Johnson B, Dunlap E. Bongs and blunts: notes from a suburban marijuana subculture. *J Ethn Subst Abuse.* 2005;4:81–97.

44. Gorelick DA, Heishman SJ. Methods for clinical research involving cannabis administration. In: *Marijuana and Cannabinoid Research.* Humana Press; 2006:235–253. https://doi.org/10.1385/1-59259-999-0:235.

45. Gray KM, Hart CL, Christie DK, Upadhyaya HP. Tolerability and effects of oral Δ9-tetrahydrocannabinol in older adolescents with marijuana use disorders. *Pharmacol Biochem Behav.* 2008;91:67–70.

46. Gray KM, et al. A double-blind randomized controlled trial of N-acetylcysteine in cannabis-dependent adolescents. *Am J Psychiatry.* 2012;169:805–812.

47. Greenwald MK, Stitzer ML. Antinociceptive, subjective and behavioral effects of smoked marijuana in humans. *Drug Alcohol Depend.* 2000;59:261–275.

48. Hall W, Lynskey M. Long-term marijuana use and cognitive impairment in middle age. 2016; 6:2–3.

49. Haney M. Opioid antagonism of cannabinoid effects: differences between marijuana smokers and nonmarijuana smokers. *Neuropsychopharmacology.* 2007;32:1391–1403.

50. Haney M, Bisaga A, Foltin RW. Interaction between naltrexone and oral THC in heavy marijuana smokers. *Psychopharmacology (Berl).* 2003;166:77–85.

51. Haney M, Hart CL, Ward AS, Foltin RW. Nefazodone decreases anxiety during marijuana withdrawal in humans. *Psychopharmacology (Berl).* 2003;165:157–165.

52. Haney M, Spealman R. Controversies in translational research: drug self-administration. *Psychopharmacology (Berl).* 2008;199:403–419.

53. Haney M, Ward AS, Comer SD, Foltin RW, Fischman MW. Abstinence symptoms following oral THC administration to humans. *Psychopharmacology (Berl).* 1999;141:385–394.

54. Haney M, et al. Bupropion SR worsens mood during marijuana withdrawal in humans. *Psychopharmacology (Berl).* 2001;155:171–179.

55. Haney M, et al. Marijuana withdrawal in humans: effects of oral THC or divalproex. *Neuropsychopharmacology.* 2004;29:158–170.

56. Haney M, et al. Effects of THC and lofexidine in a human laboratory model of marijuana withdrawal and relapse. *Psychopharmacology (Berl).* 2008;197:157–168.

57. Harris RT, Waters W, McLendon D. Evaluation of reinforcing capability of delta-9-tetrahydrocannabinol in rhesus monkeys. *Psychopharmacologia.* 1974;37:23–29.

58. Hart C, et al. Comparison of smoked marijuana and oral Δ 9-tetrahydrocannabinol in humans. *Psychopharmacology (Berl).* 2002;164:407–415.

59. Hart CL. Increasing treatment options for cannabis dependence: a review of potential pharmacotherapies. *Drug Alcohol Depend.* 2005;80:147–159.

60. Hart CL, Haney M, Foltin RW, Fischman MW. Alternative reinforcers differentially modify cocaine self-administration by humans. *Behav Pharmacol.* 2000;11:87–91.

61. Hart CL, Haney M, Vosburg SK, Comer SD, Foltin RW. Reinforcing effects of oral Δ9-THC in male marijuana smokers in a laboratory choice procedure. *Psychopharmacology (Berl).* 2005;181:237–243.

62. Hart CL, Haney M, Ward AS, Fischman MW, Foltin RW. Effects of oral THC maintenance on smoked marijuana self-administration. *Drug Alcohol Depend.* 2002;67:301–309.

63. Hemby SE, Co C, Koves TR, Smith JE, Dworkin SI. Differences in extracellular dopamine concentrations in the nucleus accumbens during response-dependent and response-independent cocaine administration in the rat. *Psychopharmacology (Berl).* 1997;133:7–16.

64. Hiller K, Templeton WW. Regulation of noradrenaline overflow in rat cerebral cortex by prostaglandin E2. *Br J Pharmacol.* 1980;70:469–473.

65. Ma H, et al. Blockade of effects of smoked marijuana by the CB1-selective cannabinoid receptor antagonist SR141716. *Arch Gen Psychiatry.* 2001;58:322–328.

66. Huestis MA, et al. Single and multiple doses of rimonabant antagonize acute effects of smoked cannabis in male cannabis users. *Psychopharmacology (Berl).* 2007;194:505–515.

67. Justinova Z, Tanda G, Munzar P, Goldberg SR. The opioid antagonist naltrexone reduces the reinforcing effects of Δ9-tetrahydrocannabinol (THC) in squirrel monkeys. *Psychopharmacology (Berl).* 2004;173:186–194.

68. Justinova Z, Tanda G, Redhi GH, Goldberg SR. Self-administration of Δ9-tetrahydrocannabinol (THC) by drug naive squirrel monkeys. *Psychopharmacology (Berl).* 2003;169:135–140.

69. Justinova Z, et al. Blockade of THC-seeking behavior and relapse in monkeys by the cannabinoid CB1-receptor antagonist rimonabant. *Neuropsychopharmacology.* 2008;33:2870–2877.

70. Karila L, et al. New treatments for cocaine dependence: a focused review. *Int J Neuropsychopharmacol.* 2008;11:425–438.

71. Karler R, Turkanis SA. Subacute cannabinoid treatment: anticonvulsant activity and withdrawalexcitability in mice. *Br J Pharmacol.* 1980;68:479–484.

72. Kaymakçalan Ş, Ayhan IH, Tulunay FC. Naloxone-induced or postwithdrawal abstinence signs in Δ9-tetrahydrocannabinol-tolerant rats. *Psychopharmacology (Berl).* 1977;55:243–249.

73. King L. Understanding cannabis potency and monitoring cannabis products in Europe. EMCCDA Monographs. *A Cannabis Reader: Global Issues and Local Experiences.* Vol. 1. 2008.

74. Kosten TRO', Connor PG. Management of drug and alcohol withdrawal. *N Engl J Med.* 2003;348:1786–1795.

75. Kouri EM, Pope HG. Abstinence symptoms during withdrawal from chronic marijuana use. *Exp Clin Psychopharmacol.* 2000;8:483–492.

76. Kouri EM, Pope HG, Lukas SE. Changes in aggressive behavior during withdrawal from long-term marijuana use. *Psychopharmacology (Berl).* 1999;143:302–308.

77. Ksir C, Hart CL. Cannabis and psychosis: a critical overview of the relationship. *Curr Psychiatry Rep.* 2016;18:12.

78. Lai AA, Schroeder DH. Clinical pharmacokinetics of bupropion: a review. *J Clin Psychiatry.* 1983;44:82–84.

79. Levin FR, et al. Pharmacotherapy for marijuana dependence: a double-blind, placebo-controlled pilot study of divalproex sodium. *Am J Addict.* 2004;13:21–32.

80. Levin FR, et al. Dronabinol for the treatment of cannabis dependence: a randomized, double-blind, placebo-controlled trial. *Drug Alcohol Depend.* 2011;116:142–150.

81. Levin FR, et al. A randomized double-blind, placebo-controlled trial of venlafaxine-extended release for co-occurring cannabis

dependence and depressive disorders. *Addiction*. 2013;108:1084–1094.

82. Licata SC, Rowlett JK. Abuse and dependence liability of benzodiazepine-type drugs: GABAA receptor modulation and beyond. *Pharmacol Biochem Behav*. 2008;90:74–89.

83. Lichtman AH, Fisher J, Martin BR. Precipitated cannabinoid withdrawal is reversed by Δ9-tetrahydrocannabinol or clonidine. *Pharmacol Biochem Behav*. 2001;69:181–188.

84. Lopez-Quintero C, et al. Probability and predictors of transition from first use to dependence on nicotine, alcohol, cannabis, and cocaine: results of the National Epidemiologic Survey on Alcohol and Related Conditions (NESARC). *Drug Alcohol Depend*. 2011;115:120–130.

85. Mansback R, Nicholson BM, Balster R. Failure of delta9-tetrahydrocannabinol and CP 55,940 to maintain intravenous self-administration under a fixed-interval schedule in rhesus monkeys. *Behav Pharmacol*. 1994;5:219–225.

86. Manzanares J, et al. Pharmacological and biochemical interactions between opioids and cannabinoids. *Trends Pharmacol Sci*. 1999;20:287–294.

87. Marshall K, Gowing L, Ali R, BLF. Pharmacotherapies for cannabis dependence (Review). *Cochrane Database Syst Rev*. 2014. https://doi.org/10.1002/14651858.CD008940.pub2.   www.cochranelibrary.com.

88. Martellotta MC, Cossu G, Fattore L, Gessa GL, Fratta W. Self-administration of the cannabinoid receptor agonist WIN 55,212-2 in drug-naive mice. *Neuroscience*. 1998;85:327–330.

89. Mason BJ, et al. A proof-of-concept randomized controlled study of gabapentin: effects on cannabis use, withdrawal and executive function deficits in cannabis-dependent adults. *Neuropsychopharmacology*. 2012;37:1689–1698.

90. McLean MJ, Macdonald RL. Sodium valproate, but not ethosuximide, produes use- and voltage- dependent limitation of high frequency repetitive firing of action potentials of mouse central neurons in cell culture. *J Pharmacol Exp Ther*. 1986;237:1001–1011.

91. McRae AL, Brady KT, Carter RE. Buspirone for treatment of marijuana dependence: a pilot study. *Am J Addict*. 2006;15:404.

92. McRae-Clark AL, et al. A placebo-controlled trial of buspirone for the treatment of marijuana dependence. *Drug Alcohol Depend*. 2009;105:132–138.

93. McRae-Clark AL, et al. A placebo-controlled trial of atomoxetine in marijuana-dependent individuals with attention deficit hyperactivity disorder. *Am J Addict*. 2010;19:481–489.

94. Moore BA, Budney AJ. Relapse in outpatient treatment for marijuana dependence. *J Subst Abuse Treat*. 2003;25:85–89.

95. Navarro M, et al. CB 1 cannabinoid receptor antagonist-induced opiate withdrawal in morphine-dependent rats. *Neuropharmacology*. 1998;9:3397–3402.

96. Navarro M, et al. Functional interaction between opioid and cannabinoid receptors in drug self-administration. *J Neurosci*. 2001;21:5344–5350.

97. Neumann ID, Torner L, Wigger A. Brain oxytocin: differential inhibition of neuroendocrine stress responses and anxiety-related behaviour in virgin, pregnant and lactating rats. *Neuroscience*. 1999;95:567–575.

98. Neumann ID, Wigger A, Torner L, Holsboer F, Landgraf R. Brain oxytocin inhibits basal and stress-induced activity of the hypothalamo-pituitary-adrenal axis in male and female rats: partial action within the paraventricular nucleus. *J Neuroendocrinol*. 2000;12:235–243.

99. Parale MP, Kulkarni SK. Studies with alpha-adrenoceptor agonists and alcohol abstinence syndrome in rats. *Psychopharmacology (Berl)*. 1986;88:237–239.

100. Penetar DM, Looby AR, Ryan ET, Maywalt MA, Lukas SE. Bupropion reduces some of the symptoms of marihuana withdrawal in chronic marihuana users: a pilot study. *Subst Abus Res Treat*. 2012;6:63–71.

101. Pertwee RG. Pharmacology of cannabinoid CB1 and CB2 receptors. *Pharmacol Ther*. 1997;74:129–180.

102. Pertwee RG, Ross RA. Cannabinoid receptors and their ligands. *Prostaglandins Leukot Essent Fat Acids*. 2002;66:101–121.

103. Phillips NI, Fowler LJ. The effects of sodium valproate on γ-aminobutyrate metabolism and behaviour in naive and ethanolamine-O-sulphate pretreated rats and mice. *Biochem Pharmacol*. 1982;31:2257–2261.

104. Pletcher MJ, Safford M, Sidney S, Lin F, Kertesz S. Association between marijuana exposure and pulmonary function over 20 years. *JAMA*. 2012;307:173–181.

105. Pope HG, Gruber AJ, Hudson JI, Huestis MA, Yurgelun-Todd D. Cognitive measures in long-term cannabis users. *J Clin Pharmacol*. 2002;42:4–47.

106. Ream GL, Benoit E, Johnson BD, Dunlap E. Smoking tobacco along with marijuana increases symptoms of cannabis dependence. *Drug Alcohol Depend*. 2008;95:199–208.

107. Richelson E, Souder T. Binding of antipsychotic drugs to human brain receptors focus on newer generation compounds. *Life Sci*. 2000;68:29–39.

108. Rodriguez de Fonseca F. Activation of corticotropin-releasing factor in the limbic system during cannabinoid withdrawal. *Science*. 1997;276(80):2050–2054.

109. Sim LJ, Selley DE, Xiao R, Childers SR. Differences in G-protein activation by mu- and delta-opioid, and cannabinoid, receptors in rat striatum. *Eur J Pharmacol*. 1996;307(1):97–105.

110. Solinas M, et al. Nicotinic alpha 7 receptors as a new target for treatment of cannabis abuse. *J Neurosci*. 2007;27:5615–5620.

111. Solowij N. Cognitive Functioning of long-term heavy cannabis users seeking treatment. *J Am Med Assoc*. 2002;287:1123.

112. Stahl SM, et al. A Review of the neuropharmacology of bupropion, a dual norepinephrine and dopamine reuptake inhibitor. *Prim Care Companion J Clin Psychiatry*. 2004;6:159–166.

113. Stephens RS, Roffman RA, Simpson EE. Adult marijuana users seeking treatment. *J Consult Clin Psychol*. 1993;61:1100–1104.

114. Szabo B, Siemes S, Wallmichrath I. Inhibition of GABAergic neurotransmission in the ventral tegmental area by cannabinoids. *Eur J Neurosci*. 2002;15:2057–2061.

115. Tanda G. Cannabinoid heroin activation. of mesolimbic dopamine transmission by a common μ1 opioid receptor mechanism. *Science (80-.)*. 1997;276:2048–2050.

116. Tanda G, Goldberg SR. Cannabinoids: reward, dependence, and underlying neurochemical mechanisms—a review of recent preclinical data. *Psychopharmacology (Berl)*. 2003;169:115–134.

117. Tanda G, Loddo P, Di Chiara G. Dependence of mesolimbic dopamine transmission on delta9-tetrahydrocannabinol. *Eur J Pharmacol*. 1999;376:23–26.

118. Tanda G, Munzar P, Goldberg SR. Self-administration behavior is maintained by the psychoactive ingredient of marijuana in squirrel monkeys. *Nat Neurosci*. 2000;3:1073–1074.

119. Taylor DP, et al. Pharmacology and neurochemistry of nefazodone, a novel antidepressant drug. *J Clin Psychiatry*. 1995;56(suppl 6):3–11.

120. Tirado CF, Goldman M, Lynch K, Kampman KM, Obrien CP. Atomoxetine for treatment of marijuana dependence: a report on the efficacy and high incidence of gastrointestinal adverse events in a pilot study. *Drug Alcohol Depend*. 2008;94:254–257.

121. Touriño C, Maldonado R, Valverde O. MDMA attenuates THC withdrawal syndrome in mice. *Psychopharmacology (Berl)*. 2007;193:75–84.

122. Uhde TW, Redmond DE, Kleber HD. Clonidine suppresses the opioid abstinence syndrome without clonidine-withdrawal symptoms: a blind inpatient study. *Psychiatry Res*. 1980;2:37–47.

123. UNDOC. United Nations Office on Drugs and Crime. *World Drug Report 2017. Unodc*. 2017.

124. Uvnäs-Moberg K, Ahlenius S, Hillegaart V, Alster P. High doses of oxytocin cause sedation and low doses cause an anxiolytic-like

effect in male rats. *Pharmacol Biochem Behav*. 1994;49:101–106.

125. Uylings HBM. Development of the human cortex and the concept of 'critical' or 'sensitive' periods. *Lang Learn*. 2006;56:59–90.

126. Valjent E, Mitchell JM, Besson M-J, Caboche J, Maldonado R. Behavioural and biochemical evidence for interactions between Δ9-tetrahydrocannabinol and nicotine. *Br J Pharmacol*. 2002;135:564–578.

127. Vandrey RG, Budney AJ, Hughes JR, Liguori A. A within-subject comparison of withdrawal symptoms during abstinence from cannabis, tobacco, and both substances. *Drug Alcohol Depend*. 2008;92:48–54.

128. Verberne AJM, Taylor DA, Fennessy MR. Withdrawal-like behaviour induced by inhibitors of biogenic amine reuptake in rats chronic. *THC*. 1980;267:261–267.

129. Verberne AJM, Taylor DA, Fennessy MR. Attenuation of Δ9-tetrahydrocannabinol-induced withdrawal-like behavior by Δ9-tetrahydrocannabinol. *Psychopharmacology (Berl)*. 1981;73:97–98.

130. Volkow ND, et al. Effects of cannabis use on human behavior, including cognition, motivation, and psychosis: a review. *JAMA Psychiatry*. 2016;73:292.

131. Wachtel SR, de Wit H. Naltrexone does not block the subjective effects of oral Delta(9)-tetrahydrocannabinol in humans. *Drug Alcohol Depend*. 2000;59:251–260.

132. Wegener N, Koch M. Neurobiology and systems physiology of the endocannabinoid system. *Pharmacopsychiatry*. 2009;42(suppl 1):S79–S86.

133. Weinstein AM, et al. Treatment of cannabis dependence using escitalopram in combination with cognitive-behavior therapy: a double-blind placebo-controlled study. *Am J Drug Alcohol Abuse*. 2014;40:16–22.

134. Winstock A, Lea T, Copeland J. Lithium carbonate in the management of cannabis withdrawal in humans: an open-label study. *J Psychopharmacol*. 2009;23:84–93.

135. Woods JH, Katz JL, Winger G. Benzodiazepines: use, consequences. *Pharmacol Rev*. 1992;44:151–271.

136. Zajecka JM. The effect of nefazodone on comorbid anxiety symptoms associated with depression: experience in family practice and psychiatric outpatient settings. *J Clin Psychiatry*. 1996;57(suppl 2):10–14.

57

Hallucinogens

JOHN H. HALPERN, JOJI SUZUKI, PEDRO E. HUERTAS, AND TORSTEN PASSIE

Historical Perspectives

Psychoactive substances derived from botanicals have been used ritualistically used for millennia.[64,74] Developments during the second half of the 20th century in neuroscience and in synthetic organic chemistry recast natural and synthetic intoxicants into a new biological and clinical light.[53] These chemicals, referred to improperly as "hallucinogens," alter psychoneurobiological behavior in ways both subtle and overt. The term "hallucinogen" suggests the induction of hallucinations, a symptom of psychosis well-known within clinical psychiatry, but this is not the case with most hallucinogens and some closely related substances (i.e., entactogens such as 3,4-methylenedioxymethamphetamine), which do not induce major sensory alterations. The terms "psychotomimetics" (psychosis-mimicking) and "psychedelics" have also been used. Psychotomimetic appears only rarely in the scientific literature, since, much like with hallucinogen, these substances are not primarily psychotogenic, whether mimicking or otherwise, although hallucinogens can exacerbate or contribute to worsening the mental health of those vulnerable to a formal thought disorder. The term "psychedelic," first offered by the psychiatrist Humphrey Osmond,[57] may be the most commonly used lay term for hallucinogens, and it used to be an accepted alternate descriptor in the scientific literature.

Albert Hofmann first synthesized lysergic acid diethylamide in 1938 and accidentally ingested it in 1943. Publishing on these findings heralded much research in the 1950s, when hallucinogens became the focus of intense interest in psychiatric research and stimulated the discovery of the neurotransmitter systems and their functions in the brain.[39]

More than 10,000 subjects received lysergic acid diethylamide (and other hallucinogens) in controlled research settings in studies published from 1951 to the late 1960s, resulting in more than 1000 clinical papers, dozens of books, and six international conferences on their use as aids in psychotherapy.[12,25,51,58]

A number of substances have been categorized as hallucinogens or hallucinogen-like: (1) the classical hallucinogens (e.g., mescaline, psilocybin, lysergic acid diethylamide, and dimethyltryptamine), (2) the entactogenic phenethylamines (3,4-methylenedioxyamphetamine, 3,4-methylenedioxymethamphetamine, 3,4-methylenedioxyethylamphetamine, and methylbenzodioxolylbutanamine), (3) the anticholinergic delirants (atropine, hyoscyamine, and scopolamine), and (4) dissociative anesthetics/miscellaneous (N_2O, ketamine, phencyclidine, and salvinorin A). This chapter focuses on the more commonly used classical and entactogenic hallucinogens, but will mention the other substances where appropriate or necessary.

Epidemiology

The Substance Abuse and Mental Health Services Administration's (SAMHSA's) National Survey on Drug Use and Health estimated that among Americans 12 years of age or older in 2006, close to 4 million used hallucinogens that year, with 1.1 million trying one for the first time ever, and some 35.3 million Americans have tried one at least once in their lifetime.[62] Of a total of 23.6 million persons classified with any substance abuse or dependence in 2006, 380,000 Americans 12 years of age or older were estimated to meet *Diagnostic and Statistical Manual of Mental Disorders, Fourth Edition* (DSM-IV) criteria for hallucinogen abuse or dependence.[62] SAMHSA's Warning Network data estimated that 16,408 emergency room visits for the entire United States in 2005 involved a hallucinogen (not including phencyclidine: 7535), with 10,752 for the entactogen 3,4-methylenedioxymethamphetamine and fewer than 1900 for the classical hallucinogen lysergic acid diethylamide (of a total of 1.45 million drug-related visits).[61]

Among high school students, the Monitoring the Future data have shown a continuous decline since the late 1990s in the lifetime, annual, and past-month use of hallucinogens.[44] In 2006, 8.3% of 12th graders in the United States reported lifetime use of hallucinogens, a drop from 15.1% in 1997.[44]

Taken together, these numbers indicate that the prevalence of hallucinogen use still is lower compared with other substances of abuse in the United States and is significantly lower in morbidity and mortality. The prevalence of the various hallucinogen-related disorders is not known.

Basic Pharmacology

Table 57.1 lists some of the more commonly known hallucinogens. As shown by the table, the various hallucinogens are wide-ranging

TABLE 57.1 The Common Hallucinogens (Partial List)

Class	Chemical Name	Common or Street Name	Source	Dosage	Route	Duration of Action	Major Neurobiological Target	Notes
Indolealkylamines	Lysergic acid diethylamide	LSD, Acid, Blotter	Synthesis	50–200 µg	By mouth	8–14 h	5-HT$_{2A}$ partial agonist	Distributed on small squares of blotting paper, drops of liquid, gel-caps, small pills
	Psilocybin	Magic mushrooms, Shrooms,	Psilocybe cubensis, Psilocybe azurescens, and many other subspecies, Synthesis	10–50 mg, 1–5 g dried mushroom; quite variable	By mouth	4–8 h	5-HT$_{2A}$ partial agonist	Psilocybin is converted in the body to psilocin, the actual active hallucinogen. Continued shamanic use in Mexico. Bruising of mushroom turns blue.
	Dimethyltryptamine	DMT, Yopo, Cohoba	Psychotria viridis, Anadenanthera peregrina, Mimosa hostilis, and many other natural sources, Synthesis	5–40 mg	Smoked, inhaled snuff	30–60 min	5-HT$_{2A}$ partial agonist	Continued Amazonian shamanic use
	Dimethyltryptamine + monoamine oxidase inhibitors (harmala betacarbolines)	Ayahuasca, yajé, Hoasca, Daime, "vine of the soul"	Psychotria viridis (dimethyltryptamine) + Banisteropsis caapi (monoamine oxidase inhibitor)	Variable	By mouth	2–4 h	5-HT$_{2A}$ partial agonist	Brewed as a tea; religious sacrament
	Ibogaine	Ibogaine	Tabernathe iboga	200–300 mg	By mouth	12+ h	Likely 5-HT$_{2A}$ partial agonist	Religious sacrament; long-acting metabolites may contribute to purported anti-opiate withdrawal benefits.
Phenyl-alkyl-amines	3,4,5-trimethoxyphenylethylamine	Mescaline, Peyote, San Pedro	Lophophora williamsii, Echinopsis panachoi, other cacti, Synthesis	200–500 mg, 10–20 g or 5–10 dried peyote buttons, 1 kg fresh E. pachanoi	By mouth	6–12 h	5-HT$_{2A}$ partial agonist	Religious sacrament
Entactogenic phenylalkylamine	3,4-methylenedioxymethamphetamine	MDMA, Ecstasy, X, XTC, Rolls, Molly	Synthesis	80–150 mg	By mouth	4–6 h	Serotonin release and depletion	Mildly hallucinogenic at high doses
	3,4-methylenedioxyamphetamine	MDA, Love drug, Adam	Synthesis	75–160 mg	By mouth	4–8 h	Serotonin release and depletion	
	4-bromo-2,5-dimethoxy-phenethylamine	2C-B, Nexus	Synthesis	5–30 mg	By mouth	4–8 h	Unknown	
	4-chloro-2,5-dimethoxy-amphetamine	DOC	Synthesis	1–5 mg	By mouth	4–8 h	Unknown	Has been found on blotting paper
	4-methyl-2,5-dimethoxy-amphetamine	DOM, STP	Synthesis	1–10 mg	By mouth	14–20 h	Unknown	Higher doses used in the 1960s resulted in many ER visits then.

Continued

TABLE 57.1　The Common Hallucinogens (Partial List)—cont'd

Class	Chemical Name	Common or Street Name	Source	Dosage	Route	Duration of Action	Major Neurobiological Target	Notes
Dissociative	Ketamine	Ketamine, Special K, Vitamin K, K hole,	Synthesis	25–50 mg (intramuscularly), 50–100 mg (by mouth or snorted)	Intramuscularly, by mouth, snorted	1–2 h (intramuscularly), 1–4 h (by mouth)	N-methyl-D-aspartate antagonist	Sub-anesthetic dose: lost sense of time, space, verbal skills, balance, drooling
	Dextromethorphan	DXM, Robo, DM	Synthesis	100–600 mg	By mouth	4–8 h	N-methyl-D-aspartate antagonist	
	Phencyclidine	PCP, Angel dust	Synthesis	3–10 mg	By mouth	8–24 h	N-methyl-D-aspartate antagonist	
Other	Salvinorin A	Salvia, Sally D, Diviner's sage	Salvia divinorum	250–750 mg (smoked), 2–10 g dried leaves (by mouth)	Smoked, by mouth	30–60 min (smoked), 1–3 h (by mouth)	Kappa-opioid selective agonist	Atypical hallucinogen; no longer found in the wild
	Scopolamine and atropine	Datura, Jimson weed, loco weed, Thorn apple, Angel's trumpet, belladonna, deadly nightshade	Datura stramonium, Atropa belladonna, many related species	Highly variable	By mouth	12–48 h	Competitive muscarinic acetylcholine antagonist	Plants of the Solanaceae family contain various ratios of scopolamine to atropine; blurred vision
	Muscimol (5-(aminomethyl)-3-isoxazolol)	Fly agaric, Amanita	Amanita muscaria, Amanita pantherine	1–30 g dried mushrooms	By mouth	5–10 h	Gamma-aminobutyric acid-A agonist glutamate	Shamanic use in eastern Siberia; over 600 species of agarics—easy to misidentify. Some are extremely poisonous, such as "death cap" A. phalloides; mushrooms also contain ibotenic acid—as it dries/ages, decarboxylation of ibotenic acid creates muscimol.

in dosage and duration. In general, hallucinogens exert their effects by sympathomimetic actions on the central nervous system. This activation may be due to agonist properties on different neurotransmitter-modulated brain systems that are adrenergic, dopaminergic, and, perhaps most importantly, serotonergic. The brain contains approximately 40,000 serotonergic neurons, mainly located in the dorsal raphe nucleus of the mid-brain. This tiny population of neurons maintains a widely distributed network throughout the brain, which modulates nearly every kind of brain activity.

Despite heterogeneity, most classical hallucinogens appear to exert pharmacologic action through agonist effects on 5-HT$_{2A}$/c receptors.[53] Hallucinogens have high affinity for serotonin receptors,[22,28] and genetic or pharmacologic inactivation of 5-HT$_{2A}$ receptors blocks behavioral effects in preclinical models as well as subjective effects in humans.[10,22,23,73] Rapid tolerance develops due to receptor downregulation, and repeated administration leads to markedly diminished effects within several days.[53]

It remains unclear as to whether a specific pattern of alterations of brain functioning is involved in the psychoactive effects of hallucinogens. Neurometabolic studies to date point to activation of the frontal cortex, limbic/paralimbic structures, and the right hemisphere.[24,45,60,72]

Entactogenic substances, such as 3,4-methylenedioxyamphetamine and 3,4-methylenedioxymethamphetamine, differ from classic hallucinogens by inducing a marked release of serotonin from serotonin-containing neurons and (to a lesser extent) dopamine release from dopamine-containing neurons.[71] Their neurometabolic actions show minor deactivation of cortical regions and limbic activation[24] as well as deactivation of the left amygdala.[20] The latter may be responsible for their most prominent effect: the decrease of emotional tension and anxiety.

Psychological and Biological Effects

Intoxication with hallucinogens, commonly referred to as "tripping," may induce some physiological effects that are quite subtle to observation and a wide variety of behavioral, emotional, and cognitive effects (Table 57.2).[29,42] The visual images experienced are usually not true hallucinations but rather illusions, such as the perception of geometric patterns or scenic dream-like visions appearing before closed eyes, perception of movement in stationary objects, and synesthesias. The content of visual and most emotional phenomena most often reflects the psychodynamics of the user.[47,49] Colors may appear intensified, and humans (self and others) and animals may be viewed as altered or exaggerated directly or in mirrored reflection.[70] Hallucinogens amplify affectivity and may cause significant changes of mood, with possible rapid changes from euphoria to depression or anxiety or vice versa.[68] In extreme cases, especially with higher order overdoses, psychotic-like reactions may be experienced. In short, the psychological effects of hallucinogens are highly variable and strongly influenced by the individual's psychological state at the time of ingestion (mind-set) as well as the social and physical setting.[43]

Toxicity of lysergic acid diethylamide, psilocybin, and other classical hallucinogens is very low. Overdosing leads to psychological complications to psychological crises or (rarely) psychotic symptoms. However, no case of lethal overdose is known, and there is no evidence of toxicity beyond the acute state of intoxication.[33] A recent review of the harmful consequences of drugs of abuse found that the classical (and the most used, by far) hallucinogen lysergic acid diethylamide is near the bottom in a ranking of risk to users and society.[54]

TABLE 57.2	Hallucinogen[a] Physical and Psychological Effects
INTOXICATION MAY INCLUDE A CLUSTER OF THE FOLLOWING	
Physical Effects[b]	Psychological Effects
Regular (mild to very mild): • Tachycardia • Palpitations • Hypertension or hypotension • Diaphoresis • Hyperthermia • Motor incoordination • Tremors, hyperreflexia • Altered neuroendocrine functioning Regular (mild to strong): • Mydriasis • Arousal • Insomnia Occasional: • Nausea, vomiting, diarrhea • Blurred vision • Nystagmus • Piloerection • Salivation	• Intensification and/or lability of affectivity with euphoria, anxiety, depression, and/or cathartic expressions • Dream-like state • Sensory activation with illusions, pseudo-hallucinations, hallucinations,[c] synesthesias • Altered experience of time and space • Altered body image • Increased suggestibility • Acute neuropsychological/cognitive impairments with loosening of associations, inability for goal-directed thinking, memory disturbances • Paranoid/suicidal ideation • Impaired judgment • Megalomania, impulsivity, odd behavior • Lassitude, indifference, detachment • Psychosomatic complaints • Derealization, depersonalization • Mystical experiences • Sense of profound discovery/healing

[a]Indolealkylamine and phenylalkylamine hallucinogens only (see Table 57.1)

[b]Some effects are reactionary to psychological content (e.g., increased heart rate and nausea due to anxiety), and complaints can be dependent on factors such as mindset, setting, dose, and supervision. Intoxicated individuals may also deny physical impairment and/or claim increased energy, sharpened mental acuity, and improved sensory perception

[c]A subject experiencing "pseudo-hallucinations" retains the capacity to recognize that these perceptions are transient and drug induced, as opposed to true hallucinations in which no such discernment from reality is possible

Hallucinogen Use Disorders

Hallucinogen abuse and hallucinogen dependence are organized in the DSM-IV much like most other listed substance use disorders. Both are characterized by patterns of compulsive and repeated drug use despite the knowledge of significant harm caused by this use. Hallucinogen use only almost never leads to the development of classic dependence syndromes as seen with opiates or alcohol.[55] By far the most typical pattern is for users to experiment with a few doses of a hallucinogen and then discontinue further use.[38] Users do not experience withdrawal symptoms as seen with other substances of abuse, so this symptom is not a criterion in diagnosing hallucinogen dependence. Note that tolerance rapidly increases, in general, when hallucinogens are used with frequency, which strongly limits their use on a regular basis.

Hallucinogen-Induced Disorders

The DSM-IV allows for the diagnosis of numerous substance-induced disorders. Specific to hallucinogens are hallucinogen

Diagnostic and Statistical Manual of Mental Disorders, Fourth Edition, Text Revision, Criteria (292.89): Hallucinogen Intoxication

A. Recent use of hallucinogen
B. Clinically significant maladaptive behavior or psychological changes (e.g., marked anxiety or depression, ideas of reference, fear of losing one's mind, paranoid ideation, impaired judgment, or impaired social or occupational function) that developed during or shortly after, hallucinogen use.
C. Perceptual changes occurring in a state of full wakefulness and alertness (e.g., subjective intensification of perceptions, depersonalization, derealization, illusions, hallucinations, synesthesias) that developed during, or shortly after, hallucinogen use.
D. Two (or more) of the following signs, developing during, or shortly after, hallucinogen use:
   1. Pupillary dilatation
   2. Tachycardia
   3. Sweating
   4. Palpitations
   5. Blurring vision
   6. Tremors
   7. Incoordination
E. The symptoms are not due to a general medical condition or are not better accounted for by another mental disorder.

Reprinted with permission from the *Diagnostic and Statistical Manual of Mental Disorders, Fourth Edition, Text Revision*, 2000, American Psychiatric Association.

intoxication, hallucinogen persisting perception disorder, and hallucinogen-induced psychotic, mood, anxiety, delirium, or "not otherwise specified" disorder. These disorders arise in the context of substance use and may manifest during intoxication, during withdrawal, or long after the drug has been ingested and the acute effects have subsided.[5] The diagnosis of a hallucinogen-induced psychotic, mood, anxiety, or delirium disorder is made only if the symptoms are in excess of what is expected from intoxication or withdrawal.[5]

Assessment and Treatment

Hallucinogen Intoxication

The *Diagnostic and Statistical Manual of Mental Disorders*, Fourth Edition, Text Revision (DSM-IV-TR) criteria for hallucinogen intoxication are presented in Table 57.3.

Assessment

An individual will most often present for treatment because he or she is experiencing an acute panic and/or depressive reaction (sometimes combined with temporary delusional ideation), commonly referred to as a "bad trip." Symptoms begin any time after the onset of effects and may include marked anxiety or fears of going insane.[19,66] Paranoid ideation, feelings of being manipulated, or feelings of being in a situation without any escape may also occur. Hallucinogen intoxication should be suspected when a patient or his or her friends report recent ingestion of a hallucinogen and the patient presents with a characteristic constellation of sympathomimetic findings with a clear sensorium. Because laboratory testing is generally not available in most acute settings, obtaining an accurate history and clinical examination is critical in establishing this diagnosis, and because illicit drugs often contain various substances, the actual identity of the offending substance ingested may

not be known. However, hallucinogens in general produce similar effects, which should be carefully assessed. Signs and symptoms of hallucinogen intoxication are reviewed in the previous section (see Table 57.2). Physical examination will also provide important clues that can help support the diagnosis of hallucinogen intoxication (in particular, widely dilated pupils that do not rapidly/tightly constrict to accommodate bright light). Although duration of action can vary considerably among hallucinogens, the acute reaction typically lasts less than 12–24 hours; persisting reactions will require further investigation to rule out other etiologies.

Differential Diagnosis

Because polysubstance ingestion is common, history should be sought on whether other substances were also recently consumed. Urine toxicology should also be performed, but tests for specific hallucinogens are specially ordered and results typically will not be available for a few days. Anticholinergic intoxication should be considered in individuals with a suggestive history (i.e., ingestion of jimson weed, or Datura) and findings of hyperthermia, delirium, dry mouth, urinary retention, headache, and blurred vision. Delirium due to alcohol, sedative, or hypnotic withdrawal will present not only with sympathomimetic findings, but also with confusion; seizures; tremors; and visual, auditory, or tactile hallucinations. Stimulant psychosis, a psychosis in the setting of a clear sensorium induced by chronic stimulant abuse, presents with paranoid delusions and visual or auditory hallucinations, and the stimulant abuser may report compulsive fascination with and performance of complex, stereotyped repetitive behaviors known as "punding."[17] Phencyclidine, ketamine, or dextromethorphan intoxication may present similarly to hallucinogen intoxication, but differentiates with additional symptoms, including ataxia, horizontal nystagmus, rage, erythema, amnesia, and dry skin.[8,21] Dextromethorphan intoxication will also produce a distinctive, plodding "zombie-like" gait abnormality.[9] In addition, phencyclidine overdose can prolong the toxic effects to 3 days owing to its long half-life.[3]

If mood, anxiety, and psychotic symptoms warrant clinical evaluation, then hallucinogen-induced mood, anxiety, or psychotic disorder, respectively, should be considered. Psychiatric diagnoses, including affective psychoses, schizophrenia, anxiety, and dissociative disorders, also can present with varying degrees of acute dysphoria, depersonalization, and hallucinations. Medical causes of perceptual disturbances and mental status change should be ruled out, including adverse medication reaction, metabolic disturbance, infection, dementia, stroke, seizure, central nervous system tumor, and Charles Bonnet syndrome. Collection of a careful history and physical, collateral information from family and friends, where appropriate, as well as laboratory data, will be needed for narrowing to the correct working diagnoses.

Treatment

The "talk down" (more accurately the "talk through") is usually the only intervention indicated in these situations.[69] Recommendations include placing the patient in a low-stimulus environment—that is, a quiet space with dimmed lights and minimal distractions—and providing emotional support. Arrange for a reliable sitter (a nonintoxicated family member or friend) to remain with and attend to the patient. The sitter can help keep him or her calm and oriented by providing a sympathetic presence. In addition, provide reassurance to the patient that the experience is generally nonhazardous, drug-induced, and time-limited and will resolve with full recovery. The patient should not be left alone until the effects of the drug wear off.[68]

Hallucinogens rapidly absorb in the gastrointestinal tract. Therefore, unless ingestion occurred within 30 minutes of presentation, gastric lavage is unlikely to remove additional undigested drug. The patient's mental state will invariably worsen if gastric lavage is forcefully attempted; therefore, it should be avoided.

If severe agitation does not respond to redirection and if concerns of safety remain for the patient and/or others, benzodiazepines are quite effective in reducing anxiety and panic.[3] Many authorities recommend diazepam or lorazepam as drugs of choice, by mouth if possible, but intramuscular and intravenous administrations are more effective.[15] In any case, avoid physical restraints, if possible, and limit the use of neuroleptics, since paradoxical effects have been reported with chlorpromazine,[66] and hallucinogen persisting perception disorder symptoms have been reported to worsen after receiving phenothiazines[1,65] and 5-HT$_{2A}$ antagonists such as risperidone.[2,56] Haloperidol may be considered in rare cases of severely agitated patients who require further acute interventions after benzodiazepines have not proven to be sufficient. Great caution must be exercised, however, because neuroleptics lower the seizure threshold and may also induce hypotension.[68]

Once acute symptoms subside, patients usually are able to return home accompanied by a family member or friend.[66] It is important to advise patients that subsequent ingestion of hallucinogens may precipitate similar reactions and (especially after bad trips) the risk for uncontrolled reexperience ("flashback") of some element(s) of the altered state is heightened. These flashbacks usually last for seconds, but may last longer if an actual hallucinogen (or cannabis) is re-ingested (see subsequent text). If symptoms persist for longer than 24 hours or there are accompanying severe mood or psychotic symptoms that warrant further clinical attention, hospitalization may be appropriate.[67]

Hallucinogen Abuse and Dependence
The DSM-IV-TR criteria for hallucinogen abuse are presented in Table 57.4.

Assessment
For hallucinogen abuse and dependence, evaluation and treatment should proceed in a manner similar to that for patients diagnosed with hallucinogen intoxication. Hallucinogen abuse should be diagnosed when individuals report using hallucinogens despite evidence and knowledge of related harm. Hallucinogen dependence should be considered when the pattern of use appears to be out of control, such as when using larger amounts than intended or when there is an inability to cut down on the frequency of use.[5]

Overall rates of abuse and dependence are estimated to be low compared with other substances.[44,75] In clinical settings, individuals often present as polydrug users; therefore a complete history is always needed to assess for other drug use.

Differential Diagnosis
With polydrug use being common, a differential diagnosis must always list other substance use or substance-induced disorders. In addition, a significant portion of illicit drugs sold as lysergic acid diethylamide (or some other hallucinogen) may contain other substances such as amphetamines or phencyclidine.[68] Therefore, diagnosis of amphetamine or phencyclidine abuse and dependence should be included for consideration and further data gathering. Alcohol is likely the drug that is most commonly abused comorbidly, and this should be assessed especially carefully in this population.[16] Schizophrenia, schizophreniform disorder, bipolar disorder, and schizoaffective disorder should be ruled out in these individuals

TABLE 57.4 *Diagnostic and Statistical Manual of Mental Disorders,* **Fourth Edition, Text Revision, Criteria (305.30): Hallucinogen Abuse**

A. A maladaptive pattern of hallucinogen use leading to clinically significant impairment or distress, as manifested by one (or more) of the following, occurring within a 12-month period:
 1. Recurrent hallucinogen use resulting in a failure to fulfill major role obligations at work, school, or home (e.g., repeated absences or poor work performance related to the substance use; substance-related absences, suspensions, or expulsions from school; neglect of children or household)
 2. Recurrent hallucinogen use in situations in which it is physically hazardous
 3. Recurrent hallucinogen-related legal problems
 4. Continued hallucinogen use despite having persistent or recurrent social or interpersonal problems caused or exacerbated by the effects of the substance
B. The symptoms have never met the criteria for Substance Dependence for this class of substance.

Reprinted with permission from the *Diagnostic and Statistical Manual of Mental Disorders,* Fourth Edition, Text Revision, Copyright 2000, American Psychiatric Association.

by assessing the longitudinal course of the constellation of symptoms and their temporal relation to hallucinogen ingestion.

Treatment
General principles of substance abuse and dependence treatment apply to treating these individuals.[16] Motivational interviewing, detoxification, relapse prevention, intensive outpatient counseling, and family therapies are examples of interventions that may be individualized to the person presenting. Treatment should target all other substance abuse and dependence, irrespective of whether they are thought to be contributing to the presenting disturbances. Moreover, treatment should be provided with a dual diagnosis approach, such that any underlying psychiatric disorder(s) will receive concurrent attention. No controlled trials have been conducted to evaluate the efficacy of pharmacotherapies.

Hallucinogen Persisting Perception Disorder
The DSM-IV-TR criteria for hallucinogen persisting perception disorder (i.e., flashbacks) are presented in Table 57.5.

Assessment
Diagnosis of hallucinogen persisting perception disorder requires differentiation into two kinds of phenomena. The 10th revision of the *International Statistical Classification of Diseases and Related Health Problems* (ICD-10), describes symptoms as the reemergence of fragments, scenarios, and/or altered states of consciousness and mood that are similar to those experienced during the hallucinogen intoxication. This implies a reexperience (flashback) of the initial intoxication. These flashbacks, as they are often nonspecifically called, may (in some rare cases) occur intermittently over weeks, months, or years after the hallucinogen intoxication. Some people intentionally try to induce these reexperiences (with specific music/surroundings), describing them as "free trips." Flashback episodes are short-lived (usually seconds) but may extend longer with additional cannabis intoxication. There is no documented case in the literature of a flashback leading to real danger or suicide.[41]

TABLE 57.5	*Diagnostic and Statistical Manual of Mental Disorders*, Fourth Edition, Text Revision, Criteria (292.89): Hallucinogen Persisting Perception Disorder (Flashbacks)

A. The re-experiencing, following cessation of use of a hallucinogen, of one or more of the perceptual symptoms that were experienced while intoxicated with the hallucinogen (e.g., geometric hallucinations, false perception of movement in the peripheral visual fields, flashes of color, intensified colors, trails of images of moving objects, positive afterimages, halos around objects, macropsia, and micropsia).

B. The symptoms in Criterion A cause clinically significant distress or impairment in social, occupational, or other important areas of functioning.

C. The symptoms are not due to a general medical condition (e.g., anatomical lesions and infections of the brain, visual epilepsies) and are not better accounted for by another mental disorder (e.g., delirium, dementia, schizophrenia) or hypnopompic hallucinations.

Reprinted with permission from the *Diagnostic and Statistical Manual of Mental Disorders*, Fourth Edition, Text Revision, Copyright 2000, American Psychiatric Association.

Different from flashback phenomena is the hallucinogen persisting perception disorder phenomena as described by Abraham[1] and specified in the DSM-IV. They are nearly all visual in nature (including flashes of color, geometric images, and afterimages of moving objects, or "trails"),[16] and appear to be continuous phenomena starting in the days to weeks after hallucinogen consumption. Hallucinogen persisting perception disorder is a rare disorder that may afflict individuals who, in particular, report anomalous visual disturbances (such as "floaters" or episodes of micropsia/macropsia) premorbid to hallucinogen exposure and who did eventually try lysergic acid diethylamide.[16] One web-based survey of purported hallucinogen users estimated hallucinogen persisting perception disorder prevalence at 0.17%–4.1% of users.[6]

The DSM-IV diagnostic criteria require that the individual not be intoxicated with other substances.[34] As such, urine toxicology screens should be performed routinely.

Differential Diagnosis

Hallucinogen-induced psychotic disorder should be considered in patients experiencing significant psychotic symptoms shortly after their use of hallucinogens, but it is important to note that the DSM-IV does not list a diagnosis for hallucinogen-induced *persistent* psychotic symptoms. However, very rare cases of a prolonged post-lysergic acid diethylamide psychosis have been reported but also, tellingly, have been more likely in patients with schizophrenia.[66] Psychotic disorders, including schizophrenia and bipolar disorder, should be ruled out by careful psychiatric examination and review of history. Medical causes of intermittent perceptual disturbances should also be considered, including adverse medication reaction, metabolic disturbance, migraine, temporal lobe epilepsy, ocular disease, stroke, or primary or secondary cancer of the central nervous system.

Treatment

Simple reassurance that symptoms do not reflect brain damage, and that the complained-about symptoms typically resolve over additional time, can prove tremendously effective in an anxious patient with hallucinogen persisting perception disorder. A variety

of treatments have been reported in several case series to ameliorate symptoms as well as the distress associated with hallucinogen persisting perception disorder, including the use of benzodiazepines, clonidine, haloperidol, olanzapine, carbamazepine, psychotherapy, behavior modifications, and sunglasses.[34] Some case reports note worsening hallucinogen persisting perception disorder symptoms after trials of risperidone,[2] phenothiazines,[1] and selective serotonin reuptake inhibitors.[37] Clearly, avoiding further hallucinogen use is recommended. In addition, other substances, particularly cannabis, may also trigger hallucinogen persisting perception disorder symptoms. Avoiding triggering drugs (e.g., cannabis) is an important element of treatment. Those providing treatment should consider the need for symptom relief while also remaining vigilant for benzodiazepine abuse and dependence (when such drugs are chosen for pharmacological intervention), as polysubstance abuse and dependence is common in this patient population.[16]

Hallucinogen-Induced Psychotic Disorder

The DSM-IV-TR criteria for substance-induced psychotic disorder are presented in Table 57.6.

Assessment

Hallucinogen-induced psychotic disorder is considered in individuals with recent ingestion of a hallucinogen who also present with marked psychotic symptoms and who are often lacking insight that their symptoms are related to this hallucinogen use. Although this reaction may be a more severe form of the bad trip, the diagnosis is made in the setting where a patient's psychotic symptoms are more severe than what would be expected to extend from hallucinogen intoxication. The DSM-IV lists modifiers to indicate whether hallucinations or delusions are prominent features.[5] Hallucinogen-related psychotic reactions usually end once the effects of the drug wear off.

Differential Diagnosis

Differential diagnosis includes diagnoses considered for any acute psychosis. Because toxicology screens do not routinely test for hallucinogens, obtaining a thorough history and physical examination is critical. Collateral information from families and friends will aid in narrowing the possible diagnoses. As is stressed several times earlier in this chapter, evaluation must include a careful review of the use of other substances of abuse and their frequency of ingestion, including information gained from sources other than the patient. Formal thought disorders and affective psychoses should be considered, with relevant historical information sought to help rule in or out a primary psychiatric illness for the presenting condition. Any evidence for delirium needs careful continued evaluation and management, including infection, adverse medication reaction, metabolic disturbance, central nervous system tumor, stroke, and head injury. Finally, diagnosis should be distinguished from hallucinogen persisting perception disorder, which represents a reexperiencing of the perceptual disturbances of past hallucinogen intoxication (see preceding text).

Treatment

Procedures for the treatment of recent hallucinogen intoxication should be followed as described earlier, and underlying etiologies for psychosis should be further investigated. In rare occurrences, the patient may require hospitalization, because the prolonged reaction can persist for days.

TABLE 57.6 *Diagnostic and Statistical Manual of Mental Disorders,* **Fourth Edition, Text Revision, Criteria: Substance-Induced Psychotic Disorder.**

A. Prominent hallucinations or delusions (Note: Do not include hallucinations if the person has insight that they are substance induced.)

B. There is evidence from the history, physical examination, or laboratory findings of either (1) or (2):
  1. The symptoms in Criterion A developed during or within a month of substance intoxication or withdrawal
  2. Substance use is etiologically related to the disturbance

C. The disturbance is not better accounted for by a psychotic disorder that is not substance induced. Evidence that the symptoms are better accounted for by a psychotic disorder that is not substance induced might include the following: the symptoms precede the onset of the substance use (or medication use); the symptoms persist for a substantial period of time (e.g., about a month) after the cessation of acute withdrawal or severe intoxication or are substantially in excess of what would be expected given the type or amount of the substance used or the duration of use; or there is other evidence that suggests the existence of an independent non-substance-induced psychotic disorder (e.g., a history of recurrent non-substance-related episodes).

D. The disturbance does not occur exclusively during the course of delirium.

Note: This diagnosis should be made instead of a diagnosis of substance intoxication or substance withdrawal only when the symptoms are in excess of those usually associated with the intoxication or withdrawal syndrome and when the symptoms are sufficiently severe to warrant independent clinical attention.

Code specific substance-induced psychotic disorder:
- 292.11: amphetamine (or amphetamine-like substance), with delusions
- 292.12: amphetamine (or amphetamine-like substance), with hallucinations
- 292.11: hallucinogen, with delusions
- 292.12: hallucinogen, with hallucinations

Specify:
- With onset during intoxication: if criteria are met for intoxication with the substance and the symptoms develop during the intoxication syndrome.
- With onset during withdrawal: if criteria are met for withdrawal from the substance and the symptoms develop during, or shortly after, a withdrawal syndrome.

(Reprinted with permission from the *Diagnostic and Statistical Manual of Mental Disorders,* Fourth Edition, Text Revision, 2000, American Psychiatric Association.)

Hallucinogens as Treatment Tools for Addiction?

Past research has indicated a use for lysergic acid diethylamide in the treatment of alcoholism and drug dependence.[a] This promising research collapsed under the weight of federal de-funding, decreased access to test compounds, and political hostility to research involving drugs thought to foment the public unrest of the era.[26]

In the 1980s, the indolealkylamine hallucinogen ibogaine was patented as a treatment of addiction,[50] but it has remained an underground tool in America and elsewhere, with only limited research published to date.[7,11] Ayahuasca, which contains

dimethyltryptamine, has been proposed to help those seeking recovery within the religious practices of the União do Vegetal[18] and the Santo Daime Church,[36] as well as to possibly inoculate teen members from engaging in the addictive use of drugs of abuse.[14] Similarly, anecdotal evidence exists that sacramental peyote taken within the prayer ceremonies of the Native American Church by Native Americans may assist in recovery from drug dependence and alcoholism.[31-32,35]

There is an ongoing, desperate need for effective treatments for alcoholism and other drug abuse and dependence disorders. The longstanding and continued religious use of hallucinogens suggests that some hallucinogens (combined with psychotherapeutic and sociotherapeutic procedures) may well be an effective psychopharmacologic intervention for these disorders. As research to evaluate hallucinogens for therapeutic use is no longer a major area of investigation, the few legitimate research groups in the United States and elsewhere will hopefully reevaluate hallucinogens' potential for addictions as well as continue to encourage more colleagues to return to this field. It is also hoped that future research will avoid methodological flaws, which unfortunately made the studies of the 1950s and 1960s less reliable from today's perspective.[4,32,59] Without current, clearly favorable clinical research findings, hallucinogen treatments for drug dependence hold only aging speculative promise and are not accepted for any medical indication, including for those seeking treatment for their problematic drug use.

Acknowledgments

The authors greatly appreciate the editing assistance of medical student Sean Doherty of Cardiff University School of Medicine.

References

1. Abraham HD. Visual phenomenology of the LSD flashback. *Arch Gen Psychiatry.* 1983;40:884–889.
2. Abraham HD, Mamen A. LSD-like panic from risperidone in post-LSD visual disorder. *J Clin Psychopharmacol.* 1996;16:228–231.
3. Abraham HD, McCann UD, Ricaurte GA. Psychedelic drugs. In: Davis KL, Charney D, Coyle JT, Nemeroff C, eds. *Neuropsychopharmacology: The Fifth Generation of Progress.* Philadelphia: Lippincott Williams & Wilkins; 2002:1545–1556.
4. Abuzzahab FS, Anderson BJ. A review of LSD treatment in alcoholism. *Int Pharmacopsychiatry.* 1971;6:223–235.
5. American Psychiatric Association. *Diagnostic Criteria from DSM-IV-TR.* Washington, DC: American Psychiatric; 2000.
6. Baggott MJ, Erowid E, Erowid F, Robertson LC. Prevalence of chronic flashbacks in hallucinogen users: a web-based questionnaire [Abstract]. *Presented at the 68th Annual Meeting of the College on Problems of Drug Dependence, Scottsdale, AZ, 21 June 2006;* 2006.
7. Belgers M, Leenaars M, Homberg JR, Riskes-Hoitinga M, Schellekens AF, Hooijmans CR. Ibogaine and addiction in the animal model, a systematic review and meta-analysis. *Transl Psychiatry.* 2016;6(5):e826.
8. Bey T, Patel A. Phencyclidine intoxication and adverse effects: a clinical and psychological review of an illicit drug. *Cal J Emerg Med.* 2007;8(1):9–14.
9. Boyer EW. Dextromethorphan abuse. *Ped Emerg Care.* 2004;20:858–963.
10. Canal CE, Murnane KS. The serotonin 5-HT2C receptor and the non-addictive nature of classic hallucinogens. *J Psychopharmacol.* 2017;31(1):127–143.
11. Chang Q, Hanania T, Mash DC, Maillet EL. Noribogaine reduces nicotine self-administration in rats. *J Psychopharmacol.* 2015;29(6):704–711.

[a]References 13, 4, 46, 27, 40, 48, 52, 63.

12. Cohen S. Lysergic acid diethylamide: side effects and complications. *J Nerv Ment Dis*. 1960;130:30–40.

13. Reference deleted in review.

14. Doering-Silveira E, Grob CS, de Rios MD, et al. Report on psychoactive drug use among adolescents using ayahuasca within a religious context. *J Psychoactive Drugs*. 2005;37:141–144.

15. Dribben B, Wood A. *Toxicity, hallucinogens—LSD. eMedicine article topic #2809*. 2006 http://www.emedicine.com.

16. El-Mallakh RS, Halpern JH, Abraham HD. Substance abuse: hallucinogen- and MDMA-related disorders (chapter 60). In: Tasman A, Maj M, First MB, Kay J, Lieberman JA, eds. *Psychiatry*. 3rd ed. London: Wiley; 2008:1100–1126.

17. Fasano A, Barra A, Nicosia P, et al. Cocaine addiction: from habits to stereotypical-repetitive behaviors and punding. *Drug Alcohol Depend*. 2008;96:178–182.

18. Frecska E, Bokor P, Winkelman M. The therapeutic potentials of Ayahuasca: possible effects against various diseases of civilization. *Front Pharmacol*. 2016;7(35).

19. Frosch WA, Robbins ER, Stern M. Untoward reactions to lysergic acid diethylamide (LSD) resulting in hospitalization. *NEJM*. 1965;273:1245–1239.

20. Gamma A, Buck A, Berthold T, Liechti ME, Vollenweider FX. 3,4-Methylenedioxymethamphetamine (MDMA) modulates cortical and limbic brain activity as measured by [H(2)(15)O]-PET in healthy humans. *Neuropsychopharmacology*. 2000;23:388–395.

21. Giannini AJ, Loiselle RH, Price WA. Antidotal strategies in phencyclidine intoxication. *Int J Psychiatry Med*. 1984;4:513–518.

22. González-Maeso J, Sealfon S. Hormone signaling via G protein-coupled receptors. In: DeGoot LC, Jameson JL, eds. *Endocrinology*. Amsterdam: Elsevier; 2006:177–203.

23. González-Maeso J, Yuen T, Ebersole BJ, et al. Transcriptome fingerprints distinguish hallucinogenic and nonhallucinogenic 5-hydroxytryptamine 2A receptor agonist effects in mouse somatosensory cortex. *J Neurosci*. 2003;23:8836–8843.

24. Gouzoulis-Mayfrank E, Schreckenberger M, Sabri O, et al. Neurometabolic effects of psilocybin, 3,4-methylenedioxyethylamphetamine (MDE) and d-methamphetamine in healthy volunteers. *Neuropsychopharmacology*. 1999;20:565–581.

25. Grinspoon L, Bakalar JB. *Psychedelic Drugs Reconsidered*. 2nd ed. New York: The Lindesmith Center; 1997.

26. Grob CS. Psychiatric research with hallucinogens: what have we learned? *Yearbook Ethnomedicine Consciousness Res*. 1994;3:91–112.

27. Reference deleted in review.

28. Halberstadt AL, Geyer MA. Multiple receptors contribute to the behavioral effects of indoleamine hallucinogens. *Neuropharmacology*. 2011;61(3):364–381.

29. Halpern JH. Hallucinogens, anesthetic agents, and amphetamines. *Pharm News*. 2000;7:21–29.

30. Reference deleted in review.

31. Halpern JH. Hallucinogens and dissociative agents naturally growing in the United States. *Pharmacol Ther*. 2004;102:131–138.

32. Halpern JH. Hallucinogens in the treatment of alcoholism and other addictions. In: Winkelman M, Roberts T, eds. *Psychedelic Medicine: Scientific Evidence for Hallucinogenic Substances as Treatments*. vol. 2. Westport, CT and London: Praeger; 2007:1–14.

33. Halpern JH, Pope Jr HG. Do hallucinogens cause residual neuropsychological toxicity? *Drug Alcohol Depend*. 1999;53:247–256.

34. Halpern JH, Pope Jr HG. Hallucinogen persisting perception disorder: what do we know after 50 years? *Drug Alcohol Depend*. 2003;69:109–119.

35. Halpern JH, Sherwood AR, Hudson JI, Yurgelun-Todd D, Pope Jr HG. Psychological and cognitive effects of long-term peyote use among Native Americans. *Biol Psychiatry*. 2005;58:624–631.

36. Halpern JH, Sherwood AR, Passie T, Blackwell KC, Ruttenber AJ. Evidence of health and safety in American Members of a religion who use a hallucinogenic sacrament. *Med Sci Monit*. 2008;14:SR15–SR22.

37. Hermle L, Simon M, Ruchsow M, Geppert M. Hallucinogen-persisting perception disorder. *Ther Adv Psychopharmacol*. 2012;2(5):199–205.

38. Hillebrand J, Olszewksi D, Sedefov R. *Hallucinogenic Mushrooms: An Emerging Trend Case Study*. Lisbon: European Monitoring Centre for Drugs and Drug Addiction; 2006.

39. Hintzen A, Passie T. *The Pharmacology of LSD*. Oxford, New York: Oxford University Press; 2010.

40. Reference deleted in review.

41. Holland D. *Flashback-Phänomene als Nachwirkung von Halluzinogeneinnahme*. Hannover: Hannover Medical School Dissertation; 2004.

42. Hollister LE. Effects of hallucinogens in humans. In: Jacobs BL, ed. *Hallucinogens: Neurochemical, Behavioral, and Clinical Perspectives*. New York: Raven; 1984:19–33.

43. Johnson MW, Richards WA, Griffiths RR. Hallucinogen research: guidelines for safety. *J Psychopharmacol*. 2008;22(6):603–620.

44. Johnston LD, Bachman JG, O'Malley PM. *Monitoring the Future: Questionnaire Responses from the Nation's High School Seniors, 2005*. Ann Arbor, MI: Institute for Social Research; 2006.

45. Kiehl KA. A cognitive neuroscience perspective on psychopathy: evidence for paralimbic system dysfunction. *Psychiatry Res*. 2006;142(2–3):107–128.

46. Reference deleted in review.

47. Kumar S, Soren S, Chaudhury S. Hallucinations: etiology and clinical implications. *Ind Psychiatry J*. 2009;18(2):119–126.

48. Reference deleted in review.

49. Leuner H. *Die Experimentelle Psychose*. Berlin, Heidelberg: Julius Springer; 1962.

50. Lotsof HS. *Rapid Method for Interrupting the Narcotic Addiction Syndrome*. U.S. Patent # 4,499,096;1985.

51. Malleson N. Acute adverse reactions to LSD in clinical and experimental use in the United Kingdom. *Br J Psychiatry*. 1971;118:229–230.

52. Reference deleted in review.

53. Nichols DE. Hallucinogens. *Pharmacol Ther*. 2004;101:131–181.

54. Nutt D, King LA, Saulsbury W, Blakemore C. Development of a rational scale to assess the harm of drugs of potential misuse. *Lancet*. 2007;369:1047–1063.

55. O'Brien CP. Drug addiction and drug abuse. In: Brunton L, Lazo J, Parker K, eds. *Goodman & Gillman's the Pharmacological Basis of Therapeutics*. 11th ed. New York: McGraw-Hill; 2005:607–628.

56. Orsolini L, Papanti GD, De Berardis D, Guirguis A, Corkery JM, Schifano F. The "Endless Trip" among NPS users: psychopathology and psychopharmacology in the hallucinogen-persisting perception disorder. A systematic review. *Front Psychiatry*. 2017;8:240.

57. Osmond H. A review of the clinical effects of psychotomimetic agents. *Ann NY Acad Sci*. 1957;66:418–434.

58. Passie T. *Psycholytic and Psychedelic Therapy Research: A Complete International Bibliography 1931–1995*. Hannover: Laurentius; 1997.

59. Pletscher A, Ladewig D, eds. *50 Years of LSD: Current Status and Perspectives of Hallucinogens*. New York & London: Parthenon; 1994.

60. Riba J, Romero S, Grasa E, Mena E, Carrio I, Barbanoj MJ. Increased frontal and paralimbic activation following ayahuasca, the pan-Amazonian inebriant. *Psychopharmacology (Berl.)*. 2006;186:93–98.

61. SAMHSA, Office of Applied Studies. *Drug Abuse Warning Network, 2005: National Estimates of Drug-Related Emergency Department Visits*. Rockville, MD: DAWN Series D-29, DHHS Publication No. SMA 07-4256; 2007.

62. SAMHSA, Office of Applied Studies. *Results from the 2006 National Survey on Drug Use and Health: National Findings*. Rockville, MD: NSDUH Series H-32, DHHS Publication No. SMA 07–4293; 2007.

63. Reference deleted in review.

64. Schultes RE, Hofmann A, Rätsch C. *Plants of the Gods: Their Sacred, Healing and Hallucinogenic Powers*. 2nd ed. Vermont: Inner Traditions; 2001.

65. Schwarz CJ. The complications of LSD: a review of the literature. *J Nerv Ment Dis*. 1968;146:174–186.

66. Strassman RJ. Adverse reactions for psychedelic drugs: a review of the literature. *J Nerv Ment Dis*. 1984;172:577–595.

67. Strassman RJ. Hallucinogenic drugs in psychiatric research and treatment: perspectives and prospects. *J Nerv Ment Dis*. 1995;183:127–138.

68. Tacke U, Ebert MH. Hallucinogens and phencyclidine. In: Kranzler HR, Ciraulo DA, eds. *Clinical Manual of Addiction Psychopharmacology*. Washington, DC: American Psychiatric; 2005:211–241.

69. Taylor RL, Maurer JI, Tinklenberg JR. Management of "bad trips" in an evolving drug scene. *J Am Med Assoc*. 1970;213:422–425.

70. Ungerleider JT, Pechnick RN. Hallucinogens. In: Galanter M, Kleber HD, eds. *Textbook of Substance Abuse Treatment*. Washington, DC: American Psychiatric; 1999:195–203.

71. Vollenweider FX. Brain mechanisms of hallucinogens and entactogens. *Dialog Clin Neurosci*. 2001;3:265–279.

72. Vollenweider FX, Leenders KL, Scharfetter C, Maguire P, Stadelmann O, Angst J. Positron emission tomography and fluorodeoxyglucose studies of metabolic hyperfrontality and psychopathology in the psilocybin model of psychosis. *Neuropsychopharmacology*. 1997;16:357–372.

73. Vollenweider FX, Vollenweider-Scherpenhuyzen MF, Babler A, Vogel H, Hell D. Psilocybin induces schizophrenia-like psychosis in humans via a serotonin-2 agonist action. *Neuroreport*. 1998;9:3897–3902.

74. Wasson RG. The hallucinogenic fungi of Mexico: an inquiry into the origins of the religious idea among primitive peoples. *Bot Mus Leaflets Harv Univ*. 1961;19:137–162.

75. Wright D, Sathe N, Spagnola K. *State Estimates of Substance Use from the 2004–2005 National Surveys on Drug Use and Health (DHHS Publication No. SMA 07-4235, NSDUH Series H-31). Substance Abuse and Mental Health Services Administration*. Rockville, MD: Office of Applied Studies; 2007.

58

Molecular Genetics and the Treatment of Addiction

LARA A. RAY, ANITA CSERVENKA, AND KENT E. HUTCHISON

CHAPTER OUTLINE

Overview

Substance use disorders represent complex phenotypes that result from the intricate interplay of genetic variation, neurobiological mechanisms, psychosocial variables, and environmental variables. To date, one of the least-studied factors has been genetic variation. However, basic research on the human genome is progressing at a rapid pace, and investigations of genetic factors that influence the etiology and treatment of substance use disorders are now much more common. The promise of this research is that it may help scientists optimize the success of treatments by matching specific treatments with individuals who have specific genetic vulnerabilities. The ability to match a specific treatment with an individual who is most likely to benefit from that treatment is especially exciting because, while a number of treatment alternatives exist, the overall effectiveness of these treatments is quite modest and there are currently no objective criteria that can be used to match an individual with the treatment that is most likely to be effective.

It is only a matter of time before much of the genetic variation that contributes to the risk of addiction is uncovered and, likewise, only a matter of time before clinicians begin to utilize genetic information to match individuals with the treatment that is safest and most likely to benefit them.

This chapter provides a critical review of the expanding literature with respect to molecular genetics and the treatment of addiction. First, we present a brief overview of key concepts in the genetics of addictions. Second, we provide a more extended review and discussion of pharmacogenetics and pharmacogenomics applied to addiction medicine. Recent studies of genetic differences and responses to pharmacological, and to a lesser degree psychosocial, treatments for addictions will be reviewed for various substances of abuse, including alcohol, nicotine, cocaine, and opiates. Third, we discuss practical and ethical issues in the translation of pharmacogenetics science into clinical practice. Fourth, we outline several future directions for the field of molecular genetics applied to the treatment of addictions. Finally, we present a summary and some concluding remarks.

Genetics and the Treatment of Addictions

Twin and adoption studies have suggested that approximately 50% of the variance in risk for developing alcohol dependence can be explained by genetic factors.[40,67] Likewise, studies have demonstrated that genetic factors account for a significant portion of variance in drug use, abuse, and dependence.[a] The progression from initial use to abuse or dependence for substances such as marijuana and cocaine also appears to be largely due to genetic factors.[64,65]

Just as the etiology of substance use disorders appears to be under moderate genetic control, so does the response to pharmacotherapies. Broadly speaking, evidence for heritability of medication effects in psychiatry dates as far back as 1967, when heritable variation in plasma concentration of the tricyclic antidepressants, desipramine and nortriptyline, were first shown in twin and family studies.[3,46] In addition, more recent research has documented the heritability of response to typical antipsychotics,[145] including differences in antipsychotic response among ethnic groups.[1,35]

[a]References 9, 43, 44, 66, 68, 138, 139.

As discussed in detail below, genetic factors also seem to play a role in response to pharmacotherapies, and perhaps psychosocial treatments, for substance use disorders.

After determining that genetic variation plays a substantial role in the etiology of addictive disorders and the response to treatment through family, twin, and adoption studies, the next step in genetics research often consists of identifying specific genetic variations that contribute to the etiology and response to treatment for these disorders. In many ways, research on genetics of addiction has already transitioned from establishing that genetic variables contribute to the variance in a disorder to identifying the specific genetic variables that actually contribute to the disorder.

Currently, there are two basic approaches to the identification of genetic variations that influence substance use disorders and/or treatment outcomes. The first is a hypothesis-driven approach, in which investigators develop a priori hypotheses based on what is known about the genetic variation and the neurobiology of the disorder or the mechanism of action for a specific treatment. For example, one might hypothesize that a specific genetic variation that influences the mu opioid receptor expression might also predict acute responses to alcohol[11,107] and the effects of a medication (e.g., naltrexone) that targets this receptor.[4,98,111]

In many cases, it is more common to work with a gene for which function variations have yet to be identified. In this situation, a variation on the approach described earlier is to hypothesize that a gene is related to a specific aspect of a substance use disorder or the effects of a medication and then use special analytic approaches to probe genetic variation across the entire gene. This approach is commonly known as a haplotype-based approach, and is designed to capture most of the genetic variation across the gene even when the function variations have not been identified. To that end, "tag single nucleotide polymorphisms" are often used, as they allow scientists to capture genetic variation in various loci by genotyping fewer, but informative, markers. More specifically, tag single nucleotide polymorphisms are selected on the basis of patterns of linkage disequilibrium that indicate several polymorphisms are highly correlated, in which case, instead of having to genotype all markers, scientists can identify a few that strongly predict genetic variation in a given area or locus. This approach has become increasingly accessible due to the availability of bioinformatics resources, most notably results from the International HAPMAP Project, which have been made publicly available in the user-friendly HAPMAP Project website (http://www.hapmap.org/). The next step after identifying tag single nucleotide polymorphisms for areas of interest is often to build haplotypes, which describe common patterns of DNA sequence variation. In fact, the objective of the HAPMAP Project is to develop a haplotype map of the human genome, which in turn can aid scientists in finding genes affecting health, disease, and responses to medications and environment.[36,58,136] A detailed review of haplotype-based techniques in pharmacogenetics is beyond the scope of this chapter and can be found elsewhere.[86]

Finally, a more recent approach is to conduct exploratory genome-wide analyses to identify genetic variation that influences substance use disorders or responses to medications. The genome-wide association study is currently in vogue and represents one of the most cutting-edge approaches in terms of identifying sources of genetic variation that may eventually be used to predict response to treatment. A genome-wide association study utilizes a high-density single nucleotide polymorphism array to generate data on more than one million genetic markers (e.g., using the Illumina 1 M array). This vast array of genetic data can then be analyzed in combination with a set of phenotypes. A number of reviews have been published recently on the advantages, disadvantages, limitations, and recommendations associated with this approach.[21,102,135] One obvious problem with this approach is the sheer number of statistical tests and the resulting increase in type I error that may lead to false positives. A corollary is the requirement of strict statistical corrections and the need for massive sample sizes. To date, there have been a number of genome-wide association study reports in the psychiatric genetics literature, including major depressive disorder,[12] bipolar disorder,[33] and schizophrenia,[96] but only one that involves a substance abuse disorder, namely nicotine dependence.[141] Although genome-wide association is the approach du jour and has generated much excitement in the field, it is important to note that genome-wide association studies represent a transition to even more difficult and time-consuming work. Once new genetic variations are identified, models will need to be developed and hypothesis-driven research will be needed to translate the effect of genetic variation uncovered in the genome-wide association studies regarding the effect of the genetic variations from the molecular level, to the cellular level, to the systems level, and to the behavioral level in order to understand the implications of these findings for the etiology, prevention, and treatment of substance use disorders. This translation will likely lead to new findings on as-yet unknown neuronal mechanisms that influence the development of substance use disorders and lead to new targets for pharmacotherapies as well as generate information about which individuals will be most likely to respond to those new pharmacotherapies.

Pharmacogenetics and Pharmacogenomics

Pharmacogenetics is a field of research that seeks to understand individual differences in the metabolism and efficacy of medications. As described by Vogel,[144] pharmacogenetics is the study of heritable differences in the metabolism and activity of exogenous agents, including medications and environmental toxins. Current pharmacogenetics research focuses on identifying genetic factors that account for variability in pharmacotherapy effects, in terms of both pharmacodynamics and efficacy.[28, 91] In recent years, the term pharmacogenomics has been defined[118] as the application of genomics to the study of pharmacogenetics. In brief, the distinction between the two terms refers to the methodological and theoretical approach such that pharmacogenetics investigations are generally hypothesis driven and focus on a few loci at a time. Conversely, pharmacogenomics investigations include the use of high-throughput genotyping and genome-wide association approaches to understanding genetic determinants of pharmacotherapy response. In essence, the objective of pharmacogenomics is the same as pharmacogenetics, which is to elucidate genetic variants that influence the efficacy and safety of pharmacotherapies. For simplicity, we will refer simply to pharmacogenetics in this chapter.

The field of pharmacogenetics has grown rapidly and has benefited greatly from advancements in molecular genetics tools for identifying gene polymorphisms, developments in bioinformatics and functional genomics, and new findings from the human genome project. The foremost goal of this line of research is to optimize pharmacotherapy by identifying genetic factors that predict who is more likely to respond to certain pharmacotherapies and who will not respond, thereby matching individuals to medications on the basis of genetic factors. Genetic factors can account for individual differences in medication toxicity and response in many ways. Genetic polymorphisms may lead to functional differences in medication metabolism and disposition, such as functional differences in enzyme activity or medication transporters. Alternatively, genetic polymorphisms may impact the target of a medication, such as a particular receptor. An example of the first case is a polymorphism of the *CYP2D6* gene, which is involved in the availability of specific medication-metabolizing enzymes associated with one's response to opioid painkillers, such as codeine or morphine. Individuals who are homozygous for the nonfunctional *CYP2D6* alleles were found to be resistant to the analgesic effects of opioid painkillers.[105] It is important to note that this response in poor metabolizers may be moderated by ethnicity. Specifically, individuals who carry the *CYP2D6*10* allele, which is most common among Chinese individuals, have reduced metabolism of opioid analgesics, such as codeine[146] or tramadol.[85] Furthermore, treatments such as methadone maintenance therapy can inhibit the metabolism of tramadol to *O*-desmethyltramadol by interfering with CYP2D6 activity.[20] This has important implications for therapy as those individuals receiving methadone may not experience the same degree of opioid analgesia, as those receiving other treatment, such as buprenorphine maintenance.[20] Thus both ethnic variation in allele types and treatment considerations are important when determining the potential efficacy of opioid analgesics.

On the other hand, genetic polymorphisms involved in a medication's target may also impact one's response to pharmacotherapy. For example, polymorphisms of the dopamine D4 receptor gene (*DRD4*) have been associated with differential response to antipsychotic medications.[19] For example, a recent finding suggests that for the DRD4 exon III repeat polymorphism, the 4R allele is associated with better clozapine response, but other individual single nucleotide polymorphisms (SNPs) in this study showed no association with clozapine response.[57] Similarly, when individual SNPs of DRD4 (rs1800955 and rs4646984) were analyzed, they did not show any associations with antipsychotic drug response.[101] Thus future studies may consider further exploring the efficacy of the 48-bp repeat polymorphism of the 4R allele. There is also a growing literature on the pharmacogenetics of antidepressant medications.[71] Specifically, research has suggested that the functional polymorphism of the serotonin transporter gene located in the 5′ upstream regulatory region consisting of a 44-bp insertion/deletion, which results in a long or short variant, predicts response to various selective serotonin reuptake inhibitors, including fluoxetine,[106] fluvoxamine,[131] and paroxetine.[147] Carriers of the long allele of the serotonin transporter promoter polymorphism have better clinical response to antidepressant medications compared with individuals who are homozygous for the short allele, which results in twofold decreased expression and transport activity of the receptor in vitro.[48] These results suggest that pharmacogenetics may soon inform a more targeted use of antidepressant medications. In addition to medications' efficacy, pharmacogenetics research has focused on identifying susceptibility loci contributing to adverse effect profiles and medications' toxicity, thereby enhancing the safety profile of pharmacotherapies. Next we review pharmacogenetic studies in the field of addictions to various substances of abuse.

Nicotine

Currently, there are two non-nicotine pharmacotherapies approved by the FDA for the treatment of nicotine dependence, namely bupropion hydrochloride and varenicline. In addition,

there are five FDA-approved nicotine replacement therapies, which vary mostly in terms of their delivery kinetics; these include transdermal patch, gum, lozenge, inhaler, and nasal spray. Several candidate genes have been subjected to pharmacogenetic studies, mostly those of nicotine replacement therapies and bupropion, as described in recent reviews of the pharmacogenetics of smoking cessation.[8,93,116] Specifically, pharmacogenetic studies of nicotine dependence have examined genes underlying the metabolism of nicotine, focusing primarily on the cytochrome P450 (CYP)2A6 gene (*CYP2A6*). This gene codes for the primary enzyme that converts nicotine to cotinine and cotinine to 3-hydroxycotinine. In a study of transdermal patch and nasal spray nicotine replacement therapies, at the same levels of nicotine replacement, carriers of *CYP2A6* alleles coding for a slower metabolism were found to have higher plasma nicotine concentrations following 1 week of the nicotine patch than normal metabolizers.[89] Those differences were not seen using the nasal spray, and at 6-month follow-up, slow metabolizers had higher quit rates in the transdermal patch condition, as compared with normal metabolizers.[81] A community sample of treatment-seeking nicotine-dependent patients who received transdermal nicotine therapy were also found to benefit more from the treatment if they were slow metabolizers,[63] whereas another study found that extended release transdermal nicotine therapy (24 weeks) was more effective than standard therapy (8 weeks) in slow metabolizers.[83] Other important considerations may be examining whether interactions between the *CYP2A6* gene and other genes predict quit success rates. For example, a study investigating the role of serotonergic systems in treatment response found that slow metabolizer patients with the 5-HTTL allele or HTR2A-1438GG alleles benefited more from nicotine replacement therapy, suggesting reduced levels of synaptic serotonin may be a mechanism by which slow metabolizers may show better success for smoking cessation.[143] However, the results have not been consistent, and a study found that slow metabolizers had higher relapse rates when treated with the nicotine patch,[100] whereas another study reported that nicotine replacement therapy was more effective in fast metabolizers.[17] It is important to note that findings may also depend on the treatments being tested. For example, in one study, bupropion was shown to result in 1.7 times longer abstinence in slow metabolizers than fast metabolizers.[2] More research is needed to identify the reason for discrepancies across studies, but the *CYP2A6* gene appears to be a promising target for translating personalized treatment to the clinic.

In addition, nicotinic receptor genes have been subjected to pharmacogenetic investigations. Nicotine binds to nicotinic acetylcholine receptors, which are ligand-gated ion channels for which there are several subunits. Allelic variation in the gene coding for the nicotinic acetylcholine receptor's α4 subunit (CHRNA4) has been associated with nicotine dependence.[32,84] More recent molecular work has suggested that certain single nucleotide polymorphisms in the *CHRNA4* gene are functional and related to smoking cessation during nicotine replacement therapy[56] and varenicline treatment.[119] Although promising, these findings await replication. Likewise, a series of studies have examined the role of functional genetic variation in the DRD2 in response to bupropion and nicotine replacement therapy.[60,82] Results revealed that the DRD2–141C Ins/Del genotype was associated with treatment response to bupropion, such that smokers homozygous for the Ins C allele had a more favorable response to treatment compared with those carrying the Del C allele. Conversely, regardless of nicotine replacement therapy type, those carrying the Del C allele had higher quit rates from nicotine replacement therapy compared with those homozygous for the Ins C allele.[82] Additional polymorphisms that have received attention as putative genetic moderators of smoking cessation in response to nicotine replacement therapies and bupropion include dopaminergic genes (e.g., the Val/Met single nucleotide polymorphism of the catechol-O-methyltransferase gene),[79] opioidergic genes (e.g., Asn40Asp single nucleotide polymorphism of the *OPRM1* gene),[80,117] and serotonergic genes (e.g., the serotonin transporter promoter polymorphism).[94]

Perhaps one of the more exciting new developments in the pharmacogenetics of smoking cessation is a series of genome-wide association studies of smoking cessation with bupropion and nicotine replacement therapy.[141] These studies revealed that genetic variants in quit-success were likely to alter cell adhesion, enzymatic, transcriptional, structural, and protein-handling functions. The genes identified through these genome-wide association studies had modest overlap with genes associated with addictions and memory processes. Clearly, as noted previously, there are limitations to the genome-wide association approach, and these results should be interpreted with caution until replicated in an independent sample.

Alcohol

Several studies to date have investigated genetic polymorphisms in the context of pharmacotherapies for alcohol dependence. Naltrexone, a mu-opioid receptor antagonist, is one of the very few pharmacotherapies currently approved for the treatment of alcoholism by the US Food and Drug Administration (FDA). From a pharmacogenetics perspective, there has been recent interest in the gene coding for mu-opioid receptors (*OPRM1*), as they represent a primary target of naltrexone. More specifically, studies have focused on the Asn40Asp mutation of the *OPRM1* gene, given evidence that this nonsynonymous mutation leads to an amino acid change, which in turn codes for more potent receptors. Human laboratory studies have shown that the Asp40 allele of the *OPRM1* gene is associated with greater sensitivity to the reinforcing effects of alcohol[107] and greater neural activation in the mesocorticolimbic structures following a priming dose of alcohol.[34]

In a pharmacogenetic study of naltrexone, Oslin and colleagues[98] found that the Asn40Asp allele of the *OPRM1* gene was associated with clinical response to naltrexone for the treatment of alcohol dependence. The relationship was such that individuals with at least one copy of the Asp40 variant showed lower relapse rates and longer time to return to heavy drinking when treated with naltrexone, as compared with homozygotes for the Asn40 allele.[98] These findings have been recently replicated and extended in the multisite COMBINE Study, such that carriers of the Asp40 allele of the *OPRM1* gene had better clinical response to naltrexone, in combination with medication management, as compared with homozygotes for the Asn40 allele.[4] A double-blind, placebo-controlled laboratory trial of naltrexone (50 mg) found that carriers of the Asp40 allele of the *OPRM1* gene showed significantly greater naltrexone-induced blunting of the alcohol high, as compared with individuals who were homozygous for the Asn40 allele.[111] These findings suggest that the differential clinical response to naltrexone may be due to differential blunting of alcohol-induced reward as a function of genotype and propose a mechanism for this important pharmacogenetic relationship. Nevertheless, there have been null findings regarding the association between this functional polymorphism and the efficacy of naltrexone for alcoholism[6,38,49,99] such that further work is necessary before these findings can be translated into clinical practice.

Limitations notwithstanding, the pharmacogenetics of naltrexone and the putative moderating effects of a functional single nucleotide polymorphism of the *OPRM1* gene represent an interesting line of work that is both promising and exciting from a pharmacogenetics perspective. In this case, functional variation in a gene coding for a medication (i.e., naltrexone) target, namely mu-opioid receptors, may be used to predict the efficacy of a pharmacotherapy. This case most likely represents an exception, rather than the rule, in pharmacogenetics research as most pharmacotherapies do not have such targeted neurobiological effects and the functional significance of most single nucleotide polymorphisms are not well characterized.

It is important to note, however, that ancestral background can moderate the efficacy of pharmacotherapeutic treatments. For example, the prevalence of the Asp40 allele varies by ancestral background, such that individuals of East Asian ancestry, are more likely to carry the Asp40 allele.[70] This suggests that this population may particularly benefit from naltrexone treatment. A study of Korean alcohol-dependent adults found that treatment-adherent patients who carried the Asp40 allele (G allele) took significantly longer to relapse than Asn40 homozygotes.[69] Again, the underlying mechanism of this effect may be through a reduction of reward-associated craving, as an intravenous alcohol administration study showed that individuals of East Asian descent who carried the Asp40 allele were less likely to crave alcohol when administered with naltrexone relative to placebo or those participants who were Asn40 homozygotes.[115]

Using a similar hypothesis-driven approach, a series of pharmacogenetic studies have tested the association between olanzapine, a medication that targets dopamine receptors, alcohol craving, and a polymorphism of the dopamine D4 receptor gene (DRD4 variable number tandem repeat).[52,54,55] One study found an association between the 7-repeat allele of the DRD4 variable number tandem repeat polymorphism and increased craving for alcohol after a priming dose of alcohol.[53] Another study found that olanzapine decreased craving after a priming dose of alcohol in a nonclinical sample of college drinkers.[54] Finally, results from a recent clinical trial revealed that the efficacy of olanzapine in the treatment of alcohol dependence was moderated by this genetic variation, such that individuals with at least one copy of the long allele showed greater reductions in cue-elicited craving and greater decreases in alcohol consumption during the 12-week clinical trial, as compared with individuals who were homozygous for the short allele.[55] This genetic variation has also been associated with increased activation of mesocorticolimbic regions during the presentation of alcohol cues.[34] Together these series of laboratory and clinical trials have established a relationship between a polymorphism of the DRD4, craving for alcohol in the laboratory, and response to a medication that targets dopamine receptors. Despite this intriguing relationship, much work is needed to determine whether there is clinical utility of olanzapine for treating alcohol dependence. For example, a recent 12-week clinical trial that did not examine genetic moderators of olanzapine response, suggests that despite reductions in craving and proportion of drinking days with olanzapine treatment, the cost-benefit of this medication does not currently support its clinical utility.[87]

The approach in this series of studies of olanzapine for alcoholism was theory driven and focused on intermediate phenotypes for alcoholism, in this case alcohol craving, rather than the diagnostic phenotype of alcohol dependence per se. There are important advantages to a theory-driven pharmacogenetics approach, such as the ability to answer more specific questions about the mechanisms of action of pharmacotherapies, genetic variants, and biobehavioral risk makers of complex disorders, such as alcoholism. It is notable that theory-driven approaches can be complementary to data-driven pharmacogenomics investigations, which are likely to become increasingly accessible given recent advances in DNA genotyping technology.

Topiramate, an antiepileptic medication that is a glutamatergic antagonist and γ-aminobutyric acid (GABA)ergic agonist, has also shown promise for the treatment of alcohol dependence across several studies.[10] A study of problem drinkers by Kranzler and colleagues found that topiramate was able to significantly reduce heavy drinking days compared to placebo, and in European Americans, this effect was moderated by the SNP rs2832407 in the glutamate receptor, ionotropic, kainate 1 (GRIK1) gene.[77] Specifically, CC homozygotes reduced their drinking significantly more than A allele carriers. This same gene has also been shown to be associated with the severity of topiramate-induced side effects and the topiramate serum concentration, which were both found to be higher in A allele carriers than CC homozygotes.[114] Furthermore, the findings by Kranzler and colleagues were extended in a subsequent study that suggested that the GRIK1 genotype also moderated positive expectancy of alcohol's effects and the desire to drink when patients' daily reports on these measures were examined.[75] This was followed by an analysis that indicated an interaction between genotype, expectancies, and medication, such that topiramate was less effective in CC homozygotes at reducing heavy drinking on days when more positive effects of alcohol were expected.[76] This series of studies not only showed that the GRIK1 genotype may be an important marker of topiramate's efficacy, but that the genotype is associated with cognitive processes and craving associated with alcohol use. It is notable that treatment, genotype, and cognitive processes may interact to predict heavy drinking days in problem drinkers.

Cocaine

Currently, there are no FDA-approved pharmacotherapies for the treatment of cocaine dependence; however, many recent advances have taken place in the search for medications to treat this disorder.[62,127,128] Medications such as dopamine agonists, disulfiram, the cocaine vaccine, and GABAergic treatments have all been explored, and many of them have undergone testing in phase II or phase III clinical trials.[127] For example, the cocaine vaccine, which creates an immunologic response and reduces the rewarding effect of cocaine, may be most effective at preventing relapse to cocaine use.[127] Other treatments, including GABAergic medications, such as topiramate, appear to be advantageous for treatment of comorbid alcohol and cocaine dependent patients,[61] whereas results of studies with disulfiram have been mixed.[97,104]

Associations between treatment and pharmacogenetics have recently been explored with some of these medications. One such example is with disulfiram, which is believed to inhibit the activity of dopamine β-hydroxylase (DβH), an enzyme that converts dopamine to norepinephrine.[37] Mixed findings with disulfiram may be attributed to differences in genetic variation among individuals. In a trial for disulfiram in patients with comorbid cocaine and opioid dependence, disulfiram treatment was not effective in individuals who had a variant in the DβH gene that resulted in low DβH enzyme levels.[73] Thus genotyping of individuals for this particular DβH polymorphism could determine the success of disulfiram treatment, and exemplifies the importance of pharmacogenetics in treatment of cocaine addiction. In another study

of cocaine-dependent patients, the methylene tetrahydrofolate reductase (MTHFR) gene was studied as a moderator of disulfiram response, as it is involved with global methylation, which may also be moderated by disulfiram.[132] Although disulfiram treatment was effective at reducing cocaine-positive urine samples across all individuals relative to placebo, a slightly greater efficacy was present in patients who were homozygous or heterozygous for the T allele of the MTHFR gene, suggesting that the MTHFR genotype may be used to tailor pharmacotherapy for cocaine-dependent individuals.[132] Other moderators of the disulfiram response have also been shown for the α1A-adrenoceptor (ADRA1A) gene,[129] the ankyrin repeat and kinase domain-containing 1 (ANKK1) gene, and the dopamine receptor D2 (DRD2) gene.[133] Together, these studies suggest that the efficacy of disulfiram treatment may be determined by a number of different polymorphisms in genes involved with decreased stimulation of the α1A-adrenoceptor, global methylation, and dopaminergic function.

It is important to consider that the interaction of genetic variants and treatment response is not the same across different medication types. Of interest, the DβH gene variant showed the opposite effect in a treatment trial for the cocaine vaccine, such that patients with the low-activity DβH gene displayed a reduction in cocaine-positive urine samples with treatment, but not those with the high-activity gene variant.[72] Within the same cocaine vaccine clinical trial, individuals who carried the protective A allele of the κ-opioid receptor (OPRK1) gene, which inhibits dopamine-associated reinforcement, were also significantly less likely to have cocaine-positive urines.[95]

Furthermore, topiramate, an antiepileptic drug that has shown promise for the treatment of alcohol dependence, appears to be another promising new pharmacotherapy for cocaine dependence,[130] as suggested by results from a phase II clinical trial.[59]

Over the past two decades, several pharmacotherapies have been under study for other stimulant use disorders, such as methamphetamine dependence. These clinical trials have shown the most promising results for naltrexone, methylphenidate, bupropion, and mirtazapine.[13] Unfortunately, although there have been some promising findings across these studies, there is not a clear candidate among these medications.

Opiates

Opiate addiction is treated pharmacologically through opiate agonists, antagonists, and partial agonists (for a review see Haile et al.[45]) The first medication for opioid addiction was methadone, a selective synthetic opioid agonist.[24] Buprenorphine is another synthetic opiate that functions as a partial agonist at mu-opioid receptors and an antagonist at kappa-opioid receptors.[78] Both methadone and buprenorphine are equally effective for maintenance treatment of heroin dependence.[90] Methadone and buprenorphine are metabolized by CYP3A4; however, buprenorphine is metabolized to a much lesser degree than methadone by CYP2D6. Studies have found that Caucasians who lack CYP2D6 function have a poor metabolizer phenotype, which in turn is protective against opiate dependence.[140] Nevertheless, when slow opioid metabolizers go on to develop opioid addiction, they tend to respond well to methadone treatment, whereas opioid-dependent individuals with the CYP2D6 genotype coding for the "ultra-rapid" opioid metabolism are less responsive to the withdrawal relief afforded by methadone maintenance therapy[103] and respond better to buprenorphine, which is not as significantly metabolized by CYP2D6. The case of pharmacogenetics of opioid addiction is an interesting one in that what was learned about the pharmacogenetics of responsiveness to opiates for pain management purposes (described earlier) has informed the clinical literature on the use of opiates for the treatment of opiate addiction and has ultimately led toward the optimization of pharmacotherapy for opioid dependence.

In addition to *CYP3A4* and *CYP2D6*, a number of other genes have recently been investigated as moderators of the response to methadone and buprenorphine treatment. As an example, the *OPRD1* gene, which encodes for the δ-opioid receptor, was examined as a moderator of treatment response in European American and African American opioid-dependent patients assigned to either 24 weeks of methadone or buprenorphine treatment.[22] The authors found that African American CC homozygotes, for the SNP rs678849, were more likely than T allele carriers to have opioid-negative urines if they received methadone treatment. However, of interest, the opposite effect was seen in CC homozygotes who received buprenorphine treatment, as they were more likely than the T allele carriers to have opioid-positive urines.[22] This study exemplifies that not only is genetic variation related to treatment response, but that among these two common treatments for opioid dependence, very different effects may be seen depending on genetic variation of this SNP in the *OPRD1* gene. Furthermore, the effect was present only in African American patients, which suggests that genetic variation of certain alleles may not have the same effects across different ancestral backgrounds. Another study of the *OPRD1* gene found that genetic variation at other SNPs, namely rs581111 and rs529520, interacted with buprenorphine treatment in females but not in males of European ancestry.[18] Thus sex may be another important factor in the selection of pharmacotherapies for opioid dependence.

Furthermore, the brain-derived neurotrophic factor (BDNF) has been examined for SNPs that may moderate methadone maintenance treatment because BDNF is involved with the neural plasticity that may underlie opioid-induced plasticity.[23] The authors found a haplotype consisting of six SNPs for which genetic variation was related to a greater likelihood of being a poor responder to methadone treatment. *OPRD1* and *BDNF* are just a few of many genes that have been recently explored in pharmacogenetic studies of opioid dependence, but these preliminary findings have yet to be replicated in future studies.

An Intermediate Phenotype-Driven Pharmacogenetics Approach

Recent research has increasingly recognized the heterogeneity of diagnostic phenotypes and argued for the development of more discrete and homogeneous phenotypes, or intermediate phenotypes, for psychiatric disorders of complex genetics,[41,42] including addictions.[25,50] Recently, intermediate phenotypes have been further refined as translational phenotypes, which emphasizes the role of the phenotype in translating the effect at the genetic level to the clinical level.[51] An ideal translational phenotype is one that is narrowly defined and biologically based with a plausible link to the gene as well as the clinical presentation of the disorder. The use of intermediate phenotypes for disorders of complex genetics has allowed for progress in genetic association studies, and importantly, this approach not only increases power to detect genetic effects but also allows scientists to ask different research questions about the neurobiology and mechanisms underlying disease processes and pharmacotherapy response. When applied

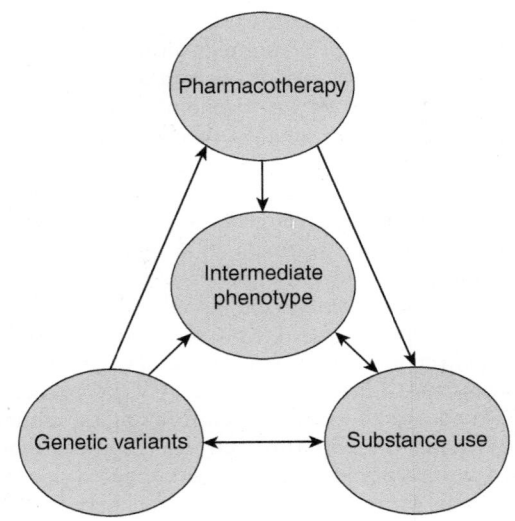

• **Fig. 58.1** An intermediate phenotype-driven pharmacogenetics model for addiction treatment.

to pharmacogenetics research, intermediate or translational phenotypes often involve examining the mechanisms of medication response that go beyond clinical outcomes. Examples of intermediate phenotypes for substance use disorders include craving for a substance, withdrawal mechanisms, substance-induced reward, reinforcing value of the substance, and response inhibition processes, to name a few.

Based on the literature on intermediate phenotypes for addictions and their potential to advance etiologic and treatment approaches to these disorders, a conceptual model that integrates translational addiction phenotypes, genetic factors, and pharmacological treatments for addictions is clearly warranted.[110] In this model, phenotypes, such as subjective responses to alcohol, represent an important translational link between genetic variations and the effects of medications and clinical outcomes. More specifically, this theoretical framework may be used to improve our understanding of pharmacotherapies for addictions in several ways (Fig. 58.1). First, intermediate phenotypes for alcoholism, such as alcohol craving and subjective responses to alcohol, have been shown to predict drinking behavior and the risk for developing alcohol use disorders.[50,53,109,121,137] Second, medications found to operate at the level of intermediate phenotypes, such as craving and subjective responses to alcohol,[92,108] may ultimately be effective in reducing drinking. In a recent example of this approach, a laboratory study found that aripiprazole increased the sedative effects of alcohol and decreased its euphoric and stimulant properties; those effects, in turn, are thought to capture the mechanisms of action of aripiprazole for alcoholism.[74] Third, genetic variants appear to underlie the expression of alcohol phenotypes such as craving[53,88,142] and subjective responses to alcohol.[47,107,122] Fourth, genetic variants associated with alcohol intermediate phenotypes may, in turn, be used to predict responses to pharmacotherapies thought to affect those phenotypes.[53,55,107,108]

In sum, we have proposed that a theory-driven pharmacogenetic approach can be used to enhance the pharmacological treatment of alcoholism.[110] This approach is interdisciplinary and translational by definition, as it integrates aspects of behavioral genetics, pharmacology, and clinical and experimental science. Focusing on theory-driven addiction intermediate phenotypes and the genetic and neurobiological factors underlying these phenotypes may help us elucidate the mechanisms of action of pharmacotherapies, as well as moderators of response. Most importantly, this approach has the potential to enhance the translation of basic science to treatment, as it connects more directly translational phenotypes and genetic variants to pharmacotherapies for addictions. The intermediate phenotype-driven pharmacogenetics model described herein offers a potentially useful framework for better understanding how addiction phenotypes and genetic factors concomitantly influence responses to pharmacotherapies. Similar approaches may be useful in optimizing psychosocial interventions by targeting more specific and narrowly defined components of the risk for substance use disorders (i.e., prevention efforts) or the clinical syndrome itself (i.e., treatment efforts).

Optimizing Psychosocial Treatments Through Genetics

Molecular genetics may also inform psychosocial treatments for substance use disorders. In a recent example of the application of behavioral genetics to optimizing treatment, Bauer and colleagues[7] reported that variation within the *GABRA2* gene, thought to increase the risk for alcoholism,[26] predicted the response to the psychosocial interventions tested in Project MATCH. Specifically, the low-risk allele was associated with more robust differences in drinking outcomes in the trial, enhancing the superiority of 12-step facilitation over cognitive behavioral therapy and motivational enhancement therapy.[7] A recent study examined the DRD4 variable number tandem repeat polymorphism, previously linked to alcohol use and cue reactivity,[53] possibly through an underlying impulsivity phenotype,[27,113] and response to a brief motivational intervention.[30] The findings suggested that heavy-drinking college students who were carriers of the long allele of the DRD4 variable-number tandem-repeat polymorphism were more impulsive and less likely to benefit from the brief motivational intervention for drinking problems. In another study, the 5-HTTLPR polymorphism in the promoter region of the serotonin transporter gene *SLC6A4* was investigated as a moderator of treatment response in problem drinking men who have sex with men.[16] The SS genotype of the *5-HTTLPR* gene has been associated with greater stress[15] and alcohol dependence.[29] A significant interaction was seen such that individuals with the SS risk genotype receiving the modified behavioral self-control therapy, which included a combination of motivational interviewing and cognitive behavioral therapy (CBT), significantly reduced their heavy drinking days compared to individuals who received a minimal treatment intervention.[16] Other risk alleles have also interacted with psychosocial treatments and impacted neural response in adolescents with cannabis use disorder. For example, youth homozygous for the C risk allele of the serotonin 2A receptor gene (5-HT-2A; rs6311) had greater brain activity following the presentation of "change talk" statements in frontal, parietal, and temporo-occipital regions, a finding that was not present in those carrying the T allele.[31] These findings point to the potential underlying mechanisms by which gene-by-psychosocial interactions may be more effective in certain individuals. In another elegant study, the interaction of computerized CBT and the SNP at codon 158 (Val158Met) in the catechol-*O*-methyltransferase (COMT) enzyme, which metabolizes dopamine in the prefrontal cortex, was investigated in cocaine-dependent individuals.[14] As the authors indicate, Val carriers have been shown to be more efficient than Met carriers on cognitive flexibility tasks, which led to the hypothesis that they would benefit more from the

computerized CBT relative to standard treatment. This hypothesis was supported because Val carriers receiving computerized CBT had a greater number of cocaine-abstinent days than patients who received standard treatment.[14] In summary, these results indicate that the assessment of genetic liability may also be important to studies of the efficacy of psychosocial interventions. More broadly, these results allude to the importance of integrating biological and psychosocial variables to capture more fully the clinical phenomenon of addiction and its treatment.

Translating Pharmacogenetic Approaches Into Practice

In anticipation of the translation of pharmacogenetic approaches into practice, issues of physicians' attitudes and training have received recent attention, particularly in the field of cessation of smoking, a highly prevalent chronic condition and public health concern. In a national mailed survey study of 2000 primary care physicians in the United States, the self-reported likelihood that physicians would offer a new test to tailor smoking cessation treatment ranged between 69% and 78% across various scenarios.[126] Describing the test as genetic versus nongenetic decreased the likelihood of physicians offering the test across all scenarios. Moreover, physicians were less likely to offer the test when the scenario indicated that the same genotypes used for treatment tailoring may identify individuals at risk for other conditions (e.g., cocaine or alcohol addiction), differed in allele frequency by race, and may also predict individuals predisposed to become addicted to nicotine.[126] The authors concluded that physicians' responses may reflect an assumption of greater complexity in genetic testing, as compared with other laboratory tests, for example. A broader survey of genetic testing in clinical practice, nonspecific to addictions, revealed that physicians serving minority patients were less likely to use, and refer for, genetic testing in their practice.[123] In short, it has been suggested that several steps are necessary to facilitate the translation of pharmacogenetics science to practice, especially in primary care, including issues such as physicians' training and experience, organizational-level policy, and infrastructure, including reimbursement for pharmacogenetic testing and protections of privacy and against discrimination.[124,125] Those practical and ethical issues warrant further attention, as they are critical to the integration of pharmacogenetic treatment strategies for addiction.

Future Directions of Molecular Genetics and Addiction Treatment

In many ways, the future impact of genetic research on addiction medicine will depend on the substance use disorder in question. For example, there are currently no medications approved for cocaine dependence but a number that have been approved for alcohol dependence. The opportunity to make progress with respect to identifying genetic variation that influences treatment effectiveness for cocaine dependence is limited by the lack of approved medications for cocaine dependence. Additional directions for future research include:

1. There is great need and opportunity to develop robust brain-based translational phenotypes for each substance use disorder, thereby examining specific mechanisms of genetic risk and therapeutics for various substances of abuse.[51] Brain-based translational phenotypes may also be informative in

investigations of pharmacotherapies for addictions as they can advance the knowledge on the neuropharmacological mechanisms of the efficacy of medications as well as help identify genetic factors that may operate at the neural level, leading to differential clinical response to a given pharmacotherapy. A recent example of this was demonstrated in a study by Schacht and colleagues who showed an interaction between naltrexone treatment and A118G and DAT1 genotypes on ventral striatum activation in response to alcohol cues in alcohol-dependent individuals.[120] Therefore, reward processing may be one of the mechanisms by which naltrexone may be effective in individuals who carry particular alleles of the *A118G* and *DAT1* genes. Thus further work examining the interactions between genetic factors and pharmacological treatments as they relate to neural activity is an important avenue of future research.

2. Genome-wide association studies with refined behavioral and brain-based phenotypes are necessary to isolate important sources of genetic variation. These initial findings of genome-wide association studies can lead to more refined genetic analyses, including custom genetic panels designed based on the more consistent findings of genome-wide association studies.

3. Laboratory-based studies of candidate medications using behavioral and brain-based translational phenotypes are needed to inform large-scale clinical trials and address more-specific and mechanistic questions regarding medications' efficacy. Specifically, these phenotypes not only enhance the power to detect genetic effects, they also allow scientists to answer more nuanced questions regarding the pathophysiology of addictive disorders and their pharmacological treatment.[112]

4. According to recent research, genotypes used to tailor the pharmacological treatment of alcohol and nicotine dependence may vary in allele frequencies across populations.[39] For instance, the Asn40Asp allele of the *OPRM1* gene, thought to predict clinical response to naltrexone for the treatment of alcoholism, has a minor allele frequency of approximately 20%–25% in individuals of European ancestry, 50% in Asians, and <5% in African Americans.[5] If treatment recommendations are to be developed based on genetic variants, careful attention to issues of allele frequency across racial and ethnic groups is essential in ensuring that appropriate recommendations are made and that the ethical principle of beneficence is upheld across populations. As discussed by Tate and Goldstein, in order to make medications more inclusive, it is critical that laboratory studies and clinical trials enroll more underrepresented racial and ethnic minority patients, as most studies have largely included individuals of European ancestry.[134] This makes it challenging to know how efficacious medications are for individuals of other ancestries. The goal of precision medicine is to provide the most effective treatments for individuals. Therefore, pharmacotherapeutic medications for alcohol or substance use disorders should be tailored to individuals based on genetic variation in alleles that show the best response to those medications. To provide the best treatment options for patients, it is essential to understand how ancestral background influences treatment response.

5. Clinical scientists need to integrate multiple pieces of information to determine which medications have promise, which genetic variables are likely to predict the effectiveness of those medications, and for which population. Clearly, much work

has yet to be done before these findings are translated into clinical practice.

6. Educating and training physicians to implement pharmacogenetic treatment strategies in clinical practice is critical to the translation of science into practice. As discussed above, much work remains to be done in the area of physicians' training and education before pharmacogenetic findings for addictions can be disseminated into clinical practice.[125,126]

Summary and Conclusions

Translational approaches such as the ones described in this chapter have the potential to inform clinical practice by identifying individuals who are more likely to benefit from a given pharmacotherapy on the basis of genetic factors. At present, efforts at optimizing pharmacotherapy according to genetic factors, often referred to as personalized medicine, remain incipient, and considerable research is required before these findings can be translated into clinical practice. Important issues such as the differential frequency of certain gene variants among various ethnic groups and the clinical significance of these differential treatment responses must be evaluated carefully in future pharmacogenetic trials and before translating these findings to clinical practice. Likewise, because the technology for high-throughput genotyping becomes increasingly accessible, the use of genomic approaches to the study of pharmacotherapy response will become more widespread, hopefully leading to more consistent findings that can be rapidly translated into clinical practice. Limitations notwithstanding, research efforts in pharmacogenetics and pharmacogenomics hold considerable promise for optimizing treatment for a host of medical and psychiatric disorders, including addiction.

References

1. Aitchison KJ, Jordan BD, Sharma T. The relevance of ethnic influences on pharmacogenetics to the treatment of psychosis. *Drug Metabol Drug Interact*. 2000;16(1):15–38.
2. Akrodou YM. CYP2A6 polymorphisms may Strengthen Individualized treatment for nicotine dependence. *Scientifica (Cairo)*. 2015;2015:491514.
3. Alexanderson B. Prediction of steady-state plasma levels of nortriptyline from single oral dose kinetics: a study in twins. *Eur J Clin Pharmacol*. 1973;6(1):44–53.
4. Anton RF, et al. An evaluation of mu-opioid receptor (OPRM1) as a predictor of naltrexone response in the treatment of alcohol dependence: results from the Combined Pharmacotherapies and Behavioral Interventions for Alcohol Dependence (COMBINE) study. *Arch Gen Psychiatry*. 2008;65(2):135–144.
5. Arias AJ, et al. Effects of opioid receptor gene variation on targeted nalmefene treatment in heavy drinkers. *Alcohol Clin Exp Res*. 2008;32(7):1159–1166.
6. Arias AJ, et al. Pharmacogenetics of naltrexone and disulfiram in alcohol dependent, dually diagnosed veterans. *Am J Addict*. 2014;23(3):288–293.
7. Bauer LO, et al. Variation in GABRA2 predicts drinking behavior in project MATCH subjects. *Alcohol Clin Exp Res*. 2007;31(11):1780–1787.
8. Berrettini WH, Lerman CE. Pharmacotherapy and pharmacogenetics of nicotine dependence. *Am J Psychiatry*. 2005;162(8):1441–1451.
9. Bierut LJ, et al. Familial transmission of substance dependence: alcohol, marijuana, cocaine, and habitual smoking: a report from the Collaborative Study on the Genetics of Alcoholism. *Arch Gen Psychiatry*. 1998;55(11):982–9888.

10. Blodgett JC, et al. A meta-analysis of topiramate's effects for individuals with alcohol use disorders. *Alcohol Clin Exp Res.* 2014;38(6):1481–1488.

11. Bond C, et al. Single-nucleotide polymorphism in the human mu opioid receptor gene alters beta-endorphin binding and activity: possible implications for opiate addiction. *Proc Natl Acad Sci U S A.* 1998;95(16):9608–9613.

12. Boomsma DI, et al. Genome-wide association of major depression: description of samples for the GAIN Major Depressive Disorder Study: NTR and NESDA biobank projects. *Eur J Hum Genet.* 2008;16(3):335–342.

13. Brensilver M, Heinzerling KG, Shoptaw S. Pharmacotherapy of amphetamine-type stimulant dependence: an update. *Drug Alcohol Rev.* 2013;32(5):449–460.

14. Carroll KM, et al. Catehol-o-methyltransferase gene Val158met polymorphism as a potential predictor of response to computer-assisted delivery of cognitive-behavioral therapy among cocaine-dependent individuals: preliminary findings from a randomized controlled trial. *Am J Addict.* 2015;24(5):443–451.

15. Caspi A, et al. Influence of life stress on depression: moderation by a polymorphism in the 5-HTT gene. *Science.* 2003;301(5631):386–389.

16. Chen AC, et al. 5-HTTLPR moderates naltrexone and psychosocial treatment responses in heavy drinking men who have sex with men. *Alcohol Clin Exp Res.* 2014;38(9):2362–2368.

17. Chen LS, et al. Pharmacotherapy effects on smoking cessation vary with nicotine metabolism gene (CYP2A6). *Addiction.* 2014;109(1):128–137.

18. Clarke TK, et al. Genetic variation in OPRD1 and the response to treatment for opioid dependence with buprenorphine in European-American females. *Pharmacogenomics J.* 2014;14(3):303–308.

19. Cohen BM, et al. Polymorphisms of the dopamine D4 receptor and response to antipsychotic drugs. *Psychopharmacology (Berl).* 1999;141(1):6–10.

20. Coller JK, et al. Inhibition of CYP2D6-mediated tramadol O-demethylation in methadone but not buprenorphine maintenance patients. *Br J Clin Pharmacol.* 2012;74(5):835–841.

21. Craddock N, O'Donovan MC, Owen MJ. Genome-wide association studies in psychiatry: lessons from early studies of non-psychiatric and psychiatric phenotypes. *Mol Psychiatry.* 2008;13(7):649–653.

22. Crist RC, et al. An intronic variant in OPRD1 predicts treatment outcome for opioid dependence in African-Americans. *Neuropsychopharmacology.* 2013;38(10):2003–2010.

23. de Cid R, et al. BDNF variability in opioid addicts and response to methadone treatment: preliminary findings. *Genes Brain Behav.* 2008;7(5):515–522.

24. Dole VP, Nyswander ME. Rehabilitation of heroin addicts after blockade with methadone. *N Y State J Med.* 1966;66(15):2011–2017.

25. Ducci F, Goldman D. Genetic approaches to addiction: genes and alcohol. *Addiction.* 2008;103(9):1414–1428.

26. Edenberg HJ, et al. Variations in GABRA2, encoding the alpha 2 subunit of the GABA(A) receptor, are associated with alcohol dependence and with brain oscillations. *Am J Hum Genet.* 2004;74(4):705–714.

27. Eisenberg DT, et al. Examining impulsivity as an endophenotype using a behavioral approach: a DRD2 TaqI A and DRD4 48-bp VNTR association study. *Behav Brain Funct.* 2007;3:2.

28. Evans WE, Johnson JA. Pharmacogenomics: the inherited basis for interindividual differences in drug response. *Annu Rev Genomics Hum Genet.* 2001;2:9–39.

29. Feinn R, Nellissery M, Kranzler HR. Meta-analysis of the association of a functional serotonin transporter promoter polymorphism with alcohol dependence. *Am J Med Genet B Neuropsychiatr Genet.* 2005;133B(1):79–84.

30. Feldstein Ewing SW, et al. Do genetic and individual risk factors moderate the efficacy of motivational enhancement therapy? Drinking outcomes with an emerging adult sample. *Addict Biol.* 2009;14(3):356–365.

31. Feldstein Ewing SW, et al. A preliminary examination of how serotonergic polymorphisms influence brain response following an adolescent cannabis intervention. *Psychiatry Res.* 2012;204(2–3):112–116.

32. Feng Y, et al. A common haplotype of the nicotine acetylcholine receptor alpha 4 subunit gene is associated with vulnerability to nicotine addiction in men. *Am J Hum Genet.* 2004;75(1):112–121.

33. Ferreira MA, et al. Collaborative genome-wide association analysis supports a role for ANK3 and CACNA1C in bipolar disorder. *Nat Genet.* 2008;40(9):1056–1058.

34. Filbey FM, et al. Differential neural response to alcohol priming and alcohol taste cues is associated with DRD4 VNTR and OPRM1 genotypes. *Alcohol Clin Exp Res.* 2008;32(7):1113–1123.

35. Frackiewicz EJ, et al. Ethnicity and antipsychotic response. *Ann Pharmacother.* 1997;31(11):1360–1369.

36. Frazer KA, et al. A second generation human haplotype map of over 3.1 million SNPs. *Nature.* 2007;449(7164):851–861.

37. Gaval-Cruz M, Weinshenker D. Mechanisms of disulfiram-induced cocaine abstinence: antabuse and cocaine relapse. *Mol Interv.* 2009;9(4):175–187.

38. Gelernter J, et al. Opioid receptor gene (OPRM1, OPRK1, and OPRD1) variants and response to naltrexone treatment for alcohol dependence: results from the VA Cooperative Study. *Alcohol Clin Exp Res.* 2007;31(4):555–563.

39. Goldstein DB, Tate SK, Sisodiya SM. Pharmacogenetics goes genomic. *Nat Rev Genet.* 2003;4(12):937–947.

40. Gordis E. Contributions of behavioral science to alcohol research: understanding who is at risk and why. *Exp Clin Psychopharmacol.* 2000;8(3):264–270.

41. Gottesman II , Gould TD. The endophenotype concept in psychiatry: etymology and strategic intentions. *Am J Psychiatry.* 2003;160(4):636–645.

42. Gould TD, Gottesman II. Psychiatric endophenotypes and the development of valid animal models. *Genes Brain Behav.* 2006;5(2):113–119.

43. Grove WM, et al. Heritability of substance abuse and antisocial behavior: a study of monozygotic twins reared apart. *Biol Psychiatry.* 1990;27(12):1293–1304.

44. Gynther LM, et al. A twin study of non-alcohol substance abuse. *Psychiatry Res.* 1995;56(3):213–220.

45. Haile CN, Kosten TA, Kosten TR. Pharmacogenetic treatments for drug addiction: alcohol and opiates. *Am J Drug Alcohol Abuse.* 2008;34(4):355–381.

46. Hammer W, Sjoqvist F. Plasma levels of monomethylated tricyclic antidepressants during treatment with imipramine-like compounds. *Life Sci.* 1967;6(17):1895–1903.

47. Haughey HM, et al. Human gamma-aminobutyric acid A receptor alpha2 gene moderates the acute effects of alcohol and brain mRNA expression. *Genes Brain Behav.* 2008;7(4):447–454.

48. Heils A, et al. Allelic variation of human serotonin transporter gene expression. *J Neurochem.* 1996;66(6):2621–2624.

49. Hernandez-Avila CA, et al. Population-specific effects of the Asn40Asp polymorphism at the mu-opioid receptor gene (OPRM1) on HPA-axis activation. *Pharmacogenet Genomics.* 2007;17(12):1031–1038.

50. Hines LM, et al. Alcoholism: the dissection for endophenotypes. *Dialogues Clin Neurosci.* 2005;7(2):153–163.

51. Hutchison KE. Alcohol dependence: neuroimaging and the development of translational phenotypes. *Alcohol Clin Exp Res.* 2008;32(7):1111–1112.

52. Hutchison KE, et al. Olanzapine reduces urge to drink after drinking cues and a priming dose of alcohol. *Psychopharmacology (Berl).* 2001;155(1):27–34.

53. Hutchison KE, et al. The DRD4 VNTR polymorphism moderates craving after alcohol consumption. *Health Psychol.* 2002;21(2):139–146.

54. Hutchison KE, et al. Olanzapine reduces craving for alcohol: a DRD4 VNTR polymorphism by pharmacotherapy interaction. *Neuropsychopharmacology.* 2003;28(10):1882–1888.

55. Hutchison KE, et al. The effect of olanzapine on craving and alcohol consumption. *Neuropsychopharmacology.* 2006;31(6):1310–1317.

56. Hutchison KE, et al. CHRNA4 and tobacco dependence: from gene regulation to treatment outcome. *Arch Gen Psychiatry.* 2007;64(9):1078–1086.

57. Hwang R, et al. Dopamine D4 and D5 receptor gene variant effects on clozapine response in schizophrenia: replication and exploration. *Prog Neuropsychopharmacol Biol Psychiatry.* 2012;37(1):62–75.

58. International HC. A haplotype map of the human genome. *Nature.* 2005;437(7063):1299–1320.

59. Johnson BA, et al. Topiramate's effects on cocaine-induced subjective mood, craving and preference for money over drug taking. *Addict Biol.* 2013;18(3):405–416.

60. Johnstone EC, et al. Genetic variation in dopaminergic pathways and short-term effectiveness of the nicotine patch. *Pharmacogenetics.* 2004;14(2):83–90.

61. Kampman KM, et al. A double-blind, placebo-controlled trial of topiramate for the treatment of comorbid cocaine and alcohol dependence. *Drug Alcohol Depend.* 2013;133(1):94–99.

62. Karila L, et al. New treatments for cocaine dependence: a focused review. *Int J Neuropsychopharmacol.* 2008;11(3):425–438.

63. Kaufmann A, et al. Rate of nicotine metabolism and smoking cessation outcomes in a community-based sample of treatment-seeking smokers. *Addict Behav.* 2015;51:93–99.

64. Kendler KS, Prescott CA. Cannabis use, abuse, and dependence in a population-based sample of female twins. *Am J Psychiatry.* 1998;155(8):1016–1022.

65. Kendler KS, Prescott CA. Cocaine use, abuse and dependence in a population-based sample of female twins. *Br J Psychiatry.* 1998;173:345–350.

66. Kendler KS, Thornton LM, Pedersen NL. Tobacco consumption in Swedish twins reared apart and reared together. *Arch Gen Psychiatry.* 2000;57(9):886–892.

67. Kendler KS, et al. A twin-family study of alcoholism in women. *Am J Psychiatry.* 1994;151(5):707–715.

68. Kendler KS, et al. The structure of genetic and environmental risk factors for common psychiatric and substance use disorders in men and women. *Arch Gen Psychiatry.* 2003;60(9):929–937.

69. Kim SG, et al. A micro opioid receptor gene polymorphism (A118G) and naltrexone treatment response in adherent Korean alcohol-dependent patients. *Psychopharmacology (Berl).* 2009;201(4):611–618.

70. Kim SG, et al. Association of functional opioid receptor genotypes with alcohol dependence in Koreans. *Alcohol Clin Exp Res.* 2004;28(7):986–990.

71. Kirchheiner J, et al. Pharmacogenetics of antidepressants and antipsychotics: the contribution of allelic variations to the phenotype of drug response. *Mol Psychiatry.* 2004;9(5):442–473.

72. Kosten TR, et al. DBH gene as predictor of response in a cocaine vaccine clinical trial. *Neurosci Lett.* 2013;541:29–33.

73. Kosten TR, et al. Pharmacogenetic randomized trial for cocaine abuse: disulfiram and dopamine beta-hydroxylase. *Biol Psychiatry.* 2013;73(3):219–224.

74. Kranzler HR, et al. Effects of aripiprazole on subjective and physiological responses to alcohol. *Alcohol Clin Exp Res.* 2008;32(4):573–579.

75. Kranzler HR, et al. GRIK1 genotype moderates topiramate's effects on daily drinking level, expectations of alcohol's positive effects and desire to drink. *Int J Neuropsychopharmacol.* 2014;17(10):1549–1556.

76. Kranzler HR, et al. GRIK1 genotype and daily expectations of alcohol's positive effects moderate the reduction of heavy drinking by topiramate. *Exp Clin Psychopharmacol.* 2014;22(6):494–501.

77. Kranzler HR, et al. Topiramate treatment for heavy drinkers: moderation by a GRIK1 polymorphism. *Am J Psychiatry.* 2014;171(4):445–452.

78. Kreek MJ, Vocci FJ. History and current status of opioid maintenance treatments: blending conference session. *J Subst Abuse Treat.* 2002;23(2):93–105.

79. Lerman C, et al. Individualizing nicotine replacement therapy for the treatment of tobacco dependence: a randomized trial. *Ann Intern Med.* 2004;140(6):426–433.

80. Lerman C, et al. The functional mu opioid receptor (OPRM1) Asn40Asp variant predicts short-term response to nicotine replacement therapy in a clinical trial. *Pharmacogenomics J.* 2004;4(3):184–192.

81. Lerman C, et al. Nicotine metabolite ratio predicts efficacy of transdermal nicotine for smoking cessation. *Clin Pharmacol Ther.* 2006;79(6):600–608.

82. Lerman C, et al. Role of functional genetic variation in the dopamine D2 receptor (DRD2) in response to bupropion and nicotine replacement therapy for tobacco dependence: results of two randomized clinical trials. *Neuropsychopharmacology.* 2006;31(1):231–242.

83. Lerman C, et al. Genetic variation in nicotine metabolism predicts the efficacy of extended-duration transdermal nicotine therapy. *Clin Pharmacol Ther.* 2010;87(5):553–557.

84. Li MD, et al. Ethnic- and gender-specific association of the nicotinic acetylcholine receptor alpha4 subunit gene (CHRNA4) with nicotine dependence. *Hum Mol Genet.* 2005;14(9):1211–1219.

85. Li Q, et al. Relationship of CYP2D6 genetic polymorphisms and the pharmacokinetics of tramadol in Chinese volunteers. *J Clin Pharm Ther.* 2010;35(2):239–247.

86. Lin E, et al. Pattern-recognition techniques with haplotype analysis in pharmacogenomics. *Pharmacogenomics.* 2007;8(1):75–83.

87. Littlewood RA, et al. Dose specific effects of olanzapine in the treatment of alcohol dependence. *Psychopharmacology (Berl).* 2015;232(7):1261–1268.

88. Mackillop J, et al. Effects of craving and DRD4 VNTR genotype on the relative value of alcohol: an initial human laboratory study. *Behav Brain Funct.* 2007;3:11.

89. Malaiyandi V, et al. Impact of CYP2A6 genotype on pretreatment smoking behaviour and nicotine levels from and usage of nicotine replacement therapy. *Mol Psychiatry.* 2006;11(4):400–409.

90. Mattick RP, et al. Buprenorphine maintenance versus placebo or methadone maintenance for opioid dependence. *Cochrane Database Syst Rev.* 2004;(3):CD002207.

91. McLeod HL, Evans WE. Pharmacogenomics: unlocking the human genome for better drug therapy. *Annu Rev Pharmacol Toxicol.* 2001;41:101–121.

92. Monti PM, et al. Naltrexone and cue exposure with coping and communication skills training for alcoholics: treatment process and 1-year outcomes. *Alcohol Clin Exp Res.* 2001;25(11):1634–1647.

93. Munafo MR, et al. Pharmacogenetics and nicotine addiction treatment. *Pharmacogenomics.* 2005;6(3):211–223.

94. Munafo MR, et al. Lack of association of 5-HTTLPR genotype with smoking cessation in a nicotine replacement therapy randomized trial. *Cancer Epidemiol Biomarkers Prev.* 2006;15(2):398–400.

95. Nielsen DA, Hamon SC, Kosten TR. The kappa-opioid receptor gene as a predictor of response in a cocaine vaccine clinical trial. *Psychiatr Genet.* 2013;23(6):225–232.

96. O'Donovan MC, et al. Identification of loci associated with schizophrenia by genome-wide association and follow-up. *Nat Genet.* 2008;40(9):1053–1055.

97. Oliveto A, et al. Randomized, double blind, placebo-controlled trial of disulfiram for the treatment of cocaine dependence in methadone-stabilized patients. *Drug Alcohol Depend.* 2011;113(2–3):184–191.

98. Oslin DW, et al. A functional polymorphism of the mu-opioid receptor gene is associated with naltrexone response in alcohol-dependent patients. *Neuropsychopharmacology.* 2003;28(8):1546–1552.

99. Oslin DW, et al. Naltrexone vs placebo for the treatment of alcohol dependence: a randomized clinical trial. *JAMA Psychiatry*. 2015;72(5):430–437.

100. Ozaki S, et al. Smoking cessation program and CYP2A6 polymorphism. *Front Biosci*. 2006;11:2590–2597.

101. Pai P, et al. Association of GRIN1, ABCB1, and DRD4 genes and response to antipsychotic drug treatment in schizophrenia. *Psychiatr Genet*. 2015;25(3):135–136.

102. Pearson TA, Manolio TA. How to interpret a genome-wide association study. *J Am Med Assoc*. 2008;299(11):1335–1344.

103. Perez de los Cobos J, et al. Association of CYP2D6 ultrarapid metabolizer genotype with deficient patient satisfaction regarding methadone maintenance treatment. *Drug Alcohol Depend*. 2007;89(2–3):190–194.

104. Petrakis IL, et al. Disulfiram treatment for cocaine dependence in methadone-maintained opioid addicts. *Addiction*. 2000;95(2):219–228.

105. Poulsen L, et al. Codeine and morphine in extensive and poor metabolizers of sparteine: pharmacokinetics, analgesic effect and side effects. *Eur J Clin Pharmacol*. 1996;51(3–4):289–295.

106. Rausch JL, et al. Initial conditions of serotonin transporter kinetics and genotype: influence on SSRI treatment trial outcome. *Biol Psychiatry*. 2002;51(9):723–732.

107. Ray LA, Hutchison KE. A polymorphism of the mu-opioid receptor gene (OPRM1) and sensitivity to the effects of alcohol in humans. *Alcohol Clin Exp Res*. 2004;28(12):1789–1795.

108. Ray LA, Hutchison KE. Effects of naltrexone on alcohol sensitivity and genetic moderators of medication response: a double-blind placebo-controlled study. *Arch Gen Psychiatry*. 2007;64(9):1069–1077.

109. Ray LA, Hutchison KE, Bryan A. Psychosocial predictors of treatment outcome, dropout, and change processes in a pharmacological clinical trial for alcohol dependence. *Addictive Disorders Treat*. 2006;5(4):179–190.

110. Ray LA, Mackillop J, Monti PM. Subjective responses to alcohol consumption as endophenotypes: advancing behavioral genetics in etiological and treatment models of alcoholism. *Subst Use Misuse*. 2010;45(11):1742–1765.

111. Ray LA, Meskew-Stacer S, Hutchison KE. The relationship between prospective self-rating of alcohol sensitivity and craving and experimental results from two alcohol challenge studies. *J Stud Alcohol Drugs*. 2007;68(3):379–384.

112. Ray LA, et al. Effects of naltrexone on cortisol levels in heavy drinkers. *Pharmacol Biochem Behav*. 2009;91(4):489–494.

113. Ray LA, et al. The dopamine D Receptor (DRD4) gene exon III polymorphism, problematic alcohol use and novelty seeking: direct and mediated genetic effects. *Addict Biol*. 2009;14(2):238–244.

114. Ray LA, et al. A preliminary pharmacogenetic investigation of adverse events from topiramate in heavy drinkers. *Exp Clin Psychopharmacol*. 2009;17(2):122–129.

115. Ray LA, et al. Pharmacogenetics of naltrexone in asian americans: a randomized placebo-controlled laboratory study. *Neuropsychopharmacology*. 2012;37(2):445–455.

116. Ray R, Schnoll RA, Lerman C. Pharmacogenetics and smoking cessation with nicotine replacement therapy. *CNS Drugs*. 2007;21(7):525–533.

117. Ray R, et al. Association of OPRM1 A118G variant with the relative reinforcing value of nicotine. *Psychopharmacology (Berl)*. 2006;188(3):355–363.

118. Rioux PP. Clinical trials in pharmacogenetics and pharmacogenomics: methods and applications. *Am J Health Syst Pharm*. 2000;57(9):887–898; quiz 899–901.

119. Rocha Santos J, et al. CHRNA4 rs1044396 is associated with smoking cessation in varenicline therapy. *Front Genet*. 2015;6:46.

120. Schacht JP, et al. Interacting effects of naltrexone and OPRM1 and DAT1 variation on the neural response to alcohol cues. *Neuropsychopharmacology*. 2013;38(3):414–422.

121. Schuckit MA, Smith TL. An 8-year follow-up of 450 sons of alcoholic and control subjects. *Arch Gen Psychiatry*. 1996;53(3):202–210.

122. Schuckit MA, Smith TL, Kalmijn J. The search for genes contributing to the low level of response to alcohol: patterns of findings across studies. *Alcohol Clin Exp Res*. 2004;28(10):1449–1458.

123. Shields AE, Burke W, Levy DE. Differential use of available genetic tests among primary care physicians in the United States: results of a national survey. *Genet Med*. 2008;10(6):404–414.

124. Shields AE, Lerman C. Anticipating clinical integration of pharmacogenetic treatment strategies for addiction: are primary care physicians ready? *Clin Pharmacol Ther*. 2008;83(4):635–639.

125. Shields AE, et al. Barriers to translating emerging genetic research on smoking into clinical practice. Perspectives of primary care physicians. *J Gen Intern Med*. 2005;20(2):131–138.

126. Shields AE, et al. Primary care physicians' willingness to offer a new genetic test to tailor smoking treatment, according to test characteristics. *Nicotine Tob Res*. 2008;10(6):1037–1045.

127. Shorter D, Domingo CB, Kosten TR. Emerging drugs for the treatment of cocaine use disorder: a review of neurobiological targets and pharmacotherapy. *Expert Opin Emerg Drugs*. 2015;20(1):15–29.

128. Shorter D, Kosten TR. Novel pharmacotherapeutic treatments for cocaine addiction. *BMC Med*. 2011;9:119.

129. Shorter D, et al. Pharmacogenetic randomized trial for cocaine abuse: disulfiram and alpha1A-adrenoceptor gene variation. *Eur Neuropsychopharmacol*. 2013;23(11):1401–1407.

130. Siniscalchi A, et al. The role of topiramate in the management of cocaine addiction: a possible therapeutic option. *Curr Neuropharmacol*. 2015;13(6):815–818.

131. Smeraldi E, et al. Polymorphism within the promoter of the serotonin transporter gene and antidepressant efficacy of fluvoxamine. *Mol Psychiatry*. 1998;3(6):508–511.

132. Spellicy CJ, et al. The MTHFR C677T variant is associated with responsiveness to disulfiram treatment for cocaine dependency. *Front Psychiatry*. 2012;3:109.

133. Spellicy CJ, et al. ANKK1 and DRD2 pharmacogenetics of disulfiram treatment for cocaine abuse. *Pharmacogenet Genomics*. 2013;23(7):333–340.

134. Tate SK, Goldstein DB. Will tomorrow's medicines work for everyone? *Nat Genet*. 2004;36(suppl 11):S34–S42.

135. Teo YY. Common statistical issues in genome-wide association studies: a review on power, data quality control, genotype calling and population structure. *Curr Opin Lipidol*. 2008;19(2):133–143.

136. The International HapMap Project. *Nature*. 2003;426(6968):789–796.

137. Tidey JW, et al. Moderators of naltrexone's effects on drinking, urge, and alcohol effects in non-treatment-seeking heavy drinkers in the natural environment. *Alcohol Clin Exp Res*. 2008;32(1):58–66.

138. Tsuang MT, et al. Genetic influences on DSM-III-R drug abuse and dependence: a study of 3,372 twin pairs. *Am J Med Genet*. 1996;67(5):473–477.

139. Tsuang MT, et al. Co-occurrence of abuse of different drugs in men: the role of drug-specific and shared vulnerabilities. *Arch Gen Psychiatry*. 1998;55(11):967–972.

140. Tyndale RF, Droll KP, Sellers EM. Genetically deficient CYP2D6 metabolism provides protection against oral opiate dependence. *Pharmacogenetics*. 1997;7(5):375–379.

141. Uhl GR, et al. Molecular genetics of successful smoking cessation: convergent genome-wide association study results. *Arch Gen Psychiatry*. 2008;65(6):683–693.

142. van den Wildenberg E, et al. A functional polymorphism of the mu-opioid receptor gene (OPRM1) influences cue-induced craving for alcohol in male heavy drinkers. *Alcohol Clin Exp Res*. 2007;31(1):1–10.

143. Verde Z, et al. Are serotonergic system genes associated to smoking cessation therapy success in addition to CYP2A6? *Pharmacopsychiatry.* 2014;47(1):33–36.

144. Vogel F. Moderne probleme der humangenetik. *Ergeb Inn Med U Kinderheilkd.* 1959;12:52–125.

145. Vojvoda D, et al. Monozygotic twins concordant for response to clozapine. *Lancet.* 1996;347(8993):61.

146. Wu X, et al. The impact of CYP2D6 polymorphisms on the pharmacokinetics of codeine and its metabolites in Mongolian Chinese subjects. *Eur J Clin Pharmacol.* 2014;70(1):57–63.

147. Zanardi R, et al. Efficacy of paroxetine in depression is influenced by a functional polymorphism within the promoter of the serotonin transporter gene. *J Clin Psychopharmacol.* 2000;20(1):105–107.

59

Physical Considerations for Treatment Complications of Alcohol and Drug Use and Misuse

GIOVANNI ADDOLORATO, ANTONIO MIRIJELLO, GABRIELE ANGELO VASSALLO,
CRISTINA D'ANGELO, ANNA FERRULLI, MARIANGELA ANTONELLI, FABIO CAPUTO,
CAROLINA MOSONI, CLAUDIA TARLI, MARIA MARGHERITA RANDO, LUISA SESTITO,
TOMMASO DIONISI, LORENZO LEGGIO, AND ANTONIO GASBARRINI

CHAPTER OUTLINE

Introduction

The effects of chronic ingestion of alcohol and other substances of abuse vary considerably and depend on the concentration and dose, together with various other factors, such as nutritional status, gender, and ethnicity. The present chapter analyzes the main medical consequences related to substance abuse, particularly abuse of alcohol, nicotine, opioids, cocaine, amphetamine, and benzodiazepines. The effects of these substances on the liver, gut, pancreas, nervous system, cardiovascular system, and endocrine system will

TABLE 59.1	Main Hepatic Features in Subjects With Substance Abuse or Dependence	
Substance	Main Feature(s)	Other Feature(s)
Alcohol	Enzyme induction; steatosis	Chronic liver disease; acute liver failure; liver cirrhosis
Nicotine	Enzyme induction	Risk factor for: gallstones; PSC; HCC
Opioids	Hepatotoxicity	High risk factor for hepatitis viruses, especially HCV
Cocaine	Hepatotoxicity	Impaired hepatic perfusion
Amphetamine	Hepatotoxicity	Chronic liver disease; acute liver failure
Benzodiazepines	Enzyme induction	Hepatotoxicity

HCC, Hepatocellular carcinoma; *HCV*, hepatitis C virus; *PSC*, primary sclerosing cholangitis.

be discussed. The link between substance abuse disorders and tumors will also be reported, as well as the relationship between substances of abuse and nutrition and body composition.

Liver

Alcohol

Alcoholic liver disease is one of the major medical complications of alcohol abuse.[259] In particular, 80% of heavy drinkers develop steatosis, 10%–35% develop alcoholic hepatitis, and approximately 10% will develop cirrhosis.[259] Steatosis represents an abnormal retention of lipids accumulated in vesicles that displace the cytoplasm of the hepatocytes. Although liver function is usually normal, if alcohol abuse continues, steatosis may progress to cirrhosis[259] (Table 59.1).

It has been suggested that 15–20 years of alcohol abuse are necessary to develop alcoholic hepatitis, which usually results in cholestasis.[259] When alcohol abuse is persistent for a long period and generally follows a regular pattern, an individual can often develop cirrhosis. Alcoholic liver disease represents the most common cause of liver cirrhosis in the Western world.[242,245] Liver damage is related to the toxicity of alcohol being linked to its metabolism via alcohol dehydrogenase. Alcohol dehydrogenase converts nicotinamide adenine dinucleotide to nicotinamide adenine dinucleotide-reduced form, which contributes to hyperuricemia, hypoglycemia, and hepatic steatosis by inhibiting lipid oxidation and promoting lipogenesis.[150] Another pathway of ethanol metabolism is the microsomal ethanol oxidizing system. The activity of its main enzyme, cytochrome P450 2E1 (CYP2E1), and its gene are increased by chronic consumption, resulting in metabolic tolerance to ethanol.[150] The activity of CYP2E1 is also associated with the generation of free radicals, with resulting lipid peroxidation and membrane damage as well as depletion of mitochondrial reduced glutathione and its ultimate precursor—methionine activated to *S*-adenosyl-*L*-methionine.[150] The involvement of free radical mechanisms in the pathogenesis of alcoholic liver disease is demonstrated by the detection of lipid peroxidation markers in the liver and the serum of alcohol-dependent individuals, as well as by experiments in alcohol-fed rodents that show a relationship

between alcohol-induced oxidative stress and the development of liver pathology.[11,16,24] In particular, oxidative stress promotes hepatocyte necrosis as well as a pro-apoptotic action via tumor necrosis factor-alpha. Furthermore, oxidative mechanisms can contribute to liver fibrosis by triggering the release of profibrotic cytokines and collagen gene expression in hepatic stellate cells.[24]

In the last years, growing evidence has suggested the role of gut microbiota in the pathogenesis of alcoholic liver disease. The dysbiosis related to chronic alcohol consumption may induce intestinal mucosal inflammation and increased gut permeability with bacterial translocation to portal blood. The exposure of liver parenchyma to lipopolysaccharides and other products of bacterial wall stimulates innate immune receptors, such as Toll-like receptors and CD14, which activate hepatic stellate and Kupffer cells, releasing proinflammatory mediators that ultimately contribute to liver damage. Quantitative and qualitative microbiota alterations contribute to hepatocyte injury, already damaged by chronic alcohol exposure.[253]

From a clinical point of view, alcohol-related damage can be present without any apparent symptoms or signs of liver disease. Otherwise, nonspecific clinical features can include nausea, vomiting, or fatigue. When liver cirrhosis is present, typical cirrhosis-related signs and symptoms can include jaundice, ascites, encephalopathy, or upper gastrointestinal bleeding.

Alcoholic hepatitis (AH) is a clinical syndrome characterized by rapid onset of jaundice and liver failure that occurs in patients with chronic alcohol abuse. The histological picture consists of ballooned hepatocytes, Mallory bodies, and lobular neutrophils. Common signs and symptoms include encephalopathy, fever, ascites, and proximal muscle loss; typically, the liver is enlarged and tender.[154]

In its milder forms, alcohol abstinence is sufficient for clinical recovery. Severe forms of AH characterized by a Maddrey discriminant function >32, could benefit from the anti-inflammatory effect of corticosteroids or pentoxifylline.[79] However, despite a number of trials and meta-analyses encouraging their use, their efficacy has recently been questioned by a recent randomized controlled trial (RCT) that failed to demonstrate any significant improvement in long-term survival.[241]

Thus absolute alcohol abstinence together with supportive treatment remains the cornerstone of treatment. Recently, early liver transplantation (orthotopic liver transplantation [OLTx]) approach has been tested in AH patients with a first episode of severe alcoholic hepatitis not responding to medical therapy. Early OLTx showed to improve long-term survival in this subset of patients.[161]

The treatment of patients with alcohol-related cirrhosis is mainly symptomatic and no other therapies are currently available. Recently, several drugs have been tested to improve survival in patients with alcohol-related cirrhosis, including antioxidants, metadoxine, therapeutic modulation of gut microbiota, nutritional support, and phosphatidylcholine. However, although some drugs have shown to be promising, none has shown a survival improvement in these clusters of patients.[17]

OLTx represents an option when liver cirrhosis is present. Survival after a liver transplantation for alcoholic cirrhosis is similar to—or even better than—that for other end-stage liver diseases.[242,259] However, several ethical concerns are still present due to the limited availability of liver donors and the risk of relapse after transplantation.[242,259] A 6-month abstinence period before listing patients is recommended to prevent unnecessary liver transplantation in patients who will spontaneously recover.[79] However, when medical urgency does not allow a 6-month waiting time (e.g., AH or severely decompensated ESLD) an urgent OLTx evaluation may proceed in selected patients.[2,161]

Independently of stage of disease, abstinence from alcohol is the cornerstone of management. Accordingly, total alcohol abstinence can improve the histology and/or survival of individuals with alcoholic liver disease[242] and the clinical outcome of all stages of alcoholic liver disease.[74] Persistent alcohol intake in patients with alcoholic cirrhosis is associated with a significant risk ratio of death[195] due to bleeding esophageal varices, infection, renal failure, and/or hepatic failure.[266] In recent decades, several medications able to reduce alcohol craving and, consequently, to increase abstinence and prevent alcohol relapse have been evaluated.[1,12] Anticraving drugs approved by National Medical Agency are naltrexone, nalmefene, acamprosate, sodium oxybate, and baclofen. Among them, baclofen represents the only anticraving medication formally tested in an RCT involving patients with alcohol use disorder (AUD) with advanced liver disease.[13,14,92] For this reason, this medication has been included in the European[79] and American[28,210] Clinical Practice Guidelines for the treatment of alcoholic liver disease.

Nicotine

Several preclinical studies suggest an influence of nicotine on the hepatic enzymatic systems. For example, the chronic exposure of rats to cigarette smoke does not alter hepatic biotransformation processes.[101]

However, in a rat model of cirrhosis, a reduction of nicotine metabolism has been observed and linked to the decreases in CYP and flavin-containing mono-oxygenase protein expression levels.[181] Clinical studies have often been performed considering both smoking and alcohol consumption. Whitehead et al.[261] evaluated a large population of 46,775 men and showed a joint effect of cigarette smoking and alcohol consumption in increasing the levels of γ-glutamyl transferase, whereas alcohol but not cigarette smoking was related to an increase of transaminases.[261] In other words, nicotine can modify the hepatic enzymatic system but not induce liver damage. Consistently, smoking does not appear to be a risk factor for cirrhosis of the liver.[31] On the other hand, a link between smoking and hepatocellular carcinoma has been suggested because constituents of cigarette smoke are hepatic carcinogens in animals.[269] Cigarette smoking has been suggested as an important risk factor for primary sclerosing cholangitis and gallstones, although in the latter case other cofactors should be taken into account, such as gender, alcohol consumption, and overweight.[31] Finally, there is growing interest in the role of nicotine in those individuals with liver disease who are undergoing surgical procedures, particularly OLTx. In one study,[77] 60% of OLTx recipients reported a lifetime history of smoking, with 15% reporting smoking post-OLTx. Of smokers who quit before OLTx, 20% reported relapse to smoking post-OLTx. This observation has been subsequently confirmed by DiMartini and colleagues,[75] who showed that individuals with alcoholic liver disease resume smoking early post-OLTx, increase their consumption over time, and quickly become tobacco dependent. Moreover, there is growing evidence that smoking cigarettes after liver transplantation is associated with a higher risk to develop de novo malignancies, particularly of the gastrointestinal and respiratory tracts.[46]

Opioids

Preclinical studies show that opioid substances, such as morphine, heroin, meperidine, and methadone at therapeutic doses, do not usually produce irreversible damage to human hepatocytes, whereas opiate doses during tolerance or abuse may be a cause of liver dysfunction.[99] However, it has also been noted that chronic use at therapeutic doses of opioids such as tramadol and, most of all, morphine for the management of chronic pain, increases liver damage via oxidative stress and induction of apoptosis.[193] Consistent with the preclinical findings, intravenous drug abusers are commonly found to have altered transaminases.[260] However, from a clinical perspective, the most important implications of opioid abuse and dependence are related to the high prevalence of hepatitis infection. In fact, over 90% of intravenous heroin addicts carry the hepatitis C virus.[236] Accordingly, a hepatitis C virus–related elevation of the liver enzyme can be present, along with several stages of liver damage leading to cirrhosis.[236] Furthermore, several extrahepatic clinical features can be present (e.g., immune suppression, collagen diseases, lymphoma, and leukemia) and included in the so-called hepatitis C virus syndrome.[236] The hepatitis B virus may hold a similar chronic and degenerative course.[236]

Finally, in patients with advanced liver disease, opioid administration could precipitate hepatic encephalopathy. Thus opioids should be used cautiously or possibly avoided in these patients.[94]

Cocaine

Animal data show cocaine-induced liver damage including periportal and portal damage and elevated transaminases.[200] In subjects using cocaine, acute hepatotoxicity and hepatocellular necrosis have been described,[100] perhaps via oxidative stress.[220] However, because cocaine is a sympathomimetic agent it could lead to acute ischemic hepatocellular injury or hypoxic hepatitis as a consequence of impaired hepatic perfusion.[38] Of interest, the concurrent use of cocaine and alcohol produces another psychoactive substance called cocaethylene and can induce significant liver damage.[29]

Amphetamine

Methylenedioxymethamphetamine (ecstasy) and amphetamine abuse can be associated with serious liver clinical features. Intoxication with amphetamine or methylenedioxymethamphetamine can be associated with severe hepatotoxicity[124] as a consequence of ischemic hepatocellular injury.[38] In addition, chronic abuse of amphetamines/methylenedioxymethamphetamine can be associated with either subclinical liver damage[127] or cholestatic chronic liver damage.[124] Histological features include confluent necrosis and ballooning degeneration in centrilobular zones.[127] The use of steroids has been suggested according to a possible immune-mediated component of amphetamine-related hepatic damage, whereas the benefit/risk ratio of OLTx for fulminant hepatic failure is still controversial.[124]

Benzodiazepines

Liver alterations can be present in individuals who are abusing benzodiazepines, especially those with a liver metabolism like diazepam and chlordiazepoxide. Subjects with benzodiazepine abuse or dependence can present with an increase of γ-glutamyl transferase, reflecting the chronic enzymatic induction.[113] With a much lower frequency, benzodiazepines such as diazepam and chlordiazepoxide can induce cholestatic hepatotoxicity by a hypersensitivity mechanism.[220] Both these drugs and other long-acting benzodiazepines with hepatic metabolism could cause excess of sedation in patients with advanced liver disease.[172] Moreover, in these patients, all classes of benzodiazepines could precipitate or aggravate hepatic encephalopathy.[13,79] Furthermore, the use of benzodiazepines needs to be evaluated carefully in those alcohol-dependent individuals with liver damage, taking into account the possibilities of both dual substance abuse (alcohol and benzodiazepines) and the need to administer benzodiazepines to treat alcohol withdrawal symptoms.

Gut and Pancreas

Alcohol

The effects of alcohol on the gastrointestinal apparatus include those on the esophagus, stomach, small bowel, colon, and pancreas. Excess alcohol ingestion at the esophageal level can induce the Mallory-Weiss syndrome due to vomiting. In the Mallory-Weiss syndrome, about 60%–80% of patients show very high alcohol consumption in the previous hours.[45] Given its strong association with alcoholism, the Mallory-Weiss syndrome is more prevalent in patients with advanced alcoholic liver disease. Furthermore, patients with advanced alcoholic liver disease have more severe bleeding and are more likely to rebleed when compared to patients with nonalcoholic cirrhosis.[185] In addition, gastroesophageal reflux is facilitated in these individuals for the existence of esophageal peristaltic dysfunction, making the development of esophagitis and/or Barrett esophagus easier.[237] A recent study revealed that 60% of alcoholic patients show alterations in the autonomic nervous system, specifically in the sympathetic system, resulting in an altered postprandial gastric emptying. This motility dysfunction could be induced by a combination of both autonomic neuropathy and direct toxicity of ethanol on smooth muscle cell contractile proteins.[73] Furthermore, alcohol can cause direct damage of the mucosa via alterations in epithelial transport, intercellular junction disorders, and impairment of the mucosal barrier.[45] Both superficial and chronic atrophic gastritis are common in alcoholics. For example, 25.8% of alcohol-dependent individuals enrolled in detoxification programs present with superficial gastritis, and 24.2% have chronic atrophic gastritis. In healthy subjects, the incidence is 10.7% for superficial gastritis and 3% for chronic atrophic gastritis.

The relationship between alcohol consumption and *Helicobacter pylori* infection is controversial. Some studies report a significantly inverse association with *H. pylori* infection, whereas others found no significant association. A recent study indicates that nondrinkers exhibit a significantly lower rate of *H. pylori* infection compared with drinkers, demonstrating a positive association.[270] More generally, it is conceivable that although mild-moderate amounts of alcohol may exert protective effects against *H. pylori* infection through a bactericidal effect or stimulation of gastric acid secretion, heavy alcohol consumption promotes colonization of the gastric mucosa by *H. pylori*.

Alcohol abuse has been implicated in peptic ulcer disease,[167] and is associated with a high risk of rebleeding, and increased mortality.[129] In alcoholic patients with a history of nonvariceal upper gastrointestinal bleeding, close follow-up and long-term proton pump inhibitor therapy are recommended.

In the small intestine, acute and chronic alcohol misuse impairs the barrier function of the gastrointestinal mucosa, resulting in increased permeability and translocation of macromolecules. Dysbiosis reported in patients with AUD is characterized by a reduced abundance of Bacteroidetes and a decreased abundance

of Proteobacteria, such that microbial alterations correlated with elevated serum endotoxin levels.[179] Small intestine bacterial overgrowth (SIBO) has been also demonstrated in individuals with chronic alcohol abuse; SIBO shows a higher prevalence in alcoholic compared to nonalcoholic subjects. These bacteria may cause mucosal damage and contribute to malabsorption (for review see Vassallo et al.[253]) Furthermore, a bidirectional pathway of communication along the microbiome-gut-brain axis exists. Neural signaling can alter the composition and function of the gut microbiota. Conversely, gut microbiota can influence neural, endocrine, and/or immune pathways, and may impact behavior, brain activity, and neurotransmitter systems, playing a role in developing and maintaining an AUD.[235]

Exposure of the mucosal side of the small intestine to alcohol inhibits the active transport of numerous macro- and micronutrients across the epithelial layer, such as folate and others. Moreover, alcohol affects the metabolism of carbohydrates and lipids in the brush border membrane of the small intestinal mucosa by damaging the villi where lactase and sucrase are located. The activities of both enzymes are reduced, which may exacerbate lactose intolerance. However, the activities of lactase and sucrase return to normal within weeks of abstinence.[204] Acute alcohol reduces impending wave motility and increases propulsive wave motility, through both a direct and indirect action on local musculature and nervous plexus; this may result in reduced transit time to the colon and diarrhea.[82] Conversely, chronic alcohol misuse may induce a reversible prolonged orocecal transit time.[18] Both abnormalities could contribute to diarrhea, as shortened transit reduces absorption while prolonged transit predisposes to bacterial overgrowth. In contrast to the organs of the upper gastrointestinal tract, the mucosa of the large bowel is exposed only to alcohol concentrations corresponding to those in the blood.[39] However, due to the low aldehyde dehydrogenase activity of the colonic mucosa, acetaldehyde accumulates in the colon and may contribute to the pathogenesis of alcohol-induced diarrhea and colon cancer. The morphology of the rectum is altered by chronic alcohol misuse; rectal biopsies often show crypt destruction, inflammation, and proliferation of epithelial cells. Abnormal cellular proliferation is the hallmark of malignant neoplasia.[202]

Given ethanol's pro-oxidant properties and its deleterious effects on gut barrier function, alcohol abuse is a potential trigger for the onset and reactivation of inflammatory bowel diseases (IBDs). Specifically, current drinkers with inactive IBD more frequently report worsening of gastrointestinal symptoms with alcohol, compared to drinkers with irritable bowel disease.[228] Pancreatitis due to alcohol abuse is a very painful and potentially fatal condition. About one-third of acute pancreatitis cases in the United States are related to alcohol, and 60%–90% of patients with pancreatitis have a history of chronic alcohol consumption. There is dose-response association between the risk of pancreatitis and the amount of alcohol (specifically, spirits) consumption, reaching an exponential correlation beyond the threshold of five drinks per day.[135,213]

Possible mechanisms involved in the pathophysiology of alcoholic pancreatitis include inhibition of secretion from acini, microtubular dysfunction, induction of oxidative stress, production of pro-inflammatory cytokines, alteration of cell permeability, increased lysosomal fragility, inhibition of apoptosis, and enhancement of necrosis.[58] Alcoholic pancreatitis is characterized by a higher risk of recurrence, progression to chronic pancreatitis, and development of diabetes mellitus, compared to pancreatitis with different etiologies. Finally, an increased risk of pancreatitis is

TABLE 59.2	Main Gastrointestinal and Pancreatic Features in Subjects With Substance Abuse or Dependence.	
Substance	Main Feature(s)	Other Feature(s)
Alcohol	Gastric and intestinal motility disorders; malabsorption; pancreatitis	Esophagitis; Mallory-Weiss syndrome; esophageal varicosities; acute and chronic gastritis; peptic ulcer disease; bacterial overgrowth; inflammatory bowel diseases (IBD); acute and chronic pancreatitis
Nicotine	Peptic ulcer disease; risk factor for pancreatic carcinoma	Gastroesophageal reflux disease; atrophic gastritis; reduced risk of developing UC; detrimental effect on CD; chronic pancreatitis; altered gut microbiota composition
Opioids	Inhibition of gastric and intestinal motility	Nausea; constipation; increased sphincter of Oddi tonicity; pancreatitis
Cocaine	Bowel ischemia	"Candy-cane" esophagus; intestinal perforations; ischemic colitis; pancreatitis
Amphetamine	Ischemic colitis; Decreased gut motility	Constipation; teeth damage
Benzodiazepines	Gastric and gut motility disorders	Vomiting; nausea; diarrhea; epigastric distress; abdominal pain; gaseous distension; dysphagia; gastroesophageal reflux

CD, Crohn disease; *UC*, ulcerative colitis.

present in individuals with acute alcohol intoxication and secondary hyperlipidemia. This hyperlipidemia, together with hemolytic anemia and the consequent increase of bilirubin, is called Zieve syndrome (Table 59.2).

Nicotine

Smoking could worsen gastroesophageal reflux disease; specifically, nicotine might be responsible for lower esophageal sphincter pressure.[238] A large case control study found a dose-response association between smoking and reflux symptoms: individuals who smoked more than 20 cigarettes daily had a significantly increased risk for reflux symptoms compared with nonsmokers. However, tobacco smoking cessation seems to improve severe gastroesophageal reflux symptoms only in individuals with normal body mass index (BMI), but not in other individuals.[183]

Epidemiological data show that cigarette smoking increases both the incidence and relapse rate of peptic ulcer disease and delays ulcer healing in humans. Nicotine may tilt the balance between aggressive and defensive factors of the gastric and duodenal mucosal integrity, favoring aggressive factors (e.g., increased gastric acid secretion, increased biliary reflux, increased susceptibility to *H*. infection, free radical exposure) and attenuating defensive factors (decreased pancreatic bicarbonate secretion, dysregulated gastrointestinal immune system, decreased blood flow in the gastrointestinal mucosa).[146] In particular, *H. pylori* infection is more common in smokers and eradication therapy is less effective. Several mechanisms could explain the association between smoking and failure of eradication of *H. pylori*: low adherence to treatment, reduced gastric mucosal blood flow, reduced effectiveness of antibiotics due to a more acidic environment which could increase non-replicative bacteria, altered protein pump inhibitor (PPI) metabolism in smokers [119].

Regarding the effects of nicotine on the gut, smoking is the only well-established environmental risk for IBDs. An increased risk for both Crohn disease and ulcerative colitis has been observed in former smokers, whereas current smoking seems to predispose to Crohn disease and protect against ulcerative colitis, as shown by a large prospective study.[114]

Various mechanisms have been considered to explain the beneficial effect of nicotine on ulcerative colitis, including effects on the epithelial mucus (increased mucin synthesis), gut motility (reduction of circular muscle activity), eicosanoid metabolism, inhibition of pro-inflammatory cytokine production, and parasympathetic nervous system.[238]

Therefore, nicotine, a major component of tobacco, has been examined as a possible pharmacological agent in the treatment of ulcerative colitis.

On the other hand, smoking has a detrimental effect on the course of Crohn disease. The reason for the opposite association with smoking status compared with ulcerative colitis is still unclear. This opposite effect could be related to several causes: smoking's immunosuppressive effects on macrophages, which might further compound any deficiency in the host response to luminal bacteria (a possible mechanism of the pathogenesis of Crohn disease); smoking-induced compositional changes of the gut microbiota; smoking-induced modification of key proteins that activate the immune response and induce inflammation; interaction of smoking with genes associated with risk for IBDs.[265]

Smoking is able to influence gut microbiota composition; specifically, gut microbial diversity in tobacco smokers is lower compared to nonsmoker controls. The changes in gut microbiota composition after smoking cessation seem to be similar to the differences observed in microbiota of obese compared to lean subjects.

Finally, epidemiological evidence shows an association between cigarette smoking and pancreatic diseases.

Smoking has been found to be a considerable risk factor for chronic pancreatitis both alone and associated with alcohol consumption; smoking accelerates the progression of pancreatic disease in a dose-dependent fashion, regardless of the level of alcohol consumption.[144]

The mechanism is perhaps mediated by signal transduction pathways in the pancreatic acinar cell, leading to enhanced levels of intracellular calcium release and thereby resulting in cytotoxicity and eventual cell death.[59] In addition, the induction of pancreatic injury by nicotine may involve the activation and expression of the proto-oncogene H-ras, which may lead to the development of pancreatic carcinoma in cigarette smokers.[59]

Opioids

Opioid-induced gastrointestinal dysfunctions are well known. In particular, nausea and vomiting are severe adverse effects of opioids.

Among individuals being treated with opioids, 8%–35% have reported nausea, whereas 14%–40% have had vomiting.[166] Opioids act at the chemoreceptor trigger zone (area postrema in the medulla), triggering emetic mechanisms mediated by the vomiting center in the medulla. By an action on mu receptors, opioids result in inhibition of gastric motility and a delay in gastric emptying, leading to gastroesophageal reflux/heartburn.[264] The inhibitory effect of opioids on the ileocecal sphincter and defecation reflexes contributes to opioid-induced constipation. Cases of severe constipation in heroin addicts leading to stercoral perforation of the colon have been described.[43] A large observational study carried out on heroin-dependent patients treated with methadone or buprenorphine showed a high prevalence of constipation and consequently, an impaired quality of life in this population.[155]

Opioids do not seem able to induce detrimental effects on the gastrointestinal mucosa. Conversely, it has been suggested that morphine protects against stress-induced gastric ulceration in a dose-dependent manner.[57] Opioids can increase sphincter tonicity and result in sphincter of Oddi dysfunction.[177] Sphincter of Oddi dysfunction may be manifested clinically by alteration of liver tests, pancreaticobiliary pain, and pancreatitis. For example, a study conducted in a group of 91 hospitalized heroin addicts evidenced hyperamylasemia in 19% of the individuals.[110] However, it also has been suggested that hyperamylasemia after heroin usually arises from sources other than the pancreas.

Cocaine

Gastrointestinal complications of cocaine abuse occur less frequently than those in the cardiovascular and nervous systems. Esophageal lesions are characterized by alternating pink and white linear bands imparting a candy-cane appearance to the mucosa. The injury produces chest pain, as well as dysphagia, odynophagia, and abdominal pain. However, when individuals with candy-cane esophagus have chest pain, myocardial ischemia should remain the first possible diagnosis.

Smoking cocaine and its alkaloid-free base crack-cocaine has been reported to induce deep gastric ulcerations, intestinal perforations, and consequently, severe gastrointestinal hemorrhage.[47]

These perforations occur in a predominantly male population of drug addicts who are 8–10 years younger than the usual group of individuals with pyloroduodenal perforations. H. pylori infection may be a contributing factor to these perforations.[97] Cocaine injected intravenously has been shown to cause bowel ischemia without evidence of thrombosis, embolism, or atherosclerosis.[89] The intestinal vasculature contains alpha-adrenergic receptors, which are stimulated by norepinephrine, leading to mesenteric vasoconstriction and focal ischemia.[97] Few cases of cocaine-induced pancreatitis have been reported; a thrombotic microangiopathy has been hypothesized to be the main pathophysiologic mechanism.[53]

The practice to swallow multiple packets filled with illicit drugs, mainly cocaine, in order to avoid controls, is increasingly widespread among "body packers." This practice may have disastrous consequences, including gastrointestinal obstruction or perforation, signs of systemic drug toxicity from a ruptured packet, or even death after rupture in 56% of cases.[246]

Amphetamines

Amphetamines act as an indirect sympathomimetic amine and may include decreased gut motility with consequent constipation (Matochik et al.,[162] Schifano et al.[219]).

As with cocaine, methamphetamines increase release of monoamines in the sympathetic nervous system, inducing splanchnic vasoconstriction and necrotizing vasculitis.[53] Cases of amphetamine-related ischemic colitis causing gastrointestinal bleeding have been described.[117]

Typically, misuse of crystal meth, the smokable form of methamphetamine hydrochloride, can have an important effect on teeth. In a few months, healthy teeth can turn grayish-brown, twist, and begin to fall out. The mechanism is due to the dry mouth caused by amphetamine sympathomimetic action, which in turn makes users thirsty and crave sugary soft drinks. The problem is aggravated by caustic substances used in the drug preparation, such as lithium and red phosphorus.[70]

Benzodiazepines

Oral benzodiazepine poisoning produces minimal effects on the gastrointestinal tract. Benzodiazepines may promote gastroesophageal reflux by reducing lower esophageal sphincter pressure.[252] Vomiting, nausea, diarrhea, epigastric distress, abdominal pain, gaseous distension, and dysphagia can occur after the administration of high doses of benzodiazepines.[105] Conversely, several studies have evidenced possible protective effects of benzodiazepines against ethanol-induced gastric mucosa damage and stress-induced gastric ulcerations for the involvement of central-type benzodiazepine receptors located in the stomach.[26] Finally, peripheral benzodiazepine receptors are expressed also in human pancreatic islets, and prolonged binding to peripheral benzodiazepine receptors may cause human beta-cell functional damage and apoptosis.[159] Recently, a positive correlation between the event of benzodiazepine poisoning and an increased risk of acute pancreatitis has been found.[147]

Nervous System

Alcohol

Alcohol abuse is often related to brain defects and associated cognitive, emotional, and behavioral impairments. Of interest, it has recently been suggested that the right hemisphere may be more vulnerable than the left to the effects of alcohol.[188] The regions particularly vulnerable to damage and dysfunction in individuals with chronic abuse are the frontal lobes, limbic system, and cerebellum.[189] The alterations of the frontal lobes in alcoholics are related to a decreased neuronal density, a reduction of the regional blood flow, reduced amplitude of event-related potentials, and a low glucose metabolism. These alterations generally determine some aberrations of emotion and personality including disinhibition, impulsivity, and antisocial trait. The alterations of the limbic system in alcoholics are related to dysfunction in the amygdala, a reduction of the hippocampal volume, and damage to the mammillary bodies of the hypothalamus. Clinical consequences include alterations in the control of major emotions, memory deficits (anterograde amnesia), and learning impairments. The alterations in the cerebellum in alcoholics are related to a reduction of the white matter volume of the vermis, a disruption of the frontocerebellar circuitry.[52] Clinical consequences include walking alterations, ataxia, and alterations of executive function.[52] Moreover, a 36% reduction in Purkinje cell number in the cerebellar vermis has been correlated to Korsakoff syndrome in alcoholics.[34] Korsakoff syndrome is characterized by anterograde and retrograde amnesia, disorientation, and impairment of

TABLE 59.3	Main Neurological Clinical Symptoms in Subjects With Alcohol Abuse or Dependence.	
Symptoms	**Area(s) Mainly Involved**	
Disinhibition, impulsivity, antisocial trait	Frontal lobes	
Control emotions altered, memory deficits, learning impairments	Limbic system	
KS: walking alterations, ataxia, executive function alterations	Cerebellum	
Polyneuropathy: nociception alteration, painful symptoms	PNS	
WKS: ocular motility disorders, ataxia, confusion, drowsiness, obtundation, pre-coma, coma	Cerebellum, thalamus, hypothalamus	

KS, Korsakoff syndrome; *PNS,* peripheral nervous system; *WKS,* Wernicke-Korsakoff syndrome.

recent memory coupled with confabulation.[20] This syndrome is often associated with Wernicke encephalopathy. The typical signs of Wernicke encephalopathy are ocular motility disorders, ataxia, and mental changes (confusion, drowsiness, obtundation, clouding of consciousness, pre-coma, or coma).[20,239] These two disorders are usually termed the Wernicke-Korsakoff syndrome and considered as a single clinical manifestation.[20] The prevalence of Wernicke-Korsakoff syndrome is 8–10 times higher in alcoholics than in the general population (12.5% and 0.8%, respectively) and is caused by thiamine (vitamin B_1) deficiency in these individuals.[239] Moreover, thiamine deficiency is probably the basis of the cause of polyneuropathy often present in alcoholics, although the pathogenesis of alcoholic neuropathy is still unclear.[133] Alcoholic peripheral neuropathy is characterized by an asymmetric polyneuropathy pattern with greater involvement of the lower extremities, via distal axonal degeneration, that involves both myelinated and nonmyelinated fibers[133] (Table 59.3).

Nicotine

Among the 4700 compounds found in tobacco smoke, many are associated with brain toxicity, including vinyl chloride, a risk factor for brain cancer. Other components are associated with negative effects on the pulmonary system, with secondary effects on the central nervous system. Several animal and human studies have demonstrated that chronic nicotine exposure induces an increase in the number of central nervous system nicotinic acetylcholine receptors.[211] Nicotinic acetylcholine receptors are highly represented in the thalamus and cerebellum. Both acute and chronic nicotine exposure can induce changes in the central nervous system. Cerebral responses to acute administration of nicotine or smoking include reduction in global brain activity; activation of the prefrontal cortex, thalamus, and visual cortex during visual cognitive tasks; and increased dopamine concentration in the ventral striatum/nucleus accumbens. Responses to chronic nicotine exposure include decreased monoamine oxidase A and B activity in the basal ganglia and a reduction in alpha-4-beta-2 nicotinic acetylcholine receptor availability in the thalamus and putamen.[227] Ultimately, nicotine is able to induce free radicals, to deplete antioxidants, and to increase markers of oxidative stress in neural cells, inflammatory response, and atherosclerosis.[227] Smoking history represents a reliable risk factor for preclinical brain changes, such as accelerated risk for incident silent brain infarct, reduction of gray matter volumes, and densities in the prefrontal cortex, in the left dorsal anterior cingulated cortex, and in the cerebellar gray matter. From a clinical perspective, it has been reported that continuous smoking is associated with an increased risk of cognitive impairment[32] and dementia.[170]

Opioids

Chronic opiate abuse can modify several neurotransmitter systems of the central nervous system. In particular, chronic opiate abuse has been associated with marked changes in the brain density of mu-opioid receptors.[168] Of interest, although methadone is used as a substitute for heroin in the treatment of opiate-dependent individuals, the long-lasting effects of these two opiates differ. Methadone administered in a maintenance regimen results in an upregulation of the mu-opioid receptors, which persists even after detoxification from opiates.[68] Conversely, postmortem analyses of chronic heroin users have shown a downregulation of the mu-opioid receptors.[90] Regarding monoamine neurotransmission, chronic opiate abuse has been associated with reduced densities in noradrenaline (α2) and dopamine (D2) receptors.[90] The effects on the dopamine system overall in opiate users are less pronounced than in stimulant users.[131] From a clinical perspective, heroin vapor inhalation induces leukoencephalopathy, or "chasing the dragon" syndrome, characterized by progressive neurological deficits such as altered levels of consciousness, spastic paraparesis, ataxia, bradykinesia, and dysarthria.[187] Intravenous injection of heroin also can induce permanent neuropathies. Rhabdomyolysis and myopathy have been attributed to toxicity and ischemia or a gluteal compartment syndrome, whereas the associated neuropathy could have been caused by compression.[182]

Cocaine

Within the central nervous system, frontal lobes represent the areas most affected by cocaine abuse.[91] For example, imaging results show volumetric deficits in multiple frontal areas in cocaine users, including the anterior cingulate and orbitofrontal cortex as well as the insula and temporal cortex.[162] Chronic cocaine users often present with poor performance on experimental and neuropsychological tasks that probe working memory function.[91] This feature is consistent with the observations that many of these compromised cognitive functions involve the dopaminergic neurons of the dorsolateral prefrontal and orbitofrontal regions.[91] In cocaine abusers, some cerebral vascular alterations have also been recognized.[182] In particular, cerebral hemorrhage and ischemic stroke have been reported. Silent ischemia has been suggested as a possible mechanism for the cerebral atrophy, and consequent encephalopathy often presents in cocaine abusers.[192] Either ischemic or hemorrhagic stroke can lead to ex novo seizures or exacerbate a preexisting seizure disorder.[143] However, seizures can also occur in the absence of vascular disorders when high blood concentrations of cocaine are present, suggesting a direct toxicity.[182] Cocaine can also induce transient movement disorders, characterized by choreoathetosis, akathisia, parkinsonian tremor, and multifocal tics, and can aggravate the symptoms of individuals with Tourette syndrome.[191] Furthermore, some cocaine abusers experience an acute severe migrainous headache, which can be attributed to either acute use or withdrawal of the drug.[72]

TABLE 59.4	Main Neurological Clinical Symptoms in Subjects With Substance Abuse or Dependence.
Substance	Neurological Features
Alcohol	Disinhibition, impulsivity, antisocial trait, control emotions altered, memory deficits, learning impairments, KS, WKS, polyneuropathy
Nicotine	Atherosclerosis, stroke vigilant, attention and memory, cognitive decline, dementia
Opioids	Neuropathies, rhabdomyolysis, myopathy, altered levels of consciousness, spastic paraparesis, ataxia, bradykinesia, dysarthria
Cocaine	Hemorrhagic stroke, ischemic stroke, encephalopathy, seizure disorder, choreoathetosis, akathisia, parkinsonian tremor, multifocal tics, Tourette syndrome symptoms, headache
Amphetamines	Ischemic stroke, hemorrhagic stroke, euphoria, enhanced energy, alertness, increase in libido, sleep deprivation, affective distress, psychiatric disorders, increased risk of depression and suicidal ideation, jerking syndrome
Benzodiazepines	Benzodiazepine withdrawal: "rebound anxiety," anxiety, apprehension, irritability, insomnia, dysphoria, tremor, palpitations, dizziness, sweating, muscle spasm, hypersensitivity to light, sound or touch body pains, headache, generalized seizure

KS, Korsakoff syndrome; *WKS*, Wernicke-Korsakoff syndrome.

Amphetamines

Methamphetamine-induced neurotoxicity involves several neurotransmitter systems, mostly by altering the function of the dopamine frontostriatothalamocortical loops.[49] Both high doses and chronic administration of methamphetamine can result in a depletion of dopamine and destruction of dopamine nerve terminals.[60] Several mechanisms have been implicated in methamphetamine-induced neurotoxicity, including production of reactive oxygen and nitrogen species, hyperthermia, and the triggering of an apoptotic cascade dependent upon mitochondria.[60] Acute effects of methamphetamine use are mediated by the sympathetic branch of the autonomic nervous system and include hypertension, tachycardia, hyperthermia, increased breathing rate, and constriction of blood vessels. Cognitive and emotional effects include euphoria, enhanced energy and alertness, a surge in productivity, and an increase in libido.[60] Chronic methamphetamine use can result in pulmonary hypertension, acute aortic dissection, myocardial infarction, and ischemic and hemorrhagic strokes. In addition, some physical and mental consequences can occur, including sleep deprivation, affective distress, psychiatric disorders, and an increased risk of depression and suicidal ideation.[60] Furthermore, methamphetamine may induce seizures, delirium, and coma, especially if used in combination with other drugs.[182] Either hemorrhagic[267] or ischemic stroke[267] may also occur. Finally, in chronic methamphetamine addicts, a transient movement disorder called "jerking syndrome" has been described. The jerking syndrome is probably caused by a basal ganglia disorder and is characterized by constant automatic involuntary choreiform movements, stereotyped dystonic facial movements, and/or chewing-gum movements.[182]

Benzodiazepines

In individuals with benzodiazepine abuse, many studies have demonstrated a downregulation of the benzodiazepine-binding sites, although the affinity is usually unchanged.[118] Symptoms of benzodiazepine withdrawal are time-limited, usually occurring for only 1 or 2 weeks after the discontinuation of the drug, but the duration varies according to the drug and the individual subject.[186] During withdrawal, the original anxiety symptoms often return in a more intense form, a phenomenon known as "rebound anxiety."[118] Rebound anxiety can include psychological and physiological symptoms such as anxiety, apprehension, irritability, insomnia, dysphoria, tremor, palpitations, mild systolic hypertension, dizziness, sweating, muscle spasm, and gastrointestinal disturbances[118] (Table 59.4).

Cardiovascular System

Alcohol

Alcohol abuse has been associated with several cardiovascular diseases, such as hypertension, cardiomyopathy, coronary artery disease, and stroke.[153] However, low-to-moderate ethanol consumption has been linked to a reduced cardiovascular risk, with a J-shaped dose-response curve. Although red wine consumption and the related compounds (i.e., polyphenols) were considered important in the so-called French paradox, alcohol itself seems to hold the major benefits.[153] On the other hand, chronic alcohol abuse induces several alterations in the cardiovascular system, including low-grade systemic inflammation, hyperuricemia, dyslipidemia, hyperhomocysteinemia, increased oxidative stress with enhanced lipid peroxidation, impaired glucose tolerance with insulin resistance, endothelial dysfunction, arterial hypertension, and alcoholic cardiomyopathy.[153,173,174,197] From a clinical point of view, all the mentioned mechanisms are able to modify the pathophysiology of atherosclerosis. Atherosclerosis is a diffuse disease, and its clinical presentation varies depending on the vascular bed in which it occurs. Moreover, long-term heavy alcohol consumption (of any beverage type) is the leading cause of a nonischemic dilated cardiomyopathy called alcoholic cardiomyopathy.[173,197] The exact pathogenesis of alcoholic cardiomyopathy is still unclear. Alcohol induces several changes in the myocardial structure by inducing myocyte loss, intracellular organelle dysfunction, and contractile protein alterations, and influencing calcium homeostasis. These changes can alter several aspects of myocyte function and, therefore, may lead to myocyte dysfunction and alcoholic cardiomyopathy. Symptoms often appear late, and the diagnosis could be difficult because the symptoms are close to those of chronic heart failure. Alcohol abstinence often results in at least partial recovery of the myocyte damage, with a consequent improvement in cardiac function. The term "holiday heart syndrome" was coined by Ettinger et al.[78] and defined as "an acute cardiac rhythm and/or conduction disturbance associated with heavy ethanol consumption in a person without other clinical evidence of heart disease and disappearing, without evident residual, with abstinence." In sum, although numerous studies have described a J-shaped or U-shaped curve to describe the relationship between alcohol intake and total and cardiovascular mortality, these studies have been observational and epidemiological

TABLE 59.5	Main Cardiovascular Features in Subjects With Substance Abuse or Dependence.
Substance	Cardiovascular Features
Alcohol	Hypertension, alcoholic cardiomyopathy, coronary artery disease, stroke
Nicotine	Atherosclerosis, hypertension, myocardial infarction, angina, sudden cardiac death, stroke
Opioids	Bradycardia/bradyarrhythmias, hypotension, pulmonary edema, endocarditis
Cocaine	Severe hyper-/hypotension
Amphetamines	Arrhythmias (supraventricular/ventricular), chest pain/myocardial infarction, acute heart failure, dilated cardiomyopathy/chronic heart failure, endocarditis
Benzodiazepines	Bradycardia, myocardial infarction (?)

in nature. Prescribing alcohol for individuals who do not drink and the use of alcohol as a cardioprotective strategy are not recommended[132] (Table 59.5).

Nicotine

Smoking is associated with an increased risk of atherosclerotic vascular disease, hypertension, myocardial infarction, unstable angina, sudden cardiac death, and stroke.[263] Acute and chronic cigarette smoking impairs nitric oxide synthase–mediated relaxation of large blood vessels. Smoked tobacco, in fact, contains high levels of free radicals and pro-oxidant agents. There is considerable evidence that cigarette smoking can result in both morphological and biochemical disturbances to the endothelium both in vivo and in cell culture systems. However, a consensus of the causal relationship between cardiovascular disorders and the consumption of smokeless tobacco has not yet been established.[104] An acute hypertensive effect has been shown, up to 90 minutes after smoking tobacco. In particular, absorbed nicotine stimulates the release of catecholamines; the subsequent activation of alpha-adrenoceptors in vascular smooth muscle cells contracts vascular tissues and elevates blood pressure. Free radicals and aromatic compounds diminish the endothelial synthesis of nitric oxide, causing impaired endothelium-dependent relaxation of arteries, which is the earliest clinical sign of endothelial dysfunction, and they injure the arterial endothelium, promoting atherogenesis.[104] The increased oxidation of low-density lipoprotein in smokers has synergetic effects to promote monocyte adhesion and monocyte migration into the subintimal space. Continued stimulation of intimal cells by oxidized low-density lipoprotein leads to the development of atherosclerosis. Smokeless tobacco use has been linked to impotence,[125] acute myocardial infarction, congestive heart failure,[205] and ischemic stroke.[95] In particular, diseases of the cardiovascular system and their final or lethal states occur three to four times more frequently than lung cancer in heavy smokers.[104]

Opioids

The cardiovascular effects of opioids are directed to the vasomotor center to increase parasympathetic activity, reduce sympathetic activity, and release histamine from mast cells. These combined effects produce bradycardia and hypotension.[151] Acute cardiac effects of opioid abuse are represented by drug-induced bradycardia.[151] The reduction in the heart rate increases the automaticity in ectopic electrical myocardial activity, leading to atrial fibrillation, idioventricular rhythm, or potentially lethal ventricular tachyarrhythmias.[151] Some opioids (such as dextropropoxyphene) have additional sodium channel-blocking effects, which further contribute to the pro-arrhythmic and myocardial depressant effects, leading to acute left ventricular dysfunction and cardiogenic pulmonary edema. Overdose of narcotic analgesics can also cause acute noncardiogenic pulmonary edema. This may be related to an anaphylactic reaction to the drug, to an increase in pulmonary capillary hydrostatic pressure resulting from pulmonary vasoconstriction induced by hypoxia, or to disruption of alveolar capillary membrane integrity. Apart from the well-described central nervous system and respiratory depressant effects, there also may be profound cardiovascular collapse or arrhythmias after narcotic analgesic overdose.[96] Chronic consequences of intravenous opioid injection include the risk of infection of the injection site, along with the risk of bacterial endocarditis, which usually affects the right-sided heart valves and may be associated with pulmonary abscess formation.[223] Because the abused drug is rapidly metabolized, the majority of arrhythmias are short-lived. Compared with abusers of other drugs, opioid abusers show a low prevalence of coronary artery disease.[158] On this point, the binding of morphine to opioid receptors before induction of an infarction in a rat model results in smaller infarcts, with protection of cardiomyocytes mediated by peripheral opioid receptors.[96] Moreover, in humans, long-term exposure to opioids is associated with decreased severity of coronary artery disease, with a decreased incidence of fatal myocardial infarctions. One possible explanation is that narcotics may decrease inflammation,[67] which is associated with atherogenesis and plaque disruption.[148]

Cocaine

Cocaine affects the cardiovascular system, predominantly via activation of the sympathetic nervous system.[96] Cocaine acts indirectly as a sympathomimetic drug inhibiting the reuptake of noradrenaline and dopamine at the sympathetic nerve terminals. Cocaine can also act through central pathways to release noradrenaline from the adrenal medulla.[56] At high doses, cocaine can impair myocyte electrical activity and contractility by blocking fast sodium and potassium channels and inhibiting calcium entry into myocytes.[176] Furthermore, cocaine has a short serum half-life of approximately 30–80 minutes, but some of its metabolites are more cardiotoxic than the parent compound.[111] Cocaethylene, for example, is formed when cocaine is taken with alcohol and has an important cardiotoxic effect.[111] The clinical symptoms related to the cocaine-induced sympathetic activation include tachycardia, vasoconstriction, unpredictable blood pressure effects, and arrhythmias, depending on the dose and the possible presence of a coexisting cardiovascular disease. Hypertension is common, but severe hypotension (due to a paradoxical central sympathetic suppression) can also occur.[176] Chest pain, myocardial ischemia, and infarction can be produced by various mechanisms, such as diffuse or local coronary artery spasms.[175] A procoagulant effect that can facilitate a thrombotic coronary occlusion can also occur by decreasing the concentrations of protein C and antithrombin III, activating platelets, and potentiating thromboxane production. Chronic use of cocaine can induce repetitive episodes of coronary spasm and paroxysms of hypertension, which may result in endothelial damage, coronary artery dissection, and subsequent acceleration of atherosclerosis. Prolonged administration of cocaine may be associated with an irreversible dilated cardiomyopathy, related to subendocardial ischemia and fibrosis and myocyte necrosis produced by exposure to excessive catecholamine concentrations or repeated episodes of myocarditis. Myocardial cellular injury can also occur in association with exposure to infectious agents or heavy metals, such as manganese, that contaminate street preparations of cocaine. A wide and unpredictable range of supraventricular and potentially lethal ventricular tachyarrhythmias can be precipitated by such a sympathomimetic stimulation. Moreover, cocaine can impair cardiac conduction, inducing a wide range of bradyarrhythmias such as sinus arrest and atrioventricular block. Sudden cardiovascular collapse may occur as a result of myocardial ischemia and infarction, arrhythmias, acute heart failure, or mechanical complications. Benzodiazepines attenuate the cardiac and central nervous system toxicity of cocaine and should be given in sedative dosages, also to manage hypertensive and cardiovascular complications, in addition to nitrates.[116] Cocaine-induced chest pain should be treated initially with oxygen, aspirin, and benzodiazepines. If the ischemia damage continues, then the use of additional vasodilators such as nitrates or phentolamine to reverse residual coronary spasm may be necessary.

Amphetamines

As a consequence of acute amphetamines intoxication, cardiovascular symptoms, including chest pain, palpitations, and dyspnea, are common.[25] Cardiovascular effects of amphetamines are similar to those induced by cocaine and include hypertension, supraventricular tachyarrhythmias, ventricular arrhythmias, myocardial ischemia and infarction, acute heart failure, chronic heart failure, and endocarditis.[96] Similar principles should be applied to the management of the cardiovascular complications associated with these recreational drugs, although the duration of treatment will vary depending on the half-life of the agent taken.

Benzodiazepines

Benzodiazepines, particularly diazepam, are usually considered primarily to exert a cardiodepressant effect, which is a consequence of a centrally mediated decrease in cardioregulatory outflow of the sympathetic nervous system.[51] On the other hand, some studies report that diazepam produces positive inotropic effects on the myocardium, which have been related to catecholamines released from sympathetic nerve terminals located in the heart.[21] Moreover, it has also been shown that diazepam potentiates the positive inotropic effect of both noradrenaline and adrenaline, as well as that of the endogenous noradrenaline-releasing agent tyramine in electrically driven right ventricular strips of rat, by directly inhibiting the enzyme cyclic nucleotide phosphodiesterase.[157] Diazepam overdose can produce cardiac sympathomimetic-like effects on atrioventricular conduction. Recently, it has been shown that peripheral-type benzodiazepine receptors are almost ubiquitous (i.e., platelets, erythrocytes, lymphocytes, and mononuclear cells) and are abundant in the cardiovascular system (endothelium, striated cardiac muscle, vascular smooth muscles, and mast cells) and in intracellular locations (mitochondria).[254] The exact function of peripheral-type benzodiazepine receptors is still unclear, but they seem to take part in some responses to trauma such as ischemia. The irreversible peripheral-type benzodiazepine receptor antagonist, SSR180575, was found to reduce the ischemia-related damage.[254] Diazepam is often found to be a substance of abuse that

can induce a myocardial infarction secondary to coronary spasm, mostly in teenagers.

Oncology

Alcohol

Excessive alcohol consumption carries a high burden of cancer morbidity and mortality.[17] A recent study estimated that the total number of alcohol attributable cancer cases was approximately 770,000 worldwide (5.5% of the total number of cancer cases); alcohol attributable cancer deaths were 480,000 (5.8% of the total number of cancer deaths), significantly increasing compared to previous studies.[201] Among the possible mechanistic pathways, the formation of acetaldehyde seems to be the most important.[123] Twenty-five percent to 80% of upper aerodigestive tract cancers are attributable to alcohol acetaldehyde. For example, individuals heterozygous for inactive ALDH2 are at increased risk for upper aerodigestive tract cancers because of the accumulation of acetaldehyde after alcohol consumption.[202] In a recent meta-analysis, the pooled relative risk (RR) for oral and pharyngeal cancers was 1.21 (95% confidence interval [CI] 1.10-1.33) for one or fewer drinks per day while 5.24 (95% CI 4.36-6.30) for four or more drinks per day.[247] Concerning colorectal cancer, the RRs were 1.21 (95% CI 1.13-1.28) for moderate alcohol consumption and 1.52 (95% CI 1.27-1.81) for heavy (≥4 drinks/day) alcohol consumption.[83]

Although the association between cirrhosis and the development of hepatocellular carcinoma is well documented, a direct correlation between ethanol consumption and the development of hepatocellular carcinoma remains debatable. Among individuals with alcoholic cirrhosis, the annual incidence of hepatocellular carcinoma is 1%–2%.[165] Similarly, although heavy alcohol consumption represents a major cause of chronic pancreatitis and a risk factor for type 2 diabetes mellitus (both of which are linked to pancreatic cancer), there is little or no support for a direct causal relationship between light and moderate alcohol use and risk of pancreatic cancer.[98]

Alcohol consumption is associated with increased risk for breast cancer in both premenopausal and postmenopausal women, regardless of the type of alcoholic beverage consumed. In 2012, an estimated 140,000 breast cancer cases and 38,000 breast cancer deaths were ascribable to alcohol consumption, even among light-drinking woman, who were affected in 18.8% of the cases and 17.5% of the deaths.[221] There is also some evidence that alcohol consumption plays a role in breast cancer recurrence, especially in postmenopausal women. It may be involved also in the development of second primary breast cancers, but the connection is less clear.[222]

The role of alcohol consumption in the etiology of lymphomas, both Hodgkin and non-Hodgkin, is still debatable.[231,249] Even for leukemias and multiple myeloma, alcohol effect has not been confirmed[208,209] (Table 59.6).

Nicotine

Cigarette smoke contains 4800 identified chemicals, including at least 61 products (e.g., benzene, polonium, polycyclic aromatic hydrocarbons, nitrosamines, and aromatic amines) able to cause cancer.[108] Moreover, tobacco components have been recognized to induce immunosuppression, which may play an important role in the development of malignant cells.[231] The unequivocal role of

TABLE 59.6   Pathways and Related Effects on the Basis of the Link Between Cancers and Substances of Abuse.

Possible Pathways Involved	Effects
Alcohol-Related Cancer	
Alcohol contacts-related local effects	Cancer of UADT, stomach, colon
Alcohol's solvent effects on tobacco and other carcinogens	Cancer of UADT, stomach, colon, pancreas
Induction of microsomal enzymes involved in carcinogen metabolism	Cancer of UADT, stomach, colon, liver, pancreas
Generation of oxygen radicals and lipid peroxidation products	Cancer of UADT, stomach, colon, liver, pancreas
Nutritional deficiency	Cancer of colon, breast, blood
Suppressed immune function	Cancer of UADT, stomach, colon, liver, pancreas, breast, NHL
Acetaldehyde-induced carcinogenesis	Cancer of UADT, stomach, colorectal, liver
Decreased hepatic retinoic acid	Cancer of liver
Iron overload	Cancer of liver
Perturbation of estrogen metabolism and response	Cancer of breast
Down-regulated BRCA1 expression	Cancer of breast
Tobacco Component-Related Cancer	
Increasing mean leukocyte counts	Cancer of lung, larynx, mouth, esophagus, bladder, pancreas, kidney, cervix uteri, stomach, breast, blood
Decreasing serum concentration of immunoglobulins	
Decreasing NK-cells	
Decreasing CD41/CD81 ratio	
Altering T-cell function	
Opioid-Related Cancer	
Decreased natural and adaptive immunity	Worsening of cancer in animal models
Cocaine-Related Cancer	
Vasoconstriction irritating to the respiratory epithelium of the nasal airway	Nasal SFT
Amphetamine-Related Cancer	
Suppresses neutrophil phagocytosis	Reduced tumor surveillance
Suppresses production of TNF-alpha and IL1	
Suppresses circulating lymphocyte numbers	
Alters T-cell function	

IL1, Interleukin-1; *NHL*, non-Hodgkin lymphoma; *NK-cells*, natural killer cells; *SFT*, solitary fibrous tumor; *TNF*, tumor necrosis factor; *UADT*, upper aerodigestive tract.

exposure. The annual number of deaths caused in the United States by smoking-related cancers was 163,700 (100,300 men and 63,400 women).[50] The risk for lung cancer among cigarette smokers increases with the duration of smoking and the number of cigarettes smoked per day. Genetic factors can also contribute. For example, it has been shown recently that a common variant in the nicotinic acetylcholine receptor gene cluster on chromosome 15q24 with an effect on smoking quantity confers a risk of lung cancer.[240] Regarding upper aerodigestive tract cancers, the risk of laryngeal cancer in smokers is on the order of 10 relative to nonsmokers and >15 for heavy smokers, and the risk seems stronger for glottic than for supraglottic neoplasms. Smokers are at a dramatically increased risk for oral carcinoma, particularly squamous cell cancer. In addition, studies have demonstrated a dose-response effect of intensity and duration of smoking[136] on this risk. Epidemiological studies report a two- to fivefold increase in the risk of esophageal cancer among smokers. A dose-response increased risk of squamous cell carcinoma of the esophagus with increased intensity and duration of smoking and a decline in risk after smoking cessation have been demonstrated repeatedly. Smoking is also responsible for a two- to threefold increased risk of adenocarcinoma of the esophagus, and risk relates to the intensity of smoking.[136] Relevant cohort and case-control studies that have examined the relationship between tobacco smoking and stomach cancer show an up to twofold increase in risk for smokers compared with nonsmokers. A positive dose-response relationship with intensity and duration of smoking was demonstrated in most studies. A large number of case-control and cohort studies have reported an increased risk for liver cancer in smokers. Smoking is associated with an approximate two- to fourfold increased risk of pancreatic cancer. The proportion of pancreatic cancer attributable to cigarette smoking was 29% in blacks and 26% in whites.[136] Furthermore, an increased risk of kidney and renal pelvis cancers has also been reported in smokers compared with nonsmokers.[136] During the last four decades, many epidemiological studies and reviews have consistently shown that cigarette smoking substantially increases the risk of bladder cancer. A positive dose-response relationship has been found with both the number of cigarettes smoked per day and the number of years smoking. Age at first exposure and cessation of cigarette smoking were inversely associated with bladder cancer risk. The role of human papillomavirus in cervical tumors in women is well known. Accordingly, recent cohort and case-control studies have investigated the association between tobacco smoking and the incidence of invasive cervical cancer, cervical intraepithelial neoplasia, and cervical cancer in situ using analyses adjusted for human papillomavirus status or restricted to human papillomavirus–positive women. In these studies, the association between tobacco smoking and cervical cancer was present and remained even after adjustment for a series of other potentially confounding factors. The association between smoking and breast cancer is constantly growing. Although not initially defined as a smoke-related cancer, recent evidence suggests a potentially casual role for active smoking on breast cancer, particularly for long-term heavy smoking and early smoking initiation. Second-hand smoking may relate to an increased risk for premenopausal breast cancer, but this connection is less clear.[206] A recent systematic review suggested an association between cigarette smoking and aggressive prostate cancer; however, with a still-to-define pathophysiology, smokers presented worse outcome after treatment and higher mortality.[71] Finally, among hematological tumors, the available literature on tobacco smoking and leukemia indicates that there is an association between tobacco smoking

cigarette smoking in causing lung cancer is one of the most thoroughly documented causal relationships in biomedical research. In the United States, from 2005 to 2009, approximately 127,000 people/year died from smoke-related lung cancer, while 36,000 people/year died from other cancers ascribable to cigarette smoke and myeloid leukemia, with an increased risk with higher intensity and longer duration of smoking. In recent years, a direct relationship between tobacco smoking and the risk of non-Hodgkin lymphoma has been suggested. Compared with those who have never smoked, current smokers had a 10%–40% higher risk of developing non-Hodgkin lymphoma. The association seemed stronger for follicular and high-grade lymphomas.[231] On the contrary, Nieters et al.[184] showed an elevated risk of Hodgkin lymphoma in relation to smoking but did not find any association between tobacco smoking and risk of non-Hodgkin lymphoma. However, the latter study was based on a small sample size.

Opioids

There are few data on this topic; the most important pertain to the immunomodulatory activities of morphine and the related potential risk of carcinogenesis.[212] Moreover, injecting opioids also exposes an individual to an indirect risk of cancer, considering the impairment of the immune system in individuals with human immunodeficiency virus/acquired immune deficiency syndrome.[13]

Some evidence suggests that opioid use is associated with an increased risk of cancers of the esophagus, stomach, larynx, lung, and urinary bladder, but further epidemiological studies are needed.[126]

Cocaine

Also in this case, few data are available. Reactive vascular lesions of the nasal septum simulating angiosarcoma have been reported in chronic cocaine abusers.[22] Cocaine that is snorted is vasoconstricting and locally irritating to the respiratory epithelium of the nasal airway. An anecdotal report also described a solitary fibrous tumor of the nasal cavity in an individual with a long-standing history of cocaine inhalation.[22]

Amphetamines

Both animal and human studies demonstrated that amphetamines, particularly methylenedioxymethamphetamine, has immunosuppressive actions that can play a role in reducing tumor surveillance. However, it is difficult to predict the impact of methylenedioxymethamphetamine-induced immunosuppression on disease susceptibility, particularly cancer onset risk.[62]

Benzodiazepines

For most benzodiazepines, results of genotoxicity and carcinogenicity tests recommended by current guidelines are difficult to retrieve.[41] In some instances, an agent for which there is inadequate evidence or no data in humans but limited evidence of carcinogenicity in experimental animals, together with supporting evidence from other relevant data, may be placed in Group 2B. On the basis of these indications, three drugs might be considered as possibly carcinogenic to humans: oxazepam, already classified by the International Agency for Research on Cancer in Group 2B, and, tentatively, midazolam and zopiclone due to sufficient evidence of carcinogenicity in experimental animals. Three other drugs—brotizolam, quazepam, and zolpidem—might be tentatively classified as probably not carcinogenic to humans (Group 4). All the other benzodiazepines, on the basis of available data, should be considered not classifiable as to their carcinogenicity to

humans (Group 3), including diazepam, doxefazepam, estazolam, prazepam, ripazepam, and temazepam.[41] A recent meta-analysis of observational studies, including 18 case-control studies and 4 cohort studies, reported that benzodiazepine use was significantly associated with an increased risk of cancer (relative risk 1.19; 95% confidence interval 1.16-1.21), with a significant dose-response relationship.[130]

Endocrinology

Alcohol

Alcohol abuse can often be associated with several endocrine disorders. Among them, the thyroid gland seems to be typically affected. Most studies have shown a reduction in peripheral thyroid hormones and/or blunted thyroid-stimulating hormone response to thyrotropin-releasing hormone in alcohol-dependent individuals.[112] Consistently, in these individuals, both ultrasound and autopsy studies have shown a significant reduction of the thyroid gland volume. Decreased thyroid hormones might result from damage to the thyroid gland or from alterations of the hypothalamic-pituitary-thyroid axis due to chronic alcohol intake. Of interest, thyroid hormone dysfunction has been associated with some behavioral features of alcohol dependence, such as the severity of withdrawal, negative mood status, and an increased risk of alcohol relapse and alcohol craving, especially in its compulsive component.[140,190] This last feature is of interest and in line with other similar findings found with other hormones and peptides able to modulate food intake, such as leptin,[115] ghrelin,[9] and insulin.[142] Alcohol-dependent individuals may show a chronic activation of the hypothalamic-pituitary-adrenal axis, with increased concentrations of cortisol during periods of heavy intake.[152] Recent abstinent alcoholics also show a blunted adrenocorticotropin response to corticotropin-releasing hormone, possibly caused by a direct pituitary effect of chronic ethanol exposure. Alcohol-dependent individuals tend to relapse more rapidly when they have smaller cortisol responses to public stress or in response to alcohol cues in a cue exposure procedure. Consistent with these data, the involvement of other stress hormones in alcoholism has been shown. For example, alcohol drinking is known to cause hyperprolactinemia in both humans and laboratory animals after acute and chronic ethanol exposure, with a consequent normalization during abstinence.[137] Accordingly, women addicted to alcohol have menstrual cycle irregularities, amenorrhea, and infertility because hyperprolactinemia is able to increase the dysfunction of the pituitary-ovarian axis, as caused directly by alcohol. Consistent with the involvement of the hypothalamic-pituitary-adrenal axis in alcohol addiction, a significant decrease in aldosterone levels during abstinence, as well as its potential role in mediating alcohol craving, has been suggested.[141] With regard to the link between alcohol and diabetes, a recent meta-analysis showed that a moderate alcohol intake was associated with a reduced risk of type 2 diabetes compared with low consumption or abstinence, whereas high consumption of alcohol was associated with an increased risk of type 2 diabetes compared with moderate consumption.[48] Chronic moderate use of alcohol has no deleterious effect on metabolic control in individuals with diabetes. The relationship between alcohol use and insulin sensitivity is J-shaped, with the lowest fasting insulin levels and the lowest insulin resistance index values in moderate drinkers and higher values in both abstainers and heavy drinkers. Finally, some sexual dysfunction also can be present in alcohol-dependent individuals. In fact, alcohol impairs testicular

TABLE 59.7	Main Endocrine Features in Subjects With Substance Abuse or Dependence.				
Substance	HPT Axis	HPA Axis	HPG Axis	Sexual Dysfunction(s)	Other(s)
Alcohol	↓ thyroid hormones ↓ TSH response to TRH	↑ Cort ↓ DXT suppression of Cort	↓ FSH, LH ↓ GnRH ↓ TESTO ↑ ESTRO	↑ mci ↓ libido ↓ fertility ↑ risk for ED	↑ PRL ↓ GH ↑ risk of diabetes
Nicotine	↓ TSH ↑ risk of thyroid dysfunction ↓ risk for thyroid cancer	↑ACTH ↑ Cort ↑ Adr & NAdr ↑ Aldo ↑ Andro ↑ DHEAS	↓ ESTRO	↑ mci ↓ fertility ↑ risk for ED ↑ menopausal symptoms	↓ PRL ↑ GH ↑ AVP ↑ Ins ↑ Ins-R ↑ renin
Opioids		↓ ACTH ↑ adrenal insufficiency ↓ circadian HPA hormone secretion	↓ LH ↓ TESTO	↓ libido ↑ risk for ED ↑ mci	↓ GH ↑ Ins ↑ glucagon
Cocaine		↑ CRH ↑ ACTH ↑ Cort	↑ FSH ↑ LH	↑ sexual feelings ↑ mci ↑ risk for ED ↑ risk for priapism	↑ PRL ↑ AVP ↓ renin
Amphetamines		↑ CRH ↑ ACTH ↑ Cort		↑ sexual desire ↑ risk for ED ↑ ejaculation latency	↓ PRL
Benzodiazepines	↓ TSH	↓ ACTH ↓ Cort	↑ TESTO ↑ 11- hydrocorticoid	↑ sexual dysfunctions ↓ libido	↓ PRL ↓ GH

ACTH, Adrenocorticotropin; *Adr*, adrenaline; *Aldo*, aldosterone; *Andro*, androstenedione; *AVP*, arginine vasopressin; *Cort*, cortisol; *CRH*, corticotropin-releasing hormone; *DHEAS*, dehydroepiandrosterone sulfate; *DXT*, dexamethasone; *ED*, erectile dysfunction; *ESTRO*, estrogen; *FSH*, follicle-stimulating hormone; *GH*, growth hormone; *GnRH*, gonadotropin-releasing hormone; *HPA axis*, hypothalamic-pituitary-adrenal axis; *HPG axis*, hypothalamic-pituitary-gonadal axis; *HPT axis*, hypothalamic-pituitary-thyroid axis; *Ins*, insulin; *Ins-R*, insulin resistance; *LH*, luteinizing hormone; *mci*, menstrual cycle irregularities; *NAdr*, noradrenaline; *PRL*, prolactin; *TESTO*, testosterone; *TRH*, thyrotropin-releasing hormone; *TSH*, thyroid-stimulating hormone.

production of testosterone as well as hypothalamic pituitary secretion of gonadotropin-releasing hormone and the two gonadotropins, follicle-stimulating hormone and luteinizing hormone. In addition, acute alcohol intoxication increases sexual desire but inhibits sexual performance. On the other hand, chronic alcohol consumption is associated with the risk of an erectile dysfunction, in a J-shaped manner, with moderate consumption conferring the highest protection and higher consumption conferring fewer benefits.[54] In alcoholic females, several gynecological problems such as gonadal dysfunction, loss of libido, and infertility are frequent. Consistently, various studies have shown that alcohol consumption increases estrogen levels in the pre-ovulation and luteal phases of the menstrual cycle[33] (Table 59.7).

Nicotine

Smoking is a risk factor for Graves hyperthyroidism, and especially for Graves ophthalmopathy, due to both a tissue hypoxia and an immune-mediated effect.[255] Consistently, the response to the treatment in individuals with ophthalmopathy is delayed and markedly poorer in smokers. Furthermore, in individuals with Graves disease, smoking may promote the development of thyrotoxicosis. Cigarette smoking has been found to be negatively associated with thyroid cancer, a feature probably due to both the lower thyroid-stimulating hormone levels that reduce thyroid cell proliferation and a smoking-related anti-estrogen effect. With regard to hypothyroidism, a meta-analysis has suggested that Hashimoto thyroiditis, postpartum thyroid dysfunction, and nontoxic goiter

are associated with smoking.[255] Smoking acutely increases the plasma levels of prolactin, adrenocorticotropin, cortisol, growth hormone, and arginine vasopressin without significant changes in thyroid-stimulating hormone, luteinizing hormone, and follicle-stimulating hormone.[128] These effects are directly proportional to the nicotine content of cigarettes. Four potential mechanisms may cause these effects: nausea induced by smoking via the stimulation of the emetic center; nicotine-stimulated cyclic adenosine monophosphate production; stress per se; and a direct effect of nicotine on the anterior pituitary or hypothalamus. In chronic smokers, however, inhibition of prolactin secretion occurs, and it depends on a nicotinic release of dopamine acting as a prolactin-inhibitory factor.[251] Chronic smoking stimulates plasma renin activity and raises plasma aldosterone levels. Higher levels of androstenedione and dehydroepiandrosterone sulfate are found in smokers. Plasma adrenaline and noradrenaline levels rise after smoking. Cigarette smoking has an antiestrogenic effect in women. This is probably due to increased production of 2-hydroxyestrogen compounds with minimal estrogenic activity.[233] Some physiological estrogen-dependent processes, such as the menstrual cycle, are affected by the risk of anovulation and the consequent decreased fertility. Menopausal symptoms such as hot flashes are experienced more commonly among smokers. Cross-sectional studies have also shown increased insulin resistance in smokers versus nonsmoking controls.[81] The reduced insulin sensitivity seen in smokers could be due to the increase in counterregulatory hormones such as growth hormone, cortisol, and catecholamines, which all raise blood glucose levels. Calcium absorption is lower in smokers than in nonsmokers, a feature probably related to the lower parathyroid hormone and serum calcitriol levels seen in smokers. An association between smoking and erectile dysfunction has also been suggested. Smokers were 1.5 times more likely than nonsmokers to have erectile dysfunction,[76] and the significant association of smoking with erectile dysfunction was strengthened as the number of cigarettes smoked increased. Smoking results in alterations of the male sex hormones and is a key cause of and contributor to erectile dysfunction. Smoking may cause erectile dysfunction by several mechanisms, including adversely affecting intrapenile blood flow caused by endothelial dysfunction. A decrease in sperm quality and a reduced response to fertility treatments have also been reported in male smokers.

Opioids

Opiate users who inject heroin, or those on methadone maintenance treatment, may exhibit adrenal insufficiency and atypical circadian patterns of hypothalamic-pituitary-adrenal hormone secretion.[80] Opiate use increases corticosteroid-binding globulins, which can mask adrenal dysfunction. During chronic administration of opioids, the acute stimulatory effect on prolactin, growth hormone, and thyroid-stimulating hormone secretion is abolished, whereas adrenocorticotropin is inhibited and luteinizing hormone remains suppressed. The inhibition of adrenocorticotropin release can be explained by the concomitant release of beta-endorphin. A lower, but substantial, percentage of individuals may develop adrenal insufficiency. This condition should be properly diagnosed and treated to avoid Addisonian crises. Growth hormone deficiency may affect an equivalent number of individuals. Methadone dose showed a significant direct correlation with increased orgasm dysfunction, both before and after adjusting for duration of treatment.[44] Heroin addiction influences sexual function negatively. Although opiate addicts often equate the drug experience with sexual orgasm, diminished libido and impaired sexual performance such as erectile dysfunction are common sequelae of chronic use. Substitution therapy by sex steroids restored libido in most men and women and improved their quality of life. A clear and significant suppression of luteinizing hormone and testosterone in virtually all males and a similar decrease in luteinizing hormone secretion with a disrupted menstrual cycle in females were found in a recent study.[69]

Cocaine

There is evidence from brain imaging studies that the pituitary gland is larger in men who abuse cocaine chronically than in controls.[169] Chronic cocaine abuse can be associated with hyperprolactinemia. Prolactin release is pulsatile. Hyperprolactinemic cocaine abusers have higher average prolactin peak heights than controls or normoprolactinemic cocaine abusers, and they have higher average prolactin levels between peaks than the other groups. Intravenous cocaine administration is usually followed by an increase in adrenocorticotropin and a subsequent increase in cortisol in male humans.[169] When cocaine was administered intranasally, a change in adrenocorticotropin was not detected, but there was a significant increase in cortisol levels.[109] Peak plasma cocaine levels were coincident with the peak increase in plasma adrenocorticotropin levels; adrenocorticotropin peak amplitude and height increased significantly after intravenous cocaine administration, and pulse frequency remained unaltered. These data are consistent with the hypothesis that the reinforcing properties of cocaine may occur as a consequence of its effects on dopaminergic neural systems, which comodulate corticotropin-releasing hormone release in the brain. Cocaine also reduces renin secretion and increases arginine vasopressin. Acute administration of cocaine intravenously or intranasally was followed by a significant increase in luteinizing hormone. Clinical effects include increases in sexual feelings and energy as well as intense euphoria. The adverse effects of cocaine on reproductive function include disorders of menstrual cycle duration and impairments in folliculogenesis, ovulation, and luteal phase adequacy. Compared with placebo, both luteinizing hormone and, to a lesser degree, follicle-stimulating hormone levels increased significantly after cocaine administration.[109] Chronic cocaine abuse is associated with erectile dysfunction, perhaps due to endothelial dysfunction.[107] Finally, several reports have associated priapism with intranasal, intraurethral, intracavernous, and topical recreational use of cocaine.[178]

Amphetamines

Cocaine- and amphetamine-regulated transcript is suggested to be involved in the regulation of the hypothalamic-pituitary-thyroid axis. Co-secretion of cocaine- and amphetamine-regulated transcript with thyrotropin-releasing hormone into the portal pituitary circulation, therefore, may have an important modulatory influence on the effect of thyrotropin-releasing hormone on pituitary hormone secretion.[84] D-Amphetamine resulted in poor prolactin suppression in normo- and hyperprolactinemic subjects. Methylenedioxymethamphetamine use can cause neurochemical, behavioral, and endocrine alterations, similar to those produced by exposure to acute stress, suggesting its possible role as a chemical stressor.[36] In humans, acute methylenedioxymethamphetamine treatment results in a rise in cortisol plasma concentrations, supporting the hypothesis of methylenedioxymethamphetamine-induced release of corticotropin-releasing hormone from the median eminence of the hypothalamus and subsequent hypothalamic-pituitary-adrenal axis and sympathetic nervous system activation. A recent study showed that amphetamine or methylenedioxymethamphetamine abusers were prone to having increased sexual desire, erectile dysfunction, and increased ejaculation latency.[35]

Benzodiazepines

Although benzodiazepines produce inconsistent effects on basal hormone secretion, they have potent effects on the inhibition of adrenocorticotropin, cortisol, thyroid-stimulating hormone, and prolactin secretion in response to stressful and pharmacological stimuli.[120] However, it is still unclear whether benzodiazepines reduce thyroid hormones. Acute diazepam administration causes stimulation of growth hormone secretion, but individuals taking this medication regularly over periods of years have an impaired growth hormone response or no response at all (tolerance). Benzodiazepines may act on the γ-aminobutyric acid (GABA)–coupled benzodiazepine receptors at the hypothalamus or other brain regions to reinforce the effects of endogenous GABA. Nevertheless, some neuroendocrine effects of benzodiazepines are mediated through actions on benzodiazepine receptors in the pituitary gland. Plasma testosterone and 11-hydrocorticoid levels are increased by benzodiazepine ligands in humans.[93] In males, testosterone modulates peripheral-type benzodiazepine receptor density in the genital tract. The peripheral-type benzodiazepine receptor density is increased in the human ovary proportional to greater

TABLE 59.8 Main Nutritional and Metabolic Features in Subjects With Substance Use Disorders.

Substance	Nutritional Features	Metabolic Features
Alcohol	Reduced BMI, reduced FM, increased ECW in light to moderate drinking Increased BMI, increased FM in binge drinking and heavy drinking	Increased REE, lower carbohydrate oxidation, higher lipid oxidation Increased energy intake
Nicotine	Reduced BMI, increased WHR	Increased lipid oxidation and lipolysis, decreased lipoprotein lipase activity
Opioids	Reduced BMI, reduced FM	Normal REE
Cocaine	Reduced BMI, reduced FM	Normal REE
Amphetamines	Loss of appetite	Indirect fat-mobilizing action, through an endogenous catecholamine release, and exercise-promoting effects, increasing EE
Benzodiazepines	Hyperphagia, enhanced palatability	Increased glycemia and alterations in insulin secretion

BMI, Body mass index; *ECW*, extracellular water; *EE*, energy expenditure; *FM*, fat mass; *REE*, resting energy expenditure; *WHR*, waist-to-hip ratio.

cell maturation and differentiation. Finally, individuals with benzodiazepine abuse can present with significant sexual dysfunctions such as erectile dysfunction,[87] including a complete loss of libido.

Nutrition and Body Composition

Alcohol

There is some controversy about the effect of ethanol on body weight and about the contribution of alcohol energy to body mass. In fact, several studies have shown a positive, a negative, or no relationship between alcohol consumption and body composition alterations. These discrepancies are at least partially related to the different sample of subjects evaluated (healthy social drinkers, alcohol abusers, or subjects affected by chronic alcoholism) (Table 59.8).

According to Cordain et al.,[64] the intake of small quantities of alcohol by social drinkers seems to have no effect on body composition or metabolism. Consistently, Addolorato et al.[4] have reported no significant modifications of body weight, fat mass, fat-free mass, or total body water in healthy social drinkers. However, although fat-free mass and fat mass were unmodified in the control group, fat mass increased in subjects drinking beer and wine and decreased in subjects who drank liquor. Fat-free mass was stable in beer and wine drinkers and increased in subjects who drank liquor. These data have been confirmed by a recent review paper.[218]

On the contrary, in a study carried out in Italy, the caloric intake from alcohol in males was related to a significant increase in body mass and in the waist-to-hip ratio value, indicating a greater body fat distribution in the intra-abdominal region,[214] which is considered as harmful fat for hypertension. On this connection, energy assumed in the form of alcoholic beverages is additive to the energy absorbed through other foods, leading to calorie overload.[268] Moreover, drinking alcohol before or with meals seems to increase food intake, enhancing the rewarding effects of food, involving, plausibly, GABA, opioid, and dopaminergic systems,[268] or enhancing the perceived palatability of foods.[268]

Other studies have found a positive correlation between alcohol intake and BMI,[65] but it could be related to several factors, including age, gender, the kind of alcoholic beverage used, and the intake patterns.[217,244] Indeed, different studies show that the amount and the intensity of drinking is positively correlated with BMI, whereas frequent light drinking is negatively correlated.[24,42,88,217,244]

The odds of overweight and obesity are higher among binge drinkers (consuming four or more drinks/day), whereas light-to-moderate drinkers (one or two drinks/day).[30] Moreover, binge drinking is associated with higher weight and an adverse body composition profile in young men, but also favorable changes in weight and body composition with exercise intervention.[103] Furthermore, a recent review shows a positive association between beer consumption and abdominal adiposity in men.[37]

On the other hand, the intake of large amounts of alcohol is associated with several nutritional disorders. Indeed, patients with AUD show lower energy intake from fat and carbohydrates, reduced appetite, and malnutrition.[257,262] Ethanol may supply, in fact, more than 50% of the dietary energy partly because of the high caloric content of ethanol (7.1 kcal/g). According to Lieber,[149] long-term consumption of up to 2000 calories/day in the form of alcohol does not produce the expected gain in body weight.

In addition, ethanol can promote a satiety effect by inhibiting gastric motility and by an anorexic effect due to the toxicity of the substance on liver function.[268]

Moreover, nutritional disorders caused by heavy alcohol intake are due to malabsorption of intestinal origin, steatorrhea, and pancreatic disorders, together with impaired hepatic metabolism of nutrients.[149] In past years, a set of studies performed in our laboratory were aimed at evaluating the effect of chronic alcohol abuse on energy metabolism and substrate oxidation in alcoholics without clinical or laboratory evidence of liver disease or malabsorption. Alcohol-dependent individuals seem to have a high resting energy expenditure, thus consuming, even at rest, more energy than social drinkers, and producing heat instead of storing energy in response to food or liquid intake as happens in normal metabolic pathways.[6] The increased resting energy expenditure in these individuals is related in part to the induction of the microsomal ethanol oxidizing system caused by chronic alcohol abuse[4,149,225] and in part to the high thermogenic effect of the ethanol.[85] Ultrastructural abnormalities of mitochondria have been shown in alcohol-dependent individuals, with formation of giant mitochondria and functional alterations characterized by increased thermogenesis with dissipation of heat.[149] A further loss of energy by thermogenesis may be related to increased catecholamine levels.[226] Chronic heavy amounts of ethanol exposure in individuals without malabsorption also produce a lower body weight with respect to control groups and induce a preferential utilization of lipids as energy substrate and a lower carbohydrate oxidation, as indicated by a significantly lower nonprotein respiratory quotient measured by indirect calorimetry assessment.[4,18] These alterations cause alcoholics to have a lower BMI and fat mass and a similar fat-free mass value with respect to controls as measured by dual-energy x-ray absorptiometry.[3,7,10] The alterations in body composition and metabolism seem to be completely reversible, at least in alcohol-dependent individuals who do not have severe alcohol-related disease, after 3 months of complete alcohol abstinence without pharmacotherapy or nutritional supplementation.[3,8] With regard to body fluid distribution, alcohol-dependent individuals show an increase in the extracellular water compartment, with a higher extracellular water/total body water ratio compared with controls.[5] The mechanism responsible for this increase remains unclear. It could be hypothesized that the increased extracellular water/total body water ratio in alcoholics is a result of an increased leak of vacuolar fluid into the interstitial space caused by endothelial damage that occurs due to ethanol-induced vasoconstriction[27] and/or a direct toxic effect of ethanol on the cellular membrane.[7] Moreover, acute ingestion of alcohol causes water diuresis due to inhibition of arginine vasopressin (AVP) release, but an anti-natriuretic effect occurs during chronic exposure, which leads to increase in sodium reabsorption by both the proximal nephron and loop of Henle that contributes to decrease potassium secretion due to a decrease sodium delivery to the distal nephron.[19]

Finally, compared with noncirrhotic subjects, alcoholics affected by liver cirrhosis, and especially those with ascites, show a more impaired nutritional status, with not only increased resting energy expenditure, preferential lipid oxidation, and a reduction in fat mass, but also a reduction in fat-free mass.[4,102,215] This could be due to the low protein intake with the diet, aggravated by ascites gastric compression and consequent anorexia, impaired enteric absorption due to portal hypertension with intestinal protein loss, and disturbance in substrate utilization.[163,215,234] Complications of liver disease such as hematemesis, encephalopathy, and sepsis also caused prolonged periods of poor oral intake. Moreover, low-grade endotoxemia facilitated by portal hypertension and gut bacterial translocation leads to increased levels of cytokines that, especially in acute alcoholic hepatitis and in decompensated liver cirrhosis, cause metabolic and nutritional abnormalities such as fever, anorexia, muscle breakdown, and wasting and altered mineral metabolism.[164]

Nicotine

Chronic nicotine administration and its withdrawal produce significant effects on body weight and food intake. Several studies have reported a significantly lower weight and BMI in cigarette smokers than in non-smokers.[19,23]

Nicotine in fact produces anorexia and promotes weight loss in humans and mice.[160]

However, the former had a significantly higher waist-to-hip ratio than the latter,[250] indicating that cigarette smoking could have harmful effects on the pattern of distribution of body fat. According to Perkins et al.,[194] an acute intake of nicotine significantly increases energy expenditure, slightly at rest, and more significantly during physical exercise. These data were recently confirmed in animal studies.[160]

Changes in body weight could be related to enhanced fat oxidation[121] and increased lipolysis and, over time, decreased lipoprotein lipase activity.[230] Moreover nicotine may alter the energy

balance through the modulation of different hypothalamic pathways. In fact, chronic exposure to the substance in mice reduces the expression of neuropeptide Y (NPY), orexigenic neuropeptide, inducing hyperphagia. It has also been proved that nicotine upregulates the expression of proopiomelanocortin (POMC), anorexigenic neuropeptide, and decreases feeding through activation of POMC neurons.[160,171] An important mediator of these effects seems to be hypothalamic AMP-activated protein kinase (AMPK), and based on this evidence, Martinez De Morentin et al. have shown that nicotine decreases hypothalamic AMPK activation, altering the parameters of energy balance.[160]

Furthermore, nicotine seems to modulate peripheral metabolism in rats increasing brown adipose tissue (BAT) thermogenesis through activation of the sympathetic nervous system.

Opioids and Cocaine

Data available in the literature focus overall on the metabolic and nutritional alterations in subjects with opioid and/or cocaine abuse and dependence. According to Santolaria-Fernandez et al.,[215] drug addicts, especially those with heavier consumption, are undernourished. A recent review by Nabipour et al. shows that opioid-dependent patients have little nutritional knowledge, have little ability to prepare food, and live in poorly placed environments. These factors contribute to their unhealthy eating behaviors.[180] Li et al. have shown that BMI is lower among more frequent heroin users, particularly heroin smokers. In fact, opiates may compete for foods in brain reward sites suppressing appetite.[145]

In particular, the risk of malnutrition in drug users seems to be multifactorial, correlating with lower caloric intake and anorexia, abnormal gastrointestinal function or metabolism, direct effects of the drug itself,[203] intensity of drug addiction and ways of administration, female gender, and disturbance of the social and familial networks.

Consistently, in a small cohort of opioid-addicted subjects evaluated before and after 4 years in a methadone maintenance program, weight loss and decreased BMI were observed in the women, whereas the men experienced an increase in BMI.[134]

Furthermore, drug dependence, especially when parenteral, is frequently complicated by infections, which are particularly harmful when affecting a previously malnourished person. Repeated infections, such as the hepatitis B virus, staphylococcal phlebitis, endocarditis, sepsis, systemic yeast infections, and so on, contribute through the enhancement of catabolism to the development of undernutrition.[215] Moreover, human immunodeficiency virus (HIV) infection may be a main cause of malnutrition (wasting syndrome) in drug addicts. Among HIV-infected individuals with a high prevalence of drug use, females have lower average weight, BMI, and fat mass than nonusers. In particular, women with heavy drug use have lower whole-body fat in both absolute and percentage amounts and higher lean mass. In a recent study, Forrester et al.[86] reported a lower weight and BMI in Hispanic men with and without HIV infection who used cocaine alone or with opiates compared with men who used only opiates or men who were HIV positive but who did not use drugs. The observed differences in BMI are not attributed to differences in reported dietary energy intake, resting energy expenditure, malabsorption, or infection with HIV or hepatitis. According to Cofrancesco et al., the only factor associated with reduced lean and fat mass is heavy illicit drug use among women, a pattern not seen in men, whereas other factors, such as HIV or hepatitis C, seem not to be associated with body composition parameters.[61] Quach et al. showed that body weight was lower among HIV-infected drug addicts than nondrug users; and that cocaine use (and not heroin) was associated with the lowest BMI among HIV-infected patients, even after adjusting for other factors such as age, race, gender, poverty, CD4+ cell count, and individual efforts to gain or lose weight.[203] Tang et al. found a lower percentage of body fat among polysubstance users of cocaine and heroin. No differences were found in BMI between cocaine addicts and heroin addicts, probably due to the fact that the effect of drug use on body mass may be related to the behavior patterns of drug users, rather than to a biological effect of the type of the drug.[232]

Finally, it is imperative to emphasize how more research is needed to better understand the causal relationship between the use of these substances and body weight status.

Amphetamines

No data are available in the literature on the nutritional status and energy expenditure in amphetamines abuse. However, several studies have shown a marked loss of appetite secondary to 3,4-methylene-dioxymethamphetamine and methamphetamine exposure, which persists for a day or more after the drug is taken.[258] Amphetamines act on hypothalamic receptors to release norepinephrine, dopamine, and serotonin, thereby increasing central nervous system activity and decreasing appetite and food intake, factors that lead to weight loss.[106]

In addition, thanks to endogenous catecholamine release, amphetamines have an indirect fat-mobilizing action,[198] and exercise-promoting effects, which increase energy expenditure.[66]

Benzodiazepines

Several previous studies have shown a trend to increased glycemia, aggravation of hyperglycemia in diabetic patients, alteration in insulin secretion, and weight gain related to insulin resistance after consumption of benzodiazepines.[a] Recently, Chevassus et al. showed that benzodiazepines, in particular clonazepam, may alter insulin secretion and insulin sensitivity after a single administration in healthy volunteers.[55] Moreover, benzodiazepines have the property of enhancing palatability through their central brain action. The effects of this action include the promotion of food consumption.[63] However, further studies are necessary to establish whether benzodiazepine abuse is correlated to changes in nutritional status and metabolic features.

References

1. Addolorato G, Abenavoli L, Leggio L, et al. How many cravings? Pharmacological aspects of craving treatment in alcohol addiction: a review. *Neuropsychobiology*. 2005;51:59–66.
2. Addolorato G, Bataller R, Burra P, et al. Liver transplantation for alcoholic liver disease. *Transplantation*. 2016;100:981–987.
3. Addolorato G, Capristo E, Caputo F, et al. The influence of chronic alcohol abuse on energy metabolism and substrate oxidation in human: evaluation of nutritional status in subjects with and without liver cirrhosis. Alcologia. *Eur J Alcohol Studies*. 1998;10:56–61.
4. Addolorato G, Capristo E, Caputo F, et al. The influence of chronic alcohol abuse on energy metabolism and substrate oxidation in human: evaluation of nutritional status in subjects with and without liver cirrhosis. Alcologia. *Eur J Alcohol Studies*. 1998;10:56–61.
5. Addolorato G, Capristo E, Caputo F, et al. Nutritional status and body fluid composition in chronic alcoholics compared with controls. *Alcohol Clin Exp Res*. 1999;23:1232–1237.
6. Addolorato G, Capristo E, Greco AV, et al. Energy expenditure, substrate oxidation and body composition in chronic alcoholism: new findings from metabolic assessment. *Alcohol Clin Exp Res*. 1997;21:962–967.
7. Addolorato G, Capristo E, Greco AV, et al. Influence of chronic alcohol abuse on body weight and energy metabolism: is ethanol consumption in excess a risk factor for obesity or malnutrition? *J Intern Med*. 1998;244:387–395.
8. Addolorato G, Capristo E, Greco AV, et al. Three months of abstinence from alcohol normalizes energy expenditure and substrate oxidation in alcoholics: a longitudinal study. *Am J Gastroenterol*. 1998;93:2476–2481.
9. Addolorato G, Capristo E, Leggio L, et al. Relationship between ghrelin levels, alcohol craving and nutritional status in current alcoholic patients. *Alcohol Clin Exp Res*. 2006;30:1933–1937.
10. Addolorato G, Capristo E, Marini M, et al. Body composition changes induced by chronic ethanol abuse: evaluation by dual energy X-ray absorptiometry. *Am J Gastroenterol*. 2000;95:2323–2327.
11. Addolorato G, Di Campli C, Simoncini M, et al. Oxygen free radical production in rat liver: dose-related effect of ethanol on perfusion injury. *Dig Dis Sci*. 2001;46:1057–1066.
12. Addolorato G, Leggio L, Abenavoli L, et al. Alcoholism Treatment Study Group. Neurobiochemical and clinical aspects of craving in alcohol addiction: a review. *Addict Behav*. 2005;30:1209–1224.
13. Addolorato G, Leggio L, Agabio R, et al. Baclofen: a new drug for the treatment of alcohol dependence. *Int J Clin Pract*. 2006;60:1003–1008.
14. Addolorato G, Leggio L, Ferrulli A, et al. Effectiveness and safety of baclofen for maintenance of alcohol abstinence in alcohol-dependent patients with liver cirrhosis: randomised, double-blind controlled study. *Lancet*. 2007;370:1915–1922.
15. Addolorato G, Leggio L, Ferrulli A, et al. Effectiveness and safety of baclofen for maintenance of alcohol abstinence in alcohol-dependent patients with liver cirrhosis: randomised, double-blind controlled study. *Lancet*. 2007;370:1915–1922.
16. Addolorato G, Leggio L, Ojetti V, et al. Effects of short-term moderate alcohol administration on oxidative stress and nutritional status in healthy males. *Appetite*. 2008;50:50–56.
17. Addolorato G, Mirijello A, Barrio P, et al. Treatment of alcohol use disorders in patients with alcoholic liver disease. *J Hepatol*. 2016;65:618–630.
18. Addolorato G, Montalto M, Capristo E, et al. Influence of alcohol on gastrointestinal motilità: lactulose breath hydrogen testing in orocecal transit time in chronic alcoholics, social drinkers and teetotaler subjects. *Hepato-Gastroenterology*. 1997;44:1076–1081.
19. Adewale A, Ifudu O. Fluid balance: kidney injury, fluid, electrolyte and acid base abnormalities in alcholics. *Niger Med J*. 2014;55:93–98.
20. Agabio R. Thiamine administration in alcohol-dependent patients. *Alcohol Alcohol*. 2005;40:155–156.
21. Akahane K, Furukawa Y, Ogiwara Y, et al. Pharmacological analysis of chrono and inotropic responses to diazepam in the isolated, blood-perfused canine atrium. *Arch Int Pharmacodyn Ther*. 1987;290:173–184.
22. Alameda F, Fontane J, Corominas JM, et al. Reactive vascular lesion of nasal septum simulating angiosarcoma in a cocaine abuser. *Hum Pathol*. 2000;31:239–241.
23. Albanes D, Jones DY, Micozzi MS, et al. Associations between smoking and body weight in the US population: analysis of NHANES II. *Am J Public Health*. 1987;77:439.
24. Albano E. Alcohol, oxidative stress and free radical damage. *Proc Nutr Soc*. 2006;65:278–290.
25. Albertson T, Walby W, Derlet R. Stimulant induced pulmonary toxicity. *Chest*. 1995;198:1140–1149.
26. Al-Mulla Hummadi YM, Najim RA, Farjou IB. Benzodiazepines protect against ethanol-induced gastric mucosal damage in vitro. *Fundam Clin Pharmacol*. 2001;15:247–254.

---

[a] References 40, 122, 138, 156, 196, 229, 271.

27. Altura BM, Altura BT, Carella A. Ethanol produces coronary vaso-spasm: evidence for a direct action of ethanol on vascular muscle. *Br J Pharmacol.* 1983;78:260–262.

28. American Association for the Study of Liver Diseases. European association for the study of the liver hepatic encephalopathy in chronic liver disease: 2014 practice guideline by the European association for the study of the liver and the American association for the study of liver diseases. *J Hepatol.* 2014;61:642–659.

29. Andrews P. Cocaethylene toxicity. *J Addict Dis.* 1997;16:75–84.

30. Arif AA, Rohrer JE. Patterns of alcohol drinking and its association with obesity: data fromo the third National health and nutrition examination survey, 1988-94. *BMC Public Health.* 2005;5:1.

31. Ashley MJ. Smoking and diseases of the gastrointestinal system: an epidemiological review with special reference to sex differences. *Can J Gastroenterol.* 1997;11:345–352.

32. Atkinson HH, Cesari M, Kritchevsky SB, et al. Predictors of combined cognitive and physical decline. *J Am Geriatr Soc.* 2005;53:1197–1202.

33. Augustyńska B, Ziółkowski M, Odrowaz-Sypniewska G, et al. Menstrual cycle in women addicted to alcohol during the first week following drinking cessation—changes of sex hormones levels in relation to selected clinical features. *Alcohol Alcohol.* 2007;42:80–83.

34. Baker KG, Harding AJ, Halliday GM, et al. Neuronal loss in func-tional zones of the cerebellum of chronic alcoholics with and with-out Wernicke's encephalopathy. *Neuroscience.* 1999;19:429–438.

35. Bang-Ping J. Sexual dysfunction in men who abuse illicit drugs: a preliminary report. *J Sex Med.* 2009;6:1072–1080.

36. Baylen CA, Rosenberg H. A review of the acute subjective effects of MDMA/ecstasy. *Addiction.* 2006;101:933–947.

37. Bendsen NT, Christensen R, Bartels E, et al. Is beer consumption related to measures of abdominal and general obesity? A systematic review and meta-analysis. *Nutr Rev.* 2013;71:67–87.

38. Bernal W, Wendon J. Acute liver failure. *N Engl J Med.* 2013;369:2525–2534.

39. Bode C, Bode JC. Effect of alcohol consumption on the gut. *Best Pract Res Clin Gastroenterol.* 2003;17:575–592.

40. Bottaï T, Cartault F, Pouget R, et al. An imidazopyridine anxiolytic alters glucose tolerance in patients: a pilot investigation. *Clin Neu-ropharmaco.* 1995;18:79–82.

41. Brambilla G, Carrozzino R, Martelli A. Genotoxicity and carcinoge-nicity studies of benzodiazepines. *Pharmacol Res.* 2007;56:443–458.

42. Breslow RA, Smothers BA. Drinking patterns and body mass index in never smokers: National Health Interview Survey, 1997-2001. *Am J Epidemiol.* 2005;161:368–376.

43. Brown CD, Maxwell F, French P, et al. Stercoral perforation of the colon in a heroin addict. *BMJ Case Rep.* 2017 (in press).

44. Brown R, Balousek S, Mundt M, et al. Methadone maintenance and male sexual dysfunction. *J Addict Dis.* 2005;24:91–106.

45. Bujanda L. The effects of alcohol consumption upon the gastroin-testinal tract. *Am J Med.* 2000;95:3374–3382.

46. Burra P, Senzolo M, Adam R, et al. Liver transplantation for alco-holic liver disease in Europe: a study from the ELTR (European liver transplant registry). *Am J Transplant.* 2010;10:138–148.

47. Carlin N, Nguyen N, DePasquale JR. Multiple gastrointes-tinal complications of crack cocaine abuse. *Case Rep Med.* 2014;2014:512939.

48. Carlsson S, Hammar N, Grill V. Alcohol consumption and type 2 diabetes meta-analysis of epidemiological studies indicates a U-shaped relationship. *Diabetologia.* 2005;48:1051–1054.

49. Cass WA. Decreases in evoked overflow of dopamine in rat stria-tum after neurotoxic doses of methamphetamine. *J Pharmacol Exp Ther.* 1997;280:105–113.

50. Centers for Disease Control and Prevention Website, https://www.cdc.gov/tobacco/data_statistics/fact_sheets/health_effects/tobacco_related_mortality/index.htm.

51. Chai C, Wang S. Cardiovascular actions of diazepam in the cat. *J Pharmacol Exp Ther.* 1966;154:271–280.

52. Chanraud S, Martelli C, Delain F, et al. Brain morphometry and cognitive performance in detoxified alcohol-dependents with preserved psychosocial functioning. *Neuropsychopharmacology.* 2007;32:429–438.

53. Chapela SP, Paz SLA, Ballestero FM. Pancreatitis induced by cocaine. *Case Rep Gastroenterol.* 2017;11:212–218.

54. Cheng JY, Ng EM, Chen RY, et al. Alcohol consumption and erec-tile dysfunction: meta-analysis of population-based studies. *Int J Impot Res.* 2007;19:343–352.

55. Chevassus H, Mourand I, Molinier N, et al. Assessment of single-dose benzodiazepines on insulin secretion, insulin sensitivity and glucose effectiveness in healthy volunteers: a double-blind, placebo-con-trolled, randomized cross-over trial. *BMC Clin Pharmacol.* 2004;4:3.

56. Chiueh CC, Kopin IJ. Centrally mediated release by cocaine of endogenous epinephrine and norepinephrine from the sympatho-adrenal medullary system of unanesthetised rats. *J Pharmacol Exp Ther.* 1978;205:148–154.

57. Cho CH, Wu KK, Wu S, et al. Morphine as a drug for stress ulcer prevention and healing in the stomach. *Eur J Pharmacol.* 2003;460:177–182.

58. Chowdhury P, Gupta P. Pathophysiology of alcoholic pancreatitis: an overview. *World J Gastroenterol.* 2006;12:7421–7427.

59. Chowdhury P, MacLeod S, Udupa KB, Rayford PL. Pathophysi-ological effects of nicotine on the pancreas: an update. *Exp Biol Med.* 2002;227:445–454.

60. Cobb Scott J, Woods SP, Matt GE, et al. Neurocognitive effects of methamphetamine: a critical review and meta-analysis. *Neuropsy-chol Rev.* 2007;17:275–297.

61. Cofrancesco Jr J, Brown TT, Luo RF, et al. Body composition, gender, and illicit drug use in an urban cohort. *Am J Drug Alcohol Abuse.* 2007;33:467–474.

62. Connor TJ. Methylenedioxymethamphetamine (MDMA, 'Ecstasy'): a stressor on the immune system. *Immunology.* 2004;111:357–367.

63. Cooper SJ. Palatability-dependent appetite and benzodiazepines: new directions from the pharmacology of GABA(A) receptor sub-types. *Appetite.* 2005;44:133–150.

64. Cordain L, Bryan ED, Melby CL, et al. Influence of moderate daily wine consumption on body weight regulation and metabolism in healthy free-living males. *J Am Coll Nutr.* 1997;16:134–139.

65. Croezen S, Visscher T, Ter Bogt N, et al. Skipping breakfast, alco-hol consumption and pshysical inactivity as risk factors for over-weight and obesity in adolescent: result of the E-MOVO project. *Eur J Clin Nutr.* 2009;63:405–412.

66. Curran HV, Robjant K. Eating attitudes, weight concerns and beliefs about drug effects in women who use ecstasy. *J Psychophar-macol.* 2006;20:425–431.

67. Czlonkowski A, Stein C, Herz A. Peripheral mechanisms of opioid antinociception in inflammation: involvement of cytokines. *Eur J Pharmacol.* 1993;242:229–235.

68. Daglish MRC, Nutt DJ. Brain imaging studies in human addicts. *Eur Neuropsychopharmacol.* 2003;13:453–458.

69. Daniell HW. Hypogonadism in men consuming sustained-action oral opioids. *J Pain.* 2002;3:377–384.

70. Davey M. *Grisly effect of One Drug: "Meth Mouth".* New York Times; 2005.

71. De Nunzio C, Andriole GL, Thompson Jr IM, et al. Smoking and prostate cancer: a systematic review. *Eur Urol Focus.* 2015;1:28–38.

72. Dhuna A, Pascual-Leone A, Belgrade M. Cocaine-related vascular headaches. *J Neurol Neurosurg Psychiatry.* 1991;54:803–806.

73. Di Ciaula A, Grattagliano I, Portincasa P. Chronic alcoholics retain dyspeptic symptoms, pan-enteric dysmotility, and autonomic neu-ropathy before and after abstinence. *J Dig Dis.* 2016;17:735–746.

74. Diehl AM. Liver disease in alcohol abusers: clinical perspective. *Alcohol.* 2002;27:7–11.

75. DiMartini A, Javed L, Russell S, et al. Tobacco use following liver transplantation for alcoholic liver disease: an underestimated prob-lem. *Liver Transpl.* 2005;11:679–683.

76. Dorey G. Is smoking a cause of erectile dysfunction? A literature review. *Br J Nurs.* 2001;10:455–465.

77. Ehlers SL, Rodrigue JR, Widows MR, et al. Tobacco use before and after liver transplantation: a single center survey and implications for clinical practice and research. *Liver Transpl.* 2004;10:412–417.

78. Ettinger PO, Wu CF, De La Cruz Jr C, et al. Arrhythmias and the "Holiday Heart": alcohol-associated cardiac rhythm disorders. *Am Heart J.* 1978;95:555–562.

79. European Association for the Study of Liver. EASL clinical practical guidelines: management of alcoholic liver disease. *J Hepatol.* 2012;57:399–420.

80. Facchinetti F, Grasso A, Petraglia F, et al. Impaired circadian rhythmicity of beta-lipotrophin, beta-endorphin and ACTH in heroin addicts. *Acta Endocrinol.* 1984;105:149–155.

81. Facchini FS, Hollenbeck CB, Jeppesen J, et al. Insulin resistance and cigarette smoking. *Lancet.* 1992;339:1128–1130.

82. Federico A, Cotticelli G, Festi D, et al. The effects of alcohol on gastrointestinal tract, liver and pancreas: evidence-based suggestions for clinical management. *Eur Rev Med Pharmacol Sci.* 2015;19:1922–1940.

83. Fedirko V, Tramacere I, Bagnardi V, et al. Alcohol drinking and colorectal cancer risk: an overall and dose-response meta-analysis of published studies. *Ann Oncol.* 2011;22:1958–1972.

84. Fekete C, Lechan RM. Neuroendocrine implications for the association between cocaine- and amphetamine regulated transcript (CART) and hypophysiotropic thyrotropin-releasing hormone (TRH). *Peptides.* 2006;27:2012–2018.

85. Flechtner-Mors M, Biesalski HK, Jenkinson CP, et al. Effects of moderate consumption of white wine on weight loss in overweight and obese subjects. *Int J Obes Relat Metab Disord.* 2004;28:1420–1426.

86. Forrester JE, Tucker KL, Gorbach SL. The effect of drug abuse on body mass index in Hispanics with and without HIV infection. *Public Health Nutr.* 2005;8:61–68.

87. Fossey MD, Hamner MB. Clonazepam-related sexual dysfunction in male veterans with PTSD. *Anxiety.* 1994;1:233–236.

88. French MT, Norton EC, Fang H, et al. Alcohol consumption and body weight. *Health Econ.* 2010;19:814–832.

89. Freudenberger RS, Cappell MS, Hutt DA. Intestinal infarction after intravenous cocaine administration. *Ann Intern Med.* 1990;113:715–716.

90. Gabilondo AM, Meana JJ, Barturen F, et al. Mu-opioid receptor and alpha(2)-adrenoceptor agonist binding-sites in the postmortem brain of heroin-addicts. *Psychopharmacology.* 1994;115:135–140.

91. Garavan H, Hester R. The role of cognitive control in cocaine dependence. *Neuropsychol Rev.* 2007;17:337–345.

92. Garbutt JC, Flannery B. Baclofen for alcoholism. *Lancet.* 2007;370:1884–1885.

93. Gavish M. Hormonal regulation of peripheral-type benzodiazepine receptors. *J Steroid Biochem Mol Biol.* 1995;53:57–59.

94. Ge PS, Runyon BA. Treatment of patients with cirrhosis. *N Engl J Med.* 2016;375:2104–2105.

95. Gerzanich V, Zhang F, West GA, et al. Chronic nicotine alters NO signaling of Ca2+ channels in cerebral arterioles. *Circ Res.* 2001;88:359–365.

96. Ghuran A, Nolan J. Recreational drug misuse: issues for the cardiologist. *Heart.* 2000;83:627–633.

97. Glauser JQueen JR. An overview of non-cardiac cocaine toxicity. *J Emerg Med.* 2007;32:181–186.

98. Go VLW, Gukovskaya A, Pandol SJ. *Alcohol and pancreatic cancer.* 2005;35:205–211.

99. Gómez-Lechón MJ, Ponsoda X, Jover R, et al. Hepatotoxicity of the opioids morphine, heroin, meperidine, and methadone to cultured human hepatocytes. *Mol Toxicol.* 1987–1988;1:453–463.

100. Gourgoutis G, Das G. Gastrointestinal manifestations of cocaine addiction. *Int J Clin Pharmacol Ther.* 1994;32:136–141.

101. Graziano MJ, Dorough HW. Effect of cigarette smoking on hepatic biotransformations in rats. *Toxicol Appl Pharmacol.* 1984;75:229–239.

102. Greco AV, Mingrone G, Benedetti G, et al. Daily energy and substrate metabolism in patients with cirrhosis. *Hepatology.* 1998;27:346–350.

103. Hagnäs MP, Jokelainen J, Cederberg-Tamminen H, et al. Alcohol consumption and binge drinking in youg men as predicotrs of body composition changes during military service. *Alcohol Alcohol.* 2016;53(3):365–371.

104. Hanna ST. Nicotine effect on cardiovascular system and ion channels. *J Cardiovasc Pharmacol.* 2006;47:348–358.

105. Harvez SC, Gilman AG, Goodman LS, et al. Hypnotics and sedatives. In: Gilman AG, Goodman LS, eds. *Goodman and Gilman's the Pharmacological Basis of Therapeutics.* New York: Macmillan; 1985.

106. Haslam D. Weight management in obesity – past and present. *Int J Clin Pract.* 2016;70(3):216–217.

107. Havranek EP, Nademanee K, Grayburn PA, et al. Endothelium-dependent vasorelaxation is impaired in cocaine arteriopathy. *J Am Coll Cardiol.* 1996;28:1168–1174.

108. Hecht SS. Tobacco carcinogens, their biomarkers and tobacco-induced cancer. *Nat Rev Cancer.* 2003;3:733–744.

109. Heesch CM, Negus BH, Keffer JH, et al. Effects of cocaine on cortisol secretion in humans. *Am J Med Sci.* 1995;310:61–64.

110. Heffernon JJ, Smith WR, Berk JE, et al. Hyperamylasemia in heroin addicts. Characterization by isoamylase analysis. *Am J Gastroenterol.* 1976;66:17–22.

111. Henning RJ, Wilson RD, Glauser JM. Cocaine plus ethanol is more cardiotoxic than cocaine or ethanol alone. *Crit Care Med.* 1994;22:1896–1906.

112. Hermann D, Heinz A, Mann K. Dysregulation of the hypothalamic–pituitary–thyroid axis in alcoholism. *Addiction.* 2002;97:1369–1381.

113. Herzberg M, Fishel B, Wiener MH. Hepatic microsomal enzyme induction and its evaluation in a clinical laboratory. *Isr J Med Sci.* 1977;13:471–476.

114. Higuchi LM, Khalili H, Chan AT, et al. A prospective study of cigarette smoking and the risk of inflammatory bowel disease in women. *Am J Gastroenterol.* 2012;107:1399–1406.

115. Hillemacher T, Kraus T, Rauh J, et al. Role of appetite-regulating peptides in alcohol craving: an analysis in respect to subtypes and different consumption patterns in alcoholism. *Alcohol Clin Exp Res.* 2007;31:950–954.

116. Hollander J. The management of cocaine associated myocardial ischemia. *N Engl J Med.* 1995;333:1267–1271.

117. Holubar SD, Hassinger JP, Dozois EJ, et al. Methamphetamine colitis: a rare case of ischemic colitis in a young patient. *Arch Surg.* 2009;144:780–782.

118. Hutchinson MA, Smith PF, Darlington CL. The behavioural and neural effects of the administration of benzodiazepine anxiolytic and hypnotic drugs. *Prog Neurobiol.* 1996;49:73–97.

119. Itskoviz D, Boltin D, Leibovitzh H, et al. Smoking increases the likelihood of Helicobacter pylori treatment failure. *Dig Liver Dis.* 2017;49:764–768.

120. Järvinen A, Rägo L, Männistö PT. Effects of central and peripheral type benzodiazepine ligands on thyrotropin and prolactin secretion. *Neuropeptides.* 1992;21:183–191.

121. Jensen EX, Fusch C, Jaeger P, Peheim E, Horber FF. Impact of chronic cigarette smoking on body composition and fuel metabolism. *J Clin Endocrinol Metab.* 1995;80:2181–2185.

122. Jing X, Wala EP, Sloan JW. The effect of chronic benzodiazepines exposure on body weight in rats. *Pharmacol Res.* 1998;37:179–189.

123. Jokoiama A, Omori T. Genetic polymorphisms of alcohol and aldehyde dehydrogenases and risk for esophageal and head and neck cancers. *Alcohol.* 2005;35:175–185.

124. Jones AL, Simpson KJ. Review article: mechanisms and management of hepatotoxicity in ecstasy (MDMA) and amphetamine intoxications. *Aliment Pharmacol Ther.* 1999;13:129–133.

125. Juenemann KP, Lue T, Luo J, et al. The effect of cigarette smoking on penile erection. *J Urol.* 1987;138:438–441.

126. Kamangar F, Shakeri R, Malekzadeh R, et al. Opium use: an emerging risk factor for cancer? *Lancet Oncol.* 2014;15:e69–e77.

127. Kamijo Y, Soma K, Nishida M, et al. Acute liver failure following intravenous methamphetamine. *Vet Hum Toxicol.* 2002;44:216–217.

128. Kapoor D, Jones TH. Smoking and hormones in health and endocrine disorders. *Eur J Endocrinol.* 2005;152:491–499.

129. Kärkkäinen JM, Miilunpohja S, Rantanen T, et al. Alcohol abuse increases rebleeding risk and mortality in patients with non-variceal upper gastrointestinal bleeding. *Dig Dis Sci.* 2015;60:3707–3715.

130. Kim HB, Myung SK, Park YC, et al. Use of benzodiazepine and risk of cancer: a meta-analysis of observational studies. *Int J Cancer.* 2017;140:513–525.

131. Kish SJ, Kalasinsky KS, Derkach P, et al. Striatal dopaminergic and serotonergic markers in human heroin users. *Neuropsychopharmacology.* 2001;24:561–567.

132. Kloner RA, Rezkalla AH. To drink or not to drink? That is the question. *Circulation.* 2007;116:1306–1317.

133. Koike H, Sobue G. Alcoholic neuropathy. *Curr Opin Neurol.* 2006;19:481–486.

134. Kolarzyk E, Pach D, Wojtowicz B, et al. Nutritional status of the opiate dependent persons after 4 years of methadone maintenance treatment. *Przegl Lek.* 2005;62:373–377.

135. Kristiansen L, Grønbaek M. Risk of pancreatitis according to alcohol drinking habits: a population-based cohort study. Becker U at al. *Am J Epidemiol.* 2008;168:932–937.

136. Kuper H, Boffetta P, Adami HO. Tobacco use and cancer causation: association by tumour type. *J Intern Med.* 2002;252:206–224.

137. Kutscher S, Heise DJ, Banger M, et al. Concomitant endocrine and immune alterations during alcohol intoxication and acute withdrawal in alcohol-dependent subjects. *Neuropsychobiology.* 2002;45:144–149.

138. Langer SZ, Arbilla S. Imidazopyridines as a tool for the characterization of benzodiazepine receptors: a proposal for a pharmacological classification as omega receptor subtypes. *Pharmacol Biochem Behav.* 1988;29:763–766.

139. Reference deleted in review.

140. Leggio L, Ferrulli A, Cardone S, et al. Relationship between the hypothalamic-pituitary-thyroid axis and alcohol craving in alcohol-dependent patients: a longitudinal study. *Alcohol Clin Exp Res.* 2008;32:2047–2053.

141. Leggio L, Ferrulli A, Cardone S, et al. Renin and aldosterone but not the natriuretic peptide correlate with obsessive craving in medium-term abstinent alcohol-dependent patients: a longitudinal study. *Alcohol.* 2008;42:375–381.

142. Leggio L, Ferrulli A, Malandrino N, et al. Insulin but not insulin growth factor-1 correlates with craving in currently drinking alcohol-dependent patients. *Alcohol Clin Exp Res.* 2008;32:450–458.

143. Levine SR, Brust JCM, Futrell N, et al. A comparative study of the cerebrovascular complications of cocaine: alkaloidal versus hydrochloride—a review. *Neurology.* 1991;41:1173–1177.

144. Lew D, Afghani E, Pandol S. Chronic pancreatitis: current status and challenges for prevention and treatment. *Dig Dis Sci.* 2017;62:1702–1712.

145. Li J, Yang C, Davey-Rothwell M, et al. Associations between body weight status and substance use among African American women in Baltimore, Maryland: the CHAT study. *Subst Use Misuse.* 2016;51:669–681.

146. Li LF, Chan RL, Lu L, et al. Cigarette smoking and gastrointestinal diseases: the causal relationship and underlying molecular mechanisms (review). *Int J Mol Med.* 2014;34:372–380.

147. Liaw GW, Hung DZ, Chen WK, et al. Relationship between acute benzodiazepine poisoning and acute pancreatitis risk: a population-based cohort study. *Medicine (Baltim).* 2015;94:e2376.

148. Libby P, Ridker PM, Maseri A. Inflammation and atherosclerosis. *Circulation.* 2002;105:1135–1143.

149. Lieber CS. Perspectives: do alcohol calories count? *Am J Clin Nutr.* 1991;54:976–982.

150. Lieber CS. The discovery of the microsomal ethanol oxidizing system and its physiologic and pathologic role. *Drug Metab Rev.* 2004;36:511–529.

151. Lipski J, Stimmel B, Donoso E. The effect of heroin and multiple drug abuse on the electrocardiogram. *Am Heart J.* 1973;86:663–668.

152. Lovallo WR. Cortisol secretion patterns in addiction and addiction risk. *Int J Psychophysiol.* 2006;59:195–202.

153. Lucas DL, Brown RA, Wassef M, et al. Alcohol and the cardiovascular system. *J Am Coll Cardiol.* 2005;45:1916–1924.

154. Lucey MR, Mathurin P, Morgan TR. Alcoholic hepatitis. *N Engl J Med.* 2009;360:2758–2769.

155. Lugoboni F, Mirijello A, Zamboni L, et al. High prevalence of constipation and reduced quality of life in opioid-dependent patients treated with opioid substitution treatments. *Expert Opin Pharmacother.* 2016;17:2135–2141.

156. Marchetti P, Trincavelli L, Giannarelli R, et al. Characterization of peripheral benzodiazepine receptors in purified large mammal pancreatic islets. *Biochem Pharmacol.* 1996;51:1437–1442.

157. Marin J, Hernandez J. Diazepam potentiates the effects of endogenous catecholamines on contractility and cyclic AMP levels in rat ventricular myocardium. *Naunyn Schmiedebergs Arch Pharmacol.* 2002;365:260–268.

158. Marmor M, Penn A, Widmer K, et al. Coronary artery disease and opioid use. *Am J Cardiol.* 2004;93:1295–1297.

159. Marselli L, Trincavelli L, Santangelo C, et al. The role of peripheral benzodiazepine receptors on the function and survival of isolated human pancreatic islets. *Eur J Endocrinol.* 2004;151:207–214.

160. Martinez de Morentin PB, Whittle AJ, Fernø J, et al. Nicotine induces negative energy balance through hypotalamic AMP-Activated Protein Kinase. *Diabetes.* 2012;61:807–817.

161. Mathurin P, Moreno C, Samuel D, et al. Early liver transplantation for severe alcoholic hepatitis. *N Engl J Med.* 2011;365:1790–1800.

162. Matochik JA, London ED, Eldreth DA, et al. Frontal cortical tissue composition in abstinent cocaine abusers: a magnetic resonance imaging study. *Neuroimage.* 2003;19:1095–1102.

163. Matos C, Parayko MK, Francisco-Ziller N, et al. Nutrition in chronic liver disease. *J Clin Gastroenterol.* 2002;35:391–397.

164. McClain CJ, Barve SS, Barve A, et al. Alcoholic liver disease and malnutrition. *Alcohol Clin Exp Res.* 2011;35:815–820.

165. McKillop IH, Schrum LW. Alcohol and liver cancer. *Alcohol.* 2005;35:195–203.

166. Mehendale SR, Yuan CS. Opioid-induced gastrointestinal dysfunction. *Dig Dis.* 2006;24:105–112.

167. Mehta AJ. Alcoholism and critical illness: a review. *World J Crit Care Med.* 2016;5:27–35.

168. Melichar JK, Hume S, Williams T, et al. Using [C-11]diprenorphine to image opioid receptor occupancy by methadone in opioid addiction: clinical and preclinical studies. *J Pharmacol Exp Ther.* 2005;312:309–315.

169. Mello NK, Mendelson JH. Cocaine's effects on neuroendocrine systems: clinical and preclinical studies. *Pharmacol Biochem Behav.* 1997;57:571–599.

170. Meyer JS, Rauch G, Rauch RA, et al. Risk factors for cerebral hypoperfusion, mild cognitive impairment, and dementia. *Neurobiol Aging.* 2000;21:161–169.

171. Mineur YS, Abizaid A, Rao Y, et al. Nicotine decreases food intake through activation of POMC neurons. *Science.* 2011;332:1330–1332.

172. Mirijello A, D'Angelo C, Ferrulli A, et al. Identification and management of alcohol withdrawal syndrome. *Drugs.* 2015;75:353–365.

173. Mirijello A, Tarli C, Vassallo GA, et al. Alcoholic cardiomyopathy: what is known and what is not known. *Eur J Intern Med.* 2017;43:1–5.

174. Mirijello A, Vassallo G, Landolfi R, et al. Alcoholic cardiomyopathy. *BMJ Case Rep.* 2013. pii: bcr2013201449.

175. Mittleman MA, Mintzer D, Maclure M. Triggering of myocardial infarction by cocaine. *Circulation.* 1999;99:2737–2741.

176. Mouhaffet A, Madu E, Satmary W, et al. Cardiovascular complications of cocaine. *Chest.* 1995;107:1426–1434.

177. Mousavi S, Toussy J, Zahmatkesh M. Opium addiction as a new risk factor of sphincter of Oddi dysfunction. *Med Sci Monit.* 2007;13:CR528–CR531.

178. Munarriz R, Hwang J, Goldstein I, et al. Cocaine and ephedrine-induced priapism: case reports and investigation of potential adrenergic mechanisms. *Urology.* 2003;62:187–192.

179. Mutlu EA, Gillevet PM, Rangwala H, et al. Colonic microbiome is altered in alcoholism. *Am J Physiol Gastrointest Liver Physiol.* 2012;302:G966–G978.

180. Nabipour S, Ayu Said M, Hussain Habil Mohd. Burden and nutritional deficiencies in opiate addiction- systematic review article. *Iran J Public Health.* 2014;43:1022–1032.

181. Nakajima M, Iwata K, Yamamoto T, et al. Nicotine metabolism in liver microsomes from rats with acute hepatitis or cirrhosis. *Drug Metab Dispos.* 1998;26:36–41.

182. Neiman J, Haapaniemi M, Hillbom M. Neurological complications of drug abuse: pathophysiological mechanism. *Eur J Neurol.* 2000;7:595–606.

183. Ness-Jensen E, Lindam A, Lagergren J, et al. Tobacco smoking cessation and improved gastroesophageal reflux: a prospective population-based cohort study: the HUNT study. *Am J Gastroenterol.* 2014;109:171–177.

184. Nieters A, Rohrmann S, Becker N, et al. Smoking and lymphoma risk in the European prospective investigation into cancer and nutrition. *Am J Epidemiol.* 2008;167:1081–1089.

185. Nojkov B, Cappell MS. Distinctive aspects of peptic ulcer disease, Dieulafoy's lesion, and Mallory-Weiss syndrome in patients with advanced alcoholic liver disease or cirrhosis. *World J Gastroenterol.* 2016;22:446–466.

186. O'Brien CP. Benzodiazepine use, abuse, and dependence. *J Clin Psychiatry.* 2005;66:28–33.

187. Offiah C, Hall E. Heroin-induced leukoencephalopathy: characterization using MRI, diffusion-weighted imaging, and MR spectroscopy. *Clin Radiol.* 2008;63:146–152.

188. Oscar-Berman M, Bowirrat A. Genetic influences in emotional dysfunction and alcoholism-related brain damage. *Neuropsychiatr Dis Treat.* 2005;1:211–229.

189. Oscar-Berman M, Marinković K. Alcohol: effects on neurobehavioral functions and the brain. *Neuropsychol Rev.* 2007;17:239–257.

190. Ozsoy S, Esel E, Izgi HB, et al. Thyroid function in early and late alcohol withdrawal: relationship with aggression, family history, and onset age of alcoholism. *Alcohol Alcohol.* 2006;41:515–521.

191. Pascual-Leone A, Dhuna A. Cocaine-associated multifocal tics. *Neurology.* 1990;40:999–1000.

192. Pascual-Leone A, Dhuna A, Anderson DC. Cerebral atrophy in habitual cocaine abusers: a planimetric CT study. *Neurology.* 1991;41:34–38.

193. Payabvash S, Beheshtian A, Salmasi AH, et al. Chronic morphine treatment induces oxidant and apoptotic damage in the mice liver. *Life Sci.* 2006;79:972–980.

194. Perkins KA, Epstein LH, Stiller RL, et al. Acute effects of nicotine on resting metabolic rate in cigarette smokers. *Am J Clin Nutr.* 1989;50:545–550.

195. Pessione F, Ramond MJ, Peters L, et al. Five-year survival predictive factors in patients with excessive alcohol intake and cirrhosis. Effect of alcoholic hepatitis, smoking and abstinence. *Liver Int.* 2003;23:45–53.

196. Petit P, Manteghetti M, Berdeu D, et al. Effects of a peripheral-type benzodiazepine on glucose-induced insulin secretion. *Eur J Pharmacol.* 1992;221:359–363.

197. Piano MR. Alcoholic cardiomyopathy: incidence, clinical characteristics, and pathophysiology. *Chest.* 2002;121:1638–1650.

198. Pinter EJ, Patee CJ. Fat-mobilizing action of amphetamine. *J Clin Invest.* 1968;47:394–402.

199. Reference deleted in review.

200. Powell CJ, Charles SJ, Mullervy J. Cocaine hepatotoxicity: a study on the pathogenesis of periportal necrosis. *Int J Exp Pathol.* 1994;75:415–424.

201. Praud D, Rota M, Rehm J, et al. Cancer incidence and mortality attributable to alcohol consumption. *Int J Cancer.* 2016;138:1380–1387.

202. Purohita V, Khals J, Serrano J. Mechanisms of alcohol-associated cancers: introduction and summary of the symposium. *Alcohol.* 2005;35:155–160.

203. Quach LA, Wanke CA, Schmid CH. Drug use and other risk factors related to lower body mass index among HIV-infected individuals. *Drug Alcohol Depend.* 2008;95:10.

204. Rajendram R, Preedy VR. Effect of alcohol consumption on the gut. *Dig Dis.* 2005;23:214–221.

205. Repetto A, Bello BD, Pasotti M, et al. Coronary atherosclerosis in end-stage idiopathic dilated cardiomyopathy: an innocent bystander? *Eur Heart J.* 2005;26:1519–1527.

206. Reynolds P. Smoking and breast cancer. *J Mammary Gland Biol Neoplasia.* 2013;18:15–23.

207. Reference deleted in review.

208. Rota M, Porta L, Pelucchi C, et al. Alcohol drinking and risk of leukemia-a systematic review and meta-analysis of the dose-risk relation. *Cancer Epidemiol.* 2014;38:339–345.

209. Rota M, Porta L, Pelucchi C, et al. Alcohol drinking and multiple myeloma risk–a systematic review and meta-analysis of the dose-risk relationship. *Eur J Cancer Prev.* 2014;23:113–121.

210. Runyon BA, AASLD Practice Guidelines Committee. Management of adult patients with ascites due to cirrhosis: an update. *Hepatology.* 2009;49:2087–2107.

211. Sabbagh MN, Lukas RJ, Sparks DL, et al. The nicotinic acetylcholine receptor, smoking, and Alzheimer's disease. *J Alzheimer's Dis.* 2002;4:317–325.

212. Sacerdote P. Opioids and the immune system. *Palliat Med.* 2006;20:9–15.

213. Sadr Azodi O, Orsini N, Andrén-Sandberg Å, et al. Effect of type of alcoholic beverage in causing acute pancreatitis. *Br J Surg.* 2011;98:1609–1616.

214. Salvagnini M, Martines D. Alcohol and nutrition: changing the risk from malnutrition to hypernutrition. *Eur J Alcohol.* 1997;9:75–76.

215. Santolaria F, Pérez-Manzano JL, Milena A, et al. Nutritional assessment in alcoholic patients. Its relationship with alcoholic intake, feeding habits, organic complications and social problems. *Drug Alcohol Depend.* 2000;59:295–304.

216. Reference deleted in review.

217. Sayon Orea C, Bes-Rastrollo M, Nunez-Corboda JM, et al. Type of alcoholic beverage and incidenze of overweight/obesity in a Mediterranean cohort: the SUN project. *Nutrition.* 2011;27:802–808.

218. Sayon-Orea C, Mertinez-Gonzales MA, Bes-Rastrollo M. Alcohol consumption and body weight: a systematic review. *Nutr Rev.* 2011;69:419–431.

219. Schifano F, Corkey JM, Cuffolo G. Smokable ("ice", "crystal meth") and smokable amphetamine-type stimulants: clinical pharmacological and epidemiological issues, with special reference to the UK. *Ann Ist Super Sanita.* 2007;43:110–115.

220. Selim K, Kaplowitz N. Hepatotoxicity of psychotropic drugs. *Hepatology.* 1999;29:1347–1351.

221. Shield KD, Soerjomataram I, Rehm J. Alcohol use and breast cancer: a critical review. *Alcohol Clin Exp Res.* 2016;40:1166–1181.

222. Simapivapan P, Boltong A, Hodge A. To what extent is alcohol consumption associated with breast cancer recurrence and second primary breast cancer?: a systematic review. *Cancer Treat Rev.* 2016;50:155–167.

223. Spijkerman IJ, van Ameijden EJ, Mientjes GH, et al. Human immunodeficiency virus infection and other risk factors for skin abscesses and endocarditis among injection drug users. *J Clin Epidemiol.* 1996;49:1149–1154.

224. Reference deleted in review.

225. Suter PM. Is alcohol consumption a risk factor for weight gain and obesity? *Crit Rev Clin Lab Sci.* 2005;42:197–227.

226. Suter PM, Hasler E, Vetter W. Effects of alcohol on energy metabolism and body weight regulation: is alcohol a risk factor for obesity? *Nutr Rev.* 1997;55:157–171.

227. Swan GE, Lessov-Schlaggar CN. The effects of tobacco smoke and nicotine on cognition and the brain. *Neuropsychol Rev.* 2007;17:259–273.

228. Swanson GR, Sedghi S, Farhadi A, et al. Pattern of alcohol consumption and its effect on gastrointestinal symptoms in inflammatory bowel disease. *Alcohol.* 2010;44:223–228.

229. Syvälahti EK, Kanto JH. Serum growth hormone, serum immunoreactive insulin and blood glucose response to oral and intravenous diazepam in man. *Int J Clin Pharmacol Biopharm.* 1975;12:74–82.

230. Sztalryd C, Hamilton J, Horwitz BA, Johnson P, Kraemer FB. Alterations in lipolysis and lipoprotein lipase in chronically nicotine-treated rats. *Am J Physiol.* 1996;270:E215–E223.

231. Talamini R, Polesel J, Spina M, et al. The impact of tobacco smoking and alcohol drinking on survival of patients with non-Hodgkin lymphoma. *Int J Cancer.* 2008;122:1624–1629.

232. Tang AM, Forrester JE, Spiedelman D, et al. Heavy injection drug use is associated with lower percent body fat in a multi-ethnic cohort of HIV-positive and HIV-negative drug users from three U.S. cities. *Am J Drug Alcohol Abuse.* 2010;36(1):78–86.

233. Tanko LB, Christiansen C. An update on the antiestrogenic effect of smoking: a literature review with implications for researchers and practitioners. *Menopause.* 2004;11:104–109.

234. Teiusanu A, Andrei M, Arbanas T, et al. Nutritional status in cirrhotic patients. *Maedica.* 2012;7(284):9.

235. Temko JE, Bouhlal S, Farokhnia M, et al. The Microbiota, the Gut and the Brain in Eating and Alcohol Use Disorders: a 'Ménage à Trois'? *Alcohol Alcohol.* 2017;52:403–413.

236. Tennant F. Hepatitis C, B, D, and A: contrasting features and liver function abnormalities in heroin addicts. *J Addict Dis.* 2001;20:9–17.

237. Teyssen S, Singer MV. Alcohol-related diseases of the oesophagus and stomach. *Best Pract Res Clin Gastroenterol.* 2003;17:557–573.

238. Thomas GA, Rhodes J, Ingram JR. Mechanisms of disease: nicotine—a review of its actions in the context of gastrointestinal disease. *Nat Clin Pract Gastroenterol Hepatol.* 2005;2:536–544.

239. Thomson AD. Mechanisms of vitamin deficiency in chronic alcohol misusers and the development of the Wernicke-Korsakoff syndrome. *Alcohol Acohol Suppl.* 2000;35:2–7.

240. Thorgeirsson TE, Geller F, Sulem P, et al. A variant associated with nicotine dependence, lung cancer and peripheral arterial disease. *Nature.* 2008;452:638–642.

241. Thursz MR, Forrest EH, Ryder S. STOPAH investigators. Prednisolone or pentoxifylline for alcoholic hepatitis. *N Engl J Med.* 2015;373:282–283.

242. Tilg H, Day CP. Management strategies in alcoholic liver disease. *Nat Clin Pract Gastroenterol Hepatol.* 2007;4:24–34.

243. Reference deleted in review.

244. Tolstrup JS, Heitmann BL, Tjonneland AM, et al. The relation between drinking pattern and body mass index, waist and hip circumference. *Int J Obes.* 2005;29:490–497.

245. Tome S, Lucey MR. Review article: current management of alcoholic liver disease. *Aliment Pharmacol Ther.* 2004;19:707–714.

246. Trabulo D, Marques S, Pedroso E. Cocaine capsules in the colon: the internal concealment of illicit drugs. *J Gastrointestin Liver Dis.* 2015;24:9.

247. Tramacere I, Negri E, Bagnardi V, et al. A meta-analysis of alcohol drinking and oral and pharyngeal cancers. Part 1: overall results and dose-risk relation. *Oral Oncol.* 2010;46:497–503.

248. Reference deleted in review.

249. Tramacere I, Pelucchi C, Bonifazi M, et al. A meta-analysis on alcohol drinking and the risk of Hodgkin lymphoma. *Eur J Cancer Prev.* 2012;21:268–273.

250. Troisi RJ, Heinold JW, Vokonas PS, Weiss ST. Cigarette smoking, dietary intake, and physical activity: effects on body fat distribution—the Normative Aging Study. *Am J Clin Nutr.* 1991;53:1104–1111.

251. Trummer H, Habermann H, Haas J, et al. The impact of cigarette smoking on human semen parameters and hormones. *Hum Reprod.* 2002;17:1554–1559.

252. Tutuian R. Clinical lead outpatient services and gastrointestinal function laboratory. Adverse effects of drugs on the esophagus. *Best Pract Res Clin Gastroenterol.* 2010;24:91–97.

253. Vassallo G, Mirijello A, Ferrulli A, et al. Review article: alcohol and gut microbiota - the possible role of gut microbiota modulation in the treatment of alcoholic liver disease. *Aliment Pharmacol Ther.* 2015;41:917–927.

254. Veenman L, Gavish M. The peripheral-type benzodiazepine receptor and the cardiovascular system. Implications for drug development. *Pharmacol Ther.* 2006;110:503–524.

255. Vestergaard P. Smoking and thyroid disorders. *Eur J Endocrinol.* 2002;146:153–161.

256. Reference deleted in review.

257. Victor M, Adams RD, Collins GH. *The Wernicke–Korsakoff Syndrome and Other Related Neurologic Disorders Due to Alcoholism and Malnutrition.* Philadelphia: FA Davis; 1989.

258. Vollenweider F, Gamma A, Liechti M, Huber T. Psychological and cardiovascular effects and short-term sequelae of MDMA ('ecstasy') in MDMA-naive healthy volunteers. *Neuropsychopharmacology.* 1998;19:241–251.

259. Walsh K, Alexander G. Alcoholic liver disease. *Postgrad Med J.* 2000;76:280–286.

260. Weller IV, Cohn D, Sierralta A, et al. Clinical, biochemical, serological, histological and ultrastructural features of liver disease in drug abusers. *Gut.* 1984;25:417–423.

261. Whitehead TP, Robinson D, Allaway SL. The effects of cigarette smoking and alcohol consumption on serum liver enzyme activities: a dose-related study in men. *Ann Clin Biochem.* 1996;33:530–535.

262. Windham CT, Wyse BW, Hansen RG. Alcohol consumption and nutrient density of diets in the Nationwide food consumption survey. *J Am Diet Assoc.* 1983;82:365–372.

263. Winniford MD. Smoking and cardiovascular function. *J Hypertens.* 1990;9:S17–S23.

264. Wood JD, Galligan JJ. Function of opioids in the enteric nervous system. *Neuro Gastroenterol Motil.* 2004;16:17–28.

265. Yadav P, Ellinghaus D, Rémy G, et al. Genetic factors interact with tobacco smoke to modify risk for inflammatory bowel disease in humans and mice. *Gastroenterology.* 2017;153:550–565.

266. Yates WR, Labrecque DR, Pfab D. The reliability of alcoholism history in patients with alcohol-related cirrhosis. *Alcohol Alcohol.* 1998;33:488–494.

267. Yen DJ, Wang SJ, Ju TH, et al. Stroke associated with methamphetamine inhalation. *Eur Neurol.* 1994;34:16–22.

268. Yeomans MR. Alchol, appetite and energy balance: is alcohol intake a risk factor of obesity? *Physiol Behav.* 2010;100:82–89.

269. Yu MC, Yuan JM. Environmental factors and risk for hepatocellular carcinoma. *Gastroenterology.* 2004;127:S72–S78.

270. Zhang Y, Eslick GD, Xia HH, et al. Relationship between alcohol consumption and active Helicobacter pylori infection. *Alcohol Alcohol.* 2010;45:89–94.

271. Zumoff B, Hellman L. Aggravation of diabetic hyperglycemia by chlordiazepoxide. *J Am Med Assoc.* 1977;237(18):1960–1961.

60

Quadruple Diagnosis: Substance Use Disorder, Comorbid Psychopathology, Human Immunodeficiency Virus Infection, and Hepatitis C Virus Infection

KARL GOODKIN, STEVEN F. KENDELL, DAENA PETERSON, LEON CUSHENBERRY, AND FRANCISCO FERNANDEZ

Introduction

Comorbid substance use disorders (SUDs) and other psychiatric disorders (dual diagnosis) in individuals who are infected with human immunodeficiency virus (HIV) and hepatitis C virus (HCV) are common. Prevalence rates of such dual diagnoses vary significantly across reported studies, ranging from 10% to 50% or more, depending on the sample assessed.[85,98] In a large cross-sectional study, up to half of the clients in an HIV-dedicated clinic carried a diagnosis of at least one psychiatric disorder, and nearly 40% also had psychoactive SUDs (other than marijuana)—with up to 12% of the latter having severe use disorder (formerly "dependence") over the prior 12 months. In a review of the area, the prevalence of co-occurring substance use and mental health disorders ranged from a low of 10%—similar to the aforementioned study—to a high of 28% among persons living with HIV,[21] and the concern for this triply diagnosed group continues to grow. A focus has grown on another triply diagnosed group—those diagnosed with an SUD, other psychiatric disorder, and HCV infection. One study of this group (n = 293) coming for an initial hepatology clinic visit showed that 93% had a current psychiatric disorder or a history of at least one psychiatric disorder, and 73% had more than two disorders, with depressive disorder being the most common (81%), followed by posttraumatic stress disorder (PTSD) (62%), SUD (58%), bipolar affective disorder (20%), and other psychotic disorders (17%).[41] Of note, SUDs are specifically associated with increased sensation seeking and impulsivity, both of which are related to high-risk behavior for HIV and HCV infection in this population. That is, unsafe sexual practices and needle sharing are greatly increased in this group. Vice versa, individuals with other psychiatric disorders may eventually develop SUDs, varying according to the specific type of disorder. SUDs contribute to psychological distress and the emergence of new psychiatric disorders, many times induced by the substance itself. Both SUDs and other psychiatric disorders manifest with impaired insight and judgment. The related ongoing change in mental status, in turn, contributes to the aforementioned HIV and HCV high-risk behaviors, including severe substance use urges, sharing of substances to facilitate immediate use, and use by injection with sharing of needles and injection paraphernalia to maximize the impact on sensation of such use. Similarly, in this setting as well, high urges to engage in sexual activity occur, sexual risk-taking discussion and precautions are neglected in favor of immediate sexual gratification, and unprotected sexual intercourse occurs (including very high-risk associated behaviors, such as trading sex for money). Given the high comorbidity between the dually diagnosed (SUDs and other psychiatric disorders), HIV infection, and HCV infection, the focus of this chapter is to examine recent data regarding the interactions between this specific form of dual psychiatric comorbidity with HIV and HCV infection, as well as other associated comorbidities, that is, HIV-associated neurocognitive disorder (HAND), morbidity, and mortality.

Nearly 37 million people are living with HIV around the world. In the United States, 1.2 million people are living with HIV, of whom 13% are unaware of their diagnosis. Regarding HCV infection, there are an estimated 3.5 million HCV-infected persons in the United States, 2.7 million in the general noninstitutionalized population,[35] plus an additional 800,000 incarcerated, institutionalized, or homeless[37]; about half of all infected people are unaware that they are infected. Among patients with chronic HCV infection, approximately one-third progress to cirrhosis, at a median time of less than 20 years. The rate of progression increases with older age, alcohol use disorder, male sex, and HIV co-infection. About 25% of people living with HIV in the United States also have HCV infection, approximately 300,000 people. A meta-analysis found that HCV/HIV co-infected patients had a threefold greater risk of progression to cirrhosis or decompensated liver disease than HCV mono-infected patients. The risk of progression is even greater in HCV/HIV co-infected patients, with low CD4+ T lymphocyte count (i.e., CD4 cell count). Although effective antiretroviral therapy (ART) appears to slow the rate of HCV disease progression in HCV/HIV co-infected patients, the rate continues to exceed that in HCV mono-infected. Whether HCV infection accelerates HIV progression remains unclear, although some antiretroviral medications (ARVs) are associated with higher rates of hepatotoxicity in patients with chronic HCV infection.

For more than a decade, the mainstay of HCV treatment had been a combination regimen of pegylated interferon and ribavirin, but this regimen was associated with a poor rate of sustained virologic response (SVR) to HCV, especially in co-infected patients. Rapid advances in HCV drug development since 2011 led to the use of new classes of direct-acting antivirals (DAAs) that target the HCV replication cycle. Recently approved DAAs are used without interferon and with or without ribavirin and have higher SVR rates, reduced pill burden, less frequent dosing, fewer side effects, and shorter durations of therapy than the earlier approved regimens, yielding a new dawn for the medical treatment of the HIV/HCV co-infected patient. These gains have yet to be applied to the care of co-infected patients with SUDs and other psychopathology.

Scope of the Problem

High rates of HIV infection have been documented in individuals with dual diagnosis. In one study of persons living with HIV with comorbid SUDs and other psychiatric disorders ($n = 1,848$), HIV prevalence was 4.7% versus only 2.4% in participants diagnosed with a SUD without another psychiatric disorder comorbidity. A cross-sectional survey of 3806 adults living

with HIV infection across four major metropolitan areas in the United States showed that nearly 75% of respondents reported occasional use of psychoactive substances, 40% reported frequent use of various psychoactive substances, and only 28% declared abstinence from all psychoactive substances.[72] In the group reporting frequent use of psychoactive substances, more were likely to be identified as heterosexual, had public health insurance, and endorsed increased symptoms of major depressive disorder (MDD)[13,72]—illustrating the impact of triple diagnosis of SUDs, other psychiatric disorders, and HIV infection. In the quadruply diagnosed with HIV and HCV co-infection, it has been reported that nearly one-third have a concomitant mental disorder—predominantly depressive—whereas approximately one-fifth have active SUDs.[114]

Substance Use Disorders (SUDs)

Intravenous substance use has long been associated with an increased prevalence of a comorbid psychiatric diagnosis— especially dysthymic disorder and MDD[2, 68]. Depressive spectrum disorders in intravenous substance-using individuals have been repeatedly linked to increased likelihood of sharing needles, syringes, and other paraphernalia, which further increases the risk of HIV and HCV transmission.[2,16,113] Stein and colleagues examined the association of depressive disorder severity (i.e., MDD, dysthymic disorder, and substance-induced mood disorder lasting at least 3 months) with substance injection risk behaviors among injecting substance users. After controlling for multiple confounding variables, including age, race, gender, number of days on which injection drugs were used, and the average number of injections per injection-day, a diagnosis of a depressive disorder was still significantly associated with injection substance use behaviors.[113]

Similarly, other data illustrate that individuals with depressive spectrum disorders are more likely to engage in unprotected sexual activity with intravenous substance-using individuals—heightening an already substantial risk of HIV and HCV transmission.[58] This same population also demonstrates increased rates of sexual abuse, which predicts depressive features, increased suicidality, and increased nonadherence to antiretroviral therapy for HIV and direct-acting antiviral (DAA) therapy for HCV, making the risk of progression and viral resistance to HIV and HCV greater in these groups.[14,73,95] Deleterious outcomes in HIV-infected intravenous substance users have been related to a variety of factors, including increased rates of HCV co-infection, decreased access to and engagement in care, diminished adherence to effective ART regimens, MDD and other depressive disorders, psychosocial stressors, and HIV-associated AIDS and non-AIDS (HANA) morbidity and mortality.[71]

Among individuals who inject substances, studies have shown that up to one-third are at risk for severe MDD, with women experiencing greater severity. Correlates of depressed mood and general distress in both men and women include perceived functional limitations, greater negative feelings regarding condom use, higher life stressor burden and impact, lower social support availability and satisfaction, higher passive, maladaptive coping strategy use, and a lower sense of empowerment with higher external locus of control. Similarly, a history of physical abuse and minority ethnicity also appear to be significant predictors of MDD among intravenous drug users of both genders who are living with HIV.[120] Methamphetamine-dependent men who have sex with men also demonstrate high lifetime rates of psychiatric disorders including major depression and anxiety disorders. Generalized anxiety disorder, specific phobia, bipolar disorder, and major depressive disorder have all been linked to higher rates of sexually transmitted infections, including gonorrhea and HIV.[108] Crystal methamphetamine use has evolved to be a major risk factor for the development of MDD and other psychiatric disorders as well as increased transmission rates of HIV infection. Naturalistic interview studies have demonstrated the wide prevalence of a cycle of severe depressed and anxious mood level in the context of methamphetamine use as well as persistent anhedonia. Almost all respondents in such studies have reported that methamphetamine was severely damaging to social relationships, resulting in increased self-isolation. In addition, methamphetamine use has been tied closely to random sexual encounters and increased numbers of sexual partners, with a decreased likelihood of condom use.[84] A better understanding of these patterns and risks is essential in developing effective prevention strategies. Alcohol use alone has been linked to multiple risk factors associated with HIV including sexually transmitted disease histories, condom nonuse, multiple sex partners, and lower HIV-related knowledge. These risks appear to increase substantially with increasing amounts of alcohol use, and individuals demonstrating abstinence from alcohol appear to have the lowest risk profile. The impact of alcohol upon these risk factors remains present even in the absence of other drug abuse.[56,87]

Psychiatric Disorders Other Than SUDs

Common mental disorders among individuals with HIV and substance abuse include adjustment disorders, sleep disorders, depressive disorders, mania, dementia, delirium, psychosis, and personality disorders.[13] A careful psychiatric assessment is necessary to engage in differential diagnostic considerations and differential therapeutics. There are three categories of mental disorders of concern in substance users living with HIV: substance-induced mental disorders, HIV-related mental disorders, and medication-related mental disorders.[13]

Psychiatric Disorders in Human Immunodeficiency Virus Infection

Depressive Spectrum Disorders

Depression is a highly general term that specifies neither level of decreased mood nor the presence of a syndromal disorder including decreased mood. Syndromal depression is a collection of symptoms that—when taken in different combinations—characterize one of the depressive spectrum disorders, including MDD, dysthymia, adjustment disorder with depressed mood, substance-induced depressive disorder, and depression due to a general medical condition. Thus the etiology and pathophysiology of the various sub-types constituting the more properly described group of depressive spectrum disorders are quite varied. MDD, specifically, is the most common mood disorder in the general population, with a 12-month prevalence of 4.7% in men and 8.5% in women.[107] MDD, also, is the most common mood disorder in people living with HIV infection, occurring at rates two to three times higher than that in the general population.[18] Commensurate with the prevalence of MDD in the general population, the MDD rate in women living with

HIV is higher than that of men. A study by Bhatia and Munjal examining the prevalence of depressive disorder in people living with HIV/AIDS undergoing ART demonstrated a 63% prevalence in females, thereby exceeding the 58.1% prevalence shown in males.[12] Furthermore, MDD severity is associated with an increased frequency of intravenous substance use and associated high-risk behaviors,[113] placing such individuals at greater risk for both HIV and HCV infection.

Despite the high rates of comorbidity between mood and SUDs, the origins of this association are not well understood. Self-medication, genetic predisposition, and psychosocial factors all may be involved.[20] Further complicating this picture, epidemiological studies note that prevalence rates differ between individuals with primary MDD and a comorbid SUD versus the prevalence of a primary SUD with comorbid MDD.[49] A study of individuals with primary MDD demonstrated a relatively low 8.5% prevalence rate for a comorbid SUD.[67] In contrast, a study of individuals with a primary SUD and comorbid MDD showed a considerably higher 20% prevalence of MDD.[48] The high prevalence of MDD in the population living with HIV speaks to the impact of inflammation in both disorders. Manifested by a potent inflammatory response, the acute stage of HIV infection involves a substantial elevation of the pro-inflammatory cytokines tumor necrosis factor α (TNF-α), interleukin-1 (IL-1), and IL-6. Of note, this potent inflammatory cytokine response has also been identified in HCV infection.[111] As an etiological component of depressive disorders, this acute increase in pro-inflammatory cytokines induces sickness behavior—a behavioral complex of responses.[76] Acting on the hypothalamus, the cytokine response induces changes in homeostatic set points resulting in fatigue and hypersomnolence, loss of appetite and subsequent weight loss, anhedonia, malaise, and neurocognitive symptoms.[115] As depicted, the similarities between sickness behavior and MDD are striking; in turn, the associated, potent inflammatory response and accompanying pro-inflammatory cytokine elevations may in fact contribute to the etiology of MDD symptoms in persons living with HIV.[102] Additional neurocognitive manifestations of the highly detrimental synergistic impact of HIV and MDD may include decreased attention and vigilance, cognitive slowing, and impaired working and episodic memory.[40] Such neurocognitive deficits may reflect the propensity for MDD to be associated with increased cerebrospinal fluid (CSF) HIV load.[61]

By means of the cytokine inducer, lipopolysaccharide (LPS), animal models of MDD also depict the impact of inflammation on behavior.[91] Although acute inflammation is essential for pathogen removal and tissue repair, the impact of unchecked chronic inflammation may be significantly destructive. As might be expected, high life-stressor burden is a significant risk factor for the development of MDD, and— of relevance here—life stressors have been shown to activate the production of pro-inflammatory cytokines[75] due, in part, to associated cortisol secretion. In turn, it has been suggested that chronic exposure to pro-inflammatory cytokines may contribute to glucocorticoid resistance[29] by means of a decrease in glucocorticoid receptor alpha (the active form of the receptor) and an increase in glucocorticoid receptor beta (a relatively inert form).[92] Such glucocorticoid resistance manifests as a decrease in the sensitivity of immune cells to glucocorticoid hormones that normally terminate the inflammatory response.[29,112] In addition to neuroendocrine function, both neurotransmitter metabolism and neuronal plasticity are affected by the impact of cytokines on pathophysiologic processes.[34] Through the stimulation of multiple signaling pathways, cytokines can activate indoleamine 2,3 dioxygenase (IDO).[35] This stimulation of IDO results in the breakdown of tryptophan (TRP), serotonin's primary amino acid precursor, into kynurenine (KYN), which converted to quinolinic acid (QUIN) in microglia, promotes glutamate release via the activation of N-methyl-D-aspartate (NMDA) receptors, an important factor in excitotoxicity.[88]

Although depressive disorders may decline in patients not infected by HIV with advancing age, this does not appear true of persons living with HIV, who are at continued risk for depressive disorders well into older age.[97] In addition, depressive disorders have been closely linked to apathy in patients living with HIV, and this apathy may reflect HIV infection of the brain. Both apathy and depressed mood are linked to suboptimal adherence to effective ART.[99] Similarly, fatigue has also been linked to depressed mood and a diagnosis of MDD,[66] with an increase in the release of pro-inflammatory cytokines, for example, TNF-α, and subsequent long-term neuroinflammation inducing fatigue in persons living with HIV.[74] Furthermore, a recent study by Barroso et al. reported that HIV-related fatigue remains the most frequent complaint of patients living with HIV,[8] and fatigue is known to be caused by pro-inflammatory cytokine release (particularly TNF-α) associated with the long-term inflammation seen in treated persons living with HIV. Depressive disorder severity has also been linked to a greater frequency of intravenous substance use and its associated high-risk behaviors.

Women appear to be a special at-risk group with regard to depressive disorders and intravenous substance use. Depressive disorder prevalence rates and severity are elevated among women who are both infected with HIV and intravenous substance users.[86] Women also frequently report a history of childhood and adult trauma and poorer quality of life scores in the context of HIV infection, despite showing some protection against neurocognitive decline with respect to their male counterparts.[123] Substance use, violence, and depressive disorders have been deemed a tripartite HIV risk among African American women, which remains an underexplored area of research. Women with a history of sexually transmitted infections (STIs) have been noted to be more likely to experience violence and depressive disorders, both individually and jointly. This described tripartite risk group is also reflective of those women having two or more sexual partners in the last 30 days as well as those having an early onset of alcohol use disorder.[63] Similarly, ARV adherence has been noted to be low in substance-using women as compared with men; however, mental health care has been shown to be significantly associated with improved adherence in this patient subgroup as opposed to their male counterparts[117]—again highlighting the need for effective psychiatric services in this at-risk group.

HIV-Associated Mania and Bipolar Affective Disorder in HIV Infection

HIV-induced mania may occur in up to 8% of late-stage patients.[38] The impulsivity and hypersexuality associated with mania exacerbates an already increased risk for HIV and HCV infections.[78,101] In addition, the considerably inflated risk of SUDs in mania further magnifies both impulsivity and high-risk behaviors.[78,80] In addition to HIV infection itself, one of its complications, cryptococcal meningitis, may also present as mania in full-blown AIDS.[23,62] The "great masquerader," syphilis, may also present with mania. It has been suggested that the CSF of patients living with HIV being evaluated for HAND should be screened using both the venereal disease research

laboratory (VDRL) and the fluorescent treponemal antibody (FTA) absorption test, since patients with a history of syphilis may lose serum reactivity in the setting of HIV infection (even when otherwise asymptomatic). Moreover, neurosyphilis itself may be asymptomatic in about 10% of cases. Corticosteroid treatment commonly used with acute presentations of *Pneumocystis carinii* pneumonia (PCP; later documented to be due to *Pneumocystis jirovecii* and now less common in the high-resource countries) in persons living with HIV carries a known risk for mania.[19] Iatrogenic mania also remains a risk with zidovudine (ZDV) therapy,[79] although ZDV (formerly azidothymidine [AZT]) is rarely used today. HIV-induced mania more frequently presents with neurocognitive impairment (NCI) in persons living with HIV and has been associated with a better response to the use of valproic acid over lithium.

Preexisting bipolar disorder in the context of HIV infection is especially problematic in that it involves cycling between depressive and manic episodes, with the complications related to decreased and increased goal-directed behavior in each phase, respectively. The manic phase of bipolar disorder increases the likelihood of psychoactive substance use and is related to increased impulsivity and sexual risk-taking behavior. One study examining the link between mania and HIV infection demonstrated that a significant majority of study participants had been sexually active in the past 6 months (75%). They disclosed engaging in high-risk sexual behaviors such as unprotected intercourse (69%), having multiple partners (39%), sex with prostitutes (24%, men only), and sex trading (10%). Severity of bipolar illness was also associated with HIV risk profile.[80]

Psychosis and Thought Disorders

Up to 30%–50% of patients living with serious mental illness (SMI) have SUDs.[100] Earlier studies by one prominent group in New York City suggested that the prevalence rate of HIV infection among persons living with SMI was variable, depending upon relevant factors in the population living with SMI, including homelessness, treatment setting and status, specific psychotic diagnosis, dual diagnosis with substance use disorders, and sampling method (open vs. anonymous).[121] Additional foci of import directly related to persons living with SMI are cognitive impairment and psychotic symptoms that impede the planned use of risk precautions for sexual activity and injection substance use—and present special difficulties to control in this population.[9] Another issue of import not addressed by the paper is the percentage of patients with co-infections—dual and triple, as mentioned earlier. HCV co-infection occurs in up to 25% of patients living with HIV in the United States. Worldwide, 10% of patients are co-infected with HIV and HBV, with an up to 20% HIV-HBV co-infection rate in Southeast Asia. The exact number of patients co-infected with HCV and HBV is unknown; in patients with chronic HBV infection, estimates of the rates of HCV co-infection vary from 9% to 30%. Finally, triple infection has been reported worldwide at a rate from 1%–7%[14]; hence, an attempt to dissect out the population living with SMI by these specific co-infection rates would be of interest.[44] In addition to the cognitive impairment associated with chronic HIV infection, acute infection may also present with psychosis.[6] New onset of psychosis can also emerge in chronically persons living with HIV, with methamphetamine use, in particular, being a significant risk factor.[124] It cannot be concluded that only the typical risk factors apply to this patient population when the factors that would be specific to patients living with SMI contributing to their risk have not been taken into account (e.g., cognitive impairment and psychotic symptom severity). Frequently, patients living with SMI are managed while experiencing chronic cognitive impairment that might impede their adherence to antipsychotic medication therapy, which can result in ongoing psychotic symptoms that can prevent them from accessing and implementing precautions for preventing these infections. Future research should aim at assessing the contributions of these factors to additional risk for these infections in SMI patients. Health providers should discuss sexual health and risk for blood-borne viral infection with SMI patients and offer HIV testing to all patients 13 to 64 years of age at least once in their lifetimes and should offer HCV testing to all adults born from 1945 through 1965 once (without prior ascertainment of HCV risk factors) in the United States. HBV screening should be offered under specific circumstances, as recommended by the Centers for Disease Control and Prevention (CDC). Ongoing risk should result in more frequent testing per CDC recommendations for these infections. Worldwide screening recommendations for these infections may be accessed through the World Health Organization.

Psychosocial Issues in Persons Living With HIV

Childhood sexual experiences have been linked as a strong predictor to psychological distress as well as risk of substance abuse and HIV transmission risk.[5,64] Among men who have sex with men (MSMs), those with a history of childhood sexual abuse were more likely to engage in high-risk sexual behaviors including unprotected receptive anal intercourse, trading sex for money or drugs, reporting HIV seropositive status, and experiencing nonsexual relationship violence.[64] In addition, when confronting this group of at-risk individuals, it is useful to distinguish between forced childhood sexual abuse and consensual childhood sexual experiences. Individuals who experienced forced sexual contact have the highest risk of these three factors as compared with the consensual group who demonstrated only increased rates of substance abuse and HIV transmission risk compared with a no-exposure group.[5] Thus, an assessment of these groups should include a discussion of patterns of risk exposure and childhood sexual exposure to better tailor interventions to the specific individual.

The role of past trauma in placing individuals at risk of HIV has also been found in large populations of women living with HIV.[58,89] Hutton identified that among women prisoners, HIV risk behaviors in the 5 years preceding incarcerations included unprotected sex (56%), injection substance use (42%), sexual intercourse with a partner who injected drugs (42%), prostitution (30%), needle sharing (30%), receptive anal sex (19%), and having more than 100 sex partners (7%). After adjusting for age, education, race, HIV serostatus, and addictive disorders, posttraumatic stress disorder was associated with the practice of receptive anal sex and prostitution and appeared to contribute to these high-risk activities.

In addition, Myers identified an association between greater frequency of severe SUDs and increasing rates of HIV infection, depressive disorders, and higher chronic disease burden among women. Similarly, severe alcohol use disorder and trauma have been associated with increased depression and social instability in this group as well.[89,110] It is important to note that both childhood trauma and depression severity appear to exacerbate ineffective and avoidant coping strategies, which may predispose this group to additional burdens of depression and disease throughout life.[110] Likewise, among nonadherent women who are prescribed effective ART, the use of cocaine and heroin and a history of SUDs decreased

the likelihood of acceptable adherence to effective ART.[28] These items taken alone or together illustrate not only the need for substance abuse programs but also the important role of sexual abuse prevention efforts and abuse treatment strategies in at-risk groups.

Other data support a high prevalence of depression and substance use disorder among persons living with HIV enrolled in methadone maintenance treatment programs or needle exchange. Depression is extremely common in these programs, and one study has estimated rates as high as 54%. Women, persons with a comorbid alcohol abuse diagnosis, and those with diminished social support were more likely to be depressed, even after controlling for age, race, education, and HIV status. Those enrolled in methadone programs showed significantly less depression than similar participants in a needle exchange program.[17]

Three predictors have been conceptualized as an stressor-support-coping model[3,43] as follows. Life stressors (especially when unpredictable, uncontrollable, and chronic) are associated with greater distress. Social support (especially if available, satisfactory, and sufficient to the situation) may have both direct and indirect effects on reducing distress, the latter by buffering the negative impact of life stressors. Passive, maladaptive coping styles such as denial, or mental or behavioral disengagement (e.g., drinking alcohol or using substances to manage a stressor) may be expected to increase distress, as has been shown in persons living with HIV.[69] In contrast, active coping strategies (e.g., taking action or reduce stressor impact, or creating a plan to cope with a stressor; positive reinterpretation and finding meaning in a stressor) may be expected to decrease distress.

Hepatitis C Virus (HCV) Infection

Another complicating factor that commonly exists in dually diagnosed individuals with HIV disease is the concurrent diagnosis of HCV infection, yielding the quadruply diagnosed. Large observational retrospective cohort studies in high-risk populations have demonstrated that approximately 25% of persons living with HIV are co-infected with HCV; the co-infected group is characterized by being older minority men more likely to acquire HIV through intravenous substance use. In addition, individuals co-infected with HIV and HCV are more likely to have a diagnosis of a depressive disorder, alcohol or substance use disorder, and a history of "hard-drug" use compared to the HIV monoinfected. Co-infected individuals are also less likely to have received effective ART during the previous year.[7]

In one study of 293 patients being seen for an initial hepatology visit, 93% had a current or past history of at least one psychiatric disorder, and 73% carried at least two psychiatric disorder diagnoses.[41] The most common disorders included depressive disorders (81%), posttraumatic stress disorder (62%), any substance use disorder (58%), bipolar affective disorder (20%), and other psychotic disorders (17%); in addition, 61 patients (21%) had AUDIT-C alcohol screening test scores indicating current, heavy alcohol use.

Neurocognitive Impairment Related to Substance Use Disorder, Other Psychiatric Disorder, HIV Infection, and HCV infection

Previous alcohol use disorder has been demonstrated to be linked with additive levels of cognitive dysfunction in populations living with HIV. Significant and synergistic interactions in the realm of reaction time (representing the domain of information processing speed) have been noted in populations living with HIV with a history of alcohol use disorder.[50] There may also be neurocognitive complications of SUDs, including effects from both recreational and prescribed use of psychoactive substances as well psychoneurotoxicity of antiretroviral medications and cancer chemotherapy.[26,57,70] Substance-induced NCI is of greatest concern regarding psychostimulant use, particularly cocaine and methamphetamine, but also is related to opioid use. Opioid use disorder is associated with NCI spanning multiple domains that may negatively affect daily psychosocial function and response to SUD treatment.[39]

Of psychiatric disorders other than SUDs, MDD is the most common in the setting of current SUDs, HIV infection, and HCV infection. It is defined, in part, by neurocognitive symptoms—that is, by impaired memory and concentration. A systematic review and meta-analysis of cognitive function assessed using the Cambridge Neuropsychological Test Automated Battery (CANTAB) battery in patients with MDD revealed significant, moderate neurocognitive deficits in executive function, memory, and attention in patients with MDD relative to controls (effect size $d = -0.34$ to -0.65). Significant, moderate deficits in executive function and attention ($d = -0.52$ to -0.61) and nonsignificant, milder deficits in memory ($d = -0.22$ to -0.54) were found to persist in remitted patients, suggesting that mild cognitive impairment (MCI) may occur separately from the episodes of MDD themselves.[104]

One of the common complications of HIV infection is NCI. Numerous studies indicate the percentage of individuals living with HIV and having any NCI during the course of their infection to be 39%–54% overall, despite greater access to effective ART,[90] with much fewer in recent studies meeting the criteria for HIV-associated dementia (HAD).[33,55,90,103] Given these prevalence rates, clinicians working with patients living with HIV must screen for signs indicating the presence of NCI regardless of the lack of any associated symptoms; in turn, with a positive screen, a referral for a formal neuropsychological evaluation to fully delineate the etiology of the NCI is indicated. An assessment for associated deficits in functional status—as indicated by a decline in activities of daily living—is also warranted, as is the development of a treatment plan geared toward improving cognition and daily life function.[54] HIV infects the brain during the initial stage of infection as part of the natural course of the infectious process and may eventually cause HIV-associated neurocognitive disorder (or HAND). HAND represents a spectrum proceeding from asymptomatic neurocognitive impairment (ANI) to mild neurocognitive disorder (MND) on to HIV-associated dementia (or HAD). Today, data show that ANI is the most common HAND condition; however, as the mildest one of the spectrum, there is frequent lack of its recognition. Likewise, MND may frequently be overlooked by the primary care provider who is not actively screening for NCI. As a whole, HAND is currently very common but less severe than it had been prior to the era of effective ART. Thus, it could be characterized as an "invisible epidemic." The criteria defining these disorders were reviewed at the Frascati Conference, where HAD was defined by standardized testing as two standard deviations (SDs) or greater below demographically corrected means on at least two neurocognitive domains. Furthermore, in HAD, NCI must be associated with at least moderate interference with activities of daily living/functional status. For MND, the cognitive impairment must be documented by a milder decrement in standardized test performance of at least 1.0 SD below demographically corrected means on at least two domains and not meet the criteria for dementia (2 SDs or greater below demographically

corrected means). This impairment must, in turn, be associated with at least mild decrements in functional status. Like MND, the newly coined condition of ANI is documented by NCI on standardized test performance of 1.0 SD below demographically corrected means on at least two domains and not meeting the HAD criteria; however, in contrast to MND, the NCI associated with ANI does not interfere with functional status. Hence, the designation of ANI is more fittingly described as a condition rather than a disorder or disease. For all of these conditions, there should be no evidence of another preexisting cause, including systemic and CNS opportunistic infections and tumors, non–HIV-associated neurological disease, metabolic causes, CNS toxicities due to prescribed medications, and potentially confounding psychiatric disorders (e.g., major depressive disorder and alcohol or SUDs). Screening tests useful for NCI in the general population, such as the Mini-Mental State Examination (MMSE) and (to a lesser extent) the Montreal Cognitive Assessment, do not perform particularly well among patients living with HIV. Disease-specific tests such as the HIV dementia scale (HDS),[96] the Modified HIV Dementia Scale (m-HDS), and the International HIV Dementia Scale (IHDS),[105] may be used but have recognized limitations as well. Thus, there is no single best screening test for HAND. Moreover, there are no US Food and Drug Administration (FDA)–approved specific treatments for HAND. Clinically, the first line generally used is the CNS-penetrating ARVs and the second line is the psychostimulants. Similarly, for HCV-associated NCI, the first-line treatment considered is the DAAs (or direct-acting antivirals).

Individuals with HIV and HCV co-infection may incur more substantial NCI than that occurring with either infection alone. Both HIV and HCV infections can deleteriously impact CNS processes. More specifically, and like HIV infection, HCV infection has been linked to increased depressive disorder rates and impairment in health-related quality of life—independent of the severity of associated liver disease and the related metabolic effects.[1] Regarding HCV infection, the direct and detrimental CNS impact of HCV infection on the domains of attention, concentration, and information processing has been well documented[27]; notably, all of these deficits are consistent with the deleterious effects, too, of HIV infection.[25] Extensive evidence attests to the impact of inflammation on the pathophysiology of all three disorders.[11,24,42,52,53]

The impact of MDD itself on neurocognitive performance in populations living with HIV should not be overlooked. Published studies are scarce as of yet, but do support the link of MDD with NCI in HIV infection.[123] Neurocognitive performance across multiple domains appears impaired on the latter group—including attention, neurocognitive flexibility, and motor speed.[46] These results illustrate the potentially synergistic combinations of neurocognitive effects that triply diagnosed individuals may experience, which are further exacerbated in the quadruply diagnosed (with HCV infection as well). Along with the need for an exquisitely high level of clinical suspicion for neurocognitive disorders in this group of patients, it is especially important to recognize their associated deleterious impact on medication adherence—not only to ART for HIV treatment but also to the DAAs used in HCV treatment, and, in turn, on mortality. Even when suppression of plasma HIV load is attained long-term and sustained virologic response (SVR) is achieved with HCV treatment, the negative impact of the associated inflammatory processes may nevertheless make themselves known clinically. Thus addressing both HIV- and HCV-induced neurocognitive deficits will likely continue to be of high importance in the dually diagnosed psychiatric patient population.

Stigma, HIV Infection, Hepatitis C Virus Infection, Substance Misuse and SUDs, and Other Psychiatric Disorders

The multiple impacts of racism in the United States are implicated as factors in the increasing rates of HIV infection among racial minority groups.[15,93] Impacts of racism within the literature have focused on problem behaviors and psychiatric disorders, including SUDs, as personal barriers to successful HIV prevention and treatment, thereby reducing the scope of the problem to the level of the individual patient within a medical framework. Current research documents the critical need to extend the focus to include the role of institutions and systems in perpetuating racial stigma through structural racism.[4,15,93,119] Erving Goffman in 1963 defined stigma as "an attribute that is significantly discrediting"—reducing individuals, groups, or people to "physical, behavioral, or social traits seen as divergent from group norms."[4] More recently, stigma has become better defined from the structural perspective—as a symptom and byproduct of social and structural inequality, organized along axes of nationality, gender, race/ethnicity, class, and sexual orientation. Thus individuals who are positioned at the intersection of social and structural forms of inequality due to their ethnoracial, gender, sexual, or class identity may also be stigmatized due to these identities as well.[a]

Social stigma as it relates to race may be a cause for increasing racial HIV disparities due to its influence on individual and structural factors. Structural factors, such as current and past practices of racism by various social institutions, combine with individual-level concerns, such as racial stereotypes, prejudice, and discrimination to compound social segregation and restrict access to limited resources.[36] Perceptions and anticipation of racial stigma can add to distrust toward providers. Decreased HIV testing in racial minorities may stem from efforts to avoid the diagnosis and the subsequent placement into a more stigmatized group. The stigma associated with sexuality and race themselves may lead to decreased intraracial and interracial social support, which is worsened when a person is known to have HIV infection. Moreover, social segregation generally leads African American men to become isolated from their communities, and this isolation is compounded by perceptions of the low acceptability of HIV infection within the African American community. The combination of loss of acceptance within one's own community and rejection by society as a whole can lead to internalized oppression and depressive disorders. Stressors induced by these forms of rejection are perceived to be mitigated by unprotected sexual intercourse with other African American men as a form of validation and the desire to counteract isolation. Furthermore, among heterosexual African American men, there have been reported links between the impacts of racial discrimination and increased high-risk sexual HIV behaviors.[4,15,36] There are well-documented studies showing that youth with the experience of racism have an increased likelihood of the use of multiple psychoactive substances compared with those without such experiences.[93] There remains a need for more research studies to further detail these relationships.

As gender and sexual minority individuals become more visible in the United States, the effects of stigma become more apparent. Gender and sexual minorities, as well as racial minorities, increase misuse of alcohol, psychoactive substances, and prescribed psychoactive medications in response to experiences laden with stigma. Individuals with multiple minority identities are at particularly increased risk for HIV infection, hepatitis C virus infection, alcohol and substance misuse and SUDs, and other psychiatric disorders, including mood disorders, anxiety disorders, and posttraumatic stress disorder.[b] Meyer[81,82] reported that gay men experiencing the effects of multiple stressors due to their minority status demonstrate increasing mental health concerns in an additive fashion. Subsequent research demonstrated that sexual and gender minority individuals experience the deleterious effects of stigma on their mental health and physical health in a manner similar to that of racial minorities. In addition, racial minority individuals who represent sexual and gender minority groups demonstrate minority-associated distress in an additive manner, leading to significantly increased levels of physical and mental illness.[81,82]

Role of SUDs and Other Psychiatric Disorders in the Treatment With and Adherence to Effective ART for HIV Infection and DAAs for HCV Infection

Previous studies examining the relationship between depressive disorders and HIV transmission have shown mixed results, but the role of depressive disorders upon adherence to effective ART has been confirmed in multiple studies on the subject.[118] A longitudinal study of persons living with HIV with dual diagnosis (comorbid SUDs and other psychiatric disorder) demonstrated several concerning results. Almost 73% of participants met criteria for MDD, which was linked, in turn, to suboptimal medication adherence.[10] It is notable that the demography of this sample was reflective of that of more recently infected persons living with HIV, as 75% were people of color, 66% self-reported sexual orientation as heterosexual, and >50% were unemployed.[10] Given that high dual psychiatric diagnosis rates are common among HIV-infected individuals, a great deal of attention has been devoted to the study of these factors and their impact on adherence in persons living with HIV. Large cross-sectional studies demonstrated that individuals with psychiatric diagnoses, including depressive disorders, generalized anxiety disorder (GAD), and panic disorder, were more likely to be less adherent to effective ART over the previous week than controls without these diagnoses. Suboptimal adherence was also associated with cocaine, amphetamine, or sedative use in the previous month, with cocaine use being the strongest predictor of low adherence in the SUD group, whereas GAD demonstrated the highest rate of suboptimal adherence among the psychiatric diagnoses. However, severe alcohol use disorder also showed the highest rate of suboptimal adherence among all psychiatric diagnoses combined—illustrating the considerable need for effective interventions with this specific disorder—one that is frequently neglected compared to other SUDs.[116] It should similarly be noted that the rate of cannabis use disorder is quite high in this patient population—partly related to the acknowledged treatment effects of cannabis to increase appetite and decrease chronic pain. However, cannabis has recently become much better recognized to carry the potential for harmful effects as well. The impact of SUDs and other psychiatric disorders on persons living with HIV is significant in that multiple studies have also linked diminished adherence rates to the direct effects of these conditions. Beyond the frequently overlooked negative impacts of alcohol and cannabis use disorders, nicotine use disorder (cigarette smoking) has also been shown to be

---

[a]References 4, 15, 31, 36, 93, 119.

[b]References 4, 7, 15, 83, 93, 94.

an independent predictor of suboptimal adherence in persons living with HIV who are receiving effective ART, who smoke at frequencies as high as 70%. It is notable that this risk of suboptimal adherence diminishes with cessation of smoking.[109] Based on available data, a history of SUDs without current use does not predict suboptimal ART adherence, which again illustrates the importance of active interventions designed to curb SUDs.

Furthermore, the presence of depressive disorders has also been linked as an independent risk factor not only to suboptimal ARV adherence but also to HIV disease progression, plasma viral load elevations, and CD4 cell count diminution. (Note that CD4 cells are directly invaded and killed by HIV and that the count of these cells in the peripheral blood is used as a laboratory marker of HIV disease progression.) These associated outcomes have been documented in a study of effective ART-treated substance users living with HIV and comprising 17% intravenous users. Depressive disorder was found in 46% of the study group during the follow-up period, with suboptimal adherence in 31%. Clinical predictors of disease progression included both higher depressive symptom scores following the initiation of effective ART and suboptimal ARV adherence, with higher depressive symptom scores remaining significant after controlling for adherence behavior.[14] Similar studies focusing on HIV-seropositive women living with HIV also found that chronic depressive disorder was a predictor of AIDS-related death, with symptoms being more severe among women in the terminal phase of their illness.[60] Of interest, mental health care has been associated with reduced mortality.[32] Other affective syndromes including bereavement and chronic grief have also been linked to disease progression in HIV-infected populations living with HIV.[45,47] Persons living with HIV who have depressive disorders and receive psychiatric treatment with antidepressants are more likely than untreated individuals to receive appropriate care for their HIV disease and increase their ARV adherence. Antidepressant therapy for treatment of depressive disorders in this population has also been demonstrated to be associated with a lower monthly cost of medical care services based upon at least one study examining merged Medicaid and surveillance data. Moreover, women and substance users engaged in treatment were most likely to receive an antidepressant response, and those receiving antidepressants achieved a 24% reduction in monthly total health care costs as compared with a depressed but untreated cohort.[106]

Risk-Taking Behaviors

Previous cross-sectional data have illustrated a close relationship between SUDs, depressive disorders, and at-risk behaviors, but a limitation of cross-sectional research is that it does not confirm causal inferences. One longitudinal study examining the relationship between depressive disorder and sexual risk behaviors in a community sample of 332 inner-city persons with SUDs reported that increasing severity of depressive disorder predicted sexual encounters with multiple partners as well as sexual encounters with known intravenous substance users.[122] Similarly, depressive disorder has been linked to greater frequency of injection risk behaviors among depressed intravenous substance users.[113]

Other studies have confirmed a link between mental health and risk-taking behaviors, controlling for SUD patterns. One study using a subset analysis of clinic clients with STIs who met the criteria for MDD[58] demonstrated that individuals with depressive disorders were more likely to trade sex for money or drugs, to have a greater number of lifetime sexual partners, and to have a higher likelihood of abusing alcohol or other substances. The

HIV risk behaviors associated with depressive disorder persisted despite control for SUDs. This emphasizes the critical need to more frequently screen for and actively treat depressive disorders in at-risk populations. Another longitudinal study reported on HIV risk behaviors and substance use among 557 Latino heroin and cocaine intravenous substance users not in treatment. Not surprisingly, this study showed a strong association between mental health and SUD variables.[77] Intravenous substance users in the study reported high rates of both depressive (52%) and anxiety disorder (37%), with concurrent alcohol intoxication in the last 30 days by 18% of participants. Those showing SUDs with multiple substances were three times more likely to share needles and cotton. Those with SUDs using multiple substances were also more likely to engage in unprotected sex.[77] These studies illustrate that prevention efforts designed to reduce HIV infection risk must address both SUDs and other psychiatric disorders in the triply diagnosed population. It might be anticipated that these results would also apply to the HCV infected as well as the HBV infected, as both are predominantly contracted through injection substance use; hence, these results may well typify the quadruply diagnosed as well.

Another impact of the presence of comorbid psychiatric disorders and SUDs has been the role associated with specific forms of psychopathology in promoting increased sexual risk-taking behaviors in youthful populations. One study examining a cohort of newly homeless youth followed longitudinally for up to 24 months demonstrated that substance use was a significant predictor of having multiple sexual partners as well as decreased condom use. It has also been associated with low body mass index and malnutrition. Moreover, the impact of depressive disorder and SUDs upon ARV adherence and HIV transmission is heightened by the consideration that dual mental disorder diagnosis increases the risk of unsafe sexual encounters —specifically among those with HIV strains identified as resistant to ARV treatment. Data from the Study of the Consequences of the Protease Inhibitor Era[22] showed that among participants taking effective ART, 60% had genotypic resistance to at least one ARV medication. In those with documented ARV medication resistance, 27% of MSMs and 11% of heterosexual men and women reported at least one episode of unprotected penile-anal or penile-vaginal intercourse over the previous 4 months. Of prominent import, up to 17% of MSMs reported unprotected intercourse with an HIV-seronegative partner or a partner of unknown HIV serostatus. Significant predictors included younger age, depressive disorder, and the use of sildenafil and alcohol. These risk factors readily allow for the development of targeted behavioral prevention interventions regardless of limitations in resources.[22]

As noted previously, the role of psychostimulant SUDs—especially with cocaine and methamphetamine—is major in determining HIV risk. Moreover, rates of methamphetamine use appear to be increasing in at-risk populations (e.g., MSMs). Furthermore, medical complications of methamphetamine use are multiple. They include hypertension, hyperthermia, rhabdomyolysis, and cerebrovascular accident.[22] In addition, comorbid methamphetamine use and HIV infection have been linked to increased likelihood of severe cognitive and movement disorders[65] as well as chronic psychosis—despite discontinuation of methamphetamine use. A large analysis of 736 enrolled participants in the EXPLORE study, who were MSMs, reported use of methamphetamine, nitrite inhalants ("poppers"), and cocaine to be linked to sexual risk behavior. Younger participants were more likely to increase their substance use over time. High-risk sexual behavior was most common during periods characterized by increased methamphetamine, popper, or inhaled cocaine use. A within-person analysis indicated that both low-frequency substance use periods (less than weekly) and frequent substance use periods were significantly associated with unprotected anal sex involving partners living with HIV or partners of unknown HIV serostatus, when compared to abstinence periods.[30] Thus, an abstinence model may be safer and more efficacious than models targeting controlled substance use outcomes. Similar data regarding alcohol use support abstinence over controlled use outcome models.[116]

Assessment of the Quadruply Diagnosed

The assessment of the quadruply diagnosed poses special difficulties, as they are more likely to manifest complex disease in all aspects of care (primary medical and mental health), including increased numbers of HIV mutations and resistance, failure to achieve an SVR after HCV treatment with DAAs, treatment-resistant MDD, posttraumatic stress disorder, as well as either ongoing SUDs or a high SUD recidivism risk. Ideally, psychiatric consultation-liaison services and psychiatric addiction subspecialty services are available to the infectious diseases clinic, so that the patient can be approached and evaluated simultaneously by practitioners of complementary but independent disciplines to gain a more "four-dimensional" understanding of his or her needs, and risk factors, so as to allow optimization of the individual patient's treatment plan. The comprehensive assessment of these individuals should include an extensive and detailed psychosocial history assessing major and minor stressful life events and their impact; social support availability, satisfaction, and sufficiency; active versus passive maladaptive coping strategy use; prior psychiatric history, and any history of trauma or physical or sexual abuse—given that all of these factors have been suggested to be significant in predicting suboptimal medication treatment adherence and disease progression of both HIV and HCV infections. In addition, a detailed SUD history, including types of substances, age at first use, frequency and route of use, triggers, and any available protective or resiliency factors is absolutely essential in providing support and guiding individuals toward appropriate mental health treatments for SUDs and other psychiatric disorders that will allow concurrent HIV and HCV treatment.[12,18,72] Of note, effective ART slows the progression of HCV-associated liver disease by preserving or restoring immune function and reducing HIV-associated immune activation and inflammation; for the majority of patients, the benefits of effective ART outweigh the concerns about possible medication-induced liver injury, and effective ART should be initiated in all HIV/HCV co-infected patients (regardless of CD4 cell count).[51]

SUD Treatment of the Quadruply Diagnosed

Many factors contribute to the delayed treatment entry of the quadruply diagnosed. These can include dropping out of care, living in unstable housing or being homeless, lack of food, lack of transportation, the complexities of the health care system, health maintenance organization-required payment authorizations, and idiosyncratic referral practices of the medical team for SUD or other psychiatric care consultations, or both. Intravenous substance users are less likely to receive effective ART than any other subgroup of patients living with HIV. Factors associated with their low access to treatment include active intravenous substance use, suboptimal engagement in health care, lack

of SUD treatment provision, recent incarceration, and lack of specific, relevant health care provider expertise.[111] Yet, effective ART is of proven utility in intravenous substance users.[51] Optimal use of ART in this patient subgroup requires that primary care providers and their clinical care sites become more actively patient-centered and have increased capacity to integrate with and/or provide opioid substitution therapies (also referred to as "medication-assisted treatment") for SUDs. It is particularly important to have access to both methadone and buprenorphine with resources to appropriately manage side effects and toxicities and to enhance ARV and DAA adherence. One study of triply diagnosed women lost to follow-up in an HIV clinic[85] evaluated a nursing outreach intervention over 3 months to assist with treatment entry. It showed that home visits to assist in making and keeping appointments, accompanying women on their initial clinic visits, and integration of care among HIV, SUD, and other mental health providers were each found to improve outcomes in access to, adherence to, and retention in care.

Longitudinal data demonstrate that both HIV-seropositive status and baseline depressive disorder status independently predicted recurrent or persistent episodes of MDD in intravenous substance users. Substance users living with HIV with baseline MDD showed a 90% rate of at least one subsequent major depressive episode over a 3-year period, and 47% experienced at least three subsequent episodes.[112] Still, less than 40% of this patient subgroup received psychiatric treatment during this time period, resulting in maintaining a high-risk group not only continuously engaging in HIV risk behaviors but also being undertreated for risk factors contributing to these same high-risk behaviors. One study examining the effects of an intensive outpatient cocaine treatment program over 9 months found that risk behavior among participants was correlated with high mental health problem severity and symptom level at intake. Over the course of treatment, risk behaviors were found to decrease significantly among individuals actively participating in the outpatient treatment program. The decrement in risk behaviors was linked to decreased substance use but did not appear to be affected by demographic variables or type or duration of treatment in this study.[115] Other potential data-driven intervention models include brief peer-delivered educational interventions. These models have been shown to be effective when compared with a standard National Institute on Drug Abuse (NIDA) HIV testing and counseling protocol for patients with cocaine use disorder.[108] Both types of treatment models have demonstrated efficacy in reducing crack cocaine use, intravenous substance use, and the number of intravenous substance-using sex partners. Patients also diagnosed with an antisocial personality disorder demonstrated less improvement than their non-antisocial personality disorder controls. Neither intervention model was shown to be effective in improving condom use,[108] which illustrates the complex nature of these risk factors and the need to have multiple intervention targets for high risk behaviors.

Methadone maintenance treatment programs are also an essential part of the treatment of quadruply diagnosed individuals. Increasing numbers of patients in methadone maintenance treatment are showing abstinence from intravenous substance use,[107] generating a successful harm reduction outcome. Methadone maintenance treatment has also been demonstrated to dramatically reduce recreational opioid use as well as related criminal activities. More recently, data support that methadone maintenance treatment can reduce incarceration rates. This would likely also result in diminution of needle sharing and of exposure to high-risk practices during incarceration.[39] In addition, opioid treatment-resistant dually diagnosed individuals show better long-term retention in methadone maintenance treatment programs than their opioid treatment responsive, dually diagnosed counterparts.[117] Buprenorphine programs centering on group activity and support also demonstrate significant roles for the treatment of the quadruply diagnosed, and involvement in either methadone or buprenorphine maintenance treatment programs is associated with improved adherence to effective ART regimens[97] and to DAA treatment for HCV infection. Buprenorphine is likewise associated with improved ARV therapy adherence,[89] although it is greatly underutilized in patients living with HIV in the United States. France appears to have the most experience with buprenorphine programs in patients living with HIV, and the data support their efficacy in this patient subgroup,[58] despite the fact that both methadone and buprenorphine have significant drug-drug interactions with the ARVs. Regarding HCV treatment, the agents oxycodone, tramadol, and fentanyl are metabolized primarily by cytochrome P450 (CYP)3A and might require dose reduction when used with the DAAs boceprevir or telaprevir. Other opioids have a reduced potential for interaction with boceprevir, telaprevir, simeprevir, faldaprevir, daclatasvir, and sofosbuvir.

Methadone is metabolized primarily via CYP3A4, and this CYP isoenzyme also is responsible for the metabolism of multiple ARVs—most notably, those in the protease inhibitor (PI) class. Consequently, drug-drug interactions and potential complications involving methadone/buprenorphine prescribed concurrently with effective ART include changes in pharmacokinetics as well other effects such as a prolonged QTc interval.[37,101] Ritonavir produces strong CYP3A4 inhibition initially, but has also been documented to induce the 3A4 iso-enzyme when administered chronically. Therefore, it is clear that clinical drug-drug interactions are difficult to predict over time and require careful monitoring. For instance, initiation of a ritonavir- or other PI-containing ARV regimen in an individual on stable methadone maintenance treatment might result in opiate toxicity and overdose due to early CYP3A4 inhibition.[92] Conversely, lopinavir (another PI) is a potent inducer of methadone metabolism, with one study finding that the combined effects of lopinavir/ritonavir administered to methadone maintenance treatment recipients included significant reductions in the methadone area under the curve (AUC) and reduction in the maximum serum concentration achieved in the setting of increased methadone oral clearance.[62] Consequently, the authors also noted increased rates of apparent opioid withdrawal in this patient subgroup, highlighting the need for careful monitoring of patients during initiation of either effective ART or methadone maintenance treatment.

Buprenorphine is also metabolized by CYP3A4, and concurrent ritonavir acutely inhibits its metabolism, producing higher levels—as with methadone.[92] However, conflicting data also demonstrate relative safety in using buprenorphine in the setting of the PIs as well as the nonnucleoside reverse transcriptase inhibitor (NNRTI) ARV class (which includes efavirenz).[80] Nevertheless, one case series of three buprenorphine/naloxone-maintained patients did report increased sedation with buprenorphine when the atazanavir/ritonavir combination was initiated, which raises the possibility that atazanavir or atazanavir/ritonavir may increase buprenorphine concentrations that would require a subsequent dose reduction.[78] The area of clinical evidence for drug-drug interactions of the ARVs with the opioids and with psychotropics used for other psychiatric disorders must be monitored on an ongoing basis.

Summary and Conclusions

In summary, the quadruply diagnosed patient presents with significant disadvantages with regard to optimizing health status. High HIV and HCV prevalence rates are seen in individuals with dual diagnoses of SUDs and other psychiatric disorders. Multiple factors may contribute to the delayed entry or premature cessation of ARV and/or DAA treatment of these patients. All patients who enter an HIV, HCV, or HIV/HCV co-infection treatment program should also be assessed systematically for SUDs and other psychiatric disorders. Individuals with dual diagnoses who are also diagnosed with HIV, HCV infection, or HIV/HCV co-infection should be referred both to SUD treatment programs and to programs offering psychopharmacological interventions coupled with individual, group, and/or family psychotherapy, as appropriate, for the other comorbid psychiatric disorder diagnosed. Drug-drug interactions between ARVs (and to a lesser extent DAAs) and recreational psychoactive substances or prescribed psychotropics can increase or decrease action of either drug. Thus special attention must be given to potential drug-drug interactions in the triply and quadruply diagnosed patient. CNS-penetrating ARVs and psychostimulant treatment may be used with comorbid neurocognitive disorder to improve neurocognitive impairment, while harm reduction approaches exemplified by opioid substitution therapies with methadone or buprenorphine can minimize the impact from concurrent opioid use disorder.

References

1. A guide to the clinical care of women with HIV/AIDS - 2005 edition. 2005.
2. Abbott PJ, Weller SB, Walker SR. Psychiatric disorders of opioid addicts entering treatment: preliminary data. *J Addict Dis.* 1994;13(3):1–11.
3. Antoni MH, Goodkin K. Host moderator variables in the promotion of cervical neoplasia–II. Dimensions of life stress. *J Psychosom Res.* 1989;33(4):457–467.
4. Arnold EA, Rebchook GM, Kegeles SM. Triply cursed': racism, homophobia and HIV-related stigma are barriers to regular HIV testing, treatment adherence and disclosure among young Black gay men. *Cult Health Sex.* 2014;16(6):710–722.
5. Arreola S, et al. Childhood sexual experiences and adult health sequelae among gay and bisexual men: defining childhood sexual abuse. *J Sex Res.* 2008;45(3):246–252.
6. Atlas A, et al. Acute psychotic symptoms in HIV-1 infected patients are associated with increased levels of kynurenic acid in cerebrospinal fluid. *Brain Behav Immun.* 2007;21(1):86–91.
7. Backus LI, Boothroyd D, Deyton LR. HIV, hepatitis C and HIV/hepatitis C virus co-infection in vulnerable populations. *AIDS.* 2005;19(suppl 3):S13–S19.
8. Barroso J, et al. Fatigue in HIV-infected people: a three-year observational study. *J Pain Symptom Manage.* 2015;50(1):69–79.
9. Batki SL. Drug abuse, psychiatric disorders, and AIDS. Dual and triple diagnosis. *West J Med.* 1990;152(5):547–552.
10. Berger-Greenstein JA, et al. Major depression in patients with HIV/AIDS and substance abuse. *AIDS Patient Care STDS.* 2007;21(12):942–955.
11. Berk M, et al. So depression is an inflammatory disease, but where does the inflammation come from? *BMC Med.* 2013;11:200.
12. Bhatia MS, Munjal S. Prevalence of depression in people living with HIV/AIDS undergoing ART and factors associated with it. *J Clin Diagn Res.* 2014;8(10):WC01–WC04.
13. Bing EG, et al. Psychiatric disorders and drug use among human immunodeficiency virus-infected adults in the United States. *Arch Gen Psychiatry.* 2001;58(8):721–728.

14. Bouhnik AD, et al. Depression and clinical progression in HIV-infected drug users treated with highly active antiretroviral therapy. *Antivir Ther.* 2005;10(1):53–61.

15. Bowleg L, et al. Racial discrimination and posttraumatic stress symptoms as pathways to sexual HIV risk behaviors among urban Black heterosexual men. *AIDS Care.* 2014;26(8):1050–1057.

16. Braine N, et al. HIV risk behavior among amphetamine injectors at U.S. syringe exchange programs. *AIDS Educ Prev.* 2005;17(6):515–524.

17. Brienza RS, et al. Depression among needle exchange program and methadone maintenance clients. *J Subst Abuse Treat.* 2000;18(4):331–337.

18. Bunmi A. *Review of Treatment Studies of Depression in HIV*; 2006. Available from: https://www.iasusa.org/sites/default/files/tam/14-3-112.pdf.

19. Capaldini L, Feldman MD. HIV/AIDS. In Feldman MD, Christensen JF, eds: *Behavioral Medicine: A Guide for Clinical Practice*, ed 3. New York, 2008, McGraw Hill.

20. Cerda M, Sagdeo A, Galea S. Comorbid forms of psychopathology: key patterns and future research directions. *Epidemiol Rev.* 2008;30:155–177.

21. Chander G, Himelhoch S, Moore RD. Substance abuse and psychiatric disorders in HIV-positive patients: epidemiology and impact on antiretroviral therapy. *Drugs.* 2006;66(6):769–789.

22. Chin-Hong PV, et al. High-risk sexual behavior in adults with genotypically proven antiretroviral-resistant HIV infection. *J Acquir Immune Defic Syndr.* 2005;40(4):463–471.

23. Chou PH, et al. *Secondary Mania Due to AIDS and Cryptococcal Meningitis in a 78-Year-Old Patient*; 2015.

24. Churchill MJ, et al. Extensive astrocyte infection is prominent in human immunodeficiency virus-associated dementia. *Ann Neurol.* 2009;66(2):253–258.

25. Clifford DB, Ances BM. HIV-associated neurocognitive disorder. *Lancet Infect Dis.* 2013;13(11):976–986.

26. Clifford DB, et al. Impact of efavirenz on neuropsychological performance and symptoms in HIV-infected individuals. *Ann Intern Med.* 2005;143(10):714–721.

27. Clifford DB, et al. The neuropsychological and neurological impact of hepatitis C virus co-infection in HIV-infected subjects. *AIDS.* 2005;19(suppl 3):S64–S71.

28. Cohen MH, et al. Medically eligible women who do not use HAART: the importance of abuse, drug use, and race. *Am J Public Health.* 2004;94(7):1147–1151.

29. Cohen S, et al. Chronic stress, glucocorticoid receptor resistance, inflammation, and disease risk. *Proc Natl Acad Sci U S A.* 2012;109(16):5995–5999.

30. Colfax G, et al. Longitudinal patterns of methamphetamine, popper (amyl nitrite), and cocaine use and high-risk sexual behavior among a cohort of san francisco men who have sex with men. *J Urban Health.* 2005;82(1 suppl 1):i62–i70.

31. Comas-Diaz L, Racial trauma recovery: a race-informed therapeutic approach to racial wounds. In: AN. Alvarez, Liang, Christopher, TH, Neville, Helen A, Ed. *The Cost of Racism for People of Color: Contextualizing Experiences of Descrimination.* Washington, D.C: American Psychological Association; 2016.

32. Cook JA, et al. Depressive symptoms and AIDS-related mortality among a multisite cohort of HIV-positive women. *Am J Public Health.* 2004;94(7):1133–1140.

33. Cysique LA, Maruff P, Brew BJ. Prevalence and pattern of neuropsychological impairment in human immunodeficiency virus-infected/acquired immunodeficiency syndrome (HIV/AIDS) patients across pre- and post-highly active antiretroviral therapy eras: a combined study of two cohorts. *J Neurovirol.* 2004;10(6):350–357.

34. Dantzer R, et al. From inflammation to sickness and depression: when the immune system subjugates the brain. *Nat Rev Neurosci.* 2008;9(1):46–56.

35. Denniston MM, et al. Chronic hepatitis C virus infection in the United States, national health and Nutrition Examination survey 2003 to 2010. *Ann Intern Med.* 2014;160(5):293–300.

36. Earnshaw VA, et al. Stigma and racial/ethnic HIV disparities: moving toward resilience. *Am Psychol.* 2013;68(4):225–236.

37. Edlin BR, et al. Toward a more accurate estimate of the prevalence of hepatitis C in the United States. *Hepatology.* 2015;62(5):1353–1363.

38. Ellen SR, et al. Secondary mania in patients with HIV infection. *Aust N Z J Psychiatry.* 1999;33(3):353–360.

39. Ersche KD, Sahakian BJ. The neuropsychology of amphetamine and opiate dependence: implications for treatment. *Neuropsychol Rev.* 2007;17(3):317–336.

40. Fellows RP, et al. Major depressive disorder, cognitive symptoms, and neuropsychological performance among ethnically diverse HIV+ men and women. *J Int Neuropsychol Soc.* 2013;19(2):216–225.

41. Fireman M, et al. Addressing tri-morbidity (hepatitis C, psychiatric disorders, and substance use): the importance of routine mental health screening as a component of a comanagement model of care. *Clin Infect Dis.* 2005;40(suppl 5):S286–S291.

42. Gill AJ, Kolson DL. Chronic inflammation and the role for cofactors (hepatitis C, drug abuse, antiretroviral drug toxicity, aging) in HAND persistence. *Curr HIV AIDS Rep.* 2014;11(3):325–335.

43. Goodkin K. Deterring the progression of HIV infection. *Compr Ther.* 1990;16(8):17–23.

44. Goodkin K. Assessing the prevalence of HIV, HBV, and HCV infection among people with severe mental illness. *Lancet Psychiatry.* 2016;3(1):4–6.

45. Goodkin K, et al. A bereavement support group intervention is longitudinally associated with salutary effects on the CD4 cell count and number of physician visits. *Clin Diagn Lab Immunol.* 1998;5(3):382–391.

46. Goodkin K, et al. Cognitive-motor impairment and disorder in HIV-1 infection. *Psychiatr Ann.* 2001;31(1):37–44.

47. Gottheil E, et al. Does intensive outpatient cocaine treatment reduce AIDS risky behaviors? *J Addict Dis.* 1998;17(4):61–69.

48. Grant BF, et al. Co-occurrence of 12-month alcohol and drug use disorders and personality disorders in the United States: results from the National Epidemiologic Survey on Alcohol and Related Conditions. *Arch Gen Psychiatry.* 2004;61(4):361–368.

49. Grant BF, et al. Prevalence and co-occurrence of substance use disorders and independent mood and anxiety disorders: results from the national epidemiologic survey on alcohol and related conditions. *Arch Gen Psychiatry.* 2004;61(8):807–816.

50. Green JE, Saveanu RV, Bornstein RA. The effect of previous alcohol abuse on cognitive function in HIV infection. *Am J Psychiatry.* 2004;161(2):249–254.

51. *Guidelines for the Use of Antiretroviral Agents in Adults and Adolescents Living with HIV.* Washington, DC: NIH; 2017.

52. Haroon E, Miller AH, Sanacora G. Inflammation, glutamate, and Glia: a Trio of Trouble in mood disorders. *Neuropsychopharmacology.* 2017;42(1):193–215.

53. Hazleton JE, Berman JW, Eugenin EA. Novel mechanisms of central nervous system damage in HIV infection. *HIV AIDS (Auckl).* 2010;2:39–49.

54. Heaton RK, et al. HIV-associated neurocognitive disorders persist in the era of potent antiretroviral therapy: CHARTER Study. *Neurology.* 2010;75(23):2087–2096.

55. Heaton RK, et al. HIV-associated neurocognitive disorders before and during the era of combination antiretroviral therapy: differences in rates, nature, and predictors. *J Neurovirol.* 2011;17(1):3–16.

56. Hendershot CS, et al. Alcohol use, expectancies, and sexual sensation seeking as correlates of HIV risk behavior in heterosexual young adults. *Psychol Addict Behav.* 2007;21(3):365–372.

57. Hestad K, et al. Neuropsychological deficits in HIV-1 seropositive and seronegative intravenous drug users. *J Clin Exp Neuropsychol.* 1993;15(5):732–742.

58. Hutton HE, et al. HIV risk behaviors and their relationship to posttraumatic stress disorder among women prisoners. *Psychiatr Serv.* 2001;52(4):508–513.

59. Hutton HE, et al. Depression and HIV risk behaviors among patients in a sexually transmitted disease clinic. *Am J Psychiatry.* 2004;161(5):912–914.

60. Ickovics JR, et al. A grief observed": the experience of HIV-related illness and death among women in a clinic-based sample in New Haven, *Connecticut. J Consult Clin Psychol.* 1998;66(6):958–966.

61. Ironson G, et al. Psychosocial factors predict CD4 and viral load change in men and women with human immunodeficiency virus in the era of highly active antiretroviral treatment. *Psychosom Med.* 2005;67(6):1013–1021.

62. Johannessen DJ, Wilson LG. Mania with cryptococcal meningitis in two AIDS patients. *J Clin Psychiatry.* 1988;49(5):200–201.

63. Johnson SD, Cunningham-Williams RM, Cottler LB. A tripartite of HIV-risk for African American women: the intersection of drug use, violence, and depression. *Drug Alcohol Depend.* 2003;70(2):169–175.

64. Kalichman SC, et al. Trauma symptoms, sexual behaviors, and substance abuse: correlates of childhood sexual abuse and HIV risks among men who have sex with men. *J Child Sex Abus.* 2004;13(1):1–15.

65. Kenedi CA, Joynt KE, Goforth HW. Comorbid HIV encephalopathy and cocaine use as a risk factor for new-onset seizure disorders. *CNS Spectr.* 2008;13(3):230–234.

66. Kennedy SH. Core symptoms of major depressive disorder: relevance to diagnosis and treatment. *Dialogues Clin Neurosci.* 2008;10(3):271–277.

67. Kessler RC, et al. The epidemiology of major depressive disorder: results from the National Comorbidity Survey Replication (NCS-R). *J Am Med Assoc.* 2003;289(23):3095–3105.

68. Kidorf M, et al. Prevalence of psychiatric and substance use disorders in opioid abusers in a community syringe exchange program. *Drug Alcohol Depend.* 2004;74(2):115–122.

69. Koopman C, et al. Relationships of perceived stress to coping, attachment and social support among HIV-positive persons. *AIDS Care.* 2000;12(5):663–672.

70. Langford D, et al. Patterns of selective neuronal damage in methamphetamine-user AIDS patients. *J Acquir Immune Defic Syndr.* 2003;34(5):467–474.

71. Lert F, Kazatchkine MD. Antiretroviral HIV treatment and care for injecting drug users: an evidence-based overview. *Int J Drug Policy.* 2007;18(4):255–261.

72. Lightfoot M, et al. Predictors of substance use frequency and reductions in seriousness of use among persons living with HIV. *Drug Alcohol Depend.* 2005;77(2):129–138.

73. Lloyd JJ, et al. The relationship between lifetime abuse and suicidal ideation in a sample of injection drug users. *J Psychoactive Drugs.* 2007;39(2):159–166.

74. Louati K, Berenbaum F. Fatigue in chronic inflammation - a link to pain pathways. *Arthritis Res Ther.* 2015;17:254.

75. Maes M, et al. The effects of psychological stress on humans: increased production of pro-inflammatory cytokines and a Th1-like response in stress-induced anxiety. *Cytokine.* 1998;10(4):313–318.

76. Maes M, et al. Depression and sickness behavior are Janus-faced responses to shared inflammatory pathways. *BMC Med.* 2012;10:66.

77. Matos TD, et al. HIV risk behaviors and alcohol intoxication among injection drug users in Puerto Rico. *Drug Alcohol Depend.* 2004;76(3):229–234.

78. Matthews AM, et al. Hepatitis C testing and infection rates in bipolar patients with and without comorbid substance use disorders. *Bipolar Disord.* 2008;10(2):266–270.

79. Maxwell S, et al. Manic syndrome associated with zidovudine treatment. *J Am Med Assoc.* 1988;259(23):3406–3407.

80. Meade CS, et al. HIV risk behavior among patients with co-occurring bipolar and substance use disorders: associations with mania and drug abuse. *Drug Alcohol Depend.* 2008;92(1–3):296–300.

81. Meyer IH. Minority stress and mental health in gay men. *J Health Soc Behav.* 1995;36(1):38–56.

82. Meyer IH. Prejudice, social stress, and mental health in lesbian, gay, and bisexual populations: conceptual issues and research evidence. *Psychol Bull.* 2003;129(5):674–697.

83. Meyer IH, Dean L. Patterns of sexual behavior and risk taking among young New York City gay men. *AIDS Educ Prev.* 1995;7(5 Suppl):13–23.

84. Mimiaga MJ, et al. Experiences and sexual behaviors of HIV-infected MSM who acquired HIV in the context of crystal methamphetamine use. *AIDS Educ Prev.* 2008;20(1):30–41.

85. Moore DJ, et al. HIV-infected individuals with co-occurring bipolar disorder evidence poor antiretroviral and psychiatric medication adherence. *AIDS Behav.* 2012;16(8):2257–2266.

86. Morrison MF, et al. Depressive and anxiety disorders in women with HIV infection. *Am J Psychiatry.* 2002;159(5):789–796.

87. Morrison TC, et al. Frequency of alcohol use and its association with STD/HIV-related risk practices, attitudes and knowledge among an African-American community-recruited sample. *Int J STD AIDS.* 1998;9(10):608–612.

88. Muller N, Schwarz MJ. The immune-mediated alteration of serotonin and glutamate: towards an integrated view of depression. *Mol Psychiatry.* 2007;12(11):988–1000.

89. Myers HF, et al. Trauma and psychosocial predictors of substance abuse in women impacted by HIV/AIDS. *J Behav Health Serv Res.* 2009;36(2):233–246.

90. Neuenburg JK, et al. HIV-related neuropathology, 1985 to 1999: rising prevalence of HIV encephalopathy in the era of highly active antiretroviral therapy. *J Acquir Immune Defic Syndr.* 2002;31(2):171–177.

91. O'Connor JC, et al. Lipopolysaccharide-induced depressive-like behavior is mediated by indoleamine 2,3-dioxygenase activation in mice. *Mol Psychiatry.* 2009;14(5):511–522.

92. Pace TW, Hu F, Miller AH. Cytokine-effects on glucocorticoid receptor function: relevance to glucocorticoid resistance and the pathophysiology and treatment of major depression. *Brain Behav Immun.* 2007;21(1):9–19.

93. Paul JP, et al. Substance use and experienced stigmatization among ethnic minority men who have sex with men in the United States. *J Ethn Subst Abuse.* 2014;13(4):430–447.

94. Pieterse AL, et al. Perceived racism and mental health among Black American adults: a meta-analytic review. *J Couns Psychol.* 2012;59(1):1–9.

95. Plotzker RE, Metzger DS, Holmes WC. Childhood sexual and physical abuse histories, PTSD, depression, and HIV risk outcomes in women injection drug users: a potential mediating pathway. *Am J Addict.* 2007;16(6):431–438.

96. Power C, et al. HIV Dementia Scale: a rapid screening test. *J Acquir Immune Defic Syndr Hum Retrovirol.* 1995;8(3):273–278.

97. Rabkin JG, McElhiney MC, Ferrando SJ. Mood and substance use disorders in older adults with HIV/AIDS: methodological issues and preliminary evidence. *AIDS.* 2004;18(suppl 1):S43–S48.

98. Rabkin JG, et al. Prevalence of axis I disorders in an AIDS cohort: a cross-sectional, controlled study. *Compr Psychiatry.* 1997;38(3):146–154.

99. Rabkin JG, et al. Relationships among apathy, depression, and cognitive impairment in HIV/AIDS. *J Neuropsychiatry Clin Neurosci.* 2000;12(4):451–457.

100. RachBeisel J, Scott J, Dixon L. Co-occurring severe mental illness and substance use disorders: a review of recent research. *Psychiatr Serv.* 1999;50(11):1427–1434.

101. Ribeiro CM, et al. Is bipolar disorder a risk factor for HIV infection? *J Affect Disord.* 2013;146(1):66–70.

102. Rivera-Rivera Y, et al. Depression correlates with increased plasma levels of inflammatory cytokines and a dysregulated oxidant/antioxidant balance in HIV-1-infected subjects undergoing antiretroviral therapy. *J Clin Cell Immunol.* 2014;5(6):1000276.

103. Robertson KR, et al. The prevalence and incidence of neurocognitive impairment in the HAART era. *AIDS.* 2007;21(14):1915–1921.

104. Rock PL, et al. Cognitive impairment in depression: a systematic review and meta-analysis. *Psychol Med.* 2014;44(10):2029–2040.

105. Sacktor N, et al. HIV-associated cognitive impairment before and after the advent of combination therapy. *J Neurovirol.* 2002;8(2):136–142.

106. Sambamoorthi U, et al. Antidepressant treatment and health services utilization among HIV-infected medicaid patients diagnosed with depression. *J Gen Intern Med.* 2000;15(5):311–320.

107. SAMHSA. National. *Survey on Drug Use and Health (NSDUH)*; 2015. Available from: www.nimh.nih.gov/health/statistics/prevalence/major-depression-among-adults.shtml. https://www.nimh.nih.gov/health/statistics/prevalence/major-depression-among-adults.shtml.

108. Shoptaw S, et al. Psychiatric and substance dependence comorbidities, sexually transmitted diseases, and risk behaviors among methamphetamine-dependent gay and bisexual men seeking outpatient drug abuse treatment. *J Psychoactive Drugs.* 2003;35(suppl 1):161–168.

109. Shuter J, Bernstein SL. Cigarette smoking is an independent predictor of nonadherence in HIV-infected individuals receiving highly active antiretroviral therapy. *Nicotine Tob Res.* 2008;10(4):731–736.

110. Simoni JM, Ng MT. Trauma, coping, and depression among women with HIV/AIDS in New York City. *AIDS Care.* 2000;12(5):567–580.

111. Stacey AR, et al. Induction of a striking systemic cytokine cascade prior to peak viremia in acute human immunodeficiency virus type 1 infection, in contrast to more modest and delayed responses in acute hepatitis B and C virus infections. *J Virol.* 2009;83(8):3719–3733.

112. Stark JL, et al. Social stress induces glucocorticoid resistance in macrophages. *Am J Physiol Regul Integr Comp Physiol.* 2001;280(6):R1799–R1805.

113. Stein MD, et al. Depression severity and drug injection HIV risk behaviors. *Am J Psychiatry.* 2003;160(9):1659–1662.

114. Taylor LE, et al. Psychiatric illness and illicit drugs as barriers to hepatitis C treatment among HIV/hepatitis C virus co-infected individuals. *AIDS.* 2002;16(12):1700–1701.

115. Tizard I. Sickness behavior, its mechanisms and significance. *Anim Health Res Rev.* 2008;9(1):87–99.

116. Tucker JS, et al. Substance use and mental health correlates of nonadherence to antiretroviral medications in a sample of patients with human immunodeficiency virus infection. *Am J Med.* 2003;114(7):573–580.

117. Turner BJ, et al. Relationship of gender, depression, and health care delivery with antiretroviral adherence in HIV-infected drug users. *J Gen Intern Med.* 2003;18(4):248–257.

118. Uthman OA, et al. Depression and adherence to antiretroviral therapy in low-, middle- and high-income countries: a systematic review and meta-analysis. *Curr HIV AIDS Rep.* 2014;11(3):291–307.

119. van Doorn N. Between hope and abandonment: black queer collectivity and the affective labour of biomedicalised HIV prevention. *Cult Health Sex.* 2012;14(7):827–840.

120. Vazquez-Justo E, Rodriguez Alvarez M, Ferraces Otero MJ. Influence of depressed mood on neuropsychologic performance in HIV-seropositive drug users. *Psychiatry Clin Neurosci.* 2003;57(3):251–258.

121. Walkup J, et al. Use of Medicaid data to explore community characteristics associated with HIV prevalence among beneficiaries with schizophrenia. *Public Health Rep.* 2011;126(suppl 3):89–101.

122. Williams CT, Latkin CA. The role of depressive symptoms in predicting sex with multiple and high-risk partners. *J Acquir Immune Defic Syndr.* 2005;38(1):69–73.

123. Wisniewski AB, et al. Depressive symptoms, quality of life, and neuropsychological performance in HIV/AIDS: the impact of gender and injection drug use. *J Neurovirol.* 2005;11(2):138–143.

124. Yeon PA, Albrecht H. Crystal Meth and HIV/AIDS: the Perfect Storm? *NEJM Journal Watch.* 2007.

61

Substance Use Stigma As a Barrier to Treatment and Recovery

JASON B. LUOMA

Introduction

Stereotypes and judgments about people with substance misuse problems are extremely prevalent and negative.[16,18,68,72] The content of these stereotypes varies, with examples including "people who use drugs are immoral," "alcoholics are unreliable," or "addicts are dangerous." These negative evaluations are held not only by those who abstain from substance use, but also by those who themselves use and abuse substances. As the criminalization of drug use has increased over recent decades in the United States, the level of negative attitudes toward drug use has also increased.[10]

Although the exact form of these stereotypes and judgments may vary across different substances and social groups, substance misuse appears to be at least as stigmatized, if not more so, as psychological disorders such as depression, schizophrenia, or borderline personality disorder.[16,18,68,72] The data about the prevalence and negativity of stigmatizing attitudes are clear; research to date on the links between these attitudes and subsequent negative outcomes for those with substance addiction is relatively sparse. Because the body of data on stigma toward the mentally ill is much broader and deeper, especially for psychotic disorders, this chapter depends somewhat on extrapolation from mental illness stigma, to substance abuse stigma.

A review of sociological and historical analyses of factors that have contributed to the stigma of substance abuse is beyond the scope of this chapter. Other authors (e.g., Read et al.[105]) have provided excellent narratives on such topics as the history of legal policy toward substance use and how larger values systems such as Puritanism contribute to stigmatization. Instead, this chapter focuses on the nature of stigma and its impact on individuals with substance abuse problems through review of scientific research and theory. In addition, we discuss implications for interventions regarding stigma, particularly in the context of the substance abuse treatment system. The chapter begins with a short review on the nature of stigma in general, followed by a focus on stigma as directed toward those using or abusing substances.

What Is Stigma?

As with most other common language terms that have been adopted by the social sciences, the concept of stigma has been difficult to narrow to a single definition. As used conventionally, stigma refers to an attribute or characteristic of an individual that identifies him or her as different in some manner from a normative standard and marks that individual to be socially sanctioned and devalued. One of the most widely cited definitions of stigma comes from Goffman,[35] who saw stigma as an "attribute that is deeply discrediting." This attribute affects the perceiver's global evaluation of the person, reducing him or her "from a whole and usual person to a tainted, discounted one" (p. 3). Another influential definition comes from Jones et al.,[54] who suggested that a stigmatized person is "marked" as having a condition considered deviant by a society. Through an attributional process, this mark is linked to undesirable characteristics that discredit the person in the minds of others. Perhaps one of the most comprehensive definitions of stigma comes from the work of Link and Phelan,[67] who define stigma as occurring when the following processes converge: (1) people distinguish and label human differences; (2) dominant cultural beliefs link labeled persons to undesirable characteristics that form a stereotype; (3) labeled persons are seen as an outgroup, as "them" and not "us"; (4) labeled persons experience status loss and discrimination that lead to unequal outcomes; and (5) this process occurs in a context of unequal power distribution, where one group has access to resources that the other group desires.

Stigma Depends on Basic Verbal/Cognitive Processes

Stigma is always in the eye of the beholder. At a psychological level of analysis, all the preceding definitions hinge on the role of the cognitive and emotional responses of the perceiver in determining who is stigmatized. Stigma emerges from some of the most basic functions of language and cognition, such as categorical, evaluative, and attributive processes.[40] As verbally able humans, a common cognitive activity is evaluating and classifying the people in our social world. This is particularly common when a lack of extensive personal experience with someone leads us to rely on cues for assigning that person to a social category, whether accurately or inaccurately. Our ability to classify according to socially defined categories is universal among language-able humans and also unique to us as a species. Just try it out for yourself. Read the following sentences and fill in the blank:

Men are _____.
Women are _____.
Alcoholics are _____.
Gays are _____.
Addicts are _____.

Were you able to fill in those blanks? Even if doing so felt uncomfortable, most people are able to provide responses that *seem* to describe the group in question. Answers may readily appear even when they are unwanted or disagreeable. Anyone who participates in a cultural/verbal system learns common stereotypes for the groups that have been defined in that culture,[26] whether they agree with them or not.

Throughout a typical day we classify people into groups based on some identifying characteristic or behavior, make judgments about what this means about them, and respond based on this judgment. Much of this process of stereotyping and responding occurs outside of our normal awareness and is harmless, even adaptive. For example, we identify the person at the checkout counter in the grocery store as a clerk and proceed to have them scan our groceries. Research has shown that stereotypes help to reduce the burden of problem solving in complex social environments (e.g., Mann and Himelein[77]). We are able to quickly develop evaluations and expectations of individuals based on their perceived membership in a group about which we have some social knowledge (i.e., stereotypes[39]). These stereotypes allow us to predict that person's behavior and act accordingly. Sometimes this is quite useful, such as when purchasing items in a grocery store. Sometimes it is less so; for example, when seeing a bumper sticker on a person's car endorsing a disliked political candidate, we may make unsavory assumptions about the driver and may be more

inclined to engage in discourteous behavior on the road. Sometimes this process is clearly harmful, for example, where culturally sanctioned stereotypes devalue certain individuals and this same process results in stigmatizing, rejecting, and even discriminatory interactions. Through this process of objectification and dehumanization, we fail to appreciate the complex, historical human being and respond to the person solely in terms of their participation in verbal categories.[42,74]

Stigmatizing Thoughts Are Resistant to Change

Stigmatizing thoughts and attributions have been shown to be difficult to change through direct intervention.[42] One reason for this may be that judgment and stereotyping are massively useful for the individual in many social situations and thus are highly prevalent and automatic, often happening without awareness. In addition, verbal/cognitive networks, once formed, tend to maintain themselves.[42] Stereotype disconfirming information that occurs during social interactions tends to be forgotten if the new material conflicts with older stereotypes.[49] People tend to infer stereotype-congruent behaviors to dispositional causes, whereas stereotype-incongruent behaviors are inferred to situational causes,[46] thus further supporting their already existing stereotypes. Even people who exhibit low levels of prejudice know the common stereotypes of stigmatized groups, and once learned, these stereotypes do not go away.[26] If a person learns new ways of thinking, the old ways of thinking do not disappear, but rather are available to reemerge if the new ways of thinking are frustrated or punished (e.g., Wilson and Hayes[144]). Thus if new stereotypes are learned about a group, these generally do not replace the old stereotypes; rather, the new learning is metaphorically layered over the old learning. The old stereotypes are still available to reemerge under situations in which the newer learning is put under strain.

Stigma Is Sustained Through Cultural Practices

Although stigmatization is a universal human phenomenon, *what* is stigmatized has been shown to vary over time and across cultures.[62] This suggests that stigma results from cultural practices that exist on the basis of their past ability to facilitate the survival of that culture,[5,145] much in the same way that genes are selected based on their contribution to the survival of a species. Cultural practices that support categorization and stereotyping facilitate membership in and favoritism toward a perceived in-group (e.g., Hilton and von Hippel[47] and Starr et al.[128]), as well as the resulting mistreatment of individuals in a perceived out-group.[132] These distinctions preserve and sustain a variety of cultural practices when they generate advantages for the in-group, even when the groups are based on arbitrary characteristics bearing no direct adaptive value. Although stigmatization is defined as the behavior of an individual, it is always generated and sustained by cultural practices that reinforce and support stigmatizing attitudes, stereotypes, and actions. Thus in order to change stigma, it is important to change both the behavior of individuals and the cultural practices that support stigma among individuals of that culture.

Types and Levels of Stigma Toward Substance Abuse

The preceding section was only a brief overview of the vast literature on stigma, stereotyping, and prejudice. In contrast, the rest of this chapter focuses specifically on stigma toward addiction and begins with a review of types and levels of stigma in relation to substance abuse. Stigma can be subdivided into various types and levels. One distinction can be made between structural and individual stigma. Structural or institutional stigma refers to macroscopic patterns of discrimination toward those with substance misuse that cannot be explained at the individual psychological level alone. This kind of stigma can be either intentional or unintentional.[15] Intentional stigma refers to the rules, policies, and procedures of private and public organizations and structures with power that consciously and purposely restrict rights and opportunities of the stigmatized group. Intentional structural stigma toward addiction would include laws and tax codes that provide inadequate levels of funding for addictions treatment compared to other health conditions or harsher sentencing laws for crack cocaine versus powder cocaine. In contrast, unintentional stigma refers to instances where rules, policies, or procedures result in discrimination, seemingly without the conscious prejudicial efforts of a powerful few.[48] Examples of unintentional structural stigma might include the lower wages and poorer benefits paid to substance abuse treatment professionals compared to other health care or mental health care workers, thus potentially resulting in poorer quality care. Another potential example of unintentional structural stigma would be the exclusion of substance abuse treatment benefits from the Mental Health Parity Act of 1997, resulting in less accessibility of addiction treatment services. This exclusion continued until 2008, when the Mental Health Parity Act of 2008 included substance use disorders.

It is conceivable that prevalent negative attitudes toward substance abuse might contribute to institutional practices that typify structural stigma. For example, prevalent attitudes that people who are addicted to substances are blameworthy and not likely to recover from addiction might make it less likely that the public would be supportive of spending a portion of their tax dollars on treatment. This phenomenon has been witnessed in a German sample who reported that during periods of economic difficulty, they would prefer to cut funding for mental illness and addiction treatment before cutting funding for physical problems.[120]

At the individual level, stigma can be broken down into two types[11,75]: public stigma and self-stigma. The most obvious form of stigma is public stigma, which refers to the reaction the general public has toward the stigmatized group. This includes stereotypes and attitudes toward the stigmatized group, as well as acts of discrimination, termed enacted stigma. For example, rejection by a friend following discovery of a person's substance abuse history, denial of a job opportunity because an employer suspects an applicant is in recovery, or disparaging remarks about people with addictive disorders would all be examples of enacted stigma. People abusing substances and those in recovery frequently encounter enacted stigma.[1,75] Enacted stigma has been clearly associated with a number of adverse outcomes in mentally ill populations.[93,95,98,99,101] Although data demonstrating direct links between encounters with enacted stigma and negative outcomes are less available in substance-misusing populations, data showing more negative social attitudes toward substance abusers than those diagnosed with schizophrenia[16,18,68,72] suggest that enacted stigma is even more severe toward those abusing substances.

The second type of individual level stigma is that of self-stigma, which refers to difficult thoughts and feelings (e.g., shame, negative self-evaluative thoughts, fear of enacted stigma) that emerge from identification with a stigmatized group and their resulting behavioral impact.[75] For example, a person with substance abuse problems or a person in recovery might avoid treatment, not apply for jobs, or avoid intimate social relationships because, as a result of self-stigma, they no longer trust themselves to fulfill these roles or fear rejection based on their substance-using identity. Among populations with serious mental illness and dual diagnoses, self-stigma has been associated with delays in treatment seeking,[61,118,130] diminished self-esteem and self-efficacy,[22,69,145] and lower quality of life.[113]

Perceived stigma is a component of self-stigma and refers to beliefs among members of a stigmatized group about the level of public stigma in society (cf. Parcesepe and Cabassa[93]). A result of perceived stigma may be that people may limit their actions (e.g., seeking treatment or acknowledging their own struggles with recovery) in an attempt to avoid stigmatization. Some data are available showing that perceived stigma may serve as a barrier to treatment adherence, at least in some groups.[127] At least one cross-sectional study of stigma in addiction[75] has generated empirical support for the conceptual distinctions between public, perceived, and self-stigma.

The Need to Study Stigma in Context

Despite the volume of available research on stereotyping, prejudice, discrimination, scapegoating, social categorization, and social deviance, the amount of stigma literature relating these processes specifically to substance abuse is quite sparse. Ahern[1] has suggested that this hole in the literature may result from the common perception that stigma and discrimination against drug users serves to deter drug use and that the possible negative effects of stigma are relatively minor compared to the deterrent value of stigmatization. A substantial body of literature from a law enforcement and criminal justice perspective views stigma as a positive form of social control that discourages illegal activity.[12,70] This literature largely ignores the potential negative effects of stigma. In contrast, most of the professional literature from mental health and recovery perspectives views stigma as negative and in need of reduction.[112] This literature seems to largely ignore the possibility that stigma might have beneficial effects in some contexts. Each of these perspectives seems to minimize the importance of context and neither seems to acknowledge the possibility that stigma may have both beneficial and harmful effects, depending on the context in which it is found.

A comprehensive scientific approach to stigma would involve examination of the phenomenon across the myriad of situations in which it occurs. Stigma is a complex phenomenon with many forms and widely varying impacts on the individual. Prior to initial drug use and throughout the developmental trajectory for addition and recovery, stigma may have various possible functions. For example, stigma may affect some individuals who are currently not using drugs by dissuading them from initial use. On the other hand, individuals who identify with marginalized populations may actually be attracted to drug use because of its marginalized status. Once a person has bypassed barriers to initial drug use, stigma could serve to further reinforce and isolate drug-using subcultures, further supporting consumption. For many, stigma serves as a barrier to entering treatment because of fear of being labeled and stigmatized by others. For others, experiences of being stigmatized and judged by others once drug use is discovered or labeled as problematic might serve as a motivator for treatment entry. The effects of stigma might change again after a person enters treatment. Individuals experiencing more self-stigma or who are more fearful of enacted stigma may stay in treatment for longer periods, perhaps benefiting more from treatment. On the other hand, the impact of self-stigma may impede recovery by reducing the motivation of substance abusers and creating negative beliefs about their ability to recover, thereby resulting in earlier relapse. Some people may be relatively unaffected by stigma, perhaps because of personal conditions that help guard against its impact (e.g., financial resources), or because they do not identify with a stigmatized group. Finally, ongoing experiences of stigma-related rejection may serve as a barrier to reengagement with healthy, non–drug-using social relationships, returning to work, or obtaining a reasonable living arrangement. This array of possibilities suggests that simple judgments about the goodness or badness of stigma may be insufficient in understanding the role of stigma in initial drug use, the development of addiction, and recovery from substance abuse. Given the potential complexities, we need a contextually situated approach to examining the effects of stigma on drug use and related outcomes in order to maximally benefit all involved.

Straying from the hypothetical scenarios described in the preceding paragraph, a study by Farrimond[31] nicely demonstrates the contextual nature of stigma's impact. Qualitative analyses of reports from tobacco smokers in the United Kingdom showed that smokers from lower socioeconomic status groups were more likely to internalize smoking-related stigma and feel badly about themselves for smoking, rather than change their behavior to avoid it. In contrast, smokers from higher socioeconomic status groups were less likely to internalize smoking-related stigma and were more likely to have the resources to change their behavior to avoid being stigmatized. The authors suggested that this finding was a partial explanation for the much higher rates of smoking found in lower socioeconomic status groups. They hypothesized that broad-scale campaigns to stigmatize smokers might reduce smoking in persons from higher socioeconomic status brackets who would work to avoid it, whereas individuals in lower socioeconomic status may not be responsive, and furthermore, that such campaigns may even impede efforts to stop smoking because of increased internalized stigma. They argued that intervention efforts promoting stigma could actually exacerbate disparities already present between higher and lower status groups.

Thus far, this chapter has outlined the nature of stigma in general, including its types and levels. It has outlined how stigma is a complex phenomenon, the effects of which vary by context. The remainder of this text is more focused specifically on what is known about the stigma of substance abuse specifically, describing its importance for those individuals with substance abuse problems, information about stigma in families and social networks of those with addiction, stigma in the treatment system, and interventions to change stigma.

The Impact of Stigma on Individuals With Substance Abuse Problems

Self-Stigma

The psychological impact of stigma on the individual can be described under the term self-stigma. Self-stigma can be defined as shame, evaluative thoughts, and fear of enacted stigma that results from an individual's identification with a stigmatized group and serves as a barrier to the pursuit of valued life goals.[74] The dominant stereotypes about stigmatized groups are widely known in a given culture. Self-stigma comes about when a person first sees himself or

herself as a member of a stigmatized group; now the negative stereotypes and biases of society that used to be about someone else apply to the self. For example, at the point when the person who misuses substances identifies himself or herself as an addict, relevant stereotypes (e.g., addicts are irresponsible) that once applied to another now apply to himself or herself. To the extent that people believe this stereotype, they are likely to impede their own chances for success, for example, by not applying to jobs that would require them to be responsible. Because the dominant stereotypes of marginalized groups are largely negative and devaluing, self-stigma may further increase the shame that often comes with addictive behavior that violates important societal and personal values and norms.

A second component of self-stigma is the fear of enacted stigma. Out of this fear of being the target of stigma a person might avoid treatment in the first place or might not get needed social support that could come from disclosing their concerns to trustworthy others. People with substance abuse widely report fear of stigma as a reason for avoiding treatment.[2,24,50,137,139] Less evidence is available for other effects of self-stigma in addiction, but self-stigma in mental illness has been associated with delays in treatment seeking,[61,118,130] diminished self-esteem/self-efficacy,[22,71,145] lower quality of life,[113] early dropout from treatment,[127] poorer social functioning over time,[100] and increased depression at follow-up.[110]

Coping and Self-Stigma

Much of the harm of self-stigma comes not only from the presence of shame, painful self-evaluations, or fear of stigmatization, but also from understandable yet costly attempts to cope with these difficult thoughts and feelings. For example, when people who identify with a stigmatized group enter situations where they perceive the potential for devaluation based on this identity,[131] they often expend energy searching for and defending against this perceived threat. The effort is taxing and distracts the individual in ways that might hinder social or intellectual performance. In a recent test of this idea, Quinn et al.[103] found that individuals with a history of mental illness who revealed this history prior to taking an intelligence test had poorer performance compared to a control group who did not relate their history of mental illness. These results are in line with more general findings on stereotype threat, that is, that people perform more poorly in situations where a specific stereotype about the group of which they are a member applies.[131] Specifically in relation to substance abuse stigma, these findings suggest that when people with a history of substance abuse problems are in a situation in which addiction-related stereotypes might apply, they may perform more poorly than they would in situations unrelated to addiction-related stigma.

People also cope with stigma by withdrawing their efforts from or disengaging their self-esteem from domains in which one's ingroup is negatively stereotyped or in which they fear being a target of discrimination. In an attempt to cope with the potential judgment, failure, or shame that might result from confirming a stereotype, a person may exert less effort in domains of living that relate to relevant stereotypes.[78] For example, a person who identifies with the stereotype that alcoholics are immoral might not engage with spiritual or religious groups out of fear that he or she might be judged by others for their moral weakness. Unfortunately, when a domain is one that might be part of living well (e.g., a steady job) and is likely to elicit thoughts of common stereotypes (e.g., "they won't hire an addict"), then disengagement from that domain (e.g., not looking for work) is likely to interfere with recovery.

Whether a stigmatizing mark can be concealed is also a relevant variable to how people cope. For example, some stigmas may be relatively concealable, such as a past felony conviction or a history of depression, whereas others may be quite difficult to conceal, such as obesity or diseases with obvious physical characteristics. For many people with substance abuse problems, their condition is concealable, whereas for others it is less so. Another way to think about concealable stigma is the distinction between "discredited" versus "discreditable" individuals.[37] For individuals with a concealable stigma, a common occurrence is deciding with whom, where, and when to disclose the stigmatizing identity. Whether disclosing a stigmatizing identity is helpful or harmful is likely to be highly dependent on context.[28] In some cases, through disclosing a stigma a person may be able to obtain social support or direct assistance from treatment agencies or health care professionals. Revealing a secret to a trusted confidant has also been shown to be related to a number of psychological benefits, including improved psychological and physical health.[57,111] On the other hand, disclosure of a stigma could result in social rejection and isolation, the loss of a job, rejection by family members, judgment from treatment professionals, or disappointment that others were not more helpful. Research on secrecy as a method for coping with the stigma of addiction is relatively scarce and what exists is somewhat crude, typically examining secrecy as a generalized tendency in response to the fear of stigma, rather than examining the patterns of disclosure and how they might interact with social context. As a general rule, the use of secrecy and withdrawal from others as a coping mechanism has been associated with negative psychosocial outcomes.[1,66,75,115] However, this general pattern should not be overgeneralized, as a recent large study of mostly minority drug users[1] found that talking with friends and family about being stigmatized and judged was associated with poorer health outcomes. One difference between the Ahern study and other studies of stigma was that Ahern specifically focused on discussions of being stigmatized, whereas most other studies examined the tendency to keep substance use a secret. This suggests that the content of what is disclosed may also affect the likelihood of a positive outcome from disclosure.

All of the coping processes described above (i.e., searching for potential threats, withdrawing efforts from valued domains, and secrecy) could be seen as forms of a broader process termed experiential avoidance. Experiential avoidance refers to the attempt to avoid, control, or reduce the frequency of difficult or painful emotions, thoughts, memories, or other private experiences.[44] Experiential avoidance overlaps with several closely related concepts, including lack of distress tolerance,[9] cognitive and emotional suppression,[142] and emotion/avoidance-focused coping.[21] As a broader pattern, experiential avoidance has been shown to contribute to a wide range of psychological and behavioral problems, including substance abuse, depression, anxiety, psychosis, and burnout, among others.[44] Because experiential avoidance has been shown to be modifiable through mindfulness and acceptance-based interventions,[34,45,140] teaching mindfulness and acceptance may be helpful in coping with stigma.

Multiple Stigmatized Identities

For a person with substance abuse problems, the stigma of substance abuse is often only one of several stigmatized identities. Each stigmatized identity is layered on top of the other, creating a dense web of ideas about the self that must be managed and responded to, depending on the social and personal contexts. For example, substance abuse disorders are highly comorbid with other psychiatric disorders,

meaning that the majority of people in treatment for drug abuse also have to contend with the stigma of mental illness.[29,58] Many people in addiction treatment are also sexual or racial minorities. They may have a stigmatized medical condition such as hepatitis or HIV. They are frequently poor or homeless, both situations that carry their own stigma. Women who abuse substances are often assumed to be promiscuous.[119] Many people with substance abuse histories also have had problems with the legal system or have been incarcerated. In addition to the stigmatization that people may experience directly from the legal system, they now have the added stigma of a prior conviction. Each additional stigmatized identity increases the chance of stigmatization. Each layer of stigmatized identity carries its own challenges that make it even harder to cope with the stigma of drug addiction.

In addition to the problem of multiple stigmas, the impact of substance abuse stigma can also compound existing social inequalities. For example, the stigma of substance abuse has disproportionately impacted the African American community in the United States, whose drug-related incarceration rate far outstrips their comparative prevalence as drug users.[143] Because many in treatment for addiction are relatively poorer, the stigma of drug abuse that tends to fall on individuals in treatment will also tend to further reduce the life chances available to those who are experiencing poverty.[31] Again, in addition to the direct effects of the stigma of addiction, stigma also tends to exacerbate the effects of already existing prejudice, marginalization, and disadvantage based on other identities.

Stigmatizing Attitudes and Behavior of Friends and Family

Supportive, cohesive, and noncritical social networks predict good outcomes in addictions treatment,[30,94,138] whereas conflict with several members of a social support network, interpersonal conflict, and isolation predict poor treatment outcomes.[87,138] People entering treatment for addictive disorders are often marginalized, with few connections to family, friends, or coworkers. Entering treatment may be a marker for having exhausted their "moral credit" with employers and families.[112] Stigma may contribute to poorer outcomes by further contributing to the disruption of social ties and increasing isolation beyond the problems created through the direct impact of addictive behavior. Some data are available that bear directly on this point. A recent study of primarily minority drug users[1] found that discrimination and stigmatizing interactions from family and friends was common and independently associated with poorer mental and physical health.

Stigma appears to degrade social networks over time. In one longitudinal study of people with mental illness, many of whom also abused substances,[65] perceptions of stigma were associated with reduction in support from nonhousehold relatives over time. Stigmatizing attitudes and behavior of friends and family may also reduce treatment adherence. A recent study of individuals taking antidepressants for depression[121] found that stigmatizing caregiver attitudes predicted premature discontinuation of treatment.

Family members of substance abusers may also experience "courtesy stigma." Courtesy stigma refers to the tendency to devalue and stigmatize people who maintain or enter relationships with those in the stigmatized group.[37] For example, in a study by Barton,[43] parents of adolescents who abused drugs reported that neighborhood children were told to stay away from their child, resulting not only in isolation for the child but also feelings of shame for the parents. Parents of substance-abusing adolescents also experienced shaming interactions when dealing with institutions such as schools, police, and the legal system. Courtesy stigma may disrupt social cohesion through contributing to struggles inside families that have a member who abuses substances. Family members may attempt to distance themselves from a substance-abusing family member in order to distance themselves from courtesy stigma and the shame that can accompany it. It may be the case that much of the behavior described in the literature as enabling or codependent may result from the family's attempt to avoid the shame of stigma[33] and maintain its identity as a normal family.

Stigma in Treatment Settings

Stigma as a Barrier to Initial Treatment Engagement

The public health implications of untreated substance abuse and dependence are enormous. Despite the proven benefits of substance abuse treatment, only a small fraction of individuals who could benefit ever enter treatment. In 2005, only about 2.3 million of an estimated 23.2 million Americans with substance abuse problems received some form of treatment.[116] Barriers to treatment entry are structural (e.g., location of facilities, lack of qualified personnel, lack of funding) and social (e.g., fear of stigma among those with substance misuse). Stigma contributes to structural barriers when people resist having substance abuse treatment facilities placed in their neighborhoods,[6,92] thereby limiting access to treatment. This is important because having to travel a longer distance to obtain addictions treatment has been associated with poorer retention.[4] The public is less interested in funding substance abuse treatment compared to treatment for other health or mental health problems,[120] contributing to long waiting lists and prohibitive cost for treatment. Stressful job conditions result in high rates of burnout and job turnover in addictions professionals,[59] resulting in less-experienced counselors and less-integrated, cohesive treatment centers.

Among the social barriers to treatment entry for addiction, probably the most common barrier cited in the literature is stigma.[a] Across numerous studies, substance-abusing individuals report fear of stigma as a reason for not seeking treatment.[2,24,50,137,139] For example, Cunningham et al.[24] examined reasons for delaying or not seeking treatment among people with alcohol abuse problems who either self-changed and were in sustained recovery, were still actively abusing, or were currently in treatment. They found that people who were either actively using or self-changed saw treatment as stigmatizing, wanted to avoid the stigma of the label "alcoholic," and reported that embarrassment and pride were barriers to seeking treatment. All three groups reported relatively similar reasons for avoiding treatment, leaving the authors to conclude that "current treatment is stigmatizing and that some alcohol abusers believe that seeking treatment would reflect negatively on them" (p. 352). A study of depressed individuals in Australia found it common to fear that others would think less of them for seeking help and that professionals would respond to them in a condescending manner.[3]

Stigma and Treatment Retention and Outcome

For individuals who are able to overcome barriers and enter treatment, the most stable predictor of positive outcome is length of time in treatment, with studies commonly finding rates of dropout in the first month of outpatient and residential treatment

exceeding 50%.[52,89,125,126] Early treatment retention is critical, as data show that early dropouts have equivalent outcomes to those who are untreated,[129] and that more time in treatment is related to better outcomes.[53,84,124] Unfortunately, stigma does not only serve as a barrier to treatment entry; stigma also appears to increase when individuals enter treatment, possibly contributing to poorer retention and thus poorer outcomes.[52,122,129] The modified labeling theory of stigma in mental illness of Link and colleagues[65] holds that stigma begins to affect people once they have officially received a label from the treatment establishment. A relatively large body of data on seriously mentally ill and dually diagnosed populations supports the hypothesis that entering treatment for a stigmatized condition can result in a labeling process that negatively affects people's engagement with treatment, psychosocial functioning, and self-concept.[22,69,145]

The data on such a stigma-labeling process are less developed in the area of addiction, but some direct data are available to support this view. For example, Semple et al.[119] found that methamphetamine abusers who had been in treatment previously reported higher levels of stigma-related rejection than those who had never been in treatment. Another survey of people in treatment for substance abuse[75] found that people with higher levels of current stigma-related rejection had more previous episodes of treatment and that this relationship remained stable even after controlling for other explanatory variables, such as current severity of addiction, demographics, secrecy coping, and current mental health. Although this evidence suggests that the impact of stigma and the rate of contact with stigmatizing experiences may increase with treatment entry, we know little about how this happens. For example, we know little about whether stigmatizing messages and rejecting experiences primarily come from nonfamily social relationships, close family, employers, media, or treatment staff. Moreover, we do not know if certain sources have greater effects than others, or whether the effect is different for individuals new to treatment versus individuals returning to treatment.

Stigmatizing Attitudes and Behavior of Professional Staff

The therapeutic alliance early in counseling has been shown to be a predictor of engagement and retention in substance abuse treatment.[86] Other data show that negative therapeutic alliances predict deterioration in substance abuse treatment.[42] Thus any actions on the part of substance abuse treatment practitioners that harm the therapeutic alliance are likely to negatively impact retention and treatment outcome among their clients. Health professionals, including addiction counselors, nurses, physicians, and support staff, have been exposed to the same cultural environment that instills stereotyped beliefs in other people. Thus whether they are aware of it or not, providers likely have internalized many of the same stigmatizing beliefs about substance abuse as others in society. Research shows that health care professionals often have moralistic, negative, and stigmatizing attitudes toward substance misuse and believe that substance-abusing individuals are unlikely to recover.[83,109,138] For example, one study of mental health support workers in the United Kingdom found that alcohol and drug addiction produced more negative responses to an attitude questionnaire than did other problems or mental illness and that individuals with alcohol and drug problems were mostly likely to be seen as unable to improve if treated.[135]

To the extent that stigmatizing attitudes are expressed by providers, they could negatively affect the alliance, thereby reducing

---

[a]References 2, 3, 24, 50, 119, 137.

retention and creating poorer outcomes. Similarly, support and non-treatment staff could create a hostile atmosphere for clients, further contributing to reduced retention. Because stigmatizing attitudes tend to have a greater impact in situations in which one group has power over another,[67] stigmatizing beliefs among health care providers may be particularly likely to negatively affect the recovery of those they are trying to help.[8] Some evidence suggests that stigmatizing interactions with providers may be more frequent than expected: one study of methamphetamine abusers found clients' inability to get along with treatment staff was a major reason for dropout,[123] whereas two surveys of consumers of mental health services found that 19%[27] and 25%[141] of consumers had experienced stigmatizing provider behavior. Data from a qualitative study of alcohol and drug abuse counselors found that counselors largely saw illicit drug use as a failing of the individual that needed to be fixed with drug treatment rather than seeing the larger context, which includes such factors as stigma. In this study, although counselors were generally aware that stigma serves as a barrier to drug treatment, they "did not perceive they as individuals and as treatment workers could perpetuate the same barriers and prejudices"[136] (p. 378).

Interventions to Reduce Stigma

Although a large body of literature on the nature of stigma exists, research on how to change stigma or how to help people with stigma is much more limited.[12,70] Interventions can target either public or self-stigma and can vary from large-scale interventions targeting the general public to focused interventions targeting high-risk or identified target populations.

Reducing Public Stigma

A number of kinds of interventions for reducing stigma in the general public have been proposed and researched. Corrigan et al.[17] proposed three strategies derived from social psychology theory for changing public mental illness stigma that could also be applied to substance abuse stigma: education, contact, and protest. Each of these approaches is reviewed below.

Educational approaches aim to provide new information about a stigmatized group and dispel negative stereotypes. Nearly all the research on education as a stigma-reduction method involves mental illness rather than substance abuse stigma. Cross-sectional research has shown that individuals who are more knowledgeable about mental illness are less likely to exhibit stigmatizing attitudes.[20,93] Whether this indicates that people who are less stigmatizing are more open to learning about mental illness, or whether education reduced stigma is unclear. A number of studies have shown short-term improvements in attitudes toward stigmatized groups as a result of educational interventions,[17,19,56,91,97] although results are sometimes inconsistent,[51] and studies have generally lacked follow-up assessments. One study that did have a follow-up showed that initial positive results were not maintained.[19] Haghighat[38] has suggested that these positive results might be a product of social desirability rather than true attitude changes. Other data suggest that education may serve to increase positive attitudes among persons who already exhibit positive attitudes but may not impact individuals with negative attitudes or may even reinforce preexisting negative biases.[7]

Recently, researchers have also begun to pay attention to the content of educational interventions for stigma reduction, especially the effects of characterizing psychiatric symptoms as caused by psychosocial events versus a disease of the brain with biological, genetic, or structural abnormalities. In general, data are not very supportive for the effectiveness of a biological/genetic message as a method for reducing stigma, and some data suggest that it may actually increase stigma. The one exception is that a biological/genetic message has sometimes been shown to reduce blame toward those with mental illness for causing their own problems, which was found in two studies[64,85] but not in a third.[103] One of these same studies showed that although a disease explanation reduced blame, it actually provoked *harsher* behavior toward a person described as mentally ill versus a psychosocial explanation.[85] Another experimental study showed that a biological explanation resulted in a less-hopeful expectation of improvement.[64] Extensive correlational research shows that genetic or biological explanations for mental illness and diagnostic labeling are related to greater perceptions of dangerousness, desire for distance, and prediction of poor prognosis.[103,107,108] For example, surveys in the United States from 1950 and 1996 showed both an increased likelihood to view mental illness as having a biological cause and also to believe that those with mental illness are dangerous.[104] In contrast, data are more reliably supportive of interventions presenting psychiatric symptoms as understandable reactions to life events (i.e., psychosocial explanations). Psychosocial explanations of mental illness have also been related to more positive attitudes toward mental illness in correlational studies.[108] Interventions promoting a psychosocial explanation have resulted in a reduction in fear of dangerousness, desire for social distance, and other negative attitudes,[64,79,88,91] although the impact has sometimes been found to vary by target group,[64] and these results have not been assessed for their long-term effects. In sum, although a small sample of data suggests that a brain disease message may reduce blame, the preponderance of existing data supports the idea that describing mental illness as a brain disease is not likely to improve stigma on a broad scale and may even lead to increased stigma of some kinds. At the current time, promoting a brain disease message as a stigma reduction method could not be considered an evidence-based practice, whereas promoting psychosocial explanations for mental illness appears to be promising, at least in these preliminary studies.

Although the data indicate that educational interventions based on efforts to characterize mental illness as a brain disease are not likely to reduce stigma, these results do not mean that more complex and nuanced approaches to stigma education that emphasize both biological and psychosocial causes, such as diathesis-stress models, might not be effective. In addition, it remains unknown whether current findings will reliably generalize to the stigma of addiction. It may also be the case that there has been an overemphasis on educational approaches predicated on the idea of information provision as a primary method for stigma reduction and that information provision is simply not a very effective way to change entrenched attitudes. Other types of interventions based on models other than information provision may be more effective in reducing stigma. Some of these models are explored in more detail below.

The second category of interventions—protest—involves attempting to suppress negative attitudes and representations of a stigmatized group through disputing the morality of holding and expressing such views or through threatening a boycott of a company's products. Research on thought suppression suggests that attempting to suppress or avoid unwanted thoughts can result in paradoxical increases in those very thoughts.[142] People who are asked to suppress thoughts about stereotyped groups can actually become more sensitized to them, resulting in unwanted intrusions of thoughts about that group and more behavioral avoidance of the stigmatized group.[76] Creating conditions that demand correct behaviors (e.g., "do not stare at the physically disabled") can also increase the physical avoidance of stigmatized persons.[63] As suggested by this basic research, most studies of protest strategies targeting attitude and behavior change in individuals have shown it to be inert.[17] In contrast, some anecdotal reports of the use of protest strategies, such as letter writing campaigns or product boycotts to get companies to remove or correct stigmatizing portrayals of mentally ill individuals in the media, have reported some success.[13] In sum, systematic confrontation and protest targeting the stigmatizing behavior of individual persons seems to be largely ineffective and may even exacerbate stigma. On the other hand, the effects of targeting corporations or organizations with organized protest campaigns have not been systematically evaluated.

Finally, contact strategies attempt to change attitudes toward stigmatized groups by creating positive social contact between members of the stigmatized group and the public. Research has shown that people who have more contact with mentally ill individuals endorse less stigma,[20,96,97] although it is unclear whether contact with mentally ill individuals decreases stigma or whether individuals with lower levels of stigma are more likely to seek contact. Contact as a strategy for reducing prejudice has long been known to be successful in research on racial prejudice.[102] Interventions based on contact have been the most consistently successful at reducing negative attitudes toward the mentally ill,[17,19] generating at least some maintenance of attitude change over time and impact on related overt behavior. The limits and exportability of this approach are still somewhat unknown, as past research has shown that there are a number of situational constraints that can make this approach difficult to implement in real-world settings.[14] Specifically, as this approach does not appear to have been tested in stigma reduction with those with substance abuse or in recovery, its putative efficacy in that area remains hypothetical.

The lack of research on stigma-reduction strategies in addiction may have to do with conflicting societal views about the usefulness and moral correctness of stigma toward substance use and substance users. In contrast with mental illness where few would argue in support of stigma, there are vocal proponents of actively stigmatizing drug use and drug users.[117] Some large-scale drug-prevention programs, such as the Montana Meth Project, which uses advertisements featuring dramatic and often violent depictions of problem drug use, appear actively designed to stigmatize drug users. The Montana program appears to be focused largely on preventing initial drug use, and some evidence suggests that this program may be effective in that aim.[55] However, as is common in the criminal justice literature, the potential impact of this campaign on individuals who are currently using illicit drugs or attempting to recover appears unexamined. Thus although these types of approaches may reduce initial drug use through increasing stigma, they may have the unintended effect of compounding stigma toward and among those who do become addicted, although further research is needed to examine this question. Thus the overall public health impact of campaigns such as the Montana Meth Project may be negative, despite the possible reduction in rates of initial drug use that may result from these stigmatization-focused programs.

Reducing Stigma in the Health Care System

Because stigma appears to increase after the person has entered the treatment system and has been labeled as a substance abuser, it

would make sense that interventions targeting the health care system and the process of entry into treatment might be particularly important in reducing the impact of stigma on those attempting to recover from drug addiction. Thus interventions targeting the prevalent stigmatizing attitudes and behaviors of health care providers and professional staff or focusing on changing organizational structures or admissions procedures might have promise in improving treatment engagement or retention. In targeting stigma in addictions specialty providers, programs designed to provide direct education about stigmatized groups or to promote contact with those in the stigmatized group do not seem very relevant, since addictions professionals already know vastly more about these topics than do average persons and have also had a great deal of contact. Because protest has not shown much promise, other interventions are needed.

One alternative intervention that has been studied is the use of mindfulness, acceptance, and values processes derived from Acceptance and Commitment Therapy.[41] Acceptance and Commitment Therapy, as applied to stigma in addictions professionals, focuses on promoting psychological acceptance of difficult thoughts and feelings that come when working with difficult clients (i.e., those most likely to be stigmatized), reducing the behavior regulating impact of the literal content of stigmatizing and evaluative thoughts (e.g., "This client is hopeless"), and helping clinicians to contact the values they bring to their work so that these values can better guide their behavior. In one pilot study of this approach,[41] Ninety licensed or certified alcohol and drug abuse counselors were randomly assigned to one-day workshops based on Acceptance and Commitment Training ($N = 30$), Multicultural Training ($N = 30$), or a control lecture about methamphetamine and MDMA (3,4-methylenedioxymethamphetamine) interventions. Stigmatizing attitudes were reduced posttraining in both active treatment groups, but only the Acceptance and Commitment Therapy condition generated lower stigmatizing attitudes at the 3-month follow-up. An additional benefit of the Acceptance and Commitment Therapy intervention is that it decreased burnout at the 3-month follow-up, suggesting that interventions targeting stigma in providers may also have the effect of reducing burnout.

Organizational interventions might also be useful in identifying and remediating stigmatizing policies and procedures. For example, an admission process walk-through[32] might be used to examine whether stigmatizing messages or behaviors occur during initial treatment engagement. These stigmatizing messages might range from the more overt (e.g., telling a client they are hopeless) to more subtle (e.g., therapists telling jokes about addicts). Admission walk-throughs could identify stigmatizing interactions that happen during potential client's first contacts with the treatment system and options for remediating these problematic interactions. The overall goal of a walk-through exercise is to identify problematic processes and improve service delivery by allowing providers and those in charge of the system of care to understand what it is like to enter the treatment system.[32] Other organizational and quality improvement interventions might also be adapted to target organizational change relating to stigma.

Empowering Those in Recovery

Another way to help participants in the addictions treatment system is to empower them to overcome the negative evaluative thoughts, shame, and fear of enacted stigma that are part of self-stigma. For substance abuse–related stigma, an uncontrolled pilot study targeting self-stigma with Acceptance and Commitment

Therapy[75] showed promising outcomes with medium to large effects across a number of variables at posttreatment. However, the intervention was delivered along with concurrent treatment, making it difficult to rule out the possibility that the observed effects were not simply the result of concurrent treatment. Other studies that have examined interventions for self-stigma in mental illness might provide some guidance for developing interventions for self-stigma in addiction.

One aspect of self-stigma is the way that fear of enacted stigma can impede recovery. One study tested an intervention that consisted of education about stigma, discussion of methods to combat and cope with stigma, and discussion about personal experiences of stigma that focused more on coping with enacted stigma than on other aspects of self-stigma. In this study, rehabilitation clubhouse members ($N = 88$) were randomly assigned to either 16 group sessions of the stigma intervention or no treatment. At a 6-month follow-up the intervention group was not significantly different from controls on any measure.

Knight et al.[59] compared a six-session group intervention based on cognitive behavioral therapy to a waitlist. The cognitive behavioral therapy intervention was developed primarily from existing manuals on the group treatment of auditory hallucinations and the group treatment of poor self-esteem. At posttreatment, effects were seen for measures of psychopathology and self-esteem, with these effects mostly maintained through follow-up. However, no effects were seen on stigma coping or empowerment measures, making it less clear whether the effects were more general therapeutic effects or had any specific impact on self-stigma.

Another group intervention for mental illness examined the impact of a 12-session group intervention (1.5 hours per group) that focused on helping individuals with first-episode psychosis to maintain an identity distinct from mental illness, promote hopefulness, minimize the impact of stigma, and help them to embrace a healthy sense of self.[81] Results of this randomized trial, comparing treatment as usual to treatment as usual plus the stigma intervention, showed that at posttreatment, the group that received the experimental intervention had improved scores on a measure of self-stigma, hopefulness, and quality of life, but not on several other scales.[82] A previous pilot study of the same intervention also showed an impact on a measure of self-stigma that the investigators termed engulfment, which refers to the tendency to allow illness and its associated stigma to entirely define the self-concept.[81]

In summary, there exist a number of promising interventions for self-stigma, with some mixed findings regarding the specificity of their effects. Now that some interventions have begun to show promising effects on stigma and related variables, future research needs to focus more on testing of specific models of change.

Stigma and the Emotion of Shame

Both of the definitions of stigma and most of the research on stigma ignore the emotional responses that are entailed in this phenomenon,[73] such as guilt, disgust, anger, and, most prominently, shame. Recently, several prominent stigma researchers called for more research into the relationship between stigma and shame.[114] Much of what has been described as characteristic of the personal experience of being stigmatized has also been described in the literature on the emotion of shame. For example, shame has been defined as an experience of "self as flawed and undesirable in the eyes of others,"[36,134] which is similar to Goffman's[35] idea of stigma as an "attribute that is deeply discrediting" that reduces a person "from a whole and usual person to a tainted, discounted

one" (p. 3). Shame is often elicited in social contexts and is associated with thoughts that one is seen as inferior or that others are condemning the self.[36] Similarly, in self-stigma people are fearful of being condemned, stigmatized, or judged by others because of their membership in the stigmatized group. Shame is also associated with cultural values, meaning that what is shameful varies according to the standards and ideals of a particular culture[62] as is what is stigmatized varies across cultures.

Shame has been called a "moral emotion,"[133] in that it is seen as relating to transgressions of the norms and values of a society. Although most authors agree that shame is a highly socially based emotion, substantial disagreement exists as to the usefulness of shame in regulating human behavior. Some authors see shame as a largely maladaptive, negative emotion, with little useful function.[134] Following similar reasoning, some therapy developers have suggested that shame should be directly targeted using shame-reduction strategies.[25,144] Other authors have suggested that shame may serve a valuable function in regulating people's behavior through limiting deviations from accepted norms.[23] Because shame can also arise when people violate their own standards and values, shame may have a role in alerting people to important deviations from their own values or self-standards[80] so that they can self-correct their behavior. Seen through this lens, attempts to directly reduce shame during treatment may actually feed the addictive cycle[74] by allowing people to continue deviant behavior or violate self-standards and values[35] without feeling the shame that would ordinarily attend those actions. At least one study[75] specifically targeted the experience of shame in addiction and showed that it could be reduced through treatment. However, in this study, although shame was reduced at posttreatment, the target of the intervention was not the reduction of shame, but rather increasing acceptance of the feeling of shame and mindfulness of stigmatizing thoughts and evaluations. Thus it may not be as helpful to try to reduce shame directly, but rather to help people change their psychological relationship to shame, so that they are more mindful and accepting of the experience.

As discussed above in reference to stigma, the context in which shame is experienced is probably extremely important in understanding its function and usefulness. In some contexts, shame may be an adaptive, although painful, emotion that highlights deviations from important values or self-standards, whereas in other contexts, shame may simply be excessive and serve no useful function. The debate over whether shame is a maladaptive or adaptive emotion will likely be resolved when more attention is paid to the specific social and psychological contexts in which shame is experienced and how people cope with and respond to shame.

Conclusions

Stigma operates at many levels. Self-stigma works within the individual to impede recovery. Structural stigma operates through the formal and informal policies and procedures of the health care and legal systems. Enacted stigma is expressed in the negative attitudes and behavior of the public. Courtesy stigma extends the impact of stigma to families and to addictions treatment professionals who are paid more poorly than professionals in other health care fields.[90] Furthermore, the stigma of substance abuse falls disproportionately on those who already experience greater societal injustice, such as racial and sexual minorities and individuals living in poverty, and who, as a result, have been denied many life opportunities. Stigma is such a broad, pervasive process that it is difficult to characterize its full impact, with any one study only able to document a small portion of its effects. Only by taking an expansive view and appreciating the effects of stigma across many contexts can we begin to see the tremendous cost of this process to the people struggling with drug and alcohol addiction and to society in general.

A broad and pervasive problem like stigma merits a comprehensive and systematic solution. Currently, research and theorizing about the impact of stigma in addiction is in its infancy. We know even less about how to reduce the burden of stigma on those who are attempting to recover from a life damaged by addiction. Anyone who has ever worked with addiction has seen its devastating effects on the lives of individuals and the immense struggle involved in living even a single day clean and sober. People attempting to climb the mountain of recovery do not need the additional burden of stigma, as their road is hard enough.

References

1. Ahern J, Stuber J, Galea S. Stigma, discrimination and the health of illicit drug users. *Drug Alcohol Depend.* 2007;88:188–196.
2. Ahmedani BK. Mental health stigma: society, individuals, and the profession. *J Soc Work Values Ethics.* 2011;8(2):4-1–4-16.
3. Barney LJ, Griffiths KM, Jorm AF, Christensen H. Stigma about depression and its impact on help-seeking intentions. *Australian N Z J Psychiatry.* 2006;40:51–54.
4. Beardsley K, Wish ED, Fitzelle DB, O'Grady K, Arria AM. Distance traveled to outpatient drug treatment and client retention. *J Subst Abuse Treat.* 2003;25:279–285.
5. Biglan A, Embry DE. A framework for intentional cultural change. *J Context Behav Sci.* 2013;2(3–4):10.1016/j.jcbs.2013.06.001.
6. Boysen GA, Vogel DL. Education and mental health stigma: the effects of attribution, biased assimilation, and attitude polarization. *J Soc Clin Psychol.* 2008;27:447–470.
7. Brener L, von Hippel W, Kippax S. Prejudice among health care workers toward injecting drug users with hepatitis C: does greater contact lead to less prejudice? *Int J Drug Policy.* 2007;18:381–387.
8. Brown RA, Lejuez CW, Kahler CW, Strong DR. Distress tolerance and duration of past smoking cessation attempts. *J Abnorm Psychol.* 2002;111:180–185.
9. Burris S. Disease stigma in US public health law. *J Law Med Ethics.* 2002;30:179–190.
10. Campbell C, Deacon H. Unravelling the contexts of stigma: from internalisation to resistance to change. *J Community Appl Soc Psychol.* 2006;16:411–417.
11. Chung YY, Shek DT. Reasons for seeking treatment among young drug abusers in Hong Kong. *Int J Adolesc Med Health.* 2008;20:441–448.
12. Corrigan P, Gelb B. Three programs that use mass approaches to challenge the stigma of mental illness. *Psychiatr Serv.* 2006;57:393–398.
13. Corrigan PW, Lurie BD, Goldman HH, Slopen N, Medasani K, Phelan S. How adolescents perceive the stigma of mental illness and alcohol abuse. *Psychiatr Serv.* 2005;56:544–550.
14. Corrigan PW, Markowitz FE, Watson AC. Structural levels of mental illness stigma and discrimination. *Schizophr Bull.* 2004;30:481–491.
15. Corrigan PW, River LP, Lundin RK, et al. Stigmatizing attributions about mental illness. *J Community Psychol.* 2000;28:91–102.
16. Corrigan PW, River LP, Lundin RK, et al. Three strategies for changing attributions about severe mental illness. *Schizophr Bull.* 2001;27:187–195.
17. Corrigan PW, Rowan D, Green A, et al. Challenging two mental illness stigmas: personal responsibility and dangerousness. *Schizophr Bull.* 2002;28:293–309.
18. Corrigan PW, Watson AC. The paradox of self-stigma and mental illness. *Clin Psychol Sci Pract.* 2002;9:35–53.
19. Corrigan PW, Watson AC. Understanding the impact of stigma on people with mental illness. *World Psychiatry.* 2002;1:16–20.
20. Corrigan PW, Watson AC. Understanding the impact of stigma on people with mental illness. *World Psychiatry.* 2002;1(1):16–20.
21. Corrigan PW. Changing mental illness stigma as it exists in the real world. *Aust Psychol.* 2007;42:90–97.
22. Crisp AH, Gelder MG, Rix S, Meltzer HI, Rowlands OJ. Stigmatisation of people with mental illnesses. *Br J Psychiatry.* 2000;177:4–7.
23. De Leersnyder J, Boiger M, Mesquita B. Cultural regulation of emotion: individual, relational, and structural sources. *Front Psychol.* 2013;4:55.
24. Dearing RL, Stuewig J, Tangney JP. On the importance of distinguishing shame from guilt: relations to problematic alcohol and drug use. *Addict Behav.* 2005;30:1392–1404.
25. Dickerson FB, Sommerville JL, Origoni AE. Mental illness stigma: an impediment to psychiatric rehabilitation. *Am J Psychiatric Rehabil.* 2002;6:186–200.
26. Dijker AJM, Koomen W. *Stigmatization, Tolerance and Repair: An Integrative Psychological Analysis of Responses to Deviance.* Cambridge University; 2007.
27. Dindia K. Going into and coming out of the closet: the dialectics of stigma disclosure. In: Montgomery BM, Baxter LA, eds. *Dialectical Approaches Studying Personal Relationships.* 1998:83–108.
28. Fals-Stewart W, O'Farrell TJ, Hooley JM. Relapse among married or cohabiting substance-abusing patients: the role of perceived criticism. *Behav Therapy.* 2001;32:787–801.
29. Farrimond HR, Joffe H. Pollution, peril and poverty: a British study of the stigmatization of smokers. *J Community Appl Soc Psychol.* 2006;16:481.
30. Ford JH, Green CA, Hoffman KA, et al. Process improvement needs in substance abuse treatment: admissions walk-through results. *J Subst Abuse Treat.* 2007;33:379–389.
31. Fulton R. *The Stigma of Substance Use: A Review of the Literature.* Toronto: Canada; Centre for Addiction and Mental Health; 1999.
32. Gifford EV, Kohlenberg BS, Hayes SC, et al. Acceptance-based treatment for smoking cessation. *Behav Therapy.* 2004;35:689–705.
33. Gilbert P. *Counselling for Depression.* Sage; 2000.
34. Gilbert P, Tarrier N. *A Biopsychosocial and Evolutionary Approach to Formulation With a Special Focus on Shame. Case Formulation in Cognitive Behavior Therapy: The Treatment of Challenging and Complex Cases.* New York, NY: Routledge/Taylor & Francis Group; 2006:81–112.
35. Goffman E. *Stigma: Notes on the Management of Spoiled Identity.* NJ: Prentice Hall; 1963.
36. Haghighat R. A unitary theory of stigmatisation: pursuit of self-interest and routes to destigmatisation. *Br J Psychiatry.* 2001;178:207–215.
37. Hamilton DL, Sherman JW. Stereotypes. *Handbook Soc Cogn.* 1994;2:1–68.
38. Hayes SC, Barnes-Holmes D, Roche B. Relational frame theory: a post-Skinnerian account of human language and cognition. *Advances in Child Development and Behavior: Academic.* 2001:101–138.
39. Hayes SC, Bissett R, Roget N, Padilla M. The impact of acceptance and commitment training and multicultural training on the stigmatizing attitudes and professional burnout of substance abuse counselors. *Behav Therapy.* 2004;35:821–835.
40. Hayes SC, Niccolls R, Masuda A, Rye AK. Prejudice, terrorism and behavior therapy. *Cogn Behav Pract.* 2002;9:296–301.
41. Hayes SC, Strosahl K, Wilson KG, et al. Measuring experiential avoidance: a preliminary test of a working model. *Psychol Rec.* 2004;54:553–578.
42. Hayes SC, Wilson KG, Gifford EV, et al. A preliminary trial of twelve-step facilitation and acceptance and commitment therapy with polysubstance-abusing methadone-maintained opiate addicts. *Behav Ther.* 2004;35:667–688.
43. Henricson C, Roker D. Support for the parents of adolescents: a review. *J Adolesc.* 2000;23:763–783.
44. Hewstone M. The "ultimate attribution error"? A review of the literature on intergroup causal attribution. *Eur J Soc Psychol.* 1990;20:311–335.

45. Hewstone M, Jaspars J, Lalljee M. Social representations, social attribution and social identity: the intergroup images of 'public' and 'comprehensive' schoolboys. *Eur J Soc Psychol.* 1982;12:241–269.

46. Hill RB. Structural discrimination: the unintended consequences of institutional processes. In: O'Gorman HJ, ed. *Surveying Social Life: Papers in Honor of Herbert H. Hyman.* Middletown, CT: Wesleyan University Press; 1988:353–375.

47. Hilton JL, von Hippel W. Stereotypes. *Ann Rev Psychol.* 1996;47:237–271.

48. Hingson R, Mangione T, Meyers A, Scotch N. Seeking help for drinking problems – a study in the Boston Metropolitan area. *J Studies Alcohol.* 1982;43:273–288.

49. Hoge MA, Morris JA, Daniels AS. *An Action Plan for Behavioral Health Workforce Development.* Cincinnati, OH: Annapolis Coalition on the Behavioral Health Workforce; 2007.

50. Holmes EP, Corrigan PW, Williams P, Canar J, Kubiak MA. Changing attitudes about schizophrenia. *Schizophr Bull.* 1999;25:447–456.

51. Hubbard RL, Craddock SG, Flynn PM, Anderson J, Etheridge RM. Overview of one-year follow-up outcomes in the drug abuse treatment outcome study (DATOS). *Psychol Addict Behav.* 1997;11:261–278.

52. Hubbard RL, Marsden ME, Rachal JV, Harwood HJ, Cavanaugh ER, Ginzburg HM. *Drug Abuse Treatment: A National Study of Effectiveness.* London: Chapel Hill; 1989.

53. Jackson TR. Treatment practice and research issues in improving opiod treatment outcomes. *Sci Pract Perspect.* 2002;1(1):22–28.

54. Keane M. Acceptance vs. rejection: nursing students' attitudes about mental illness. *Perspect Psychiatr Care.* 1991;27:13–18.

55. Kelly AE, McKillop KJ. Consequences of revealing personal secrets. *Psychol Bull.* 1996;120:450–465.

56. Kessler RC. The epidemiology of dual diagnosis. *Biol Psychiatry.* 2004;56:730–737.

57. Kimberly JR, McLellan AT. The business of addiction treatment: a research agenda. *J Subst Abuse Treat.* 2006;31:213–219.

58. Klingeman HKH. The motivation for change from problem alcohol and heroin use. *Br J Addict.* 1991;86:727–744.

59. Knight MTD, Wykes T, Hayward P. Group treatment of perceived stigma and self-esteem in schizophrenia: a waiting list trial of efficacy. *Behav Cogn Psychotherapy.* 2006;34:305–318.

60. Langer EJ, Fiske S, Taylor SE, Chanowitz B. Stigma, staring, and discomfort – novel-stimulus hypothesis. *J Exp Soc Psychol.* 1976;12:451–463.

61. Leeming D, Boyle M. Shame as a social phenomenon: a critical analysis of the concept of dispositional shame. *Psychol Psychother Theory Res Pract.* 2004;77:375–396.

62. Lewis M, Takai-Kawakami K, Kawakami K, Sullivan MW. Cultural differences in emotional responses to success and failure. *Int J Behav Dev.* 2010;34(1):53–61.

63. Lincoln TM, Arens E, Berger C, Rief W. Can antistigma campaigns be improved? A test of the impact of biogenetic vs psychosocial causal explanations on implicit and explicit attitudes to schizophrenia. *Schizophr Bull.* 2007;34:984–994.

64. Link BG, Cullen FT. Contact with the mentally ill and perceptions of how dangerous they are. *J Health Soc Behav.* 1986;27:289–302.

65. Link BG, Phelan JC. Conceptualizing stigma. *Annu Rev Sociol.* 2001;27:363–385.

66. Link BG, Phelan JC, Bresnahan M, Stueve A, Pescosolido BA. Public conceptions of mental illness: labels, causes, dangerousness, and social distance. *Am J Public Health.* 1999;89:1328–1333.

67. Link BG, Struening EL, Neese-Todd S, Asmussen S. JCP. On describing and seeking to change the experience of stigma. *Psychiatric Rehabil Skills.* 2002;6:201–231.

68. Link BG, Struening EL, Neese-Todd S, Asmussen S, Phelan JC. Stigma as a barrier to recovery: the consequences of stigma for the self-esteem of people with mental illnesses. *Psychiatr Serv.* 2001;52:1621–1626.

69. Link BG, Yang LH, Phelan JC, Collins PY. Measuring mental illness stigma. *Schizophr Bull.* 2004;30:511–541.

70. Livingston JD, Milne T, Fang ML, Amari E. The effectiveness of interventions for reducing stigma related to substance disorders: a systematic review. *Addiction.* 2012;107:39–50.

71. Luoma JB, Kohlenberg BS, Hayes SC, Bunting K, Rye AK. Reducing self-stigma in substance abuse through acceptance and commitment therapy: model, manual development, and pilot outcomes. *Addict Res Theory.* 2008;16:149–165.

72. Luoma JB, Kulesza M, Hayes SC, Kohlenberg B, Larimer M. Stigma predicts residential treatment length for substsance use disorder. *Am J Drug Alcohol Abuse.* 2014;40(3):206–212.

73. Luoma JB, Twohig MP, Waltz T, et al. An investigation of stigma in individuals receiving treatment for substance abuse. *Addict Behav.* 2007;32:1331–1346.

74. Macrae CN, Bodenhausen GV, Milne AB, Jetten J. Out of mind but back in sight – stereotypes on the rebound. *J Personality Soc Psychol.* 1994;67:808–817.

75. Macrae CN, Milne AB, Bodenhausen GV. Stereotypes as energy-saving devices: a peek inside the cognitive toolbox. *J Personality Soc Psychol.* 1994;66. 37–37.

76. Major BO'Brien LT. The social psychology of stigma. *Annu Rev Psychol.* 2005;56:393–421.

77. Mann CE, Himelein MJ. Putting the person back into psychopathology: an intervention to reduce mental illness stigma in the classroom. *Soc Psychiatry Psychiatric Epidemiol.* 2008;43:545–551.

78. Mascolo MF, Fischer KW. Developmental transformations in appraisals for pride, shame, and guilt. In: Tangney JP, Fischer K, Fischer KW, eds. *Self-conscious Emotions: The Psychology of Shame, Guilt, Embarrassment, and Pride*; 1995:64–113.

79. McCay E, Beanlands H, Leszcz M, et al. A group intervention to promote healthy self-concepts and guide recovery in first episode schizophrenia: a pilot study. *Psychiatric Rehabil J.* 2006;30:105–111.

80. McCay E, Beanlands H, Zipursky R, et al. A randomised controlled trial of a group intervention to reduce engulfment and self-stigmatisation in first episode schizophrenia. *Australian e-J Advance Mental Health.* 2007;6(3):212–220.

81. McLaughlin D, Long A. An extended literature review of health professionals' perceptions of illicit drugs and their clients who use them. *J Psychiatric Mental Health Nurs.* 1996;3:283–288.

82. Mehta S, Farina A. Is being sick really better? Effect of the disease view of mental disorder on stigma. *J Soc Clin Psychol.* 1997;16:405–419.

83. Meier PS, Barrowclough C, Donmall MC. The role of the therapeutic alliance in the treatment of substance misuse: a critical review of the literature. *Addiction.* 2005;100:304.

84. Montana Department of Justice. *Methamphetamine in Montana: A Follow-Up Report on Trends and Progress.* 2008. Retrieved June 7, 2009, from: http://www.methproject.org/documents/MT_AG_Report_Final.pdf.

85. Moos RH. Iatrogenic effects of psychosocial interventions for substance use disorders: prevalence, predictors, prevention. *Addiction.* 2005;100:595–604.

86. Moos RH, Nichol AC, Moos BS. Risk factors for symptom exacerbation among treated patients with substance use disorders. *Addiction.* 2002;97:75–85.

87. Morrison JK, Teta DC. Reducing students' fear of mental illness by means of seminar-induced belief change. *J Clin Psychol.* 1980;36:275–276.

88. O'Farrell TJ, Hooley J, Fals-Stewart W, Cutter HSG. Expressed emotion and relapse in alcoholic patients. *J Consult Clin Psychol.* 1998;66:744–752.

89. Olfson M, Motjabai R, Sampson NA, Hwang I, Kessler RC. Dropout from outpatient mental healthcare in the United States. *Psychiatri Serv.* 2009;60(7):898–907.

90. Ostaszkiewicz J, O'Connell B, Dunning T. 'We just do the dirty work': dealing with incontinence, courtesy stigma, and the low occupational status of carework in long-term aged care facilities. *J Clin Nurs.* 2016;25(17–18):2528–2541.

91. Page S. Psychiatric stigma: two studies of behaviour when the chips are down. *Can J Community Mental Health*. 1983;2:13–19.
92. Parcesepe AM, Cabassa LJ. Public stigma of mental Illness in the United States: a systematic review. *Adm Policy Mnt Health*. 2013;103:853–860.
93. Parcesepe AM, Cabassa LJ. Public stigma of mental illness in the United States: a Systematic Review. *Adm Policy Ment Health*. 2013;40(5).
94. Penn DL, Guynan K, Daily T, Spaulding WD, Garbin CP, Sullivan M. Dispelling the stigma of schizophrenia: what sort of information is best? *Schizophr Bull*. 1994;20:567–578.
95. Penn DL, Kommana S, Mansfield M, Link BG. Dispelling the stigma of schizophrenia: II. The impact of information on dangerousness. *Schizophr Bull*. 1999;25:437–446.
96. Penn DL, Martin J. The stigma of severe mental illness: some potential solutions for a recalcitrant problem. *Psychiatric Q*. 1998;69:235–247.
97. Penn DL, Ritchie M, Francis J, Combs D, Martin J. Social perception in schizophrenia: the role of context. *Psychiatry Res*. 2002;109:149–159.
98. Perlick DA, Rosenheck RA, Clarkin JF, et al. Stigma as a barrier to recovery: adverse effects of perceived stigma on social adaptation of persons diagnosed with bipolar affective disorder. *Psychiatric Serv*. 2001;52:1627–1632.
99. Perlick DA, Rosenheck RA, Clarkin JF, et al. Stigma as a barrier to recovery: adverse effects of perceived stigma on social adaptation of persons diagnosed with bipolar affective disorder. *Psychiatric Serv*. 2001;52:1627.
100. Pettigrew TF, Tropp LR. Does intergroup contact reduce prejudice? Recent meta-analytic findings. In: Oskamp S, ed. *Reducing Prejudice and Discrimination*. ; 2000:93–114.
101. Phelan JC. Geneticization of deviant behavior and consequences for stigma: the case of mental illness. *J Health Soc Behav*. 2005;46:307–322.
102. Phelan JC, Link BG, Stueve A, Pescosolido BA. Public conceptions of mental illness in 1950 and 1996: what is mental illness and is it to be feared? *J Health Soc Behav*. 2000;41:188–207.
103. Quinn DM, Kahng SK, Crocker J. Discreditable: stigma effects of revealing a mental illness history on test performance. *Personality Soc Psychol Bull*. 2004;30:803.
104. Rasinski KA, Woll P, Cooke A, Corrigan PW. Stigma and substance use disorders. In: Corrigan PW, ed. *On the Stigma of Mental Illness: Practical Strategies for Research and Social Change*. Washington, DC: American Psychological Association; 2005:219–236.
105. Read J, Haslam N, Sayce L, Davies E. Prejudice and schizophrenia: a review of the 'mental illness is an illness like any other' approach. *Acta Psychiatr Scand*. 2006;114:303–318.
106. Read J. Why promoting biological ideology increases prejudice against people labelled 'schizophrenic'. *Aust Psychol*. 2007;42:118–128.
107. Richmond I, Foster J. Negative attitudes towards people with co-morbid mental health and substance misuse problems: an investigation of mental health professionals. *J Mental Health*. 2003;12:393–403.
108. Ritsher JB, Phelan JC. Internalized stigma predicts erosion of morale among psychiatric outpatients. *Psychiatry Res*. 2004;129:257–265.
109. Rodriguez RR, Kelly AE. Health effects of disclosing secrets to imagined accepting versus nonaccepting confidants. *J Soc Clin Psychol*. 2006;25:1023–1047.
110. Room R. Stigma, social inequality and alcohol and drug use. *Drug Alcohol Rev*. 2005;24:143–155.
111. Rosenfield S. Labeling mental illness: the effects of received services and perceived stigma on life satisfaction. *Am Sociol Rev*. 1997;62:660–672.
112. Rüsch N, Angermeyer MC, Corrigan PW. Mental illness stigma: concepts, consequences, and initiatives to reduce stigma. *Eur Psychiatry*. 2005;20:529–539.
113. Rüsch N, Hölzer A, Hermann C, et al. Self-stigma in women with borderline personality disorder and women with social phobia. *J Nervous Mental Dis*. 2006;194:766.
114. SAMHSA. *Results From the 2005 National Survey on Drug Use and Health: National Findings*. Office of Applied Studies, NSDUH Series H-30, DHHS Publication No. SMA 06-4194, Rockville, MD; 2006.
115. Satel S. In praise of stigma. In: Henningfield JE, Santora PB, Bickel WK, eds. *Addiction Treatment: Science and Policy for the Twenty-First Century*. Baltimore, MD: Johns Hopkins University; 2007:147–151.
116. Scambler G. Stigma and disease: changing paradigms. *Lancet*. 1998;352:1054–1055.
117. Schober R, Annis HM. Barriers to help-seeking for change in drinking: a gender-focused review of the literature. *Addict Behav*. 1996;21:81–92.
118. Schomerus G, Matschinger H, Angermeyer MC. Familiarity with mental illness and approval of structural discrimination against psychiatric patients in Germany. *J Nervous Mental Dis*. 2007;195:89.
119. Semple SJ, Grant I, Patterson TL. Utilization of drug treatment programs by methamphetamine users: the role of social stigma. *Am J Addictions*. 2005;14:367–380.
120. Sher I, McGinn L, Sirey JA, Meyers B. Effects of caregivers' perceived stigma and causal beliefs on patients' adherence to antidepressant treatment. *Psychiatr Serv*. 2005;56:564.
121. Simpson DD, Joe GW, Brown BS. Treatment retention and follow-up outcomes in the drug abuse treatment outcome study (DATOS). *Psychol Addict Behav*. 1997;11:294–307.
122. Simpson DD, Joe GW, Brown BS. Treatment retention and follow-up outcomes in the drug abuse treatment outcome study (DATOS). *Psychol Addict Behav*. 1997;11:294–307.
123. Simpson DD. Treatment for drug abuse: follow-up outcomes and length of time spent. *Archiv Gen Psychiatry*. 1981;38:875–880.
124. Simpson DD, Sells SB. Effectiveness of treatment for drug abuse: an overview of the darp research program. *Eval Drug Treat Programs*. 1982;2(1):7–29.
125. Sirey JA, Bruce ML, Alexopoulos GS, Perlick DA, Friedman SJ, Meyers BS. Stigma as a barrier to recovery: perceived stigma and patient-rated severity of illness as predictors of antidepressant drug adherence. *Psychiatric Serv*. 2001;52:1615–1620.
126. Spears R, Manstead ASR. The social context of stereotyping and differentiation. *Eur J Soc Psychol*. 1989;19:101–121.
127. Stark MJ. Dropping out of substance abuse treatment: a clinically oriented review. *Clin Psychol Rev*. 1992;12:93–116.
128. Starr S, Campbell LR, Herrick CA. Factors affecting use of the mental health system by rural children. *Issues Ment Health Nurs*. 2002;23:291–304.
129. Steele CM, Spencer SJ, Aronson J. Contending with group image: the psychology of stereotype and social identity threat. *Adv Exp Soc Psychol*. 2002;34:379–440.
130. Tajfel H. Social psychology of intergroup relations. *Annu Rev Psychol*. 1982;33:1–39.
131. Tangney JP. Shame and guilt in interpersonal relationships. In: Tangney JP, Fischer KW, eds. *Self-conscious Emotions: The Psychology of Shame, Guilt, Embarrassment, and Pride*. ; 1995:114–139.
132. Tangney JP, Dearing RL. *Shame and Guilt*. New York, NY: The Guilford Press; 2002.
133. Tipper R, Mountain D, Lorimer S, McIntosh A. Support workers' attitudes to mental illness: implications for reducing stigma. *RCP*. 2006:179–181.
134. Treloar C, Holt M. Deficit models and divergent philosophies: service providers' perspectives on barriers and incentives to drug treatment. *Drugs: Edu Prevent Policy*. 2006;13:367–382.
135. Tuchfeld BS. Spontaneous remission in alcoholics – empirical observations and theoretical implications. *J Studies Alcohol*. 1981;42:626–641.

136. Tucker JA, Vuchinich RE, Gladsjo JA. Environmental events surrounding natural recovery from alcohol-related problems. *J Studies Alcohol*. 1994;55:401–411.

137. Twohig MP, Shoenberger D, Hayes SC. A preliminary investigation of acceptance and commitment therapy as a treatment for marijuana dependence in adults. *J Appl Behav Anal*. 2007;40:619–632.

138. Van Boekel LC, Brouwers EPM, et al. Comparing stigmatizing attitudes towards people with substance abuse disorders between the general public, GPs, mental health and addiction specialists and clients. *Int J of Social Psychiatry*. 2014;61(6):539–549.

139. Wahl OF. Mental health consumers' experience of stigma. *Schizophr Bull*. 1999;25:467–478.

140. Wenzlaff RM, Wegner DM. Thought suppression. *Annu Rev Psychol*. 2000;51:59–91.

141. White WL. *The Day Is Coming: Visions of a Recovery Advocacy Movement*. Bloomington, IL: Lighthouse Institute; 2001.

142. Wiechelt SA. The specter of shame in substance misuse. *Subst Use Misuse*. 2007;42:399–409.

143. Wilson DS. *Darwin's Cathedral: Evolution, Religion, and the Nature of Society*. University of Chicago; 2003.

144. Wilson KG, Hayes SC. Resurgence of derived stimulus relations. *J Exp Anal Behav*. 1996;66:267–282.

145. Wright ER, Gronfein WP, Owens TJ. Deinstitutionalization, social rejection, and the self-esteem of former mental patients. *J Health Soc Behav*. 2000;41:68–90.

62

Religiousness, Spirituality, and Addiction: An Evidence-Based Review

J. SCOTT TONIGAN AND ALYSSA A. FORCEHIMES

CHAPTER OUTLINE

Introduction

The 12-step model to the treatment of addiction is the most popular therapeutic model in the United States, and most adherents of the 12-step approach consider spiritual growth singular with recovery. This chapter offers a critical review and discussion of spirituality and religiousness as it has been investigated in the empirical literature on addiction. Curiously, although the 12-step model has been reported to produce outcomes relatively equivalent to more research-based therapies, for example, cognitive behavioral and motivational enhancement therapies,[42,50] and actually a superior outcome when the treatment goal is total abstinence, the underlying *stated* mechanism of this approach, spirituality, has only begun to be systematically investigated using rigorous methodologies including randomized clinical trials. It is important to acknowledge that non–12-step spiritual and religious approaches also intended to mobilize and sustain addictive behavior change have proliferated in the United States, *regardless* of the presence or absence of empirical support. A cursory Internet search using "alcoholism" and "spirituality" as key words, for example, yielded 944,000 hits. It seems that the absence of empirical support for the efficacy of spirituality in reducing substance abuse has hardly impeded its application. Furthermore, referral to Alcoholics Anonymous during and after treatment is the norm in the United States, also regardless of the therapeutic orientation of the treatment provider. In this light, the practical issue is not if treatment-seeking alcoholics ought to be introduced to spiritual models of recovery. Rather, it is vital that researchers and clinicians have a working knowledge of spiritual approaches to addiction in order to better understand the psychological and social forces and resources facing prospective clients.

This chapter is organized into three sections. Historical reticence to investigate spirituality and religiosity by addiction researchers stems, in part, from the constructs poorly understood dimensions.[23] The first section of this chapter therefore offers several working definitions of religiosity and spirituality. These definitions are intimately tied to distinct conceptual models pertaining to the role of spirituality in addiction. These models will be presented and discussed, and some attention will then be given to four psychometrically validated measures that are available to clinicians and researchers. The second section of the chapter advances the orientation that spirituality can be viewed as an outcome, a catalyst or intervention, a moderator, and as a mediational variable; in fact, the construct has been treated in each of these capacities in the empirical literature. A keen awareness of these distinctions is paramount to grasping the implications and avoiding the many pitfalls surrounding the study of alcoholism and spirituality. Third, this chapter focuses on what is currently known about Alcoholics Anonymous-related benefit, the largest and most studied of spiritual interventions. Here, special attention will be given to what is known about the importance of prescribed Alcoholics Anonymous spiritual practices in accounting for reduced drinking. The chapter will conclude with a brief summary.

Several caveats need to be voiced at the beginning of this chapter. First, the accelerating nature of empirical research in this area necessarily will result in a somewhat incomplete review. Studies now underway may offer findings that elaborate upon, clarify, or even contradict positions and interpretations offered in this chapter. Related, studies reviewed in this chapter were purposefully selected according to their scientific rigor, not because of the claims and interpretations made by study investigators. In essence, cross-sectional studies purporting to investigate causal temporal relationships were rarely selected for review. Third, it is important to stress the plasticity of spiritual and religious practices and beliefs. An individual rarely is "spiritual" in all situations with all people; nor does evidence indicate that the nature and expression of spirituality remains fixed over time. Although this plasticity is obvious and volumes have been written about it, there is a tendency nevertheless to reify spirituality as a trait construct. It is wise to remember that even prophets question, at one time or another, the depth and value of their spiritual and religious beliefs. It is also instructive to remember throughout this chapter that the measurement of this fluid and evolving construct occurred, in general, in research settings. The extent that this context influenced that measurement of spiritual beliefs and practices is unclear but certainly raises concern. Related, the very subjective nature of spiritual and religious beliefs and practices and experiences requires, at this juncture in time and technology, self-report. Legions of studies have investigated the unintended and undetected biases that arise in relation to self-report on subjective states. Beyond the scope of this chapter, we recommend that readers consult one of several excellent discussions on the reliability and validity of self-report in the areas of spirituality and religiosity.[23]

Section I

Definitions of Religiosity and Spirituality

Now the whole earth had one language and a common speech...let us go down and confuse their language so they will not understand each other...That is why it was called Babel—because there the Lord confused the language of the whole world.

GENESIS 11

The struggle of defining spirituality and religiosity makes it clear how far we have come from a universally understood language. Researchers and practitioners posit opinions on how to define these constructs; the diversity in meanings clearly echoes the confusion, disagreement, and lack of productivity described in the book of Genesis. Zinnbauer and Pargament[64] have aptly called these terms the "definitional tower of Babel." As Zinnbauer and Pargament wrote regarding those in the field who study spirituality and religion, "[We] can agree on one thing: we have never agreed about anything"[64] (p. 4). There is little disagreement that spirituality and religion are constructs deserving of research and clinical attention, but because an important first step in researching a construct is how to operationalize and measure the construct, we begin in a tumultuous place.

Definitions of religion, and particularly spirituality, have changed and evolved over the years. Once representing a single construct, these constructs are now distinct[20] and some would say even incompatible. Spirituality is increasingly defined in contrast to religion rather than as interchangeable terms.[64] The definitions are marked by explicit and implicit philosophical and theological underpinnings and thus remain vulnerable to claims that the definitions are either too broad or too narrow. Koenig[29] described religion as an expression that is institutional, formal, outward, doctrinal, authoritarian, and inhibiting, and spirituality as an expression that is individual, subjective, emotional, inward,

unsystematic, and freeing. Pargament[45] reported that religion is moving "from a broadband construct—one that includes both the institutional and the individual, and the good and the bad—to a narrowband institutional construct that restricts and inhibits human potential" (p. 3). Apparent in the polarization of these two constructs is an underlying message that is an exaltation of spirituality and a condemnation of religion.

It is common for scholars to begin manuscripts with caveats of the difficulty in defining these terms, discuss the divergent definitions, and then provide an entirely new definition altogether. Other researchers approach the complexity by simply avoiding a definition, instead asking questions such as "do you consider yourself spiritual?" or "how important is religion in your life?"[37] Although results from questions such as these contribute to our understanding of the perceived importance of religiosity and spirituality and other variables, this approach is limited in terms of not furthering our understanding of how these terms are uniquely understood and defined by participants.

It is evident that defining these constructs is difficult; however, research evidence supports the usefulness of this pursuit because of the clear connection between spirituality and religion and mental health.[31] In a recent review[32] of longitudinal studies, increased spirituality and religion seem to consistently promote a longer, happier life. For individuals with mental or physical health problems, spirituality and religion enhance pain management, improve surgical outcomes, protect against depression, provide coping resources, and reduce the risk of suicide. Although religion and spirituality are relevant to many problems dealt with by practitioners and there is a consistent link between spirituality/religiousness and physical and psychological well-being, in few areas of mental health are these issues as central as addictive behaviors.

The Relationship Between Religiosity/Spirituality and Addiction

In some sense, addiction represents the antithesis of spirituality. For example, one of the four noble truths of Buddhism is "Suffering is caused by attachment," and a central focus for followers of this tradition is to relinquish craving and clinging to things. Yet the centrality of attachment is readily apparent in the diagnosis of substance use disorders—part of the criteria for a substance use diagnosis is that a great deal of time is spent in activities necessary to obtain the substance.[3] May describes the spiritual nature of addiction as "a deep-seated form of idolatry. The objects of our addictions become our false gods. These are what we worship, what we attend to, where we give our time and energy."[35] Attachment to a substance is a futile attempt to impose direction in one's life, a direction that displaces one's prior values, meaning structures, and goals. Instead, individuals become concerned with purposeful action toward their next drink or their next high. In Tillich's[54] terminology, the substance becomes the individual's ultimate concern.

Spirituality is also central to the most influential model of recovery in the United States. The recovery program of Alcoholics Anonymous views addiction as a fundamentally spiritual problem and has promoted spirituality and religion as a central factor to recovery since 1935.[33] In the words of Bill W., the co-founder of Alcoholics Anonymous, individuals with substance abuse problems "have been not only mentally and physically ill, [they] have been spiritually sick"[1] (p. 34). The program of recovery is therefore based upon a model of prescribed spiritual practices.

In addition to the spiritual program of Alcoholics Anonymous and other 12-step programs, the literature is also quite clear that religious involvement is predictive of lower current and future rates of problem drinking. For instance, more than 80% of the nearly 100 studies on alcohol and religion reviewed by Koenig et al.[29] reported a negative association between religiosity and problems with alcohol. It seems that individuals who are more active in a religion and for whom faith occupies a central place in their lives are less likely to develop dependence on a drug. Similarly, individuals entering treatment for alcohol/drug problems tend to have very low religious involvement and are often quite alienated from organized religion.

Religiosity/Spirituality and Addiction Research: An Overview

In a review of the literature on spirituality and addiction, Cook[8] examined 265 publications in order to identify the definition of spirituality by different authors. Cook found that only 12% of the papers explicitly defined the term "spirituality," 32% offered a description of the concept of spirituality, 12% defined a related concept (such as "the spiritually healthy person"), and in 44% of the papers the term "spirituality" was left undefined. Breaking the conceptual content of the definitions into component parts, Cook classified the content of the various definitions into 13 conceptual components. Cook found that the four components that were encountered most frequently and were most central to the definition of spirituality were transcendence, relatedness, core/force/ soul, and meaning/purpose. On the basis of these components, Cook proposed the following definition:

> Spirituality is a distinctive, potentially creative and universal dimension of human experience arising both within the inner subjective awareness of individuals and within communities, so- cial groups, and traditions. It may be experienced as relationship with that which is intimately "inner," immanent and personal, within the self and others, and/or as relationship with that which is wholly "other," transcendent and beyond the self. It is experi- enced as being of fundamental or ultimate importance and is thus concerned with matters of meaning and purpose in life, truth and values[8] (pp. 548–549).

One particular conundrum, evident in Cook's[8] definition and many other definitions of spirituality, is that scholars have begun to include aspects of mental health within the definition.[23,28] If terms such as well-being and connectedness with others are con- sidered part of the definition of spirituality, there is an inherent measurement problem when examining spirituality and religious- ness in relation to positive mental health functioning. As Koenig[28] stated, "Defining spirituality in this way assures that those who are 'spiritual' will be mentally healthy, and excludes those who are mentally ill from this desirable classification" (p. 351). In addition to this classification problem, there is also a concern in terms of measurement of treatment outcome. If a client shows improve- ment in mental health, we encounter the dilemma of whether this improvement is due to an increase in spirituality or religion or whether we are simply measuring improvement in quality of life.

Koenig's[28] concern is particularly relevant to how researchers understand addiction. Addiction involves a setting apart from oneself, others, and the world—a direct opposition to spiritual- ity's emphasis of oneness with all of humanity. There is therefore a clear confound as individuals with substance use problems begin to succeed in recovery—they begin to reconnect with humanity and realign their values and goals. The use of substances offers a way to "avoid being present to oneself"[35] (p. 44). It is common

for individuals with substance use problems to report that they feel disconnected from others, and as attachment to the substance increases there is a tendency to isolate from important relation- ships. In Alcoholics Anonymous, a common term is "terminal uniqueness," describing a feeling of the alcoholic who feels an extreme uniqueness and alienation from his or her peers. Con- versely, during recovery from substances, there is a tendency for individuals to attach to a Higher Power and reaffirm important relationships.

Readers interested in further exploring the definitions and distinctions of spirituality/religiousness are encouraged to access Geppert et al.[17] These authors have compiled a priceless annotated bibliography of 1353 scholarly papers on spirituality/religiousness and addictions that are divided into 10 categories, ranging from the measurement of spirituality with attitudes about spirituality and substance use.

Conceptual Models of Spirituality and Religiousness in Addiction Research and Four Religiosity/Spirituality Measures

Although there are diverse definitions and applications of spiritual- ity/religiousness topics in addiction research, two conceptual mod- els serve as a framework for a majority of these endeavors. On one hand, the deficit model of spirituality/religiousness and addictions assumes that the process of deepening addiction involves the loss of spiritual/religious values, beliefs, and practices. Recovery, then, necessarily involves the acquisition or reestablishment of these values and beliefs. Here, the seeking of spiritual/religious values, practices, and beliefs fills an existential void created by years of sub- stance abuse. Tacit to this model is the assumption that the quest or search for spiritual/religious meaning is innate. The second model, the coping model of spirituality/religiousness and addic- tion, makes few, if any, assumptions about the etiology of sub- stance abuse and dependency. Instead, this model focuses on the potentially buffering properties of spiritual/religious practices and beliefs in avoiding relapse. Specifically, spiritual/religious practices and beliefs are interpreted to sever the linkage between aroused negative emotional states and subsequent substance use and abuse. In this regard, the coping model has explicit connections with two popular cognitive behavior–based strategies in the treatment of addiction: relapse prevention[2] and cognitive behavioral therapy.[36] Less obvious is the theoretical relationship between the coping and protective factor models in addiction research. One of the most consistent and enduring findings in spirituality/religiousness addic- tion research is the inverse relationship reported between spiritual/ religious beliefs and practices and the *development* of substance abuse.[17] Essentially, spiritual/religious practices are interpreted to buffer or attenuate processes that promote substance abuse. Pro- cesses within the coping model operate in a similar fashion, but with the key difference that spiritual/religious practices now buffer against the reestablishment of addictive behaviors.

Knowledge of these two spirituality/religiousness models offers at least two benefits. First, understanding these two models pro- vides a conceptual framework to judge, classify, and select from the plethora of spirituality/religiousness measures available to addiction researchers and clinicians. Too often, authors of spiritu- ality/religiousness measures do not explicitly identify the concep- tual basis of their respective tool. As such, spirituality/religiousness measures are frequently misused, or they fail to provide a sensitive assessment of the process under investigation. Conceptual models offer clear predictions about causal relationships, and knowledge of the different predictions of these two models offers an important second benefit. Most striking, the deficit model ultimately predicts that the failure to enlarge upon spiritual/religious practices and beliefs will result, in the long run, in relapse to substances. Some of the most explicit examples of this model and its prediction on relapse can be found in the core Alcoholics Anonymous literature.[1] The coping model of spirituality/religiousness and addictions does not lead to such a categorical prediction. Instead, failures to develop and apply spiritual/religious behaviors and beliefs may result in a continuum of adverse consequences given the absence of the presumed positive buffering effect, but alternative resources at multiple levels may offset the absence of spiritual/religious practices, for example, social networks supportive of abstinence. With this background, it is instructive to briefly review four spirituality/religiousness measures that have demonstrated psychometric properties and that are frequently encountered in the addiction literature.

Religious Beliefs and Behaviors[6] is a 13-item self-report measure with demonstrated psychometric properties. The tool yields two scales: Formal practices and God consciousness. Items in the God consciousness scale inquire about the frequency of prayer, meditation, and thoughts about God, whereas items in the Formal practices scale inquire about attendance at worship service and reading of scriptures or holy writings. Strengths of the Religious Beliefs and Behaviors measure include fast administration, availability of normative data based upon an alcohol treatment seeking sample (N = 1637), and documented sensitivity to discriminate three groups of Alcoholics Anonymous–exposed adults over time in predictable directions, for example, gains in God consciousness and Formal practices increased at a faster rate over time among adults with more Alcoholics Anonymous exposure. The Religious Beliefs and Behaviors measure does, however, have limitations. Noted by Johnson and Robinson,[23] one cannot determine from the Religious Beliefs and Behaviors measure if the behaviors of prayer and meditation occur independently of Formal practices, and findings are mixed about the ability of the Religious Beliefs and Behaviors scales to predict positive outcome.[7,26,53] The Religious Beliefs and Behaviors measure is not copyrighted and can be used free of charge.

The Brief Multidimensional Measure of Religiousness/Spirituality,[13] a 38-item self-report questionnaire, has 10 scales: Daily Spiritual practices (6 items), Values/Beliefs (2 items), Forgiveness (3 items), Private Religious practices (5 items), Religious and Spiritual Coping (7 items), Religious Support (4 items), Religious/Spiritual History (3 items), Organizational Religiousness (2 items), Religious Preference (1 item), and Overall Self-Ranking (2 items). The Brief Multidimensional Measure of Religiousness/Spirituality was a collaborative effort between the Fetzer Institute and the National Institutes of Health to construct a multifaceted measure of spirituality/religiousness that explicitly decoupled private and public spiritual/religious behaviors and practices. Widely recognized scholars developed spirituality/religiousness scales independently, often by reducing parent instruments into a brief scale. In addition to strong psychometric properties and partial normative data, the Brief Multidimensional Measure of Religiousness/Spirituality is especially useful because the manual provides the rationale, application, and psychometric citations for each scale. Based on a treatment-seeking adult sample (N = 123), half of the scales showed significant increases over a 6-month period, and the Daily Experience scale was prognostic of reductions in heavy drinking even after controlling for a number of rival explanations (e.g., Alcoholics Anonymous involvement and gender).[53]

The Spiritual Coping Questionnaire[46] is a 22-item questionnaire that measures perceived relationship to God, with the basic premise that different kinds of God relationships imply different coping mechanisms. Three relationship-coping scales have been empirically validated with Alcoholics Anonymous–exposed persons and are labeled: Cooperative (α = 0.93), Deferring (α = 0.89), and Self-directing (α = 0.91) God relationships. Items pertaining to the cooperative God relationship stress mutual exchange between a deity and individual in making choices and decisions, while the deferring style is characterized by items that endorse the release of all responsibility for decisions to a deity. Finally, the self-directed style characterizes individuals who assume all responsibility for choices and who do not seek spiritual guidance. Spiritual Coping Questionnaire scales have been attractive to 12-step researchers because of the hypothesized developmental changes in spirituality that occur among Alcoholics Anonymous members as they work through the 12 steps. Specifically, steps 1–3 have been interpreted as reflecting a deferring relationship with a Higher Power, while later steps encourage a cooperative deity relationship, for example, steps 11 and 12. To date, temporal changes in coping styles have been documented among 12-step members,[53] but the nature and pattern of these changes appear to be more complex than originally thought. In particular, longevity and participation in Alcoholics Anonymous appear to be related with shifting preferences in spiritual coping style, but actual step work was not.[19]

Purpose in Life[9] is a 20-item self-report questionnaire that uses a 7-point Likert scale (anchors: Never and Constantly). Used in a number of alcohol studies,[49,50,62] the Purpose in Life measure is used to assess the extent that one experiences life meaning. Lower scores on the Purpose in Life reflect a relative lack of current life meaning. Little support has been found for this construct predicting later substance use among outpatient and aftercare adult alcoholics,[57] and the item content measuring life meaning itself has been criticized.[23] Specifically, the Purpose in Life along with other measures of life meaning is correlated with measures of well-being and, equally important, it is problematic to determine whether experienced life meaning is the result of spiritual/religious behaviors or practices or not.

Section II

Empirical Religiosity/Spirituality Questions in Addiction Research

There are four types of research questions that can be asked about spirituality using prospective longitudinal studies. Heuristically, these questions are, (1) what *direct* effect does spirituality, or changes in spirituality, have on drinking? (intervention question); (2) what *changes* in spirituality occur as a result of trying to mobilize and sustain addictive behavior change? (dependent measure question); (3) How may spiritual/religious practices and beliefs *attenuate* or enhance receptivity to treatment, aftercare, or Alcoholics Anonymous (moderation question) and, most complex (4) how may spirituality, or changes in spirituality, statistically *explain* the direct relationship between a cause (e.g., prayer) and a desired effect (e.g., abstinence)? (mediation question). This latter question, first formally described by Baron and Kenny,[4] comprises four subquestions that focus on the temporal and causal relationships between, at a minimum, three measured variables. Fig. 62.1 highlights, with a hypothetical example pertaining to spirituality and addiction, both the ideal temporal relationship between measures and the nature of questions that must be affirmed to declare that

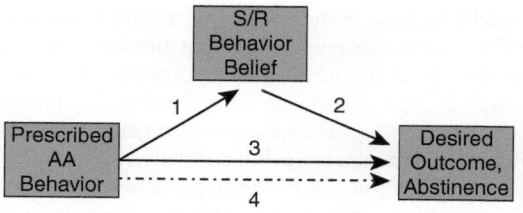

• **Fig. 62.1** Four conditions to establish statistical mediation in identifying spiritual or religious actions. Condition 1: Active ingredient, prescribed AA behavior, mobilizes S/R practice or belief. Condition 2: S/R practice effects desired outcome, increased abstinence. Condition 3: Active ingredient, prescribed AA behavior, effects desired outcome. Condition 4: Strength of pathway from prescribed AA behavior and desired outcome is significantly reduced (eliminated) when statistically controlling for S/R practice or belief. *AA*, Alcoholics Anonymous; *S/R*, spiritual/religious.

a measure, here spirituality, explains or accounts for an observed and desired effect. For the interested reader, a detailed collection of papers specific to mediation and alcoholism can be found in Huebner and Tonigan.[22]

Spirituality as an Intervention and Outcome

Investigations of spirituality/religiousness have used both cross-sectional and prospective longitudinal designs to address these empirical questions, with cross-sectional investigators frequently making the case that study findings offer insight into casual relationships. Although one-shot studies do offer some important perspectives on the correlational structure of domains of interest, a number of factors limit their value in understanding causality, not the least of which is the self-selected (and often) biased samples upon which study findings are based. As an example, Poage et al.[48] conducted a cross-sectional study of 53 Alcoholics Anonymous–exposed adults. From this volunteer convenience sample, the investigators asked if length of sobriety, spirituality, and general life contentment were associated. Consistent with predictions, Alcoholics Anonymous members with more years of sobriety reported significantly higher spirituality than Alcoholics Anonymous members with fewer years of sobriety, and spirituality and contentment were significantly and positively associated. Of interest, years of sobriety and contentment were not associated. Pointed out by the authors, however, causal linkages between these three constructs remain unclear, at best. Did spiritual growth predict the sustaining of sobriety (or vice versa)? Alternatively, years sober and age were positively related ($r = 54$) in this sample. Did the enhanced spirituality of Alcoholics Anonymous members with more sobriety, then, simply reflect the well-documented phenomenon that as we age we become more open to religious and spiritual explanations for the human experience? Although studies such as this certainly have value and should be conducted, they are generally avoided in this review because of the number of rival explanations for study findings.

With the exception of studies specifically focused on Alcoholics Anonymous (reviewed in Section III), there have been surprisingly few longitudinal studies that have investigated how, if at all, spirituality/religiousness-based interventions influence subsequent substance use. For clarity, the studies reviewed in this section are arranged according to the intensity of the spiritual/religious intervention, beginning with the studies that involved minimal or modest intervention efforts. Walker and colleagues,[61] for example, sought to determine whether intercessory prayer impacted the drinking of 40 treatment-seeking alcoholics. Consenting participants were randomized into treatment as usual, which consisted of individual and group counseling in an outpatient setting, and the other half of the sample was assigned to the intercessory prayer condition. Here, in addition to treatment as usual, volunteers prayed for the well-being and abstinence of individuals in the intercessory prayer group. No mean differences on the key measure of drinking were observed between the two groups at the 3- and 6-month follow-ups. Findings suggested that prayer by the substance abuser did predict subsequent reductions in drinking in both groups, but this finding did not consider that prayer is a prescribed Alcoholics Anonymous–related behavior and, as such, this benefit may have reflected the social benefit of Alcoholics Anonymous as much as that of prayer. Counter to investigator predictions, alcoholics who reported that family members or close friends were praying for their welfare and treatment success tended to drink more frequently at follow-up relative to those alcoholics who did not report such prayer efforts by loved ones.

Extending this line of research, Miller et al.[38] tested the efficacy of a trained and monitored spiritual guide on later substance use. Here, the spiritual intervention intentionally went beyond Judeo-Christian beliefs and practices and included such Eastern practices as meditation. In the first of two companion studies, the investigators recruited 60 inpatients from a 30-day program to receive treatment as usual or treatment as usual plus 12 sessions with a spiritual guide. The spiritual intervention consisted of 13 modules that included such topics as prayer and meditation, gratitude, guidance, acceptance, fasting, service to others, and worship. Although both intervention groups reported large pre-post gains in abstinence, no between-group differences in substance use were observed between the treatment as usual and treatment as usual + spiritual guide groups at follow-up. Also, contrary to prediction, the group receiving spiritual guidance did not report higher scores on three a priori selected measures of spiritual functioning: daily spiritual experiences (Brief Multidimensional Measure of Religiousness/Spirituality), meaning in life (Purpose in Life questionnaire), and private religious practices (Religious Beliefs and Behaviors). Not addressed in this study was whether the emphasis on 12-step attendance in treatment as usual adversely affected the discriminability of the two interventions.

A second study at the same facility was done to increase exposure to the spiritual guide intervention. Here, facility counselors delivered the spiritual guide intervention and it was embedded into the treatment as usual program.[16] In a cohort design, 40 participants received treatment as usual and the following 40 received a spiritual guide in addition to the treatment as usual. In general, findings paralleled the earlier study: no group differences in substance use at 3- and 6-month follow-ups were found, although both groups reported significant reductions across a variety of illicit drug use measures. Unlike the first study, modest between-group differences in daily spiritual experiences were found favoring the spiritual guide group at 4- and 6-month follow-ups, but this differential change in spirituality did not statistically mediate or explain increased abstinence for the spiritual guide group.

Bowen and colleagues[5] have provided tentative support for the effectiveness of Vipassana meditation in reducing substance use among incarcerated adults. Although replication via a randomized clinical trial design is highly desirable, this work represents some of the more rigorous study of the effects of spirituality that is not Judeo-Christian in origin. Specifically, they reported that an intensive 10-day Vipassana meditation program housed in a minimum-security prison resulted in significantly lower substance use and alcohol-related consequences relative to self-selected control inmates. In addition, at 3-month follow-up the inmates who participated in the Vipassana meditation also reported significantly higher optimism scores and lower levels of psychiatric problems relative to controls. The Vipassana meditation protocol consisted of long hours of silence, teaching of Buddhist principles including the Four Noble Truths, and instruction in meditation.

Spiritually Based 12-Step Therapy

Twelve-step treatment is the final spiritual intervention to be addressed in this section. Placement of this intervention in this section, separate from our review on Alcoholics Anonymous, reflects the important, albeit frequently forgotten, distinction between formal 12-step treatment and community-based 12-step programs.[5] (See Ferri et al.[12] for an example of how confusing the two can lead to erroneous conclusions.) To be sure, both 12-step entities introduce and facilitate progress through the 12 steps of Alcoholics Anonymous and strongly encourage long-term Alcoholics Anonymous meeting attendance. In this regard, both 12-step entities can be regarded as sharing a common spiritual focus—for example, 11 of the 12 steps make reference to God or a Higher Power, and spiritual concepts such as acceptance, surrender, meditation, and belief in a Higher Power are the central content of the steps.

It is the *practice* of the prescribed 12-step behaviors that most clearly distinguishes community-based Alcoholics Anonymous and formal treatment, and these differences in practice fundamentally influence both the interpretation and impact of working the 12 steps. Some of the more obvious examples of how the two 12-step entities differ include: Community-based Alcoholics Anonymous encourages sponsorship to aid an Alcoholics Anonymous neonate through the 12 steps while formal 12-step treatment offers no analog to this important sponsor-sponsee relationship. Continuing Alcoholics Anonymous meetings are led by a nonprofessional member of the group and cross talk in meetings is strongly discouraged. Just the opposite conditions are found in group-based therapy in formal 12-step treatment, with further distinctions made by the use of evidence-based treatment manuals.[60] And, finally, confrontation to accept the label of alcoholic frequently occurs in 12-step treatment (i.e., denial is a concept developed within the treatment context in response to this practice), while in community-based Alcoholics Anonymous the individuals elects if, when, and how self-labeling of "alcoholic" is appropriate. Beyond the scope of this discussion, it is also important to note that 12-step treatment shares several features incorporated within cognitive behavioral therapy.[10]

With this background, the focus of this section is to review those studies that investigated the independent effect(s) of the spiritual emphasis in formal 12-step treatment. To begin, several studies have investigated the plasticity of "Alcoholics Anonymous–specific" cognitions that are foundational to spirituality as it is expressed in 12-step programs. Morgenstern and Bates,[41] for example, reported that cognitive shifts promoted by 12-step therapists at residential and intensive outpatient treatment centers did predict later improvement, for example, commitment to abstinence, but others did not, for example, negative expectancies. Of interest, the authors also reported that severity of cognitive impairment did not influence or moderate the extent of desired cognitive shifts, yet more impaired individuals did not appear to benefit from such cognitive shifts to the extent of those who were less impaired. Likewise, using a composite measure of 12-step

disease model beliefs, Finney et al.[14,15] found modest increases among 970 veterans assigned to 12-step treatment in Alcoholics Anonymous–related cognitions during therapy, but such changes did not explain later abstinence rates. Finney also reported that 12-step therapy led to a significant pre-post gain in the percentage of individuals endorsing an alcoholic identity (7% gain).

Project MATCH was one of the largest and most rigorous prospective studies of the efficacy of 12-step therapy to mobilize spiritual/religious practices and beliefs.[49,50] At 12-month follow-up, no group differences were found in measures of drinking intensity and frequency of abstinent days between 12-step, cognitive behavioral, and motivational enhancement therapies, although 12-step therapy did have a significantly higher rate of total abstinence relative to cognitive behavioral therapy and motivational enhancement therapy at 12 months. Tonigan and Miller[56] sought to identify those aspects in the 12-step facilitation that accounted for the relative parity in increased days of abstinence and reductions in drinking intensity. No support was found for 12-step therapist emphasis upon total abstinence as an explanation for the relatively good outcomes in the 12-step condition, although these therapists did endorse the goal of abstinence more than cognitive behavioral therapy and motivational enhancement therapists did. Likewise, intended cognitive shifts in perceived powerlessness and loss of control over alcohol did occur within the 12-step treatment, but these shifts did not explain drinking outcomes at 12 months. Finally, a primary objective for the 12-step facilitation counselor was the encouragement of client spiritual development. As intended, at the end of 12 weeks of therapy, 12-step facilitation clients reported significantly higher God consciousness scores[6] relative to cognitive behavioral therapy and motivational enhancement therapy clients. Virtually no relationship, however, was found between increased God consciousness at the end of treatment and proximal abstinence 6 months after treatment, days to first drink and heavy drinking day, or 1-year total abstinence. Thus although 12-step facilitation therapists were effective in evoking increased God awareness, this increase appeared to be unrelated to subsequent increases in abstinence.

Robinson and colleagues[53] have recently reported positive findings between increased spirituality and abstinence among 12-step–treated adults (N = 123), and some of the unique features of this study warrant special attention. As background, they recruited 154 adults with alcohol use disorders who were presenting for 12-step outpatient treatment and, following consenting procedures, administered a baseline assessment that included an array of spirituality/religiousness measures along with semi-structured interviews for measuring alcohol consumption. Eighty percent of the sample was contacted and interviewed 6 months after recruitment and the assessment battery was readministered. In this naturalistic study, significant pre-post gains were reported on 5 of 10 spirituality/religiousness measures, nearly all of which were different than those measures described earlier in this section: Purpose in Life (d = 0.26), Positive religious coping (d = 0.14), Forgiveness (d = 0.24), Daily spiritual experiences (d = 0.19), and Spiritual/religious practices (d = 33). By isolating the effects of spiritual gains in predicting the presence or absence of heavy drinking at 6 months by first controlling for gender, baseline heavy drinking, and pre-post changes in Alcoholics Anonymous involvement, they found that two spirituality/religiousness measures sustained their prognostic value in predicting abstinence, gains in purpose in life, and daily spiritual experiences. This set of findings represents one of the rare examples of mediated spirituality/religiousness effects as defined by the criteria of Baron and Kenny.[4] It is not known why gains in spirituality/religiousness measures explained reductions in heavy drinking in the Robinson et al.[53] sample but not in previous investigations. Methodologically, earlier investigations used continuously scaled measures of drinking, whereas the Robinson et al. group employed a dichotomous measure of relapse to heavy drinking over the 6-month period (yes/no). Furthermore, the Robinson et al. team used spirituality/religiousness change scores despite voiced concerns that such techniques are prone to regression artifacts. Nevertheless, all investigations approached the topic of study with (1) standard recruitment and design choices, (2) psychometrically sound measures, and (3) achieved good follow-up rates.

In general, then, the weight of evidence suggests that cognitive shifts congruent with Alcoholics Anonymous ideology can be successfully mobilized in 12-step therapy. Demonstrations of such shifts have included beliefs in the disease model, endorsement of the alcoholic identity, commitment to abstinence, and a belief in a Higher Power. Applying a Scotch verdict, the relative importance of these shifts is mixed, at best, in accounting for the generally good outcomes associated with 12-step therapy. The question is not decided, however. Work by Robinson et al. offers the possibility that previous studies have employed measures that were insensitive to the processes of interest.

Religiosity/Spirituality as a Moderator in 12-Step Therapy

Propst[51] reported that the effectiveness of cognitive behavioral therapy for depression was significantly enhanced for religiously oriented individuals when spiritual matters were discussed within therapy sessions. Here, a person's spirituality/religiousness orientation moderated the effectiveness of an evidence-based approach. In the treatment of alcoholism and addictions, the moderator role of spirituality has not yielded as straightforward findings. At face value, for example, it would seem that spiritually focused treatments, for example, 12-step program, would be received more favorably and be more effective for like-minded people.

Two investigators have examined this issue within the context of a randomized clinical trial. Connors et al.[7] essentially made this prediction when they argued that self-reported religiosity of an alcoholic would moderate the effectiveness of 12-step outpatient and aftercare therapy.[49,50] The composite measure of spirituality/religiousness included responses to questions about the practice and frequency of prayer, meditation, and formal practice of religious attendance and reading of Holy Scripture. They predicted that alcoholics higher in endorsement of spirituality/religiousness would be more comfortable with the spiritual aspects of the 12-step therapy. Enhanced comfort with the 12-step model would become manifest in higher treatment retention, stronger therapeutic bond, and greater satisfaction with treatment, each of which is a positive and significant predictor of increased abstinence after treatment. On the basis of drinking outcome, no support for this matching hypothesis was found. Likewise, no support was found that comfortability with spiritual/religious beliefs and practices led to higher 12-step treatment retention, satisfaction, or therapeutic bond relative to individuals lower in spiritual/religious values.

Within the same study, Tonigan and colleagues[58] applied a more general and inclusive definition of spirituality in predicting a differential response to 12-step therapy. In particular, they computed a difference score that represented current perceived

meaning in life after subtracting the seeking of life meaning.[9] Unlike the comfortability hypothesis, they reasoned that alcoholics high in meaning seeking (but perhaps not very high on spirituality/religiousness) would find the spiritual focus of the 12-step therapy more engaging and, hence, more effective. Consistent with the work by Connors et al.,[7] no support was found for a differential response to 12-step therapy based on the general measure of clients' meaning seeking when judged by percentage abstinent days or drinking intensity for the 12 months after treatment.

Several naturalistic studies have approached the question of whether client spiritual/religious beliefs and practices moderated treatment effectiveness. Oumilettee et al.,[42] for example, made a similar prediction as Connors et al., with the key distinction that sampled alcoholics were veterans, and participants were not randomized to treatments. Here, substance abuse treatment programs were classified according to their dominant therapeutic orientation, that is, cognitive behavioral, 12-step, and milieu therapy, and matching of client characteristics and provider types was self-selective. Using similar spirituality/religiousness measures as Connors et al. (e.g., Religious Beliefs and Behaviors)[6] they, too, reported that 12-step treatment response was unrelated to baseline spirituality/religiousness status. Finally, Kaskutas et al.[26] investigated the role and influence of spiritual/religious practices and beliefs on long-term sobriety and Alcoholics Anonymous involvement among 587 men and women presenting for treatment at private and public facilities in California. Although the sampled treatment centers represented a broad spectrum of services and therapeutic orientations, nearly all encouraged 12-step attendance and included 12-step induction strategies as part of their services. At 3-year follow-up, no association was found between length of continuous sobriety and spirituality/religiousness endorsement at baseline.

Finally, Kelly et al.[27] conducted a unique single-group longitudinal 3-year study of substance-abusing adults who presented for intensive outpatient treatment ($N = 227$). Here, individuals were assessed at intake and at 1-, 2-, and 3-year follow-ups. In addition to concluding that mutual-help participation contributed to positive outcomes during the follow-up phase of the study, Kelly et al.[27] tested several prospective hypotheses about the role and influence of religious/spiritual variables in recovery.

In sum, findings from both randomized clinical trials and naturalistic studies appear to have arrived at the same conclusion, namely that spiritual/religious practices and beliefs are relatively inert in the context of being offered a spiritually based 12-step program. Contrary to predictions, then, endorsement of spiritual/religious practices and beliefs does not seem to provide an advantage to a substance abuser when they are assigned to 12-step therapy. Conversely, substance abusers who report less interest in spiritual/religious practices and beliefs do not appear to be placed at a disadvantage when assigned to 12-step therapy. It should be stressed that almost all of the studies reviewed in this section relied on self-reported spirituality/religiousness status, generally a single item asking whether one was religious, spiritual, agnostic, or an atheist. Well known, single-item responses lack reliability, and it is not clear whether more comprehensive spirituality/religiousness measures collected at the onset of 12-step treatment may offer a different picture than the one presented here. At this time, however, the limited evidence suggests that spiritual/religious beliefs and practices are relatively unimportant when determining whether or not to assign substance abusers to spiritually based 12-step therapy.

Section III

Religiosity/Spirituality and Community-Based 12-Step Programs

Few topics in addiction research generate as much controversy as the question, does community-based Alcoholics Anonymous work and how, especially as a stand-alone intervention? It is well documented that a majority of treatment-seeking adolescents and adults in the United States report exposure to community-based 12-step programs prior to entering treatment. Likewise, in a survey of treatment providers, Kelly et al.[27] Reported that a majority of treatment providers encourage Alcoholics Anonymous attendance during and after inpatient and outpatient treatment, regardless of provider therapeutic orientation. Furthermore, rates of referral to 12-step programs by treatment providers appear to be similar regardless of the nature of substance use dependency, for example, alcohol, cocaine, and opioid dependency.[19] Given the widespread acceptance of the 12-step model and approach by the clinical community in the United States, why, then, has there been such reticence, ambivalence and, at times, outright hostility by researchers about community-based Alcoholics Anonymous?

The nexus of the conflict lies in the pronouncements by Alcoholics Anonymous that alcoholism is a physical, emotional, and spiritual malady, that total abstinence is necessary for recovery, and that spiritual practices provide the foundation for sustained sobriety.[1] Disagreement, then, about Alcoholics Anonymous is rooted in ideological conflict. Derived from Judeo-Christian doctrines,[31] the 12 steps of Alcoholics Anonymous are a concise statement of the prescribed and sequential program for recovery, and the 12 traditions are the blueprint for how the fellowship of Alcoholics Anonymous ought to be conducted. Both sets of prescriptions rest upon spiritual principles, and make frequent reference to the value of prayer and meditation, and the existence of God or a Higher Power. Tonigan and colleagues[59] point to five spiritual axioms in the core Alcoholics Anonymous literature: (1) the existence of a transcendent power, (2) the need to develop a personal relationship with God, (3) a belief in mysticism, (4) daily reaffirmation of a God relationship, and (5) the belief that emotional discord signals a departure from spiritual principles. At face value, the spiritual axioms of Alcoholics Anonymous are innocuous and would likely be accepted—with perhaps minor revision—by most theologians. Likewise, the emphasis in Alcoholics Anonymous upon incorporating these spiritual axioms into daily living is not unique, but the steadfast belief in the necessity of doing so to sustain sobriety is unique to 12-step programs.

Community-Based 12-Step Programs and Abstinence

Four of five meta-analyses[11,16,30,58,59] have concluded that Alcoholics Anonymous participation is predictive of increased abstinence, although findings are mixed about improvements in other areas, for example, psychological functioning. In general, effect size estimates of Alcoholics Anonymous–related benefit range between $d = 0.18$ and $d = 0.33$, which fall into the small to moderate range of "intervention" effect. The difficulty in addressing the question of benefit solely based on community-based Alcoholics Anonymous is that most of the literally hundreds of empirical studies on Alcoholics Anonymous have been based on treatment-seeking adult samples.[11] Thus the impact of treatment often confounds investigations into the unbiased benefit of Alcoholics Anonymous. Traditionally, two

strategies have been used in an effort to isolate the influences of Alcoholics Anonymous: one statistical and the second based on conducting distal follow-ups to minimize the direct and indirect influence of formal treatment, for example, 5–10 years after treatment. Both strategies have important limitations, although both strategies have, to their credit, employed prospective designs. Statistical approaches to control for confounding treatment and self-selective factors, for example, may fail to adequately model all relevant factors. Alternatively, treatment-seeking substance abusers typically have frequent encounters with treatment over time, and is not clear how effective, if at all, distal follow-ups eliminate the influence of formal treatment on client functioning. Keeping these caveats in mind, these two approaches have tended to yield findings in agreement with those generated through the use of treatment-seeking samples, namely, that 12-step participation is helpful in reducing problematic drinking for many alcohol abusers. Interested readers should review Kelly et al.,[27] Moos and Moos,[40] Connors et al.,[7] and Kaskutas et al.[25] for exemplars.

What Spiritual Practices Predict Benefit?

Positive albeit modest associations between Alcoholics Anonymous meeting attendance and abstinence have been reported in most meta-analyses,[11,16,59] and many investigators have reported that measures of commitment to, and involvement in, prescribed Alcoholics Anonymous behaviors are even stronger and more positive predictors of increased abstinence.[19,52] Although these Alcoholics Anonymous meeting and composite measures of Alcoholics Anonymous participation have utility, they do not shed light on the relevance, if any, on the specific spiritually focused behaviors that contribute to increased abstinence. Unfortunately, given the centrality of spirituality to 12-step programs it is surprising how few of these prescribed behaviors have been isolated and studied.

A majority of Alcoholics Anonymous–exposed individuals practice the steps of Alcoholics Anonymous, and step work is routinely encouraged in Alcoholics Anonymous meetings.[58] Furthermore, in a cross-sectional study of four Alcoholics Anonymous groups it was reported that steps 1–3, typically regarded as the surrender steps, and 10–12 (maintenance steps) were discussed significantly more often than steps 4–9 (action steps).[55] Finally, in a second cross-sectional study, Horstman and Tonigan[21] reported that Alcoholics Anonymous groups that were perceived to be more supportive and expressive were also judged to endorse the practicing of the 12 steps more frequently than Alcoholics Anonymous groups perceived to be more aggressive and less supportive. Here, Alcoholics Anonymous member perceptions of the social dynamics of Alcoholics Anonymous groups were assessed using the Group Environment scale.[39] It would appear, then, that practicing of the 12 steps is common in Alcoholics Anonymous that such practice frequently focuses on those steps that endorse the existence of a benevolent deity, and that the extent that such discussion occurs in an Alcoholics Anonymous meeting is influenced by the perceived social dynamics of an Alcoholics Anonymous group.

Few studies have investigated the actual benefit associated with doing the 12 steps. Patton[47] conducted a single-group longitudinal study ($N = 769$) of individuals who had received inpatient treatment at Hazelden. Twelve months after treatment, a significant positive association was found between completing steps 6–12 and total abstinence. Likewise, to the question, "do you do step work?" a significant and positive relationship was reported between answering *yes* to this question and complete abstinence at 12-month follow-up ($r = 0.22$). In a second longitudinal study of a Hazelden sample ($N = 592$), Kammeier and Anderson[24] reported that there was no relationship between working steps 1–4 and abstinence at a 24-month follow-up, yet there was a significant and positive relationship between self-reported "step work" and total abstinence. Continuing, as part of a psychometric project, Gilbert[18] recruited 183 veterans receiving substance abuse treatment to participate in a 12-month study. Here, Gilbert reported that completing step 1 during the first 3 months postdischarge significantly and positively predicted days sober at the 6- and 12-month follow-ups. Finally, Tonigan and Miller[56] reported that, among 226 outpatients who had received treatment 3 years earlier, the number of steps completed at 3 years was significantly and negatively predictive of the amount of alcohol consumed at the 10-year follow-up. In general, then, these studies suggest that working through the steps is beneficial in reducing alcohol consumption, although it must also be acknowledged that those individuals who heed the prescription to do step work are self-selected and may be more motivated and have a better prognosis.

Progression through the 12 steps of Alcoholics Anonymous is most commonly achieved with the guidance of a sponsor, a fellow Alcoholics Anonymous member who has already completed the 12 steps. In this context, a sponsor is a spiritual mentor, and the acquisition of a sponsor signals a conscious decision to work the spiritual program of Alcoholics Anonymous. What is known about the benefits of acquiring a spiritual mentor in Alcoholics Anonymous? In a retrospective analysis of the Project MATCH study, Pagano et al.[43] reported that sponsorship led to a significant reduction in relapse rate at 1 year, for example, 60% versus 78%. Kaskutas et al.[25] have likewise reported that having a sponsor was one of the few Alcoholics Anonymous–prescribed behaviors that predicted reductions in substance abuse here in a community-based sample. Kaskutas et al.[25] have also reported findings that suggest that there may be indirect benefits associated with sponsorship, namely that Alcoholics Anonymous members with sponsors tend to have triple the rate of Alcoholics Anonymous meeting attendance than Alcoholics Anonymous members without sponsors. Given the documented advantage of continued Alcoholics Anonymous attendance to sustain long-term abstinence,[40] this indirect benefit is worthy of further study.

An emerging line of research has addressed the related question of whether helping others in 12-step programs, a prescribed spiritual activity in Alcoholics Anonymous, benefits the helper as well as the person helped. In a retrospective study of 11 Alcoholics Anonymous members with long-term sobriety, for example, Pagano et al.[44] reported that, for these Alcoholics Anonymous members, helping other alcoholics increased with time, and that such helping was felt to enhance the quality of sobriety. In a second cross-sectional study, Zemore and Kaskutas[63] reported findings similar to those of Pagano et al.[44] Specifically, Zemore and Kaskutas found that among 198 recovering alcoholics in Alcoholics Anonymous, a composite measure of helping (Sponsorship and step work) was more strongly and positively related to length of sobriety than was a composite measure of Alcoholics Anonymous involvement.

Summary and Future Directions

Religiosity and spirituality are associated with improved health-related functioning, especially with regard to mental health. As described in this chapter, the relationship between spirituality and addiction is unique and quite distinct from other mental health problems. Except in rare cases, for example, few clinicians would conclude that the onset of depression was the process of spiritual bankruptcy. In the treatment of substance abuse in the United

States, however, the dominant therapeutic model embraces this belief. As such, a majority of treatment providers will uniformly refer individuals to 12-step programs during and after treatment.

Distinctions between the religiosity and spirituality constructs are frequently blurred in addictions research, with many investigators failing to adequately define the constructs if they make any attempt at all. The point was stressed when presenting four popular measures of spirituality/religiousness constructs in this chapter that each construct is multidimensional in nature, and dimensions within each construct appear to have differential sensitivity to the effects of spiritual interventions and in predicting positive outcome(s). In this regard, investigators and practitioners need to be keenly aware of the subtle complexities in what, at first glance, appears to be self-evident and face valid measures. The measurement of meaning in life exemplifies some of these complexities. On one hand, few would argue that the belief in, and practice of, religious/spiritual behaviors can offer feelings of contentedness and purpose. However, a sense of well-being can as easily result from nonreligious/spiritual practices. General measures developed to assess changes in broadly defined spirituality are especially prone to such measurement confounding.

Strong evidence indicates that 12-step treatment is equally effective as more research-based interventions for substance abuse, including therapies that combine psychosocial interventions with pharmacotherapy, for example, naltrexone. The factors accounting for this parity, however, are only beginning to be understood. Most often, efforts to understand the role and influences of religiousness/spirituality in recovery from addiction adopt one of two conceptual models. The deficit model of spirituality has clear linkages to the 12-step spiritual paradigm and posits that the spiritual void created by addiction ultimately must be filled in order to avoid relapse. In fact, the distinction made in 12-step literature between abstinence and sobriety suggests that spiritual growth is even necessary to achieve well-being. The coping model of religiousness/spirituality is gaining popularity among addiction researchers, and some of the implications of this model were identified. Foremost, the coping model does not imply that religiousness/spirituality development is essential for recovery, but the model does posit that such growth may offer individuals the means to more positively interpret and adjust to negative affect. In this light, the coping model of religiousness/spirituality is wholly compatible and can be integrated with cognitive behavioral and relapse prevention strategies.

Religious/spiritual measures have been used as dependent, independent, moderator, and mediator variables in addiction research. Reviewed in some detail in this chapter, there is strong evidence that psychosocial interventions can produce desired shifts in religious/spiritual measures. In both 12-step and non–12-step religious/spiritual interventions, for instance, significant gains have been reported in religious/spiritual beliefs, cognitions, and practices. Such gains in clients' beliefs and practices appear to occur in both individualized and group therapy and for alcoholics and polysubstance abusers. Mostly negative findings have been reported, however, about the effectiveness of religious/spiritual interventions to produce, as independent variables, reductions in substance use. To date, efforts to assess the effectiveness of a spiritual guide[38] have not produced the desired effects on a reliable scale, and although 12-step therapy is effective it does not appear to be the result of the spiritual focus of the formal intervention. Important exceptions were identified. Work by Robinson et al.[53] using new religious/spiritual measures and with Vipassana meditation, for instance, offer promising possibilities about the use of religious/spiritual interventions in the treatment of addiction.

The consistent absence of a moderator effect in religious/spiritual research in addictions can be viewed several ways. On one hand, client-treatment matching offers an efficient way to improve treatment effects through the appropriate assignment of individuals with different characteristics to different kinds of interventions. Findings that some clients fared better in spiritually focused interventions than others would have thus provided important information. The lack of evidence for client-treatment matching, using a diverse number of religiousness/spirituality measures of client characteristics, is also good news for practitioners in the United States. Specifically, this information suggests that the assignment of clients low on religious/spiritual beliefs and practices to a spiritually based intervention does not place them at a serious disadvantage. It is estimated that about 6%–9% of the population in the United States is atheistic, and their proportional representation among alcohol and polysubstance abusers is unknown. Findings suggest that this infrequently studied group of substance abusers is not at higher risk of poorer outcomes when assigned to 12-step therapy relative to nonatheists.

The effectiveness of community-based 12-step programs as a standalone intervention is not entirely clear because of standard sampling procedures in mutual-help research. With this caveat, strongest support for the effectiveness of spiritually focused practices in Alcoholics Anonymous was found for the guidance provided by having and or being a sponsor and for completing prescribed Alcoholics Anonymous steps. Cross-sectional work indicated that encouragement to do step work is associated with Alcoholics Anonymous groups that are more cohesive and supportive and that some steps are endorsed more than other steps. Although some confidence can be placed on the findings that step work is relatively common in Alcoholics Anonymous, the findings about the conditions in which they are (or are not) stressed requires prospective study. Current prospective findings offer three relatively firm evidence-based recommendations: (1) encouragement to attend Alcoholics Anonymous meetings is important, especially during early efforts to reduce drinking; (2) encouragement to become engaged in prescribed Alcoholics Anonymous behaviors beyond that associated with simple meeting attendance increases the prospect for Alcoholics Anonymous-related benefit; (3) acquiring a sponsor reduces later relapse; and (4) religious/spiritual orientation of the client, although important, may not be important in determining whether or not to refer to Alcoholics Anonymous. Although we await replication with prospective studies, it may be the case that helping other Alcoholics Anonymous members as prescribed in the Alcoholics Anonymous literature also increases Alcoholics Anonymous-related benefit for the helper.

At the beginning of the chapter the cautionary statement was made that ongoing 12-step research funded by the National Institute on Alcohol Abuse and Alcoholism may qualify the findings and recommendations in this chapter. Currently, for example, there are at least six large-scale longitudinal studies of 12-step programs in the United States, and many of them are specifically investigating the mechanisms that account for Alcoholics Anonymous-related benefit. Clearly, findings from these studies will produce several new chapters on the narrative of the relative importance of spirituality in recovery. Also mentioned earlier, several excellent evidence-based monographs on 12-step programs in particular and spirituality in general have just been published. Perhaps the soundest recommendation that can be made is that readers interested in this topic need, over the next decade, to become actively engaged in the scholarly empirical literature that is focused on religiousness/spirituality and addictions.

References

1. AA World Services. *Alcoholics Anonymous: The Story of How Many Thousands of Men and Women Have Recovered From Alcoholism*. 4th ed. New York: Author; 2001.
2. Agorastos A, Demiralay C, Huber CG. Influence of religious aspects and person beliefs on psychological behavior: focus on anxiety disorders. *Psychol Res Behav Manag*. 2014;7:93–101.
3. American Psychiatric Association. *Diagnostic and Statistical Manual of Mental Disorders, Text Revision [DSM-IV-TR]*. 4th ed. Washington, DC: Author; 2000.
4. Baron RM, Kenny DA. The moderator-mediator distinction in social psychological research: conceptual strategic, and statistical considerations. *J Personality Soc Psychol*. 1986;51:1173–1182.
5. Bowen S, Witkiewitz K, Dillworth TM, et al. Mindfulness meditation and substance use in an incarcerated population. *Psychol Addict Behav*. 2006;20(3):343–347.
6. Connors G, Tonigan JS, Miller WR. The religious background and behavior instrument: psychometric and normed findings. *Psychol Addict Behav*. 1996;10:90–96.
7. Connors GJ, Tonigan JS, Miller WR. Religiosity and responsiveness to alcoholism treatments: matching findings and causal chain analyses. In: Longabaugh RH, Wirth PW, eds. *Project MATCH: A Priori Matching Hypotheses, Results and Mediating Mechanisms*. Rockville, MD: US Government Printing Office; 2001.
8. Cook CH. Addiction and spirituality. *Addiction*. 2004;99:539–551.
9. Crumbaugh JC, Maholick LT. *Purpose in Life Scale*. Murfreesboro, TN: Psychometric Affiliates; 1976.
10. Donovan DM, Ingalsbe MH, Benbow J, Daley DC. 12-step interventions and mutual support programs for substance use disorders: an overview. *Soc Work Public Health*. 2013;28(0):313–332.
11. Emrick CD, Tonigan JS, Montgomery HA, Little L. Alcoholics anonymous: what is currently known?. In: McCrady BS, Miller WR, eds. *Research on Alcoholics Anonymous: Opportunities and Alternatives*. New Brunswick, NJ: Rutgers Center on Alcohol Studies; 1993:41–76.
12. Ferri MMF, Amato L, Dvoli M. Alcoholics anonymous and other 12-step programmes for alcohol dependence. *Cochrane Database Syst Rev*. 2006;3:CD005032.
13. Fetzer I. *Multidimensional Measurement of Religiousness/spirituality for Use in Health Research*. Kalamazoo, MI: John E. Fetzer Institute; 1999.
14. Finney JW, Moos RH, Humphreys K. A comparative evaluation of substance abuse treatment: II. Linking proximal outcomes of 12-step and cognitive behavioral treatment to substance use outcomes. *Alcoholism: Clin Exp Res*. 1999;23:537–544.
15. Finney JW, Noyes CA, Coutts AI. Evaluating substance abuse treatment process models: I. Changes on proximal outcome variables during 12-step and cognitive behavioral treatment. *J Studies Alcohol*. 1998;59:371–380.
16. Forcehimes AA, Tonigan JS. Self-efficacy to remain abstinent and substance abuse: a meta-analysis. *Alcohol Treat Q*. 2008;26(4):480–489.
17. Geppert C, Bogenschutz MP, Miller WR. Development of a bibliography on religion, spirituality and addictions. *Drug Alcohol Rev*. 2007;26:389–395.
18. Gilbert FS. Development of a "steps questionnaire". *J Studies Alcohol*. 1991;52:353–360.
19. Greenfield BLTonigan JS. The general Alcoholic Anonymous tools of recovery: the adoption of 12-step practices and beliefs. *Psychol Addict Behav*. 2013;27(3):553–561.
20. Hill PC, Pargament KI, Hood RW, et al. Conceptualizing religion and spirituality: points of commonality, points of departure. *J Theory Social Behavior*. 2000;30(1):51–77.
21. Horstmann MJTonigan JS. Faith development in alcoholics anonymous: a study of two AA groups. *Alcohol Treat Q*. 2000;18:75–84.
22. Huebner RBTonigan JS. The search for mechanisms of behavior change in evidence-based behavioral treatments for alcohol use disorders: overview. *Alcohol Clin Exp Res*. 2007;31(S3):1S–3S.

23. Johnson T, Robinson EAR. Issues in measuring spirituality and religiousness in alcohol. In: Galanter M, Kaskutas LA, eds. *Recent Developments in Alcoholism: Alcoholics Anonymous and Spiritual Aspects of Recovery.* Vol. 18. New York: Springer; 2008:167–186.

24. Kammeier ML, Anderson PO. Two years later: posttreatment participation in AA by 1970 Hazelden patients. Paper presented at the annual meeting of Alcohol and Drug Problems Association of North America, New Orleans; 1976.

25. Kaskutas LA, Ammon L, Delucchi K, Room R, Bond J, Weisner C. Alcoholics anonymous careers: patterns of AA involvement five years after treatment entry. *Alcohol Clin Exp Res.* 2005;29(11):1983–1990.

26. Kaskutas LA, Turk N, Bond J, Weisner C. The role of religion, spirituality, and Alcoholics anonymous in sustained sobriety. *Alcohol Treat Q.* 2003;21(11):1–16.

27. Kelly JF, Stout R, Zywiak W, Schneider R. A 3-year study of addiction mutual-help group participation following intensive outpatient treatment. *Alcohol Clin Exp Res.* 2006;30:1381–1392.

28. Koenig HG. Concerns about measuring 'spirituality' in research. *J Nervous Mental Dis.* 2008;196:349–355.

29. Koenig HG, McCullough ME, Larson DB. *Handbook of Religion and Health.* Oxford University, New York. Int J Psychol Religion 2001;9:3–16.

30. Kownacki RJ, Shadish WR. Does alcoholics anonymous work? The results from a meta-analysis of controlled experiments. *Subst Use Misuse.* 1999;34(13):1897–1916.

31. Kurtz E. *Not God: A History of Alcoholics Anonymous.* San Francisco: Harper & Row; 1991.

32. Larson DB, Larson SS. Spirituality's potential relevance to physical and emotional health: a brief review of quantitative research. *J Psychol Theol.* 2003;31(1):37–51.

33. Laudet AB, Morgan K, White WL. The role of social supports, spirituality, religiousness, life meaning, and affiliation with 12-step fellowships in quality of life satisfaction among individuals in recovery from alcohol and drug problems. *Alcohol Treat Q.* 2006;24(1–2):33–73.

34. Marlatt AG, Donovan D. *Relapse Prevention: Maintenance Strategies in the Treatment of Addictive Behaviors.* 2nd ed. New York: Guilford; 2005.

35. May G. *Addiction and grace.* San Francisco: Harper Collins; 1991.

36. McHugh RK, Hearon BA, Otto MW. Cognitive behavioral therapy for substance use disorders. *Psychiatr Clin North Am.* 2010;33(3):511–525.

37. Michalak L, Trocki K, Bond J. Religion and alcohol in the U.S. national alcohol survey: how important is religion for abstention and drinking? *Drug Alcohol Depend.* 2007;87(2):268–280.

38. Miller WR, Forcehimes AA, O'Leary M, LaNoue M. Spiritual direction in addiction treatment: two clinical trials. *J Subst Abuse Treat.* 2008;35:434–442.

39. Moos RH. *Group Environment Scale Manual.* Vol. 2. Palo Alto, CA: Consulting Psychologist; 1986.

40. Moos RH, Moos BS. Sixteen-year changes and stable remission among treated and untreated individuals with alcohol disorders. *Drug Alcohol Depend.* 2005;80(3):337–348.

41. Morgenstern J, Bates ME. Effects of executive function impairment on change processes and substance use outcomes in 12-step treatment. *J Studies Alcohol.* 1999;60:846–855.

42. Ouimette PC, Finney JW, Moos RH. Twelve-step and cognitive-behavioral treatment for substance abuse: a comparison of treatment effectiveness. *J Consult Clin Psychol.* 1997;65:230–240.

43. Pagano ME, Friend KB, Tonigan JS, Stout R. Sponsoring others in alcoholics anonymous and avoiding a drink in the first year following treatment: findings from project MATCH. *J Studies Alcohol.* 2004;65:766–773.

44. Pagano ME, Zeltner B, Post S, Jaber J, Zywiak WH, Stout RL. Who should I help to stay sober?: helping behaviors among alcoholics who maintain long-term sobriety. *Alcohol Treat Q.* 2009;27(1):38–50.

45. Pargament KI. The psychology of religion and spirituality? Yes and no. *Int J Psychol Religion.* 1999;9:3–16.

46. Pargament KI, Kennell J, Hathaway W, Grevengoed N, Newman J, Jones W. Religion and the problem-solving process: three coping styles. *J Scientific Study Religion.* 1988;27(1):90–104.

47. Patton MQ. *The Outcomes of Treatment: A Study of Patients Admitted to Hazelden in 1976.* Center City, MN: Hazelden Foundation; 1979.

48. Poage ED, Ketzenberger KE, Olson J. Spirituality, contentment and stress in recovering alcoholics. *Addict Behav.* 2004;29:1857–1862.

49. Project Match Research Group. Matching alcoholism treatments to client heterogeneity: project MATCH posttreatment drinking outcomes. *J Studies Alcohol.* 1997;58:7–29.

50. Project Match Research Group. Matching alcoholism treatments to client heterogeneity: project MATCH three-year drinking outcomes. *Alcohol Clin Exp Res.* 1998;22:1300–1311.

51. Propst L. The comparative efficacy of religious and nonreligious imagery for the treatment of mild depression in religious individuals. *Cogn Therapy Res.* 1980;4(2):167–178.

52. Rice SL, Tonigan JS. Impressions of Alcoholics Anonymous (AA) group cohesion: a case for a nonspecific factor predicting later AA attendance. *Alcohol Treat Q.* 2012;30(1):40–51.

53. Robinson EAR, Cranford JA, Webb JR, Brower KJ. Six-month changes in spirituality, religiousness, and heavy drinking in a treatment-seeking sample. *J Studies Alcohol Drugs.* 2007;68(2):282–290.

54. Tillich P. *Dynamics of Faith.* New York: HarperCollins; 2001 (Original work published in 1957).

55. Tonigan JS, Ashcroft F, Miller WR. AA group dynamics and 12 Step activity. *J Studies Alcohol.* 1995;56:616–621.

56. Tonigan JS, Miller WR. AA practicing subtypes: are there multiple AA fellowships? Alcohol. *Clin Exp Res.* 2005;29(suppl 5):384 (Abstract).

57. Tonigan JS, Miller WR, Connors GJ. Meaning-seeking and treatment outcome: matching findings and causal chain analyses. In: Longabaugh RH, Wirtz PW, eds. *Project MATCH: A Priori Matching Hypotheses, Results, and Mediating Mechanisms.* US Government Printing Office; 2001.

58. Tonigan JS, Miller WR, Connors GJ. Prior alcoholics anonymous involvement and treatment outcome. In: Longabaugh R, Wirtz PW, eds. *Project MATCH Hypotheses: Results and Causal Chain Analyses. Project MATCH Monograph Series.* Vol. 8. Bethesda, MD: National Institute on Alcohol Abuse and Alcoholism; 2001:276–284.

59. Tonigan JS, Toscova R, Miller WR. Meta-analysis of the alcoholics anonymous literature: sample and study characteristics moderate findings. *J Studies Alcohol.* 1996;57:65–72.

60. Tracy K, Wallace SP. Benefits of peer support groups in the treatment of addiction. *Subst Abuse Rehab.* 2016;7:143–154.

61. Walker SR, Tonigan JS, Miller WR, Kahlich L. Intercessory prayer in the treatment of alcohol dependence. *Alternative Therapies.* 1997;3:79–86.

62. Walsberg JL, Porter JE. Purpose in life and outcome treatment for alcohol dependence. *Br J Clin Psychol.* 1994;33(Pt1):49–63.

63. Zemore SEKaskutas LA. Helping, spirituality, and alcholics anonymous in recovery. *J Studies Alcohol.* 2004;65(3):383–301.

64. Zinnbauer BJ, Pargament KI. Capturing meanings of religiousness and spirituality: one way down from a definitional tower of Babel. *Res Soc Scientific Study Religion: Res Ann.* 2002;13:23–54.

63

In Silico Models of Alcohol Kinetics: A Deterministic Approach

MARC D. BRETON

CHAPTER OUTLINE

Introduction

In recent years, the mathematical representation of physiological systems and its use in computer simulations have come of age. Initially restricted to pharmacokinetics and pharmacodynamics studies, they are now used in many different fields of medicine (e.g., diabetes and metabolic syndrome) to explore previously inaccessible metabolic markers, develop candidate treatments, and even to obtain authorization of regulatory agencies for clinical research, thereby bypassing animal testing. The field of alcohol addiction is of particular interest for such applications: it is both very developed (e.g., in modeling the dynamics of ethanol in blood or the diffusion from blood to brain tissues) and in its infancy, with only two simulation studies in the past 20 years.[3,4] In addition, it requires modeling of behavioral system and medication effects that are not yet mainstream (see Chapter 64). In this chapter, we present several published and novel models of ethanol blood distribution, leading to simulation studies linking system-level characteristics to clinical outcomes.

Mechanisms of Alcohol Intoxication

Ethyl alcohol, also known as ethanol, is the substance found in alcoholic beverages. It is a colorless liquid that mixes in all proportions with water and therefore is readily distributed throughout the body in the aqueous bloodstream after consumption. In addition, because of this water miscibility it readily crosses important biological membranes, such as the blood-brain barrier. After it reaches the brain, alcohol affects multiple molecular targets, some of which remain unknown. In particular, alcohol causes γ-aminobutyric acid (GABA) receptors to remain open longer, allowing more chloride ions to enter brain cells and, therefore, causing relaxation, sedation, and overall inhibition of brain activity. At low concentrations, alcohol sensitizes the glutamate system, which stimulates areas of the brain associated with pleasure such as the cortico-mesolimbic dopamine system. With chronic exposure to alcohol, the brain undergoes long-lasting biochemical changes including neurological adaptation of the ion channels. Alcohol is also responsible for structural changes in the brain, such as loss of neuronal mass and brain shrinkage, which, in turn, is responsible for impaired cognitive function. Of interest, the maximum quantity of alcohol consumed, such as in binge drinking, seems to be a better predictor of alcohol-related impairment. Hence, understanding the elimination process of alcohol will, to a certain degree, help us predict the extent of the neurological adaptation that takes place with chronic alcohol use.

Alcohol Metabolism

When we consume alcohol, the majority of it is absorbed from the small intestine (approximately 80%) and the stomach (approximately 20%). Generally, drinking more alcohol within a certain period of time will result in increased blood alcohol concentrations due to more alcohol being available for absorption into the bloodstream. More than 90% of the alcohol that enters the body is completely metabolized in the liver. The remaining 10% is not metabolized and is excreted in the sweat, urine, and breath. There are several routes of metabolism of alcohol in the body. The major pathways involve the liver and, in particular, the oxidation of alcohol by alcohol dehydrogenase to produce acetaldehyde, a highly toxic substance. The second step is catalyzed by acetaldehyde dehydrogenase. This enzyme converts acetaldehyde to acetic acid, a nontoxic metabolite. Acetic acid is eventually metabolized to carbon dioxide and water. Another system in the liver oxidizes ethanol via the enzyme cytochrome P450 (CYP)IIE1. This microsomal ethanol-oxidizing system seems to play a more important role at higher concentrations of ethanol.

Individual Differences in the Rate of Alcohol Metabolism

There are genetic variations in the CYPE1 enzyme system that lead to individual differences in the rate of ethanol metabolism in humans.[5] The rate of alcohol metabolism depends, in part, on the amount of metabolizing enzymes in the liver, which varies among individuals and appears to have some genetic determinants. After the consumption of one standard drink, the amount of alcohol in the drinker's blood usually peaks within 30–45 minutes. (A standard drink is defined as 12 ounces of beer, 5 ounces of wine, or 1.5 ounces of 80-proof distilled spirits, all of which contain approximately the same amount of alcohol.) The concentration of alcohol in the entire body, including the brain, is always less than that in the blood; human tissues contain a much lower percentage of water compared with the blood. However, organs having a rich blood supply, such as the brain, will quickly reach alcohol diffusion equilibrium with arterial blood. This explains why most people experience intoxication very quickly after taking a couple of drinks and then sober up rapidly as other bodily tissues with less blood supply, such as the muscle, start to absorb alcohol from the blood, meaning that less alcohol is circulating in the bloodstream.

Mathematical Modeling of the Pharmacokinetics of Ethanol

Ethanol elimination has been assumed to exhibit a zero-order metabolism, which means that a constant amount of alcohol is eliminated per unit of time regardless of blood levels. However, a number of studies have identified that elimination of ethanol follows different clearance models including first-order kinetic and a combination of zero- and first-order kinetic together. This, coupled with individual genetic differences, makes it hard to predict blood alcohol concentration based on the total amount of alcohol consumed.[13] Since the early 20th century, efforts have been directed toward the understanding of alcohol dynamics in humans and, more specifically, the blood concentration of ethanol.

Numerous models have since been devised, beginning with the early Widmark's zero-order model assuming a constant clearance rate β_0 (Equation 1) and modeling the human body as one compartment (concentration, or blood alcohol level, BAL(t) and constant volume V)[14] (Fig. 63.1):

$$\frac{\partial BAL}{\partial t} = -\beta_0 BAL + \frac{D(t)}{V} \tag{1}$$

where $D(t)$ is the dose of ethanol received. This zero-order model is still commonly used in forensic sciences for its ease of use and the relative simplicity of its structure (very few parameters, easily identifiable). Nonetheless, this oversimplification of the clearing process of ethanol is responsible for additional variability in the model coefficients, within and more importantly between subjects. It is this between-subject variability, in particular, that makes the Widmark's model ill-defined for simulation purposes.

A deeper understanding of the processes involved and novel measuring tools have allowed more precise measurement and understanding of ethanol pharmacokinetics and the development of more complex nonlinear multicompartment models.[7,9,10,12] Most of these models are compartmental—for example, they represent the human body as a set of homogeneous (i.e., the ethanol concentration is the same everywhere) compartments of specific

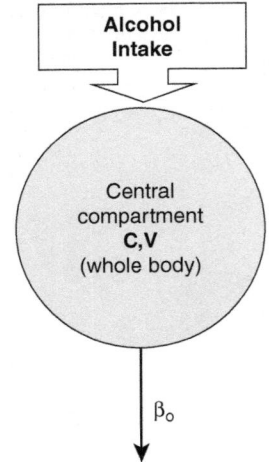

• **Fig. 63.1** Widmark's zero-order model.

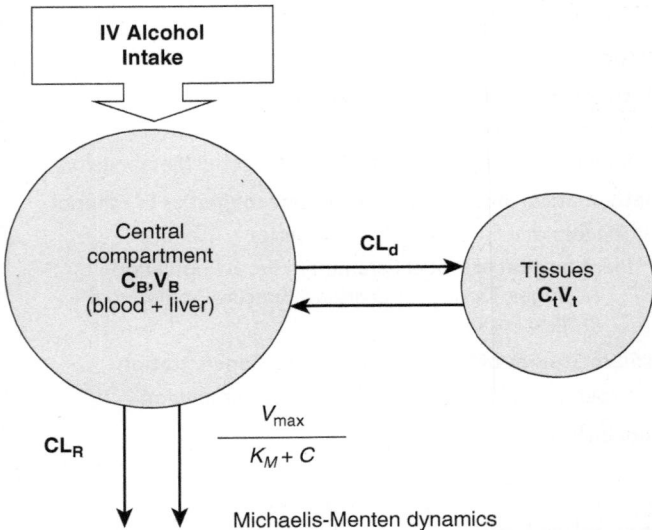

• **Fig. 63.2** Norberg's alcohol clearance model featuring Michaelis-Menten dynamics. Suitable for description of intravenous (IV) ethanol injection.

concentration and volume linked by diffusion or rate-limited pathways. The study of ethanol kinetics in vivo has led to a better representation of the ethanol-aldehyde-acetate process, leading to Norberg's model of alcohol dynamics[9] (Fig. 63.2), which introduces a Michaelis-Menten rate of alcohol clearance—a common enzyme-catalyzed, rate-limited clearance model (see Equation 2):

$$\frac{dC_B}{dt} = -(CL_R + CL_d)\,C_B - \frac{V_{max}C_B}{K_m + C_B}$$
$$\frac{dC_T}{dt} = -CL_d\,(C_T - C_B) \tag{2}$$

where C_B stands for blood ethanol concentration, C_T is the tissue concentration, CL_R is the renal clearance, and CL_d is the diffusion constant.

It is now widely accepted that alcohol clearance is a Michaelis-Menten controlled reaction—an enzyme-enhanced chemical reaction with limited supply.[6] These previously introduced models allow for a mathematical description of alcohol clearance following intravenous alcohol injection (Fig. 63.3).

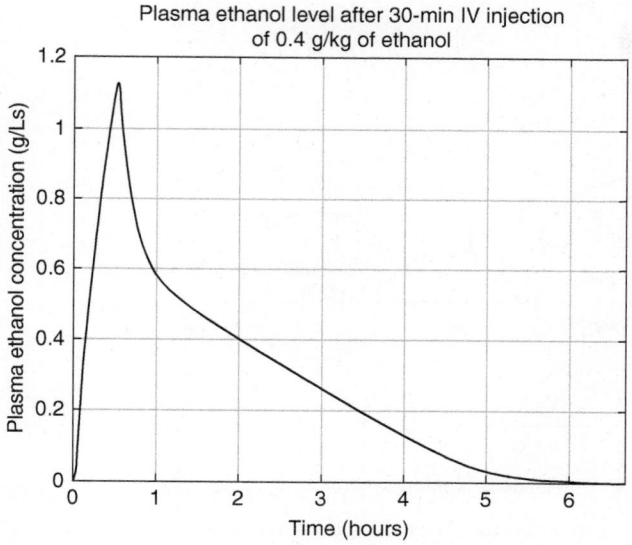

• **Fig. 63.3** Blood alcohol level following intravenous (IV) ethanol injection.

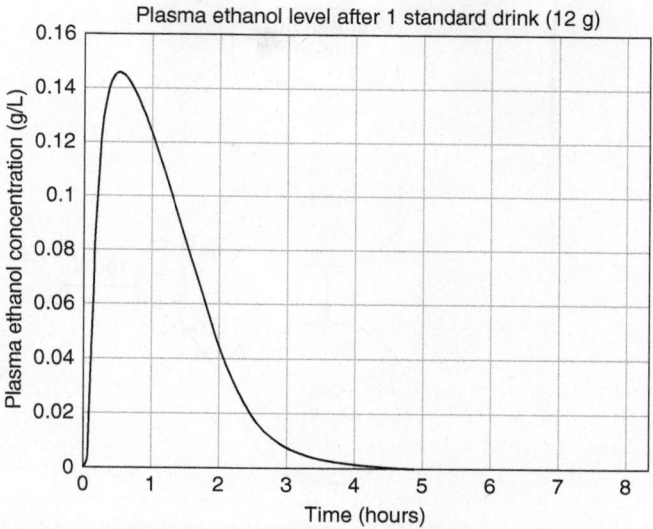

• **Fig. 63.4** Blood alcohol level following oral alcohol ingestion.

Although it is able to represent closely the clearance processes of ethanol in blood, this type of model is often unwieldy compared with the first-order Widmark's model. The larger number of parameters and the nonlinearity of the model make the parameter estimation procedure difficult and sometimes yield imprecise estimates. For example, V_{max} and K_m are often highly correlated, as are the variances of their estimates. These numerical limitations can be alleviated by proper design of clinical data collection—for example, the ethanol dose should be greater than two standard drinks, and numerous samples should be obtained at low levels. These restrictions should be supplemented by specific numerical techniques such as initialization of the minimization procedure (see the next section).[10]

However, the dynamics of orally ingested alcohol has not been well quantified. The compartmental model in Fig. 63.2 cannot reproduce the dynamics of blood alcohol level presented in Fig. 63.4. In particular, the increase in blood alcohol level after alcohol ingestion is poorly described.

This is partly due to the slow diffusion of ethanol from the gastrointestinal tract to blood; whereas with intravenous injection the total dose of ethanol is immediately present in blood and its concentration is at equilibrium after a couple of minutes, orally ingested ethanol can take much longer to percolate fully from the digestive system to blood, therefore allowing for clearance even before the full dose has transferred to the blood. Modeling this process is difficult because ethanol diffuses to the blood from both the stomach and the intestines and at different rates; the speed of gastric emptying (and, therefore, the content and amount of what is ingested with alcohol) also plays a critical role in the dynamics of absorption.

The Minimal Model of Ethanol Kinetics

Here, we present a model directly derived from the work of Norberg (see earlier) but including a two-compartment model of the gastrointestinal tract. This allows us to make use of the simplicity of Norberg modeling, keeping the model complexity to a minimum (the number of equations and parameters to estimate), while also allowing for a semi-physiological representation of ethanol absorption and clearance, ultimately leading to the possibility of simulation of ethanol ingestion and finally drinking behavior.

Fig. 63.5 presents the compartments included in the Minimal Model of Ethanol Kinetics. To properly represent oral alcohol intake, the model needs to include at least two compartments of the gastrointestinal tract: the stomach and gut. Following the minimal model approach, we do not need to add more compartments unless it is proven that the two-compartment gastrointestinal tract model is inherently insufficient. Furthermore, the processes linking these compartments include one-way diffusions from the stomach and the gut into the bloodstream (ethanol in the blood cannot diffuse back to the gastrointestinal tract). Final assumptions of the model include gastric emptying following an exponential decay with a certain half-life (e.g., 50 minutes[15]) and the proportion of gastric diffusion from the stomach W_G versus diffusion from the gut W_G (e.g., $W_S = 20\%$ vs. $W_G = 80\%$[1]).

The differential equations governing the processes depicted in Fig. 63.5 are as follows:

1. Ethanol is transported from the stomach to the gut with a rate constant k_{SG} and diffuses from the stomach into the bloodstream with a rate constant k_G:

$$\frac{\partial C_S}{\partial t} = \frac{1}{V_S W}\left(I(t) - k_S C_S - k_{SG} C_S\right) \qquad (3)$$

2. Ethanol diffuses from the gut into the bloodstream with a rate constant k_G:

$$\frac{\partial C_G}{\partial t} = \frac{1}{V_G W}\left(-k_G C_G + k_{SG} C_S\right) \qquad (4)$$

3. The total ethanol diffusion into the bloodstream is then given by the combination of diffusions from the stomach and the gut:

$$D(t) = k_G C_G + k_S C_S \qquad (5)$$

4. Michaelis-Menten clearance of ethanol from the bloodstream occurs:

$$C(t) = \frac{V_m}{K_m + BAL(t)} BAL(t) \qquad (6)$$

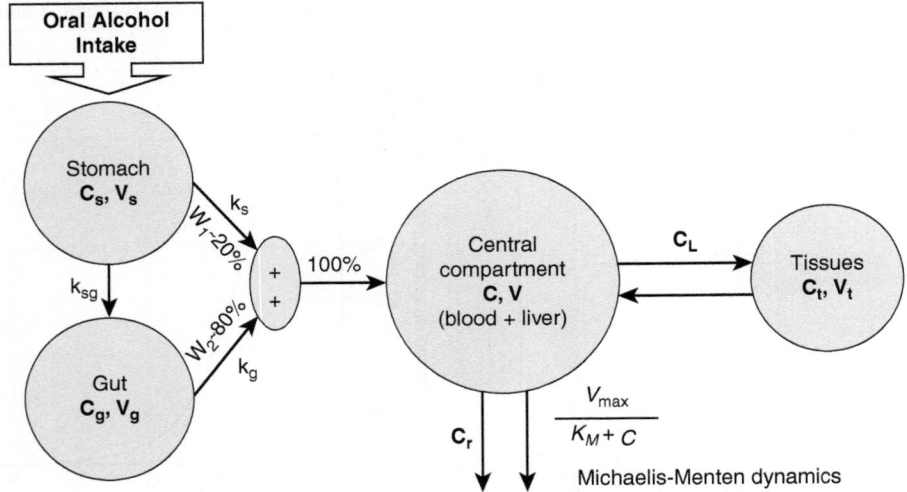

• **Fig. 63.5** The minimal model of ethanol kinetics following oral alcohol intake. The model allows the computation of the idiosyncratic Alcohol Sensitivity Index.

5. Two-way diffusion of ethanol between the bloodstream and tissues/liver occurs, including ethanol transport to the brain:

$$\frac{\partial BAL}{\partial t} = \frac{1}{V_C W}(D(t) + CL_d(TAL(t)$$
$$- BAL(t) - CL_r BAL(t) - C(t) \qquad (7)$$
$$\frac{\partial TAL}{\partial t} = \frac{CL_d}{V_T W}(BAL(t) - TAL(t))$$

Identification of Model Parameters: From Population Averages, Through Individuals' Specific Profiles, to the *In Silico* Population

Population Averages

Using the previously described model, one can fairly easily extract the population average values from the literature. In particular, parameters common to Norberg's two-compartment model can be found in the report of Norberg and colleagues.[10] Tuning of the gastric model is somehow more complex but can be done to reflect the generally admitted equilibrium between the stomach and gut of 20% versus 80% and the 50-minute half-life of gastric emptying. Although these values are sufficient to simulate the dynamics of ethanol and to extract interesting general characteristics of the addiction process, they do not reflect the large variability observed in vivo and, therefore, do not allow the study of a specific group of subjects and, *a fortiori*, a particular subject.

Subject-Specific Identification

We propose a clinical data collection based on the 20-point sampling protocol presented in Fig. 63.6. This protocol is similar to the standard profile used for determination of insulin resistance[2,8] and is modified to account for the specifics of ethanol dynamics. Under this protocol, plasma blood alcohol level samples are collected at times (t) = −30, 0, 5, 10, 15, 20, 30, 40, 50, 60, 75, 90, 120, 150, 180, 210, 240, 300, 360, and 420 minutes. Time 0 is the time of initiation of oral alcohol intake. The total amount of ingested alcohol is equivalent to three standard drinks (45 g of ethanol), and, therefore, the average blood alcohol level profile of a person would be similar to the profile presented in Fig. 63.4. The blood alcohol level measurement prior to initiation of alcohol intake provides a baseline used for calibration; denser sampling is anticipated during the expected increase in blood alcohol level, and less frequent sampling is anticipated during blood alcohol level decay.

A gradient search, simplex, or other nonlinear optimization technique is used to minimize the distance between the predicted blood ethanol concentration course of the model and the data collected as described earlier. Examples of distances include—but are not restricted to—the Euclidian norm (least square), infinite norm (maximum), and weighted least square, the most common being the Euclidian norm.

At convergence, the optimal parameters for this specific subject are fixed, and the model can be used to study the reaction of this subject to different scenarios, including some not easily reproducible in vivo (e.g., extreme/dangerous drinking).

In Silico *Population*

By repeating the procedure above on a large number of individuals, in different conditions (e.g., fasting vs. fed, with a meal or not), we can start to understand the distribution of the model parameters—their mean, bounds, spread, and correlation with each other. With such a distribution, it then becomes possible to create an entirely simulated population spanning the entire (or a chosen subset of) space of possible reactions. In turn, this population can be used for simulated trials, as described in detail in Chapter 64.

In Silico Studies of Blood Ethanol Time-Concentration

To illustrate the use of such models, we present *in silico* experiments reproducing key features of the ethanol metabolism system reported in the literature. The parameters of the Minimal Model of Ethanol Kinetics were first estimated using data available in the literature and from prior studies; then the model was applied to study the behavior of the system during simulated drinking of 1 through >10 standard drinks dispersed randomly throughout an average day.

Experimental Setting of the Computer Simulation

The computer reproduced the system behavior over 72 drinking days. The simulation of a day of drinking was based on the generation of a

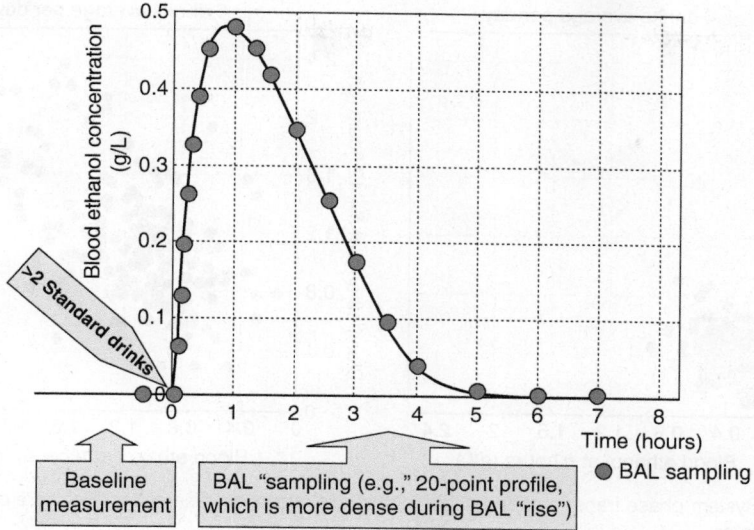

• **Fig. 63.6** Common features of a clinical testing protocol collecting data for an individual ethanol dynamics profile. The blood alcohol level (BAL) sampling can be done directly through blood samples or by using a breath analyzer.

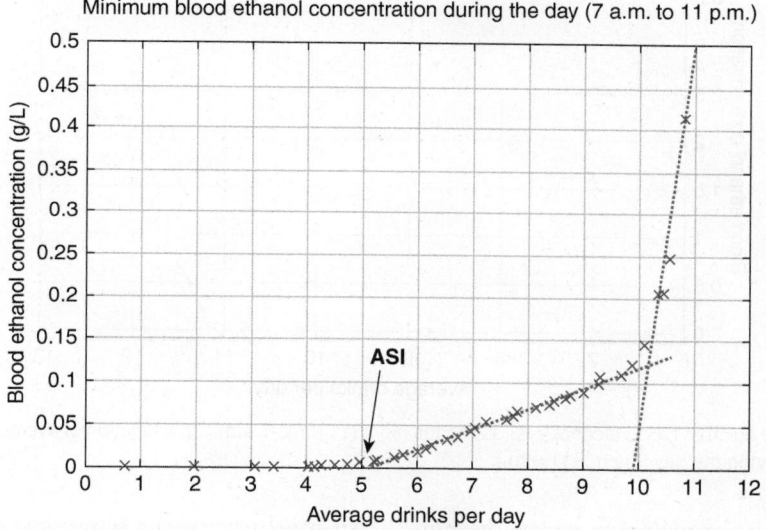

• **Fig. 63.7** Minimum blood alcohol level during daytime (7 a.m.–11 p.m.) as a function of average number of drinks per day. *ASI*, Alcohol Sensitivity Index.

typical drinking day, taking into account the given average number of drinks per day. For example, with 4 preset drinks/day on average, the computer generated a 72-day sequence of drinking days with any number of drinks (i.e., between 1 and 15) dispersed throughout each day, amounting to 4 drinks/day on average.

This was done by modeling a drinking day as a Wiener stochastic renewal process, which means that the time between drinks is a Gaussian (normal) random variable. To follow a more reasonable pattern of drinking, we also limited the drinks to be between 7 a.m. and 11 p.m.—that is, what we considered a standard daytime. The mean time between drinks was set at the ratio of the number of daytime minutes to the average number of drinks per day, and its coefficient of variation was set at 20%.

Each drink was standardized and set to be equivalent to a glass of wine—12 g of ethanol in 100 mL (3.5 oz)—consumed in 5 minutes. The simulation was run for 72 days (100,000 minutes)

in a standard human model (i.e., a weight of 70 kg). The time course of blood alcohol level was recorded for each run. The range of average drinks per day was bounded between 1 and 15. Initial settings for identifying the Minimal Model of Ethanol Kinetics were adopted from the literature: C_{max} = 0.1614 g/L, t_{max} = 47 minutes, and AUC = 0.23 g × h/L (area under the curve).[5,10,11]

Two outcome measures were analyzed from this *in silico* experiment: the minimum of blood ethanol concentration over daytime and over 24 hours. Each measure was calculated for each day between days 10 and 72, avoiding the initiation period of 9 days to allow the system to become stationary; the mean blood alcohol level was computed as well.

Fig. 63.7 presents the minimum blood alcohol level during daytime as a function of the average number of drinks per day. In other words, the line represents whether or not the blood alcohol level would ever go down to zero during the day. The computer

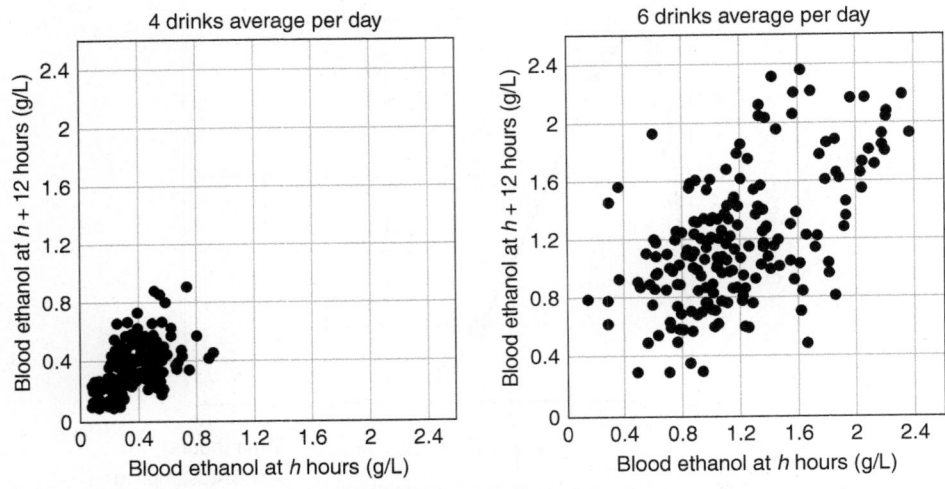

• **Fig. 63.8** System phase transition from stable to unstable dynamics indicated by Poincaré plots of the system attractor.

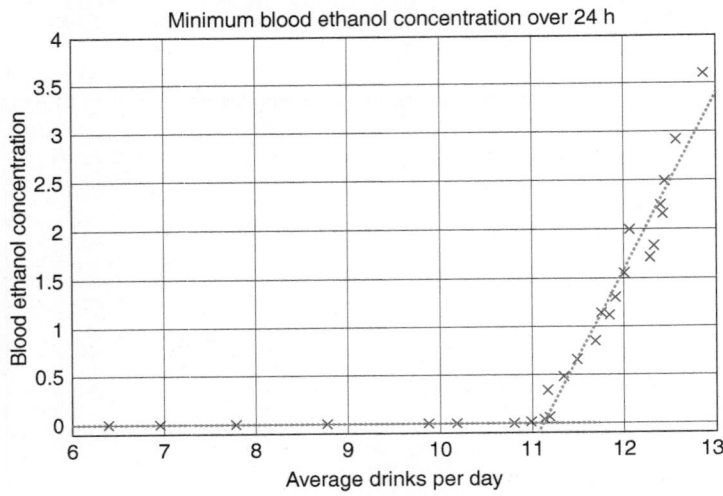

• **Fig. 63.9** Minimum blood alcohol level during the night (11 p.m.–7 a.m.) as a function of average number of drinks during the day (7 a.m.–11 p.m.).

simulation shows that with up to 5 *drinks/day on average*, the minimum blood alcohol level during daytime is zero, indicating that the system reaches its steady (sober) state at least for a while during the day. With between 5 and 11 drinks/day, there is a linear increase of the minimum blood alcohol level (slope = 0.0235, R^2 = 0.99). After 11 drinks/day, the slope of the linear relationship increases dramatically to 1.71 ($R^2 > 0.99$).

Thus the computer simulation indicates that there are two well-defined threshold points defining abrupt system changes: 5 and 11 *drinks/day on average*. The first threshold point, at 5 drinks/day, indicates the transition of zero versus nonzero daily (7 a.m.–11 p.m.) blood alcohol level minimum. This means that with 4 drinks/day or fewer, the system is still capable of metabolizing fully the ingested alcohol, whereas at 5 or more drinks/day, there is always a certain residual amount of alcohol. From a system biology point of view, this first critical point indicates a phase transition from stable to unstable system dynamics. This is well visualized by the Poincaré plots in Fig. 63.8.

As seen in Fig. 63.8, five or more drinks/day would cause metabolic perturbations, never allowing the system to come to rest; the left panel represents a sustainable system dynamics, whereas the right panel represents a system that is clearly out of control.

This computer simulation result is consistent with—and to some degree explains at a system physiology level—the generally accepted understanding of heavy drinking defined as five or more drinks/day. *It appears that this critical value is not only an empirically established threshold but also an indication of an abrupt metabolic phase transition.*

To explain the second threshold value of 11 drinks/day, we need to look at the nighttime. As presented in Fig. 63.9, the minimum blood alcohol level during the night (11 p.m.–7 a.m., which was simulated as free of drinking) reaches zero for up to 11 drinks consumed during the day (7 a.m.–11 p.m.). When the number of drinks during the day exceeds 11, the system cannot metabolize the amount of consumed alcohol even during the nighttime hours, which are free of drinking.

Thus, 11 or more standard drinks/day results in a transition of the system dynamics to a higher blood ethanol value, which never goes down to zero. Because every morning there is still residual ethanol in the bloodstream, there is a very steep rise of blood alcohol level after 11 drinks/day. This explains the abrupt change in the slope of the dependence of blood alcohol level on average number of drinks per day depicted in Fig. 63.7.

Conclusion

In summary, the Minimal Model of Ethanol Kinetics is capable of reproducing (via computer simulation)—and to some degree explaining—the well-known empirical definition of heavy drinking, that is, five or more standard drinks/day for men. The model also suggests other extreme situations, such as those that would occur with more than 11 drinks/day, which theoretically should result in a protracted cognitive impairment due to continuous alcohol intoxication.

In this computer simulation, we used average parameters of alcohol metabolism. The Minimal Model of Ethanol Kinetics will allow for the computation of such parameters for each individual. This, in turn, is expected to facilitate the tailoring of individualized treatment.

This approach can be expanded to *in silico* studies of alcohol addiction, as presented in Chapter 64. With the creation of an *in silico* population spanning the large observed variability in absorption and clearance of alcohol, it would become possible to study further drinking behavior as part of a high-order metabolic system, thereby applying long-held methods pertaining to system engineering to supplement/enhance well-known techniques used in the actual prevention/treatment of alcohol addiction. Further along, it will become possible to run preclinical testing of varied treatment strategies, as was done recently in the case of an artificial pancreas study, bypassing long-term animal studies and greatly accelerating the transition from medication development to human testing.

References

1. Cortot A, Jobin G, Ducrot F, et al. Gastric emptying and gastrointestinal absorption of alcohol ingested with a meal. *Dig Dis Sci.* 1986;31:343–348.
2. Dalla Man C, Caumo A, Basu R, et al. Minimal model estimation of glucose absorption and insulin sensitivity from oral test: validation with a tracer method. *Am J Physiol Endocrinol Metab.* 2004;287:E637–E643.
3. Derr RF. Simulation studies on ethanol metabolism in different human populations with physiological pharmacokinetic model. *J Pharm Sci.* 1993;82:677–682.
4. Duffy JC, Alanko T. Self-reported consumption measures in sample surveys: a simulation study of alcohol consumption. *J Official Statistics.* 1992;8:327–350.
5. Fraser AG, Rosalki SB, Gamble GD, et al. Inter-individual and intra-individual variability of ethanol concentration-time profiles: comparison of ethanol ingestion before or after an evening meal. *Br J Clin Pharmacol.* 1995;40:387–392.
6. Matsumoto H, Fukui Y. Pharmacokinetics of ethanol: a review of the methodology. *Addiction Biol.* 2002;7:5–14.
7. Mumenthaler MS, Taylor JL, Yesavage JA. Ethanol pharmacokinetics in white women: nonlinear model fitting versus zero-order elimination analyses. *Alcohol Clin Exp Res.* 2000;24:1353–1362.
8. Muniyappa R, Madan R, Quon MJ. *Assessing Insulin Sensitivity and Resistance in Humans.* Endotext (ed) South Dartmouth (MA): MDText.com, Inc; 2000: 2015.
9. Norberg A, Gabrielsson J, Jones AW, et al. Within- and between-subject variations in pharmacokinetic parameters of ethanol by analysis of breath, venous blood and urine. *Br J Clin Pharmacol.* 2000;49:399–408.
10. Norberg A, Jones AW, Hahn RG, et al. Role of variability in explaining ethanol pharmacokinetics. *Clin Pharmacokinet.* 2003;42:1–31.
11. Plawecki MH, Han J-J, Doerschuk PC, Ramchandani VA, O'Connor SJ. Physioloigcally based pharmacokinetic (PBPK) models for ethanol. *IEEE Trans Biomed Eng.* 2008;55(12):2691–2700.
12. Umulis DM, Gürmen NM, Singh P, et al. A physiologically based model for ethanol and acetaldehyde metabolism in human beings. *Alcohol.* 2005;35:3–12.
13. Ward RJ, Coutelle Ch. Women and alcohol susceptibility: could differences in alcohol metabolism predispose women to alcohol-related diseases? *Arch Womens Ment Health.* 2003;6:231–238.
14. Widmark EMP. *Die Theoretischen Grundlagen Und Die Praktische Verwendbarkeit Der Gerichtlich-Medizinischen Alkoholbestimmung.* Berlin: Urban & Schwarzenberg; 1932.
15. Yokrattanasak J, De Gaetano A, Panunzi S, Satiracoo P, Lawton WM, Lenbury Y. A simple, realistic, stochastic model of gastric emptying. *PLoS One.* 2016;11(4):e0153297.

64

In Silico Models of Alcohol Dependence Treatment: A Stochastic Approach

BORIS P. KOVATCHEV

CHAPTER OUTLINE

Introduction

In the past two decades, computer simulation and computer-aided design have made dramatic progress in all areas of development of complex engineering systems. A prime example is the Boeing 777 jetliner, which has been recognized as the first airplane to be 100% digitally designed, assembled, and tested preflight *in silico*, (i.e., in a computer simulation environment). This virtual design has eliminated the need for many costly experiments and accelerated immensely the development process. The final result has been impressive; the 777 s flight deck and passenger cabin received the Design Excellence Award of the Industrial Designers Society—the first time any airplane was recognized by the society.[4] There is an enormous body of literature on computer simulation methods applicable to physics, engineering, economics, biology, metabolism, aerospace, meteorology and climatology, warfare, and just about any other subject of investigation that can be described approximately by a mathematical model. The review of this literature is beyond the scope of this chapter; here we will only mention a few biomedical modeling and simulation projects that are relevant to the topic at hand—in silico prediction of the effects of alcohol dependence treatment. For example, accurate prediction of the outcome of clinical trials has been achieved using the Archimedes diabetes model.[10,11] Entelos, Inc., specializes in predictive biosimulation, introducing in its Physiolab suite in silico models for various physiological systems: cardiovascular, metabolic (diabetes), and others.[27]

These in silico models are typically based on mathematical models of the studied physiological system, which are developed from extensive data collection examining underlying physiology in sufficient detail to allow for formal modeling. The models are then used to develop algorithms and software that power up simulation experiments. According to Winsberg,[41] simulation experiments are typically classified with respect to the type of algorithm that they employ: Discretization techniques transform continuous differential equations into step-by-step algebraic expressions. Monte Carlo methods use random sampling algorithms even when there is no underlying indeterminism in the system. Cellular automata assign a discrete state to each node of a network of elements, and assign rules of evolution for each node based on its local environment in the network. In this chapter, we utilize both discretization and Monte Carlo (or generally stochastic) methods, but first we discuss three types of mathematical models of biosystems, classified according to the purpose of modeling: models to *measure*, to *simulate*, or to *control* the biosystem under consideration.

Models to Measure

The models to measure are generally simpler, allowing hidden relationships to be evaluated by estimating underlying parameters. Most of these models are compartmental; for example, they represent the human body as a set of homogeneous compartments of specific concentrations and volumes linked by diffusion or rate-limited pathways. Classic examples include the Widmark Model of Ethanol Pharmacokinetics, which offers a straightforward interpretation with a constant ethanol clearance rate and the human body modeled as one compartment,[40] and the more complex Minimal Model of Glucose Kinetics suggested by Bergman and Cobelli more than 30 years ago to measure insulin resistance in health and diabetes.[5] More recently, with the advent of the digital biology paradigm, various models to measure have been developed that address pharmacokinetics, physiology, and human behavior. Deeper understanding of the processes involved and the development of novel measuring tools have allowed for more precise measurement of ethanol pharmacokinetics and the development of more complex nonlinear models.[28–30,39] The study of ethanol kinetics in vivo has led to a better representation of the ethanol-aldehyde-acetate process via the Michaelis-Menten rate of alcohol clearance introduced by Norberg.[29] It is now widely accepted that alcohol clearance is a Michaelis-Menten–controlled reaction—that is, an enzyme-enhanced chemical reaction with limited supply.[39] These and other pharmacokinetic models are discussed in detail in Chapter 63.

Models to Simulate

The models to simulate are maximal multiparameter models that describe the complexity of the system as comprehensively as possible.[7,8] For example, the meal model of glucose-insulin dynamics is a descendant of the Minimal Model, which encompasses several metabolic subsystems including the gastrointestinal tract, renal function, hepatic glucose production, and others.[7,8] When a maximal model is built, the computer simulation of the observed biosystem becomes possible, leading to in silico trials involving virtual "subjects" rather than real people. Such in silico trials can serve as precursors, guiding expensive and time-consuming clinical investigations by outruling ineffective treatment approaches. For example, our simulator of the human metabolic system has received US Food and Drug Administration (FDA) approval and recognition for the preclinical testing of control strategies in artificial pancreas studies.[20] Using this simulator, the time for refining and safety testing of new algorithms that target the closed-loop control of diabetes has been reduced from years to several months.[19,24,31] Therefore, realistic computer simulation is capable of providing valuable information about the effectiveness, safety, and limits of various treatments. Computer simulation allows experiments with extreme situations and testing of extreme failure modes that are unrealistic in animals and clinically impossible in humans. In addition to extreme experiments, various treatment scenarios can be efficiently tested and either rejected or accepted for inclusion in future clinical experiments, which allows for rapid, comprehensive, and cost-effective clinical trial design. *We need to emphasize, however, that good* in silico *performance of a treatment does not guarantee* in vivo *performance. Computer simulation should be used only to reject inefficient treatments; it cannot confirm the efficacy of an intervention.*

Models to Control

External control of a complex technical or living system is generally achieved by control algorithms that are based on a certain mathematical representation of the system—a model to control—combined with the ability to observe the system in real time and make immediate decisions for correction of the system state. The models to control are typically simplified (frequently linearized) models that allow for rapid observation and computation of the corrective action. A prime example of medical devices that use adaptive control algorithms is the cardiac pacemaker, which in the past two decades has been incorporating automated control functions such as automatic capture and sensing control, self-adjusting rate response settings, sinus rhythm and atrioventricular conduction preference, and others.[13,17,37,42] In diabetes, successful attempts

at external closed-loop control have been made using various systems and algorithms, from cumbersome intravenous systems and implantable devices[1,33,36] to external subcutaneous control,[15,18,38] and portable "artificial pancreas."[22] Relating control to simulation, comprehensive in silico testing of control algorithms is an efficient strategy if a model to control is tested against a much more complex model to simulate. In other words, the effectiveness of a controller can be judged if it is tested in realistic in silico conditions, which can be achieved by a comprehensive simulation model.

Formal Description of Human Behavior and Social Conditioning

In the context of in silico models of alcohol dependence treatment, applicable quantitative strategies include models to measure and models to simulate. In order to build such models, a formal mathematical description of human behavior and environmental conditioning is needed. However, the behavioral and social modeling field is still quite limited. Although theoretical models based on internal somatic perception have been proposed,[3,23] their heuristic approach has not permitted their development in sufficient mathematical detail to guide data analysis. For example, the stages of change described by the Transtheoretical Model of DiClemente and Prochaska[9] refer to a stochastic sequence—of readiness to change, stage of change status, temptation, and confidence—that has consistently shown predictive and explanatory ability for clinical outcome in alcohol dependence treatment studies. However, this sequence has not been identified as stochastic and has not been formalized to the extent that would permit computerized assessment and simulation. Another example can be provided in the context of nonspecific treatment effects, such as the Hawthorne effect, which describes the tendency of an individual to change his or her behavior as a consequence of being observed or studied.[26,35] Although this effect provides evidence for the importance of environmental conditioning and external reinforcement for all stages of the progression of alcohol dependence—from acquisition of alcohol dependence, through treatment, to potential relapse—there is no formal description of environmental conditioning that would allow its inclusion in an integrated in silico model encompassing physiology, behavior, and social conditioning. Therefore, to advance the field, we have proposed a formal stochastic biobehavioral model of the sequence leading to self-regulation decision, in which the first three steps of the process were described by continuous variables, whereas the decisions at Step 4 were binary.[19] The general concept is that decisions concerning self-regulation behaviors are often based on perception and appraisal of the body's internal state. Thus the sequence preceding a certain action includes at least four sequential steps: internal condition → perception → environmental conditioning → self-regulation decision. We have applied this general framework to evaluate the relationship between self-treatment behavior and the development of hypoglycemia in diabetics,[6,12] as well as the psycho-physiological factors associated with the attention impairment experienced by those with attention-deficit/hyperactivity disorder.[21,32,34]

Combining Biology and Behavior In Silico

In this chapter, we view alcohol dependence and the response to alcohol dependence treatment as a recurrent bio-behavioral process developing in time. Such an approach captures the dynamics of sequential changes occurring during acquisition of alcohol dependence, successful treatment, or relapse. We provide a rigid

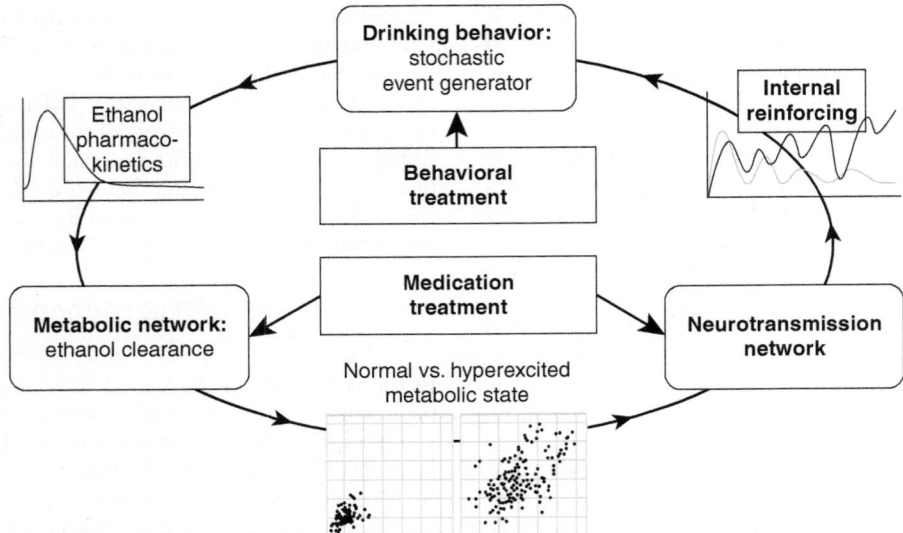

• **Fig. 64.1** Recurrent bio-behavioral process of alcohol dependence and treatment.

mathematical framework formally describing these dynamics. To do so, we first introduce a stochastic model of behavioral and social conditioning, describing the frequently random[a] effects of human behavior and social reinforcement. We then merge this stochastic model with the deterministic model of alcohol metabolism described in Chapter 63. In combination, these two models provide the background for in silico interpretation of biology and behavior in their relationship to treatment effect. To formally represent behavioral and social conditioning, we identify several sequential steps. Each step is represented by a probability distribution, and the set of these distributions across all steps regulates the feed-forward relationships of the process from internal condition to self-regulation decision. *Each person* is represented by an individual treatment-effect profile, defined as the set of transition probabilities between the sequential steps of the model specific to that person. This model serves as a stochastic behavioral generator of events, each event being a drink, which is supplied as an input to an individualized model of alcohol metabolism. In other words, the in silico experiments with alcohol dependence treatment use behavioral and social parameters that serve as generators of metabolic disturbances to the system (person), which are then processed through an individualized metabolic model, thereby allowing the formal decomposition and reconstruction of the patterns of drinking behavior and their modulation by placebo or medication treatment. We illustrate our proposed approach by re-analyzing data from a study of ondansetron for the treatment of alcohol dependence[16] and include in the model the nonspecific placebo effects that occurred before the active treatment phase of the study,[32] with a special emphasis on the highly significant differences between heavy and nonheavy drinkers observed during the study.

[a]Here we need to make a distinction between the lay and scientific understanding of randomness: scientifically, a random variable is a variable that can assume a set of values with certain probabilities comprising its distribution. For example, any constant is a random variable assuming its only value with probability 1 and all other values with probability 0. Other random variables have normal (Gaussian) distribution; others have uniform distribution, and so on. The lay understanding of randomness typically refers to uniformly distributed variables that can assume any of multiple values with equal probabilities..

Methods

Recurrent Bio-Behavioral Process of Alcohol Dependence and Treatment

Fig. 64.1 presents the general concept of the self-reinforcing recurrent bio-behavioral process, describing the progression of alcohol dependence, its remission through medication or behavioral treatment, and potential relapse.

As presented in Fig. 64.1, the system (person) is represented by several blocks (components) linked via a circular pattern of sequential steps. First, a behavioral event generator actuates system disturbances (e.g., drinks), which cause metabolic disturbances that can be different for each person, depending on his or her individual parameters of alcohol pharmacokinetics. Furthermore, when the metabolic network is subjected to recurrent stress, the intensity of stress determines whether or not a phase transition to a hyperexcited metabolic state would occur. (Metabolic phase transitions are discussed in Chapter 63.) A chronic hyperexcited metabolic state would influence the neurotransmission network, potentially leading to alcohol dependence. This in turn would result in a high degree of internal reinforcing (craving), which accelerates the behavioral event generator by triggering excessive drinking. Medication treatment would typically target the neurotransmission or the metabolic component of this recurrent process, whereas behavioral treatment would attempt to reduce the frequency of firing of the behavioral event generator. With this formal overall understanding, we now proceed to a mathematical description of the general components of the alcohol dependence process that would be used for its in silico representation and treatment evaluation: (1) a mathematical model of the human metabolic system specifically targeting ethanol kinetics; (2) a stochastic model of behavioral and social conditioning, and (3) a comprehensive population of in silico "subjects" spanning the observed in vivo interindividual metabolic and behavioral differences.

In Silico Models of Ethanol Metabolism

As presented in the Introduction, several models of ethanol metabolism exist.[28–30,40] Based on these models, we have proposed the

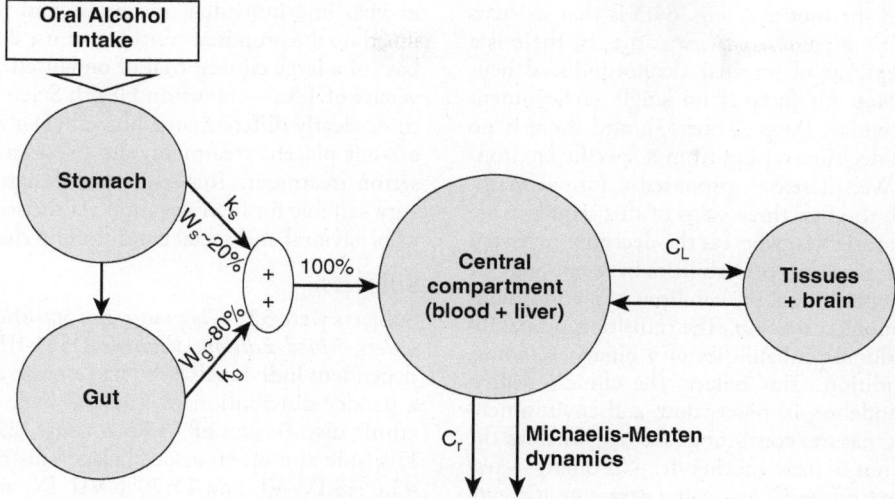

• **Fig. 64.2** The metabolic minimal model of alcohol dynamics following oral alcohol intake.

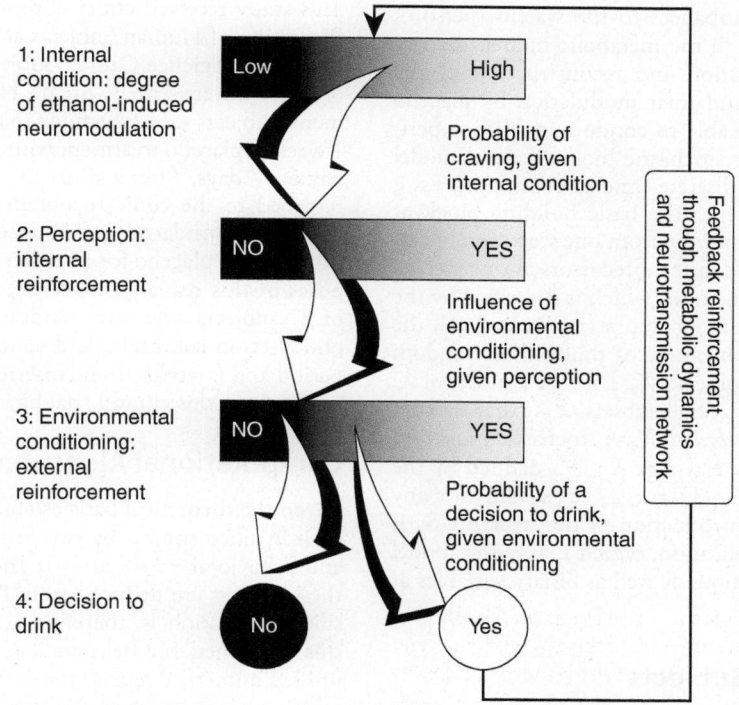

• **Fig. 64.3** Stochastic model of behavioral and social conditioning.

Minimal Model of Ethanol Dynamics (see Chapter 63). To properly represent oral alcohol intake, the model includes two previously unexplored compartments of the gastrointestinal tract—the stomach and gut (Fig. 64.2). Following the classic minimal model approach,[5] we determined that we did not need to add more compartments. Furthermore, the processes linking these compartments include one-way diffusions from the stomach and gut into the bloodstream (ethanol in the blood cannot diffuse back to the gastrointestinal tract). The assumptions of the model include gastric emptying following an exponential decay with a certain half-life (rate constants k_s and k_g) and the proportion of gastric diffusion from the stomach, W_s, versus diffusion from the gut, W_g (e.g., $W_s = 20\%$ vs. $W_g = 80\%$[30]).

The alcohol clearance is represented by a Michaelis-Menten controlled reaction, for example, an enzyme-enhanced chemical reaction with limited supply,[25,39] which has individual parameters (rate constant Cr) for each person. The mathematical details of this model and the process of its derivation and validation are discussed in Chapter 63.

Stochastic Model of Behavioral and Social Conditioning

Fig. 64.3 presents the four steps of the alcohol intake self-regulation sequence introduced earlier: internal condition → perception → environmental conditioning → self-regulation decision.

The basic idea behind the model of Fig. 64.3 is that its steps are linked by a *continuum of possible pathways*: that is, there is a variety of possible perceptions of internal alcohol-induced neuromodulation (Step 1–Step 2); there is no single environment corresponding to a perception (Step 2–Step 3), and there is no uniquely predetermined decision arising from a specific environment (Step 3–Step 4). We, therefore, proposed a formal mathematical model in which the first three steps of this sequence are described by continuous variables, whereas the decisions at Step 4 are binary. In detail, the transition probabilities between Steps 1, 2, and 3 are modeled as conditional probabilities of a continuous outcome, given a continuous condition. The transition probabilities at Step 4 are conditional probabilities of a binary outcome, given a continuous condition. This reflects the clinical reality: the level of alcohol dependence, its perception, and environmental reinforcement are, by nature, continuous factors, whereas the final decision to have or not to have another drink is binary—Yes/No. This model serves as a *stochastic behavioral generator of events*, each event being a drink that is supplied as an input to the metabolic model of Fig. 64.2. In other words, the in silico preclinical experiments use behavioral and social parameters that serve as generators of metabolic disturbances to the system (person), which are then processed through the metabolic model, thereby allowing the formal decomposition and reconstruction of the patterns of drinking behavior and their modulation by placebo or medication treatment. To be able to conduct in silico experiments, we need to describe our stochastic bio-behavioral model in algorithmic terms. We use a discrete-time stochastic process ξ that goes through sequential steps. The basic building block of such a process is the *stochastic transition* from one step to the next, that is, a transition that allows identical precursors at one step to have different consequences at the next, which is described by the following scheme: Suppose that at its Step n ($n = 1, 2, 3, 4$), the process $\xi(n)$ is described by a univariate or multivariate random variable x_n, having its values in some set X_n. Let S be a subset of X_n (we write $S \, \delta \, X_n$). A structure S_n of all subsets of X_n that satisfies certain conditions is called σ-*algebra* on X_n. A stochastic transition of the process ξ from X_n to its next stage X_{n+1} is defined by the conditional probabilities $P(\xi(n+1) = x_{n+1} \,|\, \xi(n) \in S)$ for any $x_{n+1} \in X_{n+1}$ and $S \in S_n$. The introduction of the structure S_n is a necessary mathematical complication, which makes the model capable of incorporating continuous as well as binary variables at each step.

Population of In Silico "Subjects"

Given the models in the previous sections, each person's ethanol metabolism is described via a set of several parameters $(k_s, k_g, C_r, \ldots)$, and one set of fixed values of these parameters defines the metabolism of one in silico subject. The in silico population is then derived by estimating the across-subject variance of these parameters and generating a number of parameter sets to span the metabolic diversity observed in vivo. Similarly, the behavioral and social specifics of each in silico subject are defined by an individual behavioral/social profile, for example, by his or her own set of transition probabilities $(p_1, p_2, \ldots)$ between the sequential steps of the model of Fig. 64.3 that are specific to that subject. The diversity of behaviors and social interactions of the in silico population is then described by diverse sets of transition probabilities.

Although a comprehensive population of in silico subjects can be built only by collecting extensive data spanning the observed in vivo interindividual metabolic and behavioral differences, to illustrate the proposed concepts we use data derived from the database of a large clinical trial of ondansetron conducted at the University of Texas—Houston Health Science Center. This study had three clearly differentiated phases: (1) a 7-day baseline period, (2) a 7-day placebo treatment, and (3) several weeks of active ondansetron treatment. This sequential design made the collected data very suitable for interpretation via the sequential stochastic model of behavioral and social conditioning that is conceptualized here.

Subjects

Subjects were 321 *Diagnostic and Statistical Manual of Mental Disorders, Third Edition, Revised* (DSM-III-R)[2]–diagnosed alcohol-dependent individuals, who had a mean age of 41.50 ± 1.34 years; a gender distribution of 73.81% male and 26.19% female; an ethnic distribution of 76.05% white, 22.10% black, and 1.85% Hispanic and other; a social class[14] distribution of 39.25% I–III, 49.05% IV–VI, and 11.70% VII–IX, and a mean drinking level of 8.04 ± 5.80 drinks/day in the past 90 days prior to enrollment.

Procedure

This study received ethics approval from the Committee for the Protection of Human Subjects at the University of Texas – Houston Health Science Center. Subjects were recruited by newspaper or radio advertisement in the Houston area. Following recruitment, subjects were scheduled to return to the clinic to commence 1 week of placebo treatment with an inert pill to be taken twice per day for 7 days. After a study calendar week (7–10 days), subjects returned to the clinic to obtain their randomized double-blind medication (ondansetron) in doses of 1, 4, or 16 µg/kg twice daily or matching placebo for a further period of 11 weeks. For the purposes of this reanalysis, we selected the homogeneous subgroup of 87 subjects who were randomized to the 4-µg/kg twice daily ondansetron condition, and concentrated on their initial placebo period and 6 weeks of ondansetron treatment data. The complete results from this clinical trial have been published elsewhere.[16]

Computational Algorithms

Given the theoretical basis established in this section, we identify each in silico subject by two vectors: metabolic $= (k_s, k_g, C_r, \ldots)$ and behavioral $= (p_1, p_2, \ldots)$. The limits of the space occupied by these vectors are deduced from literature and study data. The in silico population is, therefore, a population of vectors spanning this combined bio-behavioral space. Such an approach ensures unified numerical representation of physiological, behavioral, and social interactions, and enables the two-stage simulation procedure that we employ in this chapter:

- *Stage 1— behavior*: Computer-simulated idiosyncratic drinking patterns using the behavioral/social span of the vectors $(p_1, p_2, \cdots)^1, (p_1, p_2, \cdots)^2, \cdots, (p_1, p_2, \cdots)^N$. Each of these patterns would result in a decision to drink or not to drink for each in silico subject. These decisions serve as behavioral event generators, and the generated events (i.e., drinks) are supplied to initialize the metabolic simulation model. In other words, the Stochastic Model of Behavioral and Social Conditioning creates the basic building block for in silico evaluation of treatment effect—the probability of a subject having a drink at any given point in time.

- *Stage 2—metabolism*: Computer-simulated idiosyncratic alcohol intoxication patterns using the span of the metabolic vectors $(k_s, k_g, C_r, \cdots)^1, (k_s, k_g, C_r, \cdots)^2, (k_s, k_g, C_r, \cdots)^N$.

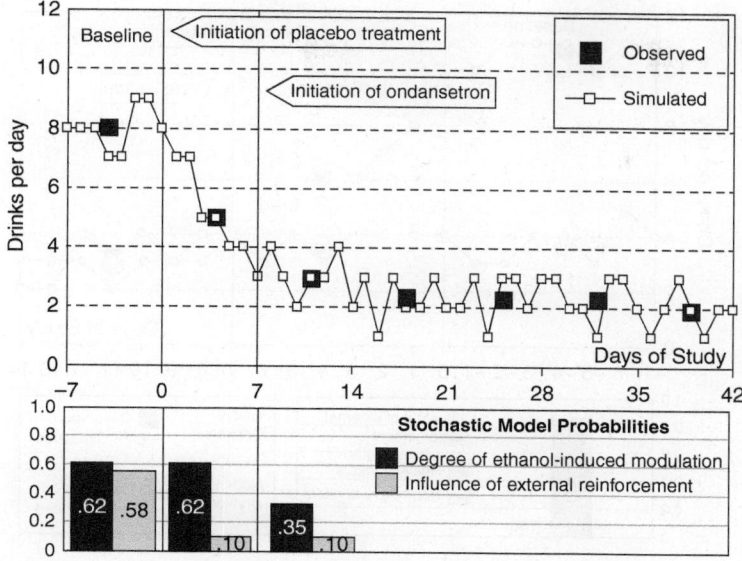

• **Fig. 64.4** Model-predicted and observed effect of placebo and ondansetron treatment.

This is done as follows: at each simulated drink for each in silico subject, this subject's metabolic model produces a specific trace in time of alcohol intoxication. The next simulated drink will come somewhere in this trace and, depending on this individual's specific metabolic and drinking behavior, will hit at different stages of alcohol clearance. If the simulated drinks are sufficiently infrequent so that this individual can fully metabolize the ingested alcohol, the system (subject) will remain in a subcritical drinking pattern; conversely, if the drinks are too frequent, the system (subject) will transit to a super-critical pattern. Metabolic patterns are discussed in detail in Chapter 63.

This simulation procedure was programmed in MATLAB, a high-level programming language widely adopted for technical computing.

Results

The following results are provided as an example of how the stochastic model can be applied.

Empirical Findings

The average number of drinks per day during the baseline period for the selected subgroup of 87 subjects was 8.01 (SD = 5.28). Thus the selected subgroup was representative of the entire study cohort, which reported an average of 8.04 (SD = 5.80) drinks/day for the 90 days prior to recruitment. During the placebo treatment period, the alcohol consumption in the selected subgroup was reduced to 5.03 (SD = 4.64) drinks/day, followed by a further gradual reduction to 1.88 (SD = 2.21) drinks/day after 6 weeks of active ondansetron treatment ($F = 56.1$, $p < 0.0001$) using repeated-measures analysis of variance. (This empirical pattern of passive and active reduction in drinking is included in Fig. 64.4.)

During the baseline period, 54 subjects (62%) in the illustrative subgroup were classified as heavy drinkers, consuming ≥5 drinks/day and ≥4 drinks/day for men and women, respectively. This classification had a significant ($F = 20.1$, $p < 0.001$) effect on the outcome from nonspecific placebo treatment: the number

of drinks per day in heavy drinkers changed from 10.70 (SD = 5.02) at baseline to 6.06 (SD = 5.31) at the end of the placebo period; in nonheavy drinkers, there was no change: 3.61 (SD = 1.06) drinks/day at baseline versus 3.65 (SD = 2.94) drinks/day at the end of the placebo period. The difference between heavy and nonheavy drinkers became negligible during the first week of active ondansetron treatment and remained negligible throughout the rest of the observation period. (The empirical patterns of these two groups are included in Fig. 64.5.)

In Silico Versus In Vivo Responses to Placebo and Ondansetron Treatment

To evaluate the closeness of in silico prediction to observed clinical outcome, we compared the computer-simulated and clinically observed patterns of treatment response. Throughout the simulation, we kept the metabolic parameters (see Fig. 64.2) of the simulated subjects constant and used the stochastic model of Fig. 64.3 to decompose the observed drinking patterns into two sections explained by different model steps:

1. The response to initial placebo treatment was attributed to the influence of study enrollment, which was modeled as a reduction of the probability for environmental conditioning (Step 3 in Fig. 64.3) from its baseline value of 0.58–0.10. Because this effect occurs relatively quickly (within a week) and no active medication was provided, no other system changes were anticipated, such as feedback downregulation through modulation of the neurotransmission system.

2. The response to ondansetron was attributed to neurotransmission changes influenced by the degree of ethanol-induced neuromodulation. This was modeled via reduction of the probability of Step 1 from its baseline value of 0.62–0.35.

Fig. 64.4 compares the results of this in silico treatment experiment to the clinically observed treatment effects. Black squares represent the empirical pattern of baseline drinking (Days −7 to 0) and the pattern of drinking reduction due to placebo (Days 1 to 7) and ondansetron treatment (Days 8 to 42). The in silico–generated pattern (black line) follows closely these empirical

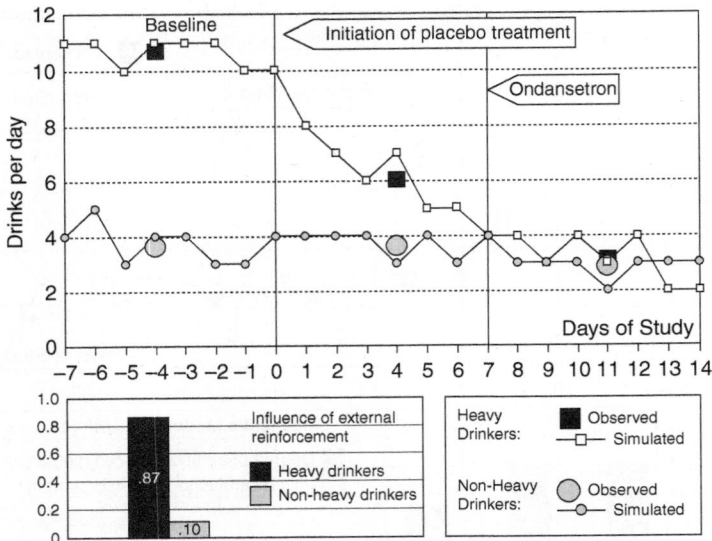

• **Fig. 64.5** Model-predicted and observed treatment effect in heavy drinkers and nonheavy drinkers.

observations, confirming that in silico experiments could provide realistic representation of treatment effect. The lower panel of the figure includes the change in environmental reinforcement probability, which is responsible for the placebo effect, and the reduction in the degree of ethanol-induced modulation describing the effect of ondansetron.

Modeling Idiosyncratic Treatment Response

The empirical results presented in the preceding text suggest highly significant differences between heavy and nonheavy drinkers in their responses to placebo treatment, followed by a regression into a common pattern of response to ondansetron. Fig. 64.5 focuses on the first three weeks of observation, where these idiosyncratic differences were most evident.[32] Following the assumption that the placebo effect is due primarily to reduced environmental reinforcement, we model the difference between these two groups of subjects via different probabilities at Step 3.

Indeed, environmental reinforcement probabilities of 0.87 and 0.10 for heavy and nonheavy drinkers allow for excellent simulated approximation of the observed empirical patterns of placebo response. (Note that the overall baseline probability of environmental reinforcement, 0.58, is the weighted sum of the probabilities in the two subject subpopulations.) As is empirically established and evident from Fig. 64.5, nonheavy drinkers (gray circles) were nonresponsive to the effect of study enrollment. In contrast, heavy drinkers (black squares) appeared to be vulnerable to environmental conditioning effects, and, therefore, their response to placebo treatment was highly significant. Furthermore, these two subject subpopulations were approximately equally responsive to the effect of medication, which explains the similarities in their patterns during the period of active ondansetron treatment. The environmental probabilities used for simulation are included in the bar graph in the lower section of Fig. 64.5.

Conclusions

The principal utility of in silico modeling efforts is threefold. First, models allow the measurement of latent factors that cannot be observed directly but that frequently predetermine the behavior of

a biosystem. A classical example is the Minimal Model of Glucose Kinetics suggested by Bergman and Cobelli almost 30 years ago to measure insulin resistance in health and diabetes.[5] Second, models allow for computer simulation and in silico studies involving virtual subjects rather than real people. Such in silico trials can serve as cost-effective precursors, guiding expensive and time-consuming in vivo investigations by ruling out ineffective treatment approaches. For example, our simulator of the human metabolic system has received FDA approval and recognition for the preclinical testing of control strategies in artificial pancreas studies.[20] Third, when a system (person) is adequately modeled, its control via engineering means becomes possible. Examples include cardiac pacemakers and, more recently, the artificial pancreas emerging as a means for control of blood glucose levels in diabetes.

The basic premise of in silico modeling of alcohol dependence is that alcohol dependence and the outcome of its treatment result from the action of a stochastic self-reinforcing bio-behavioral process, combined with each individual's metabolic specifics. In other words, the interplay between biology and behavior, which develops in a certain time frame, would trigger (with a certain probability) metabolic and neurobiological changes that in turn would reinforce uncontrolled or poorly controlled drinking behavior. Treatment would, therefore, be expected to modulate, attenuate, or reverse these changes with a certain level of probability. Such a quantitative approach has several potential advantages:

- First, the overall treatment effect can be deconstructed into meaningful steps, with each step serving as a target for a specific treatment. For example, Step 1 (internal condition) would reflect pharmacological treatment, while Step 3 (environmental conditioning) would reflect the placebo effect of study enrollment, or any type of socio-behavioral intervention. Such a decomposition of the treatment effect allows for better understanding of the time course of treatment and the relationships among the various treatment components.
- Second, the proposed model would allow for individualized treatment tailoring. For example, it appears that in heavy drinkers, environmental conditioning is a significant predictor of treatment response, whereas in nonheavy drinkers the effect of the environment is minimal. The effect of ondansetron is similar in the two groups but occurs faster in nonheavy drinkers.

- Third, one of the advantages of a model-based investigation is that separate steps can be estimated in different studies and then the results can be integrated via the model. For example, neurotransmission or physiological parameters can be evaluated in animal studies and then related to human behavior parameters. That is, the proposed concept is *species invariant*, capable of bridging results from human and animal studies.

Most importantly, the stochastic process described here serves as an event generator of behavioral disturbances (i.e., drinks), which in turn influence the internal condition. Thus the initial entry conditions for a person change with each repetition of the cycle presented in Fig. 64.1. This recurrence provides powerful tools for in silico analysis of the progression of alcohol dependence and treatment response, taking into account both biological and environmental factors.

To illustrate this concept, we conducted in silico experiments that reproduced patterns observed in a clinical trial of ondansetron. It became evident that placebo and ondansetron, as well as their interaction, contribute to the overall therapeutic response. There might, however, be other nonspecific effects that can affect clinical outcome and that we need to discover. Hence, the in silico model presented here is less developed than the metabolic models adopted for the study of diabetes. Nevertheless, this text represents an initial step to introduce the concept of in silico analysis to the area of alcohol dependence research. Because the first results appear promising and explanatory for the observed phenomena, we think that with the accumulation of data (both existing and from future clinical studies), in silico analysis would find its place in the arsenal of tools to help decipher the mechanisms that govern treatment response among alcohol-dependent individuals.

References

1. Albisser AM, Leibel BS, Ewart TG, Davidovac Z, Botz CK, Zingg W. An artificial endocrine pancreas. *Diabetes*. 1974;23:389–396.
2. American Psychiatric Association. *Diagnostic and Statistical Manual of Mental Disorders*. 3rd ed. Washington, DC: American Psychiatric; 1987.
3. Baumann LJ, Cameron LD, Zimmerman RS, Leventhal H. Illness representations and matching labels with symptoms. *Health Psychol*. 1989;8:449–469.
4. Benhabib B. *Manufacturing: Design, Production, Automation, and Integration*. Boca Raton, FL: CRC Press; 2003.
5. Bergman RN, Ider YZ, Bowden CR, Cobelli C. Quantitative estimation of insulin sensitivity. *Am J Physiol*. 1979;236:E667–E677.
6. Clarke WL, Cox DJ, Gonder-Frederick L, Julian D, Kovatchev B, Young-Hyman D. Biopsychobehavioral model of severe hypoglycemia. Self-management behaviors. *Diabetes Care*. 1999;22:580–584.
7. Dalla Man C, Raimondo DM, Rizza RA, Cobelli C. GIM, simulation software of meal glucose-insulin model. *J Diabetes Sci Technol*. 2007;1:323–330.
8. Dalla Man C, Rizza RA, Cobelli C. Meal simulation model of the glucose-insulin system. *IEEE Trans Biomed Eng*. 2007;54:1740–1749.
9. DiClemente CC, Prochaska JO. Treating addictive behaviors. In: Miller WR, ed. *Applied Clinical Psychology*. 2nd ed. New York: Plenum; 1998.
10. Eddy DM, Schlessinger L. Archimedes: a trial-validated model of diabetes. *Diabetes Care*. 2003;26:3093–3101.
11. Eddy DM, Schlessinger L. Validation of the Archimedes diabetes model. *Diabetes Care*. 2003;26:3102–3110.
12. Gonder-Frederick L, Cox D, Kovatchev B, Schlundt D, Clarke W. A biopsychobehavioral model of risk of severe hypoglycemia. *Diabetes Care*. 1997;20:661–669.
13. Haddad SAP, Houben R, Serdijn WA. The evolution of pacemakers: an electronics perspective, from the hand crank to advanced wavelet analysis. In: *Proceedings of the 3rd DISENS Symposium on Biomedical Sensors*. Delft, the Netherlands; 2005.
14. Hollingshead AB, Redlich FC. *Social Class and Mental Illness: A Community Study*. New York: Wiley; 1958.
15. Hovorka R, Canonico V, Chassin LJ, et al. Nonlinear model predictive control of glucose concentration in subjects with type 1 diabetes. *Physiol Meas*. 2004;25:905–920.
16. Johnson BA, Roache JD, Javors MA, et al. Ondansetron for reduction of drinking among biologically predisposed alcoholic patients: a randomized controlled trial. *JAMA*. 2000;284:963–971.
17. Khasnis A, Tepper D. A new pacemaker algorithm for the treatment of atrial fibrillation: results of the atrial dynamic overdrive pacing trial (ADOPT). *Cardiovasc Rev Rep*. 2003;24:532–533.
18. Klonoff DC. The artificial pancreas: how sweet engineering will solve bitter problems. *J Diabetes Sci Technol*. 2007;1:72–81.
19. Kovatchev B, Cox D, Gonder-Frederick L, Schlundt D, Clarke W. Stochastic model of self-regulation decision making exemplified by decisions concerning hypoglycemia. *Health Psychol*. 1998;17:277–284.
20. Kovatchev BP, Breton MD, Dalla Man C, Cobelli C. In Silico preclinical trials: A proof of concept in closed-loop control of type 1 diabetes. *J Diabetes Sci Technol*. 2009;3:44–55. PMCID: PMC2681269; PMID: 19444330.
21. Kovatchev BP, Penberthy JK, Robeva RS, Breton M, Cox DJ. Computational strategies in the evaluation of attention deficit/hyperactivity disorder. In: Larimer M, ed. *Attention Deficit/Hyperactivity Disorder (ADHD) Research*. New York: Nova Science; 2005.
22. Kovatchev BP, Renard E, Cobelli C, et al. Feasibility of outpatient fully integrated closed-loop control: First studies of wearable artificial pancreas. *Diabetes Care*. 2013;36:1851–1858. https://doi.org/10.2337/dc12-1965.
23. Leventhal H, Diefenbach M, Leventhal EA. Illness cognition: using common sense to understand treatment adherence and affect cognition interactions. *Cogn Ther Res*. 1992;16:143–163.
24. Magni L, Raimondo F, Bossi L, et al. Model predictive control of type 1 diabetes: an in silico trial. *J Diabetes Sci Technol*. 2007;1:804–812.
25. Matsumoto H, Fukui Y. Pharmacokinetics of ethanol: a review of the methodology. *Addict Biol*. 2002;7:5–14.
26. Mayo E. *The Human Problems of an Industrial Civilization*. New York: Macmillan; 1933.
27. Michelson S. The impact of systems biology and biosimulation on drug discovery and development. *Mol Biosyst*. 2006;2:288–291.
28. Mumenthaler MS, Taylor JL, Yesavage JA. Ethanol pharmacokinetics in white women: nonlinear model fitting versus zero-order elimination analyses. *Alcohol Clin Exp Res*. 2000;24:1353–1362.
29. Norberg A, Gabrielsson J, Jones AW, Hahn RG. Within- and between-subject variations in pharmacokinetic parameters of ethanol by analysis of breath, venous blood and urine. *Br J Clin Pharmacol*. 2000;49:399–408.
30. Norberg A, Jones AW, Hahn RG, Gabrielsson JL. Role of variability in explaining ethanol pharmacokinetics: research and forensic applications. *Clin Pharmacokinet*. 2003;42:1–31.
31. Patek SD, Breton MD, Chen Y, Solomon C, Kovatchev BP. LQG-based closed-loop control of type 1 diabetes. *J Diabetes Sci Technol*. 2007;1:834–841.
32. Penberthy JK, Cox D, Breton M, et al. Calibration of ADHD assessments across studies: a meta-analysis tool. *Appl Psychophysiol Biofeedback*. 2005;30:31–51.
33. Renard E. Implantable closed-loop glucose-sensing and insulin delivery: the future for insulin pump therapy. *Current Opin Pharmacol*. 2002;2:708–716.
34. Robeva R, Penberthy JK, Loboschefski T, Cox D, Kovatchev B. Combined psychophysiological assessment of ADHD: a pilot study of Bayesian probability approach illustrated by appraisal of ADHD in female college students. *Appl Psychophysiol Biofeedback*. 2004;29:1–18.

35. Roethlisberger FJ, Dickson WJ, Wright HA. *Management and The Worker; An Account of a Research Program Conducted by the Western Electric Company, Hawthorne Works. Chicago.* Cambridge, MA: Harvard University; 1939.

36. Santiago JV, Clemens AH, Clarke WL, Kipnis DM. Closed-loop and open-loop devices for blood glucose control in normal and diabetic subjects. *Diabetes.* 1979;28:71–84.

37. Saoudi N, Appl U, Anselme F, Voglimacci M, Cribier A. How smart should pacemakers be? *Am J Cardiol.* 1999;83:180D–186D.

38. Steil GM, Rebrin K, Darwin C, Hariri F, Saad MF. Feasibility of automating insulin delivery for the treatment of type 1 diabetes. *Diabetes.* 2006;55:3344–3350.

39. Umulis DM, Gürmen NM, Singh P, Fogler HS. A physiologically based model for ethanol and acetaldehyde metabolism in human beings. *Alcohol.* 2005;35:3–12.

40. Widmark EMP. *Die theoretischen Grundlagen und die Praktische Verwendbarkeit der Gerichtlich-Medizinischen Alkoholbestimmung.* Berlin: Urban & Schwarzenberg; 1932.

41. Winsberg E. Simulated experiments: methodology for a virtual world. *Philosophy Sci.* 2002;70:105–125.

42. Wood MA. Automated pacemaker function. *Cardiol Clin.* 2000;18:177–191.

65

Dynamic and Systems-Based Models for Evaluating Hypotheses Related to Predicting Treatment Response

SCOTT F. STOLTENBERG

Introduction

Approaches to treating alcohol dependence are heterogeneous, ranging from group therapy in 12-step programs to pharmacotherapy. Such treatment heterogeneity is a reflection of client heterogeneity that results from the complex biopsychosocial architecture underlying multiple alcoholism types with different developmental trajectories.[39]

Although each treatment approach is successful in reducing the number of drinking episodes and the amount of alcohol consumed per episode, no single treatment approach is superior to the others in all cases. One size does not fit all when it comes to treatment for alcohol dependence. If no single alcoholism treatment is equally effective for all individuals who seek treatment, is there some way to identify those who will respond best to a particular treatment? In other words, is there some way to *personalize* treatment for alcohol dependence? Although the relevant individual differences among treatment seekers have not been fully elucidated, it is likely that at least some of those relevant individual differences result from genetic variation in mechanisms crucial to etiology or to treatment response. In this sense, alcoholism treatment providers are in the same situation as much of the medical profession in the quest for personalized medicine. In addition, although there is much to anticipate about developments in the area of personalized medicine, progress has not kept pace with the clamor. As interest intensifies in personalized medicine, it seems prudent to consider the ways in which investigators will endeavor

to make sense of often conflicting empirical results in an effort to understand complex biological systems across levels of analysis from gene to physiological systems to treatment outcome. In this chapter, an approach is presented that focuses on genetic variation in neurotransmitter systems and utilizes dynamic systems modeling to better understand the contribution of genetic variation to pharmacological treatment for alcohol dependence.

The goals of this chapter are to: (1) discuss personalized treatment and pharmacogenetics as it applies to alcoholism, (2) describe the Johnson Model of individual differences in response to pharmacological treatment for alcoholism, (3) discuss a dynamic control system model developed to examine the Johnson Model, and (4) discuss the potential for the use of control systems modeling to test hypotheses regarding the pharmacogenetics of alcoholism.

Personalized Alcoholism Treatment

Substantial efforts to identify personal traits that can inform choice of alcoholism treatment have not yet borne fruit. The most notable of such efforts is Project MATCH (Matching Alcoholism Treatment to Client Heterogeneity). Project MATCH was a large, multisite psychotherapy trial that ran for over a decade and enrolled over 1700 clients.[22] It was designed to test 21 matching hypotheses by assigning clients randomly to three treatment groups—cognitive behavioral therapy, motivational enhancement therapy, or 12-step facilitation—and measuring the associations among matching characteristics and multiple alcohol outcomes across five follow-up periods.[4] Project MATCH examined both primary (alcohol involvement, cognitive impairment, gender, meaning seeking, motivation, psychiatric severity sociopathy, support for drinking, and Babor's Typology) and secondary (alcohol dependence, anger, antisocial personality disorder, interpersonal dependency, Axis I psychopathology, Alcoholics Anonymous history, readiness to change, religiosity, self-efficacy, and social functioning) matching hypotheses.[15]

Clients in each of the Project MATCH treatment conditions showed rates of improvement, as measured by drinks per drinking day and abstinent days, similar to other treatment studies.[22] Disappointingly, Project MATCH did not succeed at identifying personal traits associated with significant differences in treatment outcomes for the three alcoholism psychotherapies. Client anger, psychiatric comorbidity, and level of alcohol dependence were some of the client traits that provided limited prognostic utility.[22]

Recently, a large trial to test alcoholism-treatment matching hypotheses was conducted in the United Kingdom.[34] In the UK Alcohol Treatment Trial, investigators conducted 3- and 12-month follow-ups on clients (n = 742 at baseline) who were assigned to either motivational enhancement therapy or social behavior and network therapy. The matching hypotheses in the UK study included (1) size of social network, (2) readiness to change/negative expectancies, (3) psychiatric severity, (4) anger, and (5) degree of alcohol dependence. The investigators found no evidence for matching effects on these client characteristics to the two types of treatment studied.

Although this brief review of personalized alcoholism treatment is not exhaustive, it does provide powerful evidence that easily observable client characteristics do not appear to be useful for matching individual clients to particular psychosocial treatments. Much of the excitement regarding personalized medicine, however, has to do with a better understanding of the biological underpinnings of disease and disorder, as well as the promise of applying this understanding to improving pharmacotherapy by informed dosage practices, increased response rates, and a reduction in the number and severity of side effects. This area, known as pharmacogenetics, is the major thrust of personalized medicine and is reviewed in the next section.

Pharmacogenetics

Pharmacokinetics is an area of focus within pharmacogenetics that studies how genetic differences influence the bioavailability of an agent.[19] Individual differences in the rate of an agent's metabolism produce variability in treatment response and may be crucial in serious or fatal adverse reactions to the medication.[27] The cytochrome P450 (CYP) enzymes are located on organelles in liver cells and are one of the most studied components in agents' metabolism. Approximately 7% of Caucasians can be classified as "poor metabolizers" on the basis of their genotype at the CYP2D6 polymorphism, which is known to be involved with the breakdown of many psychotropic medications.[27] The end result of metabolizing psychotropic agents at a slower than average rate is that higher levels of the agents remain in the bloodstream, effectively raising the dose to levels that could potentially be harmful.

Pharmacodynamics is an area of focus within pharmacogenetics that studies the ways in which genetic differences in the proteins at which medications act produce individual differences in treatment response.[19] An example of pharmacodynamic research that is important to psychiatry is the examination of the association between genetic variation in the gene that codes for the serotonin transporter and the response to depression treatment with selective serotonin reuptake inhibitors. Because reuptake of serotonin from the synapse via the serotonin transporter is the primary mode for inactivating serotonin's actions and because the serotonin transporter is the primary target of selective serotonin reuptake inhibitors, it is logical to assume that genetic variation that influences serotonin transporter function would also affect efficacy of selective serotonin reuptake inhibitor treatment.

For more than a decade, the most studied genetic polymorphism in psychiatric or behavior genetics has been the so-called 5-HTTLPR insertion/deletion in the regulatory region located upstream of the structural gene that codes for the serotonin transporter.[32] A recent search on PubMed for the term "HTTLPR" resulted in over 500 hits. The polymorphism is both functional

and common, which makes it an excellent candidate for association studies. The L allele is a high-functioning allele that results in 2–3 times higher transcriptional efficiency than the S allele.[20] Recently, investigators have been using functional magnetic resonance imaging (fMRI) to study associations between the 5-HTTLPR genotype and the activity of different brain regions. Specifically, amygdala activity in response to fearful or threatening facial expressions is greater in individuals who carry at least one S allele compared with those with the LL genotype.[11] In addition, the functional connectivity between the amygdala and the prefrontal cortex is weaker in those who carry an S allele, which suggests that those individuals may be less able to dampen amygdala activity following an assessment of the potential threat.[11]

Because the serotonin transporter is the primary target of selective serotonin reuptake inhibitors, it is of interest whether the 5-HTTLPR polymorphism is associated with a different response to selective serotonin reuptake inhibitor treatment. In a recent meta-analysis of 15 studies of selective serotonin reuptake inhibitor treatment for depression including a total of 1435 subjects, the L allele was associated with better treatment outcomes.[29]

In addition to response to selective serotonin reuptake inhibitor treatment for depression, the 5-HTTLPR polymorphism is also associated with differences in the personality trait of neuroticism,[28] suicide,[2] impulse control disorders,[21] and eating disorders.[8] It is important to note that in the context of the present chapter, a meta-analysis of 17 published studies examining the association between 5-HTTLPR polymorphisms and alcohol dependence showed that the S allele was associated with an increased risk for alcohol dependence and that this association was strongest in the presence of psychiatric comorbidity.[6]

The pharmacogenetics of alcoholism presents a complicated picture with a plethora of molecular targets for both ethanol and the medications used in alcoholism treatment. An examination of the pharmacokinetics of alcohol reveals genetic variants in ethanol-metabolizing enzymes that are associated with different levels of risk for alcohol dependence and that vary across ethnic groups.[5] The well-studied enzymes in ethanol metabolism—alcohol dehydrogenase and aldehyde dehydrogenase—clearly affect the bioavailability of ethanol and a toxic by-product, acetaldehyde. Alcohol dehydrogenase converts ethanol to acetaldehyde, which is then quickly converted by aldehyde dehydrogenase to acetate. If these two conversions take place at similar rates, levels of the toxic acetaldehyde stay rather low in the blood. However, if the alcohol dehydrogenase enzyme is fast or if the aldehyde dehydrogenase enzyme is slow, toxic levels of acetaldehyde result. The medication disulfiram (Antabuse) inhibits aldehyde dehydrogenase, and when an individual drinks alcohol while taking disulfiram, severe nausea and other aversive symptoms result. This reaction is similar to the flushing response that occurs when individuals with one or two copies of a mutant version of aldehyde dehydrogenase-2 that produces a nonfunctioning version of the enzyme drink alcohol.

The pharmacodynamics of alcohol is complicated by its many targets. Ethanol facilitates the activity of γ-aminobutyric acid A (GABA$_A$) receptors, inhibits the activity of N-methyl-D-aspartate (NMDA) glutamate receptors, and, at high doses, inhibits many voltage-sensitive calcium channels. In addition, ethanol has direct influences on neurotransmission via serotonin, dopamine, and norepinephrine neurons, and modulates opioid neuropeptides.[17] The endogenous opioid system is implicated in the rewarding effects of alcohol consumption and in alcohol craving.[35] Genetic variation at these many sites of action is likely to be responsible for variation in responses to ethanol exposure.

Both Project MATCH and the UK Alcohol Treatment Trial focused solely on psychosocial therapies and excluded pharmacotherapy to simplify the designs of such large complicated studies.[4,34] Clearly, there are biologically based individual differences that are likely to influence treatment outcome. Of interest, the Project MATCH investigators have recently begun to explore how variation in specific genes may prove to be predictive of drinking behavior and of the outcome of psychosocial treatment for alcoholism.[1] A high-risk genotype of the *GABRA2* gene (A/A) was associated with less variability in treatment outcome and higher risks for drinking and heavy drinking.

The pharmacodynamics of agents used in alcoholism pharmacotherapy is also of interest. Examples of medications used for the treatment of alcoholism include opiate antagonists (e.g., naltrexone); medications that interact with glutamate (e.g., acamprosate); modulators of both glutamate and GABA systems (e.g., topiramate); agents that influence serotonin uptake (e.g., selective serotonin reuptake inhibitors); and those that modulate serotonergic function and, as a consequence, dopaminergic neurotransmission (e.g., ondansetron). There are known genetic variants for neurotransmitter system components (e.g., receptors and enzymes) in all of these systems in which medications to treat alcoholism might act.

In this section, I provide a general description of pharmacogenetics along with a more specific discussion of the pharmacogenetics of alcohol and of medications used to treat alcoholism. It is clear that there are sufficient pharmacogenetics targets to begin examining the best candidates empirically. In the next section, a pharmacogenetics theoretical model is described that takes important steps toward the goal of better understanding how genotypes can be used to identify the most effective pharmacotherapy for alcoholism treatment.

The Johnson Model

Because both the serotonin and dopamine neurotransmitter systems are intimately involved with alcoholism in ways that are complex and not yet fully understood, theoretical models focusing on the impact of genetic variation at the level of the synapse may provide a productive approach to better understanding of the individual differences in response to alcoholism treatment. Such work combines empirical data from several different areas of study, such as human alcoholism treatment trials, candidate gene association studies, and pharmacological studies with both human and nonhuman animals. Alcoholism treatment trials can provide information regarding characteristics of subjects that are predictive of treatment response or of etiological significance. Candidate gene association studies can identify allelic variants associated with different alcohol phenotypes. The best of these candidates also will produce functional differences in the physiological systems of interest and are often targets of pharmacological agents. Pharmacological studies provide evidence regarding the effects of agonists and antagonists on system function and on alcohol phenotypes. The development of theoretical models that attempt to elucidate the impact of variation at functional candidate genes on the response to pharmacological treatment for alcoholism is an important stage in a systematic approach to personalized alcoholism treatment. Johnson and Ait-Daoud[14] presented a theoretical model that was elaborated upon by Johnson[12] and that aimed at better understanding the role of genetic variation in the serotonin transporter promoter region (5-HTTLPR) and differential response to two pharmacological treatments for alcoholism

(hereafter called the Johnson Model). In this section, I provide details of this model on which a subsequent control system model was based.

The development of the Johnson Model was motivated by the desire to better understand the contribution of allelic variation at components of neurotransmitter systems to individual differences in pharmacological alcoholism treatment response.[12,14] As such, these efforts should constitute a pharmacodynamic approach because the genetic differences examined are hypothesized to influence the proteins at which the medications act.[19]

Fig. 65.1 presents the Johnson Model schematically. The main premise of the model is that relative serotonergic hypofunction, a result of efficient reuptake for individuals with the 5-HTTLPR LL genotype, produces an upregulation of serotonin-3 receptors and an enhanced urge to drink. This heightened urge to drink is the result of dopaminergic activation due to the action of serotonin at postsynaptic serotonin-3 receptors on dopaminergic neurons.

Several lines of empirical evidence led to the Johnson Model (see references in Johnson[12] and Johnson and Ait-Daoud[14]):

1. The S allele of the 5-HTTLPR polymorphism is a common variant that is dominant to the L allele and reduces serotonin reuptake by approximately one-third via a reduction in the number of serotonin transporter proteins produced (i.e., it significantly influences serotonin neurotransmission).
2. Selective serotonin reuptake inhibitors bind to the serotonin transporter and block serotonin reuptake, thereby enhancing serotonin neurotransmission.
3. Response to selective serotonin reuptake inhibitor treatment for alcoholism is better for those with late-onset alcoholism than for those with early onset alcoholism.
4. Serotonin-3 receptors are located on mesocorticolimbic dopamine-containing neurons and are involved in the rewarding effects of alcohol.
5. Ethanol potentiates the activity of serotonin-3 receptors.
6. Response to alcoholism treatment with the serotonin-3 receptor antagonist ondansetron is better for those with early onset alcoholism than for those with late-onset alcoholism.
7. Acute alcohol exposure increases serotonin function.
8. Chronic alcohol exposure decreases serotonin function.

The primary focus of the Johnson Model was to explain the observation that for individuals with early onset alcoholism (assumed to be predominantly of the LL genotype), alcoholism pharmacotherapy with ondansetron was more effective than treatment with selective serotonin reuptake inhibitors. The efficacy of ondansetron was hypothesized to be due to its presumed effectiveness at reducing the rewarding effects of alcohol (via a reduction in dopaminergic activation due to serotonin-3 antagonism). The relative effectiveness of selective serotonin reuptake inhibitor pharmacotherapy for individuals with late-onset alcoholism (assumed to be predominantly carrying one or more S alleles) was hypothesized not to be due to serotonin-3 mechanisms. Rather, individuals with late-onset alcoholism and chronic selective serotonin reuptake inhibitor treatment were hypothesized to experience an anti-rewarding effect as a result of drinking alcohol because of a long-term inhibition of dopaminergic activity.[12]

Because of the large number of components involved in the Johnson Model and the rather complex nature of the interactions among them, a systems-based model provides a platform for systematic testing of the model's hypotheses. In the next section, I use a dynamic systems-based model to examine the Johnson Model.

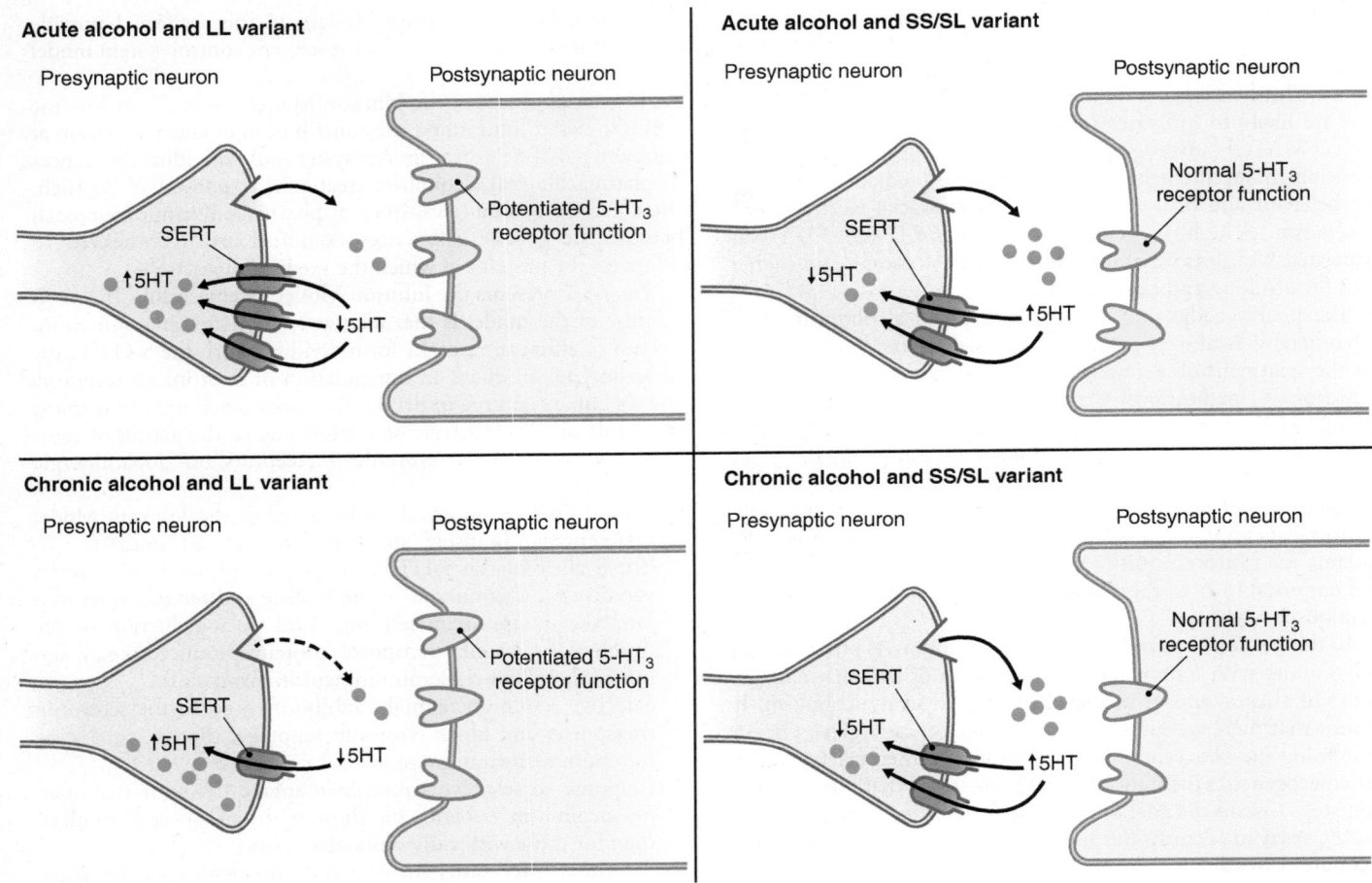

Acute alcohol and LL variant

Acute alcohol and SS/SL variant

Chronic alcohol and LL variant

Chronic alcohol and SS/SL variant

• **Fig. 65.1** The Johnson Model is a theoretical mode that has been derived from empirical observations and hypothesizes the mechanism of how variation in 5-HTTLPR genotype is associated with differences in the effectiveness of selective serotonin reuptake inhibitor and ondansetron alcoholism treatment. The LL genotype of 5-HTTLPR produces a hypodopaminergic state and potentiated serotonin-3 ($5\text{-}HT_3$) receptors on dopaminergic neurons, which results in an enhanced urge to drink. *5HT,* Serotonin; *SERT,* serotonin transporter. (Figure reprinted with kind permission from Springer Science+Business Media: Johnson and Ait-Daoud,[21] p. 335.)

A Dynamic Systems-Based Model

Although control system modeling has a relatively long history, with Wiener's influential book on cybernetics first published in 1948,[37] it has not been widely used in behavior genetic analysis. However, with an increasing focus on the mechanisms of heredity-behavior relations made possible by advances in molecular genetics and neuroscience, it seems that control system modeling is poised to catalyze significant contributions to our understanding of how genes influence behavior.

The Johnson Model is well suited for implementation as a control system model because it considers the system as a whole that can be described by the levels or rates of specified parameters.[9] Levels are sometimes referred to as "stocks" or "states" and rates as "flows." For example, in the Johnson Model, the level of serotonin in the synapse can be considered a stock and the rate of serotonin reuptake determined by 5-HTTLPR genotype can be considered a flow. Control system models are dynamic models, in that they utilize difference or differential equations to account for change over time, deriving subsequent states of the system from the current state.[9] Control system models are particularly useful

for modeling the influence of genetic differences or of pharmacological intervention on neurotransmitter system function where feedback loops are known to occur and where epistatic interaction plays a role.[31,33] It is important to keep in mind that these kinds of control system models are not intended to be exact replicas of the system being simulated. These models describe qualitative behavior of the actual system under varied parameter states that can simulate genetic variation or pharmacological manipulation. An important goal of the control system model is to help to identify leverage points—that is, components of the system that are key in controlling system function. Therefore, a complete catalog of every component of the system is not necessary. Similarly, in control system modeling there is little focus on scaling every parameter so that biological realism is obtained. On the contrary, one often works with standardized parameters so that matters of scale are de-emphasized. One is more concerned with the functional relations among the parameters than with the relative lack of biological realism.

One of the most favorable features of control system modeling using systems of differential equations is that when these equations are solvable and produce unique solutions, the toolkit of

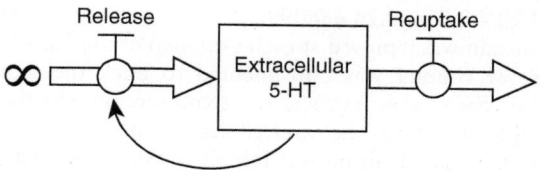

• **Fig. 65.2** A stock and flow diagram of a control system model of serotonin (*5-HT*) function. The stock of extracellular serotonin is increased by presynaptic neural activity (i.e., release) and is decreased by serotonin transporter–mediated reuptake. When extracellular levels of serotonin are above some threshold, somatodendritic autoreceptors (serotonin-1A) inhibit neural firing via a feedback mechanism. When presynaptic neural firing is enabled, terminal autoreceptors (serotonin-1B) control the serotonin release amount. The infinity sign represents an infinite reservoir for the production of serotonin.

the mathematician can be brought to bear,[33] such as fast, general-purpose differential equation solvers such as Berkeley Madonna.[38] Most importantly in the context of pharmacogenetics, one can examine the controllability of the system under study. That is, it may be possible to adjust the parameters of a system to move its functioning from an undesirable state to a desirable one.[33] In the context of the serotonin system, there is substantial empirical evidence that it is possible to manipulate system parameters either by the use of medications or by genetic techniques (e.g., constructing "knockout" lines of mice) to alter serotonin system function. Although a complete understanding of the dynamics of the serotonin system has not yet been achieved, the use of control system modeling may enable the systematic variation of parameters in silico to achieve empirically based controllability of the system. In other words, dynamic systems models such as this one may provide us with the platform on which we can build an empirically derived understanding of how to adjust system parameters with medication to move an individual's serotonin function into a desired state.

The model to test the Johnson Model[30] arose out of efforts to model presynaptic regulation of the serotonin system.[31] In that base model, presynaptic regulation of serotonin function was hypothesized to be controlled by three components, each of which varied genetically (Fig. 65.2). These components included the serotonin transporter that removes serotonin from the extracellular space via reuptake; the somatodendritic autoreceptor (serotonin-1A) that inhibits neural firing and, therefore, serotonin release; and the terminal autoreceptor (serotonin-1B) that influences the amount of serotonin released. Each of these components was hypothesized to have a high and a low functioning variant. The main outcome variable for this model of presynaptic regulation is the level of extracellular serotonin. Another outcome that can be considered is the firing rates of serotonin neurons.

As previously mentioned, the gene that codes for the serotonin transporter contains a variant in the upstream regulatory region (5-HTTLPR) that does not affect the structure of the serotonin transporter, but does affect the number of serotonin transporters produced. The S allele acts in a dominant fashion so that individuals with one or two copies (i.e., SS or SL, the low functioning variant in the model) produce fewer serotonin transporters than those homozygous for the L allele (the high functioning variant in the model).[20] The most commonly prescribed class of antidepressants, the selective serotonin reuptake inhibitors, bind to the serotonin transporter and block the transport of serotonin from the extracellular space to the intracellular space, where it can be either repackaged into vesicles for re-release or catabolized by monoamine oxidase. Lines of mice that have the structural gene for the serotonin transporter knocked out have been studied widely and have much to contribute to our understanding of pathways from gene to behavior.[7,23,24]

The serotonin-1A somatodendritic autoreceptor is a key controller of the firing of serotonin-containing neurons.[10] When levels of extracellular serotonin are elevated, the serotonin-1A receptor inhibits neural firing. This type of feedback inhibition resembles the functioning of a thermostat that sends a signal to the furnace to turn off when the room temperature exceeds some set point. Such feedback mechanisms are well modeled with control system models. A recent study reported that a single nucleotide polymorphism in the serotonin-1A gene may be functional and is associated with the response to selective serotonin reuptake inhibitor treatment for depression.[16] Both agonists and antagonists for the serotonin-1A receptor have been identified and have been used widely to study the function of the receptor. Lines of mice have been developed in which the structural gene for the serotonin-1A receptor has been knocked out. These serotonin-1A knockout mice exhibit elevated anxiety-like behaviors when compared with mice with functioning serotonin-1A genes.[26]

The serotonin-1B terminal autoreceptor controls the amount of serotonin released when neural firing occurs.[10] Therefore, the serotonin-1B receptor can be considered a second controller of serotonin release that has its effect only after the primary controller (serotonin-1A) has enabled neural firing (i.e., not inhibited firing). Both agonists and antagonists of the serotonin-1B receptor have been developed and have been used to study the function of the receptor. Lines of mice have been developed with the structural gene for the serotonin-1B receptor knocked out. These serotonin-1B knockout mice drink more alcohol and attack intruders more quickly and vigorously than do wild-type mice.[3] In addition, there is evidence in human populations that genetic variation in the serotonin-1B gene is associated with early onset alcoholism.[18]

The starting point to simulate the Johnson Model was a relatively simple control system model of presynaptic serotonin function that focused on extracellular serotonin level and rates of serotonin firing.[31] The model included three main components: the serotonin transporter, the somatodendritic autoreceptor (serotonin-1A), and the terminal autoreceptor (serotonin-1B; see Fig. 65.2). To test the Johnson Model, only the function of the serotonin transporter was varied.[30] The functioning of the two autoreceptors was held constant because these controlling system components were not part of the Johnson Model. The functioning of the serotonin transporter was modeled as having a high and a low functioning variant to correspond to the LL and S/_ (i.e., SS or SL) genotypes, respectively.

From this basic model, extensions were added to accommodate the Johnson Model (Fig. 65.3). Sixteen separate conditions were modeled that consisted of two levels of each of the following parameters: 5-HTTLPR genotype, alcoholism status, acute drinking status, ondansetron treatment status, and selective serotonin reuptake inhibitor treatment status (Table 65.1).

In the model, the flow of serotonin into the extracellular space (i.e., release) was influenced primarily by acute drinking status. In the acute drinking conditions, the release of serotonin was doubled.

In the model, reuptake was primarily dependent on serotonin transporter functioning, which was affected by 5-HTTLPR genotype and selective serotonin reuptake inhibitor treatment status and, for the LL genotype condition, chronic alcoholism status. For the LL genotype, the reuptake rate was set at 0.90, whereas for the S/_ genotype, the reuptake rate was set at 0.30. The selective serotonin reuptake inhibitor treatment condition further reduced reuptake by a multiplier, 0.20. In addition, for those with the LL genotype, chronic alcoholism further reduced the reuptake rate by a multiplier, 0.55. So, for example, the LL, chronic alcoholic on selective serotonin reuptake inhibitor treatment had a reuptake

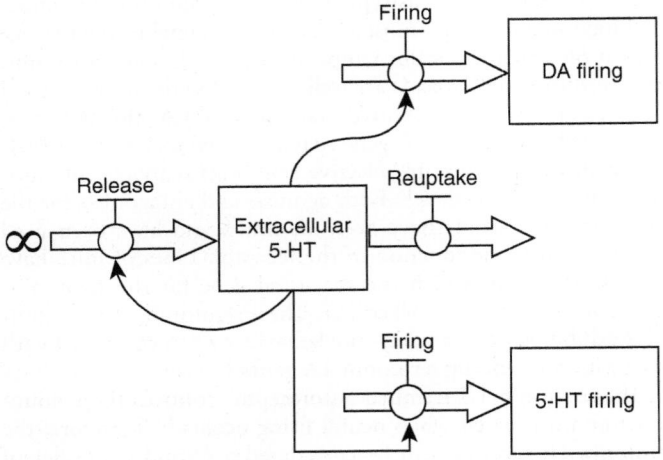

• Fig. 65.3 A stock and flow diagram of the Johnson Model. This is an extension of the basic model presented in Fig. 65.2, with additions of counters to track both dopamine (*DA*) and serotonin (*5-HT*) firing rates. Both of these firing rates are dependent on extracellular serotonin level. The infinity sign represents an infinite reservoir for the production of serotonin.

rate of 0.90 × 0.55 × 0.20 = 0.099. That is, 9.90% of the extracellular serotonin was removed at each time step of the model.

A simple counter was implemented to track the serotonin firing rate. The level of extracellular serotonin affected the serotonin firing rate. When the extracellular serotonin level exceeded a dynamic threshold, firing was inhibited (see Stoltenberg[31] for details about firing inhibition mediated by the serotonin-1A autoreceptor).

In general, the firing of dopaminergic neurons mediated by serotonin-3 receptor activation was modeled as a binary variable (i.e., either fire or not fire) with probabilities that were inversely proportional to the level of extracellular serotonin. However, when extracellular serotonin levels were very low, the probability of dopamine firing was increased, to model the potentiation or upregulation of serotonin-3 receptors. Ondansetron treatment status reduced the probability of dopamine firing by half.

One of the first steps in the modeling process subsequent to model development is model validation. It is important to test whether the model produces output that is consistent with expectations. For example, the LL genotype should produce lower levels of extracellular serotonin than the S/_ genotype because the LL genotype has relatively higher reuptake rates, which should produce a relative reduction in serotonin levels in the synapse. For the Johnson Model simulation, we can identify the S/_ genotype as the standard (i.e., 100%) and the simulation produces extracellular serotonin levels for the LL genotype that are 39% of those produced by the S/_ genotype. Similarly, modeling a selective serotonin reuptake inhibitor should produce increases in extracellular serotonin levels because selective serotonin reuptake

TABLE 65.1	Parameter Values for Conditions Tested by Stoltenberg[27]				
Condition	Genotype	Alcoholism	Drink	Selective Serotonin Reuptake Inhibitor	Ondansetron
L	0.90	1.00	0	1.00	0
LD	0.90	1.00	1	1.00	0
LA	0.90	0.55	0	1.00	0
LAD	0.90	0.55	1	1.00	0
LAO	0.90	0.55	0	1.00	1
LAOD	0.90	0.55	1	1.00	1
LAS*	0.90	0.55	0	0.20	0
LAS*D	0.90	0.55	1	0.20	0
S	0.30	1.00	0	1.00	0
SD	0.30	1.00	1	1.00	0
SA	0.30	1.00	0	1.00	0
SAD	0.30	1.00	1	1.00	0
SAO	0.30	1.00	0	1.00	1
SAOD	0.30	1.00	1	1.00	1
SAS*	0.30	1.00	0	0.20	0
SAS*D	0.30	1.00	1	0.20	0

A, Chronic alcoholism; *D*, drink condition; *L*, LL genotype; *O*, ondansetron treatment; *S*, S/_ genotype; *S**, selective serotonin reuptake inhibitor treatment.

inhibitor treatment reduces reuptake rates. In the simulation, selective serotonin reuptake inhibitor treatment for the S/_ condition raised serotonin levels to 283% of baseline. A similar increase was observed in the LL genotype condition. Ondansetron treatment should reduce dopamine firing, which it did by approximately half in both the LL and S/_ genotype conditions. Acute drinking approximately doubled extracellular serotonin levels for both genotypes. In each case, the model provided output that was consistent with expectations, which provides a measure of confidence in the model's face validity.

The Johnson Model was motivated by an interest in improving our understanding of the mechanisms by which the 5-HTTLPR polymorphism may be associated with differential outcome of alcoholism pharmacotherapy with ondansetron and selective serotonin reuptake inhibitors. One of the important results of the simulation is that the LL genotype condition shows a dramatic difference in how reinforcing alcohol drinking is under ondansetron and selective serotonin reuptake inhibitor treatment. Fig. 65.4 presents simulation data showing that under selective serotonin reuptake inhibitor treatment, alcohol drinking is more rewarding in the LL condition than it is under ondansetron treatment. Reward is operationalized as the difference in dopamine firing for the drink and no-drink conditions, such that higher levels of dopamine firing are considered more rewarding. That is, for those with the LL genotype, drinking in the selective serotonin reuptake inhibitor treatment condition is relatively more rewarding than drinking in the ondansetron treatment condition (see Fig. 65.4). It seems a reasonable interpretation that the ineffectiveness of selective serotonin reuptake inhibitor treatment for individuals with the 5-HTTLPR LL genotype is due to the reinforcing properties (i.e., capacity to activate dopaminergic neurons) of drinking. In contrast, under ondansetron treatment, drinking alcohol is not very reinforcing, which may explain the relative effectiveness of ondansetron treatment for those with the LL genotype. For those with the S/_ genotype, there is little difference in the reinforcing properties of drinking for the two treatment conditions. It may be that those with the LL genotype drink alcohol primarily for its rewarding properties, and, because ondansetron

reduces the reward of drinking, it can be an effective treatment. Because selective serotonin reuptake inhibitor treatment actually increases the rewarding effects of drinking, for those with the LL genotype, it is ineffective as a treatment. The simulation results are consistent with the Johnson Model predictions regarding ondansetron treatment.

The simulation results for the selective serotonin reuptake inhibitor treatment conditions do not lend themselves to a simple interpretation. Fig. 65.5 presents extracellular serotonin levels in both treatment conditions for both genotypes. The pattern of extracellular serotonin is similar for the LL and S/_ genotypes. Drinking raises serotonin levels across the board and, when coupled with selective serotonin reuptake inhibitor treatment, does so rather dramatically. It is worth noting that acute drinking raised serotonin to about the same level as did selective serotonin reuptake inhibitor treatment. Therefore, if an individual were to drink to increase serotonin into some target zone, the same result could be accomplished by taking a selective serotonin reuptake inhibitor. The combination of drinking and selective serotonin reuptake inhibitor treatment raises serotonin levels substantially, perhaps to levels that could be considered aversive. For the LL genotype condition, the reinforcing effects due to dopaminergic activation may outweigh such aversive feelings. Because drinking is less reinforcing for the S/_ genotype group, the elevated serotonin levels may be sufficiently aversive that drinking is reduced under selective serotonin reuptake inhibitor treatment. These data seem to fit with a craving pathway model[36] such that those with the S/_ genotype experience relief craving and those with the LL genotype experience reward craving.[30]

Such findings suggest questions that could be addressed empirically. Do individuals with the LL genotype drink primarily for alcohol's positive reinforcing effects? Do individuals with the S/_ genotype drink primarily for alcohol's negative reinforcing effects? Do individuals who drink for alcohol's positive reinforcing effects respond well to ondansetron treatment? Do individuals who drink for alcohol's negative reinforcing effects respond well to selective serotonin reuptake inhibitor treatment? Ondansetron does appear to reduce cue-induced alcohol craving[25] as well as other

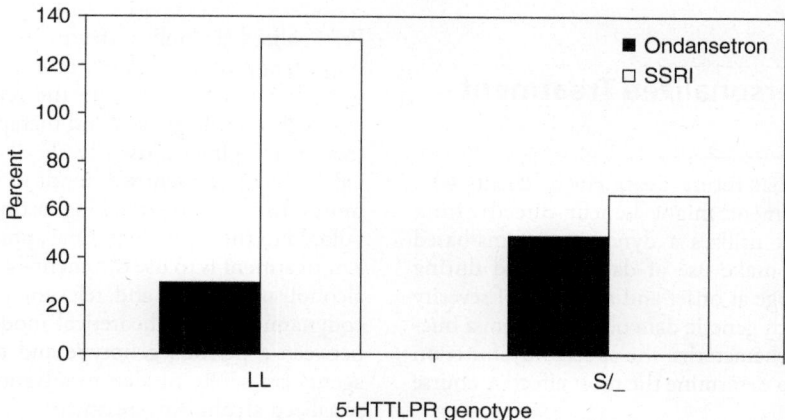

• **Fig. 65.4** The positive reinforcing effects of drinking alcohol are presented for groups defined by 5-HTTLPR genotype and treatment condition. The reinforcing effects of drinking alcohol are operationalized as the difference in dopaminergic activation between the drinking and no drinking conditions. For individuals with the LL genotype, drinking is relatively more rewarding in the selective serotonin reuptake inhibitor (*SSRI*) treatment condition than in the ondansetron treatment condition. For those with an S allele, little difference in reward is seen between the two treatment conditions.

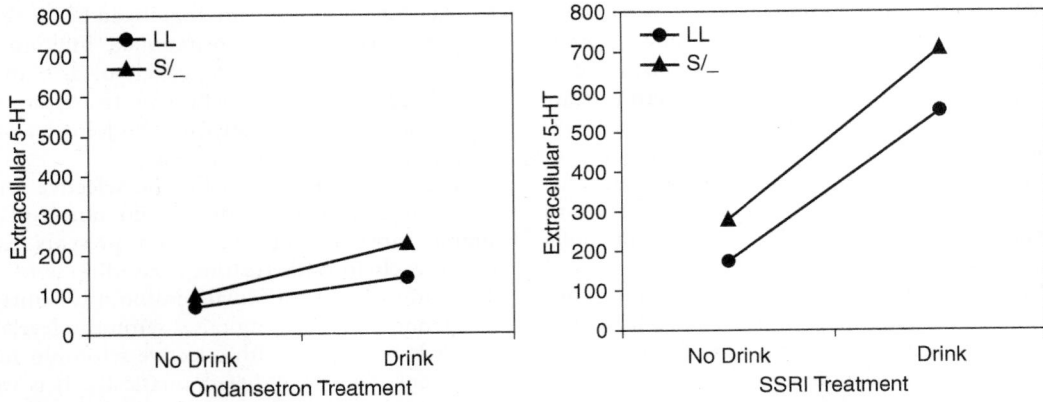

• **Fig. 65.5** Levels of extracellular serotonin (*5-HT*) across treatment and drinking conditions for groups defined by 5-HTTLPR genotype. Drinking raises serotonin levels for both ondansetron and selective serotonin reuptake inhibitor (*SSRI*) treatment, but the drinking-related increase is greater in the selective serotonin reuptake inhibitor treatment condition.

reinforcing effects of alcohol,[13] but these effects might be specific to certain genotypes or alcoholism subtypes.[13,30]

In this section, a dynamic systems-based model was described as an example of how to incorporate genetic variation into mechanistic models of alcoholism treatment. The potential for the use of such control system modeling to test and to generate hypotheses regarding alcoholism pharmacogenetics has not yet been fully realized. Models such as these enable the systematic investigation of systems that have many parameters and in which components interact, thereby making predictions difficult. Dynamic control system models are relatively easy to construct using commercially available software such as STELLA (http://www.iseesystems.com/) or Berkeley Madonna (http://www.berkeleymadonna.com/). Both of these systems enable the user to build models with graphic interfaces and do not require the user to write systems of equations. These easy-to-use software packages enable the non-mathematician to engage in theoretically stimulating model building. Increased use of such modeling is likely to catalyze an increase in our understanding of the complex genetic architecture that underlies the etiology of alcoholism and the heterogeneity of alcoholism treatment response.

Modeling and the Personalized Treatment of Alcoholism

It is reasonable to envisage that future treatment of clients who present for alcoholism treatment might benefit directly from a personalized approach that utilizes a dynamic systems-based model. Such a model could make use of data obtained during the intake interview, such as age at onset and measures of severity and comorbidity, together with genetic data obtained from a buccal cell or blood sample, to characterize the specific dysfunction related to their disorder and to determine the most effective course of treatment.

Dynamic system models enable the researcher to utilize the full toolbox developed by mathematicians for solving and manipulating differential and difference equations. One of the most important properties of such equations is that they can often be shown to be controllable. The controllability of such systems of equations is of particular interest in terms of personalized medicine. If the system is controllable, then it may be possible to adjust parameters

to move the system's current state into a desirable space. In the context of personalized alcoholism treatment, such controllability suggests that it may be possible to identify a combination of medications at specific doses that have a high probability of altering system function to, for example, reduce or eliminate the urge to drink in a particular individual. Such an approach to alcoholism treatment that is informed by biological mechanism, individual differences, and dynamic system models would be an important advance in personalized medicine.

Although the systems involved have not been characterized fully, there is no question that genetic variation plays a significant role in the effectiveness of alcoholism treatments. The use of theoretical models, such as the Johnson Model, is an important first step in an empirically based, mechanistic understanding of the pharmacogenetics of alcoholism treatment. Dynamic systems-based models are important tools for systematically investigating complex systems across levels of analysis such as individual differences in alcoholism treatment response.

Conclusions

Personalized alcoholism treatment, although not yet a reality, is an important goal for researchers and treatment providers. Currently the focus is on identifying the relevant personal characteristics that will be of diagnostic and therapeutic utility. It is thought that treatment regimens based on specific characteristics of the individual seeking treatment will result in outcomes that are more rapid, more effective, and more long-lasting than treatment regimens not tailored to the individual. One approach to personalizing alcoholism treatment is to use the client's genotype for information about alcoholism subtype and relevant pharmacokinetic and pharmacodynamic states. Theoretical models that describe the relations between a person's genotype and the action of pharmacological agents are sorely needed to advance the science underlying personalized alcoholism treatment, and the Johnson Model is a step in the right direction. The Johnson Model proposes a mechanistic explanation of differential outcomes of pharmacological alcoholism treatment based on genotype. The simulation described in this chapter advances the study of personalized alcoholism treatment by providing a platform to facilitate systematic hypothesis testing and generation. Because the systems of interest are complex and cross levels of analysis, dynamic and systems-based models are likely to be of great utility in the quest to develop a rational and systematic approach to personalized treatment for alcoholism.

Acknowledgments

This work was made possible by grants from the National Center for Research Resources (P20 RR016479) and the National Institute of Mental Health (R15 MH077654). The author thanks Dr. Parthasarathi Nag for helpful comments on an earlier version of this chapter.

References

1. Bauer LO, Covault J, Harel O, et al. Variation in GABRA2 predicts drinking behavior in project MATCH subjects. *Alcohol Clin Exp Res.* 2007;31:1780–1787.
2. Bondy B, Buettner A, Zill P. Genetics of suicide. *Mol Psychiatry.* 2006;11:336–351.
3. Crabbe JC, Phillips TJ, Feller DJ, et al. Elevated alcohol consumption in null mutant mice lacking 5-HT1B serotonin receptors. *Nat Genet.* 1996;14:98–101.
4. Del Boca FK, Mattson ME, Fuller R, Babor TF. Planning a multisite matching trial: organizational structure and research design. In: Babor TF, Del Boca FK, eds. *Treatment Matching in Alcoholism.* Cambridge, UK: University Press; 2003:15–28.
5. Edenberg HJ. The genetics of alcohol metabolism: role of alcohol dehydrogenase and aldehyde dehydrogenase variants. *Alcohol Res Health.* 2007;30:5–13.
6. Feinn R, Nellissery M, Kranzler HR. Meta-analysis of the association of a functional serotonin transporter promoter polymorphism with alcohol dependence. *Am J Med Genet B Neuropsychiatr Genet.* 2005;133:79–84.
7. Fox MA, Andrews AM, Wendland JR, Lesch KP, Holmes A, Murphy DL. A pharmacological analysis of mice with a targeted disruption of the serotonin transporter. *Psychopharmacology (Berl).* 2007;195:147–166.
8. Frieling H, Romer KD, Wilhelm J, et al. Association of catecholamine-O-methyltransferase and 5-HTTLPR genotype with eating disorder-related behavior and attitudes in females with eating disorders. *Psychiatr Genet.* 2006;16:205–208.
9. Gilbert N, Troitzsch KG. *Simulation for the Social Scientist.* Philadelphia, PA: Open University; 1999.
10. Gothert M, Schlicker E. Regulation of 5-HT release in the CNS by presynaptic 5-HT autoreceptors and by 5-HT heteroreceptors. In: Baumgarten HG, Gothert M, eds. *Serotonergic Neurons and 5-HT Receptors in the CNS.* Berlin: Springer; 1999:307–350.
11. Hariri AR, Drabant EM, Weinberger DR. Imaging genetics: perspectives from studies of genetically driven variation in serotonin function and corticolimbic affective processing. *Biol Psychiatry.* 2006;59:888–897.
12. Johnson BA. Serotonergic agents and alcoholism treatment: rebirth of the subtype concept – an hypothesis. *Alcohol Clin Exp Res.* 2000;24:1597–1601.
13. Johnson BA. Update on neuropharmacological treatments for alcoholism: scientific basis and clinical findings. *Biochem Pharmacol.* 2008;75:34–56.
14. Johnson BA, Ait-Daoud N. Neuropharmacological treatments for alcoholism: scientific basis and clinical findings. *Psychopharmacology (Berl).* 2000;149:327–344.
15. Kadden RM, Longabaugh R, Wirtz PW. The matching hypotheses: rational and predictions. In: Babor TF, Del Boca FK, eds. *Treatment Matching in Alcoholism.* Cambridge, UK: University Press; 2003:81–102.
16. Kato M, Fukuda T, Wakeno M, et al. Effect of 5-HT1A gene polymorphisms on antidepressant response in major depressive disorder. *Am J Med Genet B Neuropsychiatr Genet.* 2009;150B(1):115–123.

17. Krystal JH, Tabakoff B. Ethanol abuse, dependence, and withdrawal: neurobiology and clinical implications. In: Davis KL, Charney D, Coyle JT, Nemeroff C, eds. *Neuropsychopharmacology: The Fifth Generation of Progress.* Philadelphia, PA: Lippincott, Williams & Wilkins; 2002:1425–1443.
18. Lappalainen J, Long JC, Eggert M, et al. Linkage of antisocial alcoholism to the serotonin 5-HT1B receptor gene in 2 populations. *Arch Gen Psychiatry.* 1998;55:989–994.
19. Lerer B. Genes and psychopharmacology: exploring the interface. In: Lerer B, ed. *Pharmacogenetics of Psychotropic Drugs.* Cambridge, UK: University Press; 2002:3–17.
20. Lesch K-P. Molecular biology, pharmacology, and genetics of the serotonin transporter: psychobiological and clinical implications. In: Baumgarten HG, Gothert M, eds. *Serotonergic Neurons and 5-HT Receptors in the CNS.* Berlin: Springer; 1999:671–705.
21. Li J, Wang Y, Zhou R, et al. Association between polymorphisms in serotonin transporter gene and attention deficit hyperactivity disorder in Chinese Han subjects. *Am J Med Genet B Neuropsychiatr Genet.* 2007;144B(1):14–19.
22. Miller WR, Longabaugh R. Summary and conclusions. In: Babor TF, Del Boca FK, eds. *Treatment Matching in Alcoholism.* Cambridge, UK: University Press; 2003:207–221.
23. Murphy DL, Lerner A, Rudnick G, Lesch KP. Serotonin transporter: gene, genetic disorders, and pharmacogenetics. *Mol Interv.* 2004;4:109–123.
24. Murphy DL, Uhl GR, Holmes A, et al. Experimental gene interaction studies with SERT mutant mice as models for human polygenic and epistatic traits and disorders. *Genes Brain Behav.* 2003;2:350–364.
25. Myrick H, Anton RF, Li X, Henderson S, Randall PK, Voronin K. Effect of naltrexone and ondansetron on alcohol cue-induced activation of the ventral striatum in alcohol-dependent people. *Arch Gen Psychiatry.* 2008;65:466–475.
26. Overstreet DH, Commissaris RC, De La Garza 2nd R, File SE, Knapp DJ, Seiden LS. Involvement of 5-HT1A receptors in animal tests of anxiety and depression: evidence from genetic models. *Stress.* 2003;6:101–110.
27. Ozdemir V, Kashuba ADM, Basile VS, Kennedy JL. Pharmacogenetics of psychotropic drug metabolism. In: Lerer B, ed. *Pharmacogenetics of Psychotropic Drugs.* Cambridge, UK: University Press; 2002:157–180.
28. Sen S, Burmeister M, Ghosh D. Meta-analysis of the association between a serotonin transporter promoter polymorphism (5-HTTLPR) and anxiety-related personality traits. *Am J Med Genet B Neuropsychiatr Genet.* 2004;127:85–89.
29. Serretti A, Kato M, De Ronchi D, Kinoshita T. Meta-analysis of serotonin transporter gene promoter polymorphism (5-HTTLPR) association with selective serotonin reuptake inhibitor efficacy in depressed patients. *Mol Psychiatry.* 2007;12:247–257.
30. Stoltenberg SF. Serotonergic agents and alcoholism treatment: a simulation. *Alcohol Clin Exp Res.* 2003;27:1853–1859.
31. Stoltenberg SF. Epistasis among presynaptic serotonergic system components. *Behav Genet.* 2005;35:199–209.
32. Stoltenberg SF, Burmeister M. Recent progress in psychiatric genetics-some hope but no hype. *Hum Mol Genet.* 2000;9:927–935.
33. Stoltenberg SF, Nag P. Applying control system modelling to understand how genetic variation influences serotonin function and behavior. In: Lassau JA, ed. *Neural Synapse Research Trends.* New York, NY: Nova Science; 2007:133–171.
34. UKATT Research Team. UK alcohol treatment trial: client-treatment matching effects. *Addiction.* 2008;103:228–238.
35. van den Wildenberg E, Wiers RW, Dessers J, et al. A functional polymorphism of the mu-opioid receptor gene (OPRM1) influences cue-induced craving for alcohol in male heavy drinkers. *Alcohol Clin Exp Res.* 2007;31:1–10.
36. Verheul R, van den Brink W, Geerlings P. A three-pathway psychobiological model of craving for alcohol. *Alcohol Alcohol.* 1999;34:197–222.

37. Wiener N. *Cybernetics: or Control and Communication in the Animal and the Machine.* 2nd ed. Cambridge, MA: MIT; 1965.

38. Zahnley T, Macey R, Oster G. *Berkeley Madonna 8.0.1*; 2000. Berkeley, CA.

39. Zucker RA. Pathways to alcohol problems and alcoholism: a developmental account of the evidence for multiple alcoholisms and for contextual contributions to risk. In: Zucker RA, Boyd G, Howard J, eds. *The Development of Alcohol Problems: Exploring the Biopsychosocial Matrix of Risk. Research monograph 26.* Rockville, MD: U.S. Department of Health and Human Services; 1994:255–289.

66

Enhancing Positive Outcomes for Children of Substance-Abusing Parents

KAROL L. KUMPFER[a] AND JEANNETTE L. JOHNSON

CHAPTER OUTLINE

Introduction

Adolescent behavioral health problems are on the rise worldwide, particularly for impulse control disorders (ICDs) including substance abuse, delinquency, obesity, and HIV/sexually transmitted diseases (STDs) for genetic and environmental reasons. Contributing to these developmental issues are children growing up in families of substance abusing, depressed, highly stressed, and dysfunctional parents. Even simple things such as the diminishing number of family meals eaten together has been found to have a negative impact on adolescent's risk for substance use and negative youth development.[1,20]

Substance abuse has been a concern for many years, but recently there have been alarming rates of increasing adolescent tobacco, alcohol, and drug use worldwide, particularly in girls and women.[89] In many developed countries, adolescent legal and illegal substance use has been rising for the past 5 years.[26,25,33,51] along with concerns about youth risky consumption patterns in Europe and the United States.[11,34,35,56] In the United States, 2014 resulted in nonsignificant decreases in adolescent substance use mostly because of a decrease in marijuana use. The biggest recent increase in substance use in adolescents has been in the use of party drugs—prescription drugs, binging on alcohol, and prescription drug misuse and e-cigarettes.[73] The use of e-cigarettes is now higher than use of regular cigarettes, the use of which has decreased since 1992. Of course, teen alcohol misuse and accidents is the major cause of teen mortality. Traditional gender differences have narrowed in the United States and most countries.[89] Girls have higher rates of tobacco and alcohol use in the 8th grade; however, by 10th grade, boys generally catch up.

[a]The primary co-author, Karol L. Kumpfer at the University of Utah, was supported by Grant DA10825 from the National Institute on Drug Abuse to conduct an RCT of SFP with COAs in the United States and Canada.

The misuse of alcohol and other drugs has a significant impact on the global health and economy as well as the well-being of children and families. It is estimated that around 48% of adults worldwide use alcohol and 4.5% use illicit drugs, although only about 15% misuse alcohol and drugs.[4] The greater the consumption of alcohol, the greater the harm done.[7,148] It is of interest that Europeans have the highest amount of yearly alcohol consumption in the world: 2.5 times that of the world average.[4] Despite lower overall consumption levels in Northern European countries compared with Southern European countries, where drinking small amounts of wine with meals is common, when Northern Europeans in Nordic counties drink they display more detrimental patterns of excessive use.[111] Alcohol and other drug misuse has a wide impact on all strata of society, not just in terms of illness and disease, but also related to violence and crime rates, workplace injuries and performance, and family stability and relationship breakdown. The cost of addictions in the United States is very high and is estimated at about $2000 per person in economic costs related to lost revenue, taxes, treatment costs, criminal justice costs, fires, accidents, and other related costs.[22]

Prevalence of Children of Substance Abusers

Substance misuse by adults does great harm to both themselves and society in general. Their children are impacted as well, often negatively, because many adult substance abusers are also parents. Substance abuse is a family disease because the addict affects those who live around him or her. Parental substance abuse is a public health concern due to its high prevalence and relationship to many negative child developmental and health outcomes. Although about 10.5% of US children currently live with a parent who had a diagnosed alcohol use disorder, about 25% of US children (19 million) have been exposed to parental alcoholism at some point while growing up and about 12.7%, or 9.2 million, have been exposed to parental drug abuse.[53,154] These children might have been damaged by alcohol or drug exposure in utero or impacted by a chaotic and nonsupportive family environment.[78,100]

Children's Feelings and Beliefs About Parents' Substance Misuse

Recent studies[8,10,18] have reported on the child's perspective toward their alcohol or drug-using parents. These studies demonstrate three common themes: family role reversal with the child taking on some parental duties, keeping the family secret with a strong "Do Not Tell" message from parents, and various coping and resilience strategies such as finding supportive people outside the family, use of humor, and having goals in life.[99] These themes demonstrate the need for new approaches and interventions to support the development of children living in families where drug use is a problem. Children can feel confused and insecure when they do not understand their parents' erratic behavior and mood, which can be significantly impacted by the effect of alcohol or other drugs. Parents are often like Dr. Jekyll and Mr. Hyde—two different personalities. They tend to be more loving and humorous when using moderately, but can be anxious, paranoid, and use excessive punishment when in withdrawal from their drugs. Of course, the impact on the personality of the parent depends on the drug of choice and other mental health problems. Excessive use of stimulants can make parents more agitated and dangerous to children, whereas heroin or depressant users tend to just get sleepy and

groggy. Many children take on the parents' role for their younger siblings due to the incapacitating effects of some drugs.

Differences Between Children of Alcoholics and Children of Other Drug Abusers

There are many different combinations of substances that can be abused and patterns of parental chemical dependence that influence the lives of the children growing up in alcoholic or chemically addicted families.[72] First, the behavior surrounding the drug of choice differs. Unlike alcohol, the possession of heroin or cocaine is illegal, as is marijuana in most states. Children exposed to parents who abuse illegal drugs are also exposed to an aspect of life that children of alcoholics are not; using illegal drugs means that it is a criminal offense. The children who know about their parents' drug use must be involved in a shroud of secrecy, giving rise to a home environment that is veiled in fear, lest the authorities find out about what their parents do. Unlike alcohol, which can be consumed openly and without fear of legal reprisal (barring certain restrictions), illicit drug use/abuse requires great secrecy. For this reason, the child of an addicted parent must contend with the secretive illegal drug activity of their parent both at home and in the community. Second, unlike children of alcoholics, the AIDS epidemic directly confronts the children of addicted parents, especially if the parents are intravenous drug users. Loss of significant others due to AIDS-related illness may become more pronounced in the lives of these children. Addicted parents may have AIDS (or be HIV positive); friends of their parents may have AIDS, or babies in the community may be HIV positive. Third, the type of chemical dependence influences the type of childhood home environment, especially if the addicted parent abuses heroin or is involved with an insidious addiction to crack. Parents involved with deviant activities may invite adult friends into the home who are also involved with similar activities. The presence of adult antisocial role models is a strong possibility for children living with addicted parents. Home environment is a critically important variable in shaping cognitive skills, academic achievement, and psychosocial[55] adjustment. Deviant home environments are the source of many childhood behavioral problems.[152] Finally, the effect of the drug on the parents' behavior is profound. Methamphetamine addicts act one way, and heroin addicts another. This affects the parental role and parental behavior profoundly.

Higher Risk for Addictions

Research suggests that children of addicted parents are at 2–9 times greater risk of becoming substance abusers as adolescents or adults depending on genetic risk,[1,31,82] despite the positive and adaptive behavioral outcomes of many of these children.[56] Among adolescents, children of substance abusers misuse substances more than children whose parents are not substance abusers and escalate their use more steeply. As young adults they are more likely to be diagnosed with alcohol and drug abuse/dependence.[33] The risk for later substance misuse depends on their degree of risk factors compared with protective factors including risk factors associated with the extent of their family history of alcoholism, which includes whether one or both parents are abusers and the addiction severity, the type of alcoholism that runs in the family,[1,22,157] and the extent of their parents' antisocial behavior, health, and mental health problems. Gender differences also exist; for example, girls have increased vulnerability to the negative impact on later drug use from family environmental risks, which are high in families with substance-abusing parents.[73]

Living with a parent who abuses alcohol or other drugs can have severe effects on every aspect of a child's life, including social acceptance, mental and physical health, and school performance.[31,161] Most studies find that children of substance abusers have elevated rates of psychological symptoms.[137] Beyond risk for addictive behaviors, children of substance abusers are also at higher risk for developing emotional, behavioral, academic, criminal, and other social problems,[113,135] particularly if both parents are substance abusers, have type II alcoholism, or genetic risks such as short alleles of the serotonin transporter (5-HTTLPR) gene, and there is high stress and conflict in the family.[90] They tend to be lower on protective factors and higher on risk factors,[130] thereby increasing their risk for depression, anxiety, suicide, eating disorders, chemical dependency, teen pregnancy, and HIV.

They tend to have heightened levels of conduct problems in preschool[53] and elementary school[173] and delinquency in adolescence,[34,137] particularly if their parents also show antisocial behaviour.[146] Children of substance abusers also demonstrate elevations in impulsivity and activity level[53] as well as behavioral disinhibition,[168] leading some researchers to view them as behaviorally undercontrolled. Children of alcoholics have been found in a longitudinal study to age 23 years to employ more of a cognitive coping style and less of a decision-making coping style than children of nonalcoholic parents.[66] Similarly, children of two parents with substance use disorders tend to use aggression as a major coping style, compared with children of only one or no parents with substance abuse disorders, who use a more problem-solving, decision-making style of coping.[9] Earlier studies described children of substance abusers as higher in "difficult temperament," meaning a relatively stable trait, likely genetically linked, that led to increased emotional and behavioral liability and difficulty with behavioral control.[13] Parental alcoholism has also been linked to anxiety and depression in children,[34,151] and West and Prinz[178] have noted that children of alcoholics had higher levels of anxiety and depression than did controls in 10 of 11 published studies. Longitudinal studies up to three decades,[64] found that children of alcoholics consistently reported greater risk for stressors in the family domain of 11 life areas. In addition, they report repeated and more severe stressors into adulthood in their family.

In addition, children of substance abusers show lower academic achievement than do children whose parents are not substance abusers,[122] even in comparison with depressed children or children of divorce,[156] and they have poorer cognitive functioning in the preschool years than do children whose parents are not substance abusers.[134] Casas-Gil and Navarro-Guzman[23] have identified five variables in which school performance by children of alcoholics was poorer: intelligence, repeating a grade, low academic performance, skipping school days, and dropping out of school. Sons of male alcoholics who have many alcoholic relatives across generations have been reported to show deficits in verbal and abstract reasoning and verbal learning.[62,179] For this subgroup, Pihl and associates[142] suggested that cognitive deficits may be caused by heritable dysfunctions of the prefrontal cortex and limbic systems. However, cognitive impairments may also stem from fetal alcohol exposure,[166] high stress levels in pregnant mothers or a lack of environmental stimulation or conversely a chaotic home environment.[134] Studies[161] find that in the absence of family stress and conflict, the academic performance of boys who are children of alcoholics is similar to that of boys who are not until high school. As more thoroughly explained below, high family stress and elevated cortisol levels has been found to be related to triggering the phenotypic expression of genetic risks according to Brody and associates.[16] Hence, for both environmental and genetic reasons, children of alcoholics living with high family conflict would likely have more trouble with their academic performance.

Genetic Risks

Family, adoption, and twin studies support the heritability of addictions, which is estimated to contribute to about 40%–60% of the overall risk. This heritable influence appears not to be substance specific. For instance, children of alcoholics today are also becoming abusers of illegal and prescription drugs. Children in families with many early onset alcoholics (beginning use before 15 years of age) are at highest risk for later substance abuse or addiction because this is an indicator of type II alcoholism. Type II alcoholism is the highly heritable type of alcoholism that appears to have a heavy genetic loading as compared with type I alcoholism, which is more environmentally caused. Research suggests that about 60% of the variance in risk for an alcohol use disorder is related to genetic factors and the remaining 40% is due to environmental factors in this type of alcoholism in males.[157] However, twin and adoption studies suggest that girls are not at such a high risk. In females, only about 40% of the variance in risk for an alcohol use disorder is related to genetic factors and the remaining 60% is due to environmental factors. However, this risk increases if both biological parents are alcoholics from type II alcoholism families. Luthar and associates[118] found that similar adverse circumstances are present for children whose parents abuse illegal drugs. They concluded, however, that maternal drug abuse per se is not as damaging to children's resilience as maternal stress, depression, and anxiety disorders.[118]

Which Genes Are Involved?

Since the completion of the human genome project, there has been considerable interest in the identification of genes involved in this complex disease. Research has identified many genes that contain allelic variants associated with heritable phenotypes or characteristics that enhance vulnerability to addiction.[169] More than 1500 genes have been implicated in research to increase vulnerability to addiction. However, a meta-analysis of these studies by a Chinese research team found that only five gene pathways were involved in the four major types of drug dependency from a total of 18 statistically significant molecular pathways for single types of addiction.[112] These five pathways may underlie shared rewarding and addictive processes—that is, neuroactive ligand-signaling interaction, long-term potentiation, and the mitogen-activated protein kinase signaling pathway linked to memory and learning, and two new ones: (1) the gonadotrophin-releasing hormone signaling pathway involved in gonadotrophin secretion, and (2) stress-induced drug seeking and gap junction. They connected the five pathways into one common hypothetical molecular network for addictions. Although there are many genes involved in substance use disorder, researchers have found that the most genetically at-risk adolescents are those with one or two short alleles of the 5-HTTLPR serotonin transporter gene. They are more likely to become substance abusers,[77,129] depressed,[24] or delinquent, with lower behavioral and emotional control.[81,145] This genetic risk is not rare and is found in 40% of whites and 60% of Asians and Native Americans, making them at higher risk for substance use disorders, depression, anxiety, and behaviors disorders. The 7-repeat dopamine gene has also been linked to increase substance abuse.

Epigenetic studies of the interaction of genes and environment have found that reducing stress in genetically at-risk individuals through positive parenting can dramatically reduce the phenotypic expression of genetic vulnerability in mice[27,28] and children by 50%.[15–17] According to Uhl and associates, "The overlapping genetic vulnerability for developing dependence on a variety of addictive substances suggests large roles for 'higher order' pharmacogenomics in addiction molecular genetics."[170] Discovering the pharmacogenomics of addiction is likely to have broad implications for neurotherapeutics.

Genetic factors have been shown to influence deviant peer selection.[32] However, there is also support for interactions between genetic risk and peer influences. For example, Harden et al.[61] found that adolescents who were genetically at risk for alcohol and tobacco use were also the most vulnerable to influences from their closest friends. Park et al.[141] found that carriers of the dopamine receptor D4 long allele were more prone to alcohol dependency related to the influence of their heavy drinking sorority and fraternity friends.

Characteristics or Phenotypes of Children of Alcoholics That Increase Their Risk

Because the specific genes for addiction are only now beginning to be discovered, research has focused on identification of the phenotypes or disorders these children could inherit that increase their rates of substance abuse. Actually, genotypes do not always translate directly into phenotypes; hence, predicting later substance abuse is enhanced by monitoring the behaviors of high-risk children with many relatives who began alcohol or drug use before the age of 15 years of age.

These phenotypes or characteristics of children of substance abusers with type II alcoholism with genetic risks include higher rates of neuropsychological and limbic system deficits that include either: (1) behavioral and emotional self-regulation problems or (2) reduced executive functioning.[31] Research suggests that these two cognitive deficits are primary factors leading to reduced resilience and increase risk for addiction.[57,60]

Children of substance abusers have been reported to be genetically vulnerable to two major syndromes: (1) the overstressed youth syndrome (e.g., poor emotional regulation, difficult temperament, autonomic hyperreactivity, and rapid brain waves) and (2) prefrontal cognitive deficits in verbal and abstract reasoning and verbal learning. These cognitive deficits reduce their ability to understand that their parents' erratic behaviors are caused by drugs and not by the child's own behaviors.[120] Schuckit[157] found that alcohol smooths out the overactive autonomic nervous system stress response in children of alcoholics so that they report feeling normal for the first time in their lives. Alcohol and drugs also increase essential neurotransmitters such as dopamine, serotonin, and noradrenalin, which reduce their depression and anxiety. Hence, children of alcoholics are likely self-medicating their overreaction to stressors and depression/anxiety with alcohol and drugs. Unfortunately, the consequences of substance abuse frequently leads to increased negative consequences and more stress.

Fetal Alcohol and Drug Exposure

Of interest is that exposure to toxins like alcohol, tobacco, and other drugs in utero, appears to lead to similar neurodevelopmental deficits (e.g., prefrontal cognitive deficits and poor emotional regulation) as the genetic risks listed above. Unfortunately substance abuse by girls has been increasing dramatically since 1992;

hence, young women are attracting attention as more enter drug treatment and are mothers. They become addicted more quickly and for different reasons. They appear to be influenced more by pressures to use or by observing the use of substances by friends, peers, and family members.

The economic cost of fetal alcohol syndrome and fetal alcohol effect (FAS and FAE) is very high. Popova et al.[143] estimated that the lifetime economic costs of just one baby born with FAS in 2002 was estimated at $2 million. Chasnoff's research suggests that the damage to the brain is mostly in the last 3 months when the brain is developing rapidly. Hence, if a pregnant woman stops substance use in the last trimester, much of the brain damage can be prevented. If not, children with FAS generally have significantly reduced general intelligence, executive functioning, language-based memory, and functional communication skills, which can result in more aggression and behavioral disorders.[30] Unfortunately, more than 80% are not diagnosed appropriately when adopted or put into foster care, so they are not getting the services they need.[29]

Adolescent Drinking and Brain Development

The adolescent brain is still maturing until about 25 years. Hence high levels of drinking or drug use in adolescence can lead to brain neurotoxicity and affect cognitive development, particularly in the higher cognitive executive functioning in the prefrontal cortex. The prefrontal cortex is involved in working memory, voluntary motor behavior, impulse control, rule learning, spatial learning, planning, and decision-making (Spear[162] and White and Swartzwelder[180]). The new brain science suggests that youth who drink regularly may be delayed in brain development and not be connecting the dots about consequences that would possibly reduce their drinking in risky situations such as drinking and driving.

Two important neurotransmitter systems that undergo substantial changes during adolescence and are affected by alcohol consumption are dopamine and γ-aminobutyric acid (GABA). This damage to neurotransmitters and brain development can also affect increased depression and anxiety, and social and educational achievement. The ability to form new memories under the influence of alcohol is reduced, particularly in younger adolescents. A study of college students found that students with a history of binge drinking performed worse on memory tasks after consuming alcohol than did students without such a history.[175] Adolescents were more disrupted by ethanol in trace conditioning than adults, and adults were more disrupted by ethanol in context fear conditioning than adolescents.[63] Adolescent rats with prenatal exposure to alcohol are more impacted in fear conditioning studies than those without prenatal exposure, because of damage to hippocampal anatomy.[68]

Adolescents seem less sensitive than adults to other effects of drinking, such as impairment of motor coordination, sedation, and susceptibility to seizures during withdrawal. A study by Slawecki et al.[160] found that during adolescence an acute alcohol dose significantly altered several electroencephalography (EEG) variables in the hippocampus and other brain regions of the control animals, but not in animals that had been exposed to alcohol during adolescence. Hence, it appears they can develop a tolerance to some alcohol effects. Some positron emission tomography (PET) studies[174] suggest that the brain's recovery from dopamine depletion from substance use disorders (particularly cocaine and methamphetamine) can take up to 2 years, but luckily it can recover.

Diversity of Outcomes in Children of Substance Abusers

Although having a substance-abusing parent affects many aspects of a child's life, the degree of impact on children of substance abusers varies considerably. Although they are at higher risk, many children of substance abusers manifest few detectable or diagnosed developmental and psychological problems and do *not* develop substance use disorders.[158] The great difference in later substance use disorder rates among children of substance abusers appears related to the number of inherited phenotype risks from type II alcoholism family history and the number of type I alcoholism environmentally caused risks. In addition, girls appear to have less genetic risk than boys, but girls have slightly higher sensitivity to family environmental risks.[89,95]

The impact of parental addiction on children of substance abusers varies with degree of severity, developmental timing, and length of parental substance misuse. For example, children of active alcoholics have greater psychological distress than children of parents in recovery,[126] particularly if the parent's abuse ended early in the child's development before 6 years of age.[127] A longitudinal study by Andreas and O'Farrell[5] suggested that periods of fathers' heavier drinking patterns lead to increased children's psychosocial problems. O'Farrell and Feehan[136] found that remission after alcoholism treatment was associated with reduced family stressors, domestic violence and conflict, separation, and divorce, as well as improvement in family cohesion and caring. In addition, children were less affected by parental substance abuse if their parents had no other mental disorders.[69]

The Family

Environmental Impacts: Global Negative Impact of Childhood Adverse Experiences on Children of Substance Abusers

There has been considerable interest recently in the negative impact of early childhood adverse experiences on children's neurodevelopment and health outcomes leading to increased health care costs.[3] Parental drug abuse and alcoholism has been found, in a decade-long study by the Centers for Disease Control and Prevention (CDC) of health management organization members, to be associated with multiple adverse early childhood circumstances.[45] This same research group found that parental alcoholism and multiple childhood adverse experiences increased the risk for later adult alcoholism.[46] However, multiple childhood adverse experiences increased the risk two- to fourfold for later self-reported alcoholism, heavy drinking, and marrying an alcoholic, even without parental alcoholism. In this retrospective self-report study of over 8500 individuals, those who grew up with *both* an alcohol-abusing mother and father had the highest likelihood of childhood adverse experiences. The mean number of childhood adverse experiences for persons with no parental alcohol abuse was only 1.4, compared with about twice as many for those with an alcohol-abusing father only (2.6) or mother only (3.2). Having both parents abusing alcohol increased the risk of childhood adverse experiences almost threefold for a mean of 3.8 childhood adverse experiences. Of interest is the lack of protection from adverse experiences in the family if the mother was an alcohol abuser.

Similar adverse circumstances are present for children whose parents abuse illegal drugs.[117] These childhood adverse experiences can include exposure to frequent stressful and traumatic experiences such as abuse (emotional, physical, and sexual), neglect (emotional and physical), witnessing family violence and criminal behavior, parental divorce and separation, and parental incarceration. Hence, parental substance abuse or a family history of early onset alcoholism or drug abuse is a potent risk factor for later addiction in children.

Family Environmental Risk and Protective Factors

A growing number of family risk factors and fewer protective factors contribute to the higher rates of substance use in youth today. Worldwide, parents are spending less time parenting and supporting their children. Few parents in the United States still have a meal each day with their children, although two-thirds of children in other countries still have the main meal with their parents.[89] However, fewer children than that talk with their parents on a regular basis.[171] Living with drug-addicted caretakers, who spend about half as much time with their children as the average parents spend, increases children's stress levels.

Other research suggests that positive family functioning and parenting that reduces children's stress and cortisol levels can reduce by half genetic predispositions to a number of behavioral health disorders (substance abuse, depression, anxiety, thrill seeking, delinquency, and HIV status).[16,17] The negative impact of parental drinking on children's self-worth was mediated by family cohesion and supportive relationships, while good communication and problem-solving skills were associated with more effective parenting despite parental alcohol abuse.[39] Having a mother who is an addict or two parents who are addicted increases the risk for later developmental problems.[41] Without extended family protection and family or agency support, many children of substance abusers live in disruptive family environments. These environments are frequently characterized by family conflict, disorganization, or disrupted family rituals (meals together, bedtime rituals, holidays, and so on). The environment contributes to an already elevated sense of anxiety and stress in the children.

In families in which alcohol or other drugs are being abused, behavior is frequently unpredictable and communication is unclear. Family life is characterized by chaos and unpredictability. Behavior can range from loving to withdrawn to crazy. Structure and rules may be either nonexistent or inconsistent. Adult children of alcoholics report more parentification, instrumental caregiving, emotional caregiving, and past unfairness in their families of origin.[80]

The SEM tested Social Ecology Model of Substance Abuse Vulnerability[95] found that three factors (family cohesion, supervision and monitoring, and communication) in the family pathway were the most preventive of substance use. Unfortunately, addicted parents often fail to monitor their children's behavior. The risk for substance use associated with early pubertal maturation was found to be increased by lax parental supervision (for girls) and a family history of substance use, psychiatric problems, or crime (for boys[38]).

Not every family is affected identically. Research has shown that families that maintain certain rituals, such as holiday traditions or a Friday night pizza and movie, can help mediate the chaos of addiction. Sober parents who are able to provide stability, support, and nurturing also help to minimize confusion and strengthen children. Sometimes family life is less damaging because children rely on adaptive distancing, a technique in which the child separates from the centrifugal pull of family problems in order to maintain pursuits and seek fulfillment in life, school, and friendships.[85]

Finally, in addition to adverse circumstances within the family, parental alcoholism is also associated with elevated levels of more general negative uncontrollable life events.[34,152,163] In particular, because alcoholics are likely to have less education and lower income,[131] children of alcoholics may have fewer economic resources available to them. Consistent with their lowered socioeconomic status, children of alcoholics are more likely to report that a parent was fired from a job and that their families have financial problems.[163] Although little is known about the exposure of children of alcoholics to adverse neighborhood or school environments, their lowered socioeconomic status raises the possibility that their broader social environments may also be less than ideal.

Substance Abuse Impact on Parenting

An important, yet poorly understood, feature of drug overuse is the potential impact on parenting capacity and child health outcomes. It is known that parents who are substance users become more aggressive and/or abusive toward their child when under the influence of drugs.[184] It is estimated that 40%–80% of child maltreatment reports concern families with substance abuse issues.[35,137] Parents who use alcohol and drugs tend to be poor role models for their children, often exposing them to drug use and illegal behaviors, which may increase the risk of the children being recruited into drug use as they get older.[25] Thus parents who use alcohol or drugs have greater risk of influencing children's developmental outcomes negatively.

Although not all children are negatively impacted by their parents' use of alcohol or drugs, the task of raising a child is undoubtedly made more difficult when a parent is regularly affected by alcohol or drug use.[10] Despite federal funding and Medicaid funding for mothers' and children's residential or outpatient treatment facilities, there are still not enough treatment facilities that accept children; when they do, therapeutic programming for the children is frequently neglected. Unfortunately, there is a common notion among many substance abuse treatment programs that the parent should focus on his or her own recovery; the children are kept separated from the treatment process. This ignores the fact that the children also need preventive or therapeutic services and that improving parenting significantly reduces the parent's guilt and depression and potentially reduces their relapse.

Child Abuse Potential

The comprehensive national survey conducted by the National Center on Child Abuse and Neglect[132] found that 80% of surveyed states reported that parental substance abuse and poverty are the two major problems among child protective caseloads. Children of substance-abusing parents are three times more likely to be abused and 4 times more likely to be neglected than children from families where parents do not abuse alcohol and/or other drugs.[98] Other national studies also support these findings; between 40% and 80% of all child maltreatment cases involve parental misuse of alcohol or drugs.[35]

Compared with nonaddicted parents, addicted parents tend to neglect their children, spend about half as much time with them, and use more of a punitive and authoritarian parenting style with higher levels of corporal punishment.[101] However, these children are more often neglected rather than emotionally or physically abused. Suomi's[167] research with peer-raised monkeys suggests that neglect may be more devastating to children's brain and social/emotional development than physical punishment because neglected children feel unprotected by parents. Their levels of stress and anxiety are increased, resulting in insecurity, lack of parental bonding, and stronger peer cluster bonding; in turn, exploratory behaviors are reduced. Exploratory behaviors are needed in the development of self-control and executive functioning, but since they are reduced in stressful and anxiety-producing environments, the developmental process is perturbed.

The less-than-optimal parenting and family environments that children of alcoholics experience extend beyond the relationship between the alcoholic parent and the child. Even in infancy, deficits in mother-infant attachment have been found in families with problem-drinking fathers.[48] Moreover, parental alcoholism is associated with higher levels of parent-adolescent conflict.[12] Parental alcoholism is also associated with higher levels of exposure to family conflict and violence,[126,163] although parents are not necessarily the perpetrators of the violence.[97]

Genetic Vulnerability to Harsh Parenting in Children of Alcoholics Linked to Anger, Stress, Depression, and Negative Health Outcomes

The impact of family stress and conflict on children of alcoholics and their later drinking is complicated by genetic mediators and later environmental moderators. High levels of life stress overall is linked in adolescents to greater likelihood of alcohol use and to escalation in the quantity and frequency of their use over time.[41,66,181] However, there is less empirical support for negative affect as the mediator between stress and alcohol use in adolescents than in adults. Over time, children who receive harsh parenting develop a heightened state of vigilance for signs of anger and tend to respond with anger when they perceive anger toward themselves.[36] This negative affect leading to drinking is true only for some youths and in some contexts.[37] Anger in adolescence related to harsh parenting is associated with poorer health (e.g., autoimmune disorders, higher stress or cortisol levels, and so on) but only in youth with a genetic sensitivity to negative affect related to one or two short alleles of the serotonin transporter gene (5-HTTLPR).[153] Like the CDC's Adverse Childhood Experiences Study (ACES) results,[47] other studies found that adults reared in harsher home environments evince higher blood pressure, worse metabolic profiles, greater inflammatory activity, and higher levels of depressive symptoms than adults reared in less harsh households.[124] Hence, non-nurturing parenting leads to higher health care costs.

Resilience and Protective Factors in Children of Substance Abusers

Resilience has been defined as the achievement of competence or positive developmental outcomes under conditions that are adverse or that challenge adaptation.[121] The Resilience Framework[62] suggests that the development of resilience in high-risk children, such as children of substance abusers, is a complex transactional process between the child, his or her parents or caretakers, and their environment.

Not enough research has been conducted to understand these resilience processes. In contrast to the substantial literature on the relationship between parental alcoholism and children's psychological problems, studies have generally failed to examine the development of resilience and competent performance or positive outcomes in children of alcoholics, although some relevant work has been done on the absence of negative outcomes. Generally, these studies have sought to specify factors that protect children of alcoholics from the negative outcomes associated with parental alcoholism. For example, Werner[176] followed children of alcoholics from birth to age 18 and reported that those who did not develop serious problems had experienced fewer negative stress events, had more cuddly and affectionate infant temperaments, and had higher self-esteem and better communication skills. In a 32-year longitudinal study, Werner and Johnson[177] found that one caring adult in the child's life is a significant protective factor resulting in better adult adjustment and behavioral health.

Several studies have focused on positive family environment factors and have discovered a few protective factors or processes. Wolin and colleagues[182] found that alcoholic families who maintained consistent rituals (e.g., vacations, birthday celebrations) had children who were less likely to develop alcohol problems. Similarly, children of alcoholics whose families had higher levels of organization were less likely to initiate illegal drug use.[66]

Higher levels of family cohesion and support have also been shown to enhance outcomes for children of alcoholics. Farrell et al.[52] found that children of alcoholics showed high levels of adolescent deviance and distress when family cohesion was low, but that these effects were reduced when family cohesion was higher. Similarly, Barrera and associates[12] found that children of alcoholics in low-conflict families resembled children whose parents were not alcoholics, whereas children of alcoholics who experienced high levels of family conflict showed elevated levels of psychological distress. The notion that family cohesion and support are associated with better outcomes among children of alcoholics is consistent with the finding of Moos and Billings[126] that families in which paternal alcoholism had remitted after treatment had both higher levels of family cohesion and lower levels of psychological distress among their children. These data suggest that parental recovery may promote resilience for children of alcoholics, perhaps because the family environment also recovers. However, because these findings are from a sample of fathers who received alcohol treatment, they may not generalize to untreated families.[33]

Research has also suggested that parental supervision is an important protective factor for children of alcoholics. Curran and Chassin[41] found that consistent discipline and monitoring of their adolescents' behavior by mothers were associated with better outcomes among both children of alcoholics and children whose parents were not alcoholics. However, consistency of discipline includes monitoring and positive reinforcement and should not be taken as synonymous with punishment, which has been associated with poorer outcomes among children of alcoholics.[176]

Finally, some data point to the importance of extrafamilial influences. Ohannessian and Hesselbrock[138] found that children of alcoholics with high levels of support from friends closely resembled children whose parents were not alcoholics, whereas children of alcoholics with less peer support consumed more alcohol and had more alcohol-related problems. Thus a supportive relationship with someone outside of the family may be protective. Moreover, Jordan and Chassin[74] found that adolescent children of alcoholics who had greater involvement in positive activities outside the home were less likely to develop a substance use disorder in young adulthood. In the case of parental alcoholism, where adverse circumstances exist within the family environment, extrafamilial influences may be particularly important.

A significant protective factor to build the resiliency of children is to bolster social support networks and to increase autonomy and sense of safety. For children growing up in an unpredictable environment with parental substance abuse, improving resilience and enhancing protective factors is valuable. It seems clear that educational health care interventions presented in a supportive social environment are a useful and effective strategy for improving outcomes and enhancing health behaviors.

In summary, although little research has focused specifically on positive outcomes and competent performance among children of alcoholics, some work has been done to identify factors that predict lower levels of negative outcomes. These studies suggest that parental support and control, and family environments that are characterized by stability, cohesion, organization, and preservation of routines and rituals are associated with better outcomes. These critical family protective processes (e.g., family attachment, parental supervision and monitoring, and organization and communication) were found to be the most important protective factors of later substance use in a major cross-site study of 8500 high-risk youth funded by the Center for Substance Abuse Prevention.[166] In addition, high levels of friend support and involvement in positive activities outside the home reduce negative outcomes for children of alcoholics. Finally, it has been suggested that parental recovery from alcoholism is itself protective.

Prevention Programs Specifically for Children of Alcoholics

Most of the evidence-based programs for children from substance-affected homes identified and reviewed in the Broning and associates (2010) meta-analysis were school-based, while two were family-based and one was community-based. Most programs lasted between 8 and 14 weeks, with weekly sessions of approximately 90 minutes. Group sizes were not always reported and usually ranged from 8 to 12 children. Program content did vary, but common themes for most of the programs emerged, such as coping with emotions, problem solving, education on drugs and addiction, peer resistance, communication skills, and ways to be safe in family relations. Didactics usually included theory and practical exercises, discussion, role-play, and video material in some case.

School-Based Primary Prevention Programs

Very few prevention programs have been developed specifically for children of alcoholics.[84,182] Most prevention programs specifically for children of alcoholics are limited to school-based education programs that are relatively short in duration and conducted with small groups of students who self-identify as children of alcohol or drug abusers.[144] Although there may be many such school-based programs for children of alcoholics, according to Price and Emshoff,[144] very few of them are even described in the prevention literature and even fewer have outcome evaluations. Because of the positive research results for behavioral training models, programs for children of alcoholics are including more social competency skills training. In one of the few research-based models, Roosa and colleagues[150] found positive changes in knowledge, social support, and emotion-focused coping behavior in their 8-week, school-based program for children of alcoholics. Emshoff's[49] Students Together And Resourceful program teaches students social competency skills, and provides accurate information about alcoholism and its effects on the family. Participants reported more friends and stronger social relations, increased sense of control, and improved self-concept with less depression.

Family-Focused Prevention Programs for Children of Alcoholics and Substance Abusers

Several prevention programs for children of alcoholics and substance abusers that include a family-strengthening approach to increasing resiliency through family skills training have been developed and tested in federally funded prevention research—namely, the Strengthening Families Program[31,86] and Focus on Families.[26] Positive results have been found for the 14-session Strengthening Families Program in improving social competencies and family relationships and in reducing later tobacco, alcohol, and drug use in children of addicted parents in treatment. Moreover, this program has been culturally adapted and evaluated in separate 5-year federal phase-in designs for rural and urban African American, Latino, Asian and Pacific Islander, and Native American families.[105]

A very similar family skills training program, designed also specifically for children of alcoholics, is the 16-session Celebrating Families Program. It was tested in a quasi-experimental pilot study against a strengthening family program (SFP) and found to have as good parenting and family outcomes, but not as good child behavioral health outcomes.[100] It is currently being tested in several federal Administration for Children and Families (ACF) grants along with SFP, but outcome results are not yet analyzed. However, the providers and families do not seem to like the program as much and one state stopped implementation in favor of continuing SFP (Brook, February 2016, personal communication). Celebrating Families is much more based on Alcoholics Anonymous (AA) practices and philosophy, so possibly if parents are still in denial, they will reject Celebrating Families. In addition, the children's behaviors got worse, which resulted in a higher number of parents dropping from the program in the comparative evaluation.[100]

Community-Based Prevention Programs for Children of Alcoholics

There are very few community-based programs for children of alcoholics, but one popular one is Alateen. This self-help support program for children of alcoholics is implemented in the community through Alcoholics Anonymous. This program provides a safe environment in which children can share their feelings, experiences, and tips for surviving their parents' addictions and negative behaviors. The Cambridge and Somerville Program for Alcoholism Rehabilitation program[42] offered junior-high-age children of alcoholics or children whose parents were not alcoholics a range of after-school services at schools or in community settings. DiCicco et al.[44] found that mixing children of alcoholics and children whose parents were not alcoholics in alcohol education groups, compared with groups specifically for children of alcoholics, resulted in reduced drinking among children of alcoholics and reductions in the intention to drink in the future. Moreover, because of stigmatization issues, recruitment of children of alcoholics was easier for the basic education group than for the group that was specifically for children of alcoholics. These results suggest that prevention programs not specifically for children of alcoholics may be a valuable option for recruiting and delivering services to children of addicted or substance-abusing parents.

Family-Based Prevention and Treatment

Developmental theories support the critical role of families in child raising and suggest that supportive families are key to raising healthy children and preventing later adolescent problems. Our consumer-oriented, fast-paced society appears to have forgotten this important role for parents. Longitudinal research suggests that parents substantially impact their teens' health behaviors.[150] Although peer influence is a major reason that adolescents initiate negative behaviors, a positive family environment (e.g., family bonding, parental supervision, and communication of prosocial family values) protects youth from engaging in unhealthy behaviors, such as substance abuse, delinquency, and early or unprotected sex. These protective family factors have even a stronger influence on girls.[106]

What can be done to reduce unacceptably high levels of harmful behaviors in adolescents? Evidence-based family intervention approaches that have been found to be effective include[66]: (1) behavioral parent training (primarily cognitive/behavioral parent training); (2) family skills training (including parent training, children's skills training, and family practice time together); (3) family therapy (structural, functional, or behavioral family therapy), and (4) in-home family support. The most recent review[2,88] identified 35 family interventions. Information on these specific family interventions including program descriptions, websites, and contact information can be found at www.strengtheningfamilies.org.

Only 7 family interventions of these 35 programs met the highest level of evidence of effectiveness, or Exemplary I, which required a minimum of two randomized controlled trials with positive results implemented by at least two independent research teams with different populations.[95] These Exemplary I family programs included: Helping the Noncompliant Child, The Incredible Years, the Strengthening Families Program, Functional Family Therapy, Multisystemic Family Therapy, Preparing for the Drug Free Years, and Treatment Foster Care. A subsequent review of family interventions for substance abuse prevention for the United Nations Office of Drugs and Crime (2010) identified one other Exemplary I program—Triple P.[155] Many of these best of the best family evidence-based interventions are described in an edited book by Van Ryzin and associates.[172]

Seven programs were classified into the Exemplary II Level because they had at least one randomized controlled trial with positive prevention results. The other programs were classified primarily into the Model Level because they had only quasi-experimental research results. Some Promising Level programs were added to the list because they were programs that were based on existing proven programs, but did not yet have outcome results. Since the last expert review in 1999, additional randomized controlled trials have been conducted on existing and new family interventions; hence, this list is not complete.

The senior author developed a website for the United Nations Office of Drugs and Crime with program descriptions and contact information of all the best parenting and family programs in the world for dissemination to developing countries. So far, at least 50 high level evidence-based programs were identified from over 500 programs nominated by different governments and literature searches. A protocol for culturally adapting evidence-based family strengthening interventions has already been published from this United Nations Expert Group's work.[110]

Family-Focused Interventions for Children of Parents With Substance Use Disorders

Although a number of effective family-based approaches to substance abuse prevention have been found through expert reviews of the literature,[106,117] only a few were designed specifically for children of substance abusers and only two have been tested in randomized controlled trials—The Strengthening Families Program and Focus on Families.

The Strengthening Families Program[43,92,101] was designed by Kumpfer and colleagues in 1982 and tested specifically for children of substance abusers in outpatient methadone maintenance and mental health drug treatment centers in a National Institute on Drug Abuse randomized controlled trial testing the three different components compared to treatment as usual. The resulting Strengthening Families Program includes three 14-week sessions in parent training, children's social skills, and family relationship enhancement, followed by booster sessions every 6 months. Specific program results included improved parenting skills, confidence, and parenting efficacy, which led to a reduction in children's overt and covert aggression, hyperactivity, depression, conduct disorders, and improved social competencies. Family relationships (organization, cohesion, communication, conflict) were significantly improved. Decreases in substance use in both the parents and older children were also revealed. Moreover, this program has been culturally adapted and evaluated by independent researchers for rural and urban African American, Latino, Asian and Pacific Islander, and Native American families with positive program outcomes including a 40% improvement in recruitment and retention for culturally tailored programs.[94,104] In a National Institute on Alcoholism and Alcohol Abuse (NIAAA) randomized controlled trial (RCT) with children of alcohol abusers in Canada and the United States, positive results were found for behavioral and social outcomes in the children of alcoholics.[119] Other RCTs have reported positive program results for different age-adaptations of SFP (SFP 0-3, 3-5, 6-11, 12-16 years) in elementary school-aged rural children,[96,107] junior high school rural children,[165] and inner-city 7- to 11-year-olds.[59]

One 10-year study followed participants to the age of 22 years and found a two- to threefold reduction in lifetime diagnosis of anxiety, social phobia, depression, and personality disorders when compared with their no-treatment controls.[165] Another 10-year follow-up study of genetically at-risk African American students completing a culturally adapted version of SFP 10-14, called Strengthening African American Families (SAAF) in RCT schools, found a 50% reduction in diagnosed substance abuse, depression, anxiety, thrill seeking, and HIV status.[16,17] This human epigenetic study with humans replicated the finding with mice that nurturing parenting can dramatically reduce the phenotypic expression of substance abuse in children with risky genes.

Recently, a Cochrane Collaboration and World Health Organization meta-analysis of universal alcohol prevention programs in schools[45] found that a 7-session Strengthening Families Program for 10- to 14-year-olds[108] was twice as effective in reducing alcohol use as any other school-based intervention having at least 2 years of follow-up data. A cost-benefit analysis showed a return of $9.60 for every dollar spent by the school when they implemented the Strengthening Families Program for 10- to 14-year-olds.[164] Because of these positive results, the Strengthening Families Program has been adopted for replication and evaluation in seven countries in Europe, including four that have 1–2 years of pre- to posttest outcome results—Spain,[140] The Netherlands,[139] Sweden,[80] and the United Kingdom.[54]

The second program, Focus on Families,[26] was also developed for children of parents in methadone maintenance treatment. This program found reductions in relapse for the parents but no significant improvement in the children.[25] Zucker and associates[119a] found positive results on children's prosocial skills at a 6-month follow-up after the fathers or both parents participated in a 12-session behavioral parenting program tested with fathers arrested for drunk driving.

Two other programs have been designed for children of substance abusers and show promising preliminary nonexperimental research results—Celebrating Families and Nurturing Program for Families in Substance Abuse Treatment and Recovery. Designed to prevent child maltreatment in children of alcoholics, the 15-session Celebrating Families has been found to improve family reunification rates from 37% to 72% for children of alcoholics removed by child protective services[148] as well as to reduce the number of days to reunification. Positive changes in knowledge, coping skills, decision-making, and feelings expression were also reported for the program.[76] Using the same evaluation instruments as those used for the Strengthening Families Program, Celebrating Families reported similarly positive effects at posttest on several outcome measures: improving parenting skills, family organization, communication, and cohesion. The child outcomes were mixed, however, and only two positive child outcomes were reported (reduced depression and concentration problems). The study also reported a nonsignificant positive trend for social skills, and three negative iatrogenic effects, namely for overt and covert aggression and hyperactivity.[91] A longitudinal study is necessary, as children of substance abusers have been observed to increase their negative acting-out behaviors when their parents enter treatment. Some suggest that these children act out because they feel safer to do so. Finally, research on 170 mothers participating in the Nurturing Program[21] suggested improved parenting attitudes at posttest on the Adult-Adolescent Parenting Inventory and reduced relapse.[130]

Prevention programs not specifically designed for children of substance abusers may also be effective if they have core content demonstrated to be effective in reducing mediating factors for later substance abuse in children of substance abusers. For example, Chassin and associates[31] have discussed necessary core content for children of alcoholics that includes content that increases children's alcohol and drug awareness, social competencies, awareness of feelings, emotional and behavioral control, and reducing depression. With the exception of Zucker's intervention,[119a] most family-based programs for children of substance abusers are family skills training programs that typically include the parent training component and not children's skills training or family skills training utilizing a standard dosage between 14 and 17 sessions. Shorter programs are not as effective in attaining behavioral changes in addicted families.

Reviews of prevention programs for children of alcoholics and substance abusers[31,40,146] have expressed the need for additional research on etiology and effective prevention programming as available outcome studies are dated. Ethical and practical issues in designing, implementing, and evaluating programs for children of substance users are discussed in several publications.[b]

Core Content of Effective Family Programs

Effective family programs involve the whole family (rather than just the parents or children) in interactive, skills, or behavior change processes, rather than involving them in didactic educational lessons. The underlying psychological theories include behavioral psychology and/or family systems theory,[116] which stress the importance of the engagement process and reducing barriers to attendance through relationship building; personal invitations; provision of meals, childcare, and transportation, and sometimes, paying families for their time. Most effective programs

[b]References 39, 49, 72, 79, 87, 121, 146.

begin with sessions designed to improve positive feelings in the family through positive reframing or skills exercises stressing family strengths. Engagement in structured methods for communication and discipline techniques are also practiced once positive family feelings are increased. O'Farrell and Fals-Stewart[135] have found that behavioral couples therapy reduces domestic violence, which indirectly benefits the couple's children. Hence, behavioral couples therapy should be expanded to include children of substance abusers to improve outcomes. An affectionate parent-child bond has a protective effect on later drug use[19]; hence, therapeutic interventions that strengthen parent and child bonding are recommended, particularly when there is already stress from the generation gap or differential generational acculturation in immigrant families.

Kaminski and associates[76] at the Centers for Disease Control and Prevention have analyzed the critical core components of evidence-based family intervention programs from 77 studies of programs for 0 to 7-year-olds. Because the presence of conduct disorders in early life often precedes later delinquent, aggressive, and risky behaviors in adolescence, they reasoned that effective parenting could reverse this trend. The core components of effective parenting and family interventions are: (1) the format should include practice time for the parents with their children in the sessions with the therapists or group leaders available for coaching; (2) during family sessions, parents should be taught to interact positively with children (such as showing enthusiasm and attention for good behavior and letting the child take the lead in play activities); (3) parenting content should include increasing attention and praise for positive children's behaviors, children's normal development to make expectations realistic for children's behaviors, positive family communication including active listening and reducing criticism and sarcasm, and effective and consistent discipline including time-outs; (4) children's content should include teaching children social skills for how to get along better with parents, peers, and teachers in a more respectful manner; and (5) home practice assignments should be assigned and encouraged to improve generalization of new behaviors at home. Additional reviews of the literature on effective family strengthening approaches have also supported these findings[97,110] (Office of Juvenile Justice & Delinquency Prevention, Strengthening America's Families Web site, www.strengtheningfamilies.org; United Nations Office of Drugs and Crime Web site, www.unodc.org/unodc/en/prevention/index.html).

Effective Prevention Programs

Kumpfer and Hopkins[101] have stressed preventive approaches for prevention programs for children of alcoholics and substance abusers that include emphasizing the negative consequences of alcohol; developing in youth an increased sense of responsibility for their own success; helping them to identify their talents; motivating them to dedicate their lives to helping society rather than feeling that their only purpose in life is to be consumers; providing realistic appraisals and feedback for youth rather than graciously building up their self-esteem; stressing multicultural competence in an ever-shrinking world; encouraging and valuing education and skills training; increasing cooperative solutions to problems rather than competitive or aggressive solutions, and increasing a sense of responsibility for others and caring for others.

Research-based prevention interventions developed for other high-risk youth can also be very effective for children of alcoholics if they address risk factors for children of alcoholics (described earlier) including externalizing problems, internalizing problems, and cognitive deficits or delays. Here we summarize prevention interventions not specifically for children of alcoholics that may be capable of strengthening resilience to later alcohol and drug use among children of alcoholics, organized by their targeted risk factors.

Programs That Increase Behavioral Control and Social Competency

A number of preventive interventions have been developed that are helpful in increasing social competencies, emotional management, and behavioral control, and these may be useful for children of alcoholics who manifest conduct disorders and aggression. When applied universally in classrooms,[14,69] these programs can reduce conduct problems, promote healthier friendships with prosocial children, and hence prevent substance abuse and violence. They are effective without the children having to be identified as children of alcoholics or drug abusers. Some of the indicated prevention programs, however, do require that the teacher refer children with aggressive tendencies and conduct disorders to a pull-out group. Because of possible negative contagion and labeling effects, it is best also to include socially skilled youth in the group.

Programs to Increase Emotional Resilience, Happiness, Self-Esteem, and Humor

Research on resilience in children of alcoholics[114,178,183] suggests that hopefulness, happiness, and emotional management increase positive outcomes in children of alcoholics. Universal prevention programs that support improved mental health and resilience also help children of alcoholics. One universal, school-based resilience program is the Strengthening Families Program for 10- to 14-year-olds,[108] which was first developed in Iowa with National Institute on Drug Abuse and National Institute of Mental Health funds. It is a 7-session parent, child, and family intervention for middle school students. Because resilience studies with adult children of alcoholics have found that meaning or purpose in life is the most critical resilience factor in positive life adaptation, this new Strengthening Families Program focused the first sessions on parents supporting children in developing dreams and goals.[115] Depression is reduced by having children and their parents focus on hopefulness and positive dreams for the future. Youth are encouraged to think about their talents and the ways that they can use these talents to help others through kind acts and a productive and successful career. Positive psychology[158] suggests that feelings of well-being are more enhanced by doing kindness to others than by doing nice things for oneself. Children of alcoholics who are resilient are youth who have meaningful roles in their families to help others, or the characteristic of required helpfulness, found in resilience research. Hence, parenting and family skills training programs that teach parents to negotiate chores, create chore charts, and monitor and reward completion of chores help to increase positive self-concept and increase happiness.

Programs for Emotional Management and the Awareness of Feelings

Because children of alcoholics have a higher likelihood of having alexithymia, an inability to identify feelings, most programs for children of alcoholics focus on feelings identification training and on training parents to label feelings that the child appears to be having. This intervention may also help to promote stronger parent-child attachments.[48] Anxiety in children of alcoholics can be reduced through increased predictability of the family environment as well as the school and community environment through family strengthening prevention programs that increase family organization, family management, and expression of supportiveness and love. Children of alcoholics often do have realistic reasons to be worried about their parents' welfare, their welfare, and the stability of the family, because child abuse and neglect,[98] job loss and poverty, divorce, and parent deaths are more common.[163] Emotion-focused and problem-focused coping skills training within prevention programs for children of alcoholics[134] can help children to talk through feelings, reframe the negative aspects of the situations, create emotional distance from their fears, and develop other emotional supportive relationships with other adults. Mentoring and after-school programs can be very helpful to children of alcoholics in developing these needed supportive relationships with other caring adults. As found by Jordan and Chassin,[74] involvement in positive activities outside the home by young children of alcoholics tends to reduce the likelihood of a substance use disorder in young adults.

Programs to Increase Cognitive Resilience Characteristics

Research with children of alcoholics[72,177] has found that cognitive resilience characteristics include a conceptual understanding of the parents' disease and relationships, the capability of distancing oneself from the alcoholic parents in terms of identification, humor, and academic skills and mastery. Both traditional educational programs for children of alcoholics and community media campaigns can be used to promote these resilience factors.

Programs for Educational Interventions, Screening, and Referral

Children of substance abusers, as well as their parents, should know the results of the risk and resilience research on children of alcoholics. They need to know what signs and symptoms to watch for that might indicate that they or their children are high or low in resilience or in risk factors. Research demonstrates that children of substance abusers who are aware of their risk status drink significantly less than those who are unaware of their risk status.[84] Public media and education campaigns could be developed that will disseminate this research and allow children of substance abusers to conduct risk and resilience assessments for themselves. They need to know that a high tolerance for alcohol and being able to "drink others under the table" is not a good sign. Public education campaigns are also needed to reduce stigma and provide additional legal, social, educational, and academic supports for children of alcoholics in a nonstigmatizing environment. Parents and youth should be informed that living with an alcoholic parent can, in fact, lead to increased cognitive, behavioral, and emotional management. Increased stress-coping competencies can improve the ability of children of alcoholics to function in very stressful careers and in times of distress, thereby improving pride and self-confidence and reducing the fear of a self-fulfilling prophecy.

Summary of Recommendations for Future Research and Policy Improvements

The most obvious implication from this review points toward the need for better longitudinal research. Most studies on children of alcoholics or other drug abusers are not longitudinal; that is, they examine behavior at one point in time. From these studies, it is unclear whether we see true deficits or merely developmental delay. Longitudinal studies allow us to predict when early disorders and behavioral deviations will be transient or when they will be precursors to more severe types of maladaptive behavior. Longitudinal research would also enable us to explain specific childhood outcomes. Differences in outcome could be studied simultaneously to understand whether antecedents discovered for one outcome are specific to it or are general antecedents leading to a broad variety of outcomes. The second implication from this review is the need also to understand the characteristics of resilient children in order to apply these protective factors in our campaign messages. Researchers and helping professionals have long identified a subgroup of children who grow up in homes with alcoholic parents and seem to be relatively invulnerable to the detrimental effects of familial alcoholism. The research focusing on this subgroup is scarce. Anthony[6] suggested that there may be subgroups of children of substance abusers who, despite all odds, do, in fact, enjoy good health from birth, experience a positive environment at home, and develop rather normally into socialized, competent, and self-confident individuals. Certain individuals may be more competent in adapting to stressful living environments than others. These children are somehow able to compensate and cope with the various negative biological or environmental influences in their lives. Certain individuals may be able to manipulate their environment by choosing roles and goals in life that stabilize their developmental process and bring them the positive reinforcement they need to develop a positive self-image and, eventually, a relatively healthy life. Other individuals may be able to master the processing of incoming data and to conceptualize these data in such a way as to choose positive behaviors in life that compensate for whatever problems present. Finally, a list of policy recommendations, modified from a more extensive discussion by Chassin and associates,[31] point the way toward future social responsibility:

1. International and local national agencies and institutes should develop research programs and support the implementation of evidence-based and family-focused prevention programs for children of substance abusers.
2. Policymakers within international, federal, state, and local governments should provide adequate funds for research, field tests, and wide-scale dissemination of effective prevention approaches for children of alcohol and drug abusers.
3. National surveys should include information that assesses and evaluates precursors of substance abuse such as risk and protective factors including strength-based behaviors.
4. Research on evidence-based interventions for the prevention and treatment of substance abuse in high risk children of substance abusers should include funding for development and testing of the generic or original evidence-based interventions (EBIs) compared to culturally adapted EBIs that have been found to improve recruitment and retention of culturally diverse populations.[105]

5. To reduce the cost of dissemination of evidence-based interventions, federal and foundation funding should be provided to develop and test EBI content delivered using lower cost mass digital delivery on TV, DVDs, You Tube, computer apps, and smart phones.

6. Cost-benefit analyses should include the actually costs of program delivery in schools and not exclude the time of teachers to deliver school-based EBIs when they include staff implementation costs for family interventions. In addition, benefits to the whole family for family EBIs should be included in cost-benefit analyses, rather than just to benefit the child.

7. Legislation affecting agencies providing services to children of substance abusers should include language that specifically stipulates the importance of funding effective and evidence-based prevention approaches that include parenting and family skills training programs.

8. Future research should maintain the privacy and confidentiality of children of addicted parents enrolled in prevention, education, and intervention programs.

9. Interagency collaboration is essential if public policy related to children of substance abusers is going to shift.

10. Effective prevention programs for children of alcoholics and children of alcoholics and other addicts should start early to help prevent damage to the developing child and provide them with all the benefits for a happy and healthy life as other children have. This included reducing the use of tobacco, alcohol, and other drugs in pregnant women and educating them on the dangers of use during pregnancy.

References

1. Adger H. Children in alcoholic families: family dynamics and treatment issues. In: Abbott S, ed. *Children of Alcoholics: Selected Readings*. vol. II. Rockville, MD: National Association of Children of Alcoholics; 2000:385–395.

2. Alvarado R, Kumpfer KL. Strengthening Americas families. *Juv Justice*. 2000;7(2):8–18.

3. Anda RF, Brown DW, Dube SR, Bremner JD, Felitti VJ, Giles WH. Adverse childhood experiences and chronic obstructive pulmonary disease in adults. *Am J Prevent Med*. 2008;34(5): 396–403.

4. Anderson P, Baumberg B. *Alcohol in Europe: a Public Health Perspective*. London.

5. Andreas JB, O'Farrell TJ. Longitudinal associations between fathers' heavy drinking patterns and children's psychosocial adjustment. *J Abnormal Child Psychol*. 2007;35:1–16.

6. Anthony E. Children at psychiatric risk. *The Child in His Family*. vol. 3. New York, NY: Wiley; 1974.

7. Babor TF, Caetano R, Casswell S, Edwards G, Giesbrecht N, Graham K, et al. *Alcohol: No Ordinary Commodity. Research and Public Policy*. Oxford.

8. Bancroft A, Wilson S, Backett-Milburn K, et al. *Risk and Resilience: Older Children of Drug and Alcohol Misusing Parents*. New York: Joseph Rowntree Foundation; 2004.

9. Barco J, Reynolds M, Gao Z, Kirisci L. *Tarter R Parents' Substance Use Disorder Affects Children's Coping Styles*. San Francisco, CA.

10. Barnard M. Between a rock and a hard place: the role of relatives in protecting children from the effects of parental drug problems. *Child Fam Soc Work*. 2003;8:291–299.

11. Barnard M, McKeganey N. The impact of parental problem drug use on children: what is the problem and what can be done to help? *Addiction*. 2004;99(5):552–559.

12. Barrera Jr M, Rogosch F, Chassin L. Social support and conflict among adolescent children of alcoholics. *J Personality Social Psychol*. 1993;64:602–613.

13. Blackson TC, Tarter R, Loeber R, Ammerman R, Windle M. The Influence of paternal substance abuse and difficult temperament in fathers and sons on sons' disengagement from family to deviant peers. *J Youth Adolesc*. 1996;25:25–37.

14. Botvin G. Preventing adolescent drug abuse through life skills training: theory, evidence of effectiveness, and implementation issues. In: Hansen WB, Giles SM, Fearnow-Kenney MD, eds. *Improving Prevention Effectiveness*. Greensboro, NC: Tanglewood Research; 2000:141–154.

15. Brody GH, Beach SR, Philibert RA, et al. Parenting moderates a genetic vulnerability factor in longitudinal increases in youths' substance use. *J Consult Clini Psychol*. 2009;77:1–11.

16. Brody GH, Chen YF, Beach SR, et al. Differential sensitivity to prevention programming: a dopaminergic polymorphism-enhanced prevention effect on protective parenting and adolescent substance use. *Health Psych*. 2014;33(2):182–191.

17. Brody GH, Chen Y-f, Kogan SM, et al. Family-centered program to prevent substance use, conduct problems, and depressive symptoms in Black adolescents. *Pediatrics*. 2012;129(1):108–115.

18. Bröning S, Kumpfer K, Kruse K, et al. Selective prevention programs for children from substance-affected families: a comprehensive systematic review. *Subst Abuse Treat Prev Policy*. 2012;7:23.

19. Brook DW, Brook JS, Rubenstone E, Zhang C, Singer M, Duke MR. Alcohol use in adolescents whose fathers abuse drugs. *J Addict Dis*. 2003;22(1):11–34.

20. Buehler C, Gerard JM. Cumulative family risk predicts increases in adjustment difficulties across early adolescence. *J Youth Adoles*. 2013;42(6):905–920.

21. Camp JM, Finkelstein N. Parenting training for women in residential substance abuse treatment: results of a demonstration project. *J Subst Abuse Treat*. 1997;14(5):411–422.

22. Cartwright WS. Cost-benefit analysis of drug treatment services: review of the literature. *J Ment Health Policy Econ*. 2000;3: 11–26.

23. Casas-Gil MJ, Navarro-Guzman JI. School characteristics among children of alcoholic parents. *Psychol Rep*. 2002;90(1): 341–348.

24. Caspi A, Sugden K, Moffitt TE, et al. Influence of life stress on depression: moderation by a polymorphism in the 5-HTT gene. *Science*. 2003;301:386–389.

25. Catalano RF, Gainey RR, Fleming CB, Haggerty KP, Johnson NO. An experimental intervention with families of substance abusers: one-year follow-up of the focus on families project. *Addiction*. 1999;94(2):241–254.

26. Catalano RF, Haggerty KP, Gainey RR, Hoppe MJ. Reducing parental risk factors for children's substance misuse; preliminary outcomes with opiate-addicted parents. *Subst Use Misuse*. 1997;32(6):699–721.

27. Champagne F. *Epigenetic Influences of Social Interaction Across the Lifespan. Developmental Psychobiology. Wiley Intersci*. 2010. online publication www.interscience,wiley.com.

28. Champagne FA, Meaney MJ. Transgenerational effects of social environment on variations in maternal care and behavioral response to novelty. *Behavioral Neurosci*. 2007;111(6):1353–1363.

29. Chasnoff IJ, Wells AM, King L. Misdiagnosis and missed diagnoses in foster and adopted children with prenatal alcohol exposure. *Pediatrics*. 2015;135(2):2014–2171.

30. Chasnoff IJ, Wells AM, Telford E, Schmidt C, Messer G. Neurodevelopmental functioning in children with FAS, pFAS, and ARND. *J Develop Behavioral Pediatr*. 2010;31(3):192–201.

31. Chassin L, Carle A, Nissim-Sabat D, Kumpfer KL. Fostering resilience in children of alcoholic parents. In: Maton KI, ed. *Investing in Children, Youth, Families, and Communities: Strengths-Based Research and Policy*. Washington DC: APA Books; 2004.

32. Chassin L, Lee M, Cho Y-I, et al. Testing multiple levels of influence in the intergenerational transmission of alcohol disorders from a developmental perspective: the example of alcohol use promoting peers and m-opioid receptor M1 variation. *Develop Psychopathol.* 2012;12(24):953–967.

33. Chassin L, Pitts S, DeLucia C. A longitudinal study of children of alcoholics: predicting young adult substance use disorders, anxiety, and depression. *J Abnormal Psychol.* 1999;108:106–119.

34. Chassin L, Rogosch F, Barrera Jr M. Substance use and symptomatology among adolescent children of alcoholics. *J Abnormal Psychol.* 1991;100:449–463.

35. Child Welfare League of America [CWLA]. *State Child Welfare agency Survey.* Washington, DC: Child Welfare League of America; 2003.

36. Cicchetti D, Rogosch FA. Adaptive coping under conditions of extreme stress: Multilevel influences on the determinants of resilience in maltreated children. In: Skinner EA, Zimmer-Gembeck MJ, eds. *New Directions for Child and Adolescent Development: No. 124. Coping and the Development of Regulation.* San Francisco, CA: Jossey-Bass; 2009:47–59.

37. Colder CR, Chassin L, Lee MR, Villalta IK. (2010). Developmental perspectives: affect and adolescent substance use. In Kassel JD, ed. *Substance Abuse and Emotion.* Washington, DC: American Psychological Association; 2010:109–135.

38. Costello EJ, Sung M, Worthman C, Angold A. (2007) Pubertal maturation and the development of alcohol use and abuse. *Drug Alcohol Depend.* 2007;88:S50–S59.

39. Coyle JP, Nochajski T, Maguin E, et al. (2009). An exploratory study of the nature of family resilience in families affected by parental alcohol abuse. J Fam Issues. 2009;30(12):1606–1623.

40. Cuijpers P. Effective ingredients of school-based drug prevention programs: a systematic review. *Addict Behav.* 2002;27:1009–1023.

41. Curran P, Chassin L. A longitudinal study of parenting as a protective factor for children of alcoholic fathers. *J Studies Alcohol.* 1996;57:305–313.

42. Davis RB, Wolfe J, Orenstein A, et al. Intervening with high risk youth: a program model. *Adolescence.* 1994;29:763–774.

43. DeMarsh JP, Kumpfer KL. Family-oriented interventions for the prevention of chemical dependency in children and adolescence. In: Ezekoye S, Kumpfer K, Bukoski W, eds. *Childhood and Chemical Abuse: Prevention and Intervention.* New York: Haworth; 1985:117–151.

44. DiCicco L, Davis RB, Hogan J, MacLean A, Orenstein A. Group experiences for children of alcoholics. *Alcohol Health Res World.* 1984;8:20–24.

45. Dube SR, Anda RF, Felitti VJ, Croft JB, Edwards VJ, Giles WH. Growing up with parental alcohol abuse: exposure to childhood abuse, neglect, and household dysfunction. *Child Abuse Neglect.* 2001;25:1627–1640.

46. Dube SR, Anda RF, Felitti VJ, Edwards VJ, Croft JB. Growing up with parental alcohol abuse: adverse childhood experiences and personal alcohol abuse as an adult. *Addict Behav.* 2002;27(5): 715–725.

47. Dube SR, Fairweather D, Pearson WS, Felitti VJ, Anda RF, Croft JB. Cumulative childhood stress and autoimmune diseases in adults. *Psychosomatic Med.* 2009;71:243–250.

48. Eiden R, Leonard K. Paternal alcohol use and the mother-infant relationship. *Develop Psychopathol.* 1996;8:307–323.

49. Emshoff JG. A preventive intervention with children of alcoholics. *Prevent Human Services.* 1990;7:225–253.

50. Reference deleted in review.

51. European Monitoring Center for Drugs and Drug Addiction (EMCDDA, 2012). 2012 Annual report on the state of the drugs problem in Europe. *Portugal:Lisbon*; 2012. ISBN/ISSN:1609–6150. Found on http://www.emcdda.europa.eu/publications/annual-report/2012.

52. Farrell MP, Barnes GM, Banerjee S. Family cohesion as a buffer against the effects of problem-drinking fathers on psychological distress, deviant behavior, and heavy drinking in adolescents. *J Health Social Behav.* 1995;36:377–385.

53. Fitzgerald H, Sullivan L, Ham H, et al. Predictors of behavior problems in three-year-old sons of alcoholics: evidence for the onset of risk. *Child Develop.* 1993;64:110–123.

54. Foxcroft D, Allen D, Coombes L. Adaptation and Implementation of SFP 10–14 Years for U.K. *Abstract Submitted to Society for Prevention Research, San Antonio, May 2005.* Oxford, UK: School of Health and Social Care, Oxford Brookes University; 2005.

55. Foxcroft DR, Ireland D, Lister-Sharp DJ, Lowe G, Breen R. Longer-term Primary prevention for alcohol misuse in young people: a systematic review. *Addiction.* 2003;98(4):397–411.

56. Friese B, Grube J. *Youth Drinking Rates and Problems: A Comparison of European Countries and the United States*; 2010. Available at: http://resources.prev.org/underagedrinking_resources.html.

57. Gardner TW, Dishion TJ, Connell AM. Adolescent self-regulation as resilience: resistance to antisocial behavior within the deviant peer context. *J Abnormal Child Psychol.* 2007;36(2):273–284.

58. Reference deleted in review.

59. Grant BF. Estimates of US children exposed to alcohol abuse and dependence in the family. *Am J Public Health.* 2000;90:112–115.

60. Greenberg M. Promoting resilience in children and youth: preventive interventions and their interface with neuroscience. *Ann NY Acad Sci.* 2007;1094:139–150.

61. Harden KP, Hill JE, Turkheimer E, Emery R. Gene–environment correlation and interaction in peer effects on adolescent alcohol and tobacco use. *Behavioral Genetics.* 2008;38:339–347.

62. Harden P, Pihl R. Cognitive function, cardiovascular reactivity, and behavior in boys at high risk for alcoholism. *J Abnormal Psychol.* 1995;104:94–103.

63. Hunt PS, Barnet RC. Adolescent and adult rats differ in the amnesic effects of acute ethanol in two hippocampus-dependent tasks: trace and contextual fear conditioning. *Behav Brain Res.* 2016;298(Pt A):78–87.

64. Hussong A, Bauer D, Huang W, Chassin L, Sher K, Zucker R. Characterizing the life stressors of children of alcoholic parents. *J Family Psychol.* 2008;22(6):819–832. https://doi.org/10.1037/a0013704.

65. Reference deleted in review.

66. Hussong AChassin L. Stress and coping among children of alcoholic parents through the young adult transition. *Develop Psychopathol.* 2004;16:985–1006.

67. Reference deleted in review.

68. Jablonski SA, Stanton ME. Neonatal alcohol impairs the context preexposure facilitation effect in juvenile rats: dose-response and post-training consolidation effects. *Alcohol.* 2014;48(1):35–42.

69. Jacob T, Leonard K. Psychological functioning in children of alcoholic fathers, depressed fathers, and control fathers. *J Studies Alcohol.* 1986;47:373–380.

70. Reference deleted in review.

71. Reference deleted in review.

72. Johnson JL, Rolf JE. When children change: research perspectives on children of alcoholics. In: Collins RL, Leonard KE, Searles JS, eds. *Alcohol and the Family: Research and Clinical Perspectives.* New York, NY: Guilford; 1990:162–193.

73. Johnston LD, O'Malley PM, Miech RA, Bachman JG, Schulenberg JE. *Monitoring the Future National Survey Results on Drug Use: 1975-2014: Overview, Key Findings on Adolescent Drug Use.* Ann Arbor: Institute for Social Research, The University of Michigan; 2015.

74. Jordan L, Chassin L. *Protective Factors for Children of Alcoholics: Parenting, Family Environment, Child Personality and Contextual Supports.* San Francisco: Presented at the 106th Annual Convention of the American Psychological Association; 1998.

75. Jrapko A, Ward D, Hazelton T, Foster TL. *Family Treatment Drug Court Head Start Program: Annual Report.* San Jose, CA: Center for Applied Local Research; 2003.

76. Kaminski JW, Valle LA, Filene JH, Boyle CL. A meta-analytic review of components associated with parent training program effectiveness. *J Abnormal Child Psychol.* 2008;36:567–589.

77. Kaufman J, Yang BZ, Douglas-Palumber H, et al. Genetic and environmental predictors of early alcohol use. *Biol Psychiat.* 2007;61:1228–1234.

78. Kelley ML, Fals-Stewart W. Couple-versus individual-based therapy for alcohol and drug abuse: effects on children's psychosocial functioning. *J Consult Clin Psychol.* 2002;70:417–427.

79. Kelley ML, French A, Bountress K, et al. Parentification and family responsibility in the family of origin of adult children of alcoholics. *Addict Behav.* 2007;32(4):675–685.

80. Kimber B. Cultural adaptation and preliminary results of the strengthening families program 6–11 in Sweden. *Paper presented at Society for Prevention Research, San Antonio, TX. Department of Public Health Sciences.* Stockholm, Sweden: Karolinska Institutet; 2005.

81. Kreek MJ, Nielsen DA, Laforge KS. Genes associated with addiction: alcoholism, opiate, and cocaine addiction. *NeuroMolecular Med.* 2004;5(1):85–108.

82. Kumpfer KL. Special populations: etiology and prevention of vulnerability to chemical dependency in children of substance abusers. In: Brown BS, Mills AR, eds. *Youth at High Risk for Substance Abuse. NIDA, DHHS Pub.# (ADM) 90-1537*; 1987:1–71. Washington, DC.

83. Reference deleted in review.

84. Kumpfer KL. The strengthening families program. In: Ashery R, Robertson E, Kumpfer KL, eds. *Drug Abuse Prevention through Family Interventions, NIDA Research Monograph #177, DHHS.* Rockville, MD: National Institute on Drug Abuse; 1998. NIH Publication No. 97–4135.

85. Kumpfer KL. *Strengthening America's Families: Promising Parenting and Family Strategies for Delinquency Prevention.* A User's Guide, Prepared for the U.S. Department of Justice under Grant No. 87-JS-CX-K495 from the Office of Juvenile Justice and Delinquency Prevention, Office of Juvenile Programs US Department of Justice; 1999. Also see www.strengtheningfamilies.org.

86. Kumpfer KL. *Factors and Processes Contributing to Resilience: The Resilience Framework.* In: Glantz MD, Johnson JL, eds. *Resilience and Development: Positive Life Adaptation.* New York: Kluwer Academic/Plenum; 1999:179–224.

87. Kumpfer KL. Outcome measures of interventions in the study of children of substance abusing parents. *J Am Academy Pediatrics.* 1999;103:1128–1144.

88. Kumpfer KL (2006) *Year One (Fy '05 – '06) Evaluation Report for Celebrating Families Grant.* LutraGroup, Salt Lake City, Utah, July 15, 2006.

89. Kumpfer KL. *Family-Based Interventions for the Prevention of Substance Abuse and Other Impulse Control Disorders in Girls. Invited Spotlight Article, ISRN Addiction.* Hindawi Publishing; 2014.

90. Kumpfer KL. Middle Childhood: Strengthening Families Program 6–11. Chapter 4 in Van Ryzin M, Kumpfer KL, Fasco G, Greenberg, M. (2015) eds. *Family-Centered Prevention Programs for Children and Adolescents: Theory, Research, and Large-Scale Dissemination.* NY: Psychology Press; 2015.

91. Kumpfer KL, Alvarado R. Family strengthening approaches for the prevention of youth problem behaviors. *Am Psychologist.* 2003;58(6/7):457–465.

92. Kumpfer KL, Alvarado R, Smith P. Drug abuse prevention tools and programs. In: Coombs RH, ed. *Addiction Counseling Review: Preparing for Comprehensive, Certification, and Licensing Exams. Lahaska.* New York: Houghton Mifflin; 2004:467–486.

93. Kumpfer KL, Alvarado R, Smit P, Bellamy N. Cultural sensitivity in universal family-based prevention interventions. *Prevent Sci.* 2002;3(3):241–244.

94. Kumpfer KL, Alvarado R, Tait C, Turner C. Effectiveness of school-based family and children's skills training for substance abuse prevention among 6–8 year old rural children. *Psychol Addict Behav.* 2002;16(4):65–71.

95. Kumpfer KL, Alvarado R, Whiteside HO. Family-based interventions for the substance abuse prevention. *Subst Use Misuse.* 2003;38(11–13):1759–1789.

96. Kumpfer KL, Alvarado R, Whiteside HO, Tait C. The strengthening families program (SFP): an evidence-based, multi-cultural family skills training program. In: Szapocznik J, Tolan P, Sambrano S, eds. *Preventing Substance Abuse.* Washington DC: American Psychological Association Books; 2005:3–14.

97. Kumpfer KL, Bayes J. Child abuse and alcohol and other drug abuse. In: Jaffe JH, ed. *The Encyclopedia of Drugs and Alcohol.* New York: Macmillan; 1995:217–222.

98. Kumpfer KL, DeMarsh JP. Family environmental and genetic influences on children's future chemical dependency. In: Ezekoye S, Kumpfer K, Bukoski W, eds. *Childhood and Chemical Abuse: Prevention and Intervention.* New York: Haworth; 1985:49–91.

99. Kumpfer KL, Fenollar J, Xie J, Bluth Dellinger B. Resilience Framework: resilience and resourcefulness in the face of chronic family adversity. In: Celinski M, Gow K, eds. *Continuity versus Creative Response to Challenge: The Primacy of Resilience & Resourcefulness in Life & Therapy.* New York: Nova Science Publishers Inc; 2011:259–272.

100. Kumpfer KL, Fowler M. Parenting skills and family support programs for drug-abusing mothers. *Semin Fetal Neonatal Med.* 2007;12(2):134–142.

101. Kumpfer KL, Hopkins R. Recent advances in addictive disorders. Prevention: current research and trends. *Psychiatr Clin North Am.* 1993;16(1):11–20.

102. Reference deleted in review.

103. Reference deleted in review.

104. Kumpfer KL, Magalhães C, Xie J, Kanse S. Cultural and gender adaptations of evidence-based family interventions, Chapter 12. In: Van Ryzin M, Kumpfer KL, Fosco GM, Greenberg M, eds. *Family-based Prevention Programs for Children and Adolescents: Theory, Research, and Large-Scale Dissemination.* NY: Psychology Press; 2015:256–282.

105. Kumpfer KL, Magalhães C, Xie, J. Cultural adaptation and implementation of family evidence-based interventions (EBIs) with diverse populations. *Prev Sci.* 2017;18(6):649–659.

106. Kumpfer KL, Molgaard V, Spoth R. The strengthening families program for prevention of delinquency and drug use in special populations. In: Dev Peters R, McMahon RJ, eds. *Childhood Disorders, Substance Abuse, and Delinquency: Prevention and Early Intervention Approaches.* Newbury Park, CA: Sage; 1996.

107. Kumpfer KL, Pinyuchon M, de Melo A, Whiteside H. Cultural adaptation process for international dissemination of the strengthening families program (SFP). *Eval Health Professions.* 2008;33(2):226–239.

108. Kumpfer KL, Smith P, Summerhays JF. A wake -up call to the prevention field: are prevention programs for substance use effective for girls? *Subst Use Misuse.* 2008;43:978–1001.

109. Kumpfer KL, Whiteside HO. *Strengthening Families Program 6–11 Years: Parent, Child, and Family Skills Training Group Leaders Manuals.* Salt Lake City: LutraGroup; Utah; 2004.

110. Lambie DM, Sias SM. Children of alcoholics: implications for professional school counselling. *Professional School Counselling, Special issue Professional School Counsell Urban Settings.* 2005;8(3):266–273.

111. Leifman H. Trends in population drinking. In: Norström T, ed. *Alcohol in Postwar Europe: Consumption, Drinking Patterns, Consequences and Policy Responses in 15 European Countries.* Stockholm: National Institute of Public Health; 2002.

112. Li C, Mao X, Wei L. Genes and (common) pathways underlying drug addiction. *Comput Biol.* 2008;4(1):10–37.

113. Li C, Pentz MA, Chou C. Parental substance use as a modifier of adolescent substance use risk. *Addiction*. 2002;97:1537–1550.
114. Liddle HA, Santisteban D, Levant R, Bray J. *Family Psychology: Science-Based Interventions*. Washington DC: American Psychological Association; 2002.
115. Lloyd TJ, Hastings R. (2009). Hope as a psychological resilience factor in mothers and fathers of children with intellectual disabilities. *J Intellect Disabil Res*. 2009;53(12):957–968.
116. Lochman JE, Steenhoven A. Family-based approaches to substance abuse prevention. *J Primary Prevent*. 2002;23(1):49–114.
117. Luthar S, Cushing G, Merikangas K, Rounsaville B. Multiple jeopardy: risk and protective factors among addicted mothers' offspring. *Develop Psychopathol*. 1998;10:117–136.
118. Luthar SS, D'Avanzo H. Maternal drug abuse versus other psychological disturbances. In: Luthar SS, ed. *Resilience and Vulnerability: Adaptation in the Context of Childhood Adversities*. Cambridge UK: University Press; 2005.
119. Maguin E, Nochajski TH, De Wit DJ, Safyer A. Strengthening family program (SFP) for COAs: parenting and child behavior outcomes. [Abstract]. *Alcohol Clin Exp Res*. 2006;30(6): Supplement, P770.
119a. Maguin E, Zucker RA, Fitzgerald HE. The path to alcohol problems through conduct problems: a family-based approach to very early intervention with risk. *J Res Adolesc*. 1994;4(2):249–269.
120. Markowitz R. Dynamics and treatment issues with children of drug and alcohol abusers. In: Straussner SLA, ed. *Clinical Work with Substance-Abusing Clients*. 2nd ed. New York: Guilford; 2004: 125–145.
121. Masten A, Coatsworth D. The development of competence in favorable and unfavorable environments. *Am Psychologist*. 1998;53: 205–220.
122. McGrath C, Watson A, Chassin L. Academic achievement in adolescent children of alcoholics. *J Studies Alcohol*. 1999;60:18–26.
123. Reference deleted in review.
124. Miller GE, Chen E, Parker KJ. Psychological stress in childhood and susceptibility to the chronic diseases of aging: Moving toward a model of behavioral and biological mechanisms. *Psychol Bull*. 2011;137:959–997.
125. Reference deleted in review.
126. Moos R, Billings A. Children of alcoholics during the recovery process: alcoholics and matched control families. *Addict Behav*. 1982;7:155–163.
127. Moss H, Clark D, Kirisci L. Timing of paternal substance use disorder cessation and effects on problem behaviors in sons. *Am J Addiction*. 1997;6:30–37.
128. Reference deleted in review.
129. Munato M, Lingford-Hughes A, Johnstone E, Walton R. Association between serotonin transporter gene and alcohol consumption in social drinkers. *Am J Med Gen Part B: Neuropsychiatr Genetic*. 2005;135B:10–14.
130. Mylant ML, Ide B, Cuevas E, Meehan M. Adolescent children of alcoholics: vulnerable or resilient? *J Am Psychiatric Nurses Assoc*. 2002;18(2):57–64.
131. Natasi BK, DeZolt DM. *School Interventions for Children of Alcoholics*. New York: Guilford; 1994.
132. National center on child abuse and neglect, national child abuse and neglect data system. Reports from the states to the national center on child abuse and neglect. In: *Child Maltreatment 2001*. Washington, DC: U.S. Government Printing Office; 2003.
133. Reference deleted in review.
134. Noll R, Zucker R, Fitzgerald H, Curtis J. Cognitive and motoric functioning of sons of alcoholic fathers and controls: the early childhood years. *Child Develop*. 1992;28:665–675.
135. O'Farrell TJ, Fals-Stewart W. Behavioral couples and family therapy for substance abusers. *Curr Psychiatry Report*. 2002;4(5):371–376.
136. O'Farrell TJ, Feehan M. Alcoholism treatment and the family: do family and individual treatments for alcoholic adults have preventive effects for children? *J Studies Alcohol Suppl*. 1999;13:125–129.
137. Obot IS, Anthony JC. Mental health problems in adolescent children of alcohol dependent parents: epidemiologic research with a nationally representative sample. *J Child Adolesc Subst Abuse*. 2004;13(4):83–96.
138. Ohannessian C, Hesselbrock V. The influence of perceived social support on the relationship between family history of alcoholism and drinking behavior. *Addiction*. 1993;88:1651–1658.
139. Onrust S, Bool M. *Evaluatie van de cursus Gezin aan Bod: Nederlandse versie van het Strengthening Families Program (SFP), Evaluation Report submitted to MonZw*. Utrecht, Netherlands: Trimbos Institute; 2006 (July, 2006).
140. Orte C, March MX, Ballester L, Touza C. *Results of a family competence program adapted for Spanish drug abusing parents. Abstract submitted to Society for Prevention Research*. Palma of Majorca, Spain: University of the Balearic Islands (UIB); 2006.
141. Park A, Sher K, Todorov A, Heath A. Interaction between the DRD4 VNTR polymorphism and proximal and distal environments in alcohol dependence during emerging and young adulthood. *J Abnormal Psychol*. 2011;120:585–595.
142. Pihl R, Peterson J, Finn P. The inherited predisposition to alcoholism: characteristics of sons of male alcoholics. *J Abnormal Psychol*. 1990;99:291–301.
143. Popova S, Slade B, Bekmurdova D, Lange S, Rehn J. What do we know about the economic impact of Fetal Alcohol Spectrum Disorder? A systematic literature review. *Alcohol Alcohol*. 2011;46(4):490–497. https://doi.org/10.1093/alcalc/agr029.
144. Price AW, Emshoff JG. Breaking the cycle of addiction: prevention and intervention with children of alcoholics. *Alcohol Health Res World*. 1997;21(3):241–246.
145. Propper C, Moore GA. The influence of parenting on infant emotionality: a multi-level psychobiological perspective. *Develop Rev*. 2006;26:427–460.
146. Puttler L, Zucker R, Fitzgerald H, Bingham C. Behavioral outcomes among children of alcoholics during the early and middle childhood years: familial subtype variations. *Alcohol Clin Exp Res*. 1998;22:1962–1972.
147. Reference deleted in review.
148. Rehm J, Room R, Monteiro R, et al. Alcohol. In: Ezzati M, Lopez AD, Rodgers A, Murray CJ, eds. *Comparative Quantification of Health Risks: Global and Regional burden of Disease Due to Selected Major Risk Factors*. Geneva: WHO; 2004:959–1108.
149. Reference deleted in review.
150. Roosa M, Gensheimer L, Ayers T, Shell RA. Preventive intervention for children in alcoholic families: results of a pilot study. *Fam Relat*. 1989;38:295–300.
151. Roosa M, Sandler I, Beals J, Short J. Risk status of adolescent children of problem drinking parents. *Am J Community Psychol*. 1988;16(2):225–239.
152. Rutter M, Quinton D, Liddle C. *Parenting in two generations*: looking backwards and looking forwards. In: Madge N, ed. *Families at Risk*. London: Heinemann Educational Books; 1983:60–84.
153. Sales JM, DiClemente RJ, Brody GH, et al. Interaction between 5-HTTLPR polymorphism and abuse history on adolescent African-American females' condom use behavior following participation in an HIV prevention intervention. *Prev Sci*. 2014;15(3):257–267.
154. SAMHSA. *National Survey on Drug Use and Health*. Data Spotlight; 2012. Feb. 16, 2012 retrieved from: http://www.samhsa.gov/data/spotlight/Spot061ChildrenOfAlcoholics.pdf
155. Sanders M, Mazzucchelli T, Studman L. *Facilitator's Manual for Group Stepping Stones Triple P: For Families With a Child Who Has a Disability*, ed 2. Brisbane, Australia: Triple P International; 2015.
156. Schuckit M, Chiles JA. Family history as a diagnostic aid in two samples of adolescents. *J Nervous Mental Dis*. 1978;166(3):165–176.
157. Schuckit MA. A longitudinal study of children of alcoholics. In: Galanter M, Begleiter H, eds. *Recent Developments in Alcoholism*. vol. 9: children of alcoholics. New York, NY: Plenum; 1991:5–19
158. Sher K. *Children of Alcoholics: A Critical Appraisal of Theory and Research*. Chicago: University of Chicago; 1991.

159. Reference deleted in review.

160. Slawecki CJ, Thomas JD, Riley EP, Ehlers CL. Neonatal nicotine exposure alters hippocampal EEG and event-related potentials (ERPs) in rats. *Pharmacol Biochem Behav.* 2000;65(4):711–718.

161. Solis J, Shadur J, Burns A, Hussong A. Understanding the diverse needs of children whose parents abuse substances. *Curr Drug Abuse Review.* 2012;5(2):135–147.

162. Spear L. Modeling adolescent development and alcohol use in animals. *Alcohol Res Health.* 2000;24(2):115–123.

163. Spoth R, Guyll M, Day SX. Universal family-focused interventions in alcohol-use disorder prevention: cost-effectiveness and cost-benefit analyses of two interventions. *J Studies Alcohol.* 2002;63(2):219–228.

164. Spoth R, Shin C, Guyll M, Redmond C, Azevedo K. Universality of effects: an examination of the comparability of long-term family intervention effects on substance use across risk-related subgroups. *Prevent Sci.* 2006;7:209–224.

165. Springer JF, Sambrano S, Sale E, Nistler, M, Kasim R, Hermann, J. The National Cross-Site Evaluation of High-Risk Youth Programs: Final Report. Rockville, MD: EMT Associates, Inc. and ORC Macro, Prepared for CSAP.

166. Streissguth A, Barr H, Bookstein F, Sampson P, Olson H. The long-term neurocognitive consequences of prenatal alcohol exposure: a 14-year study. *Psychol Sci.* 1999;10:186–190.

167. Suomi SJ. Risk, resilience, and gene X environment interactions in rhesus monkeys. *Ann NY Acad Sci.* 2007;1094:52–62.

168. Tarter R. Neurobehavior disinhibition in childhood predisposes boys to substance use disorder by young adulthood: direct and mediated etiologic pathways. *Drug Alcohol Depend.* 2004;73(2):121–132.

169. Uhl GR. Molecular genetics of addiction vulnerability. *NeuroRx.* 2006;3(3):295–301.

170. Uhl GR, Drgon T, Johnson C, et al. "Higher order" addiction molecular genetics: convergent data from genome-wide association in humans and mice. *Biochem Pharmacol.* 2008;75(1):98–111.

171. UNICEF. Child poverty in perspective: an overview of child well-being in rich countries. *Innocenti Report Card.* 2007;7.

172. Van Ryzin M, Kumpfer KL, Fasco G, Greenberg M, eds. *Family-Centered Prevention Programs for Children and Adolescents: Theory, Research, and Large-Scale Dissemination.* NY: Psychology Press; 2015.

173. Vitaro F, Dobkin P, Carbonneau R, Tremblay R. Personal and familial characteristics of resilient sons of male alcoholics. *Addiction.* 1996;91:1161–1177.

174. Volkow ND, Fowler JS, Wang GJ, Swanson JM. Dopamine in drug abuse and addiction: results from brain scans and treatment implications. *Molecular Psychiatr.* 2004;9:557–569.

175. Weissenborn R, Duka T. Acute alcohol effects on cognitive function in social drinkers: their relationship to drinking habits. *Psychopharmacology.* 2003;165:306–312.

176. Werner EE. Resilient offspring of alcoholics: a longitudinal study from birth to age 18. *J Studies Alcohol.* 1986;47:34–40.

177. Werner EE, Johnson JL. The role of caring adults in the lives of children of alcoholics. *Subst Use Misuse.* 2004;39(5):699–720.

178. West MO, Prinz R. Parental alcoholism and childhood psychopathology. *Psychol Bull.* 1987;102:204–218.

179. Whipple S, Parker E, Noble E. An atypical neurocognitive profile in alcoholic fathers and their sons. *J Studies Alcohol.* 1988;49:240–244.

180. White AM, Swartzwelder HS. Age-related effects of alcohol on memory and memory-related brain function in adolescents. In: Galanter M, ed. *Recent Developments in Alcoholism, Vol. 17: Alcohol Problems in Adolescents and Young Adults: Epidemiology, Neurobiology, Prevention, Treatment.* 2005:161–176.

181. Wills TA, McNamara G, Vaccaro D, Hirky A. Escalated substance use: a longitudinal grouping analysis from early to middle adolescence. *J Abnorm Psychol.* 1996;105(2):166.

182. Wolin S, Bennett L, Noonan D, Teitelbaum M. Disrupted family rituals. *J Studies Alcohol.* 1980;41:199–214.

183. Young L. *Wednesday's Children—A Study of Child Neglect and Abuse.* New York: Dushkin/McGraw-Hill; 1964.

67

Alcohol and Substance Abuse in African Americans

WILLIAM B. LAWSON

CHAPTER OUTLINE

Introduction

Substance abuse is being increasingly appreciated for contributing to overall mortality and morbidity in the United States.[1,41] Yet, at the same time, substance use continues to be criminalized, especially for African Americans. Disparities in morbidity and mortality across ethnic groups continue to persist. Mortality rates for African Americans are about 1.6 times higher than those for whites, with much higher disparities for certain causes, such as HIV/AIDS and diabetes. A major factor in the disparities is the consequence of use of drugs of abuse. However, the problem is not simply excess of use by minorities. Disparities exist in the level of substance use and abuse but the greatest impact is from consequences resulting from the lack of access to treatment.[7]

Substance abuse is perceived as being more common among African Americans, yet that is often not the case. Among ethnic minorities, drug abuse has been shown in repeated studies to disproportionately contribute to individual, family, and societal burden. Moreover it also complicates mental disorders and contributes to the spread of chronic disorders such as HIV/AIDS and hepatitis C infection, which also disproportionately affect African Americans. African Americans have less treatment access and disproportionately face punitive interventions such as the correctional system. More needs to be done to recognize and address the misconceptions and disparities in care seen with African Americans.

Epidemiology

We and others reported that after adjustments, both African Americans and Caribbean blacks had a lower lifetime likelihood than non-Hispanic whites of having any Axis I substance abuse disorder, including alcohol abuse, alcohol dependence, drug abuse, drug dependence, and nicotine dependence.[19,66] Dr. Dan Blazer reported that "There's a perception among many individuals that African Americans as a group—regardless of socioeconomic status—tend to abuse or use drugs at higher rate and this [does not support] that."[66] He reported that young African Americans were less likely than whites to use drugs and less likely to develop substance use disorders. Another study, a 12-year longitudinal study, showed that the rates of hard drug abuse were highest among non-Hispanic whites, followed by Hispanics and then African Americans. Whites were more than 30 times likely to have cocaine-use disorder, 50 times more likely to develop opiate-use disorder, and 18 times more likely to have PCP-use disorder than blacks. Dr. Teplin, the principal investigator, noted that "Those findings are striking considering the widely accepted stereotype of African-Americans as the most prevalent abusers of hard drugs. Our findings add to the growing debate on how the war on drugs has affected African-Americans."[59] She is referring to the ongoing problem that was precipitated by the War on Drugs. African American youth are arrested for drug crimes at a rate 10 times higher than that of whites. Moreover nearly one in three black men will be imprisoned, and nearly half of black women currently have a family member or extended family member who is in prison. In addition,[61] this overrepresentation of African Americans in the correctional system has long been noted and is not helped by the misconception that African Americans are more likely to be addicts. War on Drugs policing has failed to reduce domestic street-level drug activity. The cost of drugs remains low and drugs remain widely available.[21]

The issue of cocaine use remains problematic in the African American community but has been exacerbated by correctional system involvement. Crack cocaine is more commonly used than powdered cocaine by African Americans and may be related to income, since the former is much cheaper.[35] Black males between the ages of 26 and 34 reported using crack cocaine more than any other racial and gender combination[16] and most offenders arrested for crack cocaine are black. Because African Americans make up the majority of most crack cases, they are more likely to receive the mandatory minimum prison sentencing more than any other ethnicity.[43] Drug trafficking, the availability of crack, and the Federal Anti-Drug Abuse Act led to mandatory minimum prison sentencing of dealers, which has been a controversial issue. Originally the sentencing for crack versus cocaine was 100:1, meaning the amount of crack versus the amount of powder cocaine needed to establish a mandatory minimum prison sentence.[43] Driving the disparate sentencing was the increased homicide rate in the African American community during the 1990s. Homicides increased among African Americans when crack cocaine was popular but decreased with the decline of crack cocaine and crack cocaine consumption in recent years.[16,55] It is important to note that the violence associated with crack cocaine is probably not linked to the psychopharmacological effects of the substance, as much as it is to the crack cocaine distribution in neighborhoods that are stricken with poverty and economic disadvantages, along with distribution competition.[55] Most importantly, differential sentencing did not lead to improvement in quality of life in African American communities.

Since 2000 there has been a shift in focus on eliminating the additional sentencing for crack cocaine and a shift to the use of treatment. This shift was prompted by findings that tended to show that the mandatory minimum prison sentencing was racially motivated and specifically targeted blacks.[16,43] Moreover, mandatory sentencing did not reduce the amount of drug trafficking into the United States. Instead it turned state-level offenses into federal crimes, created strain on families by imprisoning violators for long periods, and impacted minorities, resulting in vastly different sentences for equally blameworthy offenders.[31]" As noted earlier, non-Hispanic whites are now more likely to abuse hard drugs, such as cocaine or opiates, than their black counterparts, and by a substantial amount.

Racial differences have been seen in opiate use, but the increasing use in nonminorities and overall death rate have overshadowed these disparities. Major cities are experiencing hundreds of overdose deaths every year.[10] What changed about US heroin consumption to make it more dangerous? Analyses of market trends have repeatedly demonstrated a relationship between the price of an item and demand for it, and a similar relationship exists between heroin price, consumption, and associated dangers. Moreover, a major goal of drug supply control efforts is to increase the street price of a drug by shifting the supply curve; this in turn reduces the quantity demanded by consumers as the market reaches a new equilibrium.[10]

In addition there has been a shift in who is abusing opioid. Whites and Native Americans have experienced the largest increase in death rates, particularly when it comes to opioid-related fatalities. Since 2000, the rate of deaths from drug overdoses has increased 137%, including a 200% increase in the rate of overdose deaths involving opioids (opioid pain relievers and heroin). The Centers for Disease Control and Prevention (CDC) analyzed recent multiple cause-of-death mortality data to examine current trends and characteristics of drug overdose deaths, including the types of opioids associated with drug overdose deaths. During 2014, a total of 47,055 drug overdose deaths occurred in the United States, representing a 1-year increase of 6.5%, from 13.8 per 100,000 persons in 2013 to 14.7 per 100,000 persons in 2014. The rate of drug overdose deaths increased significantly for both sexes, persons 25–44 years of age and ≥55 years of age, non-Hispanic whites and non-Hispanic blacks, and in the Northeastern, Midwestern, and Southern regions of the United States. Rates of opioid overdose deaths also increased significantly, from 7.9 per 100,000 in 2013 to 9.0 per 100,000 in 2014, a 14% increase. Individuals who began using heroin in the 1960s were predominantly young men (82.8%; mean age, 16.5 years) whose first opioid of abuse was heroin (80%). However, more recent users were older (mean age, 22.9 years) men and women living in less urban areas (75.2%) who were introduced to opioids through prescription drugs (75.0%).[50] Whites and nonwhites were equally represented in individuals initiating use prior to the 1980s, but nearly 90% who began use in the last decade were white. Although the high produced by heroin was described as a significant factor in its selection, it was often used because it was more readily accessible and much less expensive than prescription opioids.[11]

Fentanyl is a synthetic and short-acting opioid analgesic, is 50–100 times more potent than morphine, and is approved for managing acute or chronic pain. Increases in fentanyl deaths were driving the increases in synthetic opioid deaths in six states.[20] Among high-burden states, all demographic groups experienced substantial increases in synthetic opioid death rates. Increases of >200% occurred among males (227%); persons aged 15–24 years (347%), 25–34 years (248%), and 35–44 (230%) years; Hispanics (290%), and persons living in large fringe metro areas (230%). The highest rates of synthetic opioid deaths in 2014 were among males (5.1 per 100,000); non-Hispanics whites (4.6 per 100,000); and persons aged 25–34 years (8.3 per 100,000), 35–44 years (7.4 per 100,000), and 45–54 years (5.7 per 100,000). Note that in contrast to public perceptions, the highest rates were NOT in African Americans. Drug overdose is now the leading cause of unintentional death nationwide, driven by increased prescription opioid overdoses.[20] Although African Americans are not the heaviest abusers nationally, drug abuse remains a problem in many communities. In San Francisco, for example, from 2010 to 2012, 331 African Americans died of accidental overdose caused by opioids (310 involving prescription opioids and 31 involving heroin). The deaths were concentrated in a small, high-poverty, central area of San Francisco and disproportionately affected African American individuals.[56] Nevertheless the news media and intervention programs have focused on non-Hispanic whites.

Racial differences in alcohol abuse have also been reported, but again African Americans are not the heaviest abusers. Compared to European Americans, African Americans report later initiation of drinking, lower rates of use, and lower levels of use across almost all age groups.[67] However, African Americans are more likely to have negative health-related and socioeconomic consequences, as is true for other drugs of abuse. African Americans are more likely than European Americans to encounter legal problems from drinking, even at the same levels of consumption.[67] African American culture is characterized by norms against heavy alcohol use or intoxication, which probably protects against heavy use but also provides within-group social disapproval.[67]

Marijuana use and consequences are complicated by cultural issues in the African American community, as are other drugs of abuse. As noted earlier, multiple studies have shown that African Americans are less likely to use cannabis.[19,66] More recent studies, however, have shown an uptick in cannabis use.[65] Part of the issue may be a result of the increasing diversity of African Americans. We reported earlier that differences exist in mental disorders and substance abuse with African Americans and Afro-Caribbeans.[19,66] Another study of noninstitutionalized Caribbeans living in the United States, Jamaica, and Guyana revealed that substance use and other physical health conditions and major depressive disorder and mania vary by national context, with higher rates among Caribbeans living in the United States, but lower rates of cannabis use. Context and generation status influenced health outcomes and drug use. The results of this study support the need for additional research to explain how national context, migratory experiences, and generation status contribute to understanding substance use and mental disorders and physical health outcomes among Caribbean first generation and descendants within the United States, compared to those remaining in the Caribbean region.[29]

Consistent with other drugs of abuse, African Americans have higher marijuana arrest rates than those for whites.[25] Arrest data in New York indicated that during the 1990s the primary focus of policing became smoking marijuana in public view. By 2000, smoking marijuana in public view had become the most common misdemeanor arrest, accounting for 15% of all NYC adult arrests and rivalling controlled substance arrests as the primary focus of drug abuse control. Moreover, most arrestees were African American or Hispanic, and they were more likely to be detained prior to arraignment, convicted, and sentenced to jail than their white counterparts.[21]

Although the benefits and safety of marijuana have been promoted in recent years, this has increased health as well as legal risks for African Americans. Heavy or chronic cannabis use is associated with a wide range of health-related conditions, such as motor vehicle injuries, cognitive impairment, chronic bronchitis symptoms, and cardiovascular diseases, which may exacerbate the disparities in health-related problems seen in African Americans.[58,65] To date, 33 states and the District of Columbia currently have passed laws broadly legalizing marijuana in some form. As the wave of state-specific policies on cannabis legalization continues to spread across the nation, they could have unintended consequences (e.g., an increase in supply or use-related problems) with lasting implications for the health and social systems of racial and ethnic minorities.[58,65]

There has been an emergence of synthetic cannabinoid use. Synthetic cannabinoid receptor agonists (SCRAs), also known as "K2" or "Spice," have drawn considerable attention due to their potential for abuse and harmful consequences. The most frequently mentioned effects were "getting high" (44.0%), "hallucinations" (10.8%), and "anxiety" (10.2%).[30] Synthetic cannabinoids (SCs) are a large, heterogeneous group of chemicals that are structurally similar to δ-9-tetrahydrocannabinol. Many are high-efficacy full agonists of the CB1 and/or CB2 cannabinoid receptors, resulting in a potent group of chemicals with a variety of negative health effects, including death. They are available to adolescents at convenience stores and smoke shops and on the Internet. However, little is known about the risk factors that contribute to eventual use of in adolescents, and no research has examined the psychiatric, personality, and substance-use risk factors that prospectively predict use. Thus far African Americans have been less likely to use SCs.[42] However, these chemicals are especially tempting for African American youth because they often test negative on screens for job applicants; positive drug screens are often a challenge for inner city African Americans seeking employment.

Preventive and Risk Factors

A risk factor is gateway drugs. The good news is the lower risk of cigarette smoking, drug use, and alcohol abuse in African American adolescents. However, we also noted an uptake in marijuana use in adolescents and the increasing legalization. Although marijuana use is common during adolescence, it can have adverse long-term consequences, with serious criminal involvement being one of them, especially in African Americans. The effects of heavy adolescent marijuana use (20 or more times) on adult criminal involvement, including perpetration of drug, property, and violent crime, as well as being arrested and incarcerated, was examined in the Woodlawn study, a longitudinal study of African Americans through the lifespan.[22] Heavy adolescent marijuana use led to drug and property crime and criminal justice system interactions, but not violent crime. The significant associations of early heavy marijuana use with school dropout, and the progression to cocaine and/or heroin use only partially account for these findings. Nevertheless, these results suggest that the prevention of heavy marijuana use among adolescents could reduce the perpetration of drug and property crime in adulthood, as well as the burden on the criminal justice system, but would have little effect on violent crime.[22]

In another study adolescent regular smokers also showed significantly higher odds of using marijuana, cocaine, and heroin, having alcohol abuse problems and any drug dependence, and abuse problems in adulthood. Educational attainment mediated most of the drug progression pathway, including cigarette smoking, marijuana, cocaine and heroin use, and drug dependence or abuse problems in adulthood, but not alcohol abusers.[54] Thus the benefits of not being early smokers in African Americans may be offset by high school dropout rates and other educational challenges.

Contextual factors are increasingly prominent in studies of illegal drug use in the United States. Studies suggest, for example, that neighborhood economic disadvantage predicts illegal drug use, and that local social disorder and unemployment rates predict the prevalence of injection drug use in metropolitan areas.[15] Preventive efforts for African Americans therefore must focus on these important socio-environmental factors that are prevalent in many African American communities. These factors extend to the health consequences of drug use. African Americans were more likely to be HIV-negative and drug free if they lived in less economically disadvantaged counties, or in communities with less criminal-justice activity (i.e., lower drug-related arrest rates, lower policing/corrections expenditures).[13]

These types of observations can be extended to alcohol use. Use of alcohol treatment may be affected by factors such as trends in public knowledge about treatment, social pressures to reduce drinking, and changes in the public financing of treatment.[9] As noted previously, within-group social disapproval also plays an important role in the lower risk of drinking in African American youth.[67]

An adverse family environment in late adolescence was found to be related to greater marijuana use in emerging adulthood. This in turn was positively associated with partner marijuana use in young adulthood, which in turn, was ultimately related to maladaptive behaviors in adulthood. An adverse family environment in late adolescence was also related to greater marijuana use in emerging adulthood, which in turn, was associated with an adverse relationship with one's partner in young adulthood. Such a negative partner relationship was related to maladaptive behaviors in adulthood. The findings suggest that family-focused interventions should be considered.[33]

Community violence, witnessing of violent crime, and victimization has been an ongoing problem in low-income African American communities. One longitudinal study examined the interrelationship among victimization, posttraumatic stress disorder (PTSD), and substance use in African Americans; victimization at ages 19, 24, and 29 was directly associated with substance use at age 36 and was also related to PTSD at age 36. PTSD, in turn, was related to substance use at age 36. This study indicated the importance of intervention for those who have been victimized, with a focus on PTSD treatment.[34] In addition, in another study, youth with greater exposure to violent victimization were 3.89 times as likely to initiate marijuana first than to initiate tobacco first. African American youth and youth with greater exposure to victimization had an increased risk of initiating marijuana before tobacco. Substance use prevention efforts should consider taking into account that marijuana use may put certain youth at risk of initiating tobacco use. Future research needs to monitor sequencing as well as risk factors for and consequences of the various patterns, particularly because marijuana use and the mixing of tobacco and marijuana use are gaining acceptability in general populations and the African American community, which historically have been at lower risk.[23]

It has been reported that African American youth are significantly more religious than white and Hispanic youth, which could explain the lower rates of drug use.[46] However, more recent studies have found that religion does, in fact, protect African American and Hispanic youth from substance abuse, but the strength of this relationship is greater for white than for non-white youth. The reasons for racial and ethnic differences in the strength of the relationship between religiosity and substance abuse are not clear. One possibility is that religiosity may be more of a cultural or group phenomenon among non-white youth, whereas among white youth it may be more of an individual factor affecting individual behavior such as substance use. Understanding the mechanisms by which religion might influence substance use and the reasons that these mechanisms may vary by race and ethnicity may provide clues to implementing effective prevention programs.[17]

Impact on the Individual

As noted previously, drug abuse adversely affects health outcome irrespective of race. African Americans, however, seem to be more adversely affected and have worse social and health care outcomes.[62] A study examined a nationally representative sample of whites, African Americans, and Latinos and predicted expenditures for each racial/ethnic group. African Americans required more expenditures because of the greater health consequences.[18,32]

The problem of increased risk of incarceration in African Americans for drug use was noted earlier in this chapter. Recent incarceration independently predicted worse health outcomes and greater use of emergency services among HIV-infected adults currently in HIV care. Options to improve the HIV continuum of care, including preenrollment for health care coverage and discharge planning, may lead to better health outcomes for HIV-infected inmates postrelease.[39]

Consistent with other studies, significant racial-ethnic disparities were seen in opioid prescriptions, with non-Hispanic African Americans being less likely to receive opioid prescription at discharge during emergency department visits for back pain and abdominal pain, but not for toothache, fractures, and kidney stones, compared to non-Hispanic whites after adjusting for other covariates. Differential prescription of opioids by race-ethnicity could lead to widening of existing disparities in health, and may have implications for a disproportionate burden of opioid abuse among whites.[52]

Experiences of discrimination in health care settings may contribute to disparities in mental health outcomes for African Americans and Latinos. Perceived discrimination in mental health/substance abuse visits was found to contribute to participants' ratings of treatment helpfulness and led to stopping treatment. The most commonly reported reasons for health care discrimination were race/ethnicity for blacks (52%) and Latinos (31%), and insurance status for whites (40%). Experiences of discrimination in mental health/substance abuse visits were associated with early treatment termination for African Americans. Experiences of discrimination are associated with negative mental health/substance abuse treatment experiences and stopping treatment, and could be a factor in mental health outcomes.[36]

A review and critique of empirical research on perceived discrimination and health suggested that there are multiple ways by which racism can affect health. Perceived discrimination is one such pathway, and this research continues to document an inverse association between discrimination and health. This pattern is now evident in a wider range of contexts and for a broader array of outcomes. Advancing our understanding of the relationship between perceived discrimination and health will require more attention to situating discrimination within the context of other health-relevant aspects of racism, measuring it comprehensively and accurately, assessing its stressful dimensions, and identifying the mechanisms that link discrimination to health.[63]

Comorbidity

For those with either an alcohol or other drug disorder, the odds of having the other addictive disorder were seven times greater than in the rest of the population. Among individuals with an alcohol disorder, 37% had a comorbid mental disorder. The highest mental-addictive disorder comorbidity rate was found for individuals with drug (other than alcohol) disorders, among whom more than half (53%) were found to have a mental disorder, with an odds ratio of 4.5. Individuals treated in specialty mental health and addictive disorder clinical settings have significantly higher odds of having comorbid disorders. Among the institutional settings, comorbidity of addictive and severe mental disorders was highest in the prison population, most notably with antisocial personality, schizophrenia, and bipolar disorders.[48]

Nearly half of the people with schizophrenia also present with a lifetime history of substance use, a rate that is much higher than the one seen among unaffected individuals. It is critically important to address this comorbidity because substance use in schizophrenic patients and others with severe mental illness is associated with poorer clinical outcomes and contributes significantly to their morbidity and mortality.[57] These disorders have greater illness burden in African Americans, so comorbidity may confer even greater health and social consequences. Most individuals with drug use disorders have never been treated, and racial and ethnic treatment disparities exist among those at high risk, despite substantial disability and comorbidity.[12]

Some evidence suggests that youth who use marijuana heavily during adolescence may be particularly prone to health problems in later adulthood (e.g., respiratory illnesses, psychotic symptoms). However, relatively few longitudinal studies have prospectively examined the long-term physical and mental health consequences associated with chronic adolescent marijuana use. A longitudinal study of African American and white young men was done to determine whether different developmental patterns of marijuana use were associated with adverse physical (e.g., asthma, high blood pressure) and mental (e.g., psychosis, anxiety disorders) health outcomes in the mid-30s. Chronic marijuana use was more strongly associated with later health problems in African American relative to white men.[5]

Often African Americans are triply diagnosed. African Americans with substance abuse are at greater risk of becoming HIV positive, especially those that are intravenous drug users. Moreover, many of these individuals also develop hepatitis C, which has been found to be very common in this population. Finally, they are at risk of being incarcerated. The higher concentration of HIV in prisons stems, in large part, from the incarceration of people who use illicit drugs. Half of the correctional population meets standard diagnostic criteria for drug dependence or abuse. Currently, >95% of incarcerated individuals will be released and reenter society, with nearly 80% being released to parole supervision. About 1 in 35 adults in the United States are under criminal justice supervision, and the number is expected to continue to increase. Specifically, the estimated HIV prevalence among individuals incarcerated in the US prison system is two to three times higher than the general population, with one in seven of people living with HIV being incarcerated each year, a figure that rises to one in five who are African American or Hispanic.[8] Although HIV testing rates in federal and state prisons are generally high, testing rates in jails are not. As a result, substance abusers who are incarcerated have a high risk of being HIV positive and unknowingly transmitting it to the larger community. Persons with HIV who return to the communities where they may lack access to health care services, including screening and early diagnosis, are likely to receive HIV treatment only after the disease has progressed to an advanced stage.[8] Moreover, with limited access to substance abuse treatment, many will return to drug use, and with high-risk sexual behavior or needle sharing, further increase the risk of disease spread to the community. Moreover, prisons are vectors for hepatitis C virus (HCV), which is more prevalent in African Americans than in any other racial group in the United States. However, African Americans are more likely than non-African Americans to be deemed ineligible for HCV treatment.[8] Rates of active and latent tuberculosis in correctional institutions remain considerably higher than those in the general population. Alcohol use disorders are also prevalent among incarcerated populations, and inmates are usually ineffectively treated or remain untreated during incarceration. Relapse to alcohol use occurs in 75%–85% of released prisoners. In summary, incarceration of those with substance abuse can be associated with an increased risk of HIV/AIDS infection when in correctional systems and abusers have a higher burden of co-occurring disease especially when they are African Americans. Untreated, these comorbid disorders have significant consequences for the health of the larger community.[8]

The interaction of stressful communities and mental disorders may contribute to the comorbidity. Jackson and associates proposed that individuals who are exposed to chronic stress and live in poor environments will be more likely to engage in poor health behaviors such as smoking, alcohol use, drug use, and overeating, because they are the most environmentally accessible coping strategies for socially disadvantaged groups.[26] These behaviors act on common biological structures and processes associated with pleasure and reward systems and alleviate, or interrupt, the physiological and psychological consequences of stress and reduce reported or measured depression and other mental disorders. Moreover African American female adolescents who reported depressive symptoms and substance use were more likely to engage in risky behavior. This population might benefit from future prevention efforts targeting the intersection of depression and substance use.[27] To conclude, comorbidity is yet another complication of substance abuse in African Americans. The co-occurrence may be yet another factor that contributes to health disparities.

Treatment

There is now little doubt that treatment can work, and it works for a variety of substances, across ethnicity groups, and in a variety of settings. Treatment programs, especially if they address cultural needs, are effective and have strong participation by ethnic minorities.[4] In addition, effective treatment can mean reductions in behaviors that increase the risk of comorbidities such as HIV, hepatitis C, and treatment resistant tuberculosis (TB).[49]

Treatment can work. Medication-assisted therapy with agents such as methadone and buprenorphine have been found to be extremely effective in preventing the complications of drug abuse including arrests, use of opiates, and criminal behavior. They have also been found to reduce the spread of AIDS, HCV, and mortality from these disorders.[8] Buprenorphine is a long-acting partial agonist that acts on the same receptors as heroin and morphine, relieving drug cravings without producing the same intense high or dangerous side effects. Unlike methadone, other opiates cannot be readily used with buprenorphine, so it is much less likely to be a drug of abuse as well. Congress passed the Drug Addiction Treatment Act, permitting qualified physicians to prescribe Schedule III–V narcotic medications for the treatment of opioid addiction. This legislation created a major paradigm shift by allowing access to opiate treatment in a medical setting rather than limiting it to federally approved opioid treatment programs. Buprenorphine was found to be effective in reducing opiate abuse and is an effective tool in AIDS prevention.[6] Moreover, African Americans were as accepting as other ethnic groups of this treatment.[66] Buprenorphine has advantages over methadone that can improve access, including less-associated stigma; fewer regulations, which permit its use outside opioid treatment programs; and lower risk of overdose. Its combination with naloxone reduces the likelihood of intravenous abuse of the medication. It can be a valuable tool in addressing the problem of adherence, since in the correctional system 85% to 90% of such persons relapse to opioid use within 1 year after release.[28] Overall, buprenorphine has been found to be effective during incarceration and for postincarceration. In parolees it showed significant declines in heroin and cocaine use, illegal activity, and in meeting *Diagnostic and Statistical Manual of Mental Disorders, Fourth Edition* (DSM-IV) criteria for opioid and cocaine dependence. Probationers/parolees reported lower frequency of illegal activities at 3 months compared to nonprobationers/parolees. Buprenorphine treatment should be made more widely available to individuals on parole/probation, as they respond as well to treatment as patients not supervised by the criminal justice system.[37] Moreover, it has been shown repeatedly to be effective in African Americans.[37]

Primary care practitioners are often called upon to differentiate between appropriate, medically indicated opioid use in pain management versus inappropriate abuse or addiction. Racial and ethnic minority populations tend to favor primary care treatment settings over specialty mental health settings. Buprenorphine has been shown to be effective in primary care settings and its use should be encouraged.[6]

Yet most individuals who have access to buprenorphine are non-white males. The lack of availability is related to a number of factors including the unwillingness of some substance abuse specialists to provide it, despite the fact that it was first introduced to increase availability of treatment by being an agent that can be prescribed in a primary care setting. Moreover, it has been shown to be effective in African American youth.[24] Unfortunately like other substance abuse treatments, it is less available for African Americans. It is not explained by disparities in health insurance coverage. Even with coverage, non-Hispanic black and Hispanic youth are less likely than non-Hispanic white youth to receive medications for opiate disorders

Nonpharmacological interventions for drug use can be effective. A review of the Cochrane Collaboration criteria was used to identify trials across multiple databases and found limited effect in reducing rearrests but significant reduction in reincarceration. Therapeutic community programs were found to significantly reduce the number of rearrests and a few determined cost effectiveness of the intervention. Differential benefits or lack of them were not reported.

Other effective programs that can reduce the treatment gap and have been shown to be effective for African Americans include the peer navigator program. In one study, improvements were seen in general health status psychological experience of physical health recovery and quality of life.[14] Integrated care has also been shown to be effective. In one such program, substance use and mental health symptoms were both reduced and there were some positive results on HIV risk behaviors.[47]

Unfortunately a significant proportion of African Americans with mental or substance abuse disorders still do not receive professional help. Part of the disparity may be related to the unwillingness of African Americans to accept treatment. In many cases, limited attention to ethnicity and sociocultural factors in health research has resulted in beliefs and assumptions that may not fit the experiences of African Americans. The significant proportion of black Americans with a mental disorder who relied on informal support alone, professional services alone, or no help at all suggests potential unmet need. However, the reliance on informal support also may be evidence of a strong protective role that informal networks play in the lives of African Americans and Caribbean blacks.[64] Effectively aiding the African American community means understanding and appreciating their internal realities.[40]

Prior research has shown that minority groups experience greater levels of disability associated with psychiatric and substance use conditions due to barriers to treatment. Treatment delays are an important part of the overall problem of service utilization and access to treatment, yet little work has been done to understand the factors associated with treatment delays among ethnic minorities.[45] Black and Hispanic youth were significantly less likely than whites to complete treatment for both alcohol and marijuana. Factors related to social context are likely to be important contributors to white-minority differences in addiction treatment completion, Increased Medicaid funding, coupled with culturally tailored services, could be particularly beneficial.[41] In another study, black adolescents reported receiving less specialty and informal care. Potential mechanisms of racial and ethnic disparities were identified in federal and economic health care policies and regulations, the operation of the health care system and provider organization, provider level factors, the environmental context, the operation of the community system, and patient level factors. Significant disparity decreases could be achieved by adoption of certain state policies and regulations that increase eligibility to public insurance.[3]

Clearly a key factor is criminal justice involvement. The incarcerated population has increased to unprecedented levels following the 1970 US declaration of war on illicit drug use. A substantial proportion of people at risk for HIV infection, including those with substance use and mental health disorders, have become incarcerated. Policing and racism have been mutually constitutive in the United States. Erosions to the Fourth Amendment to the Constitution and to the Posse Comitatus Act set the foundations for two War on Drugs policing strategies: stop and frisk and Special Weapons and Tactics (SWAT) teams. These strategies have created specific conditions that end up offering punitive approaches

to drug abuse in African American communities. War on Drugs policing strategies appear to increase police brutality targeting black communities, even as they make little progress in reducing street-level drug activity. Due to cost and lack of effectiveness, many jurisdictions are retreating from the War on Drugs.[21] Nevertheless, race and ethnicity are inconsistently addressed regarding arrests versus access to treatment. Inconsistent effects across states between the hazard of arrest and treatment engagement. Racial/ethnic minority groups may benefit from additional treatment support to reduce criminal justice involvement. It has been proposed that states should examine whether disparities exist within their treatment system and incorporate disparities reduction in their quality improvement initiatives.[2] After detention, substance abuse disorders present a continuing challenge for the community mental health system. Most stays in detention are brief (median, 15 days), and when detained youths return to their communities, a substantial proportion may need treatment. As noted above, they may also have comorbidities associated with drug abuse. Many correctional systems still do not offer effective substance abuse treatment or medication-assisted therapy such as buprenorphine or methadone, which has been shown repeatedly to be effective for substance abuse.[8]

Still many large jails and prisons do not presently have a substance abuse treatment program despite clear evidence of widespread drug and alcohol dependence problems among inmate populations. Where substance abuse treatment resources are available, administrators face difficult choices in determining which inmates will receive services. Lack of participation in treatment programs by African Americans has led to an evaluation of referral and screening systems implemented in several jails across the country. Unfortunately there are not enough treatment and diversion programs.[46] Alternatives to incarceration such as diversion programs and drug courts do work.[38,53] The result has been that more African Americans can have treatment available and avoid the revolving door of reincarceration. Moreover, such treatment also reduces the spread of HIV, which as we noted has been associated with individuals in corrections returning to the community. African Americans have been found to have less access to newer, more effective treatment approaches in mental health services.[32] The same is true for drug courts. Additional efforts such as drug courts to avoid incarceration and legislative changes making it easier for inmates to expunge criminal records if substance use or possession is the only crime would go a long way to reduce the factors that contribute to involvement in the correctional system. Most importantly, it would move the focus of drug use in African Americans from punishment to treatment.

In other studies, African Americans have reported higher levels of spirituality than Caucasians. African American participants indicated more perceived benefits of 12-step involvement, whereas Caucasians were more likely to endorse future involvement in 12-step programs. There were no outcome differences.[44] In yet another study, people with lived experiences reported their ongoing recovery as a process reliant upon (1) an intimate and personal relationship with God; and (2) engagement in certain core private religious activities, most notably prayer, reading of scripture, and listening to religiously inspired radio, television, or music. Psychiatric services serving an African American clientele with lived experience of dual diagnosis may increase effectiveness by better harnessing client religiosity to assist recovery.[60] A critical examination of black cultural traditions and the realities of inner-city living is important to consider in forming an understanding of substance abuse in this population. Research and treatment that lacks this perspective is less likely to identify key interventions for primary, secondary, and tertiary prevention. It takes the art of listening from those administering the health care system to hear and understand the cultural needs of this twice-stigmatized population—individuals who are African American as well as substance abusers.

If the racial disparities in substance abuse and outcomes are to be reduced, there needs to be a recognition of the contextual environment of African Americans, the cultural needs, the institutional barriers to access to care, and the importance of including evidence-based treatment. Moreover including such preventive measures such as spirituality is important to the process of recovery from all illnesses. Research has shown that integration of culturally specific factors such as spirituality into the treatment of substance abuse is consistently associated with better outcomes and lower rates of relapse. It can also help negate the hardships in the lives of substance abusers, which often are precursors to addiction and causes of relapse for patients in recovery.

Conclusions

Addressing the problem of drug use and abuse in the African American community has special challenges. Yet the problem must be addressed if there is going to be a genuine effort to reduce racial disparities in health. Drug abuse is clearly a problem that exacerbates the consequences of discrimination and poverty. The good news is that advances have been made in understanding the behavior and neurobiology of addiction, which has led to effective methods of detection, prevention, and treatment. These interventions work for African Americans. The challenge is to create the public and political will to shift the addiction focus to prevention and treatment, and to reduce disparities and improve treatment accessibility.

References

1. Abram KM, et al. Sex and racial/ethnic differences in positive outcomes in delinquent youth after detention: a 12-year longitudinal study. *JAMA Pediatr.* 2017;171(2):123–132.
2. Acevedo A, et al. Performance measures and racial/ethnic disparities in the treatment of substance use disorders. *J Stud Alcohol Drugs.* 2015;76(1):57–67.
3. Alegria M, et al. Disparities in treatment for substance use disorders and co-occurring disorders for ethnic/racial minority youth. *J Am Acad Child Adolesc Psychiatr.* 2011;50(1):22–31.
4. An interview with nora volkow. *Trends Pharmacol Sci.* 2015;36(4):187–188.
5. Bechtold J, et al. Chronic adolescent marijuana use as a risk factor for physical and mental health problems in young adult men. *Psychol Addict Behav.* 2015;29(3):552–563.
6. Bonhomme J, et al. Opioid addiction and abuse in primary care practice: a comparison of methadone and buprenorphine as treatment options. *J Natl Med Assoc.* 2012;104(7–8):342–350.
7. Buka SL. Disparities in health status and substance use: ethnicity and socioeconomic factors. *Public Health Rep.* 2002;117(suppl 1):S118–S125.
8. Chandler R, et al. Cohort profile: seek, test, treat and retain United States criminal justice cohort. *Subst Abuse Treat Prev Policy.* 2017;12(1):24.
9. Chartier KG, et al. A 10-year study of factors associated with alcohol treatment use and non-use in a U.S. population sample. *Drug Alcohol Depend.* 2016;160:205–211.
10. Ciccarone D, Unick GJ, Kraus A. Impact of South American heroin on the US heroin market 1993–2004. *Int J Drug Policy.* 2009;20(5):392–401.
11. Cicero TJ, et al. The changing face of heroin use in the United States: a retrospective analysis of the past 50 years. *JAMA Psychiatry.* 2014;71(7):821–826.
12. Compton WM, et al. Prevalence, correlates, disability, and comorbidity of DSM-IV drug abuse and dependence in the United States: results from the national epidemiologic survey on alcohol and related conditions. *Arch Gen Psychiatry.* 2007;64(5):566–576.
13. Cooper HL, et al. Risk environments, race/ethnicity, and HIV status in a large sample of people who inject drugs in the United States. *PLoS One.* 2016;11(3):e0150410.
14. Corrigan PW, et al. Using peer navigators to address the integrated health care needs of homeless African Americans with serious mental illness. *Psychiatr Serv.* 2017;68(3):264–270.
15. Culyba AJ, et al. Protective effects of adolescent-adult connection on male youth in urban environments. *J Adolesc Health.* 2016;58(2):237–240.
16. Fellner J. Race, drugs, and law enforcement in the United States. In: *Stanford Law and Policy Review.* 2009.
17. Freese TE, et al. Real-world strategies to engage and retain racial-ethnic minority young men who have sex with men in HIV prevention services. *AIDS Patient Care STDS.* 2017;31(6):275–281.
18. Galea S, Rudenstine S. Challenges in understanding disparities in drug use and its consequences. *J Urban Health.* 2005;82(2 suppl 3):iii5–iii12.
19. Gibbs TA, et al. Mental health of african Americans and caribbean blacks in the United States: results from the national Epidemiological survey on alcohol and related conditions. *Am J Public Health.* 2013;103(2):330–338.
20. Gladden RM, Martinez P, Seth P. Fentanyl law enforcement submissions and increases in synthetic opioid-involved overdose deaths - 27 states, 2013-2014. *MMWR Morb Mortal Wkly Rep.* 2016;65(33):837–843.
21. Golub A, Johnson BD, Dunlap E. The race/ethnicity disparity in misdemeanor marijuana arrests in New York City. *Criminol Public Policy.* 2007;6(1):131–164.
22. Green KM, et al. Does heavy adolescent marijuana use lead to criminal involvement in adulthood? Evidence from a multiwave longitudinal study of urban African Americans. *Drug Alcohol Depend.* 2010;112(1–2):117–125.
23. Green KM, et al. Racial differences and the role of neighborhood in the sequencing of marijuana and tobacco initiation among urban youth. *Subst Abus.* 2016;37(4):507–510.
24. Hadland SE, et al. Trends in receipt of buprenorphine and naltrexone for opioid use disorder among adolescents and young adults, 2001-2014. *JAMA Pediatr.* 2017.
25. Iguchi MY, et al. How criminal system racial disparities may translate into health disparities. *J Health Care Poor Underserved.* 2005;16(4 suppl B):48–56.
26. Jackson JS, Knight KM, Rafferty JA. Rafferty, Race and unhealthy behaviors: chronic stress, the HPA axis, and physical and mental health disparities over the life course. *Am J Public Health.* 2010;100(5):933–939.
27. Jackson JM, et al. Association of depressive symptoms and substance use with risky sexual behavior and sexually transmitted infections among african American female adolescents seeking sexual health care. *Am J Public Health.* 2015;105(10):2137–2142.
28. Kinlock TW, Battjes RJ, Schwartz RP. A novel opioid maintenance program for prisoners: preliminary findings. *J Subst Abuse Treat.* 2002;22(3):141–147.
29. Lacey KK, et al. Substance use, mental disorders and physical health of Caribbeans at-home compared to those residing in the United States. *Int J Environ Res Public Health.* 2015;12(1):710–734.
30. Lamy FR, et al. Increased in synthetic cannabinoids-related harms: results from a longitudinal web-based content analysis. *Int J Drug Policy.* 2017;44:121–129.

31. Lawrence A. The dope on drug sentencing: new approaches simplify sentencing, get more drug abusers treatment and save states money. *State Legis.* 2011;37(10):23–25.

32. Le Cook B, et al. Comparing methods of racial and ethnic disparities measurement across different settings of mental health care. *Health Serv Res.* 2010;45(3):825–847.

33. Lee JY, et al. An adverse family environment during adolescence predicts marijuana use and antisocial personality disorder in adulthood. *J Child Fam Stud.* 2016;25(2):661–668.

34. Lee JY, et al. Pathways from victimization to substance use: post traumatic stress disorder as a mediator. *Psychiatry Res.* 2016;237:153–158.

35. Lopes-Rosa R, et al. Predictors of early relapse among adolescent crack users. *J Addict Dis.* 2017;36(2):136–143.

36. Mays VM, et al. Perceived discrimination in health care and mental health/substance abuse treatment among blacks, Latinos, and whites. *Med Care.* 2017;55(2):173–181.

37. Mitchell SG, et al. Treatment outcomes of african American buprenorphine patients by parole and probation status. *J Drug Issues.* 2014;44(1):69–82.

38. Morgan RD, et al. Specialty courts: who's in and are they working? *Psychol Serv.* 2016;13(3):246–253.

39. Nasrullah M, et al. The association of recent incarceration and health outcomes among HIV-infected adults receiving care in the United States. *Int J Prison Health.* 2016;12(3):135–144.

40. Neighbors HW, et al. Mental health service use among older African Americans: the National Survey of American Life. *Am J Geriatr Psychiatry.* 2008;16(12):948–956.

41. NIDA. *Health Consequences of Drug Misuse.* National Institute on Drug Abuse website. https://www.drugabuse.gov/related-topics/health-consequences-drug-misuse; 2017. Accessed June 12, 2017.

42. Ninnemann AL, et al. Longitudinal predictors of synthetic cannabinoid use in adolescents. *Pediatrics.* 2017;139(4).

43. Palamar JJ, et al. Powder cocaine and crack use in the United States: an examination of risk for arrest and socioeconomic disparities in use. *Drug Alcohol Depend.* 2015;149:108–116.

44. Peavy KM, et al. A comparison of African American and Caucasian stimulant users in 12-step facilitation treatment. *J Ethn Subst Abuse.* 2016:1–20.

45. Perron BE, et al. Ethnic differences in delays to treatment for substance use disorders: African Americans, Black Caribbeans and non-Hispanic whites. *J Psychoactive Drugs.* 2009;41(4):369–377.

46. Peters RH. Referral and screening for substance abuse treatment in jails. *J Ment Health Adm.* 1992;19(1):53–75.

47. Rasch RF, et al. Integrated recovery management model for ex-offenders with co-occurring mental health and substance use disorders and high rates of HIV risk behaviors. *J Assoc Nurses AIDS Care.* 2013;24(5):438–448.

48. Regier DA, et al. Comorbidity of mental disorders with alcohol and other drug abuse. Results from the Epidemiologic Catchment Area (ECA) Study. *JAMA.* 1990;264(19):2511–2518.

49. Rich JD, et al. HIV-related research in correctional populations: now is the time. *Curr HIV AIDS Rep.* 2011;8(4):288.

50. Rudd RA, et al. Increases in drug and opioid overdose deaths--United States, 2000-2014. *MMWR Morb Mortal Wkly Rep.* 2016;64(50–51):1378–1382.

51. Reference deleted in review.

52. Singhal A, Tien YY, Hsia RY. Racial-ethnic disparities in opioid prescriptions at emergency department visits for conditions commonly associated with prescription drug abuse. *PLoS One.* 2016;11(8):e0159224.

53. Sloan FA, et al. Does the probability of DWI arrest fall following participation in DWI and hybrid drug treatment court programs? *Accid Anal Prev.* 2016;97:197–205.

54. Strong C, Juon HS, Ensminger ME. Effect of adolescent cigarette smoking on adulthood substance use and abuse: the mediating role of educational attainment. *Subst Use Misuse.* 2016;51(2):141–154.

55. Vaughn MG, et al. Is crack cocaine use associated with greater violence than powdered cocaine use? Results from a national sample. *Am J Drug Alcohol Abuse.* 2010;36(4):181–186.

56. Visconti AJ, et al. Opioid overdose deaths in the city and county of san Francisco: prevalence, distribution, and disparities. *J Urban Health.* 2015;92(4):758–772.

57. Volkow ND. Substance use disorders in schizophrenia--clinical implications of comorbidity. *Schizophr Bull.* 2009;35(3):469–472.

58. Volkow ND, et al. Effects of cannabis use on human behavior, including cognition, motivation, and psychosis: a review. *JAMA Psychiatry.* 2016;73(3):292–297.

59. Welty LJ, et al. Health disparities in drug- and alcohol-use disorders: a 12-year longitudinal study of youths after detention. *Am J Public Health.* 2016;106(5):872–880.

60. Whitley R. "Thank you God": religion and recovery from dual diagnosis among low-income African Americans. *Transcult Psychiatry.* 2012;49(1):87–104.

61. Wildeman C, Wang EA. Mass incarceration, public health, and widening inequality in the USA. *Lancet.* 2017;389(10077):1464–1474.

62. Williams DR. Miles to go before we sleep: racial inequities in health. *J Health Soc Behav.* 2012;53(3):279–295.

63. Williams DR, Mohammed SA. Discrimination and racial disparities in health: evidence and needed research. *J Behav Med.* 2009;32(1):20–47.

64. Woodward AT, et al. Use of professional and informal support by African Americans and Caribbean blacks with mental disorders. *Psychiatr Serv.* 2008;59(11):1292–1298.

65. Wu LT, Zhu H, Swartz MS. Trends in cannabis use disorders among racial/ethnic population groups in the United States. *Drug Alcohol Depend.* 2016;165:181–190.

66. Wu LT, et al. Racial/ethnic variations in substance-related disorders among adolescents in the United States. *Arch Gen Psychiatry.* 2011;68(11):1176–1185.

67. Zapolski TC, et al. Less drinking, yet more problems: understanding African American drinking and related problems. *Psychol Bull.* 2014;140(1):188–223.

68

Substance Use Disorders in Health Care Professionals

GEORGE A. KENNA, JEFFREY N. BALDWIN, ALISON M. TRINKOFF, AND DAVID C. LEWIS

CHAPTER OUTLINE

Introduction

The impact of licit (i.e., alcohol and nicotine used legally) and illicit (including nonmedical prescription) drug use, abuse, and dependence in the United States is well documented in the general population. Overall, a 2006 survey reported that an estimated 20.4 million Americans 12 years of age or older were current illicit drug users, meaning they had used an illicit drug—defined as "marijuana/hashish, cocaine (all forms), heroin, methamphetamine, hallucinogens, inhalants or psychotherapeutics used nonmedically"—during the month prior to the survey interview.[86] This estimate represents 8.3% of the population 12 years of age or older. More specifically, an estimated 5.2 million persons were current nonmedical users of prescription pain relievers, up from an estimated 4.7 million in 2005.

A recent report of abuse of prescription medication in the United States reported that many health care professionals are poorly trained to deal with alcohol or drug abuse.[84] A substantial number of patients served daily by health care professionals in various health care facilities are abusing or dependent on alcohol and or other drugs. On the other hand, the public expects health care professionals to understand the proper use of the medicines they prescribe, dispense, or administer to their patients. Just as in their patients, though, alcohol or drug use also affects the lives of a number of health care professionals.[23]

Starting in college, some health care students develop an attitude of invulnerability and immunity to addiction, fueled by their advanced understanding of the mechanisms of drug action. What begins as recreational college alcohol or drug use[73] may, for some, develop into a complicated pattern of alcohol or drug abuse or dependence intended to attain a "sense of well-being"[77] (p. 17) without an overt manifestation of intoxication or side effects. This concept of balancing drug effects, also called "titration," or "walking a chemical tightrope,"[23] refers to a practice whereby students or health care professionals use their pharmacological knowledge to balance positive and negative drug actions and reactions by "enhancing, neutralizing or counteracting specific drug effects through ingesting multiple types of drugs" [Dabney D (1997) A sociological examination of illicit prescription drug use among pharmacists. University of Florida, "An Unpublished Dissertation"].

Health care professionals have a significant responsibility that comes with the privilege of using medications to treat patients.[11,56,59,71] Although most health care professionals engage in appropriate prescribing, dispensing, and administration of medication, reports of exceptional cases often receive public attention. A North Hollywood, California, physician, for example, was charged with conspiring to distribute 406 prescriptions of hydrocodone and oxycodone over 2 months after he surrendered his license to the US Drug Enforcement Administration (DEA) in May 2008. This pain management specialist was also being investigated regarding a role that his prescriptions might have played in the deaths of six patients over the past 3 years.[121] A Virginia pharmacist was caught with hundreds of phentermine capsules when he was apprehended by law enforcement authorities,[90] and a Maryland pharmacist was trading sex for drugs.[90] Medication errors caused by substance-impaired pharmacists have been cited as posing a direct and serious threat to the public.[78] Moreover, nurses were reported to be alcohol or drug impaired while committing "dozens of errors leading to patient deaths in Illinois"[9] (p. A1).

Whether by virtue of their drug access[72] or socioeconomic status,[48] most evidence supports the notion that a small but significant proportion of health care professionals do experience personal problems with the use of alcohol and other drugs, which can result in serious consequences to themselves and to the public [Valentine N (1991) Stress, alcohol and psychoactive drug use among nurses in Massachusetts. Brandeis University, Boston, MA, "An Unpublished Dissertation"].[73,83] Not only can the economic costs of substance use disorders[27] in health care professionals be considerable,[67] but early identification is essential because patient and provider well-being may be at risk.[23] Given the increasingly stressful environment due to manpower shortages in the health care system in general,[91] alcohol or drug use and misuse among health care professionals has been projected to grow.[89] Treatment of alcohol or drug disorders by health care workers was a policy issue recognized years ago by the professional organizations,[2,5] and the Joint Commission requires hospitals to monitor and identify matters of health[52] including substance use and abuse by physicians and other health care professionals.

The aim of this chapter is to provide perhaps the most comprehensive review of the problem of drug abuse by health care professionals to date. In addition, although covered in greater detail in other chapters in this book, we also briefly discuss the behavioral signs and symptoms of addiction in health care professionals, the treatment of substance use disorders in this special subpopulation, and the prognosis of sustained recovery and efforts needed to enlighten the various health care professional programs and groups.

Epidemiology of Alcohol and Other Drug Use by Health Care Professionals

The current literature regarding the prevalence of substance use and dependence in health care professionals is limited in both its scope of generalizability and methodological rigor.[13,60] Lack of empirical data have contributed to an air of skepticism regarding the actual prevalence of substance abuse (abuse as referred to colloquially, not a *Diagnostic and Statistical Manual of Mental Disorders*, Fifth Edition[5a] [DSM-5] diagnosis) and dependence by health care professionals. In fact, evidence of the extent of medication diversion, considered to be the major source of nonprescribed drug abuse by health care professionals, is based primarily on retrospective accounts [Dabney D (1997) A sociological examination of illicit prescription drug use among pharmacists. University of Florida, "An Unpublished Dissertation"],[10,70,111] although the actual size of the diversion problem is largely unknown.[36] As a result, the prevalence of inappropriate substance abuse and chemical dependency among health care professionals is inconclusive[16,72] and, like the extent of prescription opioid drug diversion in the United States, for example, is impossible to estimate at the present time.[54] The fact that the behaviors being measured represent illegal or inappropriate behaviors compounds the problem, as it is difficult to obtain accurate estimates of sensitive variables such as substance use.[117]

A glimpse of the lack of epidemiological knowledge in the field is best illustrated by contradictory prevalence estimates found in the literature. For example, reports[18,107] have suggested that narcotic addiction in US physicians was as much as 30–100 times the rate found in the general population, but these data were based on data from Germany in the 1950s.[13,31] In addition, the lifetime estimate of combined substance abuse and dependence among health care professionals was reported by Kessler et al.[65] to be at a rate nearly equal to that of the general population, or 26%. Similarly, estimates from other studies of health care professionals have reported a lifetime prevalence of substance dependence ranging from 3% to 20%.[11,42,95,114,116] Although the literature provides limited studies of substance use by dentists, Hedge[46] has estimated that up to 15%–18% of dentists could be addicted to drugs and alcohol. In contrast to these rates, however, another report concluded that physicians were at a "greater lifetime probability of developing a substance-related disorder than the general population"[30] (p. 7).

Such statements clearly demonstrate the confusion and misinformation surrounding a meaningful discussion of alcohol or drug use by health care professionals. These generalizations have not only contributed to the uncertainty about the prevalence of substance use, but also to the confusion with regard to risk factors that contribute to substance use among health care professionals.[13] For example, although referring to pharmacists as "drugged experts"[26] (p. 102), Dabney[24] used a measure of questionable reliability and validity to assess substance use in a nationwide sample of pharmacists. Specifically, the measure assessed redundant drug use items, categorized unauthorized use of nonnarcotic medications as addictive drug use, and provided no direction to participants regarding exactly which drugs were included in each drug category.[55] Moreover, as also noted by Baldwin,[7] the frequency data reported by Dabney[24] contained no time frame for reported substance use and were, therefore, not useful in estimating the prevalence of substance use. Although Dabney[24] claimed that the onset of potentially addictive drug use in pharmacists occurred upon becoming a professional, such a conclusion was essentially impossible without longitudinal data or some specific items assessing age at the onset of regular use. The methods were strongly defended by the author[25]; however, these issues contribute to a suspect interpretation of the data.

Overgeneralizations from methodologically questionable data also exist in the limited amount of literature describing substance use by the dental profession. Except for reporting the number of disciplinary actions taken against Oregon dentists from 1979 to 1984,[20] no known empirical prevalence data for substance use had ever been reported for practicing dentists until recently.[62] However, Chiodo and Tolle,[17] drawing on nonrepresentative disciplinary action data, inaccurately concluded that dentists, like physicians, were at higher risk for substance use and abuse than the general population, and also concluded that the literature had consistently reported higher rates of chemical dependency in health care professionals, a notion unsupported by quantitative self-reported data.[62]

In a series of important analyses, McAuliffe et al.[71–75] assessed alcohol or drug use by both physicians and pharmacists, and Valentine [Valentine N (1991) Stress, alcohol and psychoactive drug use among nurses in Massachusetts. Brandeis University, Boston, MA, "An Unpublished Dissertation"] assessed alcohol or drug use by nurses. Lack of generalizability to other practitioners outside these two disciplines was a major limitation of these studies. In addition, these studies were conducted in the Northeast, where past-year alcohol or drug use has been reported to be higher than in other areas of the United States.[86] Subsequently, to address some of the methodological shortcomings of these studies, Hughes and colleagues[48] (p. 2333) compared a national sample of physician use of alcohol or drugs with that of the general population. They reported that when compared with the general population, physicians were more likely to use alcohol, benzodiazepines, and minor opioids but less likely to use street drugs such as marijuana and cocaine. Furthermore, contrary to the suggestion made by Chiodo and Tolle,[17] that the literature consistently reported disproportionately higher rates of chemical dependency in health care professionals, Hughes et al. reported that only 7.9% of physicians identified themselves as substance abusers, while the corresponding rate for the general population at that time was 15%–18%.[98] Hughes et al. also noted, however, that physicians were as likely as their age and gender peers to have experimented with illicit substances in their lifetime, an observation also affirmed more recently.[59] Although methodologically rigorous, Hughes et al. acknowledged the narrow focus of their study to physicians alone that subsequently limited their findings due to the lack of comparable national data across other similar professions. In recognition of this limitation, the authors concluded that any comparisons between physicians and other health care professionals in "similar socioeconomic strata may have yielded different results"[48] (p. 2337). Complicating these issues is stigma that accompanies alcohol or drug use in any population, which leads to underestimates of problem use.[88]

Etiology of Substance Use Disorders in Health Care Professionals

Many etiologic factors have been reported to contribute to substance use in health care professionals, such as a family history for drug or alcohol use,[21,76,104] college substance use,[6,19] or age at first alcohol or drug use[66]; psychological factors such as "pharmacological optimism,"[23,34,42,119] access to prescription medications,[42,69] self-prescribing,[19,48,72] socioeconomic status,[48] and additional factors such as gender (male), lack of religious practices,[72,123] and social influences.[66,92]

Drug Access

Drug access, and in particular easy drug access,[118] is generally recognized as a principal factor contributing to substance use by health care professionals. Certainly, studies show that access to prescription medications would explain the higher rates of use of these drugs among health professionals than in the general population.[48,60] Although research on drug use in the working population in general has been inconclusive, Mensch and Kandel[81] have suggested that drug use by workers was due less to the workplace than to the workers themselves. Clearly, however, a substantial foundation of research indicates that health care professionals are at considerable risk due to their working environment.[23,114,118] Drug access is related directly to the job of being a health care professional. As such, the working condition related to medical practice is an important contributing factor enhancing one's exposure to addicting drugs.

To illustrate this point, dentists have historically had easy access to nitrous oxide, an inhalant commonly kept in dental offices, and a known drug of abuse for dentists. Although the data are now dated (1979–1984), 7.1% of 109 impaired dentists in a study that took place in Oregon were sanctioned for abusing nitrous oxide.[20]

The authors concluded that nitrous oxide in particular posed a serious hazard for dentists. Although dentists have access to nitrous oxide for procedures, access to other drugs such as minor opioids and anxiolytic drugs is limited. For example, dentists were the only health care professional group who did not report personal use of samples; the study, nonetheless, indicated that they found other sources for addicting prescription medications.[63]

Different researchers have developed measures to assess the impact of drug access by health care professionals on drug use [Dabney D (1997) A sociological examination of illicit prescription drug use among pharmacists. University of Florida, "An Unpublished Dissertation"].[75,118] A pilot study by Trinkoff and Storr[117] suggested that easy access to drugs contributed to misuse. This was more firmly supported in a later, more extensive study of nurses ($n = 3917$), wherein the ease of access correlated positively with past-year misuse.[118] Three workplace dimensions were measured (availability, frequency of administration, and workplace controls), and, summed as an index, nurses with easy access on all dimensions were most likely to have misused prescription-type drugs (odds ratio = 4.18; 95% confidence interval [CI] 1.70–10.30). Furthermore, access continued to show the same correlation to misuse, even when knowledge of substances was also controlled in the analysis, thereby showing that access was not explained by nurses' knowledge of substances used.

In a survey study performed comparing alcohol or drug use by pharmacy and nursing students and with pharmacists and nurses, predictors of lifetime illicit drug use by pharmacists and nurses included having a family history of drug problems, greater amount of past-month alcohol use, lack of religious affiliation, and notably greater access to drugs.[60] Predictors for use of an illicit drug (any Schedule I or unprescribed drug use) by pharmacy and nursing students included a family history of drug problems, less drug access, and cigarette use in the past year. Of interest, lower drug access was a significant predictor for lifetime illicit substance use by pharmacy and nursing students, suggesting that when substances were unavailable in the workplace, students were more likely to obtain them elsewhere. Despite a reassurance of anonymity, students may also have been reluctant to admit to such behavior due to the fear of being discovered. In support of this notion, none of the students in the study reported diverting any medications from where they work, yet a greater number of pharmacy and nursing students in the same sample reported use of prescription medications than among the general population.[60] We know that various sources for drug use include the home[108] and friends [Dabney D (1997) A sociological examination of illicit prescription drug use among pharmacists. University of Florida, "An Unpublished Dissertation"], but we also know that sources include the workplace as well [Dabney D (1997) A sociological examination of illicit prescription drug use among pharmacists. University of Florida, "An Unpublished Dissertation"].

Where pharmacy students worked did not appear to be related to disproportionate drug use; however, a greater number of retail pharmacists reported illicit drug use than pharmacists in other pharmacy practice areas.[60] When parsing out comparisons of individual drugs, except for marijuana, consistent with the data from Hughes et al.[48] a higher proportion of the general population reported use of street drugs such as cocaine, hallucinogens, and inhalants. A greater number of health care professionals and students, however, reported use of drugs to which they typically had access, such as opioids and anxiolytics.[60] In sum, quantitative and qualitative studies have all demonstrated that increased drug access in an unrestrictive environment provides an important substrate permissive of drug use by health care professionals. The available studies are consistent for studies of nurses,[118] pharmacists [Dabney D (1997) A sociological examination of illicit prescription drug use among pharmacists. University of Florida, "An Unpublished Dissertation"],[72] certain types of physicians,[114] and health care professionals in general[23,83] that report drug access to be a key element leading to drug misuse and abuse in health care professionals. Efforts to restrict drug access in every setting, as well as increased vigilance to monitor drug procurement and drug disposition by clinicians who dispense from their offices, should be considered a priority.

Family History of Alcohol and Drug Use

Without a doubt, the greatest concern for health care professionals, as for the public, are alcohol use disorders.[87] Lifetime prevalence of alcohol abuse in the United States is 17.8% and alcohol dependence is 12.5%. Past 12-month prevalence of alcohol abuse is 4.7%, while alcohol dependence over the same period is 3.8%.[44] Alcohol dependence is significantly more prevalent among men, whites, and younger unmarried adults, and lifetime alcohol abuse is highest among middle-aged Americans.[44]

Twin studies of alcoholics have highlighted the possibility of genetic components of alcoholism[94] while other researchers[105] have also sought genetic markers for individuals with a positive family history for alcoholism. Studies have demonstrated that first-degree relatives (parents, siblings, or offspring) are more likely to use alcohol, become alcohol dependent, and are at substantially higher risk of developing problems with alcohol at some point during their lives.[88] Family history of alcoholism has been estimated to be approximately 38% in the United States.[43]

A retrospective review of substance use and addiction in medical students, residents, and physicians[33] suggested that the most predictive factor for alcoholism in physicians was a positive family history for alcoholism. Kenna and Wood[62] reported that significant bivariate correlations between positive family history and pattern of alcohol use (r = 0.31), as well as positive family history for drug problems and current drug use (r = 0.55), existed for physicians alone. There is the possibility that there were genuine relationships between those physicians reporting a positive family history for alcoholism and their alcohol use and between a positive family history for drug problems and drug use. Physicians are trained diagnosticians and can putatively accurately assess the presence or lack of alcohol and drug use problems by family members. These diagnoses may have led to a more accurate assessment of family members, thereby reducing measurement error in this particular group.

Numerous studies also demonstrate that first-degree relatives are at substantially higher risk of developing problems with alcohol at some point during their lives.[88] Coombs[23] proposed that the health care professions attract "people vulnerable to drug abuse because of emotional impairment due to alcoholic and emotionally abusive parents"[23] (p. 192). Several studies of dental students[12,100–102] previously speculated that many dentists perhaps come from dysfunctional families or families with a history of alcoholism or chemical dependency. Sammon et al.,[100] for example, reported that 35%–39% of students at two dental schools had an alcoholic parent or grandparent, and Sandoval et al.[101] reported that 15% of all dental students at the University of Texas had a family history of alcoholism and 17% of illicit drug use. In a more recent study, however, dentists reported the fewest family members with alcohol problems of any health care professional

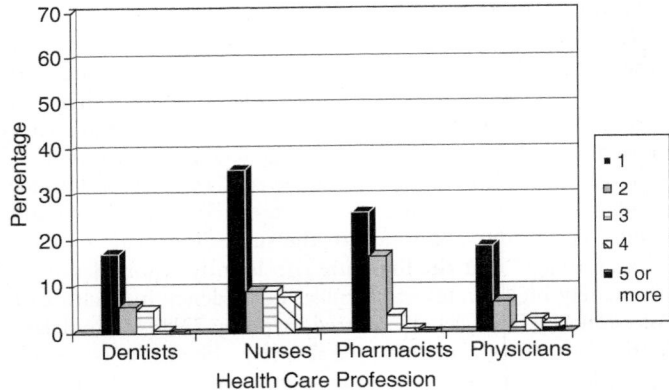

• **Fig. 68.1** Family history of alcoholism among health care professionals (*n* = 479).

group,[62] suggesting that there is little evidence that dentists are at greater risk than other health care professionals to report a family history of alcohol problems.

Several other studies have also reported high rates of positive family history for alcoholism for health care students and health care professionals as well. For example, in a comparison of chemically dependent and nondependent nurses, Sullivan[110] reported that 62% of chemically dependent nurses reported an alcoholic family member, compared with 28% for nonchemically dependent nurses. In addition, in a sample of recovering pharmacists, Bissell et al.[10] reported a positive family history for alcoholism rate of 55%–58% in recovering pharmacists, slightly higher than the 47.4% prevalence estimate reported by Kenna and Wood[59] in a survey. What of course must be considered between the two rates are the differences between the two study populations: one clinical[10] and the other population based. In college students, Tucker et al.[120] reported a positive family history for alcoholism in 28.1% in a sample of pharmacy students, and Kriegler et al.[66] established that a positive family history for alcoholism was reported by 38.3% of nursing student respondents. In a measure including eight close relatives (other studies typically included parents, grandparents, and siblings), Kenna and Wood[58] reported a positive family history for alcoholism in 46% of pharmacy students and 74.5% of nursing students surveyed.

In a follow-up study of 479 licensed health care professionals (68.7% response), researchers sought to ascertain whether positive family history for alcoholism and positive family history for drug problems were more prevalent among nurses than among dentists, pharmacists, and physicians and if an association between positive family history for alcoholism or positive family history for drug problems and current alcohol or drug use, respectively, existed.[62] Nurses reported a significantly higher prevalence of positive family history for alcoholism than other groups of health care professionals (*P* < 0.001) (Fig. 68.1), and nurses also reported a significantly higher prevalence of positive family history for drug problems than dentists and physicians (*P* < 0.01), but not pharmacists (Fig. 68.2). The study also demonstrated that positive family history for alcoholism in nursing was not associated with either amount of current alcohol use or abstinence. On the other hand, as noted previously, among physicians alone, relationships between alcohol use and positive family history for alcoholism as well as between drug use and positive family history for drug problems were significant. The results of this study support the notion that positive

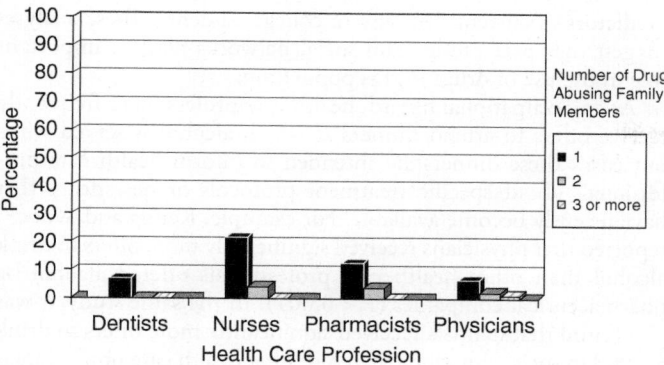

• **Fig. 68.2** Family history of drug abuse among health care professionals (*n* = 479).

family history for alcoholism and positive family history for drug problems differ across groups of health care professionals.

While speculated, no one truly understands why a significant number of people with a positive family history for alcoholism appear to select nursing as a profession. Some have suggested that the desire to go into nursing emanates from the family of origin[66] and that nurses assume parental roles taken on in childhood.[82] For example, in a study of the characteristics of chemically dependent nurses,[110] 48% indicated that while growing up, they had acted in some type of parental role compared with only 22% of nondependent nurses. In order to delineate the association between nursing and family history of alcoholism, more research into the familial dynamics or individual differences of nurses and nursing students needs to be performed.

Professional Invincibility

Many health care professionals assume that their education, intelligence and knowledge of pharmacology will provide immunity from substance-related impairment.[23] This self-deception of professional invincibility is an attitude of denial of impairment. More importantly, intervention is difficult in health care professionals as denial to the existence of a substance-related problem contributes to continued substance use, abuse, and dependence.[106,113] Hankes and Bissell[42] referred to this air of invincibility in physicians as "MDeity" (p. 890). The attitude that health care professionals are selectively immune to the pharmacological actions of addictive medications—based primarily on their knowledge of drug action—has been the subject of retrospective accounts given by many health care professionals [Dabney D (1997) A sociological examination of illicit prescription drug use among pharmacists. University of Florida, "An Unpublished Dissertation"].[23] The health care professionals may believe that their education, particularly with respect to drug titration, makes them impervious to physical or psychological dependence, or the unconsidered equivalent, drug addict. Health care professionals are good at hiding their addiction by walking a pharmacological tightrope[23]; they tend to take greater amounts and a wider variety of drugs, making them more difficult to treat.[115] Perhaps, then, it is this attitude of pharmacological invincibility that becomes the fundamental problem with substance use experimentation and addiction in health care professionals, particularly those who choose to treat themselves or who continue treatment beyond the period of illness or at dosages escalating beyond those required to circumvent tolerance.

Pharmacological Optimism

Pharmacological optimism, or the anticipated benefits of medication use, has also been suggested to be a contributing factor in the development of chemical impairment by health care professionals. In 2000, pharmaceutical companies spent 15.7 billion dollars on drug promotion that grew to almost 30 billion dollars by 2005,[29] with most of the expenditure aimed toward health care professionals.[37] Although pharmaceutical companies relentlessly directly target consumers, the impact does not compare to the decades-long indoctrination that health care professionals have received. Moreover, in view of a health care professional's training and education, familiarity with drugs is an important aspect of professional competency. Development of beliefs about the anticipated outcomes using drugs can be assumed to be a logical extension of knowledge of a drug's effect.

The literature has been inconsistent in defining pharmacological optimism. For example, one researcher defined pharmacological optimism as "a generalized positive belief about the efficacy of drugs for managing symptoms as measured by an individual's willingness to use psychoactive drugs under varying circumstances"[36] (p. 48). Although reported to be based on alcohol expectancy literature,[14] the measure developed did not assess specific beliefs about the effects of psychoactive drugs but misoperationalized the concept as a general willingness to use psychoactive drugs.[34]

A qualitative study of health care professionals suggested that pharmacological optimism was synonymous with the concept of "better living through chemistry"[23] (p. 187), which suggests that all ills can be cured with a medication. Although pharmacological optimism was one of several key factors considered to contribute to substance use and abuse by health care professionals, the author did not further define or quantitatively assess the construct.[23] Trinkoff and colleagues[119] suggested that pharmacological optimism may occur as a result of highly specialized knowledge about drugs. For example, self-administration practices by health care professionals may occur as a result of the development of attitudes and or beliefs that drugs may be the quickest route to change one's feelings and mood. Trinkoff et al. measured pharmacological optimism with the combination of access to drugs and knowledge of drugs, reporting pharmacological optimism to be significantly associated with past-year substance use, but only when access was not included in the analysis.[119]

Other researchers suggest that pharmacological optimism is more specifically based on beliefs of a drug's anticipated effect and conceptually similar to alcohol and other drug expectancies.[64] Alcohol,[14,96] marijuana, and cocaine[50,103] expectancies are beliefs about the effects of these specific drugs that develop prior to and as a result of their use and show significant variability across levels of use.

To test this theory related to prescription medications, Kenna and Wood[64] developed scales to measure pharmacological optimism and one's willingness to use drugs of abuse.[34] The authors administered a self-report cross-sectional survey to upperclassmen and graduate pharmacy and nursing students as well as comparable non–health care students (*n* = 401). The results demonstrated that although pharmacological optimism predicted unique variance in drug use over a person's willingness to use a drug, no differences were demonstrated between health care and non–health care students on pharmacological optimism, and pharmacological optimism was not associated with greater drug use by health care students. In sum, although the results support the existence of pharmacological optimism, these beliefs ultimately did not appear to facilitate drug use by health care students over and above experiential or occupational circumstances such as workplace access to substances.

Negative Proscriptions

Winick[122] proposed a theory that the incidence of substance abuse is highest in those groups in which easy drug access, role strain, and disengagement from negative proscriptions exist. Disengagement from negative proscriptions regarding substance use may be an important correlate to one's level of association with conventional institutions and subsequent risk for substance use. Although difficult to measure directly, both religiosity (internal factors) and social networks (external factors) have been hypothesized to be important conjoined factors to measure negative proscriptions. Religiosity has been hypothesized to be an internal factor that may mitigate substance use.[99] One's social network has been found to be an important external factor, linked to one's reference group, norms, and peer group choices that may promote drug use.[51] Trinkoff et al.[119] tested the utility of this theory in 3600 nurses and reported that nurses were more likely to use drugs when drug access increased, social networks contained drug users, and religiosity decreased. These data also suggest that weak attachments to negative proscriptions (low religiosity and social networks that promote drug use) and high drug access are influences related to one's drug use.

Social and Professional Influences

Social influences have been hypothesized to play a central role in models of substance initiation[39] and are considered among the strongest correlates of alcohol use and misuse.[45] Within the social influence framework, two types of social influences (active and passive) are proposed.[39] Active social influences consist of explicit offers to use drugs or alcohol that require an immediate response from the individual offered the substance and are seen as important sources for substance use initiation. Passive social influences include both social modeling and perceived peer norms. Social modeling involves observing drug or alcohol use by one's family or friends. Perceived norms are beliefs surrounding what referents consider or perceive as normal drinking or drug use that may affect both behavior and attitudes about alcohol or drug consumption. In short, these social influences are the means by which a person may gain information simply by observing another's behavior or developing a sense or misperception of what level of substance use is ongoing and acceptable by peers. It is thought that this information may influence future behaviors. For example, social modeling by family members has been hypothesized to be a risk factor in nurses.[110] Significant differences were found when comparing drinking behaviors in the families of chemically dependent and non–chemically dependent nurses; 32% of the chemically dependent nurses reported heavy drinking at home during childhood as compared with only 10% of the non–chemically dependent nurses.[110] Moreover, Dabney [Dabney D (1997) A sociological examination of illicit prescription drug use among pharmacists. University of Florida, "An Unpublished Dissertation"] reported from the qualitative arm of his study of 50 recovering pharmacists that 30% of these health care professionals were encouraged by peers and supervisors that it was acceptable to use drugs to be able to function and perform at work. Kenna and Wood[59] demonstrated that social influences, primarily active offers of drugs and to a lesser degree social modeling of drug use, were strong predictors of current drug use in college students. These analyses suggest that peer groups and social networks play an important role in the use of drugs in this population.

As an occupational hazard, health care professionals frequently receive offers to attend dinners at which alcohol is served without cost. These dinners are intended to inform health care professionals about specific treatment protocols or new drugs that have recently become available. For example, Kenna and Wood[61] reported that physicians received significantly more offers to drink alcohol than other health care professionals offered alcohol by pharmaceutical companies ($P < 0.001$). In the same study, it was also found that dentists received significantly more offers to drink alcohol in social situations than did other health care professionals ($P < 0.01$). As for prescription medications, Clark and colleagues[18] reported that physicians wrote more prescriptions for family, friends, and colleagues immediately upon receiving prescriptive authority. Although not statistically significant, these results do suggest that physicians, dentists, and potentially other health care professionals are asked to provide prescriptions or medications to friends, family, and other colleagues.

Age and Substance Use

The data from studies consistently demonstrate that older health care professionals drink significantly more alcohol than younger health care professionals, a finding that is supported by both quantitative and qualitative data in health care professionals. For example, McAuliffe et al.[71] first reported that among physicians, heavy alcohol use (five or more drinks at one time on five or more days during the past 30 days) increased with age. Moreover, heavy alcohol use by pharmacists declined only slightly after peaking at ages 31–40 years. Notably, each professional group in the McAuliffe et al. study had their own distinctive trend of heavy alcohol use across age. Drinking habits among doctors were not associated with medical specialty or type of practice but were positively related to gender (men greater than women) and to age (older were more apt to qualify as heavy drinkers than younger doctors). Hughes et al.[48] reported that physicians were more likely to report past-year alcohol use than age- and gender-matched cohorts to the general population. On the contrary, after peaking at ages 21–25 years, past-year alcohol use, binge use, and heavy alcohol use all decrease with age among US adults.[86]

Qualitative studies also report that older substance-impaired health care professionals have a tendency to be more alcohol involved than younger ones. Retrospective studies with health care professionals[111,114] suggest that younger health care professionals tend to use a greater variety of drugs in addition to alcohol than older health care professionals. For example, Talbott et al.[114] examined the substance abuse patterns and specialties in 1000 substance-impaired physicians referred for treatment in Georgia and reported that younger physicians tended to be more polydrug involved than older physicians, who tended to use alcohol alone. General population data would suggest that combined alcohol and illicit substance use peaks in the range of 18 to 25 years of age.[86] Similarly, in a study of nurses, Sullivan et al.[111] reported that alcohol was the most common drug of dependency and that women and older registered nurses tended to use alcohol alone while younger registered nurses tended to report narcotic dependency more frequently. In a study of recovering pharmacists, Bissell et al.[10] found that by the age of 49 years, the majority of pharmacists in their study abused alcohol alone.

Alcohol, Tobacco, and Other Drug Use in the Health Care Professions

Dentists

Although there is no overwhelming evidence that dentists are at a higher risk for developing alcohol dependence than the general population, alcohol use/misuse appears to be the most notable substance use problem facing dentistry. As noted previously, dentists engage in other social interactions that promote their alcohol use.[61] Nearly every major alcohol use standard assessed indicated that dentists were significantly more likely than other health care professionals surveyed to self-report use and misuse of alcohol.[62] Compared with other health care professionals, dentists reported a higher lifetime prevalence of alcohol use, significantly greater past 30-day quantity and frequency of alcohol use, greater past-year and past-month binge drinking (five or more drinks for men or four or more drinks for women at one time), as well as greater daily use. When compared with the US general population data for individuals 35 years of age or older at the time,[85] dentists reported a greater prevalence of lifetime alcohol use and past-year binge drinking.[62] These data are consistent with retrospective treatment records of 2015 health care professionals in Georgia's substance abuse treatment program in which dentists, in addition to physicians, were more likely to be exclusively alcohol dependent.[35]

Information is limited as to why alcohol use, misuse, and problems appear to be higher among dentists compared with other health care professionals. Hankes and Bissell[42] pointed out that good data regarding substance use for dentists were extremely limited; this has not changed. Putatively, causes could be linked to several risk factors previously noted in the general population, such as gender, family history, income, and social factors.[44]

Certainly, one could assume that alcohol use differences may be related to the gender imbalance of more men in the dental profession, and men report more alcohol use than women.[65] More so than in any other health care professional group surveyed,[62] male dentists (85%) outnumbered female dentists, which was consistent with American Dental Association[1] data, which reported that almost 83% of dentists were men. However, it is important to note that 74% of the physicians in the Kenna and Wood[62] study were men, and physicians reported the least amount of alcohol use of any of the professions. In addition, although there were no differences between men and women regarding regular alcohol use, analyses demonstrated no gender difference in weekly quantity and frequency of alcohol use in health care professionals in general.

One potential explanation for the increased alcohol use by dentists may be related to higher income. In other words, the use of alcohol may increase with increased incomes.[38] Previously, Hughes et al.[48] noted that the prevalence of alcohol use was greater among physicians than in the general population by virtue of their socioeconomic class and not related to the profession of medicine. Consistent with Hughes et al.,[48] lifetime prevalence and past-year binge drinking reported by physicians were higher than reported for the general population.[61,85] Although dentists did report the highest mean income of all health care professional groups, they also reported income only slightly greater than that of physicians, who reported the least amount of alcohol use of all health care professional groups. In short, dentists drank significantly more alcohol than physicians, yet dentists and physicians reported essentially the same income. Furthermore, nurses and pharmacists reported a substantially lower income than dentists and physicians

and still reported greater lifetime prevalence of alcohol use and past-year binge drinking than the general US population and physicians. The results reported by Kenna and Wood[61] support the notion that alcohol use may, indeed, vary by virtue of health care profession and independent of socioeconomic status.

As noted, social factors might significantly affect alcohol use by dentists. An underlying social structure defines and shapes a relationship between alcohol use, alcohol involvement, and group membership. One must consider that dentistry is also a business, and networking through memberships in various organizations is an important part of building a successful dental practice.[68] Kenna and Wood[61] reported that, during the past year, dentists were offered alcohol by friends and colleagues significantly more often than any of the other health care professional groups ($P < 0.01$). In addition, although nurses knew significantly more heavy drinkers or alcoholics than pharmacists and physicians did in their social networks, there was no significant difference between dentists and nurses, perhaps suggesting that a strong social interaction component, more than any other risk factor, may contribute to alcohol use and misuse by dentists.

Nurses

In 1991, Nancy Valentine's study of Massachusetts nurses led her to conclude that alcohol use by her sample was low compared with use by the physicians, pharmacists, and students in the McAuliffe et al.[72] study. More recently, however, alcohol use by nurses overall was surprisingly high given the overwhelming proportion of women compared with the other health care professional groups.[61] Nurses used less (mean use) alcohol than only dentists surveyed, but not significantly less. Although nurses reported fewer mean drinks per day than dentists, they also reported more mean monthly alcohol use than pharmacists and physicians. Moreover, although nurses reported less past-year binge drinking than the other three health care professional groups, they reported more past-year binge drinking than the general population 35 years of age or over, despite the fact that they are largely female. Results from the Kenna and Wood[61] study report higher lifetime (67%) and past-year (22%) binge rates compared with rates reported by Trinkoff and Storr[117] in a comparably sized study (54.4 and 19.3%, respectively). In a larger study performed by Trinkoff and colleagues,[118] 17% of nurses reported binge drinking during the past year ($n = 3919$). In the Kenna and Wood study,[61] 55% of nurses reported that they used alcohol on at least 4 days or more a month during the past year, and only 20.2% of nurses reported that they were nondrinkers.

Surprisingly, one of the primary substance use concerns for nurses compared with other health care professionals continues to be cigarette use. Padula[93] previously suggested that the level of smoking in the nursing profession was unacceptably high, higher than other health care professionals, and should be cause for concern within the profession. Consistent with Padula's findings, more recent research reported that past-month cigarette use by nurses was significantly greater than any other health care professional group,[59] although the past-month rate was less than half the rate reported by similarly aged peers in the general population.[85]

A significant number of nurses also report use of illicit drugs. For example, Trinkoff and Storr[117] reported significant rates for lifetime (41%) and past-year (3%) marijuana use by nurses in their study. Lifetime marijuana use self-reported by nurses in the Kenna and Wood[57] study was 57.4%, and past-year use was 4.7%, which was less than the 61% lifetime use reported by experimenters in the Sullivan et al.[111] study of nurses, but consistent with the 37.3% lifetime use reported by nurses surveyed in New York[22] and by 37% of nurses surveyed in Massachusetts [Valentine N (1991) Stress, alcohol and psychoactive drug use among nurses in Massachusetts. Brandeis University, Boston, MA, "An Unpublished Dissertation"].

Nurses also report extensive nonprescribed prescription medication use. For example, 14% of the nurses in the Kenna and Wood[57] study reported ≥61 nonprescribed medication taking episodes, which was more than any of the other professions surveyed. Lifetime nonprescribed opioid use reported by nurses ranges from 52% [Valentine N (1991) Stress, alcohol and psychoactive drug use among nurses in Massachusetts. Brandeis University, Boston, MA, "An Unpublished Dissertation"] to 45.7 %[117] to 21%.[57] In addition, when combining one or more episodes of lifetime drug or medication use, 63.6% of nurses reported use of one or more drugs,[57] which is less than rates reported by 68.6% of nurses surveyed by Trinkoff and Storr[117] and 73.7% surveyed by Valentine [Valentine N (1991) Stress, alcohol and psychoactive drug use among nurses in Massachusetts. Brandeis University, Boston, MA, "An Unpublished Dissertation"]. However, when compared with the general population, with a few exceptions (e.g., cigarettes consistently, minor differences with cocaine and hallucinogens), lifetime, past-year, and past-month substance use rates were higher among nurses.[57]

Although still high compared with the general population, one possibility for the reduced drug use among nurses over the last 20 years may be twofold. First, the mechanism for access to prescription medications in many facilities has changed a great deal. The link between access and drug use has been noted by many researchers [Dabney D (1997) A sociological examination of illicit prescription drug use among pharmacists. University of Florida, "An Unpublished Dissertation"].[23,114,117,118] In order to meet Joint Commission[53] requirements to maintain strict controls over medications to promote patient safety, most hospitals use automated machines that control and dispense medications to nurses for patients. One of the major advantages of these dispensing units is to maintain accurate counts of controlled drugs that must be verified at each shift change. Potential unauthorized access can be more readily detected. Although speculative, the automation of dispensing has probably reduced the access-prescription medication use link for many nurses. Second, the steady decline of drug use in society in general[86] is also likely an important factor in this observation.

A number of nurses in the Kenna and Wood[57] study reported iatrogenic drug exposure as they had been prescribed medications such as minor (e.g., C-III–C-IV) and major (C-II) opioids by practitioners. This finding was consistent with Valentine's [Valentine N (1991) Stress, alcohol and psychoactive drug use among nurses in Massachusetts. Brandeis University, Boston, MA, "An Unpublished Dissertation"] study that reported that prescribed drug use was much higher in nurses than other health care groups used for comparison, which led Valentine to conclude that "the path to dependence for nurses is use of drugs as a consequence of treatment under another provider's direction" [Valentine N (1991) Stress, alcohol and psychoactive drug use among nurses in Massachusetts. Brandeis University, Boston, MA, "An Unpublished Dissertation"; p. 651]. Although the issue regarding gender has generally not been considered, data suggest that there is an increased likelihood that more women than men will visit a physician and receive a prescription. In a report on the ambulatory care of patients in the United States,[15] women were 33% more likely than men to visit a doctor, even after accounting for pregnancy-associated visits. Moreover, the rate of physician's office visits for such reasons as annual exams and preventive services was 100% higher for women than men. Furthermore, prescriptive habits differed as well. Women were more likely than men to receive medications such as nonnarcotic analgesics and antidepressants. The likelihood that a group such as nurses that is predominately female would report more iatrogenic contact with various addictive substances is consistent with this notion.

Pharmacists

The data suggest that pharmacists are not more inclined than other groups of health care professionals to drink more alcohol. The mean drinks per month reported by pharmacists surveyed by Kenna and Wood[61] was 18.4, which was comparable to the rate of 21.2 drinks per month reported by McAuliffe et al. in 1991 for pharmacists.[71] One possible reason accounting for the slight difference might be attributed to the dominance of men (84%) in the McAuliffe et al. study compared with only 59% of men in the Kenna and Wood study. Twelve percent of pharmacists also reported past-month use of five or more drinks or binge drinking,[61] which was comparable to 9.3% of physicians reporting binge drinking by Hughes et al.[48]

Based on qualitative studies,[10,23] alcohol remains one of the salient drugs of choice for substance-impaired pharmacists, although it is important to note that alcohol was rarely the sole drug of choice. Bissell et al.[10] reported that only 21% of the pharmacists in their study were addicted to alcohol alone, whereas 77% were addicted to a combination of alcohol and other drugs, most always prescription medications.

As noted by Bissell et al.,[10] the combination of alcohol and prescription drugs presents a more formidable threat to pharmacists, and the pathway to addiction for most pharmacists who may become impaired is probably through polydrug use.[10] That is, alcohol in combination with medications, most notably minor opioids and anxiolytics, comprise the bulk of current substance use by pharmacists. Seldom are pharmacists addicted to just a prescription medication.[10]

Studies using varying designs suggest that pharmacists do use drugs and suffer the consequences of their use.[8] These include quantitative,[74,92] qualitative,[10,70] retrospective,[35] and combination designs [Dabney D (1997) A sociological examination of illicit prescription drug use among pharmacists. University of Florida, "An Unpublished Dissertation"]. There is currently no evidence that total lifetime or past-year drug use by pharmacists significantly exceeds that of other major groups of health care professionals or the general population.[57] Yet, pharmacists by virtue of their ease of access may be at greater risk to use prescription medications than the general population. It appears that the greatest threat to pharmacists is nonmedical opioid, stimulant, and anti-anxiety drug use due to easy availability. McAuliffe[70] initially reported what he called "nontherapeutic" opioid use by health care professionals. The health care professionals interviewed described their progression of opioid use that led to becoming addicted. A high rate of self-treatment with tranquilizers was also noted in the McAuliffe et al.[74] study that included pharmacists. Most nonprescribed opioid and anti-anxiety drug use seems to be for self-diagnosed ailments and most stimulant use is reported to be for facilitating performance, such as staying awake, performing better, and studying.[72]

As reported, lifetime stimulant use by pharmacists was 15.8%,[57] and was greater than twice the general population rate.

Access to drugs by pharmacists would most likely explain the differences in prescription medication use between the general population and pharmacists. Consistent with studies of resident physicians who gain access to prescriptive privileges at that stage of their medical career,[18,49] opioid and benzodiazepine self-treatment represented the bulk of prescription medication use by resident physicians. The majority of pharmacists who report the unauthorized use of prescription medications, not surprisingly, initially did so after leaving college.[24] Dabney reported that 40% of pharmacists surveyed had used prescription medications without a physician's authorization, and 20% reported that they had done so five or more times in their lifetime. It was proposed that diversion was the primary source for obtaining these medications,[8] and that access to medications is therefore a prerequisite to use for many pharmacists. However, as noted by Trinkoff and Storr,[117] perhaps access alone is necessary but may not be sufficient to foster the conditions that promote drug use in health care professionals. Access in a permissive environment, coupled with drug use knowledge; the lack of education of the developmental dynamics of addiction[69]; and peer, academic, or occupational influences that do not dissuade substance use, appear to be the primary factors contributing to illicit prescription medication use [Dabney D (1997) A sociological examination of illicit prescription drug use among pharmacists. University of Florida, "An Unpublished Dissertation"].[23,114, 17,119] Among other legal and ethical concerns for such behavior is the concern with self-diagnosing of their condition by pharmacists. A common theme with pharmacists who were interviewed for the Bissell et al.[10] study was that although pharmacists sought help, they often misdiagnosed their substance use problem and sought ineffectual or misplaced support and did not see, or were unable to correctly diagnose, their own addiction.

Physicians

With the exception of anxiolytics, physicians appear to be less likely than other health care professionals or the general population to use alcohol, tobacco, or other drugs.[57] For example, McAuliffe et al.[71] reported that physicians drank 20.3 drinks per month in their study and concluded that there was no reason to suspect that alcohol use by physicians differed from that by other professionals. More recently,[61] physicians reported consuming an average of only 17.9 drinks per month, which was also the lowest monthly mean total of any health care professional group. Not only was alcohol use lower than in other health care professional groups surveyed, alcohol use was lower compared with previous data reported by Hughes et al.[48] and McAuliffe et al.[71] Physicians' lifetime prevalence (92.3%) was similar to that of the general population (85.8%) as was past-year binge drinking (22.1% vs. 18.6%, respectively), although past-month binge drinking was much lower (7.7% vs. 16.2%, respectively).[61]

As noted earlier, an important social-professional contributor to alcohol use includes alcohol served by pharmaceutical companies at education seminars. A Kaiser Family Foundation[3] study of physicians found that of 2608 physicians polled, 61% received free meals, drinks, travel and tickets from pharmaceutical companies. Pharmaceutical companies are providing alcohol at continuing education seminars as a part of a marketing approach targeting practitioners.[97] Some estimate that 12% of a pharmaceutical company's marketing budget (12.5–15 billion dollars a year) is targeted at physicians.[4] Although the use of alcohol by physicians does not appear to be a problem, alcohol continues to be served by pharmaceutical companies to provide sales representatives the opportunity to engage with health care professionals and facilitate conversations regarding the use of their particular medication. Kenna and Wood[61] reported that physicians were offered alcohol by pharmaceutical companies, significantly more often than all other health care professionals.

As for other drug use, Kenna and Wood[57] reported that the prevalence of lifetime street drug use among physicians exceeded rates reported by the general population, some other health care professional groups in the study, and rates reported previously by Hughes et al.[48] For example, lifetime prevalence of marijuana use by physicians (51.9%) exceeded rates reported by the general population (31.6%), by physicians in the Hughes et al. study (35.6%), as well as rates reported by pharmacists (44.4%) and dentists (48.7%) in the Kenna and Wood[57] study. Furthermore, Kenna and Wood[57] reported that the lifetime prevalence of cocaine (17.3%) and hallucinogen (11.5%) use by physicians was the highest among health care professional groups used for comparison and higher than both the general population (11.8 and 10.1%, respectively) and the physicians surveyed (10.3 and 7.8%) by Hughes et al.[48] Results regarding past-year use of street drugs by physicians from the study of Kenna and Wood,[57] however, were consistent with data reported previously by McAuliffe et al.[72] and Hughes et al.,[48] and self-prescribed minor opioid use among physicians was far lower in the Kenna and Wood study. In addition, past-year minor opioid use (1%) was only one-eighth the rate reported by pharmacists (8.3%). On the other hand, prevalence of anxiolytic use by physicians was the highest among health care professional groups and much higher than rates reported for the general population.[85] Despite this, reported rates have been dropping. For example, past-year use by physicians was 4.8%, a rate higher than that reported by pharmacists (4.5%), nurses (3.1%), dentists (2.7%), and the general population,[57] whereas past-year use of benzodiazepines (anxiolytics) was 11.4% as reported by Hughes et al. and 9% in the McAuliffe et al. study.

In terms of onset of use, initiation of street drugs often begins in college, high school, or earlier; only opioid and anxiolytic use began during residency.[20,49] Hughes et al.[48] suggested that unsupervised opioid and anxiolytic use could contribute to substance abuse or dependence in physicians, particularly in light of the results in their study that found that physicians were more likely than age and gender peers to have used alcohol, minor opioids, and anxiolytics.

Identifying Drug Problems in Health Care Professionals

Job performance issues such as excessive absenteeism, errors, frequently changing jobs, calling in sick or offering to work overtime, frequent wasting of medication, sleeping on duty, and always giving maximum doses of medications are a few of the important behavioral signs useful in identifying substance abuse problems in health care professionals.[95] In addition, there are several symptoms of alcohol or drug abuse that coworkers may experience, such as memory blackouts, emotional lability, withdrawal from family or coworkers, depression, insomnia, slurred speech, disappearing frequently, or the odor of mouthwash or mints on their breath (Table 68.1). In fact, some of these markers may hold the key to the type of impairment. For example, unexplained work absenteeism may indicate an alcohol abuse or dependence problem, since, in addition to hangover, home is the more convenient place to store and access this drug of choice. By contrast, consistently volunteering

TABLE 68.1	Signs and Symptoms of Potential Chemical Impairment in a Coworker.

- The odor of alcohol on the breath or strong odor of mouthwash or mints to mask the alcohol.
- Hand tremor that occurs when in alcohol withdrawal (such as in the morning)
- Excessive perspiration
- Absence from work without notice, frequent absenteeism, or late for work
- Unexplained disappearance during work for long periods of time
- Sleeping or dozing off while on duty or complaints of difficulty sleeping
- Frequent bathroom breaks
- Volunteering for overtime or being at work when not scheduled to be there
- Deterioration in personal appearance
- Reports of illness, minor accidents, and emergencies
- Confusion, memory loss, and difficulty concentrating
- Heavy drug waste or drug shortages
- Inappropriate prescriptions for large narcotic doses
- Increase in medication order entry errors or sloppy recordkeeping
- Work performance that alternates between periods of high and low productivity
- Unreliability in keeping appointments and meeting deadlines
- Personality changes and mood swings

to work overtime, or arriving at work when not scheduled, provides an impaired coworker the opportunity to access controlled substances not available at home. Unfortunately, such symptoms are more easily identified with hindsight than before a coworker is identified with an alcohol or drug use disorder.

Governmental, state, local, corporate, and hospital employers use statistical analysis to monitor worker access to specific drugs performed on a periodic basis. Subsequently, at the person level, if a particular health care professional appears to consistently access controlled drugs at higher rates than peers, a more formal investigation is begun, perhaps instituting use of investigators, covertly employing video cameras or auditing the site.

The Intervention of Health Care Professionals

Data suggest that denial is often greatest for those health care professionals who are the most addicted.[42] Health care professionals often use a greater amount of drugs for longer periods, for they can go undetected by their ability to use various drugs to cover drug side effects.[23] Often the only time health care professionals are caught is through a drug audit by supervisors or internal security measures.

Probably one of the most difficult professional decisions a health care professional can make is to intervene on behalf of a coworker who has an alcohol or drug problem. Given the seriousness of dependence disease and its treatment, intervention can present problems at many levels for both individuals. Despite these difficulties, it is important to recognize that health care professionals with alcohol or drug problems in retrospect feel that an intervention probably saved their lives [Dabney D (1997) A sociological examination of illicit prescription drug use among pharmacists. University of Florida, "An Unpublished Dissertation"]. In addition, although at the time of their discovery these individuals were devastated, the reality is that after receiving treatment the majority do successfully return to work.[80]

Interventions are different for health care professionals than for others. The intervention is professionally based and focused on practice. The intervention team must recognize that the professional's identity is fused with the role they perform, and the intervention must focus on objective data from their investigation. There are potentially significant financial implications if the professional is unable to practice, so leverage during the intervention is focused on the ability to practice and on maintaining employment.[112]

There are three major reasons that early intervention and treatment for health care professionals is desirable: (1) it should lower the risk of patient care errors due to substance impairment; (2) it helps the health care professionals prevent overdose that could result in their own death, suicide or other problems from adverse drug reactions; and (3) the health care professionals may have an easier experience with drug withdrawal and less resistance to treatment. There are also advantages for health care professionals who come in for treatment on their own, as they are protected by confidentiality laws that protect their identity. In these cases, neither the employer nor the state is notified of treatment. This can protect the health care professionals from loss of privileges or licensure versus if their addiction were to become known to the Drug Enforcement Administration or state licensure boards and is a powerful incentive to engage in the recovery process. In addition, the health care professionals may be able to stay at work and not experience economic hardships that accompany forced loss of licensure due to discovery. This is not necessarily the best treatment strategy, as treatment may require work modification to restrict access to substances. Finally, if treatment is successful, the health care professionals will not be subjected to stigma associated with loss of licensure.

Once an individual's alcohol or drug problem surfaces, treatment decisions are generally tailored to his or her needs. Although a thorough discussion of the diverse treatment options are better covered elsewhere in this book, certain basic goals of treatment include matching the patient to the correct level of care, such as deciding whether someone is better suited to inpatient versus outpatient treatment,[83] are also relevant for health care professionals. Beyond placement, fundamental components of treatment include individual and group therapy, pharmacotherapy when appropriate, urine drug monitoring, and 12-step facilitation. Twelve-step programs include Alcoholics Anonymous, Narcotics Anonymous, as well as programs targeted toward health care professionals such as Caduceus, International Pharmacists Anonymous (a psychosocial support group specifically for pharmacists), International Doctors in Alcoholics Anonymous, and many others.

There is relatively little research assessing risk factors for relapse or treatment success of recovering health care professionals. In a retrospective cohort study of 292 health care professionals enrolled in the state of Washington's Physicians Health Program, only about 25% of the study population had one or more relapses.[28] The risk of relapse was significantly increased in health care professionals who had used a major opioid, had a coexisting psychiatric illness, or reported a family history of an alcohol or drug disorder. Coexisting risk factors and previous relapse significantly increased the likelihood of relapse.

For health care professionals formally referred to treatment programs, one of the keys to reentry is signing a contract that delineates what is expected by the treatment agency or wellness program. These programs are responsible for overseeing treatment plans, urine drug monitoring, and advocating for health care professionals with licensing boards. Generally, treatment is successful whether initiated by the health care professional or others. In

1988, for example, a survey examined pharmacist-assistance programs in all 50 states and the District of Columbia.[80] Although the survey reported that only 20% of impaired pharmacists in these treatment programs voluntarily disclosed their chemical use problem, just over 88% successfully completed treatment and returned to practice. More recently, McLellan et al.[79] reported on urine drug monitoring during a 5-year follow-up study of 802 physicians in 16 state Physician Health Programs. At the conclusion of the study, 81% were licensed and working. In sum, these studies suggest that the goal of returning a recovering health care professional to practice with the proper aftercare and monitoring program is realistic with a good chance of success.

Prevention and Education

What seems clear from the data presented is the need to highlight: (1) an appropriate respect for alcohol use and, in particular, misuse; (2) the dangers of self-treatment, especially with any controlled prescription medications; and (3) recognizing risk factors such as family history of alcohol or drug use that may predispose individual health care professionals to subsequent substance abuse under the right conditions as with other non–health care professionals.

That substance use rates reported by most of the studies referred to in this chapter would not be categorized as psychoactive substance abuse or dependence using criteria from the *Diagnostic and Statistical Manual of Mental Disorders, Fourth Edition, Text Revision,*[27] should not imply that health care professionals are safe from addiction. Health care professionals work in stressful positions and people outside of each profession have little connection with the specific responsibilities and demands of each. In addition, health care professionals work with medications that are efficacious when used properly but when abused may facilitate a quick progression to dependence under the proper circumstances. Self-treatment removes the opportunity for oversight of a provider for appropriateness of use. Furthermore, as qualitative and review studies have determined,[23,24,32,70] substance-related impairment often includes diverted medications. Nonprescribed substance use, no matter how infrequent and how little, is just as illegal for health care professionals[7] as it is for the general population.

Wright[123] admonished the medical profession for attempting to simply provide more substance abuse education for physicians and students, arguing that it was the type of education that was being presented that was questionable. Therefore, the quality of education with regard to medication use, be it alcohol or otherwise, cannot be stressed enough. Understanding the disease model is critical to the professional development of clinicians but does not provide the sort of preventative information necessary to sensitize one to substance use or abuse either in patients or in themselves. Education in the context of requiring health care students to attend Alcoholics Anonymous, Narcotics Anonymous, or Caduceus groups and sitting in on group counseling sessions or attending talks by health care professionals who have been alcohol and or other drug dependent as they detail their story of addiction may provide the pathways that connect theory with practice. The data would suggest that the triggers and risk factors are different for each health care profession, but the interventions and successful treatments that promote abstinence, with minor variations, are similar.

Although some suggest that stress alone does not cause addiction,[10] the added factor of medication availability may enhance risk,[23,83,117,119] as availability has been found to be a significant risk factor for many health care professional groups [Dabney D

(1997) A sociological examination of illicit prescription drug use among pharmacists. University of Florida, "An Unpublished Dissertation"].[72,117] The data suggest that the majority of the initiation of minor opioid and anxiolytic use by health care professionals occurred after college when access increased in the workplace through obtaining prescriptive authority. In a similar manner, prescription medication initiation today by adolescents is primarily from available unused medications left and forgotten in the home medicine cabinet.[109]

Universities and colleges routinely encounter the consequences of unhealthy alcohol or drug use by health care professionals but do not systematically present medical education designed to prevent these behavioral misadventures. The importance and quality of education with regard to alcohol or drug use, be it prescription medications or otherwise, cannot be stressed enough. Although there has been some progress in curriculum and faculty development in many health care professional schools, much more needs to be accomplished in terms of substance abuse education generally and the vulnerability of health care professionals specifically. It appears that medical education about substance use disorders generally is scanty at best. For example, when the physician Leadership on National Drug Policy conducted a survey of over 1500 medical students at a random sample of 15 schools, 56% responded that they had received little education about drug and alcohol abuse, and 20% said they received none.[47]

A recent successful national training project for interdisciplinary faculty development across several traditional health professions as well as allied professionals and dentistry issued a strategic plan to improve health care professional education and review progress in several health disciplines.[40] That strategic plan made recommendations to strengthen substance abuse medical education: "because of health professional's vulnerability to impairment, information about the causes, risk factors, symptoms, and treatment options for substance abuse needs to be developed further and taught to all health professionals"[41] (p. 158). The plan further acknowledges that "Chemically dependent professionals unfortunately do not readily recognize their own impairments…. Guilt and shame over past behaviors prevent health professionals from admitting their problems, seeing the difficulties that addiction has caused in their lives, and voluntarily seeking help"[41] (p. 158).

As for the curriculum, understanding the disease model is critical to the professional development of clinicians but does not provide the sort of preventative information necessary to sensitize one to substance use or abuse either in patients or in themselves. Recommendations suggest that education in the context of requiring health care students to attend Alcoholics Anonymous, Narcotics Anonymous or Caduceus groups or sitting in on group counseling sessions give them a direct sense of the power of addictive disease and the strength needed to attain and maintain recovery.

References

1. American Dental Association. *Survey Center. Who Knows? Ask the ADA Survey Center;* 2003. http://www.ada.orge/prof/resources/pubs/adanews/adanewsarticle.asp?articleid=782.
2. American Medical Association. *Resolution 113: Drug Dependencies as Diseases.* Chicago, IL: American Medical Association House of Delegates; 1987.
3. American Medical Association. *Pharmacy Group Details What Drug Reps Can Give Physicians.* Amednews.Com, 27 May 2002. 2002. http://www.ama-assn.org/sci-pubs/amnews/pick_02/prl10527.htm_add. Retrieved 17 Feb 2008.

4. American Medical Association. *Pharmaceutical marketing to physicians: free gifts carry a high price.* 2002. Amednews.Com, 10 June 2002. http://www.ama-assn.org/sci-pubs/amnews/amn_02/edsa0610.htm#rbar_add. Retrieved 17 Feb 2008.

5. American Pharmaceutical Association (APhA). Report of the American pharmaceutical association policy committee on professional Affairs. *Am Pharm NS.* 1982;22:368–380.

5a. American Psychiatric Association. *Diagnostic and Statistical Manual of Mental Disorders.* 5th ed. Washington, DC: American Psychiatric Association; 2013.

6. Baldwin D, Hughes P, Conard S, et al. Substance use among senior medical students. *J Am Med Assoc.* 1991;265:2074–2078.

7. Baldwin J. Self-medication by pharmacists: familiarity breeds attempt? *J Am Pharm Assn.* 2001;41:371.

8. Baldwin J, Thibault E. Substance abuse by pharmacists: stopping the insanity. *J Am Pharm Assn.* 2001;41:373–375.

9. Berens M. *Problem Nurses Escape Punishment.* Chicago, IL: A1: Chicago Tribune; 2000.

10. Bissell L, Haberman PW, Williams RL. Pharmacists recovering from alcohol and other addictions: an interview study. *Am Pharm NS.* 1989;29:19–30.

11. Bissell L, Skorina J. One hundred alcoholic women in medicine. An interview study. *J Am Med Assoc.* 1987;257:2939–2944.

12. Bowermaster DP. Chemical dependency: are dental students at risk? *Ohio Den J.* 1989;63:26–30.

13. Brewster J. Prevalence of alcohol and other drug problems among physicians. *J Am Med Assoc.* 1986;255:1913–1920.

14. Brown S, Goldman M, Inn A, et al. Expectations of reinforcement from alcohol: their domain and relation to drinking patterns. *J Consult Clin Psy.* 1980;48:419–426.

15. Center for Disease Control. *Utilization of Ambulatory Medical Care by Women: United States, 1997–1998. Series Report 13, No 149. 51 Pp (PHS) 2001-1720.* Washington, DC: U.S. Department of Health and Human Services; 2001.

16. Centrella M. Physician addiction and impairment – current thinking: a review. *J Addict Disease.* 1994;13:91–105.

17. Chiodo GT, Tolle SW. Chemically dependent doctors. *Gen Den.* 1997;4:532–536.

18. Clark A, Kay J, Clark D. Patterns of psychoactive drug prescriptions by house officers for non-patients. *J Med Ed.* 1988;63: 44–50.

19. Clark D, Gibbons R, Daugherty S, et al. Model for quantifying the drug involvement of medical students. *Int J Addictions.* 1987;22:249–271.

20. Clark JH, Chiodo GT, Cowan FF. Chemical dependency among dentists: prevalence and current treatment. *Gen Den.* 1988;36:227–229.

21. Cloninger CR, Bohman M, Sigvardsson S. Inheritance of alcohol abuse. *Arch Gen Psy.* 1981;38:861–868.

22. Collins RL, Gollnisch G, Morsheimer ET. Substance use among a regional sample of female nurses. *Drug Alc Dep.* 1999;55: 145–155.

23. Coombs RH. Addicted health professionals. *J Subst Misuse.* 1996;1:187–194.

24. Dabney D. Onset of illegal use of mind altering or potentially addictive prescription drugs among pharmacists. *J Am Pharm Assn.* 2001;41:392–400.

25. Dabney D. Response to Kenna (2001). *J Am Pharm Assn.* 2001;41:790.

26. Dabney D, Hollinger R. Illicit prescription drug use among pharmacists: evidence of a paradox of familiarity. *Work Occup.* 1999;26:77–106.

27. Reference deleted in review.

28. Domino KB, Hornbein TF, Polissar NL, et al. Risk factors for relapse in health care professionals with substance use disorders. *J Am Med Assoc.* 2005;293:1453–1460.

29. Donohue JM, Cevasco M, Rosenthal MB. A decade of direct-to-consumer advertising of prescription drugs. *N Engl J Med.* 2007;357:673–681.

30. Earley P. Chapter I, Substance abuse, from problem physicians: a national perspective. In: Talbott GD, Crosby LR, eds. *A Report to the Georgia Composite State Board of Medical Examiners.* 2000.

31. Ehrhardt H. Drug addiction in the medical and allied professions in Germany. *Bul Narc.* 1959;11:18–26.

32. Femino J, Nirenberg T. Treatment outcome studies of physician impairment. *R I Med.* 1994;77:345–350.

33. Flaherty J, Richman J. Substance use and addiction among medical students, residents, and physicians. *Psych Clin North Am.* 1993;16:189–197.

34. Floyd J. Nursing student's stress levels, attitudes towards drugs and drug use. *Arch Psych Nurs.* 1991;5:46–53.

35. Gallegos KV, Veit FW, Wilson PO, et al. Substance abuse among healthcare professionals. *Md Med J.* 1988;37:191–197.

36. Gebhart F. The dope on drug diversion. *Hosp Pharm Rep.* 2001;17:24–28.

37. Gellad Z, Lyles K. Direct-to-consumer advertising of pharmaceuticals. *Am J Med.* 2007;120:475–480.

38. Godfrey C, Maynard A. An economic theory of alcohol consumption and abuse. In: Chaudron CD, Wilkinson DA, eds. *Theories on Alcoholism.* Toronto, CA: Addiction Research Foundation; 1988:411–435.

39. Graham JW, Marks G, Hansen WB. Social influence processes affecting adolescent substance use. *J Appl Psy.* 1991;76:291–298.

40. Haack MR, Adger H, eds. Strategic plan for interdisciplinary faculty development. *Subst Abuse.* 2002:169–319(suppl)23:3.

41. Haack MR, Adger H, eds. *Strategic Plan for Interdisciplinary Faculty Development.* Subst Abuse; 2002:158(supp)23:3.

42. Hankes L, Bissell L. Health professionals. In: Lowinson J, Ruiz P, Millman R, Langrod J, eds. *Substance Abuse a Comprehensive Textbook.* New York, NY: Williams and Wilkins; 1992:897–907.

43. Harford TC. Family history of alcoholism in the United States: prevalence and demographic characteristics. *Br J Addiction.* 1992;87:931–935.

44. Hasin DS, Stinson FS, Ogburn E, et al. Prevalence, correlates, disability, and comorbidity of DSM-IV alcohol abuse and dependence in the United States: results from the national epidemiologic survey on alcohol and related conditions. *Arch Gen Psych.* 2007;64:830–842.

45. Hawkins JD, Catalano RF, Miller JY. Risk and protective factors for alcohol and other drug problems in adolescence and early adulthood: implications for substance abuse prevention. *Psy Bull.* 1992;112:64–105.

46. Hedge HR. Recovering alcoholic dentists, a preliminary survey. *Iowa Dent J.* 1982;68:41–42.

47. Hoffman NG, Chang AJ, Lewis DC. Medical student attitudes toward drug addiction policy. *J Addict Dis.* 2000;19:1–12.

48. Hughes P, Brandenburg N, DeWitt B, et al. Prevalence of substance use among US physicians. *J Am Med Assoc.* 1992;267:2333–2339.

49. Hughes P, Conard S, Baldwin D, et al. Resident physician substance use in the United States. *J Am Med Assoc.* 1991;265:2069–2073.

50. Jaffe AJ, Kilbey M. The cocaine expectancy questionnaire (CEQ): construction and predictive utility. *Psych Assess.* 1994;6:18–26.

51. Jessor R, Jessor SL. *Problem Behavior and Psychosocial Development: A Longitudinal Study of Youth.* New York: Academic; 1977.

52. Joint Commission on Accreditation of health care organizations. In: *Medical Standard. Oakbrook Terrace.* Vol. 2. ; 2001:6. IL.

53. Joint Commission on Accreditation of health care organizations. In: *Medical Standard. Oakbrook Terrace.* Vol. 13. ; 2002:3. IL.

54. Joranson DE, Gilson AM. Wanted: a public health approach to prescription opioid abuse and diversion. *Pharmacoepidemiol Drug Saf.* 2006;15:632–634.

55. Kenna GA. Non-narcotic analgesics: appropriate to include in a study of illicit drug use? *J Am Pharm Assoc.* 2001;41:790.

56. Kenna GA, Lewis DC. Risk factors for alcohol and other drug use by healthcare professionals. *Subst Abuse Treat Prevent Policy.* 2008;3(3):1–8.

57. Kenna GA, Wood MD. Family history of alcoholism and alcohol use in college healthcare students. Presented at the 72nd Annual Eastern Psychological Association Convention; 2001, Washington, DC.

58. Kenna GA, Wood MD. Relations between social influence factors, pharmaco-expectancy, drug use and problems in healthcare students. Presented to the 72nd Annual Eastern Psychological Association Convention; 2001, Washington, DC.

59. Kenna GA, Wood MD. Substance use by pharmacists and other health professionals. *J Am Pharm Assoc.* 2004;44:684–693.

60. Kenna GA, Wood MD. Substance use by pharmacy and nursing practitioners and students in a northeastern state. *Am J Health-System Pharm.* 2004;61:921–930.

61. Kenna GA, Wood MD. Alcohol use by healthcare professionals. *Drug Alc Dep.* 2004;75:107–116.

62. Kenna GA, Wood MD. Family history of alcohol and drug use in healthcare professionals. *J Subst Use.* 2005;10:225–238.

63. Kenna GA, Wood MD. The prevalence of alcohol, cigarette and illicit drug use and problems among dentists. *J Am Dental Assoc.* 2005;136:1023–1032.

64. Kenna GA, Wood MD. In search of pharmacological optimism: investigating beliefs about effects of drugs: a pilot study. *Addiction Res Theory.* 2008;16:383–399.

65. Kessler RC, McGonagle KA, Zhao S, et al. Lifetime and 12-month prevalence of DSM-III-R psychiatric disorders in the United States. Results from the national co-morbidity survey. *Arch Gen Psych.* 1994;51:8–19.

66. Kriegler K, Baldwin J, Scott D. A survey of alcohol and other drug use behaviors and risk factors health profession students. *J Col Health.* 1994;42:259–265.

67. LaGodna GE, Hendrix MJ. Impaired nurses: a cost analysis. *J Nurs Admin.* 1991;19:13–17.

68. Levin RP. The ABCs of increasing referrals. *J Am Dent Assoc.* 2008;139:351–352.

69. Lewis D. Doctors and drugs. *N Engl J Med.* 1986;315:826–828.

70. McAuliffe W. Non-therapeutic opioid addiction in health professionals: a new form of impairment. *Am J Drug Alc Abuse.* 1983;10:1–22.

71. McAuliffe W, Rohman M, Breer P, et al. Alcohol use and abuse in random samples of physicians and medical students. *Am J Pub Health.* 1991;81:177–182.

72. McAuliffe W, Rohman M, Santangelo S, et al. Psychoactive drug use among physicians and medical students. *N Eng J Med.* 1986;315:805–810.

73. McAuliffe W, Santangelo S, Gingras J, et al. Use and abuse of controlled substances by pharmacists and pharmacy students. *Am J Hosp Pharm.* 1987;44:311–317.

74. McAuliffe W, Santangelo S, Magnuson E, et al. Risk factors of drug impairment in random samples of physicians and medical students. *Int J Addictions.* 1987;22:825–841.

75. McAuliffe W, Wechsler H, Rohman M, et al. Psychoactive drug use by young and future physicians. *J Health Soc Beh.* 1984;25:34–54.

76. McGue M, Pickens RW, Svikis DS. Sex and age effects on the inheritance of alcohol problems: a twin study. *J Ab Psy.* 1992;101:3–17.

77. McGuffey EC. Lessons from pharmacists in recovery from drug addiction. *J Am Pharm Assoc.* 1998;38:17.

78. McGuire D. Impaired druggists pose serious threat. The Kansas City Star, 10/7/2002; 2002. http://www.kansascity.com/mld/kansascity/news/ 4226754.htm. Accessed 10 Apr 2008.

79. McLellan AT, Skipper GS, Campbell M, DuPont R. Five-year outcomes in a cohort study of physicians treated for substance use disorders in the United States. *BMJ.* 2008;237:a2038.

80. McNees GE, Godwin HN. Programs for pharmacists impaired by substance abuse: a report. *Am Pharm NS.* 1990;30:33–37.

81. Mensch B, Kandel D. Do job conditions influence the use of drugs? *J Health Soc Beh.* 1988;29:169–184.

82. Mynatt S. A model of contributing risk factors to chemical dependency in nurses. *J Psychosoc Nurs Ment Health Serv.* 1996;34:13–22.

83. Nace E. *Achievement and Addiction: A Guide to the Treatment of Professionals.* New York, NY: Brunner/Mazel; 1995.

84. National Center on Addiction and Substance Abuse at Columbia University. *Under the Counter: The Diversion and Abuse of Controlled Prescription Drugs in the U.S.* New York, NY; 2005.

85. National Household Survey on Drug Abuse Series: H-14. *Summary of Findings From the 2001 National Household Survey on Drug Abuse.* Washington, DC: Substance Abuse and Mental Health Services Administration; 2002. Office of Applied Studies, DHHS Pub. No. (SMA) 01-3549.

86. National Survey on Drug Use and Health Series: H-32. *Results From the 2006 National Survey on Drug Use and Health: National Findings.* Rockville MD: Substance Abuse and Mental Health Services Administration; 2007. Office of Applied Studies, DHHS Pub No. (SMA) 07-4293.

87. National Institute on Alcohol Abuse and Alcoholism. *Tenth Special Report to the U.S. Congress on Alcohol and Health.* Washington, DC: U.S. Department of Health and Human Services; 2000.

88. National Institute on Drug Abuse. The validity of self-reported drug use: improving the accuracy of survey estimates. *NIDA Research Monograph.* 1996;167: 247–272. Washington, DC: U.S. Department of Health and Human Services, National Institutes of Health.

89. National Pharmacy Compliance News. Pharmacist impairment. *Natl Assoc Boards Pharmacy.* 2000;7:1–4.

90. *Prince George's Co. pharmacist charged with stealing drugs 4NBC4. com.* 2008. http://www.nbc4.com/news/14983257/detail.html.

91. Nelson R. Missing persons: RN/RPH shortages taking their toll. *Hosp Pharm Rep.* 2001;15:26–27.

92. Normark JW, Eckel FM, Pfifferling JH, et al. Impairment risk in North Carolina pharmacy students. *Am Pharm NS.* 1985;25:45–48.

93. Padula CA. Nurses and smoking: review and implications. *J Pro Nurs.* 1992;8:120–132.

94. Pickens R, Svikis D, McGue M, et al. Heterogeneity in the inheritance of alcoholism. A study of male and female twins. *Arch Gen Psych.* 1991;48:19–28.

95. Pullen LM, Green LA. Identification and education: essential curriculum components for chemical dependency in nurses. *J Con Ed Nurs.* 1997;28:211–216.

96. Rather BC, Goldman MS. Drinking-related differences in the memory organization of alcohol expectancies. *Exp Clin Psychopharm.* 1994;2:167–183.

97. Razack S, Arbour L, Hutcheon R. Proposed model for interaction between residents and residency training programs and the pharmaceutical industry. *Ann Res Col Phy Surg Can.* 1999;32:93–96.

98. Robins LN, Helzer JE, Weismann MM, et al. Lifetime prevalence of specific psychiatric disorders in three sites. *Arch Gen Psych.* 1984;41:949–958.

99. Rohrbaugh J, Jessor R. Religiosity in youth. A personal control against deviant behavior. *J Personality.* 1975;43:136–155.

100. Sammon PJ, Smith TA, Cooper TM, et al. Teaching an alcohol prevention course in the dental school chemical dependency curriculum: a preliminary report. *J Den Ed.* 1991;55:30–31.

101. Sandoval VA, Dale RA, Huddleston AM. Abstract from the 67th AADS conference. *J Den Ed.* 1990;54:36.

102. Sandoval VA, Hendricson WD, Dale RA. A survey of substance abuse education in North American dental schools. *J Den Ed.* 1988;52:167–169.

103. Schafer J, Brown S. Marijuana and cocaine effect expectancies and drug use patterns. *J Consult Clin Psychol.* 1991;59:558–565.

104. Schuckit M. Biological vulnerability to alcoholism. *J Con Clin Psy.* 1987;55:301–309.

105. Schuckit M, Gold E. A simultaneous evaluation of multiple markers of ethanol/placebo challenges in sons of alcoholics and control. *Arch Gen Psych.* 1988;45:211–216.

106. Skipper GE. Treating the chemically dependent health professional. *J Addict Dis.* 1997;16:67–73.

107. Stoudemire A, Rhoads J. When a doctor needs a doctor: special considerations for the physician-patient. *Ann Int Med*. 1983;98(Part 1):654–659.

108. Substance Abuse and Mental Health Services Administration (SAMHSA). New national survey reveals drug use down among adolescents in the US-successes in substance abuse recovery highlighted. *SAMHSA News Release*. 2007.

109. Substance Abuse and Mental Health Services Administration Results from the 2006 national survey on drug use and health: national findings. Office of Applied Studies Rockville, MD. In: Series H-32, DHHS Publication No SMA 07-4293; 2007.

110. Sullivan E. Comparison of chemically dependent and nondependent nurses on familial, personal and professional characteristics. *J Stud Alcohol*. 1987;48:563–568.

111. Sullivan E, Bissell L, Leffler E. Drug use and disciplinary actions among 300 nurses. *Int J Add*. 1990;25:375–391.

112. Talbott GD. Substance abuse relapse. In: Talbott GD, Crosby LR, eds. *Problem Physicians: A National Perspective. A Report to the Georgia Composite State Board of Medical Examiners*. ; 2001. Atlanta, GA.

113. Talbott GD, Gallegos K. Intervention with health professionals. *Addict Recov*. 1990;10:13–16.

114. Talbott GD, Gallegos K, Wilson P, et al. The medical association of Georgia's impaired physician program. Prevalence of alcohol and other drug problems among physicians. *J Am Med Assoc*. 1987;257:2927–2930.

115. Talbott GD, Wright C. Chemical dependency in health care professionals. *Occup Med*. 1987;2:581–591.

116. Trinkoff AM, Eaton WW, Anthony J. The prevalence of substance abuse among registered nurses. *Nurs Res*. 1991;40:172–175.

117. Trinkoff AM, Storr CL. Incorporating auxiliary variables into probability sampling designs. *Nurs Res*. 1997;46:182–185.

118. Trinkoff AM, Storr CL, Wall MP. Prescription-type drug misuse and workplace access among nurses. *J Add Dis*. 1999;18:9–17.

119. Trinkoff AM, Zhou A, Storr CL, et al. Workplace access, negative proscriptions, job strain, and substance use in registered nurses. *Nurs Res*. 2000;49:83–90.

120. Tucker DR, Gurnee MC, Sylvestri MF, et al. Psychoactive drug use and impairment markers in pharmacy students. *Am J Pharm Ed*. 1988;52:42–46.

121. Ventura County Star July 12. *Staffer Faces Charges Tied to Doctor's Prescriptions*; 2008. http://www.venturacountystar.com/news/2008/jul/12/in-02/.

122. Winick C. A sociological theory of the genesis of drug dependence. In: Winick C, ed. *Sociological Aspects of Drug Dependence*. Cleveland, OH: CRC; 1974:3–13.

123. Wright CIV. Physician addiction to pharmaceuticals: personal history, practice setting, access to drugs, and recovery. *Md Med J*. 1990;39:1021–1025.

69

Identification and Treatment of Alcohol or Drug Dependence in the Elderly

FREDERIC C. BLOW AND KRISTEN LAWTON BARRY

CHAPTER OUTLINE

Introduction

Substance abuse and dependence are considered significant problems in society, warranting identification and treatment. However, substance misuse, abuse, and dependence in older adults are complex issues that are often not recognized and, if recognized at all, are undertreated. Substance misuse/abuse, in particular, among elders is an increasing problem. Older adults with these problems are a special and vulnerable population that can benefit from elder-specific strategies focused on their unique issues associated with alcohol and medication/drug misuse/abuse in later life. There are concerns in the field that the standard diagnostic criteria for abuse/dependence are difficult to apply to older adults, leading to underidentification and treatment. This chapter covers four major areas that can benefit both research and clinical professionals working with older adults: (1) prevalence, impact, and correlates of the substance abuse in this population; (2) screening and identification; (3) use of brief interventions to either encourage behavior change or facilitate treatment entry, if needed; and (4) treatment research and related issues.

Prevalence and Impact of Substance Use Among Older Adults

Community surveys have estimated the prevalence of problem drinking among older adults to range from 1% to 16%.[7,31,35,66] These rates vary widely depending on the definitions of older adults, at-risk and problem drinking, alcohol abuse/dependence, and the methodology used in obtaining samples. The National Survey on Drug Use and Health (2002–2003) found that, for individuals 50 years or older, 12.2% were heavy drinkers, 3.2% were binge drinkers, and 1.8% used illicit drugs.[48] Estimates of alcohol problems are much higher among health care–seeking populations, because problem drinkers are more likely to seek medical care.[51] In 2002, over 616,000 adults 55 years of age or older reported alcohol dependence in the past year (*Diagnostic and Statistical Manual of Mental Disorders, Fourth Edition, Text Revision* [DSM-IV-TR] definition): 1.8% of those 55–59 years of age, 1.5% of those 60–64 years of age, and 0.5% of those 65 years of age or older.[47] Although alcohol and drug/medication dependence are less common in older adults when compared to younger adults, the mental and physical health consequences are serious.[40] The 2011 National Survey on Drug Use and Health[20] showed a significant level of binge drinking among individuals 60 years of age or older. The authors found that 19% of the men and 13% of the women had two or more drinks a day, considered heavy or at-risk drinking. The survey also found binge drinking in individuals older than 65, with 14% of men and 3% of women engaging in binge drinking.

Medication Misuse

Misuse of medications by older adults is perhaps a more challenging issue to identify. Older adults are at higher risk than younger groups for inappropriate use of medications. Older adults use more prescriptions and over-the-counter medications than other age groups: in 2000, the average older American received over

20 prescriptions per year, often coming from an average of 4.7 therapeutic classes.[60] It is estimated that up to 33% of older adults receive psychoactive drugs with abuse potential.[58] There over 2 million serious adverse drug reactions annually, with 100,000 deaths per year. Adverse drug reactions are especially prominent among nursing home patients with 350,000 events each year.[37] A survey of social services agencies indicated that medication misuse affects 18%–41% of the older clients served, depending on the agency.[55]

Substance abuse problems among elderly individuals often occur from misuse of over-the-counter and prescription medications. Older adults who misuse prescription drugs may be different from older adults who abuse illegal substances, in that drug misuse in older adults is often unintentional.[58] For example, a recent study found that 32.1% of older participants needed assistance in proper medication use, 15.6% had difficulty recalling the purpose of one or more of their medications, 10.9% reported an incorrect dose for their medications, and 8.2% of participants took medications that were inappropriate for their symptoms.[55] Drug misuse can result from the overuse, underuse, or irregular use of either prescription or over-the-counter medications. Misuse can become abuse relatively easily. In addition, cofactors such as alcohol and/or mental health problems, white race, living in rural areas, poor health status, social isolation, and older age increase vulnerability for misusing prescribed medications.[58] Likewise, being female significantly increases vulnerability, with an estimated 2.8 million (11.0%) of US women older than 60 years of age misusing psychoactive prescription medications.[58]

Vulnerabilities for Substance Use Problems

Older adults have specific vulnerabilities for substance abuse problems due to the physical and psychological changes that accompany aging. These may include bereavement, loneliness, diminished mobility, impaired sensory capabilities, chronic pain, poor physical health, cognitive impairment, and poor economic and social supports.[59] In addition, older adults have an increased sensitivity to alcohol, over-the-counter medications, and prescription medications. The age-related decrease in lean body mass compared to total volume of fat and the decrease in total body volume increase the total distribution of alcohol and other mood-altering chemicals in the body, which increases vulnerability. In addition, central nervous system sensitivity increases with age. Liver enzymes that metabolize alcohol and certain other drugs are less efficient with aging.

Chronic pain presents as a risk factor for prescription drug misuse, specifically in older adults. Although pain reliever misuse is lower in older adults than in younger adults, rates of misuse among individuals older than 50 years of age have been reported at 1.7%. It has been found that as individuals age, their patterns of pain reliever misuse change. A primary theme emerges when considering pain reliever misuse in this population: rather than actively seeking out pain relievers, older adults are likely to report pain reliever possession originating from multiple medical doctors.[34]

A major concern in working with older adults is the interactions between alcohol and medications, particularly psychoactive medications, such as benzodiazepines, barbiturates, and antidepressants. Older adults metabolize drugs more slowly and are more sensitive to drug effects. On top of the natural slowing of the metabolism, alcohol use can interfere with the metabolism of many medications and is a risk factor for the development of adverse drug reactions.[35] A recent study found that 62.2% of older adults taking alcohol-interactive medications used alcohol in combination with their medication; 42.2% of at-risk alcohol users were taking drugs that had the potential to cause significant interactions with alcohol.[41] There are individuals for whom *any* alcohol use, coupled with the use of specific over-the-counter/prescription medications, can be problematic. For example, it was found that the use of antidepressant medications did not result in a decrease of at-risk drinking among older adults. The concerning issue is that the use of alcohol can decrease the effectiveness of antidepressant medications, and conversely, reducing the consumption of alcohol can be beneficial in reducing some of the symptoms of depression.[63] Furthermore, co-occurring psychiatric conditions including comorbid depression, anxiety disorders, and cognitive impairment can be a complication of alcohol and medication abuse in older adults.[51] It is also possible that alcohol abuse can aggravate medical problems specifically associated with aging.[35]

The medical and emotional consequences of heavy or excessive alcohol consumption have been well documented. These risks include increased risk of coronary heart disease, hypertension, dementia, depression, and insomnia.[6] However, there is now more evidence of the medical risks of moderate alcohol use for some older adults. Moderate alcohol consumption has been demonstrated to increase the risk of strokes caused by bleeding, although it decreases the risk of strokes caused by blocked blood vessels.[38] Moderate alcohol use has also been demonstrated to impair driving-related skills even at low levels of consumption and it may lead to other injuries such as falls.[50] Of particular importance to the elderly is the potential interaction between alcohol and both prescribed and over-the-counter medications, especially psychoactive medications such as benzodiazepines, barbiturates, and antidepressants, as discussed earlier. Alcohol is also known to interfere with the metabolism of medications such as digoxin, warfarin, and metformin, all medications that are commonly prescribed to older adults.[41]

Comorbidities

There are a number of physical and mental health comorbidities associated with alcohol/medication/illicit drug misuse/abuse. In working with older adults, the most difficult-to-identify symptoms are often related to mental health. Epidemiological studies have demonstrated that alcohol use in the presence of psychiatric symptoms is a common problem with wide-reaching consequences in younger age groups. There is much less research on the comorbidity of alcohol and psychiatric conditions in later life. In an early study of 216 elderly presenting for alcohol treatment, Finlayson and associates found 25% had an organic brain syndrome (dementia, delirium, amnestic syndrome), 12% had an affective disorder, and 3% had a personality disorder.[29] In a similar study, Blow and colleagues reviewed the diagnosis of 3986 Veterans Administration patients (60–69 years of age) presenting for alcohol treatment.[16] The most common comorbid psychiatric disorder was an affective disorder found in 21% of the patients. The Liverpool Longitudinal Study found a fivefold increase in psychiatric illness among elderly men who had a lifetime history of five or more years of heavy drinking.[53]

In a study of adults entering substance abuse treatment programs, 35% reported having had both internalizing and externalizing problems in the year prior to entering treatment. Older adults seem to be at greater risk of comorbid internalizing problems as these increased with age.[23]

Comorbid depressive symptoms are not only common in late life but are also an important factor in the course and prognosis of psychiatric disorders. Compared to the general adult population, alcohol consumption and problems are substantially higher in individuals with mild to moderate depression. Binge drinking also tends to be more common in individuals with comorbid depression.[2] Individuals who have co-occurring depression and alcohol abuse/dependence have been shown to have a more complicated clinical course of depression, with an increased risk of suicide and more social dysfunction than individuals with alcohol problems with no depression.[14,17] The risk of suicide is also higher in older adults with early-onset alcohol dependence.[62,64] Relapse rates for those who were alcohol dependent did not appear to be influenced by the presence of depression. Alcohol use prior to late life has also been shown to influence the treatment of late-life depression.

Sleep disorders and sleep disturbances represent another group of comorbid disorders associated with excessive alcohol use. Alcohol causes well-established changes in sleep patterns such as decreased sleep latency, decreased stage 4 sleep, and precipitation or aggravation of sleep apnea.[64] In addition there are age-associated changes in sleep patterns including increased rapid eye movement episodes, a decrease in rapid eye movement length, decrease in stages 3 and 4 sleep, and increased awakenings.

The age-associated changes in sleep can all be worsened by alcohol use and depression. Moeller and colleagues demonstrated in younger subjects that alcohol and depression had additive effects upon sleep disturbances when occurring together.[45] In addition, alcohol-dependent adults 55 years of age or older have more disturbed sleep than those younger than 55 years of age. Rates of insomnia for this age also increase with binge drinking.[21] Furthermore, sleep disturbances (especially insomnia) have been implicated as a potential etiologic factor in the development of late-life alcohol problems or in precipitating a relapse.[49] Sleep disturbance is relatively common in older adulthood. Separating out the role of alcohol or drugs and psychiatric symptomatology with the overlay of sleep issues requires time and nonjudgmental questioning to elicit the nature of the problems and to work toward positive outcomes.

Identifying Alcohol and Drug Use Problems in Older Adults

Many older individuals have unique drinking patterns and alcohol-related consequences, social issues, and treatment needs, compared to their younger counterparts.[1] Because of this, assessment, intervention, and relapse prevention planning for alcohol problems in late life are likely to require elder-specific approaches. Many older adults who are experiencing problems related to their drinking do not meet *Diagnostic and Statistical Manual of Mental Disorders, Fifth Edition* (DSM-5) criteria for alcohol use disorder.[4] Alcohol problems are typically thought to occur in persons who consume larger quantities and drink frequently. For some older individuals, any alcohol use can present problems, particularly when coupled with some psychoactive medications. DSM-5 criteria may not be appropriate for many older adults with substance use problems because people in this age group do not often experience the social or psychological consequences specified in the criteria. In addition, a lack of tolerance to alcohol may not be as appropriate an indicator of alcohol-related problems in older ages. Most DSM criteria for tolerance are based on increased consumption over time. This does not take into account physiological

changes of aging that can lead to physiological tolerance at lower levels of alcohol consumption. In addition, the physical and emotional consequences of alcohol use, as listed in the DSM-5, may not be as relevant to older adults with alcohol problems.

Table 69.1 shows some of the signs of potential problems related to alcohol use or alcohol/medication misuse in older adults. Although some of these symptoms can be applied to other conditions in older individuals, they are important markers that provide the opportunity for professionals to ask more questions and determine differential diagnoses. Given the high rate of utilization of medical services by older adults, physicians and other health care professionals can be the key to identifying those in need of brief interventions and/or treatments and providing appropriate care based clinical need.

Classification of Alcohol Use Patterns and Problems in Older Adults

There are two main methods that have been used over many years to understand alcohol problems in older adults: (1) the medical diagnostic approach and (2) the spectrum-of-use approach. Although the DSM-5 criteria do not differentiate between abuse and dependence, it is still clinically useful to think about the level of risk for individual patients depending on their age, gender, use patterns, and other characteristics. These approaches use criteria that may not always apply to older adults and can lead to under-identification of alcohol use problems in this population. These were originally described in 1990 by Atkinson[5] and have been applied in the literature since then.

The Medical Diagnostic Approach involves applying criteria for alcohol dependence to the older adult population as they are applied to younger adults. Clinicians often rely on the American Psychiatric Association's DSM-5 when making a substance use disorder diagnosis. These criteria may not apply to older adults with substance use problems because they do not often experience the social or psychological consequences specified in the criteria. For example, one criterion asks if drinking causes issues at work and/or school, which may not be applicable to retired persons with fewer familial and work obligations.[27] A lack of tolerance to alcohol may not indicate that an older adult does not have problems related to alcohol use. Moreover, DSM-5 criteria for tolerance are mostly based on increased consumption over time, which ignores the physiological changes of aging that would account

TABLE 69.1	Signs of Potential Problems Related to Alcohol and Medication/Drugs in Older Adults (Need For Differential Diagnosis)
Anxiety	Increased tolerance to alcohol
Depressed feelings	Unusual response to medications
Disorientation	New difficulties in decision-making
Excessive mood swings	Poor hygiene
Falls, bruises, burns	Poor nutrition
Family problems	Idiopathic seizures
Financial problems	Sleep problems
Headaches	Social isolation
Incontinence	

for physiological tolerance in the setting of decreased alcohol consumption.

The spectrum-of-use approach uses definitions of abstinence, low-risk use, at-risk use, and alcohol/drug dependence to help clinicians determine the types of interventions that will be most effective.[8,10]

Abstinence refers to drinking no alcohol in the previous year. Approximately 60%–80% of US older adults are abstinent.[31] If an older individual is abstinent, it is useful to ascertain why alcohol is not used. Some individuals are abstinent because of a previous problem with alcohol. Some are abstinent because of recent illness, whereas others have life-long patterns of low-risk use or abstinence. Those older adults who have a history of alcohol problems may require preventive monitoring to determine whether any new stressors could exacerbate an old pattern.

Low-risk use is alcohol use that does not lead to problems. Older adults in this category drink within recommended drinking guidelines (no more than one drink/day or seven drinks/week, never more than two drinks on any one drinking day), are able to employ reasonable limits on alcohol consumption, and do not drink when driving a motor vehicle or boat, or when using contra-indicated medications. Low-risk use of medications/drugs would generally include using medications following the physician's prescription. However, a careful check of the number and types of medications, and whether or not the patient is taking psychoactive medications, is important because medication interactions/reactions are not uncommon in older adults and the mix of medications and alcohol can be problematic. These individuals can benefit from preventive messages but may not need interventions.

Use that increases the chances that an individual will develop problems and complications is at-risk use. Persons older than 65 who drink more than seven drinks/week—one per day—are in the at-risk use category. Although they may not *currently* have a health, social, or emotional problem caused by alcohol, they may experience family and social problems, and, if this drinking pattern continues over time, health problems could be exacerbated. At-risk use can also represent those who use alcohol within healthy limits but whose use can become hazardous due to combined comorbidities and medication use.[28] Brief interventions have been shown to be useful for older adults in this group as a prevention measure. Individuals who begin to experience problems related to their risky use of substances may benefit from brief treatments.

Dependence can include preoccupation with alcohol or drugs, continued use despite adverse consequences, and physiological symptoms such as tolerance and withdrawal. Formal specialized treatments are generally used with individuals who meet the criteria for alcohol abuse or dependence and who cannot discontinue drinking with a brief intervention protocol. Nonetheless, pretreatment strategies are also appropriate for individuals with the highest problem severity. Brief interventions were recommended by the Center for Substance Abuse Treatment's Treatment Improvement Protocol on brief interventions and brief therapies for substance use disorders, for use either as a pretreatment strategy to assist individuals on waiting lists for formalized treatment programs—in the case of those who meet criteria for a disorder with no physical dependence or withdrawal—or as an adjunct to specialized treatment to assist with specific issues (e.g., completing homework for treatment groups, attendance at work, adherence to the treatment plan).[9]

Drinking Guidelines for Screening

The National Institute on Alcohol Abuse and Alcoholism and the Center for Substance Abuse Treatment's Treatment Improvement Protocol on older adults recommended that persons 65 years or older consume no more than one standard drink/day or seven standard drinks/week.[44] In addition, older adults should consume no more than two standard drinks on any drinking day.

Screening for Alcohol/Medication Problems in Older Adults

To practice prevention and early intervention with older adults, clinicians need to screen for alcohol use (frequency and quantity), drinking consequences, and alcohol/medication interaction problems. Screening can be done as part of routine mental and physical health care and updated annually, before the older adult begins taking any new medications, or in response to problems that may be related to alcohol or medication. Clinicians can obtain more accurate histories by asking questions about the recent past, embedding the alcohol use questions in the context of other health behaviors (i.e., exercise, weight, smoking, alcohol use), and paying attention to nonverbal cues that suggest the client is minimizing use (i.e., blushing, turning away, fidgeting, looking at the floor, change in breathing pattern). The "brown bag approach"—where the clinician asks the client to bring all of his/her medications, over-the-counter preparations, and herbs in a brown paper bag to the next clinical visit—is often recommended to determine medication use. This provides an opportunity for the provider to determine what the individual is taking and what, if any, interaction effect these medications, herbs, and so on, may have with each other and with alcohol.

Screening questions can be asked by verbal interview, by paper-and-pencil questionnaire, or by computerized questionnaire. All three methods have equivalent reliability, and any positive responses can lead to further questions about consequences.[12,36] Any positive responses can lead to further questions about consequences. To successfully incorporate alcohol (and other drug) screening into clinical practice with older adults, it should be simple and consistent with other screening procedures already in place.[10]

Before asking any screening questions, the following conditions are needed: (1) the interviewer needs to be empathetic and nonthreatening; (2) the purpose of the questions should be clearly related to health status; (3) the client should be alcohol free at the time of the screening; (4) the information must be confidential; and (5) the questions need to be easy to understand. In some settings (such as waiting rooms), screening instruments are given as self-report questionnaires with instructions for patients to discuss the meaning of the results with their health care providers.

The following interview guidelines can be used. For patients requiring emergency treatment or for those who are temporarily impaired, it is best to wait until their condition has stabilized and they have become accustomed to the health setting where the interview will take place. Signs of alcohol or drug intoxication should be noted. Individuals who have alcohol on their breath or appear intoxicated give unreliable responses, so consideration should be given to conducting the interview at a later time. If this is not possible, findings and conditions of the interview should be noted in the medical record. If the alcohol questions are embedded in a longer health interview, a transitional statement is needed to move into the alcohol-related questions. The best way to introduce alcohol questions is to give the client a general idea of the content of the questions, their purpose, and the need for accurate answers.[11] This statement should be followed by a description of the types of alcoholic beverages typically consumed. If necessary, clinicians may include a description of beverages that may not be considered alcoholic (e.g., cider, low alcohol beer). Determinations of consumption are based on standard drinks. A standard drink is a 12-ounce bottle of beer, a 4-ounce glass of wine, or 1½ ounces (a shot) of liquor (e.g., vodka, gin, whiskey).

Screening for alcohol use and alcohol-related problems does not always follow a standardized format. In addition, not all standardized instruments exhibit good reliability and validity when used with older adults. There are a few screening instruments that have been used effectively with older adults. The Michigan Alcoholism Screening Test (MAST) has been shown to be effective in older adult populations, but is lengthy and requires a paper form, making it difficult to perform in a busy clinical practice.[15] On the other hand, the Alcohol Use Disorders Identification Test (AUDIT) is very brief, but has not performed as well in the elderly population.[25] The Wales Integrated In-depth Substance Misuse Tool (WISSMAT) annexes can be completed by multiple health care providers, creating a broad picture of the patient in the context of substance misuse.[65] The Alcohol-Related Problems Survey (ARPS) not only identifies older people who have symptoms of alcohol abuse/dependence but also identifies those whose use places them at elevated risk due to comorbidities and medication use. This questionnaire how been shown to be easy to understand and an appropriate length according to the majority of participants who completed it.[28] In addition to quantity/frequency questions to ascertain use, the Michigan Alcoholism Screening Test-Geriatric Version (MAST-G), the Short Michigan Alcoholism Screening Test-Geriatric Version (SMAST-G), and the AUDIT are often used with older adults. Of these, the MAST-G and the SMAST-G were developed specifically for older adults. The AUDIT, developed by the World Health Organization, has been tested in a number of countries with various populations.

The MAST-G was developed at the University of Michigan[15] as an elderly alcoholism screening instrument for use in a variety of settings. The MAST-G was the first major elder-specific alcoholism screening measure to be developed with items unique to older problem drinkers. It is a 24-item scale with a sensitivity of 94.9%, specificity of 77.8%, positive predictive value of 89.4%, and negative predictive value of 88.6%. The SMAST-G is a 10-item validated form.[17]

There has been much early work validating the World Health Organizations' AUDIT in adults younger than 65 years of age in primary care settings[30,54] and some early validation in a study of older adults.[17] The AUDIT is a 10-item scale with alcohol-related information for the *previous year only*. The questionnaire is often used as a screener. The recommended cut-off score for the AUDIT has been 8, but Blow and colleagues[17] found a Cronbach's alpha reliability of 0.95, sensitivity of 0.83, and a specificity of 0.91 in a sample of older adults with a cut-off score of 7.

Broad-Based Assessment of Substance Use Problems

Clinicians can follow-up the brief questions about consumption and consequences such as those in the MAST-G and the AUDIT with more in-depth follow-up questions, where appropriate. In addition, information obtained in the brown bag approach regarding medication use will assist in making any diagnoses and brief intervention or treatment plans.

The use of validated substance abuse assessment instruments will provide a structured approach to the assessment process as well as a checklist of items that should be evaluated, with each older adult receiving a substance abuse assessment. Specialized assessments are generally conducted by substance abuse treatment program personnel or trained mental and physical health care providers.[43] Compared to mental health services, aging services, and substance abuse treatment services, health care providers have the lowest rates of positive screens for alcohol use disorders. In addition, health care providers provide less follow-up to positive screens than do other providers. It is unlikely that one treatment provider will possess the expertise to address the full spectrum of substance use, medical, psychological, and social service needs, suggesting that care coordination as well as the integration of physical and mental health care would be beneficial.[57]

Use of Brief Alcohol Interventions With Older Adults With Substance Dependence

Low intensity, brief interventions are cost-effective and practical techniques that were used as an initial approach to at-risk and problem drinkers in primary care settings and well validated through many studies in primary care[67] and emergency medicine settings.[39] In general, the results of brief intervention studies support the recommendations of the Center for Substance Abuse Treatment expert committee report[9] and the National Institute on Alcohol Abuse and Alcoholism[46] that early identification/screening and brief interventions are effective and should be a matter of routine practice in primary and other health care settings to detect patients with hazardous or harmful patterns of alcohol use. Early identification and secondary prevention of alcohol problems using straightforward, nontechnical, and nonjudgmental terms can motivate change and can have broad positive public health implications. It appears that brief interventions with one or a few sessions have the potential of reaching the largest number and broadest spectrum of individuals from diverse settings.

There had been much less attention given to the use of brief interventions with older adults. The spectrum of alcohol interventions for older adults ranges from prevention/education for persons who are abstinent or low-risk drinkers, to minimal advice or brief structured interventions for at-risk or problem drinkers, and formalized alcoholism treatment for drinkers who meet the criteria for abuse and/or dependence. It is recommended that the least intensive treatment options be explored first when working with older adults.[17] Formalized treatment is generally used with persons who meet the criteria for alcohol abuse or dependence and cannot discontinue drinking with a brief intervention protocol. Nonetheless, pretreatment brief intervention strategies can be appropriate for this population.

Brief alcohol interventions have been shown to be effective with older adults who are at-risk and with problem drinkers,[17,30] and were recommended by the Center for Substance Abuse Treatment Improvement Protocol on brief interventions and brief treatments for substance abuse. There are two main goals of brief interventions: (1) to motivate the individual to cut down or stop using, *or* (2) to motivate the individual who has more serious substance use problems to seek brief or more formalized treatment. Brief intervention with older adults should include customized feedback on screening questionnaires; discussion of where the patient's drinking falls in relation to their peers; understanding reasons for drinking; physical, psychological, and social consequences of heavier drinking;

reasons to cut down, sensible drinking limits and strategies to reach these limits, and a drinking agreement between the care provider and patient.[17] Because this population may have fewer work/family responsibilities, there may be less pressure for older adults to decrease their alcohol consumption. A harm-reduction approach can be particularly beneficial[59] in this age group. Setting drinking limits has been shown to decrease consumption regardless of the specific limit chosen and regardless of baseline drinking severity.

It has been shown that older people respond well to substance use treatment and sometimes have better outcomes than younger users.[24] Treatment should be carried out at a pace and with content that is appropriate for older populations. To help older individuals understand and integrate new information, it is often helpful to expose them to information twice (e.g., each session should begin with a brief review of the last). Intervention should take into account clients' sensory decline by incorporating simultaneous visual and audible presentation materials, enlarged print, and voice enhancers. Medications used to modify drinking should be considered with caution and take into account age- and disease-related increases in vulnerability to side effects and adverse interactions with other medications.[17]

Because many older adults with at-risk use or substance use disorders are ashamed of their use, it is crucial that interventions be nonconfrontational and supportive in nature. It is suggested that therapies include adaptive coping strategies for issues that do not include substance use. These strategies can help to reduce depressive symptoms that are often co-occurring in older adults.[42] Motivational Enhancement Therapy (MET) is also recommended because MET incorporates the supportive, empathetic, nonconfrontational style of motivational interviewing with the individualized feedback used in brief interventions.[57] MET accepts the individual where he/she is in the change process and works to elicit internal motivation for change rather than just directing the individual through the steps in the change process.

A shortcoming in intervention is that there is resistance by many physicians to integrate Brief Intervention into their practice. This may be due to lack of time or lack of education regarding addiction intervention.[26] To reduce this concern, a review of brief interventions showed that all brief interventions produced a decline in alcohol consumption (both quantity and frequency) regardless of whether a doctor or nondoctor carried out the intervention.[3] Rao found that training community nurses to implement brief intervention can be a greatly effective strategy.[52]

Mutual self-help groups can be beneficial for improvement, although there is some evidence that older adults are less engaged than younger adults when attending groups such as Alcoholics Anonymous. Being in age-segregated groups has shown to be important for engagement and retention for older adults.[57] In addition, older adults may face unique barriers to attendance such as transportation difficulties, disabilities, and so on.

By thinking of alcohol use and medication misuse as a continuum, clinicians are given flexible guidelines to work most effectively with older adults across the range of use patterns. Brief interventions can offer a step toward assisting this vulnerable group of older adults to make changes in their alcohol/medication/drug use that can have positive health benefits.

Detoxification and Withdrawal

Alcohol withdrawal symptoms commonly occur in individuals who stop drinking or markedly cut down their drinking after regular heavy use. Alcohol withdrawal can range from mild and almost unnoticeable symptoms to severe and life-threatening ones. The classical set of symptoms associated with alcohol withdrawal includes autonomic hyperactivity (increased pulse rate, blood pressure, and temperature), restlessness, disturbed sleep, anxiety, nausea, and tremor. More severe withdrawal can be manifested by auditory, visual, or tactile hallucinations, delirium, seizures, and coma. Other substances of abuse such as benzodiazepines, opioids, and cocaine have distinct withdrawal symptoms that are also potentially life-threatening. Benzodiazepine withdrawal symptoms in older adults are usually different than those seen in younger populations: in older adults, symptoms include confusion and/or disorientation rather than anxiety, insomnia, and perceptual changes.[58] Elderly individuals have been shown to have a longer duration of withdrawal symptoms, and withdrawal has the potential for complicating other medical and psychiatric illnesses.[19] There is no evidence, however, to suggest that older individuals are more prone to alcohol withdrawal or need longer treatment for withdrawal symptoms.[18,50] Because of the potential for life-threatening complications, clinicians caring for older clients who may be abusing substances need a fundamental understanding of withdrawal symptoms and the potential complications as well as when to refer clients to treatment.

New Models for Screening and Treatment

The Substance Abuse and Mental Health Services Administration's Center for Substance Abuse Treatment published the Treatment Improvement Protocol #26 titled "Substance Abuse Among Older Adults."[17] It provided recommendations from the expert panel on innovative models for screening, brief intervention, and brief treatment approaches appropriate for the older population.

Several states followed the guidelines and recommendations and implemented screening and brief intervention services where older adults can be found (at home, senior centers). Brief interventions involve offering one to five one-on-one sessions. Brief interventions for older adults with alcohol problems or risk of such problems have been implemented in a number of settings including primary care.[13] Others have implemented more formal, elder-specific treatment using brief therapy or brief treatment employing relapse-prevention models, cognitive-behavioral treatment, and self-management skills.[22] This methodology has been implemented in day treatment or outpatient settings.[55,56]

Studies of Treatment Compliance in Older Adults

Treatment outcomes research on older adults with substance use disorders has focused primarily on compliance with treatment program requirements, with an emphasis on the individuals' fulfillment of prescribed treatment activities and goals, including whether or not those in recovery returned to drinking.[5,17] The few studies that have addressed these issues in the aging population have shown that age-specific programming improved treatment completion compared with mixed-age treatment.[57]

There have been major limitations in the treatment compliance literature on older adults and few prospective studies conducted. Data issues have included a lack of drinking outcome data, failure to report on treatment dropouts, and variations in definitions of treatment completion. In addition, few prospective treatment outcome studies including sufficiently large numbers of older subjects who meet the criteria for alcohol dependence have been conducted to address the methodological limitations of prior work.

Limitations of Treatment Outcome Research

Although it is important to examine factors related to completion of treatment to have a better understanding of client characteristics for those who complete treatment—the lack of information on treatment dropouts or on short- or long-term treatment outcomes, the paucity of females in these studies, the widely varying age cutoffs for inclusion in studies, and the use of abstinence only as the outcome—it may be more useful in future studies to measure more clearly nonabstinent drinking outcomes along dimensions such as whether drinkers ever drink to the point of intoxication, binge drinking episodes, consequences over time, physical and mental health status changes, and psychological distress changes over time. Finally, testing elder-specific treatment with mixed-age treatments will help to shape the field in the future as greater percentages of adults reach older ages.

Future Trends: Impact of the Baby Boom Cohort

The use of illicit drugs is currently relatively rare in older adults. However, research suggests that the number of illicit drug users in older adulthood is likely to increase due to the aging of the Baby Boom generation.

The higher risk for alcohol and medication use in older adults, coupled with the rapid growth in this population, highlights the need for targeted intervention, treatment, and relapse prevention strategies. Demographic projections indicate that the aging of the Baby Boom generation will increase the proportion of persons 65 of age or older from 13% currently to 20% by the year 2030.[61] The extent of alcohol and medication misuse is likely to increase significantly as the Baby Boom cohort ages, due to both the growth in the older population as well as cohort-associated lifestyle differences.[18] The projected increase in the number of older adults with substance abuse problems is associated with a 50% increase in the number of older adults and a 70% increase in the rate of treatment needed among older adults.[33]

Recent studies of consumption patterns suggest that the baby boom generation, as it continues to age, could maintain a higher level of alcohol consumption than in previous older adult cohorts.[18] Rates of heavy alcohol use have been shown to be higher among baby boomers than in earlier cohorts. In addition, drug use is heightened in the baby boomer cohort. It has been shown that birth cohorts that experience high rates of drug use in youth have subsequently higher rates of use and associated problems as they age, compared to other cohorts. It is estimated that there will be a tripling in the number of older adults needing treatment for a substance abuse problem by 2020.[33] The increasing rate of problem substance use in this population may be attributed to an increase in problems related to the use of illicit drugs or nonmedical use of prescription medications.[18,32,33] Furthermore, these projections may be underestimates, as criteria used to define problem substance use may not be most appropriate for older populations. Increased substance abuse, coupled with the projected increase in the older adult population, will place increasing pressure on the treatment programs and health care resources.[55]

Older adults are a diverse population with substance use patterns that differ across individuals and groups and cover the spectrum of use patterns include abstinence, low-risk use, at-risk use, problem use, and abuse/dependence. Developing brief, cost-effective methods to work with older adults who are experiencing problems related to their use of alcohol, medications, and illicit drugs is becoming a more crucial issue in this era of changing demographic and substance use patterns. It will be the challenge for current and future clinicians, trainers, and researchers to develop methods to ensure more positive outcomes for vulnerable older citizens.

References

1. Adams WL, et al. Primary care for elderly people: why do doctors find it so hard? *Gerontol.* 2002;42(6):835–842.
2. Åhlin J, Hallgren M, Öjehagen A, Källmén H, Forsell Y. Adults with mild to moderate depression exhibit more alcohol related problems compared to the general adult population: a cross sectional study. *BMC Public Health.* 2015;15(1):542.
3. Álvarez-Bueno C, Rodríguez-Martín B, García-Ortiz L, Gómez-Marcos MÁ, Martínez-Vizcaíno V. Effectiveness of brief interventions in primary health care settings to decrease alcohol consumption by adult non-dependent drinkers: a systematic review of systematic reviews. *Prev Med.* 2015;76:S33–S38.
4. Atkinson R. Aging and alcohol use disorders: diagnostic issues in the elderly. *Int Psychogeriatr.* 1990;2(1):55–72.
5. Atkinson R. Treatment programs for aging alcoholics. In: Beresford TP, Gomberg ESL, eds. *Alcohol and Aging.* New York: Oxford University; 1995:186–210.
6. Bakhshi S, While AE. Older people and alcohol use. *Br J Comm Nurs.* 2014;19(8).
7. Barnes AJ, Moore AA, Xu H, et al. Prevalence and correlates of at-risk drinking among older adults: the project SHARE study. *J Gen Int Med.* 2010;25(8):840–846.
8. Barry K. Alcohol and drug abuse. *Fundamentals of Clinical Practice: A Textbook on the Patient, Doctor, and Society.* New York: Plenum Medical Book; 1997.
9. Barry K. *Brief Interventions and Brief Therapies for Substance Abuse.* Rockville, MD: US Department of Health and Human Services, Public Health Service, Substance Abuse and Mental Health Services Administration, Center for Substance Abuse Treatment; 1999.
10. Barry KL, Blow FC. Screening and assessment of alcohol problems in older adults. In: Lichtenberg P, ed. *Handbook of Assessment in Clinical Gerontology.* New York: Wiley; 2000.
11. Barry KL, Blow FC. Substance safety in health promotion. In: Gorin SS, Arnold J, eds. *Health Promotion in Practice.* San Francisco, CA: Jossey-Bass; 2006:329–360.
12. Barry KL, Fleming MF. Computerized administration of alcoholism screening tests in a primary care setting. *J Am Board Fam Pract.* 1990;3:93–98.
13. Barry KL, Oslin D, Blow FC. *Alcohol Problems in Older Adults: Prevention and Management.* New York: Springer; 2001.
14. Blow FC, Brockmann LM, Barry KL. The role of alcohol in late-life suicide. *Alcohol Clin Exp Res.* 2004;28(5S):48S–56S.
15. Blow FC, Brower KJ, Schulenberg JE, et al. The Michigan alcoholism screening test – geriatric version (MAST-G): a new elderly-specific screening instrument. *Alcohol Clin Exp Res.* 1992a;16:372.
16. Blow FC, Cook CA, Booth BM, et al. Age-related psychiatric comorbidities and level of functioning in alcoholic veterans seeking outpatient treatment. *Hosp Comm Psychiatr.* 1992b;43:990–995.
17. Blow FC, Gillespie BW, Barry KL, Mudd SA, Hill EM. Brief screening for alcohol problems in elderly populations using the short Michigan alcoholism screening test-geriatric version (SMAST-G). *Poster presented at the Research Society on Alcoholism Annual Scientific Meeting, Hilton Head Island, SC, June 20–25, 1998.* 1998.
18. Blow FC, Oslin DW, Barry B. Misuse and abuse of alcohol, illicit drugs, and psychoactive medication among older people. *Generations.* 2002;26(1):50 (5).
19. Brower KJ, Mudd S, Blow FC, et al. Severity and treatment of alcohol withdrawal in elderly versus younger patients. *Clin Exp Res.* 1994;18:196–201.
20. Butler JS, Coffey LE, Griffin AB. *2011 National Survey on Drug Use and Health;* 2012.
21. Canham SL, Kaufmann CN, Mauro PM, Mojtabai R, Spira AP. Binge drinking and insomnia in middle–aged and older adults: the Health and Retirement Study. *Int J Geriatr Psychiatry.* 2015;30(3):284–291.

22. Center for Substance Abuse Treatment. Substance abuse relapse prevention for older adults: a group treatment approach. *Report No. DHHS Publication No. (SMA) 05-4053*. Rockville, MD: Substance Abuse and Mental Health Services Administration; 2005.

23. Chan YF, Dennis ML, Funk RR. Prevalence and comorbidity of major internalizing and externalizing problems among adolescents and adults presenting to substance abuse treatment. *J Substance Abuse Treat*. 2008;34(1):14–24.

24. Chapman SLC, Wu LT. Epidemiology and Demography of illicit drug Use and drug Use disorders among adults aged 50 and older-*Substance Use and Older People*. Vols. 91–108; 2015.

25. Conigliaro J, Kraemer K, McNeil M. Screening and identification of older adults with alcohol problems in primary care. *J Geriatr Psychiatr Neurol*. 2000;13(3):106–114.

26. Coogle CL, Owens MG. Screening and brief intervention for alcohol misuse in older adults: training outcomes among physicians and other healthcare practitioners in community-based settings. *Commun Ment Health J*. 2015;51(5):546–553.

27. DSM-5 American Psychiatric Association. *Diagnostic and Statistical Manual of Mental Disorders*. Arlington: American Psychiatric Publishing; 2013.

28. Fink A, Morton SC, Beck JC, et al. The alcohol–related problems survey: identifying hazardous and harmful drinking in older primary care patients. *J Am Geriatr Soc*. 2002;50(10):1717–1722.

29. Finlayson RE. Prescription drug dependence in the elderly: the clinical pathway to recovery. *J Mental Health Aging*. 1998;4:233–249.

30. Fleming MF, Manwell LB, Barry KL, et al. Brief physician advice for alcohol problems in older adults: a randomized community-based trial. *J Fam Pract*. 1999;48(5):378–384.

31. Gell L, Meier PS, Goyder E. Alcohol consumption among the over 50s: international comparisons. *Alcohol Alcohol*. 2015;50(1):1–10.

32. Gfoerer JC, Pemberton MR. Substance use by older adults: estimates of future impact on the treatment system. Substance abuse and mental health services administration, Office of applied studies, Rockville, MD. In: Gurnack A, Osgood N, eds. *Treating Alcohol and Drug Abuse in the Elderly*. New York: Springer; 2002.

33. Gfroerer J, Penne M, Pemberton M, Folsom R. Substance abuse treatment need among older adults in 2020: the impact of the aging baby-boom cohort. *Drug Alcohol Depend*. 2003;69(2):127–135.

34. Gilson KM, Bryant C, Judd F. The hidden harms of using alcohol for pain relief in older adults. *Int Psychogeriatr*. 2014;26(11):1929–1930.

35. Gossop M, Moos R. Substance misuse among older adults: a neglected but treatable problem. *Addiction*. 2008;103(3):347–348.

36. Greist JH, Klein MH, Erdman HP. Comparison of computer- and interviewer-administered versions of the diagnostic interview schedule. *Hosp Commun Psychiatr*. 1987;38(12):1304–1311.

37. Gurwitz JH, et al. Incidence and preventability of adverse drug events in nursing homes. *Am J Med*. 2000;109(2):87–94.

38. Hansagi H, Romelsjo A, Gerhardsson De Verdier M, et al. Alcohol consumption and stroke mortality: 20-year follow-up of 15077 men and women. *Stroke*. 1995;26:1768–1773.

39. Havard A, Shakeshaft A, Sanson-Fisher R. Systematic review and meta-analyses of strategies targeting alcohol problems in emergency departments: interventions reduce alcohol-related injuries. *Addiction*. 2008;103(3):368–376; discussion 377–378.

40. Huang B, et al. Prevalence, correlates, and comorbidity of nonmedical prescription drug use and drug use disorders in the United States: results of the national epidemiologic survey on alcohol and related conditions. *J Clin Psychiatry*. 2006;67(7):1062–1073.

41. Immonen S, Valvanne J, Pitkälä KH. The prevalence of potential alcohol–drug interactions in older adults. *Scandinavian J Prim Health Care*. 2013;31(2):73–78.

42. Mauro PM, Canham SL, Martins SS, Spira AP. Substance-use coping and self-rated health among US middle-aged and older adults. *Addictiv Behav*. 2015;42:96–100.

43. Menninger JA. Assessment and treatment of alcoholism and substance-related disorders in the elderly. *Bull Menninger Clin*. 2002;66(2):166–183.

44. Merrick EL, Horgan CM, Hodgkin D, et al. Unhealthy drinking patterns in older adults: prevalence and associated characteristics. *J Am Geriatr Soc*. 2008;56(2):214–223.

45. Moeller FG, Gillin JC, Irwin M. A comparison of sleep EEGs in patients with primary major depression and major depression secondary to alcoholism. *J Affect Disord*. 1993;27:39–42.

46. National Institute on Alcohol Abuse and Alcoholism. *Brief Interventions for Alcohol Problems*. Alcohol Alert; No. 43. Rockville, MD: NIAAA Publications Distribution Center, P.O. Box 10686; 1999. 20849–0686.

47. Office of Applied Studies. *Summary of Findings from the 2002 National Survey on Drug Use and Health*. Rockvilled, MD: Substance Abuse and Mental Health Services Administration, Department of Health & Human Services; 2002.

48. Office of Applied Studies, US Department of Health and Human Services. The DASIS report. Older adults in substance abuse treatment: update; 2017. Available at: http://oas.samhsa.gov/2k5/olderAdultsTX/olderAdults.TX. Accessed 18 Feb 2016.

49. Oslin DW. *Alcohol Geriatric Secrets*. Philadelphia: Hanley and Belfus; 1996.

50. Oslin DW. Late-life alcoholism: issues relevant to the geriatric psychiatrist. *Am J Geriatr Psychiatry*. 2004;12(6):571–583.

51. Oslin DW. Evidence-based treatment of geriatric substance abuse. *Psychiatr Clin North Am*. 2005;28(4): 897–911.

52. Rao T. The role of community nursing in providing integrated care for older people with alcohol misuse. *Br J Commun Nurs*. 2014;19(2).

53. Saunders PA, Copeland JR, Dewey ME. Heavy drinking as a risk factor for depression and dementia in elderly men. *Br J Psychiatry*. 1991;159:213–216.

54. Schmidt A, Barry KL, Fleming MF. Detection of problem drinkers: the alcohol use disorders identification test (AUDIT). *South Med J*. 1995;88(1):52–59.

55. Schonfeld L, King-Kallimanis BL, Duchene DM, et al. Screening and brief intervention for substance misuse among older adults: the Florida BRITE project. *Am J Public Health*. 2010;100(1):108–114.

56. Schonfeld L, et al. Cognitive-behavioral treatment of older veterans with substance abuse problems. *J Geriatr Psychiatry Neurol*. 2000;13(3):124–129.

57. Schutte K, Lemke S, Moos RH, Brennan PL. Age-sensitive psychosocial treatment for older adults with substance abuse. *Substance Use Older People*. 2015:314–339.

58. Simoni-Wastila L, Yang HWK. Drug abuse and addiction in elderly. *Drug Abuse and Addiction in Medical Illness*. New York: Springer; 2012:455–465.

59. Taylor C, Jones KA, Dening T. Detecting alcohol problems in older adults: can we do better? *Int Psychogeriatr*. 2014;26(11):1755–1766.

60. Thomas CP, Ritter G, Wallack SS. Growth in prescription drug spending among insured elders. *Health Aff*. 2001;20(5):265–277.

61. U.S. Census Bureau. *Projections of the Resident Population by Age, Sex, Race, and Hispanic Origin: 1999–2100*. Washington, DC: Population Projections Program; 2000.

62. van den Berg JF, Hermes JS, van den Brink W, Blanken P, Kist N, Kok RM. Physical and mental health and social functioning in older alcohol-dependent inpatients: the role of age of onset. *Eur Addict Res*. 2014a;20(5):226–232.

63. van den Berg JF, Kok RM, van Marwijk HW, et al. Correlates of alcohol abstinence and at-risk alcohol consumption in older adults with depression: the NESDO study. *Am J Geriatr Psychiatr*. 2014b;22(9):866–874.

64. Wagman AM, Allen RP, Upright D. Effects of alcohol consumption upon parameters of ultradian sleep rhythms in alcoholics. *Adv Exp Med Biol*. 1997;85A:601–616.

65. Wallace C, Black DJ, Fothergill A. Integrated assessment of older adults who misuse alcohol. *Nurs Standard*. 2010;24(33):51–57.

66. Wang YP, Andrade LH. Epidemiology of alcohol and drug use in the elderly. *Curr Opin Psychiatr*. 2013;26(4):343–348.

67. Whitlock EP, et al. Behavioral counseling interventions in primary care to reduce risky/harmful alcohol use by adults: a summary of the evidence for the U.S. Preventive Services Task Force. *Ann Intern Med*. 2004;140(7):557–568.

70

Alcohol and Drugs of Abuse in Pregnant Women: Effects on the Fetus and Newborn, Mode of Action, and Maternal Treatment

ASHER ORNOY AND SARAH YACOBI

CHAPTER OUTLINE

Introduction

Several drugs and chemicals are known to be teratogenic to the human embryo when administered throughout pregnancy, especially during the period of organogenesis. The evidence for their teratogenicity has been shown by human epidemiologic and clinical studies as well as in studies carried out in animals such as rats, mice, rabbits, and primates. The most important disadvantage of the animal models used is the interspecies differences in toxicity and teratogenicity. These teratogenic insults occurring during embryonic life may be present immediately after birth, at infancy, or even later in life, especially if the damage involves the central nervous system.[103] Moreover, many of the insults to the central nervous system occur in the second and third trimesters of pregnancy, when most other organs have already passed the stage of active organogenesis. Briefly, the main stages of human central nervous system development are the formation of the neural folds, their closure to form the neural tube that closes completely toward the end of the fourth week post-fertilization, and the formation of the main brain vesicles during weeks 5 and 6, with the medulla, pons, and midbrain undergoing much of their active development during that time. However, the cortical plate starts to develop mainly during weeks 8–9 postfertilization, and the cerebellar cortex develops even later, mainly during the second and third trimesters of pregnancy. The cerebral cortex continues to develop actively throughout gestation and even in the early postnatal life, mainly by forming the different cortical layers, neuronal growth and sprouting, synapse formation, and myelinization. It is therefore expected that psychotropic agents such as ethanol, opioids, cannabis, and cocaine, as well as different psychotropic drugs, may affect the development of the central nervous system almost throughout the entire pregnancy.[102,103,124] Hence, such late effect will not necessarily be manifested by distinct morphological changes in the central nervous system but rather by more subtle changes in intellectual capacity, learning ability, attention span, and behavior. Often, slight pathological changes in different regions of the brain can be demonstrated by using newer brain imaging methods.

In this chapter, we discuss only the possible effects of ethanol, opiates, cannabis, and cocaine use during pregnancy on the human embryo and fetus. We survey studies concerning substance-abusing women either throughout pregnancy or following sporadic use. In addition, we discuss some animal studies, especially those related to mechanism of action. Unlike other drugs that impact the central nervous system or other organs, all drugs of abuse may affect both the mother and embryo, inducing mainly, but not exclusively, behavioral and psychiatric problems and intellectual deficits.

Effects of Maternal Alcohol (Ethanol) Consumption During Pregnancy

History of Alcohol Effects in Pregnancy

The history of maternal alcoholism and development of the offspring goes back to the Bible and to early Greek mythology. Samuel the prophet forbids Samson's mother from drinking wine during her pregnancy because she is going to give birth to an exceptional child blessed by God with special power, and the bridal couple, in Carthage, was forbidden to drink wine on the wedding night to prevent the birth of a defective child. In 1834, a report to the House of Commons (by a select committee investigating drunkenness) indicated that some of the alcoholic mothers gave birth to infants with "a starved, shrivelled and imperfect look." Later, in 1900, the earliest suspicion of the teratogenic effects of alcohol came from Sullivan, who reported an increase in the rate of abortions and stillbirths as well as increased frequency of epilepsy among live-born infants of chronic alcohol-abusing women.[67] The teratogenic effects of ethanol on human fetuses were first reported by Lemoine et al. in 1968. The authors described a common pattern of birth defects in 127 children born to alcoholic mothers in France that included growth deficiency, psychomotor retardation, low IQ, and atypical electroencephalogram.[82] Alcohol was used at the time to prevent premature labor, and its use was so widespread that if any causal correlation existed between prenatal alcohol use and birth defects, it should have been recognized and reported long before 1968. The adverse/harmful effects of alcohol use during pregnancy have been suggested for decades, and despite the numerous case reports, the implication of alcohol as a teratogen was greeted with skepticism by the medical community. Furthermore, it was rather difficult to document or diagnose formally the constellation of problems observed in these children until guidelines for fetal alcohol syndrome were established.[119]

Effects on the Developing Embryo and Fetus

Fetal Alcohol Spectrum Disorder

It is well known that alcohol in pregnancy may lead to a variety of damaging effects on the fetus. Hence, the general term for alcohol disruptive effects is fetal alcohol spectrum disorder (FASD). Basically, there seem to be several categories of prenatal exposure to ethanol related to quantity (amount of alcohol used), modality (whether continuous or binge drinking), and fetal age at exposure (whether pre- or postorganogenesis). Exposure to heavy drinking (more than 100 g of ethanol/day), which may cause the full-blown fetal alcohol syndrome (FAS), exposure to moderate drinking (between 50 and 100 g of ethanol/day), which may result in fetal "alcohol effects" (the differences between these categories are not sharp), and binge drinking-occasions with intakes of four to five drinks of ethanol (altogether more than 100 g of ethanol in each of such occasions.[28,75,92,114,138] Additional factors such as maternal age, weight, and genetic makeup of the mother and fetus play an important role. Most investigators are in agreement that binge drinking may also cause damage to the developing fetal brain.[75,104] The amount of alcohol ingested, the length of the period of alcohol use, and the developmental stage of the embryo and fetus at exposure mediate the effects of ethanol intake on the developing fetus. It is important to note that a meta-analysis of reports on the incidence of fetal malformations in moderately alcohol-abusing women during pregnancy did not show an increase in congenital defects.[86] Alcohol drinking, even in moderate amounts, also is associated with an increased risk of spontaneous abortions, especially in the first trimester of pregnancy, and with infertility in males and females.[75]

It has been demonstrated by many investigators that high alcohol consumption during pregnancy may seriously affect the embryo. The severity of the malformations ranges from FAS, which is evident in 4%–6% of infants of heavy-drinking mothers with the typical clinical picture of facial dysmorphism, mental retardation, and disruptive behavior, to minor effects, such as low birth weight, intrauterine growth retardation, a slight reduction in IQ of the infants, and an increased rate of congenital anomalies and behavioral emotional changes.[67,68,82,104,119]

Alcohol consumption during pregnancy was associated with a variety of abnormalities in the newborn. However, the more serious and specific syndrome FAS has been described only for regular/daily alcohol users. Fig. 8.2).[a] Recognition of the syndrome was made by Drs. David Smith and Kenneth Jones in 1973 based on the evaluation of eight children born to mothers who were defined as chronic alcoholics.[66] The principal features were determined as prenatal and postnatal growth deficiency, short stature, developmental delay, microcephaly, fine-motor dysfunction, and facial dysmorphism manifested by short palpebral fissures, long smooth philtrum, thin vermilion border of upper lip, and maxillary hypoplasia. In addition, there may be cleft palate, joint anomalies, altered palmar creases, and cardiac anomalies.[67] Many of these children also show disruptive behavior, such as severe ADHD, oppositional defiant disorder (ODD), conduct disorder (CD), and autism spectrum disorder (ASD)–like behavior.[110,111,151] Many of them also need appropriate medication for their disrupted behavior. The above-described facial dysmorphism tends to improve with the advancement in age of the affected individuals.

[a] References 4, 37, 67, 84, 114, 119, 138.

Anomalies of Organs Other Than the Brain

Alcohol is known to affect not only the central nervous system but also organs that are developmentally related to central nervous system derivatives, including those developmentally dependent on neural crest cells like the craniofacial complex and the heart.

Orofacial Clefts

A number of reports addressed potential correlation between alcohol consumption and oral clefts. However, effect estimates were often unstable due to numbers of the cases studied. In a case-control surveillance study, Meyer et al.[96] collected 5956 live-born infants with cleft palate, cleft lip, or both. Based on the maternal report of alcohol use during the first 4 months of pregnancy, the authors failed to link low levels of alcohol use and oral clefts. Even the highest level of alcohol consumption (three or more drinks per week, three or more drinks per drinking day, and maximum daily consumption of five or more drinks) did not result in a higher number of infants born with a cleft than did the use of less than one drink per week or less than one drink per drinking day. In addition, folic-acid–supplemented multivitamins used by some of the women did not modify the association between oral clefts and ethanol consumption.[96] Contradictory results were reported by Romitti et al.[123] based on the data from the National Birth Defects Prevention Study. The authors found a weak correlation between average periconceptional alcohol consumption and all orofacial clefts (combined and isolated clefts). A moderate link was identified for multiple clefts and for Pierre-Robin syndrome. Estimates for this latter phenotype, however, were based on small numbers, reflecting the study criteria to exclude cases of known etiology. An increased risk of orofacial clefts was observed among infants born to binge-drinking (five or more drinks per occasion) mothers exposed in the first trimester of pregnancy. Maternal binge drinking may be particularly harmful, since it results in a greater peak of blood ethanol concentration and, therefore, a prolonged alcohol exposure.[32] In contrast, Bell et al.[10] in their recent review and meta-analysis of 33 studies (from 737 publications) did not find any increase in oral clefts, with odds ratios near 1.00.

Cardiac Anomalies

There is sparse literature dealing with the effects of alcohol abuse in pregnancy on cardiac anomalies. It is accepted that about one-third of children with alcohol embryopathy will also have congenital cardiac problems. Krasemann and Klingebiel[79] retrospectively reviewed electrocardiographic and echocardiographic data of all patients with clinical signs of alcoholic embryopathy between the years 1976 and 2003. Electrocardiographic and echocardiographic measurements often showed slightly altered values in individuals with alcoholic embryopathy, resulting in the conclusion that alcohol abuse during pregnancy as a primary toxin can lead to minor cardiac abnormalities, even without structural congenital cardiac defects.[79] Conotruncal cardiac defects are among the more common serious cardiac anomalies following periconceptional use of alcohol,[19,137] but the extent of their increase following alcohol use in pregnancy is in debate.

Reduced Fetal Growth

Intrauterine growth restriction is a well-known feature of alcohol embryopathy. There is a growing mass of data demonstrating postnatal long-term height and weight deficits among children born to ethanol-using women. Furthermore, Covington et al.[29] found a moderating effect of maternal age on children's weight at age 7, as children born to women over 30 years of age at the time of birth had significantly lower weight compared with those born to younger women.[29] Nykjaer et al.[100] found that alcohol drinking, mainly in the first trimester of pregnancy, is associated with reduced birth weight and increased prematurity.

Behavioral and Developmental Changes

1. Attention-deficit/hyperactivity disorder (or ADHD): Alcohol is considered one of the risk factors for ADHD, independently of prenatal nicotine exposure or other familial-hereditary risk factors. One study showing a positive correlation between alcohol and ADHD included 26 prenatally alcohol-exposed children. Of the 24 children followed up, 10 were diagnosed with ADHD, two with Asperger syndrome, and one with mild mental retardation. The severity of the disorder correlated in a linear pattern with the amount of alcohol used by the mother during pregnancy. This effect was reversible, since discontinuation of alcohol consumption by the 12th week resulted in normally developed children. Moreover, consumption of less than one alcoholic drink per day in the last 3 months of pregnancy, despite heavier drinking earlier, did not result in increased rate of ADHD, learning disabilities, or cognitive impairment at the age of 14 years.[101]

It has been difficult to define and characterize developmental risks associated with binge drinking or moderate drinking in pregnancy,[50] and some studies have failed to demonstrate an association between alcohol exposure and sustained attention performance in school-aged children.[13]

2. Intellectual impairment: Alcohol in pregnancy may affect intellectual ability, which, together with attention span and behavior, is considered a higher function of the cerebral cortex. Children with the complete FAS generally have different degrees of mental retardation, occasionally moderate to severe retardation. Studies in 7-year-old school children following prenatal exposure to moderate amounts of alcohol show a decrement of 7 points in IQ.[140] Binge drinking was also associated with poorer achievements at school compared to children of nondrinking mothers.[127] On the other hand, drinking relatively low amounts of alcohol (1-2 drinks/week) did not result in any increased risk of cognitive or behavioral difficulties.[74]

3. Cerebellar changes: Alcohol may affect the cerebellum. In the human cerebellum, Purkinje cell migration is completed and dendritic outgrowth begins around gestational week 26, extending to the third trimester of pregnancy. Consequently, a period of enhanced vulnerability of Purkinje cells to binge alcohol exposure in humans would be predicted near the end of the second trimester and may extend over the first half of the third trimester.[52] Cerebellar developmental disorders and disproportionate reduction in the anterior cerebellar vermis have been identified by magnetic resonance imaging (MRI) in children who were exposed prenatally to alcohol during each trimester of pregnancy.[117] Decreased cerebellar growth and decreased cranial-to-body growth in fetuses of alcohol-abusing mothers were also observed on fetal ultrasound performed in the 18th week of gestation.[57] If the mothers stopped drinking at the beginning of pregnancy, cerebellar growth was normal.

Mechanisms of Alcohol Teratogenicity

The exact mechanism(s) of the teratogenic effects of alcohol on the developing embryo and fetus are not yet well established. However, the extent of damage depends on the dose, duration, and developmental stage at exposure. Different mechanisms have been offered to explain the teratogenic effects of alcohol on the developing embryo. They stem from results of different experimental studies and include the following: (1) increased oxidative stress;

(2) disturbed metabolism of glucose, protein, lipid, and DNA; (3) epigenetic changes; and (4) effects on neurons: impaired neurogenesis and increased cellular apoptosis, especially of neural crest cells.

Oxidative Stress

One process implicated is an alteration in the reduction-oxidation reaction status in the central nervous system. This hypothesis was supported by studies demonstrating that ethanol mediated changes in the production and/or activity of endogenous antioxidants in various organs, including the cerebellum and placenta.[61,72,104]

Oxidative stress has been increasingly recognized as one of the mechanisms underlying ethanol toxicity. Ethanol can induce oxidative stress directly by formation of free radicals, which react with different cellular compounds, or indirectly by reducing intracellular antioxidant capacity, such as decreased glutathione peroxidase levels. The levels of oxidative stress markers were studied in placental villous tissue following 2 hours of ethanol perfusion.[72] The results demonstrated a significant increase in oxidative stress, primarily involving the nitric oxide pathway in the trophoblast and DNA damage in the villous stromal cells. Alcohol-induced oxidative stress was also found to increase lipid peroxidation and damage protein and DNA.

Disturbed Metabolic Pathways: Prostaglandin Synthesis

Alcohol is known to affect prostaglandins, hence influencing fetal development and parturition. When mice were treated with aspirin (a prostaglandin synthesis inhibitor) prior to alcohol exposure, aspirin pretreatment reduced by 50% the alcohol-induced malformations in comparison with mice treated with aspirin after alcohol exposure.[120]

Effects on Neurons

Several studies in rats and mice have shown that in utero exposure to alcohol caused structural defects in the hippocampus, cerebellum, and neural crest cells, with increased cell death.[21,61,118] Similar changes in the brain of affected children were also described.

Epigenetic Changes

Epigenetic changes manifested by changes in gene expression, DNA methylation, histone modification, and changes in micro RNA have been observed in children with FASD.[142] Recently, Laufer at al.[81] have found changes in DNA methylation in six children with FASD. These DNA methylation changes, observed in DNA obtained from buccal swabs, are influenced by sex and medication exposure. Masemola et al.[93] studied the methylation of DNA samples obtained from blood or buccal cells in 73 children with FAS compared to 50 control children, and they found, by using pyrosequencing, hypomethylation at *KvDMR1* and *PEG3 DMR* genes, which are maternally imprinted loci. Changes in DNA methylation are responsible for changes in gene expression, which might induce a variety of long-term behavioral and molecular changes in the brain. Similar epigenetic changes were also observed in mouse models of FASD.

In light of these different mechanisms of action, it is reasonable to presume that alcohol-induced teratogenicity is probably the result of injuries caused by several mechanisms.[25,105]

Prevention and Treatment

Prevention

Because the diagnosis of FAS in young children is often difficult, the first challenge is identification and follow-up of children at risk. The second challenge is to prevent this disorder by preventing alcohol drinking. Unfortunately, there are only a few reports demonstrating success in reducing drinking of alcohol in pregnancy, and these reports even declined from 1995 to 1999. The rate of binge drinking apparently remained stable, and chronic heavy drinking remained unchanged, suggesting that the education programs were not effective. Preventing alcohol abuse must therefore start with educational programs in schools and later during academic studies. Prevention programs need to be addressed primarily toward high-risk individuals and groups.[65]

Treatment During Pregnancy

Assuming that oxidative stress is one of the major routes of ethanol-induced damage, it is reasonable to supplement with antioxidants in an effort to attenuate this damage. Antioxidants, such as vitamin C, vitamin E, folic acid, beta-carotene, and flavonoids can be supplemented by food, therefore reversing other nutritional deficits common among this population.[28] However, to our knowledge, only a few, if any, such programs exist.

Treatment of the Child With Fetal Alcohol Spectrum Disorder

There is no effective treatment for children with FASD. However, treatment of the behavioral and emotional symptoms as well as special educational methods are helpful in improving the neurobehavioral function of the affected children. Stimulants can be used for the treatment of ADHD, inducing improvement in more than 80% of the children with ADHD. Aggression and defiant behavior can best be treated with low doses of risperidone or other neuroleptics. These can be given even in children treated with stimulants (i.e., methylphenidate, dextroamphetamine, and so on) because of ADHD symptoms.[111]

Lactation

Because alcohol is transferred to human milk, reaching levels similar to those in maternal serum, women drinking high amounts of alcohol should refrain from nursing their infants. Moreover, nursing infants suckle lower amounts of alcohol-containing milk. If nursing mothers drink only small-to-moderate amounts of alcohol, they should wait 2–3 hours before nursing their infants.[128] In infants fed on milk from mothers who drank heavily, the sleep patterns of their nursing infants were disturbed.[95]

Prevention and Treatment of Alcohol-Exposed Pregnant Animals

Alcohol-exposed C57BL/6 J mice were injected twice with 2.9 g/kg, 4 hours apart, of EUK-134 (a potent synthetic superoxide dismutase plus catalase mimetic) on their ninth day of pregnancy. EUK-134 supplementation induced a notable reduction in cell death of the apical ectodermal ridge of the newly forming limb buds in ethanol-exposed embryos and reduced the forelimb malformations by about half (67.3%–35.9%).[23]

Further support for the efficiency of antioxidants in attenuating the teratogenic effects of alcohol consumption throughout pregnancy comes from Wentzel et al.,[148] who studied the effects of 5% vitamin E added to food on the outcome of ethanol-exposed rat pregnancies, showing a reduced rate of malformed or dead fetuses, but no change in the alcohol-induced reduction of body weight.

Animal Models for Alcohol-Induced Embryopathy

The growth spurt of the human brain is mainly during the third trimester of pregnancy, continuing into postnatal life. In rats, the brain growth spurt takes place almost entirely in the postnatal period. Therefore, rats must be exposed to alcohol during the equivalent periods of the brain development in humans, which is in the early postnatal life.[91] The reduced Purkinje cell number demonstrated by Goodlett et al.[52] supports the contention that a significant amount of pathological loss of postmitotic Purkinje cells occurs, yet it is dependent on the time of alcohol exposure. Hamre and West[56] found in newborn rats that postnatal days 4–6 were the most sensitive period for cerebellar Purkinje and granule cell loss following binge alcohol exposure.[56]

Alcohol exposure of pregnant rats, equivalent to all three trimesters of human pregnancy, was shown to reduce cerebellar Purkinje cell numbers compared with the group that was exposed only in the third or first and second trimesters equivalent. In contrast, exposure to alcohol in the third trimester equivalent yielded a decrement in the olfactory bulb mitral cell numbers as compared with other timing groups (first or second trimester).[56,91]

Similar results were demonstrated by Ramadoss et al.,[117] utilizing an ovine model to determine the critical period of vulnerability of fetal Purkinje cells following prenatal alcohol abuse, mimicking a human binge pattern during the first and third trimesters of pregnancy. In these animals, unlike the rat model, the entire brain development occurs in utero. They found that the fetal cerebellar Purkinje cells are sensitive to alcohol throughout gestation.[117] The short- and long-term effects of ethanol were studied by Dembele et al.[31] in 7-day-old and 3-month-old rats following alcohol exposure. They found that prenatal ethanol exposure led to hypothalamic oxidative stress persisting into adult life and being significantly higher among the group of older rats, implying long-term damage of ethanol consumption during pregnancy.[31]

In a meta-analysis of 22 studies using different strains of rats and one study on mice, Chotro et al.[24] found in 18 of 22 studies that prenatal exposure to ethanol increased ethanol intake among the offspring. The four remaining studies failed to show any effect whatsoever, a result interpreted and explained as the age of testing, 120 days and over.[24] Simpson et al.[132] have shown that alcohol exposure in rats decreased fetal body weight and bone length and delayed skeletal ossification. These effects persisted postnatally, leading to growth plate abnormalities and decreased skeletal maturity scores at 2–4 weeks of age. FAS-like craniofacial malformations were demonstrated by Rogers et al.[122] following treatment of pregnant C57 BL/6 J mice with methanol on GD-7 during gastrulation. These malformations included anophthalmia, microphthalmia, holoprosencephaly (in varying degrees), and ear and jaw malformations.[122] The involvement of ethanol in cardiac anomalies was also studied in rats. Alcohol administration during pregnancy reduced cardiac mass and depressed function, evidently, due to microstructural changes of the myocytes, even when affected animals reached adulthood.[79]

The exposure of *Xenopus laevis* frog embryos to alcohol during gastrulation has shown that alcohol competes with retinoic acid retinaldehyde dehydrogenase 2, interfering with retinoic acid signaling pathway.[77] Thus interference in such an early phase in this important pathway may explain many of the observed injuries in FASD. Whether this mechanism is also operating in humans is as of yet unknown, but we have to remember that the damaging effects of alcohol are not confined only to the early phases of embryonic development, as initiation of alcohol ingestion in the second half of pregnancy is also teratogenic in humans.

Recently, epigenetic changes have been described in the brains of mice exposed in utero to alcohol. Specific changes were observed in the PTEN/P13K/AKT/mTOR pathway, which is responsible for alterations in cell adhesion and proliferation, inducing long-lasting changes in cortical regions of the brain.[81]

Conclusions

Maternal alcohol ingestion in pregnancy may have deleterious effects on the central nervous system and other organs of the developing embryo and fetus, depending on the dose and duration and on the developmental stage of the embryo at exposure. These embryotoxic effects of alcohol were observed in many animal species. It is therefore important to reduce alcohol drinking during pregnancy to a minimum. However, as of today, it is still difficult to define the minimal dose that will affect the developing embryo and the exact dose-response relationship. Animal studies are helpful in understanding the pathogenesis of FASD but do not help in the delineation of the exposure level that may be safe in pregnancy.

Heroin-Dependent Mothers in Pregnancy

Pregnant mothers who are heroin dependent often belong to one of the following three categories: (1) women treated with opiates (i.e., methadone and in recent years also buprenorphine or naltrexone) and who carefully follow the treatment regimen, (2) women treated with opiates but who on occasion also use heroin or other street drugs, and (3) women addicted to heroin or other opiates and who hence use heroin, depending on availability. These women also have periods without drugs, a fact that may result in withdrawal symptoms in the mother and the fetus. In many cases, these mothers also use other psychotropic drugs such as benzodiazepines, phenothiazines, or barbiturates. Rarely, they may also use cocaine. Many of these women also smoke cigarettes and/or ingest different amounts of ethanol (alcohol). Moreover, they often do not seek medical care and suffer from medical neglect even during pregnancy. The addicted mothers are at increased risk for various acute and chronic serious infections, such as hepatitis B, hepatitis C, and HIV.[103]

Relation Between Substance Abuse and Attention-Deficit/Hyperactivity Disorder

Several studies have found an association between ADHD and substance abuse. The prevalence of substance abuse is therefore much higher among persons with ADHD, which was found to be common among opioid (heroin) abusers.[149] It is more difficult to treat opioid-dependent individuals with ADHD than it is to treat those without it.[149] Moreover, stimulant treatment of adolescents with ADHD can effectively reduce the rate of substance abuse.[76,149] In addition, there seem to be specific differences between drug abusers with and without ADHD. Drug abusers with ADHD report an earlier start to using the substances; their substance abuse is more severe, and they may also need treatment for their ADHD to achieve abstinence. Similar types of genetic polymorphism to genes related to dopamine metabolism have been found among individuals with ADHD and those who are heroin dependent. For example, several investigators have shown in heroin-dependent individuals, or those with other substance abuse, a polymorphism to the catechol-*O*-methyl transferase gene, to the dopamine D4 receptor, or to the mu-opioid receptor gene.[78,131] Similar gene polymorphism was also observed in individuals with ADHD.

Effects of Heroin and Opiates on the Fetus and Newborn

Although several reports of children with congenital anomalies born to heroin-dependent mothers have been published, there is no consistent pattern of anomalies, and heroin is not considered to be a teratogenic agent and, in contrast to cocaine, is not considered to cause intrauterine fetal bleeding or placental abruption.[a] However, heroin (and opiate) use during pregnancy is associated with increased prematurity, low birth weight, small head circumference, and increased neonatal and perinatal mortality. Withdrawal symptoms may also develop in 40%–80% of the newborns; a high incidence of sudden infant death syndrome during the first year of life was also described, although this is subject to some debate.[70] The use of methadone during pregnancy seems to be much safer for the developing embryo and fetus, with relatively few side effects, but withdrawal symptoms are frequent in the offspring of methadone-treated mothers to the same extent as with heroin.

Effects on Postnatal Development

Developmental delay, as well as behavioral and emotional problems, was often encountered in children born to opiate-dependent mothers using heroin or methadone during pregnancy.[b] Some investigators have demonstrated an improvement of the developmental scores in these children with the advancement of age, but others have not. A high proportion of children demonstrated inattention, hyperactivity, aggressiveness (ADHD), and lack of social inhibition.[c]

The environment in which a child is raised seems to be one of the most important factors that determine his or her developmental outcome. In children born small for their gestational age, the parental socioeconomic status influences the development, especially during the early years of life, with children in families from lower socioeconomic status failing to show developmental recovery. In fact, the relative impact of the clinical and biological factors of these children seems to be overshadowed by the family factors.[146] A similar phenomenon was described repeatedly in very-low-birth-weight infants, where the major factors affecting cognitive development of the children were the home environment and their neurological status.[15]

In studies describing the development of children born to heroin-dependent mothers, often there may be many confounding factors influencing the results. They are often influenced by the fact that they suffer from significant neglect. Therefore the outcome is the result of interaction between in utero exposure to heroin and the postnatal environment. Hence it is important in evaluating the outcome of these children to compare them with relevant controls.[102,107–109]

We had the opportunity to study the developmental outcome of children born to heroin-dependent mothers who were either raised at home or sent for adoption (or foster homes) immediately after birth or at a very young age.[102,107–108] Because there is evidence of a correlation between socioeconomic status and cognitive functioning of children, and most adoptions are into middle or high socioeconomic status environments, adoption should have a positive effect on cognitive functioning.[15,16,125] Indeed, most adopted children score in the normal range on assessment of cognitive and emotional development. This enabled us to isolate the prenatal effects of heroin on neurobehavioral development from the postnatal possible impact of environmental deprivation, which is so common in families of drug addicts.

Comparison groups were composed of children born to heroin-dependent fathers; children with severe environmental deprivation born to nonaddicted parents of low socioeconomic status; and a group of normal, age-matched children. About 400 children from 6 months to 12 years of age were studied.[102,107–109]

A lower birth weight and a shorter gestation were recorded for children born to heroin-dependent mothers and, to a lesser degree, for children born to heroin-dependent fathers when compared with the other groups. The head circumference and height at examination were lower for children born to heroin-dependent mothers raised at home in comparison with controls. There was no difference in the weight at examination among the different groups of children.

Intellectual Developmental Outcome

We have found that children of preschool age born to heroin-dependent fathers, thereby not being exposed in utero to heroin, function as poorly as children born to heroin-dependent mothers. However, paternal drug use in and of itself did not have a more deleterious effect on school-age children than parental low socioeconomic status, and children born to nonaddicted parents who had environmental deprivation performed even less well than children born to heroin-dependent fathers or to mothers with nonaddicted fathers. Finally, when children of preschool-age born to heroin-dependent mothers were adopted at a young age and hence raised in a stable environment, their intellectual function was similar to that of control children. These results show that in utero exposure to heroin per se does not affect the cognitive ability of preschool-age children, and that most harm to those children is caused by their unstable postnatal environment because the mother is a heroin addict. However, there was a high rate of children with behavioral problems among those born to heroin-dependent mothers when the children were raised at home.[107]

We then studied similar groups of children aged 6–12 years who attended regular school.[102,108] At that age, the children born to heroin-dependent mothers had a very high rate (54%) of inattention and hyperactivity (ADHD). The rate of ADHD was reduced to 24% in the heroin-exposed adopted children, whereas 24% of those born to drug-dependent fathers (and not exposed to heroin) had ADHD. It is important to add that 21% of the children with environmental deprivation had ADHD, whereas none of the control children had it, as evidenced from the abbreviated Conner's Questionnaire. We also studied their arithmetic and reading abilities and found that they were poor in the children born to heroin-dependent fathers, in those born to heroin-dependent mothers when children were raised at home, and in the children with environmental deprivation. However, the adopted children at that age had slightly lower cognitive abilities compared with controls, although the difference was not statistically significant. Their arithmetic and reading abilities were also lower.

---

[a]References 36, 86, 87, 121, 136, 139, 143.
[b]References 36, 86, 87, 121, 136, 139, 143.
[c]References 20, 37, 102, 107–109, 129.

Because it is possible that the high incidence of inattention, hyperactivity, and behavioral disorders found in the children in our study is related to a high incidence of ADHD among their parents who were therefore prone to substance abuse more than the general population, we used the Wender-Utah questionnaires to assess for maternal ADHD. We indeed found a high rate of ADHD among drug-dependent mothers. However, there was no correlation with the rate of ADHD in their children, implying that in utero heroin exposure is responsible, at least partially, for the high rate of ADHD among the heroin-exposed children, whether raised at home or adopted. This is in line with other studies showing a high rate of ADHD among the offspring of heroin-dependent parents.[76,149]

We also studied the development of these groups of children at 12–17 years of age. The findings were similar to those observed in children at school age, with a high rate of ADHD and learning and behavioral problems in the heroin-exposed children. Moreover, adolescents born to heroin-dependent mothers who were raised at home performed less well than adolescents with environmental deprivation, implying that heroin might have affected some of the higher cortical functions that are related to learning abilities and attention span. In that context, we should mention that other investigators[126,135] have found that exposure to multiple risk factors is associated with poor developmental outcomes. Therefore in utero heroin exposure and postnatal poor environment may have a multiple and long-lasting deleterious effect.

The beneficial effects of a good postnatal environment on the intellectual and behavioral outcome of children born to heroin-dependent mothers emphasize the importance of the social and educational services for improving the outcome of children of drug-dependent parents, as well as of children from low socioeconomic status families.

Polymorphisms in dopaminergic and serotonergic genes such as *DAT1*, *5HTTLPR*, *D4DR4*, and *MAO-A* have been linked to ADHD and also to susceptibility to opiate addiction. We investigated[106] in opiate-addicted parents and their children the rate of ADHD and genetic markers that could predict susceptibility to ADHD and/or opiate addiction. A total of 64 heroin-addicted, methadone-maintained parents and their 94 children who had or had not been exposed prenatally to opiates were studied. DNA was extracted from mouthwash and assessed for genetic polymorphism for six polymorphic sites of four different genes. Study subjects also filled a variety of questionnaires assessing the rate of ADHD in the parents and children, and the children's Intelligence Quotient (IQ). Children of opiate-dependent mothers had a higher rate of ADHD compared to children of the opiate-dependent fathers, without correlation with the presence of ADHD in their parents, demonstrating again that intrauterine exposure to heroin increases the rate of ADHD. Opiate-dependent parents have a high risk of being carriers of most risk alleles examined, except DRD4EX3 (allele7). There was no difference whether the addicted parents did or did not have ADHD. From these studies, it seems that serotonergic and dopaminergic risk alleles seem to be related mainly to opiate dependence with no effect on the occurrence of ADHD. Hence people carrying those polymorphisms are susceptible to opioid addiction and not necessarily to ADHD.

Because in many cases where the mother is drug dependent it is expected that the father will be addicted as well, it is important to mention that children born to drug-dependent fathers were also shown to be at risk for developmental problems as well as for ADHD, further demonstrating the importance of the postnatal environment. Sowder and Burt[135] found that children born to

heroin-dependent fathers were at high risk for early school behavioral and learning problems. Similarly, children born to drug-free parents of a similar underprivileged environment and low socioeconomic status were also at risk for early school problems, but to a lesser extent. These results are similar to our findings in school-age children. Herjanic et al.[62] found slow mental development in 44% of children born to heroin-dependent fathers. By age 12, conduct disorders and behavioral problems were common among these children. Behavioral problems, attention deficit disorder, and ADHD were also described in the offspring of cocaine-using mothers.[149] Thus whenever both parents are addicted, their children seem to be at higher risk than when only the mother is addicted.

Treatment of the Pregnant Mother

The most common approach for treating opiate addicts, whenever weaning is unsuccessful, is methadone treatment.[18,39] Because it is not accepted to wean pregnant women from heroin, methadone is the preferred treatment in pregnancy. The daily doses vary and range from 10–20 mg up to 100 mg or even more, according to individual needs. Pregnancy outcome in women who are on strict methadone treatment throughout the entire pregnancy and attend antenatal care seems to be good, with very little long-term effects on the infants except neonatal abstinence symptoms that are common and necessitate transfer to neonatal special care units.[18,102] However, there seems to be no correlation between the presence of withdrawal symptoms and developmental outcome, even in children born to heroin-dependent mothers.[107] Although methadone treatment during pregnancy seems to be relatively safe, more recent studies show that women treated with methadone have similar complications of pregnancy as those that are heroin dependent, although to a lesser degree.[22] Relatively low amounts of methadone are transferred to milk and therefore women on methadone maintenance can nurse their infants.[26]

In the last few years, there have been two additional successful approaches to treatment, using either buprenorphine (an opiate with agonist-antagonist properties) or naltrexone (an opiate antagonist) in low, intermediate, or high doses. In some cases, buprenorphine was administered through slow-release implanted devices.[64] Both of these methods are successful in maintaining normal pregnancy outcomes, but they do not seem to be superior to methadone in terms of maternal retention of treatment.[94] However, it is possible that these new modes of therapy are superior to the traditional methadone treatment for the fetus, as prematurity, fetal weight at birth, withdrawal symptoms, and other pregnancy complications were apparently lower than with methadone maintenance.[17,30] However, in one study[144] of 25 children born to heroin-addicted mothers who were treated with buprenorphine, there was a higher rate of inattention and memory problems at 5 and 6 years compared to controls. The few data that exist on the specific effects of naltrexone on the developing fetus seem to be reassuring.[64]

Lactation

Because heroin and other opiates are transferred to human milk, reaching relatively high levels, women using heroin or other opiates might be advised to refrain from nursing their infants, depending on the dose.[128] This is because of the depressive effects of large amounts of opiates on the central nervous system, including the possibility of causing respiratory depression in the suckling infants. As stated above, nursing is permitted in women treated with methadone, depending on the daily dose. Both naltrexone and buprenorphine are excreted in human milk but lactation is permitted, depending on the dose.

Animal Models for Heroin- and Opiate-Induced Fetal Damage

There are not too many studies on the effects of heroin on pregnancy in animals. This stems from the fact that in the absence of structural anomalies following exposure to heroin and opiates in experimental animals, it is difficult to use animal models that mimic the behavioral changes observed in men.[65] However, several studies were carried out on pregnant mice and rats, demonstrating functional and pathological changes in various parts of the brain in the offspring.[58,63,70,134] Such studies have used in pregnant rats osmotic mini-pumps with opiates or opiate antagonists-buprenorphine, naloxone, and methadone-demonstrating changes in mu-opioid receptor G protein in the offspring, with male offspring showing more sensitivity than female offspring.[63] Slotkin et al.[134] found in mice that administration of heroin during pregnancy causes changes in the hippocampal cholinergic neurons of the offspring, as it induced a deficit in muscarinic cholinergic receptor-induced translocation of protein kinase C gamma. These authors also demonstrated changes in adenylyl cyclase, the latter changes also occurring in the cerebellum, where there are only few cholinergic neurons. Changes in signaling proteins distal to neurotransmitter receptors were proposed by the authors as a general mechanism related to several neuroteratogens.[134] Whether these changes are relevant to the human situation is currently unknown.

Of special interest is the fact that grafting of neural progenitor cells into the hippocampus of these mice offspring at adulthood reversed the behavioral deficits observed in non-treated, heroin-exposed mice[71].

Conclusions

Heroin exposure in utero seems to have little effect on the intellectual ability of young children if they are raised in a supportive environment. However, it induces a high rate of ADHD, which seems to be attributed to the direct effect of heroin on the fetal brain as well as to genetic and environmental factors. Moreover, ADHD and opiate addiction share several common issues like similar genetic polymorphism and the relation to the dopaminergic brain systems. We should try to improve the home environment of the children born to heroin-dependent mothers and thus minimize the damaging effects of maternal drug addiction. It is important to develop adequate social and educational services to improve the outcome of children of drug-dependent parents as well as of children from low socioeconomic status families. Appropriate treatment of children with ADHD might reduce the rate of addiction to drugs in general and to opiates specifically.

Mothers Using Cannabis (Marijuana, Hashish) During Pregnancy

Cannabis

The cannabis plant has been cultivated for centuries and its leaves used as a source of recreational drugs. The dried leaves and flowering parts of the cannabis plant are known in different parts of the world by a variety of names, including Indian hemp and marijuana. The extract of the plant is termed hashish. Although many active compounds with various effects are found in the cannabis plants, the primary active agent is delta-9-tetrahydrocannabinol. This agent has been used recently for increasing appetite and controlling nausea. The main recreational use of cannabis is by smoking.[41–47,55,58] The use of cannabis in pregnancy is quite common; in meconium analyses from about 1000 newborns in Barcelona, Spain, traces of cannabis were found in 5.3% of the newborns. By this method it is possible to detect cannabis use only starting from the second trimester of pregnancy; hence the true percentage of use is apparently even higher.[90]

Delta-9-tetrahydrocannabinol is known to cross the placenta and may therefore affect the developing fetus.[14] Women who smoked relatively large numbers of marijuana cigarettes during pregnancy may have impaired fetal growth and hence lower-than-normal birth weight with differences from controls of about 100 g. A continuous use of marijuana during pregnancy is also associated with lower gestational age at birth of about 1 week. Both phenomena seem to be dose related. Hayatbakhsh et al.[29] found after adjusting for confounders such as cigarette smoking, alcohol consumption, and so on, that marijuana smoking decreased fetal weight, and increased preterm labor and postnatal problems, which necessitated admission to the neonatal intensive care units. Similar findings were observed by other investigators but there are also studies that showed no damaging effects of marijuana use when following adjustment to various confounders. A meta-analysis of reports available through 1996 did not find a significant association between maternal cannabis use and birth weight when the possible effects of cigarette smoking were controlled.[34] There seems to be no increase in the rate of major congenital anomalies associated with the smoking of even large numbers of marijuana cigarettes. There is no effect of marijuana use during pregnancy on subsequent childhood growth or pubertal development.[43,46]

Heavy exposure during pregnancy has been associated with increased behavioral and psychiatric disorders in adulthood.[39] This is due mainly to the interference of cannabinoids with the endocannabinoid system in different phases of brain development, affecting various neurotransmitters interfering with the modulation of neuronal proliferation, migration, and differentiation.

Marijuana smoking is known to increase the content of carbon monoxide in the blood much more than regular cigarette smoking.[128] Hence, one of the suggested mechanisms for the possible negative effect of marijuana on fetal growth focuses on the relatively large increases in carboxyhemoglobin generated by smoking marijuana.[150] This effect reduces the oxygen-carrying capacity of the maternal blood, impairs the release of oxygen from hemoglobin in the tissues, and indirectly impairs fetal oxygenation. Placental blood flow also may be reduced by the increase in maternal heart rate and blood pressure that may accompany marijuana smoking. Delta-9-tetrahydrocannabinol may also, after its transplacental passage, decrease fetal heart rate.

In several case-control studies, marijuana smoking was associated with an increased rate of gastroschisis and cardiac ventricular septal defect but not with neural tube defects.[140] There is no pattern of anomalies associated with cannabis use. We should remember that women using cannabis also often use alcohol and smoke cigarettes.

Neonatal Effects

Increased tremulousness, altered visual response to light stimulus, withdrawal-like crying, and alteration in neonatal sleep pattern have been reported in newborn infants of marijuana-smoking mothers.[2]. As with other signs of abstinence following maternal use of psychotropic agents, these findings usually diminish within several weeks.

Postnatal Developmental and Behavioral Effects

Several investigators reported withdrawal-like symptoms and alteration of sleep pattern in the neonates born to mothers using marijuana during pregnancy. However, it is unknown whether it is the marijuana or other substances they used during pregnancy. The studies on long-term developmental follow-up of children born to mothers using cannabis during pregnancy are mostly negative, with no long-term effects of marijuana on intellectual abilities.[65] In a series of studies performed by Fried et al.,[41-46] prenatally marijuana-exposed children were followed until school age. The children antenatally exposed to marijuana had, up to 4 years of age, a slight delay on cognitive testing due to some impairment in brain executive functions, especially verbal and memory abilities. It is interesting to note that similar findings were reported by these authors following cigarette smoking in pregnancy but not after exposure to low amounts of alcohol.[45] Although these children were reexamined at 60 and 72 months of age, the language delay of the prenatally marijuana-exposed children disappeared, while in the children prenatally exposed to cigarette smoke it did not.[46] Goldshmid et al.[51] examined children born to 218 mothers who smoke marijuana during pregnancy, 79 of them who smoke more than one joint per day. The offspring of these 79 mothers had, at 14 years, lower scores on the Wechsler intelligence test, especially on the reading and composite scores, implying possible long-term effects of marijuana on learning.

Lactation

Delta-9-tetrahydrocannabinol and its metabolites are concentrated in breast milk and absorbed by the nursing baby.[113] Although specific adverse effects have not been identified, one author recommends that breastfeeding be discontinued if marijuana is being used by the mother.[25,128] The American Academy of Pediatrics lists marijuana among drugs of abuse that should not be ingested by nursing mothers.[26]

Animal Studies

Several animal studies have shown teratogenic effects of marijuana, producing limb, digit, and neural tube closure defects in rats, while others were negative.[49] Pregnant hamsters injected with marijuana extract or resin had an increased incidence of malformed offspring, and high doses of a marijuana extract induced neural tube closure defects and phocomelia in rabbits.[48]

Animal studies with delta-9-tetrahydrocannabinol itself have produced similar conflicting results. No teratogenic effects were noted in several studies in rats, hamsters, or chimpanzees.[54] The inconsistent results of these studies may be explained by the use of different doses and different methods of administration.

Conclusions

The use of cannabinoids during pregnancy does not seem to have significant teratogenic effects. However, there does seem to be dose-dependent effects on fetal growth, early delivery, and perinatal complications, and apparently also on learning and behavior. Hence it is advisable to refrain from the use of cannabinoids during pregnancy.

Mothers Using Cocaine in Pregnancy

Historical Background

Cocaine is an alkaloid extracted from the leaves of the plant *Erythroxylum coca*. It was first isolated by Friedrich Gaedcke, a German chemist, in 1855, and has a long history of medical and recreational use. Cocaine causes transient euphoria through the well-documented biochemical stimulation of the dopaminergic system, apparently by inhibiting the dopamine transporters; however, the mechanism of the lasting and inheritable effects of cocaine is known only partially.[5,115]

For thousands of years, coca has been used in South America for special medical purposes and as a general stimulant, and remains one of the commonly used medicines in different areas of Peru and Bolivia. Cocaine was the first effective local anesthetic, and when its danger became obvious and substitutes were available, especially in the 1930s, its medical use declined.[55] The use of coca in pre-Hispanic America is confirmed by archeological and artistic sources (sculptures, ceramics, fabrics, and pictures). Diffusion of these pieces of evidence, historical and geographical, seems to point to the fact that coca was a strong, central element in the union of the different cultures of the continent.[38]

The Aymara Indians of the Andes Mountains were the first to consume coca, which was reserved in the beginning for priests and princes in religious ceremonies, extending later to the common people. Coca and cocaine were used once more in the 19th century. In 1870, Angelo Mariani brought to the market a kind of wine based on coca extract, with a great success. A competitive drink was produced by Pemberton in the United States, named Vin Francais Cola.

Cocaine was used medically for the treatment of asthma and hay fever, was officially agreed upon by the famous scientific societies in America, and was finally abandoned.[2]

In 1559, the Italian neurologist Mantegazza was the first to try out the remedy on himself, advocating the use of coca as an internal medicine. In psychiatry, cocaine was used in patients with melancholia, exhaustion (physical and psychic), and cachexia, and later as a substitution therapy for morphine addicts. Cocaine was first used in 1884 as a local anesthetic agent, first in eye surgery and later applied in dentistry and minor surgery. Among other indications, cocaine was aimed to treat asthma, pregnancy vomiting, and cramping pains.[141] Nowadays, cocaine is used mainly for recreational purposes. However, chronic users may develop addiction, dependency, and tolerance to cocaine.

Effects of Cocaine on the Embryo and Fetus

Cocaine is a small molecule, largely un-ionized at physiological pH; therefore it readily crosses the placental barrier, and because of a lower pH in the fetal blood, it flows readily from the maternal into the fetal blood. Due to low levels of esterases in the fetus, it is only slowly metabolized. By causing vasoconstriction, cocaine can induce fetal brain ischemia. As described in several studies, cocaine abuse during pregnancy was able to induce premature birth, lower birth weight, more respiratory distress, bowel and cerebral infarctions, reduced head circumference, and increased risk of seizures.[73]

From the mid-1980s into the early 1990s, numerous reports raised concerns referring to the possible teratogenic effects of cocaine abuse in pregnancy on the embryo and fetus. Most observations included congenital anomalies, especially of the central nervous system, limbs, urogenital and gastrointestinal systems, growth retardation, microcephaly, central nervous system infarction, seizures, cortical atrophy and cysts, intraventricular hemorrhage, and sudden infant death.[116]

More recent studies, however, did not find any clear association between prenatal cocaine exposure and an increased rate of major congenital anomalies. Behnke et al.[9] studied the rate of major anomalies in 272 offspring of 154 mothers using cocaine or crack during pregnancy in comparison with 154 control infants, and found no difference between the groups in the rate of congenital anomalies. However, they found decreased birth weight, birth length, and head circumference among the cocaine-exposed infants and an increased rate of prematurity. Similarly, Bauer et al.[7] investigated the association between prenatal exposure to cocaine and the medical condition of the newborn infants. The observations demonstrated a decrease in birth weight (536 g), body length (2.6 cm), and head circumference (1.5 cm) among cocaine-exposed newborns, who were also born about 1.2 weeks earlier. Although relatively frequent among the exposed children, the central and autonomic nervous system symptoms attributed to cocaine effects were usually transient. These authors, too, did not find an increased rate of congenital malformations among the cocaine-exposed infants.[7] Thus if an increase in major anomalies exists, especially in urinary tract anomalies and those resulting from vascular disruption, it is small. There may be, however, an increase in prenatal cerebral hemorrhages and infarctions, increased intrauterine fetal death, as well as placental abruptio and infarcts.[53] Moreover, an increase in the rate of necrotizing enterocolitis in the offspring of cocaine-using mothers is explained by as one of the well-known vasospastic effects of cocaine.[89]

Developmental Outcome

To assess the impact of cocaine exposure of the fetus on neonatal auditory information processing ability, Potter et al.[88] used habituation and recovery of the head-turning toward an auditory stimulus (across the three phases of the procedure). Their results exhibited a response pattern that is consistent with a slower speed of auditory information processing, implying that cocaine is a neuroteratogenic agent during the newborn period. Similarly, in a prospective longitudinal study of 154 mothers using cocaine during pregnancy, Eyler et al.[35] observed in their neonates, while using blinded developmental examinations, fewer alert periods and less alert responsiveness, implying a reduced state of regulation, especially when cocaine was used in the third trimester of pregnancy.

Studies on the later postnatal cognitive development of children who were prenatally exposed to cocaine report, however, on contradictory results, and the majority of studies did not find a deleterious effect of cocaine alone on the intellectual abilities of the children. Assessing the possibility of an independent link between the levels of prenatal cocaine exposure and developmental test scores (after controlling for the confounding variables: alcohol, cigarettes, and marijuana), Frank et al.[40] failed to find any significant interaction between prenatal exposure to cocaine or cigarettes on the Bayley Scales of Infant Development. In a later study, when analyzing cocaine exposure in pregnancy and IQ scores, they failed to find a distinct negative effect of cocaine on global or specific cognitive competence in preschool-age children.[40]

Singer et al.[133] studied the cognitive abilities at 4 years of age of 190 children prenatally exposed to cocaine in comparison with 186 nonexposed children who demonstrated environmental deprivation. There was no difference between the groups, and both had lower-than-average full-scale IQ scores. However, differences between the groups were found in several subscales of the Wechsler Preschool and Primary Scale of Intelligence-Revised (the psychometric test used by the investigators). These differences were in visual spatial skills, general knowledge, and arithmetic skills, where the cocaine-exposed children performed less well in comparison with the nonexposed. The results of this study, which were very similar to our findings in prenatally heroin-exposed children,[79,80] clearly demonstrate the importance of the environment for early cognitive development.

One important additional negative effect of cocaine exposure was implied by Noland et al.,[98] showing in school-age children a higher rate of commission errors on the Continuous Performance Task and suggesting that cocaine-exposed children had difficulty maintaining a good attention span. A study by Bada et al.[3] on adolescents exposed in utero to cocaine alone or cocaine and other drugs in comparison with those who were not exposed found a high rate of attentional problems (ADHD) as observed from the Child Behavior Checklist. They, along with Eiden et al.,[33] also found that good home environments might have a protective role in reducing the rate and severity of the behavioral problems. These findings are similar to our findings in children who were born to heroin-dependent mothers but had good home environment— that is, adoption at a young age attenuated the neurobehavioral problems in the children.[107,108]

Brain MRI studies have shown that cocaine may induce cerebral and cerebellar changes. Akyuz et al.[1] compared the MRI brain morphometry of 11 heroin-exposed children to 10 controls at 8–10 years of age. The cocaine-exposed children had a smaller brain volume, the main differences being observed in the cortical gray matter, thalamus, and putamen. Similar findings were also observed at 13–15 years of age. Liu et al.[88] compared the brain MRI studies of 20 adolescents exposed in utero to cocaine to those of 20 nonexposed, 13- to 15-year-olds and also found thinner prefrontal cortex in the exposed children. In this study, impulsivity was correlated with smaller thalamus. However, the functional implications of these volumetric brain changes are as of yet unknown.

Effects of Gender

Beeghly et al.[8] found that in utero cocaine-exposed girls scored lower on language-related tasks than boys at 6 years but not at 9 years of age. Bendersky et al.[11] found that in utero cocaine-exposed 5-year-old girls were less likely to engage in aggressive behavior than similarly exposed boys. The results suggest that gender may be a risk factor among children who have been prenatally exposed to cocaine for some cognitive developmental processes and a protective factor for problematic social behavior.

Mechanisms of Action

Despite more than two decades of research, the mechanism underlying cocaine-induced brain damage is still under debate.[60] Speculation on the mechanism of action of cocaine runs basically in two directions: cocaine-induced transient hypertension and vasoconstriction that damages the placenta, inducing placental infarctions with partial or complete abruption[12,145] or increased oxidative stress.[104,152] Because the first mechanism is now under debate, we expand mainly on the second mechanism.

The mechanism of increased oxidative stress induced by cocaine was apparently first proposed by Zimmerman et al.[152] However, in their study, the addition of antioxidants to the cocaine-treated mice did not prevent the occurrence of neural tube defects, possibly casting some doubt on this proposed mechanism.

Other more recent studies, however, suggest that oxidative stress is an important mechanism of cocaine teratogenesis. The offspring of cocaine-injected, pregnant rats showed low levels of nitric oxide in the brain on the first two postnatal days; these returned to normal on the fourth day. Thiobarbituric acid–reactive species content in the hippocampus of cocaine-injected rats was, however, increased during days 1–4, showing an oxidative stress–related increase in lipid peroxidation. Prenatal cocaine-injected rats demonstrated, at day 25, significant learning impairment in the water-maze test as compared with nontreated rats, and had increased thiobarbituric acid–reactive species in their brain. This demonstrates that learning in the treated rats causes higher oxidative stress in the brain, possibly related to their impaired learning ability.[6] It can therefore be summarized that oxidative stress is playing an important and significant role in cocaine-induced disruption of the central nervous system.

To understand further whether cocaine-induced oxidative stress also causes apoptosis, Poon et al.[115] monitored the oxidative stress and apoptotic effects in human neuronal progenitor cells exposed to cocaine during culture. The results showed a significant increase in oxidative stress at 48 hours, followed by cell death at 72 hours. Thus whenever the antioxidant capacity is compromised (e.g., in fetuses or in old age), the cocaine-induced damage may be higher.

Lipton et al.[84,85] investigated whether cocaine-induced constriction of the umbilical/ placental vessels that induce significant changes in uterine and placental blood flow also causes oxidative stress. They found that following a single prenatal injection of cocaine in pregnant rats, there was a reduction in the levels of reduced glutathione and of reduced α-tocopherol in the fetal brains. In addition, there was an elevation of the oxidized form of α-tocopherol. As for oxidized glutathione, a rise was found in the fetuses at the ovarian extreme, where the greatest degree of vasoconstriction was demonstrated, and a decrease in the fetuses at the cervical extreme, where cocaine-induced vasoconstriction is the least. The authors speculate that cocaine-induced vasoconstriction causes increased oxidative stress, thus tying both mechanisms of action. They also show the important role of oxidative stress in the teratogenic mechanism.[84]

Following animal and in vitro studies, an additional mechanism has been proposed: alteration of proliferation and differentiation of neuronal precursor cells.[63,82] In a neural progenitor cell line exposed to cocaine, Lee et al.[82] found that cocaine downregulates the expression of the cyclin A genes, thus reducing neuronal proliferation. This was apparently caused by the cocaine-induced oxidative stress. Indeed, in their rat model, cimetidine, a cytochrome P450 (CYP) inhibitor, counteracted the down-inhibition of cyclin A and restored proliferation. These studies, too, demonstrated the role of oxidative stress in cocaine-induced damage.

Prevention and Treatment

Home Intervention Programs for Children Prenatally Exposed to Cocaine

Regardless of drug exposure, children living in poverty are at risk of cognitive delays. Children from low-income families exhibit intellectual declines as toddlers and preschoolers. Indeed, home intervention programs or adoption at a young age yielded higher

cognitive scores among drug-exposed infants.[107,108] Schuler et al.[130] studied the effect of home intervention programs on the infants' developmental outcome among a group of inner-city residents with low socioeconomic status. They found that home intervention led to higher scores on the Bayley Scales of Infant Development, mainly of the Mental Developmental Index. These developmental scores, however, declined during the first postnatal 18 months.[130]

To determine the relation between prenatal cocaine exposure and children's standardized cognitive tests at age 4, Frank et al.[40] assessed 91 children using the Wechsler Preschool and Primary Scale of Intelligence-Revised or the Wechsler Intelligence Scale for Children, Third Edition (WISC-III). Unlike other widespread assumptions relating to the disabling effects of prenatal cocaine exposure on the cognitive abilities of preschool children, Frank et al. strengthened results of other studies, claiming that exposure during pregnancy does not negatively affect the global or specific cognitive functions.[40] They also suggested that children known as being prenatally exposed to cocaine benefit from the early intervention and preschool program. Moreover, increased resilience of cocaine-addicted parents reduced the severity of the behavioral problems in adolescents prenatally exposed to cocaine.[3]

Intervention Programs for the Mothers

Intervention for cocaine-using mothers during pregnancy should use programs similar to those used in nonpregnant women. The dropout rate from such programs was significantly lower than in nonpregnant women, implying, as was also found for the treatment of pregnant women dependent on other drugs, that pregnancy may be a good time for prevention of further use of substances that may cause addiction.[147]

Lactation

Because cocaine and metabolites are transferred to human milk, reaching relatively high levels, women using cocaine should be advised to refrain from nursing their infants, depending on the dose. However, if there is only occasional use, then refraining from breastfeeding for about 24 hours following intake is sufficient.[128]

Studies in Animals

One of cocaine's important actions is to block the reuptake of dopamine, serotonin, and norepinephrine. In a rat model prenatally exposed to cocaine, Keller and Sntyder-Keller[73] examined the extracellular fluid levels of dopamine, serotonin, and metabolites and found changes in their levels compared with controls, together with long-term behavioral abnormalities. These changes subsided with the advancing age of the rats, similar to the behavioral changes that are observed in the offspring of cocaine-using mothers.

Investigating in utero cocaine-exposed rhesus monkey offspring, Paul et al.[112] found that two-thirds of controls and only one-fourth of exposed subjects demonstrated clear evidence of reversal learning (i.e., the ability to adapt to the new environmental contingencies in a seemingly simple way). Zimmerman et al.[118] demonstrated that in mice, cocaine caused vasodilation in the fetal vasculature and an increased the rate of neural tube defects, hypoplastic prosencephalon, and microcephaly. The administration of the antioxidants 2-oxothiazolidine-4-carboxylate and α-phenyl-N-t-butyl significantly reduced cocaine-induced vasodilation; however, it did not prevent neural tube defects.[152] Cocaine's vasoconstrictive property on the uterine and placental vasculature is enabled by its potential to increase catecholamine levels (especially norepinephrine) via inhibition of its reuptake. However, He and Lidow[83] found that the cocaine-induced vasoconstriction of the uteroumbilical and fetal brain vessels in the rhesus monkey does not seem to be the main cause of the cerebral damage, and that cocaine damages the fetal brain by a different mechanism. They examined the possible correlation between high levels of the cocaine metabolite benzoylecgonine, a potent vasoconstrictor, and cocaine-induced abnormal brain lamination and found that benzoylecgonine did not induce any brain damage, whereas cocaine did.

Lipton et al.[84] found that cocaine can differentially reduce dopamine and glial-derived neurotrophic factor levels, depending upon the location of the fetus in the uterus. The extent of dopamine depletion was in correlation with the extent of cocaine-induced restriction of uterine blood flow, as indicated by additional studies.[84]

A survey of studies in nonhuman primates indicates that prenatal cocaine exposure interferes with structural and biochemical development of the brain, consequently resulting in postnatal and adulthood behavioral deficits. Differences in the outcome between various models of prenatal cocaine exposure are likely to reflect the route, dose, gestational period, and daily pattern of cocaine use. This fact is most relevant to studies in human populations with cocaine abuse.[83]

Conclusions

The use of cocaine during pregnancy interferes with fetal weight gain, and increases the rate of premature labor and of stillbirth. It does not seem to increase the rate of major congenital anomalies, although some increase in the rate of urinary anomalies and of anomalies related to vascular disruption cannot be excluded. Cocaine may cause fetal cerebral hemorrhage and infarcts as well as placental abruption and bleeding. Cocaine seems to increase the rate of ADHD and other behavioral problems in the offspring and increase the rate of learning difficulties.

References

1. Akyuz N, Kekatpure MV, Liu J, et al. Structural brain imaging in children and adolescents following prenatal cocaine exposure: preliminary longitudinal findings. *Dev Neurosci.* 2014;36(3–4):316–328. 2014.
2. Appleboom T. Consumption of coca in history. *Verh K Acad Geneeskd Belg.* 1991;53:497–505.
3. Bada HS, Bann CM, Whitaker TM, et al. Protective factors can mitigate behavior problems after prenatal cocaine and other drug exposures. *Pediatrics.* 2012;130(6):e1479–e1488.
4. Banerjee TS, Middleton F, Faraone SV. Environmental risk factors for attention-deficit hyperactivity disorder. *Acta Pediatrica.* 2007;96:1269–1274.
5. Barik S. The thrill can kill: murder by methylation. *Mol Pharmacol.* 2007;71:1203–1205.
6. Bashkatova V, Meunier J, Vanin A Maurice T. Nitric oxide and oxidative stress in the brain of rats exposed in utero to cocaine. *Ann NY Acad Sci.* 2006;1074:P632–P642.
7. Bauer CR, Langer JC, Shankaran S, et al. Acute neonatal effects of cocaine exposure during pregnancy. *Arch Pediatr Adolesc Med.* 2005;159:824–834.
8. Beeghly M, Martin B, Rose-Jacobs R, et al. Prenatal cocaine exposure and children's language functioning at 6 and 9.5 years: moderating effects of child age, birth weight, and gender. *J Pediatric Psychol.* 2006;31:98–115.
9. Behnke M, Eyler FD, Garvan CW, et al. The search for congenital malformations in newborns with fetal cocaine exposure. *Pediatrics.* 2001;107:E74.
10. Bell JC, Raynes-Greenow C, Turner RM, et al. Maternal alcohol consumption during pregnancy and the risk of orofacial clefts in infants: a systematic review and meta-analysis. *Paediatr Perinat Epidemiol.* 2014;28:322–332.
11. Bendersky M, Bennett D, Lewis M. Aggression at age 5 as a function of prenatal exposure to cocaine; gender and environmental risk. *J Pediatric Psychol.* 2006;31:71–84.
12. Bingo N, et al. Teratogenicity of cocaine in humans. *J Pediatrics.* 1987;110:93–96.
13. Boyd TA, Ernhart CB, Greene TH, et al. Prenatal alcohol exposure and sustained attention in the preschool years. *Neurotoxicol Teratol.* 1991;13:49–55.
14. Blackard C, Tennes K. Human placental transfer of cannabinoids. *N Engl J Med.* 1984;311:797.
15. Bradley RH, Corwyn RF. Socio-economic status and child development. *Annu Rev Psychol.* 2002;53:371–399.
16. Brodzinsky DM, Smith DW, Brodzinsky AB. *Children's Adjustment to Adoption: Developmental and Clinical Issues.* Thousand Oaks, CA: Sage; 1998.
17. Brogly SB, Saia KA, Walley AY, et al. Prenatal buprenorphine versus methadone exposure and neonatal outcomes: systematic review and meta-analysis. *Am J Epidemiol.* 2014;180(7):673–686.
18. Burns L, Mattick RP, Lim K, Wallace C. Methadone in pregnancy: treatment retention and neonatal outcomes. *Addiction.* 2006;102:264–270.
19. Carmichael SL, Shaw GM, Yang W, Lammer EJ. Maternal periconceptional alcohol consumption and risk for conotruncal heart defects. *Birth Defects Res Clin Mol Teratol.* 2003;67:875–878.
20. Carroll KM, Rounseville BJ. History and significance of childhood attention deficit disorder in treatment-seeking cocaine abusers. *Comprehensive Psychiatr.* 1993;34:75–82.
21. Cartwright MM, Smith SM. Increased cell death and reduced neural crest cell numbers in ethanol-exposed embryos: partial basis for the fetal alcohol syndrome phenotype. *Alcohol Clin Exp Res.* 1995;19:378–386.
22. Chen CY, Lien YT, Yeh HH, et al. Comparison of adverse obstetric outcomes and maternity hospitalization among heroin-exposed and methadone-treated women in Taiwan. *Int J Drug Policy.* 2015;26:191–198.
23. Chen SY, Dehart DB, Sulik KK. Protection from ethanol-induced limb malformations by the superoxide dismutase/catalas mimetic, EUK-134. *FASEB J.* 2004;18:1234–1236.
24. Chotro MG, Arias C, Laviola G. Increased ethanol intake after prenatal ethanol exposure: studies with animals. *Neurosc Biobehav Rev.* 2007;31:181–191.
25. Cohen-Kerem R, Koren G. Antioxidants and fetal protection against ethanol teratogenicity I. Review of the experimental data and implications to humans. *Neurotoxicol Teratol.* 2003;25:1–9.
26. Committee on Drugs, American Academy of Pediatrics. The transfer of drugs and other chemicals into human breast milk. *Pediatrics.* 2001;108:776–789.
27. Cook PS, Petersen RC, Moore DT, et al. Alcohol, tobacco, and other drugs may harm the unborn. *Govt Rep Announcements Index (GRA&I).* 1991;(15).
28. Coriale G, Fiorentino D, Di Lauro F, et al. Fetal Alcohol Spectrum Disorder (FASD): neurobehavioral profile, indications for diagnosis and treatment. *Riv Psychiatr.* 2013;48:356–369.
29. Covington CY, Nordstrom-Klee B, Ager J, et al. Birth to age 7 growth of children prenatally exposed to drugs. A prospective cohort study. *Neurotoxicol Teratol.* 2002;24:489–496.
30. Davids E, Gastpar M. Buprenorphine in the treatment of opioid dependence. *Eur Neuropsychopharmacol.* 2004;14:209–216.
31. Dembele K, Yao XH, Chen L, et al. Intrauterine ethanol exposure results in hypothalamic oxidative stress and neuroendocrine

alterations in adult rat offspring. *Am J Physiol Regul Integr Comp Physiol.* 2006;291:R796–R802.

32. DeRoo LA, Wilcox AJ, Drevon CA, et al. First-trimester maternal alcohol consumption and the risk of infant oral clefts in Norway: a population-based case-control study. *Am J Epidemiol.* 2008;168:638–646.

33. Eiden RD, Godleski S, Colder CR, Schuetze P. Prenatal cocaine exposure: the role of cumulative environmental risk and maternal harshness in the development of child internalizing behavior problems in kindergarten. *Neurotox Teratol.* 2014;44:1–10.

34. English DR, Hulse GK, Milne E, et al. Maternal cannabis use and birth weight: a meta-analysis. *Addiction.* 1997;92:1553–1560.

35. Eyler FD, Behnke M, Colon M, et al. Birth outcome from a prospective, matched study of prenatal crack/cocaine use: II. Interactive and dose effects on neurobehavioral assessment. *Pediatrics.* 1998;101:237–241.

36. Fajemirokun-Odudeyi O, Sinha C, et al. Pregnancy outcome in women who use opiates. *Eur J Obststr Geynecol Reprod Biol.* 2006;126:170–175.

37. Farran DC. Effects of intervention with disadvantaged and disabled children: a decade review. In: Meisels SJ, Shorikoff JP, eds. *Handbook of Early Childhood Intervention.* Cambridge, MA: University Press; 1990:501–539.

38. Fierens E. Archeological and artistic sources of coca consumption in pre-hispanic America. *Verh K Acad Geneeskd Belg.* 1991;53:463–485.

39. Fisher G. Treatment of opioid dependence in pregnant women. *Addiction.* 2000;95:1141–1144.

40. Frank DA, Jacobs RS, Beeghly M, et al. Levels of prenatal cocaine exposure and scores on the Bayley scales of infant development: modifying effects of caregivers, early intervention, and birth weight. *Pediatrics.* 2002;110:1143–1152.

41. Frank DA, Jacobs RS, Beeghly M, et al. Levels of cocaine exposure and 48-month IQ: importance of preschool enrichment. *Neurotox Teratol.* 2005;27:15–28.

42. Fried PA, James DS, Watkinson B. Growth and pubertal milestones during adolescence in offspring prenatally exposed to cigarettes and marihuana. *Neurotoxicol Teratol.* 2001b;23:431–436.

43. Fried PA, O'Connell C, Watkinson B. 60 and 72 months follow up of children prenatally exposed to marijuana, cigarettes and alcohol: cognitive and language assessment. *J Dev Behav Pediatr.* 1992;13:383–391.

44. Fried PA, Smith AM. A literature review of the consequences of prenatal marihuana exposure. An emerging of a deficiency in aspects of executive function. *Neurotoxicol Teratol.* 2001a;23:1–11.

45. Fried PA, Watkinson B. 12-and 24-month neurobehavioral follow up of children prenatally exposed to marijuana, cigarettes and alcohol. *Neurotox Teratol.* 1988;10:305–313.

46. Fried PA, Watkinson B. 36-and 48-month neurobehavioral follow up of children prenatally exposed to marijuana, cigarettes and alcohol. *J Dev Behav Pediatr.* 1990;11:49–58.

47. Fried PA Watkinson B, Willan A. Marijuana use during pregnancy and decreased length of gestation. *Am J Obstet Gynecol.* 1984;150:23–27.

48. Gerber WF, Schramm LC. Effect of marihuana extract on fetal hamsters and rabbits. *Toxicol Appl Pharmacol.* 1969;14:276–282.

49. Gianutsos G, Abbatiello ER. The effect of prenatal cannabis sativa on maze learning ability in the rat. *Psychopharmacologia.* 1972;27:117–122.

50. Gladstone J, Nulman I, Koren G. Reproductive risks of binge drinking during pregnancy. *Reprod Toxicol.* 1996;10:3–13.

51. Goldschmidt L, Richardson GA, Willford JA, et al. School achievement in 14-year-old youths prenatally exposed to marijuana. *Neurotoxicol Teratol.* 2012;34(1):161–167.

52. Goodlet R, Eilers AT. Alcohol-induced Purkinje cell loss with a single binge exposure in neonatal rats: a stereological study of temporal windows of vulnerability. *Alcohol Clin Exp Res.* 1997;22:738–744.

53. Gratacos E, Torres PJ, Antolin E. Use of cocaine during pregnancy. *N Engl J Med.* 1993;329:667.

54. Grilly DM, et al. Observations on the reproductive activity of chimpanzees following long-term exposure to marihuana. *Pharmacology.* 1974;11:304–307.

55. Grinspoon L, Bakalar JB. Coca and cocaine as medicines: an historical review. *J Ethnopharmacol.* 1981;3:149–159.

56. Hamre KM, West JR. The effects of the timing of ethanol exposure during the brain growth spurt on the number of cerebellar Purkinje and granule cell nuclear profiles. *Alcohol Clin Exp Res.* 1993;17:610–622.

57. Handmaker NS, Rayburn WF, Meng C, et al. Impact of alcohol exposure after pregnancy recognition on ultrasonographic fetal growth measures. *Alcohol Clin Exp Res.* 2006;30:892–898.

58. Hatch EE, Bracken MB. Effect of marihuana use in pregnancy on fetal growth. *Am J Epidemiol.* 1986;124:986–993.

59. Hayatbakhsh MR, Flenady VJ, Gibbons KS, et al. Birth outcomes associated with cannabis use before and during pregnancy. *Pediatric Res.* 2012;71(2):215–219.

60. He N, Lidow MS. Cerebral cortical abnormalities seen in a nonhuman primate model of prenatal cocaine exposure are not related to vasoconstriction. *NeuroToxicology.* 2004;25:419–432.E.

61. Heaton MB, Paiva M, Mayer J, et al. Ethanol – mediated generation of reactive oxygen species in developing rat cerebellum. *Neurosci Lett.* 2002;334:83–86.

62. Herjanic BM, Barredo HV, Herjanic M, et al. Children of heroin addicts. *Int J Addiction.* 1979;14:919–931.

63. Hou Y, Tan Y, Belcheva MM, et al. Differential effects of gestational buprenorphine, naloxone and methadone on mesolimbic mu opioid and ORL1 receptor G protein coupling. *Brain Res Dev Brain Res.* 2004;151:149–157.

64. Hulse GK, O'Neil G, Arnold-Reed DE. Methadone maintenance vs. implantable naltrexone treatment in the pregnant user. *Int J Gynecol Obstetr.* 2004;85:170–171.

65. Hutchings DE, Dow-Edwards D. Animal models of opiate, cocaine and cannabis use. *Clin Perinatol.* 1991;18:1–22.

66. Jones KL. From recognition to responsibility: Josef Warkany, David Smith, and the fetal alcohol syndrome in the 21st century. *Birth Defects Res (Part A).* 2003;67:13–20.

67. Jones KL, Smith DW. Recognition of the fetal alcohol syndrome in early infancy. *Lancet.* 1973;3:999–1001.

68. Jones KL, Smith DW, Ulleland CN, et al. Pattern of malformations in offspring of chronic alcoholic mothers. *Lancet.* 1973;1:1267–1271.

69. Jutras-Aswad D, DiNieri JA, Harkany T, Hurd YL. Neurobiological consequences of maternal cannabis on human fetal development and its neuropsychiatric outcome. *Eur Arch Psychiatry Clin Neurosci.* 2009;259(7):395–412.

70. Kandall SR, Gaines J. Maternal substance use and subsequent sudden infant death syndrome (SIDS) in offspring. *Neurotoxicol Teratol.* 1991;13:235–240.

71. Katz S, Ben-Hur T, Ben-Sahaanan TL, et al. Reversal of heroin neurobehavioral teratogenicity by grafting of neural progenitors. *J Neurochem.* 2008;104:38–49.

72. Kay HH, Tsoi S, Grindle K, et al. Markers of oxidative stress in placental villi exposed to ethanol. *J Soc Gynecol Investig.* 2006;13:118–121.

73. Keller Jr RW, Sntyder-Keller A. Prenatal cocaine exposure. *Ann NY Acad Sci.* 2000;909:217–232.

74. Kelly YJ, Sacker A, Gray R, et al. Light drinking during pregnancy: still no increased risk for socioemotional difficulties or cognitive deficits at 5 years of age? *J Epidemiol Community Health.* 2012;66(1):41–48.

75. Kesmodel U, Wisborg K, Olsen SF, et al. Moderate alcohol intake in pregnancy and the risk of spontaneous abortions. *Alcohol.* 2002;37:87–92.

76. Kolpe M, Carlson GA. Influence of attention – deficit/hyperactivity disorder symptoms on methadone treatment outcome. *Am J Addict.* 2007;16:46–48.

77. Kot-Lebovich H, Fainsod A. Ethanol induces embryonic malformations by competing or retinaldehyde dehydrogenase activity during gastrulation. *Dis Models Mech.* 2009;2:295–305.

78. Kotler M, Cohen H, Segman R, et al. Excess dopamine D4 receptor (DRD4) exon III 7 repeat allele in opioid dependent subjects. *Mol Psych.* 1997;2:251–254.

79. Krasemann T, Klingebiel S. Influence of chronic intrauterine exposure to alcohol on structurally normal hearts. *Cardiol Young.* 2007;17:185–188.

80. Laufer BI, Kapalanga J, Castellani CA, et al. Associative DNA methylation changes in children with prenatal alcohol exposure. *Epigenomics.* 2015;7:1259–1274.

81. Laufer BI, Chater-Diehl EJ, Kapalanga J, Singh SM, Long-term alterations to DNA methylation as a biomarker of prenatal alcohol exposure: from mouse models to human children with fetal alcohol spectrum disorders. *Alcohol.* 2017;60:67–75.

82. Lee CT, Chen J, Hayashi T, et al. A mechanism for the inhibition of neural progenitor cell proliferation by cocaine. *PLoS Med.* 2008;10(6):e117. 5.

82. Lemoine P, Haroussesear H, Borteyro V, et al. Les enfants de parents alcooliques: anomalies observees a propos de 127 cas. *Archive Franc Pediatr.* 1968;25:830.

83. Lidow MS. Consequences of prenatal cocaine exposure in nonhuman primates. *Develop Brain Res.* 2003;147:23–36.

84. Lipton JW, Gyawali S, et al. Prenatal cocaine administration increases glutathione and alpha-tocopherol oxidation in fetal rat brain. *Develop Brain Res.* 2003;147:77–84.

85. Lipton JW, Vu TQ, Ling Z, et al. Prenatal cocaine exposure induces an attenuation of uterine blood flow in the rat. *Neurotoxicol Teratol.* 2002;24:143–148.

86. Little BB, Snell LM, Klein VR, et al. Maternal and fetal effects of heroin addiction during pregnancy. *J Reproductive Med.* 1990;35:159–162.

87. Little BB, Snell LM, Knoll KA. Heroin abuse during pregnancy: effects on perinatal outcome and early childhood growth. *Am J Human Biol.* 1991;3:463–468.

88. Liu J, Lester BM, Neyzi N. Regional brain morphometry and impulsivity in adolescents following prenatal exposure to cocaine and tobacco. *JAMA Pediatr.* 2013;167(4):348–354.

89. Lopez SL, Taeusch HW, Findlay RD, Walther FJ. Time of onset of necrotizing enterocolitis in newborn infants with known prenatal cocaine exposure. *Clin Pediatr.* 1995;34:424–429.

90. Lozano J, Garcia-Algar O, Marchei E, et al. Prevalence of gestational exposure to cannabis in a Mediterranean city by meconium analysis. *Acta Pediatrica.* 2007;96:1734–1737.

91. Maier SE, Miller JA, Blackwell JM, West JR. Fetal alcohol exposure and temporal vulnerability: regional differences in cell loss as a function of the timing of binge-like alcohol exposure during brain development. *Alcohol Clin Exp Res.* 1999;23:726–734.

92. Martinez-Frias ML, Bermejo E, Rodriguez-Pinilla E, Frias JL. Risk for congenital anomalies associated with different sporadic and daily doses of alcohol consumption during pregnancy: a case control study. *Birth Defects Res (part A).* 2004;70:194–200.

93. Masemola ML, van der Merwe L, Lombard Z, et al. Reduced DNA methylation in the PEG3DMR and KvDMR1 lici in children exposed to alcohol in utero: south African Fetal Alcohol Syndrome cohort study. *Front Genet.* 2015;6:85–97.

94. Mattick RP, Kimber J, et al. Buprenorphine maintenance versus placebo or methadone maintenance for opioid dependence. *Cochrane Database Syst Rev.* 2008;16(2):CD002207.

95. Mennella JA, Garcia-Gomez PL. Sleep disturbances after acute exposure to alcohol in mothers' milk. *Alcohol.* 2001;25:153–158.

96. Meyer KA, Werler MM, Hayes C, et al. Low maternal alcohol consumption during pregnancy and oral clefts in offspring: the slone birth defects study. *Birth Defects Res (Part A).* 2003;67:509–514.

97. Murawski NJ, Moore EM, Thomas JD, Riley EP. Advances in diagnosis and treatment of fetal alcohol spectrum disorder. From animal models to human studies. *Alcohol Res.* 2015;37:97–108.

98. Noland JS, Singer LT, Short EJ, et al. Prenatal drug exposure and selective attention in preschoolers. *Neurotoxicol Teratol.* 2005;27:429–438.

99. Nygaard E, Moe V, Slinning K, Kristine B. Walhovd Longitudinal cognitive development of children born to mothers with opioid and polysubstance use. *Ped Res.* 2015;78:330–335.

100. Nykjaer C, Alwan NA, Greenwood DC, et al. Maternal alcohol intake prior to and during pregnancy and risk of adverse birth outcomes: evidence from a British cohort. *J Epidemiol Community Health.* 2014;68(6):542–549.

101. O'Callaghan FV, O'Callaghan M, Najman JM, et al. Prenatal alcohol exposure and attention, learning and intellectual ability at 14 years: a prospective longitudinal study. *Early Hum Dev.* 2007;83:115–123.

102. Ornoy A. The effects of alcohol and illicit drugs on the human embryo and fetus. Emphasis on developmental studies. Invited review. *Isr J Psychiatry.* 2002;39:120–132.

103. Ornoy A. The impact of intrauterine exposure versus postnatal environment in neurodevelopmental toxicity: long term neurobehavioral studies in children at risk for developmental disorders. *Toxicol Lett.* 2003;140/141:171–181.

104. Ornoy A. Embryonic oxidative stress as a mechanism of teratogenesis with special emphasis on diabetic embryopathy. *Reproductive Toxicol.* 2007;24:31–41.

105. Ornoy A, Ergaz Z. Alcohol abuse in pregnant women: effects on the fetus and newborn, mode of action and maternal treatment. A review. *Int J Environ Res Public Health.* 2010. *www.mdpi.com/journal/ijerph.*

106. Ornoy A, Finkel –Pekarsky V, Peles E, Adelson M, Schreiber S, Ebstein RP. ADHD risk alleles associated with opiate addiction: study of addicted parents and their children. *Ped Res.* 2016. [In press].

107. Ornoy A, Michailevskaya V, Lukashov I, et al. The developmental outcome of children born to heroin dependent mothers, raised at home or adopted. *Child Abuse Neglect.* 1996;20:385–396.

108. Ornoy A, Segal J, Bar-Hamburger R, et al. The developmental outcome of school age children born to heroin-dependent mothers: importance of environmental factors. *Dev Med Child Neurol.* 2001;43:668–675.

109. Ornoy A, Segal J, Greenbaum C, Bar-Hamburger R. The development of children from birth to early school age born to drug dependent mothers. *World Pediatrics Child Care.* 2001;8:29–40.

110. Ornoy A, Weinstein-Fudim L, Ergaz Z. Prenatal factors associated with autism spectrum disorder (ASD). *Reprod Toxicol.* 2015;56:155–169.

111. Ozsarfati J, Koren G. Medication used in the treatment of disruptive behavior in children with FASD – a guide. *J Popul Ther Clin Pharmacol Therapeut.* 2015;22:e59–e67.

112. Paul MG, Gillan MP, Allen RR, et al. Effects of chronic in utero exposure to cocaine on behavioral adaptability in Rhesus monkey offspring when examined in adulthood. *Ann NY Acad Sci.* 2000;914:412–417.

113. Perez-Reyes M, Wall ME. Presence of delta-9-tetrahydrocannabinol in human milk. *N Engl J Med.* 1982;307:819–820.

114. Polygenis D, Wharton S, Malmberg C, et al. Moderate alcohol consumption during pregnancy and the incidence of fetal malformations: a meta-analysis. *Neurotoxicol Teratol.* 1998;20:61–67.

115. Poon HF, Abdullah L, Mullan MA, et al. Cocaine-induced oxidative stress precedes cell death in human neuronal progenitor cells. *Neurochem Int.* 2007;50:69–73.

116. Potter SM, Zelazo PR, Stack DN, et al. Adverse effects of fetal cocaine exposure on neonatal auditory information processing. *Pediatrics.* 2000;105:E40.

117. Ramadoss J, Lunde ER, Chen WJA, et al. Temporal vulnerability of fetal cerebellar purkinje cells to chronic binge alcohol exposure: ovine model. *Alcohol Clin Exp Res.* 2007;31:1738–1745.

118. Randall CL. Alcohol as a teratogen: a decade of research in review. *Alcohol Alcohol Suppl.* 1987;1:125–132.

119. Randall CL. Alcohol and pregnancy: highlights from three decades of research. *J Stud Alcohol.* 2001;62:554–561.

120. Randall CL, Anton RF. Aspirin reduces alcohol-induced prenatal mortality and malformations in mice. *Alcohol Clin Exp Res.* 1984;8:513–515.

121. Rivers RPA. Neonatal opiate withdrawal. *Arch Dis Child.* 1986;61:1236–1239.

122. Rogers JM, Brannen KC, Barbee BD, et al. Methanol exposure during gastrulation causes holoprosencephaly, facial dysgenesis, and cervical vertebral malformations in C57BL/6 J Mice. *Birth Defects Res (Part B).* 2004;71:80–88.

123. Romitti PA, Sun L, Honein MA, et al. Maternal periconceptional alcohol consumption and risk of orofacial clefts. *Am J Epidemiol.* 2007;166:775–785.

124. Sadler TW, ed. *Langman's Medical Embryology.* 7th ed. Williams & Wilkins; 1995:374–412.

125. Sameroff AJ. Models of developmental risk. In: Zeanah CH, ed. *Handbook of Infant Mental Health.* 2nd ed. New York: Guilford; 2000:3–19.

126. Sameroff AJ. Developmental systems and psychopathology. *Develop Psychopathol.* 2000;12:367–399.

127. Sayal K, Heron J, Draper E, et al. Prenatal exposure to binge pattern of alcohol consumption: mental health and learning outcomes at age 11. *Eur Child Adolesc Psychiatry.* 2014;23(10):891–899.

128. Schaefer C, Peters P, Miller R, eds. *Drugs during Pregnancy and Lactation. Treatment Options and Risk Assessment.* 2nd ed. Elsevier; 2007:530–531. 797–807.

129. Schubiner H, Tzelepis A, Isaacson JH, et al. The dual diagnosis of attention-deficit/ hyperactivity disorder and substance abuse: case reports and literature review. *J Clin Psychiatry.* 1995;56:146–150.

130. Schuler ME, Nair P, Kettinger L. Drug – exposed infants and developmental outcome : effects of a home intervention and ongoing maternal drug use. *Arch Pediatr Adolesc Med.* 2003;157:133–138.

131. Shi J, Hui L, Xu Y, et al. Sequence of variation in the mu – opioid receptor gene (OPRM1) associated with human addiction to heroin. *Hum Mut.* 2002;19:459–460.

132. Simpson ME, Duggal S, Keiver K. Prenatal ethanol exposure has differential effects on fetal growth and skeletal ossification. *Bone.* 2005;36:521–532.

133. Singer LT, Minnes S, Short E, et al. Cognitive outcomes of preschool children with prenatal cocaine exposure. *J Am Med Assoc.* 2004;291:2448–2456.

134. Slotkin TA, Seidler FJ, Yanai J. Heroin neuroteratogenicity: targeting adenylyl cyclase as an underlying biochemical mechanism. *Brain Res Dev Brain Res.* 2001;132:69–79.

135. Sowder BJ, Burt MR. Children of addicts and non-addicts. A comparative investigation in five urban sites. In: *Addicted Parents and Their Children, Two Reports.* Rockville, MD: National Institute of Drug Abuse; 1980.

136. Steinhausen HC, Blattman B, Pfund F. Developmental outcome in children with intrauterine exposure to substances. *Eur Addict Res.* 2007;13:94–100.

137. Strandberg-Larsen K, Skov-Ettrup LS, Gronbaek M, et al. Maternal alcohol drinking pattern during pregnancy and the risk for an offspring with an isolated congenital heart defect and in particular a ventricular septal defect or an atrial septal defect. *Birth Defects Res A Clin Mol Teratol.* 2011;91:616–622.

138. Streissguth AP, Barr HM, Sampson PD. Moderate prenatal alcohol exposure: effects on child IQ and learning problems at age 7.5 years. *Alcohol Clin Exp Res.* 1990;14:662–666.

139. Sumner GS, Mandoki MW, Matthews-Ferrari K. A psychiatric population of prenatally cocaine-exposed children. *J Am Acad Child Adolesc Psychiatry.* 1993;32:1003–1006.

140. Torfs CP, Velie EM, Oechsli FW, et al. A population-based study of gastroschisis: demographic, pregnancy, and lifestyle risk factors. *Teratology.* 1994;50:44–53.

141. Tricot JP. Cocaine: half a century of therapeutic use (1880–1930). *Verh - K Acad Geneeskd Belg.* 1991;53:487–496.

142. Ungerer M, Knezovich J, Ramsay M. In Utero alcohol exposure, epigenetic changes, and their consequences. *Alcohol Res.* 2013;35:37–46.

143. Van Baar AL. Development of infants of drug dependent mothers. *Child Psychol Psychiatry.* 1990;31:911–920.

144. Wahlsten VS, Sarman I. Neurobehavioural development of preschool-age children born to addicted mothers given opiate maintenance treatment with buprenorphine during pregnancy. *Acta Paediat.* 2013;102:544–549.

145. Webster WS, Brown-Wooddman ODC. Cocaine as a cause of congenital malformations of vascular origin: experimental evidence in the rat. *Teratology.* 1990;41:689–697.

146. Weiglas-Kuperus N, Baerts W, Smirkovsky M, et al. Effects of biological and social factors on the cognitive development of very low birth weight children. *Pediatrics.* 1993;92:658–665.

147. Weisdorf T, Parran Jr TV, Graham A, et al. Comparison of pregnancy – specific interventions to a traditional treatment program for cocaine-addicted pregnant women. *J Subst Abuse Treat.* 1999;16:39–45.

148. Wentzel P, Rydberg U, Eriksson UJ. Antioxidative treatment diminishes ethanol-induced congenital malformations in the rat. *Alcohol Clin Exp Res.* 2006;30:1752–1760.

149. Wilens TE. Attention deficit/hyperactivity disorder and the substance use disorders: the nature of the relationship, subtypes at risk and treatment issues. *Psych Clinic North Am.* 2004;27:283–301.

150. Wu TC, Tashkin DP, Djahad B, Rose JE. Pulmonary hazards of smoking marijuana as compared with tobacco. *N Engl J Med.* 1988;318:347–351.

151. Yolton K, Cornelius M, Ornoy A, et al. Exposure to neurotoxicants and the development of attention deficit hyperactivity disorder and its related behaviors in childhood. *Neurotoxicol Teratol.* 2014;44:30–45.

152. Zimmerman EF, Potturi RB, Resnick E, Fisher JE. The role of oxygen free radicals in the cocaine-induced vascular disruption in mice. *Teratology.* 1994;49:192–201.

71

Forensic Issues

MICHAEL H. GENDEL AND LAURENCE M. WESTREICH

Introduction

Forensic psychiatry is the branch of psychiatry that addresses the intersection of psychiatry and the law. In the practice of medicine, psychiatry, and a variety of other clinical professions, legal or forensic issues are commonly encountered. Confidentiality, for instance, is a key legal and ethical concern in general medical and psychiatric practice but is subject to special treatment in certain addiction treatment settings, which may result in the federal confidentiality statute coming into play. It is important in the clinical practice of addiction medicine and psychiatry to be aware than this statute supersedes state confidentiality laws, broadly defines the confidential doctor/agency–patient/client relationship, and outlines sanctions for violating the statute, which could include loss of federal funding or special tax status for the agency in question. This chapter addresses the range of forensic issues that are relevant for practicing physicians, psychiatrists, and addiction specialists and may be of interest to a wide variety of health care professionals and scientists. Working in forensic environments is, essentially, practicing forensic medicine. For instance, in the preceding example concerning confidentiality, managing the special confidentiality requirements for certain patients or clients with addictive illness requires forensic expertise and knowledge of the federal confidentiality statute and its implications. Furthermore, physicians frequently venture into the forensic realm when they are asked to give opinions about disability, whether a patient can give informed consent for treatment, or whether an intoxicated individual could form the specific intent to commit a crime. Assessing fitness for duty in a physician with alcoholism or comorbid addiction and mood disorder and addressing the relevant regulatory (licensing board) issues, opining about the meaning of a positive drug screen in a medical review officer role, and treating addiction in correctional settings are other examples of the enormous scope of forensic situations in psychiatric and other medical practice. Needless to say, working with attorneys in many contexts and testifying in a court of law are forensic activities commonly encountered in medicine.

Because forensic issues flow from the law, not medicine, many doctors are uncomfortable with the concepts and demands of working at the clinical/forensic intersection. Physicians frequently see forensic issues as intrusive in their work rather than protective of their patients, and many do their best to avoid the courtroom. The authors encourage the reader to cultivate interest in the dynamic body of statutes, courts, and cases that constitute the law; familiarity will breed comfort. From the opposite vantage point, although the law has long addressed problems of mental illness, especially the law regarding criminal responsibility, it has been slow to recognize addictive illness, which until relatively recently was seen as moral weakness or depravity. At least some of this problem has to do with the voluntary element in drug use.[9] Courts and lawmakers are obviously not immune to biased societal attitudes toward individuals with addictive disease; nor are they educated about the nature of such illness.

In this chapter, we have chosen to organize the material according to the forensic context, including civil, criminal, and regulatory environments, and to first review some of the essential differences between the style of thinking and nature of practice in forensic contexts compared with the usual clinical thinking in medical practice. In addition, the authors have chosen to include new and emerging areas of forensic interest, in part to underscore the dynamic nature of this field.

The Forensic Evaluation Process

There are two essential differences in performing any evaluation in a forensic context when compared with performing a clinical examination, be it determining whether someone is disabled, competent to make a will, or criminally responsible. Because the findings and opinions in forensic evaluations are meant to be communicated to another party, confidentiality is limited, although obtaining a release of information for that party is often advisable, depending on the context. In addition, the purpose of the examination is to evaluate and reach conclusions regarding the referral questions, not to provide medical care to the examinee. It is not a doctor–patient relationship in the usual sense. Because an examinee often expects both help and at least a measure of confidentiality, both of these differences should be communicated to the examinee at the outset. Even after such advisement, examinees often lapse into looking upon the physician as a helper, so the physician should be alert to signs of this and be prepared to remind the examinee about the context. It is equally important for examiners to be watchful for signs that they want to help the examinee. Examiners also should carefully consider their feelings about and reactions to the examinee, which if left unattended could interfere with being neutral and objective. If the examiner develops doubts as to whether the examinee is competent to understand or agree to the conditions of examination, the report should reflect how this was assessed and the conclusions reached.

There are other technical differences between forensic evaluations and clinical evaluations. Because of the need to answer specific and complex questions, forensic evaluations often take more time than clinical evaluations and may require several interviews. Consider an examination in which a psychiatrist is asked to opine whether, due to hallucinogen intoxication, a criminal defendant was able to form the specific intent to commit a capital crime. Reviewing all relevant documents such as police investigative records and medical records will be an essential task. Incomplete review of documents will undermine the authority of a forensic evaluation. Collateral information is frequently necessary, often from several sources. In assessing whether or not a physician is alcohol dependent, speaking to his or her spouse, employer, and office and hospital staff will be helpful. Forensic reports should be quite detailed, specifically addressing the referral questions in the context of a complete report, including all the data from the examination. This requires that the referral questions be accurately understood by the examiner. This in turn necessitates spending as much time as necessary communicating with the referring party— a court, lawyer, regulatory board, or employer—and making sure that all relevant documents are in the examiner's possession.

Medical and Legal Terminology and Reports of Evaluation

Encountering words that sound like clinical terms but are in fact legal terms is a common situation in forensic work. Other words may be "terms of art" within the legal system and cannot be defined. The forensic examiner must learn about and consider the legal

framework. For instance, in Colorado, the Medical Practices Act, the law that regulates medical practice, lists "habitual intemperance" as unprofessional behavior for a physician.[50] Habitual intemperance, a 19th-century expression used in many laws created in that era, is not in the Fifth Edition of the *Diagnostic and Statistical Manual of Mental Disorders* (DSM-5).[4] Is it the equivalent of a substance use disorder, or a certain severity of substance use disorder? The forensic examiner cannot actually answer these questions without a legal definition. Asking for such a definition from the lawyers involved in the case is always a good step; the evaluator would be told, in this case, that it is a term of art. The examining physician may be unable to say whether their clinical diagnosis meets the standard for this term. The answer may be left to a fact finder, which in the legal system is a judge or jury. The term "disability" appears in the same Colorado statute referenced above. The state may act against a license on the basis that the physician has a disability. Again, this term is legal rather than medical in its meaning, referring to a condition that would meet the statutory requirement for unprofessional conduct. Now the examiner has the complex task of sorting out whether habitual intemperance is a disability, whether a DSM-5-defined substance use disorder is a disability, and the relationship between clinical disability and disability under the statute.

In writing reports, physicians should discuss the relationship of a diagnosis or other clinical term to the legal terms used under that statute, regulation, bylaw, or definition in question. For instance, in the preceding example concerning the term "disability", if a substance-related disorder is found, the report should review how the diagnosis was reached, sort out the relationship of the clinical and legal terms, and acknowledge any outside sources of information used to understand the legal terms, in the process of answering the referral questions.

Working With Attorneys: Testimony

Due to space limitations, the authors give only a brief introduction to these topics. The reader is referred to forensic psychiatry texts or other works for this information.[80,85] In these areas, the need for neutrality and objectivity, necessary in all forensic work, is paramount. The "hired gun," a medical evaluator who will testify favorably for any side, regardless of the facts, is anathema to the medical profession. The American Academy of Psychiatry and the Law has published ethics guidelines[2]; these should be reviewed carefully by physicians anticipating these activities. Remaining neutral may be harder than one imagines because of doctors' natural wish to be helpful to whomever is asking for their opinion. One must keep in mind that it is actually helpful for an attorney to hear an opinion unfavorable about his or her client or case. In court, even the appearance of advocacy or subjectivity is deadly to the credibility of the medical expert witness. Ultimately, credibility is the only currency of the medical expert. A corollary of this principle is that the attorney representing the opposing side in an adversarial proceeding has a duty to attack the credibility as well as the opinions of the medical expert. Although it is not easy to remain neutral and objective in the face of such attack, it is easier if one conceptualizes it as part of the job.

Psychiatrists and other physicians, as opposed to forensic psychiatrists, may testify only occasionally, so that lessons learned once may be forgotten before the next occasion arises. The authors recommend that physicians consult their forensic colleagues, forensic texts, and the attorneys involved in the case for help in orienting or reorienting themselves to the demands of testimony, be it in court or in deposition.

Compulsion and Responsibility

In all of the legal environments discussed later in this chapter, the psychiatrist may be asked to discuss the voluntary element involved in all substance use and what it means and implies about the character, reliability, credibility, and responsibility of the addicted individual. Kalivas and Volkow[39] have written that understanding addiction must involve understanding why addicted persons continue to be vulnerable to relapse even after extended abstinence and understanding their difficulty in curbing drug-seeking behavior even in the face of serious adverse consequences.[39] The authors will not attempt to review here the many recent advances in understanding of the neurobiology of addiction, as this subject is covered elsewhere in this book. However, a brief review is warranted because the neurobiology may shed light on forensic issues insofar as addiction is associated with the impaired ability to choose abstinence. Generally, as Kalivas and Volkow,[39] and Hyman[36] have argued, the brain circuitry involved in motivation is reorganized and reoriented by repeated use of addictive compounds. Drugs of abuse cause dopamine release in the reward circuitry more powerfully than do the natural reinforcers of behavior, such as food and sex, much less than the everyday reinforcers such as relationships and other enjoyable or rewarding activities.[97] Thus addicted individuals find that drugs of abuse and their cues become more salient than any other source of motivation. Over time, the potent release of dopamine in the reward pathways in response to drugs of abuse becomes attenuated,[98] rendering the brain less sensitive to any motivational stimulus. The drug user then seeks the lost euphoric response and remains less motivated by any other rewarding activity. In addition, an "antireward" system, mediated by the extended amygdala[38,41] and factors involved in the stress response, causes severe dysphoria when the drug effect wears off. At that point, the addict is motivated to use the drug to seek transient relief from discomfort. In the later stages of addictive drug use, altered dopamine and glutaminergic function in regions of the prefrontal cortex that control self-regulation, inhibitory control, and decision making,[29,97] make it more difficult to choose to refrain from drug use even in the presence of a genuine wish to stop.[97] These conditions help to explain relapse among those who have faced severe adverse consequences of drug use, and the tenacious nature of the illness.

Bonnie[9] discussed issues concerning an addict's ability to choose whether or not to use drugs. He rightly pointed out that one can resist a compulsion, and that having a hard choice and having no choice are profoundly different conditions. Although the "voluntariness" of drug-seeking behavior may be altered by addiction due to the neurobiological vulnerabilities of addicts, drug use is not involuntary. Limited volition and lack of volition are fundamentally different. Bonnie explored issues of the addict's responsibility for becoming addicted, for behaviors caused by addiction, and for sustaining sobriety after diagnosis and treatment. In his analysis, staying sober is the clearest responsibility. Whether or not his view of responsibility for relapse comports with the science of how the brain is enduringly altered by addictive experience, the fact that in some populations the realistic threat of adverse consequences of relapse decreases relapse rates underscores the pragmatism of the concept of responsible choice.

The addiction psychiatrist who is interested in the legal framework for considering these issues should be familiar with landmark judicial decisions in landmark cases. The United States Supreme Court has ruled in three such cases. *Robinson v. California*[79] held that it was unconstitutional to convict a person for being an addict

because to do so would be to punish him for having a disease, in violation of the Eighth Amendment, which prohibits cruel and unusual punishment. But what about behavior caused by or related to addictive illness? Is that punishable? In *Powell v. Texas*,[76] the high court ruled that an extension or broad reading of *Robinson* would not hold. Powell was convicted of public drunkenness, and argued that this was a symptom of a disease, alcoholism, and that he was powerless to control it. The Court ruled that Powell could not be found criminally responsible for being an alcoholic but could be found responsible for being drunk in public. The majority of the justices decided that although Powell was an alcoholic, he did not experience an "irresistible compulsion" that he was "utterly unable to control." Bonnie wrote that the justices in *Powell* were cautious about accepting that conditions that impair volition (such as kleptomania and pyromania) could excuse criminal conduct, and were reluctant to constitutionalize addiction as a justification for such behavior; to do so would "unsettle the law of criminal responsibility." Ironically, this case represented Powell's 100th conviction for public drunkenness. (Criminal responsibility is discussed further, below.)

Montana v. Egelhoff[62] is a more recent landmark case. Egelhoff was convicted of murder even though he argued that his blood alcohol level of 0.36% rendered him incapable of the mental state required for conviction of the crime. The Montana criminal code excluded consideration of voluntary intoxication in determining the mental state of a defendant. The Montana Supreme court overturned the trial court, arguing that "all relevant evidence" should be considered when evaluating whether Egelhoff acted "knowingly and purposefully," the mental state required for conviction. The United States Supreme Court upheld the ruling of the lower court, not the Montana Supreme Court. Although four-fifths of the states permitted the use of information about intoxication in addressing whether a defendant had the mental capacity to form the specific intent to commit a given crime, the Court noted that under well-established common law, voluntary intoxication did not excuse committing a crime. The Court held that general acceptance of taking intoxication into consideration when determining mental state did not make such consideration fundamental. (See below for a discussion of diminished capacity.)

In the future, the neurobiology of choice, volition, and motivation will be better worked out, which will lead to even more spirited discussion of these matters in the courts and in forensic psychiatry. It is wise for all the physicians involved in addiction medicine to keep up with these developments. It will be a challenge to weigh and understand the significance of the effects of illness on behavior and responsibility for that behavior.

Civil Matters

Involuntary Commitment

State and federal laws govern involuntary commitment of a psychiatric patient and/or addicted individual, although there is considerable variation from state to state. Grounds for civil commitment are usually that the individual has a mental disease that is causing dangerousness to self or others or grave disability. Because substance use disorders are mental illnesses according to the psychiatric nomenclature, they qualify as a "mental disease" that causes dangerousness or grave disability. However, there is state-to-state variability in this, as well as variable interpretation of the involuntary commitment statute in a given state over time. Furthermore, some states have separate involuntary commitment laws specific to alcohol and/or drug problems. Those states also may require that an individual committed under such a statute be treated in a facility approved and designated by the responsible state agency. Such a facility need not be a psychiatric hospital. When addictive illness is comorbid with another psychiatric disorder that is also a cause of the dangerousness or disability, civil commitment to a psychiatric facility is appropriate. It is essential for psychiatrists and other physicians to familiarize themselves with the range of statutory obligations and conditions for civil commitment in the jurisdiction in which they practice, including the regulations and case law in situations in which addictive disorder is the mental disease. In states with such laws, familiarity with specific commitment statutes for alcohol or drugs (and in some states it is only one or the other) is similarly necessary.

Civil Competencies

There are many areas in which a psychiatrist may be asked to evaluate whether someone is competent. These include competence to sign into a hospital voluntarily, to consent to other surgical procedures, to sign a contract, and to make a will, among others. Addictive disorders can impair these competencies. Impairment is characteristically caused by problems with cognition or judgment related to intoxication, withdrawal, persistent cognitive problems caused by substance use, or the combined impairment of these functions linked to the addiction and a co-occurring psychiatric illness. In determining competence, one must know the criteria for competence for the particular act in question. It is wise to ask the attorney or court requesting the evaluation to provide the examining psychiatrist with a copy of the statute or case that defines the competence. If the examiner finds that the examinee is not competent, the report should be accompanied by an explanation of how the substance-related illness was diagnosed, how specific symptoms resulted in the compromise of competence, and which criteria for competence are compromised by those symptoms.

Disability

Eligibility for disability benefits and eligibility for protections under disability laws are the two areas covered in this section. The reader should note that "disability" is another word with a meaning that differs across contexts, in this case even across forensic contexts.

If an individual is covered by private disability insurance, the meaning of disability is defined by the policy. The evaluating physician should review that definition and be clear about the criteria before rendering an opinion.[55] Criteria can include being unable to perform all duties of the job or able to perform only one or more duties. The policy may cover disability for a specific job, say, transplant surgeon, or although the examinee is a transplant surgeon the policy may cover only the more general job of physician. In the latter circumstance, even if the physician could no longer work as a transplant surgeon as a result of addictive illness, the examiner could find the doctor disabled under the policy only if the doctor could no longer work in any field of medicine as a physician. In some policies, the coverage is job specific for a period of time, and then general. Some disability carriers do not ask the evaluating physician to render an opinion about disability (a legal adjudication regarding whether they have met policy criteria for being found disabled) but rather ask for an opinion about impairment (a medical conclusion about loss of function).[55] If rendering an opinion that an examinee with a substance-related

disorder (or additional other mental disorder) is impaired, the evaluator should describe how the diagnosis was reached, note the symptoms present, and illustrate how the symptoms cause loss of specific functions. If rendering an opinion about disability, one must add an account of the job duties affected by this impairment and address the policy criteria for disability. In looking at these questions, a physician could consider whether the claimant is disabled by active addiction, the need to obtain treatment, the need to pursue recovery activities so extensive as to preclude work, the need to recuperate and convalesce, or the need to handle a specific stressor.[17] Disability companies may be reluctant to consider the risk for relapse as relevant to disability and prefer to address only here-and-now impairments and restrictions related to active disease or treatment. If the examiner believes that relapse is a major clinical risk and danger, it is vital to explain this in detail. For instance, one study of resident anesthesiologists addicted to the parenteral use of fentanyl found that when, after treatment, they returned to the operating room, death was a first symptom of relapse in an extraordinarily high number of cases[51] (although subsequent studies cast doubt on this finding[18,72,87]). It has thus been argued that this specific pattern of addiction renders an anesthesiologist permanently disabled from operating room practice. The authors note that many disability companies stress that losing one's license to practice one's profession, even if due to illness, does not necessarily imply that the professional is disabled.

Because both other psychiatric disorders and medical disorders often complicate addictive illness, the presence of such illness should be noted in disability-related examinations. How each disorder affects the other (for an excellent discussion of this, see Weiss[101]) and the ways in which functional impairment and limitations are produced (or not) are essential aspects of such a discussion.

Social Security provides disability benefits through Social Security Disability Insurance and Supplemental Security Income. The criteria for a finding of disability are specified in the Social Security regulations but will not be reviewed in this chapter (see Metzner and Buck[55]) because substance-related disorders alone do not qualify someone for compensation in this system. The Contract with America Advancement Act of 1996 abolished substance use disorders as a cause of disabling impairment. If an individual suffers from other psychiatric or medical disorders and also from addictive disease, he or she may qualify, but only if he or she would continue to be disabled upon stopping the use of substances.[55] In the same way, in the absence of another psychiatric or medical condition, an individual is not eligible for disability benefits under the Veterans Administration for an addictive disorder alone.[6] The reason for this exclusion relates to a United States Supreme Court ruling concerning a Veterans Administration case in which the alcoholic drinking was determined to be willful misconduct, and willful misconduct disqualifies someone for such benefits under Veterans Administration regulations.[93]

Protections from workplace discrimination for disabled persons are offered by the Americans with Disabilities Act of 1990 (ADA).[5] The statute defines a covered disability as one that substantially limits one or more major life activities as a result of illness. The ADA protections require an employer to offer reasonable accommodation to a qualified (disabled) individual in performing his or her basic job functions unless such accommodation would impose undue hardship on the employer.[26] Individuals with addictive disorders may be covered under the ADA, but only in a limited and specific manner. The ADA differentiates alcohol and illegal drugs, and protects those addicted to them differently.[102] Individuals with alcohol dependence are protected under the ADA, but in order for those addicted to illegal drugs to be protected they must be in or have completed treatment for addiction and must not be currently using such drugs. The ADA only protects those addicted to legal but controlled substances if they are under the care of a licensed health care professional. An addict's posing a danger to the safety of others (or possibly oneself) is not covered under the ADA. Courts have issued contradictory opinions as to whether the employee is protected in cases when performance problems or workplace misconduct is clearly causally related to the addictive disorder. Performance problems caused by using alcohol away from work may not be protected.[7] Recent case law has limited the ADA protections afforded to those with substance use disorders.[102] Although it is settled law that preemployment drug tests are not considered medical tests under the ADA[24] and can therefore can be used by employers to screen out drug using job applicants, a recent Federal Court case[23] differentiated between licit and illicit drugs in these preemployment drug tests. The defendant employers lawfully tested their job applicant for drugs, but denied him a job offer based on a positive result for a prescribed medication. The court found that this action violated the ADA, since the drug test was not in fact for an illegal drug. Employers must therefore carefully distinguish between drugs used illegally, which are a basis for exclusion from job offers, and similar drugs which are used with a legitimate prescription.

Professional Liability

Issues in the prescribing of addictive compounds to a variety of patients and in the management of addicted individuals can give rise to malpractice claims and litigation. The most common allegations in such litigation include that prescribing addictive medication led to the death or suicide of a patient or to the patient developing an addictive illness, or that failure to assess and diagnose addictive illness led to inappropriate prescribing or inappropriate monitoring of addictive medications. Most of these claims involve the prescribing of opioids or benzodiazepines. Less commonly such suits allege failure to recognize alcohol dependence or to consider the risks of cross-addiction. Cross-addiction is sometimes narrowly conceptualized as a person addicted to one drug becoming addicted to another substance. However, a more common cross-addiction problem is relapsing on one's drug of choice because of exposure to another drug of abuse. Litigation also arises out of the alleged failure to obtain informed consent concerning the addictive characteristics of medications prescribed for a variety of conditions and the ensuing risk of developing addictive illness.[7]

Suicide is the most frequent precipitant for malpractice claims against psychiatrists and is not an uncommon source of claims for other medical practitioners who treat addictions and other mental disorders. Those with addictive illness, alone or with co-occurring other psychiatric conditions, are at significantly increased risk for suicide. Obviously, attempted suicide also is commonly associated with substance intoxication. Substance-related disorders and depression commonly co-occur because addiction causes depression, depression heightens the risk for addiction, or they exist independently and affect each other. Because addiction also affects the social and occupational arenas, morbidity and losses further enhance suicide risk. Clearly, managing suicide risk is an integral part of the job for anyone treating substance-related disorders.

Strategies for managing chronic nonmalignant pain in a person with an opioid or other addictive disorder remain controversial, as is the related question of the frequency with which pain patients develop addictive illness when treated with opioids.[13] All pain patients should be assessed for substance-related disorders and for risk factors for developing such disorders. Assessing the patient, discussing risks with the patient, and documenting one's reasoning about the risks and benefits of the prescribed treatment are all central to the management of liability risk in these cases.

The forensic assessment of alleged medical negligence requires being familiar with the standard of care concerning the medical practice at issue. Given that malpractice cases involving the management and treatment of addiction may also include questions on a wide range of subjects, such as the treatment of a co-occurring psychiatric illness, the appropriateness of prescribing and following the use of addictive substances, or the meaning of toxicology or autopsy findings in a person with an addictive disorder, it is necessary for the medical expert to know the relevant standards of care, including the presence of controversies and other unsettled areas of clinical protocol. It is vital for medical experts to be clear to referring parties as to the areas and limits of their expertise.

Confidentiality

The federal confidentiality statute (42 CFR, Part 2) was intended to guarantee that an individual who voluntarily seeks treatment for addictive illness is not subject to a penalty that someone who does not seek treatment for the same condition would not suffer—that penalty being loss of confidentiality concerning the addictive condition.[26] Although this law specifically addresses alcohol or drug treatment programs that receive federal funding (such as federal tax-exempt status), it is prudent to consider that it applies to all treatment and evaluation settings. The law greatly restricts communication about such a client or patient without a signed, written release of information. A few examples of communication permitted by the statute include when there is a need to address a life- or health-threatening medical emergency, report a crime committed in the program setting or in which treatment personnel are victims, report child abuse, or respond to a court order (among other conditions). Note that a subpoena is not a court order and is not an exception to the statute. The authors recommend consulting with an attorney knowledgeable about 42 CFR, Part 2, if treatment records are subpoenaed; responding to a subpoena without contesting it has been the source of successful litigation alleging violation of confidentiality. Under the statute, patients may rescind their release of information at any time, except when their treatment is a condition of parole or probation. The law presents many complexities that require interpretation in the context of each treatment situation. When does a person acquire the status of "patient" for whose protection the law provides? At the point of referral, the first phone call, or the first visit? This is only one of the myriad questions that may arise given the breadth and complexity of the law. The structure of each program, agency, or other practice environment may be sufficiently unique that legal consultation is necessary to understand the implications of this statute. Other issues may arise because of conflict between the federal statute and various state laws. Generally, federal law supersedes state law in confidentiality unless state law is more restrictive. Sorting out a program's or a physician's risks and responsibilities requires careful thought and often legal input. For a more extensive discussion of 42 CFR, see Brooks.[10]

Another law that protects the privacy of patient information is the Health Insurance Portability and Accountability Act of 1996 (or HIPAA), promulgated by the United States Department of Health and Human Services. This law applies to a variety of health care providers, including addiction treatment programs, if they electronically transmit individually identifiable patient information. However, because the confidentiality requirements are stricter in 42 CFR, Part 2, the authors will not address the HIPAA in this chapter.

Duty to Protect or Warn

A physician's or psychiatrist's duty to warn or protect a specific person whose safety has been threatened by a patient may be in conflict with other legal and ethical requirements of medical practice, such as protecting the confidentiality of the threatening patient. That the patient has an addiction neither alters the essence of this duty nor makes the conflict easier to resolve. This duty originated with *Tarasoff*, a California Supreme Court decision.[91] Although this ruling has evolved in California, it is the basis of similar laws or case law in most states. The duty to warn is usually met by notifying the threatened person or the police of the patient's threat to harm; the duty to protect also may be met by involuntary commitment of the patient. Because law and case law vary so considerably between states, physicians and program personnel should be knowledgeable about the duty as it applies in the jurisdictions in which they practice. A major difference in the manner in which warnings should be given when the threatening patient is in addiction treatment, versus other psychiatric or medical treatment, is that under 42 CFR, Part 2, the notification to the threatened person or to law enforcement should not reveal that the patient has a substance-related disorder.

Child Custody

Child custody proceedings are at best adversarial and at worst a vitriolic environment. Even when divorce is first raised, in the hope to gain leverage or advantage, one parent may threaten the other that his or her real or alleged substance abuse will damage rights to child custody. It is not unusual for these questions to be raised in the custody proceedings, and addiction experts are frequently retained to evaluate such cases. In practice, courts vary considerably in how much weight they give to a mere history of an addiction in a parent. Many courts have ruled that a parent who has obtained appropriate help for his or her addiction and/or can demonstrate recovery or abstinence is not disadvantaged. On the other hand, the court will want to know the evaluator's opinion as to whether or not the parent has such a condition, his or her degree of insight, whether he or she has had appropriate treatment, the outcome of treatment, the prognosis, and so on. In addition, the evaluator should address the impact of the substance-related disorder on—and its interaction with—other medical and psychiatric illness. The court may ask for the evaluator's treatment recommendations. The evaluator also should be prepared to discuss the question of whether a child has been harmed or neglected by an addicted parent and the likelihood of this occurring in the future. The standard used by the courts in these proceedings is the parent's ability to attend to the best interests and safety of the child or children.[40] Occasionally addiction clinicians are asked to administer a court-ordered monitoring program for a custodial parent who misuses, or is accused of misusing, addictive substances. The clinician should assist the court in drafting that plan, but in the final analysis, the clinician must accommodate the final court order, rather than the other way around. The essential elements of a child custody drug and alcohol monitoring program

include a definition of the relevant substances, a workable and effective testing protocol, and a selection of random, scheduled, or for-cause testing or some combination thereof. It is important to note that each monitoring program must contain a carefully structured definition of the consequences of a positive or missed test. In protecting the best interests of the child, the consequences of a positive or missed test usually include the immediate transfer of the child to a safe environment. This most commonly involves the person who receives the positive test result—usually a physician monitoring the testing—notifying the other parent, or the other parent's attorney, of the positive test result.

Criminal Matters

Competence to Stand Trial

Competence to stand trial in a criminal matter is related to the current mental state of the individual charged with a crime, not to his or her state of mind at the time of the crime's commission. Neither intoxication from a substance of abuse nor withdrawal from such a drug is likely to impair such competence because these conditions would have resolved long before the pretrial process. Nevertheless, accused persons have been known to come to their competence evaluation severely intoxicated in hopes of being found incompetent. Some examples of substance-related conditions that can impact competence include enduring toxic states (such as an amphetamine- or hallucinogen-induced psychotic disorder, which may last for weeks), other persistent conditions (which may last months or longer), and brain injury caused by drug use.

Dusky v. United States[20] is the landmark United States Supreme Court case that defines incompetence to proceed in a criminal matter. It is utilized in all states with minor variations. *Dusky* states, "The test must be whether he [the defendant] has sufficient present ability to consult with his attorney with a reasonable degree of rational understanding and a rational as well as a factual understanding of the proceedings against him." The competence evaluator must examine carefully the current mental condition of the examinee, asking very specific questions about his or her comprehension of the legal process and assessing the ability to work rationally with the attorney in his or her defense. To determine a defendant's knowledge of the legal process, forensic examiners frequently ask defendants to recite and discuss the charges against them and the job of the various players in the courtroom. In determining their ability to cooperate with their attorney, it is useful to ask how they decide what is pertinent to discuss with their attorney and how they manage their relationship with their attorney when there is divergence about the best way to defend the case. It is also key to determine how accurately the defendant understands the possible outcomes of various legal strategies in the case. In all cases where the examiner finds incompetence, the written report and subsequent testimony should note the diagnosis and symptoms and describe the manner by which the symptoms interfere with competence criteria in *Dusky*. The examiner also should recommend any treatment that might restore competence and the likelihood of restoration. Because—as noted above—substance-related disorders only lead to incompetence proceeding under narrow conditions, it is especially important to explain how and why the condition continues to affect the accused, which will require knowledge of the toxicity of the drug responsible for the disorder and/or the nature of the brain injury associated with the use of that substance.

Sanity and Diminished Capacity

The question of sanity in a criminal case has to do with the state of mind of the defendant at the time of commission of the criminal act, not with his or her mental state at the time of trial. The insanity defense has its roots in the common law of England, which recognized that under specific circumstances a mentally ill person should not be held responsible for a criminal act. In the majority of states in the United States, the definition of insanity applies to defendants who, as a result of mental disease or defect, are unable to know or understand the nature and quality of their criminal act or are incapable of distinguishing right from wrong in relation to that act. This test is referred to as the M'Naghten Standard, named after the defendant in an 1843 case in England.[61] M'Naghten is a cognitive standard, referring to what a defendant fails to know and understand. Several states use both the cognitive test and a volitional test. The volitional arm is often modeled after the standard published by the American Law Institute.[3] This volitional test considers that defendants can avoid criminal responsibility if they were, as a result of mental disease or defect, unable to conform their behavior to the requirements of the law. In most cases and jurisdictions, substance use of any kind, even when the defendant has a substance use disorder, is not an allowable defense under an insanity plea in a criminal case. Most courts have found that voluntary ingestion of a substance of abuse does not excuse criminal behavior. That drugs of abuse and addictive illness can impair volition, however, may be relevant in states with a volitional arm in the law that governs the insanity defense. Clearly, it is imperative that forensic examiners know the laws in the state or states in which they practice so that they know exactly the applicable definition(s) of insanity, including the conditions that are excluded as arguments. When in doubt, the examiner should request that the referring court or attorney give him or her a copy of the relevant laws and cases.

A few specific clinical situations involving substance use may be relevant to sanity even under a strict cognitive test, such as involuntary intoxication, in which the defendant was poisoned or tricked into using a drug that resulted in criminal behavior. Another example is when a criminal act was committed during a withdrawal delirium. In a few states, a persistent drug-induced psychosis may be an admissible factor in an insanity defense. *People v. Kelly*[75] is a California case in which Kelly attempted to kill her mother after recent exposure to mescaline and a long history of hallucinogen use. She believed that her mother was "with the devils." She had a previous history of persistent psychotic states related to drug use and remained psychotic for several months after she attempted to kill her mother. The court ruled: "We hold that such a temporary psychosis which was not limited merely to periods of intoxication…and which rendered defendant insane under the M'Naghten test constitutes a settled insanity that is a complete defense to the offense here charged." In other states, in lower courts, cases similar to *Kelly* have not been opened to the insanity defense. *Kelly* also referred to "settled psychosis" and brain damage; brain damage due to addiction under certain circumstances may be used in an insanity defense.[40] *Kelly* also termed Kelly's mental condition as one of "pathological intoxication," further confusing an already puzzling concept.[73] "Pathological" or "idiosyncratic" intoxication is a state in which an individual undergoes a strange and previously unfamiliar reaction to drug exposure. There are a few jurisdictions in which the occurrence of pathological intoxication has qualified a criminal defendant to use the insanity defense.

Diminished capacity is another important legal concept in the domain of criminal responsibility; it is a partial defense, and, as in *Egelhoff* (see section "Compulsion and Responsibility"), voluntary ingestion of a substance of abuse may be considered relevant. This defense applies only in cases in which a conviction requires proving that the defendant had the specific intent to commit the crime, meaning that the defendant had to deliberate or harbor the thought of the specific crime. Specific-intent crimes include first- and second-degree murder, as opposed to most felonies, which require proving only general intent for conviction. If upon examination a forensic evaluator finds, and the fact finder—the judge or jury—agrees, that due to ingestion of a drug of abuse a defendant could not form the specific intent to commit second-degree murder, then the accused can only be found guilty of the lesser charge of manslaughter. Like the insanity defense and most other matters considered in this chapter, the diminished capacity (or "diminished responsibility") defense varies between jurisdictions. In fact, California has abolished the diminished capacity defense and replaced it with the concept of diminished actuality.[78,98,100] Under this structure, the issue thus becomes whether a defendant actually formed specific intent, not whether he or she had the capacity to do so. A psychiatrist or other forensic evaluator cannot opine on the question of what actually happened; this is a question that can be addressed only by the finder of fact. The evaluator may still testify about the state of mind of the accused and the effects of drug use on his or her mental state. This may provide some information for the fact finder about specific intent. Knowing current state law is again necessary for psychiatrists and other forensic evaluators involved in evaluating someone in which such a defense is being considered.

In alcoholic blackouts, there is anterograde amnesia for some or all events that transpired during a drinking experience. In typical cases, the individuals are described by others as behaving purposefully, but they cannot recall their actions. Controversy about whether blackouts should be considered under the concept of diminished capacity rests on the issue of whether or not the individual experiencing the blackout is capable of forming criminal intent. The blackout syndrome certainly occurs, and memory loss is an essential feature, but whether or not behavior performed during a blackout is intentional is not clear.[32,52]

Imperfect self-defense is another construct in which substance use may be relevant in a criminal defense. The essential element is that the defendant believes, incorrectly, that he or she was in danger and the criminal act was thus believed to be in self-defense to prevent bodily harm or injury. Consider a person who kills another because of such a belief—a paranoid delusion caused by chronic stimulant dependence. If persuaded that this were the case, a court might find such a defendant guilty of manslaughter rather than murder.

Sentencing

The sentencing phase of a criminal trial is another arena in which a court may hear expert testimony about substance use and addiction, although it is difficult to predict whether this testimony will be seen as aggravating or mitigating. Consider a vehicular homicide case in which at sentencing the addiction expert presents information about the defendant's severe sedative dependence and how sincere and successful the accused has been in subsequent recovery since the homicide. The defense may call the expert in hopes that the jury will think about a lesser sentence but find the jury members irate that the defendant did not responsibly seek treatment before anyone was killed, and thus be inclined toward a harsher sentence. Similarly, in death penalty cases, it may be difficult to predict whether testimony about drug or alcohol use or addiction will be viewed as aggravating or mitigating by a judge or jury. The ability of the expert witness to communicate effectively is of paramount importance in this phase of a criminal trial.

Pregnancy, Harm to the Fetus, and Child Abuse

In alarming developments, pregnant women have been successfully prosecuted for harming their fetuses by abusing drugs. Laws enabling such prosecution are becoming more common [Adams]. As of 2014, the only states in which such prosecutions have been upheld are South Carolina and Alabama.[1,25] The first two South Carolina cases are instructive. In *Regina McKnight v. State of South Carolina*,[48] McKnight's stillborn child's blood contained cocaine metabolites. She was charged with homicide by child abuse and sentenced to a 20-year jail term. In *Cornelia Whitner v. State of South Carolina*,[104,105] Whitner's child was taken from her care after testing positive for cocaine metabolites. Whitner was prosecuted under South Carolina's child neglect statute for having exposed her fetus and subsequent child to cocaine. She was sentenced to a jail term of 8 years. The Supreme Court of South Carolina upheld these decisions upon appeal. The United States Supreme Court denied *certiorari*—that is, declined to review either case on further appeal. This was despite numerous national professional organizations, such as the American Academy of Addiction Psychiatry and the American Psychiatric Association, having filed amicus briefs on behalf of *McKnight*. However, in 2008 the Supreme Court of South Carolina reversed the *McKnight* decision based on the ineffective assistance of counsel.[89]

In *Whitner*, the potential harm to the fetus was considered to be information that she should have considered to be "...well documented and in the realm of public knowledge...." Thus, the court considered Whitner "on notice that her conduct in utilizing cocaine during pregnancy constituted child endangerment," as if knowledge could be expected to serve as the antidote to addictive drug use. The Court in *McKnight* reasoned similarly, finding that she had the requisite criminal intent to kill her child (defined as "the person causes the death of a child under the age of eleven while committing child abuse or neglect, and the death occurs under circumstances manifesting an extreme indifference...to human life"[83]). To our knowledge, the defense of these and similar cases has not involved the argument that criminal intent was marginal or absent as a result of the addiction. It is also counterintuitive to believe that addicted pregnant women have had the intent to harm their fetuses, any more than pregnant women who consume alcohol or nicotine, the most common drug-related causes of fetal harm. The successful prosecution of these cases followed from the interpretation that the South Carolina child abuse and neglect statutes applied to the unborn. McKnight pointed to sections of those statutes that addressed harm due to corporal punishment and/or abandonment, which could only apply to children. The Court considered whether "this demonstrates that the statute was clearly intended to apply only to children. However, section 16-3-85(B) [of the statute] also defines harm as inflicting or allowing to be inflicted on the child physical injury ... and failing to supply the child with adequate health care ... Either of these provisions may clearly be applied to an unborn child. Accordingly, given the language of the statute, and this Court's prior opinions defining

a child to include a viable fetus, we find the plain language of the statute does not preclude its application to the present case."

An interesting twist on such prosecutions is *Lovill v. Texas*, in which Lovill, a pregnant probationer in treatment for cocaine addiction, experienced relapse, thereby violating her probation. The state of Texas decided to incarcerate her in order to protect her fetus, although such probation violations are typically treated with less-restrictive actions. This action was reversed on appeal.[46] The Court of Appeals ruled that the prosecution represented a violation of Lovill's 14th Amendment protection against sex discrimination: "The evidence shows (1) that Lovill was treated differently than others who violated the terms of their probation but were not pregnant, and (2) that her pregnancy was a motivating factor in the decision to prosecute."

There are many criticisms of these decisions and similar prosecutions across the country. In most cases, there is a strong argument that science does not support the reputed harm attributed to drugs of abuse such as cocaine. Ironically, similar charges have not been brought against women who use the two drugs of abuse that are most closely associated with fetal harm, alcohol and nicotine, although such prosecutions are possible under most of these laws. (In a Wisconsin case a woman was prosecuted for alcohol use during pregnancy, but this case was dismissed.[30]) As was argued in a similar case in Maryland[16] following *Robinson*, addiction is a disease, not subject to punishment and not cured by self-discipline or health warnings. Criminal penalties are likely to result in harm to newborns by virtue of separating them from their mother. Perhaps most important, it is likely that once it is known that mothers will be prosecuted under these conditions, they will avoid seeking medical care during pregnancy, including treatment for addictive illness or the many causes of fetal and maternal morbidity. Thus mothers will be deterred from seeking care for themselves and their fetuses, their medical care and health will be undermined, and the very children intended to be protected by these legal actions will experience greater endangerment.[84] These recent decisions are important lessons in how, even in relatively well-informed contemporary times, the legal system can act on biased presuppositions and endanger the very individuals it is trying to protect. These cases also underscore the importance of the legal and medical/psychiatric communities communicating about such legal movements so that they can be addressed through the work of professional organizations serving as *amici*. Adams[1] has provided a recent review of the history, cases, and legal and social arguments related to these laws.

Addiction in Criminal Populations

A great majority, up to 95% in some studies, of individuals in prisoner populations have some form of addictive illness.[40,42] Estimates from 2004 found that half of prisoners in federal and state prisons met criteria for drug abuse or dependence.[63] More than half of state and federal prisoners reported being under the influence of drugs or alcohol at the time of their criminal offense.[12] These findings raise the important question of the relationship between substance use and criminality. Of course, this is a broad subject in which there are opposing views. One idea is that criminals become involved with drugs along with other criminal activities and that incarceration is the correct punishment.[86] Another analysis argues that drug-abusing individuals commit crimes related to and caused by their addiction. A corollary of the latter analysis is that treatment is the only remedy for criminal behavior caused by addictive illness; punishment is less likely to remedy such behavior. Studies that show decreased criminal recidivism following addiction treatment support this point of view.[31,99] These ideas also have given rise to the development of alternatives to incarceration such as drug courts (discussed below) and similar diversion programs. Court-ordered, coerced addiction treatment has been found to be effective.[57]

Despite the fact that so many prisoners have addictive disorders and that their crimes were committed while they under the influence, only about 40% of state and federal prisons provided on-site addiction treatment in 1997.[90] Only about one-third of state and one-fourth of federal inmates reported receiving drug or alcohol treatment in that year.[37]

Standards for correctional mental health care have been published by The National Commission on Correctional Health Care in 1999 and the American Psychiatric Association in 2000. The principle behind these recommendations is that the same level of mental health services should be provided to each individual in the criminal justice system as is available in the community.[56] The situation in correctional addiction treatment falls short of this target.

Among the many kinds of treatment programs offered in correctional settings, the most successful are residential programs,[74] including therapeutic communities,[103] which require 6–24 months to complete. The most successful groups in terms of success with criminal recidivism are those individuals who complete a therapeutic community treatment in prison and, upon release from incarceration, enter a community-based residential therapeutic community or other aftercare.[60] Jails and prisons also utilize less-intensive programs, especially for those who reside in the general population of prisoners (as opposed to higher security levels or protective custody), which may engage a prisoner up to 4 hours a day—short-term programs in which the goal is to motivate inmates to obtain addiction treatment in the community when released, that is, group and individual therapies modeled after outpatient community treatment. Twelve-step programs are generally available, although in many jails and prisons not widely so—that is, there are few meetings, and they may not be available throughout the facility. Twelve-step programs are often problematic to utilize in correctional settings because of their emphasis on openness and honesty, whereas in most other prison venues the "convict code" ("don't rat on another inmate") and the need for protecting oneself physically and emotionally rule inmate behavior. It is important to underscore that most correctional programming for the treatment of substance use disorders consists of self-help groups such as 12-step meetings and educational groups, rather than clinical, therapeutic, and pharmacotherapeutic interventions.[92] Standards for the treatment of substance use disorders in correctional settings have been articulated[53,54,67] but may not be employed. Similarly, standards for detoxification are included in these guidelines, but the availability of this care is not uniform,[63] which unfortunately leads to morbidity and mortality in correctional settings.

In addition, there is a high rate of comorbid psychiatric illness among criminal offenders with addiction problems. However, there are few treatment programs in jails and prisons for this population. In correctional settings, there is a long history of bifurcation between the systems that address addiction problems and those that treat mental illness. The paucity of programming for comorbid conditions in part reflects this legacy. Another problem is that therapeutic communities and other residential programs in correctional settings are psychologically stressful because of their emphasis on one-to-one confrontational techniques. This makes it troublesome to tolerate, if not contraindicated, for inmates with moderate-to-severe mental illnesses. More intensive psychiatric services and modified therapeutic community techniques are necessary for this population.[22]

Drug Courts

Drug courts have taken hold in the popular imagination: one newspaper story reported that as an addicted woman graduated from a drug court program, "Prosecutors and public defenders applauded when she was handed her certificate; a policewoman hugged her, and a child shouted triumphantly, 'Yeah, Mamma!'[21]" Although such optimism is encouraging, the drug court model deserves a rigorous evaluation. The diversion of nonviolent drug offenders to drug courts is increasingly popular and, as defined by the United States Department of Justice, "…(integrates) substance abuse treatment, sanctions, and incentives with case processing to place nonviolent drug-involved defendants in judicially supervised rehabilitation programs."[19]

Engendered in the late 1980s as the crack cocaine epidemic overwhelmed US jails and prisons, drug courts have evolved as collaborations between the justice system and addiction treaters— collaborations based on the ability of the two camps to speak and understand the other's professional language. Studies reveal that the high up-front cost of drug courts often—but not always—pay off in terms of improved outcomes for addicts and benefits to society, economic and otherwise. Challenges to the drug court model include the obvious bias to help addicts who commit crimes over other addicts who do not, objections to a government mandate for participation in quasi-religious programs such as Alcoholics Anonymous, inadequate data on the overall economic benefits of drug courts, and a philosophical concern about providing punishment for relapse.

Formal drug courts first arose in Judge Stanley Goldstein's 1989 Miami Circuit Court in response to the huge numbers of cocaine-linked offenders flooding the local jails. The prevailing ethos in the late 1980s was a simplistic response to addiction best exemplified by Nancy Reagan's 1982 recommendation that people should "just say no"[43] to drugs. It quickly became apparent to the court that addicted offenders responded well to the treatment services offered, and made quantifiable gains in terms of reduced criminal activity, educational strides, employment, and stabilized family interactions.

By establishing similar drug court dockets within their courts, judges around the country quickly followed Miami's lead, integrating to various degrees drug law enforcement with addiction treatment. By 2007, all 50 states had active drug courts, with 1932 judges serving on a total of 1662 drug courts nationwide, and with 386 more drug courts in the planning stages.[11]

The concept of therapeutic jurisprudence, which came to fruition in the late 1980s, was defined as "the study of the extent to which substantive rules, legal procedures, and the roles of lawyers and judges produce therapeutic or antitherapeutic consequences for individuals involved in the legal process."[35] This paradigm shift for the legal system was matched by a similar shift in the drug treatment system, an acceptance of the role of coercion in the treatment of addicted individuals:

Addicts need not be internally motivated at the outset of treatment in order to benefit from it. Indeed, addicts who are legally pressured into treatment may outperform voluntary patients, because they are likely to stay in treatment longer and are more likely to graduate.[82]

Unlike the judicial coercion inherent in civil commitment proceedings, entrance into a drug court system necessitates a choice by the addicted offender. He or she may choose to accept the legal consequences of the crime, a choice some make in order to avoid treatment. In many circumstances, the drug treatment entails a longer time under judicial supervision than the threatened jail sentence.

The US Government Accountability Office (GAO) conducted a 2005 meta-analysis of adult drug courts,[95] in which they evaluated 23 programs and found demonstrable reductions in criminal recidivism, although less clear results for actual reductions in drug use. This was confirmed in a 2012 study.[59] The GAO study clearly demonstrated the financial benefits of the drug courts. Generally, the drug court model costs substantially more than the non–drug court model. However, the authors conclude that reductions in recidivism would more than compensate for this increased upfront cost. Another study reached similar conclusions.[8]

Sentencing in drug courts will involve orders to maintain sobriety, attend treatment and support groups, and participate in tissue screening, as well as other requirements that are essentially clinical in their thrust. Addiction specialists are often asked to evaluate criminal offenders related to such sentencing issues. As in other areas of the law that make use of the concept of therapeutic jurisprudence—mental health courts and parental psychiatric evaluation in child-custody disputes—it behooves the addiction specialist to become familiar and comfortable with the actors and institutions of the legal system.

Regulatory Matters

Impairment and Fitness to Practice

The word "impairment" is used quite differently across the literature, and verbiage about impaired professionals. It is sometimes used to refer to having an addictive illness, recovering from an addictive illness, or having an illness that can cause impairment. The authors define it as the inability to practice the profession with sufficient skill and safety to the clientele of that profession due to illness or injury.[27] The illness may be addictive, other psychiatric, or medical, including comorbidities of the three categories. Note that by this definition, having the illness, even if it impairs functioning outside of work, does not constitute impairment. Impairment should be distinguished from deficiencies of knowledge and skill to practice the profession, which have to do with competence. Impairment does not imply incompetence, and incompetence does not imply impairment. Psychiatrists and addiction specialists are often asked by professional licensing boards—regulatory boards that operate based on regulatory laws of the states in the United States—to evaluate practitioners to determine whether they are safe to practice. This raises the question of impairment and the practitioner's fitness for duty, concepts that are related.[6] Professions controlled by regulatory/licensing authorities include most medically related professions (medicine, nursing, dentistry, pharmacy, veterinary medicine, and podiatry) through their boards, attorneys through boards or the state supreme courts, and commercial and private pilots through the Federal Aviation Administration, among others. Each of these agencies has laws, regulations, and policies unique to them; physicians and others performing evaluations for such agencies must become familiar with them individually. For instance, the Federal Aviation Administration has specific ways of defining addictive illness as it applies to commercial pilots; working from the *Diagnostic and Statistical Manual of Mental Disorders* will not suffice.

Impairment, as defined here, usually occurs in the late stages of addictive illness, at least among professionals. Professionals tend to be strongly identified with their profession, and their self-esteem is quite tied to work performance. As a result, even when other areas of life—family, marriage, emotions, and health—are suffering as a result of an addiction, the professional will protect the sanctity of the workplace until the illness is completely out of control. A corollary of this analysis is that by the time impairment occurs, the professional's life—and not just his or her career—is in danger.

When addictive illness causes impairment, it is usually related to symptoms of cognitive dysfunction, emotional liability, impaired judgment, erratic behavior, or a combination thereof. Interference with these functions may be caused by the neurological consequences of substance intoxication, an acute or sustained withdrawal syndrome, or damage to other organs that secondarily affects brain function (e.g., severe liver disease in chronic alcoholism). Chronic exposure to drugs of abuse also causes personality changes, especially irritability, reduced tolerance of frustration and ambiguity, and impulsivity—the psychotoxicity of extended substance exposure. Evaluating fitness for duty requires understanding the nature of the work that the professional is either fit or unfit to practice. In the report, the evaluator should connect the diagnosis to the symptoms, to the bearing of those symptoms on mental and physical functioning, to the relationship between any loss of function and its impact on the duties of the job in question. The report also should discuss treatment for the addiction (and/or the degree to which recovery and abstinence have been achieved), the prognosis, and the best strategies for monitoring the professional in the future. The interplay of the addictive illness with other psychiatric and medical conditions also should be addressed, along with how this might affect work function. Treatment and prognosis of all potentially impairing illnesses should be discussed because the regulatory authority will be concerned about both the present and future safety of the professional's clientele.

"Monitoring" is a technical term referring to how professionals are followed once their condition is known. Monitoring activities support but do not substitute for treatment. In fact, the success of physicians with addictive disorders, defined in terms of rates of recovery and rates of returning to or maintaining professional practice,[18,49] may be largely due to the systematic monitoring that they receive. Monitoring activities typically consist of periodic clinical assessment, random tissue testing for alcohol and drugs (and other laboratory testing for markers of addictive illness), and repeated contact with outside sources of information such as spouse, therapist, treatment program, and the professional's workplace. In the United States and Canada, those doctors with addictive disorders (and other illnesses) are monitored by physician health programs, a variation on the theme of peer assistance programs that are involved with many of the other professions. From profession to profession and from state to state, there is much variability in these programs in terms of the illnesses that they address, their structure, their relationship to the regulatory (licensing) authority, and the laws that govern that authority. Most peer assistance programs provide at least some degree of confidentiality from the licensing board, but only with the consent of the board. Addiction specialists involved in evaluating a professional's fitness for duty should be knowledgeable about the capabilities of the peer assistance program of that profession.

Every physician and other addiction specialist who treats or evaluates professionals should be familiar with the laws that govern the profession, especially as applied to any duties that they may have to report an addicted professional to the licensing authority and whether that report is immune from liability.[81] Taking the example of the Medical Practices Act, which governs physicians in Colorado,[50] the condition of being addicted to alcohol or drugs is classified as unprofessional conduct. All physicians have a duty to report unprofessional conduct to the Board of Medical Examiners. Colorado law, however, provides a reporting exception for a physician involved in treating physicians with mental health problems, including addictions. However, there is an exception to the exception if the treating physician thinks that the physician-patient is not safe to practice. If a doctor makes a report about another physician to the medical board, the doctor is immune from liability, assuming that the action was taken in good faith.

When working with professionals, addiction psychiatrists and other addiction specialists may work in roles other than forensic evaluator, but all roles require knowledge and facility in the forensic world. For instance, working as a treating psychiatrist, especially if treating in the rubric of a professional's participation in a monitoring program or license stipulation, requires understanding the limitations on the confidentiality of the treatment and the specific reporting responsibilities that come with that role. Other possible roles include that of medical directors of monitoring programs, which are embedded in specific legal and regulatory contexts and must be well understood for the program to be effective.

For all addiction specialists working with professionals, it is essential for them to understand the psychology, culture, mores, demands, and realities of that profession: that physicians do not function well as patients,[27] that lawyers often reject the concept of illness as a factor affecting their behavior, that commercial pilots deny weaknesses, and that astronauts believe that they must be perfect in all dimensions, are extremely relevant to evaluating, assessing, and monitoring these professionals.

Tissue Testing

Testing various body tissues for drugs of abuse is a standard practice in the regulation and monitoring of professionals and other workers when public safety is at risk. Commercial pilots, for instance, are randomly tested for drugs and alcohol; the Federal Aviation Administration prohibits pilots from using intoxicants, including legal ones such as alcohol, within 12 hours of flying. Other professionals are routinely required to undergo such testing if they are known to have an addictive illness. In 1988, the United States Department of Health and Human Services published guidelines[94] mandating a drug-free workplace for federal employees. These guidelines also have served as the model for employment policies and practices in private industry. Preemployment screening, random testing, and testing for cause are the common types of testing. Working with government or private industry, an addiction specialist may serve in a clinical role, evaluating individuals found positive on testing, or in a medical review officer role, ensuring that the process of drug testing and the interpretation of the results are appropriate.[88] Medical review officer work requires knowledge of the techniques and procedures of tissue testing so that false positives and false negatives can be distinguished from accurate results. Urine is the tissue that is most commonly screened; all tissues have their advantages and disadvantages. The important variables include the ease of obtaining the sample; ease of tampering with, contaminating, or substituting the sample; length of the window of detection; and likelihood that brief drug exposure could be found in the tissue. Besides urine, sweat (via a skin patch), blood, nails, and hair are the most commonly tested.[96]

Sports

Although the absolute numbers of athletes troubled by addictive illness may seem too small to warrant discussion in this chapter, the types of drugs used and abused in athletic communities are sufficiently different, and how the relevant institutions are responding to these problems are sufficiently important, to merit discussion. Furthermore, the precedents set in this domain may well presage how other arenas of society approach these problems.

Differentiating between addictive responses to substances and the voluntary use of substances for performance enhancement is an important role for the addiction specialist working for a sports organization. Although the categories of "addiction" and "cheating" may seem clear a priori, the two interact in multiple and subtle ways. For instance, the anabolic androgenic steroids are unlikely to engender classic withdrawal and tolerance unless they are taken in massive supraphysiologic doses; some athletes do take them in such doses. Although most sports organizations now classify stimulants as performance-enhancing substances, the stimulants can be used as part of an addictive diathesis, or, more commonly for the elite athlete, their use can evolve from performance enhancing to addictive.

Addiction specialists who understand the legal and procedural framework of modern sports programs can function in one of three separate roles. First, they can work as a medical review officer, whose essential role is overseeing drug testing and verifying the validity of the results. Second, they can work as a treating clinician with a well-defined and transparent reporting obligation. Third, they can develop and administer employee assistance programs for a team or within a particular sport. In all these roles, the combination of addiction and forensic knowledge allows the physician or the professional to produce accurate and helpful case formulations and treatment recommendation. As in other workplaces, the medical review officer must understand the complexities of drug and alcohol testing within the context of the particular industry and federal law, especially the Americans with Disability Act (or ADA).[71] In a sports organization, however, the medical review officer must, in addition, understand the science of testing for the specific drugs used illicitly,[34] the culture and demographics of the program participants, and some specifics about the sport itself. For instance, the medical review officer must schedule the timing of testing before or after competition in order to provide an accurate assessment of any drug use actually taking place, while considering the convenience and dignity of the athletes. Testing for stimulants before a competition is less useful than testing during or after the competition, since illicit users take the substances just before the game or event. As a matter of fairness to athletes with legitimate medical or psychiatric conditions, there is a need for occasional therapeutic use exemptions.[33] The therapeutic use exemption allows an athlete to use a banned substance after an appropriate diagnostic assessment, legitimate prescription, and ongoing monitoring. Psychostimulants for the treatment of attention-deficit disorder (ADD) and attention-deficit/hyperactivity disorder (ADHD) are the most common class of medications for which athletes request a therapeutic use exemption. The addiction specialist working in the sports environment must fashion a plan that allows the person with ADD or ADHD to use appropriately prescribed medication while denying an exemption to individuals who are merely using the medications to improve their athletic performance. In addition, the therapeutic use exemption program must contemplate other potentially therapeutic uses for banned substances, such as testosterone for testicular deficiency, diuretics for hypertension, and opioids for pain. Major sports organizations, including the Olympics,[15] the National Collegiate Athletic Association,[65] the National Football League,[68] Major League Baseball,[47] the Professional Golf Association,[77] and the National Hockey League,[69] have processes for evaluating therapeutic use exemption requests.

In addition to drug and alcohol misuse, athletes and those associated with elite sports are vulnerable to problems with gambling,[6a] and clinicians may be called upon to evaluate, treat, and monitor these individuals. As with substance addiction, the evaluating clinician should avoid advocacy or criticism of the evaluee, and rather focus on the—admittedly sparse—body of psychiatric knowledge surrounding compulsive gambling.[4]

Addiction psychiatrists and other addiction specialists can serve as treating physicians for athletes; a good understanding of forensic issues is important even in this clinical context. Even without any reporting responsibility, the clinician should be aware of the high visibility of elite athletes in the public consciousness: individual courts,[70] the US Congress,[44] and private investigative bodies[58] may request—or subpoena—information about the treatment of such individuals.

Treating an athlete for an addictive disorder, or any substance use, requires that the clinician understand the profound pressures and stresses that affect the athlete. In addition to the rewards of fame and sometimes money that elite athletic performance can bring, the family dynamics of these individuals can be quite disturbing and counterintuitive to the clinician. The desires of family members for material success and celebrity treatment can drive the athlete to behavior that he or she would not otherwise have considered, especially if the financial rewards of peak performance can put food on the table for an otherwise indigent family.

More significant than financial rewards, however, is the internal driving force that the athlete may feel. If one's core value from a very early age is to win at any cost, boundaries often become fluid. Athletes at the elite level are not paralyzed by worry about hurting themselves, or they would not be elite athletes. In 1995, a sports medicine specialist informally posed the following question to 198 Olympic-level athletes:

> If I had a drug that was so fantastic that if you took it once, you would win every competition you would enter, from the Olympic decathlon to the Mr. Universe Contest, for the next five years. But it had one minor drawback: It would kill you five years after you took it. Would you still take it?

More than half of the athletes acknowledged that they would take the drug.[14] So, taking a chance on a performance-enhancing drug might not be a great leap, given the single-minded determination that these athletes have in their emotional repertoire.

For athletes—elite or otherwise—the rationale for allowing a treating psychiatrist or other physician to report relapse to a regulatory authority may appear less convincing than for commercial airline pilots or physicians. For professional athletes, labor unions may necessitate that any monitoring protocol be negotiated under the rules of the National Labor Relations Board.[70] As with any other impaired professional who is part of a monitoring program, the burden falls on the treating physician to make sure that the patient is well aware of the reporting obligations, his or her options for having treatment elsewhere, and the right to withdraw permission for reporting.

The clinician who decides to manage an employee assistance program has different and more complicated obligations than the treating clinician or the medical review officer. The administrator must fashion a program that delivers good care to athletes, functions well from the perspective of management, and conforms to mandates from all applicable laws. An understanding of the sport's culture, and close liaison with coaches, medical staff, and athletic trainers, will ensure that the employee assistance program functions as well as possible in an inherently difficult environment. As is the case with employee assistance programs in other industries, the limits of confidentiality must be spelled out as clearly as possible.

As in all forensic work, the addiction specialist must be prepared to justify clinical and administrative decisions on the basis of evidence-based clinical care and respect for the applicable legal or procedural framework.

Conclusions

There is a broad array of forensic contexts and considerations that present themselves to physicians and other health care providers interested in addictive illness. The contexts range from civil to criminal to regulatory, and within each are complex conceptual problems that must be addressed by the practitioner. This requires mastery of the clinical and scientific elements unique to addictive disease and their intersection with the specific forensic environment. That intersection is approached through unifying principles: neutrality in examination and reporting; addressing multifaceted confidentiality issues; distinguishing clinical from forensic terms; understanding and respecting legal definitions and the institutions from which they flow; working with attorneys and courts to gain sufficient knowledge and comprehension of the forensic questions to be answered; and carefully attending to the policies, statutes, and regulations that define the parameters of the forensic work to be done. The legal realm is not a comfortable one for most medical and psychiatric practitioners; the authors suggest that becoming familiar with this territory and asking for expert consultation when needed will allow those interested in or specializing in addictive illness to enrich their professional experience.

References

1. Adams K. Chemical endangerment of a fetus: societal protection of the defenseless or unconstitutional invasion of women's rights? *Ala L Rev.* 2014;65:1353.
2. American Academy of Psychiatry and the Law. *Ethics Guidelines for the Practice of Forensic Psychiatry*, 2005. http://www.aapl.org/ethics.htm.
3. American Law Institute. *Model penal code, Sec.* 1955;401(1):1 (Tent. Draft No. 4).
4. American Psychiatric Association. *Diagnostic and Statistical Manual of Mental Disorders.* 5th ed. Arlington, VA: American Psychiatric Association; 2013.
5. *Americans with Disabilities Act. 42 USC§§ 12101 et seq.* 1990.
6. Anfang SA, Faulkner LR, Fromson JA, et al. The American Psychiatric association's resource document on guidelines for psychiatric fitness-for-duty evaluations of physicians. *J Am Acad Psychiatry Law.* 2005;33:85–88.
6a. Associated Press. Pete Rose banned for life: Giamatti says he bet on games; appeal possible in year. *The Los Angeles Times* 24 Aug 1989. Print.
7. Beckson M, Bartzokis G, Weinstock R. Substance abuse and addiction. In: Rosner R, ed. *Principles and Practice of Forensic Psychiatry.* London: Arnold; 2003.
8. Bhati AS, Roman JK, Chalfin A. *To Treat or Not to Treat: Evidence of the Prospects of Expanding Treatment Drug-Involved Offenders.* Washington, DC: Justice Policy6 Center, The Urban Institute; 2008.

9. Bonnie RJ. Responsibility for addiction. *J Am Acad Psychiatry Law.* 2002;30:405–413.

10. Brooks MK. Legal aspects of confidentiality of patient information. In: Lowinson JH, Ruiz P, Millman RB, et al., eds. *Substance Abuse, a Comprehensive Textbook.* Baltimore: Williams & Wilkins; 2005.

11. Bureau of Justice Assistance (BJA). Drug court clearinghouse/drug court activity update. 2007. http://spa.american.edu/justice/documents/1956.pdf.

12. Bureau of Justice Statistics. *Substance Abuse and Treatment: State and Federal Prisoners, 1997.* U.S. Dept of Justice NCJ 172871; 1999. http://www.ojp.usdoj.gov/bjs/.

13. Burglass ME. Forensics. In: Lowinson JH, Ruiz P, Millman RB, et al., eds. *Substance Abuse: A Comprehensive Textbook.* 3rd ed. Baltimore: Williams & Wilkins; 1997.

14. Carpenter L. Poor sports: risking livelihood and reputation, some stars don't play by the rules. *The Washington Post.* 2007. http://www.washingtonpost.com/wp-dyn/content/article/2007/07/28/AR2007072801369_pf.html. Accessed 31 Dec 2008.

15. Sports CBS. *Game of Shadows Authors Subpoenaed.* CBS News; 2006, Saturday. http://www.cbsnews.com/stories/2006/05/06/sportsline/main1596031.shtml. Accessed 31 Dec 2008.

16. *Cruz v. Maryland.* WL 6152524 (Md. App.). 2005.

17. Dilts SL, Gendel MH. Substance use disorders. In: Goldman LS, Myers M, Dickstein LJ, eds. *The Handbook of Physician Health.* Chicago: American Medical Association; 2000.

18. Domino KB, Hornbein TF, Polissar NL, et al. Risk factors for relapse in health care professionals with substance use disorders. *J Am Med Assoc.* 2005;293:1453–1460.

19. Drug Courts Program Office. *About the Drug Courts Program Office: FS 000265.* U.S. Department of Justice; 2000.

20. *Dusky v. United States,* 362 U.S. 402 (1960)

21. Eckholm E. Courts give addicts a chance to straighten out. *New York Times.* 2008.

22. Edens JF, Peters RH, Hills HA. Treating prison inmates with co-occurring disorders: an integrative review of existing programs. *Behav Sci Law.* 1997;15:439–457.

23. EEOC v. Grane Healthcare Co. and Ebensburg Care Center, LLC, d/b/a Cambria Care Center, CV No. 3:10-250 (W. Dist. Pa. Mar. 6, 2014).

24. Equal Employment Opportunity Commission http://www.eeoc.gov/policy/docs/medfin5.pdf, Accessed 3/3/2016.

25. Fentiman LC. Rethinking addiction: drugs, deterrence, and the Neuroscience Revolution. *U Pa J.L Soc Change.* 2011;14(233):237–238.

26. 42 U.S.C. §290 dd-2 and 42 Code of Federal Regulations, Part 2.

27. Gendel MH. Treatment adherence among physicians. *Prim Psychiatry.* 2005;12:48–54.

28. Reference deleted in review.

29. Goldstein RZ, Volkow ND. Dysfunction of the prefrontal cortex in addiction: neuroimaging findings and clinical implications. *Nat Rev Neurosci.* 2011;12:652–669.

30. Goodman E. Troubled pregnant women turn to the system-aand the system turns against them. *Miami Herald.* 1990.

31. Gossop M, Trakeada K, Sterward D, et al. Reductions in criminal convictions after addiction treatment: 5-year follow-up. *Drug Alcohol Depend.* 2005;79:295–302.

32. Granacher RP Jr. Commentary: alcoholic blackout and allegation of amnesia during criminal acts. *J Am Acad Psychiatry Law.* 2004;32:371–374.

33. Green GA. Doping control for the team physician: a review of drug testing procedures in sport. *Am J Sports Med.* 2006;34:1690–1698.

34. Hatton CK. Beyond sports-doping headlines: the science of laboratory tests for performance-enhancing drugs. *Pediatr Clin North Am.* 2007;54:713–733.

35. Hora P, Schma W, Rosenthal J. Therapeutic jurisprudence and the drug court movement: revolutionizing the criminal justice system's response to drug abuse and crime in American. *Notre Dame Law Rev.* 1999;74:439–555.

36. Hyman SE. Addiction: a disease of learning and memory. *Am J Psychiatry.* 2005;162:1414–1422.

37. Inciardi J, McBride D, Rivers J. *Drug Control and the Courts.* vol. 3. Thousand Oaks, CA: SAGE; 1996.

38. Jennings JH, Sparta DR, Stamatakis AM, et al. Distinct extended amygdala circuits for divergent motivational states. *Nature.* 2013;496:224–228.

39. Kalivas PW, Volkow ND. The neural basis of addiction: a pathology of motivation and choice. *Am J Psychiatry.* 2005;162:1403–1413.

40. Kermani DJ, Castaneda RC. Psychoactive substance use in forensic psychiatry. *Am J Drug Alcohol Abuse.* 1996;22:17–19.

41. Koob GF, Le Moal M. Plasticity of re- ward neurocircuitry and the 'dark side' of drug addiction. *Nat Neurosci.* 2005;8:1442–1444.

42. Kouri EM, Pope HG, Powell KF, et al. Drug use history and criminal behavior among 133 incarcerated men. *Am J Drug Alcohol Abuse.* 1997;23:413–419.

43. Loizeau PM. *Nancy Reagan: The Woman Behind the Man.* New York: Nova History; 2004.

44. Los Angeles Times. *Congress Wants to Talk to Clemens, McNamee;* 2008.

45. Reference deleted in review.

46. Lovill Appeal. http://www.13thcoa.courts.state.tx.us/opinions/docket.asp?FullDate=20081222. Accessed 25 Aug 2010

47. Major League Baseball/Major League Baseball Player Association Press release (April 11, 2008) MLB, players association modify joint drug agreement

48. McKnight v. State, SC Sup Ct No.25585 (2003).

49. McLellan AT, Skipper GS, Campbell M, et al. Five year outcomes in a cohort study of physicians treated for substance use disorders in the United States. *BMJ.* 2008;337:a2038.

50. Medical Practices Act. *Colorado Revised Statutes.* §§ 12-36-117. (amended 1995).

51. Menk EJ, Baumgarten RK, Kingsley CP, et al. Success of reentry into anesthesiology training programs by residents with a history of substance abuse. *J Am Med Assoc.* 1990;263:3060–3062.

52. Merikangas J. Commentary: alcoholic blackout – does it remove Mens Rea? *J Am Acad Psychiatry Law.* 2004;32:375–377.

53. Metzner J. Standards for health services in jails. *National Commission on Correctional Health Care.* 2008:103–105, 106–108, 177–184.

54. Metzner J. Standards for health services in prisons. *National Commission on Correctional Health Care.* 2008:103–105, 106–108, 177–184.

55. Metzner JL, Buck JB. Psychiatric disability determinations and personal injury litigation. In: Rosner R, ed. *Principles and Practice of Forensic Psychiatry.* London: Arnold; 2003.

56. Metzner JL, Dvoskin JA. Psychiatry in correctional settings. In: Simon RI, Gold LH, eds. *Textbook of Forensic Psychiatry.* Washington, DC: American Psychiatric Publishing; 2004.

57. Miller NS, Flaherty JA. Effectiveness of coerced addiction treatment (alternative consequences): a review of the clinical research. *J Subst Abuse.* 2000;18:9–16.

58. Mitchell GJ, DLA Piper US LLP. *Report to the Commissioner of Baseball of an Independent Investigation into the Illegal Use of Steroids and Other Performance Enhancing Substances by Players in Major League Baseball;* 2007. http://files.mlb.com/mitchrpt.pdf. Accessed 14 Dec 2008..

59. Mitchell O, Wilson D, Eggers A, MacKenzie D. Assessing the effectiveness of drug courts on recidivism: a meta-analytic review of traditional and non-traditional drug courts. *J Crim Justice.* 2012;40:60–71.

60. Mitchell O, Wilson D, MacKenzie D. Does incarceration-based drug treatment reduce recidivism? A meta-analytic synthesis of research. *J Exp Criminol.* 2007;3:353–375.

61. M'Naghten's Case, 8 Eng. *For Rep.* 1843;718:722.

62. Montana v. Egelhoff, 116 S.Ct. 2013 (1996).

63. Mumola C, Karberg J. *Drug Use and Dependence, State and Federal Prisoners, 2004*. Bureau of Justice Statistics Special Report, NCJ 213530. Washington, DC: U.S. Department of Justice, Office of Justice Programs; 2006.

64. National Basketball Association. http://www.nba.com/news/sternpc_070724.html. Accessed 3/4/16.

65. National Collegiate Athletic Association. http://www.ncaa.org/wps/ncaa?ContentID=481. Accessed 03 Nov 2008.

66. National Collegiate Athletic Association. http://www.ncaa.org/health-and-safety/sport-science-institute/mind-body-and-sport-gambling-among-student-athletes. Accessed 3/5/16.

67. National Commission on Correctional Health Care. *Standards for Mental Health Services in Correctional Facilities*; 2015:113–114.

68. National Football League. http://sports.espn.go.com/espnmag/story?section=magazine&id=3636294. Accessed 13 Dec 2008.

69. National Hockey League. http://www.nhl.com/nhlhq/cba/drug_testing072205.html. Accessed 05 Nov 2008.

70. National Labor Relations Board. http://www.nlrb.gov/. Accessed 14 Dec 2008.

71. Olympics. http://www.wada-ama.org/en/World-Anti-Doping-Program/Sports-and-Anti-Doping-Organizations/International-Standards/International-Standard-for-Therapeutic-Use-Exemptions/. Accessed 15 Jun 2010.

72. Oreskovich MR, Caldeiro RM. Anesthesiologists recovering from chemical dependency: can they safely return to the operating room? *Mayo Clin Proc.* 2009;84:576–580.

73. Pandina RJ. Idiosyncratic alcohol intoxication: a construct that has lost its validity?. In: Schlesinger LB, ed. *Explorations in Clinical Psychopathology: Clinical Syndromes with Forensic Implications*. Springfield, IL: Charles C. Thomas; 1996.

74. Pelissier B, Wallace S, O'Neil JA, et al. Federal prison residential drug treatment reduces substance use and arrests after release. *Am J Drug Alcohol Abuse.* 2001;27:315–337.

75. People v. Kelly. 10 Cal.3d 565, 516 P.2d 875, 111 Cal. Rptr. 171.

76. Powell v. Texas, 392 U.S. 514 (1968).

77. Professional Golf Association Tour. *Anti-Doping Program Manual*; 2008:27–32.

78. Resnick PJ, Noffsinger S. Competency to stand trial and the insanity defense. In: Simon RI, Gold LH, eds. *Textbook of Forensic Psychiatry*. Washington, DC: American Psychiatric Publishing; 2004.

79. Robinson v. California, 370 U.S. 660 (1962).

80. Rosner R, ed. *Principles and Practice of Forensic Psychiatry*. London: Arnold; 2005.

81. Sadoff RL, Sadoff JB. The impaired health professional: legal and ethical issues. In: Bluestone H, Travin S, Marlowe DB, eds. *Psychiatric-Legal Decision Making by the Mental Health Practitioner: The Clinician as de Facto Magistrate*. New York: Wiley; 1994.

82. Satel S. *Drug Treatment, the Case for Coercion*. Washington, DC: AEI; 1999.

83. S.C.Code Ann For. §16–3–85(A).

84. Sikich K. Peeling back the layers of substance abuse during pregnancy. *DePaul J Health Care L.* 2005;369.

85. Simon RI, Gold LH, eds. *The American Psychiatric Association Text-Book of Forensic Psychiatry*. 2nd ed. Washington, DC: American Psychiatric Publishing, Inc; 2010.

86. Sinha R, Easton C. Substance abuse and criminality. *J Am Acad Psychiatry Law.* 1999;27:513–523.

87. Skipper GE, Campbell MD, DuPont RL. Anesthesiologists with substance use disorders: a 5-year outcome study from 16 state physician health programs. *Anesth Analg.* 2009;109:891–896.

88. Smith DE, Glatt W, Tucker W, et al. Drug testing in the workplace: integrating medical review officer duties into occupational medicine. *Occupational Med.* 2002;17:79–90.

89. State v. McKnight 661 S.E.2d 354 (S.C. 2008).

90. Substance Abuse and Mental Health Services Administration. *Office of Applied Studies. Substance abuse Treatment in Adult and Juvenile Correctional Facilities*; 2000. http://www.oas.samhsa.gov/UFDS/CorrectionalFacilities97/hilite_m.htm. Accessed 25 Aug 2010.

91. Tarasoff v. Regents of the University of California, 17 Cal 3d 425 (1976).

92. Taxman FS, Perdoni M, Harrison L. Drug treatment services for adult offenders: the state of the state. *J Substance Abuse Treat.* 2007;32:239–254.

93. Traynor and McKelvey v. Turnage, Vol. 485 U.S. 539 (1988).

94. United States Department of Health and Human Services. *The Mandatory Guidelines for Federal Workplace Drug Testing Programs: Final Guidelines*. Washington, DC: U.S. Department of Health and Human Services; 1988.

95. United States Government Accountability Office. *Adult Drug Courts, Evidence Indicated Recidivism Reductions and Mixed Results for Other Outcomes*. Report to Congressional Committees, GAO-05-219. 2005.

96. Verebey KG, Meehan G, Buchan BJ. Diagnostic laboratory: screening for drug abuse. In: Lowinson JH, Ruiz P, Millman RB, et al., eds. *Substance Abuse, a Comprehensive Textbook*. 4th ed. Philadelphia: Lippincott Williams & Wilkins; 2005.

97. Volkow ND, Koob GF, McLellan AD. Neurobiologic advances from the brain disease model of addiction. *N Engl J Med.* 2016;374:363–371.

98. Volkow ND, Tomasi D, Wang GJ, et al. Stimulant-induced dopamine increases are markedly blunted in active cocaine abusers. *Mol Psychiatry.* 2014;19:1037–1043.

99. Wald HP, Flaherty MT, Pringle JL. Prevention in prisons. In: Ammerman RT, Ott PJ, Tarter RE, eds. *Prevention and Societal Impact of Drug and Alcohol Abuse*. Mahwah, NJ: Lawrence Erlbaum Associates; 1999.

100. Weinstock RW, Leong GB, Silva JA. California's diminished capacity defense: evolution and transformation. *Bull Am Acad Psychiatry Law.* 1996;24:347–366.

101. Weiss R, Collins D. Substance abuse and psychiatric illness. *Am J Addict.* 1992;1:93–99.

102. Westreich LM. Addiction and the Americans with disabilities act. *J Am Acad Psychiatry Law.* 2002;30:355–363.

103. Wexler H, Falkin GP, Lipton DS, et al. Outcome evaluation of a prison therapeutic community for substance abuse treatment. In: Leukefeld C, Tims FD, eds. *Drug Abuse Treatment in Prisons and Jails*. Rockville, MD: U.S. Department of Health and Human Services; 1992.

104. Whitner v. State, SC Sup Ct No. 24468.

105. Whitner v. South Carolina, 492 SE 2nd 777 (SC 1997).

72
Disability and Addiction

QIANA L. BROWN

CHAPTER OUTLINE

Introduction

The terms substance use disorders (which include both drug and alcohol use disorders) and addiction are sometimes used synonymously among professional and lay populations. However, there are important distinctions to consider. Substance use disorders, as characterized by the *Diagnostic and Statistical Manual of Mental Disorders, Fifth Edition* (DSM-5), can range from mild to severe, and are a cluster of symptoms that can be cognitive, behavioral, and physiological in nature, indicating continued use of substances despite significant drug-related problems.[7] Addiction, as defined by the National Institute on Drug Abuse, is a chronic, relapsing brain disease consisting of compulsive drug seeking and use regardless of harmful consequences, and is equivalent to a severe substance use disorder as defined by the DSM-5.[71,72] Addiction, unlike substance use disorders, is not an actual diagnosis according to the DSM-5.[7,71] However, in this chapter, substance use disorders and addiction are used interchangeably.

Substance use disorders affect the body and brain on multiple levels and may have long-term disabling effects on the ability to function independently and meet the demands of daily living.[a] The very nature of substance use disorders (e.g., seeking/using drugs despite harmful consequences) overlaps with the definition of disability—"a physical or mental impairment that substantially limits one or more major life activities"—as defined by the Americans with Disabilities Act Amendments Act of 2008.[3] However, many people with substance use disorders are denied the protections of the Americans with Disabilities Act due to the Act's exclusionary criteria of this population.[95] For example, the Americans with Disabilities Act excludes from its definition of disability people who are currently engaged in the illegal use of drugs (i.e., not in recovery) defined as drug use not under the supervision of a licensed health care provider, and not under the provisions of federal law.[8] This population is also prohibited from receiving disability entitlements provided by the Social Security Administration through Supplemental Security Income and Social Security Disability Insurance.[29,60] Individuals in recovery (i.e., not engaging in the illegal use drugs) are covered. However, the varying definitions of what qualifies as "in recovery" often make the process of obtaining benefits or protections difficult.[60] Some of the current policies governing entitlements and protections for people with disabilities raise fundamental concerns about civil rights, equality, and fairness for people affected by substance use disorders, both those in recovery and those currently using. These policies reflect varying understandings of what it means to have a disability. Given that disability is a legal and administrative term, as well as a medical one, this variation is not surprising.[60]

Discrimination Protections for Persons With Disabilities

Rehabilitation Act of 1973, Title V, Section 504

Historically, the legal protections for people with disabilities that are now in place began in 1973 in Title V of the Rehabilitation Act of 1973, Section 504.[60,79] Section 504 titled "Nondiscrimination Under Federal Grants and Programs," protected both persons who were currently addicted and those in recovery under federal law. Specifically, the act stipulated that any organization receiving federal funds could not discriminate against people who were currently addicted to drugs or alcohol or in recovery from either condition.[60,79]

---

[a]References 30, 36, 38, 60, 61, 66, 92, 93.

Americans With Disabilities Act

The Rehabilitation Act of 1973 was a significant milestone that recognized the need to protect the rights of those with disabilities. It was, however, not comprehensive, so lobbying continued on the part of people with disabilities and their advocates. Their efforts bore fruit, and the Americans with Disabilities Act was enacted on July 26, 1990.[8,60] The primary objective of the Americans with Disabilities Act is to extend maximum opportunity for full community participation to persons with disabilities in both public and private sectors of the United States. The Americans with Disabilities Act prohibits employment discrimination on the basis of disability in both private and public sectors, extending the protections of the Rehabilitation Act of 1973 beyond federally funded and conducted activities. In particular, the Americans with Disabilities Act applies to private employment, all publicly funded services, and public accommodations and services managed by private organizations.[60]

When the Americans with Disabilities Act was passed, protections for people who use illicit drugs that were present in Section 504 of the Rehabilitation Act of 1973 were dropped. Anyone who is currently engaged in the illegal use of drugs is not considered a qualified person with a disability under the Americans with Disabilities Act. However, persons who have completed or are participating in a supervised rehabilitation program and are no longer using illegal drugs are protected.[8,60] The implication is that an individual who is addicted to heroin, for example, must be abstinent from the use of heroin to qualify for the protections afforded by the Americans with Disabilities Act.[60]

Many individuals who are impaired because of their addiction are unable to perform one or more major life activities. Therefore, at least one of the three criteria for disability as defined by the Americans with Disabilities Act has been met.[60] The statute is particularly important for many people with substance use disorders who also have co-occurring mental health disorders. This population often faces difficulties in finding and holding jobs, in part because of the stigma attached to both addiction and mental health disorders.[43,60] However, disabling psychiatric illnesses that meet any of the three criteria for disabilities are considered qualified disabilities under the Americans with Disabilities Act, whereas addiction is not.[60]

In addition to the Americans with Disabilities Act's exclusion of those currently using illegal drugs, the act has several barriers that are of concern to the substance use disorders services and treatment community and to individuals with these disorders who wish to claim protection under the Act.[60] As noted earlier, people with substance use disorders who are not currently using illicit drugs can claim protection from employment discrimination under the Americans with Disabilities Act. However, the meaning of "current use" is vague. Some court decisions have been equivocal about when recovery begins, requiring a period of active stability of, for example, 6 months, to be considered in recovery, and therefore eligible for the Americans with Disabilities Act protections.[60,95] Employees who have alcoholism or who use illegal drugs must meet the same standards other employees are held to, even if their unsatisfactory behavior is attributable to their use of substances.[8,60] Finally, employees must not pose a "direct threat" to others because of their substance use—a term that, like "current" use, has been debated frequently in litigation.[60,95]

Protections against discrimination for people who actively use drugs and alcohol are influenced by current law and can change depending on case law rulings.[60] Several key decisions narrowed the focus of the Americans with Disabilities Act's protections and increased the barriers that individuals who are disabled or impaired must overcome to obtain equal opportunities in the United States. Restrictive case law necessitated passage of the Americans with Disabilities Act Amendments Act of 2008 to reaffirm Congress's original intent.[60]

Key Case Law for the Americans With Disabilities Act, 1990

Interpretation of the Americans with Disabilities Act is established through trial law as individual cases are considered; therefore, the rights afforded to people who are in recovery and those who are actively using are often determined in an administrative law hearing or through precedents established by court cases.[60] The Americans with Disabilities Act offers technical definitions of disability and delineates the applications of and exceptions to these definitions. Nevertheless, the US judicial system has the authority to interpret the act and to determine the extent to which a particular impairment qualifies as a disability.[60]

Raytheon v. Hernandez

Raytheon v. Hernandez[60,78] was a case that explored the extent to which employers can classify substance use disorders–related behaviors as workplace misconduct rather than behaviors related to the substance use disorder.[60] This case eventually appeared before the Supreme Court, and the decisions from *Raytheon v. Hernandez* may have an impact on how the Americans with Disabilities Act protections are applied to people in recovery from substance use disorders.[60] Joel Hernandez applied for a position at Raytheon in 1994. He had previously worked for Raytheon (at that time Hughes Missile Systems) from 1966 to 1991. During his employment, he had experienced on-the-job challenges related to substance use disorders, but treatment efforts supported by his company were unsuccessful. One day Mr. Hernandez came to work with alcohol and cocaine in his system, which his employers confirmed through a drug test. Mr. Hernandez was offered the option to resign or face termination. He resigned.[60]

After 2 years in recovery from his substance use disorder, Mr. Hernandez applied for a position doing the same work he had been doing before his resignation, submitting letters from his church and his Alcoholics Anonymous sponsor with his application. The company had a no-rehire policy for ex-employees who had been terminated because of workplace misconduct, and Mr. Hernandez did not get the job. Mr. Hernandez surmised that he was being discriminated against because of his substance use disorder history. The Equal Employment Opportunity Commission supported his claim of discrimination and granted him permission to sue Raytheon for violating his rights under the Americans with Disabilities Act.[31,60]

The case was heard by the US District Court in Arizona, which ruled in favor of Raytheon. Mr. Hernandez then appealed to the Ninth District Court of Appeals, which reversed the lower court's ruling.[31,60] Raytheon appealed the Ninth Circuit Court's decision, and the case was eventually argued before the Supreme Court of the United States on October 8, 2003, and decided on December 2, 2003.[60,78] The Supreme Court upheld the ruling of the Arizona District Court in favor of Raytheon, stating that Mr. Hernandez was not passed over because of his substance use disorder history and, therefore, was not the object of disparate treatment because of his disability, as he claimed in his arguments.[60]

The opinion of the Supreme Court, as delivered by Justice Thomas, was that "Petitioner's [Raytheon's] proffer of its neutral no-rehire policy plainly satisfied its obligation under McDonnell Douglas [a previous decision] to provide a legitimate, nondiscriminatory reason for refusing to rehire respondent."[60,78] The opinion of the Court found that there was insufficient evidence to prove that Raytheon did not rehire Mr. Hernandez because of his substance use disorder history. In effect, the ruling allowed Raytheon to characterize Mr. Hernandez's behavior on the day he came to work under the influence of alcohol and cocaine as workplace misconduct rather than as behavior consistent with a treatable substance use disorder.[16,31,32,60,94]

The Sutton Trilogy

The "Sutton Trilogy" refers to three rulings issued by the US Supreme Court in Spring 1999. These cases addressed how the possibility of devices, medication, or even unconscious neuropsychological phenomena that mitigate a disabling condition can affect a person's disability status.[60,65] The first case, *Sutton v. United Air Lines, Inc.*, found that twin sisters with severe myopia that could be corrected to 20/20 vision with glasses were not protected under the Americans with Disabilities Act because the glasses mitigated the disability by improving their vision.[60,88] The second case, *Albertson's Inc. v. Kirkingburg*, found that Mr. Kirkingburg, a truck driver who was blind in one eye, was not protected under the Americans with Disabilities Act because he had developed the ability to compensate automatically for his lack of depth perception.[4,60] His compensation mitigated his disability. The third case, *Murphy v. the United States Postal Service, Inc.*, found that Mr. Murphy, a mechanic also required to drive a truck who was dismissed because his blood pressure did not meet Department of Transportation's health guidelines, was not protected by the Americans with Disabilities Act because, when medicated, his high blood pressure was near normal; in addition, he could still work as a mechanic, so he was not considered disabled.[60,69]

In these three examples, mitigating factors included such things as medications, corrective lenses, and even neuropsychological phenomenon, all of which reduced the severity of the impairment. Recovery may be viewed as mitigation for people with substance use disorders, but a history of drug addiction still carries a significant burden of social stigma. People with substance use disorder histories may still require the Americans with Disabilities Act's protections, even though their technical impairment has been mitigated.[32,60]

Americans With Disabilities Act Amendments Act of 2008

The Americans with Disabilities Act Amendments Act of 2008, which was signed into law on September 25, 2008, and became effective on January 1, 2009, amended the Americans with Disabilities Act of 1990 to redefine the term "disability."[60] This change marks a broader interpretation of, and coverage for, individuals with a disability. The Americans with Disabilities Act Amendments Act of 2008 overturned the mitigating-measures holding of *Sutton v. United Air Lines* (1999), which had been applied to deprive many individuals with disabilities of the Americans with Disabilities Act's protections.[27,60] A key purpose of the Act was to

reinstate the "broad scope of protection" Congress intended to be available.[8,60] The new law clarifies that the effects of mitigating measures, such as hearing aids and prosthetics, could not be used in weighing how a person's disability affects life activities.[28,60] The 2008 legislation also overturned the restrictive interpretation of substantially limits, often narrowly interpreted by court rulings.[27] These changes now create an easier path for establishing that a person has a disability within Americans with Disabilities Act guidelines, and for a disabled person to seek protection under this Act. Passage of the legislation also extends protections to people with disabilities not immediately evident in the workplace, such as those of the immune, digestive, and neurological systems. These changes still, however, exclude those with current substance use disorders from qualifying as disabled, arguably in a discriminatory way.[95]

History of Entitlements for People With Disabilities and the Place for People With Substance Use Disorders

In the past, Supplemental Security Income and Social Security Disability Insurance programs provided monetary assistance as well as medical benefits to individuals with substance use disorders because substance abuse was considered a qualifying impairment.[60] The level of oversight and scrutiny of Supplemental Security Income/Social Security Disability Insurance recipients with substance use disorders was much higher compared with that of other beneficiaries. In particular, a referral monitoring agency was enlisted by the Social Security Administration to ensure that Supplemental Security Income recipients with substance use disorders were compliant with treatment. People with substance use disorders did not receive their own entitlement checks. Instead, the checks were sent monthly to a representative payee, who disbursed the funds. The benefits were not to exceed 3 years.[60]

There were problems associated with this method of organizing benefits for individuals with substance use disorders. At one point, the number of people with substance use disorders receiving disability benefits increased by more than 500% in a 4-year period, and the Social Security Administration found it difficult to establish whether recipients were in treatment.[60] One study found that the rates of rehabilitation and returns to work were very low. In addition, there was evidence that representative payees were allowing income to be used to purchase drugs.[44,60]

Under the Clinton Administration, enactment of the Contract with America Advancement Act of 1996 (PL 104–121) made important changes that affected people with substance use disorders.[44,60] In particular, the Social Security Administration terminated payments for Social Security Disability Insurance and Supplemental Security Income on the basis of addiction alone.[60] When someone has a co-occurring disabling condition and an active substance use disorder, the Social Security Administration must currently determine whether the disability being claimed is the result of a medical condition or the result of the effects of active drug use. The disability must be present even if consumption of alcohol and drugs has ceased.[60] This determination is made by theoretically removing the limitations resulting from the substance use disorder and then deciding whether the remaining limitations from other impairments would still be disabling. Only after such an analysis can a determination of disability be made.[60,82] This situation points to the complexities in classifying addiction as a disability.[60]

Before PL 104–121, people with substance use disorders who received Supplemental Security Income and Social Security Disability Insurance for at least 2 years were eligible to receive Medicaid (for Supplemental Security Income) and Medicare (for Social Security Disability Insurance).[60,82] A significant amount of federal funds for substance use disorder treatment flowed to the states through the two programs. With the new legislation, determination of benefits is now made by the states, and states vary to a considerable degree in how they fund substance abuse treatment.[10,60] Some states fully cover a course of treatment, whereas others only partially reimburse substance abuse treatment.[60]

The clinical and social effects of the decision to eliminate Supplemental Security Income and Social Security Disability Insurance benefits for substance use disorders in 1996 are substantial for people with substance use disorders who are now ineligible for this resource.[60] Although the problems inherent in the previous legislation were removed by eliminating the entitlement, an important issue remains: The substantial prevalence of people with substance use disorders and co-occurring mental illnesses[b] creates a challenge for the Social Security Administration. For example, it is difficult to make materiality determinations if the agency cannot separate the functional limitations that each condition imposes.[60] There is no evidence in the scientific literature that indicates whether and how the limitations from substance use disorders can be completely separated from the limitations of a mental health condition when both are present.[60] This paradox calls into question the reliability and validity, or lack thereof, in the disability determination process when people with co-occurring disorders apply for disability benefits; many cases may remain undetermined or delayed in the decision-making process. In the meantime, a person who is truly disabled may not be able to gain access to the resources that he or she needs to make a recovery that would help improve quality of life and potentially reduce costs to society.[60]

Policy, Treatment, and Medical Coverage

People with disabilities who also have current substance use disorders tend to enter drug treatment at a much lower rate than those without co-occurring disabilities.[59,60] Some barriers to care include lack of transportation, difficulty with physical access to the treatment center, and limited knowledge among treatment providers about the special needs of people with disabilities.[9,59,60] Two important policies that have implications for treatment and medical coverage for people with substance use disorders (and mental health conditions) are the Paul Wellstone and Pete Domenici Mental Health Parity and Addiction Equity Act of 2008, and the 2010 Patient Protection and Affordable Care Act.[37] On October 3, 2008, the Paul Wellstone and Pete Domenici Mental Health Parity and Addiction Equity Act of 2008 (usually referred to as the Parity Act) was signed into law.[37] The Parity Act requires covered health plans to provide the same financial terms, conditions, and requirements for mental health and substance use disorder benefits as provided medical/surgical conditions.[37,60] The Affordable Care Act extended the Parity Act to apply to individual health insurance markets (as opposed to only group plans), and requires the coverage of substance use disorder and mental health services as essential health benefits.[37] There is overwhelming evidence that substance use disorders take a great toll on the lives of individuals, their families, and their communities.

Numerous studies have demonstrated the disabling neurological, physiological, and genetic dimensions of addiction, and the effectiveness of treatment. The 2008 Parity Act and the 2010 Affordable Care Act affirmed these findings.

Substance Use Disorders and Comorbid Disability

Drug and alcohol use disorders (collectively referred to as substance use disorders) are associated with adverse health and mental health conditions. If a person has discontinued drug use, the source of a disabling condition is immaterial to the protections provided by the Americans with Disabilities Act and eligibility for benefits from the Social Security Administration.[60] Disabling conditions that are protected under the Americans with Disabilities Act can include infectious diseases and psychological illnesses, as well as substantial physical impairment.[60] This section describes the association between disability and different classes of drugs of abuse, with details about neurological, physical, sensory, and functional impairment from each class. Prenatal substance use and associated disability and consequences are also discussed.

Alcohol

Alcohol use disorder accounts for a high proportion of disability in the United States and globally.[34,81] There is extensive literature on the many disabling conditions, to include physical and mental health conditions associated with alcohol misuse use and disorders.[c] Alcohol use disorder can harm most of the body's organs, including the liver, the immune system, the cardiovascular system, and the skeletal system.[2,47,60]

Injury

Alcohol use is a leading risk factor for intentional and unintentional injury.[21,34,50,81,80] In addition, a significant proportion of disability-adjusted life years (DALYs) from injuries, in the United States and globally, is attributable to alcohol use.[21,80] Alcohol-related injuries and their circumstances are wide ranging to include, but not limited to, falls, automobile crashes, and fires.[1] There is a positive association between alcohol consumption and injury (i.e., the more a person drinks, the higher the risk for injury), especially among frequent heavy drinkers and binge drinkers.[1] The increased risk for injury due to alcohol stems from impairments in cognitive capacity, physical coordination, and performance, in addition to increased risk-taking behavior associated with drinking.[1]

In a literature review that examined the role of substance abuse in the cause of injury for patients using physical rehabilitation services, Hubbard and colleagues found that up to 79% of rehabilitation patients had alcohol-related traumatic injuries and that 35% of automobile injuries, 55% of motor vehicle deaths, 40% of drownings, and 30% of noncommercial airplane crashes were related to alcohol. Up to 72% of patients with head injuries from car crashes had positive blood alcohol levels; and males were more than twice as likely as females to have positive blood alcohol levels at the time of head injury.[52,60] Drinking or intoxication is also associated with up to 79% of spinal cord injuries.[52,60] Furthermore, a retrospective cohort study of medical claims data on patients with alcohol- or drug-related primary or secondary diagnosis by Miller and colleagues estimated the excess risk of medically treated and

---

[b]References 23, 26, 40, 41, 42, 44, 47, 60.

[c]References 1, 2, 21, 29, 34, 41, 47, 81.

hospitalized nonoccupational injury for people younger than age 65 with medically identified substance abuse. They found that people who were medically identified as abusing substances had a higher risk of injury in a 3-year period. People who abused alcohol and drugs were almost four times as likely as controls to be hospitalized for an injury during the 3-year period, and the risk of injury was substantially higher for female than male users of substances.[60,67]

Liver Disease

Alcohol consumption is causally related to liver disease (e.g., cirrhosis),[1,80] and accounts for nearly a third of liver cirrhosis worldwide.[81] Risk of liver disease is positively related to alcohol consumption[1] and varies by race and gender.[34] For example, a higher proportion of men than women have alcohol-related cirrhosis[34,81]; however, women may be more susceptible to the cumulative effects of alcohol on the liver.[1] In addition, Hispanic-white males have higher age-adjusted mortality rates from liver cirrhosis than non-Hispanic white males, non-Hispanic black males, Hispanic-black males, and females.[34] There are three forms of alcoholic liver disease: fatty liver, which is usually reversible with abstinence; alcoholic hepatitis, characterized by persistent liver inflammation; and cirrhosis, characterized by progressive scarring of liver tissue.[60,87] More than one type of liver disease can be present at the same time. Individuals with both cirrhosis and alcoholic hepatitis have a death rate of more than 60% over a 4-year period, with most deaths occurring within the first 12 months of diagnosis.[14,60,67] Alcohol initially causes liver injury by generating harmful metabolites, and continuing alcohol use exacerbates the initial injury. Chronic alcohol use leads to inflammation and weakens the ability of the liver to repair itself. It also leads to increased fibrogenesis, a major source of cirrhosis.[60,87]

Neurological and Social Functioning

Alcohol-related limitations in neuropsychiatric and social functioning contribute to a significant proportion of disability.[1,41,47,80,81] Neurological complications from alcohol can lead to substantial long-term disabling conditions. Lasting cognitive impairment in people with alcoholism can be direct, through brain damage from long-term alcohol exposure, or indirect, as a result of head trauma, central nervous system infection, hepatic failure, or nutritional deficiency. Direct neurological consequences of long-term alcohol use include Wernicke-Korsakoff syndrome, Marchiafava-Bignami syndrome, and central pontine myelinosis. Wernicke syndrome, in which decreased attentiveness, alertness, and memory are usually accompanied by disordered eye movements and ataxia, is often followed by Korsakoff psychosis, a lasting amnestic disorder.[1,60] Marchiafava-Bignami syndrome and central pontine myelinosis are related to damage to the myelin sheath of neurons in the corpus callosum and pons, respectively.[14,60,83] Studies have shown that alcohol also directly damages the cerebrum sufficiently to cause dementia.[14,60]

A study by Hasin and colleagues, using data from wave 1 (2002–2003) of the National Epidemiological Survey on Alcohol and Related Conditions, further highlights the relationship between alcohol use disorders and poor social and mental functioning. Hasin and colleagues measured the prevalence, correlates, disability, and comorbidities associated with alcohol abuse and dependence in the United States. When adjusted for sociodemographic characteristics and other disorders, alcohol abuse was associated with lower social functioning (e.g., limitations due to emotional problems) and role emotional functioning (e.g., role impairment related to emotional problems). Alcohol dependence was associated with lower social and role emotional functioning, as well as with poorer mental health; and disability increased with severity of alcohol dependence.[47,60] Results were similar in the National Epidemiological Survey on Alcohol and Related Conditions-III (2012–2013), such that after adjusting for sociodemographic characteristics and psychiatric comorbidity, people with alcohol use disorder had lower social and role emotional functioning and poorer mental health than people without alcohol use disorder; and disability generally increased with severity of alcohol use disorder.[41]

Immune System

Alcohol use disorder can lead to impaired immune response, which can increase vulnerability to certain diseases. Genetic factors may also contribute to individual vulnerability to reduced immune functioning related to alcohol consumption.[1] Autoimmune-related diseases associated with alcohol consumption (e.g., alcoholic liver disease) can be life-threatening.[1] Alcohol-related immunodeficiency can also exacerbate diseases and health conditions such as pneumonia, tuberculosis, and organ damage—particularly in the liver.[1] Furthermore, people who abuse alcohol, compared to those who do not, are more susceptible to infections like septicemia, empyema, lung abscesses, cellulitis, and meningitis.[1]

Cardiovascular System

Chronic heavy drinking is a leading cause of cardiovascular illnesses such as cardiomyopathy, coronary heart disease, high blood pressure, arrhythmias, and stroke.[1,60] In alcoholic cardiomyopathy, long-term heavy drinking can enlarge the heart and impair its ability to contract. Symptoms of cardiomyopathy include shortness of breath and insufficient blood flow to the rest of the body. Women may have a greater risk than men of developing alcoholic cardiomyopathy. The condition may be at least partially reversible with abstinence.[14,60] Some studies report potential benefits of light to moderate drinking in relation to cardiovascular diseases. However, these benefits are off-set at higher drinking levels and by irregular heavy drinking, which are associated with increased morbidity and mortality.[1,80,81]

An association between heavy alcohol consumption and increased blood pressure has been observed in more than 60 studies in diverse cultures and populations.[2,60] Heavy drinking can disrupt the heart rhythm both acutely (during an episode of drinking) and chronically (during long-term use). Intoxication can cause certain types of arrhythmia in both those with alcoholism and otherwise healthy individuals. Sudden death attributable to arrhythmia is one of the causes of mortality in people with alcoholism with or without preexisting heart disease. Such deaths often occur during periods of abstinence, suggesting that arrhythmias are more likely to develop during alcohol withdrawal.[2,14,60,83]

Skeletal System

Epidemiologic studies have found a significant association between alcohol consumption and bone fracture risk. In addition to the increased risk of accidental injury from impaired gait and balance, people with alcoholism may also have a generalized decrease in bone mass. Heavy drinking may lead to osteoporosis, characterized by severe back pain, spinal deformity, and increased risk of wrist and hip fractures.[2,14,60,83]

Drugs of Abuse

Drug use disorders are associated with increased disability and comorbidity,[26,33,42] some of which are detailed in this section.

There are several drugs of abuse and drug classes.[7,72] This section provides an overview of a few and related disability.

Cocaine

Cognitive deficits are of the many disabling factors associated with cocaine use. People who abuse cocaine often exhibit lasting cognitive deficits even after cessation of use.[13,60,77] In a study comparing 20 people in recovery who chronically abused with controls matched for age and education, O'Malley and colleagues used a series of standardized neuropsychological assessment procedures to assess cognitive impairment. They found that people who abused cocaine were 35% more likely than the control group to score in the impaired range of the neuropsychological screening exam. Those who abused cocaine also performed more poorly on tests for abstract thinking and reasoning and verbal memory. Neuropsychological performance was directly related to the severity of cocaine abuse, suggesting that cocaine played a direct role in affecting cognitive functioning.[60,77] Cognitive deficits from cocaine are often related to perfusion abnormalities or changes of blood flow in the brain.[13,36,60] A study by Browndyke and colleagues showed the relationship between cognitive performance and the magnitude of perfusion abnormality. Their findings indicated significant regional perfusion abnormalities among people who abused cocaine relative to controls, and substantial deficits in neuropsychological functioning for people who abused cocaine.[13,60]

Heroin

Injection drug users, as well as noninjection drug users are at risk for consequences associated with heroin use.[46,56,91] For example, in an epidemiological study conducted in Baltimore, Maryland, that identified three classes of heroin and cocaine users—crack/nasal-heroin users, polysubstance users, and heroin injectors—found that crack smoking/nasal heroin users had lower odds of hepatitis C virus than heroin injectors, but these groups did not differ on HIV status.[46] The lack of significant difference on HIV status between these two groups highlights a potential equal risk for disability regardless of route of administration. Other risk factors associated with infectious diseases and potential disability varied by route of administration. For example, polysubstance users had more than a 2.5 times higher odds of sharing needles as compared to those who injected heroin; and the odds of high-risk sex behaviors were 2.5 times higher among crack smoking/nasal heroin users as compared to polysubstance users.[46]

Methamphetamine

Methamphetamine use is associated with physical, cognitive, and psychiatric deficits.[22,49,64,73–76] For example, the prevalence of ADHD was higher among people with methamphetamine use disorder compared to those without methamphetamine use disorder.[75] Physical impairments like neck and back injuries were commonly reported among methamphetamine users.[49] In addition, long-term methamphetamine use is associated with impaired performance on a number of cognitive tasks, including verbal memory and motor function, manipulation of information, abstract reasoning, and task-shifting strategies.[60,75] The cognitive impairment observed in people who abuse methamphetamine may also be related to abnormalities of frontal lobes of the brain.[22] Chung and colleagues reported that decreased gray-matter densities and glucose metabolism in the frontal region of the brain were correlated with impaired frontal executive functions in people who abuse methamphetamine.[22,60] Executive functions are necessary for goal-directed behavior and come into play when adapting to

change, in planning for the future, and in abstract thinking. In a study comparing people who abuse methamphetamine with healthy subjects, Chung and colleagues used diffusion tensor imaging to describe the differences in frontal white-matter integrity and assessed differences in frontal executive functions with the Wisconsin Card Sorting Test. They found that frontal white matter was compromised in people who abuse methamphetamine and that these people showed more errors in the Wisconsin Card Sorting Test relative to healthy subjects. They also noted that the neurotoxic effect of methamphetamine on frontal white matter may be less prominent in women than in men, possibly because of estrogen's neuroprotective effect.[22,60]

3,4-Methylenedioxymethamphetamine ("Ecstasy" or "Molly")

3,4-Methylenedioxymethamphetamine (also known as Ecstasy or Molly) and related compounds have serious acute and chronic toxic effects that resemble those seen with other amphetamines. Neurotoxicity to the serotonergic system in the brain can also cause permanent physical and psychiatric problems, including confusion, depression, and impaired memory.[55,60,73] The brains of people who used Ecstasy/Molly over a long term, when examined while free of the drug, have abnormally low levels of serotonin and its metabolites in the cerebrospinal fluid and other significant alterations of neurotransmitter functioning. Among this population there is upregulation of serotonin receptors during abstinence, in response to the decrease in serotonin release caused by the action of the drug. Electroencephalographic studies show changes similar to those seen in aging and dementia and a change in response to auditory stimuli. The prolactin and cortisol responses to stimulation of the serotonin system were reduced in the people who used Ecstasy/Molly. These changes persisted for up to a year or more after the last use of the drug.[55,60]

The demonstrated neurotoxic effects of Ecstasy/Molly on the serotonin system may be associated with a variety of mental health and behavioral problems that outlast the actual drug experience by months or years. These problems are quite varied, but they all involve functions in which serotonin is known to play an important role.[60] Some persistent problems include impaired verbal and visual memory, decision-making, information processing, logical reasoning, and simple problem solving, as well as greater impulsivity and lack of self-control, recurrent paranoia, hallucinations, depersonalization, flashbacks, and psychotic episodes.[55,60] In addition, past-year Ecstasy/Molly use is associated with anxiety and personality disorders.[57]

Inhalants

The term *inhalants* is typically used in reference to a wide range of substances to include solvents, aerosols, gases, and nitrites, which are primarily inhaled and rarely taken by other routes of administration.[70] Long-term abuse of solvents, for example, can cause damage to most organ systems, including the central and peripheral nervous systems and hepatic, renal, pulmonary, and cardiovascular systems. Solvent abuse can also affect bone marrow formation and lead to anemia. Cognitive effects include confusion, forgetfulness, and irritability.[15,60] The psychiatric and neurological sequelae of chronic solvent abuse are serious and potentially irreversible.[15,60]

To measure the consequences of long-term exposure to inhaled solvents, Yücel and colleagues reviewed neuroimaging and neuropsychological studies, examining chronic toluene misuse in humans. They found that toluene preferentially affects white-matter structures and periventricular/subcortical regions in the brain. They hypothesized that the lipid-dependent distribution and pharmacokinetic properties of toluene would likely explain the pattern of abnormalities, as well as the common symptoms and signs of toluene encephalopathy. The commonly observed neuropsychological deficits such as impairments in processing speed, sustained attention, memory retrieval, executive function, and language are also consistent with white-matter pathology.[60,96]

Anabolic Steroids

The abuse of androgenic anabolic steroids can cause high blood pressure, heart attacks, and liver cancer.[54,60] Long-term use of anabolic steroids may cause a range of adverse cardiovascular effects, some of which may be irreversible, including cardiomyopathy, dyslipidemia, and other atherosclerotic effects, hypertension, myocardial ischemia, and arrhythmias.[54,60] Anabolic steroids are capable of increasing vascular tone, arterial tension, and platelet aggregation and may give rise to atherothrombotic phenomena.[60,84] Although there are few reports of ischemic stroke related to anabolic steroid abuse, Santamarina and colleagues reported a case of a 26-year-old male amateur athlete who had a posterior territory ischemic stroke, whose only known significant risk factor was nonmedical use of stanozolol, an anabolic steroid.[60,84]

Neuroendocrine effects from anabolic steroid abuse are associated with infertility and depression.[54,60] In a study of the long-term side effects of high doses of self-administered anabolic steroids, Bonetti and colleagues observed 20 male bodybuilders who voluntarily self-administered anabolic steroids. The participants were tested every 6 months over 2 years. Physical examinations, and hematological, metabolic, and endocrine tests were performed, as well as semen analysis, hepatic and prostate ultrasounds, and echocardiographic evaluations. Long-term adverse effects observed included lower fertility and sperm counts and impaired lipid profiles associated with increased cardiovascular risk.[11,60]

More rarely, the long-term use of orally active anabolic steroids can have adverse hepatic effects, ultimately resulting in hepatocellular adenomas or carcinomas, although these hepatic effects are often reversible. In vitro studies have shown that concentrations of anabolic steroids comparable with those likely present in many people who abuse steroids can cause apoptosis in human endothelial and neuronal cell lines, as well as apoptotic death of myocardial cells in rat models, suggesting the possibility of irreversible neuropsychiatric toxicity, as well as a mechanism for the cardiovascular effects already noted. Steroid abuse also appears to be associated with a range of potentially prolonged psychiatric effects, including dependence syndromes, mood syndromes, and progression to other forms of substance abuse.[54,60]

Prescription Medications

Drugs classified as prescription medications have become a major category of abused substances. For example, the high prevalence of nonmedical prescription opioid use and associated morbidity and mortality are major public health problems.[25] For example, in 2014, more than 10 million people in the United States reported nonmedical use of prescription opioids. Underlying this epidemic is the association between increasing rates of opioid prescribing and increasing opioid-related morbidity and mortality.[25]

Sedative-hypnotic medications, which include benzodiazepines, barbiturates, and nonbenzodiazepine anxiolytics, are generally prescribed to treat insomnia or anxiety. In current practice, the term "sedative-hypnotic" often refers to benzodiazepines (e.g., diazepam and lorazepam). Neuropsychiatric effects of prolonged sedative-hypnotic abuse include deficits in memory, motor coordination, visuospatial learning, processing speed, and verbal learning. These phenomena have been difficult to study because some of the cognitive difficulties may result from sedation while others result from inattention or abnormally high plasma levels. However, meta-analyses have demonstrated that these effects can occur even after drug discontinuation. After drug discontinuation, cognition improves but may not return to the baseline level of function.[18,60]

Prescription stimulants, such as dextroamphetamine and methylphenidate (which are often prescribed to treat ADHD), are classified as controlled substances with a high potential for dependence or abuse when used outside of appropriate medical supervision.[18,60] With long-term use, stimulants may cause insomnia, irritability, aggressive behavior, and psychosis. Medical complications of acute intoxication with stimulants include altered mental status, autonomic instability (e.g., hyperthermia), seizures, or development of serotonin syndrome.[18,60] Methylphenidate and dextroamphetamine have been associated with cerebral arteritis, renal necrotizing vasculitis, and systemic and pulmonary hypertension.[18,60,86,89]

Prenatal Substance Use: Associated Disability and Consequences

Prenatal substance use and associated disability can affect both mother and child. For example, tobacco, alcohol, and marijuana are the most commonly used substances among pregnant and reproductive age women who may become pregnant,[39,58] and are preventable causes of adverse health outcomes for both mother and baby.[d] Adverse outcomes associated with prenatal alcohol use include, but are not limited to, fetal alcohol syndrome,[45,63] spontaneous abortion, neurodevelopment problems, and pre- and post-natal growth deficits.[39] Prenatal tobacco use is associated with pre-term and low birth-weight deliveries and infant mortality.[35] Likewise, prenatal marijuana use is associated with low birth-weight, poor school achievement, and impaired neurodevelopment and executive functioning.[5,6,17,48,85]

Opioid and other illicit drug use disorders are also problematic among pregnant women, and can lead to increased risk for disability.[12,19,20,53] For example, sex trade (a risk factor for disabling infectious diseases) and psychiatric comorbidity were prevalent among pregnant women in treatment for cocaine and opioid use disorders.[12,19,20] In this sample, both sex trade and psychiatric comorbidity were associated with higher odds of sexually transmitted infections,[19] which have potential implications for long-term disability.

Conclusions

Substance use disorders are disabling, comorbid conditions associated with significant impairment of major life activities. However, the legal and administrative concepts of disability and what people experience as disabling conditions are sometimes disparate. The political climate can substantially affect the help that people with substance use disorders can expect from federal, state, and local agencies. Policies regarding disability should make every effort to

---

[d]References 5, 17, 24, 45, 48, 51, 62, 63, 68, 85, 90.

create equitable conditions for people with substance use disorders, and help eliminate the stigma associated with these health conditions.

Acknowledgments

My work on this project was supported by the National Center for Advancing Translational Sciences, Clinical and Translational Science Awards Program via a career development award from the New Jersey Alliance for Clinical and Translation Science (grant KL2TR003018 [P.I. Qiana L. Brown]), the National Institute on Drug Abuse grant T32DA031099 (P.I. Deborah Hasin, PhD), and TrendologyIT Corporation. I also acknowledge Dr. Charlene Le Fauve for writing the original version of this chapter, published in 2011 in the first edition of *Addiction Medicine*, and for offering me the opportunity to revise and update the chapter for the current edition of this book.

References

1. 10th special report to the U.S. *Congress Alcohol and Health: Highlights from Current Research*. U.S. Department of Health and Human Services; 2000.
2. 10th Special Report to the U.S. Congress on alcohol and health, medical consequences of alcohol abuse. *Alcohol Res Health*. 2000;24:27–31.
3. *ADA Amendments Act of 2008, Pub. L. No. 110-325*. 2008. %3ci%3e%3ca href=https://www.congress.gov/110/plaws/publ325/PLAW-110publ325.pdf. Accessed 9 February 2016.
4. Albertsons, Inc. v. Kirkingburg (1999) 527 U.S. 555.
5. Alpar A, Di Marzo V, Harkany T. At the Tip of an Iceberg: prenatal marijuana and its possible relation to neuropsychiatric outcome in the Offspring. *Biol Psychiatr*. 2015.
6. American College of Obstetricians Gynecologists Committeeon Obstetric Practice, Committee Opinion No. 637. Marijuana Use during pregnancy and Lactation. *Obstet Gynecol*. 2015;126(1):234–238.
7. American Psychiatric Association. Substance-related and addictive disorders. In: *Diagnostic and Statistical Manual of Mental Disorders*. American Psychiatric Association; 2013.
8. Americans with Disabilities Act of 1990, Pub. L. No. 101-336. %3ci%3e%3cahref=http://library.clerk.house.gov/reference-files/PPL_101_336_AmericansWithDisabilities.pdf. Accessed 7April 2016.
9. Bachman SS, Drainoni ML, Tobias C. Medicaid managed care, substance abuse treatment, and people with disabilities: review of the literature. *Health Soc Work*. 2004;29(3):189–196.
10. Bada HS, et al. Impact of prenatal cocaine exposure on child behavior problems through school age. *Pediatrics*. 2007;119(2):e348–e359.
11. Bonetti A, et al. Side effects of anabolic androgenic steroids abuse. *Int J Sports Med*. 2008;29(8):679–687.
12. Brown QL, et al. The impact of homelessness on recent sex trade among pregnant women in drug treatment. *J Substance Use*. 2012;17(3):287–293.
13. Browndyke JN, et al. Examining the effect of cerebral perfusion abnormality magnitude on cognitive performance in recently abstinent chronic cocaine abusers. *J Neuroimaging*. 2004;14(2):162–169.
14. Brust JC. Neurologic complications of substance abuse. *J Acquir Immune Defic Syndr*. 2002;31(suppl 2):S29–S34.
15. Byrne A, et al. Psychiatric and neurological effects of chronic solvent abuse. *Can J Psychiatry*. 1991;36(10):735–738.
16. Calsyn RJ, et al. Recruitment, engagement, and retention of people living with HIV and co-occurring mental health and substance use disorders. *AIDS Care*. 2004;16(suppl 1):S56–S70.
17. Calvigioni D, et al. Neuronal substrates and functional consequences of prenatal cannabis exposure. *Eur Child Adolesc Psychiatr*. 2014;23(10):931–941.
18. Caplan JP, et al. Neuropsychiatric effects of prescription drug abuse. *Neuropsychol Rev*. 2007;17(3):363–380.
19. Cavanaugh CE, Hedden SL, Latimer WW. Sexually transmitted infections among pregnant heroin- or cocaine-addicted women in treatment: the significance of psychiatric co-morbidity and sex trade. *Int J STD AIDS*. 2010;21(2):141–142.
20. Cavanaugh CE, Latimer WW. Recent sex trade and injection drug use among pregnant opiate and cocaine dependent women in treatment: the significance of psychiatric comorbidity. *Addictiv Disorders Their Treat*. 2010;9(1):32–40.
21. Cherpitel CJ. Focus on: the burden of alcohol use--trauma and Emergency outcomes. *Alcohol Res Curr Rev*. 2013;35(2):150–154.
22. Chung A, et al. Decreased frontal white-matter integrity in abstinent methamphetamine abusers. *Int J Neuropsychopharmacol*. 2007;10(6):765–775.
23. Clark HW, et al. Policy and practice implications of epidemiological surveys on co-occurring mental and substance use disorders. *J Subst Abuse Treat*. 2008;34(1):3–13.
24. Coleman-Cowger VH, et al. Smoking cessation during pregnancy and postpartum: practice patterns among obstetrician-gynecologists. *J Addict Med*. 2014;8(1):14–24.
25. Compton WM, Jones CM, Baldwin GT. Relationship between nonmedical prescription-opioid Use and heroin Use. *New Engl J Med*. 2016;374(2):154–163 10p.
26. Compton WM, et al. Prevalence, correlates, disability, and comorbidity of DSM-IV drug abuse and dependence in the United States: results from the national epidemiologic survey on alcohol and related conditions. *Archiv Gen Psychiatr*. 2007;64(5):566–576.
27. Congressional Record House Page H605. June 25, 2008. U.S. Government Printing Office; 2008.
28. Congressional Record Senate Page S6282 June 26, 2008. 2008, U.S. Government Printing Office.
29. Contract with America Advancement Act of 1996, Pub. L. No. 104-121, 110 Stat. 8508. 1996.
30. De Alba I, Samet JH, Saitz R. Burden of medical illness in drug- and alcohol-dependent persons without primary care. *Am J Addict*. 2004;13(1):33–45.
31. de Miranda J. Locked Out of the workplace. *Behav Healthcare Tomorrow*. 2003;12:16–21.
32. de Miranda J. Addiction as a disability. *NAADD Rep*. 2004;7(1).
33. Delker E, Brown Q, Hasin D. Epidemiological studies of substance dependence and abuse in adults. *Curr Behav Neurosci Rep*. 2015;2(1):15–22.
34. Delker E, Brown Q, Hasin DS. Alcohol consumption in Demographic Subpopulations. *Alcohol Res Curr Rev*. 2016;38(1):e1–e9.
35. Dietz PM, et al. Infant morbidity and mortality attributable to prenatal smoking in the U.S. *Am J Prev Med*. 2010;39(1):45–52.
36. Ernst T, et al. Cerebral perfusion abnormalities in abstinent cocaine abusers: a perfusion MRI and SPECT study. *Psychiatry Res*. 2000;99(2):63–74.
37. Federal Register, Final rules under the Paul Wellstone and Pete Domenici Mental Health Parity and Addiction Equity Act of 2008; technical amendment to external review for multi-state plan program. Final rules. Office of the Federal Register, National Archives and Records Service, General Services Administration; distribution by the Supt. of Docs., U.S. Govt. Print. Off. [etc.]: United States. p. 68239-68296; 2013.
38. Feltenstein MW, See RE. The neurocircuitry of addiction: an overview. *Br J Pharmacol*. 2008;154(2):261–274.
39. Floyd RL, et al. The clinical content of preconception care: alcohol, tobacco, and illicit drug exposures. *Am J Obstet Gynecol*. 2008;199(6 suppl 2):S333–S339.
40. Grant BF, et al. Prevalence and co-occurrence of substance use disorders and independent mood and anxiety disorders: results from the National Epidemiologic Survey on Alcohol and Related Conditions. *Arch Gen Psychiatry*. 2004;61(8):807–816.

41. Grant BF, et al. Epidemiology of DSM-5 alcohol Use disorder: results from the national epidemiologic survey on alcohol and related conditions III. *JAMA Psychiatr*. 2015;72(8):757–766.

42. Grant BF, et al. Epidemiology of DSM-5 drug Use disorder: results from the national epidemiologic survey on alcohol and related conditions-III. *JAMA Psychiatr*. 2016;73(1):39–47.

43. Greenbaum PE, Foster-Johnson L, Petrila A. Co-occurring addictive and mental disorders among adolescents: prevalence research and future directions. *Am J Orthopsychiatry*. 1996;66(1):52–60.

44. Gresenz CR, Watkins K, Podus D. Supplemental Security Income (SSI), disability insurance (DI), and substance abusers. *Community Mental Health J*. 1998;34(4):337–350.

45. Hankin JR. Fetal alcohol syndrome prevention research. *Alcohol Res Health*. 2002;26(1):58.

46. Harrell PT, et al. Latent classes of heroin and cocaine users predict unique HIV/HCV risk factors (English). *Drug Alcohol Depend*. 2012;122(3):220–227.

47. Hasin DS, et al. Prevalence, correlates, disability, and comorbidity of DSM-IV alcohol abuse and dependence in the United States: results from the National Epidemiologic Survey on Alcohol and Related Conditions. *Archiv Gen Psychiatr*. 2007;64(7):830–842.

48. Hayatbakhsh MR, et al. Birth outcomes associated with cannabis use before and during pregnancy. *Pediatr Res*. 2012;71(2):215–219.

49. Herbeck D, Brecht ML, Pham A. Racial/ethnic differences in health status and morbidity among adults who use methamphetamine. *Psychol Health Med*. 2013;18(3):262–274.

50. Hingson RW, Zha W. Age of drinking onset, alcohol use disorders, frequent heavy drinking, and unintentionally injuring oneself and others after drinking. *Pediatrics*. 2009;123(6):1477–1484 8p.

51. Holtrop JS, et al. Smoking among pregnant women with Medicaid insurance: are mental health factors related? *Maternal Child Health J*. 2010;14(6):971–977.

52. Hubbard JR, Everett AS, Khan MA. Alcohol and drug abuse in patients with physical disabilities. *Am J Drug Alcohol Abuse*. 1996;22(2):215–231.

53. Jones HE, et al. Clinical care for opioid-using pregnant and postpartum women: the role of obstetric providers. *Am J Obstetr Gynecol*. 2014;210(4):302–310.

54. Kaiser Family Foundation. *State Mandated Benefits: Mental Health Parity*; 2008. http://www.statehealthfacts.org/comparereport.jsp?rep=1&cat=7. Accessed 2 June 2009.

55. Kalant H. The pharmacology and toxicology of "ecstasy" (MDMA) and related drugs. *CMAJ (Can Med Assoc J)*. 2001;165(7):917–928.

56. Keen 2nd L, et al. Injection and non-injection drug use and infectious disease in Baltimore City: differences by race. *Addictiv Behav*. 2014;39(9):1325–1328 4p.

57. Keyes KM, Martins SS, Hasin DS. Past 12-month and lifetime comorbidity and poly-drug use of ecstasy users among young adults in the United States: results from the National Epidemiologic Survey on Alcohol and Related Conditions. *Drug Alcohol Depend*. 2008;97(1–2):139–149.

58. Ko JY, et al. Prevalence and patterns of marijuana use among pregnant and nonpregnant women of reproductive age. *Am J Obstet Gynecol*. 2015;213(2):201.e1–201.e10.

59. Krahn G, et al. Access barriers to substance abuse treatment for persons with disabilities: an exploratory study. *J Subst Abuse Treat*. 2006;31(4):375–384.

60. Le Fauve CE. Disability and addiction. In: Johnson BA, ed. *Addiction Medicine: Science and Practice*. New York, NY: Springer; 2011:1459–1486.

61. Li CS, Sinha R. Inhibitory control and emotional stress regulation: neuroimaging evidence for frontal-limbic dysfunction in psychostimulant addiction. *Neurosci Biobehav Rev*. 2008;32(3):581–597.

62. Li Q, et al. Detection of alcohol use in the second trimester among low-income pregnant women in the prenatal care settings in Jefferson County, Alabama. *Alcohol Clin Exp Res*. 2012;36(8):1449–1455.

63. Maier SE, West JR. Drinking patterns and alcohol-related birth Defects. *Alcohol Res Health*. 2001;25(3):168.

64. McKetin R, et al. The profile of psychiatric symptoms exacerbated by methamphetamine use. *Drug Alcohol Depend*. 2016.

65. McMahon BT, West SL, Hurley JE. Who is a person with a disability under the ADA? Mitigating circumstances, the US Supreme Court, and the case of diabetes. *J Vocational Rehabil*. 2006;24(3):177–182.

66. Mertens JR, et al. Medical and psychiatric conditions of alcohol and drug treatment patients in an HMO: comparison with matched controls. *Arch Intern Med*. 2003;163(20):2511–2517.

67. Miller TR, Lestina DC, Smith GS. Injury risk among medically identified alcohol and drug abusers. *Alcohol Clin Exp Res*. 2001;25(1):54–59.

68. Mund M, et al. Smoking and pregnancy--a review on the first major environmental risk factor of the unborn. *Int J Environ Res Public Health*. 2013;10(12):6485–6499.

69. Murphy v. *United Parcel Service, Inc*. 527 U.S. 516; 1999. http://www.law.cornell.edu/supct/html/97-1992.ZS.html. Accessed 2 June 2009.

70. National Institute on Drug Abuse. *Drug Facts: Inhalants*; 2012.

71. National Institute on Drug Abuse. *The National Instute on Drug Abuse*. Media guide; 2014.

72. National Institute on Drug Abuse. *Drugs, Brains, and Behavior: The Science of Addiction*; 2014.

73. National Institute on Drug Abuse Research and Reports Series. Methamphetamine abuse and addiction. (nd). http://drugabuse.gov/ResearchReports/Methamph/Methamph.html. Accessed April 11, 2016.

74. Nordahl TE, Salo R, Leamon M. Neuropsychological effects of chronic methamphetamine use on neurotransmitters and cognition: a review. *J Neuropsychiatry Clin Neurosci*. 2003;15(3):317–325.

75. Obermeit LC, et al. Attention-deficit/hyperactivity disorder among chronic methamphetamine users: Frequency, persistence, and adverse effects on everyday functioning. *Addictiv Behav*. 2013;38(12):2874–2878 5p.

76. Okita K, et al. Emotion dysregulation and amygdala dopamine D2-type receptor availability in methamphetamine users. *Drug Alcohol Depend*. 2016.

77. O'Malley S, et al. Neuropsychological impairment in chronic cocaine abusers. *Am J Drug Alcohol Abuse*. 1992;18(2):131–144.

78. Raytheon Co. v. Hernandez, 540 U.S. 44 (2003). %3ci%3e%3ca href=http://www.law.cornell.edu/supct/html/02-749.ZO.html. Accessed 29 June 2016.

79. Rehabilitation Act of 1973, §791, 29 U.S.C. §504. 1973.

80. Rehm J, et al. Global burden of disease and injury and economic cost attributable to alcohol use and alcohol-use disorders. *Lancet (London, England)*. 2009;373(9682):2223–2233.

81. Room R, Babor T, Rehm J. Alcohol and public health. *Lancet (London, England)*. 2005;365(9458):519–530.

82. Rosenbaum S, Teitelbaum J. The Americans with disabilities act: implications for managed care for persons with mental illness and addiction disorders. *Behavioal Health Issue Brief Series*. 1999:1–35.

83. Saitz R, et al. Medical disorders and complications of addiction. In: Graham AW, et al., ed. *Principles of Addiction Medicine*. Chevy Chase. MD: American Society of Addiction Medicine; 2003.

84. Santamarina RD, et al. Ischemic stroke related to anabolic abuse. *Clin Neuropharmacol*. 2008;31(2):80–85.

85. Saurel-Cubizolles MJ, Prunet C, Blondel B. Cannabis use during pregnancy in France in 2010. *BJOG*. 2014;121(8):971–977.

86. Schteinschnaider A, et al. Cerebral arteritis following methylphenidate use. *J Child Neurol*. 2000;15(4):265–267.

87. Seth D, et al. Direct effects of alcohol on hepatic fibrinolytic balance: implications for alcoholic liver disease. *J Hepatol*. 2008;48(4):614–627.

88. Sutton v. United Air Lines, Inc. 527 U.S. 471 (1999). http://www.law.cornell.edu/supct/html/97-1943.ZS.html. Accessed 2 June 2009.

89. Syed RH, Moore TL. Methylphenidate and dextroamphetamine-induced peripheral vasculopathy. *J Clin Rheumatol*. 2008;14(1):30–33.

90. Terplan M, Cheng D, Chisolm MS. The relationship between pregnancy intention and alcohol use behavior: an analysis of PRAMS data. *J Subst Abuse Treat.* 2014;46(4):506–510.

91. Theodorou S, Haber PS. The medical complications of heroin use. *Curr Opin Psychiatry.* 2005;18(3):257–263.

92. Vengeliene V, et al. Neuropharmacology of alcohol addiction. *Br J Pharmacol.* 2008;154(2):299–315.

93. Volkow ND, Li TK. Drugs and alcohol: treating and preventing abuse, addiction and their medical consequences. *Pharmacol Ther.* 2005;108(1):3–17.

94. Wasserman DA, Havassy BE, Boles SM. Traumatic events and post-traumatic stress disorder in cocaine users entering private treatment. *Drug Alcohol Depend.* 1997;46(1–2):1–8.

95. Westreich LM. Addiction and the Americans with disabilities act. *J Am Acad Psychiatr Law.* 2002;30(3):355–363.

96. Yucel M, et al. Toluene misuse and long-term harms: a systematic review of the neuropsychological and neuroimaging literature. *Neurosci Biobehav Rev.* 2008;32(5):910–926.

73

The Homeless

DAVID E. POLLIO, KARIN M. EYRICH-GARG, AND CAROL S. NORTH

Introduction

Understanding the composition and needs of the homeless represents a major challenge for all researchers and providers, not least for a group endeavoring to present a chapter summarizing available knowledge about this complex population. Starting with seemingly simple questions, such as defining homelessness, and moving to much more complex questions, such as treatment and other interventions for this population with multiple needs and problems, numerous interrelated issues must be considered. Complicating this discussion, existing research studies share limited methodological commonalities, often making direct comparisons of the findings from the diverse endeavors speculative at best.

Despite these challenges, the purpose of this chapter is to conceptualize the homeless as a population and discuss population prevalence; to detail rates of substance use and abuse, other mental illness and medical risk factors, and comorbidities; and to identify service models that have been demonstrated effective. Conceptually, this task begins with the complex issue of identifying just what is meant by a homeless population and understanding how different inclusion criteria led to very different prevalence estimates and identified characteristics of the population. Following the discussion of the definition of homeless population, given the disproportionate rates of substance use disorders relative to housed populations, the next task is to understand the issues surrounding substance use and disorders, including general estimates of all substances combined and those specific to individual substances. Once substance use and misuse have been presented, it becomes important to understand rates of other psychiatric and other medical illnesses, especially the remarkably high rates of psychiatric comorbidities. This chapter will conclude by discussing treatment needs and reviewing the increasingly available evidence for the effectiveness of specific types of interventions.

Before beginning this examination of homelessness, it is important to note a few caveats. This chapter focuses almost exclusively on homeless adults, specifically single homeless adults. The length constraints of a single chapter preclude discussion of various subpopulations, such as homeless children, runaway and homeless adolescents, single women with children, or homeless families. Furthermore, except where those issues have specific relevance for individual-level risk factors, this chapter does not investigate structural and economic causes for homelessness. A broader consideration of homelessness as an economic or social phenomenon would need to include discussions around housing availability and affordability, extreme poverty, social inequalities, and the impact of policy decisions on rates of homelessness.

Homelessness

Historical Context

Multiple historical events have been linked with current conceptualizations of homelessness, including such disparate populations as those created by the 16th-century Elizabethan Poor Law, colonization of the North American continent, and itinerant workers in the late 19th century.[104] For example, Elizabethan Poor Laws were the first attempt to provide service for landless and homeless poverty populations. In the 19th century, discussions of homelessness often focused on itinerant workers, or "hobos." Historically, homelessness has not necessarily been identified as a "problem." Wright[104] points out that various descriptions of the homeless, some as recently as the 1950s and 1960s, have romanticized the lives of hobos and migrant workers. However, starting with changes in the population from the time of deinstitutionalization in the 1960s, there is a general consensus that homelessness has emerged as a serious and increasingly important social issue,[3,9,34,97,104] and that this issue is closely interrelated with substance use and abuse and other psychiatric illness.[2,59]

It is also important to consider the conduct of research on this population from a historical perspective. Although there are no doubt exceptions, early research on homelessness (for the sake of the current discussion, operationalized as published prior to 1970) was generally ethnographic or even anecdotal in method. Seminal works, such as those by Whyte,[102] Gans,[32] and Liebow,[44] focused on the complex interactions among small groups of urban dwellers. Although more recent reexamination of these works demonstrates the significance of illicit substances in the lives of these "streetcorner" groups,[44] questions of "how many" or prevalence of these disorders were not addressed in these studies.

The 1970s and 1980s witnessed an explosion of research on homelessness, with more than 500 published articles and books listed on the subject in those two decades.[88] Unfortunately, most of this research was also methodologically flawed, presenting population descriptions incorporating a convenience sample, services-limited research consisting of program descriptions, or nonrandomized studies comparing different interventions.[52,88] It was not until the late 1980s that leaders in the field called for research to move beyond demographic descriptions to conduct more complete and methodologically sophisticated research[55,96] addressing complex epidemiologic issues.[94]

In the last two decades, numerous methodologically sound cross-sectional studies have concluded that addiction and other psychiatric disorders are disproportionately prevalent in the homeless population. Unfortunately, because of sampling-related issues emanating from varied definitions applied to the problem of homelessness, changes in the population over time, and the lack of an acceptable national sample, our subsequent discussions of homelessness and associated comorbidities represent at best an incomplete snapshot of the problem. Thus answers to the specific questions of how many (e.g., What is the prevalence of psychiatric illness in the homeless population?) vary with these methodological differences, even among studies deemed methodologically adequate for most purposes. Given this situation, we present ranges of likely prevalence estimates rather than provide specific figures of undeterminable validity.

Operationalizing Homelessness

Historically, homeless samples in research studies have often been limited to service-using populations, especially individuals using services directed to homeless populations, such as overnight shelters. General consensus, however, is that this subset captures only a segment of the homeless population that may not be representative of the larger homeless population.[28] Perhaps the most commonly accepted definition of homelessness is that of the 1987 Stewart B. McKinney Homeless Assistance Act,[49] which defines a homeless person as:

(1) an individual who lacks a fixed, regular, and adequate nighttime residence and (2) an individual who has a primary nighttime residence that is (a) a supervised, publicly or privately operated shelter designed to provide temporary living accommodations, (b) an institution that provides a temporary residence for individuals intended to be institutionalized, or (c) a public or private place not designed for or ordinarily used as a regular sleeping accommodation for human beings.

Understanding differences among specific definitions of homelessness requires consideration of a number of factors. These factors include what personal circumstances are considered homeless (e.g., inclusion of individuals doubled up/marginally housed versus only counting individuals literally without housing), how long one must be homeless to be included (one night vs. a longer spell), and whether one self-identifies or is identified by some external criteria as homeless. Currently, operational definitions of homelessness have focused either on individuals who are literally homelessness or those marginally housed. Definitions of literal homelessness include not only those found in shelter settings, following the definition in the McKinney Act,[49] but also individuals sleeping on the streets and in other locations not considered appropriate housing (e.g., subways, abandoned properties). Definitions of literal homelessness vary both in duration and in the types of nonhousing locations included.[28,61] Inclusion of marginally housed individuals broadens the definition of homelessness to include individuals with precarious housing situations such as those living in single room occupancy buildings and staying with others without paying rent, and has been used to provide broader estimates of the lifetime prevalence of homelessness.[45] Most recently, researchers have identified an additional dimension to measuring homelessness with given definitions that may affect estimates of population prevalence. Eyrich-Garg and colleagues[28] have discussed differences between subjective (self-identified) and objective (identified by others) determinations of homelessness, and have demonstrated significant differences in risk patterns among samples of heavy-drinking women identified with different methods of determining homelessness.

As discussed in the preceding text, the many definitions of homelessness emerging from variations on an array of elements comprising this concept are destined to yield inconsistent sample characteristics and prevalence estimates. Because there is no unified definition of homelessness, there can be no single gold standard for determining the status of homelessness of individuals, and, therefore, it should be understood that in the remainder of this chapter, the relevant research to be reviewed necessarily consists of work derived from samples based on a variety of nonuniform definitions of homelessness from different perspectives. Although we are careful to identify both definitions of homelessness and the resulting types of samples included in specific studies (and to present critiques of current estimates in part based on this limitation), readers are encouraged to pay attention to these issues and remain cognizant of how these choices can subtly or even dramatically influence estimates of homelessness prevalence and observed characteristics of the population being studied.

Population Size Estimates

A number of methodological and conceptual issues must be considered in answering the question, how many homeless people are there? Similar to the complexities described around defining homelessness discussed in the previous section, issues requiring explication in interpreting estimations of population size include considerations of the sampling source and measurement methods (e.g., agency-based versus epidemiologic samples, neighborhood vs. urban area vs. national samples, point vs. recent or lifetime prevalence estimates vs. incidence).

Early prevalence estimates of homeless populations consisted of cross-sectional point prevalence estimates projected from samples counted at one or more overnight shelters. In one of the more thorough studies of this type, Burt and Cohen[11] estimated that there were 194,000 adult users of homeless shelters and soup kitchens in cities of 100,000 or more in a given week in 1987. Although basing their estimate on national shelter numbers represented a methodological improvement on previous estimates, because their estimate excluded multiple other sources of homeless people (e.g., soup kitchens, unsheltered locations), it was generally considered a substantial underestimate. Other commonly discussed population estimates (e.g., census enumeration) attempted to determine the size of homeless populations on a given night using single enumeration methods. However, we agree with an assertion made by Burt and Cohen[11] and endorsed by many others that these single-night estimations are also likely to miss substantial proportions of the literally homeless population, and thus represent significant undercounts. Populations underrepresented include the literal homeless (particularly those sleeping in hidden locations, such as in abandoned buildings) and those housed for single nights or for short spells. For these reasons, we will not further consider single-night estimates here.

Perhaps the best of the prevalence estimates emerge from the seminal work on homelessness of Burt et al.[10] Using data from the 1996 National Survey of Homeless Assistance Providers and Clients (a survey of a variety of providers for two, 1-month periods) and extrapolating from previous estimations, they were able to arrive at reasonable estimates of how many service-using individuals were homeless on a given day or week, and estimating the total number of homeless individuals (both accessing and not accessing services) for the same periods. Readers wishing to understand more about how these estimates were reached are invited to explore the details of the various methods and estimates provided in this work.[10]

In examining the various estimates, the best defensible figures of homeless service users who were homeless at the time of receipt of services were approximately between 440,000 and 840,000 in a given week and between 260,000 and 460,000 on a given night (including adults and children) in the National Survey of Homeless Assistance Providers and Clients.[10] Using their methods for estimating the proportion of individuals not using services, Burt and colleagues argued that between 1.4 and 2.1 million adults were homeless in a given year. This number is not out of line with other estimates for approximately the same time period.[22] More recently, using multiple enumeration strategies, the "Homelessness Counts" report gave a higher estimation of around 750,000 on a given night.[58] It is important to note that in estimating lifetime prevalence, a telephone household survey found that 6.5% of adults had experienced a spell of literal homelessness at some time in their lives, and that 3% had been homeless within the past year,[45,46] numbers far greater than any of the previous estimates.

An ongoing debate in the homelessness arena is the accuracy of these population estimates over time and their applicability to current population size and generalizability across locations. In terms of current population estimates, a relative consensus holds that the size of the homeless population increased in the 1980s[76] and that the population size has remained stable or grown since. However, as the National Alliance to End Homelessness has pointed out,[58] consistent enumerations are lacking beyond the flawed census attempts in 1990 and 2000,[48] and, therefore, any discussions around changing size of the population are more speculative than factual. Thus the estimates presented here, while representing best available evidence, cannot be considered precise or even necessarily accurate. In terms of generalizability of findings across locations, Culhane and colleagues[50] have used administrative records from homeless service providers to attempt to examine population size across multiple jurisdictions. Their results, although representing the state of the art, point out once again the difficulties in estimating population size, as they find rates ranging from 0.1% to 2.1% in different cities of the overall population on a yearly basis using approaches similar to those applied in administrative records data collection.

Although discussions of overall population size over time have been inconsistent at best and lacking at worst, some persuasive evidence points to recent changes in the composition of those who are homeless. North and colleagues,[61] using three comparable representative samples each examined a decade apart within a single urban environment, noted significant increases in substance use and mood disorders among homeless cohorts over time. Their findings suggest that the homeless population may be changing, and that some of the differences found across studies are likely attributable to changing characteristics of the population rather than simply variation created by use of different sampling strategies and study of different environments. Furthermore, they argued that observed changes in the population over time may represent unintended consequences of changes in national policy.

Chronic Versus Short Term

Efforts to understand the composition of the homeless population require examination of linked issues of duration of homelessness and number of spells of homelessness that have long received considerable attention in the homelessness literature and have focused efforts to help this population toward specific subgroups with distinct characteristics. Currently, much of the federal policy is aimed at addressing the chronic homeless population. Classifications of homelessness generally break the population into some variation of three not-always-distinct groups: crisis/first-episode, episodic, and chronic.[1,7,10,42,71,103] Estimates of proportions for the chronic subgroups vary from almost half falling into the chronic category[11] to less than one-fourth[7,10] and as low as 10%.[22] Caton and colleagues[13] examined predictors of remaining homelessness over 18 months in a cohort of newly homeless individuals, finding that shorter duration of homeless spells was associated with employment, no history of substance treatment or incarceration, and younger age. These observed differences indicate that these subgroups are distinct, with the additional implication that they may have differing treatment needs.

A Critique

Careful readers will note that much of this discussion of the homelessness population has included repeated cautions about the role of methodological issues in shaping the findings, including the definition of homelessness, sampling methods (e.g., service-using vs. non–service-using samples), and evolution of the population over time, to name only a few. Although numerous articles, books, and governmental reports have debated each of these issues separately and together, a broad conclusion from this literature is that it collectively yields only a vague understanding of the size and composition of the homeless population. We echo numerous other writers in noting the frustrations and complexities of integrating a large, methodologically flawed body of information that has been unable to describe this multifaceted population coherently or precisely. Much more could be written, including similar discussions of proportions of the population falling into various demographic subgroupings, but all would be marred by this same general critique. Given the focus of this chapter on substance use disorders and associated psychiatric and medical risk factors, we now move away from this general discussion of the homeless population to the central task of examining substance use disorders and comorbidities.

Substance Use Disorders

Association Between Substance Use Disorders and Other Risk Factors and Homelessness

Before launching a discussion of rates of risk factors in the homeless population, it is important to address the relationships of substance use disorders and other risk factors associated with homelessness. Generally, an implicit assumption in the popular literature holds that the disproportionate findings of these risk factors in the homeless population indicate that substance use and abuse/dependence and other mental illness cause these individuals to become homeless. However, evidence on onset of homelessness and psychiatric disorders has called into question this assumption.

Research on the causal nature of psychiatric disorders on homelessness has, in fact, concluded that the association between these factors is not simply unidirectional. O'Toole and colleagues[68] found evidence for changes in alcohol and drug abuse patterns after first onset of homelessness, including escalating use for some individuals and diminished use among others. North and colleagues[63] compared the relative timing of onsets of substance use disorders and other psychiatric disorders with first episode of homelessness and found that the proportion of homeless individuals with onset of their illnesses prior to the onset of their first episode of homelessness was similar to the proportion of a national community sample with onset of illness before an age comparable to that of the homeless sample's age at first homelessness. Earlier assumptions of direct unidirectional causality from psychopathology, to homelessness have largely been abandoned by the experts who now argue that there are also multiple indirect effects related to having a psychiatric disorder that may not only increase individual risk for entering homelessness but also create barriers to exiting homelessness.[4,31,68,100]

Prevalence Rates

When we use the term "substance use disorder," we are referring to substance abuse or substance dependence as defined in the *Diagnostic and Statistical Manual of Mental Disorders* (DSM; editions III, III-R, IV, IV-TR, or 5 depending on when the research was conducted). Meeting diagnostic criteria for either alcohol use disorder or for any specific drug use disorder (e.g., cocaine use disorder, cannabis use disorder, opioid use disorder) qualifies one for a diagnosis of substance use disorder.

There is a general scientific consensus that the prevalence of substance use disorder is disproportionately high in the homeless population. According to epidemiologic studies, the lifetime prevalence of substance use disorder is estimated to be in excess of two-thirds of homeless people.[40,79] Women range between 31% and 63%, and men between 71% and 75%,[62,79,91,92] Systematic shelter-selected samples (e.g., 30) yield similar lifetime prevalence rates. The current (12-month) prevalence of substance use disorder is estimated to be somewhere between 38% and 52%.[61,79]

One study[61] found that substance use disorders accounted for most of all lifetime psychiatric disorders among a representative sample of homeless people. A lifetime psychiatric diagnosis was detected in 88% of men and 69% of women, and a lifetime substance use disorder was identified in 84% of men and 58% of women.

Alcohol and Drug Use Disorder Comorbidity

The overlap between alcohol use disorders and drug use disorders is considerable in the homeless population. Approximately 61% of homeless women with lifetime alcohol use disorder also report a history of lifetime drug use disorder,[92] and approximately 40% of men and women who report a history of lifetime drug use disorder also report a history of lifetime alcohol use disorder.[91,92] A substantial proportion of the homeless population meets criteria for both alcohol and other drug use disorders. Approximately 36%–42% of homeless people meet lifetime criteria for both alcohol and other drug use disorders.[61,79] Somewhere between 29% and 33% of women meet lifetime criteria for both alcohol and other drug use disorders,[79,92] and approximately 38% of men meet lifetime criteria for both types of disorders.[79] Approximately 18% of homeless people meet current (12-month) criteria for both alcohol and other drug use disorders.[79]

Many homeless people with substance use disorders also have at least one other psychiatric disorder. Epidemiological studies have shown that of homeless people with lifetime alcohol use disorder, 32%–38% meet diagnostic criteria for a lifetime nonsubstance psychiatric disorder.[62] Of men with a lifetime nonsubstance psychiatric disorder, 60% meet diagnostic criteria for lifetime alcohol use disorder and 24% meet diagnostic criteria for lifetime drug use disorder.[62] Of women with a lifetime nonsubstance psychiatric disorder, 46% meet diagnostic criteria for lifetime alcohol use disorder and 20% meet criteria for lifetime drug use disorder.[62]

Alcohol Use Disorder

Prevalence Rates

Alcohol use disorders are highly prevalent in the homeless population, ranging from approximately 53%–63% according to epidemiological studies of lifetime rates.[40,61,79] Lifetime prevalence ranges from 17% to 40% in women and 56% to 68% in men.[62,91,92] Most individuals who meet criteria for lifetime alcohol use disorder also meet criteria for current alcohol use disorder.[79,91,92] Current-year prevalence rates for the disorder among homeless populations are estimated to be between 39% and 42%,[61,79] approximately 32% in women and 41%–50% in men.[79,91,92]

Studies comparing prevalence rates of lifetime and current (6-month) alcohol use disorder between homeless persons and housed groups have found significantly higher alcohol use disorder rates among the homeless.[40] However, this finding may not generalize to particular homeless subgroups. For example, lifetime rates of alcohol use disorder do not appear to differ between first-time, nonmentally ill shelter-seekers and persons applying for government assistance.[14] Shelter-using, mentally ill women have been found to have higher current (6-month) rates of alcohol use disorder than their housed, mentally ill female counterparts[15]; however, no significant difference was detected in the current (6-month) rates of alcohol use disorder between shelter-using, mentally ill men and housed, mentally ill men.[16] The literature indicates that excessive alcohol use is a strong discriminator between homeless and housed families. For instance, single female parents who were homeless reported a history of using alcohol excessively 23 times more frequently than single female parents who were housed.[5]

Other Drug Use Disorders

Overall Prevalence Rates

As with alcohol use disorder, drug use disorder is overrepresented in homeless populations. Lifetime prevalence of drug use disorder is estimated between 31% and 58%.[40,61,79] According to North and colleagues,[61] drug use disorders in the homeless population have increased significantly in prevalence over the past two decades. Women's lifetime rates range between 23% and 51%, and men's lifetime rates range between 40% and 61%.[61,79,91,92] Current (12-month) prevalence of drug use disorder is estimated to be between 31% and 38%,[61,79] approximately 32%–35% for women and 18%–38% for men.[61,79,91,92] Current (12-month) prevalence among shelter-using mentally ill women appears to be in line with these estimates,[15] but shelter-using mentally ill men appear to have a substantially higher prevalence of drug use disorder (77%).[16]

Drugs of Choice

The literature is clear that the drug associated with the highest rates of abuse and dependence among the homeless is cocaine. Cocaine use disorder has grown substantially in the homeless population through the 1990s and 2000s.[61] Lifetime cocaine use disorder prevalence rates range from 16% to 40% for women and from 37% to 46% for men.[61,79,91,92] Current (12-month) cocaine use disorder rates are approximately 26%–29% for women and 24%–33% for men.[61,79]

The drug with the second highest abuse/dependence rate is cannabis. During the mid-1980s, cannabis appeared to be the most prevalent drug of abuse (8% for women and 7% for men) in the homeless population,[62] but that has changed. Lifetime cannabis use disorder prevalence estimates range between 7% and 28% for women and 30% and 37% for men.[61,79,91,92] Current (12-month) prevalence of cannabis use disorder is approximately 8%–12% for women and 10%–16% for men.[61,79]

Stimulant, opioid, and sedative use disorders have estimated lifetime prevalence rates between 3% and 10%.[61,79] Current (12-month) prevalence is similar for stimulant, opioid, and sedative use disorders.[61,79]

Some differences emerge for subgroups of the homeless population. First-time shelter-seeking men appear to have lifetime prevalence rates of cocaine (33%), cannabis (32%), and heroin (11%) use disorders that are similar to those of their housed counterparts.[14] First-time shelter-seeking women, however, have elevated prevalence of cocaine (40%) and heroin (23%) but not cannabis (22%) use disorders, when compared with their housed counterparts.[14]

Injection Drug Use

In this brief section, we present information on a particular type of drug ingestion—injection drug use. Note that we discuss use (as opposed to drug abuse/dependence) and that this use may or may not be part of a drug use disorder. Injection drug use is important to mention apart from diagnosis because sharing works (e.g., needles) is a risk factor for contracting and spreading HIV. Many cities view needle-sharing as such a problem that they fund needle-exchange programs in which people can exchange their used needles for sanitary ones free of charge.

Epidemiological studies have found that 22% of the homeless population has a lifetime history of injection drug use, with 10% of men and 5% women injecting within the past year. The relative proportions of injection drugs of choice were heroin (94%), cocaine (58%), stimulants (45%), other opiates (20%), sedatives (19%), and hallucinogens (7%). Sex and age appear to play a role in the likelihood of injection drug use. In one study of severely mentally ill homeless people, rates of injection drug use across study recruitment sites ranged from 16% to 26% for men and 6% to 8% for women.[93] Younger persons in this subpopulation (e.g., under the age of 45) were more likely than older persons to have injected drugs at some point in their lives.[93]

Looking Forward

Substance use disorders among the homeless have been studied for many years now. Research needs to continue to identify shifts in the abuse/dependence of popular substances. It is not yet known whether the recently documented trends of increasing oxycodone abuse in the general substance abuse treatment-seeking population[12] and methamphetamine abuse observed in the general population[89] are also reflected in the homeless population.

Nonsubstance Psychiatric Disorders

Besides substance abuse, other psychiatric illness is an important issue to examine in homeless populations because of its prevalence, its relationship to homelessness, and its implications for service use and outcomes (for both homelessness and psychiatric illness). It can compromise a person's economic situation (e.g., psychiatric care costs, medication costs, inability to work), medical status (reducing ability to care for oneself), and social status (in terms of family and friendships).

Mood Disorders

Major depression is the most prevalent nonsubstance disorder in the homeless population. The lifetime prevalence of major depression is estimated to be between 18% and 21%,[61,40] with greater prevalence found among women (around 25%)[92] compared with men (around 18%).[91]

Major depression can be challenging to assess and difficult to interpret in homeless populations. North and colleagues[63] studied the relationship between ambient weather and same-day assessments of major depression in homeless people using a structured diagnostic interview. They found that men were more likely to meet diagnostic criteria for major depression when the weather was cold and wet. Yet, this difference was not detected among women, who are often allowed to spend days in the shelters (probably because most of them have children) while men are thrust out into the day's weather each day. North and colleagues concluded that the symptoms of major depression can be difficult to separate from the "miseries of homelessness," including hardships of exposure to inclement weather, especially for men. It is possible that the methods used to measure major depression in many epidemiological studies do not distinguish between the major depression that people typically present with in psychiatric treatment settings and emotional distress and disillusionment among homeless people coping with the extraordinary hardships of being homeless (physical and mental discomforts, hunger, fatigue, social isolation, demoralization, lack of privacy, and the presence of danger). If this is the case, then the standard treatments for major depression (e.g., medication, talk therapy) may not be appropriate for distressed homeless people as with clinically depressed treatment populations. Treatments for major depression are likely to be ineffective for ameliorating the situational distress and misery of homelessness that may be difficult to differentiate from major depression.

Instead of using a systematic diagnostic instrument to provide diagnosis of major depression according to DSM criteria (e.g., the Diagnostic Interview Schedule, the Composite International Diagnostic Interview, or the Structured Clinical Interview for DSM), many studies use proxies such as symptom screens, measures of distress or depressed mood, or distinctions of "clinical caseness." Studies based on such nondiagnostic measures have asserted that almost three-fourths (73%) of homeless samples can be defined as having clinically significant emotional distress or clinical caseness for some sort of depressive-like syndrome,[77] and approximately one-third of epidemiological and first-time shelter-user samples (ranging from 33% to 37%) have been reported to have "extreme distress."[77,94] As we stated before, being homeless can make one extremely stressed and unhappy. Even diagnostic instruments may overrepresent distress as major depression in this population, but they are far less likely than nondiagnostic screening tools to fall into this error. We suspect that high rates, such as 73%, for emotional distress/clinical caseness are a result of inadvertent capturing of the agonies of homelessness and their obfuscation with diagnostic syndromes.

The next mood disorder we will discuss is bipolar disorder. Breakey and colleagues[62] estimated the lifetime prevalence of bipolar disorder in homeless populations of the mid-80s to be around 7%–8% for both women and men. Another epidemiological study of homelessness estimated the lifetime prevalence of bipolar disorder to be around 11%.[40] A study conducted in the early 2000s[61] estimated lifetime rates of bipolar disorder to be around 9%.

Anxiety Disorders

Anxiety disorders, including panic disorder, generalized anxiety disorder, and posttraumatic stress disorder, are prevalent in the homeless population as well. One epidemiological study estimated the lifetime prevalence of any anxiety disorder for shelter users to be around 39% and the 6-month prevalence to be around 22%.[29] However, prevalence estimates of these disorders have been lower in more recent epidemiological studies. Similar to our discussion of the challenges of diagnosing major depression in the homeless population, it can be difficult to diagnose anxiety disorders correctly in this population. Real threats of violence, theft, lack of food, and a need to avoid the police in some cities (for fear of being arrested for vagrancy) understandably generate anxiety for many homeless people. This situational anxiety can be difficult to distinguish from symptoms of psychiatric disorders such as panic disorder and generalized anxiety disorder.

Posttraumatic stress disorder appears to be the most prevalent anxiety disorder among homeless people. Lifetime prevalence of posttraumatic stress disorder is estimated to be around 20% for all homeless people[61]—34% for homeless women[92] and 18% for homeless men.[91] Current (12-month) prevalence is estimated to be slightly less (15%).[61]

Panic disorder is typically the next most prevalent anxiety disorder in studies of homeless populations. The lifetime prevalence of panic disorder in the homeless population is estimated to be around 8%–9%[40,61]—3% in women[92] and 5% in men.[91] Current (both 6-month and 12-month) prevalence of panic disorder appears to be slightly less overall (5%) but very similar when reported separately by sex (women: 3%; men: 4%).[40,91,92]

Generalized anxiety disorder is the last anxiety disorder we will discuss. Lifetime rates of generalized anxiety disorders range from 7% to 14%.[40,61,91,92] Current (both 6-month and 12-month) prevalence rates of the disorder appear to be slightly lower, ranging from 5% to 11%.[40,6140,91,92]

Psychotic Disorders

When asked to conjure up an image of a homeless person, most people imagine someone who is severely mentally ill. They think of someone who is psychotic (hearing voices and seeing images that do not exist) and who talks to or yells at imaginary others, such as someone with schizophrenia. Systematic research shows, however, that a very small percentage of the homeless population fits this description. Contrary to anecdotal evidence, psychotic disorders, most often represented by schizophrenia, are not nearly as prevalent as the news media's sensationalistic presentation of them in the homeless population. Epidemiological studies have estimated the lifetime prevalence of schizophrenia to be between 4% and 17%.[40,61,62,65] First-time homeless shelter–using men have reported a prevalence estimate within this range: 8%.[94]

Personality Disorders

The most consistently measured personality disorder in the homeless literature is antisocial personality disorder. The prevalence of antisocial personality disorder appears to be remarkably, disproportionately high among homeless populations. Epidemiological data show that between 16% and 20% of the homeless population meet criteria for the lifetime disorder[29,61] with approximately 10% of women and 25% of men qualifying for the diagnosis.[91,92] Some researchers[66] have argued that meeting criteria for antisocial personality disorder can be a functional and adaptive, survival pattern of behavior in the context of homelessness rather than a strictly pathological phenomenon. Therefore, they would argue that using the diagnosis in the homeless population is culturally insensitive. North et al.[67] refuted this argument, contending that the onset of adult antisocial personality disorder almost always occurs prior to the onset of homelessness and correlates with childhood conduct symptoms, and, in their analysis, the rates of antisocial personality disorder did not decline significantly when they removed criterion symptoms related to homelessness from the algorithms. They concluded that although homelessness may exacerbate the manifestations of antisocial personality disorder, it is a valid diagnosis in this population.

Other personality disorders have received generally less attention in the scientific literature. A pioneering study in the 1980s by Bassuk and colleagues[6] examined rates of DSM-III–diagnosed personality disorders in sheltered homeless families. In this study, an astounding 71% of homeless mothers in their sample met diagnostic criteria for at least one personality disorder. Diagnoses provided by psychiatrists yielded the following prevalence rates of various personality disorders: dependent (24%), atypical (10%), borderline (6%), narcissistic (4%), antisocial (4%), passive-aggressive (4%), mixed (4%), schizoid (3%), and histrionic (1%). The authors of the study were quick to point out that Axis II diagnoses are less reliable than Axis I diagnoses and that many external environmental factors (e.g., poverty, racism, and sexism) may play a role in determining observable features masquerading as personality traits in this population barraged by extraordinary stressors.

Overall Prevalence Rates

According to a major epidemiological study conducted in the early 2000s,[61] 49% of homeless people have a lifetime history of at least one nonsubstance disorder, most of which is accounted for by major depression. This means that (1) half of the homeless population does not have any history of nonsubstance disorder and (2) of those with a lifetime history of nonsubstance disorder, very few have chronic and persistent severe mental illness (e.g., schizophrenia, bipolar disorder). We exclude major depression from chronic and persistent severe mental illness (see reference 83 for definitions).

The Roles of Sex and Race in Psychiatric Disorders Among the Homeless

A common theme among the psychiatric disorders in the homeless population is differences in findings by sex and race. Homeless Caucasian women have been found to have a greater prevalence of schizophrenia, major depression, and bipolar, panic, generalized anxiety, and posttraumatic stress disorders than homeless women of color.[65] This indicates that the homeless women of color may have less major psychiatric illness than homeless Caucasian women. Although we cannot determine causality, these data lend support to ideas that racism, oppression, social inequities, and social injustices may play a proportionately greater role in the homelessness of women of color.

The prevalence of cocaine, opioid, and amphetamine use disorders is greater among homeless men than among homeless women, and more homeless women have alcohol and cannabis use disorders, major depression, and schizophrenia compared with homeless men.[62,79]

Medical Illness

Medical illness is also disproportionately overrepresented in the homeless population. Life on the streets and in the shelter system can be dangerous, stressful, and hazardous to one's health. It can be difficult to locate a free place to shower and wash one's clothes to maintain proper hygiene; this makes it difficult to prevent as well as treat illness. Few homeless people have health insurance and can take preventive health care measures (perhaps, in part, because of competing immediate demands such as food and shelter). Many may wait for health conditions to become urgent or emergent before seeking medical attention and then use emergency rooms rather than regular outpatient services for treatment.[36]

We cannot state that all medical problems in the homeless population are the direct result of homelessness. Housed low-income populations often have poor health as well. This poor health can be attributed to a variety of factors including poor diet, lack of preventive health care, and lack of exercise. Medical problems among those who are low-income and become homeless are generally problems that are well known to be associated with circumstances of extreme poverty and other associated social problems. It is, however, likely that being homeless exacerbates the health problems that are already endemic in these populations.

HIV/AIDS

HIV/AIDS has recently begun to receive increased attention in homeless populations. The prevalence of HIV/AIDS among the homeless and marginally housed populations has been estimated to be between 10% and 15% in San Francisco,[8] 6% and 19% among the mentally ill homeless in New York City,[26,95] and 16% among soup kitchen attendees in New York City.[47] One study[23] found that people with HIV/AIDS in Philadelphia were three times as likely to be homeless as people without the infection. Another study[90] found that homeless injection drug users had a greater prevalence of HIV than housed injection drug users (19% vs. 11%).

Risk for engaging in risky sexual behaviors, which increase one's chances of contracting HIV, is increased in association with intoxication with alcohol and other drugs in homeless populations as in other populations.[30] Because many homeless people, particularly women, trade sex for food, clothing, drugs, or a place to stay, they are at heightened risk for contracting the virus.[101] Homeless people, especially those who are most transient, may not have a reliable place to store their works; therefore, they are more likely than others to borrow injection equipment[21,33] or visit a shooting gallery.[33] This places them at even greater risk for contracting the virus.

Infectious Diseases

People who experience homelessness may be exposed to or carry infectious diseases. One study of people using soup kitchen services in New York City[47] found high rates of hepatitis B virus exposure (21%), hepatitis B carrier (6%), hepatitis C seropositive (19%), and syphilis exposure (15%).[17,86] The Centers for Disease Control and Prevention (CDC) reported the rate of tuberculosis among the homeless to be 6.5% in 1997.[17]

Services for the Homeless

Following the considerations presented above, the treatment of homeless individuals requires attention to a variety of interrelated treatment needs. A general consensus in the treatment literature is that information sought to identify specific treatment needs must address issues around housing, psychiatric and medical illness, employment and economic factors, family[72] and social supports,[27] and contextual elements such as availability and accessibility of services.[10] It is equally clear from both the services literature and the review of risk factors presented in this chapter that individual treatment requires attention to these multiple needs.

Research has further identified a series of barriers that complicate delivery of services to homeless individuals. These include suspicions harbored by homeless individuals about the consequences of receiving treatment,[43] "hang out" or "street" groups that discourage treatment engagement,[73] and disjuncture between professionally assessed needs versus those perceived by the homeless individual.[19,64]

Despite the complex needs identified in this chapter and the multiple factors complicating service delivery, it is possible to make some general statements about what constitutes effective treatment for this population. Perhaps most simply, there is a positive association between amount of service use and the achievement of favorable outcomes.[a] A second consistent finding is that achievement of a broad variety of outcomes requires effective matching of needs to services, as well as integration of care.[b] A third finding is that coordination of intensive services with transitions to housing increases the likelihood of positive outcomes.[24,25,75,81,105]

Research on effective treatment for homeless individuals has generally focused on the development and testing of intervention models. Although an in-depth discussion of services research is beyond the scope of this chapter, examining existing intervention models provides insight into effective approaches and can help point to opportunities for individual treatment and broader service responses. The past decade has seen the development and testing of a variety of effective models of intervention for homeless populations. Perhaps the most promising of these models is the Housing First approach to permanent housing.[69,98,99] This model, which combines immediate noncontingent housing and supportive services, has been demonstrated to have relatively substantial effect sizes in increasing housing stability and other associated outcomes.[60] It is important to note that Housing First services have also been shown to be equally effective as treatment-first approaches in outcomes around drug and alcohol use over time.[69] In a comparison of permanent housing with assertive community treatment and intensive case management, although all three service types did better than their various comparison conditions (generally treatment as usual, which in most instances was case management), permanent housing was shown to have greater effect sizes for housing outcomes than assertive community treatment or intensive case management.[60]

A number of other models have demonstrated promise through either clinical trials or quasi-experimental designs for homeless populations with mental illness. The "critical time intervention" by Susser and colleagues[25,37] demonstrated significant gains in housing stability relative to usual services; Assertive Community Treatment demonstrated superior housing and mental health outcomes to case management[20,57]; a psychiatric rehabilitation model demonstrated a wide variety of housing and psychiatric outcomes relative to standard treatment[87]; and intensive case management demonstrated moderate effect sizes relative to case management.[18] Examining costs associated with outcomes,[80] noted that innovative programs tend to be more expensive than usual services, but challenged his readers to examine his findings in light of the value that society places on these marginalized members.

In the literature on services for homeless populations, addiction treatment is often not the primary focus of the intervention. As we have already noted, housing first is eponymous—it aims to get individuals into housing first regardless of other behaviors (primarily addiction-related ones). Thus the findings from these type of interventions generally focus extensively on housing outcomes, often concluding that housing-first approaches do equally well as their comparison groups in addiction-related outcomes (cf. reference 99). Generally, research on services for addiction in homeless populations focuses on either dually diagnosed populations[35]

or on including substances in integrated models.[70] One effective model for homelessness that incorporates a contingency management intervention paired with abstinence-based housing demonstrated positive and housing-related outcomes.[53,84]

Conclusions

In summing up knowledge on homelessness, substance use and abuse, other psychiatric and medical illness, and available services, some very broad conclusions can be made. The homeless population is a substantial one in terms of size, particularly with consideration of longer assessment periods. Although spells of homelessness for a majority of the population identified are relatively short-term, the substantial minority of individual spells that are chronic present complex challenges in service provision.

In terms of substance use and abuse, all psychiatric disorders have a disproportionate prevalence in the homeless population, regardless of sampling or assessment methods. The primary drugs of abuse are cocaine (in various forms, but especially crack cocaine), alcohol, and marijuana; and the proportion of the homeless population with addictions appears to be increasing in recent decades. However, despite popular assumptions, addiction does not appear to have a simple direct causal relationship with homelessness, rather it appears to have indirect effects contributing to the likelihood of becoming homeless. Furthermore, it appears that homelessness has a similar indirect effect on the likelihood of substance use and abuse.

There appears to be a disproportionate prevalence of psychiatric (especially substance use disorders) and other medical illness in this population. However, even including the disproportionate prevalence of psychiatric and medical illness among the homeless, the majority do not have a non–substance-related psychiatric diagnosis, and the most common category of psychiatric malady (outside of the highly prevalent substance abuse) is not a severe and persistent mental illness such as schizophrenia, but rather major depression or some homelessness-related phenotypic variant of depression related to the miseries of homelessness. Furthermore, these psychiatric and other medical disorders in homeless populations appear to occur almost exclusively as comorbidities with addictive disorders.

Generally effective services for homeless populations must be intensive in nature, matched closely with assessed and perceived needs, effectively addressing barriers to care (especially lack of coordination across providers), and providing intensive services at key transitional times. A number of effective models have been demonstrated to yield favorable housing outcomes relative to comparison conditions, including Housing First, Assertive Community Treatment, Intensive Case Management, Critical Time interventions, and psychiatric rehabilitation.

In concluding this review, we return to the ongoing methodological issues that have consistently plagued the field and, therefore, complicated this chapter. At best, the research applied to discuss this population has limited consistency, in large part due to difficulties in the methodological designs of existing research studies. Important issues such as changes to the population over time, differences among locations such as cities (particularly around transience), and the interrelationship of the individual-level risk factors with economic and policy factors all remain understudied and may significantly impact our understanding of homeless individuals. What is required to address these issues is methodologically sophisticated, longitudinal research that incorporates multiple sites, consistent sampling and multiple levels of data (individual, social, environmental), and complex modeling congruent with the data sophistication.

---

[a]References 39, 54, 56, 74, 75, 85.
[b]References 18, 35, 38, 41, 51, 70, 82.

References

1. Arce A, Vergare M. Identifying and characterizing the mentally ill among the homeless. In: Lamb HR, ed. *The Homeless Mentally Ill: A Task Force Report of the American Psychiatric Association*. Washington, DC: American Psychiatric Association; 1984:75–90.
2. Bachrach LL. What we know about homelessness among mentally ill persons: an analytical review and commentary. *Hospital Commun Psychiatr*. 1992;43:45–464.
3. Badiago S, Raoult D, Brouque P. Preventing and controlling emerging and reemerging transmissible diseases in the homeless. *Emerg Infect Dis*. 2008;14(9):1353–1359.
4. Balshem H, Christensen V, Tuepker A, et al. *A Critical Review of the Literature Regarding Homelessness Among Veterens*. Washington, DC: Department of Veterans Affairs (US); 2011.
5. Bassuk EL, Buckner JC, Weinreb LF, et al. Homelessness in female-headed families: childhood and adult risk and protective factors. *Am J Public Health*. 1997;87:241–248.
6. Bassuk EL, Rubin L, Lauriat AS. Characteristics of sheltered homeless families. *Am J Public Health*. 1986;76(9):1097–1101.
7. Bray RM, Dennis ML, Lambert EY. *Prevalence of Drug Use in the Washington DC Metropolitan Area Homeless and Transient Population: 1991*. Rockville, MD: NIDA; 1993.
8. Bucher JB, Thomas KM, Guzman D, Riley E, Dela Cruz N, Bangsberg DR. Community-based rapid HIV testing in homeless and marginally housed adults in San Francisco. *HIV Med*. 2007;8:28–31.
9. Burt MR, Aron LY, Douglas T, Valente J, Lee E, Iwen B. Homelessness: programs and the people they serve. In: *Summary Report*. Washington, DC: The Urban Institute; 1999.
10. Burt MR, Aron LY, Lee E. *Helping America's Homeless*. Washington, DC: Urban Institute; 2001.
11. Burt MR, Cohen BE. *America's Homeless: Numbers, Characteristics and the Programs that Serve Them*. Washington, DC: Urban Institute; 1989.
12. Carise D, Dugosh KL, McLellan AT, Camilleri A, Woody GE, Lynch KG. Prescription oxycontin abuse among patients entering addiction treatment. *Am J Psychiatry*. 2007;164(11):1750–1756.
13. Caton CLM, Dominguez B, Schanzer B, et al. Risk factors for long-term homelessness: findings from a longitudinal study of first-time homeless single adults. *Am J Public Health*. 2005;95(10):1753–1759.
14. Caton CLM, Hasin D, Shrout PE, et al. Risk factors for homelessness among indigent urban adults with no history of psychotic illness: a case-control study. *Am J Public Health*. 2000;90:258–263.
15. Caton CLM, Shrout PE, Dominguez B, Eagle PF, Opler LA, Cournos F. Risk factors for homelessness among women with schizophrenia. *Am J Public Health*. 1995;85:1153–1156.
16. Caton CLM, Shrout PE, Eagle PF, Opler LA, Felix A, Dominguez B. Risk factors for homelessness among schizophrenic men: a case-control study. *Am J Public Health*. 1994;84:265–269.
17. Centers for Disease Control and Prevention. In: *Reported Tuberculosis in the United States, 1997*. Atlanta, GA: CDC; 1998.
18. Clark C, Rich AR. Outcomes of homeless adults with mental illness in a housing program and in case management only. *Psychiatr Serv*. 2003;54:78–83.
19. Cohen C, Onserud H, Monaco C. Outcomes for the mentally ill in a program for older homeless persons. *Hospital Commun Psychiatr*. 1993;44:650–656.
20. Coldwell CM, Bender WS. The effectiveness of assertive community treatment for homeless populations with severe mental illness: a meta-analysis. *Am J Psychiatr*. 2007;164:393–399.
21. Corneil TA, Kuyper LM, Shoveller J, et al. Unstable housing, associated risk behavior, and increased risk for HIV infection among injection drug users. *Health Place*. 2006;12:79–85.
22. Culhane DP, Dejowski E, Ibanez J, Needham E, Macchia I. Public shelter admission rates in Philadelphia and New York City: implications for sheltered population counts. *Housing Policy Debate*. 1994;5(2):107–140.
23. Culhane DP, Gollub E, Kuhn R, Shpaner M. The co-occurrence of AIDS and homelessness: results from the integration of administrative databases for AIDS surveillance and public shelter utilization in Philadelphia. *J Epidemiol Community Health*. 2001;55:515–520.
24. De Vet R, van Lutjelaar MJA, Brilleslijper-Kater SN, Vanderplasschen W, Beijersbergen MD, Wolf JRLM. Effectiveness of case management for homeless persons: a systematic review. *Am J Public Health*. 2013;103(10):e13–e26.
25. Dixon LB, Holoshitz Y, Nossel I. Treatment engagement of individuals experiencing mental illness: a review and update. *World Psychiatry*. 2016;15(1):13–20.
26. Empfield M, Cournos F, Meyer I, et al. HIV seroprevalence among homeless patients admitted to a psychiatric inpatient unit. *Am J Psychiatr*. 1993;150:47–52.
27. Eyrich KM, Pollio DE, North CS. Differences in social support between short-term and long-term homelessness. *Social Work Res*. 2003;27(4):222–231.
28. Eyrich-Garg KM, Callahan O'Leary C, Cottler L. Subjective versus objective definitions of homelessness: are there differences in risk factors among heavy drinking women? *Gend Issues*. 2008;25(3):173–192.
29. Fischer PJ, Shapiro S, Breakey WR, Anthony JC, Kramer M. Mental health and social characteristics of the homeless: a survey of mission users. *Am J Public Health*. 1986;76:519–523.
30. Forney JC, Lombardo S, Toro PA. Diagnostic and other correlates of HIV risk behaviors in a probability sample of homeless adults. *Psychiatr Serv*. 2007;58(1):91–99.
31. Fountain J, Howes S, Marsden J, Taylor C, Strang J. Drug and alcohol use and the link with homelessness: results from a survey of homeless people in London. *Addiction Res Theory*. 2003;11(4):245–256.
32. Gans HJ. *The Urban Villagers*. New York: Free; 1962.
33. German D, Davey MA, Latkin CA. Residential transience and HIV risk behaviors among injection drug users. *AIDS Behav*. 2007;11:S21–S30.
34. Goldman HH. Deinstitutionalization and community care. *Harvard Rev Psychiatr*. 1998;6:219–222.
35. Gonzalez G, Rosenheck R. Outcomes and service use among homeless persons with serious mental illness and substance abuse. *Psychiatr Serv*. 2002;53:437–446.
36. Henry R, Richardson JL, Stoyanoff S, et al. HIV/AIDS health service utilization by people who have been homeless. *AIDS Behav*. 2008;12:815–821.
37. Jones K, Colson PW, Holter MC, et al. Cost-effectiveness of critical time intervention to reduce homelessness among persons with mental illness. *Psychiatr Serv*. 2003;54:884–890.
38. Kertesz SG, Larson MJ, Cheng DM, et al. Need and non-need factors associated with addiction treatment utilization in a cohort of homeless and housed urban poor. *Med Care*. 2006;44(3):225–233.
39. Kertesz SG, Mullins AN, Schumacher JE, Wallace D, Kirk K, Milby JB. Long-term housing and work outcomes among treated cocaine-dependent homeless persons. *J Behav Health Serv*. 2007;34(1):17–33.
40. Koegel P, Burnam MA, Farr RK. The prevalence of specific psychiatric disorders among homeless individuals in the inner city of Los Angeles. *Archiv Gen Psychiatry*. 1988;45:1085–1092.
41. Koegel P, Sullivan G, Burnam A, Morton S, Wenzel S. Utilization of mental health and substance abuse services among homeless adults in Los Angeles. *Med Care*. 1999;37(3):306–317.
42. Kuhn R, Culhane DP. Applying cluster analysis to test a typology of homelessness by patterns of shelter utilization: results from the analysis of administrative data. *Am J Community Psychol*. 1998;12(2):207–232.
43. Lam JA, Rosenheck R. Street outreach for homeless persons with serious mental illness: is it effective? *Med Care*. 1999;37(9):894–907.
44. Liebow E. Tally's corner. In: *Little*. Boston, MA: Brown; 1967.
45. Link B, Phelan J, Bresnahan M, Stueve A, Moore R, Susser E. Lifetime and five-year prevalence of homelessness in the United States: new evidence on an old debate. *Am J Orthopsychiatry*. 1995;65(3):347–354.

46. Link B, Susser E, Stueve A, Phelan J, Moore R, Struening E. Lifetime and five-year prevalence of homelessness in the United States. *Am J Public Health.* 1994;84:1907–1912.

47. Magura S, Nwakeze PC, Rosenblum A, Joseph H. Substance misuse and related infectious diseases in a soup kitchen population. *Subst Use Misuse.* 2000;35(4):551–583.

48. Martin E. Assessment of S-night enumeration in the 1990 census. *Eval Rev.* 1992;16(4):418–438.

49. McKinney Act (1987) (P.L. 100–77, sec 103(2)(1), 101 sat. 485).

50. Metraux S, Culhane D, Raphael S, et al. Assessing homeless population size through the use of emergency and transitional shelter services in 1998: results from the analysis of administrative data from nine US jurisdictions. *Public Health Rep.* 2001;116:344–352.

51. Metraux S, Marcus SC, Culhane DP. The New York–New York housing initiative and use of public shelters by persons with severe mental illness. *Psychiatr Serv.* 2003;54:67–71.

52. Milburn NG, Watts RJ, Anderson SL. An analysis of current research methods for studying the homeless: final report. In: *Institute for Urban Affairs and Research.* Howard University; 1984.

53. Milby J, Schumacher J, Wallace D, Freedman MJ, Vuchinich RE. To house or not to house: the effects of providing housing to homeless substance abusers in treatment. *Am J Public Health.* 2005;95(7):1259–1265.

54. Miller ER, Paschall KW, Azar ST. Latent classes of older foster youth: prospective associations with outcomes and exits from the foster care system during the transition to adulthood. *Children Youth Serv Rev.* 2017;79:495–505.

55. Morrisey J, Dennis D. *Homelessness and Mental Illness: Toward the Next Generation of Research Studies.* Washington DC: National Institute on Mental Health; 1990.

56. Morse GA, Calsyn RJ, Allen G. Helping homeless mentally ill people: what variables mediate and moderate program effects? *Am J Community Psychol.* 1994;22:661–683.

57. Morse GA, Calsyn RJ, Klinkenberg WD, et al. An experimental comparison of three types of case management for homeless mentally ill persons. *Psychiatr Serv.* 1997;48:497–503.

58. National Alliance to End Homelessness. *First Nationwide Estimate of Homeless Population in a Decade Announced.* Washington DC: NAEH; 2007.

59. National Coalition for the Homeless. *Substance Abuse and Homelessness*; 2009.

60. Nelson G, Aubry T, Lafrance A. A review of the literature on the effectiveness of housing and support, assertive community treatment, and intensive case management interventions for persons with mental illness who have been homeless. *Am J Orthopsychiatry.* 2007;77(3):350–361.

61. North CS, Eyrich KM, Pollio DE, Spitznagel EL. Are rates of psychiatric disorders in the homeless population changing? *Am J Public Health.* 2004;94(1):103–108.

62. North CS, Eyrich KM, Pollio DE, Spitznagel EL. Are rates of psychiatric disorders in the homeless population changing? *Am J Public Health.* 2004;94(1):103–108.

63. North CS, Pollio DE, Smith EM, Spitznagel EL. Correlates of early onset and chronicity of homelessness in a large urban homeless population. *J Nervous Mental Dis.* 1998;186:393–400.

64. North CS, Smith EM. A systematic study of mental health services utilization by homeless men and women. *Soc Psychiatry Psychiatr Epidemiol.* 1993;28:77–83.

65. North CS, Smith EM. Comparison of white and nonwhite homeless men and women. *Soc Work.* 1994;39:639–647.

66. North CS, Smith EM, Spitznagel EL. Is antisocial personality a valid diagnosis among the homeless? *Am J Psychiatry.* 1993;150(4):578–583.

67. North CS, Smith EM, Spitznagel EL. Is antisocial personality disorder a valid diagnosis among the homeless? *Am J Psychiatry.* 1993;150:578–583.

68. O'Toole TP, Gibbon JL, Hanusa BH, Freyder PJ, Conde AM, Fine MJ. Self-reported changes in drug and alcohol use after becoming homeless. *Am J Public Health.* 2004;94(5):830–835.

69. Padgett DK, Gulcur L, Tsemberis S. Housing first services for people who are homeless with co-occurring serious mental illness and substance abuse. *Res Social Work Pract.* 2006;16(1):74–83.

70. Palepu A, Gadermann A, Hubley AM, et al. Substance use and access to health care and addiction treatment among homeless and vulnerably housed persons in three Canadian cities. *PLoS One.* 2013;8(10):e75133.

71. Phelan JC, Link BG. Who are "the homeless?" reconsidering the stability and composition of the homeless population. *Am J Public Health.* 1999;84:1907–1912.

72. Polgar M, North CS, Pollio DE. Family support for homeless individual adults. *J Social Distress Homeless.* 2006;15:273–293.

73. Pollio DE. Group membership as a predictor of service use related behavior for persons "on the streets". *Res Social Work Pract.* 1999;9(5):575–592.

74. Pollio DE, North CS, Thompson S, Paquin JW, Spitznagel EL. Predictors of achieving stable housing in a mentally ill homeless population. *Psychiatr Serv.* 1997;48(4):258–260.

75. Pollio DE, Spitznagel EL, North CS, Thompson S, Foster DA. Service use over time and achievement of stable housing in a mentally ill homeless population. *Psychiatr Serv.* 2000;51:1536–1543.

76. Quigley JM, Raphael S, Smolensky E. Homeless in America, homeless in California. *Rev Economics Statistics.* 2001;83(1):37–51.

77. Ritchey FJ, LaGory M, Fitzpatrick KM, Mullis J. A comparison of homeless, community-wide, and selected distressed samples on the CES-Depression Scale. *Am J Public Health.* 1990;80:1384–1386.

78. Reference deleted in review.

79. Robertson MJ, Zlotnick C, Westerfelt A. Drug use disorders and treatment contact among homeless adults in Alameda county, California. *Am J Public Health.* 1997;87:221–228.

80. Rosenheck R. Cost-effectiveness of services for mentally ill homeless people: the application of research to policy and practice. *Am J Psychiatry.* 2000;157:1563–1570.

81. Rosenheck R, Dennis D. Time-limited assertive community treatment for homeless persons with mental illness. *Archiv Gen Psychiatry.* 2001;58:1073–1080.

82. Rosenheck R, Morrissey J, Lam J, et al. Service system integration, access to services, and housing outcomes in a program for homeless persons with severe mental illness. *Am J Public Health.* 1998;88(110):1610–1615.

83. Schinnar AP, Rothbard AB, Kanter R, Jung YS. An empirical literature review of definitions of severe and persistent mental illness. *Am J Psychiatry.* 1990;147:1602–1608.

84. Schumacher JE, Mennemeyer ST, Milby JB, Wallace D, Nolan K. Costs and effectiveness of substance abuse treatment for homeless persons. *J Mental Health Policy Economics.* 2002;5:33–42.

85. Schumacher JE, Milby JB, Caldwell E, et al. Treatment outcome as a function of treatment attendance with homeless persons abusing cocaine. *J Addict Dis.* 1995;14(4):73–85.

86. Schwartz KB, Garrett B, Alter MJ, Thompson D, Stradthee SA. Seroprevalence of HCV infection in homeless families in Baltimore. *J Health Care Poor Underserved.* 2008;19(2):1049–2089.

87. Shern DL, Tsemberis S, Anthony W, et al. Serving street-dwelling individuals with psychiatric disabilities: outcomes of a psychiatric rehabilitation clinical trial. *Am J Public Health.* 2000;90:1873–1878.

88. Shinn M, Burke P, Bedford S. *Homelessness: Abstracts of the Psychological and Behavioral Literature, 1967–1990.* Washington, DC: American Psychological Association; 1990.

89. Shrem MT, Halkitis PN. Methamphetamine abuse in the United States: contextual, psychological, and sociological considerations. *J Health Psychol.* 2008;13(5):669–679.

90. Smereck GA, Hockman EM. Prevalence of HIV infection and HIV risk behaviors associated with living place: on-the-street homeless drug users as a special target population for public health intervention. *Am J Drug Alcohol Abuse.* 1998;24:299–319.

91. Smith EM, North CS, Spitznagel EL. A systematic study of mental illness, substance abuse, and treatment in 600 homeless men. *Ann Clin Psychiatry.* 1992;4:111–120.

92. Smith EM, North CS, Spitznagel EL. Alcohol, drugs, and psychiatric comorbidity among homeless women: an epidemiologic study. *J Clin Psychiatry.* 1993;54:82–87.

93. Susser E, Betne P, Valencia E, Goldfinger SM, Lehman AF. Injection drug use among homeless adults with severe mental illness. *Am J Public Health.* 1997;87:854–856.

94. Susser E, Conover S, Struening EL. Problems of epidemiologic method in assessing the type and extent of mental illness among homeless adults. *Hospital Community Psychiatry.* 1989;40:261–265.

95. Susser E, Valencia E, Conover S. Prevalence of HIV infection among psychiatric patients in a New York City men's shelter. *Am J Public Health.* 1993;83:568–570.

96. Tessler R, Dennis D. *A Synthesis of NIMH Funded Research Concerning Persons Who Are Homeless and Mentally Ill.* Washington, DC: National Institute on Mental Health; 1989.

97. Testa M, West SG. Civil commitment in the United States. *Psychiatry.* 2010;7(10):30–40.

98. Tsemberis S, Eisenberg RF. Pathways to housing: supported housing for street-dwelling homeless individuals with psychiatric disabilities. *Psychiatr Serv.* 2000;51:487–493.

99. Tsemberis S, Gulcar L, Nakae M. Housing first, consumer choice and harm reduction for homeless individuals with a dual diagnosis. *Am J Public Health.* 2004;94(4):651–656.

100. Vangeest JB, Johnson TP. Substance abuse and homelessness: direct or indirect effect? *Ann Epidemiol.* 2002;12:455–461.

101. Wenzel SL, Tucker JS, Elliott MN, Hambarsoomians K. Sexual risk among impoverished women: understanding the role of housing status. *AIDS Behav.* 2007;11:S9–S20.

102. Whyte WF. *Street Corner Society.* Chicago: University of Chicago; 1943.

103. Wong YI, Piliavin I. A dynamic analysis of homeless-domicile transitions. *Soc Probl.* 1997;44(3):408–423.

104. Wright JD. *Address Unknown: The Homeless in America.* New York: Aldine de Gruyter; 1989.

105. Wright JD, Devine JA. Factors that interact with treatment to predict outcomes in substance abuse programs for the homeless. *J Addict Dis.* 1995;14(4):169–181.

74

Opening New Vistas in Basic and Preclinical Addiction Research

RAINER SPANAGEL

A Retrospective View on the Hallmarks of Neurobiological Alcohol and Drug Abuse Research

What were the major achievements in the past in neurobiologically oriented alcohol and drug abuse research? This can only be answered by a very personal view. I would like to illustrate this in terms of the hallmarks of alcohol research. In 1940, Curt Paul Richter[80] reported that laboratory rats voluntarily consume alcohol, although with high individual variability. This discovery marked the beginning of animal research in the study of alcohol. Furthermore, this observed variability in alcohol intake provided the basis for the generation of alcohol-preferring and nonpreferring rat and mouse lines, eight of which have been genetically

selected since 1960.[26] Thousands of studies on alcohol drinking in rodents have been conducted subsequently, permitting the deciphering of the genetic and neurochemical basis of alcohol reinforcement. Studies of alcohol self-administration in laboratory animals remain crucial to the development of medication in the field of alcohol research, and the predictive value of these models is demonstrated by the fact that all available pharmacotherapies (e.g., naltrexone and acamprosate)[98] have been based on animal work of this nature. The same is true for any other drug of abuse—without appropriate animal models only little progress would have been made in the field of addiction research. In fact, most of the animal models (e.g., intravenous self-administration of heroin and cocaine) provide excellent face and construct validity.[86]

In terms of construct validity, the discovery of the brain reinforcement system by James Olds in 1954[70]—one of the outstanding experimental psychologists of the last century—ultimately provided the key to understanding the neuroanatomical correlates underlying alcohol and drug reinforcement. Again, knowledge derived from animal work on the neuroanatomical and functional aspects of alcohol and drug reinforcement has been systematically translated to humans by means of neuroimaging techniques.[116]

The foundation for understanding the neurochemical substrates of alcohol and drug reward[1] was laid by the three research teams in 1973 responsible for identifying the first opioid receptors.[74,93,104] In the hunt for the endogenous ligands, John Hughes and Hans Kosterlitz[40] then identified the first opioids in the brain only 2 years later, and called them enkephalins. However, it took almost two decades until the molecular cloning of the first opioid receptors was achieved.[27,49] These studies not only promoted opioid research in general, but also represented key discoveries for subsequent alcohol and drug abuse research. Similarly, the isolation of Δ^9-tetrahydrocannabinol in 1964 by the group of Ralph Mechoulam[29] marked the beginning of cannabinoid research. The brain targets of tetrahydrocannabinol remained unidentified until 1988, when a seminal paper by the group of Allyn Howlet[16] identified a G-protein–coupled receptor as the target of natural cannabinoids. It was followed immediately by the molecular cloning of the cannabinoid receptor 1[60] and by the identification of the first endogenous ligand of the cannabinoid receptor, an arachidonic acid derivative termed anandamide.[17] These key discoveries led to one of the most active fields of research in neurobiology. But the real surprise came from the discovery of the role of the endocannabinoid system in reward processes and in the neurobiology of addictive behavior. Both the endocannabinoids and the cannabinoid receptor appear to be crucial in opioid, alcohol, psychostimulant, and nicotine addiction and it can be foreseen that within the next 10 years we will have effective treatments on the market targeting various components of the endocannabinoid system.[82]

In addition to endocannabinoids, endogenous opioid systems are thought to induce the pleasurable and rewarding effects of alcohol and other drugs of abuse, and thereby constitute ideal targets for treatment.[96] The first description of opioid receptor blockade by means of naltrexone, and the resultant reduction of voluntary alcohol consumption in rats[2] marked the starting point of the development of relapse medication in alcohol research. A decade later, the first reports on the clinical efficacy of naltrexone in alcohol-dependent individuals were published[71,117] and a recent meta-analysis of 24 randomized controlled trials that included a total of 2861 subjects demonstrates that naltrexone decreased the relative risk of relapse compared to placebo by a significant 36%.[101] A further milestone in medication development was the finding that a functional polymorphism of the μ-opioid receptor gene may predict response to naltrexone.[72] Although this finding has been replicated recently,[3] no final judgement on this pharmacogenetic discovery will be possible for several years. Nevertheless given that our century is dominated by the belief that personalized medicine will power further biomedical developments, the study of Oslin et al. has already marked this shift in paradigms. Despite the promise of pharmacogenetics to identify treatment responders, there have so far been very few success stories in all of medicine.

New Vistas in Neurobiological Alcohol and Drug Abuse Research

Addictive behavior is the result of cumulative responses to drug exposure, the genetic make-up of an individual, and the environmental perturbations over time. This very complex drug × gene × environment interaction, which has to be seen in a lifespan perspective, cannot be studied by a reductionistic approach. Instead, a systems-oriented perspective in which the interactions and dynamics of all endogenous and environmental factors involved are centrally integrated, will lead to further progress in alcohol and drug abuse research.[96] My future perspective adheres to a systems biology approach such that the interaction of a drug with primary targets within the brain is fundamental to an understanding of the behavioral consequences. As a result of the interaction of a drug with these targets, alterations in gene expression and synaptic plasticity take place that either function as protective mechanisms or lead to long-lasting alteration in neuronal network activity. As a subsequent consequence, drug-seeking responses ensue that can finally lead via complex environmental interactions to an addictive behavior (Fig. 74.1). This systems biology approach opens up new vistas in addiction research on the genetic (see Section "New Vistas on the Genetic Level"), molecular (see Section "New Vistas on the Molecular Level"), synaptic (see Section "New Vistas in Alcohol- and Drug-Induced Synaptic Plasticity"), neuronal network (see Section "New Vistas on Neuronal Network Activity"), and finally on the behavioral level (see Section "New Vistas on Studying Alcohol- and Drug-Related Behaviors").

New Vistas on the Genetic Level

Genetics of Addictive Behavior

A large body of genetic epidemiological data strongly implicates genetic factors in the etiology of addictive behavior. In the following I focus mainly on smoking behavior, as progress in genetics is most pronounced in the field of nicotine addiction. The data from family, adoption, and twin studies strongly support a genetic influence on the initiation and maintenance of smoking.[102,103] Two general scientific human approaches to identify candidate genes are genetic linkage analysis and genetic association studies including genome-wide association studies. Despite the success of linkage approaches in unravelling the genetic antecedents of disease, the findings with respect to smoking behavior have been disappointingly inconsistent. However, a variety of plausible candidate genes have been examined for associations with smoking behavior. Most of these studies have focused on genetic variations in relevant neurotransmitter pathways and/or nicotine-metabolizing enzymes or neuronal nicotinic receptors. Despite the large number of studies published on the association between specific candidate genes and smoking behavior, one has to conclude from the existing literature that the evidence for a contribution of a specific gene to smoking behavior is rather small.

Genome-Wide Association Studies in Addiction Research

Genome-wide association studies employing a high number (500,000+) of single nucleotide polymorphisms across the genome have been conducted in a variety of complex disorders and have been shown to be a successful tool in identifying underlying susceptibility genes (for all published genome-wide association studies see: www.genome.gov/26525384). Several genome-wide association studies have recently also been conducted on smoking behavior phenotypes. These studies have used sample sizes of up to 11,000 cases[106] and have implicated a number of novel genes in nicotine addiction[2] and smoking cessation, as well as known candidate genes.[8,10,21,106,111] Especially, in conjunction with several candidate gene studies,[85,87] evidence has been accumulated that genes encoding nicotinic acetylcholine receptor proteins are associated with multiple smoking phenotypes.[1] In particular, the nicotinic acetylcholine receptor subunit genes CHRNA3, 4 and 5, as well as CHRNB4 are associated with nicotine addiction. Although the robust association of the nicotinic acetylcholine receptor subunit genes investigated with smoking-related phenotypes is an apparent success story of genetic epidemiology, the respective variations seem to exert no relevant influence on smoking cessation probability in heavy smokers in the general population.[11] These data suggest that the corresponding nicotinic acetylcholine receptor single nucleotide polymorphisms are relevant to the development of chronic smoking behavior but might not influence abstinence and relapse behavior. Although this is somewhat discouraging regarding the usability of genetic determinants of susceptibility to nicotine addiction as predictors of smoking cessation, it highlights the importance of taking this highly interesting phenotype explicitly into account in future studies.[11] In conclusion, genome-wide association approaches as discussed here offer great promise for detecting candidate genes for the development of chronic smoking behavior and relapse, respectively. However, the demonstration of a causal relationship of a specific genotype with a pathological phenotype is difficult, if not impossible, to achieve in humans.

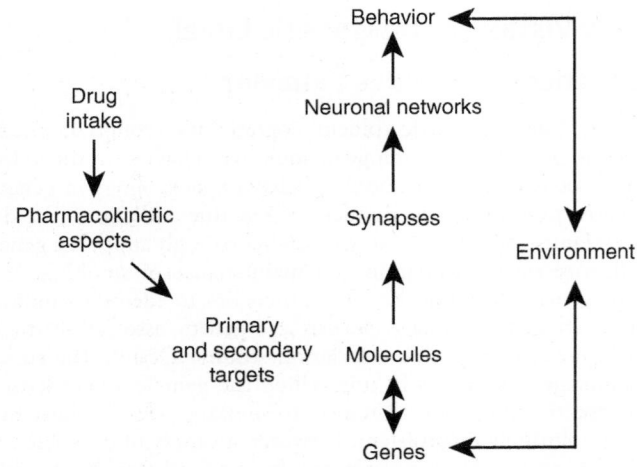

• **Fig. 74.1** This scheme shows a systems approach toward a better understanding of the acute and chronic effects of a drug. The future perspective described here directly follows this approach. Thus future advances on the genetic level, drug-receptor interaction, drug-induced synaptic plasticity, neuronal network activity, and behavioral analysis are described.

Forward Genetics in Preclinical Addiction Research

Animal Models as the Basis for Forward Genetic Approaches

Animal studies using intravenous self-administration in rodents represent a powerful method to functionally validate candidate genes deriving either from human genome-wide association study approaches or from gene expression profiling studies in animals. Intravenous self-administration is commonly used as an animal model for studying nicotine intake as it offers face validity from various perspectives; for example, there is good concordance between the nicotine concentrations in plasma of human cigarette smokers and of rats in intravenous self-administration studies.[92] Furthermore, genetic differences have been reported because various strains of rats show different latencies to acquire nicotine self-administration behavior.[91] Thus studies on the acquisition of intravenous self-administration will help to elucidate the genetic vulnerability of the development of chronic smoking behavior in humans.

Major progresses in animal models for addictive behavior also allow now the study of compulsive nicotine-seeking behavior and relapse.[97] The most common procedure to study nicotine-seeking behavior—which can be considered as the motivational component of nicotine craving and relapse—is the reinstatement model.[13] In this model, intravenous self-administration of nicotine paired with conditioned cues has to be acquired at first. This is followed by a nicotine-free period where the animals undergo extinction (i.e., allowing the animal to perform the operant response without programmed consequences). Finally, in response to previously conditioned cues reinstatement can be tested. If instead of extinction training protracted abstinence is applied, responsiveness to conditioned cues progressively increases over the first weeks of abstinence (i.e., the animals remain in their home cage for at least 1 month without any further conditioning)—a phenomenon called incubation.[35] In summary, reinstatement of drug-seeking behavior as well as the incubation of this behavior following protracted abstinence has become the gold standard to measure craving and relapse in animals.

Alterations in Gene Expression in Drug-Exposed Animals

Microarray studies have revealed that chronic exposure of nicotine increases expression of genes involved in regulation of food intake and energy expenditure as well as it coregulates multiple neurotransmitter systems and pathways involved in protein modification/degradation in rat brain.[45,118] Our knowledge on how these changes in gene expression contribute toward nicotine addiction is substantially limited because nicotine was administered passively in these studies, which do not mimic the situation observed in smokers. No previous study has identified the effects of nicotine in active self-administering animals on brain regions and performed gene expression profiles of such regions. However, we know from a key publication by Jacobs et al.[42] that active drug consumption during intravenous self-administration is a crucial psychological factor directing long-term genomic responses in the brain, especially in the nucleus accumbens shell. Therefore, it will be crucial to establish gene expression profiles in a triad design from animals that actively self-administer nicotine in direct comparison to yoked nicotine and saline control animals. These kinds of studies usually result in a huge database on gene expression profiles in animals and it will be essential to combine this genomic information with datasets deriving from human genetic studies by a convergent translational genomics approach.

Convergent Translational Genomics Approach for Addictive Behavior

Convergent translational genomics approaches integrate genomic information (e.g., from microarray analysis) from animal models with a candidate gene or genome-wide association study approach in humans. Especially the explanatory power of genetic findings is enhanced by such a convergent approach[9] and as a result a priority gene list for functional validation is obtained. Recently a convergent translational genomics approach was successfully applied to alcohol addiction.[108] In this study, genome-wide association study data from a huge case-control sample for alcoholism were combined with massive information from gene expression profiling in alcohol addicted rats. The genome-wide association studies produced approximately 100 single nucleotide polymorphisms with nominal $p < 10^{-4}$. These, together with 20 additional single nucleotide polymorphisms from genes showing differential expression in rats, were genotyped in a large replication sample. Fifteen single nucleotide polymorphisms showed significant association (two single nucleotide polymorphisms met genome-wide significance) with the same allele as in the genome-wide association studies. Eight of the 15 genes derived from the animal data, demonstrating that relevant genes would have been lost by a mere genome-wide association study approach.[108] In response to this study, the Integrative Neuroscience Initiative on Alcoholism has announced that one of their major aims is to integrate animal data into data obtained from studies in humans with alcoholism (www.scripps.edu/cnad/inia/structure.html). In summary, this novel translational tool results in a priority gene list that has to be functionally validated.

Reverse Genetic Approaches for the Functional Validation of Candidate Genes

Reverse genetics are used to assess the role of a candidate gene in a specific behavior, for example, in nicotine self-administration. The most common reverse genetic approach is the generation of a conventional mouse knockout model and its subsequent behavioral analysis. However, the generation of a conventional knockout model is time consuming, cost-intensive, and has no tissue specificity, and because the gene is ablated early in development, numerous compensatory mechanisms may ensue. Through more advanced techniques such as Cre/loxP and tetracycline-inducible systems, a gene of interest can be expressed or inactivated in a tissue-specific and time-controlled manner.[30] Although those conditioned knockout models are of very high value for the neuroscience community they still do not provide a good rational for large-scale functional validation of candidate genes because there is still an enormous effort to generate those model. As an alternative, the use of viral vectors for gene delivery offers many advantages for rapid functional validation studies. In particular, the advent of adeno-associated virus vectors carrying cDNA for—or short hairpin RNA against—specific genes allows for the first time the rapid bidirectional manipulation of gene function.[51]

New Vistas on the Molecular Level

Hallmarks in drug abuse research were the discoveries of endogenous primary target systems. Thus drugs of abuse act on specific receptors, channels, or transporters within the brain to produce their psychoactive and reinforcing effects: for example, opiates act mainly on μ-opioid receptors,[61] cannabis products such as Δ^9-tetrahydrocannabinol act mainly on cannabinoid receptor 1 receptors,[16] nicotine acts on the nicotinic acetylcholine receptor,[1] psychostimulants such as cocaine act mainly via monoaminergic transporters,[38] and hallucinogens such as lysergic acid diethylamide act via the serotonin-2A receptor[34]—to name the primary targets of the most important drug classes. However, how does alcohol affect the functions of the central nervous system—are there any primary sites of action?

Primary Targets of Alcohol in the Central Nervous System

It is only recently that a shift from the so-called lipid theory (i.e., the primary targets of ethanol are membrane lipids) to the protein theory (i.e., the primary targets of ethanol are membrane proteins, especially receptors) took place.[73] Into the 1990s, different lipid theories postulated that alcohol acts via some perturbation of the membrane lipids of central nervous system neurons. In particular, effects on membrane fluidity and disordering of the bulk lipid phase of membranes was originally an attractive hypothesis of alcohol action because it provided a possible mechanism by which alcohol could affect membrane proteins, such as ion channels, via an action on membrane lipids.

There are clear limitations to the lipid theory. First, effects of alcohol on membrane disorder are generally measurable only at alcohol levels well above the pharmacological range (>500 mg/dL blood alcohol levels); these levels are close to the LD_{50} of ethanol in humans.[3] Significant effects of membrane disordering on protein function are even more difficult to envision at pharmacologically relevant alcohol concentrations. For example, at very high intoxicating blood alcohol levels associated with loss of consciousness (~300 mg/dL), there would be only one alcohol molecule per approximately 200 lipid molecules.[73] Second, membrane effects induced by alcohol concentrations exceeding the pharmacological range can be mimicked by an increase in temperature of just a few tenths of a degree Celsius,[73] which clearly does not produce behavioral signs of alcohol intoxication or appreciably alter the function of membrane proteins such as neurotransmitter-gated ion channels. Therefore, the reported effects of alcohol on membrane fluidity and organization seem to be a purely biophysical

phenomenon without any relevance for the pharmacological central nervous system effects of alcohol. Taking even more refinements of the lipid theory into consideration[73] it remains unlikely that membrane lipids are the primary targets of alcohol.

The protein theory predicts that alcohol acts specifically on membrane proteins such as receptors and ion channels. The main reason for a shift toward the protein theory comes from findings that alcohol—at concentrations in the 10–20 mM range—directly interferes with the function of several ion channels and receptors.[4] In a key publication, David Lovinger and colleagues[58] showed that N-methyl-D-aspartate function was inhibited by ethanol in a concentration-dependent manner over the range of 5–50 mM, a range that also produces intoxication. The amplitude of the N-methyl-D-aspartate–activated current was reduced 61% by 50 mM ethanol. What is more, the potency for inhibition of the N-methyl-D-aspartate–activated current by several alcohols is linearly related to their intoxicating potency. This suggests that ethanol-induced inhibition of responses to N-methyl-D-aspartate receptor activation may contribute to the neural and cognitive impairments associated with intoxication.[58] But how can ethanol directly interfere with N-methyl-D-aspartate receptor function?

The N-methyl-D-aspartate receptor is a ligand-gated ion channel with a heteromeric assembly of NR1, NR2 (A-D), and NR3 subunits. The NR1 subunit is crucial for channel function, the NR2 subunits contain the glutamate binding site, and the NR3 subunits have some modulatory function on channel activity, especially under pathological conditions. Electrophysiological studies show that ethanol interacts with domains that influence channel activity,[120] suggesting that residues within transmembrane domains may be involved. In the search for a possible binding site of alcohol at the N-methyl-D-aspartate receptor, several site-directed mutagenesis studies were performed and putative binding sites in the transmembrane 3 and 4 of the NR1 and NR2A subunit, respectively, were identified.[37,78,79,83,95]

It is not yet possible to directly measure the binding of an ethanol molecule to the N-methyl-D-aspartate receptor by means of physical methods because ethanol is a small molecule with low binding energy being efficient only in the mid-millimolar range. These pharmacological characteristics preclude a direct assessment of an ethanol protein binding site. However, with the discovery of the LUSH protein in the fruit fly *Drosophila melanogaster* it became possible to model how transmembrane residues can form a specific protein-binding pocket for ethanol. The high-resolution crystal structures of LUSH in complex with a series of short-chain alcohols were obtained by the team of David Jones in 2003.[53] The structure of LUSH reveals a specific alcohol-binding site. LUSH exists in a partially molten globule state. The presence of ethanol at pharmacologically relevant concentrations <50 mM shifts the conformational equilibrium to a more compact state,[12] demonstrating that ethanol induces a conformational change of the binding protein—an important requirement for a functional binding site. A group of amino acids form a network of concerted hydrogen bonds between the protein and the ethanol molecules provide a structural motif to increase alcohol-binding affinity at this site. This motif seems to be conserved in a number of mammalian ligand-gated ion channels, and it is therefore suggested that the alcohol-binding site in LUSH represents a general model for putative alcohol binding sites in proteins such as the N-methyl-D-aspartate receptors.

Taken together it has been demonstrated over the last 20 years that ethanol acts directly on the N-methyl-D-aspartate receptor. However, direct interactions have been also described with γ-aminobutyric acid A receptor, serotonin-3, glycine and nicotinic acetylcholine receptors, as well as with several ion channels such as L-type Ca^{2+} channels, where concentrations as low as 1 mM produce alterations in the function of these receptors and ion channels.[96,115] This modern view on selective primary targets of alcohol in the central nervous system has so far not been implemented well into the general knowledge of drug abuse researchers and neuroscientists. Actually, most researchers still consider alcohol as a "dirty drug" with an undefined mode of action. In the future it will therefore be important to better define the putative binding sites for ethanol in the central nervous system. In particular, the findings on LUSH have to be translated to the mammalian brain.

Agonist-Directed Trafficking of Receptor Stimulus—A Key for Understanding Drug Action

A gain of knowledge in structural biology will not only be essential to define the molecular mode of action of the ethanol molecule but also for other drugs of abuse. This is best exemplified by the mode of action of lysergic acid diethylamide on the serotonin-2A receptor. The demonstration that lysergic acid diethylamide and other hallucinogenic compounds elicit their psychoactive effects via serotonin-2A receptor activation has generated a fundamental paradox in a way that not all serotonin-2A receptor agonists exhibit hallucinogenic activity. Indeed, nonhallucinogenic compounds such as lisuride and ergotamine share significant structural similarities and comparable agonist activities at this receptor,[24] but they lack psychoactive properties. This pharmacological paradox has been resolved recently by demonstrating that hallucinogenic versus. nonhallucinogenic compounds, although acting at the same binding site, elicit different patterns of signaling that are responsible for their different behavioral activities.[34] But how can such a divergent effect been explained in view of the standard pharmacological model of G-protein–coupled receptor activation. The ternary complex model postulates a conformational change from an inactive to an active state following agonistic activation.[48] However, both theory and experimental evidence suggest that G-protein–coupled receptors adopt multiple conformations when activated by different agonists.[6,32] Thus an advanced model of agonist-directed trafficking of receptor stimulus has recently been proposed by Kenakin.[48] This expanded version of the ternary complex model posits that different receptor agonists stabilize distinct conformations that preferentially recruit and activate specific signaling pathways.[48,113] The fact that serotonin-2A agonists can activate different signaling pathways is consistent with such an expanded version of the ternary complex model because it explains how distinct cellular responses could be produced by agonists acting at the same binding sites. Paradoxical effects on the receptor level have been also observed with other drugs of abuse (e.g., opioids); progress in structural biology and the application of the new concept of agonist-directed trafficking of receptor stimulus will not only be helpful for a better understanding of the molecular action of alcohol and drugs of abuse but will be also important for gaining better insight into the molecular processes underlying drug-induced synaptic plasticity.

New Vistas in Alcohol- and Drug-Induced Synaptic Plasticity

A ubiquitous property of all synapses is their ability to undergo activity-dependent changes in synaptic plasticity that can be studied most effectively using electrophysiological methods in brain slices. Because these slices only remain viable for several hours, the cellular mechanisms underlying the first few hours of long-term potentiation and long-term depression are the best understood. It has been suggested that synaptic plasticity within the mesolimbic dopaminergic system and associated limbic structures, including the extended amygdala, becomes manifest following drug exposure.[46] Some key publications on drug-induced adaptations in the mesolimbic system have revealed that glutamatergic synapses on dopamine neurons in the ventral tegmental area in particular undergo plastic changes following administration of drugs of abuse including ethanol.[84,112]

By increasing synaptic strength,[112] facilitating long-term potentiation,[57] or blocking long-term depression,[44] drugs of abuse augment the responsiveness of dopamine neurons to glutamate and ultimately promote enhanced dopamine release in brain areas such as the nucleus accumbens and the prefrontal cortex.[33] Drug-induced synaptic strengthening in dopamine neurons in the ventral tegmental area is associated with changes in alpha-amino-3-hydroxy-5-methylisoxazole-4-propionic acid (AMPA) receptor subunit composition.[5] Incorporation of the AMPA receptor subunit GluR1 promotes drug-induced synaptic strengthening, probably through the formation of highly conductive, Ca^{2+} permeable GluR1 homomeric AMPA receptors,[20] whereas insertion of GluR2-containing receptors reverts it.[59] Synaptic recruitment of GluR1 subunits and the resultant synaptic potentiation require the activation of N-methyl-D-aspartate receptors.[20] These synaptic changes in dopamine neurons are thought to be related to the development of drug-induced reinforcement processes[46] (see also Engblom et al.[25]).

In conclusion, drug-induced synaptic plasticity has been found in the ventral tegmental area—nucleus accumbens projection as well as in other brain areas of the extended amygdala. However, the generally held view that these cellular adaptations underlie drug reinforcement is based on purely associative findings. Direct experimental evidence for the behavioral significance of these drug-induced synaptic changes involving glutamate receptors is still lacking. Only in vivo electrophysiology in conditional mouse models that selectively lack, for example, N-methyl-D-aspartate receptors in dopaminergic neurons will provide a clear answer as to whether AMPA/ N-methyl-D-aspartate receptor–induced synaptic strengthening of dopamine neurons within the ventral tegmental area serves as a cellular model for the induction of drug reinforcement. It will be important also to know whether these drug-induced synaptic changes modulate neuronal network activity. For answering this question, multielectrode recording and ultra-high-field imaging in rodents will be useful.

New Vistas on Neuronal Network Activity

Multielectrode Recording to Reveal Neuronal Network Activity Underlying Alcohol- and Drug-Related Behavior

An increasing number of laboratories now have the capability to simultaneously monitor the extracellular activity of more than 100 single neurons in freely moving animals. This paradigm, known as multielectrode recording, is revolutionizing systems neuroscience by enabling the visualization of the function of entire neural circuits.[69]

So far, only a few studies have used this technique in freely moving animals in order to correlate drug-related behavior with neuronal activity. Janak et al.[43] used multielectrode recording within the shell of the nucleus accumbens during operant alcohol self-administration, and found that different, but overlapping, populations of neurons in the nucleus accumbens mediate each event occurring along the temporal dimension of a single trial performed to obtain ethanol reward. These data suggest that the nucleus accumbens plays a crucial role in linking conditioned and unconditioned internal and external stimuli with motor plans in order to allow ethanol-seeking behavior to occur. In a recent study, multielectrode recording was used to determine the effects of ethanol on neuronal firing and network patterns of persistent activity in prefrontal cortex neurons.[110] The results of this study show that ethanol inhibits persistent activity and spike firing of prefrontal cortex neurons, and that the degree of ethanol inhibition may be influenced by dopamine D1 receptor tone. Ethanol-induced alterations in the activity of deep-layer cortical neurons may therefore underlie the disruptive effects of alcohol on cognitive functions supported by these neurons.

These few examples demonstrate that multielectrode recording in freely moving animals may prove a powerful future approach in understanding alterations of neural network activity during the course of long-term alcohol consumption. Application of this technique to investigate the transition from drug-seeking behavior to more compulsive behavior would be particularly valuable.[86,119] Such studies would need to be performed over a long period; however, with repeated measures being taken over several weeks or even months, and data handling and analysis would be further limiting factors.

Animal Brain Imaging to Identify the Neuroanatomical and Neurochemical Substrates of Addictive Behavior

Brain imaging in small laboratory animals such as mice and rats is restricted because the brain sites of interest are very small compared to those of the human brain and measurements can be performed in anesthetized animals only. Use of a comfortable head restraint device in well-trained conscious monkeys; however, enables the performance of imaging and the assessment of conditioned drug responses.[39] Recent progress in ultra-high-field imaging up to 17 T now allows brain imaging in rodents with a good resolution (<100 m). Spectroscopy and pharmacological magnetic resonance imaging provide particularly powerful tools for the study of the progression of alcohol and drug consumption toward addictive behavior. The advantage of animal neuroimaging is that a subject can be studied repeatedly over a long period, allowing the investigation of neuronal network activity in the transition phase from controlled to compulsive behavior.

One important application for future studies in laboratory animals is glutamate spectroscopy. Pfeuffer and colleagues[75] demonstrated as long ago as 1999 that at least 18 metabolites, including glutamate and γ-aminobutyric acid, can be quantified in the adult rat brain using [^{1}H] nuclear magnetic resonance spectroscopy at 9.4 T. In vivo detection and quantification of glutamate in the rat brain, as well as regional differences in signal intensities, have been also demonstrated by others.[62] High-field spectroscopy provides superior peak separation, allowing the direct measurement of glutamate in different brain areas of small laboratory animals, providing an ideal tool for noninvasive longitudinal tracking of neurometabolic plasticity within the glutamatergic systems accompanying alcohol and drug withdrawal, abstinence, and relapse.

The most promising approach however, is the in vivo mapping of functional connectivity in neurotransmitter systems using pharmacological magnetic resonance imaging. Schwarz and colleagues[88,89] have pioneered the application of functional connectivity studies to pharmacological challenges. In their studies, analysis of the pharmacological magnetic resonance imaging responses to various drugs revealed specific structures for functionally connected brain regions that closely reflect known pathways in the neurotransmitter systems targeted by these drugs.[88,89] These studies therefore demonstrate that the hemodynamic responses observed following a pharmacological challenge are closely related to drug-specific changes in neurotransmission. This novel approach can be used to study the impact of pharmacological or genetic manipulation on functional connectivity. This application has already been used to study the disruption of drug-induced functional connectivity by a dopamine D3 antagonist. The strongest modifications of functional connectivity by dopamine D3 blockade occurred in nigrostriatal connections.[90] This approach is also being applied to current alcohol research. The progression of alcohol drinking toward a habit-like behavior, as studied in terms of alteration in nigrostriatal connectivity of brain sites, is being studied in a long-term alcohol self-administration paradigm using a 9.4 T scanner. The working hypothesis is that the nigrostriatal pathway may be involved in the habit-forming properties of alcohol and other drugs of abuse.[18,28,31,97] More precisely, a neuroanatomical principle of striatal organization is that ventral domains, including the nucleus accumbens, exert control over dorsal striatal processes that are mediated by so-called spiraling, striato-nigro-striatal circuitry. Chronic administration of drugs of abuse may lead to alterations in this serial connectivity, and drug-seeking habits—a key characteristic of addictive behavior—are triggered as a result.[4] Functional connectivity studies with good resolution conducted in a high-field scanner provide a tool for proving this attractive hypothesis of alcohol/drug-induced alterations of striato-midbrain-striatal serial connectivity and will be very helpful to understand the neurobiology of drug-related behaviors such as drug-seeking and relapse.

New Vistas on Studying Alcohol- and Drug-Related Behaviors

Reconsolidation of Alcohol- and Drug-Related Memories

Relapses contribute considerably to the maintenance of addiction and are a major challenge in the treatment of addictive diseases. One fundamental problem in the treatment of drug addiction is the ability of drug-associated environmental cues to evoke drug-seeking behavior leading to relapse even after years of abstinence. Consistent with the long-lasting risk of relapse, several recent studies indicate that long-term memory formation and development of drug addiction are sharing common neural circuitries and molecular mechanisms.[41,47] Thus understanding learning and memory processes in the addicted brain is an important key for understanding the persistence of addiction and it is reasonable to hypothesize that selective disruption of drug-related memories might help to prevent relapses.

Several earlier studies have shown that newly acquired memories are initially labile but then are stabilized through a process called memory consolidation.[22,63] Within the first minutes to hours this process is susceptible to interference. Following this stabilization period the consolidation theory proposes that memories, once stored, are resistant to interference.[63] In contrast to this idea, Misanin and colleagues[66] proposed that reactivation of a consolidated memory trace returns it to an unstable state again. More than 30 years later, Nader et al.[67,68] confirmed this assumption in a fear-conditioning paradigm with targeted infusions of the protein synthesis inhibitor anisomycin into the lateral and basal nuclei of the amygdala—sites known to play an important role in fear learning—after retrieving previously conditioned fear memories. This study demonstrated that infusion of anisomycin shortly after memory reactivation produced amnesia on later tests, whereas anisomycin application in the absence of reexposure to the conditioned cue left the memory intact.[68] Thus reactivation of a consolidated memory can return into a labile state in which the memory trace has to undergo reconsolidation for which, like consolidation, new protein synthesis is required. Subsequently, further evidence for the reconsolidation theory and its dependence on renewed protein synthesis has been provided.[15,23,67] In particular, antagonism of the N-methyl-D-aspartate subtype of glutamate receptor has been shown to be effective in disruption of memory reconsolidation,[55,77,107,109] likely because of the crucial role of these receptors in learning and memory. Furthermore, given the fact that adrenal stress hormones activate adrenergic receptors in the amygdala and that the basolateral amygdala is essential for fear memory,[63] it is suggested that the release of norepinephrine within the amygdala is of importance for reconsolidation processes. Indeed, infusion of the nonselective beta-adrenergic antagonist propranolol into the amygdala of rats shortly after the reactivation period of a previously acquired fear association impaired the fear expression on a long-term test.[14] Very recently, this finding was translated to humans in a randomized and double-blind placebo-controlled design. In volunteers, oral administration of propranolol before memory reactivation erased the behavioral expression of the fear memory 24 hours later and prevented the return of fear.[50] This key finding has important implications for the treatment of persistent and self-perpetuating memories in individuals with not only anxiety disorders but also drug addiction.

The reconsolidation hypothesis was also tested in regard to drugs of abuse. In the laboratory of Barry Everitt, rats were examined in a cocaine self-administration paradigm in which a conditioned stimulus was presented during each self-administered cocaine infusion. The conditioned reinforcing properties of the conditioned stimulus were tested subsequently by measuring their ability to support the acquisition of a new instrumental drug-seeking response of lever pressing in the absence of the primary drug reinforcer. Thus the rats were exposed to a brief test session in which a nose-poke resulted in presentation of the conditioned stimulus, but an infusion of saline instead of cocaine. This session was sufficient to reactivate the previously formed conditioned stimulus-drug association and render it sensitive to disruption, since an infusion of anisomycin into the basolateral amygdala immediately after reactivation subsequently impaired the acquisition of the new response.[56] Furthermore, a single reactivation-dependent infusion of an antisense oligonucleotide targeting Zif268—an immediate-early gene (also known as EGR1, NGFI-A, and Krox24) that is significantly upregulated in the basolateral amygdala following self-administered cocaine[105]—into the amygdala, 24 hours prior to testing resulted in a long-lasting disruption of the ability of a drug-associated stimulus to act as a conditioned reinforcer.[54] These results demonstrate that addictive drug memories undergo reconsolidation in a manner similar to that of fear memories. This key publication was followed by several

other studies demonstrating disruption of the reconsolidation of cocaine-, heroin-, and morphine-related memories with various pharmacological manipulations and behavioral paradigms.[a] Disruption of alcohol-associated memories was also very recently tested in animals trained to self-administer orally alcohol, during which each self-administered alcohol drop a conditioned stimulus was presented. The protein synthesis inhibitor anisomycin and the noncompetitive N-methyl-D-aspartate receptor antagonist MK-801 were given after retrieval of alcohol-related memories to test whether these memories undergo a protein synthesis- and N-methyl-D-aspartate receptor-dependent reconsolidation. In addition, acamprosate as an abstinence-promoting agent that is widely used in the treatment of alcohol addiction, was administered. Although the primary site of action is still not known, it has been demonstrated that acamprosate dampens a hyper-glutamatergic state in the alcohol-dependent brain and thereby reduces the risk of relapse.[97,98] Due to this interference with the glutamatergic system it is hypothesized that acamprosate may also have an impact on the memory reconsolidation processes. With these experiments, evidence was provided that alcohol-associated memories can also become unstable and liable to disruption after their reactivation. Thus both the protein synthesis blocker anisomycin as well as the N-methyl-D-aspartate receptor antagonist MK-801 given immediately after reexposure of animals to alcohol-paired conditioned stimuli impaired the ability of the conditioned stimuli to induce alcohol-seeking behavior in subsequent test sessions, whereas acamprosate had no impact on reconsolidation processes (von der Goltz et al., unpublished results). These findings demonstrate that the administration of anisomycin and MK-801 specifically disrupted reconsolidation, as the administration of these agents without the reactivation of the conditioned stimulus-alcohol-related memory had no effect on the responsiveness of the animals to the alcohol-paired conditioned stimulus during alcohol-seeking tests. Finally, reactivated alcohol-related memories as well as other reactivated reward-related memories are also susceptible to interference with beta-adrenergic blockade by propranolol.[19]

In conclusion, it was shown that alcohol- and drug-associated memories can be disrupted pharmacologically after their reactivation by both protein synthesis inhibition and N-methyl-D-aspartate receptor antagonism. These findings have important clinical implications, because they show that it is possible to selectively reduce long-lasting drug-associated memories. Hence, the disruption of drug-related memory reconsolidation may be an effective treatment strategy for the reduction of relapse. These findings should be rapidly translated into alcoholics, smokers, and illicit drug users, as pharmacological manipulations before memory reactivation was shown to prevent the return of fear.[50] Either propranolol or ketamine treatment before memory reactivation in addicted individuals would be a promising starting point.

Summary

In this chapter I have given a personal retrospective view on the hallmarks of neurobiological alcohol and drug abuse research and have then discussed new approaches and challenges in the addiction field.

In terms of future genetic work I have highlighted the application of convergent translational genomics approaches. This novel bioinformatic tool has already been successfully applied to

---

[a]References 7, 36, 56, 65, 81, 114.

alcohol addiction.[108] It allows the integration of genetic information from animal and human studies thereby enhancing the explanatory power of genetic findings and it will be essential to define candidate genes for alcohol- and drug-related phenotypes. Most importantly, candidate genes have to be functionally validated. Two reverse genetic strategies for the functional validation of candidate genes have been proposed here: the use of conditional mouse models and the application of virus-mediated gene transfer. Following this validation process genetic risk profiles can be defined for alcohol- and drug-taking behavior.

On a molecular level, the interaction of a drug with primary targets (e.g., receptors) within the brain has been discussed. In this context the concept of agonist-directed trafficking of receptor stimulus was highlighted for a future key to understand the consequences of drug-receptor interactions and subsequent signaling transduction.

On the synaptic level, new concepts were discussed with regard to drug-induced synaptic plasticity. Alterations on the synaptic level can modulate neuronal network activity, which can be studied by means of multielectrode recording or ultra-high-field imaging in small rodents. A systems biology approach will then be helpful to integrate data sets obtained on the genetic, molecular, synaptic, and neuronal network level in order to understand addictive behavior.

Finally, the most burning question relates to new options for the treatment of addictive behavior. Instead of having discussed new potential antirelapse compounds (for review see Kreek et al.,[52] Preti,[76] Siu and Tyndale,[94] and Spanagel and Kiefer[98]), I have highlighted the *possibility* of disrupting reconsolidation of alcohol- or drug-related memories as a new approach to treat our clients.

References

1. Albuquerque EX, Pereira EF, Alkondon M, et al. Mammalian nicotinic acetylcholine receptors: from structure to function. *Physiol Rev.* 2009;89:73–120.
2. Altshuler HL, Phillips PE, Feinhandler DA. Alteration of ethanol self-administration by naltrexone. *Life Sci.* 1980;26:679–688.
3. Anton RF, Oroszi G, O'Malley S, et al. An evaluation of mu-opioid receptor (OPRM1) as a predictor of naltrexone response in the treatment of alcohol dependence: results from the combined pharmacotherapies and behavioral interventions for alcohol dependence (COMBINE) study. *Arch Gen Psychiatry.* 2008;65:135–144.
4. Belin D, Everitt BJ. Cocaine seeking habits depend upon dopamine-dependent serial connectivity linking the ventral with the dorsal striatum. *Neuron.* 2008;57:432–441.
5. Bellone C, Luscher C. Cocaine triggered AMPA receptor redistribution is reversed in vivo by mGluR-dependent long-term depression. *Nat Neurosci.* 2006;9:636–641.
6. Berg KA, Maayani S, Goldfarb J, et al. Effector pathway-dependent relative efficacy at serotonin type 2A and 2C receptors: evidence for agonist-directed trafficking of receptor stimulus. *Mol Pharmacol.* 1998;54:94–104.
7. Bernardi RE, Lattal KM, Berger SP. Anisomycin disrupts a contextual memory following reactivation in a cocaine-induced locomotor activity paradigm. *Behav Neurosci.* 2007;121:156–163.
8. Berrettini W, Yuan X, Tozzi F, et al. Alpha-5/alpha-3 nicotinic receptor subunit alleles increase risk for heavy smoking. *Mol Psychiatry.* 2008;13:368–373.
9. Bertsch B, Ogden CA, Sidhu K, et al. Convergent functional genomics: a Bayesian candidate gene identification approach for complex disorders. *Methods.* 2005;37:274–279.
10. Bierut LJ, Madden PA, Breslau N, et al. Novel genes identified in a high-density genome wide association study for nicotine dependence. *Hum Mol Genet.* 2007;16:24–35.
11. Breitling LP, Dahmen N, Mittelstrass K, et al. Smoking cessation and variations in nicotinic acetylcholine receptor subunits alpha-5, alpha-3, and beta-4 genes. *Biol Psychiatry.* 2009;65(8): 691–695.
12. Bucci BK, Kruse SW, Thode AB, et al. Effect of n-alcohols on the structure and stability of the Drosophila odorant binding protein LUSH. *Biochemistry.* 2006;45:1693–1701.
13. Crombag HS, Bossert JM, Koya E, et al. Context-induced relapse to drug seeking: a review. *Philos Trans R Soc Lond B Biol Sci.* 2008;363:3233–3243.
14. Debiec J, LeDoux JE. Disruption of reconsolidation but not consolidation of auditory fear conditioning by noradrenergic blockade in the amygdala. *Neuroscience.* 2004;129:267–272.
15. Debiec J, LeDoux JE, Nader K. Cellular and systems reconsolidation in the hippocampus. *Neuron.* 2002;36:527–538.
16. Devane WA, Dysarz FA, Johnson MR, et al. Determination and characterization of a cannabinoid receptor in rat brain. *Mol Pharmacol.* 1988;34:605–613.
17. Devane WA, Hanus L, Breuer A, et al. Isolation and structure of a brain constituent that binds to the cannabinoid receptor. *Science.* 1992;258. 1946–1194.
18. Dickinson A, Wood N, Smith JW. Alcohol seeking by rats: action or habit? *Q J Exp Psychol.* 2002;55:331–348.
19. Diergaarde L, Schoffelmeer AN, De Vries TJ. Beta-adrenoceptor mediated inhibition of long-term reward-related memory reconsolidation. *Behav Brain Res.* 2006;170:333–336.
20. Dong Y, Saal D, Thomas M, et al. Cocaine-induced potentiation of synaptic strength in dopamine neurons: behavioral correlates in GluRA(-/-) mice. *Proc Natl Acad Sci USA.* 2004;101:14282–14287.
21. Drgon T, Montoya I, Johnson C, et al. Genome-wide association for nicotine dependence and smoking cessation success in NIH research volunteers. *Mol Med.* 2009;15:21–27.
22. Dudai Y. The neurobiology of consolidations, or, how stable is the engram? *Annu Rev Psychol.* 2004;55:51–86.
23. Duvarci S, Nader K. Characterization of fear memory reconsolidation. *J Neurosci.* 2004;24:9269–9275.
24. Egan CT, Herrick-Davis K, Miller K, et al. Agonist activity of LSD and lisuride at cloned 5HT2A and 5HT2C receptors. *Psychopharmacology (Berl.).* 1998;136:409–414.
25. Engblom D, Bilbao A, Sanchis-Segura C, et al. Glutamate receptors on dopamine neurons control the persistence of cocaine seeking. *Neuron.* 2008;59:497–508.
26. Eriksson K. Genetic selection for voluntary alcohol consumption in the albino rat. *Science.* 1968;159:739–741.
27. Evans CJ, Keith Jr DE, Morrison H, et al. Cloning of a delta opioid receptor by functional expression. *Science.* 1992;258:1952–1955.
28. Everitt BJ, Robbins TW. Neural systems of reinforcement for drug addiction: from actions to habits to compulsion. *Nat Neurosci.* 2005;8:1481–1489.
29. Gaoni Y, Mechoulam R. Isolation, structure and partial synthesis of an active constituent of hashish. *J Am Chem Soc.* 1964;86:1646–1647.
30. Gavériaux-Ruff C, Kieffer BL. Conditional gene targeting in the mouse nervous system: insights into brain function and diseases. *Pharmacol Ther.* 2007;113:619–634.
31. Gerdeman GL, Partridge JG, Lupica CR, et al. It could be habit forming: drugs of abuse and striatal synaptic plasticity. *Trends Neurosci.* 2003;26:184–192.
32. Ghanouni P, Gryczynski Z, Steenhuis JJ, et al. Functionally different agonists induce distinct conformations in the G protein coupling domain of the beta 2 adrenergic receptor. *J Biol Chem.* 2001;276:24433–24436.
33. Giorgetti M, Hotsenpiller G, Ward P, et al. Amphetamine-induced plasticity of AMPA receptors in the ventral tegmental area: effects on extracellular levels of dopamine and glutamate in freely moving rats. *J Neurosci.* 2001;21:6362–6369.

34. González-Maeso J, Weisstaub NV, Zhou M, et al. Hallucinogens recruit specific cortical 5-HT(2A) receptor-mediated signaling pathways to affect behavior. *Neuron.* 2007;53:439–452.

35. Grimm JW, Hope BT, Wise RA, et al. Neuroadaptation. Incubation of cocaine craving after withdrawal. *Nature.* 2001;412:141–142.

36. Hellemans KG, Everitt BJ, Lee JL. Disrupting reconsolidation of conditioned withdrawal memories in the basolateral amygdala reduces suppression of heroin seeking in rats. *J Neurosci.* 2006;26:12694–12699.

37. Honse Y, Ren H, Lipsky RH, et al. Sites in the fourth membrane-associated domain regulate alcohol sensitivity of the NMDA receptor. *Neuropharmacology.* 2004;46:647–654.

38. Howell LL, Kimmel HL. Monoamine transporters and psychostimulant addiction. *Biochem Pharmacol.* 2008;75:196–217.

39. Howell LL, Wilcox KM. Functional imaging and neurochemical correlates of stimulant self-administration in primates. *Psychopharmacology (Berl).* 2002;163:352–363.

40. Hughes J, Smith TW, Kosterlitz HW, Fothergill LA, Morgan BA, Morris HR. Identification of two related pentapeptides from the brain with potent opiate agonist activity. *Nature.* 1975;258:577–580.

41. Hyman SE, Malenka RC, Nestler EJ. Neural mechanisms of addiction: the role of reward-related learning and memory. *Annu Rev Neurosci.* 2006;29:565–598.

42. Jacobs EH, Spijker S, Verhoog CW, et al. Active heroin administration induces specific genomic responses in the nucleus accumbens shell. *FASEB J.* 2002;16:1961–1973.

43. Janak PH, Chang JY, Woodward DJ. Neuronal spike activity in the nucleus accumbens of behaving rats during ethanol self-administration. *Brain Res.* 1999;817:172–184.

44. Jones S, Kornblum JL, Kauer JA. Amphetamine blocks long-term synaptic depression in the ventral tegmental area. *J Neurosci.* 2000;20:5575–5580.

45. Kane JK, Konu O, Ma JZ, et al. Nicotine coregulates multiple pathways involved in protein modification/degradation in rat brain. *Brain Res Mol Brain Res.* 2004;132:81–91.

46. Kauer JA, Malenka RC. Synaptic plasticity and addiction. *Nat Rev Neurosci.* 2007;8:844–858.

47. Kelley AE. Memory and addiction: shared neural circuitry and molecular mechanisms. *Neuron.* 2004;44:161–179.

48. Kenakin T. Ligand-selective receptor conformations revisited: the promise and the problem. *Trends Pharmacol Sci.* 2003;24:346–354.

49. Kieffer BL, Befort K, Gaveriaux-Ruff C, et al. The delta-opioid receptor: isolation of a cDNA by expression cloning and pharmacological characterization. *Proc Natl Acad Sci USA.* 1992;89:12048–12052.

50. Kindt M, Soeter M, Vervliet B. Beyond extinction: erasing human fear responses and preventing the return of fear. *Nat Neurosci.* 2009;12:256–258.

51. Klugmann M, Szumlinski KK. Targeting Homer genes using adeno-associated viral vector: lessons learned from behavioural and neurochemical studies. Kelley AE (2004) Memory and addiction: shared neural circuitry and molecular mechanisms. *Neuron.* 2008;44:161–179.

52. Kreek MJ, LaForge KS, Butelman E. Pharmacotherapy of addictions. *Nat Rev Drug Discov.* 2002;1:710–726.

53. Kruse SW, Zhao R, Smith DP, et al. Structure of a specific alcohol-binding site defined by the odorant binding protein LUSH from Drosophila melanogaster. *Nat Struct Biol.* 2003;10:694–700.

54. Lee JL, Di Ciano P, Thomas KL, et al. Disrupting reconsolidation of drug memories reduces cocaine-seeking behaviour. *Neuron.* 2005;47:795–801.

55. Lee JL, Everitt BJ. Appetitive memory reconsolidation depends upon NMDA receptor-mediated neurotransmission. *Neurobiol Learn Mem.* 2008;90:147–154.

56. Lee JL, Milton AL, Everitt BJ. Cue-induced cocaine seeking and relapse are reduced by disruption of drug memory reconsolidation. *J Neurosci.* 2006;26:5881–5887.

57. Liu QS, Pu L, Poo MM. Repeated cocaine exposure in vivo facilitates LTP induction in midbrain dopamine neurons. *Nature.* 2005;437:1027–1031.

58. Lovinger DM, White G, Weight FF. Ethanol inhibits NMDA-activated ion current in hippocampal neurons. *Science.* 1989;243:1721–1724.

59. Mameli M, Balland B, Lujan R, et al. Rapid synthesis and synaptic insertion of GluR2 for mGluR-LTD in the ventral tegmental area. *Science.* 2007;317:530–533.

60. Matsuda LA, Lolait SJ, Brownstein MJ, et al. Structure of a cannabinoid receptor and functional expression of the cloned cDNA. *Nature.* 1990;346:561–564.

61. Matthes HW, Maldonado R, Simonin F, et al. Loss of morphine-induced analgesia, reward effect and withdrawal symptoms in mice lacking the mu-opioid-receptor gene. *Nature.* 1996;383:819–823.

62. Mayer D, Zahr NM, Sullivan EV, et al. In vivo metabolite differences between the basal ganglia and cerebellum of the rat brain detected with proton MRS at 3T. *Psychiatry Res.* 2007;154:267–273.

63. McGaugh JL. Memory – a century of consolidation. *Science.* 2000;287:248–251.

64. McGaugh JL. The amygdala modulates the consolidation of memories of emotionally arousing experiences. *Annu Rev Neurosci.* 2004;27:1–28.

65. Milekic MH, Brown SD, Castellini C, et al. Persistent disruption of an established morphine conditioned place preference. *J Neurosci.* 2006;26:3010–3020.

66. Misanin JR, Miller RR, Lewis DJ. Retrograde amnesia produced by electroconvulsive shock after reactivation of a consolidated memory trace. *Science.* 1968;160:554–555.

67. Nader K, Hardt O. A single standard for memory: the case for reconsolidation. *Nat Rev Neurosci.* 2009;10:224–234.

68. Nader K, Schafe GE, Le Doux JE. Fear memories require protein synthesis in the amygdala for reconsolidation after retrieval. *Nature.* 2000;406:722–726.

69. Nicolelis MA, Ribeiro S. Multielectrode recordings: the next steps. *Curr Opin Neurobiol.* 2002;12:602–606.

70. Olds J, Millner P. Positive reinforcement produced by electrical stimulation of septal area and other regions of the rat brain. *J Comp Physiol Psychol.* 1954;47:419–426.

71. O'Malley SS, Jaffe AJ, Chang G, et al. Naltrexone and coping skills therapy for alcohol dependence. A controlled study. *Arch Gen Psychiatry.* 1992;49:881–887.

72. Oslin DW, Berrettini W, Kranzler HR, et al. A functional polymorphism of the mu-opioid receptor gene is associated with naltrexone response in alcohol-dependent patients. *Neuropsychopharmacology.* 2003;28:1546–1552.

73. Peoples RW, Li C, Weight FF. Lipid vs. protein theories of alcohol action in the nervous system. *Annu Rev Pharmacol Toxicol.* 1996;36:185–201.

74. Pert CB, Snyder SH. Opiate receptor: demonstration in nervous tissue. *Science.* 1973;179:1011–1014.

75. Pfeuffer J, Tkac I, Provencher SW, et al. Toward an in vivo neurochemical profile: quantification of 18 metabolites in short-echo-time (1)H NMR spectra of the rat brain. *J Magn Reson.* 1999;141:104–120.

76. Preti A. New developments in the pharmacotherapy of cocaine abuse. *Addict Biol.* 2007;12:133–151.

77. Przybyslawski J, Sara SJ. Reconsolidation of memory after its reactivation. *Behav Brain Res.* 1997;84:241–246.

78. Ren H, Honse Y, Peoples RW. A site of alcohol action in the fourth membrane-associated domain of the N-methyl-D-aspartate receptor. *J Biol Chem.* 2003;278:48815–48820.

79. Ren H, Salous AK, Paul JM, et al. Mutations at F637 in the NMDA receptor NR2A subunit M3 domain influence agonist potency, ion channel gating and alcohol action. *Br J Pharmacol.* 2007;151:749–757.

80. Richter CP, Campbell KH. Alcohol taste thresholds and concentrations of solution preferred by rats. *Science.* 1940;91:507–508.

81. Robinson MJ, Franklin KB. Effects of anisomycin on consolidation and reconsolidation of a morphine-conditioned place preference. *Behav Brain Res.* 2007;178:146–153.

82. Rodriguez de Fonseca FR, Schneider M. The endogenous cannabinoid system and drug addiction: 20 years after the discovery of the CB1 receptor. *Addict Biol.* 2008;13:143–146.

83. Ronald KM, Mirshahi T, Woodward JJ. Ethanol inhibition of N-methyl-D-aspartate receptors is reduced by site-directed mutagenesis of a transmembrane domain phenylalanine residue. *J Biol Chem.* 2001;276:44729–44735.

84. Saal D, Dong Y, Bonci A, et al. Drugs of abuse and stress trigger a common synaptic adaptation in dopamine neurons. *Neuron.* 2003;37:577–582.

85. Saccone SF, Hinrichs AL, Saccone NL, et al. Cholinergic nicotinic receptor genes implicated in a nicotine dependence association study targeting 348 candidate genes with 3713 SNPs. *Hum Mol Genet.* 2007;16:36–49.

86. Sanchis-Segura C, Spanagel R. Behavioural assessment of drug reinforcement and addictive features in rodents: an overview. *Addict Biol.* 2006;11:2–38.

87. Schlaepfer IR, Hoft NR, Collins AC, et al. The CHRNA5/A3/B4 gene cluster variability as an important determinant of early alcohol and tobacco initiation in young adults. *Biol Psychiatry.* 2008;63:1039–1046.

88. Schwarz AJ, Gozzi A, Reese T, et al. In vivo mapping of functional connectivity in neurotransmitter systems using pharmacological MRI. *Neuroimage.* 2007;34:627–636.

89. Schwarz AJ, Gozzi A, Reese T, et al. Functional connectivity in the pharmacologically activated brain: resolving networks of correlated responses to d-amphetamine. *Magn Reson Med.* 2007;57:704–713.

90. Schwarz AJ, Gozzi A, Reese T, et al. Pharmacological modulation of functional connectivity: the correlation structure underlying the phMRI response to d-amphetamine modified by selective dopamine D3 receptor antagonist SB277011A. *Magn Reson Imaging.* 2007;25:811–820.

91. Shoaib M, Schindler CW, Goldberg SR. Nicotine self-administration in rats: strain and nicotine pre-exposure effects on acquisition. *Psychopharmacology (Berl).* 1997;129:35–43.

92. Shoaib M, Stolerman IP. Plasma nicotine and cotinine levels following intravenous nicotine self-administration in rats. *Psychopharmacology (Berl).* 1999;143:318–321.

93. Simon EJ, Hiller JM, Edelmann I. Stereospecific binding of the potent narcotic analgesic (3H)-Etorphine to rat homogenate. *Proc Natl Acad Sci USA.* 1973;70. 1974–1949.

94. Siu EC, Tyndale RF. Non-nicotinic therapies for smoking cessation. *Annu Rev Pharmacol Toxicol.* 2007;47:541–564.

95. Smothers CT, Woodward JJ. Effects of amino acid substitutions in transmembrane domains of the NR1 subunit on the ethanol inhibition of recombinant N-methyl-D-aspartate receptors. *Alcohol Clin Exp Res.* 2006;30:523–530.

96. Spanagel R. Alcoholism – a systems approach from molecular physiology to behavior. *Physiol Rev.* 2009;89:649–705.

97. Spanagel R, Heilig M. Addiction and its brain science. *Addiction.* 2005;100:1813–1822.

98. Spanagel R, Kiefer F. Drugs for relapse prevention of alcoholism – 10 years of progress. *Trends Pharmacol Sci.* 2008;29:109–115.

99. Spanagel R, Pendyala G, Abarca C, et al. The circadian clock gene Period2 alters the glutamatergic system and thereby modulates alcohol consumption. *Nat Med.* 2005;11:35–42.

100. Spanagel R, Weiss F. The dopamine hypothesis of reward: past and current status. *Trends Neurosci.* 1999;22:521–527.

101. Srisurapanont M, Jarusuraisin N. Opioid antagonists for alcohol dependence. *Cochrane Database Syst Rev.* 2000;3:CD001867. https://doi.org/10.1002/14651858.CD001867.pub2.

102. Sullivan PF, Kendler KS. The genetic epidemiology of smoking. *Nicotine Tob Res.* 1999;2(suppl 1):S51–S57; discussion S69–S70.

103. Sullivan PF, Neale BM, van den Oord E, et al. Candidate genes for nicotine dependence via linkage, epistasis, and bioinformatics. *Am J Med Genet B Neuropsychiatr Genet.* 2004;126:23–36.

104. Terenius L. Stereospecific interaction between narcotic analgesics and a synaptic plasma membrane fraction of rat cerebral cortex. *Acta Pharmacol Toxicol.* 1973;32:317–320.

105. Thomas KL, Arroyo M, Everitt BJ. Induction of the learning and plasticity-associated gene Zif268 following exposure to a discrete cocaine-associated stimulus. *Eur J Neurosci.* 2003;17:1964–1972.

106. Thorgeirsson TE, Geller F, Sulem P, et al. A variant associated with nicotine dependence, lung cancer and peripheral arterial disease. *Nature.* 2008;452:638–642.

107. Torras-Garcia M, Lelong J, Tronel S, et al. Reconsolidation after remembering an odor-reward association requires NMDA receptors. *Learn Mem.* 2005;12:18–22.

108. Treutlein J, Cichon S, Ridinger M, et al. Genome-wide association study of alcohol dependence. *Arch Gen Psychiatry.* 2009;66:773–784.

109. Tronson NC, Taylor JR. Molecular mechanisms of memory reconsolidation. *Nat Rev Neurosci.* 2007;8:262–275.

110. Tu Y, Kroener S, Abernathy K, et al. Ethanol inhibits persistent activity in prefrontal cortical neurons. *J Neurosci.* 2007;27:4765–4775.

111. Uhl GR, Liu QR, Drgon T, et al. Molecular genetics of nicotine dependence and abstinence: whole genome association using 520,000 SNPs. *BMC Genet.* 2007;8:10–17.

112. Ungless MA, Whistler JL, Malenka RC, et al. Single cocaine exposure in vivo induces long-term potentiation in dopamine neurons. *Nature.* 2001;411:583–587.

113. Urban D, Clarke WP, von Zastrow M, et al. Functional selectivity and classical concepts of quantitative pharmacology. *J Pharmacol Exp Ther.* 2006;320:1–13.

114. Valjent E, Corbillé AG, Bertran-Gonzalez J, et al. Inhibition of ERK pathway or protein synthesis during reexposure to drugs of abuse erases previously learned place preference. *Proc Natl Acad Sci USA.* 2006;103:2932–2937.

115. Vengeliene V, Bilbao A, Molander A, et al. Neuropharmacology of alcohol addiction. *Brit J Pharmacol.* 2008;154:299–315.

116. Volkow ND, Li TK. Drug addiction: the neurobiology of behaviour gone awry. *Nat Rev Neurosci.* 2004;5:963–970.

117. Volpicelli JR, Alterman AI, Hayashida M, et al. Naltrexone in the treatment of alcohol dependence. *Arch Gen Psychiatry.* 1992;49:876–880.

118. Wang J, Gutala R, Hwang YY, et al. Strain- and region-specific gene expression profiles in mouse brain in response to chronic nicotine treatment. *Genes Brain Behav.* 2008;7:78–87.

119. Wolffgramm JHeyne A. From controlled drug intake to loss of control: the irreversible development of drug addiction in the rat. *Behav Brain Res.* 1995;70:77–94.

120. Wright JM, Peoples RW, Weight FF. Single-channel and whole-cell analysis of ethanol inhibition of N-methyl-D-aspartate-activated currents in cultured mouse cortical and hippocampal neurons. *Brain Res.* 1996;738:249–256.

APPENDIX 1

National Institute on Drug Abuse (NIDA): Medications to Treat Opioid Use Disorder*

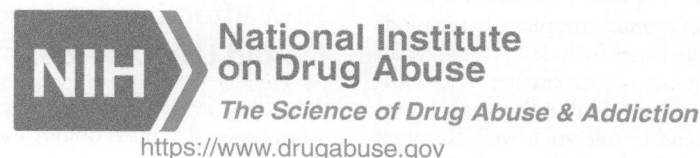

National Institute on Drug Abuse

The Science of Drug Abuse & Addiction

https://www.drugabuse.gov

OUTLINE

Overview

An estimated 2.1 million people in the United States had a substance use disorder related to prescription opioid pain medicines in 2016. However, only a fraction of people with prescription opioid use disorders receive specialty treatment (17.5% in 2016).[97] Overdose deaths linked to these medicines were five times higher in 2016 than in 1999.[84] There is now also a rise in heroin use and heroin use disorder as some people shift from prescription opioids to their cheaper street relative; 626,000 people had a heroin use disorder in 2016, and more than 15,000 Americans died of a heroin overdose in 2016.[85,97] Besides overdose, consequences of the opioid crisis include a rising incidence of infants born dependent on opioids because their mothers used these substances during pregnancy,[79,102]

and increased spread of infectious diseases, including HIV and hepatitis C virus (HCV), as was seen in 2015 in southern Indiana.[19]

Effective prevention and treatment strategies exist for opioid misuse and use disorder but are highly underutilized across the United States. An initiative of the Secretary of Health and Human Services (HHS)[105] began in 2015 to address the complex problem of prescription opioid and heroin use. In 2017, HHS announced five priorities for addressing the opioid crisis:

1. improving access to treatment and recovery services
2. promoting use of overdose-reversing drugs
3. strengthening our understanding of the epidemic through better public health surveillance
4. providing support for cutting-edge research on pain and addiction
5. advancing better practices for pain management

Effective medications exist to treat opioid use disorder: methadone, buprenorphine, and naltrexone. These medications could help many people recover from opioid use disorder, but they remain highly underutilized. Less than half of private-sector treatment programs offer medications for opioid use disorders, and of patients in those programs who might benefit, only a third actually receive it.[55] Overcoming the misunderstandings and other barriers that prevent wider adoption of these treatments is crucial for tackling the problem of opioid use disorder and the epidemic of opioid overdose in the United States.

How Do Medications to Treat Opioid Use Disorder Work?

Opioid Agonists and Partial Agonists (Maintenance Medications)

Studies show that people with opioid use disorder who follow detoxification with complete abstinence are very likely to relapse, or return to using the drug.[4] Although relapse is a normal step on the path to recovery, it can also be life-threatening, raising the risk for a fatal overdose.[22] Thus an important way to support recovery from heroin or prescription opioid use disorder is to maintain abstinence from those drugs. Someone in recovery can also use medications that reduce the negative effects of withdrawal and

---

*Last updated June 2018.

cravings without producing the euphoria that the original drug of abuse caused. For example, the US Food and Drug Administration (FDA) recently approved lofexidine, a nonopioid medicine designed to reduce opioid withdrawal symptoms. **Methadone** and **buprenorphine** are other medications approved for this purpose.

Methadone is a synthetic *opioid agonist* that eliminates withdrawal symptoms and relieves drug cravings by acting on opioid receptors in the brain—the same receptors that other opioids such as heroin, morphine, and opioid pain medications activate. Although it occupies and activates these opioid receptors, it does so more slowly than other opioids and, in an opioid-dependent person, treatment doses do not produce euphoria. It has been used successfully for more than 40 years to treat opioid use disorder and must be dispensed through specialized opioid treatment programs.

Buprenorphine is a *partial opioid agonist*, meaning that it binds to those same opioid receptors but activates them less strongly than full agonists do. Like methadone, it can reduce cravings and withdrawal symptoms in a person with an opioid use disorder without producing euphoria, and patients tend to tolerate it well. Research has found buprenorphine to be similarly effective as methadone for treating opioid use disorders, as long as it is given at a sufficient dose and for sufficient duration.[65] The FDA approved buprenorphine in 2002, making it the first medication eligible to be prescribed by certified physicians through the Drug Addiction Treatment Act. This approval eliminates the need to visit specialized treatment clinics, thereby expanding access to treatment for many who need it. In addition, the Comprehensive Addiction and Recovery Act (CARA), which was signed into law in July 2016, temporarily expands eligibility to prescribe buprenorphine-based drugs for medication-assisted treatment (MAT) to qualifying nurse practitioners and physician assistants through October 1, 2021. Buprenorphine has been available for opioid use disorders since 2002 as a tablet and since 2010 as a sublingual film,[92] and the FDA approved a 6-month subdermal buprenorphine implant in May 2016. This formulation is available to patients stabilized on buprenorphine and will eliminate the treatment barrier of daily dosing for these patients. (Also see "What Are Misconceptions About Maintenance Treatment?")

Opioid Antagonists

Naltrexone is an *opioid antagonist*, which means that it works by blocking the activation of opioid receptors. Instead of controlling withdrawal and cravings, it treats opioid use disorder by preventing any opioid drug from producing rewarding effects such as

euphoria. Its use for ongoing opioid use disorder treatment has been somewhat limited because of poor adherence and tolerability by patients. However, in 2010, an injectable, long-acting form of naltrexone (Vivitrol), originally approved for treating alcohol use disorder, was FDA-approved for treating opioid use disorder. Because its effects last for weeks, Vivitrol is a good option for patients who do not have ready access to health care or who struggle with taking their medications regularly.

Each medication works differently, therefore a treatment provider should decide on the optimal medication in consultation with the individual patient and should consider the patient's unique history and circumstances.

How Effective Are Medications to Treat Opioid Use Disorder?

Abundant evidence shows that methadone, buprenorphine, and naltrexone all reduce opioid use and opioid use disorder–related symptoms, and they reduce the risk of infectious disease transmission as well as criminal behavior associated with drug use.[100] These medications also increase the likelihood that a person will remain in treatment, which itself is associated with lower risk of overdose mortality, reduced risk of HIV and HCV transmission, reduced criminal justice involvement, and greater likelihood of employment.[100]

Methadone

Methadone is the medication with the longest history of use for opioid use disorder treatment, having been used since 1947. A large number of studies (some of which are summarized in the graph below) support methadone's effectiveness at reducing opioid use. A comprehensive Cochrane review in 2009 compared methadone-based treatment (methadone plus psychosocial treatment) to placebo with psychosocial treatment and found that methadone treatment was effective in reducing opioid use, opioid use-associated transmission of infectious disease, and crime.[24,54,65,87,108,117] Patients on methadone had 33% fewer opioid-positive drug tests and were 4.44 times more likely to stay in treatment compared to controls.[65] Methadone treatment significantly improves outcomes, even when provided in the absence of regular counseling services[64,54,88]; long-term (beyond 6 months) outcomes are better in groups receiving methadone, regardless of the frequency of counseling received.[42,89]

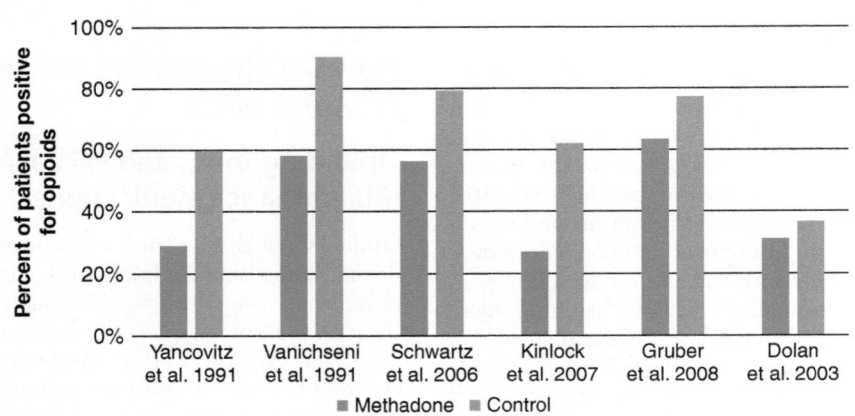

Opioid use with or without methadone treatment.

Buprenorphine

Buprenorphine, which was first approved in 2002, is currently available in two prescription forms: alone (Probuphine, Sublocade, and Bunavail) and in combination with the opioid receptor antagonist naloxone (Suboxone, Zubsolv). Both formulations of buprenorphine are effective for the treatment of opioid use disorders, although some studies have shown high relapse rates among patients tapered off buprenorphine compared to patients maintained on the drug for a longer period.[30]

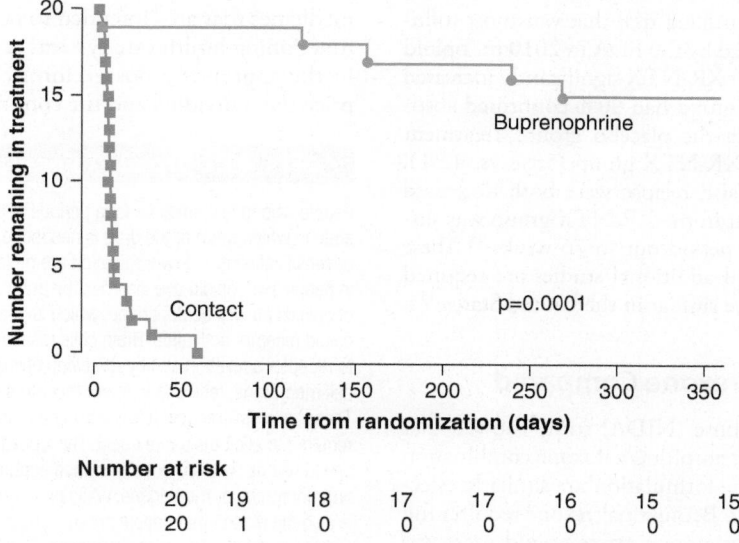

Number at risk							
20	19	18	17	17	16	15	15
20	1	0	0	0	0	0	0

From Kakko J, Svanborg KD, Kreek MJ, Heilig M. One-year retention and social function after buprenorphine-assisted relapse prevention treatment for heroin dependence in Sweden: a randomised, placebo-controlled trial. *Lancet Lond Engl.* 2003;361(9358):662-668.

A Swedish study compared patients maintained on 16 mg of buprenorphine daily to a control group that received buprenorphine for detoxification (6 days) followed by placebo.[51] All patients received psychosocial supports. In this study, the treatment failure rate for placebo was 100% versus 25% for buprenorphine. More than two opioid-positive urine tests within 3 months resulted in cessation of treatment, so treatment retention was closely related to relapse. Of patients not retained in treatment, there was a 20% mortality rate.

Meta-analysis determined that patients on doses of buprenorphine of 16 mg per day or more were 1.82 times more likely to stay in treatment than placebo-treated patients and that buprenorphine decreased the number of opioid-positive drug tests by 14.2% (the standardized mean difference was −1.17).[35,51,65]

To be effective, buprenorphine must be given at a sufficiently high dose (generally, 16 mg per day or more). Some treatment providers wary of using opioids have prescribed lower doses for short treatment durations, leading to failure of buprenorphine treatment and the mistaken conclusion that the medication is ineffective.[62,65]

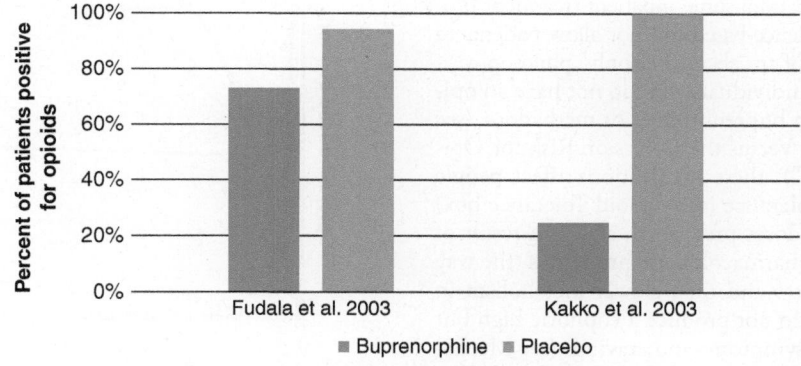

Opioid use with or without buprenorphine treatment.

Methadone and Buprenorphine Compared

Methadone and buprenorphine are equally effective at reducing opioid use. A comprehensive Cochrane review comparing buprenorphine, methadone, and placebo found no differences in opioid-positive drug tests or self-reported heroin use when treating with methadone or buprenorphine at medium-to-high doses.[65]

Notably, flexible dose regimens of buprenorphine and doses of buprenorphine of 6 mg or less are less effective than methadone at keeping patients in treatment, highlighting the need for delivery of evidence-based dosing regimens of these medications.[65]

Naltrexone

Naltrexone was initially approved for the treatment of opioid use disorder in a daily pill form. It does not produce tolerance or withdrawal. Poor treatment adherence has primarily limited the real-world effectiveness of this formulation.[75] As a result, there is insufficient evidence that oral naltrexone is an effective treatment for opioid use disorder.[70] Extended-release injectable naltrexone (XR-NTX) is administered once monthly, which removes the need for daily dosing. Although this formulation is the newest form of medication for opioid use disorder, evidence to date suggests that it is effective.[57,75]

The double-blind, placebo-controlled trial that was most influential in getting XR-NTX approved by the FDA in 2010 for opioid use disorder treatment showed that XR-NTX significantly increased opioid abstinence. The XR-NTX group had 90% confirmed abstinent weeks compared to 35% in the placebo group. Treatment retention was also higher in the XR-NTX group (58% vs. 42%), whereas subjective drug craving and relapse were both decreased (0.8% vs. 13.7%).[58] Improvement in the XR-NTX group was sustained throughout an open label period out to 76 weeks.[98] These data were collected in Russia, and additional studies are required to determine if effectiveness will be similar in the United States.[45]

Buprenorphine and Naltrexone Compared

A National Institute on Drug Abuse (NIDA) study showed that once treatment is initiated, a buprenorphine/naloxone combination and an extended release naltrexone formulation are similarly effective in treating opioid use disorder. Because naltrexone requires full detoxification, initiating treatment among active opioid users was more difficult with this medication. However, once detoxification was complete, the naltrexone formulation had an effectiveness similar to that of the buprenorphine/naloxone combination.

What Are Misconceptions About Maintenance Treatment?

Because maintenance medications (methadone and buprenorphine) are themselves opioids and can produce euphoria in people who are not dependent on opioids, many people have assumed that this form of treatment simply substitutes a new substance use disorder for an old one. This belief has unfortunately hindered the adoption of these effective treatments. In the past, even some inpatient treatment programs that were otherwise evidence-based did not allow patients to use these medications, in favor of an "abstinence only" philosophy.

Although it is possible for individuals who do not have an opioid use disorder to get high on buprenorphine or methadone (see "What Is the Treatment Need Versus the Diversion Risk for Opioid Use Disorder Treatment?"), these medications affect people who have developed a high tolerance (see Opioid Tolerance box) to opioids differently. At the doses prescribed, and as a result of their pharmacodynamic and pharmacokinetic properties (the way they act at opioid receptor sites and their slower metabolism in the body), these medications do not produce a euphoric high but instead minimize withdrawal symptoms and cravings (see Mechanisms of Opioid Dependence box). This makes it possible for the patient to function normally, attend school or work, and participate in other forms of treatment or recovery support services to help them become free of their substance use disorder over time.

The ultimate aim can be to wean off the maintenance medication, but the treatment provider should make this decision jointly with the patient and tapering of the medication must be done gradually. It may take months or years in some cases. Just as body tissues require prolonged periods to heal after injury and may require external supports (e.g., a cast and crutches or a wheelchair for a broken leg), brain circuits that have been altered by prolonged drug use and substance use disorder take time to recover and benefit from external supports in the form of medication. In cases of serious and long-term opioid use disorder, a patient may need these supports indefinitely.

In 2005, methadone and buprenorphine were added to the World Health Organization's list of essential medicines, defined as medicines that are "intended to be available within the context of functioning health care systems at all times in adequate amounts, in the appropriate dosage forms, with assured quality, and at a price the individual and the community can afford."[114,115]

• BOX A1.1 Opioid Tolerance

People who take opioids for long periods of time typically develop *tolerance*, a state in which more of the drug is needed to produce the same effect. Receptor desensitization and downregulation are molecular processes that cause tolerance. In people with opioid use disorder, the brain is continually exposed to high levels of opioids as well as dopamine, which is released in the reward circuit following opioid receptor activation. Brain cells respond to this by reducing their response to receptor activation and by removing opioid and dopamine receptors from the cell membrane, resulting in fewer receptors that can be activated by the drug.[3,112] These mechanisms result in a lessened response to the drug, so higher doses are required to elicit the same effect. This opioid tolerance is the reason that people with opioid use disorder do not experience euphoric effects from therapeutic doses of buprenorphine or methadone, while people without opioid use disorder do.[44,110] It is also the reason that people are at increased risk of overdose when relapsing to opioid use after a period of abstinence: They lose their tolerance to the drug without realizing it, so they no longer know what dose of the drug they can safely tolerate.

• BOX A1.2 Mechanisms of Opioid Dependence

The sustained activation of opioid receptors that results from opioid use disorder and causes tolerance also causes withdrawal symptoms when the opioid drugs leave the body. Drug withdrawal symptoms are opposite to the symptoms caused by drug taking. In the case of opioids, they include anxiety, jitters, and diarrhea.[56] Avoidance of these negative symptoms is one reason that people keep taking opioids, and in the early stages of treatment, medications such as methadone and buprenorphine reduce withdrawal symptoms.

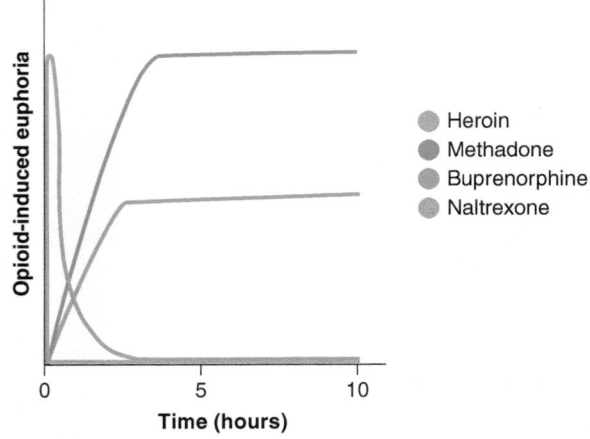

Legend:
● Heroin
● Methadone
● Buprenorphine
● Naltrexone

Opioid receptor activity. Heroin (*red line*) activates opioid receptors fully and quickly. Methadone (*blue line*) is also a full agonist, but the activation is much slower and longer lasting. Buprenorphine (*green line*) activates the receptors partially, with a similar time course to methadone. Naltrexone (*purple line*) is an opioid receptor. (Data from Cruciani RA, Knotkova H, eds. *Handbook of Methadone Prescribing and Buprenorphine Therapy.* New York: Springer-Verlag; 2013, and Brunton LL, Lazo JS, Parker KL, eds. *Goodman & Gilman's: The Pharmacological Basis of Therapeutics.* 11th ed. New York: McGraw Hill Medical; 2011.)

What Is the Treatment Need Versus the Diversion Risk for Opioid Use Disorder Treatment?

Like other opioid medications, buprenorphine and methadone are sometimes diverted and misused. However, most data suggest that the majority of buprenorphine and methadone misuse (use without a prescription) is for the purpose of controlling withdrawal and cravings for other opioids and not to get high. Among all opioid agonist medications, methadone and buprenorphine together make up 15% of diversion reports, while oxycodone and hydrocodone are responsible for 67%.[106] Naltrexone, an opioid antagonist used to treat opioid addiction, does not cause euphoric effects and is not a diversion risk.

Diversion Risk of Buprenorphine

Both buprenorphine and buprenorphine/naloxone formulations can interfere with the effects of full opioid agonists, such as heroin, and can precipitate withdrawal in individuals with opioid dependence. Two US surveys of people with opioid use disorder found that a majority of those who used illicit buprenorphine reported that they used it for therapeutic purposes (i.e., to reduce withdrawal symptoms, reduce heroin use, and so on).[6,86] Ninety-seven percent reported using it to prevent cravings, 90% to prevent withdrawal, and 29% to save money.[86] Illicit use of buprenorphine decreased as individuals had access to treatment.[86] The minority proportion of people who use buprenorphine illicitly to get high (ranging from 8% to 25%)[17,86] has been shown to decrease over time, which could suggest that people abandon this goal after they experience the drug's blunted rewarding effects.[17] Indeed, patients in treatment for opioid use disorder rarely endorse buprenorphine as the primary drug of misuse.[16]

Although there is some risk associated with misuse of buprenorphine, the risk of harms, such as fatal overdose, is significantly lower than risks associated with use of full agonist opioids (oxycodone, hydrocodone, heroin).[44,91] Overdoses and related deaths do occur but are usually the result of combination with other respiratory depressant drugs such as benzodiazepines or alcohol. Emergency department (ED) visits involving buprenorphine increased from 3161 in 2005 to 30,135 visits in 2010 as availability of the drug increased (buprenorphine was first approved in 2002); but ED visits for buprenorphine remain significantly less common than those for other opioids.[14] Fifty-two percent, or 15,778 visits (see left bar chart below), were related to nonmedical use in 2010; 59% of these visits involved additional drugs (see right bar chart below).[94,96]

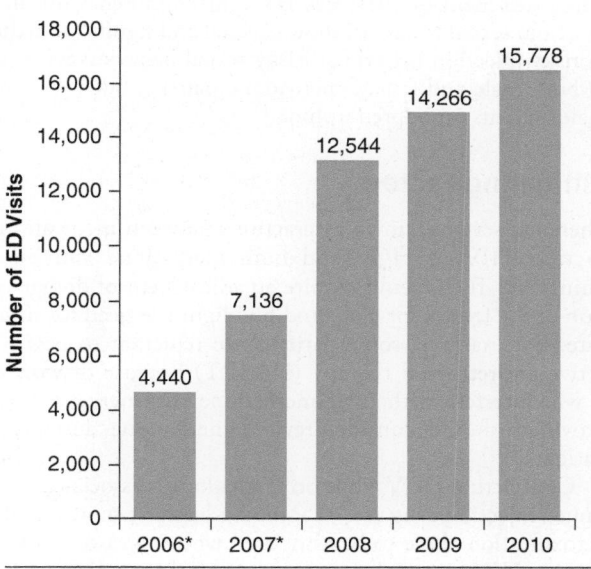

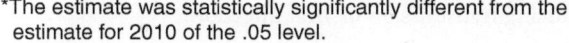

*The estimate was statistically significantly different from the estimate for 2010 of the .05 level.

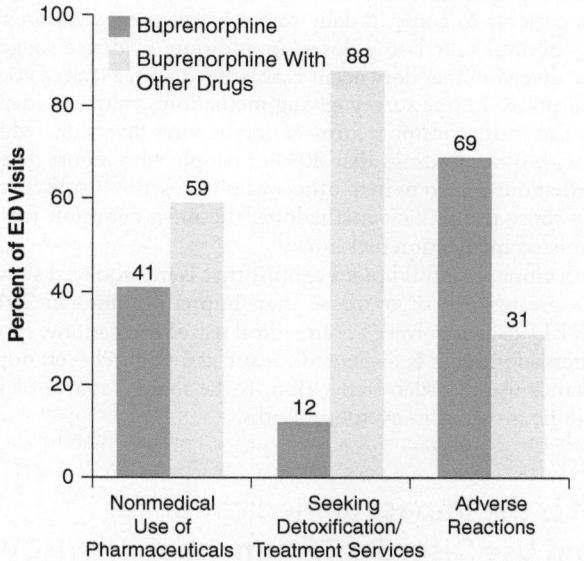

Emergency department (ED) visits involving buprenorphine increased as drug availability increased, but ED visits for buprenorphine are far less common than those for other products. (From 2006 to 2010 SAMHSA Drug Abuse Warning Network [DAWN] and 2010 SAMHSA Drug Abuse Warning Network [DAWN].)

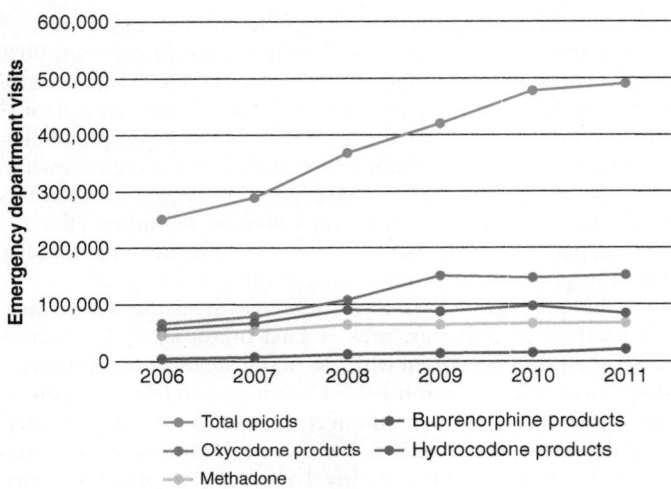

Opioid-related emergency department visits. (From Center for Behavioral Health Statistics and Quality [CBHSQ]. *Drug Abuse Warning Network: 2011: Selected Tables of National Estimates of Drug-Related Emergency Department Visits.* Rockville, MD: Substance Abuse and Mental Health Services Administration; 2013.)

Diversion Risk of Methadone

Methadone diversion is primarily associated with methadone prescribed for the treatment of pain and not for the treatment of opioid use disorders. Opioid treatment programs are required to maintain and implement a diversion control plan; they typically require patients to come in daily to receive their medication and strictly monitor take-home doses. In addition, evidence suggests that the diversion that does occur is associated with a lack of access to medication. In one survey, giving methadone away was identified as the most common form of methadone diversion, which aligns with other findings that 80% of people who report diverting methadone did so to help others who misused[25,47] substances. Among those using illicit methadone, the most common reason was a missed medication pick-up.

Methadone, as a full opioid agonist that is metabolized slowly, poses a greater risk of overdose than buprenorphine. In 2010, 65,945 ED visits involved[94] nonmedical use of methadone. However, methadone that is dispensed for use as a pain reliever, not as a substance use disorder medication, is the main[15] source of the methadone involved in overdose deaths.

What Is the Impact of Medication for Opioid Use Disorder Treatment on HIV/HCV Outcomes?

Injection drug use is still a primary driver of the HIV/AIDS epidemic around the world.[68] A recent example is the small community of Austin, Indiana, where 170 new HIV infections occurred in the 8 months between November 2014 and June 2015 among people misusing the prescription opioid pain reliever oxymorphone (Opana) via injection.[19] People who inject drugs frequently share their needles and other injection equipment, enabling viruses such as HIV and HCV to spread between people.

Medications for opioid use disorder treatment can reduce transmission of HIV and HCV by reducing risk behaviors in people who inject drugs and can improve HIV- and HCV-related outcomes by treating those not engaged in injection opioid use who might otherwise transition to injection, linking those with HIV/HCV infection to appropriate treatment,[78,82] and improving adherence to HIV/HCV treatment.[5,63] These improvements depend on accessibility of medications for opioid use disorder to people who need it and coordinating medication delivery with HCV/HIV screening and treatment.

Treatment with methadone or buprenorphine is associated with reduced injection drug use risk behaviors. Meta-analyses have shown a reduction in risk behaviors including a 32% to 69% reduction in illicit opioid use, a 20% to 60% reduction in injection drug use, and a 25% to 86% reduction in sharing of injection equipment.[39,40] Treatment with extended-release naltrexone also reduced HIV-risk behaviors compared to placebo.

Methadone and buprenorphine treatment are also associated with lower HCV infection rates in young adults who inject drugs, whereas other treatments and detoxification alone are not.[103] Methadone treatment is associated with low rates of contracting HCV overall,[74] with mathematical modeling suggesting that it can prevent 22.6 new HCV infections per 100 treated people who engaged in injection drug use, per year.[2,81] Methadone treatment also reduces both HIV risk behaviors and HIV infection, with better outcomes for people who inject drugs who are in treatment (3.5% contracting HIV vs. 22%), and better outcomes for longer treatment duration and for continuous (vs. interrupted) treatment.[36,43,69]

A study comparing the effects of methadone and buprenorphine treatment on HIV risk from injection behaviors and HIV risk from sexual behaviors showed equal and significant reductions in risky injection behaviors. Risky sexual behaviors were reduced in both male and female methadone patients but were higher in male patients on buprenorphine.[113]

Mitigating Factors

There are several known interactions between medications used to treat HIV or HCV and both methadone and buprenorphine.[11,60] These could require an adjustment of dosage or revision of the treatment plan, and highlight the need for integrated care. For example, some patients are reluctant to begin highly active antiretroviral therapy (HAART) because of worries that it will interfere with their methadone treatment, so treatment providers should consider revised methadone doses for these patients.[60]

Contracting HCV while on methadone is associated with continued injection drug use.[119] Some studies have shown methadone detoxification alone to be associated with increased rates of contracting HIV, so ongoing treatment with this medication is key to reducing transmission of viral infection.[61]

Possibility of Dual Therapeutic Potential

One recent report demonstrates the potential of buprenorphine to counteract a neuroinflammatory process that is involved in HIV-associated neurocognitive disorders, suggesting that buprenorphine could potentially be simultaneously therapeutic for opioid use disorder and HIV.[13,32] Opioid use disorder medications are also associated with increased adherence to HAART for the treatment of HIV.[5,63] Some providers hesitate to treat HCV in people who inject drugs, but a naltrexone implantation clinic showed rates of sustained virologic response in their patients that were comparable to clinics treating non-injection-drug-using patients.[46]

How Is Opioid Use Disorder Treated in the Criminal Justice System?

Opioid use disorders are highly prevalent among criminal justice populations. According to data from the US Department of Justice, approximately half of state and federal prisoners meet criteria for substance use disorder.[72] Even so, there has been reticence in criminal justice settings to using methadone, buprenorphine, and naltrexone to treat opioid use disorder. In national surveys, utilization of these medications is very low in criminal justice settings, including drug courts,[66] jails,[31] and prisons.[76] Thus opioid use disorder goes largely untreated during periods of incarceration, and opioid use often resumes after release.

A former inmate's risk of death within the first 2 weeks of release is more than 12 times that of other individuals, with the leading cause of death being a fatal overdose.[8] Overdoses are more common when a person relapses to drug use after a period of abstinence due to loss of tolerance to the drug. One study found a reduction in postincarceration deaths from overdose among individuals who had received medication for opioid use disorder in correctional facilities.[41] Untreated opioid use disorders also contribute to a return to criminal activity, reincarceration, and risky behavior contributing to the spread of HIV and hepatitis B and C infections (see https://www.drugabuse.gov/publications/medications-to-treat-opioid-addiction/what-impact-medication-opioid-use-disorder-treatment-hivhcv-outcomes[118]).

The World Health Organization's Guidelines for the Psychosocially Assisted Pharmacological Treatment of Opioid Dependence recommends that incarcerated individuals should receive adequate health care and that "opioid withdrawal, agonist maintenance, and naltrexone treatment should all be available in prison settings, and prisoners should not be forced to accept any particular treatment."[116]

Many states currently do not offer appropriate access to or utilize medications to treat opioid use disorder among arrestees or inmates,[31,34] even though research has shown many benefits of incorporating MAT into criminal justice treatment programs. Inmates who receive buprenorphine treatment prior to release are more likely to engage in treatment after their release than inmates who participate in counseling only.[38] Participants who engage in methadone treatment and counseling in prison are more likely to enter community-based methadone treatment centers after their release (68.6%) than those receiving only counseling (7.8%) or those in counseling and referred to a treatment center (50%).[54]

In one study, inmates who began buprenorphine treatment while incarcerated engaged in post-release treatment sooner, averaging 3.9 days after release, compared to 9.2 days for participants referred to treatment post-release.[118] They were also likely to stay in treatment longer if they were initiated in treatment prior to release (20.3 weeks on average) than if they began treatment after their release (13.2 weeks).[118]

Inmates who participate in methadone treatment and counseling while in prison are less likely to test positive for illicit opioids at 1 month following their release (27.6%) compared to those who only receive counseling (62.9%) and those who receive counseling and a referral to a treatment center (41%).[54]

A randomized controlled trial was published in 2016, comparing prison-initiated extended-release naltrexone (XR-NTX) treatment to standard counseling protocols for prevention of opioid relapse. During the treatment phase, relapse was significantly lower in the group receiving XR-NTX (43% vs. 64%). The XR-NTX group also experienced no overdose events, while there were seven overdose events in the control group.[59]

A survey of community correction agents' views on using medications to treat opioid use disorder showed that more favorable attitudes toward medication use are associated with greater knowledge about the evidence base for these medications and greater understanding of opioid use disorder as a medical disorder.[71] Organizational linkage between correctional stakeholders and community treatment providers, along with training sessions, can be an effective way to change perceptions and increase knowledge about the efficacy of these medications, and can increase the intent within correctional facilities to refer individuals with opioid use disorder to treatment that incorporates medications.[34]

A mechanism to reduce recidivism and divert nonviolent offenders from traditional jail and prison settings is the drug treatment court model, which provides treatment services in combination with judicial supervision.[10] Still, resistance to medications persists even in this area of the criminal justice system; a survey published in 2013 reported that 50% of drug courts did not allow agonist treatment for opioid use disorder under any circumstances.[66] In 2015, the Office of National Drug Control Policy announced that state drug courts receiving federal grants must not: (1) deny any appropriate and eligible client for the treatment drug court access to the program because of their use of FDA-approved medications that is in accordance with an appropriately authorized prescription; or (2) mandate that a drug court client no longer use medications as part of the conditions of the drug court if such a mandate is inconsistent with a medical practitioner's recommendation or prescription.[95]

Is Medication to Treat Opioid Use Disorder Available in the Military?

Rates of prescription opioid misuse are higher among service members than among civilians.[73] Survey results suggest that drug use among returning soldiers is often a coping strategy to treat arousal symptoms of posttraumatic stress disorder.[90] Returning military personnel also experience higher rates of chronic pain and related medical use of opioid pain relievers compared to the civilian population. These data collectively suggest an unmet need for the assessment, management, and treatment of both chronic pain and opioid use disorder in this population.[101]

The Veterans Health Administration (VHA) acknowledges that treatment with opioid agonists (methadone or buprenorphine) is the first-line treatment for opioid use disorder and recommends it for all opioid-dependent patients. Notably, a 2015 revision of treatment guidelines for the US Department of Veteran Affairs and US Department of Defense shifted toward allowing these medications as a treatment option for active duty military members.[107] Still, only about a quarter of patients with an opioid use disorder treated at VHA facilities receive medication. Barriers to opioid agonist medication among VHA providers include lack of perceived patient interest, stigma toward the patient population, and lack of education about opioid agonist treatment.[37]

In the past, lack of insurance coverage for opioid agonist medications was a barrier for use among active duty military; however, as of 2013, TRICARE included coverage for these medications, and a 2016 modification of TRICARE regulation included provisions for expanded coverage of opioid use disorder treatment.[104] This expanded coverage removed annual and lifetime limitations on substance use disorder treatment allowed for office-based opioid treatment, and established opioid treatment programs as a newly recognized category of institutional provider under TRICARE.

What Treatment Is Available for Pregnant Mothers and Their Babies?

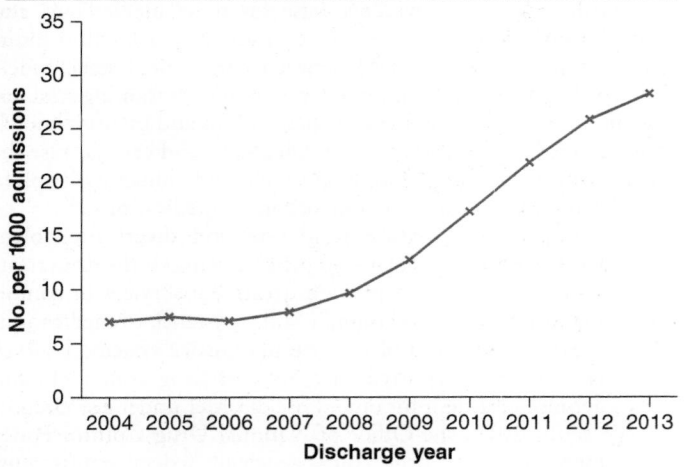

Admissions for the neonatal abstinence syndrome. (From Tolia VN, Patrick SW, Bennett MM, et al. Increasing incidence of the neonatal abstinence syndrome in U.S. neonatal ICUs. *N Engl J Med.* 2015;372[22]:2118–2126.)

Paralleling the large recent increases in opioid use, use disorder, and overdose, the incidence of babies born dependent on opioids (neonatal abstinence syndrome, or NAS) as a result of the mother's opioid use during pregnancy has also greatly increased.[102] Incidence of NAS rose nearly fivefold between 2000 and 2012[79]; this increase was associated with increases in the prescription of opioids to pregnant women for pain, which doubled between 1995 and 2009.[28,80]

Untreated opioid use disorder during pregnancy can have devastating effects on the fetus. The fluctuating levels of opioids in the blood of mothers who are misusing opioids expose the fetus to repeated periods of withdrawal,[52] which can also harm the function of the placenta and increase the risk of:
- fetal growth restriction[52]
- placental abruption[52]
- preterm labor[52]
- fetal convulsions[52]
- intrauterine passage of meconium[52]
- fetal death[99]

In addition to these direct physical effects, other risks to the fetus include:
- untreated maternal infections such as HIV[26]
- malnutrition and poor prenatal care[93]
- dangers conferred by drug-seeking lifestyle, including violence and incarceration[93,99]

Methadone and Buprenorphine as the Standard of Care for Opioid Use Disorder in Pregnancy

To lessen the negative effects of opioid dependence on the fetus, treatment with methadone has been used for pregnant women with opioid use disorder since the 1970s and has been recognized as the standard of care since 1998.[26,99] Recent evidence, however, suggests that buprenorphine may be an even better treatment option.[9]

Both methadone and buprenorphine treatment during pregnancy:
- stabilize fetal levels of opioids, reducing repeated prenatal withdrawal[9,52]
- improve neonatal outcomes[93]
- increase maternal HIV treatment to reduce the likelihood of transmitting the virus to the fetus
- link mothers to better prenatal care[26,93,99]

A meta-analysis showed that, compared to single-dose methadone treatment, buprenorphine resulted in:
- 10% lower incidence of NAS
- shorter neonatal treatment time (an average of 8.4 days shorter)
- lower amount of morphine used for NAS treatment (an average of 3.6 mg lower)
- higher gestational age, weight, and head circumference at birth[9]

Data from the NIDA-funded Maternal Opioid Treatment: Human Experimental Research study show similar benefits of buprenorphine.[50] Still, methadone is associated with higher treatment retention than buprenorphine.[9] Divided dosing with methadone has been explored as a way to reduce fetal exposure to withdrawal periods, and recent data show low levels of NAS in babies born to mothers treated with divided doses of methadone.[67] Larger comparison studies are needed to determine if split methadone dosing for opioid use disorders in pregnancy is associated with better outcomes.

NAS still occurs in babies whose mothers have received buprenorphine or methadone, but it is less severe than it would be in the absence of treatment.[29] Research does not support reducing maternal methadone dose to avoid NAS, as this may promote increased illicit drug use, resulting in increased risk to the fetus.[52]

Mother's buprenorphine treatment during pregnancy benefits infants. (From Jones HE, Kaltenbach K, Heil SH, et al. Neonatal abstinence syndrome after methadone or buprenorphine exposure. *N Engl J Med.* 2010;363[24]:2320–2331.)

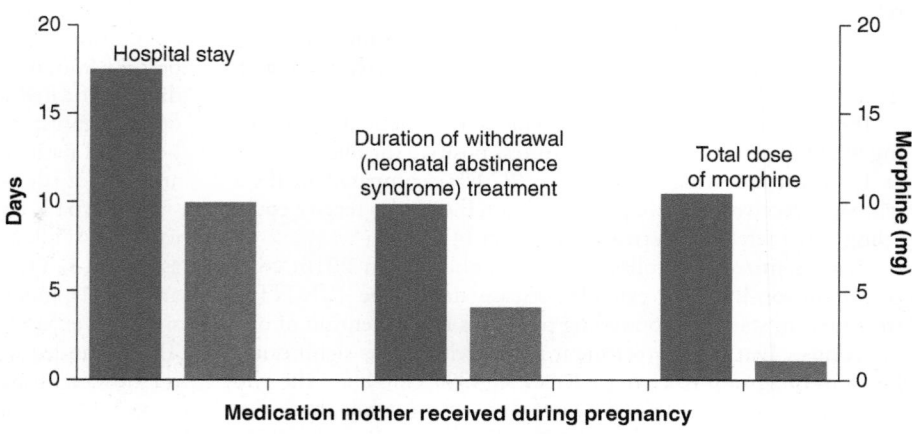

How Much Does Opioid Treatment Cost?

Although the price for opioid treatment may vary based on a number of factors, recent preliminary cost estimates from the US Department of Defense for treatment in a certified opioid treatment program (OTP) provide a reasonable basis for comparison[104]:

- methadone treatment, including medication and integrated psychosocial and medical support services (assumes daily visits): $126.00 per week or $6,552.00 per year
- buprenorphine for a stable patient provided in a certified OTP, including medication and twice-weekly visits: $115.00 per week or $5,980.00 per year
- naltrexone provided in an OTP, including drug, drug administration, and related services: $1,176.50 per month or $14,112.00 per year

To put these costs into context, it is useful to compare them with the costs of other conditions. According to the Agency for Healthcare Research and Quality, annual expenditures for individuals who received health care are $3,560.00 for those with diabetes mellitus and $5,624.00 for kidney disease.[1]

It is also important to remember the costs associated with untreated opioid use disorders, including costs associated with:

- criminal justice
- treating babies born dependent on opioids
- greater transmission of infectious diseases
- treating overdoses
- injuries associated with intoxication (e.g., drugged driving)
- lost productivity

The amount paid for treatment of substance use disorders is only a small portion of the costs these disorders impose on society. An analysis suggested that the total costs of prescription opioid use disorders and overdoses in the United States was $78 billion in 2013. Of that, only 3.6%, or about $2.8 billion, was for treatment.[33]

Is Naloxone Accessible?

Naloxone is an opioid antagonist that can reverse an opioid overdose. Naloxone access increased between 2010 and 2014, with[111]:

- more than three times the number of local sites providing naloxone (from 188 to 644)
- nearly three times the number of laypersons provided naloxone kits (from 53,032 to 152,283)
- a 94% increase in states (from 16 to 30), including Washington, DC, with at least one organization providing naloxone
- more than 2.5 times the number of overdose reversals reported (from 10,171 to 26,463)

Naloxone prescriptions dispensed from retail pharmacies increased nearly 12-fold between the fourth quarter of 2013 and the second quarter of 2015.[49]

Most states have passed laws to widen the availability of naloxone for family, friends, and other potential bystanders of overdose.

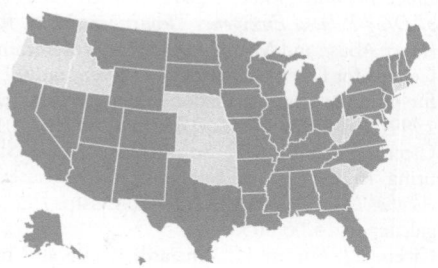

Prescription by Standing Order Authorized
43 states have a standing order to authorize non-medical personnel to issue naloxone (as of 7/2017)

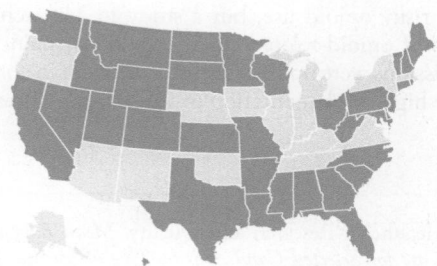

Prescribers Immune from Liability
34 states have laws to protect naloxone prescribers from civil and criminal liability (as of 7/2017)

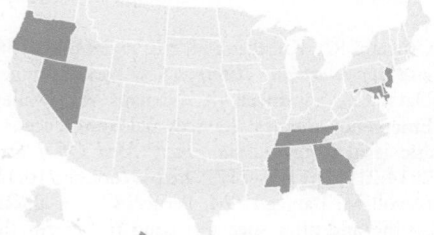

Good Samaritan Law Protects Against Arrest
10 states have Good Samaritan Laws that prevents a person who calls 911 from arrest for drug possession, drug paraphernalia possession, and probation/parole violation (as of 12/2016)

Variation in state naloxone and Good Samaritan laws as of October 24, 2017.

Naloxone has become widely used by emergency medical providers, with all 50 states and the District of Columbia, Guam, and Puerto Rico certifying and approving emergency medical service personnel at the paramedic level to administer naloxone. One step further, emergency medical technicians (EMTs) were explicitly permitted to administer naloxone in 12 of these 53 jurisdictions (23%—California, Colorado, District of Columbia, Massachusetts, Maryland, New Mexico, North Carolina, Ohio, Oklahoma,

Rhode Island, Virginia, and Vermont) as of November 2013. Because non-paramedic EMTs are typically the first and sometimes only source of emergency care, providing authorization and training for them to administer naloxone is a promising strategy to reduce overdose deaths.[21]

After a naloxone training session, most police officers reported that it would not be difficult to use naloxone at the scene of an overdose (89.7%) and that it was important that other officers be trained to use naloxone (82.9%).[83]

Effects of Naloxone Distribution

Overdose education and naloxone distribution (OEND) has been shown to increase the reversal of potentially fatal overdoses; one study showed opioid overdose death rates to be 27% to 46% lower in communities where OEND was implemented.[109] Among 4926 people who used substances and participated in OEND in Massachusetts, 373 (7.6%) reported administering naloxone during an overdose rescue,[23] with few differences in behavior between trained and untrained overdose rescuers. A naloxone distribution study in San Francisco reported that 11% of participants used naloxone during an overdose; of 399 overdose events where naloxone was used, 89% were reversed.[27] Brief education is sufficient to improve comfort and competence in recognizing and managing overdose.[7] Prospective studies are needed to determine the optimal level of training and whether naloxone rescue kits can meet the standard for becoming available over the counter.[23]

In a probabilistic analysis, naloxone distribution programs were shown to prevent overdose deaths, increase quality-adjusted life years (QALYs), and be highly cost-effective. Naloxone distribution was predicted to prevent 6% of overdose deaths, 1 for every 227 naloxone kits distributed. Cost effectiveness, under markedly conservative predictions, was measured to be $14,000.00 per QALY, well within the standard favorable range of cost-benefit ratios (under $50,000.00 per QALY).[18]

Critics of naloxone distribution have claimed that it could lead to an increase in risky opioid use, but a study in Massachusetts showed that rates of opioid-related emergency department visits and hospital admissions were not significantly different in communities with low or high implementation of OEND programs.[109]

References

1. Agency for Healthcare Research and Quality. *Mean Expenses per Person with Care for Selected Conditions by Type of Service: United States, 2014. Medical Expenditure Panel Survey Household Component Data*; 2016. https://meps.ahrq.gov/mepsweb/survey_comp/household.jsp. Accessed May 11, 2017.
2. Alavian SM, Mirahmadizadeh A, Javanbakht M, et al. Effectiveness of methadone maintenance treatment in prevention of hepatitis C virus transmission among injecting drug users. *Hepat Mon.* 2013;13(8):e12411. https://doi.org/10.5812/hepatmon.12411.
3. Allouche S, Noble F, Marie N. Opioid receptor desensitization: mechanisms and its link to tolerance. *Front Pharmacol.* 2014;5:280. https://doi.org/10.3389/fphar.2014.00280.
4. Bart G. Maintenance medication for opiate addiction: the foundation of recovery. *J Addict Dis.* 2012;31(3):207–225. https://doi.org/10.1080/10550887.2012.694598.
5. Batki SL, Gruber VA, Bradley JM, Bradley M, Delucchi K. A controlled trial of methadone treatment combined with directly observed isoniazid for tuberculosis prevention in injection drug users. *Drug Alcohol Depend.* 2002;66(3):283–293.
6. Bazazi AR, Yokell M, Fu JJ, Rich JD, Zaller ND. Illicit use of buprenorphine/naloxone among injecting and noninjecting opioid users. *J Addict Med.* 2011;5(3):175–180. https://doi.org/10.1097/ADM.0b013e3182034e31.
7. Behar E, Santos G-M, Wheeler E, Rowe C, Coffin PO. Brief overdose education is sufficient for naloxone distribution to opioid users. *Drug Alcohol Depend.* 2015;148:209–212. https://doi.org/10.1016/j.drugalcdep.2014.12.009.
8. Binswanger IA, Stern MF, Deyo RA, et al. Release from prison—a high risk of death for former inmates. *N Engl J Med.* 2007;356(2):157–165. https://doi.org/10.1056/NEJMsa064115.
9. Brogly SB, Saia KA, Walley AY, Du HM, Sebastiani P. Prenatal buprenorphine versus methadone exposure and neonatal outcomes: systematic review and meta-analysis. *Am J Epidemiol.* 2014;180(7):673–686. https://doi.org/10.1093/aje/kwu190.
10. Brown RT. Systematic review of the impact of adult drug-treatment courts. *Transl Res J Lab Clin Med.* 2010;155(6):263–274. https://doi.org/10.1016/j.trsl.2010.03.001.
11. Bruce RD, Moody DE, Altice FL, Gourevitch MN, Friedland GH. A review of pharmacological interactions between HIV or hepatitis C virus medications 42 and opioid agonist therapy: implications and management for clinical practice. *Expert Rev Clin Pharmacol.* 2013;6(3):249–269. https://doi.org/10.1586/ecp.13.18.
12. Brunton LL, Lazo JS, Parker KL, eds. *Goodman & Gilman's: The Pharmacological Basis of Therapeutics.* 11th ed. New York: McGraw Hill Medical; 2011.
13. Carvallo L, Lopez L, Che F-Y, et al. Buprenorphine decreases the CCL2-mediated chemotactic response of monocytes. *J Immunol Baltim Md.* 1950. 2015;194(7):3246–3258. https://doi.org/10.4049/jimmunol.1302647.
14. Center for Behavioral Health Statistics and Quality (CBHSQ). *Drug Abuse Warning Network: 2011: Selected Tables of National Estimates of Drug-Related Emergency Department Visits.* Rockville, MD: Substance Abuse and Mental Health Services Administration; 2013.
15. Centers for Disease Control and Prevention (CDC). Vital signs: risk for overdose from methadone used for pain relief - United States, 1999-2010. *MMWR Morb Mortal Wkly Rep.* 2012;61(26):493–497.
16. Cicero TJ, Ellis MS, Surratt HL, Kurtz SP. Factors contributing to the rise of buprenorphine misuse: 2008-2013. *Drug Alcohol Depend.* 2014;142:98–104. https://doi.org/10.1016/j.drugalcdep.2014.06.005.
17. Cicero TJ, Surratt HL, Inciardi J. Use and misuse of buprenorphine in the management of opioid addiction. *J Opioid Manag.* 2007;3(6):302–308.
18. Coffin PO, Sullivan SD. Cost-effectiveness of distributing naloxone to heroin users for lay overdose reversal. *Ann Intern Med.* 2013;158(1):1–9. https://doi.org/10.7326/0003- 4819-158-1- 201301010-00003.
19. Conrad C, Bradley HM, Broz D, et al. Community outbreak of HIV infection linked to injection drug use of Oxymorphone-Indiana, 2015. *MMWR Morb Mortal Wkly Rep.* 2015;64(16):443–444.
20. Cruciani RA, Knotkova H, eds. *Handbook of Methadone Prescribing and Buprenorphine Therapy.* New York: Springer-Verlag; 2013.
21. Davis CS, Southwell JK, Niehaus VR, Walley AY, Dailey MW. Emergency medical services naloxone access: a national systematic legal review. *Acad Emerg Med Off J Soc Acad Emerg Med.* 2014;21(10):1173–1177. https://doi.org/10.1111/acem.12485.
22. Davoli M, Bargagli AM, Perucci CA, et al. Risk of fatal overdose during and after specialist drug treatment: the VEdeTTE study, a national multi-site prospective cohort study. *Addict Abingdon Engl.* 2007;102(12):1954–1959. https://doi.org/10.1111/j.1360-0443.2007.02025.x.
23. Doe-Simkins M, Quinn E, Xuan Z, et al. Overdose rescues by trained and untrained participants and change in opioid use among substance-using participants in overdose education and naloxone distribution programs: a retrospective cohort study. *BMC Public Health.* 2014;14:297. https://doi.org/10.1186/1471-2458-14-297.

24. Dolan KA, Shearer J, MacDonald M, Mattick RP, Hall W, Wodak AD. A randomized controlled trial of methadone maintenance treatment versus wait list control in an Australian prison system. *Drug Alcohol Depend.* 2003;72(1):59–65.

25. Duffy P, Mackridge AJ. Use and diversion of illicit methadone – under what circumstances does it occur, and potential risks associated with continued use of other substances. *J Subst Use.* 2014;19(1-2):48–55. https://doi.org/10.3109/14659891.2012.734539.

26. Effective medical treatment of opiate addiction. National Consensus Development Panel on Effective Medical Treatment of Opiate Addiction. *JAMA.* 1998;280(22):1936–1943.

27. Enteen L, Bauer J, McLean R, et al. Overdose prevention and naloxone prescription for opioid users in San Francisco. *J Urban Health Bull N Y Acad Med.* 2010;87(6):931–941. https://doi.org/10.1007/s11524-010-9495-8.

28. Epstein RA, Bobo WV, Martin PR, et al. Increasing pregnancy-related use of prescribed opioid analgesics. *Ann Epidemiol.* 2013;23(8):498–503. https://doi.org/10.1016/j.annepidem.2013.05.017.

29. Fajemirokun-Odudeyi O, Sinha C, Tutty S, et al. Pregnancy outcome in women who use opiates. *Eur J Obstet Gynecol Reprod Biol.* 2006;126(2):170–175. https://doi.org/10.1016/j.ejogrb.2005.08.010.

30. Fiellin DA, Schottenfeld RS, Cutter CJ, Moore BA, Barry DT, O'Connor PG. Primary care-based buprenorphine taper vs maintenance therapy for prescription opioid dependence: a randomized clinical trial. *JAMA Intern Med.* 2014;174(12):1947–1954. https://doi.org/10.1001/jamainternmed.2014.5302.

31. Fiscella K, Moore A, Engerman J, Meldrum S. Jail management of arrestees/inmates enrolled in community methadone maintenance programs. *J Urban Health Bull N Y Acad Med.* 2004;81(4):645–654. https://doi.org/10.1093/jurban/jth147.

32. Fitting S, Zou S, El-Hage N, et al. Opiate addiction therapies and HIV-1 Tat: interactive effects on glial $[Ca^{2+}]i$, oxyradical and neuroinflammatory chemokine production and correlative neurotoxicity. *Curr HIV Res.* 2014;12(6):424–434.

33. Florence CS, Zhou C, Luo F, Xu L. The economic burden of prescription opioid overdose, abuse, and dependence in the United States, 2013. *Med Care.* 2016;54(10):901–906. https://doi.org/10.1097/MLR.0000000000000625.

34. Friedmann PD, Wilson D, Knudsen HK, et al. Effect of an organizational linkage intervention on staff perceptions of medication-assisted treatment and referral intentions in community corrections. *J Subst Abuse Treat.* 2015;50:50–58. https://doi.org/10.1016/j.jsat.2014.10.001.

35. Fudala PJ, Bridge TP, Herbert S, et al. Office-based treatment of opiate addiction with a sublingual-tablet formulation of buprenorphine and naloxone. *N Engl J Med.* 2003;349(10):949–958. https://doi.org/10.1056/NEJMoa022164.

36. Gibson DR, Flynn NM, McCarthy JJ. Effectiveness of methadone treatment in reducing HIV risk behavior and HIV seroconversion among injecting drug users. *AIDS Lond Engl.* 1999;13(14):1807–1818.

37. Gordon AJ, Kavanagh G, Krumm M, et al. Facilitators and barriers in implementing buprenorphine in the Veterans Health Administration. *Psychol Addict Behav J Soc Psychol Addict Behav.* 2011;25(2):215–224. https://doi.org/10.1037/a0022776.45.

38. Gordon MS, Kinlock TW, Schwartz RP, Fitzgerald TT, O'Grady KE, Vocci FJ. A randomized controlled trial of prison-initiated buprenorphine: prison outcomes and community treatment entry. *Drug Alcohol Depend.* 2014;142:33–40. https://doi.org/10.1016/j.drugalcdep.2014.05.011.

39. Gowing L, Farrell MF, Bornemann R, Sullivan LE, Ali R. Oral substitution treatment of injecting opioid users for prevention of HIV infection. *Cochrane Database Syst Rev.* 2011;8:CD004145. https://doi.org/10.1002/14651858.CD004145.pub4.

40. Gowing LR, Hickman M, Degenhardt L. Mitigating the risk of HIV infection with opioid substitution treatment. *Bull World Health Organ.* 2013;91(2):148–149. https://doi.org/10.2471/BLT.12.109553.

41. Green TC, Clarke J, Brinkley-Rubinstein L, et al. Postincarceration fatal overdoses after implementing medications for addiction treatment in a statewide correctional system. *JAMA Psychiatry.* 2018. https://doi.org/10.1001/jamapsychiatry.2017.4614.

42. Gruber VA, Delucchi KL, Kielstein A, Batki SL. A randomized trial of 6-month methadone maintenance with standard or minimal counseling versus 21-day methadone detoxification. *Drug Alcohol Depend.* 2008;94(1-3):199–206. https://doi.org/10.1016/j.drugalcdep.2007.11.021.

43. Hallinan R, Byrne A, Amin J, Dore GJ. Hepatitis C virus incidence among injecting drug users on opioid replacement therapy. *Aust N Z J Public Health.* 2004;28(6):576–578.

44. Highlights of Prescribing Information: SUBOXONE®; 2017. https://www.suboxone.com/content/pdfs/prescribing-information.pdf. Accessed May 11, 2017.

45. Jackson H, Mandell K, Johnson K, Chatterjee D, Vanness DJ. Cost-effectiveness of injectable extended-release naltrexone compared with methadone maintenance and buprenorphine maintenance treatment for opioid dependence. *Subst Abuse.* 2015;36(2):226–231. https://doi.org/10.1080/08897077.2015.1010031.

46. Jeffrey GP, MacQuillan G, Chua F, et al. Hepatitis C virus eradication in intravenous drug users maintained with subcutaneous naltrexone implants. *Hepatol Baltim Md.* 2007;45(1):111–117. https://doi.org/10.1002/hep.21470.

47. Johnson B, Richert T. Diversion of methadone and buprenorphine by patients in opioid substitution treatment in Sweden: prevalence estimates and risk factors. *Int J Drug Policy.* 2015;26(2):183–190. https://doi.org/10.1016/j.drugpo.2014.10.003.

48. Johnson B, Richert T. Diversion of methadone and buprenorphine from opioid substitution treatment: a staff perspective. *J Psychoactive Drugs.* 2014;46(5):427–435. https://doi.org/10.1080/02791072.2014.960109.

49. Jones CM, Lurie PG, Compton WM. Increase in naloxone prescriptions dispensed in US retail pharmacies since 2013. *Am J Public Health.* 2016;106(4):689–690. https://doi.org/10.2105/AJPH.2016.303062.

50. Jones HE, Kaltenbach K, Heil SH, et al. Neonatal abstinence syndrome after methadone or buprenorphine exposure. *N Engl J Med.* 2010;363(24):2320–2331. https://doi.org/10.1056/NEJMoa1005359.

51. Kakko J, Svanborg KD, Kreek MJ, Heilig M. 1-year retention and social function after buprenorphine-assisted relapse prevention treatment for heroin dependence in Sweden: a randomised, placebo-controlled trial. *Lancet Lond Engl.* 2003;361(9358):662–668. https://doi.org/10.1016/S0140-6736(03)12600-1.37.

52. Kaltenbach K, Berghella V, Finnegan L. Opioid dependence during pregnancy. Effects and management. *Obstet Gynecol Clin North Am.* 1998;25(1):139–151.

53. Kandall SR, Doberczak TM, Jantunen M, Stein J. The methadone-maintained pregnancy. *Clin Perinatol.* 1999;26(1):173–183.

54. Kinlock TW, Gordon MS, Schwartz RP, O'Grady K, Fitzgerald TT, Wilson M. A randomized clinical trial of methadone maintenance for prisoners: results at 1-month post-release. *Drug Alcohol Depend.* 2007;91(2-3):220–227. https://doi.org/10.1016/j.drugalcdep.2007.05.022.

55. Knudsen HK, Abraham AJ, Roman PM. Adoption and implementation of medications in addiction treatment programs. *J Addict Med.* 2011;5(1):21–27. https://doi.org/10.1097/ADM.0b013e3181d41ddb.

56. Kosten TR, George TP. The neurobiology of opioid dependence: implications for treatment. *Sci Pract Perspect.* 2002;1(1):13–20.

57. Krupitsky E, Nunes EV, Ling W, Gastfriend DR, Memisoglu A, Silverman BL. Injectable extended-release naltrexone (XR-NTX) for opioid dependence: long-term safety and effectiveness. *Addict Abingdon Engl*. 2013;108(9):1628–1637. https://doi.org/10.1111/add.12208.

58. Krupitsky E, Nunes EV, Ling W, Illeperuma A, Gastfriend DR, Silverman BL. Injectable extended-release naltrexone for opioid dependence: a doubleblind, placebo-controlled, multicentre randomised trial. *Lancet Lond Engl*. 2011;377(9776):1506–1513. https://doi.org/10.1016/S0140-6736(11)60358-9.

59. Lee JD, Friedmann PD, Boney TY, et al. Extended-release naltrexone to prevent relapse among opioid dependent, criminal justice system involved adults: rationale and design of a randomized controlled effectiveness trial. *Contemp Clin Trials*. 2015;41:110–117. https://doi.org/10.1016/j.cct.2015.01.005.44.

60. Maas B, Kerr T, Fairbairn N, Montaner J, Wood E. Pharmacokinetic interactions between HIV antiretroviral therapy and drugs used to treat opioid dependence. *Expert Opin Drug Metab Toxicol*. 2006;2(4):533–543. https://doi.org/10.1517/17425255.2.4.533.

61. MacArthur GJ, Minozzi S, Martin N, et al. Opiate substitution treatment and HIV transmission in people who inject drugs: systematic review and metaanalysis. *BMJ*. 2012;345:e5945.

62. MacDonald K, Lamb K, Thomas ML, Khentigan W. Buprenorphine maintenance treatment of opiate dependence: correlations between prescriber beliefs and practices. *Subst Use Misuse*. 2016;51(1):85–90. https://doi.org/10.3109/10826084.2015.1089905.

63. Malta M, Strathdee SA, Magnanini MMF, Bastos FI. Adherence to antiretroviral therapy for human immunodeficiency virus/acquired immune deficiency syndrome among drug users: a systematic review. *Addict Abingdon Engl*. 2008;103(8):1242–1257. https://doi.org/10.1111/j.1360-0443.2008.02269.x.

64. Mattick RP, Breen C, Kimber J, Davoli M. Buprenorphine maintenance versus placebo or methadone maintenance for opioid dependence. *Cochrane Database Syst Rev*. 2014;(2):CD002207. https://doi.org/10.1002/14651858.CD002207.pub4.

65. Mattick RP, Breen C, Kimber J, Davoli M. Methadone maintenance therapy versus no opioid replacement therapy for opioid dependence. *Cochrane Database Syst Rev*. 2009;3:CD002209. https://doi.org/10.1002/14651858.CD002209.pub2.

66. Matusow H, Dickman SL, Rich JD, et al. Medication assisted treatment in US drug courts: results from a nationwide survey of availability, barriers and attitudes. *J Subst Abuse Treat*. 2013;44(5):473–480. https://doi.org/10.1016/j.jsat.2012.10.004.

67. McCarthy JJ, Leamon MH, Willits NH, Salo R. The effect of methadone dose regimen on neonatal abstinence syndrome. *J Addict Med*. 2015;9(2):105–110. https://doi.org/10.1097/ADM.0000000000000099.

68. Metzger DS, Donnell D, Celentano DD, et al. Expanding substance use treatment options for HIV prevention with buprenorphine-naloxone: HIV Prevention Trials Network 058. *J Acquir Immune Defic Syndr*. 1999. 2015;68(5):554–561. https://doi.org/10.1097/QAI.0000000000000510.

69. Metzger DS, Woody GE, McLellan AT, et al. Human immunodeficiency virus seroconversion among intravenous drug users in and out-of-treatment: an18-month prospective follow-up. *J Acquir Immune Defic Syndr*. 1993;6(9):1049–1056.

70. Minozzi S, Amato L, Vecchi S, Davoli M, Kirchmayer U, Verster A. Oral naltrexone maintenance treatment for opioid dependence. *CochraneDatabase Syst Rev*. 2011;4:CD001333. https://doi.org/10.1002/14651858.CD001333.pub4.

71. Mitchell SG, Willet J, Monico LB, et al. Community correctional agents' views of medication-assisted treatment: examining their influence on treatment referrals and community supervision practices. *Subst Abuse*. 2016;37(1):127–133. https://doi.org/10.1080/08897077.2015.1129389.

72. Mumola CJ, Karberg JC. *Bureau of Justice Statistics Special Report: Drug Use and Dependence, State and Federal Prisoners, 2004*. U.S. Department of Justice, Office of Justice Programs; 2006. https://www.bjs.gov/content/pub/pdf/dudsfp04.pdf. Accessed May 11, 2017.

73. National Institute on Drug Abuse. *Substance Abuse in the Military*. https://www.drugabuse.gov/publications/drugfacts/substance-abuse-inmilitary. Published March 1, 2013. Accessed May 11, 2017.

74. Nolan S, Dias Lima V, Fairbairn N, et al. The impact of methadone maintenance therapy on hepatitis C incidence among illicit drug users. *Addict Abingdon Engl*. 2014;109(12):2053–2059. https://doi.org/10.1111/add.12682.

75. Nunes EV, Krupitsky E, Ling W, et al. Treating opioid dependence with injectable extended-release naltrexone (XR-NTX): who will respond? *J Addict Med*. 2015;9(3):238243. https://doi.org/10.1097/ADM.0000000000000125.

76. Nunn A, Zaller N, Dickman S, Trimbur C, Nijhawan A, Rich JD. Methadone and buprenorphine prescribing and referral practices in US prison systems: results from a nationwide survey. *Drug Alcohol Depend*. 2009;105(1-2):83–88. https://doi.org/10.1016/j.drugalcdep.2009.06.015.

77. Oliva EM, Trafton JA, Harris AHS, Gordon AJ. Trends in opioid agonist therapy in the Veterans Health Administration: is supply keeping up with demand? *Am J Drug Alcohol Abuse*. 2013;39(2):103–107. https://doi.org/10.3109/00952990.2012.741167.

78. Otiashvili D, Piralishvili G, Sikharulidze Z, Kamkamidze G, Poole S, Woody GE. Methadone and buprenorphine-naloxone are effective in reducing illicit buprenorphine and other opioid use, and reducing HIV risk behavior--outcomes of a randomized trial. *Drug Alcohol Depend*. 2013;133(2):376–382. https://doi.org/10.1016/j.drugalcdep.2013.06.024.

79. Patrick SW, Davis MM, Lehmann CU, Lehman CU, Cooper WO. Increasing incidence and geographic distribution of neonatal abstinence syndrome: United States 2009 to 2012. *J Perinatol Off J Calif Perinat Assoc*. 2015;35(8):650–655. https://doi.org/10.1038/jp.2015.36.

80. Patrick SW, Dudley J, Martin PR, et al. Prescription opioid epidemic and infant outcomes. *Pediatrics*. 2015;135(5):842–850. https://doi.org/10.1542/peds.2014-3299.

81. Peles E, Schreiber S, Rados V, Adelson M. Low risk for hepatitis C seroconversion in methadone maintenance treatment. *J Addict Med*. 2011;5(3):214–220. https://doi.org/10.1097/ADM.0b013e31820e13dd.

82. Perlman DC, Jordan AE, Uuskula A, et al. An international perspective on using opioid substitution treatment to improve hepatitis C prevention and care for people who inject drugs: structural barriers and public health potential. *Int J Drug Policy*. 2015;26(11):1056–1063. https://doi.org/10.1016/j.drugpo.2015.04.015.

83. Ray B, O'Donnell D, Kahre K. Police officer attitudes towards intranasal naloxone training. *Drug Alcohol Depend*. 2015;146:107–110. https://doi.org/10.1016/j.drugalcdep.2014.10.026.

84. Rudd RA, Aleshire N, Zibbell JE, Gladden RM. Increases in drug and opioid overdose deaths-United States, 2000-2014. *MMWR Morb Mortal Wkly Rep*. 2016;64(5051):1378–1382. https://doi.org/10.15585/mmwr.mm6450a3.

85. Rudd RA, Seth P, David F, Scholl L. Increases in drug and opioid-involved overdose deaths - United States, 2010-2015. *MMWR Morb Mortal Wkly Rep*. 2016;65(5051):1445–1452. https://doi.org/10.15585/mmwr.mm655051e1.

86. Schuman-Olivier Z, Albanese M, Nelson SE, et al. Self-treatment: illicit buprenorphine use by opioid-dependent treatment seekers. *J Subst Abuse Treat*. 2010;39(1):41–50. https://doi.org/10.1016/j.jsat.2010.03.014.

87. Schwartz RP, Highfield DA, Jaffe JH, et al. A randomized controlled trial of interim methadone maintenance. *Arch Gen Psychiatry*. 2006;63(1):102–109. https://doi.org/10.1001/archpsyc.63.1.102.

88. Schwartz RP, Kelly SM, O'Grady KE, Gandhi D, Jaffe JH. Randomized trial of standard methadone treatment compared to initiating methadone without counseling: 12-month findings. *Addict Abingdon Engl*. 2012;107(5):943–952. https://doi.org/10.1111/j.1360-0443.2011.03700.x.

89. Sees KL, Delucchi KL, Masson C, et al. Methadone maintenance vs 180-day psychosocially enriched detoxification for treatment of opioid dependence: a randomized controlled trial. *JAMA.* 2000;283(10):1303–1310.

90. Shipherd JC, Stafford J, Tanner LR. Predicting alcohol and drug abuse in Persian Gulf War veterans: what role do PTSD symptoms play? *Addict Behav.* 2005;30(3):595–599. https://doi.org/10.1016/j.addbeh.2004.07.004.

91. Soyka M. New developments in the management of opioid dependence: focus on sublingual buprenorphine-naloxone. *Subst Abuse Rehabil.* 2015;6:1–14. https://doi.org/10.2147/SAR.S45585.

92. Substance Abuse and Mental Health Services Administration. *Medication-Assisted Treatment for Opioid Addiction in Opioid Treatment Programs. Treatment Improvement Protocol (TIP) Series 43.* Substance Abuse and Mental Health Services Administration; 2005. https://www.ncbi.nlm.nih.gov/books/NBK64164/pdf/Bookshelf_NBK64164.pdf. Accessed May 11, 2017.

93. Substance Abuse and Mental Health Services Administration, *Center for Behavioral Health Statistics and Quality (CBHSQ). The DAWN Report: 40 Emergency Department Visits Involving Buprenorphine.* Substance Abuse and Mental Health Services Administration; 2013. http://archive.samhsa.gov/data/2k13/DAWN106/sr106-buprenorphine.pdf. Accessed May 12, 2017.

94. Substance Abuse and Mental Health Services Administration. *Drug Abuse Warning Network, 2011: National Estimates of Drug-Related Emergency Department Visits.* https://www.samhsa.gov/data/sites/default/files/DAWN2k11ED/DAWN2k11ED/DAWN2k11D. Published May 2013. Accessed May 12, 2017.

95. Substance Abuse and Mental Health Services Administration. *Grants to Expand Substance Abuse Treatment Capacity in Adult and Family Drug Courts: Request for Applications (RFA) No. TI-15-002;* 2015. http://www.samhsa.gov/sites/default/files/grants/doc/ti-15-002.doc.

96. Substance Abuse and Mental Health Services Administration. *Clinical Guidelines for the Use of Buprenorphine in the Treatment of Opioid Addiction: A Treatment Improvement Protocol TIP 40.* Substance Abuse and Mental Health Services Administration; 2004. https://www.ncbi.nlm.nih.gov/books/NBK64245/pdf/Bookshelf_NBK64245.pdf. Accessed May 11, 2017.

97. Substance Abuse Center for Behavioral Health Statistics and Quality. *Results from the 2016 National Survey on Drug Use and Health: Detailed Tables. SAMHSA.* https://www.samhsa.gov/data/sites/default/files/NSDUHDetTabs-2016/NSDUH-DetTabs-2016.htm. Published September 7, 2017. Accessed March 7, 2018.

98. Syed YY, Keating GM. Extended-release intramuscular naltrexone (VIVITROL®): a review of its use in the prevention of relapse to opioid dependence in detoxified patients. *CNS Drugs.* 2013;27(10):851–861. https://doi.org/10.1007/s40263-013-0110-x.

99. The American College of Obstetricians and Gynecologists, The American Society of Addiction Medicine. *Opioid Use and Opioid Use Disorder in Pregnancy.* The American College of Obstetricians and Gynecologists; 2017. https://www.acog.org/Clinical-Guidance-and-Publications/Committee-Opinions/Committee-on-Obstetric-Practice/Opioid-Use-and-Opioid-Use-Disorder-in-Pregnancy. Accessed March 30, 2018.

100. The American Society of Addiction Medicine. *Advancing Access to Addiction Medications.* http://www.asam.org/docs/defaultsource/advocacy/aaam_implications-for-opioid-addiction-treatment_final.

101. Toblin RL, Quartana PJ, Riviere LA, Walper KC, Hoge CW. Chronic pain and opioid use in US soldiers after combat deployment. *JAMA Intern Med.* 2014;174(8):1400–1401. https://doi.org/10.1001/jamainternmed.2014.2726.

102. Tolia VN, Patrick SW, Bennett MM, et al. Increasing incidence of the neonatal abstinence syndrome in U.S. neonatal ICUs. *N Engl J Med.* 2015;372(22):2118–2126. https://doi.org/10.1056/NEJMsa1500439.

103. Tsui JI, Evans JL, Lum PJ, Hahn JA, Page K. Association of opioid agonist therapy with lower incidence of hepatitis C virus infection in young adult injection drug users. *JAMA Intern Med.* 2014;174(12):1974–1981. https://doi.org/10.1001/jamainternmed.2014.5416.

104. U.S. Department of Defense, Office of the Secretary. TRICARE; Mental Health and Substance Use Disorder Treatment. Federal Register. https://www.federalregister.gov/documents/2016/09/02/2016-21125/tricare-mental-health-and-substance-use-disorder-treatment. Published September 2, 2016. Accessed May 11, 2017.

105. U.S. Department of Health and Human Services, Office of the Assistant Secretary for Planning and Evaluation. Opioid Abuse in the U.S. and HHS Actions to Address Opioid-Drug Related Overdoses and Deaths. ASPE. https://aspe.hhs.gov/pdf-report/opioid-abuse-us-and-hhs-actions-address-opioid-drug-related-overdoses-and-deaths. Published November 23, 2015. Accessed May 11, 2017.

106. U.S. Department of Justice Drug Enforcement Administration, Office of Diversion Control. *National Forensic Laboratory Information System (NFLIS) 2013 Annual Report.* https://www.nflis.deadiversion.usdoj.gov/DesktopModules/ReportDownloads/Reports/N FLIS2013AR.

107. U.S. Department of Veteran Affairs. *A/DoD Clinical Practice Guideline for the Management of Substance Use Disorders;* 2015. https://www.healthquality.va.gov/guidelines/MH/sud/VADoDSUDCPGRevised22216.pdf.

108. Vanichseni S, Wongsuwan B, Choopanya K, Wongpanich K. A controlled trial of methadone maintenance in a population of intravenous drug users in Bangkok: implications for prevention of HIV. *Int J Addict.* 1991;26(12):1313–1320.

109. Walley AY, Xuan Z, Hackman HH, et al. Opioid overdose rates and implementation of overdose education and nasal naloxone distribution in Massachusetts: interrupted time series analysis. *BMJ.* 2013;346:f174.

110. Walsh SL, June HL, Schuh KJ, Preston KL, Bigelow GE, Stitzer ML. Effects of buprenorphine and methadone in methadone-maintained subjects. *Psychopharmacology (Berl).* 1995;119(3):268–276.

111. Wheeler E, Jones TS, Gilbert MK, Davidson PJ, Centers for Disease Control and Prevention (CDC). Opioid overdose prevention programs providing naloxone to laypersons – United States, 2014. *MMWR Morb Mortal Wkly Rep.* 2015;64(23):631–635.

112. Williams JT, Ingram SL, Henderson G, et al. Regulation of μ-opioid receptors: desensitization, phosphorylation, internalization, and tolerance. *Pharmacol Rev.* 2013;65(1):223–254. https://doi.org/10.1124/pr.112.005942.

113. Woody GE, Bruce D, Korthuis PT, et al. HIV risk reduction with buprenorphine-naloxone or methadone: findings from a randomized trial. *J Acquir Immune Defic Syndr.* 2014;66(3):288–293. https://doi.org/10.1097/QAI.0000000000000165.

114. World Health Organization. *Proposal for the Inclusion of Methadone in the WHO Model List of Essential Medicines.* World Health Organization; 2004. http://www.who.int/substance_abuse/activities/methadone_essential_medicines.pdf. Accessed May 11, 2017.

115. World Health Organization. *Guidelines for the Psychosocially Assisted Pharmacological Treatment of Opioid Dependence.* World Health Organization; 2009. http://www.who.int/substance_abuse/publications/opioid_dependence_guidelines.pdf. Accessed May 11, 2017.

116. World Health Organization. *Proposal for the Inclusion of Buprenorphine in the WHO Model List of Essential Medicines;* 2004. https://www.who.int/substance_abuse/activities/buprenorphine_essential_medicines.pdf. Accessed May 11, 2017.

117. Yancovitz SR, Des Jarlais DC, Peyser NP, et al. A randomized trial of an interim methadone maintenance clinic. *Am J Public Health.* 1991;81(9):1185–1191.

118. Zaller N, McKenzie M, Friedmann PD, Green TC, McGowan S, Rich JD. Initiation of buprenorphine during incarceration and retention in treatment upon release. *J Subst Abuse Treat.* 2013;45(2):222–226. https://doi.org/10.1016/j.jsat.2013.02.005.

119. Zhou W, Wang X, Zhou S, et al. Hepatitis C seroconversion in methadone maintenance treatment programs in Wuhan, China. *Addict Abingdon Engl.* 2015;110(5):796–802. https://doi.org/10.1111/add.12836.

APPENDIX 2

TIP 63: Medications for Opioid Use Disorder

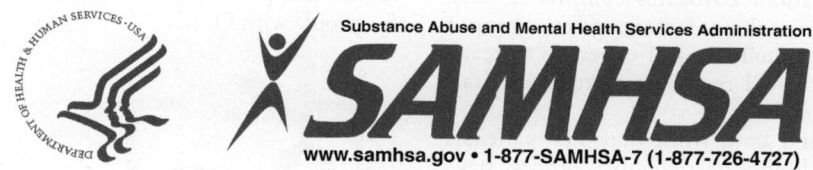

Substance Abuse and Mental Health Services Administration

SAMHSA

www.samhsa.gov • 1-877-SAMHSA-7 (1-877-726-4727)

Executive Summary

For Healthcare and Addiction Professionals, Policymakers, Patients, and Families

The Executive Summary of this **Treatment Improvement Protocol** provides an overview on the use of the three US Food and Drug Administration–approved mediations used to treat opioid use disorder—methadone, naltrexone, and buprenorphine—and the other strategies and services needed to support recovery.

TIP Navigation

Part 1: Introduction to Medications for Opioid Use Disorder Treatment
    For healthcare and addiction professionals, policymakers, patients, and families

Part 2: Addressing Opioid Use Disorder in General Medical Settings
    For healthcare professionals

Part 3: Pharmacotherapy for Opioid Use Disorder
    For healthcare professionals

Part 4: Partnering Addiction Treatment Counselors with Clients and Healthcare Professionals
    For healthcare and addiction professionals

Part 5: Resources Related to Medications for Opioid Use Disorder
    For healthcare and addiction professionals, policymakers, patients, and families

OUTLINE

Foreword

The Substance Abuse and Mental Health Services Administration (SAMSA) is the US Department of Health and Human Services agency that leads public health efforts to advance the behavioral health of the nation. SAMHSA's mission is to reduce the impact of substance abuse and mental illness on America's communities.

The Treatment Improvement Protocol (TIP) series fulfills SAMHSA's mission by providing science-based best-practice guidance to the behavioral health field. TIPs reflect careful consideration of all relevant clinical and health service research, demonstrated experience, and implementation requirements. Select nonfederal clinical researchers, service providers, program administrators, and patient advocates comprising each TIP's consensus panel discuss these factors, offering input on the TIP's specific topic in their areas of expertise to reach consensus on best practices. Field reviewers then assess draft content.

The talent, dedication, and hard work that TIP panelists and reviewers bring to this highly participatory process have helped bridge the gap between the promise of research and the needs of practicing clinicians and administrators to serve, in the most scientifically sound and effective ways, people in need of behavioral health services. We are grateful to all who have joined with us to contribute to advances in the behavioral health field.

Elinore F. McCance-Katz, MD, PhD
Assistant Secretary for Mental Health and Substance Use
SAMHSA

A. Kathryn Power, MEd
Acting Director
Center for Substance Abuse Treatment
SAMHSA

Frances M. Harding
Director
Center for Substance Abuse Prevention
SAMHSA

Paolo del Vecchio, MSW
Director
Center for Mental Health Services
SAMHSA

Daryl W. Kade, MA
Director
Center for Behavioral Health Statistics and Quality
SAMHSA

Executive Summary

The goal of treatment for opioid addiction or opioid use disorder (OUD) is remission of the disorder leading to lasting recovery. Recovery is a process of change through which individuals improve their health and wellness, live self-directed lives, and strive to reach their full potential.[18] This Treatment Improvement Protocol (TIP) reviews the use of the three US Food and Drug Administration (FDA)–approved medications used to treat OUD—methadone, naltrexone, and buprenorphine—and the other strategies and services needed to support recovery for people with OUD.

Introduction

Our nation faces a crisis of overdose deaths from opioids, including heroin, illicit fentanyl, and prescription opioids. These deaths represent a mere fraction of the total number of Americans harmed by opioid misuse and addiction. Many Americans now suffer daily from a chronic medical illness called "opioid addiction" or OUD (see the Glossary in Part 5 of this TIP for definitions). Healthcare professionals, treatment providers, and policymakers have a responsibility to expand access to evidence-based, effective care for people with OUD.

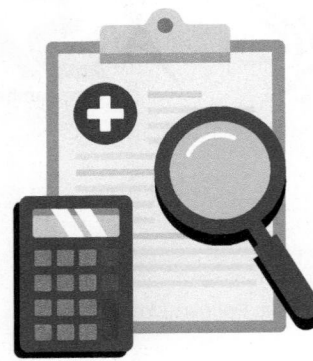

Estimated cost of the OPIOID EPIDEMIC was **$504 BILLION** in 2015.[5]

An expert panel developed the TIP's content based on a review of the literature and on their extensive experience in the field of addiction treatment. Other professionals also generously contributed their time and commitment to this project.

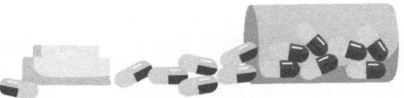

An estimated **1.8M AMERICANS** have OUD related to opioid painkillers; **626K** have heroin-related OUD.[3]

The TIP is divided into parts so that readers can easily find the material they need. Part 1 is a general introduction to providing medications for OUD and issues related to providing that treatment. Some readers may prefer to go directly to those parts most relevant to their areas of interest, but everyone is encouraged to read Part 1 to establish a shared understanding of key facts and issues covered in detail in this TIP.

Following is a summary of the TIP's overall main points and brief summaries of each of the five TIP parts.

Overall Key Messages

Addiction is a chronic, treatable illness. Opioid addiction, which generally corresponds with moderate to severe forms of OUD, often requires continuing care for effective treatment rather than an episodic, acute-care treatment approach.

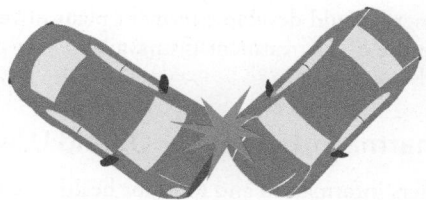

OPIOID OVERDOSE caused **42,249 DEATHS** nationwide in 2016—this exceeded the number caused by motor vehicle crashes.[4,15]

General principles of good care for chronic diseases can guide OUD treatment. Approaching OUD as a chronic illness can help providers deliver care that helps patients stabilize, achieve remission of symptoms, and establish and maintain recovery.

Patient-centered care empowers patients with information that helps them make better treatment decisions with the healthcare professionals involved in their care. Patients should receive information from their healthcare team that will help them understand OUD and the options for treating it, including treatment with FDA-approved medication.

Patients with OUD should have access to mental health services as needed, medical care, and addiction counseling, as well as recovery support services, to supplement treatment with medication.

The words you use to describe OUD and an individual with OUD are powerful. The TIP defines, uses, and encourages providers to adopt terminology that will not reinforce prejudice, negative attitudes, or discrimination.

There is no "one size fts all" approach to OUD treatment. Many people with OUD benefit from treatment with medication for varying lengths of time, including lifelong treatment. Ongoing outpatient medication treatment for OUD is linked to better retention and outcomes than treatment without medication. Even so, some people stop using opioids on their own; others recover through support groups or specialty treatment with or without medication.

The science demonstrating the effectiveness of medication for OUD is strong. For example, methadone, extended-release injectable naltrexone (XR-NTX), and buprenorphine were each found to be more effective in reducing illicit opioid use than no medication in randomized clinical trials, which are the gold standard for demonstrating efficacy in clinical medicine.[9,11-13] Methadone and buprenorphine treatment have also been associated with reduced risk of overdose death.[1,6,8,16,21]

This does not mean that remission and recovery occur only through medication. Some people achieve remission without OUD medication, just as some people can manage type 2 diabetes with exercise and diet alone. But just as it is inadvisable to deny people with diabetes the medication they need to help manage their illness, it is also not sound medical practice to deny people with OUD access to FDA-approved medications for their illness.

Medication for OUD should be successfully integrated with outpatient and residential treatment. Some patients may benefit from different levels of care at different points in their lives, such as outpatient counseling, intensive outpatient treatment, inpatient treatment, or long-term therapeutic communities. Patients treated in these settings should have access to OUD medications.

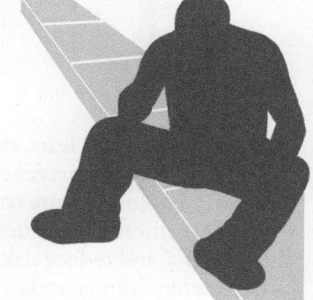

2.1 MILLION people in the United States ages 12 and older have OUD involving PRESCRIPTION OPIOIDS, HEROIN, or both in 2016.[3]

Patients treated with medications for OUD can benefit from individualized psychosocial supports. These can be offered by patients' healthcare providers in the form of medication management and supportive counseling and/or by other providers offering adjunctive addiction counseling, recovery coaching, mental health services, and other services that may be needed by particular patients.

Expanding access to OUD medications is an important public health strategy.[8] The gap between the number of people needing opioid addiction treatment and the capacity to treat them with OUD medication is substantial. In 2012, the gap was estimated at nearly 1 million people, with about 80% of opioid treatment programs (OTPs) nationally operating at 80% capacity or greater.[10]

Improving access to treatment with OUD medications is crucial to closing the wide gap between treatment need and treatment availability, given the strong evidence of effectiveness for such treatments.[10]

Data indicate that medications for OUD are cost-effective and cost-beneficial.[2,14]

Content Overview

The TIP is divided into parts to make the material more accessible according to the reader's interests.

Part 1: Introduction to Medications for Opioid Use Disorder Treatment

This part lays the groundwork for understanding treatment concepts discussed later in this TIP. The intended audience includes:

- Healthcare professionals (physicians, nurse practitioners, physician assistants, and nurses)
- Professionals who offer addiction counseling or mental health services
- Peer support specialists
- People needing treatment and their families
- People in remission or recovery and their families
- Hospital administrators
- Policymakers

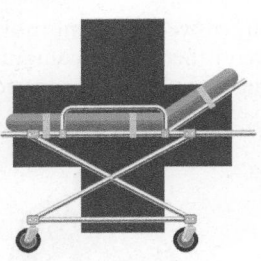

OPIOID-RELATED **EMERGENCY DEPARTMENT** visits nearly doubled from 2005-2015.[20]

In Part 1, readers will learn that:
- Increasing opioid overdose deaths, illicit opioid use, and prescription opioid misuse constitute a public health crisis.
- OUD medications reduce illicit opioid use, retain people in treatment, and reduce risk of opioid overdose death better than treatment with placebo or no medication.
- Only physicians, nurse practitioners, and physician assistants can prescribe buprenorphine for OUD. They must get a federal waiver to do so.
- Only federally certified, accredited OTPs can dispense methadone to treat OUD. OTPs can administer and dispense buprenorphine without a federal waiver.
- Any prescriber can offer naltrexone.
- OUD medication can be taken on a short- or long-term basis, including as part of medically supervised withdrawal and as maintenance treatment.
- Patients taking medication for OUD are considered to be in recovery.
- Several barriers contribute to the underuse of medication for OUD.

Part 2: Addressing Opioid Use Disorder in General Medical Settings

This part offers guidance on OUD screening, assessment, treatment, and referral. Part 2 is for healthcare professionals working in general medical settings with patients who have or are at risk for OUD.

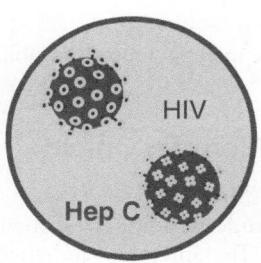

OPIOID ADDICTION is linked with significant **MORBIDITY** and **MORTALITY** related to HIV and hepatitis C.[19]

In Part 2, readers will learn that:
- All healthcare practices should screen for alcohol, tobacco, and other substance misuse (including opioid misuse).
- Validated screening tools, symptom surveys, and other resources are readily available; this part lists many of them.
- When patients screen positive for risk of harm from substance use, practitioners should assess them using tools that determine whether substance use meets diagnostic criteria for a substance use disorder (SUD).
- Thorough assessment should address patients' medical, social, SUD, and family histories.
- Laboratory tests can inform treatment planning.

- Practitioners should develop treatment plans or referral strategies (if onsite SUD treatment is unavailable) for patients who need SUD treatment.

Part 3: Pharmacotherapy for Opioid Use Disorder

This part offers information and tools for healthcare professionals who prescribe, administer, or dispense OUD medications or treat other illnesses in patients who take these medications. It provides guidance on the use of buprenorphine, methadone, and naltrexone by healthcare professionals in:
- General medical settings, including hospitals.
- Office-based opioid treatment settings.
- Specialty addiction treatment programs, including OTPs.

In Part 3, readers will learn that:
- OUD medications are safe and effective when used appropriately.
- OUD medications can help patients reduce or stop illicit opioid use and improve their health and functioning.
- Pharmacotherapy should be considered for all patients with OUD. Opioid pharmacotherapies should be reserved for those with moderate-to-severe OUD with physical dependence.
- Patients with OUD should be informed of the risks and benefits of pharmacotherapy, treatment without medication, and no treatment.
- Patients should be advised on where and how to get treatment with OUD medication.

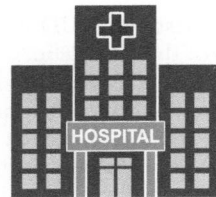

OPIOID-RELATED inpatient hospital stays **INCREASED 64%** nationally from 2005-2014.[20]

Part 4: Partnering Addiction Treatment Counselors With Clients and Healthcare Professionals

This part recommends ways that addiction treatment counselors can collaborate with healthcare professionals to support client-centered, trauma-informed OUD treatment and recovery. It also serves as a quick guide to medications that can treat OUD and presents strategies for clear communication with prescribers, creation of supportive environments for clients who take OUD medication, and ways to address other common counseling concerns when working with this population. In Part 4, readers will learn that:
- Many patients taking OUD medication benefit from counseling as part of treatment.
- Counselors play the same role for clients with OUD who take medication as for clients with any other SUD.
- Counselors help clients recover by addressing the challenges and consequences of addiction.
- OUD is often a chronic illness requiring ongoing communication among patients and providers to ensure that patients fully benefit from both pharmacotherapy and psychosocial treatment and support.
- OUD medications are safe and effective when prescribed and taken appropriately.

- Medication is integral to recovery for many people with OUD. Medication usually produces better treatment outcomes than outpatient treatment without medication.
- Supportive counseling environments for clients who take OUD medication can promote treatment and help build recovery capital.

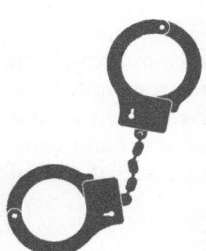

OPIOID ADDICTION is linked with high rates of **ILLEGAL ACTIVITY** and **INCARCERA-TION.**[17,21]

Part 5: Resources Related to Medications for Opioid Use Disorder

This part has a glossary and audience-segmented resource lists to help medical and behavioral health service providers better understand how to use OUD medications with their patients and to help patients better understand how OUD medications work. It is for all interested readers. In Part 5, readers will learn that:

- Practice guidelines and decision-making tools can help healthcare professionals with OUD screening, assessment, diagnosis, treatment planning, and referral.
- Patient- and family-oriented resources provide information about opioid addiction in general; the role of medication, behavioral and supportive services, and mutual-help groups in the treatment of OUD; how-to's for identifying recovery support services; and how-to's for locating medical and behavioral health service providers who specialize in treating OUD or other SUDs.

References

1. Auriacombe M, Fatséas M, Dubernet J, Daulouède JP, Tignol J. French field experience with buprenorphine. *Am J Addict.* 2004;13(Suppl. 1):S17–S28.
2. Cartwright WS. Cost-benefit analysis of drug treatment services: review of the literature. *J Ment Health Policy Econ.* 2000;3(1):11–26.
3. Center for Behavioral Health Statistics and Quality. *Key Substance Use and Mental Health Indicators in the United States: Results from the 2016 National Survey on Drug Use and Health.* Rockville, MD: Substance Abuse and Mental Health Services Administration; 2017.
4. Centers for Disease Control and Prevention. *Drug Overdose Death Data* [Webpage]. 2017. Retrieved January 9, 2018, from www.cdc.gov/drugoverdose /data/statedeaths.html.
5. Council of Economic Advisers. *The Underestimated Cost of the Opioid Crisis.* Washington, DC: Executive Office of the President of the United States; 2017.
6. Degenhardt L, Randall D, Hall W, Law M, Butler T, Burns L. Mortality among clients of a state-wide opioid pharmacotherapy program over 20 years: risk factors and lives saved. *Drug Alcohol Depend.* 2009;105(1–2):9–15.
7. Department of Health and Human Services, Office of the Surgeon General. *Facing Addiction in America: The Surgeon General's Report on Alcohol, Drugs, and Health.* Washington, DC: Department of Health and Human Services; 2016.
8. Gibson A, Degenhardt L, Mattick RP, Ali R, White J, O'Brien S. Exposure to opioid maintenance treatment reduces long-term mortality. *Addiction.* 2008;103(3):462–468.
9. Johnson RE, Chutuape MA, Strain EC, Walsh SL, Stitzer ML, Bigelow GE. A comparison of levomenthol acetate, buprenorphine, and methadone for opioid dependence. *N Engl J Med.* 2000;343(18):1290–1297.
10. Jones CM, Campopiano M, Baldwin G, McCance-Katz E. National and state treatment need and capacity for opioid agonist medication assisted treatment. *Am J Public Health.* 2015;105(8):e55–e63.
11. Krupitsky E, Nunes EV, Ling W, Illeperuma A, Gastfriend DR, Silverman BL. Injectable extended-release naltrexone for opioid dependence: a double-blind, placebo-controlled, multicenter randomized trial. *Lancet.* 2011;377(9776):1506–1513.
12. Lee JD, Friedmann PD, Kinlock TW, et al. Extended-release naltrexone to prevent opioid relapse in criminal justice offenders. *N Engl J Med.* 2016;374(13):1232–1242.
13. Mattick RP, Breen C, Kimber J, Davoli M. Buprenorphine maintenance versus placebo or methadone maintenance for opioid dependence. *Cochrane Database Syst Rev.* 2014;(2):1–84.
14. McCollister KE, French MT. The relative contribution of outcome domains in the total economic benefit of addiction interventions: a review of first findings. *Addiction.* 2003;98(12):1647–1659.
15. National Safety Council. *NSC motor vehicle fatality estimates.* 2017. Retrieved October 31, 2017, from www.nsc.org/NewsDocuments/2017/12-month -estimates.pdf.
16. Schwartz RP, Gryczynski J, O'Grady KE, et al. Opioid agonist treatments and heroin overdose deaths in Baltimore, Maryland, 1995–2009. *Am J Public Health.* 2013;103(5):917–922.
17. Soyka M, Träder A, Klotsche J, et al. Criminal behavior in opioid-dependent patients before and during maintenance therapy: 6-year follow-up of a nationally representative cohort sample. *J Forensic Sci.* 2012;57(6):1524–1530.
18. Substance Abuse and Mental Health Services Administration. Recovery and recovery support [Webpage]. 2017. Retrieved November 17, 2017, from www.samhsa.gov/recovery.
19. Wang X, Zhang T, Ho WZ. Opioids and HIV/HCV infection. *J Neuroimmune Pharmacol.* 2011;6(4):477–489.
20. Weiss AJ, Elixhauser A, Barrett ML, Steiner CA, Bailey MK, O'Malley L. *Opioid Related Inpatient Stays and Emergency Department Visits by State, 2009–2014. HCUP Statistical Brief No. 219.* Rockville, MD: Agency for Healthcare Research and Quality; 2017.
21. World Health Organization. *Guidelines for the Psychosocially Assisted Pharmacological Treatment of Opioid Dependence.* Geneva, Switzerland: WHO Press; 2009.

TIP Development Participants

Expert Panelists

Each Treatment Improvement Protocol's (TIP's) expert panel is a group of primarily nonfederal addiction-focused clinical, research, administrative, and recovery support experts with deep knowledge of the TIP's topic. With the Substance Abuse and Mental Health

Services Administration's (SAMHSA's) Knowledge Application Program (KAP) team, they develop each TIP via a consensus-driven, collaborative process that blends evidence-based, best, and promising practices with the panel's expertise and combined wealth of experience.

TIP Chair

Robert P. Schwartz, MD
Medical Director/Senior Research Scientist
Friends Research Institute
Baltimore, MD

TIP Expert Panelists

Sarah Church, PhD
Executive Director
Montefiore Medical Center
Wellness Center at Waters Place
Bronx, NY

Diana Coffa, MD, FM
Associate Professor
University of California School of Medicine
Family Community Medicine
San Francisco, CA

Zwaantje Hamming, MSN, FNP-C, CARN-AP
La Familia Medical Center
Santa Fe, NM

Ron Jackson, MSW, LICSW
Affiliate Professor
University of Washington School of Social Work
Seattle, WA

Hendree Jones, PhD
Professor and Executive Director
Horizons Program
Chapel Hill, NC

Michelle Lofwall, MD, DFASAM
Medical Director
University of Kentucky College of Medicine—Straus Clinic
Associate Professor of Behavioral Science and Psychiatry
Faculty in UK Center on Drug and Alcohol Research
Lexington, KY

Shannon C. Miller, MD, DFASAM, DFAPA
(ad hoc panelist)
Director, Addiction Services
Veterans Affairs Medical Center
Cincinnati, OH

Charles Schauberger, MD
Obstetrician-Gynecologist
Gundersen Health System
La Crosse, WI

Joycelyn Woods, MA, CMA
Executive Director
National Alliance for Medication Assisted Recovery
New York, NY

SAMHSA's TIP Champion

Melinda Campopiano von Klimo, MD
Senior Medical Advisor
Center for Substance Abuse Treatment
SAMHSA
Rockville, MD

Scientific Reviewers

This TIP's scientific reviewers are among the foremost experts on the three medications discussed in this TIP to treat opioid use disorder. Their role in the collaborative TIP development process was to help the KAP team include current, accurate, and comprehensive information and instructions about the use of each of these medications.

Buprenorphine

David A. Fiellin, MD
Professor of Investigative Medicine and Public Health
Yale University School of Medicine
New Haven, CT

Naltrexone

Joshua D. Lee, MD, MSc
Associate Professor
Department of Population Health
Division of General Medicine and Clinical Innovation
NYU Langone Health
New York, NY

Methadone

Andrew J. Saxon, MD
Professor
Department of Psychiatry and Behavioral Sciences
University of Washington School of Medicine Director
Center of Excellence in Substance Abuse Treatment and
    Education
Veterans Affairs Puget Sound Health Care System
Seattle, WA

Field Reviewers

Field reviewers represent each TIP's intended target audiences. They work in addiction, mental health, primary care, and adjacent fields. Their direct front-line experience related to the TIP's topic allows them to provide valuable input on a TIP's relevance, utility, accuracy, and accessibility.

William Bograkos, MA, DO, FACOEP, FACOFP
Adjunct Professor
Center for Excellence in the Neurosciences
University of New England (UNE)
Clinical Professor of Medical Military Science
Family Practice and Emergency Medicine, UNE
Biddeford, ME

Meg Brunner, MLIS
Librarian
Alcohol and Drug Abuse Institute
University of Washington
Seattle, WA

Kathryn Cates-Wessell
Chief Executive Officer
American Academy of Addiction Psychiatry
East Providence, RI

Mary Catlin, BSN, MPH, CIC
Public Health Nurse
Alcohol and Drug Abuse Institute
University of Washington
Seattle, WA

Kelly J. Clark, MD, MBA, DFASAM
President
American Society of Addiction Medicine
Rockville, MD

Marc Fishman, MD
Assistant Professor
Johns Hopkins University School of Medicine
Psychiatry/Behavioral Sciences Expert Team
Baltimore, MD

Katherine Fornili, DNP, MPH, RN, CARN
Assistant Professor
University of Maryland School of Nursing
Baltimore, MD

Adam Gordon, MD, MPH, FACP, FASAM, CMRO
Associate Professor of Medicine and Advisory Dean
University of Pittsburgh School of Medicine
Pittsburgh, PA

Ellie Grossman, MD
Instructor in Medicine
Cambridge Health Alliance
Somerville Hospital Primary Care
Somerville, MA

Kyle Kampman, MD
Professor
Department of Psychiatry
Perelman School of Medicine
University of Pennsylvania
Center for Studies of Addiction
Philadelphia, PA

Janice Kauffman, MPH, RN, CAS, CADC-1
Vice President of Addiction Treatment Services
North Charles Foundation, Inc.
Director of Addictions Consultation
Department of Psychiatry
Cambridge Health Alliance
Assistant Professor of Psychiatry
Harvard Medical School
The Cambridge Hospital
Cambridge, MA

Jason Kletter, PhD
President
Bay Area Addiction Research and Treatment President
California Opioid Maintenance Providers
San Francisco, CA

William J. Lorman, JD, PhD, MSN, PMHNP-BC, CARN-AP
Vice President and Chief Clinical Officer
Livengrin Foundation, Inc.
Bensalem, PA

Megan Marx-Varela, MPA
Associate Director
The Joint Commission—Behavioral Health Care Accreditation
Oakbrook Terrace, IL

Alison Newman, MPH
Continuing Education Specialist
Alcohol and Drug Abuse Institute
University of Washington
Seattle, WA

David O'Gurek, MD, FAAFP
Assistant Professor
Family and Community Medicine
Lewis Katz School of Medicine
Temple University
Philadelphia, PA

Yngvild Olsen, MD, MPH, FASAM
Medical Director
Institutes for Behavior Resources, Inc./Recovery Enhanced by Access to Comprehensive Healthcare (REACH) Health Services
Baltimore, MD

Shawn A. Ryan, MD, MBA, ABEM, FASAM
President & Chief Medical Offcer
BrightView
Cincinnati, OH

Paul Stasiewicz, PhD
Senior Research Scientist
Research Institute on Addictions
State University of New York-Buffalo
Buffalo, NY

Kenneth Stoller, MD
Director
Broadway Center for Addiction at the Johns Hopkins Hospital
Assistant Professor of Psychiatry and Behavioral Sciences
Johns Hopkins University Baltimore, MD

Mishka Terplan, MD, MPH, FACOG
Professor Department of Obstetrics and Gynecology
Division of General Obstetrics and Gynecology
Virginia Commonwealth University
Richmond, VA

Christopher Welsh, MD
Associate Professor of Psychiatry
University of Maryland Medical Center
Baltimore, MD

George E. Woody, MD
Professor of Psychiatry
Department of Psychiatry Center for Studies of Addiction
University of Pennsylvania's Perelman School of Medicine
Philadelphia, PA

Publication Information

Acknowledgments

This publication was prepared under contract number 270-14-0445 by the Knowledge Application Program (KAP) for the Center for Substance Abuse Treatment, Substance Abuse and Mental Health Services Administration (SAMHSA), US Department of Health and Human Services (HHS). Suzanne Wise served as the Contracting Officer's Representative, and Candi Byrne served as KAP Project Coordinator.

Disclaimer

Public Domain Notice

Electronic Access and Copies of Publication

This publication may be ordered or downloaded from SAMHSA's Publications Ordering webpage at https://store.samhsa.gov. Or, please call SAMHSA at 1-877-SAMHSA-7 (1-877-726-4727) (English and Español).

Recommended Citation

Substance Abuse and Mental Health Services Administration. *Medications for Opioid Use Disorder.* Treatment Improvement Protocol (TIP) Series 63, Executive Summary. HHS Publication No. (SMA) 18-5063EXSUMM. Rockville, MD: Substance Abuse and Mental Health Services Administration, 2018.

Originating Office

Quality Improvement and Workforce Development Branch, Division of Services Improvement, Center for Substance Abuse Treatment, Substance Abuse and Mental Health Services Administration, 5600 Fishers Lane, Rockville, MD 20857.

Nondiscrimination Notice

HHS Publication No. (SMA) 18-5063EXSUMM
Published 2018

APPENDIX 3

The ASAM National Practice Guideline for the Use of Medications in the Treatment of Addiction Involving Opioid Use*

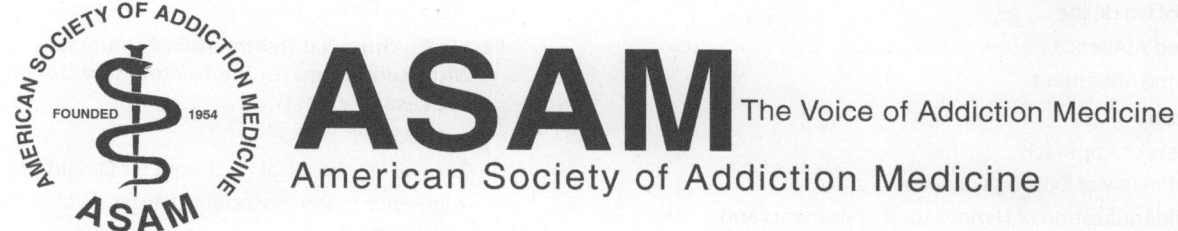

ASAM — The Voice of Addiction Medicine

American Society of Addiction Medicine

Guideline Committee Members *(alpha order)*†

Sandra Comer, PhD
Chinazo Cunningham, MD, MS
Marc J. Fishman, MD, FASAM
Adam Gordon, MD, MPH, FASAM
Kyle Kampman, MD, *Chair*
Daniel Langleben, MD
Ben Nordstrom, MD, PhD
David Oslin, MD
George Woody, MD
Tricia Wright, MD, MS
Stephen Wyatt, DO

ASAM Quality Improvement Council *(alpha order)*

John Femino, MD, FASAM
Margaret Jarvis, MD, FASAM, *Chair*
Margaret Kotz, DO, FASAM
Sandrine Pirard, MD, MPH, PhD

Robert J. Roose, MD, MPH
Alexis Geier-Horan, *ASAM Staff*
Beth Haynes, *ASAM Staff*
Penny S. Mills, MBA, ASAM, *Executive Vice President*

Special External Reviewer

Michael M. Miller, MD, FASAM, FAPA

Treatment Research Institute Technical Team Members *(alpha order)*

Amanda Abraham, PhD
Karen Dugosh, PhD
David Festinger, PhD
Kyle Kampman, MD, *Principal Investigator*
Keli McLoyd, JD
Brittany Seymour, BA
Abigail Woodworth, MS

*From Kampman K, Jarvis M. American Society of Addiction (ASAM) national practice guidelines for the use of medications in the treatment of addiction involving opioid use. *J Addict Med.* 2015;9(5):358–367.
†Disclosure information for Guideline Committee Members, the ASAM Quality Improvement Council, and External Reviewers is available respectively in Appendices III, IV, and V.

OUTLINE

Executive Summary

Purpose

The American Society of Addiction Medicine (ASAM) developed this National Practice Guideline for the Use of Medications in the Treatment of Addiction Involving Opioid Use to provide information on evidence-based treatment of opioid use disorder. (Hereafter, in this document, this National Practice Guideline will be referred to as "Practice Guideline.")

Background

Opioid use disorder is a chronic, relapsing disease, which has significant economic, personal, and public health consequences. Many readers of this Practice Guideline may recognize the term "opioid use disorder" as it is used in the *Diagnostic and Statistical Manual of Mental Disorders, Fifth Edition* (DSM-5), developed by the American Psychiatric Association; others may be more familiar with the term "opioid dependence," as used in the previous edition of the DSM.[7]

The ASAM defines addiction as "a primary, chronic disease of brain reward, motivation, memory, and related circuitry," with a "dysfunction in these circuits" being reflected in "an individual pathologically pursuing reward and/or relief by substance use and other behaviors." In this context, the preferred term by ASAM for this serious bio-psycho-social-spiritual illness would be "addiction involving opioid use." ASAM views addiction as a fundamental neurological disorder of "brain reward, motivation, memory, and related circuitry," and recognizes that there are unifying features in all cases of addiction, including substance-related addiction and nonsubstance-related addiction. It is clear that a variety of substances commonly associated with addiction work on specific receptors in the nervous system and on specific neurotransmitter systems. Specific pharmacological agents used in the treatment of addiction exert their effects via their actions on specific receptors. Hence, the medications used in the treatment of addiction have specific efficacy based on their own molecular structure and the particular neurotransmitters affected by that medication. Medications developed for the treatment of addiction involving opioid use may have benefits in the treatment of addiction involving an individual's use of other substances. For instance, naltrexone, which is approved by the US Food and Drug Administration (FDA) for the treatment of opioid dependence using DSM, Fourth Edition (DSM-IV) terminology, is also FDA-approved for the treatment of alcohol dependence as per the DSM-IV guidelines.[8]

The ASAM recognizes that research is yet to be done to confirm the specificity of its conceptualization of addiction as a medical and a psychiatric illness. Both the American Medical Association (AMA), as noted in various policy and position statements, and the International Classification of Diseases (ICD), recognize addiction as both a medical and a psychiatric disorder.[111,171] ASAM encourages clinicians, researchers, educators, and policy makers to use the term "addiction" regardless of whether the patient's condition at a given point in its natural history seems to more prominently involve opioid use, alcohol use, nicotine use, or engagement in addictive behaviors such as gambling. Given the widespread North American application of the DSM's categorization of disorders, this Practice Guideline will, for the sake of brevity and convention, use the term "opioid use disorder."

According to the 2013 National Survey on Drug Use and Health (NSDUH), 4.5 million individuals in the United States were current (past month), nonmedical users of prescription opioids. Nonmedical use of opioids and other prescription drugs constitute hazardous and risky behavior that should be discouraged given the potential that unauthorized use of such substances has for harm (to the user). Medication therapy related to opioids focuses not only on nonmedical use but also on an attempt to treat the medical illness, addiction. The 2013 NSDUH further found that 1.9 million persons in America met DSM-IV criteria for opioid use disorder associated with their use of prescription opioids, and that more than 0.5 million additional individuals have met DSM-IV criteria for opioid use disorder associated with their use of heroin.[146]

Opioid use is associated with increased mortality. The leading causes of death in people using opioids for nonmedical purposes are overdose and trauma.[50] The injection route use (intravenous or even intramuscular [IM]) of opioids or other drugs increases the risk of being exposed to HIV, viral hepatitis, and other infectious agents.

Scope of Guideline

This Practice Guideline was developed for the evaluation and treatment of opioid use disorder and for the management of opioid overdose. The medications covered in this guideline are mainly, but not exclusively, those that have been FDA-approved for the treatment of opioid dependence, as defined in prior versions of the DSM, and not necessarily the most recent version of the manual, the DSM-5.[151] DSM-5 combined the criteria for opioid abuse and opioid dependence from prior versions of the DSM in its new diagnosis of opioid use disorder: therefore, pharmacological treatment may not be appropriate for all patients along the entire opioid use disorder continuum. In a study comparing opioid dependence from DSM-IV and opioid use disorder from DSM-5, optimal concordance occurred when four or more DSM-5 criteria were endorsed (i.e., the DSM-5 threshold for moderate opioid use disorder).[42] Other medications have been used off-label to treat opioid use disorder (clearly noted in the text); however, the Guideline Committee has not issued recommendations on the use of those medications. As a final note related to references to medications, whether FDA-approved or off-label, cost and/or cost effectiveness were not considerations in the development of this Practice Guideline.

Intended Audience

This Practice Guideline is primarily intended for clinicians involved in evaluating patients and providing authorization for pharmacological treatments at any level. The intended audience falls into the broad groups of physicians; other healthcare providers (especially those with prescribing authority); medical educators and faculty for other healthcare professionals in training; and clinical care managers, including those offering utilization management services.

Qualifying Statement

This ASAM Practice Guideline is intended to aid clinicians in their clinical decision-making and patient management. The Practice Guideline strives to identify and define clinical decision-making junctures that meet the needs of most patients in most circumstances. Clinical decision-making should involve consideration of the quality and availability of expertise and services in the community wherein care is provided. In circumstances in which the Practice Guideline is being used as the basis for regulatory or payer decisions, improvement in quality of care should be the goal. Finally, prescribed courses of treatment contained in recommendations in this Practice Guideline are effective only if the recommendations, as outlined, are followed. Because lack of patient understanding and adherence may adversely affect outcomes, clinicians should make every effort to promote the patient's understanding of, and adherence to, prescribed and recommended pharmacological and psychosocial treatments. Patients should be informed of the risks, benefits, and alternatives to a particular treatment, and should be an active party to shared decision-making whenever feasible. Recommendations in this Practice Guideline do not supersede any federal or state regulation.

Overview of Methodology

This Practice Guideline was developed using the RAND Corporation (RAND)/University of California, Los Angeles (UCLA) Appropriateness Method (RAM)—a process that combines scientific evidence and clinical knowledge to determine the appropriateness of a set of clinical procedures. The RAM is a deliberate approach encompassing review of existing guidelines, literature reviews, appropriateness ratings, necessity reviews, and document development. For this project, ASAM selected an independent committee to oversee guideline development, to participate in review of treatment scenarios, and to assist in writing. ASAM's Quality Improvement Council, chaired by Margaret Jarvis, MD, oversaw the selection process for the independent development committee, referred to as the Guideline Committee.

The Guideline Committee comprised 10 experts and researchers from multiple disciplines, medical specialties, and subspecialties, including academic research, internal medicine, family medicine, addiction medicine, addiction psychiatry, general psychiatry, obstetrics/gynecology, pharmacology, and clinical neurobiology. Physicians with both allopathic and osteopathic training were represented in the Guideline Committee. The Guideline Committee was assisted by a technical team of researchers from the Treatment Research Institute (TRI) affiliated with the University of Pennsylvania, and worked under the guidance of Dr. Kyle Kampman who led the TRI team as Principal Investigator in implementing the RAM.

Summary of Recommendations
Part 1: Assessment and Diagnosis of Opioid Use Disorder
Assessment Recommendations
(1) First clinical priority should be given to identifying and making appropriate referral for any urgent or emergent medical or psychiatric problem(s), including drug-related impairment or overdose.

(2) Completion of the patient's medical history should include screening for concomitant medical conditions, including infectious diseases (hepatitis, HIV, and tuberculosis [TB]), acute trauma, and pregnancy.

(3) A physical examination should be completed as a component of the comprehensive assessment process. The prescriber (the clinician authorizing the use of a medication for the treatment of opioid use disorder) may conduct this physical examination him/herself, or, in accordance with the ASAM Standards, ensure that a current physical examination is contained within the patient medical record before a patient is started on a new medication for the treatment of his/her addiction.

(4) Initial laboratory testing should include a complete blood count, liver function tests, and tests for hepatitis C and HIV. Testing for TB and sexually transmitted infections should also be considered. Hepatitis B vaccination should be offered, if appropriate.

(5) The assessment of women presents special considerations regarding their reproductive health. Women of childbearing age should be tested for pregnancy, and all women of childbearing potential and age should be queried regarding methods of contraception, given the increase in fertility that results from effective opioid use disorder treatment.

(6) Patients being evaluated for addiction involving opioid use, and/or for possible medication use in the treatment of opioid use disorder, should undergo (or have completed) an assessment of mental health status and possible psychiatric disorders (as outlined in the ASAM Standards).

(7) Opioid use is often co-occurring with other substance-related disorders. An evaluation of past and current substance use and a determination of the totality of substances that surround the addiction should be conducted.

(8) The use of marijuana, stimulants, or other addictive drugs should not be a reason to suspend opioid use disorder treatment. However, evidence demonstrates that patients who are actively using substances during opioid use disorder treatment have a poorer prognosis. The use of benzodiazepines and other sedative hypnotics may be a reason to suspend agonist treatment because of safety concerns related to respiratory depression.

(9) A tobacco use query and counseling on cessation of tobacco products and electronic nicotine delivery devices should be completed routinely for all patients, including those who present for evaluation and treatment of opioid use disorder.

(10) An assessment of social and environmental factors should be conducted (as outlined in the ASAM Standards) to identify facilitators and barriers to addiction treatment, and specifically to pharmacotherapy. Before a decision is made to initiate a course of pharmacotherapy for the patient with opioid use disorder, the patient should receive a multidimensional assessment in fidelity with the ASAM Criteria: Treatment Criteria for Addictive, Substance-Related, and Co-occurring Conditions (the "ASAM Criteria"). Addiction should be considered a bio-psycho-social-spiritual illness, for which the use of medication(s) is but only one component of overall treatment.

Diagnosis Recommendations

(1) Other clinicians may diagnose opioid use disorder, but confirmation of the diagnosis by the provider with prescribing authority, and who recommends medication use, must be obtained before pharmacotherapy for opioid use disorder commences.

(2) Opioid use disorder is primarily diagnosed on the basis of the history provided by the patient and a comprehensive assessment that includes a physical examination.

(3) Validated clinical scales that measure withdrawal symptoms, for example, the Objective Opioid Withdrawal Scale (OOWS), the Subjective Opioid Withdrawal Scale (SOWS), and the Clinical Opioid Withdrawal Scale (COWS), may be used to assist in the evaluation of patients with opioid use disorder.

(4) Urine drug testing during the comprehensive assessment process, and frequently during treatment, is recommended. The frequency of drug testing is determined by a number of factors including the stability of the patient, the type of treatment, and the treatment setting.

Part 2: Treatment Options

(1) The choice of available treatment options for addiction involving opioid use should be a shared decision between clinician and patient.

(2) Clinicians should consider the patient's preferences, past treatment history, and treatment setting when deciding between the use of methadone, buprenorphine, and naltrexone in the treatment of addiction involving opioid use. The treatment setting described as level 1 treatment in the ASAM Criteria may be a general outpatient location such as a clinician's practice site. The setting described as level 2 in the ASAM Criteria may be an intensive outpatient treatment or partial hospitalization program housed in a specialty addiction treatment facility, a community mental health center, or another setting. The ASAM Criteria describes level 3 or level 4 treatment, respectively, as a residential addiction treatment facility or hospital.

(3) The venue in which treatment is provided is as important as the specific medication selected. Opioid treatment programs (OTPs) offer daily supervised dosing of methadone, and increasingly of buprenorphine. In accordance with the Federal law (21 CFR §1306.07), office-based opioid treatment (OBOT), which provides medication on a prescribed weekly or monthly basis, is limited to buprenorphine. Naltrexone can be prescribed in any setting by any clinician with the authority to prescribe any medication. Clinicians should consider a patient's psychosocial situation, co-occurring disorders, and risk of diversion when determining whether OTP or OBOT is most appropriate.

(4) OBOT may not be suitable for patients with active alcohol use disorder or sedative, hypnotic, or anxiolytic use disorder (or who are undergoing treatment for addiction involving the use of alcohol or other sedative drugs, including benzodiazepines or benzodiazepine receptor agonists). It may also be unsuitable for persons who are regularly using alcohol or other sedatives, but do not have addiction or a specific substance use disorder related to that class of drugs. The prescribing of benzodiazepines or other sedative-hypnotics should

be used with extreme caution in patients who are prescribed methadone or buprenorphine for the treatment of an opioid use disorder.

(5) Methadone is recommended for patients who may benefit from daily dosing and supervision in an OTP, or for patients for whom buprenorphine for the treatment of opioid use disorder has been used unsuccessfully in an OTP or OBOT setting.

(6) Oral naltrexone for the treatment of opioid use disorder is often adversely affected by poor medication adherence. Clinicians should reserve its use for patients who would be able to comply with special techniques to enhance their adherence, for example, observed dosing. Extended-release injectable naltrexone reduces, but does not eliminate, issues with medication adherence.

Part 3: Treating Opioid Withdrawal

(1) Using medications for opioid withdrawal management is recommended over abrupt cessation of opioids. Abrupt cessation of opioids may lead to strong cravings, which can lead to continued use.

(2) Patients should be advised about risk of relapse and other safety concerns from using opioid withdrawal management as standalone treatment for opioid use disorder. Opioid withdrawal management on its own is not a treatment method.

(3) Assessment of a patient undergoing opioid withdrawal management should include a thorough medical history and physical examination, focusing on signs and symptoms associated with opioid withdrawal.

(4) Opioid withdrawal management in cases in which methadone is used to manage withdrawal symptoms must be done in an inpatient setting or in an OTP. For short-acting opioids, tapering schedules that decrease in daily doses of prescribed methadone should begin with doses between 20 and 30 mg per day, and should be completed within 6–10 days.

(5) Opioid withdrawal management in cases in which buprenorphine is used to manage withdrawal symptoms should not be initiated until 12–18 hours after the last dose of a short-acting agonist such as heroin or oxycodone, and 24–48 hours after the last dose of a long-acting agonist such as methadone. A dose of buprenorphine sufficient to suppress withdrawal symptoms is given (this can be 4–16 mg per day) and then the dose is tapered. The duration of the tapering schedule can be as brief as 3–5 days or as long as 30 days or more.

(6) The use of combinations of buprenorphine and low doses of oral naltrexone to manage withdrawal and facilitate the accelerated introduction of extended-release injectable naltrexone has shown promise. More research will be needed before this can be accepted as standard practice.

(7) The Guideline Committee recommends, based on consensus opinion, the inclusion of clonidine as a practice to support opioid withdrawal. Clonidine is not FDA-approved for the treatment of opioid withdrawal, but it has been used extensively off-label for this purpose. Clonidine may be used orally or transdermally at doses of 0.1–0.3 mg every 6–8 hours, with a maximum dose of 1.2 mg daily to assist in the management of opioid withdrawal symptoms. Its hypotensive effects often limit the amount that can be used.

Clonidine can be combined with other non-narcotic medications targeting specific opioid withdrawal symptoms such as benzodiazepines for anxiety, loperamide for diarrhea, acetaminophen or nonsteroidal anti-inflammatory medications (NSAIDs) for pain, and ondansetron or other agents for nausea.

(8) Opioid withdrawal management using anesthesia UROD is not recommended due to high risk for adverse events or death. Naltrexone-facilitated opioid withdrawal management can be a safe and effective approach, but should be used only by clinicians experienced with this clinical method, and in cases in which anesthesia or conscious sedation are not being employed.

Part 4: Methadone

(1) Methadone is a treatment option recommended for patients who are physiologically dependent on opioids, able to give informed consent, and who have no specific contraindications for agonist treatment when it is prescribed in the context of an appropriate plan that includes psychosocial intervention.

(2) The recommended initial dose for methadone ranges from 10 to 30 mg, with reassessment in 3–4 hours, and a second dose not to exceed 10 mg on the first day if withdrawal symptoms are persisting.

(3) The usual daily dosage of methadone ranges from 60 to 120 mg. Some patients may respond to lower doses and some patients may need higher doses. Dosage increases in 5- to 10-mg increments applied no more frequently than every 7 days (depending on clinical response) are necessary to avoid over sedation, toxicity, or even iatrogenic overdose deaths.

(4) The administration of methadone should be monitored because unsupervised administration can lead to misuse and diversion. OTP regulations require monitored medication administration until the patient's clinical response and behavior demonstrates that the prescribing of nonmonitored doses is appropriate.

(5) Psychosocial treatment, although sometimes minimally needed, should be implemented in conjunction with the use of methadone in the treatment of opioid use disorder.

(6) Methadone should be reinstituted immediately if relapse occurs, or when an assessment determines that the risk of relapse is high for patients who previously received methadone in the treatment of opioid use disorder, but who are no longer prescribed such treatment.

(7) Strategies directed at relapse prevention are an important part of comprehensive addiction treatment and should be included in any plan of care for a patient receiving active opioid treatment or ongoing monitoring of the status of their addictive disease.

(8) Switching from methadone to another medication for the treatment of opioid use disorder may be appropriate if the patient experiences intolerable side effects or is not successful in attaining or maintaining treatment goals through the use of methadone.

(9) Patients switching from methadone to buprenorphine in the treatment of opioid use disorder should be on low doses of methadone before switching medications. Patients on low doses of methadone (30–40 mg per day or

less) generally tolerate transition to buprenorphine with minimal discomfort, whereas patients on higher doses of methadone may experience significant discomfort in switching medications.

(10) Patients switching from methadone to oral naltrexone or extended-release injectable naltrexone must be completely withdrawn from methadone and other opioids before they can receive naltrexone. The only exception would apply when an experienced clinician receives consent from the patient to embark on a plan of naltrexone-facilitated opioid withdrawal management.

(11) Patients who discontinue agonist therapy with methadone or buprenorphine and then resume opioid use should be made aware of the risks associated with opioid overdose, and especially the increased risk of death.

Part 5: Buprenorphine

(1) Opioid-dependent patients should wait until they are experiencing mild to moderate opioid withdrawal before taking the first dose of buprenorphine to reduce the risk of precipitated withdrawal. Generally, buprenorphine initiation should occur at least 6–12 hours after the last use of heroin or other short-acting opioids, or 24–72 hours after their last use of long-acting opioids such as methadone.

(2) Induction of buprenorphine should start with a dose of 2–4 mg. Dosages may be increased in increments of 2–4 mg.

(3) Clinicians should observe patients in their offices during induction. Emerging research, however, suggests that many patients need "not" be observed and that home buprenorphine induction may be considered. Home-based induction is recommended only if the patient or prescribing physician is experienced with the use of buprenorphine. This is based on the consensus opinion of the Guideline Committee.

(4) Buprenorphine doses after induction and titration should be, on average, at least 8 mg per day. However, if patients are continuing to use opioids, consideration should be given to increasing the dose by 4–8 mg (daily doses of 12–16 mg or higher). The FDA approves dosing to a limit of 24 mg per day, and there is limited evidence regarding the relative efficacy of higher doses. In addition, the use of higher doses may increase the risk of diversion.

(5) Psychosocial treatment should be implemented in conjunction with the use of buprenorphine in the treatment of opioid use disorder.

(6) Clinicians should take steps to reduce the chance of buprenorphine diversion. Recommended strategies include frequent office visits (weekly in early treatment), urine drug testing, including testing for buprenorphine and metabolites, and recall visits for pill counts.

(7) Patients should be tested frequently for buprenorphine, other substances, and prescription medications. Accessing Prescription Drug Monitoring Program (PDMP) data may be useful for monitoring.

(8) Patients should be seen frequently at the beginning of their treatment. Weekly visits (at least) are recommended until patients are determined to be stable. There is no recommended time limit for treatment.

(9) Buprenorphine taper and discontinuation is a slow process and close monitoring is recommended. Buprenorphine tapering is generally accomplished over several months. Patients should be encouraged to remain in treatment for ongoing monitoring past the point of discontinuation.

(10) When considering a switch from buprenorphine to naltrexone, 7–14 days should elapse between the last dose of buprenorphine and the start of naltrexone to ensure that the patient is not physically dependent on opioids before starting naltrexone.

(11) When considering a switch from buprenorphine to methadone, there is no required time delay because the addition of a full mu-opioid agonist to a partial agonist does not typically result in any type of adverse reaction.

(12) Patients who discontinue agonist therapy and resume opioid use should be made aware of the risks associated with an opioid overdose, and especially the increased risk of death.

Part 6: Naltrexone

(1) Naltrexone is a recommended treatment in preventing relapse in opioid use disorder. Oral formula naltrexone may be considered for patients in whom adherence can be supervised or enforced. Extended-release injectable naltrexone may be more suitable for patients who have issues with adherence.

(2) Oral naltrexone should be taken daily in 50-mg doses, or three times weekly in two 100-mg doses followed by one 150-mg dose.

(3) Extended-release injectable naltrexone should be administered every 4 weeks by deep IM injection in the gluteal muscle at a set dosage of 380 mg per injection.

(4) Psychosocial treatment is recommended in conjunction with treatment with naltrexone. The efficacy of naltrexone use in conjunction with psychosocial treatment has been established, whereas the efficacy of extended release injectable naltrexone without psychosocial treatment "has not" been established.

(5) There is no recommended length of treatment with oral naltrexone or extended-release injectable naltrexone. Duration depends on clinical judgment and the patient's individual circumstances. Because there is no physical dependence associated with naltrexone, it can be stopped abruptly without withdrawal symptoms.

(6) Switching from naltrexone to methadone or buprenorphine should be planned, considered, and monitored. Switching from an antagonist such as naltrexone to a full agonist (methadone) or a partial agonist (buprenorphine) is generally less complicated than switching from a full or partial agonist to an antagonist because there is no physical dependence associated with antagonist treatment and thus no possibility of precipitated withdrawal. Patients being switched from naltrexone to buprenorphine or methadone will not have physical dependence on opioids and thus the initial doses of methadone or buprenorphine used should be low. Patients should not be switched until a significant amount of the naltrexone is no longer in their system, about 1 day for oral naltrexone or 30 days for extended-release injectable naltrexone.

(7) Patients who discontinue antagonist therapy and resume opioid use should be made aware of the increased risks associated with an opioid overdose, and especially the increased risk of death.

Part 7: Psychosocial Treatment in Conjunction With Medications for the Treatment of Opioid Use Disorder

(1) Psychosocial treatment is recommended in conjunction with any pharmacological treatment of opioid use disorder. At a minimum, psychosocial treatment should include the following: psychosocial needs assessment, supportive counseling, links to existing family supports, and referrals to community services.

(2) Treatment planning should include collaboration with qualified behavioral healthcare providers to determine the optimal type and intensity of psychosocial treatment and for renegotiation of the treatment plan for circumstances in which patients do not adhere to recommended plans for, or referrals to, psychosocial treatment.

(3) Psychosocial treatment is generally recommended for patients who are receiving opioid agonist treatment (methadone or buprenorphine).

(4) Psychosocial treatment is recommended in the treatment of pregnant women with opioid use disorder.

(5) Counseling and testing for HIV should be provided in accordance with state law. Tests for hepatitis B and C and liver function are also suggested. Hepatitis A and B vaccination is recommended for those whose hepatitis serology is negative.

(6) Urine drug testing may be used to detect or confirm suspected opioid and other drug use with informed consent from the mother, realizing that there may be adverse legal and social consequences of her use. State laws differ on reporting substance use during pregnancy. Laws that penalize women for use and for obtaining treatment serve to prevent women from obtaining prenatal care and worsen outcomes.

(7) Pregnant women who are physically dependent on opioids should receive treatment using methadone or buprenorphine monoproduct rather than withdrawal management or abstinence.

(8) Care for pregnant women with opioid use disorder should be comanaged by an obstetrician and an addiction specialist physician. Release of information forms need to be completed to ensure communication among healthcare providers.

(9) Treatment with methadone should be initiated as early as possible during pregnancy.

(10) Hospitalization during initiation of methadone and treatment with buprenorphine may be advisable due to the potential for adverse events, especially in the third trimester.

(11) In an inpatient setting, methadone should be initiated at a dose range of 20–30 mg. Incremental doses of 5–10 mg are given every 3–6 hours, as needed, to treat withdrawal symptoms.

(12) After induction, clinicians should increase the methadone dose in 5- to 10-mg increments per week. The goal is to maintain the lowest dose that controls withdrawal symptoms and minimizes the desire to use additional opioids.

(13) Twice daily dosing is more effective and has fewer side effects than single dosing but may not be practical because methadone is typically dispensed in an outpatient clinic.

(14) Clinicians should be aware that the pharmacokinetics of methadone are affected by pregnancy. With advancing gestational age, plasma levels of methadone progressively decrease and clearance increases. Increased or split doses may be needed as pregnancy progresses. After child birth, doses may need to be adjusted.

(15) Buprenorphine monoproduct is a reasonable and recommended alternative to methadone for pregnant women. Whereas there is evidence of safety, there is insufficient evidence to recommend the combination buprenorphine/naloxone formulation.

(16) If a woman becomes pregnant while she is receiving naltrexone, it is appropriate to discontinue the medication if the patient and doctor agree that the risk of relapse is low. If the patient is highly concerned about relapse and wishes to continue naltrexone, she should be informed about the risks of staying on naltrexone and provide her consent for ongoing treatment. If the patient wishes to discontinue naltrexone, but then reports relapse to opioid use, it may be appropriate to consider treatment with methadone or treatment with buprenorphine.

(17) Naloxone is not recommended for use in pregnant women with opioid use disorder except in situations of life-threatening overdose.

(18) Mothers receiving methadone and buprenorphine monoproduct for the treatment of opioid use disorders should be encouraged to breastfeed.

Part 9: Special Populations: Individuals With Pain

(1) For all patients with pain, it is important that the correct diagnosis be made and that a target suitable for treatment is identified.

(2) If pharmacological treatment is considered, non-narcotic medications such as acetaminophen and NSAIDs should be tried first.

(3) Opioid agonists (methadone or buprenorphine) should be considered for patients with active opioid use disorder who are not under treatment.

(4) Pharmacotherapy in conjunction with psychosocial treatment should be considered for patients with pain who have opioid use disorder.

(5) Patients on methadone for the treatment of opioid use disorder will require doses of opioids in addition to their regular daily dose of methadone to manage acute pain.

(6) Patients on methadone for the treatment of opioid use disorder and who are admitted for surgery may require additional short-acting opioid pain relievers. The dose of pain relievers prescribed may be higher due to tolerance.

(7) Temporarily increasing buprenorphine dosing may be effective for mild acute pain.

(8) For severe acute pain, discontinuing buprenorphine and commencing on a high-potency opioid (such as fentanyl) is advisable. Patients should be monitored closely and additional interventions such as regional anesthesia should also be considered.

(9) The decision to discontinue buprenorphine before an elective surgery should be made in consultation with the attending surgeon and anesthesiologist. If it is decided that buprenorphine should be discontinued before surgery, this should occur 24–36 hours in advance of surgery and restarted

postoperatively when the need for full opioid agonist analgesia has passed.

(10) Patients on naltrexone will not respond to opioid analgesics in the usual manner. Therefore, it is recommended that mild pain be treated with NSAIDs, and moderate to severe pain be treated with ketorolac on a short-term basis.

(11) Oral naltrexone should be discontinued 72 hours before surgery and extended-release injectable naltrexone should be discontinued 30 days before an anticipated surgery.

Part 10: Special Populations: Adolescents

(1) Clinicians should consider treating adolescents who have opioid use disorder using the full range of treatment options, including pharmacotherapy.

(2) Opioid agonists (methadone and buprenorphine) and antagonists (naltrexone) may be considered for treatment of opioid use disorder in adolescents. Age is a consideration in treatment, and Federal laws and US FDA approvals need to be considered for patients under age 18.

(3) Psychosocial treatment is recommended in the treatment of adolescents with opioid use disorder.

(4) Concurrent practices to reduce infection (e.g., sexual risk reduction interventions) are recommended as components of comprehensive treatment for the prevention of sexually transmitted infections and blood-borne viruses.

(5) Adolescents may benefit from treatment in specialized treatment facilities that provide multidimensional services.

Part 11: Special Populations: Individuals With Co-occurring Psychiatric Disorders

(1) A comprehensive assessment including determination of mental health status should evaluate whether the patient is stable. Patients with suicidal or homicidal ideation should be referred immediately for treatment and possibly hospitalization.

(2) Management of patients at risk for suicide should include reducing immediate risk; managing underlying factors associated with suicidal intent; and monitoring and follow-up.

(3) All patients with psychiatric disorders should be asked about suicidal ideation and behavior. Patients with a history of suicidal ideation or attempts should have opioid use disorder, and psychiatric medication use, monitored.

(4) Assessment for psychiatric disorder should occur at the onset of agonist or antagonist treatment. Reassessment using a detailed mental status examination should occur after stabilization with methadone, buprenorphine, or naltrexone.

(5) Pharmacotherapy in conjunction with psychosocial treatment should be considered for patients with opioid use disorder and a co-occurring psychiatric disorder.

(6) Clinicians should be aware of potential interactions between medications used to treat co-occurring psychiatric conditions and opioid use disorder.

(7) Assertive community treatment should be considered for patients with co-occurring schizophrenia and opioid use disorder who have a recent history of, or are at risk of, repeated hospitalization or homelessness.

Part 12: Special Populations: Individuals in the Criminal Justice System

(1) Pharmacotherapy for the continued treatment of opioid use disorders, or the initiation of pharmacotherapy, has been shown to be effective and is recommended for prisoners and parolees regardless of the length of their sentenced term.

(2) Individuals with opioid use disorder who are within the criminal justice system should be treated with some type of pharmacotherapy in addition to psychosocial treatment.

(3) Opioid agonists (methadone and buprenorphine) and antagonists (naltrexone) may be considered for treatment. There is insufficient evidence to recommend any one treatment as superior to another for prisoners or parolees.

(4) Pharmacotherapy should be initiated a minimum of 30 days before release from prison.

Part 13: Naloxone for the Treatment of Opioid Overdose

(1) Naloxone should be given in case of opioid overdose.

(2) Naloxone can and should be administered to pregnant women in cases of overdose to save the mother's life.

(3) The Guideline Committee, based on consensus opinion, recommends that patients who are being treated for opioid use disorder and their family members/significant others be given prescriptions for naloxone. Patients and family members/significant others should be trained in the use of naloxone in overdose.

(4) The Guideline Committee, based on consensus opinion, recommends that first responders such as emergency medical services personnel, police officers, and firefighters be trained in and authorized to administer naloxone.

Abbreviations and Acronyms

AA Alcoholics Anonymous
ACT assertive community treatment
AIDS acquired immunodeficiency syndrome
ASAM American Society of Addiction Medicine
CBT cognitive behavioral therapy
CDC Centers for Disease Control and Prevention
COWS Clinical Opioid Withdrawal Scale
DATA 2000 Drug Addiction Treatment Act of 2000
DEA Drug Enforcement Administration
DSM-III Diagnostic and Statistical Manual of Mental Disorders, Third Edition
DSM-IV Diagnostic and Statistical Manual of Mental Disorders, Fourth Edition
DSM-5 Diagnostic and Statistical Manual of Mental Disorders, Fifth Edition
ECG electrocardiogram
EMS emergency medical services
FDA US Food and Drug Administration
HBV hepatitis B virus
HCV hepatitis C virus
HIV human immunodeficiency virus
IDU injection drug use
IM intramuscular
IV intravenous
NA Narcotics Anonymous
NAS neonatal abstinence syndrome
NSAIDs nonsteroidal anti-inflammatory drugs
NSDUH National Survey on Drug Use and Health
OBOT office-based opioid treatment

OOWS Objective Opioid Withdrawal Scale
OTP opioid treatment program
PMDP prescription drug monitoring program
RCT randomized clinical trial
RAM RAND/UCLA Appropriateness Method
SAMHSA Substance Abuse and Mental Health Services Administration
SMART self-management and recovery therapy
SOWS Subjective Opioid Withdrawal Scale
TB tuberculosis
UROD ultra-rapid opioid detoxification

National Practice Guideline Glossary

Abstinence: Intentional and consistent restraint from the pathological pursuit of reward and/or relief that involves the use of substances and other behaviors. These behaviors may involve, but are not necessarily limited to, gambling, video gaming, spending, compulsive eating, compulsive exercise, or compulsive sexual behaviors.[111]

Abuse: This term is not recommended for use in clinical or research contexts. Harmful use of a specific psychoactive substance. When used to mean "substance abuse," this term also applies to one category of psychoactive substance-related disorders in previous editions of the *Diagnostic and Statistical Manual of Mental Disorders* (DSM). While recognizing that "abuse" is part of past diagnostic terminology, ASAM recommends that an alternative term be found for this purpose because of the pejorative connotations of the word "abuse."[111]

Addiction: Addiction is a primary, chronic disease of brain reward, motivation, memory, and related circuitry. Dysfunction in these circuits leads to characteristic biological, psychological, social, and spiritual manifestations. This is reflected in an individual pathologically pursuing reward and/or relief by substance use and other behaviors.

Addiction is characterized by inability to consistently abstain, impairment in behavioral control, cravings, diminished recognition of significant problems with one's behaviors and interpersonal relationships, and a dysfunctional emotional response. Like other chronic diseases, addiction often involves cycles of relapse and remission. Without treatment or engagement in recovery activities, addiction is progressive and can result in disability or premature death.[111]

Addiction specialist physician: Addiction specialist physicians include addiction medicine physicians and addiction psychiatrists who hold either a board certification in addiction medicine from the American Board of Addiction Medicine, a subspecialty board certification in addiction psychiatry from the American Board of Psychiatry and Neurology, a subspecialty board certification in addiction medicine from the American Osteopathic Association, or certification in addiction medicine from the American Society of Addiction Medicine.[118]

Adherence (see also Compliance): To "adhere" is "to cling, cleave (to be steadfast, hold fast), to stick fast" (Webster's Dictionary). Adherence is a term that health professionals have been using increasingly to replace the term "compliance." Both terms have been used, sometimes interchangeably, to refer to how closely patients cooperate with, follow, and take personal responsibility for the implementation of their treatment plans. The terms are often used with the more narrow sense of how well patients accomplish the goal of persistently taking medications, and also refer more broadly to all components of treatment. Assess-ment of patients' efforts to accomplish the goals of a treatment plan is essential to treatment success. These efforts occur along a complex spectrum from independent proactive commitment, to mentored collaboration, to passive cooperation, to reluctant partial agreement, to active resistance, and to full refusal. Attempts to understand factors that promote or inhibit adherence/compliance must take into account behaviors, attitudes, willingness, and varying degrees of capacity and autonomy. The term "adherence" emphasizes the patient's collaboration and participation in treatment. It contributes to a greater focus on motivational enhancement approaches that engage and empower patients.[111]

Adolescence: The American Academy of Pediatrics categorizes adolescence as the totality of three developmental stages—puberty to adulthood—which occur generally between 11 and 21 years of age.[71]

Agonist medication: See Opioid agonist medication.

Antagonist medication: See Opioid antagonist medication.

ASAM Criteria dimensions: The ASAM Patient Placement Criteria use six dimensions to create a holistic biopsychosocial assessment of an individual to be used for service planning and treatment. Dimension one is acute intoxication or withdrawal potential. Dimension two is biomedical conditions and conditions. Dimension three is emotional, behavioral, or cognitive conditions or complications. Dimension four is readiness for change. Dimension five is continued use or continued problem potential. Dimension six is recovery/living environment.[111]

Assertive community treatment: An evidence-based, outreach-oriented, service delivery model for people with severe and persistent mental illnesses that uses a team-based model to provide comprehensive and flexible treatment.[13]

Clinician: A health professional, such as a physician, psychiatrist, psychologist, or nurse, involved in clinical practice, as distinguished from one specializing in research.[111]

Cognitive behavioral therapy: An evidence-based psychosocial intervention that seeks to modify harmful beliefs and maladaptive behaviors, and help patients recognize, avoid, and cope with the situations in which they are most likely to misuse drugs.[149]

Co-occurring disorders: Concurrent substance use and mental disorders. Other terms used to describe co-occurring disorders include "dual diagnosis," "dual disorders," "mentally ill chemically addicted" (MICA), "chemically addicted mentally ill" (CAMI), "mentally ill substance abusers" (MISA), "mentally ill chemically dependent" (MICD), "concurrent disorders," "coexisting disorders," "comorbid disorders," and "individuals with co-occurring psychiatric and substance symptomatology" (ICOPSS). Use of the term carries no implication as to which disorder is primary and which secondary, which disorder occurred first, or whether one disorder caused the other.[111]

Compliance (see also Adherence): "To comply" is "to act in accordance with another's wishes, or with rules and regulations" (Webster's Dictionary). The term "compliance" is falling into disuse because patient engagement and responsibility to change is a goal beyond passive compliance. Given the importance of shared decision-making to improve collaboration and outcomes, patients are encouraged to actively participate in treatment decisions and take responsibility for their treatment, rather than to passively comply.[111]

Concomitant conditions: Medical conditions (e.g., HIV, cardiovascular disease) and/or psychiatric conditions (e.g., depression, schizophrenia) that occur along with a substance use disorder.[120]

Contingency management: An evidence-based psychosocial intervention in which patients are given tangible rewards to reinforce positive behaviors such as abstinence. Also referred to as motivational incentives.[149]

Dependence: Used in three different ways: physical dependence is a state of adaptation that is manifested by a drug class-specific withdrawal syndrome that can be produced by abrupt cessation, rapid dose reduction, decreasing blood level of the drug, and/or administration of an antagonist; psychological dependence is a subjective sense of need for a specific psychoactive substance, either for its positive effects or to avoid negative effects associated with its abstinence; and one category of psychoactive substance use disorder in previous editions of the DSM, but not in DSM-5.[111]

Detoxification: Usually used to refer to a process of withdrawing a person from a specific psychoactive substance in a safe and effective manner. The term actually encompasses safe management of intoxication states (more literally, "detoxification") and of withdrawal states. In this document, this term has been replaced by the term Withdrawal Management.[111]

Failure (as in treatment failure): This term is not recommended for use in clinical or research contexts. Lack of progress and/or regression at any given level of care. Such a situation warrants a reassessment of the treatment plan, with modification of the treatment approach. Such situations may require changes in the treatment plan at the same level of care or transfer to a different (more or less intensive) level of care to achieve a better therapeutic response and outcome. Sometimes used to describe relapse after a single treatment episode—an inappropriate construct in describing a chronic disease or disorder. The use of "treatment failure" is therefore not a recommended concept or term to be used.[111]

Harm reduction: A treatment and prevention approach that encompasses individual and public health needs, aiming to decrease the health and socioeconomic costs and consequences of addiction-related problems, especially medical complications and transmission of infectious diseases, without necessarily requiring abstinence. Abstinence-based treatment approaches are themselves a part of comprehensive harm reduction strategies. A range of recovery activities may be included in every harm reduction strategy.[111]

Induction (office and home): The phase of opioid treatment during which maintenance medication dosage levels are adjusted until a patient attains stabilization. Buprenorphine induction may take place in an office-based setting or home-based setting. Methadone induction must take place in an opioid treatment program (OTP).[152]

Illicit opioid (nonmedical drug use): Use of an illicit drug or the use of a prescribed medicine for reasons other than the reasons intended by the prescriber, for example, to produce positive reward or negative reward. Nonmedical use of prescription drugs often includes use of a drug in higher doses than authorized by the prescriber or through a different route of administration than intended by the prescriber, and for a purpose other than the indication intended by the prescriber (e.g. the use of methylphenidate prescribed for attention-deficit/hyperactivity disorder [ADHD] to produce euphoria rather than to reduce symptoms or dysfunction from ADHD).[6]

Maintenance treatment(s): Pharmacotherapy on a consistent schedule for persons with addiction, usually with an agonist or partial agonist, which militates against the pathological pursuit of reward and/or relief and allows remission of overt addiction-related problems.

Maintenance treatments of addiction are associated with the development of a pharmacological steady state in which receptors for addictive substances are occupied, resulting in relative or complete blockade of central nervous system receptors such that addictive substances are no longer sought for reward and/or relief. Maintenance treatments of addiction are also designed to militate against the risk of overdose. Depending on the circumstances of a given case, a care plan including maintenance treatments can be time-limited or can remain in place lifelong. Integration of pharmacotherapy via maintenance treatments with psychosocial treatment generally is associated with the best clinical results. Maintenance treatments can be part of an individual's treatment plan in abstinence-based recovery activities or can be a part of harm reduction strategies.[111]

Moderation management: Moderation management (MM) is a behavioral change program and national support group network for people concerned about their drinking and who desire to make positive lifestyle changes. MM empowers individuals to accept personal responsibility for choosing and maintaining their own path, whether moderation or abstinence. MM promotes early self-recognition of risky drinking behavior, when moderate drinking is a more easily achievable goal.[116]

Motivational interviewing:

(1) Layperson's definition: A collaborative conversation style for strengthening a person's own motivation and commitment to change.

(2) Practitioner's definition: A person-centered counseling style for addressing the common problem of ambivalence about change.

(3) Technical definition: A collaborative, goal-oriented style of communication with particular attention to the language of change. It is designed to strengthen personal motivation for and commitment to a specific goal by eliciting and exploring the person's own reasons for change within an atmosphere of acceptance and compassion.[111]

Naloxone challenge: Naloxone is a short-acting opioid antagonist. Naloxone challenge is a test in which naloxone is administered to patients to evaluate their level of opioid dependence before the commencement of opioid pharmacotherapy.[152,170]

Naltrexone-facilitated opioid withdrawal management: This is a method of withdrawal management. It involves the use of a single dose of buprenorphine combined with multiple small doses of naltrexone over a several day period to manage withdrawal and facilitate the initiation of treatment with naltrexone.[136]

Narcotic drugs: Legally defined by the Controlled Substances Act in the United States since its enactment in 1970. The term "narcotic" is broad and can include drugs produced directly or indirectly by extraction from substances of vegetable origin, or independently by means of chemical synthesis, or by a combination of extraction and chemical synthesis. The main compounds defined as narcotics in the United States include opium opiates, derivatives of opium and opiates, including their isomers, esters, ethers, salts, and salts of isomers, esters, ethers (but not the isoquinoline alkaloids of opium), poppy straw and concentrate of poppy straw, coca leaves, cocaine, its salts, optical and geometric isomers, and salts of isomers and ecgonine, its derivatives, their salts, isomers, and salts of isomers. Any compound, mixture, or preparation which contains any quantity of any of the substances referred to above.[54]

Neuroadaption: See "Tolerance" for the definition.

Office-based opioid treatment (OBOT): Physicians in private practices or a number of types of public sector clinics can be authorized to prescribe outpatient supplies of the partial opioid agonist buprenorphine. There is no regulation per se of the clinic site itself, but of the individual physician who prescribes buprenorphine.[111]

Opiate: One of a group of alkaloids derived from the opium poppy (*Papaver somniferum*), with the ability to induce analgesia, euphoria, and, in higher doses, stupor, coma, and respiratory depression. The term excludes synthetic opioids.[170]

Opioid: A current term for any psychoactive chemical that resembles morphine in pharmacological effects, including opiates and synthetic/semisynthetic agents that exert their effects by binding to highly selective receptors in the brain where morphine and endogenous opioids affect their actions.[6]

Opioid agonist medication: Opioid agonist medications pharmacologically occupy opioid receptors in the body. They thereby relieve withdrawal symptoms and reduce or extinguish cravings for opioids.[111]

Opioid antagonist medication: Opioid antagonist medications pharmacologically occupy opioid receptors in the body, but do not activate the receptors. This effectively blocks the receptor, preventing the brain from responding to opioids. The result is that further use of opioids does not produce euphoria or intoxication.[111]

Opioid intoxication: A condition that follows the administration of opioids, resulting in disturbances in the level of consciousness, cognition, perception, judgment, affect, behavior, or other psychophysiological functions and responses. These disturbances are related to the acute pharmacological effects of, and learned responses to, opioids. With time, these disturbances resolve, resulting in complete recovery, except when tissue damage or other complications have arisen. Intoxication depends on the type and dose of opioid, and is influenced by factors such as an individual's level of tolerance. Individuals often take drugs in the quantity required to achieve a desired degree of intoxication. Behavior resulting from a given level of intoxication is strongly influenced by cultural and personal expectations about the effects of the drug. According to the International Classifications of Diseases, Tenth Revision (ICD-10), acute intoxication is the term used for intoxication of clinical significance (F11.0). Complications may include trauma, inhalation of vomitus, delirium, coma, and convulsions, depending on the substance and method of administration.[170]

Opioid treatment program (OTP): A program certified by the United States, Substance Abuse and Mental Health Services Administration (SAMHSA), usually comprising a facility, staff, administration, patients, and services, that engages in supervised assessment and treatment, using methadone, buprenorphine, L-alpha acetyl methadol, or naltrexone, of individuals who are addicted to opioids. An OTP can exist in a number of settings including, but not limited to, intensive outpatient, residential, and hospital settings. Services may include medically supervised withdrawal and/or maintenance treatment, along with various levels of medical, psychiatric, psychosocial, and other types of supportive care.[152]

Opioid treatment services (OTS): An umbrella term that encompasses a variety of pharmacological and nonpharmacological treatment modalities. This term broadens understanding of opioid treatments to include all medications used to treat opioid use disorders and the psychosocial treatment that is offered concurrently with these pharmacotherapies. Pharmacological agents include opioid agonist medications such as methadone and buprenorphine, and opioid antagonist medications such as naltrexone.[111]

Opioid use disorder: A substance use disorder involving opioids. See Substance Use Disorder.

Opioid withdrawal syndrome: Over time, morphine and its analogs induce tolerance and neuroadaptive changes that are responsible for rebound hyperexcitability when the drug is withdrawn. The withdrawal syndrome includes craving, anxiety, dysphoria, yawning, sweating, piloerection (gooseflesh), lacrimation (excessive tear formation), rhinorrhea (running nose), insomnia, nausea or vomiting, diarrhea, cramps, muscle aches, and fever. With short-acting drugs, such as morphine or heroin, withdrawal symptoms may appear within 8–12 hours of the last dose of the drug, reach a peak at 48–72 hours, and clear after 7–10 days. With longer-acting drugs, such as methadone, onset of withdrawal symptoms may not occur until 1–3 days after the last dose; symptoms peak between the third and eighth day and may persist for several weeks, but are generally milder than those that follow morphine or heroin withdrawal after equivalent doses.[170]

Overdose: The inadvertent or deliberate consumption of a dose much larger than that either habitually used by the individual or ordinarily used for treatment of an illness, and likely to result in a serious toxic reaction or death.[111]

Patient: As used in this document, an individual receiving alcohol, tobacco, and/or other drug or addictive disorder treatment. The terms "client" and "patient" sometimes are used interchangeably, although staff in nonmedical settings more commonly refer to "clients."[111]

Physical dependence: State of physical adaptation that is manifested by a drug class-specific withdrawal syndrome that can be produced by abrupt cessation, rapid dose reduction and/or decreasing blood level of a substance and/or administration of an antagonist.[152]

Psychosocial treatment: Any nonpharmacological intervention carried out in a therapeutic context at an individual, family, or group level. Psychosocial interventions may include structured, professionally administered interventions (e.g., cognitive behavior therapy or insight-oriented psychotherapy) or nonprofessional interventions (e.g., self-help groups and nonpharmacological interventions from traditional healers).[13]

Precipitated withdrawal: A condition that occurs when an opioid agonist is displaced from the opioid receptors by an antagonist. It is also possible for a partial agonist to precipitate withdrawal.[170]

Recovery: A process of sustained action that addresses the biological, psychological, social, and spiritual disturbances inherent in addiction. This effort is in the direction of a consistent pursuit of abstinence, addressing impairment in behavioral control, dealing with cravings, recognizing problems in one's behaviors and interpersonal relationships, and dealing more effectively with emotional responses. Recovery actions lead to reversal of negative, self-defeating internal processes and behaviors, allowing healing of relationships with self and others. The concepts of humility, acceptance, and surrender are useful in this process. (Note: ASAM continues to explore, as an evolving process, improved ways to define Recovery.)[111]

Relapse: A process in which an individual who has established abstinence or sobriety experiences recurrence of signs and symptoms of active addiction, often including resumption of the pathological pursuit of reward and/or relief through the use of substances and other behaviors. When in relapse, there is often disengagement from recovery activities. Relapse can be triggered by exposure to rewarding substances and behaviors, by exposure to environmental cues to use, and by exposure to emotional stressors that trigger heightened activity in brain stress circuits. The event of using or acting out is the latter part of the process, which can be prevented by early intervention.[111]

Sedative, hypnotic, or anxiolytics: This class of substances includes all prescription sleeping medications and virtually all prescription antianxiety medications. Nonbenzodiazepine antianxiety medications, such as buspirone and gepirone, are not included in this class because they are not associated with significant misuse.[160]

Sobriety: A state of sustained abstinence with a clear commitment to and active seeking of balance in the biological, psychological, social, and spiritual aspects of an individual's health and wellness that were previously compromised by active addiction.[111]

Spontaneous withdrawal: A condition that occurs when an individual who is physically dependent on an opioid agonist suddenly discontinues or markedly decreases opioid use.[158]

Stabilization: Includes the medical and psychosocial processes of assisting the patient through acute intoxication and withdrawal to the attainment of a medically stable, fully supported, substance-free state. This often is done with the assistance of medications, although in some approaches to detoxification, no medication is used.[152]

Substance use disorder: Substance use disorder is marked by a cluster of cognitive, behavioral, and physiological symptoms indicating that the individual continues to use alcohol, tobacco, and/or other drugs despite significant related problems. Diagnostic criteria are given in the DSM-5. Substance use disorder is the new nomenclature for what was included as substance dependence and substance abuse in the DSM-IV.[6]

Tolerance: A decrease in response to a drug dose that occurs with continued use. If an individual is tolerant to a drug, increased doses are required to achieve the effects originally produced by lower doses. Both physiological and psychosocial factors may contribute to the development of tolerance. Physiological factors include metabolic and functional tolerance. In metabolic tolerance, the body can eliminate the substance more readily, because the substance is metabolized at an increased rate. In functional tolerance, the central nervous system is less sensitive to the substance. An example of a psychosocial factor contributing to tolerance is behavioral tolerance, when learning or altered environmental constraints change the effect of the drug. Acute tolerance refers to rapid, temporary accommodation to the effect of a substance after a single dose. Reverse tolerance, also known as sensitization, refers to a condition in which the response to a substance increased with repeated use. Tolerance is one of the criteria of the dependence syndrome.[170]

Withdrawal management: Withdrawal management describes services to assist a patient's withdrawal. The liver detoxifies, but clinicians manage withdrawal.[118]

Introduction

Purpose

The American Society of Addiction Medicine (ASAM) developed the National Practice Guideline for the Use of Medications in the Treatment of Addiction Involving Opioid Use (the "Practice Guideline") to provide information on evidence-based treatment of opioid use disorder. This guideline is intended to assist clinicians in the decision-making process for prescribing pharmacotherapies and psychosocial treatments to patients with opioid use disorder.

Specifically, the Practice Guideline helps in the following:
(1) Identifies current practices and outstanding questions regarding the safe and effective use of medications for the treatment of opioid use disorder.
(2) Uses a methodology that integrates evidence-based practices and expert clinical judgment to develop recommendations on best practices in opioid use disorder treatment.
(3) Presents best practices in a cohesive document for clinicians' use to improve the effectiveness of opioid use disorder treatment.

Background on Opioid Use Disorder

Opioid use disorder is a chronic, relapsing disease, which has significant economic, personal, and public health consequences. Many readers of this Practice Guideline may recognize the term "opioid use disorder" as it is used in the *Diagnostic and Statistical Manual of Mental Disorders, Fifth Edition* (DSM-5) developed by the American Psychiatric Association; others may be more familiar with the term "opioid dependence," as used in previous editions of the DSM.

The ASAM defines addiction as "a primary, chronic disease of brain reward, motivation, memory, and related circuitry," with a "dysfunction in these circuits" being reflected in "an individual pathologically pursuing reward and/or relief of withdrawal symptoms by substance use and other behaviors." In this context, the preferred term by ASAM for this serious bio-psycho-social-spiritual illness would be "addiction involving opioid use." ASAM views addiction as a fundamental neurological disorder of "brain reward, motivation, memory, and related circuitry," and recognizes that there are unifying features in all cases of addiction, including substance-related addiction and nonsubstance-related addiction. It is clear that a variety of substances commonly associated with addiction work on specific receptors in the nervous system and on specific neurotransmitter systems. Specific pharmacological agents used in the treatment of addiction exert their effects via their actions on specific receptors. Hence, the medications used in the treatment of addiction have specific efficacy based on their own molecular structure and the particular neurotransmitters affected by that medication. Medications developed for the treatment of addiction involving opioid use may have benefits in the treatment of addiction involving an individual's use of other substances. For instance, naltrexone (US Food and Drug Administration [FDA]), for the treatment of opioid dependence using DSM, Fourth Edition (DSM-IV) terminology, is also FDA-approved for the treatment of alcohol dependence, as per the DSM-IV guidelines.

The ASAM recognizes that research is yet to be done to confirm the specificity of its conceptualization of addiction as a medical and a psychiatric illness (note: the International Classification of Diseases-10 [ICD-10], and the American Medical Association in various policy and position statements recognize addiction as both a medical and a psychiatric disorder). ASAM encourages clinicians, researchers, educators, and policymakers to use the term "addiction" regardless of whether the patient's condition at a given point in its natural history appears to more prominently involve opioid use or alcohol use, nicotine use, or engagement in addictive behaviors such as gambling. Given the widespread North American application of the DSM's categorization of disorders, this Practice Guideline will for the sake of brevity and convention, use the term "opioid use disorder."

Epidemiology

According to the 2013 National Survey on Drug Use and Health (NSDUH),[146] 4.5 million individuals were current nonmedical users of prescription opioids (past month) and 1.9 million individuals met DSM-IV criteria for abuse or dependence of prescription opioids. In addition, the NSDUH reported that 289,000 people were current (past month) users of heroin and 517,000 met DSM IV criteria for abuse or dependence in 2013. The rate of prescription opioid use for nonmedical purposes was 1.7% in persons 12 years and older. However, the rate of prescription opioid use among youth aged 12–17 declined from 3.2% in 2002 and 2003 to 1.7% in 2013.

It is important to note that nonmedical use of prescription opioids has been shown to be associated with the initiation of heroin use. In a study pooling data from the NSDUH from 2002 to 2012, the incidence of heroin use was 19 times greater among individuals who reported prior nonmedical use of prescription opioids compared to individuals who did not report prior nonmedical prescription opioid use.[117]

Mortality and Morbidity

Opioid use is associated with increased mortality. The leading causes of death in people using opioids for nonmedical purposes are overdose and trauma.[50] The number of unintentional overdose deaths from prescription opioids has more than quadrupled since 1999.[127]

Opioid use increases the risk of exposure to HIV, viral hepatitis, and other infectious agents through contact with infected blood or body fluids (e.g., semen) that results from sharing syringes and injection paraphernalia, or through unprotected sexual contact. Similarly, it increases the risk of contracting infectious diseases such as HIV/AIDS and hepatitis because people under the influence of drugs may engage in risky behaviors that can expose them to these diseases.[50]

It is notable that injection drug use (IDU) is the highest-risk behavior for acquiring hepatitis C virus (HCV) infection and continues to drive this epidemic. Of the 17,000 new HCV infections in the United States in 2010, more than half (53%) involved IDU. In 2010, hepatitis B virus (HBV) infection rates were estimated to be 20% higher among people who engaged in IDU in the United States.[123]

Scope of Guideline

This Practice Guideline was developed to assist in the evaluation and treatment of opioid use disorder. Although there are existing guidelines for the treatment of opioid use disorder, none have included all of the medications used for its treatment at present. Moreover, few of the existing guidelines address the needs of special populations such as pregnant women, individuals with co-occurring psychiatric disorders, individuals with pain, adolescents, or individuals involved in the criminal justice system.

Overall, the Practice Guideline contains recommendations for the evaluation and treatment of opioid use disorder, opioid withdrawal management, psychosocial treatment, special populations, and opioid overdose.

(1) Part 1: Contains guidelines on the evaluation of opioid use disorder

(2) Part 2: Provides recommendations regarding treatment options

(3) Part 3: Describes the treatment of opioid withdrawal

(4) Parts 4–6: Provide guidelines on medications for treating opioid use disorder

(5) Part 7: Describes psychosocial treatment used in conjunction with medications

(6) Parts 8–12: Provide guidelines for treating special populations and circumstances

(7) Part 13: Describes the use of naloxone in treating opioid overdose

Included and Excluded Medications

The medications covered in this guideline include the following:

(1) Methadone (Part 4)

(2) Buprenorphine (Part 5)

(3) Naltrexone in oral and extended-release injectable formulations (Part 6)

(4) Naloxone (Part 13)

All of these medications act directly upon the opioid receptors, particularly the mu-subtype. Methadone is a mu-receptor agonist; buprenorphine is a partial mu-receptor agonist; and naltrexone is an antagonist. Naloxone is a fast-acting antagonist used to reverse opioid overdose, a condition that may be life-threatening. Because of the differing actions of these medications at the receptor level, they can have very different clinical effects during treatment.

Other medications show promise for the treatment of opioid use disorder; however, there is insufficient evidence at this writing to make a full analysis of their effectiveness. For example, whereas not FDA-approved for opioid withdrawal syndrome in the United States, it is recognized that clonidine, an alpha-2 adrenergic agonist, has been in use in clinical settings for 25 years. Lofexidine (known as BritLofex, Britannia Pharmaceuticals) is approved for treating opioid withdrawal use in the United Kingdom. Because of their long history of off-label use in the United States, clonidine and buprenorphine are described for opioid withdrawal syndrome in this Practice Guideline. Again, there are other off-label medications for withdrawal management in the treatment of opioid use disorder (e.g., tramadol) that have been excluded from this guideline because there is insufficient evidence to make a full analysis of their effectiveness or consensus recommendations for their use at this time.

The ASAM recognizes that withdrawal management and withdrawal management medications could be potential topics for future guideline development. ASAM will regularly review its published guidelines to determine when partial or full updates are needed. The emergence of newly approved medications and new research will be considered as part of this process. It is also recognized that ASAM may develop guidelines or consensus documents on topics addressed in this Practice Guideline (e.g., urine drug testing). If that occurs before any update to this Practice Guideline, it is to be assumed that the recommendations in the latter documents will take precedence until this Practice Guideline is updated.

Intended Audience

This Practice Guideline is intended for all clinicians, at any level, involved in evaluating for, and/or providing, opioid use disorder treatment in the United States. The intended audience falls into the following broad groups:

(1) Physicians involved in the assessment, diagnosis, and treatment of opioid use disorder. General practice physicians (including family practitioners, pediatricians, obstetricians,

and gynecologists) are often first-line providers of medical care related to opioid use disorder and are a key audience for the guideline.

(2) Clinicians involved with the completion of health assessments and delivery of health services to special populations.

(3) Clinicians involved in making an initial assessment and offering psychosocial treatments in conjunction with medications to treat opioid use disorder.

(4) Clinical case managers responsible for clinical care support, coordination of health-related and social services, and tracking of patient adherence to the treatment plan.

Qualifying Statement

The ASAM Practice Guideline is intended to aid clinicians in their clinical decision-making and patient management. It strives to identify and define clinical decision-making junctures that meet the needs of most patients in most circumstances. The ultimate judgment about care of a particular patient must be made together by the clinician and the patient in light of all the circumstances presented by the patient. As a result, situations may arise in which deviations from the Practice Guideline may be appropriate. Clinical decision-making should involve consideration of the quality and availability of expertise and services in the community wherein care is provided.

In circumstances in which the Practice Guideline is being used as the basis for regulatory or payer decisions, improvement in quality of care should be the goal. Finally, prescribed courses of treatment contained in recommendations in this Practice Guideline are effective only if the recommendations, as outlined, are followed. Because lack of patient understanding and adherence may adversely affect outcomes, clinicians should make every effort to engage the patient's understanding of, and adherence to, prescribed and recommended pharmacological and psychosocial treatments. Patients should be informed of the risks, benefits, and alternatives to a particular treatment and should be shared parties to decision-making whenever feasible. Recommendations in this Practice Guideline do not supersede any federal or state regulation.

Methodology

Overview of Approach

These guidelines were developed using the RAND/UCLA Appropriateness Method (RAM)—a process that combines scientific evidence and clinical knowledge to determine the appropriateness of a set of clinical procedures.[64] This process is particularly appropriate for these guidelines for two reasons. First, there are very few randomized clinical trials directly comparing the approved medications for the treatment of opioid use disorder. Second, evidence supporting the efficacy of the individual medications reflects varying years of research and varying levels of evidence (e.g., nonrandomized studies, retrospective studies). The randomized clinical trial (RCT) is the gold standard for evidence-based medicine. When data are lacking from RCT, other methods must be used to help clinicians make the best choices. In addition, these guidelines are unique in that they include all three of the medications approved at present by the FDA in multiple formulations, and they address the needs of special populations such as pregnant women, individuals with pain, adolescents, individuals with co-occurring psychiatric disorder, and individuals in criminal justice. Such special populations are often excluded from RCTs, making the use of RCT data even more

difficult. The RAM process combines the best available scientific evidence combined with the collective judgment of experts to yield statements about the appropriateness of specific procedures that clinicians can apply to their everyday practice.

The ASAM's Quality Improvement Council (QIC) was the oversight committee for the guideline development. The QIC appointed a Guideline Committee to participate throughout the development process, rate treatment scenarios, and assist in writing. In selecting the committee members, the QIC made every effort to avoid actual, potential, or perceived conflicts of interest that may arise as a result of relationships with industry and other entities among members of the Guideline Committee. All QIC members, committee members, and external reviewers of the guideline were required to disclose all current related relationships, which are presented in Appendixes III, IV, and V.

The Guideline Committee comprised 10 experts and researchers from multiple disciplines, medical specialties, and subspecialties, including academic research, internal medicine, family medicine, addiction medicine, addiction psychiatry, general psychiatry, obstetrics/gynecology, and clinical neurobiology. Physicians with both allopathic and osteopathic training were represented in the Guideline Committee. The Guideline Committee was assisted by a technical team of researchers from the Treatment Research Institute (TRI) affiliated with the University of Pennsylvania, and worked under the guidance of Dr. Kyle Kampman who led the TRI team as Principal Investigator in implementing the RAM.

The RAM process is a deliberate approach encompassing review of existing guidelines, literature reviews, appropriateness ratings, necessity reviews, and document development. The steps are summarized in the flow chart in "Exhibit 1: Methodology."

Task 1: Review of Existing Guidelines

Review of Existing Clinical Guidelines

All existing clinical guidelines that addressed the use of medications and psychosocial treatments in the treatment of opioid use disorders including special populations (e.g., pregnant women, individuals with pain, and adolescents), and that were published during the period from January 2000 to April 2014, were identified and reviewed. In total, 49 guidelines were identified and 34 were ultimately included in the analysis. See "Appendix I" for a list of the guidelines that were reviewed. The included guidelines offered evidence-based recommendations for the treatment of opioid use disorder using methadone, buprenorphine, naltrexone, and/or naloxone.

The majority of existing clinical guidelines are based on systematic reviews of the literature including appropriateness criteria used in the RAM. Therefore, the aim of this exercise was not to re-review all of the research literature, but to identify within the existing clinical guidelines how they addressed common questions or considerations that clinicians are likely to raise in the course of deciding whether and how to use medications as part of the treatment of individuals with opioid use disorder.

Analysis of Clinical Guidelines

On the basis of the previously reviewed existing clinical guidelines, an analytic table was created and populated to display the identified key components. This table served as the foundation for development of hypothetical statements. The hypothetical statements were sentences describing recommendations derived from the analysis of the clinical guidelines.

Preparation of Literature Review on Psychosocial Interventions

A review of the literature on the efficacy of psychosocial treatment delivered in conjunction with medications for the treatment of opioid use disorder was conducted. This review was partially supported by funding from the National Institute on Drug Abuse (NIDA). Articles were identified for inclusion in the review through searches conducted in two bibliographic databases (e.g., PsycINFO and PubMed) using predefined search terms and established selection criteria. Titles and abstracts were reviewed for inclusion by two members of the research team.

To increase the overall relevance of the review, the search was limited to articles in the 6-year period from 2008 to the present. In the event that the article reflected a secondary analysis of data from a relevant study, the original study was included in the literature review. In addition, findings from three prominent systematic reviews (i.e., 2007 review on psychosocial interventions in pharmacotherapy of opioid dependence prepared for the Technical Development Group for the World Health Organization, "Guidelines for Psychosocially Assisted Pharmacotherapy of Opioid Dependence," and two 2011 Cochrane reviews examining psychosocial and pharmacological treatments for opioid withdrawal management and psychosocial interventions combined with agonist treatment) were summarized.[4,5,55]

The literature search yielded 938 articles. The titles and abstracts were reviewed to determine if the study met the inclusion/exclusion criteria, and those that did not (*n* = 787) were removed. The remaining 151 articles were then reviewed for inclusion, and 27 articles were ultimately retained for use in the literature review, as the others did not meet the predetermined inclusion/exclusion criteria. These articles, along with the relevant systematic reviews of the literature, are described in the literature review in the next section.

Task 2: Identification of Hypothetical Statements and Appropriateness Rating

RAND/UCLA Appropriateness Method

The first step in the RAM is to develop a set of hypothetical statements, which were derived from the guideline analysis and literature review described in the previous section, for appropriateness rating.

The analysis and literature review generated a list of 245 hypothetical statements that reflected recommended medical or psychosocial treatment. Each member of the Guideline Committee reviewed the guideline analysis and literature review, and privately rated 245 hypothetical clinical statements on a nine-point scale of "appropriateness." In the context of this Practice Guideline, the meaning of appropriateness was defined as:

> *A statement, procedure or treatment is considered to be appropriate if the expected health benefit (e.g., increased life expectancy, relief of pain, reduction in anxiety, improved functional capacity) exceeds the expected negative consequences (e.g., mortality, morbidity, anxiety, pain) by a sufficiently wide margin that the procedure is worth doing, exclusive of cost.*

An appropriateness score of 1 meant that the statement was "highly inappropriate." An appropriateness rating of 9 meant that the statement was "highly appropriate." These appropriateness statements were meant to identify a lack of consensus in existing guidelines and research literature.

Guideline Committee Meeting

Upon completion and collection of the individual Guideline Committee member ratings, 201 of the 245 hypothetical statements were identified as meeting the criteria for consensus. The remaining 44 statements had divergent ratings. On September 15, 2014, the Guideline Committee met in Washington, District of Columbia, to discuss the hypothetical clinical statements. At this meeting, the committee came to consensus on the hypothetical statements. After the meeting, the information gathered was used to revise several of the statements; and the Guideline Committee was asked to re-rate the revised statements.

Literature Review

A supplementary literature review was also conducted to identify relevant studies that might resolve statements that had resulted in divergent ratings during the Guideline Committee meeting. Information relating to the vast majority of these divergent ratings was subsequently found within the existing guideline data set, and consequently included in the first draft of the Practice Guideline.

For the topics and questions for which answers were not found in the existing guideline data set, a full literature review was conducted. The topics and questions for which no further clarification was found in the literature were considered "gaps" that require additional research before inclusion in this guideline. These gaps in the literature were: urine drug testing; patients using marijuana; the safety of delivering injectable naltrexone doses to patients with high metabolism every 3 weeks; and the safety of adding full agonists to treatment with buprenorphine for pain management.

Creation and Revision of Guideline Outline

All the identified appropriate/uncertain hypothetical statements and supporting research were incorporated into an outline defining each specific section to be included in the final Practice Guideline. The draft outline, review of existing guidelines, and literature review were all sent to the Guideline Committee members for review and discussion during two web teleconferences and through private communication. Two teleconferences were held to ensure full participation from members of the Guideline Committee.

Task 3: Comparative Analysis, Review, and Necessity Rating

Committee Review and Rating

The Guideline Committee then re-rated the 211 "appropriate" hypothetical statements for necessity. When rating for necessity, the Guideline Committee members were asked to adhere to the following guidance:

A statement was considered necessary when all the following criteria were met:

(1) It would be considered improper care not to provide this service.
(2) Reasonable chance exists that this procedure and/or service will benefit the patient. (A procedure could be appropriate if it had a low likelihood of benefit, but few risks; however, such procedures would not be necessary.)
(3) The benefit to the patient is of significance and certainty. (A procedure could be appropriate if it had a minor but almost certain benefit, but it would not be necessary.)

Necessity is a more stringent criterion than appropriateness. If a procedure is necessary, this means that the expected benefits outweigh the expected harms (i.e., it is appropriate), and that they do so by such a margin that the physician must recommend the service. Of course, patients may decline to follow their physician's recommendations.[64]

Of the 211 rated statements, 184 hypothetical statements met the criteria for being both appropriate and necessary, and were incorporated in the guideline.

Final Draft Outline

The final draft outline highlighted hypothetical statements that had been determined to rise to the level of necessity.

Task 4: Drafting the National Practice Guideline

Draft and Review

A first draft of the Practice Guideline was created using the Guideline Committee's recommendations resulting from supporting evidence and the appropriateness and necessity ratings discussed above. The first draft of the Practice Guideline was sent to the Guideline Committee for review and electronic comment. During a subsequent teleconference in January 2015, the Guideline Committee discussed the comments received via first review. Revisions were made to the draft, which went again through subsequent reviews by the Guideline Committee and the ASAM Quality Council throughout February and March 2015.

Task 5: External Review

External Review

The ASAM sought input from ASAM members—patients and caregiver groups, stakeholders including experts from criminal justice system, government agencies, other professional societies, and hospitals and health systems. ASAM also made the document and a qualitative review guide available to ASAM members and the general public for a one week period of review and comment. The final draft Practice Guideline was submitted to the ASAM Board of Directors in April 2015.

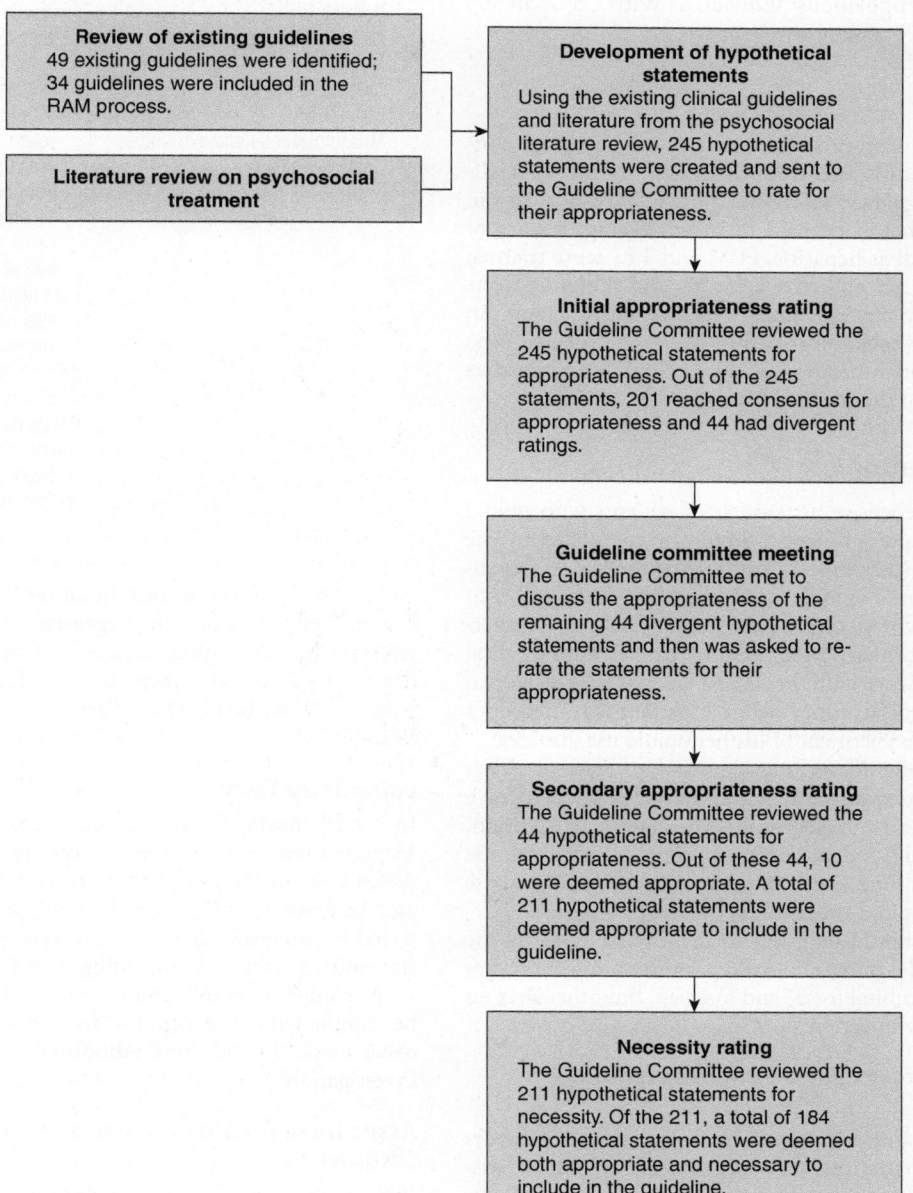

Review of existing guidelines
49 existing guidelines were identified; 34 guidelines were included in the RAM process.

Literature review on psychosocial treatment

Development of hypothetical statements
Using the existing clinical guidelines and literature from the psychosocial literature review, 245 hypothetical statements were created and sent to the Guideline Committee to rate for their appropriateness.

Initial appropriateness rating
The Guideline Committee reviewed the 245 hypothetical statements for appropriateness. Out of the 245 statements, 201 reached consensus for appropriateness and 44 had divergent ratings.

Guideline committee meeting
The Guideline Committee met to discuss the appropriateness of the remaining 44 divergent hypothetical statements and then was asked to re-rate the statements for their appropriateness.

Secondary appropriateness rating
The Guideline Committee reviewed the 44 hypothetical statements for appropriateness. Out of these 44, 10 were deemed appropriate. A total of 211 hypothetical statements were deemed appropriate to include in the guideline.

Necessity rating
The Guideline Committee reviewed the 211 hypothetical statements for necessity. Of the 211, a total of 184 hypothetical statements were deemed both appropriate and necessary to include in the guideline.

Exhibit 1: Methodology

Part 1: Assessment and Diagnosis of Opioid Use Disorder

Comprehensive Assessment

The ASAM *Standards of Care for the Addiction Specialist Physician* (the "ASAM Standards") describe the importance of comprehensive assessment. Although the assessment process is ongoing for the patient with substance use disorder, a comprehensive assessment is "a critical aspect of patient engagement and treatment planning" and should be conducted during the initial phase of treatment.[118]

The assessment is not necessarily the first visit; it is critical, however, to determine emergent or urgent medical problems. Patients with opioid use disorder often have other physiological or psychiatric conditions that may complicate their treatment. These concomitant medical and psychiatric conditions may need immediate attention and require transfer to a higher level of care (see "Part 11: Special Populations: Individuals With Co-occurring Psychiatric Disorders.")

Medical History

The patient's medical history should include screening for concomitant medical conditions and routine identification of medications, allergies, pregnancy, family medical history, and so on. Particular attention should be paid to the following: history of infectious diseases such as hepatitis, HIV, and TB; acute trauma; psychiatric, substance use, addictive behavior, and addiction treatment history; and any previous history of pharmacotherapy. An intake of the patient's social history and assessment of readiness for change including identification of any facilitators and barriers are also components of the medical history.

Physical Examination

As part of the comprehensive assessment of patients with opioid use disorder, a physical examination should be completed by the prescriber him/herself (the clinician authorizing the use of a medication for the treatment of opioid use disorder), another member of the clinician's health system, or the prescribing physician. Furthermore, the responsible clinician should assure that a current physical examination (in accordance with the ASAM Standards) is contained within the patient medical record before a patient is started on a new medication for the treatment of his/her opioid use disorder.

The examination should include identifying objective physical signs of opioid intoxication or withdrawal. See Table 1 for a list of common signs of intoxication or withdrawal. In addition, the examination should evaluate objective signs of substance use disorders. See Table 2 for a list of physical signs of substance use disorders (including opioid use disorder).

Special attention should be given to identifying IDU by the presence of new or older puncture marks. Common injection sites are inside the elbow (cubital fossa) and forearm, but other sites on the extremities may be injection sites.

Assessment and History Considerations Specific to Females

Use of contraception and determination of pregnancy are factors in choosing treatment options for women with opioid use disorder. Contraception and reproductive health are topics of discussion within the assessment process of female patients who are considering opioid use disorder treatment. Clinicians and female

TABLE A3.1	Common Signs of Opioid Intoxication and Withdrawal.
Intoxication Signs	**Withdrawal Signs**
Drooping eyelids	Restlessness, irritability, anxiety
Constricted pupils	Insomnia
Reduced respiratory rate	Yawning
Scratching (due to histamine release)	Abdominal cramps, diarrhea, vomiting
Head nodding	Dilated pupils
	Sweating
	Piloerection

TABLE A3.2	Objective Physical Signs in Substance Use Disorders.
System	**Findings**
Dermatologic	Abscesses, rashes, cellulitis, thrombosed veins, jaundice, scars, track marks, pock marks from skin popping
Ear, nose, throat, and eyes	
Mouth	
Cardiovascular	
Respiratory	Pupils pinpoint or dilated, yellow sclera, conjunctivitis, ruptured eardrums, otitis media, discharge from ears, rhinorrhea, rhinitis, excoriation or perforation of nasal septum, epistaxis, sinusitis, hoarseness, or laryngitis
Musculoskeletal and extremities	
Gastrointestinal	
	Poor dentition, gum disease, abscesses
	Murmurs, arrhythmias
	Asthma, dyspnea, rales, chronic cough, hematemesis
	Pitting edema, broken bones, traumatic amputations, burns on fingers
	Hepatomegaly, hernias

patients should keep in mind that fertility increases as treatment becomes effective. Case management plans may need to include referral to gynecological services for female patients. An in-depth discussion of the treatment of opioid use disorder in pregnant women is described later in "Part 8: Special Populations: Pregnant Women."

Laboratory Tests

Initial lab testing should include hepatitis C and HIV testing. Hepatitis serology and vaccination are recommended. Hepatitis A and B testing and vaccination should be offered when appropriate. As above, women of childbearing potential and age should be tested for pregnancy. Tuberculosis testing and testing for sexually transmitted infections, including syphilis, may be considered.

A complete blood count and liver function study should be conducted to screen for liver dysfunction, infection, and other medical conditions. Abnormal results may require further investigation.

Assessment for Mental Health Status and Psychiatric Disorder

Patients being evaluated for opioid use disorder, and/or for possible medication use in the treatment of opioid use disorder, should undergo an evaluation of possible co-occurring psychiatric disorders. During the assessment process and physical examination, it is important for the clinician to assess for mental health status consistent with the ASAM Standards.

In the ASAM Standards, I.1 indicates that the physician "assures that an initial comprehensive, multicomponent assessment is performed for each patient, either by performing it her/himself or by assuring it is conducted in full or in part by another qualified professional within the system in which she/he is working." A thorough medical and psychiatric history and family history is indicated as a component of this same standard. Patients who are determined as exhibiting urgent or emergent psychiatric conditions, or who are psychiatrically unstable and represent a danger to themselves or others, should be referred to the appropriate level of care for their safety and the safety of others. Further specialty evaluation may be warranted depending on severity of indicators for psychiatric instability. Indicators of psychiatric instability or disorder include acute suicidal or homicidal ideation, acute psychosis, and delirium.

Assessment for Alcohol and Substance Use and Treatment History

A careful evaluation of current and past use of alcohol and drugs, including nonmedical use of prescription medications, is required to diagnose opioid use disorder. Because opioid use disorder may co-occur with other use disorders, the evaluator should assess frequency and quantity of use.

Completing a history of opioid drug use with a patient who has been identified as using opioids should focus on the following:
(1) type and amount of opioid(s) used recently;
(2) route of administration;
(3) last use;
(4) treatment history; and
(5) problems resulting from drug use.

The amount of drug being consumed will impact the likelihood and severity of withdrawal symptoms when the drug is stopped, so it is useful to obtain an estimate of the amount used (each time and number of times per day).

Prescription Drug Monitoring Programs (PDMPs) offer information about prescription opioid use. They can serve as important resources for clinicians' use in completing full patient clinical assessments of opiate and other controlled substance use history, and it is recommended that they be utilized. It is recognized, as detailed in "Exhibit 2: Prescription Drug Monitoring Programs," that there is variation across states in terms of the level of operation of these programs, the extent of their data sharing across states, and state requirements for their use before prescribing controlled substances.

In addition, a history of outpatient and inpatient treatment for alcohol and other substance use disorders should be collected. Clinicians should ask for information about the type and duration of treatment and outcomes.

Assessment for Co-Occurring Alcohol and Substance Use

Opioid use disorder often co-occurs with alcohol and other substance use disorders. Therefore, evaluation of co-occurring alcohol and substance use is recommended.

Clinicians should assess signs and symptoms of alcohol or sedative, hypnotic, or anxiolytic intoxication or withdrawal. Alcohol or sedative, hypnotic, or anxiolytic withdrawal may result in seizures, hallucinosis, or delirium, and may represent a medical emergency. Likewise, concomitant use of alcohol and sedatives, hypnotics, or anxiolytics with opioids may contribute to respiratory depression.

Patients with significant co-occurring substance use disorders, especially severe alcohol or sedative, hypnotic, or anxiolytic use, may require a higher level of care.

An evaluation of past and current substance use should be conducted, and a determination as to whether addiction involving other substances or other behaviors is present. For instance, the regular use of marijuana or cannabinoids, tobacco or electronic nicotine delivery devices, or other drugs should not be a reason to suspend medication use in the treatment of addiction involving opioid use. Concurrent use of other drugs or active engagement in other addictive behaviors should lead to consideration of other treatment plan components for the patient. The presence of co-occurring substance use disorders should provoke a re-evaluation of the level of care that is in place for psychosocial treatment, along with pharmacological therapy. In most cases, co-occurring drug use will not represent a medical emergency. In such cases, patients can be treated for both their opioid use disorder and co-occurring alcohol or substance use disorders. However, ongoing use of other drugs may lead to poorer treatment outcomes. Evidence does demonstrate that individuals who are actively using other substances during opioid use disorder treatment have a poorer prognosis.[66,99,128]

The Guideline Committee cautioned against excluding patients from treatment for their opioid use disorder because they are using marijuana or other psychoactive substances that do not interact with opioids, and that are not prescribed by their physician. Whereas there is a paucity of research examining this topic, evidence demonstrates that patients under treatment have better outcomes than those not retained under treatment.[82,108]

Suspension of opioid use disorder treatment may increase the risk for death from overdose, accidents, or other health problems. However, continued use of marijuana or other psychoactive substances may impede treatment for opioid use disorder; thus, an approach emphasizing cessation of all unprescribed substances is likely to result in the best results. Further research is needed on the outcomes of patients in opioid use disorder treatment who are continuing the nonmedical use of psychoactive substances.

Assessment for Tobacco Use

Tobacco use should be queried, and the benefits of cessation should be promoted routinely with patients presenting for evaluation and treatment of opioid use disorder. Several studies have demonstrated that smoking cessation improves long-term outcomes among individuals receiving treatment for substance use disorders.[15,129,157]

Assessment of Social and Environmental Factors

Clinicians should conduct an assessment of social and environmental factors (as outlined in the ASAM Standards) to identify facilitators and barriers to addiction treatment and specifically to pharmacotherapy. Before a decision is made to initiate a course of pharmacotherapy for the patient with opioid use disorder, the patient should receive a multidimensional assessment in fidelity with the ASAM Criteria: Treatment Criteria for Addictive, Substance-Related, and Co-occurring Conditions (the "ASAM Criteria"). The ASAM Patient Placement Criteria uses six dimensions to create a holistic biopsychosocial assessment of an individual to be used for service planning and treatment. Dimension one is acute intoxication or withdrawal potential. Dimension two is biomedical conditions and conditions. Dimension three is emotional, behavioral, or cognitive conditions or complications. Dimension four is readiness for change. Dimension five is continued use or continued problem potential. Dimension six is recovery/living environment.[111]

The use of medications for the patient with addiction involving opioid use can be appropriate across all levels of care. Pharmacotherapy is not a "level of care" in addiction treatment, but one component of multidisciplinary treatment. Whereas medication as a standalone intervention has been utilized in North America and internationally, ASAM recommends that the use of medications in the treatment of addiction be part of a broad bio-psycho-social-spiritual intervention appropriate to the patient's needs and to the resources available in the patient's community. Addiction should be considered a bio-psycho-social-spiritual illness, for which the use of medication(s) is but only one component of overall treatment.

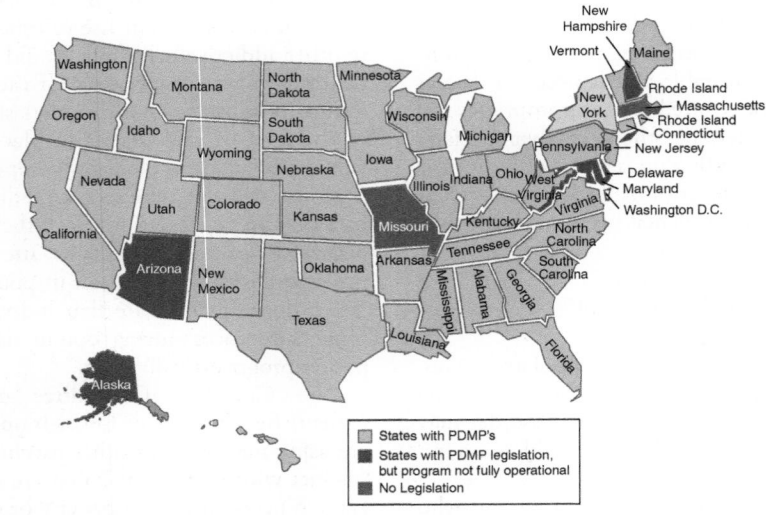

Exhibit 2: Prescription Drug Monitoring Programs

Diagnosing Opioid Use Disorder

Opioid use disorder is primarily diagnosed on the basis of the history provided by the patient and a comprehensive assessment that includes a physical examination. Corroborating information reported by significant others can be used to confirm the diagnosis, especially when there is lack of clarity or inconsistency in information. Other clinicians may make a diagnosis of opioid use disorder; however, provider confirmation of the diagnosis is required before medications are prescribed. This is discussed further in later parts that address specific medications.

DSM-5 Criteria for Diagnosis

The diagnosis of opioid use disorder is based on criteria outlined in the DSM-5. The criteria describe a problematic pattern of opioid use leading to clinically significant impairment or distress. There are a total of 11 symptoms and severity is specified as either mild (presence of 2–3 symptoms), moderate (presence of 4–5 symptoms) or severe (presence of 6 or more symptoms) within a 12-month period. Opioid use disorder requires that at least two of the following 11 criteria be met within a 12-month period: (1) taking opioids in larger amounts or over a longer period of time than intended; (2) having a persistent desire or unsuccessful attempts to reduce or control opioid use; (3) spending excess time obtaining, using, or recovering from opioids; (4) craving for opioids; (5) continuing opioid use causing inability to fulfill work, home, or school responsibilities; (6) continuing opioid use despite having persistent social or interpersonal problems; (7) lack of involvement in social, occupational, or recreational activities; (8) using opioids in physically hazardous situations; (9) continuing opioid use in spite of awareness of persistent physical or psychological problems; (10) tolerance, including need for increased amounts of opioids or diminished effect with continued use at the same amount—as long as the patient is not taking opioids under medical supervision; and (11) withdrawal manifested by characteristic opioid withdrawal syndrome or taking opioids to relieve or avoid withdrawal symptoms—as long as the patient is not taking opioids under medical supervision.

More detail about diagnosing opioid use disorder is available in the American Psychiatric Association: *Diagnostic and Statistical Manual of Mental Disorders, Fifth Edition*. Arlington, VA, American Psychiatric Association, 2013.

Withdrawal Scales

There are a number of useful opioid withdrawal scales that can assist the clinician in evaluating patients with opioid use disorder by identifying and quantitating the severity of opioid withdrawal symptoms. The Objective Opioid Withdrawal Scale (OOWS), which relies on clinical observation, is useful in measuring and documenting the objectively measurable symptoms of opioid withdrawal. The Subjective Opioid Withdrawal Scale (SOWS) records the patient's rating of opioid withdrawal on a 16-item scale.[74]

Finally, the Clinical Opioid Withdrawal Scale (COWS) includes 11 items, and contains signs and symptoms of opioid withdrawal, which are both objective and subjective in nature.[74]

Urine Drug Testing

Urine drug testing, or other reliable biological tests for the presence of drugs, during the initial evaluation and frequently throughout treatment, is highly recommended. There are a variety of toxicology tests available, some with greater and lesser reliability and validity. The person who is interpreting these labs should be very familiar with the methodology and the reliability. There is little research on the optimal frequency of testing. The recommendations given below are based on the consensus opinion of the Guideline Committee. The frequency of drug testing will be determined by a number of factors, including the stability of the patient, the type of treatment, the treatment setting, and the half-life of drugs in the matrix being tested. Patients will likely require more testing early in treatment or during periods of relapse. Patients participating in office-based treatment with buprenorphine may be tested at each office visit. Patients participating in treatment for opioid use disorder at Opioid Treatment Programs (OTPs) are mandated by the Federal law[30] to receive a minimum of eight drug tests per year, but may be tested more frequently based on clinical need. More detailed information on drug testing is contained in "Drug Testing: A White Paper of the American Society of Addiction Medicine."[10]

Opioids are detectable in the urine for 1–3 days after use. A negative urine test combined with no history of withdrawal may indicate a lack of physical dependence. However, a negative urine test does not rule out opioid use, disorder, or physical dependence. Urine testing is also helpful to identify use of other psychoactive substances.

Summary of Recommendations

Assessment Recommendations

(1) First clinical priority should be given to identifying and making appropriate referral for any urgent or emergent medical or psychiatric problem(s), including drug-related impairment or overdose.

(2) Completion of the patient's medical history should include screening for concomitant medical conditions including infectious diseases (hepatitis, HIV, and TB), acute trauma, and pregnancy.

(3) A physical examination should be completed as a component of the comprehensive assessment process. The prescriber (the clinician authorizing the use of a medication for the treatment of opioid use disorder) may conduct this physical examination him/herself, or, in accordance with the ASAM Standards, ensure that a current physical examination is contained within the patient medical record before a patient is started on a new medication for the treatment of his/her addiction.

(4) Initial laboratory testing should include a complete blood count, liver function tests, and tests for hepatitis C and HIV. Testing for TB and sexually transmitted infections should also be considered. Hepatitis B vaccination should be offered, if appropriate.

(5) The assessment of women presents special considerations regarding their reproductive health. Women of childbearing age should be tested for pregnancy, and all women of childbearing potential and age should be queried regarding methods of contraception, given the increase in fertility that results from effective opioid use disorder treatment.

(6) Patients being evaluated for addiction involving opioid use, and/or for possible medication use in the treatment of opioid use disorder, should undergo (or have completed) an assessment of mental health status and possible psychiatric disorders (as outlined in the ASAM Standards).

(7) Opioid use is often co-occurring with other substance-related disorders. An evaluation of past and current substance use and a determination of the totality of substances that surround the addiction should be conducted.

(8) The use of marijuana, stimulants, or other addictive drugs should not be a reason to suspend opioid use disorder treatment. However, evidence demonstrates that patients who are actively using substances during opioid use disorder treatment have a poorer prognosis. The use of benzodiazepines and other sedative hypnotics may be a reason to suspend agonist treatment because of safety concerns related to respiratory depression.

(9) A tobacco use query and counseling on cessation of tobacco products and electronic nicotine delivery devices should be completed routinely for all patients, including those who present for evaluation and treatment of opioid use disorder.

(10) An assessment of social and environmental factors should be conducted (as outlined in the ASAM Standards to identify facilitators and barriers to addiction treatment, and specifically to pharmacotherapy). Before a decision is made to initiate a course of pharmacotherapy for the patient with opioid use disorder, the patient should receive a multidimensional assessment in fidelity with the ASAM Criteria. Addiction should be considered a bio-psycho-social-spiritual illness, for which the use of medication(s) is but only one component of overall treatment.

Diagnosis Recommendations

(1) Other clinicians may diagnose opioid use disorder, but confirmation of the diagnosis by the provider with prescribing authority and who recommends medication use must be obtained before pharmacotherapy for opioid use disorder commences.

(2) Opioid use disorder is primarily diagnosed on the basis of the history provided by the patient and a comprehensive assessment that includes a physical examination.

(3) Validated clinical scales that measure withdrawal symptoms, for example, the OOWS, SOWS, and the COWS, may be used to assist in the evaluation of patients with opioid use disorder.

(4) Urine drug testing during the comprehensive assessment process, and frequently during treatment, is recommended. The frequency of drug testing is determined by a number of factors, including the stability of the patient, the type of treatment, and the treatment setting.

Areas for Further Research

(1) More research is needed on best practices for drug testing during the initial evaluation and throughout the entire treatment process.

(2) Further research is needed on evidence-based approaches for treating opioid use disorder in patients who continue to use marijuana and/or other psychoactive substances.

(3) Whereas research indicates that offering tobacco cessation is a standard for all medical care, more research is needed before specific evidence-based recommendations can be made.

Part 2: Treatment Options

Introduction

Once the diagnosis of opioid use disorder has been established, and it has been determined that the patient is medically and psychiatrically stable, the next task is to decide on a course of treatment. Potential treatments include withdrawal management in conjunction with psychosocial treatment, or psychosocial treatment combined with one of three medications: methadone, buprenorphine, or naltrexone (oral or extended-release injectable formulations). Withdrawal management alone can be the first step, but is not a primary treatment for opioid use disorder and should "only" be considered as a part of a comprehensive and longitudinal plan of care that includes psychosocial treatment, with or without medication-assisted therapy.

The choice among available treatment options should be a shared decision between the clinician and the patient. There are a number of factors to consider in deciding what treatment to choose. Among the first considerations are the priorities of the patient, for instance: Is the patient open to pharmacotherapy? What type of treatment setting does the patient prefer? Does the patient understand the physical dependence aspects of treatment medication? A patient's past experiences with treatment for opioid use disorder should be considered as well. Of course, above all, evidence supporting the potential efficacy and safety of the various treatments is critically important.

For most patients with opioid use disorder, the use of medications (combined with psychosocial treatment) is superior to withdrawal management (combined with psychosocial treatment), followed finally by psychosocial treatment on its own. This is true for both agonist and partial agonist, and antagonist medications. Evidence suggests that methadone maintenance treatment is superior to withdrawal management alone and significantly reduces opioid drug use.[107]

Further, mortality is lower in patients on methadone, as compared to those not undergoing treatment.[50] Methadone also lowers the risk of acquiring or spreading HIV infection.[162,124] In clinical studies, evidence favors buprenorphine, compared to no treatment, in decreasing heroin use and improving treatment retention.[82,98] Finally, evidence supports the efficacy of both oral naltrexone and extended-release injectable naltrexone versus placebo for the treatment of opioid use disorder.[40,92,154]

Pharmacotherapy Options

The medications covered in this guideline are mainly those that have been approved by the FDA for the treatment of opioid dependence as defined in prior versions of the DSM-III and DSM-IV, and "not necessarily" the definition contained in the current version of the manual, the DSM-5. DSM-5 combined "opioid abuse" and "opioid dependence" criteria from prior versions of the DSM and included them in the new definition of "opioid use disorder." As a result, pharmacologic treatment may not be appropriate for all patients along the entire opioid use disorder continuum. In a study comparing opioid dependence from DSM-IV and opioid use disorder from DSM-5, optimal concordance occurred when four or more DSM-5 criteria were endorsed (i.e., the DSM-5 threshold for moderate opioid use disorder).[42]

The medications discussed in this Practice Guideline all have ample evidence supporting their safety and efficacy. It is recognized that other medications have been used off-label to treat opioid use disorder, but with some exceptions (clearly noted in the text) the Guideline Committee has not issued recommendations on the use of these medications. Cost-efficacy was not a consideration in the development of this Practice Guideline.

Each medication will be discussed in detail in subsequent sections:

(1) Methadone (mu-agonist) for opioid use disorder treatment and withdrawal management (Part 4).

(2) Buprenorphine (partial mu-agonist) for opioid use disorder treatment and withdrawal management (Part 5).
(3) Naltrexone (antagonist) for relapse prevention (Part 6).
(4) Naloxone (antagonist) to treat overdose (Part 13).

The only medication that is "not" FDA-approved for the treatment of opioid use disorder that will be covered in this Practice Guideline is the use of the alpha-2 adrenergic agonist, clonidine, for the treatment of opioid withdrawal (see "Part 3: Treating Opioid Withdrawal").

Key outcomes in evaluating the efficacy of the various pharmacotherapies include: decreased mortality, abstinence from opioids, and retention in treatment. In regards to these key outcomes, there is some evidence supporting the relative efficacy of one medication over another, but in many cases, there are no good-quality studies comparing the relative benefits of one medication over another. As noted above, there is strong evidence supporting the superiority of methadone over drug-free treatment for reducing mortality, reducing opioid use, and promoting treatment retention.[138]

Efficacy Considerations

Treatment Setting

In accordance with US Federal laws and regulations derived from the Harrison Act and Congressional exceptions to that 1914 law, the venue in which treatment for opioid use disorder is provided is as important a consideration as is the specific medication selected (methadone vs. buprenorphine vs. naltrexone).[75] Federal and state-licensed OTPs offer daily supervised dosing of methadone. OTPs are state and federally regulated to dispense opioid agonist treatment. An increasing number of such highly regulated programs also offer the option of daily supervised dosing of buprenorphine.

In accordance with Federal law 21 CFR §1306.07, office-based opioid treatment (OBOT), which provides authorization of medication via regular outpatient prescriptions filled in a retail pharmacy like any other prescription medication, is available for buprenorphine, but not for methadone. Physicians in private practices, or various other types of private and public sector clinics, can be authorized to prescribe outpatient supplies of the partial opioid agonist buprenorphine. This flexibility to provide OBOT is discussed more in "Part 5: Buprenorphine." There are no regulations regarding facilities themselves, but rather of the individual physician who prescribes buprenorphine (see "Part 5: Buprenorphine" for physician qualifications associated with OBOT).

Naltrexone can be prescribed in any setting by any clinician with the authority to prescribe any medication. It is not listed among federal or state-controlled substances schedules, and there are no regulations of facilities or prescribers for the use of naltrexone in the treatment of opioid use disorder (such that there are for OTP and OBOT).

It is recommended that the clinician consider a patient's psychosocial situation, co-occurring disorders, and opportunities for treatment retention versus risks of diversion when determining whether OTP or OBOT is most appropriate.

Pharmacology

Differences in efficacy may also arise from differences in pharmacology; whereas methadone is a full agonist at the mu-opioid receptor and produces higher levels of physiological dependence; buprenorphine is a partial agonist with less physiological dependence. There are few studies comparing the relative efficacy of methadone versus buprenorphine in reducing opioid use. Likewise, evidence supports the efficacy of naltrexone for relapse prevention compared to a placebo control.[40,93] There is an absence of studies that compare treatment using either oral naltrexone or extended-release injectable naltrexone versus agonist treatment with either methadone or buprenorphine.

Contraindications and Precautions

The following section describes the major indications, contraindications, and precautions for methadone, buprenorphine, and naltrexone. This section is a summary and is not an exhaustive description of medication information. (Refer to Table 3 below for a summary of contraindications and precautions.)

Methadone

Methadone is frequently used to manage withdrawal symptoms from opioids and is recommended for pharmacological treatment of opioid use disorder (see "Part 4: Methadone").

Methadone is "contraindicated" for the following conditions:
(1) Patients with known hypersensitivity to methadone hydrochloride.

(2) Patients experiencing respiratory depression (in the absence of resuscitative equipment or in unmonitored settings).
(3) Patients with acute bronchial asthma or hypercapnia (also known as hypercarbia).
(4) Patients with known or suspected paralytic ileus.

Methadone should be used with "caution" for the following conditions:
(1) Patients with decompensated liver disease (e.g., jaundice, ascites) due to increased risk of hepatic encephalopathy.
(2) Patients with respiratory insufficiency.
(3) Patients with concomitant substance use disorders, particularly patients with sedative, hypnotic, or anxiolytic use disorders. Interactions between methadone and hypnotics, sedatives, or anxiolytics may be life-threatening.
(4) Patients with concomitant psychiatric diagnoses that impair their ability to maintain daily attendance at an OTP.
(5) Patients with low levels of physical dependence to opioids should be started with low doses of methadone.

TABLE A3.3   Contraindications and Precautions for Pharmacotherapy Options.

Medication	Contraindications	Warnings and Precautions
Methadone	Hypersensitivity Respiratory depression Severe bronchial asthma or hypercapnia Paralytic ileus	Cardiac conduction effects Diversion and misuse are possible Physical dependence Respiratory depression when used in association with CNS depressants including alcohol, other opioids, and illicit drugs Head injury and increased intracranial pressure Liver disease Respiratory insufficiency Concomitant substance use disorders Co-occurring psychiatric disorders Drug interactions with medications metabolized by cytochrome P450 enzymes principally CYP34A, CYP2B6, CYP2C19, and to a lesser extent by CYP2C9 and CYP2D6 drugs coadministered with methadone should be evaluated for interaction potential
Buprenorphine (all formulations)	Hypersensitivity	Diversion and misuse are possible Physical dependence Respiratory depression when used in association with CNS depressants including alcohol, other opioids, and illicit drugs Precipitated withdrawal if used in patients physically dependent on full agonists opioids before the agonist effects have worn off Neonatal withdrawal has been reported after use of buprenorphine during pregnancy Not recommended for patients with severe hepatic impairment May cause sedation
Naltrexone (oral and injectable formulations)	Hypersensitivity reactions to naltrexone, or for injectable previous hypersensitivity reactions to polylactide-co-glycolide, carboxymethylcellulose, or any other constituent of the diluent Patients currently physically dependent on opioids, including partial agonists Patients receiving opioid analgesics Patients in acute opioid withdrawal	Vulnerability to overdose Injection site reactions associated with injectable naltrexone Precipitated opioid withdrawal Risk of hepatotoxicity Patient should be monitored for the development of depression and suicidality Emergency reversal of opiate blockade may require special monitoring in a critical care setting Eosinophil pneumonia has been reported in association with injectable naltrexone Administer IM injections with caution to patients with thrombocytopenia or a coagulation disorder

IM, Intramuscular.

Significant "medication interactions" to consider before starting methadone are as follows:

(1) Methadone may prolong the QT interval and should be used in caution with other agents that may also prolong the QT interval. These include class I or class III anti-arrhythmic drugs, calcium channel blockers, some anti-psychotics, and some antidepressants.

(2) Methadone is metabolized through the cytochrome P450 enzyme pathway. Many agents interact with this pathway including alcohol, anticonvulsants, antiretrovirals, and macrolide antibiotics.

Buprenorphine

Buprenorphine is a partial opioid agonist and mixed opioid agonist–antagonist. It is usually provided in a formulation that includes naloxone. Buprenorphine is recommended for pharmacological treatment of opioid use disorder (see "Part 5: Buprenorphine").

Buprenorphine is also an effective treatment for opioid withdrawal with efficacy similar to methadone, and much superior to clonidine in opioid withdrawal management.[20,35,97]

Although one trial did find that longer courses of buprenorphine with gradual tapering were superior to rapid tapering for withdrawal,[137] there is insufficient evidence on outcomes to make recommendations on buprenorphine taper duration.

Buprenorphine is "contraindicated" for the following conditions:

(1) Patients with hypersensitivity to buprenorphine or any component of the formulation.

(2) Patients with severe liver impairment are not good candidates for office-based treatment with buprenorphine. (Patients with hepatitis C infection who do not have severe liver impairment may, however, be considered for buprenorphine.)

Buprenorphine should be used with "caution" for the following conditions:

(1) Patients in whom hepatitis has been reported, particularly in patients with previous hepatic dysfunction. A direct comparison of the effects of buprenorphine and methadone, however, showed no evidence of liver damage during the initial 6 months in either treatment groups.[134] Monitoring liver function in patients at increased risk for hepatotoxicity may be considered.

(2) Patients who, at present, have an alcohol use or sedative, hypnotic, or anxiolytic use disorder.

(3) Patients with hypovolemia, severe cardiovascular disease, or taking drugs that may exaggerate hypotensive effects. Buprenorphine may cause hypotension, including orthostatic hypotension and syncope.

Significant "medication interactions" to consider before starting buprenorphine include the following:

(1) Alcohol and sedatives, hypnotics, or anxiolytics may enhance the central nervous system depressive effect of buprenorphine.

(2) Buprenorphine is metabolized to norbuprenorphine primarily by cytochrome CYP3A4; therefore, potential interactions may occur when buprenorphine is given concurrently with agents that affect CYP3A4 activity. The concomitant use of buprenorphine with CYP3A4 inhibitors (e.g., azole antifungals such as ketoconazole, macrolide antibiotics such as erythromycin, and HIV protease inhibitors) should be monitored and may require dose reduction of one or both agents.[27,144,173]

Naltrexone

Naltrexone is recommended for pharmacological treatment of opioid use disorder (see "Part 6: Naltrexone"). Naltrexone is an opioid antagonist that blocks the effects of opioids. It is a pharmacotherapy option used to treat opioid use disorder and prevent relapse after detoxification. Naltrexone causes immediate withdrawal symptoms (precipitated withdrawal) in a person with active physical dependence on opioids. There are oral and extended-release injectable formulas of naltrexone. Oral naltrexone, if taken daily, is most effective in patients who are highly motivated or legally mandated to receive treatment, and/or when taking the medication is closely supervised. Conversely, the efficacy of oral naltrexone for the treatment of opioid use disorder is often adversely affected by poor medication adherence.[114] Clinicians may want to reserve using oral naltrexone for patients who are able to comply with special techniques to enhance their adherence, for example, observed dosing. An extended-release injectable naltrexone formulation is available, which may overcome the adherence limitations of the oral formulation. This formulation requires a once-monthly injection.

Naltrexone is "contraindicated" under the following conditions:

(1) Patients with hypersensitivity reactions to naltrexone.

(2) Patients who have previously exhibited hypersensitivity to naltrexone, polylactide-coglycolide, carboxymethyl-cellulose, or any other components of the diluent (for extended-release injectable naltrexone).

(3) Patients with current physical dependence on opioids, including partial agonists.

(4) Patients with current physiologic opioid dependence.

(5) Patients in acute opioid withdrawal.

(6) Any individual who has failed the naloxone challenge test (see "Glossary") or has a positive urine screen for opioids.

Naltrexone should be used with "caution" under the following conditions:

(1) All patients should be warned of the risk of hepatic injury and advised to seek medical attention if they experience symptoms of acute hepatitis. Hepatic injury is a concern if very high doses are used, for example, 200–300 mg per day. Use of naltrexone should be discontinued in the event of symptoms and/or signs of acute hepatitis. Cases of hepatitis and clinically significant liver dysfunction were observed in association with naltrexone exposure during the clinical development program and in the postmarketing period. Transient, asymptomatic hepatic transaminase elevations were also observed in the clinical trials and postmarketing period.

(2) Patients with liver impairment should complete liver enzyme tests before and during treatment with naltrexone to check for additional liver impairment.

(3) Patients who experience injection site reactions should be monitored for pain, redness, or swelling. Incorrect administration may increase the risk of injection site reactions. Reactions have occurred with extended-release injectable naltrexone.

(4) Patients with co-occurring psychiatric disorders should be monitored for adverse events. Suicidal thoughts, attempted suicide, and depression have been reported.

Significant "medication interactions" with naltrexone are as follows:

(1) Naltrexone should not be used with methylnaltrexone or naloxegol.

(2) Naltrexone blocks the effects of opioid analgesics because it is an opioid antagonist.

(3) Glyburide may increase serum concentration of naltrexone. Monitor for increased toxicity effects of naltrexone.

Summary of Recommendations

(1) The choice of available treatment options for addiction involving opioid use should be a shared decision between the clinician and the patient.

(2) Clinicians should consider the patient's preferences, past treatment history, and treatment setting when deciding between the use of methadone, buprenorphine, and naltrexone in the treatment of addiction involving opioid use.

The treatment setting described as level 1 treatment in the ASAM Criteria may be a general outpatient location such as a clinician's practice site. The setting as described as level 2 in the ASAM Criteria may be an intensive outpatient treatment or partial hospitalization program housed in a specialty addiction treatment facility, a community mental health center, or another setting.

The ASAM Criteria describes level 3 or level 4 treatment, respectively, as a residential addiction treatment facility or hospital.

(1) The venue in which treatment is provided is as important as the specific medication selected. OTPs offer daily supervised dosing of methadone, and increasingly of buprenorphine. In accordance with Federal law (21 CFR §1306.07), OBOT, which provides medication on a prescribed weekly or monthly basis, is limited to buprenorphine.[9] Naltrexone can be prescribed in any setting by any clinician with the authority to prescribe any medication. Clinicians should consider a patient's psychosocial situation, co-occurring disorders, and risk of diversion when determining whether OTP or OBOT is most appropriate.

(2) OBOT may not be suitable for patients with active alcohol use disorder or sedative, hypnotic, or anxiolytic use disorder (or who are in the treatment of addiction involving the use of alcohol or other sedative drugs, including benzodiazepines or benzodiazepine receptor agonists). It may also be unsuitable for persons who are regularly using alcohol or other sedatives, but do not have addiction or a specific substance use disorder related to that class of drugs. The prescribing of benzodiazepines or other sedative-hypnotics should be used with extreme caution in patients who are prescribed methadone or buprenorphine for the treatment of an opioid use disorder.

(3) Methadone is recommended for patients who may benefit from daily dosing and supervision in an OTP, or for patients for whom buprenorphine for the treatment of opioid use disorder has been used unsuccessfully in an OTP or OBOT setting.

(4) Oral naltrexone for the treatment of opioid use disorder is often adversely affected by poor medication adherence. Clinicians should reserve its use for patients who would be able to comply with special techniques to enhance their adherence, for example, observed dosing. Extended release injectable naltrexone reduces, but does not eliminate, issues with medication adherence.

Areas for Further Research

More research is needed to compare the advantages of agonists and antagonists in the treatment of opioid use disorder. Whereas methadone, buprenorphine, and naltrexone are all superior to no treatment in opioid use disorder, less is known about their relative advantages.

Part 3: Treating Opioid Withdrawal

Background

Opioid withdrawal syndrome refers to the wide range of symptoms that occur after stopping or dramatically reducing the dose of opioid drugs after heavy and prolonged use. For short-acting opioids such as heroin and oxycodone, symptoms usually emerge within 12 hours of the last opioid use, peak within 24–48 hours, and diminish over 3–5 days. For long-acting opioids such as methadone, withdrawal symptoms generally emerge within 30 hours of the last methadone exposure and may last up to 10 days. Although distressing, opioid withdrawal syndrome is rarely life-threatening. However, abrupt discontinuation of opioids is not recommended because it may precipitate withdrawal, lead to strong cravings, and result in relapse to drug use.

Symptoms of opioid withdrawal may include any of the following:

(1) Muscle aches
(2) Increased tearing
(3) Runny nose
(4) Dilated pupils
(5) Piloerection
(6) Agitation
(7) Anxiety
(8) Insomnia
(9) Sweating
(10) Yawning
(11) Abdominal cramping
(12) Nausea
(13) Vomiting
(14) Diarrhea

Opioid withdrawal generally results from the cessation or a dramatic reduction in the dose of opioids, which is referred to as spontaneous withdrawal. Opioid withdrawal can also be precipitated when a patient who is physically dependent on opioids is administered an opioid antagonist such as naloxone or naltrexone, or an opioid partial agonist such as buprenorphine. Signs and symptoms of precipitated withdrawal are similar to those of spontaneous withdrawal, but the time course is different and symptoms may be much more severe. Review of postmarketing cases of precipitated opioid withdrawal in association with treatment with naltrexone has identified cases with symptoms of withdrawal severe enough to require hospital admission, and in some cases, management in the intensive care unit.[76,131]

The timing of maximal precipitated withdrawal usually occurs in the following scenarios:

(1) Within 1 minute for intravenously administered naloxone.
(2) Several minutes after IM naloxone.
(3) Up to 90 minutes after sublingual buprenorphine.
(4) Up to several hours after extended-release injectable naltrexone.[62]

The duration of the withdrawal depends on the half-life and dose of the partial agonist or antagonist. Naloxone-precipitated withdrawal typically lasts for 30–60 minutes, whereas buprenorphine- or naltrexone-precipitated withdrawal may last for several days. The ability to accurately assess patients for opioid withdrawal is important to avoid precipitated withdrawal when introducing antagonists and partial agonists for relapse prevention.

Withdrawal management can make withdrawal from opioids more comfortable. Given the high rate of relapse, opioid withdrawal management is not considered an effective treatment of opioid use disorder on its own.[86]

If withdrawal management alone, or withdrawal management followed by psychosocial treatment alone is proposed, the patient should be informed of the estimated risks of subsequent relapse, including the increased risk for death, as compared to treatment with opioid agonists. Withdrawal management is not necessary or recommended for patients being referred for treatment with methadone or buprenorphine.

Assessment of Patient for Opioid Withdrawal

Assessment of a patient undergoing opioid withdrawal should include a thorough medical history and physical examination focusing on signs and symptoms associated with opioid withdrawal. There are various scales available to assess opioid withdrawal. Objective signs, when present, are more reliable, but subjective withdrawal features can also be sensitive measures of opioid withdrawal. These scales may be used to measure opioid withdrawal symptoms during the initial assessment to make the diagnosis of opioid withdrawal. In addition, clinicians can assess the effectiveness of withdrawal management by repeating these scales intermittently as they treat withdrawal symptoms.

Objective Opioid Withdrawal Scale (OOWS) is an objective measure in which the clinician checks for 13 signs of opioid withdrawal (e.g., yawning, perspiration).[74]

Clinical Opioid Withdrawal Scale (COWS) is a clinical assessment for 11 medical signs and symptoms of opioid withdrawal (e.g., gastrointestinal distress).[166]

Subjective Opioid Withdrawal Scale (SOWS) is a measure of 16 subjective symptoms of withdrawal, in which the patient rates their experience on a 5-point scale (e.g., "I feel restless").[74]

Opioid withdrawal management may occur in either inpatient or outpatient settings. There is a lack of evidence to determine the relative safety of inpatient versus outpatient withdrawal management. Inpatient withdrawal management has higher rates of completion compared to outpatient withdrawal management; however, there is no demonstrable difference in relapse among inpatient versus outpatient withdrawal management.[48]

Medications in Opioid Withdrawal

For the management of opioid withdrawal, two main strategies have evolved. The first involves the provision of gradually tapering doses of opioid agonists, typically methadone or buprenorphine. The other strategy is the use of alpha 2 adrenergic agonists (clonidine) along with other non-narcotic medications to reduce withdrawal symptoms. Both strategies have advantages and disadvantages. Using tapering doses of opioid agonists has been shown to be superior to clonidine in terms of retention and opioid abstinence. However, the use of nonopioid medications may be the only option available to clinicians in some healthcare settings and may also facilitate the transition of patients to opioid antagonist medications and help prevent subsequent relapse. Recently, researchers have begun to investigate the use of combinations of buprenorphine and low doses of oral naltrexone to rapidly detoxify patients and facilitate the accelerated introduction of extended-release injectable naltrexone.[136] Although these techniques seem promising, more research will be needed before these can be accepted as standard practice.

Withdrawal Management With Opioid Agonists

Methadone and buprenorphine are both recommended in the management of opioid withdrawal and have comparable results in terms of retention and opioid abstinence. Withdrawal management with methadone must be done in an OTP or inpatient setting. Methadone tapers generally start with doses in the range of 20–30 mg per day, and are completed in 6–10 days.

Buprenorphine withdrawal management can be done either in an outpatient or an inpatient setting. None of the available forms of buprenorphine, including the buprenorphine mono products (Suboxone, Zubsolv, and Bunavail), are specifically US FDA-approved for withdrawal management, but may be used for this purpose. None of the products have shown superiority over another for this purpose. In the remainder of this section, the term buprenorphine refers to the monotherapy and combination formulations.

Buprenorphine is a partial mu-opioid receptor antagonist with a higher affinity for the mu-receptor than most full agonists such as heroin and oxycodone. Therefore, it is important that buprenorphine should not be started until a patient is exhibiting opioid withdrawal to avoid precipitated withdrawal. Usually buprenorphine is not started until 12–18 hours after the last dose of a short-acting agonist such as heroin or oxycodone, and 24–48 hours after the last dose of a long-acting agonist such as methadone. A dose sufficient to suppress withdrawal symptoms is achieved (4–16 mg per day) and then the dose is tapered. The duration of the taper can be as brief as 3–5 days or as long as 30 days or more.

Studies examining the relative efficacy of long- versus short-duration tapers are not conclusive, and the Guideline Committee was unable to reach a consensus on this issue. Physicians should be guided by patient response in determining the optimum duration of the taper.

Withdrawal Management With Alpha-2 Adrenergic Agonists

Because opioid withdrawal results largely from over-activity of the brain's noradrenergic system, alpha-2 adrenergic agonists (clonidine, lofexidine) have a long history of off-label use for the treatment of opioid withdrawal in the United States. Lofexidine is approved for the treatment of opioid withdrawal in the United Kingdom. Clonidine is generally used at doses of 0.1–0.3 mg every 6–8 hours, with a maximum dose of 1.2 mg daily. Its hypotensive effects often limit the amount that can be used. Clonidine is often combined with other non-narcotic medications targeting specific opioid withdrawal symptoms such as benzodiazepines for anxiety, loperamide or bismuth-salicylate for diarrhea, acetaminophen or nonsteroidal anti-inflammatory medications (NSAIDs) for pain, various medications for insomnia, and ondansetron for nausea. Other agents in the same pharmacological family as clonidine, such as guanfacine (available in the United States) and lofexidine (available in many other countries) can be used off-label as safe and effective agents in the management of opioid withdrawal.

Anesthesia-Assisted Withdrawal Management

Anesthesia-assisted opioid detoxification or ultra-rapid opioid detoxification (UROD) uses large doses of naloxone to precipitate acute opioid withdrawal in the patient who is under general anesthesia. Patients are anesthetized, then intubated and mechanically ventilated. A diuretic is used to enhance excretion of the opioid. Patients experience mild withdrawal symptoms for about 6 days after awakening from anesthesia, compared with similar withdrawal symptoms on a 20-day methadone taper.[39,90]

The ASAM recommends against the use of UROD in the treatment of opioid withdrawal and stated these same recommendations in a policy statement.[11] ASAM's position is in accordance with other guidelines. Serious complications including cardiac arrest and death have been reported with anesthesia-assisted withdrawal management.[73] The Centers for Disease Control and Prevention issued a warning in 2013 about severe adverse events including death from anesthesia-assisted withdrawal management.[31] Furthermore, a systematic review of five randomized trials concluded that the lack of benefit, potential serious harms, and costs of heavy sedation or anesthesia do not support its use.[68]

Summary of Recommendations

(1) Using medications for opioid withdrawal management is recommended over abrupt cessation of opioids. Abrupt cessation of opioids may lead to strong cravings, which can lead to continued use.

(2) Patients should be advised about risk of relapse and other safety concerns from using opioid withdrawal management as standalone treatment for opioid use disorder. Opioid withdrawal management on its own is not a treatment method.

(3) Assessment of a patient undergoing opioid withdrawal management should include a thorough medical history and physical examination focusing on signs and symptoms associated with opioid withdrawal.

(4) Opioid withdrawal management in cases in which methadone is used to manage withdrawal symptoms must be done in an inpatient setting or in an OTP. For short-acting opioids, tapering schedules that decrease in daily doses of prescribed methadone should begin with doses between 20 and 30 mg per day, and should be completed in 6–10 days.

(5) Opioid withdrawal management in cases in which buprenorphine is used to manage withdrawal symptoms should not be initiated until 12–18 hours after the last dose of a short-acting agonist such as heroin or oxycodone, and 24–48 hours after the last dose of a long-acting agonist such as methadone. A dose of buprenorphine sufficient to suppress withdrawal symptoms is given (this can be 4–16 mg per day) and then the dose is tapered. The duration of the tapering schedule can be as brief as 3–5 days or as long as 30 days or more.

(6) The use of combinations of buprenorphine and low doses of oral naltrexone to manage withdrawal and facilitate the accelerated introduction of extended-release injectable naltrexone has shown promise. More research will be needed before this can be accepted as standard practice.

(7) The Guideline Committee recommends, based on consensus opinion, the inclusion of clonidine as a recommended practice to support opioid withdrawal. Clonidine is not US FDA-approved for the treatment of opioid withdrawal, but it has been extensively used off-label for this purpose. Clonidine may be used orally or transdermally at doses of 0.1–0.3 mg every 6–8 hours, with a maximum dose of 1.2 mg daily to assist in the management of opioid withdrawal symptoms. Its hypotensive effects often limit the amount that can be used. Clonidine can be combined with other non-narcotic medications targeting specific opioid withdrawal symptoms such as benzodiazepines for anxiety, loperamide for diarrhea, acetaminophen or NSAIDs for pain, and ondansetron or other agents for nausea.

(8) Opioid withdrawal management using anesthesia UROD is not recommended due to high risk for adverse events or death. Naltrexone-facilitated opioid withdrawal management can be a safe and effective approach, but should be used only by clinicians experienced with this clinical method and in cases in which anesthesia or conscious sedation are not being employed.

Areas for Further Research

(1) Further research is needed to evaluate the efficacy and safety of alpha-2 adrenergic and other nonopioid medications that are being used off-label for withdrawal management. These nonopioid medications may have use in transitioning patients onto antagonists for relapse prevention.

(2) Further study is needed on other methods to accelerate the withdrawal process and facilitate the introduction of antagonists.

(3) More research is needed to make recommendations on the optimal duration of a buprenorphine taper.

(4) More research is needed to evaluate the safety of inpatient as compared to outpatient withdrawal management.

(5) More research is needed to compare the effectiveness of short versus long tapers with buprenorphine withdrawal management.

Part 4: Methadone

Background

Methadone (Dolophine or Methadose) is a slow-acting opioid agonist. Methadone is an effective treatment for opioid withdrawal management and the treatment of opioid use disorder. Methadone is taken orally so that it reaches the brain slowly, dampening the euphoria that occurs with other routes of administration while preventing withdrawal symptoms. Methadone has been used since the 1960s to treat heroin addiction and remains an effective treatment option. Many studies have demonstrated its superiority to using abstinence-based approaches.[107] Methadone is only available through approved OTPs, where it is dispensed to patients on a daily or almost daily basis in the initial stages of treatment. Federal and state laws allow take-home doses for patients who have demonstrated treatment progress and are judged to be at low risk for diversion.

Patient Selection and Treatment Goals

Treatment with methadone at an OTP is recommended for patients who have opioid use disorder, are able to give informed consent, and have no specific contraindications for agonist treatment. Treatment with methadone has the following four goals:

(1) To suppress opioid withdrawal.
(2) To block the effects of illicit opioids.
(3) To reduce opioid craving and stop or reduce the use of illicit opioids.
(4) To promote and facilitate patient engagement in recovery-oriented activities including psychosocial intervention.

Precautions
Arrhythmias
Patients should be informed of the potential risk of arrhythmia when they are dispensed methadone. It is recommended to get a history of structural heart disease, arrhythmia, or syncope. In addition, the clinician should assess the patient for other risk factors for QT-interval prolongation. An electrocardiogram (ECG)

should be considered when high doses of methadone (over 120 mg per day) are being employed, there is a history of prolonged QT interval, or the patient is taking medications known to prolong the QT. However, there is no research on the use of ECG data for improving patient outcomes.

Course of Treatment

Induction

Initial dosing depends on the level of physical dependence. Consequently, induction varies widely. In a recent publication prepared by ASAM's Methadone Action Group, the recommended initial dose ranges from 10 to 30 mg, with reassessment in 2–4 hours when peak levels have been reached.[17]

Given the risk of overdose in the first 2 weeks, tolerance is an important safety consideration. Federal law mandates that the initial dose cannot exceed 30 mg and not exceed 40 mg in 1 day.[30]

Dosing

Methadone has a long half-life and care must be taken to avoid too rapid dose increases during the first 1–3 weeks of treatment so as to avoid increasing the dose before the full effect of the last dose has been realized. Dosing should be based on patients achieving goals of treatment, can vary widely between patients, and doses do not correlate well with blood levels. Trough and peak plasma levels of methadone (or methadone blood levels) may be used in addition to clinical evaluation to assess the safety and adequacy of a patient's dose, particularly in patients who seem to be rapid metabolizers and may need a split dose.[57,58,96,101,152] A relatively low dose of methadone (e.g., <30 mg per day) can lessen acute opioid withdrawal, but is often not effective in suppressing craving and blocking the effects of other opioids. Most patients fare better on methadone doses between 60 and 120 mg per day, which typically creates sufficient tolerance to minimize a euphoric response if patients self-administer additional opioids.

A relatively low dose of methadone (e.g., <30 mg per day) can lessen acute withdrawal, but is often not effective in suppressing craving and blocking the effects of other opioids. Though a few patients respond to a maintenance dose of 30–60 mg per day, most patients fare better if their initial 30–40 mg per day dose is gradually raised to a maintenance level of 60–120 mg per day, which typically creates sufficient tolerance to minimize a euphoric response if patients self-administer additional opioids. Multiple randomized trials have found that patients have better outcomes, including retention in treatment, with higher doses (80–100 mg per day) than lower doses.[140,141] Though not well studied, doses above 120 mg per day are being used with some patients as blockade of opioid effects is becoming increasingly more difficult due to the increased purity of heroin and strength of prescription opioids.[59]

Adverse Effects

Higher methadone doses may be associated with increased risk of adverse effects, including prolongation of the QT interval and other arrhythmias (torsades des pointes), which in some cases have been fatal.[59] The US FDA issued a safety alert for methadone regarding these cardiac events.[159]

Clinicians, in consultation with patients, may need to consider the relative risk of adverse events due to QT prolongation with methadone as compared to the risk of morbidity and mortality of an untreated opioid use disorder.[38] Changing to buprenorphine or naltrexone maintenance should be considered when risks of QT

prolongation are high as they do not seem to significantly prolong the QT.

Psychosocial Treatment

Because opioid use disorder is a chronic relapsing disease, strategies specifically directed at relapse prevention are an important part of comprehensive outpatient treatment and should include drug counseling and/or other psychosocial treatments. However, there may be instances when pharmacotherapy alone results in an excellent outcome.

Family involvement in treatment provides strong support for patient recovery; and family members also benefit. The concept of "family" should be expanded to include members of the patient's social network (as defined by the patient), including significant others, clergy, employers, and case managers.

Monitoring Treatment

Federal and state-approved OTPs dispense methadone and supervise administration. Treatment should include relapse monitoring with frequent testing for alcohol and other relevant psychoactive substances. Testing for methadone and buprenorphine is recommended to ensure adherence and detect possible diversion.

Length of Treatment

The optimal duration of treatment with methadone has not been established; however, it is known that relapse rates are high for most patients who drop out; thus long-term treatment is often needed. Treatment duration depends on the response of the individual patient and is best determined by collaborative decisions between the clinician and the patient. Treatment should be reinstituted immediately for most patients who were previously taking methadone and have relapsed or are at risk for relapse.

Switching Treatment Medications

Switching from methadone to other opioid treatment medications may be appropriate in the following cases:
(1) Patient experiences intolerable methadone side effects.
(2) Patient has not experienced a successful course of treatment on methadone.
(3) Patient wants to change and is a candidate for the alternative treatment.

Transfer of medications should be planned, considered, and monitored. Particular care should be taken in reducing methadone dosing before transfer to avoid precipitating a relapse. If the patient becomes unstable and appears at risk for relapse during the transfer of medications, reinstating methadone may be the best option.

Switching to Buprenorphine

Patients on low doses of methadone (30–40 mg per day or less) generally tolerate the transition to buprenorphine with minimal discomfort; whereas patients on higher doses of methadone may find that switching causes significant discomfort. Patients should be closely monitored during such a switch because there is a risk that stable methadone patients may become unstable when changing to buprenorphine.

To minimize the risk of precipitated withdrawal, it is recommended that physicians use careful initial dosing followed by rapid titration up to an appropriate maintenance dose. Because of concern that sublingually absorbed naloxone could increase the risk of precipitated withdrawal, treatment initiation with buprenorphine monoproduct is recommended for patients transitioning from methadone and any other long-acting opioid. Patients should be experiencing mild to moderate opioid withdrawal before the switch. This would typically occur at least 24 hours after the last dose of methadone, and indicates that sufficient time has elapsed for there to be minimal risk that the first dose of buprenorphine will precipitate significant withdrawal. Moderate withdrawal would equate to a score greater than 12 on the COWS.[166]

An initial dose of 2–4 mg of buprenorphine should be given and the patient should be observed for 1 hour. If withdrawal symptoms improve, the patient can be dispensed two additional 2- to 4-mg doses to be taken as needed. The prescribing doctor should contact the patient later in the day to assess the response to dosing. The likelihood of precipitating withdrawal on commencing buprenorphine is reduced as the time interval between the last methadone dose and the first buprenorphine dose increases.

Switching to Naltrexone

Patients switching from methadone to oral naltrexone or extended-release injectable naltrexone need to be completely withdrawn from methadone and other opioids before they can receive naltrexone. This may take up to 14 days, but can typically be achieved in 7 days.[163] A naloxone challenge (administration of 0.4–0.8 mg naloxone and observation for precipitated withdrawal) may be useful before initiating treatment with naltrexone to document the absence of physiological dependence and to minimize the risk for precipitated withdrawal (see "Glossary" for more on naloxone challenge).

Summary of Recommendations

(1) Methadone is a treatment option recommended for patients who are physiologically dependent on opioids, able to give informed consent, and who have no specific contraindications for agonist treatment when it is prescribed in the context of an appropriate plan that includes psychosocial intervention.

(2) The recommended initial dose ranges for methadone are from 10 to 30 mg, with reassessment in 3–4 hours and a second dose not to exceed 10 mg on the first day if withdrawal symptoms are persisting.

(3) The usual daily dosage of methadone ranges from 60 to 120 mg. Some patients may respond to lower doses and some may need higher doses. Dosage increases in 5–10-mg increments applied no more frequently than every 7 days (depending on clinical response) are necessary to avoid over-sedation, toxicity, or even iatrogenic overdose deaths.

(4) The administration of methadone should be monitored because unsupervised administration can lead to misuse and diversion. OTP regulations require monitored medication administration until the patient's clinical response and behavior demonstrate that the prescribing of nonmonitored doses is appropriate.

(5) Psychosocial treatment, though sometimes minimally needed, should be implemented in conjunction with the use of methadone in the treatment of opioid use disorder.

(6) Methadone should be reinstituted immediately if relapse occurs, or when an assessment determines that the risk of relapse is high for patients who previously received methadone in the treatment of opioid use disorder, but who are no longer prescribed such treatment.

(7) Strategies directed at relapse prevention are an important of comprehensive addiction treatment and should be included in any plan of care for a patient receiving active opioid treatment or ongoing monitoring of the status of their addictive disease.

(8) Switching from methadone to another medication for the treatment of opioid use disorder may be appropriate if the patient experiences intolerable side effects or is not successful in attaining or maintaining treatment goals through the use of methadone.

(9) Patients switching from methadone to buprenorphine in the treatment of opioid use disorder should be on low doses of methadone before switching medications. Patients on low doses of methadone (30–40 mg per day or less) generally tolerate transition to buprenorphine with minimal discomfort, whereas patients on higher doses of methadone may experience significant discomfort in switching medications.

(10) Patients switching from methadone to oral naltrexone or extended-release injectable naltrexone must be completely withdrawn from methadone and other opioids, before they can receive naltrexone. The only exception would apply when an experienced clinician receives consent from the patient to embark on a plan of naltrexone-facilitated opioid withdrawal management.

(11) Patients who discontinue agonist therapy with methadone or buprenorphine and then resume opioid use should be made aware of the risks associated with opioid overdose, and especially the increased risk of death.

Areas for Further Research

(1) Further research is needed to assess the effectiveness of added psychosocial treatment to treatment with methadone in OTP or inpatient settings. Treatment with methadone generally includes some psychosocial components.

However, it is unclear whether added psychosocial treatment improves patient outcomes.

(2) Research is needed to evaluate the use of ECG in treatment with methadone in preventing adverse events.

Part 5: Buprenorphine

Background

Buprenorphine is recommended for the treatment of opioid use disorder. Buprenorphine relieves drug cravings without producing the euphoria or dangerous side effects of other opioids. In addition to its pharmacological properties, an important feature of buprenorphine is its ability to be prescribed in office-based treatment settings. The US FDA approved buprenorphine in 2002, making it the first medication eligible to be prescribed by certified physicians through the Drug Addiction Treatment Act of 2000 (DATA 2000). Through DATA 2000, physicians may apply for waivers to prescribe certain narcotic schedule III, IV, or V medications, including buprenorphine, from their office settings. This provision of the act expands accessibility of community-based treatment options and mitigates the need to receive treatment through more specialized, and often less available, OTPs. However, buprenorphine may also be administered in an OTP setting with structure and administration requirements identical to those for methadone.

Formulations of Buprenorphine

For this Practice Guideline, recommendations using the term "buprenorphine" will refer generally to both the buprenorphine only and the combination buprenorphine/naloxone formulations. When recommendations differ by product, the type of product will be described. The monoproduct (generic name buprenorphine) will be referred to as "buprenorphine monoproduct." The combination product will be referred to as "combination buprenorphine/naloxone."

This Practice Guideline recommends using combination buprenorphine/naloxone for withdrawal management and treatment of opioid use disorder, with the exception of treatment for pregnant women. (Buprenorphine monoproduct is recommended for pregnant women, because naloxone in the combination product is not recommended for use by pregnant women.) (See "Part 8: Special Populations: Pregnant Women.")

Combination buprenorphine contains naloxone (an opioid antagonist), which is included to discourage intravenous misuse of buprenorphine. If a patient who is physically dependent on a full agonist opioid injects buprenorphine/naloxone, the naloxone will induce withdrawal symptoms. These withdrawal symptoms are averted when buprenorphine/naloxone is taken sublingually as prescribed.

A combination product of buprenorphine and naloxone (Suboxone, Zubsolv, Bunavail) is taken sublingually or in a buccal film. The US FDA-approved generic forms of buprenorphine/naloxone sublingual tablets and buprenorphine monoproduct provide a broader array of treatment options. The ratio of buprenorphine to naloxone in Suboxone is 4 : 1, and a variety of dose sizes are available (e.g., 2/0.5, 4/1, 8/2). Other formulations of buprenorphine/naloxone (Zubsolv, Bunavail) have different bioavailability and have different buprenorphine/naloxone dose strengths. The approved doses of Zubsolv and Bunavail are bioequivalent to the doses of Suboxone discussed in this guideline. Bioequivalence information and charts are contained in Appendix II.

All information provided in this section is based on dosages for the generic equivalents of buprenorphine/naloxone sublingual tablets and buprenorphine sublingual tablets. Because of the possibility of slight differences in bioavailability between the different formulations of buprenorphine, patients switching from one form of buprenorphine to another should be monitored for adverse effects.

Patient Selection and Treatment Goals

Buprenorphine is an effective treatment recommended for patients who have opioid use disorder, are able to give informed consent, and have no specific contraindications for agonist treatment. Treatment with buprenorphine has the following four goals:
(1) To suppress opioid withdrawal.
(2) To block the effects of illicit opioids.
(3) To reduce opioid craving and stop or reduce the use of illicit opioid.
(4) To promote and facilitate patient engagement in recovery-oriented activities including psychosocial intervention.

There is ample evidence for the efficacy of buprenorphine for the treatment of opioid use disorder.[126] The risk of lethal overdose in an opioid-tolerant individual on buprenorphine is substantially less than that associated with the use of other opioid medications such as methadone. This is due to the ceiling effects of buprenorphine across a wide range of doses. Consequently, buprenorphine has been approved for OBOT.

Precautions

Alcohol or Sedative, Hypnotic, or Anxiolytic Use

Some studies have shown potential adverse interactions between buprenorphine and sedatives. Therefore, patients with opioid use disorder and concurrent alcohol, sedative, hypnotic, or anxiolytic use disorders should receive more intensive monitoring during office-based treatment with buprenorphine to minimize the risk of adverse events. Alternatively, patients with these co-occurring disorders may be better treated in a setting with greater supervision such as an OTP.

Course of Treatment

The DATA 2000[9] allows physicians who are trained or experienced in opioid addiction treatment to obtain waivers to prescribe certain schedule III, IV, or V narcotic drugs in the Controlled Substances Act, for the treatment of opioid dependence in their office practices or in a clinic setting. Both buprenorphine monoproduct and combination buprenorphine/naloxone are approved by the US FDA for the treatment of opioid dependence and can be used in settings outside of an OTP. Physicians who wish to prescribe buprenorphine monoproduct or combination buprenorphine/naloxone for the treatment of opioid use disorder or withdrawal management must qualify for a waiver under DATA 2000. Physicians with approved DATA 2000 waivers are not confined to the office-based setting. Physicians with DATA 2000 waivers may treat opioid addiction with approved buprenorphine products in any outpatient practice settings in which they are otherwise credentialed to practice and in which such treatment would be medically appropriate. This flexibility for place of services is referred to as OBOT. Physicians who qualify for DATA 2000[9] waivers are initially limited in the number of patients they can treat, but after 1 year may apply for a waiver to treat more (see "Exhibit 4: Physician Qualifications for OBOT").

Exhibit 4: Physician Qualifications for OBOT

To qualify for a DATA 2000 waiver, a physician must hold a current, valid state medical license and a drug enforcement agency (DEA) registration number. In addition, the physician must meet at least one of the following criteria outlined by the US Department of Health and Human Services, Substance Abuse, and Mental Health Services Administration:
(1) The physician holds a subspecialty board certification in addiction psychiatry from the American Board of Medical Specialties.
(2) The physician holds an addiction certification from the ASAM. (ASAM certification was taken over by the American Board of Addiction Medicine [ABAM] in 2007.)
(3) The physician holds a subspecialty board certification in addiction medicine from the American Osteopathic Association.
(4) The physician has, with respect to the treatment and management of opioid-addicted patients, completed not less than 8 hours of training (through classroom situations, seminars at professional society meetings, electronic communications, or otherwise) that is provided by the ASAM, the American Academy of Addiction Psychiatry, the American Medical Association, the American Osteopathic Association, the American Psychiatric Association, or any other organization that the Secretary determines is appropriate for purposes of this subclause.

(5) The physician has participated as an investigator in one or more clinical trials leading to the approval of a narcotic drug in schedule III, IV, or V for maintenance or detoxification treatment, as demonstrated by a statement submitted to the Secretary by the sponsor of such approved drug.

(6) The physician has such other training or experience as the state medical licensing board (of the state in which the physician will provide maintenance or detoxification treatment) considers to demonstrate the ability of the physician to treat and manage opioid-addicted patients.

(7) The physician has such other training or experience as the Secretary considers to demonstrate the ability of the physician to treat and manage opioid-addicted patients. Any criteria of the Secretary under this subclause shall be established by regulation. Any such criteria are effective only for 3 years after the date on which the criteria are promulgated, but may be extended for such additional discrete 3-year periods as the Secretary considers appropriate for purposes of this subclause. Such an extension of criteria may only be effectuated through a statement published in the Federal Register by the Secretary during the 30-day period preceding the end of the 3-year period involved.

More detailed information can be found at the website: http://buprenorphine.samhsa.gov/waiver_qualifications.html

Induction

The buprenorphine monoproduct and Suboxone film are the only medications approved by the US FDA for induction. However, other forms of the combination product have been used by clinicians in patients addicted to short-acting opioids without other complications. Because of concern that sublingually absorbed naloxone could increase the risk of precipitated withdrawal, treatment initiation with buprenorphine monoproduct is recommended for patients transitioning from methadone and any other long-acting opioid, and patients with hepatic impairment.

Buprenorphine has a higher affinity for the mu-opioid receptor compared to most full opioid agonists. Because buprenorphine is a partial mu-agonist, the risk of overdose during buprenorphine induction is low. However, buprenorphine will displace full agonists from the receptor with resultant reduction in opioid effects. Thus, some patients may experience precipitated withdrawal if insufficient time has elapsed since their last dose of opioids.

Patients should wait until they are experiencing mild to moderate opioid withdrawal before taking the first dose of buprenorphine to reduce the risk of precipitated withdrawal. Generally, buprenorphine initiation should occur at least 6–12 hours after the last use of heroin or other short-acting opioids, or 24–72 hours after their last use of long-acting opioids such as methadone. The use of the COWS can be helpful in determining if patients are experiencing mild to moderate withdrawal.[166] A COWS score of 11–12 or more (mild to moderate withdrawal) is indicative of sufficient withdrawal to allow a safe and comfortable induction onto buprenorphine.

Induction within the clinician's office is recommended to reduce the risk of precipitated opioid withdrawal. Office-based induction is also recommended if the patient or physician is unfamiliar with buprenorphine. However, buprenorphine induction may be done by patients within their own homes.[69]

Home-based induction is recommended only if the patient or prescribing physician is experienced with the use of buprenorphine. The recommendation supporting home induction is based on the consensus opinion of the Guideline Committee.

Dosing

At Induction

The risk of precipitated withdrawal can be reduced by using a lower initial dose of buprenorphine. It is recommended that induction start with a dose of 2–4 mg, and that the patient is observed for signs of precipitated withdrawal. If 60–90 minutes have passed without the onset of withdrawal symptoms, then additional dosing can be done in increments of 2–4 mg. Repeat of the COWS during induction can be useful in assessing the effect of buprenorphine doses. Once it has been established that the initial dose is well tolerated, the buprenorphine dose can be increased fairly rapidly to a dose that provides stable effects for 24 hours and is clinically effective.

After Induction

On average, buprenorphine doses after induction and titration are usually at least 8 mg per day. However, if patients are continuing to use opioids, consideration should be given to increasing the dose by 4–8 mg (daily dose of 12–16 mg or higher). The US FDA approves dosing to a limit of 24 mg per day, and there is limited evidence regarding the relative efficacy of higher doses. In addition, the use of higher doses may increase the risk of diversion.

Adverse Effects

Buprenorphine and combinations of buprenorphine and naloxone are generally well tolerated. Side effects reported with these medications include headache, anxiety, constipation, perspiration, fluid retention in lower extremities, urinary hesitancy, and sleep disturbance. Unlike treatment with methadone, QT-interval prolongation does not seem to be an adverse effect associated with treatment with buprenorphine.

Psychosocial Treatment

Psychosocial treatment is recommended for all patients. The types and duration of psychosocial treatment will vary, and the topic is discussed further in "Part 7: Psychosocial Treatment in Conjunction With Medications for the Treatment of Opioid Use Disorder."

Monitoring Treatment

Patients should be seen frequently at the beginning of their treatment. Weekly visits (at least) are recommended until patients are determined to be stable. The stability of a patient is determined by an individual clinician based on a number of indicators which may include abstinence from illicit drugs, participation in psychosocial treatment and other recovery-based activities, and good occupational and social functioning. Stable patients can be seen less frequently but should be seen at least monthly.

Accessing PDMP data is advisable to check for other medications that the patient may be receiving. Due to the variation in state PDMP laws, clinicians are encouraged to be familiar with the legal requirements associated with PDMPs and prescribing of controlled substances in their state (see "Exhibit 2" in "Part 1: Assessment and Diagnosis of Opioid Use Disorder"). In addition, objective measurement of body fluids for the presence of buprenorphine and illicit drugs of misuse is recommended.

Urine drug testing is a reasonably practical and reliable method to test for buprenorphine and illicit drugs. However, other reliable biological tests for the presence of drugs may be used. It is recommended that patients be tested often and that testing should be done for buprenorphine, substances such as heroin and marijuana, and prescription medications including benzodiazepines, prescription opioids, and amphetamines. How often and exactly what drugs should be tested for to optimize treatment has not been definitively established and is a topic that should be researched further (please see "Drug Testing: A White Paper of the American Society of Addiction Medicine" for detail on types of drug testing).[10]

Clinicians should take steps to reduce the chance of diversion. Diversion has been reported with buprenorphine monotherapy and combination buprenorphine/naloxone.[172]

Strategies to reduce the potential of diversion include: frequent office visits, urine drug testing including testing for buprenorphine and metabolites, observed dosing, and recall visits for pill counts. Patients receiving treatment with buprenorphine should be counseled to have adequate means to secure their medications to prevent theft. Unused medication should be disposed of safely.[121]

Length of Treatment

There is no recommended time limit for treatment with buprenorphine. Buprenorphine taper and discontinuation is a slow process and close monitoring is recommended. Buprenorphine tapering is generally accomplished over several months. Patients and clinicians should not take the decision to terminate treatment with buprenorphine lightly. Factors associated with successful termination of treatment with buprenorphine are not well described, but may include the following:

(1) Employment, engagement in mutual help programs, or involvement in other meaningful activities.
(2) Sustained abstinence from opioid and other drugs during treatment.
(3) Positive changes in the psychosocial environment.
(4) Evidence of additional psychosocial supports.
(5) Persistent engagement in treatment for ongoing monitoring past the point of medication discontinuation.

Patients who relapse after treatment has been terminated should be returned to treatment with buprenorphine.

Switching Treatment Medications

Buprenorphine is generally tolerated well by patients.

Switching from buprenorphine to other opioid treatment medications may be appropriate in the following cases:

(1) Patient experiences intolerable side effects.
(2) Patient has not experienced a successful course of treatment in attaining or maintaining goal through the initially chosen pharmacotherapy option.
(3) Patient requires a greater level of supervision or services than office-based buprenorphine offers.
(4) Patient wants to change and is a candidate for treatment.

Switching to Naltrexone

Buprenorphine has a long half-life; 7–14 days should elapse between the last dose of buprenorphine and the start of naltrexone to ensure that the patient is not physically dependent on opioids before starting naltrexone. It may be useful to conduct a naloxone challenge (see "Glossary") before starting naltrexone to demonstrate an absence of physical dependence.

Recently, investigators have begun to evaluate newer methods of rapidly transitioning patients from buprenorphine to naltrexone using repeated dosing over several days with very low doses of naltrexone along with ancillary medications.[105]

Although the results are promising, it is too early to recommend these techniques for general practice, and the doses of naltrexone used may not be readily available to most clinicians.

Switching to Methadone

Transitioning from buprenorphine to methadone is less problematic because the addition of a full mu-opioid agonist to a partial agonist does not typically result in any type of adverse reaction. There is no time delay required in transitioning a patient from buprenorphine to treatment with methadone.

Summary of Recommendations

(1) Opioid-dependent patients should wait until they are experiencing mild to moderate opioid withdrawal before taking the first dose of buprenorphine to reduce the risk of precipitated withdrawal. Generally, buprenorphine initiation should occur at least 6–12 hours after the last use of heroin or other short acting opioids, or 24–72 hours after their last use of long-acting opioids such as methadone.
(2) Induction of buprenorphine should start with a dose of 2–4 mg. Dosages may be increased in increments of 2–4 mg.
(3) Clinicians should observe patients in their offices during induction. Emerging research, however, suggests that many patients need "not" be observed and that home buprenorphine induction may be considered. Home-based induction is recommended only if the patient or prescribing physician is experienced with the use of buprenorphine. This is based on the consensus opinion of the Guideline Committee.
(4) Buprenorphine doses after induction and titration should be, on average, at least 8 mg per day. However, if patients are continuing to use opioids, consideration should be given to increasing the dose by 4–8 mg (daily doses of 12–16 mg or higher). The US FDA approves dosing to a limit of 24 mg per day, and there is limited evidence regarding the relative efficacy of higher doses. In addition, the use of higher doses may increase the risk of diversion.
(5) Psychosocial treatment should be implemented in conjunction with the use of buprenorphine in the treatment of opioid use disorder.
(6) Clinicians should take steps to reduce the chance of buprenorphine diversion. Recommended strategies include frequent office visits (weekly in early treatment), urine drug testing including testing for buprenorphine and metabolites, and recall visits for pill counts.
(7) Patients should be tested frequently for buprenorphine, other substances, and prescription medications. Accessing PDMP data may be useful for monitoring.
(8) Patients should be seen frequently at the beginning of their treatment. Weekly visits (at least) are recommended until patients are determined to be stable. There is no recommended time limit for treatment.
(9) Buprenorphine taper and discontinuation is a slow process and close monitoring is recommended. Buprenorphine tapering is generally accomplished over several months. Patients should be encouraged to remain in treatment for ongoing monitoring past the point of discontinuation.
(10) When considering a switch from buprenorphine to naltrexone, 7–14 days should elapse between the last dose of buprenorphine and the start of naltrexone to ensure that the patient is not physically dependent on opioids before starting naltrexone.

(11) When considering a switch from buprenorphine to methadone, there is no required time delay because the addition of a full mu-opioid agonist to a partial agonist does not typically result in any type of adverse reaction.

(12) Patients who discontinue agonist therapy and resume opioid use should be made aware of the risks associated with an opioid overdose, and especially the increased risk of death.

Areas for Further Research

Further research is needed to evaluate the safety and efficacy of buprenorphine induction conducted in the patient's own home, although current research supports this practice in select cases.

Part 6: Naltrexone

Background

Naltrexone is a long-acting opioid antagonist that may be used to prevent relapse to opioid use. Naltrexone blocks the effects of opioids if they are used. Naltrexone is available in oral (ReVia, Depade) and extended-release injectable (Vivitrol) formulations.

Formulations of Naltrexone: Oral Versus Extended-Release Injectable

Most studies that found oral naltrexone effective were conducted in situations in which patients were highly motivated, were legally mandated to receive treatment, and/or taking the medication under the supervision of their family or significant others. A meta-analysis of 1158 participants in 13 randomized trials compared treatment with oral naltrexone to either placebo or no medication for opioid use disorder.[115]

The evidence generated from these trials was limited by poor adherence and high dropout rates. Oral naltrexone was more efficacious than placebo in sustaining abstinence in three trials in which patients had external mandates (e.g., legal requirements) and were monitored in adhering to daily doses of the medication.[3,115]

An extended-release injectable naltrexone formulation is available for patients with difficulty adhering to daily medication. This formulation requires an injection once per month. Extended-release injectable naltrexone has been found to be more efficacious than placebo for opioid dependence in randomized trials, although the trials were limited by high dropout rates of about 45% observed at 6 months.[93] One trial found naltrexone to be efficacious in patients with more than one substance use disorder and using more than one drug (heroin and amphetamines), which is a drug combination common in patients with opioid use disorder.[156]

Patient Selection and Treatment Goals

Oral naltrexone and extended-release injectable naltrexone are efficacious treatments recommended for patients who have an opioid use disorder, are able to give informed consent, and have no specific contraindications for agonist treatment.

The 1-month protection from relapse after a single dose may make it particularly useful in preventing overdoses and facilitating entry into longer-term treatment if given to prisoners shortly before re-entry or to patients who are discharged from general hospitals after being detoxified in the course of treatment for medical or surgical problems.

Treatment with naltrexone generally has the following four goals:

(1) To prevent relapse to opioids in patients who have already been detoxified and are no longer physically dependent on opioids.

(2) To block the effects of illicit opioids.

(3) To reduce opioid craving.

(4) To promote and facilitate patient engagement in recovery-oriented activities including psychosocial intervention.

Oral Naltrexone

Because oral naltrexone has high rates of nonadherence and the potential for overdose upon relapse, this treatment is best for candidates who can be closely supervised and who are highly motivated. There is a risk of opioid overdose if the patient ceases naltrexone and then uses opioids. Groups that may benefit from oral naltrexone include employed patients, those who have been using drugs for only a short time (e.g., younger patients), and those under threat of legal sanctions.

Extended-Release Injectable Naltrexone

Extended-release injectable naltrexone is also an efficacious treatment for opioid use disorder. It may be especially useful for patients who have contraindications to, or who failed pharmacotherapy with buprenorphine and methadone; patients confined to drug-free environments such as prison or inpatient rehabilitation; patients living in areas where agonist treatment is not available; individuals who are highly motivated and are willing to taper off their current agonist therapy; or patients who simply do not want to be treated with an agonist. Because it is US FDA-approved for the treatment of alcohol use disorder, it may be well suited for patients with co-occurring opioid and alcohol use disorders.

Precautions

Risk of Relapse and Subsequent Opioid Overdose

Patients maintained on naltrexone will have diminished tolerance to opioids and may be unaware of the consequent increased sensitivity to opioids if they stop taking naltrexone. Patients who discontinue antagonist therapy should be made aware of this phenomenon. If the patient stops naltrexone and resumes use of opioids in doses similar to those that were being used before the start of treatment with naltrexone, there is risk of an opioid overdose. This is due to the loss of tolerance to opioids and a resulting misjudgment of dose at the time of relapse.[143] A similar dynamic occurs in patients who detoxify with no meaningful follow-up treatment, or those who drop out of methadone or buprenorphine maintenance.

Course of Treatment

Induction

Before administering naltrexone, it is important that the patient has been adequately detoxified from opioids and is no longer physically dependent. Naltrexone can precipitate severe withdrawal symptoms in patients who have not been adequately withdrawn from opioids. As a general rule, patients should be free from short-acting opioids for about 6 days before starting naltrexone, and free from long-acting opioids such as methadone and buprenorphine for 7–10 days. A naloxone challenge can be used if it is uncertain whether the patient is no longer physically dependent on opioids. In the naloxone challenge, naloxone hydrochloride (a shorter-acting injectable opioid antagonist) is administered and the patient is monitored for signs and symptoms of withdrawal. A low-dose oral naltrexone challenge has been used as an alternative.

Dosing

"Oral naltrexone" can be dosed at: 50 mg daily or three times weekly dosing with two 100-mg doses followed by one 150-mg dose. Oral naltrexone seems to be most useful when there is a support person to administer and supervise the medication. A support person may be a family member, close friend, or an employer.

"Extended-release injectable naltrexone" can be given every 4 weeks by deep intramuscular (IM) injection in the gluteal muscle at a set dosage of 380 mg per injection. Whereas the injection interval is generally every 4 weeks, some clinicians have administered the medication more frequently (e.g., every 3 weeks). There is no objective evidence supporting the safety or efficacy of this practice, however, and the Guideline Committee did not endorse it. More research is needed on safe dosing intervals for long-acting injectable naltrexone.

Special consideration should be made in naltrexone dosing for incarcerated groups. Re-entry into the community after imprisonment is a high-risk period for relapse to opioid misuse and overdose. Therefore, extended-release injectable naltrexone dosing before re-entry may serve to prevent relapse and overdose. A similar situation may apply to individuals leaving detoxification with no meaningful follow-up treatment, or to persons who have been detoxified in the course of medical or surgical treatment and who leave the hospital with no immediate relapse prevention follow-up therapy.

Adverse Effects

Naltrexone, both oral and extended-release injectable, is generally well tolerated. Apart from opioids, it does not typically interact with other medications. Most common side effects in random order can include insomnia, lack of energy/sedation, anxiety, nausea, vomiting, abdominal pain/cramps, headache, cold symptoms, joint and muscle pain, and specific to extended-release injectable naltrexone injection site reactions. To reduce injection site reactions in obese patients, a longer needle size may be used.[128]

Psychosocial Treatment

Psychosocial treatment is recommended and its efficacy is established when used in combination with naltrexone. Extended-released injectable naltrexone has not been studied as a standalone therapy without psychosocial treatment (for more recommendations regarding psychosocial treatment, see "Part 7: Psychosocial Treatment in Conjunction with Medications for the Treatment of Opioid Use Disorder").

Monitoring Treatment

Patients should be seen frequently at the beginning of their treatment. Weekly or more frequent visits are recommended until patients are determined to be stable. The stability of a patient is determined by an individual clinician based on a number of indicators which may include abstinence from illicit drugs, participation in psychosocial treatment and other recovery-based activities, and good occupational and social functioning. Stable patients can be seen less frequently, but should be seen at least monthly.

Accessing PDMP data is advisable to check for use of other prescription medications. In addition, objective measurement of body fluids for the presence of drugs of misuse is recommended.

Urine drug testing is a reasonably practical and reliable method to test for illicit drugs. However, other reliable biological tests for the presence of drugs may be used. It is recommended that patients be tested often and that testing should be done for substances such as heroin and marijuana, and prescription medications including benzodiazepines, prescription opioids, and amphetamines. How often and exactly what drugs should be tested for to optimize treatment has not been definitively established and is a topic that should be researched further.[6]

Length of Treatment

Data are not available at present on the recommended length of treatment with oral naltrexone or extended-release injectable naltrexone. Duration of treatment depends on the response of the individual patient, the patient's individual circumstances, and clinical judgment.

Switching Treatment Medications

Switching from naltrexone to other opioid treatment medications may be appropriate in the following cases:
(1) Patient experiences intolerable side effects.
(2) Patient has not experienced a successful course of treatment in attaining or maintaining goal through the initially chosen pharmacotherapy option.
(3) Patient wants to change medications and is a candidate for alternative treatment.

Transfer of medications should be planned, considered, and monitored. Switching from an antagonist such as naltrexone to a full agonist (methadone) or a partial agonist (buprenorphine) is generally less complicated than switching from a full or partial agonist to an antagonist because there is no physical dependence associated with antagonist treatment. Patients being switched from naltrexone to buprenorphine or methadone will not have physical dependence on opioids and thus the initial doses of methadone or buprenorphine used may be less. Patients should not be switched until a significant amount of the naltrexone is no longer in their system—about 1 day for oral naltrexone or 30 days for extended-release injectable naltrexone.

Summary of Recommendations

(1) Naltrexone is a recommended treatment in preventing relapse in opioid use disorder. Oral formula naltrexone may be considered for patients in whom adherence can be supervised or enforced. Extended-release injectable naltrexone may be more suitable for patients who have issues with adherence.
(2) Oral naltrexone should be taken daily in 50-mg doses, or three times weekly in two 100-mg doses followed by one 150-mg dose.
(3) Extended-release injectable naltrexone should be administered every 4 weeks by deep IM injection in the gluteal muscle at a set dosage of 380 mg per injection.
(4) Psychosocial treatment is recommended in conjunction with treatment with naltrexone. The efficacy of naltrexone use in conjunction with psychosocial treatment has been established, whereas the efficacy of extended-release injectable naltrexone without psychosocial intervention "has not" been established.
(5) There is no recommended length of treatment with oral naltrexone or extended-release injectable naltrexone. Duration depends on clinical judgment and the patient's individual

circumstances. Because there is no physical dependence associated with naltrexone, it can be stopped abruptly without withdrawal symptoms.

(6) Switching from naltrexone to methadone or buprenorphine should be planned, considered, and monitored. Switching from an antagonist such as naltrexone to a full agonist (methadone) or a partial agonist (buprenorphine) is generally less complicated than switching from a full or partial agonist to an antagonist because there is no physical dependence associated with antagonist treatment and thus no possibility of precipitated withdrawal. Patients being switched from naltrexone to buprenorphine or methadone will not have physical dependence on opioids and thus the initial doses of methadone or buprenorphine used should be low. Patients should not be switched until a significant amount of the naltrexone is no longer in their system—about 1 day for oral naltrexone or 30 days for extended-release injectable naltrexone.

(7) Patients who discontinue antagonist therapy and resume opioid use should be made aware of the increased risks associated with an opioid overdose, and especially the increased risk of death.

Areas for Further Research

(1) Further research is needed to test the relative efficacy of extended-release injectable naltrexone as compared to agonist treatment.

(2) Further research is needed on optimal withdrawal management to initiate treatment with naltrexone and minimize the risk of precipitated withdrawal.

(3) Further research is needed about the safety and efficacy of administering extended-release injectable naltrexone every 3 weeks for individuals who metabolize naltrexone at higher rates.

Part 7: Psychosocial Treatment in Conjunction With Medications for the Treatment of Opioid Use Disorder

Background

Psychosocial treatment can help patients manage cravings, reduce the likelihood of relapse, and assist them in coping with the emotional and social challenges that often accompany substance use disorders. Psychosocial treatment is available in a variety of outpatient and inpatient settings, but the majority of studies have focused on outpatient treatment. Psychosocial treatment is provided using a variety of approaches in various milieus, including social skills training; individual, group, and couples counseling; cognitive behavioral therapy; motivational interviewing; and family therapy. Determining level of need and best approach to psychosocial treatment is individualized to each patient. In accordance with ASAM policy, mutual help compliments professional treatment, but is not a substitute for professional treatment.[12]

Goals of Psychosocial Treatment for Opioid Use Disorder

Although psychosocial treatment options vary, common therapeutic goals are to:

(1) modify the underlying processes that maintain or reinforce use behavior;

(2) encourage engagement with pharmacotherapy (e.g., medication compliance); and

(3) treat any concomitant psychiatric disorders that either complicate a substance use disorder or act as a trigger for relapse.

Components of Psychosocial Treatment for Opioid Use Disorder

Psychosocial treatment is recommended in conjunction with any/all pharmacological treatment for opioid use disorder. At a minimum, the psychosocial treatment component of the overall treatment program should include the following:

(1) assessment of psychosocial needs;
(2) supportive individual and/or group counseling;
(3) linkages to existing family support systems; and
(4) referrals to community-based services.

More structured psychosocial treatment may be offered, and may potentially include more intensive individual counseling and psychotherapy, more specific social needs assistance (e.g., employment, housing, and legal services), and case management.

Efficacy of Psychosocial Treatments in Opioid Use Disorder

There is evidence of the superiority of some psychosocial treatments over others, particularly contingency management (CM) and cognitive behavioral therapy (CBT). A 2008 meta-analysis compared the 2340 participants who received one of the following interventions: CM, relapse prevention, CBT, and CBT combined with CM. Participants receiving any psychosocial treatment had better outcomes than participants who did not. Contingency management and the combined CM and CBT intervention produced better outcomes than the other interventions.[56]

Other potentially useful psychosocial treatments include, but are not limited to, the following:

(1) behavioral couples counseling;
(2) cognitive behavioral coping skills training;
(3) community reinforcement approach;
(4) contingency management/motivational incentives; and
(5) motivational enhancement.

Most recommendations for psychosocial treatments are not correlated with any specific pharmacological approach. Many patients have been shown to experience improved outcomes after receiving psychosocial treatment, in both individual and group formats, from a variety of approaches. Ancillary drug addiction counseling and mutual-help programs are generally considered beneficial.

Mutual Help Programs

Although not considered by ASAM to be a psychosocial treatment on its own, mutual help is an ancillary service that may be effective. Mutual-help programs may include 12-step programs such as Alcoholics Anonymous (AA), Narcotics Anonymous (NA), and Methadone Anonymous (MA). Other mutual-help groups include Self-Management and Recovery Therapy (SMART), and Moderation Management. Many providers recommend mutual-help programs, but there is anecdotal information to suggest that some of these programs may be less acceptable to patients receiving medications for opioid use disorder.

Adherence to Psychosocial Treatment Within Overall Treatment

Clinicians should determine the optimal type of psychosocial treatment to which to refer patients based on shared decision-making with the patient and in consideration of the availability and accessibility of area resources. Collaboration with qualified behavioral health providers is one way for clinicians to determine the type of psychosocial treatment that would best fit within a patient's individualized treatment plan. The ASAM Standards describe in standards III.1 and III.2 the role of the clinician in coordinating care and providing therapeutic alternatives. Key concepts within these standards speak to the importance of patient education about alternatives, shared decision-making in selection of therapeutic services, and the incumbent responsibility of the clinician to assure through the treatment planning and treatment management processes to assure that psychosocial treatment is being received and that the patient is progressing towards mutually agreed upon goals. Renegotiated treatment plans should be established when patients do not follow through with psychosocial treatment referrals and/or that it is determined that the treatment plan goals are not being advanced.

Psychosocial Treatment and Treatment With Methadone

Psychosocial treatment is generally recommended for patients in treatment with methadone (see "Part 4: Methadone," subsection "Patient Selection and Treatment Goals").

Studies have found that psychosocial treatment in conjunction with methadone pharmacotherapy improves treatment effectiveness. The addition of psychosocial treatment has been associated with improved retention and reduced opioid use. A meta-analysis in 2011 found that psychosocial treatment improved withdrawal management outcomes.[4]

Some research, however, suggests the lack of efficacy in adding psychosocial treatment to treatment with methadone alone. Analyses of specific psychosocial treatments, including contingency management, did not show significant benefit over agonist medication alone.[56]

This analysis, however, did not examine the effect of existing psychosocial treatments given during the course of treatment with methadone. Instead, the meta-analysis measured the effect of added psychosocial treatments.

Psychosocial Treatment and Treatment With Buprenorphine

Clinicians who are prescribing buprenorphine should consider providing or recommending office-based or community-based psychosocial treatment. There is some research evidence that the addition of psychosocial treatment improves adherence and retention in treatment with buprenorphine[23,86,133]; however, these findings are mixed.[5,60,61,155,165] It is recommended that clinicians offer patients psychosocial treatment early in their treatment with buprenorphine.

Effective therapies may include the following:
(1) cognitive behavioral therapies;
(2) contingency management;
(3) relapse prevention; and
(4) motivational interviewing.

Psychosocial Treatment and Treatment With Naltrexone

Psychosocial treatment is a recommended component of the treatment plan that utilizes the pharmacological therapy of naltrexone. In fact, extended-release injectable naltrexone's efficacy was established only when used in combination with psychosocial

treatment. Conversely, extended-release injectable naltrexone's efficacy has not been tested as a standalone treatment without a psychosocial component. There are, however, limited data available on long-term outcomes.

Summary of Recommendations

(1) Psychosocial treatment is recommended in conjunction with any pharmacological treatment of opioid use disorder. At a minimum, psychosocial treatment should include the following: psychosocial needs assessment, supportive counseling, links to existing family supports, and referrals to community services.
(2) Treatment planning should include collaboration with qualified behavioral healthcare providers to determine the optimal type and intensity of psychosocial treatment and for renegotiation of the treatment plan for circumstances in which patients do not adhere to recommended plans for, or referrals to, psychosocial treatment.
(3) Psychosocial treatment is generally recommended for patients who are receiving opioid agonist treatment (methadone or buprenorphine).
(4) Psychosocial treatment should be offered with oral and extended-release injectable naltrexone. The efficacy of extended-release injectable naltrexone to treat opioid use disorder has not been confirmed when it has been used as pharmacotherapy without accompanying psychosocial treatment.

Areas for Further Research

(1) Further research is needed to identify the comparative advantages of specific psychosocial treatments.
(2) Further study is needed to evaluate the effectiveness of psychosocial treatment in combination with specific pharmacotherapies.
(3) More research is needed on which concurrent psychosocial treatments are most effective for different patient populations and treatment settings including primary care.
(4) Further research is needed on which psychosocial treatments are suitable for addition to buprenorphine or treatment with naltrexone, which can be delivered in primary care settings.

Part 8: Special Populations: Pregnant Women

Background

Many of the medical risks associated with opioid use disorder are similar for both pregnant and nonpregnant women; however, opioid use disorder carries obstetrical risks for pregnant women. Several obstetrical complications have been associated with opioid use in pregnancy, including preeclampsia, miscarriage, premature delivery, fetal growth restriction, and fetal death.[41] It is difficult to establish the extent to which these problems are due to opioid use, withdrawal, or co-occurring use of other drugs.

Other factors that may contribute to obstetrical complications include concomitant maternal medical, nutritional, and psychosocial issues.

Pregnant women with opioid use disorder are candidates for opioid agonist treatment if a return to opioid use is likely during pregnancy. Methadone is the accepted standard of care for use during pregnancy. Buprenorphine monoproduct is a reasonable and recommended alternative to methadone for pregnant women.

There is insufficient evidence to recommend the combination buprenorphine/naloxone formulation, though there is evidence of safety.

Assessment of Opioid Use Disorder in Pregnant Women

As is the case for any patient presenting for assessment of opioid use disorder, the first clinical priority should be to identify any emergent or urgent medical conditions that require immediate attention. Diagnosing emergent conditions can be challenging because women may present with symptoms that may be related to overdose and/or a complication in pregnancy.

A comprehensive assessment including medical examination and psychosocial assessment is recommended in evaluating opioid use disorder in pregnant women. The clinician should ask questions in a direct and nonjudgmental manner to elicit a detailed and accurate history.

Medical Examination

Physical Examination

A physical examination should be conducted for pregnant women who are presenting with potential opioid use disorder. The examination should include identifying objective physical signs of opioid intoxication or withdrawal. The objective physical signs for patients, including pregnant women, are described in "Part 1: Assessment and Diagnosis of Opioid Use Disorder." Obstetricians and gynecologists should be alert to signs and symptoms of opioid use disorder. Pregnant women with opioid use disorder are more likely to seek prenatal care late in pregnancy, miss appointments, experience poor weight gain, or exhibit signs of withdrawal or intoxication. Positive results of serologic tests for HIV, hepatitis B, or hepatitis C may also indicate opioid use disorder. On physical examination, some signs of drug use may be present, such as puncture marks from intravenous injection, abscesses, or cellulitis.

Laboratory Tests

Routine prenatal laboratory tests should be performed. Women who use opioids intravenously are at high risk for infections related to sharing injection syringes and sexually transmitted infections. Therefore, counseling and testing for HIV should be provided, according to state laws. Tests for hepatitis B and C and liver function are also suggested. Hepatitis A and B vaccination is recommended for those whose hepatitis serology is negative. Urine drug testing may be used to detect or confirm suspected opioid and other drug use, but should be performed only with the patient's consent and in compliance with state laws. State laws differ in terms of clinicians' reporting requirements of identified drug use to child welfare services and/or health authorities. Laws that penalize pregnant women for substance use disorders serve to prevent women from obtaining prenatal care and treatment for opioid use disorder, which may worsen outcomes for mother and child. According to the American Congress of Obstetricians and Gynecologists (ACOG) 2014 Toolkit on State Legislation, mandatory urine drug testing is considered an unfavorable policy that does not support healthy pregnancy outcomes.[6] Routine urine drug testing is not highly sensitive for many drugs and results in false-positive and negative results that are misleading and potentially devastating for the patient. ACOG suggests that even with patient consent, urine testing should not be relied upon as the sole or valid indication of drug use. They suggest that positive urine screens should be followed with a definitive drug assay. Similarly, in a study conducted on pregnant women in Florida, where there is mandatory reporting to health authorities, study authors identified that compliant clinician reporting of drug misuse was biased by racial ethnicity and socioeconomic status of the pregnant woman. It was their conclusion that any state that regulates for mandatory urine testing and reporting do so based on medical criteria and medical necessity of such testing.[34]

Imaging

Confirmation of a viable intrauterine pregnancy by sonography is often required before acceptance into an OTP that is tailored specifically to pregnant women. Imaging is also useful for confirmation of gestational age.

Psychosocial Assessment

Research has found that the majority of women entering treatment for opioid use disorder have a history of sexual assault, domestic violence, and/or come from homes where their parents used drugs. Therefore, it is important to obtain a psychosocial history when evaluating pregnant women for opioid use disorder.

Opioid Agonist Treatment in Pregnancy

Decisions to use opioid agonist medications in pregnant women with opioid use disorder revolve around balancing the risks and benefits to maternal and infant health. Opioid agonist treatment is thought to have minimal long-term developmental impacts on children relative to harms resulting from maternal use of heroin and prescription opioids. Therefore, women with opioid use disorder who are not in treatment should be encouraged to start opioid agonist treatment with methadone or buprenorphine monotherapy (without naloxone) as early in the pregnancy as possible. Furthermore, pregnant women who are on agonist treatment should be encouraged not to discontinue treatment while they are pregnant.

Treatment Management Team

Pregnancy in women with opioid use disorder should be co-managed by an obstetrician and an addiction specialist physician. Release of information forms need to be completed to ensure communication among healthcare providers.

Opioid Agonists Versus Withdrawal Management

Pregnant women who are physically dependent on opioids should receive treatment using agonist medications rather than withdrawal management or abstinence as these approaches may pose a risk to the fetus. Furthermore, withdrawal management has been found to be inferior in effectiveness over pharmacotherapy with opioid agonists and increases the risk of relapse without fetal or maternal benefit.

Methadone Versus Buprenorphine

The discussion and decision for medication should be reviewed with the patient and documented in her chart. For women who are pregnant or breastfeeding, opioid agonist treatment with methadone or buprenorphine is seen as the most appropriate treatment, taking into consideration effects on the fetus, neonatal abstinence syndrome, and impacts on perinatal care and parenting of young children.

Methadone is the accepted standard of care for use during pregnancy; however, buprenorphine monoproduct is a reasonable alternative and also has some advantages over methadone. Infants born to mothers treated with buprenorphine had shorter hospital stays (10 vs. 17.5 days), had shorter treatment durations for neonatal abstinence syndrome (NAS) (4.1 vs. 9.9 days), and required a lower cumulative dose of morphine (1.1 vs. 10.4 mg) compared to infants born to mothers on treatment with methadone.[83] However, in this trial, mothers treated with buprenorphine were more likely to drop out of treatment compared to mothers treated with methadone.

Combination Buprenorphine/Naloxone

There is some evidence suggesting that buprenorphine/naloxone is equivalent in safety and efficacy to the monoproduct for pregnant women.[49,167] At present, however, this evidence is insufficient to recommend the combination buprenorphine/naloxone formulation in this population. The buprenorphine monoproduct should be used instead.

Naltrexone in Pregnancy

If a woman becomes pregnant while she is receiving naltrexone, it is appropriate to discontinue the medication if the patient and doctor agree that the risk of relapse is low. If the patient is highly concerned about relapse and wishes to remain on naltrexone, it is important to inform the patient about the risks of staying on naltrexone and obtain consent for ongoing treatment. If the patient discontinues treatment with naltrexone and subsequently relapses, it may be appropriate to consider methadone or treatment with buprenorphine.

Naloxone in Pregnancy

The use of an antagonist such as naloxone to diagnose opioid use disorder in pregnant women is contraindicated because induced withdrawal may precipitate preterm labor or fetal distress. Naloxone should be used only in the case of maternal overdose to save the woman's life.

Methadone Induction

Conception While in Treatment With Methadone

Conceiving while on methadone has been associated with better drug treatment outcomes compared to women who initiate methadone during pregnancy. Pregnant women in treatment with methadone before conception who are not in physical withdrawal can be continued on methadone as outpatients.

Timing of Treatment in Pregnancy

Treatment with methadone should be initiated as early as possible during pregnancy to produce the most optimal outcomes. Longer duration of treatment with methadone is associated with longer gestation and higher birth weight.[28]

There is insufficient evidence of teratogenic effects in pregnancy. NAS occurs while under treatment with methadone, but is easily treated if all parties are aware that it is likely to occur. The NAS risk to the fetus is significantly less than the risk of untreated opioid dependence. Data collected on exposure in human pregnancies are complicated by confounding variables including drug, alcohol, and cigarette use; poor maternal nutrition; and an increased prevalence of maternal infection.

The optimum setting for initiation of therapy has not been evaluated in this population. Hospitalization during initiation

of treatment with methadone may be advisable due to the potential for adverse events (e.g., overdose and adverse drug interactions), especially in the third trimester. This is also an ideal time for the woman to be assessed by a social worker and case manager, and initiate prenatal care if it has not been initiated earlier.

In an inpatient setting, methadone is initiated at a dose range from 10 to 30 mg. Incremental doses of 5–10 mg are given every 3–6 hours as needed to treat withdrawal symptoms, to a maximum first day dose of 30–40 mg. After induction, clinicians should increase the methadone dose in 5–10 mg increments per week, if indicated, to maintain the lowest dose that controls withdrawal symptoms and minimizes the desire to use additional opioids.

Buprenorphine Induction

Initiation or induction of buprenorphine may lead to withdrawal symptoms in patients with physical dependence on opioids. To minimize this risk, induction should be initiated when a woman begins to show objective, observable signs of moderate withdrawal, but before severe withdrawal symptoms are evidenced. This usually occurs 6 hours or more after the last dose of a short-acting opioid, and typically 24–48 hours after the use of long-acting opioids. Hospitalization during initiation of treatment with buprenorphine may be advisable due to the potential for adverse events, especially in the third trimester.

Drug dosing is similar to that in women who are not pregnant (see "Part 5: Buprenorphine" for more information).

Dosing of Opioid Agonists During Pregnancy

Methadone Dosing

In the second and third trimester, methadone doses may need to be increased due to increased metabolism and circulating blood volume. With advancing gestational age, plasma levels of methadone progressively decrease and clearance increases.[91,122,147,168] The half-life of methadone falls from an average of 22–24 hours in nonpregnant women to 8.1 hours in pregnant women.[153] As a result, "increased" or split methadone doses may be needed as pregnancy progresses to maintain therapeutic effects. Splitting the methadone dose into two 12-hour doses may produce more adequate opioid replacement in this period. There is frequent misconception that doses of methadone should decrease as pregnancy progresses; however, data refute this misconception. The risk and severity of NAS are not correlated with methadone doses taken by the mother at the time of delivery and tapering of dose is not indicated.[37,109] After birth, the dose of methadone may need to be adjusted.

Buprenorphine Dosing

The need to adjust dosing of buprenorphine during pregnancy is less than that of methadone. Clinicians may consider split dosing in patients who complain of discomfort and craving in the afternoon and evening.

Breastfeeding

Mothers receiving methadone and buprenorphine monoproduct for the treatment of opioid use disorders should be encouraged to breastfeed. Naltrexone is not recommended for use during breastfeeding.[163]

Specialty advice should be sought for women with concomitant medical or substance use disorders. Contraindications or precautions in breastfeeding include the following:
(1) HIV-positive mothers.
(2) Mothers using alcohol, cocaine, or amphetamine-type drugs.

Guidelines from the Academy of Breastfeeding Medicine encourage breastfeeding for women treated with methadone who are enrolled in methadone programs.[2] Some of the benefits include improved maternal–infant bonding and favorable effects on NAS.[1,16] It is not clear whether the favorable effects of breastfeeding on NAS are related to the breast milk itself or the act of breastfeeding.[16,100] In a study of buprenorphine and breastfeeding, it was shown that the amount of buprenorphine metabolites secreted in breast milk are so low that they pose little risk to breastfeeding infants.[81]

Summary of Recommendations

(1) The first priority in evaluating pregnant women for opioid use disorder should be to identify emergent or urgent medical conditions that require immediate referral for clinical evaluation.
(2) A medical examination and psychosocial assessment is recommended when evaluating pregnant women for opioid use disorder.
(3) Obstetricians and gynecologists should be alert to signs and symptoms of opioid use disorder. Pregnant women with opioid use disorder are more likely to seek prenatal care late in pregnancy, miss appointments, experience poor weight gain, or exhibit signs of withdrawal or intoxication.
(4) Psychosocial treatment is recommended in the treatment of pregnant women with opioid use disorder.
(5) Counseling and testing for HIV should be provided in accordance with state law. Tests for hepatitis B and C and liver function are also suggested. Hepatitis A and B vaccination is recommended for those whose hepatitis serology is negative.
(6) Urine drug testing may be used to detect or confirm suspected opioid and other drug use with informed consent from the mother, realizing that there may be adverse legal and social consequences of her use. State laws differ on reporting substance use during pregnancy. Laws that penalize women for use and for obtaining treatment serve to prevent women from obtaining prenatal care and worsen outcomes.
(7) Pregnant women who are physically dependent on opioids should receive treatment using methadone or buprenorphine monoproduct rather than withdrawal management or abstinence.
(8) Care for pregnant women with opioid use disorder should be comanaged by an obstetrician and an addiction specialist physician. Release of information forms need to be completed to ensure communication among healthcare providers.
(9) Treatment with methadone should be initiated as early as possible during pregnancy.
(10) Hospitalization during initiation of methadone and treatment with buprenorphine may be advisable due to the potential for adverse events, especially in the third trimester.
(11) In an inpatient setting, methadone should be initiated at a dose range of 20–30 mg. Incremental doses of 5–10 mg are given every 3–6 hours, as needed, to treat withdrawal symptoms.
(12) After induction, clinicians should increase the methadone dose in 5- to 10-mg increments per week. The goal is to maintain the lowest dose that controls withdrawal symptoms and minimizes the desire to use additional opioids.
(13) Twice-daily dosing is more effective and has fewer side effects than single dosing, but may not be practical because methadone is typically dispensed in an outpatient clinic.
(14) Clinicians should be aware that the pharmacokinetics of methadone are affected by pregnancy. With advancing gestational age, plasma levels of methadone progressively decrease and clearance increases. Increased or split doses may be needed as pregnancy progresses. After child birth, doses may need to be adjusted.
(15) Buprenorphine monoproduct is a reasonable and recommended alternative to methadone for pregnant women. Whereas there is evidence of safety, there is insufficient evidence to recommend the combination buprenorphine/naloxone formulation.
(16) If a woman becomes pregnant while she is receiving naltrexone, it is appropriate to discontinue the medication if the patient and doctor agree that the risk of relapse is low. If the patient is highly concerned about relapse and wishes to continue naltrexone, she should be informed about the risks of staying on naltrexone and provide her consent for ongoing treatment. If the patient wishes to discontinue naltrexone, but then reports relapse to opioid use, it may be appropriate to consider treatment with methadone or treatment with buprenorphine.
(17) Naloxone is not recommended for use in pregnant women with opioid use disorder except in situations of life-threatening overdose.
(18) Mothers receiving methadone and buprenorphine monoproduct for the treatment of opioid use disorders should be encouraged to breastfeed.

Areas for Further Research

Further research is needed to establish the safety of buprenorphine or the combination of the buprenorphine/naloxone for use in pregnancy.

Part 9: Special Populations: Individuals With Pain

Background

The occurrence of acute and chronic pain among patients with an opioid use disorder is not uncommon. Because of the current epidemic of nonmedical prescription drug use, it is critical to know how to manage pain safely and effectively. There are three general situations (listed below), each of which will be addressed separately, in which patients with opioid use disorder could be treated for pain:
(1) Pain in patients with an untreated and active opioid use disorder
(2) Pain in patients under opioid use disorder treatment with opioid agonists
(3) Pain in patients under opioid use disorder treatment with naltrexone

General Considerations for All Patients With Pain

For all patients with pain, it is important that the correct diagnosis of pain etiology be made and that a suitable treatment be identified. Nonpharmacological treatments have been shown to be effective for pain (e.g., physical therapy) and may be considered.

If pharmacological treatment is considered, then non-narcotic medications such as acetaminophen and NSAIDs should be tried first. Adjunctive medications including anticonvulsants may be useful. Tricyclic antidepressants or combined norepinephrine-serotonin reuptake inhibitors may also be used.

Pain Management in Patients Using Opioids

Opioid agonists (methadone or buprenorphine) may be considered for patients with an active opioid use disorder who are not undergoing treatment. Both methadone and buprenorphine have analgesic effects. Transition to opioid agonist treatments can help comanage pain and opioid use disorder.

Methadone and Pain Management

Patients prescribed methadone for opioid use disorder treatment should receive pain management in the same way as other patients in consultation with a pain specialist.

Acute and Chronic Pain Control

Because of the tolerance associated with daily methadone dosing, the usual dose of methadone may be inadequate for pain control. Patients in treatment with methadone will require doses of opioids in addition to their regular daily dose of methadone to manage acute pain.[79] However, in some cases, the tolerance associated with daily methadone dosing may result in the need for higher doses of narcotic analgesics.[132,135] Methadone patients who have chronic pain should optimally be treated in consultation with a pain specialist.

Buprenorphine and Pain Management

Acute Pain Control

Although it is a mu-opioid partial agonist, buprenorphine does have analgesic properties. Temporarily increasing buprenorphine dosing or dividing the dose may be effective for acute pain management.

Patients' pain may not be adequately addressed with buprenorphine and may require a full agonist. In situations when a full opioid agonist is needed for pain control, patients may be taken off buprenorphine and switched to a full opioid agonist until analgesia is no longer necessary. This may occur when patients undergo elective surgery. However, there are data to suggest that the discontinuation of buprenorphine is unnecessary and that adequate analgesia may be possible by simply adding non-narcotic and narcotic analgesics to the patient's baseline buprenorphine dose.[161]

For severe acute pain, discontinuing buprenorphine is advisable, and then commencing a high-potency opioid (such as fentanyl) in an attempt to over-ride the partial mu-receptor blockade of the buprenorphine is recommended. Patients should be monitored closely because high doses of a full agonist may be required. As the buprenorphine's partial blockade dissipates, the full agonist effect may lead to oversedation and respiratory depression. Additional interventions such as regional anesthesia should also be considered.

Chronic Pain Control

Buprenorphine may be adequate for chronic pain control in many patients with opioid use disorder and other types of chronic pain. Chronic opioid therapy, especially at high doses, may heighten

pain sensitivity.[125] There is some evidence suggesting that patients experiencing significant pain on high doses of full agonist opioid pain relievers experience improved pain control when transitioned to buprenorphine.[46] Split dosing of buprenorphine should be considered for patients with pain.

Considerations for Buprenorphine in Surgery

Discontinuation of buprenorphine is not recommended before elective cesarean section as it creates the potential for fetal withdrawal. For other elective surgeries in which buprenorphine is discontinued, the last dose of buprenorphine is usually delivered 24–36 hours before the anticipated need for analgesia. The buprenorphine is then restarted after a period of time after the discontinuation of full opioid agonists. Short-acting opioids should be given during or after surgery and titrated to maintain proper analgesia. In cases in which the buprenorphine cannot be stopped abruptly, pain control may be achieved with full opioid agonists added to the buprenorphine, but the doses may need to be increased to overcome the receptor blockade produced by buprenorphine.[26,103,110] The decision to discontinue buprenorphine before an elective surgery should optimally be made in consultation with the attending surgeon and anesthesiologist.

Naltrexone and Pain Management

Patients on naltrexone will not respond to opioid analgesics in the usual manner. Mild pain may be treated with NSAIDs. Ketorolac may be prescribed for moderate to severe pain, but its use should be time-limited due to higher risk of gastritis.

Emergency pain control options in patients taking naltrexone include the following:

(1) regional anesthesia;
(2) conscious sedation with benzodiazepines or ketamine; and
(3) nonopioid options in general anesthesia.

Considerations for Naltrexone in Surgery

Oral naltrexone should be discontinued at least 72 hours before elective surgery if pain management using opioids is anticipated. Extended-release naltrexone should be stopped at least 30 days before surgery, and oral naltrexone may be used temporarily. The surgical team should be aware of the use of naltrexone. Patients should be off opioids for 3–7 days before resuming naltrexone (oral or extended-release formulations). A naloxone challenge may be used to confirm that opioids are no longer being used.

Summary of Recommendations

(1) For all patients with pain, it is important that the correct diagnosis be made and that a target suitable for treatment is identified.
(2) If pharmacological treatment is considered, non-narcotic medications such as acetaminophen and NSAIDs should be tried first.
(3) Opioid agonists (methadone or buprenorphine) should be considered for patients with active opioid use disorder who are not under treatment.
(4) Pharmacotherapy in conjunction with psychosocial treatment should be considered for patients with pain who have opioid use disorder.
(5) Patients on methadone for the treatment of opioid use disorder will require doses of opioids in addition to their regular daily dose of methadone to manage acute pain.

(6) Patients on methadone for the treatment of opioid use disorder and who are admitted for surgery may require additional short-acting opioid pain relievers. The dose of pain relievers prescribed may be higher due to tolerance.

(7) Temporarily increasing buprenorphine dosing may be effective for mild acute pain.

(8) For severe acute pain, discontinuing buprenorphine and commencing on a high-potency opioid (such as fentanyl) is advisable. Patients should be monitored closely and additional interventions such as regional anesthesia should also be considered.

(9) The decision to discontinue buprenorphine before an elective surgery should be made in consultation with the attending surgeon and anesthesiologist. If it is decided that buprenorphine should be discontinued before surgery, this should occur 24–36 hours in advance of surgery and restarted postoperatively when the need for full opioid agonist analgesia has passed.

(10) Patients on naltrexone will not respond to opioid analgesics in the usual manner. Therefore, it is recommended that mild pain be treated with NSAIDs and moderate to severe pain be treated with ketorolac on a short-term basis.

(11) Oral naltrexone should be discontinued 72 hours before surgery and extended-release injectable naltrexone should be discontinued 30 days before an anticipated surgery.

Areas for Further Research

Further research is needed to examine whether the discontinuation of buprenorphine before elective surgery is necessary. Studies on whether it is possible to provide adequate analgesia by adding full agonist opioid analgesics to the patient's baseline buprenorphine dose are needed.

Part 10: Special Populations: Adolescents

Background

The American Academy of Pediatrics categorizes adolescence as the totality of three developmental stages—puberty to adulthood—which occur generally between 11 and 21 years of age.[71] Young people within this age group—adolescents—present for treatment with a broad spectrum of opioid use disorder severity and with co-occurring medical and psychiatric illness. Consequently, physicians will need to respond with a full range of treatment options, including pharmacotherapy. However, limited evidence exists regarding the efficacy of opioid withdrawal management in adolescents.[112] Pharmacological therapies have primarily been developed through research with adult populations.[113]

The treatment of adolescents with opioid use disorder presents many unique medical, legal, and ethical dilemmas that may complicate treatment. Given these unique issues, adolescents with opioid use disorder often benefit from services designed specifically for them. Furthermore, the family should be involved in treatment whenever possible.

Confidentiality in Treatment

One issue that may be of particular importance to consider in the treatment of adolescents is confidentiality.

Adolescents have reported that they are less likely to seek substance use disorder treatment if services are not confidential.[65] Confidential care, particularly with respect to sensitive issues such as reproductive health and substance use, has become a well-established practice.[72,164] This is a subject of complexity as it is an area governed by both Federal and state laws. Moreover, defined age ranges of "adolescence" vary. A myriad of clinical and legal responsibilities may be evoked if confronted by a young person's request for confidentiality. More than half of the states in the United States, by law, permit adolescents less than 18 years of age to consent to substance use disorder treatment without parental consent. State law should also be consulted. An additional reference source in decision-making regarding the implications on coordination of care, effectiveness of treatment without parental communication, and more are fully discussed in a publication of the Substance Abuse and Mental Health Services Administrations (SAMHSA), Center for Substance Abuse Treatment, Treatment Improvement Protocol (TIP) #33.[150]

Pharmacotherapy Options for Adolescents

Opioid agonists (methadone and buprenorphine) and antagonists (naltrexone) may be considered for treatment of opioid use disorder in adolescents. However, efficacy studies for these medications have largely been conducted in adults.

This recommendation is based on the consensus opinion of the Guideline Committee. There are virtually no data comparing the relative effectiveness of these treatments in adolescents.

Opioid Agonists: Methadone and Buprenorphine

Agonist medications are indicated for the treatment of patients who are aged 18 years and older. The Federal code on opioid treatment—42 CFR § 8.12—offers an exception for patients aged 16 and 17, who have a documented history of at least two prior unsuccessful withdrawal management attempts, and have parental consent.[148]

Efficacy Research on Agonists and Partial Agonists in Adolescents

There are no controlled trials evaluating methadone for the treatment of opioid use disorder in adolescents under the age of 18. Descriptive trials support the usefulness of treatment with methadone in supporting treatment retention in adolescent heroin users.[80] The usefulness of treatment with buprenorphine has been demonstrated in two RCTs. Studies have, however, not included adolescents under the age of 16.[106,169]

Buprenorphine is not US FDA-approved for use in patients less than 16 years old. Buprenorphine is more likely to be available in programs targeting older adolescents and young adults. No direct comparison of the efficacy of buprenorphine versus methadone has been conducted in adolescent populations.

Opioid Antagonist: Naltrexone

Naltrexone may be considered for young adults aged 18 years and older who have opioid use disorder. Naltrexone does not induce physical dependence and is easier to discontinue. Oral naltrexone may be particularly useful for adolescents who report a shorter duration of opioid use. Extended-release injectable naltrexone is administered monthly and can be delivered on an outpatient basis. There is only one small case series that demonstrated the efficacy of extended-release injectable naltrexone in adolescents.[63] The safety, efficacy, and pharmacokinetics of extended-release injectable naltrexone have not been established in the adolescent population.

Psychosocial Treatment for Adolescents

Psychosocial treatment is recommended in the treatment of adolescents with opioid use disorder. Recommended treatments based on the consensus opinion of the Guideline Committee include family intervention approaches, vocational support, and behavioral interventions to incrementally reduce use. Holistic risk-reduction interventions, which promote practices to reduce infection, are particularly important in the prevention of sexually transmitted infections and blood-borne viruses. Treatment of concomitant psychiatric conditions is also especially important in this population. Adolescents often benefit from specialized treatment facilities that provide multiple services.

Summary of Recommendations

(1) Clinicians should consider treating adolescents who have opioid use disorder using the full range of treatment options, including pharmacotherapy.
(2) Opioid agonists (methadone and buprenorphine) and antagonists (naltrexone) may be considered for treatment of opioid use disorder in adolescents. Age is a consideration in treatment, and Federal laws and US FDA approvals need to be considered for patients under age 18.
(3) Psychosocial treatment is recommended in the treatment of adolescents with opioid use disorder.
(4) Concurrent practices to reduce infection (e.g., sexual risk-reduction interventions) are recommended as components of comprehensive treatment for the prevention of sexually transmitted infections and blood-borne viruses.
(5) Adolescents may benefit from treatment in specialized treatment facilities that provide multidimensional services.

Areas for Further Research

(1) More studies are needed to examine the efficacy of pharmacotherapy for adolescents with opioid use disorder. Due to the few clinical trials in adolescents, most of the current recommendations are based on research with adults.
(2) More research is needed to identify which psychosocial treatments, alone and in combination with pharmacotherapy, are best suited for use with adolescents.

Part 11: Special Populations: Individuals With Co-Occurring Psychiatric Disorders

Background

Co-occurring psychiatric disorders are common among individuals who have opioid use disorder. Epidemiological studies have demonstrated a higher prevalence of substance use among people with psychiatric disorders relative to the general population.[24]

Reasons for the association between psychiatric and substance use disorders are not known. One hypothesis is that the dual diagnoses result from risk factors that are common to both disorders. A shared genetic vulnerability has been proposed to explain dysregulation in dopamine and glutamate systems in schizophrenia and substance use disorders.[33,94]

Another hypothesis is that people with psychiatric disorders are more likely to use drugs as a method of self-medication.[22,89,102]

Co-occurring psychiatric disorders should not bar patients from opioid use disorder treatment. The presence of the following common psychiatric disorders should be evaluated in patients presenting with possible opioid use disorder:
(1) Depression
(2) Anxiety
(3) Personality disorders
(4) Post-traumatic stress disorder.

Assessment of Psychiatric Co-occurrence

The assessment of psychiatric disorders is critical when attempting to place patients in the appropriate treatment.

Hospitalization may be appropriate for patients with severe or unstable psychiatric symptoms that may compromise the safety of self and others. An initial patient assessment should determine whether the patient is stable. Patients with suicidal or homicidal ideation should be referred immediately for treatment and possibly hospitalization. Patients should also be assessed for signs or symptoms of acute psychosis and chronic psychiatric disorders.

An assessment including medical history, physical examination, and an assessment of mental health status and/or psychiatric disorder should occur at the beginning of agonist or antagonist treatment (see "Part 1: Assessment and Diagnosis of Opioid Use Disorder"). Reassessment using a detailed mental status examination should occur after stabilization with methadone, buprenorphine, or naltrexone.

Co-occurring Psychiatric Disorders and Suicide Risk

Psychiatric disorders are strongly associated with suicide. More than 90% of patients who attempt suicide have a major psychiatric disorder.[70] In cases where suicide attempts resulted in death, 95% of patients had a psychiatric diagnosis.[51]

Management of a suicidal patient should include the following:
(1) Reduce immediate risk
(2) Manage underlying factors associated with suicidal intent
(3) Monitor and follow-up

Considerations With Specific Psychiatric Disorders

Depression or Bipolar Disorder

Antidepressant therapy may be initiated with pharmacotherapy for opioid use disorder for patients with symptoms of depression. Patients presenting with mania should be evaluated to determine whether symptoms arise from the bipolar disorder or substance use. Patients with bipolar disorder may require additional psychiatric care, hospitalization, and/or treatment with prescription mood stabilizers.

All patients with depression, including bipolar disorder, should be asked about suicidal ideation and behavior. Patients with a history of suicidal ideation or attempts should have their medication use monitored regularly. This includes medications for the treatment of opioid use disorder and psychiatric medications.

Schizophrenia

Antipsychotic therapy may be initiated with pharmacotherapy for opioid use disorder for patients with schizophrenia or other psychotic disorder. Coadministration of antipsychotic medications with agonist pharmacotherapy or use of long-acting depot formulations of antipsychotic medications is an option to consider in patients with histories of medication nonadherence.

All patients with schizophrenia should be asked about suicidal ideation and behavior. Patients with a history of suicidal ideation or attempts should have their medication use monitored regularly. This includes medications for the treatment of opioid use disorder and psychiatric medications.

For patients with schizophrenia and concomitant opioid use disorder who have a recent history of, or are at risk of repeated hospitalization or homelessness, assertive community treatment (ACT) should be considered. ACT is designed to provide treatment, rehabilitation, and support services to individuals who are diagnosed with severe psychiatric disorders, and whose needs have not been well met by more traditional psychiatric or psychosocial services. The efficacy of ACT has had mixed results on substance use disorder outcomes, but has shown benefit in preventing homelessness.[25,51,78] When ACT or another intensive case management program is unavailable, traditional case management can be helpful to patients who are unable to manage necessary, basic tasks.

Co-occurring Psychiatric Disorders and Agonist Treatment

Pharmacological and conjunctive psychosocial treatments should be considered for patients with both an opioid use disorder and a psychiatric disorder. Actively suicidal patients are not good candidates for any opioid treatment.

Methadone

Methadone for the treatment of opioid use disorder has been found to reduce psychiatric distress in a few weeks. Psychotherapy has been found useful in patients who have moderate to severe psychiatric disorders.

Buprenorphine

Psychiatrically stable patients are good candidates for buprenorphine. Patients with depression who are receiving treatment with buprenorphine require a higher level of monitoring.

Co-occurring Psychiatric Disorders and Antagonist Treatment

Psychiatrically stable patients are good candidates for treatment with oral naltrexone or extended-release injectable naltrexone. There are little data, however, regarding the relative efficacy of these medications in opioid-dependent patients with co-occurring psychiatric disorders. The once-monthly injections of extended-release injectable naltrexone may be especially useful in patients with a co-occurring psychiatric disorder, who may not be able to adhere well to daily dosing. Patients should be closely observed for adverse events as some patients have reported suicidal ideation, suicide attempts, and depression.

Summary of Recommendations

(1) A comprehensive assessment including determination of mental health status should evaluate whether the patient is stable. Patients with suicidal or homicidal ideation should be referred immediately for treatment and possibly hospitalization.
(2) Management of patients at risk for suicide should include the following: reducing immediate risk; managing underlying factors associated with suicidal intent; and monitoring and follow-up.

(3) All patients with psychiatric disorders should be asked about suicidal ideation and behavior. Patients with a history of suicidal ideation or attempts should have opioid use disorder, and psychiatric medication use, monitored.
(4) Assessment for psychiatric disorder should occur at the onset of agonist or antagonist treatment. Reassessment using a detailed mental status examination should occur after stabilization with methadone, buprenorphine, or naltrexone.
(5) Pharmacotherapy in conjunction with psychosocial treatment should be considered for patients with opioid use disorder and a co-occurring psychiatric disorder.
(6) Clinicians should be aware of potential interactions between medications used to treat co-occurring psychiatric disorders and opioid use disorder.
(7) Assertive community treatment should be considered for patients with co-occurring schizophrenia and opioid use disorder, who have a recent history of, or are at risk of, repeated hospitalization or homelessness.

Part 12: Special Populations: Individuals in the Criminal Justice System

Background

A substantial proportion of persons in prisons, jails, drug courts, probation, parole, and who are criminally involved have opioid use disorder and related problems. A lifetime history of incarceration is common among intravenous drug users; 56–90% of intravenous drug users have been incarcerated previously.[84]

The United States leads the world in the number of people incarcerated in Federal and state correctional facilities. There are, at present, more than 2 million people in American prisons.

Approximately one-quarter of those people held in US prisons have been convicted of a drug offense.[85]

Continued drug use is common among prisoners, and many individuals initiate intravenous drug use while in prison.[18, 25]

Prison drug use is particularly risky because of the environment. The high concentration of at-risk individuals and general overcrowding can increase the risk of adverse consequences associated with drug use, including violence, drug-related deaths, suicide, and self-harm.[139]

Drugs and sterile injection equipment is rare and sharing needles is common, leading to a high risk of spreading HIV and hepatitis C. Discharge from prison is often associated with opioid overdose and death. Consequently, it is important to identify and implement effective treatments for prisoners and probationers/parolees.

For the purposes of this Practice Guideline, a prison is to be differentiated from a jail. At the most basic level, the fundamental difference between jail and prison is the length of stay for inmates. Jails are usually run by local law enforcement and/or local government agencies, and are designed to hold inmates awaiting trial or serving a short sentence. Prison terms are of longer duration. Anyone incarcerated, regardless of sentence term, should be continued on opioid treatment.

Effectiveness of Pharmacotherapy

Pharmacotherapy for the treatment of opioid use disorder among prisoners has been shown to be effective. Most evidence for the effectiveness of pharmacotherapy for the treatment of opioid use disorder among prisoners has been derived from treatment with methadone. However, there is some evidence supporting the use of buprenorphine and naltrexone in this population.[44]

Methadone

Treatment with methadone has been shown to have a number of beneficial effects in inmates with opioid use disorders. Prisoners with opioid use disorder treated with methadone inject a lesser amount of drugs.[18,47,52,77]

Prisoners treated with methadone used less drugs after release and were more likely to participate in community-based addiction treatment.[19] Treatment with methadone lowered the rate of reincarceration during the 3-year period following first incarceration.[19,29]

Buprenorphine

Although less extensively studied, in some early trials, buprenorphine has also been associated with beneficial effects in prisoners with opioid use disorder. A RCT comparing buprenorphine and methadone among male heroin users who were newly admitted to prison showed that treatment completion rates were similar, but that buprenorphine patients were significantly more likely to enter community-based treatment after release.[104] In a more recent trial, buprenorphine initiated in prison was also associated with a greater likelihood of entering community treatment.[67] However, buprenorphine was diverted in some cases. Although promising, more research needs to be done to establish the effectiveness of in prison treatment with buprenorphine.

Naltrexone

Extended-release injectable naltrexone is the newest, and consequently least studied, medication for the treatment of prisoners and parolees. It has been shown to be effective for the treatment of opioid dependence in some early trials; however, there are no published studies evaluating the effectiveness of extended-release injectable naltrexone for the treatment of opioid use disorder in prisoners. In one small pilot trial involving parolees with prior opioid use disorder, 6 months of treatment with extended-release injectable naltrexone was associated with fewer opioid-positive urine drug screens and a reduced likelihood of reincarceration.[43] There are no studies establishing effectiveness of extended-release injectable naltrexone for persons in prison, or comparing it to either methadone or buprenorphine. Further research is needed in this area.

Treatment Options

All adjudicated individuals, regardless of type of offense and disposition, should be screened for opioid use disorder and considered for initiation or continuation of medication for the treatment of opioid use disorder. For incarcerated individuals, it should be initiated a minimum of 30 days before release, and aftercare should be arranged in advance.[119]

Methadone and Buprenorphine

Methadone or treatment with buprenorphine that is initiated during incarceration and to be continued after release is recommended for inmates with opioid use disorder without contraindications to these two medications. There is limited research comparing methadone and buprenorphine. In one trial, outcomes after release were similar; however, there was a problem with diversion of buprenorphine.[104]

Naltrexone

Extended-release injectable naltrexone may be considered for prisoners with opioid use disorder. However, there are little data about efficacy in prison populations. Extended-release injectable naltrexone should be considered for patients with opioid use disorder, with no contraindications, before their release from prison. Whether or not extended-release injectable naltrexone is superior to buprenorphine or methadone for the treatment of prisoners with opioid use disorder is unknown.

Summary of Recommendations

(1) Pharmacotherapy for the continued treatment of opioid use disorders, or the initiation of pharmacotherapy, has been shown to be effective and is recommended for prisoners and parolees regardless of the length of their sentenced term.
(2) Individuals with opioid use disorder who are within the criminal justice system should be treated with some type of pharmacotherapy in addition to psychosocial treatment.
(3) Opioid agonists (methadone and buprenorphine) and antagonists (naltrexone) may be considered for treatment. There is insufficient evidence to recommend any one treatment as superior to another for prisoners or parolees.
(4) Pharmacotherapy should be initiated a minimum of 30 days before release from prison.

Areas for Further Research

Further research is needed on the effectiveness of pharmacotherapy in prisoner populations.

Part 13: Naloxone for the Treatment of Opioid Overdose

Introduction

Death from opioid overdose is a growing epidemic in the United States. Poisoning deaths involving opioid analgesics have more than tripled in the United States since 1999.[36]

Unintentional poisoning (primarily due to drug overdose) is now the leading cause of injury-related death among Americans aged 25–64, having surpassed motor vehicle accidents in 2009.[32] Patients who overdose on opioids are in a life-threatening situation that requires immediate medical intervention. Naloxone is a mu-opioid antagonist with well-established safety and efficacy that can reverse opioid overdose and prevent fatalities. As well, naloxone can and should be administered to pregnant women in cases of overdose to save the mother's life.

As of December 15, 2104, a total of 27 states (NM, NY, IL, WA, CA, RI, CT, MA, NC, OR, CO, VA, KY, MD, VT, NJ, OK, UT, TN, ME, GA, WI, MN, OH, DE, PA, and MI) and the District of Columbia amended their state laws to make it easier for medical professionals to prescribe and dispense naloxone, and for lay administrators to use it without fear of legal repercussions.[95] State laws generally dictate various levels of prescriptive authority and generally speaking discourage the prescription of drugs to an individual other than the intended recipient, third-party prescription, or to a person the physician has not examined to be used in specific scenarios to assist others (prescription via standing order).

Patients and Significant Others/Family Members

Patients who are being treated for opioid use disorder, and their family members or significant others, should be given prescriptions for naloxone. Patients and family members/significant others should be trained in the use of naloxone in overdose. The practice of coprescribing naloxone for home use in the event of an overdose situation experienced by the patient or by any others in the household is endorsed by ASAM in a public policy statement and by SAMHSA in its toolkit on opioid overdose.[14,145]

Individuals Trained and Authorized to Use Naloxone

Until recently, administration of naloxone for the treatment of opioid overdose was only recommended for hospital personnel and paramedics. However, efforts are underway to expand the use of naloxone for the treatment of overdose to other first responders, including emergency medical technicians, police officers, firefighters, correctional officers, and others who might witness opioid overdose such as addicted individuals and their families. The primary issues to be considered in this Practice Guideline include the safety and efficacy of naloxone for the treatment of opioid overdose by first responders and bystanders, and the best form of naloxone to use for this purpose.

Safety and Efficacy of Bystander Administered Naloxone

Although there is ample evidence supporting the safety and efficacy of naloxone for the treatment of opioid overdose,[21,36,87] less is known about the effectiveness of naloxone used by other first responders and bystanders. Naloxone has been shown to be effective when used by paramedics.[45,88] There are no trials specifically evaluating the effectiveness of naloxone when administered by nonmedical first responders such as police officers and firefighters.

There have been a number of nonrandomized studies evaluating the effectiveness of community-based overdose prevention programs that include the distribution of naloxone to nonmedical personnel. In a comprehensive review of these trials, Clark et al.[36] concluded that bystanders (mostly opioid users) can and will use naloxone to reverse opioid overdose when properly trained, and that this training can be done successfully through these programs. The authors acknowledge that the lack of randomized controlled trials of community-based overdose prevention programs limits conclusions about their overall effectiveness. SAMHSA supports the use of naloxone for the treatment of opioid overdose by bystanders in their Opioid Overdose Prevention Toolkit.[145]

Routes of Administration

Naloxone is marketed in vials for injection and in an autoinjector for either IM or subcutaneous (SC) use. The US FDA-approved autoinjectors were designed to be used by a patient or family member for the treatment of opioid overdose. There is not yet an US FDA-approved intranasal formulation – there are only kits made available to deliver the injectable formulation intranasally. Despite the intranasal formulation's current lack of US FDA approval, it is being used off-label by first responders.

Although there are some data from head-to-head trials suggesting that IM naloxone may be superior to intranasal naloxone, there are few studies comparing the superiority of naloxone by route of administration, including intranasal, IM, or intravenous. The present available intranasal naloxone formulation is not dispensed in a preloaded syringe and this may affect its usefulness.[130] More research is needed to definitively assess the relative effectiveness of injectable vs. intranasal naloxone. In addition, the development of a more convenient administration device for intranasal naloxone could improve the effectiveness of this form of naloxone.

Summary of Recommendations

(1) Naloxone should be given in case of opioid overdose.
(2) Naloxone can and should be administered to pregnant women in cases of overdose to save the mother's life.
(3) The Guideline Committee, based on consensus opinion, recommends that patients who are being treated for opioid use disorder and their family members/significant others be given prescriptions for naloxone. Patients and family members/significant others should be trained in the use of naloxone in overdose.
(4) The Guideline Committee, based on consensus opinion, recommends that first responders, for example, emergency medical services personnel, police officers, and firefighters, be trained in and authorized to administer naloxone.

Part 14: Areas for Further Research

Although this Practice Guideline is intended to guide the assessment, treatment, and use of medications in opioid use disorder, there are areas where there was insufficient evidence to make a recommendation. Further research is needed to compare the advantages of different medications for different patient groups, especially with the emergence of new treatments. The recommended areas of future research are outlined below and presented in the order they were introduced in the guideline.

Assessment and Diagnosis of Opioid Use Disorder (Part 1)

(1) More research is needed on best practices for drug testing during the initial evaluation and throughout the entire treatment process.
(2) Further research is needed on evidence-based approaches for treating opioid use disorder in patients who continue to use marijuana and/or other psychoactive substances.
(3) Whereas research indicates that offering tobacco cessation is a standard for all medical care, more research is needed before specific evidence-based recommendations can be made.

Treatment Options (Part 2)

(1) More research is needed to compare the advantages of agonists and antagonists in the treatment of opioid use disorder. Whereas methadone, buprenorphine, and naltrexone are all superior to no treatment in opioid use disorder, less is known about their relative advantages.

Opioid Withdrawal Management (Part 3)

(1) Further research is needed to evaluate the efficacy and safety of alpha-2 adrenergic and other nonopioid medications that are being used off-label for withdrawal management. These nonopioid medications may have use in transitioning patients onto antagonists for relapse prevention.

(2) Further study is needed on other methods to accelerate the withdrawal process and facilitate the introduction of antagonists.

(3) More research is needed to make recommendations on the optimal duration of a buprenorphine taper.

(4) More research is needed to evaluate the safety of inpatient as compared to outpatient withdrawal management.

(5) More research is needed to compare the effectiveness of short versus long tapers with buprenorphine withdrawal management.

Methadone (Part 4)

(1) Further research is needed to assess the effectiveness of added psychosocial treatment to treatment with methadone in OTP or inpatient settings. Treatment with methadone generally includes some psychosocial components. However, it is unclear whether added psychosocial treatment improves patient outcomes. Research is needed to evaluate the use of ECG in treatment with methadone in preventing adverse events.

Buprenorphine (Part 5)

(1) Further research is needed to evaluate the safety and efficacy of buprenorphine induction conducted in the patient's own home, although present research supports this practice in select cases.

Naltrexone (Part 6)

(1) Further research is needed to test the relative efficacy of extended-release injectable naltrexone as compared to agonist treatment.

(2) Further research is needed on optimal withdrawal management to initiate treatment with naltrexone and minimize the risk of precipitated withdrawal.

(3) Further research is needed about the safety and efficacy of administering extended-release injectable naltrexone every 3 weeks for individuals who metabolize naltrexone at higher rates.

Psychosocial Treatment in Conjunction With Medications for the Treatment of Opioid Use Disorder (Part 7)

(1) Further research is needed to identify the comparative advantages of specific psychosocial treatments.

(2) Further study is needed to evaluate the effectiveness of psychosocial treatment in combination with specific pharmacotherapies.

(3) More research is needed on which concurrent psychosocial treatments are most effective for different patient populations and treatment settings including primary care.

(4) Further research is needed on which psychosocial treatments are suitable for addition to buprenorphine or treatment with naltrexone, which can be delivered in primary care settings.

Special Populations: Pregnant Women (Part 8)

(1) Further research is needed to establish the safety of buprenorphine or the combination of the buprenorphine/naloxone for use in pregnancy.

Special Populations: Individuals With Pain (Part 9)

(1) Further research is needed to examine whether the discontinuation of buprenorphine before elective surgery is necessary. Studies on whether it is possible to provide adequate analgesia by adding full agonist opioid analgesics to the patient's baseline buprenorphine dose are needed.

Special Populations: Adolescents (Part 10)

(1) More studies are needed to examine the efficacy of pharmacotherapy for adolescents with opioid use disorder. Due to the few clinical trials in adolescents, most of the present recommendations are based on research with adults.

(2) More research is needed to identify which psychosocial treatments, alone and in combination with pharmacotherapy, are best suited for use with adolescents.

Special Populations: Individuals in the Criminal Justice System (Part 12)

(1) Further research is needed on the effectiveness of pharmacotherapy in prisoner populations.

References

1. Abdel-Latif ME, Pinner J, Clews S, et al. Effects of breast milk on the severity and outcome of neonatal abstinence syndrome among infants of drug-dependent mothers. *Pediatrics*. 2006;117:e1163–e1169.

2. Academy of Breastfeeding Medicine Protocol Committee, Jansson L. ABM clinical protocol #21: guidelines for breastfeeding and the drug-dependent woman. *Breastfeed Med*. 2009;4:225–228.

3. Adi Y, Juarez-Garcia A, Wang D, et al. Oral naltrexone as a treatment for relapse prevention in formerly opioid-dependent drug users: a systematic review and economic evaluation. *Health Technol Assess*. 2007;11:1–85, iii–iv.

4. Amato L, Minozzi S, Davoli M, et al. Psychosocial and pharmacological treatments versus pharmacological treatments for opioid detoxification. *Cochrane Database Syst Rev*. 2011:CD005031.

5. Amato L, Minozzi S, Davoli M, et al. Psychosocial combined with agonist maintenance treatments versus agonist maintenance treatments alone for treatment of opioid dependence. *Cochrane Database Syst Rev*. 2011:CD004147.

6. American Congress of Obstetricians and Gynecologists. *Pregnant Women and Prescription Drug Abuse, Dependence and Addiction. Toolkit on State Legislation*. ACOG; 2014.

7. American Psychiatric Association. *Diagnostic and Statistical Manual of Mental Disorders: DSM-5*. Washington, DC: American Psychiatric Association; 2013.

8. American Psychiatric Association. *Diagnostic and Statistical Manual of Mental Disorders: DSM-IV*. Washington, DC: American Psychiatric Association; 1994.

9. American Psychiatric Association. *Diagnostic and Statistical Manual of Mental Disorders: DSM-III*. Washington, DC: American Psychiatric Association; 1980.

10. American Society of Addiction Medicine. *Drug Testing: a White Paper of the American Society of Addiction Medicine*; 2013. Available at: http://www.asam.org/docs/default-source/policy-policy-statements/drug-testing-a-white-paper-by-asam.pdf?sfvrsn¼0.

11. American Society of Addiction Medicine. *Policy Statement on Rapid and Ultra Rapid Opioid Detoxification*; 2005. http://www.asam.org/docs/publicly-policy-statements/1rod-urod-rev-of-oadusa-4-051.pdf?sf vrsn=0.

12. American Society of Addiction Medicine. *Public Policy Statement on the Relationship Between Treatment and Self Help: a Joint Statement of the American Society of Addiction Medicine, the American Academy of Addiction Psychiatry, and the American Psychiatric Association*; 1997. http://www.asam.org/docs/publicy-policy-statements/1treatment-and-self-help-joint-12-971.pdf?sfvrsn=0.

13. American Society on Addiction Medicine. *The ASAM Standards of Care for the Addiction Specialist Physician*; 2014. Available at: http://www.asam.org/docs/default-source/practice-support/quality-improvement/asam-standards-of-care.pdf?sfvrsn=10.

14. American Society of Addiction Medicine. *Public Policy Statement on the Use of Naloxone for the Prevention of Drug Overdose Deaths*. http://www.asam.org/docs/default-source/publicy-policy-statements/1naloxone-rev-8-14.pdf?sfvrsn=0. Accessed January 31, 2015.

15. Baca CT, Yahne CE. Smoking cessation during substance abuse treatment: what you need to know. *J Subst Abuse Treat.* 2009;36:205–219.

16. Ballard JL. Treatment of neonatal abstinence syndrome with breast milk containing methadone. *J Perinat Neonatal Nurs.* 2002;15:76–85.

17. Baxter LE, Sr Campbell A, Deshields M, et al. Safe methadone induction and stabilization: report of an expert panel. *J Addict Med.* 2013;7:377–386.

18. Bertolote J, Fleischmann A, De Leo D, et al. Psychiatric diagnoses and suicide: revisiting the evidence. *Crisis.* 2004;25:147–155.

19. Bertram S GA. *Views of Recidivists Released After Participating in the N.S.W. Prison Methadone Program and the Problems They Faced in the Community*. Sydney, Australia: Department of Corrective Services; 1990.

20. Bickel WK, Stitzer ML, Bigelow GE, et al. A clinical trial of buprenorphine: comparison with methadone in the detoxification of heroin addicts. *Clin Pharmacol Ther.* 1988;43:72–78.

21. Boyer EW. Management of opioid analgesic overdose. *N Engl J Med.* 2012;367:146–155.

22. Bradizza CM, Stasiewicz PR, Paas ND. Relapse to alcohol and drug use among individuals diagnosed with co-occurring mental health and substance use disorders: a review. *Clin Psychol Rev.* 2006;26:

23. Brigham GS, Slesnick N, Winhusen TM, et al. A randomized pilot clinical trial to evaluate the efficacy of Community Reinforcement and Family Training for Treatment Retention (CRAFT-T) for improving outcomes for patients completing opioid detoxification. *Drug Alcohol Depend.* 2014;138:240–243.

24. Brooner RK, King VL, Kidorf M, et al. Psychiatric and substance use comorbidity among treatment-seeking opioid abusers. *Arch Gen Psychiatry.* 1997;54:71–80.

25. Brunette MF, Mueser KT. Psychosocial interventions for the long-term management of patients with severe mental illness and co-occurring substance use disorder. *J Clin Psychiatry.* 2006;67(suppl 7):10–17.

26. Bryson EO. The perioperative management of patients maintained on medications used to manage opioid addiction. *Curr Opin Anaesthesiol.* 2014;27:359–364.

27. BUNAVAIL [package insert]. Raleigh, NC: BioDelivery Sciences International, Inc. Revised June 2014.

28. Burns L, Mattick RP, Lim K, et al. Methadone in pregnancy: treatment retention and neonatal outcomes. *Addiction.* 2007;102:264–270.

29. Canada ARCRBCS. *Institutional Methadone Maintenance Treatment: Impact on Release Outcome and Institutional Behaviour. Ottawa, ON, Canada*. Available at: http://198.103.98.138/text/rsrch/reports/r119/r119_e.pdf.

30. Center for Substance Abuse Treatment. *Federal Guidelines for Opioid Treatment*. Rockville, MD: Substance Abuse and Mental Health Services Administration; 2013. http://dpt.samhsa.gov/pdf/FederalGuidelinesforOpioidTreatment5-6-2013revisiondraft_508.pdf.

31. Centers for Disease Control. Deaths and severe adverse events associated with anesthesia-assisted rapid opioid detoxification: New York City, 2012. *Morbidity and Mortality Weekly*; 2013. Available at: http://www.cdc.gov/mmwr/preview/mmwrhtml/mm6238a1.htm.

32. Centers for Disease Control. *Injury Prevention and Control: Data and Statistics (WISQARS)*. Available at: http://www.cdc.gov/injury/wisqars/.

33. Chambers RA, Bickel WK, Potenza MN. A scale-free systems theory of motivation and addiction. *Neurosci Biobehav Rev.* 2007;31:1017–1045.

34. Chasnoff IJ, Landress HJ, Barrett ME. The prevalence of illicit-drug or alcohol use during pregnancy and discrepancies in mandatory reporting in Pinellas County. *Florida N Engl J Med.* 1990;322:1202–1206.

35. Cheskin LJ, Fudala PJ, Johnson RE. A controlled comparison of buprenorphine and clonidine for acute detoxification from opioids. *Drug Alcohol Depend.* 1994;36:115–121.

36. Clarke SF, Dargan PI, Jones AL. Naloxone in opioid poisoning: walking the tightrope. *Emerg Med J.* 2005;22:612–616.

37. Cleary BJ, Donnelly J, Strawbridge J, et al. Methadone dose and neonatal abstinence syndrome-systematic review and meta-analysis. *Addiction.* 2010;105:2071–2084.

38. Cohen SP, Mao J. Concerns about consensus guidelines for QTc interval screening in methadone treatment. *Ann Intern Med.* 2009;151:216–217; author reply 218–219.

39. Collins ED, Kleber HD, Whittington RA, et al. Anesthesia-assisted vs buprenorphine- or clonidine-assisted heroin detoxification and naltrexone induction: a randomized trial. *J Am Med Assoc.* 2005;294:903–913.

40. Comer SD, Sullivan MA, Yu E, et al. Injectable, sustained-release naltrexone for the treatment of opioid dependence: a randomized, placebo-controlled trial. *Arch Gen Psychiatry.* 2006;63:210–218.

41. Committee on Health Care for Underserved Women, American Society of Addiction Medicine. ACOG Committee Opinion No. 524: Opioid abuse, dependence, and addiction in pregnancy. *Obstet Gynecol.* 2012;119:1070–1076.

42. Compton WM, Dawson DA, Goldstein RB, et al. Crosswalk between DSM-IV dependence and DSM-5 substance use disorders for opioids, cannabis, cocaine and alcohol. *Drug Alcohol Depend.* 2013;132:387–390.

43. Coviello DM, Cornish JW, Lynch KG, et al. A multisite pilot study of extended-release injectable naltrexone treatment for previously opioid-dependent parolees and probationers. *Subst Abus.* 2012;33:48–59.

44. Cropsey KL, Villalobos GC, St Clair CL. Pharmacotherapy treatment in substance-dependent correctional populations: a review. *Subst Use Misuse.* 2005;40:1983–1999, 2043–2048.

45. Dahan A, Aarts L, Smith TW. Incidence, reversal, and prevention of opioid-induced respiratory depression. *Anesthesiology.* 2010;112:226–238.

46. Daitch D, Daitch J, Novinson D, et al. Conversion from high-dose full-opioid agonists to sublingual buprenorphine reduces pain scores and improves quality of life for chronic pain patients. *Pain Med.* 2014;15:2087–2094.

47. Darke S, Kaye S, Finlay-Jones R. Drug use and injection risk-taking among prison methadone maintenance patients. *Addiction.* 1998;93:1169–1175.

48. Day E, Strang J. Outpatient versus inpatient opioid detoxification: a randomized controlled trial. *J Subst Abuse Treat.* 2011;40:55–66.

49. Debelak K, Morrone WR, O'Grady KE, et al. Buprenorphine + naloxone in the treatment of opioid dependence during pregnancy-initial patient care and outcome data. *Am J Addict.* 2013;22:252–254.

50. Degenhardt L, Randall D, Hall W, et al. Mortality among clients of a state-wide opioid pharmacotherapy program over 20 years: risk factors and lives saved. *Drug Alcohol Depend.* 2009;105:9–15.

51. Dixon LB, Dickerson F, Bellack AS, et al. The 2009 schizophrenia PORT psychosocial treatment recommendations and summary statements. *Schizophr Bull.* 2010;36:48–70.

52. Dolan KA, Shearer J, White B, et al. Four-year follow-up of imprisoned male heroin users and methadone treatment: mortality, re-incarceration and hepatitis C infection. *Addiction.* 2005;100:820–828.

53. Dolan KA, Wodak AD, Hall WD. Methadone maintenance treatment reduces heroin injection in New South Wales prisons. *Drug Alcohol Rev.* 1998;17:153–158.

54. Drug Enforcement Administration. *Drugs of Abuse: A DEA Resource Guide.* 2011. Available at: http://www.dea.gov/pr/multimedia-library/publications/drug_of_abuse.pdf.

55. Drummond D, Perryman K. *Psychosocial Interventions in Pharmaco- therapy of Opioid Dependence: A Literature Review.* London: St George's University of London, Division of Mental Health, Section of Addictive Behaviour; 2007.

56. Dutra L, Stathopoulou G, Basden SL, et al. A meta-analytic review of psychosocial interventions for substance use disorders. *Am J Psychiatry.* 2008;165:179–187.

57. Eap CB, Bourquin M, Martin J, et al. Plasma concentrations of the enantiomers of methadone and therapeutic response in methadone maintenance treatment. *Drug Alcohol Depend.* 2000;61:47–54.

58. Eap CB, Buclin T, Baumann P. Interindividual variability of the clinical pharmacokinetics of methadone: implications for the treatment of opioid dependence. *Clin Pharmacokinet.* 2002;41:1153–1193.

59. Ehret GB, Voide C, Gex-Fabry M, et al. Drug-induced long QT syndrome in injection drug users receiving methadone: high frequency in hospitalized patients and risk factors. *Arch Intern Med.* 2006;166:1280–1287.

60. Fiellin DA, Barry DT, Sullivan LE, et al. A randomized trial of cognitive behavioral therapy in primary care-based buprenorphine. *Am J Med.* 2013;126:74.e11–74.e17.

61. Fiellin DA, Pantalon MV, Chawarski MC, et al. Counseling plus buprenorphine-naloxone maintenance therapy for opioid dependence. *N Engl J Med.* 2006;355:365–374.

62. Fishman M. Precipitated withdrawal during maintenance opioid blockade with extended release naltrexone. *Addiction.* 2008;103:1399–1401.

63. Fishman MJ, Winstanley EL, Curran E, et al. Treatment of opioid dependence in adolescents and young adults with extended release naltrexone: preliminary case-series and feasibility. *Addiction.* 2010;105:1669–1676.

64. Fitch K BS, Bernstein SJ, Aguilar MD, et al. The Rand/UCLA appropriateness method user's manual. *Rand Corporation.* 2001.

65. Ford CA, Millstein SG, Halpern-Felsher BL, et al. Influence of physician confidentiality assurances on adolescents' willingness to disclose information and seek future health care. A randomized controlled trial. *J Am Med Assoc.* 1997;278:1029–1034.

66. Ghitza UE, Epstein DH, Preston KL. Nonreporting of cannabis use: predictors and relationship to treatment outcome in methadone maintained patients. *Addict Behav.* 2007;32:938–949.

67. Gordon MS, Kinlock TW, Schwartz RP, et al. A randomized controlled trial of prison-initiated buprenorphine: prison outcomes and community treatment entry. *Drug Alcohol Depend.* 2014;142:33–40.

68. Gowing L, Ali R, White JM. Opioid antagonists under heavy sedation or anaesthesia for opioid withdrawal. *Cochrane Database Syst Rev.* 2010:CD002022.

69. Gunderson EW, Wang XQ, Fiellin DA, et al. Unobserved versus observed office buprenorphine/naloxone induction: a pilot randomized clinical trial. *Addict Behav.* 2010;35:537–540.

70. Gvion Y, Apter A. Suicide and suicidal behavior. *Public Health Rev.* 2012;34:1–20.

71. Hagan J, Shaw J, Duncan P, eds. *Bright Futures: Guidelines for Health Supervision of Infants, Children, and Adolescents. Pocket Guide.* 3rd ed. Elk Grove Village, IL: American Academy of Pediatrics; 2008.

72. Hallfors DD, Waller MW, Ford CA, et al. Adolescent depression and suicide risk: association with sex and drug behavior. *Am J Prev Med.* 2004;27:224–231.

73. Hamilton RJ, Olmedo RE, Shah S, et al. Complications of ultra-rapid opioid detoxification with subcutaneous naltrexone pellets. *Acad Emerg Med.* 2002;9:63–68.

74. Handelsman L, Cochrane KJ, Aronson MJ, et al. Two new rating scales for opiate withdrawal. *Am J Drug Alcohol Abuse.* 1987;13:293–308.

75. Harrison Narcotic Act of 1914, Pub. L. No. 63-223, 38 Stat. 785, repealed by Comprehensive Drug Abuse Prevention and Control Act of 1970, Pub. L. No. 91-513, 84 Stat. 1236 (codified as amended at 21 U.S.C. §§ 801–971).

76. Hassanian-Moghaddam H, Afzali S, Pooya A. Withdrawal syndrome caused by naltrexone in opioid abusers. *Hum Exp Toxicol.* 2014;33:561–567.

77. Heimer R, Catania H, Newman RG, et al. Methadone maintenance in prison: evaluation of a pilot program in Puerto Rico. *Drug Alcohol Depend.* 2006;83:122–129.

78. Himelhoch S, Lehman A, Kreyenbuhl J, et al. Prevalence of chronic obstructive pulmonary disease among those with serious mental illness. *Am J Psychiatry.* 2004;161:2317–2319.

79. Hines S, Theodorou S, Williamson A, et al. Management of acute pain in methadone maintenance therapy in-patients. *Drug Alcohol Rev.* 2008;27:519–523.

80. Hopfer CJ, Khuri E, Crowley TJ, et al. Adolescent heroin use: a review of the descriptive and treatment literature. *J Subst Abuse Treat.* 2002;23:231–237.

81. Ilett KF, Hackett LP, Gower S, et al. Estimated dose exposure of the neonate to buprenorphine and its metabolite norbuprenorphine via breastmilk during maternal buprenorphine substitution treatment. *Breastfeed Med.* 2012;7:269–274.

82. Johnson RE, Eissenberg T, Stitzer ML, et al. A placebo controlled clinical trial of buprenorphine as a treatment for opioid dependence. *Drug Alcohol Depend.* 1995;40:17–25.

83. Jones HE, Kaltenbach K, Heil SH, et al. Neonatal abstinence syndrome after methadone or buprenorphine exposure. *N Engl J Med.* 2010;363:2320–2331.

84. Jurgens R, Ball A, Verster A. Interventions to reduce HIV transmission related to injecting drug use in prison. *Lancet Infect Dis.* 2009;9:57–66.

85. Justice Policy Institute. *Substance Abuse Treatment and Public Safety*; 2008. Available at: http://www.justicepolicy.org/images/upload/08_01_rep_drugtx_ac-ps.pdf.

86. Katz EC, Brown BS, Schwartz RP, et al. Transitioning opioid-dependent patients from detoxification to long-term treatment: efficacy of intensive role induction. *Drug Alcohol Depend.* 2011;117:24–30.

87. Kelly AM, Kerr D, Dietze P, et al. Randomised trial of intranasal versus intramuscular naloxone in prehospital treatment for suspected opioid overdose. *Med J Aust.* 2005;182:24–27.

88. Kerr D, Kelly AM, Dietze P, et al. Randomized controlled trial comparing the effectiveness and safety of intranasal and intramuscular naloxone for the treatment of suspected heroin overdose. *Addiction.* 2009;104:2067–2074.

89. Khantzian EJ. The self-medication hypothesis of addictive disorders: focus on heroin and cocaine dependence. *Am J Psychiatry.* 1985;142:1259–1264.

90. Kienbaum P, Scherbaum N, Thurauf N, et al. Acute detoxification of opioid-addicted patients with naloxone during propofol or methohexital anesthesia: a comparison of withdrawal symptoms, neuroendocrine, metabolic, and cardiovascular patterns. *Crit Care Med.* 2000;28:969–976.

91. Kreek MJ. Methadone disposition during the perinatal period in humans. *Pharmacol Biochem Behav.* 1979; 11(suppl):7–13.

92. Krupitsky E, Nunes E, Ling W, et al. Injectable extended-release naltrexone for opioid dependence: a double-blind, placebo-controlled, multicentre randomised trial. *Lancet.* 2011;377:1506–1513.

93. Krupitsky E, Nunes EV, Ling W, et al. Injectable extended-release naltrexone for opioid dependence: a double-blind, placebo-controlled, multicentre randomised trial. *Lancet.* 2011;377:1506–1513.

94. Krystal JH, D'Souza DC, Gallinat J, et al. The vulnerability to alcohol and substance abuse in individuals diagnosed with schizophrenia. *Neurotox Res.* 2006;10:235–252.

95. Law Atlas Map. *Public Health Law Research Law Atlas Web site.* http://www.lawatlas.org/query?dataset=laws-regulating-administration-of-nal oxonexc.

96. Leavitt SB, Shinderman MD, Maxwell S, et al. When 'enough' is not enough: new perspectives on optimal methadone maintenance dose. *Mount Sinai J Med.* 2000;67:404–411.

97. Ling W, Amass L, Shoptaw S, et al. A multi-center randomized trial of buprenorphine-naloxone versus clonidine for opioid detoxification: findings from the national institute on drug abuse clinical trials network. *Addiction.* 2005;100:1090–1100.

98. Ling W, Charuvastra C, Collins JF, et al. Buprenorphine maintenance treatment of opiate dependence: a multicenter, randomized clinical trial. *Addiction.* 1998;93:475–486.

99. Lions C, Carrieri MP, Michel L, et al. Predictors of non-prescribed opioid use after one year of methadone treatment: an attributable-risk approach (ANRS-Methaville trial). *Drug Alcohol Depend.* 2014;135:1–8.

100. Liu AJ, Nanan R. Methadone maintenance and breastfeeding in the neonatal period. *Pediatrics.* 2008;121:106–114.

101. Loimer N, Schmid R. The use of plasma levels to optimize methadone maintenance treatment. *Drug Alcohol Depend.* 1992;30:241–246.

102. Lybrand J, Caroff S. Management of schizophrenia with substance use disorders. *Psychiatr Clin North Am.* 2009;32:821–833.

103. Macintyre PE, Russell RA, Usher KA, et al. Pain relief and opioid requirements in the first 24 hours after surgery in patients taking buprenorphine and methadone opioid substitution therapy. *Anaesth Intensive Care.* 2013;41:222–230.

104. Magura S, Lee JD, Hershberger J, et al. Buprenorphine and methadone maintenance in jail and post-release: a randomized clinical trial. *Drug Alcohol Depend.* 2009;99:222–230.

105. Mannelli P, Peindl KS, Lee T, et al. Buprenorphine-mediated transition from opioid agonist to antagonist treatment: state of the art and new perspectives. *Curr Drug Abuse Rev.* 2012;5:52–63.

106. Marsch LA, Bickel WK, Badger GJ, et al. Comparison of pharmacological treatments for opioid-dependent adolescents: a randomized controlled trial. *Arch Gen Psychiatry.* 2005;62:1157–1164.

107. Mattick R, Breen C, Kimber J, et al. Methadone maintenance therapy versus no opioid replacement therapy for opioid dependence. *Cochrane Database Syst Rev.* 2009: CD002209.

108. Mattick RP, Breen C, Kimber J, et al. Methadone maintenance therapy versus no opioid replacement therapy for opioid dependence. *Cochrane Database Syst Rev.* 2009: CD002209.

109. McCarthy JJ, Leamon MH, Willits NH, et al. The effect of methadone dose regimen on neonatal abstinence syndrome. *J Addict Med.* 2015;9:105–110.

110. McCormick Z, Chu SK, Chang-Chien GC, et al. Acute pain control challenges with buprenorphine/naloxone therapy in a patient with compartment syndrome secondary to McArdle's disease: a case report and review. *Pain Med.* 2013;14:1187–1191.

111. Mee-Lee D, Shulman GD, Fishman MJ, et al., eds. *The ASAM Criteria: Treatment Criteria for Addictive, Substance-Related, and Co-occuring Conditions.* 3rd ed. The Change Companies; 2013.

112. Minozzi S, Amato L, Bellisario C, et al. Detoxification treatments for opiate dependent adolescents. *Cochrane Database Syst Rev.* 2014;4:CD006749.

113. Minozzi S, Amato L, Bellisario C, et al. Maintenance treatments for opiate-dependent adolescents. *Cochrane Database Syst Rev.* 2014;6:CD007210.

114. Minozzi S, Amato L, Vecchi S, et al. Oral naltrexone maintenance treatment for opioid dependence. *Cochrane Database Syst Rev.* 2006:CD001333.

115. Minozzi S, Amato L, Vecchi S, et al. Oral naltrexone maintenance treatment for opioid dependence. *Cochrane Database Syst Rev.* 2011:CD001333.

116. Moderation Management. *What is moderation management?* Available at: http://moderation.org/whatisMM.shtml. Accessed February 2, 2015.

117. Muhuri PK, Gfroerer JC, Davies MC. *Associations of Nonmedical Pain Reliever Use and Initiation of Heroin Use in the US.* Rockville, MD: Center for Behavioral Health Statistics and Quality Data Review; 2013.

118. National Alliance on Mental Illness. *Psychosocial Treatments.* 2014. Available at: https://http://www.nami.org/Learn-More/Treatment/Psychosocial-Treatments. Accessed February 2, 2015.

119. National Commission on Correctional Health Care. *Standards for Opioid Treatment Programs in Correctional Facilities.* NCCHC; 2004. http://www.ncchc.org/standards.

120. National Institute on Drug Abuse. *Principles of Drug Addiction Treatment: A Research-Based Guide.* Bethesda, MD: National Institute on Drug Abuse; 2009.

121. National Institutes of Health. *Buprenorphine Sublingual. What Should I Know About Storage and Disposal of This Medication?* 2012. Available at: http://www.nlm.nih.gov/medlineplus/druginfo/meds/a605002.html-storage-conditions.

122. Nekhayeva IA, Nanovskaya TN, Deshmukh SV, et al. Bidirectional transfer of methadone across human placenta. *Biochem Pharmacol.* 2005;69:187–197.

123. Nelson PK, Mathers BM, Cowie B, et al. Global epidemiology of hepatitis B and hepatitis C in people who inject drugs: results of systematic reviews. *Lancet.* 2011;378:571–583.

124. Newman RG, Whitehill WB. Double-blind comparison of methadone and placebo maintenance treatments of narcotic addicts in Hong Kong. *Lancet.* 1979;2:485–488.

125. Pade PA, Cardon KE, Hoffman RM, et al. Prescription opioid abuse, chronic pain, and primary care: a Co-occurring Disorders Clinic in the chronic disease model. *J Subst Abuse Treat.* 2012;43:446–450.

126. Parran TV, Adelman CA, Merkin B, et al. Long-term outcomes of office-based buprenorphine/naloxone maintenance therapy. *Drug Alcohol Depend.* 2010;106:56–60.

127. Paulozzi LJ, Zhang K, Jones CM, et al. Risk of adverse health outcomes with increasing duration and regularity of opioid therapy. *J Am Board Fam Med.* 2014;27:329–338.

128. Preston KL, Silverman K, Higgins ST, et al. Cocaine use early in treatment predicts outcome in a behavioral treatment program. *J Consult Clin Psychol.* 1998;66:691–696.

129. Prochaska JJ, Delucchi K, Hall SM. A meta-analysis of smoking cessation interventions with individuals in substance abuse treatment or recovery. *J Consult Clin Psychol.* 2004;72:1144–1156.

130. Robinson A, Wermeling DP. Intranasal naloxone administration for treatment of opioid overdose. *Am J Health Syst Pharm.* 2014;71:2129–2135.

131. Ruan X, Chen T, Gudin J, et al. Acute opioid withdrawal precipitated by ingestion of crushed embeda (morphine extended release with sequestered naltrexone): case report and the focused review of the literature. *J Opioid Manag.* 2010;6:300–303.

132. Rubenstein RB, Spira I, Wolff WI. Management of surgical problems in patients on methadone maintenance. *Am J Surg.* 1976;131:566–569.

133. Ruetsch C, Tkacz J, McPherson TL, et al. The effect of telephonic patient support on treatment for opioid dependence: outcomes at one year follow-up. *Addict Behav.* 2012;37:686–689.

134. Saxon AJ, Ling W, Hillhouse M, et al. Buprenorphine/naloxone and methadone effects on laboratory indices of liver health: a randomized trial. *Drug Alcohol Depend.* 2013;128:71–76.

135. Scimeca MM, Savage SR, Portenoy R, et al. Treatment of pain in methadone-maintained patients. *Mt Sinai J Med.* 2000;67:412–422.

136. Sigmon SC, Bisaga A, Nunes EV, et al. Opioid detoxification and naltrexone induction strategies: recommendations for clinical practice. *Am J Drug Alcohol Abuse.* 2012;38:187–199.

137. Sigmon SC, Dunn KE, Saulsgiver K, et al. A randomized, double-blind evaluation of buprenorphine taper duration in primary prescription opioid abusers. *J Am Med Assoc Psychiatry.* 2013;70:1347–1354.

138. Soyka M, Apelt S, Lieb M, et al. One-year mortality rates of patients receiving methadone and buprenorphine maintenance therapy: a nationally representative cohort study in 2694 patients. *J Clin Psychopharmacol.* 2006;26:657–660.

139. Stover H, Michels II. Drug use and opioid substitution treatment for prisoners. *Harm Reduct J.* 2010;7:1–7.

140. Strain EC, Bigelow GE, Liebson IA, et al. Moderate- vs high-dose methadone in the treatment of opioid dependence: a randomized trial. *J Am Med Assoc.* 1999;281:1000–1005.

141. Strain EC, Stitzer ML, Liebson IA, et al. Dose-response effects of methadone in the treatment of opioid dependence. *Ann Intern Med.* 1993;119:23–27.

142. Strang J, Gossop M, Heuston J, et al. Persistence of drug use during imprisonment: relationship of drug type, recency of use and severity of dependence to use of heroin, cocaine and amphetamine in prison. *Addiction.* 2006;101:1125–1132.

143. Strang J, McCambridge J, Best D, et al. Loss of tolerance and overdose mortality after inpatient opiate detoxification: follow up study. *Br Med J.* 2003;326:959–960.

144. SUBOXONE [package insert]. Richmond, VA: Reckitt Benckiser Pharmaceuticals Inc. Revised April 2014.

145. Substance Abuse and Mental Health Services Administration. *Opioid Overdose Prevention Toolkit - Updated 2014*; 2014. Available at: http://store.samhsa.gov/product/Opioid-Overdose-Prevention-Toolkit-Updated-2014/SMA14-4742.

146. Substance Abuse and Mental Health Services Administration. *Results from the 2013 National Survey on Drug Use and Health: Summary of National Findings.* Rockville, MD: Substance Abuse and Mental Health Services Administration; 2014.

147. Substance Abuse and Mental Health Services Administration. *Treatment Improvement Protocol Series 2: Pregnant, Substance-Using Women. Rockville, MD: Substance Abuse and Mental Health Services Administration*; 1995.

148. Substance Abuse and Mental Health Services Administration. *Federal Guidelines for Opioid Treatment, 2013 revision, draft.* Available at: http://www.dpt.samhsa.gov/pdf/FederalGuidelinesforOpioidTreatment5-6-2013revisiondraft_508.pdf.

149. Substance Abuse and Mental Health Services Administration. *Treatment Improvement Protocol Series 42: Substance Abuse Treatment for Persons with Co-Occuring Disorders.* Rockville, MD: Substance Abuse and Mental Health Services Administration; 2008.

150. Substance Abuse and Mental Health Services Administration. *Treatment Improvement Protocol Series 33: Treatment for Stimulant Use Disorders.* Rockville, MD: Substance Abuse and Mental Health Services Administration; 1999.

151. Substance Abuse and Mental Health Services Administration. *Drug Addiction Treatment Act, full text. 2000.* Available at: http://buprenorphine.samhsa.gov/fulllaw.html.

152. Substance Abuse and Mental Health Services Administration. *Treatment Improvement Protocol Series 45: Detoxification and Substance Abuse Treatment.* Rockville, MD: Substance Abuse and Mental Health Services Administration; 2006.

153. Swift RM, Dudley M, DePetrillo P, et al. Altered methadone pharmacokinetics in pregnancy: implications for dosing. *J Subst Abuse.* 1989;1:453–460.

154. Syed YY, Keating GM. Extended-release intramuscular naltrexone (VIVITROL(R)): a review of its use in the prevention of relapse to opioid dependence in detoxified patients. *CNS Drugs.* 2013;27:851–861.

155. Tetrault JM, Moore BA, Barry DT, et al. Brief versus extended counseling along with buprenorphine/naloxone for HIV-infected opioid dependent patients. *J Subst Abuse Treat.* 2012;43:433–439.

156. Tiihonen J, Krupitsky E, Verbitskaya E, et al. Naltrexone implant for the treatment of polydrug dependence: a randomized controlled trial. *Am J Psychiatry.* 2012;169:531–536.

157. Tsoh JY, Chi FW, Mertens JR, et al. Stopping smoking during first year of substance use treatment predicted 9-year alcohol and drug treatment outcomes. *Drug Alcohol Depend.* 2011;114:110–118.

158. Types of withdrawal. *Bupproactice Web site.* Available at: http://www.buppractice.com/node/4818.

159. US Food and Drug Administration. *Information for Healthcare Professionals Methadone Hydrochloride: Text Version.* Available at: http://www.fda.gov/Drugs/DrugSafety/PostmarketDrugSafetyInformationfor-PatientsandProviders/ucm142841.htm. Accessed January 12, 2015.

160. US Food and Drug Administration. *Sleep disorder (sedative-hypnotic) drug information.* 2015; Available at: http://www.fda.gov/drugs/drug-safety/postmarketdrugsafetyinformationforpatient-sandproviders/ucm101557.htm.

161. Vadivelu N, Mitra S, Kaye AD, et al. Perioperative analgesia and challenges in the drug-addicted and drug-dependent patient. *Best Pract Res Clin Anaesthesiol.* 2014;28:91–101.

162. Vanichseni S, Wongsuwan B, Choopanya K, et al. A controlled trial of methadone maintenance in a population of intravenous drug users in Bangkok: implications for prevention of HIV. *Int J Addict.* 1991;26:1313–1320.

163. VIVITROL [package insert]. Waltham, MA: Alkermes, Inc. Revised July 2013.

164. Weddle M, Kokotailo PK. Confidentiality and consent in adolescent substance abuse: an update. *Virtual Mentor.* 2005;7(3).

165. Weiss RD, Potter JS, Fiellin DA, et al. Adjunctive counseling during brief and extended buprenorphine-naloxone treatment for prescription opioid dependence: a 2-phase randomized controlled trial. *Arch Gen Psychiatry.* 2011;68:1238–1246.

166. Wesson DR, Ling W. The Clinical Opiate Withdrawal Scale (COWS). *J Psychoactive Drugs.* 2003;35:253–259.

167. Wiegand SL, Stringer EM, Stuebe AM, et al. Buprenorphine and naloxone compared with methadone treatment in pregnancy. *Obstet Gynecol.* 2015;125:363–368.

168. Wolff K, Boys A, Rostami-Hodjegan A, et al. Changes to methadone clearance during pregnancy. *Eur J Clin Pharmacol.* 2005;61:763–768.

169. Woody GE, Poole SA, Subramaniam G, et al. Extended vs short-term buprenorphine-naloxone for treatment of opioid-addicted youth: a randomized trial. *J Am Med Assoc.* 2008;300:2003–2011.

170. World Health Organization. *Guidelines for the Psychosocially Assisted Pharmacological Treatment of Opioid Dependence.* Department of Mental Health, Substance Abuse and World Health Organization; 2009.

171. World Health Organization. *The ICD-10 Classification of Mental and Behavioural Disorders: Clinical Descriptions and Diagnostic Guidelines.* Geneva: World Health Organization; 1992.

172. Yokell MA, Zaller ND, Green TC, Rich JD. Buprenorphine and buprenorphine/naloxone diversion, misuse, and illicit use: an international review. *Curr Drug Abuse Rev.* 2011;4:28–41.

173. ZUBSOLV [package insert]. Morristown, NJ: Orexo US, Inc. Revised December 2014.

Appendices

Appendix I: Clinical References Reviewed

Baltimore Buprenorphine Initiative. *Clinical Guidelines for Buprenorphine Treatment of Opioid Dependence in the Baltimore Buprenorphine Initiative.* Baltimore, MD; 2011.

Bell J, Kimber J, Lintzeris N, et al. *Clinical Guidelines and Procedures for the Use of Naltrexone in the Management of Opioid Dependence.* Commonwealth of Australia: National Drug Strategy; 2003.

Bell J. *The Role of Supervision of Dosing in Opioid Maintenance Treatment.* London: National Addiction Centre; 2007.

Brooking A. *Guidelines for the Management of Opiate Dependent Patients at RCHT.* Royal Cornwall Hospitals, NHS; 2010.

Chou R, Cruciani RA, Fiellin DA, et al. Methadone safety: a clinical practice guideline from the American Pain Society and College on Problems of Drug Dependence, in collaboration with the Heart Rhythm Society. *J Pain.* 2014;15(4):321–337.

Chou R, Weimer MB, Dana T. Methadone overdose and cardiac arrhythmia potential: findings from a review of evidence for an American Pain Society and College on Problems of Drug Dependence Clinical Practice Guideline. *J Pain.* 2014; 15(4):338–365.

Committee on Health Care for Underserved Women and the American Society of Addiction Medicine. Opioid abuse, dependence, and addiction in pregnancy. 2012; Committee Opinion Number 524.

Department of Health (England) and the Devolved Administrations. *Drug Misuse and Dependence: UK Guidelines on Clinical Management.* London: Department of Health (England), the Scottish Government, Welsh Assembly Government and Northern Ireland Executive; 2007.

Federal Bureau of Prisons Clinical Practice Guidelines. *Detoxification of Chemically Dependent Inmates.* Washington, DC: 2009.

Ford A. *WPCT Guidelines—Methadone and Buprenorphine in the Management of Opioid Dependence. Prescribing Guidelines for the Young Person's Substance Use Service—SPACE.* Worchester: NHS; 2009.

Ford C, Halliday K, Lawson E, Browne E. *Guidance for the Use of Substitute Prescribing in the Treatment of Opioid Dependence in Primary Care.* London: Royal College of General Practitioners; 2011.

Gowing L, Ali R, Dunlap A, Farrell M, Lintzeris N. *National Guidelines for Medication-Assisted Treatment of Opioid Dependence.* Commonwealth of Australia; 2014.

Handford C, Kahan M, Lester MD, & Ordean A. *Buprenorphine/Naloxone for Opioid Dependence: Clinical Practice Guideline.* Canada: Centre for Addiction and Mental Health; 2012.

Hanna, M. *Supporting Recovery from Opioid Addiction: Community Care Best Practice Guidelines for Buprenorphine and Suboxone1.* USA: Community Care Behavioral Health Organization; 2013.

Henry-Edwards S, Gowing L, White J, et al. *Clinical Guidelines and Procedures for the Use of Methadone in the Maintenance Treatment of Opioid Dependence.* Commonwealth of Australia: National Drug Strategy; 2003.

Hudak ML, Tan RC. The committee on drugs, & the committee on fetus and newborn. Neonatal drug withdrawal. *Pediatrics.* 2012;129(2):e540–560.

Johnston A, Mandell TW, Meyer M. *Treatment of Opioid Dependence in Pregnancy: Vermont Guidelines.* Burlington, VT; 2010.

Lintzeris N, Clark N, Muhleisen P, et al. *Clinical Guidelines: Buprenorphine Treatment of Heroin Dependence.* Commonwealth of Australia: Public Health Division; 2003.

The Management of Substance Use Disorder Working Group. VA/DoD Clinical Practice Guideline for management of substance use disorders (SUDs). Version 2.0; 2009.

Ministry of Health. *New Zealand Clinical Guidelines for the Use of Buprenorphine (with or without Naloxone) in the Treatment of Opioid Dependence.* Wellington: Ministry of Health; 2010.

Ministry of Health. *Practice Guidelines for Opioid Substitution Treatment in New Zealand 2008.* Wellington: Ministry of Health; 2008.

Nicholls L, Bragaw L, Ruetsch C. Opioid dependence treatment and guidelines. *J Manag Care Pharm.* 2010;16(suppl 1b):S14–S21.

Stephenson D. *Guideline for Physicians Working in California Opioid Treatment Programs. California Society of Addiction Medicine.* San Francisco, CA: CSAM Committee on Treatment of Opioid Dependence; 2008.

Substance Abuse and Mental Health Services Administration. An introduction to extended-release injectable naltrexone for the treatment of people with opioid dependence. *Advisory.* 2012;11(1):1–8.

Substance Abuse and Mental Health Services Administration. *Addressing Viral Hepatitis in People With Substance Use Disorders. Treatment Improvement Protocol (TIP) Series 53.* HHS Publication No. (SMA) 11-4656. Rockville, MD: Substance Abuse and Mental Health Services Administration; 2011.

Substance Abuse and Mental Health Services Administration Center for Substance Abuse Treatment. *Clinical Guidelines for the Use of Buprenorphine in the Treatment of Opioid Addiction. Treatment Improvement Protocol (TIP) Series 40.* DHHS Publication No. (SMA) 04-3939. Rockville, MD: Substance Abuse and Mental Health Services Administration; 2004.

Substance Abuse and Mental Health Service Administration Center for Substance Abuse Treatment. *Detoxification and Substance Abuse Treatment. Treatment Improvement Protocol (TIP) Series 45.* DHHS Publication No. (SMA) 06-4131. Rockville, MD: Substance Abuse and Mental Health Services Administration; 2006.

Substance Abuse and Mental Health Service Administration Center for Substance Abuse Treatment. *Medication-Assisted Treatment for Opioid Addiction in Opioid Treatment Programs. Treatment Improvement Protocol (TIP) Series 43.* HHS Publication No. (SMA) 12-4214. Rockville, MD: Substance Abuse and Mental Health Services Administration; 2005.

Substance Abuse and Mental Health Services Administration. *Quick Guide for Physicians Based on Tip 40: Clinical Guidelines for the Use of Buprenorphine in the Treatment of Opioid Addiction. Treatment Improvement Protocol (TIP) Series 40.* DHHS Publication No. (SMA) 05-4003. Rockville, MD: Substance Abuse and Mental Health Services Administration; 2005.

The College of Physicians and Surgeons of Ontario. *Methadone Maintenance Treatment Program Standards and Clinical Guidelines.* 4th ed. Toronto, Ontario; 2011.

Verster A, Buning E. *Methadone Guidelines.* Amsterdam, Netherlands: Euro-Meth; 2000.

Vermont Department of Health. *Vermont Buprenorphine Practice Guidelines.* Burlington, VT; 2010.

Weimer MB, Chou R. Research gaps on methadone harms and comparative harms: findings from a review of the evidence for an American Pain Society and College on Problems of Drug Dependence Clinical Practice Guideline. *J Pain.* 2014;15(4):366–376.

World Health Organization, Department of Mental Health, Substance Abuse and World Health Organization. *Guidelines for the Psychosocially Assisted Pharmacological Treatment of Opioid Dependence.* World Health Organization; 2009.

Appendix II: Bioequivalence Information and Charts

Bioequivalence of Suboxone (Buprenorphine and Naloxone) Sublingual Tablets and Suboxone Sublingual Film

Patients being switched between Suboxone (buprenorphine and naloxone) sublingual tablets and Suboxone sublingual film should be started on the same dosage as the previously administered product. However, dosage adjustments may be necessary when switching between products. Not all strengths and combinations of the Suboxone sublingual films are bioequivalent to Suboxone (buprenorphine and naloxone) sublingual tablets as observed in pharmacokinetic studies. Therefore, systemic exposures of buprenorphine and naloxone may be different when patients are switched from tablets to film, or vice-versa. Patients should be monitored for symptoms related to over-dosing or under-dosing.

In pharmacokinetic studies, the 2 mg/0.5 mg and 4 mg/1 mg doses administered as Suboxone sublingual films showed comparable relative bioavailability to the same total dose of Suboxone (buprenorphine and naloxone) sublingual tablets, whereas the 8 mg/2 mg and 12 mg/3 mg doses administered as Suboxone sublingual films showed higher relative bioavailability for both buprenorphine and naloxone compared to the same total dose of Suboxone (buprenorphine and naloxone) sublingual tablets. A combination of one 8 mg/2 mg and two 2 mg/0.5 mg Suboxone sublingual films (total dose of 12 mg/3 mg) showed comparable relative bioavailability to the same total dose of Suboxone (buprenorphine and naloxone) sublingual tablets.

Switching Between Suboxone (Buprenorphine and Naloxone) Sublingual Film and Suboxone Sublingual Tablets

Because of the potentially greater relative bioavailability of Suboxone sublingual film compared to Suboxone (buprenorphine and naloxone) sublingual tablets, patients switching from Suboxone (buprenorphine and naloxone) sublingual tablets to Suboxone sublingual film should be monitored for over-medication. Those switching from Suboxone sublingual film to Suboxone (buprenorphine and naloxone) sublingual tablets should be monitored for withdrawal or other indications of under-dosing. In clinical studies, pharmacokinetics of Suboxone sublingual film were similar to the respective dosage strengths of Suboxone (buprenorphine and naloxone) sublingual tablets, although not all doses and dose combinations met bioequivalence criteria.

Switching Between Suboxone Sublingual Tablets or Films and Bunavail Buccal Film

The difference in bioavailability of Bunavail compared to Suboxone sublingual tablet requires a different dosage strength to be administered to the patient. A Bunavail 4.2/0.7 mg buccal film provides equivalent buprenorphine exposure to a Suboxone 8/2 mg sublingual tablet. Patients being switched between Suboxone dosage strengths and Bunavail dosage strengths should be started on the corresponding dosage as defined below:

Suboxone Sublingual Tablet Dosage Strength	Corresponding Bunavail Buccal Film Strength
4/1 mg buprenorphine/naloxone	2.1/0.3 mg buprenorphine/naloxone
8/2 mg buprenorphine/naloxone	4.2/0.7 mg buprenorphine/naloxone
12/3 mg buprenorphine/naloxone	6.3/1 mg buprenorphine/naloxone

Dosage and Administration of Zubsolv

The difference in bioavailability of Zubsolv compared to Suboxone tablet requires a different tablet strength to be given to the patient. One Zubsolv 5.7/1.4 mg sublingual tablet provides equivalent buprenorphine exposure to one Suboxone 8/2 mg sublingual tablet. The corresponding doses ranging from induction to maintenance treatment are:

Induction Phase: Final Sublingual Buprenorphine Dose	Maintenance Phase: Corresponding Sublingual Zubsolv Dose
8 mg buprenorphine, taken as: • One 8 mg buprenorphine tablet	5.7/1.4 mg Zubsolv, taken as: • One 5.7 mg/1.4 mg Zubsolv tablet
12 mg buprenorphine tablet, taken as: • One 8 mg buprenorphine tablet AND • Two 2 mg buprenorphine tablets	8.6 mg/2.1 mg Zubxolv, taken as: • One 8.6 mg/2.1 mg Zubsolv tablet
16 mg buprenorphine, taken as: • Two 8 mg buprenorphine tablets	11.4 mg/2.9 mg Zubsolv1, taken as: • One 11.4/2.9 mg Zubsolv1 tablet

Switching Between Zubsolv Sublingual Tablets and Other Buprenorphine/Naloxone Combination Products

For patients being switched between Zubsolv sublingual tablets and other buprenorphine/naloxone products, dosage adjustments may be necessary. Patients should be monitored for over-medication as well as withdrawal or other signs of under-dosing.

The differences in bioavailability of Zubsolv compared to Suboxone tablet requires that different tablet strengths be given to the patient. One Zubsolv 5.7/1.4 mg sublingual tablet provides equivalent buprenorphine exposure to one Suboxone 8/2 mg sublingual tablet.

When switching between Suboxone dosage strengths and Zubsolv dosage strengths, the corresponding dosage strengths are:

Suboxone Sublingual Tablets (Including Generic Equivalents)	Corresponding Dosage Strength of Zubsolv Sublingual Tablets
One 2 mg/0.5 mg buprenorphine/naloxone sublingual tablet	One 1.4 mg/0.36 mg Zubsolv sublingual tablet
One 8 mg/2mg buprenorphine/naloxone sublingual tablet	One 5.7 mg/1.4 mg Zubsolv sublingual tablet
12 mg/3 mg buprenorphine/naloxone, taken as: • One 8 mg/2 mg sublingual buprenorphine/naloxone tablet AND • Two 2 mg/0.5 mg sublingual buprenorphine/naloxone tablets	One 8.6 mg/2.1 mg Zubsolv sublingual tablet
16 mg/4 mg buprenorphine/naloxone, taken as: • Two 8 mg/2 mg sublingual buprenorphine/naloxone tablets	One 11.4 mg/2.9 Zubsolv sublingual tablet

Appendix III: Guideline Committee Member Relationships With Industry and Other Entities

Guideline Committee Member	Employment	Consultant	Speakers Bureau	Ownership/ Partnership/ Principal	Personal Research	Institutional, Organizational, or Other Financial Benefit	Salary	Expert Witness	Other
Sandra D. Comer, PhD	Columbia University and NYSPI New York, NY Professor of Neurobiology	• J&J • AstraZeneca • Salix • Cauarus • Pfizer • Mallincrodt	None	None	• Reckitt Benckiser[a] • Omeras[a] • Medicinova[a]	None	None	None	None
Chinazo Cunningham, MD, MS	Albert Einstein College of Medicine, Yeshiva University Bronx, NY	None	None	None	None	None	None	None	Quest Diagnostics[a]
Marc Fishman, MD, FASAM	Maryland Treatment Centers Baltimore, MD Medical Director	• CRC Health Group, Advisory Board • NY State JBS/ SAMHSA Youth Opioid Addiction Project • University of Maryland	None	Maryland Treatment Centers[a]	• Alkermes US World Meds[a] • NIDA[a]	None	Maryland Treatment Centers[a]	Board of Physician case reviews	None
Adam Gordon, MD, MPH, FASAM	University of Pittsburgh and VA Pittsburgh Healthcare System	None	None	None	None	None	None	None	None
Kyle Kampman, MD, TRI (Chair and Principal Investigator)	University of Pennsylvania VAMC Philadelphia, PA Professor of Psychiatry/Staff Physician	None	None	None	Braeburn Pharma	None	None	None	None
Daniel Langleben, MD	University of Pennsylvania Philadelphia, PA Associate Professor	None	None	None	Alkermes	None	None	None	None

Continued

Guideline Committee Member	Employment	Consultant	Speakers Bureau	Ownership/ Partnership/ Principal	Personal Research	Institutional, Organizational, or Other Financial Benefit	Salary	Expert Witness	Other
Benjamin Nordstrom, MD, PhD	Dartmouth College Hanover, NH Associate Professor of Psychiatry Director of Addiction Services	None	None	None	None	None	None	None	None
David Oslin, MD	Director, Addiction Psychiatry Fellowship University of Pennsylvania Medical Center Philadelphia, PA Associate Professor of Psychiatry Associate Chief of Staff, Behavioral Health	None	None	None	Department of Veteran Affairs, State of Pennsylvania	None	None	None	None
George Woody, MD	Perelman School of Medicine University of Pennsylvania Philadelphia, PA Professor, Department of Psychiatry	RADARS Scientific Advisory Board[a]	None	None	• Alkermes[a] • Reckitt Benckiser[a] • Fidelity Capital[a]	None	NIDA[a]	• U.S. Attorney's Office and DEA, Philadelphia[a] • Pennsylvania Bureau of Professional and Occupational Affairs[a]	None
Tricia E. Wright, MD, MS	University of Hawaii John A. Burns School of Medicine Honolulu, HI Assistant Professor	None	None	None	None	None	None	None	None
Stephen A. Wyatt, DO	Carolinas Healthcare System Medical Director, Addiction Medicine Charlotte, NC	None	None	None	None	None	None	None	None

The above table presents the relationships of Guideline Committee Members during the past 12 months with industry and other entities that were determined to be relevant to this document. These relationships are current as of the completion of this document and may not necessarily reflect relationships at the time of this document's publication. A person is deemed to have a significant interest in a business if the interest represents ownership of 5% or more of the voting stock or share of the business entity, or ownership of $10,000 or more of the fair market value of the business entity; or if funds received by the person from the business entity exceed 5% of the person's gross income for the previous year. A relationship is considered to be modest if it is less than significant under the preceding definition. No financial relationship for which there is no monetary reimbursement.

[a]Indicates significant relationship.

Appendix IV: ASAM Quality Improvement Council (Oversight Committee) Relationships With Industry and Other Entities

Oversight Committee Member	Employment	Consultant	Speakers Bureau	Ownership/ Partnership/ Principal	Personal Research	Institutional, Organizational, or Other Financial Benefit	Salary	Expert Witness	Other
John Femino, MD, FASAM	Meadows Edge Recovery Center North Kingstown, RI Medical Director	Inflexxion[a] Dominion Diagnostics[a]	None	None	None	None	None	None	None
Margaret Jarvis, MD, FASAM, Chair	Marworth/Geisinger Health System Waverly, PA Medical Director of Marworth	None	None	U.S. Preventive Medicine	None	None	Geisinger Health System[a]	Preston vs. Alpha Recovery Centers	Royalties-addiction article
Margaret Kotz, DO, FASAM	University Hospitals of Cleveland Cleveland, OH Case Medical Center Medical Director, Addiction Recovery Services Professor of Psychiatry and Anesthesiology Case Western Reserve University School of Medicine	None	None	None	None	None	None	None	None
Sandrine Pirard, MD, MPH, PhD	Johns Hopkins Bayview Medical Center Baltimore, MD Psychiatrist	None	None	None	None	None	None	None	None
Robert Roose, MD, MPH	Sisters of Providence Health System Holyoke, MA CMO, Addiction Services	None	None	None	None	None	None	None	None

The above table presents the relationships of the ASAM Quality Improvement Council (Oversight Committee) during the past 12 months with industry and other entities that were determined to be relevant to this document. These relationships are current as of the completion of this document and may not necessarily reflect relationships at the time of this document's publication. A person is deemed to have a significant interest in a business if the interest represents ownership of 5% or more of the voting stock or share of the business entity, or ownership of $10,000 or more of the fair market value of the business entity; or if funds received by the person from the business entity exceed 5% of the person's gross income for the previous year. A relationship is considered to be modest if it is less than significant under the preceding definition. No financial relationship pertains to relationships for which there is no monetary reimbursement.

[a]Indicates significant relationship.

Appendix V: External Reviewer Relationships With Industry and Other Entities

External Reviewer	Representation	Employment	Consultant	Speakers Bureau	Ownership/ Partnership/ Principal	Personal Research	Institutional, Organizational, or Other Financial Benefit	Salary	Expert Witness	Other
B. Steven Bentsen, MD, DFAPA	Value Options	Beacon Health Options Regional Chief Medical Officer	None	None	None	None	Beacon Health Options- Medical Director[a]	None	None	None
Melinda Campoppiano, MD	Substance Abuse Mental Health Services Administration (SAMHSA)	SAMHSA Medical Officer Chooper's Guide Managing Partner	None	None	None	None	None	None	None	None
Timothy Cheney	Faces and Voices of Recovery (FAVOR)		• FAVOR • Floridians for Recovery • Maine Harm Reduction Coalition • C4 Recovery Solutions[a]	None	None	None	None	None	None	None
H. Westley Clark, MD	Individual Reviewer	Santa Clara University Dean's Executive Professor, Public Health Program	None	None	None	None	None	None	None	None
Kelly Clark, MD, MBA, FASAM, DFAPA	Individual Reviewer- ASAM Board Member	Clean Slate Addiction Treatment Centers	• Grunenthal US • Behavioral Health Group (BHG)[a] • Clean Slate[a]	None	• CVS Caremark • Clean Slate[a]	None	None	BHG[a] Clean Slate[a]	None	None
Itai Danovitch, MD	Individual Reviewer– ASAM State Chapter Leader	Cedars-Sinai Medical Center Chairman, Dept of Psychiatry	None	None	None	None	None	None	None	None

Name	Organization	Title							
Karen Drexler, MD	U.S. Department of Veterans Affairs	Department of Veterans Affairs Deputy National Program Director- Addictive Disorders	None	None	None	None	None	None	None
Michael Fingerhood, MD	Individual Reviewer	Johns Hopkins University Associate Professor of Medicine	None	None	None	None	None	None	None
Kevin Fiscella, MD, MPH	National Commission on Correctional Health Care (NCCHC)	University of Rochester Professor, Family Medicine, Public Health Science	None	None	None	None	None	None	None
Rollin M. Gallagher, MD, MPH	Individual Reviewer	Philadelphia VA Medical Center National Program Director for Pain Management	None	None	None	None	None	None	None
D. Ray Gaskin Jr., MD FASAM	Individual Reviewer- Georgia Chapter President	Self-employed Physician	• Reckitt Benckiser • Orexo	None	None	None	None	None	- None
Stuart Gitlow, MD, MPH, MBA, FAPA	Individual Reviewer- President, ASAM	Self-employed Physician	Orexo Medical Director (January-June 2014)[a]	None	None	None	None	None	None
Dennis E. Hagarty, MSN, RN, CARN-AP, LCAS	International Nurses Society on Addiction (IntNSA)	Charles George VAMC	None	None	None	None	None	None	None'
Henrick J. Harwood	National Association of State Alcohol and Drug Abuse Directors, Inc. (NASADAD)	NASADAD Deputy Executive Director	None	None	None	None	None	None	None

Continued

External Reviewer	Representation	Employment	Consultant	Speakers Bureau	Ownership/ Partnership/ Principal	Personal Research	Institutional, Organizational, or Other Financial Benefit	Salary	Expert Witness	Other
Frank P. James, MD, JD	Optum/UBH	United HealthCare Associate Medical Director	None	None	None	None	None	None	None	None
Hendree Jones, MD	Individual Reviewer	University of North Carolina Executive Director/Professor OB/GYN	None	None	None	None	None	None	None	None
Miriam Komaromy, MD	Individual Reviewer	University of New Mexico, Echo Institute Associate Director, Echo Institute	None	None	None	None	None	None	None	None
Mark L. Kraus, MD, FASAM, DABAM	Individual Reviewer- ASAM Board Member	Franklin Medical Group, PC Asst. Clinical Professor of Medicine, Yale University School of Medicine; Chief Medical Officer, Connecticut Counseling Centers	• BioDelivery Services, International; • Indivior/ Reckitt Benckiser; • PCM Healthcare	• Biodelivery Services International; • Indivior/ Reckitt Benckiser; • PCM Healthcare ASAM; Coalition on Physician Education on Substance Use Disorders	None	None	None	None	Defendant physician on regarding proper scope of practice	None
Joshua D. Lee, MD MSc	Individual Reviewer	NYU School of Medicine Associate Professor/Physician	None	None	None	Alkermes; Reckitt Benckiser[a]	None	None	None	None
David Mee-Lee, MD	Individual Reviewer	The Change Companies Senior Vice-President	None	None	None	None	None	None	None	None

Continued

Name	Role	Affiliation								
Frances R. Levin, MD	American Psychiatric Association (APA)—Council on Addiction Psychiatry	Columbia University Kennedy Leavy Professor of Psychiatry at CUMC	GW Pharmaceuticals	None	None	US World Med	None	None	None	None
Petros Levounis, MD	Individual Reviewer	Rutgers NJ Medical School Chair, Department of Psychiatry	None	None	None	None	None	None	None	None
Sharon Levy, MD	American Academy of Pediatrics (AAP)	Boston Children's Hospital Director, Adolescent Substance Abuse Program	None	None	None	None	None	None	None	None
Michelle Lofwall, MD	Individual Reviewer-Past President, ASAM Kentucky Chapter	University of Kentucky Associate Professor, Behavioral Science and Psychiatry	• PCM Scientific (Reckitt Benckiser) • CVS Caremark	None	None	Braeburn Pharmaceuticals	None	None	None	None
Ed Madalis, LPC	Geisinger Health Plan	Geisinger Health Plan Lead Behavioral Health Coordinator	None	None	None	None	None	None	None	None
Steven C. Matson, MD	Individual Reviewer— ASAM Ohio Chapter President	Nationwide Children's Hospital Chief, Division of Adolescent Medicine, Associate Professor of Pediatrics	None	None	None	None	None	None	None	None
Michael Miller, MD, FASAM, FAPA	Individual Reviewer	Medical Director Herrington Recovery Center	Curry Rockefeller Group	• Alkermes • BDSI	None	None	None	• Braeburn Pharma • BDSI	None	None
Ivan Montoya	National Institute for Drug Abuse (NIDA)	NIDA Deputy Director, DPMC	None	None	None	None	None	None	None	None
Douglas Nemecek, MD, MBA	CIGNA	CIGNA Chief Medical Officer- Behavioral Health	None	None	None	None	None	None	None	None

External Reviewer	Representation	Employment	Consultant	Speakers Bureau	Ownership/ Partnership/ Principal	Personal Research	Institutional, Organizational, or Other Financial Benefit	Salary	Expert Witness	Other
Yngvild Olsen, MD	Individual Reviewer—ASAM Maryland Chapter President	Institutes for Behavior Resources, Inc. Medical Director	None	CORE REMS	None	Friends Research Institute	None	Institutes for Behavior Resources, Inc.[a]	None	None
David Pating, MD	Individual Reviewer	Permanente Medical Group Chief, Addiction Medicine, Kaiser SFO	None	None	None	None	None	None	None	None
Ashwin A. Patkar, MD	Individual Reviewer	Duke University Medical Center Professor of Psychiatry and Community and Family Medicine	• Reckitt Benckiser • BDSI • Cubist • Titan Pharma • Braeburn Pharm	BDSI, Alkermes	Generys Biopharma	• PI Forest Research Institute • Co-I NIDA and SAMHSA grants • PI Titan Pharmaceuticals[a]	None	None	None	None
Jeffrey Quamme, MD	Individual Reviewer	Connecticut Certification Board Executive Director	None	None	None	None	None	None	None	None
John A. Renner, Jr., MD	American Psychiatric Association (APA)—Council on Addiction Psychiatry	VA Boston Healthcare System Associate Chief of Psychiatry	National Institute on Drug Abuse, Clinical Trials Network	None	None	None	• Department of Psychiatry Boston University Center • Psychiatric Assoc, Consultant and Council on Addiction Psychiatry • Academy of Addiction Psychiatry Consultant & Board of Trustees	VA Boston Healthcare System[a]	None	None

Name	Organization	Role/Position									
Robert L. Rich, Jr., MD, FAAFP	American Academy of Family Physicians (AAFP)	Community Care of the Lower Cape Fear Medical Director/Reviewer	None	None	None	None	None	None	Community Care of the Lower Cape Fear	None	None
A. Kenison Roy III, MD	Individual Reviewer - ASAM Board Member	Biobehavioral Medicine Company, LLC Owner/Medical Director	Orexo, Biobehavioral Sciences, Inc. (BDSI)	• Orexo • BDSI • Alkermes	Addiction Recovery Resources, Inc.**	None	None	None	None	None	None
Albert A. Rundio, Jr., PhD	International Nurses Society on Addictions (IntNSA)	Drexel University Associate Dean for Post-Licensure Nursing Programs and CNE	None	None	None	None	None	None	None	None	None
Edwin Salsitz, MD	Individual Reviewer	Mount Sinai Beth Israel Physician	None	None	None	None	None	None	None	None	None
Andrew J. Saxon, MD	American Psychiatry Association (APA)—Council on Addiction Psychiatry	Department of Veterans Affairs Director, Center of Excellence in Substance Abuse Treatment and Education	None	None	None	• NIDA CTN grant[a] • Alkermes	None	None	None	None	None
Ian A Shaffer, MD	Healthfirst	Executive Medical Director & VP	None	None	None	None	None	None	None	None	None
Dominique Simon	Allies in Recovery	Allies in Recovery Director	None	None	None	None	None	None	None	None	None
Sandra Springer, MD	Individual Reviewer	Yale School of Medicine Associate Professor of Medicine	None	None	None	NIH-funded Research[a]	None	None	None	None	Free drug and placebo from Alkermes
Knox Todd, MD, MPH	American College of Emergency Physicians (ACEP)	MD Anderson Cancer Center Professor and Chair of Emergency Medicine	Kaleo, Inc.	None	None	None	Depomed, Inc.	None	None	None	None

Continued

External Reviewer	Representation	Employment	Consultant	Speakers Bureau	Ownership/ Partnership/ Principal	Personal Research	Institutional, Organizational, or Other Financial Benefit	Salary	Expert Witness	Other
Howard Wetsman, MD	Individual Reviewer- ASAM Board Member	Self-employed Chief Medical Officer	None	None	• Wetsman Forensic Medicine LLC dba Sagenex Labs • Rush Medical • Idea Breeder LLC • Tres Amigos LLC • Keystone Acquisition LLC	None	None	None	None	None
Amanda Wilson, MD	Individual Reviewer	Clean Slate Addiction Treatment Centers President and CEO	None	None	Clean Slate Centers, Inc.[a]	None	None	Clean Slate Centers, Inc.[a]	None	None
Celia Winchell	Food and Drug Administration (FDA)	Medical Team Leader Food and Drug Administration	None	None	None	None	None	None	None	None

The above table presents the relationships of invited external reviewers during the past 12 months with industry and other entities that were determined to be relevant to this document. These relationships are current as of the completion of this document and may not necessarily reflect relationships at the time of this document's publication. A person is deemed to have a significant interest in a business if the interest represents ownership of 5% or more of the voting stock or share of the business entity; or ownership of $10,000 or more of the fair market value of the business entity; or if funds received by the person from the business entity exceed 5% of the person's gross income for the previous year. A relationship is considered to be modest if it is less than significant under the preceding definition. No financial relationship pertains to relationships for which there is no monetary reimbursement.

[a]Indicates significant relationship.

An entry followed by *f* indicates figure, by *t* table, and by *b* box.